YO-AKK-427

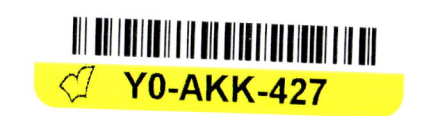

SURGERY

Principles and Practice

Contributors

William E. Adams
J. Garrott Allen
W. A. Altemeier
James Barrett Brown
Robert Bruce Brown
Harvey R. Butcher, Jr.
Isidore Cohn, Jr.
David Y. Cooper
Oliver Cope
W. R. Culbertson
Robert D. Dripps
William S. Dye
William T. Fitts
Minot P. Fryer
John H. Gibbon, Jr.
Lawrence M. Haas
Oscar P. Hampton, Jr.
James D. Hardy
*Henry N. Harkins**
Paul V. Harper, Jr.
John M. Howard
Julian Johnson
Ormand C. Julian
Stanley F. Katz
Jack Lapides
K. Alvin Merendino
Francis D. Moore
Carl A. Moyer
Thomas F. Nealon, Jr.
Michael Newton
Lloyd M. Nyhus
Erle E. Peacock, Jr.
Robert G. Ravdin
Mark M. Ravitch
Fred C. Reynolds
Jonathan E. Rhoads
Paul S. Russell
Karl F. Schroeder
William H. Sweet

* *Deceased* August 12, 1967.

SURGERY

Principles and Practice

JONATHAN E. RHOADS, M.D., D.SC. (MED.)
*John Rhea Barton Professor of Surgery, School of Medicine,
University of Pennsylvania, Philadelphia*

J. GARROTT ALLEN, M.D.
*Professor of Surgery, Stanford University Medical School;
Attending Surgeon, Stanford University
Medical Center, Stanford*

HENRY N. HARKINS, M.D., PH.D.
*Late Professor of Surgery, University of Washington
School of Medicine, Seattle*

CARL A. MOYER, M.D.
*Formerly Bixby Professor of Surgery, Washington University
School of Medicine, St. Louis*

Fourth Edition

---

758 Illustrations

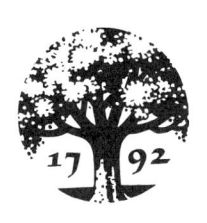

J. B. Lippincott Company
Philadelphia and Toronto

Fourth Edition

Copyright © 1970, by J. B. Lippincott Company

Copyright © 1957, 1961, 1965, by J. B. Lippincott Company

This book is fully protected by copyright and, with the exception of brief excerpts for review, no part of it may be reproduced in any form, by print, photoprint, microfilm, or any other means, without the written permission of the publishers.

Distributed in Great Britain by
Blackwell Scientific Publications,
Oxford and Edinburgh

Library of Congress Catalog Card Number
72-109953

Printed in the United States of America

Dedicated to

Alfred Blalock
Frederick A. Coller
Lester R. Dragstedt
Dallas B. Phemister
Isidor S. Ravdin

Henry Nelson Harkins
(1905-1967)

Preparations for this revision were initiated in early 1967 when the publishers informed the editors that the demand for the third edition had increased over that for the second edition. Dr. Henry Harkins met with the other editors and with Mr. Walter Kahoe of the Lippincott Company in May, 1967. After a further exchange of correspondence, the decision was made to plan a fourth edition.

Dr. Harkins suffered a serious heart attack while attending the annual summer outing of the Department of Surgery at the Medical School of the University of Washington—the department that he had organized and had headed from 1948 to 1966 as its first chairman. His death occurred the following day, August 12, 1967.

Dr. Harkins had collected and set aside much material for the fourth edition, which the other editors have drawn upon freely. The chapters that he had written personally have, for the most part, required very little revision. Therefore, and in accordance with the original agreement among the editors, his name has been carried in this edition with a footnote indicating the date of his death. While he could not participate in the actual redrafting of the material, his contributions to the book remain very extensive and very fundamental.

The loss of Henry N. Harkins to surgical education in its broadest sense has been most keenly felt by the other three editors of this textbook. Each of us loved him as an individual and admired him as a surgeon and a scholar.

A broad outline of many of the roles he played in surgery appeared in *The Transactions of the American Surgical Association,* Vol. 75, page 412, 1967. It was prepared by his longtime friend and colleague, his successor as chairman of the Department of Surgery at the University of Washington, Dr. Alvin K. Merendino.

Contributors

WILLIAM E. ADAMS, M.D., F.A.C.S.
Raymond Professor Emeritus of Surgery, University of Chicago; Assistant Director, American College of Surgeons

J. GARROTT ALLEN, M.D.
Professor of Surgery, Stanford University Medical School; Attending Surgeon, Stanford University Medical Center, Stanford, California

W. A. ALTEMEIER, M.D., F.A.C.S.
Christian R. Holmes Professor of Surgery and Chairman, Department of Surgery, University of Cincinnati and the University of Cincinnati Medical Center, Cincinnati, Ohio

JAMES BARRETT BROWN, M.D., F.A.C.S.
Professor of Clinical Surgery, Washington University School of Medicine, St. Louis, Missouri

ROBERT BRUCE BROWN, Vice Admiral, M.C., U.S.N. (Ret.)
Past Surgeon General, U.S. Navy

HARVEY R. BUTCHER, JR., M.D.
Professor of Surgery, Washington University School of Medicine, St. Louis, Missouri

ISIDORE COHN, JR., B.S., M.D., M.Sc. (Med.), D.Sc. (Med.), F.A.C.S.
Professor and Chairman, Department of Surgery, Louisiana State University School of Medicine; Surgeon-in-Chief, L.S.U. Surgical Division, Charity Hospital of Louisiana, New Orleans, Louisiana

DAVID Y. COOPER, M.D.
Professor of Surgical Research, University of Pennsylvania School of Medicine, Philadelphia, Pennsylvania

OLIVER COPE, M.D.
Emeritus Professor of Surgery, Harvard Medical School; Board of Consultation, Massachusetts General Hospital, Boston, Massachusetts

W. R. CULBERTSON, M.D.
Associate Professor of Surgery, University of Cincinnati and the Cincinnati General Hospital

ROBERT D. DRIPPS, A.B., M.D.
Professor and Chairman, Department of Anesthesia, University of Pennsylvania School of Medicine, Philadelphia, Pennsylvania

WILLIAM S. DYE, M.D., M.S., F.A.C.S.
Clinical Professor of Surgery, University of Illinois College of Medicine; Attending Surgeon, Presbyterian-St. Luke's Hospital, Chicago, Illinois

WILLIAM T. FITTS, JR., M.D., F.A.C.S.
Professor of Surgery, University of Pennsylvania School of Medicine; Chief, Surgical Division B, Hospital of the University of Pennsylvania, Philadelphia, Pennsylvania

MINOT P. FRYER, M.D., F.A.C.S.
Professor of Clinical Surgery, Washington University School of Medicine, St. Louis, Missouri

JOHN H. GIBBON, JR., M.D., F.A.C.S., F.R.C.S. (Hon.)
Emeritus Professor of Surgery, Jefferson Medical College, Philadelphia, Pennsylvania

LAWRENCE M. HAAS, M.D.
Instructor in Orthopedic Surgery, Washington University School of Medicine, St. Louis, Missouri

OSCAR P. HAMPTON, JR., M.D., F.A.C.S.
Assistant Director, Trauma Activities, American College of Surgeons; Associate Professor of Clinical Orthopedic Surgery, Washington University School of Medicine, St. Louis, Missouri

JAMES D. HARDY, B.A., M.S. (Chem.), M.D.
Professor and Chairman, Department of Surgery, University of Mississippi School of Medicine; Surgeon-in-Chief, Hospital of the University of Mississippi, Jackson, Miss.

HENRY N. HARKINS, M.D., Ph.D.
Late Professor of Surgery, University of Washington School of Medicine; formerly Consultant in Surgery, King County, Seattle Veterans Administration, Bremerton Naval, Children's Orthopedic and Madigan General Hospitals

Contributors

PAUL V. HARPER, JR., M.D.
Professor, Department of Surgery, University of Chicago

JOHN M. HOWARD, M.D.
Professor of Surgery, Hahnemann Medical College, Philadelphia, Pennsylvania

JULIAN JOHNSON, M.D., D.Sc. (Med.), F.A.C.S.
Professor of Surgery, University of Pennsylvania School of Medicine, Philadelphia, Pennsylvania

ORMAND C. JULIAN, M.D., Ph.D., F.A.C.S.
Professor of Surgery, University of Illinois College of Medicine; Attending Surgeon and Chairman, Division of Surgery, Presbyterian-St. Luke's Hospital, Chicago, Illinois

STANLEY F. KATZ, M.D.
Instructor in Orthopedic Surgery, Washington University School of Medicine, St. Louis, Missouri

JACK LAPIDES, A.M., M.D., F.A.C.S.
Professor of Surgery, University of Michigan Medical School; Chief of Urology Services of University of Michigan Medical Center and Affiliated Hospitals

K. ALVIN MERENDINO, M.D., Ph.D. Surgery (Minn.)
Professor and Chairman, Department of Surgery, University of Washington School of Medicine, St. Louis, Missouri

FRANCIS D. MOORE, M.D., S.D.(Hon.), LL.D. (Hon.), M.Ch. (Hon.), F.R.C.S. (Hon.), F.R.C.S. (Ed.) (Hon.)
Moseley Professor of Surgery, Harvard Medical School; Surgeon-in-Chief, Peter Bent Brigham Hospital, Boston, Massachusetts

CARL A. MOYER, M.D., F.A.C.S.
Formerly Bixby Professor of Surgery, Washington University School of Medicine, St. Louis, Missouri

THOMAS F. NEALON, JR., M.D.
Director of Surgery, St. Vincent's Hospital and Medical Center of New York; Professor of Clinical Surgery, New York University School of Medicine

MICHAEL NEWTON, M.D. (Penn.), M.A., M.B., B.Ch. (Cantab), F.A.C.S., F.A.C.O.G.,
Clinical Professor of Obstetrics and Gynecology, Pritzker School of Medicine, Division of Biological Sciences, University of Chicago; Attending Staff, Chicago Lying-in Hospital; Director, American College of Obstetricians and Gynecologists, Chicago, Illinois

LLOYD M. NYHUS, M.D., F.A.C.S.
Warren H. Cole Professor and Head of Department of Surgery, the Abraham Lincoln School of Medicine, University of Illinois College of Medicine, Chicago, Illinois

ERLE E. PEACOCK, JR., M.D., F.A.C.S.
Professor and Chairman, Department of Surgery, University of Arizona College of Medicine, Tucson, Arizona

ROBERT G. RAVDIN, M.D., F.A.C.S.
Professor of Surgery, University of Pennsylvania School of Medicine, Philadelphia, Pennsylvania

MARK M. RAVITCH, M.D.
Professor of Surgery, University of Pittsburgh School of Medicine; Surgeon-in-Chief, Montefiore Hospital of Pittsburgh

FRED C. REYNOLDS, M.D., F.A.C.S.
Professor of Orthopedic Surgery, Washington University School of Medicine, St. Louis, Missouri

JONATHAN E. RHOADS, B.A., M.D., D.Sc. (Med.), LL.D. (Hon.), D.Sc. (Hon.), F.A.C.S.
John Rhea Barton Professor and Chairman, Department of Surgery; Director of the Harrison Department of Surgical Research of the University of Pennsylvania School of Medicine, Philadelphia, Pennsylvania

PAUL S. RUSSELL, M.D.
John Homans Professor of Surgery, Harvard Medical School; Visiting Surgeon at the Massachusetts General Hospital

KARL F. SCHROEDER, M.D.
Instructor, Section of Urology, Department of Surgery, University of Michigan Medical School, Ann Arbor, Michigan

WILLIAM H. SWEET, M.D., D.Sc., F.A.C.S.
Professor of Surgery, Harvard Medical School; Chief, Neurosurgical Service, Massachusetts, General Hospital, Boston, Massachusetts

Preface to the Fourth Edition

The objectives of this textbook are set forth rather fully in the Preface to the first edition, which is reprinted herewith. The philosophy on which the editors have proceeded in their educational and scientific work is set forth in considerably greater detail in Chapter 1. We have been very much gratified with the acceptance of the first three editions of the book and it was for this reason that it has been revised. The objectives of the revision have been to introduce new material which has developed since the third edition went to the printer and to provide references to important work which has appeared since that time.

A number of new authors have contributed to the book, but we have carried forward the original intention to try to restrict the authorship to as small a group as we could, without sacrifice of competence. We believe this leads to a more homogeneous and a more useful text and, while this policy has led to contributions from many geographic areas, authors have been selected strictly on the basis of their competence and interest, and affiliations with particular schools have never been a consideration in their selection.

Two completely new chapters have been introduced because the fields have grown in importance. The first of these is entitled "The Molecular Attack on Cancer" and has been written by Dr. Robert G. Ravdin, Professor of Surgery, University of Pennsylvania School of Medicine, and member of the Task Force on Breast Carcinoma, National Cancer Institute. The second chapter is entitled "Tissue and Organ Transplantation" and has been prepared by Dr. Paul H. Russell, Homans Professor of Surgery at Harvard University, who has contributed extensively to both the theory and practice of organ transplantation. The chapter, "Military Surgery," previously written by Dr. John Howard and Dr. I. S. Ravdin, has been carried forward, since Dr. Ravdin became disabled, by Dr. Howard and Admiral Robert B. Brown, who recently retired as surgeon-general of the United States Navy. We believe his contributions, coming from another branch of the service, have added significantly to the breadth of this chapter. The section on "Physiology of the Pituitary and Adrenal Glands" has been rewritten and updated by Dr. David Y. Cooper, Professor of Surgical Research, University of Pennsylvania School of Medicine. Dr. Harkins' chapters have been changed as follows: The chapter on Hernia has been left as nearly intact as possible. Only minor revisions were found necessary by Dr. J. Garrott Allen. The chapter on Wound Healing was revised and updated by Dr. Carl Moyer. The chapter on Shock has been largely rewritten by Dr. Jonathan Rhoads, retaining a number of valuable sections from the original. The chapter on Tumors of the Colorectum has been prepared in this edition by Dr. Isidore Cohn, Jr., Professor and Chairman of the Department of Surgery at Louisiana State University in New Orleans. The chapter on the Stomach and Duodenum has been revised by Dr. Lloyd Nyhus, Warren H. Cole Professor and Chairman of the Department of Surgery at the University of Illinois, and co-author with Dr. Harkins, of works on this and other subjects. The chapter on the Anorectum has been revised by Dr. Carl Moyer.

In view of the large amount of historical material presented in the individual chapters, where it seemed more relevant to the material presented to the student, we decided to omit the special chapter, "History of Surgery," in order to save the considerable amount of space which a thorough treatment of this area requires.

As in the preface to the earlier editions, each editor has a number of acknowledgments he wishes to make. First, however, they wish jointly to thank Mrs. Henry Harkins for her great help in sorting and making available those of Dr. Harkins' papers which he had accumulated for this edition and for intensive help to the other editors in organizing revisions and corrections during the summer of 1968.

Again the editors wish to thank the publishers for their wholehearted cooperation and especially Mr. Walter Kahoe, vice-president of the J. B. Lippincott Company, who has shepherded the book through each publication, and

Mr. Stuart Freeman, who has borne the brunt of solving the innumerable problems connected with an undertaking of this kind. As counselors and expediters, they have contributed greatly to the result. Our special thanks go to Miss Naomi Coplin of the Medical Department at Lippincott, who has devoted countless hours to transforming the manuscripts into a book.

Dr. Allen wishes to express his appreciation to Mrs. Lesley Harding and Mrs. Helene Smith for secretarial work and to his wife, Kathryn Allen, without whose cooperation and assistance in organization of material, typing and proofreading, his chapters could not have been revised.

Dr. Jonathan Rhoads wishes to acknowledge his debt to those who assisted him in the preparation of his contributions to this and earlier editions of this text and to reaffirm his appreciation of their help as expressed in the preface to the first edition, which is reprinted immediately following this page. These debts accumulate with successive editions and as responsibilities are transferred with the commitment of successive secretaries to matrimony. The fourth edition brought substantially increased responsibilities to this office as the office of the senior editor; therefore, special acknowledgment is due Miss Irene Dudrick and Mrs. Ina Brown for their work on the fourth edition.

Dr. Howard Reber contributed important material on the excretory functions of the pancreas and Dr. Stanley J. Dudrick and Dr. Douglas W. Wilmore have contributed much new knowledge in the field of intravenous alimentation, which is reflected in the chapter on Nutrition. Dr. William M. Parkins, Professor of Surgical Research at the University of Pennsylvania School of Medicine, has helped a great deal in the revision of the Chapter on Shock.

Preface to the First Edition

The original reason for the writing of this textbook of Surgery was the idea that there was need for a surgical textbook that included to a greater extent the physiologic, biochemical, pathologic and anatomic bases of surgical practice. Each of the editors shared this view. A number of avenues of approach were considered, namely: the revision of an outdated text, the collection of a number of monographs covering the major surgical specialties, and the compilation of an entirely new textbook. The last approach was finally adopted because of the belief that it was the simplest way of providing the medical student with a background knowledge of anatomy, pathology, physiology and biochemistry so as to enable him to develop acumen in the diagnosis of surgical lesions; facility in the preoperative, operative and postoperative care of patients; and an understanding of the principles, aims and methods of conduct of the more important operations. More of the thought leading to the production of this book is set forth in the first chapter entitled, "Surgical Philosophy."

Our objectives, in addition to those listed above, were:

1. The provision in one volume of an introduction to general surgery and the surgical specialties (gynecology, neurosurgery, orthopedics, pediatric surgery, thoracic surgery and urology), excepting only ophthalmology and otorhinolaryngology, believing they are better presented in separate treatises.

2. The writing of the text in such a way as to lead the student to realize that surgical practice is not standardized or perfected, with the hope that by so doing research would be stimulated and open-mindedness fostered.

3. To emphasize that which is important in contemporary surgery, and more especially in the fields of cardiac, vascular and military surgery, even at the expense of omitting some of the rarer conditions and the finer points included in more compendious texts.

4. To emphasize the things that most doctors need to know about surgery rather than the more detailed points of technic that the surgeon uses. However, because we feel that one cannot understand surgery without some exposition of the central act—the operation—the text contains descriptions of several of the more important procedures with emphasis on technical principles rather than on minute details.

5. To cover the physiologic bases of surgical practice in such a way that the surgical resident, while learning technic by actual observation and experience, will find the book a useful reference in matters of nonoperative care, fluid therapy, shock, blood transfusion, nutrition and so forth.

6. To place some emphasis on what surgery has to offer, therapeutically, based on the prognosis of various conditions with and without the exercise of existent operative procedures.

Although the result of such an effort always falls short of the aspirations which lead one to undertake the task, we hope that the objectives have been realized sufficiently to justify the expenditure of time and effort.

We have concentrated responsibility for the text in the hands of as few persons as we could, without sacrifice of firsthand knowledge of the subjects covered. Thus, the four editors have undertaken about one half of the book. For the remaining half, we have called upon individuals of special competence in their respective fields, but with a broad scientific point of view, who are at the same time individuals with a gift for exposition. In an effort to obtain a cross section of surgical thought in the United States, one editor was selected from the West Coast, one from the East Coast, and two from the central part of the United States. The selection of contributors will also show a broad geographic distribution. The average age of the editors, when the book was begun in 1953, was 45 and at its completion in 1956, 48. In an effort to give the book as much cohesion and uniformity as possible, each chapter has been gone over by several of the editors, and insofar as possible this has been done at joint meetings where free discussion of differences of opinion was possible.

It should be emphasized that every effort was made to make this book a common effort of the many individuals who contributed to it. Each of the editors has contributed more than the others in some particular direction. Dr. Allen has written the largest number of chapters. Dr. Harkins has made the most exhaustive study of the proofs. Dr. Moyer had the most to do with organizing the original group and arranged for the largest number of the contributors. Dr. Rhoads kept in touch with the publisher and interrupted the active lives of the other editors to hold meeting after meeting, some for a few hours, some for as long as 12 days. Therefore, the arrangement of the names of the editors in the frontispiece is an alphabetical one. Should this text undergo subsequent editions, the editors plan a re-arrangement in the order of their names, for it is hoped that the text will not come to be known by the name of a specific individual. It is desirable that such a text be moderated and maintained as a joint venture, presenting fairly and as nearly as possible the current teachings and practices in the ever-changing field of surgery.

The fact that the book has been produced without an editor-in-chief has undoubtedly increased the burdens of the publisher. To Mr. Walter Kahoe, Medical Director of the J. B. Lippincott Company, our special thanks are due. We are also grateful to Ellis Bacon, formerly Vice President of the J. B. Lippincott Company, and to Stanley A. Gillett, Production Editor of the Medical Department, who has carried so great a load in the production of the book. We also wish to express appreciation to Mr. T. A. Phillips and to Dr. Morris Fishbein for an early interest and discussions.

Dr. J. Garrott Allen wishes to acknowledge the tireless efforts, in particular, of Miss Reecie Hodgson for her assistance in the preparation and the typing of his portion of this textbook of surgery, and also to Miss Wendy Kemp, Miss Lola Tucker, and Mrs. Carol Kemp for their generous secretarial services when the load became too heavy. This author is indebted to Miss Gladys McHugh for her suggestions and resourcefulness in the layout of a number of illustrations which she prepared for his portion of the text.

Dr. Henry N. Harkins is grateful to all those in his department who helped him with this work, but particularly to Miss Jessie Phillips and Mrs. Helen Halsey, who did all the new art work in his chapters; to his colleague, Dr. Lloyd M. Nyhus for much help; to members of his resident staff who helped with the proof: Drs. Paul W. Herron, John E. Jesseph, Thomas W. Jones, George I. Thomas, John K. Stevenson, and Roy R. Vetto; and especially to his administrative secretary, Mrs. Eleanore B. Ploger, whose intelligent and capable assistance was of help during all phases of the work.

Dr. Carl A. Moyer wishes to acknowledge the secretarial services of Mrs. Carmen Woelfle, Mrs. Mary Ann Sexauer and Miss Carol Hobbs.

Dr. Jonathan E. Rhoads wishes to acknowledge the aid of Drs. Lawrence C. Blair, John P. Dodds, William G. B. Graham, John Helwig, Jr., Paul G. Koontz, Jr., and Robert J. Reed, III, who as fourth-year medical students helped with the manuscript, references and illustrations and gave valuable advice regarding the method of presentation on the basis of their recent and current learning experience. Miss Edna Hill is credited with the drawings in his chapters and most of them in the chapters of Drs. Hampton and Fitts, Dr. Johnson, and Dr. Newton. Mr. R. L. Chapman, Mr. Robert J. Lucas and Miss Mildred M. Stelling performed most of the photographic work for these chapters. He is grateful to Dr. Eugene P. Pendergrass, Dr. Philip J. Hodes and Dr. Lawrence A. Post for radiologic illustrations, particularly in the chapters on the biliary tract and the pancreas. Dr. J. Russell Elkinton was helpful with illustrative material for the chapter on Fluid and Electrolytes; Dr. H. T. Enterline supplied illustrative material from the laboratory of surgical pathology; and Dr. John W. Thomas provided bibliographic assistance and helped prepare the section on iron metabolism. He is indebted to a former secretary, Mrs. Jane R. Lohmeyer, and to Miss Florence Conway for help in typing. He is most indebted to his present secretary, Miss Jeanette B. Mager, who has carried the brunt of the preparation of his manuscripts and much of the organizational work for the book.

THE EDITORS

Contents

1. **Surgical Philosophy** — 1
   Jonathan E. Rhoads, J. Garrott Allen, Henry N. Harkins and Carl A. Moyer

   The Field of Surgery — 1
   Historical Development of Surgery — 1
   Relation of Surgery to Medicine — 2
   Obligations of the Surgeon Beyond Patient Care — 3
   The Art of Surgery — 5
   Opportunities for Surgical Training — 5
   The Place of the Healing Arts in Society — 6
   The Effect of Decreasing Availability of the Primary Physician on the Need of the Specialist for Breadth of Medical Knowledge — 7

2. **Wound Healing** — 8
   Henry N. Harkins and Carl A. Moyer

   Introduction — 8
   Historical — 8
   Types of Healing — 8
   Physiology of Wound Healing — 10
   General Factors in Wound Healing — 12
   Local Factors in Wound Healing — 14
   Technical Factors in Wound Healing — 17
   Healing of Special Tissues — 24
   New Developments in the Study of Wound Healing — 27

3. **Applied Surgical Bacteriology** — 34
   W. A. Altemeier and W. R. Culbertson

   Classification of Bacteria Important in Surgery — 34
   Consideration of Effects of Pathogenic Bacteria in Surgery — 42
   Resistance of the Host to Bacterial Invasion — 44

4. **Surgical Infections** — 48
   W. A. Altemeier and W. R. Culbertson

   General Considerations — 48
   Primary and Secondary Bacterial Contamination and Infection — 50
   Methods of Diagnosis of Surgical Infections — 51
   Treatment of Surgical Infections — 52
   Classification of Wound Infections — 58

xiv   Contents

5. **Fluid and Electrolytes** 75
   Carl A. Moyer and Jonathan E. Rhoads

   Clinical Group 1-a Sodium Normal With Water Deficit 82
   Clinical Group 1-b Sodium Excess Either With Water Normal or Water Deficit . . 82
   Clinical Group 2-a Sodium Normal With Water Excess (Simple Water Intoxication) 83
   Clinical Group 2-b Sodium Deficit With Water in Excess 83
   Clinical Group 2-c Sodium Deficit With Water Normal 84
   Clinical Group 3-a Combined Sodium With Water Deficits 84
   Clinical Group 4-a Excess Sodium and Excess Water 86
   Acidosis and Alkalosis 86
   Cation Abnormalities 88
   Exchanges of Water, Sodium, Potassium and Chloride Occurring in Normal Man
     Between the Individual and His External Environment 88
   Internal Exchanges of Water, Sodium, Potassium and Chloride in Normal Man
     Across the Walls of the Alimentary Tract 89
   Examples of Abnormal Losses and Intakes of Water and Electrolytes in Surgical
     Patients 90
   Methods for Suspecting and Quantitating the Deficits or the Surpluses of Water,
     and Abnormalities of Concentration of Sodium, Chloride and Potassium Ions . 91
   Maintenance of Water and Electrolyte Equilibrium 95
   The Patient With Hyposthenuria 97
   The Patient With Salt-Losing Kidneys 97
   The Patient With the Lower Nephron Syndrome 97
   The Diabetic Patient Undergoing Surgical Procedures 98
   The Relations of Respiration to Acid-Base Balance 98

6. **Nutrition** 101
   Jonathan E. Rhoads

   Protein Nutrition 101
   Estimations of Probable Protein Deficits 104
   Carbohydrate and Fat 107
   Routes of Alimentation 108
   Intravenous Hyperalimentation 111
   Nutritional Role of Blood and Plasma 112
   Diabetes 112
   Vitamins 113
   Iron 116
   Obesity 118

7. **Shock** 121
   Henry N. Harkins and Jonathan E. Rhoads

   Introduction 121
   Definitions 122
   History 122
   Etiology 124
   Accompanying Factors 127
   Irreversibility 130
   Diagnosis 132

7. Shock—(*Continued*)
Therapy: Experimental Approaches 135
Clinical Treatment 137

8. Blood Transfusions and Related Problems 149
J. Garrott Allen

Developmental Interrelations of Surgery and the Discovery of the Circulation, Transfusion, Hemostasis and Shock 149
Practical Aspects and Precautions in Blood Transfusions 156
The Nature of Blood Transfusion Reactions 167
The Single Transfusion and Its Multiple Hazards 175
Special Transfusions 176
Abnormal Bleeding in the Surgical Patient 191

9. The Principles of Isotope Technics in Surgery 202
Paul V. Harper

Physical Properties 202
Isotopic Radiation Measurements 203
Practical Considerations 204
Applications 205

10. Neoplastic Disease—General Considerations 209
Carl A. Moyer and Jonathan E. Rhoads

Neoplasms 209
Certain Practical Considerations in Cancer Surgery 216
Hereditary Factors in Cancer 222

11. The Molecular Attack on Cancer 224
Robert G. Ravdin

Hormones 226
Radioisotopes 227
Cytotoxic Agents 228

12. The Assessment of Operative Risk 232
Carl A. Moyer

13. Anesthesia 244
Robert D. Dripps

Premedication 244
Management of the Drug-Dependent Patient 246
Inhalational Anesthesia 247
Intravenous Anesthesia 251

13. Anesthesia—(*Continued*)

Conduction Anesthesia	252
Spinal Anesthesia	253
Epidural Anesthesia	255
Muscle Relaxants	256
Respiratory Problems Associated With Unconsciousness	260
Anesthetic Management of the "Poor Risk" Patient	261
Anesthesia for Battle Casualties	264
Special Anesthetic Technics	264
Unusual Complications of Anesthesia	266
Fire and Explosion Hazards	267
Postanesthetic Observation Room (Recovery Room)	268
Mechanical Ventilation of the Lungs	269

14. Operative Surgical Care ... 275
James D. Hardy

Preoperative Preparation	275
The Operating Suite	276
Final Preparation	277
The Operation	280
Emergence from Anesthesia and Immediate Recovery Room Care	289

15. Nonoperative Surgical Care ... 293
Carl A. Moyer

Introduction	293
Section 1. General Considerations	293
Section 2. Fever	300
Section 3. Postoperative Pain	307
Section 4. Gas Therapy	315
Section 5. Postoperative Urinary Retention and Oliguria	317
Section 6. Postoperative Jaundice	321
Section 7. Edema	321
Section 8. Nausea and Vomiting	326
Section 9. Headache; Care of Mouth and Skin	327
Section 10. Symptomatic Psychoses	328

16. The Endocrine and Metabolic Basis of Surgical Care ... 337
Francis D. Moore

Recovery—The Reaction of Survival	337
Clinical Metabolic Management	348
Summary	357

17. Burns and Cold Injury ... 360
Carl A. Moyer

Burns	360
Classification	360

17. Burns and Cold Injury—(*Continued*)

Historical Considerations	363
Burn Shock	364
General Therapeutic Principles of Wound Care	373
Burn Sepsis	374
Other Disturbances Associated With Burns	385
Results of Treatment	393
Cold Injury	398

18. Radiation Injury From Local or Total Body Exposure   403
J. Garrott Allen

Considerations in Radiation Exposure in Whole Body Injury	403
Injury from Local or Portal Irradiation	421
Latent Consequences of Ionizing Irradiation from Atomic and Thermonuclear Bombs	432
Protection of Personnel	432
Genetic Effects of Irradiation	432
Laser-Maser Radiation	433

19. Tissue and Organ Transplantation   435
Paul S. Russell

Transplantation Technics	435
Terminology	436
The Rejection Reaction	436
Donor Organ Availability	443
Clinical Transplantation	443
Transplantation in the Future	447

20. Fractures and Dislocations: General Considerations   448
Oscar P. Hampton, Jr. and William T. Fitts, Jr.

Fracture Maxims	448
Definitions	448
Healing of Fractures	450
Diagnosis of a Fracture	451
Priority of Injury	453
Complications of Fractures	454
Objectives of Management of Fractures	459
Emergency Splinting of Fractures	460
Methods of Management of Fractures	463
Open Fractures	467
Fractures in Children	471
Pathologic Fractures	473
Plaster of Paris	473
Rehabilitation	477

21. Fractures and Dislocations of the Upper Extremity ... 478
Oscar P. Hampton, Jr. and William T. Fitts, Jr.

Fractures and Dislocations About the Shoulder ... 478
Fractures of the Shaft of the Humerus ... 487
Fractures and Dislocations About the Elbow ... 490
Fractures of the Shaft of the Bones of the Forearm ... 502
Fractures and Dislocations About the Wrist ... 507

22. Fractures and Dislocations of the Lower Extremity ... 518
Oscar P. Hampton, Jr. and William T. Fitts, Jr.

Fractures and Dislocations About the Hip ... 518
Fractures of the Shaft of the Femur ... 527
Fractures of the Distal End of the Femur ... 533
Dislocation of the Knee ... 534
Internal Derangements of the Knee ... 535
Fractures of the Patella ... 539
Fractures of the Proximal End of the Tibia ... 540
Fractures of the Shafts of the Bones of the Leg ... 543
Fractures of the Shaft of the Fibula With an Intact Tibia ... 549
Fractures and Dislocations of the Ankle ... 550
Fractures of the Bones of the Foot ... 555
Dislocations of the Foot ... 560

23. Fractures and Dislocations of the Spine, the Pelvis, the Sternum and the Ribs ... 562
Oscar P. Hampton, Jr. and William T. Fitts, Jr.

Fractures and Dislocations of the Spine ... 562
Fractures of the Pelvis ... 569
Fractures of the Sternum ... 571
Fractures of the Ribs ... 571

24. Principles of Hand Surgery ... 574
Erle E. Peacock, Jr.

Introduction ... 574
Soft Tissue Injuries Exclusive of Nerves and Tendons ... 574
Soft Tissue Infections ... 577
Nerves ... 578
Tendons ... 580
Bones and Joints ... 583
Compound Wounds ... 585
Secondary Reconstruction of the Hand ... 585
Joints ... 592
Disease and Congenital Deformity ... 592
Tumors ... 595
Rehabilitation and Disability ... 596

25. Military Surgery ... 599
John M. Howard and Robert B. Brown

Function of a Combat Medical Service ... 599
Organization of a Combat Medical Service ... 599
Wounding Agents ... 601
Wound Ballistics ... 601
Problems Related to the Management of Combat Wounds Caused by Specific Ordnance ... 603
The Battle Wound ... 605
Resuscitation and Evacuation ... 609
Regional Surgery: Principles of Surgery ... 617
Specific Complications ... 637
Principles of Management of Atomic Casualties ... 642
Submarine Medicine ... 645
Chemical Warfare ... 646
Arctic Medicine ... 646

26. Skin and Subcutaneous Tissues ... 649
Carl A. Moyer and Jonathan E. Rhoads

Introduction ... 649
Benign Tumors of the Skin ... 652
Malignant Tumors of the Skin ... 664

27. Breast ... 668
J. Garrott Allen

Embryology ... 668
Anatomy ... 668
Inflammatory Diseases ... 670
Benign Tumors ... 671
Cancer ... 674
Attempts to Improve Survival Results ... 703
The Male Breast ... 709
Prognostic Considerations ... 710

28. Thyroid, Thymus and Parathyroids ... 714
Oliver Cope

The Thyroid Gland ... 714
    Pathogenesis of Goiter ... 715
    Hyperthyroidism ... 716
    Nodular Goiter ... 720
    Thyroiditis ... 722
    The Normal Gland ... 723
    Suggestions About the Investigation of the Patient ... 723
    Pointers on Surgical Technic ... 726
The Thymus Gland ... 727
    Surgical Anatomy ... 727

28. Thyroid, Thymus and Parathyroids—(Continued)

Pathologic Physiology	727
Status Thymicolymphaticus	727
As a Seat of Tumor	728
As an Instigator of Myasthenia Gravis	728
The Parathyroid Glands	729
Introduction	729
History	729
Hypoparathyroidism	731
Hyperparathyroidism	731
Pathophysiology	732
Anatomic Pathology	733
Diagnosis	735
Treatment	737

29. Section I: Physiology of the Pituitary and Adrenal Glands — 748
David Y. Cooper

Introduction	748
Physiology and Biochemistry	748
Response in Surgical Stress	762
Diagnosis of Adrenal and Pituitary Insufficiency	764
Pathologic Changes Caused by Excess of Adrenal Steroids or ACTH	764

29. Section II: Pituitary and Adrenal Glands — 766
J. Garrott Allen

Pituitary Gland	766
Adrenal Gland	774

30. Esophagus — 795
K. Alvin Merendino

Anatomy and Physiology	795
Foreign Bodies	797
Benign Stricture	799
Spontaneous Rupture of the Esophagus	800
Esophageal Diverticula	802
Reflux Esophagitis (Peptic Esophagitis)	804
Cardiospasm	807
Tumors of Esophagus	810

31. Stomach and Duodenum — 819
Henry N. Harkins and Lloyd M. Nyhus

Introduction	819
Peptic Ulcer	829
Carcinoma of the Stomach	844
Hypertrophic Pyloric Stenosis	851

31. Stomach and Duodenum—(*Continued*)

Operative Procedures on the Stomach 852
Late Complications of Gastric Surgery: The Postgastrectomy Syndrome . . . 856
Miscellaneous Surgical Diseases of the Stomach and the Duodenum 860

32. Liver, Gallbladder and Bile Passages 880
Jonathan E. Rhoads

Introduction 880
Anatomic Considerations 881
Physiologic Considerations 883
Tumors of the Gallbladder and the Extrahepatic Bile Ducts 886
Hemobilia 886
Acute Cholecystitis 887
Perforation of the Gallbladder With Abscess, Peritonitis or Biliary Fistula . . 888
Chronic Calculous Cholecystitis and Chronic Noncalculous Cholecystititis . . 890
Diagnosis of Common Duct Stone and Other Indications for Choledochostomy . 895
The Jaundiced Patient 899
The Prognostic Significance of Obstructive Jaundice 900
Preparation of the Jaundiced Patient for Operation 902
Standard Operative Procedures on the Gallbladder and the Extrahepatic Biliary Passages 904
Pathologic Conditions of the Liver Parenchyma With Notes Regarding Surgical Therapy 910

33. Pancreas 916
Jonathan E. Rhoads

Anatomy 916
Physiology 917
Acute Pancreatitis 920
Postoperative Pancreatitis 924
Chronic Pancreatitis and Chronic Relapsing Pancreatitis 925
Unusual Associations of Acute Pancreatitis With Other Conditions 928
Trauma 928
Islet Cell Tumors 929
Pancreaticoduodenal Cancers 930
Cysts 939
Benign Solid Tumors 942
Pancreatic Heterotopia 942
Metabolic Effects of Total Pancreatectomy 942

34. Spleen 947
J. Garrott Allen

Historical Note 947
Anatomy 948
Physiology 949
Splenic Function, Hyperfunction and Dysfunction 950

34. Spleen—(Continued)

Auto-immune Diseases Benefited by Splenectomy	953
Diseases of the Spleen	959
Inherited Diseases Benefited by Splenectomy	965
Splenic Tumors	973
Technic of Splenectomy	974
Splenic Transplantation in Classical Hemophilia A	977

35. Mesentery, Splanchnic Circulation and Mesenteric Thrombosis 980
J. Garrott Allen

Anatomic Consideration of the Mesentery and the Splanchnic Circulation	980
Diseases of the Mesentery	990
Mesenteric Thrombosis	991

36. Portal Hypertension and Ascites 996
J. Garrott Allen

Definition and Diagnosis	996
Anatomic Causes of Portal Hypertension	997
Pathogenesis of Ascites in Portal Hypertension	1000
The Natural History of Patients With Esophagogastric Varices	1003
Diagnosis	1004
General Evaluation of Patients With Portal Hypertension	1007
Tests of Liver Function	1008
Evaluation by Histology Examination (Liver Biopsy)	1010
Complications	1011
Indications for Operation and Selection of Patients	1012
Management of the Patient With the Bleeding Varix	1014

37. Appendicitis, Peritonitis, and Intra-Abdominal Abscesses 1022
J. Garrott Allen

Section I: Appendicitis and the Acute Abdomen — 1022

Introduction	1022
Nonperforative Acute Appendicitis	1028
Perforative Acute Appendicitis	1033
Appendicitis in Pregnancy	1038
Recurrent Appendicitis	1039
Removal of the Normal Appendix in the Course of Other Intra-abdominal Operations	1039
Complications of Acute Appendicitis	1039
Mortality from Appendicitis	1041
Tumors of the Appendix	1043
Abdominal Pain	1043
Differential Diagnosis of Appendicitis	1045

Section II: Peritonitis and Intra-abdominal Abscesses — 1049

The Peritoneum	1049
Subdivisions of the Abdominal Cavity	1049
Acute Peritonitis	1050
Chronic Peritonitis	1056
Intra-abdominal Abscesses	1058

38. Anatomy and Physiology of the Small Bowel and Colon, and Intestinal Obstruction 1066
J. Garrott Allen

Anatomy 1066
Physiology 1067
Diagnosis of Intestinal Obstruction 1074
Clinical Features 1088
Treatment 1092

39. Small Bowel and Colon 1103
J. Garrott Allen

Congenital Disorders of the Intestinal Tract Afflicting Adult Patients 1103
Trauma of the Small Bowel and the Colon 1106
Inflammatory Diseases of the Small Bowel and the Colon 1111
Tumors of the Small Bowel 1135
Pseudomembranous Enterocolitis 1137

40. Tumors of the Colorectum 1140
Isidore Cohn, Jr.

Benign Tumors: Polyps 1140
Benign Tumors: Rarer Lesions 1146
Premalignant Lesions of the Colon 1148
Malignant Tumors 1153
Malignant Tumors: Rarer Lesions 1170

41. Anorectum 1174
Henry N. Harkins, revision by Carl A. Moyer

Definition 1174
General Considerations 1174
Anatomy 1175
Diagnosis 1181
Clinical Conditions 1181

42. Hernia 1204
Henry N. Harkins, revision by J. Garrott Allen

Introduction 1204
Historical Considerations 1205
Definition, Diagnosis, Incidence and Prognosis 1205
The Hernia Problem Today 1208
Subsidiary Problems in the Field of Hernia 1235
Aids to Repair 1239
Rarer Hernias: Treatment and Glossary of Terms 1243

43. Cardiac Surgery . . . 1259
Julian Johnson

Congenital Cardiac Lesions . . . 1259
Acquired Heart Disease . . . 1282
Open Cardiac Surgery Under Direct Vision . . . 1294
Cardiac Resuscitation . . . 1295

44. Peripheral Vascular Surgery . . . 1298
Ormand C. Julian and William S. Dye

Arterial Surgery . . . 1298
    Introduction . . . 1298
    Acute Arterial Occlusion . . . 1298
    Arterial Trauma . . . 1305
    Chronic Occlusive Arterial Disease . . . 1315
    Renal Artery Disease . . . 1327
    Arterial Insufficiency Affecting the Brain . . . 1330
    Visceral Arteriosclerosis . . . 1332
    Buerger's Disease—Thromboangiitis Obliterans . . . 1334
    Angiospastic Conditions . . . 1336
    Arterial Aneurysm . . . 1339
Surgery of the Venous System . . . 1353
    Introduction . . . 1353
    Varicose Veins of the Lower Extremity . . . 1353
    Thrombophlebitis . . . 1358
    Syndrome of Superior Vena Cava Obstruction . . . 1362
    Acute Thrombosis of the Subclavian Vein (Effort Thrombosis) . . . 1363

45. Lung . . . 1371
K. Alvin Merendino

Anatomic Considerations . . . 1371
Physiologic Considerations . . . 1373
Thoracic Trauma . . . 1376
Lung Abscess . . . 1381
Bronchiectasis . . . 1383
Empyema . . . 1386
Certain Fungal Diseases . . . 1389
Trachea . . . 1391

46. Pulmonary Tuberculosis . . . 1393
W. E. Adams

Pathology . . . 1394
General Considerations . . . 1395
Indications for Surgical Therapy . . . 1395
Operative Procedures . . . 1396
Results of Surgery . . . 1399

47. Carcinoma of the Lung and Tumors of the Thorax 1402
John H. Gibbon, Jr. and Thomas F. Nealon, Jr.

Tumors of the Lung 1402
Tumors of the Mediastinum 1410
Tumors of the Thoracic Wall 1412

48. Tumors of the Head and the Neck 1415
Erle Peacock, Jr.

Eyelids 1415
Ear 1417
Face 1417
Nose, Paranasal Sinuses and Nasopharynx 1419
Lips 1421
Oral Cavity and Tongue 1423
Mandible 1426
Salivary Glands 1428
Larynx 1431
Neck 1432
Palliative Care 1435

49. Principles of General Plastic Surgery 1437
James Barrett Brown and Minot P. Fryer

Skin Grafting and Deep Burns 1437
Cleft Lip and Cleft Palate 1450
Deformities and Inflammatory Diseases of the Jaws 1456
Reconstruction of the Jaw 1462
Compound Facial Injuries 1462
Facial Paralysis 1469
Deformities of the Ear 1476
Deformities of the Eyelids 1477
Salivary Glands 1479
Congenital Wryneck 1480
Industrial and Farm Injuries 1480
Hypospadias 1481
Repair of Surface Defects of the Feet 1481
Use of Silicone, Teflon, Polyvinyl Alcohol and Di-Isocyanate as Prostheses in Reconstructive Surgery 1482

50. Pediatric Surgery 1491
Mark M. Ravitch

General Considerations 1491
Head and Neck 1494
Thorax 1499
Gastrointestinal Tract 1506

51. Gynecology ... 1534
Michael Newton

History and Examination ... 1534
Congenital Abnormalities ... 1535
Displacements of the Uterus and Pelvic Relaxation ... 1536
Diseases of the Lower Genital Tract ... 1542
Disease of the Cervix ... 1549
The Upper Genital Tract ... 1556
Tumors of the Upper Genital Tract ... 1558
Menstrual Disorders ... 1568
Fertility ... 1571
Infertility ... 1572
Endometriosis ... 1574
Ectopic Pregnancy ... 1576

52. Urology ... 1580
J. Lapides and Karl F. Schroeder

Introduction ... 1580
Renal Physiology ... 1585
Diuretics ... 1596
Renal Function Tests ... 1598
Renal Function in Disease ... 1599
Acute Renal Failure ... 1599
Chronic Renal Failure ... 1602
Hypertension ... 1602
Obstructive Urinary Tract Disease ... 1603
Urinary Tract Infections ... 1614
Neoplasms of the Genitourinary Tract ... 1620
Calculous Disease ... 1625
Traumatic Lesions ... 1627
Physiology of Urinary Transport and Micturition ... 1633
Congenital Anomalies ... 1643

53. Orthopedics (Nontraumatic) ... 1657
Fred C. Reynolds, Lawrence M. Haas, and Stanley F. Katz

Development of the Skeleton ... 1657
Composition of Bone ... 1658
Composition of Cartilage ... 1659
The Metabolism of Bone and Cartilage ... 1659
Response of Bone to Injury ... 1660
The Fate of Bone Grafts ... 1667
Deossification of the Skeleton ... 1667
Scurvy ... 1671
Other Metabolic Diseases of Bone ... 1672
Inborn Errors of Metabolism ... 1674
Developmental Abnormalities ... 1680
Orthopedic Treatment of Paralytic Disorders ... 1695
Cerebral Palsy ... 1698

53. Orthopedics (Nontraumatic)—(*Continued*)

Myelodysplasia	1700
Scoliosis	1700
Infections in Bone	1703
Degenerative Disease of Joints	1717
Upper Extremity Pain	1723
Bone Tumors	1728
Tumors of the Soft Tissue	1735
Common Foot Problems	1735
Low Back Pain	1739

54. Surgery of the Nervous System ... 1755
William H. Sweet

Diseases Affecting the Central Nervous System	1755
Diseases Affecting the Peripheral Nervous System	1799
Neurosurgical Operations on Normal Tissues to Relieve Disease Elsewhere	1800
Diseases Affecting the Autonomic Nervous System	1807
Conclusion	1808

55. Mathematical Analysis of Surgical Data ... 1810
Harvey R. Butcher, Jr.

Population Sampling	1811
Means and Rates	1812
Analysis of Measurements	1815
Mortality Data	1817

Bibliographic Index ... 1825

Subject Index ... 1837

Chapter 1

JONATHAN E. RHOADS, M.D., J. GARROTT ALLEN, M.D.,
HENRY N. HARKINS, M.D., AND CARL A. MOYER, M.D.

Surgical Philosophy

THE FIELD OF SURGERY

Surgery is a form of service to man. It is a body of knowledge and experience developed by man to meet human needs in certain fields and has come to be entrusted to a group of individuals who have devoted themselves more or less successfully to acquiring this requisite body of knowledge and experience.

Its boundaries and those of internal medicine are more distinct in the popular mind than in practice. The practitioner of internal medicine generally abstains from performing formal operations and by doing so has more time which he can devote, if he will, to the study of diagnostic problems, for consideration of psychosomatic difficulties encountered by his patients, and for study of advances in the basic sciences or to clinical investigation.

A number of years ago one of our senior surgeons made the statement that internal medicine was becoming more and more surgical in its outlook, and, in all fairness, one must add that in the last third of the twentieth century, general surgery has become more and more steeped in medicine and the basic medical sciences.

There is no more basic objective for the surgeon than the precept of the late John B. Deaver who said that a surgeon must be a medical man and something more—not something less.

Anyone who enters the field of surgery to escape from the rigorous mental discipline required to think straight in medicine is likely either to fail or, worse, do a great amount of harm.

HISTORICAL DEVELOPMENT OF SURGERY

The place of surgery in the whole of medicine and in our general social structure gains perspective from its historical development. The writings of Hippocrates (5th century, B.C.) reveal much valuable knowledge about the treatment of fractures, drainage of abscesses and the management of wounds. Surgery and medicine were practiced by the same people in his day. Many of the concepts in the Oath of Hippocrates are valid today, and one cannot consider the philosophy of medicine and surgery without coming back to it.

Much that the Greeks knew was utilized during Roman times largely by Greek physicians. Few Romans became physicians. Even the greatest, Galen, was a Greek by birth. Medical knowledge apparently grew very little until the Renaissance, when artists and sculptors began the study of anatomy, and Vesalius wrote *De Humani Corporis Fabrica* (1543). During the long centuries that intervened, medical care had become a function of the clergy, and it was not until the Church ordered the monks not to operate that they started having their barbers do it. Thus there grew up a group of barber-surgeons, the best of whom devoted themselves to surgery.

In England, there was a brief period in the early 16th century when the surgeons were associated with the physicians, but later in the 16th century Henry VIII granted a charter to the Guild of Barbers and Surgeons, and, despite various attempts to break away, the surgeons remained organized with the barbers until 1745. The distinction is still perpetuated in England where a surgeon is addressed as Mr. Smith while a physician is referred to as Dr. Smith.

In the United States and in other countries of the Western Hemisphere this distinction has not been made. For many years all medical men performed both medical and surgical services.

During the middle of the 19th century, the

development of anesthesia, antisepsis and asepsis greatly increased the range and the effectiveness of surgery, and this has been further extended by the development of roentgenology, the development of transfusion, of parenteral nutrition (including water and electrolytes) and by antibiotics. Concomitantly, a great group of surgical specialties and subspecialties has developed. Today, the danger of overspecialization is often spoken of, but the probability is that the future will bring more rather than less specialization. The antidote to the danger envisioned appears to be a training period which includes a broad background in medicine and general surgery and some continued contact with these fields throughout the whole of one's professional life.

RELATION OF SURGERY TO MEDICINE

Surgery is very much a part of medicine in the broad sense. The fact that "medicine" is used to denote the whole field covered by the school of medicine in a university and also in a narrow sense, to denote the department of that school which teaches internal medicine, is often a source of confusion.

Certain common usages of the word "surgery" carry by implication such a slur on the profession that they cannot pass unnoticed. The British use the word as synonymous with the office of a practitioner. This usage has no place in the American language and therefore will not be commented upon. However, a common Americanism is to say that on such and such a date the patient was taken to surgery —meaning that the patient had an operation performed. The phraseology is vaguely reminiscent of taking sheep to the slaughter, but our basic objection to it is the implication that the operation constitutes all or most of what the surgeon has to contribute. This may apply to the "ghost surgeon" but not to the more creditable representatives of the profession.

Surgery is a body of knowledge not only of operative technics but also of human anatomy (gross, microscopic and ultramicroscopic), biochemistry, biophysics, genetics, physiology, pharmacology, pathology, microbiology and immunology, medicine and psychology (to mention only some of its components). This knowledge helps to determine from careful consideration of the patient's history and physical findings what laboratory aids are needed, and on the basis of these to establish the diagnosis or probable diagnosis. One must decide whether or not there is a worthwhile chance of helping the patient by operative intervention and if so when it should be done. Only on the basis of such preoperative study can one make proper decisions at operation about what should be done. More and more mathematical technics must be used in converting these data into valid decisions. It is in recognition of this factor that a chapter on mathematical analysis of surgical data is included in this book. The surgical responsibility then continues into the postoperative period for days or weeks, providing for the patient's recovery, averting and/or combating complications and endeavoring to restore the patient to complete health or to obtain for him the most in rehabilitation that his condition permits.

Obviously, the surgeon cannot do all these things alone. He must function as a member of a team helping to coordinate the services of clinical pathologists, radiologists, nurses, surgical house officers, social workers, rehabilitation experts and many others for the welfare of the patient.

Why, one may ask, must the surgeon concern himself with all this? Should not the job of coordination be left to the internist? In some cases the internist or general medical man can do a very good job of it. In other clinics, major shares of responsibility in preoperative and postoperative care are carried by anesthesiologists. Basically, however, a surgeon assumes the greatest responsibility for the patient when he operates on him. The responsibility as a rule is no less when he counsels against operation. The responsibility is of such a personal nature that it can hardly be escaped. Too often it involves life itself. A surgeon needs all the help he can get, but if things go badly when they need not go badly, the patient and the patient's family will hold him responsible, whether it be for his own acts or failure to act or for the performance of others involved in the case.

The division of responsibility between the medical man and the surgeon may be difficult. Usually, agreement is reached on diagnostic probabilities and on the indications for operation. Then it is generally best for the primary responsibility to shift to the surgeon during the operative and the postoperative periods. Thus, the surgeon is in the position of a consultant up to the immediate preoperative period—the internist then becomes a consultant, usually until the patient is well enough to leave the hospital. This policy is supported by a broad experience which indicates (probably without statistical proof) that the surgeon who follows his patient carefully before and after operation achieves better results than one who acts solely during the period of the operation itself.

Recently, a group of general surgeons became so alarmed by the development of subspecialties that they proposed a special organization partially to protect the general surgeon from the inroads of men in narrower fields. Already we have the vascular surgeon, the thoracic surgeon, the neurosurgeon, the gynecologist, the urologist, the plastic surgeon, the proctologist, etc. There is no way to predict how far this process may go. It is dependent on the size of medical units. Thus, a 100-bed hospital will do well to support men in 2 or 3 of these specialties. The 1,000-bed teaching hospital probably can support most of them. What then would be possible in a 10,000-bed hospital, if such came into being? Who can say that a man who devotes 90 per cent of his time to hernia cases might not gain experience and be able to evaluate methods that would permit him to excel in this field? Another might concentrate on abdominoperineal resections, another on gastric resections, et cetera.

It is obviously important that talent be on hand at operations to cope with unexpected findings and occurrences and especially to recognize things outside the narrowly specialized field. It is here that breadth of training appears to be an essential to safe surgery and safe medicine.

Therefore, young men entering surgery should avail themselves of broad training and education, even though they have definite plans for going into a highly specialized field.

OBLIGATIONS OF THE SURGEON BEYOND PATIENT CARE

The Oath of Hippocrates not only binds the physician to restrict his relations with patients to the care of illness or injury and to eschew social entanglements, particularly of a sexual character, but it also contains some less widely known provisions for the perpetuation of medical knowledge.

The physician was to care for his teacher as for a member of his own family and he was obligated to pass on his knowledge to the children of his teacher if they want to study medicine.

The practicing physician uses almost entirely knowledge that has been transferred to him, and he often receives payment for his services without much thought of his debt to the past. If he contributes nothing either to the transfer of old knowledge to those who must succeed him or to the discovery of new knowledge through experience or experiment, he is purely a parasite in his relations with his profession. He may still be a useful member of society as a purveyor of medical knowledge to the consumer, but he adds nothing to the continuity or progress of his profession.

The term "doctor" means teacher. The physician is expected to teach his patients things selected from his store of knowledge which will be of benefit to them. He should take time to do so.

He should also teach what he can to his younger colleagues and share with colleagues of all ages information which is of value for their patients. In this obligation which medicine has accepted from the time of Hippocrates it has set itself off from most fields of human endeavor where advantageous knowledge is too often restricted for the benefit of an individual, a corporation or some other special group.

While it is not given to every surgeon to make important new contributions to the science of surgery, it is the opportunity of nearly every surgeon to participate in the transfer of knowledge to others and especially to younger colleagues.

This habit may well begin in medical school and surely should be established during hospital training. As the individual becomes more senior he should still reserve time to do it, remembering that what he has to give them will be the more appreciated and often better remembered.

Such contributions by the surgeon, whether they be great or small, are not limited by place or type of practice. A practitioner in even the smallest community may be presented with the opportunity to make a contribution of consequence. Such an opportunity was presented to William Beaumont by the accident to his patient, Alexis St. Martin. This occurred under the most primitive conditions, yet the positive and persistent approach to the situation by Beaumont led to a truly great contribution to knowledge.

Particularly in surgery much depends on clinical experience. Through a proper transfer of knowledge, the experience of one surgeon may prevent others from making mistakes that cost the lives or impair the welfare of patients. When a surgeon or a physician speaks of his experience, he includes in the term knowledge which has come to him not only from his successful cases but also from his failures. Therefore, it is a serious obligation to pass on that which he has learned to the other members of his profession. This may be done by presenting case reports or analyses of series of cases to local or national medical societies and, if they prove to be of sufficient value, by publishing them in appropriate medical journals.

The further elucidation of clinical observations generally requires laboratory technics. The surgeon has certain peculiar advantages as an investigator which should be borne in mind. He is in intimate contact with patients and, if he is alert to the potentialities of modern laboratory methods, he is in a key position to see significant problems which are susceptible of solution. He may then be able to draw experts in the laboratory sciences into the study or to seek their advice in applying appropriate laboratory technics himself.

Furthermore, he has access to patients, and the decision of whether and when to try a new method or a new drug in these patients is frequently his. The moral issues raised by this situation are important ones. The obligation of the surgeon is primarily to his individual patient. He must not subject his patient to an unnecessary risk, even with the ultimate objective of benefiting thousands of other people, without full understanding by and consent of the patient. The availability of individuals clearly succumbing to disease, who have more to gain than to lose by the trial of something new, does much to bridge the gap which otherwise would exist between what is good for the individual and what is good for others. Here, as everywhere in surgery, the Golden Rule is the best guide to conduct.

These vistas broaden as the fields of organ transplantation evolve, for not only is the welfare of the recipient a matter of legal and ethical concern but so also is that of the donor. Formulations of firm guidelines in these and perhaps other areas, especially when nonpaired vital organs are to be transplanted, require agreement as to when the donor is dead, because the sooner the organ can be transplanted, the better the chance for its survival.

The surgeon alone has the opportunity of applying new operative technics. Furthermore, he has the unique opportunity of seeing and feeling internal lesions in the living patient. He also has certain opportunities to make physiologic observations at the time of operation and often to obtain biopsy material for histologic and biochemical study.

His technical skills open certain doors in animal experimentation, particularly where survival experiments are desirable. From the time of John Hunter (1728-1793) nearly all the great surgical investigators have leaned heavily on a variety of species of animals to try out their ideas and perfect their technics before applying them to man.

Surgery, like all medicine, is an applied science, and the greater portion of the investigative work done by surgeons will consist in so-called applied research. However, the surgical investigator should not be blind to the opportunities he has of contributing to basic knowledge either in the clinic or the laboratory, and a number of contributions to fundamental biologic information have come from surgeons. Furthermore, as Sir John Bruce has pointed out, Lister's demonstration of the value of antiseptics not only revolutionized clinical surgery but for the first time made survival experiments in animals practical. Thus a new technic of immense value in physiology, pharmacology and experimental pathology was made available. Other technics developed largely by surgeons, which have opened new possibilities in basic science, have been the heart-lung apparatus of Gibbon and long-term total parenteral alimentation (*see* Chap. 6).

It should be emphasized that in clinical investigation more is generally to be learned from the careful study of a few cases than from the more casual review of long series.

Studies of great scientific contributions have shown that the years from 25 to 35 are the most productive. In medicine this means that a man's best contributions are often made during his period of study and training.

Today the surgeon has an additional responsibility: engagement in the development of solutions to the problem of distribution of medical care to all segments of the population. With the growth of specialization, medical care has become concentrated in large urban communities, and in rural America the population to physician ratio has steadily risen, often to impossible heights. For example, in urban Michigan there is one physician to about 800 people; in rural upper Michigan, one to 2,000—and steadily getting worse.

THE ART OF SURGERY

In one's pursuit of science in surgery one must not become oblivious to the fact that surgery is an art as well as a science. The art is thought of often as the manual dexterity which a surgeon must possess or acquire to do his work. This is a very important aspect but not the whole of it. It also includes much of the decision-making process which goes on constantly at the operating table. Differing degrees of skill in this field account for one man frittering away time on unimportant minutiae while another man abridges a procedure at the expense of thoroughness, and a third man strikes a proper balance by taking time to do what is important thoroughly, without wasting it to achieve perfection in minutiae that are meaningless for the welfare of the particular patient.

A third and important aspect of the art of surgery lies in the field of talking to patients and their families. This is a most complicated art. What is said should depend on a host of perceptions of the patient's fears, of his doubts, of his past relationships with the surgeon and with other doctors. It is colored by the seriousness of the illness and the obstacles in the mind of the patient in the way of accepting treatment. It is necessarily colored by the surgeon's age, how well known he is in the community and how he is regarded in the patient's mind. The same surgeon at 30 may need a 10-minute exposition of facts to create the same degree of acceptance for a needed cholecystectomy that he could convey to the patient 20 years later in a sentence or two. Success in this field is again partly native ability and partly acquired skill.

One of the most important prerequisites to success in acquiring this skill is a strong enough desire for such skill to make one strive continuously to improve it. One must spend time in listening to patients and to their relatives and in trying to perceive and to understand their reactions. Considerable native modesty and a strong liking for people are most helpful. It is also extremely important to know something of one's self. When one's inner hackles rise in irritation or anger it is time to turn one's attention inward and to try to understand the why and the wherefore before giving vent to such feelings in remarks to the patient. While this brief discussion of the art of surgery is far from complete, perhaps it will convey some concept of what is involved.

Finally, if the surgeon is to do his utmost to advance his profession, he should endeavor to make opportunities for his younger colleagues to develop. This may require some self-denial on his part, some risk of being superseded in this field or that. If he is convinced that he is backing able and rightly motivated younger men, he should make some sacrifices and accept these risks.

OPPORTUNITIES FOR SURGICAL TRAINING

One purpose of setting forth our views about the obligations of surgeons in a textbook planned primarily for medical students is to provide a background for certain comments about the selection of training by those who contemplate specializing in this field.

How does one become a surgeon? How does he know a good residency opportunity from a poor one? If possible, select a medical school where the surgical department is interested in research as well as in teaching. If possible, obtain an internship in the best teaching hospital you can—be it medical, rotating or surgical in nature. Criteria that have proved useful in estimating the value of a hospital for internship are the following:

Ordinarily, the intern should have major

responsibility in writing the orders for the patient's care. Rounds should be made regularly by the visiting staff with the house officers.

Do your utmost to be helpful on your hospital assignments. The unpopular assignments are often the ones where good performance will stand out most and be most appreciated.

So far as possible, steer clear of those institutions where the house is divided against itself but try to get an assistant residency in a teaching hospital. Most men are happier in a residency system that does not require progressive elimination of the fit by the more fit. The old pyramidal system which eliminates men at the end of each year may lead to competition but at the same time is apt to produce poor working relationships and bitter disappointments.

It is a good rule during one's training period, as well as in the years that follow, to participate in at least one good scientific society meeting each year.

Finally, measure your chiefs by the standards discussed above. One who takes not only an interest but an active responsibility in helping his men another step up the ladder and has been successful in doing so generally affords a much better association than a man of the "take you and leave you" type, no matter how brilliant.

It is often said that those who can, do and those who can't, teach. The basic criticism is one from which surgery has so far nearly escaped. The teachers of surgery are nearly always selected from highly competent performers, and many of the best performers in surgery play key roles in teaching. Pressures have been increasing to change this pattern by selecting for teaching appointments men whose clinical finesse is attested only by board certification and whose claim to distinction is largely in related fields. We believe that the student desiring to enter surgery in general does well to seek out a department that is distinguished for its performance in clinical surgery as well as for its research contributions.

Monetary advantages during the training period should not be given primary consideration. It is usually wiser to emerge from a first-class training program in debt than to avoid the debt by accepting less than the best training opportunities for which one can qualify.

THE PLACE OF THE HEALING ARTS IN SOCIETY

Today the healing arts are the subject of close scrutiny by government officials and by the rank and file of voters. There are proponents and opponents of so-called "socialized medicine." The terminology employed by its proponents has placed those who are opposed to state or corporation controlled medical care in the position of being considered antisocial. Nothing could be further from the truth. No matter how it is practiced, medicine and its branches are basically social in their attitudes. Medicine is for society—not for society as an organization but for each and every individual composing it. Thus, we would not want medical care used as a tool of the state—for instance, to be turned off or on for political minorities; but there is never any question that the job of the doctor is to help the sick and the injured and this he must do whatever the framework in which he practices.

A considerable degree of independence of thought, judgment and action must be the surgeon's if he is to perform his essential functions. This independence may be threatened in the future by economic pressures, and we shall have to depend on those in the profession who will put patient welfare ahead of financial security or so-called professional advancement to demonstrate the value to the patient of such independence and thereby guard against the dangers of any systems which would suppress it.

The doctors of the past often were paid little or not at all. The doctors of the present are required to perform a major tax-collecting job for the Federal Government, and the doctors of the future may be, for the most part, salaried civil servants. Despite the overtones of the last designation, the relationship of the physician to his patient can still probably be about as good as the doctor makes it, provided that he does not start "taking his profit in leisure."

Future events seldom develop in exactly the way one foresees, and it is the judgment of the editors that the possibility of changes in medical organization should not deter any rightly motivated young man from going into surgery.

THE EFFECT OF DECREASING AVAILABILITY OF THE PRIMARY PHYSICIAN ON THE NEED OF THE SPECIALIST FOR BREADTH OF MEDICAL KNOWLEDGE

Some of the factors which have tended to decrease the availability of the primary physicians were discussed by one of us a few years ago in the Journal of Medical Education.* They include: the growth in the population; the slow growth in the numbers of graduates from medical schools; the greater attraction of other fields of graduate education due, in part, to subsidization in the form of graduate fellowships; the sharp increase in intramural "residency" positions in large centers; the demands of the military services; the growth of full time faculties which devote major time and energy to research; and the decreasing willingness of physicians to work very long hours in a society working 40 hours a week or less. All of these factors and others appear to have reduced the *night* doctor/patient ratio very seriously—that is, the number of physicians who will respond at night to a sudden patient need, particularly if that need is undefined.

The effect of this trend is most keenly felt in rural and sylvan communities and in city slums. One of us (C. M.) has studied this situation at first hand in upper Michigan since 1965. The paucity of physicians practicing in the slums and in rural and sylvan communities of this nation leaves millions of inhabitants without primary medical care. This is exemplified by what has happened along Highway M28 in upper Michigan. Forty years ago, four physicians practiced in four of the five villages located along 40 miles of this highway. Now there is no physician in any of these hamlets. The doctor's office nearest the 7,600 people living in these communities today is between 25 and 50 miles away. One may say, "That is not far in an automobile, they can get to a doctor 50 miles away more quickly today than they could get to one 5 miles away 40 years ago." All well and good, but—can they get a doctor when they get there—wherever it might be? Surrounding them are small cities located on or near the shoreline of Lake Superior, in which there are now only 43 grossly overworked, one might say overwhelmed, physicians serving more than 90,000 inhabitants. Among this medical service body there is *not one* internist, pediatrician, anesthesiologist, obstetrician, gynecologist, urologist or neurologist. Under such circumstances the surgeon's relationship to the internist, pediatrician, and anesthesiologist is inconsequential and his medical responsibilities to the community become vastly broadened.

Not only is there a dearth of specialists but there is a relative lack of generalists. In such a situation much can be salvaged if those specialists who do practice in the area are broadly knowledgeable in medicine as a whole and able to recognize pathology outside of their own fields and to help the patient to get the care essential to his needs.

While the dearth of specialists does not occur in our medical centers, even in these localities there is a dearth of generalists or primary physicians. This is reflected in an increasing demand for self-referred initial appointments in the offices of surgeons in the big cities. Those specialists who insist on a physician referral often obtain them only to find that no true doctor-patient relationship exists between the overworked practitioner who has lent his name to the referral and the patient in question.

Thus, in a day of progressive specialization of knowledge and skills, there is a rising pressure from the public for broad competence and understanding of disease. Those who would prepare themselves to take care of patients should take this trend into consideration during their course work and training periods, especially if they would serve in the geographic areas of greatest need.

* Rhoads, J. E.: J. Med. Ed., 36(12) P-12:171, 1961.

CHAPTER 2

HENRY N. HARKINS,* M.D.

Wound Healing†

A thorough knowledge of wound healing will lead to a more intelligent practice of our art as well as to greater perfection in it.—MONT REID.

Introduction
Historical
Types of Healing
Physiology of Wound Healing
General Factors in Wound Healing
Local Factors in Wound Healing
Technical Factors in Wound Healing
Healing of Special Tissues
New Developments in the Study of Wound Healing

INTRODUCTION

A knowledge of wound healing is the central core of the science of surgery; in fact, surgery is dependent upon wound healing for its very existence.

The healing of a wound is a wondrously complex thing. It includes: (1) the awakening of mitotic activity and ameboid motion of basal epithelial cells and their manufacturing of an ordered sulfide-bridged macromolecular system that is impervious to water, gases and ions—the keratin layer; (2) the reactivation of inactive fibroblasts in proximity to the wound, their proliferation in the vicinity of the wound, and their production of monomer collagen and important components of ground substance, such as the acid polysaccharides; (3) the extracellular polymerization of proto or monomer collagen and the arrangement of the collagen so formed into an intricate reticular system of fibrils and fibers; and (4) the cessation of all of these processes when tissue continuity has been re-established, in which process cellular contact inhibition seemingly plays a very important role.

HISTORICAL

The history of the study of wounds is indeed the history of surgery itself. A well-known incident is when Ambroïse Paré (1510-1590), one of the greatest army surgeons of all time, ran out of the boiling oil then used to treat battle wounds. He had to treat the wounds without it and was satisfied with the results. This was an important turning point in surgical history. Paré's appreciation of the principle of avoiding harmful interference with natural forces is epitomized by the inscription on his statue: *"Je le pansay, Dieu le guarist"* (I treated him, God healed him).

Many of the major contributions of William S. Halsted (1852-1922) had to do with wound healing. In more recent times the contributions of Harvey (1929) and of Howes and Harvey (1935) are important.

TYPES OF HEALING

Healing of wounds can be divided into 3 types (Fig. 2-1): (1) Healing by *first intention* (*per primam intensionem: primary union*). This involves healing of an aseptic, accurately closed, incised wound. In instances of primary union granulation tissue approaches the irreducible minimum. (2) Healing by *second intention* (*granulation*). This involves a defect which is first covered by granulation tissue and then closed by contraction and with secondary ingrowth of epithelium. Another way of stating this is that healing occurs by granulation in wounds where primary union fails

* Deceased.
† Revised by J. E. Rhoads and Carl A. Moyer.

A. FIRST INTENTION (Primary union)

1. Clean incision
2. Early suture
3. "Hairline" scar

B. SECOND INTENTION (Granulation)

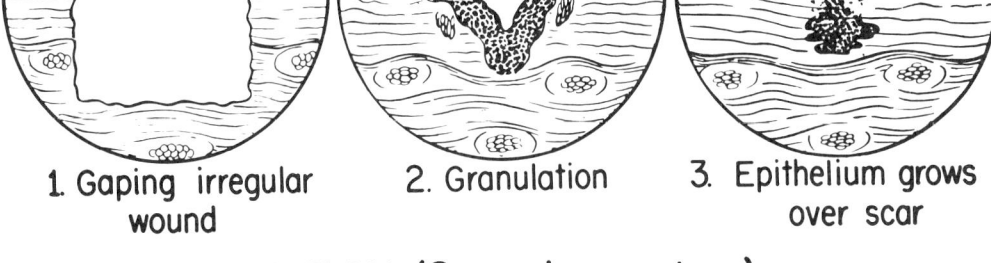

1. Gaping irregular wound
2. Granulation
3. Epithelium grows over scar

C. THIRD INTENTION (Secondary suture)

1. Wound
2. Granulation
3. Closure with wide scar

FIG. 2-1. Chronologic course of wound healing by first, second and third intention. In the final stage of second-intention healing it is to be noted that the underside of the epithelium is smooth and not serrated as normally. In the healing by second intention, the important role of contraction, which occurs in the patient in 3 dimensions and in the illustrations (B-2 and B-3) in 2, is shown. Contraction also plays a role in third-intention healing (C-2 and C-3). According to Gillman, Penn, Bronks and Roux (1955), the skin islands shown under the epithelium in B-2 and C-2 are typical of this phase of early healing. In C-3 an early phase is shown. Later the granulation tissue will be incorporated as a wide fibrous scar.

because of excessive trauma or tissue loss, infection, or because the wound surfaces have not been brought together. An example is a third-degree burn which heals without grafting. The concept of Gillman, Penn, Bronks and Roux (1955) is to be considered—that in the healing of wounds by second intention (Fig. 2-1-B) the epithelium plays a greater role in the early stages than according to the classic concept. (3) Healing by *third intention (secondary suture)*. If a deep wound has either not been sutured primarily, or later breaks down and then is sutured or resutured several days later when granulations are present, two apposing granulating surfaces are brought together. The result is a wider and deeper scar than is the case with healing by first intention. Examples are wounds that are deliberately left open for 4 or 5 days before secondary suture (see Chap. 25, Military Surgery) or the secondary suture of a dehisced wound.

In discussing the different types of healing, one must consider the effect of the character of the wound. The healing of a superficial or flat wound such as an abrasion, superficial burn or irradiation injury involves, in the main, regeneration of the epithelium and the keratin layer of the skin without granulation. The closed incised wound heals with little granulation and little epithelial regeneration. The healing of any open wound such as a laceration, avulsion, deep burn, or open fracture devolves importantly upon three processes: (1) epithelial proliferation; (2) granulation, including collagen production; and (3) wound contraction. The amount of eventual scar is a direct function of the amount of *collagen* that is formed during healing.

PHYSIOLOGY OF WOUND HEALING

The various responses elicited by a wound present a complicated yet orderly sequence of events. The relative intensity and duration of the different phases in this sequence depend on the type of wound, the presence or the absence of infection, and whether healing is by first, second or third intention. Recent reviews of the physiology of wound healing include those of van den Brenk (1956), Gillman and Penn (1956), Jackson (1958), Cuthbertson (1959), Connell and Rousselot (1959), Hoover and Ivins (1959), Jacob and Houck (1959), McMinn (1960), Dunphy (1960), and Van Winkle (1967).

Phase 1. Initial Productive or Substrate Phase (about 5 days). This phase is also termed the lag, autolytic, catabolic or inflammatory phase. During this phase there is an outpouring of tissue fluids, accumulation of leukocytes and mast cells, and an ingrowth of capillary buds and fibroblasts, and the pH of the wound drops to acidic levels. The fibroblasts arise predominantly by proliferation of locally resident connective tissue cells, rather than from precursor cells recruited from the blood stream (Grillo and Potsaid, 1961; Grillo, 1963). Hadfield (1963) pinpoints this origin to perivascular sheaths, with the corollary that vascularity and supply of fibroblasts are directly related. Damaged cells are catabolized. During this phase the coapted tissues can be separated with little force. During the later part of this phase, as Dunphy and Udupa (1955), and Shetlar, Lacefield, White and Schilling (1959) have shown, there is a rapid increase in hexosamine content of the wound and of other positive signs of the presence of acid polysaccharides. The relationships between adenosine 5-metaphosphate hexosamine, methionine and mucopolysaccharides has been discussed by Udupa, Woessner and Dunphy (1956), Edwards and Udupa (1957), and Reynolds, Codington and Buxton (1958). Metachromasia reaches a peak about the 5th or 6th day when the first chemical and histologic evidence of collagen fibers develops (Fig. 2-2).

Menkin (1940, 1950) has studied the first or "inflammatory" phase of wounds from the standpoint of substances produced by injured cells. These can be *summarized* as follows:

1. Leukotaxine: A substance that increases the permeability of capillary walls and causes diapedesis of leukocytes. This substance differs from histamine in that it does not cause a fall in general blood pressure. (Kátó and Gözsy, 1956. Kahlson, Nilsson, Rosengren and Zederfeldt, 1960, have reported on wound healing as dependent on the rate of histamine formation.)

2. Leukocytosis-promoting factors (thermolabile and thermostable components) (LPF)

3. Necrosin

4. Pyrexin

5. Leukopenic factors (leukopenin and the leukopenic factor)
6. Glucose
7. Possibly a growth-promoting factor

Menkin studied these different factors and separated them into discrete, although not chemically pure, fractions. The number of these substances indicates the complexity of the inflammatory process. This complexity is attested by the multiple symptomatology, so well expressed by Celsus (25 B.C.-A.D. 45): *"Notae vero inflammationis sunt quatuor: rubor et tumor, cum calore et dolore."*

Phase 2. Collagen or Second Phase (from about the 6th day until healing is complete). This phase is also called the proliferative or anabolic phase. As collagen forms there is a prompt decline in metachromasia (a histochemical test for the free sulfate groups attached to the polysaccharides) and in hexosamine content of the wound. At the same time there is a parallel rise in collagen content and tensile strength of the wound.

Dunphy and Udupa have reported an alteration in these chemical changes in scorbutic guinea pigs. In such instances the productive phase is greatly extended, and there is no collagen phase. The concentration of mucopolysaccharides rises progressively, reaching levels per gram of tissue by the 12th to the 14th day far in excess of that observed in normal wounds about the 5th day. That this material is abnormal is evidenced by the fact that it does not stain metachromatically. These authors concluded:

It appears that in ascorbic acid deficiency the building blocks of wound healing are produced plentifully in the productive phase, but an important key to synthesis of collagen is lacking.

This key has been somewhat defined by Ross and Benditt (1961 and 1964) among others. In the absence of vitamin C monomer collagen is not secreted by the fibroblast and the ribosomes of the wound fibroblasts are not in their normal paired order. In other words, scurvy evidently interrupts intracellular collagen synthesis at the ribosomal level.

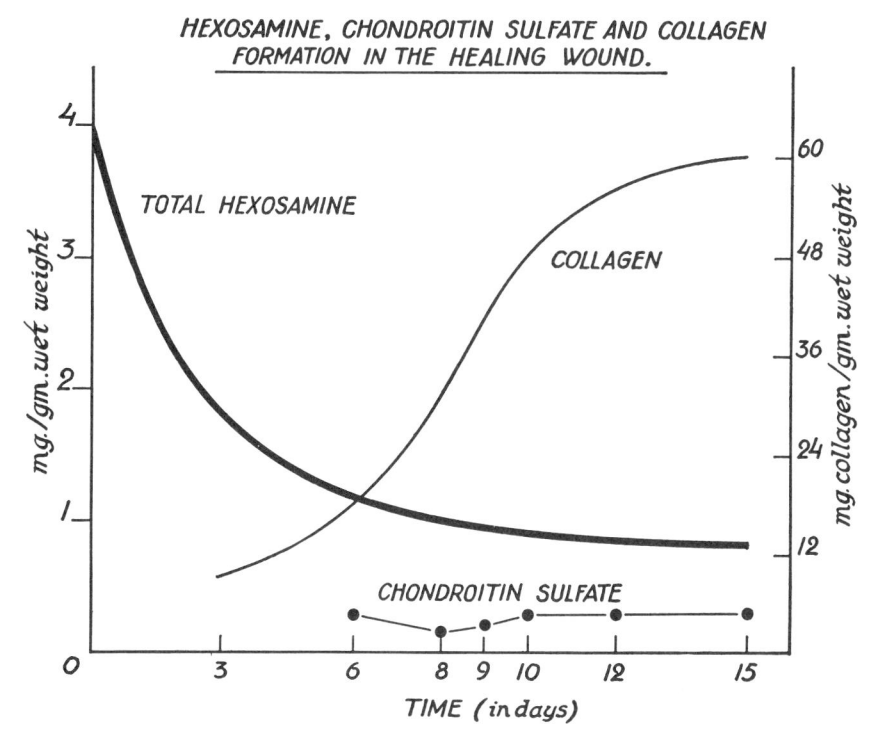

Fig. 2-2. Relative chemical composition of the healing wound with reference to (1) hexosamines; (2) the specific mucopolysaccharide, chondroitin sulfate; and (3) collagen. (Dunphy, J. E.: Ann. Roy. Coll. Surg. Eng., 26:82)

The role of the fibroblast in wound healing has recently been reviewed by Van Winkle (1967).

In the literature the experimental evidence indicating the need for ascorbic acid is consistent except in regard to the site of action.

Thompson, Ravdin and Frank found significant delay in the healing rate of test wounds in dogs prepared by a low protein diet and plasmaphoresis. These animals were severely hypoproteinemic.

In contrast with this, Andrews, Morgan and Jurkiewicz (1956) did not find much of a change.

In dogs rendered hypoproteinemic by the same technic as that used by Thompson, Ravdin and Frank (1938), Rhoads, Fliegelman and Panzer (1942) found that wound healing proceeded normally if gum acacia was given intravenously on the day the test wound was made, suggesting that the interference was related to the edema factor rather than a matter of "protein building blocks."

This hypothesis is supported by studies of proto or monomer collagen and collagen. It is known that the monomer collagen fibers are salt-linked to form collagen. Studies of Schiller bands and Liesegang rings in the ground substance of healing wounds indicate that collagen is laid down in ground substance in which the cations line up in layers and the anions (chloride) line up in other layers. The distance from one anion layer to the next is about 20,000 Å, the distance between one cation band and the next is about the same. These observations suggest that ordered ionic concentrational separations in the ground substance of cations from anions might well be the factor determining polymerization of monomer collagen and the organization of collagen fibrils and fibers into coordinate systems such as dermis, tendon, etc.

These bands and rings are well developed in human healing wounds and young scars, and in smooth scars the arrangement is regular. On the other hand, in fresh hypertrophic scars some of which become keloids the band arrangements are random—that is, they are skewed with respect to each other and not parallel.

In longitudinal wounds made immediately medial to the knee joint, thick scars usually develop. Samples of these have shown disturbance of the pattern of the bands and their corresponding collagen fibrils.

This organization of collagen takes place outside of the cell and must obey physical laws, the genetic laws ceasing to operate at the point at which the protocollagen is extruded from the cell.

It seems likely that edema fluid could interfere with this physical process and prevent the normal and orderly organization of the collagen on which the strength of the wound depends.

Thus, it is probable that mild to moderate hypoproteinemia need not interfere with wound healing, whereas hypoproteinemia of a degree which permits edema can be a very adverse factor.

GENERAL FACTORS IN WOUND HEALING

There are both general and local influences which affect the healing of a wound. At one extreme is a clean sharp laceration of the skin of the face in a healthy young adult; at the other is a dirty ragged wound of the foot in an elderly diabetic with poor circulation and nutrition. Between these two extremes many factors determine the course of healing. These will now be considered under the separate headings of general and local factors in wound healing, realizing, of course, that to some extent these factors overlap. Also, it should be recognized that the normal rate of healing in a perfectly healthy patient is the optimum rate that can be attained. There is no known method by which healing can be forced beyond this normal rate (Zintel, 1946). Efforts to accelerate healing beyond the normal rate have been generally unavailing at the clinical level (Zintel, 1946). Some acceleration has been reported with the use of "royal jelly," and recently Hunt and Dunphy* reported acceleration for open wounds in the rat by use of a 45 to 50 per cent oxygen environment.

The normal rate of healing of an open wound is a single valued function of the natural logarithm of the perimeter (Andrews, Morgan and Jurkiewicz, 1956). The slope of

---

* Hunt, T. K., and Dunphy, J. E.: Personal communication, 1969.

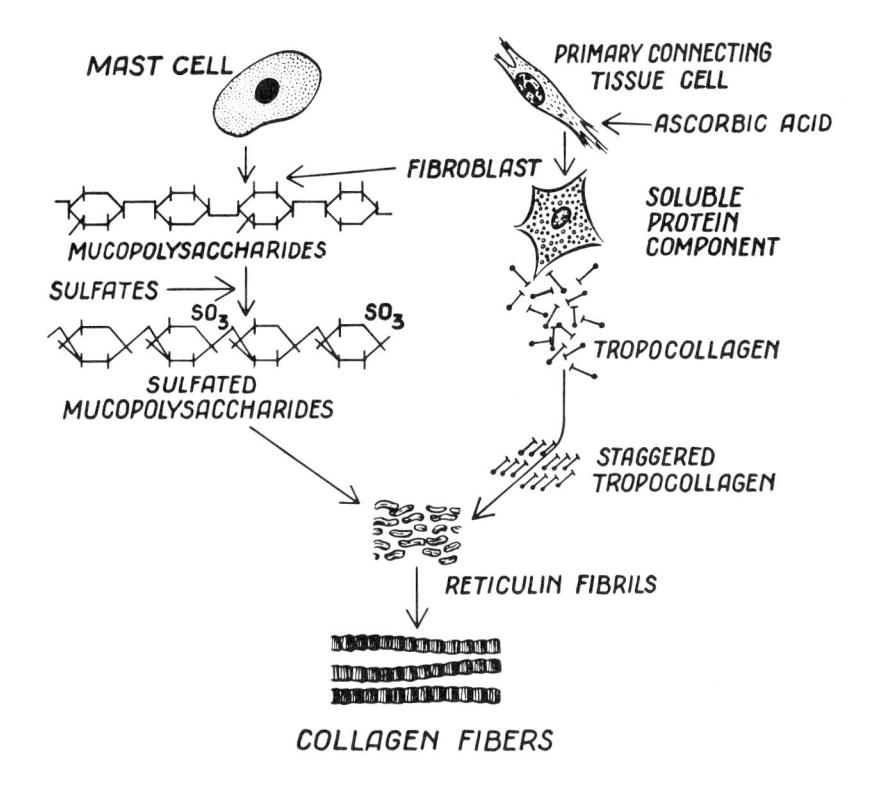

FIG. 2-3. A hypothetical model of some of the factors which contribute to the formation of collagen in the healing wound. (Adapted from Dunphy.)

the curve is steeper with excisions or avulsions than it is with burn wounds. In their experiments the rate of healing of a particular type of wound appeared to be all-or-none. With infection or severe ascorbic acid deficit (scurvy) the slope of the healing curve was zero; with the termination of the infection or ascorbic acid deficiency the normal healing slope for the particular wound was attained immediately.

Recent studies relating to an early accelerating effect of *parenterally* administered cartilage extracts in rats (Prudden, Gabriel and Allen, 1963), to a very slight but statistically significant accelerating effect of *locally* applied cartilage powder on granulating wounds in rats (Sabo, Oberlander and Enquist, 1964) and orally administered zinc salts (Pories *et al.*, 1967) may seem to dispute this "negativistic" view. However, many other "wound-accelerating" substances have been reported over the past 30 years, only to fade into oblivion. The philosophical question arises as to whether any control healing rate, e.g., exposure to room air, no matter how scientifically contrived, truly represents "normality" in the sense used by Zintel.

Table 2-1 summarizes the effects of general factors on wound healing.

In summary, besides ascorbic acid deficit (scurvy) and rare genetic blood coagulation defects, the influences of general factors on wound healing are relatively inconsequential to the surgery of man, notwithstanding all of the varied claims to the contrary made during the earlier decades of the twentieth century. It might be said that, given twenty days of life, as long as the man has not scurvy the wound will heal if it be properly closed and uninfected, regardless of the general condition

Wound Healing

TABLE 2-1. GENERAL FACTORS IN WOUND HEALING

Vitamins	C (*ascorbic acid*)	*Absolutely essential to wound healing. No collagen production at scorbutic levels*
	Fat soluble	No demonstrable effect of deficits
	B complex	No demonstrable effect of deficits, possibly excepting wet beriberi.
Genetic factors	Genetic coagulation defects	Slow healing with hemophilia and lack of factor 13. Slow and abnormal healing with Danlos's syndrome.
Anemia		No significant influence per se down to Hb levels of 4.0 Gm.% and lower in congenital hemolytic, chronic secondary (blood loss) anemias and large burns.
Protein deficiency		*No demonstrable effects* on rate of epithelialization or wound contraction With severe deficits, serum albumin below 1.5 Gm.% or less, induced by plasmapheresis and starvation, gain in wound strength and regeneration of parenchymatous organs such as the liver is slowed or stopped.
Amino acid deficits		No fully established influences on healing of wounds in man as yet demonstrated. Lack of sulfur-containing amino acids in the diet slows gain of tensile strength in wounds of hairy animals and fowl.
Age		In old age rate of gain of tensile strength may be slower than in youth; fractures heal slower in the aged.
Endocrine		No established effects on wound healing.
Minerals		Zinc deficit may slow wound contraction.
Chronic diseases		Active rheumatoid arthritis, lupus erythematosus, myositis ossificans, periarteritis nodosa, thromboangiitis obliterans are considered to interfere with wound healing on clinical grounds.

of the patient. The local factors over which the surgeon has immediate control are the important ones from the standpoint of wound healing. If an attended wound fails to heal, it should be ascribed to local factors rather than to general ones, provided that scurvy and rare blood dyscrasias and severe starvation and protein deficiency are all ruled out.

LOCAL FACTORS IN WOUND HEALING

Vascularity

All of the physicochemical factors in wound healing depend on an adequate, even increased, blood supply. Weiber (1964) has studied the vascularization of healing wounds in experimental animals with radioactive ^{24}Na. His observations indicate that vascularization progresses successively during the first 5 days, i.e., during the so-called lag period, and then gradually decreases but is still 50 per cent higher than in intact tissue as late as on the 13th day.

Clearly there can be *no wound healing in the absence of blood flow*. No cell can grow and work without food. In the care and closure of any wound all measures to ensure blood flow to the wound wall are the sine qua non of wound surgery. These are: (1) Effect hemostasis by closing the bleeding vessel without including other tissue in the ligature or fulguration. (2) Do not undercut skin within 3 to 5 mm. of the undersurface of the dermis. (3) Coapt without tension. (4) Should an encircling bandage be needed to dress the wound it must be elastic and the pressure it exerts on the wound should not cause capillary blanching or distal venous stasis. (5) Do not closely shave the areolar tissue from fascial layers such as the rectus sheath, fascia of the external oblique, etc., blood flow to the overlying tissue would be cut.

Pressure and Tension

Pressure and tension upon a wound must be minimal for best healing. They interfere with blood flow to the wound wall and in addition are capable of altering the chemical organization of collagen and disrupting lymph flow.

Distraction and Interposition

Distraction of wound walls by fluid (serum), blood clots (hematoma), or foreign bodies such as large pieces of gel foam increases the time requisite for collagen bridging between opposing wound walls and increases the probability of wound infection. Meticulous hemostasis and apposition of wound walls by suture and avoidance of the use of masses of hemostatic crutches are the essentials for avoiding distraction.

Infection

It can truly be said that nothing but devascularization is as inimical to wound healing as is infection. No infected wound heals at all! The only way to prevent infection is to keep bacteria out of the wound or remove them if they are there—aseptic technics and débridement are the bases of the prevention of infection. The parenteral administration of a wide spectrum bacteriocidal antibiotic such as cephalothin (Keflin) during débridement and closure of wounds and for one to three days after closure appears to be effective in preventing invasive infections.

Trauma

A cleanly cut incised wound will heal more rapidly (healing by first intention) than an irregular ragged undébrided wound (healing by second or third intention). Similarly, an operative wound with much traumatic damage due to rough handling of tissues, prolonged pressure and tearing action of retractors, mass ligatures with large necrotic portions of tissue distal to the ligature, numerous plugs of necrotic tissue from electrocoagulation ("the tombstones of the coagulator"—Stevenson and Reid, 1947) will not "heal kindly." This necrotic tissue must be destroyed before final wound healing is accomplished, as in a bombed city the rubble must be hauled away before rebuilding can be completed. The catabolic and destructive phase of the inflammatory process is exaggerated with prolongation of the initial "lag" period before the collagen or anabolic and proliferative phase of wound healing can take over, even though these two phases of wound healing can overlap to some extent. As a consequence, even in the absence of infection, local edema and serum production and possibly a general febrile reaction are more apt to occur. Furthermore, the necrotic tissue itself, as well as the local reaction it produces, affords a highly favorable environment for the proliferation of bacteria which are present in essentially all wounds.

Suture Material

The suture materials most commonly used include plain catgut, chromic catgut, silk, cotton, nylon and steel wire. Steel wire has the objections that it is difficult to handle and is difficult to remove if an incision has to be reopened but it has the advantage that in infected wounds it not only maintains the integrity of the wound as well as or better than silk but also is seldom extruded. Catgut, silk and cotton, and nylon and tantalum and steel wire form a spectrum in this particular order. Plain catgut is the most rapidly absorbed, which is advantageous in some respects (if it is not accomplished before Phase 3 of the general metabolic response to injury, see above), but at the same time it produces the most reaction. Tantalum and steel are imbedded in the tissues forever but at the same time produce the least reaction.

The studies of Postlethwait, Schauble, Dillon and Morgan (1959) on plain and chromic catgut, silk, cotton, wire, nylon, Ramie, Nymo, Dacron and Teflon considered not only tissue reaction, tensile strength of the wound and tensile strength of the knot but also fraying tendency of the thread. Teflon received a high rating except from the standpoint of fraying, while Dacron's main shortcoming was the tendency of its knots to slip.

Certain suture materials may produce sensitivity reactions. This complication is most common with catgut (Kraissl, Kesten and Cimiotti, 1938) and nylon.

While proper recognition should be given to the tissue factors in wound healing as supplying *strength* to the wound, the obvious but often neglected importance of the *sutures themselves* should not be forgotten in this regard. Adamsons and Enquist (1963) quantitated these two items in guinea pigs. Up to 45 days postincision, all wounds were stronger with the sutures in place than with the sutures removed, but the difference in tensile strength became progressively less. Also, the wound with sutures in place became as strong as the unwounded controls by the 9th day and exceeded them thereafter. The wound with sutures removed was 80 per cent as strong as unwounded tissue by the 9th day and even stronger than unwounded tissue by the 45th day. In scorbutic animals the relative importance of the sutures at a given day was even greater.

The role of suture materials in the development of wound infection has been recently studied by Alexander, Kaplan and Altemeier (1967). Monofilament suture of any type is superior to multifilament sutures of any type in contaminated wounds. They concluded that only multifilament sutures and plain catgut are unsuitable for closing contaminated wounds.

Antiseptics and Chemicals

Antiseptics and chemicals may destroy bacteria but also tend to injure the body cells lining the wound. With their injudicious use, not only is wound healing impaired but also infection may be more apt to occur.

Farhat, Miller and Musselman (1959) and Rath and Enquist (1959) reported that triethylenethiophosphoramide (Thio-TEPA) does not delay wound healing in cats. On the other hand, Farhat, Amer, Weeks and Musselman (1958) found that mechlorethamine hydrochloride (nitrogen mustard) did interfere with such healing, but possibly no more than did the accompanying malnutrition induced by administration of the drug.

Foreign Bodies

Aside from sutures, it is now fashionable, particularly in orthopedic and vascular surgery, but to some extent in all branches of the art, to place a variety of foreign bodies in the tissues. Largely because of the pioneer work of Venable, Stuck and Beach (1937) who introduced vitallium, an alloy which is essentially nonreactive in the body, these foreign bodies (vitallium, stainless steel, nylon, Orlon, Vinyon "N," Teflon, Dacron, Ivalon, Lucite, Marlex—Usher and Wallace, 1958—etc.) do not produce much foreign body reaction, but they still are to be used with caution. Pieces of dead bone, tendon, muscle, and detached portions of intestine with mucous membrane are gross examples of *autogenous* foreign bodies that should not be purposelessly left in wounds.

One type of foreign body which caused considerable reaction in many wounds until about 1950, when its use was discontinued, is talcum (hydrous magnesium silicate). Talcum was used to facilitate putting on sterile rubber gloves. It entered into wounds not only from the outside of the gloves but also from frequent puncture of a finger of the gloves. Then the sweat-talc suspension in the glove finger would leak into the wound. Talcum leads to granuloma formation, as first described by Antopol (1933). The talc, being relatively insoluble, remains in the tissues almost indefinitely and is recognized by double refractility with polarized light.

Even though talcum is no longer used for surgical gloves, the late results of talc granulomata are still coming to hospitals throughout the country for fistulas, chronic sinus tracts and especially intestinal obstruction associated with intestinal adhesions.

To obviate the dangers of talc granulomata, a treated powder derived from corn starch, Biosorb®, was introduced. At first it was believed that this would entirely eliminate foreign-body reactions. More recent reports of starch granulomas have shown that there is still a danger of foreign-body granulomata, even with the use of starch powders (Lee, Collins and Largen, 1952; Wise, 1955; Sneierson and Woo, 1955; McAdams, 1956; Hyden and McClellan, 1959; and Radke, Nyhus and Bell, 1961. Wise summarized his experiments in this regard as follows:

The starch caused less scarring and cellular reaction than talc, but more than occurred in controls in which no powder was used. In these experiments, starch was still visible in tissue sections 60 days after operation. Starch glove powder is preferable to talc, but is not entirely innocuous, and should be used as sparingly as possible. The surgeon should use as little powder as possible on his hands, and wash off all powder from rubber gloves before starting to operate.

This knowledge of the effect of foreign bodies, such as talcum or starch, on wound healing is the basis for the recommendations concerning washing of powder off surgical gloves (p. 280, Chap. 14, Operative Surgical Care).

TECHNICAL FACTORS IN WOUND HEALING

Such factors are largely related to the local factors discussed above but are also dependent on the technical aims of the operation and on the general condition of the patient. The technic should be selected with a proper judgment as to the entire situation involved and not with a consideration of only one factor. Thus, drainage of joints must be decided upon not only from the standpoint of permitting blood to escape but also from that of the dangers of allowing infection to get in.

INCISIONS

A properly planned incision is fundamental to the performance of any surgical operation. From the practical standpoint a balance must be obtained between the desire to make a wound that will heal as soon as possible and at the same time one that will permit as ready access to the place of operation as possible. Generally speaking, surgical incisions are more often made too short than too long. The statement that a wound heals crosswise rather than lengthwise is true to a large degree. At the same time, an unnecessarily long incision involves more general trauma to the patient and more operative time is consumed in its closure.

Incisions on the surface of the body should be planned to follow certain dynamic "wrinkle lines" on the skin. As Kraissl (1951) pointed out, these lines are in many parts of the body at variance with "Langer's lines" (1861) with which they are often confused. Langer's lines are the result of a study of the static forces acting on the puncture wounds of the skin of a cadaver, whereas the wrinkle lines are produced by the dynamic forces acting on the skin of a living person. In general, the wrinkle lines run perpendicular to the action of the underlying muscles upon which they are dependent for their formation. Kraissl also pointed out that scars may become adherent to the underlying tissue and consequently they will interfere least with body mechanics if placed transversely across muscles and joints in the wrinkle lines. The scar then simply

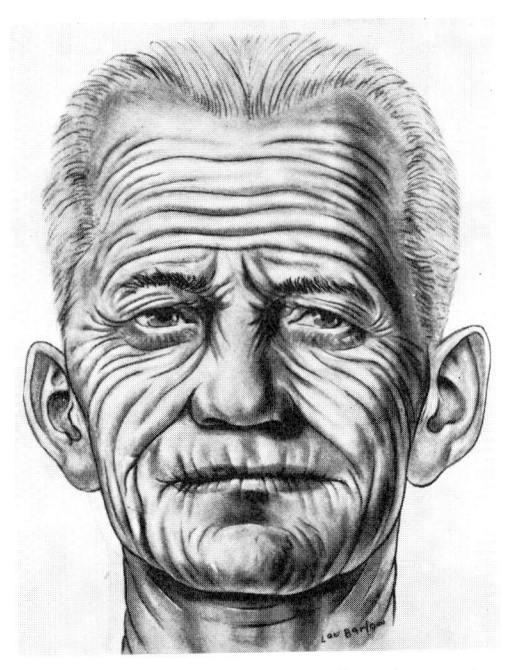

Fig. 2-4. Exaggerated drawing of normal face wrinkles. (Kraissl, C. J.: Plast. Reconstr. Surg., 8:5)

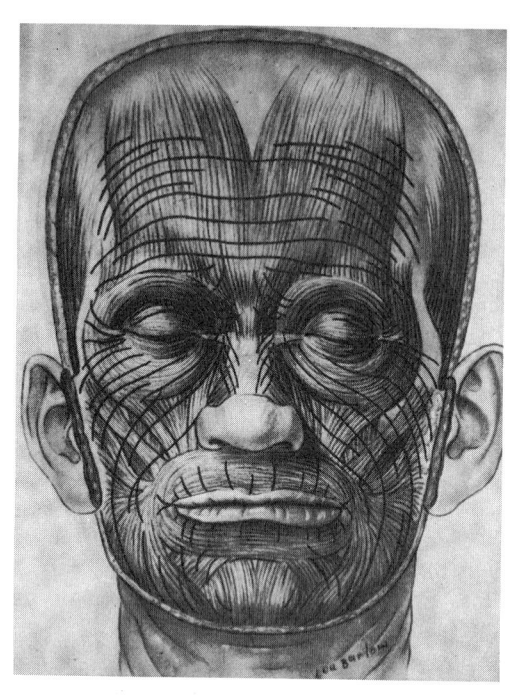

Fig. 2-5. The black lines in this figure are tracings of the wrinkles shown in Figure 2-4 superimposed upon the muscles of facial expression. Note that these wrinkle lines uniformly are at right angles to the direction of contraction of the muscles. (Kraissl, C. J., and Conway, H.: Surgery, 25:596)

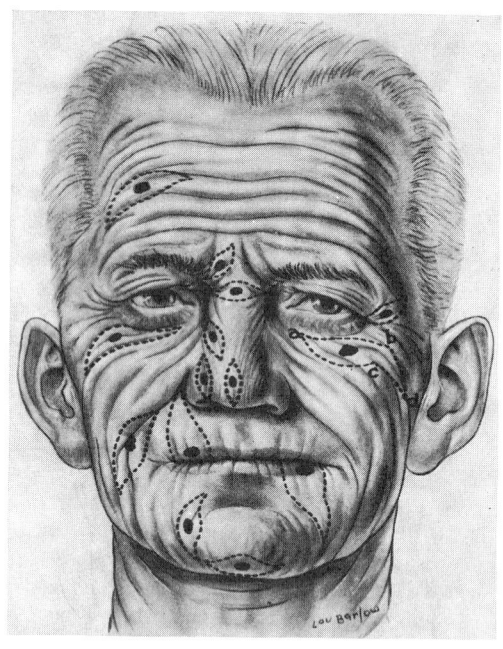

Fig. 2-6. Diagram of suggested lines of excision to allow the ultimate scar to fall in normal wrinkles. (Kraissl, C. J., and Conway, H.: Surgery, 25:598)

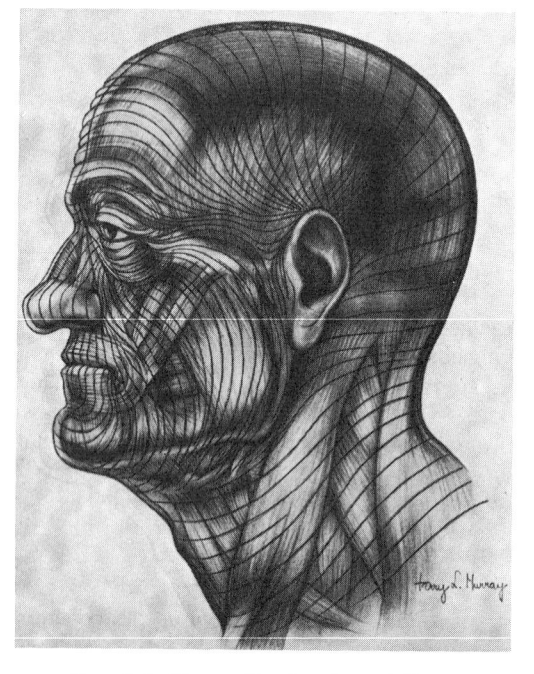

Fig. 2-7. Composite drawing of lines on the side of the head and the face superimposed on the muscles. (Kraissl, C. J.: Plast. Reconstr. Surg., 8:8)

becomes an exaggeration of the normal physiologic perpendicular strands of connective tissue. In excising a lesion on the skin (warts, moles, tumors, etc.) incisions should be planned to have the resultant scars fall in the wrinkle lines (Metzger, 1957); whenever possible tubes, flaps and free grafts should be planned in a similar manner. Representative diagrams of the wrinkle lines according to Kraissl and Conway (1949) and Kraissl (1951) are shown in Figures 2-4 to 2-9.

It is currently accepted that incisions parallel with the wrinkle lines give a better cosmetic and functional result. Berard, Woodward, Herrmann and Pulaski (1964) have made the situation more complicated. They found that incisions placed parallel with the wrinkle lines in rats were significantly thicker and weaker than those placed perpendicularly. However, the long-term result in humans would still favor the parallel incision!

Other rules concerning the placing of inci-

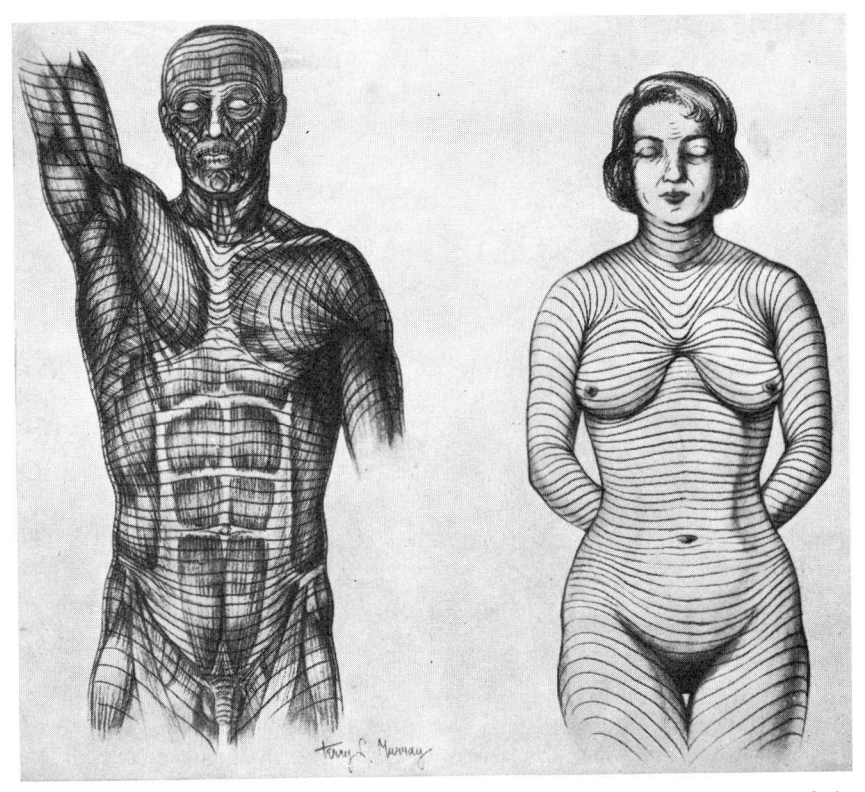

Fig. 2-8. Comparative lines on the thorax and the abdomen of the male and the female. The difference in pattern is due to the gravitational action of the mammary glands. (Kraissl, C. J.: Plast. Reconstr. Surg., 8:11)

sions are as follows: On the chest these should be placed parallel with the ribs. When incising an intercostal space, the incision should hug the superior border of the rib below because the neurovascular bundle is adjacent to the inferior border of the rib above. Abdominal incisons must be planned not only for the most probable operation but also so that if additional lesions necessitating more exposure are discovered, extension of the original incision can be accomplished most readily. For this purpose, horizontal or vertical incisions near the umbilicus can be lengthened in the desired direction with the greatest facility. In other instances, as when a McBurney (right lower quadrant muscle-splitting) incision is made for possible appendicitis and signs of perforated peptic ulcer are discovered, it may be preferable to close the McBurney incision and make a separate epigastric incision rather than to extend the original wound. Additional practical advice concerning the clinically important subject of placement of skin incisions is given by Courtiss, Longacre, de Stefano, Brizio and Holmstrand (1963). These authors correlate the deep muscle pull and skin wrinkle lines as being connected by collagenous septa. De Vito (1965) has also reviewed the subject.

Careful consideration of underlying nerves, blood vessels, muscles and other structures is important in planning incisions. Thus, a long vertical abdominal incision will paralyze most of the muscular structure between it and the midline. For this reason, short transverse (or midline vertical of any length) abdominal incisions are preferable, since they cut the fewest important nerves in the abdominal wall.

Anatomic Dissections

The student of anatomy has learned to dissect out the structure he is attempting to expose, at the same time preserving important ("named") nerves, arteries, etc., in the region. The surgeon must do the same except

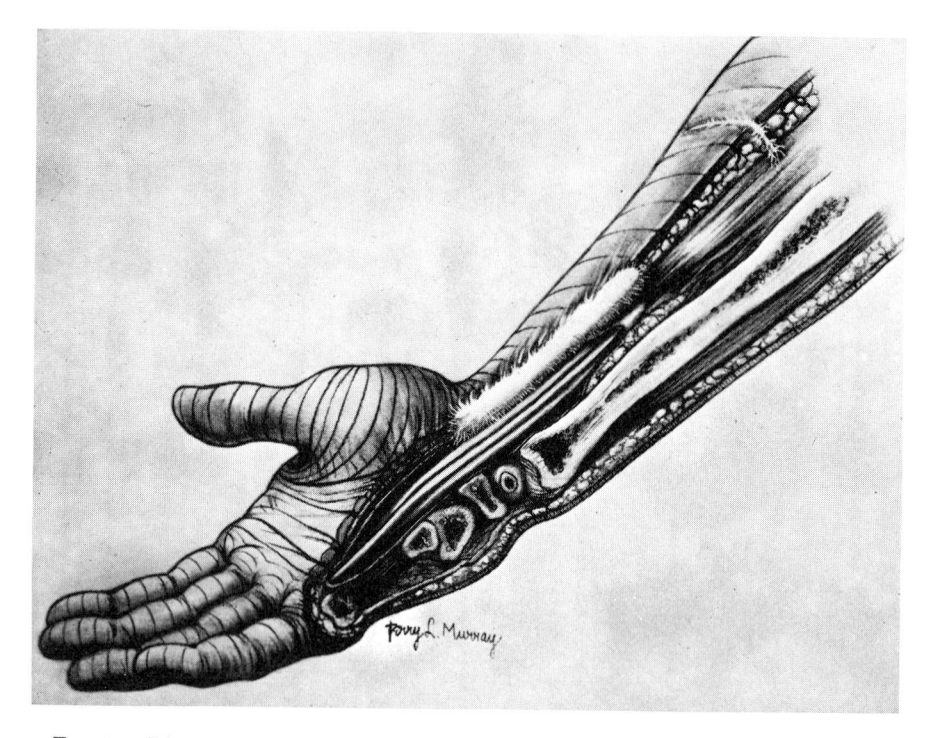

FIG. 2-9. Diagrammatic representation of transverse scar as compared with vertical scar on forearm. A transverse scar shown proximally, which is parallel with the skin lines, may become adherent to muscle without interference with function, but the vertical scar shown at the wrist, which cuts across the skin lines, splints the action of the muscle and the tendon and causes skin contraction because of muscular forces acting on it. (Kraissl, C. J.: Plast. Reconstr. Surg., 8:24)

that his dissection should be no wider than necessary and should also preserve the minute and "unnamed" blood supply. An example is the freeing of the external oblique aponeurosis in performing a herniorrhaphy: this structure should be freed no more than necessary to obtain exposure of the underlying structures and the eventual apposition of the edges of the aponeurosis on closure. To do more is to deprive the aponeurosis of part of its blood supply and create unnecessary open tissue spaces in which hematomas might form and infections might develop.

LIGATURES AND SUTURES

Some of the differentiating characteristics of absorbable and nonabsorbable sutures have already been considered under "Local Factors in Wound Healing." Sutures may be of various types (Fig. 2-10). In general, fine suture material inserted as atraumatically as possible and without strangulation of tissue is a desirable aim. Halsted (1913) epitomized this as follows:

I believe that the tendency will always be in the direction of exercising greater care and refinement in operating, and that the surgeon will develop increasingly a respect for tissues, a sense which recoils from inflicting unnecessary insult to structures concerned in the process of repair. . . . Healing is menaced when the circulation of the tissues to be united is impaired.

As shown in Figure 2-11, sutures that are placed too tightly cause tissues to become necrotic and tend to pull out, thus defeating their original purpose. Not only should the sutures be tied without excessive tension, but when they are inserted, the skin (or other edges to be approximated) should not be held tightly with the forceps. Stevenson and Reid (1947) go so far as to state: "Skin edges should never be picked up with hemostats or

1. Continuous   2. Blanket   3. Subcuticular

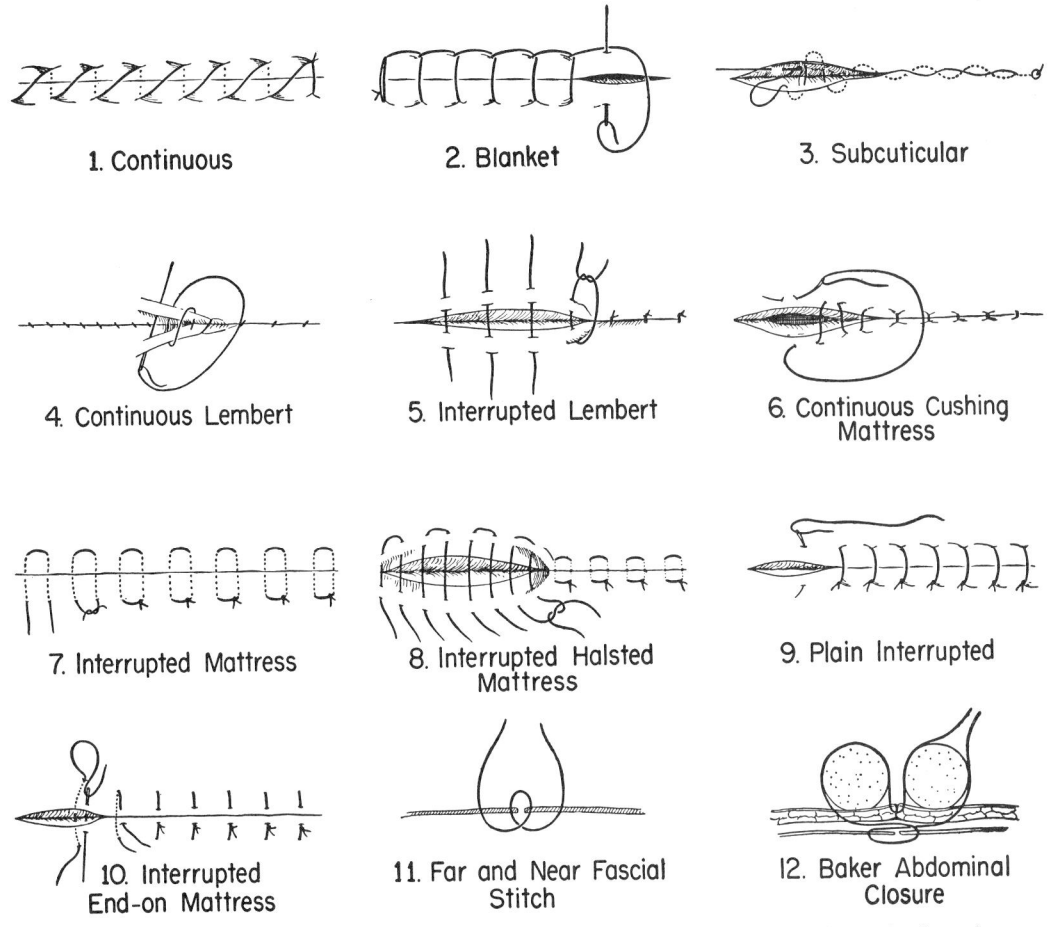

4. Continuous Lembert   5. Interrupted Lembert   6. Continuous Cushing Mattress

7. Interrupted Mattress   8. Interrupted Halsted Mattress   9. Plain Interrupted

10. Interrupted End-on Mattress   11. Far and Near Fascial Stitch   12. Baker Abdominal Closure

Fig. 2-10. Types of sutures commonly used. Types 4, 5 and 8 are utilized on the intestine; Types 3 and 10 on the skin; Type 11 on the fascia; and Type 12 on the entire thickness of the abdominal (or thoracic) wall. The other sutures depicted have more general applications.

smooth forceps unless one intends to cut off the part that has been contused."

The use of "stay" sutures, either alone or to supplement a layer-by-layer closure, particularly of abdominal wounds, is advocated by many surgeons. Such sutures should also be placed without excess tension (Holman and Eckel, 1941).

HEMOSTASIS

This all-important element of surgical technic is too significant to be taken for granted. Hemostasis is of importance for 3 reasons: (1) it prevents blood loss and shock; (2) in a bloodless field one can dissect with greater accuracy; and (3) hemostasis helps to prevent postoperative hematomas.

DRAINAGE OF WOUNDS

Drains may be classified according to whether they are placed prophylactically, to prevent the accumulation of fluids in a fresh wound, or therapeutically, to permit the escape of fluids that have already accumulated. They may be also classified as to whether they are to drain off air (as from the pleural cavity in a patient with tension pneumothorax), pus (as from a perirectal abscess), blood (as from under a widely undermined abdominal wall flap in a fat person), or secretions (as from the region of the pancreas after partial pancreatectomy). In some instances, a single drain may be placed to provide egress for more than one of these types of collections (as drainage of both blood and bile following certain biliary

Wound Healing

tract operations, or both air and pus following acute rupture of a lung abscess).

In modern surgery drains are still placed for the removal of air, pus, blood, or secretions. However, drainage for pus and for bleeding may be avoided more often than in the past and for different reasons. Most abscesses still require the placing of a temporary drain after incision. In infections of the peritoneal cavity, if operation is performed early (e.g., generalized peritonitis after perforation of a peptic ulcer), it is not considered mandatory to drain the peritoneal cavity and was not so even before the use of antibiotics. However, as advocated by Coller and Valk (1940) it is recommended that after closure of the peritoneum and the fascia in cases of peritonitis, the superficial part of the wound be drained for several days.

The harmful effects of using even soft drains must be considered. Not only will blood, etc., drain out, which is helpful, but bacteria may travel down the drains. In addition, the

FIG. 2-11. The harmful effects of sutures that are too tight. (A) Too tight sutures and too big bites with ligatures. (A^1) Result 10 days later: necrosis of ligatured material, pulling out of sutures, necrosis and edema, etc. (B and B^1) Normal tension and result in 10 days. (Reid, M. R.: New Eng. J. Med., 215:756)

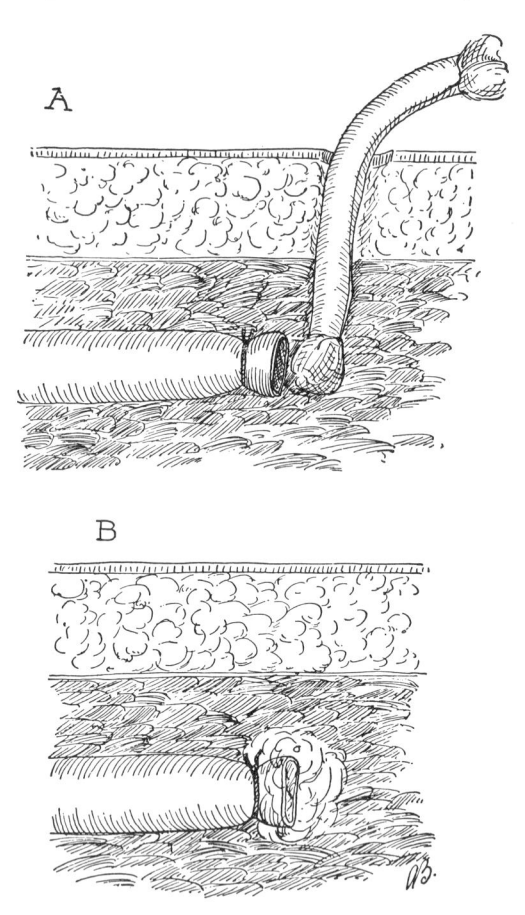

FIG. 2-12. A possible harmful effect of drains: (A) Showing how a drain removes the plastic exudate and invites infection by capillarity from the skin surface. (B) Showing plastic exudate about vessel when no drain is inserted. (McNealy, R. W.: Aneurysms. *In*: Lewis-Walters' Practice of Surgery. Vol. 12. Hagerstown, Md., Prior)

fibrinoplastic exudate (Fig. 2-12), which may be beneficial, is apt to be removed by drains.

Wilder (1955) stated that

A safe rule is: Use drains whenever an abnormal collection of fluid is encountered, be it contaminated, or infected material, blood, bile, or lymph, exudate or transudate; or whenever such an accumulation is anticipated. Avoid drains in joint spaces or in similar areas where excess reaction is detrimental to function.

Most drains are made of soft rubber (Penrose drains); in the neighborhood of tendons, large vessels, etc., only soft drains should be used, otherwise necrosis of these vital structures may result. Pitts (1954) showed that in rats drains made of Teflon (polytetrafluorethylene) function better and produce fewer adhesions than rubber drains. Rigid drains have an indication when suction is to be applied, particularly with an air vent producing a "sump" type of drain (Fig. 2-13) of the type popularized by Chaffin. Sump drains of rubber or stainless steel are used more widely now than formerly. *Drains should not be placed across tendon sheaths* in the foot or the hand lest the tendon become fixed and useless.

WOUND CLOSURE

Wound closure involves a final examination of the wound as to adequacy of hemostasis, a decision as to drainage, and a utilization of the type of sutures most applicable to the particular wound in the particular patient at hand. In all wounds inadequate or improper closure may result in wound disruption, but in the case of abdominal wounds the additional problem of evisceration is ever present. First heralded by the appearance of a *watery* blood-stained discharge on the dressings, disruption may lead to evisceration so rapidly that the first finding is that of warm coils of intestine protruding from the wound and even lying on the bed beside the patient. To prevent this catastrophe, particularly in persons with general or local factors (see above) predisposing to poor wound healing, all of the technical ability of the surgeon is called into play. Adequate bites of the fascial layers with special attention to preserving their circulation is paramount, along with a vigorous attempt to control the predisposing factors to poor healing. Coapt but do not strangulate.

DRESSINGS

As stated in Chapter 14, dressings are usually applied to wounds. All draining and discharging wounds are usually dressed. Some surgeons, however, do not apply dressings to sutured wounds that are not expected to drain. Dressings have 4 main functions: (1) protection, (2) absorption, as of drainage, (3) compression and (4) stabilization. Compression is still considered applicable for prevention of

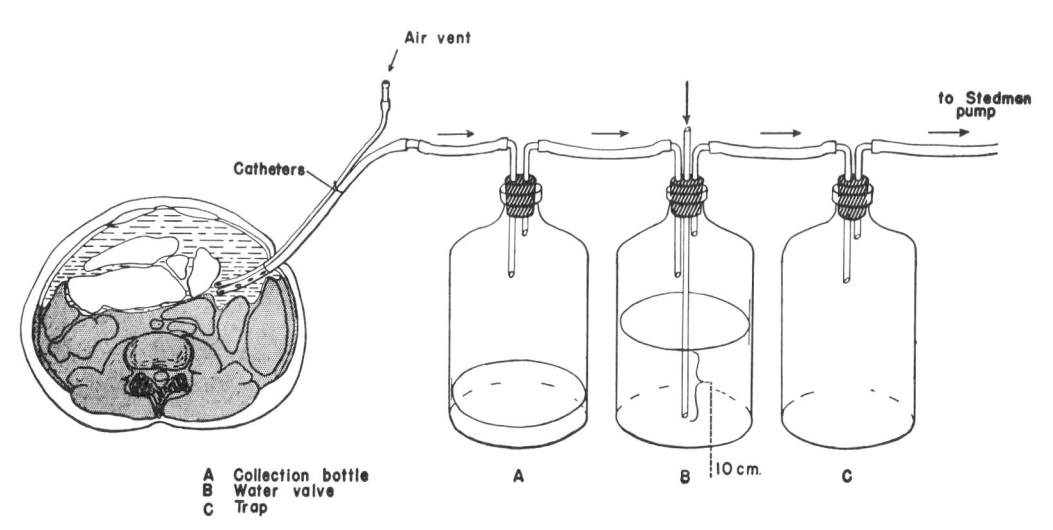

FIG. 2-13. Diagram of application of sump drain in abdominal surgery. The air vent usually has a gauze sponge loosely wrapped around the end of the catheter. (Scott, O. B., and Harkins, H. N.: West. J. Surg., 59:619)

hematoma formation in "dead" spaces left in some wounds such as following a radical mastectomy for carcinoma of the breast. Even in such instances more aggressive means of eliminating the dead space, such as removable apposing sutures, followed by sump drainage may be preferable. On the other hand, compression may interfere with circulation, especially if considerable inflammatory swelling occurs under a compression dressing. Most surgeons no longer consider compression applicable for preventing inflammatory swelling and exudation from wounds of a type such as a thermal burn. In many instances, particularly with wounds of the extremities, a well padded splint or plaster cast is advisable to help stabilize and immobilize the wound during the early part of the healing period.

HEALING OF SPECIAL TISSUES

Many aspects of wound healing are the same, irrespective of the special tissue involved, while others are different in each case. Some of the special features of healing are discussed below.

Skin and Mucous Membrane

Epithelium shows a strong tendency to spread out and cover defects by both migration and multiplication of cells. At the same time, the farther epithelium has to travel from its original source, the thinner it is apt to become. Furthermore, the longer it takes to cover a defect, the more granulation tissue will form, and the greater will be the scar contraction. Healing by epithelization is more properly a "pushing" in rather than a "pulling" in or contraction as far as the epithelium itself is concerned. On the skin this results in deforming scars or webs; in the intestinal tract it may result in stricture formation. When scar skin spreads out to cover a granulating surface (healing by second intention, Fig. 2-1) it does not develop the wavy rete mucosum, the internal surface of the rete mucosum being more or less flat. This flatness increases the chances of separation of the rete mucosum from the cutis vera, especially from oblique blows, and explains why a large section of apparently well-healed scar epithelium may occasionally be raised up with a hematoma beneath it following a relatively trivial injury.

A rule may be stated that tissue is intended to be covered by either skin or mucous membrane which may be exposed to the air (ectodermal or entodermal layer), or by a layer of serosa which may not be exposed to the air (mesodermal layer). Examples of the former are the skin, the pharynx and the intestinal tract. Examples of the latter are the peritoneum, joint endothelium and the vascular intima. When trauma disrupts this continuity, the rule is broken, and scar tissue will result; the more scar tissue the greater the delay. Graham (1952) has expressed this as far as the skin is concerned by his alliteration: "Scab or skin." In the early stages of a flat wound when either a scab (in abrasions) or eschar (in burns) is present, skin grafting may be delayed. However, once the scab or eschar separates, usually in less than 3 weeks, skin grafting must be done promptly over any granulations that are present.

In the intestinal tract, an example of the observance of the rule against exposing the serosa to air is the following: Formerly all terminal ileostomies were fashioned by bringing the end of the loop of ileum about 2 to 3 cm. above the skin level, and consequently leaving a corresponding length of serosa exposed to the air. During the ensuing weeks, or months, the mucosa and the skin would tend to grow out over the serosa, finally joining so that no more serosa was exposed, and the "law" expressed in the previous paragraph was obeyed. During this "maturaton" process considerable scar tissue resulted, and certain remote effects, such as diarrhea, may have been related to the resulting serositis (Figs. 2-14 and 2-15). Dragstedt, Dack and Kirsner (1941) attacked this problem by placing a dermatome skin graft over the exposed serosa.

The principle of immediate mucous-membrane-to-skin suture of ileostomies was first introduced by Strauss, Friedman and Bloch (1924) and extended by Brooke (1952) and by Crile and Turnbull (1954). This avoids the lengthy and artificial "maturation" process formerly resulting in much scar tissue. The principle has also been extended to colostomies. The Brooke technic involves turning down the distal half of the ileostomy stump over the proximal half and suturing the mucosal end immediately to the skin margin. Crile and Turnbull accomplished this by re-

Healing of Special Tissues

ILEOSTOMY

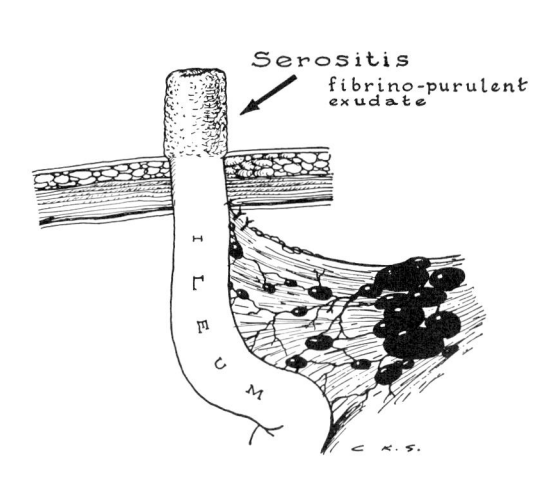

FIG. 2-14. Serositis of an exposed ileostomy with secondary inflammatory hypertrophy of the lymph glands in the mesoileum. (Crile, G., Jr., and Turnbull, R. B., Jr.: Ann. Surg., 140:461)

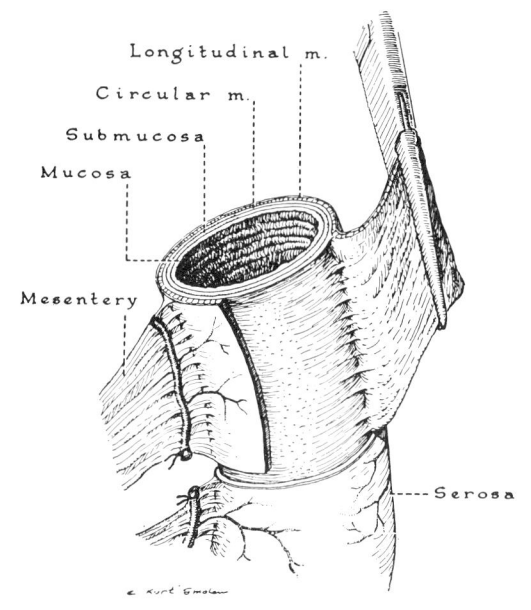

FIG. 2-16. The technic of removing the seromuscular coat from the distal half of the ileostomy. (Crile, G., Jr., and Turnbull, R. B., Jr.: Ann. Surg., 140:461)

moving the outer seromuscular coat from the distal half of the ileostomy stump and then turning down the still attached mucosa over the proximal portion and suturing it immediately to the skin margin (Figs. 2-16 and 2-17). Since most modern ileostomies are made shorter, our current technic is more nearly like that of the original Strauss technic (1924) in which nothing is turned back and the ileostomy—primarily sutured—is almost flush with the level of the skin.

Peculiarly, a healed union between intesti-

MATURATION OF ILEOSTOMY

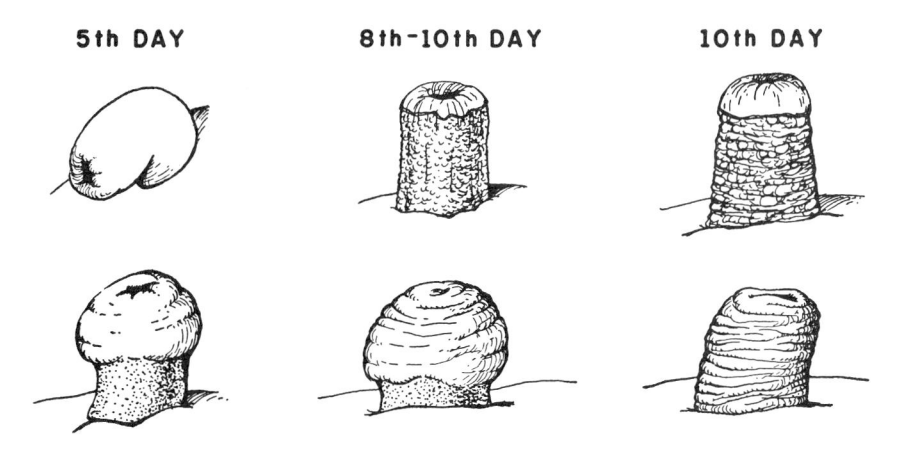

5th DAY   8th-10th DAY   10th DAY

4th TO 6th WEEKS

FIG. 2-15. The usual protracted course of maturation of an ileostomy with a serosal surface exposed to the air. (Crile, G., Jr., and Turnbull, R. B., Jr.: Ann. Surg., 140:461)

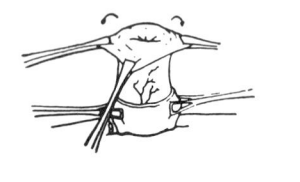

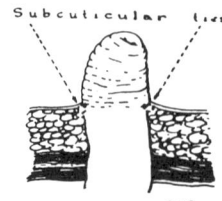

FIG. 2-17. Eversion of the submucosal-mucosal layer over the ileostomy (Crile-Turnbull technic). (Crile, G., Jr., and Turnbull, R. B., Jr.: Ann. Surg., 140:461)

nal mucosa and skin is never attained. They merely coapt but do not unite and may be separated easily by minor trauma, producing more scar tissue each time a separation occurs.

GASTROINTESTINAL TRACT

Not only must the mucosa not have to bridge too great a gap, but for strength the all-important submucosa must be approximated along with the rest of the muscular layer in intestinal suture. Approximation of the serosa, with or without inversion, is also advisable, this being done with the same row of sutures that approximates the submucosa. The importance of the submucosa in intestinal suture was first demonstrated by Halsted (1887) when he stated: "Each stitch should include a bit of the submucosa. A thread of this coat is much stronger than a shred of the entire thickness of the serosa and muscularis. . . . For us [it is] the most important coat."

NERVOUS SYSTEM

Generally speaking, nerve cells do not regenerate. Nerve fibers usually will regenerate if the cell remains intact and if they themselves are postganglionic, but not if they are preganglionic.

MUSCLE

Muscle tissue is generally considered to be so specialized that it will not regenerate after injury but will be replaced by fibrous tissue.

CARTILAGE

Since cartilage gets its nutrition, in part at least, from the joint fluid, joint wounds, even when drained, should be closed so that the cartilage is not exposed to air; furthermore, drainage is seldom advisable for other reasons. The biologic survival and growth of cartilage grafts, as opposed to the healing of cartilage in its natural locations, has been discussed by Schatten, Bergenstal, Kramer, Swarm and Siegel (1958).

BONE

Repair of bone occurs by osteoblastic growth from the periosteum and by creeping substitution of callus and of dead or transplanted bone. Thus, bone goes through a third phase of healing in addition to the productive and collagen phases, namely, a maturation or organizing differentiation (see Chap. 53, Orthopedics).

TENDON

Since tendons are made up of parallel collagenous bundles, their repair involves a regrowth of these bundles, usually mixed with more or less connective tissue scar.

BLOOD VESSELS

When a blood vessel is injured, new tissue may arise theoretically from 3 sources: longitudinal ingrowth from the vessel walls, centripetal growth from the surrounding and supporting tissues about the vessel, and from the centrifugal deposition of platelets, fibrin and cells from the blood stream. The first two of these sources are the most important. In the case of long previous prosthetic vascular grafts, the second is the most important. In the case of arteral homografts, the elastic tissue layer serves as a barrier to the further ingrowth of tissue from the periarterial tissues so that the other mechanisms must play a role, the elastic tissue of the graft serving to give strength in the meantime. Sauvage and Wesolowski (1955) showed that longitudinal ingrowth of fibrous tissue seldom occurs into arterial homografts for more than 2 cm. from each anastomotic line. This implies that, except near the ends, a long arterial homograft with intact elastic layer presents essentially a nonviable surface to the blood stream. These authors concluded that "the healing of arterial grafts is the same as that of other tissues that do not regenerate specialized elements." (See Chap. 44, Peripheral Vascular Surgery.)

The usual types of vascular suture are shown in Figure 2-18. The continuous over-and-over (Carrel) is the most frequently used, while the continuous everting mattress (Bla-

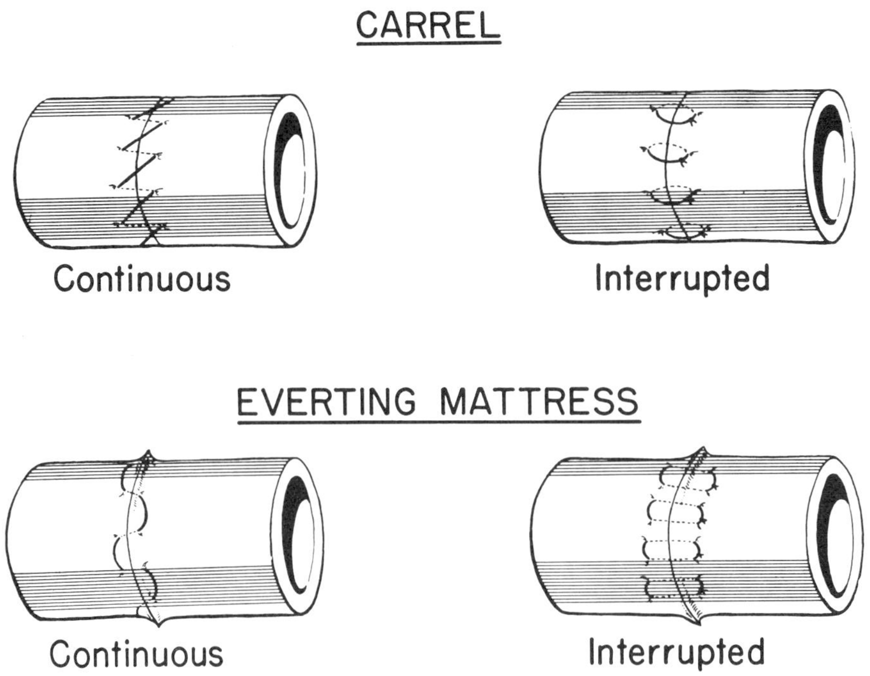

CARREL

Continuous   Interrupted

EVERTING MATTRESS

Continuous   Interrupted

FIG. 2-18. Suture methods for use on blood vessels. The end-on coaptation (Carrel) method has the advantage of rapidity of performance but the disadvantage of placing considerable material in the lumen. The everting mattress, either continuous (Blalock) or interrupted (Jaboulay), method of intima-to-intima approximation has the advantage of placing little suture material in the lumen. (Sauvage, L. R., and Harkins, H. N.: Bull. Johns Hopkins Hosp., 91:279)

lock) is used when an intima-to-intima approximation is desired, as in suturing veins, in which the blood flow is slower and the danger of thrombosis is greater.

NEW DEVELOPMENTS IN THE STUDY OF WOUND HEALING

Progress in this field of surgical research is fundamental to all surgery. While it is impossible to compartmentalize such research, advances are being made along the following three fronts. The studies mentioned are intended as a rough indication of the advances being made rather than as a comprehensive review of the subject.

HOMOGRAFTS

Autografts (from the same individual) of tissues or of organs are successfully utilized daily. Homografts (from another individual of the same species) are generally successful only if the donor is an identical twin. Apparent successes of certain homografts, as an arterial homograft implanted into the aorta to replace a thrombosed segment, are of benefit to the patient because the homograft serves as a fibrous tissue framework for ingrowth of new autogenous tissue, not because the graft survives as viable tissue. Heterografts (from another species) do not survive.

One aspect of homografting that has aroused interest is the "second-set" phenomenon. A second set of homografts taken from the same donor and transplanted to the same host sloughs more rapidly than the first set of homografts (Medawar, 1944). This observation indicates an acquired immunity and would fit in with the observations of Lehrfeld, Taylor and Converse (1954, 1955) on the relation of survival time to implantation time of second set homografts. The cogent observation of Varco, MacLean, Aust and Good (1955) of a successful homotransplantation of skin in a patient with agammaglobulinemia offers strong support for the acquired immunity theory. When a homograft does *not* take, its rejection is accompanied by an early and uniform development of multiple thromboses in the recipient bed to which a skin homograft has been transplanted (Conway and Stark, 1955). As Dempster (1955) pointed out, one must consider not only the response of the host to the homograft but also the response of the homograft, if viable, to the host tissues.

There have been so many recent studies on the subject of homograft immunity that only a few key references can be given here (Billingham and Medawar, 1953; Andresen, Monroe, Squire, Hass and Madden, 1957; Edgerton, Peterson and Edgerton, 1957; Peer, Bernhard, Walker, Bagli and Christensen, 1957; Rapaport and Converse, 1957, 1958; Andresen and Monroe, 1958; Arguedas and Pérez-Tamayo, 1958; Braunwald and Hufnagel, 1958; Cannon, Terasaki and Longmire, 1958; Converse, Ballantyne and Woisky, 1958; Fisher, Axelrod, Fisher, Lee and Calvanese, 1958; Hubay and Holden, 1958; Kamrin, 1958, 1959; Kay, 1958; Kelly, Good and Varco, 1958; Mariani, Martinez, Smith and Good, 1958; Marino and Benaim, 1958; Markowitz and Schwartz, 1958; Martinez, Smith, Aust, Mariani and Good, 1958; Peer, Bernhard and Walker, 1958; Stark, 1958; Martinez, Smith, Shapiro and Good, 1959; Meeker, Condie, Weiner, Varco and Good, 1959; Terasaki, Cannon and Longmire, 1959).

For further information on organ transplantation see Chapter 19.

RELATION OF STRESS TO WOUND HEALING

The early belief of a few that ACTH and cortisone would make all men alike as far as take of homografts is concerned was not sustained. However, such hormones and related stress do have some effect on wound healing. Howes, Plotz, Blunt and Ragan (1950) showed that very large doses of cortisone inhibit normal wound healing. Chassin, McDougall, Stahl, MacKay and Localio (1954) reported that while nonspecific stress of sufficient magnitude results in depression of the bursting pressure of standard laparotomy incisions in rats, such stress does not have this effect in adrenalectomized rats maintained on fixed doses of aqueous adrenal cortex extract. Montgomery and Green (1954) reported that tissue culture extracts applied locally will completely reverse cortisone inhibition of wound healing. Extending this into the realm of patients, Biström (1955) reported 7 patients with destructive inflammation who presented definite aggravation of symptoms after cortisone therapy. The inflammatory symptoms abated temporarily during therapy but were replaced by severe destructive changes, with increased inflammatory symptoms after cessation of cortisone therapy. This author concluded that "the examples given should serve as a warning against the uncritical use of cortisone."

Moltke (1955) studied the effects of another gland of internal secretion on wound healing, by utilizing the Sandblom-Petersen-Muren tensiometer to study healing wounds in guinea pigs. Moltke came to the following conclusions: (1) The wounds of thyroidectomized guinea pigs possess the same tensile strength as those of intact controls. (2) Thyroxine inhibits wound healing in intact as well as in thyroidectomized guinea pigs. (3) Thyrotropic hormone inhibits wound healing only in intact guinea pigs, whereas it does not appear to alter the normal course of healing in thyroidectomized guinea pigs.

Other recent work involves a study of the effect of a previous wound on the healing of a second wound. Sandblom and Muren (1954) have shown the need for careful controls in such experiments because even the change in cutaneous circulation following depilation for one wound may affect the rate of healing of the other wound. Savlov and Dunphy (1954) made observations which indicate that local factors are most important in determining the effect of preliminary local and distant incisions. Wounds of the abdomen made 15 days after wounds on the backs of rats did not show any greater tensile strength on the third day than 3-day abdominal wounds of a control group on which no previous wounding had been made. A summation of such an effect could not be demonstrated by multiple wounding on the back before an abdominal wound. On the other hand, 15-day-old abdominal wounds that were opened and resutured revealed a significant increase in tensile strength on the third day after exposure.

Raventos (1954) studied another type of stress, namely, total body exposure to ionizing radiation (500 r.). Irradiated mice showed a significant retardation of wound healing from the 6th through the 11th day after wounding, but not thereafter.

BIBLIOGRAPHY

Abt, A. F., and Von Schuching, S.: Aging as a factor in wound healing. Arch. Surg., 86:627-632, 1963.

Adamsons, R. J., and Enquist, I. F.: The relative importance of sutures to the strength of healing wounds under normal and abnormal conditions. Surg., Gynec., Obstet., 117:396-401, 1963.

Alexander, J. W., Kaplan, J. Z., and Altemeier, W. A.: Role of suture materials in the development of wound infection. Ann. Surg., 165:192, 1967.

Andresen, R. H., Monroe, C. W., Squire, F. H., Hass, G. M., and Madden, D. A.: Types of host-graft interactions. Proc. Inst. Med., Chicago, 21:329, 1957.

Andresen, R., and Monroe, C. W.: Elimination of inflammation to homografts by transfusions of donor's blood cells. Proc. Cent. Soc. Clin. Research, 31:9, 1958.

Andrews, R. P., Morgan, H. C., and Jurkiewicz, M. J.: The relationship of dietary protein to the healing of experimental burns. S. Forum, 6:72-75, 1956.

Anson, G. (1748): Cited by Localio, Casale and Hinton (see reference below), 1943.

Antopol, W.: Lycopodium granuloma; its clinical and pathologic significance, together with a note on granuloma produced by talc. Arch. Path., 16:326-331, 1933.

Arguedas, J. M., and Pérez-Tamayo, R.: The pattern of wound healing of skin autografts and skin homografts in the rat. Surg., Gynec., Obstet., 106:671-678, 1958.

Berard, C. W., Woodward, S. C., Herrmann, J. B., and Pulaski, E. J.: Healing of incisional wounds in rats: The relationship of tensile strength and morphology to the normal skin wrinkle lines. Ann. Surg., 159:260-270, 1964.

Billingham, R. E., and Medawar, P. B.: "Desensitization" to skin homografts by injections of donor skin extracts. Ann. Surg., 137:444-449, 1953.

Biström, O.: The injurious effect of cortisone on destructive inflammation. Acta chir. scandinav., 109:200-202, 1955.

Borgström, S., and Sandblom, P.: Suture technic and wound healing. Ann. Surg., 144:982-990, 1956.

Botsford, T. W.: Tensile strength of sutured skin wounds during healing, Surg., Gynec., Obstet., 72:690-697, 1941.

Braunwald, N. S., and Hufnagel, C. A.: Modification of homotransplantation by growth in tissue culture. Surgery, 43:501-509, 1958.

Brooke, B. N.: Management of an ileostomy including its complications. Lancet, 2:102-104, 1952.

Cannon, J. A., Terasaki, P. I., and Longmire, W. P.: Induction of tolerance to homografts by nonspecific pooled blood. A.M.A. Arch. Surg., 76:769-773, 1958.

Celsus: Book III, cited by Menkin (see reference below), 1940.

Chassin, J. L., McDougall, H. A., Stahl, W., MacKay, M., and Localio, S. A.: Effect of adrenalectomy on wound healing in normal and in stressed rats. Proc. Soc. Exp. Biol. Med., 86:446-448, 1954.

Coller, F. A., and Valk, W. L.: The delayed closure of contaminated wounds: a preliminary report. Ann. Surg., 112:256-270, 1940.

Connell, J. F., Jr., and Rousselot, L. M.: New concepts in the treatment of surgical wounds. Am. J. Surg., 97:429-433, 1959.

Converse, J. M., Ballantyne, D. L., Jr., and Woisky, J.: The vascularization of skin homografts and transplantation immunity. Ann. N.Y. Acad. Sci., 73:693-697, 1958.

Conway, H., Sedar, J., and Stark, R. B.: Observations on the development of circulation in skin grafts. X. Effect of sodium salicylate on homologous skin grafts. Plast. Reconstr. Surg., 15:56-60, 1955.

Conway, H., and Stark, R. B.: Homologous skin graft used as a life-saving expedient to promote thrombosis of a bleeding wound in a patient with hemophilia. Plast. Reconstr. Surg., 13:446-450, 1954.

Courtiss, E. H., Longacre, J. J., de Stefano, G. A., Brizio, L., and Holmstrand, K.: The placement of elective skin incisions. Plast. Reconstr. Surg., 31:31-44, 1963.

Crile, G., Jr., and Turnbull, R. B., Jr.: The mechanism and prevention of ileostomy dysfunction. Ann. Surg., 140:459-466, 1954.

Cuthbertson, A. M.: Contraction of full thickness skin wounds in the rat. Surg., Gynec., Obstet., 108:421-432, 1959.

Dempster, W. J.: Personal communication, July 20, 1955.

Dettinger, G. B., and Bowers, W. F.: Tissue response to Orlon and Dacron sutures: a comparison with Nylon, cotton, and silk. Surgery, 42:325-335, 1957.

DeVito, R. V.: Healing of wounds. S. Clin. N. Am., 45:441-459, 1965.

Dragstedt, L. R., Dack, G. M., and Kirsner, J. B.: Chronic ulcerative colitis: summary of evidence implicating *vacterium necrophorum* as etiologic agent. Ann. Surg., 114:653-662, 1941.

Du Noüy, P. le C.: Cicatrization of wounds. III. The relation between the age of the patient, the area of the wound and the index of cicatrization. J. Exp. Med., 24:461-470, 1916.

Dunphy, J. E.: On the nature and care of wounds. Ann. Roy. Coll. Surg. Eng., 26:69-86, 1960.

———: The fibroblast—a ubiquitous ally for the surgeon. New Eng. J. Med., 268:1367-1377, 1963.

Dunphy, J. E., and Udupa, K. N.: Chemical and histochemical sequences in the normal healing of wounds. New Eng. J. Med., 253:847-851, 1955.

Dunphy, J. E., Udupa, K. N.: and Edwards, L. C.: Wound healing: a new perspective with particular reference to ascorbic acid deficiency. Ann. Surg., 144:304-317, 1956.

Ebeling, A. H.: Cicatrization of wounds. XIII. The temperature coefficient. J. Exp. Med., 35:657-659, 1922.

Edgerton, M. T., Peterson, H. A., and Edgerton, P. J.: The homograft rejection mechanism. Arch. Surg., 74:238-244, 1957.

Edwards, L. C., Pernokas, L. N., and Dunphy, J. E.: The use of a plastic sponge to sample regenerating tissue in healing wounds. Surg., Gynec., Obstet., 105:303-309, 1957.

Edwards, L. C., and Udupa, K. N.: Autoradiographic determination of S^{35} in tissues after injection of Methionine–S^{35} and sodium sulfate–S^{35}. J. Biophys. Biochem. Cytol., 3:757-766, 1957.

Erici, I.: Effect of environmental temperature on the rate of wound healing. Acta chir. scandinav., 112:346-347, 1956.

Farhat, S. M., Amer, N. S., Weeks, B. S., and Musselman, M. M.: Effect of mechlorethamine hydrochloride (nitrogen mustard) on healing of abdominal wounds. Surgery, 76:749-753, 1958.

Farhat, S. M., Miller, D. M., and Musselman, M. M.: Effect of triethylenethiophosphoramide (Thio-TEPA) upon healing of abdominal wounds. Arch. Surg., 78:729-731, 1959.

Fisher, B., Axelrod, A. E., Fisher, E. R., Lee, S. H., and Calvanese, N.: The favorable effect of pyridoxine deficiency of skin homograft survival. Surgery, 44:149-167, 1958.

French, J. E., and Benditt, E. P.: Observations on the localization of alkaline phosphatase in healing wounds. Arch. Path., 57:352-356, 1954.

Gillman, T., and Penn, J.: Studies on the repair of cutaneous wounds. Mediese Bydraes, 2:121-186, 1956.

Gillman, T., Penn, J., Bronks, D., and Roux, M.: A re-examination of certain aspects of the histogenesis of the healing of cutaneous wounds: a preliminary report. Brit. J. Surg., 43:141-153, 1955.

Gouws, F., Silbermann, O., and MacKenzie, W. D.: The effect of 17-Ethyl-19 Nortestosterone (Nilevar) on healing of experimental wounds. Canad. J. Surg., 1:362-365, 1958.

Graham, J. E.: Personal communication, 1952.

Grillo, H. C.: Origin of fibroblasts in wound healing: An autoradiographic study of inhibition of cellular proliferation by local x-irradiation. Ann. Surg., 157:453-467, 1963.

Grillo, H. C., and Gross, J.: Studies in wound healing. III. Contraction in vitamin C deficiency. Proc. Soc. Exp. Biol. Med., 101:268-270, 1959.

Grillo, H. C., and Potsaid, M. S.: Studies in wound healing: IV. Retardation of contraction by local x-irradiation, and observations relating to the origin of fibroblasts in repair. Ann. Surg., 154:741-750, 1961.

Grillo, H. C., Watts, G. T., and Gross, J.: Studies in wound healing. I. Contraction and the wound contents. Ann. Surg., 148:145-152, 1958.

Hadfield, G.: The tissue of origin of the fibroblasts of granulation tissue. Brit. J. Surg., 50:870-881, 1963.

Halsted, W. S.: Circular suture of the intestine: an experimental study. Am. J. Med. Sci., 94:436-461, 1887.

———: Ligature and suture material: The employment of fine silk in preference to catgut and the advantages of transfixion of tissues and vessels in control of hemorrhage. J.A.M.A., 60:1119-1126, 1913.

Harrison, J. H.: Synthetic materials as vascular prostheses. I. A comparative study in small vessels of Nylon, Dacron, Orlon, Ivalon sponge and Teflon; II. A comparative study of Nylon, Dacron, Orlon, Ivalon sponge and Teflon in large blood vessels with tensile strength studies. Am. J. Surg., 95:3-15, 16-24, 1958.

Harrison, J. H., Swanson, O. S., and Lincoln, A. F.: A comparison of the tissue reactions to plastic materials. Arch. Surg., 74:139-144, 1957.

Hartzell, J. B., Winfield, J. M., and Irvin, J. L.: Plasma vitamin C and serum protein levels in wound disruption. J.A.M.A., 116:669-674, 1941.

Harvey, S. J.: The velocity of the growth of fibroblasts in the healing wound. Arch. Surg., 18:1227-1240, 1929.

Holman, C. W., and Eckel, J. H.: Prevention of wound disruption with through-and-through silver wire stay sutures. Surg., Gynec., Obstet., 72:1052-1055, 1941.

Hoover, N. W., and Ivins, J. C.: Wound debridement. Arch. Surg., 79:701-710, 1959.

Howes, E. L., and Harvey, S. C.: The clinical significance of experimental studies on wound healing. Ann. Surg., 102:941-946, 1935.

Howes, E. L., Plotz, C. M., Blunt, J. W., and Ragan, C.: Retardation of wound healing by cortisone. Surgery, 28:177-181, 1950.

Hubay, C. A., and Holden, W. D.: The effect of the properdin system upon first and second set homografts. Surg., Gynec., Obstet., 107:311-316, 1958.

Hume, D. M.: Discussion of paper by Murray, Merrill and Harrison (see reference below), 1958.

Hyden, W. H., and McClellan, J. T.: Glove powder granuloma in peritoneal cavity. J.A.M.A., 170:1048-1050, 1959.

Jackson, D. S.: Some biochemical aspects of fibrogenesis and wound healing. New Eng. J. Med., 259:814-820, 1958.

Jacob, R., and Houck, J. C.: A chemical description of inflammation and repair. Surg., Gynec., Obstet., 109:85-88, 1959.

Kahlson, G., Nilsson, K., Rosengren, E., and Zederfeldt, B.: Wound healing as dependent on rate of histamine formation. Lancet, 2:230-233, 1960.

Kamrin, B. B.: The use of globulins as a means of inducing acquired tolerance to parabiotic union. Ann. N.Y. Acad. Sci., 73:848-861, 1958.

———: Successful skin homografts in mature non-littermate rats treated with fractions containing Alpha-globulins. Proc. Soc. Exp. Biol. Med., 100:58-61, 1959.

Káto, L., and Gözsy, B.: Role of histamine and leucotaxin in function of cellular defense mechanism. Am. J. Physiol., 184:296-300, 1956.

Kay, G. D.: Homologous skin grafts—factors affecting survival and a report illustrating prolonged survival. Canad. J. Surg., 2:60-67, 1958.

Kelly, W. D., Good, R. A., and Varco, R. L.: Anergy and skin homograft survival in Hodgkin's disease. Surg., Gynec., Obstet., 107:565-570, 1958.

Kobak, M. W., Benditt, E. P., Wissler, R. W., and Steffee, C. H.: The relation of protein deficiency to experimental wound healing. Surg., Gynec., Obstet., 85:751-756, 1947.

Kraissl, C. J.: The selection of appropriate lines for

elective surgical incisions. Plast. Reconstr. Surg., 8:1-28, 1951.

Kraissl, C. J., and Conway, H.: Excision of small tumors of the skin of the face with special reference to the wrinkle lines. Surgery, 25:592-600, 1949.

Kraissl, C. J., Kesten, B. M., and Cimiotti, J. G.: The relation of catgut sensitivity to wound healing. Surg., Gynec., Obstet., 66:628-635, 1938.

Kredel, F. E., Harkins, H. N., and Harkins, W. D.: Toxicity of heavy water. Proc. Soc. Exp. Biol. Med., 32:5-6, 1934.

Langer, K. (1861): Cited by Kraissl, C. J. (see reference above), 1951.

Lee, C. M., Jr., Collins, W. T., and Largen, T. L.: A reappraisal of absorbable glove powder. Surg., Gynec., Obstet., 95:725-737, 1952.

Lehrfeld, J. W., Taylor, A. C., and Converse, J. M.: Relation of survival time to implantation time of second set skin homografts in the rat. Proc. Soc. Exp. Biol. Med., 86:849-851, 1954.

⸺: Observations on second and third set skin homografts in the rat. Plast. Reconstr. Surg., 15:74-76, 1955.

Leriche, R., and Haour, J. (1921): Cited by Localio, Casale and Hinton (see reference below), 1943.

Localio, S. A., Casale, W., and Hinton, J. W.: Wound healing—experimental and statistical study. Internat. Abstr. Surg., 77:369-375, 457-469, 1943; Surg., Gynec., Obstet., 77:243-249, 376-378, 481-492, 1943.

Löfström, B., and Zederfeldt, B.: Effects of induced hypothermia on wound healing, an experimental study in the rabbit. Acta chir. scandinav., 112:152-159, 1956.

⸺: Wound healing after induced hypothermia. II. An experimental investigation of the importance of intravascular aggregation of blood cells. Acta chir. scandinav., 113:272-281, 1957.

Long, C. N. H.: A discussion of the mechanism of action of adrenal cortical hormones on carbohydrate and protein metabolism. Endocrinology, 30:870-883, 1942.

Lund, C. C., and Crandon, J. H.: Human experimental scurvy and the relation of vitamin C deficiency to postoperative pneumonia and to wound healing. J.A.M.A., 116:663-668, 1941.

Lundgren, C., Muren, A., and Zederfeldt, B.: Effect of cold-vasoconstriction on wound healing in the rabbit. Acta chir. scandinav., 118:1-4, 1959.

McAdams, G. B.: Granulomata caused by absorbable starch glove powder. Surgery, 39:329-336, 1956.

McMinn, R. M. H.: The cellular anatomy of experimental wound healing. Ann. Roy. Coll. Surg. Eng., 26:245-260, 1960.

Mariani, T., Martinez, C., Smith, J. M., and Good, R. A.: Immunological tolerance to male skin isografts in female mice. Proc. Soc. Exp. Biol. Med., 99:287-289, 1958.

Marino, H., and Benaim, F.: Experimental skin homografts. Am. J. Surg., 95:267-273, 1958.

Markowitz, A. S., and Schwartz, S. D.: Secondary rejection phenomenon elicited by primary homograft in pretreated rats. Proc. Soc. Exp. Biol. Med., 99:753-754, 1958.

Martinez, C., Smith, J. M., Aust, J. B., Mariani, T., and Good, R. A.: Transfer of acquired tolerance to skin homografts in mice. Proc. Soc. Exp. Biol. Med., 98:640-641, 1958.

Martinez, C., Smith, J. M., Shapiro, F., and Good, R. A.: Transfer of acquired immunological tolerance of skin homografts in mice joined in parabiosis. Proc. Soc. Exp. Biol. Med., 102:413-417, 1959.

Mason, M. L.: Wound healing. Illinois Med. J., 78:523-529, 1940.

Medawar, P. B.: The behaviour and fate of skin autografts and skin homografts in rabbits. J. Anat., 78:176-199, 1944.

Meeker, W., Condie, R., Weiner, D., Varco, R. L., and Good, R. A.: Prolongation of skin homograft survival in rabbits by 6-mercaptopurine. Proc. Soc. Exp. Biol. Med. 102:459-461, 1959.

Meleney, F. L.: Infection in clean operative wounds: a nine year study. Surg., Gynec., Obstet., 60:264-276, 1935.

Menkin, V.: Dynamics of Inflammation: An Inquiry into the Mechanism of Infectious Processes. New York, Macmillan, 1940.

⸺: Newer Concepts of Inflammation. Springfield, Ill., Thomas, 1950.

Metzger, J. T.: Cosmetic closure of simple lacerations. Delaware Med. J., 29:255-261, 1957.

Moltke, E.: Wound healing influence by thyroxine and thyrotrophic hormone. A tensiometric study (21665). Proc. Soc. Exp. Biol. Med., 88:596-599, 1955.

Montgomery, P. O'B., and Green, C.: Reversal of cortisone inhibition of wound healing by tissue culture media. Proc. Soc. Exp. Biol. Med., 86:657-660, 1954.

Moore, F. D.: Bodily changes in surgical convalescence. I. The normal sequence—observations and interpretations. Ann. Surg., 137:289-315, 1953.

Murray, J. E., Merrill, J. P., and Harrison, J. H.: Kidney transplantation between seven pairs of identical twins. Ann. Surg., 148:343-359, 1958.

Ogilvie, R. R., and Douglas, D. M.: Collagen synthesis and preliminary wounding. Brit. J. Surg., 51:149-153, 1964.

Paré, Ambroïse: Cited by Garrison, F. H.: An Introduction to the History of Medicine. ed. 4. Philadelphia, Saunders, 1929.

Peacock, E. E., Jr.: The effects of acid extract of collagen, cold neutral solutions of collagen, and reconstituted collagen fibrils on wound healing in normal and protein-depleted rats. Surg., Gynec., Obstet., 113:329-338, 1961.

Peer, L. A., Bernhard, W. G., and Walker, J. C., Jr.: Full-thickness skin exchanges between parents and their children. Am. J. Surg., 95:239-245, 1958.

Peer, L. A., Bernhard, W. G., Walker, J. C., Jr., Bagli, V. J., and Christensen, J. A.: Behavior of skin switch homografts between parents and infants. Plast. Reconstr. Surg., 20:273-280, 1957.

Pitts, F. W.: Comparative study of the Penrose drain and drains of Teflon. Proc. Soc. Exp. Biol. Med., 85:404-406, 1954.

Pories, W. J., Henzel, J. H., Rob, C. G., and Strain, W. H.: Acceleration of wound healing in man with zinc sulfate given by mouth. Lancet, 1:121-124, 1967.

Postlethwait, R. W., Schauble, J. F., Dillon, M. L., and Morgan, J.: Wound healing. II. An evaluation of surgical suture material. Surg., Gynec., Obstet., 108:555-566, 1959.

Prudden, J. F., Gabriel, O., and Allen, B.: The acceleration of wound healing. Arch. Surg., 86:157-161, 1963.

Prudden, J. F., Nishihara, G., and Ocampo, L.: Studies on growth hormone. III. The effect on wound tensile strength of marked postoperative metabolism induced with growth hormone. Surg., Gynec., Obstet., 107:481-482, 1958.

Radke, H. M., Nyhus, L. M., and Bell, J. W.: Starch granuloma; The problem of surgical glove powder. Northwest Med., 60:283-284, 1961.

Rapaport, F. T., and Converse, J. M.: Observations on immunological manifestations of the homograft rejection phenomenon in man: the recall flare. Ann. N.Y. Acad. Sci., 64:836-841, 1957.

———: The immune response to multiple-set skin homografts: an experimental study in man. Ann. Surg., 147:273-280, 1958.

Rath, H., and Enquist, I. F.: The effect of Thio-TEPA on wound healing. Arch. Surg., 79:812-814, 1959.

Raventos, A.: Wound healing and mortality after total body exposure to ionizing radiation. Proc. Soc. Exp. Biol. Med., 87:165-167, 1954.

Reid, Mont R.: Some considerations of the problems of wound healing. New Eng. J. Med., 215:753-766, 1936.

———: Introductory statement, cited by Caulfield, P. A., and Madigan, H. S.: Wound healing. Northwest Med., 54:918-919, 1955.

Reynolds, B. L., Codington, J. B., and Buxton, R. W.: Wound healing: a study of the response of injured tissues to the coenzyme adenosine 5-monophosphate. Surgery, 44:33-42, 1958.

Rhoads, J. E., Fliegelman, M. T., and Panzer, L. M.: The mechanism of delayed wound healing in the presence of hypoproteinemia. J.A.M.A., 118:21-25, 1942.

Rosen, H., Geever, E. F., Berard, C. W., and Levenson, S. M.: Effect of deuterium oxide on wound healing, collagen and metabolism of rats. New Eng. J. Med., 270:1142-1149, 1964.

Ross, R., and Benditt, E. P.: A comparison of the ultrastructure sequences in normal versus scorbutic wounds. Fed. Proc., 20:164, 1961.

———: Wound healing and collagen formation. IV. Distortion of ribosomal patterns of fibroblasts in scurvy. J. Cell. Biol., 22:365, 1964.

Sabo, J., Oberlander, L., and Enquist, I. F.: The effect of cartilage powder on granulating wounds in diabetic animals. Surg., Gynec., Obstet., 119:559-562, 1964.

Sandberg, N.: Granulation tissue hydroxyproline in the rat after inhibition of histamine formation. Acta chir. scandinav., 127:22-34, 1964a.

———: Enhanced rate of healings in rats with an increased rate of histamine formation. Acta chir. scandinav., 127:9-21, 1964b.

Sandblom, P.: The tensile strength of healing wounds, an experimental study. Acta chir. scandinav. (Supp.), 89:1-108, 1944.

Sandblom, P., and Muren, A.: Differences between the rate of healing of wounds inflicted with short time interval. I. Cutaneous incisions. Ann. Surg., 140:449-458, 1954.

Sandblom, P., Petersen, P., and Muren, A.: Determination of the tensile strength of the healing wound as a clinical test. Acta chir. scandinav., 105:252-257, 1953.

Sauvage, L. R., and Wesolowski, S. A.: The healing and fate of arterial grafts. Surgery, 38:1090-1131, 1955.

Savlov, E. D., and Dunphy, J. E.: Mechanisms of wound healing: comparison of preliminary local and distant incisions. New Eng. J. Med., 250:1062-1065, 1954.

———: The healing of the disrupted and resutured wound. Surgery, 36:362-370, 1954.

Schatten, W. E., Bergenstal, D. M., Kramer, W. M., Swarm, R. L., and Siegel, S.: Biological survival and growth of cartilage grafts. Plast. Reconstr. Surg., 22:11-28, 1958.

Schauble, J. F., Chen, R., and Postlethwait, R. W.: A study of the distribution of ascorbic acid in the wound healing of guinea pig tissue. Surg., Gynec., Obstet., 110:314-318, 1960.

Schilling, J. A., Joel, W., and Shurley, H. M.: Wound healing: a comparative study of the histochemical changes in granulation tissue contained in stainless steel wire mesh and polyvinyl sponge cylinders. Surgery, 46:702-710, 1959.

Schilling, J. A., and Milch, L. E.: Fractional analysis of experimental wound fluid. Proc. Soc. Exp. Biol. Med., 89:189-192, 1955.

Shetlar, M. R., Lacefield, E. G., White, B. N., and Schilling, J. A.: Wound healing: glycoproteins of wound tissue. I. Studies of hexosamine, hexose, and uronic acid contents. Proc. Soc. Exp. Biol. Med., 100:501-503, 1959.

Sisson, R., Lang, S., Serkes, K., and Pareira, M. D.: Comparison of wound healing in various nutritional deficiency states. Surgery, 44:613-618, 1958.

Sneierson, H., and Woo, Z. P.: Starch powder granuloma: a report of two cases. Ann. Surg., 142:1045-1050, 1955.

Stark, R. B.: Current concepts of the hemoplastic enigma. Bull. N.Y. Acad. Med., 34:561-577, 1958.

Stevenson, J. M., and Reid, M. R.: The fundamental principles of surgical technic. In Bancroft, F. W., and Wade, P. A.: Surgical Treatment of the Abdomen. Philadelphia, Lippincott, 1947.

Strauss, A. A., Friedman, J., and Bloch, L.: Colectomy for ulcerative colitis. S. Clin. N. Am., 4:667-686, 1924.

Terasaki, P. I., Cannon, J. A., and Longmire, W. P.: Antibody response to homografts. I. Technic of lymphoagglutination and detection of lymphoagglutinins upon spleen injection. Proc. Soc. Exp. Biol. Med., 102:280-285, 1959.

Thompson, W. D., Ravdin, I. S., and Frank, I. L.: Effect of hypoproteinemia on wound healing. Arch. Surg., 36:509, 1938.

Udupa, K. N., Woessner, J. F., and Dunphy, J. E.: The effect of methionine on the production of mucopolysaccharides and collagen in healing wounds of protein-depleted animals. Surg., Gynec., Obstet., 102:639-645, 1956.

Usher, F., and Wallace, S. A.: Tissue reaction to plastics. Arch. Surg., 76:997-999, 1958.

van den Brenk, H. A. S.: Studies in restorative growth processes in mammalian wound healing. Brit. J. Surg., 43:525-550, 1956.

Van Winkle, W., Jr.: The fibroblast in wound healing. Surg., Gynec., Obstet., 124:369, 1967.

Varco, R. L., MacLean, L. D., Aust, J. B., and Good, R. A.: Agammaglobulinemia: An approach to homovital transplantation. Ann. Surg., 142:334-345, 1955.

Venable, C. S., Stuck, W. G., and Beach, A.: The effects on bone of the presence of metals; based upon electrolysis: an experimental study. Ann. Surg., 105:917-938, 1937.

Watts, G. T., Grillo, H. C., and Gross, J.: Studies in wound healing. II. The role of granulation tissue in contraction. Ann. Surg., 148:153-160, 1958.

Weiber, A.: Studies of the vascularization of healing wounds with radioisotopes. Bull. Soc. Internat. Chir., 23:171-182, 1964.

Whipple, A. O., and Elliott, R. H. E., Jr.: The repair of abdominal incisions. Ann. Surg., 108:741-756, 1938.

Wilder, J. R.: Atlas of General Surgery. St. Louis, C. V. Mosby, 1955.

Williamson, M. B.: The Healing of Wounds. New York, McGraw-Hill, 1957.

Williamson, M. B., and Fromm, H. J.: Excretion of sulfur during healing of experimental wounds. Proc. Soc. Exp. Biol. Med., 87:366-368, 1954.

Wise, B. L.: The reaction of the brain, spinal cord and peripheral nerves to talc and starch glove powders. Ann. Surg., 142:967-972, 1955.

Zederfeldt, B.: Studies on wound healilng and trauma. Acta chir. scandinav. (Supp.), 224:1-85, 1957.

Zintel, H. A.: The healing of wounds. S. Clin. N. Am., 26:1404-1415, 1946.

Three monographs on wound healing include:

Allgöwer, M.: The Cellular Bases of Wound Repair. Springfield, Ill., Charles C Thomas, 1956.

Hartwell, S. W.: The Mechanisms of Healing in Human Wounds: A Correlation of the Clinical and Tissue Factors Involved in the Healing of Human Surgical Wounds, Burns, Ulcers, and Donor Sites. Springfield, Ill., Charles C Thomas, 1955.

Williamson, M. B.: The Healing of Wounds. New York, McGraw-Hill, 1957.

An excellent biological-clinical correlation of the status of wound healing is given by Dunphy in his Shattuck Lecture (Dunphy, J. E.: The fibroblast—a ubiquitous ally for the surgeon. New Eng. J. Med., 268:1367-1377, 1963).

CHAPTER 3

W. A. ALTEMEIER, M.D., AND W. R. CULBERTSON, M.D.[*]

Applied Surgical Bacteriology

Classification of Bacteria Important in Surgery
Consideration of Effects of Pathogenic Bacteria in Surgery
Resistance of Host to Bacterial Invasion

The application of bacteriologic knowledge and technics to surgery provides the surgeon with information valuable in the prevention, the diagnosis and the treatment of infections seen in surgical practice. Historically, surgery has advanced largely through contributions made to it by the various basic sciences—Philosophy, Anatomy, Pathology, Physiology, Bacteriology and Biochemistry—each adding to its development. Bacteriology has given to surgery aseptic and antiseptic technics, methods of more accurate diagnosis, and effective means of preventing and treating many surgical infections. The expanding horizons of surgery have often been and still are dependent upon the development of special methods of overcoming the hazards of postoperative infections.

Before the era of bacteriology, all wounds, both accidental and planned, became infected. The developing infections were classified as (1) benign, with "laudable pus," or (2) malignant, with "hospital gangrene" and a high mortality. With the advent of the bacteriologic era, the germ concept of infections was established, and antiseptic and aseptic technics were developed. These advances permitted the rapid expansion and the technical development of modern surgery. Without the control of bacteria and infection, this technical development would have been impossible.

[*] From the Department of Surgery, University of Cincinnati College of Medicine and the Cincinnati General Hospital, Cincinnati, Ohio.

During the past two and a half decades, many physicians and students had assumed that there were no longer any problems in the prevention or the control of surgical infections since a wide selection of antibacterial agents was available. This belief was erroneous. Many of the old problems persisted, and new ones arose with the introduction of each new antibacterial agent.

Therefore, surgical bacteriology has maintained its position of relative importance in clinical surgery. While it is true that we have means of controlling many infections, it is also true that bacteriologic studies and sensitivity tests are more important than ever for the successful utilization of these means. It is very questionable whether or not there are fewer infections now than 15 years ago, and many of the infections encountered now are more complex and difficult to treat. The number of specimens of pus submitted to clinical bacteriology laboratories for culture is much greater now than it was then. In addition, there are occurring recently an increasing number of severe and often fatal infections which are produced by bacteria that have acquired resistance to most or all of the available antibiotic agents. Moreover, recent investigations have shown that antibiotic therapy used under some circumstances for the prevention or the treatment of an infection may actually cause another which then becomes an *iatrogenic* infection.

CLASSIFICATION OF BACTERIA IMPORTANT IN SURGERY

A great host of microorganisms may contaminate wounds, but the various types which produce surgical infections are fortunately more limited. Strictly speaking, the infecting

Classification of Bacteria Important in Surgery

agents are not all bacterial, others being spirochetal, fungal, parasitic and viral.

The more important of these may be classified as follows:

I. Aerobic bacteria
  1. Gram-positive cocci
      A. Staphylococcus
          a. aureus
          b. albus
          c. citreus
      B. Streptococcus
          a. hemolyticus
          b. nonhemolyticus
          c. viridans
      C. Pneumococcus
  2. Gram-negative cocci
      A. Neisseria gonorrhoeae
      B. Neisseria catarrhalis
  3. Gram-positive bacilli
      A. Bacillus anthracis
      B. Corynebacterium diphtheriae
      C. Diphtheroid bacilli
      D. Mycobacterium tuberculosis
  4. Gram-negative bacilli
      A. Escherichia coli
      B. Aerobacter aerogenes
      C. Proteus
      D. Pseudomonas aeruginosa
      E. Alcaligenes faecalis
      F. Klebsiella pneumoniae
      G. Serratia marcescens
      H. Salmonella typhosa
      I. Hemophilus influenzae
      J. Hemophilus ducreyi
II. Micro-aerophilic bacteria
  1. Gram-positive cocci
      A. Streptococcus
          a. hemolyticus
          b. nonhemolyticus
III. Anaerobic bacteria
  1. Gram-positive cocci
      A. Streptococcus
  2. Gram-positive bacilli
      A. Clostridia
          a. tetani
          b. welchii (perfringens)
          c. novyi
          d. septicum
          e. histolyticum
          f. sordellii
          g. sporogenes
  3. Gram-negative Bacteroides
      A. melaninogenicus
      B. funduliformis
IV. Spirochaeta
V. Higher microorganisms
  1. Actinomyces
  2. Blastomyces
  3. Coccidioides
  4. Sporotrichum
  5. Candida albicans
  6. Aspergillus niger
  7. Endamoeba histolytica
VI. Viruses

The bacteria of greatest importance in acute surgical infections are the *pyogenic bacteria*. The term "pyogenic" (pus forming) is usually applied to the staphylococcus, streptococcus, pneumococcus, gonococcus and meningococcus. Sometimes it is applied to the colon bacillus and *Ps. aeruginosa* and other bacteria. The tubercle bacillus, although not considered a pyogenic bacterium, may produce typical thick creamy pus in "cold" abscesses.

The *Staphylococci* occurring in surgical infections may be classified into various subgroups on the basis of their cultural characteristics or their lysis by specific bacteriophages. As grown in culture, the *Staphylococcus* may be designated as *aureus, albus* or *citreus*, depending upon the color of its colonies. This organism is a normal inhabitant of the human skin and the nasopharynx, and it may be found in wounds as a pathogen or as a contaminant. In fact, it is often difficult to determine whether the organism isolated from many areas of infection represents a pathogenic or a saprophytic strain. A *Staphylococcus* which is hemolytic, coagulase positive, mannitol-positive and of the *aureus* variety is usually pathogenic. In addition, the *80-81, 77, 42B* or *U.C.18* bacteriophage types have been shown not only to be virulent varieties but also to have an unusual epidemiologic potential.

Bacteriophage typing is a means of further classification of this organism. When the pathologic strains are subjected to lysis by specific bacteriophaging, recognition of epidemic and hospital strains is facilitated. Strains may be responsible for local epidemics occurring in newborn nurseries, geriatric wards and surgical and medical wards in hospitals. These strains are likely to have antibiotic patterns of resistance to the majority

36   Applied Surgical Bacteriology

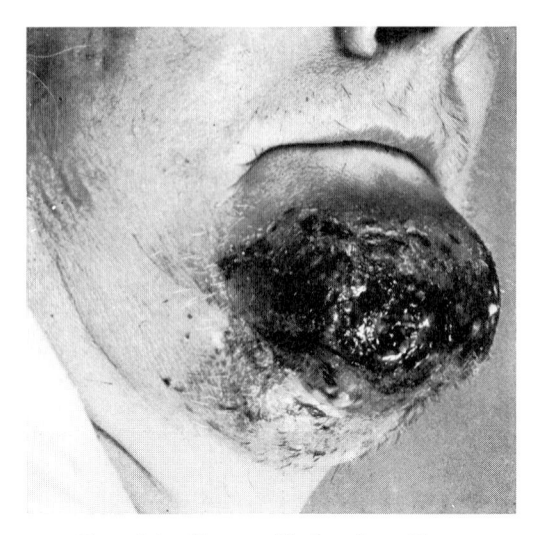

FIG. 3-1. 65-year-old female with carbuncle of chin of 1 week's duration caused by hemolytic *Staphylococcus aureus*. No evidence of involvement of underlying mandible. Multiple draining sinuses and extensive necrosis of overlying skin are prominent.

of agents used. Their ability to spread from personnel to patient or from patient to patient requires particular attention to effective isolation methods and meticulous hygienic and aseptic technics.

Pathogenic staphylococci usually cause rapid necrosis and suppuration, forming thick, creamy and odorless pus. Their infections display a tendency to remain localized as an abscess, which eventually heals after drainage. The favorable outcome which followed staphylococcal infection led to the old term of "laudable pus." On the other hand, strains of staphylococci may be very virulent and may produce serious or fatal invasive infections, such as septicemia and pyemia in which the organisms are circulated in the blood stream. The tendency of staphylococcic infections to remain localized is thought to be related to the production of an enzyme coagulase which produces thrombosis of vessels.

The *aerobic Streptococcus* may occur as one of several types; *hemolytic, nonhemolytic,* or *viridans*. Its strains may be normal inhabitants of the oral cavity, the upper respiratory tract, the vaginal tract, or the gastrointestinal tract. Virulent strains are prone to produce serious, invasive and rapidly developing infections which spread to involve wide areas of tissues. Necrosis may be produced, but there is much less tendency to form pus, the exudate usually being watery in character. The *Streptococcus* is regularly or frequently the etiologic agent in erysipelas, scarlet fever, acute tonsillitis, cellulitis, osteomyelitis (infrequent), septicemia, mastoiditis, lymphangitis, and many other infections. The tendency of streptococcic infection to spread has been attributed to the production of streptokinase which initiates fibrinolysis.

The *Pneumococcus* may be associated with infections of the lung and the pleura, septicemia, osteomyelitis, meningitis and sinusitis. Pneumococcic infections of the lung may be followed by empyema. The pus in such cases, although thin at first, rapidly becomes thick, creamy, mucoid, and contains much clotted fibrin. The *Pneumococcus* may also cause primary peritonitis in children and occasionally acute pyogenic arthritis.

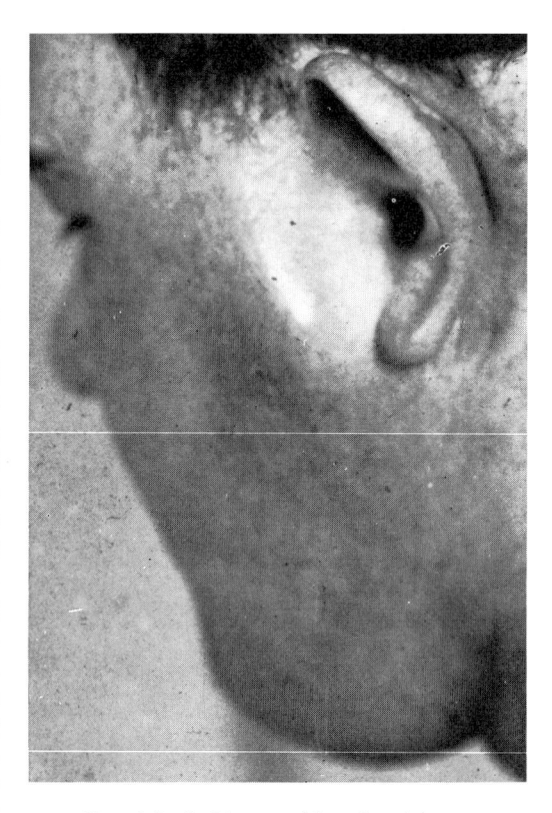

FIG. 3-2. A 24-year-old male with acute purulent parotitis and parotid abscess caused by hemolytic *Staphylococcus aureus*.

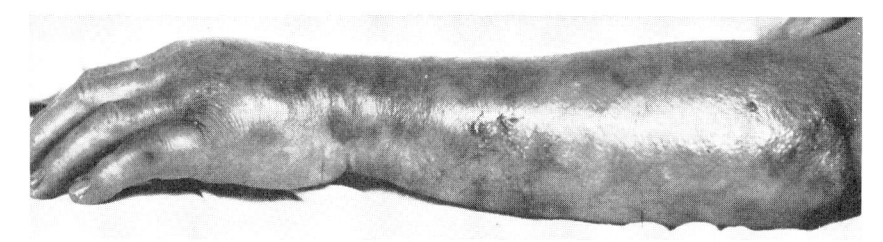

FIG. 3-3. Severe hemolytic streptococcal cellulitis of arm and hand secondary to infection of small burn. Note bronze appearance of skin and diffuseness of process with no signs of localization. Patient's temperature reached 105°. Three blood cultures were positive.

The *Neisseria gonorrhoeae* or *Gonococcus* is a gram-negative coccus which does not occur as a normal inhabitant in man. In the usual infection, it grows in the urethra, the seminal vessels, the prostate, or the epididymis in the male, and in the urethra, the cervix, or the fallopian tubes and the peritoneum in the female. However, it may occur elsewhere, as in infections of the conjunctiva. The infection produced by the gonococcus is customarily localized to the genitourinary tract, causing severe inflammation of the mucosal surface with production of a thin purulent discharge. Occasionally, the organism may become vigorously invasive and cause meningitis, arthritis (sometimes of a temporomandibular joint), septicemia, or endocarditis.

The *Neisseria catarrhalis* (*Micrococcus catarrhalis*) is also a gram-negative coccus and is frequently a normal inhabitant of the nasopharynx. It may cause disease by producing meningitis, conjunctivitis and occasionally septicemia or meningitis.

Bacillus anthracis is an aerobic gram-positive bacillus which causes anthrax. It is of historical interest because it was the first organism found to be the cause of a specific disease. Anthrax is primarily a disease of animals, but it may produce serious infection in man, either as a result of local subcutaneous invasion or as a pneumonialike infection.

Anthrax still occurs sporadically in this country as an occupation-related disease in workers dealing in imported hair for the production of felt cloth. Another potential source of this infection has been occasional epidemics developing in herds of cattle.

Corynebacterium diphtheriae (*Bacillus diphtheriae*) is the cause of a serious toxemia in man. The organisms are gram-positive and may be present in large numbers in localized surface lesions, usually in the upper respiratory tract where a thick membrane forms which may cause respiratory obstruction and death when it becomes dislodged. However, superficial wounds of the skin may become infected with the organisms, particularly among the inhabitants of desert regions. The organism secretes a powerful exotoxin which is absorbed readily from the surface wound and produces serious systemic manifestations, especially myocardial damage.

In the *Corynebacterium* group are also included the *"diphtheroid" bacilli*. These organisms are not sufficiently virulent to produce disease by themselves but are frequently of importance as secondary contaminants in infections due to other organisms.

The gram-positive group also includes the

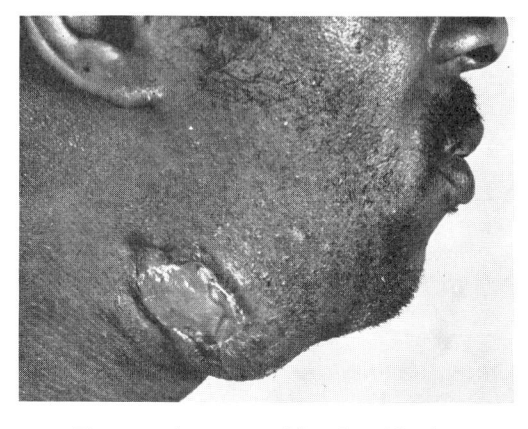

FIG. 3-4. A 25-year-old male with ulcerative tuberculous lymphadenopathy of 4 months' duration. Diagnosis proved by biopsy and culture.

bacillus of tuberculosis, *Mycobacterium tuberculosis*. This organism classically retains staining by the "acid-fast" technic. It produces disease of the respiratory tract, causing necrosis of lung tissue with caseation and cavitation. In addition, it may cause infection of skin, bones, lymph nodes and intestinal tract, with the formation of slowly progressive, chronic, infiltrative abscesses containing thick creamy pus and necrotic tissue in the walls of the abscesses. Characteristically, soft tissue abscesses produced by it near the body surface are devoid of the local signs of inflammation and are referred to as "cold abscesses."

The gram-negative bacillary group of bacteria includes a number of organisms of surgical import. These have become of increasing consequence since the discovery of penicillin, the use of which has often permitted secondary or superimposed infections by gram-negative bacilli during treatment, particularly by strains of *Ps. aeruginosa, Proteus vulgaris, Aerobacter aerogenes* and *E. coli*. Characteristically, they are of lesser virulence than the gram-positive pyogenic cocci, but they play an important part in the etiology of many mixed bacterial infections, such as peritonitis, putrid empyema, infected burns, urinary tract infections, postoperative cellulitis, wound infections, etc. More infrequently, they may produce monobacterial infections, such as ascending cholangitis, meningitis, urinary tract infections and septicemia.

Escherichia coli is very widespread in nature, particularly within the intestinal tracts and the excretions of man and animals. The organism appears in the intestinal tract of infants shortly after birth and remains there throughout life, usually without harmful effects. *E. coli* is of surgical interest as a partial cause of many mixed infections, including appendicitis, cholecystitis, peritonitis and infected burns, but the usual designation of the unaided activities of *E. coli* as the cause of appendiceal peritonitis is not justified or founded upon fact. The organism has little native virulence for animals when injected intraperitoneally, unless a foreign body or substance to delay its absorption is also inoculated. However, when grown and inoculated with other types of bacteria intraperitoneally, a mixed and virulent peritonitis can be produced. Frequently, it is possible to inject intravenously more than 2,500 million *E. coli* into the marginal ear vein of rabbits with no demonstrable harmful effects.

To *E. coli* has been falsely assigned also the responsibility for the putrid odor of appendiceal peritonitis. It has been shown that this organism when grown on sterile pus does not produce a foul odor, since its enzymes apparently cannot attack native protein. The principal and important causes of this foul odor are anaerobic bacteria of the *Bacteroides*, the *Clostridia*, or the anaerobic *Streptococcus* groups.

Aerobacter aerogenes is customarily a saprophyte found in the intestinal tract of man. It may become virulent and of pathologic significance in a manner similar to *E. coli*. *A. aerogenes* can cause urinary tract infections alone or in association with other bacteria; it can be associated with other organisms as causative agents in peritonitis and wound infections; and occasionally it may cause serious septicemia.

Proteus is usually also a nonpathogenic inhabitant of the intestinal tract, but it may cause infection alone or in synergism with other bacteria. It is seen most commonly in infections such as fecal peritonitis, urinary tract infections, infected burns, postoperative infections of abdominal or perineal wounds, or septicemia. At times, it may assume significant virulence and invade the blood stream to produce a secondary or superimposed infection. The latter complication may develop as the result of newly assumed virulence during intensive antibiotic treatment with the various antibacterial agents.

Salmonella typhosa (the typhoid bacillus) produces disease in the human being primarily after its invasion of the gastrointestinal tract (typhoid fever). This is followed by invasion of the lymphoid tissue of the gastrointestinal tract and early dissemination in the blood stream. Hemorrhage into the intestine or perforation of the intestinal wall with secondary peritonitis may complicate the course of typhoid fever (see Chap. 37, Appendicitis, Peritonitis and Intra-abdominal Abscesses). As patients with typhoid fever are usually very ill, perforation must be detected early if the patient is to be saved by operation and closure of the opening. Frequent visits with a close watch for changes in abdominal rigidity are necessary. As in other ill patients, pain may not be as pronounced as in perforated peptic ulcer. Localized infection may occur later in the disease in the form of acute and chronic osteomyelitis, periostitis, pyelitis, or cholecystitis. Chronic infection may persist after subsidence of symptoms, and a carrier state may result. Wound infections may also be caused by the typhoid bacillus, particularly after cholecystectomy for the removal of the gallbladder in a carrier patient.

Klebsiella pneumoniae may produce severe pneumonia in a man and may also cause other infections such as sinusitis, empyema, pulmonary abscess, septicemia, or meningitis.

Alcaligenes faecalis is a saprophytic inhabitant of the gastrointestinal tract under normal circumstances, but it may occur in human infections as the primary etiologic agent or as a secondary invader. It has been found to be the cause of septicemia on occasions, but most frequently it is found in cases of peritonitis due to fecal contamination and occasionally is responsible for urinary tract infections.

Pseudomonas aeruginosa or *Bacillus pyocyaneus* is found frequently as a secondary infecting agent of wounds. Usually it is encountered as part of a mixed infection, particularly in large wounds containing necrotic material or consisting of large granulating defects. This bacterium is an important etiologic agent of troublesome infections of the eye, the external and the internal auditory canals, and burns. Its presence is indicated by the development of a greenish or bluish discoloration of the wound discharges and by its peculiar musty odor. Occasionally, it may assume marked virulence and in such cases produce severe invasion and life-endangering infections.

As with *Escherichia coli*, the *Pseudomonas aeruginosa* often occurs in association with other organisms, particularly the *Staphylococcus*. Symbiotic and synergistic effects of these in association may produce a more invasive infection than either is likely to do alone. Septicemia complicating burns or secondary peritonitis may be very difficult to manage and may be fatal. Meningitis caused by *Ps. aeruginosa* likewise has a high mortality. Purulent material produced by it is usually thick and blue-green in color. Further characterization of various strains of *Pseudomonas* is possible by specific bacteriophage typing.

Serratia marcescens and related bacteria of the para colon group have recently assumed importance in hospital-acquired infections, particularly those related to continuous intravenous therapy or respiratory tract infections developing in debilitated or elderly postoperative patients.

Hemophilus influenzae is another gram-negative bacterium which may be found in the nose and the throat of healthy individuals. Pathogenically, it may produce sinusitis, pneumonitis, suppurative pleurisy, otitis media, or occasionally a particularly serious type of meningitis in children.

Micro-aerophilic organisms, especially the *Streptococci*, occasionally may assume importance in surgical lesions. They may be present as etiologic agents in certain chronic infections, such as chronic burrowing ulcer or chronic cutaneous progressive gangrene. At times, they may produce severe acute infections with septicemia, as in puerperal sepsis, meningitis, brain abscess, or osteomyelitis. When first isolated, they are often strictly anaerobic, but after 2 subcultivations they become micro-aerophilic in their oxygen requirements. They are isolated with difficulty and may be missed with ordinary methods of bacterial cultivation.

The *nonhemolytic micro-aerophilic Streptococcus* has been found in cutaneous gangrenous lesions of the skin, peritonitis, intra-abdominal abscess and empyema.

The *hemolytic micro-aerophilic Streptococcus* has been found most frequently in chronic burrowing infections of the neck, the axillary, the perineal and the popliteal regions.

The *anaerobic Streptococcus* is also a serious invader of the human body and is encountered in various infections, such as peritonitis, lung abscess, putrid empyema, tubo-ovarian abscess, septic abortion, puerperal sepsis, or symbiotic infections. Purulent material produced by it is usually foul smelling, thick, and grayish in color. Because of its strict anaerobic requirements, frequently this organism is not isolated or identified as an etiologic agent in many surgical infections. When exposed to the air at room temperature for periods of 5 or 10 minutes or longer, the organism may die and will not grow on artificial media. In addition, if only aerobic methods of cultivation are used the organism will be overlooked. The presence of highly motile organisms in mixed culture will often obscure anaerobic *Streptococci* through their overgrowth. Although there is little or no evidence of native virulence of the anaerobic *Streptococci* for experimental animals, recent experimental work has demonstrated unquestionably their virulence and pathogenicity for man.

The pathogenic microorganisms of the anaerobic gram-positive group which are of surgical significance include the causative agents of tetanus and gas gangrene. *Clostridium tetani* is a gram-positive sporulating anaerobe which is commonly found in the feces of animals, particularly the horse. It is also found in manured or pastured soil. As an infecting agent of wounds, *Cl. tetani* may produce the disease of tetanus through the effect of its powerful exotoxin. Absorption and distribution of this toxin affect the central nervous system and the neuromuscular end-organs to produce the typical signs and symptoms of tetanus. The local wound infected by the tetanus bacillus has no changes which are specific for this type of infection. The organism does not invade the body but remains localized in the wound. It requires very strict anaerobic environment for its growth; consequently, infection by it may occur as a complication of any deep penetrating wound. Its growth is also facilitated by the presence of necrotic material in the wound.

Cl. welchii, Cl. novyi, Cl. septicum, Cl. histolyticum and *Cl. sordellii* are anaerobic gram-positive spore-forming bacteria commonly found in the intestinal tracts of animals and man and in fertilized soil and wool clothing. Individually, or in various combinations, these organisms may cause the dreaded infectious complication of wounds known as gas gangrene. They require the presence of necrotic tissue for their growth, and the development of infection by them is aided by the presence of foreign bodies. They may cause destruction of adjacent and intact tissues by toxin production, thrombosis of vessels and mechanical effects of gas and edema. In military and civilian practice, gas gangrene may complicate crushing injuries, compound fractures, or fracture dislocations involving muscle masses. The infections produced by these bacteria are characteristic and serious, with severe toxemia, wet gangrene and a high mortality rate. The gas formation may be demonstrated by feeling crepitation or by roentgenogram, but it does not invariably occur.

The *Bacteroides* are pleomorphic, anaerobic, gram-negative bacilli which occasionally produce serious infections in wounds. Also, they may be of importance in such infections as fecal peritonitis, retroperitoneal cellulitis, pilonidal abscesses, or perineal abscesses. Septicemia and metastatic abscess formation can occur. The *Bacteroides melaninogenicus* may produce infections, usually in association with the anaerobic *Streptococcus*. Its growth in tissues is associated with grayish or black discoloration of the tissues, a gray exudate and a putrid odor.

The higher phylogenetic orders of microorganisms of surgical importance include the *Actinomyces*, which are the cause of actinomycosis and usually are anaerobic fungi. They may be found as nonpathogenic inhabitants of the oral cavity of man and animal. When they produce disease, they cause a chronic burrowing suppurative process which develops granulomatous lesions. Liquefaction and suppuration may occur with sinus formation and discharge of purulent material containing the characteristic sulfur granules. The usual pathogenic strain of *Actinomyces* is the *A. israelii*. Of less importance are the *Nocardia* which are aerobic fungi assigned to this group. *N. asteroides* is occasionally the cause of disease which is clinically similar to actinomycosis. *N. madurae* is one of the causes of mycetoma or madura foot.

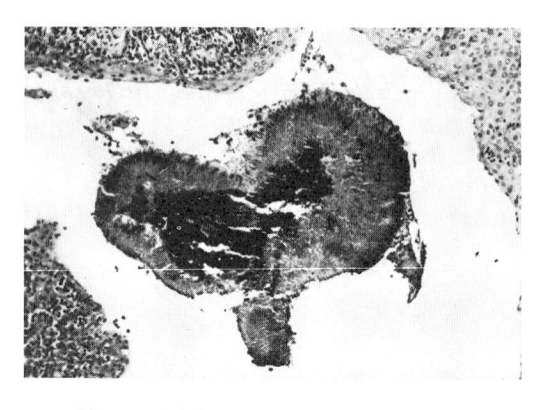

Fig. 3-5. Microscopic appearance of *Actinomyces* colony in tonsillar tissue.

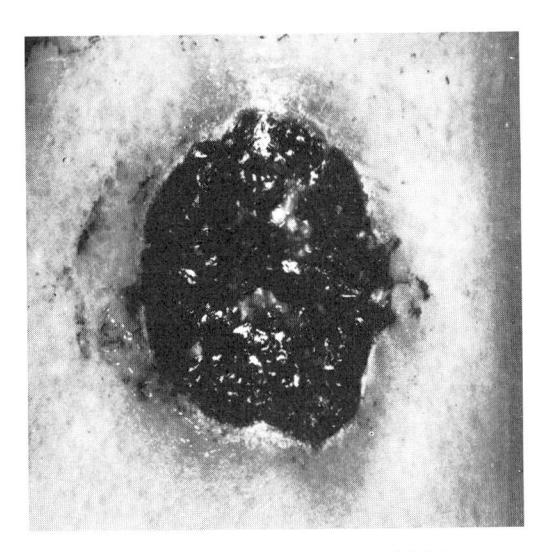

FIG. 3-6. An 81-year-old male with blastomycotic ulcer of left leg of 5 months' duration. Diagnosis made by demonstrating *Blastomyces* in discharge at margin of wound by hanging-drop technic.

Blastomyces dermatitidis is a fungus pathogenic for man, which produces a very serious infection originating either as a skin surface lesion or as a pulmonary pneumonitis. The cutaneous lesion develops as a chronic, progressive, wartlike lesion composed of multiple intradermal abscesses containing the organism. It may advance to general dissemination with involvement of the lungs, bone, the kidneys and the brain. The pulmonary type is usually a fatal pneumonitis associated with cavitation.

Coccidioidal granuloma is caused by the *Coccidioides immitis*. This is usually a pulmonary infection, although there may be an involvement of the skin by nodular, ulcerative, or granulomatous lesions and, occasionally, of any parts of the body.

Sporotricha are widely distributed in nature and usually are saprophytic. However, *Sporotrichum schenckii* may cause granulomatous infections of a chronic nature with indolent ulcerations of the skin. These may progress to involve muscle, bone, or lung tissue.

Histoplasma capsulatum produces an infection in man ranging from a slight illness lasting a few days to acute and fulminating fatal disease. The organism may invade the blood stream. A pneumonia refractory to all available antibiotics is one form the disease may take. It may also produce hepatomegaly, lymphadenopathy, anemia and leukopenia.

Infections produced by *Candida albicans* are usually superficial and mild, since this organism is not vigorously invasive. The common site is the mouth, where the infection is known as thrush or mycotic stomatitis. Antibiotic therapy has permitted an increased number of pulmonary and intestinal infections by this agent, many of which have become difficult to control. Invasive moniliasis is increasing in incidence and has become another hazard to patients with severe burns, during intensive antibiotic therapy for other infectious agents. Meningitis and pneumonitis caused by *C. albicans* may be fatal.

Members of the *Aspergillus* group have been responsible upon rare occasions for chronic surface infections in man and occasionally for the formation of mycetoma. *Aspergillus niger* may produce cutaneous ulcerations which are chronic, mildly suppurative and covered by a black crust typical of the organism's growth.

Some *viral* infections are of surgical importance. Included are the filtrable viruses that can cause lymphopathia venereum. The initial lesion is a small ulcer of the genitalia following inoculation by sexual contact. Involvement of the lymphatics may lead to spread to the genital organs and the rectum. The resulting proctitis may cause stricture formation and obstruction requiring surgical intervention.

The *virus* causing homologous serum jaundice is transmitted from one individual to another by the injection of blood or blood products or by accidental inoculation through the medium of contaminated needles or similar objects. The virus is active in the blood of 1 in 200 to 1 in 500 donors, dependent on the geographic area and the methods of screening involved. Pooled human plasma increases the risk of infection. Previous experimental work indicated that the storage of plasma in the liquid state for 6 months at temperatures of 32° C. or modified pasteurization procedures would inactivate this virus. Recent studies, however, have indicated that this method may not be fully effective.

The incubation period is usually about 3 months but ranges from 3 weeks to 6 months. The virus causes a form of hepatitis of varying severity, generally associated with jaundice (see Chap. 8, Blood Transfusions and Related Problems).

Historically, rabies was one of the more dramatic viral infections whose infectious nature was discovered by Pasteur. This infection is transmitted by the bite of rabid animals and, fortunately, occurs rarely in human beings in this country.

Spirochetes of surgical importance include the *Treponema pallidum*, *T. macrodentium* and *T. microdentium*. The first may produce chronic ulcerations of primary syphilis or granulomatous lesions of tertiary syphilis, and these must be considered frequently in differential diagnosis of surgical lesions. The *T. macrodentium* and *microdentium* may contribute to the development of foul-smelling cervical or mouth infections or human-bite infections.

Transitional and "L-forms." Bacteria usually appear in the rigid form of a bacillus, a coccus, or a vibrio. Not infrequently, however, aberrant or pleomorphic forms may occur in blood cultures, freshly isolated cultures from pathologic material, and old laboratory cultures. These aberrant forms vary from dwarf cells to giant bodies and may be quite irregular in their outline, bearing no resemblance morphologically or culturally to the conventional parent form. Currently, these are referred to as "L-forms" ("L" standing for Lister Institute).

However, these transitional stages are capable of reversion to the parent bacillary form when cultivated under appropriate media and conditions. Under antibiotic therapy, the conventional bacterial forms have occasionally been noted to change to the transitional stages of the "L-forms." When antibiotic therapy was interrupted, patients have been noted to suffer a recurrence of fever and illness associated with reappearance of the bacillary form of the organism in the blood or lesion.

CONSIDERATION OF EFFECTS OF PATHOGENIC BACTERIA IN SURGERY

Origin and Spread of Infections

Infection is the result of the entrance, the growth and the metabolic activities of microorganisms in tissues. *Surgical* infections differ from *medical* infections in 2 principal manners: (1) the infected area or primary focus is unlikely to resolve spontaneously, producing suppuration, necrosis, gangrene, prolonged morbidity, death, or other serious effects if untreated; and (2) excision, incision and/or drainage must be possible. In addition, surgical infections are often *polymicrobic* and invasive, with rapid growth and spread of bacteria into the surrounding tissues or systems. In contrast, medical infections are usually *monomicrobic*, diffuse, and associated with little or no tissue reaction but a marked systemic response.

The point of bacterial entrance through the skin or the mucous membrane of the body is known as the *portal of entry*. The cutaneous surfaces and the mucous membranes of the human body are normally intact. Although often contaminated with bacteria, they are normally resistant to the invasion of microorganisms. Bacteria cannot invade these surfaces normally except through injuries produced by trauma or some other physical, chemical, or metabolic factor that decreases the local resistance of the tissues and favors the growth of bacteria.

Obstruction to the flow of fluid excretions or secretions through tubular structures such as the ureter, the common bile duct, the intestine and the appendix usually enhances local bacterial growth and invasion of tissues by microorganisms. In some instances, however, highly virulent bacteria may penetrate the mucous membrane without trauma, such as the typhoid, the dysentery and the tubercle bacilli, or the *T. pallidum*. In others, the bacteria will be unable to produce infection in that they will be destroyed or inhibited by the natural defenses of the body.

The period between contamination of tissues and the onset of infection is known as the *incubation period*. After invasion of the physiologic interior, bacteria may grow and produce a variety of inflammatory reactions. Their toxins may cause hyperemia, edema, increased capillary permeability, cellular infiltration, thrombosis, clot lysis and tissue liquefaction, suppuration, spontaneous bleeding or necrosis.

The reaction of the tissues locally to the growth and the products of bacterial metabolism produces the *local* signs and symptoms of infection. The reaction of tissues or organs distant to the primary focus or of the body as a whole may produce *general* signs and symptoms of the infection. *Regional* spread through adjacent tissues or neighboring lymphatics may also occur.

When infection occurs, it usually starts as a *cellulitis*, a diffuse inflammatory process without suppuration which is characterized by edema, redness, pain and interference with function. Cellular infiltration of the tissues by red blood cells, leukocytes, histiocytes and macrophages occurs. *Suppuration* often follows and is the result of local liquefaction of tissue with the formation of pus, known as an *abscess*. The abscess is usually walled off by an area of inflammatory reaction which produces induration about the abscess and a softening at the center of the lesion. Cellulitis in varying degrees usually extends beyond the abscess's area of induration.

Bacterial proteolytic enzymes aid in the process of tissue liquefaction. Many bacteria produce *proteinases* which are capable of breaking down proteins. *Collagenase* is one of these which favors the liquefaction of collagen and the dissemination of infection along or even through fascial barriers. *Hyaluronidase* presumably favors the spread of bacterial toxins through alteration of the ground substances.

The hemolytic *Streptococcus* may produce a fibrinolysin, an enzyme which dissolves fibrin and makes it difficult for the body to ward off streptococcal infections.

Septic thrombosis of adjacent blood vessels frequently occurs and contributes to the local destruction and liquefaction of tissues. Small abscesses, areas of cutaneous gangrene, or infectious gangrene of entire extremities may be the result of septic thrombosis.

Thrombophlebitis of veins adjacent to infections may have additional effects. Septic emboli may be dislodged from the area of primary infection and gain their way into the circulating blood stream. The hemolytic *Staphylococcus*, in particular, produces a coagulase which clots small vessels and favors spread by septic embolization. Occasionally, other organisms demonstrate the propensity for producing thrombophlebitis. The Bacteroides group and their "L" forms, in particular, have been shown to have this ability; and some strains have been found to produce heparinase.

The dissemination of microorganisms by a distributing focus results in either a bacteremia or a septicemia. In a *bacteremia* the primary focus distributes bacteria once or intermittently, resulting in their transient appearance in the blood. When it distributes organisms more or less constantly, their continued presence in the blood stream is known as a *septicemia*. The old concept suggested that the actual growth or reproduction of bacteria within the circulating blood stream was a septicemia in contrast with a bacteremia in which the microorganisms found it impossible to reproduce in the circulating blood. The newer concept indicates that the difference is in the rate of dissemination from the distributing focus, it being more or less constant in a septicemia and intermittent or single in a bacteremia. Remember that any bacterium discharged into the circulation makes a complete circuit in the blood stream about every 23 seconds and, in doing so, runs the gamut of such hostile forces as circulating antibodies, polymorphonuclear leukocytes, macrophages and histiocytes of the reticuloendothelial system. It is possible to inject intravenously as many as 2,500 million bacteria in 2 cc. of culture media and to note the progressive disappearance of the bacteria from the blood stream by serial blood cultures. Usually within 2 to 6 hours the bacteria will have been completely removed, and negative blood cultures will result.

Virulent microorganisms distributed from a *primary focus* to distant organs or tissues may set up *metastatic* infections which in turn may become *secondary* or *tertiary* distributing *foci*. Under the circumstances, the signs of invasive infection with positive blood cultures may have a cyclic sequence.

Bacteria may be carried away from the area of infection in the lymph fluid and distributed to regional areas through the *regional lymphatics or lymph nodes*. In doing so, they may cause an inflammatory reaction in the lymph vessels known as *lymphangitis*, and in the regional lymph nodes known as *lymphadenitis*. The latter may be suppurative or nonsuppurative, depending upon the resistance of the organism and the host.

Gangrene or necrosis may result in areas of

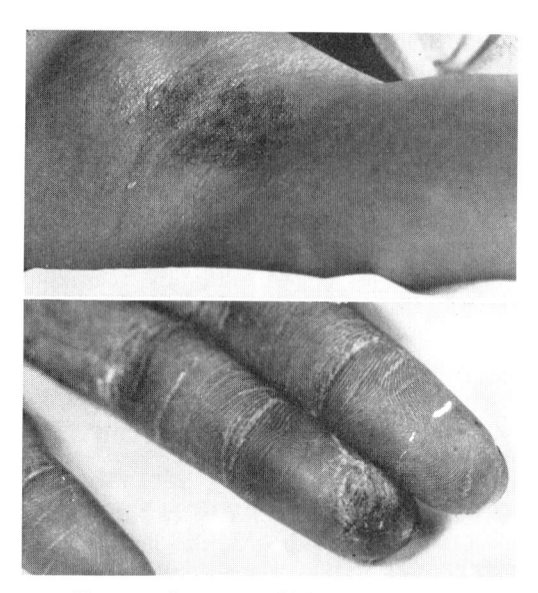

FIG. 3-7. A 30-year-old female with ulceration of 4th finger, lymphangitis and suppurative axillary lymphadenopathy. Diagnosis of tularemia proved by culture of ulceration and pus aspirated from abscess.

infection produced by necrotizing bacterial enzymes, thrombosis of nutrient vessels, bacterial action, or ischemia resulting from the tourniquet effect caused by marked swelling of the tissues incident to infection.

Uncontrolled infections may become *chronic* and may be characterized by excessive fibrosis, sinus or fistulous tract formation, variable alterations in the local and general physiology, continued fever, anemia, sequestration of bone, fascia or tendon, contractures, limitation of function, or cosmetic disfigurement.

Thus infection may *subside spontaneously, remain localized, extend to regional or distant areas,* or *become chronic.* If the infections do extend, they do so by direct extension, lymphatic spread, venous spread or, rarely, arterial spread. Direct extension is most common, with spread by way of the subcutaneous tissues, muscles, vessel planes, or tendon sheaths. They may also spread diffusely through cavities such as the peritoneal or the thoracic cavities.

RESISTANCE OF THE HOST TO BACTERIAL INVASION

The power of resistance of a patient to bacterial infection is a complex physiologic phenomenon which is generally referred to as his *resistance* or *immunity*. The development of any infection is the result of failure of the dynamic interplay of the various factors of resistance to oppose successfully the number and the virulence of the contaminating microorganisms.

Unfortunately, resistance, immunity and their opposite, susceptibility, are *relative* and *not absolute*. Degrees of resistance exist which may be modified by a number of factors. Absolute immunity is rare, but there are isolated instances in nature in which large inoculations of microorganisms virulent to one species will not produce significant infections in other species.

In a clinical sense, host resistance is a broad concept, representing the summation of many forces and influences in the defense mechanism which controls the relationship between the host and the parasite. An understanding of the factors that control and promote host resistance is a major responsibility of all surgeons. The basis of the treatment of infections rests essentially upon *promoting* the measures that fortify the resistance of the patient, and even the administration of antibiotic agents, which serves to control the growth of the invading parasite, cannot effect a cure without the occurrence of an adequate immune response.

Resistance or immunity of the host may be classified as *local, regional,* or *general*.

LOCAL RESISTANCE

Local resistance is accomplished initially by the intact barrier of the skin and the mucous membranes which is generally impermeable to bacteria. However, this barrier may be penetrated or weakened by the effects of nonbacterial disease or trauma. Occasionally, as in the case of the spirochete of syphilis, the microorganisms may possess innate ability to penetrate the cutaneous or mucous surfaces. When the surface membranes have been broken down, permitting bacterial invasion, many other local defense mechanisms are alerted. The number, the type and the effectiveness of these depend somewhat on the tissue invaded and its vascularity. Concurrently, the phenomenon of local resistance occurs in the form of septic inflammation. This process is generally purposeful, serving to localize, destroy, or remove the invading bacteria. This inflammatory response is characterized by increased *local heat, redness, swelling* and *tenderness*, as originally noted by Celsus. Later, John Hunter added another characteristic, *interference with function*.

The increased heat and redness reflect an increase in the local blood supply to the area, with the enhancement of local defense by more oxygen and nutrition, as well as the later supply of the products which are part of general immunity.

When local pain develops in an infected area, involuntary splinting of the affected part may reduce the discomfort, decrease the dissemination of the infection and permit the tissues to localize and heal the involved area.

The swelling which develops is the result of a series of local resistance factors. One of the early changes is caused by injury to the cellular membranes which increases the vascular permeability and permits the extravasation of fluid into the intercellular spaces, with the formation of an effusion. This effusion has definite antibacterial properties, and its character often varies with the type of infecting organism. Leukocytes, which have the ability to ingest and destroy many types of bacteria, migrate into the areas of edema and aid in the formation of an inflammatory exudate, the toxins and other bacterial products which may evoke different changes in areas of infection. The local lymphatics may become blocked by plugs of fibrin, venous capillaries may become thrombosed, fibrin precipitated, bacterial proteins trapped locally, and *granulation tissue* formed to create a *pyogenic membrane* or *barrier*. Either as a membrane for a surface wound or as a retaining wall about an inflammatory process, granulation tissue is a great natural protective device.

Local immunity may also be enhanced by the occurrence of a previous or recent inflammation in the same area. The effect is probably nonspecific, which in some manner potentiates a more rapid and effective mobilization of defenses to a renewed insult. It was a common observation in the preantibiotic era that the creation of a colostomy, with the associated regional soiling, protected the patient from the dangers of spreading peritonitis when a resection of the colon was performed several weeks later.

REGIONAL RESISTANCE

The second major line of defense which is elaborated by the host is a regional one. When local barriers have been overcome by the infection, spreading cellulitis or lymphangitis may occur. This extension then places the greatest burden of regional defense on the lymphatic system. With the progression of inflammation there is a great outpouring of plasma proteins, fluids and cellular elements, facilitated by bacterial spreading factors such as hyaluronidase. The rate of lymph flow, increasing greatly as extracellular pressure rises in the areas of swelling, achieves the purpose of removing waste products and cellular debris from a focus of high metabolic activity. Invading bacteria quickly appear in the regional lymph stream as though the accelerated flow washes away the organisms from the site of infection. As a consequence, the lymph vessels may become inflamed, producing the clinical picture of lymphangitis which always signifies a potentially serious process. The lymphatic pathways are filtered by the lymph nodes, which usually are located in well-defined anatomic areas along the course of major arteries and veins. When taxed beyond their capacity to react or when overwhelmed by the infection, the regional lymph nodes may become permanently damaged or permit the invasion of the blood stream, with resultant *septicemia*.

The lymph nodal system serves at least two basic purposes: (1) *filtration* of infecting bacteria and cellular debris, and (2) the *production of specific antibodies* against the invading bacteria. The first of these is accomplished by the macrophages of the reticuloendothelial system which line the sinusoids of the lymph gland and there engulf the particles brought to it by the flow of lymph.

The second purpose, production of specific antibodies, is understood less clearly. In experimental animals it has been shown that the regional nodes are an important site of the production of specific immune antibodies to a localized antigenic stimulus. The origin of the lymphoid cell that produces specific antibodies is undecided, but logically the same element that filters out the bacteria might be expected to produce these antibodies. Once formed, the specific antibodies travel from the node into the general circulation for wide distribution.

If lymphatic stasis continues and becomes chronic, its harmful effects may lower the resistance of the involved tissues. Chronic lymphedema may seriously impair resistance to bacterial infection, and a vicious cycle may develop, characterized by recurrent attacks of inflammation and increasing lymphatic damage.

General Resistance

General resistance pertains to the protection afforded by antibodies which are continually circulated throughout the body in some quantity but may, upon proper stimulus, be increased significantly.

The general factors which play an important role in the over-all pattern of resistance may be natural or acquired, specific or nonspecific. *Natural immunity* refers to general resistance which is inherent, congenital, or acquired in some unknown way. Natural and nonspecific factors of general immunity include age, sex, race, individual variations, nutrition, climate and associated metabolic diseases.

Infants have inadequate resources to develop natural immunity or have not had specific stimulation for the formation of general antibodies. Therefore, they have an increased susceptibility to infection and must depend upon passive immunity acquired transplacentally from the mother. This passive immunity disappears in about 6 months and should be replaced by active general immunity.

Natural immunity may be dependent in some circumstances on nutrition, but it is not usually affected by acute processes. In long-term chronic illness associated with inadequate or unbalanced dietary replacement, there is a severe decrease in host resistance to infection.

Severe metabolic disturbances may influence a patient's resistance. In uncontrolled diabetes there is often a marked decrease in general immunity. Because of the damage to peripheral arteries in this disease, there may be a diminished local resistance to add to the over-all hazard. Other metabolic diseases which adversely influence general immunity include portal cirrhosis, vitamin deficiency states, leukopenia, multiple myeloma and Addison's or Cushing's diseases.

Specific immunity is largely dependent upon specific humeral factors which include antitoxins, bacteriolysins, agglutinins and precipitins. The evidence suggests that the gamma globulin fraction of the plasma contains and stores specific bacterial antibodies. In conjunction with local measures of defense the antigen-antibody response assumes great importance in controlling spreading infections.

Antibodies resulting from infection or reaction to antigens in patients confer *acquired immunity* which is lasting or permanent. *Passive immunity* follows the administration of serum containing preformed antibodies. Specific active immunity, once developed, remains more or less permanent against the particular strain of infecting parasite and confers on the host the greatest degree of serologic protection.

The specific antibodies are carried in the gamma globulin fraction of the blood stream. In recent years the fractionation of plasma proteins on a large scale has become feasible; and *gamma globulin*, made from pools of plasma representing many donors, may contain a wide spectrum of immune substances useful for the prevention or the amelioration of specific diseases.

For in-vivo antibody-antigen reactions, *complement* is a necessary element, particularly in the lysis of bacteria. In some patients with infections it has been found that there is a complement deficiency in the blood. Recent investigations have uncovered a serum protein fraction called *properdin*, a serum protein which is essential for the proper function of complement and the antigen-antibody reaction.

An understanding of the various factors concerned with host resistance is a major responsibility of every surgeon. The physiologic process of wound healing is intimately associated with resistance, and a very valuable support to resistance lies in the intelligent care of the injured or infected area to ensure prompt and complete healing. Although much is known about the resistance of the host to the invasion of microorganisms, there are still many gaps in our knowledge which must be filled in before the mechanisms of immunity will be clearly understood.

Hospital-Acquired and Iatrogenic Infections. Recently, world-wide attention has been focused on the causes of postoperative and other hospital infections. Increasing emphasis has been placed on the fact that a significant number and variety of surgical infections may actually be caused by physicians or their treatment and therefore are classified as *iatrogenic*. It is important to realize that the opportunities for the development of infection in hospitalized patients are many and varied. The mechanisms and the routes of contamination are well understood, but the factors of actual infection may be obscure. Antibiotic therapy has increased the complexity of this problem and has created a number of new problems, one of which has been an increased incidence of iatrogenic postoperative infections by antibiotic-resistant bacteria and other microorganisms. Moreover, the extension of surgery to an ever-increasing number of debilitated and aged patients, the use of various drugs and other methods of treatment, such as steroid therapy, extensive x-ray therapy, cancer chemotherapy, etc., have provided surgeons with a large group of patients who are more susceptible to infections. These have required considerable supportive therapy by the use of intravenous injections, blood transfusions, antibiotic preoperative bowel preparation, tracheostomy, indwelling urinary catheters and the like, any of which may in turn be the mechanism of an increased incidence of life-threatening infection.

Some forms of treatment in use now for the postoperative control of patients who have undergone organ transplantation from other patients or animals suppress the white blood cell count and produce a secondarily increased susceptibility to severe and often fatal infection. The success of organ and tissue transplantation operations may be related to iatrogenic infections secondary to the use of these "immunosuppressive drugs."

In a similar manner, some cancer chemotherapeutic agents in use now may suppress the white blood cell count and increase susceptibility to infection.

BIBLIOGRAPHY

Altemeier, W. A.: Bacteriology of war wounds. Internat. Abstr. Surg. *In* Surg., Gynec., Obstet., 75:518-533, 1942.

———: The pathogenicity of the bacteria of appendicitis peritonitis. Ann. Surg., 114:158-159, 1941.

———: Postoperative infections. S. Clin. N. Am., 25: 1202-1228, 1945.

Altemeier, W. A., and Wulsin, J. H.: Natural resistance to infection. *In* Progress In Surgery. Karger, Basel, 1960.

Balch, H. H.: Nutrition and resistance to infection. Ann. Surg., 147:423, 1958.

Churchill, E. D.: The American surgeon, A.U.S. Surg., Gynec., Obstet., 84:529-539, 1947.

Editorial: The ward dressing. Lancet, 2:565, 1941.

Editorial: Surgical bacteriology. Am. Surgeon, 25: 713-714, 1959.

Fleming, A.: Bacteriological examination of wounds. *In* Bailey, H.: Surgery of Modern Warfare. Vol. 1. Chap. 16. Baltimore, Williams & Wilkins, 1941.

Hare, R.: Sources of hemolytic streptococcal infection of wounds in war and in civil life. Lancet, 1:109-112, 1940.

Meleney, F.: Bacterial synergism in disease processes, with a confirmation of the synergistic bacterial etiology of a certain type of progressive gangrene of the abdominal wall. Ann. Surg., 94:961-981, 1931.

———: Bacteriological and surgical principles in management of surgical septicemia. Internat. Abstr. Surg. *In* Surg., Gynec., Obstet., 65:513-521, 1938.

Meleney, F. L., and Whipple, A. O.: Statistical analysis of study of prevention of infection in soft part wounds, compound fractures and burns with special reference to sulfonamides. Surg., Gynec., Obstet., 80:263-296, 1945.

Price, P. B.: Bacteriology of normal skin: new quantitative test applied to study of bacterial flora and disinfectant action of mechanical cleansing. J. Infect. Dis., 63:301-318, 1938.

Redeker, A. G., Hopkins, C. E., Jackson, B., and Peck, B.: A controlled study of the safety of pooled plasma stored in the liquid state in 30-32 C for six months. Transfusion, 8:60-64, 1968.

Reid, M. R.: Some considerations of problems of wound healing. New Eng. J. Med., 215:753-766, 1936.

Thomas, D. C., Hill, E. O., Culbertson, W. R., and Altemeier, W. A.: Development of new bacteriophages for staphylococcal typing. Surg. Forum, 10: 334, 1960.

CHAPTER 4

W. A. ALTEMEIER, M.D., AND W. R. CULBERTSON, M.D.*

Surgical Infections

General Considerations
Primary and Secondary Bacterial Contamination and Infection
Methods of Diagnosis of Surgical Infections
Treatment of Surgical Infections
Classification of Wound Infections

Infections of surgical significance may occur spontaneously, develop in wounds after trauma, or arise in remote areas of the body as postoperative complications. Spontaneous infections, such as acute appendicitis and acute cholecystitis, will be discussed elsewhere in the text. While many infections, such as pneumonia and pyelocystitis, may develop during the postoperative state in tissues or organs remote from the region of an operative area, most surgical infectious lesions are the result of the growth of bacteria introduced through a portal of entry caused by some type of trauma.

When infections develop in wounds resulting from accidental injury, violence, or planned operative procedures, they may have a profound effect on mortality, morbidity and the final result of the injury or the operation. Death, loss of limb, or disability which may be prolonged or permanent may result. The complication of infection, particularly in large wounds, almost certainly increases the period of morbidity after operation, since infection, the greatest enemy of wound healing, produces further destruction of tissue and suppresses the process of healing. Tissue destroyed by infection is usually replaced by scar tissue which may affect cosmetic appearance as well as function.

In recent years considerable attention has been focused throughout the world on the incidence of postoperative wound and other hospital-acquired infections produced by antibiotic-resistant bacteria. The number of infections has apparently increased, and this trend has been ascribed to such factors as indiscriminate antibiotic prophylaxis, overconfidence in the effectiveness of these agents, a disregard of important operating room principles and technics, discontinuation of the principle of isolation, and a continuing and progressively active reservoir of antibiotic-resistant and virulent bacteria in the hospital environment.

The problem of hospital infection, just as with other wound infections, is a double problem—one of contamination and one of effect of the various factors that provoke its actual development.

GENERAL CONSIDERATIONS

The primary essential for the development of infection within wounds is the growth of bacteria. Experience and experimental work have shown that all injuries resulting in penetration of the skin or the mucous membrane are associated with contamination of the wounded tissues by microorganisms of various types. Some may be highly virulent, others less so, and still others saprophytic. Even clean surgical wounds which heal *per primam* are contaminated by airborne microorganisms. Their presence in wounds may or may not be followed by infection, depending upon certain factors that influence the growth of bacteria and determine not only the development of any septic process but also its characteristics. These factors include the following:

1. The virulence, the types and the numbers of contaminating bacteria
2. Devitalized tissue within the wound
3. The presence of foreign bodies

---

* From the Department of Surgery, University of Cincinnati College of Medicine and the Cincinnati General Hospital, Cincinnati, Ohio.

4. The nature, the location and the duration of the wound

5. The local and general immunity response of the individual

6. The type and the thoroughness of treatment

7. The general condition of the patient

The number and the types of contaminating bacteria have long been known to increase the probability and the severity of wound infection, and the premise that infection is the unfavorable result of the equation of dose multiplied by virulence and divided by resistance still holds. However, it must be remembered that the mere presence of virulent bacteria in a wound does not make infection of that wound a certainty. The evidence indicates that the physiologic state of the tissues within the wound before and after treatment is more important than the presence of bacteria per se. The synergistic or cumulative activity of the bacteria present may also determine to a large extent the nature and the severity of the infection.

Unhealthy, irritated or dead tissue in wounds invites and supports the growth of virulent and nonvirulent organisms, since it has limited or little power of resistance to their growth and action. Conversely, *healthy* tissue fortunately possesses a remarkable capacity to kill bacteria or withstand their effects.

Foreign bodies, particularly those of organic composition or contamination, carry large numbers of bacteria into wounds and further the probability of infection through their local irritative action on the tissues. It must be remembered that suture material buried within a wound may act as a foreign body and therefore must be used intelligently, just enough being employed to approximate live tissues and obliterate "dead pockets" as much as possible (see Chap. 2, Wound Healing).

The type of wound is also an important factor. Extensive wounds containing large amounts of devitalized tissues, especially muscle, fascia and bone, furnish excellent culture media for bacteria. Injuries of the thigh or the buttocks may severely damage a pound or more of muscle, and these greatly devitalized masses may become severely infected. Wounds produced by crushing and associated with heavy contamination are frequently multiple and are characterized by extensive tissue destruction, severe shock and early virulent infection.

The location of the wound is another significant consideration. Not only are the various tissues known to have different powers of local resistance to infection, but the resistance of these tissues also varies with their location in the body. For example, lacerations of the face and the neck are prone to heal kindly unless they are in communication with the mouth and the pharynx, while wounds of the perineum practically always become infected to some degree.

The multiplicity of severe wounds in one person may so compromise the treatment that adequate débridement of one or more of the wounds is not possible. Because of associated severe shock, hemorrhage, or wounds of the chest or the head, the local treatment of wounds necessarily assumes a minor role in relation to the general treatment of the patient. If the period of time required for the successful general treatment exceeds 6 to 8 hours, often infection will have occurred before local definitive treatment can be started.

The immunity response of the individual may be local, regional or general, as has been discussed previously. *Local immunity* depends somewhat on the type of tissue, especially its vascularity. The term is used mostly to describe the local resistance which an area develops after fighting off an infection so that the same organisms can no longer invade, at this point at least, though they may still get a foothold in some other part of the body. After a consideration of the available evidence, Topley concluded that "it is possible to induce an immunity which is confined to the neighborhood of the treated area, and is not shared by the body as a whole."

The resistance of the body ordinarily is largely due to a *general immunity*. The possession of such immunity is specific and resides in the body as a whole, although the protein, particularly the globulin fraction of the plasma, and the cells of the so-called reticuloendothelial system are primarily involved in the mechanisms of immunity. A third and important factor in resistance is the protective action of the lymph nodes. The development of leukocytosis during infections is also a manifestation of resistance. *Natural immunity* refers to resistance inherent or at least obtained in some unknown spontaneous way or congenitally. *Acquired immunity,* on the other hand, is the result of defenses built up in fighting a previous infection. *Artificial immunity* is a similar defense obtained, however, by passive or active immunization. Of the two, the latter is especially important in the prevention of tetanus.

Treatment influences the development of infection more than most physicians realize. Of primary importance is the surgical excision or removal of all dead or devitalized tissue and foreign bodies within the wound, preferably within 4 to 6 hours after injury in order to remove any potential pabulum for bacterial growth. Of almost equal importance, however, is the prevention of the development of devitalized tissue during the postoperative state. Impairment of the local blood supply by damage to or ligation of large vessels, by displaced fractures, by pressure of hematomas, by tourniquets or ill-applied and ill-fitting casts, or by increased subfascial tension due to edema, hemorrhage or sutures, decreases local resistance of tissues and favors the development of infection.

The alteration of the "normal" bacterial flora of patients by antibiotic agents may suppress sensitive microorganisms and permit the emergence of resistant and virulent forms. The latter may then become invasive and pathogenic.

The physical condition of the patient is an important predisposing factor to infection, and dehydration, shock, malnutrition, exhaustion, uncontrolled diabetes and anemia may lower his resistance sufficiently to permit bacterial invasion.

PRIMARY AND SECONDARY BACTERIAL CONTAMINATION AND INFECTION

Bacterial contamination of wounds may be either primary or secondary, depending upon the time when bacteria are carried into the wound. Contamination occurring at the time of or within a few hours of injury is considered primary, while that occurring 24 hours or more after trauma is secondary. The *infection* caused by these methods is likewise designated as *primary* and *secondary*.

Primary Contamination. The sources of primary contamination include the patient's skin or hair, clothing, various foreign bodies carried into the wound, such as wood splinters, the missile, soil, pieces of glass, etc., and discharges from various tracts including the upper respiratory, the genital, or the gastrointestinal. The more common types of bacteria associated with primary contamination and infection include staphylococci, enterobacilli such as *E. coli, B. proteus* and the Clostridia of gas gangrene and tetanus.

Secondary contamination may be caused by contact or by airborne spread. It emanates primarily from the respiratory tract of the patient or other persons in his vicinity, particularly those treating or observing his wound. Other sources include unsterile dressings, the fingers of anyone touching the wound, dust of the operating room or the hospital ward, and contaminated dressings, instruments, or utensils. Care should be exercised in the dressing of wounds to prevent cross-contamination and secondary infection. These precautions include the wearing of the mask, the avoidance of touching the wound with the bare fingers, and the avoidance of using any instruments, material, or dressings which are not sterile.

Primary infection tends to disappear at variable rates in different wounds, depending on the type of infection, the severity of the wound and the presence of sloughs, sequestra or foreign bodies.

Secondary Infection. Primary infection is gradually replaced, often during the second week, by the stage of secondary infection caused chiefly by the pyogenic cocci, especially the hemolytic *Staphylococcus aureus* and *Streptococcus hemolyticus* and to a lesser extent by *B. pyocyaneus, E. coli* and *Proteus vulgaris.*

Hare and Fleming believed that the hemolytic *Streptococcus* was the most important agent in secondary infection, but it has been our experience at the Cincinnati General Hospital that the hemolytic *Staphylococcus aureus* is both more prevalent and more important.

It is interesting to recall that Lord Lister laid great stress on airborne infections, but until very recently their importance has been underestimated or overlooked. Unless strict precautions are taken, secondary or cross infections are bound to occur in a surgical ward. The longer a wound is allowed to remain open, the greater is the chance for secondary contamination and infection.

METHODS OF DIAGNOSIS OF SURGICAL INFECTIONS

Accurate and prompt methods of diagnosis of surgical infections are more important now than ever, the discovery and general use of antibiotics notwithstanding. The reasons for this continued importance of early and accurate diagnosis will be discussed in detail later.

The diagnostic methods useful in determining the location and the nature of surgical infections include the following:

1. **A careful history and physical examination,** coupled with a general knowledge of surgical infections and their etiology, may lead to the presumptive diagnosis of the lesion and the causative organism. For example, the early diagnosis of acute hematogenous osteomyelitis can be made entirely upon the history and the physical examination long before positive x-ray findings are present. In addition, we know that approximately 80 to 88 per cent of such cases are caused by the hemolytic *Staphylococcus aureus*, and that approximately 99 per cent are caused by some form of gram-positive cocci. In this manner it is possible to make a presumptive diagnosis of the lesion and the etiologic agent early in the course of the infection when antibiotic therapy will give the best results.

2. **Laboratory data,** such as red blood counts, hemoglobin, white blood counts, differential counts and urinalysis, are important sources of information which aid in differential diagnosis. Of particular importance in many patients with severe infections is the physician's recognition of the presence of diabetes by urinalysis and blood sugar determinations, because of the susceptibility of diabetics to infection and the difficulty in controlling the combined diseases. Generally speaking, patients with infections exhibit varying degrees of leukocytosis, and valuable information regarding the nature and the course of the infection can be gained from serial counts. Every patient with a surgical infection of moderate or greater severity should have complete blood counts daily for 3 days and then at least twice weekly thereafter until the infection is well under control.

A study of circulating leukocytes in the blood may be very helpful in the diagnosis of surgical infections. Many infections produce only slight or moderate increases in the total count which may not be particularly useful in establishing a specific diagnosis. Differential counts frequently are useful in arriving at a diagnosis; the shift to the left in suppurative infections, the relative lymphocytosis of tuberculosis, the eosinophilia of certain mycotic infections, and the toxic granulation of the cells are examples of the value of differential counts. Overwhelming infection may be associated with absence of elevation or even a reduction of the total white cell count. Other surgical infections may be associated with very high total white blood cell counts (leukemoid response), and examples are pneumococcal peritonitis, retroperitoneal phlegmon, septicemia, suppurative pancreatitis, etc.

White blood cell counts are an important part of the initial workup of patients with surgical infections and a valuable means of assessing the progress of treatment thereafter. Infections caused by hemolytic bacteria such as the *Streptococcus hemolyticus* or *Cl. welchii* may produce profound anemia.

3. **Special procedures,** such as roentgen examinations, are of considerable aid in the localization of the infection and its spread.

4. **Infectious exudates** should be obtained whenever possible from the area of infection by swab or aspiration for *examination*, 4 general procedures being possible.

Direct observation of the pus to detect its color, consistency, odor and other physical characteristics is often of great diagnostic help to the experienced surgeon.

Direct microscopic examination of a smear stained by the Gram stain, acid-fast, or other technics may yield immediate information regarding the type or general types of microorganisms present. It may also show the types of leukocytes predominant in the wound.

Culture of the pus under aerobic, microaerophilic and anaerobic conditions may indicate the specific organism or organisms causing the infection. Cultures made of infectious material should be placed *immediately* into appropriate media and then into the incubator for cultivation. Every effort should be made to do this rather than keep the material overnight in an icebox or at room temperature which favors drying of the specimen and death of all but the hardiest organisms, which unfortunately are often not the true pathogens.

Examination of a wet preparation of the exudate, treated with 15 per cent sodium hydroxide solution, under a cover glass or by the hanging-drop technic may demonstrate the presence of yeast or fungi.

In obscure infections in which there is no purulent exudate, material aspirated by needle and syringe from cellulitic areas or areas of suspected infection may establish the diagnosis and indicate the infecting agent by examination of the smear and culture.

5. **Culture of the blood** also can provide diagnostic information. This may be the only manner of identifying the etiologic agent when pus is not available for culture or when the primary focus is hidden, obscure, or silent. Whenever possible, the blood cultures should be taken as close to the onset of a chill as possible, or when the temperature is rising rapidly.

6. **Biopsy of the lesion** in granulomatous infections, particularly tuberculous, syphilitic or mycotic, gives material for microscopic examination which may be of great value in arriving at a definite diagnosis in difficult cases.

Other special diagnostic procedures that may be used include *agglutination tests* made with the patient's serum and *skin tests* made with various antigens. The latter may be used as aids in establishing the diagnosis of lesions such as lymphopathia venereum, tuberculosis, blastomycosis, histoplasmosis and coccidioidomycosis.

7. **Bacteriophage Typing.** Bacteriophage typing may be useful in the identification of different strains of the *Staphylococcus* and the *Pseudomonas*. This technic may also provide information on the virulence and the epidemic potential of these bacteria, particularly the *Staphylococcus*.

TREATMENT OF SURGICAL INFECTIONS

Great advances have been made during the past 70 years in the prevention and the control of surgical infections, particularly during the last 15 years. Today it is routinely possible to prevent infection in planned operative wounds, an achievement which is one of the great milestones of surgery. In addition, considerable progress has been made in preventing or attenuating infection in accidental wounds or wounds of violence. The outlook of surgical patients with established lesions or operations performed in contaminated fields has become vastly improved. Many of the surgical infections commonly seen can now be controlled effectively in conjunction with operative intervention when indicated. However, there are still many surgical lesions of microbial etiology which are refractive to any known form of chemotherapy.

Prophylaxis

In addition to directing treatment toward overcoming the various factors that predispose to the development of surgical infections, such as early excision of devitalized tissue, removal of foreign bodies, preservation of blood supply, and immobilization of injured extremities, other means of preventing infections are available.

Antibiotic agents may be used to considerable advantage, but the indications for their use in civilian surgical practice are considerably more limited than those generally practiced. Their indiscriminate or blind use is to be discouraged.

1. In contaminated wounds of violence and burns, adequate débridement often cannot be accomplished, and devitalized tissue and bacteria may remain to cause infection. The systemic administration of an agent such as penicillin is indicated and usually will inhibit the growth of hemolytic streptococcal infections and prevent infection by this organism. There is no definite evidence that systemic antibiotic therapy also reduces the incidence of other invasive infections produced by the staphylococcus, *Bacillus pyocyaneus, Escherichia coli, Aerobacter aerogenes* and other gram-negative bacilli. There is some clinical evidence to indicate that excessive doses may *increase* the probability of secondary bacterial invasion in patients with burns or other severe trauma.

2. In elective procedures performed through or in contaminated areas such as the gastrointestinal, the respiratory, or the genitourinary tracts, prophylactic therapy may be useful. Here, again, unavoidable contamination of the

wound by pathogenic bacteria occurs in such numbers that development of infection becomes a real probability unless the patient has the added defense of prophylactic antibiotic treatment.

3. The use of antibiotics is warranted in an effort to prevent infection in patients who have associated derangements of the urinary tract or require indwelling catheters as part of their surgical care.

4. It is also indicated in patients with pre-existing valvular heart disease who receive injuries or require elective surgical procedures in the oral or pharyngeal cavities. The well-known relationship of the initiation of subacute bacterial endocarditis under these circumstances warrants the use of penicillin or sulfadiazine as prophylaxis against this dreaded complication.

5. Prophylactic antibacterial treatment should be considered in patients requiring emergency operative surgical treatment in the presence of associated but unrelated infections, such as tonsillitis.

6. For elective preoperative preparation of the gastrointestinal tract, selected antibiotics administered orally prior to operation reduce both the numbers and the virulence of intestinal organisms that may accidentally contaminate the required operative wound.

7. In elderly people with pre-existing pulmonary disease who require essential operative treatment antibiotics may be useful in controlling existing subclinical infection or postoperative complications. If this is done, great care should be exercised because of the danger of precipitating an antibiotic-resistant infection as a complication in such patients.

The prophylactic application of antibacterial agents in circumstances other than these is usually unwarranted and potentially dangerous. The routine use of such agents in clean surgical procedures may lull the physician into a feeling of false security that infection will not occur. Such treatment may partially abort a developing infection or mask its usual and recognizable clinical signs long enough to permit serious and extensive damage to occur before its diagnosis. Some "masked infections" may even become lethal without the appearance of clinical signs diagnostic of virulent infection.

Moreover, the indiscriminate prophylactic use of antibacterial agents is causing sensitivity of an increasing percentage of the population to the various antibiotics. This may be dangerous or even fatal. It also denies the patient the benefit of that antibacterial agent in the future, should he need it. It is also possible for antibiotics used prophylactically to cause serious superimposed or secondary infections by resistant bacteria such as staphylococci or fungi which may be more serious than those to be prevented. Finally, antibiotic agents may be harmful to the patient as a result of toxicity, overdosage, or idiosyncrasy.

SEROTHERAPY may be useful to a limited degree in prophylaxis. The two surgical infections which may be considered in this regard are gas gangrene and tetanus. Experimentally and clinically, prophylactic serotherapy against gas gangrene has been found to be without benefit for practical purposes, and its use is not recommended.

IMMUNITY AGAINST TETANUS is of great value and is an essential part of the treatment of all accidental wounds.

Passive immunity can be produced by the hypodermic injection of tetanus antitoxin as soon after the injury as possible. The usual patient who is seen within 24 hours after injury should receive 1,500 units of tetanus antitoxin after proper skin-testing has shown no sensitivity to horse serum in the antitoxin. Recently it has been recommended that the prophylactic dose of tetanus antitoxin be increased to a minimum of 5,000 units. In our experience at the Cincinnati General Hospital, a dose of 1,500 units is adequate, provided that it is given shortly after injury and certainly within 24 hours. If the wound is large and grossly contaminated, or if the patient has co-existing diabetes mellitus, the dose should be 3,000 or more units. If the patient is seen more than 24 hours after injury, the dose should be doubled for each 24 hours of elapsed time up to a maximum dose of 12,000 units. Under circumstances of delayed definitive treatment of the wound or manipulations of the injured area, passive immunity should be maintained by the injection of 1,500 units of tetanus antitoxin repeated in 7 days. Patients who show evidence of sensitivity to horse serum may be given passive immunity by the use of homologous hyperimmune gamma globulin prepared from hyperimmunized human donor's blood. The average adult will maintain apparently adequate passive protection for at least 3 weeks by an intramuscular injection of 5 units per kilogram. This gamma globulin must be given intramuscularly and cannot be given intravenously.

Active immunity against tetanus can be attained by 2 or 3 injections of tetanus toxoid at intervals of 3 to 6 weeks, followed by a booster injection at the time of injury. Individuals who have this active basic immunity do not require *antitoxin* in the prophylaxis of tetanus, but can be protected by reactivation of the immunity by injection of a booster dose of toxoid after injury.

THERAPY OF ESTABLISHED INFECTIONS

Factors and Principles To Be Observed. As a result of the numerous advances in the field of antibacterial therapy during the past 25 years, the outlook of surgical patients with established infections has become much improved. Experience has shown that successful treatment of surgical infections depends largely upon the physician's observance of certain factors or principles.

1. He must realize that the use of the newer antibiotic agents is adjunctive to the employment of old and established surgical principles.

2. Antibiotic agents used properly can produce profound effects in the prevention and the control of infections, but when used improperly their clinical effects may be limited, incomplete or absent.

3. He must recognize that early diagnosis is of great importance in the control of surgical infections, affecting morbidity, mortality and function. If the diagnois is established early when infections are in the diffuse or cellulitic stage, antibacterial therapy is most apt to produce a prompt and rapid control of the invasiveness with either complete and spontaneous resolution of the infection or minimal complications. This is due to 2 factors. The capillary circulation is intact and can deliver adequate doses of the antibacterial agent throughout the zone of infection. There is also greater susceptibility of the bacteria to the antibiotics while they are rapidly proliferating. However, if the diagnosis is made late, the infectious process usually has become more established, and either local necrosis or abscess formation has occurred, or systemic invasion has developed. If the blood supply to an area is impaired or destroyed, insufficient concentrations of antibiotics are carried to the area of infection. In those cases in which the infection has become disseminated before a diagnosis has been made, with the production of metastatic abscess or secondary infectious complications in remote areas, the control of the infection is considerably more difficult.

For the most efficient control of surgical infections, not only must the diagnosis be early, but it must be accurate and complete. The necessity of a correct clinical diagnosis as well as an evaluation of the patient's condition for intelligent treatment is obvious. This implies the recognition of the existence and the site of metastatic abscess or other complications. Failure of the elevated temperature and other general signs of infection to recede within 72 hours of the start of antibacterial therapy and other treatment generally implies the co-existence of a neighboring abscess, one or more complicating metastatic infections, resistance of the infecting bacteria to the antibiotic in use, or the development of vegetative endocarditis. This emphasizes the wisdom of re-evaluating the patient's disease and his treatment every 72 hours if a satisfactory response has not been obtained.

The importance of obtaining information regarding the infecting microorganism is increasing. Such information can be obtained by the immediate examination of stained smears of the pus and by culture of exudate obtained by incision and drainage or aspiration with needle and syringe from the actual site of infection (see p. 52). Biopsy of the lesion is often very helpful in establishing the nature of the infection, particularly in chronic infection of a specific nature, such as tuberculosis, syphilis and actinomycosis.

Errors in Diagnosis. In this regard it must be kept in mind that errors in diagnosis can be made very easily by accepting the report of the laboratory on cultures made of surface lesions. Such positive cultures may actually represent contaminants or secondary invaders, not the true pathogens which may be much more difficult to cultivate. This trend is of clinical significance, since it re-emphasizes the necessity of sound clinical diagnosis.

The selection of the proper chemotherapeutic agent is extremely important in the

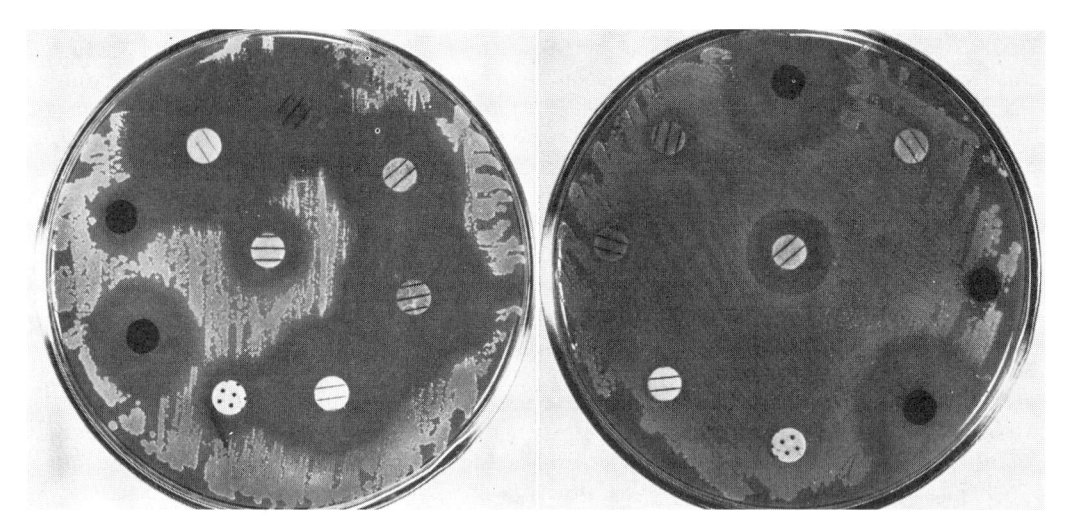

Fig. 4-1. (*Left*) Disk sensitivity studies on strain of hemolytic *Staphylococcus aureus* which is sensitive to penicillin, erythromycin, tetracycline, Oxytetracycline, chlortetracycline, chloramphenicol, bacitracin and neomycin. (*Right*) Disk sensitivity studies on strain of hemolytic *Staphylococcus aureus* which is sensitive to erythromycin, bacitracin and neomycin but resistant to tetracycline, oxytetracyline, chlortetracycline, penicillin and streptomycin. It is slightly sensitive to chloramphenicol.

modern control of surgical infections. The choice of an antibiotic effective for the particular etiologic agent in any given case is obviously desirable. Whenever possible the selection should be made on the basis of data resulting from studies of the gram-stained smears, cultures of exudates obtained from the lesions and sensitivity tests. Also, whenever possible one agent should be used instead of a shotgun mixture of 3 or 4. If no infectious exudate can be obtained, or if no local lesion is demonstrable in a patient with a severe systemic infection, the selection of the antibacterial agent must be made necessarily on a presumptive diagnosis until the nature of the causative organism is determined. Such a procedure is necessarily blind.

It is important to realize that there is considerable variation in natural bacterial resistance within strains of bacteria. Consequently, the haphazard selection of an antibiotic agent which presumably should be effective for a given etiologic agent may yield an uncertain result or a failure. Many strains of bacteria in our environment, particularly in hospitals, are gradually acquiring resistance to various antibiotics. For example, only 25 to 50 per cent of the strains of hemolytic *Staphylococcus aureus* are still sensitive to penicillin, and sensitivity tests are particularly important in the management of infections caused by it.

SENSITIVITY STUDIES are of considerable value in the selection of the antibiotic agent or agents of choice for the treatment of a given infection (Fig. 4-1). Sensitivity determinations may be done in the laboratory by the serial dilution tube method or the disk method, using commercially prepared disks. The latter method is considerably less accurate than the former but is the only one that is available for general clinical use. Although not infallible, this method gives information on a qualitative basis valuable for clinical use, and it is sufficiently simple for any laboratory employing a technician trained in bacteriology. In our experience there generally has been good correlation between the results of in-vitro sensitivity tests, as determined by the serial dilution tube method, and the clinical responses obtained.

In the treatment of serious mixed infections produced by a variety of gram-positive and gram-negative aerobic and anaerobic bacteria, it may be advisable to select 2 antibacterial agents for treatment of such conditions as acute septic peritonitis, intra-abdominal abscess, perinephritic abscess, urinary tract infections and various types of wound infections.

56   Surgical Infections

Usually, aqueous penicillin G and one of the broad-spectrum group such as chloramphenicol, tetracycline, chlortetracycline, oxytetracycline, declomycin or streptomycin are selected. There is some test-tube evidence that antagonism may occur between two or more antibiotics which may decrease their effectiveness, but fortunately there is no significant evidence of this antagonism existing in vivo. There is also some in-vitro evidence that synergism or increased antibacterial power occurs with the use of combinations of some of the agents such as penicillin and streptomycin.

It is advisable to *repeat cultures and sensitivity tests* at weekly intervals in severe prolonged infections because of the possibility of acquired bacteria resistance or development of secondary infections. Apparently, bacteria may acquire resistance to all of the antibiotic agents in varying degrees except polymyxin B and neomycin. Occasionally, suppression of sensitive bacteria in mixed infections by antibiotics may permit other bacteria normally of lesser virulence to become invasive and to invade the blood stream, the meninges or some other tissue system. Infections produced in this manner are known as *superinfections* or *superimposed infections*, and they might be overlooked unless repeated cultures are taken.

ADEQUATE DOSAGE implies the use of the antibiotic agent in doses sufficiently large to produce antibacterial concentrations in the blood and intercellular fluids and tissues for a period of time long enough to permit the natural defense mechanism of the body to dispose of the inhibited but often still viable bacteria. The majority of the agents exert only a bacteriostatic effect which is greatest on actively growing and reproducing bacteria. In the case of some of the antibiotics, particularly penicillin, the evidence suggests that progressively large doses have an increasingly greater clinical effect and at times a bactericidal action.

TIME ELEMENT. Antibiotic treatment should be started as promptly as possible after injury. Its use may keep any infection localized, at-

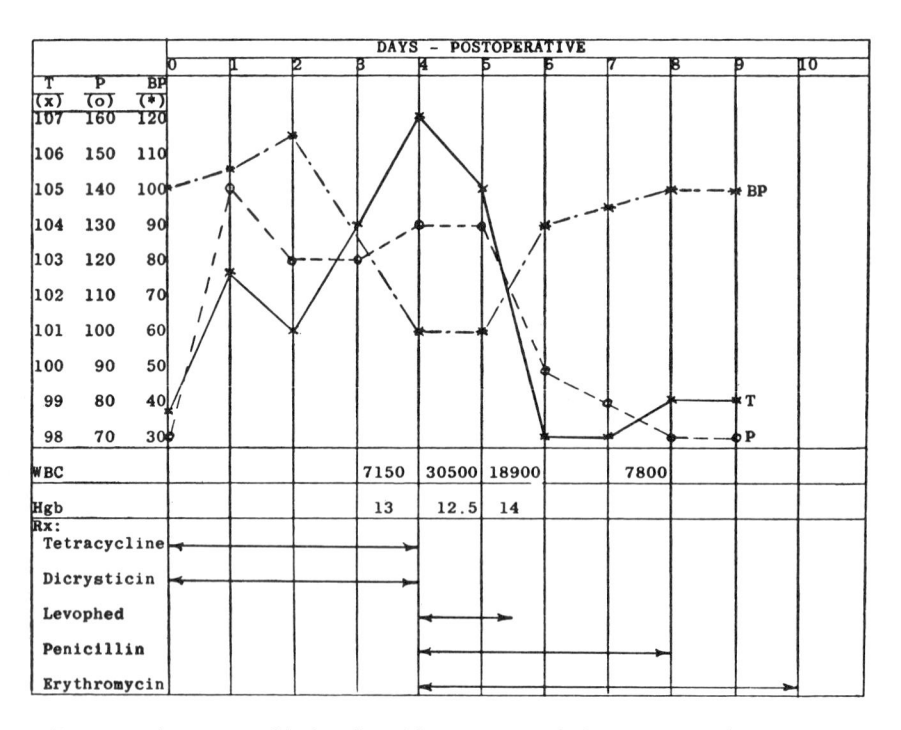

FIG. 4-2. A 14-year-old female with severe staphylococcal pseudomembranous enterocolitis developing 4 days after gastrectomy as a complication of tetracycline therapy. Note high fever, fall in blood pressure and WBC of 30,500 associated with infection. Excellent response to erythromycin and Levophed.

tenuated, or dormant. In established infections early antibiotic therapy gives a better chance of producing rapid and prompt control of invasiveness. Late treatment usually results in a more limited or delayed effect, and complications are more numerous, including local necrosis, abscess formation or systemic invasion (Fig. 4-2).

METHOD OF ADMINISTRATION. This is worthy of some discussion. The systemic administration of antibiotics is generally by the parenteral or oral routes, depending upon the agent used and various other factors. *Local application* of chemotherapeutic agents to wounds is seldom indicated. In traumatic shock the absorption of antibiotics from the gastrointestinal tract or muscular areas may be retarded. Consequently, the intravenous administration of aqueous penicillin G or other antibiotics is recommended during traumatic shock to guarantee rapidly an adequate blood and fluid concentration.

The timing of surgical intervention with antibiotic therapy is of special importance. Necessary operative procedures should not be delayed unless the patient's condition is too poor to withstand anesthesia and surgery. On the other hand, care should be taken to perform necessary operative procedures after the start of antibiotic treatment if possible and before the development of bacterial resistance. In general, the principles of operative treatment of surgical infection have not been changed significantly by modern chemotherapy. (See Fig. 4-3.) In serious infections such as septic peritonitis secondary to perforated appendicitis or peptic ulcer, best results have been obtained by the parenteral administration of antibiotics preoperatively and as soon as possible after the patient has been seen. This rapidly produces a bacterial-inhibiting concentration at the site of the infection, retards the progress of the infection and makes unnecessary the local application of antibiotics within the peritoneal cavity.

Supportive treatment is valuable in the management of many patients with surgical infections. Obvious local and general physiologic derangements are frequently overlooked or disregarded in present-day practice. If they are not corrected, the full therapeutic effect of the antibacterial agent will not be obtained.

Untoward reactions following the administration of antibiotic agents have been shown to be of 3 general types: toxic reactions related to the amount of the drug given, sensitivity

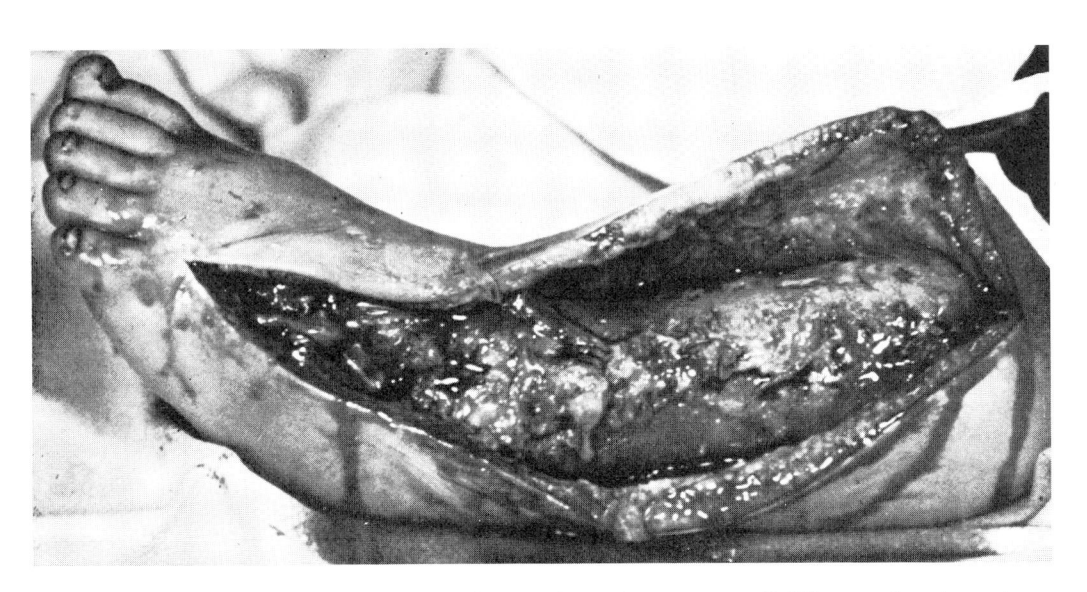

FIG. 4-3. A 2-year-old boy with extensive purulent subcutaneous cellulitis secondary to acute osteomyelitis of lower end of tibia and ruptured subperiosteal abscess caused by hemolytic *Staphylococcus aureus*. Note creamy pus. There was an associated septicemia. Although moribund when this picture was taken, the patient recovered. Without timed surgical intervention with emergency incision and drainage, the patient would have died before adequate antibiotic effect.

reactions due to idiosyncrasy or sensitization of the patient, or secondary inflammations or ulcerations produced by superimposed infections. Each of the agents has been shown to be capable of producing one or more of these types of reaction. Those produced by overdosage can be readily prevented or controlled. Those secondary to *sensitization* of the host are becoming more and more important, particularly in the case of penicillin. Many patients, some of whom were sensitized during the misuse of penicillin, are now deprived of its benefits and apparently will be hereafter.

IDIOSYNCRASY. Certain of the antibiotic and chemotherapeutic agents (chloramphenicol and the sulfonamides in particular) are capable of producing severe depression of the bone marrow, probably on the basis of an idiosyncrasy. When medications having this possibility are used, repeated and regular blood cell counts during their administration are indicated to monitor the bone marrow response.

As more antibiotics have been developed the choice between those to which the offending organism is sensitive is more and more dictated by the relative safety of the drugs.

Secondary or superimposed infections caused by the suppression of susceptible microbial agents and overgrowth of those resistant to the antibiotic administered have become of increasing importance. The most severe form has been the pseudomembranous enterocolitis which has developed in some cases, usually after the use of chlortetracycline, oxytetracycline, tetracycline or neomycin, although it has been noted occasionally after other forms of antibacterial therapy, and even in the absence of such treatment. Fortunately, these severe and potentially fatal infections can be treated successfully by methicillin, erythromycin or chloramphenicol. If they are associated with septic shock, hypotension and urinary suppression, active supportive treatment is also recommended, including the intravenous administration of norepinephrine and large doses of steroids. (See Chap. 7 on Shock.)

Specific serotherapy with biologic antigens or antitoxins is of limited use in surgery for the control of established infections. Vaccines or suspensions of bacteria killed by heat or chemicals occasionally are of great value in the management of infections resistant to all other forms of therapy. As the result of numerous advances in the field of antibiotic therapy during the past 10 years, the antisera have assumed lesser importance in the control of infections. Their use in established infections is probably limited to the antitoxins of tetanus and gas gangrene and will be discussed elsewhere in the text.

Occasionally, specific staphylococcal bacteriophage may also be used to advantage.

CLASSIFICATION OF WOUND INFECTIONS

Infections may be monomicrobic or polymicrobic, depending upon the presence of one or more varieties of infecting bacteria. Many *early infections* of wounds are pyogenic, the staphylococcus being the most frequent cause, the streptococcus the next. Mixed infections by aerobic and anaerobic, gram-negative and gram-positive bacteria may also occur, particularly in extensive wounds with retained dead tissue. Anaerobic cellulitis, clostridial myositis (gas gangrene), wound diphtheria, tetanus, anthrax and rabies are less frequent lesions.

The following is a brief classification of infections that may develop in wounds:

1. Staphylococcal
2. Streptococcal
   A. Aerobic
   B. Micro-aerophilic
   C. Anaerobic
3. Gram-negative bacillary
4. Mixed
5. Clostridial
6. Tetanus
7. Diphtheritic
8. Rabies
9. Mycotic
   A. Actinomycotic
   B. Blastomycotic
   C. Coccidioidomycotic
   D. Sporotrichotic
10. Miscellaneous
    A. Anthrax
    B. Granuloma inguinale
    C. Lymphopathia venereum
    D. Histoplasmosis

Classification of Wound Infections

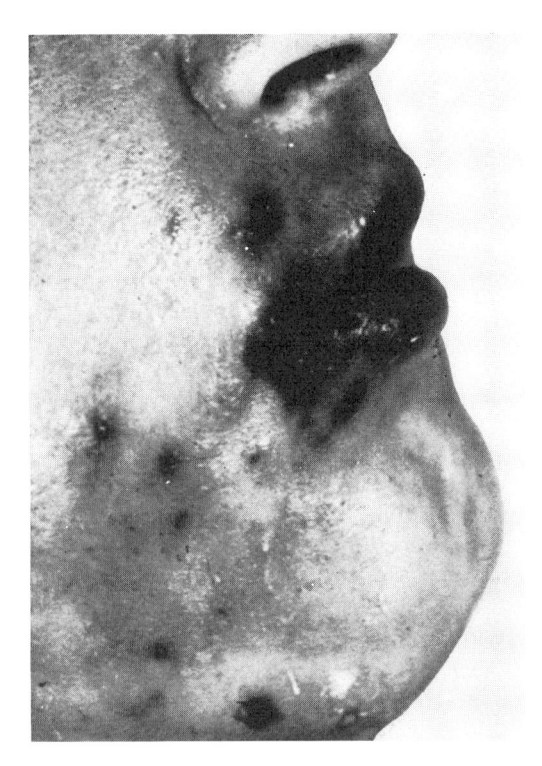

FIG. 4-4. A 33-year-old female with severe staphylococcal cellulitis of face and early carbuncle formation about lips, thrombosis of the external jugular vein, septic embolic pneumonitis and hemolytic *Staphylococcus aureus* septicemia. Recovery with penicillin therapy.

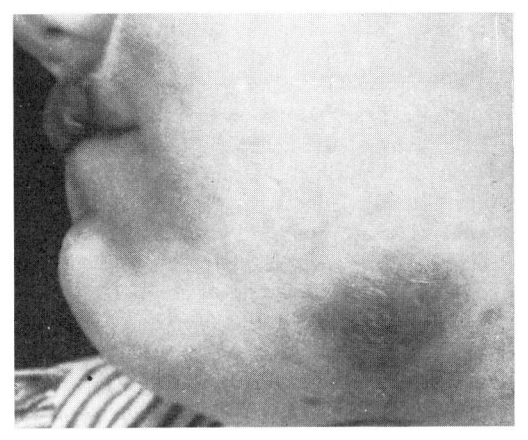

FIG. 4-5. Infected laceration of lip with purulent lymphadenopathy and cervical abscess caused by hemolytic *Staphylococcus aureus*.

STAPHYLOCOCCAL INFECTIONS

Staphylococcal infections are usually localized and are characterized by an area of cellulitis and erythema which subsequently may undergo central necrosis or abscess formation with thick, creamy, odorless, and yellowish or reddish-yellow pus.

The hemolytic *Staphylococcus aureus*, which liquefies gelatin and produces a locally necrotizing toxin, is the most important variety of staphylococcus. The coagulation of plasma by its enzyme, coagulase, favors the development of thrombosis and thrombophlebitis in the adjacent veins and is generally indicative of the pathogenicity of that particular strain. The symptoms of staphylococcal infection include swelling, erythema, and local pain which is throbbing and often synchronous with the heart beat. Fever and leukocytosis are usually present. The process may become invasive and complicated by lymphangitis, lymphadenitis, or thrombophlebitis. As a distributing focus it may produce a bacteremia and broadcast bacteria through the blood stream.

Staphylococcal infections that patients acquire during hospitalization may be particularly serious. Such infections are nearly always caused by a highly virulent staphylococcus which is resistant to most of the commonly used and available antibiotic agents. They may be characterized in some instances by a sudden onset, high fever and a fulminating course. They may have epidemic potentiality as manifested by persistent recurrences of less serious but equally refractive infections lasting for many months or years and by spread to other members of the families with whom they come in contact. Typing of the staphylococci associated with hospital-acquired infections by specific bacteriophage has revealed that the organisms responsible are one of three or four types, the most common ones being the 80-81 and the 77 strains.

The successful management of such infection necessarily require the careful observance of established surgical principles and asepsis, meticulous selection of the proper antibiotic agent, general supportive care and active stimulation of immunity.

Folliculitis, furuncles and carbuncles are types of local staphylococcal infection of the skin and the subcutaneous tissues which usually begin spontaneously as infections of hair follicles and progress to produce small areas of induration of varying size with central necrosis. These lesions occur most frequently on the back of the neck, the face, the axillae, the groins, the buttocks and the fingers.

Treatment. The treatment of established staphylococcal infections is definitely influenced by early accurate diagnosis and consists of rest, heat, elevation of the infected area, adequate surgical drainage when pus has formed, and antibiotic therapy. Acute spreading processes should not be traumatized by incision or otherwise until the invasive characteristics have been brought under control. When pus or necrotic tissue develops in *localized* infections, its removal is extremely important for healing.

Infected wounds should be reopened with a hemostat at the point of maximum pain, swelling, or fluctuation, followed by removal of all skin sutures to enlarge the size of the cavity. In abscesses developing without reference to a wound, drainage is advocated by an adequate incision made over the area in such a manner as to avoid disfiguring scars, disabling contractures, or injury to important structures. Drainage of the wound is facilitated by fine-mesh gauze laid loosely in the cavity to keep the wound edges separated. Care should be taken not to pack the gauze tightly into the wound and thereby interfere with free drainage. The drain may be removed within 48 to 72 hours and may or may not be replaced, depending on the existing circumstances.

Antibiotic therapy should be started promptly, preferably before operation, so that a bacteriostatic concentration is produced in the blood stream to inhibit any bacteria distributed by operative manipulation. *Aqueous sodium or potassium penicillin G in doses of 500,000 units every 8 to 12 hours is the agent of choice.* As an alternative method penicillin may also be administered effectively as a mixture of 300,000 units of procaine penicillin and 100,000 units of aqueous penicillin G every 12 to 24 hours until the infection is definitely under control. Erythromycin in doses of 100 to 200 mg. every 6 hours orally is likewise effective. The drugs of second choice include chloramphenicol, tetracycline, oxytetracycline and chlortetracycline in doses of 250 to 500 mg. every 4 to 6 hours. Declomycin and vancomycin may also be of great value in the control of these infections. In severe or fulminating cases with septicemia, aqueous crystalline penicillin G may be administered in doses of 100,000 to 200,000 units every 3 hours or 500,000 units intramuscularly every 6 to 8 hours. One of the broader-spectrum antibiotics may be used if the organism is resistant to penicillin. Bacitracin is also effective, but its administration should be controlled by daily urinalysis to detect any evidence of nephrotoxicity.

Recognition of penicillinase-producing strains of staphylococci and the attendant resistance to penicillin G may not be possible until sensitivity studies are completed. If the staphylococcal infection is "hospital-acquired" or happens as a part of an in-hospital epidemic, it is more than likely that the organism is not sensitive to the basic penicillins. In this circumstance, the empiric use of the biosynthesized penicillins is indicated, particularly if the infection is life-endangering or occurs in debilitated patients. Sodium oxacillin (in oral divided doses of 3 to 4 Gm. daily) or methicillin (in parenteral divided doses of 4 to 6 Gm. daily) are indicated in such circumstances.

STREPTOCOCCAL INFECTIONS

Streptococcal infections are produced most frequently by the aerobic *Streptococcus hemolyticus*, although some are caused by the *Streptococcus nonhemolyticus*, the *Streptococcus viridans*, the *Streptococcus anaerobicus*, or the micro-aerophilic Streptococcus.

Lesions caused by the aerobic *Streptococcus hemolyticus* characteristically are invasive and run a rapid course initially. They may develop within 12 to 48 hours after injury, or as late as 7 to 14 or more days. The incidence of infection by this organism in open wounds increases with the duration of the wound as a result of secondary contamination. In its early stages the process is usually one of diffuse inflammation with cellulitis, lymphangitis, lymphandenitis, or extension along fascial planes in deep wounds. There is little tendency to form abscesses, but gangrene of the overlying skin or thin watery pus may result. Invasion of the blood stream is frequent, and this complication should be recognized early to minimize the distribution of virulent bacteria throughout the body. Bacteremia is suggested by the development of chills, high fever, rapid thready pulse, prostration and other signs of toxemia.

Surgical scarlet fever may occur infrequently in a postoperative wound in association with the hemolytic streptococcus. The lesion is characterized by spreading cellulitis with redness, swelling, and frequently bullous formation in and about the margins of the wound. A typical scarlatiniform eruption may occur 2 to 4 days after injury or operation, starting at the wound and spreading peripherally. The local lesion may be very severe, but the general reaction may not be.

Erysipelas, also produced by the hemolytic streptococcus, may occur about small wounds, usually about the face and the neck. After an incubation period of 1 to 3 days, it is usually ushered in by chills, high fever, rapid pulse and severe toxemia. It is characterized by a spreading cellulitis with raised, irregular, indurated margins. Its appearance is characteristic, and its course is often self-limited in 4 to 8 days.

Hemolytic streptococcal gangrene (Figs. 4-6 and 4-7) occasionally follows some relatively minor injury in the extremities and is an epifascial, spreading, subcutaneous gangrene with thrombosis of the nutrient vessels and slough of the overlying skin. At the onset it is associated with pain and marked swelling at the site of wounds, chills, elevation of the temperature to 101° to 104° F., tachycardia, toxemia, marked prostration, and a rapidly spreading, painful cellulitis. The overlying skin of the diffusing cellulitis shows bullous formation and a peculiar patchy and coalescing necrosis. Hemolytic streptococci, often in pure culture, may be found in the fluid aspirated from the bullae or areas of subcutaneous slough.

Necrotizing fasciitis is an infection which involves the epifascial tissues of an operative area, laceration, abrasion, or puncture wound. It may either spread rapidly over large areas of the body or remain dormant for 6 or more days before beginning its rapid spread. In those cases which we have seen, the hemolytic staphylococcus or the hemolytic streptococcus has been found. Undermining of the skin is marked, and gangrenous changes in the skin may occur late or be absent. High fever, de-

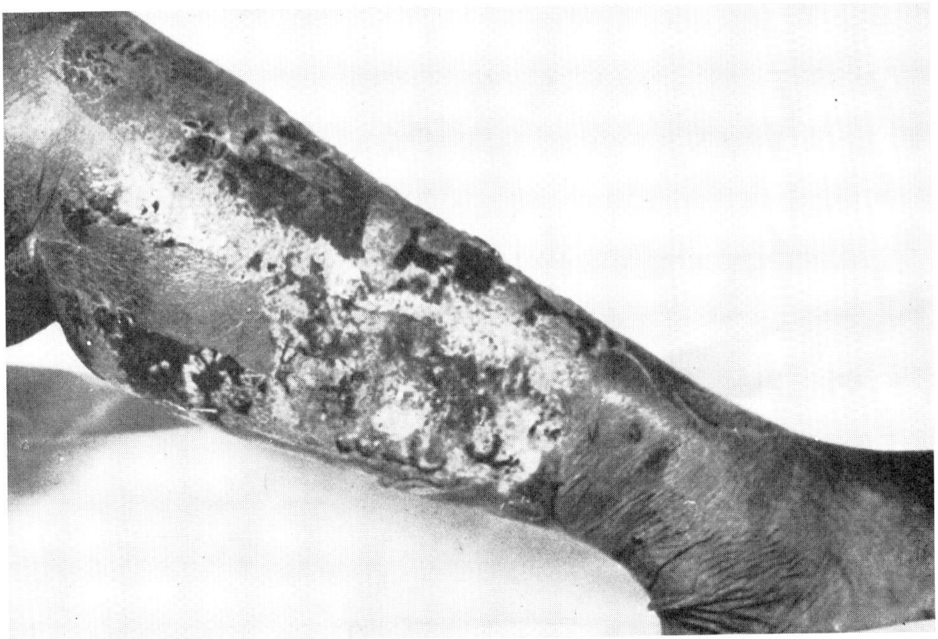

FIG. 4-6. Acute streptococcal gangrene of lower leg caused by *Streptococcus hemolyticus*. This lesion followed a slight injury to the ankle area. Note residual bullae and marked gangrene of skin.

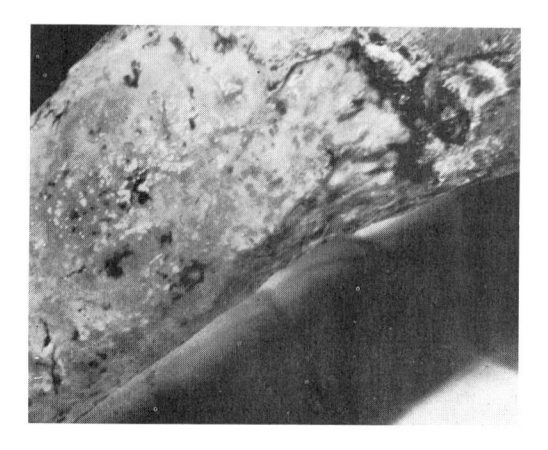

FIG. 4-7. Chronic progressive cutaneous gangrene of leg with extensive ulceration. Note gangrenous margin of ulcer where micro-aerophilic nonhemolytic *Streptococcus* and hemolytic *Staphylococcus aureus* were demonstrated.

hydration, anemia, marked leukocytosis and, occasionally, jaundice occur. The process may become chronic and may be characterized by multiple draining sinuses connected with areas of necrotic underlying fascia.

The treatment of hemolytic streptococcal infections consists of the preliminary control of their invasive characteristics by antibiotic therapy, rest and hot applications, followed by surgical drainage if abscesses or cutaneous gangrene develop. Penicillin, erythromycin, sulfadiazine, or one of the broad-spectrum antibiotics is very effective, but penicillin is usually the agent of choice in doses essentially the same as those described earlier for the treatment of staphylococcal infections. Operative treatment should be delayed until the invasive qualities of the infection have been controlled. Free drainage of collections of pus should be done along with the removal of necrotic tissue, infected hematomas, or foreign bodies. After incision, the wound is left open for further drainage and healing by granulation. The topical application of antibiotics in such wounds is unnecessary. If suppurative thrombophlebitis exists, proximal ligation or excision of the involved vein should be considered.

In hemolytic streptococcal gangrene emergency drainage with longitudinal incision is often necessary as early as possible. It is important to make long incisions through and beyond the gangrenous area as an emergency measure without attempting to wait for control of the invasiveness by antibiotic therapy, in contrast with the usual treatment for streptococcal cellulitis. After operation the wound is treated by rest, elevation of the part if possible, and application of moist compresses. The removal of slough by sharp dissection without bleeding during subsequent dressings is possible. Before and after operation antibiotic therapy, preferably with aqueous penicillin, should be given in adequate amounts as in other aerobic streptococcal infections.

Streptococcal Fasciitis. As soon as the diagnosis of streptococcal fasciitis is established, drainage by long incisions made throughout the entire area of involvement should be made as described for hemolytic streptococcal gangrene. The skin and the subcutaneous tissues should be separated from the deep fascia. Involved necrotic fascia should be excised completely and the wound covered with fine-mesh gauze. When adequate granulations have developed, skin grafting usually is necessary.

In many streptococcal infections, general supportive therapy consisting of the intelligent administration of adequate fluid and electrolytes is very important. Daily blood transfusions may be helpful, but care must be taken not to overload the heart and produce pulmonary edema. Frequent examinations for metastatic infectious complications are necessary, and any that may have developed is treated according to its individual location and characteristics.

Micro-aerophilic Streptococci. Infections caused by micro-aerophilic streptococci develop and progress more slowly as a rule. Two illustrative examples are chronic burrowing ulcer and chronic progressive cutaneous gangrene. Chronic burrowing ulcer is an infrequent lesion caused by a micro-aerophilic hemolytic streptococcus and is characterized by the progressive extension of burrowing sinus tracts through the underlying tissues. Invasion and penetration of fascia, bone, muscle, peritoneum, meninges or brain have been noted. The sinus tracts usually become lined with indolent granulation tissue. General signs of infection associated with this are minimal, a low-grade fever and marked pain being likely to appear during the acute exacerbations of the lesions.

The treatment of choice consists of the radical incision and drainage of the sinus tracts throughout their entire extent, or radical excision of the sinuses in association with antibiotic therapy. Penicillin, erythromycin, bacitracin, chloramphenicol, or one of the broad-spectrum agents may be used. Antibiotic treatment without surgical treatment is inadequate.

Chronic progressive cutaneous gangrene (known also as Meleney's synergistic gangrene) may complicate operations for purulent infections of the chest or the peritoneal cavity. It is caused by the synergistic action of a micro-aerophilic nonhemolytic streptococcus and an aerobic hemolytic staphylococcus. After an incubation period of 7 to 14 days after operation for a wound involving the gastrointestinal, the genitourinary, or the respiratory tracts, the surrounding skin becomes tender, red and edematous, particularly about stay sutures. The appearance of the lesion is characteristic. A wide area of bright-red cellulitis develops about a central purplish area which widens, becomes gangrenous and finally ulcerates. The base of the ulcer is covered with dirty infected granulation tissue, and the margin is purplish black, slightly undermined and very painful.

This ulceration is slowly progressive, and ultimately it may denude larger areas and cause death unless treated adequately. Systemic manifestations at first are slight, but in neglected cases profound derangements in physiology may develop, with wasting of the muscles, low-grade fever, anemia and chronic septic shock.

Local excision of gangrenous margins or other conservative methods usually fail to check this process. Radical excision of the ulcerated lesion and its gangrenous borders is indicated, along with systemic antibiotic treatment with penicillin G or erythromycin. There is some evidence that bacitracin is particularly valuable in the treatment of this condition.

During treatment of patients with chronic progressive cutaneous gangrene with penicillin the hemolytic staphylococcus may disappear and be replaced by a strain of *Proteus sp.* In some instances, a synergism between *Proteus sp.* and nonhemolytic and micro-aerophilic streptococcus can exist primarily to cause the lesion.

Anaerobic streptococcal infections may occur as either acute or chronic lesions. In the acute type, they may occur with or without bacteremia, particularly in wounds that involve or penetrate the genital, the intestinal or the respiratory tracts. Metastatic abscesses in distant regions such as the brain may develop. These infections, which usually progress more slowly than other streptococcal infections, are characterized by the development of marked induration, foul-smelling and thick pus, extending necrosis of the involved tissues and progression along fascial planes or in muscle.

Streptococcal myositis is an infrequent type of anaerobic streptococcal infection. It is associated with massive involvement of muscle, local pain and generalized toxemia. Discoloration, edema, and crepitation of the muscle is characteristic, and a foul odor is generally apparent. Differentiation of streptococcal from clostridial myositis is its more pronounced cutaneous erythema, discolored muscle which is still viable and reactive to stimuli, the different odor, and the demonstration of vast numbers of streptococci in gram-stained smears of the exudate.

The management of anaerobic streptococcal infections is dependent upon early diagnosis, operative treatment, antibiotic therapy and supportive treatment. Abscesses, areas of fasciitis, or infected groups of muscle should be incised and drained promptly, and ulcers showing phagedenic progression should be excised. Antibiotic therapy is of considerable benefit, and penicillin is the agent of choice in doses somewhat larger than those recommended for aerobic streptococcal infections. From 100,000 to 200,000 units of aqueous crystalline penicillin G every 2 to 3 hours or 500,000 units every 6 to 8 hours usually will suffice to bring the invasive qualities of the infection under control. Bacitracin or the broader-spectrum antibiotics are alternate choices.

GRAM-NEGATIVE BACILLARY INFECTIONS

Infections may be produced by gram-negative bacteria of the gastrointestinal, the urinary, or the genital tracts. *Escherichia coli,*

64 Surgical Infections

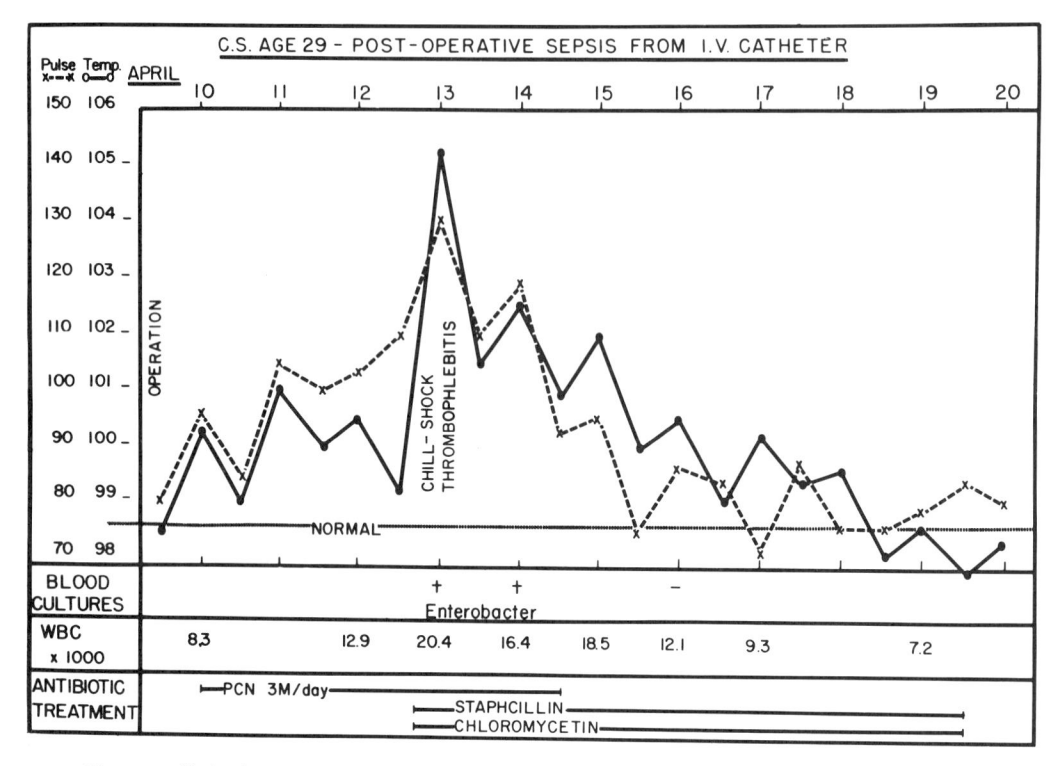

FIG. 4-8. "Third Day Fever," with gram-negative bacteremia caused by continuous intravenous infusion, with acute thrombophlebitis, chills, fever, and arterial hypertension.

Pseudomonas aeruginosa, Proteus vulgaris and *Salmonella typhosa* are examples of organisms capable of causing wound infections. Invasive lesions with bacteremia may occur. Often these gram-negative bacilli are relatively nonvirulent, but in the presence of such factors as necrotic tissue, general debility, or cortisone therapy, they may produce serious infections. Organisms of this group, particularly *Pseudomonas aeruginosa*, have become the chief cause of infectious death associated with severe burns. A relatively long incubation period is also characteristic of postoperative wound infections by these bacilli.

The treatment of these lesions is dependent upon incision and drainage of abscesses, excision of necrotic tissue, and antibiotic therapy based upon in-vitro sensitivity tests. Chloramphenicol has been particularly useful in these infections. Polymyxin B and sodium colistimethate and (Coly-Mycin) are recommended for infections produced by *Ps. aeruginosa*. A recently developed antibiotic, garamycin, is showing promise in the control of established gram-negative bacillary infection and is exceptionally valuable in the treatment of those due to *Pseudomonas aeruginosa*.

Bacteroides infection occasionally occurs as a monomicrobial infection whose outward manifestation may be thrombophlebitis without apparent cause. Unimpressive pulmonary or pelvic infection often precedes the development of venous thrombosis in these patients, and pulmonary infarction due to embolus may be the presenting finding. Persistent bacteremia or septicemia from the infected clot requires operative ligation of the involved vein and prolonged antibiotic therapy with sulfonamides or tetracycline for effective control.

Septicemia due to various species of gram-negative bacilli has become an increasing threat to hospitalized patients in the last 10 years. This progressive increase is probably related to an increase in major trauma and to iatrogenic factors including continuous intravenous administration, tracheostomy wounds and their care, respiratory assistance therapy, steroid therapy, and intensive or excessive antibiotic therapy (Fig. 4-8). The mortality rate from this form of septicemia remains high at about 60 per cent.

MIXED OR SYNERGISTIC INFECTIONS

A large and miscellaneous group of infections with a polymicrobic etiology are found in surgical practice, particularly in association with injuries or operations on the gastrointestinal, the respiratory, or the genitourinary tracts. Symbiosis of aerobes and anaerobes may exist and determine the characteristics of the lesions. The bacterial toxins and enzymes usually cause a necrotizing and suppurative infection, beginning in the wound and extending along fascial and areolar tissues. Cellulitis, abscesses, necrosis and bacteremia may develop. Examples of mixed infections include deep infections of the neck, human-bite infections, putrid empyema, peritonitis and nonclostridial cellulitis.

Human-bite infections (morsus humanus) are usually severe and occur when a human being voluntarily bites another or strikes a blow with his hand which is cut by the teeth of the intended victim. The wound is usually a puncture wound through the various levels of tissue which supports the growth of the mouth organisms contaminating the tissues. A mixture of bacteria is usually found consisting of aerobic nonhemolytic streptococci, anaerobic streptococci, *Bacterium melaninogenicum*, spirochetes or staphylococci. In our experience spirochetes have never been found alone in these infections, but they are associated with the more severe lesions. If the original bite wound is treated by limited or inadequate surgical measures, evidence of inflammation appears within the first 1 to 3 days after injury and progresses steadily thereafter. Swelling, redness, pain, and limitation of motion develop and are followed by fever which is usually moderate but may be as high as 105° F. Systemic reaction is occasionally profound, and the appearance of the local infection soon becomes alarming. Granulation tissue forming within the wound becomes shaggy, gray, cyanotic and edematous and exudes a thick, foul, purulent material. Progressive necrosis extends through the tissues, particularly the areolar ones.

The prevention of infections of this type is the most effective form of treatment. Adequate excision of the wound, as soon as the patient is seen, followed by immobilization and antibiotic therapy, usually with penicillin, is the most effective means of preventing human-bite infections. When tendons are severed by human bites, primary tenorrhaphy should not be attempted. When infection has become established, radical decompression of the infected area and tissue planes by incision is extremely important, accompanied by antibiotic therapy.

Crepitant (nonclostridial) cellulitis is a mixed infection which is usually seen as a complication of wounds of the perineum, abdominal wall, buttocks, hip, thorax, or neck which have been contaminated by discharges from the intestinal, the genitourinary, or the respiratory tracts. When it occurs in the region of the perineum or inguinal area, its spread is often beneath Scarpa's fascia into the abdominal wall and flank. It is caused by bacteria other than the clostridia, no single type of etiologic agent being found consistently. Those associated with this process include strains of the coliform group, the anaerobic Bacteroides group such as *Bacterium melaninogenicus* and *Bacillus thetoides* and the anaerobic streptococci. The areolar and fascial tissues usually become necrotic and develop a putrid odor similar to that of an appendiceal abscess. Progressive gangrenous changes in the skin occur as a result of thrombosis of the nutrient vessels. As the process extends, toxemia usually becomes evident, with dehydration, fever, a weak and thready pulse, prostration, and elevation of W.B.C. to 20,000 or more.

Prompt surgical decompression of all involved areas by multiple incisions is imperative to control this process. Aqueous penicillin G in doses of 200,000 to 1,000,000 units every 3 to 4 hours is recommended along with one of the broad-spectrum antibiotics in doses of 500 mg. Supportive therapy may be lifesaving. These infections are serious, but the prognosis is good for patients treated promptly and adequately. After the infection has been controlled and healthy granulation tissue has developed, skin-grafting is usually necessary to cover the large residual cutaneous defects.

CLOSTRIDIAL INFECTIONS

Clostridial cellulitis is a serious, crepitant, septic process of subcutaneous, retroperito-

66 Surgical Infections

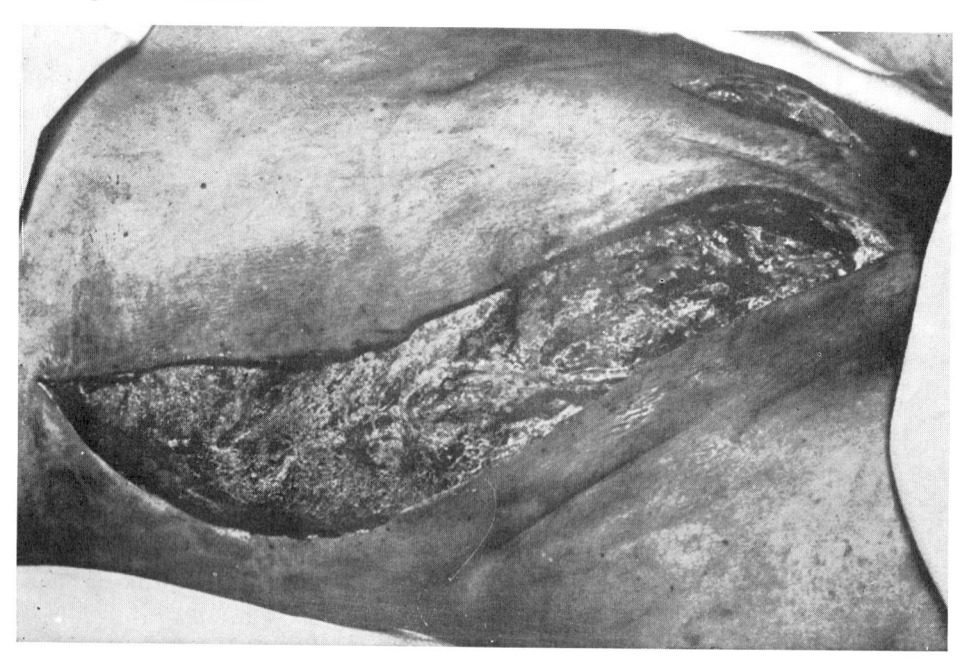

FIG. 4-9. A 50-year-old male with acute crepitant cellulitis of abdominal wall caused by mixed infection arising in a left inguinal hernioplasty wound made for the repair of a strangulated hernia. Spread was rapid and beneath Scarpa's fascia.

neal, or other areolar tissues which is caused by one or more of the clostridia. *Clostridium welchii* is the chief agent. However, other bacteria are usually present. It is characterized by an emphysematous cellulitis which spreads rapidly along fascial planes and is to be differentiated from clostridial myositis by the absence of invasion of living muscle.

Pain about a wound is usually the first symptom, and it may precede any obvious swelling, erythema, or crepitation of the overlying skin by several days. A gray or reddish-brown, seropurulent or putrid discharge may develop as the infection progresses. Slough of the areolar and fascial tissues occurs, associated with thrombosis of the neighboring vessels and finally extensive gangrene of the overlying skin.

The systemic effects may be slight, moderate or severe. Compared with clostridial myositis or true gas gangrene, the fever, tachycardia, leukocytosis and anemia are more moderately altered. Clostridial cellulitis is a serious disease but does not have the high mortality of clostridial myositis if treated promptly. Prompt surgical decompression of all involved areas by extensive multiple incisions is indicated in the treatment of this condition. The incisions should be made to extend through the area of involvement into the adjacent normal tissues. The skin flaps are elevated superficial to the fascia, and any portions of necrotic fascia present should be excised. Antibiotic treatment is similar to that described for nonclostridial cellulitis, although, in our experience, the tetracycline agents have been most efficacious, both experimentally and clinically. Antibiotic therapy should be started preoperatively and continued until all evidence of local or systemic invasiveness of the infection has disappeared. Supportive therapy is likewise important. Inspection of the involved area should be made every 24 or 48 hours and careful search made for areas of spread which are prone to develop.

Clostridial myositis is a spreading or localized gangrenous infection of muscle caused by one or more clostridia. It is usually a mixed infection which involves muscle primarily and is characterized by spreading infectious gangrene, profound toxemia and a rapidly fatal course, unless treated properly. Injuries of the extremities or the buttocks associated with devitalized, torn or contami-

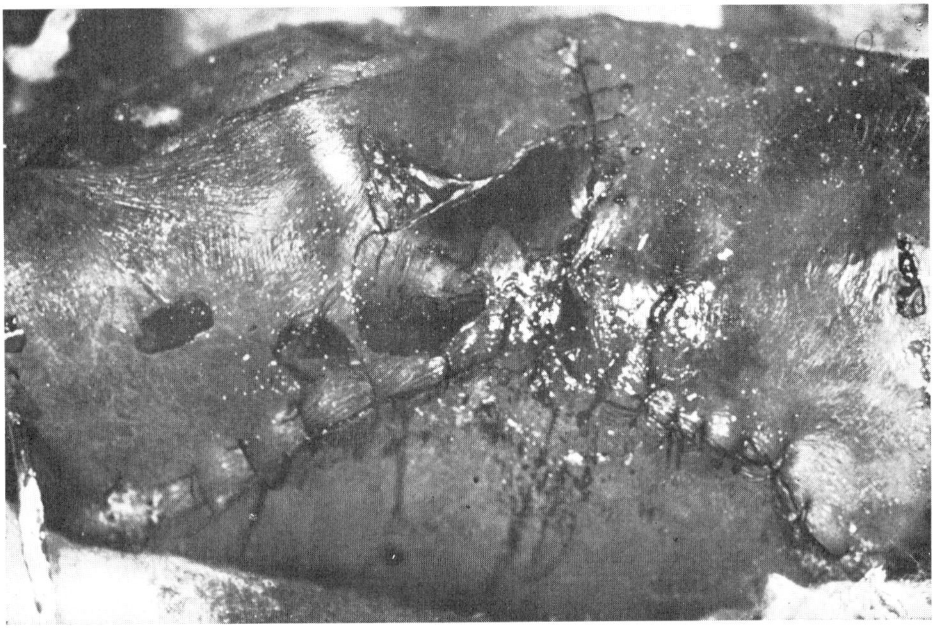

Fig. 4-10. Far-advanced gas gangrene of leg in patient 3 days after débridement and closed reduction of compound fracture of tibia and fibula. Note marked swelling, necrosis of skin, brownish watery discharge, and herniation of muscle through relaxing incision. Amputation was necessary because of irreversible gangrenous changes.

nated muscle are prone to develop this type of infection. Interference with the main blood supply to a limb or a muscle group, the presence of foreign bodies, delay in surgical treatment, or improper surgical care are important predisposing factors. Crepitation of the tissues produced by gas occurs in most cases, particularly in those produced by *Clostridium welchii* and *Cl. septicum*. A great variety of anaerobes have been found in this infection, chiefly *Cl. welchii, Cl. novyi, Cl. sordellii* and *Cl. septicum*. The infection may be confined to a muscle or spread rapidly to involve a single group of muscles, an entire limb, or the torso. In other instances, edema may occur without gas, and with still others, rapid digestion and dissolution of tissue with moderate edema but no gas. The saccharolytic clostridia ferment the muscle sugar to produce acid and gas, and the proteolytic clostridia digest muscle to liquefy it. Gaseous infiltration, edema, and rapid liquefaction of the tissues may exist in the same wound. Soluble toxins diffuse into adjacent tissues, causing further destruction and thrombosis of the vessels or are absorbed into the circulation to produce marked toxemia, septic shock, damage of the liver, the heart and the kidneys, profound anemia, prostration and death.

Pain is the earliest symptom of clostridial myositis, appearing in the first 24 hours after injury and caused principally by the rapid infiltration of the tissues by fluid and gas. The patient may develop a peculiar grayish pallor, listlessness, weakness, profuse sweating, prostration and breathlessness. A striking pallor of the face develops. Anorexia is a fairly constant finding, and vomiting is not uncommon. The mental state is one of apathy and indifference to the seriousness of his condition; stupor, delirium and coma may occur later. A rapid and feeble pulse may follow the onset of pain. Circulatory collapse, which may be abrupt, progressive and severe, may develop. Fever is not a reliable index of the severity of the infectious process, varying considerably, and frequently is less than 101° F. A low temperature, a very rapid pulse and hypotension are indicative of a grave prognosis.

The skin overlying the lesion is at first white and tense, and the infected muscle visible in the wound becomes dark red, soft and swollen. It frequently herniates into the wound and discharges a brown, watery, foul-smelling exudate containing many bacteria and red blood cells but a paucity of leukocytic cells. The overlying skin becomes dusky or bronze in appearance, and vesicles filled with dark-red fluid may appear and coalesce. The distal portion of the limb involved becomes edematous, engorged, discolored, cold and finally obviously gangrenous. Laboratory data usually show a marked reduction in the number of red corpuscles, with counts ranging between 1 and 2 million per cm., low hemoglobin levels of 30 to 40 per cent, and relatively low leukocytic counts not exceeding 12,000 to 15,000 cells per mm.[3] in many instances.

The early diagnosis of gas gangrene may be difficult because large dressings, casts or splints used for the treatment of the injury may mask the progress of the infection until a far-advanced process is present. Continued pain at the site of a wound containing injured muscle; a rapid and easily compressible pulse; varying degrees of fever; toxemia in association with spreading edema; a thin, brown, watery, malodorous discharge; crepitation; herniation of discolored muscle which does not bleed or contract; and typical discolorations of the skin in the regions of the wound—these are diagnostic signs. Infiltrating gas may be detected early by the experienced observer through auscultatory percussion or by serial roentgenograms.

It is important to explore surgically and without delay any wound in which the presence of clostridial myositis is suspected. Early and adequate operation is the most effective means of treating established gas gangrene; no other form of treatment, including chemotherapy and serotherapy, replaces it. Radical incision through the skin and the fascia to decompress the muscle compartments and to permit excision of all devitalized and infected muscles is imperative. If the diagnosis is made when gangrenous changes implying death of the extremity and permanent loss of function have occurred, open amputation of the guillotine type should be performed, supplemented by drainage of any infected fascial compartments and excision of any devitalized muscle remaining above the line of amputation.

Intensive antibiotic therapy is recommended in conjunction with surgery, consisting of tetracycline, oxytetracycline, or chlortetracycline in doses of 500 mg. intravenously every 6 to 8 hours. Aqueous crystalline penicillin G in large doses of 1 million units intramuscularly every 3 hours or chloramphenicol in doses of 500 mg. every 6 to 8 hours may also be used but apparently are not as effective.

Supportive therapy is of marked importance for maintaining fluid and electrolyte balance and for correcting the derangements in physiology produced by this infection. Frequent blood transfusions of whole blood are of value in correcting the severe hemolytic anemia and decreased blood volume associated with this infection, provided that prompt surgical and antibiotic therapy have also been instituted.

TETANUS

Etiology. Tetanus, also known as lockjaw or trismus, is another very serious wound infection. It is caused by the growth of *Clostridium tetani* and its generation of a potent toxin within the wound. The toxin diffuses through the adjacent skeletal muscles, acting on the neuromuscular end organs and causing a state of local tonic contraction (local tetanus). It is also distributed by the circulating blood or lymph to susceptible cells in the cord, the medulla and the motor end organs of the skeletal muscles, resulting in trismus, risus sardonicus, opisthotonos, rigidity of the abdominal muscles, spasm of the skeletal muscles of the extremities, and generalized clonic convulsions precipitated by external stimuli (generalized tetanus).

The incubation period varies from 4 to 21 or more days, the usual being 6 to 10. In general the severity of the disease decreases as the incubation period increases. A prodromal period follows the incubation period and is characterized by stiffness of jaw muscles, headache, restlessness, yawning, and twitches of pain in the region of the wound.

Pathology. In generalized tetanus, the *active stage* usually begins within 12 to 24 hours after onset of the prodromal period and is characterized by tonic spasms of the skeletal muscles. Trismus of the jaw may be extreme, and spasms of the facial musculature may produce a grimace or facial distortion.

Opisthotonos with retraction of the head may be caused by tonicity of the spinal group of muscles. Extreme irritability occurs, and the slightest irritation sets up clonic spasms which may involve the musculature of the entire body, including the diaphragm. Between clonic attacks, the tonic spasm is maintained. During clonic contractions, the pain is intense, the pulse is rapid, and sweating and salivation are profuse. The leukocytic count is usually 12,000 to 15,000, with a relative polymorphonuclear leukocytosis.

During the *terminal stage*, the fever becomes greater, the pain more severe, and urinary retention may occur. There is seldom any stupor, and mental clarity persists to the end. Death is usually due to the respiratory arrest occurring during a convulsion, to asphyxia, to an exhausting toxemia, or to poisoning by barbiturates used to control the convulsive seizures.

The diagnosis of tetanus is usually not difficult, particularly when the disease is seen in the third stage or period of convulsions.

Treatment. The successful management of established tetanus depends particularly on early diagnosis and prompt adequate treatment. Severe symptoms do not necessarily indicate a fatal outcome. The main objectives of treatment are the prevention of additional toxin from reaching the central nervous system, removal of the source of toxin, adequate sedation of the patient to control convulsions, and maintenance of adequate respiration. An initial intravenous dose of 50,000 units of tetanus antitoxin is given immediately after a preliminary skin test has shown the patient not to be sensitive to horse serum. An additional injection of 40,000 units of tetanus antitoxin may also be given intramuscularly. If the skin test is positive, rapid desensitization is carried out to permit the injection of a therapeutic dose. The tissues around the site of injury may be infiltrated with 10,000 units of antitoxin. Also, a single dose of 10,000 to 20,000 units of antitoxin may be injected intrathecally by lumbar puncture; 5,000 units of antitoxin may be injected daily until the disease is obviously under control.

Whenever possible, local excision or incision of the wound should be done 1 hour later under anesthesia with intravenously administered Pentothal Sodium. Removal of any foreign bodies or infected granulation tissues should be included. Thereafter, the cleansing care of the wound is the same as that given for the average granulating wound.

The patient is placed in bed in a darkened, quiet room in order to reduce the number of external stimuli to a minimum. A nurse or a physician should be in constant attendance for the prompt recognition of respiratory arrest and the immediate institution of appropriate treatment for its correction. We have seen a patient with severe tetanus, who had been carried successfully through 11 seizures of respiratory arrest, die during his 12th seizure when the nurse left him unattended for 15 minutes.

The control of convulsive seizures is difficult. Barbiturates or paraldehyde may be administered orally, rectally or intramuscularly. Our preference is the administration of a very dilute solution of Pentothal Sodium (0.5 to 1.0 Gm. per 1,000 ml. by continuous drip in physiologic saline or glucose solution administered at the rate of 20 to 25 drops per minute). In addition, a syringe of 2.5 per cent Pentothal Sodium solution is kept in constant readiness for the emergency intravenous injection of a few ml. should convulsive respiratory arrest occur. In our experience the immediate injection of a few ml. of 2.5 per cent of Pentothal solution to a patient with a generalized convulsion and respiratory arrest is usually followed by prompt resumption of spontaneous breathing within 30 to 45 seconds. Of course, artificial respiration should be instituted.

Curarelike drugs may be given to aid in the control of the convulsive seizures. Mephenesin in a 1 or 2 per cent solution may be given in amounts sufficient to meet the patient's individual requirements. The initial dose is usually 0.5 to 1.0 Gm. Thereafter, 0.2 to 1.0 Gm. per hour may be necessary. Individual requirements vary greatly. Mephenesin and other curarelike drugs may be toxic or dangerous and must be used cautiously. In addition, they may not have any beneficial effect on the course of tetanus.

Tracheotomy may be considered, and oxygen therapy should be available for use if indicated. Excessive saliva should be removed by a soft rubber catheter connected to a suction pump which is kept at the bedside.

Tongue blades covered with gauze may be held in place between the teeth to prevent laceration of the tongue. Adequate fluid, electrolyte and caloric intake should be maintained.

Antibiotic therapy is of no value in the treatment of established tetanus except for its control of associated wound infections or for its effect on pulmonary complications. None of the antibiotics presently available has any influence on the tetanus toxin per se or its effect.

Diphtheritic Infection

Wounds occasionally become infected by the Klebs-Löffler bacillus and develop either an acute ulceration and cellulitis, with infiltration of the skin and the subcutaneous tissues about the wound, or a chronic indolent ulceration of an open wound which fails to heal. In the acute form, the systemic symptoms may be severe. A typical diphtheritic membrane adheres to the surface of the wound, and its removal results in bleeding. If paralysis of the facial muscles, cardiac arrhythmia, or respiratory difficulty occurs in a patient with a wound covered by a gray adherent membrane, a diagnosis of surgical diphtheria should be considered until proved otherwise. The diagnosis is proved by demonstrating the organisms in stained smears and by recovering them in cultures from the wound.

The treatment consists of isolation of the patient, injection of diphtheria antitoxin, and administration of penicillin or one of the broad-spectrum antibiotics.

Rabies

Etiology. Rabies is an infection caused by a virus which is inoculated into the host by means of a bite by another animal. The disease produced is a fatal encephalitis resulting from passage of the neurotropic virus along the nerve axis cylinders to the central nervous system. Infection most frequently follows a bite by a dog but has been reported after bites by other animals, including horses, cattle, cats, squirrels and bats.

The incubation period varies almost directly with the distance of the injury from the brain and may cover from 2 weeks to several months, usually being 30 to 40 days. In the prodromal phase, the infected individual shows nonspecific malaise, but this is followed by an excitement phase in which there is the characteristic paralysis of the muscles of swallowing. Since attempts to swallow precipitate severe paroxysms of coughing, the victim becomes maniacal when he sees a glass of water. Hence the term hydrophobia.

Treatment of established rabies is unsuccessful, and prophylaxis is the only means of control for this infection. Following a bite by a suspected animal the local wound should be meticulously débrided and cleansed. The animal responsible for the injury should be carefully examined and impounded for 14 days. If the animal cannot be identified, or if it should develop rabies within the observation period, antirabies vaccine should be given immediately. Because of the very short incubation period in injuries of the face and the neck, it is probably wise to begin immunization immediately after such a bite and discontinue the treatment when the animal proves to be free from disease. It must be kept in mind that the injection of rabies vaccine is not without danger, since encephalitic paralysis may follow its use.

Mycotic Infections

Actinomycosis is a surgical infection caused by *Actinomyces bovis*. This fungus may also be found growing noninvasively in the pharynx of man and some mammals. It is probable that invasion is always preceded by local surface injury which may be unrecognized.

When infection develops, it is characterized by the development of nodular granulomatous areas which subsequently suppurate and discharge pus through sinus tracts. The purulent discharge characteristically contains "sulfur granules" which are masses of lightly entwined mycelial filaments. The infection is a chronic process which typically burrows through adjacent tissues and does not spread by way of the regional lymphatics.

The clinical forms of actinomycosis may be classified into 3 types:

1. The cervicofacial variety, which is seen most frequently originating near the mandible as a hard, moderately tender, inflammatory nodule. It progresses to suppuration with central necrosis and fistulous tract formation.

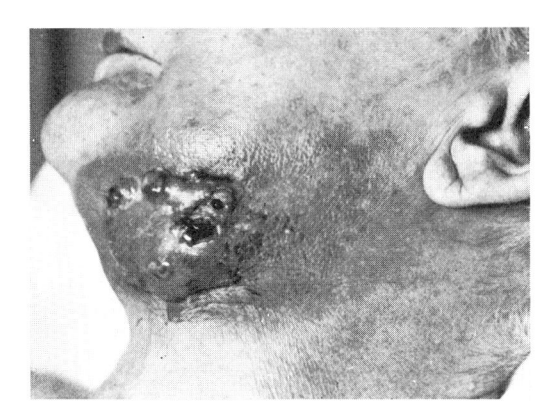

FIG. 4-11. Cervicofacial actinomycosis caused by *Actinomyces bovis*. Marked induration, discoloration of adjacent skin, and multiple sinuses apparent. Sulfur granules were identified in discharge from sinuses, and the organism was cultured anaerobically.

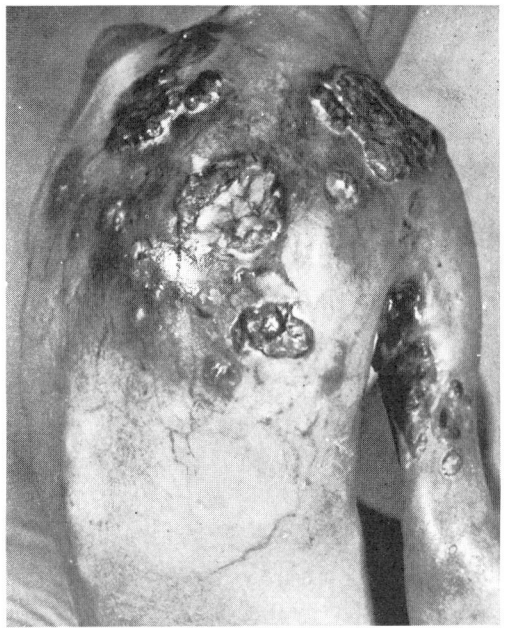

FIG. 4-12. An 11-year-old female with far-advanced actinomycosis of thoracic type. Note characteristic discoloration of skin, granulomatous granulation tissue and marked emaciation.

Peripheral extension develops with similar nodules undergoing the same course.

2. The thoracic form of the infection may be well advanced before it is recognized. Its early symptoms are nonspecific and are similar to any chronic pulmonary infection. As the disease advances, its burrowing nature becomes apparent by the involvement of pleura and ribs. Far-advanced cases may develop cutaneous fistulae.

3. The abdominal variety may be confused with cases of appendiceal abscess or carcinoma of the cecum, even at the operating table. Persistent cutaneous abdominal fistulae may develop. The diagnosis is usually made by demonstration of the actinomycotic colonies in hanging-drop preparations, in biopsies, or in cultures.

Treatment of actinomycotic infections has become impressively more successful since the introduction of the various chemotherapeutic agents. Indicated surgical operative treatment by incision and drainage of abscesses or excision, if practical, must be accompanied and followed by a prolonged course of treatment (4 to 6 months) with chemotherapeutic agents, preferably penicillin and sulfadiazine.

Blastomycosis is another of the mycotic infections that is due to yeastlike organisms. Subsequent to local inoculation a painless papule develops and persists until it ulcerates. The ulceration has a characteristic appearance, with multiple small daughter abscesses along the advancing margin. There may occur some degree of central healing of the ulcer as it increases in diameter.

The course of blastomycosis is one of relatively slow progression while the infection remains localized. As the disease extends, distant metastases develop most often in the lungs or bone. When systemic spread has occurred, the prognosis of a patient with this infection is very grave.

The treatment of blastomycosis confined to the cutaneous surface is radical excision of the involved area followed by skin grafting. Large doses of sodium or potassium iodide may be given as a systemic medication in the control of the infection. Many other forms of treatment have been used with minimal degrees of success. These include x-ray therapy, arsenicals and topical antiseptics.

Hydroxystilbamidine isethionate has shown some promise in the treatment of this condition. Amphotericin B is the most effective antibiotic in all forms of this infection, but requires careful administration and supervision.

Coccidioidomycosis is an infection caused by the fungus *Coccidioides immitis*. The most frequent type is a pulmonary infection, since the life cycle of the organism includes a sporulating stage in which it may be blown about in dust and thereby inhaled by man. The clinical picture of this infection in the chronic form resembles that of tuberculosis. An acute fulminating type is recognized in which there is an overwhelming respiratory infection which may end in death within 2 months. In the chronic form granulomatous lesions of the lung occur and may be controlled by the patient's resistance. This form of the disease progresses, with the occurrence of skin lesions, chronic granulomatous nodules, or spread to the bones or brain. Diagnosis is accomplished by demonstration of the organism in smears of sputum or local discharges and by examination of biopsied material. Skin sensitivity test may be useful in establishing the diagnosis.

Amphotericin B is an effective antibiotic in the early form of this infection, but is less valuable in the chronic stages. The other principles of treatment are based on supportive measures to encourage development of body defenses and resistance against the organism. Recent experimental evidence suggests that a vaccine for this infection may be possible. Aside from drainage of abscesses, operative surgical treatment is usually of little value (see Chap. 45, Surgery of the Lung).

Sporotrichosis. *Sporothrix schenckii* is the etiologic agent of sporotrichosis. This rare disease results from inoculation of the organisms into a small wound, usually of the hand or the foot. Ulceration with nodular lymphangitis develops along the course of the lymphatics draining the area of the wound. Secondary ulcerations of the nodules may also develop. These findings in the disease may be limited to the regional area, since systemic invasion is rare.

Treatment is usually successful with the use of large doses of potassium iodide (150 to 200 drops per day of a saturated solution). If iodide treatment is not successful, amphotericin B or hydroxystilbamidine may be used.

Anthrax, formerly known as "woolsorter's disease," was the first infectious disease proved to be caused by a bacterial agent, *Bacillus anthracis*, by Robert Koch in 1877. Initially, the disease is characterized by the development of small red macules which occur in individuals who handle animals or animal products. These macules, representing the portal of entry, become vesicles. As the disease progresses, satellite vesicles occur. The primary lesion becomes necrotic, and a black eschar forms in the center. The cutaneous lesion is usually not painful, but regional lymphadenopathy, which follows, often results in localized pain and tenderness. Septicemia may occur. The general symptoms of malaise, fever and prostration develop in proportion to the stage and the severity of the infection.

A separate form of the disease may arise after infection of the victim by inhalation of these bacteria. This form is rapidly progressive and usually fatal, since the first manifestation may be septicemia with or without pneumonia.

The mortality rate in the cutaneous form of the infection in the untreated cases was approximately 25 per cent, and approximately 100 per cent in the septicemic variety.

Modern antibiotic treatment has profoundly influenced these mortality rates. Anthrax, particularly the cutaneous variety, responds rapidly to the administration of penicillin, and the tetracyclines and chloramphenicol have been reported to be similarly effective.

Granuloma inguinale is a venereal disease seen most frequently in the tropics but occasionally in all climates, particularly in the vicinity of seaports. It is caused by the bacterium, *Donovania granulomatis*, which is a gram-negative organism having a well-defined capsule and usually found intracellularly, particularly in large mononuclear cells. The incubation period, following inoculation, may vary from a few days to as long as 3 months. This is followed by the appearance of an indolent dirty ulcer on the scrotum, the penis or the groin which is slowly progressive. The associated odor is easily recognized by experienced physicians. The causative organism may be seen in smears of the exudate or in histologic section of the edge of the ulcer.

Treatment of this infection with streptomycin, the tetracyclines, or chloramphenicol is usually followed by prompt improvement.

Lymphopathia venereum is another of the venereal diseases and it is caused by a filtrable virus. Although its incidence is higher in the tropics, it is found throughout the world. The infection occurs in both males and females but is more likely to persist and cause secondary complications in the female. Non-white patients are affected more frequently than white.

The infection, usually contracted by sexual intercourse, is manifested initially by a small genital ulceration which may heal slowly. Associated systemic manifestations are those of malaise, fever, which is usually low-grade, and often signs of meningeal irritation. Spread to the regional lymph nodes results in their marked enlargement and occasionally in suppuration. The disease may subside and lapse into a stage of apparent quiescence. After months or years, the process may lead to rectal stricture and associated intestinal obstruction due to fibrosis or contracture of the anogenital lymphatics, particularly in women. Diagnosis is suggested by positive skin test with Frei antigen.

In the acute infectious stage, apparent benefit in the control of the disease has been obtained by the use of chloramphenicol and the tetracyclines. In the late or cicatricial stage, these antibiotics are of no direct value, and abdominoperineal resection may become necessary.

Due to the reaction in the tissues surrounding the rectum, this operation is apt to be considerably more hazardous and difficult in this condition than in early carcinoma of the rectum. If a preliminary colostomy is done, the reaction may subside to some extent after several months, facilitating the resection at a second stage.

Histoplasmosis is a granulomatous infection whose etiologic agent is the fungus *Histoplasma capsulatum*. Exposure and subclinical infection as manifest by positive skin reaction and chest x-ray changes are very common, particularly in the midwestern states of the U.S.A. The clinical picture of established infection by this organism is either subacute with chronic granulomatous ulceration of the oropharynx or acute with extensive pneumonic pulmonary involvement. The subacute form progresses to involve regional lymph nodes and in the severe state leads to intestinal ulceration and invasion of the bone marrow.

Diagnosis may be difficult because of the clinical resemblance to many of the granulomatous processes and requires demonstration of *H. capsulatum* by culture or biopsy of lymph node, bone marrow, or ulcer. Treatment with amphotericin B of patients in the acute and the subacute stages is very successful. This effective but toxic antibiotic is recommended in doses of 0.25 to 1.0 mg. per kilogram per day given by slow intravenous drip.

Moniliasis is most often an infection of the alimentary tract or the female genitourinary tract by the yeast *Monilia albicans*. The usual mild infection produces flat creamy white patches in the mouth, particularly in infants, or a vaginitis with such patches on the labia, the vagina, or the cervix in adult females, particularly in diabetic or pregnant women. Iatrogenic factors may permit overgrowth under the influence of antibiotic therapy which encourages the emergence of this yeast in a virulent and invasive form.

In severely debilitated patients, the infection may produce bronchitis, pneumonia, meningitis, endocarditis, or it may invade the blood stream with fatal results.

Satisfactory management of the milder mucous membrane involvement by this organism results from topical application of gentian violet or nystatin. Iodide therapy is indicated when there is pulmonary involvement. In meningitis or endocarditis caused by this organism, amphotericin B may be used.

BIBLIOGRAPHY

Altemeier, W. A.: Prevention and control of infections in hospitals. Hospitals, Vol. 37, May 16, 1963.

Altemeier, W. A.: Symposium on hospital acquired staphylococcus infections. Part III. Recommendations for control of epidemic spread of staphylococcal infections in surgery. Ann. Surg., 150:774-778, 1959.

Altemeier, W. A., Coith, R., Sherman, R., Logan, M. A., and Tytell, A.: Toxoid immunization of experimental gas gangrene. A.M.A. Arch. Surg., 65:633-640, 1952.

Altemeier, W. A., and Culbertson, W. R.: Acute nonclostridial crepitant cellulitis. Surg., Gynec., Obstet., 87:206-212, 1948.

———: The prevention and control of surgical infections. S. Clin. N. Am., 35:1645-1661, 1955.

———: Prophylactic antibiotic therapy. A.M.A. Arch. Surg., 71:2-6, 1955.

Altemeier, W. A., Culbertson, W. R., and Gonzalez,

L. L.: Clinical experiences in the treatment of tetanus. A.M.A. Arch. Surg., 80:977-985, 1960.

Altemeier, W. A., Culbertson, W. R., Sherman, R., Cole, W., Elstun, W., and Fultz, C. T.: Critical re-evaluation of antibiotic therapy in surgery. J.A.M.A., 157:305-309, 1955.

Altemeier, W. A., and Furste, W. L.: Gas gangrene. Internat. Obstr. Surg. In Surg., Gynec., Obstet., 84:507-523, 1947.

Altemeier, W. A., and Garth, T.: The treatment of tetanus. In Current Therapy. sect. 1. pp. 48-50. Philadelphia, W. B. Saunders, 1956.

Altemeier, W. A., Giuseffi, J., and Stevenson, J.: Wound infections. In Surgery of Trauma. pp. 80-101. Philadelphia, J. B. Lippincott, 1953.

Altemeier, W. A., Hummel, R. F., and Hill, E. O.: Staphylococcal enterocolitis following antibiotic therapy. Ann. Surg., 157:847-858, 1963.

Altemeier, W. A., and Largen, T.: Antibiotic and chemotherapeutic agents in infections of the skeletal system. J.A.M.A., 150:1462-1468, 1952.

Altemeier, W. A., and Sherman, R.: The use of antibiotics and antisera in the treatment of acute injuries. J. Kentucky M.A., 55:428-433, 1954.

Altemeier, W. A., and Wulsin, J. H.: Antimicrobial therapy in injured patients. J.A.M.A., 173:527-533, 1960.

Culbertson, W. R., Altemeier, W. A., Gonzalez, L. L., and Hill, E. O.: Studies on the epidemiology of postoperative infection of clean operative wounds. Ann. Surg., 154:599-610, 1961.

Dowling, H. F., Lepper, M. H., and Jackson, G. G.: The clinical significance of antibiotic resistant bacteria. J.A.M.A., 157:327-331, 1955.

Edsall, G.: Active immunization tetanus. New Eng. J. Med., 241:18-26, 60-70, 99-107, 1949.

Hare, R., and Willits, R. E.: Bacteriology of recently inflicted wounds with special reference to hemolytic streptococci and staphylococci. Canad. M.A.J., 46:23-30, 1942.

Hill, E. O., Altemeier, W. A., and Culbertson, W. R.: An appraisal of methods of testing bacterial sensitivity to antibiotics. Ann. Surg., 148:410-428, 1958.

Larrey, D. J.: Memoirs of Military Surgery. vols. I & II. Paris, Cushing, 1812-1814.

MacLennan, J. D.: Anaerobic infections of war wounds in Middle East. Lancet, 2:63-66, 94-99, 123-126, 1943.

Meleney, F.: Differential diagnosis between certain types of infectious gangrene of skin with particular reference to hemolytic streptococcus gangrene and bacterial synergistic gangrene. Surg., Gynec., Obstet., 56:847-867, 1933.

———: Zinc peroxide in treatment of micro-aerophilic and anaerobic infections, with special reference to group of chronic, ulcerative burrowing, non-gangrenous lesions of abdominal wall apparently due to micro-aerophilic hemolytic streptococcus. Ann. Surg., 101:997-1011, 1935.

Miles, A. A., et al.: Hospital infection of war wounds. Brit. M. J., 2:855 and 895, 1940.

Pulaski, E. J.: Medical progress. New Eng. J. Med., 249:890-897, 932-938, 1953.

———: Surgical Infections: Prophylaxis, Treatment, Antibiotic Therapy. Springfield, Ill., Charles C Thomas, 1953.

Reid, M. R.: Infections in surgery. Internat. Abstr. Surg. In Surg., Gynec., Obstet., 69:107-109, 1939.

Report of Committee: Measures to combat antibiotic-resistant infections in hospitals. Bull. Am. Coll. Surgeons, 44:73-79, 1959.

Williams, R. E. O., and Shooter, R. A.: Infection in hospitals, epidemiology and control. Ed. 1. 1963, Davis, Philadelphia.

CHAPTER 5

CARL A. MOYER, M.D., AND JONATHAN E. RHOADS, M.D.

Fluid and Electrolytes

Exchanges of Water, Sodium, Potassium and Chloride Occurring in Normal Man Between the Individual and His External Environment

Internal Exchanges of Water, Sodium, Potassium and Chloride in Normal Man Across the Walls of the Alimentary Tract

Examples of Abnormal Losses and Intakes of Water and Electrolytes in Surgical Patients

Methods for Suspecting and Quantitating the Deficits or the Surpluses of Water, and Abnormalities of Concentration of Sodium, Chloride and Potassium Ions

The Patient With Hyposthenuria

The Patient With Salt-Losing Kidneys

The Patient With the Lower Nephron Syndrome

The Diabetic Patient Undergoing Surgical Procedures

The Relations of Respiration to Acid-Base Balance

The Comatose Patient

The subject of water and electrolyte balance has been obscured by a long series of efforts to establish short cuts. It is not a simple subject but rather one that requires careful study and thought. The body ordinarily meets its water and electrolyte requirements through response to thirst and hunger.

In the rat, Richter[15, 16] has demonstrated a selective thirst for calcium-containing solutions in parathyroidectomized rats and for hypertonic salt solutions in adrenalectomized rats. Animals whose sweats contain sodium chloride possess the sense of salt hunger when in need of salt. Salt-starved cattle will force their way through strong fences and travel long distances for salt. Man possesses this sense feebly or not at all. However, hunger and appetite lead to the ingestion of a varied diet, which usually contains the requirements for electrolytes.

The body, having received sufficient water, salt and other elements by satisfying thirst and hunger, then provides a rather constant internal environment for its constituent cells and their enzymes. This is accomplished primarily by the kidney, but heart, liver, lungs, adrenals and other factors play important roles.

The great importance of this subject in surgery lies in the frequency with which normal processes are changed by certain of the diseases for which surgical treatment is required, and by operation and conditions obtaining during the preoperative and the postoperative periods.

In this chapter we will not consider at length electrolytes such as magnesium, phosphate, etc., about which relatively little is known and which do not constitute such important problems in the general run of surgical patients.

Calcium and phosphorus metabolism will be considered in the section on the parathyroid gland. Bicarbonate is considered under respiratory acidosis and alkalosis.

Even after eliminating these large fields, it is clear that water and electrolyte balance is far from a simple subject, and attempts to simplify it usually have led to faulty thinking and, as a result, to inadequate care of those patients who most need help. These attempts at simplification have gone in two directions. First is the compounding of stock solutions, such as so-called physiologic saline solution, Ringer's solution, Hartmann's solution, etc., with all further thought being in terms of milliliters of this solution. Second is the measurement of concentrations of ions without regard to the volume in which such concentrations are distributed. This has led to the use of erroneous formulas for calculating electrolyte requirements from concentration figures.

It is proposed to review briefly some physiologic functions of water and sodium salts and normal exchanges of water, sodium, chloride and potassium, with emphasis on normal requirements. Next, examples of abnormal losses and intakes encountered in surgical patients will be given. Third, mention will be made of the available methods of suspecting and quantitating the deficits or surpluses of these substances. On the basis of these sections a method of caring for the water, sodium, potassium and chloride requirements of patients with competent kidneys will be presented. Finally, 5 special problems will be considered: (1) the patient with hyposthenuria; (2) the patient with the salt-losing kidney; (3) the patient with the lower nephron syndrome; (4) the diabetic patient undergoing surgical procedures; (5) the effect of respiration on blood pH; and (6) the comatose patient.

The first scientific application of biologic chemistry to medical therapeutics occurred in the field of fluid and electrolytes. During a cholera epidemic in London in 1830, the chemist, O'Shaughnessy, analyzed the bloods of a number of victims of the disease and reported the following:

To the Editor of *The Lancet*[14]
Sir,—Having been enabled to complete the experimental inquiries on which I have for some time back been engaged in Newcastle upon Tyne, I beg you will have the kindness to give insertion to the annexed outlines of the results I have obtained:

1. The blood drawn in the worst cases of the cholera, is unchanged in its anatomical or globular structure.
2. It has lost a large proportion of its water, 1,000 parts of cholera serum having but the average of 860 parts of water.
3. It has lost also a great proportion of its NEUTRAL saline ingredients.
4. Of the free alkali contained in healthy serum, not a particle is present in some cholera cases, and barely a trace in others.*
5. Urea exists in the cases where suppression of urine has been a marked symptom.
6. All the salts deficient in the blood, especially the carbonate of soda, are present in large quanties in the peculiar white dejected matters.*

* The blood and dejected substances were obtained in one analysis, from the same patient, and the blood was drawn half an hour after the evacuation occurred.

There are other results of minor consequence to which I will not at present allude, neither shall I on this occasion offer any observation on the practical influence to which my experiments may lead. In a few days a detailed report shall be published, in which the mode of analysis, etc., will be minutely described. It will be found, I regret to say, in every essential particular, to contradict that recently given by Hermann. All my experiments, however, have been publicly performed, and can be authenticated by numerous witnesses, a precaution I thought it necessary to adopt, lest it might be supposed that I impugned, without sufficient foundation, the accuracy of the Moscow professor.

May I add, that until the publication of my report, I shall deem the suspension of discussion on the results now introduced as a matter of personal courtesy and obligation.

I am, Sir,
Your obedient servant,
W. B. O'Shaughnessy, M.D.
London, 29 December, 1831.

Within 6 months after this publication, a general practitioner in Leith (Scotland), T. Latta, put this knowledge to practical therapeutic use. Latta's report of this experience, with the giving as much as 16 quarts of a saline solution, intravenously, during 24 hours, to persons dying of the cholera, has in it such vivid and accurate descriptions of many of the clinical signs of extracellular fluid volume deficiency, including shock, that parts of his report are used here to introduce the subject of fluid and electrolytes. Actually, no better writing on certain phases of the subject can be found anywhere.

(Latta's first article, *The Lancet*)[10]
Documents Communicated by the Central Board of Health, London, Relative to the Treatment of Cholera by the Copious Injection of Aqueous and Saline Fluids Into the Veins.

Letter from Dr. Latta to the Secretary of the Central Board of Health, London, affording a View of the Rationale and Results of his Practice in the Treatment of Cholera by Aqueous and Saline Injections. Leith, May 23, 1832. (Excerpt from letter)

So as soon as I learnt the result of Dr. O'Shaughnessy's analysis, I attempted to restore the blood to its natural state, by injecting copiously into the larger intestines warm water, holding in solution the requisite salts, and also administered quantities from time to time by the mouth, trusting that the power of absorption might not be altogether lost, but by these means I produced, in no case, any permanent benefit, but, on the contrary, I thought the tormina, vomiting, and purging, were much aggravated thereby, to the further reduction of the little remaining strength of the patient; finding thus that such, in common with all the ordinary means in use, was either useless or hurtful, I at length resolved to throw the fluid immediately into the circulation. In this, having no precedent to direct me, I proceeded with much caution. The first subject of experiment was an aged female, on whom all the usual remedies had been fully tried, without producing one good symptom; the disease, uninterrupted, holding steadily on its course. She had apparently reached the last moments of her earthly existence, and now nothing could injure her—indeed so entirely was she reduced, that I feared I should be unable to get my apparatus ready ere she expired. Having inserted a tube into the basilic vein, cautiously—anxiously, I watched the effects; ounce after ounce was injected, but no visible change was produced. Still persevering I thought she began to breathe less laboriously, soon the sharpened features, and sunken eye, and fallen jaw, pale and cold, bearing the manifest impress of death's signet, began to glow with returning animation; the pulse, which had long ceased, returned to the wrist; at first small and quick, by degrees it became more and more distinct, fuller, slower, and firmer, and in the short space of half an hour, when six pints had been injected, she expressed in a firm voice that she was free from all uneasiness, actually became jocular, and fancied all she needed was a little sleep; her extremities were warm, and every feature bore the aspect of comfort and health. This being my first case, I fancied my patient secure, and from my great need of a little repose, left her in charge of the hospital surgeon; but I had not been long gone, ere the vomiting and purging recurring, soon reduced her to her former state of debility. I was not apprised of the event, and she sunk in five and a half hours after I left her. As she had previously been of a sound constitution, I have no doubt the case would have issued in complete reaction, had the remedy, which already had produced such effect, been repeated.

Not having by me the number of *The Lancet* containing Dr. O'Shaughnessy's analyses, I adopted that of Dr. Marcet,* only allowing a smaller proportion of saline ingredients. This I now find to be considerably less than natural according to the more recent analyses. I dissolved from two to three drachms of muriate of soda and two scruples of the subcarbonate of soda in six pints of water, and injected it at a temperature of 112° Fah. If the temperature is so low as a hundred, it produces an extreme sense of cold, with rigors; and if it reaches 115°, it suddenly excites the heart, the countenance becomes flushed, and the patient complains of great weakness. At first there is but little felt by the patient, and symptoms continue unaltered, until the blood, mingled with the injected liquid, becomes warm and fluid; the improvement in the pulse and countenance is almost simultaneous, the cadaverous expression gradually gives place to appearances of returning animation, the horrid oppression at the praecordia goes off, the sunken turned-up eye, half covered by the palpebrae, becomes gradually fuller, till it sparkles with the brilliancy of health, the livid hue disappears, the warmth of the body returns, and it regains its natural colour,—words are no more uttered in whispers, the voice first acquires its true cholera tone, and ultimately its wonted energy, and the poor patient, who but a few minutes before was oppressed with sickness, vomiting and burning thirst, is suddenly relieved from every distressing symptom; blood now drawn exhibits on exposure to air its natural florid hue.

Such symptoms, so gratifying both to the sick and the physician, must never allow the latter to relax in his care—the utmost vigilance is still necessary. At first the change is so great that he may fancy all is accomplished, and leave his post for a while. The diarrhoea recurring, he may find his patient, after the lapse of two or three hours, as low as ever.

I have already given an instance where deficiency in quantity was the cause of failure which I will now contrast with one in which it was used freely. A female, aged 50, very destitute, but previously in good health, was on the 13th instant, at four A.M., seized with cholera in its most violent form, and by half-past nine was reduced to a most hopeless state. The pulse was quite gone, even in the axilla, and strength so much exhausted, that I had resolved not to try the effects of the injection, conceiving the poor woman's case to be hopeless, and that the failure of the experiment might afford the prejudiced and the illiberal an opportunity to stigmatize the practice, however, I at length thought I would give her a chance, and in the presence of Drs. Lewins and Craigie, and Messrs. Sibson and Paterson, I injected one hundred and twenty ounces, when like the effects of magic, instead of the pallid aspect of one whom death had sealed as his own, the vital tide was restored, and life and vivacity returned! but diarrhoea recurred and in three hours she again sunk. One hundred and twenty ounces more were injected with the same good effect. In this case 300 ounces (10

---

* The exact composition of the Marcet solution used by Latta cannot be determined. The concentration of sodium chloride in it was about 0.4–0.55 per cent and that of the sodium subcarbonate ($NaHCO_3$ or Na_2CO_3) 0.1–0.25 per cent.

liters) were so used in twelve hours, when reaction was completely re-established and in forty-eight hours she smoked her pipe free from distemper.

During the past decade, observations made upon unanesthetized, healthy men and women, depleted of sodium salts and water by prolonged duodenal intubation, have established the fact that Latta accurately depicted the signs and symptoms of what is now called "extracellular fluid deficit or depletion."

Relatively small variances in the body's content of water and salts are attended by profound illness and even death. For each fixed cell in the normal human body there are approximately 2×10^{13} molecules of water and 5×10^{10} sodium ions, located extracellularly, exclusive of the water and the salts in the blood. An acute reduction in number of extracellular water molecules per body cell to 1.33×10^{13} and extracellular sodium ions to 3.3×10^{10} per cell completely incapacitates normal man and often is accompanied by renal failure and shock. An acute simultaneous reduction of extracellular water molecules per cell to 1×10^{13} and sodium ions to 2.5×10^{10} kills dogs.

The chemical reasons for the lethality of salt and water deficits are still obscure. However, the subjection of animals and men to measured deficits of salt and water, and the examination of the responses of dehydrated man before, during and after combined salt and water deficits have been corrected have provided some physiologic insight into the problem. The induction of a combined sodium salt and water deficit in man, in such a fashion as not to change the proportion of the salt to water left in the body (the serum sodium concentration is unchanged), is associated with a decrease in the volume of the plasma amounting to a difference, plus or minus, of 4.5 per cent of the original for each 1 mEq. Na+ deficit and 7 ml. water deficit per kilo of body weight.[8]

The rate of change of plasma volume per mEq. Na+ and 7 ml. of water does not decrease as the deficits grow, even should they attain the point of producing complete physical incapacity and profound hypotension— e.g., B.P. 40/0. (See Figures 5-1 and 5-2.)

This occurs, although the plasma protein concentration almost doubles, and with it, the

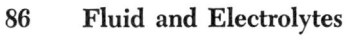

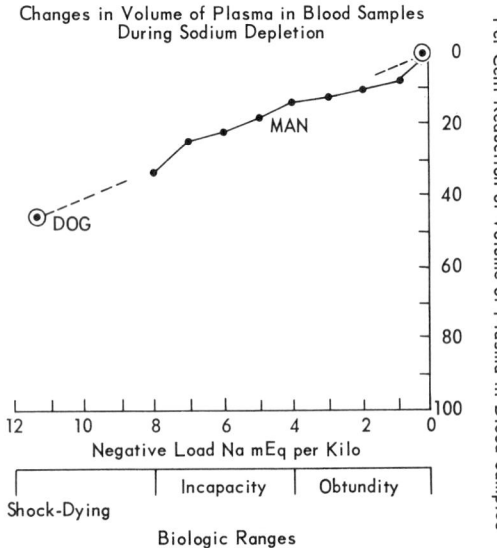

FIG. 5-1. Mean changes in the plasma volumes of blood samples from 5 normal and 5 alcoholic men and women, and from 3 dogs during depletions of sodium salts.[8] Graphs 5-1 and 5-3 have Cartesian coordinates. The curves move to the left because the changes are related to progressive deficits of sodium.

intravascular oncotic pressure. In other words, the numbers of sodium ions and water molecules in the extracellular space are very important determinants of the plasma volume, *and the blood volume is not sustained by a rising serum protein concentration in the face of combined losses of sodium and water from the body.*

Recently Moyer and others (1967) have been able to relate changes in plasma volume to water and sodium loads separately. Within limits, the plasma volume changes about 75 ml. per liter of water loading and 1,150 ml. per equivalent weight (23 grams) of sodium load. This means that the plasma volume of a person losing 2 liters of water and 0.5 equivalent of sodium through diarrhea will decline about 150 + 575, or 725 ml.

It is easy to see why the removal of Na salts from the body, proportionately faster than water, is attended by a rate of decrease of plasma volume that is practically the same as it is when both sodium salts and water are removed simultaneously at the rates proportional of 1 mEq. Na to 7 ml. H_2O.[2] Indubit-

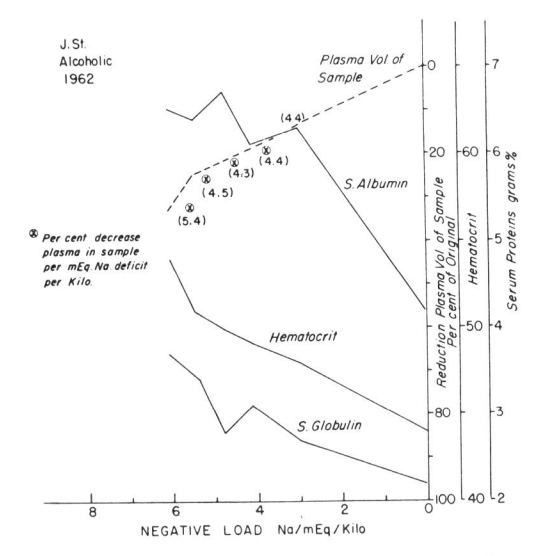

FIG. 5-2. Hematocrit, concentrations of serum albumin and globulin, and plasma volumes of blood samples of an alcoholic man during depletion of sodium salts.[8]

ably then, the number of extracellular-extravascular sodium ions is a most important determinant of the volume of the plasma in man. These observations and conclusions agree with those made by Gregersen,[3] Maddock and Coller.[4]

This does not imply that the concentration of plasma proteins and oncotic pressure are not important determinants of plasma volume under conditions other than absolute sodium deficiency. Hypoproteinemic cirrhotics and nephrotics, with larger than normal plasma volumes when recumbent, manifest about 4 times the decline in blood volume when they stand that normal persons do.[6] However, remarkable accommodations to low oncotic pressures in the plasma have been observed by human beings. Some cases of complete analbuminemia without hyperglobulinemia have been discovered, and these persons have normal plasma volumes, no edema and lead long normal lives.[3] These are rare genetic abnormalities.

Although, in man, hypotension, severe oliguria, rapidly rising blood urea nitrogen, low glomerular filtration rate and slow renal plasma flow are regularly produced by sodium depletions varying between 4 and 8 mEq. Na per Kg. of original body weight, the hypotension and other manifestations of shock cannot be ascribed to the oligemia alone. Sodium deficits varying between 4 to 8 mEq. per Kilo are associated with oligemias varying between 12 and 24 per cent of the original blood volumes, respectively. Oligemias of 12 to 20 per cent, when induced by hemorrhage, are not attended by hypotension, tachycardia, physical weakness or renal insufficiency in unanesthetized, healthy, recumbent men or women. In the case of the sodium deficit, illustrated in Figure 5-3, hypotension, both orthostatic and recumbent, tachycardia, great weakness and oliguria attended an oligemia that did not exceed 14 per cent.

There is other evidence that the shock associated with sodium deficiency is not oligemic in origin. (See Chap. 17, Burns.) With burns larger than 50 per cent of body surface, the treatment of burn-shock with lactated-Ringer's solution alone is associated with

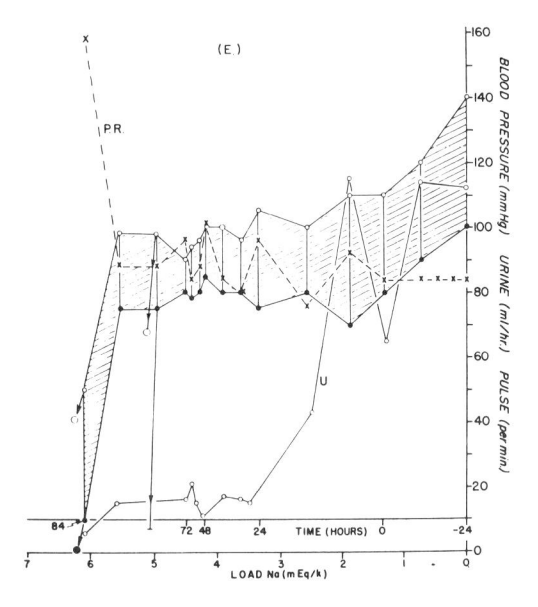

FIG. 5-3. Blood pressure, pulse rate and rate of excretion of urine during transduodenal sodium depletion or negative sodium loading. The graph has standard Cartesian coordinates. The onset of orthostatic tachycardia is designated by lines consisting of arrows starting upward at the recumbent pulse line (dashed between Xs), and orthostatic hypotension by solid lines dropped from the systolic (solid line connecting solid black circles) lines of the graph. The rate of excretion of urine is designated by open circles connected by a solid line.[8]

rises in the hematocrit of as much as 33 per cent—e.g., 48 to 64, indicating a decline in blood volume of approximately 25 per cent, while concomitantly rates of urine excretion as high as 60 ml. per hour, clear sensoria, normal blood pressures and a sense of well-being by the patient are attained. In other words, many of the signs of burn-shock disappear as sodium salts and water are being given, while the blood volume may be falling concomitantly as much as 20 per cent.

In other words, evidence is gradually being collected which indicates that shock attending sodium deficits is a phenomenon that is not completely relatable to oligemia. What are the effects of sodium deficit on other biologic processes that might have some bearing on clearing up the problem?

Besides inducing oligemia, sodium deficit is attended by hypometabolism. Sodium deficits in normal, nonalcoholic man, varying between 4 and 8 mEq. per Kg.[1], are associated with drops in resting consumptions of oxygen of 20 to 34 per cent.[8] The oxygen consumptions of slices of various tissues devoid of circulation decrease as sodium salts are removed from them.[7, 17] How a reduction in number of sodium ions about cells effects this hypometabolism is unknown; nonetheless, it could be an important factor in the genesis of shock associated with any sodium depletion, as well as that induced by a slow or recurrent hemorrhage.

During 1962, 1963 and 1964, the giving of lactated-Ringer's solution (Na^+ 130 to 134 mEq./L.), in addition to giving back the blood removed from the animal, was found to effect recovery in more than 85 per cent of the animals; whereas, returning only the blood removed during the hemorrhage causing the shock effects recovery in only 50 per cent of animals[5] (see Table 5-1).

Obviously, the sodium ion, in addition to being an important determinant of the plasma volume, and thereby of blood volume, is an important determinant of the rates of cellular metabolism in man and animals and of recovery from prolonged hemorrhagic shock (dog).

A more extensive exposition of the roles played by sodium and water in the regulation of plasma volume and the treatment of burn and hemorrhagic shock is to be found in reference 12.

All of the other cations (H^+, Ca^{++}, K^+, Mg^+), the anions (Cl^-, HCO_3^-, HPO_4^-, SO_4^{--}, plasma protein) and the body solvent (water molecules themselves) play important physiologic roles. The most important of these will be listed subsequently.

Because the abnormalities of fluids and electrolytes are often very complex, the use of some practical scheme for diagnoses should be used, in order that the proper treatments and chemical determinations may be selected for a particular case. The schema outlined in Table 5-2 (p. 81) is functional and simple.

The schema particularly emphasizes the physiologic roles played by sodium salts and water, singularly and in combination. Some of the physiologic consequences of a deficiency of sodium have been described. The consequences of sodium deficit, as well as excess, are modified by the direction taken by the water content of the body during the development of the abnormality of sodium. Conversely, the abnormalities induced by changes in water content of the body are modified by

TABLE 5-1. THE RESULTS OF TREATING CONTROLLED CANINE HEMORRHAGIC SHOCK
(Modified Wiggers' Preparation)

METHOD OF TREATMENT	NUMBER TREATED	NUMBER DYING	NUMBER SURVIVING	PROPORTION SURVIVING
1. Shed blood only	24	12	12	.50
2. Shed blood plus lactated-Ringer's solution* (pH 8.5)	9	3	6	.67
3. Lactated-Ringer's solution alone† (pH 8.5)	20	10	10	.50
4. Lactated-Ringer's solution plus ½shed blood (pH 8.5)	8	1	7	.87

* Volume lactated-Ringer's solution equaled volume of shed blood.
† Volume of lactated-Ringer's solution equaled the plasma plus 4 times the red blood cell volume removed.

TABLE 5-2. DIAGNOSES OF ABNORMALITIES OF FLUID AND ELECTROLYTES

Clinical Group of Electrolyte and Water Abnormalities (Group)	(1) Numbers of (Na+) Sodium Ions in Body	(2) Numbers of Water Molecules in Body	(3) Serum Na Concentrations	(4) Proton Concentration pH of Blood	(5) Serum Ionic Concentrations Other Than +Na
1. a. b.	Normal Excess	Deficit Normal or Deficit	Increased only		
2. a. b. c.	Normal Deficit Deficit	Excess Excess Normal	Decreased only	Metabolic Acidosis or Alkalosis or Respiratory Acidosis or Alkalosis	Hypo- or Hyper- kalemia, calcemia, magnesemia, chloremia, proteinemia, phosphatemia, etc.
3. a.	Deficit	Deficit	Variable: may be Increased, Normal, Decreased		
4. a.	Excess	Excess	Variable: may be Increased, Normal, Decreased		

the directions and the extents of the concomitant changes in bodily content of sodium taking place subsequently or concomitantly. For instance, a simultaneous gain in body sodium and water, proportional to 1 mEq. Na:7 ml. H$_2$O* is associated with gain in weight—some edema and plethora and hypoproteinemia—but no real illness until the plethora becomes so great as to produce congestive heart failure. However, the addition of sodium to the body, in relation to water in the proportion of 1 mEq. Na+ to 1.2 ml. H$_2$O ($\cong$ 5% NaCl), in relatively small quantity (200 ml. of 5% NaCl), is attended quickly by fever, hypermetabolism, thirst, and mental agitation and aberrations. The death that attends a sufficient accretion of sodium, under these circumstances, is from respiratory failure—not heart failure. To illustrate further, a gain of body water and sodium in the proportion of any number of ml. H$_2$O to 0 mEq. Na produces water gain, while sodium content is unchanged (water gain > 0 : salt gain = 0). This is associated with headache, disturbances of vision, rising intracranial pressure, and when enough water is gained, there are epileptiform convulsions that may be fatal. Should water be gained while sodium is being lost, convulsions and shock tend to occur simultaneously.

It is self-evident that the pH and ionic concentrations that may attend the various combinations of sodium and water abnormalities may vary. They may increase, remain normal or decrease somewhat independently of the body's content of sodium and water.

In view of the fact that means of measuring easily and accurately the body's functional content† of water and sodium are still lack-

* Normal ratio of Na to water in extracellular fluid.

† The sodium and the water in the intestinal tract during ileus, in the peritoneal cavity containing ascites, in the fluid constituting the swelling of all injured tissues are physiologically nonfunctional. They do not serve to maintain blood volume or any other general physiologic purpose. Yet, these adventitious nonfunctional fluid spaces constitute functional volumes of distribution for such things as tritium, deuterium and radioactive sodium and inulin, thiocyanate and radioactive sulfate and, consequently, without exercising special precautions and making certain mathematical assumptions, one cannot measure the functional water volume and sodium mass of the body of ill persons with any degree of certainty.

ing, the history and certain aspects of the physical examination must be correlated with laboratory data, in order to ascertain tentatively the character of the bodily fluid and electrolyte status. The more important anamnestic features, physical signs and laboratory data pertinent to the more frequent types of fluid and electrolyte disturbances in surgical patients are listed below.

CLINICAL GROUP 1-a
SODIUM NORMAL WITH WATER DEFICIT

Basic cause: loss of water from body as vapor through skin and lungs, or as water through kidneys, while little sodium is being excreted by the kidneys or the sweat glands and no, or insufficient, water is being drunk or given.

Etiologic Factors

Anything that reduces or abolishes a person's capacity or will to drink, such as unconsciousness, disorientation, great weakness or paralysis, and aposia.

Anything that abolishes or curtails normal vasopressin secretion and the facultative reabsorption of water by the kidney—e.g., diabetes insipidus, head injuries, operations upon the pituitary or structures near it.

Physical Signs and Symptoms

Thirst, if patient is fully conscious
Dry mucous membranes and injection of the conjunctiva
Skin hot and flushed
Fever, hypermetabolism and disorientation in the previously oriented
Coma and deep breathing
Death from respiratory failure

Shock does not appear until death is imminent. The pulse is bounding and full, and the blood pressure is normal until then.

Blood volume does not decrease significantly. Plasma volume decreases only on an average of 75 ml. for every liter of water lost without sodium.

Urine flows are minimally 15 to 20 ml. per hour, but they may be faster than 200 ml. per hour, even just before death, if suppression of the secretion of vasopressin is the cause of the trouble.

Laboratory Signs

Serum sodium concentration—*Elevated*
Serum chloride—*Elevated*

The illness is roughly proportional to the elevation of serum sodium concentration.

With serum Na above 170 mEq./L., there is stupor or coma, and fever of about 40° C. or higher, and there is danger of immediate death.

The serum protein concentrations and the hematocrit are in the high range of normal, because the plasma volume does not decline more than 6 to 10 per cent before death.

The BUN is not much elevated in cases in which pituitary dysfunction is the cause.

Treatment

The need is for WATER. A certain means of delivering it is to give 5 per cent dextrose solution intravenously, gauging the speed and volume of administration on the nature of the illness, and rate of change and level of the serum sodium.

Vasopressin and adrenocorticoids are usually needed in cases of acute postoperative or post-traumatic dysfunction of the posterior pituitary.

CLINICAL GROUP 1-b
SODIUM EXCESS EITHER WITH WATER-NORMAL OR WATER-DEFICIT

Etiologic Factors

Iatrogenic factors predominate; the giving of hypertonic (3 to 5%) saline solutions to persons with normal kidneys, or the administration of slightly hypertonic solutions of sodium salts, such as 0.9 per cent NaCl solution or Ringer's solution, as the only fluid intake to patients with abnormal renal function, are the most frequent causes.

During anesthesia, and for 1 or 2 days after major operations, the renal handling of isotonic saline is often abnormal.

When isotonic saline alone is given to a normal person, the kidneys excrete a urine containing sodium in concentrations of 180 to 260 mEq. Na/L. By doing this, the kidneys "distill" some water from the 155 mEq. Na/L. saline given, making up for the loss of water vapor insensibly through skin and lungs. During and for a time after major operations, the kidneys do not do this. Instead, they usually excrete urine containing sodium in lower concentrations than 155 mEq./L.[13] Consequently, whereas hyperosmolarity does not follow the giving of isotonic saline as the only fluid to normal persons, it often follows the giving of only isotonic saline to a person during the immediate postoperative period.

Physical Signs and Symptoms

Thirst, fever, disorientation, hypermetabolism, plethora, rarely convulsions

Laboratory Signs

Serum sodium concentration increased
Serum chloride elevated
Hematocrit and plasma proteins—low normal or subnormal
Urine flow, usually in normal range, 20 to 50 ml./hour—rarely higher

Treatment

Stop giving salt and *give water*, as for Group 1-a.

CLINICAL GROUP 2-a
SODIUM NORMAL WITH WATER EXCESS (SIMPLE WATER INTOXICATION)

Etiologic Factors

Iatrogenic causes predominate; however, the stage is set for it by the antidiuresis stimulated by stimuli other than the normal one of water deficit with increasing osmolar concentration. Such things as severe emotional disturbances, pain, trauma, neoplasia and drugs, such as morphine and barbiturates, may set the stage for it, because these are frequently associated with antidiuresis.

Its cause is clearly the retention of water drunk or given in excess of the amount requisite for the maintenance of normal salt concentrations in the body. Normally, should more water (not containing any sodium) be drunk or given than needed, the secretion of antidiuretic substances into the blood stops, and the kidneys excrete the water very rapidly —up to 600 to 1,000 ml. per hour (see Fig. 15-2, p. 319). However, for as long as a week after an operation, during pain and emotional stress, and with some cancers, the secretion of antidiuretic substances is kept up, although its normal stimulus is completely lacking. Under these circumstances, an intake or input of water larger than 1 to 1½ liters a day will lead to water retention, barring, of course, accelerated losses of water insensibly from fever, through burned skin and hyperpnea.

Of course, the administration of vasopressin for diabetes insipidus does the same thing. In fact, the first cases of water intoxication recognized as such were patients with diabetes insipidus treated with vasopressin who continued to drink 4 to 10 liters of water a day after treatment with pitressin was begun— habit was the stimulus to drinking in such cases.

It also, fairly regularly, attends transurethral resection of the prostate gland, because of the rapid entrance into the opened veins and tissues of the nonelectrolyte-containing fluid used to distend the bladder. Decreases of serum sodium from 136 mEq./L. to 112 mEq./L. have occurred from this mechanism during a transurethral prostatic resection lasting 1 hour.

Physical Signs and Symptoms

Salivation, headache, nausea, vomiting, nervous irritability, increased intracranial pressure, hypertension, convulsions

Laboratory Signs

Sodium concentration reduced; serum chloride concentration decreased

Treatment

Withhold water until serum sodium concentration is normal.
Convulsions are an indication for giving enough hypertonic saline to stop them; 3 per cent NaCl 100 to 200 ml. by vein is usually enough.

CLINICAL GROUP 2-b
SODIUM DEFICIT WITH WATER IN EXCESS

Etiologic Factors

The drinking of water or the giving of 5 or 10 per cent dextrose in water in excess of its insensible loss and urinary secretion during intestinal obstructions, generalized peritonitis, acute fulminant thrombophlebitis and after serious trauma, such as large burns, and fractures of the pelvis or femora, before the sodium deficit related to the swelling of the injured part has been treated adequately are the most frequent causes. The trauma, as well as the sodium deficits, sets the stage for water retention (Group 2-a, this chapter). Other causes are: (1) The drinking of water or the giving of 5 per cent dextrose in water, in excess of the water lost insensibly in the sweat and in the urine, while the person sweats profusely. (Sweat contains sodium chloride.) (2) The giving of large enemata of water, and the irrigation of indwelling gastric tubes with water, especially among the weak and the elderly. They are more likely to hold the enemata for a relatively long time before expelling them. During the retention of the water in the colon, salts enter the water in the bowel while some water is absorbed into the body.

PHYSICAL SIGNS AND SYMPTOMS

"Low salt syndrome": weakness, apathy and hypometabolism; in addition, hypothermia occurs when the sodium deficit is severe and there is no infection or other cause for fever, such as myocardial infarct.

Orthostatic hypotension occurs with moderate sodium deficits, and recumbent hypotension, tachycardia, oliguria, and azotemia attend sodium deficits of 4 to 8 mEq. per Kg. Muscle cramps and abdominal cramps are complained of occasionally.

LABORATORY SIGNS

Serum sodium concentration decreased; chloride concentration decreased

Elevation of hematocrit; rising BUN or N.P.N. (prerenal azotemia)

Plasma volume is distinctly subnormal with sodium deficits of 4 to 8 mEq. per Kg. Plasma volume declines, on an average, 1.15 liters for every equivalent of net sodium loss[12] (23 grams of sodium, i.e., 58 grams of sodium chloride).

TREATMENT

Give an appropriate isotonic saline solution intravenously *and withhold water.*

Hypertonic saline is rarely needed (only for convulsions).

CLINICAL GROUP 2-c
SODIUM DEFICIT WITH WATER NORMAL

ETIOLOGIC FACTORS

Same as for Group 2-b above. This is a rare condition and is a transitional phase leading to 2-b above.

The *Physical Signs and Symptoms*, the *Laboratory Signs* and *Treatment* are the same as for Group 2-b.

CLINICAL GROUP 3-a
COMBINED SODIUM AND WATER DEFICITS

This group of fluid and electrolyte imbalances is the one most frequently encountered by surgeons. It attends all types of trauma within minutes of sufferance of the injury; it accompanies protracted hemorrhage and hemorrhagic shock; it follows vomiting and diarrhea and fistulous drainages; it attends and follows rapid decompression of the obstructed urinary bladder and the correction of total ureteral obstructions; it is prone to occur during the overzealous use of diuretics; it is practically a constant attendant of ileus of all types; it occurs with great speed, during minutes, with occlusion of such veins as the portal and the vena cava above the diaphragm; it also occurs with anaphylaxis and severe acute drug reactions.

Although it is the most frequently occurring of all fluid and electrolyte disturbances, its existence and magnitude often are not recognized. The reason for this is the false assumption that sodium and water deficits are always attended by declining or lower-than-normal concentrations of serum sodium.

Serum sodium concentrations do not fall significantly, and, under certain circumstances, they may even rise, while lethal sodium and water deficits are generated by such things as rapidly reforming or forming ascites, hemorrhage, massive contusional injuries of soft parts, burns, ileus, acute occlusions of large venous systems, giant urticaria and fulminant diarrhea. With the exception of diarrhea, in all of the other circumstances, the cause of the sodium and water deficit is invisible, and the magnitude of the losses is not appreciated. The magnitudes of the losses of sodium salts and water into the intestine with ileus are tabulated in Chapter 38 (Intestinal Obstruction). As much as 7 liters of extracellular fluid have been observed to move into the legs and the thighs of a man in 6 hours after ligation of the vena cava; 2 liters into the wall of the intestine after 10 minutes of occlusion of the portal vein; 3 liters into the skin in 30 minutes during the development of giant urticaria; 23 liters into and through a burn covering 1.2 M^2 during 12 hours; and 2.5 to 5 liters into nonfunctional extracellular tissue spaces during 2 hours of hemorrhagic shock.

In all cases such as this, the serum sodium concentration does not decline significantly *unless* the person drinks water or is given water with some sodium-free solute, intravenously. *Body cells do not give up their water to the extracellular space in appreciable quantity during the genesis of acute combined sodium and water depletions.* This was discovered by Tappeiner[18] almost a century ago. He measured the mass of water in the serum and in the red blood cells of persons and animals dead of burns and found the serum impoverished of water, while the red blood cells contained their normal amount. Then he asked the question, "Why have not the water-rich cells given up water to the water-impoverished serum?" Consequently, unless water is drunk or given, while sodium salts and water are sequestered in or lost from the body, the sodium concentration will not fall significantly during the genesis of acute sodium depletion, and the surgeon, falsely believing that it will, will leave injured men go to untimely deaths for want of a few bottles of salt water.

If the serum sodium concentration cannot serve as a dependable diagnostic yardstick in such cases, how does one make the diagnosis of sodium and water deficit? First, one must appreciate that the swelling of all injured parts produces sodium and water deficit in all uninjured tissues; their extracellular salts and water are sucked up by the injured swelling members; that the same is true for rapidly reforming ascites, the filling of part of thoracic cage with fluid after pneumonectomy, and the collection of fluid in the intestine during ileus. The remaining bases of diagnosis consist of recognizing the physical signs of sodium depletion.

PHYSICAL SIGNS AND SYMPTOMS

Weakness, somnolence (excepting in the alcoholic, in whom excitement and mania often exist with sodium deficit), oliguria and often tachycardia are associated with moderate deficits. Anuria, stupor, tachycardia and slow venous filling and hypotension occur with severe deficits.

The normal tissues do not show signs of shrinkage for hours, even though, functionally, almost lethal sodium deficits may exist. That is to say, the tongue does not get soft, the skin does not lose turgor, the eyeballs do not sink or soften for hours. Consequently, these signs are of little worth for the detection of the acute extracellular fluid volume deficits associated with trauma and other rapid internal translocations of sodium salts and water.

LABORATORY SIGNS

A rising or elevated hematocrit and plasma protein concentration regularly attend sodium salt and water deficits.

The serum sodium is usually normal for many hours, unless large volumes of water are drunk or injected intravenously as 5 or 10 per cent dextrose.

A falling sodium concentration, coupled with a steady hematocrit, while glucose in water or a solute diuretic in water is being given intravenously is a sign of this sort of sodium depletion.

TREATMENT

The treatment consists of administering an isotonic solution of sodium salts appropriate to the status of the pH of arterial blood, and the chloride bicarbonate concentrations of serum. Usually, lactated-Ringer's solution is an appropriate solution, because the pH of arterial blood and the bicarbonate and chloride concentrations are most often normal. During hemorrhagic or traumatic shock a severe life-endangering metabolic acidosis may exist. In such cases 1.25 per cent $NaHCO_3$ may be used intravenously to start the correction of the sodium deficit.

CLINICAL GROUP 4-a
EXCESS SODIUM AND EXCESS WATER

Etiologic Factors

This group of electrolyte and water imbalances is now encountered relatively rarely in surgical patients. The predominant cause of this group of disorders is the administration of solutions of sodium salts in any quantity larger than that lost renally, cutaneously (sweat) and enterally.

Peculiarly, the rate of renal excretion of sodium salts is directly proportional to the body load, with the rate of excretion relative to load being not faster than 0.1 of the load (excess above normal) per hour. This ratio is called the velocity quotient. This means that, should a person having the high velocity quotient of excretion of sodium of 0.1 of the load per hour be given isotonic sodium chloride intravenously at the rate of 50 mEq. of sodium per hour for 9 hours, at the end of the 9th hour about 270 mEq. of sodium of the 450 given would still be in the body; and, after the passage of 15 more hours, at least 60 of the 450 would still not have been excreted. Should the same amount of sodium be given the 2nd day at the same rate, at the end of the 2nd 24 hours, about 90 mEq. of the sodium given the previous 2 days would still be in the body. The prolongation of this process for 7 days would effect a significant excess of sodium salts and water in the body. Among persons with velocity quotients of excretion of sodium chloride of about 0.05 of the load per hour—and there are many such among the elderly and the malnourished—generalized edema would be produced by such practices in 4 to 5 days.

This sort of thing is prone to happen whenever the outmoded and ill-conceived practice of alternating a bottle of glucose and a bottle of saline is used for intravenous alimentation preoperatively and postoperatively.

Physical Signs and Symptoms

Pitting edema, puffiness of eyelids and acceleration of enteral drainage, such as gastric and duodenal, and diarrhea are the main signs of moderate excesses of sodium salts and water. Large excesses are occasionally accompanied by all the signs of congestive heart failure.

A swollen edematous gastric wall is peculiar to a combined sodium and water excess. The small intestine does not become edematous with simple sodium and water loads, and the colon relatively little (C.A.M.). A swollen edematous stomach is not a sign of lack of gastric decompression but a sign of too much saline, preoperatively. The unobstructed stomach of any mammal can be rendered massively edematous by the administration of isotonic sodium chloride or Ringer's solution in a few hours.

Laboratory Signs

Hypoproteinemia is characteristic. Most of the acute hypoproteinemias occurring preoperatively and postoperatively are related solely to acute positive loads of sodium salts. The hematocrit also falls, but less rapidly than the concentration of plasma proteins.

The changes in serum sodium concentration are variable. There is no change when 1 mEq. of sodium and 7 ml. of water are gained concomitantly; the serum Na^+ falls when more than 7 ml. of water are gained, while 1 mEq. of Na is gained. The serum sodium rises when less than 7 ml. of water are gained with each mEq. of sodium.

Treatment

Stop giving sodium salts and give glucose in water, in quantity enough to provide a volume equal to the insensible loss of 600 to 1,000 ml. daily plus one half the estimated volume of sweat during hot weather. Occasionally, diuretics are indicated.

ACIDOSIS AND ALKALOSIS

Acidosis and alkalosis often attend fluid and electrolyte imbalances. Acidosis or proton excess (arterial blood pH less than 7.3) has many causes. A pulmonary ventilation inadequate to effect the expulsion of carbon dioxide from the body at the rate it is being formed leads to an increase in the concentration of carbonic acid and, in turn, an excess of hydrogen ions (protons) in body fluids. At the same time, the base bicarbonate concentration in serum rises, because of the shift of bicarbonate out of and chloride into red blood cells. Consequently, the bicarbonate concentration of serum or plasma increases, while the pH decreases. This is called "respiratory acidosis."

Metabolic acidosis is a consequence of the accumulation of anions other than the bicarbonate anion in the body, such as chloride, lactate, pyruvate, dihydrogen phosphate and sulfate. These anions displace the bicarbonate anion, reducing the serum base bicarbonate concentration and decreasing pH. Obviously, metabolic acidosis may be associated with many and varied physiologic aberrations: lactic acid acidosis with hypoxia and shock, chloride acidosis with the ingestion of ammonium and calcium chlorides and with the administration of large quantities of Ringer's solution or of 0.9 per cent NaCl while renal function is inadequate, acetoacetic and beta-hydroxy pyruvic acidosis with starvation and diabetes, and phosphate and sulfate acidosis with renal insufficiency.

If sodium ions and chloride ions are given in equivalent amounts as in 0.9 per cent sodium chloride solution, the effect is to dilute the bicarbonate which probably accounts for Van Slyke's term "dilution acidosis." Normal plasma contains approximately 140 mEq. of sodium but only 100 mEq. of chloride. If physiologic saline solution containing 155 mEq. of each is added, it increases the chloride concentration more than it does the sodium concentration and tends to lower the pH. With normal kidneys the body is able to correct for a considerable excess of chloride by excreting it with NH_3, but, if larger amounts are to be given or if kidney function may be impaired it won't. For this reason sodium bicarbonate or lactate solution should be substituted for one third of the sodium chloride in the repair solution when large quantities of sodium containing solutions are needed. (See Chap. 17, Burns and Cold Injury.)

The symptoms of acidosis per se are few, being only breathlessness with slight exertion, and anorexia. The signs vary with the severity and the nature of the acidosis. As respiratory acidosis (CO_2 retention) deepens and CO_2 tensions rise above 77 mm. Hg, respiration becomes slower and shallower. Hyperpnea rarely is seen. The person shows all of the signs of a deepening general anesthesia progressing from excitement to coma, and finally respiratory arrest. (Carbon dioxide was used by Hickman in 1817 to effect general anesthesia in dogs.) Respiratory acidosis is an occasional cause of failure to recover from general anesthesia and always must be suspected as a cause of respiratory arrest during or after anesthesia, or after the administration of soporifics or narcotics to old, asthmatic, emphysematous or very debilitated persons.

Conversely, metabolic acidosis is associated with a deepening of breathing until the pH of arterial blood falls below 7.0, and then breathing becomes shallower as the pH drops more, and it finally stops when the pH reaches $\cong$ 6.7. With metabolic acidosis, the signs of anesthesia are absent or few, unless the acidosis is attended by large sodium and potassium deficits (diabetic acidosis). The accurate diagnosis of acidosis requires the measurement of CO_2 tension and the pH of arterial blood, together with the serum base bicarbonate and chloride concentrations.

The treatment of acidosis varies with its cause: assisted breathing is the only effective way to treat respiratory acidosis (see Chap. 13, Anesthesia). Chloride acidosis should be treated by stopping the administration of excess chloride and, at times, base bicarbonate 1.25 to 2.5 per cent $NaHCO_3$ may be indicated, the more especially when a chloride acidosis accompanies a sodium deficit, such as that produced by pancreatic fistulous drainage or ileostomy diarrhea. The bases of treatment of diabetic acidosis are glucose and insulin and base bicarbonate and potassium phosphate in addition. Lactacidosis is treated most properly by abolishing anoxia: oxygen for pneumonia, blood for hemorrhage, sodium salts and water for sodium deficit shock, and assisted breathing for anoxic anoxia related to the great muscular weakness of myasthenia gravis, and the like. Occasionally, a proton acceptor, such as T.H.A.M. (Tris [Hydroxymethyl] Aminomethane) may be used. The administration of $NaHCO_3$ is relatively ineffective for treating lactacidosis, as long as the cause of lactic acid accumulation, such as anoxia, continues. It is contraindicated for respiratory acidosis.

Alkalosis is rarely seen in surgical patients today. Respiratory alkalosis attendant upon willful overbreathing is rare. Emotionally unstable patients or patients in an excitement stage as they emerge from anesthesia will occasionally exhibit it. Metabolic alkalosis is caused mainly by the prolonged vomiting of acid gastric juice by a person whose pylorus is obstructed, the ingestion of sodium bicarbonate in large quantity, prolonged gastric drainage, and potassium deficiency.

The signs and the symptoms of alkalosis per se are few and feeble. Muscle cramps and irritability are practically all.

Diagnosis requires the measurement of arterial P-CO$_2$ and pH, and serum base bicarbonate and potassium concentrations.

The treatment of alkalosis again depends on its cause: rebreathing into a bag or breathing 5 per cent CO$_2$ in air for respiratory alkalosis; NaCl 0.9 per cent for the base chloride deficit of profuse acute vomiting; potassium chloride or phosphate for the alkalosis associated with potassium deficit attendant upon prolonged vomiting, diarrhea, large villous adenomata of the large bowel, tumors of the adrenal cortex, and the prolonged and ill-regulated administration of adrenal corticoids; and cessation of the ingestion of sodium carbonate or bicarbonate in cases in which these salts are being taken in excess.

CATION ABNORMALITIES

Hypocalcemia

Circumoral numbness and itching are the first symptoms of hypocalcemia. Later, muscle cramps and carpopedal spasms may be experienced. Trousseau's and Chvostek's signs are manifestations of the muscular and nervous hyperirritability of hypocalcemia.

The predominant causes of hypocalcemia are: parathyroprivia, pancreatitis, large deep burns, and phagedenic infections such as necrotizing fascitis. Lack of mobilization of calcium from bones is the cause of the hypocalcemia of hypoparathyroidism, and very rapid deposition of calcium into the area of injury is the cause in the other conditions.

Administrations of calcium lactate, orally, and calcium gluconate, intravenously, are adequate measures for the treatment of acute hypocalcemia. The treatment of chronic hypocalcemia is more complex. This as well as *hypercalcemia* is discussed in Chapter 28, Thyroid, Thymus and Parathyroids.

Magnesium Deficit

Magnesium deficiency is rare but may attend long-standing diarrheas and alcoholism with delirium tremens. The symptoms are similar to those of hypocalcemia. Magnesium sulfate, intramuscularly, is used to treat it.

Hypopotassemia

Hypopotassemia is characterized by weakness, hyperreflexia with moderate deficits, and absent tendon reflexes with severe deficits. Adynamic ileus and symptomatic psychoses are regularly associated with it. The ECG may show flattening or inversion of T-waves, prolongation of QT intervals, depression of ST segments, and appearance of U-waves. This is commonly attended by an alkalosis, which will, however, respond to the administration of an ammonium chloride solution but the alkalosis will recur until the potassium deficit is at least partially corrected.

Hyperpotassemia

Hyperpotassemia is usually characterized by electrocardiograph changes, including spiking elevation of T-waves, depression of ST segments, and conduction defects. It seldom occurs except in renal failure, and the uremic patient may lapse into coma. When the potassium concentration gets up between 8 and 12 mEq./L., it is likely to produce cardiac arrest with immediate death. This is, at times, the terminal event in uremia.

We will now consider the questions: (1) How does one categorize the fluid and electrolyte status of a sick person who is presented to the surgeon for the first time? (2) How does one approach the treatment of a fluid and electrolyte imbalance? (3) How does one maintain fluid and electrolyte balance during and after an operation?

One cannot approach these problems without a knowledge of water and ion exchanges between the organism and the environment under normal and abnormal circumstances.

EXCHANGES OF WATER, SODIUM, POTASSIUM AND CHLORIDE OCCURRING IN NORMAL MAN BETWEEN THE INDIVIDUAL AND HIS EXTERNAL ENVIRONMENT

An adult man ingests about 1,000 ml. of water in liquid form daily and derives an additional 1,000 ml. from solid foods, partly as water and partly as a result of the oxidation of carbohydrates and fat. Of this amount, only about 200 ml. normally is excreted in the stools.

About 400 to 800 ml. is lost as water vapor from the respiratory passages and the skin, without gross perspiration—the so-called insensible loss. The balance, in this example 1,000 to 1,400 ml., is lost as urine. Clearly, all of these figures are susceptible to marked variation to meet sweating, enforced fluid restriction, etc.

The average sodium chloride intake has been found to be 5 or 6 Gm., providing about 100 mEq. of each of these ions. Loss in the stool is normally small, and excretion is largely in the urine. Loss through skin is dependent upon rate of sweating. The sodium exchange follows a pattern similar to that of chloride. Potassium intake probably varies more widely with the diet but can be thought of as about 20 mEq. per day.

A striking difference between the body's management of sodium and potassium occurs in the kidney. Here, cessation of sodium intake is followed very soon by a marked decrease in excretion so that the sodium store in the body is conserved. However, a cessation in the intake of potassium is not followed quickly by a corresponding decrease in its excretion—the kidney continuing to excrete about 10 mEq. per day for a long period. On the other hand, in the event of an abnormally high intake of potassium, excretion of this ion by the kidneys is very rapid compared with the rate with which an excess of sodium chloride is excreted.

INTERNAL EXCHANGES OF WATER, SODIUM, POTASSIUM AND CHLORIDE IN NORMAL MAN ACROSS THE WALLS OF THE ALIMENTARY TRACT

In this section, we are not considering the rapid molecular exchanges between capillaries and tissues demonstrable by heavy water or isotopes, but are concerned with the major moieties secreted into the alimentary tract which may be lost by fistulae or aspiration through tubes. These moieties are largely reabsorbed so that under normal conditions they do not represent an exchange with the environment. Some authors prefer to regard them as actual body tissues not in the cellular sense

TABLE 5-3. NORMAL RANGE OF ELECTROLYTE CONCENTRATIONS IN ADULT HUMAN PLASMA

ELECTROLYTE	CONCENTRATION (mEq./L. OF PLASMA)
Sodium	134–144
Potassium	3.5–5.3
Chloride	98–105
Calcium	4.5–5.7
	(9–11.4 mg. %)
Inorganic phosphate	2.7–4.4
(as phosphorus)	(4.6–7.6 mg.%)
Total carbon dioxide	23–29
(as bicarbonate)	(51–64 vol. %)

but as functional entities like the extracellular fluid from which these moieties are derived.

To the water ingested is added per 24 hours: as saliva, 500 ml.; as gastric juice, 1,200 ml.; as bile, 600 ml.; as pancreatic juice, 1,200 ml.; as succus entericus, 2,000 ml.* Thus, a total of 8,000 ml. of water or potential water enters the gastrointestinal tract per 24-hour period. This constitutes over 11 per cent of the body weight and over half of the extracellular water. Not all of this is in the gastrointestinal tract at any one time. Rather, there is a constant turnover of much smaller amounts. Absorption of water probably begins in the upper small bowel and assumes some importance in the distal ileum. However, it occurs especially rapidly in the right half of the colon, so that normally only about 200 ml. is excreted from the body in the feces.

Measurements of chloride concentration in gastric and small intestinal juices have averaged about 100 mEq./L. The total daily excretion of hydrochloric acid by the stomach is of the order of 120 mEq. in the normal adult but may be considerably higher in some individuals, especially those with duodenal ulcer. Normally, this is compensated for beyond the pylorus by the alkalinity of the juices entering the alimentary tract. Movement of chloride out of the intestine is said to proceed more rapidly than bicarbonate or sodium but not as rapidly as water.

The concentration of potassium in gastric and intestinal drainage ranges from 4 to 14 mEq./L. The higher levels may be expected in intestinal obstruction and diarrhea. Absorp-

---

* All of these figures are cited as representative approximations for an adult man.

TABLE 5-4. AVERAGE ELECTROLYTE CONTENT OF ORAL AND GASTROINTESTINAL SECRETIONS[5]

SUBJECTS	SECRETION	NA (mEq./L.)	K (mEq./L.)	CA (mEq./L.)	CL (mEq./L.)
Healthy, young adults	Resting saliva	44	20.4	6.5	
Healthy, young adults	Overnight gastric	49	11.6	3.6	
Preoperative patients	Gastric	66.5	13.7		100.6
Resections	Gastric	136	5.3		98
Surgical patients	Small bowel	111.3	4.6		104.2
Surgical patients	Ileostomy (recent)	129.4	11.2		116.2
Surgical patients	Ileostomy (adapted)	46	3.0		21.4
Surgical patients	Bile	148.9	4.98		100.6
Surgical patients	Pancreas	141.1	4.6		76.6

tion is believed to parallel that of sodium and chloride, and the level in the plasma is maintained at 3.5 to 5 mEq./L. Most of the body potassium is within the cells, whereas most of the body sodium and nearly all of the chloride is outside the cells. The principal intracellular anion is phosphate. See Table 5-3 for normal serum electrolyte values and Table 5-4 for representative values for certain other body fluids.

EXAMPLES OF ABNORMAL LOSSES AND INTAKES OF WATER AND ELECTROLYTES IN SURGICAL PATIENTS

WATER

Vomiting is encountered in pyloric obstruction, intestinal obstruction, as a reflex phenomenon after anesthetics, after various drugs, as a response to intracranial lesions, as a psychogenic phenomenon and under innumerable other circumstances. The water losses can easily amount to 2,000 ml. in 24 hours, and often a large residual collection will remain in the stomach which, for practical purposes, is lost to the body.

Diarrhea may lead to extreme losses. The classic example comes not from surgical experience but in cholera where the "rice water" stools may carry off extracellular fluid at rates of from 10 to 40 L. per day. Patients with ulcerative colitis will not infrequently lose from 2 to 8 L. of extracellular fluid in the stools per day. Pseudomembranous enteritis has been observed to produce losses as high as 11 L. in a 24-hour period.[1]

Sweating during a prolonged operation may account for a loss of a liter or more of fluid containing 20 to 80 mEq. of NaCl per liter, but the omission of blankets and other impediments to heat loss, such as hot humid air in the operating rooms, has tended to reduce this loss. Patients with heat exhaustion are sometimes admitted to surgical wards after depletions of 4 to 5 liters of extracellular fluid through sweating. Before the days of air-conditioned operating rooms, the surgeon himself not infrequently lost 2,500 ml. during a long summer operating schedule (as judged by weight changes).

Biliary fistulae and T-tube drainage may account for losses of 1,000 to 1,500 ml. per day.

Pancreatic fistulae usually drain more modest amounts, since they probably do not, as a rule, drain the whole pancreas. Potentially they could cause losses of a liter or more per day.

Salivary fistulae are seldom important as a cause of fluid loss in a patient who can swallow.

Intestinal Fistulae. A direct corollary of the finding that very large amounts of extracellular fluid enter the upper intestinal tract is that huge losses occur if a fistula opens from this area to the outside of the body. In one such case developing after failure of an anastomosis in the jejunum, Walker[19] collected up to 4 L. per day with a 24 hour loss by all routes of over 40 per cent of the total chloride ion calculated to be in the extracellular space. Prior to the development of suitable methods for replacement therapy, such cases were invariably fatal.

Lower in the intestinal tract, however, the body may tolerate fistulae quite well. Thus, colostomy and ileostomy are established surgical procedures, and the patients do well, although some of those with ileostomy require a period of adjustment during which intravenous replacement therapy is essential. Partial obstruction of an ileostomy stoma is especially dangerous, because of the profuse ileostomy drainage that attends it. As much as 11 liters of extracellular fluid has been lost because of this in a single day!

Suction Drainage of the Alimentary Tract. This method, introduced by Wangensteen and Paine in 1933,[20] has been of inestimable value in surgery in preventing distention and many of its consequences. However, it does constitute a fistula, and occasionally as much as 5,000 ml. will drain out of the body within 24 hours. If appropriate replacement therapy is not provided, the method is capable of doing more harm than good.

Hemorrhage, whether operative or due to gastrointestinal ulceration, results in a reduction of the water and sodium salt contents of the body. Losses of blood into the gastrointestinal tract through bleeding esophageal varices and gastric and duodenal ulcers often exceed 1,500 ml. in 24 hours.

Injury. The adsorbtion of water and ions by physically, thermally, or chemically injured tissues and consequent edematous swelling of injured tissue constitute one of the commonest and most important abnormal losses of water and *extracellular* ions among surgical patients. With fractures of the pelvis or femora as much of 4 to 6 liters of extracellular fluid is removed from the uninjured parts of the body and sequestered in the injured parts, thereby dehydrating the body core and effecting within it all of the physiologic derangements that attend the same losses of extracellular fluid through diarrhea, vomiting, or fistulae (external losses). The same phenomenon occurs in the adsorption of water and ions into the tissues about an incision, into the walls of bowel bathed in the spill from a ruptured duodenal ulcer, into burned skin, and into regions in and about an infection. With a deep burn covering a square meter of body surface the *loss* of extracellular fluid into the injured skin amounts to 6 to 14 liters within 12 hours after the injury.

IRRIGATING FLUIDS AND ION LOSS

The use of hypotonic or saltless irrigating fluids through tubes extending into the body can produce notable ion losses. When water is used for this purpose, a loss of ions always results. Thus, multiple water enemas may produce hypochloremia, hyponatremia and symptoms of water intoxication.

Likewise, the irrigation of tubes used for suction from the stomach and the small intestine with water carries away the ions found in these organs. In fact, repeated irrigation of the stomach with 200 ml. of tap water every 20 minutes is a very effective method of reducing a hyperchloremia and has been used for this purpose. Unfortunately, the concentration of chloride ion in the water after a 20-minute stay in the stomach is quite variable from one individual to another, so that fairly frequent measurements of the effects are necessary.

Sodium chloride, 0.9 per cent, or better yet a balanced solution such as that recommended by Hartmann,[9] should be used for irrigation of suction tubes, and water and ice should not be permitted by mouth in patients on Wangensteen suction, unless special provision is made to compensate for the ion losses.

Temporary ion losses into subcutaneous infusions of 5 per cent dextrose or other nonelectrolyte in water may in the debilitated and malnourished lead to shock and even death. For this reason solutions of nonelectrolytes should not be given subcutaneously and the more especially to infants.

Selective ion losses can be brought about by the ingestion of ion exchange resins if the alimentary tract is functioning.

METHODS FOR SUSPECTING AND QUANTITATING THE DEFICITS OR THE SURPLUSES OF WATER, AND ABNORMALITIES OF CONCENTRATION OF SODIUM, CHLORIDE AND POTASSIUM IONS

The diagnosis of fluid balance disturbances is based on history and physical examination; quantitation usually requires laboratory methods. Without suspicion based on history and a general knowledge of the nature of fluid exchanges and routes of loss, as well as the physical examination, the laboratory tests may not be done.

Another good rule to follow in fluid therapy is: if a patient is alive with his total deficit, he should be out of immediate danger when it is half corrected and probably when it is only one third corrected.

Therefore, it is seldom essential to know exactly the water deficit, but it is essential to know that the patient is suffering from a shortage rather than an excess of body fluid and to have some general idea of the magnitude of the probable change. Furthermore, if one is going to replace water, it is extremely important to know whether chloride (or sodium) concentration is low or normal. If it is already low or normal, the administration of water (5 or 10% glucose in water) without simultaneous salt administration is dangerous in the patient in shock.

The problem of detecting abnormalities of ionic concentration is simply solved today with the modern instrumentation and automated chemical analytic technics that are available in large hospitals and will be available soon even in hospitals of 50 to 75 beds. The admission blood work on every incoming sick surgical patient should include the determination of the serum concentrations of sodium, potassium, bicarbonate and chloride and, additionally, in the very sick, and especially in cases of coma and shock, a blood urea nitrogen, a blood sugar and an arterial blood pH. If the blood sample is drawn in the emergency room or admitting office, the laboratory reports can be available within the hour.

The detecting and quantitating of abnormalities of volume of water and quantities of the rapidly exchangeable or functional masses of the ionic constituents of the body is much more difficult.

Actually, the quantitation of the functional volumes of water and quantities of ions in a sick person is still essentially impossible, except in a very few institutions with special computerized laboratory facilities capable of solving the complex differential equations necessary for the calculation of the functional quantities of water and ions from the slopes of the disappearance curves of specific trace materials introduced into the blood stream. Until such capability has become widespread, detection of the variance, and ascertainment of the magnitude of such variance from the normal in functional water and ion quantities in a given case must be approached on clinical bases.

As illustrated earlier in this chapter, the physiologic effects of sodium depletion—namely, hypometabolism, oligemia, hyperproteinemia, polycythemia, renal insufficiency and, ultimately, shock—may attend water, sodium, chloride and HCO_3 ionic depletions in which no change in the concentrations of Na^+, Cl^- and HCO_3^- occurs. This signifies that the numbers of water molecules and ions per unit of cell surface or mass are important determinants of cell function even though there is *no* change of the concentrations of water or ions in the extracellular environment.

To be sure, the measurement of the volumes of distribution of deuterium or tritium is now relatively simple with mass spectrometric and radioisotopic technics, and, seemingly, the determination of the quantity of water in a given patient is not beyond the capabilities of many hospital laboratories. The same can be said for the determination of the volumes of distribution of inulin, thiocyanate, sulfate and radioactive sodium, which constitutes approximations of the actual volumes of distribution of sodium and chloride in the body. These data, together with the simultaneous determination of Na^+, Cl^- and HCO_3^- concentrations in plasma, constitute bases for the calculation of the total quantities of these ions in the ground substance (extracellular space). Often, however, the *biologically functional quantities of water and ions in the ground substance of the body core cannot be ascertained* by these methods. Take, for example, the badly contused patients with fractures of the pelvis and femora and in shock: in him the measured volumes of distribution of water, sodium and chloride will be normal—*but the water, the sodium, the chloride, the calcium and magnesium in the edematous, swollen pelvic structures and thighs have been removed from the uninjured parts, and the extracellular space of the uninjured core tissues is deficient in water and extracellular ion numbers.* That is to say, biologically the functional masses of water and extracellular ions of the body core are in deficit while the total or gross mass of

Methods for Suspecting and Quantitating Deficits or Surpluses

water and ions in the body is normal. They are maldistributed because of the injury.

The same situation often exists in the patient with acute ascites, ileus, acute thrombophlebitis with rapid massive swelling of the legs, burns, or peritonitis, and in the elderly edematous cardiac or hypertensive treated vigorously with powerful modern diuretics.

In brief: although the measurement of the volumes of distribution of appropriate materials can provide data permitting the assessment of the actual quantities of water and ions in the normal body, it cannot provide the bases for the ascertainment of their biologically active moieties in a given surgical case. The data can be valuable but the user of them must have a broad knowledge of fluid balance and much clinical experience to employ them meaningfully and safely.

How is one to ascertain the functional volume of water and masses of extracellular ions in a given case? First, the history is important: (1) Has there been external loss of water and salt through diarrhea, vomiting, sweating, the rapid and open decompression of a chronically obstructed ureter or bladder, the prolonged administration of chorthiazides or other powerful diuretics or fistulous drainage? (2) Has there been translocation of extracellular fluid into the intestine from mechanical or adynamic ileus, into various body cavities or tissues from contusional, thermal, chemical or bacterial injury and obstruction of great veins or arteries, or translocation into the skin from allergens, manifested by giant hives and generalized cutaneous vesicular or bullous dermatitis?

If there is a history of external loss or translocation of extracellular components and sodium salts have not been given or taken, one can be practically sure that biologically functional deficits of extracellular ions do exist and a biologically functional deficit of water likely exists.

If the concentration of sodium in the serum is normal or high in such cases, water volume deficit certainly coexists with the mass ion deficits; if hyponatremia coexists, the functional water volume rarely may be normal or even supernormal instead of deficient.

The physical examination also is important. Functional deficits of sodium salts of 2.5 to 4.0 mEq. per kilo of body weight in man are attended by weakness, apathy and urine flows usually of less than 40 ml. per hr. Deficits of 4.0 to 8 mEq. per kilo are associated with decreasing pulse pressures, orthostatic hypotension, great weakness and urine flows of 10 to 20 ml. per hour and, occasionally, tachycardia and shock. Deficits greater than 8 mEq. per kilo are universally attended by recumbent hypotension, severe oliguria (10 ml. or less) or anuria, total physical incapacity, distant heart sounds and soft pulse (all put together —shock).

With slowly developed sodium or extracellular fluid volume deficits, skin turgor is decreased, eyeballs sink in their sockets and muscle plasticity replaces muscle turgor. These signs are often absent with rapidly developed life-endangering translocational deficits of extracellular fluid following burns, ruptured peptic ulcers, acute fulminant thrombophlebitis, massive fractures and the like.

The physical signs of acidosis, alkalosis, potassium and calcium deficits have been treated earlier in this chapter.

Clearly the ultimate test of a suspicion of fluid imbalance is a test of therapy appropriate to the ionic concentrational status of the individual—a bioassay, so to speak.

The following cases illustrate this.

Case 1. Male, age 75, weight 50 kilos with a history of vomiting for 5 days. He is found in bed stuporous. Examination: Patient is semicomatose, eyeballs are sunken and soft, blood pressure is 80/20, pulse is 100 per minute, heart sounds are distant. Laboratory data available 45 minutes after admission are: serum Na 130, K 4.2, Cl 84, HCO_3 34 mEq./L., BUN 100 mg.%. Diagnosis: Water deficit with sodium and chloride deficits and slight base bicarbonate excess. Treatment: Initial, 0.9 per cent NaCl or Ringer's solution with 0.25 M dextrose/liter.

Estimate of Na deficit: 4 to 8 mEq./kilo (stupor, tachycardia, hypotension) or 50 × 4 = 8 = 200 to 400 mEq. Na deficit = 1.5 to 3 liters of 0.9 per cent NaCl or mEq. Ringer's solution.

After giving 1.5 to 2 liters the serum analyses are repeated: the data are Na 134, K 3.6, HCO_3 32. Blood pressure is 130/80, the pulse is 84, and the patient is fully conscious and feels well lying down. He has passed 100 ml. of urine in 3 hours, but on elevating the head of the bed to 45° he becomes dizzy, the pulse rises to 94, and blood pressure falls to 90/60.

Diagnosis now is: Residual sodium salt and water deficits and in addition K^+ deficit with residual base bicarbonate excess.

Treatment now: 0.9 per cent NaCl or Ringer's solution with 40 mEq. KCl per mEq. liter. Amount given during next 6 to 10 hours: 1.5 to 2 liters, after which serum Na is 136, K is 4.0, HCO_3 is 30, blood pressure is 130/86, pulse is 74, the patient can stand and walk unaided and he says that he feels well.

Problem now is maintenance of fluid balance.

Case 2. Male, age 83, weight 80 kilos. History: Unable to move his bowels for 2 days; lower abdominal pain; no vomiting. The abdomen is distended and peristalsis is absent. B.P. is 100/20, pulse is 90, serum Na is 144, K is 5.4, Cl is 108, HCO_3 is 26 mEq./L. BUN is 30 mg.%.

Diagnosis: Water and sodium deficits with normal ion concentrations.

Again the estimated Na deficit is 4 to 8 mEq./kilo or 320 to 640 mEq., approximately the amounts contained in 2.5 to 5 liters of Ringer's with lactate or acetate containing 130 mEq. Na^+ per liter.

Initial treatment: Lactated Ringer's solution 1.0 to 1.5 liters rapidly. Patient is now awake, pulse is 90, blood pressure is 110/70. X-ray films taken at this time show liquid filled loops of colon from 14 to 20 cm. in diameter filling the whole of the abdomen.

Sigmoidoscopy was performed in the left lateral Sims's position; sigmoid volvulus was discovered and decompressed of 6 liters of liquid feces. Estimate now of total water and salt needs: 3 to 4 more liters of lactated Ringer's solution given more slowly, in toto, 4 to 5.5 liters being given.

The method of approaching the therapy of translocational deficits of sodium salts and water is illustrated in Chapter 17, Burns and Cold Injury. No meaningful approximation of the need for salt and water in any case of translocational water and salt deficit can be completed for 12 to 24 hours after injury while the injured tissues still take up a great part of the salts and water given parenterally. The aim is: keep the injured individual alive and secreting urine at rates of 20 to 50 ml. an hour *without* significantly increasing central venous pressure.

In any case of dehydrational shock requiring the rapid parenteral administration of fluids the venous pressure proximal to the zone of injury needs to be measured every quarter hour in order not to induce plethoric circulatory overload. An indwelling catheter is also needed for repeated measurement of the rate of urine flow. The rate of administering repair solutions to the severely injured should be such as to provide urine flows of 25 to 50 ml. per hour and normal venous pressures. Other valuable rules are:

(1) After one has considerable assurance that the patient is well out of danger of death from dehydration or ion deficits, it is wise to approach full repletion slowly, the more especially if he has become adjusted to his deficiencies through a long illness.

(2) If urinary output is above 20 ml. per hour and increases substantially with the infusion, mild aberrations in the carbon dioxide combining power may be neglected, as the normal kidneys will make the correction if they have ample water, sodium and chloride to excrete. On the other hand, if the base bicarbonate is very low, say 10 mEq./L., some sodium should be given without equivalent chloride. This is usually provided as 1.25 to 2.5 per cent sodium bicarbonate or M/6 sodium lactate solution (166 mEq./L.).

In a case of metabolic acidosis with an arterial pH of 7.2 and a bicarbonate of 14 mEq./L., about one liter of 1.25 per cent sodium bicarbonate will be needed. Here again, administration of one half the amount is prudent, and subsequent administration should be based on repeat bicarbonate and blood pH determinations.

(3) In patients with vomiting or in those who have lost large amounts of gastric juice by suction drainage, the carbon dioxide combining power may be high, say 38 mEq./L. Unless signs of tetany or impending tetany are present (Chvostek or Trousseau signs), it is probably best to see if the carbon dioxide level will return toward normal after the salt and water deficits are restored. If it does not, the plasma potassium concentration should be investigated and, if low, potassium administration should be started (see below). In rare cases alkalosis persists after restoration of

sodium, chloride and potassium concentrations and total amounts to normal. In these cases, ammonium chloride may be given intravenously, as suggested by Zintel and his associates,[21] if one is certain that the elevation of carbon dioxide is not due to respiratory acidosis. Arterial pH must be determined before administering ammonium chloride, especially in aged people.

Surpluses of water, sodium and chloride usually have been dealt with by withholding the material or materials present in excess. Water and sodium loss often has been accelerated by the administration of one of the mercurial diuretics, such as Mercuhydrin* (adult dose, 1 ml. ampule containing 39 mg. of organically combined mercury and 48 mg. of theophylline), which has the property of inhibiting reabsorption of water and sodium by the kidney tubules.

Another method is to induce sweating by external heat—a method occasionally used by jockeys and athletes to meet maximum weight criteria.

Another method is to introduce hypertonic solutions into the duodenum, preferably between 2 occluding balloons (using a 3-lumen tube). This induces a prompt outpouring of digestive juices which may be aspirated and replaced by more hypertonic glucose. While the effectiveness of the method has been demonstrated experimentally, it has not been applied generally in practice. Still another possible method is the induction of diarrhea with cathartics.

It is obvious that these methods remove ions as well as water, so that if any of them is used, the ionic loss must be taken into consideration.

Hyperchloremia and hypernatremia can be considered together. They rarely occur in conscious persons if the kidneys are normal and are not under the influence of excess adrenal steroids and then only in response to overdoses of salt. When a severe hypernatremia (160 mEq./L.) and hyperchloremia (> 115 mEq./L.) are discovered, they can be corrected by gastric lavage, 200 ml. of tap water being instilled through a tube and left in the stomach 20 minutes, then aspirated and replaced with another 200 ml. and so forth. The rate of chloride withdrawal is inconstant but probably can be as rapid as 50 mEq. per hour, so that it is well to recheck the chloride level after 4 hours of treatment. Colonic irrigations with water are effective. However, before these methods are used one must be sure that sodium deficit does not coexist. If it does, the proper treatment is glucose in water 5 per cent intravenously, and not gastric or colonic lavage with water.

Potassium. Because most of the body potassium is intracellular, one cannot calculate probable deficits of potassium as for the extracellular electrolytes. If plasma potassium concentrations are normal, only maintenance doses of potassium salts are given. If plasma potassium is reduced, 50 mEq. of potassium in excess of maintenance requirements may be given daily in 5 or 10 per cent glucose intravenously or as a 5 per cent solution orally until the potassium level is restored to normal.

In the administration of potassium it must be recalled that small absolute increments in potassium from 4 to 8 or 10 mEq./L. threaten death by cardiac standstill. Therefore, hypertonic solutions should not be used, administration should be slow (not over 20 mEq./hour), and one should have established a satisfactory urine output (at least 30 ml./hour) before its administration.

In the anuric patient, potassium is usually high, and in uremia it may rise to 6, 8, or 10 mEq., producing electrocardiographic changes and eventually cardiac standstill (Fig. 5-4 C). Under such circumstances one can remove potassium by in-vivo dialysis (artificial kidney), provided that the solution against which it is dialyzed contains little or no potassium. It can be removed by the ingestion of suitable ion exchange resins prepared so as to take up potassium. Furthermore, the rate of release of intracellular potassium in the body can be reduced by feeding protein-sparing foods, such as carbohydrate and fat, to minimize the breakdown of body proteins for nutritional purposes.

MAINTENANCE OF WATER AND ELECTROLYTE EQUILIBRIUM

The maintenance of water and electrolyte equilibrium is somewhat easier than the correction of existing abnormalities but sometimes requires more attention because it covers a

---

* Sodium salt of meralluride with theophylline.

96 Fluid and Electrolytes

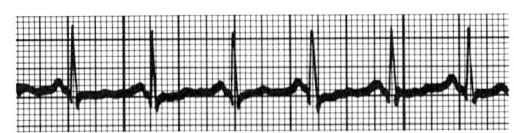

FIG. 5-4, A. Lead II—Normal.

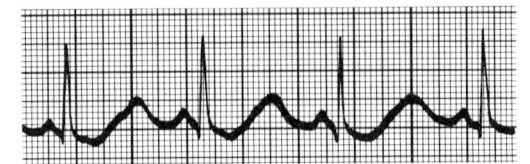

FIG. 5-4, B. Lead II—Hypokalemia. A.B. K+ = 2.7 mEq./L. Note: Depression of ST segment, widening of QT interval, T-wave not lowered in this example, and U-wave superimposed on T-wave.

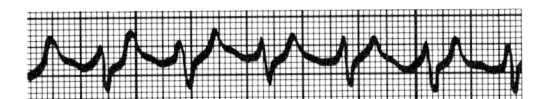

FIG. 5-4, C. Lead II—Hyperkalemia. R.S. Before dialysis K = 7.5 mEq./L. Note: Widened QRS complex, absence of P-waves, peaked T-waves, and depressed ST segments.

longer time period. One can keep a record of intake by mouth, by vein and by any other route which may be employed and a simultaneous record of the output of urine, vomitus, gastrointestinal drainage, etc. Such a record includes volume and description of whatever is given as 1,000 ml. of 5 per cent glucose or 600 ml. of M/6 sodium lactate solution. The output record states the volume of the urine, the vomitus, etc., in ml. and also should state the volume of the stool if it is liquid.

Furthermore, the patient can be weighed on admission and serially thereafter. A litter type scale is needed for bed patients. Short-term changes in weight are largely due to water that has entered or left the body. Thus, if the 2nd or the 3rd determinations of chloride, carbon dioxide and potassium reveal levels within the normal range and the urine volume is up to 1,000 ml. per day, usually the patient may be carried for 48 to 72 hours by calculating his requirements on the following assumptions:

1. That insensible loss of water will amount to 600 ml. per day plus an additional 1,000 ml. if the environmental temperature is above 90° F. or there is fever of 2 to 4 degrees Fahrenheit or 39° C. and over.

2. That a urine volume of 1,000 to 1,500 ml. will be adequate.

3. That, barring abnormal external, and dislocational losses, 60 mEq. of sodium, 50 of chloride and 12 to 15 of lactate or ½ liter of Ringer's with lactate will cover urinary excretion of these ions (5 Gm. of sodium chloride or 3.5 Gm. of sodium chloride and 1.5 Gm. of sodium bicarbonate).

4. That 20 mEq. of potassium added to the dextrose in water will cover the urinary excretion of potassium (1.5 Gm. of potassium chloride).

5. That vomitus and gastrointestinal drainage will have an average content of about 120 mEq. of sodium and 100 mEq. of chloride and not more than 10 mEq. of potassium per liter.

The daily maintenance dose is then calculated as follows: To the measured abnormal losses of water for the preceding 24 hours (vomitus, diarrhea, gastrointestinal suction drainage) is added 2,500 ml. to determine the amount of water to be administered. For every liter of abnormal loss from the gastrointestinal tract 140 mEq. of sodium, 100 mEq. of chloride and 20 to 30 mEq. of lactate or bicarbonate should be given. If we assume abnormal losses of 500 ml., the patient will need 2,100 to 2,600 ml. containing 120 mEq. of sodium, 100 of chloride and 20 of lactate or acetate or bicarbonate. One liter of lactated Ringer's solution will provide these ion requirements. An additional 1,000 ml. of dextrose (5 or 10%) to which has been added 20 mEq. of potassium chloride usually will complete the potassium and water needs.

Whatever system is used, the important point is that it should be flexible so that one is not obliged to give chloride instead of bicarbonate or lactate in order to administer a given quantity of sodium and that one can vary the potassium intake independently of either sodium or chloride. It is better to give potassium in solutions of glucose whenever it is feasible to do so.

If one has available 0.85 per cent sodium chloride (approximately 150 mEq./L.) and 5 per cent glucose, M/6 sodium lactate (166 mEq./L.) and 1.2 per cent potassium chloride (approximately 150 mEq./L.) and 5 per cent glucose in water, it becomes a typical problem in arithmetic to calculate how many milliliters of each must be used to provide, say—

    3,000 cc. water
    100 mEq. sodium
    22 mEq. potassium
    92 mEq. chloride
    30 mM. lactate

Answer: approximately
    200 ml. M/6 sodium lactate
    500 ml. 0.85% sodium chloride
    150 ml. 1.2% potassium chloride
    2,150 ml. 5% glucose in water

Today the maintenance of fluid balance is readily effected with commercial solutions such as Ringer's with lactate or acetate, 5 and 10 per cent dextrose in distilled water, and ampules of potassium chloride or phosphate containing 20 and 40 mEq. that can be readily added to the glucose solutions. At least every 10 liters of total water exchange it is wise to repeat the determinations of sodium, chloride, carbon dioxide and potassium in the plasma. In the average patient this is every 72 hours, but in one with large abnormal losses it will be at least every 24 hours. When the abnormal losses have stopped, and the patient has resumed normal water and food intake, the chemical determinations can be omitted, but it is still wise to chart the intake and the output until one is sure that the patient can maintain himself.

THE PATIENT WITH HYPOSTHENURIA

Especially in patients with hypertension, chronic obstructive uropathy and arteriosclerosis, the kidneys frequently lose their capacity to concentrate urine. When specific gravity becomes fixed at 1.010, 3 times as large a urine volume is required to remove a given quantity of solute as when the specific gravity is 1.030. Therefore, such patients require a larger urine output than the normal patient—possibly 2,000 ml. or more.

Recognition of this fact makes it possible to effect the improvement of many patients who appear, on the basis of rising urea levels in the blood, to be going into uremia. Formerly, many such patients were given up.

So long as the urine volume will respond to increases in water intake, there is hope that they can be salvaged. Usually additional quantities of 5 per cent glucose or 10 per cent glucose are most effective, and only basal requirements for sodium salts are necessary. Sodium, chloride, bicarbonate and especially potassium levels should be watched carefully in such patients, and the intake of these ions should be adjusted promptly to assist the impaired kidneys in maintaining homeostasis. Fluid intakes for such patients may be pushed up to 4,000 to 5,000 ml. unless pulmonary edema develops or edematous retention occurs.

Basal rales per se are not interpreted as pulmonary edema. If one does precipitate pulmonary edema, all intravenous therapy must be stopped, and an immediate venesection should be carried out with removal of 250 to 1,000 ml. of blood.

THE PATIENT WITH SALT-LOSING KIDNEYS

A small group of patients, especially after the release of a chronic partial obstruction of the ureter or bladder or both, have diminished tubular resorption of sodium and chloride ions. They tend to develop hypochloremia and hyponatremia and will require larger than average amounts of sodium chloride, especially if the urine volume is high. The response in some of these patients is better if hypertonic solutions are given (e.g., 2% or 3% sodium chloride solution).

THE PATIENT WITH THE LOWER NEPHRON SYNDROME

Whether precipitated by transfusion reaction, crush, chemical poisons ($HgCl_2$, uranium salts) or other trauma, the pathologic features of this syndrome are similar. There is extensive degeneration and sloughing of tubular epithelium. This is followed after 10 to 14 days by regeneration if the patient survives. Anuria or severe oliguria is the rule during the early part of his course. If urine formation is resumed, as it is when the tubular epithelium regenerates, the urine volume increases gradually to normal amounts and then increases further so that a marked diuresis may occur. The newly regenerated organ for a time has little power of salt retention and is, for the time being, a salt-losing kidney. Therefore, the diuresis may result in serious depletion of body sodium and chloride, and a number of patients have died because of inadequate replacement at this time.

During the period of anuria, water intake should be restricted to 700 to 1,000 ml. per day, preferably by mouth. No electrolytes should be given unless there are large external losses through diarrhea, vomiting, or enteral tube drainage, and especially no potassium. Body proteins should be spared by a liberal intake of fat and carbohydrate (butter and sugar on bread or crackers). It is preferable to give no protein or protein derivatives.

The blood urea nitrogen and creatinine and potassium concentrations should be determined at frequent intervals, usually once a day, and if the potassium level rises to 6 mEq./L. or above, electrocardiographic tracings should be made at still more frequent intervals. If characteristic changes develop (Fig. 5-4 C), strenuous efforts should be made to remove potassium. If an artificial kidney is not available, peritoneal dialysis may be used or an ion exchange resin with avidity for potassium may be given by mouth, provided that the alimentary tract is functioning.

One of the wisest young surgeons the author has known was the one who transferred his anuric patient on the 3rd day of her anuria to an institution where an effective artificial kidney was available, rather than waiting until it was clear that dialysis would be necessary. If one waits until it is clear that the patient cannot recover without this aid, frequently it is too late.

THE DIABETIC PATIENT UNDERGOING SURGICAL PROCEDURES

Infection and inflammation have long been known to make diabetes mellitus more severe. Therefore, it is not surprising that diabetic patients undergoing operation often have an increase in their insulin requirement if they remain on their usual diets. However, when food intake is interrupted, they may go into insulin shock. When insufficient insulin and carbohydrate are provided, acetone, diacetic acid and β-oxybutyric acid are formed and excreted in the urine with basic ions, principally sodium. This reduces the carbon dioxide combining power and tends to lower the pH of the blood. As has been stated already, this may require sodium lactate or bicarbonate as well as sodium chloride for correction.

At the time of operation and during the early postoperative period, it is rarely possible to regulate the diabetic surgical patient accurately (e.g., to keep his fasting blood sugar between 80 and 140 mg./100 ml. and his urine free of acetone bodies). The attempt usually fails in its objectives and is often attended by bouts of insulin shock. It is far wiser to avoid insulin shock and to avoid ketosis and its attendant losses of basic ions and temporarily to abandon the third objective of keeping the blood sugar below 150. If one resolves to permit the blood sugar to remain in a high range, it is not difficult to achieve the other two objectives. About 1.5 Gm. of glucose is usually needed to cover one unit of insulin. The author gives 2 Gm. of glucose with each unit of insulin. Only regular insulin is used, and the insulin is actually added to each flask of glucose solution when patients are receiving parenteral solutions. Rarely a patient may require more glucose than 2 Gm. per unit of insulin.

The amounts of glucose and insulin must be increased sufficiently to prevent ketosis, as shown by testing the urine for acetone and diacetic acid. A check, daily at first, is also kept on the carbon dioxide combining power of the plasma in case of losses of base with β-oxybutyric acid which is not usually analyzed in the urine.

If such infusions of glucose and insulin are given rapidly, it has been stated that the insulin effect has outlasted the glucose, with resultant insulin shock. At slow rates of infusion, this has not been a problem, but if it ever should arise, additional glucose without insulin should be given.

THE RELATIONS OF RESPIRATION TO ACID-BASE BALANCE

One of the factors affecting acid-base equilibrium in the body is carbon dioxide which dissolves in water to form carbonic acid (H_2CO_3). This is in equilibrium in the body with base, chiefly sodium with which it forms (reversibly) sodium bicarbonate ($NaHCO_3$).

Carbon dioxide is being formed constantly in the body by oxidation of foodstuffs and is being excreted constantly as carbon dioxide in expired air.

Anything that slows this process of excretion, be it respiratory obstruction, emphysema, pulmonary fibrosis (silicosis, pulmonary hypertension), or depressed respiratory reflexes, as during anesthesia or heavy narcosis, leads to an accumulation of carbon dioxide in the blood and plasma. This lowers the blood pH and increases the carbonic acid level in the body more rapidly than the base bicarbonate level rises.

As most laboratories determine plasma carbon dioxide without equilibration, one has the confusing situation that an elevated carbon dioxide content may be due to retarded respiratory excretion of carbon dioxide resulting in respiratory acidosis or it may mean that there is a relative excess of base bicarbonate in the plasma—a situation which represents an alkalosis (metabolic alkalosis).

Respiratory acidosis and metabolic acidosis are readily distinguished today. All that is needed is a blood pH, the bicarbonate ion concentration in plasma and the tension of carbon dioxide in the alveolar air or arterial blood.

Clinically, however, if the respiratory tract is organically normal and if respiratory function is normal, there is little chance of serious variance between carbon dioxide and carbon dioxide combining power. A high level signifies metabolic alkalosis and a low one metabolic acidosis.

Through a series of mechanisms, the body tends to use respiration to help regulate the blood pH when metabolic changes disturb it. Thus, in metabolic acidosis with blood pHs between 7.3 and 6.8 or 6.9, respirations are deep (Kussmaul breathing), which tends to blow carbon dioxide off and raise the pH. Conversely, in metabolic alkalosis, respirations tend to be shallow which results in carbon dioxide retention and lowering of the high pH.

THE COMATOSE PATIENT

It will be noted that the end stage of several of the electrolyte imbalances is coma. If the patient is comatose when first seen, how does one decide whether or not this is due to electrolyte imbalance? The respirations may be deep and frequent, pointing to acidosis. The patient may have a positive Chvostek's sign, muscular twitchings or irritability, suggesting alkalosis. The breath may smell of ketone bodies, suggesting diabetic acidosis.

The possible role of metabolic aberrations in the causation of the coma can be assessed chemically by carrying out the following determinations on plasma:

Urea nitrogen
Carbon dioxide combining power
Chloride
Sodium
Potassium
Sugar

If there is any likelihood that abnormal respiration is a primary etiologic factor and not compensatory, a blood pH is important.

If coma is associated with metabolic acidosis, the carbon dioxide combining power will be low, as in diabetic acidosis. If it is due to respiratory acidosis, the carbon dioxide combining power will be high (see below). If the coma is due to uremia, the urea nitrogen usually will be above 100 mg. per 100 ml.

If the primary abnormality is a potassium deficiency, the potassium concentration usually will be low. The authors have not seen real coma from hypopotassemia alone, but deep stupor does occur. Likewise, they have not seen unconsciousness in respiratory alkalosis (blowing off CO_2 by hyperventilation) unless important metabolic changes are also present.

A low blood pH with a normal or elevated HCO_3^- signifies respiratory acidosis, and a high blood pH with a normal or low HCO_3^- signifies respiratory alkalosis.

Respiratory acidosis is a common cause of coma among elderly asthmatics and persons with incapacitating emphysema, especially when they are given morphine, meperidine or large doses of barbiturates—drugs that reduce the respiratory center's sensitivity to carbon dioxide, permitting carbon dioxide tensions to build up in the body above 77 mm. Hg tension, at which level CO_2 becomes anesthetic.

REFERENCES

1. Allen, J. G.: Personal communication.
2. Bennhold, H., Peters, H., and Roth, E.: Ueber einen Fall von kompletter Analbuminaemie

ohne wesentliche klinische Krankheitszeichen. Verh. Deutsch. Ges. Inn. Med. 60:630, 1954.
3. Cizek, L. J., Semple, R. E., Huang, K. C., and Gregersen, M. I.: Effect of extracellular electrolyte depletion on water intake in dogs. Am. J. Physiol., 164:415, 1951.
4. Coller, F. A., and Maddock, W. G.: Study of dehydration in humans. Ann. Surg., 102:947-960, 1935.
5. Dillon, J., and Butcher, H. R., Jr.: Treatment of Hemorrhagic Shock (Wiggers Type) with Blood Alone, Buffered Saline Alone, and Buffered Saline Followed by Blood. (Unpublished—Presented at the National Academy of Sciences, National Research Council, Symposium on the Use of Buffered Saline Solutions in the Management of Hemorrhagic Hypovolemia, May 2, 1964, Washington, D. C.).
6. Eisenberg, S.: Postural changes in plasma volume in hypoalbuminemia. Arch. Int. Med., 112:544, 1963.
7. Gore, M. B., and McIlwain, H.: Effects of some inorganic salts on the metabolic response of sections of mammalian cerebral cortex to electrical stimulation. J. Physiol., 117:471, 1952.
8. Grayson, T. L., White, J. E., and Moyer, C. A.: Oxygen consumptions; concentrations of inorganic ions in urine, serum and duodenal fluid, hematocrits, urinary excretions; pulse rates and blood pressure during duodenal depletions of sodium salts in normal and alcoholic man. Ann. Surg., 158:840, 1963.
9. Hartmann, A. F., Perley, A. M., Basman, J., Nelson, M. F., and Asher, C.: Further observations on metabolism and clinical uses of sodium lactate. J. Pediat., 13:696-723, 1938.
10. Latta, Thomas: Documents communicated by the Central Board of Health, London, relative to the treatment of cholera by the copious injection of aqueous and saline fluids into the veins. The Lancet, No. 2, 1832.
11. Moore, F. D.: Determination of total body water and solids with isotopes. Science, 104:157, 1936.
12. Moyer, C. A., and Butcher, H. R.: Burns, shock and plasma volume regulation. C. V. Mosby, St. Louis, 1967.
13. Moyer, C. A., Coller, F. A., Bryant, L., Iob, V., Vaughan, H., Kalder, N. B., and Berry, R. E. L.: Some effects of an operation, anesthesia and composition of parenteral fluids upon the excretion of water and salt. Southern Surg., 15:218, 1949.
14. O'Shaughnessy, W. B.: Experiments on the blood in cholera. London, Lancet, Vol. 1, 1832.
15. Richter, C. P.: Increased salt appetite in adrenalectomized rats. Am. J. Physiol., 115:155-161, 1936.
16. Richter, C. P., and Eckert, J. F.: Increased calcium appetite of parathyroidectomized rats. Endocrinology, 21:50-54, 1937.
17. Takagi, G., and Tsukada, Y.: Sodium ions and tissue metabolism, some metabolic peculiarities of brain tissues. Nature, 180:707, 1957.
18. Tappeiner, von H.: Ueber Veranderungen des Blutes und der Muskelin nach ausgedehnten Hautverbrennungen, Centralbl. med. Wiss. 31:385, 1881.
19. Walker, J., Jr.: Fluid and electrolyte replacement for the surgical patient. S. Clin. N. Am., 29:1849-1858, 1949.
20. Wangensteen, O. H., and Paine, J. R.: Treatment of acute intestinal obstruction by suction with a duodenal tube. J.A.M.A., 101:1532-1539, 1933.
21. Zintel, H. A., Rhoads, J. E., and Ravdin, I. S.: The use of intravenous ammonium chloride in the treatment of alkalosis. Surgery, 14:728, 1943.

Chapter 6

JONATHAN E. RHOADS, M.D.

Nutrition

Introduction
The Key Role of Protein in Nutrition
   Hypoproteinemia—Significance and Effects
   Estimation of Probable Protein Deficits
      Significance of the Catabolic Response to Injury and Operation
Carbohydrate and Fat
Routes of Alimentation
Intravenous "Hyperalimentation"
Nutritional Role of Blood and Plasma
Diabetes
Vitamins
Iron
Obesity

Prior to 1940, nutrition was thought of chiefly in its relation to internal medicine, as in the management of diabetes and vitamin deficiencies. As other advances permitted an enlargement in the scope of surgical operations, it became increasingly evident that nutritional factors could often play a decisive role in the recovery of patients from surgical procedures. It was Ambroise Paré who made the famous statement: "Man dresses the wound, God heals it." It is evident that wound healing involves the formation of new tissue, and new tissue requires "building stones," whether they are supplied from other tissues or from currently ingested food. As the materials used in repair are basically protein in nature, it is not surprising to find that proteins occupy a central position in the nutrition of surgical patients, and that carbohydrates and fats are of value largely because of their protein-sparing qualities.

Several of the vitamins have specific roles in surgery, notably vitamin K (see Chap. 32, Liver, Gallbladder and Bile Passages), vitamin C, thiamine and probably others of the B group. Vitamin D has a specific usefulness in hypoparathyroidism, and vitamin E has been recommended in the treatment of Peyronie's disease and in the treatment of Dupuytren's contracture, although its effectiveness in these conditions does not as yet rest on firm proof.

The subject of mineral nutrition leads us directly into the field of the electrolytes, which will be considered separately, and, therefore, it will be omitted from this chapter. An exception is iron metabolism, which is considered in a later section of this chapter.

In the field of nutrition, it is a fair generalization to say that it is easier to demonstrate changes due to a deficiency of a specific food component than it is to demonstrate benefit from an amount larger than what is termed the normal requirement. In fact, it is generally doubtful whether excesses of any specific food components are definitely useful over a long period. However, temporary increases above the usual requirement may hasten restoration of accumulated deficits.

PROTEIN NUTRITION

Applying this principle to the field of protein nutrition, we find that if an animal is maintained on a protein-deficient regimen, a series of changes, which have received considerable study, occur. The animal usually will adapt himself to a moderately low protein intake, but if the intake is very low, e.g., 1 per cent of the diet, he will go into negative nitrogen balance, putting out more nitrogen in the urine than he takes in. As this process goes forward, there will be a concomitant diminution in blood volume out of proportion to the loss in body weight and a decrease in plasma protein concentration. As a rule, the plasma albumin component will go down more rapidly than the globulin component, and this often leads to a reversal of the normal albumin-globulin ratio.

Hypoproteinemia

With the decline in serum protein concentration, there is of course a corresponding decline in the colloid osmotic pressure of the plasma.

Nutrition

This permits water and electrolytes to accumulate outside the blood vessels. While this change also occurs gradually, at a serum protein level of the order of 5.0 to 5.5 Gm. per 100 ml. or at an albumin level of about 2.5 Gm. per 100 ml., edema is likely to become grossly demonstrable in dependent areas, such as the ankles. If pressure for 10 seconds or so with the finger leaves a dent, edema is spoken of as pitting, and this state usually represents an increase in the weight of the leg in the amount of 8 to 10 per cent or more. Similarly, a circular dent left on the abdominal wall by the examining stethoscope is suggestive of edema. The extracellular fluid increases gradually, though its appearance as detected clinically may seem rather abrupt. Therefore, it is a mistake to speak of a critical level of serum protein or serum albumin at which edema forms.

Plasma colloid osmotic pressure is by no means the only factor in edema. Increased venous pressure produces edema by increasing the capillary pressure at the venous end of the loop so that less fluid is drawn back into the circulation at that level. Salt intake is another factor that affects edema formation, and renal function plays an important role. Jones and Eaton (1933) were the first to call attention to what they called postoperative edema due to the excessive administration of sodium chloride after operation. Jones, Eaton and White (1934) showed that the hypoproteinemic patient is susceptible to an excess of salt intake, and it has been shown that edema can be produced by the administration of sodium chloride solutions alone in man as well as in experimental animals (Coller et al., 1944).

As suggested by Jones and Eaton and also by Ravdin (1938) the edema is not confined to the extremities but may involve the visceral tissues also and thus be a factor in failure of gastroenterostomy stomas to function after gastric operations. Here, a local-traumatic factor accentuates the edema. The picture of the nonfunctioning gastroenterostomy stoma was reproduced in the dog by Mecray, Barden and Ravdin (1937) by lowering the serum protein with a low protein diet and repeated plasmapheresis and carrying out a simple gastroenterostomy. X-ray studies showed a marked delay in gastric emptying so that the gastric emptying time was almost inversely propor-

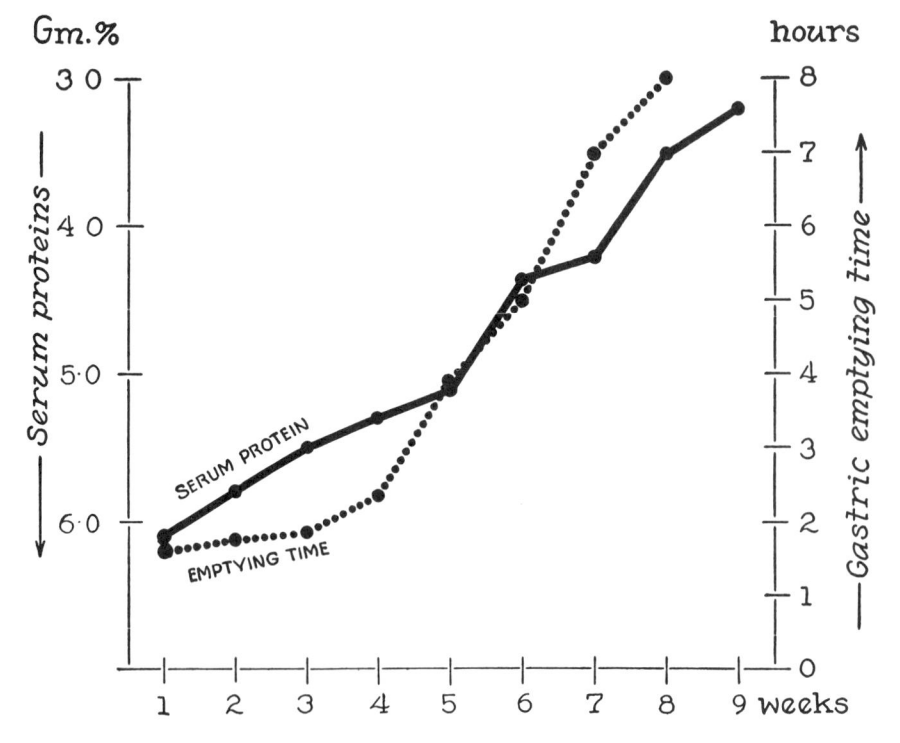

FIG. 6-1. Serum proteins and gastric emptying time. Mean values for 8 dogs.

tional to the serum protein level (Fig. 6-1). Extending their studies to dogs that had had a gastroenterostomy carried out many months earlier and finally to normal dogs, they demonstrated that hypoproteinemia retarded gastric emptying and also retarded the movement of a water barium meal from the pylorus to the cecum.

A serendipitous finding in this study was the marked frequency of wound rupture, suggesting interference with wound healing. Subsequent studies by Thompson, Ravdin and Frank (1938) confirmed the observation that hypoproteinemia resulting from a low protein diet and plasmapheresis interferes with the healing of laparotomy wounds in the dog. Histologic evidence indicated that this was due to a failure or delay in fibroplasia. Whether this effect is due to the edema or to a lack of "building stones" in hypoproteinemic animals never has been completely settled. A later study by Rhoads, Fliegelman and Panzer (1942) showed that in hypoproteinemia produced by the administration of acacia this change did not occur and, furthermore, that if a dog was previously rendered hypoproteinemic, fibroplasia would proceed normally if acacia was given at the time the test wounds were made. This, of course, suggests that the colloid osmotic relationships are the important thing. However, it is also possible that plasma expanders may release some plasma protein from the circulation for other uses.

Other studies showed that fracture healing in the dog could be interfered with by hypoproteinemia, as judged by the appearance of calcification on x-ray examination after a Gigli saw transection of the ulna (Fig. 6-2).

Since a decrease in blood volume usually has been reported with hypoproteinemia, it is not surprising to find that the hypoproteinemic animal is hypersusceptible to hemorrhagic shock. This was demonstrated by Ravdin, McNamee, Kamholz and Rhoads (1944) in a study in which it was found that the animal rendered hypoproteinemic by plasmapheresis could withstand only about 60 per cent as much hemorrhage per kilogram as the normal.

One of the most interesting effects of hypoproteinemia is that on resistance to infection. Knowledge in this field was greatly enriched by Dr. Paul Cannon who showed in the experimental animal that certain specific anti-

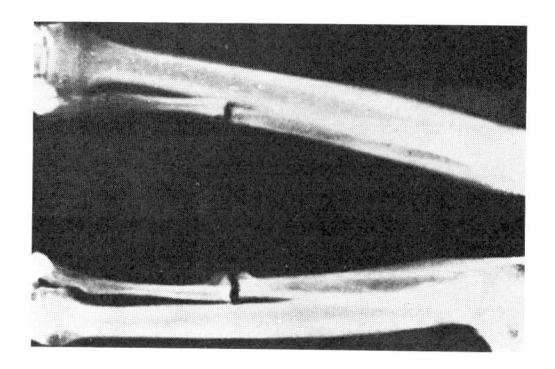

Fig. 6-2. (*Top*) Roentgenogram of Gigli saw fracture of hypoproteinemic dog after 40 days. (*Bottom*) Similar fracture of the opposite ulna of the same dog after 39 days when plasma protein levels were normal. Note increase in callus production. (Rhoads, J. E., and Kasinskas, W.: The influence of hypoproteinemia on the formation of callus in experimental fracture. Surgery, 11:38-44)

bodies form more slowly in the presence of hypoproteinemia. The response to a typhoid antigen was studied in man by Matthew Wohl (1949), who confirmed this work by finding that in hypoproteinemic patients the rise of the antibody titer is much slower after injections of the typhoid H antibody.

Gell (1948) studied antibody formation in undernourished men in the German Ruhr in 1946, using a group of normal subjects as controls. He used 32 cases of malnutrition from the Barmen Municipal Hospital, 25 civilian prisoners from the Siegburg jail, and 16 subjects in a good state of nutrition as controls. All were given injections of 3 antigens for which preformed immunity could not be present. The antigens used were tobacco mosaic virus, avian red blood cells, and a saprophytic vibrio, which failed to produce demonstrable agglutinins. He summarized the results for the first two in Table 6-1.

Although these data indicated a significant superiority of the controls over the undernourished persons at all periods and for both antigens, Gell emphasized the following points in his conclusions:

(1) The extremely severe degree of undernutrition from which the test subjects were suffering —severe enough to render active life impossible;

TABLE 6-1. PERCENTAGES OF SERUMS GIVING AGGLUTINATION*

	WITH AVIAN CELLS			WITH TOBACCO MOSAIC		
	Before	3 Weeks	Second	Before	3 Weeks	Second
25 Prisoners	8.0	60.0	60.0	0.0	52.0	48.0
32 Patients	6.3	37.5	65.5	0.0	53.1	31.3
16 Controls	0.0	81.3	87.5	0.0	93.7	93.7

* Gell, P. G. H.: Discussion on nutrition and resistance to infection. London, Proc. Roy. Soc. Med., 41:323, 1948.

and (2) in spite of this, the comparatively small differences between these literally famished subjects and the controls in first-class condition; (3) the significant fact that there actually was not any widespread epidemic disease in Germany after World War II. These points taken together suggest that undernutrition does not play as large a part in widespread epidemics as is generally supposed.

Without going into further detail, it is evident that the protein-deficient patient is at a great disadvantage. He is often hypovolemic. His resistance to hemorrhagic shock is decreased, and his resistance to infection may be decreased. Wound healing is likely to be delayed if hypoproteinemia is severe, and the disturbance in gastrointestinal motility may interfere with the resumption of normal nutrition, especially following a gastroenterostomy.

Unfortunately, the same group of patients who are often deprived of the use of the gastrointestinal tract for several days after operation are the ones who commonly have had digestive disturbances and consequently have developed serious nutritional deficits before operation. The extent of the deficits that individuals develop before operation is not known accurately, although it is, of course, not uncommon to find patients with gastrointestinal malignant lesions who have lost 20, 40, 60 or more pounds in weight since the onset of symptoms.

ESTIMATIONS OF PROBABLE PROTEIN DEFICITS

If hypoproteinemia has actually developed, it is safe to assume that a substantial nutritional deficit has developed unless there has been a rapid expansion of the extracellular space with solutions containing sodium. This is based on the difficulty of producing hypoproteinemia of any degree in experimental animals. A dog on a 1 per cent protein diet requires about 15 plasmaphereses in a 3-week period to carry him down to edema level. At each bleeding, hemorrhage is carried to or close to the point of air hunger—the blood citrated and the cells separated and returned in a saline suspension.

In some patients, weight loss may be a valuable index. In others, the dietary history may be helpful (e.g., a patient may have been put on a meat-free diet or a low protein diet by a physician who may not have been sufficiently mindful of the effects of the low protein intake). It is probable that the measurement of the total number of grams of circulating plasma protein will give a more sensitive indication of protein loss than would the serum protein concentration alone. It has been stated that the estimation of the total number of grams of circulating albumin is an even more sensitive index.

It should be emphasized that a normal serum protein concentration by no means rules out the possible existence of substantial protein deficits which may have serious significance for the patient undergoing extensive operation or a complicated postoperative course. This can be suspected in some patients if a careful dietary history is taken. Muscular wasting is an important physical sign of protein deficiency.

PREOPERATIVE PROTEIN LOSS

Some of the more acute losses of protein occurring before operation in surgical patients are shown in Table 6-2, and it is to be remembered that a considerable additional loss of protein is apt to occur during operation in the form of hemorrhage (Bockus, 1949; Cuthbertson, 1936; Fine and Gendel, 1940; Hirshfeld et al., 1944; Howard et al., 1944). Unquestionably there are additional losses as the result of tissue trauma, leakage of plasma from the circulation in the form of serum, or sequestration of plasma and possibly of cells in the local area of in-

TABLE 6-2. NITROGEN LOSSES IN VARIOUS TYPES OF SURGICAL PATIENTS BEFORE OPERATION*

ILLNESS	N LOSS IN GRAMS	TIME IN DAYS
Bleeding peptic ulcer—Bockus (1949)	90.72	5
Thermal burn—Hirshfeld et al. (1944)		
Surface oozing	7.84	1
Total nitrogen loss	30.88	1
Small bowel obstruction—Fine and Gendel (1940)	11.04	1
Long bone fractures—Cuthbertson (1936)	137.00	10
Long bone fractures—Howard et al. (1944)	190.00	Variable number of weeks

* Rhoads, J. E.: Supranormal dietary requirements of acutely ill patients. J. Am. Dietet. A., 29:897-903, 1953.

flammation. The losses due to hemorrhage alone have been measured by a number of writers, and a group of such figures have been compiled in Table 6-3.

POSTOPERATIVE PROTEIN LOSS

After operation, the picture is a complex one. Not only is there a continuing loss of protein during a period when the intake may be quite restricted, but the loss is enhanced by a phenomenon known as the catabolic response to injury. The first attempt to quantitate this response in patients was made by Cuthbertson and his collaborators (1936), who studied the metabolism of patients following fractures of the long bones. Their observations were confirmed by John Eager Howard (1944) and others in this country. In general, it was found that there was an increase in the output of nitrogen in the urine for a period of 10 days or so following fractures. This resulted in a negative nitrogen balance on ordinary diets containing 3.4 Gm. to 9.4 Gm. of nitrogen. When the dietary protein intake was increased to 11.6 Gm. of nitrogen and to 14.0 Gm. of nitrogen per day, the output rose also, and the patient remained in negative balance for a period in the neighborhood of 10 days. There are many ways of demonstrating this catabolic loss of nitrogen. Dr. George Whipple (1938) noted it

TABLE 6-3. NITROGEN LOSSES (DUE TO BLOOD LOSS) IN VARIOUS TYPES OF SURGICAL PATIENTS DURING OPERATION (BASED ON 3 GM. OF NITROGEN PER 100 CC. OF BLOOD)*

OPERATION	NUMBER OF PATIENTS	NITROGEN LOSS IN GRAMS *Minimum*	*Average*	*Maximum*
Radical mastectomy				
Coller et al. (1944b)	4	15	24	31.5
Thyroidectomy				
Coller et al. (1944b)	8	3	12	21
Abdominoperineal resection				
Coller et al. (1944b)	12	6	12	21
Gastric operations (complicated)				
Coller et al. (1944b)	3	9	18	24
Operations involving body surfaces				
Coller et al. (1944b)	3	13.5	36	42
Pneumonectomy				
Miller, Gibbon and Allbritten (1949)	16	21	57	108
First-stage thoracoplasty				
Miller, Gibbon and Allbritten (1949)	10	12	22.5	60

* Rhoads, J. E.: Supranormal dietary requirements of acutely ill patients. J. Am. Dietet. A., 29:897-903, 1953.

followed chloroform poisoning in dogs and in a number of other conditions (see Chap. 15, Nonoperative Surgical Care).

SIGNIFICANCE OF THE CATABOLIC RESPONSE TO INJURY AND OPERATION

The significance of this phenomenon has been the subject of much speculation among surgical physiologists. Those of one school of thought view it as a teleologic mechanism by which the body gets rid of excess protein at a time when this may be harmful. Others view it as an attempt on the part of the body to mobilize large quantities of tissue nitrogen, possibly because of a specific need for certain moieties of the protein molecule, as for instance a particular amino acid. If one accepts the first viewpoint, one withholds protein, or at least does not push it, and accepts a negative nitrogen balance for a period of several days following the injury. If one believes in the second hypothesis, one would be led to augment protein intake in order to provide materials to enable the body to prolong its responses for a greater period than is possible from its own stores.

TABLE 6-4. NITROGEN LOSSES IN VARIOUS TYPES OF SURGICAL PATIENTS AFTER OPERATION*

ILLNESS	N LOSS IN GRAMS	TIME IN DAYS
Herniotomy (Brunschwig et al., 1942)	18.0	10
Subtrochanteric osteotomy (Howard et al., 1944)	65.0†	14
Gastric resection (Riegel et al., 1947)	54.0	5
Cholecystectomy (Brunschwig et al., 1942)	114.0	10
Gastric resection (Brunschwig, et al., 1942)	175.0	10
Acute appendicitis (Peritonitis) (Brunschwig et al., 1942)	49.0	10
Repair perforated peptic ulcer (Brunschwig et al., 1942)	136.0	10
Radical mastectomy (Brunschwig et al., 1942)	15.0	10

* Rhoads, J. E.: Supranormal dietary requirements of acutely ill patients. J. Am. Dietet. A., 29:897-903, 1953.
† Average of 3.

Experimental data are available in the case of the liver that suggest that it is the mobilization of the body's protein stores that is important. Hepatic injury produced by a standard chloroform anesthesia in the dog is better tolerated, in terms of histologic evidence of degeneration and necrosis, if the animal concomitantly receives an irritating subcutaneous injection of sodium ricinoleate capable of initiating a catabolic response. It would seem in this experimental setup that the liver injured by chloroform was actually benefited as a result of the catabolic phenomena induced by injury to subcutaneous tissue and muscle caused by the injection of sodium ricinoleate or some other irritating material.

The extent of the catabolic response in a variety of surgical conditions is presented in Table 6-4. It is evident that much more protein and protein-sparing food are required to achieve nitrogen equilibrium in the patient following extensive operation than would be the case in the normal individual.

For the normal adult male of 70 Kg., the Food and Nutrition Board recommends a daily allowance of 65 Gm. of protein; and 55 Gm. for the normal adult woman of 58 Kg. It is considered that this provides a sufficient excess to cover ordinary variations in the character of the food protein and in the activity of the individual. It does not provide for pregnancy, for lactation or for growth of the young individual. The Food and Nutrition Board has estimated that the allowance of almost 1 Gm. per Kg. of body weight per day provides protein in almost double the amount of the minimal requirement. To be compared with this is the figure of 130 Gm. of protein, arrived at by Riegel and her co-workers (1947) for gastrectomy patients during the first 5 postoperative days. To obtain balance on this allowance, a relatively high caloric allowance was provided of the order of 2,100 calories or 30 calories per kilogram. These figures were average and do not provide excess for individual variation. Thus it would appear that the postgastrectomy patient has at least 3 times the protein requirement of the normal. After smaller operations, however, the change is less marked. For instance, after herniorrhaphy there is relatively little excess nitrogen catabolism.

While the above considerations are of help in thinking of the more difficult nutritional problems, they must be mixed with much common sense when dealing with the average surgical patient. The many patients requiring minor surgical procedures and the more moderate major ones present no nutritional problem other than the provision of a normal intake, such as they might enjoy away from the hospital. Even for those patients who have a considerable accumulated nutritional deficit and must look forward to several days after operation before food is permitted by mouth, a complicated nutritional regimen is seldom required. In most instances, if moderate support is provided, they can be expected to take sufficient food by mouth within 5 to 7 days after operation and to go into positive balance and correct any deficiencies that may have developed. However, such patients are losing body nitrogen during the postoperative period, and it may well be advantageous to provide for their needs by the intravenous route even when this is not essential for recovery (*see* section on parenteral hyperalimentation).

Some authors have recommended 100 Gm. of glucose and 100 Gm. of protein hydrolysate per day by vein as a compromise regimen. This mixture provides only 800 calories; therefore, it is inadequate for an adult on any long-term basis. Whether or not it will be adequate for nitrogen balance on a short-term basis will depend on the manner in which the individual mobilizes his own tissues. If he mobilizes fat in sufficient quantities, it may be perfectly adequate. If, on the other hand, he does not and mobilizes more protein instead, 100 Gm. of protein and 100 Gm. of carbohydrate do not constitute a satisfactory diet.

Elman has reported that the patient receiving no protein loses no more nitrogen on 100 Gm. of glucose than when a larger amount is given. However, the studies of Zollinger and Ellison (1950) indicated that, with a steady nitrogen intake, increases in carbohydrate to provide higher caloric intakes are accompanied by a substantial rise in nitrogen retention.

CARBOHYDRATE AND FAT

The surgeon's interest in carbohydrate and fat is concerned primarily with its effect in sparing proteins by supplying calories (see discussion in the section on proteins). A certain amount of carbohydrate is necessary, even if the body is able to provide ample fat from its stores for caloric requirement. If some carbohydrate is not supplied, acetone bodies will be formed and will carry off a portion of the alkali reserve, resulting in acidosis; 100 Gm. of carbohydrate a day are ordinarily more than sufficient to provide for this requirement. It should be remembered that children are probably more susceptible to the development of acidosis by this mechanism than are adults.

It is not entirely certain that fat can be replaced in the diet by carbohydrate on an isocaloric basis. There is evidence that with extremely low fat diets the total number of calories must be increased. Some evidence has been presented indicating that growth can proceed at a more rapid rate if some fat is provided in the diet. Practically speaking, a fat-free diet, or even one very low in fat (less than 10 per cent of the calories), is very unpalatable. Within a fairly wide range, however, carbohydrate and fat can be substituted for each other to provide calories and to spare proteins.

The bearing of high fat diets on the development of atherosclerosis has received much study. It has long been known that a number of disease conditions that are commonly associated with hypercholesterolemia are also associated with a high incidence of atherosclerosis and its complications. Atherosclerosis can be produced prematurely in some species by feeding a high cholesterol diet. Because of the ease with which the body produces cholesterol, it has not been sufficient to lower the cholesterol intake if one wishes to lower the blood cholesterol level. However, the blood cholesterol level generally can be reduced if the total fat intake is curtailed drastically.

Machella and his associates found that patients kept on a diet rich in protein and carbohydrate and free of fat during therapy for ulcerative colitis developed remarkably low serum cholesterol levels. Accordingly, they undertook a study (Mellinkoff, Machella and Reinhold, 1950) in which patients with a variety of gastrointestinal conditions were placed on a synthetic fat-free diet consisting of protein hydrolysate and Dextri-Maltose. This diet, which supplied from 2,200 to 4,000 calories a day was supplemented with vitamins and iron and was maintained for periods up to 55 days. They found that the patients were maintained in a satisfactory stage of nutrition and health and noted an average decrease of 85 (5 to 169) milligrams of cholesterol per 100 ml. of serum in 15 days. They further noted that a significant decrease occurred within 5 days of starting this diet, and that the cholesterol level returned to the former level within 8 days of resuming a normal diet. If they added moderate amounts of fat, a significant decrease (to 96 mg.%) still occurred. They concluded that a palatable diet which is high in proteins and carbohydrate and low in fat will maintain a reduced serum cholesterol concentration.

The extensive studies of Keys and his associates (1950) have indicated that those population groups in Western Europe whose average dietary provides about 20 per cent of the calories as fat have a far lower incidence of coronary occlusion than exists in the United States, where studies indicate that about 40 per cent of the calories of the diet are provided as fat. Keys's studies show further that the population groups on the lower fat intake generally have lower cholesterol levels in the blood.

The interrelationship between dietary fat, serum cholesterol and the complications of atherosclerosis with its possible effects on the incidence of vascular disease is demanding more attention. Although the evidence to date is not unequivocal, it is highly suggestive that elevated serum cholesterol levels are undesirable and should be reduced in patients with coronary artery disease, diabetes mellitus and some peripheral vascular diseases (Meltzer et al., 1958). Current studies reveal that the greatest and most practical cholesterol-decreasing regimen is one in which the total fat is reduced along with a reduction in the saturated fatty acids and replaced with unsaturated fatty acids, such as those found in plant foods (Beeson et al., 1959; Meltzer et al., 1958). It is emphasized that unsaturated fatty acids should not be used as a supplement but as a substitute for other dietary fatty acids. Kuo (1967) has correlated serum lipid levels with dietary intake of soluble carbohydrates in certain patients.

ROUTES OF ALIMENTATION

Now that we have considered some of the unfortunate consequences and dangers of hypoproteinemia and the amount of protein needed under a variety of circumstances, we next must consider the means at our disposal for supplying these needs. It must be emphasized again and again that the alimentary canal, if normal or only moderately impaired, is the best route for alimentation. The other routes are utilized only when the oral route is contraindicated for some particular reason, such as persistent vomiting, recent operation upon the gastrointestinal tract, severe diarrhea, etc. Generally speaking, in postoperative patients, it is wise to wait until peristaltic sounds return before using the oral route.

Rectal Route

The rectal route, although used extensively in the past (clysters), is seldom used today, but it is still a very practical route for the administration of water and isotonic sodium chloride solution. Tap water or isotonic sodium chloride solution dripped through a small catheter at a pressure of not more than 20 to 40 cm. of water ordinarily can be absorbed in amounts up to a liter or so every 12 hours. The addition of glucose to the water or saline solution retards absorption and, according to the studies of Ebeling (1933), very little glucose is absorbed. For a more detailed consideration of this subject, the reader is referred to Edsal and Miller (1902) and Rhoads et al. (1939).

Jejunostomy

Allen (1941) recommended jejunostomy as a preliminary procedure in malnourished patients requiring extensive operation. The use of this method has not been uniformly successful in the hands of the author, due to the fact that instillation of food directly into the jejunum will often set up a diarrhea. A variation of the jejunostomy suggested by Ravdin and implemented by Abbott and Rawson (1937) consists of placing a double lumen tube in the stomach before operation. One lumen is connected to a single tube which, during the course of a gastric operation, can be moved through the gastroenterostomy and allowed to go well down into the jejunum below the gastrojejunostomy. The tube may be passed either through the nose or the mouth, as originally suggested by the authors, or it may be brought out through the gastric wall and through the abdominal wall like the tube in a Stamm gastrostomy. The limitations of this method are influenced by the tolerance of the jejunum for food that has not been prepared in the stomach.

Studies indicate that one of the functions of the stomach, in addition to storage, is to dilute hypertonic foods to or almost to isotonicity (Ravdin et al., 1943). Thus, when a large load of 50 per cent glucose was placed in the stomach of the dog, the highest glucose concentrations obtained in duodenal samples were 5.3 per cent and those in the jejunum were of the order of 2.4 per cent. In general, hypertonic materials introduced into the jejunum draw in a lot of fluid immediately. This may produce local pain, as in the "dumping syndrome" (see Chap. 31, Stomach and Duodenum), or it may set up a diarrhea (Machella, 1948, 1949). At times, this may be controlled with paregoric, but on other occasions the feeding mixture will have to be decreased in amount or stopped.

The response of the small bowel to direct feeding through a tube is difficult to predict—one patient accepting a substantial liquid diet and another responding with hypermotility and diarrhea. In general, isotonic mixtures are better tolerated and hypertonic mixtures less well tolerated. A general diet, such as patients with normal gastrointestinal tracts eat, can be homogenized with a Waring blender, and experience indicates that such a mixture is often better tolerated via the jejunostomy than more nearly synthetic diets. It is often helpful to start the feedings off slowly—perhaps 800 or 1,000 calories per day, divided into 30 to 40 parts—and then to build the amount up to the desired levels as rapidly as tolerated. Two cautions should be borne in mind. First, an occasional patient will retain too much salt so that the serum sodium concentration should be monitored; second, the Waring blends are not easily soluble, so that it is important to rinse the tube with water after each feeding to prevent the lumen from becoming blocked with successive layers of insoluble materials.

If natural foods are blended in large quantities to be held for later use, it must be kept in mind that this product, if it is not promptly pasteurized and refrigerated properly, will soon be teeming with bacteria. Homogenized milk, taken directly from half pint containers and supplemented with ascorbic acid, sometimes makes a most adequate jejunostomy feeding.

The drip method of administration will often be attended by diarrhea sooner or later.

Parenteral Routes

We are left with the parenteral routes for the majority of patients who cannot take feedings by mouth, and of these the intravenous route is certainly the most versatile and probably the safest if one has access to pyrogen-free fluids.

Nutrients Suitable for Intravenous Administration

Glucose is readily administered by vein in concentrations from 5 to 50 per cent; 5 per cent glucose solution is about isotonic. Weaker solutions may be given provided that the total osmotic pressure of the solution is made up with sodium chloride or some other substance suitable for intravenous injection. If this is not done, the hypotonic solution may produce hemolysis of red blood cells.

Fructose. Intravenous fructose also has been proposed and has certain advantages. In experiments carried out by Rosenthal and his associates (1953), at a moderately rapid infusion rate about 6 per cent less sugar was spilled when using invert sugar (glucose and fructose in equal parts) than when using glucose. Infusions at rates of 1.5 Gm./Kg. per hour resulted in the liberation of a considerable amount of lactate which may be measured in the blood stream but so far has not been shown to be definitely injurious. At times very rapid rates of infusion have produced hyperpnea.

Protein may be given either in the form of amino acid mixtures or in the form of hydrolyzed protein. Protein hydrolysates may be prepared either by acid hydrolysis, which destroys tryptophan, or by enzymatic hydrolysis. A common preparation results from the enzymatic hydrolysis of a mixture of casein and animal pancreas. If acid hydrolysis is used, it is essential to replace the tryptophan and tyrosine in appropriate amounts so that the resulting material will have the effect of a so-called whole or complete protein.

It is now well documented that omission of an essential amino acid from the feeding mixture results in a practically complete wasting of the rest of the material. Furthermore, all of the essential constituents must be given at approximately the same time. Thus, if an incomplete protein is fed in the morning and the moiety required to complete it is not fed until evening, most of both feedings will be lost in the form of increased nitrogen in the urine.

Ethyl alcohol is another preparation that may be administered intravenously. If there is any doubt as to whether the available ethyl alcohol is adulterated, it may be safest to use absolute alcohol, diluted to a concentration of 10 per cent or less. It is, of course, unnecessarily expensive as much of the cost of absolute alcohol is due to the expense incurred in eliminating residual water. The alcohol provides 7 calories per gram. Its pharmacologic actions are well known, although it should be emphasized that it sometimes seems to function as an excellent sedative, especially in older people who often tolerate barbiturate sedatives poorly.

Where a serious effort is being made to achieve caloric as well as nitrogen balance in the postoperative patient, a mixture of 5 per cent alcohol, 5 per cent glucose and 5 per cent protein hydrolysate can be very useful. Two liters of such a solution provide in the neighborhood of 1,500 calories and, when supplemented by an additional liter of 10 per cent glucose, often will provide a sufficient caloric intake. Such solutions are definitely hypertonic and will produce excessive thrombosis in some individuals at the site of injection. However, if the injection site is changed once every 12 to 24 hours, the majority of individuals will tolerate it.

At present, glucose, fructose, sorbitol, hydrolyzed protein (or amino acid mixtures) and ethyl alcohol comprise our principal repertory for parenteral alimentation.

STAGES IN THE DEVELOPMENT OF INTRAVENOUS FEEDING

Only minor amounts of food substances can be successfully given by the subcutaneous intraperitoneal or intramedullary routes. Therefore, this section will be devoted to the intravenous route.

Methods for injecting fluids into veins had been developed by Richard Lower of Oxford by 1662, only 34 years after Harvey's description of the circulation of the blood in *De Motu Cordis* appeared in 1628. French workers are said to have applied the method to the transfusion of blood in the following year. Sir Christopher Wren, the architect of St. Paul's Cathedral, is credited with having been the first to use it for the administration of drugs in animals. By 1670 a monograph had been published in Holland entitled *Clysmatica Nova*, giving detailed instructions not only for the transfusion of blood from man to man but "ex animali in homines" (from animals to man!). The use of the intravenous infusion could not have been successful until the work of Pasteur and Lister established sterilization. It further required the recognition of the role of dead bacterial products as pyrogens (Seibert, 1923-24) and the application of this knowledge by others to make the method widely acceptable on an elective basis. At a clinical level, parenteral nutrition has developed through the following phases:

1. The administration of isotonic aqueous solutions of glucose, fructose or invert sugar within volume limits safe for most postoperative patients—usually 3 liters of 5 per cent solution yielding 600 calories.

2. The attempt to give hypertonic solutions in peripheral veins to augment the calorie intake. These often included protein hydrolysates. Ten per cent solutions were usually practical but 15 per cent solutions caused excessive thrombosis of veins at the common injection sites in one third of cases, in the author's experience.

3. The search for nutrients yielding more than four calories per gram. This led to trials of ethyl alcohol, which yields 7 calories per gram, and of neutral fats, which provide 9 calories per gram but must be emulsified very thoroughly to avoid fat embolism.

4. The endeavor to increase the volume of the solution, depending on diuretics to remove the excess water before it accumulated in the body to a harmful degree. This proved possible and effective but required very careful monitoring.

INTRAVENOUS HYPERALIMENTATION

The most recent development to receive extensive trial has been the use of concentrated solutions of monosaccharides and hydrolyzed protein, avoiding thrombosis by central administration into large veins in which the passing volume of blood effects very prompt dilution to isotonic concentrations. This is usually achieved by a percutaneous puncture of the subclavian vein with a No. 18 gauge needle through which is passed an intracath about 14 inches long so that the end lies in the midportion of the superior vena cava. A strict aseptic technic as thorough as that used in the operating room is observed. The wound of entrance is protected by an antibiotic ointment covered with a sterile dressing which is carefully changed every 2 or 3 days, and, after cleansing, additional antibiotic ointment is applied. Wilmore and Dudrick (1969) have found it possible with this procedure, to avoid infection and to use the same catheter continuously for 2 to 4 weeks. Utilizing 20 to 30 per cent concentrations of solutes and 3 liters per day in the adult, they have given 2,500 to 3,200 calories per day and the equivalent of 100 to 150 grams of protein in the form of a fibrin hydrolysate. The vitamin complement used in man and the mineral allowance usually administered is shown in Table 6-5. The amounts particularly of sodium chloride and of potassium chloride are adjusted according to the patient's needs as estimated by measurement and analysis of fluids lost from the body and by measurement of serum sodium, potassium chloride and bicarbonate (see Dudrick et al., 1969).

This work was based on the demonstration by Dudrick, Wilmore and Vars (1966) that beagle puppies could be reared from the age of about 12 weeks to maturity on such a regimen and that their weight curve and length and height measurements increased as rapidly as littermate controls fed isocalorically by mouth. The opportunity to induce weight gain in a human baby on a purely parenteral regimen presented itself in 1967 and excellent weight gain, growth and development were achieved (Dudrick and Wilmore, 1968).

If water retention occurs, the regimen generally does not have to be stopped or even relaxed if one utilizes diuretics. Chlorthiazide (Diuril) in a dose of 250 mg. every 12 hours by vein is usually adequate for this purpose, but we have also used Mannitol, Thiomerin and ethacrynic acid (Rhoads et al., 1965).

TABLE 6-5. COMPOSITION OF DAILY AVERAGE ADULT NUTRIENT SOLUTION*

Water	2500–3500 mL.	Vitamin A	5,000–10,000 U.S.P. units
Protein Hydrolysates (Amino acids)	100–130 Gm.	Vitamin D	500–1,000 U.S.P. units
Nitrogen	12–20 Gm.	Vitamin E	2.5–5.0 I.U.
Carbohydrate (Dextrose)	525–750 Gm.	Vitamin C	250–500 mg.
Calories	2500–3500 Kcal	Thiamine	25–50 mg.
Sodium	125–150 mEq	Riboflavin	5–10 mg.
Potassium	75–120 mEq	Pyridoxine	7.5–15 mg.
Magnesium	4–8 mEq	Niacin	50–100 mg.
		Pantothenic acid	12.5–25 mg.

Calcium and phosphorus are added to the solution as indicated.

Iron is added to the solution, given intramuscularly in depot form as iron-dextran, or given via blood transfusion as indicated.

Vitamin B_{12}, vitamin K, and folic acid are given intramuscularly or added to the solution for intravenous administration as indicated.

Trace elements such as zinc, copper, manganese, cobalt, and iodine are added only after total intravenous therapy exceeds one month. Alternatively, one unit of plasma twice a week has been given to provide required amounts of trace elements.

* Dudrick, S. J., Wilmore, D. W., Vars, H. M., and Rhoads, J. E.: Ann. Surg., 169:974, 1969.

With these regimens there is sometimes some spill of dextrose in the urine, but this has not been of sufficient magnitude to impair significantly the overall nutritional effect.

When the first and the second editions of this book were written, it was only occasionally that a patient who could take nothing by mouth was brought into positive nitrogen balance by parenteral means. The gains made by using diuretics and giving larger volumes were noted in the third edition.

Now it is possible to achieve positive calorie balance and nitrogen balance in nearly all patients with protein deficits by using central vein administration of concentrated nutrient solutions. Rigid aseptic and antiseptic technics are essential, but clinical results have been striking when such a regimen has been fully implemented. The rate of wound healing has, we believe, been markedly accelerated toward the normal.

The accomplishment of the strongly positive N balance as compared with bare equilibrium has resulted in a new era in supportive care. Patients gain weight, indolent wounds fill with healthy granulations, fistulas often close and the patients quickly begin to look healthier and to act more normally in a behavioral sense.

The catabolic response to injury has proved to be a relative rather than an absolute influence and in nearly all patients it has been possible to induce a positive balance within 48 to 72 hours. The concept that fat is essential has not been supported by the studies referred to above. F.D.A. approval for fat emulsions for I.V. use were withdrawn in 1967 except under very special circumstances and American manufacturers stopped their production. This necessitated a change in the protocol for one of the canine experiments. With isocaloric substitutions of glucose, the growth curve was unchanged. Thus, in the presence of an excess of carbohydrate and protein, an otherwise well balanced diet is effective over a period of many weeks without fat.

Fat emulsions for administration in man are available outside the United States and are widely used in Europe. Where available and if tolerated by the particular patient, such emulsions may form a part of the regimen outlined above. Usually, the dose is limited to 500 ml. of 15 per cent emulsion per day. For a fuller discussion of the advantages and disadvantages of intravenous infusion of fat emulsions, see the 3rd edition of this book, pp. 114-115.

NUTRITIONAL ROLE OF BLOOD AND PLASMA

The role of plasma proteins and whole blood in nutrition deserves consideration here. Whipple and his associates (Pommerenke *et al.*, 1935) showed that a dog could be maintained by giving it intravenous dog plasma as the sole source of protein (the dogs received nonprotein caloric supplements by mouth). It was believed as the result of additional studies on phlorizinized dogs that the protein actually could be converted to various body proteins without being broken down all the way to amino acids. Allen and his associates have demonstrated more recently that dog plasma permits normal growth of puppies receiving nonprotein foods by mouth (see Chap. 8, Blood Transfusions). In spite of this finding, most experts in the field of nutrition do not recommend plasma for its nutritional value, believing that its conversion to other body proteins is slow and that the plasma itself is too expensive. Blood is considered to be even less suitable, because it takes a long time for protein in red cells to be converted to other proteins, if indeed this conversion takes place to any appreciable extent. However, in spite of this, blood and plasma do provide for the blood volume deficit which is so regularly seen in hypoproteinemic patients. At present we have no safe substitute for the erythrocyte as a carrier of oxygen. Thus, in the face of a critical anemia either whole blood or erythrocytes suspended in saline must be used. For the correction of blood volume deficits one has several choices (see Chapter 7, Shock). For chronic or subacute protein deficits one now has the choice of employing either oral supplements or intravenous hyperalimentation (see section above). The role of plasma and its fractions in the restoration of certain clotting factors and in supplying certain immune substances is discussed in Chapter 8 (Blood Transfusions).

DIABETES

Any full discussion of the problems of diabetic management is, of course, beyond the scope of this book. It is of interest, however, that surgical operations, while they may accentuate diabetes and call for a temporary increase in the insulin requirement, may also have a steadying influence on the so-called "brittle" or unstable diabetic, making him easier to handle for a period. Because the insulin requirement is unpredictably affected by operation and by some of the diseases for which operation is carried out, particularly those of an inflammatory nature, it is in general unwise to attempt a precise regulation of diabetes near the time of operation. The objects of diabetic management should then be: (1) to prevent ketosis and (2) to prevent insulin shock. A normal blood sugar level and freedom from glycosuria should not be objectives during the acute period. Therefore, diabetic management during such an acute period may be reduced in the opinion of the author to the administration of enough insulin to abolish ketosis, and of sufficient glucose concomitantly to prevent hypoglycemia. In the author's experience this is accomplished most safely by administering the insulin intravenously with the glucose solution, thus starting the glucose concomitantly with the insulin, even though the initial blood sugar is exceedingly high. Plasma carbon dioxide determinations are most valuable and, if the level is low, it should be corrected. Correction may be achieved by the abolition of ketosis and the administration of isotonic sodium chloride solution in suitable amounts, but if the bicarbonate is below 20 millimols per liter, the author prefers the direct method of giving sixth molar sodium lactate or bicarbonate in appropriate amounts in addition to the other measures (see Chap. 5, Fluid and Electrolytes).

Schecter and his associates (1941) demonstrated marked reductions in plasma volume in 8 patients with diabetic coma. Such patients may need whole blood or plasma transfusions quite as urgently as the other elements of therapy alluded to above, and this should be considered at the time of admission of all patients in diabetic coma.

VITAMINS

In considering the requirements of surgical patients for the various accessory food substances, attention must be focused principally on those for which storage is quite limited, as is the case with most of the water-soluble vitamins, and on those for which a conditioned deficiency may develop over a period of time in patients with surgical diseases, such as vitamin K.

THE FAT-SOLUBLE VITAMINS

Vitamin A

While a vitamin A deficiency, if fully developed, might be harmful to many surgical patients, the chance of such a deficiency developing is relatively small. The precursor of the vitamin, carotene, is fairly widely distributed in the average American diet and, as a rule, patients have an ample store of the vitamin capable of lasting them many weeks. Vitamin A has been recommended in large doses in the treatment of plantar warts. The status of this therapy is not well established, as these lesions sometimes come and go rather unpredictably without treatment.

Vitamin D

Vitamin D, another of the fat-soluble vitamins, is of course as important to infants and children who happen to be in surgical wards as it is for those in pediatric wards. This is particularly true of orthopedic patients who may be kept in a hospital for many weeks or months without exposure to sunlight. In the normal adult, however, vitamin D deficiency does not seem to be a problem of much practical importance. Considerable effort has been expended at different times to obtain faster fracture healing by the administration of additional amounts of vitamin D. However, there is no clear evidence that it effects more rapid healing of fractures. Overdosage of vitamin D can produce a complex toxic picture characterized by significant changes in renal, vascular and nervous systems.

Vitamin D does have a special role in surgery in patients suffering from hypoparathyroidism. As a rule, hypoparathyroidism comes about as a result of the removal of the parathyroid tissue during thyroidectomy, or during surgical operations on the parathyroids themselves. Vitamin D with large doses of calcium lactate or calcium gluconate may be given by mouth on a chronic basis and are quite effective in restoring the serum calcium level to normal. The usefulness of vitamin D in this group of patients is mentioned in the chapter on the parathyroid. The usual dosage for this purpose is 50,000 to 200,000 units per day or 10 to 50 times the dosage usually employed for the correction of rickets.

Vitamin E

Vitamin E, a third fat-soluble vitamin, was identified in animal studies as being necessary for normal reproduction. While it has been administered fairly widely among patients, its field of usefulness is apparently quite limited. It has been reported to be helpful in Peyronie's disease, and some individuals have given it to patients with both Dupuytren's contracture and Peyronie's disease. In some of the early cases, it seems to have arrested the development of the process, but this is a clinical impression rather than a well-controlled observation.

Vitamin K

Vitamin K is a nutrient of exceptional interest to surgeons. Its existence was postulated by Dam (1934) when a group of chicks which he was feeding on synthetic diets developed a hemorrhagic tendency. He suggested that the diet was deficient in a fat-soluble substance required by the animal for normal coagulation. While his original observations were made in 1929, he did not publish the discovery of the new accessory food factor until 1934. The hemorrhagic condition in the chicks was shown to be due to a deficiency in prothrombin. Later, H. P. Smith and his co-workers (Warner, Brinkhous and Smith, 1938) established the relationship of the new vitamin to hypoprothrombinemia resulting from obstructive jaundice.

It was A. J. Quick who first showed in 1934 and 1935 that the hemorrhagic tendency, so long known to develop in patients with obstructive jaundice, was due to a prothrombin deficiency. In man, the hypoprothrombinemia is due to a conditioned deficiency. Sufficient vitamin K is formed by intestinal microorganisms to supply the requirements of most individuals. However, bile salts which lower surface tension and assist in the emulsification of fats are lacking from the intestine in obstructive jaundice. As shown by Greaves and Schmidt, bile salts are necessary for the absorption of the naturally occurring forms of vitamin K. Hence, their absence results in a deficiency of vitamin K. If the deficiency of prothrombin is to be treated orally, it is important to give either a water-soluble form of the vitamin or to give bile salts in suitable quantities to assist in its absorption. Therefore, it is not the failure of the biliary system to excrete bile, but the failure of the bile (specifically, the bile salts) to reach the intestine, that leads to hypoprothrombinemia. This explains the fact that patients with external biliary fistula may develop a hemorrhagic tendency even though they are not icteric. It also explains the fact that patients may develop a hemorrhagic tendency with incomplete common duct obstruction. It has long been known that decrease in the concentration of bile salts in the bile is one of the earliest indications of liver damage. Therefore, it seems reasonable to explain this last group of patients on the basis that they are excreting bile pigments in adequate amounts but failing to excrete bile salts in adequate amounts.

Vitamin K was, perhaps, the first of the vitamins to be found in multiple forms and is still, perhaps, the only vitamin for which a synthetic substitute is more potent than the naturally occurring forms. Vitamin K_1 in the form found naturally in alfalfa and other green vegetables has the long phytyl radical found in chlorophyll and is of relatively heavy molecular weight and of low solubility in water. The central nucleus of K_1, 2-methyl-1, 4-naphthoquinone (menadione), is more effective per milligram than is K_1 itself and is slightly more soluble in water. Some of the derivatives of this product are considerably more soluble in water and may easily be given by parenteral injection in doses of 5, 10, or 20 mg. every 4 hours until prothrombin has returned to safe levels or risen to a maximum.

Early studies showed that not all patients with hypoprothrombinemia responded to vitamin K, and there is now a body of evidence that indicates that prothrombin is synthesized to a large extent in the liver, and that, if liver damage is sufficiently pronounced, hypoprothrombinemia will develop despite large doses of vitamin K. Allen (1943) has found the prothrombin response useful as a test of liver function.

However, in the hypoprothrombinemia produced by Dicoumarol, there is a relatively normal level of accelerator globulin and a reduced level of prothrombin. When administered intravenously in doses of 25 mg. a fine emulsion of vitamin K_1 in an aqueous medium appears to have a mass action effect against Dicoumarol and can be very valuable in patients who have received excessive doses or have had excessive responses to Dicoumarol. Also, it has been given intramuscularly in doses up to 50 mg. The response after intravenous administration is very rapid, often being well marked with ½ to 1 hour. The effect may be rather transient, necessitating the administration of additional doses, often at 4- or 6-hour intervals until the prothrombin concentration is stabilized at satisfactory levels. Failure to check the prothrombin at short time intervals can easily lead to the view that no response has been obtained, because the prothrombin may have fallen back to the original level in 12 hours or so if Dicoumarol is still active in the body.

Asteriadon-Samartzis and Leiken (1958), among others, demonstrated that large doses of water-soluble vitamin K led to increased bilirubin in newborn babies at all birth weights and that vitamin K, given intravenously in doses of 25 mg., had no effect in full-term babies but did increase bilirubin in premature infants. In the latter, its oral administration also could be followed by a rise in bilirubin. Because of the danger of kernicterus, vitamin K should not be used in excessive doses in the newborn nor in mothers about to deliver.

The Water-Soluble Vitamins

Thiamine. One of the most important of the water-soluble vitamins is thiamine. Its effects are tied up so much with the effects of riboflavin and nicotinic acid deficiency and possibly of other B component deficiencies that it is exceedingly difficult to be sure which of these substances is having a particular effect. In its extreme forms B_1 deficiency produces the clinical picture of beriberi with peripheral neuritis, anorexia, changes in the electrocardiogram, and eventually interference with cell metabolism. The requirement for thiamine is low, of the order of 1 to 2 mg. a day in normal adults. It may be doubled by fever or hyerpthyroidism. In thyroid storm, when the temperature is high, the requirement can possibly go up as much as 4-fold. Therefore, the usual custom of giving 5, 10, or 20 mg. per day should provide enormous excesses of this vitamin. So far as we know, these excesses are harmless, but their utility never has been demonstrated. It has been postulated that, when circulation to an extremity or some other local area of the body is very poor, there may be an advantage in supplying the vitamin at higher concentrations. However, this remains rather hypothetical.

Anorexia and miscellaneous pains simulating peripheral neuritis are frequently treated with thiamine and other members of the B complex. Their specific usefulness remains uncertain, except where a specific deficiency exists.

Folic acid will induce a remission in patients with folic acid deficiency anemia. Unfortunately its use in persons with pernicious anemia will effect remission of the anemia but has no therapeutic effect on the neural lesions (postero lateral sclerosis) of pernicious anemia. These can be prevented only by the use of B_{12}.

Pantothenic Acid. Another vitamin of the B group, pantothenic acid, has been shown to have an unusual influence on resistance of animals to cold stress. When given very large doses, rats could swim in cool or cold water for significantly increased periods of time, and, according to Ralli (1952) in doses of 10 Gm. a day it increased, to some extent, the tolerance of young men to immersion in extremely cold water. The significance of these findings remains obscure, but such experiments stand squarely in the way of the generalization that an excess of vitamins above the ordinary requirement is of no use. Inositol, pyridoxine, and the other members of the B group are commonly included in polyvitamin therapy, particularly for liver disease, although their importance in man under various conditions has not been completely studied as yet.

Vitamin C is of special interest to surgical patients because of its influence on wound healing. Early records of scurvy occurring among men on sailing ships refer to the fact that wounds long healed would sometimes break down. Wolbach (1932) and others confirmed the fact that a vitamin C deficiency reduces the healing strength of wounds. While the ordinary requirement is, perhaps, 50 to

Nutrition

TABLE 6-6. RECOMMENDED DAILY DIETARY ALLOWANCES*†

	AGE YEARS	VITAMIN A I.U.	THIAMINE MG.	RIBOFLAVIN MG.	NIACIN (MG. EQUIV.‡)	ASCORBIC ACID MG.	VITAMIN D I.U.
Men	25	5,000	1.4	1.7	18	60	..
	45	5,000	1.3	1.7	17	60	..
	65	5,000	1.2	1.7	14	60	..
Women	25	5,000	1.0	1.5	13	55	..
	45	5,000	1.0	1.5	13	55	..
	65	5,000	1.0	1.5	13	55	..
Pregnant		6,000	1.1	1.8	15	60	400
Lactating		8,000	1.5	2.0	20	60	400
Infants	2/12–6/12	1,500	0.4	0.5	7	35	400
	7/12–1	1,500	0.6	0.6	8	35	400
Children	1–3	2,000	0.6	0.7	8	10	400
	4–6	2,500	0.8	0.9	11	40	400
	7–9	3,500	1.1	1.2	14	40	400
	10–12	4,500	1.3	1.3	17	40	400
Boys	13–15	5,000	1.5	1.5	19	50	400
	16–19	5,000	1.6	1.6	19	60	400
Girls	13–15	5,000	1.2	1.4	16	50	400
	16–19	5,000	1.2	1.5	14	50	400

* The allowance levels are intended to cover individual variations among most normal persons as they live in the United States under usual environmental stresses. (Adapated from Cooper, L. F., Barber, E. M., Mitchell, H. S., and Rynbergen, H. J.: Nutrition in Health and Disease, Philadelphia, Lippincott, 1968.)

† Food and Nutrition Board, National Research Council Recommended Daily Dietary Allowances, Revised 1968.

‡ Niacin equivalents include dietary sources of the vitamin itself plus 1 mg. equivalent of each 60 mg. of dietary tryptophan.

100 mg. of ascorbic acid a day, very large doses such as 1,000 mg. a day are required to evoke any excretion of the vitamin during the first 2 days after a severe thermal burn (Lund). (See Chap. 2, Wound Healing.)

Recommended Daily Dietary Allowances. Obviously, the requirements of the various vitamins for health and growth are rather difficult to state. The Food and Nutrition Board in its "Recommended Daily Dietary Allowances" (1968) has backed the values shown in Table 6-6. However, in patients who are ill, it is considered that higher vitamin intakes are safer and probably useful. A special committee of the Food and Nutrition Board on therapeutic nutrition was formed to study this problem and, as a result of its deliberations, therapeutic formulas were proposed. These were thought of as possibly advantageous in patients who may have an increased need for vitamins for short periods of time. The values given are shown in Table 6-7.

Undoubtedly, vitamins are being given in a very wasteful manner. Patients who are on parenteral feedings for only a day or two probably need no vitamin supplement. Those who are on parenteral feedings for 3 to 5 days or more should receive thiamine and the B complex vitamins and vitamin C. The indications for vitamin K are special ones, and vitamins A, D and E are not required in surgical patients as a general rule.

IRON

One is often faced with problems in disturbed iron metabolism in surgery in conditions such as malnutrition, hemorrhage, malignant disease, chronic infection, hemolytic anemia, hemosiderosis from repeated transfusions, and diseases of the upper gastrointestinal tract and the liver. Our knowledge of the essential role of iron in cellular function has been increased by a number of extensive studies, and the reader is referred to these for a more detailed discussion of the subject (Drabkin, 1951; Granick, 1947; Gubler,

TABLE 6-7. VITAMIN REQUIREMENTS DURING ILLNESS OR INJURY*

	MODERATE ILLNESS OR INJURY	SEVERE ILLNESS OR INJURY
Thiamine (mg.)	2	10
Riboflavin (mg.)	2	10
Nicotinic acid (mg.)	20	100
Pantothenic acid (mg.)	18	40
Pyridoxine hydrochloride (mg.)	2	40
Folic acid (mg.)	1.5	2.5
Vitamin B$_{12}$ (mcg.)	2	4
Ascorbic acid (mg.)	75	300†
Vitamin A, I.U.	5000	5000‡
Vitamin D, I.U.	400	400‡
Vitamin K (mg.)	2	20‡§

* Adapted from "Therapeutic Nutrition With Special Reference to Military Situations," National Academy of Sciences, National Research Council, Jan., 1951.
† Up to 1,000 mg./day may be needed to cause excretion of the vitamin in a severely burned patient.
‡ Not needed in short-term therapy unless specific deficiency exists.
§ Dose for severe and resistant hypoprothrombinemia may be much higher.

1956; Hahn, 1948; Schultz, 1940; Wintrobe, 1952).

Iron plays an essential role because of its widespread distribution in hemoglobin, myoglobin and in fundamental enzyme systems such as cytochrome, catalase and peroxidase. In this way, it is indispensable for the transport and the utilization of oxygen.

The body of the average adult contains approximately 4.5 Gm. of iron, of which 60 to 70 per cent is in hemoglobin, 3 to 5 per cent in myoglobin, 0.1 per cent in essential enzyme systems, 0.1 per cent in transport in the serum, and the remainder in storage mainly in the liver, bone marrow and the spleen.

Metabolism of iron differs from that of the other electrolytes and elements in the manner in which iron is absorbed and excreted. Reutilization of iron liberated by normal disintegration of red blood cells supplies most of the iron needed for hemoglobin synthesis. The remainder is derived from storage iron, and a small fraction from recently absorbed iron. About 28 mg. is released daily, and most of this is utilized over and over again. As a result, only 0.6 to 1.5 mg. need be absorbed from the diet each day; 0.5 to 1.5 mg. is excreted daily in urine, bile, sweat and feces, which is derived entirely from the desquamation and the disintegration of cells.

McCance and Widdowson (1937) first noted that the intestines regulate the amount of iron absorbed. According to this hypothesis, called the "mucosal block theory," and given considerable experimental support by the work of Granick (1947), and Hahn (1948), the mucosal cells of the duodenum and the jejunum absorb iron in the ferrous ionic form. It is oxidized to the ferric state and combines with a protein acceptor, apoferritin, to yield ferritin, one of the storage forms of iron. When the mucosal cells become saturated, they form a barrier to further absorption until this supply is utilized. This mechanism maintains iron absorption at the fairly constant rate of 0.6 to 1.5 mg. a day when the individual is in a healthy state. However, if the need for iron is increased, the degree of absorption may be increased 5 to 15 times. Following an acute massive hemorrhage in a previously healthy person, this response does not occur for 6 or 7 days. This suggests that the body stores must first be utilized by accelerated hemopoiesis before the intestinal mucosa will respond to a reduced hemoglobin level (Gubler, 1956; Hahn, 1943). In chronic states of iron deficiency, the degree of iron absorption is increased in spite of an adequate or even excessive iron store (Dubach et al., 1948). In response to whatever the body needs may be, the ferritin in the mucosal cell releases iron in the ferrous form. It enters the blood stream, is oxidized again to the ferric state and combines with a specific B$_1$-globulin called siderophilin. By this means it is transported by the blood to the tissues for storage and utilization.

Of the total iron circulating in the blood 0.1 per cent is contained in plasma, and 99.9 per cent is in the hemoglobin of red cells. The normal whole blood content of iron is 40 to 50 mg./100 ml. and the normal serum iron level is 100 to 110 mcg./100 ml. The total iron-binding capacity (TIBC) of the serum is 300 to 350 mcg./100 ml. when siderophilin is completely saturated, and normally it is about one third saturated.

The serum iron level is lowered in iron

deficiency anemia and raised in certain other types of anemia and in conditions of iron overload. Therefore, the measurement of serum iron levels and the total and unsaturated iron-binding capacity (UIBC) are of importance. In cases of iron need, as in iron deficiency and chronic hemorrhage, the total capacity to bind iron increases, and the degree of saturation decreases markedly. On the other hand, an excess of iron in the storage depots, as in transfusional hemosiderosis, is associated with a decrease in the total iron-binding capacity and a marked increase in the degree of saturation. In infection and malignant disease the total iron-binding capacity and the serum iron are decreased, which results in a slightly decreased degree of saturation.

Iron is stored in the tissues as ferritin, mainly in the liver, bone marrow and the spleen. Some of it is released for synthesis of heme compounds as the need arises. When the capacity to store iron as ferritin is exceeded in conditions of iron overloading, it is stored as hemosiderin and can be detected microscopically with appropriate iron stains.

Due to the re-utilization of iron released from hemoglobin breakdown and the very small amount excreted, the daily requirement for a normal male is 0.8 to 1.0 mg. a day, and about twice that amount for a female. Since only 2 to 10 per cent of the oral iron intake is absorbed, the minimal daily requirement must be increased as shown in Table 6-8.

TABLE 6-8. RECOMMENDED DAILY DIETARY ALLOWANCE OF IRON*

	IRON (MG.)
Man (70 Kg.) or 154 lbs.	10
Woman (58 Kg.) or 128 lbs.	18
Pregnancy (latter half)	18
Lactation	18
Children	
1–6 months	10
7–12 months	15
1–3 years	15
4–6 years	10
7–9 years	10
10–12 years	10
Over 12 years	18

*Food and Nutrition Board, National Research Council Recommended Daily Dietary Allowances, Revised 1968.

For patients who cannot take iron by mouth, iron dextran solutions containing 50 mg. of iron per ml. can be given by deep intramuscular injection. Some of the parenteral iron preparations are quite irritating. Rare serious reactions have been reported.

OBESITY

Obesity is perhaps the commonest nutritional disease in 20th-century America. For the most part, it is due to overeating and lack of activity and will respond to dietary restriction and additional exercise. However, there are extreme cases in which weights rise to 300 to 600 pounds and dietary restriction is not accomplished even after much effort. The mechanisms by which ingested carbohydrate and fat are partitioned between stored fat and circulating dextrose are not completely understood. Some individuals feel well if they are moderately overweight and weak and lethargic if they diet.

There is a general correlation between marked obesity and elevated blood lipids and between increasing weight in an adult and blood lipids. Likewise, there is some correlation between high blood lipids, particularly cholesterol, and atherosclerosis. Certain individuals are characterized by a positive correlation between serum cholesterol concentration and the intake of soluble carbohydrates (Kuo, P. T., et al., 1967). It can be important for them to keep the latter low.

While surgical procedures often result in temporary weight loss, and some, such as total gastrectomy, often result in permanent weight loss, it is rare that surgical procedures have been employed to induce weight loss.

The procedure employed for this purpose by Troncelliti* consisted in sidetracking the greater part of the small bowel leaving a defunctionalized loop connected distally for drainage. Such a loop can be re-established as a functional part of the alimentary tract at a second operation should indications arise to do so. Troncelliti's patients weighed up to 500 pounds before operation and some have lost more than 200 pounds. The procedure is not without some risk and is still under study. (See Chapter 38, p. 1073.)

*Troncelliti, M. A.: Personal communication, 1969.

REFERENCES

Abbott, W. O., and Rawson, A. J.: A tube for use in the postoperative care of gastroenterostomy cases, J.A.M.A., 108:1873, 1937.

Allen, A. W., and Welch, C. E.: Jejunostomy for relief of malfunctioning gastroenterostomy. Surgery, 9:163, 1941.

Allen, J. G.: The diagnostic value of prothrombin response to Vitamin K therapy as a means of differentiating between intrahepatic and obstructive jaundice; collective review. Int. Abstr. Surg., 76:401, 1943.

Asteriodin-Somartzis, E., and Leikin, S.: Relation of Vitamin K to hyperbilirubinemia. Pediatrics, 21:397-402, 1958.

Beeson, P. B., Muschenheim, C., Castle, W. B., Harrison, T. R., Ingelfinger, F. J., and Bondy, P. K.: Year Book of Medicine. 1959-1960 Series. p. 687. Chicago, 1959.

Bockus, H. L.: Gastroenterology. Philadelphia, W. B. Saunders, 1949.

Brunschwig, A. D., Clark, D. E., and Corbin, N.: Symposium on abdominal surgery: postoperative nitrogen loss and studies on parenteral nitrogen nutrition by means of casein digest. Ann. Surg., 115:1091, 1942.

Coller, F. A., Campbell, K. N., Vaughn, H. H., Iob, V., and Moyer, C. A.: Postoperative salt intolerance. Ann. Surg., 119:533-541, 1944a.

Coller, F. A., Crook, C. E., and Iob, V.: Blood loss in surgical operations. J.A.M.A., 126:1, 1944b.

Cuthbertson, D. P.: Further observations on the disturbance of metabolism caused by injury, with particular reference to the dietary requirements of fracture cases. Brit. J. Surg., 23:505, 1936.

Dam, H.: Hemorrhages in chicks reared on artificial diets; new deficiency disease. Nature, 133:909, 1934.

Drabkin, D. L.: Metabolism of the hemin chromoproteins. Physiol. Rev., 31:345, 1951.

Dubach, R., Callender, S. T. E., and Moore, C. V.: Studies in iron transportation and metabolism; absorption of radioactive iron in patients with fever and anemias of varied etiology. Blood, 3:526-540, 1948.

Dudrick, S. J., Wilmore, D. W., and Vars, H. M.: Total intravenous feeding and growth in puppies. Fed. Proc., 25:481, 1966.

Dudrick, S. J., Wilmore, D. W., Vars, H. M., and Rhoads, J. E.: Can intravenous feeding as the sole means of nutrition support growth in the child and restore weight loss in an adult? An affirmative answer. Ann. Surg., 169:974, 1969.

Dumm, M. E., and Ralli, E. P.: The critical requirements for pantothenic acid by the adrenalectomized rat. Endocrinology, 43:283, 1948.

Ebeling, W. W.: Absorption of dextrose from the colon. Arch. Surg., 26:134, 1933.

Edsal, D. L., and Miller, C. W.: Study of two cases nourished exclusively per rectum; with a determination of absorption nitrogen metabolism and intestinal putrefaction. Tr. Coll. Physicians, Philadelphia, 24:225, 1902.

Fine, J., and Gendel, S.: Plasma transfusion in experimental intestinal obstruction. Ann. Surg., 112:976, 1940.

Food and Nutrition Board, National Research Council: Recommended Daily Dietary Allowances, revised 1958. Publication No. 589.

Frazier, W. D., and Ravdin, I. S.: The use of vitamin B_1 in the preoperative preparation of the hyperthyroid patient. Surgery, 4:680, 1938.

Gell, P. G. H.: Discussion on nutrition and resistance to infection. Proc. Roy. Soc. Med., 41:323, 1948.

Granick, S.: Iron and porphyrin metabolism in relation to red blood cells. Ann. N. Y. Acad. Sci., 48:657, 1947.

Gubler, C. J.: Absorption and metabolism of iron. Science, 123:87, 1956.

Hahn, P. F.: Metabolism of iron. Fed. Proc., 7:493, 1948.

Hahn, P. F., et al.: Radioactive iron absorption by gastrointestinal tract; influence of anemia, anoxia, and antecedent feeding distribution in growing dogs. J. Exp. Med., 78:169, 1943.

Hirshfeld, J. W., Williams, H. H., Abbott, W. E., Heller, C. G., and Pilling, M. A.: Significance of nitrogen loss in exudate from surface burns. Surgery, 15:766, 1944.

Howard, J. E., Parson, W., Stein, K. E., Eisenberg H., and Reidt, V.: Studies on fracture convalescence: I. Nitrogen metabolism after fracture and skeletal operations in healthy males. Bull. Johns Hopkins Hosp., 75:156, 1944.

Jones, C. M., and Eaton, F. B.: Postoperative nutritional edema. Arch. Surg., 27:159, 1933.

Jones, C. M., Eaton, F. B., and White, J. C.: Experimental postoperative edema. Arch. Int. Med., 53:649-674, 1934.

Keys, A. B., Brozek, J., Henschel, A., Mickelson, O., and Raylor, H. L.: The Biology of Human Starvation. vol. 2. p. 1006. Minneapolis, Univ. Minnesota Press, 1950.

Kuo, P. T., Feng, L., Cohen, N. N., Fitts, W. T., and Miller, L. D.: Dietary carbohydrates in hyperlipemia. Am. J. Clin. Nutr., 20:116, 1967.

Lehr, H. B., Rhoads, J. E., Rosenthal, O., and Blakemore, W. S.: The use of intravenous fat emulsions in surgical patients. J.A.M.A., 181:745-749, 1962.

McCance, R. A., and Widdowson, E. M.: Absorption and secretion of iron. Lancet, 2:680, 1937.

Machella, T. E.: The mechanism of the postgastrectomy "dumping" syndrome. Tr. Am. Clin. Climat. A., 60 (1948), 206-231, (1949).

Mecray, P. M., Barden, R. P., and Ravdin, I. S.: Nutritional edema; its effect on gastric emptying time before and after gastric operations. Surgery, 1:53, 1937.

Mellinkoff, S. M., Machella, T. E., and Reinhold, J. G.: The effect of a fat-free diet in causing low serum cholesterol. Am. J. Med. Sci., 220:203, 1950.

Meltzer, L. E., Bockman, A. A., and Berryman, G. H.: A means of lowering elevated blood cholesterol levels in patients with previous myocardial infarction. Am. J. Med. Sci., 236:595, 1958.

Miller, B. J., Gibbson, J. H., Jr., and Allbritten, F. F., Jr.: Blood volume and extracellular fluid changes during thoracic operations. J. Thoracic Surg., 18: 605, 1949.

Pommerenke, W. T., Slavin, H. B., Kariher, D. N., and Whipple, G. H.: Dog plasma protein by vein utilized in body metabolism of dog. J. Exper. Med., 61:261, 283, 1935.

Ralli, E. P.: The effect of certain nutritional factors on the reactions produced by acute stress in human subjects. Recent Advances in Nutrition Research. Nutritional Symposium Series 5, 78, Aug., 1952.

Ravdin, I. S.: Factors involved in the retardation of gastric emptying after gastric operations. Pennsylvania M. J., 41:695, 1938.

Ravdin, I. S., Johnston, C. G., and Morrison, P. J.: Comparison of concentration of glucose in the stomach and intestines after intragastric administration. Proc. Soc. Exp. Biol. Med., 30:955, 1933.

Ravdin, I. S., McNamee, H. G., Kamholz, J. H., and Rhoads, J. E.: Effect of hypoproteinemia on susceptibility to shock resulting from hemorrhage. Arch. Surg., 48:491, 1944.

Rhoads, J. E., Fliegelman, M. T., and Panzer, L. M.: The mechanism of delayed wound healing in the presence of hypoproteinemia. J.A.M.A., 118:21-25, 1942.

Rhoads, J. E., and Lehr, H. B.: Intravenous nutrition with fat emulsions (Presented before Fifth International Congress on Nutrition, Session on Lipids: Man II 9/3/60, Washington, D. C.).

Rhoads, J. E., Rawnsley, H. M., Vars, H. M., Crichlow, R. W., Nelson, H. M., Spagna, P. M., Dudrick, S. J., and Rhoads, J. E., Jr.: The use of diuretics as an adjuvant in parenteral hyperalimentation for surgical patients with prolonged disability of the gastrointestinal tract. Bull. Soc. Int. Chir., 1:59-70, 1965.

Rhoads, J. E., Stengel, A., Riegel, C., Cajori, F. A., and Frazier, W. D.: Absorption of protein split products from chronic isolated colon loops. Am. J. Physiol., 125:707, 1939.

Riegel, C., Koop, C. E., Drew, J., Stevens, L. W., and Rhoads, J. E.: The nutritional requirements for nitrogen balance in surgical patients in the early postoperative period. J. Clin. Invest., 26:18, 1947.

Rosenthal, O., Stainback, W. C., Rhoads, J. E., and Engelberg, J.: The utilization of invert sugar and glucose following intravenous administration to postoperative patients. S. Forum, 3:585-589, 1953.

Schecter, A. E., Wiesel, B. H., and Cohn, C.: Peripheral circulatory failure in diabetic acidosis and its relationship to treatment, Am. J. Med. Sci., 202: 364, 1941.

Schultz, M. O.: Metallic elements and blood formation. Physiol. Rev., 20:37, 1940.

Scott, S. M., and Vars, H. M.: Response of animals with biliary fistula, bile duct occlusion, or chloroform intoxication to parenteral fat feeding. S. Forum, 5:350-354, 1955.

Seibert, F. B.: Fever producing substances found in some distilled water. Am. J. Physiol., 67:90, 1923-4.

Thompson, W. D., Ravdin, I. S., and Frank, I. L.: Effect of hypoproteinemia on wound disruption. Arch. Surg., 36:500, 1938.

Warner, E. D., Brinkhous, K. M., and Smith, H. P.: Bleeding tendency of obstructive jaundice, Proc. Soc. Exp. Biol. Med., 37:628, 1938.

Warren, R., and Rhoads, J. E., Hepatic origin of the plasma-prothrombin observations after total hepatectomy in the dog. Am. J. Med. Sci., 198:193, 1939.

Whipple, G. H.: Protein production and exchange in the body, including hemoglobin, plasma protein, and cell protein. Am. J. Med. Sci., 196:609, 1938.

Wilmore, D. W., and Dudrick, S. J.: Growth and development of an infant receiving all nutrients exclusively by vein. J.A.M.A., 203:860, 1968.

———: Safe long term venous catheterization. Arch. Surg., 98:256, 1969.

Wintrobe, M. M.: Clinical Hematology. Philadelphia, Lea & Febiger, 1952.

Wohl, M. G., Reinhold, J. G., and Rose, S. B.: Antibody response in patients with hypoproteinemia. Arch. Int. Med., 83:402, 1949.

Wolbach, S. B., and Howe, P. R.: Intercellular substances in experimental scorbutus. Arch. Path. & Lab. Med., 1:1-24, 1936.

Zollinger, R. M., and Ellison, E. H.: Nutrition in surgical patients. GP, 2:37, 1950.

CHAPTER 7

HENRY M. HARKINS,* M.D., AND
JONATHAN E. RHOADS, M.D.

Shock

Introduction
Definitions
History
Etiology
   Experimental Studies
   Initiating Factors
Accompanying and Perpetuating Factors
Irreversibility
Diagnosis
Therapy: Experimental Approaches
Clinical Treatment
Summary

INTRODUCTION

In its broader sense, shock includes all states in which there is a progressive decompensation of the transport mechanisms serving body cells generally.

These mechanisms are the airways, alveolar membranes, the lesser circulation, the heart, the systemic circulation, the capillary walls, interstitial fluid, and perhaps the cell walls.

If the blockage to the ingress of oxygen and the egress of carbon dioxide is in the respiratory tract, it is called anoxic or hypoxic shock. If it results from failure of the heart to circulate blood rapidly enough, it is called cardiac shock. If it is due to a lack of sufficient blood to pump, it is called hypovolemic shock, and it is this form of shock which is of particular importance in surgical patients and will be the central concern of this chapter.

Interference with the exchange of oxygen and other metabolites from the capillaries to the living cells is not a well defined entity, as a systemic condition, but may enter into the complex picture known as septic shock.

Relaxation of vascular tone due to changes in sympathetic nervous regulation, as seen in fainting, affects the distribution of the circulating blood and is especially a phenomenon of man related to his erect posture. Treatment is mainly to return him to a recumbent position in which his long axis is parallel to level ground (or better, a partially head-down position).

Interference with the sympathetic nervous mechanisms can also be caused by drugs such as morphine, which profoundly alters the capacity of normal volunteers to withstand the tilt-test (Drew, Dripps and Conroe, 1946).

Shock is a general phenomenon and the term is not used to describe localized circulatory disturbances such as ischemia of the foot due to atherosclerosis in the femoral artery. This is not to say that a localized disturbance of the circulatory system may not be severe enough to cause shock in the true general sense and examples of this will be cited later.

Septic shock, or its experimental counterpart, endotoxin shock, may not seem to fall very neatly into this classification, and to what extent it may be an actual intracellular poisoning is probably unknown. It is clear from clinical observation that it may reduce peripheral resistance, with a lowering of blood pressure, and may produce fever with an increase in oxygen requirement and a corresponding increase in the need to remove carbon dioxide. Eventually it leads to oxygen debt, decreased cardiac output and death.

Crowell and Smith (1964) measured various forms of shock in terms of oxygen debt per Kg. of body weight and found that, if this accumulates to 120 cc. per Kg., the process was usually irreversible even when vigorous treatment was instituted at that point.

* Deceased.

There is no doubt that as shock progresses, a point comes beyond which recovery is impossible even though the patient is still alive and has not necessarily even lost consciousness. The surgical problem is to devise and institute treatment which in proportion to the physical insult will shift the point of irreversibility to the advantage of the patient.

Thus, the average experimental animal or patient can survive approximately twice as large an area of burn with treatment as with none. If, in contrast to quantifying the extent of the injury, one defines the injury in terms of the oxygen deficit, treatment may appear to be unavailing. This line of thought, however, would miss the fact that the treatment, instituted early, could prevent the oxygen deficit from rising to critical levels. In this chapter, therefore, we are more interested in evaluating treatment in terms of the extent of the injury as seen clinically rather than in biochemical terms.

DEFINITIONS

The evolution of ideas concerning shock is shown by the following definitions:

"Shock is a species of functional concussion by which the influence of the brain over the organ of circulation is deranged or suspended."—Travers (1826).

"A manifestation of a rude unhinging of the machinery of life."—Gross (1850).

"Peripheral circulatory failure resulting from a discrepancy in the size of the vascular bed and the volume of intravascular fluid."—Minot and Blalock (1940).

"A progressive vasoconstrictive oligemic anoxia."—Harkins (1940).

"Wound shock may be defined broadly as the clinical manifestations of an inadequate volume of circulating blood accompanied by physiologic adjustments of the organism to a progressive discrepancy between the capacity of the arterial tree and the volume of blood available to fill it."—Simeone (1953).

"Hypovolemic shock is an acute reaction to a rapidly reduced volume of circulating blood."—J. Garrott Allen (1955).

"A state of profound depression of the vital processes of the body. . . . The total blood volume is reduced. . . . Shock occurs as a result of extensive wounds, hemorrhage, crushing injuries . . . etc."—Webster's New International Dictionary of the English Language, ed. 2, Unabridged (1959).

"Shock—conceived broadly—is a decompensation of the transport mechanism serving body cells generally." (Rhoads, 1969).

Because of the rapid nature of the development of the hypovolemic shock syndrome, it is less often encountered in nonsurgical patients. An exception to this may be the sudden loss of large amounts of plasma-like fluid into the lungs in certain instances of pneumonia (Andrews and Harkins, 1937).

Definition by example may be helpful. The following patient seen over 25 years ago before the use of adequate blood replacement was recognized is illustrative:

J. J., a college student aged 21 years, was run over one morning by a truck, and both legs were severely crushed. He became temporarily unconscious but was able to talk on the way to the hospital. Three broken bones were easily set; there was no visible bleeding, and after taking a sedative he felt well enough to smile and appeared to be on the road to recovery. In the afternoon, however, he became restless; his face showed an anxious expression, with pallor; his pulse became weak and rapid, his skin cold and clammy and his breathing labored and shallow, he sank into coma despite a 500 ml. blood tranfusion and, toward evening, died.

This boy died of shock. Such injuries are accompanied by large concealed hemorrhages possibly of 1 to 3 liters of blood with additional movement of large amounts of interstitial fluid. It is generally said that it takes withdrawal of more than 20 per cent of the blood volume to cause a reduction in blood pressure in recumbent men who were previously normal. The same presumably applies to loss of whole blood or plasma during surgical operations, as a result of burns, and following other types of trauma.

HISTORY

The history of shock can be divided into 2 periods. The first, or qualitative period, includes the years up to about 1930, during which the physiologic and pathologic changes accompanying shock were demonstrated and correlated. During this first period there was a beginning awareness of the advisability of blood

FIG. 7-1. Diagrammatic representation of classical hindquarter weight comparison experiment of Blalock and of Phemister following unilateral traumatic shock.

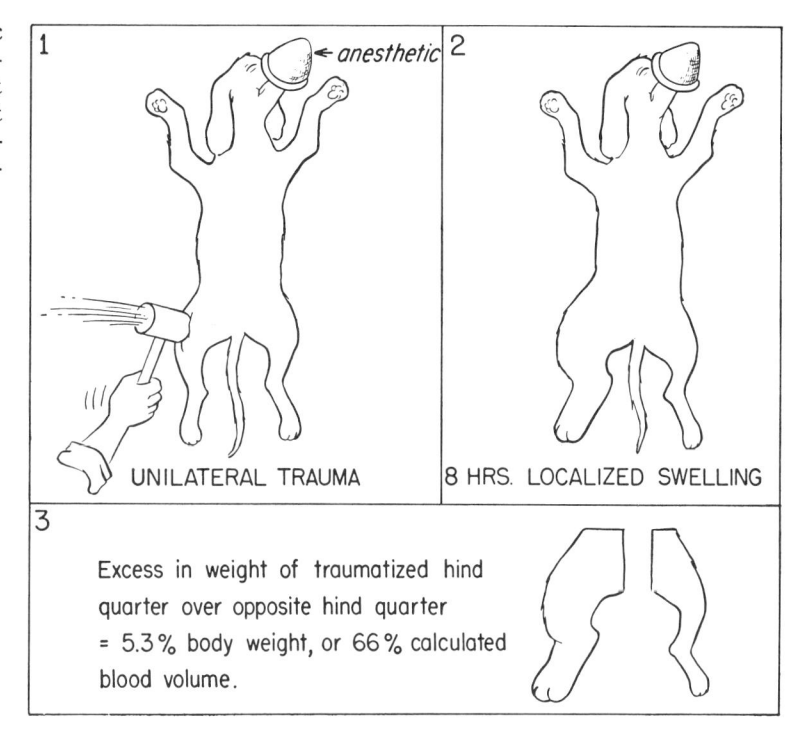

1 ← anesthetic 2

UNILATERAL TRAUMA | 8 HRS. LOCALIZED SWELLING

3 Excess in weight of traumatized hind quarter over opposite hind quarter = 5.3% body weight, or 66% calculated blood volume.

transfusions, but this awareness was more qualitative than quantitative and usually was satisfied by giving one pint.

The publications of Blalock (1930) and of Phemister (Parsons and Phemister, 1930), working independently, can be selected arbitrarily as ushering in the second or quantitative period in the history of shock. These authors applied mechanical trauma to one hind limb of anesthetized dogs so that shock and death resulted. At necropsy there was extensive swelling of the traumatized limb, and the amount of swelling as measured by hind-quarter amputation and comparison of the weight of the traumatized and opposite untraumatized limbs was essentially enough to account for death of the animal (Fig. 7-1). This quantitative observation was based on a further comparison of this weight difference with the amount of bleeding necessary to cause death in dogs of similar size. Finally, the excess fluid which was present in the swollen limb was found to be a mixture of extracellular fluid, blood and plasma and was not just water.

The whole modern blood and plasma bank program is based on the quantitative concept brought out by these papers. Next to the conquest of pain (by anesthesia) and of infection (by antisepsis, asepsis and by antibiotics) one of the greatest advances in surgery has been the advance in the control of surgical and traumatic shock. It is of great historical interest that this same experiment later performed by Blalock and by Phemister was reported by Cannon and Bayliss in 1919. Because of the terrific number of casualties occurring in the Allied Troops in World War I, a Joint Commission headed by two of the leading physiologists of the world, Walter B. Cannon of Harvard, representing the United States, and William M. Bayliss of London, representing Great Britain, performed the 1919 experiment. On the basis of their interpretation of this jointly performed experiment, they concluded that local fluid loss could not be the major factor in the production of shock. Because of the authority of these two great men, this view held sway until 1930 when Blalock and Phemister showed that a simple error had been made in setting up the terms of the experiment and that, when correctly performed, the logical conclusion follows that fluid loss is a major factor in the production of shock. This incident is recited, not to cast doubt on the experimental abilities of these two workers in the 1917-1919 Joint Commission on Shock (the writer of these pages (H. N. H.) believed them to be two of the greatest physiologists of all time), but rather to point out the hazard of blindly accepting an authoritarian statement which held back progress in the understanding of shock for over half of the period between the two world wars.

ETIOLOGY

Hypovolemic Shock—Experimental Studies on Etiology

Acute hemorrhage is the most direct cause of hypovolemia and, hence, of shock. Small hemorrhages are easily compensated for by normal individuals, but a sudden loss of 7 to 10 per cent of the circulating blood frequently causes faintness when the erect position is abruptly assumed. Blood pressure may not drop much until 20 per cent of the blood volume is removed if the individual remains in the supine position. Pulse rate may actually slow rather than accelerate under these conditions (Shenkin et al., 1944).

Dehydration is a direct cause of loss of blood volume. As set forth in Chapter 5, Moyer et al. (1967) believe that within normal limits the loss of 1 L. of water from the body reduces blood volume by about 75 ml.

Hyponatremia is a much more important factor in reducing blood volume. Moyer and associates found that the loss of 100 mEq. of Na resulted in a blood volume reduction of 115 ml. in an average adult.

Hypoproteinemia predisposed to shock in dogs, as demonstrated in the experiments of Ravdin, McNamee, Kamholz and Rhoads (1944).

Any of these last three factors, or a combination of them, may constitute a predisposing factor for hemorrhagic shock.

The role of pain and fear, in short, of sympathetic stimulation—was emphasized by Walter Cannon (1915). Freeman (1933) measured the effect of these factors on peripheral blood flow and on plasma volume by plethysmography. He later showed that the sympathectomized dog could withstand hypotension better than could the normal, but that such animals bled smaller amounts in reaching the predetermined B.P. level.

Also, he showed that fatal shock could be induced in dogs by a prolonged intravenous infusion of epinephrine (Freeman, Freedman and Miller, 1941). It was Freeman's thesis that, with severe vasoconstriction in peripheral areas, sufficient anoxia would develop in these tissues to cause incompetency of capillary walls (Landis, 1928) and losses of fluid from the circulation.

The use of a constant low B.P. end point as a shock model gained popularity through the studies of Jacob Fine and his associates (Fine, 1954). When a major artery such as the femoral is connected to a reservoir set at a height corresponding to a central arterial pressure of 30 mm. of mercury, the animal pumps blood into the reservoir until his arterial pressure is reduced to this level. As additional fluid and plasma protein are mobilized from body stores, additional increments may be pumped into the reservoir. After an hour or two, as shock develops, the animal is automatically transfused from the reservoir—but never enough to raise the blood pressure above 30. Eventually all of the blood will run back from the reservoir, but the animal will die anyway (the phenomenon of irreversibility). Reservoir blood remaining after a stated interval of time (e.g., 2 hours) or after a 30 per cent uptake may be rapidly retransfused in order to obtain percentage mortality rates suitable for experimental study.

This technic has the advantage over bleeding a fixed percentage of body weight, in that it compensates for pre-existing hypovolemia. However, in Freeman's experiments it did not compensate for loss of the sympathetic nervous system, and one can hypothesize that it may not compensate for variations in the responsiveness of the sympathetic systems of different individuals.

Suffice it to say that, although controlled hemorrhagic hypotension is a most useful experimental procedure for the study of shock, great caution must be exercised in applying what is learned in the laboratory, by its use, to shock-like states encountered in clinical practice.

Tourniquet shock results when arterial flow and venous return to one or more limbs is occluded for a period of several hours and the tourniquet is then removed. Death ensues. Fluid loss into the ischemic limb is probably sufficient to account for it.

Pounding of tissues without producing gross hemorrhage (Fig. 7-1) may also produce fatal shock. A variant of this technique is "drum shock" produced by tumbling a rat, whose legs are taped, inside a drum rotating on its axle.

INITIATING FACTORS

Clinical conditions in which shock may occur are primarily surgical but may include certain medical conditions. Essentially, they include situations in which the blood volume may be lowered rapidly, particularly by loss of whole blood or plasma, or loss of water containing sodium ions.

1. "HEMORRHAGIC SHOCK"—e.g., externally from a lacerated vessel, or internally into a free cavity, as from a ruptured spleen or ectopic pregnancy. An example of fatal postoperative intraperitoneal hemorrhage treated 30 years ago is shown in Figure 7-2. (See also the review of shock by Harkins, 1941.) Extensive retroperitoneal hemorrhage is another condition which, when encountered at operation or necropsy, was, according to Cushman (1953), "usually . . . reported as an uncommon and puzzling condition in which loss of blood had not been suspected."

It has been stated that hemorrhage and shock are separate entities because the former is not accompanied by hemoconcentration while the latter is. As shown in Figure 7-3, this is not a differentiating factor, and the extent of hemoconcentration merely depends on the proportions of blood cells and plasma lost and upon the adjustments that the body is able to make after the loss. To show how at one time it was erroneously believed that hemorrhage and shock are completely discrete, the following quotation is taken from Gross (1882):

In shock [in contradistinction to hemorrhage], the same effect [death] may happen, and yet the body be literally surcharged with blood, not a single drop, perhaps, having been spilled in the accident causing the fatal result.

2. "TRAUMATIC SHOCK"—e.g., crushed thigh after automobile accident (see case history, p. 122). In such instances the loss is of whole blood, interstitial fluid and also of some plasma. In 1937, Harkins and Roome presented 10 clinical traumatic cases with quantitative measurements of the injured parts indicating that the "concealed hemorrhage" pres-

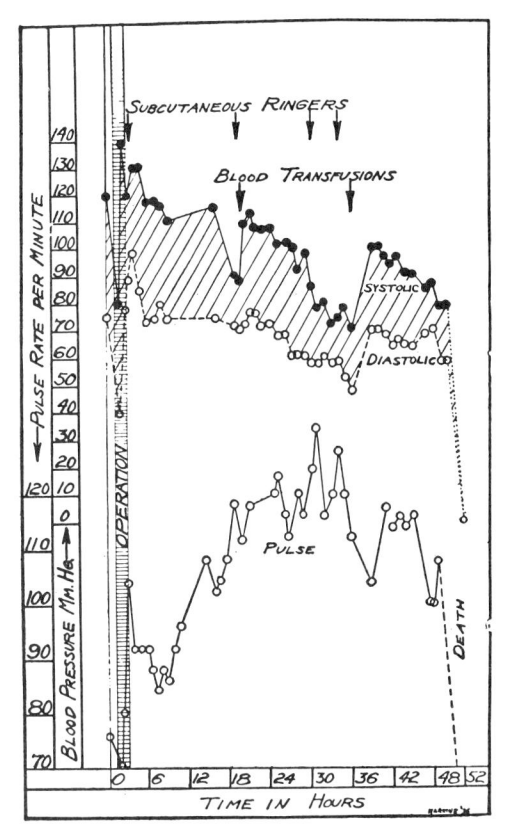

FIG. 7-2. Inadequacy of observation of fall in blood pressure in diagnosis of shock due to hemorrhage. In this patient with malignancy of the head of the pancreas, marked jaundice, and postoperative bleeding into the peritoneal cavity, treated before the days of vitamin K, it is seen that the fall in blood pressure was not a perfect guide to the seriousness of the condition until shortly before death. The increase in pulse rate was a much better guide early, but its late improvement was deceiving. (Harkins, H. N.: Surgery, 9:268)

ent was (1) far greater than casual inspection would indicate and (2) large enough to be of definite significance as a causative factor in the resultant shock.

3. "SURGICAL OR OPERATIVE SHOCK." Such cases are in the main a variety of hemorrhagic shock. Formerly, surgical shock was chiefly attributed by many authors to the reflex phenomena that follow handling of intestines. Now it is generally recognized that underestimated blood loss at the time of operation is the usual

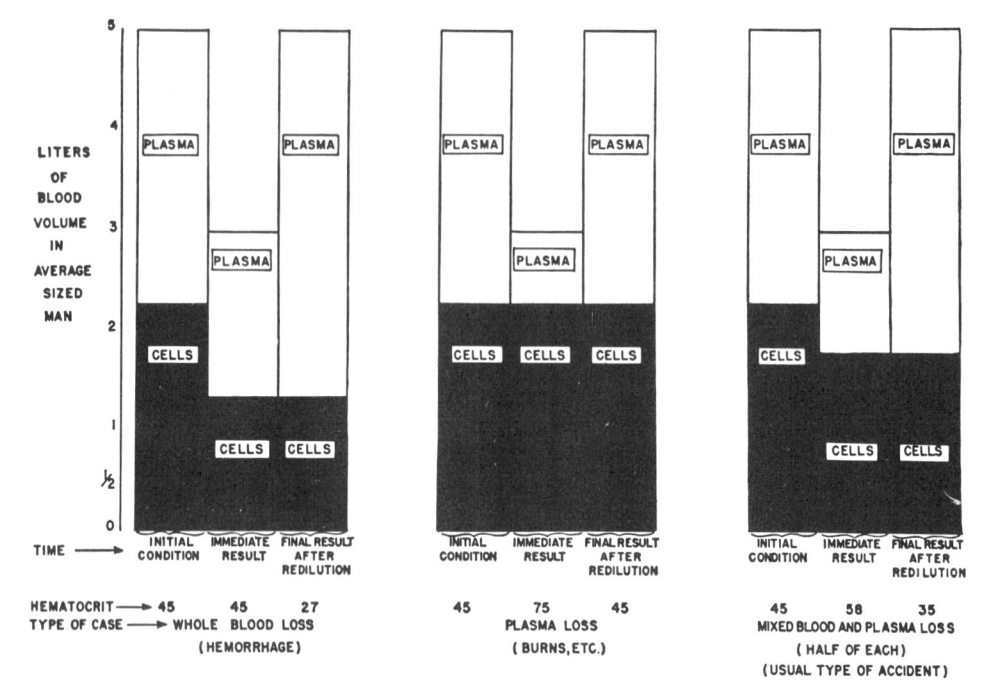

CHART DEMONSTRATING SIX POSSIBLE RESULTS IN SHOCK CASES AND THE FALLACY OF USING HEMOCONCENTRATION AS THE ONLY GUIDE TO TREATMENT

FIG. 7-3. Hemoconcentration and shock. The variability in blood concentration in various types of shock is shown graphically. The chart demonstrates the fallacy of using hemoconcentration as the only guide to treatment. (Harkins, N. H.: Survey, 9:258)

causative factor. Gatch and Little (1924) determined the blood loss during surgical operations by testing the sheets, sponges, etc., and found it greater than was anticipated (mastectomy, 710 ml.; nephrectomy, 816 ml.; laminectomy, 672 ml., etc.). They advised the transfusion of as much as 3 liters of blood to counteract the blood loss attending operation.

Coller and Maddock (1932) confirmed Gatch's observations and concluded:

In general, the operator is surprised to find the blood loss as high as calculated, since he does not think of the gauze sponge as absorbing much blood. . . . It is probable that most surgeons underestimate the amount of blood lost, especially in operations . . . in which wide areas of the body are uncovered with many small points of hemorrhage, control of which is attempted by gauze packing.

One patient upon whom radical mastectomy was performed under nitrous oxide-oxygen anesthesia lost 1,272 ml. of blood.

In patients with tuberculosis subjected to thoracoplasty, Allbritten, Lipshutz, Miller and Gibbon (1950 found not only that such individuals were admitted with a low blood volume to begin with (hence, a "predisposing factor" to shock was present), but that they lost considerable blood with each stage of the thoracoplasty. The blood loss from a single stage of the procedure was as much as 1,407 ml. (as determined by weighing the sponges) or 1,558 ml. (as determined in the patient by the dye method). This important subject has been analyzed with exactly the same conclusions by Coller, Crook and Iob (1944), Bonica and Lyter (1951), Engberg (1956), Borden (1957), Williams and Parsons (1958), and Cáceres and Whittembury (1959). Ditzler and Eckenhoff (1956) reported that controlled hypotension definitely reduces blood loss in standard surgical procedures. Thus the average total blood loss in the controlled hypotension cases as opposed to control patients was as follows: radical dissections of the neck, 910 and 1,415 ml., respectively; radical dissection within the pelvis 1,870 and 2,805 ml., respectively.

4. "BURN SHOCK." (See Chap. 17, Burns, and also Chap. 8, Blood Transfusions and Related Problems.)

5. MISCELLANEOUS CAUSES OF SHOCK. These include intestinal strangulation (Barnett, Truett, Williams and Crowell, 1963), release of a tourniquet that has been in place for several hours, mesenteric vascular occlusion, bile peritonitis, freezing, acute pancreatitis, certain acute pneumonias, irritant war gas (e.g., phosgene [carbonyl chloride, $(COCl_2)$]) poisoning, etc. Concomitant water and salt loss is commonly considered to be a cause of shock but must be fairly severe to produce it in the absence of other factors (see Chap. 5, Fluid and Electrolytes).

ACCOMPANYING AND PERPETUATING FACTORS

If one accepts hypovolemia as the primary disturbance in the surgical types of shock, one may list other changes as secondary to the reduced blood volume. Table 7-1 lists a series

TABLE 7-1. ACCOMPANYING PATHOLOGIC PHYSIOLOGIC FACTORS IN HYPOVOLEMIC SHOCK

1. Decreased cardiac output
2. Decreased peripheral blood flow
3. Fall in peripheral arterial pressure
4. Fall in central venous pressure
5. Sympathetic overactivity
6. Vasoconstriction
7. Lowered urinary output
8. Hypocapnia
9. Hypoxia
10. Decreased metabolism
11. Lactacidemia
12. Parenchymatous tissue damage

of pathologic physiologic changes that are dependent upon the hypovolemia and may disappear once the hypovolemia is corrected. In the early phases of shock, while the cardiac output is still only moderately reduced, the heart rate is usually normal, at least if the patient is lying down. Later, when the hypovolemia has advanced to such a degree that the cardiac output is much increased, tachycardia or even bradycardia may ensue. Shenkin and associates (1944) studied human volunteers following bleeding of 1 liter or more.

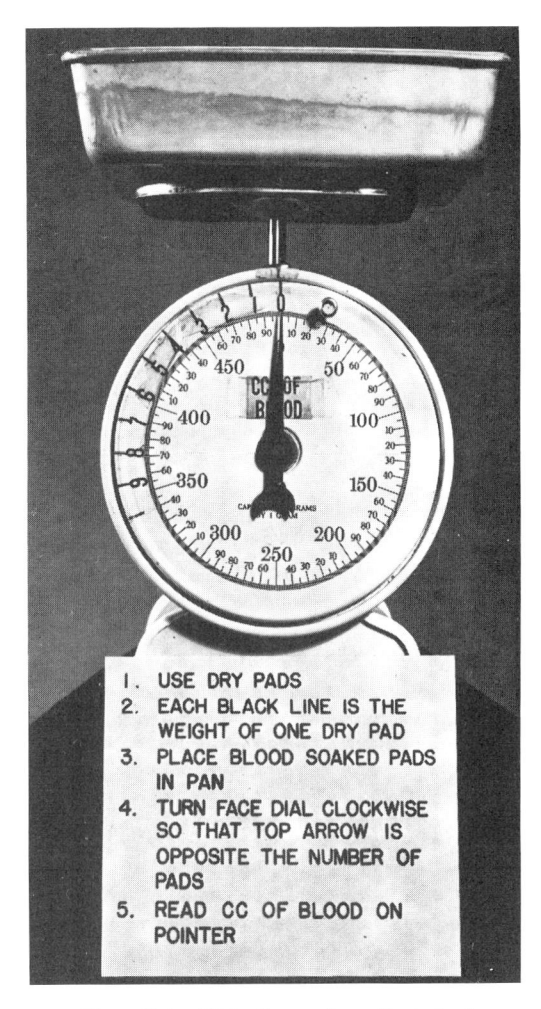

FIG. 7-4. Diabetic scale adjusted for weight of dry sponges, with a metal instrument pan (8 by 8 by 2 in.) fastened to the weighing platform. (Dr. H. C. Saltzstein, Detroit)

They observed that in the recumbent position, the pulse rate and blood pressure tended to remain normal, whereas, if the patient became erect, the blood pressure fell, and the pulse became rapid in early cases and slow in patients with severe symptoms. On the other hand, even when recumbent, almost all the subjects demonstrated a significant fall in cardiac output as determined by ballistocardiographic tracings. These authors concluded:

that the slowing of the pulse was more common than acceleration greatly surprised us. In subjects first seen after the event, the hemorrhage could never have been diagnosed from the pulse rate. ... The old concept that acute hemorrhage can be readily diagnosed by a rapid pulse and a low blood pressure is erroneous.

As stated above, bradycardia may occur early. However, tachycardia is generally considered to be characteristic of shock and, when it occurs, results from a reflex cardiac mechanism according to Marey's law, whereby it is activated by the lowered arterial pressure.

Additional factors include the increased sympathico-adrenal activity brought on reflexly by the carotid sinus and aortic reflexes and by direct action of the excitement associated with the injury. The heart rate may not be as closely associated with the degree of shock as is the blood pressure and, furthermore, bradycardia may occur in the terminal stages of fatal shock. The relationship of some of these factors was correlated by Zweifach, Lee, Hyman and Chambers (1944).

Reasons for not depending too much on a blood pressure fall alone in the diagnosis of shock, particularly at the operating table, are as follows: (1) It is generally a late sign, especially in the horizontal position. (2) A compensatory hypertension may result, especially in the young patient (Howard, 1953). (3) Anesthesia hypercapnia may induce such vasoconstriction as to mask the shock hypotension. (4) The anesthetist may have given vasospastic drugs which also may mask the shock hypotension.

In their interesting studies of a Wiggers-type preparation, Schenk, Camp, Kjartansson and Pollock (1964) pointed out that this "bleed-wait-reinfuse" type of experiment has few clinical parallels. Furthermore, they showed that, with relatively smaller hemorrhages in dogs, yet with a 40 per cent reduction in blood volume, homeostatic mechanisms maintained the arterial blood pressure and the blood flow in the renal and the coronary arteries at the same time that there was a marked shift of flow away from the hind limb somatic area.

The spleen contracts when shock due to hemorrhage occurs. This contraction represents a protective mechanism, the spleen serving as a blood reservoir in case of accident. In dogs (Lewis, Werle and Wiggers, 1942) the amount of contraction may be over 50 per cent of the control volume, but in human beings it is unlikely that it often exceeds 100 ml., the spleen being relatively smaller in the human patient.

The lack of blood in the vascular bed is contributory to the decreased cardiac output. As the cardiac output decreases, the peripheral blood flow tends to decrease also, and this tendency is accentuated by peripheral vasoconstriction. A fall in blood pressure, particularly in young patients, may be a late occurrence and hence is a relatively poor early diagnostic sign of shock. So long as the blood pressure is maintained at reasonable levels despite the decreased cardiac output, the vasopressor activity must not only be intact but possibly exaggerated. The vasoconstriction that exists in hypovolemic shock may be considered as practically maximal. Therefore, vasoconstrictor agents such as ephedrine, Neosynephrine, epinephrine, and even levorotatory norepinephrine should not be depended upon for definitive treatment, and reliance upon them may delay the introduction of appropriate fluid replacement. Watts (1956) found a significant rise in blood epinephrine levels (up to 37 μg/L.) during hemorrhagic shock in dogs. In fact, use of the vasoconstrictors to treat hypovolemic shock has been shown to be deleterious, especially to the kidney, and to reduce blood volume further by inducing a flux of plasma out of the blood stream.

Associated with the early decrease in cardiac output coupled with vasoconstriction during this period, the volume flow of blood shows a marked early decrease. Gesell (1919 a, b) studied the effects of hemorrhage and of intestinal trauma on the volume flow of blood through the submaxillary gland of the dog. He found that a decrease in blood volume of less than 10 per cent produced by hemorrhage may elicit a decreased flow of blood through the submaxillary gland of more than 60 per cent even though accompanied by a rise in blood pressure. Changes of similar nature and degree were produced by intestinal manipulation. Gesell and Moyle (1922) found that hemorrhage produces a similar decrease in blood flow through the striated muscle of the dog. Sometimes the early decrease in minute volume flow can be detected by determining how long it takes finger pressure pallor on the skin of the patient to return to the color of the surrounding skin. The decrease in minute volume flow also applies to the coronary arteries (Edwards, Siegel and Bing, 1954).

The hypocapnia present in shock is a result of reflexly stimulated overbreathing. The hypoxia, decreased metabolism and accompanying lactacidemia together are results of the decreased circulation. One of the effects of anoxia is to increase capillary permeability. Landis (1928) showed by quantitative experiments on single capillaries of the frog mesentery that, immediately after a 3-minute period of oxygen lack, fluid filters through the capillary wall at approximately 4 times the normal rate. The increased permeability of the wall permitted also the passage of protein, thus reducing the effective osmotic pressure of the plasma proteins in these particular experiments to almost one half their normal value.

Metabolic acidosis (Artz and Fitts, 1962) is an important feature in severe shock. This factor may be treated by sodium bicarbonate (Smith and Moore, 1962), or by tris hydroxymethyl aminomethane (THAM) which supposedly elevates the intracellular as well as the extracellular pH (Nelson, Poulson, Lyman and Henry, 1963; Selmonosky, Goetz and State, 1963). In both instances, however, such treatment alone is not sufficient to relieve the shock syndrome.

McClure, Hartman, Schnedorf and Schelling (1939) pointed out that anoxic anoxia occurring during general anesthesia, particularly with nitrous oxide, is apt to produce tissue damage. Not only will this increase the tendency to shock but also it may leave permanent cerebral damage. These authors cited the instance of a girl who previously had done well in school and, after having a tooth pulled under some difficulty with nitrous oxide alone, did very poorly in school. Instances of prolonged cardiac arrest in which the patient lives but his mind remains cloudy are also examples of the same effects of anoxia, in this case both anoxic and stagnant anoxia (see list below). An increased body temperature also disturbs the balance between the body's demand for oxygen and the supply thereof, and in cases of marked hyperthermia with the increased demand involved, additional oxygen may have to be given to the patient. The importance of an adequate airway is always paramount. These authors classified anoxia into 4 types, as follows:

1. *Anoxic anoxia*—due to inadequate oxygen reaching the lungs

2. *Anemic anoxia*—due to lack of, or inactivation of, hemoglobin, decreasing its capacity to take up oxygen

3. *Stagnant anoxia*—due to retardation of the circulation and transportation of oxygen

4. *Histologic anoxia*—due to drugging of the tissue cells so that they cannot utilize the available oxygen

Finally, parenchymatous tissue damage, which is the cumulative consequence of all the above-mentioned changes, is the harbinger of irreversibility. All treatment of shock should be aimed at preventing such parenchymatous tissue damage by correcting deficits in the blood volume and, hence, improving the circulation before irreversibility occurs.

Electrolyte changes are numerous (many of these are discussed in Chapter 17, Burns, and Chapter 5, Fluid and Electrolytes). The cellular destruction accompanying shock results in a liberation of potassium, with resultant high serum levels of this cation. In tourniquet shock in rats, the potassium content of muscle was reported to drop to 10 per cent of the normal value (Ravin, Denson and Jensen, 1954). At the same time the serum concentration rose from 5.7 to 11.5 mEq./L. The serum sodium fell only slightly, while the calcium and magnesium values rose. The alterations in the adrenal cortex are appreciable; Harkins and Long (1945) found a decrease in adrenal total cholesterol to only 30 per cent of the control value in 6 hours following burn shock in rats. It is significant that previous hypophysectomy entirely abolished this response. At the same time, the plasma amino nitrogen level became 4 times the control value. Changes in the blood hormonal concentrations are considered in Chapter 16, The Endocrine and Metabolic Basis of Surgical Care.

Secondary effects of shock include a predisposition to other conditions such as acute peptic ulcer of the Curling's type (see Chap. 17, Burns), lower nephron anuria, pulmonary embolism, possibly acute enterocolitis, and possibly infections in general (see p. 142, ed. 3). Some of the aspects of the "crush syndrome" appear to be related to shock and to immunologic hemolytic transfusion reactions. These three syndromes are also related to postoperative renal shutdown. Crush syndrome was described by Bywaters and Beall (1941) and was studied especially in Great

Britain during World War II as a result of the bombing catastrophes in London. Patients with crush syndrome usually have been buried or pinned down for several hours by beams or debris impinging on a limb. In the same year, Bywaters and Delory attributed the condition, with its accompanying oliguria, to deposits in the kidneys of myohemoglobin from the damaged muscle. While a true crush syndrome may exist, in many instances the supposed syndrome is merely hypovolemic shock with inadequate fluid replacement because of underestimated blood loss into the crushed tissues or is an instance of reaction to mismatched blood.

IRREVERSIBILITY

Investigation of the phenomenon of irreversibility in shock early pointed to the liver. Shorr, Zweifach and Furchgott (1950) implicated the liver as the critical organ. By study of depressor and exicitatory activity on the microcirculation of the rat mesentery, these authors concluded that an excitatory principle was released from the kidneys early in hypotension and then a vasodepressor material appeared which either was made in the liver or which the normal liver removed and the damaged liver permitted to accumulate. Later, workers in the same laboratory described this depressor substance as ferritin.

Other workers investigating the role of the liver reached other conclusions.

Parkins, Ben and Vars (1955, 1957) produced shock by inflating a balloon in the lower thoracic aorta. This left the heart, lungs, brain and forelimbs well supplied with blood but lowered the blood pressure in the hepatic artery, the splanchnic circulation and the hind limbs to approximately 16 mm. Hg. This produced shock in 120 minutes in the normothermic animal, which was fatal and was irreversible by the therapy applied.

They repeated the experiment, adding a supply of arterial blood through the hepatic portal vein. To avoid adding to blood volume, a like amount of blood was concomitantly removed from the body. This maneuver did not protect the animals, but ice cold saline applied to the small intestine to decrease the metabolism did prolong survival and lower mortality to a degree greater than could be accounted for by the general body cooling produced. They concluded that the intestinal tract was the critical organ in the processes leading to irreversibility.

Richard Lillehei (1957) compared animals in hemorrhagic shock, with and without added blood supply for the superior mesenteric artery, and also concluded that the intestinal tract was critical in dogs. Bounous, Hampson and Gurd (1964) took up the study of irreversibility in dogs and showed that, after a critical period of hypotension in the dog, transfusion might restore total blood flow through the superior mesenteric artery to the normal range without restoring the microcirculation. This was demonstrated by measuring the uptake of radioactive rubidium 86 in the bowel wall and mucosa.

Work by Bounous, Hampson and Gurd (1964) indicates that the hemorrhagic lesions found in the intestine of the dog in severe shock may be explained by chemical rather than by mechanical (intravascular coagulation) or bacterial (endotoxin) causes. These authors utilized a technic employing ^{32}P to label in vivo the nucleotides of intestine and liver to study the visceral damage which follows the ischemic anoxia of hemorrhagic shock in the dog. Samples of intestine and liver taken after ^{32}P injection, during a control period and following reinfusion of blood, showed profound depression of oxidative phosphorylation and nucleotide synthesis in the intestinal mucosa in irreversible shock. The time curves of the specific activity of inorganic phosphorus in the intestine, together with gross and microscopic observations, provided a sequential study of hemodynamic alterations and of the development of hemorrhagic enteritis.

The following summarizes the principal observations of the McGill group:

1. The metabolic deterioration in the mucosa of the intestine appears to reach an irreversible stage before the appearance of detrimental alterations in the hemodynamics of the intestine itself.

2. The metabolic depression renders the mucosal cells susceptible to permeation by intraluminal proteolytic enzymes such as trypsin. The characteristic hemorrhagic enteritis of late shock in the dog is produced by this mechanism.

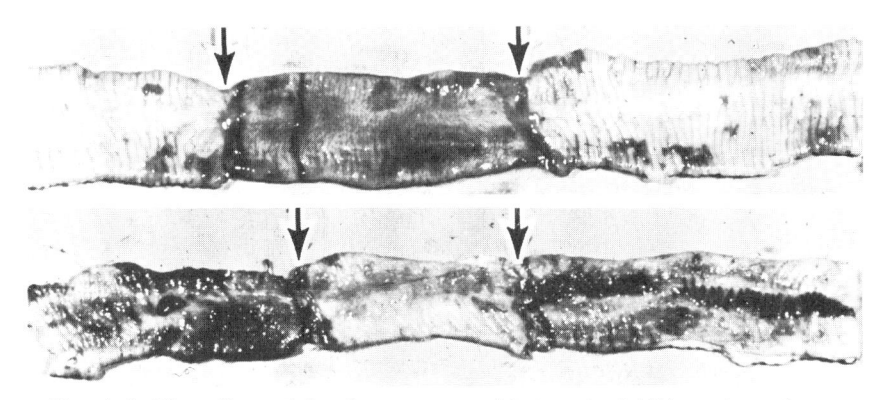

FIG. 7-5. The effect of local treatment with trypsin inhibitor (area between arrows) on the development of hemorrhagic lesion in the ileum: (*Top*) Segment instilled with trypsin. (*Bottom*) Segment instilled with Trasylol. (Bounous, G., Hampson, L. G., and Gurd, F. N.: Ann. Surg., 160-661)

3. Hemorrhagic enteritis is prevented by inactivating intraluminal tryptic ferments by means of a protease inhibitor aprotinin (Trasylol). (See Fig. 7-5.)

4. The inactivation of trypsin in the presence of intraluminal stool has no favorable effect upon the development of the metabolic depression in the mucosa. However, when Trasylol application is combined with lavage of the bowel to remove stool, the metabolic deterioration is delayed.

5. The advent of the severe metabolic depression in the intestinal mucosa is conditioned not only by low blood flow for a critical time interval but also by the direct contact with intestinal content other than trypsin.

6. The intestinal mucosa in late shock undergoes an alteration in its normal function as a barrier. The breakdown of the barrier is not dependent upon the prior development of hemorrhagic enteritis. Therefore, the serious consequences of a loss of barrier function might quite conceivably develop in species in which the trypsin induced hemorrhagic enteritis is not ordinarily a feature of shock, such as in man.

In summary, the experimental evidence indicates that, in the dog at least, hemorrhagic shock develops by first reducing cardiac output. The splanchnic circulation is reduced (perhaps preferentially); the supply of metabolites to the mucosa falls below a critical level, at which time autodigestion by proteolytic enzymes in the lumen begins. Presumably, this permits the absorption of endotoxins, adding the elements of septic shock to an already dire situation. Beyond a certain point, replacement of the lost blood or restoration of normal circulating volume cannot restore the damage to the intestinal mucosa in time to prevent death.

It is easy to hypothesize that there are many other dynamic equilibria in the body maintained metabolically which permit other deleterious occurrences to take place if the circulation becomes inadequate for an appreciable length of time. The experiments of Weinberger, Gibbon and Gibbon showed that 6 minutes of anoxia could produce blindness in the cat, and 8 minutes, early death. Tourniquet shock in a limb probably has some similar mechanism.

Hypothermia, as Parkins' group, as well as many others, have shown, slows the rate at which damage is done—presumably by lowering the reaction rate at which critical chemical (including enzymatic) processes occur. Thus, with local hypothermia to the canine intestine, Parkins (1955) was able to increase the tolerance of dogs for occlusion of the distal thoracic aorta from less than 60 minutes to over 120 minutes, and Wolfson *et al.* (1965) were able to increase the tolerance of dogs (and later of monkeys) to interruption of the circulation by ventricular fibrillation to 60 minutes and more, by moderate general hypothermia plus preferential cooling of the brain.

DIAGNOSIS

GENERAL FACTORS

The diagnosis of shock is based chiefly on the following:

1. **Recognition of the possibility of shock** when etiologic factors are present, such as hemorrhage, crushed limb, burns, intestinal strangulation, etc.
2. **Observation of the symptoms and the signs of shock**—pallor, cold sweat, cold extremities, contracted superficial veins evidenced by actual "grooves" (Berne, 1962), anxious expression, weak pulse, thirst, etc.

TESTS AND MEASUREMENTS

The following procedures are useful and sometimes permit the recognition of impending shock before it is evident clinically. These include: (a) the determination of blood loss; (b) the measurement of blood volume; (c) the use of the tilt test; and (d) the monitoring of central venous pressure.

Determination of Blood Loss

Rains (1955) studied 4 methods of measuring blood and fluid loss at operation: (1) sponge weighing, (2) sponge washing and hemoglobin determination, (3) weighing the patient, and (4) blood volume estimation (Evans blue). All of these methods have advantages and disadvantages. This author also pointed out that one third of each unit of blood to be administered represents citrate solution. Furthermore, since some of the blood is left in the bottle or tubing "one finds that just over half a pint of blood is given when one thinks one has given a patient a pint of blood."

LeVeen and Rubricius (1958) reported the use of a continuous, automatic, electronic method for determining operative blood loss, as did Rustad (1963a).

The Rustad-Ohlin "perdometer" (Rustad, 1963b) represents an automatic recorder of blood loss at operation based on hemoglobin loss analysis.

At the hospital of one of the writers of this chapter (H.M.H.) it is routine to measure the blood loss at major operations by weighing the sponges and laparotomy pads and comparing such weight with a control dry weight. The amount of blood in the suction bottle, etc., is added, and a running total figure is written in large letters on a blackboard on the wall within view of the surgeon. In another column the amount of blood administered is similarly totaled, and an attempt is made in extensive operations to keep the total of the second column at least equal to that of the first column. Further details of technic are given in the papers by Baronofsky, Treloar and Wangensteen (1946), Gross (1949), and Saltzstein and Linkner (1952), and in Chapter 8, Blood Transfusion. A useful scale for measuring the blood in sponges is shown in Figure 7-4.

Determination of Blood Volume

Measurements of this parameter are more nearly accurate the earlier in the course of shock they are recorded (Gregersen and Rawson, 1959). Irrespective of the method used—Evans blue, i.e., T-1824; other dye tests (Henegar, 1963); RISA, tagged ^{51}Cr red cells (see Albert, 1963); tagged ^{32}P red cells; or certain items of commercial equipment that are designed for these purposes and are useful (Williams and Fine, 1961; Fine, 1963a; Greep, Litwin and Nardi, 1963)—the methods must be used with judgment. In the later stages of shock, because of increased diffusibility into all tissue spaces, and also because of possible "sequestration" of slowly circulating or non-circulating red cells, blood volume measurements become less and less accurate. During the intermediate period, such determinations are of value, depending on the knowledge and the judgment of the surgeon who interprets the data. Reeve and Vincent (1962) presented a good review of blood volume measurements.

The "Tilt Test"

This was first suggested by Duncan, et al. (1944) and later developed as a practical test by Green and Metheny (1947). This test brings out *latent* arterial hypotension which does not demonstrate itself early in shock patients—probably because most patients with injuries or conditions severe enough to produce shock are examined when they are lying down—by tilting the head end of the patient up. Tachycardia of varying degrees at certain angles of tilt is roughly proportional to the amount of blood lost. This test is especially useful in cases of massive upper, or lower, gastrointestinal hemorrhage. The test has been modified as the "L-test," involving an arterial blood pressure rise (more than 10 mm. Hg in 30 seconds being considered as positive) if the legs of the supine patient are elevated abruptly to the vertical position (Greene, 1958).

Monitoring of Central Venous Pressure (CVP)

This determination, recognized as adding certain information that measurement of peripheral arterial pressure (PAP) and pulse rate do not provide, should be considered as an addition to the surgeon's armamentarium, not as a substitute for observation of the latter two parameters. It has become standardized, partly because of the stimulation of cardiac surgeons. The term "central" signifies that the catheter tip must be in the true central venous system. This location is such that peripheral venous constriction and intervening venous valves cannot interfere with transmission of the right atrial pressure directly to the venous catheter.

Because of variations in stage of shock and unrelated disease, peripheral venous pressure may vary widely in its correlation with the CVP and hence be of limited clinical value. The peripheral venous pressure, usually higher, may be *less than* the CVP by as much as 10 to 20 cm. of H_2O.

Methodology of CVP Determination. Central venous pressure is measured with a vinyl catheter, inserted through a jugular, brachial, or cephalic vein in the antecubital fossa into the subclavian vein (or innominate or vena cava or right atrium, Cohn and Luria, 1964) and connected with a 3-way stopcock to a saline manometer. A brisk excursion with respiration should be evident, and readings are determined in the supine patient from the level of the right atrium (usually 6 cm. below the level of the sternal notch). Normal values are difficult to define, since their relationship to peripheral arterial pressure and dynamic responses to intravenous therapy must be taken into consideration, but generally they can range from 6 to 17 cm. H_2O above the center of the heart (level of the right atrium) in the supine position, but more generally the midnormal range is 9 to 12 cm. H_2O.

Wilson, Grow, Demong, Prevedel and Owens (1962) and most others prefer monitoring the superior vena cava for two reasons: (1) less danger of thrombophlebitis and (2) less interference by abdominal distention. A third advantage might be added, namely, that if during an operation the abdominal vena cava needs to be compressed, the CVP readings can still be made if the catheter is in the upper cava. The superior vena caval readings are elevated only about 2 cm. by ventilatory support with positive pressure, so this factor does not serve as an objection to the superior approach. Muller (1963) also uses the superior approach through the jugular vein. Still others use the brachial or cephalic; in such instances the catheter should be long enough to extend into the superior vena cava. The intravenous catheter should not be left in place for longer than 48 hours to avoid thromboembolic complications.

Use of CVP determinations in shock should be dynamic, with continuous monitoring, rather than static, with a single measurement (Johnson, 1964). The chief value is not in single readings (normal 6 to 15 cm. H_2O), but in the rise in CVP with intravenous therapy, indicating a danger of fluid "overload." Correlation with observation of distention of neck veins and presence of pulmonary rales, and with arterial blood pressure readings is essential. To give an example, a low CVP (0 to 6 cm. H_2O) in a patient in shock with associated low arterial blood pressure suggests *hypovolemia*, and intravenous treatment is indicated. If the CVP remains low, such treatment is continued, and the fluid may be injected more rapidly. If the CVP then approaches normal (e.g., 6 to 8 cm. H_2O), yet arterial hypotension persists, the intravenous treatment is continued but is given more slowly. If the CVP becomes markedly elevated, blood volume expanders are discontinued irrespective of whether the arterial blood pressure remains low or has returned to normal (McGowan and Walters, 1963). A significantly elevated and rising CVP (15 to 20 cm. H_2O and above) indicates "overload," and blood volume expanders would be dangerous. In the latter instance, attention should more properly be directed to other causes of persisting low arterial blood pressure and use of appropriate treatment, possibly including digitalization of the heart.

Blood volume expanders may be used to bring the CVP continuously up to 15 cm. H_2O

134 Shock

DIAGRAMS
HEMORRHAGIC SHOCK PROCEDURES IN DOGS

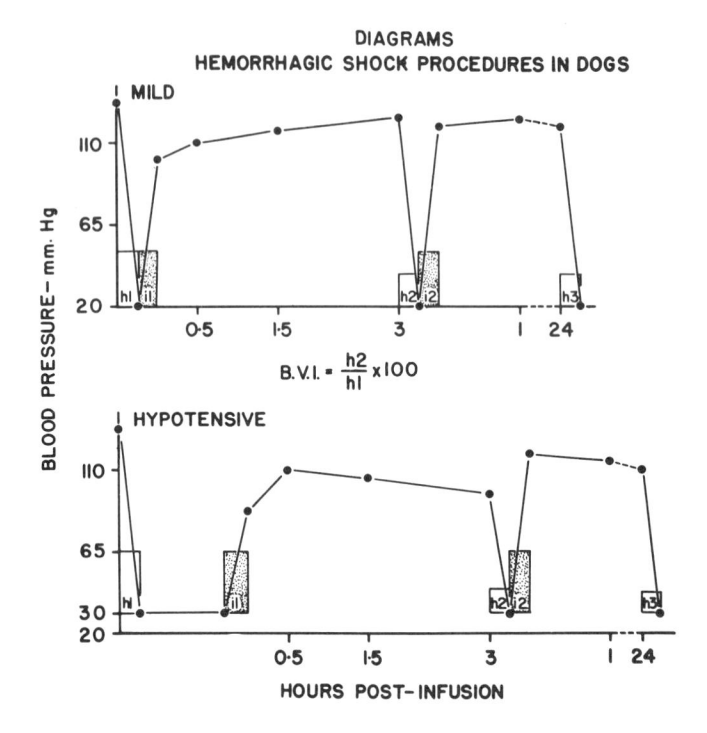

[Figure: Two graphs of BLOOD PRESSURE — mm. Hg vs HOURS POST-INFUSION. Top graph labeled MILD with pressures 110, 65, 20 and time points 0.5, 1.5, 3, 24. Middle label: B.V.I. = $\frac{h2}{h1} \times 100$. Bottom graph labeled HYPOTENSIVE with pressures 110, 65, 30, 20 and same time points.]

FIG. 7-6. Two procedures for producing hemorrhagic shock in dogs for the comparative testing of therapeutic agents such as blood, plasma, dextrans, gelatines, etc. In the "mild" procedure (*top*), bleeding is carried out at 4 ml./Kg./min. until the arterial blood pressure falls to 20 mm. of mercury. The material to be tested is then infused at the same rate, starting immediately. The volume given is the same as the amount of blood removed, unless otherwise noted. After 3 hours the animal is again bled at the same rate to the same blood pressure end point. The ratio of the second hemorrhage to the first is called the bleeding volume index.

In the "hypotensive" hemorrhagic shock procedure, (*bottom*), the blood pressure is lowered, by bleeding, to 30 mm. of mercury and maintained at that level for 1 hour by additional withdrawals (or infusions) of blood before reinfusion with the test material. If the second bleeding is quantitatively replaced with the material to be tested, a third bleeding can be carried out 24 hours later to the same blood pressure end point, as shown in the figure. (Modified from Parkins, W. M., Perlmutt, J. H., and Vars, H. M.: Surg. Forum, 3:421, 1952)

(Berne, 1963). If the heart is enlarged or known myocardial disease is present, a lower level is preferable. Also, if the level of 15 cm. is attained rapidly, this may be because of too short a time for stabilization of the "plasticity" factor of even the large veins. Reexamination of the level will obviate this influence. Longerbeam, Bloch, Manax and Lillehei (1964) summarize the case by stating, "It is our feeling that carefully determined central venous pressures are more important than blood volume determinations in guiding fluid therapy."

An additional indication for CVP monitoring is the case of arterial hypotension in which a differential diagnosis must be made between hypovolemic shock and some other condition. Thus, in "septic" shock the earlier it can be established that the CVP is normal and rises readily with the administration of even a small amount of expander, the less the danger of overload (Hallin, 1963). In a series of 93 patients studied by Altemeier and Cole (1958) with so-called "septic" shock, the most common postmortem finding was pulmonary edema which they attributed to overloading of the circulation.

Despite enthusiasm for observation of CVP in shock, the surgeon should not forget the long-proved usefulness of the PAP (peripheral arterial pressure). Central venous pressure determinations have their particular usefulness, it seems, as a guide to therapy rather than as a means of diagnosis of shock.

THERAPY: EXPERIMENTAL APPROACHES

The evaluation of treatment in clinical shock is generally unsatisfactory because it is rare to find comparable injuries in comparable subjects. Therefore, students have turned to anesthetized animals and particularly to inbred strains of rodents to study burn shock and to dogs to study hemorrhagic shock.

In a very rational approach to the subject, Parkins (1953) bled healthy dogs at a constant rate of 4 ml. per Kg. per minute to a blood pressure end point of 20 mm. Hg and replaced the blood with an equal volume of a solution to be tested, infused at the same rate. He then waited 3 hours. At the end of this time, bleeding was repeated to the same blood pressure end point. The relationship between the amount of blood removed at the second hemorrhage and the amount of the original bleeding was expressed as a percentage (Fig. 7-6). Thus, autotransfusion yielded a bleeding volume index of 95 per cent. (Other sample results are shown in Table 7-2.)

A second protocol used by Parkins was similar to this except that the end point was 30 mm. Hg and, instead of immediate replacement, hypotension at 30 mm. Hg was maintained for 1 hour before replacement.

Using these two technics, Parkins compared the efficacy of whole blood, dog plasma, dextran, albumin, and various gelatin preparations (Table 7-2). Included in the comparison was 0.9 per cent NaCl solution. Previously, Parkins et al. (1952) had employed twice and three times the volume of saline that had been removed as blood. Using these amounts, he achieved a bleeding volume index only a little below that achieved with one volume of dog plasma.

Attempts to give the saline by mouth were unsuccessful unless the first portion was given by vein. Thus, if an amount equivalent to the blood loss was given by vein and the second and third volumes given into the stomach, the results were about the same as

TABLE 7-2. COMPARISON OF BLEEDING VOLUME INDICES*

	PROCEDURE I (3 HRS.)		PROCEDURE II (3 HRS.)	
INFUSION FLUID	No. OF Dogs	BLEEDING VOLUME INDEX (per cent)	No. OF Dogs	BLEEDING VOLUME INDEX (per cent)
1. Whole blood (autogenous)	6	96	5	72
2. Fluid gelatin 3%	11	83	5	67
3. Saline 0.9%	6	54	5	12
4. Untreated	6	17	—	—
5. Gelatin (P-20) 6%	5	84	—	—
6. Gelatin (P-180) 6%	5	65	—	—
7. Plasma (dog)	7	70	5	46
8. Albumin (human) 5%	5	88	3	59
9. Oxypolygelatin 5%	5	78	4	34
10. Dextran (C.S.C.) 6%	5	87	5	53

* After Parkins, W. M., Perlmutt, J. H., and Vars, H. M. (1952)

when all three volumes were given by vein. After one hour of hypotension, however, the results of saline administration were much poorer.

Hypertonic sodium chloride was not employed in hemorrhagic shock in dogs, but McCarthy (1953) utilized it in rats subjected to superficial burns under anesthesia. He tried concentrations form 0.9 to 3.6 per cent and found the optimum for survival to be about 1.4 per cent. However, thermal burns produce a particular need for sodium (Fox, 1944 Moyer and associates—see Chapter 17, Burns). The latter reported that the withdrawal of 1 liter of water from normal man reduced blood volume an average of 45 ml. and that the withdrawal of one equivalent of sodium (the amount in 58.5 grams of sodium chloride) reduced blood volume 1,150 ml. Thus, dehydration, especially if there is an accompanying sodium loss, has a tremendous effect on blood volume and hence presumably on susceptibility or resistance to hypovolemic shock.

Plasma protein loss, as in dogs rendered severely hypoproteinemic by a low protein diet and plasmapheresis, also increases susceptibility to hemorrhagic shock (Ravdin, MacNamee, Kamholz and Rhoads, 1944).

The capacity of man to shift plasma protein in or out of the circulation in accordance with the need of the individual was brought out in the experiments of Barker, Elder, Walker and Vars (1952). These investigators administered 1 liter of a modified gelatin preparation intravenously to normal volunteers and to volunteers from whom 1,000 ml. of blood had just been withdrawn. Blood volume measurements were made serially, as well as measurements of the concentration of the gelatin. The rate of departure of the gelatin from the circulation was only moderately faster in unbled recipients, but the bled recipients retained virtually the whole increment in blood volume of 1000 ml., whereas the increment of 1000 ml. given to the unbled volunteers disappeared very rapidly. It seems probable from these experiments that the serum protein moved into the circulation as the gelatin left in the bled subjects, whereas it moved out and then came back in the unbled subjects.

The Role of Drugs in the Treatment of Shock

The role of drugs in the treatment of shock has given rise to much discussion. Morphine, which was a mainstay of an earlier generation of physicians, should be used sparingly if at all, in the light of evidence that it interferes with the control of the circulation during changes in position.

Epinephrine was shown to be capable of producing shock, albeit in doses above physiologic levels (Freeman et al., 1941).

The concept of using vasorelaxants or sympatholytic agents came from the French school, and the use of chlorpromazine was recommended. This drug, however, has a very complicated pharmacodynamic action. Nickerson and Gourzis (1962) proposed the use of dibenzyline (phenoxybenzamine hydrochloride), which reduced the function of the alpha receptors of the sympathetic nervous system.

Lillehei proposed the use of cortisone in a dosage range far beyond that which had been employed in earlier experiments and reported favorable results in septic shock. We have found little other evidence that administered adrenocortical hormones are helpful in a person with functioning adrenal glands; however, the evidence is overwhelming that the adrenalectomized individual is most susceptible to shock and cannot withstand even mild insult without the aid of adrenal steroids or high sodium chloride supplements or both (Swingle, et al., 1933). Therefore, in a patient with Addison's disease, adrenal steroids are the mainstay of treatment and the dosage needs to be sharply increased during periods of stress.

The beneficial effects of catecholomines, norepinephrine especially, on the myocardium must be considered.

It was conceived that a drug that had similar effects on the myocardium but acted as a relaxant for arterioles peripherally might be beneficial. Isoproterenol is such a drug. Johnson and Parkins (1966) tested this drug in dogs in whom flow measurements were being made with electromagnetic flowmeters at the root of the aorta, the superior mesenteric artery and one renal artery.

The flows were sharply reduced as hemorrhage approached shock levels. At this point, administration of isoproterenol increased the circulation as measured in the superior mesenteric artery. However, simple intravenous infusion of 40 ml. Kg. of 0.9 per cent NaCl solution produced far greater improvement.

Thus, as far as *hypovolemic shock* is concerned, the role of drugs is very small and the logical treatment is to increase the circulating volume with whole blood, blood plasma, albumin, a plasma expander, a balanced salt solution, or simple sodium chloride and water in a concentration of about 0.9 per cent.

Endotoxin shock is well portrayed in Chapters 3 and 4 and will be considered here only briefly from the standpoint of differential diagnosis. Excellent work on this subject has been reported by Selkurt (1959); Gans and Krivit (1960); Schayer (1960); Hinshaw, et al., (1960; 1961); Vesell, Palmerio and Frank (1960); Gilbert (1962); Marston (1962); Longerbeam, et al. (1962); Fiorica and Funkhouser (1963); and Sherman and Noyes (1963).

Endotoxin "shock" is the laboratory prototype of septic shock. The release of an endotoxin from gram-negative organisms is in the form of a high molecular weight phospholipid polysaccharide complex (Spink, 1960). Major blood volume changes are not necessary for endotoxin shock to occur (MacLean, 1962), in contradistinction to true hypovolemic shock.

It should be emphasized that many of the studies of endotoxin shock are based on observations of the effect of intravenous injections of endotoxins rather than on absorption from infected foci in the body. While endotoxins may possibly play an exacerbatory role in true hypovolemic shock, the condition of pure endotoxin shock is essentially a separate one.

In the case of septic shock, intravenous fluids are not so clearly superior to the use of drugs as they are in hypovolemic shock. As of 1969, many clinicians would be likely to try large doses of cortisone (1,000 mg. every 3 to 4 hours) as a supplement to building up blood volume as high as possible without raising central venous pressure above 15 cm. of water, in any patient with septic shock who was not doing well.

CLINICAL TREATMENT

The treatment of shock is urgent and should be carried out before irreversible changes supervene. Even more urgent, however, are preservation of an adequate airway, control of sucking wounds of the chest, and control of rapid hemorrhage.

The following are regularly part of the standard treatment of shock:

Fluid Replacement

In the selection of a replacement fluid to be transfused into the circulation, one must have assurance (1) that it is sterile and pyrogen free; (2) that the risk of its carrying a virus (particularly that responsible for serum hepatitis) has been minimized; (3) that it is not so hypotonic with respect to erythrocytes to cause hemolysis, and (4) that it will not adversely increase the viscosity or seriously decrease the oxygen-carrying capacity of the blood.

In progressive shock it is apt to be the heart which eventually fails. There is a calculable ratio between the work of the heart and the amount of oxygen delivered to the tissues. The work is defined by the cardiac output and the mean pressure against which it is pumped. The oxygen delivered is a function of the cardiac output and the mean A-V oxygen difference. For practical purposes, oxygen is measured in the arterial circulation and in mixed venous blood. Strictly speaking, this permits a possible error, in that the blood returning to the heart through the coronary sinus might have a different composition from the mixed venous blood.

If the peripheral resistance is raised, as by epinephrine, the work of the heart is increased. If the viscosity of the blood is raised, as by increase in the hemoglobin above 15 Gm. per cent, the work of the heart is increased. If, in compensating for blood loss with plasma, saline, or some plasma expanders such as dextran, the hemoglobin is lowered, the viscosity falls; however, more blood needs to be pumped in order to carry sufficient oxygen to the tissues and, therefore, severe anemia should be avoided.

If there is an abnormal tendency to aggregation of erythrocytes (so-called sludging), resistance to pumping through small capillaries presumably is increased.

If tissue metabolism is increased by fever, shivering or excessive thyroid hormone, the work of the heart is increased also—there is simply more work to do.

Although, in the treatment of hemorrhage, plasma may be substituted for whole blood until the hematocrit falls to one third of the normal level, it is believed that in the treatment of shock the hemoglobin is best kept in the range of 11 to 14 Gm. per 100 ml. or close to this range.

PLASMA VOLUME EXPANDERS

Gelatin was introduced by British workers in 1915 and received a limited trial in World War I.

It was further perfected in 1940-1955 and an acceptable product known as P-20 Gelatine was produced. The viscosity tended to be higher than that of plasma or albumin. It was solid at 68°F. but liquid at or near body temperature. The need to warm it before use made it undesirable for field use and, if reserved for emergency use in a hospital, it had to be kept in a warm closet.

Oxypolygelatine and Modified Fluid Gelatine remain fluid at room temperature but probably have only marginal advantages. Low molecular weight gelatin is readily made by continuing the process of hydrolysis by which P-20 is made. It remains liquid but the smaller molecules leave the circulation more quickly, so that it does not meet the criteria that one-half remain in the circulation for 12 hours.

The small molecule gelatine (under the name of Rheomacrodex) has found a special role because of its capacity to reduce viscosity of blood (C. Gelin: 1955, 1956, 1957, 1959, 1962). This may be an important feature when "sludging" of the blood, as studied by M. Knisely (1951, 1961), occurs in shock or shock-like states. It is possible that micro-agglutinations of red cells may actually occlude certain capillaries temporarily, potentially interfering with the proper distribution of blood in tissues.

Polyvinlypyrrolidine, the plasma volume expander developed in Germany during World War II, is an effective agent but has the disadvantage of not being entirely excreted. The possible longterm effect within the body has not been established, and it seems undesirable to use a product for which this question is unanswered, when there are other alternatives. The dog reacts poorly to it, so that other species are preferable for experimental studies.

Dextran is a form of dextrose polymerized by the microorganism *Leuconostoc mesenteroides* and then hydrolyzed to an appropriate molecular size. It was first prepared in England but really developed as a plasma expander in Sweden. A number of molecular sizes have been tried. It is effective as a plasma volume expander and does not give many reactions. Unfortunately, patients may develop a hemorrhagic tendency if a number of units are given. Up to 1,000 ml. of 6 per cent dextran have been found safe and most patients will accept 2,000 cc. before a bleeding tendency becomes manifest.

Serum albumin is good but expensive. It is a blood derivative rather than a substitute. It is discussed in the chapter on Blood, as is human plasma stored for 6 months at 32°C.

In summary, it seems fair to say that, in most clinical situations, balanced salt solutions (0.6% NaCl, 0.3% Na HCO$_3$) plus suitable whole blood will do about as much in the treatment of hypovolemic shock as any combination of liquids. The delay encountered in crossmatching of blood derivatives makes it still worthwhile to keep a stock of 6 per cent dextran or gelatin available for emergency use in hospitals.

DRUGS

In some instances, antibiotics may help control the problematical bacterial factors which may be present in shock. Generally speaking, administration of corticoids may produce the other effects of these substances more certainly than the control of shock. Frank, H. A., et al. (1955) reported that while the output of corticosteroids in the adrenal veins of dogs suffering from hemorrhagic shock tended to be reduced as compared with the levels before the induction of shock, there was no correlation between the extent of reduction and the fate of the animal. ACTH is usually not helpful because the patient's own stress reaction is already stimulating the adrenal cortex to its full capacity, so that adding more ACTH would be like "whipping a tired horse." In fact, Hechter et al. (1955) studied the corticosteroid output in adrenal veins of "normal" dogs before and after exogenous ACTH administration and found no significant increase. They concluded that "the conditions of the experiments provided maximum endogenous stimulation." Hume and Nelson (1955) reported that the increase in adrenal venous blood corticosteroid secretion following hemorrhage did not occur in hypophysectomized dogs.

Steenburg, Lennihan and Moore (1956) observed an early and substantial (4-fold in 4 hours) increase in the free serum 17-hydroxycorticoids after major operation in man. This level was higher than that produced by maximal doses of ACTH over similar periods of time. The level of 17-hydroxycorticoids seemed to be an index of the timing and the intensity of adrenal response to injury, whereas the urinary excretion of total steroid provided a more suitable index of the duration of this response. The excretion of 17-hydroxycorticoids was proportionate to the extent of trauma; that of 17-ketosteroids was not a suitable index in this regard.

Smith and Moore (1962), in their excellent study of 15 cases of refractory hypotension in man, found that the intravenous administration of corticosteroids in large doses failed to produce improvement in any one of these patients. Longerbeam et al. (1964) found that their best results in the treatment of endotoxin shock in dogs were produced by either 25 ml./Kg. of plasma or 2 Gm./Kg. of Rheomacrodex in 5 per cent dextrose in water, combined with 50 mg./Kg. of hydrocortisone.

HEAT

The application of external heat is usually harmful, but conservation of normal body heat is helpful. The recovery rate from experimental shock in mice was found by Bergman and Prinzmetal (1945) to be greatest at a room temperature of 68°F. and to be progressively less at temperatures higher or lower than this figure (Fig. 7-7).

ANALGESICS AND SEDATIVES

Analgesic drugs should be given only for actual pain, not for restlessness, and should be administered intravenously, the initial dosage being from one half to two thirds that usually employed hypodermically. Sedatives,

FIG. 7-7. Effect of environmental temperature on mortality in burn shock. Each point represents 20 to 26 mice, etherized and scalded up to the head at 65° C. for 10 seconds, kept in rooms at various constant temperatures. The range of environmental temperatures for optimal survival is 65° to 71° F. (Redrawn from Bergman, H. C., and Prinzmetal, M.: Arch. Surg., 50:202)

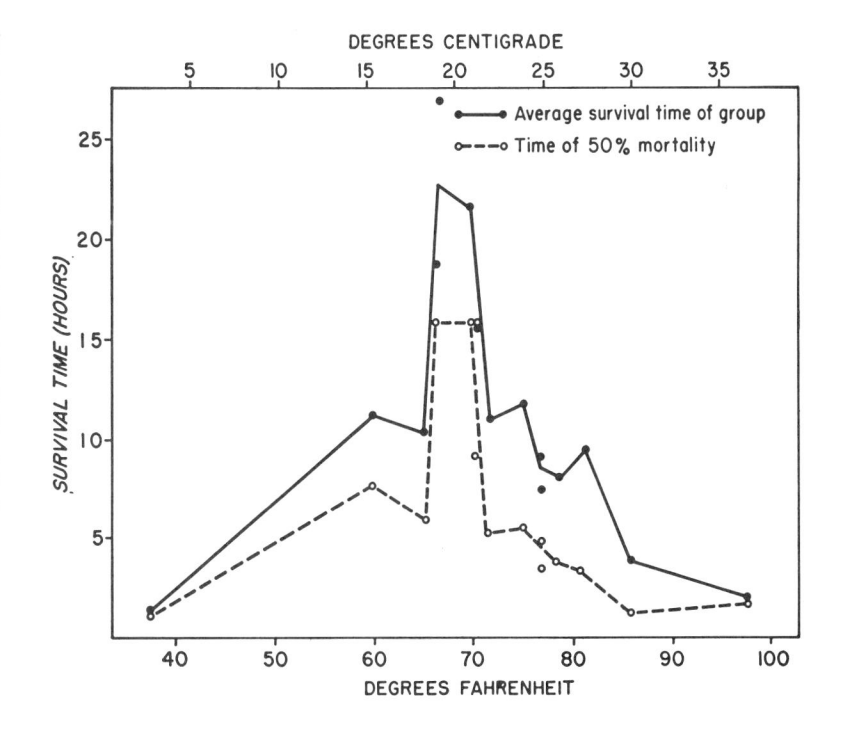

such as the barbiturates, are of little value and may be harmful in large amounts or even in normal therapeutic doses.

The danger of giving repeated doses of subcutaneous morphine to men with shock from war wounds was emphasized by Beecher (1944) in the African Theater of World War II. When shock is severe enough to prevent ready absorption of the morphine it becomes pooled in the subcutaneous tissues, and morphine poisoning follows the absorption of the accumulated doses when the patient receives blood replacement therapy. For these reasons, morphine given to patients in shock should be by the intravenous route and should not exceed gr. ⅙ (10 mg.) as an initial dose.

In addition to the dangers of overdosage of analgesics and sedatives, there is a definite possibility of overdosage of anesthetic agents in the shock patient (see Chap. 13, Anesthesia, and Chap. 25, Military Surgery).

Reports continue to appear concerning the benefits of certain sedative agents in shock. These should be approached with caution. Hershey, Guccione and Zweifach (1955) reported a beneficial action of pretreatment with chlorpromazine following graded hemorrhage in the rat; Overton and De Bakey (1955) used the dog for their studies. The application of this preliminary work to human patients awaits further studies. Sensitivity to these drugs must also be considered.

OXYGEN

Maintenance of an adequate airway for ready inhalation of air is mandatory. As Fitts (1955) stated, the priority of treatment in injury is as follows: (1) airway; (2) sucking wound of the thorax; (3) hemorrhage; (4) shock.

Supplemental oxygen may be tried and should be continued if it improves the color, lowers the pulse rate or otherwise benefits the patient. In all patients with shock, especially in those with multiple injuries, definite attention should be paid to the airway (Kinney and Wells, 1962).

Developments in the use of hyperbaric oxygenation are perhaps apropos to the future treatment of shock (Boerema, 1961; Illingworth states, 1961; Cowley et al., 1964). The possibility that hyperbaric oxygen might be of value is indicated by the observation of Guyton and Crowell (1961) that, in hemorrhagic shock in dogs, recovery bore a relationship to the depression of over-all oxygen consumption during the hypotensive period. Bounous, Hampson and Gurd (1964) corroborated this by the observation that, in animals that had reached the irreversible stage, the total oxygen consumption did not recover to preshock levels following reinfusion. Favorable results in the treatment of endotoxin shock in dogs with hyperbaric oxygen have been reported by Evans et al. (1964). The clinical value of this method has, however, not been clearly established.

POSITION OF THE PATIENT

Elevation of the foot of the bed to relieve shock—the opposite of the tilt test which is used to test for shock—is useful as a *temporary* measure. Caution must be employed in using this maneuver with the obese patient (because of interference with movement of the diaphragm), (2) in patients with peripheral arterial disease (because of danger of permanent ischemic changes in the feet due to reduction in local arterial blood flow), or (3) for prolonged periods of time because of actually increased danger of mortality from shock (Weil and Whigham, 1965).

SUMMARY OF TREATMENT IN HYPOVOLEMIC SHOCK

The prime factor in the treatment of oligemic shock is to restore the blood volume to normal levels, starting at the earliest possible moment. As Howard (1955) stated, "Never give up." Also, as Moore (1963 b) said, "Any case of hypotension in association with surgical trauma should be assumed to be due to blood loss until proven otherwise." Other measures, while useful, should not be utilized as an excuse to avoid or postpone this main element in the treatment.

It is always important to be sure that, in each instance, the case with supposedly "irreversible" shock is not in fact a matter of incorrect diagnosis or inadequate therapy.

A number of papers have in the past argued in favor of the intraarterial route of administration as opposed to the intravenous route in shock treatment. It is now generally agreed that the intravenous route is suitable and that no practical advantage is conferred by the intraarterial route. Indeed, the latter is unsafe for fluids requiring dilution. Concentrated solutions may damage tissues in the part supplied by the artery even though the solution would be well tolerated if mixed with the circulating blood returning to the heart.

Auxiliary Treatment in Septic Shock

Septic shock is characteristically accompanied by signs of infection: elevation of temperature, and, often, chills. Therefore, one or more polyvalent antibiotics should be started immediately and a blood culture taken in the hope of isolating living organisms whose sensitivity to specific antibiotics can be determined.

Elevations of temperature cause a marked increase in metabolism (8 per cent per 1°F. of elevation). A marked rise in temperature places a special strain on the heart and the embarrassed circulation. For this reason, it has been the practice of the author to apply hypothermia to the patients to force the temperature down to 101° or lower. If this is to be effective, it is necessary to use sufficient sedation to prevent shivering.

Summary

Frank shock is characterized by abnormally low blood pressures. Hypovolemic shock is characterized at an earlier stage by coolness of the extremities as compared with the proximal parts of the body. The demarcation of the zone of skin temperature change is quite sharp and moves centrally as hypovolemia increases.

Shock should be anticipated rather than awaited. A person suspected of developing shock may show a drop in blood pressure when changed from a lying to a standing position—a useful test in some patients who can stand briefly.

Actual blood volume measurements should be made when there is serious doubt.

Treatment should be prophylactic to the extent possible. Whether prophylactic or therapeutic, replacement therapy in hypovolemic shock should consist of balanced saline solution (0.9 per cent NaCl if balanced saline is not available), and properly matched, properly prepared whole blood.

Plasma stored 6 months at 32°C., serum albumin, dextran, gelatin prepared for intravenous use, etc., are useful to amplify blood volume but add almost nothing to oxygen-carrying capacity. They are more expensive than balanced salt solution.

The principal indications for their use have been either the unavailability of suitable blood or the finding of an abnormally high hematocrit. In persons who were previously in good health, balanced salt solutions can usually be pushed to the point of correcting the hematocrit. This, of course, adds to the interstitial fluid a larger amount than it does to the intravascular fluid. Therefore, in older individuals and persons with edema, this author believes that the colloid solutions are indicated when the hematocrit is too high for whole blood to be indicated.

If the kidneys are working, urinary output, collected by indwelling catheter and measured hourly, is a fine indicator of the adequacy of treatment. Hourly output should be 30 ml. or above. The central venous pressure is the best warning of overtreatment and, in general, should not be elevated above 15 cm. of water.

If the central venous pressure rises without restoration of renal function, the patient is in serious trouble. The trouble may be with the heart, and digitalization may improve the situation. If the blood pressure is back to normal levels, or above, the trouble may well be with the urinary tract. The indwelling catheter should be checked for patency and placement. A diuretic such as mannitol in 25 to 50 gram doses by vein may improve urinary function.

Shock treatment probably has not been pushed to the ultimate limits of possible usefulness unless the early signs of pulmonary edema have appeared. Thus—while at the same time, pulmonary edema is very dangerous and should be avoided—one does not necessarily stop supporting blood volume at a central venous pressure of 15 cm. if the arterial blood pressure has not reached at least low normal levels. Here again, colloid has a specific role; human albumin in concentrated form (25 per cent) is especially useful when hypoalbuminemia is present.

Finally, cortisone or hydrocortisone may be added particularly in septic shock. If used, large doses appear logical on the basis of animal experimentation.

The role of sympatholytic agents is not well enough defined to permit recommendation for clinical use in the treatment of shock. At a stage of hypovolemic shock, when central circulation is maintained by peripheral constriction, they are believed to be definitely dangerous.

BIBLIOGRAPHY

Albert, S. N.: Blood volume: a review. Anesthesiology, 24:231-247, 1963.

Allbritten, F. F., Jr., Lipshutz, H., Miller, B. J., and Gibbon, J. H., Jr.: Blood volume changes in tuberculous patients treated by thoracoplasty. J. Thoracic Surg., 19:71-79, 1950.

Allen, F. M.: Physical and toxic factors in shock. Arch. Surg., 38:155-180, 1939.

Allen, J. Garrott: Personal communication. June, 1955.

Altemeier, W. A., and Cole, W.: Septic shock, Ann. Surg., 143:600-607, 1956.

———: Nature and treatment of septic shock. Arch. Surg., 77:498-507, 1958.

Andrews, E., and Harkins, H. N.: "Surgical shock" factors in pneumonia. Ann. Int. Med., 10:1503-1507, 1937.

Artz, C. P., and Fitts, C. T.: Replacement therapy in shock. J. Trauma, 2:358-369, 1962.

Aub, J. C.: Toxic factor in experimental traumatic shock. New Eng. J. Med., 231:71-75, 1944.

Baker, R. J., Shoemaker, W. C., Suzuki, F., Freeark, R. J., and Strohl, E. L.: Low molecular weight dextran therapy in surgical shock. Arch. Surg., 89:373-389, 1964.

Balch, H. H.: The effect of severe battle injury and of posttraumatic renal failure on resistance to infection. Ann. Surg., 142:145-163, 1955.

Baltch, A., and Bunn, P. A.: Studies of the properdin system in normal humans, in infections and in malignant blood dyscrasias, using the phage technique for its measurement. J. Clin. Invest., 37:876, 1958.

Baratz, R. A., and Ingraham, R. C.: Capillary permeability during hemorrhagic shock in the rat. Proc. Soc. Exp. Biol. Med., 89:642-644, 1955.

Barnett, W. O., Truett, G., Williams, R., and Crowell, J.: Shock in strangulation obstruction: mechanisms and management. Ann. Surg., 157:747-758, 1963.

Baronofsky, I. D., Treloar, A. E., and Wangensteen, O. H.: Blood loss in operations: a statistical comparison of losses as determined by the gravimetric and colorimetric methods. Surgery, 20:761-769, 1946.

Baue, A. E., Johnson, D. G., and Parkins, W. M.: Blood flow and oxygen consumption with adrenergic blockade in hemorrhagic shock. Am. J. Physiol., 211:354, 1966.

Beecher, H. K.: Delayed morphine poisoning in battle casualties. J.A.M.A., 124:1193, 1944.

Bergentz, S-E., and Nilsson, I. M.: Effect of trauma on coagulation and fibrinolysis in dogs. Acta chir. scand., 122:21-29, 1961.

Bergman, H. C., and Prinzmetal, M.: Influence of environmental temperature on shock. Arch. Surg., 50:201-206, 1945.

Berne, C. J.: Diagnosis of compensated hypovolemic shock (compensated acute hypovolemia). Am. J. Surg., 103:412-414, 1962.

———: Discussion of paper by Hallin (1963).

Bing, R. J., and Ramos, H.: The role of the heart in shock. J.A.M.A., 181:871-873, 1962.

Blalock, A.: Experimental shock: the cause of the low blood pressure produced by muscle injury. Arch. Surg., 20:959-996, 1930.

———: Acute circulatory failure as exemplified by shock and hemorrhage. Surg., Gynec. Obstet., 58:551-566, 1934.

Blattberg, B., and Levy, M. N.: Properdin titers of dogs surviving hemorrhagic hypotension. Proc. Soc. Exp. Biol. Med., 104:155, 1960.

Boerema, I.: An operating room with high atmospheric pressure. Surgery, 49:291-298, 1961.

Bonica, J. J., and Lyter, C. S.: Measurement of blood loss during surgical operations. Am. J. Surg., 81:496-502, 1951.

Borden, F. W.: Loss of blood at operation. California Med., 87:91-97, 1957.

Bounous, G., Hampson, L. G., and Gurd, F. N.: Cellular nucleotides in shock: relationship of intestinal metabolic changes to hemorrhagic enteritis and the barrier function of intestinal mucosa. Ann. Surg., 160:650-668, 1964.

Bywaters, E. G. L., and Beall, D.: Crush injuries with impairment of renal function. Brit. M. J., 1:427-432, 1941.

Bywaters, E. G. L., and Delory, G. E.: Myohaemoglobinuria. Lancet, 1:648, 1941.

Cáceres, E., and Whittenbury, G.: Evaluation of blood losses during surgical operations. Surgery, 45:681-687, 1959.

Cannon, W. B.: Bodily Changes in Pain, Hunger, Fear, and Rage. New York, Appleton, 1915.

Cannon, W. B., and Bayliss, W. M.: Note on muscle injury in relation to shock. Report of Shock Committee, Medical Research Committee, No. 26, 19-23, March, 1919. Cited by Blalock (1930).

Catchpole, B. N., Hackel, D. B., and Simeone, F. A.: Coronary and peripheral blood flow in experimental hemorrhagic hypotension treated with l-norepinephrine. Ann. Surg., 142:372-381, 1955.

Chien, S.: Role of sympathetic nervous system in surviving acute hemorrhage. Am. J. Physiol., 206:21-24, 1964.

Clark, J. H., Nelson, W., Lyons, C., Mayerson, H. S., and De Camp, P.: Chronic Shock: The problem of reduced blood volume in the chronically ill patient. Ann. Surg., 125:618-646, 1947.

Cohn, I., Jr.: Strangulation obstruction—Thirty fistula studies. S. Forum, 6:344-347, 1956.

Cohn, J. N., and Luria, M. H.: Studies in clinical shock and hypotension: the value of bedside hemodynamic observations. J.A.M.A., 190:891-896, 1964.

Coller, F. A., Crook, C. E., and Iob, V.: Blood loss in surgical operations. J.A.M.A., 126:1-5, 1944.

Coller, F. A., and Maddock, W. G.: Dehydration attendant on surgical operations. J.A.M.A., 99: 875-880, 1932.

Cowley, R. A., Attar, S., Esmond, W., and Blair, E.: The Utilization of Hyperbaric Oxygenation in Hemorrhagic Shock in Dogs. In: Boerema, I., Brummelkamp, W. H., and Meijne, N. G. (eds.); Clinical Application of Hyperbaric Oxygen: Proceedings of the First International Congress, Amsterdam, September, 1963. Amsterdam, Elsevier, 1964.

Crowell, J. W., Bounds, S. H., and Johnson, W. W.: Effect of varying the hematocrit ration on the susceptibility to hemorrhagic shock. Am. J. Physiol., 192:171-174, 1958.

Crowell, J. W., Ford, R. G., and Lewis, V. M.: Oxygen transport in hemorrhagic shock as a function of the hematocrit ratio. Am. J. Physiol., 196: 1033-1038, 1959.

Crowell, J. W., and Guyton, A. C.: Evidence favoring a cardiac mechanism in irreversible hemorrhagic shock. Am. J. Physiol., 201:893-896, 1961.

Crowell, J. W., and Smith, E. E.: Oxygen deficit and irreversible hemorrhagic shock. Am. J. Physiol., 206:313-316, 1964.

Culbertson, W. R., Elstun, W., Cole, W., and Altemeier, W. A.: Bacterial studies in irreversible hemorrhagic shock. Arch. Surg., 79:185-189, 1959.

Cushman, G. F.: Subperitoneal hemorrhage. California Med., 78:11-16, 1953.

deAlvarez, R. R., Nyhus, L. M., Merendino, K. A., Harkins, H. N., and Zech, R. K.: Tissue necrosis associated with intravenous norepinephrine administration. Am. Surg., 23:619-635, 1957; J.A.M.A., 165:1878, 1957.

Ditzler, J. W., and Eckenhoff, J. E.: A comparison of blood loss and operative time in certain surgical procedures completed with and without controlled hypotension. Ann. Surg., 143:289-293, 1956.

Drawhorn, C. W., and Howard, J. M.: Clinical evaluation of "Dextraven," a dextran of high molecular weight. U. S. Armed Forces M. J., 6:1576-1580, 1955.

Drew, J. H., Dripps, R. D., and Conroe, J. H.: Clinical studies on morphine. II. The effect of morphine upon the circulation of man and upon the circulatory and respiratory response to tilting. Anesthesiology, 7:44, 1946.

Duncan, G. W., Sarnoff, S. J., and Rhode, C. M.: Studies on effects of posture in shock and injury. Ann. Surg., 120:24-33, 1944.

Edwards, W. S., Siegel, A., and Bing, R. J.: Studies on myocardial metabolism. III. Coronary blood flow, myocardial oxygen consumption and carbohydrate metabolism in experimental hemorrhagic shock. J. Clin. Invest., 33:1646-1661, 1954.

Egdahl, R. H.: Pituitary-adrenal response following trauma to the isolated leg. Surgery, 46:9-21, 1959.

——: The differential response of the adrenal cortex and medulla to bacterial endotoxin. J. Clin. Invest., 38:1120-1125, 1959.

Egdahl, R. H., Melby, J. C., and Spink, W. W.: Adrenal cortical and body temperature responses to repeated endotoxin administration (24944), Proc. Soc. Exp. Biol. Med., 101:369-372, 1959.

Engberg, H.: Blood loss in operations: A practical colorimetric method. Acta. chir. scand., 111:235, 1956.

Erlanger, J., and Gasser, H. S.: Studies in secondary traumatic shock. III. Circulatory failure due to adrenalin. Am. J. Physiol., 49:345-376, 1919.

Evans, W. E., Darin, J. C., End, E., and Ellison, E. H.: The use of hyperbaric oxygen in the treatment of endotoxin shock. Surgery, 56:185-192, 1964.

Fåhraus, R.: The suspension stability of the blood. Physiol. Rev. 9:241-274, 1929.

Fine, J.: The Bacterial Factor in Traumatic Shock. Springfield, Ill., Charles C Thomas, 1954.

——: Relation of bacteria to the failure of blood volume therapy in traumatic shock. New Eng. J. Med., 250:889-895, 1954.

——: Host resistance to bacteria and to bacterial toxins in traumatic shock. Ann. Surg., 142: 361-371, 1955.

——: Traumatic shock. S. Clin. N. Am., 43:597-608, 1963a.

——: Irreversible shock. New Eng. J. Med., 268: 108, 1963b.

——: Septic shock. J.A.M.A., 188:427-432, 1964.

Fine, J., Frank, E. D., Ravin, H. A., Rutenberg, S. H., and Schweinburg, F. B.: The bacterial factor in traumatic shock. New Eng. J. Med., 260: 214-220, 1959.

Finnerty, F. A., Jr., Buchholz, J. H., and Guillaudeu, R. L.: Blood volumes and plasma protein during levarterenol-induced hypertension. J. Clin. Invest., 37:425-429, 1958.

Fiorica, V., and Funkhouser, G. E.: Dose-dependent responses to endotoxin in the dog. Proc. Soc. Exp. Biol. Med., 113:889-892, 1963.

Fitts, W. T., Jr.: Postgraduate Course on Preoperative and Postoperative Care. 41st Annual Clinical Congress, American College of Surgeons, Chicago, November 2, 1955.

Fogelman, M. J., and Wilson, B. J.: A different concept of volume replacement in traumatic hypovolemia. Am. J. Surg., 99:694-701, 1960.

Fox, C. L., Jr.: Oral sodium lactate in the treatment of burn shock. J.A.M.A., 124:207-212, 1944.

Frank E., Fine, Jr., and Pillemer, L.: Serum properdin levels in hemorrhagic shock. Proc. Soc. Exp. Biol. Med., 89:223-225, 1955.

Frank, E. D., Kaufman, D., Korman, H., Schweinburg, F., Frank, H. A., and Fine, J.: Effect of antibiotics on hemodynamics of hypovolemic septic shock. Am. J. Physiol., 182:166-176, 1955.

Frank, H. A., Frank, E. D., Korman, H., Macchi, I. A., and Hechter, O.: Corticosteroid output and adrenal blood flow during hemorrhagic shock in the dog. Am. J. Physiol., 182:24-28, 1955.

Freeman, N. E.: Decrease in blood volume after prolonged hyperactivity of the sympathetic nervous system. Am. J. Physiol., 103:185-202, 1933.

Freeman, N. E., Freedman, H., and Miller, C. C.: The production of shock by the prolonged con-

tinuous injection of adrenalin in unanesthetized dogs. Am. J. Physiol., 131:545-553, 1941.
Gans, H., and Krivit, W.: Effect of endotoxin shock on the clotting mechanism of dogs. Ann. Surg., 152:69-76, 1960.
Gatch, W. D., and Little, W. D.: Amount of blood lost during some of the more common operations. J.A.M.A., 83:1075-1076, 1924.
Gelin, L-E.: Macrodex in burns. International Surgical Society Travel Club Meeting. Lund, Sweden, August 4, 1955.
———: Studies in anemia of injury. Acta chir. scand., [Supp.] 210:130, 1956.
———: Intravascular aggregation and capillary flow. Acta chir. scand., 113:463-465, 1957.
———: The significance of intravascular aggregation following injury. Bull. Soc. Int. Chir., 18:4-19, 1959.
———: Rheologic disturbances and the use of low viscosity dextran in surgery. Rev. Surg., 19:385-400, 1962.
Gelin, L-E., and Löfström, B.: A preliminary study on peripheral circulation during deep hypothemia: Observations on decreased suspension stability of the blood and its prevention. Acta chir. scand., 108:402-404, 1955.
Gelin, L-E., Sölvell, L., and Zederfeldt, B.: Plasma volume expanding effect of low viscous dextran and Macrodex. Acta chir. scand., 122:309-323, 1961.
Gesell, R.: Studies on the submaxillary gland. III. Some factors controlling the volume-flow of blood. Am. J. Physiol., 47:438-467, 1919a.
———: Studies on the submaxillary gland. IV. A comparison of the effects of hemorrhage and of tissue-abuse in relation to secondary shock. Am. J. Physiol., 47:468-506, 1919b.
Gesell, R., and Moyle, C. A.: On the relation of blood volume to tissue nutrition. II. The effects of graded hemorrhage on the volume-flow of blood through the striated muscle of the dog. Am. J. Physiol., 61:412-419, 1922.
Gilbert, R. P.: Endotoxin shock in the primate. Proc. Soc. Exp. Biol. Med., 111:328, 1962.
Green, D. M., and Metheny, D.: The estimation of acute blood loss by the tilt test. Surg., Gynec. Obstet., 84:1045-1950, 1947.
Greene, B. A.: Cardiac output and total peripheral resistance in anesthesiology: Clinical applications. J.A.M.A., 166:1003-1010, 1958.
Greenfield, L., and Blalock, A.: Effect of low molecular weight dextran on survival following hemorrhagic shock. Surgery, 55:684-686, 1964.
Greep, J. M., Litwin, S. B., and Nardi, G. L.: Comparative study of new device for measuring blood volume. Arch. Surg., 86:164-169, 1963.
Gregersen, M. I., and Rawson, R.: Blood volume. Physiol. Rev., 39:307-342, 1959.
Gross, R. E.: A scale for rapid measurement of blood which is lost in surgical sponges. J. Thoracic Surg., 18:543-545, 1949.
Gross, S. D.: System of Surgery, 1850, cited by Mann, F. C.: Bull. Johns Hopkins Hosp., 25:205-212, 1914.
———: System of Surgery. ed. 6. vol. 1. p. 412. Philadelphia, H. C. Lea's Son & Co., 1882.
Gurd, F. N.: A symposium on shock. J. Trauma, 2:353-423, 1962.
Gurd, F. N., and Gardner, C. McG.: Reappraisal of the treatment of hemorrhagic shock. Am. J. Surg., 89:725-729, 1955.
Guyton, A. C.: Textbook of Medical Physiology. ed. 2. Philadelphia, W. B. Saunders, 1961.
Guyton, A. C., and Crowell, J. W.: Dynamics of the heart in shock. Fed. Proc., 20:51-60, 1961.
Haber, M. H., Brown, W. T., and Schneider, K. A.: Ischemic necrosis of multiple organs in prolonged shock. J.A.M.A., 183:1107-1109, 1963.
Hakstian, R. W., Hampson, L. G., and Gurd, F. N.: Pharmacological agents in experimental hemorrhagic shock. Arch. Surg., 83:335-347, 1961.
Hall, C. E., and Hall, O.: Protection against tourniquet shock afforded by parabiosis. Proc. Soc. Exp. Biol. Med., 90:230-232, 1955.
Hallin, R. W.: Continuous venous pressure monitoring as a guide to fluid administration in the hypotensive patient. Am. J. Surg., 106:164-172, 1963.
Hammond, W. G., Vandam, L. D., Davis, J. M., Carter, R. D., Ball, M. R., and Moore, F. D.: Studies in surgical endocrinology. IV. Anesthetic agents as stimuli to change in corticosteroids and metabolism. Ann. Surg., 148:199-211, 1958.
Hampson, L. G., Scott, H. J., and Gurd, F. N.: A comparison of intra-arterial and intravenous transfusion in normal dogs and in dogs with experimental myocardial infarction. Ann. Surg., 140:56-66, 1954.
Hardaway, R. M.: The role of intravascular clotting in the etiology of shock. Ann. Surg., 155:325-338, 1962.
Hardaway, R. M., Brune, W. H., Geever, E. F., Burns, J. W., and Mock, H. P.: Studies on the role of intravascular coagulation in irreversible hemorrhagic shock. Ann. Surg., 155:241-250, 1962.
Hardaway, R. M., and Johnson, D. G.: Influence of fibrinolysin on shock. J.A.M.A., 183:597-599, 1963.
Hardaway, R. M., and McKay, D. G.: Disseminated intravascular coagulation: a cause of shock. Ann. Surg., 149:462-470, 1959a.
———: Intravascular thrombi and the intestinal factor of irreversible shock. Ann. Surg., 150:261-265, 1959b.
———: The syndromes of disseminated intravascular coagulation. Rev. Surg., 20:297-328, 1963.
Hardaway, R. M., Neimes, R. E., Burns, J. W., Mock, H. P., and Trenchak, P. T.: Role of the canine spleen in irreversible hemorrhagic shock. Ann. Surg., 156:197-203, 1962.
Hardy, J. G., Morris, G. C., Jr., Yow, E. M., Haynes, B. W., Jr., and De Bakey, M. E.: Studies on the role of bacteria in irreversible hemorrhagic shock in dogs Ann. Surg., 139:282-286, 1954.
Harkins, H. N.: Experimental burns. I. The rate

Bibliography 145

of fluid shift and its relation to the onset of shock in severe burns. Arch. Surg., 31:71-85, 1935.

———: Physical factors in surgical shock. Nord. med., 6:1112-1115, 1940.

———: Recent advances in the study and management of traumatic shock. Surgery, 9:231-294, 447-482, 607-655, 1941.

———: Sodium therapy of experimental tourniquet shock. Am. J. Physiol., 148:538-545, 1947.

Harkins, H. N., and Long, C. N. H.: Metabolic changes in shock after burns. Am. J. Physiol., 144:661-668, 1945.

Harkins, H. N., and Roome, N. W.: Concealed hemorrhage into tissues and its relation to traumatic shock. Arch. Surg., 35:130-139, 1937.

Hechter, O., Macchi, I. A., Korman, H., Frank, E. D., and Frank, H. A.: Quantitative variations in the adrenocortical secretion of dogs. Am. J. Physiol., 182:29-34, 1955.

Henegar, G. C.: The importance of blood volume determination in surgical patients. S. Clin. N. Am., 43:187-199, 1963.

Hershey, S. G., Guccione, I., and Zweifach, B. W.: Beneficial action of pretreatment with chlorpromazine on survival following graded hemorrhage in the rat. Surg., Gynec. Obstet., 101:431-436, 1965.

Hinshaw, L. B., Vick, J. A., Carlson, C. H., and Fan, Y. L.: Role of histamine in endotoxin shock. Proc. Soc. Exp. Biol. Med., 104:379-381, 1960.

Hinshaw, L. B., Vick, J. A., Wittmers, L. E., Worthen, D. M., Nelson, D. L., and Swenson, O. P.: Changes in total peripheral resistance in endotoxin shock. Proc. Soc. Exp. Biol. Med., 108:24-27, 1961.

Hoitink, A. W. J. H.: Treatment of acute fatal hemorrhage by injection of artificial blood substitutes. Surg. Gynec. Obstet., 61:613-622, 1935.

Hopkins, R. W., Sabga, G., Bernardo, P., Penn, I., and Simeone, F. A.: The significance of posttraumatic and postoperative oliguria. Arch. Surg., 87:320-330, 1963.

Hopkins, R. W., and Simeone, F. A.: Trimethaphan camsylate in hemorrhagic shock. Arch. Surg., 89:365-372, 1964.

Howard, J.: Experiences with shock in the Korean Theater. In: Tr. Third Conf. on Shock and Circulatory Homeostasis, 1953. New York, Macy, 1954.

———: Postgraduate Course on Preoperative and Postoperative Care. 41st Annual Clinical Congress, American College of Surgeons, Chicago, November 1, 1955.

Howard, J. M., Ebert, R. V., Bloom, W. L., and Sloan, M. H.: The present status of dextran as a plasma expander. Am. J. Surg., 97:593-596, 1959.

Howard, J. M., Teng, C. T., and Loeffler, R. K.: Studies of dextrans of various molecular sizes. Ann. Surg., 143:369-372, 1956.

Hoxworth, P. I., Haesler, W. E., Jr., and Smith, H., Jr.: The risk of hepatitis from whole blood and stored plasma. Surg., Gynec. Obstet., 109:38-42, 1959.

Hume, D. M., and Nelson, D. H.: Adrenal cortical function in experimental shock, measured by adrenal venous blood corticosteroid secretion. Nav. M. Res. Inst. Res. Rep., 13:167-176, 1955.

Illingworth, C. F. W., Smith, G., Lawson, D. D., Ledingham, I. M., Sharp, G. R., Griffiths, J. C., and Henderson, C. I.: Surgical and physiological observations in an experimental pressure chamber. Brit. J. Surg., 49:222-227, 1961.

Johnson, D. G., and Parkins, W. M.: Effects of isoproterenol and levarterenol on blood flow and oxygen use in hemorrhagic shock. Arch. Surg., 92:277-286, 1966.

Johnson, H. D.: Venous pressure: its physiology and pathology in haemorrhage, shock, and transfusion. Brit. J. Surg., 51:276-281, 1964.

Kinney, J. M., and Wells, R. E., Jr.: Problems of ventilation after injury and shock. J. Trauma, 2:370-385, 1962.

Knisely, M. H.: An annotated bibliography on sludged blood. Postgrad. Med., 10:15-24, 80-93, 1951.

———: The settling of sludge during life. Acta anat., 44 (suppl. 41):1-64, 1961.

Koletsky, S., and Gustafson, G. E.: Tourniquet shock in rats; reversibility in the terminal phase. Am. J. Physiol., 178:229-232, 1954.

Koletsky, S., and Klein, D. E.: Reversibility of tourniquet shock with massive saline therapy. Am. J. Physiol., 182:439-442, 1955.

Laborit, H., and Huguenard, P.: L'hibernation artificielle chez le grand choqué. Presse méd., 61:1029-1030, 1953.

Landis, E. M.: Micro-injection studies of capillary permeability. III. The effect of lack of oxygen on the permeability of the capillary wall to fluid and to the plasma proteins. Am. J. Physiol., 83:528-542, 1928.

Lansing, A. M., Stevenson, J. A. F., and McLachlin, A. D.: The use of vasopressor agents in the treatment of shock. J. Trauma, 2:386-398, 1962.

Lepley, D., Jr., Weisfeldt, M., Close, A. S., Schmidt, R., Bowler, J., Kory, R. C., and Ellison, E. H.: Effect of low molecular weight dextran on hemorrhagic shock. Surgery, 54:93-103, 1963.

LeVeen, H. H., and Rubricius, J. L.: Continuous, automatic, electronic determinations of operative blood loss. Surg., Gynec. Obstet., 106:368-374, 1958.

Levenson, S. M., Einheber, A., and Malm, O. J.: Metabolic aspects of shock. J.A.M.A., 181:874-877, 1962.

Lewis, R. N., Werle, J. M., and Wiggers, C. J.: The behavior of the spleen in hemorrhagic hypotension and shock. Am. J. Physiol., 138:205-211, 1942.

Lillehei, R. C.: The prevention of irreversible hemorrhage shock in dogs by controlled cross perfusion of the superior mesenteric artery. Surg. Forum, 7:6-11, 1957.

Lillehei, R. C., and Macbean, L. D.: The intestinal factor in irreversible endotoxin shock. Ann. Surg., 148:513, 1958.

Longerbeam, J. K., Bloch, J. H., Manax, W. G., and Lillehei, R. C.: The treatment of irreversible shock. Hektoen Gold Medal Scientific Exhibit, A.M.A. Meeting, San Francisco, June 21-25, 1964.

Longerbeam, J. K., Lillehei, R. C., Scott, W. R., and Rosenberg, J. C.: Visceral factors in shock. J.A.M.A., 181:878-883, 1962.

MacLean, L. D.: Shock due to sepsis—a summary of current concepts of pathogenesis and treatment. J. Trauma, 2:412-423, 1962.

Maloney, J. V., Smythe, C. M., Gilmore, J. P., and Handford, S. W.: Intra-arterial and intravenous transfusion: a controlled study of their effectiveness in the treatment of experimental hemorrhagic shock. Surg., Gynec. Obstet., 97:529-535, 1953.

Marston, A.: The bowel in shock: the role of mesenteric arterial disease as a cause of death in the elderly. Lancet, 2:365-370, 1962.

McCarthy, M. D., and Newlin, N.: Range of efficacy of sodium chloride solution in treating severe thermal injury in the rat. J. Lab. Clin. Med., 41:416-420, 1953.

McClure, R. D., Hartman, F. W., Schnedorf, J. G., and Schelling, V.: Anoxia: a source of possible complications in surgical anesthesia. Ann. Surg., 110:835-850, 1939.

McGowan, G. K., and Walters, G.: The value of measuring central venous pressure in shock. Brit. J. Surg., 50:821-826, 1963.

Millican, R. C.: S^{35}-plasma and erythrocyte distribution in tourniquet-shocked mice. Am. J. Physiol. 179:513-519, 1954.

———: Tourniquet shock in mice: comparison of serum and saline therapy administered early and late after injury. Am. J. Physiol., 183:187-192, 1955.

Millican, R. C., Tabor, H., Stohlman, E. F., and Rosenthal, S. M.: Traumatic shock in mice: acute hemodynamic effects of therapy. Am. J. Physiol., 170:187-195, 1952.

Minot, A. S., and Blalock, A.: Plasma loss in severe dehydration, shock and other conditions as affected by therapy. Ann. Surg., 112:557-567, 1940.

Moore, F. D.: Metabolic Care of the Surgical Patient. Philadelphia, W. B. Saunders, 1959.

———: Shock and surgical trauma. J.A.M.A., 185:1047, 1963a.

———: Irreversible shock, New Eng. J. Med., 268:108, 1963b.

Moyer, C. A.: Personal communication, July 12, 1964.

Moyer, C. A., Coller, F. A., Iob, L. V., Vaughan, H. H., and Marty, D.: A study of the interrelationship of salt solutions, serum and defibrinated blood in the treatment of severely scalded, anesthetized dogs. Ann. Surg., 120:367-376, 1944.

Muller, W. H., Jr.: Discussion of paper by Hallin, 1963.

Nelson, R. M., Poulson, A. M., Lyman, J. H., and Henry, J. W.: Evaluation of tris(hydroxymethyl)-aminomethane (THAM) in experimental hemorrhagic shock. Surgery, 54:86-92, 100-103, 1963.

Nickerson, M.: Epinephrine and norepinephrine. Tr. Second Conf. on Shock and Circulatory Homeostasis, 1952. New York, Macy, 1953.

Nickerson, M., and Gourzis, J. T.: Blockade of sympathetic vasoconstriction in the treatment of shock. J. Trauma, 2:399-411, 1962.

Overton, R. C., and De Bakey, M. E.: Experimental observations on the influence of hypothermia and autonomolytic drugs in hemorrhagic shock. Paper given before Annual Congress, American College of Surgeons, November 2, 1955.

Palmerio, C., Zetterstrom, B., Shammash, J., Euchbaum, E., Frank, E., and Fine, J.: Denervation of the abdominal viscera for the treatment of traumatic shock. New Eng. J. Med., 269:709-716, 1963.

Parkins, W. M., Perlmutt, S. H., and Vars, H. M.: Modified fluid gelatin as plasma volume expander in hemorrhagic hypotensive dogs. S. Forum (1952), 3:421, 1953.

———: Dextran, oxypolygelatine, modified fluid gelatine as replacement fluids in experimental hemorrhage. Am. J. Physioi., 173:403, 1953.

Parkins, W. M., Ben, M., and Vars, H. M.: Tolerance of temporary occlusion of the thoracic aorta in normothermic and hypothermic dogs. Surgery, 38:38, 1955.

———: General and differential hypothermia (intraperitoneal) in prevention of ischemic shock and paraplegia following temporary occlusion of the thoracic aorta. Surg. Forum, 7:337, 1957.

Parsons, E., and Phemister, D. B.: Haemorrhage and "shock" in traumatized limbs: an experimental study. Surg., Gynec. Obstet., 51:196-207, 1930.

Pearson, W. T., Johnston, G. S., and Murphy, G. P.: Hemodynamic changes from low molecular weight dextran. Arch. Surg., 88:999-1002, 1964.

Peterson, C. G., and Haugen, F. P.: Hemorrhagic shock and the nervous system. Am. J. Surg., 106:233-242, 1963.

Pillemer, L., Blum, L., Lefrow, I. H., Ross, O. A., Todd, E. W., and Wardlaw, A. C.: The properdin system and immunity: I. Demonstration and isolation of a new serum protein, properdin, and its role in immune phenomena. Science, 120:279-285, 1954.

Rains, A. J. H.: Experience in the measurement of blood- and fluid-loss at operation. Brit. J. Surg., 43:191-196, 1955.

Raker, J. W., and Rovit, R. L.: The acute red blood cell destruction following severe thermal trauma in dogs. Surg., Gynec. Obstet., 98:169-176, 1954.

Ravdin, I. S., McNamee, H. G., Kamholz, J. H., and Rhoads, J. E.: Effect of hypoproteinemia on susceptibility to shock resulting from hemorrhage. Arch. Surg., 48:491-492, 1944.

Ravin, H. A., Denson, J. R., and Jensen, H.: Electrolyte shifts and electrocardiographic changes during tourniquet shock in rats. Am. J. Physiol., 178:419-426, 1954.

Reeve, T. S., and Vincent, P. C.: Factors controlling blood volume: a review. Aust. New Zeal. J. Surg., 32:152-156, 1962.

Rosenthal, S. M.: Experimental chemotherapy of burns and shock. IV. Production of traumatic shock in mice; V. Therapy with mouse serum and sodium salts. Pub. Health Rep., 58:1429-1436, 1943.

Rothstein, D. A., Rosen, S., Markowitz, A., and Fuller, J. B.: Ferritin and antiferritin serum treatment of dogs in irreversible hemorrhagic shock. Am. J. Physiol., 198:844-846, 1960.

Rustad, H.: Measurement of operative blood loss. Acta chir. scand., 125:14-18, 1963a.

———: Measurement of blood-loss during surgery. Lancet, 1:1304, 1963b.

Saltz, N. J.: The effect of ganglionic blockade on survival after tourniquet shock. Arch. Surg., 81:618-623, 1960.

Saltzstein, H. C., and Linkner, L. M.: Blood loss during operations. J.A.M.A., 149:722-725, 1952.

Saltzberg, A. M., and Evans, E. I.: Blood volumes in normal and in burned dogs: a comparative study with radioactive phosphorus tagged red cells and T-1824 dye. Ann. Surg., 132:746-759, 1950.

Sayman, W. A., and Allen, J. G.: Blood, plasma and expanders of plasma volume in the treatment of hemorrhagic shock. S. Clin. N. Am., 39:133-143, 1959.

Sayman, W. A., Gauld, R. L., Star, S. A., and Allen, J. G.: Safety of liquid plasma—A statistical appraisal. J.A.M.A., 168:1735-1739, 1958.

Schayer, R. W.: Relationship of induced histidine decarboxylase activity and histamine synthesis to shock from stress and from endotoxin. Am. J. Physiol., 198:1187-1192, 1960.

Schenk, W. G., Jr., Camp, F. A., Kjartansson, K. B., and Pollock, L.: Hemorrhage without hypotension: an experimental study of aortic flow distribution following minor hemorrhage. Ann. Surg., 160:7-13, 1964.

Schmutzer, K. J., Raschke, E., and Maloney, J. V., Jr.: Intravenous l-norepinephrine as a cause of reduced plasma volume. Surgery, 50:452-457, 1961.

Schweinburg, F. B., and Fine, J.: Resistance to bacteria in hemorrhagic shock. II. Effect of transient vascular collapse on sensitivity to endotoxin. Proc. Soc. Exp. Biol. Med., 88:589-591, 1955.

Schweinburg, F. B., Yashar, Y., Aprahamian, H. A., Davidoff, D., and Fine, J.: Resistance to bacteria in hemorrhagic shock. I. Decline in phagocytosis-promoting capacity of serum in shock. Proc. Soc. Exp. Biol. Med., 88:587-589, 1955.

Scott, R., Jr., Howard, J. M., Shorr, E., Lawson, N., and Davis, J. H.: Circulatory homeostasis following massive injury: studies of vasodepressor and vasoexcitatory substances in the circulating blood. Ann. Surg., 141:504-509, 1955.

Seeley, S. F., and Nelson, R. M.: Intra-arterial transfusion. Int. Abstr. Surg., 94:209-214, 1952.

Selkurt, E. E.: Intestinal ischemic shock and the protective role of the liver. Am. J. Physiol., 197:281-285, 1959.

Selmonosky, C. A., Goetz, R. H., and State, D.: The role of acidosis in the irreversibility of experimental hemorrhagic shock. J. Surg. Res., 3:491-496, 1963.

Serkes, K. D., Lang, S., and Pareira, M. D.: Efficacy of plasma and dextran compared to saline for fluid replacement following tourniquet shock. Surgery, 45:623-633, 1959.

———: Response of acutely starved and chronically undernourished rats to saline therapy following tourniquet shock. Proc. Soc. Exp. Biol. Med., 103:12-16, 1960.

Shenkin, H. A., Cheney, R. H., Govons, S. R., Hardy, J. D., Fletcher, A. G., Jr., and Starr, I.: On the diagnosis of hemorrhage in man: a study of volunteers bled large amounts. Am. J. Med. Sci., 208:421-436, 1944.

Sherman, R. T., and Noyes, H. E.: Lethality studies of the blood of irreversibly shocked dogs. J. Surg. Res., 3:409-411, 1963.

Shires, T., Coln, D., Carrico, J., and Lightfoot, S.: Fluid therapy in hemorrhagic shock. Arch. Surg., 88:688-693, 1964.

Shorr, E.: Tr. Second Conf. on Shock and Circulatory Homeostasis, 1952. New York, Macy, 1953.

Shorr, E., Zweifach, B. W., and Furchgott, B. F.: The role of hepatorenal vasotropic principles in experimental shock. In: Green, D. (ed.): Research in Medical Science. pp. 301-326. New York, Macmillan, 1950.

Simeone, F. A.: Wound shock. In: Bowers, W. F. (ed.): Surgery of Trauma. Philadelphia, J. B. Lippincott, 1953.

Smith, L. L., and Moore, F. D.: Refractory hypotension in man—is this irreversible shock?: clinical and biochemical observations, New Eng. J. Med. 267:733-742, 1962.

Smith, L. L., Muller, W., and Hinshaw, D. B.: The management of experimental endotoxin shock. Arch. Surg., 89:630-636, 1964.

Soffer, A.: Therapy of syncope. J.A.M.A., 154:1177-1179, 1954.

Spink, W. W.: The pathogenesis and management of shock due to infection. Arch. Int. Med., 106:433-442, 1960.

Spink, W. W., and Vick, J. A.: Endotoxin shock and the coagulation mechanism: modification of shock with epsilon-aminocaproic acid. Proc. Soc. Exp. Biol. Med., 106:242-247, 1961.

Stead, E. A., Jr.: Fainting. Am. J. Med., 13:387-388, 1952.

Steenburg, R. W., Lennihan, R., and Moore, F. D.: Studies in surgical endocrinology; II. The free blood 17-hydroxycorticoids in surgical patients; their relation to urine steroids, metabolism and convalescence. Ann. Surg., 143:180-209, 1956.

Swingle, W. W., Pfiffner, J. J., Vars, H. M., Bott, P. A., and Parkins, W. M.: The function of the adrenal cortical hormone and the cause of death from adrenal insufficiency. Science, 77:58, 1933.

Thomas, J. E., and Rooke, E. D.: Fainting, Proc. Mayo Clinic, 38:397-410, 1963.

Thorsén, G.: The use of dextrans as infusion fluids. Surg., Gynec. Obstet., 109:43-52, 1959.

Topete, A., Huizar Lara, H., Trinidad Pulido, J. T., and Diaz Caro, G.: New findings in the coronary-encephalic perfusion in depressed surgical cases. J. Thorac. Cardiov. Surg., 40:161-171, 1960.

Travers, B.: An inquiry concerning irritation, London, 1826. Cited by Mann, F. C.: Bull. Johns Hopkins Hosp., 25:205-212, 1914.

Veal, J. R., Russell, A. S., and Stubbs, D.: Intra-arterial transfusions: indications and technic. Am. Surgeon, 18:1150-1159, 1952.

Vesell, E. S., Palmerio, C. F. P., and Frank, E. D.: Serum lactic dehydrogenase activity in experimental endotoxic shock. Proc. Soc. Exp. Biol. Med., 104: 403-405, 1960.

Vick, J. A.: Vasodilator therapy of shock. J. Clin. Invest., 43:279-284, 1964.

Vick, J. A., and Spink, W. W.: Supplementary role of hydralazine in reversal of endotoxin shock with metaraminol and hydrocortisone. Proc. Soc. Exp. Biol. Med., 106:280-283, 1961.

Vowles, K. D. J., Barse, F. E., Bovard, W. J., Couves, C. M., and Howard, J. M.: Studies of coronary and perpiheral flow following hemorrhagic shock, transfusion and l-norepinephrine. Ann. Surg., 153:202-208, 1961.

Wadström, L. B.: Effect of trauma on plasma lipids; an experimental study on the rat. Acta chir. scand., 115:409-416, 1958.

Watts, D. T.: Arterial blood epinephrine levels during hemorrhagic hypotension in dogs. Am. J. Physiol., 184:271-274, 1956.

Weale, F. E.: A simplified theory of shock: the fundamental role of the myocardium. Lancet, 1:973-976, 1963.

Webb, W. R., and Jackson, J.: Blood pressure and urinary responses to increasing concentrations of norepinephrine in sequential hemorrhage. J. Surg. Res., 1:85-90, 1961.

Weil, M. H., Udhojl, V. N., and Allen, K. S.: The head-down position in treatment of shock. Surg. Gynec. Obstet., 116:669-672, 1963.

Weil, M. H., and Whigham, H.: The head-down (Trendenlenburg) position for treatment of "irreversible" hemorrhagic shock. Ann. Surg., 162: 905, 1965.

Weinberger, L. M., Gibbon, M. H., and Gibbon, J. H., Jr.: Temporary arrest of the circulation to the central nervous system. I—Physiologic effects. Arch. Neurol. Psychiat., 43:615-634, 1940.

Wiggers, H. C., and Ingraham, R. C.: Hemorrhagic shock: definition and criteria for its diagnosis. J. Clin. Invest., 25:30-36, 1946.

Wiggers, H. C., Roemhild, F., Goldberg, H., and Ingraham, R. C.: The influence of prolonged vasoconstriction on the transition from impending to irreversible hemorrhagic shock. Fed. Proc., 6:226-227, 1947.

Williams, J. A.: and Fine, J.: Measurement of blood volume with a new apparatus. New Eng. J. Med., 264:842-848, 1961.

Williams, W. T., and Parsons, W. H.: The indications for blood volume determinations in major surgical procedures. Surg., Gynec. Obstet., 106: 435-440, 1958.

Wilson, J. N., Grow, J. B., Demong, C. V., Prevedel, A. E., and Owens, J. C.: Central venous pressure in optimal blood volume maintenance. Arch. Surg., 85:563-578, 1962.

Wilson, R. F.: Jablonski, D. V., and Thal, A. P.: The usage of Dibenzyline in clinical shock. Surgery, 56:172-183, 1964.

Wolfman, E. F., Jr., Neill, S. A., Heaps, D. K., and Zuidema, G. D.: Donor blood and isotonic salt solution: effect on survival after hemorrhagic shock and operation. Arch. Surg., 86:869-873, 1963.

Wolfson, S. K., Jr., Inouye, W. Y., Kavanian, A., Icoz, M. V., and Parkins, W. M.: Preferential cerebral hyopthermia for circulatory arrest. Surgery, 57:846, 1965.

Zweifach, B. W.: Tissue mediators in the genesis of experimental shock. J.A.M.A., 181:866-870, 1962.

Zweifach, B. W., Lee, R. E., Hyman, C., and Chambers, R.: Omental circulation in morphinized dogs subjected to graded hemorrhage. Ann. Surg., 120:232-250, 1944.

CHAPTER 8

J. GARROTT ALLEN, M.D.

Blood Transfusions and Related Problems

Developmental Interrelations of Surgery and the Discovery of the Circulation
Practical Aspects and Precautions in Blood Transfusions
The Nature of Blood Transfusion Reactions
The Single Transfusion and Its Multiple Hazards
Special Transfusions
   Serum Hepatitis and the Australia (Au) Antigen
Abnormal Bleeding in the Surgical Patient

The development of blood transfusion is one of the most fascinating stories in the history of medicine. It is of special significance to surgery, for the evolution of the circulation, transfusion, hemostasis, and shock are much of the warp and woof of the fabric of modern surgery. In essence, present-day blood and plasma replacement is the inevitable result of scientific studies in many fields.

DEVELOPMENTAL INTERRELATIONS OF SURGERY AND THE DISCOVERY OF THE CIRCULATION, TRANSFUSION, HEMOSTASIS AND SHOCK

The story of transfusion is that of the scientific method itself. While the discovery of the circulation was prerequisite to its experimental and clinical trial, the developments in immunology and coagulation 250 years later were essential to its success and general usage. The interval between the first transfusion and its mature development demanded careful attention to hemostasis if operative surgery was to take advantage of the advances which anesthesia, immunology, and microbiology made possible after the mid-portion of the 19th century.

To recount, as often done, the fables and the folklore of transfusion history is to ignore or to relegate to an inferior position the wealth of historical facts which have accrued through nearly 2,000 years.

THE DISCOVERY OF THE CIRCULATION

The concepts of the circulation required no less than 1200 years of recorded history to emerge from its Galenic shackles before it could assume a sound scientific footing. The writings of Aristotle (384-322 B.C.) are among the first to be cited in this epic. He studied the movement of blood in the chick embryo and believed that the arteries connected with the veins through pores in the septum of the heart. He believed that the heart was the source of body heat and the seat of the soul, that expansion of the heart was the result of boiling blood heated within the heart, and that the heart was the all-important organ to the body, as well as to the vessels.

Erasistratus (330-245 B.C.), an early Greek physiologist, described the auriculoventricular valves, but unfortunately assigned to the liver the role that Aristotle credited to the heart. He introduced a second misconception, long perpetuated, that the arteries carried air rather than blood.

Both Aristotle and Erasistratus believed that the arteries communicated with the veins through pores in the intraventricular septum. Their views might well seem to be reaffirmed, were Aristotle and Erasistratus to witness today an operation for the closure of a septal defect in the heart. It is possible that in their limited dissections they encountered a septal defect and, failing to find such obvious communications between the right and the left chambers of the heart in the vast majority, postulated the invisible pores to account for the passage of blood from the right ventricle to the left.

Some of the views credited to each of these men may have been in some measure those of Galen (A.D. 130-200) because of the difficulties often entailed in the course of translations. Therefore, there is a moderate degree of uncertainty expressed among scholars as to some of the interpretations attributed to the ancient Greeks. Harvey quotes Aristotle as writing

. . . the blood of animals pulsates within their veins (meaning the arteries) and by the pulse is sent everywhere simultaneously . . . thus do all the veins pulsate together and by successive strokes, because they all depend upon the heart; and, as it is always in motion, so are they likewise always moving together, but by successive movement.

A similar but not identical view also was expressed by Erasistratus, but it was the Galenic view that the pulse was a function of respiratory motion which was to prevail for more than 1200 years.

Galen had to limit his prodigious numbers of dissections to animals, especially to apes. He taught Erasistratus' belief "that the blood is prepared in the liver and is thence transferred to the heart to receive its proper form and last perfection" (Payne, 1896). To him, blood ebbed to and fro in the veins and the arteries, passing from side to side through the porous intraventricular septum as suggested by Aristotle. Galen believed that arteries distributed both air and blood through the body and that in some manner air was derived from the lungs, whereas Erasistratus conceived the arteries to contain "nothing but spirits" (air); hence, they were named "arteria" from the Latin. Born in Pergamon, Mysia, Galen later migrated to Rome via Alexandria, bringing with him many of the concepts of Greek medicine.

Harvey and De Motu Cordis. History often discloses serious injustice in science—perhaps Galen was such a victim. He must have appeared to Harvey as an unusually strong opponent, for his work had been brought to England less than a century in advance of Harvey's times and hence likely was then under critical review. Thomas Linacre (1460-1524) translated Galen from Greek into Latin in England; Linacre was the first president of the Royal College of Physicians of London. Harvey's attack upon Galenic doctrines and Galen's students and admirers was relentless, dissecting as it were, truth from fantasy, logic from confusion, and candor from "divine expression." However mild Harvey is depicted by some, there is little evidence of fear as to the correctness of his own scientific conclusions or of any reservation or concern for reprisal to be found in his vigorous writings:

Good God! how should the mitral valves prevent the regurgitation of air and not of blood? I do not see how he (Galen) can deny that the great artery is the very vessel to carry the blood, when it has attained its highest term of perfection for distribution to all parts of the body. Or would he perchance still hesitate, like all who come after him, even to the present hour, because he did not perceive the route by which the blood was transferred from the veins to the arteries, as I have already said, of the intimate connection between the heart and the lungs? And it plainly appears that this has puzzled the anatomists no little when, in their dissections, they found the pulmonary artery and left ventricle full of thick, black, and clotted blood, and felt themselves compelled to affirm that the blood made its way from the right to the left ventricle by transudating through the septum of the heart. But this fancy I have already refuted. A pathway for the blood must therefore be prepared and thrown open, and being once exposed, no further difficulty will, I believe, be experienced by anyone in what I have already proposed in regard to the pulse of the heart and the arteries, viz., the passage of the blood from the veins to the arteries and its distribution to the whole of the body by means of these vessels.

In *De Motu Cordis*, Harvey clearly postulated a peripheral communication between the small arteries and the veins based on observations made upon the comb of the young cock, the ears of white rabbits, the wings of the bat, the tails of tadpoles, the fins of fish, and other more primitive forms of animal life. He assumed that the arteries delivered blood to the tissues, flowing through a structureless parenchyma to enter the venous side of the circulation. However, Harvey, an Aristotelian devotee, could not bring himself to refute the latter's concept that the heart was the source of body heat.

Capillaries. The anatomic demonstration of the capillary circulation was to come from the microscopic observations of Marcello Malpighi (1628-1694) in 1661. This practicing clinician and professor of medicine is said by some to have used a compound microscope, whether the one invented by Zacharias and Hans Janssen about 1590 or the much improved Drebbel version made about the same time is unknown to me. Others say that he used the simple microscope of von Leeuwenhoek (1632-1723) invented before 1673. In any case, the microscope allowed Malpighi to describe the capillaries, though he misinterpreted blood corpuscles as fat cells. In letters to his mathematician friend, Borelli, is contained his first description of the capillary circulation. Malpighi wrote:

Hence, it was clear to the senses that blood flowed away along tortuous vessels and was not poured into spaces, but was always contained within tubules, and that its dispersion is due to the multiple winding of these vessels.

His studies were greatly extended by Leeuwenhoek, beginning in 1668.

The Pulmonary Circulation. Recognition of the pulmonary circulation in 1553 is to be found in the writings of Michael Servetus (1509-1553), as student prosector and contemporary of Vesalius. By nature, Servetus was a dissenter and nonconformist, if not a heretic. He decried with contempt the formalities of religion of his day, advocating simplicity and an ungarnished Christianity. This same spirit prevailed upon Servetus in his scientific attitudes, especially as applied to Galen; interestingly, his friend and colleague, Vesalius, the father of gross anatomy, discredited much of Galen's anatomy, though perhaps with less malice.

Servetus recognized the pulmonary circuit and emphatically denied Galen's concept of septal pores as the means of transit for blood from the right ventricle to the left. This unfortunate soul, like Vesalius, was to come to an untimely end, the result of his religious fervor and fanaticism. A copy of Servetus' *Christianismi Restituto*, which also contained his views on the pulmonary circulation, fell into the hands of his one-time friend, Calvin, in Geneva. Through the latter's influence, Servetus was condemned. Calvin seems to have cunningly mobilized the opposing forces of the Reform movement and of the Catholic Church against Servetus. Brought to trial in Geneva, imprisoned but escaped, he was burned in effigy with 5 bales of his book, April 17, 1553. Subsequently recaptured and tried, he was sentenced to death by slow burning at the stake, carried out at noon, October 27, 1553. With all but 2 copies of *Christianismi Restituto* devoured in the flames of April 17, there is little reason to believe that Harvey was aware of the contributions of Servetus, and his failure to acknowledge Servetus is no surprise.

In *Christianismi Restituto* were Servetus' comments on the pulmonary circuit:

The vital spirit has its source in the left ventricle of the heart, the lungs aiding most essentially in its production. . . . The right ventricle of the heart communicates to the left. This communication, however, does not take place through the septum, partition, or midwall of the heart, as is commonly believed, but by another admirable contrivance, the blood being transmitted from the pulmonary artery to the pulmonary vein by a lengthened passage through the lungs, in the course of which it is elaborated and becomes a crimson color. It is finally attracted by diastole and reaches the left ventricle of the heart. Moreover, it is not simply air, but air mingled with blood that is returned from the lungs to the heart through the pulmonary vein. . . . It is in the lungs that the mixture of blood with inspired air takes place, and it is in the lungs, not in the heart, that the crimson color of the blood is acquired. To conclude, the septum or middle portion of the heart, seeing that it is without vessels or special properties, is not competent to permit and accomplish the communication and elaboration in question, although it may be that some transudation occurs through it.

TRANSFUSION DEVELOPMENTS

One of the natural outgrowths of Harvey's discovery was to be the first documentation of blood transfusion by Richard Lower (1631-91) carried out in dogs at Gresham College in Oxford late in February of 1665. Sir Christopher Wren (1632-1723) experimented earlier with the intravenous infusion of ales, wines and drugs as a method of administration of drugs while at Oxford and is credited by many as having also infused blood. The latter activity seems to be unconfirmed. Lower, in publishing his observations in the *Transactions of the Philosophical Society*, December 17, 1666, recognized transfusion to have its greatest potential value in the replacement of blood lost in hemorrhage.

His successful demonstration of transfusion in dogs on November 14, 1666, before the Royal Society (newly formed at Oxford in 1662) proved the feasibility of transfusion and its value in hemorrhage. About this event, Dr. Samuel Pepys recorded in his Diary of that date: "This did give occasion to many pretty wishes, as the blood of a Quaker to be let into an Archbishop, and such like." Lower, himself, did not deny the importance of his observation, writing,

At least, it is a comfort to our Nation and credit to our fame that Harvey became pre-eminent by first demonstrating that blood circulated inside the body. That this circulation could be extended outside the body was first discovered by me.

Unfortunately, the freedom with which dogs may be transfused without resort to crossmatch or typing, in sharp contrast with man, was not to be recognized until 250 years later. Thus, the excellent results of Lower obtained on dogs were doomed from the start so far as human transfusion was concerned. Jean Baptiste Denis (1630-1695) administered transfusions of human blood to 3 patients in 1667, but his 3rd patient died with all the symptoms of an acute transfusion reaction and its attendant shock. Charged by the patient's wife of murdering her husband, Denis was tried and eventually exonerated in the French courts, but not without the wise decree prohibiting further trial of human transfusions unless sanctioned by the Faculty of Medicine of Paris. A decade later, similar action was taken by Parliament and soon thereafter by papal and governmental decree in Italy.

More than 125 years elapsed until John Blundell (1790-1877), a London obstetrician, once again gave human transfusions and once again with disastrous result in 1818. Five of his 10 patients died; his work is said by some to have served to reawaken interest and to reopen the subject of transfusion, but certainly there was no great tendency to resume its use.

Blood Typing. As William Harvey set in order the knowledge of the circulation, so Karl Landsteiner (1868-1943) accomplished the same for the field of blood transfusion immunology. Examining bloods of various members of his laboratory, he was able from this limited experience to recognize 3 blood types (A, B and O) in 1900. In this publication he emphasized the importance of blood typing preliminary to transfusion. Decastello and Sturli described the 4th and rarest type, AB, in 1902. Landsteiner provided the classification which is the international nomenclature used today. Within the intervening 40 years of his study, Landsteiner described cold agglutinins, the M and the N factors, the Rh factors and their significance, as well as certain other minor types and agglutination irregularities. His subject matter and accomplishments deserve no less recognition than those of Harvey. More recently the Rhesus systems, the system of "H" substances, and the Lewis (Le) system have been elucidated. The revised classification by Wiener (1967) serves as a useful guide (see Table 8-3, A and B) and compares his with that of Fisher-Race (British).

Crossmatching. Ludwig Hektoen (1863-1951) re-emphasized in 1907 the need for selecting donors according to blood type, and in 1908 Epstein and Ottenberg devised the slide method for the detection of incompatible mixtures of blood. To Ottenberg must also go the credit for the first large-scale use of blood typing in the selection of donors for patients to be transfused, reporting with Kaliski in 1913 the transfusion of blood to 128 patients with only 3 deaths, and these he proved to be fatalities from mismatched blood. They observed agglutination of the donors' cells by the patients' serum to be more important "to avoid than the reverse." Thus developed the concept of "major" and "minor" fields of agglutination in transfusion crossmatchings, as well as the concept of the "universal donor" (Type O) and the "universal recipient" (Type AB).

Anticoagulants in Transfusion. Lower described the use of defibrinated blood in his transfusions among dogs in 1665 and pointed out that coagulation presented one of the most serious problems in blood transfusion. Braxton-Hicks, encountering hemorrhage in his obstetric practice, introduced sodium phosphate as an anticoagulant to facilitate blood transfusion, but its toxicity prevented its general acceptance.

The role of the calcium ion in blood coagulation needed to be elucidated before transfusions were to become practical, even though typing and crossmatching procedures would eliminate most incompatibilities. By precipitating blood calcium with sodium oxalate, Arthrus and Pages in 1890 were able to prevent coagulation in vitro. Schmidt in 1895 was unable to accept the Arthrus and Pages explanation for the anticoagulant action of oxalate, because he noted that sodium citrate added to blood had the same anticoagulant effect without altering the concentration of calcium in blood. Sabbatini in 1903 explained this seeming discrepancy, demonstrating the action of citrate as one in which the calcium ion is firmly bound but not precipitated. In this bound state, calcium was incapable of participating in blood coagulation.

Lewisohn, Agote, Hustin, and Weil, each working independently, in 1914 and 1915 suggested the use of sodium citrate as an anticoagulant adequate for blood transfusion purposes. Lewisohn's contributions continued for more than 10 years, logically answering each of the many objections raised, and finally established sodium citrate as an anticoagulant useful and safe in the preparation for blood transfusion. Citrate remains the basic anticoagulant of choice today and has eliminated the need for haste in transference of blood from donor to recipient. To Lewisohn (1875-1965) belongs the credit for the recognition and the development of the usefulness of citrate in blood transfusion.

Citrate-phosphate-dextrose has been suggested as another anticoagulant. It is claimed to extend the life of the red cell, but subsequent results have been conflicting. It has some theoretic advantages but few, if any, that can be realized practically (Orlina and Josephson, 1969). It may be harmful to use.

Hemostasis. One of the benevolent influences of the "transfusion failures" after Lower's 17th-century experiments was the continuing emphasis for improvements in technics for operative hemostasis. If surgery was to take advantage of the opportunities to be afforded by the mastery of anesthesia and operative asepsis 200 years later, careful hemostasis was essential. Recognizing the importance of hemostasis was not new. For centuries it was proposed that amputation be carried out in the gangrenous or necrotic portions of limbs where bleeding would not occur, or that *en masse* ligation of the vessels be employed at the time of amputation.

Archigenes (A.D. 48-117) and Celsus (circa A.D. 25) recommended the use of the ligature as early as A.D. 100, and compression bandages were applied by the early Greeks. However, as a technic for hemostasis, compression bandages were of little value until the tourniquet or garrot technic was introduced in 1674 by Morel. Both linen and catgut were employed as ligature material by the ancients and were mentioned so frequently in the early writings as to mask the exact identity of their origins.

Cautery, too, was used at an early date in the control of hemorrhage and certainly was in general use at the time of Hippocrates and Galen and later was advocated in the writings of John de Vigo (1460-1520) to whom Paré referred (Paget, 1899).

At Tourin in 1537, Ambroise Paré (1510-1590) exhausted his supply of boiling oil used for hemostasis and the general wound care before he could treat the large numbers of wounded soldiers assigned to him. Thus he was forced to treat the remaining casualties with a medicament comprised of egg yolk, oil of roses and turpentine. Fearing that all the latter group might die before morning for the want of boiling oil, he arose early to visit them:

where beyond my expectation, I found that those to whom I had applied my digestive medicament had but little pain, and their wounds were without inflammation or swelling, having rested fairly well that night; the others, to whom the boiling oil was used, I found feverish, with great pain and swelling about the edges of their wounds. Then I resolved never more to burn cruelly poor men with gunshot wounds.

To Paré belongs the credit for recognizing that the treatment of wounds with cautery was harmful. But it was not until 15 years later that he abandoned the searing cautery as a means of hemostasis in amputation. The occasion was his military journey to Danvilliers in 1552, where he reports that he drew forth the vessels with bullet forceps, ligated them *en masse* and amputated above the line of demarcation. Thereby the surgical use of ligature was rediscovered.

Through the ages, materials for ligature have included many items: among them were linen, catgut, "animal sinews," strips of doeskin, silk, and cotton. Joseph Baron Lister (1827-1912), originally a student of colloidal chemistry under Sir Thomas Graham (1805-1869) and later entering surgery, revived the use of catgut. Lister invented the chromicizing process in 1876 and was the first to use it. By chromicizing catgut, he hoped to prolong its effectiveness in tissue on one hand and, at the same time, to avoid its unnecessary persistence when ligatures no longer served a useful purpose.

William Stewart Halsted (1852-1923), a great admirer of German aseptic technic and of the operative meticulousness of the Swiss surgeon, Theodor Kocher (1841-1917), was among the first to emphasize the principles of hemostasis in this country. Halsted, like Kocher, favored the use of silk ligatures and despaired of catgut. Doubtless, catgut was a troublesome product in that day, but in his condemnation of it, Halsted overlooked or failed to appreciate the biologic principles which were always so much a part of Lister's investigations. Perhaps more to the point are the principles of careful hemostasis and the gentle handling of tissues, for these have not changed—the quality of suture material has.

Hemostatic instruments, beginning with the bullet forceps, were developed shortly after the invention of firearms, but otherwise were slow to come into extensive general use. Centuries later, Physick, Liston, Péan, Kocher, Halsted and many others designed or made contributions to the various types of hemostats, some of which bear their names and are still in use today. Samuel Harvey's account of *The Story of Hemostasis* and Halsted's excellent review of surgery in general, related in his 1920 *The Operative Story of Goitre*, afford a pleasant evening's reading for the student of surgery who is searching for or seeking out the "genetics and mutations" of his professional heritage. In these two tracts are told the stories of many of the men and their accomplishments in the long search to overcome the hazards and the fears of operative hemorrhage.

Historical developments in respect to shock and its relationship to hemorrhage, hemostasis, and transfusions are not easily explained, for one of the curious failures in the historical trails left by the surgeon and the physician alike was their inability to understand that hemorrhage was the chief cause of operative or hemorrhagic shock. For 500 years can be found written evidences of many shots striking the target circle but never once quite hitting the "bull's-eye." While all recognized the important association of shock and hemorrhage, the concepts of hidden, internal, or sequestered hemorrhages and/or of plasma loss did not receive serious consideration until the 1930's. In such patients, shock seemed to have occurred without hemorrhage or at least with less bleeding than was realized. This reason, more than any other, clouded the issue and delayed its understanding. The choice and the derivation of the word "shock" (Fr. *choque*: the phenomenon following a blow, impact, or collision, especially as applied to combat injuries) to define the patient's condition, is, to a certain extent, a misinterpretation of its nature and of the patient's response. Much of its earlier meaning yet remains, and it is a term all too frequently abused by the medical profession and the laity alike even today.

As recently as 1923, Walter Cannon (1871-1945), in a monograph entitled *Traumatic Shock*, presented data of his own as well as referring extensively to those of others, especially to Keith and to Gasser on shock. All of these reports had demonstrated conclusively that a diminished circulating blood volume was a constant finding in traumatic shock and frequently this was also accompanied by a rise in the hematocrit reading and acidosis; nonetheless, the cardinal point (hypovolemia and its resultant reduction of organ perfusion), while acknowledged and extensively discussed, failed to impress Cannon and others of its all-important role in the genesis of hemorrhagic, burn, or traumatic shock.

Cannon agreed with O. H. Robertson that the transfusion of compatible blood was the most effective treatment of shock but did not emphasize the singular importance of hypovolemia and its resultant poor tissue perfusion as its cause. He wrote in his preface, "because of its mysterious onset and nature, traumatic shock has long suggested problems of unusual clinical and scientific interest . . . it has remained an enigma." Toxemias and neural reactions continued to cloud the ultimate and basic disturbance, even at the present time.

Out of the experimental studies of Phemister and of Blalock in the late 1920's and the early 30's was to emerge the true significance of the role of hypovolemia in shock of traumatic, hemorrhagic, or burn origin. The experimental observations of these two men were soon to be confirmed and the soundness of treatment with blood and/or plasma to be documented thoroughly by the military experiences of World War II.

Thus from the cumulative observations, beginning 400 years ago with Paré, Servetus, Harvey and Lower and revived 300 years later by the works of Landsteiner, Lewisohn, Robertson, Cannon, Phemister, Blalock and many others, evolved the knowledge and the background which were to provide the present-day indications and status of one of our greatest therapeutic pillars: the proper use of blood transfusion and allied substances. If one man's contributions in this field are to be singled out above all others, they would seem to be those of Karl Landsteiner. Because of his brilliance and keenness of insight, his contributions must stand abreast of those of all time.

Glycerolized Frozen Blood. One important new development in blood preservation is the use of glycerolized frozen blood (Tullis et al., 1958; Haynes et al., 1960; O'Brien and Watkins, 1960; and Huggins, 1964). Such blood, collected in acid-citrate-dextrose solution and stored at −80° C. for 5 years and longer, showed less deviation of the oxyhemoglobin saturation curve than blood stored by conventional methods at 4° C. beyond 7 days. Frozen blood also can be used for pump priming and transfusion in cardiovascular surgery (see Chap. 41, Cardiac Surgery).

"Frozen blood" refers to washed packed cells, and is thus essentially free of isologous plasma and of platelets. Of the seven methods presently under clinical trial, the method of Huggins (1964) appears the most promising. It depends upon a simplified technic in which the red-cell mass is suspended in a solution of glycerol with a final molarity of 5.4 moles per liter (50%, weight per volume). The glycerol does not penetrate the cells, and it is thought to exert its protective action against hemolysis (1) by minimizing the formation of sharp ice crystals within the cells, (2) by preventing the increase of intracellular and extracellular electrolytes that normally would occur and tend to cause the cells to imbibe water during thawing and (3) to minimize the alterations of lipid complexes, especially within the cell and its membrane.

Diluting or washing of the red-cell mass with nonelectrolyte solutions (8% glucose and 1% fructose) results in clumping or agglomeration of the red cells because of the low ionic concentration. At these low ionic concentrations, Coombs-positive (p. 160) erythrocytes were observed because the cells became coated with the B_1C component of complement as well as with beta and gamma globulin. After disaggregation by the agglomerated cells, beta globulin may still coat the red cells, yielding still a Coombs-positive cell but of the non-immune type. This may be prevented by adding disodium ethylenediaminetetraacetate (disodium edetate; Na EDTA—Mollison and Polly, 1964), thereby eliminating the false-positive Coombs test; 0.3 per cent of disodium EDTA is added to the glycerolized solutions.

After these storage conditions the temperature is elevated, and the agglomerated mass is resuspended in ACD solution with 85 to 95 per cent cell recovery. It is centrifuged once to remove any cellular fragments and free hemoglobin. It should be used within a day or two. The older the blood when frozen, the shorter is its post-transfusion survival time.

The chief advantage of this process is that it makes possible the long-term storage of the rare types of blood. It is, however, a transfusion of red cells, devoid of the additional advantages of whole blood.

A note of caution in regard to the use of frozen glycerolized packed red cells was stated by Valeri and Henderson (1964). They observed that when deglycerolized, thawed red cells were resuspended in a 5 per cent solution of human albumin and transfused, hemoglobinuria with or without acute renal insufficiency occurred in about 40 per cent of patients. This reaction was not a serious one when hypovolemic hypotension was not the reason for transfusion but, when it was, the consequences were severe in some patients. By contrast, they failed to observe these reactions when deglycerolized, thawed red cells were resuspended in autologous plasma. The reasons for these differences are not known.

Finch et al. (1969), for more than 13 years have been studying the life-extending possibilities of the addition of adenosine triphosphate (ATP) to citrated blood and to packed red cells. The added ATP may prove useful, but is not without some risk.

Cadaver Blood. In March of 1930, S. S. Yudin of the Sklifassovsky Institute in Moscow performed the first transfusion of cadaver blood to a patient. Since that time, such transfusions have been done extensively in Russia and have been redescribed recently in the American literature by Petrov of Moscow. When such blood is collected within 6 hours after death, the oxygen-carrying capacity is the same as that of ACD blood collected from live donors, and bacterial contamination presents no insurmountable problem. The expiration date is approximately the same as ordinary ACD blood—21 days. Usually, no anticoagulant is needed because, after death, blood remains in a fluid state, either because of fibrinolysis or because of the depletion of fibrinogen by the deposition of fibrin along the surfaces of the vessel walls. Since embalming is among the funeral rites practiced in this country and entails removal of blood, which is washed down the drain, this is a source of blood that could represent a substantial increase in the quantities available currently (Kevorkian and Bylsma, 1961; Swan and Schechter, 1962). Unlike cadaveric organ transplantation, cadaver blood is not a popular source for transfusion in the United States.

Cadaver blood transfusion offers the only possibility for the administration of the 2 to 4 liters of blood obtained with only one crossmatch procedure required and, in addition, the only possibility that such a large volume of blood may be given with no greater risk of transmitting serum hepatitis than is entailed in the administration of the usual one 500-ml. unit of blood.

Autotransfusions. Emergency autotransfusions have been employed where blood is not available and where the cause of hypovolemic shock is hemorrhage into the patient's chest or abdomen (Brown and Debenham, 1931). The use of this type of autotransfusion continues to be reported when blood otherwise is not available (Lamm, 1963).

Jehovah's Witnesses, for religious reasons, may refuse transfusion in spite of its lifesaving value in a situation where it might otherwise cure the patient of his disease or injury. Recently, the use of autotransfusion has been found to be acceptable by some patients of this sect. Therefore, in these patients the liberal use of dextran, plasma, or albumin, and the return of the patient's own blood may make possible an extensive operation under conditions acceptable to the patient.

The U.S. Supreme Court rendered a decision in 1965 holding that, if blood is deemed life-sparing to a minor whose parents hold these religious convictions, blood may be given by court order. However, the court also held that an adult member of such sects (i.e., Jehovah's Witnesses, etc.) who chooses to refuse transfusions may not be compelled to accept transfusion, regardless of the envisioned consequences to the patient.

PRACTICAL ASPECTS AND PRECAUTIONS IN BLOOD TRANSFUSIONS

Although blood transfusion became a practical possibility with Landsteiner's discovery of blood groups, nearly 15 years were to elapse before the general use of transfusions was to receive serious consideration. Even then, its development was to be slow; each point of theory or practice was to be debated extensively but to the ultimate advantage and safety of the patient. From this sound approach was to emerge one of the important improvements in the general care of the patient, especially the surgical patient. It was well after 1930 before transfusions were to be employed as procedures other than those of last resort or desperation.

For 40 years (1900-1940), only 4 blood types or groups were considered as being of consequence. In 1940, Landsteiner and colleagues, particularly Levine, introduced a secondary series of blood groups, the Rh groups. The Rh groups were destined to explain many of the hemolytic transfuson reactions not accountable on the basis of Landsteiner's initial discoveries of 1900. The term "blood group" applies to the identity of

TABLE 8-1. ISO-AGGLUTINOGENS AND ISO-HEMAGGLUTININS OF THE MAJOR BLOOD GROUPS

BLOOD GROUP INTERNATIONAL	CELLS CONTAIN ISO-AGGLUTINOGENS	SERUM OR PLASMA CONTAINS ISO-HEMAGGLUTININS	APPROX. % OF POPULATION (U.S. WHITE)
O	None	ab (Anti-A and Anti-B)	40–45
A	A	b (Anti-B)	40
B	B	a (Anti-A)	10–15
AB	A & B	o (Neither Anti-A nor Anti-B)	5

cellular antigens—i.e., the ABO groupings, the Rh groupings and the family groupings. Typing applies primarily to the act of determining blood groups and is no longer used as a noun synonymous with blood groups.

BLOOD GROUPS

Blood Groups AB, A, B and O. The standard nomenclature identifying major blood groups is that of Landsteiner, which is now employed internationally. Its advantage over the Moss or the Jansky numerical classification is that the International nomenclature is descriptive of the iso-agglutinogen and iso-agglutinin composition of each blood group (Table 8-1).

It is clearly evident from this table that 4 factors are concerned in establishing any blood group. Two of these, factors A and B, may be present on the red cells and are referred to as *iso-agglutinogens*. Two may be present in the serum, *a* and *b*, and are termed *agglutinins*. Blood groups are known by the cellular agglutinogens they contain and not by their serum iso-agglutinin. Thus, blood whose cells bear only iso-agglutinogens A is known as Group A, and blood cells whose iso-agglutinogens contain only B are known as Group B blood. Cells containing both iso-agglutinogens A and B belong to Group AB, and those containing neither iso-agglutinogens A or B are referred to as Group O.

Serum iso-agglutinin *a* will coat or be adsorbed upon erythrocytes containing iso-agglutinogen A, causing them to clump and/or to hemolyze. For this reason, serum containing only the iso-agglutinin *a* is antagonistic to cellular agglutinogen A; therefore, this serum is known as *Anti-A*. The same holds for serum containing only iso-agglutinin *b*, which agglutinates the cellular iso-agglutinogen B. This serum is known as *Anti-B* serum. Serum containing both iso-agglutinogens A and B is known as Anti-A and Anti-B. Sera containing neither iso-agglutinins *a* or *b*, of course, are not antagonistic to erythrocytes of any of the 4 major blood groups. Thus, Group A blood is incompatible with Group B blood because the serum of Group B contains iso-agglutinogen Anti-A, and vice versa; whereas, Group AB erythrocytes are compatible with the sera of all 4 blood types, as its serum contains neither the Anti-A nor the Anti-B agglutinins.

Blood Groups or Types. These are established by determining the presence or the absence of agglutination when whole blood of the unknown group is mixed separately with Anti-A serum and Anti-B serum (Table 8-2).

H Substances. The ABO groups are inherited, with the blood groups of the individual depending upon two out of three allelic genes, "A, B and O." The Mendelian scheme can be extended to include the inheritable subgroups of A and B. The "O" gene was believed

TABLE 8-2.

ANTI-A SERUM	ANTI-B SERUM	UNKNOWN BLOOD UNDER TEST
Serum containing only Iso-agglutinin *a*	Serum containing only Iso-agglutinin *b*	Blood Group or Cell Type Indicated (International)
Agglutination	Agglutination	AB
Agglutination	No agglutination	A
No agglutination	Agglutination	B
No agglutination	No agglutination	O

to represent the absence of "*A* and *B*" genes and the only difference was that the antibody to the "*O*" character did not appear on the cells. This view, too, had to be modified when Witebsky and Klendshoj (1941) showed that the reagents in the secretions of AB individuals inhibit the anti-"*O*" reagents, and Watkins and Morgan (1955) found similar effects in homozygous AA or BB individuals. These reagents are known as ANTI-H reagents and the red-cell antigens they detect and the substances in these secretions that inhibit these agglutinins are called *H* substances, which are thought to be the product of a separate gene system, *Hh*, inherited independently of the ABO system. It is believed that the capacity to secrete *A*, *B*, or *H* substances is controlled by a pair of allelic genes, *Se* and *se*. Since *SeSe* and *Sese* are dominants, these combinations are secretors, whereas the homozygous *sese* are nonsecretors of A, B and/or H substances.

The Lewis or Le^a Substance. The Lewis groups were first detected by Mourant (1946) and their association with the ABO system was elaborated upon by Grubb (1948) and later by Ceppellini (1955). Individuals can be divided into four groups: (1) secretors of A, B, or H, Le^a and Le^b, which constitutes about 70 per cent of the Caucasian population; (2) those who secrete Le^a but not A, B, H or Le^b, and constitute about 20 per cent of the population; (3) those who secrete A, B or H but not Le^a or Le^b; (4) a very rare group, comprising those who secrete neither A, B, H nor Le^a nor Le^b. Differences in the carbohydrate and amino acid contents determine each blood group. These difficult subjects are carefully summarized by Mollison (1967), from whom these brief comments are taken.

The Rh Factors or Groups. Six different cell characteristics are identifiable in the Rh system. These are designated as Rh$_o$, rh', rh'', Hr$_o$, hr', and hr'', respectively; or by the British corresponding nomenclature of D, C and E, and *d*, *c* and *e*. However, these do not refer to the potential number of combinations of Rh groups which total 27 possibilities.

The erythrocytes of every person must contain at least one member of each of these 3 pairs of antigens. The red cells of some individuals may contain 4, 5 or even 6, so that the number of combinations possible is rather large.

Leukocyte Grouping. Although methods for establishing leukocyte groups with, at least in some instances, almost the same precision as blood groups have been recognized (Payne, 1957, 1964; Van Rood *et al.*, 1963, 1967, among others), their general usefulness did not become apparent until the need for understanding transplantation antigens arose. Twelve leukocyte antigens have been identified thus far and more may be expected to be found. The important cell is the small lymphocyte.

Leukocyte antigens can be important in platelet transfusions, because the leukocyte antigens may also be present on platelets. Thus, in sensitized patients with thrombocytopenia, only patients who are leukocyte-compatible with respect to the transfusions have normal recovery and survival time.

At least two and possibly more platelet antigens are known to exist but their clinical applications are not yet developed. Also, a number of antibodies exist; some are complement-fixing antibodies, and these are 7S. Five that do not fix complement are 19S.

Morrison and Mollison (1966) and Shulman *et al.* (1961) reported upon a rare but serious complication of blood transfusions—posttransfusion purpura. This condition develops 6 or 7 days after transfusion and appears to be caused by a platelet isoantibody. It is suggested that part of the antibody produced in response to Pl^{A1} platelet antigen cross reacts with a structurally similar antigen on autologous platelets, resulting in thrombocytopenia. The condition is troublesome though rarely fatal, and may be amenable to corticoids; cases thus far reported have all occurred in multiparous women 40 years or older, and after a blood transfusion.

Minimum Routine Blood Typing for Clinical Safety in Transfusions. Opinions differ as to the extent that routine typing procedures should be carried out. Most clinicians feel greater security when the commonly occurring subgroups as well as major groups of both donor and recipient have been identified. Those engaged in blood banking feel more secure with fewer routines for typing than does the patient's physician, who may not be as experienced in the field of blood banking.

Probably somewhere between these two views lies a practical solution that would be acceptable to both. Although a committee of the National Research Council (1963) has stated that "The only antigens for which routine testing should always be performed in donors and recipients are A, B, and D (Rh$_o$)," this does not provide the degree of protection to the patient to be transfused that is presently possible and feasible. There is a variant of D (Rh$_o$) which is designated as D^u and at times must be tested for. A blood which is negative for D may still be positive for D^u; therefore, before a blood can be considered as being negative for D, it must also be shown to be negative for D^u.

Starzl et al. in 1964 found that in homo-transplantations of kidney the patterns of acceptance by the recipients were not particularly jeopardized when the ABO blood groups of the donor and the recipient were different except when recipient presensitization had occurred in an Rh-negative patient.

In testing erythrocytes for the Rh antigens the author prefers to examine cells for the presence of Rh$_o$, rh' and rh", using the corresponding antisera—Anti-Rh$_o$ (Anti-D), Anti-rh' (Anti-C) and Anti-rh" (Anti-E). Of these three, the most important is D or Rh$_o$, as it is most frequently antigenic and is encountered most commonly. It is advisable to examine for the presence of C and E also (Table 8-3, A and B).

Testing for the presence of c, d and e antigens (Hr$_o$, hr' hr") with each respective antisera is not performed by all blood banks, although within the past few years these procedures have been readily available.

The production of Rh antibodies is stimulated in the patients receiving an Rh antigen which their blood does not contain. Sensitization generally occurs by one of two mechanisms or both. Either the Rh negative patient receives an Rh positive blood transfusion and thereby is stimulated to produce antibodies to the Rh antigen given, or the patient is an Rh negative mother bearing an Rh positive fetus whose red cells manage to enter the maternal circulation and stimulate the production of maternal Rh antibodies. The initial transfusion of Rh positive blood in an unsensitized Rh negative patient causes no reaction. However, Rh positive blood administered again several weeks later can induce serious or fatal hemolytic transfusion reactions. The following case report and the data presented in Figure 8-1 illustrate this point more vividly than is usually encountered today.

A 35-year-old married female was admitted in January, 1944, with bleeding from ulcerative colitis. Four daily transfusions were administered for anemia. Under medical management, her colitis symptoms subsided, and she improved. Forty-three days after this series of transfusions, she was given a single transfusion of blood for mild persistent anemia with the expectation of discharge to home the following day. Severe chill and symptoms of an acute hemolytic reaction near the termination of her transfusion developed. Jaundice and anemia followed the next day.

TABLE 8-3, A. COMPARATIVE NOMENCLATURES

RH SYSTEM	CDE SYSTEM
Rh$_o$	D*
rh'	C
rh"	E
Hr$_o$	d
hr'	c
hr"	e

* It is unfortunate that in the CDE designation Rh$_o$ does not correspond to C rather than to D.

TABLE 8-3, B. TEST SERUM AND USUAL RH TYPING

CELL TYPE	(ANTI-D) ANTI-RH$_o$	(ANTI-C) ANTI-RH'	(ANTI-E) ANTI-RH"	APPROXIMATE % WHITE
rh (cde)	—	—	—	15.0
rh' (Cde)	—	+	—	1.0
rh" (cdE)	—	—	+	0.7
rh'rh" (CdE)	—	+	+	0.02
Rh$_o$ (cDe)	+	—	—	1.5
Rh$_o$' (CDe)	+	+	—	54.0
Rh$_o$" (cDE)	+	—	+	14.5
Rh$_o$' Rh$_o$" (CDE)	+	+	+	13.2

160   Blood Transfusions and Related Problems

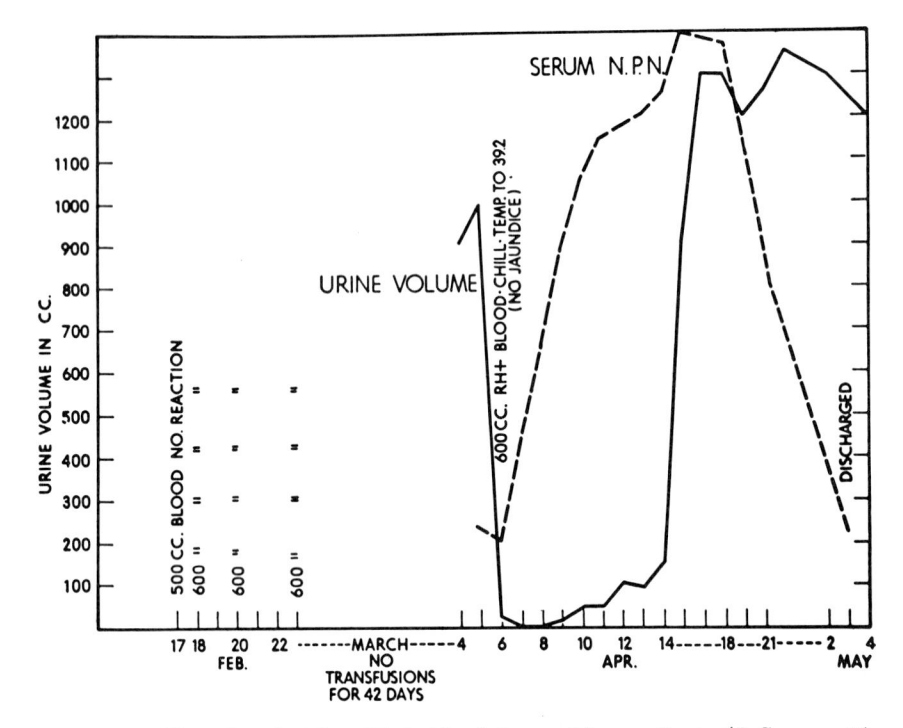

FIG. 8-1. Hazards of giving Rh+ blood to an Rh— patient. (A.C., age 35, 321275 ulcerative colitis Rh— Type O, one child L and W, no miscarriages.) The oliguric state with renal azotemia with near fatality in an Rh negative patient sensitized to Rh positive blood in 1944, as demonstrated by chart. The 4 transfusions administered over a 7-day period in February of that year were examined subsequently and proved to be Rh positive. Accidents such as this one occurred in many institutions and forced the inclusion of Rh typing as a part of the standard routine in the preparation of blood for any and all recipients.

Slowly, she recovered. Finally, she was discharged 6 weeks later (Fig. 8-1).

Rechecking of the last donor disclosed his blood to be Rh positive and the blood of the patient to be Rh negative (later identified as Rh_o negative and D^u negative). The 4 preceding donors were recalled and proved to be Rh positive also. Further encouragement to adapt Rh determinations as routine for the bloods of all donors and recipients was not necessary thereafter.

Hence, a female patient always should receive blood from a donor of the corresponding blood group and of the corresponding Rh group if she is or has been pregnant or is or will be of the childbearing age.

However, in the male who has not *before* been transfused, under emergency situations only, the administration of an Rh positive blood to an Rh negative recipient may be condoned when appropriate Rh negative blood is not available or when suitable typing facilities are not at hand. Rh negative women who never have been pregnant and are beyond the childbearing age fall into this same category. It should be remembered that subsequent transfusion of Rh positive blood a few weeks later may lead to serious hemolytic reactions. Wiener (1967) has recommended the Rh classification types as shown in Table 8-4, which simplifies the understanding of the Rh and anti-Rh classifications.

The Coombs' Antiglobulin Test has been most helpful in the recognition of Rh antibodies in Rh negative patients, thereby alerting the physician to potential trouble. The Coombs' serum reacts *only with coated* cells. Coated or sensitized red cells occur at times from autosensitization and are found in cer-

TABLE 8-4. THE 18 "STANDARD" RH-HR BLOOD TYPES*

RH BLOOD TYPE	REACTIONS OF RBC WITH Anti-hr'	Anti-hr"	RH-HR SUBTYPE Designation	Binary Code No.†
rh	+	+	rh	00011
rh'	+	+	rh'rh	01011
	−	+	rh'rh'	01001
rh"	+	+	rh"rh	00111
	+	−	rh"rh"	00110
rh_y	+	+	rh_yrh	01111
	−	+	rh_yrh'	01101
	+	−	rh_yrh"	01110
	−	−	rh_yrh_y	01100
Rh_o	+	+	Rh_o	10011
Rh_1	+	+	Rh_1rh	11011
	−	+	Rh_1Rh_1	11001
Rh_2	+	+	Rh_2rh	10111
	+	−	Rh_2Rh_2	10110
Rh_z	+	+	Rh_zRh_o	11111
	−	+	Rh_zRh_1	11101
	+	−	Rh_zRh_2	11110
	−	−	Rh_zRh_z	11100

* No comparable table employing the C-D-E notations is available.
† For the binary code number the order of the blood factor is taken as follows: **Rh$_o$, rh', rh", hr', hr"**.
After Wiener, A.S.: J.A.M.A., 199:985, 1967.

tain hemolytic diseases. The Coombs' serum is believed to react under these in-vitro conditions because this Antihuman Serum adds a second coat to the already in-vivo coated red cells, making them more susceptible to agglutination. This coating or sensitivity occurs in vivo generally but is not sufficient to induce agglutination when tested in vitro against ordinary sera. The Coombs' globulin, which will not react with erythrocytes unless they are already coated in vivo, thus acts as a booster in such reactions and makes possible the detection of sensitized or coated erythrocytes not otherwise found by laboratory methods.

Two kinds of Coombs' tests have been devised. They are known as the Direct and the Indirect Tests.

The Direct Coombs' Test is a diagnostic procedure, designed to pick up coated red cells that have been coated or sensitized by the patient's own serum when it possesses some antibody for an antigen contained on his erythrocytes. Therefore, it is a diagnostic test for unusual autohemolytic diseases and is especially useful in the recognition of erythroblastosis and certain of the hemolytic anemias, especially "splenic" anemia, and to assist in the avoidance or the explanation of hemolytic transfusion reactions. It should be requested when these conditions are suspected.

The Indirect Coombs' Test is essentially a crossmatch, wherein an attempt is made to determine whether the donor's red cells when given to the recipient are coated or sensitized by an unusual antibody contained in the donor's serum which is not otherwise recognizable and will react with an antibody in the patient's serum. Therefore, one orders a direct Coombs' test when one wishes diagnostic assistance as to the nature of the hemolytic reaction within his patient. An indirect Coombs' test is requested when one suspects that the patient's plasma may contain some unusual antibody that may antagonize the erythrocytes of a prospective donor.

The indirect Coombs' test is particularly valuable when the patient's serum is Rh negative to *d* but not to *c* or *e*. An Rh negative D donor whose C and E antigens have not been established may be recognized by the indirect Coombs' test, and then further subtyping is carried out. The indirect Coombs' test is indicated in patients receiving repeated transfusions which may have sensitized the patient to erythrocytic antigens of potential donors. The indirect test is also indicated in patients with so-called "splenic" anemia. Indeed, to provide the patient with the greatest safety in his transfusions, an indirect Coombs' test always should be performed, but often the amount of work and time consumed does not make so broad a usage possible in many blood banks.

Undoubtedly, more blood antigens will be identified and found to play an important etiologic role in some transfusion reactions. Four of the more common ones are discussed below.

Other Blood Antigens

COLD AGGLUTININS. These were first described by Landsteiner and Levine in 1926 and represent the phenomenon of autoagglutinins. The erythrocytes of an individual become agglutinable by his own plasma or serum at temperatures less than that of body heat. Landsteiner demonstrated that after thorough washing of erythrocytes when cold agglutinins existed, the cells could be resuspended in the plasma of an individual free of cold agglutinins without agglutination taking place upon lowering the ambient temperature. Thus he proved that cold agglutinins were real and not an artifact.

Cold agglutinins are said to be present in a higher percentage among Negro donors than among Caucasians. They are also frequently present in patients with Raynaud's disease, paroxysmal hemoglobinuria, cirrhosis, in severe anemia, hemolytic anemias, and in fact in an almost unending list of chronic diseases.

Two clinical facts are important and practical with reference to cold agglutinins. First, if blood typing is carried out in a cool room, the blood being typed can show agglutination against both Anti-A and Anti-B sera due to the presence of cold agglutinins rather than to an incompatibility with the specific typing serum. Thus, a Group O, a Group A, or a Group B donor could be identified erroneously as Group AB. The blood of all individuals, when agglutinated by both Anti-A and Anti-B serum, may be re-examined at 37° C. for the presence of cold agglutinins, thereby eliminating this source of typing error. This procedure is a relatively simple one. It is readily feasible, also, as only about 5 per cent of the Caucasian population normally have Group AB blood.

The second deleterious effect of cold agglutinins is the ability of the chilled blood of a donor with erythrocytic cold agglutinogens to be agglutinated in the course of transfusion in a patient whose plasma contains cold agglutinins, causing a hemolytic reaction. Cold agglutinins were seldom a factor of concern prior to the introduction of blood banking wherein blood is refrigerated before use. Most blood was administered, before 1940, very shortly after its withdrawal from the donor and without cooling. Its temperature was more nearly that of body heat. In a normal individual whose serum possesses cold agglutinins, the administration of chilled blood may result in a transient rise in temperature, a chill and mild to moderate hemolysis of little consequence. However, in the critically ill individual, a similar reaction is less well tolerated and may cause a severe enough reaction in some patients to be disastrous. The practice of administering cold blood is generally employed, except where the patient is known to possess cold agglutinins. Under these conditions, it is advised that the donor's blood be brought slowly to 37° C. under thermometer control, and administered while maintaining heat.

FAMILY GROUPS OR ANTIGENS. Other blood antigens also are recognized as capable of producing antibodies in the plasma of patients whose blood cells do not contain them. Three of these appear to be of clinical importance. They are the Kell, the Luther, and the Duffy factors, so termed because they were first described in patients bearing these respective names. The Kell antigen may be demonstrated by anti-Kell serum; those cells not reacting with anti-K serum are labeled k cells. Those reacting with anti-K serum are called K. The Duffy and the Luther factors are less well defined, but similar anti-Duffy or anti-Luther serum antibodies can be developed.

Transfusion Safeguards and the Common Sources of Transfusion Accidents and Their Prevention. The central and practical point relative to the safety of blood transfusions depended upon the development and the general availability of highly reactive and reliable typing serum. Excellent typing sera did not become generally available until after 1940. Thus, even after the contributions of Landsteiner, the introduction of crossmatching by Ottenberg and the development of citrate as an anticoagulant by Lewisohn, reliable typing sera were still a quarter of a century away.

Mistakes in blood group identification can be largely reduced to those related to or caused by human error. To a lesser or greater extent, probably these limitations always will impose a slight degree of hazard in blood transfusion, regardless of what checks and counterchecks are employed. The most important of these errors or hazards appear to arise from fatigue and vexations of blood bank personnel, however careful they may be. The physician, concerned with the safety of his own patient, must recognize that an unreasonable attitude on his part toward the blood bank serving the needs of his patients will almost certainly increase unwittingly the frequency of human error. This result is exactly what he wishes to avoid; the safety of all patients is jeopardized —not merely those of the dominant complainer, as one error tends to generate another in chain-reacting fashion. The blood bank should be able to function with the element of human error usually less than 0.05 per cent. Unfortunately, errors in the range of 0.1 per cent, or greater, still persist in many blood banks throughout the country.

The dictum of *primum non nocere*, yes—always! but this ideal when applied to the use of blood transfusions involves not only the risk entailed in the preparation of the transfusion itself but also the recognition on the part of the physician or the surgeon that unwillingness to employ blood when needed often subjects his patient to a much greater hazard. All things considered, many physicians continue in the practice of "too little and too late," failing to appreciate fully the patient's blood requirements, particularly in the field of trauma and in the course of extensive operations.

Errors do not arise in the blood bank alone. The house staff, the attending physician and the nursing staff also contribute to the total hazard involved. So far as errors attributable to the blood bank are concerned, the most important is faulty identification of the blood group—of either the donor or the recipient, or both. When blood groups are identified properly, the occurrence of serious or fatal reactions attributable to the blood bank are essentially abolished. The all-important concern of the blood bank is to be certain that the blood groups of the donor and the recipient correspond, or at least the combination of the donor's groups is not affected adversely by the patient's serum or plasma, and that the blood issued for the patient is actually the one that has been typed and crossmatched for the particular patient.

At present the crossmatching of the donor cells with those of the patient is of secondary importance, if a high titer and active typing sera are employed. Nonetheless, the crossmatch of both major and minor fields has not lost its usefulness and always should be carried out. It serves as a check on blood typing and assures one that labeling errors have not occurred.

There are two important sources of typing errors. First is the use of low-potency typing serum, or of serum that has lost its initial potency either from bacterial contamination or age. This is prevented by checking at least once a week the potency of typing sera on hand. Typing sera should be maintained under refrigeration. The second error is of human origin and relates to the faulty recording of properly typed bloods, improper identification of Anti-A or Anti-B typing sera, or the accidental placing of the donor cells in his own serum in crossmatching rather than in the serum of the recipient. These errors may be prevented by typing twice the bloods of the recipient and the donor—performed independently by 2 different persons—and the independent recording of the identification of the blood groups concerned.

The house staff or personnel administering the blood may introduce errors of another kind. Unwittingly, he may administer to the wrong patient the blood that he takes from the blood bank. This error may be largely avoided by limiting the blood which the physician may take from the blood bank at any one time to blood for only one patient and by writing in bold lettering on its label the name of the patient for whom it is intended and his blood group, as well as that of the donor. The physician's second error is the inadequate identification of the recipient's blood sample which he brings to the blood bank in requesting his transfusion. The author has been both surprised and terrified by the frequency with which the full name of the recipient and, indeed his diagnosis, will correspond exactly to that of another patient hospitalized at the same time. Therefore, in requesting the transfusion, recording the patient's name on the transfusion requisition is not enough; the requisition should bear his hospital unit number as well. Third, if irregular antibodies or sensitization are suspected, it is up to the physician to communicate his suspicions to the blood bank. Direct Coombs' testing should be the physician's responsibility to request; indirect Coombs' crossmatch is the joint responsibility of the blood bank and the physician. There remains a fourth source of potential error on the part of the physician in that he may draw from several patients samples of blood to be typed and crossmatched, unwittingly mixing his requisition slips with the sample submitted to the blood bank. In our experience, this has proved the smallest source of transfusion error and may be avoided if the person drawing the blood sample fills out each requisition individually at the patient's bedside at that time.

The National Institutes of Health established certain minimum standards for the safe preparation and preservation of blood for transfusion purposes. (Technical Methods and Procedures of the Am. Assn. of Blood Banks, 1953). These have been adopted by the American Association of Blood Banks and endorsed by the American College of Surgeons. (Minimum Standards for Blood Transfusions Outlined, 1956; Strumia et al., 1963). In the final analysis, the safety of transfusion is a summation of the joint efforts of the attending physician, all hospital personnel concerned with patient care, as well as those in the blood bank, and of the quality of the methods, the materials used, and particularly the quality of the donor population. We shall never be able to employ transfusion with complete safety; we can only hope that the accidents will be few and far between.

Crossmatching Principles. The matching of the donor's red cells with the patient's serum and the patient's cells with the donor's serum serves as a final check upon the correctness of the typing of both the blood donor and the patient, as well as the identity of both donor and recipient. As mentioned above, this procedure was more important in the days prior to the development of reliable high-titer Anti-A and Anti-B typing sera. Nonetheless, crossmatching should be carried out if at all possible. These procedures continue in our hands to reveal an occasional error in labeling of a blood type or indicate a blood of mistaken identity. However, it seldom discloses any abnormalities other than those resulting from the mixing of major groups of incompatible bloods. It will not identify incompatibilities of the Rh systems, the D^u variant, the Kell, the Duffy, the Luther or other factors. Specific antisera are needed for each of the latter.

In general, 3 types of crossmatching procedures are employed. The first and most generally used is the *saline* crossmatch, wherein a saline suspension of donor and recipient cells is mixed respectively with recipient and donor sera. The second technic, and considered by many to be more nearly accurate than the saline crossmatch, is the *gross* crossmatch. It tests only the compatibility of the donor's cells with the recipient's serum; but this is the all-important aspect of compatibility. A 4 per cent saline suspension of red cells is mixed directly with an equal volume of the recipient's serum. The final mixture, usually about 1 ml., is centrifuged at 1,000 r.p.m. for a period of 3 minutes and then agitated gently. An incompatibility is revealed by the presence of agglutinated clumped cells; the compatible reaction is revealed by the uniform suspension of all cells throughout the serum.

THE HIGH-PROTEIN CROSSMATCH is the third method and was introduced to overcome the problem of "blocking" antibodies. These are the incomplete antibodies affecting the Rh system which are not detected in saline suspensions. However, clumping of incompatible Rh bloods may occur when serum, plasma or albumin are present in sufficient concentrations. The high-protein crossmatch, wherein 30 per cent bovine albumin is used as the fluid for suspension of the red cells being tested, has been recommended and adopted for general use. However, with passage of time, the high-protein crossmatch has not proved its ability to replace entirely saline crossmatch.

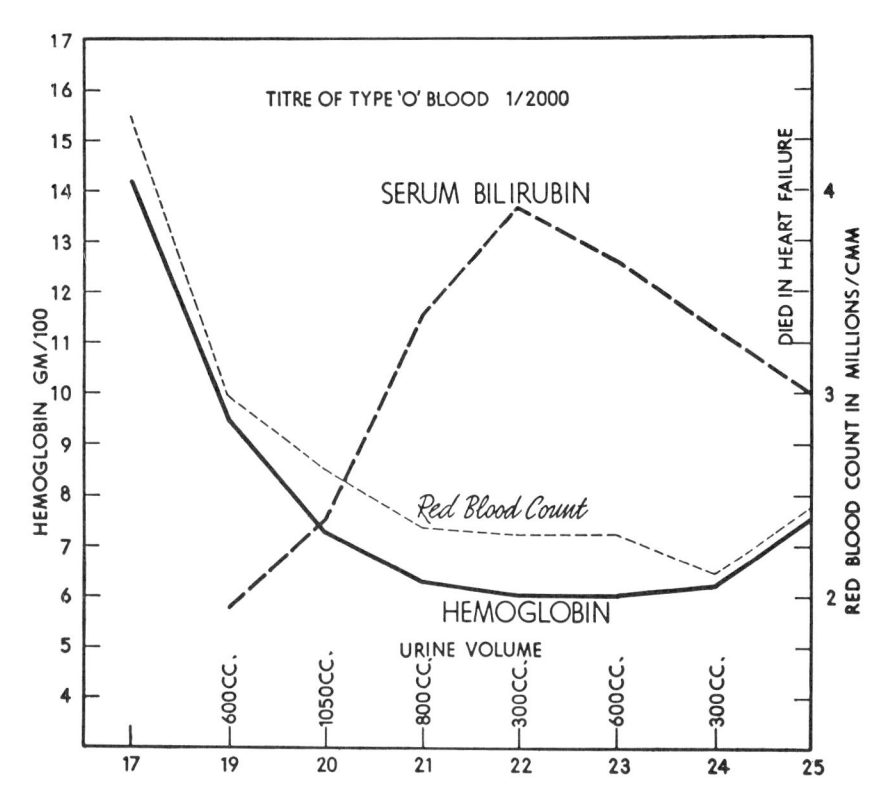

Fig. 8-2. Hazards of using universal type O blood. (D.C., age 73, 385410, Wt. 77.4 Kg. Type A Rh+.) The rare but distinct risk of group O blood administered to a patient of another blood group when the iso-agglutinin titer of group O is excessive, as illustrated graphically by the acute decline in the red cell count and hemoglobin concentration with concurrent development of icterus. This is the so-called "minor" field or crossmatch wherein the incompatibility is that of the donor's serum for the patient's cells. Note that in spite of the severe degree of hemolysis, the daily urine volume was moderately good. This is in contrast with the oliguric or anuric states which follow reactions wherein the cells of the donor are incompatible with the serum of the recipient (compare with data in Fig. 8-1).

The author prefers both crossmatching procedures for each patient.

The all-important aspect of crossmatching by any procedure is that the donor cells be compatible with the patient's serum. This is usually known as major field crossmatch.

The Universal Donor. Since the days of Ottenberg, the fact has been known that the Group O donor may give blood to recipients of any of the 4 major blood groups; he is known as the "universal" donor. His erythrocytes containing neither agglutinogens A nor B, obviously cannot be attacked by the patient's agglutinins a and/or b. However, it will be recalled that the Group O donor's plasma contains both agglutinins a and b. Usually, this is of little consequence, for as his blood is administered to the recipient, his iso-agglutinins a and b are rapidly diluted throughout the patient's circulation and cause no important hemolysis. Occasionally, however, the iso-agglutinin titers of a and b in a Group O donor's blood are very high and can induce severe hemolysis of the patient's cells should he be of another blood group. A case in point follows:

A 76-year-old man was operated upon in July, 1946, for a carcinoma of the rectum. A Miles procedure was performed by the author without difficulty. Because of an uncorrected anemia, 3 blood transfusions were administered during the day of operation. Certainly 2 were all he needed.

The first 2 transfusions were AB Rh positive and compatible with the patient's own type. The 3rd blood was administered late in the day and was given in the hope that an improved blood count, over the preoperative one, would result. As no other AB bloods were available, a Type O Rh positive blood was administered without incident until it was noted a few hours later that the urine contained an abundance of hemoglobin. The following day the patient's color was deeply icteric and for 48 hours no urine was secreted (Fig. 8-2).

Beginning with the 4th day, urine flow returned, and the high bilirubin levels (28 mg.%) receded. Slowly his general course began to improve, but his erythrocyte count was now 1,800,000 per cm. ml., and his hemoglobin determination was 5.6 Gm. per cent. On the 8th day, without previous warning, he suddenly expired from acute left heart failure.

Rechecking of the blood types of the 3 donors and the patient assured their correctness. Then the Type O donor sample was titered and found to be in excess of 1:2096, or a titer 10 to 20 times the maximum allowed. That this transfusion was not immediately fatal is in itself surprising, but it must also be admitted that this hemolytic reaction posed a threat to this 76-year-old man which might have been much less harmful to a younger and more vigorous patient. Autopsy disclosed no special cause for his acute heart failure.

As the Group O donor constitutes 40 to 45 per cent of the Caucasian population, his usefulness is an invaluable asset in times of catastrophe and emergency, especially if his titer is known. Crosby and Akeroyd employed Group O Rh positive blood of low titer in the Korean War, administering as much as 10 to 30 units of blood without regard to the recipient's blood group. Subsequent transfusions administered a week or two later should be group specific Rh negative blood. Thus, the administration of Rh positive Group O blood should not be employed electively other than in Rh positive patients, for it may cause trouble at a later date should it be necessary to administer Group O Rh positive blood under emergency circumstances.

Rh "Vaccination." The active Rh_o (D) antibody produced by the mother is the cause of Rh hemolytic disease of the newborn in subsequent pregnancies. When the formation of active Rh_o (D) antibody was prevented, Rh hemolytic disease of the newborn was not observed in the subsequent pregnancy.

When the postpartum mother receives an injection with passive Rh_o (D) antibody, the mother's antibody response to the foreign Rh_o (D) positive fetal cells is suppressed. The injected product is the immunoglobulin G fraction of plasma. This material has been shown to be effective in preventing the formation of antibodies to the Rh_o (D) factor in Rh_o (D) and D^u-negative women if administered within 72 hours of delivery or miscarriage.

The mother must be Rh_o (D) negative and D^u negative and display absence of Rh_o (D) prior to and at the time of delivery. The infant's blood should be Rh_o positive or D^u positive, show ABO compatibility, and display a negative direct antiglobulin test for cord red cells. The mother must not already be immunized to the Rh_o (D) factor. These are tests that must be performed before the "vaccine" can be safely administered. The product has been approved for routine clinical use under these conditions.

Clinical studies to date indicate that the "vaccine" effectively prevents Rh_o (D) hemolytic disease of the newborn (Ascari *et al.*, 1968).

The universal recipient is a Group AB patient whose cells contain iso-agglutinogens A and B. His plasma contains neither iso-agglutinins Anti-A nor Anti-B. He may receive blood from donors of any blood group, since his plasma is not capable of agglutinating cells containing antigens A or B. Therefore, this recipient is designated as the "universal" recipient. However, it must be remembered that only about 5 per cent of recipients have blood of the AB variety.

In general, if AB blood is not available for a Group AB patient but Group A and Group O bloods are, Group A has the advantage over Group O because the plasma of the Group A donor has only one agglutinin, Anti-B, whereas that of the Group O donor has both Anti-A and Anti-B. If Group O blood is to be used in emergency cases, it should be predetermined that this blood is Rh_o and D^u negative and of low titer Anti-A and Anti-B. Group O bloods not meeting these specifications should be used only in last resort or as packed cells.

Witebsky has shown that the addition of two polysaccharide substances to human blood is useful in the partial neutralization, respectively, of Anti-A and Anti-B agglutinins in plasma. These polysaccharides are obtained from animal tissues; they are highly purified and essentially nonantigenic. When added to Group O blood, they tend to neutralize the Group A and B antibodies in its plasma and may be used whenever it is necessary under emergency conditions to give blood to a recipient whose type is not yet established, particularly when the Anti-A and Anti-B titer of the Group O donor blood is not known. The disadvantage of these polysaccharides contained in transfused blood is that they tend to elevate the titers of Anti-A and Anti-B agglutinins in the recipient, and in the pregnant patient it is possible that this response may aggravate and possibly contribute to the incidence of erythroblastosis foetalis.

THE NATURE OF BLOOD TRANSFUSION REACTIONS

Until 1935, only three types of transfusion reactions were recognized. They were classified as hemolytic, pyrogenic and allergic. As further experience has accumulated, additional untoward manifestations have been recognized as resulting from certain reactions from the transfusions of blood. Many of these relate directly or indirectly to the larger volumes of blood replacement employed in extensive operative surgery in the fields of cancer, heart surgery and trauma; all are related to the prolonged storage of blood. They include post-transfusion hepatitis, circulatory overload, potential citrate intoxication, leukopyrogens, and the growth of bacteria under prolonged periods of refrigeration, as well as the increases in serum potassium as blood ages or hemolyzes; also, acute hemolytic reactions from autohemolysis or from the presence of unusual family groups to which either the donor or the patient is sensitized. The importance of a normal pH in bank blood has been emphasized by McLaughlin, Nealon and Gibbon (1960), and others.

Excess acidity of stored bank blood may lead to cardiac arrest. The extent and the seriousness of such acidity has not been recognized sufficiently in the past.

Hemolytic Reactions

Hemolytic transfusion reactions may or may not be of importance. Stated otherwise: some hemolytic reactions are serious; some are not. Hemolytic reactions are always a source of concern to the clinician, and their origin always must be determined as soon as possible. Only when the cause is known can proper treatment be implemented and the importance of the reaction be assessed.

Common to all hemolytic reactions usually is the early but transient occurrence of hemoglobinemia and hemoglobinuria and, a few hours later, an increase in serum bilirubin and usually clinical icterus. Ordinarily, hemoglobinuria can be detected only within the first urine sample after the reaction has occurred, as free circulatory hemoglobin is soon converted to bilirubin. Hemoglobinemia will be detected only if the serum is examined early and for the same reason. Whether or not acute and pronounced anemia occurs depends upon the extent of hemolysis; in extensive hemolytic reactions, severe anemia may develop (see case report on p. 165). The effect of the hemolytic reaction upon renal function, particularly urine secretion, depends upon its cause and kind. In general, hemolytic reactions are one of two varieties: rapid hemolysis of aged (14 to 28 days) donor blood, or the hemolysis of mismatched blood. The latter is a serious threat to the life of the patient and his renal function.

Causes of Less Serious Types of Hemolytic Reactions.

Aged blood, 14 to 21 days or older: The "life" span of the normal erythrocyte, freshly drawn and transfused without delay to the normal recipient of the same blood groups, is approximately 120 days. However, the length of life span rapidly falls off as blood ages in vitro under blood-banking conditions. The residual life span of erythrocytes of a 2-week unit of blood may be less than 1 week, even when transfused into a recipient of the same blood groupings, including subtypes. If several units of aged blood are transfused within a day or two, physiologic hemolysis of the donors' erythrocytes may proceed at a rate sufficiently rapid to produce hemoglobinuria, to elevate materially the serum bilirubin levels and cause extensive clinical icterus, especially in patients with liver disease. Transfusion icterus of this origin is generally unimportant except that the beneficial effects of such transfusions upon the patient's anemia is short-lived and renal failure may occur if the patient is hypotensive. Urine flow generally is not affected appreciably. However, the diagnosis as to the origin of the hemolytic reaction is one made by exclusion. All typing and crossmatchings must be rechecked and found satisfactory before the conclusion can be justified that hemolysis is due to outdated erythrocytes.

IMPAIRED HEPATIC BILIRUBIN EXCRETION. As the liver is the prime organ of bilirubin clearance, impaired hepatic excretion of bilirubin of any origin may result in an increased retention of serum bilirubin. If icterus is already present, it is obvious that the patient cannot clear his plasma of his own erythrocytic breakdown products. Thus, after the transfusion of relatively aged blood, an increase in clinical icterus and of the serum bililrubin level is observed so frequently as to be the rule rather than the exception. The larger the number of transfusions of properly matched bloods the icteric patient receives, the greater the post-transfusion icterus is likely to be. The extent of the increase in icterus is likely to be greater when aged bloods are given to patients with normal liver function and when Group O bloods are administered when the recipient is of another blood group.

THE HIGH AGGLUTININ TITER UNIVERSAL DONOR. The results of hemolysis, this time the destruction of the patient's cells, can be more serious (see p. 165 and Fig. 8-2). The use of Group O Rh positive blood whose titer is low, as Crosby and Akeroyd found, rarely causes icterus when the recipient is of another blood group, even when administered in large quantities, unless the recipient suffers from a high degree of impairment in his bilirubin clearance or the blood was old.

COLD AGGLUTININS. When the patient's serum has a high titer of cold agglutinins, the administration of chilled blood usually incites hemolysis of donor cells containing this antigen. As pointed out on page 162, this is an agglutinative and/or hemolytic reaction which may be prevented by warming the donor's blood slowly (several hours) to 37° C. before transfusion and by selection of donors free of cold agglutinins and leukocyte-poor blood. Hemolytic reactions from cold agglutinins are not generally as severe as those following the transfusion of the incompatibility of the major AB, A, B and O groups or of an Rh positive blood given to a sensitized Rh negative patient. On the other hand, the patient with cold agglutinins appears to acquire this antigen-antibody phenomenon in many instances in association with serious disease, if he does not possess it by inheritance. In the critically ill patient, any reaction is likely to be tolerated poorly and can contribute to, if not occasionally cause, his death.

Hemolytic Reactions From Mismatched Blood. The administration of mismatched blood was undoubtedly one of the most commonly encountered causes of acute hemolysis following blood transfusion prior to about 1940. It should be encountered rarely today. Certainly this accident should occur with a frequency less than 1 in 5,000 to 10,000 transfusions if proper precautions are observed assiduously. In the carefully controlled blood bank, errors of this origin are those of the "irreducibility of human error" (p. 163). Unfortunately, most blood banks do not function this well. The doctor's alarm index to suspected transfusion reactions is good for all concerned, for the early diagnosis of hemolytic reactions of mismatched bloods is of the greatest importance. It is incumbent upon the attending physician, the house officers and the nursing staff to report such reactions to the blood bank at once so that their nature can be established and the most effective method of treatment implemented immediately. When any transfusion reaction occurs, the transfusion should be discontinued immediately. *Any residual blood in the transfusion equipment should be returned immediately with the transfusion set to the blood bank for analysis.* Too often, the residual blood is discarded or allowed to stand for many hours before returning; not only is valuable time lost but the trail becomes too cold to track down the cause.

Certain clinical features are very suggestive that a hemolytic transfusion reaction may, or may not have arisen from the trans-

TABLE 8-5. SIGNS AND SYMPTOMS SUGGESTING INCOMPATIBLE BLOOD TRANSFUSION REACTION

IMMEDIATE (FIRST FEW MINUTES)	INTERMEDIATE (20 MINUTES TO 2 HOURS)	DELAYED (2 HOURS TO 24 HOURS)
	A. Patient awake	
1. Acute anaphylaxis	1. Pain in lumbar area	1. Chills and fever
2. Acute dyspnea and/or asthma, usually with cyanosis	2. Chills and fever. Urticaria	2. Hemoglobinemia and hemoglobinuria are likely overlooked unless checked for within the first 2 to 4 hours
3. Peripheral vascular collapse	3. Restlessness and hypotension	3. Oliguria, often followed by anuria in less than 24 hours
4. Hemoglobinemia	4. Hemoglobinemia	4. Anemia and icterus
5. Hemoglobinuria	5. Hemoglobinuria	
	B. Patient anesthetized	
1. Cyanosis	1. Fever	
2. Hypotension	2. Hemoglobinemia and hemoglobinuria	
3. Hemoglobinemia and hemoglobinuria		

fusion of mismatched blood. However, these symptoms are not to be considered as diagnostic, as some of them may also occur from a hemolytic reaction of other cause, in the so-called pyrogeneic reactions and from blood that is either hemolyzed or bacteriologically contaminated. These symptoms and signs which are suggestive of mismatched blood may be classified as immediate, intermediate and delayed.

The earlier and the more serious the reaction, the more disastrous the consequences are likely to be (Table 8-5).

Treatment procedures employed in seriously incompatible blood transfusion reactions should have some degree of priority. But no form of treatment is as effective as the prevention of the transfusion of mismatched bloods.

1. Discontinue transfusion at once but do not remove the needle in the patient's vein, as peripheral vascular collapse usually makes impossible the reintroduction of a needle into a vein. This creates unnecessary delay in treatment and may necessitate a venous cut-down in order to institute intravenous fluids.

2. Institute immediately an intravenous infusion of 10 per cent glucose in water to induce diuresis. To this should be added, as soon as obtainable, an ampule of sodium lactate containing 4.48 Gm. or 40 mEq. to ensure immediate alkalinization of urine. An acid urine favors the precipitation of an acid hematin and possibly hemoglobin in the renal tubules. If peripheral collapse is present, a second intravenous infusion of glucose is started to which has been added the contents of an ampule containing 4 mg. of norepinephrine. Sufficient volumes of 10 per cent glucose in water to induce a diuresis cannot be administered as rapidly as necessary if the glucose solution also contains norepinephrine. The quantity of norepinephrine given needs to be regulated carefully and therefore to be administered separately.

3. If respiratory difficulty occurs, particularly a severe asthmatic attack, 25 mg. of ephedrine sulfate should be administered intravenously especially when peripheral collapse is present. Should the blood pressure be normal, 50 mg. of this drug may be administered intramuscularly.

4. Nasal oxygen should be instituted promptly if cyanosis is present.

5. Analgesia and occasionally sedation may be required. Generally, 7.5 mg. of intravenously administered morphine sulfate for the 70 Kg. patient produces an effective analgesia.

6. A 30 ml. sample of the patient's blood is withdrawn as soon as practical and centrifuged to check for the presence of hemoglobinemia. Sufficient blood is obtained to resubmit

the patient's blood to the blood bank for checking and identity of blood groups. Also a portion is sent to the clinical laboratory for analysis of the nitrogen as well as urea nitrogen determinations; these 2 chemical determinations provide baseline data for subsequent comparisons should renal function be seriously impaired within the days to follow.

7. The donor's blood should also be rechecked and cultured for bacterial growth.

8. An indwelling catheter is placed in the urinary bladder to provide a means for the hourly measurement of urine flow and the early detection of hemoglobinuria. The importance of the hourly record of the urinary output cannot be overemphasized. A patient may secrete as much as 1,000 ml. of urine within the first 6 hours after his transfusion reaction, only to develop complete renal shutdown thereafter. Consequently, if urine volume is measured on a 24-hour schedule, 18 hours or more may elapse before renal shutdown is detected. This information bears directly upon the subsequent volumes and characteristics of the fluids to be administered intravenously or by mouth. (See Chap. 52, Urology, the section on Acute Renal Failure.) Hourly records are essential.

9. Avoid the infusion of electrolytes, except when their need is demonstrated by reliable chemical data.

10. Hemodialysis may be required on one or more occasions until recovery occurs.

Fresh Versus Aged Blood

The date of expiration of ACD blood refrigerated at 2° to 6° C. is usually considered to be about 21 days after it is drawn. While blood aged for this period is satisfactory for many transfusion purposes, changes that can be harmful do occur, which should encourage the use of shorter time limits for refrigeration storage. As mentioned on page 167, the younger the blood, the longer the survival of the transfused red cells in the recipient. The older the blood the higher the concentration of free hemoglobin and the higher the concentration of plasma potassium.

Glycolysis in the erythrocytes diminishes, and formation of ATP is said to be impaired as blood ages. The result is that metabolic acidosis occurs in vitro in the blood to be administered to the patient who, if suffering from acute hypovolemic shock, is already in a mild to severe degree of metabolic acidosis for reasons of impaired tissue perfusion or glycolytic metabolism. The degree of acidosis in aged blood may be lessened with the use of citrate-phosphate-dextrose as a substitute for acid-citrate-dextrose (ACD).

ATP appears to increase the survival time of erythrocytes, but when added to blood and used repeatedly, it may cause renal damage.

Hyperkalemia. One of the features of aging blood is the diffusion of potassium into plasma from the erythrocytes. Diffusion of this ion continues at a fairly steady rate from the cells of citrated blood, from the moment they are withdrawn until they are given. As potassium in blood is largely an intracellular erythrocyte cation, plasma potassium levels are higher in hemolyzed blood. It is a safe assumption that the greater the degree of hemolysis of refrigerated blood, the greater the concentration of potassium in its plasma. Also, plasma potassium may increase to as much as 10 times the normal level by diffusion alone, with little or no evidence of concurrent hemolysis. Concentration of potassium in citrated blood, stored under refrigeration with little or no evidence of hemolysis, may reach levels as high as 35 to 40 mEq. per liter (Melrose and Wilson, 1953).

The diffusion of potassium into the plasma of aging blood occurs at a slower rate when glucose is added to the citrate solution into which blood is drawn. There is some evidence that the addition of glucose to the hyperkalemic plasma of aged blood can drive potassium back into the cells, but thus far the addition of glucose to outdated blood has not proved to be a practical technic in blood banking practices.

The possibility that potassium intoxication will result from the transfusion of large volumes of aged blood is difficult to determine. Melrose and Wilson were unable to detect any significant changes in electrocardiographic tracings attributable to potassium intoxication when aged blood with elevated potassium concentration in the plasma was administered. It should be remembered that the increase in serum potassium levels of the patient under abnormal conditions is largely at the expense of his intracellular potassium and often is associated with a depletion of intracellular protein. It may be that hyperkalemia from blood transfusion in the nondepleted patient is tolerated better in man than is generally believed.

Although many deaths, including those from cardiac arrest, occur in the course of the use of massive transfusions, the relationship between these deaths and hyperkalemia from blood is not established. Again, the excellent results obtained by Crosby and Akeroyd are to be cited, for in their use of massive transfusions of blood (10 to 30 pints per patient) in the Korean war, the chief source of their Rh positive Group O blood was blood drawn in this country, flown to Korea, in which the agitation of the blood in flight should be expected to favor an accelerated hemolysis and hyperkalemia. No suggestion of potassium intoxication was reported among the recipients.

Aged blood administered intra-arterially has the benefit of greater dilution by its passage through the peripheral circulation before reaching the heart and the coronary circulation than when administered by the intravenous route. This suggestion in principle is doubtless correct, but until it can be shown that the elevated serum potassium concentration of this origin in the nondepleted recipient is definitely harmful, this consideration is not sufficient to advocate use of the intra-arterial route of transfusion. Arterial transfusions carry certain special hazards which seemingly are not compensated for by any demonstrated superiority over blood administered at the same rate by vein (Maloney *et al.*, 1953). Among the reported hazards of intra-arterial blood is arterial damage, with gangrene of the extremity peripheral to the arterial puncture, as well as the need for greater technical skill in the introduction of the intra-arterial needle; the latter introduces the hazard of delay as well as that of arterial injury. Although certain other theoretical considerations have been advocated for the intra-arterial route of administration of blood in the patient in peripheral collapse, such as reducing the hazard from air embolus, should this occur, and the reported greater ease with which the artery may be entered in shock, the author does not recommend or employ this route for ordinary blood administration.

Acidosis and Cardiac Arrest. The acidosis from the ACD blood transfused, plus that which the patient already suffers because of impaired perfusion, along with the additional hazard of diminished free calcium ion due to the binding of free calcium by the citrate contained in the transfusions, set the stage for cardiac arrest. This threat can be reduced in part by the administration of 1 Gm. of calcium chloride or calcium gluconate after every 2nd or 3rd transfusion when blood is being given rapidly (Adams *et al.*, 1944; Bunker *et al.*, 1955; Nealon *et al.*, 1963).

McLaughlin, Nealon and Gibbon (1960) presented an ingenious technic to remove excessive potassium and ammonium from bank blood prior to transfusion. This method may help in solving the problem of such excess in instances of blood subjected to prolonged storage, but to date it has not gained wide usage.

Bacterial Contamination. Another hazard of aged blood is that certain of the gram-negative bacterial contaminants, when present, may reach fairly luxuriant growth by the 21st day of refrigerated storage. Whereas, by the 10th day their growth and endotoxic products are minimal and may be tolerated, the same blood may cause a fatality if allowed to incubate at 2° to 6° C. for 18 to 21 days.

Thus, the arguments that 21-day-old blood is as useful as 5- to 10-day-old blood similarly stored is theoretically sound but can be spurious. From the standpoint of patient care, the number of man-made errors and the chemical changes that occur are enough greater in the use of 21-day-old blood compared with 5- to 10-day-old blood, that, when possible, we should try to administer most transfusions before the 10th day.

Those blood banks preparing plasma from out-dated blood will find it advantageous to declare blood available for plasma production by the 10th day and to separate the plasma from the cellular elements as soon thereafter as possible.

Deficiencies in the factors of blood coagulation in aged blood are seldom a contraindication for blood transfusion, except for hemophilia and Christmas disease in which the administration of whole freshly drawn blood, rapidly frozen plasma from freshly drawn blood, or antihemophilic globulin and Factor IX are often of value. Deficiency or absence of fibrinogen, whether from fibrinolysis or extensive intravascular coagulation (usually both) can best be treated by the administration of purified fibrinogen in 6- to 12-gram quantities or more. To supply the same amount from whole blood, about 6 to 10 units would be required and would overload the circulation. When platelets are needed, transfusions of platelet concentrates may be useful temporarily. Whole blood transfusion is of little value for this purpose.

Of the clotting factors that are relatively stable in blood up to the 21st day of storage, fibrinogen (Factor I), prothrombin (Factor II), proconvertin (Factor VII) and plasma thromboplastin component (Factor IX) are known to retain satisfactory activity under the usual conditions of blood storage. Platelets and antihemophilic globulin (Factor VIII) are not. Ac-globulin (Factor V) is moderately unstable in refrigerated blood.

What then has fresh blood to offer that cannot be supplied by 10- to 20-day-old blood? Primarily antihemophilic globulin and Ac-globulin. Platelets are present to a limited extent in fresh blood but not enough can be supplied in whole blood without the risk of circulatory overload. There may be other clotting factors, yet to be discovered, that may give more evidence that fresh blood has merits sufficiently superior to that of older blood to make its use more desirable.

Pyrogenic Reactions

Febrile reactions occur in association with the administration of any intravenous fluids, including blood and plasma. They have been recognized as long as transfusions have been employed. Halsted, in 1883, describing a transfusion given in the treatment of monoxide poisoning, remarked: "the usual post-transfusion recurrence lasted for half an hour."

Seiver demonstrated that certain nonpathogenic bacteria often multiply in distilled water and cause fever when injected into animals.

A second common source of pyrogens are the chemical contaminants in intravenous tubing, glassware or unclean needles. Now that most blood banks employ disposable administration sets, pyrogenic reactions have largely disappeared.

Allergic Reactions

Urticarial or allergic reactions are characterized by the appearance of hives and occasionally by attacks of angioneurotic edema and asthma. The exact mechanism of this phenomenon is not clearly understood. Occasionally, a patient, sensitive to a particular food or drug, will display urticarial or allergic reactions when the donor has eaten a food recently or is under a drug therapy to which the patient is sensitive. For example, the donor may have eaten tomatoes or shrimp recently, or he may be under sulfonamide therapy to which the patient is sensitive. Then the recipient may develop urticaria, angioneurotic edema or an acute asthmatic attack.

Reactions of this type usually occur in less than 1 per cent of the patients transfused with either blood or plasma. The administration of calcium gluconate is often beneficial if given promptly. In more severe reactions, especially asthmatic attacks, corticoids, antihistaminics and/or ephedrine sulfate may be administered. In general, reactions of this type are more troublesome than serious.

Circulatory Overload

Circulatory overload from excessive transfusion is seldom seen in surgical patients undergoing an operation. This does not imply that the circulation cannot be overloaded. The volume of blood lost at operation or in trauma is underestimated much more often than it is overestimated; therefore, overload is seldom encountered under these conditions. Circulatory overload is observed more commonly in the course of preoperative transfusions where an attempt is made to correct anemia or hypoproteinemia with blood and/or plasma being administered either too rapidly or in too large a volume at one time. However, it is remarkable that even under these circumstances this complication seldom occurs. Its failure to do so is excellent testimony to the ability of the vascular system to compensate for the increase in blood volume if fluids are not administered too rapidly and if cardiopulmonary reserve is reasonable. Usually, little if any increase in plasma volume can be detected 6 hours after the administration of a liter of plasma, serum albumin or dextran. The water in transfused blood or plasma is lost from the circulation fairly rapidly, either by diffusion into the extravascular spaces or via the kidney as urine. Overload from plasma transfusions is less likely to be encountered than from blood, because the transfused red cells remain within the circulation. The transfusion of blood is tolerated best in patients with anemia, provided that they are without marginal cardiovascular reserve; the increase in total blood volume probably is compensated in part by the rapid disappearance of plasma and water from the circulation.

The symptoms of circulatory overload are primarily those of left-sided heart failure with pulmonary congestion and/or edema. This complication can be rapidly fatal if not recognized promptly and treated appropriately. Its treatment may consist of the intravenous administration of digitalis preparations in patients with marginal cardiovascular function. It may be necessary also to perform phlebotomy promptly. But first one should apply the usual blood pressure tourniquets to 3 of the 4 extremities, elevating the constricting pressure to about halfway between the systolic and diastolic pressures. By rotating one tourniquet to the unconstricted extremity once every 20 minutes, no extremity remains occluded for more than 1 hour at a time.

Central venous pressure monitoring is a great help in avoiding circulatory overload.

Abnormal Bleeding

Abnormal bleeding is occasionally a disastrous complication of blood transfusions. Its pathogenesis is by no means clearly understood, although certain disorders in coagulation can be detected in some patients. The importance of such a defect probably varies from patient to patient. This is principally a complication of transfusions administered during operation and is seen more frequently under hypothermic than under normothermic conditions.

The clinical pattern is frightening indeed. The exposed surfaces suddenly begin to ooze blood from even the minutest of vessels. Death may occur in a few hours in spite of any treatment.

Although abnormal bleeding of this type usually is encountered more frequently in patients receiving massive transfusions in the course of an operative procedure, occasionally it is observed when only 1 or 2 transfusions have been administered. Characteristically, the blood is unusually dark in spite of the administration of oxygen in seemingly adequate quantities or of the type of anesthesia employed. The blood appears less viscid than usual and clotting appears to be delayed. As puddles of blood accumulate in the tissues or on drapes, coagulation usually takes place. Coagulation will not take place at all if the fibrinogen has been destroyed. Once this condition occurs, the continued administration of blood seems to be more harmful than beneficial; the author prefers to change to plasma but for no well-documented reason. Continued effort at hemostasis appears to be essentially hopeless, for the bleeding points are so numerous as to preclude satisfactory results by the ligature technic.

Blood samples examined under these conditions usually disclose more than one type of clotting disorder. The platelet count is usually at near thrombocytopenic levels (10,000 to 50,000 per cu. mm.). Prothrombin activity also may be depressed sharply, and in some patients the circulating heparinlike anticoagulant may be found (Pifer et al., 1956).

Another of the more important disorders is an increased tendency of the fibrin clots to undergo lysis. The enzyme responsible for lysis appears to be similar to, if not identical with, that normally present in the activated fibrinolytic (plasmin) system. Fibrinolysin normally exists as a relatively inactive substance; its precursor is abundantly present in plasma and is known as profibrinolysin. Although it is normally activated at all times, its rate of activation in the course of thrombin generation or fibrin formation is accelerated. In the highly active fibrinolytic state, fibrinogen and, to some extent, prothrombin are attacked as well as fibrin. Therefore, fibrinogen and prothrombin deficiencies also may exist along with thrombocytopenia.

There is also normally present an inhibitor of fibrinolysin known as antifibrinolysin (antiplasmin). An increasing fibrinolytic activity may result then from two mechanisms: There may be an actual increase in the rate at which fibrinolysin is activated, or fibrinolysin may accumulate because it is not destroyed by its inhibitor antifibrinolysin, or both.

The inhibitor apparently is produced by the liver. In far-advanced liver disease, the loss of the inhibitor appears to account for some of the fibrinolytic states described. The prostatic secretions contain the fibrinolytic enzyme or a similar enzyme whose properties affect fibrin, fibrinogen and prothrombin in a manner indistinguishable from that of fibrinolysin. Abnormal bleeding from the prostatic bed is often from the fibrinolysin of prostatic origin but is mistaken for poor mechanical hemostasis. General hemorrhagic states characterized by lysis of both fibrinogen and fibrin were first observed by the author in 1949 in patients with metastatic prostatic carcinoma irrespective of surgical operations. A number of others have reported similar cases. In general, such patients are encountered infrequently.

The hemorrhagic complication of abruptio placenta is one illustration of a highly activated fibrinolytic system (Schneider, 1952). Also, fibrinogen may disappear completely from the circulation. Fibrinogen is exhausted by the formation of multiple small thrombi throughout the circulation, caused by the introduction of thromboplastic juices of placental origin entering the circulation spontaneously under these conditions. It is possible to coagulate experimentally all of the fibrinogen within the circulation over a period of 15 minutes or less without fatal embolism. Minute quantities of fibrin can be demonstrated in the capillary bed of the liver, the lungs and the kidneys. Platelets are trapped in these thrombi and probably account for the acute thrombopenia. The plasma remaining is essentially circulating serum and has considerable increase in fibrinolytic activity.

Although the mechanism that excites fibrinolytic activity in transfusions at operation is not precisely known, it may be due to the entrance of thromboplastic substances into the circulation, either from the operative bed or from an unrecognized transfusion reaction with release of thromboplastic materials.

Fibrinolysis should be suspected if a sample of blood drawn from the patient either should not clot at all or clot quickly and lyse within 5 to 10 minutes. If 1 ml. of the patient's blood is mixed with 1 ml. of normal blood (proved with another ml. of the same normal blood that it is capable of clotting) the mixture of the patient's and the control blood should lyse in part or completely in 30 minutes at 37° C.

This type of acute fibrinogen deficiency is generally caused by an increased clotting tendency in the patient. It is best to administer heparin 50 ml. initially and then as a slow drip to prevent the patient's blood from clotting fibrinogen as it is administered. This is another example of treating a clotting syndrome with a hemorrhagic agent. Fatal pulmonary emboli have been occasionally observed when fibrinogen is administered without protection against further intravascular clotting by the use of heparin.

The above considerations would seem to contraindicate the use of EACA (epsilon-aminocaproic acid), though its use is still continued by some.

The all-important feature of this type of abnormal bleeding in the surgical patient receiving blood is its self-limiting nature. Consequently, prompt and heroic measures with reference to the administration of these agents are imperative. If they prove to be effective, the patient will recover, and hemorrhage is unlikely to recur. The surgeon should check with the anesthesiologist to make certain that adequate calcium gluconate has been administered in the course of transfusions to obviate the possibility of citrate intoxication, though hemorrhage from this cause rarely occurs before cardiac arrest.

CITRATE INTOXICATION

On repeated occasions during the past 50 years, warnings have been issued that toxic concentrations of citrate occasionally occur following the use of citrated blood or plasma transfusion. Abnormal bleeding, hypotension and other difficulties relative to the depletion of the calcium ion have been suggested. The earlier advocates of this view were answered readily by the studies of Lewisohn from 1915 to 1923. Within the next 25 years, however, when more extensive elective or traumatic surgery had been made possible by the liberal use of citrated blood and plasma, it was not so easy to deny that citrate intoxication did occur in the occasional patient.

In 1944, a study of all patients receiving transfusions in which the amount of citrate ranged from 7.6 to 40.0 Gm. disclosed no evidence that bleeding attributable to citrate had occurred (Allen et al.). This study was followed by an experimental study by Adams et al. on dogs. They demonstrated that dogs given large doses of sodium citrate would develop tetany very rapidly and die unless extra sources of calcium ion were made available, but hemorrhage was not noted except during the agonal state. Tetany appeared before coagulation was retarded and proved to be an excellent indication as to when calcium gluconate therapy should be instituted in their studies, but only when the animals were under light or no general anesthesia. With deep anesthesia tetany was absent.

Practically, these observations led to routine administration of 1 Gm. of calcium gluconate after the 2nd or the 3rd transfusion during surgery involving rapid blood loss and entailing rapid infusion of citrated blood as replacement therapy (see below). One precaution is necessary; the calcium gluconate must be administered through a separate venous infusion set; if added to the blood transfusion, coagulation of the blood in the transfusion container occurs. No evidence of calcium intoxication has been observed with this regimen.

Although it is doubtful that calcium gluconate so administered prevents the occasional hemorrhage associated with blood transfusion, it may be useful in reducing toxic effects of excessive citrate, and the author has continued its use. As late as 1955, reports continued to indict citrate intoxication (Bunker et al.), but a review of the data published disclosed that only infrequent attempts were made at calcium replacement in patients receiving massive transfusions in brief periods of time. Better results can be achieved if severe calcium depletion is prevented by the intermittent administration of calcium gluconate to prevent citrate intoxication and if reasonable attempts at surgical hemostasis are carried out so that less blood is needed.

It is possible that patients under hypothermic anesthesia or with severe liver disease may detoxify citrate at a much slower rate than normal. However, in the author's experience (1944-1946), with the administration of 1 Gm. of calcium gluconate for each 2 to 3 transfusions administered no suspicion of the occurrence of citrate intoxication in any of our patients has arisen. Confirmation of this has been reported by Bunker et al. (1962).

THE SINGLE TRANSFUSION AND ITS MULTIPLE HAZARDS

In 1954 the author drew attention to some of the hazards that may arise from a single transfusion to the adult patient (Jennings and Allen). The case reports on pages 159 and 165 illustrate 2 types of hazards; still another, which ended fatally, is shown by the following case episode.

A 61-year-old man was admitted to the hospital on January 26, 1953, having been in a coma for one day. Eighty days previously, in his community hospital, he had been operated upon for appendicitis and peritonitis. During the operation, one transfusion of whole blood was administered. His postoperative course was a stormy one, as he was a severe diabetic.

At the time of admission to another institution, he was deeply icteric. The abdomen was soft, normal peristaltic sounds were heard, and the blood pressure was 70/58 mm. of mercury. Laboratory studies disclosed a leukocyte count of 16,750 with a hemoglobin level at 10.5 Gm./100 ml. of blood. Emergency treatment was instituted immediately; it consisted of plasma, glucose and saline administration, as well as norepinephrine. The patient did not respond and succumbed a few hours later.

From the autopsy examination it was concluded that the cause of death was acute necrosis of the liver, presumably from homologous serum hepatitis. Histologic examination showed that only a few scattered islands of parenchymal cells remained. There was no evidence of bile duct obstruction.

For some years there has been a very conscious effort on the part of some hospitals to reduce the numbers of blood transfusions for each patient by the substitution of plasma or dextran and, at times, even balanced salt solution. Many patients who formerly received 1 or 2 transfusions now receive plasma or balanced salt solution without blood. We find also that we are able to limit the quantity of blood given in 36 to 37 per cent of our patients to 1 transfusion when heretofore these same patients would have been exposed to the hazards of 2 to 3 transfusions. Thus we are replacing a higher proportion of blood loss with substitutes rather than with blood itself. Because the hazards of transfusions and the possible errors entailed tend to be the sum of the numbers of transfusions given, it is better a patient receive 1 transfusion than 2, 2 than 4, etc.

The condemnation of the single transfusion applies primarily to patients in whom no strong indication for blood transfusion exists, and in whom no attempt is made to use plasma volume expanders as a substitute for blood, a case such as is illustrated above. At present the tendency to condemn the use of single transfusions in adult patients is warranted only when the evidence is clear that a substitute would have served equally well. It is probable that single transfusions, when administered properly, should be more nearly one third of all transfusions than the 10 to 15 per cent currently considered as the maximum acceptable. It follows that any institution attempting to minimize the numbers of transfusions given will thereby increase the percentage of the total patients transfused who receive but a single unit of blood, a commendable rather than deplorable trend.

It is inevitable, and also appropriate, that as one tries to restrict the numbers of blood transfusions given, the numbers of single transfusions will increase—i.e., those who currently receive 2 to 4 units of blood will more likely receive only 1 unit, supplemented with a plasma expander. The risk of serum hepatitis from 5 units of blood is essentially 5 times that from a single unit, but this relationship does not continue to the 8th or the 9th unit of blood given, for reasons not known (Allen and Sayman, 1962).

These remarks are not intended as an indictment of blood transfusion when blood is needed, for if this is the surgeon's response, he immediately becomes the victim and the source of another important abuse of blood transfusion—that of administering too little and too late. The risk entailed in multiple transfusions in the treatment of hypovolemic shock, while increasing at an arithmetical rate, is accepted much more readily, provided that every reasonable precaution in the administration of blood has been observed.

There is little reason to transfuse patients whose hemoglobin concentration is 10 grams, and in some cases 7 grams of Hg (Gm.%) is well tolerated, provided that blood volume is normal and anemia is chronic. In theory, at least, and as shown experimentally by Wise et al. (1958), 4 grams per cent of hemoglobin is tolerated in acutely bled dogs, as long as plasma volume is adequate to maintain good organ perfusion. Whenever the patient's condition permits, iron therapy is preferable to whole blood transfusions, if acute restoration of hemoglobin is not required. When a major operation is contemplated, and iron therapy is not feasible or practical, the patient's hemoglobin should be raised to 12-14 Gm. per cent, before operation, and sustained at these levels during operation, maintaining also normal blood volume.

The risk of icteric serum hepatitis from a single transfusion of blood from prison and Skid Row donors is at least 10 times that from a volunteer or family type donor. Rises in transaminase levels without icterus are 35 to 70 times more frequent when the donor blood is from Skid Row or prison than they are with blood from the volunteer or family source (Cohen and Dougherty, 1968).

The adult patient receiving the isolated 500 ml. transfusion is by no means restricted to surgical patients alone. Many patients with iron deficiency anemia are given the single transfusion on medical and surgical services when suitable preparations of iron in conjunction with a diet adequate in proteins, vitamins and calories would serve equally well. Although there always will remain a small risk in blood transfusion, the physician is in a much more defensible position when such accidents occur in patients in whom the question of need for blood cannot be challenged.

SPECIAL TRANSFUSIONS

Under certain circumstances it may be desirable to administer "washed" red cell concentrates, platelet transfusions, freshly prepared citrate transfusions, in some instances "direct" transfusions wherein no anticoagulant is employed, autotransfusions, exchange transfusions, and blood for extracorporeal circulation.

Exchange Transfusions

Such transfusions are limited principally to 3 general types of situations: (1) when the patient's hemoglobin has been rendered incapable of carrying oxygen; (2) to eliminate or reduce as far as possible the abnormally sensitized blood cells of the infant suffering from erythroblastosis foetalis; and (3) excessive volume of operative blood loss in the surgical patient, so that the replacement volume assumes exchange proportions in an attempt to sustain life by supporting the blood volume until hemorrhage is under control and the vital signs become stabilized.

Exchange transfusions may have some value

in patients in hepatic coma, as reported by others, but the author has experienced no success in this procedure.

Erythroblastosis foetalis was first explained on a rational basis by Landsteiner and developed by Levine, his pupil, in a series of papers. They attributed this disease to Rh positive cells which enter the mother's circulation from the fetus, she having Rh negative blood and being vulnerable. It has been presumed with good evidence that the blood antigen is the Rh positive red cell of the infant in most instances and that, in the course of pregnancy, small quantities of the infant's blood enter the maternal circulation by one means or another. The production of Rh antibodies is thereby stimulated in the Rh negative mother. These maternal antibodies then pass freely across the placental barrier, inducing hemolysis of the infant's red cells and other serious disorders.

Erythroblastosis foetalis is treated by means of exchange transfusions as soon after birth as the diagnosis is made. The purpose of blood exchange in this disease is to remove the infant's own red cells which are sensitized to the maternal anti-Rh antibodies that have been transmitted across the placental barrier. The use of exchange transfusions in this disease has reduced effectively the incidence of kernicterus, although jaundice alone probably is not responsible for the damaged basal nuclei often associated with this disease. Exchange transfusions where severe hydroptic changes have occurred prenatally have little to offer. The diagnosis of impending erythroblastosis is anticipated by a detection of a rise in anti-Rh titer in the maternal blood. Other antigens are also believed to be responsible occasionally for this disease in some patients.

If treatment is to succeed, exchange transfusions should be started within the first hours of infant life. Into the umbilical vein is threaded a polyethylene catheter, and the exchange is carried out by repeatedly withdrawing 20 ml. of the infant's blood and replacing this with 20 ml. of donor blood until from 300 to 500 ml. have been transferred. The donor considered best suited is an Rh negative individual of the same blood group who has no Rh antibodies. Intermittently, calcium gluconate is administered to prevent possible citrate intoxication (p. 175). In some instances, repetition of the exchange may be necessary on several occasions during the first day or two. Usually, the umbilical vein can be re-entered, but should it be thrombosed by that time, a femoral vein may be used.

Monoxide poisoning is the other usual reason for the use of exchange transfusions. In this instance, as in other types of hemoglobin poisoning affecting the oxygen-carrying capacity of red cells, the immediate problem is to provide compatible donor cells in sufficient quantity to meet oxygen transport needs. No problem of isosensitization exists in these patients. In many instances, the prompt administration of 2 or 3 units of blood in monoxide poisoning is all that is necessary. In the course of their administration, bloodletting can be instituted to avoid circulatory overload. Because of the extreme urgency, the use of Group O Rh negative blood without resorting to typing may be necessary in many instances. Usually, if the transfer of 40 to 50 per cent of the patient's estimated blood volume in monoxide or similar types of poisoning does not prove to be beneficial, further exchange is likely to be fruitless.

Hyperbaric oxygen therapy at 3 atmospheres, if available, may be very useful. At 3 atmospheres pressure, O_2 displaces CO from monoxyhemoglobin.

Direct Transfusions

A "direct" transfusion, as opposed to an "indirect" one, refers to the rapid intravascular transfer of blood from the donor to the recipient without the use of an anticoagulant. This, of course, is the type of transfusion used early and was one of the reasons why blood transfusion was such a formidable procedure prior to the citrate era. Any specific merit that this procedure has over the more deliberate and carefully planned citrated transfusion is sharply limited, if indeed a benefit actually does exist other than in the hemophilic patient.

Many clinicians believe that direct transfusion has certain beneficial properties in the treatment of patients with abnormal bleeding that are not possible with freshly prepared citrated blood or plasma. The available facts do not support this contention, except for the treatment of hemophilia, assuming that the citrated blood is less than a day or two in age.

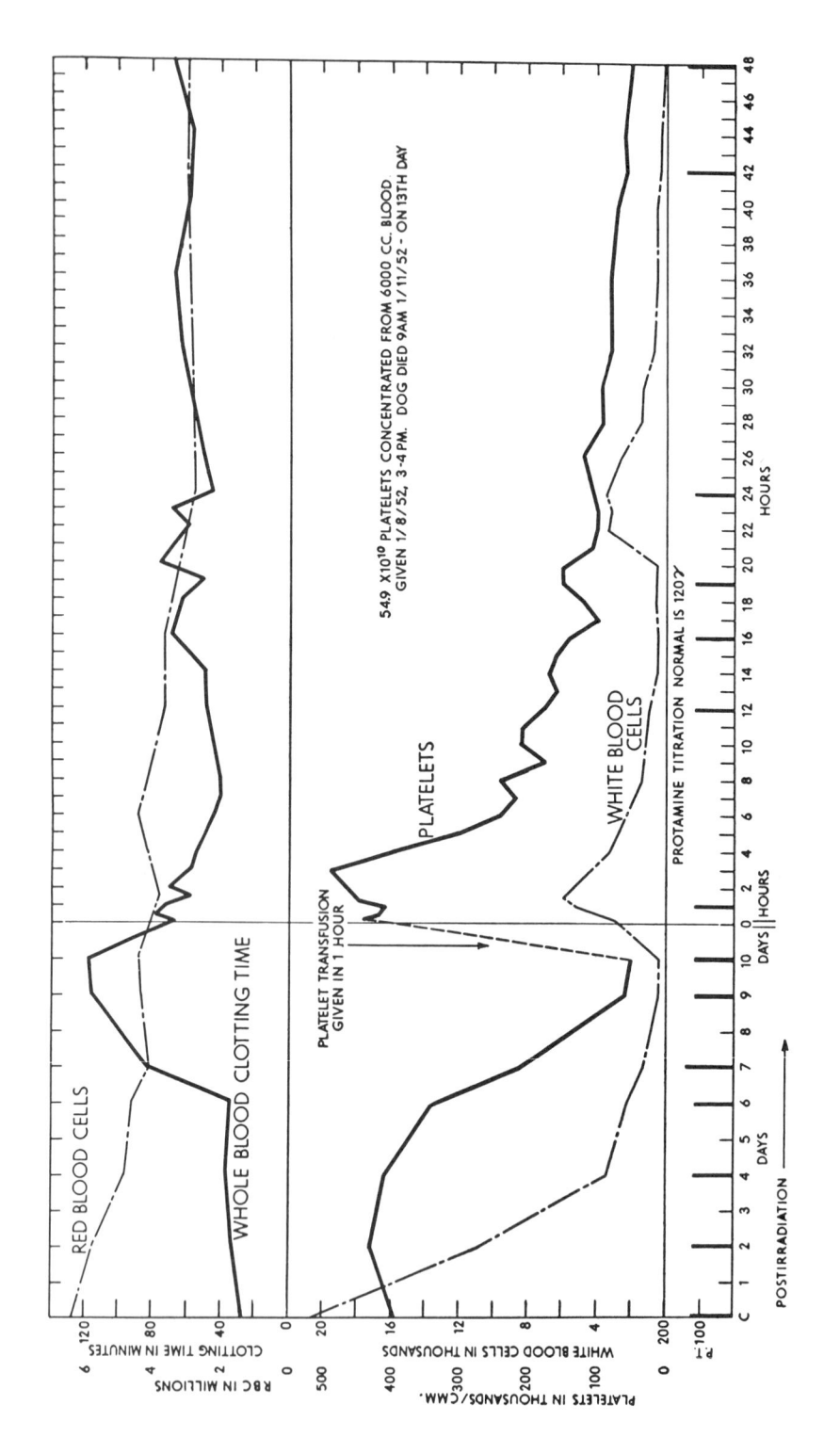

Fig. 8-3. Platelet transfusion. Illustrating the rapid declines in platelet count after platelet transfusions. Animals were rendered thrombocytopenic by total body radiation.

Of greater importance is the fact that the in-vivo turnover times are so rapid that their beneficial effect is evanescent (Fig. 8-3) in many of the clotting disorders.

The in-vitro stability of the more important clotting factors in citrated blood under refrigeration is shown in Table 8-9, page 194.

Autotransfusions

Since 1929, many obstetricians have advised their patients to contribute blood to the hospital blood bank a few days before delivery in order that they may receive their own particular blood as a transfusion should it be needed at the time of delivery. This practice obviated the need for concern about special Rh and other blood group problems as the patient often needed no more than the one unit of blood she donated (Farrar, 1929; Weekes et al., 1960).

Langston (1963) suggested extending the use of this procedure to elective surgical operations in patients in whom the moderate blood loss anticipated could be returned as a single transfusion a few days later. There is ample evidence that if the patient's blood is near normal at the time he makes his autodonation, in 24 hours or sooner his circulation is well adjusted and stable. Thus, it is possible to avoid not only problems in blood grouping but others as well, especially serum hepatitis. This procedure is sound and probably should be exploited more than it has been. Of all single-unit transfusions, this is the one that should cause the least difficulty, if any.

Packed and/or Washed Red Cells

Under certain circumstances, it may be advisable to administer "packed" red cells. The unit of blood is centrifuged, its plasma withdrawn, and only the red cell mass is transferred. Several units of transfused packed red cells will permit the rapid correction of anemia with only about half of the volume entailed when whole blood is given. However, the use of packed cells in this connection overlooks the fact that transfused plasma diffuses rapidly from the circulation of the recipient when whole blood is given. Plasma is of considerable nutritive value, whereas red cells are metabolized very slowly (see below). In essence, the patient retains the transfused red cells for days to weeks, whereas plasma in transfusions leaves the circulation in a matter of hours. Thus the patient performs his own plasmaphoresis and thereby packs the transfused red cells himself. One should remember that packed red cell transfusions are nearly twice as effective in blood volume expansion as compared with whole blood. Therefore, if the circulation is not to be overloaded, only half the volume of packed cells should be transfused when compared with whole blood. The use of red cell concentrates in the patients with cardiac disease suffering from severe anemia does have definite advantages over that of whole blood. Undoubtedly, anemia under these conditions is corrected more safely by the administration of red cell transfusions. Not only are smaller volumes required but red cell concentrates carry a minimum of sodium chloride. Some maintain that fewer pyrogenic reactions occur following transfusions of red cells than when whole blood is given; at best, these data show only a minor difference in rates of reactions and are not observed consistently or generally in most patients.

Most advocates of transfusion of red cell suspensions believe it to be the treatment of choice for anemia when the blood volume is normal. However, unless the anemia cannot be treated otherwise by appropriate medication, or its rapid correction is essential before surgery can be undertaken safely, the use of transfusions under these conditions carries in addition to the risk of errors incurred in typing and crossmatching the unpreventable hazard of transmission of serum hepatitis. Hence, in the decision to employ blood transfusions for the correction of anemia alone, whether as packed red cells or whole blood, the risk of transfusion hazards must be weighed carefully against the benefits expected, the needs of the patient, and the possibility that these needs can or cannot be met satisfactorily by alternative procedures (iron, liver, vitamin B_{12} and a sound diet). Of the 3 case reports included in this chapter (pp. 159, 165 and 175) illustrating the hazards of blood transfusion, 2 were employed for the correction of anemia alone. In retrospect, both patients could have been treated conservatively with greater safety.

If the anemia can be treated only by trans-

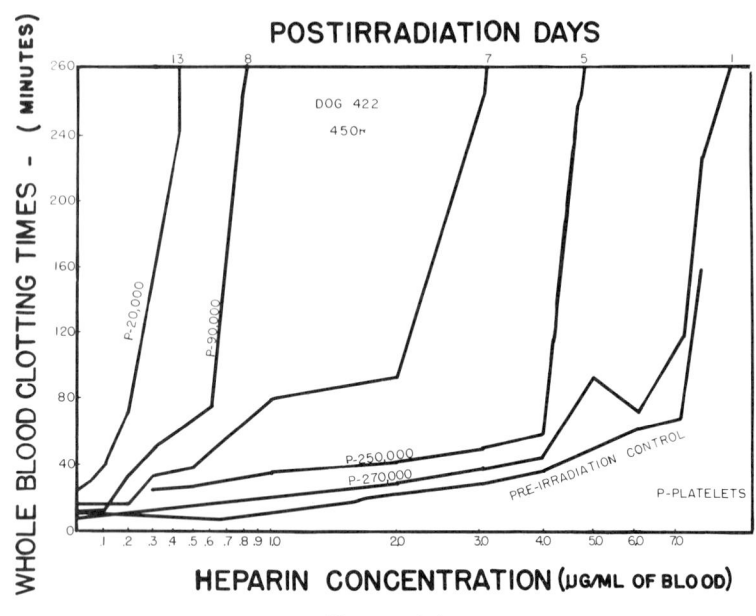

FIGURE 8-4

fusion or with greater safety—for many patients this is the case—blood transfusion as packed red cells or whole blood should be used without hesitation. On the other hand, the use of the "cosmetic" transfusion carries too great a risk to warrant its use. This risk does not exist when conservative therapy and a little patience will do equally well or better. The cosmetic transfusion constitutes one of the major abuses of blood transfusion.

Transfusion for Extracorporeal Circulation and Other Forms of Perfusion

In order to prevent coagulation by the use of citrate as the anticoagulant in extracorpo-

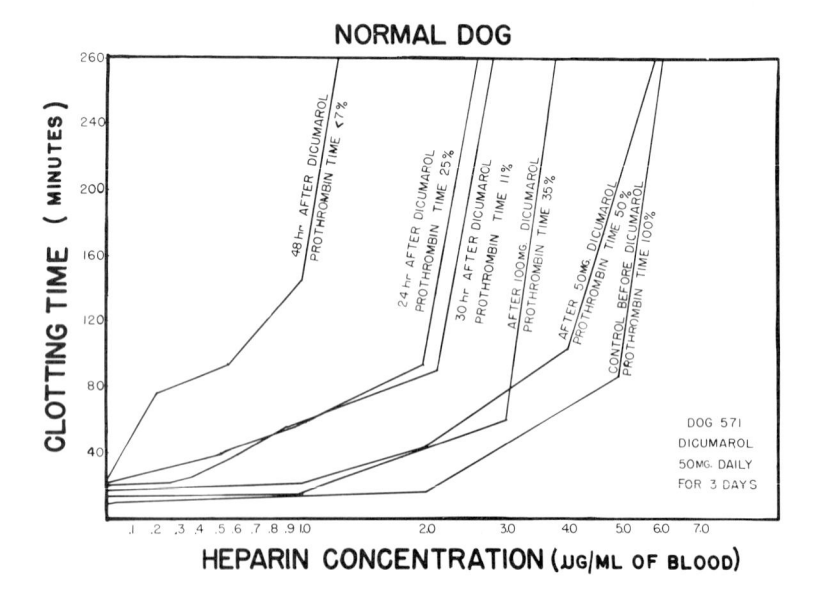

FIGURE 8-5

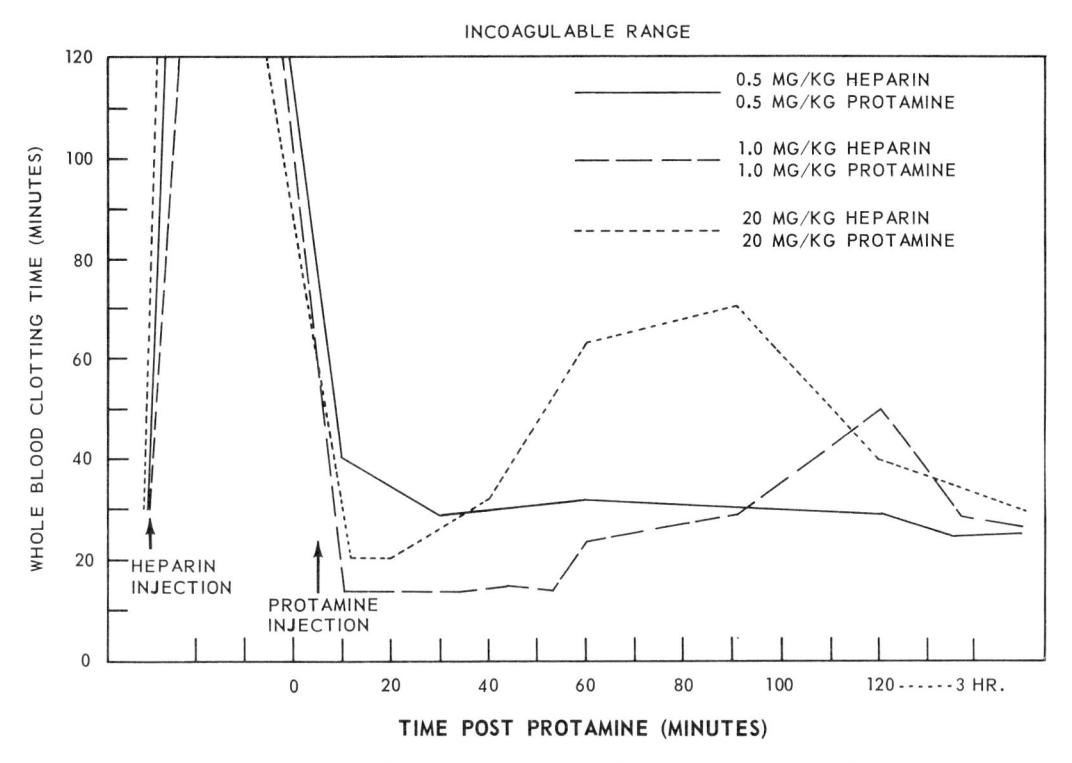

FIG. 8-6. Duration of protamine activity and its relation to various levels of intravenous heparinization in dogs (Oct., 1948).

real circulation procedures, the amounts required would result in fatal citrate intoxication. Therefore, heparinized blood must be used for these procedures. Because of heparinase in blood, the long-term storage of heparinized blood is not safe, if indeed it is feasible. Blood is usually drawn into a solution of 1,250 to 2,500 units of heparin per 500 ml. of blood not longer than 1 or 2 days prior to the planned procedure. Twice these values are used for similar volumes of plasma.

Heparin may be neutralized readily by the intravenous administration of protamine sulfate at the end of the procedure. Two variables are often overlooked that, if taken into account, would afford more effective neutralization of heparin by protamine and less hemorrhage from heparin. First, platelets are excellent antiheparins and, as such, the anticoagulant effectiveness of the same dose of heparin is increased in linear fashion as the concentration of platelets decreases (Fig. 8-4). A similar effect is also noticed in severe prothrombin deficiency (Fig. 8-5).

When circulating heparin is neutralized by the formation of heparin protaminate, the protamine moiety is metabolized more rapidly than heparin so that there may be a return of enough free heparin to give rise once again to troublesome bleeding (Fig. 8-6). As mild-to-moderate thrombocytopenia may develop in the course of extracorporeal circulation, these patients may become more sensitive to heparin; consequently, the small amounts of residual heparin freed as the more rapid metabolism of protamine occurs may, in the presence of postperfusion thrombocytopenia, cause abnormal bleeding (Allen, 1950).

Some prefer the use of up to 50 per cent volume low molecular weight dextran added to the heparinized blood for purposes of pump-priming. This kind of dextran reduces the rate of red cell sedimentation and thereby may facilitate the perfusion of tissues.

PLATELET TRANSFUSIONS

Platelet transfusions can be prepared which permit the transfusion of platelet concentrates. Many units of fresh blood are needed to accumulate sufficient platelets for transfusion purposes if the resulting platelet concentrates are to elevate the platelet count in thrombocytopenic patients (Dillard et al., 1951). Unfortunately, the increased thrombocyte level achieved is transient, lasting for only a day or two (Fig. 8-3). In the author's opinion, platelet transfusions present interesting opportunities for physiologic studies, and they offer essential therapeutic assistance in the preparation of the thrombocytopenic patient for splenectomy necessitated by hypersplenism. Once the diagnosis of idiopathic thrombocytopenia is made, there may be greater safety to the patient in prompt splenectomy than in delaying until platelet concentrates can be prepared. In some patients platelet concentrates may be better delayed until after splenectomy and transfused if the platelet count does not rise promptly and if bleeding continues.

Platelet transfusions in the bleeding patient who suffers from thrombocytopenic purpura of other origin, i.e., leukemia, aplasia of marrow, etc., are also of therapeutic value (Fig. 8-3).

Fibrinogen Transfusion

In afibrinogenemia, whether congenital or acquired, or from acute fibrinolysis, the transfusion of the fibrinogen (Cohn Fraction I) offers an immediate means for the restoration of the plasma fibrinogen concentration and effectively controls hemorrhage of this origin for short periods of time (see p. 173, Abnormal Bleeding). Because of the high incidence of serum hepatitis, fibrinogen transfusions should be used only when in the clinical judgment of the surgeon the potential advantages outweigh the risk.

Plasma Transfusion

Its Development, Use and Problems in the Treatment of Hypovolemic Shock. Although serum transfusions in the treatment of hypovolemic shock had been employed prior to the turn of the century, the need for serum or plasma as a substitute for blood transfusion did not receive serious attention prior to World War I. Abel, Rowntree and Turner demonstrated that healthy dogs withstood great losses of blood when they were infused quickly with plasma. Rous and Wilson reported that rabbits could be bled to a hemoglobin concentration of 20 per cent of the initial level when plasma infusions were given as replacement. They pointed out that at slightly lower hemoglobin concentrations, death occurred with regularity. They did not believe that death was due to lack of oxygen-carrying power but rather to the inability to maintain "blood bulk," which we now call blood volume. Today these conclusions may appear as an oversimplification. Most agree that a blood loss of more than 15 per cent of the calculated total from acute hemorrhage in man requires that a major portion of the replacement therapy be in the form of whole blood transfusion rather than as plasma therapy. Nonetheless, most agree that in the absence of available blood for transfusion, pooled plasma, 10 per cent low molecular weight dextran, and 6 per cent albumin are the safest and most effective blood substitutes currently available (see Chap. 7, Shock).

Plasma Preparation. Ward urged the use of plasma as a substitute for blood transfusion in the treatment of shock late in World War I. He believed that the risk of blood transfusion remained too high and that suitable donors and typing facilities were seldom available when such emergencies developed. He believed that plasma always should be on hand and would serve as a substitute until blood transfusion could be prepared and carried out safely.

Rous and Wilson maintained that the loss of fluid from the tissues and the organs was as important as the loss of blood per se, "a fact long known to the physiologist." However, it was recognized by these investigators that replacement of intravascular fluid had little to offer unless the fluid was one bearing colloids. The failure of replacement therapy when it consisted of glucose, saline and/or of Ringer's solution was correctly attributed to its rapid departure from the vascular bed to the tissues or to its rapid loss in the urine, the latter escape of such fluids being of much less consequence than loss into the tissues.

The basic discoveries relating to the important distinction between colloid-bearing fluids as opposed to crystalloids were those made by Starling in 1896 and by Claude Bernard as early as 1859. To Starling belongs the credit for first having demonstrated that the crystalloids of blood (plasma) and water pass very rapidly into the extravascular spaces and tissues in contrast with the colloids of plasma. The latter were shown to escape much more slowly. In consequence, Starling concluded that there exists normally a difference between the osmotic pressure of circulating protein-bearing plasma and that of "nonprotein" extravascular or interstitial fluid, which is often referred to as "effective colloid osmotic pressure." He believed that this phenomenon tended to draw water into vessels from the tissues. At the arteriolar end of the capillaries, the blood pressure being higher than the effective colloid osmotic pressure, water and crystalloids tend to enter the extravascular spaces. On the venous side, the effective colloid osmotic pressure exceeds that of blood pressure so that reversal of flow occurs; thus, fluid normally enters and leaves the circulation at a homeostatic rate.

Although more recent developments indicate the diffusion or fluid exchange to be more complex, Starling's observations have lost none of their original importance. With his observations available as common knowledge at the time of World War I, it should come as no surprise that artificial colloid-bearing fluids should have been employed more extensively in the clinical treatment of shock among the wounded soldiers than plasma, whose properties, availability and large scale preparation were yet to be developed.

The interest in plasma as a blood substitute was revived about 1940, but its usefulness was hampered to some extent because of the iso-agglutinin titer of unpooled plasma. Type-to-type plasma was originally used by many. The delay in plasma administration incurred by the time required for typing aborted any benefits that plasma might have. All acknowledged that a transfusion of properly typed blood could be prepared within the same period of time and had the advantage that it accomplished complete replacement.

With the advent of World War II, once again interest in plasma as a blood substitute came into the foreground. Its stability was well recognized, and this afforded the great advantage of indefinite storage, particularly if lyophilized (Florsdorf and Mudd, 1935). Drying of plasma lent itself well to large-scale plasma production for several reasons. If bacterial contamination of the donors' blood occurred, this was of little consequence, for if the lyophile process was carried out promptly, bacterial growth could not occur. Plasma dried by this process could be reconstituted readily and was available for instant use. The goal of stock-piling for emergencies was now a reality. Further encouragement came with the demonstration by Levinson and Cronheim (1940) that, by pooling the plasma from many donors, the risk of encountering a high iso-agglutinin from any one donor was minimized by virtue of dilution in the sum total of the pool. Pooling had the additional advantage in that it greatly facilitated the commercial production of plasma. The result was the preparation of some 15 million units of lyophilized pooled plasma in this country for military use during World War II. Pools consisted generally of the plasma from 300 to 400 donors. The liberal use of this product undoubtedly played an important part in the reduction of mortality among soldiers surviving long enough to be reached, transfused and evacuated for more definitive care (see Chap. 25, Military Surgery). However, the plasma story was not to end here, for already the serious complication of serum hepatitis was becoming evident.

Icteric Serum Hepatitis. This complication, previously mentioned for blood transfusion, formerly was of much more serious consequence for pooled plasma. The presence of this virus in the carrier donor may possibly be detected by testing for the presence of the Australian antigen. Because the blood of one carrier goes to only one recipient when the donor's blood is transfused as such, only one recipient is exposed. The hazard for pooled plasma proved to be of much more serious consequence because the plasma from one donor carrying the virus contaminates the entire plasma pool and exposes all of its recipients to the disease. The virus carrier rate among healthy donors appears to be about 1 donor among every 15 to 40 if skid-row and prison donors comprise 30 to 40 per cent of the donor population used. The attack rate among recipients of blood or plasma containing virus appears to be approximately of the order of 25 per cent. It is obvious that many of the recipients of an infected pool of plasma will contract serum hepatitis; the larger the number of recipients, the greater

TABLE 8-6. OBSERVED ATTACK RATES AMONG NORMAL RECIPIENTS OF ICTEROGENIC MATERIAL FROM INDEPENDENT POOLS

AUTHOR*	ICTEROG. AGENT	VOL. ADMIN. ML.	No. RECIP.	No. CASES	ATTACK RATE %
Murray (1954)	Plasma	1-2	100+	—	53
Gordon (1944)	Conval. Serum	5	165	79	48
Ministry of Health (1943)	Conval. Serum	5	14	6	43
McNalty (1938)	Conval. Serum	5	82	26	38
Jervis (1942)	Conval. Serum	5	80	23	30
Murray (1954)	Pooled Blood	1-2	75	17	23

* Numbers in parentheses indicate dates.

TABLE 8-7. OBSERVED ATTACK RATES AMONG ISOLATED SUBGROUPS OF NORMAL RECIPIENTS OF 0.02 ML. ALIQUOTS FROM COMMON LOTS OF POOLED ICTEROGENIC PLASMA*

No. RECIP. IN SUBGROUPS	CASES OF SERUM HEPAT.	ATTACK RATES, SUBGROUPS %
\multicolumn{3}{c}{LOT No. 335}
26	6	23.1
64	15	23.4
65	17	26.2
65	15	23.1
68	21	30.9
74	17	23.0
76	18	23.7
82	21	25.6
84	20	23.8
87	15	17.2
144	34	23.6
182	35	19.2
210	51	24.3
1,227	285	23.2
\multicolumn{3}{c}{LOT No. 338}
63	8	12.7
70	11	15.7
75	12	16.0
76	8	10.5
80	13	16.2
85	11	12.9
449	63	14.0

* Note the distinct differences in attack rates among recipients of Lot 335 contrasted with those shown under Lot 338.

will be the number of cases. Actual attack rates among the recipients of a single pool of virus-infected plasma were 10 to 70 per cent, whereas that for blood alone ranges between 0.5 to 1.0 per cent (Allen et al., 1953). There are specific attack rates for specific lots or pools of plasma (Table 8-6). More convincing evidence is shown in the follow-up studies by Sawyer et al. (1944) on the outbreaks of serum hepatitis following the administration of 2 batches of the serum-containing yellow fever vaccine to 2 groups of military recruits in the winter of 1942 (Table 8-7). But there is no indication that the susceptibility of patients to a particular batch of plasma is altered because of race, sex, or blood groups. The infant and the child may be more susceptible than the adult, but the most impressive association is the increase in frequency of hepatitis observed after transfusion among patients with pre-existing liver disease.

After the war, it became increasingly evident that hepatitis of this origin often carries a morbidity of weeks to months and in a few instances of years' duration and is accompanied by a mortality rate ranging between 5 and 50 per cent, increasing sharply in the older patient. There was nothing else to do but abandon the use of plasma except as an emergency fluid to be used where no other fluid was available, until some method to eradicate this hazard could be developed.

The serum hepatitis problem is made even more difficult because of the prolonged incubation period. Usually, 2 to 4 and even 6 months elapse from the time of exposure to the time of onset of symptoms. Moreover, about 10 to 20 times more patients develop anicteric hepatitis than develop icteric hepatitis. Usually, the shorter the period of incubation, the more severe the attack, but exceptions to this generalization are numerous.

Serum hepatitis was first described by Lürmann in 1883. A vaccine for smallpox was prepared by pooling human lymph obtained from vesicles; this was pooled and stored in glycerine; 191 of 1,293 persons vaccinated developed the disease. Several other outbreaks of icteric hepatitis of this origin were reported prior to World War II, particularly during the 1930's when pooled immune serum was employed in the treatment of various infectious and contagious diseases. In the early stages of World War II, yellow fever vaccine was prepared, using pooled plasma or serum as a stabilizing agent. Over 32,000 of those vaccinated were reported to have developed serum hepatitis believed due to the yellow fever vaccine prepared by this method. This complication immediately disappeared as soon as plasma was removed from the vaccine.

The emergency conditions of World War II undeniably made necessary the continued use of pooled plasma. The numbers of cases of hepatitis arising from the virus in pooled plasma in World War II never will be known, for one of the common diseases of wartime conditions is infectious hepatitis. No means of distinguishing between these two diseases exists, although usually in infectious hepatitis, the incubation period is about 3 weeks. Whether they represent two separate diseases or the same disease acquired by different portals of entry is still debated, especially as the Au antigen can now be tested for.

In lyophilizing, freezing, or refrigerating of pooled plasma, the preservation of the hepatitis virus, should it be present, is clearly augmented. Conversely, storing plasma in the liquid state at room temperature inevitably leads to its deterioration. The rate at which virus activity deteriorates upon standing in a liquid cell-free medium increases exponentially as the ambient temperature is elevated. In general, for each 10° C. increase in temperature, the time required to achieve the same extent of virus inactivation is reduced by 50 per cent or more. Contrariwise, for each 10° the temperature is reduced, the storage time required to achieve comparable virus inactivation by the storage technic should be doubled (Arrhenius and Van't Hoff). These are very conservative estimates. Data are now available from several sources relating to time and temperature storage of liquid pooled plasma and its safety. These can be applied in general to this important problem, thereby materially assisting in the achievement of safety (Table 8-8).

All evidence currently available, with the

TABLE 8-8. APPROXIMATE RELATIONSHIPS BETWEEN THE DURATION OF STORAGE TIME FOR VIRUS INACTIVATION AND VARIOUS TEMPERATURES EMPLOYED

VIRUS AGENT	AMBIENT STORAGE TEMPERATURE DEGREES CENTIGRADE	APPROXIMATE TIME REQUIRED FOR INACTIVATION	EXTENT OF INACTIVATION
		Minutes	
Bacteriophage (Virus T5)	63.4	480	Complete
	69.5	50	Complete
	73.0	15	Complete
Serum Hepatitis	60.0	600	Complete
	60.0	240	Incomplete
		Days	
	31.6	180	Complete
	26.0	180	Nearly complete
	20.0	180	Incomplete

COMMENTS. At the 31.6° C. employed here, the average temperature stability of plasma proteins in sodium citrate is remarkably good with reference to the use of plasma as a substitute for blood or as an intravenous source of protein administered for nutrition. However, this plasma is not useful in providing the proteins concerned with coagulation; only freshly prepared plasma or blood should be used in these latter and unusual circumstances.

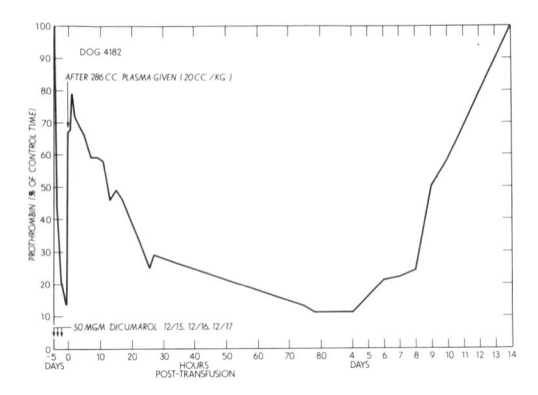

FIG. 8-7. Effect of plasma transfusion on dicumarolized dog. Shows rapid rate at which transfused prothrombin concentrates are consumed. Similar turnover rates for transfused platelets are shown in Figure 8-3 and are found for fibrinogen (actually for fibrinogen the rate is even more rapid). To keep pace with the demands of the clotting constituents by transfusions of concentrates is difficult and soon becomes impossible if the normal mechanisms do not take over soon.

exception of Redeker's work (1968), suggests that 6-month storage at a mean temperature of 31.6° C. produces a pooled plasma essentially free from the risk of transmitting icteric serum hepatitis. No cases of clinical hepatitis have been known to occur at these temperatures when properly controlled.

As the stability of plasma prepared from citrated blood is remarkably good, plasma can be stored under these conditions for several years without concern of deterioration (Fig. 8-7). However, plasma collected in A.C.D. (glucose) solution is much less stable but still serviceable if administered between 6 and 24 months of age. In both instances, however, the proteins concerned with blood coagulation lose their activity sufficiently rapidly so that plasma is not suited for the correction of coagulation defects.

TRANSAMINASE VALUES. Subclinical hepatitis has been associated with rises in SGPT and SGOT values, occurring within a few weeks to a few months after transfusion. The inference is that such rises indicate anicteric or subclinical hepatitis. The basic issue is, what is the clinical significance of these increases, in the absence of other evidence of hepatocellular disease, or of evidence of latent development of chronic hepatitis? This question becomes especially relevant when it is realized that 20 to 70 per cent of patients receiving whole blood transfusions may display positive SGPT and SGOT values within the usual period of incubation time for serum hepatitis (Cohen and Doughtery, 1968).

The flocculation tests, which include the transaminase measurements, depend largely upon increases in the plasma levels of immunoglobulins (IgA, IgG and IgM) and upon the serum levels of lipoproteins (Bevan, Taswell and Gleich, 1968). While these increases in immunoglobulins are nonspecific, when they become elevated over their previous levels after transfusion, as noted by many, the question arises as to their clinical significance and causes. If we accept the thesis that such increases reflect serum hepatitis of consequence when found in patients receiving blood, we compromise dangerously the proper indications for transfusion, as well as the welfare of the patient.

Most patients, in whom there is a post-transfusional rise in transaminases without clinical evidence of hepatitis, are unaware of illness; a few may experience some ease of fatigability. The transaminase values, in the icteric and in the anicteric patient, may remain elevated for weeks, months and even years, with no clinical evidence that the patient has chronic hepatitis.

Redeker and Hopkins (1968) reported that, among 120 patients studied, 12 patients receiving pooled plasma in a large general hospital developed rises in transaminase values, and four of the twelve were also icteric. Post-transfusional liver biopsies were claimed to show pathologic evidence of viral hepatitis, but there were no pretransfusion biopsies made for comparison. There seems little reason to question the diagnosis of their cases, but considerable reason to question their relevance. The sources of their plasma were two licensed commercial laboratories, one using exclusively Skid Row donors, and at least half of the donors from the second source were from similar high-risk sources. No records were available from the major laboratory as to the temperature and duration of storage to which each pool involved had been exposed. Thus, the significance of the Redeker studies remains in doubt. Unless precautions are strictly observed, disaster is to be expected (Allen, 1962), as Redeker and Hopkins found. The Division of Biologics Standards of the National Institutes of Health has not required that these precautions be a part of the minimal standards for plasma production for licensure of blood banks.

AUSTRALIA ANTIGEN. This antigen, discovered by Allison and Blumberg (1961), was given its name because the serum from an Australian Aborigine reacted with the sera of two hemophiliac patients who had been transfused many times. The antigen is referred to as the Au antigen, an abbreviation for *Au*stralia.

Alter and Blumberg (1966) detected the presence of antibody from the sera of patients who had received many transfusions. Blumberg et al. (1967) tested different populations against the Au antigen and found it only rarely present in North Americans and Europeans (about 1 in 800 of those tested). It was quite common in the sera of persons from tropical areas—1 to 20 per cent.

It was observed in many patients with acute leukemia who had been transfused, in patients with lepromatous leprosy, and in patients with Down's disease. Leukemic patients would ordinarily have been transfused frequently; patients with Down's disease are subject to coprophagia when institutionalized; but it is not clear how patients with lepromatous leprosy would come in contact with the antigen.

The association of this antigen with transfusion hepatitis was confirmed by Blumberg (1967), Okochi and Minamaki (1968), and Prince (1968). The studies of both Prince and Blumberg have been extensively reported in 1969 as well.

Levene, Blumberg et al. (1969) and Wright et al. (1969) by Ouchterlony's technic, observed the Au antigen reaction to be present in patients with both short- and long-term incubation periods for serum hepatitis. However, Prince was unable to detect the presence of the Au antigen in patients with

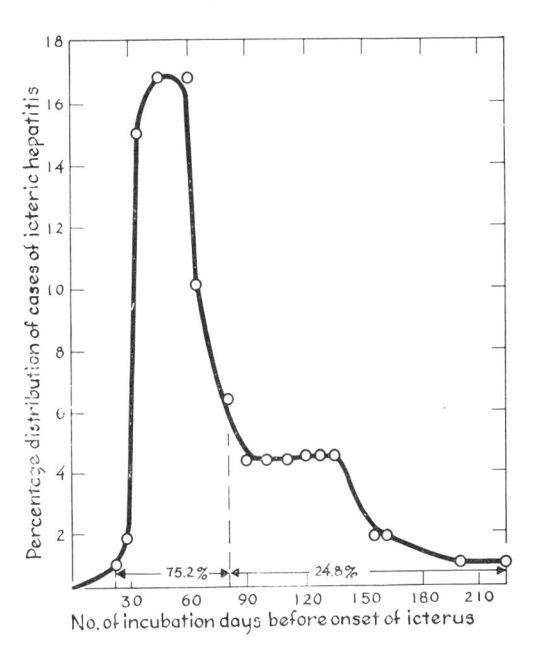

FIG. 8-8. Distribution of cases of serum hepatitis according to the day of onset of icterus. Note that 75 per cent occurred before the end of the third month. (Allen, J. G.: Immunization against serum hepatitis from blood transfusion. Ann. Surg., 160:752, 1964)

short-term incubation periods for serum hepatitis. He found it only in the long-term incubation cases. Krugman et al. also (1969) reported finding the Au antigen only among his long-term patients. These are sharp differences in excellent laboratories, and the reasons for them are not evident. Probably Prince's antigen is different from Blumberg's Au antigen. Time will tell.

If, however, the Au antigen is positive only in the long-term incubation cases, this will not be an effective screening test for serum hepatitis because of the incubation period, for essentially ¾ of the patients receiving blood will have developed clinical icterus by the 75th day (see Fig. 8-8). On the other hand, if this test is positive in both short- and long-term cases of icteric serum hepatitis, it should be of great help in donor selection. Sixty per cent of cases with long-term hepatitis seem to be detected, and in a little less than 50 per cent of the short-term cases the antigen has been recognized.

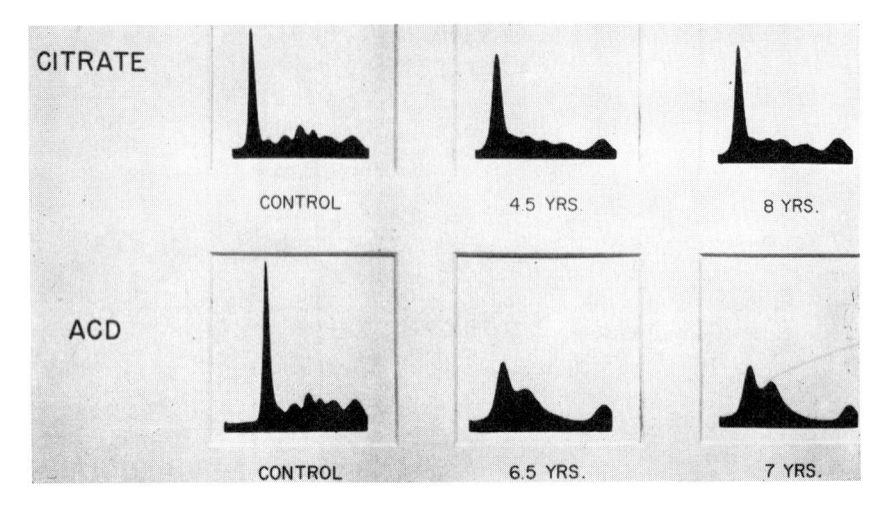

FIG. 8-9. Comparison of electrophoretic patterns. Reveals greater stability of plasma proteins when plasma is drawn in sodium citrate than in acid citrate dextrose (ACD). Note that there is a distinct difference in electrophoretic patterns. Plasma proteins are less stable in pooled plasma anticoagulated with acid-citrate-dextrose (ACD) than when anticoagulated with sodium citrate alone.

At present, a far more reliable way to reduce sharply the incidence of serum hepatitis is to stop the use of commercial blood!

The Au antigen appears from a few days to 2 to 7 weeks in advance of the development of symptomatic hepatitis, and it disappears about the time the disease has reached its peak, clinically and symptomatically.

IMMUNITY AND SERUM HEPATITIS. In 1964, Allen reported that it was possible to immunize against serum hepatitis in man, using the principle of active-passive immunization. Krugman, in 1967, reported similar findings. In neither case, however, was it possible to determine the duration of the immunity obtained. Both studies must be considered experimental and not as indicating that extensive clinical trials should yet be undertaken unless further small clinical trials yield similar results.

Intravenous Plasma for the Correction of Hypoproteinemia and Protein Depletion. Surgical patients whose pathology prevents or seriously interferes with the oral intake or absorption of food often present important systemic disorders in nutrition which increase the surgical risk over and above that presented by the local pathology. These nutritive disorders are likely to involve depletion of body fat, carbohydrate and protein reserves as well as those of minerals, vitamins and body water (see Chap. 6, Nutrition). Mineral, water and vitamin deficiencies are easy to correct by the parenteral administration of each according to estimated needs. However, if the patient cannot eat or assimilate enough food to meet the total caloric and protein requirements, operative mortality as well as morbidity are likely to be increased.

Correction of hypoproteinemia can be accomplished fairly rapidly by the infusion of plasma daily (Allen et al., 1950). Usually, 3 to 7 days of a liter of plasma, given in divided doses, will restore safely the normal concentration of plasma proteins in most patients (Figs. 8-9, 8-10).

If the benefits of plasma transfusion were limited only to those of improving the oncotic relationships of the circulation in depleted patients, its administration on this basis alone could be justified. Fortunately, plasma serves as an excellent source of protein nutrition as well as a substitute for blood (Stemmer et al., 1956). A state of strongly positive nitrogen balance exists under plasma therapy and the patient's general condition likewise usually improves. Admittedly, plasma and glucose alone do not supply the desired daily caloric

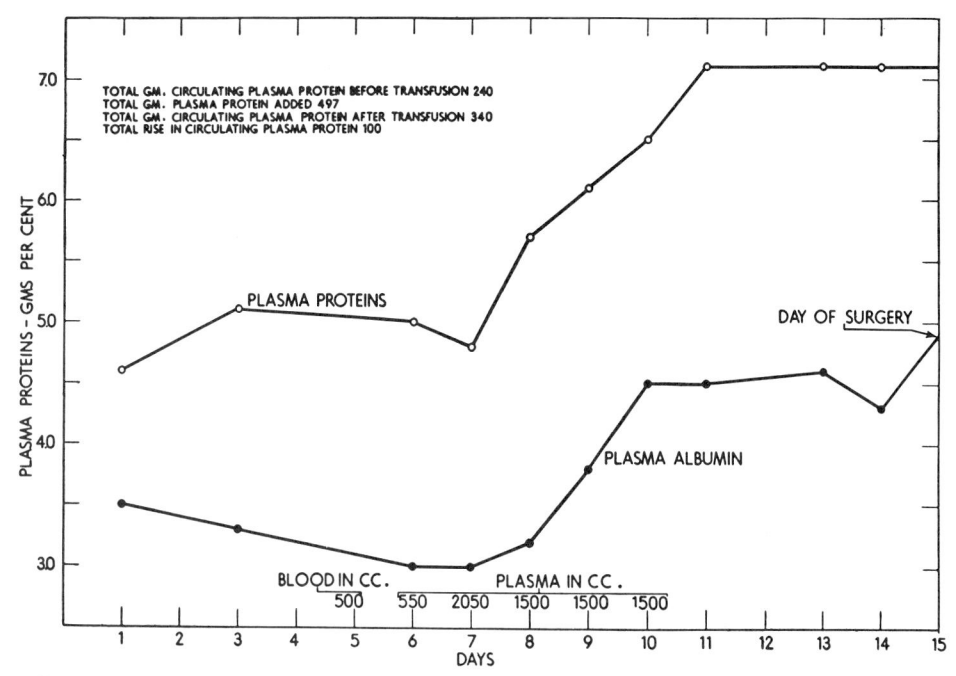

FIG. 8-10. Illustrates response of hypoproteinemia when plasma is given in volumes of 1,000 to 1,500 ml. in divided daily dosages. R.A. 398635. Gastroenterocolic fistula. Weight loss 13.5 Kg.

intake, but in many cases the correction of hypoproteinemia by plasma transfusion and the restoration of the normal hemoglobin values with blood assist materially in the preparation and in the tolerance of the patient for operation. This regimen is not the final answer to the correction of malnutrition, but it does serve as well if not better than any other parenteral feeding currently available. Plasma is used more rapidly than originally believed possible.

It has been demonstrated that littermate pups grow at least as well with intravenous plasma as their only source of protein over a 3-month period as do their sisters and brothers fed the same amount of protein by mouth (horse meat and liver). These results are illustrated in Figure 8-11.

The concentration of the calcium and potassium ions in plasma is governed partly by their being bound to some extent to plasma proteins. In the protein-depleted patient, occasionally the serum levels of these ions may be reduced simply because the extent of hypoproteinemia is so severe as to reduce the quantity of these ions that can be bound. In a few such patients, the administration of calcium or potassium salts will not correct existing deficiencies, presumably because there is insufficient plasma protein to hold these ions within the circulation. If the protein deficits can be corrected by any means, calcium and potassium are retained more easily. The reverse also appears to be true: namely, that protein repletion is difficult if not impossible to accomplish without the presence of potassium, calcium, magnesium, and possibly other trace elements. Proteins fed orally or given by vein as plasma contain both calcium and potassium. Usually, the correction of hypoproteinemia automatically corrects any existing potassium or calcium deficiency unless there are other continuing losses of these minerals.

PLASMA SUBSTITUTES have been employed longer than plasma itself in the treatment of hypovolemic shock. They are "standby fluids" until blood transfusions can be prepared. Among the first was gum acacia, introduced by Bayliss (1917) and used extensively in World

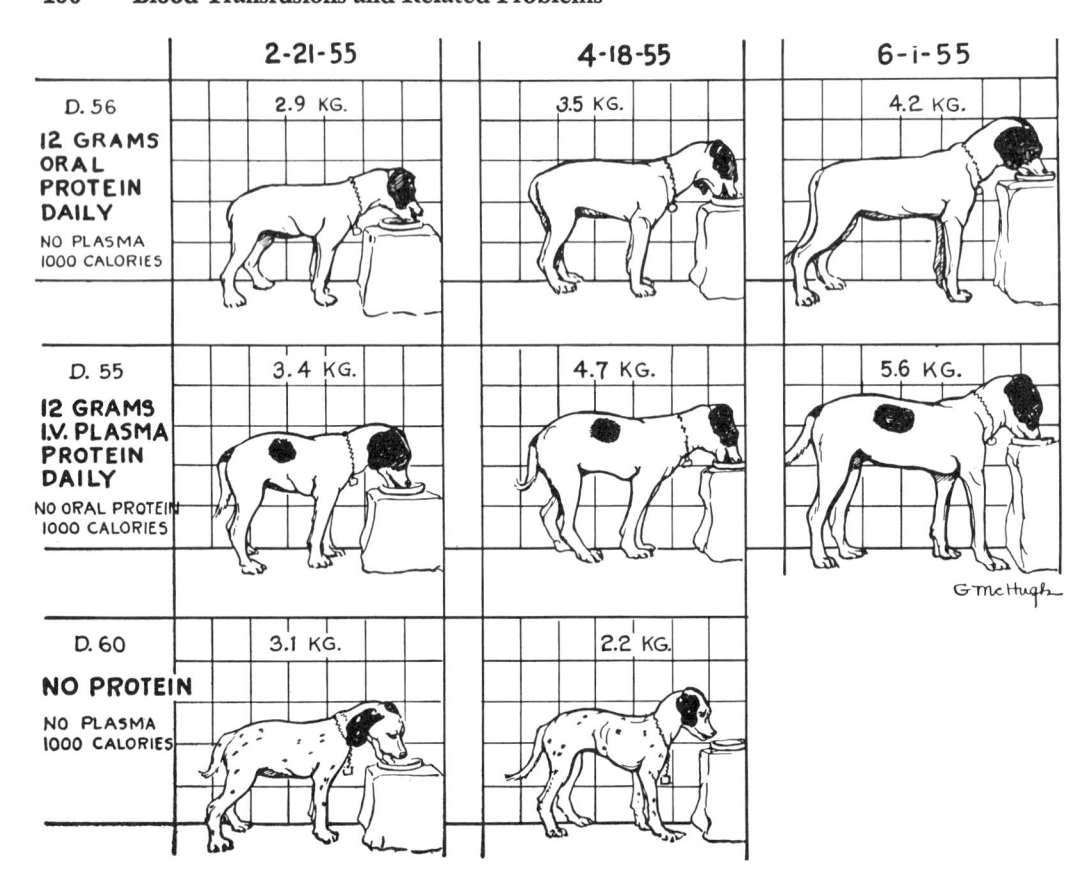

	2-21-55	4-18-55	6-1-55
D. 56 12 GRAMS ORAL PROTEIN DAILY NO PLASMA 1000 CALORIES	2.9 KG.	3.5 KG.	4.2 KG.
D. 55 12 GRAMS I.V. PLASMA PROTEIN DAILY NO ORAL PROTEIN 1000 CALORIES	3.4 KG.	4.7 KG.	5.6 KG.
D. 60 NO PROTEIN NO PLASMA 1000 CALORIES	3.1 KG.	2.2 KG.	

FIG. 8-11. These are exact tracings of littermate animals receiving the same amount of daily protein for a 99-day study period. In one case, 12 Gm. as horsemeat and liver was administered by mouth. The pup receiving its daily 12 gm. of protein as intravenously administered plasma with no oral protein grew in height and gained equally well in weight with its littermate on oral protein. Total daily calories were the same. (Tracings were made directly from the photographic negatives; all photographs were made at 114 cm. distance between camera lens and pup. (Ann. Surg. 144:349-355)

War I. Later its use was abandoned because of its retention within the body, where it appeared to concentrate within the reticuloendothelial system and the liver. Much of it appeared to remain permanently.

Oxypolygelatin also has been extensively used and is a valuable plasma volume expander. Unlike some of the heterologous sera or plasma tried earlier, gelatin as now prepared is nonantigenic and appears to display no harmful effects. It is stable in liquid form but does tend to gel at cooler temperatures. This feature has presented a difficult problem in the military services. Gelatin is largely excreted in the urine over a period of several days and may be metabolized slowly, but to an extent unimportant to nutrition. Gelatin sustains the colloidal properties of the circulation for about the same period of time as plasma or serum albumin when given in equivalent amounts.

Dextran was developed and used extensively as a substitute for plasma by the Germans during World War II. The dextrans are a series of polysaccharides with a broad spectrum of molecular weights, ranging from a few thousand to a half million. Those most useful for plasma volume expansion are selected from that portion of the spectrum corresponding to that of the plasma proteins in molecular weight. The wide range of molecular weights lends certain theoretical advantages to dextran in that it is possible to select the range which best suits the needs envisioned. Low molecular weight dextran, mean values of 40,000, has received increased attention recently because it tends to reduce sludging in patients in hypovolemic shock (Schwartz, 1964, and Shoemaker, 1963). It has also been used fairly extensively in open heart surgery to minimize the numbers of blood transfusions required to prime the pump when using extracorporeal circulation, as well as to reduce the viscosity of blood and thereby enhance tissue perfusion. However, Perkins *et al.* (1964) report that at equal concentrations, the effects of low molecular weight dextran are less upon red cell aggregation and agglutination, except in open heart surgery where in very high concentrations these effects are greater, than those of the high molecular weights generally available.

One of the complications from the administration of 2 or more units of dextran is an increased tendency to bleed and for this reason most have recommended that the volumes of dextran in the average adult patient not exceed 1,200 ml. It appears to enhance bleeding by interaction with the antihemophilic globulin (Factor VIII), to some extent by the removal of fibrinogen, and it may also coat platelets and reduce the efficiency of, and the participation in coagulation. Additional disturbances have been reported and, because the clotting factors are interdependent, when one is affected directly, the action of several others may be secondarily disturbed. While this agent is a very useful substitute for blood or plasma within the limits suggested, it should be used with caution.

About 80 per cent of infused dextran is excreted in the urine over a period of 3 to 4 days. The rate of urinary excretion is less for dextrans of higher molecular weights. The remainder is metabolized and exhaled as CO_2 over a period of 3 to 4 weeks. None remains permanently within the body.

Polyvinylpyrrolidone or PVP is a polymer of formaldehyde. This agent was also developed by the Germans and used extensively during World War II as a plasma substitute. Much of the infused PVP is excreted in the urine. That which remains within the body seems to remain indefinitely. Eosinophilic amorphous deposits have been described as appearing in a number of the tissues of the body many months after the infusion. These deposits provoke little if any reaction, and their significance is not known. For these reasons, PVP is looked upon by most with less favor than gelatin or dextran as substitutes for plasma at this time.

A state of abnormal bleeding has been observed in a few patients when large volumes of dextran, PVP, or gelatin have been administered. It is rarely observed when volumes less than a liter have been given: for this reason it is currently recommended that not more than a liter be administered to any one adult patient.

SERUM ALBUMIN is the most valuable of all plasma substitutes. It serves not only the needs of oncotic pressure supplied by plasma equally well or better, but it is also metabolized poorly (Gimbel *et al.*, 1950).

Fortunately, serum albumin will withstand 10 hours of heating at 60° C. which kills the hepatitis virus. Its great drawback is cost; only about 40 per cent of serum albumin present in plasma is recoverable by commercial processing at this time. With the exception of platelets, fibrinogen and cryoglobulins, the remainder of the protein fractions of plasma are not suited to transfusion purposes.

Serum albumin can be prepared salt-poor and administered intravenously as 6 per cent solution if desired. Because of its smaller molecular weight, it should be diluted adequately with normal saline in the treatment of hypovolemic shock lest it cause the circulation to imbibe water at the expense of extravascular water. It may be given as a 25 per cent solution as a dehydrating agent when this function is desirable to accomplish; in this capacity circulatory overload must be guarded against.

ABNORMAL BLEEDING IN THE SURGICAL PATIENT

Hemostasis was the first of the 4 historic accomplishments in surgery essential to the performance of safe operating procedures. Since recorded history, control of surgical bleeding was directed along mechanical lines,

Initial Reaction

Thrombokinase Formation

Release of intracellular thromboplastic factors ── activates (Ca^{++})* ── prothrombokinase accelerator globulins in plasma ── → Thrombokinase

| Platelet Agglutination and Lysis, Cellular Damage

Factor V — Accelerator Globulin
Factor VIII — Antihemophiliac Globulin
Factor IX — Christmas Globulin
Factor X — Stewart Globulin
Factor XII — Hageman Factor Globulin

Intermediate Reactions

A. Thrombin Formation

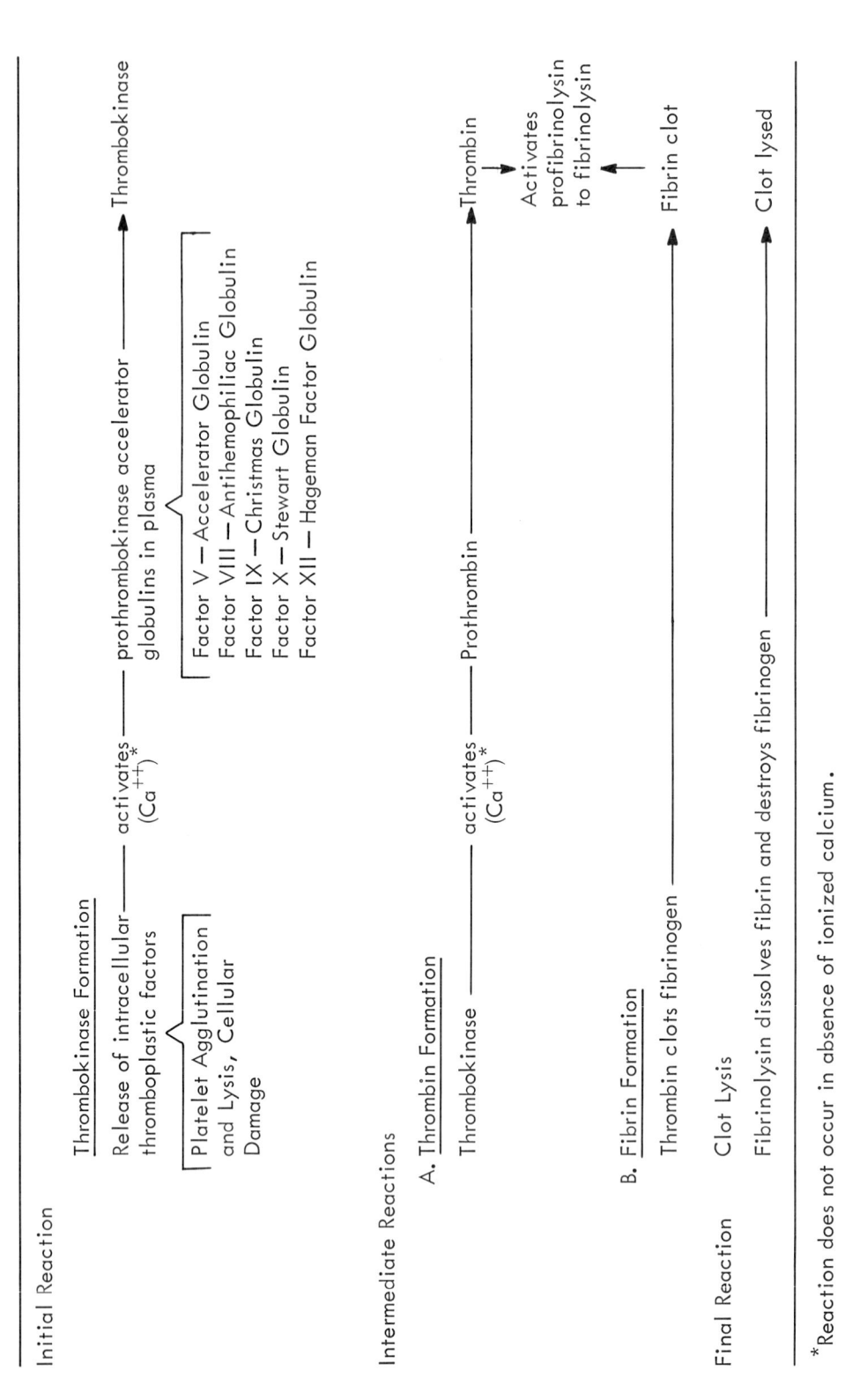

Thrombokinase ── activates (Ca^{++})* ── Prothrombin ──→ Thrombin

→ Activates profibrinolysin to fibrinolysin ←

B. Fibrin Formation

Thrombin clots fibrinogen ────────────────→ Fibrin clot

Final Reaction Clot Lysis

Fibrinolysin dissolves fibrin and destroys fibrinogen ──────→ Clot lysed

*Reaction does not occur in absence of ionized calcium.

FIG. 8-12. The dynamics of coagulation.

which included cautery, styptics, tourniquets, packs, ligature and hemostats. We did not learn that mechanical hemostasis is only a temporary measure unless it is followed by the active processes involved in blood coagulation. Since the beginning of the modern era in 1831, coagulation has appeared to be a highly complex phenomenon. Gradually, these processes have been better understood as it became possible to isolate each factor after its discovery and to test it in isolated systems. However, we still lack a great amount of fundamental information because in-vivo coagulation is concerned primarily with circulating whole blood and, until we understand how each of the isolated factors functions within whole blood, we will not understand either abnormal bleeding or abnormal coagulation.

We tend to forget that the circulating blood is in a state of equilibrium—constantly clotting and constantly lysing in order to preserve its fluidity and the "integrity" of the microcirculation and at the same time to maintain its ability to seal several vessels by local clotting without introducing generalized thrombosis. In brief, the normal clotting mechanism permits the proper balance to be struck between abnormal clotting and abnormal bleeding—*homeostatic hemostasis*.

In Figure 8-12 is shown schematically the general interactions that eventually form a fibrin clot. There is also shown the *dissolution of the clot* by the activation of profibrinolysin to fibrinolysin (proplasmin to plasmin).

The precursors of all three stages are proenzymes that, at slow but definite rates, are transformed to their respective active enzymes. Otherwise, in the absence of platelets, etc., and of prothrombin there should be no evidence of spontaneous petechial bleeding, spontaneous bleeding from prothrombin deficiency, or spontaneous bleeding in the classical hemophiliac patient, simply because there is a congenital deficiency of factor VIII (antihemophiliac globulin, AHG). The whole system appears to be accelerated in response to trauma, but when there are serious deficiencies in one or more of the proenzymes, clot or fibrin formation may be seriously retarded, so that injury of even the most miniscule vessel can represent a serious hemorrhagic threat.

In hemorrhages associated with fibrinolysin (plasmin), there may be a more rapid conversion of profibrinolysin to fibrinolysin as observed in some cases of abruptio placenta and other mechanisms that may induce extensive coagulation within the microcirculation. In others there appears to be an increased production of profibrinolysin and, hence, according to the Mass Law, more is converted to active fibrinolysin, as in some cases of carcinoma of the prostate. In still others, there may be diminished production of antifibrinolysin, as in some patients with advanced liver disease so that the normal rate of fibrinolysin is unopposed; and finally, fibrinogen levels may be congenitally deficient or consumed at rates that exceed the body's capacity to produce it. Except for the congenital deficiencies of fibrinogen production, the accelerated fibrinolytic process is generally of relatively short action—6 to 48 hours—when adequately treated.

The components of the clotting system and their locations of functions and interactions are shown in Table 8-9. Some caution is indicated in these interpretations, as these data were accumulated from the interactions of separate systems, which are the only means the chemist has available to him. The physician, on the other hand, must deal with these same interactions in whole blood or plasma circulating in the vascular system. In most instances, the observations of the chemist and the physician will coincide, but there may be some observations in the "purified" systems that have less relevance to whole blood systems shown in Table 8-9.

Most causes of surgical hemorrhage are related to faulty mechanical hemostasis. Some means to control bleeding from such causes are listed in Table 8-10. In Table 8-11 are shown some of the simple diagnostic procedures the surgeon himself can perform as preliminary measures until more precise laboratory data can be obtained. Guide-lines for the selection of interim diagnostic and therapeutic measures are given in Table 8-12.

In general, the reasons for operative and postoperative bleeding fall into two distinct categories. The most common is failure to secure surgical hemostasis by mechanical methods; consequently, bleeding either continues or is re-established within the first 12 hours of operation. In addition, there may

TABLE 8-9. CLOTTING FACTORS (PLASMATIC OR EXTRACELLULAR FACTORS) BY ENTITIES AND PRESENT TREATMENT OF DEFICIENCY

FACTOR NO.	IDENTITY	NORMAL RANGE	ACTS IN STAGE OF	DEFICIENCY	TREATMENT	DOSAGE
I.	Fibrinogen	150–300 mg.% plasma	Fibrin formation	Congenital Acquired afibrinogenemia (acute fibrinolysis)	Fibrinogen concentrate Epsilon aminocaproic acid (EACA), possibly also fibrinogen	4-8 grams as needed 4-6 grams and then 1 gram per hour (oral or I.V.)
II.	Prothrombin	7 mg.% plasma, or 300–350 units/ml	Thrombin formation	Vit. K. malabsorption Liver function impaired Congenital hypoprothrombinemia Dicumarol-induced	Water soluble vitamin K Water soluble vitamin K Water soluble vitamin K Vitamin K₁ Oxide	5-25 mg. orally or I.V. Response rapid and good Response slow and often poor 20-50 mg. Slowly I.V. or orally Response excellent 4-6 hours
III.	Thrombokinase	Minimal	Thrombin formation			
IV.	Calcium ion	10 mg.% plasma 50% ionized	Thrombokinase formation and thrombin formation	Only in rapidly administered citrated blood transfusions	Calcium gluconate or calcium chloride	1 gram slowly, intravenously (may need to repeat)
V.	Accelerator globulin or Labile Factor or Proaccelerin	Activity = "80–100% normal"	Thrombokinase formation	Congenital: "Parahemophilia," familial	Fresh Blood Transfusion? Cryoglobulins	
VI.	(a misnomer)*					
VII.	Prothrombin-conversion accelerator	5 mg.% plasma; activity = "80–100% normal"	Thrombokinase formation only in extrinsic system; together with tissue thromboplastin and calcium ion converts inactive factor X to active factor X	Congenital. Females more commonly affected than males	Fresh Blood? Cryoglobulins	

VIII.	Antihemophiliac globulin	(2–4 mg.% plasma); activity = "80–100% normal"	Thrombokinase formation Factor VII not required for intrinsic coagulation	Classical hemophilia: sex-linked disease in males	Cryoprecipitated AHG	Multiple infusion each day, usually 5-6 units for each infusion, until wound is healed
IX.	Christmas Factor	80–100% "normal"	Thrombokinase formation	Congenital. Like true hemophilia but a different gene	No specific therapy	
X.	Stuart Factor	80–100% "normal"	Thrombokinase formation	Congenital. Very rare	No specific therapy	Seldom present serious clinical problems
XI.	Rosenthal's Factor	80–100% "normal"	Thrombokinase formation	Congenital. Very rare	No specific therapy	
XII.	Hageman Factor	Less than 1 mg.% plasma	Thrombokinase formation	Congenital. Very rare	No specific therapy	
XIII.	Fibrin-stabilizing Factor		Fibrin formation	Congenital. Very rare	No specific therapy	

* This term is not ordinarily used, since it applies to the active form of factor V.

[195]

TABLE 8-10. COMMONLY USED MEANS TO ASSIST IN OBTAINING MECHANICAL HEMOSTASIS WHEN CLOTTING FACTORS ARE NORMAL

Tourniquet, where applicable
Digital pressure until other measures can be used
Transfixion sutures
Electrocoagulation
Dry gauze packs
Gelfoam and Oxycel
Locally applied vasoconstrictors
Topical thrombin and chemical styptics
Local acrylic adhesives

---

be delayed hemorrhage caused by infected wounds in which the clots may lyse and the vessels may be eroded, or the ligatures may be loosened or digested. Neither of these causes of bleeding is necessarily due to an abnormality in the physiology of the clotting mechanism, though this possibility is not thereby inevitably excluded.

Abnormal bleeding occasionally occurs for a variety of reasons, though for the most part the causes encountered are thrombocytopenia, hypoprothrombinemia, hypofibrinogenopenia (acute fibrinolysis) and congenital hemophilia of the classic variety. These 4 deficiencies, aside from patients in whom blood coagulation has been intentionally delayed by the use of anticoagulants, comprise the vast majority of conditions in which abnormal bleeding is encountered during and immediately after operation.

However, the number of isolated factors normally participating in blood coagulation continues to increase by new discovery. Some of these may be responsible for abnormal bleeding. Deficiencies in some of these may play only a minor role in the clotting mechanism. Some are known by several names, and

TABLE 8-11. SIMPLE EMERGENCY DIAGNOSTIC PROCEDURES USEFUL IN ESTABLISHING CAUSES OF PHYSIOLOGIC DEFECTS WHEN ABNORMAL BLEEDING OCCURS

Whole Blood Clotting Time
  Significantly prolonged in
    Classical hemophilia
    Profound thrombin deficiency
    Excesses of heparin
  Mildly increased in
    Deficiencies of Factors VI, VII, IX, X, XI and XII

Clot Lysis Time
  In fibrinolytic disorders, clots may form rapidly but lyse promptly.
  If fibrinogen is absent, no clot may form.
    To test:
      Add about an equal volume of normal blood as a source of fibrinogen.

Prothrombin Time
  Normal in all disorders but prothrombin-deficiency disorders, except when considerable excesses of heparin are present

Thrombin Generation Time
  Delayed, in any deficiency of thrombokinase phase of coagulation as well as in prothrombin deficiency. (Not very useful in emergency situations)

Platelet Count
  Important to perform. If platelets can be seen on blood smear in several fields, thrombocytopenia is not likely a problem.

Protamine Titration
  Useful to determine whether heparin is the cause of bleeding
  Crude estimates can be obtained by serial dilutions of patient's blood with isotonic saline: 50% saline, 60%, 70%, 80% and 90% saline.
  Protamine neutralizes heparin in vitro on a 1.3 mg. to 1.0 mg. ratio.

TABLE 8-12. ESTABLISHED ANTIHEMORRHAGIC AGENTS AND CONDITIONS IN WHICH THEY MAY BE EFFECTIVE

ANTIHEMORRHAGIC AGENT	CAUSE OF BLEEDING
Fresh Whole Blood Transfusion	Classical hemophilia (Possibly effective in "parahemophilia") (Remote possibility in deficiencies of Factors IX, X, XI, XII, XIII)
Platelet concentrates	Platelet deficiency
Cryoprecipitated AHG	Classical hemophilia
Fibrinogen	Acute fibrinolytic activity
Vitamin K	Prothrombin deficiency
Vitamin K_1 oxide	Rapid correction of prothrombin deficiency induced by dicumarol or its derivatives
Protamine sulfate	Heparin May need to repeat dosage (Often there is concurrent thrombocytopenia, and platelet transfusion may also be helpful.)

for the most part their roles in the clotting of whole blood are not well understood. The stability of function of these factors in ACD stored blood (4° C. up to 21 days) is shown in Table 8-13. Aside from deficiencies of Factor VIII (antihemophilic globulin) and possibly of Factor V (AC globulin), the other factors are sufficiently stable that ACD blood may be used for temporary replacement. However, it should be recalled that the turnover rates of many of these factors are relatively rapid and that, unless transfusions are repeated, abnormal bleeding may return if the patient cannot generate the factor himself. The preferred treatment by transfusion for these deficiencies is shown in Table 8-14. The importance of platelet transfusions and of administration

TABLE 8-14. PREFERRED TREATMENT BY TRANSFUSION FOR FACTOR DEFICIENCIES

Fresh plasma or whole blood: Factors V and VIII
Fresh serum: Factors VII and X
Stored Blood (20-30 days): Factors I, II,* III, IV, VI, IX, X, XI, XII, XIII

* Assuming no response from vitamin K.

TABLE 8-13. STABILITY OF FUNCTION IN ACD BLOOD STORED AT 4° C. UP TO 21 DAYS

Factor I	—Fibrinogen	Stable
Factor II	—Prothrombin	Stable
Factor III	—Thrombin	—
Factor IV	—Calcium ion	—
Factor V	—Proaccelerin, AC globulin (labile factor)	Possibly inadequate
Factor VI	—Hypothetical—may not exist	Unstable and harmless
Factor VII	—Proconvertin, SPCA (stable factor)	Adequate
Factor VIII	—Antihemophilic globulin, AHG	Rapidly inactivated in stored blood
Factor IX	—Christmas factor, PTC	Stable
Factor X	—Stuart factor	Stable
Factor XI	—Plasma prothrombin antecedent, PTA	Stable
Factor XII	—Hageman	Stable
Factor XIII	—Fibrin-stabilizing	—

of purified fibrinogen has been discussed.

Despite the physiologic and biochemical identity of some of these factors, replacement of them by transfusion does not always control bleeding satisfactorily. It is better that the surgeon first consider that his mechanical hemostasis has been inadequate; if assured that this is not the cause, a quick survey of the platelet count, the whole blood clotting time, the prothrombin time, the fibrinogen level, and the fibrinolytic activity should be performed. No special laboratory is necessary for these simple surveys, with the possible exception of the prothrombin time. They may be carried out by the surgeon or one of his assistants as soon as the tendency for abnormal bleeding is observed. If the platelets are present in a blood smear, they are usually adequate in number; if the whole blood clotting time is less than 10 minutes, congenital hemophilia usually does not exist; if the clot remains firm when incubated in the warmth of one's pocket for 30 minutes, acute fibrinolytic disorders are likely not the cause of abnormal bleeding; and if a firm clot forms in the course of performing a whole blood clotting time, adequate fibrinogen is usually present. The level of prothrombin activity is not revealed by any of these simple tests, but the administration of 50 mg. of vitamin K_1 oxide may be used empirically as a therapeutic trial until the laboratory can perform this particular test. If the deficiencies are more esoteric than these, it is unlikely that the cause can be determined for some hours, and highly specialized laboratory procedures are required. While it is seldom that the calcium ion is sufficiently depressed in the course of the administration of citrated blood to cause hemorrhage, it should be remembered that when other deficiencies co-exist, such as thrombocytopenia and hypoprothrombinemia, one of the complications of citrate intoxication may be abnormal bleeding. This may be corrected by the administration of calcium gluconate or calcium chloride. Other causes of abnormal bleeding are toxemias and, of course, transfusions of mismatched blood.

The management of abnormal bleeding has been discussed by many and is reviewed in the *Annals of the New York Academy of Sciences* (July 9, 1964) in a symposium entitled "Bleeding in the Surgical Patient."

In general, the field of blood and allied problems is one of continuing change and advancement. The student and the practitioner of surgery will find it to his own advantage as well as to that of his patient to keep himself informed of these developments, to pursue them with an open mind and to employ them in his practice with caution and restrained judgment.

REFERENCES

Abel, J. J., Rowntree, L. G., and Turner, B. B.: Plasma removal with return of corpuscles (plasmapheresis). J. Pharmacol. Exp. Ther., 5:625, 1914.

Adams, W. E., Thornton, T. F., Jr., Allen, J. G., and Gonzalez, D. E.: The danger and prevention of citrate intoxication in massive transfusions of whole blood. Ann. Surg., 120:656, 1944.

Allen, J. G.: Abnormal bleeding. Argonne National Laboratory, Progress Report No. ANL-4474, 1950.

———: Immunization against serum hepatitis from blood transfusion. Ann. Surg., 160:752, 1964.

Allen, J. G., Clark, D. E., Thornton, T. F., Jr., and Adams, W. E.: The transfusion of massive volumes of citrated whole blood in man: clinical evidence of its safety. Surgery, 15:824, 1944.

Allen, J. G., Enger, W., Brandt, M. B., and Phemister, D. B.: Use of blood and plasma in correction of protein deficiencies in surgical patients. Am. Surg., 131:1, 1950.

Allen, J. G., Inouye, H. S., and Sykes, C.: Homologous serum jaundice and pooled plasma—attenuating effect of room temperature storage on its virus agent. Ann. Surg., 138:476, 1953.

Allen, J. G., and Sayman, W. A.: Serum hepatitis from transfusions of blood—epidemiologic study. J.A.M.A., 180:1079, 1962.

Ascari, W. Q., Allen, A. E., Baker, W. J., and Pollack, W.: Rho (D) immune globulin (human): Evaluation in women at risk of Rh immunization. J.A.M.A. 205:71, 1968.

Bayliss, W. H.: Arch. med. belg., 70:793, 1917 (Quoted by Rous and Wilson).

Bevan, G., Taswell, H. F., and Gleich, G. J.: Serum immunoglobulin levels in blood donors implicated in transmission of hepatitis. J.A.M.A., 203:38, 1968.

Blumberg, B. S., Gerstley, B. J. S., Hungerford, D. A., London, W. T., and Sutnick, A. I.: A serum antigen (Australia antigen) in Down's syndrome, leukemia, and hepatitis. Ann. Int. Med., 66:925, 1967.

Braxton-Hicks, J.: On transfusion and new mode of management. Brit. Med. J., 2:151, 1868.

Brown, A. L., and Debenham, M. W.: Autotransfusion: Use of blood from hemothorax J.A.M.A., 96:1223, 1931.

Bunker, J. P., Bendixen, H. H., and Murphy, A. J.: Hemodynamic effects of intravenously administered sodium citrate. New Eng. J. Med., 266:372, 1962.

Bunker, J. P., Stetson, J. B., Coe, R. C., Grillo, H. C., and Murphy, A. J.: Citric acid intoxication. J.A.M.A., 157:1361, 1955.

Ceppelini, R., Dunn, L. C., and Turri, M: An interaction between alleles at the Rh locus in man which weakens the reactivity of Rh⁰ Factor (D^u). Proc. Nat. Acad. Sci., 41:283, 1955.

Cohen, S. N., and Dougherty, W. J.: Transfusion hepatitis arising from addict blood donors. J.A.M.A., 203:139, 1968.

Crosby, W. H., and Akeroyd, J.: Some immunologic results of large transfusions of Group O blood in recipients of other blood groups. Blood, 9:103, 1954.

Decastello, A., and Sturli, A.: Ueber die Isoagglutinine im Serum gesunder und kranker Menschen. München med. Wschr., 49:1090, 1902.

Denis, Jean Baptiste: Extrait d'une lettre de M. Denis (professeur de philosophie et de mathématiques) touchant la transfusion du sang. J. des Scavans, 86 (Mar. 9), 1667; 123, 178 (April 2), 1667. (See Roussel, J.: Transfusion of Human Blood by the Method of Roussel. Translated by Guiness, C. H. C., London, 1877.)

Dillard, G. H. L., Brecher, G., and Cronkite, E. P.: Separation, concentration, and transfusion of platelets. Proc. Soc. Exp. Biol. Med., 78:796, 1951.

Farrar, L. K. P.: Auto blood transfusion in gynecology Surg., Gynec. Obstet., 49:454, 1929.

Flosdorf, E. W., and Mudd, S.: An improved procedure and apparatus for preservation in lyophile form of serum and other biologic substances. J. Immun., 29:389, 1935.

Giles, J. P., McCollum, R. W., Berndtson, L. W. Jr., and Krugman, S.: Viral hepatitis: Australia/SH antigen and Willowbrook MS-2 strain. New Eng. J. Med., 281:119, 1969.

Gimbel, N. S., Riegel, C., and Glenn, W. W. L.: Metabolic and cardiovascular studies of prolonged intravenous administration of human serum albumen. J. Clin. Invest., 29:998, 1950.

Grubb, R.: Correlations between Lewis blood group and secretor character in man. Nature (London), 162:933, 1948.

Halsted, W. S.: Ligature and suture material. J.A.M.A., 60:1119, 1913.

———: The operative story of goitre. Johns Hopkins Hosp. Rep., 19:71, 1920; Surgical Papers by William Stewart Haltsted. vol. 2, second printing, Baltimore, Johns Hopkins Press, 1952.

———: Surgical Papers. vol. 1, second printing, p. 4, Baltimore, Johns Hopkins Press, 1952.

Harvey, S. C.: The History of Hemostasis. New York, Hoeber, 1929.

Harvey, William: Exerciata Anatomica De Motu Cordes et Sanguinis, 1628.

Haynes, L. L., Tullis, J. L., Pyle, H. M., Sproul, M. T., Wallach, S., and Turville, W. C.: Clinical experiences with the use of glycerolized frozen blood. J.A.M.A., 173:1657, 1960.

Hektoen, L.: Iso-agglutination of human corpuscles. J.A.M.A., 48:1739, 1907.

Huggins, C. E.: Frozen blood. Ann. Surg., 160:643, 1964.

Jennings, F. L., and Allen, J. G.: Diagnostic problems; presentation of a case. J.A.M.A., 156:1498, 1954.

Jones, H. W., and Mackmull, G.: The influence of James Blundell on the development of blood transfusion. Ann. M. Hist., 10:242, 1928.

Kevorkian, J., and Bylsma, G. W.: Transfusion of postmortem human blood. Am. J. Clin. Path., 35:413, 1961.

Lamm, H.: Emergency autotransfusion before laparotomy. J.A.M.A., 185:1043, 1963.

Landsteiner, K.: Zur Kenntniss der antifermentativen, lytischen und agglutinierenden Wirkungen des Blutserums und der Lymphe. Zbl. Bakt., 27:357, 1900.

Landsteiner, K., and Levine, P.: On the Cole agglutinins of human serum. J. Immun., 12:441, 1926.

Landsteiner, K., and Wiener, A. S.: An agglutinable factor in human blood recognized by immune sera for Rhesus blood. Proc. Soc. Exp. Biol. Med., 43:223, 1940.

Langston, H. T., Milles, G., and Dalessandro, W.: Further experiences with autogenous blood transfusions. Ann. Surg., 158:333, 1963.

Levene, C., and Blumberg, B. S.: Additional specificities of Australia antigen and the possible identification of hepatitis carriers. Nature (London), 221:195, 1969.

Levine, P.: The pathogenesis of erythroblastosis fetalis; a review. J. Pediat., 23:656, 1943.

Levine, P., and Katzin, E. M.: Iso-immunization in pregnancy and the varieties of isoagglutinins observed. Proc. Soc. Exp. Biol. Med., 45:343, 1940.

Levinson, S. O., and Cronheim, A.: Suppression of iso-agglutinins and the significance of this phenomenon in serum transfusions. J.A.M.A., 114:2097, 1940.

Lewisohn, Richard: Blood transfusion—50 years ago and today. Surg., Gynec. Obstet., 101:362, 1955.

Lister, J.: On the catgut ligature, in The Collected Papers of Joseph, Lord Lister. vol. 2. Oxford, London, 1909.

Lower, Richard: De Transfusione Sanguinis, 1665-66, and Tractus de Corde, 1669, tr. by Hollingsworth, M. W.: Ann. M. Hist., 10:213, 1928.

Lürmann of Bremen: Eine Icterusepidemie. Berl. klin. Wschr., 22:20, 1885 (Quoted by Hirsch, A.: Handbook of Geographical and Historical Pathology, tr. by C. Creighton, London, New Sydenham Soc., 3:420, 1886.

McLaughlin, E. D., Nealon, T. F., Jr., and Gibbon, J. H., Jr.: Treatment of bank blood by resins. J. Thorac. Cardiov. Surg., 40:602, 1960.

Maloney, J. V., Jr., Smythe, C. McC., Gilmore, J. P., and Handford, S. W.: Intra-arterial and intravenous transfusion: a controlled study of their effectiveness in the treatment of experimental hemorrhagic shock. Surg., Gynec. Obstet., 97:529-539, 1953.

Malpighi, Marcello: De Pulmonibus Observationes Anatomicae. In a letter to Borelli, tr. Foster, Lane Lectures on the History of Physiology, London, Cambridge, 1901.

Melrose, D. G., and Wilson, A. O.: Intra-arterial

transfusion: the potassium hazard. Lancet, 1:1266, 1953.

Minimum Standards for Blood Transfusions Outlined: Bull. Am. Coll. Surg. March-April, 1956.

Mollison, P. L.: Blood Transfusions in Clinical Medicine. Ed. 4. Philadelphia, F. A. Davis, 1967.

Morrison, F. S., and Mollison, P. L.: Posttransfusion purpura. New Eng. J. Med., 275:243, 1966.

Mourant, A. E.: A "new" human blood group antigen of frequent occurrence. Nature (London), 158:237, 1946.

Nealon, T. F., Jr, Ching, N. P. H., and Gibbon, J. H., Jr.: Prevention of citrate intoxication during exchange transfusions. J.A.M.A., 183:459, 1963.

O'Brien, T. G., and Watkins, E., Jr.: Gas-exchange dynamics of glycerolized frozen blood. J. Thorac. Cardiov. Surg., 40:611, 1960.

Okochi, K., and Minamaki, S: Australia antigen and serum hepatitis. Vox Sang., 15:374, 1968.

Orlina, A. R., and Josephson, A. M.: Comparative viability of blood stored in R.C.D. and C.P.D. Transfusion, 9:62, 1969.

Ottenberg, R., and Kaliski, D. J.: Accidents in transfusion, their prevention by preliminary blood examination. J.A.M.A., 61:2138, 1913.

Paget, Stephen: Ambroise Paré and His Times: 1510-1590, New York, Putnam, 1899.

Payne, J. H.: Harvey and Galen. Lancet, 2:1133, 1896.

Perkins, H. A., Rolfs, M. R., McBride, A., and Roe, B.: Low molecular weight dextran in open heart surgery. Transfusion, 4:10, 1964.

Petrov, B. A.: Transfusion of cadaver blood. Surgery, 46:651, 1959.

Pifer, P. W., Block, M. A., and Hodgkinson, C. P.: Thrombocytopenia and hemorrhage in hemolytic blood transfusion reactions. Surg., Gynec. Obstet., 103:129, 1956.

Prince, A. M.: Relation between SH and Australia antigens. New Eng. J. Med., 280:617, 1969.

———: Antigen detected in blood during incubation period of serum hepatitis. Proc. Nat. Acad. Sci., 60:814, 1968.

Redeker, A. G., Hopkins, C. E., Jackson, B., et al.: A controlled study of the safety of pooled plasma stored in the liquid state at 30-32 C for six months. Transfusion, 8:60, 1968.

Rous, P., and Wilson, G. W.: Fluid substitutes for transfusion after hemorrhage. J.A.M.A., 70:219, 1918.

Sabbatani, L.: Action antagoniste entre le citrate trisodique et le calcium. Mosso's Arch. ital. biol., 36:416, 1901.

Sawyer, W. A., Meyer, K. F., Eaton, M. D., Bauer, J. H., Putnam, P., and Schwentker, F. F.: Jaundice in army personnel in western region of the United States and its relations to vaccination against yellow fever. Am. J. Hyg., 39:337, 1944.

Schmidt, A.: Weitere Beiträge zur Blutlehre. Weisbaden, Bergmann, 1895.

Schneider, C. L.: Rapid estimation of plasma fibrinogen concentration and its use as a guide to therapy of intravascular defibrination. Am. J. Obstet. Gynec., 64:141, 1952.

Schwartz, S. I., Shay, H. P., Beebe, H., and Rob, C.: Effect of low molecular weight dextran on venous flow. Surgery, 55:106, 1964.

Seiver, F. B.: Fever-producing substances found in some distilled waters. Am. J. Physiol., 67:90, 1923, and 71:621, 1925.

Servetus, Michael: Christianismi Restituto, Vienna, 1553, Tr. in part by Williams, G. A.: Ann. Med. Hist., 10:287, 1928.

Shoemaker, W. C.: Effect of high and low viscosity dextran upon plasma and red cell volumes. Arch. Surg., 87:355, 1963.

Skundina, M. G., and Rusakov, A. V. (1934): Cited by Petrov (1959).

Starling, E. H.: On the absorption of fluids from the connective tissue spaces. J. Physiol., 19:312, 1896.

Starzl, T. E., Marchioro, T. L., Holmes, J. H., Hermann, G., Brittain, R. S., Stonington, O. H., Talmage, D. W., and Waddell, W. R.: Renal homografts in patients with major donor-recipient blood group incompatibilities. Surgery, 55:195, 1964.

Stemmer, E. A., Head, L. R., and Allen, J. G.: Comparative growth rates of litter mate puppies maintained on oral protein with those on the same quantity of protein as daily intravenous plasma for 99 days as only protein source. Ann. Surg., 144:349-355, 1956.

Strumia, M. M., Crosby, W. H., Gibson, J. G., 2nd, Greenwalt, T. J., and Krevans, J. R. (eds.): General principles of blood transfusion. Transfusion, 3:303, 1963.

Swan, H., and Schechter, D. C.: The transfusion of blood from cadavers: A historical review. Surgery, 52:545, 1962.

Technical Methods and Procedures of the American Association of Blood Banks: Minneapolis, Burgess, 1953.

Topley, W. W. C., and Wilson, G. S.: Topley and Wilson's Principles of Bacteriology and Immunology, rev. by Wilson, G. S., and Miles, A. A., ed. 3, London, Arnold, 1946.

Tullis, J. L., Ketchell, M. M., Lyle, H. M., Pennell, R. B., Gibson, J. G., II, Tinch, R. J., and Driscoll, S. G.: Studies on the in vivo survival of glycerolized and frozen human red blood cells. J.A.M.A., 168:399, 1958.

Valeri, C. R., and Henderson, M. E.: Recent difficulties with frozen glycerolized blood. J.A.M.A., 188:1125, 1964.

Ward, G. R.: Transfusion of plasma. Brit. Med. J., 1:301, 1918.

Weekes, L. R., Stone, E., and McCann, C.: Plea for autotransfusion. Obstet. Gynec., 16:715, 1960.

Wiener, A. S.: Elements of blood group nomenclature with special reference to the Rh-Hr blood types. J.A.M.A., 199:985, 1967.

Wise, W., Head, L. R., Morris, M., and Allen, J. G.: Physiological effects of acute anemia produced by serial hemorrhages. Surg. Forum, 8:18, 1958.

Witebsky, E., and Klendshoj, N. C.: The isolation of an O specific substance from gastric juice of secretors and carbohydrate-like substances from gastric juice of nonsecretors. J. Exp. Med., 73:655, 1941.

Wright, R., McCollum, R. W., and Klatskin, G: Australia antigen in acute and chronic liver disease. Lancet 2:117, 1969.

Yudin, S. S.: Transfusion of cadaver blood. J.A.M.A., 106:997, 1936.

CHAPTER 9

PAUL V. HARPER, M.D.*

The Principles of Isotope Technics in Surgery

Physical Properties
Isotopic Radiation Measurements
Practical Considerations
Applications

The contribution made to surgery by isotopic methods is difficult to separate from that made to biology and medicine as a whole, and no effort to do so will be made in the present discussion. Rather, certain of the physical properties of the radioactive isotopes and their radiations will be presented, together with the general methods by which these properties may be utilized in the study and the treatment of surgical disease.

PHYSICAL PROPERTIES

An isotope, or more properly nuclide, may be defined as a unique nuclear species with a definite mass, charge, and energy content, though it occupies the same place in the Periodic Table as other isotopes of the same element. For the most part, the artificial radioactive isotopes with which we are largely concerned are indistinguishable chemically from the naturally occurring stable isotopes, and in biologic systems they behave in a manner identical to the corresponding stable element. This property is the basis of the tracer method, in which the isotopic label may be detected and measured by virtue of its radioactivity.

By definition, radioactive isotopes disintegrate eventually, emitting a variety of radiations and usually giving rise to elements differing from the original ones. This process occurs at random at faster or slower rates for different isotopes. The average time required for half of a given number of atoms to disintegrate is characteristic of the isotope and is called the half life. This may vary with different isotopes from a fraction of a microsecond to many billion years. For practical purposes, in biologic work a half life of at least 12 hours is desirable, although some studies have been done with 20-minute carbon 11.

The unstable radioactive nuclei may be divided into two principal classes: (1) those containing an excess of neutrons (formed by neutron bombardment or fission) and (2) those deficient in neutrons (formed by cyclotron bombardment). Most of the elements have isotopes in both classes. The number of protons in the nucleus is, of course, fixed by the atomic number of the element. Isotopes containing a neutron surplus disintegrate by beta decay, converting one of the excess neutrons to a proton, emitting in the process an ordinary negative electron or beta particle. Often this is accompanied by one or more gamma rays. The gamma rays are rather energetic monochromatic photons, representing transitions between energy levels inside the nucleus. On the other hand, the beta particles have a continuous energy distribution from zero to a maximum value and an average value of about one third of the maximum. Some of the gamma radiation is absorbed by orbital electrons, which then appear as ejected monoenergetic "conversion" electrons along with the beta particles.

Neutron-deficient isotopes decay in an exactly analogous manner, except that they emit positrons, or positive electrons, instead of beta particles. The positrons, after losing their energy by collision, combine with ambient electrons and are annihilated, giving rise to two photons of 512,000 electron volts energy each, traveling in exactly opposite directions. This process is used in positron scanning, in which detectors placed on opposite sides of

* Professor, Department of Surgery, University of Chicago.

a source can detect specifically these simultaneous annihilation photons. This method of detection eliminates all but those disintegrations which can be viewed by both detectors along the line joining them and thus producing what is essentially electronic collimation for the radiation to be detected.

An alternative mode of decay in this class of isotope is called electron capture, which occurs when the neutron-deficient nucleus captures an orbital electron from the inner, or K, shell (thus the term "K-capture"), converting one of the nuclear protons to a neutron. This leaves the resulting atom in an ionized state, in which it emits the characteristic fluorescent x-rays.

The various alternative modes of decay which may be possible for an isotope are usually not observed, as one mode is overwhelmingly more probable than the others. However, in a few isotopes, in particular ^{64}Cu, the relative probabilities are of the same order of magnitude, and this isotope decays by electron capture 42 per cent, beta decay 39 per cent and positron decay 19 per cent.

A number of the heavier isotopes, which are intrinsically less stable, decay by emission of monoenergetic alpha particles (helium nuclei).

In using an isotope for tracer work, it is usually necessary to use chemical quantities which are negligibly small compared with those in the system under study. In this application it is often desirable to use isotopic preparations, which are referred to as "carrier free"; that is, the only atoms of the element present are those of the radioactive isotope. Radioactive phosphorus, for instance, may be prepared from normal phosphorus by neutron bombardment by the reaction ^{31}P (n,γ) ^{32}P, in which the radioactive isotope is obtained mixed with a rather large quantity of inert or carrier ^{31}P. It also may be prepared by neutron bombardment of sulfur (^{32}S [n,p] ^{32}P). The resulting phosphorus in this case may then be separated from the sulfur chemically, uncontaminated with stable ^{31}P.

For detailed information concerning any particular isotope, the student is referred to the standard compilations of nuclear data, which are extremely useful, although not always entirely up to date.[1-3]

ISOTOPIC RADIATION MEASUREMENTS

The detection of isotopic radiation is easily accomplished with relatively simple, inexpensive and reliable electronic equipment. The classic Geiger-Mueller counter tube consists of a cylindrical cathode surrounding a fine wire anode in a gaseous atmosphere. When ionizing radiation enters the sensitive volume of such a tube, the resulting electrons are strongly accelerated toward the anode, producing by collision an increasing cascade of similar electrons that finally reach the anode and cause a large voltage pulse, which is recorded. The larger positive ions move more slowly toward the cathode, and for a significant length of time following a pulse they act as a shield between the anode and the cathode, during which times the tube is dead. The Geiger counter thus detects individual ionizing events so long as they do not occur too rapidly. The counting efficiency for various types of isotopic radiation is variable. Any beta particle that enters the sensitive volume gives rise to a count, while a gamma ray has to be absorbed in the gas of the tube or in the wall with ejection of a secondary electron before it triggers the counter. Thus, the gamma counting efficiency of a Geiger tube is quite low, of the order of 1 per cent. A great variety of such tubes are available for different applications, with thick walls, thin walls, thin windows for counting weak beta radiation and flow counters in which the sample is placed within the tube itself, or where the sample in gaseous form is actually mixed with the counting gas.

When a Geiger tube is operated at a lower voltage, the electrons formed are collected as before on the anode but do not form cascades extending through the tube. Thus, while the recorded pulses are smaller, about one tenth of 1 per cent of the Geiger pulses, there is much less dead time limitation. The size of the pulse is proportional to the amount of ionization caused by the incident radiation, and for this reason such a device is called a proportional counter. An alpha particle pulse in a proportional counter is much greater than a beta or gamma pulse because of the much greater ionization produced and may be distinguished easily by this means.

Instead of counting individual pulses, the total ionization current created in the gas of the tube by the incident radiation may be measured. Such a device is called an ionization chamber. These have been designed for a variety of different applications, and the fundamental unit of radiation dosage, the roentgen, is based on such measurements. Ionization chambers usually are used in connection with intense radiation fields in therapeutic work, while counters are used in analytic and tracer work.

A very sensitive and efficient method of counting ionizing events is based on the properties of certain crystalline materials or phosphors to emit light quanta when exposed to ionizing radiation. These light quanta or scintillations are counted by a photomultiplier tube. The principal advantage of this method in gamma counting is a counting efficiency of 20 per cent to 50 per cent, which reduces the amount of isotope necessary to produce the detectable counting levels, especially in external survey in localization work. In beta counting, the liquid scintillation method, in which the sample and the phosphor are dissolved in a common solvent that then is viewed by photomultiplier tube, greatly increases the efficiency of counting soft beta rays such as of ^{14}C and ^{3}H, which are both extremely valuable tracer elements in biologic work. This method is nondestructive, so that after counting, the sample is still available for chemical or biologic analysis.

PRACTICAL CONSIDERATIONS

Production, sale, possession and disposal of all reactor-produced isotopes is under control of Federal statutes, which define the conditions of safety under which isotopes may be used. Most institutions using isotopes have committees that are responsible for radiation hazards, approval of isotope projects, etc., and a health physics department responsible for enforcing decisions of these committees.

DANGERS

The dangers of using isotopes fall into several categories. The accidental ingestion of long-lived isotopes which are not excreted rapidly is probably the most serious hazard. This is particularly well exemplified in the case of the radium dial painters.* Alpha emitters or high energy beta emitters are particularly dangerous in this connection, especially in bone-seeking isotopes such as ^{90}Sr and plutonium. The permissible body load for various isotopes may be found in the Bureau of Standards Hand Book 52, and in the Second Report (1961) of the Federal Radiation Council.

Radiation exposure from handling beta and gamma emitters must be limited to tolerable levels—by adequate shielding, by reducing exposure time or by using long instruments and relying on inverse square attenuation of the radiation. Low level contamination with radioactive isotopes, although often not a health hazard, can distort counting and survey measurements and must be strictly avoided.

In general, the clinical use of isotopes in children and in pregnant women should be avoided. This is particularly true of radioiodine. It has been definitely shown that modest doses of radiation to the thyroid gland in children (200 r-700 r) give rise to a substantial incidence of thyroid carcinoma. This dose level could easily be achieved by careless use of ^{131}I "tracer" studies.

A brief table is appended, giving pertinent physical constants of some representative isotopes, to illustrate the characteristics of the various types of isotopic radiation, nuclear reactions, shielding requirements, etc.

QUANTITATIVE CONSIDERATIONS

Tracer Level. The quantity of isotope required for any given application depends both on the isotope and the application. In tracer work, it is desirable to use a counting rate that is large compared with the cosmic ray background, and for statistical accuracy at least 1,000 counts should be recorded which gives a standard deviation of ± 3 per cent. Thus, with a background of 20 counts/min., the sample should count 200 counts/min., and sufficient counts will be recorded in 5 to 10 minutes. Assuming a counting efficiency of 20

---

* A series of cases of bone sarcoma occurred in individuals employed to paint figures on the dials of watches. Small amounts of radioactive materials had been added to the paint in order to make the figures visible at night.

per cent, which is reasonable for a thin-window beta counter or scintillation gamma counter, this means that the sample for counting should contain at least 5×10^{-4} microcuries (1 microcurie = 3.7×10^4 disintegrations per second). If a sample contains too much activity for counting, it may be placed at a distance from the counter, or absorbing material (usually aluminum) may be interposed between the sample and the counter.

A standard sample of uranium, radium or some other long-life isotope should be counted with each series of experimental samples to control changes in sensitivity of the counter; or, alternatively, a standard may be made using the isotope in question, and the counts expressed as per cent of the standard, thus automatically correcting for decay.

Therapeutic Level. In considering the quantity of isotope for use as a diffuse radiation source in tissue, it is necessary to calculate the amount of energy absorbed by the tissue from the radiation traversing it, since this is the basis for radiation dosage measurements. (The unit of absorbed dose of radiation, the rad, is 100 ergs absorbed per gram of tissue, equivalent roughly to an exposure of 1 roentgen). This is easily done for beta ray emitters, since practically all the emitted energy is absorbed within a few millimeters of its point of origin. The radiation dosage produced in tissue by the complete disintegration of 1 microcurie/Gm. depends on the energy of the radiation and the average life of the isotope. For ^{32}P the value is 730 rad; for ^{131}I, 120 rad. These calculations represent ideal distributions. For irregular distributions such as those obtained by the infiltration of radioactive colloidal material into tumors, the effective radiation dosage is much less, and to accomplish the same result the amount of isotope must be increased many times.

Energy absorbed from gamma radiation and from beta radiation is essentially the same in its biologic effects. On the other hand, the relative biologic efficiency (RBE) of alpha particles in tissue is many times greater in terms of energy absorbed.

The use of a gamma emitter in tissue in diffuse or discrete sources requires much more isotope than a beta emitter to produce the same radiation dosage, as most of the energy released leaves the neighborhood of the source. The radiation dosage calculations here depend on the average life of the isotope, the energy of the radiation and the absorption constants in tissue for the radiation. While straightforward, the dosage calculations are somewhat involved. The available data on radium and radon can serve as a model for many of these calculations. In general, from 10 to 100 millicurie quantities of isotope are required in this type of use.

When gamma emitters are substituted for radium teletherapy units, the quantity required is immensely greater, being measured in kilocuries.

APPLICATIONS

Tracer Level. The application of isotope methods in surgical diagnosis is principally in the fields of selective localization and measurements of phyisologic and chemical compartments.

For practical purposes, specific localization is limited to thyroid tissue. Here injected or ingested ^{131}I in a carrier-free state will localize to a considerable extent in the thyroid gland or in functioning thyroid metastases. Very sensitive survey methods using scintillation crystal gamma detectors and focused lead collimators have been devised in connection with mechanical scanning and recording equipment, so that the size and the shape of the thyroid gland, for instance, may be delineated quite accurately and distant metastases located accurately. Astatine, the higher homologue of iodine, will give somewhat similar localization, as will ^{99m}Tc as TcO_4^- which resembles perchlorate both in chemical structure and physiologic behavior.

Localization of radioisotopes in a variety of regions in the body for organ visualization is accomplished by making use of various physiologic functions. Radioactive material in colloidal form is removed from the blood stream by the reticuloendothelial system, permitting visualization of the liver, spleen, and bone marrow. With short lived agents such as ^{113m}I and ^{99m}Tc, which deposit little energy in the tissues, the available photon flux for organ visualization approaches to within a factor of 100 what is used in diagnostic radiology, so that defects can be made out in these organs with reasonable reliability. Damaged red cells tagged with chromium, mercury, or technetium localize in the spleen, and radioactive dye (Rose Bengal) is secreted into the biliary system. A variety of agents are secreted in the urine or are fixed in the renal parenchyma, permitting studies of renal function as well as rough anatomic studies. Agents that remain in the vascular system such as tagged albumin permit studies of blood pools for placental localization or demonstration of pericardial effusion. Rapid localization of alkali metal isotopes, potassium, rubidium and cesium, in the myocardium permits visualization of myocardial infarcts. Extracellular space tags are particularly useful in localizing brain tumors because they are excluded from normal brain tissue but penetrate into the tumor. A recent development is the introduction of radioactive microemboli into the circulation to demonstrate the path of blood flow, following pulmonary embolus.

The use of isotopic methods for studying fluid spaces differs little from similar chemical methods. A quantity of tagged material is injected intravenously, and, after mixing has been completed in the compartment in question, determination of the dilution of the isotope is made, and the size of the compartment may be calculated by knowing the quantity of isotope given. Serum albumin tagged with ^{131}I, red cells tagged with ^{32}P or ^{51}Cr, give blood-volume values more or less identical with those obtained by tagging the albumin with Evans blue or the red cells with carbon monoxide. In some cases the differences in analytic methods result in a more expeditious determination.

However, the isotope methods go beyond the chemical methods by permitting chemical spaces or pools, as well as volumes, to be determined. For instance, after injecting intravenously a millimol of sodium with a "specific activity" of 100,000 counts/sec. per millimol, the serum, after mixing, is found to contain 25 counts/sec. per millimol of sodium. It then is said that the injected sodium has been diluted by the sodium pool, which consists consequently of 4,000 millimol. Other body fluid elements may be studied in this way. Potassium, carbonate and water have suitable isotopes for use of this type in human patients. Chlorine does not have a suitable isotope, but bromine has been substituted in these circumstances. Naturally occurring potassium is slightly radioactive, so that with special shielding and using large scintillation crystals, the total potassium in the body may be measured with about 5 per cent accuracy in 15 minutes.

When pursued in detail, studies of this sort become very complex, since, in fact, they involve transient, rather than steady state measurements. In most cases, correction for excretion must be made, and the ions under study exist in several physical compartments rather than one, with varying exchange rates between the compartments. The mathematical analysis of such systems rapidly becomes impracticable, and often they are best studied by using hydrodynamic or electronic models. In general, this is true of many biochemical systems, such as the plasma phosphate, urine phosphate, organic phosphate, bone phosphate, phospholipid system, or the plasma iodine, urine iodine, thyroid iodine, plasma protein bound iodine system.

A number of transient phenomena of medical and surgical interest may be studied using isotopes. Curves showing the rate of uptake of radioiodine by the thyroid may be made by external survey of the gland. The life of the red cell may be determined by tagging it with radioactive iron or chromium. The circulation in the extremities, for instance, may be studied by watching the change in counting rate over the leg following injection of radioactive sodium intravenously. Radioisotopes have been used extensively for cardiac output studies in a manner similar to the method using dye curves, and various cardiac shunts may be demonstrated using isotopic methods.

Therapeutic Level. Isotopes have been used in a variety of ways in radiotherapy. These may be classified as (1) *teletherapy*, in which long-lived gamma emitters such as ^{60}Co or ^{137}Cs are substituted for radium to produce an intense gamma ray beam; (2) *brachytherapy*, in which small sources are implanted in tissue to produce the desired radiation fields; and (3) in the use of *diffuse sources* such as ^{32}P, ^{131}I and ^{90}Y spread evenly through the tissues or injected into cavities. Surgical applications are limited to the use of brachytherapeutic devices and the attempts to produce diffuse sources by the injection of radioactive colloidal material.

TABLE 9-1. PRINCIPAL PHYSICAL CONSTANTS OF SOME REPRESENTATIVE ISOTOPES

K indicates K-Capture. Energies of particles and photons are given in MEV (million electron volts). E_{max} indicates maximum energy, $\bar{E}$ indicates average energy. HVL (half value layer) figures are approximate. Abbreviations for nuclear reactions: ^{23}Na (n,γ) ^{24}Na means Sodium 23 absorbs 1 thermal neutron, emits 1 gamma ray and becomes Sodium 24.

			RADIATION CHARACTERISTICS							
			PARTICLES			PHOTONS				
				TISSUE			HVL CM.			
ISO-TOPE	MODE OF DECAY	HALF LIFE	E_{max}	$\bar{E}$	Range mm.	HVL mm.	MEV	Tissue	Lead	PRODUCTION	USE
^{14}C	$\beta-$	5720 y	.155	.050	.2	—	—	—	—	^{14}N(n,p)^{14}C	Tracer studies
^{24}Na	$\beta-, \gamma$	14.9 h	1.39	.54	6.4	.85	2.76 1.38	14	1.3	^{23}Na(n,γ)^{24}Na	Tracer studies
^{32}P	$\beta-$	14.3 d	1.71	.695	8.1	1.3	—	—	—	^{32}S(n,p)^{32}P ^{31}P(n,γ)^{32}P	Tracer studies Bone-marrow irradiation
^{55}Fe	K	2.91y	—	—	—	—	.0065	.032	—	^{54}Fe(n,γ)^{55}Fe	Tracer studies
^{60}Co	$\beta-, \gamma$	5.3 y	.31	.10	.8	.09	1.17 1.33	11	1.0	^{59}Co(n,γ)^{60}Co	Tracer studies Brachytherapy Teletherapy
^{74}As	K $\beta-, \gamma$ $\beta+$	17.5 d	1.4 $\beta-$ .95$\beta+$				.596 .635 .51*	7.8	.42	^{74}Ge(d,n)^{74}As	Positron Scanning
^{90}Y	$\beta-$	2.54d	2.18	.89	11	1.48	—	—	—	^{89}Y(n,γ)^{90}Y Daughter of ^{90}Sr	Brachytherapy Interstitial therapy
^{99m}Tc		6.0 h	.14	.014	—	—	.140	4.6	.02	Daughter of 2.8d ^{99}Mo	Scanning
^{131}I	$\beta-, \gamma$	8.0 d	.61	.205	2.1	.25	.365	7.0	.25	Fission of uranium	Tracer studies Diffuse source Brachytherapy
^{125}I	K, γ	60 d	—	—	—	—	.027	2	.002	Daughter of ^{125}Xe	Tracer studies
^{198}Au	$\beta-, \gamma$	2.69d	.97	.32	3.9	.36	.411	7.2	.32	^{197}Au(n,γ)^{198}Au	Brachytherapy Diffuse source
^{222}Rn	α	3.85d	5.48	5.48	41.1μ	—	—	—	—	Daughter of Natural Ra	Brachytherapy (with decay products)

Radium needles and radon seeds, which have been used for many years, are gradually being supplanted by the various isotopes with their more flexible radiation characteristics and more general availability. Much attention has been directed toward reducing the exposure hazard to the operator, since it is clear that, in addition to causing local damage, exposure to radiation induces leukemia. This has been accomplished by using isotopes emitting softer gamma radiation than radium and radon. This softer gamma radiation behaves in tissues in a manner similar to that of the familiar radium gamma radiation, but it is much more easily shielded by lead (see Table 9-1). Additional efforts along these lines include fixing sources in threads or tapes and drawing them rapidly into the tumor from a shielded container, thus avoiding prolonged exposure to the operator. Fine polyethylene tubing has also been used to form implants, which are later filled with appropriate isotopes in solution. These brachytherapeutic methods are extremely flexible, and by using them it is possible to produce many types of extremely well-localized radiation fields of any desired intensity.

The efficacy of diffuse beta ray sources in tissue has been amply demonstrated by the experience with radioactive iodine in the treatment of diseases of the thyroid gland. The thyroid tissue may be essentially destroyed with a relatively small dose of isotope without resultant damage to the surrounding tissue. Attempts have been made to reproduce in tumors the even distribution of isotope responsible for these effects by the injection of radioactive colloidal materials such as ^{198}Au, Cr^{32}PO$_4$, ^{90}Y(OH)$_3$ and ^{90}YF$_3$. These materials have been used clinically by injection into the prostate and the parametrium, where they move about in the lymphatics much as any other colloidal material. It has been found impossible to achieve more than a patchy distribution of isotope in a given volume of tissue by such local infiltration technics, and the high hopes first held out for this application have not been achieved.

The treatment of pleural effusion and ascites due to tumor by the injection of the above materials into the affected cavity has met with some success, but again the isotope is deposited in irregular patches on the cavity walls and does not produce an even radiation dosage to the cavity wall.

Certain special applications have been made of strong radioactive sources to destroy local areas of tissue. The implantation of strong (10-15 millicurie) radon seeds or the use of a number of ^{90}Y sources implanted into the hypophysis has accomplished destruction of this gland without serious damage to surrounding structures.

It is our feeling at the present time that the place of isotopes in the diagnosis and the study of disease is quite secure. However, many of the therapeutic methods presently available will have to undergo considerable evolution before their value is established. The student can expect to encounter many advances and changes within the next few years.

REFERENCES

1. Nuclear Data Sheets. National Academy of Sciences, National Research Council, Washington, D.C. (Published bi-monthly).
2. Lederer, C. M., Hollander, J. M., and Perlman, I.: Table of Isotopes. John Wiley & Sons, New York, 1967.
3. Sullivan, W. H.: Trilinear chart of Nuclides (Atomic Energy Commission). U.S. Government Printing Office, Washington 25, D.C.
4. Federal Radiation Council—Second Report, September, 1961.

CHAPTER 10

CARL A. MOYER AND JONATHAN E. RHOADS

Neoplastic Disease—General Considerations

Neoplasms
Practical Considerations in Cancer Surgery
Hereditary Factors in Cancer

NEOPLASMS

DEFINITIONS

Neoplasms are nonconformist cellular populations no longer dedicated to the purposes of the organism as a whole. In contrast with normal cellular populations, ontogenetically grouped to form organs that remain fixedly related to one another and are integratively functional, neoplastic cells do not form organs, are not fixedly related to other cells, and function physiologically as relatively independent uncontrolled elements. They are separated behavioristically into the benign and the malignant types.

Benignity implies local noninvasive growth; and malignancy, invasive growth and metastasis transplantation of cells with secondary growth at other sites in the body). The assignation of benignity or malignancy to particular neoplasms rests upon knowledge gained by the observation of the growth and the functional characteristics of other neoplasms of similar appearance in comparable locations in other individuals. The designation of benignancy or malignancy to some tumors can be made with certainty, e.g., xanthomas and keloids are benign, while Ewing's tumor, adenocarcinoma of the stomach and squamous carcinoma of the lung are malignant. However, the classification of some tumors is often impossible without knowledge of that tumor's behavior in the individual harboring it. Carcinoids of the appendix and the colon, leiomyomas, chondromas and juvenile melanomas fall into this category.

Malignancy does not always connote metastatic propensity in the individual tumor, but a tumor type that never metastasizes is regarded as benign. Medulloblastomas and glioblastomas of the brain are considered as malignant, although they metastasize with extreme rarity; they are malignant because of their local invasiveness and because metastasis has been known to occur. One of the important basic characteristics of malignant cells is a decrease in the adhesiveness of one cell to the next. This was originally demonstrated by Coman (1944) and in general differentiates malignant tumors from benign tumors as well as from normal tissue. It may be demonstrated in tissue cultures and by appropriate methods in tissues as they come from the body.

ETIOLOGY

The primary etiologic factors involved in the inception of neoplasms in man are still unknown. Presumptively, something happens to the constitution of nuclear material of a cell, rendering it no longer obeisant to regulation of its growth. Although the primary cellular genesis of neoplasia is unknown, it can be induced by a variety of agents. These may be classified as mechanical, infectious, chemical and physical (chiefly, ionizing radiation). The long exposure of skin to ultraviolet light may induce cutaneous carcinomata, as does the repeated exposure to x-rays. Long exposure to x-radiation leads to leukemia in some individuals, radium ingestion to osteogenic sarcomas and, in rats, radioiodine to carcinomas of the thyroid. Long exposure to certain aniline dyes promotes carcinomas of the bladder. Butter yellow (a dye) induces hepatic carcinomas in animals, while arsenic, chromates and pitchblende promote the development of carcinomas of the lung in man. Viruses are known to incite many types of tumors, benign and malignant in many animals, and neoplasms in plants; coal tars, human scrotal cancer; heat and infrared rays, kangri cancer; and cigarette tars, cutaneous carcinomas of mice and rabbits and probably carcinomas of the lung in man.

Epidemiologic study has pointed to asbestos as an etiologic factor in cancer. The tiny fibers enter the respiratory tract and the alimentary tract and have been identified in the peritoneum. A number of such fibers plus a fibrous reaction to them constitute an "asbestos body." Due to its use in wallboard, pipe insulation, and brake linings asbestos is very widely distributed wherever civilized man lives. Those who work with it have 8 times the usual incidence of lung cancer, 3 times the incidence of stomach cancer, 3 times the incidence of large bowel cancer as compared to the general population of the United States. In the case of lung cancer, cigarette smoking appeared to be a cofactor in all cases encountered so far, in the sample studied. There were 25 cases of mesothelioma which had arisen in this sample.*

As of the date of writing, virus etiology has not been proved for any human cancer, but Koprowski, Ponten, Jensen, Ravdin, Moorehead and Saksela exposed human cell lines derived from normal human tissue with SV 40, a simian virus capable of inducing renal carcinoma in the green monkey and have found that the growth characteristics in vitro are those of malignancy. Later, in-vivo experiments were done in man, and brief periods of invasive growth occurred before the homograft rejection phenomenon set in.

These experiments are cited as additional evidence that a virus etiology may well be demonstrated yet for at least some malignancies in man.

GROWTH FACTORS

The growth of neoplasms, both benign and malignant, often appears to be unsteady in

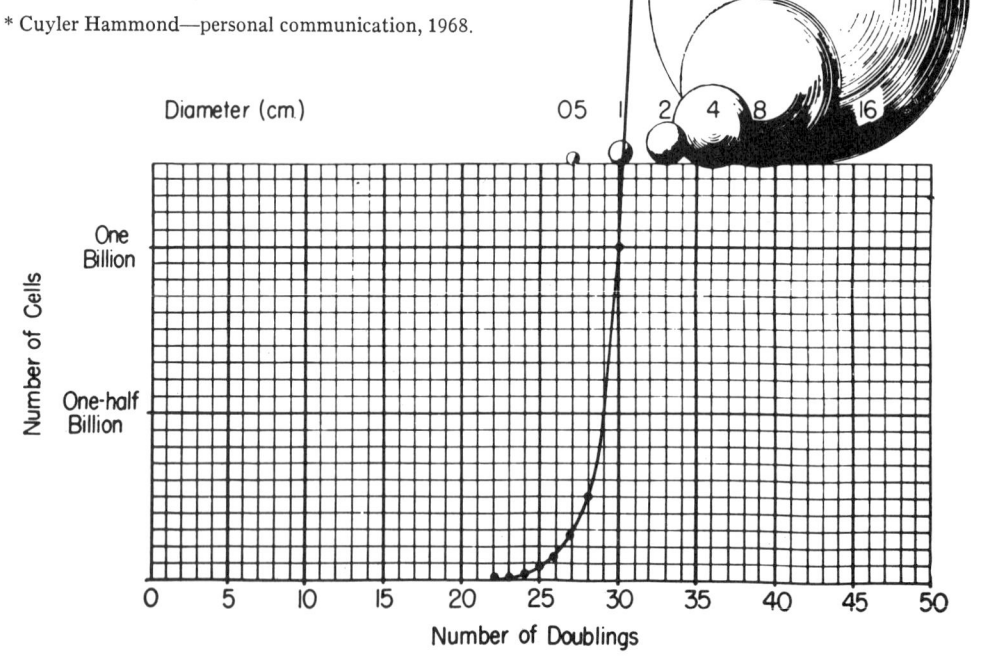

* Cuyler Hammond—personal communication, 1968.

FIG. 10-1. Diagrammatic illustration of the theoretical exponential growth rate of neoplasms demonstrates the relationship of the size of the neoplasm relative to its age. (Collins, V. P., et al.: Am. J. Roentgenol., 75:988).

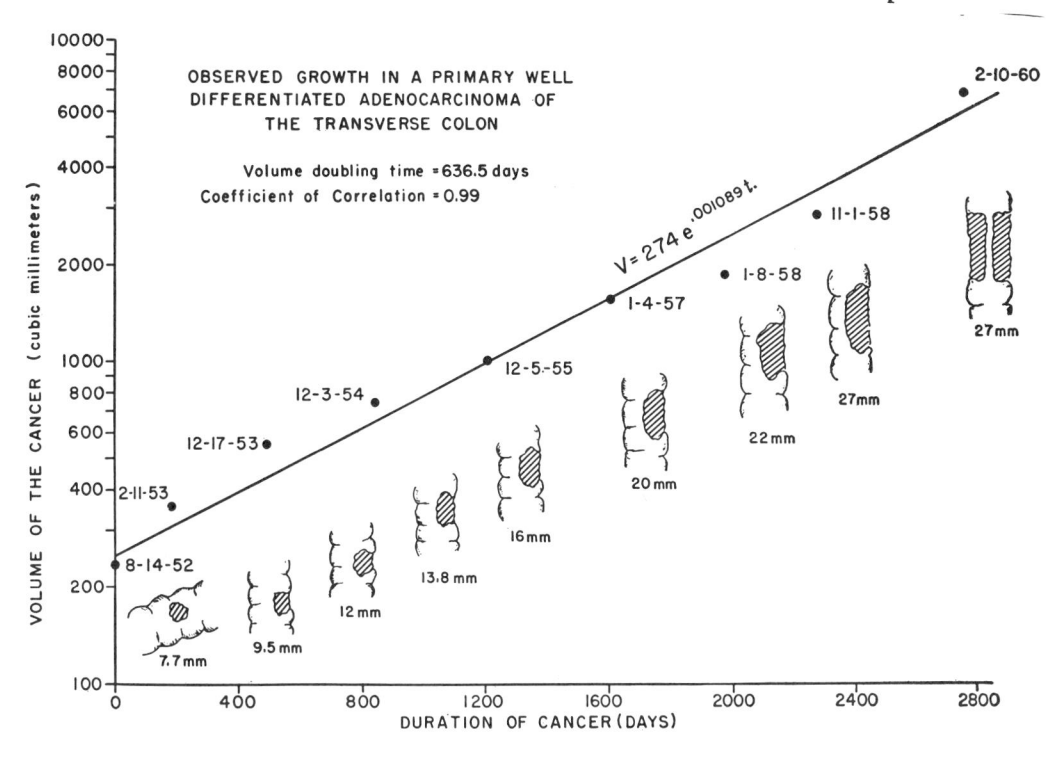

FIGURE 10-2. Observed growth in a primary well differentiated adenocarcinoma of the transverse colon. Volume doubling time = 636.5 days. Coefficient of Correlation = 0.99. $V = 274\, e^{.001089\, t}$

rate and occasionally even retrogresses. The growth rate of visible or palpable tumors rarely approaches the theoretical maximal growth rate, which may be expressed as: $X = 2^{(y-1)}$. In this formula, X represents the number of cells, and y the number of division time intervals. Should there be no biologic restrictions upon neoplastic growth, a cancer cell of 1,000 cu. micron size (10 × 10 × 10 microns) with a division time interval of 1 month would grow into a mass of about 4 cu. cm. in 31 months, 268 cu. cm. in 37 months, and 9,400 cu. cm. in 42 months! Peritoneal metastases of anaplastic carcinomas of the stomach may almost attain such a rate of growth. At celiotomy, nodules varying in size from the barely visible to 0.5 cm., tagged with silk sutures, become masses from 2 to 10 times larger in 1 or 2 months. The principle of exponential growth as applied to neoplasm is illustrated in Figure 10-1. Obviously, whatever the rate of growth of a tumor may be, at least two thirds of the life span of a tumor has transpired before it attains to a visible size, assuming that the minimal visible diameter is 4 mm. and the diameter attainable before it kills the host is 12 to 20 cm.

The rate of growth of an adenocarcinoma in a human colon is shown in Figure 10-2. The observed rate of growth of this one colonic cancer during 7 years, in a person judged to be an "impossible" surgical risk because of pulmonary and myocardial infarcts, hypertension, diabetes, advanced arteriosclerosis and obesity, indicates that it doubled in size about every 636 days. The time required by a neoplasm to double its size has been termed the doubling time. So far few measurements of the doubling times of human tumors have been made. Some of them made so far of pulmonary metastases, the sizes of which may be determined roentgenographically, are from embryonal carcinomas of the testis, 11 to 40 days; from carcinomas of the breast, 28 to 184 days; from carcinomas of the rectum, 49 to 123 days; and from one carcinoma of the esophagus, 164 days (Collins et al.).

There are local and general factors which tend to limit the growth rate of neoplasms. The generally accepted local factors are: vascularity, fibroplasia, and lymphatic and vascular resistance to invasion. Many tumors are said to grow away from their blood supply. Such tumors are prone to undergo avascular necrosis. Hodgkin's sarcoma, leiomyosarcoma and astrocytomas often demonstrate this phenomenon.

Within many neoplasms a relatively avascular fibroplasia encases the neoplastic cells into small nests. Presumptively, such encasements interfere with the growth of neoplasms as a whole.

The propensity for entry into lymphatics and veins varies a great deal from neoplasm to neoplasm. Arteries (except pulmonary arteries) are peculiarly resistant to invasion. Malignant brain tumors have little tendency to invade the blood vessels of the brain or the lymphatics in the meninges (the brain itself contains no lymphatics), while the chorioepithelioma and primary renal parenchymal carcinomas invade veins readily. The carcinomas of the intestinal tract invade both the lymphatics and the veins, and squamous cell carcinomas of the lip invade lymphatics regularly but veins rarely. The reasons for these differences in propensity of invasion of lymphatics and blood vessels are not adequately explained.

The known general factors limiting neoplastic growth are hormonal and nutritional. Reduction of the rate of growth and even retrogression of carcinomas of the breast may attend the administration of estrogenic or androgenic substances, the ablation of ovarian hormones by oophorectomy, and the removal of the adrenal or pituitary glands. The growth of prostatic carcinoma may be stayed for a time by castration, the administration of estrogen or hypophysectomy.

Although protein, carbohydrate or fat starvation has practically no detectable effect upon the growth of neoplasms in man, functional deficits of accessory foodstuffs sometimes do. The folic acid antagonists, such as Aminopterin, reduce the growth rates of a number of neoplasms such as lymphosarcoma, Hodgkin's sarcoma and leukemia but do not destroy them.

The growth of some malignant neoplasms may be reduced significantly by such diverse substances as arsenic (Fowler's solution), urethane (ethyl carbamate), toxins of streptococci and *Bacillus prodigiosus* (Coley's toxin or fluid), viruses and nitrogen mustard. Some individual tumors among the seminomas, the lymphomas and the basal cell carcinomas can be destroyed completely by x-radiation, while the irradiated contiguous normal tissue cells about the neoplastic ones remain viable. However, there are other neoplasms that are so tough that normal cells about them are killed before the majority of the neoplastic cells are affected by the irradiation. Leiomyosarcomas, adenocarcinomas of the stomach and the rectum, chondrosarcomas and melanocarcinomas are examples of this type of radiation-resistant tumor. In addition, many neoplasms are made up of cellular populations having remarkably different individual capacities to withstand radiation. Some cells of these neoplasms die while their normal neighbors live on, and others still live after such heavy radiation that their normal companions are destroyed. Carcinomas of the breast, some ovarian cancers, squamous cell cancers of the esophagus and the buccal mucosa, papillary cancers of the thyroid, and astrocytomas often exemplify this type of behavior after radiation.

Symptoms and Signs

The symptoms and signs of neoplasms are extremely variable. However, the formulation of some generalizations regarding them can be made. In general the signs and symptoms of cancer may be divided into 5 categories that are related to the biologic behavior of the neoplasm: (1) those related to expansive growth, (2) those related to infiltrative growth and metastasis, (3) those relatable to avascular necrosis and/or ulceration, (4) those attributable to the peculiar physiologic activities of neoplasms, and (5) those related to destruction of the tissue in which the neoplasm grows. There are only a relatively few neoplasms that give rise to symptoms and signs attributable to the physiologic or biochemical activities of the neoplasm. In man most of these appear to originate in the endocrine glands or gonads (see Table 10-1).

The frequency of the association of the signs with these specific neoplasms in Table 10-1 varies much. With the starred entities, the neoplasm and the signs are associated very frequently, while in the case of the others they are not. In other words, the unstarred entities

TABLE 10-1. PHYSIOLOGICALLY FUNCTIONAL NEOPLASMS

LOCUS	TYPE	SIGNS
Hypophysis	Adenoma, basophilic	Cushing's syndrome; "pituitary basophilism"
	Adenoma, eosinophilic* or mixed (rarely carcinoma in adults)	Gigantism (prepubertal) Acromegaly (postpubertal)
Thyroid	Adenoma*	Hyperthyroidism
Parathyroid	Adenomas and carcinomas of all types excepting oxyphil*	Hyperparathyroidism
Pancreas	Islet cell adenoma* Islet cell carcinoma	Hyperinsulinism
Adrenal medulla	Pheochromocytoma*	Episodic hyperadrenalism and hypertension
Adrenal cortex	Cortical adenoma and cortical carcinoma	Cushing's syndrome
	Cortical carcinoma* in women and children	Adrenal virilism and adrenogenital syndrome
Testis	Chorio-epithelioma*	Gynecomastia
	Leydig cell tumors* (interstitial cell)	Precocious puberty, the "infant Hercules"
	Sertoli cell (very rare)	Feminization
Ovary	Arrhenoblastoma	Masculinization
	Fibroma	Meigs' syndrome
	Granulosa and theca cell*	Precocious puberty, postmenopausal bleeding, menstrual irregularities
Intestine (mainly)	Malignant carcinoid	Flushing spells, pulmonic stenosis, tricupsid insufficiency, cyanosis
	Sarcoma	Hypoglycemia and signs thereof
Thorax and abdomen (mainly)	Choriocarcinomatous* teratoma (very rare)	Prepubertal uterine bleeding

* These neoplasms are very frequently associated with the signs indicated. The others listed—only occasionally associated.

TABLE 10-2. SIGNS ATTRIBUTABLE TO EXPANSIVE GROWTH

LOCUS	SIGNS
Skin and subcutaneous tissues, including mouth, breast, testes, penis and anus	Visible and palpable mass
Superior mediastinal, extratracheal	Occlusion of trachea—dyspnea and wheezing; occlusion of esophagus—dysphagia; occlusion of great cephalad veins—cyanosis and swelling of head and arms
Trachea and bronchi	Cough, dyspnea and obstructive atelectasis
Gastrointestinal tract	Signs of obstruction: esophagus—dysphagia stomach—vomiting intestine—abdominal distention, intestinal colic, obstipation
Common hepatic and common bile ducts	Jaundice and elevated serum alkaline-phosphate
Urinary tract, ureter, prostate	Ureteral colic (rare) and hydronephrosis, prostatism
Eustachian tube	Impaired hearing ("plugged-up ear")
Bone	Pain and directly or roentgenographically visible masses and defects
Intracranial	Headache; nerve and tract conduction deficits or palsies; signs of increased intracranial pressure
Spinal cord and cauda equina	Pain and paralyses, disturbance of bladder and bowel function
Liver	Hepatomegaly
Spleen	Splenomegaly

TABLE 10-3. CLINICAL SIGNS ATTRIBUTABLE TO NECROSIS OF THE TUMOR

Locus	Signs
All loci	Signs of tissue death: 1. Fever 2. Leukocytosis 3. Elevation of sedimentation rate 4. Anorexia, malaise
Visible loci	Ulceration
Intestinal tract, including biliary system	1. Micro- and macro-intestinal hemorrhage, leading to anemia with its signs such as weakness, dyspnea on exertion, etc. 2. Signs of inflammation, especially with esophageal and colonic neoplasms manifest by intra-abdominal inflammatory pain often mimicking cholecystitis, appendicitis and pancreatitis
Lung	Signs of cavitation and inflammation imitating bronchopneumonia and viral pneumonias, pulmonary abscesses, and pulmonary tuberculosis
Urinary tract: renal pelvis, ureter, bladder	Hematuria and pyuria
Uterus, corpus and cervix	Intermenstrual and postmenopausal bleeding and vaginal discharges

often exist without signs of physiologic overactivity. Peculiarly, carcinomas of the thyroid are accompanied only very rarely by signs of hyperthyroidism.

Expansive Growth. The signs of neoplastic growth associated with expansiveness are the most protean (see Table 10-2). However, they may be sorted out into a fairly orderly array because they are peculiar to the function and the location of the organ wherein the tumor is located. Clearly, expansive growth of tumors within or near the skin, or in the mouth and the anus will produce visible and palpable lumps. In the respiratory, the gastrointestinal, the biliary, the urinary and the cerebral spinal conductive tracts expansive tumor growth may lead to obstruction of the tract. In fact, the signs of neoplasms in these places are frequently related to obstruction. The expansive growth of tumors within rigid cavities, such as the skull and the spinal canal, blocks conduction over nerve fibers and may lead to a multiplicity of paralyses as well as pain. In brief, the expansive growth of tumors leads in man to palpable and visible lumps, the signs and symptoms of the obstruction of tubed structures, and disturbances of the nerve supply of parts of the body.

Necrosis of the tumor is especially prone to provide some of the early signs of cancer when it originates within the skin or the epithelium of the respiratory tract, the wall of the intestine, the cervix uteri, or the genitourinary tract (see Table 10-3). In other words, cancers arising in parts of the body that lead to the external environment will often first make themselves known by signs and symptoms of inflammation secondary to necrosis or ulceration of the tumor. With partial death of cancers of skin, lips, tongue, pharynx, larynx, penis and anus, ulceration often occurs. The ulcer supports bacterial growth, and inflammation is thereby stimulated, leading to redness, heat, pain, swelling, and impairment of function. Necrotic tumors of the bronchi also ulcerate, and the peritumorous inflammation mimics pneumonia, tuberculosis or pulmonary abscess. By virtue of this secondary bacterial inflammatory component of partially necrotic cutaneous, mucosal and pulmonary cancers, frequently the antibiotics will relieve the infection, and often the lesion will subside remarkably, and occasionally the ulcer will even heal. For this reason any ulcer within the above structures requires a biopsy before the possibility of cancer can be reasonably dismissed. A favorable response to antibiotics is not a sign that the lesion is not neoplastic.

Necrosis of tumors within the gastrointestinal tract accounts in part for carcinomas of the stomach masquerading as peptic ulcers and carcinomas of the right colon mimicking appendicitis and cholecystitis. Many a gallbladder and appendix have been removed because of symptoms and signs arising from an ulcerated carcinoma of the right colon, while at the same time the cancer has been missed. Similarly, many a cancer of the stomach has been left to grow for months before a surgeon is consulted because the gastric ulcer healed symptomatically and even roentgenographically when the patient was placed on an ulcer regimen.

Partially necrotic tumors within parenchymatous organs, such as the liver, the spleen, the kidney, the bone marrow and the retroperitoneal region constitute one of the causes of the so-called "fever of undetermined origin." Tumors encased within the body may give rise to fever, leukocytosis and an elevated sedimentation rate even as the dead cardiac muscle cells within a cardiac infarct do. Actually these signs of localized tissue death may be the sole early signs of tumor within the liver, the spleen or the kidney.

Bleeding and Anemia. Necrosis of the tumor also leads to bleeding and consequently, at times, to anemia. Slowly bleeding carcinomas of the stomach and the right colon are especially prone to produce a secondary anemia; and this secondary anemia, together with its attendant exertional dyspnea, ease of fatigue, and weakness, may constitute the sole presenting signs of these cancers. Unfortunately, this anemia, together with its signs, sometimes responds favorably to the administration of salts of iron. Consequently, some cancers of the stomach and the colon are permitted to grow until signs other than those of anemia appear, because the patient takes iron-containing nostrums or, what is worse, the physician prescribes iron for the secondary anemia without examining the gastrointestinal tract with the proper " 'scopes" and appropriate roentgenologic methods.

Occasionally, neoplasms give rise to massive gastrointestinal bleeding. Necrotic leiomyosarcomas of the stomach and the duodenum, ulcerating carcinomas on the lesser curvature of the stomach, and the rare carcinomas of the duodenum and the jejunum may bleed profusely. Cancers of the renal pelvis, the bladder, the uterus and the cervix are also prone to bleed. Hematuria and bloody intermenstrual vaginal discharges must be considered as of neoplastic origin unless specific diagnostic procedures contradict this view.

In summary, the tendency of tumors to die in part and to ulcerate may lead to a number

TABLE 10-4. CLINICAL SIGNS OF INFILTRATIVE GROWTH

Locus	Signs
Nerves in region:	
1. Parotid	Paralysis of the facial nerve
2. Thyroid (carcinoma)	Recurrent laryngeal nerve palsy and fixation of thyroid to contiguous structures
3. Apex of thoracic cavity and axilla (Pancoast's tumor and metastatic axillary carcinomas)	"Brachial plexus" pain and palsies and fixation of palpable tumors
4. Pancreas (carcinoma of body of pancreas and retroperitoneal malignant neoplasms)	Pain over lower dorsal and upper lumbar spine
5. Pelvis (carcinoma of cervix and rectum)	Lumbosacral plexus pain
Lymphatics	Lymphedema, chylous ascites or chylothorax and hydrothorax
Veins	Venous occlusive edema and nonchylous ascites or pleural effusion
Breast	Fixity of the skin to the tumor or of tumor to muscle
Cervix	Thickening of palpable ligamentous support

of signs such as fever and leukocytosis, anemia secondary to the seepage of blood, massive gastrointestinal hemorrhage and localized signs of inflammation mimicking benign gastric ulcer, appendicitis, cholecystitis, sinusitis, and so forth.

Infiltrative Growth. The infiltrative growth of malignant tumors gives rise to signs that in the main are related to the invasion of nerves (pain), the blocking of the low pressure fluid conduits, the veins and the lymphatics and the bronchi (edema, ascites and hydrothorax, and atelectasis), and the fixation of normally mobile structures, such as the cervix and the skin (see Table 10-4). Nerve invasion with its unremitting, demoralizing pains is especially prone to attend neoplasms growing in organs located near the major nerve plexuses: for example, the invasion of the brachial plexus by cancers in the apex of the lung and in the axillary lymph nodes, and the infiltration of the lumbosacral plexus by carcinomas in the rectum, the cervix and the iliac lymph nodes. Generally, the signs of infiltrative growth are signs of incurability, some mammary cancers excepted.

The neoplastic signs attributable to destruction of the host tissues, excepting panhypopituitarism, are frequently signs of incurability (see Table 10-5). Table 10-6 provides a cursory summary of this brief discussion of the clinical manifestations of neoplasia.

TABLE 10-5. CLINICAL SIGNS OF DESTRUCTION OF HOST TISSUE

Locus	Signs
Bone	Pathologic fractures
Liver	Hepatic insufficiency
Bone marrow	Aplastic anemia, neutropenia and thrombocytopenia
Pituitary	Panhypopituitarism
Brain and spinal cord	Palsies and anesthesia
Adrenals	Addison's disease

MODES OF SPREAD

As implied in various parts of this chapter, the spread of malignant neoplasms, which is the major factor in incurability, takes place contiguously by infiltration of surrounding structures and by metastasis through veins, arteries (rarely) and lymphatics. Within serous cavities, especially the peritoneal, spread through the cavitary serous fluid is known to take place—e.g., cancer of the stomach to the pelvis (Blumer's shelf). Metastasis via perineural lymphatics is a dire mode of spread: cancer possessing this propensity to a high degree, such as adenocarcinoma of the lung, pancreas or stomach, has a comparatively low rate of cure. Severe pain is a frequent consequence.

CERTAIN PRACTICAL CONSIDERATIONS IN CANCER SURGERY

A number of problems confronting the surgeon who cares for patients with cancer or suspected cancer are common to many types of the disease. Some of these will be considered here. Breast cancer (see Chap. 27) will serve to illustrate these points.

One is confronted first with the case only suspected of having cancer. What are the minimal criteria for doing a biopsy? Should this be a wedge or a chip biopsy, or should it always be an excision biopsy? Is a needle biopsy ever justified? If so, when?

What are the chances of spreading cancer by doing an incomplete biopsy? What are the chances of a sampling error (i.e., missing the cancer) by doing a limited biopsy, a needle biopsy, or a biopsy before a dominant lump is found? How reliable is the gross appearance of the lesion as a basis for diagnosis? How reliable is frozen section? Will waiting for a paraffin section reduce the chances of cure if malignancy is present?

These are questions which arise in connection with establishing a diagnosis of malignancy in many areas in which cancer may be suspected.

In more advanced cancer one must answer other questions. Is the patient operable in the sense that he can stand an exploratory operation and biopsy? Is the tumor resectable in the sense that all gross tumor can be removed completely? There follow many additional questions about the absolute efficacy of alternative methods of treatment, such as roentgen therapy; the relative efficacy of radiation as compared with attempted surgical excision as compared with no treatment at all, in various stages of advancement of the tumor.

In the cancers that are incurable by present

Table 10-6. Signs of Neoplasia

Neoplastic Location	Normal Function	Signs Due to Expansion	Necrosis or Inflammation	Signs Due to Infiltration	Destruction of Host Tissue
Brain		+++ Headache and palsies		+ Pain	+ Palsies, etc.
Endocrine glands	+++	+ Tumor		+ Recurrent nerve palsy ca. thyroid	
Lung		+++ Cough and atelectasis	++ Pneumonia, hemoptysis	+ Brachial plexus pain, pleural effusion	
Gastrointestinal tract		+++ Intestinal and gastric obstruction	++ Inflammation, anemia, hemorrhage	+ Ascites	
Biliary tract		+++ Jaundice			
Urinary tract		++ Prostatism	+++ Hematuria, pyuria		
Female genital tract		+ Tumor	+++ Intermenstrual bleeding, vaginal discharge, ulceration	+ Lumbosacral plexus pain	
Bone		+ Pain	++ Inflammation mimicking osteomyelitis		+++ Pathologic fracture
Bone marrow					+ Panhematopenia
Liver		+++ Tumor			+ Hepatic insufficiency
Spleen		+++ Tumor			
Skin and breast		+++ Tumor	++ Late ulceration	+ Fixation to skin or chest	

+ Present
++ Marked
+++ Very marked

methods, one must evaluate the results of therapy in terms of symptomatic relief, as well as in terms of life expectancy.

Such considerations bring one face to face with the philosophical problem of whether a physician has an obligation to prolong life into a period of uselessness, pain and slow dissolution in the face of a prognosis which appears on the best evidence to be hopeless.

What answers can be provided to these questions? In many instances, rather little factual material has been assembled on which answers can be based. Therefore, the following are based in part on clinical experience and opinion.

In the realm of diagnosis, a definite basis should exist for doing a biopsy for malignancy. Occasionally, this is based on suspicion of a generalized or widespread disease, such as a bone marrow biopsy in leukemia, but generally it is based on palpation of an abnormal lump or of abnormal consistency in otherwise normal tissues.

Improved radiologic methods for finding small tumors in breasts occasionally provide the principal indication for the excision of an area also. The use of the thermograph may lead to a suspicion of certain areas in which nothing abnormal is palpated, but at present experience with it is seldom a sufficient basis for action in the absence of other confirmatory findings.

In the absence of such localizing evidence, random biopsies are valueless unless they turn out to be positive, and this occurs but seldom. Furthermore, the healing of such biopsy wounds leaves areas of induration and scarring which may interfere with accurate palpation of the area for months and sometimes for years, thus diminishing the chance of discerning significant changes at subsequent examination.

In all breast lesions, except very advanced ones, and where possible in most other lesions suspected malignancy, excision biopsy should be practiced rather than incision or chip biopsy. Wedge or chip biopsies are of limited value when negative, and needle biopsies in general cannot be relied upon at all if they are negative. It is essential in doing a biopsy to avoid an error in sampling. With all hard-to-feel lumps near the surface of the body, local infiltration anesthesia should be avoided, if possible, as it often makes it impossible to identify the lesion by touch during the operation. Of course, regional nerve blocks at a distance from the lesion do not have this drawback.

Tumors of hollow viscera usually cannot be subjected to excision biopsy without undertaking a major resection (see Chap. 31, Stomach and Duodenum). Even when an intraluminal approach is used (e.g., proctoscopic examination of rectum), only a chip or partial biopsy is possible in many instances, but many a polyp which appeared to be benign in the portions removed by the biopsy forceps has revealed carcinoma when the entire specimen reached the pathologist. (See Chap. 33, Pancreas, regarding the problems of pancreatic biopsy.)

The reliability of frozen section diagnosis can be high in the breast (90 to 95% correct), though it is closely approached by the examination of the gross appearance of the cut surface of the lesion. However, it is not as good as the histologic diagnosis of the paraffin section. What evidence is available would indicate that when the pathologist is in doubt after examination of the frozen section, a delay of 2 to 5 days in carrying out a definitive cancer operation should be permitted so that examination of the paraffin section can be done. Such a delay does not result in a demonstrably worse prognosis. Such cases are usually early cases, however, and it has been argued that the 5-year survival rate should be better than average rather than about the same. Furthermore, the increased psychic trauma to the patient caused by staging the operation is an important consideration.

In certain other areas the value of the frozen section is less, e.g., polyps of the colon, and in still other areas its value is nil unless certain positive findings happen to exist. This is especially true in the examination of lymph nodes where little is certain on frozen section, unless the node is invaded by evident metastatic carcinoma.

It is not too much to hope that eventually means will be developed for producing sections of tissue suitable for definitive microscopic examination within a few minutes, but with present methods one must know when to rely on frozen section diagnosis and when not to. The use of the cryostat with differential staining is an important advance in this regard.

Turning toward the other end of the spectrum in carcinoma, when is a cancer so advanced as to make a radical attempt to remove it not worthwhile? In breast carcinoma, this problem was studied carefully by Haagensen and Stout (1943), who set up criteria of nonoperability by correlating preoperative findings with 5-year postoperative survival. Even though the series included about 700 cases, the subgroups were in some instances small, and some of the conclusions reached have had to be modified (1951). No comparable study has been achieved for cancer in any other site with the possible exception of the cervix uteri.

How serious a mistake is it to do a radical mastectomy even though it violates a criterion of nonoperability as evidenced by the study of Haagensen and Stout? Mortality, morbidity and the chances of increasing the spread or the rate of growth of unremoved tumor are all factors to be considered.

In their review of clinical experience, Boyd, Enterline and Donald (1954) report an operative mortality of 0.2 per cent for radical mastectomy. The risk to life, then, is small if available safeguards are employed during operation and the postoperative period. Disability is marked for 1 to 4 months. Residual disability is slight for the activities in which most American women engage. There are also the economic factors, but it is doubtful that irradiation therapy is much less expensive than operative treatment, and there remain psychological factors. The removal of a breast for a tumor is a heavy blow to face, but is it worse than living with the tumor visibly and palpably growing and ultimately often ulcerating? And, is it worse than prolonged x-ray therapy with its attendant "radiation" illness and local radiation reactions?

The late Dr. Eldridge L. Eliason frequently said, "In this country a person cannot be condemned to death without a fair trial." Certainly, in all borderline cases, it is better to attempt radical treatment when the operative mortality is low. However, there are cases which are clearly beyond help, and the surgeon should avoid embarking on an operation if it is a useless gesture.

The degree of palliation offered by operation in incurable cancer is a moot point. In breast cancer, it is doubtful if it offers any more for the patient with distant metastases than x-ray therapy. In colon cancer, it has been thought that liver metastases grew more slowly after surgical eradication of the primary tumor. The above is a clinical impression neither supported nor contradicted to the author's knowledge by statistically significant data. It seems improbable that removal of a primary in the colon actually decreases the growth rate of established liver metastases. However, its removal should halt the seeding of the liver with fresh metastases. Many of the liver metastases appear to be well localized or somewhat encapsulated and may grow very slowly. At least, metastases in the liver are essentially sterile, while the original colon growth is always infected.

Brunschwig (1947, 1954), who has been a strong advocate of radical surgery in advanced cancer, has been able to report significant numbers of 5-year survivors among persons who have what are generally considered "hopeless" cancers, especially of the cervix uteri and the rectum. An interesting discussion of the problems and various types of procedures of the "supraradical" nature is presented by Fisher (1954).

Miscellaneous Palliative Cancer Operations

In addition to attempts at resection, there are many other palliative operations carried out in cancer patients. Many of these are side-tracking procedures for relief of obstructions in hollow viscera. Examples are tracheostomy for carcinoma of the larynx, gastrostomy for carcinoma of the esophagus, gastro-enterostomy for carcinomas obstructing the pyloric area, entero-enterostomy, ileocolostomy, et cetera. Cholecystojejunostomy or choledochojejunostomy may relieve jaundice due to neoplastic obstructions low in the common bile duct. Similar shunting procedures are used in the urinary tract. It is hard to evaluate these methods of treatment fairly. Gastrostomy, for relief of obstruction of the esophagus by carcinoma, has been followed by an average survival of only 3 months in some series. Unfortunately, some of these patients develop pain from the advance of the malignancy, whereas they probably would have died painlessly from inanition if left alone. In arriving at final decisions in such situations, it is generally wise to have the appropriate members of the patient's family and a consultant share the responsibility for the decision.

Neurosurgery has made a great contribution to the palliative treatment of cancer by developing methods of interrupting the sensory pathways for pain with minimal interference with other modalities of sensation, or by destroying so-called association pathways. These procedures are discussed in Chapter 54, Surgery of the Nervous System.

Cancer Statistics

To evaluate the published experience of other physicians is nowhere more important than in the field of malignant disease. The pitfalls are numerous. To illustrate, a report may state that the 5-year cure rate after subtotal gastric resection for gastric cancer is 30 per cent. This statement does not tell one the following things:

How was cure judged at 5 years: by survival, by letter follow-up, by physical examination, or by physical examination plus x-ray studies of the gastrointestinal tract and the chest? Most careful authors now use the terms "5-year survival" or "5-year survival without clinical evidence of recurrence."

Does the 30 per cent relate to all of the hospital's admissions with carcinoma of the stomach, to all admissions on the entire surgical service of the hospital, to all admissions to a particular surgeon's service, to all operable cases in one of the above categories, to all such cases that were resectable, to all that were resected without leaving gross tumor behind, or to all that were resected and found to have no lymph node metastases?

One can think of other variables that might be important. For instance, with breast cancer, the incidence of axillary metastases at the time patients seek treatment has been much higher among indigent patients than among private patients.

In order to compare or combine different series, it is necessary to know how the statistics were compiled. Usually, it is best to report the 5-year survivals as a percentage of all patients in which the diagnosis was well established, admitted to an institution or, at least, to a service. The criteria for including or excluding cases should be stated in some detail. The 5-year survivals may then also be related to the total number operated upon, the total number resected with the hope of cure, the total number without lymph node metastases, etc. A good reference on the subject is Johnson (1955). (See Chap. 55 on surgical statistics.)

Prophylactic Surgery in the Field of Cancer

It is now reasonably well established that certain lesions are potentially malignant. In some cases, the lesion is a benign tumor or ulcer, which it is believed may undergo malignant transformation. In other situations, some pathologists oppose the concept of transformation and maintain that those lesions which are malignant in their late stages were always malignant, even though at the earlier stage they were grossly indistinguishable from a benign lesion. In both groups of patients having potentially malignant though probably benign tumors, it is desirable to remove the lesions if the price in terms of operative mortality, disability (both temporary and permanent) and psychological factors is not too high.

Examples in which such removal is generally considered worthwhile, except where special contraindications exist, are nodules in the thyroid gland, especially if they appear to be solitary, polyps of the rectum and the colon, and chronic sores on the lip, the tongue, or the buccal mucous membrane. An example in which the price is generally considered too high is the following:

Morbidity statistics would seem to indicate that nearly 30 per cent of cancer in women would be eliminated if the uterus and the breasts were removed after the woman had her family and had attained the age of 38 to 40 years. The mortality of the two simple mastectomies would be very low—perhaps about 0.1 per cent; the mortality of the total hysterectomy in healthy individuals at that age should be under 0.8 per cent—so that the total risk would be of the order of 1.0 per cent or less if proper safeguards were observed carefully. It is reported that in 1959 5.4% of deaths among women were due to cancer in one of these loci. There should be little permanent disability as pectoral muscles could be left intact, and the axillary lymphatics would be left intact or nearly intact. Why then is it not done? There are several reasons:

(1) The individuals who would die of the procedure would lose 35 to 40 years of expected life, including 10 to 20 years when they were of especial importance as mothers, whereas deaths due to cancer would be distributed at all ages. (2) Some of those who waited until cancer developed could still be saved by operation at that time (though this factor has already been taken into consideration in the mortality figures). (3) Such treatment involves considerable expenditure of both time and money, especially if one considers the several months of feeling below par after discharge from the hospital. (4) Probably the real reasons are the psychological ones. Breasts are too much a part of a woman's total being to be dispensed with lightly. It is possible that, in a different psychological climate, this factor might change (remember the Amazons), but this does not appear probable here

and now. Practically, since current surgical practice does not include these procedures on a purely prophylactic basis, the surgeon who began them might have difficulty in defending himself legally, even though he had acted in accordance with his best judgment.

Preventive surgery presents its own special problems. Superficially, at least, it is in contradiction of Sydenham's famous adage, *"Primum non nocere"* (First, do no harm). In preventive surgery, the harm is done first, and the benefits accrue to the survivors later. The same is true of some phases of preventive medicine as in the early poliomyelitis vaccine experiences of 1955.

The advisability of preventive surgery must be determined by mathematical analysis of experience—in other words, by statistics. In many fields, we do not have experience recorded in ways which permit analysis. What does one need, for instance, to determine whether or not one should advise a patient with a questionable gastric ulcer to have an immediate gastric resection rather than to wait 3 to 4 weeks for a trial of medical treatment? One needs a long series of such patients treated by the alternate case method in which all patients in each half of the series are followed to the time of death and the average months of life for patients in the 2 groups is compared.

Because of the lack of such data and the long time required to obtain them, one looks for more expedient methods. One interesting method depends on only 5 factors: (1) operative mortality when the lesion is benign; (2) the proportion who have or would develop malignancy in the ulcer; (3) the proportion of those who would not come to gastric resection eventually, either for carcinoma or intractability; (4) the 5-year survival rate of those with carcinoma who were operated upon without delay; and (5) the 5-year survival rate for those with carcinoma who are not operated on until lack of response to a trial of medical treatment or other evidence suggested carcinoma.

Let us pick some statistics from the literature and see how far we can get in a concrete example. The mortality of gastric resection for benign lesions as obtained by combining the statistics of Walters *et al.* (1952), Lahey and Marshall (1952), Druckerman *et al.* (1953), Priestley *et al.* (1954), and Wallensten and Gothman (1953) was about 2 per cent.

The incidence of gastric ulcers which proved to be malignant is at least 10 per cent, according to Ransom (1947) and Ravdin and Horn (1953). The percentage of those responding to medical treatment who eventually come to gastric resection is estimated by Smith and Jordan (1948) and by Marshall (1953) at 20 per cent.

The 5-year survival rate for patients with gastric carcinoma has long been given as 5 per cent and will be taken at 8 per cent on the basis of Ransom (1953). In 2 series, Lampert, Waugh and Dockerty (1950) and Ransom (1947), the 5-year survival rate for patients with gastric carcinoma after resection for "undiagnosed" gastric ulcer was over 40 per cent.

The cost in lives lost unnecessarily is the mortality which was 2 per cent multiplied by the patients who would escape operation entirely if not operated upon prophylactically. Of 100 patients with doubtful ulceration of the stomach, experience indicates that 10 will have cancer and 20 will have intractable ulcers. This leaves 70 who would escape operation if it were delayed. Thus, the cost of a policy of prophylactic resection would be seen to be $.02 \times 70 = 1.4$ per cent or 14 per thousand.

Offsetting this is the difference between the 5-year survival rate for carcinomas operated on prophylactically (S_1) and the 5-year survival rate for carcinomas operated on after the diagnosis had become apparent (S_2) multiplied by the number who have carcinoma (C). Expressed mathematically, this is $(S_1 - S_2)C$, or $(40 - 8).10 = 3.2$ or 32 per thousand. Thus, in the example given, preventive surgery would appear to save over twice as many lives as it cost.

When one considers the many other variables, such as the number dying of the cancer after 5 years, the tendency of patients who have had one cancer to develop another, the fact that the months the patient with cancer would live before diagnosis became definite are lost by the unfortunate person without cancer who dies of operation and other factors that the thoughtful student will consider, this is not a very wide margin. However, if the operative mortality could be reduced to 0.5 of 1.0 per cent, the advantage becomes about 9 to 1. This shows that preventive surgery is for the good-risk patient rather than the poor-risk one, and that greater reduction in operative mortality rates could extend the indications for prophylactic surgery further. This example is cited partly to point up how complicated these issues are and partly to indicate a more quantitative approach to the answers.

HEREDITARY FACTORS IN CANCER

Although familial tendency toward cancer is regularly sought for in taking medical histories, most statistically sophisticated studies provide either no basis for such a view or at most indicate that family background is a weak factor.

The studies of Douglas Murphy in carcinoma of the uterus (1952) and carcinoma of the breast (1959) are pertinent.

A recent study of heredity of cancer by a study of unselected twins is of value in this connection. Harvald and Hauge established satisfactory contact with 6,893 pairs of twins born in Denmark between 1870 and 1910. These were separated into monozygous and dizygous groups and a third group in which this was considered to be undetermined.

Coincidence between twins was determined both for the same site and for different sites in the 2 series. There was no significant difference between the 2 series when all sites were considered. The observed site specific concordance was 8 among 164 monozygous and 9 among 340 dizygous twins, and the authors concluded that even if a large series should show a significant difference, it would be a weak factor as compared with others.

The surgery of cancer has become a major preoccupation of many surgeons. However, it is not expected that the ultimate solutions will be found by surgical means. Pending the development of what might be called a satisfactory molecular attack on cancer, surgery is the most effective means of treating most early forms of malignancy. Some estimates of the 5-year survival rates for cancer originating in some of the common loci are presented in Table 10-7.

In addition to the survivors at the 5-year

TABLE 10-7. ESTIMATED 5-YEAR SURVIVAL RATES OF COMMON CANCERS

LOCUS	FIVE-YEAR SURVIVAL (All patients receiving definitive treatment) PER CENT
Breast	
Without axillary metastases	70
With axillary metastases	30
Lip	80
Tongue	25
Stomach	
Resectable without gross residual tumor	25
Resectable without node metastases	50
Rectum (and rectosigmoid)	40
Cervix—over-all	45
Stage 0	95
Stage I	80
Stage II	50
Stage III	25
Stage IV	10
Uterus	
Limited to uterus	70
Spread beyond uterus	20
Thyroid	65
Lung (resectable)	10
Skin	95

level, much is accomplished in prolongation of life and alleviation of symptoms by palliative procedures.

BIBLIOGRAPHY

Boyd, A. K., Enterline, H. T., and Donald, J. G.: Carcinoma of the breast: a surgical follow-up study. Surg., Gynec., Obstet., 99:9-21, 1954.

Brunschwig, A.: Radical Surgery in Advanced Abdominal Cancer. Chicago, Univ. Chicago Press, 1947.

————: Total and anterior pelvic exenteration: report of results based upon 315 operations. Surg., Gynec., Obstet., 99:324-330, 1954.

Collins, V. P., Loeffler, R. K., and Tivey, H.: Am. J. Roentgenol., 76:988, 1956.

Coman, D. R.: Decreased mutual adhesiveness, a property of cells from squamous cell carcinomas. Cancer Res., 10:625-629, 1944.

Druckerman, L. J., Weinstein, V. A., Klingenstein, P., and Colp, R.: Duodenal ulcer treated by subtotal gastrectomy with and without vagotomy. J.A.M.A., 151:1266, 1953.

Fisher, B.: Editorial: supraradical cancer surgery. Am. J. Surg., 87:155-159, 1954.

Fitts, W. T., Dexheimer, F. R., and Schor, S. S.: Carcinoma of the Breast. *In* Blakemore, W. S., and Ravdin, I. S.: Current Perspectives in Cancer Therapy. Chap. 22. pp. 189–196. New York, Hoeber, 1966.

Haagensen, C. D., and Stout, A. P.: Carcinoma of the breast; criteria of operability. Ann. Surg., 118:859, 1943.

———: Carcinoma of the breast; results of treatment. Ann. Surg., 134:151-172, 1951.

Hammond, E. Cuyler: Personal communication, 1968.

Johnson, R. E.: Editorial: deceptive associations in clinical data. Ann. Surg. 141:567-571, 1955.

Koprowski, H., Ponten, J., Jensen, J., Ravdin, R. G., Moorehead, P., and Saksela, E.: Transformation of cultures of human tissues injected with Simian Virus No. 40. J. Cell. Comp. Physiol., 59:81-292, 1962.

Lahey, F. H., and Marshall, S. F.: The surgical treatment of peptic ulcer. New Eng. J. Med., 246:115, 1952.

Lampert, E. G., Waugh, J. M., and Dockerty, M. B.: Incidence of malignancy in gastric ulcer believed preoperatively to be benign. Surg., Gynec., Obstet., 91:673, 1950.

Marshall, S. F.: The relation of gastric ulcer to carcinoma of the stomach. Ann. Surg., 137:891, 1953.

Murphy, D. P.: Heredity in Uterine Cancer. Cambrige, Mass., Harvard University Press 1952, Commonwealth Fund Publication. XI: 128.

Murphy, D. P., and Abbey, Helen: Cancer in Families: A study of the relatives of 200 breast cancer probands, Cambrige, Mass., Harvard University Press, 1959. (Commonwealth Fund Publication)

Priestley, J. T., Walters, W., Gray, H. K., and Waugh, J. M.: Annual report on surgery of stomach and duodenum for 1953. Proc. Mayo Clin., 29:638, 1954.

Ransom, H. K.: Cancer of the stomach. Surg., Gynec., Obstet., 96:275, 1953.

———: Subtotal gastrectomy for gastric ulcer: a study of end results. Ann. Surg., 126:633, 1947.

Ravdin, I. S., and Horn, R. C.: Gastric ulcer and gastric cancer. Ann. Surg., 137:904, 1953.

Smith, F. H., and Jordan, S. M.: Gastric ulcer: a study of 600 cases. Gastroenterology, 11:575, 1948.

Wallensten, S., and Gothman, L.: An evaluation of the Billroth I operation for peptic ulcer. Surgery, 33:1, 1953.

Walters, W., Gray, H. K., Priestley, J. T., and Waugh, J. M.: Report on surgery of the stomach and duodenum for 1950. Proc. Mayo Clin., 27:39, 1952.

CHAPTER 11

ROBERT G. RAVDIN, M.D.

The Molecular Attack on Cancer

It has long been the dream of the biologic scientist to develop pharmacologic agents that would destroy (preferably), or cause regression or, at least, arrest the growth of abnormal cells in patients suffering from neoplastic disease, without causing significant injury to normal body tissues.

Historically, comparable expectations have been gradually realized in relation to infectious disease. Even when such diseases were leading causes of death, and control was limited to isolation and quarantine, the use of quinine and cinchona alkaloids for malarial infestation had been empirically developed by American aborigines, and remained for centuries the sole effective treatment for this major world-wide health problem. This limited but useful armamentarium was expanded by the introduction of arsenicals in the treatment of syphilis by Ehrlich, by the discovery of Prontosil by Domagk in 1932, by the development of penicillin by Alexander and Fleming in 1939, and by the investigations of Waksman on various compounds produced by actinomyces strains, in particular streptomycin and neomycin. It is notable that these advances were also essentially empirical, with the utility of the agents being well established before their mechanisms of action were even partially understood.

The control of infectious disease has proceeded in an even more significant direction— the elaboration of means to promote host resistance to the infectious agent and thereby take advantage of the powerful mechanisms of defense against extraneous invaders, which have been developed during the evolutionary process. Since Jenner's courageous demonstration of the protective value of prior cowpox infection against subsequent exposure to smallpox, an increasing number of infectious diseases have been brought under control by this essentially chemical technic of the stimulation of production of globulins tailored to steric fit of endotoxins and cell membranes, and sensitization of phagocytic cells to the recognition of extraneous organisms, presumably by a comparable mechanism. It is noteworthy that these methods are the only available approaches to virus diseases (excepting large viruses such as lymphogranuloma, which are perhaps more comparable to Rickettsia); it is also noteworthy, and somewhat discouraging, that, with the possible exception of rabies, these measures are of no value against established viral infection.

Expectation of the control of neoplastic disease based on an analogy to infectious processes has some attractive aspects:

1. It is clear that in the majority of instances cancer is not a localized disease, but a disseminated one. In many instances, the dissemination appears to arise from a particular focus; surgical or radiotherapeutic attack is based on the possibility of ablating the focus and its environs before systemic dissemination has occurred. In other cases, the disease is evidently multifocal, as in leukemia, most lymphomas, alveolar carcinoma of the lung, and cholangiolar hepatoma. Here ablation is doomed to failure, being technically impossible, or involving entire vital organ systems. In addition, consideration of the growth rate of cells in a given locally arising neoplasm suggests that metastases occur often within a relatively few cell generations, well before the primary tumor has attained a size at which a diagnosis can be established. In such a situation, the surgeon may perform a useful function in dealing with a mechanical problem arising from the primary, such as bowel obstruction, but is helpless with respect to the underlying disease process. This is comparable to drainage of a focus of infection or resection of a pulmonary segment containing a tuberculous cavitation. The procedure is of value

provided that the disease is not further disseminated, or that host mechanisms can deal with, or be assisted by chemical means in dealing with, the residual infestation.

2. There is increasing evidence that some tumors are induced by infectious agents of a viral nature. A large number of such tumors are known in vertebrates: Peyton Rous's chicken sarcoma (the first of the solid tumors), Shope's rabbit papilloma, Bittner's mammary cancer, Lucke's frog renal tumor, a variety of mouse leukemias, and many others of recent demonstration (Dmochowski, 1959). Infection with polyoma virus leads to the development of a considerable variety of tumors in mice, hamsters, and guinea pigs (Burnet, 1964). In man, the situation is not so clear, probably to no small degree because the current methodology is not applicable to man. Viruses of known or probable oncogenicity have not been isolated from human tumors. Highly suggestive transformation of human cells in tissue culture exposed to SV-40 virus, a known oncogenic agent in lower mammals, has been observed by Jensen et al. (1964) and by Enders, and implantation of these cells in human volunteers by the former group has resulted in invasive growth prior to immune rejection. It is not improbable therefore that viral infection plays a significant role in some human cancer.

3. In some instances, particularly with respect to tumors of endocrine or reproductive system origin, malignant human cells are not so undifferentiated as to have lost their responsiveness to normal humoral growth control mechanisms. In these systems, the nature of such control is to some extent understood, and manipulations can be performed to take advantage of them. Control is obviously exerted over normal growth and reparative processes in the body, such as liver regeneration or bone remodeling, but how this is accomplished is a complete engima. Nonetheless, arrest and regression of certain tumors can be effected by physiologic means inherent in the host. The fascinating observations of the Fishers are pertinent in this connection, indicating that disseminated tumor cells can remain (be held?) dormant in the livers of mice for substantial portions of the animal's life, to become activated into establishing gross colonies by maneuvers that interfere with liver function. The fact that host alteration stimulates these cells to growth lends support to the concept that some host mechanism is inhibiting them.

Analogies between control of malignant and of infectious disease have also troublesome drawbacks:

1. Extraneous infectious agents differ significantly from mammalian cells in both metabolic mechanisms and cell membrane structure. An agent toxic to bacteria and innocuous to mammalian tissue is therefore considerably more likely to be found than is one that will selectively damage only an aberrant species, as distinct from similar but normal species, of mammalian cell. Extensive work has been done in an attempt to delineate metabolic processes that distinguish cancer cells; no qualitative differences have been found. Cancer cells may show depletion of enzyme systems characterizing their tissue of origin, and quantitative differences in synthetic or respiratory enzymes or pathways of substrate metabolism. Such, for example, is Warburg's observation of the preferential use of anaerobic pathways of glycolysis in many tumors regardless of the availability of oxygen. But such relatively minor differences have proved to be exceedingly difficult to exploit effectively. Most of the cytotoxic agents that can be used in cancer treatment—and radiation, as well—appear to operate at the level of replication of DNA, an obvious requirement of neoplastic tissue, but hardly a distinctive property.

2. Assuming that infectious agents such as viruses, proviruses, and the like, are involved in human cancers, such infection is clearly established prior to diagnosis, a situation that is not amenable to definitive therapy in the known infectious viral diseases. To be sure, the malignant diseases run a very much longer course, giving a greater opportunity for therapeutic measures to take effect; on the other hand, the hypothesized infectious agent presumably has become so firmly fixed to the cell genome that it is not recoverable by any known means and can no longer be considered an extraneous agent.

3. Host immune mechanisms, so important in the control of infectious disease, have never been unequivocally demonstrated in human cancers, or indeed for any autochthonous tumor (Furth, 1963). An exception is the

rather remarkable demonstration of immune response developed to methyl-cholanthrene-induced "spontaneous" tumor (Prehn and Main, 1957), leading to rejection of subsequently implanted methyl cholanthrene sarcomas from the same animal after amputation of the limb bearing the primary, though not to the destruction of the primary itself. It has been suggested that the erythema and round cell infiltration seen so prominently around some tumors such as inflammatory carcinoma of the breast are manifestations of host response, but the notoriously unfavorable course of this tumor in particular does not lend much hope to tumor control simply by enhancement of immune mechanisms. "Spontaneous" regression is an uncommon but well documented event which does point to some type of host process destructive to autonomous growth; certain tumor types (melanoma, carcinoma of kidney) comprise a far greater proportion of known instances of regression than expected from their frequency in the tumor spectrum and may be characterized by the development of recognizable antigens, though this has not been demonstrated. Burnet's idea (Burnet, 1964) that the immune mechanism is far too elaborate to have been evolved for the purpose of dealing with extraneous infection alone and is, in fact, designed to deal with continually appearing maverick cells from the host itself, is a very provocative concept. It follows, however, that clinically apparent tumors have circumvented the immune process and cannot be controlled by it. It is notable that many chemical carcinogens, as well as radiation, suppress immune responses. This is also true in varying degrees of almost all cytotoxic chemotherapeutic agents. If means were available for measuring tumor cell populations with any degree of precision, it is not inconceivable that under some circumstances chemotherapeutic treatment could be shown to accelerate tumor growth.

Whatever the future may hold in enhancing, revising, or replacing these speculations, the molecular attack on cancer has begun and is not without some limited successes. In experimental systems, using transplantable tumors, chemicals are to all intents curative in many instances. These results are unfortunately not transposable to autochthonous tumors in the human, possibly because such tumors are generally better established (i.e., of longer duration, better adapted to environment), possibly because minor histoincompatibility factors operate even within closely inbred strains to assist chemicals in the suppression of transplanted tumors.

HORMONES

Observation on the control of cancer (of the breast) by alteration in hormonal environment was made originally by Beatson, in 1896, who reported significant regression of mammary tumors in some oophorectomized patients. This apparent dependence of some mammary cancers on estrogen for active growth has been amply confirmed both in the human and experimental systems. (This should be distinguished from the effect of estrogen as a tumor *inducer*, which has been shown for certain experimental systems using both virus and chemical carcinogens as co-promoters, but not in the human, where the increased incidence of breast cancer in the nulliparous and the decreased incidence in women receiving estrogen for postmenopausal osteoporosis suggests an opposite effect.) Subsequently, it has been shown that a number of different hormonal manipulations lead to regression of human breast cancer in 15 to 30 per cent of cases; these include the administration of androgens, estrogens, progestational compounds, adrenal corticoids, and even steroidal structures of no visible physiologic effect, as well as the ablation of the ovaries, adrenals, and pituitary (Kennedy, 1965). Control by these means is temporary; when effective, it is of the order of 10 to 14 months. But these agents are not mutually exclusive and may be used sequentially with a reasonable chance of a second period of regression when the utility of the first selected treatment is exhausted. The mechanism of action at the cell level is completely unknown. A few generalizations can be drawn from this confused and often paradoxical picture:

1. Oophorectomy is not effective in postmenopausal women, but it is by far the treatment of choice in the premenopausal.

2. Androgens and estrogens affect predominantly the same group of tumors rather than separate groups. Both agents are substantially more likely to be effective in women with rela-

tively slow growing tumors and in patients whose disease does not involve parenchymal viscera such as liver, lung, or cerebrum (osseous metastasis is not unfavorable), and the probability of remission increases linearly for both agents with the number of years that have elapsed since menopause, being well under 10 per cent in women within a year of menopause or castration at the time of onset of therapy, and upwards of 40 per cent in women more than ten years from menopause.

3. Adrenalectomy and hypophysectomy are essentially equivalent procedures, working best in women between the ages of 45 and 65, with relatively slow growing tumors, and with known response to previous castration or androgen administration, and poorly in the very young, patients with liver metastases, and patients with rapidly disseminated or progressing disease (Joint Committee, J.A.M.A. 1961).

4. There is apparently a period of about two years from the manifestations of the need for systemic therapy in the life history of many breast cancers, during which the tumor is responsive to its environment, and after which, presumably due to dedifferentiation, the tumor becomes unresponsive or "autonomous."

In fact, the most useful area for hormonal management of malignancy stems from Huggins' report on castration in patients with prostatic cancer. Here, in well over two thirds of patients, regression of prostatic cancer is induced by orchiectomy or administration of estrogen, the former method being preferable, since estrogen administration has led to serious cardiovascular complications (Veterans Adm., Surg. Gynec. Obstet. 1967). Control is exerted for several years in most instances. Since, in contrast to breast cancer, osseous metastases of prostatic cancer are characteristically osteoblastic, bone healing is difficult to interpret on x-ray films, but the diminution of the gland itself, of acid phosphatase levels, and of node metastases when present, are clear indications of actual regression.

It is now well established that in about 30 per cent of patients endometrial carcinoma will respond by regression to high doses of progestational compounds. Adrenal corticoids induce remission in acute leukemia of childhood and occasionally in lymphosarcomas. The use of suppressive doses of thyroid to inhibit the output of pituitary thyrotropins in the management of follicular and papillary tumors of the thyroid is not so firmly established. However, theory and the weight of clinical evidence support this concept, and it is strongly espoused by most clinicians interested in this field. The rodent thyroid cancer induced by thiouracil is by far the clearest model experimental system of the development of cancer in a target organ by hormonal stimulation. This tumor is initially responsive to hormonal environment—continual exposure to, or withdrawal of, the trophic hormone—and it eventually develops autonomy (Money and Rawson, 1950).

There is real prospect that, as more is learned about the control of growth in various organ systems by humoral agents other than those now recognized as hormones, clinical application in this presently narrow field will be expanded. The work of Szent-Gyorgi (1963) on growth promoters and inhibitors is of interest in this regard.

RADIOISOTOPES

The use of cellular enzymatic processes to concentrate radioisotopes, thereby permitting large doses of radiation to be delivered to a biochemically specified tissue, has achieved striking if numerically limited success in the treatment of differentiated tumors of the thyroid gland with iodine isotopes, in particular ^{131}I. Such tumors may retain the properties of the tissue of origin, concentrating and storing iodine, though uncommonly to the degree of normal tissue itself. In this case, after ablation of the normal thyroid tissue by surgical means or by the use of the iodine isotope, the metastatic implants may take up enough ^{131}I to lead to cell destruction by this β-ray source (the γ emissions, which are used for external counting, are not responsible for the effective tissue irradiation). When concentration is present but weak, it may be stimulated by exogenous thyrotropin or by endogenous thyrotropin resulting from induced myxedema. By no means can all thyroid tumors be so treated, nor in any given patient are all the metastatic deposits necessarily equally efficient in concentration of iodine. That the method can be used at all is a remarkable instance of the contribution of biochemistry to medicine.

Other radioactive elements have been explored for comparable use with little success. ^{32}P localizes in bone, but to a lesser degree in areas bearing metastases than elsewhere. Some apparent control of bone pain has been obtained in a few instances in several metastatic tumor types; the method is of very limited use. Isotopic sulfur localizes in cartilage, but not to a degree that leads to effective radiation levels. Colloidal boron, which emits radiation on exposure to neutrons, has been administered intra-arterially to patients with brain tumors, where, after crossing the disturbed blood-brain barrier in the tumor area, it is deposited to localize radiation when the patient is treated with a neutron source. At present, localizing radiation sources are vastly more useful in diagnostic scanning of a variety of organs, since the differential uptake is more characteristic of the normal tissue than of the tumor that displaces it.

CYTOTOXIC AGENTS

A considerable number of chemical agents that function as cell poisons have been employed in the palliative treatment of disseminated tumors, and a vastly greater number have been screened against experimental tumors in an attempt to discover molecular structures that will differentially injure malignant cells to a greater extent than normal cells (Goldin et al., 1966; Skipper et al., 1964). In general, three approaches have been made to the development of such agents: (1) the empirical approach, in which organic compounds of various configurations or of biologic origin are tested in screening systems in vivo, in mammalian cell culture, or even against bacteria; nitrogen mustard and the numerous antibiotics were so discovered; (2) a rational approach based on designing substances to interfere with defined metabolic reactions of importance to cell proliferation; from such work come the fluorinated pyrimidines and other antimetabolites, in particular antifolics; (3) the chemical modification approach, in which substances with known but limited activity are employed as models for the construction of a series of compounds of comparable configuration in the hope that one of these will prove to be more damaging to malignant cells, or (what is the same thing) relatively less toxic to normal cells. The series of alkylating agents following nitrogen mustard are the result of such efforts. A series of such compounds are compared by the determination of *therapeutic index*, a ratio between the dose of drug producing a given per cent of tumor inhibition or of cure in a given in-vivo system, and the dose proving lethal to a given proportion of animals, such as the LD_{50}.

Alkylating agents, of which the prototype is nitrogen mustard, are characterized by the presence of two or more short carbon chains containing a functionally active group capable of attachment to amines, sulfhydryl groups, and the like. These groups are generally either chlorethyl amines or ethylene imines. The various alkylating agents differ in the remainder of the molecule which functions as a carrier and modifies the reactivity of the alkylating function. These compounds alkylate virtually any extra- or intracellular constituents containing the appropriate functional groups, in particular proteins, but in low concentration they produce profound effects on nucleic acids, and their physiologic effects may well be mediated by binding across the DNA helix, the simplest explanation of the necessity for more than one alkylating function in the molecule (Lawley and Brookes, 1967). Generally comparable in clinical activity, they have definite usefulness in chronic leukemias, lymphosarcomas, and carcinoma of the breast and ovary, and produce infrequent and rather short remission in a variety of other tumors. Remission in advanced breast cancer occurs in about 30 per cent of cases, for about 6 months, and in approximately half of ovarian cancers for an average of 10 months. Dosage regimens are limited by the marked toxicity to white cells and thrombocyte precursors in the bone marrow.

Nitrogen mustard itself remains the treatment of choice in advanced Hodgkin's disease, and in the local management of malignant serous effusion by direct installation, where, at least in the chest, its effect is probably due largely to the induction of a chemical pleuritis. ThioTEPA and chlorambucil are simpler to manage by virtue of being less irritating and producing less nausea and vomiting, and the latter agent can be given orally. ThioTEPA has been extensively explored as an adjuvant to definitive surgery in breast cancer, given at the time of radical mastectomy, by a cooperating group of surgical centers. In this instance, the drug may deal either with cells disseminated by manipulation at the time of surgery, or with subclinical undetectable implants outside of the operative field, as opposed to the extensive mass of disease that must be attacked when metastases become manifest. Preliminary results from this study indicate that in at least some groups of women coming to radical mastectomy, especially premenopausal women with axillary node involvement, salvage is improved. Cyclophosphamide is one of the few alkylators with a spectrum of activity in animal tumors differing from nitrogen mustard, and the clinical advantage that it does not cause thrombocytopenia. It may be the agent of choice in breast cancer.

Phenylalanine mustard also has a somewhat different activity spectrum; designed originally in the expectation that the aromatic amino acid carrier would be concentrated by melanomas producing pigment, this agent has not proved to function in this way, but it is nevertheless the most widely employed for regional perfusion, in particular for melanoma. This technic, explored extensively by Creech and associates, has been used in appropriate instances to isolate the tumor-bearing area, exposing it to a high concentration of a rapidly fixing cytotoxic agent while limiting the amount of drug reaching the remainder of the body and thereby curtailing toxicity. Of value in the treatment of melanoma in the extremity, both in the presence of established satellite nodules and probably prophylactically, and in some instances of sarcoma, the method is unfortunately not of general applicability because of the wide dissemination of most malignant disease.

The antimetabolites represent the most ingenious application of biochemistry to the cancer problem. A number of antimetabolites were developed by Wooley two decades ago, but most of these interfered with processes of such general importance (viz. respiration) that their toxicity was prohibitive. Farber introduced antifolics in the 1940's, the first of the clinically useful compounds. Amethopterin, or methotrexate, is a strikingly effective compound in acute leukemia of children, and has proved apparently curative in about half of the cases of choriocarcinoma in the female at the five-year mark, with significant regression for lesser periods in many more. The latter tumor is curious in the sense that it is of fetal rather than maternal origin, and in this instance host rejection reactions may well enhance the cytotoxic effects. Spontaneous regression is by no means unknown. Choriocarcinoma of the testis in the male is not nearly so sensitive, and is never cured by methotrexate.

Heidelberger's synthesis of 5-fluorouracil has represented a great advance in the chemical management of malignancy.[9] Stemming from the observation that uracil is selectively concentrated in rodent hepatomas and utilized for DNA synthesis, this agent closely counterfeits the normal metabolite and differs only in the substitution of a fluorine atom for hydrogen at the site where a methyl group must eventually be substituted to synthesize thymine. 5-Fluorouracil interferes competitively with several metabolic processes but most prominently, after its elaboration to the nucleoside, with the enzyme thymidylic synthetase. Because this inhibition is so marked and its result so lethal (the "thymidineless death" of Seymour Cohen) the fluorodeoxyuridine has been synthesized directly for therapeutic trial, but its superiority over fluorouracil itself has not been demonstrated, and it is vastly more expensive. Fluorouracil is the only agent of significant effectiveness in the treatment of gastrointestinal malignancy. About 20 per cent of cases of colon carcinoma showed definite regression, most commonly when the disease is locally recurrent and less so when there is liver involvement. A smaller but significant number of patients with gastric and pancreatic carcinoma also show response, and approximately the same proportion of mammary carcinomas are sensitive to this agent as are sensitive to alkylating agents.

The evolution of dosage regimens for the systemic administration of fluorouracil points up an interesting and perplexing problem in clinical chemotherapy. Early regimens required that the drug be given in 5-day courses repeated at approximately 6-week intervals. These regimens were deliberately taken to significant toxicity, not only to bone marrow but also to the mucosal lining of the gastrointestinal tract (as is characteristic of antimetabolites in general), resulting in a significant incidence of gram-negatve septicemia and, even in the most experienced hands, some lethal outcome. Toxicity was considered essential to the production of maximum therapeutic benefit. Recent clinical studies indicate that far less stringent programs, in particular, administration once a week, produce essentially equivalent results. Fluorouracil and comparable agents are classified as "cycle specific": their action appears to be exerted only during the relatively short portion of the mitotic cycle when DNA is being synthesized. For a cell population that is out of phase, it therefore seems paradoxical that exposure to an agent of this type for brief widely spaced intervals can produce any visible effect at all. The entire question of growth kinetics of solid tumors and its relation to chemotherapeutic treatment is just beginning to be explored.

Antimetabolites by their nature are not suitable agents for perfusion, because exposure to the agent must be of considerable duration. For that very reason, however, continuous infusion to maintain a relatively constant therapeutic level is a highly attractive idea, promulgated most vigorously by Sullivan. Especially when the blood supply to the tumor is accessible and effectively an end-artery, a high concentration of drug can be obtained in the tumor area while there is considerable dilution of the drug in the total blood volume. This method is applicable for tumors of the oropharynx via the external carotid, for both primary and metastatic liver tumors via the hepatic arteries and perhaps for tumors of the cervix via the hypogastric arteries. Both methotrexate and fluorinated pyrimidines have been used, the latter agents, judging from current usage, being generally more effective. Toxicity is greatly diminished and the technic is limited mainly by the restricted number of tumors to which it is applicable and technical considerations relevant to the placement and maintenance of the catheters (Brennan et al., 1963).

Antibiotics are the third great class of cytotoxic agents. These varied substances are grouped together by virtue of their biologic origin, being quite diverse chemically. Most of them are produced by actinomyces and other fungi (actinomycin, streptonigrin, mitomycin, puromycin); others are produced by bacteria, and the group also includes the periwinkle alkaloids (vincaleukoblastin and vincristine). These substances are extremely toxic in minute quantities, and at least some of them fix irreversibly to vital active configurations in chromosomes or ribosomes. For this reason, actinomycin and puromycin have been of greater value in biochemical investigation at the molecular level than in cancer therapy. Actinomycin is the only one of these agents in wide use clinically for solid tumors. It is of significant value in Wilms's tumor (Fernbach and Martyn, 1966) and childhood sarcomas, in choriocarcinoma of the female when such tumors are resistant to methotrexate, and, in combination with the latter drug, in choriocarcinoma of the testis. It does not seem improbable that continued exploration of substances of biologic origin, many of which have markedly unusual structures, will uncover some highly promising leads.

The following generalizations may be made about cytotoxic agents:

1. At effective levels some host toxicity is often produced by the agent because of the narrow margin between tumor sensitivity and the sensitivity of the most susceptible of the normal host tissues.

2. With very few exceptions, the agents are palliative only, producing regression for a limited number of months, and should not therefore be employed in asymptomatic patients, regardless of the extent of metastatic involvement, unless vital organ systems are clearly threatened.

3. Regardless of the completeness of observed remission, which is not uncommonly total, almost all tumors will eventually escape from control and become totally refractory to any given agent. At this point, persistence with the drug can only lead to toxicity without any expectation of benefit, and will prevent the employment of some other agent when there is one available.

4. Bone marrow is for all categories of cytotoxic drugs the site of limiting toxicity, and, where substantial volumes of marrow have been destroyed by irradiation and/or tumor replacement, dosage regimens suitable for the "standard" patient must be curtailed. This is also true for the debilitated patient

and patients with poor nutrition or those who are immediately postoperative.

In spite of the limitations of the molecular attack on cancer in its current state, the accomplishments are not inconsiderable. Well over two decades elapsed between the discoveries of Salvarsan and Prontosil, in the attack on considerably simpler problems. In a comparable period, a wide variety of anticancer agents have become available and a considerably greater number of leads developed which should result in more effective chemotherapeutic agents and technics of administration (Burchenal, 1963).

REFERENCES

Brennan, M. J., Talley, R. W., Drake, T. H., Vaitkevicius, V. K., Poznanski, A. K., and Brush, B. E.: 5-Fluorouracil treatment of liver metastases by continuous hepatic artery infusion via Cournand catheter. Ann. Surg., 158:405-417, 1963.

Burchenal, J. H.: Some problems basic to cancer research with particular reference to chemotherapy. Cancer Res., 23:1186-1190, 1963.

Burnet, M.: Immunologic factors in process of carcinogenesis. Brit. Med. Bull., 20:154-158, 1964.

Dmochowski, L.: Viruses and tumors. Bact. Rev., 23:18-40, 1959.

Eddy, B. E., Stewart, S. E., Stanton, M. F., and Marcotte, J. M.: Induction of tumors in rats by tissue culture preparations of SE polyoma virus. J. Nat. Cancer Inst., 22:161-171, 1959.

Fernbach, D. J., and Martyn, D. T.: Role of dactinomycin in improved survival of children with Wilms' tumor. J.A.M.A., 195:1005-1009, 1966.

Furth, J.: Influence of host factors on growth of neoplastic cells. Cancer Res., 23:21-34, 1963.

Goldin, A., Serpick, A. A., and Mantel, N.: Commentary: Experimental screening procedures and clinical predictability value. Cancer Chemother. Rep., 50:173-218, 1966.

Heidelberger, C., and Ansfield, F. J.: Experimental and clinical use of fluorinated pyrimidines in cancer chemotherapy. Cancer. Res., 23:1226-1243, 1963.

Jensen, F., Koprowski, H., Pagano, J., Ponteu, J., and Ravdin, R. G.: Autologous and homologous implantation of human cells transformed in vitro by simian virus 40. J. Nat. Cancer Inst., 32:917-937, 1964.

Joint Committee on Endocrine Ablative Procedures in Disseminated Mammary Carcinoma: Adrenalectomy and hypophysectomy in disseminated mammary carcinoma. J.A.M.A., 175:787-791, 1961.

Kennedy, B. J.: Hormone therapy in advanced breast cancer. Cancer, 18:1551-1557, 1965.

Lawley, P. D., and Brookes, P.: Interstrand cross-linking of DNA by disfunctional alkylating agents. J. Molec. Biol., 25:143-160, 1967.

Money, W. L., and Rawson, R. W.: The experimental production of thyroid tumors in the rat exposed to prolonged treatment with thiouracil. Cancer, 3:321-335, 1950.

Prehn, R. T., and Main, Z. M.: Immunity to methylcholanthrene induced sarcomas. J. Nat. Cancer Inst., 18:769-778, 1957.

Skipper, H. E., Strabel, F. M., Jr., and Wilcox, W. S.: Experimental evaluation of potential anticancer agents. XIII. On criteria and kinetics associated with "curability" of experimental leukemias. Cancer Chemother. Rep., 35:1-111, 1964.

Szent-Gyorgi, A., Hegyeli, A., and McLaughlin, J. A.: Cancer chemotherapy: A possible new approach. Science, 140:1391-1392, 1963.

Veterans Administration Co-operative Urologic Research Group: Treatment and survival of patients with cancer of prostate. Surg. Gynec. Obstet., 124:1011-1017, 1967.

CHAPTER 12

CARL A. MOYER, M.D.

The Assessment of Operative Risk

Intuition based upon personal experience and the observation of a patient's total reaction are important for judging operative risk.

Ideally, the assessment of operative risk should be approached as a statistical problem, and the risk expressed as the probability of dying during an operation and convalescence. However, the statistical approach demands accurate data pertaining to the effects of many factors such as age, starvation, heart disease, etc., upon the operative risk. These data are practically nonexistent. Furthermore, the risk attending practically all operations performed upon a random population has undergone remarkable reduction during the past half-century (Table 12-1). Obviously, because of these factors the accurate assessment of the operative risk for an individual case is impossible today. All we can do is guess. Therefore, the sole purpose of the discussion to follow is to enable the reader to make a better guess than he could before reading it as to the risk that an individual takes when submitting to an operative procedure.

The factors ostensibly affecting the operative risk are: the anatomic site, the magni-

TABLE 12-1, A. CHANGE IN OPERATIVE RISK
(Between 1916 to 1938 and 1948 to 1953)

OPERATION	1916–1945 TIME PERIOD	OPERATIVE MORTALITY PER CENT	1948–1953 TIME PERIOD	OPERATIVE MORTALITY PER CENT
Choledochostomy	1916–1938	16	1948–1952	2
Thyroidectomy for toxic goiter	1920	5–8	1953	1
Closure of perforated peptic ulcer	1935	41	1949	7
Correction of obstructions of small intestine	1928	37	1950–1953	8
Esophagectomy for cancer	1933	55	1952	16
Partial gastric resection for duodenal ulcer	1936–1945	4	1952	2
Surgical therapy of hepatic wounds	1934	62	1953	10
Surgical therapy of colonic wounds	1941	62	1953	14
Radical mastectomy	1925	1	1952	0.2

The combined unit surgical mortality rate of the above procedures between 1916–1945 was 34.1%, while it was 7.6% between 1948–1953. The 1948–1953 rate was only 22% of the 1916–1948 rate.

TABLE 12-1, B. OPERATIVE RISK
1948–1962

OPERATION	TIME PERIOD	OPERATIVE MORTALITY PER CENT
Correction of obstructions of small intestine	1948–1958	11–12%
Surgical therapy of hepatic injuries	1955–1962	14%
Simple stab wounds	1955–1962	3.4%
Blunt trauma	1955–1962	30%

TABLE 12-2. OPERATIVE MORTALITY RELATIVE TO THE ANATOMIC SITE

	OPERATION	MORTALITY RANGE PER CENT	MORTALITY MEAN PER CENT	TIME PERIOD
Group I				
Heart	Mitral commissurotomy	6–11.5		1949–1953
	Cardiopulmonary bypass	28		1956–1959
	Ball valve replacement cardiac valves	16–26	21	1961–1964
Esophagus	Thoracic esophagectomy	13–37.5		1948–1953
	Repair of congenital atresia and fistulae	42–68		1944–1953
Brain	Resection of infiltrating tumors of brain (astroblastoma, glioblastoma, and medulloblastomas)	25–45		1946–1953
Group II				
Gallbladder	Cholecystectomy	0.0– 1.8	0.4	1948–1952
Stomach	Partial gastrectomy for duodenal ulcer	0.8– 1.9		1945–1952
Breast	Radical mastectomy	0.0– 1.8		1935–1952
Colon	Colectomy	4.6– 7.7	5.7	1948–1952
	Radical resection of the rectum	0.0–11.7	6.9	1948–1952
Group III				
Esophagus	Resections of upper esophagus for carcinoma	24		1943–1954
	Resections of lower esophagus for carcinoma	7		1943–1954
Group IV				
Stomach	Closure of perforation of peptic ulcer	16.6 (gastric)		1948–1952
Duodenum	As above	2.7 (duodenal)		1948–1952

tude of the procedure, the age of the person, the character of the disease, the duration of the illness, the metabolic state of the individual, the technic employed to perform an operation, the quality of ancillary medical care and anesthesia.

To be sure, there are others such as emotional state, insanity, the duration of anesthesia and soporific and analgesic drugs. However, they will not be discussed because their influence cannot be assessed.

The locus of an operative procedure plays an important role in the risk attending an operation. Operations performed upon the heart, the thoracic esophagus and the brain are more risky than those performed upon the gallbladder, the stomach, the appendix, the lung or the breast. Even the location of the disease within a single organ affects risk; the operative death rate is higher with resections of upper esophageal carcinoma than it is with resection of lower lesions (Table 12-2).

The risk attending a surgical procedure upon an organ or within an anatomic cavity tends to be directly related to the magnitude of the procedure: a higher mortality rate obtains with a resection of the entire stomach than it does with a resection of a part of it. This and other examples of the influence of the magnitude of the operation upon operative risk are tabulated in Table 12-3.

The comparison of gross operative mortality rates among the aged and the young leads to this generalization: aging increases the operative risk. J. and J. C. Mithoefer[10] found during 1952 and 1953 a gross operative mortality rate of 8.3 per cent among 240 individuals aged over 70 years and a rate of 1.9 per cent among 1,073 persons less than 70 years old. Between 1948 and 1952 Cole[3] noted

234 The Assessment of Operative Risk

TABLE 12-3. OPERATIVE MORTALITY RELATIVE TO MAGNITUDE OF THE PROCEDURE

	OPERATION	MORTALITY RANGE PER CENT	MORTALITY MEAN PER CENT	TIME PERIOD
Stomach	Partial gastrectomy for carcinoma	6.7–13.6	..	1940–1952
	Total gastrectomy for carcinoma	20 –35.7	..	1947–1952
Colon	Appendectomy	0.1– 0.45	..	1943–1953
	Colectomy (exclusive of rectum)	4.6– 7.7	5.7	1948–1952
	Radical resection of rectum	0.0–11.7	6.9	1948–1952
Lung	Segmental resection	0.9	..	1949–1953
	Lobectomy	0.0– 2.3	2.1	1948–1952
	Pneumonectomy	12.2–27.7	16.5	1948–1952
Biliary Ducts	Cholecystectomy	0.0– 1.8	0.4	1948–1952
	Cholecystectomy and choledochostomy	0.0–10	2.0	1948–1952
	Choledochoplasty	2.3– 8.3	3.7	1948–1952
Liver	Repair hepatic injury only	4.8	..	1939–1962
	Repair hepatic injury and injuries to one or more other organs	11–85	24	1939–1962

gross operative mortality rates of 2.07 per cent and 5.1 per cent among 2,577 persons under 60 and 1,099 over 60 years of age, respectively. However, after comparing the operative mortalities pertinent to the old and the young obtaining during and after specific operations one is led to conclude that the effect of aging upon the operative risk is variable. The risk attending some operations is the same for the aged and the younger persons (Table 12-4, B),

TABLE 12-4, A. OPERATIVE RISK AND AGE

OPERATION	AGE	MORTALITY PER CENT	NUMBER IN SERIES	TIME PERIOD	P OLD = YOUNG
Closure of perforated peptic ulcer	20–39	5	41		
	40–59	15.6	64	1935–1941	0.01
	60–79	40.0	28		
Radical surgery for cancer of mouth and neck	Under 60	1.0	105	1948–1952	0.001
	Over 60	11.5	121		
*Cholecystectomy with and without choledochostomy	Under 70	1.18	513	1944–1951	0.01
	Over 70	5.7	70		
Radical resection of rectum for cancer	Under 60	0.0	53	1948–1952	0.01
	Over 60	11.7	62		
	(Over 70	16	82)	1955–1958	...
†Gastrectomy for duodenal ulcer	Under 40	1.3	77		
	Over 40	7.9	240	1940–1950	0.05
	(Over 70	23	35)		
Pneumonectomy	Under 60	12.2	49	1948–1952	0.01
	Over 60	27.2	18		
Resection abdominal aortic aneurysm	Under 60	5	444	1953–1964	0.001
	60-69	11	723		
	(70-90	12	282)		

* Between 1948 and 1952 Cole found no significant difference between individuals less than and over 60 years (see Table 12-4, B, Cholecystectomy).
† At variance with Cole's later finding (see Table 12-4, B, Gastrectomy for peptic ulcer).

TABLE 12-4, B. OPERATIVE RISK AND AGE
(From Cole—Operability in young and aged)

OPERATION	AGE	MORTALITY PER CENT	NUMBER IN SERIES	TIME PERIOD	P OLD = YOUNG
Esophagectomy for cancer	Under 60	29.4	17	1948–1952	0.4
	Over 60	41.9	31		
Colectomy	Under 60	4.6	43	1948–1952	0.6
	Over 60	7.7	26		
Radical mastectomy	Under 60	0	122	1948–1952	..
	Over 60	0	67		
Cholecystectomy	Under 60	0	169	1948–1952	>0.1
	Over 60	1.8	54		
Thyroidectomy	Under 60	0	287	1948–1952	..
	Over 60	0	44		
Herniorrhaphy	Under 60	0.3	313	1948–1952	0.3
	Over 60	1.5	68		
Partial gastrectomy for cancer	Under 60	5.8	34		
	Over 60	2.8	36	1948–1952	0.5
	(Over 70	31	45)*		
	Under 40	17.7	17	1940–1950	0.7
	Over 40	13.2	59		
Partial gastrectomy for peptic ulcer	Under 60	1.5	67	1948–1952	0.6
	Over 60	0.0	24		

* Herron et al.: Ann. Surg., 152:686, 1960.

while it is distinctly lower for the younger in others (Table 12-4, A).

The probabilities that the death rates attending the operations in Table 12-4, A, are the same among the older and the younger are so small as to permit the assumption that there is very small likelihood of chance accounting for the observed variances in mortality between the young and the old. Therefore, one may conclude that the operative risk attending the operations listed in Table 12-4, A, is greater for the aged than for the young. However, such is not the case for the operations listed in Table 12-4, B; the probabilities that the operative mortalities are the same among the old and the young are so large as to permit the conclusion that the risk attending the operations in Table 12-4, B, is the same for the old and the young.

Obviously, one cannot formulate a gener-

TABLE 12-5. CHANGING RELATIONSHIP OF OPERATIVE RISK TO AGE

OPERATION	AGE	MORTALITY PER CENT		
			1941	1951
Cholecystectomy	10–60		4.0	1.1
	61 and older		16.6	5.7
	Difference		12.6	4.6
		1928	1927–1931	1940–1949 5th decade only
Appendectomy for simple and complicated appendicitis	0–60	0.4	4.1	0.7 (274)
	61 and older	54	24.0	4.5 (88)
	Difference	53.6 (Fitch)	19.9 (Boland)	3.8 (Wolff)

The Assessment of Operative Risk

TABLE 12-6. AGE AND MORTALITY

	BURNS				OTHER OPERATIONS*		
	Mortality %†				Mortality %		
Area injured % body surface	Age 0–60	Age 60+	Difference	Operations‡	Age 0–60	Age 60+	Difference
5	0.005	2	..				
10	0.1	10	..				
15	1	35	34	2	1	11.5	10.5
20	2	60	58	4	5.8	2.8	
25	4	88	84				
30	8	95	87	1	10	40	30
35	16	98	82	3	12	27	15

* Arranged in order of mortality comparable with burns of persons 0–60 years old.
† Minimal death expectancies derived from probit analysis of thermal injuries in Dallas, Texas, between 1945 and 1952.
‡ Operation: (1) closure perforated peptic ulcer, (2) radical surgery for cancer of mouth and neck, (3) pneumonectomy, (4) partial gastrectomy for cancer.

alization pertinent to the influence of aging upon operative mortality. The rapidity with which the operative mortality rates attending certain operations upon the elderly and the young have approached or are approaching one another (Table 12-5) indicates that aging likely has little inherent effect upon one's capacity to live during an operation and the convalescence after it, provided that the time requisite for phyisologic recovery postoperatively is not prolonged. A cursory search for possible reasons for the lack of difference between the operative mortalities among the young and the old attending such major physically deforming operations as colectomy, radical mastectomy and partial gastrectomy (1948-1952), while a difference exists between the mortalities of the 2 age groups following lesser physically deforming operations such as closure of perforated peptic ulcers and radical surgery of the mouth and the neck, is highly suggestive that the time requisite for physiologic recovery is more important than the anatomic magnitude of the procedure in determining the relative capacity of an aged individual to live after an operation. In other words, of 2 operations effecting equal physical and physiologic deformations, that one producing the physiologic deformation of shortest duration will be the one least likely to be attended by a higher operative mortality among the aged.

This thesis is supported by the following observations: (1) A higher mortality exists among the aged after those operations that are especially prone to be followed by suppuration and other complications (closure of perforated peptic ulcer, radical resection of the rectum, and radical surgery of the mouth and the neck). (2) The same operative mortality exists among young and old after operations seldom attended by complications (mastectomy, thyroidectomy, herniotomy and partial gastrectomy). (3) Burns which usually are followed by a longer period of physiologic deformation than any operative procedure listed in Tables 12-4, A and B, are associated with a discrepancy between the mortality rates among old and young greater than that attending any operation (Table 12-6).

In other words, the old person is as capable as the young one of withstanding an operation having a short period of physiologic upset, but he is less capable of taking in stride one with a prolonged period of physiologic derangement. Another way to say the same thing is a paraphrase of one of Mithoefers' conclusions: An increased operative fatality rate among the aged when it exists is not dependent upon old age itself but is relatable to the lack of tolerance of the aged to complications and misdirected therapy.

These observations and surmises concerning the relationship of operative risk to age provide a basis for the expectation that surgeons may well abolish the influence of age

The Assessment of Operative Risk

Operative risk and disease are related. Partial gastrectomy, esophagectomy, and thyroidectomy performed for cancer are more risky than partial gastrectomy for duodenal and gastric ulcers, esophagectomy for benign esophageal stricture, and thyroidectomy for thyrotoxicosis. The comparative mortalities are listed in Table 12-7.

It might well be argued that the disease, cancer, is not the direct cause of this phenomenon, but rather that the greater age of the cancerous person, his poorer nutrition, and the wider extent of the operation for cancer are. These may be the real causes, but there is no objective evidence that they are. So until data are collected to prove or disprove this argument it needs be said that a particular operation performed for cancer carries a higher risk than it does when performed for another disease.

...upon operative risk by learning how to shorten the postoperative period of physiologic deformation, how to reduce further the frequency of complications, and how to avoid the use of misdirected therapy.

TABLE 12-7. OPERATIVE MORTALITY RELATIVE TO THE DISEASE OF THE ORGAN

OPERATION	MORTALITY PER CENT	NUMBER OF CASES
Partial gastrectomy (Kurzweg) 1940–50		
for: carcinoma of stomach	13.64	176
gastric ulcer	5.26	152
duodenal ulcer	6.25	320
Partial gastrectomy (Cole) 1948–52		
for: carcinoma of stomach	4.3	70
duodenal and gastric ulcers	1.1	91
Thyroidectomy		
for: carcinoma (1924–52)	8.5	64
toxic goiter (1928–29)	0.5 to 2	over 100
Esophagectomy and primary anastomosis (Burford) 1948–53		
for: chemical strictures	0.0	30
peptic esophagitis	2.4	41
carcinoma	20.0	98

TABLE 12-8. INFLUENCE OF DURATION OF ILLNESS UPON OPERATIVE MORTALITY

OPERATION	DURATION OF ILLNESS	MORTALITY	
		1940–1944	1945–1949
Closure of perforated peptic ulcer	0–12 hours	21.6%	3.8%
	12 or more	45.5%	18.7%
		1934–1951	
Reduction of intussusception, or resection for	0–24 hours	1.5% (66)	
	0–48	3.4% (89)	
	Longer than 48	25.6% (27)	
		1930–1935	
Appendectomy (all types of appendicitis—simple and complicated)	0–6 hours	0.0% (219)	
	6–12	1.0% (578)	
	13–18	1.0% (204)	
	19–36	4.4% (1,004)	
	37–72	5.4% (930)	
	72 plus	8.0% (578)	
		1936	
Appendicitis, complicated by rupture, peritonitis, etc. (appendectomy and drainage of abscesses)	0–12 hours	1.8% (212)	
	12–24	2.4% (411)	
	24–36	3.0% (134)	
	36–48	8.1% (296)	
	48–72	8.6% (221)	
	72–96	10.5% (86)	
	5 days plus	14.2% (225)	

TABLE 12-9. INFLUENCE OF SUPPURATION UPON OPERATIVE RISK

OPERATION	MORTALITY PER CENT	NUMBER IN SERIES	SOURCE AND TIME
1. Appendectomy			
A. For: acute local appendicitis	1.7	1340	St. Thomas Hospital
appendicitis with local abscess	8.0	189	London
appendicitis with generalized peritonitis	21.1	226	1920–1929
B. For: appendicitis without peritonitis	0.45	2160	Seneque
appendicitis with generalized peritonitis	4.4	253	1934–1953
C. For: acute local appendicitis	0	288	Babcock 1951–1955
	0.2	441	Campbell 1953–1956
appendicitis with local abscess	0	39	Campbell 1953–1956
perforated appendicitis with peritonitis	1.8	113	Babcock 1951–1955
	7.2	69	Campbell 1953–1956
2. Cholecystectomy			
For: uncomplicated acute cholecystitis	6.5	..	
acute cholecystitis with walled-off perforation	15.0	90	Pines 1942–1952
acute cholecystitis with free perforation	23.3		
3. Resection of small intestine			
For: nongangrenous bowel	7	14	
gangrenous nonperforated	31	32	Bollinger 1953
gangrenous perforated	40	15	
4. Pneumonectomy			
For: tuberculosis			
A. Before streptomycin	66	6	Efskind
B. With streptomycin	6	90	1946–1953

There is much to the saying that the longer the lapse of time between the onset of illness and the operation to correct it, the greater the surgical risk. The direct relationship between operative risk and procrastination is especially apparent in a number of diseases with inflammatory components. The association of risk with time in a number of such disease entities is shown in Table 12-8. By virtue of the direct relationship of time-lapse to perforation of the gallbladder with cholecystitis and gangrene of the intestine with intestinal obstructions Parts 2 and 3 of Table 12-9 are also illustrative of the increase in operative risk with increase in time between the onset of the disease and the operation.

Although for some time great emphasis has been placed upon the influence of the metabolic state of the individual upon his capacity to withstand surgical therapeusis, remarkably little human data is available for the quantitative assessment thereof. Although everyone agrees that individuals ill with adrenal cortical insufficiency, uncontrolled diabetes or myxedema are "poor operative risks," one cannot find data that might permit the formulation of an idea of how much these metabolic diseases increase risk. A rough idea of the influence exerted by two metabolic dyscrasias—myasthenia gravis and thyrotoxicosis—may be drawn from the figures presented in Table 12-10.

Because suppuration induces appreciable metabolic alterations, the relationship of operative risk to suppuration may well be considered as an example of the relationship of metabolic state to operative risk. The development of local or general peritonitis increases

TABLE 12-10. INFLUENCE OF METABOLIC STATE UPON OPERATIVE MORTALITY

OPERATION	MORTALITY PER CENT	NUMBER IN SERIES	TIME PERIOD
Superior Mediastinal Exploration			
Removal of benign			
(A) mediastinal tumors	1–3		1945–1950
Removal of thymus			
(B) or thymic tumors from persons	16.6	12	1946–1953
having myasthenia gravis	33.0	12	1953
Subtotal Thyroidectomy			
For: (A) nontoxic goiter	1	900	1895
(B) toxic goiter	3–12	+1000	1920

the postoperative mortality rate significantly, although the influence it bears is less today than it was 30 years ago. Compare parts (A) and (B) of Section 1, Table 12-9.

Malnutrition in general and more especially "protein depletion" and vitamin deficiencies are imputed to exert relatively enormous effects on operative risk. To be sure, animals are poor operative risks when so starved as to be barely alive, or so subjected to repeated plasmaphoresis as to be so ill that some die without being operated upon, but extreme states such as these are rarely seen among men, women, or children in the United States.

Without a doubt, the administration of vitamin K to jaundiced persons has reduced materially the operative hazard of choledochostomy. A statement such as this and applicable to all operations cannot be made with equal surety for the administration of vitamins A, B, C, D, or E to the malnourished person.

Although the imputation to starvation and more especially to protein-starvation of a major detrimental influence upon operative risk is logical and is supported by some experimental work performed upon animals other than man, the human evidence in support of this belief is practically nonexistent. However, human starvation effecting a loss of weight so as to reduce the individual to below 80 per cent of normal is attended by diarrhea in 20 to 50 per cent of men and a mortality up to 10 per cent among those having the flux. Obviously, the performance of surgery upon starved individuals should carry a greater risk for that reason alone. However, the experiences of American and European military physicians in Japanese prisoner-of-war camps during World War II were such as to indicate that even severe starvation has relatively little influence upon operative risk. In Gottlieb's words:[6]

An interesting observation is that men who in ordinary times would be considered very poor surgical risks because of their emaciation, amebiasis, and vitamin deficiencies responded very well under surgery. In fact, most of them sat up and asked for rice in about 36 hours. There were no cases of pulmonary embolism. Excellent results were obtained in abdominal surgery even though there was very little asepsis. There was no postoperative peritonitis, very little abdominal distention, and no stitch abscesses appeared.

Apparently, the deleterious effects of caloric and protein starvation and vitamin deficiencies upon one's capacity to live during and after an operation are not as remarkable or as general as many supposed them to be. For this reason delay of indicated operations should not be based upon need to improve nutrition and especially when the malnutrition has a surgically remedial intestinal lesion at the bottom of it.

This statement must not be construed as an argument for the reduction of attention to improving a starved individual's nutritional status before and after operating upon him. Nonetheless, it may well be used as an argument for an immediate attack upon such lesions as pyloric and intestinal obstructions, enteral fistulas and the placement of grafts on burns.

That severe anemia increases operative hazard is well established through animal experimentation and clinical observations. Such a dogmatic statement cannot be made in regard to the effect of hypoproteinemia alone, notwithstanding many positive statements to the contrary.

The operative risk attending an operation is in part dependent upon the technical manner with which the operation is performed. Table 12-11, A, illustrates this point.

TABLE 12-11, A. OPERATIVE MORTALITY RELATIVE TO TECHNIC EMPLOYED TO PERFORM A PROCEDURE

OPERATION	MORTALITY PER CENT	NUMBER IN SERIES
Partial gastrectomy (Kurzweg)* 1940–50		
with an antecolic gastrojejunostomy	10.5	210
with a retrocolic gastrojejunostomy	5.8	398
Polya	9.8	275
Hofmeister	4.6	326
Drainage of Subphrenic Abscess (Ochsner and DeBakey) 1938		
Extraperitoneal	10.8	67
Transpleural	36.2	394
Transperitoneal	35.1	327
Prefrontal Lobotomy (W. Freeman) 1936–52		
Transcranial	3.6	624
Transorbital	1.7	1239
Closure of Perforated Peptic Ulcer (Donhauser) 1935–51		
Closure without drainage of peritoneal cavity	3.2	61
Closure with drainage (nonsuction) of peritoneal cavity	20.3	54

* Partial gastrectomy for carcinoma, and peptic ulcers of stomach and duodenum. The use of the various technics, so far as can be determined, was applied randomly in the treatment of carcinoma and ulcer.

Much attention has been placed upon the so-called pulmonary-cardiac status as an important determinant of risk. However, as more surgical experience is gained upon persons suffering from pulmonary and cardiac ills, the less important as a risk factor does pulmonary-cardiac disease become. In fact, excepting the existence of angina pectoris, malignant hypertension, repeated or recent myocardial infarction, physically disabling pulmonary emphysema and uncontrolled cardiac failure, the pulmonary-cardiac status changes operative risk very little. The Mithoefers[10] studied 240 aged individuals who were classified as poor or good cardiopulmonary risks preoperatively and found no significant difference in operative mortality between the 2 groups. This led them to the conclusion that cardiopulmonary disease, when unaccompanied by angina pectoris, has no apparent influence upon the surgical mortality among the aged.

Cardiopulmonary disease, however, may influence the mortality rates after some operations. De Bakey has shown that the coexistence of heart disease and hypertension adversely affects the mortality rate associated with resections of abdominal aortic aneurysms (Table 12-11, B).

TABLE 12-11, B. THE INFLUENCE OF HEART DISEASE AND HYPERTENSION ON OPERATIVE MORTALITY ASSOCIATED WITH RESECTIONS OF ABDOMINAL AORTIC ANEURYSMS*

	NUMBER OF PATIENTS	NUMBER OF OPERATIVE DEATHS	PER CENT
Heart disease and hypertension present	342	55	16
Heart disease and hypertension absent	465	14	3

* De Bakey, Ann. Surg., 160:622, 1964.

The mortality rates in the last decade associated with operations for major arterial disease vary with the stage, type and site of the arterial disease (Table 12-11, C).

Advanced renal and hepatic insufficiency reduces the chance of living after an operation. The postoperative mortality rate attending portacaval shunting for bleeding esophageal varices was 3 to 5 times higher for those individuals having serum albumin concentrations less than 3 Gm. per cent or cephalin flocculations of 3+ to 4+, or B.S.P. retentions greater than 10 per cent, or ascites that did

TABLE 12-11, C. OPERATIVE MORTALITY ASSOCIATED WITH OPERATIONS FOR ANEURYSMAL AND OCCLUSIVE VASCULAR DISEASE

OPERATIONS TO CORRECT	TIME PERIOD	NUMBER IN SERIES	MORTALITY PER CENT
Aneurysms of the thoracic aorta	1954–1956[1]	15	33
	1951–1956[2]	68	34
Aneurysms of abdominal aorta			
a. Not ruptured	1953–1957[3]	85	26
	1958–1961[3]	85	11
	1955–1962[4]	66	15
	1958–1962[5]	791	9
	1962–1964[5]	533	5
b. Ruptured	1955–1962[4]	55	59
	1953–1961[6]	76	58
	1953–1964[5]	117	35
Aortic iliac occlusions	1953–1958[7]	448	2.7
Femoral popliteal occlusions	1953–1958[7]	353	1.0

[1] Ellis, Surg., Gynec. & Obstet., 106:179-192, 1958.
[2] Cooley, Am. Surg., 22:1043-1051, 1956.
[3] Voorhees, Surg., Gynec. & Obstet., 117:355-358, 1963.
[4] Cannon, Am. J. Surg., 106:128-143, 1963.
[5] De Bakey, Ann. Surg., 160:622, 1964.
[6] Stallworth, Ann. Surg., 155:711-720, 1962.
[7] De Bakey, Ann. Surg., 148:306, 1958.

not disappear with medical treatment, than it was for those persons having serum albumin above 3 Gm. per cent, cephalin flocculations of 1+ to 2+, B.S.P. retention less than 10 per cent, and ascites that disappeared with medical therapy.[9] Blakemore's[2] experience was similar to Linton's. Both Linton and Blakemore found that the mere existence of ascites, the level of serum bilirubin and the prothrombin time were no indicators of the operative risk attending portacaval shunting for bleeding esophageal varices or portal hypertension.

The anesthetic agent employed to perform an operative procedure often has been incriminated as a very important risk factor. The anesthetic risks associated with the administration of 9 agents or combinations thereof are listed in Table 12-12.[1] More than 60 per cent of anesthesias were performed by nurse anesthetists and residents. Clearly, today anesthesia carries relatively little of the burden of the total operative risk. Only with operations bearing little risk, such as herniorraphy, appendectomy, thyroidectomy and the like, is the anesthetic risk a highly important factor.

A gross idea of the relative importance of

TABLE 12-12. ANESTHESIA AND OPERATIVE RISK*

AGENT	ANESTHESIA DEATH RATE PER CENT	NUMBER IN SERIES
Nitrous oxide	0.0190	26,200
Thiopental	0.0430	14,000
Thiopental and nitrous oxide	0.0400	43,000
Thiopental and/or nitrous oxide with "curare"	0.1280	38,100
Cyclopropane	0.0188	37,100
Cyclopropane—"curare"	0.0833	2,400
Ether	0.0390	171,300
Ether—"curare"	0.4000	2,000
Ethylene	0.0068	29,200

* Beecher and Todd, Ann. Surg., 140:2, 1954.

anesthetic risk in the total picture of operative risk can be gained from Beecher and Todd's[1] figures listed below:

CAUSE OF DEATH (PRIMARY)	NUMBER	MORTALITY	RATE
Patient's disease	6325	1:95	1%
Surgical error	1428	1:420	0.23%
Anesthesia, primary and contributory	385	1:1560	0.06%

Clearly, surgical errors in diagnosis, judgment and technic contribute 4 times as much as anesthesia to operative risk. This statement is in part unfair to anesthesia because when the calculation of the relative contributions of surgical error and anesthesia is based upon death

TABLE 12-13. INFLUENCE OF QUALITY OF NURSING UPON OPERATIVE RISK*

OPERATION	MORTALITY PER CENT	NUMBER	P
Pneumonectomy			
Poor nursing	29.6	91	P:G
Good nursing	11.8	68	0.1
Lobectomy			
Poor nursing	7.5	13	P:G
Good nursing	3.5	28	0.5

* Brea, Buenos Aires, 1944–52.

attributable to anesthesia alone, surgical error is found to contribute 6 times as much as anesthesia to the operative risk.

The quality of nursing and general hospital services, and the capacity of the surgeon are very important risk factors, though data supporting this statement is remarkably scarce. Table 12-13 shows presumably the effect of quality of nursing upon operative risk. The mortality rate attending pneumonectomy is considerably higher with "poor" nursing than it is with "good" nursing, but the mortality

TABLE 12-14.

Formula for Adjusted χ^2 (chi square)

$$\chi^2 = \frac{[(ad - bc) - N/2]^2 N}{(a + b)(c + d)(a + c)(b + d)}$$

Treatment Series	Living	Dead	
I	a	b	a + b
II	c	d	c + d
	a + c	b + d	a + b + c × d = N

a—number patients living } of Treatment
b—number patients dead } Series I
c—number patients living } of Treatment
d—number patients dead } Series II

Table of Values of Probabilities for Adjusted Chi Square (χ^2)
One Degree of Freedom from Table IV*

If χ^2 =	.000157	.000628	.00393	.0158	.0642	.148	.455	1.074
Then P =	.99	.98	.95	.90	.80	.70	.50	.30

If χ^2 =	1.642	2.706	3.841	5.412	6.635	10.827
Then P =	.20	.10	.05	.02	.01	.001

Example:

Treatment Series		Living	Dead	
I	Albumin: <3.0 gm.	a 1	b 5	6
II	>3.0 gm.	c 63	d 6	69
		64	11	75

Calculation of example:

$$\text{Adj. } \chi^2 = \frac{[(1 \times 6) - (5 \times 63) - 75/2]^2 \, 75}{(1 + 5)(63 + 6)(1 + 63)(5 + 6)} =$$

$$\text{Adj. } \chi^2 = \frac{[(6 - 315) - 38\,^2] \, 75}{6 \times 69 \times 64 \times 11} = 18.9, \therefore P = <.001$$

Conclusion: Individuals having portacaval shunts for bleeding esophageal varices who have serum albumin concentrations above 3 grams per cent do not die postoperatively with the same frequency that persons having serum albumin concentrations below 3 grams per cent do.

* From Fisher, R. A., and Yates, F.: Statistical Tables for Biological, Medical and Agricultural Research. London, Oliver, 1939.

associated with lobectomy is not significantly higher. Data should be gathered to permit an assessment of the parts played by the surgeon and the hospital in operative risk. It may well be that the surgeon, or he who calls himself one, may be in some hospitals the major factor in the total picture of surgical risk.

Although this discussion of operative risk is sketchy and brief, it should be adequate to permit this statement: the accurate assessment of operative risk is impossible today and can be no more than a guess at best.

In a number of tables in this chapter there is a column designated "P." "P" represents the probability or the chance that if one condition exists, a "given" result will occur. Thus, a "P" value of 0.05 means that if 100 tests were run, one could expect the "given" result 95 times. The numbers in these columns were derived from calculations of chi square (x^2) using the formula of Table 12-14 and the Fisher and Yates table which is also included in Table 12-14 for the conversion of the (x^2's) to probabilities (P's).

The sample calculation of a chi square in Table 12-14 uses figures taken from Linton's article.[9]

The hypothesis tested in this way may be simply stated: "The outcome of the operation is the same regardless of the value of the variable"—the variable being such things as age of patient, sex, type of operation, etc. The derivation of a probability (P) larger than 0.05 indicates that under the conditions of the test the hypothesis stated above is conventionally acceptable and the more especially should the P be greater than 0.1.

The utility of statistical methods in evaluating the merits and the demerits of various forms of treatment, and the influence of varied factors upon the outcome of different ills and operations is now unquestioned. The medical student should look upon his mastery of the elements of statistics as an invaluable part of his education for the actual practice of medicine. He must be able to evaluate critically the claims made for the effectiveness of drugs and operations, and to do this he needs a working knowledge of statistical methods and of experimental design.

REFERENCES*

1. Beecher, H. K., and Todd, D. P.: A study of the deaths associated with anesthesia and surgery. Ann. Surg., 140:2-34, 1954.
2. Blakemore, A. H.: Portocaval shunting for portal hypertension. Surg., Gynec. Obstet., 94:443-454, 1952.
3. Cole, W. H.: Operability in the young and aged. Ann. Surg., 138:145-157, 1953.
4. Fisher, R. A., and Yates, F.: Statistical Tables for Biological, Medical and Agricultural Research. London, Oliver, 1939.
5. Gibbon, J. H., et al.: Cancer of the lung; an analysis of 532 consecutive cases. Ann. Surg., 138:489-501, 1953.
6. Gottlieb, M. L.: Impressions of a P.O.W. medical officer in Japanese concentration camps. U.S. Naval Med. Bull., 46:663-675, 1946.
7. Hill, A. B.: Principles of Medical Statistics. ed. 5. New York, Oxford University Press, 1950.
8. Johnson, P. O.: Statistical Methods in Research, New York, Prentice-Hall, 1949.
9. Linton, R. L.: Selection of patients for portacaval shunt. Ann. Surg., 134:433-443, 1951.
10. Mithoefer, J., and Mithoefer, J. C.: Studies of the aged; surgical mortality. A.M.A. Arch. Surg., 69:58-65, 1954.
11. Nemir, P., Jr.: Intestinal obstruction. Ann. Surg., 135:367-375, 1952.
12. Sparkman, R. S., and Fogelman, M. J.: Wounds of the liver. Ann. Surg., 139:690-719, 1954.
13. Sweet, R. H.: Total gastrectomy by the transthoracic approach. Ann. Surg., 138:297-310, 1953.
14. Young, M., and Russell, W. T: Appendicitis: A Statistical Study. Spec. Rep. Ser. 233, Med. Res. Council, Great Britain, 1939.

* The items listed here (but not referred to in the text) have been selected for their excellent bibliographies and comparative statistics concerning the entities named in the titles.

CHAPTER 13

ROBERT D. DRIPPS, M.D.

Anesthesia

Premedication
Inhalational Anesthesia
Intravenous Anesthesia
Conduction Anesthesia
Spinal Anesthesia
Epidural Anesthesia
Muscle Relaxants
Respiratory Problems Associated With Unconsciousness
Anesthetic Management of the "Poor Risk" Patient
Anesthesia for Battle Casualties
Special Anesthetic Technics
Unusual Complications of Anesthesia
Fire and Explosion Hazards
Postanesthetic Observation Room (Recovery Room)
Mechanical Ventilation of the Lungs

Among his professional achievements a physician should have the ability to administer an anesthetic and to supervise intelligently a patient under the influence of that anesthetic. Practical skill in anesthesia can be acquired only in the operating room through personal experience, but certain principles can be set down as guides toward that experience. Some of these will be presented in this chapter. Others can be found in a monograph published by the author and his associates (1967).

The signs and the stages of general anesthesia are described in current pharmacologic texts and should be reviewed by the student. These guides to progressive degrees of narcosis are most accurate for ether. However, familiarity with the basic pharmacologic properties of the other general anesthetic agents permits a reasonable estimate of the depth of anesthesia with these substances. Technical aspects of anesthesia will not be considered.

PREMEDICATION

Premedication refers to the use of drugs prior to the administration of an anesthetic, chiefly to decrease anxiety and to provide a smoother induction of, maintenance of, and emergence from anesthesia. Although most anesthetists use barbiturates or narcotic analgesics for premedication, other drugs such as the phenothiazines and the tranquilizers have been prescribed. Data in support of such use of these substances have been meager.

Before considering the effectiveness of drugs in reducing apprehension, one must recognize how much tranquility can result from an anesthetist's preoperative visit. Egbert and colleagues (1963) compared the calming effect of a properly conducted preoperative visit with that provided by a placebo or pentobarbital (2 mg./kg.) given intramuscularly one hour before operation. Fifty-eight per cent of patients in whom sedatives were omitted and 61 per cent receiving pentobarbital, neither group having had a preoperative visit by an anesthetist, claimed to be nervous on interview just prior to induction of anesthesia. On the other hand, nervousness existed in only 40 per cent of those who did have a preoperative visit from an anesthetist during which discussion concerned the patient's condition, the time of operation, the nature of the anesthetic, and the events of the next day. Therefore, factors other than drugs favorably affect preoperative psychologic preparation. Instruction, suggestion and encouragement are useful nonpharmacologic antidotes to anxiety and tension. A similar approach to the relief or the avoidance of postoperative pain resulted in a marked reduction of postoperative narcotic requirements.

The physical condition of the patient partially determines whether a premedicant is needed and if so in what quantity. The more ill, the more elderly, the less robust and active the patient, the less are sedatives and analgesics indicated. A degree of physical and mental depression already exists in such individuals.

Finally, it should be emphasized that the production of drowsiness or sleepiness by a drug does not guarantee the absence of apprehension. For many frightened individuals, relief of anxiety comes only with oblivion. Some pediatric anesthetists desire children below the age of 5 years to be sound asleep on arrival in the operating room area, but this need rarely be the goal of preanesthetic medication in adults.

Narcotic Analgesics. Morphine, in the usual doses of 8 to 10 mg. intramuscularly, reduces anxiety and tension in patients prior to operation, although perhaps not quite to the same extent as secobarbital. Its general depressant action is of value in children with congenital cyanotic heart disease, often decreasing the right to left shunt and lessening arterial hypoxia. If pain is present before operation, morphine is one of the drugs of choice, or if weak general anesthetic agents such as nitrous oxide, or nonanalgesic drugs such as halothane or thiopental are selected, preoperative use of narcotics provides a smoother maintenance of anesthesia. It is this pain-relieving property which in all probability minimizes the incidence of restlessness or excitation during emergence from general anesthesia, particularly after cyclopropane. Morphine's respiratory depressant action is useful in converting the tachypnea caused by trichloroethylene or to a lesser extent halothane to a slower, more efficient type of respiration.

Unfortunately, morphine may have undesirable side-effects. It can prolong the awakening from general anesthesia, since it has a long duration of action when given intramuscularly or subcutaneously. Its stimulant effect on smooth muscle may cause spasm of the sphincter of Oddi or of the ureters. Colicky pain, often relieved by atropine but nearly always abolished by a narcotic antagonist, may result from either of these effects. Bronchiolar constriction may develop in patients with asthma. Constipation and urinary retention may be annoying. Hypotension follows the use of morphine more frequently than after other narcotic analgesics. When given before cyclopropane, morphine tends to prevent or reverse the rise in cardiac output often seen with this agent in the absence of a preanesthetic narcotic. Its respiratory depressant action, more evident during cyclopropane and thiopental anesthesia, may increase intracranial pressure through retention of carbon dioxide and subsequent cerebral vasodilation. While this can be undesirable in patients with intracranial pressure already elevated, the effect can be abolished through adequate pulmonary ventilation.

Meperidine (Demerol) in doses of 50 to 100 mg. intramuscularly is commonly used for premedication, despite a high incidence of dizziness, dysphoria and nausea. The drug increases biliary ductal pressure and depresses respiration in the same fashion as does morphine. Tachycardia occasionally occurs, posing a problem in differential diagnosis.

The recent introduction of fentanyl (Sublimaze), an ultra-short-acting, powerful narcotic analgesic, has been of interest, since one now has an analgesic whose action begins to lessen within an hour. This is of use in preventing prolonged depression in the postoperative period.

Barbiturates. Pentobarbital and secobarbital are the barbituric acid derivatives used most frequently to relieve apprehension before operation. They may be administered orally or intramuscularly to adults—doses of 100 to 200 mg.—and in doses of 2 mg./lb. for infants and children. These drugs have minimal depressant action on respiration and circulation. Patients receiving either barbiturate for premedication usually awaken more promptly from a general anesthetic than if a narcotic had been given, but the incidence of emergence excitation tends to be higher, presumably because of greater awareness of pain.

Phenothiazines. At least ten different phenothiazine derivatives have been recommended for premedication. These substances were recommended because of sedative, antiarrhythmic, local anesthetic, antihistaminic and antiemetic properties. Most often these drugs are combined with a barbiturate or a narcotic, since dysphoria and restlessness may follow their use alone. In combination, greater sedation is anticipated. Although some speak of synergism or potentiation, mere addition of effect seems to be sufficient to explain the results noted. Most thoughtful clinicians doubt the value of routine adminstration of these compounds for this purpose, preferring to treat nausea and vomiting actively should such symptoms require therapy after operation. The ability of phenothiazines to prevent or minimize shock due to blood loss or trauma through an adrenergic blocking action has theoretic appeal but has proved to be difficult to document. With the availability of blood transfusions, hemorrhagic shock is so uncommon that attempts at routine preoperative prophylaxis do not seem to be necessary. Chlorpromazine has essentially been abandoned for preanesthetic purposes because of an unacceptable incidence of arterial hypotension. Tachycardia is an occasional sequel, particularly of promazine.

Rectal Premedication. Two decades ago tribromoethanol, given rectally, was popular for sedation prior to operation, but today it is used infrequently. Its tendency to produce hypotension, the possibility of hepatic or renal damage, and, most important, the relative uncontrollability of drug absorption have contributed to this decline. Thiopental, 15 to 20 mg./lb. in a 10 per cent solution, instilled into the rectum, has succeeded tribromoethanol as the agent of choice for nervous children prior to operation, but this technic is uncommon for adults.

Anticholinergic Drugs. The excessive respiratory tract secretions concomitant with ether demanded the use of some type of parasympatholytic drug prior to anesthetization. Atropine achieved considerable popularity for this purpose during the first half of this century, particularly preceding the open-drop administration of ether. With better vaporizers and more skilled personnel, secretions have become less of a problem with ether, and still less with most of the newer general anesthetics such as halothane and methoxyflurane. Despite a lessened need, atropine or a similar substance continues to be given as an antisialogogue by most anesthetists. The onset of this effect is within 10 to 15 minutes of intramuscular injection, and the duration about 90 minutes for the standard 0.4 to 0.6 mg. dose. The vagal blocking action of such an amount is small and is of briefer duration, lasting perhaps no more than 45 minutes.

Sudden and profound reduction in the pulse rate may occur during anesthesia and operation. Cessation of cardiac action may even result. When this is caused by increased vagal activity, as with increased ocular pressure, the injection of multiple doses of succinylcholine, or after traction on intra-abdominal structures such as the mesentery, the uterus, or the gallbladder, the intravenous injection of atropine often promptly restores cardiac rate and arterial pressure toward normal. If the anesthetic is cyclopropane, atropine should be injected slowly and in amounts less than 0.4 mg., lest disturbing ventricular rhythms develop. One cannot count on the prophylaxis of these events by the usual doses of atropine given intramuscularly prior to operation.

The drying effect of scopolamine is superior to that of atropine but the drug is less effective than atropine in preventing reflex bradycardia during general anesthesia, particularly in children. Its sedative action is so marked that some anesthetists use it as the sole premedicant. Occasionally, patients become restless or disoriented after scopolamine, and the incidence of emergence excitement appears to be greater after its administration. The excitation may be related to an antianalgesic effect described by Dundee, Nicholl and Moore (1961). Scopolamine is given intramuscularly as a rule in doses of 0.4 to 0.6 mg.

MANAGEMENT OF THE DRUG-DEPENDENT PATIENT

Alcoholism. The acutely intoxicated person is not difficult to manage under general anesthesia, the anesthetic essentially adding to the depressant effects of alcohol. However, inhalational anesthesia may be awkward in the chronic alcoholic. One notes tolerance to the anesthetics, as well as to drugs such as paraldehyde, chloral hydrate and barbiturates. The excitement stage can be prolonged and overdosage occurs with surprising ease. It should also be realized that alcoholics frequently show serious impairment of liver function. Finally, alcohol reduces myocardial contractile force, a fact not generally appreciated.

Barbiturate Dependency. Many individuals take barbiturates, and a high index of suspicion serves the anesthetist well. An accurate history on dosage may be difficult to elicit even when one has determined drug use. Unfortunately, induction of anesthesia may reveal some resistance to CNS depressants in these individuals, but the real problem for the chronically dependent user of barbiturates can be a serious withdrawal syndrome if barbiturates are withheld after operation. Such patients become agitated and weak, exhibit tremors, hyperreflexia, nausea and vomiting, and may hallucinate. Progression of symptoms results in convulsions and hypotension. Administration of the abused drug should be continued during hospitalization of drug-dependent persons.

Narcotic Addiction. A narcotic addict requiring anesthesia and operation is easily managed if maintained on his usual drug dosage. The exact dose may be difficult to determine because of the varying purity and strength of the illicit preparation the addict has been taking. Fortunately, experience at the Addiction Research Center in Lexington, Kentucky indicates that as little as one half of the total daily dose will maintain the average addict, so that there is a considerable margin for error. Usually it is wise to suppress abstinence symptoms until postoperative convalescence has been completed.

The "cured" narcotic user should not be given a narcotic for premedication and after operation should receive nonaddicting analgesics such as methotrimeprazine or pentazocine for pain.

Users of LSD. An adult acutely intoxicated with LSD will be quieted nicely by as little as 100 mg. of pentobarbital intramuscularly. The long-term effects of LSD as they affect general anesthesia are unknown at present.

Marihuana. No problems have yet been described nor are serious ones anticipated for the anesthetic management of patients whose drug abuse is limited to marihuana.

INHALATIONAL ANESTHESIA

GASEOUS AGENTS

Nitrous Oxide. Of the inhalational agents this drug causes the least disturbance to normal bodily function if it is given with a concentration of oxygen equal to or exceeding that in room air (21%). The onset of and the emergence from anesthesia is rapid. Nitrous oxide is a weak anesthetic, but its lack of potency can be overcome in several ways. Preanesthetic medication with narcotics can be provided in doses larger than are used for the more powerful inhalational anesthetics.

Nitrous oxide is also frequently combined with the intravenous injection of a short-acting barbiturate. The inability of the latter to provide analgesia is overcome by the ability of nitrous oxide to interrupt afferent impulses, and the two drugs supplement one another. Another combination includes nitrous oxide, thiopental and a "curare" drug, the last being added to provide muscular relaxation. Finally, volatile liquid anesthetics such as halothane or methoxyflurane are frequently added in small amounts. For the patient in profound shock, nitrous oxide alone in concentrations of as low as 50 per cent has proved to be capable of providing an adequate depth of anesthesia for many surgical procedures. This susceptibility to narcosis of the patient in shock is discussed in the section on the anesthetic management of battle casualties.

A recent combination of anesthetics built around nitrous oxide has been termed *neuroleptanesthesia*. A combination of a neuroleptic, or tranquilizer, and a powerful narcotic analgesic is added to nitrous oxide to achieve a balanced form of anesthesia. The technic originated in Europe after Janssen synthesized several members of the tranquilized butyrophenone series, droperidol and haloperidol, and the newer narcotic analgesics, fentanyl and phenoperidine. A 50:1 mixture of droperidol and fentanyl is commercially supplied in the United States in the form of Innovar. In favor of this combination is the apparent absence of toxic effects on the liver, kidneys, and heart. Droperidol produces a degree of alpha-adrenergic blockade, thus affording moderate protection against catecholamine-induced ventricular arrhythmias. The postoperative course of patients bothered by incisional pain and the discomfort of drainage tubes is more acceptable because, although consciousness returns within minutes, drowsiness and a certain indifference to discomfort persist. This state is undesirable following short operations or those associated with minimal discomfort. Rarely extrapyramidal reactions occur 10 to 24 hours after anesthesia. These respond promptly to the administration of diphenhydramine (Benadryl), atropine, benztropine (Cogentin), or small doses of barbiturates.

During the induction of anesthesia with nitrous oxide, the alveolar concentration of oxygen is increased because nitrous oxide leaves the pulmonary capillaries much more rapidly than does oxygen. At the termination of anesthesia the opposite process occurs, and the outward diffusion of nitrous oxide lowers the alveolar partial pressure of oxygen by about 10 per cent during the first few minutes after nitrous oxide–oxygen anesthesia is concluded and the patient has begun to breathe room air. It is possible and desirable to prevent hypoxia from occurring by supplying additional oxygen during this period.

In a similar fashion, the increased alveolar partial pressure of nitrous oxide which occurs when the gas is breathed will cause it to diffuse into the hollow structures of the body until it approaches equilibrium with the inspired tension. This phenomenon can lead to distention of the gastrointestinal tract, provided only that both open ends are closed. A pneumothorax will also increase in volume, as will any other closed air pockets—for example, cysts of the lung or the kidney, air injected for pneumoencephalography, or air behind the ear drum.

The principal limitation then of nitrous oxide is its lack of anesthetic potency. This fact explains several of its dangers and drawbacks, namely, the potential hazards of asphyxia, "diffusion anoxia," and unintentional overdosage with such adjuvants as narcotics, barbiturates, and myoneural blocking drugs. On the other hand, its nonflammability, lack of irritant actions, pleasant smell and marked analgesic properties have emphasized its value as a benign basal anesthetic upon which the actions of a variety of more potent, volatile anesthetic agents and muscle relaxants can be superimposed.

Cyclopropane. This drug offers a rapid, smooth induction and emergence from anesthesia, easy controllability and, since it is potent, it can be given with a high concentration (60 to 80%) of inspired oxygen.

Atropine or scopolamine is used before cyclopropane anesthesia in order to reduce mucus secretion and to counteract the parasympathomimetic properties both of cyclopropane and of certain narcotics which may be used for preanesthetic sedation. The likelihood of reduced alveolar ventilation is increased after narcotic administration, as is a tendency toward reduction in cardiac output. The reduction in ventilation is annoying if it is desired to have the patient breathe spontaneously, and it may provoke the appearance of cardiac arrhythmias (discussed below). On the other hand, the respiratory effects of a narcotic will be advantageous if the aim is (for example in intrathoracic operations) to control the respiration by artificial means. Neuromuscular blockers are used as adjuvants to obtain adequate skeletal muscular relaxation with a lighter plane of anesthesia for certain operative procedures, although cyclopropane itself is usually sufficiently potent when combined with controlled respiration to provide adequate relaxation. Induction of anesthesia wth a rapidly acting barbiturate is common practice.

Cyclopropane is relatively benign with regard to the cardiovascular system, except for its effect on cardiac ryhthm. The *blood pressure* is usually little affected by concentrations causing surgical anesthesia, provided that respiratory efficiency is not diminished; the modest elevation which is frequently observed is believed to be caused by a direct central autonomic action of cyclopropane itself. The increase in pressure can be augmented by respiratory acidosis, anoxia, or surgical stimulation. At concentrations causing respiratory arrest, blood pressure is maintained better with cyclopropane than with other general anesthetic agents. An immediate decrease in blood pressure occasionally seen at the conclusion of cyclopropane anesthesia usually is due to the sudden decrease in an abnormally elevated plasma carbon dioxide tension. Both cyclopropane and hypercarbia stimulate the sympathetic nervous system, and the mechanism involved in postcyclopropane hypotension may be similar to that which follows the discontinuation of an intravenous infusion of norepinephrine. Therapy consists of the intravenous administration of fluids, elevation of the lower extremities and, occasionally, injection of a vasopressor. *Cardiac rate* tends to be either normal or somewhat slow during surgical anesthesia under cyclopropane, usually 60 to 70 beats per minute; bradycardia is especially evident if morphine is used for premedication. The reduction in cardiac rate is largely attributable to an increase in cardiac vagal activity. *Cardiac output* in intact men and animals does not begin to diminish until deep anesthesia (plane 3 or lower) is attained, but when administered following premedication with morphine, cyclopropane causes bradycardia and a reduction in output.

A variety of cardiac arrhythmias may occur during the administration of cyclopropane. The two most commonly noted are A-V nodal rhythm and ventricular extrasystoles. Both increase in incidence with increasing depth of anesthesia, even when the pCO_2 is maintained at normal levels by means of respiratory assistance. When respiratory acidosis is permitted to occur, the incidence of ventricular arrhythmias increases further. The retention of carbon dioxide causes an increase in sympathetic nervous activity affecting the heart, resulting in turn in a liberation of norepinephrine within the myocardium and specialized conducting tissue. In addition, cyclopropane in some manner "sensitizes" the heart to the actions of norepinephrine and the other catecholamines. These two effects combine to result in the emergence of ventricular rhythms.

In the absence of exogenous sources of catecholamines, cyclopropane does not cause ventricular fibrillation in man. Apparently, the endogenous rate of catecholamine liberation in normal man is insufficient. However, it is well to avoid the use of cyclopropane in conditions such as thyrotoxicosis and pheochromocytoma where either the catecholamine liberation rate or the sensitivity of the tissues to catecholamines is enhanced.

Proper therapy of an arrhythmia consists in correcting any known causes; anti-arrhythmia drugs should be avoided unless a change to another anesthetic is precluded for some reason. In the latter situation, lidocaine (50 to 100 mg.) given intravenously over the course of 1 to 2 minutes will frequently cause reversion to a normal sinus rhythm. Lidocaine apparently acts by reducing the excitability of the specialized conducting tissues of the heart.

Volatile Liquids

Ether is irritating to the respiratory tract. Its unskilled administration may be followed by increased secretions in the respiratory tract, swallowing of ether-laden mucus, and by nausea and emesis in the postoperative period. During its administration by the open-drop technic, anoxia and carbon dioxide retention are likely to occur, particularly if thick layers of gauze are used on the mask, if the gauze becomes saturated with expired water vapor or if a flow of 300 to 400/ml. per minute of oxygen is not added under the mask. A prolonged period of induction is often observed. Attempts to hurry the induction may be accompanied by cough, excessive secretions, laryngospasm and excitement. These sequelae are not inevitable and occur less commonly as experience with the drug increases.

Ether stimulates the sympathetic nervous system. Blood sugar increases through mobilization of liver glycogen. Cardiac rate and output tend to rise, in part, at least, as the result of mobilization of norepinephrine and, to a lesser extent in man, epinephrine. In patients with extensive resection of the sympathetic chain, ether may produce circulatory depression, even in relatively light planes of anesthesia, since the protective or buffering mechanism against the direct cardiac and vascular depression of ether has been reduced. Smooth muscle is relaxed, and for this reason ether is preferred to such parasympathetic stimulants as cyclopropane or thiopental for patients with bronchial asthma and allergic phenomenon.

Ether acts synergistically with the antidepolarizing or competitive blocking muscle relaxants such as *d*-tubocurarine or gallamine. Therefore, smaller doses of these relaxants are indicated during ether anesthesia. Through a variety of mechanisms ether tends to stimulate respiration, and respiratory acidosis is less common following its administration than when thiopental or cyclopropane has been given. This is particularly true if opiates are omitted from preanesthetic medication. If hypoxia is avoided there is little evidence that ether damages the liver.

Ether is a versatile anesthetic whose safety has been proved by the countless uneventful instances of its use, even by unskilled persons and with rudimentary equipment. On the other hand, it is flammable, irritating to breathe, and slow in the onset and the disappearance of its actions. For these reasons, it has declined in favor as volatile anesthetics with more desirable properties have been introduced. It retains a place in pediatric anesthesia, wherever spontaneous respirations are to be encouraged, and in locations where sophisticated anesthesia equipment is lacking.

Halothane. It was considered dangerous to use drugs with fluorine in them until it was realized that some hydrocarbons containing fluorine were among the most stable in organic chemistry. Therefore, fluorinated compounds were studied as anesthetics, primarily because some of them could be made nonflammable. Halothane—$CF_3CHClBr$—has created considerable interest during the last few years. Because it fails to mobilize norepinephrine in man to the degree characteristic of cyclopropane or ether, it can cause profound hypotension unless the inspired concentration is controlled within fairly narrow limits. Current practice suggests that induction concentrations rarely should exceed 3 to 4 per cent, with maintenance at the 0.5 to 1.5 per cent level. As a rule, these concentrations are attained with special apparatus or with such vaporizers as a copper kettle.

Price has concluded that there is no single or predominant cause for the circulatory depression produced by halothane. The combination of central autonomic inhibition, ganglionic blockade, and suppression of the peripheral actions of the sympathetic transmitter norepinephrine effectively rob the sympathetic compensatory mechanisms of their efficacy and permit an unantagonized, direct suppression of cardiac and peripheral vascular smooth muscle.

Despite hypotension, some observers regard the patient's condition as excellent, pointing to a full pulse and warm dry skin which is often of good color. Certainly, within reason, a given level of low arterial blood pressure is less important than is the mechanism underlying the reduction. The prognosis, for example, is more grave with hypotension produced by histamine than at the same level of pressure resulting from the injection of acetylcholine. Capillary circulation is better preserved in vital areas in the latter set of circumstances. In the absence of respiratory acidosis, cardiac arrhythmias are rare during anesthesia.

Respiration is depressed by all anesthetic concentrations of halothane. The drug obtunds laryngeal and pharyngeal reflexes to a marked degree, relaxes the masseter muscles and inhibits salivation. Laryngospasm, bronchospasm and coughing are all inhibited. Bronchiolar dilation is produced.

Halothane appears to be a poor analgesic, at least during the first 20 to 30 minutes of administration. The drug is more soluble in tissues than are most anesthetics, with solubility in fat being quite marked. This contributes to the slow elimination of halothane. Awakening is frequently accompanied by vasoconstriction of skin vessels, a grayish pallor of the skin and shivering. Postoperative nausea and vomiting are not common.

Halothane increases bromsulphalein retention no more than do cyclopropane or diethyl ether. However, hepatic damage following the use of halothane has been reported.

Characteristically, there is a delay between exposure to halothane and the appearance of symptoms, ranging from 5 days to nearly 3 weeks. Women are affected more frequently than men. The onset of the disease is heralded by fever, anorexia, nausea and vomiting. Occasionally, a rash is present. Leukocytosis and increased levels of serum glutamic-oxalacetic transaminase are found almost invariably; the cephalin-cholesterol flocculation test is positive, as is the test for thymol turbidity. Death occurs rapidly in about half the cases; those who recover apparently do so completely. The outstanding pathologic feature in all reported cases is extensive hepatocellular necrosis, predominantly centrolobular in location. Treatment consists of exchange transfusions and the use of large doses of ACTH and cortisone, together with general supportive measures.

The question of the possible role of halothane in the causation of liver disease is vexed by the possibility that the reported cases represent either infectious or serum hepatitis, and that they would have occurred even if halothane had not been given. The postanesthetic incidence of hepatitis is almost vanishingly small, and a cause-effect relationship is correspondingly difficult to establish.

Some believe that massive hepatic necrosis represents sensitization to a second or third administration of halothane. These individuals are not in favor of repeating halothane unless the indications for its administration are overwhelming. This is not often the case.

Methoxyflurane (Penthrane). Methoxyflurane is also a fluorinated anesthetic agent (CH_3–O–CF_2–CCl_2H). The saturated vapor pressure of this drug at room temperature is only 22 to 25 mm. of mercury and the saturation concentration 3 per cent. This is the maximum concentration that can be achieved unless the ambient temperature is raised. The effective anesthetic concentrations are well below the explosive and flammable ranges.

Because of the high blood/gas solubility coefficient, induction with methoxyflurane is slow, and most clinicians overcome this fault by giving thiopental intravenously, together with the administration of nitrous oxide and oxygen. Another factor that tends to slow the rate of induction is the uptake of methoxyflurane by the rubber in the breathing circuit. With a fresh gas flow of 3 liters per minute approximately half the vapor added to the system is taken up by rubber during the first five minutes! The effect diminishes with time but is still substantial at the end of an hour. Emergence is slow for the same reason and is made even slower by the marked solubility of methoxyflurane in fat. The clinician attempts to counter this by terminating the administration of methoxyflurane at least 30 to 40 minutes before the termination of a prolonged operation.

The muscular relaxation produced is excellent in many patients, although in achieving this one must expect a certain degree of hypotension, occasionally a major decrease in arterial pressure. The early abolition of spinal reflex activity has been advanced as one cause for the muscular relaxation produced by this anesthetic.

Methoxyflurane depresses myocardial contractile force and cardiac output is progressively reduced with increasing depth of anesthesia. Data on the response of peripheral vessels are meager, although a slight reduction in forearm blood flow has been reported. The effects on autonomic ganglionic transmission have not been studied, and liberation of catecholamines is purported not to be excessive. The pulse rate does not change a great deal, the usual trend being toward diminution. Methoxyflurane sensitizes the heart to catecholamines, but to a lesser extent than cyclopropane. "Spontaneous" ventricular arrhythmias develop rarely, being far less common than after cyclopropane.

The drug is a potent respiratory depressant. Tidal volumes decrease, as does respiratory rate. There is some disagreement on the analgesic potency of methoxyflurane. The alleged analgesia, reported to be present in the first few postoperative hours, may reflect rather the slow elimination following prolonged exposure.

Methoxyflurane does not appear to alter liver function to a greater degree than the other commonly used inhalation anesthetics, but this aspect has not been thoroughly investigated. Recent publications have called attention to a syndrome suggesting a renal tubular lesion with diuresis and lack of responsiveness to vasopressin. In some instances evidence of renal damage persisted for many months. In desperately ill patients who are given methoxyflurane, recovery may be accompanied by shivering, and for this reason oxygen demand is increased. Nausea and vomiting occur, possibly to a lesser degree than after cyclopropane or ether.

Trichloroethylene (Trilene, Trimar). This agent is used to produce analgesia for vaginal delivery, cystoscopy and other minor procedures. Because it is nonexplosive, it is also useful for major operations that do not require muscular relaxation or profound depth of anesthesia. The drug has several interesting properties. If administered in too high a concentration, it causes an increase in respiratory rate up to 50 to 60 per minute. Nausea and vomiting are not common following its administration. Because of its low volatility, open-drop administration is difficult. Therefore, the drug is given by means of a specially constructed inhaler or via a standard gas machine. Volatilization with nitrous oxide and oxygen is currently popular. A closed system with soda lime absorption of expired carbon dioxide cannot be used, since the drug decomposes in the presence of heat to form toxic or irritant products.

INTRAVENOUS ANESTHESIA

Thiopental (Pentothal) and methohexital (Brevital) are the drugs most frequently given intravenously to produce unconsciousness for surgical operations. The outstanding advantage of these substances for the patient is the smooth induction afforded. Excitement is absent, as are the unpleasant buzzing, roaring, and sinking feelings experienced during induction with inhalational agents. Their chief usefulness is for induction of anesthesia, for brief operations, or in combination with nitrous oxide for procedures not requiring muscular relaxation. Should relaxation be necessary a "curare"-like drug must be added. If large doses of either substance are used and if the anesthetist attempts to obtain deep planes of anesthesia, hypotension and tachycardia may develop.

The barbituric acid derivatives do not block sensory pathways as readily as do most anesthetics. Afferent impulses from the operative site can reach the brain more readily than when inhalational anesthetics are used. Therefore, in response to surgical manipulations, reflex spasm of the vocal cords or the abdominal muscles may occur. In attempting to treat or prevent these reactions the anesthetist may add more and more drug until dangerous degrees of respiratory and cardiovascular depression result. Therefore, there are certain disadvantages to the use of these substances for operations in which reflex stimulation is undesirable. To combat this pharmacologic weakness, the analgesic action of nitrous oxide is combined with the sedative quality of the barbiturates as has been described.

Intravenous anesthetics differ from inhalational agents in that once the injection is finished there is practically nothing that can be done to facilitate the removal of the drug. The temporal course of anesthetic effects from induction and rapidly deepening narcosis to gradual emergence depends almost entirely upon progressive redistribution of these drugs within the body. Metabolic degradation or excretion within the duration of the ordinary anesthetic administration is negligible except in the case of methohexital.

The most important property of the rapidly acting barbiturates is that they are capable of penetrating all perfused organs and tissues of the body without delay. For this reason their uptake by a given tissue depends only upon the local blood flow and the concentration of the drug in arterial blood. Because they are relatively well perfused, the viscera, including the brain, receive the bulk of any given dose of a rapidly acting barbiturate. The brain alone receives about one tenth of the dose within the first 40 seconds following an intravenous injection. As time passes, the relatively poorly perfused areas of the body (muscle, skin, connective tissue, fat and skeleton) come gradually to equilibrium with the blood stream content of barbiturate, with the result that concentrations in the various viscera decline progressively. For the brain, the barbiturate level diminishes to about half its peak in 5 minutes, and to only a tenth by half an hour following the injection. Recovery of consciousness usually occurs within this period following the administration of an ordinary induction dose.

With regard to technic, the drugs can be administered intravenously either by intermittent injection or by continuous infusion. For intermittent injection, a 2.5 per cent aqueous solution is ordinarily used in preference to stronger solutions, which are more irritating. Care must be exercised to prevent intra-arterial injection or extravasation, which may result in tissue necrosis. One way of avoiding this complication is to inject only into a freely running intravenous infusion or to use dilute solutions (2.5% or less). Higher concentrations cause ischemia by producing vascular occlusion. The injury results from actions of the drugs themselves and not their alkalinity. Sympathectomy or heparinization diminishes the degree of narcosis, but intra-arterial injections of vasodilator drugs appear to be ineffective. No completely reliable therapy is known.

CONDUCTION ANESTHESIA

Regional or Local Anesthesia

Isolation of a discrete area of the body by infiltration or block of individual nerves with a local anesthetic agent should theoretically disturb vital functions least of all of the anesthetic methods. In practice this is true for many patients, and often pain relief for operations on seriously ill individuals can be obtained with little added strain. However, this statement must be qualified. Intra-abdominal manipulations, when only block of the abdominal wall has been performed, may be attended by a reflex decrease in blood pressure and unpleasant subjective reactions such as pain, nausea and vomiting. The pathways of this reflex are ill-defined. Occasionally, atropine will reverse the untoward signs and symptoms, suggesting that at least part of the response is parasympathetic in origin. Injection of large amounts of a local anesthetic or unusual sensitivity to the drug may be followed by serious hypotension, convulsions, loss of consciousness, or disturbance in cardiac conduction. The absorption of epinephrine, used to prolong the action of the anesthetic solution, may increase cardiac work beyond the capacity of the coronary arteries to supply blood, and evidences of coronary arterial insufficiency may occur.

Treatment of Systemic Reactions. Convulsions and cardiovascular and respiratory collapse are the complications most to be feared. Immediate therapy must have as its goal reversal of these events. Prevention of cerebral hypoxia is of paramount importance. Convulsions increase cerebral metabolism to the point where oxygen demand may exceed its supply. In addition, further hypoxia may be caused by impairment of ventilation during the convulsion. Treatment should be with a rapidly acting barbiturate given intravenously; frequently as little as 25 to 50 mg. of thiopental will suffice.

If ventilation is inadequate, immediate oxygenation must be restored. The mouth and the pharynx should be cleared of obstructing material. Then the head is extended maximally in order to prevent the tongue from obstructing the airway. If equipment is available, artificial ventilation with bag and mask and oxygen may be performed. Otherwise, mouth-to-mouth respiration should be begun immediately. The physician should close the patient's nose and breathe forcefully into the open mouth. If this is successful, the chest wall will be seen to rise. After the patient's lungs have been inflated, passive expiration is allowed. Arterial hypotension should be treated with intravenously administered fluids and pressor drugs until normal pressure has been restored.

Despite these objections, local anesthesia remains of great value for operations on the head, the neck, the extremities, the trunk surface and certain mucosal areas. The cardinal principle in the safety of this method lies in the use of the smallest volume of the lowest concentration of drug which permits satisfactory pain relief. Too frequently, perhaps because of lack of skill or unfamiliarity with the properties of the local anesthetics, surgeons and anesthetists inject large volumes of highly concentrated solutions. Signs of overdosage often result. A 0.25 or 0.5 per cent concentration of procaine provides adequate pain relief during infiltration anesthesia, and the custom of using a 2 per cent solution subjects the patient to an unnecessary hazard of overdosage. For block of individual nerve roots such as the brachial plexus a stronger solution is needed.

A rough guide to the relationship of the safe volume of procaine and its concentration is as follows:

Concentration (%)	Total Volume (ml.)
0.5	200
1	100
2	30

Lidocaine (Xylocaine) is currently popular for local anesthesia, primarily because it spreads more readily through tissues. It has also proved to be useful in doses of 50 to 100 mg. intravenously in the treatment of ventricular arrhythmias occurring during general anesthesia.

SPINAL ANESTHESIA

Spinal anesthesia is chosen most often for operations performed in the perineal area, the groin and the lower extremities. It is likewise excellent for intra-abdominal operations where the combination of muscular relaxation, contracted bowel, quiet breathing and lack of venous congestion is difficult to surpass. Even though supplemental general anesthesia is required in most cases, the patients are more alert and appear to have less "hangover" postoperatively. It is useful for the patient with a full stomach and for muscular patients or alcohol addicts who usually require excessive quantities of general anesthetics. Patients with metabolic or renal disturbances seem to fare well with this technic.

The average duration of anesthesia with commonly used drugs is 60 minutes with procaine, 120 minutes with tetracaine and 180 minutes with dibucaine, but the range is considerable and unpredictable. Duration of anesthesia can be lenghtened somewhat by increasing the concentration of anesthetic agent in the injected solution, more by the addition of a vasoconstrictor drug to the anesthetic solution, and essentially indefinitely through use of continuous spinal anesthesia.

The effect of a pressor drug in the subarachnoid space is to retard the rate of removal of the local anesthetic. Analysis of the cerebrospinal fluid for local anesthetic drugs shows a higher level following the use of epinephrine. This results in a greater amount of the drug being initially available for entrance into a nerve root and offers at least some explanation for the prolongation of anesthesia. Although the additional duration of anesthesia resulting from the use of a vasoconstrictor is statistically significant in a group of patients, prediction of duration for a given individual is not possible.

Local anesthetics are usually injected into the subarachnoid space between the conus medullaris and the terminal portion of the subarachnoid space, in order to avoid injury to the spinal cord. In the adult, therefore, the injection is ordinarily made through one of the vertebral interspaces between the 2nd and the 5th lumbar levels. Obviously, upward diffusion of the anesthetic agent must take place in order to obtain extensive sensory blockade, and the topography of the anesthetized area depends on the extent of this diffusion. The upward passage of an anesthetic agent in the subarachnoid space depends on a multitude of factors, among them being the position of the patient, the specific gravity of the injected solution, the natural curvature of the spine, movements or coughing of the patient, and the size of the subarachnoid space. The last appears to be increased by anything that raises intra-abdominal pressure, viz., pregnancy at term, obesity, ascites, a large ovarian cyst and the like.

Two *immediate sequelae* of spinal anesthesia must be anticipated: (1) a decrease in arterial blood pressure; and (2) respiratory inadequacy if motor block extends high into the thorax.

A spinal anesthesia results in arteriolar dilatation in those vascular beds to which sympathetic afferent fibers have been blocked. A blockade of tonic constrictor impulses to veins can cause decreased venous tone, postarteriolar pooling of blood, and diminished venous return to the heart. This will contribute to a decrease in systolic pressure by reducing stroke volume and cardiac output. Compensatory reflexes effect vasoconstriction in unanesthetized areas. The position of the patient (head-up tilt, prone-jackknife) or the presence of packs and retractors in the abdominal cavity or weight of the gravid uterus on the great veins may also compromise venous return and produce arterial hypotension. These changes may not be as great in the young individual whose vessels may have considerable autonomy and who may have increased ability to compensate for regional sympathetic blockade. Hypotension may occur when a spinal anesthetic is given in the presence of hypovolemia. The final circulatory status will depend, then, upon the relative contributions of each of the above variables.

A rational approach to the prevention or the therapy of the hypotension caused by spinal anesthesia may be derived from a consideration of the mechanisms already discussed. Decreased venous return may be restored toward normal by elevation of the legs; one may wrap the legs in elastic bandages prior to the administration of a spinal anesthetic in order to prevent pooling in this area. The rapid infusion of intravenous fluids will fill a dilated vascular bed and result in a more adequate venous return. Sympathomimetic amines may be given intramuscularly 5 minutes before the local anesthetic is injected into the subarachnoid space to minimize hypotension, or intravenously once hypotension has developed. A variety of drugs has been used, and each has its proponents. Ephedrine, phenylephrine, hydroxyamphetamine and methoxamine have all proved to be of value.

The pressor amine restores arteriolar and venous tone to normal or prevents its decrease during sympathetic blockade. Cardiac output is elevated by augmentation of venous return. Most agents increase cardiac contractile force by a direct action. Mephentermine has been shown to restore a low arterial blood pressure to normal by increasing cardiac output if the latter had been low during the spinal anesthetic. If, on the other hand, a normal cardiac output is present in the face of hypotension, the drug elevates the arterial blood pressure by increasing total peripheral resistance.

During the first half hour of spinal anesthesia the anesthetist must be constantly on the alert to ascertain how high motor paralysis has extended. It may be as long as 50 minutes before the anesthetic has become "fixed" and the level constant. Signs of impending respiratory paralysis are diminution of thoracic respiration with increasing diaphragmatic excursions, whispering followed by loss of spoken voice, dilatation of the alae nasi, and use of the accessory muscles of respiration. A failing respiration during spinal anesthesia calls for immediate use of artificial ventilation rather than drug therapy, inasmuch as the failure is related to motor nerve block and cannot be influenced by centrally acting respiratory stimulants.

Neurologic complications may follow lumbar puncture, injection of a local anesthetic agent into the subarachnoid space, or such unrelated factors as improper positioning of the patient during the operative procedure.

Trauma occurring during a lumbar puncture can involve the ligaments, the periosteum, the annulus fibrosis, the perivertebral plexus of veins, the meninges, the nerve roots or the spinal cord. Leakage of cerebrospinal fluid can result in headache or visual and auditory symptoms (syndrome of decreased intracranial pressure). The *cauda equina syndrome* may follow a spinal anesthetic. Inasmuch as the nerves involved are those exposed to the highest concentration of local anesthetic, the lesion may be attributed to a direct toxic action of the drug on nervous tissue. Indeed, it is possible consistently to demonstrate tissue changes in experimental animals following the subarachnoid injection of supraanesthetic concentrations of local anesthetic drugs. The signs and the symptoms of the cauda equina syndrome consist of a loss of control of the sphincters of the bladder and the bowel and in varying degrees of sensory and motor disturbance in the lower extremities. Recovery may occur slowly or not at all. Another grave complication is *chronic progressive adhesive arachnoiditis* in which there is progressive proliferation of the pia-arachnoid. Eventually, the subarachnoid space may be completely obliterated, and circulation to the spinal cord seriously compromised. This entity often begins with involvement of the lumbosacral cord and progresses to thoracic, phrenic and bulbar dysfunction, resulting in death.

Bacterial contamination may result in septic meningitis. Contamination with disinfectants or detergents has been proposed as a mechanism for the production of severe neurologic complications, but whether sufficient material can gain access to the subarachnoid space to be harmful is still in dispute.

If spinal anesthesia is given to patients with pre-existing neurologic disease, sequelae are more apt to occur. If faulty sterilization of the drugs, the needles and the syringes used for this method is permitted, an increased number of complications will be noted. *But if the technic of lumbar puncture is refined, if foreign material such as talcum powder applied to gloves or skin antiseptics does not contaminate the subarachnoid space, and if all drugs are autoclaved,* spinal anesthesia is an exceptionally safe and useful method. The author and his associates have followed patients to whom spinal anesthesia was given, not only during the immediate postoperative period but also for 6 to 60 months after operation. Of approximately 9,300 patients, 89 per cent have been followed in this fashion. Not a single instance of adhesive arachnoiditis has been found during this study. Indeed, no patient appears to have suffered permanent neurologic damage of any consequence. Instances of persistent numbness, backache, pain or weakness were reported, but on examination these proved to be trivial or minor in nature. We believe that spinal anesthesia is a particularly useful method, and one which has suffered unjustly because of fear of medicolegal consequences. However, consciousness during an operation is frequently unpleasant, with fear, nausea, vomiting and pain among the undesirable aspects. The management of spinal anesthesia must be carried out with skill and understanding. Supplementation of the block with intravenous barbiturates and nitrous oxide is often essential. If no additional general anesthesia is provided, the patient must be reassured constantly and given adequate psychological support.

EPIDURAL ANESTHESIA

Epidural anesthesia is an extensive block anesthesia produced by injecting a local anesthetic into the epidural space. With this technic sensory anesthesia extending as high as the chin can be produced. A single dose of the local anesthetic may be administered or a continuous technic may be used.

Epidural anesthesia possesses most of the advantages of spinal anesthesia with many of its disadvantages. Its main advantage lies in the fact that the subarachnoid space is not entered. Thus, headache and other neurologic sequelae of spinal anesthesia are prevented. Segmental anesthesia is more predictable with epidural anesthesia. Difficulty in technic probably constitutes the chief disadvantage of epidural anesthesia. The second major disadvantage is the large amount of drug which must be employed, for systemic absorption of the agent may be significant. The somnolence often seen when lidocaine is used may be due to this. The effects on circulation and respiration are similar to those produced by spinal anesthesia inasmuch as the mechanism involved (sympathetic and motor blockade) is the same in both instances. The inability to block discomfort with visceral manipulation is also present. A final disadvantage is the latent period between the injection and the onset of anesthesia.

MUSCLE RELAXANTS

The most important action of the muscle relaxant drugs is to interfere with the passage of impulses from the motor nerve to skeletal muscle. This takes place at the nerve-muscle junction, a zone composed of motor nerve terminals and a specialized section of the muscle cell membrane called the end-plate. Although there is anatomic discontinuity between nerve and muscle, the gap is bridged by the chemical transmitting agent, acetylcholine. As the result of motor nerve activity acetylcholine is released from the nerve terminals at the cell membrane of muscle. A phenomenon known as depolarization accompanies this; a negative electrical potential develops at the end-plate. When this reaches a certain magnitude a wave of depolarization in the muscle cell is produced, and the muscle contracts. Acetylcholine is destroyed in a fraction of a second by the enzyme cholinesterase, and a restorative process begins, culminating in the return of the muscle to its precontractile state.

This natural process can be interrupted by preventing acetylcholine from reaching the receptor area of the muscle cell membrane. *d*-Tubocurarine is believed to produce muscular paralysis in this way. The hypothesis is: *d*-tubocurarine blocks the action of the chemical transmitter through combination with receptors usually occupied by acetylcholine. Gallamine (Flaxedil) and dimethyl-tubocurarine (Metubine) act in similar fashion. These drugs are currently called nondepolarizing relaxants.

The characteristics of a nondepolarization block are: (1) absence of fasciculaltions; (2) reversal of the block by acetylcholine, or anticholinesterase agents; (3) "fade" in the response of the muscle fibers after both single impulses and tetanic stimulation, the fade after tetanus being more obvious; and (4) after a tetanic stimulus, a brief increase in the response to a single stimulus, termed post-tetanic facilitation (Fig. 13-1).

The useful depolarizing drugs are decamethonium (Syncurine) and succinylcholine (Anectine, Scoline, Quelicin, suxamethonium). The initial action of these drugs resembles that of acetylcholine; depolarization of the end plate occurs; muscle contraction is produced and may appear as fine twitching or fibrillating movements called fasciculations. There may even be a major degree of contracture of most of the body's skeletal muscles, occasionally followed by aching and soreness after operation, a response most marked after use of succinylcholine. At this time the characteristics of the depolarization block (also termed Phase I block) are: (1) fasciculations; (2) potentiation of the block by acetylcholine and anticholinesterases; (3) height of twitch and response to tetanic stimulation, both sustained; and (4) absence of post-tetanic facilitation (Fig. 13-1). Continuation of depolarization of the end plate was orignally believed to be the cause of the relaxation seen with these drugs, and no doubt this is responsible for the initial effect. However, there is now evidence that there can be gradual repolarization of the end plate with neuromuscular block persisting because of a decrease in the sensitivity of the end plate to acetylcholine. As this occurs there is gradual change in the block so that it has the characteristics of, but is not identical with, a nondepolarizing block. The terms desensitization block, Phase II, or dual block have been used to describe the new pattern. The change in pattern occurs more frequently and earlier after use of succinylcholine than had been recognized previously. Katz and his associates aver that dual block will develop fully after a total dose of 3.0 mg./kg. of suc-

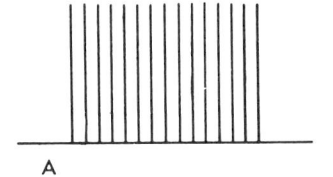

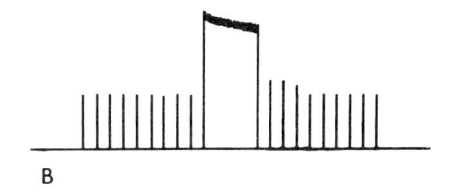

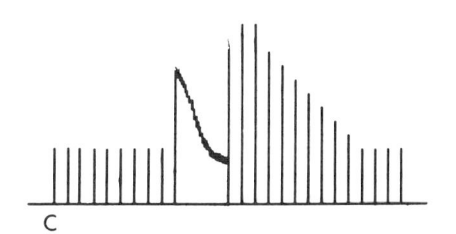

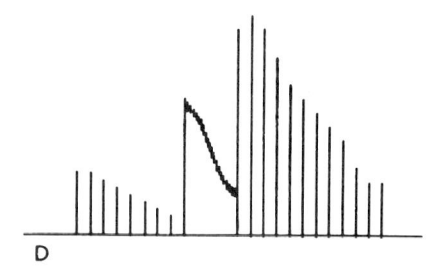

FIG. 13-1. Diagrammatic representation of adduction of the thumb to a supra-maximal stimulus applied to the ulnar nerve. A. Control: no block of myoneutral junction is present. B. Phase I block with succinylcholine: tetanus is sustained and there is no post-tetanic facilitation. C. Phase II block with succinylcholine: there is fade on tetanus, and post-tetanic facilitation is present. D. Nondepolarizing block with d-tubocurarine: there is slight fade of the twitch response, fade with tetanus, and marked post-tetanic facilitation. (Dripps, R. D., Eckenhoff, J. E., and Vandam, L. D.: Introduction to Anesthesia. ed. 3. Philadelphia, W. B. Saunders, 1967)

cinylcholine given intermittently or by continuous intravenous infusion. However, the exact dose necessary, the time course over which it must be given, and the degree of tachyphylaxis observed are questions not yet completely resolved.

In addition to an action at the nerve-muscle junction, the muscle relaxants can reduce transmission of impulses at the preganglionic and postganglionic endings in the autonomic nervous system. This has been demonstrated most clearly for *d*-tubocurarine, which depresses transmission at synapses in the sympathetic ganglia with a resultant decreased contractility of blood vessels. The tachycardia observed after administration of gallamine probably is caused by postganglionic vagal blockade. Both types of muscle relaxant are alleged to minimize the reflex circulatory and respiratory effects of intra-abdominal or intrathoracic manipulation, although the evidence is not convincing. Succinylcholine has a mild sympathetic ganglionic stimulant property, an effect partially responsible for the rise in blood pressure sometimes observed. It also can cause increased vagal tone, probably through an action in the brain. This may cause rather marked bradycardia, particularly after repeated doses have been given intravenously.

D-TUBOCURARINE

Following the intravenous injection of *d*-tubocurarine, block of the nerve-muscle junction is noted during the first passage of the drug through the circulation. The explanation for the rapidity of action is twofold: (1) a close spatial relationship between capillaries and the muscle end-plate, so that there is a short distance for diffusion from plasma to end-plate; (2) a special affinity for the end-plate for *d*-tubocurarine.

The passage of *d*-tubocurarine through the

body can be divided into three phases. During the first phase plasma levels decrease with a half-time of 5 to 6 minutes because of distribution throughout the extracellular fluid. At this time there is a dynamic equilibrium between drug in solution and drug bound to plasma proteins. In some patients, apparently, d-tubocurarine is more strongly bound to albumin than in others. Such individuals might appear to be resistant to the muscle relaxant.

During the second phase, the drug disappears from the extracellular fluid with a half-time of about 45 minutes. After 45 minutes a second injection of half the original dose gives the same effect as the total initial dose. There are two explanations for this. Within a given time about one third of the drug is excreted in the urine, while about two thirds move into some area designated as tissue compartment. This phase lasts for 2 to 3 hours and can be termed the phase of redistribution. Muscle proteins may form part of the pool into which d-tubocurarine disappears. The liver apparently does not accumulate a substantial amount.

The third phase consists of destruction of that portion of d-tubocurarine in the tissue reservoir reached during the second phase. Destruction apparently proceeds with a half-time of approximately 3½ hours. Destruction accounts for about two thirds of the total amount injected. This probably accounts for the prolonged duration of action of d-tubocurarine noted after large doses of the drug. The role of the liver in the process of destruction is unknown, as are the mechanism and the end-products.

Succinylcholine

Serum cholinesterase hydrolyzes succinylcholine. Enzymatic activity increases with a rising concentration of the relaxant, and, as the drug concentration declines, enzymatic activity slows until it becomes negligible. The rate of hydrolysis by esterase is rapid, as much as 70 per cent of an injected dose being destroyed within 1 minute.

There are two types of serum cholinesterase in man, each of which behaves differently toward succinylcholine. The type present is genetically determined. The rarer form, occurring in at least 4 per cent of the white population, is called atypical esterase. The normal esterase is quite active at concentrations of succinylcholine which are too low to induce an activity of atypical esterase. Furthermore, the action of succinylcholine lasts much longer in a person with atypical esterase than in one with the normal variety. A lowering of esterase levels occurs in liver disease and malnutrition. This decrease is probably a sign of a general reduction in protein synthesis, since other enzymes and albumin are also reduced.

Since serum cholinesterase can act only while succinylcholine is in the blood stream, this enzymatic activity is of importance only for a short period. Its contribution is primarily to regulate the amount of the relaxant which reaches the end-plate during the first phase of distribution. Termination of action of succinylcholine is probably caused by dilution, that is, diffusion from the end-plate into the interstitial fluid.

The pathway of destruction or hydrolysis for succinylcholine is biphasic, first to succinylmonocholine and then to choline. The first phase occurs with great rapidity. Succinylmonocholine, a weak neuromuscular blocking agent, is then degraded into choline and succinic acid at a slower speed. The liver contains an enzyme specific for the hydrolysis of succinylmonocholine. Only about 2 per cent of the injected succinylcholine appears to be unchanged in the urine.

Gallamine and Decamethonium

These drugs do not appear to be metabolized in the mammalian organism. The major portion of the quantity injected can be recovered in the urine. Nevertheless, the usual onset and duration of action must depend upon a process of redistribution.

Antagonism

Neostigmine (Prostigmin) and edrophonium (Tensilon), both anticholinesterases, may reverse the neuromuscular block produced by some of the relaxants. This reversal is most likely to occur when d-tubocurarine or gallamine has been used. Presumably, the anticholinesterase, in preventing the destruction of acetylcholine, permits this chemical transmitter to accumulate and to restore neuromuscular conduction.

The dose of neostigmine usually is 1.0 mg. and should rarely exceed 4.0 mg. It must be combined with atropine in 0.6 to 1.0 mg. doses intravenously to minimize the muscarinic actions of neostigmine. Anticholinesterases might fail to re-establish transmission if end-plate receptors have lost their sensitivity to acetylcholine, if there is unusual fixation of blocking agent to receptor, or if excessive acetylcholine is formed and a secondary acetylcholine block is produced. Under any of these circumstances, persistence in the administration of the anticholinesterase will prolong the block.

RESPIRATORY EFFECTS OF RELAXANTS

All of the muscle relaxants can reduce the minute volume of respiration or produce apnea through neuromuscular blockade. At the end of an operation this effect should have disappeared. Unfortunately, this does not always happen, and inadequate ventilation or apnea may persist into the postoperative period for varying lengths of time. Prolonged respiratory depression can be minimized by attention to such details as the following:

A history of unexplained muscle weakness should make one wary of all relaxants. Increased reactivity to the relaxants occurs in patients with myasthenia gravis and with carcinoma, particularly of the lung. Advanced hepatic or renal disease also demands cautious use of these drugs. Cachectic, malnourished individuals often tolerate relaxants poorly, perhaps because of reduced protein synthesis, and a lowered serum cholinesterase, perhaps because of associated electrolyte abnormalities. Low serum levels of potassium or calcium and acid-base imbalance may be associated with increased reactivity to relaxants. The antibiotics neomycin and streptomycin can produce neuromuscular block. This action can summate with that of the relaxants. An additive action may also occur with some of the relaxants and histamine, large doses of narcotics, barbiturates, and such ganglionic blocking substances as trimethaphan (Arfonad) or hexamethonium.

POSTOPERATIVE RESPIRATORY INADEQUACY

At the end of operation, an appraisal should be made of the degree of residual respiratory muscle blockade. If the patient is sufficiently conscious, he should be asked to raise his hand or head or to tighten his fist. Inability to do this indicates that the respiratory muscles too may still be affected by the drugs used. If the patient cannot cooperate, several methods of assessment are available. These are based on the fact that a patient may seem to breathe adequately until an extra effort is required of his muscles. This leads to a false sense of security by supervisory personnel. However, if a major degree of blockade persists, the patient will be unable to meet this demand. In the first method, the patient's nose and mouth can be occluded by the anesthetist's fingers and hand. The vigor of the response to complete respiratory tract obstruction so produced permits one to gauge the strength of respiratory muscular contraction. In any patient thus tested, 100 per cent oxygen should be breathed beforehand. This test establishes the reserve of the muscles of respiration which is needed to overcome obstruction, to cough and to take the deep breaths necessary to inflate all parts of the lung fully.

A more sophisticated and quantitative technic is that described by Bendixen and his colleagues. This is termed the inspiratory force measurement. A Y-piece is connected to the anesthesia mask or the endotracheal tube; one arm is attached to a manometer or a pressure transducer; the other is left open. At the end of expiration the open end is occluded, and the negative pressure developed during inspiration is read on the manometer. Again, oxygen is given to the patient beforehand. Airway occlusion is limited to 20 to 30 seconds. If at least 15 mm. of mercury pressure cannot be developed, the patient has insufficient ventilatory reserve and must be observed very closely.

If apnea is present at the end of operation, factors other than the effect of muscle relaxants must be considered, such as low arterial carbon dioxide tension and continued reflex inhibition of respiration by an inflated cuff on a tracheal tube.

Excessive depth and rate of artificial ventilation, whether provided by manual compression of the breathing bag or by machine, can reduce arterial carbon dioxide tension to a point where spontaneous respiration ceases. The pressure used for inflation of the lungs may stimulate Hering-Breuer stretch receptors which exert an inhibitory effect on the respiratory center via the vagus nerves. The combination of these factors might result in an apnea which can be interpreted erroneously as resulting from prolonged action of muscle relaxants. Treatment consists of decreasing the frequency and the depth of pulmonary ventilation so that carbon dioxide concentration in arterial blood is restored to normal, and the rhythmic discharge of the respiratory center (decreased by low carbon dioxide and inhibitory reflexes) is re-established. One should not diminish ventilation of the lungs for a period long enough for hypoxia or hypercapnia to develop.

The presence of a tracheal tube, particularly with an inflated cuff, may cause persistent apnea. The reflex pathway for this is not clear, but deflation of the cuff or withdrawal of the tube may remove the inhibitory stimulus and permit resumption of spontaneous breathing.

Another cause of postoperative respiratory inadequacy is the respiratory depressant effect of opiates used to supplement anesthesia. Should this appear to be a likely explanation, one of the opiate antagonists may be of value.

The most essential element of treatment is to ensure that the oxygen and carbon dioxide tensions of the patient's blood are kept within normal limits. This requires minute-to-minute attention and endless patience. However, it constitutes the most important therapeutic measure and is the one most frequently neglected. Patients with pulmonary disease are particularly difficult to manage. In a patient with severe emphysema the preoperative level of carbon dioxide in the blood may be high, and difficulty may be experienced in restarting respiration unless relevant laboratory data are available. Without adequate laboratory facilities, the clinician cannot determine when the carbon dioxide tension of the blood is abnormal. Nor can he estimate accurately the degree of oxygenation of blood leaving the lungs. Analyses of arterial blood samples for pH, pCO_2, and pO_2 are vital in the guidance of therapy for these patients.

RESPIRATORY PROBLEMS ASSOCIATED WITH UNCONSCIOUSNESS

Unconsciousness carries with it the threat of certain respiratory difficulties which must be anticipated constantly and treated promptly. These potential hazards exist in every unconscious individual whatever the cause of the unconsciousness. Thus the problem may complicate any type of general anesthesia, as well as such medical ills as narcotic poisoning, diabetic coma, uremia, or cranial injuries. It is unfortunate that so many physicians are unfamiliar with the management of these respiratory abnormalities and permit inadequate breathing to persist when often simple measures would suffice to correct them. Therefore, it is stressed that the following discussion is not limited solely to the management of the anesthetized patient but applies equally to any comatose person.

Air must be allowed to move in and out of the lungs freely with movement of the thoracic cage and the diaphragm. Obstruction to this movement of air causes increased work on the part of the respiratory muscles, asphyxia of a degree dependent upon the degree of obstruction, and carries with it the threat of sudden death due to exhaustion, or medullary damage if obstruction becomes complete.

Recognition of Respiratory Obstruction

A disparity between the activity of the thorax, the muscles of respiration and the volume of air moved suggests obstruction of the air passages. This may be noted by watching or feeling the chest, the abdomen and the neck and holding the palm of the hand in front of the nose and the mouth. If the air current perceived by the palm is less than the activity of the respiratory muscles indicate that it should be, a diagnosis of obstruction is reasonable. The sounds of breathing also have diagnostic import. "Noisy" breathing is "obstructed breathing." The nature of the sound may localize the site of obstruction, with stertor or snoring indicating soft tissue block (e.g., tongue, epiglottis) and stridor or crowing implicating glottic spasm. If the degree of obstruction is sufficient, cyanosis will occur.

Treatment of Respiratory Obstruction

If obstruction of the soft tissues exists, a number of maneuvers may be of value. The patient should be placed prone or in the lateral position, since the tongue tends to fall back and block the passage of air when an individual lies on his back. The mandible can be moved up and out by fingers placed behind the angles of the jaw. This movement carries the tongue forward and tends to reduce soft tissue block of the mouth and the pharynx. If the mouth can be opened, the tongue can be grasped with gauze or a forceps, or a suture can be placed through the tongue and mild traction exerted. By pulling the tongue forward toward the lips the pharynx may be freed of obstruction. Artificial metal or rubber airways may be inserted in the mouth to hold the tongue forward; rubber tubes may be passed through the nose into the posterior pharynx. Finally, an endotracheal tube may be placed or a tracheostomy performed.

INADEQUATE VENTILATION

The unconscious patient may have such depression of the respiratory center or poor tone of the respiratory muscles that the volume of air moved is not sufficient for alveolar ventilation. Then artificial respiration must be provided. This can be accomplished manually by the Holger Nielsen technic if the patient is prone, or by compression of the chest anteriorly if he is supine. Mouth-to-mouth, or mouth-to-nose breathing can be used. If as a result of artificial respiration the patient's color remains good, room air will suffice. If cyanosis is noted, 100 per cent oxygen should be used. Should support of respiration be required for hours or days, a concentration of 50 per cent oxygen may avoid signs and symptoms of oxygen toxicity. Mechanical resuscitators may be applied when they become available, but valuable time must not be lost in searching for them.

ANESTHETIC MANAGEMENT OF THE "POOR RISK" PATIENT

The term "risk" involves an estimate of prognosis. A consideration of the factors that influence the final outcome of a given case suggests that "estimating the risk" is frequently approached improperly. To designate the "risk" accurately would necessitate foreknowledge of such variables as the reliability of the suture material, the fallibility of asepsis, the availability of drugs, the responsibility of those in charge of postoperative nursing care, and a host of other aspects which cannot always be assessed for each patient by the anesthetist or the surgeon. A patient anesthetized by a medical student and operated upon by a junior surgeon has less of a chance than would the same patient in the hands of an experienced anesthesiologist and a senior surgeon. In the latter case the patient's condition has not changed, but the likelihood of survival has been increased materially. Likewise, the patient's prognosis is more favorable if the personnel responsible for his care are not tense and overworked. Again, the patient's condition remains the same, but the risk is less. The success or failure of a given procedure often depends upon many things that have little to do with the patient's physical condition.

The above is perhaps an academic discussion. Obviously, there are patients who, for a variety of reasons, are less likely to survive anesthesia and operation than others. Such patients are encountered among candidates for emergency, as well as for less urgent operations. Their anesthetic management will be considered first, in general terms.

Many an anesthetic or surgical accident could have been avoided had a careful appraisal of a patient's problems been made and appropriate corrective measures instituted prior to operation. Too often, for example, the medical work-up of a seriously ill patient or one deemed an "emergency" is inadequate. The very seriousness of the patient's condition creates an atmosphere of tension in which logical analysis is replaced by hurried decision, and attention to detail is subordinated to a cursory survey. The history is glossed over, physical examination is limited, and laboratory data are minimal. The operating room is prepared in haste, the patient is anesthetized hurriedly, and troubles which could have been avoided present themselves in rapid succession.

If the above be true for emergency situations it is at least as pertinent when time is of less concern. Thoroughness of work-up, careful appraisal of systems other than those involved by the primary surgical conditions and efforts designed to correct abnormalities of these systems form the backbone of an intelligent preoperative regimen. Such measures ease the anesthetist's burden significantly. Often the patient is classified as "poor risk" from the anesthetic standpoint solely because of inadequate preparation for the operation. The more seriously ill the patient is to begin with, the more important these principles become. Certain examples may be illustrative.

The patient with intestinal obstruction poses problems of anesthesia, many of which can be minimized by preoperative preparation. Aspiration of intestinal contents into the respiratory tract is prone to occur during induction of anesthesia or during surgical manipulation of the distended bowel. The higher the point of obstruction, the greater is the hazard. In the presence of gastric dilation and atony stomach contents may pour into the pharynx at any time and be aspirated into the lungs. The best solution to this problem is preoperative decompression and drainage of the stomach and the distended bowel. The time spent in preparing the patient with bowel obstruction for operation is obviously important to the patient's safety and reduces considerably the problems presented to the anesthetist and the surgeon. Since suction-drainage cannot empty the entire intestinal tract, the anesthetist must continue to be aware of this problem. If general anesthesia is selected, there is much to be said in favor of rapid intubation of the trachea with a cuffed tube. Intubation can also be accomplished under topical anesthesia of the mucous membrane of the upper respiratory tract while the patient is still conscious. Spinal anestheisa has been recommended because, among other virtues, it does not impair laryngeal and tracheal reflexes. However, it must be realized that many patients with intestinal obstruction have depression of all reflexes. They may be semistuporous because of dehydration and loss of electrolytes among other reasons, and aspiration of intestinal contents into the lungs is not unlikely even if the operation be conducted during local anesthesia. In addition, these patients have difficulty maintaining an adequate circulation. Spinal anesthesia may precipitate severe hypotension unless blood volume and electrolyte balance have been restored toward normal.

A second example is the patient with chronic suppuration in the respiratory tract. Administration of inhalational anesthesia to an individual with a considerable amount of purulent material in the tracheobronchial tree is difficult because of the following:

1. The exudate in the bronchioles or bronchi tends to block access of the anesthetic to the alveoli.

2. For the same reason adequate oxygenation and elimination of carbon dioxide may be less likely.

3. A smooth plane of anesthesia is difficult to maintain, since frequent aspiration of the respiratory passages is required.

4. Spread of contaminated material throughout the lung fields may occur with change of position, compression of the lung by the surgeon, and because of loss of the cough reflex.

5. There tends to be greater irritability of reflexes in the respiratory passages with more secretions, coughing and cyanosis likely.

These problems are reduced in degree by such preoperative measures as postural or bronchoscopic drainage, inhalation of aerosols, use of antibiotics, use of positive-pressure breathing and elimination of smoking. Many days may be required before the patient with advanced bronchiectasis becomes "relatively dry," but the chances of a fatal outcome or of undesirable postoperative sequelae are reduced for each day that such prophylaxis is carried out. The anesthetist can contribute further to safety by frequent aspiration of the trachea and the bronchi during anesthesia, and by having the patient awake at the conclusion of the operation so that he can rid himself of secretions by coughing.

In the cases just discussed it has been pointed out that a lowered mortality and morbidity rate may be achieved by adequate preoperative care. However, there are some patients whose condition is such that they cannot be greatly improved before operation. Under these circumstances the anesthesiologist must select that method which will interfere least with the abnormalities already present. The individual with coronary arterial disease falls into this group. In this type of patient the essential problems are to prevent an increase in cardiac work, or a decrease in coronary arterial flow with a consequent disparity between the metabolic requirements of the cardiac muscle and the available supply of oxygen.

There is no single satisfactory approach to the anesthetic management of these patients, particularly if an intra-abdominal operation is planned. The following suggestions are recommended:

1. Assurance through personal contact that the anesthetist is aware of the patient's particular problem. This relieves a great source of anxiety on the part of the patient who frequently worries lest those concerned with his care be not completely familiar with his cardiac disability.

2. Adequate sedation prior to operation. The mental stress of a trip to the operating room is understandable, and attacks of angina pectoris or coronary insufficiency may be precipitated by such an emotional crisis if proper sedation has not been achieved.

3. Smooth induction of anesthesia. A stormy induction with the likelihood of struggling, respiratory obstruction, anoxia, and retention of carbon dioxide is hazardous for a heart whose blood supply is marginal. Since this blood supply in all probability cannot be increased in the normal fashion by coronary artery dilation, further demand for blood secondary to increased cardiac work should be avoided.

4. Maintenance of blood pressure. A reduction in mean arterial blood pressure will reduce the amount of blood flowing through the coronary arteries if there cannot be compensatory dilation. Although during hypotension work of the heart against peripheral resistance may be reduced, one cannot be certain that the demand for oxygen will be lowered sufficiently to be met by the decreased supply.

5. Administration of oxygen. The value of this procedure is self-evident.

Regional anesthesia is thought by some to be the safest form of pain relief for patients with coronary arterial disease. We prefer inhalational anesthesia to unsupplemented regional anesthesia for the following reasons: Under local anesthesia the patient is conscious and aware of the sight, the sounds and the odors of the operating room. This is not calculated to provide mental calm unless large amounts of sedatives are provided. Furthermore, despite satisfactory anesthesia of the abdominal wall, intra-abdominal manipulations are often accompanied by severe pain, nausea, vomiting, dyspnea and a lowered blood pressure. The decrease in blood pressure has been ascribed by some to a reflex inhibition of the sympathetic nervous system, with diminished venous return to the heart and a lowered cardiac output. The pain, frequently substernal, and the subjective feeling of shortness of breath, have been attributed to a reflex reduction in coronary arterial blood flow, although evidence on this point is not conclusive.

If there is virtue in urging the patient with coronary arterial disease to live quietly, avoid stress and strain and adjust his way to a calmer existence, it seems unwise to subject this same individual to the mental and physical upset occasioned by an operation performed under local anesthesia, when a *properly administered* general anesthetic can abolish the mental disquiet and minimize the untoward effects of intra-abdominal traction.

A second type of patient whose problems must be solved during the anesthesia is the individual with mitral stenosis, a history of heart failure, who has a complicating surgical illness or is ready for obstetric delivery. Where the location of operation permits their use, spinal or epidural anesthesia has much to recommend it for these patients. Both methods produce a circulatory response which might be termed a bloodless phlebotomy. Vasomotor fibers to arterioles and venules are blocked in varying numbers according to the level of anesthesia. Venous pressure decreases, and blood is pooled in the peripheral circulation, largely in the legs. This is obviously an advantage to the patient with incipient pulmonary edema. However, for mitral commissurotomy, general anesthesia is used. Here the selection of drug seems to be unimportant. Of greatest concern is maintenance of an extraordinarily light plane of anesthesia, lest major depression of blood pressure result.

Positioning of the cardiac patient on the operating table is important. It is wise to test preoperatively the effects of the position required. Should the patient complain of additional dyspnea or should blood pressure be reduced as the unanesthetized individual is placed in the surgical position it may become necessary to modify the operative approach. The head-down jackknife and lateral positions are difficult for the cardiac patient to tolerate. In some of these individuals pulmonary edema can be precipitated by assumption of even the horizontal supine position. These people can be operated upon in the semi-Fowler position. This is of great importance when the myocardial weakness is combined with the elevated diaphragm and respiratory embarrassment of a full-term pregnancy. Under no circumstances should the orthopneic patient be placed flat after induction of general anesthesia merely because he is asleep and cannot complain of dyspnea.

ANESTHESIA FOR BATTLE CASUALTIES

Until shock is corrected the severely wounded soldier is inordinately susceptible to narcosis, regardless of the agent or the technic selected. Prior to anesthesia he presents a picture of apathy and depression. He appears to be already partially narcotized. In such a patient even small amounts of central nervous depressant drugs evoke a response out of proportion to the size of the dose administered. Each war has accented this fact. The prolonged postoperative sleep of these patients tends to support this contention.

The guiding principle in the administration of anesthesia to any patient is use of the least amount compatible with the surgical requirements. The susceptibility of the serious battle casualty to anesthesia enables one to provide satisfactory working conditions with 50 to 60 per cent nitrous oxide in oxygen in many such patients. This concentration may not produce even minimal surgical anesthesia in normal individuals; but if satisfactory results can be obtained, the shocked patient has been spared the consequences of a more potent depressant. In the severely wounded marked hypotension may follow even first plane anesthesia with ether. It must be administered with caution. An intravenous injection of 25 to 50 mg. of thiopental may reduce blood pressure profoundly. This drug must be given slowly and in small amounts until the patient's tolerance is established. In the recent conflict in Viet Nam both halothane and methoxyflurane have proved useful. Spinal anesthesia probably has little place in the management of the seriously wounded. Regional and local anesthesia are of value.

Regardless of the method finally selected, certain problems of the seriously wounded will affect the casualty's response to the stress of anesthesia and operation. These reactions must be anticipated and treatment begun promptly. As the patient is moved from the resuscitation unit to the operating room his blood pressure may fall markedly. Motion appears to have an adverse effect on the circulation of these patients as though compensation had been maintained by a delicate balance, almost any alteration of which proves to be upsetting. If hypotension does not follow this degree of activity, it may occur as the patient is placed in position on the operating table. Constant awareness of this possibility and treatment with parenteral fluids or pressor drugs may prevent disasters.

SPECIAL ANESTHETIC TECHNICS

Controlled or Deliberate Hypotension

The deliberate reduction of arterial pressure in an effort to produce a relatively bloodless field for operation is being re-explored. This is a challenging concept and one worthy of careful study, since its successful application might minimize the need for blood transfusions, reduce the incidence of transfusion reactions, improve the result of certain operative procedures by lessening bleeding and decrease operating time.

There can be little doubt that capillary oozing can prolong an operation, if not actually prevent its successful conclusion. However, bleeding from larger vessels can be severe, even during deliberate hypotension, and unless this blood is replaced as it is lost the result may lead to irreversible hypotension. Postoperative hemorrhage, although not reported frequently, is always a possibility as the pressure-head returns toward normal following operation. There is danger lest this procedure be attempted in instances in which perfectly satisfactory results can be obtained otherwise. Neurosurgical, plastic and radical procedures for eradication of malignancy are the most likely operations for trial of the method.

A number of methods are available for the intentional reduction of blood pressure. The primary principle is dilatation of the vascular bed with pooling of blood in the venous reservoirs. This may be achieved by block of the vasomotor outflow with epidural or spinal anesthesia, by ganglionic blocking agents such as hexamethonium salts or by trimethaphan, a drug which dilates blood vessels peripherally, blocks ganglia and may liberate histamine.

A controllable technic upon which we rely includes a combination of halothane, increased airway pressure, pentolinium (Ansolysen) and tilt, e.g., head up. All four can be varied as indicated to provide greater or lesser hypotension.

The successful use of deliberately produced arterial hypotension will depend on whether nutrition for the heart, the brain and the liver can be maintained during the period of low blood pressure. The kidney apparently will survive reasonable insults. Therefore, the clinicians electing this procedure must be able to predict which patient will tolerate it. Most observers agree that young, healthy subjects can withstand reduced blood pressure satisfactorily. Most also agree that older subjects with sclerotic vessels and previous histories of coronary, cerebral or renal insufficiency are poor candidates.

Induced Hypothermia

Deliberate reduction of body temperature during anesthesia and operation offers advantages to certain types of patients. Such patients include those scheduled for open heart operations, grafting of aortic aneurysms or other procedures that involve prolonged interruption of blood supply to tissues, and patients with uncontrolled hyperthyroidism, marked degrees of fever or anoxia. The purpose of hypothermia is to reduce metabolism so that tissues may better tolerate reduction in blood supply or may no longer require excessive oxygenation. Oxygen consumption is reduced by about 50 per cent when a body temperature of 78° F. (25.6° C.) is reached.

Cooling is unpleasant for a conscious subject, and the majority of patients are anesthetized lightly prior to reduction of their temperature. The anesthetic agents or technics do not appear to be of great importance so long as adequate pulmonary ventilation is provided. Since the heat production associated with shivering makes hypothermia more difficult to achieve, muscle relaxants may be used. The technics of cooling vary from surface application of cold to the direct cooling of blood as it passes from an arterial cannula through coils immersed in ice water back to a vein. Specially constructed blankets are also available which contain coils through which circulates a refrigerant. The patient lies between two layers of coils. Immersion of the trunk and extremities in cold water is also used. The rate of cooling is relatively slow for adults—several hours being required to decrease rectal temperature from normal to 30° C. with surface cooling. Children may be cooled more rapidly.

Many physiologic alterations accompany hypothermia. Cardiac output is reduced, blood pressure declines, and pulse rate falls. As part of the general depression of tissue activity and reactivity, respirations become inadequate. If this is not treated, respiratory acidosis may develop. Cardiac irritability increases, and ventricular fibrillation may occur. The cause of this apparent increase in myocardial irritability is unknown. Conduction of impulses in the nervous system is reduced by cooling. Blood viscosity increases. Hemoglobin tends to hold on to oxygen more tenaciously at low temperatures. The solubility of all gases increases so that much more oxygen and carbon dioxide, for example, are dissolved than at normal body temperature. The same holds true for anesthetic gases and vapors.

The length of time which tissues can survive absence of all blood supply has not yet been determined for man at varying body temperatures. However, it is known in dogs, that the liver will tolerate only 20 minutes of complete ischemia at normal temperatures, while 60 minutes is permissible at a temperature of 27° C. Similar data are being obtained for the brain, the heart, the gastrointestinal tract and the kidney.

The effect of differential cooling on the survival of the brain in laboratory animals has been studied. Striking prolongations of the period of anoxia without demonstrated residual damage were obtained by lowering the temperature. The technic may be useful in neurosurgery and in operations which can be performed only when the blood supply to tissues must be interrupted for relatively prolonged periods of time, e.g., thoracic aortic grafting, or resection of the liver. Hypothermia also deserves study as a method of anesthesia for substandard patients.

Hypnosis

Hypnosis has been re-explored recently as an adjuvant to anesthesia. Even enthusiasts agree that its role is limited, but with proper training in technic, an anesthetist can either induce anesthesia or provide total anesthesia in certain selected patients.

Hypnosis involves the uncritical acceptance of ideas by the subject from the operator and requires an exaggerated state of suggestibility. About 10 to 20 per cent of the population can respond sufficiently so that total anesthesia is possible. Children above the age of 5 or 6, anxious to explore new things, and with an ability to create a fantasy, are often good subjects. The procedure is time-consuming and, if a deep trance is to be provided for an operation, rehearsal of each step of the procedure is believed to be desirable. Constant reinforcement during operation is usually required.

Hypnosis has certain potential dangers. It may uncover critical problems or internal repressions in a patient's background which, when brought to the surface, cause a serious threat to the individual's mental balance. An anesthetist should not use the technic for psychotherapy lest lack of knowledge of psychodynamics result in tragic consequences.

UNUSUAL COMPLICATIONS OF ANESTHESIA

The administration of anesthesia involves the avoidance and the treatment of all types of complications which may be inherent in the patient, the agents employed, the technic of application, or the supportive measures used. A number of these complications have been discussed in other sections of this chapter. Those listed here have occurred with sufficient frequency or have sufficient potential to warrant mention.

Injuries to the Eyes

Careless application of a face mask, certain positions of the patient on the operating table (e.g., face down), the anesthetic agent employed and the activities of the surgeon in cleansing the skin about the face may predispose the patient to ocular injury. Open technics with liquid anesthetics are particularly liable to result in conjunctivitis or corneal abrasions, while large masks pressing on the orbits have been known to produce intraocular injuries and to give rise to reflex vagal activity.

In general, the best precaution against injury is to keep the eyelids closed. The procedure of eliciting a corneal reflex to determine depth of anesthesia is not a good one because of the possibility of abrading the cornea. It may be necessary to approximate the lids with Scotch tape or adhesive, particularly during long operations, to keep the eyes closed. Instillation of a 5 per cent boric acid ophthalmic ointment will prevent drying of the corneas in the deeper planes of anesthesia. The eyes should be inspected at the conclusion of anesthesia. Should injury have occurred, ophthalmologic consultation is indicated. Simple conjunctivitis is treated best by irrigations with saturated solutions of boric acid. Corneal abrasions are not only painful but may progress to inflammation of the uveal tract if untreated. If treated early with antibiotics locally, abrasions often begin to re-epithelialize within 24 hours.

Injuries to Nerves

Peripheral nerves can be damaged during anesthesia by overstretching between two points of fixation, pinching between unyielding structures, or direct pressure, mainly because the patient is unable to complain, and the protective action of muscle tone is lacking. The nerves most commonly injured are those which are placed superficially: the brachial plexus, the ulnar nerve, the common peroneal and the radial.

The nerves forming the brachial plexus have two points of fixation: one centrally at the transverse processes of the cervical vertebrae, and the other peripherally at the point of attachment to the tissues of the arm. Excessive separation of these two points may stretch the nerves, and nerve palsies may ensue. The presence of several natural anatomic fulcrums, such as the scaleni muscles which can compress the plexuses against the first rib, the attachment of the pectoralis minor muscle to the coracoid process of the scapula around which the plexus is stretched in hyperabduction of the arm, and the rounded head of the humerus provide additional possibilities for stretch. The use of a shoulder brace improperly applied to the soft tissues of the cervical triangles may not only act as an artificial fulcrum but also compress the brachial plexus against the underlying structures. Lastly, the plexus may be pinched between the scalene muscles and the first rib or between the clavicle and the first rib with downward displacement of the shoulder.

To avoid these brachial plexus injuries one must bear the possibility in mind constantly and avoid extremes of position of the head and the arm. Should a palsy result after operation, a careful neurologic examination must be made as a base line for future improvement, and measures for restoration of function must be begun. The latter include proper support of the weakened muscles and physiotherapy. In the case of severe injuries, restitution of normal function may not take place until 6 months or a year have elapsed.

The ulnar and the common peroneal nerves and to lesser degree the radial nerves are superficial structures liable to be compressed against bone by outer pressure or stretched around bony eminences. Again, certain operating positions will predispose these nerves to injury, and they are more apt to occur in debilitated patients where the subcutaneous protective layer of fat is absent. If the latter occur, treatment is the same as that described for brachial plexus palsies.

FIRE AND EXPLOSION HAZARDS

In comparison with the other hazards of anesthesia, explosions occur so infrequently as to be almost insignificant. However, the emotional factors involved in an anesthetic explosion make it a dreaded disaster.

Fires and explosions are combustive processes differing merely in the speed of the reaction and the magnitude of the forces released. Three elements are necessary for the production of combustion: (1) a combustible substance; (2) a supporter of combustion, oxygen, from whatever source; and (3) a source of ignition.

All hydrocarbons are subject to decomposition by heat. Several burn readily or explode when in proper mixture with air, oxygen or nitrous oxide. The volatile liquids and gases used in anesthesia may be classified as follows:

1. The vapors of divinyl ether, diethyl ether, ethyl chloride, ethylene and cyclopropane will explode violently under suitable conditions. Trichloroethylene vapor is not flammable either in oxygen or air at ordinary temperatures; however, phosgene and dichloracetylene may be liberated if the trichloroethylene vapor is heated. Chloroform vapor will not ignite but will liberate phosgene if heated. Halothane and methoxyflurane are not flammable.

2. Oxygen and nitrous oxide are not explosible but support combustion. Explosions have occurred with nitrous oxide alone, presumably because of the presence of explosive contaminants derived from the anesthetic machine.

It is impractical to memorize the flammable ranges for the various anesthetics in air, nitrous oxide and oxygen. The general order of magnitude of the flammable ranges for anesthetics is: 1.7 per cent to 37 per cent in air; 1.4 per cent to 40 per cent in nitrous oxide; and 1.8 per cent to 85 per cent in oxygen. The anesthetic concentrations of flammable gases lie within these ranges.

PREVENTION

Measures for the prevention of explosions will be discussed under the heading of the three conditions necessary for combustion.

The Combustible Substances

1. **Avoidance.** Agents or methods which do not carry the hazard of explosibility should be used whenever possible in situations involving the use of x-rays, the cautery, flame, etc.

2. **Storage of Agents and Care of Equipment.** Cylinders and containers of volatile liquids should be stored in well-ventilated places at a safe distance from radiators, steam pipes and other sources of heat. Oxidizing substances (oxygen, nitrous oxide) should be separated from reducing substances (the hydrocarbons).

The Presence of Substances That Support Combustion

1. **Dilution With Air or Inert Gases.** Since the explosive range of the flammable agent is narrower in air than with oxygen or nitrous oxide, the explosion hazard may be reduced by administering anesthetics with the minimal effective or safe concentrations of oxygen or nitrous oxide. This increased safety from fire must be weighed against the physiologic advantages of the higher tensions of oxygen in inspired mixtures. "Open" ether may be ad-

ministered with relative safety in the presence of the cautery or x-ray equipment provided that the container, the mask and the material saturated with the agent are removed at a time when sparking or heating is apt to occur.

2. **Closed System Technic.** The closed system of administering anesthetics confines the explosive mixture to the apparatus and the patient's respiratory tract save when leaks occur or the reservoir bag is emptied. Thus the hazard of ignition from exogenous sources such as sparks is lessened, but there remains a greater likelihood of injury to the patient in the event of an explosion.

Sources of Ignition

1. **Obvious sources** of ignition such as flames, cigarettes and matches should be banned from anesthetizing locations (anesthesia rooms, operating room, corridors and storage places).

2. **Electrical wiring and equipment** when installed in anesthetizing locations should conform to the specifications advised by the National Electrical Codes and National Board of Fire Underwriters, although the Underwriters occasionally appear unreasonable to the author.

3. **Static sparks** probably constitute the greatest danger as sources of ignition. Since they may be generated in so many different ways, they are difficult to control. There can be no accumulation of static electricity if all objects present are isoelectric, i.e., at the same electrical potential. The chief means of achieving isoelectric conditions is the grounding of all objects and persons within the "hazardous area." A list of preventive measures is appended.

A. Equipment

a. Floors in anesthetizing locations should provide a path of moderate electrical conductivity for grounding purposes. Too low a resistance may permit electrocution if faulty wiring is present. Too high a resistance may prevent run-off of static charge and, hence, an increased likelihood of sparking.

b. Furniture, equipment and operating tables should make contact with the ground via metal or conductive rubber contacts.

c. Woolen blankets are prohibited in anesthetizing locations, and mattresses and cushions should be conductive.

B. Activity of Personnel

a. Breaking connections on anesthetic apparatus should be carried out with both parts held by the anesthetist to maintain isoelectric conditions.

b. Persons other than the anesthetist should keep away from maximal and dangerous accumulation points of combustible substances. These are (1) the patient's respiratory tract and (2) the anesthetic machine.

c. Personnel should wear shoes with conductive soles or with conductive strips. Silk, wool, rayon or sharkskin may be worn if in contact with the skin.

C. Other Measures

a. Cautery and high-frequency equipment. If the cautery is used during operations, it should be beyond a 2-foot radius from the head of the patient, provided that there is a suitable intervening barrier and ventilation about the head.

b. Humidification. A film of moisture may serve as a means of dissipating electrical charges. This is especially important in dry climates or in winter.

POSTANESTHETIC OBSERVATION ROOM (RECOVERY ROOM)

From the standpoint of anesthesia the most critical period in a patient's postoperative course is that of the first few hours after operation. During this time the unconscious or semiconscious patient is dependent upon others for his well-being. Even the individual who has received regional anesthesia and is in control of his faculties may require prompt attention for circulatory or other abnormalities. A specially staffed and specially equipped room should be available for the care of these patients. This room should be immediately adjacent to the operating suite, for if a patient has to be transported for any distance the purpose of the room is defeated in the interim. The facilities in such an area should include oxygen and suction outlets, solutions for parenteral administration, laryngoscopic and bronchoscopic equipment, and an assortment of drugs which might be required for the treatment of various respiratory or circulatory emergencies.

If space is limited the following patients, at least, should be admitted to the recovery room: (1) any patient who has spinal anesthesia and has had significant circulatory or respiratory insufficiency; (2) any patient who has been given general anesthesia and is not oriented as to time and place; (3) any patient whose immediate postanesthetic condition concerns the anesthetist; (4) an outpatient who has received general anesthesia and needs to recover prior to departing from the hospital.

During the recovery room stay blood pressure, pulse and respiratory rate should be recorded at regular intervals. Bodily temperature should be determined in infants, and in other patients if changes in temperature are suspected. A careful physical examination of the chest should be made on patients who have a rapid respiratory rate, who have respiratory obstruction and are cyanotic, orthopneic or dyspneic. For example, pneumothorax may be found after thoracolumbar sympathetic resections, renal, thyroid, or intrathoracic operations. Atelectasis may occur at any time during or after anesthesia. Pulmonary edema may occur in patients with myocardial disease, respiratory obstruction, or after pneumonectomy. Appropriate therapeutic measures for these sequelae should be instituted promptly.

The average patient who has had general anesthesia may be dismissed from the postanesthetic observation room if he can obey simple commands (i.e., "open your eyes," "stick out your tongue"). The discharge of other patients will depend upon improvement in the primary reason for their admission. Frequently, the chief criterion for dismissing a patient from the recovery room will be the clinical judgment of the attending anesthetist and surgeon.

MECHANICAL VENTILATION OF THE LUNGS

A number of factors have contributed to improvement in design and increased use of mechanical ventilators. In the operating room, an increased awareness that gas exchange is frequently deficient during general anesthesia and operation, the development of modern anesthetic technics which diminish or eliminate spontaneous breathing, the need for greater freedom of the hands of the anesthetist during surgical procedures, and the advent of intrathoracic operations have all played a role. Elsewhere in the hospital, ventilators support the individual with weakness or paralysis of respiratory muscles (as in the bulbar poliomyelitis or myasthenia gravis), central nervous system depression (as after drugs or intracranial injury), chest wall trauma, restriction of diaphragmatic movement (as with abdominal distention or obesity); and they are used to improve the gas exchange in instances of severe lung disease, carbon dioxide retention, hypoxia, and increased work of breathing.

Action of the Mechanical Ventilator

A mechanical ventilator is a device for changing the pressure within the patient's airway in a cyclic fashion so that gas moves in and out of the lungs. This can be accomplished by raising the airway pressure either by direct application of positive pressure to the airway or by lowering the ambient pressure around the patient's chest. With both technics pressure in the airway is greater than that surrounding the body, and the patient's lungs fill with gas and then empty.

To produce pressure changes in the lungs and thorax, a source of energy is required. The energy may be contained in a tank of compressed air or oxygen, or may originate in a bellows or piston device driven by a compressed gas or an electric motor.

The action of a mechanical ventilator may be divided into four phases: inspiration; changeover from inspiration to expiration; expiration; changeover from expiration to inspiration.

Inspiration. During inspiration there is an interrelationship between the flow rate of gas into the lungs, the volume of gas delivered to the lungs, the pressure in the alveoli, and the pressure at the mouth. The interrelationship among these factors is determined by the characteristics of the patient's lungs. Only one of these factors is determined primarily by the ventilator—either pressure at the patient's mouth or flow rate into the lungs. Consequently, ventilators may be described as pressure generators or flow generators. Pressure generators exert a constant pressure throughout the inspiratory phase, and the flow patterns, volumes, and pressure changes in the lungs result from the effects of this pressure (Fig. 13-2). Flow generators produce either a

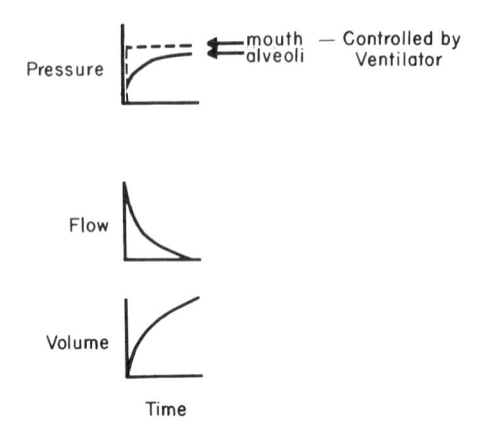

FIG. 13-2. Pressure generator. See text for explanation. (Dripps, R. D., Eckenhoff, J. E., and Vandam, L. D.: Introduction to Anesthesia. ed 3. Philadelphia, W. B. Saunders, 1967)

constant flow through inspiration (Fig. 13-3, A) or what is called a half-cycle sine wave with flows increasing to maximum halfway through inspiration, then decreasing (Fig. 13-3, B). Gas volumes and pressures result from the effects of this flow pattern on the lung.

End of Inspiration. Cycling at the end of inspiration occurs after a preset period of time, when a preset pressure is reached, or when a fixed volume has been delivered from the machine.

Expiration. During expiration flow, pressure, and volume interact as during inspiration, with the ventilator again primarily controlling pressure or flow. Expiration usually occurs by allowing the patient's airway to open to the atmosphere, utilizing the elastic recoil of the lungs and chest wall. Some ventilators can exert a negative pressure during some or all of the expiratory phase.

End of Expiration. The changeover from expiration to inspiration occurs at some preset time or may be initiated by the spontaneously breathing patient whose inspiratory effort triggers the inspiratory phase of the ventilator.

ADVERSE EFFECTS

Pressure applied to the patient's airway via a ventilator may adversely affect the circulatory system and lung structure. The cardiovascular effects include interference with venous return to the heart, lowered cardiac output, and arterial hypotension. The basis for these changes is the transmission of raised airway pressure to the pleural cavity and resulting compression of intrathoracic veins, together with reduction in the effectiveness of the "thoracic pump." The healthy individual can compensate readily for these effects on the cardiovascular system, essentially by vasoconstriction. The patient who is hypovolemic or unable to increase vasomotor tone may become hypotensive.

The degree of hypotension is proportional to the amount of pressure applied and to the duration of its application. The lower the mean airway pressure throughout the respiratory cycle, the less is cardiac output reduced. Low mean pressure may be achieved by use

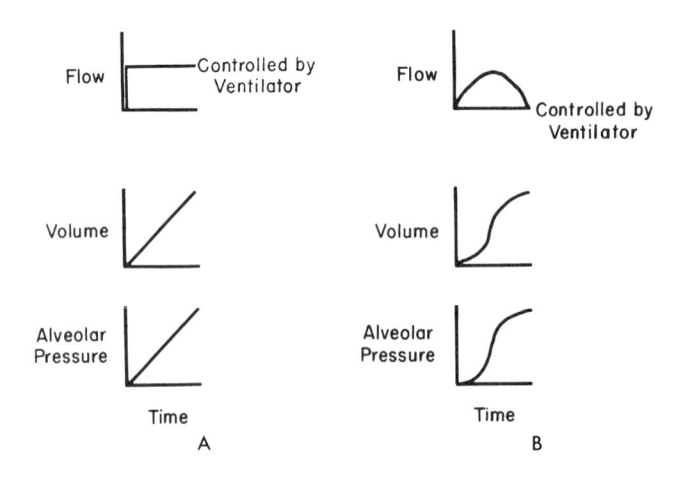

FIG. 13-3, A and B. Flow generator. See text for explanation. (Dripps, R. D., Eckenhoff, J. E., and Vandam, L. D.: Introduction to Anesthesia. ed 3. Philadelphia, W. B. Saunders, 1967)

of low peak pressures and slow inflation rates, keeping inspiration shorter than expiration, avoiding prolonged pressure plateaus, seeking minimal resistance to expiration, and using negative pressure during expiration.

Raised airway pressure may damage the lung, particularly if high pressure is applied for more than a moment. If, because of uneven ventilation, high pressure is exerted on one lung area and lower pressure on another, this unevenness may predispose to alveolar rupture. One must realize that the pressures observed on the ventilator dials are those applied to the airway at the mouth and do not indicate pressure at the alveoli.

Amount of Ventilation

Elimination of carbon dioxide by a patient on a mechanical ventilator is best determined by frequent measurement of the arterial pCO_2 and pH. The volume of ventilation necessary depends only upon the patient's metabolic rate (CO_2 production) and the physiologic dead space (anatomic and alveolar); both are frequently increased in a patient requiring mechanical ventilation. Ventilation of nonperfused lung and perfusion of underventilated or nonventilated lung increase alveolar dead space (e.g., low cardiac output, low blood volume, low arterial pressure, atelectasis, pneumonia, pulmonary emphysema, and pulmonary embolism). Dead space ventilation may be as much as 80 per cent of the tidal volume. The ratio of V_D/V_T in normal man is about 0.3. It rises in patients on ventilators, and its course is regarded by some as of greater prognostic value than x-rays, physical examination, or alveolar-arterial (A-a) gradients. Metabolic rate is increased by fever, increased muscular activity (shivering, restlessness, work of breathing, convulsions), and increased release of epinephrine (apprehension, hypercapnia, hypoxia). Hence predictions of ventilatory volumes, by the Radford nomogram for instance, are usually in error. They can only be used as a guide to initial volumes provided, and their use usually results in underventilation. Fortunately, both physiologic dead space and metabolic rate can be measured in these patients.

Hyperventilation is readily achieved in patients with normal lungs receiving mechanical ventilation but is rarely harmful. However, the reduction of cerebral blood flow caused by an arterial pCO_2 below 20 mm. of mercury may lead to cerebral hypoxia, and the danger is probably greater in elderly patients with cerebral arteriosclerosis.

Along with determination of blood gases, tidal volume and minute ventilation should be measured frequently. Estimation of the volume of gas delivered to the patient can be made only by measurement of the expired volume. Dials or spirometers recording during the inspiratory phase reflect merely the volume delivered to the patient because of leaks. With measurement of tidal volume and peak positive airway pressure, an estimate of total compliance can be made. A decrease in compliance suggests air-space collapse, pneumonia, interstitial edema, and, when a pressure-limited ventilator is used, lessened ventilation.

Amount of Oxygen

Oxygenation is best monitored by arterial pO_2 measurements, although ear oximetry can be used. Elevation of inspired oxygen above that in room air is usually necessary because of the maldistribution of ventilation and shunting that exist in most patients requiring ventilator assistance. One must, however, consider the possibility of pulmonary oxygen toxicity. Inhalation of 80 to 100 per cent oxygen by normal indviduals for more than 14 to 16 hours is followed by chest pain and other suggestions of tracheobronchial "irritation." With a Pauling-type paramagnetic oxygen analyzer, one should determine the concentration of oxygen being delivered from the ventilator. The lowest concentration needed to bring pAO_2 to 90 to 100 mm. of mercury should be selected.

Patients who are continuously ventilated with the same low tidal volumes (up to 400 to 500 ml. for an average adult male) may show a progressive reduction in arterial pO_2 for the first 90 minutes or so. Whether the reduction in arterial pO_2 represents primary alveolar collapse, as some believe, or alveolar collapse secondary to airway obstruction with subsequent alveolar gas absorption, as others contend, is not yet clear. The tendency toward hypoxemia can be compensated for to a considerable extent by periodic hyperinflation (high pressure sustained for about 10 seconds). Another prophylactic measure is to ventilate with a higher than normal tidal volume, e.g. 750 to 1,000 ml., in such a fashion that there is hardly a pause between the end of expiration and the beginning of the next inspiration. The latter precaution is to avoid absorption of alveolar gas by blood during a prolonged pause.

Use of Mechanical Ventilators

Volumes and Flow Patterns. Several problems arise as one attempts to provide optimal ventilating volumes and flow patterns. It is convenient to think of mechanical ventilators in two groups: those in which the pressure exerted by the apparatus is determined beforehand, i.e., pressure preset or pressure limited; and those in which the volume delivered is determined beforehand, i.e. volume preset or volume limited. The pressure-limited apparatus delivers a variable volume and the volume-limited device exerts a variable pressure.

With a *pressure-limited machine*, the volume of gas delivered decreases as resistance increases or compliance declines or both. The pressure limit is rapidly reached and ventilatory volumes are reduced. The duration of inspiration decreases and the short, rapid inspirations are not effective in ventilating alveoli. Such an apparatus can usually compensate for leaks, although if the leak is large and the ventilator terminates inspiration only when a certain pressure is reached, cycling may never occur. Therefore frequent measurements of expiratory volumes and frequent readjustments of cycling pressure and inspiratory flow rates are necessary with this type of ventilator.

A *volume-limited ventilator* is capable of building up great pressure to overcome resistance or decreasing compliance, or both. It will increase pressure automatically to deliver a constant tidal volume. Safety pressure valves are placed in the inspiratory circuit of volume-limited ventilators. Since inspiration ends after a certain volume has been delivered from the apparatus or after a certain time for inspiration, this apparatus will not automatically compensate for a leak.

In the use of a mechanical ventilator, flow rate, pressures, volume, and time should be planned so that pulmonary ventilation is maximally effective and adverse effects are minimal. In a person with normal lungs, many patterns of ventilation can be used. In the patient with pulmonary disease, two ventilatory patterns are widely recommended. One involves use of low flow rates and a long inspiratory period so that turbulence and pressure in the airway are reduced and large tidal volumes are delivered through the narrowed air passages. The second pattern is that of "sine-wave" flow. Pressure and volume continue to increase while closed air passages are being opened and gas is being distributed. This pattern is alleged to approximate most closely that of normal spontaneous breathing. With both patterns expiration should be longer than inspiration.

During expiration a rapid decrease in airway pressure may result in bronchial collapse and air trapping. Resistance to expiration will lessen this tendency.

Humidification. Normally, inspired air is warmed and humidified as it passes through the nasal cavities. Adequate humidification and warming of the inspired air is necessary for proper function of the respiratory tract mucosa. The secretions produced by the goblet cells and glands of the mucosa are a mixture of water, polysaccharide, and protein with a certain viscosity so that there is optimal function of the cilia and protection of the epithelial cells. If the nasal passages are by-passed by mouth breathing, by an endotracheal tube or a tracheostomy, or if the moisture content of the inspired air is low relative to the temperature, the inspired gas becomes saturated by the water from these secretions and the mucosa in an attempt to make up the deficit in humidity. The result will be increased viscosity of the mucus, poor ciliary function, retained secretions, blocked air passages, and finally infection. The importance of humidification of inspired air delivered by a ventilator is thus apparent.

Various types of equipment can be used in an attempt to saturate air reaching the trachea with water vapor at body temperature. The bubbler jar delivers gas to the patient 21 per cent saturated at body temperature and is therefore satisfactory for use only with a nasal catheter or a face mask. It should not be used with an endotracheal tube or tracheostomy. Diverting the gas through a sintered bronze disk to increase the area of contact with water or heating the water jar and bubbling gas through it will raise the relative humidity

The inspired air may be directed through a container of water heated *to* body temperature. At the exit from the humidifier unit, the humidity deficit has been eliminated, but as air passes through delivery tubes there is a decrease in temperature and water is deposited within the tubes. Air reaches the patient at less than body temperature and the patient must warm and humidify the air once again. Units have been designed to heat air *above* body temperature to compensate for the temperature drop in the delivery tube and so deliver saturated gas at body temperature to the proximal airway. With this system condensation of water may result in obstruction to air flow, and elimination of heat loss may be followed by hyperthermia.

Humidifiers are meant to saturate air with water molecules. Nebulizers, on the other hand, suspend, in the air, water particles made up of many molecules. These devices direct a rapid flow of gas over an orifice connected to a reservoir or drip water onto a metal plate which is vibrating at an ultrasonic frequency. Nebulizers using the capillary-jet principle produce particles of water with the majority between 0.001 micron and 5 microns in size. The ultrasonic nebulizer produces particles between 0.8 and 1 micron in size. The output of the nebulizers does not need to be warmed, as the particles of water in suspension can easily give up water molecules to overcome the humidity deficit arising when inspired air is warmed to body temperature. A particle size of 0.5 to 1.5 micron is most effective in avoiding fallout in the delivery tubes and upper airway and allowing deposition of particles in the terminal bronchioles and alveoli.

Water Retention. A positive water balance resulting in interstitial pulmonary edema, with consequent difficulty in ventilation and oxygenation and attendant increased work of breathing, is not uncommon in patients being mechanically ventilated for more than a day or so. The onset may be relatively sudden; its etiology is unknown, but may be related to inappropriate ADH secretion. A dramatic improvement follows administration of a diuretic. Careful, daily attention to the patient's weight and urinary output are necessary to detect fluid retention before it has progressed too far. Interestingly enough, no elevation in venous pressure has been reported with the development of the interstitial pulmonary edema; there is no evidence of cardiac failure, nor do the lungs sound "wet" by auscultation.

Weaning from the Ventilator. The weaning of a patient from a mechanical ventilator is sometimes difficult. Dyspnea is a common complaint at this time because of patient adjustment to low pCO_2, high pO_2 and deep lung inflations with adaptation of stretch receptors while undergoing mechanical ventilation. Obviously the psychological problem in removing a patient from a ventilator that has been his respiratory support for a long period is a major one. Increased dead space and shunting, decreased compliance, increased carbon dioxide production, and decreased muscle strength increase the problem.

Weaning should begin as soon as possible to diminish the progressive muscle weakness that arises from inactivity. Patient-cycled respirations with a gradual increase in the amount of effort required to initiate inspiration can be used to increase muscle tone. Weaning is likely to be unsuccessful unless the patient's vital capacity is greater than twice the predicted normal tidal volume. It is unwise to begin the process until the vital capacity is more than 10 ml./kg. Initial periods of three to four minutes off the ventilator every half hour should be gradually increased. Supplemental oxygen must be administered. The entire weaning process may be a lengthy one, and careful monitoring of the patient's general condition as well as of ventilatory volumes and blood gases throughout this period is essential.

Infection. The delivery tubing, valves, and humidifiers of ventilators are important potential sources of infection. Numerous types of pathogenic bacteria and fungi have been cultured from these within the first 24 hours of their use. *Pseudomonas aeruginosa* in particular is found in the warm, moist environment of the humidifier. Daily change and gas sterilization of tubes, valves, and humidifiers is strongly recommended.

REFERENCES

Adriani, J., and Morton, R. C.: Drug dependence: important considerations from the anesthesiologist's viewpoint. Anesth. Analg., 47:472, 1968.

Dripps, R. D., and Vandam, L. D.: Long-term follow-up of patients who received 10,098 spinal anesthetics. J.A.M.A., 156:1486-1491, 1954.

Dripps, R. D., Eckenhoff, J. E., and Vandam, L. D.: Introduction to Anesthesia. Philadelphia, W. B. Saunders, ed. 3, 1967.

Dundee, J. W., Nicholl, R. M., and Moore, J.: Alterations in response to somatic pain associated with anesthesia. VIII: The effects of atropine and hyoscine. Brit. J. Anaesth., 33:565-571, 1961.

Egbert, L. D., Battit, G. E., Turndorf, H., and Beecher, H. K.: The value of the preoperative visit by an anesthetist. J.A.M.A., 185:553-555, 1963.

Katz, R. L., Wolf, C., and Papper, E. M.: The nondepolarizing neuromuscular blocking action of succinylcholine in man. Anesthesiology, 26:784, 1963.

Parkins, W. M., Jensen, J. M., and Vars, H. M.: Brain cooling in the prevention of brain damage during periods of circulatory occlusion in dogs. Ann. Surg., 140:284-287, 1954.

CHAPTER 14

JAMES D. HARDY, M.D.

Operative Surgical Care

The operation will remain the central act of the surgical experience. This is true for the patient, the surgeon and all supporting personnel. The operation involves comprehensive planning. It imposes an immediacy of realism that can be virtually unique in medical practice. The dimensions of the "operation" range from the physiology of blood gas values to the anatomic symmetry of a perfect anastomosis.

PREOPERATIVE PREPARATION

While nonoperative surgical care is discussed elsewhere in this volume, certain preoperative measures merit repetition here. First, the general requirements involved in a careful workup of any hospitalized patient apply with special force to a patient who is to undergo a major operation. He must be not only capable of withstanding the technical procedure itself but also of surviving the increased metabolic demands and deranged organ function of the early postoperative period. For example, the patient in chronic renal failure would usually survive the operation itself, but he might well die of uremia in the late postoperative period. Likewise, the patient with severe impairment of liver or lung function may go through the operative procedure fairly well, only to slide into irreversible hepatic or pulmonary insufficiency hours or days later. Thus it is essential that the functional reserves of vital visceral organs be estimated accurately by history, physical examination and appropriate laboratory tests. Any deficiencies, whatever their natures, will be taken into account by the surgeon as he decides whether or not an operation should be performed and, if so, what type of operation is most likely to correct successfully the pathologic lesion which exists. Most patients with heart disease who are not in acute failure and have not had a myocardial infarction in the past 6 months represent acceptable operative risks for necessary operations. It is advisable to secure an electrocardiogram, a chest roentgenogram, a complete blood count, a urinalysis, and measurements of the blood urea nitrogen and fasting blood sugar levels in most older patients who are to undergo a major operation.

OPERATIVE PERMIT

During the course of the preoperative evaluation the surgeon will have discussed with the patient and perhaps members of his family the nature of the condition for which an operation is proposed, the operation that is planned and the probable prognosis. The patient himself need not be offered the total implications of his disease when he probably harbors, say, a malignant tumor. Nevertheless, some close relative should be given the complete known truth and the probable diagnosis, however unfavorable the latter may be. Furthermore, either the signed operative permit itself or the history should reflect the information given the patient and his family prior to the operation so that the consent he gives is "informed" to the extent feasible. It is advisable to have the signed permission read so as to give the surgeon a degree of freedom to proceed according to his judgment if some unexpected condition is disclosed at operation.

PREOPERATIVE ORDERS

The purpose of the preoperative orders is to render the patient as safe and as ready as possible for the operation that is planned. The primary essential is that the stomach be empty, for otherwise it would be hazardous to anesthetize the patient lest he vomit and aspirate some of this material into the lungs. Beyond this requirement, certain other orders of general applicability are valuable in preparing for operation. General preoperative orders follow:

1. Nothing by mouth (after a given time which is at least 4 hours prior to the hour for anesthesia induction).

2. Sedation to provide rest the night preceding operation.

3. Prepare (shave) proposed operative site.

4. Insert nasogastric tube and/or indwelling urinary catheter (if indicated).

5. Saline enema if indicated and especially if operation involves pelvic structures. (For operations on the colon itself special cleansing measures are employed [Chap. 39].)

6. Draw blood and cross-match with number of bottles of blood indicated, depending on type of operation (see Chap. 8).

7. Initiate intravenous fluids if operation is to be delayed beyond the morning hours.

8. Atropine and sedation in appropriate dosage on call from operating room (see Chap. 13).

Beyond these general orders which apply to most patients who are scheduled for a major operation, various additional measures will be required for particular operations.

THE OPERATING SUITE

The operating theater occupies a special position in the planning and the orientation of most hospitals. It is here that the coordinated efforts of many types of personnel are brought to bear so as to achieve an area in which the most complex modern surgical procedures can be performed with adequate supporting personnel and with minimal risk of infection. The activities carried on in the operating suite are supervised jointly by the surgeon, the anesthesiologist and the nursing personnel. In most hospitals the surgical staff sets the various standards of procedure which will prevail in the operating suite. The nursing personnel are importantly responsible for the day-to-day execution of these standards, and this segment of the administration is exerted through the operating suite supervisor. This applies especially with regard to cleanliness, to the wearing of the proper garments, to rigid sterilization of all materials to be used for operations and to monitoring traffic in the operating suite. The operating room nurses may be responsible administratively to the hospital director, but they are responsible professionally to the surgeon.

ZONES OF OPERATING SUITES

It is useful to consider 3 zones of increasingly rigid precautions in achieving an aseptic operation. The outer zone is represented by areas within the operating suite but still outside the rooms in which operations are actually performed. This outer zone of the general operating suite should be restricted to persons actually having to do with the conduct of activities within this area. In most instances persons entering the operating suite will first exchange street clothes and shoes for scrub suits and for other shoes worn only in this area. However, in the interests of more efficient function, at times these rules are relaxed to permit the pathologist, for example, to enter in covering garments to gain information and to render a frozen section diagnosis. The middle zone is represented by that portion of the operating room itself that does not actually involve the sterile operative field. At this point all personnel will have donned scrub suits, special shoes or shoe covers, and clean caps and masks. Thus the "floor" or "circulating" nurse wears cap, mask and scrub gown, but she does not don a sterile gown and gloves. Finally, the inner zone is represented by the operative field where all participants don sterile gowns and gloves, all instruments and sponges are sterile, and every effort is made to preserve completely aseptic technic.

There is considerable variation from one hospital to another with regard to the type of clothing to be worn in the outer zone of the operating suite. Most hospitals require that street clothes be replaced with a scrub suit and that street shoes be either removed or covered with clean paper, rubber or fabric. Admittedly, good results with a relative absence of postoperative wound infections are achieved in hospitals where a less rigid attitude exists regarding apparel to be worn by persons entering the operating suite and even the operating room. Nevertheless, the better institutions constantly strive for perfection, and the maximum precautions consistent with the practical circumstances should be observed in every hospital.

An infected case, as for example the patient whose abscess is to be drained, is usually placed at the end of the day's schedule of clean operations. Special measures will be employed to kill any bacteria which may have been liberated into the air of the room. Ultraviolet light is often used for this purpose, but liquid disinfectants for floor and walls will suffice. In addition, the linens, the gloves, the gowns, the caps and the masks used with the infected case are deposited in a special container placed in the infected operating room itself, and these are handled separately from the linens used for clean cases.

FINAL PREPARATION

As the patient arrives in the operating room certain final preparations and measures are completed. Although equipment for special procedures such as operative cholangiography or cardiopulmonary by-pass will have been requested previously, the surgeon or his assistants now check again to make certain that these requirements are ready. The availability of blood for transfusion is again determined, and appropriate roentgenograms are placed in the lighted viewbox. All laboratory or necessary data of any type must be available. A few words from the surgeon at this time are very reassuring to the patient, and following this exchange the operation should proceed promptly.

While these activities are proceeding, the medical students or other visiting and properly clad personnel may discuss the case with members of the surgical team. However, such discussion should not be held within earshot of the patient. Even the most secure and optimistic individual may be upset by listening to potential problems which may not even be related to his particular case.

Anesthesia

The preparations for anesthetization should not be hurried except under extreme emergency circumstances where death is imminent unless massive hemorrhage can be controlled or respiratory embarrassment relieved. An orderly procedure will provide for all needed equipment, adequate routes for intravenous infusions, and an empty stomach to prevent serious vomiting with possible pulmonary aspiration. In general, the arms should be used

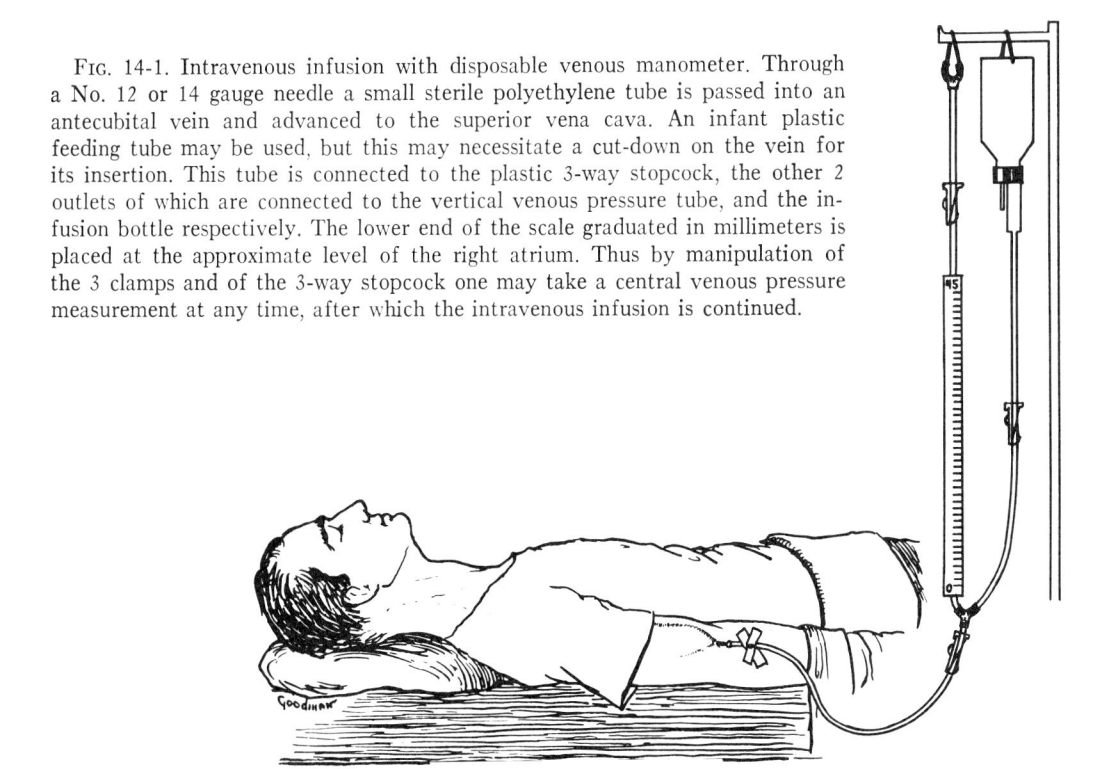

Fig. 14-1. Intravenous infusion with disposable venous manometer. Through a No. 12 or 14 gauge needle a small sterile polyethylene tube is passed into an antecubital vein and advanced to the superior vena cava. An infant plastic feeding tube may be used, but this may necessitate a cut-down on the vein for its insertion. This tube is connected to the plastic 3-way stopcock, the other 2 outlets of which are connected to the vertical venous pressure tube, and the infusion bottle respectively. The lower end of the scale graduated in millimeters is placed at the approximate level of the right atrium. Thus by manipulation of the 3 clamps and of the 3-way stopcock one may take a central venous pressure measurement at any time, after which the intravenous infusion is continued.

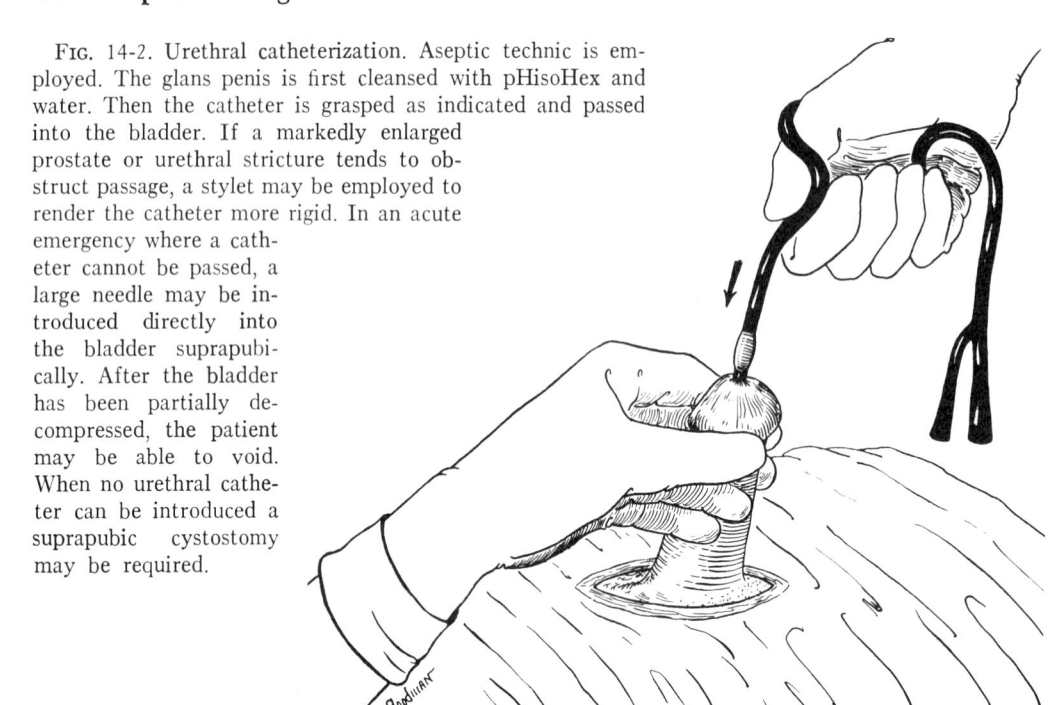

Fig. 14-2. Urethral catheterization. Aseptic technic is employed. The glans penis is first cleansed with pHisoHex and water. Then the catheter is grasped as indicated and passed into the bladder. If a markedly enlarged prostate or urethral stricture tends to obstruct passage, a stylet may be employed to render the catheter more rigid. In an acute emergency where a catheter cannot be passed, a large needle may be introduced directly into the bladder suprapubically. After the bladder has been partially decompressed, the patient may be able to void. When no urethral catheter can be introduced a suprapubic cystostomy may be required.

for intravenous infusions. The subsequent development of thrombophlebitis in the arms is not often a serious problem, but thrombophlebitis in the legs is often serious and sometimes fatal. Furthermore, deliberate steps and movements, with vocal encouragement, will reassure the anxious patient whose preoperative medication may have provided less than optimal sedation.

During the operation the surgeon and the anesthesiologist will inform each other of any circumstance or condition which could influence the welfare of the patient or the course of the procedure. In addition to the induction of anesthesia and the infusion of blood and other fluids as needed, the anesthesiologist frequently assumes responsibility for such ancillary activities as the use of hypothermia or the over-all performance of the pump oxygenator for cardiopulmonary by-pass. Where it is appropriate, he will monitor the electroencephalogram, the electrocardiogram, the blood pressure and the respiratory parameters in the given case. Special apparatus for monitoring the intra-arterial pressure or the central venous pressure (Fig. 14-1) may be attended by the anesthesiologist or his assistant. Finally, data taken at the operating table, such as arterial or intracardiac pressure measurements, may be recorded immediately on the permanent anesthesia record form by the anesthesiologist.

There is an increasing and proper tendency for the anesthesiologist to request that a member of the surgical team stand by during the actual induction. Such a physician is available to monitor the pulse, to assist with equipment or with positioning of the patient's head, or even to perform closed chest cardiac massage in the unlikely event that hypoxia or noxious reflexes should precipitate hypotension and cardiac arrest. Then this physician may insert a needed urinary catheter after the patient has been anesthetized (Fig. 14-2).

Once the patient has been anesthetized and his general condition is considered to be satisfactory, he is placed in the position which will afford an optimal operative approach to the offending organ or lesion. As soon as he has been "turned," as to a lateral decubitus position, his blood pressure will be checked again, since the mere turning of an anesthetized patient from one position to another may cause a serious drop in the blood pressure. This may be due to a reduced effective blood volume, to hypoxia or to an embarrassment of cardiac activity. Bony prominences must be protected from undue or prolonged pressure, which can produce nerve damage or actual skin necrosis. Blankets, cotton wadding, or doughnuts of soft material will usually suffice. Once the positioning is satisfactory, the patient must be secured in the proper position. In the lateral position, straps or adhesive tape may be used to prevent the patient from falling off the operating table, again with proper protection of superficial nerves and pressure points. If the patient is supine, the arms are preferably placed at his side, to avoid trauma to the brachial plexus and to give members of the surgical team more freedom of movement. However, a disadvantage of this arm position is that it is difficult for the anesthesiologist to check the intravenous needle or catheter if this becomes necessary.

Setting Up the Operating Room

The Nurse's Role. The entrance of the patient into the operating room and the preparations for anesthetization are paralleled by industrious activity on the part of the nursing staff. All persons entering the operating room now wear caps and masks and proper scrub suits, except the patient himself, who wears the usual hospital gown. One nurse wears sterile gloves and gown, and she is "setting up" by placing sterilized instruments, sponges and other materials in proper order on sterile tables. She is termed the "scrub nurse," the "suture nurse" or the "instrument nurse." Another nurse wears a cap and a mask but not a sterile gown and gloves. She is the "circulating nurse" who takes packs of sterile materials from the shelves and opens the outer covering so as to preserve the sterility of the contents, as she carefully hands them to the suture nurse as needed. The "circulator" or "floor" nurse will later place used sponges in piles and count them. These 2 nurses remain in the room throughout the operation.

In recent years there has been a growing tendency to utilize technicians for scrub nurses, since graduate nurses are in such short supply. However, the graduate nurse has a much more comprehensive understanding of the importance of special drugs that may be needed during the course of the operation, and she has a more general knowledge of medicine. Thus a technician performs a specialized service in handing the proper instruments and other materials to the surgeon as they are asked for. The circulating nurse performs a much broader function in that she must know special instruments that are needed and special drugs that may be required. The contributions which the suture nurse and the circulating nurse make toward the success of the operation are considerable, and they are important members of the first-class surgical team. The editors of this textbook join the author in asserting that the patient deserves the best possible "suture nurse" when a difficult, hazardous or novel procedure is being performed by the surgeon. Almost always such persons are trained and registered nurses who have supplemented their education with a substantial experience in this highly specialized work. To provide less is to take advantage of the unconsciousness of the patient who would not choose to effect a small economy at so critical a link in the chain on which his welfare depends.

Sterilization of Materials

Most linens and instruments employed for aseptic operations are sterilized by heat. All cloth materials must be freshly laundered, folded and packaged loosely enough to permit sterilizing steam heat to penetrate into the deepest part of each package. The packaging also should be designed to protect the linens from contamination after sterilization and to allow their easy removal and transfer from packages to sterile tables. Packages of linen, including sheets, gowns and sponges should be approximately 12 × 12 × 20 inches in size or smaller. They should be placed in double-layered cloth (muslin) wrappers and autoclaved. Large packages of linen require 2 double-layered cloth (muslin) wrappers and are autoclaved at 250° F. for 30 minutes. Blue, gray or green cloth material is more restful on the eyes and more suitable for photography during operation than is white material. Rubber gloves must be cleaned carefully and placed in double-layered cloth (muslin) envelopes, then placed in double-layered cloth (muslin) and autoclaved at 250° F. for 15 minutes. The sterilized gloves should be kept overnight before being used. Water, normal saline solution and other solutions used in the operating room should be autoclaved in flasks with loosely applied caps at 250° F. for 20 minutes. Needles, scalpel blades and scissors may be autoclaved. All metal instruments must be scrupulously clean, free of corrosion, oiled (and all excess oil wiped away) and tested for ease of operation before being sterilized in open trays or pans. Glove powder is prepared in small individual paper packages containing just enough powder for one person's hands, enclosed in the glove package and autoclaved with the gloves at 250° F. for 15 minutes. Various compounds, including starch, are suitable, but talc is avoided because it acts as an irritant to raw surfaces (see Chap. 2, Wound Healing, and Chap. 37, Appendicitis, Peritonitis and Intra-abdominal Abscesses). A similarly packaged liquid lubricant "Bio-sorb" has been substituted for the powder in many hospitals, and thus the inevitable dust particles associated with the use of powder are avoided. The powder on the gloves themselves is carefully washed away in the hand basin, after the gloves have been donned but before the operation begins. The water is then replaced.

Caps and masks are laundered and often sterilized by autoclaving in muslin bags that may be fitted into suitable covered metal containers and kept ready for use. The scrubbing brushes and fingernail cleaners are cleaned thoroughly, packed in cans and autoclaved at 250° F. for 30 minutes. These items are kept in convenient shelves or tables in the scrub-up room.

Certain equipment, such as a current type of cardiac pacemaker, is sterilized most appropriately with ethylene oxide gas. Then the equipment must not be used for 8 hours because of the irritant effect that residual gas might have on body tissue.

The Operating Room

The operating room is cleaned after each use. A room that is in service daily is readily maintained in suitable condition for major aseptic surgery, but rooms seldom used may be more difficult to keep in operating condition. The operating rooms should be so designed that they can be cleaned easily and quickly. As far as possible they should be kept free of dirt by minimizing traffic in the room, by filtering the air intake and by cleaning floors, walls, ceilings and fixtures several hours before the rooms are to be used. Persons with furuncles or serious respiratory infections should not enter the operating room.

THE OPERATION

After the operating room has been set up and the patient anesthetized and properly positioned, the first assistant proceeds with the preparation of the skin of the patient in the proposed field of operation, according to the surgeon's preference. A commonly employed routine is that of first scrubbing the skin thoroughly with pHisoHex or Septisol soap and water and then removing the soap with brilliantly colored tincture of Zephiran. The colored solution outlines unmistakably the extent of the skin preparation for reference in the draping of the patient.

Meanwhile, the surgeon and the other assistants don caps and masks, clean their fingernails and proceed to scrub their hands and forearms for 10 minutes. The object of this procedure is to eliminate as far as possible the bacteria from the skin of the hands and the arms. Perhaps needless to say, the hands of all operating room personnel should be kept as clean as possible at all times, and septic dressings should always be handled with rubber gloves or with instruments. The fingernails should be neither too long nor clipped too short, but of such a length and shape as conform to the fingertip. Nail polish must be removed with acetone or other nail-polish remover.

The routine of "scrubbing" is as follows. All rings and bracelets are removed. A clean cloth cap is taken from the container and put on so as to cover as much of the hair as possible. It should be drawn down to the level of the brows in front (so as to absorb perspiration), to the ears on both sides and as far as possible down the back of the head to prevent loose hair and dandruff from falling into the wound. Incidentally, all participants in surgical operations should wash their hair after getting a haircut to remove the numerous segments of hair that result from such a procedure. Next, a clean gauze mask is removed from the container and is secured in place over nose, mouth and chin by tying the strings over and behind the head. If eyeglasses are to be worn, the upper margin of the mask may be molded to fit tightly against the nose and the cheeks, either with a malleable metal strip that is inserted into a slot in the mask or with a strip of adhesive tape, in order to prevent fogging of the glasses. It is essential that the operating room cap and mask be applied correctly and comfortably before beginning to scrub hands and arms.

The sterile containers of brushes and fingernail cleaners are opened before starting the scrubbing procedure. First, the hands are washed with ordinary soap, and the fingernails are cleaned. The running water in the scrubbing sink is regulated to a comfortably warm temperature. At this time it is preferable to use one of the available antiseptic detergent preparations containing hexachlorophene (pHisoHex) or one of the organic iodine complex antiseptic detergent combinations for hand and arm scrubbing purposes. The time of beginning the scrubbing procedure is observed on a clock, so placed as to be viewed easily during the procedure. The surgeon's and the assistants' hands and arms are washed thoroughly with running water and the antiseptic detergent up to a level of about 2½ inches above the elbows. After rinsing hands and arms in the running water, a sterile brush is removed from the container; after wetting the brush and the arms thoroughly with water, antiseptic detergent is applied to the wet brush and, beginning with the hands and the fingers, both hands and arms are scrubbed up to a level of 2 inches above the elbows for 10 minutes by the clock. A procedure should be established so that it becomes a method whereby the entire skin surface of the hands and the arms is scrubbed completely each time. More time is spent scrubbing the fingernails and the creased areas of the hands and the wrists than is spent on the forearms and the elbows. The first assistant carries out his hand-scrubbing technic after he has finished the preparation of the skin of the patient; if he had done so previously, he now changes into another sterile gown and a second pair of sterile gloves. If the hands or the arms touch unsterile things at any time after the scrubbing has been started, the entire 10-minute period of scrubbing should be repeated. Even with the excellent antiseptic detergents available for hand-scrubbing purposes in surgical operating rooms, it is unwise and unsafe to designate a total period for hand-scrubbing routine of less than 10 minutes. When antiseptic detergents are used it is unnecessary and undesirable to rinse off completely the antiseptic detergent after finishing the 10-minute period of scrubbing. Instead, a film of the antiseptic detergent is left on the hands and the arms, which are carefully blotted dry with sterile towels.

Next, a sterile gown is put on. The gown must be unfolded completely before putting it on, and it must be donned with great care to avoid contaminating its outside surface. Usually, the gown is tied at the surgeon's back by the unsterile circulating operating room nurse. Sterile vests which tie in front and keep the back as well as the front of the operator sterile are used over the gown in some hospitals. However, it is important to be aware of the fact that the backs of such vests may become contaminated without the wearers' being aware of it. The hands are powdered from a small sterile individual packet of glove powder ("Bio-sorb," an especially prepared starch powder containing a minute amount of magnesium oxide), following which sterile gloves are put on (Fig. 14-3). The glove powder in the individual packet should be exactly enough to powder the hands of one person, and the excess of powder should be kept away from the sterile operating room supplies. A moistened towel on a convenient unsterile table will catch much of this powder if it is applied with the hands held just above the towel. The sterile rubber gloves are inspected carefully to be certain that they are free from perforations or patches. Excess powder should be washed from the gloves (see Chap. 2, Wound Healing), and then the gloved hands are folded in a sterile towel until the operation begins.

The operative field may have been prepared completely by the first assistant, as noted above. If not, the sterile preparation of the patient's skin is done by the surgeon from a sterile tray that holds a sponge forceps, gauze sponges and a small basin or basins containing an antiseptic solution or solutions, as preferred. The surgeon touches only the handle of the sponge forceps with which he picks up one of the sterile sponges, soaks it with the organic iodine-complex or other solution and gently and methodically scrubs the skin over an area several square inches larger than the area of sterilized skin proposed for the field of operation. This sterile preparation requires

282   Operative Surgical Care

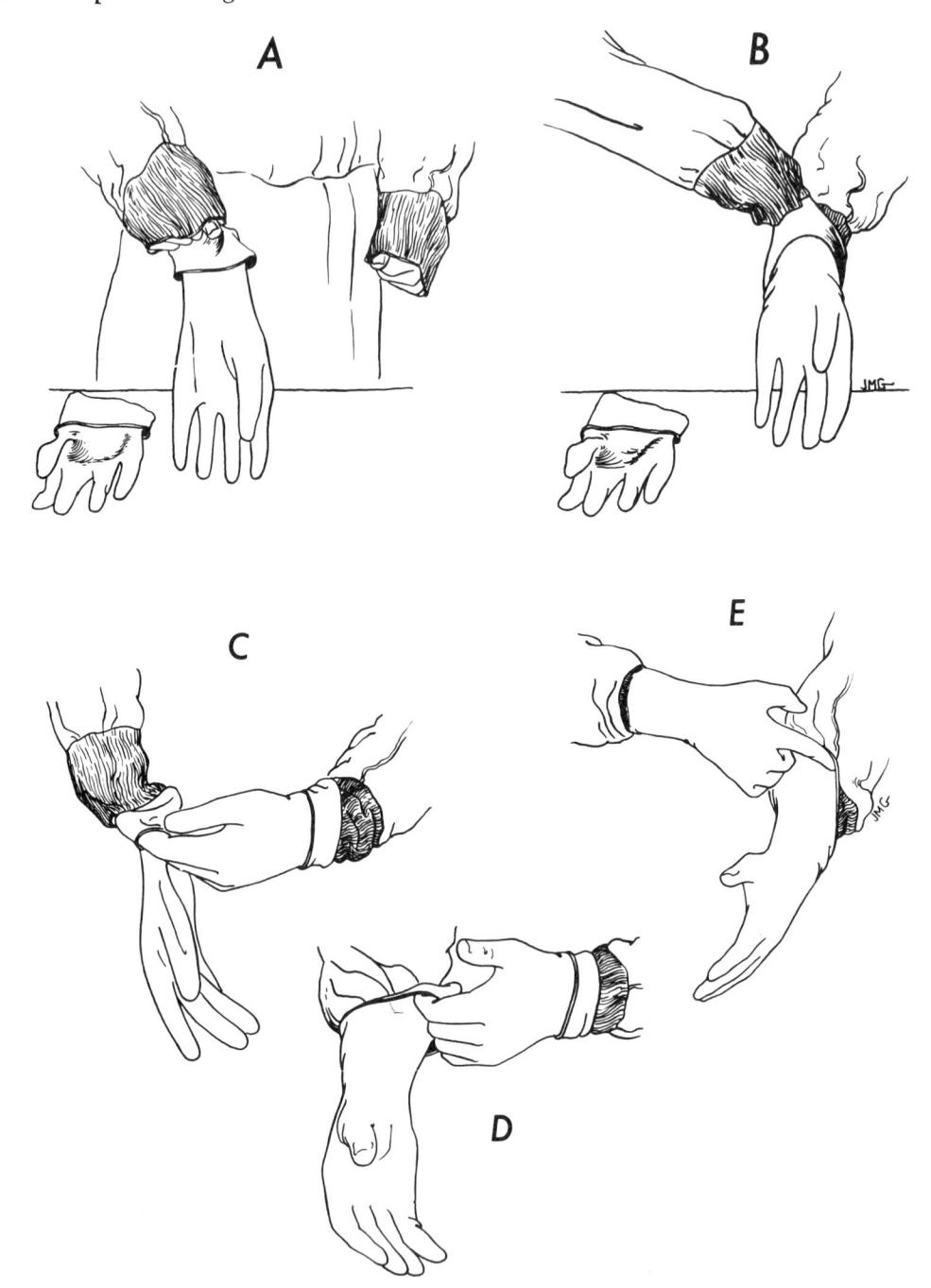

FIG. 14-3. Gloving technic. Self-gloving maneuvers.

several minutes, and a number of sponges are used to make several applications of the antiseptic to the skin in the area of sterile preparation. Following this, the sponge stick and the preparation solution basin are discarded. Larger or more complicated fields of operation require a proportionally longer period of time for the preparation of the skin. As noted, the material used for "sterilizing" the skin varies from hospital to hospital. Actually, the skin

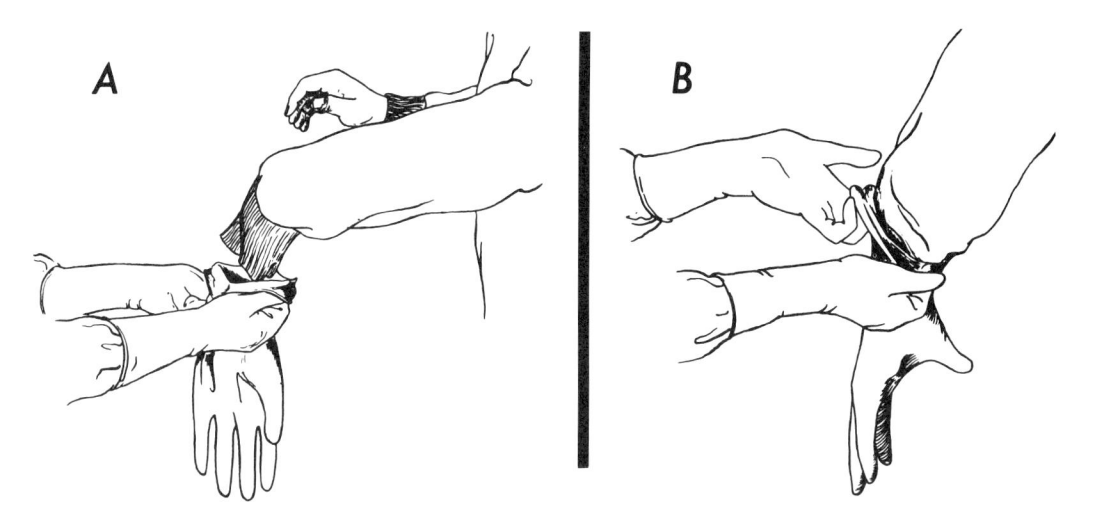

FIG. 14-3 (*Continued*). Gloving technic, by nurse.

is not sterilized, but the bacterial flora is greatly reduced.

When the proposed field of operation has been prepared (i.e., shaved, cleaned and painted with antiseptic solution) the surgeon applies sterile drapes about the proposed field of operation. The size of the patient's skin surface exposed in the draped field should not be larger than necessary for the proposed operation, but it should include enough skin surface for possible extension of the initial incision or for additional incisions if they should become necessary during the course of the procedure (Fig. 14-4). This exposed skin may then be covered with a sterile adherent transparent plastic film or surrounded with towels. Then suitable large sterile drapes are placed so as to provide a wide sterile area around the zone of operation, leaving only an aperture for the exposure of sufficient sterilized skin for the proposed site of operation. The sterile instrument tray is moved into the draped sterile field, and suitable operating room lights are directed on the proposed site of operation. For most major procedures the light should come into the surgical incision from at least two separate sources, and the light beams must be focused to give a uniform lighting over the field of operation. An auxiliary source of electric power should be available for the operating room illumination in case of failure of the main electrical power service.

The surgeon and the assistants, capped, masked, scrubbed, gowned and gloved, now assume their positions around the sterile operative field, and it is time for the incision to be made. The presence in the operating room of persons not actually involved in the operation, such as students or visiting physicians, is permitted in some hospitals but not in others. If permitted, these persons should remain well away from the operative field until members of the surgical team have taken their positions. Thereafter, the visitors, properly garbed, may carefully approach the operating table, but they must be very certain not to contaminate any part of the inner sterile zone which embraces the operating team and the operative field itself.

THE INCISION

The skin is usually incised with a scalpel. The subcutaneous tissue and the musculature may be divided with a cold scalpel or with an electro-scalpel. The incisions commonly employed for various operations are shown in Figure 14-5. Bleeding points are grasped with fine hemostats as rapidly as they appear, and these vessels are occluded by ligature or electrocautery. The rapid cauterization of small vessels substantially shortens an operation such as radical mastectomy or portacaval shunt, where a very large number of bleeding points may be encountered. Regardless of the method used, bleeding points should be

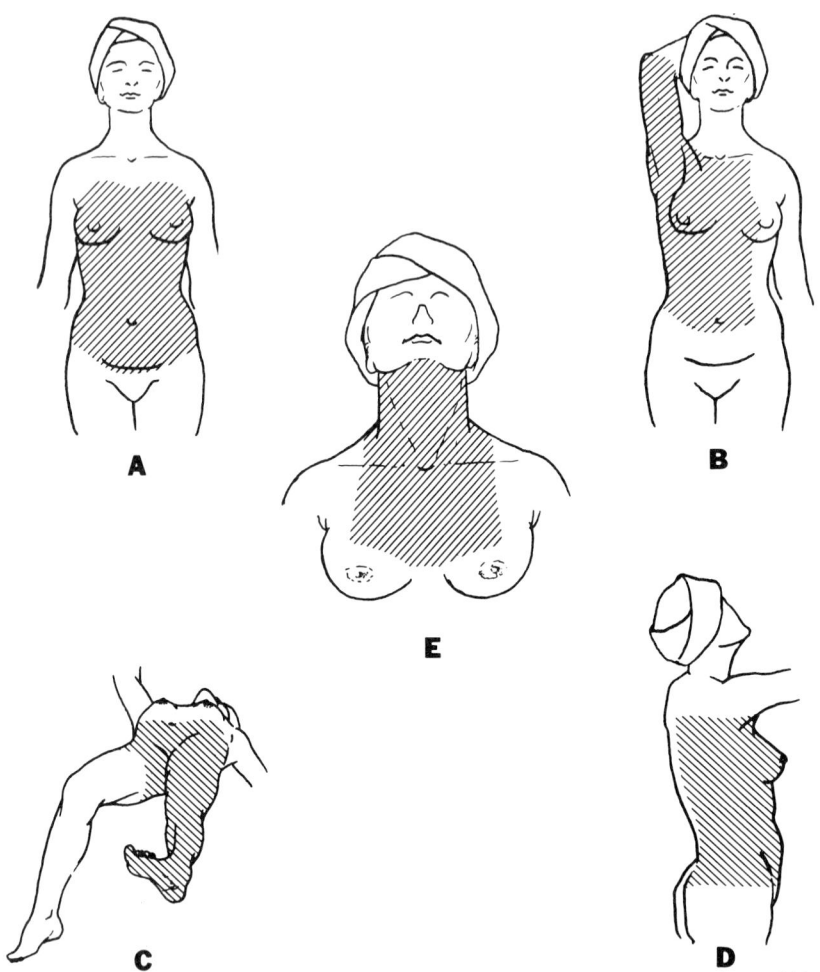

Fig. 14-4. Extent of sterile field preparation for representative operations. (A) Abdominal exploration. (B) Right radical mastectomy. (C) Left leg procedures, entire circumference prepared. (D) Nephrectomy. (E) Thyroidectomy.

controlled at once to minimize loss of the patient's own blood and the consequent need for the transfusion of homologous blood. A blood transfusion should not be given unless clearly required, but it should not be withheld when needed to prevent hypotension. Thus, the experienced surgeon will insist upon physiologic control at all times. With modern anesthesia and technics of blood replacement, there is rarely a need for haste with the operation. In fact, the patient in a critical condition may actually be managed more effectively with the endotracheal tube in place and his lungs well ventilated with pure oxygen than might be achieved elsewhere in the hospital. If the condition of the patient is momentarily precarious or otherwise unsatisfactory, the surgeon will usually delay further dissection until the anesthesiologist has improved the blood volume and/or cardiopulmonary efficiency. All dissection should be performed with the least possible trauma to tissues. This is accomplished best with sharp dissection, and with an adequate incision which reduces the need for excessively strong retraction (Fig. 14-6). If the incision is of adequate size, if lighting is satisfactory, and if anesthesia is sufficient to produce relaxation, adequate exposure is achieved readily.

Conversation unrelated to the operation

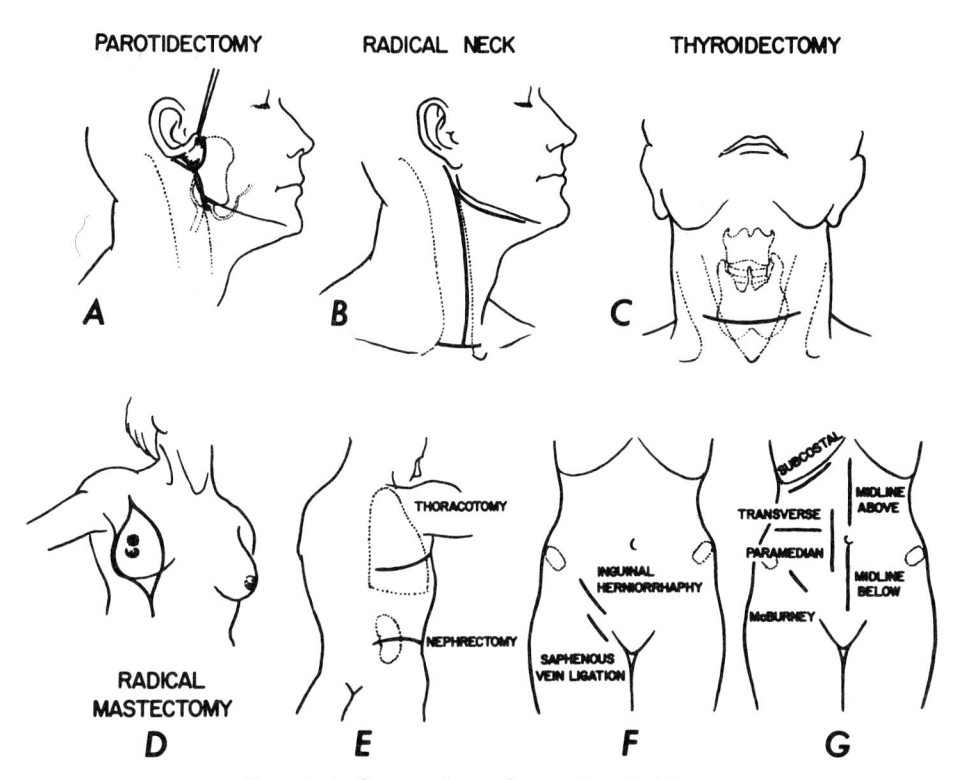

FIG. 14-5. Commonly used operative incisions.

increases the risk of bacterial contamination of the air and should be suppressed. Actually, it has been shown repeatedly that the bacterial count of operating room air declines during the night when the room is not in use but rises abruptly with the activity involved in beginning the schedule of operations the next day. However, the author believes that the operation should be an effective teaching exercise, within the limits of the safety for the patient, and that appropriate comments concerning the technic, the pathologic lesions found and management are justified. Thus, the general tone of the operation should be one of purposeful, disciplined progression without needless delay. Sponging of blood is achieved by blotting accurately and firmly once or twice, not by brushing the raw surface, which causes trauma. The sponges employed may be either wet or dry. One advantage of using dry sponges of uniform size is that by subsequent weighing of these sponges the blood loss can be approximated, taken together with the volume of blood aspirated with the suction and an estimate of any lost on the drapes.

GENERAL EXPLORATION AND MANAGEMENT OF PATHOLOGIC LESION

Immediately upon entering the peritoneal cavity the surgeon will establish the presence of the pathologic lesion suspected preoperatively, but then he will make a systematic survey of the other viscera to exclude additional lesions. If special measurements such as intravascular pressures are taken, these may be communicated to the anesthesiologist, who immediately records these values on the permanent anesthesia sheet.

Adequate exposure of the pathologic lesion and surrounding tissues greatly facilitates subsequent maneuvers. Good exposure is made more difficult to achieve by inadequate anes-

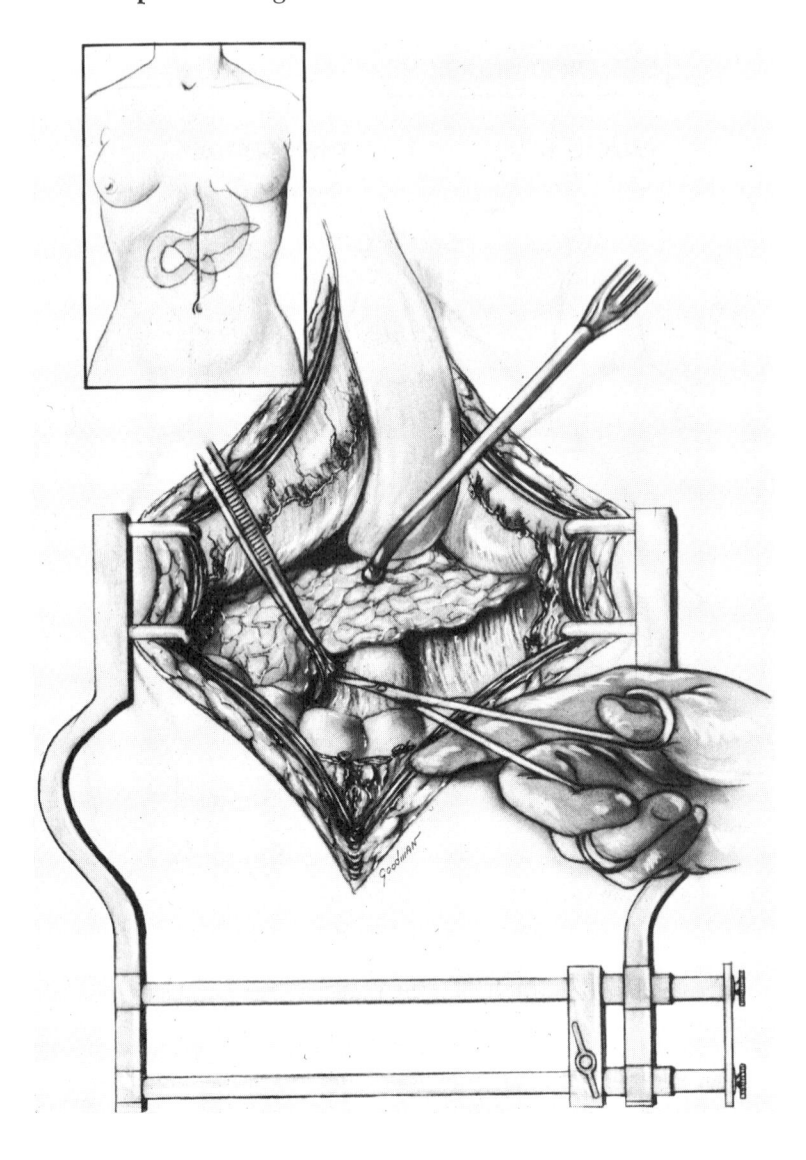

FIG. 14-6. Methods of operative exposure. The stomach is retracted cephalad with a Deaver retractor. The lateral margins of the wound are held apart with a self-retaining retractor. The peritoneum along the inferior or caudal margin of the pancreas is elevated with forceps and divided with scissors, while the suction tip is held nearby to aspirate blood as required to maintain good visualization of the point of dissection.

thesia and relaxation, an improperly placed incision or one of inadequate length, or by obesity. The thick panniculus of the abdominal wall and the thick fat in the mesentery and in the retroperitoneal spaces all serve to increase the difficulties of exposure. These fat deposits also hinder the efforts of the anesthesiologist to maintain optimal pulmonary ventilation, and fat-soluble anesthetic agents accumulate and later delay recovery from the anesthesia. Furthermore, the fat cells are fragile, have a poor blood supply and readily disintegrate into oil, and this increases the risk of postoperative infection.

Hypoxia

The greatest hazard to the patient under general anesthesia is that he cannot protect himself from hypoxia. This hypoxic state may be due to a number of factors, individually or in various combinations. Inadequate pulmonary ventilation is an ever-present hazard. This can produce hypoxia or hypercapnia or both. Excessive dosage of the anesthetic agent may result in defective cellular metabolism, both in the myocardium and elsewhere. A reduced blood volume may result in diminished tissue oxygenation despite excellent pulmonary ventilation. Tissue hypoxia results in anaerobic metabolism which gives rise to metabolic acidosis, which in turn may reduce myocardial contractile strength. The increasing clinical use of arterial blood pH and gas analyses during and following operation permits more rapid correction of related metabolic derangements. For example, an arterial blood pH of 7.21 reflects acidosis that may be due either to carbon dioxide retention or to tissue hypoxia or both. If the pCO_2 of arterial blood is markedly elevated, respiratory acidosis probably exists, and pulmonary ventilation must be improved promptly. If the pCO_2 is normal or reduced, the acidosis is metabolic in origin and should be treated with sodium bicarbonate plus other measures to improve the cardiac output and tissue perfusion. The most common causes of hypotension are inadequate blood volume, inadequate oxygenation, respiratory acidosis, or excessive doses of drugs used for anesthesia. Of course, adrenocortical insufficiency is responsible for shock upon occasion, and other complications such as myocardial infarction, cerebral thrombosis, pulmonary embolism or bacteremia may cause shock.

Hemorrhage

It has been remarked that if it were not for the bleeding, everybody would operate. This is of course a facetious statement, but it does contain a large kernel of truth. The prevention and the control of hemorrhage is certainly the most immediate consideration in operations which border on or involve important vessels. Venous ooze or even fairly brisk venous bleeding will often cease on compression of the vessel for a period of several minutes, though in many instances the defect in the wall of the vein must be exposed and closed with fine suture material. In contrast, most systemic arterial bleeding must be controlled by direct suture or by ligation of the vessel. If serious hemorrhage has occurred or appears to be imminent, certain precautions must be taken at once to avoid losing physiologic control with possible cardiac arrest. First, firm compression of the site of bleeding is established to stop or to reduce the rate of blood loss. Second, adequate amounts of compatible blood are secured and given as needed. Third, maximum use of assistants, of exposure and of lighting is achieved, to gain access to and obtain control of the vessel both proximal and distal to the site of hemorrhage. Fourth, the compression is then carefully released to permit exposure and visualization of the vessel wall defect, which is now closed with fine silk sutures. If the hemostasis appears to be the best that can be secured but is still less than completely satisfactory, drainage of the wound is advisable both to alert the attendants to continuing or renewed bleeding postoperatively and to minimize hematoma formation.

Assessment of What Has Been Accomplished

At the close of the operation the surgeon will review the situation in his mind and decide whether the pathologic state has been corrected satisfactorily. At times there is a temptation to stop short of achieving a completely adequate result, with the unfortunate consequence that the postoperative course may be complicated, and full rehabilitation of the patient thereby may not be attained. If the operation is to be performed at all, and if the patient's condition is good and there is no reason for haste, the maximum that can be achieved safely should be achieved at the time of the operation. For example, a complete cancer operation should be performed if such is indicated, rather than a limited operation with the hope that no metastases exist in the surrounding tissues and lymph nodes.

Closing the Wound

The time of wound closure is an especially important one in preventing postoperative complications. Having decided that the pathologic condition has been managed satisfactorily and that no other significant correctible lesions remain within the abdomen, the surgeon asks for a sponge count. He will himself have checked for any sponges left in the abdomen or the hemithorax, since he knows that he will be held legally responsible for a retained sponge regardless of whether the nurses' sponge count is signed out as correct or not. Actually, if a sponge is left in the patient and a lawsuit results, the surgeon, all assistants, the nurses and the hospital may be sued as having joint responsibility. If it appears that the "missing" sponge cannot be found, a proper x-ray is taken in the operating room at once, for all sponges to be used in a body cavity or any other deep operation should contain a radiopaque marker. While the sponge count is being taken, the surgeon will make a last brief survey for the adequacy of hemostasis and to remove any materials or secretions which might result in infection. Of course, any spillage of bile or gastric juice would have been aspirated quickly at the time that the spillage occurred, followed by gentle irrigation of the area with isotonic saline solution to effect the removal of still further amounts of the material. The instillation of antibiotics is employed by many surgeons (including the author) if a portion of the alimentary tract has been opened or if a major vascular operation has been performed, and at this time the question of drainage is decided.

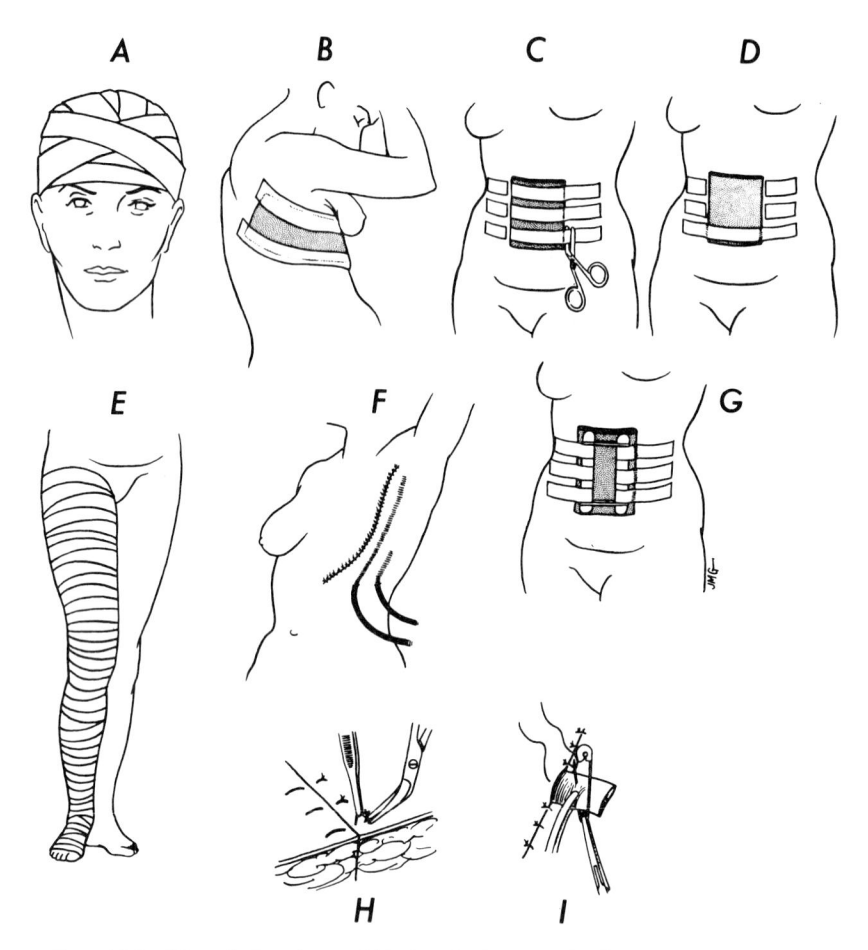

FIG. 14-7. Wound dressings. (A) Head dressing held in place by passing bandage low over the brow and below the occiput. (B) Thoracotomy. (C) Removal of abdominal dressing without removing the adhesive tape. (D) New abdominal dressing secured by adhesive tape placed over previously applied tape. (E) Leg wrapping from toes upward to groin. (F) Catheter suction drainage beneath large skin flaps, as after radical mastectomy. The commercially available plastic suction sets are convenient and usually effective. (G) Montgomery straps to hold bulky dressing in place but permit ready replacement. The 2 tongue-depressor blades are held together with a rubber band placed at each end. (H) Removal of skin sutures. (I) Sterile safety pin placed through a rubber dam or Penrose drain to prevent its retraction into the wound. The loose skin suture will be tied down when the drain is removed to provide an improved cosmetic result.

Virtually all thoracotomy wounds are drained with underwater seal drainage, and some abdominal operations require drainage. For example, most surgeons drain the gallbladder bed following cholecystectomy, and many drain the right upper quadrant following gastric resection if a duodenal stump closure is judged to be less than optimal. The drain is brought out through a separate stab wound, in most instances, but at times it is brought out through the main incision. Following radical mastectomy, radical neck dissection or radical groin dissection, small catheters are placed beneath the skin flaps and connected to continuous suction (Fig. 14-7).

By this point the nurses will have announced that they are ready to take the sponge count, and the surgeon or a member of the team carefully counts with the nurse to ensure accuracy. The instruments should also be counted, but it is surprising how seldom an instrument is left in the thoracic or peritoneal cavities. The wound is closed with different types of suture materials, depending on the routine of the individual surgeon. It has been the general experience that careful wound closure with almost any type of suture material of adequate size gives satisfactory results. The important features are the avoidance of hematomas, of contamination which may lead to infection, of excessive tissue strangulation with mass ligatures, and of defective suture placement which does not result in the apposition of the fascial layers in the correct manner. Thus, the most common causes of postoperative wound separation are hematoma formation, tissue necrosis, infection, faulty wound closure, malnutrition, or the presence of excessive intra-abdominal pressure as a result of intestinal distention, ascites or continuous coughing and straining.

The type of wound dressing used varies with the operation and whether or not drainage was employed. Facial wounds are usually not covered with dressings. Where considerable drainage is anticipated, a bulky dressing with good absorptive capacity is applied (Fig. 14-7). If little or no drainage is expected, there is an increasing tendency to use minimal dressings and to remove even these when the wound has dried postoperatively, leaving the skin sutures exposed to the air.

EMERGENCE FROM ANESTHESIA AND IMMEDIATE RECOVERY ROOM CARE

The period during which the patient is awakening from anesthesia is a critical one. He may still be unable to protect himself from hypoxia or the aspiration of vomitus, and the closest observation is essential.

POSTOPERATIVE ORDERS

The postoperative orders are usually written while the patient is still in the operating room or just as he arrives in the recovery room. The basic orders include directions regarding the frequent taking of the vital signs—blood pressure, pulse rate, respiratory rate and body temperature. An analgesic is ordered to be given in moderate dosage as necessary to relieve pain, but excessive sedation is carefully avoided. It is preferable to give multiple small doses of opiates as necessary rather than to give large doses. Most patients should receive nothing by mouth for some time postoperatively, and an intake-output record should be kept. Directions should be given to ensure deep breathing and coughing. In this connection, a small intratracheal plastic catheter may be inserted through which 2 ml. of saline solution or a mucolytic agent is injected periodically to stimulate the patient to cough (Fig. 14-8). This is frequently as effective as nasotracheal suction and is far more acceptable to the patient. If he should be unable to void, eventually he will need to be catheterized. However, catheterization should be avoided unless the indications are clear and significant. In addition to these routine orders, those pertinent to the given operation must be recorded, such as the connection of various tubes to the proper drainage bottles. Specific antibiotic therapy may be indicated. An operation around the head and the neck can result in oropharyngeal or laryngeal obstruction, requiring immediate tracheostomy, and thus the tracheostomy tray should be on hand. Finally, the nurses should always be encouraged to call the surgeon at once if they are worried about the patient's condition. It is not essential that they diagnose the exact problem, since if they are not satisfied with the general condition of the patient a person with greater experience should be called to examine him.

290 Operative Surgical Care

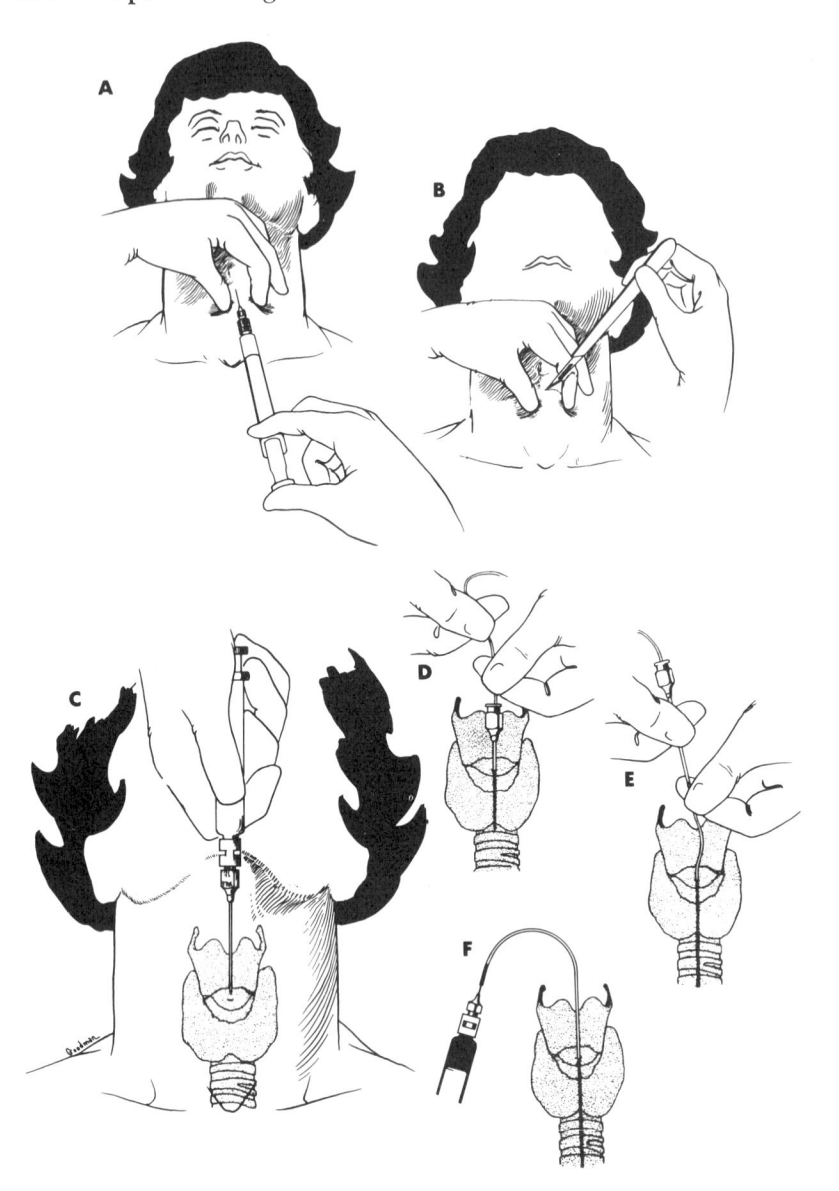

FIG. 14-8. Insertion of intratracheal catheter. First, the skin is anesthetized and then it is nicked with a sharp knife. A needle of sufficient size is passed through the cricothyroid membrane, and through this needle is inserted a small plastic catheter which is secured in place in the trachea. The catheter is used for instillation of mucolytic agents or simple saline solution to stimulate the cough reflex. The secretions so raised must be coughed out or aspirated with nasotracheal suction.

At the time the orders are being written, a brief operative note is recorded in the clinical chart, and thereafter a formal operative note is dictated while the details are fresh in the memory. The pathologic lesion or anatomic variations found and the operation performed should be outlined, along with basic sketches of the lesion and the procedure when appropriate. A simple diagram is often more effective in presenting the operation than is descriptive material (Fig. 14-9). Negative findings relative to other organs, such as the absence of gallstones or uterine fibroids, should also be recorded.

The advantages of keeping the patient in the recovery room are several. First, he is observed closely by the nurses and other personnel who are specially trained and have the experience to recognize physiologic derangements before they have reached a stage where salvage of the situation may be difficult. Second, most of the materials that may be required for the management of unanticipated complications are on hand or can be secured

FIG. 14-9. Simple diagrammatic sketches. It is frequently helpful to strengthen the operative and other clinical notes with simple diagrams.

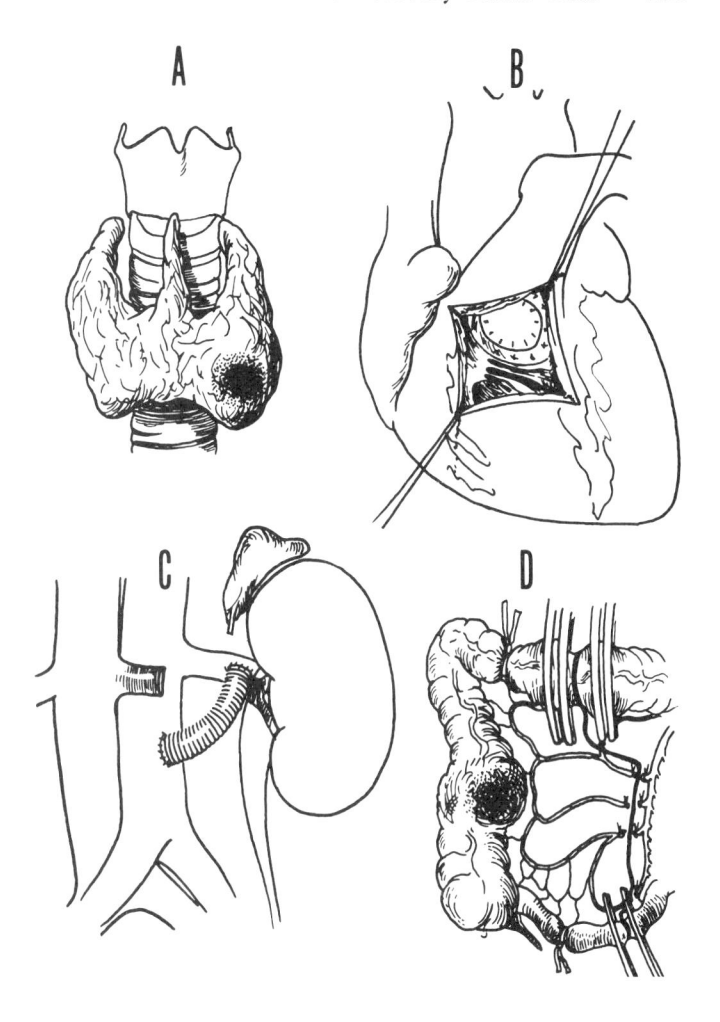

quickly. Third, if the patient should need to be returned to the operating room for the reoperation that is occasionally necessary, such as to stop continuing hemorrhage, this is carried out more readily if he is still in the recovery room or the intensive care unit. During the period of observation in the recovery room the metabolic impact of the operation can be assessed, and it can be determined whether or not the patient can return safely to his room without private duty nurses in full attendance.

The principal complications to be guarded against in the recovery room and the intensive care unit are, again, circulatory and pulmonary in nature. The lingering effects of the anesthetic agent or relaxing drugs, or excessive sedation, or the pulmonary aspiration of vomitus are the most frequent causes of defective pulmonary ventilation. Additional problems such as atelectasis or pneumothorax may also develop. The routine use of arterial blood gas and pH measurements has vastly improved the prevention or management of serious transoperative and postoperative respiratory insufficiency. The most common cause of arterial hypotension is a reduction in circulating blood volume, due either to unreplaced transoperative deficit or to continuing but perhaps concealed hemorrhage. If there is bleeding from the wound, the question arises whether the hemorrhage derives from an open vessel or from generalized ooze secondary to a coagulation defect. In general, if the clotting time and the platelet count are normal, the bleeding is from an open vessel. The majority of postoperative "bleeding diatheses" fall into this category of unligated vessels. The hypertensive patient is especially apt to exhibit postoperative bleeding from even very small arteries. Often the wound hemorrhage is due to a small skin vessel which is readily exposed under local anesthesia and ligated.

The management of the hypotensive patient with limited cardiopulmonary reserve can be especially demanding. If the relatively low blood pressure is due to acute myocardial failure rather than to inadequate blood volume, digitalization and not blood transfusion will constitute the treatment of choice. Adequate urine formation reflects a stable circulation, in most instances. If the hourly urine output is good, the systolic blood presssure of from 90 to 100 mm. Hg in the previously hypertensive patient may still be temporarily adequate. However, if oliguria exists and the blood pressure is low, a measurement of a central venous pressure should be made. If the central venous pressure is normal or low, blood transfusion should be continued until the arterial blood pressure has risen or a rise in the central venous pressure indicates adequate blood replacement. Hemorrhage into the thorax is readily detected by roentgenogram and thoracentesis, but hemorrhage into the undrained abdomen can be extremely difficult to detect.

The stage of convalescence begins when the condition of the patient has fully stabilized in the postoperative period.

BIBLIOGRAPHY

Altemeier, W. A.: Prevention and control of infections in hospitals. Hospitals, 37:62, 1963.

Artz, C. P., and Hardy, J. D. (eds.): Complications In Surgery and Their Management. ed. 2, Philadelphia, W. B. Saunders, 1967.

Bernard, H. R., Cole, W. R., Gravens, D. L., and Monsour, V.: Effect of meteorological conditions on airborne bacteria in operating rooms. Surgery, 54:1095, 1963.

Blowers, R., and Wallace, K. R.: Environmental aspects of staphylococcal infection acquired in hospitals. III. Ventilation of operating rooms—bacteriological investigation. Am. J. Pub. Health, 50:484, 1960.

Cantlin, V. L.: O. R. nursing is a professional specialty. Nurs. Outlook, 8:376, 1960.

Douglas, D. M.: Operating-theatre design. Lancet, 2:163, 1962.

Ford, C. R., and May, L. K.: Bacterial ecology of the operating room suite. Arch. Surg., 85:290, 1962.

Ginsberg, F.: What can be done about M.D.'s who violate aseptic practice? Mod. Hosp., 93:114, 1959.

Hart, D., and Nicks, J.: Ultraviolet radiation in the operating room. Intensities and bactericidal effects. Arch. Surg., 82:449, 1961.

Radigan, L. R., and King, R. D.: A technique for the prevention of postoperative atelectasis. Surgery, 47:184, 1960.

CHAPTER 15

C. A. MOYER, M.D.

Nonoperative Surgical Care

Introduction
General Considerations
Fever
Postoperative Pain
Gas Therapy
Postoperative Urinary Retention and Oliguria
Postoperative Jaundice
Edema
Nausea and Vomiting
Headache; Care of Mouth and Skin
Symptomatic Psychoses

Introduction

The initial chapter of this book emphasizes the fact that surgery must include the total care of the surgical patient and that the operation is only a part of it. This chapter will present a number of common measures employed for the benefit of surgical patients outside the operating room. These are aimed at reducing mortality, reducing morbidity and shortening convalescence and making the physical and the psychological burdens of the surgical illness easier for the patient to bear. Many methods employed in special fields of surgery will be left to the appropriate chapters addressed to these special fields.

Section 1. General Considerations

PATIENT REACTION

An operation performed today is often preceded and followed by many distressing maneuvers not employed a half century ago. To the laymen, for instance, ignorant of the nature of modern medical diagnostic methods, the placing of the electrodes and the taking of the record for an electrocardiogram is often a harrowing experience. "My God! I thought they were going to electrocute me!" was once thrown at me by an ill man whom I in haste had not apprised of his coming medical nightmare.

The taking of blood for the hemogram requires "only a little stick"! But who is there who takes pleasure from a stick, no matter how small, unless he be psychopathic? The drawing of larger samples of blood for "blood chemistries" requires larger sticks, and the sight of one's own life-blood being drained from him is unnerving.

A measure of the psychological trauma of the procedures entering into the care of a person while undergoing a gastrectomy is illustrated by the story told me by a farmer. What follows is his tale—not told as well as he did—after he learned that I was a doctor.

I had gone to the clinic to see about my stomach hurtin' two to three times. They'd taken some exer rays which didn't hurt none but were some scary! They darkened up the room as dark as a moonless night and told me to drink some stuff I couldn't see or taste from a beer-mug. While I was drinking this stuff that felt like some slaked lime I drank once, a fella was a punchin' on my stomach and running a board up and down in front of me. So he finds a right sore spot and says, "There it is." So I thinks, "I got a cancer!" They have me lie on a shiny table that's as hard as cement and cold—them city boys must have air conditionin'! After a while they let me go. I go back to the clinic frettin' about cancer! I wait about three hours when a doc tells me I have one of those stomach ulcers and not to worry. He'd give me medicine to heal it. That's what they told Jim Dyer when he took sick, and he died in three months. When he was embalmed tweren't a free piece of innard in him and his belly almost a-busting with water. I know! I was there! So I goes home and takes the medicine like Doc say to, only it don't do me no good! I began puking. It took me two weeks to get up enough gumption to go back—and then I really didn't all by myself because Harry, my boy, carries me and I so weak I couldn't help myself, I just let him.

They take me into the hospital right off and in ten minutes they took my clothes. I hoped they wouldn't lose them because they were the only clothes I had fittin' to bury me in and I didn't want Ma spendin' the milk money just to buy clothes to cover a good-for-nothin' corpse.

Well, they shooed Harry and Ma out and went to work. First, a fresh lookin' little thing a-comes and without sayin' nothing grabs my ear and—wham!—I'd thought the dangdest biggest horse fly that ever growed had a-bit my ear! I found out next day she was taken' my blood to count. Then a young studying doctor comes in and asks me a whole lot of questions that weren't especially fittin'. 'Twas in a way a-pesterin' of a sick man. All I wanted was to be alone a while to get used to the smells and the strange quarters. You know not even dumb chickens like new places! They really don't! They'll a-quit layin' for a week when you move 'em off'n the roost they're used to.

So I answered his question mostly "No" cause I found that's easiest 'cause if you say "Yes" to anything then it's "When?" and "Where?" and "What did you do for it?" He leaves and comes back shortly with a small syringe like the one I use to give the shoats the cholery vaccine. He wraps a rubber tube around my arm, a-pullin' the hair, and wipes it with cold alcyhol and then jabs a needle in! All the while tellin' me nothin' he's about. That needle must have been used to puncture a tin can! It felt like a scorpion sting. Even though I have blood-veins like a fresh cow's udder—it was plain he was tryin' to stick one of them—he couldn't stick the needle in. So he draws that needle out and it's plain why it wouldn't stick into the vein, caught in the skin-hole like it had a fish hook on the end. The next needle he tried must have been new—it went right in. Then he drawed out four of them syringes full of blood and I knew I didn't have much more of that stuff to give to anybody!

After that I was let rest for about two hours and in comes an older young doctor who asks me the same questions and looks me all over. He goes, and in comes another with a nurse and a panful of ice and a little rubber hose in it. Though that hose looked little it felt as big as an irrigation pipe going through my nose. The nose wasn't made to push tubes through. Anyway he carefully pushes this tube through my nose and I felt like my head was a-bustin' till it got in back of my throat and I suddenly feel like throwin' up which I do easy (and I do!) and out my mouth comes the tube and I feel like a bull bein' led around by his nose! Back he pulls the tube and down he tries to push it quicklike. Oh! It goes down the wrong way and I can't stop coughin' and chokin'. After what seems like an hour I play out and he gets it into my stomach. They hook it up to some bottles after fastening it to my nose. I rest for a while; then that little hose evidently kicks a little because I feel like vomitin' again.

Then this doctor comes back with a nurse and bottles. They hang these on a stand that leans over so I'm sure it'll fall. I've never liked leaning things since Pa's leaning haystack fell over on me as a kid and I near died before they dug me out. Well, Doc sticks my vein easy, he tested the needle for hooks, and they hook the bottle-tube to it and tie my arm to a board and the board to the bed. I never thought that stuff would ever get in. I was a-feared to move because the nurse told me as she left, "Don't move or the needle will come out." I wasn't goin' to move a whisker. I'd been stuck enough for one day.

Well, my elbow ached, my shoulder ached, and my rump ached before that fluid got in; in fact, they didn't ache all at once but took turns achin'.

I wear this tube in my stomach and drink and eat, so they told me, through my veins for two days then more exer rays. And after they was took the older young doctor came with an older one I'd never seen and he says to me, Mr. Beiner, you need a part of your stomach taken out so you can eat. You have a gastric ulcer blocking off your stomach." "Thank you," I says very polite like; feelin' like I'd like to crawl in a hole under the barn like Shep did when he was a-dyin'. I knew now—I just knew! I had a cancer like Jim Dyer—and I sees him again—open at the undertaker's.

Well, I signs so's they can cut as they like and the next morning they takes me to the surgery, they calls it. Before I go the nurse gives me a shot that feels cool like ice in hot weather and before I know it I feel sleepy and don't give a dangish, and I don't recall none until somebody covers my mouth and nose with a little rubber feed bag and in no time at all I see flashes that look like lightnin' and there comes a-roaring sound like those jet planes flyin' low and then I just floats off—

When I wake up my belly hurts like it was a-fire, my mouth feels like I been drunk for a week, and I can't hardly talk for my throat being sore. I knew the stomach wasn't in the throat but until the studyin' doctor told me that the throat was sore from a tube to get wind into me while I was being cut, I thought they'd maybe taken all my eating machinery out.

The next day in comes the old doctor with the young ones and he asks a few questions and says, "Dave," he says, "we're going to get you up!" "When, next month?" says I. "No, Mr. Beiner—right now." "Is he crazy?" I thought! I hadn't heard of this early perambulatin' they expect of you these days. My father had his breach fixed about forty years back and he laid in bed in the hospital for two straight weeks. Finest rest he ever had with everybody waitin' on him hand and foot. Better than stayin' in the Jefferson Hotel. I expected that too but, though I had a goodly portion of my stomach cut out yesterday, up I go! No rest! They pry me from my bed, my head swims and I almost black-out. I suppose that's good because when I fully come to, my belly is hurtin' like everything where it was cut, but up I get! I've always liked gettin' out of bed, I almost always feel so good I pound my chest a little. This was one time that I got up and wanted to pound Doc, not my chest. I didn't because I was sure if I tried it the stitchin'd tear loose. I am sure being able to contain my feelin's saved me from bustin' my stitches trying to lick those doctors. I'm sorry I felt that way! 'Twasn't really a fittin' feeling to have, but who wouldn't feel that way after expectin' a rest but getting only a real passle of sufferin' and being hauled out of the bed a-hurtin' like I'd never hurt before. It's not that I'd never suffered because I've had two felons and real bad piles that had to be lanced.

In fact, that there penicillin they'd shot into my rump for ten days was worse'n the piles. I never knew a man's rump could look like a worn-out pin cushion until I looked at it with the shavin' mirror Harry brought me after he saw me all a-whiskered-up like a mangy old he-goat.

Well, the next few days go all right. I knew now what to expect! Bein' stuck! A-lyin' still like a stove-poker! Gettin' up a-hurtin' and wearin' the little hose that wasn't botherin' much until my ear began to ache and my throat felt scratchy at the back. Finally they pull it out! On it was stuck the worst lookin' stuff you'd ever want to see. I'd never seen nothin' like it and I've seen a heap of sights.

They give me a little water to drink, and I never knew water'd taste so good. It even tasted better'n than that I remember drinkin' while puttin' up hay in August. Next day I get a little mush to eat. It tasted good but I got filled up so quick I couldn't eat half of it. Oh! I thought—"did they take out so much stomach I can never eat a square meal again?" I worry all day about that and finally ask the resident, as they call one of them young doctors, about it. He tells me the stomach needs a little stretchin' and then I can eat a *small* meal again. I didn't like that "small-meal" sayin' but I felt better and almost quit worrying.

About ten days after they cut me I hear a rattling and in comes a young doc pushing a table on rollers that were almost square—that's what made it rattle so. A nurse seemed to be riding on the front of it. My, how these young ones make light of things! Playing around sick people like they were kids! No, they were not playing, it only looked that way with my imaginin'.

They come to my bed; off come the bed clothes I was lying under right proper, because the night shirt they give me that mornin' had been shrunk so, exposin' my privates in plain view of that young nurse who had no weddin' ring on! Then off came the sticky-tape. It had been taken off before but didn't bother much the first time because the hair they'd shaved off my belly had not growed yet, but this time it seemed like the hair had growed into the tape because when he pulled it off I almost went off the bed!

Then out came a scissors and Doc told me he was going to take the stitches out. I bet that'll hurt—everything else they've did to me had! So I grit my teeth, begin to sweat, my heart pounds away—and out comes the first stitch. Well! that was the first thing that didn't hurt! I thought that was only luck and bet to myself that the next one would make up for it! No, it didn't either. Well, at least there were two things that didn't need sufferin'—the taking of the stitches and the urine analysis, they call it! Giving them the water for that was the only simple pleasure I had in two weeks in the hospital!

But after all, these doctors are wonderful! Here I am now, feelin' fit as a tom-cat! Eatin' greens and all and even takin' a little nip now and then when Ma's away visiting her kinfolk in St. Lewi. I hadn't been able to take one for three years because it burned so after. I can work or walk all day now and I feel like 40 'stead of the 66 I am!

This tale embraces some of the mental trials imposed upon a person by a major operative procedure. Although our capacity to save the lives of persons having surgically remediable ills is remarkably greater today than it was a half century ago, the mental trial of surgery is no less for the individual today than it was and, in fact, it may even be somewhat increased by our complex methods.

However, basically, today's lower mortality rates are appreciated widely enough to take some of the terror out of most operations.

What can be done to minimize the psychological upsets connected with an operation?

Obviously, a high regard for the feelings of the sick person is of first importance. He is usually apprehensive of surgery itself and is ignorant of the many protective and therapeutic details accompanying it. Therefore, no painful act should be performed on his body without telling him of the necessity for it. Not to do so serves to raise his fear and may at times lead him to believe that he is being used for experiment without his knowledge. Only the very young, the very old, and the mortally ill are insensitive to the sanctity of the body, and a sick person clings to the primary biologic urge not to be hurt or exposed without knowing why.

His capacity, too, to stand mental trial and physical suffering without losing the will to live is remarkably enhanced by the presence of kind, truthful, conscientious and knowledgeable men and women, whether they be orderlies, nurses, or physicians.

His questions should be answered without evasiveness. Occasionally, the only truthful answer must be given in the form, "I really don't know until we have examined the tissues," and questions about the character of a tumor or the cause of many ailments must be answered in this way. After the operation fewer questions will be asked, seemingly because the sick person senses what is really wrong.

Sometimes a moribund patient seems to be dimly aware of the approaching end but prefers to know it, as it were, obliquely. The physician usually can follow suit and need not state directly what the patient prefers to know indirectly.

The signs of approaching death become familiar to the medical man all too soon in his career. Fear is not commonly one of these signs. In fact, the energy required to give vigorous expression to fear is rarely found in the dying. More often the picture is like that which Shakespeare gives of the dying Falstaff:

He parted even just between twelve and one, even at the turning of the tide: for after I saw him fumble with the sheets, and play with flowers, and smile upon his finger's end, I knew there was but one way; for his nose was as sharp as a pen and 'a babbled of green fields. . . . 'A bade me lay more clothes on his feet: I put my hand into the bed, and felt them, and they were as cold as any stone; then I felt to his knees, and so upward, and upward, and all was as cold as any stone.

When we ask their help, the priest, the rabbi and the minister serve the religious well in time of trial. Often the man of religion quiets the fears of the one to be operated upon more rapidly and surely than drugs, reassurance or the psychiatric consultant.

PREVENTION OF COMPLICATIONS

The prevention of postoperative complications begins before operation, continues during operation and is renewed immediately afterward and carried on until the patient has recovered.

Before anesthesia and before abdominal operations, it is desirable to have the stomach empty. This is usually accomplished by stopping ordinary intake 8 to 12 hours before anesthesia. It may require emptying by tube. For most upper abdominal operations and for others in which a gastric or intestinal tube is to be used after operating it is best to insert such a tube before operation. This controls distention of the stomach which occasionally occurs during anesthetization and can seriously interfere with exposure of other upper abdominal organs if such distention does develop.

Likewise, the patient should void before coming to the operating room; and for most lower abdominal operations (appendectomy and groin hernia excepted) an indwelling catheter should be inserted and the bladder emptied before operation.

For some procedures enemas are most important. Their routine use does not deserve the emphasis once laid upon it, but it is undesirable for the colon to be distended with either feces or gas at the time of laparotomy. The deleterious effect of enemas on electrolyte balance can be largely avoided by using physiologic saline solution.

Preoperative medication is discussed in the anesthesia chapter (and in this chapter, page 298); specific preparation of the bowel with antibiotics, the preparation of suitable blood for the patient, corrective measures for anemia and other deficiencies, diagnostic measures and assessment of risk are covered elsewhere and will not be reiterated here.

After laparotomy, provision must be made for appropriate monitoring of the patient's vital signs. Until consciousness is regained, this should be done in the recovery room. Later, it requires observing and recording blood pressure, pulse and respiratory rate usually every one half hour for 4 hours and then every hour for 12 hours. Temperature should be taken initially and at least every 4 hours for the first few days.

Monitoring of urinary tract function must begin in about 12 hours from the standpoint of bladder distention. In other situations, the hourly output of urine should be measured with the help of an indwelling catheter from the time of operation or admission (see p. 317).

The management of water and electrolyte intake are covered in Chapter 5; nutritional considerations in Chapter 6; the requirement for sedatives in this chapter; psychological disturbances in this chapter; the prevention of embolism in Chapter 4; adynamic ileus on page 310, and a brief statement on wound management follows.

It cannot be emphasized too strongly that the success of a surgical service lies more in the prevention of complications than in their treatment.

Excellence in both prevention and in the early recognition and the prompt treatment of complications is the earmark of a fine surgical service. Differences between the good and the excellent are more apt to be found in this area of endeavor than in the operation itself.

WOUND MANAGEMENT

Wound infection is probably the most common problem to deal with in postoperative surgical patients. Special infections such as tetanus are discussed by Dr. Altemeier and Dr. Culbertson in Chapter 4 and will not be considered again here.

INCIDENCE. The incidence of infection occurring in clean surgical wounds within 4 weeks was found to average 3.4 per cent in the 5 university hospitals studying the use of ultraviolet radiation in the operating rooms. The range was from 1.3 per cent to 5.7 per cent.

With contaminated wounds, it is higher and of course varies with the degree of contamination but does not approach 100%.

Other wounds are infected to start with. These include traumatic wounds clinically infected before treatment is begun and wounds made for the drainage of abscesses or other established infections within the body.

It is believed that most wound infections are determined in the operating room. Their prevention is discussed in detail in Chapter 14, Operative Surgical Care. However, we believe that wounds can be infected afterward, at least during the first 4 or 5 days. It is difficult to control the sources of contamination, at the patient's bed, as well as in the operating room. Therefore, the original gauze dressing should not be removed for 5 days unless there is a clear indication for doing so. The 5-day interval is based, in part, on animal studies in which contaminated material was applied to sutured wounds at varying intervals after incision and suture had been carried out under sterile conditions. Infections occur up to the 4th day but seldom afterward. Also 5 days is a frequent interval selected for the removal of some sutures.

In most hospitals, the "knife and fork" technic is used to keep the wound sterile. The gauze, the instruments and other materials to be brought into contact with the wound are heat-sterilized. The physician contaminates the handles of the instruments when he lifts them from the cover in which they have been autoclaved and stored, but does not touch nor otherwise contaminate the other ends which are used to apply new sterile gauze to the wound surface. If the wound is drained with the usual metal safety pin through the outside end of the drain as a radiopaque marker, the same instruments (thumb forceps, scissors and hemostat) may be used to split the end of a gauze dressing and insinuate the edges of the gauze between the safety pin and the skin or to remove sutures. Once the instruments have touched the patient, his drain, or his old dressings, they are potentially contaminated so far as other patients are concerned and may not be used to reach back into a cannister of sterile dressings without contaminating it.

In modern practice, all sterile supplies are wrapped in small individual packages suitable for a single dressing, and any surplus is resterilized before further use.

The theory of the gauze dressing is that it acts much like the cotton plug in the neck of Pasteur's culture flask, permitting air and water vapor to pass freely but filtering out microorganisms. While the usual dressing is probably not a reliable filter, it serves to prevent contact contamination and to absorb moisture from the wound surface and permit it to evaporate. If such a dressing becomes wet, it is no longer a barrier to the ingress of microorganisms.

In the case of infected wounds or those that become infected, aseptic precautions are still as important as for a clean wound because the hospital situation is one in which it is very easy for a virulent strain of organisms to be widely spread and superimposed on an existing infection—sometimes with dire results. The dressing of an infected wound imposes a further obligation on those attending the patient —that of not becoming contaminated themselves. To this end gloves (disposable plastic) should be worn in removing dressings, and the latter should be conveyed directly into disposable containers (liners) in which they will be incinerated. Bed linen must be sterilized before reuse.

The problem has so many ramifications that patients with infected wounds are more and more being treated in isolation areas with the same rigid technics employed for isolation of the epidemic contagious diseases.

The negative aspect of such isolation is that it takes so long to see a patient that visits are reduced in frequency with resulting delays in appreciating changes in his condition. Beyond this are a whole chain of unpleasant psychological effects.

Thus a middle course is often to isolate patients with epidemic or virulent infections but to use less rigorous methods (use of gloves during dressings and careful disposal of soiled dressings) for patients with less dangerous infections such as those due to colon bacilli after bowel resection. After all, both uninfected patients and attending personnel have regular bowel movements nearly every day.

A major duty of the surgeon caring for the wound is to recognize infection when it occurs (see section on wound pain in this chapter).

MEDICATION FOR RELIEF OF PAIN AND ANXIETY

The soporific drugs help in allaying fears. Amytal Sodium, 0.06 to 0.3 Gm.; pentobarbital sodium, 0.1 to 0.2 Gm.; Seconal, 0.1 Gm. (sodium 5-allyl-5-(1-methylbutyl)barbiturate); and chloral hydrate, 1 to 2 Gm., are effective and widely used for this purpose. Scopolamine, 0.25 to 1 mg., also has the capacity to render most individuals less sensitive to their surroundings and much less apprehensive of danger and pain. The need for these drugs is especially acute on the night preceding and on the day of the operation.

The dictates of humanity require that the person having physical pain before an operation be relieved of the consciousness of his pain. For this purpose the analgesics, morphine (0.014 Gm.) and Demerol (0.050-0.150 Gm.) are remarkably effective. The patient who has peripheral circulatory failure, whatever be its cause, and pain should be given the analgesic intravenously. The intravenous dosage of most drugs usually given subcutaneously, such as morphine and Demerol, is one half to two thirds of the subcutaneous dosage with at least 5 ml. of liquid vehicle. Meperidine (Demerol) is often very effective in pain due to distention of hollow viscera. In most other situations 100 mg. of Demerol is less effective than 10 mg. of morphine sulfate, in the author's experience.

Although the soporifics and the analgesics are very beneficent drugs, their use at times poses unexpected and disturbing problems. Few situations are more discomfiting than to have everything and everyone prepared to begin an operation and then to have the anesthetist say: "I am afraid to start the anesthesia because the blood pressure is 60/20." The surgical resident says, "It wasn't low when I took it this morning; it was 160/90." Has the patient suffered a myocardial infarct? Is he bleeding internally? Is he dehydrated? Has he suffered an acute massive collapse of the lung? Is he about to die? These are some of the questions raised immediately. Whereas 5 minutes ago there was certainty, now there is only uncertainty and consternation.

The commonest cause of acute preoperative preanesthesia hypotension, especially among the elderly and the starved, is preoperative soporific-analgesic idiosyncrasy or overdosage. The combination of morphine and barbiturate is somewhat more prone to induce hypotension than is the combination of Demerol and barbiturate. (See Chap. 13, Anesthesia.)

Should acute preoperative hypotension occur, the operation should be delayed whenever possible. When a delay of the operation jeopardizes the life of the patient, a vasopressor agent may be employed. Ephedrine hydrochloride 0.03 to 0.12 Gm., or phenylephrine (Neosynephrine) 0.005 to 0.01 Gm., are effective and safe. The physiologic action of norepinephrine (Arterenol) does not differ significantly from that of ephedrine. Ephedrine's vasopressor action is effected largely by its inhibition of the enzyme which normally destroys norepinephrine. In effect, the giving of ephedrine provides the person a higher titer of his own norepinephrine.

Besides hypotension, unwanted actions of morphine and the barbiturates are respiratory depression and hypothermia.

Demerol, atropine and to a lesser degree scopolamine inhibit sweating. This action favors hyperthermia especially during hot weather and febrile illness. This complication is occasionally lethal, especially in hot operating and recovery rooms and especially among children having suppurative processes (see Heat Stroke in this chapter).

The preoperative general care of the surgical patient other than that directed toward the amelioration of psychological stimuli and pain is directed toward providing him with optimum conditions for recovery. It is aimed at the prevention of complications and therefore constitutes a major part of the preventive medical aspect of surgery.

ASPIRATIONAL PNEUMONITIS

One of the gravest dangers attendant upon anesthesia is the aspiration of vomitus into the lungs. The pulmonary aspiration of gastric juice with or without food particles in it induces a fulminant, necrotizing chemical pneumonitis. In effect, the living lung becomes acutely inflamed and edematous, and the bronchial secretions are increased, adding further to the hypoxia and promoting atelectasis. Aspiration of intestinal juice into large segments of lung is often lethal in 36 hours and sometimes within 30 minutes. The aspiration into small segments may be followed by bronchopneumonia and pulmonary abscesses especially when food particles are inhaled with the juice.

Ensuring an empty stomach before an anesthetic is given and keeping it empty during the operation obviate the danger of aspirational pneumonitis. In the absence of esophageal, pyloric or intestinal obstruction or ileus, an empty stomach *usually* is attained by merely withholding all but liquid foods for 12 hours, all liquid foods for 6 to 8 hours, and water for 4 hours preoperatively. Occasionally, the application of this rule will not secure an empty stomach. Actually, the only way to be reasonably sure of an empty stomach before an operation is to aspirate it through a tube.

The placement of an inlying gastric tube before anesthesia is begun should be mandatory for all major intra-abdominal operations excepting pelvic. However, even with pelvic operations, nephrectomy and appendectomy, trouble with postoperative ileus and gas pains is reduced remarkably by ensuring an empty stomach with the use of an inlying gastric tube before and during the operation.

The placement of a tube into the stomach should precede gastrectomy by at least 8 hours, and in cases of pyloric obstruction by 24 or more hours. The use of the long and the short intestinal tubes for intestinal obstructions and ileus is discussed in Chapter 38.

The use of cuffed intratracheal tubes for intratracheal anesthesia prevents aspiration during operations.

COMPLICATIONS OF GASTRIC INTUBATION

The indwelling gastric and intestinal tubes are mixed blessings. Occasionally, their use is attended by two complications rarely lethal but often crippling, namely, cicatricial laryngeal and esophageal stenosis. Pain in the throat radiating up behind the ear, earache and dysphonia (indications of laryngeal inflammation) and heartburn or low substernal and epigastric discomforts (indicative of lower esophageal inflammation) appearing while the intestinal tube is being worn are indications for its immediate removal and inspection. Should *bloody mucus* be found upon the tube, a tube should not be reinserted. If the illness requires further use of gastric or intestinal decompression it should be effected through a gastrostomy or a jejunostomy; fortunately, this is rarely needed.

Necrosis of the ala nasae may attend the wearing of an indwelling gastric tube. This complication is attributable to the ignorance of the person securing the tube to the face. The tube never should be secured while lying in the nasolabial groove or over the lateral aspect of the nose and being directed upward toward the eye, since the acute bend of the tube about the ala nasae compresses it.

The irrigation of gastric and intestinal tubes with water to maintain their patency may induce fluid balance disturbances. Water introduced into the stomach or the intestine, if not removed immediately, will be attended by the rapid movement of salts from the plasma into the water in the lumen of the intestine (see Chap. 38, Intestinal Obstruction). As the fluid is removed subsequently through the tube, it withdraws with it salts that would not have been lost from the body if water had not been instilled into the gut. In the process the water in the plasma previously holding the withdrawn salts is redistributed throughout the body, and the osmolar concentration of the body's fluids is reduced. The physiologic consequences of fluid changes attending the repeated instillation of water into the gastrointestinal tract and its subsequent withdrawal through tubes are a decreasing plasma volume, a decreasing interstitial fluid volume, an increasing intracellular water volume and a decreasing osmolar concentration. These changes may lead ultimately to peripheral circulatory failure coupled with water intoxication.

The rate of loss of potassium from the body of a person wearing an indwelling gastric or intestinal tube also is increased by irrigating the tubes with water or a solution containing no potassium.

If a tube must be irrigated, and this is usually necessary to ensure continuous patency, the use of Ringer's solution will prevent the development of the above disturbances of fluid balance associated with irrigating indwelling intestinal tubes with water.

Section 2. Fever

ETIOLOGY

The predominant causes of the postoperative fever are: (1) infection within the wound, (2) infection within the urinary tract, (3) pulmonary complications, (4) thrombophlebitis and (5) increased osmolar concentration secondary to a lack of water or a salt-excess (see Chap. 5, Fluid and Electrolytes). Less common causes are: (1) drug reactions (e.g., allergic-penicillin, etc.; specific-atropine), (2) malarial relapse, (3) central neurologic disturbances, (4) bacterial enterocolitis and (5) factitial factors such as the heating of the thermometer with hot liquids, radiators, matches, lighters or friction *et alia*, (6) deep abscesses, (7) peritonitis, (8) septicemia and (9) empyema.

WOUND INFECTION

Diagnosis. With such a variety of factors to consider, the search for the cause of any postoperative fever must be orderly. The wound must be examined first. Yet it is often difficult and sometimes impossible after a single examination to be sure of infection in a wound. To some degree, all the classic signs of infection—redness, heat, tenderness, swelling—are present in the primary stage of healing of a thoroughly healthy and uninfected wound. Even the systemic signs of an infection—leukocytes and fever—may be stimulated by the very small amounts of sterile dead tissues inescapably left within the wound. A single examination, therefore, is seldom enough, and repeated examinations are required to disprove the existence of a wound infection.

Clearly, repetitive examination of the wound is often required to determine the existence of an infection within it unless pathognomonic signs of a wound infection exist. These pathognomonic signs are: drainage of fluid containing numerous bacteria from the wound, fluctuation, erysipelas, necrosis of skin (phlegmonous erysipelas), vesiculation, and with clostridial infections rapidly expanding crepitus or crepitus associated with physical prostration and a tachycardia greater than that compatible with the height of the fever (see Chap. 4, Surgical Infections).

The aim of the repetitive examination of a wound in which infection is suspected is to determine whether the heat, the redness, the swelling and the tenderness are increasing or decreasing. Increasing or spreading heat, redness, swelling and tenderness indicate the probable existence of infection, and diminishing heat, redness, swelling, or tenderness indicate its nonexistence or biologic control. The comparison of one portion of the wound with another often makes the diagnosis and localizes the area to be opened.

Treatment. As soon as the diagnosis of a wound infection can be made with reasonable certainty the wound is opened at the point of maximum tenderness and swelling down to the subcutaneous fascia. Of course, aseptic precautions must be exercised. A sample is collected immediately for smearing and bacterial culturing (see Chap. 3, Applied Surgical Bacteriology). The depth of the wound is then inspected and probed gently. Free drainage should be maintained by introducing one end of a suitable drain. Wet dressings such as gauze saturated with sterile 0.9 per cent sodium chloride solution often are helpful in preventing the secretions from the wound from forming a dry coagulum which may interfere with free drainage. If the probe passes freely beneath the wound or if the tissue in its depths is shaggy, avascular and gray, suggesting one of the more serious types of infection, the entire wound should be laid open and packed loosely with fine meshed cotton or linen gauze.

Failure to open an infected wound widely may lead to loss of the patient's life. In the case of laparotomy wounds, the peritoneum and the deep fascia are left intact except for the purpose of draining a subjacent intraabdominal abscess.

The use of antibiotics has complicated the picture of wound infections. The local and systemic signs of a wound infection arising while these drugs are being administered often are remarkably delayed in their appearance and are attenuated. At times a near-fatal wound infection is attended by so few local signs that it is overlooked until the wound opens and drains spontaneously.

ACTH and the corticoids also may inhibit the development of the local and general signs of a wound infection and render the detection of suppuration difficult. Rapid physiologic deterioration occurring in a postoperative patient receiving corticoids or ACTH in whom no signs of a pulmonary, otitic, or urinary infection can be found, is sufficient indication for opening of the wound. It may be closed should no infection be found.

Diabetics and especially those who have peripheral neuropathy often respond peculiarly to a wound infection. They may manifest little fever, slight leukocytosis, little pain, tenderness, redness or warmth of the wound even though much pus be contained in it: swelling there is and little else. However, the diabetes "goes out of control" regularly with infection, the glycosuria increases, and acetone bodies appear in the urine, though the amount of insulin given previously was adequate to prevent both. In other words, a diabetic who has been stabilized postoperatively and then goes out of control probably has developed an infection somewhere in the wound, the lung or the urinary tract, and the possible location of it in the wound cannot be excluded because of lack of the classic signs of an infection about the incision.

After the wound has been examined a search always is made for the other possible causes of postoperative fever. The chest is percussed, the character of the breath sounds carefully auscultated in order to determine their qualities and the presence of concomitant adventitious sounds such as rales, ronchi or rubs. The type of breathing is observed, and the position of the trachea is determined. In addition, the relative intensity and quality of the aortic and the pulmonary second sounds are to be noted. Gallop rhythm, especially along the left border of the sternum, and cardiac irregularities are to be looked for. The quality of the apex beat and the size of the heart also are important.

PULMONOCARDIAC DISTURBANCES

The pulmonocardiac disturbances commonly associated with fever are: atelectasis (collapse of the lung) due either to bronchial obstruction, which is common, or less often to compression, congestive atelectasis (acute nonobstructive massive collapse of lung), pneumonitis (bacterial or from aspiration of gastrointestinal contents), pleuritis, acute cardiac failure, pulmonary embolism and myocardial infarct. Obviously, *roentgenograms of the chest and electrocardiograms* are invaluable for the detection and the analysis of a postoperative pulmonocardiac complication.

Brief descriptions of the characteristics of some of the above-named possible causes of postoperative fever follow.

Bronchial Obstructive Atelectasis. USUAL ORIGIN. Inspissated mucus; foreign bodies (teeth, dentures and food particles) are less frequent causes.

GENERAL COURSE OF THE ILLNESS. Tachycardia, tachypnea and fever often occur practically simultaneously. Cyanosis is an inconstant sign, but when present it indicates that a rather large segment of lung is unaerated and that a significant quantity of blood is flowing through its pulmonary arteriovenous circuit, having much the effect of a right-to-left cardiac shunt. The administration of oxygen does not abolish the cyanosis, though it may reduce it somewhat. Dyspnea is experienced only when a large segment of the lung is airless.

The trachea and the mediastinum tend to shift toward the atelectatic lung. Obviously, tracheal and mediastinal shift will be slight or undetectable with a unilateral slight or a bilateral atelectasis of equal extent. The respiratory excursion of the chest is limited and lags on the involved side. Breath sounds are diminished in intensity (distant) and tend to be bronchial in character over atelectatic segments in contact with the chest wall. Obviously, should the atelectasis occur solely within the hilar segments, the upper lobes, the lingular segment of the left upper lobe, or only in small portions of lung in contact with the chest wall, abnormalities of quality and character of breath sounds may not be detectable. For this reason atelectasis cannot be excluded as a cause of postoperative fever on the basis of absence of auscultatory or percussional signs, and roentgenographic studies are necessary. The roentgen signs of obstructive atelectasis are opacification of lung, homolateral shift of mediastinum and trachea, accentuation of bronchovascular markings, and limitation of motion of the diaphragm.

Rales, rhonchi and wheezes almost always accompany obstructive atelectasis.

TREATMENT OF OBSTRUCTIVE ATELECTASIS. This is directed toward the removal of the obstruction, permitting air to enter the lung again. The methods used consist of increasing the activity of the patient, deep breathing exercises, coughing, tracheal aspiration, bronchoscopy and loosening restrictive binders.

Increased activity of the patient may be obtained by having him roll from side to side in bed or getting him out of bed to walk. With the assumption of physical activity, coughing is often stimulated, and the atelectasis may disappear with great rapidity. However, this method of treating atelectasis is rarely effective when the atelectasis is extensive or accompanied by numerous rhonchi.

Coughing can be rendered more effective by supporting the thoracic or abdominal wound. A pillow held tightly over the wound by grasping it at the ends and pressing it about the body provides an effective external splint, permitting a much more effective cough.

If neither activity nor coughing will clear the bronchial tree, *aspiration of the trachea* is required. This may be done blindly by use of a suction apparatus.

A lubricated catheter is passed through a nostril, and the tip is advanced to the epiglottic region. The passage of the length of catheter spanning the distance between the tip of the nose and a mastoid process will place the tip near the epiglottis. Then while the patient's head is tipped backward with the chin held forward, the catheter is advanced quickly *while the patient inspires deeply*. The entry of the catheter into the trachea will be attended by a fit of coughing. Then the top of the trap connected to suction is stoppered rapidly and intermittently with the thumb or the forefinger. Next, the catheter is advanced, while the trap is being alternately opened and closed. The intermittent aspiration is kept up until secretions are not obtainable. Then the examination of the chest is repeated. Should remarkable improvement be found, bronchoscopy may not be necessary. However, should little or no improvement be found, bronchoscopy should be done.

Often *bronchoscopic aspiration* is indicated without antecedent attempts to clear the atelectasis with increased activity, coughing and tracheal aspiration. It is indicated as the primary therapeutic step in cases of massive collapse of one lung or bilateral extensive atelectasis, atelectasis secondary to aspiration of a foreign body, and atelectasis associated with hypotension, disorientation, stupor, or coma, paralysis of intercostal and abdominal musculature, or profound weakness. Skillful bronchoscopy is safe and without much actual pain and has so much potential benefit that one should not hesitate to employ it as a therapeutic measure for atelectasis. At times a tracheostomy is required to permit the repeated aspiration of mucus in order to keep the airway unobstructed. This is especially applicable to the treatment of atelectasis occurring after crushing injuries of the chest, severe facial-cervical burns, pulmonary aspiration, and among those persons who have obstructive atelectasis and are very weak or have far-advanced chronic pulmonary diseases such as pulmonary fibrosis and emphysema.

Associated measures to be taken in conjunction with and subsequent to the above methods of treating obstructive atelectasis are: (1) the giving of a wide-spectrum antibiotic; (2) the discontinuance of use of any drug having an atropinelike action, such as scopolamine, atropine, tincture of belladonna, and Demerol, as these drugs increase the viscosity of the bronchial secretions, making them more difficult to expel; (3) the avoidance of drugs which depress the cough reflex, such as opium, codeine, morphine, Dilaudid, Pantopon, etc.; (4) the use of a route other than the intravenous for the administration of needed water and electrolytes. When fluids are given intravenously while atelectasis exists they tend to increase it or at least delay its resolution. For unknown reasons, fluids given orally, subcutaneously, or rectally apparently are less prone to do so; (5) agents which increase the fluidity of the bronchial secretions may be given. Potassium iodide does so. In addition, certain surface-tension-reducing agents have been shown to effect dissipation of mucus within the respiratory tract. Their effectiveness in the prevention and the after-treatment of atelectasis has been established. These are usually given in a solution which is volatilized as a mist and inhaled (2-ethylhexyl sulfate 1/8% with 1/10% sodium iodide in water, and pancreatic dornase are among those currently used).

Oxygen therapy has a limited usefulness in the treatment of bronchial obstructive atelectasis as a supportive measure before and during bronchial aspiration. A lung filled with oxygen becomes atelectatic far more rapidly than one filled with air. Consequently, the giving of oxygen after tracheobronchial aspiration may retard recovery, especially when the secretions are copious. However, it should be given with air-hunger or cyanosis.

Compressional atelectasis attends internal encroachment upon the lung space by fluid or air within the thoracic cavity or by fluid, air or distended viscera within the peritoneal cavity. It is attended by the same physical signs as obstructive atelectasis, except that the breath sounds may be accentuated occasionally and bronchial in character since the bronchus to the atelectatic lung is open. Deviation of the mediastinum and the trachea either does not occur or is in the direction away from the disease. Circumferential binding of the abdomen with tape or a Scultetus binder is a frequent cause of compressional atelectasis. Fatal compressional atelectasis with pulmonocardiac failure is easily produced by circumferentially binding the abdomen of an anesthetized dog. The application of a circumferential abdominal dressing to an anesthetized person may be a grave surgical error.

TREATMENT OF COMPRESSIONAL ATELECTASIS. This consists of the removal of the cause, e.g., thoracentesis, drainage of empyema, drainage of subphrenic abscess, the relief of meteorism, paracentesis, and removal of abdominal binders and circumferentially bound dressings.

For many years the administration of 7 to

20 per cent carbon dioxide in oxygen was recommended for the treatment of bronchial obstructive and compressional atelectasis. It is no longer recommended.

The *antibiotics* are valuable adjuncts in the therapy of all forms of atelectasis and postoperative pneumonitis. Purulent tracheobronchitis and bronchopneumonia frequently attend or follow atelectasis. The organisms vary, with pneumococci, streptococci and staphylococci predominating. Consequently, a broad-spectrum antibiotic is best (see Chap. 3, Surgical Bacteriology).

Postoperative Pneumonia. Before the nature of bronchial obstructive atelectasis was known "ether pneumonia" was presumed to be the cause of postoperative pulmonary troubles. However, it is now known that ether does not produce pneumonia. Today primary lobular and lobar pneumonias occur rarely after operations, and the appearance of lobular pneumonia postoperatively now indicates most likely that the aspiration of gastrointestinal fluid has taken place or that bronchial obstructive atelectasis has occurred, is developing or clearing.

TREATMENT of postoperative lobular pneumonia depends somewhat upon the nature and the quantity of the bronchial secretions and upon the organisms found in the sputum. Copious tenacious secretions require the use of bronchial aspiration in addition to the giving of a wide-spectrum antibiotic. Since incomplete saturation of the pulmonary venous blood is characteristic of lobular pneumonia, the giving of oxygen is often an important part of its therapy.

Congestive Atelectasis. The air-containing space of lung may be encroached upon by blood contained within the pulmonary capillaries. Occasionally, the encroachment is so great as to render large parts of the lung essentially airless. The condition is called congestive atelectasis. It follows rapid decompression (extrusion from a pressurized airplane at very high altitudes), and occurs spontaneously among persons suffering from severe kyphosis and is then usually called pulmonocardiac failure. Congestive atelectasis occasionally occurs during or after an operation when it may be called acute postoperative nonobstructive massive collapse of the lung.

The signs of congestive atelectasis are a fulminant fever, hypotension, a cyanosis that cannot be cleared by administering pure oxygen, forceful expiratory abdominal breathing, limitation of costal breathing, tachycardia, and severe oliguria or anuria. Viewed through a bronchoscope, the bronchi are seen to be wide open during inspiration and partially or completely collapsed during expiration. Pulmonary roentgenograms may show nothing amiss, and often thoracic auscultation and percussion are not particularly abnormal until shortly before death.

No effective treatment is known. Digitalis, transfusions, phlebotomy, bronchoscopic aspiration, assisted forced breathing are all ineffective. A compression chamber should be tried; practically everything else has been tried and has failed.

Other postoperative intrathoracic complications attended by fever are pulmonary embolism (see Section on Thrombophlebitis), fat embolism, mediastinitis and pleuritis (see section on Pain).

FAT EMBOLISM

Fat embolism most often follows fractures and contusional trauma; however, it occurs rarely after mastectomy, the removal of arterial emboli, spinal and other osseous fusions, and celiotomy. The clinical picture, though often confusing, may be very clear-cut. Characteristically, a person who is recovering from an accident or an operation in fine fashion becomes short of breath, then febrile and disoriented, hypotensive with a fast small pulse, oliguric and finally comatose. The discovery of petechiae over the neck and the anterior axillary folds, the anterior chest and the inner aspect of the thighs when coupled with the above clinical picture practically clinches the diagnosis. The demonstration of globules of fat in urine and saliva and seeing them in the retinal vessels add much to the credibility of the diagnosis.

The treatment of fat embolism is poorly developed. It consists of the cessation of oral feeding, the control of the pyrexia with aspirin and tepid sponge baths, the treatment of peripheral circulatory failure with transfusions of blood, and the maintenance of fluid balance. Peltier[6] recommends that heparin not be used, but Hillman[3] does not agree. Peltier believes that it accelerates the release of free fatty acids. At present heparin is recommended.

AIR EMBOLISM

Air embolism, though not attended by fever and a very rare surgical complication, is one of the most feared complications of intracranial and intracardiac surgery, hepatectomy, thyroidectomy and pulmonary operations. It may account for more of the unsolved operative deaths than was suspected heretofore. The syndrome varies from one of fulminating circulatory failure to that of coma and death after a completely lucid interval. The rapid entry of 200 to 600 ml. of air through the systemic veins into the right heart may kill by turning the blood in the right heart to a bloody froth which cannot be pumped effectively. The opening of sigmoid venous sinuses in the skull and the transection of thyroid veins while the patient is in the head-up position, and transection of the hepatic veins while the patient is in the head-down position occasionally lead to the massive right heart type of air embolism. However, it may occur through these same vessels without regard to the position of the patient. Tachycardia, acute hypotension, cyanosis and crunchy heart sounds are its signs. The most direct form of treatment is aspiration of the right ventricle; it has been tried with some reports of success.

Air entering the pulmonary veins with thoracentesis or pulmonary operations or from the previously opened isolated left ventricle kills without foaming the blood in the heart. A small volume of air, 4 to 10 ml., entering the coronary and the cerebral circulations may kill. Acute, irreversible respiratory arrest, acute cardiac standstill and failure to recover from anesthesia are variants of left-side cardiac or pulmonary venous air embolization in anesthetized animals. No effective therapy is known, but if hyperbaric conditions can be imposed very promptly, this should be done to decrease the size of the bubbles and to increase the solubility of the gases in the body water. The emphasis must be on prevention.

THYROID STORM OR CRISIS

Fever may have peculiar connotations when it follows thyroidectomy and craniotomy. Before the discovery that the thioureas and iodine could effect the complete remission of Graves's disease, the performance of thyroidectomy for thyrotoxicosis was followed regularly by fever, and in some cases the fever was fulminant and, together with other metabolic disturbances, killed. The whole train of events was called a thyroid storm or crisis. Storm it was and still is: fulminant fever, mania, tachycardia up to 200 beats per minute, vomiting, diarrhea, coma and death. Among the aged occasionally it is relatively quiet, the fever being relatively small, and the mania absent. It is exceedingly rare after thyroidectomy today but it is still to be seen. It occasionally follows the administration of [13]I in therapeutic doses to thyrotoxicotics, the performance of any operative procedure upon them before they have been given the thioureas, and the delivery of a child or the sufferance of an accident by untreated thyrotoxic persons.

Treatment. The treatment consists of: (1) the control of the fever by sponging the torso and the legs with tepid alcohol, placing ice bags and packs to head, axillae and chest, and the giving of aspirin (0.6 to 1.0 Gm.) every 2 hours until the rectal temperature taken at intervals of 15 to 30 minutes is 100° F. or less; (2) the provision of carbohydrate and water by intravenously infusing a cooled solution of 10 or 15 per cent dextrose in water (2,500 to 4,000 ml.); (3) raising the oxygen tension of the air breathed with a good oxygen tent; (4) quieting the mania with Seconal (0.1 to 0.2 Gm.) or Pentothal Sodium intravenously; (5) digitalizing if signs of cardiac failure appear with lanatoside C (Cedilanid) 1.0 to 1.6 mg. intravenously; and (6) providing adrenal cortical support, especially if the eosinophil numbers exceed 30 to 50 per/cm., with cortisone 100 mg. every 6 hours.

POSTCRANIOTOMY FEVER

Hyperpyrexia occasionally attends or follows craniotomy. Hypophysectomy and the resection of craniopharyngiomas are frequently followed by fever. Formerly, disruption of the function of the temperature-regulating center was implicated as the cause. However, increased osmolar concentration is recognized now as one of the causes of postcraniotomy hyperpyrexia. When it is the cause the serum sodium concentration is found to be remarkably elevated, occasionally reaching 180 mEq./liter. Presumptively, an acute insufficiency of secretion of antidiuretic hormone permits the reduction of the renal tubular facultative absorption of water while the renal tubular absorption of electrolytes is enhanced by the operative stimulation of the adrenal cortex. The result is retention of solutes and loss of large amounts of water through the kidneys and an elevation of the osmolar concentration of body fluids. This is sufficient to induce fever.

Treatment. The treatment of fever attributable to hyperosmolarity by the discovery of a serum sodium concentration above 155 mEq. when it was normal preoperatively is easily effected by giving water rectally and orally, 5 per cent dextrose in water intravenously. Care must be exercised lest too much water be given. For this reason the serum concentrations of sodium should be performed at hourly intervals while the water is being administered.

Some postcraniotomy fevers are not attributable to hyperosmolarity, infection, or other febrile general postoperative complications. Such need not be treated unless they exceed 104° F. (40° C.) or persist for longer than a day. Giving aspirin (acetylsalicylic acid) 0.65 to 1.0 Gm. every 4 hours and/or sponging the body with tepid water or 70 per cent alcohol usually will control nonspecific neurogenic fevers.

Heat Stroke

Heat stroke is an occasional cause of a very high fever postoperatively. Thyroid storm, intracranial disturbances and extreme elevations of osmolar concentration (serum sodium of 170 mEq./liter or above) and heat stroke are the main causes of fever above 108° F. (42° C.).

Heat stroke is attributable to an environmental heat overload and is especially likely to occur during the first days of a hot spell. A febrile illness, lack of water, physical exertion, alcoholism, anesthesia, debility, and nonfunctioning sweat glands secondary to diabetic neuropathy and drugs such as atropine predispose one to it. Unless treated vigorously, it soon kills.

Classically, heat pyrexia or stroke consists of a rapidly mounting fever in a person having dry hot skin. He is first apathetic, then stuporous, and then comatose. Early, he is flushed, has visibly full pulses with a wide pulse pressure and exaggerated heart sounds. Later, he becomes ashen gray, has small pulses, low blood pressure and becomes anuric. Occasionally, signs of acute cardiac collapse may be found late in the illness.

Treatment. Although the pathogenesis of heat stroke is unknown, it can be treated successfully if the treatment is begun early and conducted vigorously. Reduction of the fever by immersing the person in a bathtub filled with water and ice is the basic step. After the rectal temperature falls to 100° F. (38° C.) the patient is placed upon a bed, and the rectal temperature is determined continuously with a thermistor or thermocouple or frequently with a thermometer. If the temperature begins to rise he is covered with wet sheets and fanned. Should the temperature fall below 96° F. (36° C.) he is covered with a blanket. Sponge bathing and fanning are inferior to immersion in ice water for the primary control of heat stroke. Speed is of utmost importance.

When peripheral circulatory failure persists after reducing the temperature to normal, appropriate intravenous fluids are given. Lactated Ringer's solution is suitable until a specific choice of fluids can be made upon receiving the necessary laboratory reports. While the fluid is being given, careful watch for signs of acute heart failure must be exercised. Should signs of heart failure appear, digitalization with Cedilanid is indicated. Before digitalization is begun the serum potassium should be known and the digitalization must be effected slowly if serum potassium is below 4.2 mEq./L.

Occasionally, heat stroke may develop during an operation. F. L., aged 6, on a day with a maximum temperature of 96° F. developed appendicitis and a preoperative temperature of 38.6° C. She was given 1/300 gr. of atropine a half hour before being anesthetized with ether and heavily covered with drapes in a hot operating room (31° C.). The surgeon, upon placing his fingers within the abdomen, noted great warmth and asked that the rectal temperature be taken—it was 41.6° C. The appendix was removed quickly, the wound closed, and the temperature was reduced by immersion in ice water. However, 6 hours later the child died. Necropsy demonstrated only widespread petechial hemorrhages. Extreme hyperpyrexia may be quickly lethal. One must be particularly aware of the great hazard an operation holds for a dehydrated, atropinized person subjected to high environmental temperatures.

Such cases often are complicated by convulsive movements or twitchings, the so-called ether convulsions (see Chap. 13, Anesthesia).

HYPOTHERMIA

At ordinary hospital temperatures (20 to 30° C.) noniatrogenic hypothermia is not dangerous per se. It is a rather frequent complication of morphine and barbiturate overdosage, ileostomy and colostomy diarrhea, profuse fistulous drainage, enteral aspiration and pyloric obstruction with vomiting. Of course, simple exposure to cold is a likely cause. Briefly, exposure to cold, extracellular fluid volume deficit, and overdosage with morphine and barbiturates are the main causes. Treatment is simple: warm surroundings for exposure hypothermia; saline solutions for dehydrational hypothermia; and withholding the drugs and warming for drug hypothermia.

Section 3. Postoperative Pain

Pain is a fearsome sensation. Adequacy of stimulus varies in different tissues. The application of a hot rod to the skin, a tooth, the cornea, or the parietal peritoneum is painful, while its application to muscle, fat, mucosa of the stomach or the intestine and the visceral peritoneum is not painful. An incision is exquisitely painful in skin, barely discernible in fat, nondiscernible in muscle, moderately painful in tendon or fascia, exquisitely painful in periosteum, and not felt in intestine. Incision into or acute localized pressure upon a mixed nerve is agonizing.

ETIOLOGY

The possible causes of postoperative pain are relatively few: namely, inflammation, pressure, tension and ischemia. Pains stimulated by pressure, tension, ischemia and inflammation have somewhat similar characters: they are steady, aggravated by motion and may be throbbing. Only that pain associated with intermittent increases in tension is truly and regularly intermittent. The pains of ureteral and intestinal colics are of this type; they come and go as the peristalses (pressure changes) in these structures come and go.

SITE

The commonest site of postoperative pain is the wound. All wounds are somewhat painful for 48 to 72 hours; however, normal incisional pain is not severe. Therefore, severe pain in a wound at any time signifies infection, undue pressure and tension, ischemia about the wound or of the wounded member; or the reference of pain to the wound. The phenomenon of reference of pain to the wound is especially important during the immediate postoperative period. The pain of myocardial infarct, pulmonary infarct, gastric dilatation, and vesical dilatation are frequently referred to a healing abdominal incision. Consequently, the search for the cause of unusual pain ostensibly located in an abdominal wound needs to be thorough and ofttimes extensive.

PAIN OF ISCHEMIA

Pain in a hand, a foot, an arm, a leg, or the head contained within a cast or an enveloping dressing is often ischemic in origin and demands immediate attention. Testing the painful part distal to the cast or the bandage for arterial pulses, speed of capillary flow and sensation is mandatory before an analgesic is prescribed. The speed of capillary flow can be gauged roughly by pressing upon the skin or the base of fingernail or toenail, and noting the rate of return of blood-color after the removal of pressure. A slow return of color indicates impairment of blood flow through the arteries to the part. Pressure upon nerves quickly blocks conduction in them so that parts distal to the point of pressure become hypesthetic or anesthetic. Consequently, testing the finger or toe pads with a pin is also an important part of the examination of all and more especially of the painful extremities contained in casts or encircling bandages. A slow capillary flow or a change in the sensation of a part are sufficient indications for splitting, spreading or otherwise loosening the cast and, if necessary, its removal. They are always indications for the removal of the encircling dressing, including materials used to line the cast. Gangrene, Volkmann's ischemic contracture, neural palsies and pressure sores are dire consequences of failure to remove or at least to loosen tight casts and bandages promptly.

Although capillary flow and sensibility of the distal parts of an extremity may be normal, the pain in a leg or an arm still may be ischemic in origin. The cast or the bandage may be pressing upon bony prominences. Should this be the case and the cast or the bandage is not loosened or fixed, a pressure sore will form. The pain of the localized ischemia preceding a pressure sore usually is sharply localized to the part bearing the pressure and disappears when the skin under the pressure point becomes anesthetic from pressure. Failure to recognize this may lead the physician to leave the cast or dressing alone until too late.

Incisional pain is stimulated most frequently by wound infections and faulty technic of wound closure and dressing, and adherence of the dressing to the wound. The signs of wound infections have been discussed. Tying cutaneous sutures tightly is followed by a painful wound wherever it is located. However, wounds of the chest wall and the upper abdomen are especially painful when closed with tightly tied sutures; every breath hurts.

The aim of wound closure is coaption without tension. Tight sutures about muscle fibers kill them; they turn fascia and tendon into a gluey liquid and widen the holes through the skin, leaving unsightly scars.

Meticulous adherence to the principles of wound closure and dressing, namely, coapt but do not strangulate and bind it not so tightly as to impair the venous or arterial flow of blood, or conduction in nerve, ensure minimally painful wounds. Tightly sutured wounds must be suffered, but the error need not be repeated (see Chap. 2, Wound Healing).

WOUND DISRUPTION

A sudden short-lived stabbing or burning pain in an abdominal wound brought on by coughing, sneezing, or movement never should be passed over lightly. It is indicative of disruption of the incision. Should such a pain occur, the dressing must be removed and the wound inspected. The seepage of a serosanguineous fluid from an abdominal wound at any time is indicative of disruption or infection and the more especially disruption after a sudden sharp short-lived effort pain. Some of this fluid should be collected for culture and some smeared and stained. Should the fluid contain very few or no organisms, it may be inferred that disruption of the wound has most likely taken place and that it should be opened further in an operating room, and the disrupted layers reapproximated. Should this not be done, spontaneous evisceration may follow the next cough, hiccough or movement. Bowel, especially small intestine, may catch in an incomplete disruption and become obstructed. The least life-endangering consequence of nonclosure of a deep fascial disruption of an abdominal wound is an incisional hernia. All of these consequences of disruption may be prevented by reclosure of the wound in layers, or en masse with strong through-and-through heavy malleable wire or monofilic nylon sutures.

THE PROBLEM OF NONINCISIONAL ABDOMINAL PAIN

Postoperative abdominal pain not restricted to the wound confronts the surgeon with two very perplexing problems, namely, what is the cause of the pain and what is its significance? For example, 36 hours after the performance of a resection of the ascending colon and an ileotransverse colostomy, the patient complains of intermittent epigastric pains. Are these pains merely a phase in the restitution of functional peristalsis, the so-called normal postoperative gas pains, or do they signify the existence of a mechanical intestinal obstruction? Or 15 hours after a splenectomy for idiopathic thrombocytopenic purpura we are presented with a febrile person having a distended silent abdomen, complaining of constant deep upper abdominal pain and pain in the left supraclavicular region and the mid-back. Do these pains have as their cause: a traumatic necrosis of the tail of the pancreas, an infection beneath the left hemidiaphragm, a normal abacterial nonchemical inflammatory reaction secondary to the physical trauma of the operation, a thrombosis of the portal vein, an embolus lodged in the lower lobe of the left lung, or a myocardial infarct?

Clearly, the picture is often so confusing as to prevent the formulation of a specific diagnosis. Consequently, the questions that the surgeon needs to answer soon are: shall I operate again now? Shall I wait and watch? What laboratory and roentgen examinations should be performed to permit me the maximum exercise of judgment?

In general, painful intra-abdominal postoperative complications which can be corrected by surgical intervention fall into 3 categories: (1) peritonitis with the leakage of the contents of hollow organs into the peritoneal cavities or fascial planes, (2) the obstruction of hollow viscera, (3) the impedance of the flow of blood to abdominal organs.

Postoperative abdominal pains not amenable to correction by surgical procedures may have as their origin: myocardial infarct, pulmonary infarct, pneumonia, post-traumatic sterile inflammation, and infections within the genitourinary tract.

Surgical intervention is indicated should the complication be amenable to correction by an operation and is not indicated should the illness fall into the second category. Would the postoperative patient respond to the above-named troubles as the patient who has not been operated upon does, the differentiation of the surgically significant pain from the nonsurgically significant would be relatively easy. However, the postoperative patient often does not respond to any of the above jeopardies to his life in the manner that a person who has not been operated upon does. The pain of a myocardial infarct after a celiotomy does not always have an upward and left arm radiation but may be strictly abdominal. Free leakage of the contents of the stomach, the duodenum and the jejunum into the peritoneal cavity postoperatively is often unattended by abdominal muscle spasm greater than that associated with an abdominal wound without complications; likewise, the tenderness is often relatively slight. The same insult to the peritoneum of a person who has not been operated upon is attended almost immediately by a spastically rigid abdominal musculature and great tenderness. The reason for the paucity of local response to peritonitis postoperatively is unknown. However, the person receiving cortisone or ACTH may react to a peritoneal inflammation just as a person often does during the immediate postoperative period, the response being abnormally small. It is known that the secretion of corticoids during and for a short time after an operation is remarkably enhanced. Perhaps this increase is sufficient to produce the inhibition of response to peritonitis postoperatively. Many a physician arguing that the patient he had operated upon could not have peritonitis because little tenderness and muscle spasm existed has had his argument refuted and his pride punctured by the pathologist's irrefutable revelations in the autopsy room.

Similarly, complete mechanical intestinal obstruction during the immediate postoperative period often lacks the gurgles, the tinkles and the rushes coincident with cramps characteristic of the intestinal obstructions occurring at other times.

The excruciating pain so frequently experienced with interference with blood flow to abdominal viscera may be lacking postoperatively even though the arterial and venous blood flow to the entire small intestine be occluded by volvulus, thrombi or emboli. How then does one go about the process of differentiating the surgically correctable from the nonsurgically correctable origin of abdominal pain postoperatively?

Shock rarely supervenes quickly in the case of complications that cannot be corrected by operations except with myocardial and pulmonary infarcts. Consequently, in instances in which pain and shock are joined, an electrocardiogram and a roentgenogram of the chest and the abdomen become very important parts of the examination of a patient who suffers from abdominal pain postoperatively.

The determination of the concentration of red cells with a hematocrit, a red blood cell count or a hemoglobin determination is very important. Progressive hemoconcentration means a rapid plasma loss and in a previously stable patient is indicative of peritonitis or intestinal obstruction. Therefore, it is usually an indication for reoperation. In addition, volvulus, venous vascular occlusions and pancreatitis are often attended by hemoconcentration, while myocardial and pulmonary infarcts, bronchopneumonia and genitourinary infections and obstructions rarely are.

The white blood count is of relatively little differential diagnostic importance. Leukocytosis and a shift to the left occur regularly during the immediate postoperative period—complications or not.

The search of a clean voided or better a catheterized specimen of urine for white blood cells, bacteria and albumin is the only relatively certain means of detecting an infection within the urinary tract.

Should the operation antecedent to the pain have been performed upon the biliary tract or near it, for instance, gastrectomy, the urine should be tested for the presence of bilirubin. Occlusion of the common or the hepatic ducts by ligature is soon followed by the excretion of bile in the urine. The Gmelin and the fuming nitric acid tests are satisfactory screening tests for bile in urine.

Abdominal pain coupled with tenderness or pain in the costovertebral angle or flank following an operation within the pelvis or in proximity to the abdominal ureter such as resections of the ascending, the descending and the sigmoid colons, resections of the aorta and the iliac arteries, ligation of the vena cava, and lumbar sympathectomy are sufficient indication for a pyelographic examination. One or both ureters may have been ligated or injured.

The determination of serum amylase or diastase concentrations do not always have the customary significance. Moderate elevations are not infrequent following a variety of upper abdominal operations. They may indicate postoperative pancreatitis but they may not! The author knows of 3 cases of intestinal gangrene in which the serum amylase concentration was very high, in one case being 3,600 Somogyi units. Very high serum amylase or lipase levels are indications for reoperation. They signify a surgically remediable situation.

All the while the aforementioned examinations are being conducted the person is to be examined and observed repeatedly. Pulse rate, blood pressure, rectal temperatures, the amount of abdominal tenderness and spasm are to be determined and recorded repeatedly. Postoperative abdominal pain with increasing tachycardia, a narrowing pulse pressure, or falling systolic and diastolic pressures with progressive hyperpyrexia and deterioration of general physiologic state coupled with absence of electrocardiographic signs of myocardial infarct and lack of electrocardiographic and roentgen signs of pulmonary infarct usually constitute sufficient reason for surgical re-entry of the abdominal cavity; almost certainly a postoperative surgical catastrophe has taken place, and the surgeon must make an attempt to correct it. Many an untimely death is attributable to postoperative procrastination.

However, few situations tax the judgment of the surgeon more severely than such a crisis in a postoperative patient. He must weigh all the risks and the probabilities as accurately as possible. Paracentesis may be indicated. In general, he will do well not to re-enter a closed abdomen without objective evidence of an intra-abdominal catastrophe. However, on the other hand, he must guard against any unwillingness to face the possibility that he has made a technical error. The treatment of postoperative complications productive of abdominal pain needs to fit the cause.

PAIN OF POSTOPERATIVE ILEUS

Ileus is a common cause of abdominal pain postoperatively, and the determination of cause is especially difficult because mechanical intestinal obstruction arising during the immediate postoperative period is often unattended by intestinal colic (see Chap. 38).

The causes of postoperative ileus fall into two groups: mechanical and adynamic, and the adynamic is divisible into 3 categories: vascular, chemical, of which hypokalemia is most common, and reflex.

Ileus is treated best by prevention. Mechanical ileus can be partially prevented by the avoidance of technical errors both of omission and of commission that predispose toward postoperative obstruction. Especially important in this connection is the avoidance of talc as a glove powder (see Chap. 38, Intestinal Obstruction). Even the hydrolyzed starch now used can produce granulomas, and gloves should be rinsed thoroughly before touching the viscera. Adynamic or paralytic ileus is likewise reduced by gentle handling of the viscera at operation but cannot be entirely avoided. The pain arises chiefly from distention, and a major factor in this distention is air that traverses the esophagus during swallowing or abnormal breathing. Therefore, prevention can be accomplished by continually aspirating the stomach by suction siphonage through a nasogastric tube by the method of Wangensteen and Paine.

Such tubes are uncomfortable, and judgment is required to decide when to remove the tube and discontinue gastric drainage.

The use of a cloth tape measure placed around the patient's abdomen and left there permits frequent measurements with little or no disturbance to the patient. Serial measurements of girth may then be recorded at regular intervals. If there is a marked increase when the nasogastric tube is clamped off for a few hours, it is usually too soon to remove it and suction should be resumed.

Audible peristalsis is a useful guide, but not infrequently this returns before the period of ileus is over.

If prevention has not been employed or has failed and distention supervenes, the possibility of mechanical obstruction becomes a problem. Logically, one proceeds to an x-ray examination. Because of various practical considerations, most surgeons first attempt to reduce the distention by suction siphonage through a gastric tube or sometimes through a long intestinal tube, and by the use of enemas which should be either small in volume and stimulating (e.g., 4 ounces of milk and 4 ounces of molasses) or contain salt in physiologic amounts if given in the customary volume of about 1 liter (large enemas without salt can contribute to water intoxication). If these are unsuccessful, we recommend x-ray examination before resorting to drugs.

Prostigmine methyl sulfate, starting in dose of one fourth to one half milligram, is of some use in adynamic ileus. It should not be used in mechanical obstruction. Its action is primarily on the small bowel. It is customary to give it every 4 hours for several doses, but the interval may be shorter.

The large bowel responds often to small doses of pitressin, especially if given immediately after an enema has been administered. Side-effects may be alarming, with increased pain and a cold sweaty countenance and may be dangerous. It is generally unwise to use it in persons with impaired hearts or hypertension. The initial dose should not exceed one half an ampule hypodermically.

The effect of both of these drugs occurs mainly within 20 minutes of the time of administration. Pitressin has been used by one of us (J. E. R.) under close observation and not as a running order. Another (C. A. M.) never uses drugs for the treatment of ileus.

PLEURISY

After operations on parts of the body other than the thorax, pleuritis and myocardial infarction are common causes of postoperative chest pain. Pleuritic pain is rhythmic and synchronous with breathing. Deep breathing and coughing accentuate it. A rub is almost always audible in the region of the pain. Generally, pleuritis is a manifestation of an inflammatory lesion of the lung in contact with parietal pleura such as a localized aspirational pneumonitis, pulmonary infarct or lobar pneumonia. Consequently, roentgenograms of the chest and meticulous examination of the extremities for signs of thrombophlebitis, and of the sputum for pneumococci are necessary in attempting the discovery of the cause of the pleurisy. Pleuritic pain is usually short-lived, and analgesics readily control it, while appropriate specific medications such as antibiotics and anticoagulants are given to treat the cause of the pulmonary lesion.

POSTOPERATIVE MYOCARDIAL INFARCTION

Postoperative myocardial infarct is especially prone to follow amputations for ischemic gangrene of the foot and the leg. Peripheral circulatory failure attending or following an amputation is often traceable to a myocardial infarct. Should the infarct take place while the person is anesthetized it is painless, and when it occurs while the patient is under the influence of analgesics and soporifics the retrosternal pain and oppression may be lacking or so slight as to be readily disregarded by patient and physician. Consequently, obscure weakness, fever, anterior chest pains, tachycardia, cardiac irregularities and shock postoperatively are indications for electrocardiography.

MEDIASTINITIS

Retrosternal pain may be indicative of mediastinitis when associated with fever and dyspnea after esophageal diverticulectomy, esophagectomy, pneumonectomy, gastroscopy, esophagoscopy, the removal of foreign bodies from the main stem bronchi or the trachea and the esophagus, and rarely after thyroidectomy. Mediastinitis was a highly fatal complication before the sulfonamides and the antibiotics were discovered. Today it is not, if its existence is detected and if appropriate operative measures are taken to control it.

POSTOPERATIVE DYSPNEA

Dyspnea, the consciousness of needing to breathe, has a number of important connotations postoperatively: (1) partial obstruction of the trachea or the bronchus; (2) stiffening of the lung with edema (pulmonary edema) or blood (congestive atelectasis) or obstruction of a bronchus (obstructive atelectasis); (3) the reduction of pulmonic volume by extrapulmonic intrathoracic air (pneumothorax), similarly located fluid (pleural effusion and empyema), or elevation of the diaphragm by ascites, meteorism, abdominal obesity, or tight abdominal binders; (4) muscular weakness (shock, myasthenia gravis and adrenal insufficiency); and (5) acidosis.

Airway Obstruction

Often after operations upon the tongue and the neck dyspnea is attributable to obstruction of the airway. In particular after thyroidectomy dyspnea may be caused by partial obstruction of the airway within the larynx by paralysis of the vocal cords or laryngeal edema, tracheal obstruction from tracheal ring collapse or pressure from a hematoma (hemorrhage); or by acute cardiac failure or acute hypoparathyroidism. All but hypoparathyroidism pose an immediate threat to life. Consequently, post-thyroidectomy dyspnea is a real danger signal and dictates immediate steps to determine its genesis. Inspection of the wound is first. A tense swollen neck is indicative of *hemorrhage* with tracheal or pharyngeal compression and requires *immediate opening* of the wound because arterial bleeding is the predominant cause of strangulating peritracheal and retropharyngeal hemorrhage and it leaves little time between the onset of dyspnea and death.

The breathing with tracheal obstruction is characteristic. It is audibly labored with retraction of the supraclavicular and the intercostal spaces during inspiration. Finding the pharyngeal airway obstructed or the vocal cords edematous or in the cadaveric position indicates the need for tracheostomy. It is to be performed at the bedside should the patient be severely dyspneic or unconscious. In the meantime, should the dyspnea be severe, the insertion of a pharyngeal airway and the administration of helium and oxygen usually will relieve the dyspnea *but not the necessity for tracheostomy*. Attempting to ride out partial laryngeal obstruction from paralyzed vocal cords invites disaster. Acute fulminant pulmonary edema is prone to occur, and before tracheostomy can be done the patient may be dead. Tracheostomy bears little risk to life, while asphyxia and pulmonary edema attendant upon laryngeal obstruction do.

Bronchoscopy is requisite for viewing the size of the tracheal lumen and is the only means of ascertaining the existence of tracheal ring collapse. Immediate tracheostomy is the treatment for tracheal collapse. The tracheal rings will soon stiffen, and the tracheostomy tube may be removed and the wound permitted to close, often within a week.

Dyspnea is rarely the first sign of parathyreoprivia to be appreciated. Failure to find an organic cause of post-thyroidectomy dyspnea raises the probability that hypoparathyroidism is its cause and dictates the ascertainment of the serum calcium level and search for Chvostek's and Trousseau's signs. The treatment of parathyreoprivia is discussed in Chapter 28.

CARDIAC FAILURE

Signs and Symptoms

Dyspnea may be the first sign of acute cardiac failure. Cardiac failure is a relatively infrequent postoperative complication. When it occurs it usually presents the picture of "acute cardiac collapse" rather than that of "congestive failure." Consequently, it resembles hemorrhagic shock or peripheral circulatory failure of the hypovolemic type. However, its differentiation from hematogenic shock, though usually easy, is occasionally very difficult.

The differentiation of postoperative acute cardiac failure or collapse from surgical shock depends largely upon the detection of signs of pulmonary congestion and cardiac dilatation. They appear with or soon after the beginning of acute cardiac failure, while with hemorrhagic shock they are absent or appear very late, and then in lesser degree. The measurement of venous pressure is also helpful. It is high with cardiac failure and low or normal with shock.

The signs of pulmonary congestion are dyspnea, labored breathing, rales and venous distention, most easily observed in the cervical veins although inconstant and late in appearance. The detection of left ventricular cardiac dilatation is more difficult, especially in the obese and emphysematous patient. When the physical signs of dilatation can be elicited they are diffuseness of the apical beat, shift of the point of maximum impulse to the left of the midclavicular line, and gallop rhythm.

The point of maximal impulse may be shifted toward the left by dorsal scoliosis, right pleural effusion or pneumothorax or left bronchial obstructive atelectasis. Consequently, the careful examination of the spine and the pulmonary fields is requisite to the interpretation of finding the cardiac impulse to the left of its normal position.

Gallop rhythm or three-sound rhythm has varied significance. A distinct three-sound rhythm, LUBB-dup-da, may be heard in normal persons with slow pulse rates. The third sound, the -da, disappears with a little exercise. It has no pathologic significance. True gallop rhythms do not disappear with exercise and they exist with tachycardia. They have the varied cadences of a galloping horse: da-LUBB-dup, da-LUBB-dup (presystolic gallop); LUBB-dup-da, LUBB-dup-da (protodiastolic gallop); or lubb-dup-DA, lubb-dup-DA (summation gallop). The discovery of any of the true gallop rhythms is very helpful; it means that the heart is dilated, and heart failure is imminent or exists.

Left ventricular dilatation is best determined by roentgenogram. Frontal and left anterior thoracic oblique projections are the most useful. A rounding of the apex and a widening of the transverse cardiac diameter relative to the transverse diameter of the chest, and backward displacement of the cardiac shadow are the frontal and left anterior oblique signs of left ventricular dilatation. Cardiac hypertrophy without significant dilatation is not readily apparent roentgenographically. Acute postoperative cardiac collapse or failure is often associated with abnormal cardiac rhythms, such as the ectopic tachycardias of auricular fibrillation and flutter, and extreme sinus tachycardia. Peripheral circulatory failure is rarely associated with disturbances of rhythm other than simple sinus tachycardia. The definitive determination of type of disturbance in cardiac rhythm existing in a patient requires electrocardiography. The differential signs of acute heart failure and shock are listed in Table 15-1.

Such signs as mottled cyanosis of the trunk, cold extremities, small peripheral pulses, hypotension, oliguria or anuria, sweating, slight fever and psychic disturbances are common to acute cardiac failure and shock alike and consequently have no differential diagnostic significance.

TREATMENT

The treatment of acute postoperative cardiac failure varies somewhat with the stage and the rate of development. Venesection has a place in the treatment of the acute fulminant form and the late stage of the nonfulminant type with pulmonary edema. For example: F.H., male aged 67 years, and hypertensive was catheterized at 2:30 P.M. to measure residual urine. About 5 minutes after the catheterization he was found struggling for breath, cyanotic, losing consciousness, and with gurgling breathing. Within 3 minutes venous occlusive tourniquets were placed on arms and thighs, and the antecubital veins were opened through incisions which he did not feel even though no anesthetic was used. At first blood dripped slowly from the transected veins, then the flow gradually quickened, and as it did breathing became less laborious, cyanosis

TABLE 15-1

Symptom or Sign	Acute Heart Failure or Acute Cardiac Collapse	Hypovolemic Shock
Dyspnea	Prominent	Slight or absent
Orthopnea	Prominent	Absent
Circulation time	Slow	Within normal limits
Rales	Prominent feature	Rare excepting preterminally
Heart size	Large	Normal
Maximum impulse	Outside midclavicular line	Usually within midclavicular line
Apical impulse	Diffuse	Sharply localized
Apical gallop	Often present	Absent
Cardiac arrhythmias	Frequent, especially auricular fibrillation	Rare excepting sinus tachycardia
Venous pressure	Often elevated	Infrequently elevated, is often low
Roentgenogram		
Frontal	Rounded apex	
	Increased transverse diameter	Normal apical contour
	Prominent hilar vascular shadows	Normal or faint hilar vascular shadows
Left ant. oblique	Filling of retrocardiac space	Retrocardiac space normal
ECG	Left axis deviation	Normal axis
	Ectopic rhythms	Sinus tachycardia

began to clear, and when the blood flowed a stream, consciousness returned. Then the tourniquets were removed, pressure dressings were placed over the antecubital incisions, and a digitalis glucoside was given. That evening he walked about the ward unmindful of his proximity to death 4 hours earlier. Admittedly, such a dramatic response is seldom seen.

Venesection is rarely required for less fulminant and lesser degrees of cardiac collapse without extensive pulmonary edema. Venous occlusive tourniquets, the pressure breathing of oxygen, and cardiac glucosides usually control the milder situations rapidly. A diuretic leading to a loss of sodium as well as of water such as chlorothiazide is most useful, but its use must be monitored carefully by serial determinations of serum sodium.

Because the nature of the cardiac abnormality that underlies acute postoperative cardiac failure is rarely ascertainable before digitalization, lanatoside C (Cedilanid) is most satisfactory. It acts quickly and disappears rapidly from the body, thereby minimizing the danger of overdosage. For adults the initial digitalizing dose of lanatoside C is 1.0 to 1.6 mg. parenterally. The intravenous route is used whenever there is pulmonary edema and one is reasonably certain that myocardial infarct is absent. The intramuscular route is used for acute cardiac failure without pulmonary edema.

The treatment of cardiac collapse with postoperative myocardial infarct almost defies description. Oxygen by mask, heparin, papaverine 0.1 to 0.2 Gm. every 4 to 6 hrs. and atropine 0.3 to 0.4 mg. every 6 hrs. subcutaneously are recommended. With pronounced or progressive pulmonary edema, rotating venous occlusive tourniquets or cautious venesection may be used. With pronounced signs of peripheral circulatory failure and severe oliguria or anuria and few signs of pulmonary edema the careful transfusion of blood may help. According to some internists digitalization is indicated only rarely. Because myocardial infarction is often painless postoperatively, an electrocardiogram should be performed before digitalizing a person showing signs of cardiac collapse during or after an operation. As with diabetic coma, the treatment of postinfarctional cardiac collapse demands the artistry and the experience that an internist is best able to provide.

Before undertaking rapid digitalization of any patient, the serum potassium concentration should be known. Digitalization in the face of low serum potassium levels is very hazardous and requires utmost care and skill. Consult a medical text.

Dyspnea of Weakness

Persistent dyspnea and weakness after thyroidectomy is occasionally ascribable to myasthenia gravis which is occasionally associated with thyrotoxicosis. When persistent dyspnea and weakness are accompanied by difficulty in swallowing and speaking, and the rapid fatigue of used muscles, including a drooping of the upper eyelids, myasthenia gravis should be considered as a possible cause. Rapid fatigue of muscles upon repetitive motion of an extremity and progressive weakness and slurring of speech with sustained speaking are rather peculiar to this disease. Should these signs be demonstrable, neostigmine (1 mg.) intramuscularly may be given. Any improvement tends to confirm the diagnosis.

Section 4. Gas Therapy

OXYGEN

Increasing the partial pressure of oxygen in the inspired air increases the rate with which pulmonary arterial blood is oxygenated and reduces the mass of gaseous nitrogen in solution within the body.

The primary action of oxygen therapy is the augmentation of the rate of oxygenation of pulmonary arterial blood. This action is of clinical significance for patients with abnormally incomplete oxygenation of the peripheral arterial blood. The main causes of incomplete oxygenation of the peripheral arterial blood are: patchy atelectasis, bronchopneumonia, pulmonary fibrosis, hypopnea, pulmonary edema, incomplete obstructions of the trachea or the major bronchi and severe reductions of the residual air such as attend removal of lungs. Oxygen therapy for these conditions usually will serve to improve the saturation of the systemic arterial blood if it is below normal. Oxygen therapy should be tried whenever the signs of anoxic hypoxia appear. The signs of hypoxia are: exertional dyspnea, tachycardia, fever, changes in psyche, such as euphoria, disorientation, delirium, convulsions and coma. These are more important signs of indication for the institution of oxygen therapy than is peripheral cyanosis. Often peripheral cyanosis may be lacking, even though the individual is suffering from a severe hypoxic hypoxia. Indications that oxygen therapy is effective in a particular patient are: the reduction of the pulse rate, improvement in sensorium, and the relief of breathlessness and restlessness when it is given.

Oxygen therapy has often been recommended for the treatment of peripheral circulatory failure. It is doubtful that it is particularly valuable in the treatment of the circulatory anoxia that attends shock, excepting when anoxic anoxia exists with it. When in doubt, oxygen may be given, but its use never should be accepted as a substitute for specific therapy such as transfusions of blood or other fluids.

The giving of oxygen in high concentrations may be accomplished with the use of oxygen tents, nasal catheters and the oronasal Boothby mask. The administration of oxygen with a tent or through a nasal catheter will effect increases in the oxygen tension of alveolar air to about 300 mm. Hg pressure. Alveolar partial pressures of oxygen above 400 mm. Hg can be obtained with the use of the oronasal Boothby mask or the administration of oxygen through an endotracheal tube attached to a special respiratory apparatus or anesthesia machine. The choice of the way the oxygen is given depends upon what needs to be accomplished. The nasal catheter route is usually adequate for the administration of oxygen to individuals who are not comatose and do not have high body temperatures. The oxygen tent is superior to the nasal catheter for patients who have hypoxic hypoxia and hyperpyrexia. The oxygen tent, besides increasing the oxygen in the inspired air, serves as an air-conditioning mechanism. The oronasal mask route of administration is especially applicable whenever the anoxia is particularly severe and ileus with meteorism exists.

The breathing of tensions of oxygen above

500 mm. Hg pressure is at times beneficial to individuals suffering from ileus and meteorism, partially by virtue of the denitrogenating action of breathing high concentrations of oxygen. Inspiring pure oxygen for an hour or two denitrogenates the body because though only oxygen is breathed in, nitrogen, oxygen and carbon dioxide are breathed out. Since more than two thirds of the gas in the intestines of an individual suffering from meteorism is made up of nitrogen, the denitrogenation of the body attendant upon the breathing of pure oxygen serves to reduce the meteorism (see Chap. 38). This action of high oxygen therapy has been well substantiated by Fine.

There is some danger attendant upon the administration of pure oxygen through tight-fitting masks or through endotracheal tubes for periods of time longer than 4 to 6 hours. The breathing of pure oxygen for long periods promotes a hemorrhagic pneumonia. This has been termed oxygen poisoning. It can be prevented by breaking the administration of pure oxygen every 3 to 4 hours for 5 minutes.

The danger of oxygen poisoning is not the only one attendant upon the administration of pure oxygen The giving of pure oxygen to individuals is capable of inciting respiratory arrest in persons who by reason of their illness or drugs given to them have lost their respiratory sensitivity to carbon dioxide and whose breathing, therefore, is being maintained in part by the anoxic drive of breathing. Patients who have been given morphine and short-acting barbiturates, emphysematous asthmatics and comatose persons tend to have respiratory centers that are insensitive to carbon dioxide and are prone to reduce their rate and depth of breathing when given oxygen to breathe. With the decline in pulmonary ventilation attendant upon the receipt of oxygen, carbon dioxide is retained in their bodies, and the pH of their blood falls. As the carbon dioxide tension builds up their respiration slows and ultimately stops. Carbon dioxide is a respiratory depressant in individuals whose respiratory mechanisms have lost their sensitivity to it.

Because of the danger of respiratory depression attendant upon the administration of oxygen the institution of oxygen therapy to all comatose, emphysematous, asthmatic and drugged patients should be conducted under the watch of a physician for at least 30 minutes to 1 hour, and the respiratory rate and pulse rate should be determined and charted every 15 minutes for at least 3 hours.

The administration of high oxygen tensions to individuals who have large amounts of tenacious secretions in their tracheal-bronchial tree predisposes them to the development of obstructive atelectasis. The occlusion of a major bronchus of an animal breathing air is not attended by collapse of the lung for 24 to 72 hours. However, the obstruction of the bronchus of an animal breathing oxygen is followed by collapse of the obstructed segment of lung within 3 or more hours. Because of the enhancement of atelectasis by oxygen breathing in the presence of bronchial obstruction, the clearance of the airways of secretions becomes a very important part of oxygen therapy.

CARBON DIOXIDE THERAPY

For many years from 5 to 10 per cent carbon dioxide in oxygen was administered for 3 to 5 minutes every hour or two of the operative day to stimulate breathing. Today it is used very infrequently for this purpose. The administration of 5 per cent carbon dioxide in oxygen is valuable as a temporary therapeutic measure for the control of carpopedal spasms, due to tetany resulting from respiratory alkalosis, and hiccoughs. It is also valuable occasionally for the treatment of the acute nonoligemic hypotension which sometimes follows a prolonged anesthesia with cyclopropane. Seemingly, some of the acute hypotensions which attend the recovery from cyclopropane anesthesia are attributable to hypocapnia. Sometimes children who have been relieved of severe partial obstructions of the upper airways by tracheostomy or intubation stop breathing soon after the obstruction is relieved while breathing air or oxygen. Sometimes 5 per cent carbon dioxide in oxygen will maintain the breathing of such children.

HELIUM

From 30 to 50 per cent helium in oxygen is a valuable gas mixture for the temporary relief of local partial obstructions of the major air passages. The effort required to move air through a narrowed larynx, trachea or bronchus is reduced significantly by the helium. The administration of helium in oxygen must be considered only as a temporary expedient before the correction or the removal of the obstruction of the trachea or the bronchi. It is without value in the treatment of obstructions of the minor air passages.

HYPERBARIC OXYGENATION

Pure oxygen at sea level is injurious if breathed continuously over a long period (24 hours or more).

If the pressure is to be increased further, it must be used for shorter intervals. At 3 atmospheres absolute, 1 hour 3 times a day appears to be safe.

The established indications for hyperbaric oxygenation are two, but many others are under study, and some of them may be established in the near future.

According to Brummelkamp, Hoogendijk and Boerema, hyperbaric oxygenation appears to favor the recovery of patients with gas bacillus infections. This has been substantiated in animal studies by H. G. Kelley and W. G. Pace,[5] but according to the latter, it was not helpful in tetanus in animals.

The second established indication is carbon monoxide poisoning. Here it relieves the hypoxia to some extent by increasing the dissolved oxygen in the plasma, and it also hastens the exchange of oxygen for the carbon monoxide bound to the hemoglobin in the erythrocytes.

Hyperbaric condition has a theoretic usefulness in air embolism—theoretic because most such cases seen on a surgical service culminate in death too quickly to apply the method. Its efficacy in treating the bends (caisson disease) is established, but high pressures up to 7 or 8 atmospheres are sometimes necessary to relieve the symptoms, followed by slow decompression. Air is the usual medium for this purpose, and pure oxygen is to be avoided because at such high pressures of oxygen, hemorrhagic pneumonia is to be expected, and convulsions may supervene even at lower pressures.

The use of hyperbaric conditions for the treatment of local ischemia—feet, myocardium, brain, poorly vascularized tubes, grafts, etc., is under study, as is its use during cardiac operations on tiny children requiring cardiac bypass. While some encouragement has been taken from the studies of Sir Charles Illingworth and Prof. I. Boerema[1,2] and their colleagues as well as from the work of others, it appears to be premature to say that this modality has an established place except for "the bends," for carbon monoxide poisoning, and probably for the control of gas bacillus infections.

Section 5. Postoperative Urinary Retention and Oliguria

URINARY RETENTION

Overfilling of the bladder, the incapacity to urinate in the horizontal position, obstructive uropathy, and operative disturbances of the nerves or the position of the bladder are the prominent causes of postoperative urinary retention. A distention of the bladder with urine while the patient is anesthetized or deeply depressed with opiates or barbiturates, or unconscious for other reasons renders the smooth muscle of the bladder practically incapable of contracting. This might well be termed "acute decompensation of the bladder." Peculiarly, many normal young men are unable to void while lying in bed. Many postoperative urinary retentions that occur among middle-aged and elderly men can be traced to an incomplete obstruction of the bladder neck or the urethra by prostatic hypertrophy or stricture.

After combined abdominoperineal resections of the sigmoid colon and the rectum, perineorrhaphy and hysterectomy, difficulty with the passage of urine is commonplace. At one time these difficulties were ascribed to the interference with the nervous outflow to the bladder. However, some authors believe that retroposition of the bladder and descent of the base of the bladder are partly responsible for the difficulty in the passage of urine following combined abdominoperineal resections of the sigmoid colon and the rectum.

Treatment of postoperative urinary reten-

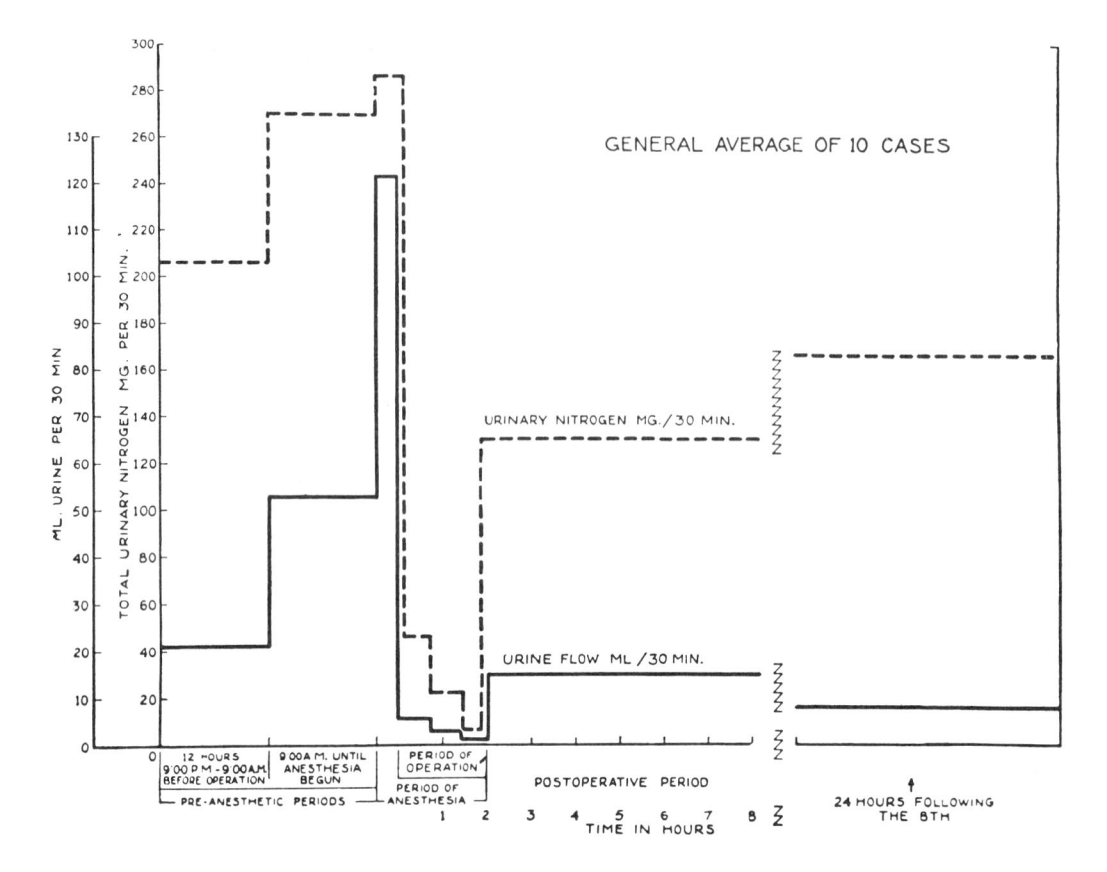

FIG. 15-1. Rates of excretion of urine and urinary nitrogen by man before, during and after ether anesthesia and various operations. Graphic representation of data of Pringle, Maunsell and Pringle (published in the British Medical Journal, September 9, 1902), showing the remarkable reduction of urea excretion and urinary flow during the operation and the immediate postoperative period. (Moyer, C. A.: Surgery, 27:199, 1950)

It must not be inferred that the anesthetic agent is the only factor influencing the changes in renal function during and immediately after an operation. Practically all of the soporific and analgesic drugs used preoperatively and postoperatively exert an antidiuretic influence. (Bibliographic references pertaining to the above statement are to be found in Smith, H. W.: *The Kidney*. Oxford University Press, New York, 1951, pp. 283, 444, 445, 446)

In addition to the antidiuretic influences exerted by the soporific, analgesic and anesthetic agent employed to permit the operation, both the painful sensory stimuli attendant upon the operation and bodily movements, such as breathing and rolling about before the wound is well along the road to healing, lead to antidiuresis (Theobald, G. W., and Verney, E. B.: J. Physiol., 83:341, 1935). The nature of the surgical illness is important also; obstructive jaundice in man is attended by a remarkable inhibition of water-diuresis. (Abe, S.: Tohoku J. Exp. Med. 17:174, 1931)

Of course, oligemia incident to the loss of blood and the sequestration of extracellular fluid in the tissues injured during the operation are determinants of the degree of functional renal incapacity attendant upon an operation. However, though oligemia may be prevented by the transfusion of blood and a balanced saline solution, renal function is disturbed during and for a time after major operations by nervous stimuli, drugs and the anesthetic agent.

Section 5. Postoperative Urinary Retention and Oliguria

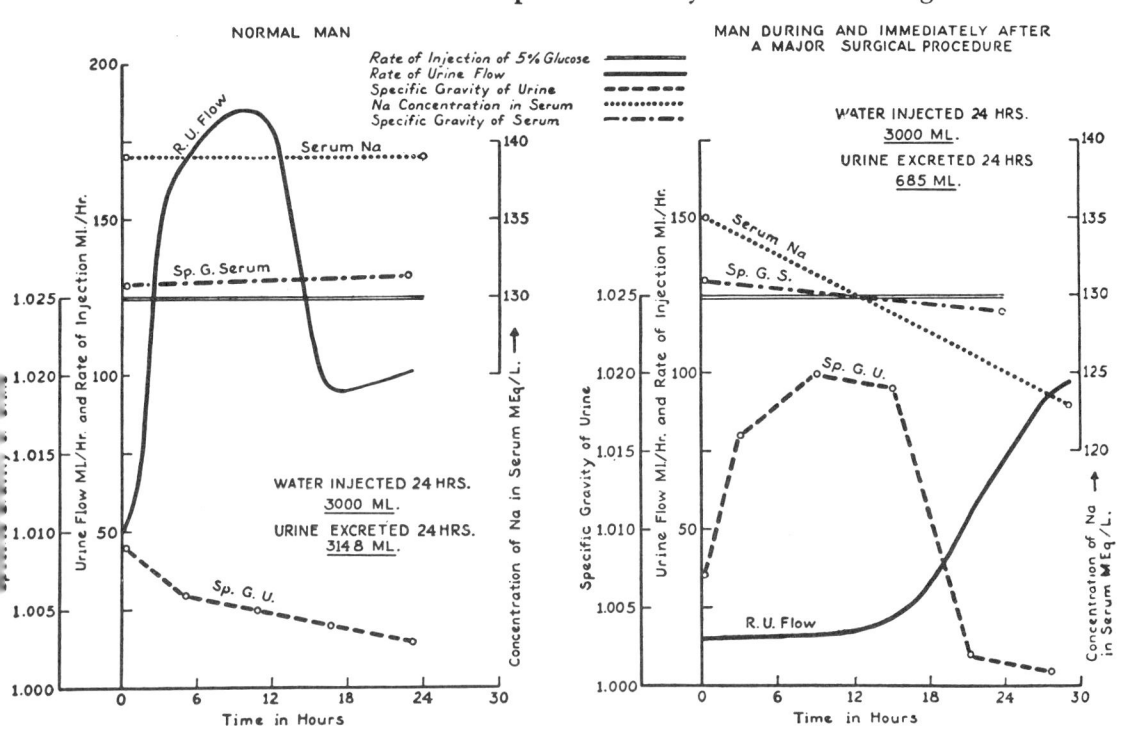

FIG. 15-2. Responses to intravenous 5 per cent glucose in distilled water. Graphic representation of data of Coller, et al. (*Left*) Response of a normal adult to the intravenous injection of 5 per cent dextrose in water, 125 ml. per hour for 24 hours. The urine flow accelerates rapidly and for a time exceeds the rate of injection, the urinary specific gravity falls, while the serum specific gravity and sodium change little, and at the end of the injection the urine excreted exceeded the volume of water given.

(*Right*) Typical response of man to the intravenous injection of 5 per cent dextrose in water, 125 ml. per hour for 24 hours, after a major operative procedure such as a combined abdominoperineal resection of the rectum, choledochostomy and gastrectomy. The urine flow accelerates slowly and does not exceed the rate of injection; the serum sodium concentration and the specific gravity of serum fall; the specific gravity of the urine rises for a time and then belatedly falls, and only 685 ml. of urine is excreted, while 3,000 ml. of dextrose solution was given. (Moyer, C. A.: Surgery, 27:201)

tion consists of first having the individual stand or sit upon the toilet and attempt to urinate. Should he be unable to do so, a small catheter is passed, and the urine is withdrawn. If the volume of urine exceeds 700 to 800 ml. the catheter should be left in place for 24 to 36 hours and connected to a continuous drainage system to permit the bladder musculature to recover from the stretching. Should smaller amounts of urine be obtained, the catheter is withdrawn, and from 4 to 6 hours later the individual is encouraged to empty the bladder.

If the catheter is left indwelling for more than 24 hours the urinary tract should be protected from infection to the extent afforded by an antibacterial drug (see Chap. 52, Urology).

OLIGURIA

Mechanical obstruction of the urinary tract, neurogenic disturbances of micturition, changes in renal function attendant upon endocrine, hemodynamic and fluid balance alterations singly or in combination may give rise to postoperative oliguria.

Because obstruction of the flow of urine by ureteral ligation and vesical obstruction from prostatic hypertrophy and sphincteric dysfunction may be the cause of oliguria or anuria postoperatively, catheterization is the first diagnostic step. (See Chap. 52, Urology, for a full discussion of obstructive uropathy.)

Actually, even though obstructive uropathy be lacking, slight oliguria is to be expected after major operative procedures. Some of the changes in the rates of renal excretion of water and urea during the induction of anesthesia, the operation and the postoperative period are shown in Figure 15-1. These observations are more than sixty years old. Notice the remarkable slowing of the rates of excretion of water and urea during the operation and the time taken for recovery. Stewart and Rourke were the first to study the alterations in the rates of renal excretion of water and salts associated with anesthesia and surgery. Many others have corroborated their discoveries. An operation greatly reduces the capacity of man to excrete water without sodium for 1 to 5 days (Fig. 15-2).

The degree of reduction in the rate of excreting a load of water attendant upon a major operation is readily secured in normal persons by injecting pitressin while infusing dextrose in water. (See Chap. 29.)

Such observations lend credence to the theory that operative pituitary stimulation is responsible for at least a portion of the postoperative oliguria. This theory is better supported by the observations of Theobald that traumatic inhibition of water diuresis does not occur in a dog after removal of the hypophysis. The inhibition of water diuresis attributable to the antidiuretic effect of an operation will not induce anuria or rates of urine flow less than 400 ml. per day. Slower rates of excretion of urine postoperatively must have additional cause. However, inhibition of water diuresis is an important cause of minor postoperative oligurias and is often so pronounced as to fix the flow of urine at rates of 450 to 800 ml. daily for hours and even days postoperatively. During the time that the operative inhibition of water diuresis exists attempts to break it by infusing glucose in water intravenously are prone to fail and are dangerous because the retained water reduces the osmolar concentration of the body's fluids and may precipitate water intoxication.

As stated above, urine flows of less than 400 ml. a day cannot be ascribed to operative inhibition of water excretion alone, because 400 ml. daily is the slowest urine flow attainable by the maximal enhancement of the facultative absorption of water by the distal renal tubular cells in normally hydrated adults. Consequently, the excretion of less than 400 ml. of urine per day at any time during a postoperative or post-traumatic period should immediately prompt a search for other causes of oliguria such as oligemia, obstructive uropathy, extracellular fluid volume deficit, osmolar dilution (water intoxication) and organic renal disease. Oligemia is the most frequent cause of the postoperative excretion of less than 400 ml. daily. Large incompletely replaced operative losses of blood and translocational losses of extracellular fluid are the main causes of postoperative oligemia. The signs and symptoms of hemorrhagic shock and dehydration are covered in Chapters 7, 8 and 5, respectively. Clearly, whenever signs of oligemia are found in an oliguric patient the oliguria is properly treated by correcting the oligemia by appropriate measures—blood transfusion for whole blood lack and lactated Ringer's solution for interstitial fluid volume translocation or external loss.

Postoperative anuria—the absence of urine flow—is a manifestation of shock, complete ureteral occlusion, a transfusion reaction, organic occlusion of the blood flow through the kidneys by emboli or thrombi, acute cardiac failure or the removal of the only functioning kidney.

No definitive treatment except renal transplant exists for the nephrectomy type of anuria. Ureteral catheterization and ureteral lavage have effected remarkably rapid corrections of anuria attributable to ureteral obstruction by crystals of sulfonamides or creatine. Ureteral catheterization alone has done the same thing for ureterolithiac obstructive anuria. The transfusion of blood has corrected many an anuria associated with hemorrhagic peripheral circulatory failure, and the infusion of sodium salt solutions has done the same for anurias attendant upon extracellular fluid volume deficit (dehydrational) shock.

The treatment of an anuria persisting after the correction of oligemic shock, after transfusion reactions, and after the removal of obstruction is discussed in Chapter 52, Urology.

Section 6. Postoperative Jaundice

Jaundice that develops during the immediate postoperative period is mainly related to one of two causes—obstruction of the extrahepatic biliary ducts or a hemoglobin overload usually due to a breakdown of erythrocytes. A steadily increasing jaundice appearing after cholecystectomy and difficult gastric resections usually means that the common hepatic or the common duct has been encircled by a ligature or cut off and tied. Acholic feces and the absence of bile in duodenal drainage are characteristic of it. The jaundice of porphyrin overload accompanies fulminant wound infections and the more especially those caused by certain anaerobes such as *Cl. histolyticum*, the hemolytic streptococci and staphylococci and the tranfusion of much aged blood during the operation. The differentiation of jaundice appearing during the first postoperative week is relatively easy. Duodenal drainage will serve to differentiate the obstructive from the porphyrin-overload type. The lack of the existence of signs of a fulminant infection distinguishes the transfusional from the infectional porphyrin overload variety.

The treatments are obvious: For the obstructive jaundice the obstruction must be removed. This requires that an operation be done as soon as the condition of the patient permits it. For that associated with infection, drain and débride and give antibiotics. For the transfusional no treatment is needed; it will disappear in a few days and serial serum bilirubins will usually show the beginning of a decline within 2 or 3 days.

Section 7. Edema

Edema, the swelling of a part of the body with fluid, has many causes: increased venous pressure, decreased arterial blood flow, decreased intravascular oncotic pressure (serum albumin deficiency), decreased lymph flow, dependency, immobility, physical trauma, infection, excessive sodium intake, cardiac failure and toxins.

VENOUS OCCLUSIVE EDEMA

Edematous swelling associated with increased venous pressure attends venous thrombosis, the application of tight encircling bandages and casts, the ligation of major veins and the obstruction of veins by neoplastic invasion or encirclement.

During the developmental phase venous occlusive edema is accompanied by some blueness of the swollen member; it is tender and painful and is firm and relatively nonpitting. Just prior to measurable subsidence, the swelling softens and pits deeply.

THROMBOPHLEBITIS

Edema is often the first sign of thrombophlebitis. Acute thrombophlebitis is an inflammatory disease of veins: the intima swells and in places disappears, the media swells and is infiltrated with wandering cells and lymphocytes, the adventitia becomes edematous, and the perivenous lymphatics are irregularly occluded. Blood clots within the lumen, and the thrombus is attached with more or less fixity to the intimally denuded vein wall. Thrombophlebitic edema varies remarkably in degree: usually it is slight when the superficial veins such as the saphenous and the cephalic are afflicted alone. It also may be slight and attended with little pain or tenderness even when the deep veins are extensively thrombosed (phlebothrombosis). However, thrombophlebitic edema may develop with remarkable rapidity and to an alarming extent. The collection of about 8 L. of edema fluid in the thighs and the legs has been observed to take place in 24 hours in a case of bilateral phlegmasia cerulea dolens.

The other signs and symptoms of thrombophlebitis also vary greatly in degree and character. The extremity may become very painful, tender and diffusely violaceous and develop bloody blebs on the digits and the dorsums of hand or foot (phlegmasia cerulea dolens), indicating a grave prognosis because few cases of phlegmasia cerulea dolens recover. It may be painful, tender and gray-white (phlegmasia alba dolens), or be practically painless, slightly tender and be normally colored (phlebothrombosis). Movement of the part may be impossible because of pain (phlegmasia dolens) or practically unrestricted (phlebothrombosis). The systemic manifestations vary from a very transient mild fever and tachycardia and slight illness to chills and very high fever, oligemic shock from sequestration of extracellular fluid within the zone of thrombosis, and the severe respiratory and circulatory disturbances of pulmonary embolization.

Chills and high fever with thrombophlebitis are indicative of thrombophlebitis purulenta, a thrombophlebitis complicated with bacterial invasion and break-up of the clot. These bacterially laden clot-fragments enter the circulation and are disseminated especially to the lungs where they are prone to produce septic pulmonary infarcts.

Tenderness is practically always elicitable in the afflicted part. Gentle dorsiflexion of the foot (Homan's sign), pressure upon the gastrocnemius-soleus and the anterior tibial muscles, and the application of a blood pressure cuff about the thigh with a pressure of 60 mm. Hg generates pain in cases of thrombophlebitis of the leg.

The arterial pulses are reduced and may even be practically obliterated during the early stages of phlegmasia cerulea and alba dolens. Presumably this is initiated by reflex arterial spasm, because blocking of the sympathetic nerves to the part restores the pulses.

Thrombophlebitis is not the only peripheral affliction attended by swelling, color changes, pain and tenderness in the leg. Consequently, the differential diagnosis is often difficult. Rupture of the tendon of the plantaris muscle, myositis, acute lymphadenitis and angiitis, and acute arterial thromboses produce many of the physical signs that thrombophlebitis does.

The treatment of thrombophlebitis is empirical. The therapeutic measures now in use are: rest and elevation, elastic bandaging, hot fomentations, blocking the sympathetic nerves, ligation and transaction of veins, the administration of the anticoagulants (heparin and Dicumarol), and thrombectomy.

Rest is universally applicable. Lumbar sympathetic nerve block is especially useful in the treatment of phlegmasia alba and cerulea dolens; it frequently relieves the pain, often restores arterial pulses and seemingly hastens the disappearance of the edema.

Venous ligation and transection proximal to the thrombosis is indicated for all cases of thrombophlebitis purulenta. Vena-caval ligation is preferable to ligation of the iliac or the common femoral veins whenever the thrombosis purulenta involves the common femoral, the external iliac or the hypogastric veins, because the disabling sequelae of vena-caval ligation apparently are fewer than those which follow interruption of the common femoral or the iliac veins. In women the ovarian veins should be ligated as well as the vena cava in treating pelvic thrombophlebitis purulenta. Ligation and transection of the saphena magna at its point of entry into the femoral is a very effective way of treating thrombophlebitis limited to the saphenous vein. Persons having varicose veins frequently develop thrombophlebitis within the saphena magna postoperatively. In purulent thrombophlebitis in an extremity very wide drainage of the superficial veins which contain pus should be done promptly in addition to the other measures.

The anticoagulants are being given now for all forms of thrombophlebitis excepting the purulent variant. Although their effectiveness is variable and still cannot be defined accurately for a given case, there is equivocal evidence that the use of these drugs has reduced the frequency of massive pulmonary embolization and has shortened the period of swelling and pain.

Before giving Dicumarol, the prothrombin time or concentration must be performed because a prothrombin deficiency may be present before the drug is given, and should the recommended initial dose of Dicumarol be given to a prothrombin-deficient patient a lethal intracranial or other hemorrhage may occur.

For the treatment of thrombophlebitis in a person with a normal prothrombin concentration the dosage of Dicumarol is 300 mg. during the first day, 200 mg. the second, and 100 mg. the third, provided that the prothrombin time does not exceed 2 to 3 times normal. Should the prothrombin time be close to 2 to 3 times normal, the dose for that day is reduced or omitted. The therapeutic aim is the maintenance of the prothrombin time at 2 to 3 times normal until signs and symptoms of the thrombophlebitis have been absent for a week or more.

The antidote for Dicumarol is Phytonadione 25 mg. i.v. This dose often restores prothrombin time to normal within 1 or 2 hours but it may need to be repeated, as its effect often expires before that of the Dicumarol. The anticoagulant effect of Dicumarol is not exerted fully for 24 to 36 hours after the first dose has been given. Whenever an immediate anticoagulant action is wanted, heparin will fill the need. Heparin should be given in the aqueous form in doses about 25 to 50 mg. i.v. every 4 hours. Controlled clotting times serve as the basis for dosage regulation; the clotting time of the patient's blood should be kept about twice as long as that of the control 4 hours after the preceding dose was given. After one is assured that the dosage of 25 mg. every 4 hours keeps the clotting time about twice normal, 25 mg. is given every 4 hours, and the clotting time is determined only once a day.

The antidote for heparin is: protamine sulfate 50 mg. i.v.; it may need to be repeated. A single dose of this drug usually counteracts the effects of heparin.

Elastic bandaging of the leg alone is a very important part of the treatment of thrombophlebitis. Bandages should be worn for 2 to 3 months after all signs of the disease disappear. Elastic bandages or stockings should not be placed or worn above the knee because they become constricting bands about the knee when the leg is flexed, tending to promote rather than ameliorate swelling of the foot and the leg. Thrombectomy is being practiced for the severer forms of thrombophlebitis. See Chapter 44.

The frequency of postoperative thrombophlebitis in the veins of the leg may be reduced somewhat by avoiding saphenous venoclysis during an operation and the preambulant postoperative period, by taking care that the straps binding the patient to the operating table are applied carefully and not too tightly, by binding the legs of persons having varices with elastic bandages before, during and after the operation, and by early active motion of the legs and the feet.

EDEMA FOLLOWING PLANTARIS TENDON RUPTURE

Plantaris tendon rupture occurs suddenly, usually as the person quickly places his weight upon an extended leg while the foot is held in an extreme equinus position, as when getting out of a high hospital bed. With the rupture the person usually falls to the floor. Synchronously, a sharp stabbing pain is felt in the calf of the leg. The leg swells, and great tenderness is immediately elicitable over the upper part of the body of the gastrocnemius muscle. Dorsiflexion of the foot is painful. Within 4 to 24 hours, ecchymosis usually appears along the Achilles tendon. Elastic bandaging of the foot and the leg so as to limit dorsiflexion of the foot while walking constitutes adequate treatment.

TRAUMATIC MYOSITIS EDEMA

Postoperative myositis is not rare. It occurs as the convalescent patient begins to walk freely in footwear having heels lower than those customarily worn. It might be called the carpet-slipper syndrome. Women who have long worn only high-heeled shoes are especially prone to suffer from carpet-slipper myositis. Homan's sign is positive; the leg and the foot are often visibly edematous; and the calf muscles are tender. All these signs subside with a day of rest and the use of their high-heeled shoes when walking is resumed.

EDEMA OF LYMPHADENITIS

Acute lymphadenitis without visible superficial lymphangitis occasionally gives rise to a tender edema of the arm or the leg. Exploration of the femoral veins of 39 people presumed to have thrombophlebitis, because all of the signs of thrombophlebitis existed, turned up 8 cases in which blood flowed freely in the superficial femoral and saphenous veins, and no clots could be aspirated from them. In every such case the inguinal lymph nodes were much enlarged, and the periglandular and the perifemoral venous tissues were edematous. No sign of superficial lymphangitis existed preoperatively. Acute lymphadenitis should be suspected as the cause of swelling of an extremity whenever the lymph nodes of the groin or the axilla are *enlarged, matted together* and *tender*. In the author's experience acute postoperative inguinal lymphadenitis without signs of superficial lymphangitis is especially prone to follow vaginoperineal repair, hemorrhoidectomy and herniotomy. Dermatophytosis on the feet is sometimes the cause of femoral and inguinal lymphadenitis.

ARTERIAL OCCLUSIVE EDEMA

The swelling of a leg or an arm that follows the interruption of blood flow through its major arteries is very hard and painful. The muscles within the zone of deficient blood flow are tense and do not contract. Consequently, free active or passive motion of the parts moved by these muscles cannot be effected. Passive motion is very painful. The differentiation of thrombophlebitis from acute incomplete arterial occlusion is often extremely difficult and occasionally is impossible without repeated examination and the ascertainment of the course of events: the loss of sense perception practically clinches the diagnosis of arterial occlusion. Restoration of arterial flow by the methods discussed in Chapter 44 constitutes the only means of preventing loss of the part. Arteriography is often necessary to differentiate arterial occlusive edema from the others.

HYPOSMOTIC EDEMA

Hyposmotic or hypoalbuminemic edema is readily pittable and with changes of position shifts rapidly from one part of the body to another, collecting about the eyes and in the hollow of the back when the person is dorsally recumbent, and flowing into the legs and the feet when he sits or stands. It is especially prone to occur in the aged, the starved, the cirrhotics and the nephritics. It may be increased by giving sodium salts. The administration of plasma or salt-free albumin temporarily reduces it. Prolonged control can be effected only by dietary measures, the feeding of sufficient protein and other foods to meet the caloric needs and to repay the deficits, and the giving of only that amount of sodium chloride necessary to prevent the low-salt syndrome. In the absence of enteral losses of salt, from 500 to 1,000 mg. of sodium chloride daily is usually enough.

LYMPHATIC OBSTRUCTIVE EDEMA

The painless swelling of the hand and the arm after radical mastectomy and of the leg after inguinal node resections has often been attributed to lymphatic obstruction. Injection of sky-blue dye into the superficial cutaneous lymphatic network of the swollen member readily differentiates lymphatic block swelling from other types. Lymphatic obstructive edema is attended by superficial lymphangiectasis while the others, excepting that associated with erysipelas, are not. Elevation of the arm, massage and active motion while the arm and the hand are encased in elastic bandages constitute its treatment. Lymphangiograms made following the injection of the lymphatics with radiopaque material shows the terminations of the dilated lymphatics at the margin of the dissection following radical mastectomy.[4]

POSTFIXATION EDEMA

The resumption of walking or sitting after long confinement to bed or after having a part encased in a cast is regularly followed by swelling of the legs or the casted arm. It is practically painless, is readily pitted and subsides rapidly upon elevating the part above the trunk. It is easily treated by the application of elastic bandages until full restoration of function is attained.

SALT-OVERLOAD EDEMA

The administration of more sodium salts than are needed to make up for fistulous, sweat, diarrheal, gastric and renal losses frequently leads to generalized postoperative edema. Salt-overload edema is frequently mistaken for hypoalbuminemic edema, because the serum albumin concentration falls as the edema grows. The case (B.G.W.) tabulated on page 325 illustrates this.

Salt-overload edema is readily differentiated from hypoalbuminemic edema by withholding all sodium salts for 48 to 72 hours; the serum protein deficiency edema does not subside remarkably within this short time when salt is withheld, while salt-overload edema does, and

Case: B. G. W., Male, Age 56 Years

	Weight	Hb.	Serum Albumin
Preoperative	67.5 K	13.1	4.7
Postoperative (partial gastrectomy)			
Day 1 } 27 Gm. NaCl daily	66.9	12.3	4.9
Day 3 } 3 liters of 0.9% NaCl i.v. daily	71.4	11.1	2.7
Day 4 } 3 liters of 5% dextrose i.v. daily	68.0	...	3.5
Day 5 }	66.3	12.8	4.4

Postoperative Day, 3: edema + to + + of hands, feet, legs, eyelids and back.
By the 5th postoperative day the edema was gone.

as it does the serum albumin level rises rapidly. Withholding salt generally constitutes adequate therapy. Diuretics may be used to hasten resolution in cases of massive saline overloads.

EDEMA DUE TO CARDIAC DECOMPENSATION

Edema attributable to cardiac failure is a rarity postoperatively. When it does occur, the associated dyspnea, orthopnea, and signs of pulmonary and hepatic congestion serve to differentiate it readily from other types of edema.

PULMONARY EMBOLUS AND PULMONARY INFARCT

Pulmonary embolus and pulmonary infarct are major postoperative worries; the gastrectomy was well done, the wound has healed per primam, the man is eating well and has high spirits, he strains at stools—and dies before he can be moved from the bathroom floor. Fortunately, most pulmonary emboli are not so deadly. Pulmonary emboli usually are blood clots detached from the veins of the leg or the pelvis. They rarely arise from clots within the veins of the arm or the right auricle or ventricle. Pulmonary infarct does not attend the lodgement of all pulmonary emboli; many a pulmonary embolus does not so occlude a pulmonary arterial branch as to kill a piece of lung. Pulmonary infarct signifies pulmonary parenchymal arterial obstructive necrosis. The signs of pulmonary embolus and infarct differ appreciably. The signs and symptoms of pulmonary embolus vary from extreme dyspnea, shock, retrosternal oppression and quick death to a mild transient dyspnea and apprehension. The lungs are usually clear to auscultation and roentgenogram. The pulmonary second sound may be accentuated.

Pulmonary infarct adds to the above signs and symptoms of embolus: leukocytosis, fever, pleurisy, dark blood-stained sputum, and auscultatory and roentgen signs of pulmonary consolidation.

The treatment of pulmonary embolus and infarct is changing. Today the giving of the anticoagulants as described in the section on thrombophlebitis and the ligation of veins either alone or combined are recommended. If venous ligational therapy is selected, both superficial femoral veins or the vena cava should be tied, because the source of the embolus cannot be determined with any degree of certainty, and the thrombi are so often bilateral. Interruption of the common femoral veins should not be performed, because persistent edema, varicosities and stasis ulcers follow interruption of the common femoral veins with remarkable regularity while they very seldom follow interruption of the superficial femoral vein.

After ligation of veins the anticoagulants should be given, excepting when there are specific contraindications to their use, e.g., prolonged clotting time, low prothrombin concentration, hemorrhage, hepatitis, or cirrhosis.

Ligations of the vena cava must be done caudal to the renal veins. It results in rather severe swelling of the legs which abates with the passage of time. Presumably, this occurs as collateral channels dilate. Heparin may be important in limiting the early swelling. Several authors have substituted point approximation of the anterior wall of the inferior vena cava to its posterior wall at intervals of about 3 mm. from one side to the other by stitching or special clamps. This connects the cava into a series of small channels which prevent the passage of large clots yet may permit fluid blood to pass.

The early experience with this has been good, but it is still too early to evaluate fully its merits relative to those of the simpler ligations.

Section 8. Nausea and Vomiting

Nausea is the sensation of needing to empty the stomach. Its causes are many: emotions, overdosage or idiosyncrasy to drugs, cardiac failure, uremia, obstructions of the cystic duct, the common duct, the ureters and the digestive tract, enteritis, pneumonia, pain, great fatigue, acidosis, adrenal cortical insufficiency, etc. Vomiting supposedly initiated by the "vomiting center" usually follows nausea. Obviously, nausea and vomiting alone cannot serve as important differential signs of illness. However, they have more limited connotations postoperatively.

Some nausea and vomiting may be considered as temporary accompaniments of the process of normal recovery from anesthesia. However, protracted postoperative nausea and vomiting indicate that something is seriously amiss.

GASTRIC DILATATION

Acute gastric dilatation or atony is one of the serious postoperative causes of protracted nausea and vomiting; unrelieved, it may be lethal in only an hour or two. Often the vomiting attending acute gastric atony or dilatation is effortless; the vomitus simply pours out of the mouth without retching. The vomitus is foul, dark, and contains altered blood. Tachycardia, prostration and hypotension often accompany it. Remarkably, little pain is usually suffered. Thirst may be insatiable. The epigastrium bulges and tympanites extends far up into the left thoracic cavity. Erect scout films of the abdomen show a very large gastric gas bubble and elevation of the left leaf of the diaphragm. Roentgen examination is not requisite to diagnosis. In any case of protracted nausea and vomiting gastric suction should be instituted: the rapid aspiration of 2 or more liters of gas and dark, foul fluid from the stomach is sufficient to establish the diagnosis of acute gastric atony.

In most cases acute gastric dilation has no demonstrable organic obstructive lesion of the stomach or intestine for its genesis. It frequently complicates operations within the chest and upon the spine as well as central nervous troubles such as strokes and acute psychosis. However, in some instances its cause may be unsuspected cicatricial pyloric or duodenal stenoses; pyloric tumors; intestinal obstruction from bands, herniae and congenital anomalies; and obstruction of the efferent stoma of a gastrojejunostomy. Hypokalemia alone at times is capable of inciting and maintaining a gastric atony, as are diabetic acidosis, acute adrenal insufficiency and uremia. Hyperextension of the spine in a cast or on a frame, retroperitoneal hemorrhage, and ureterolithotomy or catheterization may be followed by gastric atony.

Regardless of etiology, the initial treatment of gastric dilatation is: (1) the immediate emptying of the stomach (proved by irrigation with clear return) and institution of continuous gastric suction and its maintenance for 36 to 48 hours (the appropriate period of time required for the regaining of function by the stretched stomach) and (2) the restoration of fluid balance with the administration of requisite salts, e.g., potassium salts for hypokalemia, and sodium salts for deficit of extracellular fluid. These are lifesaving measures (see Chap. 5, Fluid and Electrolytes).

While the gastric aspiration and fluid therapy are being conducted search must be made for signs of intestinal obstruction while constantly bearing in mind the relative paucity of symptoms of intestinal obstruction during the early postoperative period.

EMETIC DRUGS

Other associates of postoperative nausea and vomiting, namely, ileus, cardiac failure and infections, have been discussed. Drug overdosage or idiosyncrasy is a more prominent cause of postoperative nausea now than it was 30 years ago; then digitalis, morphine, belladonna, hyoscine, barbiturates and potassium iodide constituted practically the entire gamut of the occasionally nauseating and emetic medicaments given postoperatively. Today the list is much longer and includes vitamins, sulfonamides, antibiotics, Demerol, spasmolytics such as Banthine and dicyclamine hydrochloride, and the protein hydrolysates. Iatrogenic nausea and emesis are often coupled with cutaneous signs of a drug reaction. Except in the case of such drugs as provide specific signs of toxicity, e.g., digitalis, morphine, atropine and scopolamine, ascribing postoperative nausea and vomiting to drugs is justified largely by the exclusion of possible organic and metabolic causes, by the time relationships of the nausea to the dosage schedule and to subsidence of the nausea when the drugs are stopped. The withdrawal of drugs or the giving of chlorpromazine (Thorazine) or barbiturates without ruling out gastric atony, ileus, uremia, hypokalemia, etc., as possible causes of the nausea and vomiting is ill-conceived and dangerous in practice. However, whenever mechanical and biochemical causes for nausea and vomiting can be excluded, the discontinuance of drugs and the giving of tranquilizers may be warranted.

PROJECTILE VOMITING

Projectile vomiting is a phenomenon peculiar to increased intracranial pressure and is associated with such abnormalities as intracranial tumors, encephalitis, meningitis, head injuries and water intoxication. Characteristically, it is neither preceded by nor attended with nausea. It occurs suddenly, and the ejection of the vomitus may be so forceful as to propel it many feet. Obviously, the occurrence of projectile vomiting at any time dictates the need for a neurologic and an ophthalmoscopic examination and the determination of the serum sodium concentration. See Chapter 54, Surgery of the Nervous System, for the treatment of increased intracranial pressure and meningitis and Chapter 5, Fluid and Electrolytes for the treatment of water intoxication.

HICCOUGH

Hiccough (singultus) was a rather frequent postoperative trouble 20 years ago. Today it is rare. Hiccoughs occur in conjunction with peritonitis, subphrenic abscesses, empyema, uremia, gastric dilatation, ileus, anxiety and other illnesses. It tends to occur periodically and consequently is not dangerous ordinarily. However, occasionally it may last for days and exhaust the patient physically. Ordinarily, some measure of control may be effected with gastric emptying and lavage of the stomach with an alkaline saline solution, sedation, and changing the position of the patient. Occasionally, conduction over the phrenic nerve or nerves needs to be blocked with a long-acting local anesthetic such as lidocaine in order to provide the patient with some relief. However, even this may not do so; the person hics with the intercostal musculature after the phrenic nerves are blocked.

Obviously, the surest treatment is that which corrects the associated disease. The primary surgical significance of hiccough is the implication that something that does or may soon endanger life exists, prompting the surgeon to search for the signs of such entities as subphrenic abscess, empyema, uremia, gastric atony, ileus and acidosis. Hiccoughs occasionally are the earliest sign of their presence.

Vagal pressure, breathing 5 per cent carbon dioxide, breathing into a bag, tickling the nose with a feather and the feet with a pin will often stop them. Hiccoughs are a cause of wound disruption.

Section 9. Headache; Care of Mouth and Skin

Headache is a frequent complaint following spinal anesthesia. The leakage of spinal fluid through the site of puncture of the dura is presumed to be its cause. It is aggravated by sitting, standing, coughing or sneezing. The avoidance of the upright position for 3 to 5 days usually controls it.

Some severe postoperative headaches are

merely the signs of caffeine withdrawal. Patients who were in the habit of drinking 3 to 10 cups or more of coffee a day before they were operated upon frequently complain of severe, throbbing frontal headaches during the postoperative period of fasting. These are quickly relieved by giving caffeine sodium benzoate or a cup of coffee.

Headache and blurring of vision may be the first sign of water intoxication. However, most of the postoperative headaches other than those which follow spinal anesthesia cannot be attributed to any specific biochemical disturbance. Aspirin, codeine, or other weak analgesics control them readily.

CARE OF THE MOUTH

Preoperative and postoperative oral cleanliness is important. The mouth should be looked upon as a part of the operative field during esophagectomy and gastrectomy. Consequently, meticulous cleanliness of the oral cavity should be attained before these operations are undertaken. Whenever possible badly decayed teeth should be removed before the operation is performed; however, this is often impossible. Nevertheless, even in the worst cases of dental caries a fair degree of oral cleanliness can be obtained with a dental prophylaxis or the extensive use of toothbrush and a foaming toothpaste for 3 to 5 days before the operation is performed.

Postoperatively, the maintenance of oral cleanliness is a very important part of nursing. A dry, dirty mouth may lead to surgical parotitis, and the pulmonary aspiration of bits of filth is prone to lead to lung abscesses.

CARE OF THE SKIN

The care of the skin consists of keeping it clean and dry and preventing localized ischemia. A bedsore or decubitus ulcer is evidence for poor care of the skin. Constant dryness is often very difficult to obtain. The febrile individual may sweat a great deal. Copious sweating requires frequent bathing, massaging and powdering of the skin, especially of the back. Any patient who is incontinent of urine requires the insertion of an indwelling catheter in order to keep the skin of the buttocks, the back and the legs dry. The unconscious patient and paraplegic, and the weak and the aged need to be turned in bed every 1 to 2 hours to prevent ischemic necrosis of the skin overlying the sacrum and the bony prominences such as the ischial tuberosity, the greater trochanters of the femurs, the shoulders and the elbows. The uses of an alternating pressure pneumomotor mattress and lambskin are often helpful also.

Herpes simplex, or fever blisters, occasionally are a complication of surgery. Their resolution can be hastened materially by coating them with a clear nail polish or tincture of benzoin.

The pruritic rashes that appear following operative procedures are usually attributable to the antiseptic applied to the skin preoperatively, or to medicaments given internally. The determination of the cause of the postoperative rash is usually relatively simple; the antiseptic rashes are limited to the area to which the material was applied while the drug sensitivity rashes are more generalized. Usually the removal of the cause terminates the rash. Washing the skin with alcohol and soap and water will serve to remove the antiseptic. Discontinuance of the antibiotics or such medications as iodides, bromides and penicillin and the giving of pyribenzamine and codeine is usually all that is required to control the symptoms and the rash. However, occasionally the sensitivity reaction is so severe as to require the administration of ACTH, cortisone, prednisone, prednisolone or epinephrine to obtain relief.

If exfoliative dermatitis is threatened, corticoids should be begun early, as this complication was formerly often fatal and still is in some instances.

Section 10. Symptomatic Psychoses

Today surgeons and internists alike largely disregard the psychological abnormalities associated with the ills they meet and the treatments they apply, in spite of the emphasis placed upon the symptomatic psychoses during the 19th century. Evidently, we look upon the symptomatic psychoses as "normal" behavior among the ill and consequently disregard them just as we are prone to disregard the normal leg, tooth, or heart.

However, the symptomatic psychoses (Bonhoeffer's terminology) are important signs of organic illness, especially during the postoperative period, because they often constitute the earliest manifestations of trouble. Although an operation or its complications may be the factor that relights or precipitates a functional psychosis such as a manic depression or schizophrenia, this discussion of psychoses will be limited to the symptomatic group.

CLASSIFICATION

I. Nutritional
   Origin
   1. Elemental
      Potassium deficiency
      Sodium deficiency
      Hypocalcemia
      Bromide excess
      Lead excess
   2. Water
      Water deficit with hyperosmolarity
      Water excess with hyposmolarity
   3. Organic foodstuffs
      Vitamin deficiency
         Nicotinic acid
         Thiamine
      Protein intoxication
      Hypoglycemia
   4. Gases
      Hypoxia
         Circulatory
         Respiratory
II. Complex Metabolic
   1. Uremia without hypertension
   2. Uremia with hypertenison
III. The Pharmacopsychoses
   1. Anesthetics
   2. Ethyl alcohol
      Delirium tremens
      Korsakoff's syndrome
      Wernicke's syndrome
   3. Barbiturates
   4. Lysergic acid and its derivatives
IV. Endocrinopathic
   1. Hyperthyroidism
   2. Hypothyroidism
   3. Hypoparathyroidism (calcium deficiency)
   4. ACTH and cortisone
   5. Acute adrenal cortical insufficiency
V. Septic Traumatic
   1. Acute septic
   2. Chronic septic
   3. Cranial traumatic
   4. Burn psychosis

DELIRIUM

Delirium is the term usually used to describe some of the psychotic manifestations of the symptomatic psychoses. It connotes much more than mental confusion and is distinct from the dementias, the affective disorders and stupor. Essentially, delirium consists of: (1) disorders of perception manifested as visual, auditory and tactile hallucinations; (2) disturbances of interpretation: namely, illusions and delusions; (3) psychomotor abnormalities, predominantly of the overactive type; (4) and evidence of stimulation of the sympathetic nervous system.

The clinical signs of delirium are:

1. Signs of stimulation of the sympathetic system: tachycardia, mild fever and sweating
2. Disturbances of perception: hallucinations
3. Disturbances of interpretation: delusions and illusions
4. Abnormalities of somatic motor activity: perseveration, iteration, overtalkativeness, tremors, restlessness, picking at bedclothes (carphology), convulsions
5. Disturbances of affect such as uncontrolled laughter, weeping, or moaning
6. Alterations of mood from euphoria to abject fear and violent temper
7. Disturbances in sensorium varying between coma and transient disorientation in place and time

The signs of sympathetic overactivity may be the earliest signs of delirium, especially among thyrotoxicotics. The sweating of delirium predominantly occurs on the face, the hands and the feet, though at times the whole body is drenched with sweat. The fever is usually mild, rarely above 101° F., excepting in those deliria attending infections, head injuries, hyperosmolarity, and thyroid storm when it may reach lethal heights of 108° to 112° F.

The disturbances of perception are hallucinations (*the perception of animate and inanimate objects or their relationships which have no realistic basis*). The visual and auditory forms predominate. Their characters often change frequently: one minute the delirious one is being trampled by a herd of giant mice, the next he is being eaten by a single pigmy ant, the next he is being scolded and whipped by a 10-headed grandfather, and 20 minutes later is cowering beneath the bedclothes, holding his ears because jet bombers are buzzing him. Unpleasant or horrifying hallucinations stimulate motor reactions which may be violently combative or evasive or loudly vocal. Some of the illusions of delirium are pleasant and are accompanied by tranquility: God speaks as a father to a favorite son, or the bed floats among vividly colored hanging gardens to the accompaniment of a well-ordered mélange of the music of Strauss, Beethoven, Debussy, Gershwin, and Handel. Ofttimes some components of hallucinations are remembered with remarkable tenacity.

The disturbances of interpretation are practically indistinguishable from those of perception. The difference between a hallucination and an illusion or delusion is lack of an external environment stimulus: the hallucination has no apparent real stimulus, while the illusion and the delusion have.

A delirious person looking out of a window in Kansas at the sky and saying "We're sailing on a beautifully calm sea" is suffering an illusion, and if after being told that he is not at sea and nowhere near a ship or water he persists in the belief that he is at sea he is *deluded*. However, the same statements made by a man in a completely darkened, windowless room would indicate that he is suffering hallucinations. However, this man may have heard the Sisters' raiments as they passed his doors rustling as does the quiet sea. The hallucination then becomes an illusion.

The relationship of delirium to the illness varies; at times it appears before the other signs of illness, at others with them, and occasionally after the crisis. Peculiarly, the sick person is often delirious at night and soporous during the day. The passage of delirium usually is heralded by profound sleep and leaves a weak, easily fatigued, emotionally unstable, despondent or complaining, whining patient who may be hypersensitive to odors, light and noise and he may be uncooperative.

During the delirium the patient is apt to injure and occasionally to destroy himself by jumping from a window or throttling himself with the bedclothes or venetian blind cords. Constant physical restraint often aggravates the motor activity of delirium.

At one time physicians believed that characteristic forms of deliria were associated with specific disease entities. We do not. However, there are certain differences between the compositions of the total pictures of the symptomatic psychoses that permit an initial presumptive determination of the possible causes of an observed postoperative symptomatic psychosis.

A careful history of the person's illness, a meticulous examination of the patient's hospital record, including the nurses' notes, and intelligent examinations of the patient will serve to determine the cause of most symptomatic psychoses among surgical patients.

The major categories of postoperative symptomatic psychoses are the septic, the traumatic and the nutritional. Within these categories, the acute septic, the cranial traumatic, elemental deficiencies and circulatory hypoxia (shock) are the most frequent. Space does not permit more than a cursory description of the clinical aspects of the postoperative symptomatic psychoses.

NUTRITIONAL PSYCHOSES

Potassium Deficit

The onset of the psychoses associated with potassium deficit is preceded by the history of or the actual observation of the loss of body fluids through diarrhea, vomiting and fistulous drainage, or the administration of ACTH, cortisone or diuretics without the administration of supplemental potassium.

The physical signs associated with it are: weakness, atonic musculature, ileus, and flattening and inversion of T-waves on the electrocardiogram.

The neurologic signs are: hyperactive tendon reflexes with mild deficits, and hypoactive to absent tendon reflexes and motor paralysis with the severe deficits.

The psychotic behavior is characterized by a mild delirium with overtalkativeness, iteration, confabulation and wakefulness. Vacillating disorientation in time and space is seen often.

Sodium Deficits (Extracellular Fluid Volume Deficits)

The abnormal psychotic behavior associated with sodium deficit is also preceded by a story of evidence of loss of body fluids through diarrhea, vomiting, fistulous drainage, profuse sweating, and trauma such as fractures of the femur, burns and peritonitis.

The physical signs associated with it are: weakness, tachycardia, softening of the pulse, varying degrees of hypotension, shrunken tissues, soft muscles, and subnormal temperatures in the absence of infection. The tendon reflexes tend to be hypoactive. Apathy and somnolence progressing to coma are the major psychic manifestations. Disorientation, hallucinations, illusions, or delusions are extremely infrequent.

Hypocalcemia

This is generally preceded by a recently performed thyroidectomy, removal of a parathyroid adenoma, or associated with severe, acute pancreatitis or prolonged diarrhea. Tachycardia, muscle spasms brought on by exercise or occlusion of the arterial blood flow, and hyperactive reflexes manifested by such signs as Chvostek's, are the predominant physical signs.

Psychic manifestations are paresthesia, circumoral numbness, itching of the nose, apprehension, and increased sensitivity to noise and bright lights. There is no delirium, although often the individual may manifest hysterical behavior.

Bromide Excess

Persons suffering from brominism are occasionally to be seen on the surgical services, especially for the treatment of injuries and chronic ulcers of the lower extremities. There is usually a history of taking a "nerve medicine" and of headache.

The physical signs are an acneiform eruption upon the face and the body, occasional ulcers of the extremities, coldness of the extremities and fetid breath. There are no neurologic signs. Sleepiness, slowness of speech and mental detachment are the main psychic manifestations.

Lead Poisoning

Persons suffering from acute plumbism are occasionally subjected to celiotomy because of the severe colicky abdominal pain that may attend acute lead poisoning. Plumbism has been mistaken for acute mechanical intestinal obstruction, intussusception, appendicitis, cholecystitis and ruptured peptic ulcer.

A history of chewing painted furniture and woodwork usually can be obtained from parents of children having lead colic, and a story of working with lead paints or lead-containing insect poisons, storage battery salvaging or battery casing burning is sometimes obtained from adults. There may be abdominal signs of acute intestinal obstruction. Anemia, basophilic stippling of the red cells, constipation, lead line on the gums, and motor nerve paralysis, predominating in the muscles used most, such as the antebrachial and the leg muscles (wrist drop and foot drop, respectively), are signs of plumbism. Kernig's sign and convulsions often develop in children.

The mental picture varies from depression to violent mania. Delirium occurs, especially among children.

Water Deficit With Hyperosmolarity

This occasionally follows cranial injury and intracranial operative procedures, especially resections of craniopharyngiomas and pituitary tumors.

Under other circumstances an incapacity to drink water usually precedes the onset of the syndrome. Thirst is a prominent symptom until consciousness is lost. Fever, dry mucous membranes, high urinary specific gravity and a serum sodium above 155 mEq./L. constitute the main physical aspects. Disorientation and hyperactivity are the early psychic signs and violent delirium a late accompaniment.

Water Excess With Hyposmolarity

A story can usually be obtained of vomiting, diarrhea or injury, coupled with the avid drinking of water. Muscle cramps, blurring of vision, and headache are the main symptoms.

Physical signs are: practically no sodium salts in the urine, increased cerebral spinal fluid pressure, and a serum sodium concentration below 130 mEq./L. Apprehension, restlessness, mild delirium and epileptiform convulsions among the young are the psychic manifestations.

Nicotinic Acid Deficit (Pellagra)

This occurs mainly in individuals who have been unable to eat or have followed a very poor diet, such as cornbread, fat pork and molasses. The early physical signs are a fiery red erythema of skin exposed to sunlight, diarrhea and anorexia. Later, sharkskin and beefy redness and soreness of the tongue appear. The neurologic signs of acute deficits, such as those precipitated by an operation, are cogwheel rigidity, and grasping and sucking reflexes. Irritability, insomnia, slow reactions, poor memory and delirium constitute the psychosis. This is part of the syndrome of pellagra (dermatitis, diarrhea, dementia and death).

Thiamine Deficit (Dry Beriberi)

Alcoholism, a polished rice diet, or inability to eat are its main causes. The predominant sign is generalized muscular tenderness, which in the leg is especially prominent upon squatting. Signs of congestive heart failure may appear. The neurologic picture is made up of paresthesia, hyperesthesia, loss of superficial cutaneous senses, diminution of tendon reflexes and very rarely flaccid paralysis such as foot drop. Neurasthenias, irritability, failure of memory and confusion of thought, sleeplessness, increased sensitivity to noise and pain are the predominant psychic features.

Protein Intoxication

One type of protein intoxication has all of the features of water deficit with hyperosmolarity. It attends the forced feeding of protein to individuals who by reason of weakness or physical or mental incapacity are unable to drink enough water to counter the increased need for water imposed by the large protein loads. The physical and psychic signs are those of water deficit.

The other form of protein intoxication appears among cirrhotics and individuals who have had portacaval or rarely splenorenal venous shunts performed upon them. There is usually physical evidence of cirrhosis such as esophageal varices and splenohepatomegaly and laboratory evidence of hepatic insufficiency. Failure of memory, lack of care of person, loss of inhibitions, and depression are early signs, and delirium and coma the late ones. A decreased rate of ammonia catabolism is held to account for some cases.

Hypoglycemia

Of course, this occurs most frequently among individuals taking insulin. However, surgically it may follow gastrectomy, the more especially total gastrectomy. Also, it is occasionally seen following the termination of a prolonged period of intravenous alimentation with concentrated glucose solutions. Hypoglycemia may also occur in cases of pancreatic islet cell tumors (see Chap. 33, Pancreas). Profuse sweating, tremors, incoordination, slurring of speech, apprehension, and inability to communicate with others precede convulsions or coma. For a brief time interval between incapacity to speak and coma, the person gives evidence with eye movements that he is conscious of his trouble and of what is going on about him.

Hypoxia

Oligemic shock, injuries to the chest, and the removal of lungs are the predominant causes of circulatory and anoxic hypoxia in surgery (see Chap. 7, Shock). The main physical signs are breathlessness, Cheyne-Stokes type breathing, and signs of shock. Cyanosis is rare excepting in the presence of anoxic anoxia. Psychic variances with mild anoxia are euphoria, deterioration of judgment and incoordination (a picture of moderate drunkenness). Delirium is common with severe hypoxia. Surgically, one of the important signs of hypoxia is delay or failure to recover from anesthesia. If fever is present with the hypoxia, the danger from it is enhanced. In such cases the reduction of the fever becomes a very important part of the treatment of the hypoxia.

COMPLEX METABOLIC PSYCHOSES

Uremia

The symptomatic psychosis associated with uremia is extremely variable. However, the variability of the picture may be reduced by separating the uremias without hypertension from those with hypertension. The psychologic manifestations differ: with uremia without hypertension the picture is one of apathy, sleeplessness, reduction of spontaneous movement, and coma without delirium; in the case of uremia with hypertension there are restlessness, twilight states, fits and delirium. The picture of uremia with hypertension is often that of a major psychosis.

PHARMACOPSYCHOSES

Anesthesia
(See Chap 13, Anesthesia)

Alcohol

The alcoholic psychoses are especially troublesome in surgery because they are prone to appear after injuries or operations. There are 3 types of alcoholic psychoses that the surgeon may see: (1) delirium tremens, (2) alcoholic hallucinations and (3) Korsakoff's psychosis.

Delirium tremens appears after the cessation of the imbibition of alcohol. It is one of the commonest, if not the commonest, symptomatic psychosis seen on the surgical wards of charity hospitals. Incoordination, coarse tremors of all extremities, sleeplessness, agitation, and a highly active delirium with remarkably vivid visual and auditory hallucinations make up the picture.

Alcoholic hallucinations are a complication of chronic active alcoholism. Although the person is well oriented and has clear senses, his actions speak for distrust, suspicion and jealousy. These overt reactions are attributable to auditory hallucinations. Persons suffering from alcoholic hallucinations are especially troublesome on large wards because of their tendency to seemingly unprovoked combativeness.

The signs of **Korsakoff's psychosis** are the loss of memory for recent events and remarkable confabulation. The loss of memory for recent events is often striking in that one may be greeted by such a person upon seeing him for the second time within a matter of minutes by, "Hi, Doc. I have been looking for you all day. Why don't you come and see me more often?" While the condition is usually chronic, it occasionally begins with a delirious episode after an operation or injury.

Barbiturates

The barbiturate symptomatic psychosis is divisible into two types: the chronic and the acute.

The chronic type is associated with muscle tremors, ataxia, nystagmus, vertigo, poor memory, thick speech and episodic hallucinations. All of these signs may be aggravated upon withdrawing the drug.

The acute intoxication is associated with hypotension, hypothermia, and stupor progressing to coma. The stupor may be preceded by a short phase of delirium. In brief, the acute intoxication has many of the aspects of general anesthesia.

ENDOCRINOPATHIC PSYCHOSES

Hyperthyroidism and Hypothyroidism
(See Chap. 28, Thyroid, Thymus and Parathyroids)

Hyperparathyroidism
(See Hypocalcemia, Calcium Deficits, this chapter)

ACTH and Cortisone

The psychotic picture varies from euphoria to severe depression. Delirium is rare.

Acute Adrenocortical Insufficiency

Anorexia, vertigo, vomiting and weakness are the main objective complaints. Hypotension is often detectable. Disorientation in time and place, especially during the night, with remembrance of the abnormal behavior during lucid intervals, may take place (Chap. 29).

SEPTIC PSYCHOSES

The septic symptomatic psychoses are very interesting because a number of psychic manifestations often appear before the systemic signs of illness do. Restlessness, oversensitivity to noise and light, decreased emotional control, inability to concentrate, talkativeness, euphoria and vivid dreams often precede the systemic signs of illness. At times the psychic behavior disturbance does not appear until after the crisis or subsidence of the fever or infection. In general, though, the symptomatic psychoses and the illness are associated temporally. During the febrile illness the septic psychoses may assume all of the aspects of a violent delirium. Among children the delirium may be interrupted by epileptic seizures. With the subsidence of the delirium, a period of postinfection neurasthenia or depression occasionally occurs. Frequently, the postinfection depression is not preceded by delirium. Malaise, headache, weakness, fatigue, emotional instability, episodic frightening hallucinations, and despondency with depression, or uncooperativeness with complaining and whining are the main signs of postinfection depression.

CRANIAL TRAUMATIC PSYCHOSIS

The cranial traumatic symptomatic psychoses are increasing in number. Automobile accidents constitute the main cause. Occasionally, hyperosmolarity is the precipitating factor, and at other times it is alcoholism. However, contusional injury to the brain itself is presumed to be the predominant underlying organic disturbance. Besides the alcoholic psychosis, the cranial traumatic seems to have the longest duration of the symptomatic psychoses.

The signs and symptoms run the gamut from facetiousness to delirium and coma.

SITUATIONAL, CONTINUOUS PAIN

Penetrating peptic ulcers, chronic active pancreatitis and burns are especially prone to be attended by situational symptomatic psychoses, although with burns the septic factor may be predominant. Persons suffering from penetrating peptic ulcers and chronic active pancreatitis occasionally go berserk, throwing chairs and the like through windows, and injuring themselves by running head-on into walls. During the psychotic episodes they may attempt self-destruction. The psychotic behavior of a person during the first day following a severe burn is seemingly primarily attributable to hypoxia (shock) because it usually disappears as the signs of shock do. Later, the abnormal psychic behavior ascribable to various nutritional disturbances may make their appearances, and later after a dressing change or two has been performed, the burned person becomes a detached, despondent, crying, uncooperative physical wreck. With burns delirium is rare after the first week unless uncontrolled sepsis occurs.

TREATMENT OF PSYCHOSES

The treatment of the symptomatic psychoses needs to be varied according to the biochemical and nutritional disturbance attending it.

The delirium of many patients quickly subsides with the institution of specific treatment of the underlying biochemical or bacterial cause (see Table 15-2). However, many, such as the cranial traumatic, the alcoholic and the situational, cannot be treated specifically and require symptomatic care, according to the following rules of general treatment:

1. Continuous attendance upon a delirious patient by physicians, nurses, trained attendants, or intelligent relatives is mandatory.

2. All drugs that may even remotely abet or promote the delirium, such as barbiturates, analgesics (excepting in the case of pain), atropine, hyoscine, salicylates, bromides, ACTH and cortisone (excepting in adrenocortical insufficiency and delirium tremens), are to be avoided or withdrawn slowly.

3. *Fresh* paraldehyde (10 to 15 ml. in fruit juice orally or in 50 to 100 ml. of water rectally) is a satisfactory sedative, as is also chloral hydrate. The amount of sedative given should not be so great as to abolish all signs of delirium or excitement, because to do so requires so much drug as to endanger life.

4. Place the patient in quiet and well-lighted surroundings to as to reduce the intensity of hallucinatory reactions.

5. All the while, strict attention must be paid to the pulse rate, temperature and blood pressure as well as the intake of fluid and the output of urine. An indwelling catheter is necessary for the latter.

6. Circulatory collapse may appear suddenly and requires alert and energetic treatment such as transfusions of blood and plasma, or saline solutions and vasopressor agents for shock, and digitalization for acute heart failure.

7. The delirious patient should be per-

Section 10. Symptomatic Psychoses 335

TABLE 15-2. TREATMENT OF SYMPTOMATIC PSYCHOSES

TYPE	TREATMENT
Potassium Deficiency	KCl or K_2HPO_4 (0.2 to 0.4%), 2–4 Gm./L. of 10% dextrose intravenously, provided that the patient is not anuric
Sodium Deficiency (with normal osmolarity)	Hartmann's solution (Ringer's lactate) when pH of serum is normal or below normal. NaCl 0.9% with or without NH_4Cl 0.6 to 1.1% for Na+ deficit with alkalosis
Hypocalcemia	Calcium gluconate 10% solution, 20–120 ml. intravenously
	Calcium lactate 10–40 Gm. daily orally
	Vitamin D, but no milk or cheese in diet because of phosphate content
	Occasionally, dihydrotachysterol or parathormone may be required for a short time
Bromide Excess	Sodium chloride 10–20 Gm. daily
Delirium Tremens	Cortisone or metacorten as for adrenal insufficiency
	I.V. fluids containing glucose and sodium chloride
Lead Excess (Plumbism)	For colic: calcium gluconate i.v., atropine
	For psychosis: sodium citrate 12 Gm. orally daily (Consult toxicologic text for use of B.A.L., etc.)
Water Deficit (with hyperosmolarity)	Water orally or rectally, 5% dextrose in water i.v. and subcutaneously
	Also, give pitressin, aqueous 2–10 I.U. (0.1 to 0.2 ml.) every 4 hours i.m. *if hyperosmolarity is associated with acute postoperative diabetes insipidus*
Water Excess (with hyposmolarity)	Withhold water if extracellular fluid volume is normal or above normal
	Administer i.v. 3.0 to 5.0% NaCl if extracellular fluid volume is subnormal* and the person is alkalotic or M/2 or molar sodium lactate should there be an extracellular fluid volume deficit and acidosis
	Reduce the dosage or discontinue pitressin if it is being used
Vitamin Deficiency	
Nicotinic Acid	Niacin 50 mg. orally t.i.d. or nicotinamide 100 mg. daily parenterally
Thiamine	Thiamine 2–6 mg. t.i.d. orally or 15–25 mg. daily parenterally
	Watch especially for signs of acute heart failure and digitalize should its signs appear
Protein Intoxication	
With Hyperosmolarity	As for water deficit (see above)
With Normal Osmolarity	Reduce dietary protein to 40–60 Gm. daily
Hypoglycemia	25% glucose i.v. for hypoglycemic shock, convulsions or coma
	For postgastrectomy hypoglycemia remove free sugar from the diet and raise the protein in it to 120–150 Gm. daily taken in 5 to 6 meals
Hypoxia	Reduce accompanying fever if present
Circulatory	
Oligemic Shock	Blood, plasma and saline solutions (see Chap. 7, Shock)
Vasoparalytic	Vasopressor agents (see Chap. 7, Shock)
Acute Cardiac Failure	(See page 314, this chapter)
Respiratory	Oxygen
Uremia	(See Chap. 52, Urology)
Hyperthyroidism	(See Thyroid Storm, this chapter)
Hypothyroidism	(See Chap. 28)
Hypoparathyroidism	(See above, Hypocalcemia)
ACTH and Cortisone	Reduce dosage or discontinue
Acute Adrenal Insufficiency	Cortisone 20–100 mg. daily or prednisone 5–10 mg. with sodium and potassium salts
Septic	Appropriate antibiotics and surgery and control of hyperpyrexia and hypoxia if present
Situational	Morphine i.v. for severe pain
	Gentleness in care of the injured

* See Chap. 5, Fluids and Electrolytes, for Dangers.

mitted to be up and about unless he is physically incapable of safe walking. Restraints often excite the delirium; therefore, they should be used with care.

8. Whenever coma occurs meticulous attention must be paid to the maintenance of the full patency of the airway. When necessary, an intratracheal tube may be inserted. Usually this may be done without difficulty. Rarely, a tracheostomy may be needed. Secre-

tions must be removed from the airway regularly by suction. Aminophylline will often serve to abolish Cheyne-Stokes breathing. Artificial control of body temperature with sponge bathing and ice packs may be necessary. Atropine should not be given, because it thickens secretions and disturbs temperature regulation by inhibiting sweating. The maintenance of fluid and electrolyte balance and parenteral feedings are very difficult problems in the comatose patient.

Since symptomatic psychoses may be difficult to differentiate from other psychoses, psychiatric consultation is frequently necessary.

REFERENCES

1. Brummelkamp, W. H., Hoogendijk, J. L., and Boerema, I: Treatment of anaerobic infections (clostridial myositis) by drenching the tissues with oxygen under high atmospheric pressure. Surgery, 49:299-302, 1961.
2. Brummelkamp, W. H., Boerema, I, and Hoogendijk, J. L.: Treatment of clostridial infection with hyperbaric oxygen drenching—A report of 26 cases. Lancet, 1:235-238, 1963.
3. Cobb, C. A., Jr., LeQuire, V. S., Gray, M. E., and Hillman, J. W.: Therapy of traumatic fat embolism with intravenous fluids and heparin. Surg. Forum, 9:751-756, 1958.
4. Denese, C., and Howard, J. M.: Postmastectomy edema. Surg., Gynec. Obstet. (In press)
5. Kelley, H. G., and Pace, W. G.: Treatment of anaerobic infections in mice with hyperpressure oxygen. Surgical Forum, 14:46-47, 1963.
6. Peltier, L. E.: An appraisal of the problem of fat embolism. Int. Abst. Surg., 104:313-322, 1957.
7. Postoperative Wound Infections: The influence of ultraviolet irradiation of the operating room and of various other factors. Suppl. Ann. Surg., 160: 1964.

CHAPTER 16

FRANCIS D. MOORE, M.D.

The Endocrine and Metabolic Basis of Surgical Care

RECOVERY—THE REACTION OF SURVIVAL

Severe injury is a challenge long familiar to the evolving vertebrate species. Incurred with or without an anesthetic, physical injury brings in its wake a train of internal adjustments that favor recovery. The fittest survive, yet the surgeon must know what the patient is doing for himself if he is to help when survival is threatened. Herein lies the importance of metabolic measurement and physiologic understanding in surgery.

Evolutionary development has produced a complex multivisceral adjustment as the initial response to physical injury and its inevitably attendant period of starvation. Surgical metabolism is thus strictly Darwinian in its origin. The obvious survival value of endocrine and metabolic adjustments after injury helps us to study, analyze and remember them and permits of little other interpretation.

These responses fall into 3 large groups:
1. Healing of the Wound
2. Immunologic Defense Against Bacterial Invasion
3. Systemic Metabolic Adjustments to Injury and Starvation

These three reactions are clearly interrelated. The systemic alteration in protein metabolism, for example, yields new building blocks for the wound in healing; at the same time, it raises the relative priority for globulin synthesis, so important in antibody production. Despite such overlap and interaction of bodily changes, their description is simplified, and understanding aided, by considering them separately.

Healing of the wound occurs by cellular synthesis and the production of new intercellular matrix collagen; these alterations of fibroplasia and surface coverage are considered in Chapter 2 of this book. *Defense against bacterial invasion* is found in antibody synthesis and cellular proliferation in response to the challenge of tissue injury and bacterial invasion; the host response is as important as the bacterial threat; these problems are dealt with in Chapter 3. *The systemic responses to injury and surgery* and to volume-reduction, acid-base challenge and starvation will occupy the principal body of this chapter. Knowledge of these responses has grown very rapidly in the last 50 years, and particularly so in the last 20 years, as modern biochemical technics have been applied to the phenomena of surgical recovery.

In addition to these normal endocrine and metabolic responses to trauma, there are many bodily changes imposed by the injury itself when it is severe. These are to be understood also, if the surgeon is to treat the patient effectively.

While it seems to be quite obvious that "the surgeon must know what the patient is doing for himself, if he is to help," several examples of the detailed operation of this rule serve to illustrate this point.

An Example From Early Blood Loss. The patient is bleeding and has low blood pressures as he enters the Emergency Ward; therefore, a norepinephrine drip is commenced. In point of fact, a previously normal person suffering hypotension and blood loss will produce within himself a higher level of norepinephrine (and a near-maximal vasoconstriction) in the blood than can be produced by a slow intravenous infusion. What the patient needs here is not reduplication of his normal catechol amine response but restoration of blood volume (see Chap. 7).

Examples From Transcapillary Refill. The patient seems to be bleeding severely, although there is no outward show of blood loss: blood pressure is low, flow is poor; the hematocrit has not changed, so no transfusion is given. Actually, the passage of time is required for the transcapillary refill which lowers the hematocrit by increasing plasma volume. Urgent need for blood transfusion can coexist with a normal hematocrit, and blood should be given. Later, when transcapillary refilling is complete, a low hematocrit signifies a large plasma volume and, often, a normal blood volume; delayed or tardy transfusion is potentially dangerous in the elderly patient or the cardiac.

An Example From Acid-Base Balance. The patient has been seriously injured, and no urine is being formed; renal acidosis is mounting; therefore, the patient is given large amounts of sodium bicarbonate to combat acidosis. In point of fact, renal acidosis is an "addition acidosis." It is associated with excessive amounts of water and salt in the body, and the addition of sodium bicarbonate is dangerous. For many years it was the cause of fatal outcome in acute renal failure. The patient would do much better with a low molecular weight crystalloid such as mannitol which might provide an osmotic diuresis in the early phases; later on, his acidosis should be combated by dialysis (see Chap. 5).

An Example From Abnormal Hydration. The patient has just been operated upon and is not taking any water by mouth; he is making urine and sweating; it is assumed that he must need a lot of water. Therefore, he is given a large intravenous infusion of dextrose in water. Actually, the freshly postoperative patient does not excrete water normally; this antidiuresis is accentuated by hypovolemia and certain anesthetic agents. A large water load will not be excreted normally, hypotonicity will develop, and in the end acute water intoxication results (see Chap. 15).

An Example From Oxygen Diffusion and Metabolism. The patient has suffered severe crushing trauma to the chest. He is cyanotic; therefore, he is put in an oxygen tent. In point of fact, after crushing chest trauma, although oxygen uptake is often abnormal because of pulmonary edema, ventilation is importantly restricted because of an unstable rib cage. An oxygen tent will do little for the arterial oxygen tension. Instead, the chest cage should be stabilized and the airway opened to positive pressure by tracheostomy or endotracheal intubation, and respiration assisted (see Chap. 13).

An Example From Calorie and Nitrogen Provisions. The patient has just been operated upon, and he is not eating anything; it is assumed that he must be starving, losing nitrogen and burning fat, suffering a caloric deficit. Therefore, he is given large infusions of carbohydrate, nitrogen, fat, water and salt. Actually, the intravenous provision of calories and nitrogen in the early postoperative period has no demonstrable effect on the welfare of the patient other than the sparing of body fat oxidation. The nitrogen provided as amino acids or protein hydrolysate is largely excreted in the urine as urea. The patient is hampered by prolonged intravenous infusions and swamped with unnecessary water carrying in foodstuffs that are poorly utilized. The addition of an osmotic diuretic to provide high urine volumes merely compounds this meddlesome treatment by the loss of electrolyte. In point of fact, acute short-term starvation is well borne by the traumatized person. Meddlesome alimentation, either enteral or parenteral, adds little during the early period.

An Example From Corticosteroid Treatment. The patient has been on cortisone for 3 months for his ulcerative colitis. He is going to have a colectomy. His adrenals need buildup, and cortisone is dangerous! So the hormone is stopped, he is given 1 day of ACTH, operated upon and passes into severe hypotension. The proper sequence here is based on the fact that 7 to 10 days of ACTH therapy are needed to restore adrenals inhibited by 3 months of cortisone; either this should be done, or the cortisone should be maintained across the operation and stopped, with ACTH coverage, during later convalescence (see Chap. 29).

TRAUMATIC STIMULI TO BODILY CHANGE

Physical injury is not a monovalent or pure stimulus to the human body. Injury involves many modalities which vary in severity and in the immediacy of their threat to survival. These traumatic stimuli may be considered as falling into 3 groups.

1. At the extremely *mild* end of the scale are to be listed such stimuli as apprehension, short-term starvation, normal anesthetic procedure and minor tissue trauma. These are

experienced in minor injury and minor surgery. Metabolic and endocrine changes are minimal; the surgeon's treatment need depart little from the patient's ordinary daily routine. The avoidance of meddlesome interference and of strong systemic medication are important to success.

2. In the *mid-range* of traumatic stimuli to endocrine and metabolic change are a number of more severe events, the foremost of which is acute blood loss. In most healthy adults, the acute loss of blood from the venous side of the circulation (over a period of 10 to 30 minutes) of 25 per cent of the blood volume produces a significant reduction in blood pressure and tissue perfusion. Likewise, in this middle range of traumatic stimuli are severe pain, continued contamination, and physicochemical injury to the skin or serous surfaces, such as occurs in burns and perforations of the viscera. Also in this group are more extensive cross-sectional tissue traumata, such as extensive visceral resections and multiple fractures, and fluid losses as in intestinal obstruction, vomiting or diarrhea. The injuries and the stimuli in this group seem to be the severest to which the survival process has tuned the vertebrate organism. Survival is the rule, and the surgeon's therapy can still be simple and direct: prompt volume restoration is the most important single item.

At the extremes of life, or in the presence of visceral disease of heart, lungs, liver, kidneys or brain, even this middle range of trauma is severely life-threatening. It will overcome the body's ability to respond and defend itself unless the surgeon's treatment is prompt and perfectly adapted to the needs and the capacity of the patient. This middle range of traumatic stimuli occupies the major attention of civilian and military surgeons concerned with the metabolic care of illness.

3. In the *most severe* group of traumatic stimuli are those due to anoxia, local or general death of tissue, and prolonged failure of tissue perfusion. These include suffocation (whether ventilatory or circulatory), hypercapnia, respiratory or metabolic acidosis, tissue necrosis (burns and crush), advancing invasive infection and above all (providing a final common pathway to death) prolonged deficiency of blood flow to the brain, the heart and other viscera.

This third group of stimuli are those to which the unaided human body has no adequate response or defense. These are the forms of trauma which can now be treated effectively. It is to the treatment of these patients that the military surgeon devotes virtually his entire attention in the severely wounded, and for these the civilian surgeon spends his anxious nights in the operating room, or at the bedside. Here is where perfect metabolic understanding and aggressive surgery are vital to success.

MEDIATORS FROM THE WOUND TO THE
BODY AS A WHOLE

Viewing the patient with a fractured femur, it is obvious enough that he has a local injury. Looking now at his metabolism and finding an increased level of cortisone and norepinephrine in the blood, of aldosterone in the urine, a decreased urinary sodium:potassium ratio (with inability to excrete base), an increased excretion of nitrogen, an inability to unload administered water, a tendency to metabolic alkalosis, a decreased oxygen tension in the arterial blood with a markedly decreased carbon dioxide tension—viewing all of these things, it is not quite so evident as to what mediates the local injury from the leg to the body as a whole.

The mediators that translate local injury into a systemic response may be grouped under two headings: those that involve the endocrine glands primarily, and those that do not. In the first group, normal hormones are the messengers; in the second group, biochemical deterioration is itself the messenger. The responses of the first group—those of normal hormones—are for the most part "favorable to survival." These are the normal Darwinian responses. The responses of the second group—biochemical deterioration—are for the most part compensations to severe tissue injury, the messengers themselves (acidosis, anoxia) are unfavorable, and the response they elicit is often inadequate. We will consider the mediators or pathways under these two headings.

Endocrine Activity After Tissue Injury.
ADRENAL CORTEX—GLUCOCORTICOIDS. A turning point in the history of surgical metabolism occurred in the middle 1940's, with the realization (arising in several minds inde-

pendently) that the adrenal cortex responds characteristically to severe injury, and that certain of the metabolic events of injury resemble those of an adrenal discharge. Several facts are of outstanding interest. First, the vertebrate organism with both adrenals removed and no replacement given is totally unable to withstand even the simplest of traumatic stimuli; in the years before cortical hormone treatment, even acute appendicitis was almost uniformly fatal in the patient with Addison's disease. Second is the fact that injury produces a readily detectable increase in the level of free and bound cortisol in the blood, and of its reduced and conjugated metabolites in the urine; there is an associated decrease in the lymphocytes and eosinophils of the circulating blood. An increase in ACTH in the blood can be demonstrated, and this entire response (if the injury is mild) is abated by spinal cord section above the injury.

It is evident that this is a complex neuroendocrine adaptation involving an afferent nervous pathway, central pathways from the hypothalamus to the anterior pituitary, and finally efferent endocrine pathways involving adrenocorticotropic hormone, cortisol and its metabolites, and the response elicited by these in the peripheral tissues. Altering these are the various rates at which the liver reduces the hormones, and at which the kidney excretes them.

Important as this response is, it does not account for all of post-traumatic metabolism, nor can the pharmacologic production of this endocrine discharge mimic the surgical sequence in trauma and recovery.

ADRENAL CORTEX—ALDOSTERONE. Of more recent description, but of equal significance, is the response of the adrenal cortex in producing electrolyte-active hormones such as aldosterone, as a particular response to acute volume reduction. This chain of command seems to involve at least three alternative and overlapping modes of activation. One is a neuroendocrine pathway involving ACTH, and essentially the same as that producing cortisol and its metabolites; ACTH is a very strong stimulus to the production of aldosterone. An alternative pathway exists, not involving the pituitary, and involving a substance tentatively identified as "glomerulotrophin," which stimulates the zona glomerulosa of the adrenal cortex and is active even in patients who have had the pituitary removed. A third pathway involves a direct stimulus of the adrenal cortex by angiotensin. This material is produced in the blood by enzymatic alteration of renin which in turn is secreted in response to decreased perfusion pressure in the juxtaglomerular apparatus of the kidney.

The "salt-retainer," therefore, represents a complicated feedback mechanism by which the kidney, subjected to inadequate blood flow, secretes a blood-pressure-raising hormone which effects the conservation of body sodium and thus extracellular and plasma volume. This is a strongly pressor effect.

These responses, together with those of the adrenal medulla, indicate clearly that the vertebrate organism possesses a special mass of tissue on each side of the spine including the kidney (its excretory functions), the juxtaglomerular apparatus, the glomerular blood supply, the adrenal cortex and the adrenal medulla, which together give the organism an integrated response to acute volume reduction and circulatory inadequacy. Much of surgical metabolism and surgical therapy is devoted to the understanding, the accommodation and the modification of responses in these two neighboring masses of tissue: the adrenal glands and the kidney.

ADRENAL MEDULLA—CATECHOL AMINES. Evidence for the activation of the adrenal medulla and associated nerve synapses throughout the body, both producing catechol amines, has long been found in pulse and perfusion changes after hemorrhage; and more recently in the documentation of increased blood levels of catechol amines (both epinephrine and norepinephrine) in blood. After bilateral total adrenalectomy there is no remaining source for epinephrine. Evidently this substance (which has a positive inotrophic effect on the heart and a glycogenolytic effect on the liver, as well as producing mild vasoconstriction) is produced only in the adrenal medulla. In sharp contrast, norepinephrine (which is predominantly a vasoconstrictor pressor amine) seems to be produced in nerve synapses throughout the body. It is difficult to demonstrate any alteration in blood norepinephrine levels following bilateral total adrenalectomy.

Over the past 50 years (since Dr. Cannon's

work) much consideration has been given to the survival value and the teleologic meaning of these substances, so active after injury. It is noteworthy that all of the adrenal hormones —glucocorticoids, aldosterone and catechol amines—are harmful if given at high doses for prolonged periods. Of the three, norepinephrine, is the most hazardous.

It is also noteworthy that these adrenal hormones work together. In adrenal insufficiency the catechol amines alone do not restore the circulation or produce survival. *The presence of cortisol and its metabolites is essential to the biologic action of the catechol amines.* Thus, the adrenal cortex and the adrenal medulla exist anatomically together and have an integrated effect on the circulation, even though the chemical configuration of their two hormones is quite different.

POSTERIOR PITUITARY—ANTIDIURETIC HORMONE. The fourth and most clearly documented of the normal endocrine responses to injury is the production of increased amounts of antidiuretic hormone in the blood, with an associated alteration in the ability of the kidneys to achieve free water clearance. By this is meant that the kidney under the influence of the hormone is unable to produce a urine containing more water per unit solute than is found in the glomerular filtrate. Recent evidence strongly confirms the previous supposition that this metabolic effect, so peculiar to injury and hemorrhage, is due to a direct action of antidiuretic hormone on the distal renal tubule. This polypeptide is evidently produced in the midbrain, stored in the posterior pituitary and acts primarily on the water reabsorptive sites in the distal renal tubule. Like aldosterone and the catechol amines, it is active at catalytic concentrations (i.e., $10^{-9}M$). Acting as a normal response to volume reduction and tissue injury (as well as to hypertonicity), antidiuretic hormone (ADH) is not in itself harmful; indeed, it conserves water to the patient's advantage. But, as in the introductory example quoted, it prevents the excretion of excess amounts of water ingested or injected. Therefore, if the surgeon mistakenly gives water in excess of actual requirements, severe water-logging and hemodilution result because of this otherwise helpful endocrine response.

MISCELLANEOUS ENDOCRINE ACTIVITY. In addition to these well-documented changes, nearly all of the endocrine glands have been implicated at one time or another in the response to injury. It has been considered by some that the increased caloric turnover is due to direct stimulation of the thyroid; conclusive evidence on this point is lacking. Decreased gonadal function has been noted after severe injury; amenorrhea and abnormal hair growth are observed in the female, with decreased libido and decreased excretion of androgenic hormones in the male. While these evidences are unquestioned, they appear for the most part to be the result of starvation and caloric inadequacy rather than injury per se. Alterations in the amount of insulin or glucagon in the blood have been thought to be responsible for the hyperglycemia seen after injury. Current evidence suggests that this hyperglycemia is in large part the result of catechol amine stimulation of liver glycogenolysis.

Biochemical Activity After Tissue Injury. In sharp contrast with the above normal neuroendocrine activations are the biochemical deteriorations which carry the direct message of local injury to the body as a whole. For the most part these are deleterious in their action, and they arouse a whole variety of responses and compensations. They will be described only briefly here, though later they figure very prominently in treatment.

PRIMARY DAMAGE TO THE CENTRAL NERVOUS SYSTEM. Loss of cerebral function, loss of consciousness, loss of vision, loss of swallowing and coughing reflexes, as well as peripheral vasodilatation, are the result of direct injury to the brain or the spinal cord. These impair the ability of the patient to cooperate, to respire, ventilate and maintain normal circulation.

COMPROMISE OF THE AIRWAY. Defects in airway patency arise all the way from upper airway obstruction (as produced by injuries to the nose and the throat) to more subtle defects affecting the volume of alveolar ventilation, the diffusion of gases across the alveolar membrane, or the stability of the diaphragm and the chest cage. In all, the essential component lost is the normal ratio of perfusion to ventilation. Both hypoxia and hypercapnia bring in their wake a variety of systemic deteriorations independent of the endocrine activity they arouse. Hypoxia produces lacticacidosis, alterations in cellular permeability and finally tissue death. Hypercapnia produces a fall in pH which interferes with the normal reponse of the heart and the blood vessels to catechol amines. Cardiac arrhythmias occur terminally in both anoxia and hypercapnia and are most common in respiratory failure (anoxia plus hypercapnia) to which drugs (such as anesthetics) have been added; low flow states such as shock greatly potentiate this sequence.

PROLONGED DEFICIENCY OF FLOW AND SHOCK. The term "shock" has become almost meaningless because of the confusion between blood pressure and tissue perfusion on the one hand and volume-reduction versus intoxication on the other. The important component so damaging to the patient is *tissue anoxia through lack of perfusion*, bringing in its wake the gradual death of tissues. The tissues of the body vary in their ability to withstand hypoxia; the temperature of any anoxic tissue is likewise a critical factor in its survival. When the tissues that die are brain or heart, the patient dies.

Man can survive prolonged periods of low flow and tissue perfusion if restoration of blood volume and flow occur before the heart and the brain are damaged. This is in sharp contrast to the dog where, because of bacterial processes, shock becomes irreversible long before any severe damage is externally discernible or measurable in brain or heart. Because of man's ability to withstand prolonged flow-deficiency, recovery is often followed by pathologic changes in certain organs which, while severely damaged, are not immediately necessary for life. The kidney leads the list among these; renal failure is the commonest sequela of recovery from prolonged deficiency of blood flow.

INFECTION. Severe infection is both a stimulus and a mediator for metabolic change. High fever, the production of bacterial toxins, and the loss of large amounts of protein and salt through exudate are the three most prominent modalities by which infection in a local area produces a systemic deterioration. One or all of these aspects in combination will produce bloodstream invasion, prolonged deficiency of blood flow, and death. Treatment depends upon accurate chemotherapy for the particular organism, plus such surgical measures as external drainage, exteriorization, amputation or removal.

STARVATION is a remarkably dynamic factor in surgical metabolism, changing day by day. After injury most patients are totally starved for periods from a few hours to a week. If the patient comes to his injury or operation with normal body composition, this short-term starvation seems to produce few ill-effects. Minor losses of fat are well borne, and minor losses of nitrogen are repaired quickly when refeeding begins. The provision of vitamins and minerals is helpful, but even these can be dispensed with over the short-term. If, by contrast, post-traumatic starvation is prolonged for more than a week, or if it is accompanied by severe infection so that catabolic changes and oxidative energy requirements are increased, then the starvation state per se becomes a critical factor in survival. This dynamic situation demands close attention by the surgeon. For a surgical patient who has been starving for 3 or 4 days and will soon be eating, little attention need be paid to calories, fat, protein, nitrogen, vitamins, electrolytes, or minerals. But as each day or week passes, their provision becomes progressively more urgent, the acceptable margin for error more narrow, and the price of deficiency more devastating. (See also Chap. 6, Nutrition.)

Death from starvation is death from bronchopneumonia; late starvation takes its final toll through interference with normal muscular function, the loss of coughing and expectoration, the loss of deep respiration, and the accumulation of bacterial products in the bronchial tree. The final result of starvation is not some mysterious metabolic or endocrine defect but is instead accumulative bronchopneumonia and death.

Metabolic Changes in Injury and Recovery. It remains now to describe the metabolic changes observed and the principles of treatment that are based upon them. The metabolic changes themselves are often spectacular, sometimes subtle, and in most cases but poorly understood in terms of their precise activation. In nearly all instances the metabolic changes have multiple modalities of activation, just as the trauma itself has multiple pathways by which it affects the body.

NITROGEN BALANCE is altered by injury in

a drastic but predictable way. If the trauma is mild, and starvation is brief, urinary nitrogen excretion rate is essentially unchanged from the preoperative state; alterations in intermediary metabolism are few; the negative balance results wholly from starvation and is quickly wiped out as feeding is restored. In more severe injury, absolute urinary nitrogen excretion rate is increased, even though no intake is given.

Where absolute urinary nitrogen excretion rate is increased despite the lack of intake, there is no question but what a catabolism of body protein is involved. There is no "storehouse" for small molecular-weight nitrogen compounds or protein in the body. There is no "depot" protein as there is fat and carbohydrate. This catabolism of protein comes from skeletal muscle, as reflected in an early increased rate of creatinine excretion after injury and a long-continued excretion of creatine, an abnormal urinary product in the male. This catabolic period lasts from 3 days to a month or more, depending upon circumstances. Where trauma is severe, starvation long, and infection marked, very severe catabolic destruction of body tissues amounting to 20 to 30 Gm. of nitrogen (120 to 180 Gm. protein) per day occurs. If this post-traumatic catabolic period lasts too long, it finally takes a severe toll in muscular strength and produces the respiratory disorders also characteristic of very prolonged starvation. These are failure of ventilation and cough, leading finally to accumulative bronchopneumonia with many areas of atelectasis and pulmonary suppuration, and death. This pulmonary pathway to death, characteristic of late starvation, is produced much more rapidly in the post-traumatic period when intense catabolism is added to the erosion of the body cell mass ordinarily produced rather slowly by simple starvation.

This post-traumatic catabolism is followed in the normal sequence of convalescence by a "turning-point" phase as ingested food is utilized more efficiently, and the absolute urinary nitrogen excretion rate is cut back sharply even without significant changes in intake. Then, as intake is increased, there is a prolonged period of anabolism associated with increased muscular strength and finally leading to socio-economic rehabilitation. Much research has been devoted to the dynamics of catabolism, while the details of anabolism have attracted less attention. The normal human subject will anabolize protein at a rate of approximately 3 to 7 Gm. of nitrogen per 70 kg. of body weight per day. This anabolic rate will go on for weeks or months after severe illness or starvation, finally ceasing when the genetically determined cellular mass of the body is restored. These are very brisk anabolic rates and rival those observed in the growing child.

As mentioned above, catabolic nitrogen after injury comes mostly from skeletal muscle. Later in anabolism it is largely restored to skeletal muscle, and this restoration is responsible for the remarkable gain in muscular strength, vigor and effectiveness that is observed in late convalescence. Most of the nitrogen lost after trauma is excreted in the urine as urea; as mentioned above, there is a transient increase in the excretion of creatine and creatinine. During anabolism creatinine excretion falls to a low level, reflecting the smaller body cell mass of the body. Creatine excretion ceases. Urea remains as the predominant urinary nitrogen-carrier.

Circulating dissolved proteins such as albumin and globulin undergo minor changes during this catabolic sequence. Hypoalbuminemia in surgical patients is usually dilutional in nature. A true albumin deficiency occurs only in very large starvation with waterloading or in severe liver disease. The priorities for synthesis of albumin, globulin and hemoglobin are very high, and even after prolonged post-traumatic starvation remarkably normal concentrations are observed, and good antibody function is frequently noted.

It is a common misapprehension that failure to heal a wound is the inevitable result of a negative nitrogen balance. Nothing could be farther from the case. On a busy surgical service, serving either a civilian or a military population, about two thirds of the wounds or surgical incisions heal to tensile integrity (permitting removal of sutures, resumption of function, and restoration of weight-bearing) during the nitrogen-negative phase. By the same token, fractures heal quite well during a period of negative calcium and phosphorus metabolism. Indeed, one might state the enigma the other way: normal catabolic effects in the organism appear to be associated with normal wound healing. Even in such diseases as carcinoma of the esophagus where starvation has been prolonged, normal wound healing will occur so long as the patient comes to operation with normal extracellular chemical values, avoidance of water-loading, and adequate vitamin provisions. Of all the Darwinian responses in surgical metabolism, none is more effective for survival than the ability of the starving organism to heal a wound. Ascorbic acid appears to be the only exogenous substance required; and even this may have been provided previously and stored in the organism, at least for periods up to a month.

Therefore, it can truly be said that "the nutritional objective of the early postoperative period is a scaphoid abdomen": avoidance of distention is more important than early feeding. Likewise, the objective of subsequent feeding in convalescence is to let the patient regain muscular strength and socio-economic rehabilitation, as well as normal sexual and reproductive function.

POTASSIUM is lost in the urine, after injuries, in amounts up to 70 mEq. on the first day, thereafter decreasing (in the absence of potassium intake) to 20 to 30 mEq./day, and finally after many days to values as low as 10 mEq./day. This cellular cation is lost along with the nitrogen of the body cell mass; as in the case of nitrogen, potassium is lost chiefly from skeletal muscle. The K:N ratio of the negative balance is that of very acute catabolism, suggesting loss of cellular water and salt faster than protein matrix; the result is a K:N ratio far above the tissue level of 3 mEq./Gm. The K:N ratio of the early negative balance is as high as 25 to 30 mEq./Gm. The implication of these changes is clearly that the body cell mass loses electrolyte and water before it loses matrix. Later on, during anabolism these same cells (largely muscle) appear to load electrolyte and water a little sooner and a little faster than they reconstruct matrix. Potassium balance becomes positive long before nitrogen balance. This is most clearly seen in a burned patient who is able to take food after the 3rd or 4th day; potassium balance is achieved readily, but nitrogen balance requires many weeks.

The course of serum potassium concentration bears little relation to balance. After acute trauma, particularly with anoxia or hypercapnia, there is a tendency to hyperkalemia. This may occur during the period of most acute potassium loss and with normal urine outputs; similarly, very severe hypokalemia can be produced in the presence of very minor losses of potassium by the occurrence of metabolic alkalosis. It is for this reason that the terms "potassium deficiency" and "hypokalemia" should not be regarded as synonymous. "Deficiency" of a substance should refer to its lack in the body; a low concentration in the blood (hypo-emia) may or may not coexist with a deficiency. This same paradoxical relationship between body stores and plasma concentration is noted with respect to several other substances, particularly magnesium and sodium.

SODIUM AND CHLORIDE. These extracellular ions are conserved after injury or operation. There is a reduced excretion rate in the urine, of both substances, but sodium excretion is reduced to a greater extent than chloride. This sodium conservation results in the maintenance of an effective extracellular volume, and its onset is largely related to volume changes. Sodium conservation begins immediately after operation in most cases, but in some individuals it may be delayed a day or two. If it occurs immediately, it is frequently of short duration but very intense, with the urinary sodium-excretion rate reduced from the normal range of 100 to 150 mEq./day to the range of 0.1 to 1.0 mEq./day. This latter is to be compared with the urinary sodium-excretion rate, in early starvation, of 80 to 100 mEq./day. This conservation is often followed by a "sodium-release phenomenon" with a sudden increase in sodium excretion and considerable diuresis. If, on the other hand, sodium conservation is slow to begin, commencing on the 2nd or the 3rd days after trauma (and despite normal blood volume) it may persist for many days or weeks. It is difficult to predict which type of pattern will occur, although sudden massive trauma in the healthy male tends to produce the early type of sodium conservation with early diuresis, whereas in depleted individuals (or those with visceral disease of heart or liver) a more gradual but very prolonged sodium conservation is characteristic.

If sodium is administered in any quantity during a period of sodium conservation, three important results obtain. First, the absolute urinary sodium excretion rate is increased: it may be as high as 30 to 50 mEq./day on intakes of 150 mEq./day during periods of strong electrolyte conservation and aldosterone activity. Second, so long as sodium conservation persists a positive sodium balance will ensue, the magnitude of which is a function primarily of the intake. If no intake is provided and urinary sodium conservation is marked, the situation is produced of an essentially zero balance on zero intake. This "no flux" situation is seen in patients with heart disease (in whom sodium conservation is extremely marked) when they are managed without sodium administration. Third, the decreased ability to excrete cation and base (as $NaHCO_3$) tends to produce a mild metabolic alkalosis and makes any alkalotic threat (gastric juice loss, citrate administration) more alkalinizing. As a general rule, the clinical objective of management after trauma should be zero balance of sodium, except in those instances in which losses or redistribution of interstitial fluid should be replaced.

The tendency to retain chloride after surgery is not as marked as is the case with sodium. The result is a gain in sodium greater than in chloride. This is in part responsible for the tendency of postoperative patients to become slightly alkalotic with an acid urine.

Excretion of sodium and chloride is related to effective circulating blood and extracellular volume, more than to any other single component of the post-traumatic state. This is dealt with in greater detail below.

Coincident with these changes in sodium excretion there is a consistent tendency after injury and operations for the serum sodium concentration to be lowered to the range of 130 to 135 mEq./L. One might predict that retention of sodium would raise the serum sodium concentration; quite the reverse is the case. Those patients who show the most marked restriction of urinary sodium excretion will often be those in whom the serum sodium concentration is most markedly lowered. Anomalous sodium penetration into cells accounts for only a small fraction of this hyponatremia, whereas water retention plays the predominant role.

WATER. The tendency to retain water after injury or operation takes the form of diminished urine volume which in the early post-traumatic phase may be of high specific gravity. This also manifests itself by decreased excretion of a given water load: there is an inability of the kidney to respond by diuresis to large water infusions. If too much water is given, there is a tendency to dilute all serum constituents, producing a fall, particularly of red blood cells, protein and sodium. All these changes can and will occur in the presence of a normal glomerular filtration rate; if the latter is reduced, of course they are accentuated.

Changes in the total body water are not marked after closed soft-tissue trauma; there simply is not time or flux sufficient to make a noticeable change if treatment is well-adapted to the needs of the patient. The normal male total body water is about 55 per cent of body weight; the female, 50 per cent. Although total body water does not change markedly in ordinary circumstances, there is a consistent tendency for the extracellular fraction (normally 20 to 25% of body weight) to enlarge; this is due in part to water retention, new water production by fat oxidation and, in some instances, a demonstrable change in cell permeability. In burns or massive tissue injury, body water changes are great and commence with a rapid rise under treatment, later falling with diuresis. In all forms of tissue injury there is a local accumulation of extracellular fluid as traumatic edema. This accumulates at the expense of the plasma volume and requires plasma replacement to maintain plasma and blood volume in an effective range.

PLASMA PROTEIN. The postoperative conservation of water and salt produces no consistent protein dilution if excessive administration is avoided. If large amounts of water are given, there is a significant post-traumatic fall in the concentration of sodium and protein. If large amounts of sodium are given, the sodium-concentration fall is not so great, but the drop in serum protein concentration is greater.

GLUCOSE. There is a rise in blood sugar after trauma, persisting from 1 to 2 days, depending on the magnitude of the trauma. This is associated with the virtually complete exhaustion of liver glycogen and, depending on the renal threshold, by the spilling of sugar in the urine. The hydrolysis of protein results, by deamination, in the formation of carbohydrate just as the hydrolysis of glycogen results in the formation of sugars; the hydrolysis of fat produces free fatty acids. The carbon fragments from all three sources feed into the energy mechanism to provide support for body heat and work. The elevated blood sugar after injury reflects gluconeogenesis at a rate faster than the oxidative mechanism can dispose of it.

FAT: ENERGY REQUIREMENTS AND ENERGY SOURCES. Of all these energy sources for the starving patient, none can equal the oxidation of body fat that occurs after major trauma. In starvation the fat-loss rate is about 75 Gm./day. After moderately extensive surgery this is from 100 to 150 Gm./day, and after massive trauma the fat-oxidation rates appear to run as high as 300 Gm./day. A rapid fat oxidation persists for only a few days after closed soft-tissue trauma, and then, as oral intake is resumed and endogenous substrates form a lesser fraction of the energy supply, the patient remains for many days or weeks in zero fat balance, neither gaining nor losing body fat. Then, late in convalescence, and long after anabolic protein resynthesis has begun, restoration of body fat slowly occurs. This rapid oxidation of fat emphasizes the need for new sources of energy on the part of the organism struggling to maintain life processes during starvation after severe injury.

The three fundamental determinants of the total energy requirement in the postoperative surgical patient (or the patient after injury) appear to be his temperature, the presence or the absence of infection, and a third factor relating to the rate of evaporative water-loss. As far as is known at present, alterations in thyroid hormone level in the blood are not responsible for these alterations.

In the presence of high fever, energy metabolism is increased. Carbon output exceeds carbon intake; the energy source is obviously within the body. Total caloric requirement, oxygen consumption and substrate excretion are all increased. This takes the form of an increased oxygen requirement and carbon dioxide production. An increased excretion of nitrogen in the urine is a by-product only to the extent that protein constitutes the substrate. It has been demonstrated that the metabolic increase is not a linear function of the patient's temperature. When invasive sepsis is a component of the hyperthermic state, then the increase in energy turnover is out of proportion to the body temperature. By contrast, in patients who are terminally ill, high fever may be associated with a normal or low oxygen consumption, an event of apparently dire prognosis suggesting that the metabolic machinery cannot keep up with the demand imposed upon it.

Evaporative loss of water from the body is another component in total energy turnover. If this is increased (particularly in instances where it is increased from the skin, as in the late burn with a granulating surface) then each quantum of water evaporated has a cooling effect and imposes an obligatory energy utilization to maintain normal body temperature. If temperature is increased, then this stimulatory effect of evaporative water loss becomes very marked. Fuel must be burned at excessive rates to maintain temperature despite the evaporative cooling. Both in man and animals it has been possible to reduce the caloric requirement materially by covering open burned areas with an impermeable membrane. At the present time there is no simple way of judging the total energy turnover of a patient in terms of calories per day, except by indirect calorimetry. By this method it is also possible to determine the respiratory quotient and to approximate the substrate being burned. In the starving patient after the first few days, the respiratory quotient is approximately 0.7, and most of the substrate being burned is fat. Every kilogram of fat burned yields slightly more than a liter of water of oxidation. This is added to the total body water and, in the presence of a marked antidiuretic state, further compounds the dilutional hyponatremia.

The interplay of these various factors, the role of water gain or loss in energy metabolism, the effect on energy requirements of infection, and the utilization of diet or intravenous feedings remains an important horizon of advancing knowledge in surgical care today. At the basis of any such advance is the clear identification of those phases after injury when outside sources of energy make little contribution to the patient's welfare, as contrasted with those phases or stages of convalescence wherein such provision is essential to survival. As in all other adjustments to the conditions of injury, the Darwinian process can go just so far and no farther.

ACID-BASE REGULATION. Among the most spectacular metabolic challenges thrust upon the surgical patient are the metabolic and respiratory alterations in concentration of hydrogen ion in the blood and the extracellular fluid. Tissue anoxia (whether circulatory or ventilatory) produces a severe metabolic acidosis due to the incomplete combustion of carbohydrate and the accumulation of lactic acid. This lacticacidemia far outstrips the associated increase in pyruvate, indicating that this accumulation is due to anaerobiosis rather than failure of aerobic oxidation in the oxalacetic step of the Krebs cycle. For this reason the lactate:pyruvate ratio has acquired meaning in surgical metabolism. It is one of several peripheral biochemical indices of low flow states and is of importance in understanding therapy.

If there is ventilatory impairment, hypercapnia results, and this respiratory component further compounds the acidosis. As pH falls below 7.20, the myocardium becomes progressively less responsive to catechol amines; there is progressive deterioration of the circulation, refractory to transfusion. Finally, the heart stops; this is regarded as "cardiac arrest" or "irreversible shock," depending on the happenstance circumstance (and the theory of the bystanders). It is the typical lethal sequence in prolonged hypoxic acidosis.* This pathway —low blood flow in body tissues, with superadded ventilatory impairment—is one of the most important terminal mechanisms in surgical injury in man.

A commoner and more benign acid-base alteration in surgical patients is post-traumatic alkalosis. This consists of very mild anoxia (arterial oxygen tensions in the range of 80 to 100 mm./Hg with saturation between 90 and 95%), associated with hypocapnia (carbon dioxide tensions falling to the range of 25 to 30 mm./Hg due to hyperventilation).

* Both ether anesthesia and hypocapnia likewise produce mild degrees of lacticacidemia.

This hyperventilation is produced as a response to the anoxia itself or by other factors such as pain and apprehension. In mild pulmonary injury, the diffusible carbon dioxide is lost readily, but oxygen exchange is imperfect due to shunting, yielding this frequent combination of mild anoxia with continuing respiratory alkalosis. If, in addition, the patient is ventilated by automatic devices (which tend further to lower the carbon dioxide tension of the blood) or if the patient is given blood preserved with citrate (which in effect constitutes a sodium bicarbonate load), then a mixed metabolic and respiratory alkalosis is produced which can become so severe as a pH of 7.65. In a recently studied series of patients, this mild anoxia with mixed respiratory and metabolic alkalosis was, surprisingly, the commonest acid-base abnormality seen in surgical patients. This continued alkalosis does not seem to hurt the patient, except possibly by interfering with the delivery of oxygen to the tissues by a shift in the oxyhemoglobin dissociation curve.

There are many other types of acid-base imbalance in surgery, most particularly hypokalemic alkalosis or the chronic acidosis that is seen in renal failure or diabetes. In all instances, there are renal and respiratory responses which must be understood as a basis for therapy. The renal response to chronic metabolic acidosis consists in the excretion of urine of low pH, high titratable acidity and high ammonia content. All three of these renal responses are rate-limited and, thus, are ineffective over short periods of time. In the surgical patient who is severely injured or anoxic any acid load presented to the body must be managed by the blood and cellular buffers; hypocapnia represents an additional defense. For the acutely injured patient, any further defense against this acidotic threat must come from the surgeon's treatment.

The Primacy of Volume Maintenance. Before turning to therapy, we should note the constantly recurring theme throughout the foregoing: acute volume reduction as a stimulus to endocrine, metabolic and biochemical change.

The slang term "volume reduction" has come into wide use recently because of physiologic interest in volume-regulatory and volume-receptor phenomena. An example is the strong stimulus to aldosterone production and sodium conservation resulting from a 500 ml. venesection: how does the body sense this and mediate the response? What stimulates the juxtoglomerular apparatus?

The term "volume reduction" refers to a reduction in the effective circulating volume—of blood, plasma or extracellular fluid. All three of them are closely interrelated, since the effective volume of extracellular fluid supports the plasma volume across the capillary. Used in these various contexts the term may be quite confusing. When it is applied to an individual patient it is usually reasonably clear. Prolonged or severe reduction in the volume of the extracellular fluid from diarrhea, vomiting, ileostomy malfunction, or pancreatic fistula, with an elevated hematocrit and a low plasma volume, quite clearly indicates volume reduction due primarily to alterations in extracellular fluid volume communicated across the capillary and "felt" as a low plasma volume and hence a low blood volume. Acute or chronic blood loss in the form of hemorrhage, loss of red cells by hemolysis, or loss of effective circulating volume through central defects of the heart and the great vessels, may likewise be referred to as "volume reduction," in this instance referring primarily to the blood volume as a whole.

In any of these instances, lowered rates of tissue perfusion are produced. The lowered tissue perfusion results in increased levels of catechol amines, aldosterone, corticosteroids and antidiuretic hormone in the blood, as noted previously; biochemical deterioration is likewise produced in low perfusion, including lacticacidosis, hypercapnia and finally irreversible cellular damage when volume reduction is prolonged.

Simple loss of blood volume produces a transcapillary refill from the interstitial phase that requires 20 to 40 hours to reach completion. If shock itself has not resulted, and blood pressure has been maintained, then the transcapillary refill finally restores the total volume lost (the sum of losses of plasma and red blood cells), resulting in a great expansion of the plasma volume, a low peripheral concentration of erythrocytes, a gradual restoration of the circulation, and clear subsidence of all the endocrine-metabolic responses called forth by the original hemorrhage. This innate homeostatic response to acute blood volume loss is one of the most basic of the Darwinian survival processes witnessed daily by the surgeon. It is another adaptive change resulting when volume is threatened, challenged or compromised.

If the blood loss is more acute, more severe, or more prolonged, it then brings in its train not only endocrine activity, lacticacidosis and transcapillary refill but also decreased glomerular filtration rate, anuria, azotemia, decreased coronary blood flow, myocardial ischemia, cerebral ischemia and finally death.

One may make out a strong case to suggest that, from an evolutionary point of view, acute volume reduction is the most significant traumatic stimulus. It evokes a multicellular and multivisceral response throughout the body, but its first defense lies in two masses of highly specialized tissue on each side of the spine.

As mentioned before, this renal-adrenal mass is concerned with the maintenance of normal effective, circulating volume in the injured or challenged vertebrate.

CLINICAL METABOLIC MANAGEMENT

It is not the purpose of the author in this chapter to describe in detail all of surgical care as regards the treatment of body fluid abnormalities, nutritional deficiencies, burns, heart failure, renal failure or shock. Many of these are detailed elsewhere in this text. Instead, it is our purpose to outline therapeutic categories which exemplify the basis of surgical care and indicate their endocrine and metabolic background.

Normal Convalescence After Uneventful Clean Surgery

After moderately extensive surgery, with temporary interruption of gastrointestinal function, maintenance of asepsis, and freedom from infection, the Darwinian sequences do most of the surgeon's job for him. The patient will look after himself if given a chance. Only a few therapeutic details need to be considered in an otherwise healthy person. The general program is one of early diet and ambulation and minimum meddling. An intravenous infusion need not be given at all if the patient can take some fluids by the next morning. If the patient is elderly or has visceral disease, then the addition of a small water infusion will maintain better renal function. If oral intake must be procrastinated for 24 hours or more, then lung, skin and urine losses will produce a mild dehydration, well-borne by young, healthy people. But this is not a good practice in elderly folk or in others in whom renal functional impairment will result. In any event, fat oxidation and the antidiuretic tendency reduce the amount of water that need be given, and it is rarely necessary to give more than 1,000 to 1,500 ml./day. Of course, hyperpnea, fever and extrarenal loss alter this situation drastically.

Some surgeons feel that sodium chloride should not be given at all during this period; others, that a small amount should be administered. The onset of sodium conservation after surgery is variable, and there is no great choice between the two alternatives. All are agreed that the intravenous or oral administration of large amounts of sodium (150 to 250 mEq.) in the early postoperative days will result in excessive sodium accumulation in the body with a tendency to hypoproteinemia and edema. Of course, pathologic renal or extrarenal losses increase the need for sodium.

The use of potassium is unnecessary unless the outlook is for a prolonged absence of oral intake. If such persists over 3 days, the use of intravenous potassium (40 mEq./day as KCl) is advisable until feeding starts.

Oral diet should be advanced as peristalsis and the passage of feces or flatus permit. When a gastrointestinal anastomosis has been done, it is our general aim to have the patient at the level of 500 calories and 5 Gm. of protein (oral) by the 5th day. When there is no anastomosis and an insignificant peritoneal reaction, advancement may be more rapid. When there is any delay, distention, tenderness, or fever, the diet should be held up until clinical signs of digestive function are propitious. Lack of diet at this stage will not interfere with wound healing or recovery; distention may be the forerunner of wound dehiscence or pulmonary complications. The nutritional objective at this stage of surgical convalescence is indeed a scaphoid abdomen.

POST-TRAUMATIC STARVATION; DEPLETION; INTRAVENOUS FEEDING

The administration of an adequate diet as soon as feasible after surgery is a first rule of surgical care. Its most common abuse arises from the unjustified assumption that the administration of caloric intake immediately after surgical operation will somehow alter or reverse the metabolic processes which follow surgery, and that such reversal is desirable. The premature administration of calories by mouth or by tube to a patient whose gastrointestinal tract is not yet functioning produces gastric distention and vomiting. The results are decreased diaphragmatic excursion, discomfort, distention and, at the worst, aspiration pneumonia. For this reason a realistic appraisal of the need for food and its acceptance by the patient after surgery is of front-rank importance.

A patient who in the first 3 days after surgery needs or requires very little in the way of caloric or nitrogen intake, by a week or two after surgery literally craves intake, and an intake of calories and nitrogen in a well-balanced oral diet is an indispensable condition for final recovery. Hunger, the presence of audible peristalsis and the anal expulsion of swallowed air are the most important signals for dietary advancement. When, late in convalescence, diet cannot be taken because of gastrointestinal disease, one must weigh carefully the possible usefulness of gastrostomy, jejunostomy, or high caloric intravenous feedings with glucose, alcohol, amino acids and fat. When tube feedings are used, adequate water intake must be provided. In all circumstances, an adequate supply of vitamins is essential.

The administration of glucose intravenously kills hunger; in a patient in whom the transfer to oral intake is to be made, it is important to omit the "morning intravenous" and give warm, appetizing tasty fluids and soft solids.

The ratio of calories to nitrogen in the intake acquires importance because protein synthesis will not occur in the absence of an adequate caloric intake. The calorie:nitrogen ratio is defined as the ratio of nonprotein calories to protein nitrogen in the diet. A normal resting individual consumes a calorie:

nitrogen ratio of about 200 (2,400 calories and 12 Gm. nitrogen/day). As convalescence progresses, the calorie:nitrogen ratio required for anabolism decreases progressively until at about the 7th day after operation such as cholecystectomy, prostatectomy, gastrectomy, pneumonectomy, a calorie:nitrogen ratio of 150, or even less, will suffice for beginning anabolism. An example would be found in a caloric intake of 1,200/day with 8 Gm. of nitrogen. As oral intake later increases the calorie:nitrogen ratio will naturally increase to about 200, where anabolism is most satisfactory. A proper calorie:nitrogen ratio is very difficult to provide intravenously but can be done via an indwelling caval catheter, with hypertonic glucose, fat and amino acids or polypeptide protein digests. These will support anabolism once acute catabolic processes have abated or waned.

Prolonged caloric lack produces bodily depletion and cachexia, a special compositional, endocrine and metabolic syndrome very common on a surgical ward both in preoperative as well as postoperative patients. As used here, the word "depletion" denotes cachexia due to starvation of a variety of causes, the most common causes in surgery being late post-traumatic starvation as well as preoperative patients with gastrointestinal carcinoma, intestinal obstruction of other sources, chronic sepsis, ulcerative colitis, regional enteritis and long-standing obstructing duodenal ulcer.

Common to all these conditions is loss of tissue, both lean and fat, loss of energy and loss of muscular effectiveness. There is a loss of muscle mass and of fat which is quite obvious to the onlooker, and it is noticeable to the patient, not only when looking in the mirror but when trying to carry out muscular exertion. Much teaching on this subject has been devoted to the identification of "deficits"; the syndrome of depletion includes several important "excesses."

In the "deficit" column should be included fat and muscle mass. This lack of muscle mass means that the total body protein, as well as the total body potassium, magnesium, sulfate and other intracellular ions is low. But the most important muscular deficit, as mentioned previously, is experienced in respiratory effort and cough-clearing of the bronchial tree.

The most significant "excesses" are those of water and extracellular salt, of which sodium has been studied most extensively. These patients have too much water and sodium in their body composition, both in relative and in absolute terms. As fat disappears, the relative proportion of the body which is water rises because of its inverse compositional relationship. In addition, patients with chronic depletion show a marked antidiuretic tendency and will retain most of the water they are able to drink. Since they frequently are unable to take solid foods but still have access to liquids, the accumulation of water is very marked. Therefore, the body compositional defect can be summarized as "too little fat and too little muscle, with too much water, too much of which is extracellular water, and too much sodium."

In depletion of many causes, the serum concentrations of sodium and potassium show an interesting inverse relationship to the body content. The serum potassium tends to be high (4.5 to 5.5 mEq./L.) despite the obvious depletion of body cellular mass and, therefore, potassium. The serum sodium concentration tends to be low (125 to 135 mEq./L.) despite the measurable excess of body sodium.

Surgery in this depleted condition can be carried out successfully, and wound healing often is remarkably good—as, for example, in carcinoma of stomach and pancreas. For success, the patient should come to surgery (1) dry (i.e., with minimal edema or ECF expansion), (2) with normal osmotic and oncotic pressure, (3) in normal acid-base balance and (4) with a store of liver glycogen.

Blood-volume changes in late depletion have been the source of much misunderstanding: the concept has become current that such patients have low volumes because of their low hematocrits. In our experience such has not been the case unless hemorrhage has been a significant feature of the disease process itself. In the absence of significant blood loss (carcinoma of the esophagus, the stomach, the left colon), the typical picture is a low red cell mass and a high plasma volume, the latter especially marked if edema is present. Blood volume is normal or high even for ideal weight. The hazards of indiscriminate overuse of preoperative transfusion of whole blood are obvious; cell suspensions have a place.

After operation these depleted patients rebuild their body stories with great readiness if they are given food and are able to absorb it. The depleted patient's tissues are "thirsty" for nitrogen. A very low calorie:nitrogen ratio will suffice for positive nitrogen balance in these patients. If they are operated on with gentleness and care, with vitamins provided and infection avoided, the postoperative course is most gratifying.

When dietary advancement cannot occur, and prolonged intravenous feeding is necessary, certain general rules are helpful. These are:

1. Frequent check of the patient's weight.
2. Weight gain means water accumulation and is undesirable.
3. Sudden weight loss of more than 500 Gm. means dehydration and is undesirable. The only exception is when high fever is present and catabolic weight loss is greatly accelerated.
4. A weight loss of 150 to 250 Gm./day should be expected as evidence of the fat oxidation inevitable until anabolism is established.
5. Total water intake should equal losses by all routes, allowing for renal output of 1,000 ml.
6. Total salt intake (Na, Cl, K) should balance all losses accurately, allowing for daily urine excretion of 40 mEq. of each ion. Do not try to replace daily urine losses of Na and Cl quantitatively!
7. Maximum carbohydrate intake is desirable to lessen nitrogen losses in the chronic situation, so long as the carbohydrate is utilized and intense glycosuria is avoided. From 50 to 150 Gm. of glucose is given easily (200 to 600 calories). By caval catheter much larger amounts may be used.
8. Intravenous amino acids are useful in the chronic situation so long as calorie:nitrogen ratios in the 200 range are obtainable. It is much easier to give nitrogen than the calories adequate to support protein synthesis from that nitrogen.
9. Intravenous fat and alcohol can be used to provide additional calories.
10. At least one whole blood transfusion should be given each week to provide whole protein and red cells.
11. Need for additional blood, plasma or albumin is determined by blood volume and serum protein concentration (see Chap. 8).

Water Administration

The fact that the postoperative patient does not excrete water normally signifies that he should not be given more water than he can lose. If he does not go to surgery in a dehydrated state, his water administration in the first few days should correspond to a summation of his losses. In the normal afebrile adult male, evaporative loss (lungs and skin) is about 750 ml./day; the urinary loss the first day is about 500 ml., and the second day about 750 ml. For this reason, amounts of electrolyte-free water totaling between 1,000 and 1,500 ml. on the first day are quite adequate. If there is some electrolyte loss through the gastrointestinal tract, the addition of a moderate amount of salt to this water (for example, 75 mEq. of sodium and a like amount of chloride) is well-tolerated by the patient, and a transient positive sodium balance will not harm him.

The female tends to have lesser rates of lung and skin loss, and in the adult female these may not total much more than 500 ml./day if afebrile.

The administration of too much electrolyte-free water produces plasma hypotonicity recognized by low sodium, low chloride, low serum protein and a washed-out appearance of the patient. The extreme of this overwatered scale is water intoxication, cerebral edema, coma and convulsions. The administration of inadequate water in a patient with high insensible losses or large extrarenal losses from the gastrointestinal tract produces appearances which are familiar as desiccation-dehydration, consisting of apathy, lethargy, thirst, a dry, coated tongue, loss of skin turgor, and a glassy expression.

The factors which most rapidly increase the loss of water by lungs and skin are fever and rapid respirations. A patient with a fever of 103° who is breathing rapidly with his mouth open will lose as much as 2,000 ml. of water a day through his lungs. An educated guess as to his losses must be made; if the situation is critical, daily weights should be taken.

The most accurate check of water metabolism in the postoperative patient is provided by his daily weight fluctuation. Because of the loss of nitrogen and the oxidation of fat, we expect the postoperative patient to lose from 150 to 350 Gm./day for the first few days until anabolism becomes established again.

The adjustment of water therapy to requirements is carried out best by accurate measurement of water losses, an educated guess as to evaporative loss and, in troublesome problems, the use of frequent measurement of body weight. When extrarenal loss, or prolonged starvation, is a part of the picture, water intake and output records are essential.

PLASMA HYPOTONICITY, THE LOW SODIUM SYNDROMES AND EXTRARENAL LOSS

A low serum sodium concentration (115 to 125 mEq./L., or less) denotes a sick patient: if preoperative, it carries a bad prognosis for the outcome of surgery; if postoperative, it suggests that convalescence is far from complete; if there has been blood loss, blood pressure is poorly maintained.

There is usually a multiple causation in the production of a low serum sodium, but in any given instance one mechanism usually predominates. The *accumulation of water*, accentuated by antidiuretic mechanisms is the commonest cause. Also important are lack of adequate caloric intake, loss of sodium from the body through either renal or extrarenal losses and, in some instances, disease of liver, kidney, heart or adrenals. The surgeon should seek out the predominant cause of the low serum sodium concentration, since certain causes are remediable, and, when remedied, convalescence is accelerated.

The possibility that the patient has been given too much water may be checked by history, by his weight and by the presence of edema. Current water intake should be restricted markedly, and, when water has been overadministered and serum sodium is low, minimal water administration for a day or two, permitting the patient to blow off water by lungs and lose it by kidney, is a reasonable procedure. The administration of 1,000 ml. of 10 per cent mannitol daily for 3 days will remove a significant amount of water.

Excessive *urinary* loss should be sought out. The urine should be analyzed for its sodium content very early in the course. If, in the presence of a low serum sodium concentration, the urine sodium concentrations is higher than 30 mEq./L., one may be confident that either renal or adrenal disease exists.* In such a case the patient's care requires daily urine sodium analyses and (unlike the urine from a normal kidney) accurate salt replacement; hormone therapy should be carried out if adrenal function is found to be low.

If it is discovered that the patient's urine sodium concentration is appropriately low, and if no edema is present (so that renal-adrenal mechanisms as well as the excessive accumulation of water are unlikely) one is left with plasma hypotonicity as a complication either of *visceral disease* or *caloric starvation*. The presence of heart failure, liver disease, unhealed wounds and starvation tends to produce plasma hypotonicity. The administration of moderate amounts of hypertonic saline (300 ml. of 3% of sodium chloride) is carried out cautiously for a few days, the infusion being given every other day, to observe the response. In occasional instances, the sodium concentration will start upward with a good water diuresis and gradual mending of the plasma hypotonicity. However, if such does not occur, it is dangerous to continue hypertonic saline administration, since further edema production will be the result.

If the patient is receiving a very low caloric intake but his surgical convalescence otherwise is progressing satisfactorily, it is safe to give one or two infusions of hypertonic saline and then concentrate on caloric intake, confident that as caloric intake increases serum sodium concentration will return to normal. The administration of adequate calories alone will occasionally restore the serum sodium concentration. An explanation of this is lacking, but one may assume that it requires energy at the cell surface to exclude sodium from the cell.

Finally, there are those hypotonic syndromes associated with *extrarenal* salt loss such as vomiting, diarrhea, intestinal or pancreatic fistulas. If the loss is very high in

* This test should be based on an overnight collection, taken when no sodium is being given intravenously.

sodium concentration (pancreatic juice sometimes runs as high as 185 mEq./L.), it is not remarkable that loss of 1 or 2 liters produces drastic reduction in the serum sodium concentration with lowering of the extracellular volume and, in some cases, a shocklike state, with hemoconcentration. When the sodium concentration of the lost fluid is lower, as, for instance, in gastric or duodenal contents, other events must take place for this loss to lower the serum sodium concentration. As mentioned in the preceding section, the three most common complications are (1) the administration of excessive amounts of electrolyte-free water, (2) the accumulation of sodium-free water by the lysis of cell material and the release of cellular water, and (3) caloric starvation with the accumulation of the water of oxidation of fat. Therefore, the treatment of extrarenal losses of salt must take into consideration all these factors, as well as replacement of external loss (using hypertonic saline) and the regulation of acid-base balance.

Hypoproteinemia

The commonest cause of hypoproteinemia in surgical patients is the overadministration of salt and water; the best step is prevention. If overadministration has occurred, and hypoproteinemia results, the steps to take must be balanced carefully between avoidance for a few days of much fluid therapy, the use of diuretic agents, or the use of concentrated albumin. A nice choice between these depends upon the cardiac reserve, the ventilatory capacity and the renal function of the patient.

Starvation alone, without water-and-salt loading, is remarkable for the preservation of normal serum protein and oncotic pressure, even though body protein is markedly depleted. Chronic and acute parenchymatous liver disease are important causes of hypoalbuminemia. If operation must be done, concentrated albumin is of use as temporary passive support of the albumin concentration. Loss of protein-rich exudates, as well as loss of nitrogen and whole protein in the form of diarrheal disease (such as ulcerative colitis), is an additional cause of hypoproteinemia that must be treated by the intravenous administration of whole protein, such as plasma or albumin. Hypoproteinemia does not respond to the infusion of amino acids; synthetic processes are little accelerated by the provision of amino acid substrates.

Low Flow States and Shock

Prolonged deficiency of blood flow to tissues and organs constitutes a most important circulatory cause of metabolic deterioration in surgery. Diagnosis of the cause of such a low flow state is an essential preliminary to treatment and is dependent upon the pathologic situation whether bullet wound, peritonitis, ruptured ectopic pregnancy, or undrained abscess. Restoration of lost volume is of course the first priority; if there is no response, further steps are essential. An orderly sequence should be followed. A few general guidelines can be drawn.

The treatment of hypotension, refractory to blood transfusion, falls into 3 stages or "echelons" as follows:

1. One must be assured that volume restoration has indeed been adequate. Measurement of blood volume at the bedside is helpful in this regard, but normal blood volumes are sometimes inadequate, particularly in the face of gram-negative sepsis. Criteria of return to normal effective blood volume are found in the restoration of normal tissue perfusion (skin color and blanching) and oxygenation, as well as the return of urine output. Failing these, more blood must be given. One can guard against overreplacement of blood volume by continuous measurement of the right atrial or central venous pressure via an indwelling cannula led to a water manometer. If venous pressure is elevated, but blood pressure still low, one should consider pericardial disease, pulmonary embolism, myocardial disease and the need for digitalization.

2. If volume has been restored and the low flow state (refractory hypotension with peripheral tissue anoxia) remains obdurate, one next corrects the evidences of physiologic and biochemical deterioration which, in and of itself, promotes the hypotensive state. Some of these can be treated "blindly" in the midnight emergency, without reference to precise measurement. When available, such measurements should be made. The measurement of arterial blood gases, including the hydrogen ion concentration, will show clearly the need for the administration either of fixed base such as sodium bicarbonate or an organic

buffer such as Tris. It is possible for this step alone to reverse the refractory nature of hypotension. The administration of adrenocorticosteroids with or without catechol amines can be carried out over short periods of time without hazard. Response is usually disappointing. However, the finding of many eosinophils present in the peripheral blood smear in the face of shock is virtually diagnostic of adrenal insufficiency, in which case small amounts of steroids will completely reverse the situation.

3. Finally, sepsis alone may cause a prolonged flow-deficiency, and this sepsis in turn may result from the anaerobic conditions of previously oligemic shock. For this reason multiple blood cultures, aggressive antibiotic therapy, and above all surgical drainage or exteriorization of purulent collections are essential.

Before any of these can be effective the surgeon must give careful thought again to *diagnosis*. Only for the laboratory theoretician does shock exist in the abstract; in the patient it is always highly specific, important in its detail and traceable to tissue pathology. Is the low flow state due to peripheral circulatory collapse from hypovolemic causes? Or is this peripheral collapse the result of some quite specific normovolemic lesion? Examples would be bilateral pneumothorax, mediastinal emphysema, pulmonary embolus, pericardial effusion, bloodstream infection—all common causes of hypotension refractory to transfusion and erroneously referred to as "irreversible shock."

ACUTE POST-TRAUMATIC RENAL INSUFFICIENCY: PREVENTION AND TREATMENT

The tissues of the body can be arranged in approximate order of their sensitivity to prolonged anoxia, whether this oxygen lack is of circulatory or ventilatory origin. The brain is the most sensitive, and the heart the next: when these two organs are damaged beyond repair, death ensues. The kidney is the third most vulnerable, but it has a special aspect with relation to survival: namely, that complete destruction of the kidneys, or even their bilateral removal, does not produce death immediately. Thus, after prolonged low flow with poor tissue perfusion, the kidney is severely damaged but remains in the body, in the circulation and unable to achieve its excretory capacity. The anatomic lesion thus produced is acute tubular necrosis. Essential to the production of this condition is a low flow state plus the presentation to the kidney, during its vasoconstricted phase, of a nephrotoxic substance, usually a haem pigment or porphyrin breakdown product.

The prevention of this condition lies in the prevention of the low flow state. The giving of adequate blood transfusion early, the replacement of body fluid losses, and carrying patients to operation with normal body chemistry are all-important in the prevention of renal damage. Once the hypotension has occurred with a threat to the extremely vulnerable renal tubular cell (which receives its arterial supply only after it has passed through the glomerulus), there are several things that can be done to help the kidney. First is the presentation of a slow but continuous load of an osmotic diuretic such as mannitol. Urea is also effective, but because of the fact that it is back-diffused in the proximal renal tubule, it is not quite as active as an osmotic diuretic. The function of mannitol in this situation is primarily to maintain a flow of water down the renal tubule. Just why this should help such a kidney is not wholly clear; there are some who think that the mere filling of this tubule with obligatory water held there by a nonreabsorbed crystalloid solute prevents its collapse with damage to the cells around it. Other more subtle effects are possible, such as the withdrawing into the tubular lumen of toxic substances, or the maintenance in solution within the tubular lumen of porphyrin breakdown products. An additional effect of mannitol in this situation is the maintenance of a high glomerular filtration rate. It has now been shown that an infusion of mannitol can increase glomerular filtration rate even in the face of a continued low blood volume. Mannitol is usually infused as a 10 per cent solution giving about 1,000 ml. over the course of 3 hours. There is some evidence that continued mannitol administration over a period of several days produces histologic changes in the renal tubular cell though there is recent animal evidence that this change does not alter renal function.

Of equal importance in the oliguric patient

is the demonstration that he does not suffer from ureteral obstruction or direct damage to the kidney. The retrograde pyelogram, with or without an intravenous pyelogram, is an essential part of the initial handling of such patients.

The management of established renal failure is beyond the scope of this chapter. But an understanding of post-traumatic starvation is fundamental to proper management. The gain of calories through oxidation of fat, the release of new endogenous water and its excretion, the effect of pulmonary water loss on serum tonicity, and the release of potassium to the extracellular fluid are all features of post-traumatic metabolism which are especially important in renal failure. The use of hemodialysis, with or without pressure filtration, the use of peritoneal dialysis, and such simple measures as gastrointestinal suction have all resulted in an increased survival rate.

POTASSIUM LOSS AND ALKALOSIS

The loss of potassium for a few days after surgery is ordinarily well tolerated, if not unduly prolonged: the serum potassium remains normal or becomes slightly elevated. If loss is longer in duration (i.e., no oral intake with continued renal and fecal loss) then potassium is easily given in small amounts.

Such ease of treatment is not the case if the patient is also losing gastrointestinal hydrogen ion and is developing a "subtraction" metabolic alkalosis. Such an example is commonly found in surgery for pyloric obstruction. The potassium concentration drops precipitously after operation; the aldosterone-like effects of operation have produced retention of sodium (with an acid urine) and loss of potassium with a resultant severe exacerbation in alkalosis and a lowering of the serum potassium due both to the alkalosis and to the increased rate of potassium excretion.

This clinical and chemical syndrome is characterized by fever, lethargy, distention and absent peristalsis with a high bicarbonate, low potassium, normal sodium and a low chloride in the plasma. Typical pH values are 7.52 to 7.56. Electrocardiographic changes are marked and constitute a valuable warning sign and therapeutic guide, even though they are not a direct index of the serum potassium concentration.

If the patient is alkalotic prior to surgery, the most important step is prevention of hypokalemia by administration of potassium and correction of the alkalosis prior to surgery. The administration of a 1 per cent ammonium chloride solution in the amount of 500 to 1,000 ml. suffices to lower the bicarbonate approximately 4 to 8 mM./L. in a normal-sized adult. Such therapy (plus KCl at 80 to 160 mM./day) should be continued until normal acid-base balance is restored, preferably before operation. Then, after operation, potassium chloride therapy should be resumed until acid-base balance, dietary intake and serum potassium are shown to be maintained and normal.

OTHER ACID-BASE CHALLENGES; LOW-FLOW ACIDOSIS WITH HYPERCAPNIA

Post-traumatic alkalosis is the most common acid-base defect seen on a general surgical ward. It is due to a combination of hyperventilation with hypercapnia (often caused by a mild continuing ventilatory anoxia) with superimposed oxidation of the transfused sodium citrate to sodium bicarbonate. Aiding and abetting both of these mechanisms is the aldosterone effect, which, initiated by the same volume-reduction that caused the giving of transfusions in the first place, interferes with the excretion of sodium bicarbonate in an alkaline urine. Treatment is usually unnecessary; such patients sometimes have such a severe alkalosis that it interferes with normal tissue oxygenation; lacticacidemia results.

Of far greater importance are the acidoses. The treatment of renal acidosis, diabetic acidosis and acidosis due to chronic pulmonary insufficiency is beyond the scope of this chapter, though they are major problems in surgical care.

By far the most dangerous acidosis is the mixed hypoxic and respiratory acidosis resulting from poor tissue perfusion with super-added pulmonary disease. In most instances the low tissue perfusion exists initially with good or supernormal ventilation and a mild oxygen desaturation. A common combination is a normal or slightly low pH, with a mounting lactate level (3 to 12 mM./L.) and a hypocapnia (pCO_2 25 mm./Hg) as indicator of the hyperventilation. This might be described as ventilatory compensation for hypoxic acidosis. That the compensation is not adequate is indicated by the persistently low pH at 7.30 to 7.35. This is a common situation seen in patients in shock in the emergency ward, in the intensive care unit and after extensive surgical operations. The anesthetist regularly produces hypocapnia with bag-breathing or assisted ventilation. It is evident at a glance that the hypocapnia (which can be reversed in just a few breaths) is the only thing that is holding this pH up at presentable levels. As soon as the carbon dioxide tension crosses the line of 40 mm./Hg (as, for example, with return to room air after ventilation under anesthesia) the pH will fall. Then, if there is any true ventilatory defect as is seen with the recently operated chest, pneumothorax, atelectasis or acute obliterative pneumonitis, and the pCO_2 rises across the 50 or 60 intercept, then arterial blood pH falls rapidly and dangerously.

This mounting acidosis, now due to the superimposition of hypercapnia on a low perfusion lacticacidosis, interferes with myocardial function to a remarkable degree. The heart will not respond to catechol amines in an acid environment; circulatory deterioration becomes a "vicious cycle" as acidosis mounts in the low flow state. The terminal event is a prolonged hypotensive period, refractory to blood transfusion. The heart rate, initially so rapid as to interfere with cardiac output, progressively slows down. In its initial slowing it may mislead the surgeon who believes that the worrisome tachycardia has now departed and that the patient is returning to a more normal heart rate. A glance at the reticulated mottling in the skin, the sluggish cerebral responses, and the poor urine output will suffice to show him that this slowing of the heart is due to the fact that the heart is no longer responding to the challenge of its fluid environment; and it is failing to respond because of the acidosis in which the myocardial fibers are bathed. The heart slows; the ventricular complexes become spread. The S-T segment becomes lowered, as evidence of subendocardial ischemia, and finally a cardiac arrest occurs as the terminal event. Such an arrest is difficult or impossible to resuscitate.

Therapy of this train of events depends entirely upon an understanding the physiologic and biochemical sequence. Proper ventilation, proper volume-restoration, the use of organic buffers, assisted ventilation, dialysis and intra-arterial transfusion all have their place in specific cases. Though often referred to as "shock," it is quite evident that the pathogenic mechanisms involved are far more subtle than low blood volume or pressure alone. This is a challenge for which the Darwinian survival mechanism has evolved no proper solution. Surgical therapy is challenged to the utmost, and survival is attained only when treatment is prompt and accurate.

POST-TRAUMATIC PULMONARY INSUFFICIENCY

With improved methods for the treatment of low-flow states, prolonged hypotension and renal failure, there is emerging a *pulmonary lesion* as the cause of death in those severely injured patients who later die. It is estimated in both the civilian and military that, of late deaths after severe injury and an established low-flow state, about one third are due to direct visceral injury (brain or heart), about one third are due to blood-stream invasion with pathogenic gram-negative bacilli, and about one third are due to progressive pulmonary insufficiency.

The pathogenesis of this pulmonary lesion is multiple and may be divided into those agencies which arrive at the lung via the circulation and those which arrive via the airway. Bloodborne pathogenic factors include fluid overload, over-transfusion, multiple small emboli from diffuse intravascular coagulation, platelet emboli, emboli of particulate matter from intravenous infusions, bacteremia from septic wounds, and vasoactive substances (such as serotonin) affecting the pulmonary circulation. Agencies which damage the lungs via the airway include particularly traumatic wet lung, the aspiration of gastric contents, the introduction of bacteria and excessive drying by premature tracheostomy or improper management of endotracheal intubation and most particularly the pulmonary toxicity of oxygen.

Patients who develop severe pulmonary problems after injury characteristically pass through four phases: an initial phase of acute injury with prolonged inappropriate hyperventilation with hypocapnia and borderline oxygenation; a second phase of recovery from the initial injury with improved circulation but with increasing evidences of pulmonary insufficiency characterized by inability to oxygenate on high administered oxygen tensions; the third phase, following the institution of tracheostomy and often characterized by increasing pulmonary shunt; and finally a fourth phase, in which death occurs by cessation of the heart beat in a hypoxic and acidotic fluid environment.

Inability to oxygenate on high inspired oxygen tension is characteristic of pulmonary veno-arterial admixture or "physiologic shunt." This is due to the passage of large amounts of blood (up to 50% of cardiac output) through bronchopulmonary segments that are not ventilated. The primary cause of this shunt is to be found in fluid-filled alveoli, some small areas of atelectasis (though atelectasis is not a common feature of this pathology) and in the greatly thickened blood-air barrier seen under electron microscopy.

The causes of this change in the blood-air barrier include any agency that produces pulmonary edema and an alteration in the alveolar lining cells. Most prominent among these is oxygen. The administration of 100 per cent oxygen to human subjects for 12 hours or more results in increasing oxygen desaturation. In experimental animals death ensues at 30 to 50 hours with a typically progressive veno-arterial admixture, pulmonary shunting, and the development of a hyaline membrane. The loss of the normal surface lining of the alveoli, with its surface-tension-lowering effect is but one feature of the pathologic physiology of this syndrome. It nonetheless appears to account for the loss of pulmonary compliance and some of the difficulty in ventilation.

A most effective approach to this syndrome is its prevention through the careful use of intravenous fluids, and the avoidance of premature tracheostomy or prolonged high oxygen tensions in the airway. Unlike patients with posttraumatic renal insufficiency who arrive at the hospital with the kidney lesion fully developed and pose a therapeutic problem in its most severe form, most injured patients arrive with pulmonary tissue still intact. The prevention of this lesion is extremely effective and with an increasing understanding of its cause it should disappear almost completely from the surgical scene, leaving behind only those patients in whom direct pulmonary injury or overwhelming infection causes a pulmonary death.

SUMMARY

In no other field of medical work are normal physiologic mechanisms more important to survival than in the recovery of surgical patients. These are normal responses to injury, the Darwinian product of epochs of vertebrate evolution. Modern surgical care in all its aspects is based on a growing knowledge of biochemistry and metabolism in the patient threatened by physical injury, volume-reduction, acid-base imbalance and starvation. Study of this field of biochemistry and metabolism is the first step in surgical education, and its practice is the basis of much that is done both at the operating table and at the bedside.

BIBLIOGRAPHY

Albright, F.: Cushing's syndrome: its pathological physiology, its relationship to the adrenogenital syndrome, and its connection with the problem of the reaction of the body to injurious agents ("alarm reaction" of Selye). Harvey Lecture, 38:123, 1942-1943.

Barry, K. G., Mazze, R. I., and Schwartz, F. D.: Prevention of surgical oliguria and renal-hemodynamic suppression by sustained hydration. New Eng. J. Med., 270:1371, 1964.

Cannon, W. B.: Bodily Changes in Pain, Hunger, Fear and Rage. New York, Appleton, 1915.

Coller, F. A., Campbell, K. N., Vaughan, H. H., Iob, L. V., and Moyer, C. A.: Postoperative salt intolerance. Ann. Surg., 119:533, 1944.

Cuthbertson, D. P.: Observations on the disturbance of metabolism produced by injury to the limbs. Quart. J. Med., N.S. 1:233, 1932.

Dagher, F. J., Lyons, J. H., Ball, M. R., and Moore, F. D.: Hemorrhage in normal man. II. The effects of mannitol on plasma volume and body water dynamics following acute blood loss. Ann. Surg., 163:505, 1966.

Dudley, H. A., Boling, E. A., Lequesne, L. P., and Moore, F. D.: Studies on antidiuresis in surgery: effects of anesthesia, surgery and posterior pituitary antidiuretic hormone on water metabolism in man. Ann. Surg., 140:354, 1954.

Franksson, C., Gemzell, C. A., and von Euler, U. S.: Cortical and medullary adrenal activity in surgical and allied conditions. J. Clin. Endocr., 14:608, 1954.

Gamble, J. L.: Chemical Anatomy, Physiology and

Pathology of Extracellular Fluid. Cambridge, Mass., Harvard University Press, 1952.

Gold, N. I., Smith, L. L., and Moore, F. D.: Cortisol metabolism in man: observations of pathways, pool sizes of metabolites and rates of formation of metabolites. J. Clin. Invest., 38:2238, 1959.

Hammond, W. G., Aronow, L., and Moore, F. D.: Studies in surgical endocrinology. III. Plasma concentrations of epinephrine and nor-epinephrine in anesthesia, trauma and surgery, as measured by a modification of the method of Weil-Malherbe and Bone. Ann. Surg., 144:715, 1936.

Howard, J. E.: Protein metabolism during convalescence after trauma. Recent studies. Arch. Surg., 50:106, 1945.

Hume, D. M.: The role of the hypothalamus in the pituitary adrenal cortical response to stress. J. Clin. Invest., 28:790, 1949.

———: The neuro-endocrine response to injury: present status of the problem. Ann. Surg., 138:548, 1953.

Ingle, D. J., Ward, E. O., and Kuizenga, M. H.: The relationship of the adrenal glands to changes in urinary non-protein nitrogen following multiple fractures in the force-fed rat. Am. J. Physiol., 149:510, 1947.

Kinney, J. M., and Moore, F. D.: Carbon balance. A clinical approach to energy exchange. Surgery, 40:15, 1956.

LeQuesne, L. P., and Lewis, A. A. G.: Postoperative water and salt retention. Lancet, 1:153, 1953.

Lister, J., McNeill, I. F., Marshall, V. C., Plzak, L. F., Jr., Dagher, F. J., and Moore, F. D.: Transcapillary refilling after hemorrhage in normal man: basal rates and volumes; effect of norepinephrine. Ann. Surg., 158:698, 1963.

Litwin, M. S., Panico, F. G., Rumini, C., Harken, D. E., and Moore, F. D.: Acidosis and lacticacidemia in extracorporeal circulation: the significance of perfusion flow rate and the relation to preperfusion respiratory alkalosis. Ann. Surg., 149:188, 1959.

Litwin, M. S., Smith, L. L., and Moore, F. D.: Metabolic alkalosis following massive transfusion. Surgery, 45:805, 1959.

Lown, B., Black, H., and Moore, F. D.: Digitalis, electrolytes and the surgical patient. Am. J. Cardiol., 6:309, 1960.

Lyons, J. H., Jr., and Moore, F. D.: Posttraumatic alkalosis: incidence and pathophysiology of alkalosis in surgery. Surgery, 60:93, 1966.

Merrill, J. P., Levine, H. D., Somerville, W., and Smith, S., III: Clinical recognition and treatment of acute potassium intoxication. Ann. Int. Med., 33:797, 1950.

Moore, F. D.: Bodily changes in surgical convalescence. I. The normal sequence—observations and interpretations. Ann. Surg., 137:289, 1953.

———: Hormones and Stress. Endocrine Changes After Anesthesia, Surgery and Unanesthetized Trauma in Man. *In* Recent Progress in Hormone Research. New York, Acad. Press, 13:511, 1957.

———: Metabolism in trauma. The meaning of definitive surgery. The wound, the endocrine glands and metabolism, Harvey Lectures, Series 52, 1956-1957. New York, Acad. Press, p. 74, 1958.

———: Common patterns of water and electrolyte change in injury, surgery and disease. New Eng. J. Med., 258:277, 325, 377, 427, 1958.

———: Metabolic Care of the Surgical Patient. Philadelphia, W. B. Saunders, 1959.

———: Volume and tonicity in body water (Baxter Lecture). Surg., Gynec. Obstet., 114:276, 1962.

———: Tris buffer, mannitol, and low viscous dextran. Three new solutions for old problems. Surg. Clin. N. Am., 43:577, 1963.

———: The effects of hemorrhage on body composition. (Annual Discourse, Mass. Med. Soc.). New Eng. J. Med., 273:567, 1965.

Moore, F. D., and Ball, M. R.: The Metabolic Response to Surgery. Springfield, Charles C Thomas, 1952.

Moore, F. D., Dagher, F. J., Boyden, C. M., Lee, C. J., and Lyons, J. H.: Hemorrhage in normal man: I. The distribution and dispersal of saline infusions following acute blood loss (clinical kinetics of blood volume support). Ann. Surg., 163:485, 1966.

Moore, F. D., Haley, H. B., Bering, E. A., Jr., Brooks, L., and Edelman, I. S.: Further observations on total body water. II. Changes of body composition in disease. Surg., Gynec. Obstet., 95:155, 1952.

Moore, F. D., Lyons, J. H., Pierce, E., Morgan, A. P., Drinker, P., MacArthur, J., and Dammin, G.: Post-Traumatic Pulmonary Insufficiency. Pathophysiology and Prevention of Respiratory Failure after Surgical Operations, Trauma, Hemorrhage, Burns and Shock. Philadelphia, W. B. Saunders, 1969.

Moore, F. D., Olesen, K. H., McMurrey, J. D., Parker, H. V., Ball, M. R., and Boyden, C. M.: The Body Cell Mass and Its Supporting Environment. Body Composition in Health and Disease. Philadelphia, W. B. Saunders, 1963.

Moore, F. D., Steenburg, R. W., Ball, M. R., Wilson, G. M., and Myrden, J. A.: Studies in surgical endocrinology. I. The urinary excretion of 17-hydroxycorticoids, and associated metabolic changes, in cases of soft tissue trauma of varying severity and in bone trauma. Ann. Surg., 141:145, 1955.

Moyer, C. A.: Acute temporary changes in renal function associated with major surgical procedures. Surgery, 27:198, 1950.

Rabelo, A., Brady, M. P., Litwin, M. S., and Moore, F. D.: A comparison of several osmotic agents in hydropenic and hydropenic-DOCA-pitressin-treated dogs. J. Surg. Res., 5:237, 1963.

Rabelo, A., Litwin, M. S., Brady, M. P., and Moore, F. D.: A comparison of the effects of diuretic agents in the dog after acute hemorrhage. Surg., Gynec. Obstet., 115:657, 1962.

Rhoads, J. E.: Protein nutrition in surgical patients; collective review. Int. Abstr. Surg., 94:417, 1952.

Roberts, K. E., Randall, H. T., Sanders, H. L., and Hood, M.: Effects of potassium on renal tubular reabsorption of bicarbonate. J. Clin. Invest., 34:666, 1955.

Skillman, J. J., Olson, J. E., Lyons, J. H., and Moore, F. D.: The hemodynamic effect of acute blood loss in normal man, with observations on the effect of the Valsalva maneuver and breath holding. Ann. Surg., 166:713, 1967.

Skillman, J. J., Lauler, D. P., Hickler, R. B., Lyons, J. H., Olson, J. E., Ball, M. R., and Moore, F. D.: Hemorrhage in normal man: Effects on renin, cortisol, aldosterone and urine composition. Ann. Surg., 166:865, 1967.

Smith, L. L., and Moore, F. D.: Refractory hypotension in man: is this "irreversible shock"? Clinical and biochemical observations. New Eng. J. Med., 267:733, 1962.

Smith, L. L., Williamson, A. W. R., Livingstone, J. B., Butterfield, D. E., and Moore, F. D.: The effect of acute addition acidosis on experimental hemorrhagic hypotension. S. Forum, 9:43, 1959.

Steenburg, R. W., Lennihan, R., and Moore, F. D.: Studies in surgical endocrinology. II. The free blood 17-hydroxycorticoids in surgical patients; their relation to urine steroids, metabolism and convalescence. Ann. Surg., 143:180, 1956.

Walker, W. F., Reutter, F. W., Zileli, M. S., Friend, D., and Moore, F. D.: Effects of infusion of norepinephrine on blood hormone levels, electrolytes and water excretion in man. J. Surg. Res., 1:272, 1961.

Walker, W. F., Zileli, M. S., Reutter, F. W., Shoemaker, W. C., Friend, D., and Moore, F. D.: Adrenal medullary secretion in hemorrhagic shock. Am. J. Physiol., 197:773, 1959.

Wilson, G. M., Edelman, I. S., Brooks, L., Myrden, J. A., Harken, D. E., and Moore, F. D.: Metabolic changes associated with mitral valvuloplasty. Circulation, 9:199, 1954.

CHAPTER 17

C. A. MOYER, M.D.

Burns and Cold Injury

Classification
Historical Considerations
Burn Shock
Therapeutic Principles
Burn Sepsis
Other Disturbances Associated With Burns
Results of Treatment

CLASSIFICATION

Before the discovery of the principles of cutaneous grafting the care of those injured by heat devolved largely upon doctors of physic, the equivalent of the internist of today, and during the latter part of the 19th century much of the treatment was by the dermatologist. The discoveries that led to reconstructive surgery were the primary forces finally effecting the entry of the surgeon as the therapist of thermal and radiational injury.

Burns were once classified into 7 categories or degrees. Today some still employ a 4-degree classification, but lately a simpler one is being adopted. The 4-degree classification is:

    1st degree—erythema
    2nd degree—death of epidermis while viable epidermal appendages remain within the dermis
    3rd degree—death of the epidermis and all of its appendages in the dermis
    4th degree—carbonification of the part.

The classification more recently advanced by surgeons is:

    Partial-thickness cutaneous injury
    Full-thickness cutaneous injury

Figure 17-1 shows the older and the newer classifications diagrammatically.

Often one is unable to determine for weeks whether a burn or a scald is a partial-thickness or a full-thickness cutaneous injury. It has been said that blistering denotes partial thickness; in truth, it is a good sign of partial-thickness injury should the person have been scalded, but it is often misleading should the injury have been caused by more than a momentary contact with hot metal, glowing coals, or flaming clothing. Under the latter circumstances the epidermal temperatures tend to rise above 100° C., and steam blisters may form while at the same time the dermis and all the epidermal appendages are killed. In other words, blistering may occur with a full-thickness injury. However, blistering after contact with hot water usually signifies that those parts of the hair follicles and the sweat glands lying below the superficial dermal capillaries are viable, and from them the epithelium will regenerate: a partial-thickness injury. The formation of blisters within or about a thermal cutaneous injury 12 or more hours after the exposure to heat is a sign of an infection within the dermis. Such belatedly formed blisters often contain cocci, either staphylococci or streptococci, or both.

The retention of tactile and superficial pain sensibility (pin prick) and capillary pressure blanching in an area of burn are indicative of a partial-thickness injury. The combination of loss of tactile and pain sense to pin prick, the absence of pressure-blanching, the loss of cutaneous pliability, and visibility of small veins through translucent burned skin are indicative of a very deep partial or full-thickness burn or scald. However, a burn having all of the characteristics of a partial-thickness one, when first seen, may turn out subsequently to involve the whole thickness of the epidermis and its appendages, with infection and other factors operating after the heat load has been dissipated, thus converting a partial-thickness into a full-thickness injury.

In a few words, the depth of a burn or a scald cannot be estimated accurately for days or even weeks after the injury; and the estimation of the depth of the burn soon after its sufferance often can be no more than an in-

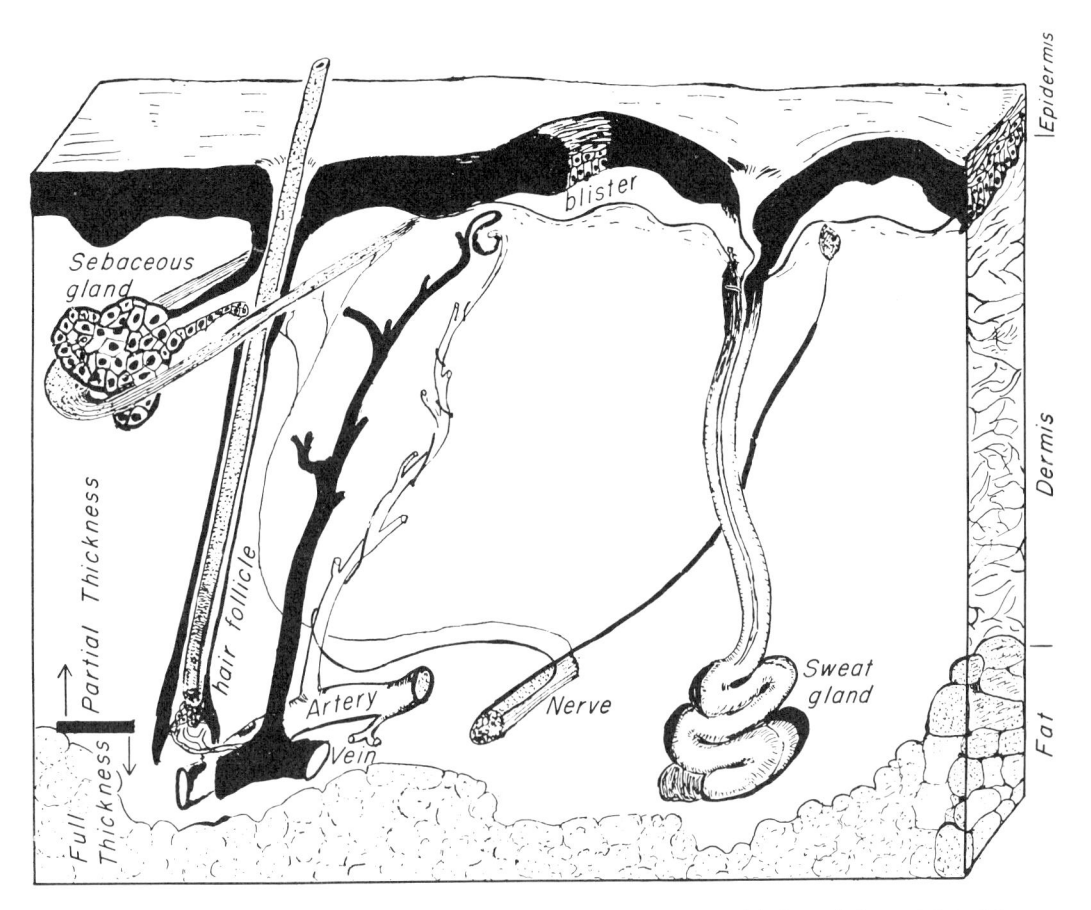

Fig. 17-1. The area of the skin is about 0.25 square meters at birth, and from 1.5 to 1.9 square meters in adults. A standard formula for the calculation of surface area in man is as follows: surface area in square centimeters = kilo-weight$^{0.425}$ × centimeter height$^{0.725}$ × 71.84.

The skin is primarily divisible into: (1) a superficial cellular ectodermal derivative, the epidermis and its appendages (sweat glands, hair follicles and sebaceous glands) and (2) a mesodermal derivative, the dermis. These two layers are underlaid by a layer of adipose tissue of variable thickness. The skin's thickness (epidermis and dermis) varies from 0.5 mm. over the eyelids and the ears to 3 to 6 mm. on the soles and the palms. The entire organ, exclusive of the fat layer, constitutes from 14 to 17 per cent of a lean adult's weight. In other words, it is one of the largest organs of the body. The thickness of the epidermis, exclusive of that on the palms and the soles, which is very thick (0.5 to 0.8 mm.), varies between 60 and 120 microns (0.06 to 0.12 mm.). A remarkably tough organ for all its thinness!

The cellular layer of the epidermis is overlaid by a fibrous macromolecular membrane, the stratum corneum. It is about 40 to 60 μ thick over most of the body and is composed of keratin fibers about 30 angstroms in diameter, surrounded by a lipid monolayer. The stratum corneum is remarkably impervious to water, water vapor, and diatomic gases such as oxygen and nitrogen. Only 5 to 10 ml. of water pass through a square meter of the lipified keratin membrane per hour under a vapor pressure gradient of 26 to 35 mm. Hg. Removal of the lipid from the stratum corneum is attended by a 30-to 60-fold increase in the rate of flux of water through it.

Delipification destroys the water-vapor-holding function of the stratum corneum, rendering the whole skin no more resistant to the passage of water vapor than a sheet of Whatman No. 2 filter paper or a piece of woman's nylon hose. Dehydrated but fully lipified human skin effects so little resistance to the passage of diatomic gases that, with a pressure gradient of

(*Continued*)

telligent guess. If, with the passage of 2 to 15 weeks of time, a burn heals from the base without grafting, it was a partial-thickness injury. If the injured skin, the eschar, separates or is separable from the living tissue below the dermis, exposing fat, muscle, or bone, the injury was a full-thickness one.

The amount of heat needed to cause a full-thickness injury to the skin of man is remarkably small. Water at 85° C. will kill the whole skin in 10 seconds.[11, 21] The chemical changes within the cells of the skin accompanying heating just capable of killing it are unknown.[2, 34] Skin just killed by heat takes up the dyes employed by histologists in a fairly normal fashion for a day or two, and then the nucleoli, the chromatin granules and the nuclei disintegrate. However, the activity of a number of the enzymes involved in the Krebs cycle, namely, succinic dehydrogenase and fumarase, decreases markedly in thermally injured skin very soon after the burn and long before any microscopic cellular changes have taken place.[5] The taking of multiple minute biopsies from burned skin and staining sections of them with tetrazolium dyes promises an earlier objective differentiation between partial and full-thickness burns than is now possible.

The formulation of therapeutic technics directed toward the reversal of heat injury to cells and extracellular macromolecules, such as collagen, must await the time when the chemical changes associated with the heating of skin are known specifically and in detail. Until that day arrives, the primary objective of the treatment of the wound itself is—*above all, do no harm*. This adage has not always been followed in the recent past. Although the intellectual attitudes of Aristotle and Galen presumably have been our guides for centuries, they have been peculiarly ineffectual determinants of the therapy of burns and scalds. Sophisticated witchcraft better characterizes many of the past practices used in the treatment of the wound than does scientific objectivity. Often there has been practically no subjection of impressions regarding the supposed efficacy of a particular medicament or physical act to

---

FIG. 17-1 (*Continued*)
1 atmosphere, a mole of air passes through a square meter of dehydrated skin in 3 minutes. Upon rehydration, this skin is then so resistant to the passage of air that 150 days must pass before a mole of air will have passed through it while a pressure gradient of 1 atmosphere is maintained. In other words, the skin's resistance to the passage of water through it is lipid-dependent, while its resistance to the passage of diatomic gases is hydration-dependent.

Were it not for the remarkable water-holding capacity of the stratum corneum, man could not live in air: vaporizational heat loss would be too great!

The dermis is from 5 to 10 times the thickness of the epidermis.

The epidermis contains no lymphatic or blood capillaries. These structures are contained especially within the superficial part of the dermis, and about the hair papillae, sweat glands, sebaceous glands and arrectores pilorum muscles. The capillaries are relatively few in the skin, numbering only 16 to 65 per square millimeter, while in skeletal muscle they number from 1,000 to 2,000. However, the skin contains numerous arteriolar venous shunts that constitute special structures, the cutaneous neuromyo-arterial glomera, that are important in regulating the radiational heat transfer from the body. When fully open, they are capable of shunting one fifth to one sixth of the resting cardiac output from the arterial to the venous system without passage of the blood through true capillaries.

The structures affected in the old classification of burns are as follows:

First degree: (erythema) minor reversible damage to the epidermis with dilatation of the superficial dermal capillaries.

Second degree: epidermal necrosis; variable dermal necrosis, but leaving viable deep parts of the epidermal appendages (hair follicles and sweat glands).

Third degree: complete epidermal and dermal necrosis (no viable epidermal appendages left).

The simpler classification lumps the older first and second orders into "partial thickness" and changes the term third degree to "full thickness."

The anatomic connotations of the simple classification are self-evident.

The main structural components of the skin, excepting the lymphatics, are shown in this semischematic scale figure. The divisional level between partial and full-thickness injuries is shown in the left lower corner.

controlled experiment, though the steps requisite to the conduct of controlled experiment have been known for more than 7 centuries (Roger Bacon: 1214-1294).

HISTORICAL CONSIDERATIONS

A historical outline* of the therapeutic practices directed toward the treatment of the burn wound during the 19th and the 20th centuries shows how far past therapeutic practices have strayed from the primary aim of *do no harm*.

The treatment of the thermal wound underwent a remarkable change about 1868. Listerism (antisepsis) then seized the minds of physicians. Consequently, one may divide the treatment of burns into two periods—one before Listerism and the other after.

The prevention of putrefaction was attempted before bacteria were discovered to be its cause. A mixture of mercuric chloride and lime water (aqua phagoedenical) was placed on burns in 1835, and even earlier concentrated silver nitrate was recommended. The idea of coagulating the wound arose, and the application of escharotics such as 10 per cent silver nitrate was begun about 1831. Tannic acid in water was employed for the same purpose in 1858, and turpentine in 1866.

The use of a pliable film as a dressing to exclude the "harmful" air was adopted fairly widely on the Continent about 1830 when compound tincture of benzoin was used. In 1858 a mixture of castor oil and collodion was praised, the more especially because the film produced was transparent—*voilà* the modern Aeroplast.

The idea that the burn wound serves as a source of toxins gave rise to the wet dressing. A solution containing sodium and calcium chlorides was recommended by Lisfranc (1835); and Carron oil (a saturated solution of calcium hydroxide in linseed oil) gained so much favor after 1850 that it is used even today.

The bath was begun in 1845, using cold water to draw out the "caloric."† Oils and waxes have been placed on burns at least since Roman times—olive oil, the oil of flax (linseed oil), lard, tallow and beeswax are still used.

The idea that wounds healed the better if the raw area was fed by applying foodstuffs to it led to the application of flour in 1829, because of its high content of "animal gluten," and molasses (treacle) in 1847.

The dry cotton wool dressing was introduced into England from the United States, presumably via Charleston, S. C., between 1827 and 1831. Fine linen (gossamer) had long been placed upon the burns of the well-to-do. Syme[31] extolled the virtues of dry cotton wool in 1833, especially when applied "with a firm degree of pressure"—the pressure dressing.

The exposure of the wound long had been practiced on the Continent but had lost favor during the early 1800's. During the antiseptic, or post-Lister period, no new ideas regarding the care of the wound were introduced, but the emphasis changed. The dry cotton wool pressure dressing employed widely in England, Germany and France between 1830 and 1867 was superseded by a cotton dressing steeped in medicaments poisonous to bacteria and man alike. Physicians caring for burned individuals seemingly became bacteria-slayers and pus-eradicators who considered little that they might also eradicate the man as well as the bacteria.

Phenol first came into favor in 1867, a 14 per cent solution in olive oil. This concentration of phenol kills unburned skin: what did it do to partial-thickness burns? Though the local and the general toxic propensities of phenol were soon recognized, a phenol-containing dressing was highly recommended as late as 1946.

The virtues of a saturated solution of boracic acid were extolled (1876) because it was cheap. It is still poured on dressings, even though it has been known to have poisoned man; toxicologically, bacteria seemingly tolerate it better than human beings.

Iodoform, soon recognized as a readily absorbable local and systemic poison, came along in 1887 and it is still to be found on the dressing carts of hospitals.

Picric acid, a more lethal agent, was dumped and sprayed upon burns after 1901. As recently as 15 years ago, I had the opportunity of seeing an instance of acute picric acid poisoning attributable to the application of Bute-

---

*Constructed from bibliographical references on burns and scalds in the Am. J. Med. Sci., Lancet, J.A.M.A., and Arch. Dermat. Syph. (Vols. 1 to current).

†Caloric—the old term for heat that was supposed to stay in the burned area until withdrawn.

sin picrate to a partial-thickness burn of the chest of a young man. The dressing had been applied by a recent graduate of a medical school.

The soluble sulfonamides superseded picric and boracic acids as locally applied bacteria-killers in 1938, and the biologic antibiotics such as penicillin and neomycin have won out over the sulfonamides since 1943.

The impervious dressing idea was extended after 1867; a combination of varnish, linseed oil, lead protoxide (litharge) and salicylic acid was compounded in 1881. It excluded air, kept the wound greased, killed organisms, and the salicylic acid separated the living tissue from the dead (chemical débridement). Gutta-percha was praised in 1887. During World War I the English and the French almost came to blows over the priority rights to a paraffin dressing.

During the impetus of atomic fear Aeroplast has been born, although Edenbuizen's[6] experiments performed during the 1860's showed clearly that mammals cannot be covered over more than 30 per cent of the body's surface with materials impervious to water vapor, such as gum arabic or linseed oil, without endangering life. In addition, such dressings soon become the outer covering of a large abscess. In spite of this, the search still goes on for an easily applied spray-on dressing material. Should one be discovered that is not toxic and has the physical properties of epidermis, permitting the normal radiation of heat and the staying of the passage of bacteria, water and salts as normal epidermis does, a significant contribution to the treatment of burns will be made. The likelihood of doing this, before much more is known about the skin, is rather remote. To our knowledge such a product is not available yet.

After 1925 the escharotics were raised from the dead. Tannic acid was reintroduced in 1925 when the modern medical tongue extolled it most fluently and persuasively. Somewhat belatedly (1942) it was found to possess few of the virtues claimed for it. In reality it is deadly: it is capable of converting a partial- to a full-thickness injury, it produces an impervious eschar that encloses infection, and it poisons the liver. During the late 1930's it was combined with 10 per cent silver nitrate, an agent long known to be inimical to healing of a wound.

The effects of therapeutic faddism upon the mortality attending thermal injury is shown in part in the plot of the burn mortality rates between 1833 and 1933 in the Glasgow Royal Infirmary (Fig. 17-2). The mortality rate between 1898 and 1910 was 3 times what it had been between 1853 and 1868.

BURN SHOCK

The human being burned or scalded to the extent of more than 70 per cent of the body's surface is in danger of certain death. Fifty years ago a burn covering 65 per cent of the

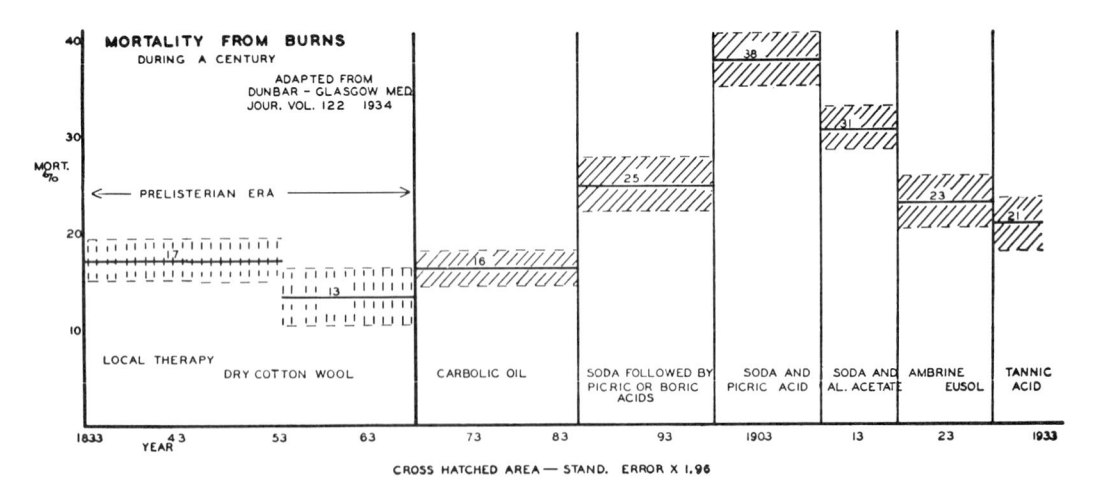

Fig. 17-2. Mortality from burns during a century.

body was with few exceptions fatal within 5 days. Today, one so burned has about 4 chances in 10 of recovering from his injury. Most of this therapeutic advance is attributable to the discovery of the physiologic deformations that follow the injury and the methods of grafting skin successfully.

The notation of the similarity of appearance and mode of death of victims of cholera and fire by Buhl (1855)[3] led to the occasional administration of a solution of sodium chloride to burned individuals after 1850. The efficacy of a saline solution in reversing much of the illness attending cholera had been discovered by Latta[15] in 1831. Later, Tappeiner[32] found the blood of men dead of burns to have a much smaller proportion of water than normal blood. After experimenting with burned rabbits he surmised the water of the blood to have entered the burned tissue because the latter became edematous. It was he who first suggested that the transfusion of serum be employed in the treatment of the systemic illness attending burns and scalds.

Soon thereafter Lesser[16] found the mass of flowing red cells reducible by burning—the mass of red cells recoverable from animals by perfusion of the circulatory system was remarkably diminished after a large burn. Upon discovering that oligocythemia attended thermal injury he suggested that the transfusion of whole blood be entertained as a therapeutic measure.

In brief, most of the basic discoveries ultimately leading to the present treatment of burn shock had been made before 1880.

The general acute physiologic disturbances attending a thermal injury are at least 6 in number: hydrational, circulatory, hematologic, metabolic, endocrine and immunologic.

It is now rather generally agreed that extracellular fluid volume depletion in the unburned tissues and in the blood by virtue of the movement of portions of their extracellular fluid into the edema and blister fluids of the burned parts is the major factor in the genesis of burn shock. This makes the shock attending burns differ somewhat from that attendant upon hemorrhage. With hemorrhagic shock the reduction in the volume of the blood, the oligemia per se, is a most important factor. With burn shock, in addition to the oligemia attendant upon the reduction of the mass of circulating red blood cells and the intravascular extracellular fluid (plasma) volume, the extravascular extracellular fluid volume of the unburned tissues is also reduced; this adds a cellular metabolic factor to the shock. Sodium depletion of vascularly isolated tissues reduces their oxygen consumptions; slight diaphoretic sodium depletion of normal human beings insufficient to produce any great impairment of the person's circulation or work capacity lowers their oxygen consumptions. Sodium depletion of rats and man (see Fig. 17-3) of degree insufficient to lower their blood pressures reduces their metabolisms by as much as 25 per cent and the more especially when sodium depletion is attended by osmolal dilution which is often the situation with burns. In addition, sodium depletion is attended by a rise in the respiratory quotient from 0.72-0.74 to 0.78-0.82. This means that protein, and possibly carbohydrate (glycogen), constitute a greater part of the source of energy during fasting and sodium depletion than they do during fasting and sodium sufficiency. Sodium depletion also affects renal function peculiarly. In a normal man the depletion of about 20 per cent of the body's sodium during 4 days is associated with a 40 to 50 per cent decline in the glomerular filtration rate even when renal blood flow remains near normal.

In other words, with burn shock in which sodium depletion of the unburned parts of the body plays a role, a number of peculiarities that distinguish it from hemorrhagic oligemic shock are to be expected. Furthermore, the direction of treatment only toward the restitution of the plasma and red blood cell volumes with colloid-containing solutions or blood disregards the physiologic importance of extravascular sodium depletion.

Recently, during the examination of the efficacy of lactated Ringer's solution (pH 8.2) in the treatment of burn shock associated with very large burns, observations were made that indicate that extravascular sodium deficiency is the major cause of burn shock and that oligemia is a minor cause.

In this study, which was performed upon human beings with burns covering more than 30 per cent of their bodies,* no glucose solu-

---
* Burn areas that healed in 21 days *were not counted.*

366 Burns and Cold Injury

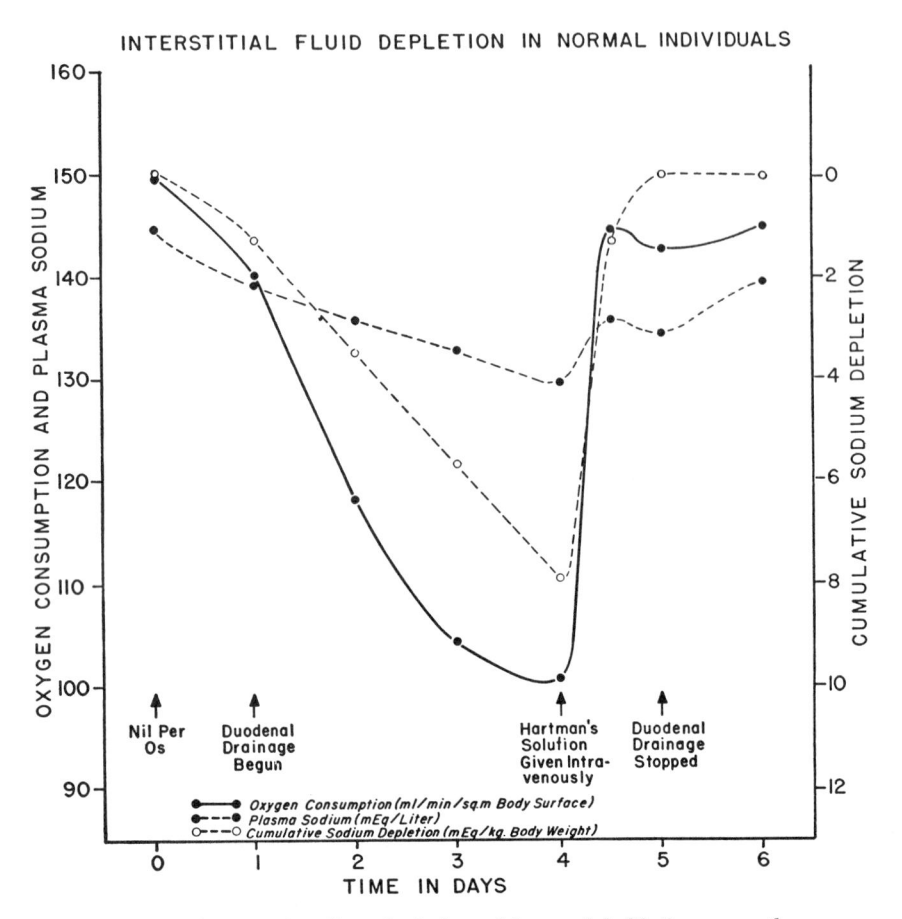

FIG. 17-3. Influence of sodium depletion with osmolal dilution upon the oxygen consumptions of normal men.

tion, no plasma, no dextran, no blood (except for 500 ml. in 1 case, that of D.W.), no solute diuretic, and no water was given during the treatment of shock. No pooled or stored plasma, no dextran, and no solute diuretic was given to anyone at any time during convalescence. There was not a death from shock. There was not a case of renal insufficiency, although, in 2 cases, the hemoglobin concentration in the first 50 ml. of urine excreted after starting treatment exceeded 500 mg. per cent. Pulmonary edema did not occur, although gains in body weight during 48 hours varied between 10 to 42 per cent (see Table 17-1).

Venous pressures were measured hourly during the intravenous infusion of the lactated Ringer's solution. Only in the case of L.S. (85% full-thickness burn) did it rise above normal and then for only an hour. Upon slowing the rate of the infusion, it quickly returned to normal.

The correlation of the changes in hematocrits in these cases with rates of flow of urine (Table 17-2) and signs of shock, such as apathy, disorientation, nausea, vomiting, tachycardia and weakness, demonstrated that recovery from anuria, disorientation, nausea, vomiting and weakness *occurred while the hematocrits rose* significantly in 6 cases out of 10. Assuming that red cells were not being added to the circulation in significant numbers from bone marrow and other places, an assumption that is warranted, because all studies of burned animals (Lesser's being the first) show the opposite, one may conclude that *recovery from burn-shock was effected by the*

TABLE 1. PERCENTILE CHANGES IN BLOOD VOLUME AND WEIGHT GAIN DURING TREATMENT OF BURN SHOCK WITH RINGER'S LACTATE; CALCULATED FROM HEMATOCRITS

CASE AND AGE	SIZE OF DEEP BURN PER CENT B.S.	H_1 HEMATOCRIT AT BEGINNING TREATMENT	H_2 MAXIMUM HEMATOCRIT DURING TREATMENT AT TIME URINE FLOW WAS 25 ML. AN HOUR OR MORE AND SIGNS OF SHOCK WERE ABSENT	CHANGE IN BLOOD VOLUME IN PER CENT OF VOLUME AT START OF SALINE INFUSIONS: $\frac{H_2 - H_1}{H_2} \times 100 =$ % CHANGE IN B.V.	WEIGHT GAIN DURING SHOCK TREATMENT— PER CENT OF BODY WEIGHT
D. H./25	40	50	62	19% decrease	10
W. G./24	30	49	57	14% decrease	8.3
L. T./64	40	61	60	no change	18
S. H./10	65	54	64	15% decrease	24
W. H./4 da.	60	65	45	44% increase	42
L. Bo./6	60	48	45	7% increase	14.5
D. S./57	80	65	64	no change	12
C. St./24	75	50	63	20% decrease	—
L. S./18	85	58	65	10% decrease	26
D. W./25*	70	58	66	12% decrease	18

* H_1 taken as 58 one hour after the transfusion of 500 ml. of blood; consequently, the calculated change in blood volume in this case applies to the time interval between the 6th and the 36th postburn hours.

infusion of lactated Ringer's solution in 6 of 10 cases while hematocrits were rising and oligemia was increasing. In this series of cases, the percentile changes in blood volume, calculated from changes in hematocrits that occurred while recovery from burn shock was effected with lactated Ringer's solution, are tabulated in Table 17-1. Only in 2 cases—one a child 4 days old (W.H.), and the other a child of 6 years (L.Bo.)—did the hematocrit and the oligemia decrease significantly during recovery from burn shock; in 2 cases (L.T. and D.S.) the hematocrit did not change, and in the other 6 cases it increased significantly, indicating that decreases in blood volume of from 7 to 20 per cent took place while all signs of shock disappeared.

The lack of correlation between the physical incapacity manifest by the burned individuals treated with lactated Ringer's solution and the high hematocrits indicative of increasing oligemia is illustrated in Figure 17-4. This photograph of a young man with deep burns covering 50 per cent of the body was taken 18 hours and 30 minutes after the infusion of the saline solution was begun; 8,825 ml. had been given intravenously during 14 hours when the intravenous catheter was removed and full dependence placed upon the drinking of a hypotonic saline solution. He had drunk 1,400 ml. of this before the photograph was taken. He had eaten a good breakfast at 8:30 A.M., when the hematocrit was 58 (it was 49 when treatment was begun). He ate most of a regular diet lunch at 1:00 P.M., when the hematocrit was 60. The photograph was taken at 2:00 P.M., when the hematocrit was 62. He sat up unaided and was not faint or dizzy.

These observations and correlations prove that oligemia is not the sole cause of burn shock and, indeed, indicate that it may be only a minor causative factor, the more especially with burns smaller than 50 per cent of body surface, because fair restoration of physical capacity, sense of well-being, renal function, and vascular sufficiency were attainable in severely burned human beings by providing only extracellular salts and water in amounts

TABLE 17-2

Case		0	3	6	9	12	15	18	21	24	27	30	33	36	39	42	45	48	51	54	57	60	Deep Burn* % B.S.	Wound Treatment
D.H.	UV/h	+	35		22	25	50					34		55		45							40	AgNO$_3$ wet dressing
	Hct	50	58			58		60	62			60					52		41					
W.G.	UV/h	47	35	95	136	88	113	85	120	73	105	150											30	Oleic acid
	Hct	49 55	57			50		51									53							
L.T.	UV/h	+	37				34			33			28		23			36		36			40	Oleic acid
	Hct	61	67				60								53			53						
S.H.	UV/h	O						58 68	85	70		51 43	40 40 38										65	AgNO$_3$ wet dressing
	Hct	54					60		64						55					52				
W.H.	UV/h	O	10	22		15		27		23			32			40				35		35	60	AgNO$_3$ wet dressing
	Hct	65 64	61			50		45		41			40										
L.Bo.	UV/h	+ 18		24				25			16			21		55		44			44		60	Locke's bath
	Hct	48				53		45						38	39					39		34	
D.S.	UV/h	O	66 53	35			15 30	14	44 22	10		24 30	20										80	Oleic acid
	Hct	65	64					62										62						
C.St.	UV/h	O		53				94		23			45			52		31		50			75	AgNO$_3$ wet dressing
	Hct	50	53		56					62								63						
L.S.	UV/h	O	41	21	27 26	43	35	40 46		50			73 78	82	90 71								85	AgNO$_3$ wet dressing
	Hct	58 56	55		58 62	65				62		60	60					51						
D.W.	UV/h	O	45		34				35			59		61			60			54		59	70	AgNO$_3$ wet dressing
	Hct	51	58		61							66			64					57				

UV/h — urine flow, ml. per hour,   + — very slow urinary excretion before treatment
Hct — Peripheral hematocrit   O — anuria before treatment
All cases were adults except W.H. (4 days old), L.Bo.(6 years old) and S.H. (10 years old)

*Minor injuries (burns that healed in 21 days) are excluded from the area estimates

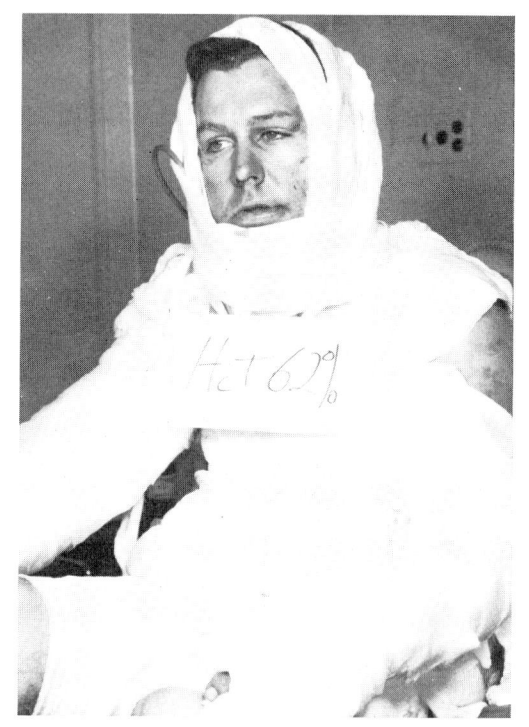

FIG. 17-4. Case D. H. (40% burn). The photo was taken 18 hours and 30 minutes after the treatment of shock with lactated Ringer's solution was begun.

that, in most instances, did not effect appreciable reductions in hematocrits.

They further indicate that much of the physiologic derangement making up burn shock is related to direct cellular effects of sodium deficit in unburned tissues and not to a reduction of minute volume flow of blood secondary to oligemia. For, if this was not true, how could one account for such happenings, as in another case (L.S.) with deep burns covering 85 per cent of the body? He was in profound shock with a hematocrit of 58, and, after 20,900 ml. of lactated Ringer's solution had been given intravenously during 30 hours, the hematocrit was 60. However, when the hematocrit was 60, there were no clinical signs of shock, and the cardiac output was a normal 4.84 liters per min. with a C.I. of 2.66 L. min.$^{-1}$ M^{-2}. If oligemia was the cause of the shock manifested with a hematocrit of 58, he should have been no better 30 hours later when the hematocrit was 60 and the oligemia no less. This is not surprising—cardiac output and minute volume flow of blood do not decrease significantly in recumbent man until total blood volume has been reduced one third or the venous blood volume has been reduced 50 per cent. In this case, even should 20 per cent of the red cells have been sequestered or destroyed during the burning, while his normal hematocrit was 45 per cent, the oligemia represented by the hematocrit of 58 would just be attaining a level that might produce peripheral circulatory insufficiency. The variable in the case is not oligemia; it is the mass of sodium salts and water in the *extravascular compartment*. The oligemia was unaltered by the addition of sodium to the body, but shock disappeared. Therefore, the shock must have been related to the extravascular sodium deficit in unburned tissues and not to the oligemic intravascular sodium deficit, which was not altered by the treatment.

BUFFERED SALINE SOLUTIONS IN TREATMENT OF BURN SHOCK

During the past decade well-controlled investigations upon burned anesthetized animals[28] and accidentally burned human beings[20, 38] have demonstrated the effectiveness of buffered saline solutions in the treatment of burn shock. As stated previously, the giving of colloid-containing solutions alone or in combination with the buffered saline solutions has not effected demonstrable improvement in the effectiveness of treatment of burn shock over that attainable with the buffered saline solutions alone, *excepting in cases of badly burned children in which there has been a delay of 4 to 6 hours in treatment of shock*. In such cases of belatedly treated children the giving of a colloid-containing solution such as plasma or serum, in addition to the buffered saline solution, significantly increased the victims' chances of survival over that of similarly burned and belatedly treated children given buffered saline solution only.[20]

Should shock be mild or impending, the buffered saline solution (90 to 120 mEq.Na/L.) may be given as a drink; 4 to 5 Gm. of table salt and 1½ Gm. of baking soda (NaHCO$_3$) or sodium citrate dissolved in a quart or a liter of iced water is well taken and is effective in preventing the subsequent appearance of shock, water intoxication and acidosis, provided that it is retained by the patient.

In cases of profound burn shock, nausea and vomiting follow the drinking of anything; evidently, the stomach does not function properly. Consequently, in cases such as these, *no attempt at oral administration of saline should be made;* instead, the buffered saline solution *must be given intravenously* until the shock has been largely overcome; then the oral solution may be used. Hartmann's solution (lactated Ringer's solution pH 8.2) or a saline-bicarbonate solution are superior to any other saline solution for the intravenous treatment of profound burn shock, especially in children, because chloride acidosis does not attend their giving, while it almost always does the administration of large amounts of 0.9 per cent NaCl or unmodified Ringer's solution. (See Chap. 5, Fluid and Electrolytes.)

The giving of the salt solution should be stopped as soon as the burned person begins to eat, a normal flow of urine is established, and the shock period (24 to 36 hours) is passed. Rarely, the wounds continue to weep large quantities of fluid for longer than 24 to 36 hours; in such cases some saline solution should be given orally in addition to food and water until the rapid transudation stops.

Vasoconstrictors and Hydrocortisone in Treatment of Burn Shock

The vasoconstrictors such as ephedrine and norepinephrine have no place in the treatment of burn shock. On the contrary, hydrocortisone may be occasionally very important. The adrenal cortical hormones play an important role in the treatment of shock in persons burned while taking corticoids, burned while chronically addicted to alcohol,* or suffering from thyrotoxicosis or subclinical adrenocortical insufficiency. A burned person in shock who does not respond well to saline or plasma therapy, especially if alcoholic or taking adrenal cortical hormones, should be given 100 to 150 mg. of hydrocortisone intravenously after blood and urine samples have been taken for the ascertainment of the concentration of blood

---

* "Chronic alcholics" behave after trauma as if they suffered from adrenal insufficiency; the concentrations of corticoids in their blood increase very little or not at all after an injury or an operation that, when experienced by normal persons, is followed by an increase in concentration of these substances in the blood of 2- to 5-fold their pre-injury levels.[35]

and urinary corticoids, and eosinophil numbers. A few such doses of corticoids do not constitute any known physiologic hazard to a badly burned person whose adrenals are sufficient, but not giving them to a burned person with insufficient adrenals is catastrophic.

Colloids in Treatment of Burn Shock

Before 1940, the treatment of burn shock consisted of the administration of 0.9 per cent sodium chloride intravenously in relatively small quantities of 1.5 to 3 liters per 24 hours and the transfusion of whole blood in amounts rarely larger than 500 ml. With the development of blood banks during the early 1940's, large quantities of plasma became available. Because it had been realized that fairly large quantities of plasma proteins were lost in burn blisters and into edematous burned tissues, large quantities of plasma were soon being given to very badly burned persons. With the giving of these large amounts of plasma, as much as 50 ml. per kilo of body weight, the mortality from burn shock dropped significantly (see Table 17-7). However, the functional significance of the colloids—serum albumin and serum globin and the carbohydrate polymer dextran—in the treatment of burn shock are still not clear. In untreated, mortally scalded anesthetized animals the plasma protein concentration often rises significantly (1 to 2 Gm.%) before the animal dies. However, in similarly injured animals treated with sodium bicarbonate or sodium lactate buffered sodium chloride or Ringer's solutions (150 mEq.Na/L.) the serum protein concentration usually declines from 1 to 3 Gm. per cent. The addition of species-specific serum in quantities sufficient to maintain the serum proteins of animals treated with the saline solutions did not measurably improve their biologic response to the injury; they died as soon as those treated with the buffered saline solutions alone. However, these experiments may have been too extreme to test the efficacy of colloid in the treatment of burn shock. Earlier, Rosenthal and associates[28] had found that colloid-containing solutions were no more effective in treating burn shock in mice than were the same solutions without colloid in them.

The effects of raising the plasma colloid concentration in sodium-depleted animals are peculiar: all of 40 rats died when acutely depleted of 20 to 24 per cent of their original extracellular fluid while their plasma colloid concentrations were being raised 2 to 4 Gm. per cent with human albumin or acacia; while none of 60 rats died after being depleted of 22 to 26 per cent of their extracellular fluid when no colloid was given to them.[25] Increasing the concentration of albumin in blood changes its characteristics of flow in glass capillaries. The addition of from 1 to 3 Gm. per cent of human albumin to human blood completely changes the relationship of the flowing hematocrit to the static hematocrit in tubes smaller than 200 μ. With normal concentrations of albumin in blood the flowing hematocrit is always lower than the static hematocrit in tubes smaller than 200 μ, but with 1 to 3 added grams of albumin or acacia, the flowing hematocrit becomes higher than the static, and when it does the rate of flow of the blood driven by a constant pressure through the tube declines precipitously. The lower the static hematocrit of the blood, the smaller is the amount of added albumin needed to reverse the relationship of the flowing to the static hematocrit. In other words, the addition of albumin to blood (raising the concentration of albumin) disrupts laminar flow in small tubes and greatly increases the resistance to flow through them. Whether this takes place in the small blood vessels of living mammals is not yet known, but the intense congestion of the lungs, the livers and the spleens, the enormously dilated hearts, the inordinately high hematocrits for the degrees of ECF volume depletion, and the bloody pleural effusions of rats dying with sodium deficiency and supernormal concentrations of albumin or acacia in their bloods, suggest that this phenomenon may take place in small blood vessels as well as in glass tubes.

Recently, various dextrans, when given intravenously in small and large but not in intermediate amounts, have been found to produce massive edema and erythema of paws, snout, ears, genitalia and feet of unanesthetized rats. Antihistamines have no effect on the phenomenon.[13]

In brief, we do not as yet know enough about the physiologic and physical functions of the serum proteins or of the dextrans to use them intelligently in the treatment of burn shock *excepting in the treatment of belatedly treated, badly burned children for whom the addition of serum and plasma to the saline therapy is known to improve the chances of recovery from shock.*

BLOOD TRANSFUSION IN THE TREATMENT OF BURN SHOCK

For a time we believed that the hemolytic destruction of red blood cells and the entrapment of blood in the capillaries of thermally injured tissues played a definite role in genesis of burn shock. This belief was engendered by the discovery that transfusion of both a buffered saline solution and whole blood was the only way that anesthetized dogs, scalded by 30-seconds immersion of the hind legs and the torso up to their scapulae into water at 80° C., could be saved from dying of shock. Actually, the reduction of the circulating red cell mass may amount to one third of the original red cell mass within 1 day after a fire burn of one half of the body's surface.[8] However, Wilson[38] has collected data that indicate that the transfusion of blood is not requisite for the successful treatment of burn shock in man, provided that sodium chloride-sodium bicarbonate or lactate solutions and water are given by appropriate routes and in sufficient quantities. We have since confirmed Wilson's observations in 17 persons, 10 with burns covering 50 to 70 per cent, and 7 covered by burns over 70 to 90 per cent of their body surfaces. Shock was treated successfully with lactated Ringer's solution alone, and no renal failure occurred. However, the transfusion of whole blood or washed red blood cells is important in treating the severely burned person whenever the postburn anemia appears. Postburn anemia occasionally becomes manifest with large deep scalds and burns between the 2nd and the 4th days after the injury. The transfusion of red blood cells then in sufficient quantities to maintain a normal hemoglobin, red count, or hematocrit prevents postburn anemia, and keeps tachycardia at a minimum.

SHOCK TREATMENT BY FORMULA

A number of formulas have been used during the past 20 years as guides for the fluid therapy of burns. Those still extant are modifications of the Evans formula: to wit, the fluids needed during the first 24 hours after a burn are: 1 ml. of plasma, plasma substitute or whole blood and 1 ml. of 0.9 per cent NaCl per kilo for each 1 per cent of body burned, and in addition enough 5 per cent dextrose in water to balance the insensible and urinary losses of water. One half of the estimated fluid is to be given during the first 8 hours, and one quarter of it during each of the 2 succeeding 8-hour periods.

These formulas, like all the others that preceded them, are now relatively useless. Since it was first propounded almost 20 years ago it has been learned that the need for colloid-containing solutions such as blood, plasma, or plasma substitutes in treating burn shock is much smaller than Evans believed it to be. In addition, slightly hypotonic glucose containing buffered salines are now known to be physiologically superior to 0.9 per cent NaCl for the treatment of burn shock. Furthermore, when these slightly hypotonic buffered salines are used there is no need for the 5 per cent glucose in water.

In addition, it has been learned that burns covering less than 20 per cent of the body infrequently produce shock except among infants and very old people. Consequently, if fluid therapy is based on the Evans formula, it will usually lead to indiscriminate overtreatment of persons whose burns cover less than 20 per cent of the body. This means that if the Evans or other formulas are used indiscriminately, about 80 per cent of the burns treated in hospitals in the United States could be overtreated, because 70 per cent of all the burned persons treated in American hospitals have injuries covering 5 to 20 per cent of the body surface. Actually, considering only burns that are judged to be truly serious, namely, those covering 15 to 100 per cent of the body, only 55 per cent of them require more than a liter or two of orally taken buffered saline for supportive fluid therapy, because about 45 per cent of such serious burns cover only 15 to 24 per cent of the body, and shock has never been a major threat to life with burns of this size (see Table 17-7).

Another criticism of the formula is that it may lead to insufficient saline therapy of very large partial-thickness injuries. Large partial-thickness injuries involving the head, the neck, or the genitalia and the perineum swell very rapidly and greatly and may be attended, especially in children, with losses of extracellular fluid that are far larger than the saline replacement recommended in the formulas.

The amounts of interstitial fluid, plasma and analgesics needed to treat burn shock must be gauged by the individual's physiologic response to the physician's ministration. Formulary regulation of the therapy of burn shock is a manifestation of biologic naïveté. *Variance,* not constancy, is characteristic of the reactions of a population parameter to a change in environment. A burn of 30 per cent of the body's surface will be unattended by shock in a few individuals, moderate shock in many, and severe peripheral circulatory failure in some. To give all the same treatment would result in overtreatment of some, adequate therapy of some, and insufficient ministration to others.

Gauging therapy entirely on the basis of the rate of flow of urine disregards the variability of response of the kidneys of traumatized individuals to the administration of fluids. Rarely, some hurt men may excrete as much as 20 ml. of urine per hour while suffering from shock, while others will excrete very little, though they are not in shock. When nature has cast a man, she throws that mold away.

To regulate treatment upon the basis of the hematocrit is improper. Often recovery from burn shock occurs while the hematocrit rises (see Table 17-2).

The repetitive examination of all vital signs while the person is being treated is the only means of regulating therapy to the needs of the individual. The signs of greatest value to the assessment of the therapy of a burned person are: the rate and the character of the pulse; the physical attitude assumed; the sensibility to the injury; hiccoughing and vomiting; the rate of flow of urine; the frequency of drinking; the rate and the character of breathing; the blood pressure; the mental reaction and attitudes, and venous pressure. To illustrate:

Case: a boy of 8 burned over one half of his body by having his clothing catch on fire
First Examination—1 hour after injury
  Pulse 76—and full
  Attitude—quiet and apprehensive, says he has little pain
  Orientation—normal

Respiration—30 per minute, of normal depth
Blood pressure—142/70, venous pressure normal
Urine—catheterized specimen, red, albumin ++
Vomiting—none
Hiccoughing—none
Thirsty and drinking often
SECOND EXAMINATION—2 hours after injury
Pulse—100, bounding
Attitude—threshing about and crying
Orientation—lost
Respiration—16 and deep
Blood pressure—112/40, venous pressure normal
Urine flow in 1 hour, 2 ml. of red albumin-containing urine
Vomiting—once, blood-tinged fluid
Drinking—none
The supportive therapy has been inadequate. The rate at which the lactated Ringer's (Hartmann's) solution is being given needs to be increased.
THIRD EXAMINATION—2 hours and 45 minutes after the injury
Pulse—120, bounding
Attitude—quiet
Orientation—partial return
Respiration—25 and less deep
Blood pressure—90/50, venous pressure normal
Urine flow—15 ml. in 45 minutes, less red, albumin ++
Vomiting—none
Asks for drink
The treatment has changed things for the better, although the pulse rate has quickened, and the blood pressure has fallen. The rate of the infusion is maintained.
FOURTH EXAMINATION—4 hours after injury
Pulse—120, full
Attitude—fidgety and complains of smarting pain
Orientation—normal
Respiration—30
Blood pressure—110/80, venous pressure normal
Urine flow—30 ml. in 1 hour and 15 minutes, albumin +
Vomiting—none
Drinking—buffered saline solution frequently
The individual is now safely alive for the time being and the infusions are slowed.
6 HOURS AFTER INJURY—all signs unchanged, rate of infusion maintained
8 HOURS AFTER INJURY—breathing has speeded, venous pressure has risen, and a few rales are heard—the rate of infusion is to be reduced or stopped and only the buffered saline solution is given to him orally.

GENERAL THERAPEUTIC PRINCIPLES OF WOUND CARE

The primary aim of treatment of the burn wound is the effective substitution for the lost physiologic functions of the thermally injured or killed skin until such time that the skin regenerates or a permanent epidermal surface has been restored by skin grafting. Skin is known to serve 3 biologic functions: (1) It is an effective barrier to bacterial invasion of the body; (2) its stratum corneum constitutes a most effective corporeal barrier to the outward and inward passage of water, water vapor, hydrated ions and diatomic gases, and (3) it is a very important thermoregulatory organ in all sweat-producing mammals.

Besides these 3 known functions, there are indications that the dermis plays a role in iron metabolism,[23] and that the epidermis may be an important organ in which chemical degradation of steroid hormones takes place.

In devising means of substituting for cutaneous functions, 3 general surgical dicta need be obeyed, namely:

1. Place nothing upon the wound having local or general toxic properties. This includes soaps and antiseptic detergents such as pHisoHex.

2. Provide for the free egress of pus if it forms.

3. Exclude from the injured part the bacteria carried by fomites, air, dressers and attendants.

Burned people still die of infections arising within the area of injury in spite of the use of antibiotics and special efforts to maintain asepsis. However, with burns covering less than 20 per cent of the body, infection of the burn wound now rarely causes death. Before the antibiotics and the sulfonamides were discovered, streptococcic wound infections, known as burn erysipelas, caused an appreciable number of deaths among persons having small as well as large burns. Today, burn erysipelas is effectively prevented by giving penicillin, 50,000 to 300,000 units, 3 or 4 times daily. However, with burns covering more than 25 per cent of the body, infection is the most important cause of death. Pathogenic strains of micrococci, especially *Staphylococcus aureus, Pseudomonadaceae, Enterobacteriaceae, (Escherichiae* and *Proteae) Parvobacteriaceae* (Bacteroides) and *Lactobacteriaceae* (*Streptococcus faecalis*) and *Streptococcus hemolyticus* (alpha viridans and beta pyogenes) are the predominant invaders of burn wounds. Excepting for the hemolytic streptococci, no satisfactory prolonged control of these organisms has yet been attained with antibiotics when they colonize burn wounds. The specific reasons for this are not apparent; the development of resistant strains of organisms while antibiotics are being given is one of the important factors; yet many others are likely to play parts such as the peculiarities of the tissue response to bacteria in a burned person, one of which is responsible for the actual growth of separate colonies of bacteria in the living tissue beneath burned skin with no cellular responses about the bacterial colonies.

Tetanus is still a threat with every burn. Give a booster dose of toxoid to those known to have been actively immunized and hyperimmune human antitetanus serum to those who are not. The amount given is determined by the size of the burn and the environment of the injury. A person who rolls or lies upon earth during or after a burn is given a larger dose. A large burn that has had contact with earth or earth-soiled clothing is a massive injury as far as the danger of tetanus is concerned.

BURN SEPSIS

The signs of the birth of serious sepsis within a thermal wound are: an inordinately painful wound later than 24 hours after the accident, appreciable swelling of the burned part for longer than 72 hours, wetting through of the occlusive dressing, blistering of the unburned skin adjacent to the wound, lymphangitis, painful lymphadenitis, ileus, and the general signs of sepsis, including shock. With and after the separation of the eschar the lack of visible evidence of a rim of epithelization about the edges of the wound, bleeding, and the formation of "pyogenic" crusts (crusts with pus beneath them) are the main local signs of a biologically significant infection. Pink, nonedematous granulation tissue with a rim of newly grown epithelium about it signifies a relatively "uninfected" wound even though pathogenic bacteria may be found upon it.

Cleansing, free drainage, and inhibition of bacterial growth without interfering with reparative processes are the principles of treating infected burns. Cleansing and effecting free drainage may be accomplished with the repeated application and removal of thick compresses wet with an 0.5 per cent aqueous solution of silver nitrate. The cloth must be exposed to air to permit evaporation at the external surface of the wet dressing. This moves bacteria from the wound surface into the dressing by capillary action. The covering of a wet dressing with an impervious cloth or plastic merely makes a fine incubator for organisms. The dressings are changed every 6 to 12 hours until the infecting organisms practically disappear from the wound and general signs of sepsis disappear. A dry sheet or blanket or an electric blanket must cover the wet dressings in order to reduce vaporizational heat loss. The changing of an exposed wet dressing effects a continuous gentle scrub of the wound.

Recently, it has been discovered that thick cotton gauze dressings, properly applied, kept continuously wet with an 0.5 per cent aqueous solution of silver nitrate (29.4 mEq. Ag^+/L.), and changed once or twice daily, effect bacteriostasis of many species of bacteria on human burn wounds at all stages.[23] However, on burn wounds, they are not bacteriostatic for Paracolon species, Klebsiella and Aerobacter species, and a number of saprophytic organisms culturable from normal human skin. Nonetheless, they have been highly bacteriostatic for *Staphylococcus aureus*, hemolytic streptococci, and in many cases, for *Pseudomonas aeruginosa* and *E. coli*. This has been so even when the silver-nitrated dressings have been applied after the wounds have been widely infected and heavily colonized by these bacteria. The rate of shedding organisms into a bath containing 450 liters of Locke's solution from a unit area of a deep burn wound treated with 0.5 per cent silver nitrate from the beginning varies between 1/100th and 1/1,000,000th of the rate obtaining from a unit of burn surface treated with occlusive dressings, continuous saline

TABLE 17-3. EFFECT OF 0.5 PER CENT AgNO₃ ON THE GROWTH OF BACTERIA ON A BURN WOUND

CASE (HARTFORD BURN CENTER)	TREATMENT	BACTERIA M² HOUR FROM THE WOUND MINIMUM	MAXIMUM	PER CENT OF BODY SURFACE BURN DEEP PARTIAL THICK-NESS*	FULL THICK-NESS†	TOTAL
R. N.	Exposure and saline bath	1.0×10^9	2.25×10^{11}	15	60	75
L. Br.	Exposure and saline bath	2.0×10^{11}	4.5×10^{11}	5	40	45
W. B.	Exposure and saline bath	2.0×10^9	1.5×10^{11}	20	60	80
S. H.	AgNO₃ & saline bath	4.5×10^5	4.5×10^7	30	35	65
N. K.	AgNO₃ & saline bath‡	1.0×10^6	4.0×10^7	10	36	46
D. W.	AgNO₃ & saline bath	$<3.0 \times 10^5$	1.0×10^7	40	35	75

* Deep partial-thickness burns are classified as those epithelizing between the 20th and the 100th post-burn days *without grafting*. Areas epithelized within 20 days of the injury are *not* counted as a burn wound.
† Requires autografting for wound closure.
‡ Treated with occlusive dressings for 8 days before AgNO₃ was begun. Eschar was colonized with *Ps. aeruginosa, Staph. aureus*, β hem. strep., Paracolon, Aerobacter, *E. coli, Proteus mirabilis*, Bact. anitratum, and anaerobes, when AgNO₃ treatment was started.

baths or with exposure (no dressing) (see Table 17-3). Functional bacteriostasis can also be effected with mafenide (Sulfamylon) cream, silver sulfadiazine, and silver nitrate 0.5 per cent, containing 1 gram of a tetracycline-nystatin mixture per liter (Mysteclin F).

Although 0.5 per cent silver nitrate is effective as a bacteriostatic agent in vivo on burn wounds, and in vitro on agar and in broth, nothing is known about the actual chemical state of the silver or its concentration, or the molecular mode of action involved in the process of its bacteriostatic or bactericidal action in vivo.

The forms of silver that have been tested against *Ps. aeruginosa* and *Staph. aureus*, cultured from burn wounds, and have been found to possess bacteriostatic activity against both organisms in low, but higher than oligodynamic concentrations, are: AgNO₃, AgCl, Ag₂O, Ag₃C₆H₅O₇, AgC₂H₃O₂, a number of Ag proteinates and colloidal silver.

An aqueous solution of AgNO₃ (29.4 mEq./L.) does *not* significantly inhibit the growth of epithelium.

Split skin grafts 0.2 to 0.3 mm. thick, cut into pieces 1 to 4 sq. cm. and placed on granulating wounds, so grow that 20 pieces with a total area of about 80 sq. cm. proliferate and cover with epidermis a granulating area of about 400 sq. cm. in 14 to 20 days, while the entire wound is continuously covered by dressings wet with 0.5 per cent AgNO₃.

Nonetheless, the margin between the concentration of AgNO₃ that is noninjurious to skin and that which is injurious is narrow. Dressings wet with 1 per cent AgNO₃, and placed upon newly regenerated epidermis of a burn, have *killed* the new, but solid, epidermis in *36 hours*, converting a closed to a shallow, open wound. This same wound healed again in 8 days after the concentration of AgNO₃ in the dressing was reduced to 0.5 per cent. For this reason, the dressings used must be thick; they must be changed at least once daily, and oftener if the humidity of the ambient air is low, and must be kept continuously wet with the 0.5 per cent solution of AgNO₃, in order that the concentration of silver nitrate at the wound-dressing interface shall not reach cutaneously lethal levels for protracted periods of time. This is especially true whenever the dressing covers skin grafts or newly regenerated epidermis.

In order that 0.5 per cent silver nitrate effect bacteriostasis on a burn wound, certain conditions must be met.

The dressing that acts as the vehicle of delivery of the silver salt to the burn wound must contain no impediment to capillarity or diffusion and must be so thick that it holds a large volume of solution, and it must be in contact with the wound everywhere.

To these ends, a satisfactory dressing consists of 6 to 8 layers of 4-ply,* 9-inch dressing gauze,† thoroughly wet with solution before its application, and closely coapted to the wound surface by spiralled elastic wrappings of 2 thicknesses of 6- to 12-inch wide stockinette cut-on-bias. This dressing complex is kept dripping or almost dripping wet by the addition of 0.5 per cent $AgNO_3$ every 3 to 4 hours between the daily changes of dressing.

The thick gauze dressing must not contain any cotton batting, cotton lint or paper filling. Such dressings have been tried and have been found to become soggy, lumpy masses that do not permit the free flow of $AgNO_3$ from dressing to wound by diffusion and the free movement of bacteria and exudate from the wound surface into the dressing by capillarity.

This dressing will not deliver $AgNO_3$ to the dermal and the subdermal parts of the wound nor remove bacteria or exudate from it by capillarity, *unless the wound is free of grease or ointment bases and is not covered by dead epidermis with its impervious keratin covering*. Failure to remove grease that may have been put on as a first-aid measure, as well as the epidermis covering blisters and nonblistered, deeply burned skin, before applying the silver-nitrated dressing renders the silver bacteriostatically ineffective—it can't get to the bacteria.

It goes without saying that the removal of eschar, as soon as possible, is also an important maneuver for securing bacteriostasis on the burn wound with $AgNO_3$ or with anything else. Bacteria may grow in the depths of the eschar, and the more deeply they are situated in the thermally killed tissue, the less likely will it be that bacteriostatic concentrations of agent can be effected about them. The eschar can be removed completely from the whole of a deep partial and full-thickness burn covering more than 70 per cent of the body in 20 days, *without anesthesia,* without measurable loss of blood, and without removing any viable cutaneous remnants*. The technics are simple: every day, during the change of dressings, the edges of the entire wound are gently probed with a grooved dissector or the blade of a flat forcep held horizontally with the smooth surface against the wound surface at the juncture of visibly pink margin of the wound with the eschar. The instrument is pushed toward the center of the eschar and, if a local cleavage is effected, the instrument is pushed until it meets high resistance or produces pain. The roof of the tunnel so made is cut with a scissors and the maneuver is repeated. The strips and pieces of eschar so made are then stripped off. *Pain or bleeding are the stop signs*. Immersion of the patient in a temperature-controlled (35.5 to 36.5° C.) sterile bath of modified Locke's solution† for 2 to 6 hours, 1 to 3 times a week, facilitates the separation and the removal of eschar and also permits quantitative assessment of the degree of bacteriostasis being effected.

The dressings must be changed at least once a day. When the dressings are not completely changed for 3 to 4 days after grafts are emplaced, graft survival and bacteriostasis are poor under the silver-nitrated dressings. Until it was learned that stamp grafts devoid of grease and oil cohere with a force of 10 to 30 Gm. of water pressure per square centimeter within an hour after being applied to a clean surface of a full-thickness burn, fear of displacing the grafts led to covering them with fine-meshed gauze before applying the silver-

---

* Bauer and Black.

† Kerlix gauze is not satisfactory as the material constituting the body of the dressing. It coapts poorly to the wound surface and therefore does not serve as a proper transfer vehicle.

* An analgesic, such as morphine, is given.

† Preparation of modified Locke's solution:
To avoid precipitation of some of the salts, 2 stock solutions are first prepared and then added to water to make the final solution.

Solution A (Gm./L.)		Solution B (Gm./L.)	
NaCl	175.5	$NaHCO_3$	73.3
KCl	9.0	$NaH_2PO_4 \cdot H_2O$	3.8
$CaCl_2 \cdot 2H_2O$	11.1		
$MgCl_2 \cdot 6H_2O$	9.13		

Add 1 volume of A, followed by 1 volume of B, to 23 volumes of water.

Burn Sepsis

RELATIONSHIP OF HEAT LOSS TO VAPORIZATIONAL (INSENSIBLE) WATER LOSS

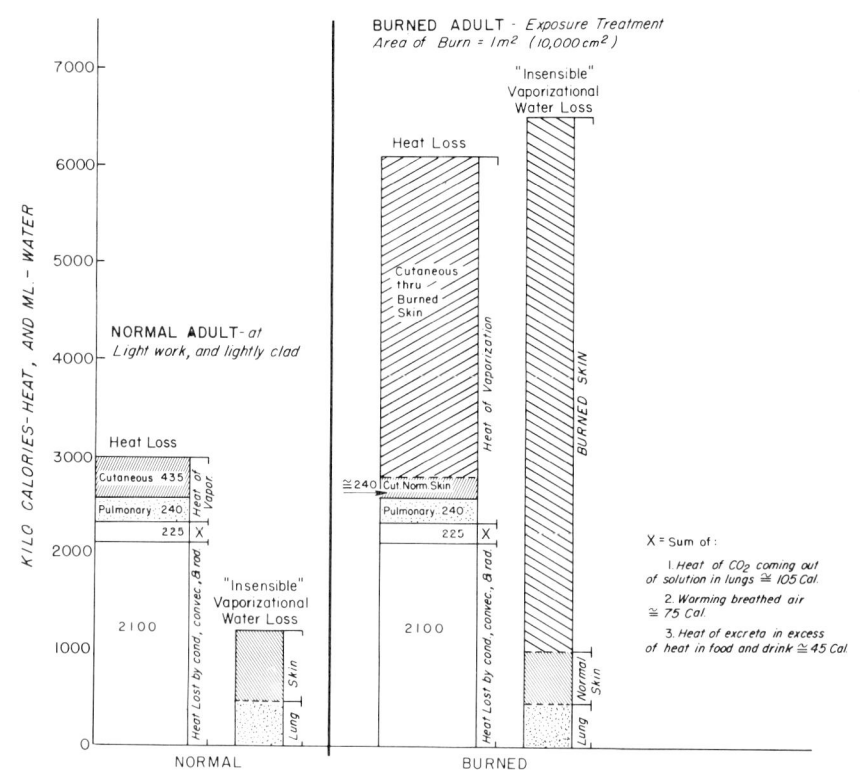

FIG. 17-5. Graph, showing the relationships of vaporizational heat loss to other modes of heat loss and insensible water loss: *(left)* a normal adult and *(right)* an adult bearing a burn covering a square meter of the body. The wound was exposed to air at a temperature of 28° to 38° C. and with a relative humidity of 25 to 40 per cent.

The insensible loss of water from the burned person so treated was measured during 4 days. The vaporizational heat loss was calculated as follows: grams insensible loss × 0.575 = Calories heat loss. This is fully permissible because the surface temperature of the burned skin was always higher than the temperature of the air of the room. Consequently, all of the heat required to maintain the mean thermal energy of the water molecules remaining in the body after the evaporative escape of those possessing high energies must have come from the human body and could not have come from the air, because heat is not transferable from the colder to the warmer object, in accord with the second law of thermodynamics.

nitrated coarse gauze, and to leaving all in place for 3 to 4 days. After recognizing the magnitude of coherence of the grafts, the fine-meshed gauze graft covering was discarded, and the dressing was changed daily. With this technic, a graft take and survival of less than 90 per cent is rare.

During 10 years of study of burned animals and man, acceleration of vaporizational heat loss through the burned skin has been established as a major cause of the hypermetabolism that attends thermal trauma under the environmental conditions obtaining with extant methods of burn treatment.[4, 18, 22] Figure 17-5 illustrates this. A number of possible substitutive and restorative means of reducing vaporizational heat loss through the burned skin have been tried and found to be therapeutically inapplicable for various reasons; these are summarized in Table 17-4.

The first substitutive measure that was tried was the continuous bath with Locke's solution containing phosphate. A 600-liter, stainless steel bathtub with built-in automatic heat controls and a high-speed microfilter system was constructed. Patients with full-thickness burns covering 30 to 90 per cent of the body were placed in the bath upon being admitted to the hospital and were kept in it until the eschar was all off or until sepsis developed. While in the bath, the burned persons were comfortable. They moved the burned parts freely and painlessly. They ate well and did not lose weight. Basal metabolic rates were near normal. The eschar came off rapidly, bloodlessly and painlessly. They needed no narcotics or soporifics. Fluid balance was maintained without the oral or intravenous administration of salts other than those contained in the food they ate. However, invasive infections occurred with *Ps. pyocyanea* and other organisms insensitive to antibiotics, most notably *Proteus mirabilis* and *morganii*. These infections developed in the bath and after removal from it while skin grafting was being done (skin grafts could not be applied when the patient was in the bath). The numbers of organisms in the bath were astronomical within a day or two after the burned person was placed in it, although the bath solution was being filtered through microfilters in series with a high capacity ultra-

TABLE 17-4

MEANS OF REDUCING WATER FLUX THROUGH BURNED SKIN		REASON FOR BEING UNSATISFACTORY
1. Substitutive measures:	(a) Covering the burn or burned person's body with water-impermeable plastics, spray-on films, and cotton dressings wet with Locke's solution	Maceration of eschar with diffuse bacterial colonization, and putrefactive destruction of the eschar and subcutaneous panniculus; sepsis
	(b) Continuous bath in modified Locke's solution	Rapid diffuse bacterial colonization of eschar followed by putrefactive destruction of all tissue down to the enveloping fascia of muscles and periosteum; and sepsis. The rate of production of organisms in 1 square meter of burned skin with the patient in the bath reached the astronomical levels of about 2.5×10^{11} organisms per square meter per hour*
2. Restorative measures:	(a) Impregnating eschar with oleic acid†	Condensation of dead dermis into a thin transparent elastic gel (0.3 mm. thick) under which bacteria grew, forming confluent abscesses with destruction of subcutaneous panniculus
	(b) Impregnating top of eschar with petroleum jelly, lanolin, mineral oil‡	Maceration of eschar and rapid, diffuse bacterial colonization and destruction of eschar with conversion of partial-deep to full-thickness injuries
	(c) Coating eschar with low-melting-point paraffins‡	Formed films that cracked and lost much of their effectiveness; in addition, bacterial colonization and destruction of the eschar occurred

* These things could not be prevented by: rapid filtration and sterilization of the bath solution with ultraviolet light or organic iodophores while a burned person was in the bath. Changing the bath solution every 3 to 4 hours, all 450 liters of it, did not prevent them either.
† Stops only the capillary flux of water through eschar.[24]
‡ Stops both capillary flux of water and water vapor flux through eschar.[24]

violet liquid sterilizer, and drainage and renewal of the bath solution was performed every 4 hours. The mean number of organisms per milliliter of bath solution within an hour after changing the bath solution was nearly 1×10^6. The inclusion of a concentration of nonabsorbable iodophore in the bath solution that quickly sterilized it, after pouring a liter of a 24-hour broth culture of *Ps. pyocyanea* into it, when a patient was not in the bath, effected only a fleeting reduction (1 hour) of the growth of Pseudomonas and other bacteria when a burned person was in it.

The Locke's solution bath did demonstrate a number of things, namely: (1) Burn wounds are painless at all stages when covered with an isotonic balanced salt solution having the ionic composition of plasma except for protein. (2) Electrolyte and water balance disturbances that occur with burns treated by exposure to air or dry dressings do not occur while the patient is in the bath. (3) The bath reduced the vaporizational and other losses of heat, and the person maintained body weight by eating a regular diet while burns covered as much as 60 per cent of the body. (4) Burn eschar could be removed painlessly and bloodlessly without the use of general anesthetics or an operating room.

However, inability to control the growth of pathogenic bacteria in the bath and on the wound obviated all these benefits, and the only thing that was accomplished was to abolish suffering for the time the patient lived before dying of sepsis in the bath, or for the time that the wound was being cleaned of dead tissue before grafting was begun. When grafting was started, the patient had to be removed from the bath, and then pain and suffering began.

Nevertheless, these experiences did lead the way to the development of the methods now being used to prevent sepsis, to remove the eschar without anesthesia and bleeding, to prevent burn-starvation, and to practically free the burned person of pain throughout convalescence. The Locke's solution bath is now a facet, but not a major part, of the burn therapy; it is used to hasten eschar separation, to ascertain the number of bacteria growing on a burn wound, and to provide painless exercise of burned extremities, preventing joint immobilization and disuse atrophy of muscles.

During investigations of factors controlling the rate of movement of water through human skin, dermal capillarity was discovered to be the mechanism responsible for the very rapid outpouring of water and salts through a burn.[24] Further research disclosed that adding lipids, including fatty acids, to bared dermis would stop the capillary transfer of water and salt through it, and would convert a wet, opaque eschar into a dry translucent one in 24 to 48 hours. After ascertaining these facts from work with human skin taken from fresh cadavers and amputated extremities, oleic acid was sprayed on burns devoid of epithelium in an attempt to restore cutaneous impermeability to water. It produced translucent eschars over full-thickness burns in 24 to 48 hours, slowed the rapid capillary transit of water (Fig. 17-6) and salt through the burn, produced a painless wound, and did not convert superficial partial to full-thickness injuries. However, bacteria grew in the elastic-gel eschar produced by the fatty acid, and invasive infections occurred, negating the metabolic and other benefits effected by the conversion of water-permeable eschar to a water-impermeable one.

Clearly, the growth of pathogenic bacteria in the burned tissue, and their invasion of the body as a whole, constituted the main difficulty that had to be surmounted if excess vaporizational heat loss was to be stopped by practicable means. The silver-nitrated wet dressing accomplished this while it simultaneously reduced insensible water loss to metabolically sustainable levels and thereby served to prevent burn-inanition.

In order that the wet dressings may prevent burn-inanition, *the person so wetly dressed must be covered with a layer or two of dry cotton sheeting or blanket,* in order to minimize evaporation from, and the loss of heat through, the dressing. This, these dry top coverings do, regardless of their mesh, by a number of mechanisms.

First, they reduce conductive and convective loss of heat from the body by confining convection currents generated at the surface of the wet dressing by the thermal agitation associated with evaporation, and by blocking those convection and other air currents exist-

380 Burns and Cold Injury

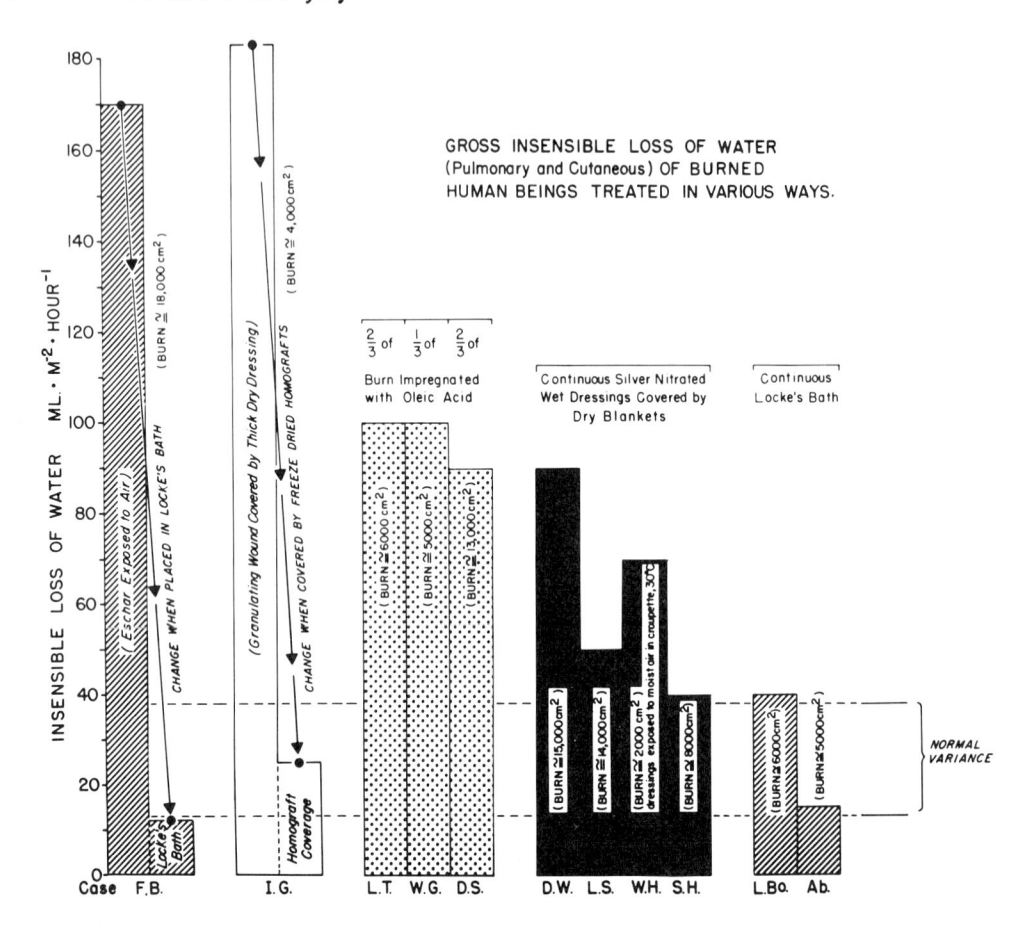

FIG. 17-6. Graphic presentation of data pertaining to the insensible losses of water by 11 burned patients while being treated in various ways.

ing within the room from the surface of the relatively good heat-conductive wet dressing.

Second, the dry covering establishes a heat reservoir between it and the wet dressing (Fig. 17-7). From this reservoir, heat is available for the vaporization of water at the interface between the wet dressing and the air under the covering.

Third, the dry blanket serves as a barrier to the convective removal of water vapor from the surface of the wet dressing. The rate of evaporation from an open beaker is reduced by half, by merely interposing a single layer of filter paper or coarse Marlex fabric between the general air reservoir and the air immediately covering the surface of water contained in the beaker.

Fourth, the dry blanket, by virtue of its having a lower thermal conductivity than water, serves to reduce conductive loss of heat from the body. Taking the thermal conductivity of the wet gauze dressing to be that of water at 35° C., and assuming the outer surface to be exposed to air, the wet gauze dressing, 2 cm. thick and having the thermal gradient as measured on the burned body, would conduct 2,500 calories of heat from body to air at 29° C. per square meter per day. The interposition of a dry blanket of cotton, 2 mm. thick, with the thermal gradient as measured and shown in the graph (Fig. 17-7), would conductively transfer to the air above it only 800 calories per square meter per day.

Clearly, the outer layer of the dressing must be dry, in order that the dressing maximally conserve body heat.

Theoretically, covering the wet dressing with a water-impervious sheet would serve to

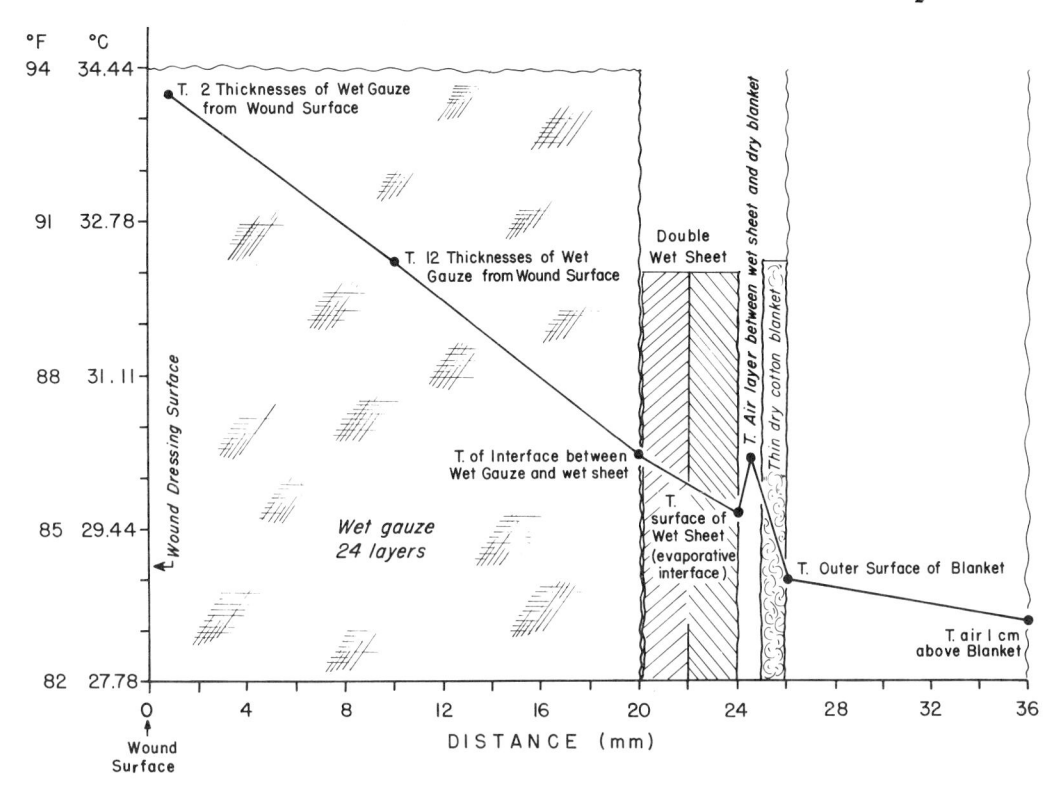

FIG. 17-7. A graphic representation of the thermal gradients in a wet dressing 2 cm. thick covered by 2 thicknesses of wet cotton sheet and 1 thickness of a dry cotton blanket. The temperature of the surface of the wound was 34.5° C. and that of the air in the room was 28° C.

The air trapped between the wet sheet and the dry blanket is warmer than the outer surface of the wet sheet. In some cases, the temperature of this trapped air-layer has been found to be as much as 3° C. higher than that of the outer surface of the wet sheet. As long as the temperature of this trapped air is higher than that of the surface of the wet sheet from which evaporation takes place, the heat of vaporization comes from the air layer and not from the person's body. However, let the blanket become wet, and the wetly dressed burned person soon complains of being cold. The reasons for this are obvious. When this happens, the air at the evaporative surface becomes colder than the surface of the wet dressing, and as a result the heat of vaporization must now come from the body. (See also caption, Fig. 17-5.) In addition, the wet-dressing surface also becomes exposed to convection currents, which remarkably hasten evaporation and heat loss.

abolish vaporizational and other losses of heat through the dressing. However, this procedure has several disadvantages: (1) It serves to reduce the concentration of silver nitrate in the dressing, because the silver salt is being precipitated at the dressing-wound interface continuously. Consequently, unless some evaporation of water from the dressing is permitted, the concentration of silver nitrate in the dressing cannot be maintained by merely wetting it every 2 to 4 hours with 0.5 per cent $AgNO_3$, and its maintenance would require very frequent changes of the entire dressing. (2) The water-impervious covering much reduces the transfer of bacteria into the dressing by stopping the capillary flow of liquid from wound surface toward the outer surface of the dressing. (3) A burned person senses heat deficit acutely, but senses heat excess poorly. Consequently, covering large burned surfaces with a dressing impervious to water vapor is dangerous, as proved by Edenbuizen[6] many years ago.

TABLE 17-5. THE RELATIONSHIP OF THE DURATION OF HOSPITALIZATION AND OF THE MAGNITUDE OF WEIGHT LOSS TO THE METHOD USED IN TREATING DEEP BURNS

CASE AGE (YRS.) PER CENT B.S. BURN*	NUMBER OF DAYS IN HOSPITAL	NUMBER OF DAYS IN HOSPITAL PER CENT B.S. BURN	BODY WEIGHT (LBS.) PREBURN MINIMUM AND AT DISCHARGE	TEMPORAL ORDER OF TREATMENTS
				OCCLUSIVE DRESSINGS
J. M. 29 27%	132	5	145 117 139	Occlusive dressings Surgical débridement§
D. P. 14 30%	111	3.7	92 70 —	Occlusive dressings Locke's bath Surgical débridement
H. C. 32 18%	39	2.1	— — —	Occlusive dressings Surgical débridement
M. A. 63 30%	110	3.7	135 94 —	Locke's bath Occlusive dressings No surgical débridement
H. S. 51 40%	59	1.5	162 134 (Died)	Occlusive dressings Locke's bath Occlusive dressings Surgical débridement
CONTINUOUS 0.5 PER CENT SILVER-NITRATED DRESSINGS				
M. K. 66 46%	119	2.6	93 84 90.5	Occlusive dressings AgNO₃ dressings Intermittent Locke's bath No surgical débridement
S. S. 54 30%	60	2.0	150 142 143	AgNO₃ dressings Intermittent Locke's bath No surgical débridement
S. H. 11 65%	143	2.2	96 90.5 91	AgNO₃ dressings Intermittent Locke's bath No surgical débridement
D. W. 25 70%	115	1.6	218 190† 167‡ 176	AgNO₃ dressings Intermittent Locke's bath No surgical débridement
R. W. 5 31%	70	2.3	35 35 35	Occlusive dressings Surgical débridement AgNO₃ dressings Intermittent saline bath
A. P. 34 60%	58	0.9	160 142 144	Occlusive dressing over Nitrofurazone ointment AgNO₃ dressings Intermittent Locke's bath No surgical débridement

* Wounds that healed in 21 days are not counted in the surface estimate.
† Before gastrectomy.
‡ After gastrectomy.
§ Surgical débridement—excision of eschar during general anesthesia down to vascular tissue. Significant hemorrhage always occurs.

Where is there proof that the wet dressings, insulated from room air by dry sheets or blankets, reduce the net rate of heat loss from a burned person, and thereby serve to minimize the patient's caloric needs? The fact that persons with deep burns covering 30 to 50 per cent of the body, eating no more than a regular hospital diet, and even as little as 1,900 calories a day, do not lose significant amounts of weights during as much as 100 days of convalescence, is evidence (see Table 17-5). Other evidences are the normal basal oxygen consumptions of burned patients measured while the burn wounds covered as much as 65 per cent of the body. Direct proof can be obtained only with the use of total body calorimetry. However, the fact that basal oxygen consumptions of badly burned patients are near normal, and they either lose relatively small amounts of weight, or actually gain weight, during convalescence from deep burns covering up to 50 to 60 per cent of the body is evidence enough to permit the conclusion that *properly constructed, applied and attended dressings, kept wet continuously with 0.5 per cent AgNO₃, effect reductions of the net heat loss and insensible water loss from burned human beings that are sufficient to reduce the caloric and water needs of the burned person close to the range of normal.* To be sure, the reduction of bacterial growth on the wound effected by the AgNO₃ may play a role in the reduction of the postburn hypermetabolism, but it could not effect this, should the dressing not effect a significant net reduction of the accelerated heat loss that is related to the destruction of cutaneous impermeability to water by the epidermal denudation of the dermis or the disappearance of lipids from the keratin after burning.

Although the silver-nitrated dressings benefit the burned patient, they are dangerous. The biologic dangers of the 0.5 per cent AgNO₃ wet dressings are theoretically four: argyria, metal toxicity, depletion of body salts and necrobiosis. Argyria is only cosmetically disfiguring. It has not occurred in any case regardless of the size or the depth of injury when the silver-nitrated dressings have not covered the mouth. In 1 case out of 15, there appears to be slight argyria (as yet not proved by biopsy) limited to a burn wound of the thigh that epithelized during the time the AgNO₃ dressings were being used on the burned lips and chin and the patient was swallowing some of the dressing liquid. None of the other burn wounds that covered at least 75 per cent of the body show any evidence of argyria; they all healed with and without skin grafting while 0.5 per cent AgNO₃ was applied to them for 130 days. In other words, argyria is a very remote possible consequence of treating burns with 0.5 per cent AgNO₃. Evidently silver does not gain access to the circulation in quantity sufficient for argyria when the silver is applied to the burn wound at any stage.

That argyria does not occur with significant frequency after the continuous use of dressings wet with 0.5 per cent AgNO₃ means that the general toxic potential of silver nitrate as used is nonexistent, because even the deposition of enough silver in the body to produce pronounced generalized argyria produces no detectable physiologic disturbance of the affected organs or of the general health.

Depletion of body salts has occurred with the use of the silver-nitrated dressing. This is readily explicable and was anticipated, *but the speed of depletion* of the body of sodium salts by the dressing was not expected because the burn wound was thought to have a poor exchange surface at least for a few days after the injury.

The mechanism of salt abstraction from the body by the dressing is simple: the solution in the dressing is hypotonic (29.4 mEq. AgNO₃/L.) and the solute composition of the solution in the dressing is much different from that in the body. In addition, with ion exchange between Ag⁺NO₃⁻ and cation ⁺-Cl⁻, HCO₃⁻, CO₃⁻ and protein⁻ at the wound surface and in the bare dermis or exposed tissue, cation-NO₃ and very slightly soluble or insoluble silver salts are formed, tending to deplete the body of anions relatively more rapidly than of cations. However, the first mechanism appears to be the most important.

The salt depletions seen thus far are all explicable on the basis of dressing hypotonicity alone. Biologically dangerous sodium and chloride deficits with osmolar dilution occur in children with large burns within a matter of a few hours after applying the hypotonic silver-nitrated dressings to the fresh burn. It also occurs, but less rapidly, in adults, while the dressing covers 2,500 to 15,000 sq.

cm. of eschar or granulating burn wound when the oral intake of salt and sodium lactate is too small. Potassium depletion occurs much more slowly, presumably because the K^+ diffusion gradient from the body into the dressing is at most only 5 mEq./L., while that of NaCl is at least 20 times as large. However, K^+ deficit may occur with full-thickness burns covering more than 30 per cent of the body surface within 3 to 10 weeks after the burn, unless adequate K^+ supplements are given. One case ended fatally because potassium supplements were not given and the signs of potassium deficit were not recognized until postmortem review of the case. Since this unfortunate experience, individuals with full-thickness burns covering more than 70 per cent of the body surface have been brought through the whole of a postburn convalescence without K^+ depletion by properly supplementing the diet with potassium salts. Calcium depletion has occurred with *very large, deep burns,* even during the oral administration of 7.2 gm. of calcium lactate daily.

Magnesium and phosphate deficits have also occurred, and the diets of persons treated with $AgNO_3$ wet dressings need supplements of magnesium and phosphate.

The danger of sodium chloride depletion associated with the use of the silver-nitrated dressing is so immediate that the dressing should not be used without very frequent monitoring of serum sodium, chloride and bicarbonate. During the acute phase these analyses must be done every *2 to 4 hours* in cases of infants and children with burns covering more than 10 per cent of body surface and every *6 to 12 hours* in cases of adults with burns covering more than 20 per cent. This frequency of monitoring must be kept up until adequate oral supplementation is possible, and then it may be reduced to once daily. *Obviously, microchemical analytic methods must be used, or red blood cell deficits from the blood sampling will soon become a serious problem, especially in infants and children.*

Methemoglobinemia has also been seen with the silver-nitrated wet dressing when the burn harbors nitrate splitting bacteria in large numbers. The production of nitrite from nitrate is responsible.

Human gamma globulin fairly effectively controls infections with *P. aeruginosa* in burned laboratory animals,[14] though its effectiveness in human beings has not been completely established. Some measure of control of the growth of many organisms can be effected by coverage repeatedly, if necessary, of the open burn wound with living homografts taken from fresh cadavers. Within an hour after covering even bacteria-laden, pale, bleeding, edematous granulation tissue with living cutaneous homografts, the wound often becomes almost free of bacteria. The biologic mechanisms concerned in this are not known. To date no effective method has been devised for treating the massively infected, large, wet eschars of large full-thickness burns. We have attempted their excision with the immediate onlay of homografts while the patient was being given very large quantities of a broad-spectrum antibiotic and penicillin intravenously, but the sepsis continued and all 3 of the persons so treated died.

Treatment with the 0.5 per cent silver-nitrated dressing has also proved to be ineffective when applied to large, deep burns that are already invasively infected by *P. aeruginosa* and anaerobic spore-forming organisms.

Vaccines or hyperimmune human sera against *P. aeruginosa* are being developed. Some of them give promise of providing means of controlling pyocyaneus sepsis in burned human beings.

When this chapter was first written, the specific recommendation was made that from 200,000 to 1,200,000 units of penicillin be given daily for at least 5 days after the burn. Some persons believe that such specific recommendation cannot be made now because of the growing body of evidence that the "prophylactic administration of antibiotics" is without general merit and that what it does is to ensure that the bacterial flora of the burn wound is free of hemolytic streptococci but covered with penicillin-resistant strains of other organisms, most notably the staphylococci. The above statements are almost certainly true for the topically applied antibiotics, but it is questionable whether one may similarly indict the giving of penicillins, especially the newer broad-spectrum forms, to a burned person for at least a few days after a burn. We believe that some form of penicillin should be given parenterally for at least 5 days after a burn because it prevents invasive lethal streptococcic infections. After an invasive streptococcal infection develops within a burn wound the antibiotics are peculiarly ineffective at times. Of course, the antibiotics must be used for an actual infection in a burn wound; and insofar as it is possible to do, the antibiotics used should be those to which the bacteria are known to be sensitive.

The immediate excision of full-thickness injuries has been practiced sporadically for more than 50 years. Weidenfeld[37] began it in Vienna as a means of preventing "toxemia." It is performed readily without deep general anesthesia at any time up to the 5th day. The mode of its application in his words is:

With a thin transplantation knife (Thiersch knife) the eschar is cut away from the underlying tissue. One cuts so deeply that the underlying tissue bleeds, for only by this sign is one able to judge when sound tissue is reached. One needs recognize that the thickness of the eschar varies in an irregular manner and cut accordingly. . . . The undertaking of this procedure causes the patient only slight pain by virtue of the fact that the eschar is anesthetic and the subcutaneous tissues are scarcely sensible. Bleeding, however, is remarkable and one must conduct the process with foresight so that the patient is not inordinately weakened therby.[37]

During World War II the procedure was reborn but has been practically abandoned again except for localized deep electrical burns. However, someday it may serve a useful function, especially in the treatment of small obviously deep burns, such as electrical; many surgical procedures have had to suffer a number of deaths and resurrections before finding acceptance.

OTHER DISTURBANCES ASSOCIATED WITH BURNS

The general care of the badly burned patient rests upon the physician's ability to recognize and treat a multiplicity of physiologic and biochemical disturbances.

Hydrational Disturbances

The hydrational disturbances associated with burns may be classified as early and late primary and secondary changes. Of the early primary disturbances the movement of extracellular fluid into the injured tissues and blisters is very important. This movement of interstitial fluid into the damaged tissues and blisters reduces the interstitial fluid mass in the uninjured tissues and blood. The fluid in the injured area has a lower content of protein than plasma but a higher content than nonvisceral lymph. It can be looked upon as a thin plasma.

The loss into the injured parts of fluid from the uninjured parts through blistering, edematous swelling and weeping proceeds with great rapidity and can well be life-endangering within an hour after an extensive partial-thickness burn or scald.[28]

The *intracellular fluid mass* of the uninjured tissues *does not move* across the cell membrane into the interstitial space to "buffer" the reduced volume of interstitial fluid. This was observed by Tappeiner[32] during the late 1870's after an analysis of the water content of the plasma and the red cells of men following fatal burns. He found the content of water in plasma to be remarkably reduced (one fifth to one third) while at the same time the content of water in red cells was normal. These observations led him to write, "Why do the still water-rich cells not give up water to the water-poor serum?" Subsequent observations of Painter[12] show that intracellular fluid does not move out of body cells when extracellular fluid is lost into injured parts. In other words, the fluid-rich cells do not give up fluid to the impoverished extracellular compartment of the uninjured core of the injured animal. Consequently, one must provide extraneous extracellular fluid for the seriously burned because there is no immediately available source of it within the body. In a physiologic sense a burn is somewhat like cholera: the normal parts of the body have lost extracellular fluid into and through the lumen of the gut with cholera and into and through the injured tissue with thermal injury.

Hyperkalemia often occurs with severe burns within an hour or two after the injury. The hyperkalemia is attributable to the egress of potassium from the injured cells (skin and red cells) and oliguria. At times the potassium concentration reaches "toxic" levels,[30] and hyperkalemia has been implicated as a possible cause of burn death since 1902.[36] Definite evidence is lacking regarding its actual contribution to the death of burned human beings, though it undoubtedly is a factor in death of burned rodents. However, the avoidance of potassium should be practiced during the acute phase of illness, the first 48 hours; fruit juices and meat broths should not be given.

Lactacidosis occasionally attends profound burn shock.

Later and especially during the phase of the open wound hypokalemia and sodium deficit may occur, especially when the silver-nitrated wet dressing is used. This appears to be related to the rapid loss of potassium and sodium through exudation and diffusion into hyposmotic wet dressings.

The early secondary hydrational disturbances are hypo-osmolality and acidosis. Both of these are often iatrogenic. The administration of more than 3 or 5 liters of water orally or 5 per cent glucose in water intravenously during the first 20 hours after a burn is often attended by the retention of much of this water in the body and the dilution of all the body's solutes. The rapid reduction of the sodium concentration from normal to 120 to 125 mEq. per liter may precipitate the convulsive phase of water intoxication and anuria, especially in children. Hyponatremia is a very dangerous complication of the silver-nitrated wet dressing.

Early postburn acidosis is usually a chloride or dilutional acidosis. It arises whenever large quantities of noncolloid- or colloid-containing saline solution made only of chloride of Na or mixtures of chlorides of Na, K, Ca and Mg are given to a severely sodium-depleted organism before renal function is established. Briefly, this chloride acidosis arises because the concentration of bicarbonate buffer in the blood and extracellular fluid is reduced by the body's retention of the solution containing only chloride anions (see Chap. 5, Fluid and Electrolytes).

Postburn dilutional or chloride acidosis does not occur to a dangerous extent when sodium bicarbonate containing Ringer's or sodium lactate or acetate containing Ringer's solutions are given because they sustain the oliguric burned body's base bicarbonate concentration —the bicarbonate-containing solution doing it directly and the lactate-acetate-containing ones doing it indirectly by virtue of the catabolic degradation of, the acetate and the levorotatory form of the lactate anion.

Another secondary hydrational disturbance of burns is hypernatremia. It is especially prone to attend the daily forced feeding of burned children with large quantities (180 to 300 Gm.) of protein.[7] Serum sodium concentrations higher than 170 mEq./L., body temperatures over 39° C., and disorientation and coma have been observed to follow the forced feeding of high protein diets to burned human beings.

Metabolic Disturbances

The changes in metabolism that attend thermal injuries of mammals are an initial hypometabolism and a subsequent hypermetabolism. Both of these alterations are the greater the larger the injury. The hypometabolic period lasts for only 24 to 48 hours. Then it is followed by the period of hypermetabolism that lasts until the wounds are healed (see Fig. 17-8). With full-thickness burns, the hypermetabolism increases abruptly when the eschar is removed and an open wound is produced. The mechanisms concerned with the initial hypometabolic period have not been fully elucidated. Extracellular fluid volume deficit amounting to 20 per cent of the normal volume produced by depleting a normal human being of interstitial fluid by duodenal drainage is attended by a reduction of that individual's resting oxygen consumption amounting to 20 to 35 per cent. During the time that the metabolism is decreasing, the attendant oligemia is within the range of that which when produced by blood-letting is attended by no gross physiologic changes other than orthostatic hypotension. The hypermetabolism that supersedes the initial period of hypometabolism is in large part, barring a serious infection, related to the increased rate of loss of water vapor through the burned skin and later through the open wound. The most superficial layers of normal epidermis, and most importantly the stratum corneum, have the remarkable property of staying the movement of water vapor through the skin.[24] Although the water vapor pressure is high in a mammal (40 to 44 mm. of mercury per square cm.), normal epidermis permits only the passage of from 200 to 400 ml. of water as water vapor through the nonsweating skin of an

FIG. 17-8. T—total metabolism (O$_2$ consumption). V—vaporizational heat loss. The scales for the total and vaporizational heat loss are so constructed that 100 Calories of total metabolism is equivalent to 25 Calories of heat of vaporization because in the normal rat vaporizational heat loss is about 25 per cent of the total.

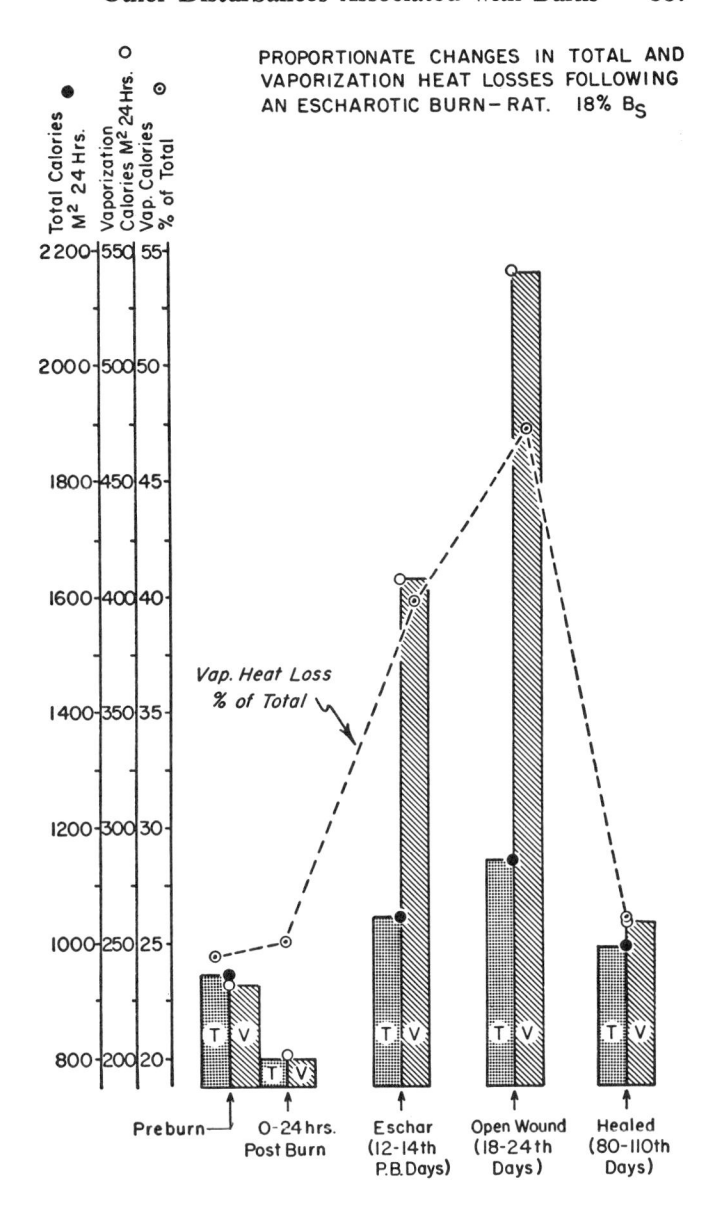

PROPORTIONATE CHANGES IN TOTAL AND VAPORIZATION HEAT LOSSES FOLLOWING AN ESCHAROTIC BURN—RAT. 18% B$_S$

adult daily. Caldwell and others have demonstrated that the hypermetabolism of the burned rat is practically entirely related to the increased heat loss secondary to the increased rate of movement of water vapor through the eschar as well as the open wound (see Figs. 17-8 and 17-6). Every gram of water lost from the body as water vapor represents the loss of a little more than one half of a kilocalorie of heat. The daily caloric expenditure by a severely burned man may reach 5,000 to 7,000 kilocalories daily. Caldwell and others have recently demonstrated that the maintenance of the temperature of the air over the burn 2° to 6° C. higher than the temperature of the surface of the wound, or the coverage of the wound with a dressing impervious to water vapor, or the immersion of the body in warm Locke's solution, remarkably reduces the postburn hypermetabolism.

Neither the hypometabolic nor the hypermetabolic postburn periods are dependent on thyroid function. They are not modified by thyroprivia when the burned animals' am-

TABLE 17-6. THE RELATIONSHIP OF BLOOD TRANSFUSION, GENERAL ANESTHESIA AND NUMBER OF SKIN GRAFTINGS TO THE METHOD USED IN TREATING DEEP BURNS

TREATMENT	CASE AGE (YRS.) AREA OF BURN, PER CENT B. S.	BLOOD TRANSFUSED FOR DÉBRIDEMENT AND SKIN GRAFTING —ML./%B. S. BURN	TOTAL VOLUME OF BLOOD TRANSFUSED FOR DÉBRIDEMENT AND SKIN GRAFTING, AND OTHER REASONS AS DESIGNATED	HEMATOCRIT AT DISCHARGE	NO. OF GENERAL ANESTHESIAS	NO. OF SKIN GRAFTING PROCEDURES	OUTCOME AND COMMENTS
Oc. Dr.	J. M. 29 27%	185	5,000 S. D. and S. G.	40	14	3	Lived
Oc. Dr., L. Ba.	D. P. 14 30%	117	3,500 S. D. and S. G.	41	15	2	Lived
Oc. Dr.	H. C. 32 18%	222	4,000 S.D. and S. G.	40	10	3	Lived Profuse bleeding occurred during and after débridement.
L. Ba., Oc. Dr.	M. A. 53 30%	50	1,500 D., S. D. and S. G.	40	2	9	Lived
L. Ba., Oc. Dr.	H. S. 51 40%	238	9,500 D., S. D. and S. G.	35	12	3	Died of sepsis after wounds were covered with autografts.

N. K. 66 46% S. S. 54 30% S. H. 11 65% D. W. 25 70%	0 0 15 0	0 0 1,000 D. and S. G. (9,500) (All for bleeding Curling's ulcer)	30 40 21 40	0 0 1 2*	4 3 9 8	Lived (Diabetic and hypertensive) Lived Lived (Religion: Jehovah's Witness) Lived Surgical débridement of hands is no longer practiced.
0.5% AgNO₃ Wet dressing and intermittent Locke's bath						
R. W. 5 31%	0 (while in H. B. U.)	(2,000) (for treatment of shock and S.D. before transfer to H. B. U.)	39	1†	9	Lived *E. coli* bacteremia prompted transfer to H. B. U.
A. P. 34 60%	0	(1,000) (for treatment of shock before transfer to H. B. U.)	39	2†	3	Lived Burns covered with nitrofurazone were badly infected.

* One for gastrectomy, one for débridement of hands.
† Before transfer.

Abbreviations: H. B. U. —Hartford Burn Unit
S. G.   —Skin grafting
Oc. Dr. —Occlusive dressing
L. Ba.   —Locke's bath
D.   —Débridement with aid of bath without anesthesia
S. D.   —Surgical débridement: excision of eschar during general anesthesia down to vascular tissue. Significant hemorrhage always occurs.

[389]

bient temperatures are kept between 24° and 30° C.[4]

CIRCULATORY DISTURBANCES

The circulatory changes attending thermal injuries are local and general. Within the thermally injured though still living tissues, red blood cells pack the widely dilated capillaries, and they flow only intermittently and slowly. This type of blood flow in capillaries is called stasic flow. The arterioles in the viable zone of injury are widely dilated and do not react to neural or hormonal stimuli until the wounds have been healed for a month or more.[27] Within the lethally injured tissues blood flow stops, the capillaries being more or less destroyed, and thrombi fill the veins and the arteries.

The circulatory abnormalities in the unburned tissues may be classified as primary and secondary. The primary alterations are evidently at least in part cardiac in origin. With large thermal injuries in dogs cardiac output declines more than can be accounted for on the bases of oligemia and venous pressures (cardiac inflow). In such animals the cardiac output increases upon giving digitalis.[10] The secondary effects, such as diminished volume flow of blood, soft pulse, etc., are related to oligemia (see Chap. 7, Shock), and possibly to other factors such as the cellular metabolic effects of sodium depletion and bacterial toxins.

Later, usually after the 10th postburn day, high-output cardiac failure often makes its appearance. The larger the burn, the more surely does it occur. Reduced peripheral resistance appears to be the cause. Digitalization takes care of it.

HEMATOLOGIC DISTURBANCES

The hemic abnormalities associated with burns are (1) an immediate hemolysis, (2) a delayed hemolysis, (3) a faster than normal coagulation of the blood, (4) leukocytosis and (5) anemia.

Hemolysis occurs rapidly during the sufferance of the burn due to the direct action of heat on the blood in the capillaries beneath the burned surface and slowly for a week thereafter. The magnitude of the immediate hemolysis is directly proportional to the area of injury and its depth: as much as 6 Gm. of free hemoglobin per 100 ml. of plasma has been found in venous blood within 5 minutes after the immersion of two thirds of an anesthetized animal in water of 80° C. for 3 minutes. Hemolysis of the blood in burned men was first found by Lichtheim.[17] The delayed hemolysis seemingly affects red cells partially injured but not completely hemolyzed by heat during the sufferance of injury.

The origins of the anemia that often follows large, deep burns are not really known. It is not measurably controlled by giving iron and vitamin B_{12}. Until the mechanisms producing it are known all that can be done to control it is to treat it by the transfusion of packed red cells or whole blood.

The severe anemia that attends large burns is related mainly to infection. Uninfected burn wounds do not bleed during changes of dressing, and in the absence of infection red blood cells are produced at such rates that, with the relatively small blood losses that come with taking grafts using the Castroviejo instrument, the red blood cell concentration of the burned person is well maintained throughout convalescence from deep burns covering 30 to 50 per cent of the body without the transfusion of blood (see Table 17-6).

However, as stated above, anemia does attend very large *full-thickness burns*, namely, those covering more than 40 per cent of body surface, but, in the absence of serious infection, its treatment requires the transfusion of relatively little blood (see Table 17-6). In such cases serum iron and extracellular iron in bone marrow may practically disappear, although ferrous sulfate is given in seemingly adequate quantity. The reticulocyte count may also be low. In such cases, after the administration of iron parenterally, the reticulocyte count rises 3- to 4-fold in a week. The dermis may play an important role in iron metabolism, because this peculiar anemia does not attend burns covering up to 75 per cent of the body surface unless large amounts of dermis are destroyed.

ENDOCRINE DISTURBANCES

The endocrinal disturbances known to accompany burns are few in number. There is evidence of adrenocortical hyperfunction for a few days after a burn: the eosinophil numbers decrease precipitously and may almost reach zero. For 4 to 7 days the urinary secretion of 17-ketosteroids is supernormal or high normal, and then they decrease, becoming low normal; the urinary secretion of cortin increases and remains high for weeks.

There is no evidence that thyroid function is significantly altered by burns.

Pituitary growth hormone is found in increased concentration in the bloods of all badly burned patients during convalescence.[26]

Immunologic Disturbances

Burn toxins have long been thought to play a part in the production of burn sickness. Ever since the last quarter of the 19th century, a part of burn illness has been ascribed to the absorption of toxic substances from the thermally injured tissues.

The lack of illness attending uninfected large burns, when electrolyte disturbances and negative thermal loading are prevented, indicates that specific burn toxins or antigens, other than bacterial, do not exist (Fig. 17-9).

Respiratory Disturbances

Obstruction of the airway from elevation of the base of the tongue by swelling of the floor of the mouth, by pharyngeal and laryngeal edema, and pulmonary edema are particularly dangerous complications of burns. Life-endangering pharyngeal and laryngeal edema obstructing breathing are especially prone to occur soon after deep burns of the face and the neck. Should tracheostomy not be performed in such cases, pulmonary edema will soon kill the patient; partial inspiratory obstruction of the trachea or the larynx, whatever its cause, is a sure way to pulmonary edema. Consequently tracheostomy is a very important early step in the treatment of deep burns of the head and the neck whenever the free flow of air through the upper airway is seriously impaired or very large quantities of sputum are being raised after the inhalation of noxious gases of combustion.

Pulmonary injury followed by pulmonary edema is a rather frequent complication of burns suffered within buildings or other confined spaces. The hot air or flames themselves do not injure the lung, because the water vapor generated in the upper air passages so cools the hot air that by the time it reaches the upper trachea it is no longer hot enough to injure tissue. Tracheobronchial and pulmonary injury associated with burns is caused by the inhalation of the many noxious gases associated with combustion of various building materials, furnishings and contents. Among these gases are nitric oxide and sulfur dioxide. Tracheostomy is indicated for this chemi-

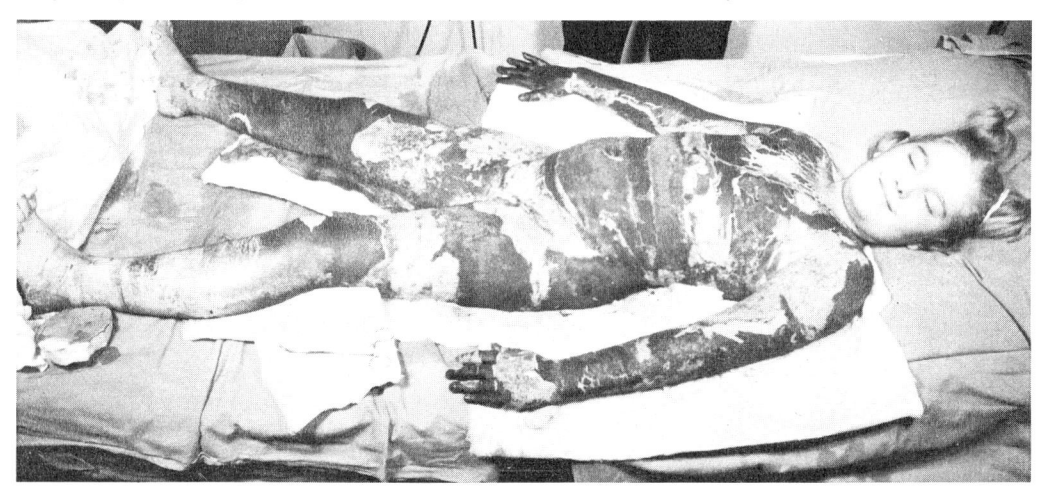

Fig. 17-9. The facial expression of this 11-year-old girl (S. H.), 20 days after sustaining a deep clothing-fire burn covering 60 per cent of the body, makes manifest her sense of physical well-being. Full-thickness eschar has been removed from the upper thighs, the lower abdomen, the lower chest and part of both shoulders and arms. Full-thickness eschar still covers most of the abdomen, the midchest, the right midthigh and the left arm below the elbow. She is now well and without major deformity.

cal tracheobronchitis. The tracheostomy reduces the dead air space, lowers the respiratory resistance offered by the inflamed airway above the tracheotomy and permits the direct clearing of the trachea and the bronchi of the secretions coming from the distal bronchial tree that at times are so copious as literally to drown the patient unless direct suction aspiration of the trachea can be done through a tracheostomy. *However, tracheostomy should not be performed just because the face and the neck have been burned!* A tracheostomy is another site for the origin of lethal infections in burned persons. One must carefully weigh potential benefit against risk.

Miscellaneous Disturbances

Should the burned individual survive the period of burn shock with its associated dangers of attendant and subsequent renal insufficiency, and occasional acute myocardial failure, his illness used to be marked by manifold nutritional problems, infection and psychic disturbances.

For a few years over-emphasis was placed upon fighting the negative nitrogen balance by pouring progressively larger masses of protein into the organism through tubes placed in the stomach. As much as 300 Gm. of protein per diem has been recommended.[33] However, it was soon learned that a forced high protein diet led to trouble; a peculiar illness having many of the characteristics of diabetes was produced occasionally, and an illness characterized by progressive fever, hypernatremia, disorientation, and elevated blood concentrations of amino acid and nonprotein nitrogen attended the forced feeding of suspensions of partially digested or native proteins.[7]

Obviously, the care of a burned person constitutes one of the most difficult and complex duties that a surgeon can undertake. The problems he may face are many more than those sketchily considered here.

Delirium tremens and the illnesses caused by the withdrawal of morphine, heroin or barbiturates are often met because the drug addict and the alcoholic are especially prone to suffer severe burns from bed fires. Acidosis is prone to occur in the severely burned child. Hypocalcemia occasionally bedevils the course of the burned person from the 2nd to the 4th weeks after injury.

Cardiac failure, myocardial infarct, pulmo-

Table 17-7

| | Expected Mortality ||||
| | Therapy (Ages 0-60) ||||
Per Cent of Body Surface	None (1902)	Plasma (1946-50)	Buffered Saline (1950-54)	Buffered Saline and AgNO$_3$ Dressing (1964-65)
12- 24	7.4	7.3	3	3
25- 34	11.5	13	5.5	4
35- 44	72.0	44	24	18
45- 54	90	69	44	25
55- 64	94	87	68	40
65- 74	100	96	86	58
75- 84	100	100	92	65
85- 94	100	100	99	80
95-100	100	100	100	85

nary infarct, acute gastrointestinal hemorrhage, the perforation of acute peptic ulcers (Curling's ulcer), venous thrombosis, gas gangrene, tetanus, encrustative pyoderma, surgical erysipelas, sensitivity reactions, especially to the antibiotics, abortion and infectious hepatitis will be encountered among burned and scalded people. In brief, the surgeon who undertakes the care of a burned man truly needs to be a physician in the broadest sense.

Little need be said about the treatment of the more frequent nonbacterial complications of burns. Vomiting needs to be treated with gastric intubation, because when it occurs soon after the burning, it is so often a sign of acute gastric dilatation.

Curling's Ulcer. Although wound bacteriostasis with silver nitrate and control of negative thermal loading have almost abolished many of the complications of burns, acute duodenal ulcer (Curling's ulcer) still occurs. However, this is not as dangerous as it was. Celiotomy may be performed through unhealed burn without complication. Even incised dermis devoid of epidermis will heal per primam when primarily closed by sutures and covered with 0.5 per cent $AgNO_3$ wet dressings. This is interesting biologically—the healing of thermally injured but not killed dermis can proceed without its normal epithelial covering.[23]

RESULTS OF TREATMENT

Inasmuch as the assessment of one's accomplishments is a most important part in the being of a surgeon, the inclusion in a surgical text of a basis for the assessment of one's treatment of burned and scalded individuals is deemed proper. The comparison of one's results with those of others without regard for the character or the size of the injuries or the ages of those treated is worthless. The relationship between the size of the injury and the mortality rate of burns and scalds in 1902 and 1964-65 is shown in Table 17-7. A cursory study of the table shows that there has been definite improvement in the effectiveness of burn therapy from a mortality standpoint during the last 50 years. However, the mortality rate attending injuries covering 5 to 20 per cent and 75 to 100 per cent of the body's surface during 1902 and 1950 are essentially alike —the former being good in both instances, the latter poor in both instances. However, remarkable advance has been made in the treatment of burns and scalds covering 40 to 60 per cent of the body's surface during the past decade.

Surgeons who deal largely with burned children have experienced lower mortality rates than others caring mainly for adults of all ages. As a consequence thereof they who deal with burned children have unjustifiably used their better gross mortality statistics as arguments for the superiority of therapeutic quirks. The remarkably deleterious effect of aging upon an individual's capacity to recover from a thermal hurt is readily seen in Table 17-8. The mortalities associated with burns and scalds of various sizes in persons of different ages is practically identical in England and the United States. The 1902 and the 1946-50 columns of Tables 16-7 and 16-8 are based on the Weidenfeld and Zumbusch[37] statistics, and a burn population of 382 seriously burned individuals who were treated in the United States between 1946 and 1954, respectively.

In order quickly to assess one's capacity to treat burns all one needs do is derive the sum of the expected mortalities with the use of Table 17-8 and compare it with the actual number of deaths in the series. Treated a certain way, the expected chance of death from a burn or a scald for an individual depends upon his age and the size of his injury.

TABLE 17-8

	MORTALITY (%)		
AREA INJURED (% BODY SURFACE)	AGES 2-60 (BASE 1946-50)	$AgNO_3$ (BASE 1964-65)	AGES 61-85 (BASED ON 1946-50 STATISTICS)*
5	0	0	5
10	0	0	10
15	1	0.2	54
20	2	0.5	92
30	10	4.0	98
40	30	16	99
50	54	25	100
60	78	40	100
70	93	56	100
80	99	65	100
90	100	80	100
100	100	85	100

* This will undoubtedly change much during the next few years.

The extent to which epidermal regeneration has taken place upon dermal remnants as long as 3.5 months after the burn with the production of fairly normal noncicatrized skin, and the remarkable propensity of stamp grafts to effect the same when placed upon subcutaneous fat under the bacteriostatic wet dressings, have shown the need for a more precise and meaningful method of classifying thermal injuries. Burn wounds that, when kept nearly free of pathogenic bacteria, heal within 21 days have no serious biologic connotation. They are not physically incapacitating for longer than a fortnight. The shock that may attend them is easy to treat solely with lactated Ringer's solution. All of the eschar separates spontaneously as brown, tough scales after epidermal regeneration, leaving no permanent scar or deformity. Deeper burns that heal from the base of the wound between the 21st and the 120th postburn days are much more important biologically because they incapacitate for a much longer period of time, and, in addition, the removal of the top dead layer of the dermis, which has been converted into an elastic gel by heat, needs to be done manually as soon as possible in order to prevent bacterial denaturation of the living dermis beneath. However, these injuries, when not infected, heal with little scar and practically no contracture after eschar removal, and no grafts are needed. It is only the deeper subdermal burns that lead to serious scarring and more or less permanent disablement. However, the subdermal burn which does not kill the whole of the subcutaneous adipose tissue still does not lead to disfigurement or permanent disability when resurfaced with even very thin partial thickness cutaneous autografts.

The classification here proposed (see Table 17-11) has prognostic as well as scientific usefulness. The mapping of the proportions of the various types of injury and the correlation of these with the mode of injury and the type

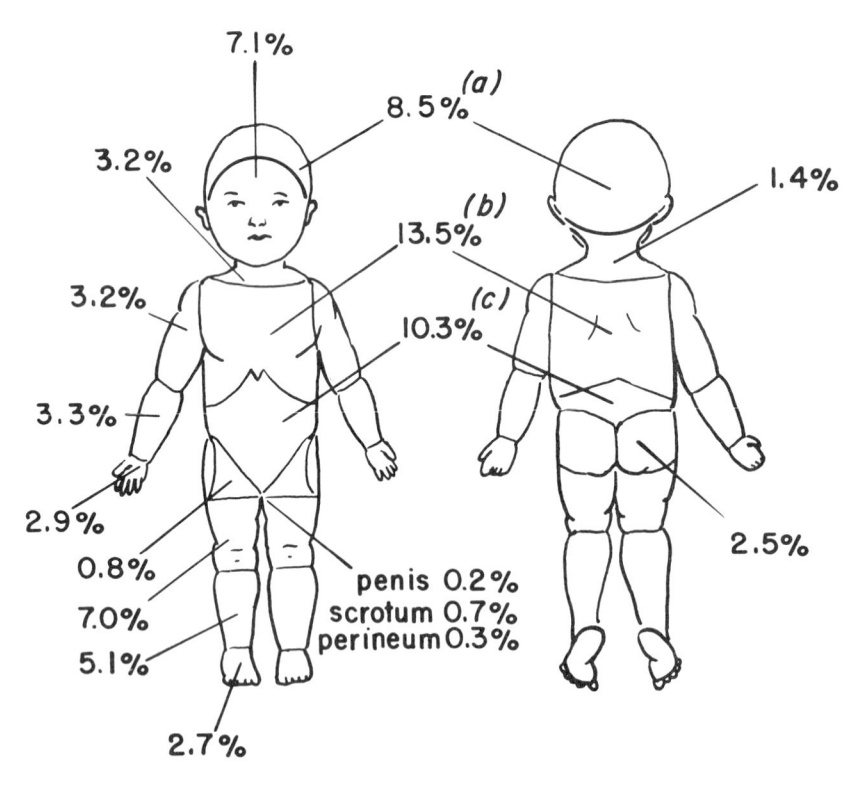

Fig. 17-10. Child, age 1 year. Surface areas of the parts of the body (%). (*a*) Entire scalp; (*b*) entire upper trunk, front and back; (*c*) entire lower trunk, front and back.

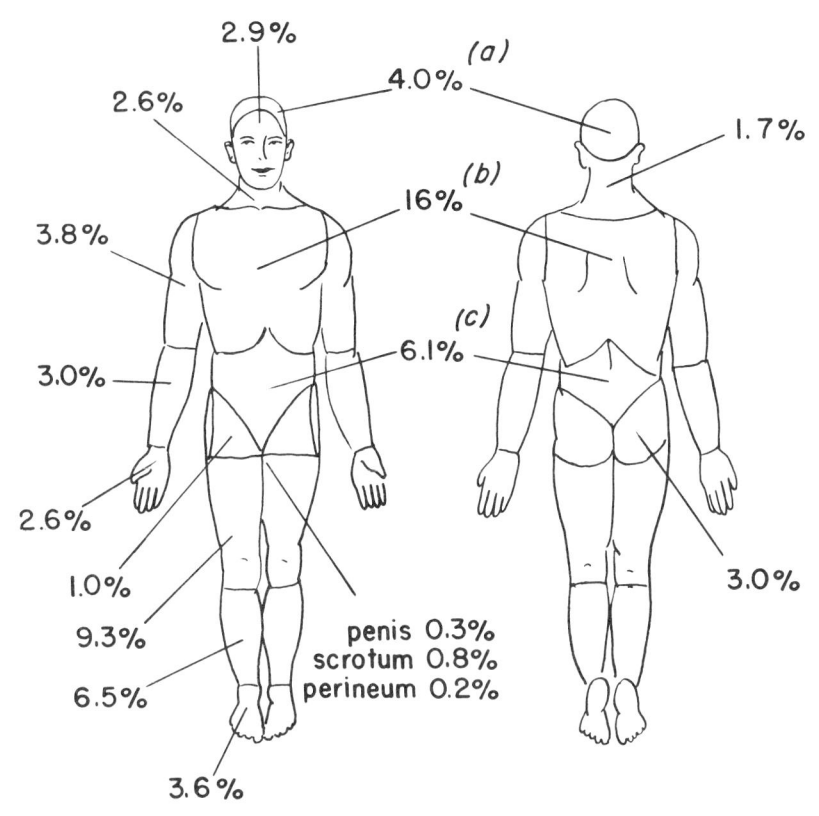

FIG. 17-11. Adult. Surface areas of the parts of the body (%). (a) Entire scalp; (b) entire upper trunk, front and back; (c) entire lower trunk, front and back.

Percentages shown on figure:
- 2.9% (top of head, front)
- 2.6% (side of head, front)
- 4.0% (a) Entire scalp
- 1.7% (back of head)
- 3.8% (upper arm, front)
- 16% (b) entire upper trunk
- 3.0% (forearm)
- 6.1% (c) entire lower trunk
- 2.6% (hand)
- 1.0%
- 9.3% (thigh)
- 6.5% (lower leg)
- penis 0.3%
- scrotum 0.8%
- perineum 0.2%
- 3.0% (back of leg)
- 3.6% (foot)

of treatment used can provide a means of measuring the relative merits of various local treatments, as well as a better insight into causes of burn deformity. Obviously, a particular thermal injury cannot be fully classified in this manner with any *degree of certainty* until all the wound has been resurfaced with epidermis spontaneously or with autografts, or a necropsy has been performed.

The meaningful use of this classification for the above-stated purposes requires a more precise means of gauging the area of injury than the "Rule of Nines" or the modified Berkow method provides. Dividing the body surface into smaller regions such as those recommended by Meeh affords sufficiently precise area definitions for the meaningful use of the proposed classifications. Figures 17-10 and 17-11 were constructed from Meeh's data. The use of this table or these figures is simple, provided that proper photographs have been taken at appropriate times, or overlay-tracings of the burn wounds have been made on the 14th, the 21st and later postburn days.

The Meeh data (Table 17-9) is of special interest in view of the dependence of mortality upon the size of the burn. A burn of both legs and thighs is as large (40%) as one covering the entire trunk, head, neck, and one upper arm. A burn of the entire head, neck, upper extremities and entire chest (½ of trunk) involves only 40 per cent of the body's surface, while one spread over the abdomen to the belt line (⅓ of trunk) and the entire lower extremities excepting the feet covers about 50 per cent. The relationship of surface area to body mass varies much with age. Consequently, the calculation of surface area from weight must take the patient's age in consideration (Table 17-10).

Figures 17-10 and 17-11 are diagrammatic representations of Table 17-9.

The treatment of thermal injury is a major health problem in the United States today.

TABLE 17-9. SURFACE AREAS OF THE PARTS OF THE BODY (SQUARE CM. AND %) (MODIFIED) FROM VON MEEH, K.: Z. BIOLOGIE 15:425-458, 1879)

PART OF BODY	CHILD OF 1 YEAR % B.S.	CHILD OF 1 YEAR SQUARE CM.	ADULT (18-66 YEARS) % B.S.	ADULT (18-66 YEARS) SQUARE CM.
One wrist and hand	2.9	149	2.6	503
One arm	3.2	171	3.8	732
One forearm	3.3	171	3.0	582
Back of neck	1.4	73	1.7	298
Front of neck	3.2	170	2.6	496
Scalp	8.5	475	4.0	787
Face	7.1	377	2.9	548
Upper trunk	13.5	719	16	3,060
Lower trunk	10.3	450	6.1	1,177
One ileopectineal fossa	0.8	42	1.0	236
Both buttocks	5	267	6.0	1,183
Perineum	0.3	15	0.2	47
Scrotum	0.7	38	0.8	174
Penis	0.2	11	0.3	66
One thigh	7	369	9.3	1,770
One leg	5.1	274	6.5	1,246
One ankle and foot	2.7	178	3.6	690

TABLE 17-10. CHANGING RELATIONSHIP OF SURFACE AREA TO BODY MASS WITH AGE (GROWTH). (VIERORDT)[34]

AGE	TOTAL SURFACE AREA (SQUARE METERS)	SURFACE AREA (SQUARE CM.) PER KG. OF BODY WEIGHT
1 day	0.2599	812
6 months	0.4381	626
1 year	0.5181	575
2 years	0.6028	533
4 years	0.7020	495
7 years	0.8552	450
10 years	1.0092	412
12 years	1.1505	386
14 years	1.3676	354
25 years	1.8936	301

Roughly 6,000 hospital beds are occupied the year around by the burned and the scalded. Almost as many people die of thermal injuries as die of all neoplasms of the head and the neck. Someday the existence of our nation may depend upon the capacity of the American physician to treat burns. Burns are a greater danger to modern armies and population than are wounds from missiles. Dresden lost 250,000 residents in one night's incendiary bombing of that city. What will new atomic bombs do? Burns accounted for about one third of the deaths in Hiroshima.

The reconstructive surgery related to burns is discussed in Chapter 49.

REFERENCES

1. Bekkum, van, D. W., and Peters, R. A.: Change in enzymatic process in burns. Quart. J. Exp. Physiol., 36:127-137, 1951.
2. Beloff, A., and Peters, R. A.: Influence of moderate temperature burns upon proteinase of skin. J. Physiol., 103:461, 476, 1945.
3. Buhl: Mittheilungen aus der Pfeufer'schen Klinik: Epidemische Cholera. Z. Rationelle Med. (Henle and Pfeufer), 6:1-105, 1855.
4. Caldwell, F. T., Jr., Osterholm, J. L., Sower, N. D., and Moyer, C. A: Metabolic response to thermal trauma of normal and thyroprivic rats at three environmental temperatures. Ann. Surg., 150:976-988, 1959.
5. Cruickshank, C. N. D., and Hershey, F. B.: The effect of heat on the metabolism of guinea pig's ear skin. Ann. Surg., 151:419-430, 1960.
6. Edenbuizen, M.: Beitrage zur Physiologie der Haut. Z. Rationelle Med. (Henle and Pfeufer), 17:35, 1863.
7. Engel, F. L., and Jaeger, C.: Dehydration with hypernatremia, hyperchloremia and azotemia complicating nasogastric tube feeding. Am. J. Med., 17:196-204, 1954.
8. Evans, E. I., and Bigger, I. A.: The rationale of whole blood therapy in severe burns. Ann. Surg., 122:693-705, 1945.
9. Evans, E. I., and Butterfield, W. J. H.: Stress response in severely burned; interim report. Ann. Surg., 134:588-613, 1951.

TABLE 17-11. FUNCTIONAL CLASSIFICATION OF BURNS

Class		
I	Epidermal	Heals within 14 days
II	Superficial dermal	Heals between 14th and 21st postburn days
III	Intradermal	Epidermal resurfacing effected by growth of epidermis out of the base of wound (not the margin) after the 21st postburn day. This may take place in significant amounts as late as the 120th postburn day under the silver-nitrated dressings.
IV	Subdermal	Spontaneous epidermal resurfacing takes place only from the margins of the wound; cutaneous autografts are needed.
	Divisions of Subdermal Burn	
	IV-A—Intra-adipose	Subcutaneous fat constitutes the wound base.
	IV-B—Fascial	Fascial covering of muscles, tendon or periosteum constitute the base of the wound.
	IV-C—Musculoskeletal	The base of the wound is muscle bare of fascia or bone devoid of periosteum.

Significant scarring and contracture follow epithelial resurfacing by spontaneous regeneration of the wound margins or grafting, only in Class IV, divisions B and C, when the continuous silver-nitrated dressing is used.

Clearly, area estimates of these various classes of burns in any particular case can be made only during necropsy, or after healing is complete.

10. Fozzard, H. A.: Myocardial injury in burn shock. Submitted for publication to Annals of Surgery.
11. Henriques, F. C.: Studies of thermal injury. Arch. Path., 43:489-502, 1947.
12. Holmes, J. H., and Painter, E. E.: Role of extracellular fluid in traumatic shock in dogs. Am. J. Physiol., 148:201, 1947.
13. Kato, L., and Gozsy, B.: Kinetics of edema formation in rats as influenced by critical doses of dextran. Am. J. Physiol., 199:657, 660, 1960.
14. Kefalides, N. F., Arana, J. A., Bazan, A., and Stastny, P.: Clinical evaluation of antibiotics and gamma globulin in septicemias following burns. In Proc. First International Congress on Reseach in Burns, Washington, D. C., 1960.
15. Latta, Thomas: Documents communicated by the Central Board of Health, London, relative to the treatment of cholera by the copious injection of aqueous and saline fluids into the veins. Lancet, 2:274, 1831-32.
16. Lesser, von, L.: Ueber Todesursachen bei Verbrennungen. Virchows Arch. path. Anat., 79:248-310, 1880.
17. Lichtheim: Ueber periodische Hämoglobinurie. Samml. Klin. Vorträge, 134:1147-1168, 1878.
18. Lieberman, Z. H., and Lansche, J. M.: Effects of thermal injury on metabolic rate and insensible water loss in the rat. Surg. Forum, 7:83, 1957.
19. Lindberg, R. B., Brame, R. E., Moncrief, J. A., and Mason, A. D., Jr.: The development of a prophylactic treatment for preventing burn infection. I. Use of Sulfamylon cream on burned rats. Army Surgical Research unit, Annual Reseach Progress Report, Section 50, June 30, 1964.
20. Markley, K., et al.: Clinical evaluation of saline solution therapy in burn shock. J.A.M.A., 161:1465-1473, 1956.
21. Moritz, A. R., Henriques, F. C., Jr., Dutra, F. R., and Weisiger, J. R.: Studies of thermal injury. Arch. Path. 43:466-488, 1947.
22. Moyer, C. A.: The metabolism of burned mammals and its relationship to vaporizational heat loss and other parameters. Research in Burns. Amer. Inst. Biol. Sci., 9:113-120, 1962.
23. Moyer, C. A., Brentano, L., Gravens, D. S., Margraf, H. W., and Monafo, W. W., Jr.: The treatment of large human burns with 0.5 per cent silver nitrate solution. Arch. Surg., 90:812, 1965.
24. Moyer, C. A., Dillon, J. S., and Butcher, H. R., Jr.: Function of human skin in relation to its macromolecular structure. Arch. Surg., 92:222, 1966.
25. Moyer, C. A., and Nissan, S.: Alterations in the basal oxygen consumptions of rats attendant upon three types of dehydration. Ann. Surg. (Suppl.), 154:51-64, 1961.
26. Parker, M., Monafo, W. W., Jr., and Moyer, C. A.: Unpublished data.
27. Ricker, G., and Regendanz, P.: Virchows Arch. path. Anat., 231:1, 1921.
28. Rosenthal, S. M.: Experimental chemotherapy of burns and shock. U. S. Pub. Health Rep., 58:513-522, 1943.
29. Rosenthal, S. R., Hartney, J. B., and Spurrier, W. A.: The "toxin-antitoxin" phenomenon in burns and injury. J.A.M.A., 174:957-965, 1960.
30. Rosenthal, S. M., and Tabor, H.: Electrolyte

changes and chemotherapy in experimental burn and traumatic shock and hemorrhage. Arch. Surg., 51:244-252, 1945.
31. Syme, James: Principles of Surgery. ed. 3. London, Baillière, Tindall & Cox, 1842.
32. Tappeiner, von, H.: Ueber Veränderungen des Blutes und der Muskeln nach ausgedehnten Hautverbrennungen. Centralbl. med. Wissenschaften, 31:385, 1881.
33. Taylor, F. H. L., Levenson, S. M., Davidson, C. S., Browder, N. C., and Lund, C. C.: Problems of protein nutrition in burned patients. Ann. Surg., 118:215-224, 1943.
34. Vierordt, H.: Anatomische, Physiologische, und Physikalische Daten und Tabellen. ed. 3. p. 52. Jena, Fischer, 1906.
35. Weichselbaum, T. E., Margraf, H. W., and Moyer, C. A.: Unpublished data.
36. Weidenfeld, St.: Ueber den Verbrennungstod. Arch. Dermat. Syph., 61:322, 1902.
37. Weidenfeld, St., and Zumbush, L. V.: Weitere Beitrage zur Pathologie und Therapie schwerer Verbrennungen. Arch. Dermat. Syph., 76:163-184, 1905.
38. Wilson, B., and Stirman, J. A.: Initial treatment of burns. J.A.M.A., 173:509-516, 1960.

Cold Injury

One of the enigmas of cold injury is the genesis of one of its forms—immersion foot. It follows long subjection of an extremity, especially when wet, to temperatures of 4° to 6° C. These temperatures are obviously above freezing. Because the freezing points of cells and body fluids are slightly below 0° C., how could freezing be the cause of such an injury as trench foot or immersion foot? Recently, human skin has been found to be a molecular hydrate system that, in a thermodynamic sense, is similar to a solution of methane in water,[8] and to the hydrate systems in the leaves of frost-sensitive plants, such as corn. Ice crystals form in growing corn leaves at a temperature of 40° F., and it forms in, and even plugs up, large gas mains carrying water-wet methane at a temperature of 65° F. It is possible, then, that ice crystals form in skin and other intracutaneous tissues, such as nerves and blood vessels, at temperatures significantly above the freezing point of water or tissue fluids.

Freezing does not kill a cell or damage macromolecular structures, such as dermal collagen, by expansional breaking of cell membranes or organic macromolecules. Instead, solute hypertonicity, attendant upon the exclusion of ions from the crystal lattice of ice, appears to be the cause of cell death and the denaturation of proteins in solution during slow freezing. It might be said that the slow formation of ice crystals within cellular and noncellular macromolecular fiber systems kills the cells, and denatures fibrous proteins, by pickling them in a strong brine made by the exclusion of ions from the intracellular and extracellular ice.

This would account for the fact that cells are not damaged by very rapid freezing, such as occurs when they are immersed in liquid nitrogen, because, in this case, the salt ions are not extruded from the ice crystals, whereas they are when the cells are frozen slowly.

Cold injury may be classified as follows:
1st degree—pernio or chilblain
2nd degree—immersion or trench foot
   a. mild
   b. moderate
   c. severe
   d. gangrenous
3rd degree—frostbite or frost gangrene
   a. superficial
   b. total (complete)

Although one form of cold injury—frostbite or frost gangrene—develops many of the grossly visible features of a burn, such as blisters and eschar, cold injury differs significantly from a burn. The cold injury is often followed by vasomotor, neural and muscular sequelae that are more or less permanent and may be disabling—while burns are not.

Although the formation of ice crystals, with the exclusion of ions from the crystal lattice, is the major cause of the tissue damage inflicted by cold, movement of the frozen part, when it is cryo-rigid, has a remarkably exacerbating effect on the amount of gangrene that follows thawing of the part. Rigidly frozen hamsters, revived by warming, did not develop frost gangrene of the extremities, unless the parts were moved or otherwise injured while the animals were still rigid from the cold.[9] This has therapeutic significance.

Intravascular thrombosis also plays a part in the genesis of frost gangrene. The frostbite that heals or can be resurfaced with split-skin grafts, after sloughing of the eschar, is an injury relatable, in the main, to cellular and extracellular fibrous tissue injury without thrombosis of the main vessels to the member, while that injury which is followed by complete dry gangrene of the part has a significant vascular thrombotic component.

The manifestations of cold injury and treatment of the various forms are included in Table 17-12. In cases of the gangrenous form of immersion foot and of frostbite, the cold lesion is not sharply demarcated but fades off proximally, passing progressively from 2nd degree, phase "c," through "b" and "a," and the 1st degree injury, before normal tissue is to be encountered. In the Arctic, the supply of readily available water for warming the frozen part is often limited, and the treatment of a large number of casualties requires other more available means. During the Russo-Finnish War, the Finns used their traditional bath houses, the saunas, for rapid warming of frostbite, employing air temperatures of 120° to 145° F. Such a structure can be made readily from a tent heated with a large primus stove or an oil drum stove, fired with oil or brush. The knowledge of the therapeutic propriety of rapid warming for frostbite has been accepted only recently in English-speaking countries; it has been common knowledge among the Finns and the Northern Swedes at least since 1939 (Russo-Finnish War), and presumably for centuries before that. It was used by my Scandinavian grandfather to treat me for frostbite during the winter of 1914. Treatment by slow warming or rubbing with snow is condemned. It is damaging, besides being worthless. It has been said that no amputation of a frozen part should be performed, no matter how bad it looks, until probing demonstrates openings into joints or the frozen part sloughs. This is correct for toes and fingers that maintain a fairly normal volume after the period of edema, but a finger or toe that becomes shrunken and mummified should be removed at the mummificational demarcation. If such digits are not removed, they may remain in place for a month or two and materially slow convalescence. The anticoagulants, vasolytic drugs, intravenous alcohol and procaine have been used in treating frostbite. How beneficial one or all of these things are is not known. Sympathectomy is useful for the symptomatic treatment of disabling vasomotor sequelae of cold injury. It is useless for the treatment of chronic pernio. The references have been selected to provide the student access to basic and clinical research on the subject. The subject titles indicate the research fields.

Shock attends the rewarming of large frostbites because of the rapidity of swelling and blistering which accompany rewarming. In the case of an inebriated man rendered cryorigid and hypothermic (rectal temperature 26° C.) after exposure to temperatures lower than 22° below zero Fahrenheit for 11 hours, 8.5 liters of lactated Ringer's solution during 2 hours' warming at 106° F. in a Hubbard tank were needed in order to maintain a palpable pulse and a detectable blood pressure. He recovered with only the loss of the terminal phalanges of a few digits.

REFERENCES

1. Blair, J. R., Schatzki, R., and Orr, R. D.: Cold injury sequelae. Paper presented at AMA Annual Meeting, Section on Military Medicine, 1956.
2. Burton, A. C., and Edholm, P. G.: Man in a Cold Environment. London, Edward Arnold and Co., 1955.
3. Hedblom, E. E.: Polar Manual. ed. 2. p. 58. Bethesda, Maryland, U.S. Naval Medical School, 1961.
4. Kreyberg, L.: Development of acute tissue damage due to cold. Physiol. Rev., 29:156, 1949.
5. Macy Foundation Conferences on Cold Injury. New York, Josiah Macy, Jr., Foundation, (Edited by Ferrer, Irene), 1951, 1952, 1954, 1956.
6. Meryman, H. L.: Tissue freezing and local tissue injury. Physiol. Rev., 37:233, 1957.
7. Mills, W. J., Jr., Whaley, R., and Fish, W.: Experience with rapid rewarming and ultrasonic treatment. Alaska Med., 2:1, 1960; 3:28, 1961.
8. Moyer, C. A., Dillon, J. S., and Butcher, H. R., Jr.: Function of human skin in relation to its

TABLE 17-12

Cold Damage	Phase	History	Symptoms and Signs	Treatment	Residua: General	Residua: Particular
1st degree Pernio or chilblain	a.	Fairly prolonged exposure of thinly clad or unclad legs or exposed face to air at temperatures below 20° F. (−7° C.)	Pruritic, painful erythema. Small, clear blisters may appear 12 to 48 hours after the exposure	Put on clothes, such as long thermal underwear and a wool face helmet, when going out into the cold	Atrophy of dermis, livedo reticularis (inconstant) and sensitivity to cold	*Chronic pernio* Ulcers of the skin, often mistaken for stasis ulcers appearing after many attacks of acute pernio. At first, the ulcers appear during winter and heal during summer. Later the ulcers do not heal during summer, and excision and resurfacing with skin grafts are needed to eradicate them
2nd degree Immersion or trench foot	a.	Prolonged exposure of wet feet and legs to temperatures between 30° and 40° F., the afflicted part does not become rigid. Upon removing the shoe and legging or boot, the foot is noted to be white, and it swells so rapidly that the well-fitted shoe or boot cannot be put on again	Edema; transitory anesthesia; hyperemia after warming; anhidrosis	Opiates for pain; warm feet rapidly in water at temperature of 98° to 100° F. (37° to 38° C.)		Pain and hyperhidrosis, especially with any exposure to cold
	b.		As for "a" and, additionally, muscle weakness	Elevate legs to minimize edema		Long, persisting vasomotor disorders and neuritis (nerve damage)
	c.		As for "a" and "b" and, additionally, hyaline degeneration of muscle and wallerian degeneration of nerves (paralysis)	Wrap in *elastic* bandages; ambulate only after swelling is gone; avoid exposure to cold		Years of pain, weakness, paresthesia and anesthesia, vasomotor instability
	d.		Gangrene	With only gangrene of skin, skin grafting; otherwise amputation		If resurfacing is possible, the residua are the same as for "c"

Cold Damage	Phase	History	Symptoms and Signs	Treatment	Residua
3rd degree Frostbite or frost gangrene	a.	Exposure to air or liquids at temperatures below 0° C. (32° F.)	Plasticity or rigidity of the part, depending on degree of solidification, pallor and anesthesia. Erythema, pain, edema and blistering appear after warming. The blisters contain a fluid that clots and has a protein concentration less than that of plasma. At times, it may be bloody	Rapid warming in water at temperature of 110° to 112° F. (43° to 44° C.). *Avoid all movement*, palpitation or other manipulation of the part until it is completely thawed and at least attains room temperature. Skin grafting after spontaneous separation of eschar	Tissue loss (skin and appendages), scars, stiff joints, abnormal nails, cystic defects in the phalanges near the joint surfaces. Vasomotor instability, hyperhidrosis and more or less permanent sensitivity to cold, characterized by severe pain and a Raynaud-like phenomenon upon exposure to a degree of cold that is not uncomfortable to a normal part or person
	b.	As for "a" and, in addition, there is often a history of walking on the frozen foot, of using the frozen hand or of vigorous rubbing of the ear, the hand or the foot while frozen		Amputation after joints open up or become infected or true mummification occurs	Loss of part

macromolecular structure. Arch. Surg., 92:222, 1966.
9. Smith, A. U.: Frostbite in golden hamsters revived from body-temperatures below 0° C. Lancet, 2:1255, 1954.
10. Ungley, A. C.: The immersion foot syndrome. Adv. Surg., 1:209, 1949.
11. White, J. C.: Immersion foot syndrome following exposure to cold. New Eng. J. Med., 228: 211, 1943.

CHAPTER 18

J. GARROTT ALLEN, M.D.

Radiation Injury from Local or Total Body Exposure

CONSIDERATIONS IN RADIATION EXPOSURE IN WHOLE BODY INJURY

Many of the physical properties of ionizing radiation are discussed in Chapter 9, The Principles of Isotope Technics in Surgery. In total body exposure, it is important to delineate clearly the type of ionizing rays to which the individual has been exposed and to define the quantities of radiation received and the methods for protection and possible methods of treatment. Such factors as energy equivalents, penetration, duration of exposure and tissue sensitivity are among the essential considerations in estimating biologic effects. These qualities in turn depend upon the nature of radiations emitted, the source or sources involved, and the rates and the amounts of exposure.

It is almost 25 years since the first atomic bomb dropped in Japan. Almost all of our knowledge of this subject has been gained since that event.

Radioactive Decay Products

Unstable elements emit one or more of several forms of energy; some are particle radiations, because they have mass, and some are not. Mass is determined by the numbers of neutrons and protons in the nucleus. More than 30 particles of the nucleus are now recognized.

Certain definitions are necessary to appreciate the concepts and the nature of the hazards of irradiation, the characteristics of its injury, and the possible means for protection of the individual against irradiation exposures.

Isotopes. An isotope is one of the several masses that atoms of a particular chemical element may display. Isotopes of most elements are stable and not radioactive. A *radioisotope* is an unstable atom of an element that, on a random basis, emits bits of matter or bursts of electromagnetic energy until this energy is exhausted and the isotope then becomes a stable one. *Radionuclide* is synonymous with the term radioisotope and is preferred because the word "nuclide" emphasizes that the properties that distinguish one isotope from another of the same element reside in the differences in the nucleus.

Ionizing Radiations. Alpha rays (particulate radiation) are positively charged helium nuclei, mass 1.672×10^{-24} Gm., which move at high speed in air for distances of 2.7 cm. to 8.6 cm., depending upon their energy. They are large particles and are stopped readily by a sheet of paper, transmitting their energies to their absorber and producing various chemical changes in it.

Beta rays are electrons, and they have a small mass, 8.999×10^{-28} Gm. They travel at much higher speeds than alpha rays and are more penetrating, though their mass is only 1/1,800 of alpha particles. They penetrate thin layers of tissue and are stopped by 2 mm. thickness of brass or 1 mm. of lead. They are identical with cathode rays except for origin, beta rays coming from radioisotopic decay and cathode rays from a heated cathode of a vacuum tube in a strong electric field. Many beta-emitting isotopes concurrently also give off gamma rays (electromagnetic radiation), which are very penetrating. The ratio of beta radiation to gamma radiation is a constant for a given radioisotope and is sustained throughout the decay of the isotope. Consequently, measurement of the quantity of penetrating gamma rays given off by a nuclide is an indication of the amount of beta radiation which it emits. Thus it is that the residual beta radiation is computed from measurement of gamma radiation.

Gamma rays travel at the speed of light; they are photons with electromagnetic energy and have neither mass nor charge. They are identical in nature with x-rays but are distinguished from x-rays because of their different source, gamma rays coming from radioactive elements and x-rays from the bombardment of various metals by fast electrons in a vacuum.

The neutron has a mass identical with that of the proton but has no charge. Those which travel slowly are known as *thermal neutrons*; those which travel at high speeds are known as *fast neutrons*. In the bombardment of nuclei with neutrons, slow, or thermal, neutrons are absorbed by the target atoms, rendering their nuclei unstable, and some of these nuclei become radioactive, emitting their characteristic radiations.

Energy Measurement of Ionizing Irradiation. *Electron volts* are expressed as million electron volts. One *mev* is the energy that an electron would acquire if, starting from rest, it were to be attracted to a 1 million volt electrode bearing a positive charge.

We also measure in several ways the quantities of ionization the target receives. Among these are:

PHYSICAL UNITS

Curie: A unit quantity of any radionuclide in which 3.7×10^{10} disintegrations per second occur, which is equal to the disintegration of 1 gram of radium per second.

Microcurie: One millionth of a curie.

Picocurie: A millionth of a millionth of a curie. This term replaces the formerly used "micromicrocurie."

Roentgen Unit: That amount of gamma or x-radiation necessary to ionize 1 cc. of dry air under standard conditions.

Rad: A unit measurement of absorbed radiation applying to all forms of ionizing radiation; 1 rad is 100 ergs of energy per gram of absorbing matter. For gamma radiation of moderate energy, the rad and the roentgen units are essentially equal and are terms that are often used interchangeably.

BIOLOGIC UNITS

REM: Roentgen equivalent in man, which is that amount of a particular type and energy of radiation that, when absorbed in man, produces the same effect as 1 roentgen or 1 rad in man.

RBE: Relative biologic efficiency for a given type and energy of radiation is the dose of gamma rays necessary to produce the same biologic effect as a unit of the dose of the energy in question. Roughly, the RBE for beta rays is 1; for slow or thermal neutrons, 5; 10 for fast neutrons; and 20 for alpha particles.

LET: Linear energy transfer is the rate at which a particle of radiation loses its energy as it moves through the absorbing medium. The shorter the distance of penetration before all energy is absorbed, the higher is the rate of energy transfer per unit length of travel, assuming transferable energy to be equal.

Natural radioactivity occurs in all elements with atomic weights above 209 or whose atomic numbers are greater than 83. Artificial radioactivity has been achieved for all elements in the Periodic Table, though not all isotopes created by neutron or electron bombardment are radioactive. The characteristics of artificial radioactivity vary tremendously with the element involved. Half-lives range from milliseconds to millions of years. A radioactive element in the course of disintegration loses by expulsion a nuclear particle from its agitated unstable nucleus, thus allowing the residual components to settle down and become a stable atom of another element with a smaller mass. The decrease in radioactivity for a quantity of a radioactive element is exponential. For a particular atom, the loss of the nuclear particle is instantaneous.

Revised international identification for chemical isotopes has been adopted by the World Health Organization (1964), and is as shown:

$_7N_2^{14}$ 14 indicates mass number
      7 indicates atomic number
      2 indicates atoms/molecule

Mass number is the only one required in most instances. Thus, instead of N^{14}, we now have ^{14}N.

THERMONUCLEAR RADIATION

Fission bombs release their power from the energies made available by the cleavage of unstable heavy elements of high atomic numbers in the Periodic Table, principally uranium 235 and plutonium 238. Absorption of an extra neutron by a radioactive atom which is already unstable renders it drastically so. The nuclear cleavage of these heavy atoms results in the formation of radioactive isotopes of atoms in the intermediate range of the Periodic

Considerations in Radiation Exposure in Whole Body Injury

TABLE 18-1. SOME POTENTIALLY HAZARDOUS PRODUCTS OF FISSION AND FUSION

\multicolumn{4}{c}{FISSION}	\multicolumn{2}{c}{FUSION}
ISOTOPE	HALF-LIFE	ISOTOPE	HALF-LIFE	ISOTOPE	HALF-LIFE
Strontium 90	28 yrs.	Lanthanum 140	40 hrs.	Hydrogen 3	12.8 yrs.
Cesium 137	30 yrs.	Barium 140	13 days	Carbon 14*	5,760 yrs.
Iodine 131	8 days	Niobium 95	35 days		
Strontium 89	54 days	Zirconium 9	65 days		

* (Secondary: derived from neutron bombardment of atmospheric nitrogen.)

Table. Fusion devices in the low-yield range derive their explosive force from nuclear fission, which gives rise to amounts of radioactive products roughly proportional to their explosive yield. Usually, the major portion of energy released by a thermonuclear device is from nuclear fusion of hydrogen nuclei forming helium and tritium. Because very high temperatures and pressures are necessary to initiate fusion, a fusion bomb is detonated by a fission device of sufficient yield to provide the necessary temperature and pressure. Consequently, certain amounts of high-speed gamma rays and neutrons are released in the explosion of thermonuclear devices. The principle products of fission and of fusion devices that are potential hazards to health are shown in Table 18-1.

In addition, the large release of neutrons by either fusion or fission induces secondary radioactivity in other environmental structures and substances: water, earth's surface, towers, buildings, etc. Most prominent among these are listed in Table 18-2.

TABLE 18-2. SECONDARILY INDUCED RADIOACTIVITY

ISOTOPE	HALF-LIFE
Iron 59	47 days
Manganese 54	310 days
Silicon 31	2.6 hrs.
Chlorine 38	37 min.
Sodium 24	14.7 hrs.

To these isotopes or nuclides should be added those elements in the body which may become radioactive when exposed to neutron bombardment in the explosion of a nuclear bomb (Table 18-3).

TABLE 18-3. POTENTIALLY RADIOACTIVE BODY ELEMENTS

ISOTOPE	HALF-LIFE
^{45}Ca	164 days
^{47}Ca	5 days
^{49}Ca	9 min.
^{41}Ca	120,000 yrs.
^{42}K	12.5 hrs.
^{198}Au (from teeth)	2.7 hrs.

In a general way, the radioactivity induced among the elements in the body, including ^2H, ^{24}Na and ^{14}C, are unimportant considerations because the distance that gamma radiation travels exceeds that of neutrons, and high-speed gamma rays do not induce radioactivity in nuclei that they strike. Therefore, when a victim is beyond the reach of neutrons, he may still be within the range of lethal radiation from high-energy gamma radiation, though he does not become radioactive. Although every atomic nucleus struck by a neutron is transformed into a new isotope, only some of these are rendered radioactive or remain so. For example, only 0.2 per cent of oxygen atoms are of the type that are rendered radioactive and the half-life of these is very short, all being inactive in less than 15 minutes. On the other hand, every sodium atom in the body is available for neutron activation. Thus, measurements of the degree of radioactivity that may be present in the body immediately after an acute neutron exposure are of assistance in estimating the degree of exposure that the victim may have received.

Irradiation injury and sickness consequent to an airburst of a 20-megaton thermonuclear device are of no biologic significance because the killing power from heat and blast extends

TABLE 18-4. MILES FROM GROUND-ZERO OF OCCURRENCE OF CERTAIN FATALITY FROM INITIAL EFFECTS AMONG UNPROTECTED PERSONS (AIR BURST OF FUSION DEVICE)

Weapon Yield (Kilotons)	Height of Typical Air Burst in Miles	Certain Fatality in Miles		
		Blast	Thermal	Initial Nuclear Radiation
1	0.13	0.39	0.29	0.51
20	0.35	1.06	0.90	0.82
400	0.95	2.87	3.67	0.94
1,000	1.29	3.90	5.73	1.04
3,000	1.87	5.62	9.25	0
5,000	2.21	6.67	11.72	0
10,000	2.79	8.40	16.05	0
20,000	3.51	10.59	22.1	0

From Russell, P. W., and Kimbrel, L. G.: Estimates of the kill probability in target area family shelters. J.A.M.A., 180:25, 1962.

considerably beyond that from direct radiation. As shown in Table 18-4, the distance that certain death from heat among the unprotected extends is 25 to 50 times greater than that from direct ionizing radiation. This is not true with fission bombs wherein the maximum obtainable blast and heat effects are infinitely less than the "unlimited" power of the fusion devices.

Magnitude of Injuries in Urban Areas. Some concept and perspective of the magnitude of potential disasters from a thermonuclear attack on areas in the United States are gained from published portions of the Holifield Committee hearings by Sidel et al. (1963). If the Boston area were hit by two 10-megaton bombs and one 8-megaton bomb, each appropriately located, the magnitude in loss of human life would be enormous. (See Table 18-5.)

Estimation of the remaining numbers of physicians is more difficult because they tend to concentrate in urban areas. In the theoretical Boston attack, Sidel estimates that of the 6,560 physicians in the area, 640 would be uninjured, 2,380 killed the first day, 2,470 would die from their injuries later, and 1,070 would be injured but would survive. In this model, each surviving physician would be obliged to treat 730 injured patients. Even so, these data may be a little too conservative as larger yielding bombs are developed, but the example shown here suggests that the enormous problems the bombs created in Hiroshima and in Nagasaki in 1945 were minor compared with the destructive forces of modern weapons.

The effect of distance upon certain kill from blast and heat among unprotected persons exposed to a 20-megaton thermonuclear bomb is illustrated graphically in Figure 18-1. Because the radius of lethal direct or initial irradiation is exceeded by that of blast and heat, the radiation problem is that produced by fallout and that to which persons entering the close-in area are exposed because of secondarily induced radioactivity. Thus, with an air burst of a 20-megaton bomb, most of the human population within a 10-mile radius will die, though not all will be killed immediately. Blast shelters may be useful if they are 10 miles or more beyond ground zero, but fallout

TABLE 18-5. ESTIMATE OF CASUALTIES IN METROPOLITAN AREA AFTER HYPOTHETICAL 28-MEGATON ATTACK

Target Area	Population 1950 Census	No. Killed First Day	No. Fatally Injured	No. Surviving Injured	No. Uninjured
Boston metropolitan area	2,875,000	1,052,000	1,084,000	467,000	272,000

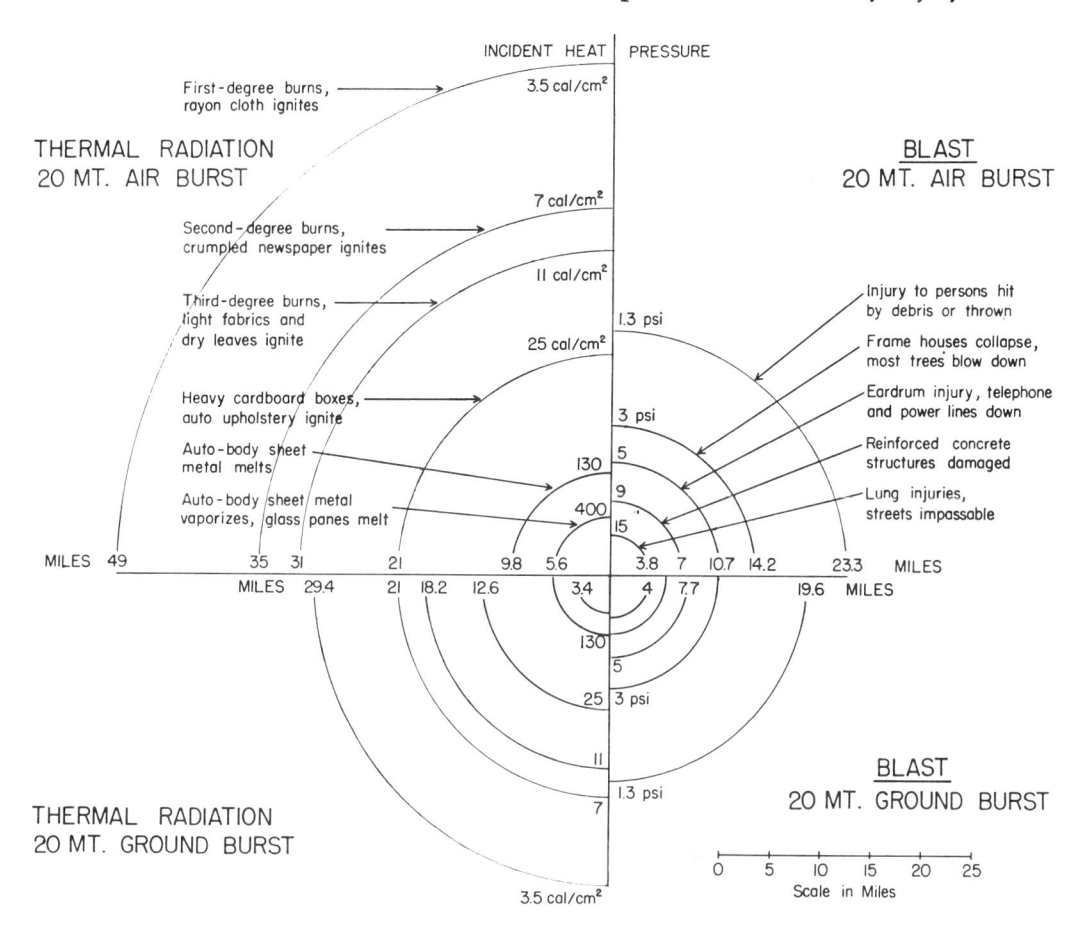

Considerations in Radiation Exposure in Whole Body Injury 407

FIG. 18-1. Effects of the detonation of a 20-megaton fusion bomb as a function of distance from ground zero. *Upper right quadrant*: blast effect at indicated distances for an air burst, in terms of pounds per square inch of overpressure and corresponding physical effects. *Lower right quadrant*: similar relations, but at reduced distances for a ground burst. *Upper left quadrant*: thermal effects at indicated distances for an air burst, in terms of calories per square centimeter of incident radiation and corresponding physical effects. *Lower left quadrant*: similar relations, but at reduced distances for a ground burst. (Ervin, F. R., Glazier, J. B., Aronow, S., Nathan, D., Coleman, R., Avery, N., Shohet, S., and Leeman. C.: Human and ecologic effects in Massachusetts of an assumed thermonuclear attack on the United States, N. Eng. J. Med. 266, 1127)

shelters will be useless this near. At 15 miles the blast effect and fire may not be fatal if those surviving can escape the flying debris carried by the shock waves, including human bodies and fragments thereof. Blast may kill directly by instantaneous increases of pressures that rise 15 to 20 pounds per square inch above atmospheric pressure. Since most housing is totally destroyed with instantaneous rises of 5 pounds per square inch, most persons inhabiting them would be crushed or killed by debris. Tertiary effects from blast, shock and wind up to 20 miles or more from ground zero will account for some casualties.

Thermal energy is released in two pulses. The first is a brief ultraviolet flash that is not seriously hazardous except to the eyes. The second is that of infrared light and accounts for 35 per cent of the bomb's energy. Up to 20 miles, an exposed person would have 2nd-degree burns, igniting most of his flammable clothing, which produces 3rd-degree burns. An unprotected glance at the fireball from a 20-megaton device 40 miles away will produce blindness.

Viewed in another way, there is a 50-50 chance that one may survive the shock wave of a 20-megaton air burst if one is in a reinforced surface level shelter about 5 miles from the epicenter. If he is in ordinary urban housing 9 to 10 miles from the epicenter, he has a 50-50 chance of survival. If he is in the open, he may have a 50-50 chance of survival of heat and blast as close as 12 miles or as far as 16 to 18 miles if the air is clear. At best, the above estimates are crude and subject to considerable error. Then, too, the effects of blast and heat may be modified considerably for an air burst by the local terrain, the energy yield of the device, and its altitude when exploded.

There are still isolated accidents that occur with injury, primarily from whole-body ionizing radiation. In addition, whole-body radiation has been employed as an immunosuppressive mechanism in preparing patients for homotransplantation and occasionally in the treatment of malignant disorders of the blood. Tolerance for total radiation varies considerably from one species to another and is also affected within a species by the duration of the administration of the dose—i.e., as a single dose or as subacute cumulative doses. Examples of LD 50 to 100 tolerances for single dose whole-body exposure to ionizing radiation are shown in Table 18-6.

TABLE 18-6. LD 50 TO 100 WITHIN 30 DAYS AFTER TOTAL BODY EXPOSURE WITHOUT PROTECTION

Man	250 to 500 r (estimated)
Dog	200 to 350 r (established)
Rabbit	800 to 950 r (established)
Rat	500 to 800 r (established)
Mouse	600 to 750 r (established)

Fallout Radiations. Fallout presented no serious problem in the Hiroshima and the Nagasaki shots because of the relatively small bombs exploded in air, but in the test shot at Almagordo it did. This shot was detonated from a tower and hence was essentially a surface burst. From studies of fallout, blast, and heat from subsequent tests, it has been learned that fallout is maximal with surface burst and that the effects of blast and heat are much less than in an air burst where the radius of destruction from heat and blast exceeds considerably that of the initial release of ionizing radiation.

Fallout radiations may be classified as 3 in kind:

1. *Local or near-in fallout* consists of nearby structures and debris in which secondary radioactivity has been induced by the primary neutron source released from the bomb burst. These are the larger fragments that fly through the air and the larger particles that are deposited downwind for a distance of a few miles to several hundred miles. This area of contamination is oval to cigar-shaped, 10 to 75 miles wide and usually 50 to 500 or more miles long, depending upon the velocity of wind and air movement. This is usually the most serious kind of fallout because of its intensity and because it occurs within minutes to a few hours; hence there has been little time for significant decay of some of the important radionuclides created by the initial burst (Table 18-7).

TABLE 18-7. CALCULATED RADIATION EXPOSURE 110 MILES AWAY FROM DETONATION OF THE THERMONUCLEAR EXPLOSION OF MARCH 1, 1954 (LAPP)

5 to 12 hours	1,000 r
12 to 24 hours	625 r additional
24 to 48 hours	545 r additional
2 days to 1 week	815 r additional
1 week to 1 month	720 r additional
1 month to 1 year	840 r additional
	4,545 r in the first year

2. *Intermediate or tropospheric fallout* consists of smaller dust particles, usually a micron to a few micra in diameter. They enter the troposphere which extends outward 7 to 10 miles from the earth's surface but not into the stratosphere (10 miles or more). In the troposphere these particles circle the earth usually in a band not wider than 20 to 30° beyond the latitude of the initial burst. There is little

tendency for such bands to cross the equator, and they tend to be widest in the temperate zones. Usually, the tropospheric fallout is complete within a few days to approximately 2 to 3 weeks. Rain and snow facilitate fallout from the troposphere, so that on earth "hot" areas may occur. This type of fallout can present a health hazard because of concentrations of material deposited locally before sufficient decay in radioactivity has occurred.

3. *Long-term or stratospheric fallout* consists of dust particles, usually less than one tenth of a micron in diameter, that rise 50,000 to 150,000 feet, where they remain for months and years. This delay greatly reduces the radiation fallout hazard because much of the radiation activity has been dissipated before these particle re-enter the troposphere to be precipitated gradually, or more hastily if snow and rain should occur.

Thus the problems from irradiation in a thermonuclear bomb burst of the 10- to 20-megaton varieties are largely those of secondarily induced radiation, to be contended with either as fallout that may be global in area, or as directly acquired environmental radioactivity which is largely limited to the distance traveled by the primarily released neutrons, usually less than 10 miles from the hypocenter. Because the area of lethal environmental irradiation from thermonuclear devices of these yields is not as great as that of either blast or heat, the problem associated with local primary environmental irradiation is only to determine how soon such an area can be reoccupied. The fallout problems are different in that they concern not only external irradiation but exposure also from food that is consumed later. Irradiation as a hazard is greatly reduced if the device is exploded 3½ miles above the earth's surface. At this distance, the amount of neutron and gamma radiation that reaches the ground is sublethal and may indeed be very little (FitzSimons, 1960). The penetrating power of neutrons is less than that of the high-energy gamma radiation released.

Federal Radiation Council Recommendations. The Federal Radiation Council, established in 1959 by Presidential order, has provided in a series of recommendations the information necessary to form our present concepts on prevention and treatment of radiation injury (Terry and Chadwick, 1964). The Council suggests the term "Radiation Protection Guide" (RPG) to supplement and to redefine the concepts embraced under the phrase "Maximum Permissible Dose." RPG was introduced to correct the growing impression that a dose of radiation less than the maximum permissible dose was harmless, when in reality "There is no level of radiation exposure below which there can be absolute certainty that no harmful effects will occur to at least a few individuals when sufficiently large numbers of people are exposed. . . . Any dose chosen as a standard will involve some risk of injury in exposed populations." But, as Terry is quick to point out, we must and always do balance risk against gain, often intuitively, for seldom can such judgment be quantitated, as in this instance where the health of total populations must be considered along with the health of the individual. Moreover, numerical values for radiation protection standards are not fixed and immutable. The LD 50 for man receiving nearly instantaneous total body exposure of gamma radiation is between 240 and 260 r or REM, for similar groups of people. It is probably also true that the LD 99 to 100 for man is not twice the LD 50 as indicated in the table below but rather that the amount of exposure exceeds that of LD 50 by no more than 20 per cent—i.e., 300 r when LD 50 is 250 r. Some data from man and an abundance from mammalian experiments are available confirming this statement (Table 18-8).

Biologic tolerance does not vary this much, but the physical aspects of a burst of ionizing radiation including backscatter, the exact locations of people from a point source, and the duration of primary exposure as well as of secondary radiation are more complex, and more difficult to determine as well as to measure or calculate. It is probable that the true LD 50 for the same exposure time in the same environment does not vary by more than 10 REM, with the exception of children, who are usually a little more sensitive. In Table 18-8 are rough estimates of human responses to short-term effects of total body irradiation. These data assume primary initial radiation as well as secondary environmental radiation; hence, rather wide ranges are shown.

The more rapidly the irradiation exposures are acquired, the lower is the LD 50 dose. For example, the LD 50 for the dog, under the

TABLE 18-8. PROBABLE SHORT-TERM EFFECTS OF ACUTE WHOLE-BODY IRRADIATION

ACUTE DOSE	PROBABLE EFFECTS
0 to 50	No obvious effect, except possibly minor blood changes
80 to 120	Vomiting and nausea for about 1 day in 5–10% of exposed persons; fatigue but no serious disability.
130 to 170	Vomiting and nausea for about 1 day, followed by other symptoms of radiation sickness in about 25% of persons; no deaths anticipated.
180 to 220	Vomiting and nausea for about 1 day, followed by other symptoms of radiation sickness in about 50% of persons; no deaths anticipated.
270 to 330	Vomiting and nausea in nearly all persons on 1st day, followed by other symptoms of radiation sickness; about 20% deaths within 2–6 wk. after exposure; survivors convalescent for about 3 mo.
400 to 500	Vomiting and nausea in all persons on 1st day, followed by other symptoms of radiation sickness; about 50% deaths within 1 mo.; survivors convalescent for about 6 mo.
550 to 750	Vomiting and nausea in all persons within 4 hr. after exposure, followed by other symptoms of radiation sickness; up to 100% deaths; few survivors, convalescent for about 6 mo.
1,000	Vomiting and nausea in all persons within 1–2 hr.; probably no survivors.
5,000	Incapacitation almost immediately; all persons dead within 1 wk.

(Ervin, F. R., et al.: Human and ecologic effects in Massachusetts of an assumed thermonuclear attack on the United States. New Eng. J. Med., 266, 1127, 1962)

circumstances that prevailed in my laboratory, proved to be 220 rads when given in 90 minutes, but when this same dosage scale was administered over a 48-hour period and everything else remained the same, LD 50 increased nearly 50 per cent. But there is a limit to the time factors.

If we assume a uniform fallout distribution over a 4,000 square mile area (40 × 100 miles) after an air burst of a 20-megaton thermonuclear device, the cumulative gamma radiation 3 feet above ground level is so great that there is little chance of an individual's escaping without fatal exposure from environmental irradiation (Table 18-9). The only protection presently possible is an adequate fall-out shelter. If one can get to it and remain in it until ambient radiation in the local or near-in fallout area is of little consequence, one may escape with little somatic damage. From this table it would appear that two kinds of information are necessary before one can decide that it is safe to leave one's shelter. The first is in which direction is the shortest distance to safe ground—i.e., away from downwind and hence out of the close-in fallout

TABLE 18-9. CUMULATIVE GAMMA-RAY DOSE AT 3 FEET ABOVE GROUND LEVEL AT INTERVALS AFTER DETONATION OF A 20-MEGATON BOMB, ASSUMING UNIFORM FALLOUT OVER 4,000 SQUARE MILES

INTERVAL	DOSE DURING INTERVAL r	CUMULATIVE DOSE FROM 1 HR. AFTER DETONATION r
1–2 hr.	2,500	2,500
2–3 hr.	1,250	3,750
3–4 hr.	800	4,550
4–5 hr.	550	5,100
5–10 hr.	1,500	6,600
10–24 hr.	1,550	8,150
2d day	950	9,100
3d day	500	9,600
4th day	300	9,900
5th day	225	10,125
6th day	175	10,300
7th day	120	10,420
2d wk.	535	10,955
3d wk.	285	11,240
4th wk.	140	11,380
2d mo.	220	11,600
3d mo.	100	11,700
4th mo.	60	11,760
5th mo.	40	11,800
6th mo.	25	11,825
6th–12th mo.	60	11,885
2d yr.	20	11,905
3d yr.	6	11,911
4th yr.	3	11,914

(Ervin, op. cit., p. 1134)

area. The second, because it is assumed that one already has had some exposure, is what is the maximum dosage that a person can tolerate between his shelter and safe ground and how can he know what this may be. Most agree that it would not be safe to leave a shelter until the amount of exposure is less than 10 r per hour and that an area of essentially no exposure can be reached in less than 10 hours. Travel will be slow, and thus a mile an hour is probably maximum speed. Of course, this is a very substantial exposure, but under emergency circumstances it may be a risk that one must take. Brucer (1962) discusses this problem and a means for providing a crude electroscope, which may be of some assistance in determining when people in a fallout shelter may leave:

When a plastic pocket comb is run through the hair, it develops sufficient static charge to pick up small pieces of paper. This static charge leaks off, and the piece of paper will drop in about 15 seconds.

Radiation, including the radiation from fallout, produces sufficient ionization so that the comb loses its charge and the paper falls off in a shorter time. In a field of about 10 roentgens (r) per hour of radiation (not enough to take an x-ray picture), the pocket comb does not keep the charge long enough to even pick up a piece of paper. (Or, if the pocket comb has attracted the piece of paper, about 10 r per hour of radiation will cause the charge to leak off and the piece of paper will drop.)

Try it. Take a cigarette butt or a piece of facial tissue. Tear off about a quarter inch square. Run a plastic pocket comb through your hair once. Long hair is better than short hair. Female hair is better than male hair. (In this one particular case a cat is even better than a wife.) The cigarette paper will stick to the comb and will stay up, even with mild shaking, for about 15 seconds. If this were in a field of radiation of about 10 r per hour, the paper would drop from the comb immediately. With only normal, ever-present background radiation, the paper stays stuck to the comb for about 15 seconds.

This is not an accurate measure. It is not really 10 r per hour. Depending on the size of the comb, its composition (nylon doesn't work as well as bakelite), the amount of moisture in the air, the amount of background radiation, and a thousand others factors, the time can change anywhere from a few seconds to a half minute. But the citizen is not completely helpless. He can estimate whether there is or is not an appreciable amount of radiation.

The half-thickness principle in radiation protection applies to the exponential absorption of gamma irradiation and is the thickness of shielding necessary to reduce the intensity of this form of irradiation by 50 per cent of its initial value. To cut irradiation exposure by a factor of 1,000 of its outside intensity requires 10 half-thicknesses (Table 18-10).

Another principle taken advantage of is the half-life decay in relation to measured time (Table 18-11).

TABLE 18-10. THICKNESS OF MATERIAL REQUIRED TO REDUCE GAMMA IRRADIATION FROM FALLOUT

MATERIAL	HALF-THICKNESS (REDUCTION BY FACTOR OF 2)	TEN HALF-THICKNESS (REDUCTION BY FACTOR OF 1,000)
Wood	8.8 inches	7 feet 4 inches
Water	4.8 inches	4 feet
Earth	3.3 inches	2 feet 9 inches
Concrete	2.2 inches	1 foot 10 inches
Steel	0.7 inches	7 inches
Lead	0.3 inches	3 inches

TABLE 18-11

MEASURED EXPOSURE		HALF-LIFE DECAY	
24 hours after blast	10 r	50% decay or 5 r in 20 hrs.	
1 week after blast	10 r	2 weeks	5 r
1 month after blast	10 r	2 months	5 r

Ionizing radiations from fallout debris will include alpha and beta particles, gamma and x-rays, and neutrons, which vary greatly in their ability to penetrate shielding materials or tissues. Detailed specifications for appropriate shelters have been published by Civil Defense authorities. The radioisotopes or nuclides that may be produced in fallout and the organ each tends to affect most are shown in Table 18-12.

It is the isotopic yield from tropospheric and stratospheric fallout that is of global consequence. It is of less immediate consequence,

TABLE 18-12. PRINCIPAL RADIONUCLIDES PRODUCED BY FISSION ARRANGED IN ORDER OF INCREASING HALF LIVES*

NUCLIDE	HALF-LIFE	RAYS EMITTED	CRITICAL ORGAN
Lanthanum 140	1.7 days	Beta, gamma	G.I. tract and liver
Molybdenum 90	2.8 days	Beta, gamma	Kidney
Iodine 131	8.1 days	Beta, gamma	Thyroid
Barium 146	12.8 days	Beta, gamma	Whole body
Praseodymium 143	13.7 days	Beta	Bone
Cerium 141	33.0 days	Beta, gamma	Liver
Niobium 95	53.0 days	Beta	Bone
Strontium 89	35.0 days	Beta, gamma	Whole body
Yttrium 91	61.0 days	Beta	Bone
Zirconium 95	65.0 days	Beta, gamma	Whole body
Cerium 144	282.0 days	Beta, gamma	Bone
Ruthenium 106	1.0 yr.	Beta	Kidney
Strontium 90	28.0 yrs.	Beta	Bone
Cesium 137	30.0 yrs.	Beta, gamma	Muscle
Carbon 14	5,568 yrs.	Beta	Whole body
Technetium 99	2×10^5 yrs.	Beta	Kidney
Cesium 135	3×10^6 yrs.	Beta	Muscle
Iodine 129	1.7×10^7 yrs.	Beta, gamma	Thyroid

* Alpha radiation not included.
(Aronow, S.: A glossary of radiation terminology. New Eng. J. Med., 266:1145, 1962)

but eventually it may become a hazard to public health days to months later. For specific guidance, the nuclides radium 226, iodine 131, strontium 90, strontium 89 and cesium 137 are included among those under surveillance by the United States Public Health Service.

Iodine I 131 is probably the most serious hazard to human health of the radionuclides in fallout. Because 80 per cent of fallout occurs within 48 hours, most of ^{131}I has not had time to decay before it is ingested by cattle grazing on plants upon which it and other radionuclides may have fallen. This presents a health hazard because cow's milk is the major component of the diets of infants and children. More of this nuclide is ingested if the area has not been washed by rain. Additional ^{131}I may be absorbed by inhalation, and a little more may be obtained by eating fresh unwashed vegetables. But fresh milk is the real threat because ^{131}I appears in milk within a matter of hours after the ingestion of forage crops upon which it has fallen. The processing and the marketing of milk are designed to bring the product to the consumer within 2 to 4 days, a period of time that allows for little decay in radioactivity. In the case of other dairy products, with the possible exception of cottage cheese, cream and ice cream, the processing time before marketing is sufficient to permit essentially the complete decay of ^{131}I—i.e., 40 days.

Because infants and children consume larger volumes of milk than adults, the dose of ^{131}I is much greater for the very young. Within 24 hours about 30 per cent of the initially ingested quantity of ^{131}I appears in the normal thyroid gland irrespective of age. In a 1-year-old child, the normal thyroid gland weighs 2 Gm. Thus, his gland will be exposed to 10 times the concentration in the adult, whose gland normally weighs about 20 Gm. Hence, the amount of ^{131}I that may enter the thyroid of a child can present serious hazards, among them the increased incidence of carcinoma of this gland (Clark, 1955).

The ^{131}I risk can be largely avoided by breast feeding, assuming that the vegetables that the mother eats have been washed and that she is not drinking fresh cow's milk, or by feeding the child processed milk 40 days old or older. Once exposed, the administration of 1.0 mg. of stable iodine daily to children and 5.0 mg. daily to adults will reduce in a few days the ^{131}I accumulation in the thyroid to about 20 per cent of its initial value. Also, the addition of thyroid extract may be helpful in reducing thyroid activity and favoring the release of ^{131}I. Both these measures should be applied on an individual basis rather than to the population as a whole.

Cesium 137, strontium 90 and strontium 89 constitute the other major radionuclides thus far thought to be ingested in significant amounts. ^{137}Cs and ^{90}Sr are activated from stable nuclides distributed in most foods; therefore, exposure to these radionuclides cannot very well be avoided at the present time unless the food is protected against neutron irradiation. ^{137}Cs, with a radioactive half-life of 30 years, is a gamma and beta emitter and is distributed primarily in muscle, where its biologic half-life is about 110 days. Its levels in man, eating caribou and reindeer meat when these animals have fed in fallout areas, have been reported as excessively high. ^{90}Sr, a slow beta emitter with a half-life of 28 years, behaves metabolically as calcium. It is estimated by the Federal Radiation Council that in fallout irradiation to the marrow, 50 per cent is from ^{90}Sr, and about 80 per cent of bone irradiation is from this radionuclide. ^{89}Sr is a beta-gamma emitter with a half-life of 54 days and is distributed throughout the body. Most data to date indicate that about 90 per cent of whole body and genetically significant exposure to fallout irradiation experienced by the present generation is from ^{131}I, ^{95}Zr-Nb, ^{140}Ba-La, ^{137}Cs, ^{90}Sr and ^{89}Sr. The United States Public Health Service at present samples milk from hundreds of stations, each representing a different geographic area in this country and abroad, for purposes of maintaining a monthly analysis of the content in milk of iodine 131, cesium 137, barium 140, strontium 89 and strontium 90 (see Table 18-12).

The Federal Radiation Council (May, 1963) proposed the following guides to apply to peacetime nuclear operation where controlled release of radioactivity to the environment is possible. These daily intakes are averaged over a year's time and at the present time are considered as an acceptable health risk for large general populations for a lifetime.

Iodine 131*	100 picocuries a day or 36,500 picocuries a year.
Strontium 90	200 picocuries a day or 73,000 picocuries a year.
Strontium 89	2,000 picocuries a day or 730,000 picocuries a year.

NATURE OF EXTERNALLY ACQUIRED WHOLE-BODY IRRADIATION

Acute Irradiation Syndrome

Much more can be said of the pathogenesis of total body radiation injury than can be said of its treatment. The clinical picture of victims of an atomic explosion differ primarily from that induced by excessive radioisotope therapy in that the onset of symptoms in the latter case may not develop for weeks, as exposure from radionuclides usually is cumulative and not instantaneous. Also, in atomic disaster most of the surviving casualties suffer from thermal and flash burns, lacerations and fractures, as well as radiation. Otherwise, when the latent symptoms of radiation appear, they are similar in nature and largely reflect the physical character and quantity of the exposure encountered.

Most of the observations on total body injury from ionizing radiation are based upon the reactions of different species of animals studied under controlled conditions. There is considerable variation from one species to another with regard to the magnitude of the lethal dose by single exposure, but the lethal exposure within any given species varies only to a slight extent. Data on man are accumulating and suggest that his response is remarkably predictable from the observations and the data obtained from the dog given whole-body x-ray.

The most complete clinical and pathologic report on radiation injury in man is that of Hempelmann, Lisco and Hoffman (1952). From what is known of the Japanese disaster and of the Los Alamos accident, the LD 50 single and brief exposure to total body radiation for man is probably within the range of

---

*The guide for ^{131}I is set for the most susceptible —infants and young children. For adults the guide for this radionuclide could be 10 times greater, or 365,000 picocuries a year.

240 to 260 rads. Because the response of the dog to total body radiation is so similar to that observed in man, and the LD 50 values are probably comparable, the presentation and the discussion that follow are derived primarily from observations and data obtained upon the dog.

Symptomatology. In case of a severe exposure from an atomic burst, nausea, vomiting and occasionally diarrhea may occur within minutes after exposure. These symptoms are transient, lasting usually less than 24 hours. This course of events usually does not occur, except in the near-lethal or lethal range of radiation exposure. However, the onset of early nausea and vomiting does not necessarily forecast a fatal outcome, although it is true that most of the fatally radiated will display these two symptoms within the first few hours (see Table 18-8).

Anorexia, nausea, vomiting and diarrhea develop in lethal and near-lethal radiation exposure between the 5th and the 20th days. This time there is adequate explanation, although that which is known may not represent the entire picture. By the time of onset of these complaints, there is extensive desquamation and superficial ulceration of the gastrointestinal tract, with bleeding. Edema and petechial bleeding into these organs are also present in varying degrees and are associated with engorgement of the lymph nodes by blood as distinguished from hemorrhage. These blood-filled nodes appear to represent the filtration of the blood-filled lymphatic circulation. Interestingly, the spleen, with little or no lymphatic circulation, is atrophied and relatively free of blood and hemorrhage.

As the radiation syndrome progresses, weakness, anorexia and fever become prominent features. These are explained to some extent by malnutrition and infection, but they also appear in irradiated germ-free animals. Weakness may continue for several months to years after fever and infection have disappeared. Characteristic of all serious total body exposure is pancytopenia (Fig. 18-2).

When the patient becomes ill from radiation, his tolerance to infection, physical exertion and other forms of stress is reduced sharply. Minor wounds and surgical procedures at the height of radiation effects may assume major significance. This point is well illustrated in Figure 18-2, wherein a radiated dog, as late as 55 days after total body exposure, developed a fever of unknown origin. A sharp reduction in the formed elements of the blood occurred and was associated with anorexia, weight loss and listlessness. At the time of onset of fever, the animal was believed to have recovered. Following transfusion and antibiotic therapy, recovery was complete. Similar observations frequently have been made by Evans, wherein he noted that otherwise nonfatal injuries, administered to dogs given sublethal exposure of total body x-ray, had a cumulative effect, with death occurring in more than 75 per cent of animals observed.

Leukopenia, curiously, does not reflect accurately the susceptibility of the individual to

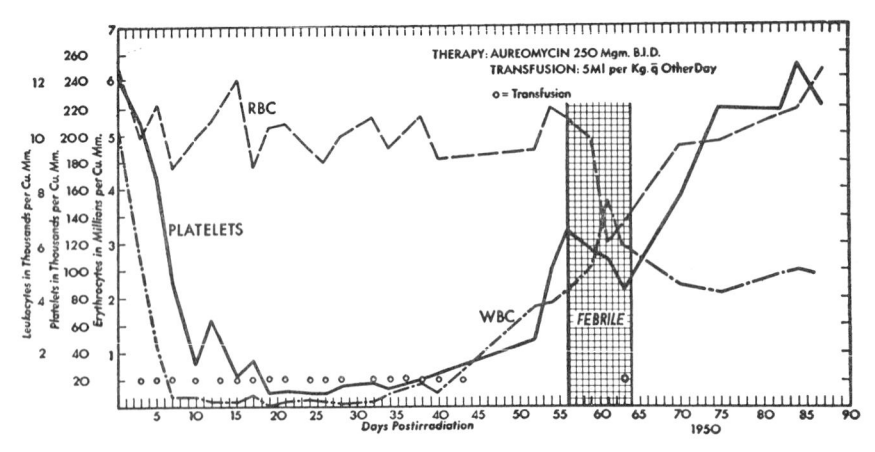

Fig. 18-2. Note unfavorable influence of infection and fever upon blood count as late as 2 months after heavy total body x-radiation exposure in dog.

325 R TOTAL BODY X-RADIATION CONTROLS AND TRANSFUSIONS

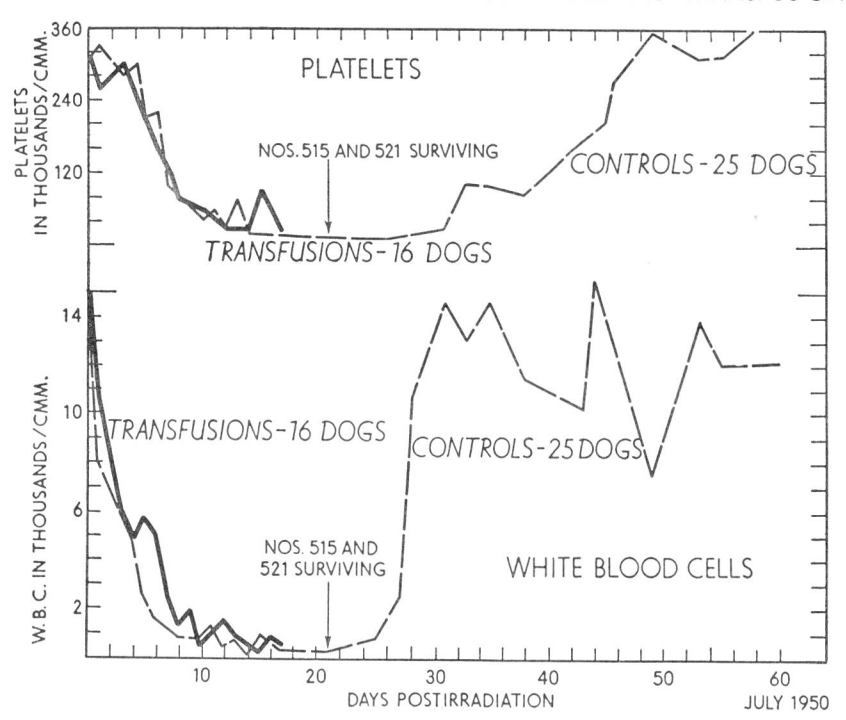

FIG. 18-3. Thrombocytopenia and leukopenia as they usually develop in range of an exposure of LD 50 or greater. Note that there is no numerical distinction between the degree of leukopenia and thrombopenia among those which die from those which survive.

infection, nor does the leukocyte count determine which individual will survive. It is possible that there may exist certain qualitative differences in the remaining leukocytes of two individuals whose leukocyte counts are equally suppressed but from different quantities of radiation exposure. The leukocyte count in the near-lethal range is just as suppressed as when the exposure range has been lethal (Fig. 18-3). It may be that the intensity of leukopenia is even quantitatively the same, and that death in one and not in the other is the result of other factors that occur with higher dosages. On the other hand, it must be admitted that an individual who maintains a near-normal leukocyte count almost surely will survive his exposure.

Anemia always develops in the total body-radiated individual who receives a near-lethal exposure, provided that he survives 7 to 10 days. Among the several factors contributing to anemia are: blood loss through hemorrhage, aplasia of the marrow, sequestration of blood by lymph nodes which filter the engorged lymphatic circulation, and possibly hemolysis. Histologically, myelopoiesis is completely inactive by the end of the 1st week in near-lethal exposure. Evidence of regeneration does not reappear until the 3rd to the 4th week. Because the life of the circulating red cell is long (3 to 4 months), it is apparent that an accelerated rate of red cell destruction or anemia from blood loss or both must take place if one is to account for the rapid onset of anemia in the absence of blood loss. The red cell count also is the last of the circulating formed elements to return to normal concentration. It appears likely that the anemia of radiation has a dual pathogenesis which is biphasic in nature. The initial or early phase appears to be more the result of blood loss than of hemolysis. The second phase is due to the lingering aplasia or hypoplasia of bone marrow.

In spite of the extent of anemia, there is little evidence that its prevention or correction is of value unless severe hypoxia develops. Iron, B_{12}, or liver extracts as therapeutic measures give no evidence of benefit in the refractory or aplastic phase. Transfusions appear to increase the rate or the extent of abnormal bleeding, if for no other reason than that more blood is available to be disposed of by hemorrhage or to be leaked into the lymphatic circulation. There may be an increased rate of reactions to blood transfusion after total body radiation. In the dog, at least, the reactions cannot be predicted on the basis of matching. Immediately following transfusion reactions, the blood in a small percentage of animals may become incoagulable (Cronkite and Brecher, 1952; Allen et al., 1952).

Hemorrhage is probably the most obvious disorder in the individual receiving total body radiation, but it is not the most important. Its time of onset and intensity vary in accordance with the severity of exposure as well as within members of the same species identically exposed. In man and in the dog, bleeding about the teeth and the mouth and from the gastrointestinal tract are commonly observed after the 1st week when exposure has been within the near-lethal range. Petechial bleeding and ecchymoses are generously distributed over the body surface. Although the skin is the most common site of hemorrhage, evidence of bleeding may be found in any organ of the body. Hemorrhage into the lungs, the myocardium and the central nervous system frequently occurs and occasionally is fatal in itself. Otherwise, the spectacular abnormal bleeding associated with total body radiation is more often a troublesome nursing problem than a fatal complication. If the individual survives, bleeding ceases spontaneously between the 3rd and the 4th weeks after exposure and before the peripheral platelet count is increased appreciably.

The pathogenesis of radiation hemorrhage is complex and poorly understood. The most consistent finding is thrombocytopenia which, in the near-lethal range, develops without fail and is full-blown by the 8th to the 10th day. The platelet count remains near zero for 3 to 4 weeks; then it begins to recover slowly, reaching maximal values by the 6th to the 7th week (Figs. 18-2 and 18-4).

The clotting time is prolonged between the

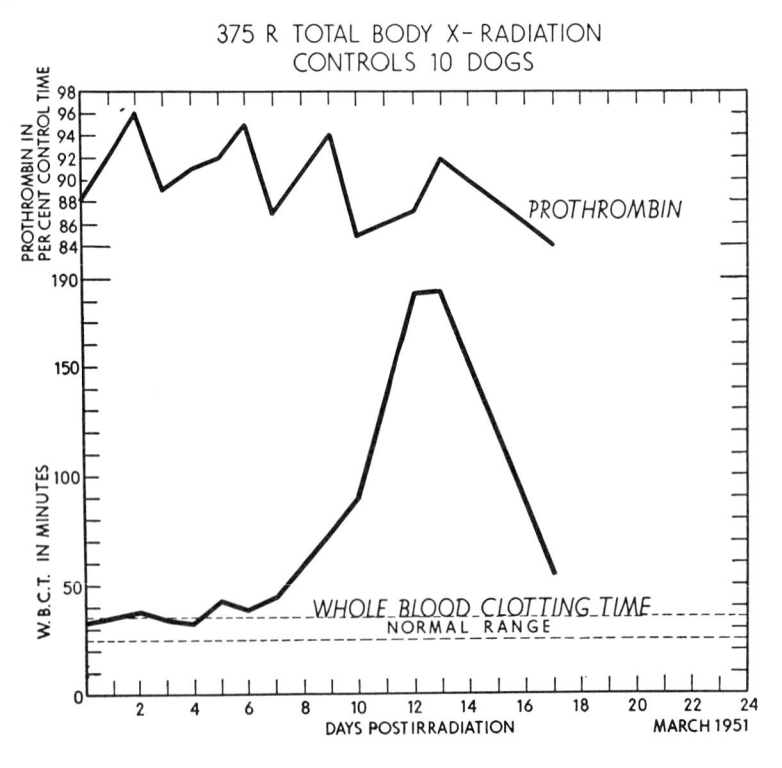

FIG. 18-4. Note abnormality of whole blood clotting time which can be detected by careful technic. Compare with Figure 18-3, and it will be noted that the clotting abnormality returns to normal before the platelet count begins to rise.

**450 R TOTAL BODY X-IRRADIATION HEAD SHIELDED
SURVIVALS-15 DOGS AND NONSURVIVALS-5 DOGS**

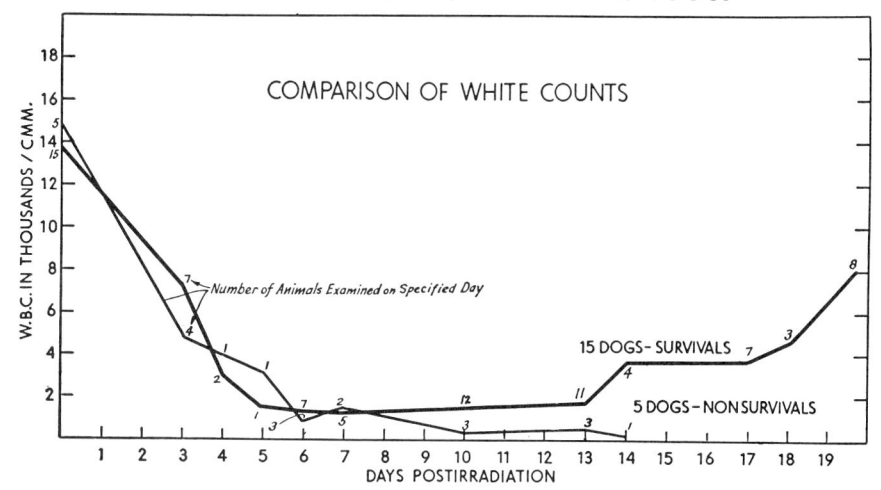

FIG. 18-5. Comparison of peripheral white cell counts in head-shielded animals, showing little difference in total residual counts among those which died from those which survived. The leukocyte response to single exposures of total body x-radiation offers no reliable clue as to prognosis.

7th and the 18th days (Fig. 18-5). To what extent the clotting abnormality is related to thrombocytopenia is not established. Certain features suggest these abnormalities to be unrelated, at least in part. For example, the clotting time may be increased before or after the onset of severe thrombocytopenia. Also, the clotting time always returns to normal or near-normal before recovery of platelet count can be detected. In the bloods of some animals a clotting inhibitor can be detected; the nature of this anticoagulant is unknown but probably is not heparin as commercially known. In some radiated animals, "heparin" or heparinoid substances can be detected and also in the course of blood transfusion where its occurrence may be the result of transfusion reactions.

Prothrombin and other clotting activities are not sufficiently altered in themselves to explain abnormal bleeding other than the retardation of the first phase of coagulation, inherent in thrombocytopenia from any cause.

The concentration of plasma fibrinogen is increased after irradiation. Because of systemic and local infections, so frequently encountered in the irradiated subject, this increase in fibrinogen concentration is to be expected, but it also occurs in germ-free animals after similar dosage of irradiation.

Vascular damage is suggested by petechial bleeding, and this appears to be related primarily to the thrombocyte count because it is largely prevented by platelet transfusions (Cronkite and Brecher, 1952; Allen et al., 1952). Transfused platelets with elevation of the platelet counts to normal levels do not abolish the increased clotting time.

Effective treatment of radiation hemorrhage at the LD 100 range is not yet devised. Blood transfusions and the control of infection have been suggested frequently as effective agents. An analysis of such reports discloses no important evidence in support of these contentions after severe radiation. There is ample proof that the liberal use of antibiotics has no beneficial effect upon the hemorrhagic tendency (Allen et al., 1952). Also, the spectrum of clinical bleeding in species subject to this complication of radiation is not reduced in germ-free animals. The LD 50 in germ-free animals after irradiation is no less than that of their brothers living in their normal environment.

In exposure less than LD 100, antibiotics appear to be beneficial to some extent, but this is less than might be expected or hoped for.

Infection. An array of evidence exists to demonstrate a reduced tolerance of the radiated individual to infection, but the control or the prevention of infection makes an unimpressive mark upon the mortality rate from radiation injury. Nevertheless, the control of infection is important to the welfare of the individual, as well as to the community, in the control and the prevention of epidemics following in the wake of disaster. The efforts which have been expended in these directions are probably more fruitful than is now apparent, for they have demonstrated that causes of death more subtle than either hemorrhage or infection undoubtedly exist. These are yet to be identified.

When interpreting the harmful effects of ionizing radiation in terms of immunity, it must be remembered that the immunity of the host and the virulence of the invading organism are measured largely in terms of one another. In the case of radiation injury, infection is not due to any increase in the virulence of the organism but to the increased susceptibility of the host to invasion and to his inability properly to isolate and destroy organisms once they enter the circulation. The ease with which bacteria may gain portals of entrance is not only the result of ulcerations, abrasions and burns immediately incident to an atomic explosion but also of the desquamation, the ulceration and/or the punctate hemorrhages so commonly noted in the gastrointestinal and the respiratory tracts in the late stages of intense radiation injury (1 to 4 weeks after exposure).

Similarly, once such organisms enter the blood stream, they are relatively unopposed by the natural forces of immunity. Leukocytes are nearly absent; the few remaining appear to be biologically inert. The antibody titer of the serum is reduced markedly. The lymph nodes are devoid of lymph follicles and lymphocytes, and the lymph channels convey blood extravasated from the microcirculation. The lymph nodes thereby become filters of blood, enlarged with erythrocytes, which may be interpreted erroneously as hemorrhagic.

Impairment of antibody production following total body radiation was observed by Hektoen as early as 1916. Subsequent investigators have confirmed his observations repeatedly. Because of the variety of bacterial flora to which the individual is exposed, the passive transfer of antibodies, for the present, may be impractical in view of the comparatively rapid turnover of protein. There is no evidence that the daily administration of gamma globulin or plasma materially improves survival rate, but neither is there evidence that in fatal exposures bacterial causes of death are important —to wit, the germ-free studies.

That total body radiation may act symbiotically with local radiation effects is supported by the following observation: Sikov and Lofstrom (1960) found that the amount of oncolysis produced by localized roentgen irradiation can be increased substantially by administering a small increment of total body irradiation. This increased oncolysis could be partially simulated by administering plasma from previously irradiated animals in conjunction with irradiation of the tumor. This phenomenon was interpreted as indicating the presence of a possible substance in the plasma following total body irradiation which may be involved in the synergism.

Treatment. The observations and the experimental approach to the problem of prevention and treatment of total body radiation injury have been along 3 lines: (1) preconditioning prior to exposure, (2) shielding in part or *in toto* at the time of exposure and (3) attempts at treatment administered after total body exposures.

Effective postexposure treatment is the ultimate hoped for, but to date it is nonexistent. While some degree of benefit has been derived from the use of transfusions combined with antibiotic therapy, it is biologically insignificant. Transfusions alone have given no evidence of any improved survival rate among dogs (Fig. 18-6). The negative results with this therapy tend to reduce the need for blood. This is important because, should the need be there, it would come at a time when donors would be scarce. Even those who can be transfused have little or no assurance that the liberal use of blood will be of value, unless the need for blood is in the treatment of hypovolemic shock in minimally irradiated victims.

Transfusions of leukocytes have been employed to treat radiation injury, but to date they too have been ineffective. One of the unusual features of an open and infected wound following an LD 50 or greater total body exposure is the absence of pus due to the severe leukopenia that develops. No leukocytes —no pus; thus one of the cardinal signs of local infection under ordinary conditions is missing after total body radiation.

The mechanism of death from total body exposure to ionizing radiation is unknown. Undoubtedly, both hemorrhage and infection may play a part and at times may be the actual cause of death; but the prevention of either or both is not sufficient statistically to alter mortality among an exposed population.

Protection by shielding portions of the myelopoietic system has been demonstrated as an effective means of survival. Shouse et al. in 1931 reported that shielding as little as one vertebra in dogs materially altered survival rate.

This phenomenon has been studied extensively by Jacobson and collaborators. They found that exteriorization of the spleen and its shielding doubled the tolerance for exposure to ionizing radiation. Moreover, when shielding is carried out, the usual delay in erythropoiesis is greatly shortened, and aplasia may not occur. Evidence of beginning marrow regeneration is detectable within a few days in contrast with several weeks required by the unshielded controls. Using homogenates of embryonic spleen injected intraperitoneally, Jacobson has been able to induce a similar beneficial reaction after total body radiation but only when the homogenates were administered within the first few hours following exposure. In this same connection, it is of interest that the benefits continue if the animal whose spleen has been shielded during radiation is subjected to splenectomy only a few hours later. Marrow transplants appear promising (see below).

"Preconditioning" of animals prior to total body exposure has been studied extensively by many, particularly Patt (1949). On the theory that radiation is due to oxidation of water with resultant free radicals responsible for much of the injury, he has attempted to overcome this potential hazard by the administration of cysteine and similar compounds prior to exposure. This amino acid is a reducing agent by virtue of its sulfhydryl component. When cysteine was administered in advance of exposure, the tolerance of mice

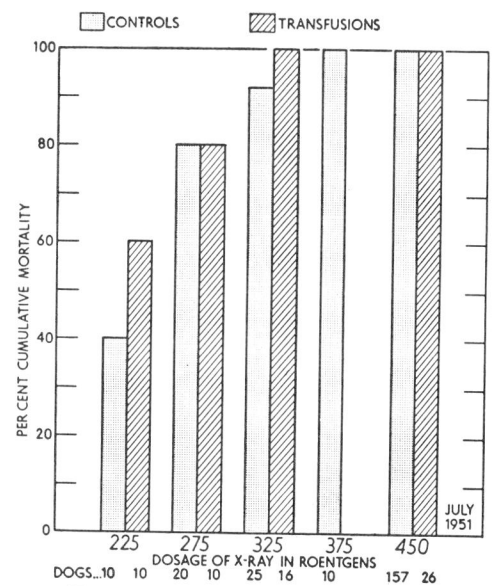

FIG. 18-6. Data indicating the lack of any general or pronounced benefit over untransfused controls from blood transfusion, administered 3 times a week to dogs after total body exposures to x-radiation, ranging from 225 to 450 r.

was increased from 550 to 1,000 r. Such a degree of benefit has not been observed by all investigators.

Anoxia or hypoxia also affords some degree of protection when employed just before radiation exposure. Hypoxia has been induced by direct oxygen deprivation as well as by the administration of compounds which compete more successfully for hemoglobin than does oxygen. Cyanide, para-aminopropriophenone and similar compounds have been tried with substantial benefit, but only when employed in advance of exposure (Storer and Coon, 1950). In another interesting series of experiments, Patt employed refrigeration following exposure of frogs to lethal body radiation. As long as the frogs remained under refrigeration (often for months), they remained, so far as could be determined, in good health. However, once removed from the refrigerator and returned to normal temperatures, the syndrome of radiation injury appeared, and the animals died.

To date, the effects of total body radiation within the lethal range have proved to be irreversible. If full knowledge as to the reason for the protective action of pretreatment and/or shielding were at hand, possibly more promising leads than those in the past could be pursued with better results. Whereas preconditioning and/or shielding are important accomplishments, the fact remains that in the event of catastrophic exposure, the therapy will be largely of the postradiation variety (Fig. 18-7).

Bone Marrow Grafts and Bone Marrow Transfusions. There is evidence that autologous bone grafts may be able to support temporarily the essential myeloplastic activities in an animal otherwise lethally exposed to ionizing whole body irradiation until his own marrow activity takes over (Alpen and Baum, 1958). It is possible that, because the immune response is effectively suppressed in whole body radiation, homologous bone grafts might serve a useful purpose for the critical weeks necessary for the victim's marrow to resume its functions. Indeed, Andrews (1962) concluded that the transfusion of adult homologous marrow given 4 of the Yugoslavian victims "probably produced a functioning but temporary graft." This view is not impressively supported by the data presented, nor were the clinical courses materially altered from those which might have occurred spontaneously. The concept of homologous grafts to serve temporarily seems to be sound, but that this practice can be useful remains to be established. Some have reported that the infusion of homogenates of embryonal spleen and marrow causes widespread deposition of thrombi in the microcirculation. The usefulness of homologous marrow transfusions and grafts in whole-body irradiation remains to be proved in mammals, including man. Autologous grafts do appear to be effective in irradiation injury, and isogenic marrow transfusions in the treatment of other forms of hypoplastic anemia in man have been successful in 3 of 5 times (Mills *et al.*, 1964; Thomas *et al.*, 1964). The apparently successful transplanting of marrow in patients has been claimed recently (1968).

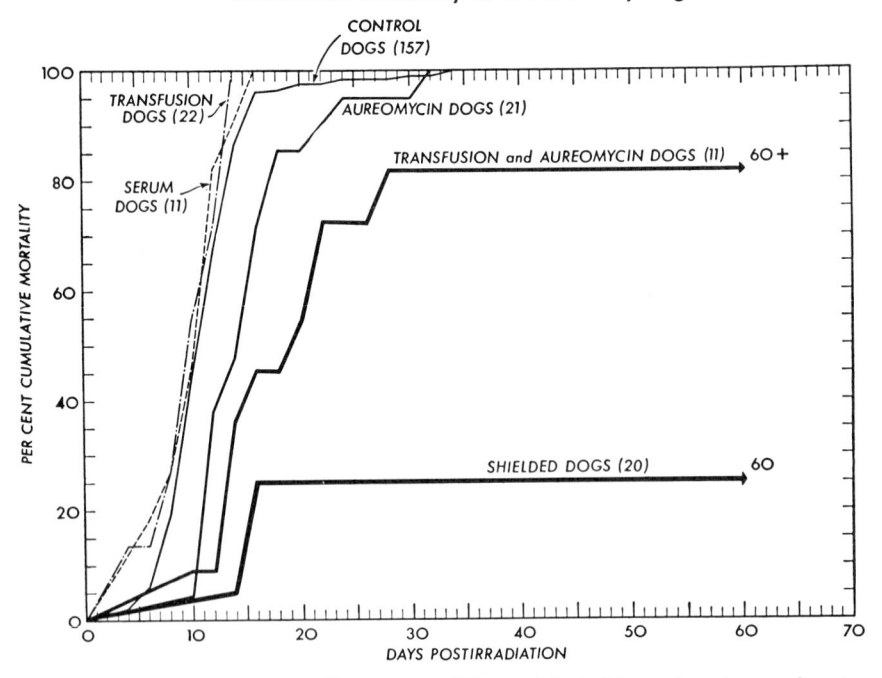

FIG. 18-7. Cumulative mortality curves of dogs subjected to various types of postradiation treatment. Included for comparison are the data obtained from head-shielding. The 450 r x-ray exposure is about 100 r above the LD 100 for this laboratory.

INJURY FROM LOCAL OR PORTAL IRRADIATION

Portal Radiation and Tolerance. X-ray machines currently employed in treatment include the 10-kv. machine used by the dermatologist, the 80- and the 250-kv. machine employed by the radiologist for therapy. Two-million volt x-ray generators are currently in use in many hospitals, and linear accelerators generating 6 million volts are employed by some. Betatrons of various designs for electron generation range upward from 30 million volts. More recently the proton beam of the cyclotron has been under test in the treatment of malignant disease after boron is introduced into the tissue to be treated. The proton beam produces neutrons from the localized interstitial boron, and these in turn radiate the area concerned.

Because the needs of the patient vary widely according to the sensitivity and location of the tumor under treatment, the radiotherapist must adjust the energies of his x-rays and electrons accordingly. This problem is complex and for the most part is regulated by variations in voltage aided by a variety of filters interposed between the energy source and the patient.

The limiting factor in portal radiation therapy is primarily the tolerance of adjacent normal tissues and secondarily the systemic response of the patient to his treatment. The patient's local and systemic responses determine the amount of allowable radiation exposure. The third and equally important consideration is the radiosensitivity of the tumor or tissue in question. Some tumors are very sensitive, but all ranges of sensitivity and resistance are encountered. Some are extremely sensitive and respond well for a while, only to become increasingly resistant in time. Moreover, the magnitude of the dose of radiation that can be administered with the second, the third or the fourth course of therapy without engendering harm is reduced sharply. Thus, a tumor which cannot be totally ablated by the first course of treatment is not likely to be curable later on by radiation therapy. The malignant lesions responding to the highest percentage rates of cure are those of the skin and the cervix. They are often curable by the first series of exposures given under appropriate conditions. Basal and early squamous cell carcinomas generally are most amenable to this form of therapy, especially if less than 2 cm. in diameter. The malignant melanoma of the skin, on the other hand, is highly resistant to any form of radiation therapy. A sound understanding as to why some tumors are radiosensitive and others are resistant could prove to be of incalculable value.

Improved technics and improved x-ray equipment whereby exposure of the patient to unnecessary radiation in diagnostic procedures can be minimized are presented in the "Report of the Medical X-Ray Advisory Committee on Public Health Considerations in Medical Diagnostic Radiology (X Rays)" (1967).

Cellular Damage From Portal or Local Radiation. By no means is it possible at this time to define accurately or completely the effects of ionizing radiation upon the living cell. On the other hand, this is a subject of much study for many years, and its ultimate solution is basic to improvement in radiotherapy and to the prevention and the treatment of radiation injury in general.

Cellular changes or their death are functions of many variables, particularly dosage, time of exposure (single or multiple exposures) and the relationship of mitotic division to the time or the occasion at which the cell is radiated.

Dosage to tissue or to an organ is not uniformly distributed among cells, nor is the intensity of exposure constant for all cells within the same field. For example, if the concentration of the sulfur or calcium ion within one cell is elevated from that of another, the dosage in the former cell or tissue is significantly over that of the latter, even though the intensity of the energy output of the extracorporeal source of radiation is the same. For this reason the tissue immediately adjacent to bone is said to receive an exposure 60 per cent greater than the dose received by cells at distances of 1 mm. or more away from bone with 200-kv. x-ray (Martin *et al.*, 1931). These differences tend to be canceled out when one considers larger quantities of exposed tissue—i.e., a gram or more. Cellular dosage and damage then become a statistical concept wherein the total exposure of the individual cell is lost in the "crowd."

Most radiobiologists believe that certain acute chemical changes occur within the radiated cell, but that these changes are essentially limited to the immediate electronic path of the electron entering or traversing the cell. This concept is not unlike the demonstrated or measured ionizing effects of particular radiation measured by the Wilson cloud chamber technic on photographic plates.

The chemical changes induced along the course or track of the bombarding electron in protoplasm are not well understood. Within the past decade, most studies have centered about the possibilities that the initial or primary effect was one of ionization of intracellular or "protoplasmic" water, and that the resultant products are at least as devastating as any direct physical effect which may also occur. It is probable that the amount of chemical toxins produced by ionized water along the immediate path of the electron particle is very great, but its pathway is submicroscopic. Thus, any of the chemical disturbances in a cell damaged by one electron traversing it are likely to be diluted rapidly in terms of the total intracellular protoplasm present.

The biologic effects upon the cell are considered to be principally two in kind. One is the influence of the particle or ray upon the state of chromosomal activity or cellular division. The more active cellular division is, the greater the retarding influence of radiation upon its reproduction. The greatest retardation to cellular division is obtained when radiation is delivered just prior to its division. Any increased metabolic activity increases the sensitivity to the effects of irradiation; tolerance is increased by hypoxia and hypometabolic states in many, if not all, species. It is this effect which the radiotherapist desires to exploit in the treatment of malignant disease. The second effect is more specific and is the induction of chromosomal rearrangement with the result that mutant strains occur as demonstrated by the classic researches of Mueller many years ago.

The cellular changes induced by ionization do undergo substantial repair. It has been demonstrated at slow rates of radiation that cellular repair may be able to keep pace reasonably well with the damages inflicted, at least for a while (Gray, 1955). Similar dosages, given rapidly, can be fatal. It becomes quite apparent that the biologic response of the cell to ionizing radiation is a function of many variables; some of these are known and well established, others are not.

Reaction of the body to ionizing radiation depends upon the physical quality of the ray, the dosage administered, the extent of the body exposed, the systemic or general reaction encountered, and the susceptibility of that portion irradiated. Because of the wide variety of exposure technics required in the treatment of human disease, the character of radiation injury assumes different patterns under different circumstances.

Local radiation, applied externally, is capable of producing acute and/or latent injury and serious sequelae, as well as systemic disturbances in the course of appropriate treatment. The systemic manifestations encountered in portal therapy differ from local reactions in regard to symptomatology, nature of the insult, its time of onset and host resistance.

Systemic Reactions to Local Irradiation. Radiation sickness is the term generally applied to the syndrome of headache, anorexia, nausea, vomiting and diarrhea which occasionally develops in the course of portal therapy. If proper therapy is applied and administered over periods of time which are now well established by experience, these reactions are seldom of serious consequence. They are to be expected if sufficient carcinocidal radiation is to be administered to many patients. Radiation sickness of this type is a self-limiting disease. When the syndrome is full blown, its symptoms may necessitate permanent abandonment of the planned program of radiation therapy, or its interruption with a period of rest before resumption. In other patients, some modification of the therapeutic program, mild sedation and reassurance may relieve the patient sufficiently to permit completion of treatment without interruption.

Local Reactions to Externally Administered Radiation. When radiation therapy is employed, it is inevitable that some degree of damage, however slight, will occur to the normal tissue exposed in the region under treatment. This is a fundamental fact to be considered in all forms of radiotherapy and, more than most other practical considerations, the threshold of damage of normal tissues or their tolerance to radiation determines the type of radiation therapy most appropriate and the quantity to be employed.

Radiotherapy is successful and the usual treatment of choice when the diseased tissue or organ is readily responsive to an exposure which provokes little damage or disorder in the surrounding normal tissue organs. If a substantial differential in radio-insensitivity between the tumor and the adjacent normal tissue included in the field of exposures does not exist, radiation is not the treatment of choice nor is it likely to serve a very useful purpose without inducing harm or at least carrying considerable risk. On the other hand, when the diseased tissue or the organ or the agent responsible for the pathology does respond to doses of radiation which are not harmful to normal adjacent structures, then radiotherapy is the treatment indicated, provided that a better form of treatment does not exist.

Carcinocidal Radiation Without Serious Local Injury. The goal of radiation therapy is to deliver to the diseased part, often a malignancy, the largest possible percentage of the total radiation which the normal tissues adjacent to the structures under treatment will tolerate very well. To this end, the radiotherapist strives to employ radiation of sufficient energy so that the skin and the underlying normal tissues receive the smallest possible percentage of radiation which does not also reach the depth of the diseased part under treatment. This may be accomplished by one or both of the following principles and technics:

External radiation may be directed to the deep-seated radiosensitive tumor from multiple portals, using the most energetic radiation suited for the particular circumstance. This practice assures penetration to the proper depth with as little extra and superficial exposure as is possible to any one adjacent area or portal of entry. The larger the percentage of ineffective penetration, the more heavily radiated will be the overlying normal structures and the smaller will be the dose delivered to the target depth. Thus in low-energy radiation, which means smaller percentages of depth penetration, the higher will be the exposure of superficial structures when it is necessary to achieve a carcinocidal dose to deeper tissues. To whatever extent the normal tissues are exposed above and beyond the exposure of the deep-seated tumor, that is the extent to which any inherent differential in sensitivity between the tumor and the normal tissue is lost. Hence, with low-energy gamma or x-radiation, the effectiveness of radiotherapy is correspondingly diminished, and the likelihood of injury to superficial structures is correspondingly increased if an adequate depth dose is to be given.

How can a larger percentage of radiation therapy be delivered to a deep-seated tissue with the least injury to normal structures? Developmentally, the first principle to be employed was to increase the tumor dosage and to lessen skin or superficial damage by the practice of alternating the portals of external exposure. It is as though one were to move the external source along the rim of a wagon wheel with the beam of radiation always directed toward its hub—the site of the tumor. Thus, radiation to the peripherally located areas or normal tissue is correspondingly reduced; that of the axis or center is increased. Lead shielding of adjacent normal tissue by carefully placing such shields in different external locations each day of treatment so that a different external area or portal of entry is used to gain depth exposure has permitted much higher dosages to be delivered to the more centripetally located tumor site.

Continuous rotation or rotational therapy is carried out by some; this is an improvement upon the more laborious and less well controlled technic of portal therapy. Rotational therapy is accomplished by rotating continuously the source of radiation 360° about the patient, placing the patient so that his tumor is located equidistant from the rotating source. In others the same is accomplished by rotating the patient continuously through a complete circle with the source remaining stationary. The results obtained by either rotational technic are similar. The chief factor in determining whether the source or the patient shall be rotated is whether the size of the source permits rotation.

A second and equally useful principle devised to increase the percentage of the total exposure to the tumor above that which is delivered to the skin and the superficial areas is accomplished by the use of more energetic radiation, often referred to as supervoltage radiation. Here again, two approaches are possible; they are generally employed in combination. First is the selection of the most energetic form of electromagnetic radiation practical to meet the patient's requirements. The second is the use of filtration. As most sources of such radiation emit a spectrum of wave lengths and energies, a portion of which has little or no penetrating power, these rays can be removed by the interposition of appropriate filters interposed between the external energy source and the surface of the patient. Filtration plays a more important role in low-energy radiation where the percentage of penetration is small. The alpha particles of radium are completely removed by the interposition of a thickness of a single sheet of paper. They present no problem for radium, as any container used effectively removes them. External beta rays are readily removed by the use of copper and/or aluminum filters; their elimination from the total dosage delivered to the skin is most important to the patient's safety. Although beta rays generally penetrate little more than the external or more superficial layers of the skin, the extent to which these rays do penetrate is just that much increase in skin exposure; hence, that much reduction in the quantity of the more penetrating gamma or x-radiation that can be administered without harm to the interposed normal structures.

Even with ordinary x-rays, the skin may receive a considerably higher percentage of electromagnetic (gamma or x-ray) radiation than does the underlying tumor. More favorable relationships between the amount of radiation delivered to the tumor compared with that delivered to the skin have been obtained by increasing the energy or the penetrating powers of electromagnetic radiation. The greater their energy, the higher will be the proportion of the total dose reaching the skin, which will also reach the tumor depth. "Softer" gamma or x-radiations which are capable only of penetrating the skin and the superficial normal tissue and not the tumor are largely removed by filtration. There is a limit beyond which these practices cannot be extended, for there remains the principle that the quantity of radiation, light or heat diminishes at an exponential rate with the square of the distance from their sources.

Local Injury From External Radiotherapy. Because normal tissue is damaged to varying degrees by radiotherapy, one must expect and accept within limits a certain amount of tissue injury if therapeutic or carcinocidal radiation is to be given. This damage the surgeon is likely to term "radiation injury"; the radiotherapist calls it "radiation reaction." In most instances where gamma or x-radiation is to be used, the damage to normal tissue is of little permanent or important consequence. In few patients, permanent damage to normal structures is the price known in advance, if treatment is to be successful, especially in malignant disease.

The following are some of the reactions and injuries to be expected from carcinocidal radiation, externally applied:

Skin reaction is a function of skin exposure and is not an indication of dose delivered to deep-seated tumors. On the other hand, cutaneous reaction should not pass unobserved, whether high- or low-energy radiation therapy is employed.

Erythema is the first reaction to appear with low-energy radiation. If sufficient gradients of radiation are administered to the skin, erythema progresses to desquamation, to superficial necrosis and to deep necrosis. Of the various qualities of radiation administered as a single dose, needed to produce the minimal erythema reaction, are the following approximate values as measured on the skin with back scatter:

Radium	1,000 r
250-kv. x-ray with 0.5 mm. copper filter	670 r
80-kv. x-ray (unfiltered)	360 r

As the intensity of external radiation is increased, the site at which the maximum dosage is delivered tends to move to deeper levels within the patient. This results from a phenomenon known as "forward scatter." For example, a 2-million volt x-ray source delivers the maximum dosage below the skin surface; it can produce destruction of the subcutaneous tissue and muscle with latent fibrosis without inducing any skin reaction. High-energy ray or particle radiation of this or greater magnitudes (supervoltage), delivered to the proximal surface of the arm, a theoretical example or model, may produce no demonstrable skin reaction at the portal of skin entry. Yet necrosis of muscle, subcutaneous tissue and skin at the portal of exit may occur due to the forward movement of the site of maximum dosage. Consequently, with the high-energy sources, the erythema reaction, so useful an indicator of dosimetry 30 years or more ago when only moderate radiation energies were possible, no longer serves as a valid indicator of exposure, especially when supervoltage radiotherapy is used.

Erythema desquamation and superficial necrosis under proper radiation therapy are to be expected in many circumstances as part of the consequences of treatment. These will heal. Pigmentation usually occurs in carcinocidal dosages of these magnitudes and may or may not diminish or disappear over a matter of months.

Loss of skin appendages—hair and sweat glands particularly—is the rule in the skin at the sites employed for ordinary radiation administered in carcinocidal dosages. Telangiectasia also occurs occasionally and is a permanent cutaneous disorder in many patients given carcinocidal radiation. Occasionally it is unavoidable. If this is cosmetically a handicap, such skin often may be removed later and a graft applied.

None of these unpleasant results is a contraindication to carcinocidal radiation therapy, provided that the dosage to be delivered is essential to the cure or the relief of a disease which is not otherwise amenable to less hazardous forms of treatment.

Wound healing is delayed when sufficient radiation has been administered. In acute but comparatively low doses (400 r or less) little change from the normal pattern of events is noted, once the victim seems on the way to recovery. More commonly encountered in surgical patients are the larger carcinocidal exposures. Under these circumstances, the healing process is impaired. Surgical incisions heal poorly if for no reason other than that the blood supply in radiated tissue is markedly impaired. It is likely that other disturbances also exist which interfere with healing. Impaired wound healing is most apparent after the 4th to 6th month and is important in the consideration of operation when preoperative x-irradiation of the lesion has been given.

Skin necrosis and its latent complications at times represent unnecessary overexposure. In a few patients, however, the risk even of this complication is warranted, should the potential and ultimate achievement of tumor necrosis appear to be possible.

An example of unnecessary skin and subcutaneous fibrosis, musculature contractures and radiation-induced squamous cell carcinoma is illustrated in Figure 18-8. The hands and the feet of this 17-year-old girl, a concert pianist of promise, were treated for psoriasis by unmonitored x-radiation administered in a doctor's office by a technician without supervision. Repetition of treatment was carried out once a week over a 3½-year period. Dosimetry and other details have not been made available to the author. Ultimate amputation of both feet and of portions of the hands and the fingers was necessary. No relief of the radiation contractures and fibrosis, involving the tendons and the joints, as well as the skin, was possible. Total disability of these structures persisted, with moderate to severe degrees of flexion deformity and fixation resulting. The end result was a permanently and totally disabled patient at the age of 25, the mother of 4 children, whose psoriasis continues as before. Already, 3 squamous cell carcinomas have been removed.

Necrosis often follows incisions in the radiated skin and necessitates grafting or excision with closure by rotation or mobilization of flaps of full thickness nonradiated skin. So frequently is this a bad sequela of surgery performed in areas of heavily radiated skin that time and hospital costs are often saved the patient if the radiated area to be incised is also excised at the same time.

The crystalline lens and probably the cornea also are very sensitive to ionizing radiation. If exposed to a few hundred roentgen units, the latent development of cataract is a good possibility. However, not all lens opacities so produced progress to permanent cataracts. Cataract formation has been observed among scientists exposed to external radiation accidentally or incidentally. In the treatment of lesions about the face, particularly in the region of the orbit, every precaution should be taken to avoid injury to the eye. In malignant lesions, permanent damage to the eye may be unavoidable if radiotherapy offers potential benefit or cure and its usage is to be effective. This hazard should be explained to the pa-

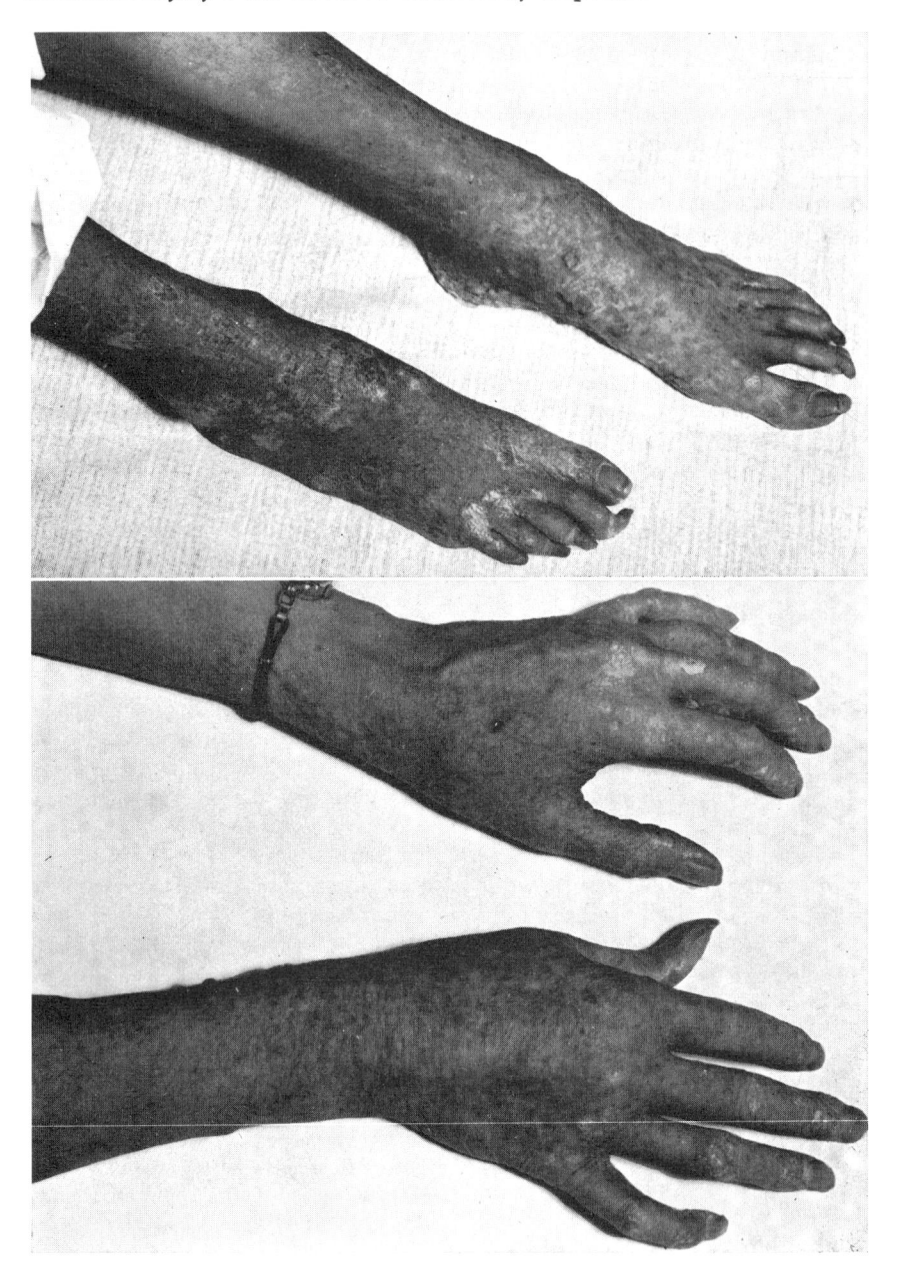

FIG. 18-8. Hands and feet 7 years after termination of an unknown amount of "soft" x-radiation in treatment of psoriasis. Fibrosis of skin and subcutaneous tissue with flexor deformities is evident. Note hyperkeratosis of skin which, along with avascularity, later necessitated amputation of both feet and some fingers. Multiple cutaneous carcinoma also developed.

tient and the immediate family before embarking upon treatment.

Necrosis of bone is a complication occasionally encountered from external radiation. This potential should be considered in planning the therapeutic dosage to be employed whenever intensive bone exposure is likely to occur. Fractures of the rib, the clavicle and the head of the humerus from aseptic necrosis have been observed in the course of therapy delivered in the postoperative treatment of carcinoma of the breast. In the growing child, the possibility of growth arrest of epiphyseal plates must be considered whenever more than 600 r are expected to be delivered to such areas. Aseptic necrosis of the head of the femur as well as the sacrum can occur among patients receiving radiotherapy for carcinoma of the uterus or the cervix, whether administered as radium therapy or x-radiation.

Gastrointestinal. Radium- or x-ray-induced necrosis of the adjacent sigmoid colon or the bladder is another occasional complication of radiotherapy for pelvic cancer. This does not appear to be avoidable in many patients when supravoltage radiation is given. As the radiotherapist becomes more bold in his therapy—which he must, if he is to improve his results for cancer beyond the skin and the squamous epithelial derivatives—he must not be surprised that he, at the same time, is bound to induce greater injury and more frequently in normal tissue. The trouble comes when the exchange of some radiation injury for a better chance for a cure is not acknowledged by the radiotherapist.

Pneumonitis and occasionally *pulmonary fibrosis* are, respectively, relatively early and comparatively latent complications in some patients under external radiotherapy for carcinoma of the breast. In the adequate roentgen treatment of the chest wall and mediastinum in cases with breast cancer, irradiation injury can scarcely be avoided if treatment is to be effective. This is the price of irradiation therapy. Lesser doses are essentially useless. Pneumonitis probably is observed more frequently than any radiation reactions other than those of the skin. Should intensive radiotherapy be necessary, pneumonitis of some degree may not be avoidable. Antibiotics are most useful in the prevention or the control of infection during its acute phases.

The avoidance, or the treatment with benefit, of minor degrees of pulmonary fibrosis with cortisone is claimed to be useful, but this has not been borne out. The development of other therapeutic methods to minimize radiation fibrosis of the lungs and other organs is under exploration. Irradiation fibrosis of the lung may progress, with enough loss of lung function to produce development of a pulmonary cripple and, indeed, end in death.

Radiation nephritis can be serious, leading in a year or longer to obliterative endarteritis of the microvasculature of the kidney and an irreversible nephritis. This is seen more frequently when higher doses of radiotherapy are given in the region of the kidneys.

Cancer Caused by Irradiation. Radiation is second to surgical extirpation as the most effective form of therapy in the overall cancer therapy program now available; on the other hand, it is one of the more dependable means we have for the production of cancer, including man. As with all cancer, the nature of its pathogenesis is not understood. Radiation-induced cancer is usually the result of excessive radiation therapy, but it is also an occupational hazard, and a latent consequence of total body irradiation.

Squamous carcinoma of the skin has already been alluded to in the case report on page 425. Many physicians using the fluoroscope indiscriminately in the developmental early years of radiotherapy, prior to a knowledge of its hazard, eventually died of metastatic squamous carcinoma, particularly those arising from the skin of the hands. This complication was also observed fairly commonly among orthopedic surgeons employing fluoroscopic control without protection, for the realignment of fractures.

Leukemia. Aside from cutaneous cancers among radiologists, there is radiation-induced leukemia. The incidence of leukemia among all physicians is said to be about twice that of the population at large. March (1944) reports the incidence of leukemia to be 0.53 per cent among 26,788 physicians where the cause of death was known. Among the causes of death in 175 radiologists, the incidence of leukemia reached 4.57 per cent. This is an attack rate of about 10 times that of all physicians and approximately 20 times that of the population at large.

Warren and Lombard (1966) report a decrease in the incident rate of leukemia among medical personnel working with diagnostic and therapeutic x-ray procedures. This beneficial effect is attributed to the more careful attention given to radiation and radiation equipment. However, Warren and Meisner (1965) report chromosomal changes in leukocytes of patients receiving x-ray therapy, which serves to emphasize the need for caution against any unnecessary exposure.

Lung Cancer. One of the associated causes of lung cancer has long been believed to be the inhalation by miners of airborne radioactive dust of isotopes of lead, bismuth, polonium, thallium, thorium and possibly of other elements. Wagoner *et al.* (1964) observed 11 cases of lung cancer among uranium workers who had worked in underground mines 5 to 12 years; whereas in a study of nonuranium workers in the same area, who were ethnically similar and in the same age group, only 1 case was observed—a P value of <0.01. The relation between the incidence of cancer and the quantity of exposure has not yet been studied. These data are reminiscent of the earlier reports at Schneeberg and Joachimsthal where the miners were exposed principally to radon gas and its daughter products.

Thyroid Cancer. Recently, data have been presented which suggest that carcinoma in the thyroid in children and young adults may follow the radiation of the gland in infancy or early childhood. Duffy and Fitzgerald reported in 1950 that, in 10 of 18 patients in the age group of 18 years or younger, radiation to the thymus had been administered some time between the 4th and the 16th months of life. Simpson *et al.* (1955) surveyed 1,400 of 1,722 children who had received x-ray therapy to the thymus between the years 1926 and 1951. The number of cases of thyroid cancer was markedly higher in the treated group than in either untreated siblings or the population at large.

Clark (1955) uncovered a history of thymic radiation in 3 of 13 children under the age of 15 whom he observed for carcinoma of the thyroid. However, a careful check with parents and their physicians established that the remaining 10 had received radiation to the neck in the treatment of cervical adenitis, enlarged tonsils, adenoids, sinusitis, peribronchitis and pertussis. Thus, in all his cases, radiation to the neck, including the thyroid area, was administered when very young. The total roentgen dosage ranged from 210 to 725 r. Of the 13 patients, 12 were girls. It is now known that as little as 50 rem to the thyroid can be carcinogenic.

Data that Hempelmann (1960) presents disclose the incidence of expected and observed cancer among 2,350 children, 90 per cent of whom have been traced, whose thymic glands were irradiated in infancy, to be significantly higher than among their untreated siblings (Table 18-13).

Hanford *et al.* (1962) reported their observations in patients receiving 500 to 1500 r to the neck in the region of the thyroid for nonmalignant disease. Their study covered the years between 1920 and 1950. There were 458 patients in the entire group. One hundred and ninety-one of these patients could be traced and examined for 10 years or longer. The expected incidence of thyroid cancer among 191 unexposed individuals would be less than 1 case. However, in this group they observed 8 cases—more than 8 times the expected rate of the untreated sibling population. The report of Socolow *et al.* (1963) is of interest. They found an increased incidence of thyroid cancer among survivors of the Hiroshima and the Nagasaki bombings who were less than 1,399 meters from the hypocenter and therefore received 200 rads or more unless individually shielded (Report of the United Nations Scien-

TABLE 18-13. EXPECTED AND OBSERVED CANCER INCIDENCE IN NEW YORK CHILDREN TREATED FOR THYMIC ENLARGEMENT AND IN UNTREATED SIBLINGS*

TYPE	TREATED CHILDREN EXPECTED	TREATED CHILDREN OBSERVED†	UNTREATED SIBLINGS EXPECTED	UNTREATED SIBLINGS OBSERVED
All cancers	3.6	21	4.3	6
Leukemia	0.9	9	1.1	0
Thyroid cancer	0.06	8	0.1	0

* Hempelmann, L. H.: The delayed effects of whole-body radiation. Bernard B. Watson (ed.). Operations Research Office, Johns Hopkins Press, 1960. Page 38.
† Includes only cancers diagnosed as such by original pathologist.

TABLE 18-14. CASES OF THYROID CANCER ACCORDING TO DISTANCE FROM THE HYPOCENTER IN HIROSHIMA AND NAGASAKI IN ADULT HEALTH STUDY POPULATION (1958-1961)

	LESS THAN 1,399 METERS FROM HYPOCENTER	1,400–2,000 METERS FROM HYPOCENTER	3,000–5,000 METERS FROM HYPOCENTER	NOT EXPOSED†
No. of cases	14*	2	3	2

* $P < 0.001$.
† Not exposed group consisted of those more than 10,000 meters from the hypocenter.

tific Committee on the Effects of Atomic Radiation, 1962). Table 18-14 summarizes their findings.

Reports indicate that the rate of breast cancer is 3 times that expected, as in Hiroshima, after repeated fluoroscopy and after treatment of mastitis by x-ray, (see Chap. 27, Breast).

Bone Cancer. Osteogenic sarcoma, chondrosarcoma and fibrosarcoma have been reported by Hatcher (1945), Cahan *et al.* (1948) and by others in association with externally administered roentgen irradiation. While these tumors are uncommon complications, their occurrence does argue against the use of radiation in the treatment of benign tumors which could be excised surgically without difficulty and with good results.

Reactions From Internally Administered Radiation. With the advent of isotope therapy in recent years, the potential hazard of overexposure from internal radiation becomes a problem with which to reckon. In general, radioactive isotopes such as ^{131}I, ^{32}P, or ^{198}Au have sufficiently short half-lives as to present little danger from chronic effects when properly used. They are capable, in excessive dosages, of producing acute radiation damage, especially aplasia of the marrow, and even death. Excessive ^{131}I can ablate thyroid function; in some patients this may be the desired result (see Chap. 28, Thyroid, Thymus and Parathyroids).

Chronic effects of the administration of isotopes that have long half-lives and are retained within the body present other problems. Most prominent of these isotopes are the so-called "bone seekers." Within less than 2 decades of the discovery of radium, its soluble salts were administered parenterally or orally for numerous diseases. Salts of thorium X and radium were the usual isotopes prescribed. Administration by inhalations of radon and thoron "gases" was also commonly practiced.

Unfortunately, because the early results for some of these diseases were interpreted as beneficial, such therapy was continued. It was only 20 to 30 years ago that toxic manifestations began to be apparent, particularly in patients receiving the bone-seeking salts of thorium, mesothorium and radium. To be included in this same group are the "dial painters" who touched the thorium X-containing paint brushes to their lips to draw out a fine brush point. The latent bone changes included necrosis, malignant disease and blood dyscrasias. These findings were first reported by Blum in 1924 and more extensively by Martland and Hoffman. By 1932, radium for internal administration was removed from the *New and Nonofficial Remedies* of the American Medical Association (Looney *et al.*, 1955).

Hatcher, Looney, Marinelli and others point out that hundreds and perhaps thousands of individuals in the United States were given radium or thorium salts orally or parenterally 40 or more years ago. They and others have examined many of these individuals and found them to be unaware that they carried radium or thorium deposits in their skeletal system. The hematologic findings also were neither striking nor diagnostic in most of these patients. Thirty-eight patients in Looney's series received radium salts therapeutically, and 6 had been employed as "radium" dial painters. Osseous lesions were readily demonstrated in many by roentgenograms. A general correlation existed between the amount of residual thorium and the frequency and the severity of osseous lesions observed. Bone sarcomas were observed in 6 patients in this series; all 6 probably received radiothorium and/or mesothorium. None was believed to have received radium alone.

TABLE 18-15. AVERAGE DOSES TO SELECTED ORGANS FOR VARIOUS AGES IN RADS PER MICROCURIE ADMINISTERED FOR DIAGNOSTIC TESTS EMPLOYING RADIOACTIVE ISOTOPES*

Organ	Radionuclide	Route of Administration	Newborn rads/microcurie	1 Yr. rads/microcurie	5 Yr. rads/microcurie	10 Yr. rads/microcurie	15 Yr. rads/microcurie	Standard Man rads/microcurie
Liver	$Na_2H^{32}PO_4$	Intravenous	0.55	0.17	0.10	0.06	0.04	0.03
	Colloidal ^{198}Au	Intravenous	0.49	0.20	0.12	0.08	0.05	0.04
	Cobalt 57-labeled Vitamin B_{12}	Oral	1.5	0.68	0.41	0.28	0.21	0.16
	Cobalt 58-labeled Vitamin B_{12}	Oral	2.3	1.2	0.76	0.54	0.42	0.33
	Cobalt 60-labeled Vitamin B_{12}	Oral	30.0	15.0	10.0	6.9	5.3	4.2
Spleen	$Na_2H^{32}PO_4$	Intravenous	0.55	0.17	0.10	0.06	0.04	0.03
	Colloidal ^{198}Au	Intravenous	0.49	0.20	0.12	0.08	0.05	0.04
	$Na_2^{51}CrO_4$ "altered" red cell	Intravenous	0.49	0.16	0.10	0.05	0.04	0.04
Bone and marrow	$Na_2H^{32}PO_4$	Intravenous	0.55	0.17	0.10	0.06	0.04	0.03
Thyroid	$Na^{131}I$	Oral	32.0	10.0	4.3	3.1	1.7	1.3
	$Na^{125}I$	Oral	19.0	6.1	2.6	1.8	1.0	0.82
	$Na^{132}I$	Oral	1.2	0.40	0.17	0.12	0.07	0.05
Kidney	Chlormerodrin	Intravenous	0.66	0.22	0.14	0.09	0.07	0.06
	Hippuran ^{131}I	Intravenous	0.01	0.004	0.003	0.002	0.001	0.001
	Hippuran ^{125}I	Intravenous	0.002	0.0006	0.0004	0.0002	0.0002	0.0002

* Seltzer, R. A., Kereiakes, J. G., and Saenger, E. L.: Radiation exposure from radioisotopes in pediatrics. New Eng. J. Med., 271: 84, 1964.

Although the hazard from persistent radiation of bone-seeking radioactive isotopes is now well recognized and assiduously avoided in industry and medicine, the total problem or the ultimate end-result is not yet clear or evident. A similar potential and possibly uncontrollable hazard exists from the radioactive fallout of strontium 90 in the event of atomic disasters and to a lesser extent from strontium 89. Kowalewski and Rodin (1964) reported the induction of bone tumors in all rats in which they injected 6 doses of 0.7 μc of strontium 89 per gram of body weight.

Exposure From Use of Tracer Doses of Isotopes. Average doses to selected organs for various ages of patients administered radioactive isotopes for diagnostic purposes are shown in Table 18-15. Clearly, quantities of specific organ exposures in infants and children range up to 30 times that for the adult. The significance of the much greater localization of activity in specific organs tends to be masked by the lower doses of total body irradiation that these data imply; nonetheless, the amount of total body irradiation per microcurie of radionuclide administered is up to 20 times that for the "standard" man (Seltzer et al., 1964).

MANAGEMENT OF WOUNDS ACUTELY CONTAMINATED WITH RADIONUCLIDES

Cuts, skin puncture wounds and abrasions may occur among those working with radioactive isotopes, whether in the laboratory or in industry, wherein the agent responsible for the break in the dermal layers is contaminated with one or more isotopes. The worker with an open wound may be peculiarly exposed to radiation should he come into contact with a radioactive isotope at a time when the wound is capable of absorption of isotopes and the infliction of local and/or systemic radiation injury. Contamination of open wounds by radionuclides in event of atomic warfare with the tens or hundreds of thousands of casualties would present a real problem. The seriousness of this problem depends upon the nature of the irradiation, the solubility of the isotope and the quantity absorbed. However, local injuries may occur from fallout caught in abrasions as well as on the skin surface. This occurred among the crew of the *Fortunate Dragon* in 1954, 110 miles away from the bomb blast.

Wounds contaminated by fallout deserve special attention, which in principle may take one or more of several courses: local débridement or excision; prompt irrigation with agents which will bind a soluble isotope and hold it in the local area until it can be removed; or the contaminant may be dissolved so that it can be removed more easily by careful irrigation. Once the isotope has entered the body, it may be desirable to accelerate its rate of excretion, if possible.

The choice of treatment most useful to the patient depends upon the character of the isotope(s) involved, the extent of contamination and the relative importance of the injury to any permanent functional or cosmetic defect that might be necessary should surgical excision of one type or another be required.

Local Treatment. While the scrubbing of a wound will remove most bacteria, it does not follow that simple mechanical cleansing will necessarily remove radioisotopes, even from the unabraded surface. (Finkel and Hathaway, 1956.) Certain special precautions are necessary. Shaving of hair from the skin should be delayed until after "decontamination" has been accomplished satisfactorily, lest uncontaminated abrasions or cuts become contaminated from surrounding skin, and to that extent compound the seriousness of the problem already presented.

Arterial tourniquet may be applied promptly should the wound be on an extremity and the isotope be a soluble one. This procedure is not without the usual hazards of any tourniquet (necrosis or nerve injury) and is to be employed only when all precautions against the dangers of prolonged applications of tourniquets are borne fully in mind. Tourniquet should be used only when appropriate decontamination can be accomplished within less than an hour after its application.

Washing or irrigation should be more extensive than in the usual case of the ordinary wound. One of the detergents (sodium alkyl sulfonate, for example) is more useful than soap, as some detergents are more effective than soap in the formation of insoluble salts with many isotopes.

Nonsoluble isotopes contaminating the skin and the wound may not be absorbed for a matter of hours or days. When contamination is from an isotope of low solubility, a tourniquet is applied upon arrival at the doctor's office, and irrigations with a 1 per cent solution of sodium citrate is begun. Citrate is used as the irrigating fluid as a number of the heavy metals, including uranium, form soluble salts with citrate and hence may be washed away harmlessly. Many of these same metals also form soluble chelates with EDTA (ethylenediamine tetra-acetate) which is an alternate irrigating solution that may be used. Citrate is the less hazardous of the two, and more likely to be available.

In a few instances, cautery of an inconspicuous small area of skin or tissue may be employed with the aim of coagulating the blood and the lymph flow in the area, preventing or delaying absorption until the area can be excised; 8 normal concentrated hydrochloric acid or 14 normal nitric acid are suitable for this purpose, if the injured area is suitable for such treatment. Although both of these acids are available in most laboratories, it is the physician—not the scientist—who should decide as to the appropriateness of their use, and only the physician should employ them.

Then the usual surgical débridement is undertaken. The tissue removed is to be saved for monitoring and analyzing for its isotope content. Débridement may entail sacrifice of adjacent normal tissue if this is an important consideration to the potential of latent effects of residual isotope. This obviously is of greater concern in young patients than in the elderly and is also modified by the half-life of the isotope concerned and whether it probably will be retained in the body, e.g., radium, thorium and strontium 90.

General Treatment. Consultation with a competent health-physicist is imperative in any event. If the radioisotope is one likely to be absorbed, the patient should be admitted to a hospital equipped for metabolic studies and isotope measurements in tissue, blood, urine, and feces.

To bind certain of the heavy metal radioactive isotopes, intravenously administered calcium disodium edetate may be helpful. This fairly nontoxic compound forms soluble chelates with yttrium, lanthanum, iron, cobalt, zinc, cadmium, lead, nickel, copper, plutonium and thorium, which are excreted unchanged in the urine. The earlier this calcium-and-sodium-containing edathamil can be administered, the greater its benefits may be. The tetrasodium salt of EDTA should not be used as it may bind calcium and induce tetany.

LATENT CONSEQUENCES OF IONIZING IRRADIATION FROM ATOMIC AND THERMO-NUCLEAR BOMBS

As the follow-up studies on the survivors of Hiroshima and Nagasaki continue, it is evident that there appears to be an accelerated rate of aging among the proximally exposed individuals (Anderson, 1965). Among 286 adolescent children, all of whom were in utero at the time of bombing, the age at menarche and the degree of epiphyseal closure in the wrist were determined. Differences were found by Burrow et al. (1965), and these differences related to the distance the mother was from the hypocenter at the time the bomb was dropped. Lisco and Conrad (1967), in a 10-year cytogenetic study of blood lymphocytes of Marshall Islanders, reported chromosome-type aberrations in 23 of 43 exposed persons. Half the aberrations are of the exchange type. An unexpectedly large number of acentric fragments, but no exchange-type aberrations, appear in a few unexposed people on the same island.

The most consistent finding in the exposed Marshall Islanders was the diminished head-circumference, especially in those in the third trimester at the time of exposure. In many experiments, premature aging and an increase in the incidence of cancer have been observed. Life expectancy is generally reduced. As the human studies continue, it appears that the complications, whether from external exposure or internal exposure to radiation as the result of atomic or hydrogen bomb explosions, rise with age.

Warren and Meisner (1965) concluded that therapeutic irradiation produces chromosomal aberration which can be assessed by analysis of lymphoid cells from peripheral blood during therapy. The incidence of such changes increased with the amount of irradiation received. Most of these changes cease after termination of irradiation therapy, though in 5 per cent they were detectable for 30 years, particularly aberrations of chromosomes 1 and 2.

PROTECTION OF PERSONNEL

Because of the potential hazards to personnel engaged in the practice of radiotherapy as well as diagnostic radiology, certain minimum standards are essential. Many useful suggestions have been published by the International Commission on X-ray and Radium Protection. In the United States, the National Bureau of Standards *Handbook 41* (*X-ray Protection*) and its *Handbook 23* (*Radium Protection*) have been carefully compiled and should be consulted for details.

Technics for lessening unnecessary exposure to x-rays in diagnostic radiology have been described by the Medical X-ray Advisory Committee to the U.S. Department of Health, Education and Welfare (1967).

The outstanding feature of radiation injury to patients or personnel is the large percentage of instances wherein evidence of serious damages does not appear until many years have elapsed after the initial exposure. This applies to gamma and x-radiation as well as to poisoning from the ingestion of radium and other of the "bone seeker" radioactive isotopes.

Little (1968) summarizes most of the foregoing material in Figure 18-9, which simply implies that the less exposure the better.

GENETIC EFFECTS OF IRRADIATION

Largely from the mutagenic effects of irradiation in the *Drosophila* and in barley, three assumptions are made about mutagenic irradiation. First, ionizing radiations may cause mutations of both genes and chromosomes. Second, the occurrence rate of mutations is a linear function of the irradiation dose the organism receives. And, third, the mutagenic effects are cumulative in many species but not necessarily in all. It is the last assumption that, if it holds true for man as for fruit flies, causes concern—deep concern—for future generations, considering the likelihood of an increasing exposure to fallout, particularly inhaled or ingested, to diagnostic and therapeutic radiologic measures and to radioactive isotopes used or produced in industry. To date, there appears to be little evidence that we have begun to approach the limits of tolerance from fallout, but it should also be clear that the current concept regarding "maximal permissible dose," as redefined by the Federal Radiation Council, is only as sound as experimental and clinical evidence to date permits. We know too little of x-radiation mutagenesis in man to feel very secure as to the possible magnitude of our problem, particularly as further exposures accumulate.

It is perhaps well to end this chapter, as we began, with Terry's statement of 1962: "There is no level of radiation exposure below which there can be absolute certainty that harmful effects will not occur to at least a few individuals when sufficiently large numbers of people are exposed." The balance to be struck is between total safety in an uncertain future, and the short-term and the long-range gains expected from the use of ionizing irradiation. There is no exact or clear answer yet in sight and, while the benefits of therapeutic and diagnostic radiology are unquestioned, it seems equally certain that future testing of nuclear devices will continue for some time to come and will add to the cumulative effects of ionizing radiation. It is better to reduce exposure from all sources whenever and wherever this is possible.

LASER-MASER RADIATION

Inasmuch as this chapter is confined to the subject of ionizing radiation, it is not appropriate to discuss the development of laser radiation and its biologic effects. However, the reader should be alerted to the possible hazards to health resulting from the use of such radiation and the means of control. The January-February, 1965, issue of "Federation Proceedings" (The Federation of American Societies for Experimental Biology) includes an addendum entitled "Biologic Effects of Laser Radiation" dealing with all aspects of this new development in radiation therapy.

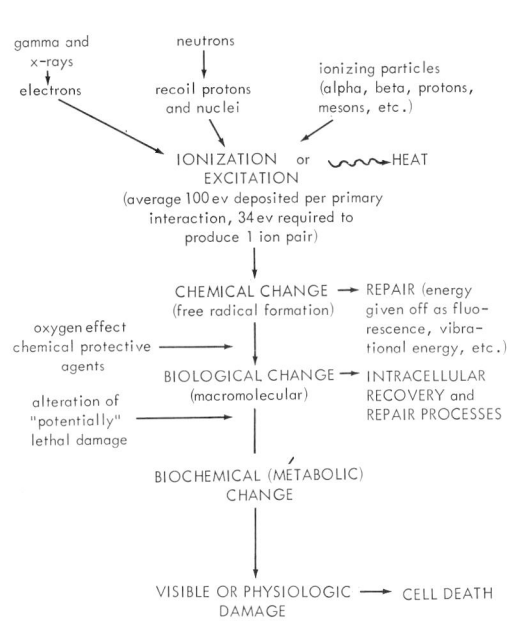

FIG. 18-9. Development of radiation injury in cells. (Little, J. B.: New Eng. J. Med., 278:369, 1968)

REFERENCES

Allen, J. G., Basinger, C. E., Landy, J. J., Sanderson, M. H., and Enerson, D. E.: Blood transfusion in irradiation hemorrhage. Science, 115:523, 1952.

Alpen, E. L., and Baum, S. T.: Modification of x-radiation lethality by autologous marrow infusion in dogs. Blood, 13:1168, 1958.

Anderson, R. E.: Aging in Hiroshima atomic bomb survivors. Arch. Path., 79:1, 1965.

Andrews, G. A.: Criticality accidents in Vinca, Yugoslavia, and Oak Ridge, Tennessee. J.A.M.A., 179:191, 1962.

Blum, T.: Osteomyelitis of mandible and maxilla. J. Am. Dent. A., 11:802, 1924.

Brucer, M.: When do you leave a fallout shelter? J.A.M.A., 180:144, 1962.

Burrow, G. N., Hamilton, H. B., and Hrubec, Z.: Study of adolescents exposed in utero to the atomic bomb, Nagasaki, Japan. J.A.M.A., 192:97, 1965.

Cahan, W. G., Higinbotham, N. L., Stewart, F. W., and Coley, B. L: Sarcoma arising in irradiated bone Cancer, 1:3, 1948.

Clark, D. E.: Association of irradiation with cancer of the thyroid in children and adolescents. J.A.M.A., 159:1007, 1955.

Conrad, R. A., and Hiching, A.: Medical findings in Marshallese people exposed to fallout. J.A.M.A., 192:113, 1965.

Cronkite, E. P., and Brecher, G.: Tr. Fifth Conf. on

Blood Clotting and Allied Problems. pp. 171-212. New York, Macy, 1952; Allen, J. G.: *ibid.*, pp. 213-246.

Duffy, B. J., Jr., and Fitzgerald, P. J.: Thyroid cancer in childhood and adolescence: report on 28 cases. Cancer, 3:1018, 1950.

Finkel, A. J., and Hathaway, E. A.: Medical care of wounds contaminated with radioactive materials. J.A.M.A., 161:121, 1956.

Gray, L. H.: Biopysical basis:physical basis of the action of radiation on living materials. *In* Carling, E. R., Windeyer, B. W., and Smithers, D. W.: Practice in Radiotherapy. London, Buterworth, 1955.

Hanford, J. M., Quimby, E. H., and Frantz, V. K.: Cancer arising many years after radiation therapy. J.A.M.A., 181:404, 1962.

Hatcher, C. H.: Development of sarcoma in bone subjected to roentgen or radium irradiation. J. Bone Joint Surg., 27:179, 1945.

Hektoen, L.: Further studies on the effects of roentgen rays on antibody production. J. Infect. Dis., 22:28, 1918.

Hempelmann, L. H., Lisco, H., and Hoffman, J. G.: The acute radiation syndrome: a study of 9 cases and a review of the problem. Ann. Int. Med., 36:282, 1952.

Hoffman, F. L.: Radium (mesothorium) necrosis. J.A.M.A., 85:961, 1925.

International Commission on X-Ray and Radium Protection: Recommendations of the Internat. Comm. on Radiological Protection and the Internat. Comm. on Radiological Units (Handbook 47). Washington, D. C., National Bureau of Standards, 1950.

Jacobson, L. O., Simmons, E. L., Marks, E. K., and Gaston, E. O.: Further studies on recovery from irradiation. J. Lab. Clin. Med., 37:683, 1951.

Kowalewski, K., and Rodin, A. E.: Strontium[89]-induced bone tumour in the rat. Canad. J. Surg., 7:204, 1964.

Lapp, R. E.: Radioactive fall-out. III. Bull. Atomic Scientist, 11:206, 1955.

Lisco, H., and Conrad, R. A.: Chromosome studies on the Marshall Islanders exposed to fallout radiation. Science, 157:446, 1967.

Little, J. B.: Cellular effects of ionizing radiation. New Eng. J. Med., 278:308, 1968.

Looney, W. B., Hasterlik, R. J., Brues, A. M., and Skirmont, E.: A clinical investigation of the chronic effects of radium salts administered therapeutically (1915-1931). Am. J. Roentgenol., 73:1006, 1955.

March, H. C.: Leukemia among radiologists. Radiology, 43:275, 1944.

Marinelli, L. D., Miller, C. E., Gustafson, P. F., and Rowland, R. E.: Quantitative determination of gamma-ray emitting elements in living persons. Am. J. Roentgenol., 73:661, 1955.

Martin, H. E., Quinby, E. H., and Pack, G. T.: Calculations of tissue dosage in radiation therapy. Am. J. Roentgenol., 25:490, 1931.

Martland, H. S., and Humphries, R. E.: Osteogenic sarcoma in dial painters using luminous paint. Arch. Path., 7:406, 1929.

Mill, S. D., Kyle, R. A., Hallenbeck, G. A., Pease, G. L., and Cree, I. C.: Bone-marrow transplant in an identical twin. J.A.M.A., 188:1037, 1964.

Patt, H. M., Tyree, E. B., Straube, R. L., and Smith, D. E.: Cysteine protection against x-irradiation. Science, 110:213, 1949.

Report of the Medical X-ray Advisory Committee on Public Health Considerations in Medical Diagnostic Radiology (X Rays). U.S. Dept. of Health, Education and Welfare, Washington, D.C., Oct. 1967.

Seltzer, R. A., Kereiakes, J. G., and Saenger, E. L.: Radiation exposure from radioisotopes in pediatrics. New Eng. J. Med., 271:84, 1964.

Shouse, S. S., Warren, S. L., and Whipple, G. H.: Aplasia of marrow and fatal intoxication produced by roentgen radiation of all bones. J. Exp. Med., 53:421, 1931.

Sidel, V. W., Geiger, H. J., and Lown, B.: The physician's role in the post-attack period. New Eng. J. Med., 266:1137, 1962.

Sikov, M. R., and Lofstrom, J. E.: Contribution of plasma constituents produced following whole body irradiation on the efficacy of local radiation therapy. Am. J. Roentgenol., 84:705, 1960.

Simpson, C. L., Hempelmann, L. H., and Fuller, L. M.: Neoplasia in children treated with x-rays in infancy for thymic enlargement. Radiology, 64:840, 1955.

Socolow, E. L., Hashizume, A., Neriishi, S., and Niitani, R.: Thyroid carcinoma in man after exposure to ionizing radiation. New Eng. J. Med., 268:406, 1963.

Storer, J. B., and Coon, J. M.: The Protective Effect of Para-Aminopropiophenone Against Lethal Doses of X-irradiation, TID-365, Univ. Chicago Toxicity Lab. Quart. Progress Rep. No. 5 on Radiology, pp. 16-19, 1950.

Terry, L., and Chadwick, D. R.: Current concepts in radiation protection. Part I. J.A.M.A., 180:995, 1962.

Terry, L. L., and Chadwick, D. R.: Current concepts in radiation protection. Part II: Radioiodine intake, 1961-62. J.A.M.A., 188:343, 1964.

Thomas, E. D., Phillips, J. H., and Finch, C. A.: Recovery from marrow failure following isogenic marrow infusion. J.A.M.A., 188:1041, 1964.

Wagoner, J. K., Archer, V. E., Carroll, B. E., Holaday, D. A., and Lawrence, P. A.: Cancer mortality patterns among U. S. uranium miners and millers, 1950 through 1962. J. Nat. Cancer Inst., 32:787, 1964.

Warren, S., and Lombard, O. M.: New data on the effects of ionizing radiation on radiologists. Arch. Environ. Health, 13:415, 1966.

Warren, S., and Meisner, L.: Chromosomal changes in leukocytes of patients receiving irradiation therapy. J.A.M.A., 193:351, 1965.

Zaret, M. M.: The laser hazard. Arch. Environ. Health, 10:629, 1965.

CHAPTER 19

PAUL S. RUSSELL, M.D.

Tissue and Organ Transplantation

Much surgical effort in the past has been devoted to the removal of localized disease, the drainage of pus, and the care of wounds. The hope that lost body substance might be made good in one way or another, or that damaged organs and tissues might be renewed from outside sources, is an ancient dream. Rapid and recent developments in transplantation biology and surgery have brought this dream much nearer to reality and, indeed, there are a number of practical applications of the new "constructive surgery" which have already gained a place in the practical armamentarium of the surgeon. For some time the orthopedist and the neurosurgeon have made good use of implanted prostheses of nonliving materials. Other needs can be met to some degree by the use of nonliving tissues, such as woven fabric blood vessels or artificial cardiac valves where living tissues may not be mandatory. This chapter will deal, however, with the complex and rapidly growing field of transplantation of living tissues in which the full vitality of the component cells, including their metabolic and self-replicating potential, is a prerequisite for success.

Sporadic attempts to perform various types of transplants from animal or human donors to patients have been made for many years, but only since the early 1950's has there been a concerted attack on the obstacles that lie in the way of transplantation becoming a useful, perhaps even a major, form of treatment. These broad problems are: (a) the understanding and management of the rejection reaction that the body naturally mounts against foreign tissue, and (b) the procurement of sufficient numbers of suitable organs for use in transplantation. Since these problems go right to the heart of some of the most interesting and rapidly developing scientific work of our day, and since they involve complex clinical and ethical challenges, an unusually active collaboration of surgery with many other disciplines is required for progress in this attractive field.

TRANSPLANTATION TECHNICS

Tissues and organs may be transferred either to a recipient site that is anatomically their normal one, such as kidney to the renal fossa, with normal vascular and ureteral connections (*orthotopic* transplant), or to an anatomically abnormal site (*heterotopic* transplant). Heterotopic grafts may function quite normally, discharging their usual metabolic functions in a novel location. Thus, a donor spleen can be placed into the iliac fossa in the retroperitoneal space, with its vessels joined appropriately to the iliac vessels. Similarly the pancreas, with or without its associated duodenal loop, may perform at least its endocrine function satisfactorily in this same recipient site. The pancreatic ducts either may be ligated or can be allowed to drain into the duodenal loop which can be led to the surface (Fig. 19-1). This retroperitoneal recipient site was first used for kidney transplantation following the original lead of Kuss (1951).

Some transplanted organs, such as the heart, must occupy their natural position in order to function normally. Others, such as the liver, must be served by vascular inflow channels from normal sources. Thus liver transplants must be provided with systemic arterial inflow to the hepatic artery and also by portal venous inflow for optimal function (Corry *et al.*, p. 437) although the actual position in which the transplanted organ lies is not as restricted as for the heart (Fig. 19-2). The need for extracorporeal support of heart and lung function for cardiac transplantation is obvious. No such assistance is required for other organs

---
This work supported in part by grants No. AI-06320 and No. AM-07055 from the U.S. Public Health Service.

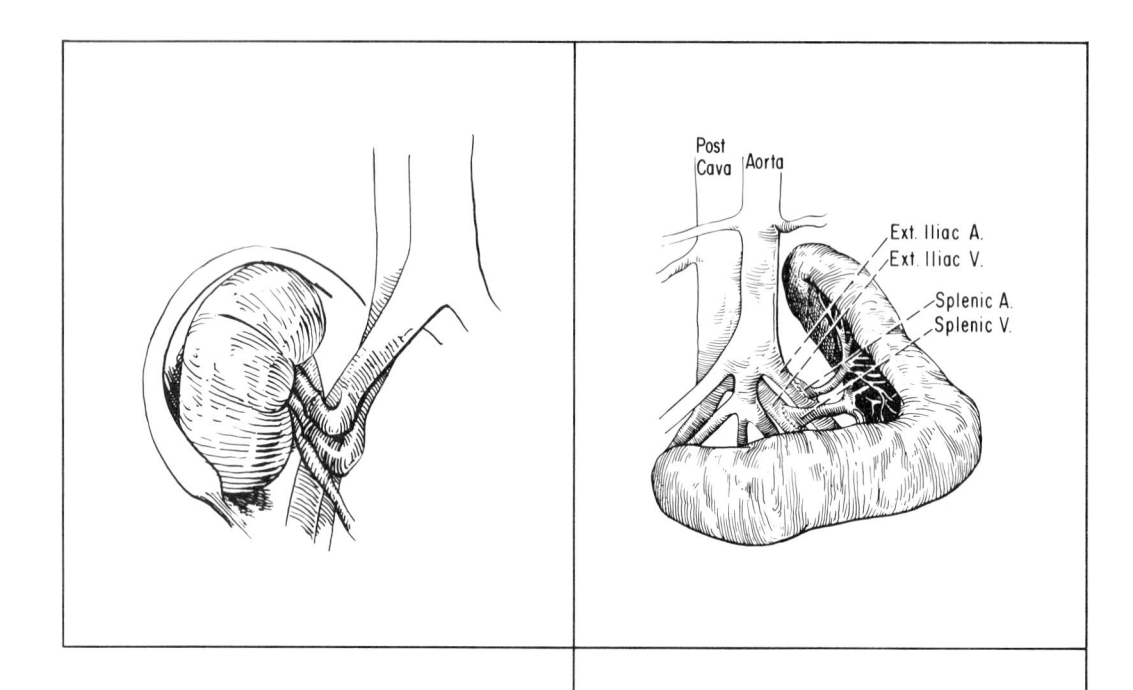

FIG. 19-1. Some examples of convenient heterotopic recipient locations for transplanted organs. The retroperitoneal position has been satisfactory for kidney, pancreas, and spleen.

although the technical demands in certain instances, such as with orthotopic liver transplantation, may require vascular shunts around the recipient site, with or without pumping, during the transplantation procedure.

TERMINOLOGY

The terminology in transplantation has undergone some fairly recent changes. Some have held to certain of the older terms, but the newer ones are steadily gaining acceptance and are recommended. (See Table 19-1.)

THE REJECTION REACTION

Description

When living grafts are transferred between adult mammals of ordinary genetic diversity within the same species they usually remain quite viable in every respect for a few days, healing into place and performing their normal functions. By the eighth to the tenth day a transplant will appear somewhat swollen and gradually becomes darker in color as blood flow within it becomes increasingly sluggish. In from 8 to 14 days almost all allotransplants have been fully rejected by normal hosts. This rejection reaction was first extensively studied by the use of skin grafts, and special attention should be drawn to the elegant and decisive experiments of P. B. Medawar in the early 1940's with skin transplants in rabbits (Medawar, 1944) (Fig. 19-3). These experiments showed with clarity that the reaction against a transplant is a specific one, in that a second transplant to a recipient from the *same donor* is met with a more rapid and violent response, the "second set reaction." Such reactions, involving accelerated reactivity on second contact, are characteristic of reactions of the *immune type*, and there is now extensive evidence that the rejection reaction is indeed an immunologic one. The specific state of immunity induced by the rejection of an organ or tissue graft is a systemic or generalized one and will remain in effect for many months. Immunity induced by dissociated cells transferred as a graft, such as blood leukocytes or bone marrow, tends to be less long lived but is no less vigorous. A particularly characteristic feature of the rejection reaction is the dense infiltrate of inflammatory cells that becomes concentrated in the graft as it is destroyed (Fig. 19-4). This cellular response is made up of a number of different types of leukocytes, with lymphoid cells predominating. In experiments making use of highly inbred strains of animals, where genetic identity can be approximated, it can be demonstrated that

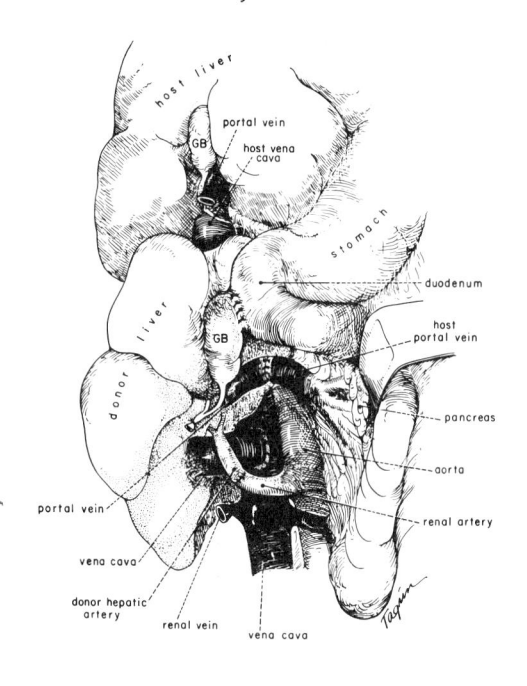

FIG. 19-2. The liver may be placed, as illustrated, in an ectopic position successfully so long as it receives vascular inflow through both portal venous and hepatic arterial channels.

sensitivity to a given donor strain of animals can be transferred from one individual to another with lymph node or spleen cells from a recipient that has rejected a transplant. Typical long-lived immunity to a transplant donor cannot be transferred with serum, even in large amounts, from sensitized recipients. Thus transplant rejection has been classified as a "delayed hypersensitivity" or cell-mediated response similar to the tuberculin reaction.

TABLE 19-1. TERMINOLOGY OF TISSUE TRANSPLANTATION

Old Terminology	New Terminology	New Adjective	Definition
Autograft	Autograft	Autologous	Graft in which donor is also recipient
Isograft	Isograft	Isogeneic	Graft between individuals identical in histocompatibility antigens
Homograft	Allograft	Allogeneic	Graft between genetically dissimilar members of same species
Heterograft	Xenograft	Xenogeneic	Graft between species

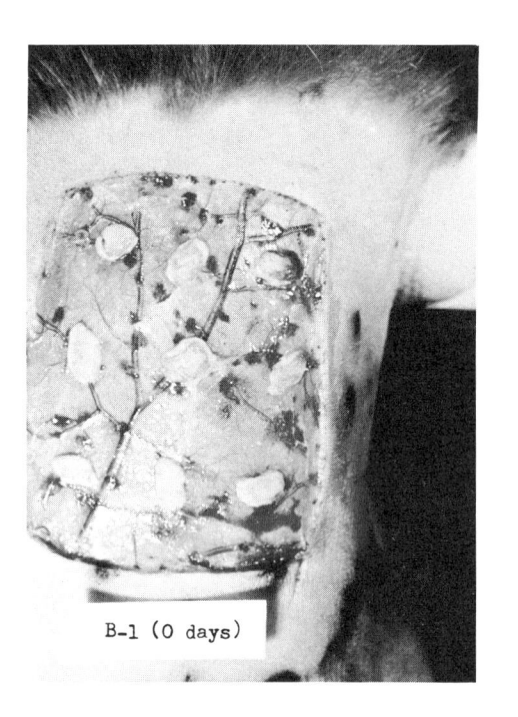

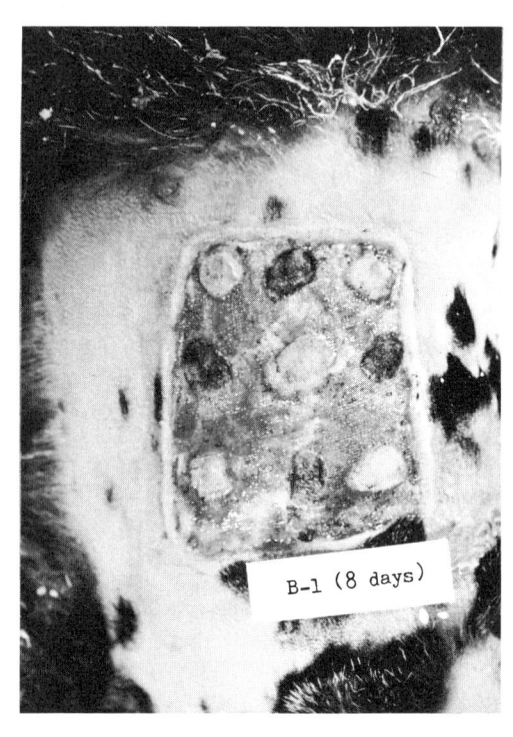

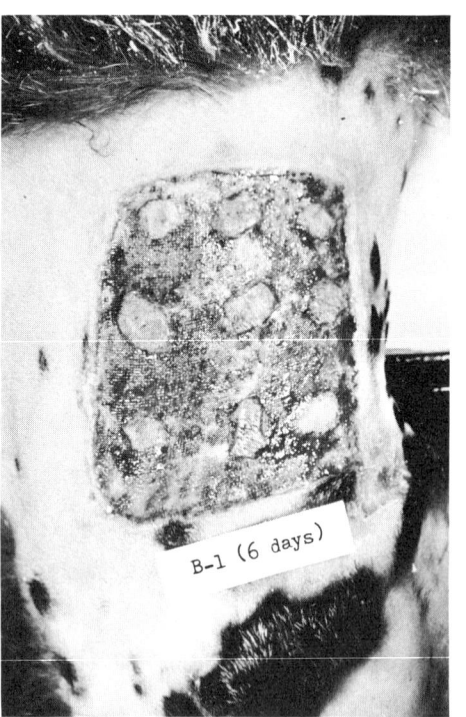

FIG. 19-3. Full thickness skin grafts on a recipient site on the lateral thoracic wall of a rabbit. Some are autologous and some allogeneic from a single unrelated donor. These photographs show the area at the time of grafting, and 6 and 8 days thereafter when the dressings were removed for inspection. At 6 days all grafts are well healed into place and are fully vascularized. By 8 days the allogeneic grafts have reached an advanced stage of rejection. They are dark, hemorrhagic and will soon be cast off as mummified scabs.

FIG. 19-4. Typical histologic appearance of a skin graft at an advanced stage of rejection (donor and recipient mouse unrelated). The donor epidermis is nonviable. The dermis of the skin graft is extensively infiltrated with leukocytes, especially of the mononuclear type.

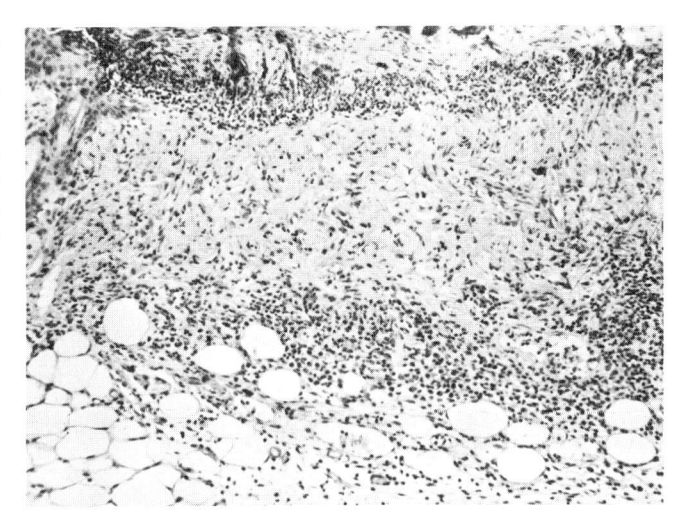

The mechanism of sensitization to the antigens in a fixed tissue graft has not been fully elucidated. Although typical immunity can apparently be induced by attaching a foreign organ of significant size, e.g., a kidney, to the vessels of a recipient through tubes by an extracorporeal circuit (Strober and Gowans, 1965), the establishment of lymphatic connections between graft and host will greatly potentiate the sensitization process. There is much to support the contention that recipient lymphoid cells find their way into a transplant, where they become specifically sensitized to the foreign antigens they encounter there. After returning, largely through afferent lymphatic channels, these cells may then set up an organized reaction in secondarily recruited cells throughout the lymphatic centers.

Recent experiments have made it clear that humoral antibodies actually are formed against the same antigenic specificities in the donor cells as are being reacted against by recipient leukocytes. Humoral antibodies were first detected by Peter Gorer and his associates (Gorer, 1942) against certain tumor transplants in animals. More recently antibodies have been demonstrated in some recipients of organ transplants by very sensitive methods. The importance of conventional humoral antibody in bringing about the destruction of organ transplants in the clinical setting is not at all clear. Experimental situations can be contrived in which humoral antibody may have very significant effects (see below). The complex serum complement system is also involved, and lowered levels of complement factors, particularly the second component ($C'2$), have been found during acute rejection reactions in patients (Austen and Russell, 1966).

In primarily vascularized organ transplants, such as the heart or kidney, the beginnings of a typical cellular infiltrate into the parenchyma of the organ can be seen on histologic examination within 12 hours. The vascular endothelium appears to be an important target for immunologic attack by humoral and cellular elements, with platelet aggregation in clusters along the linings of vessels followed by cellular infiltration of the vascular wall, and disruption of its normal laminar architecture, frequently ending in severe vascular narrowing (Fig. 19-5).

GENETICS AND CHEMISTRY OF ANTIGENS

Antigens are substances that can be recognized biologically as foreign and to which an immunologic response is generated. Where two individuals of the same species are concerned in an allogeneic combination the antigens that provoke transplant rejection are genetically determined as dominants. These antigens can be detected, in general, on all of the nucleated cells of an individual and are properly designated as *individual specific* antigens. They are to be distinguished from those antigens by which members of different species differ, the *species specific* antigens. Within several species, particularly the mouse, rat, and man, one complex locus, or series of closely placed loci on a single chromosome, appears to govern the formation of many of

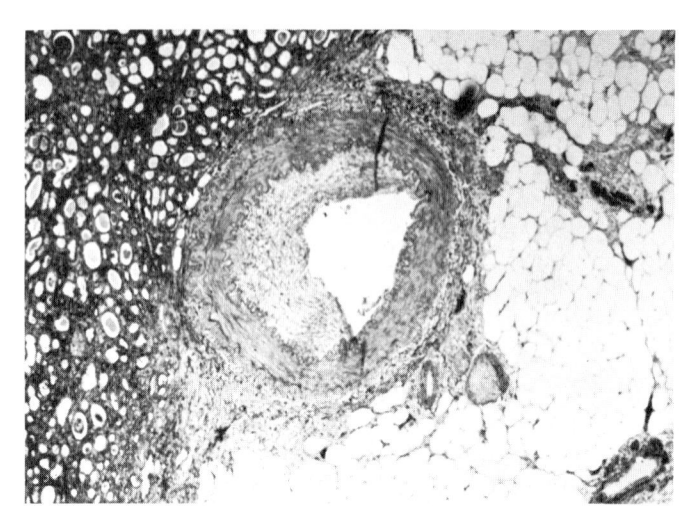

FIG. 19-5. Arteriolar constrictive lesion frequently seen in transplanted kidneys. This lesion appears to correlate with the appearance of circulating antibody to the transplant and can probably be expected as a sign of gradual rejection in any transplanted organ.

the strong transplantation antigens. A number of alleles of these genes have been shown to occur so that the number of possible combinations is great. For human beings this system of antigens has been called the HLA (human leukocyte antigen) system, so that the differences in regard to these antigens are the main factors that bring about rejection of any tissue transplanted from one human being to another. There are other genes that sponsor histocompatibility antigens apart from those of the strong HLA type. Some of these may be of considerable importance in producing rejection, but this is not yet known.

However, it is apparent that there will be many similarities between the immunology of blood grouping for transfusion and tissue typing for transplantation. It now appears that a number of transplantation antigens, perhaps as many as 12 or 15, will emerge as being of such potential importance that a transplant from a donor individual bearing any of these antigens to a healthy recipient lacking such an antigen may predictably produce a vigorous immunologic response. The avoidance of strong reactions of this type has accordingly become an important feature of clinical transplantation surgery, and knowledge of the antigens and their genetic transmission is an actively growing field.

The antigens concerned in allograft immunity have been located as residing wholly, or at least principally, on the cell membrane. Work is rapidly proceeding toward purification of these antigens from subcellular fractions and more information concerning their chemical constitutions will soon be forthcoming. At present it seems likely that at least some of the antigenic specificities of transplantation can be carried on molecules composed entirely of peptide moieties with no carbohydrate or lipid constituents (Kahan and Reisfield, 1967), although this will require confirmation.

TISSUE TYPING

As mentioned above, the identification of transplantation antigens for purposes of histocompatibility testing for transplant donor selection is of considerable practical importance (see results below). Several methods of assessing the degree of incompatibility between a recipient and a potential donor are available. Of these, three have been the most widely used.

The Normal Lymphocyte Transfer Test (NLT). This biological test yields a semiquantitative estimate of the sum of histocompatibility antigens present in the donor and absent from the recipient. The test is performed by injecting 5 million living peripheral blood lymphocytes from the intended recipient intradermally into the skin of each potential donor (Gray and Russell, 1965). As immunologically competent cells, capable of mounting a reaction against foreign antigens, these cells produce a reaction against foreign histocompatibility antigens in the skin of the potential donor. This can be read as an elevated, erythematous spot, similar to a tuberculin reaction, at about 48 hours. The potential donor whose tissues provoke the least reaction by recipient cells is preferred. The advantage of this test is that it depends upon an allograft reaction of a certain kind that can be directly observed without sensitizing the potential recipient. It does not allow actual identification of individual donor antigens, however, and is difficult to quantify accurately.

The Mixed Lymphocyte Culture Test (MLC). Lymphocytes of peripheral blood origin have been shown to react against certain antigens in tissue culture by undergoing transformation, in a few hours or days, to large blast forms. Frequent mitoses also can be observed. When cells of two patients are mixed in culture, the magnitude of their reaction to one another represents approximately the measure of the summation of histocompatibility antigens that each population of cells recognized in the other. By inhibiting blast cell transformation in the cells derived from the potential donor by certain cytotoxic agents, notably Mitomycin C, it has been possible to approach a "one way" MLC. Although difficult to quantify exactly, and lacking in information regarding the actual identity of the antigens recognized, this procedure remains of practical value as a cross-matching test.

Leukocyte Typing. As mentioned above, immunologic responses to foreign cells may include the production of humoral antibodies that are directed against the same specificities as the leukocytes comprising the cellular response. Such antibodies can be found most conveniently in some patients who have received multiple blood transfusions or in women who have had multiple pregnancies. The presence of an antibody in serum can be detected by several methods. Most commonly leukocytes are used as target cells, since they are readily available nucleated cells bearing a wide representation, perhaps all, of the histocompatibility antigens present on all cells of their donor. Sera derived in this way are virtually always directed against several antigens at once (polyspecific). This has helped to make the task of identifying all the transplantation antigens, and determining the strength of each in eliciting rejection, a lengthy and complicated one. Nevertheless, this work is now proceeding very rapidly. Tissue typing by the use of multiple serologic reagents is now regularly done in clinical transplantation, and useful information in regard to the magnitude of the rejection reaction to be anticipated can be gained in this way. The number of truly important strong histocompatibility antigens in the human population is being determined and their prevalence, or gene frequency, is being established. Much will depend upon these facts when a suitable donor organ is being selected for a given recipient in the future. It can be predicted that it will be relatively easy to find a suitable donor for some patients and much more difficult for others. Much more progress can be anticipated in this rapidly advancing field, which will be of direct relevance to clinical transplantation.

IMMUNOSUPPRESSION

The full immunologic response of a host to living foreign cells depends not only upon the receipt of antigenic stimuli through complex afferent pathways but also upon the existence of a normal population of lymphoid cells in a suitable state of readiness. Therefore many factors can influence the strength and the tempo of this response, some in a completely nonspecific way and some specifically. So far only nonspecific approaches to immunosuppression have been used in clinical transplantation.

The following is a list, doubtless incomplete, of major factors that influence the vigor of the rejection reaction:

Degree of genetic disparity
Prior sensitization
Tissue differences in antigenicity
Recipient site (anterior chamber of eye and interior of brain are examples of "privileged" recipient sites)
Immunologic enhancement
Lymphatic depression
    ablation of lymphoid tissue
    thoracic duct drainage
    whole body irradiation
    extracorporeal irradiation of the blood or lymph
Antilymphocyte serum
Acquired immunologic tolerance
Certain disease states (e.g., uremia, agammaglobulinemia)

A full discussion of each of these factors is beyond the scope of this chapter; the reader is referred to Russell and Monaco (1965) for further information. Whole body irradiation was used as an immunosuppressive treatment in clinical transplantation in the 1950's but was gradually abandoned because of its considerable dangers, even at subiethal doses, to tissues other than the lymphoid structures of the body. At about this time several chemical agents were discovered to have immunosuppressive effects. These drugs were borrowed from cancer chemotherapy, in which 6-mercaptopurine, cyclophosphamide, and others were found to have antitumor effects. The most widely used chemical immunosuppressive of this type has been an imidazole derivative of 6-mercaptopurine—azathioprine, or "Imuran." Given in doses of about 1.5 to 2.0 mg. per kilogram of body weight this drug can usually be tolerated for long periods of time with little or no depression of the peripheral white blood cell count or visible change in the lymph nodes or bone marrow. Administration of this drug is usually begun by the oral route immediately before transplantation and is continued indefinitely.

The mechanism of action of the purine analogs in producing immunosuppression is not clearly understood. It may be expected that, by interfering with DNA replication they can discourage cell division, a fundamental part of the response of lymphoid cells to antigenic stimuli. Indeed, there is some evidence that it is solely by this mechanism that immunosuppression is procured (Brent and Meadawar, 1967).

The other mainstay of current immunosuppressive treatment for clinical transplantation is cortisone or one of its derivatives. Most commonly used in prednisone. The steroids have marked anti-inflammatory effects and are particularly useful in reversing early, acute rejection reactions. Prednisone treatment is often begun at the time of transplantation or at the first clinical sign of rejection. Doses range from about 1 mg. per kilogram to much higher levels for short periods of time, and many patients bearing successful transplants are maintained on about 10 mg. of prednisone per day for extended periods.

The success of immunosuppressive therapy of this type has been truly remarkable, and many patients are able to live full lives while continuing to receive daily doses of these drugs. Nevertheless, the complications of their use, particularly in the early weeks postoperatively, have also been considerable, and in many instances even maximal doses are insufficient to overcome the advancing rejection reaction.

Newer approaches to immunosuppression are being constantly sought. Depletion of recipient lymphoid cells by thoracic duct drainage apparently has some immunosuppressive effect (Tilney and Murray, 1968) as does extracorporeal irradiation of the blood or lymph passed through a tube in a circuit through a radiation field. One of the newest approaches, not fully studied, is the use of *antilymphocyte sera* (ALS). These sera are prepared by injecting lymphoid cells from lymph nodes, thymus, spleen, peripheral blood, or lymph into a foreign species. For example, human lymph node cells are injected repeatedly into a horse. The horse develops strong antibodies in the gamma globulin fraction of its serum against the many antigens by which the species differ. High titers of antibody can be detected in the horse serum against lymphocytes from any human being by several different tests. Hemagglutinins and hemolysins against erythrocytes can also be detected, usually in high titer.

In extensive animal experiments sera of this type have been shown to have strong immunosuppressive effects allowing greatly prolonged survival of foreign transplants, particularly from allogeneic sources, but also considerable extension of survival of xenografts. The immunosuppressive capacity of these sera is largely preserved after the hemolysins are removed by adsorption with red blood cells, and the serum can be purified to some degree by separating out its gamma globulin fraction for clinical use (called by some ALG). Although the evidence currently available in regard to these sera is hopeful, much remains to be learned about them. Their mechanism of action is not well understood. Transient lymphopenia usually occurs with ALS treatment but may not be sustained in spite of continuing immunosuppression. The polymorphonuclear cell count usually remains stable or somewhat elevated. The fact that serum treatment seems to be more effective against cell-mediated immune reactions than against humoral ones opens hopeful possibilities, since much of the body's defense against bacterial invasion is by humoral antibody production.

Much remains to be done in improving the

immunosuppressive treatment that makes transplantation surgery possible.

DONOR ORGAN AVAILABILITY

When an identical twin donor is available for kidney transplantation, the biologic reasons for removing an organ from a living donor are, of course, very strong. The first long-term successes in kidney transplantation were achieved with identical twin donors, and the relative safety of a healthy young individual's sacrificing a kidney has been demonstrated. In regard to allogeneic donors also, a preference for family donors, especially when selected by histocompatibility tests, exists from the biologic point of view. Furthermore, organs from living donors can be made available at a time of election when the recipient is in optimal condition and the organ is in the best possible physiologic state. Diseases in the donor that might be transmissible to the recipient can be detected with greatest assurance in living donors. Nevertheless, the drawbacks to removing a healthy organ from a normal individual, even under the best of circumstances, are considerable. Moreover, many recipients in great need of healthy organ transplants have no potential family donors at all, and no possibility of any other than cadaver donors exists for allografts of unpaired organs. Thus, if human organs are to be used, it is imperative that they be derived from cadavers in many cases. The desirability of using cadaver organs is also great from the humanitarian point of view, but in practice there are drawbacks: the organizational arrangements for collecting organs from recently deceased donors, often in obscure locations, rarely exist; our ability to preserve such organs in a physiologically suitable state is still very rudimentary; and the awareness of people generally of the need for organ transplants and the legal machinery for making organ gifts by the potential donor during life leave much to be desired. The relationship between the number of potential donors in the population versus the number of possible recipients differs for each organ. If all the kidneys with single renal arteries (about 70 to 80 per cent) and suitable otherwise as donor organs were actually available for transplantation, current estimates are that there would probably be enough to meet the needs of the 7,000 to 9,000 patients dying of renal failure in our country each year. For patients who might receive heart transplants the number of donor hearts would, however, probably be far from sufficient. The necessity for selecting compatible donor organs complicates this picture further, since it is much more difficult to find sufficiently compatible organs for some recipients than for others.

Although progress is being made in developing improved methods of organ preservation, at present it is possible to maintain a kidney for only little more than 24 hours in an acceptable state of viability for transplantation by the most elaborate methods of perfusion with oxygenated fluid in an atmosphere of oxygen under increased pressure. Lesser periods of preservation have so far been achieved with other organs such as hearts, lungs, and livers. Only the skin is arranged architecturally in a manner that allows reliable long-term preservation in the frozen state. Agents such as glycerol and dimethyl sulfoxide, which diffuse into cells and depress the freezing point of cytoplasm, prevent the damaging effects of freezing. It has not yet been possible to arrange conditions in a manner that will permit these agents to reach the cells of vascularized parenchymatous organs, to exert their beneficial effect, and then be removed evenly from the preserved tissue successfully. Only in the case of skin, or with small bits of tissue that can be transplanted by implantation, has long-term preservation been achieved. There is great need for progress in these technics in order to make as many organs as possible available for transplantation under elective circumstances. At present the number of possible recipients far outstrips the number of readily available donors for most organs.

CLINICAL TRANSPLANTATION

Experience with transplantation of the kidney has been much more extensive than with any other organ. The requirements of the operation itself are fairly straightforward; living donors can be used in some instances, and, most important of all, patients with frankly terminal kidney failure can be maintained for extended periods by a careful program of medical management including the use of dialysis in some form.

In some clinical conditions involving a number of major organs and tissues the replacement of a single organ would retrieve an otherwise healthy individual to a vigorous state. For the present, transplantation treatment is hazardous enough so that only patients in a near terminal phase of their disease process have been selected. It has also been important to select patients in whom disease either is confined to a single organ or will be reversed when a given organ is replaced.

It may be wise to relax these restrictions to some degree in the future, should the safety and success of transplantation become more nearly assured.

KIDNEY TRANSPLANTATION

Kidney transplantation is usually performed for end stage glomerulonephritis or pyelonephritis. Concern is raised in regard to this procedure in patients with glomerulonephritis if the patient has only a brief history or if there are other reasons to believe that the process is "active." This is because there is now some evidence that the disease process can be visited upon the new kidney if it is in an active stage. Another important contraindication to transplantation is any evidence of infection in the intended recipient. Of those patients who die following transplantation, a high percentage show evidence of active infection, often in the lungs. Thus every effort is made to eliminate infection before the institution of immunosuppressive treatment which is begun at about the time of operation.

The criteria to be met and the tests usually indicated in selecting a living donor are as follows:

1. Freedom from any significant disease
2. Kidney function completely normal
   a. Creatinine clearance ⎫
   b. Urine culture   ⎬ 3 times
   c. Urinalysis   ⎭
3. Intravenous pyelogram
4. Histocompatibility and major erythrocyte blood groups
5. Emotional status and fully informed consent
6. Renal angiogram

If a living donor is to be used, adjoining operating rooms are prepared and the donor nephrectomy is carried out through a standard flank incision. The left kidney is preferred because its vessels are somewhat longer and the configuration of the right iliac vessels is such that convenient anastomosis can be made with them through a retroperitoneal incision (see Fig. 19-1). The right kidney can also be placed into the left iliac fossa and ureteral drainage established either by implanting the donor ureter into the recipient bladder by ureteroneocystostomy or by anastomosis of the donor renal pelvis directly with the recipient ureter. Bilateral nephrectomy can often be accomplished at the same operation. It is desirable to remove the patient's severely diseased kidneys if they may become a source of infection, and also as an aid to early postoperative management. It is then certain that any urine produced will be attributable to the transplanted kidney.

Prompt beginning of function of the transplant can be expected when a living donor is used and no undue delay is met in re-establishing blood supply to the organ in the recipient. When the normothermic ischemia time exceeds about 90 minutes, rapidly advancing effects of metabolic denial are to be anticipated in the form of acute tubular necrosis. For this reason some surgeons promptly perfuse donor kidneys with a cooled balanced salt solution of some kind, often containing heparin. With this protective cooling, the ischemia time can be prolonged considerably without irreversible damage to the kidney. Early urine output is often impressive in amount, sometimes reaching well over one liter per hour. Fluid management of these patients, sometimes with severe secondary effects of uremia such as pericarditis with effusion, can be a challenge. Unless the recipient has undergone previous sensitization with some of the histocompatibility antigens present in the transplant, for example by blood transfusions, there should be no evidence of rejection for at least 3 to 5 days. Sometimes rejection activity is much delayed in the presence of immunosuppressive treatment, and in occasional cases it may not be clinically apparent at all. Signs of rejection of a kidney transplant are as given in Table 19-2.

When rejection does become manifest, it may be reversible by increasing immunosuppressive treatment (as in the case illustrated

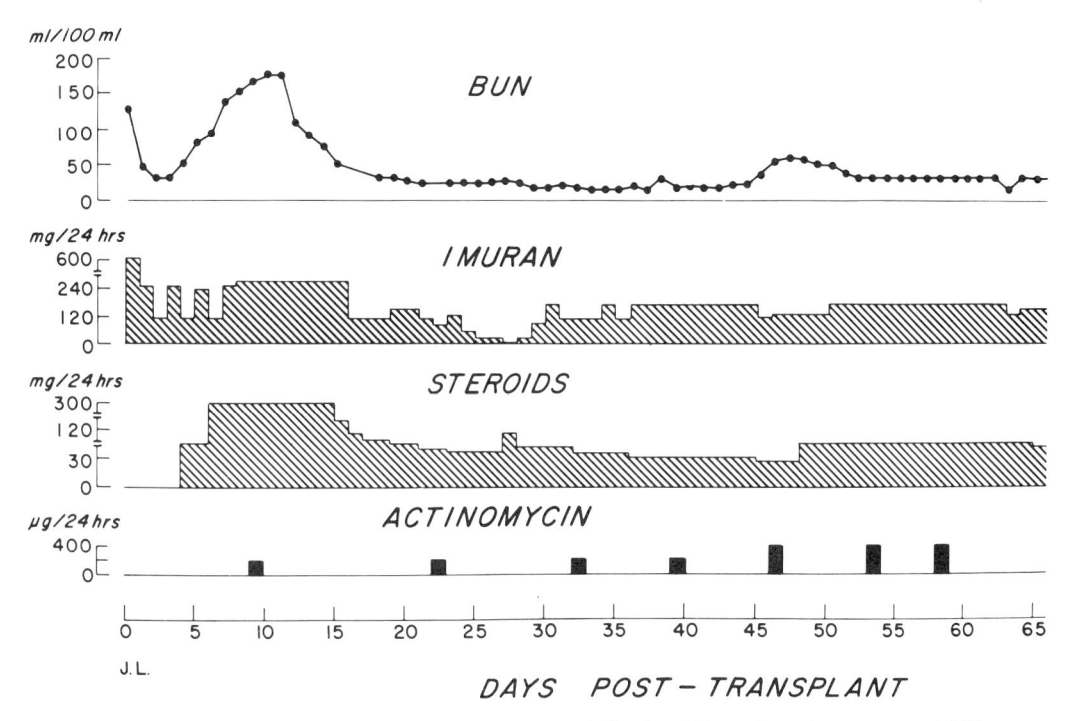

FIG. 19-6. Early postoperative course of a patient following bilateral nephrectomy and kidney transplantation from a living, related donor. A severe, early rejection reaction was observed beginning at 3 to 4 days postoperatively. This was promptly controlled by increased immunosuppressive treatment including both prednisone and Actinomycin C. A later, and much less violent rejection reaction, was seen at 45 days.

TABLE 19-2. SIGNS OF EARLY KIDNEY TRANSPLANT REJECTION

1. Fever
2. Tenderness of transplant
3. Swelling of transplant
4. Cellular casts in urine
5. Decreased renal blood flow
6. Decreased renal function
   a. Reduced urine volume
   b. Rising blood urea nitrogen and serum creatinine
   c. Reduced creatinine clearance
   d. Reduced urine sodium concentration
7. Depressed serum complement

in Fig. 19-6) or it may progress, ending in complete cessation of function of the transplant. Although it is not infrequently possible to remove the rejected transplant and support the patient on hemodialysis pending another transplant, the danger of infection during such a period is high. In addition to the commonly encountered pathogens, unusual organisms may be dangerous to patients receiving high doses of immunosuppressive treatment such as monilia, *Pneumocystis carinii*, cytomegalovirus and others.

The use of cadaver kidneys has been rapidly increasing although the success rate with organs from this source remains appreciably lower than that expected from related living donors. Less is usually known about cadaver donors concerning potentially transmissible disease, including hidden neoplasms, so that some clinics have arranged for rapid autopsy examination, including frozen sections of the major organs, while the donor organ is being harvested and cooled. As mentioned above, the capability of maintaining a kidney in a condition satisfactory for transplantation, once it is deprived of a normal circulation, is very limited. Frequently there is a period of poor perfusion before death is pronounced dur-

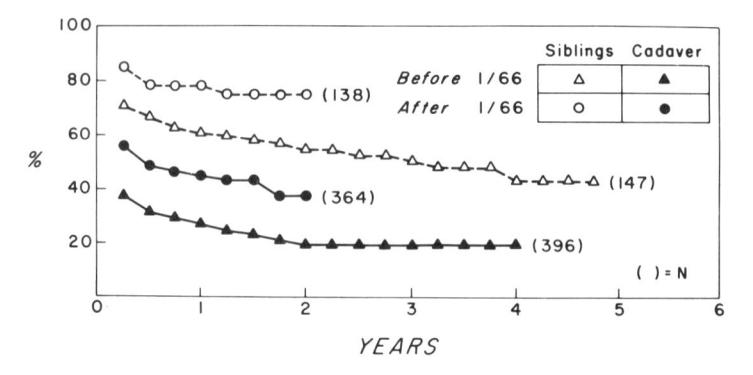

FIG. 19-7. Survival curves of transplanted kidneys in the total world experience. About half of the 2,000 transplants so far recorded were performed before January 1966 and about half since. The upper pair of curves show the improvement in survival of the recently performed transplants where living sibling donors are concerned. The lower pair of curves shows this for cadaver donors. Unrelated, and therefore less compatible, donors can be expected to involve a poorer prognosis in general than family donors.

ing which considerable damage may be done as well. Often the organ is obtained in an unknown state so that with present methods only a clinical trial reveals its potential. In the world experience about one fifth of the cadaver kidneys transplanted have never functioned in their recipients for one technical reason or another.

The most recent summary of world experience with kidney transplant survival (about 2,000 patients) from all clinics is summarized in Figure 19-7. There seems to be a distinct tendency for the patient's condition to stabilize after the first few months. Acute rejection episodes become much less common although gradual deterioration of kidney function, even to complete cessation, must be looked for. Some patients may survive for long periods of time with reduced renal function, often accompanied by hypertension of renal origin. Others remain in a state of virtually normal health except for the necessity of continuing immunosuppressive medication and of taking reasonable precautions to avoid infections.

Several attempts to treat patients in need of kidney transplants with xenografts derived from chimpanzees or baboons have been made (Reemtsma et al., 1964). Brief periods of metabolic assistance to the patient were achieved before the more violent rejection reaction, normally associated with greater genetic disparity, brought about the death of the transplants in spite of heavy immunosuppression. One young woman survived for several months after receiving both kidneys from a chimpanzee, and there was evidence that the transplants functioned for this period. This single case is of considerable interest and should not be forgotten, although the reasons for relative success in this one instance remain obscure.

OTHER ORGANS

Transplantation of the liver, lung, heart, pancreas, and skin are now being explored as possible useful forms of treatment where replacement is the only hope for the patient. Already survival of recipients for a number of months has been achieved with hearts and livers. The frequency of this outcome in a significant number of patients cannot yet be stated, although the experience with long-term survival following cadaver kidney transplantation can probably be taken as a guide.

As experience grows, transplantation of each of these organs will present its own set of problems and challenges. At present it is beyond the scope of this chapter to detail the situation with each organ as it now stands, since it must be considered to be in a frankly experimental phase.

TRANSPLANTATION IN THE FUTURE

All indications now are that the transplantation of at least certain tissues and organs will take its place as a valuable form of treatment and an important part of the armamentarium of the surgeon. Transplantation of the kidney should already be considered recognized as an impressively successful treatment under properly selected circumstances. Present developments make it seem likely that transplantation of the heart, liver, skin, and possibly certain other organs, will also earn a similar place in due course. The difficulties which have already been encountered with regard to organ availability and supply may serve as a continuing stimulus to progress in controlling rejection of transplants between species, since xenografts of some organs may be acceptable on all but immunologic, and perhaps emotional, grounds.

REFERENCES

Austen, K. F., and Russell, P. S.: Detection of renal allograft rejection in man by demonstration of a reduction in the serum concentration of the second component of complement. Ann. N. Y. Acad. Sci., 129:657, 1966.

Brent, L., and Medawar, P. B.: Cellular immunity and the homograft reaction. Brit. Med. Bull., 23:55, 1967.

Corry, R. J., Chavez-Peon, F., Miyakuni, T., and Malt, R. A.: Auxiliary partial liver transplantation in the dog. Arch. Surg., 98:799, 1969.

Gorer, P. S.: Role of antibodies in immunity to transplanted leukaemia in mice. J. Path. Bact., 54:51, 1942.

Gray, J. G., and Russell, P. S.: The lymphocyte transfer test in man. In: Histocompatibility Testing. Publication No. 1229:105. National Academy of Sciences—National Research Council, Washington, D. C., 1965.

Kahan, B. D., and Reisfeld, R. A.: Electrophoretic purification of a water soluble guinea pig transplantation antigen. Proc. Nat. Acad. Sci., 58:1430, 1967.

Kuss, R., Teinturier, J., and Milliez, P.: Quelques essais de greffes du rein chez l'homme. Mem. Acad. chir., 77:755, 1951.

Medawar, P. B.: Behavior and fate of skin autografts and skin homografts in rabbits. J. Anat., 78:176, 1944.

Russell, P. S., and Monaco, A. P.: The Biology of Tissue Transplantation. Boston, Little, Brown & Co., 1965.

Reemtsma, K., et al.: Reversal of early graft rejection after renal heterotransplantation in man. J.A.M.A., 187:691, 1964.

Strober, S., and Gowans, J. L.: The role of lymphocytes in the sensitization of rats to renal homografts. J. Exp. Med., 122:347, 1965.

Tilney, N. L., and Murray, J. E.: Chronic thoracic duct fistula: operative technic and physiologic effects in man. Ann. Surg., 167:1, 1968.

CHAPTER 20

OSCAR P. HAMPTON, JR., M.D., AND WILLIAM T. FITTS, JR., M.D.

Fractures and Dislocations: General Considerations

Fracture Maxims
Definitions
Healing of Fractures
Diagnosis of a Fracture
Priority of Injury
Complications of Fractures
Objectives of Management of Fractures
Emergency Splinting of Fractures
Methods of Management of Fractures
Open Fractures
Fractures in Children
Pathologic Fractures
Plaster of Paris
Rehabilitation

FRACTURE MAXIMS

1. The saving of life comes first: treat impending asphyxia, hemorrhage, shock and other life-endangering conditions before treating a fracture.
2. Examine the injured part for signs of vascular and nerve injuries before searching for a fracture.
3. To minimize soft tissue damage and to avoid converting a closed to an open fracture, "splint 'em where they lie."
4. Obtain roentgenograms in at least 2 planes and examine them yourself. In fractures of long bones, be certain the entire bone is visualized.
5. Open fractures are contaminated wounds. Minimize the risk of infection by adequate débridement, open drainage or closure of the wound as indicated, and immobilization.
6. One measures the end-result of treatment of a fracture by the function of the part.
7. The chief aim in the treatment of a fracture of the upper extremity is to ensure the proper functioning of the hand. Shortening and some malalignment are often acceptable.
8. The chief aim in the treatment of a fracture of the lower extremity is to ensure painless, stable weight-bearing. Malalignment must be prevented, and full length is desirable.
9. Fractures involving joints require a perfect ("cabinet-maker's") reduction to minimize future arthritis.
10. To immobilize a fracture, both the joint above and the joint below it usually must be immobilized.
11. Immediately activate all joints that are not immobilized for treatment of the fracture.
12. Throughout the treatment of a fracture, focus attention on the patient as a whole as well as on the injured part.

DEFINITIONS

A fracture is a break in the continuity of a bone. If it involves the entire cross section of the bone, it is a complete fracture; if it involves only a portion of the cross section, it is an incomplete fracture. Every fracture, therefore, is either complete or incomplete.

Every fracture is either *open** or *closed*. In an *open* fracture the wound of the fracture extends through skin or mucous membrane. Without such a wound the fracture is *closed*, i.e., does not communicate with the outside air.

Transverse, oblique and spiral are terms used to describe the direction of the line of fracture in relation to the long axis of the broken bone (Fig. 20-1).

A comminuted fracture has 2 or more communicating lines of fracture which divide the bone into more than 2 fragments.

A double fracture is present when a bone is broken at 2 levels without communicating lines of fracture. If both fractures are complete, the fracture is also a *segmental fracture*, the middle fragment being a separate segment of bone.

* The terms *compound* and *simple* have been used to indicate *open* and *closed*, respectively, until recent years.

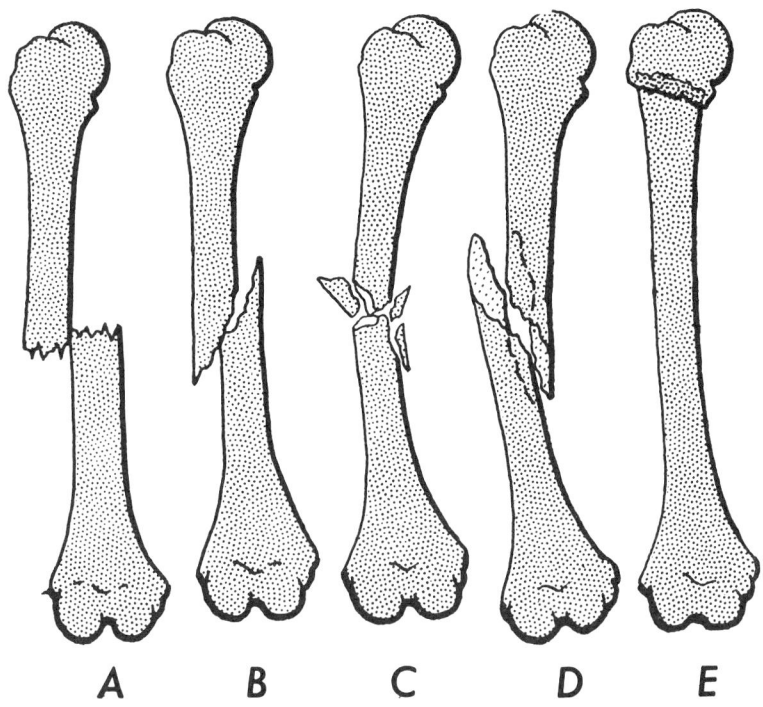

Fig. 20-1. Types of fracture, right humerus in the anteroposterior projection. (A) Transverse fracture of midshaft with medial displacement of the distal fragment. (The fragments are in poor apposition but good alignment.) (B) Oblique fracture with overriding. (The fragments are in partial apposition but good alignment.) (C) Comminuted fracture with lateral angulation (apposition is not unsatisfactory). (D) Spiral fracture with lateral angulation (both apposition and alignment are poor). (E) Impacted fracture of the neck in good apposition and alignment.

An impacted fracture is present when one fragment is driven firmly into the other. In an *impacted* fracture the fragments are usually stable.

A greenstick fracture is a form of incomplete fracture, commonly seen in the forearm of children, in which one side of the cortex breaks and the other bends as a branch of a green tree will bend.

A sprain or avulsion fracture is one in which a small piece of cortex is pulled away at the attachment of a ligament.

A depressed fracture, seen frequently in fractures of the skull and the facial bones, is one in which a fragment or fragments are in-driven.

A compression fracture is one in which the fractured bone has been compressed by another bone or bones. *Compression fractures* are seen frequently in vertebral fractures (see Fig. 23-2, p. 565).

A gunshot fracture is one produced by a bullet or other missile. For practical purposes it is always an open fracture.

A pathologic fracture occurs through an area of diseased bone such as a bone cyst or an osseous metastasis, usually as a result of minimal trauma.

March (or fatigue) fracture results presumably from lack of normal muscle protection. It may occur in soldiers who have participated in long marches, especially when the troops are poorly conditioned. It may also occur during pregnancy. The 2nd and the 3rd metatarsal bones are the most common sites of march fractures.

An epiphyseal separation is a displacement of an epiphysis and signifies an injury along the epiphyseal plate.

Dislocation signifies that a bone is "out of joint," that is, no longer in normal contact with the bone with which it articulates. Subluxation or partial dislocation is used to denote partial contact.

Nonunion of a fracture signifies that the process of healing has ended without producing bony union.

Delayed union signifies that a specific fracture has not healed in the time considered as being average for this fracture. The average time for healing of a fracture depends on many variables, and delayed union must never be considered non-union until the healing process has ceased without bony bridging.

Malunion signifies that the fracture has united with deformity sufficient to cause impairment of function or a significant cosmetic defect.

Location. In locating a fracture in the shaft of long bones, it is usually described as being in the proximal, the middle or the lower third, or at the junction of 2 of these divisions.

A fracture of one of the bony prominences of the ends of long bones is described as a fracture of that prominence by name; for example, a fracture of the olecranon, a fracture of the medial malleolus, or a fracture of the lateral condyle of the femur.

Apposition and Alignment. In describing the positions of the fragments, the terms apposition and alignment are used (Fig. 20-1). Fragments are in apposition when their ends are in contact. They are in alignment when their long axes parallel each other. Fragments may be in perfect apposition but angulated and therefore in bad alignment. They may be out of apposition but in good alignment if there is no angulation. In describing angulation, the direction of the point made by the fragments is given; for example, when fragments of the tibia and the fibula are angulated outward as in "bowlegs," they are in lateral angulation. The angulation of fragments may be lateral, medial, anterior or posterior. In describing a fracture one gives the position of the distal fragment in relation to the proximal fragment. For example, in a displaced fracture of the femoral shaft, the description might read: "There is a transverse fracture of the shaft of the femur at the junction of the middle and the lower thirds with posterior and medial displacement." This means that the *distal* fragment is posterior and medial to the *proximal* fragment.

HEALING OF FRACTURES

The healing of fractures is primarily a local phenomenon. A good blood supply to the fragments, adequate apposition of bone surfaces and adequate immobilization are the most important prerequisites for healing. Local circulatory impairment, inadequate apposition of fragments, inadequate immobilization of fragments, interposition of material between the bone ends, extensive tissue necrosis, and infection have been shown to have a profoundly adverse effect on healing. The most common sites of delayed union and nonunion—the neck of the femur, the lower shaft of the tibia and the carpal scaphoid—all have a precarious blood supply.

On the other hand, vitamin deficiencies (excepting scurvy), hypoproteinemia, osseous disease, debility and even a restricted calcium intake rarely cause an alteration in the sequence of healing of fractures, although senility and starvation may somewhat retard the rate of union. There really are no systemic causes of nonunion.

In general the healing of a wound of bone, a fracture, follows the same principles as the healing of wounds of other tissues. When a bone is broken, blood from ruptured medullary, periosteal and adjacent soft tissue blood vessels extravasates and clots so that a hematoma is formed about the fracture site. With the ingrowth of capillaries and the action of fibroblasts, the hematoma becomes organized into granulation tissue. This process is really the first stage of healing of a wound of any tissue.

In a wound of tissues other than bone (or cartilage) the fibroblastic action in the granulation tissue would continue to form mature fibrous scar. However, in a fracture, either because of the presence of bone ends in the granulation tissue or the specific action of osteoblasts upon it, the healing processes vary so that callus and eventually bone are formed to unite the fracture. Fibrous condensation of the granulation tissue takes place and then, apparently by metaplasia, areas of fibrocartilage and hyaline cartilage form in the young fibrous tissue. This seals the fragment ends together.

As the organization of the callus proceeds, the first new bone formation is seen subperiosteally at some distance from the fracture. The new bone spicules are bordered by large osteoblasts, presumably derived from the inner layer of the periosteum. This new bone forms a collar around each of the fractured segments and develops toward the fracture gap. At the same time, endosteal bone formation develops from the cells bordering the inner cortices and forms an inner core of new bone partly filling the medullary cavity and growing toward the fracture. The central area of cartilage tissue is replaced by bone as the advancing front of new bone reaches it. This latter process is similar to the endochondral ossification seen in normal growth.

The enveloping periosteal callus is usually more abundant in displaced fractures, where it acts as a scaffolding, uniting the separated fragments. The original callus is formed of rough, heavy-fibered, immature bone which is gradually replaced by more mature compact bone as the bulbous callus recedes and the new cortex and marrow cavity are formed. Fractures through bone that is primarily cancellous and flat, rather than cortical and tubular, usually show a more predominant endosteal phase with little subperiosteal new bone formation.

The exact process by which healing of a fracture is regulated is not known. Two theories have been widely advocated. These are the cellular theory (osteoblastic) and the humoral theory (physicochemical). The cellular theory holds that the osteoblast is a highly differentiated cell which has the specific function of forming bone either by actually secreting osseomucin and calcium or by secreting substances which precipitate bone-forming materials from the intercellular fluid. Experiments by Trueta suggest that the bone-forming cell, the osteoblast, comes from a vascular cell. The humoral or physicochemical theory assigns the principal responsibility for the formation of bone to the tissue fluids and not to osteoblasts.

In the present state of knowledge these theories do not influence the treatment of a fracture. Treatment is based on full recognition of the advantages of prompt, adequate and persisting reduction of the fracture so that healing processes may take place. The hematoma must become organized as the first step in the healing of a fracture. When a fracture is reduced within a few hours of injury before organization of the hematoma has begun, the healing process for the fracture has been given a good start. On the other hand, when reduction has been delayed, the manipulation of the fragment ends disrupts the healing process and, in theory, retards it. Certainly, repeated manipulations and inadequate immobilization of the fracture site may cause fresh bleeding, the formation of new granulation tissue and delayed healing. Healthy callus may never form, and the fracture may go to nonunion.

An optimum compression force across a fracture (contact-compression) appears to accelerate healing. Eggers, in experimental fractures of rats' skulls, noted an increased rate of healing when these fractures were subjected to compression forces. Whether the increased rate of healing was due to a stimulation of osteogenesis by the compression forces or was merely the result of close contact and rigid immobilization is not established. Friedenberg and French, in experiments on dogs, showed that excessive compression of fragment ends produced necrosis but that the pressure that is optimal for fracture healing is probably higher than that provided by the tone of muscles surrounding the fragments.

DIAGNOSIS OF A FRACTURE

The diagnosis of a fracture is made on symptoms reported by the patient and on physical signs and x-ray examination. Usually, but not always, a history of injury is obtained.

Symptoms

The characteristic symptoms of a fracture are (1) pain and (2) inability to use the part. Immediately following injury, a sensation of numbness may be present. After the initial numbness, pain becomes the outstanding symptom and continues with increasing severity until the fragments are immobilized. With most fractures, the patient usually is unable to use the associated part. However, with impacted or incomplete fractures, function may be impaired only slightly or not at all.

Signs

The following signs indicate a fracture: (1) localized tenderness; (2) localized swelling;

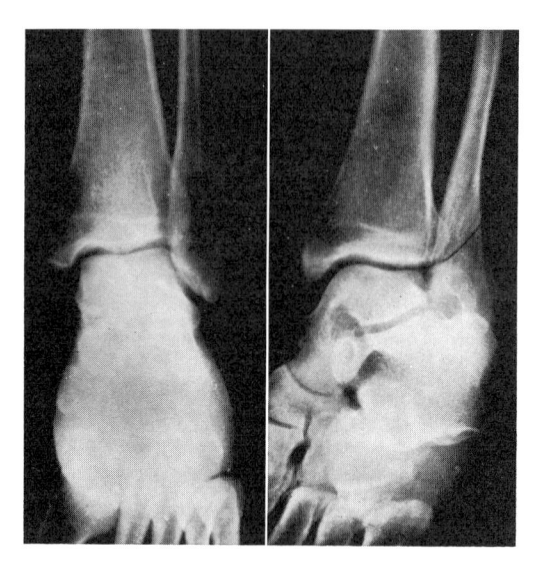

FIG. 20-2. Importance of special oblique roentgenograms in diagnosing injuries about the ankle. The standard anteroposterior view (*left*) and the standard lateral view disclosed no line of fracture. The oblique, or open mortise view (*right*) discloses an oblique fracture of the fibula.

(3) visible or palpable deformity; (4) ecchymosis; (5) protective muscle spasm; (6) false motion; (7) crepitation (audible or palpable grating of bony fragments). Obviously, the most convincing signs are motion of the bone fragments at the fracture site (false motion) and crepitation. They may be observed incidentally as the extremity is being examined, but testing for them is dangerous, as it may produce further tissue damage.

Every fracture is associated with some local soft tissue injury which may include injury to major blood vessels, peripheral nerves or tendons. The possibility of these immediate complications (see p. 455) of fracture demands that a careful and complete examination of the entire part be an integral segment of the same examination that is made to determine if a fracture is present.

As a routine in extremity injuries, the examiner must test for arterial pulsations distal to the injury (radial artery in the upper and the posterior tibial or dorsalis pedis artery in the lower extremity). Absence of the pulsation probably indicates interruption, partial or complete, of the arterial trunk of the extremity—a complication which takes precedence for treatment over the injury to the bone. If any doubt exists about the adequacy of the circulation, an arteriogram should be done to detect or rule out any arterial damage. Also as a routine, the examiner must test for the presence of nerve supply to the distal portion of the extremity. He must have the patient attempt to carry out movements of the fingers and the thumb or of the toes and test sensation of these parts. Loss of motor power in any muscle group or loss of sensation conforming to the known pattern of sensory nerve supply indicates injury to a major nerve trunk. Such a complication demands consideration as part of the entire injury and may modify the management of the fracture.

ROENTGEN EXAMINATION

The clinical diagnosis of a fracture usually must be confirmed by adequate x-ray examinations. In suspected fractures of the bones of the extremities and the spine, roentgenograms in both the anteroposterior and the lateral views must be made. Examination in 2 planes is essential, as a fracture may not be visualized in one view but may be obvious in the other (Fig. 20-2).

Roentgenograms of long bones always must include the joint above or below the injury and preferably the entire length of the bone in order that double fractures will not be overlooked.

However, routine roentgenograms in the 2 standard planes will not always visualize certain bone and joint injuries (Fig. 20-2). For example, a special oblique view is often required to demonstrate a fracture of the carpal navicular. In injuries of the cervical spine, the classic anteroposterior and lateral views may show no evidence of bone or joint injury, whereas a lateral view with the head in flexion may demonstrate a subluxation of a cervical vertebra. A special axial view is often needed to demonstrate a fracture of the patella or a fracture of the os calcis. Frequently, x-ray examination of the contralateral uninjured side for comparison is exceedingly valuable in establishing the correct diagnosis, especially in fractures about the joints in children.

The physician who is to treat the fracture

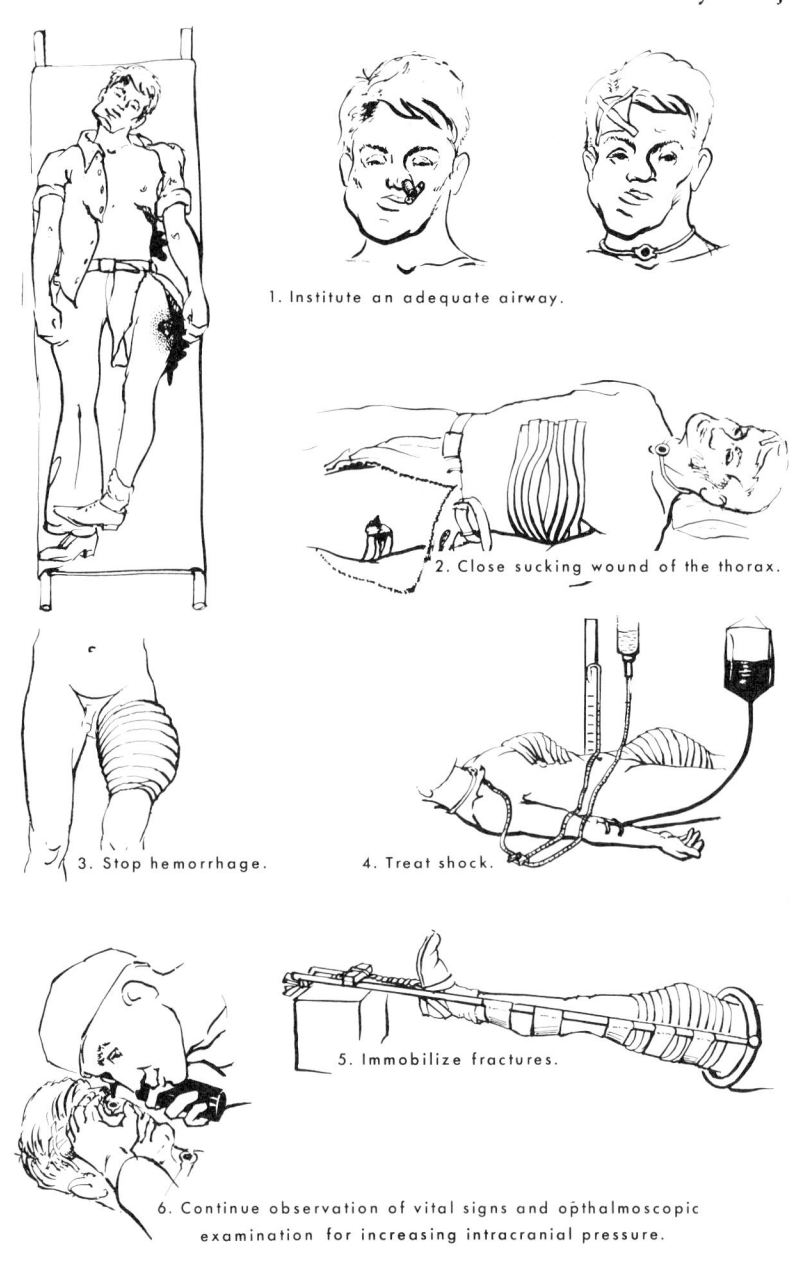

1. Institute an adequate airway.
2. Close sucking wound of the thorax.
3. Stop hemorrhage.
4. Treat shock.
5. Immobilize fractures.
6. Continue observation of vital signs and opthalmoscopic examination for increasing intracranial pressure.

Fig. 20-3. Emergency treatment of multiple injuries. Priority of injury. (See text.)

must know the views needed on x-ray examination to gain the maximum information about a fracture and *he must examine the films himself* to evaluate the problem before him. Good roentgenograms furnish information which is valuable in the selection of the method of management indicated for the fracture.

PRIORITY OF INJURY

Efforts to diagnose a fracture must not overshadow an accurate appraisal of the full effects of the injury on the patient and the injured part. These may be more important than the fracture itself. First attention always must be directed toward maintenance of an adequate airway and respiration, the control of hemorrhage and the treatment of shock, present or impending.

Consider a patient who has a cranial injury without signs and symptoms of increased intracranial pressure, a fracture of the mandible with some obstruction of the airway, an open sucking wound of the chest and an open fracture of the femur (Fig. 20-3). The patient has bled considerably and is in shock. Immediately an adequate airway is established, perhaps by an endotracheal tube or tracheostomy, and the open thoracic wound is closed by an occlusive dressing. During these procedures solutions of electrolytes and whole blood are being given intravenously as therapy for shock. A catheter is shown inserted through the subclavian vein to monitor the central venous pressure. Without signs and symptoms of increasing intracranial pressure, the head injury needs only close observation for changing neurologic signs. The open fracture of the femur receives a sterile compression dressing to the wound and adequate emergency splinting which, incidentally, is further therapy for shock. Definitive therapy and even roentgenographic visualization of the fracture of the femoral shaft must be postponed until the life-endangering injuries have been brought under control.

COMPLICATIONS OF FRACTURES

Complications of fractures may be divided conveniently into the immediate and the delayed. The immediate complications, such as hemorrhage and shock and intra-abdominal or intrathoracic injuries, may be life-endangering. The treatment of these complications takes precedence over treatment of the fracture.

IMMEDIATE COMPLICATIONS

Intra-abdominal. Fractures of the thoracic cage, the spine or the pelvis may be associated with intra-abdominal injuries. Blows to the upper abdomen which fracture the thoracic cage may rupture the spleen or the liver. Delayed splenic rupture always must be kept in mind. Fractures of the pelvis may be associated with injuries to the bladder, the urethra or the bowel (Fig. 20-4). Trauma to the pelvic region may cause only mild appearing fractures of the pelvis, yet a distended bladder may be ruptured or severe retroperitoneal bleeding may be unrecognized. Bloody urine or the inability of the patient to void immediately alerts the examiner to the possibility of severe injury to the urinary tract. Every patient with a pelvic fracture who cannot immediately void clear urine must be catheterized at once for diagnostic purposes, and

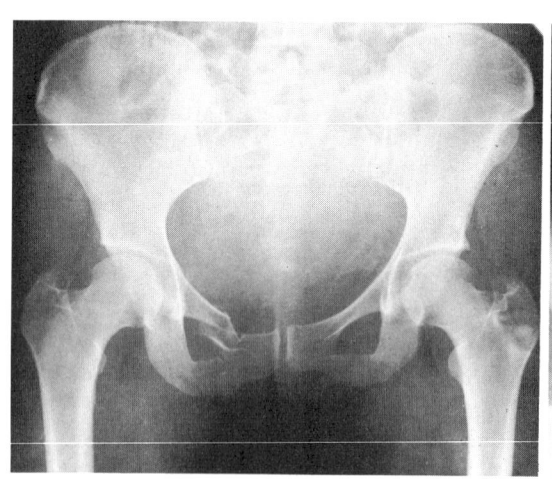

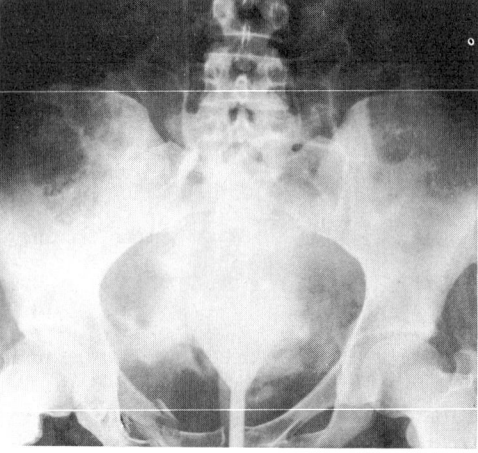

FIG. 20-4. Rupture of the bladder complicating a fracture of the pelvis with minimal displacement. (*Left*) Fractures of the pelvis with little or no displacement. (*Right*) Cystogram showing rupture of the bladder which is elevated, probably by hematoma.

usually the catheter should be left in place. Severe crushing injuries to the left side of the trunk may cause the following triad of injuries—rupture of the spleen, the left kidney and the left diaphragm. Evidence of injury to any of these organs suggests injury to the others. All of these intra-abdominal complications of fractures are life-endangering and demand first consideration.

Intrathoracic. Hemothorax or pneumothorax may result from damage to the pleura and lung by the sharp ends of broken ribs or sternum (Fig. 20-5). Severe crushing injuries may fracture multiple ribs, creating a flail segment which causes paradoxical breathing. The "flail" area of the chest wall moves in on inspiration and out on expiration and results in diminished intake of air. Traumatic rupture of the major bronchi also occasionally attends crushing thoracic injuries. All of these complications are life-endangering and take priority for treatment.

Hemorrhage and Shock. Hypovolemic or traumatic shock as a result of hemorrhage or hemorrhage plus loss of extracellular fluid into the traumatized soft tissues may accompany fractures of the extremities as well as those of the thorax, the pelvis and the spine. Loss of blood may stem from major vascular injury or merely from the broken bony fragments. It may be particularly severe in open fractures, but loss into the tissues in a closed fracture must not be underestimated. Fractures of the femoral shaft and the upper tibia are likely to result in considerable hemorrhage. The artery entering the tibia at the junction of the upper and the middle thirds is the largest nutrient artery in the body, and fractures at this level, particularly open fractures, can lead to dangerous hemorrhage. Hemorrhage and shock are life-endangering and demand immediate therapy.

Injury to Major Arteries. Any of the major arteries of the extremities may be injured or occluded by a nearby fracture (Fig. 20-6). In some instances, collateral circulation will be adequate to maintain viability of the extremity. In others, the symptoms and signs of arterial insufficiency to the distal portion of the extremity will be present. Occasionally, fractures of the femur are associated with damage to the femoral vessels; in fractures in the supracondylar area especially, popliteal vessels may be damaged by the sharp edge of the distal fragment which has been pulled posteriorly by the gastrocnemius muscle. Supracondylar fractures of the humerus, frequent in children, often cause arterial compression. Fractures and dislocations about the knee are also prone to arterial injuries.

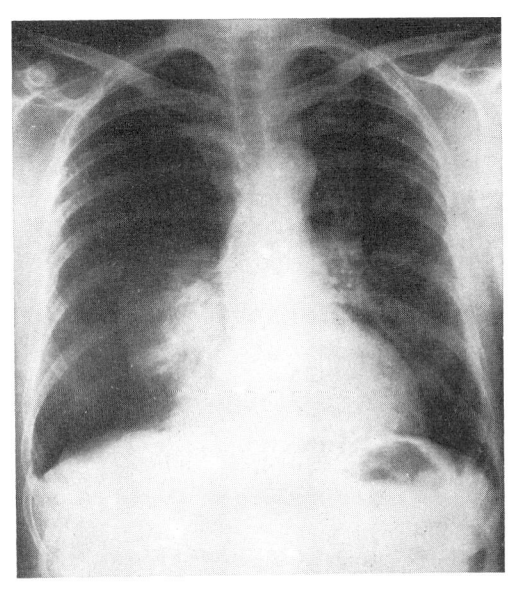

Fig. 20-5. Pneumothorax complicating fractures of the ribs. Anteroposterior roentgenograms of chest, showing complete collapse of the right lung with massive pneumothorax and slight shift of the mediastinum to the left with fractures of the ribs on the right. On admission to the hospital 16 hours before this roentgenogram was made, an admission roentgenogram showed the fractures of the ribs and only a very small pneumothorax. During the hours that followed, all of the clinical signs and symptoms of a tension pneumothorax developed. (Dr. Richard Yore)

If arterial insufficiency cannot be corrected promptly by closed manipulation, which could free an artery occluded by pressure of a displaced bone fragment, other measures must be taken immediately. An arteriogram may show the location and the nature of arterial damage. Compression by hematomas must be relieved by evacuation of blood clot and attainment of hemostasis. Arterial spasm is often diagnosed but is actually a rarity; if present, it should be treated by nerve block. A lacerated or divided artery must be repaired. An artery

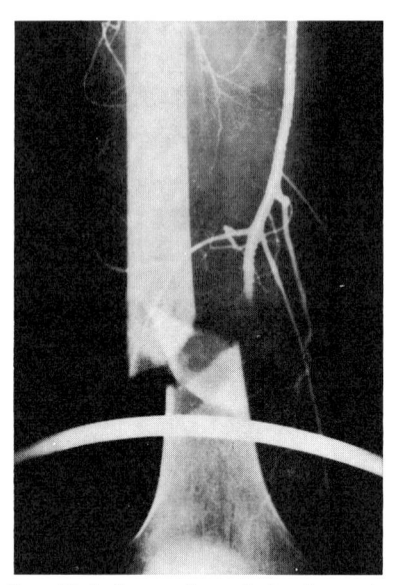

FIG. 20-6. Laceration of the femoral artery, complicating fracture of the shaft of the femur. An arteriogram demonstrates clearly the total interruption of the major arterial flow down the extremity at the level of the fracture of the femoral shaft. (Dr. James Stokes)

(Hampton, O. P., Jr.: Complications of common fractures. *In*: Harry, J. D., and Artz, C.: Complications in Surgery. Philadelphia, W. B. Saunders, 1960)

that is divided by a fracture can rarely be repaired successfully by end-to-end suture. A vascular graft is almost always necessary to repair arterial defects associated with fractures because of the extensive damage to the artery above and below the point of transection. End-to-end suture usually is attended by thrombosis if tension is used in bringing the ends together. In the extremities, venous autografts, homografts and prostheses have all been used. Venous autografts are probably the most satisfactory. When vascular repair is required, absolute fixation of the bone fragments often should be effected with an intramedullary nail, plate or screws.

Injury to Major Nerve Trunks. Fractures of the bones of the extremities may have associated major peripheral nerve injuries. These are most likely to be present when a fracture occurs at a point where the nerve trunk is normally in close approximation to the bone. Therefore the most common nerve injuries as complications of fractures are (1) the radial nerve, with fractures of the middle third of the humerus, (2) the peroneal nerve, with fractures of the proximal portion of the fibula and (3) the ulnar nerve, with fractures of the medial condyle of the humerus.

If the nerve has been merely contused, return of function may be rapid. On the other hand, if the nerve has been severed, end-to-end suture, either primarily or at a later operation, is indicated. Restoration of peripheral nerve function is often so important that it may be worthwhile to shorten the bone deliberately by excision of a portion of the fragments in order to permit end-to-end approximation of the nerve. Even with accurate suture of a severed peripheral nerve at the proper time, the eventual return of function is very likely to be incomplete.

A careful neurologic examination should be made in every injured extremity to determine if any evidence of nerve damage exists. The results of examination should be recorded before any effort at reduction of the fracture, either closed or open, so that it may be clear whether the original injury or the effort at reduction of the fracture caused damage to the nerve.

Injuries to the Spinal Cord. The seriousness of fractures of the spine is increased tremendously if the underlying spinal cord receives even the most minimal damage. Fracture-dislocations of the cervical spine are particularly likely to cause damage to the cord. Transportation of patients with suspected injuries of the spine must be carried out in such a way as to avoid or prevent further damage (see "Emergency splinting," p. 460). Early reduction of fractures or dislocations of the spine may be of utmost importance in minimizing the permanent effects of damage to the cord.

DELAYED COMPLICATIONS

Infection. Infection is not uncommon following open fractures and may follow open reduction of a closed fracture. All open fractures are contaminated and may become infected if the conditions are favorable. Such contributing factors are severe contamination, devitalized soft tissues, persisting exposure of bone, cartilage, tendon and fascia in the wound, retained foreign bodies, and poor reduction or immobilization of the fragments of bone. Clostridial myositis (gas gangrene), the most dreaded type of infection following open fractures, requires severely damaged and ischemic muscle for its development and often follows an open fracture complicated by an injury to a major artery. It is obvious, then, why thorough débridement is so important in preventing soft tissue and bone infection.

Nonunion and Delayed Union. The failure of a fracture to unite is due chiefly to local factors at the fracture site. Common sites of nonunion are the neck of the femur, the lower tibial shaft, the carpal scaphoid and the humeral shaft. These sites have in common a poor blood supply. Infection in the fracture site, interposition of soft tissues, inadequate immobilization and distraction (overpull) as part of treatment are common causes of delayed union and nonunion. Watson-Jones says, "There is only one cause of nonunion of fractures with continuous hematoma between the fragments—the cause of nonunion is inadequate immobilization."

The student must not think of a fracture in each location as having an exact time for healing, any prolongation of which means nonunion. The time required for a given fracture to heal with ideal treatment varies with many factors, known and unknown. Therefore, it is wrong to think that a fracture should be immobilized for a certain time and the immobilization then discontinued, and, if union has not occurred during that time, that nonunion has resulted. While one may properly speak of "delayed union" if the time for union goes past a theoretical average for the site involved in a given patient, nonunion is

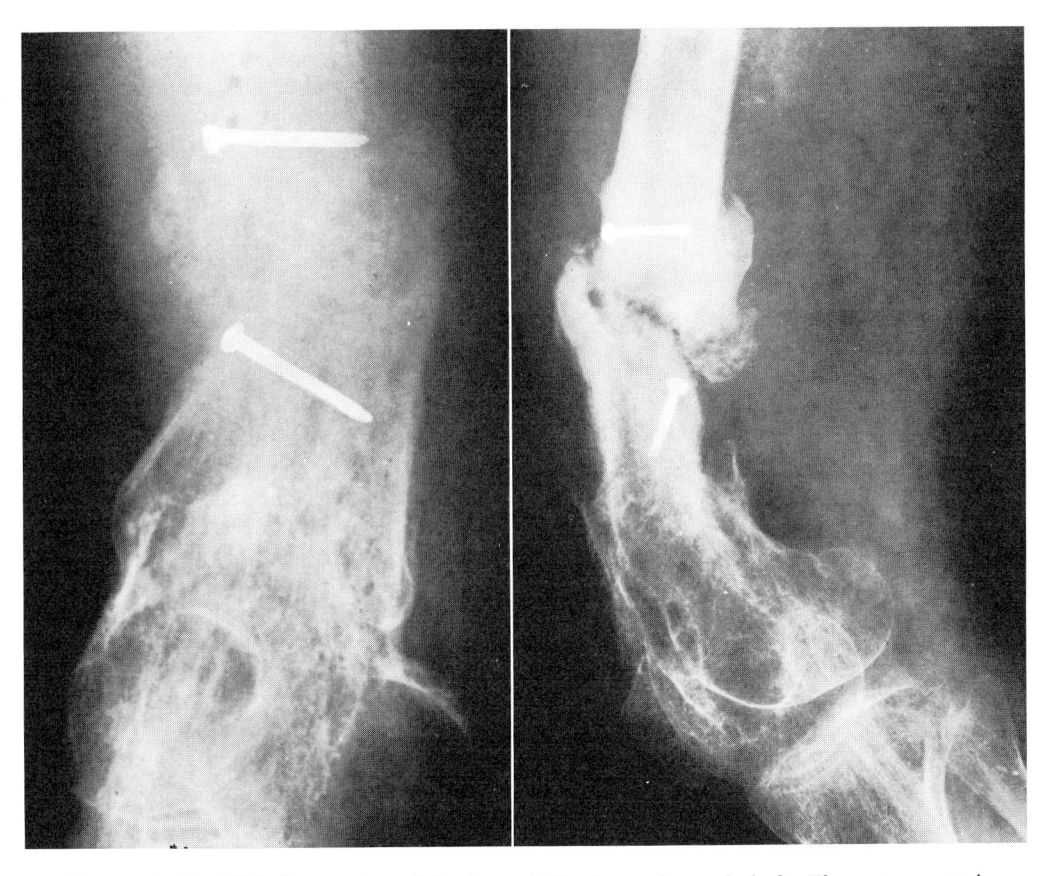

Fig. 20-7. Established nonunion of fracture of the lower femoral shaft. The anteroposterior roentgenogram (*left*) shows severe angulation, but the diagnosis of nonunion can be made only on the lateral view (*right*). When nonunion is suspected, multiple views are often necessary to make the diagnosis.

a pathologic entity that may be recognized by gross and microscopic findings at the fracture site. These changes may be noted on roentgenograms by a rounding-off and sclerosis of the fragment ends (Fig. 20-7). Once nonunion has occurred, further immobilization is to no avail.

Loss of Motion of Joints. Probably the most frequent complication of fractures is some permanent restriction of motion in the joints adjacent to the fracture. Immobilization of joints necessary for the proper management of the fractures predisposes to this complication. The older the patient, the more likely that immobilization will result in some permanent restriction of motion. Loss of motion of joints may also result from injury to the soft tissues about them with resulting scar formation, from injury to adjacent muscles, which limits their subsequent function, or from injury to the articular cartilage of the joint itself with resulting traumatic arthritis. Loss of motion of joints must be minimized by as early mobilization of them as is compatible with good management of the fracture and by as much exercise of the adjacent musculature as feasible during the period of immobilization.

Causalgia. Fractures may be associated with causalgia (post-traumatic sympathetic dystrophy, Sudeck's atrophy). An injury to a major nerve trunk of the extremity usually has occurred when causalgia develops. This condition is poorly understood. It must be treated by (1) the proper management of the fracture, (2) appropriate procedures on the sympathetic nerves and (3) general support of the patient, including recognition of the frequent emotional problems.

Ossifying Hematoma. This is an ossification in the hematoma resulting from the fracture but occurring at a distance from the area of desired bone repair. Little is known concerning its cause and prevention. Some have postulated that the combination of hematoma and damaged muscle predisposes to its formation. Not infrequently it is seen complicating dislocations of the elbow associated with fractures of the head of the radius. It is especially serious when it occurs about the elbow because it usually restricts motion of the joint. In the forearm, it may cause a bony bridge between the radius and the ulna and prevent rotation.

Volkmann's Ischemic Contracture. This is a severe fibrosis with resulting contracture of muscles which have been rendered ischemic by obstruction of the arterial flow to the extremity. It most commonly involves the musculature of the forearm and the hand as a complication of fractures about the elbow in children (see p. 490). It may develop because of unrelieved swelling about the elbow, impairing the arterial flow to the extremity as a direct result of the injury itself or because, in an effort to maintain reduction of the fragments, the elbow is immobilized in excessive flexion which causes occlusion of the arterial flow to the forearm and the hand. Volkmann's ischemic contracture is a complication that can be prevented by proper care. If allowed to develop, the results are disastrous.

Avascular Necrosis of Bone. Following injury, areas of bone may be isolated from their blood supply and die. This complication is called avascular or aseptic necrosis of bone in contrast with septic necrosis caused by infection. The process is recognized on x-ray examination by a relative increase in density of the avascular area in comparison with the surrounding bone (Fig. 20-8). Avascular necrosis is observed most frequently in the femoral head following intracapsular fractures and dislocations of the hip, injuries which severely damage the already meager blood supply of the head of the femur (Fig. 20-8). In some instances, the avascular necrosis may not appear for several years following injury. Avascular necrosis affecting the fragment deprived of its blood supply is often noted in fractures of the carpal navicular. It also may occur in the proximal fragment of a fractured talus. In general, this is an unpreventable complication.

Fat Embolism. Fat embolism following trauma is probably more common than is generally recognized. Free fat can be demonstrated in the urine of a high percentage of patients following injury. Fat embolism has been found most frequently after fractures but has also been noticed after soft tissue injuries and in certain disease states. Difference of opinion exists as to its incidence and clinical importance, and more study is

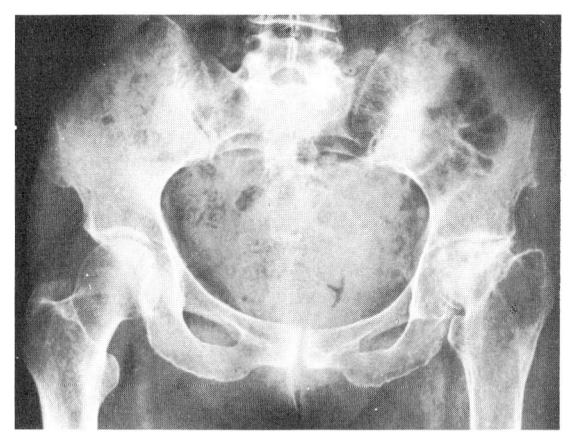

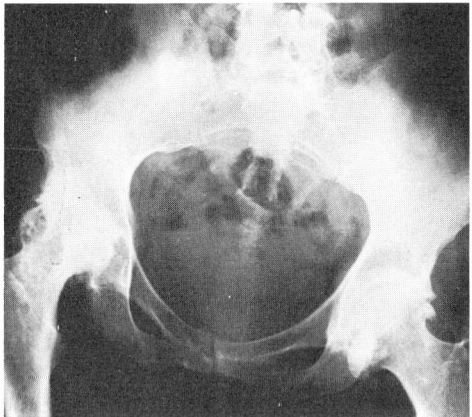

Fig. 20-8. (*Left*) Avascular necrosis of head of left femur, following fracture of the neck which united. (*Right*) Avascular necrosis of head of right femur, which developed several years after reduction of a posterior dislocation of the hip.

needed to determine its role in the complications, chiefly pulmonary, cerebral, and renal, following fracture. Symptoms and signs suggestive of pneumonia or atelectasis may result from pulmonary fat embolism and changes suggestive of cerebral trauma from cerebral fat embolism. Vigorous supportive and symptomatic treatment should be carried out. Early tracheostomy to permit excellent toilet of the tracheo-bronchial tree may be necessary. Cerebral symptoms and signs may be caused by hypoxia produced by pulmonary fat embolism and may be relieved by delivering a high concentration of oxygen to the lungs with a mechanical respirator. Blood gas determinations (pO_2, pCO_2, and pH) are useful in determining the respiratory damage caused by pulmonary fat embolism. Heparin, intravenous alcohol, and cortisone have all been advocated for treatment of fat embolism, but their efficacy has not been clearly established.

Delayed and Late Nerve Paralysis. Whereas immediate nerve injury may be caused by a tearing of a nerve (e.g., radial nerve in fractures of the humerus) or pressure on a nerve (e.g., on the peroneal nerve in fractures of the fibular neck), nerve paralysis may occur many months or years after the fracture. An outstanding example is "tardy ulnar palsy," which may develop in adult life following malunion of a fracture of the lateral condyle of the humerus in childhood. Due to lateral epiphyseal damage, growth at the elbow is limited to the medial side, with the production of a relative medial protuberance and increased carrying angle. Years later (as many as 20 or more years), ulnar palsy may result from continued stretch and trauma of movement of the ulnar nerve over the relative protuberance of the medial condyle, even though the orginal injury was a fracture of the lateral condyle.

OBJECTIVES OF MANAGEMENT OF FRACTURES

The ideal to be achieved in the management of fractures may be expressed as a solidly united fracture in perfect alignment, the bone of full length and joints freely movable by strong musculature—all having been obtained in the shortest possible period of time. These objectives really mean the rehabilitation of the patient as quickly, as possible with the patient as nearly whole as possible.

Unfortunately, in many fractures it is impossible to obtain a complete restoration of the part. For example, in some fractures, in order to obtain good contact of fragments so as to predispose to union, some shortening must be accepted. In others, particularly those about joints, the necessary immobilization to permit union of the fracture in good position may lead to some loss of motion in an adjacent joint. Necessary prolonged immobilization is likely to lead to some atrophy of the musculature of the part and it may be impossible for the patient to rebuild the muscle strength completely.

Moreover, the relative importance of each of the objectives outlined above varies with the location of the fracture. In the upper extremity, the most important objective in the management of a fracture is the maintenance or return of normal function of the hand. After the fracture has healed, stability of the fracture must be sufficient to permit the hand to function properly. While perfect alignment is desirable, union in slight angulation may be of no consequence. Certainly, the fracture may heal with some shortening without any real loss of function of the extremity.

In the lower extremity, on the other hand, stability without pain is the most important objective, but movable joints for locomotion and full length are highly desirable. In many fractures, however, mobility of the joints and full length must be sacrificed, at least partially, to ensure a solidly united fracture which will provide painless stability on weight-bearing.

The objectives in the management of fractures were well summarized by Darrach in his Presidential Address before the American Surgical Association in 1946. He listed these objectives as (1) reduction of secondary trauma to a minimum; (2) sufficient restoration of normal form to meet the requirements —this may be short of the ideal anatomic reduction; (3) immobilization of the bone fragments until healing has occurred—all joints should be mobilized immediately if their movement does not cause motion of the fragments; (4) restoration of function as early and as rapidly as possible and the atrophy of disuse minimized by the early institution of active motion; (5) sustaining of morale and physical and social rehabilitation.

Clay Ray Murray epitomized the principles of treatment of fractures in the following hypothesis:

The ideal way to treat a fracture would be to wish the fragments into place, hold them there by moral suasion and send the patient on about his business while the fracture healed. Comprehension of the implications of this hypothesis and adherence to its concept are mandatory to good fracture treatment regardless of the method used.

1. "To wish the fragments into place" would mean reduction without any additional tissue damage. It can't be done! Nevertheless, the best reduction is that most closely approximating this ideal, i.e., the earliest and gentlest reduction possible. For the same reason (prevention of secondary tissue damage) adequate first-aid care is essential to an optimum result.

2. To "hold them there by moral suasion" would mean maintenance of reduction without interfering with continued function of the associated structures. This is impossible! Nevertheless, the apparatus or method most closely approaching this ideal is best, i.e., that which provides adequate stabilization of the bone fragments coincident with minimum interference with local function throughout healing. A healed bone is of little use when the surrounding soft tissue has been ruined by overimmobilization or unnecessary disuse.

3. To "send the patient on about his business" would mean maintenance of all social, economic and other normal functions of the patient as a whole, throughout healing. This is rarely possible. However, the treatment method of choice is that which most closely approaches this ideal.

These principles cannot be taken as rules or blueprints for the treatment of fractures. Most fractures demand closed or open reduction and immobilization which must interfere with function, and for the surgeon to concentrate entirely on function in these would preclude reduction and immobilization. Other fractures require continued function of the part, even if this means accepting some bony deformity. As a rule, some compromise must be accepted. The best treatment for a fracture concentrates on the most important of the objectives at the expense of the least important.

EMERGENCY SPLINTING OF FRACTURES

Effective emergency splinting of fractures for transportation to and within a hospital is a highly significant procedure in the eventual rehabilitation of the patient. When emergency splinting is effective, the first objective outlined by Darrach—that is, the reduction of secondary trauma to a minimum—will have been achieved.

An injured part must be splinted when pain, loss of function, or deformity suggest

Emergency Splinting of Fractures

a fracture. Efforts to elicit crepitus or false motion to prove a fracture is present are dangerous. The suspicion that a fracture is present is sufficient to justify emergency splinting for transportation of the patient to a hospital for adequate x-ray examination.

The objective of emergency splinting is, of course, not reduction of the fracture but the prevention of additional damage to soft parts by fragments of bone. When fragments have been immobilized adequately, the other objectives in emergency splinting—namely, the relief of pain and the provision of comfortable and safe transportation—will have been achieved. When properly carried out, emergency splinting minimizes or prevents shock and is an important step in resuscitation of the injured.

Emergency splinting may be provided with standard or improvised splints. Standard splints, of course, are preferable but these are not always available. In such instances, vari-

Fig. 20-9. Emergency splinting. (A) Coaptation splinting with boards for fracture of the forearm. (B) Sling and circular bandage about the thorax for fracture above the forearm. (C) Fixed traction in a Thomas splint for fracture of the femur. (D) Coaptation splinting with boards of fracture of the femur. Note that the lateral board extends to the axilla and is bound to the thorax. For fractures of the leg the lateral board need extend only to the hip. (E) Inflatable splint for fractures of leg and pillow and board splints for fractures about ankle.

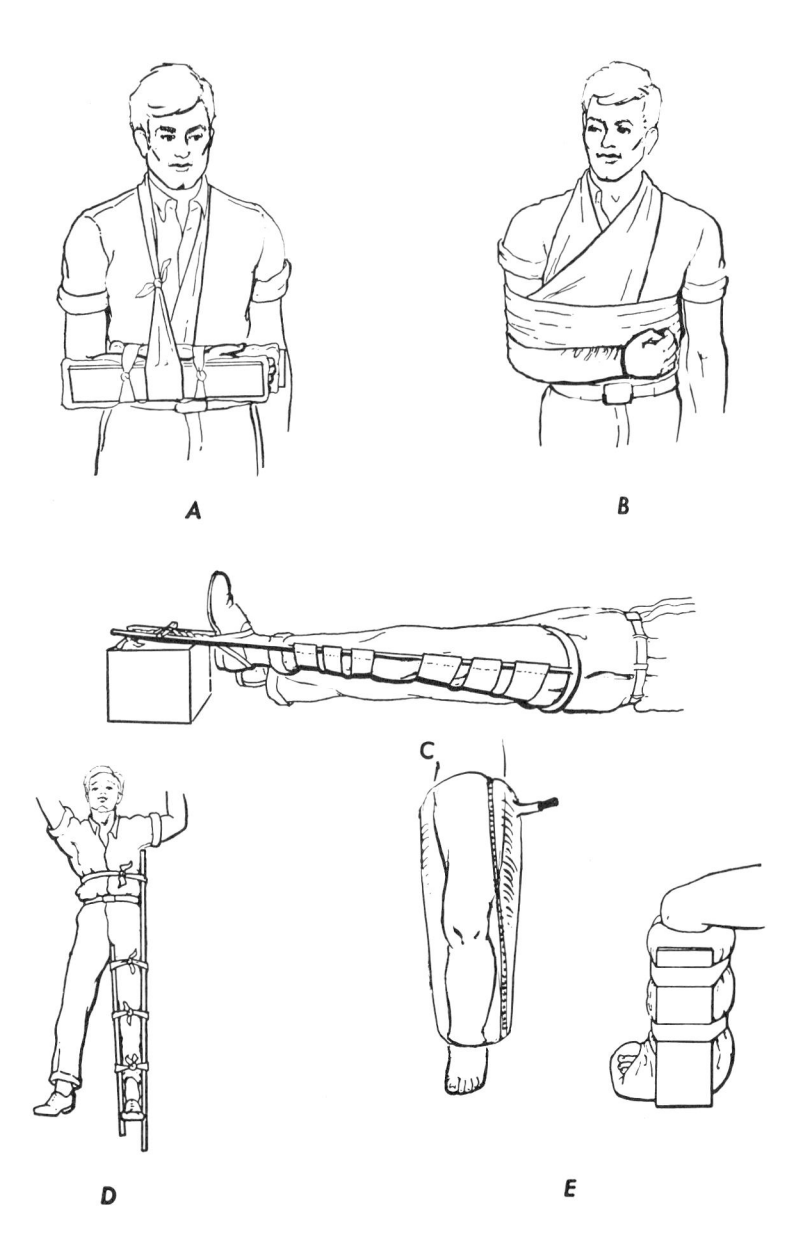

ous materials which are available may be employed to provide highly effective emergency splinting and achieve its objectives.

Effective emergency splinting is illustrated in Fig. 20-9.

UPPER EXTREMITY

Shoulder, Arm and Elbow

STANDARD. The extremity is placed in a sling, with the elbow usually at a right angle, and is bound to the chest by means of a bandage or another sling. If an injured elbow has assumed a position of extension, no attempt is made to flex it to a right angle, but the extremity is bandaged to the body with the elbow in extension.

IMPROVISED. The individual's shirt tail may be turned up and pinned to the shirt so that it serves as a sling. The extremity may then be bound to the chest with any material that is at hand.

The full-ring hinged arm traction splint is mentioned only to condemn it. It has no place in the emergency splinting of fractures of the upper extremity. This splint was given a trial during the early stages of World War II and was found to be totally unsuited for emergency splinting. It was promptly discarded and is no longer standard equipment for emergency splinting on the battlefield.

Forearm, Wrist and Hand

STANDARD. The forearm and the hand are bandaged to a board or a metal splint placed on the volar surface. The extremity is then placed in a sling with the elbow at a right angle.

IMPROVISED. As a rule the splinting will be improvised. An adequate substitute for a wood or metal splint is a magazine or even a heavy newspaper encircling the forearm and the hand and held in place with a bandage or adhesive tape. A sling is always indicated.

LOWER EXTREMITY

Standard. Traction splinting utilizing a Thomas or a hinged half-ring splint with traction being obtained by means of a hitch about the foot has been shown to be most effective for fractures of the femur. The slings on which the extremity rests may be towels, or bandages of any kind. The traction hitch is applied over the shoe if one is on the foot. Only moderate traction is desirable. The end of the splint always must be elevated sufficiently to lift the extremity so that it is entirely supported by the slings of the splint.

Recently, inflatable splints of a plastic material have become available for emergency splinting. They provide acceptable splinting for fractures below and at the knee but they are not acceptable for fractures of the femoral shaft. They should always be inflated by mouth and not by mechanical devices.

Improvised. The most common improvised splinting is obtained with board splints. For fractures of the lower two thirds of the leg and the ankle, the ideal improvised emergency splinting consists of 2 or 3 padded coaptation board splints which extend from the mid-thigh to below the foot. For injuries of the femur at any level, the knee and the upper third of the leg, the lateral board must extend to the axilla and must be bound securely to the walls of the abdomen and the chest. If the lateral board does not immobilize the hip joint, the splinting is entirely ineffective.

When board splints are applied to the lower extremity, padding must be arranged properly to protect the malleoli and the head of the fibula from painful pressure and, in the latter instance, to avoid pressure on the peroneal nerve which could cause peroneal nerve paralysis. For fractures of the bones of the leg a pillow bandaged securely about the leg, perhaps reinforced by boards extending to the mid-thigh, provides excellent emergency splinting. As a last resort when other materials are not available, the injured extremity should be tied to the uninjured counterpart.

SPINE

Cervical Spine. In suspected injuries of the cervical spine, the patient should be transported face up on a hard surface with sandbags or other heavy material placed on each side of the neck. Flexion and hyperextension of the neck must be avoided. If an appropriate neck brace is available, it should be applied.

Dorsal and Lumbar Spine. In suspected injuries of the dorsal and lumbar spine, the patient should be transported on a hard surface (a door removed from its hinges provides an excellent improvised stretcher) either face up with a small roll in the small of the back, or face downward. Flexion of the spine must be avoided. Particular care is necessary when lifting the patient on and off the support.

PELVIS

In suspected injuries of the pelvis, transportation should be provided on a hard surface with the patient on his back. Discomfort may be decreased if the thighs and the legs are tied together. If the thighs have assumed a flexed position and they cannot be extended easily, they should be kept in flexion. A record should be made as to whether the patient voids during transportation; if he does, it is important to note if the urine contains blood.

OPEN FRACTURES

On open wound should be covered promptly with a sterile dressing or the cleanest one available. If a fragment protrudes through the skin, it should be allowed to remain protruding and be covered with a sterile dressing.

In applying emergency traction splinting to the lower extremity, the amount of traction should be kept below a point which would cause the fragment to be pulled back into the wound. Information that the bone has protruded should accompany the patient in case traction inadvertently has been applied in an amount which pulled the exposed fragment back into the wound.

Massive hemorrhage may take place through the open wound. Usually the bleeding can be controlled by a compression dressing, and a tourniquet is rarely if ever needed.

METHODS OF MANAGEMENT OF FRACTURES

There are 5 general methods of management of fractures (Fig. 20-10). Every means which is available for the treatment of any given fracture may be classified as one of these 5 methods. It must be clearly understood that management of the fracture includes not only the reduction of the fracture but also the maintenance of reduction, measures designed to obtain as much mobility of joints and strength of musculature as possible, and the rehabilitation of the patient as a whole.

The 5 general methods of management of fractures are:

1. Closed reduction (or maintenance of reduction if the position is satisfactory) and immobilization, usually with a plaster cast.
2. Continuous balanced traction, usually skeletal traction, less commonly skin traction.
3. Open reduction, usually with internal fixation.
4. External skeletal fixation.
5. No immobilization (perhaps a sling or a bandage).

CLOSED REDUCTION (OR MAINTENANCE OF REDUCTION IN FRACTURES IN SATISFACTORY POSITION) AND IMMOBILIZATION

In this method of management of fractures, the fragments, if displaced, are manipulated into satisfactory apposition and alignment and held in that position by some form of immobilization, usually a plaster cast. If the position of the fragments is already satisfactory, reduction is not required, and immobilization is all that is necessary. In accordance with a fundamental rule for the splinting of fractures, the joints above and below the fracture are usually immobilized.

Efforts at closed reduction usually should be instituted promptly after the diagnosis of a fracture is made. They are most effective while the hematoma about the fracture is still liquid and before the tissues have become inelastic and water-logged from swelling. This means that closed reduction will be easier if it is carried out within 3 or 4 hours after injury.

Reduction of a fracture is almost always accomplished under general, regional or local anesthesia. Only rarely can faulty position of fragments be corrected adequately without anesthesia.

The fundamental maneuvers of a manipulative reduction are strong manual traction on the portion of the extremity distal to the fracture with equally strong counter-traction proximal to the fracture, combined with appropriate manipulation of the fragments. It is basic in closed reduction of fractures that the distal fragment be brought into approximation and alignment with the proximal fragment. When traction is slow and steady, only minimal direct manipulation of the distal fragment will be required as a rule; therefore, additional trauma to the soft tissues about the fracture will be minimal.

Closed reduction and immobilization are

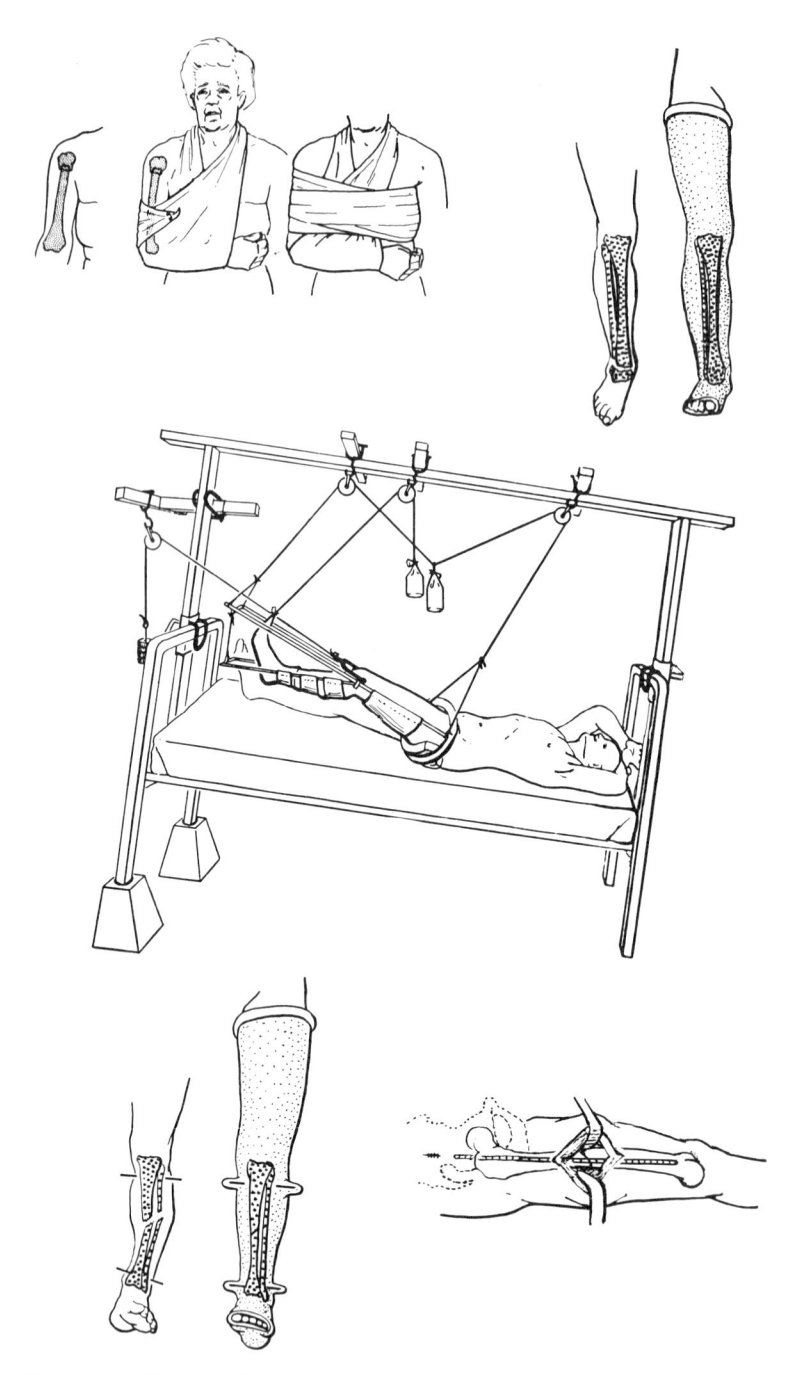

Fig. 20-10. Five methods of management of fractures. (*Top, left*) No immobilization. (*Top, right*) Closed reduction and immobilization with plaster cast. (*Center*) Continuous balanced skeletal traction. (*Bottom, left*) External skeletal fixation, Steinmann pins incorporated in a plaster cast. (*Bottom, right*) Open reduction and internal fixation with medullary nail.

usually chosen when the contour of the fracture indicates that the reduction will be so stable that it will not be lost as long as good alignment is maintained by the immobilization. Under these circumstances this is a conservative method involving a minimum risk of complications. It is the most common method of management for fractures of the extremities. It is usually the method of choice for fractures about the wrist and the ankle in adults and for practically every fracture of the long bones in children, except those of the femoral shaft.

CONTINUOUS BALANCED TRACTION

By this method, continuous traction, usually over a period of weeks, is made on the portion of the extremity distal to the fracture against the counteraction furnished by the weight of the body. As a rule, the injured extremity is suspended in a splint—for example, a Thomas splint for fractures of the shaft of the femur (Fig. 20-10).

The traction may be skin or skeletal. In skin traction, adhesive tape or moleskin is applied to the extremity, using a wooden block as a spreader just distal to the foot, as in Buck's traction. The theory of skin traction is that a weight pulling on the tape makes traction on the skin which in turn makes traction on the musculature and this in turn on the bone. In skeletal traction, pins (Steinmann pins or Kirschner wires) are drilled through a bone distal to the fracture, and traction is applied to the pin or the wire. The pin or the wire may be inserted through the distal portion of the bone which is fractured or inserted through one of the bones distal to the joint below the fracture. For example, the pin or the wire may be inserted through the tibial tubercle for continuous skeletal traction for a fracture of the femur or through the os calcis for continuous skeletal traction for fractures of both bones of the leg. Obviously, skeletal traction is more effective than skin traction because it is traction applied directly to the bone. Moreover, the hazards of slipping of the tape and of irritation and blistering beneath it are obviated.

The rationale of balanced skeletal traction for the management of fractures is that the strong continuous traction applied in the long axis of the extremity will bring the distal fragment into apposition and alignment with the proximal fragment and therefore reduce the fracture. The strapping and molding effect of the musculature surrounding the fragments aids in the reduction. It may seem unnecessary to comment that the traction must be continuous, yet, in hospitals where this method is not used regularly, one is often distressed to find hospital personnel removing the traction weight when the bed is moved or the patient turned. Such a mistake may wreck the entire course of treatment.

Continuous traction is most likely to give adequate reduction of the fracture when it is instituted relatively soon after the injury. While traction need not necessarily be provided as early as closed reduction should be attempted, it must be instituted before the fragment ends have been fixed by early healing. The quicker traction is established, the more effective it will be. This means that it should be in effect within a few days after the injury.

Enough traction should be provided to obtain reduction and then to maintain it. With this amount of traction the normal muscle tone will maintain adequate contact-compression of the fragments. Overpull (or distraction) must be avoided, as this predisposes to nonunion. The continuous traction method requires repeated roentgenograms to serve as indicators of the effectiveness of the method. Based on the findings on x-ray examination, repeated adjustments of the traction may be necessary.

Continuous balanced suspension skeletal traction has been the method of management for the great majority of battle fractures of the femoral shaft, during World War II and now during the Vietnam conflict. Until about 1950 this method was employed for the great majority of fractures of the femoral shaft in civilian injuries, and even today it is a splendid method for these injuries. However, intramedullary nailing, when applicable, is the preferred method of management for fractures of the femoral shaft in adults.

Some form of continuous traction is frequently employed for fractures of the shaft of the humerus, comminuted fractures of both bones of the leg and in selected instances of fractures of the bones of the hand and the foot.

Open Reduction, Usually With Internal Fixation

In this method, the fracture site is exposed at operation, and under direct visualization the fragment ends are brought into approximation. Usually some form of metallic internal fixation (screws, intramedullary nails, plates, malleable stainless steel wire) is employed to maintain the reduction.

Open reduction, of course, affords the most exact reduction and offers many advantages. Perfect apposition and alignment and full length are usually obtained. The excellent reduction predisposes to rapid union. Internal fixation should prevent loss of reduction.

However, there are several objections to this method. In closed fractures it converts an uncontaminated fracture into an open fracture and thereby risks infection. The operation itself adds further damage to soft tissues and bone. Moreover, with some forms of internal fixation, as a rigid plate held by screws, the plate can serve to delay union of the fragments. Some absorption of fragment ends occurs in most fractures. If so, normal tone of the surrounding musculature cannot pull the fragment ends together, if they are strutted apart by a plate and screws. In an attempt to overcome this disadvantage of rigid plating of fractures and to effect continuous contact of the fragment ends, slotted bone plates were developed to replace the rigid fixation. Although they appear to be advantageous, the relative effectiveness of slotted plates is yet to be proved. Recently, the introduction of non-slotted rigid A-O compression plates (firm compression of fragments is obtained at operation) has led to some return of popularity of the plating technic.

In summary, open reduction and internal fixation of fractures is a calculated risk affording advantages and disadvantages. The method should be selected when the former sufficiently outweigh the latter.

Open reduction is indicated as the treatment of choice for many fractures—including separated fractures of the patella and the olecranon, fractures of the neck and the trochanteric region of the femur, fractures of the shafts of both bones of the forearm in adults and, with the use of the intramedullary nail, for many fractures of the femoral shaft.

Stability of the fragments of bone sufficient to avoid the application of additional immobilization is not provided by internal fixation alone, with the exceptions of nailed fractures of the neck and the trochanteric region of the femur, intramedullary nailings of the femoral shaft and some fractures fixed with the new A-O compression plates. For practically every other form of internal fixation, a plaster cast for supplementary immobilization is required until union of the fracture has occurred. In certain fresh fractures notorious for their tendency toward nonunion, as an adjunct to the open reduction and internal fixation, autografts from the iliac crest may be added to speed union; e.g., in adults, fractures of the lower portion of the shaft of the tibia, fractures of shafts of both bones of the forearm.

External Skeletal Fixation

In this method, following closed or, at times, open reduction of the fragments, an effort is made to maintain reduction by means of strong metallic bars connected to rigid metal pins or half pins which are inserted through the skin and other soft parts into each fragment (hence, the name of the method—external skeletal fixation). A plaster cast is not used as a rule. The Rober Anderson and Stader splints are examples of the apparatus employed.

This method is not recommended. It is mentioned for completeness and to warn against it. In the hands of most surgeons it has resulted in a too high incidence of malunion and nonunion, stiffness of adjacent joints and infection along the pin tracks. Very few surgeons employ this technic today.

A method of treatment which permits classification as external skeletal fixation is the use of one or two rigid pins inserted through both the proximal and the distal fragments and, following reduction, the incorporation of the pins in a full-length plaster cast. This method has been successful in certain fractures of the shafts of both bones of the leg. It has the distinct disadvantage of potentially "holding the fragments apart" as may occur with rigid plating as described above. In addition, ring sequestra may form about the transfixion pins. This has been attributed to excessive pressure by the pins on the bone from the various movements of the plaster cast that incorporates the pins and to devitalization resulting from heat generated at the time of introduction of the pins.

No Immobilization (Perhaps a Sling or a Bandage)

In the use of this method, chiefly applicable in impacted fractures, it is recognized that displacement will not occur with motion of the part. The position of the fragments is accepted, even though it may not be ideal. Immobilization is omitted in favor of early mobilization and this really is the keynote of the method. Actually, a sling or a bandage may be employed for a short period, but these do not produce real immobilization and merely provide some relief of pain during the first few days after injury.

This method should be employed in those fractures which do not require immobilization and in which early active exercise will lead to more functional restoration of the part in a shorter period of time than would immobilization. This technic is particularly indicated in impacted fractures of the upper portions of the humerus and in undisplaced fractures of the radial head. It is applicable in many chip fractures about the hand and the foot.

Selection of a Method

Each method of management offers advantages and disadvantages and these must be weighed carefully in selecting the method of management for any given fracture. The selection of a method to be instituted is based upon several factors. Of these, the contour of the fracture as revealed by the roentgenograms is probably the most important. Others are the age and the general condition of the patient, whether the fracture is open or closed, the presence of other significant injuries, and, especially if open reduction is under consideration, the status of circulation to the soft parts, particularly the skin overlying the fracture, the equipment at hand and the experience and the ability of the surgeon.

In many fractures, one method will be employed, found to be ineffective and therefore another method must be selected. For example, Method I, closed reduction and immobilization, may be attempted for a fracture of both bones of the forearm. Postoperative roentgenograms may show a satisfactory reduction, but repeat roentgenograms a few days later may show that the fragments have slipped and are no longer in good position. Then Method III, open reduction, may be selected and the fragments stabilized in reduction by means of intramedullary fixation or slotted or compression plates held by screws. Likewise, Method II, balanced skeletal traction, may fail to reduce a comminuted fracture of the femoral shaft adequately. Then open reduction may be employed, and the fragments fixed in good position by intramedullary nailing supplemented by other forms of internal fixation if indicated.

The student of fractures, as soon as he is confronted with any given fracture, is urged to consider these 5 methods of management and select the one which best fits the requirements. Many medical students despair of acquiring a thorough knowledge of fractures because of the multiplicity of gadgets and equipment seen in the fracture room and on the wards and the varying opinions expressed in the literature concerning the treatment of many fractures. This confusion arises from too great a concern for details of treatment and too little concern for the underlying principles of management. The details of treatment and the use of a profusion of splints and gadgets should not be the primary concern of the medical student. Rather, he should concentrate on the principles involved in the selection of 1 of the 5 methods of treatment for the particular fracture with which he finds himself concerned.

OPEN FRACTURES

An open wound communicating with the fracture site adds considerably to the seriousness of the injury and complicates management of the fracture for several reasons. The hematoma from the fracture site may be lost through the wound, and this loss may retard union of the fracture. Blood loss may cause shock and seriously delay management of the fracture. The damage to soft tissues is greater in open fractures, resulting in more scarring and limiting the eventual return of function. However, the principal hazards of open fractures are those of secondary infection and failure of healing of the wound.

Infection of the wound may result in several ways. There may be a true invasive infection by bacteria, primarily or secondarily implanted in the wound. Gas gangrene is an example of such an invasive infection. More often, however, infection of the wound results from the bacterial decomposition of devitalized soft tissue and blood clot with resulting suppuration. The suppurative process may lead to further destruction of soft tissue and bone which in turn leads to more suppuration. In other instances, a true infection is not present in the beginning, but the loss of soft tissue or a gaping open wound may leave bone, fascia or tendon exposed. The superficial cortex of bone, cartilage, fascia and tendon cannot survive if they remain exposed in a wound. They soon die and serve as the nidus for wound suppuration. The end result of an open wound in which these vulnerable tissues remain exposed is wound infection.

Regardless of how and why a suppurative process develops in an open wound of a fracture, it is a most serious complication. Union of the fracture is almost always delayed and may be prevented. Massive sequestration of bone may occur. Adjacent joints may become involved and be destroyed. The infection may become so extensive as to warrant amputation as a lifesaving measure. At best, there will be slow wound healing with excessive scar formation which probably will lead to a diminished functional restoration of the part.

The objectives of management of open fractures are rapid healing of the open wound without infection and healing of the fracture in good position. It readily follows that to achieve these objectives underlying factors leading to wound infection must be overcome. The depths and the recesses of the wound must be thoroughly cleaned of foreign material and debris during the so-called contaminated period before active infection can develop in the wound. Dead and devitalized tissue, including old blood clot, must be excised surgically before it decomposes and forms pus. Those tissues which will die if they remain exposed in a wound must be covered with soft parts at the proper time. Adequate drainage must be provided for residual dead space or, if indicated, to provide a means of egress for the possible septic decomposition of bits of devitalized tissue which could not be excised.

Treatment of the Wound of Open Fractures

First-aid treatment of an open fracture is, as mentioned above, merely the application of a sterile dressing and proper splinting. Cleansing the wound with so-called antiseptics is definitely contraindicated. Protruding fragments of bone should not be replaced in the wound but should be merely covered with a sterile dressing. It follows that in applying emergency traction splinting to an open fracture of an extremity with protruding fragments only minimal traction should be employed. Of course, immediate hospitalization is indicated. Antibiotics should be administered systemically as soon as possible.

Open fractures are true surgical emergencies. They deserve investigation, appraisal and treatment in a fully equipped operating room. However, before definitive surgery is begun, several things are necessary. First, any systemic effects of hemorrhage must be overcome by whole blood transfusions and infusions of electrolyte solutions. Plasma expanders may be a temporary "stopgap" measure, but they cannot replace whole blood transfusions for the severely wounded. As soon as the general condition of the patient warrants, roentgenograms should be made. The patient must be satisfactorily anesthetized, the part surgically cleaned and prepared and the wound thoroughly examined. An appraisal of the degree of contamination of the wound and the amount of damaged tissue probably remaining in it is the basis for determining the surgical procedure that is indicated (Fig. 20-11).

In order that all devitalized tissue may be removed, exposure of the depths of the wound must be ample. As a rule the wound must be extended. These extensions are made in the direction which will afford adequate access to the depths of the wound without injury to important structures such as nerve trunks. The extension must avoid unnecessary exposure of tissues likely to die when they remain uncovered and must facilitate closure by suture. In the extremities, incisions usually are made parallel with the long axis of the limb.

In the technic of wound débridement, only the devitalized skin of wound margins should

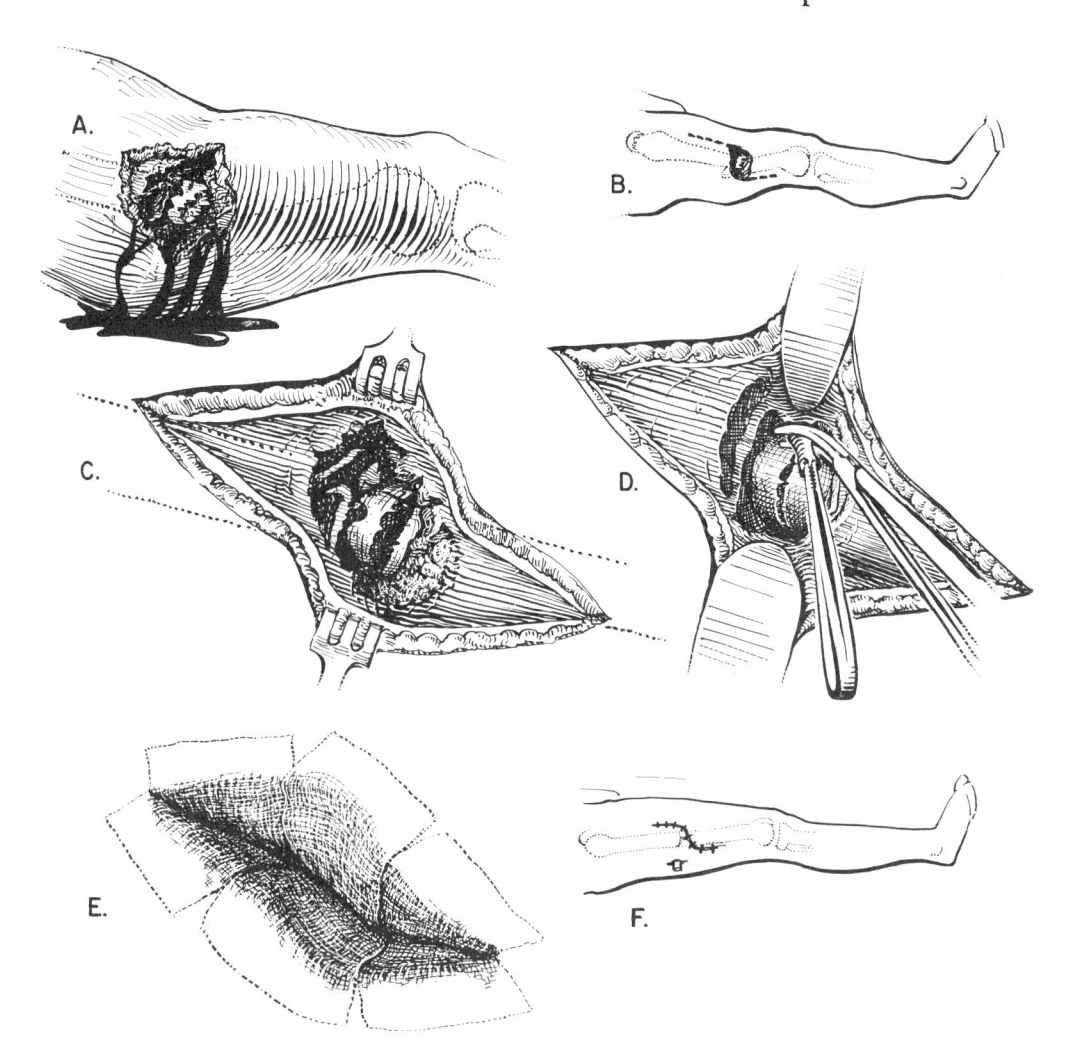

Fig. 20-11. Drawings of débridement of an open fracture. A. Open fracture of the shaft of the femur with the distal end of the proximal fragment protruding through the jagged open wound on the lateral surface of the thigh. B. The protruding bone and the exposed soft tissue are well cleaned, and any obvious tags of dead muscle are excised. Then the fragment is reduced into the depths of the wound. An important step in débridement is adequate enlargement of the wound by incision. A transverse or near-transverse wound should be enlarged by longitudinal extensions proximally and distally at opposite ends of the open wound as is illustrated by the dotted lines. Almost without exception an incision should not be made across the center of a wound so as to create a cruciate-type of wound. C. The fascia is split so as to facilitate exposure of the depths of the wound and excision of destroyed muscle tissue. D. Devitalized tags of muscle tissue are excised. Excision of muscle with scissors is highly acceptable technic, but only a knife should be used on the skin. E. Proper dressing of a wound that is to remain open with a fine mesh dry or petrolatum impregnated gauze. F. If primary suture of the wound is selected, dependent drainage for a few days through the posterolateral fascial plane as a safeguard against deep abscess formation. (Hampton, O. P., Jr.: Complications of common fractures. *In*: Hardy, J. D., and Artz, C.: Complications in Surgery. Philadelphia, W. B. Saunders, 1960)

be excised. A long incision in the fascial layer gives free access to foreign bodies and devitalized muscles, the excision of which is a major objective of wound débridement. Healthy muscle is not discolored, bleeds freely and contracts when pinched; muscle which does not meet these requirements should be excised. Foreign bodies and dirt should be removed. Thorough irrigation of the wound with a saline solution will cleanse it of small, free particles. Bleeding vessels should be ligated. Small fragments of bone completely free of soft tissue attachment should be removed; bone which has some muscular attachment should be left in place, as it is usually viable.

Closure of the wound of an open fracture by suture at the proper time is highly desirable. However, the decision to suture the wound must be based on sound surgical judgment. Much has been said about the immediate closure of the wounds of open fractures so as to convert quickly each open fracture into a closed one. Of course, an immediate successful suture of the wound is most advantageous, but an unsuccessful suture of the wound because of abscess formation or necrosis of skin margins is worse than if the wound had been left open.

In civilian surgery suture of the wound is often feasible, particularly if the time-lag after injury is not more than 4 to 6 hours, if the cleansing and the débridement of the wound have been thorough, and if closure appears to be surgically feasible without excessive tension. On the other hand, if the surgeon cannot be reasonably certain that he has rid the wound of the pabulum for sepsis, or if closure by suture would produce excessive tension likely to cause death of skin margins, then an open wound is preferable, despite its inherent hazards.

Closure of an open wound over a fracture versus the advantages of an open wound for drainage as a safeguard against deep infection (including anaerobic infection) presents a problem which may severely tax the judgment of even the most experienced surgeon. If the decision is made to leave the wound open, delayed primary closure should be performed if surgically feasible between the 3rd and the 6th days, provided that the wound is clinically clean. Delayed closure of clinically clean wounds is surgically sound, provided that dead space is obliterated or dependently drained and excessive tension is avoided. In recent years the use of continuous suction on drainage tubes brought out the dependent portions of a wound has been shown to be effective in obliterating dead space and preventing fluid collections.

Much has been written concerning the greater danger of infection in open fractures in which the wound is opened from "without-in" in comparison with those opened from "within-out." On a theoretical basis, the degree of contamination is always more in the former. Not only is foreign material more likely to be introduced into the wound but usually a greater degree of damage to the soft tissues occurs. It should be kept in mind, however, that considerable dirt and foreign material can be introduced into the wound of a fracture which is opened from within-out. For example, a child can fall on the outstretched hand so as to break both bones of the forearm in the middle third. A fragment of either the radius or the ulna may tear through soft tissues, usually on the palmar surface, and actually dig into the ground. As the child arises he may grab the injured forearm and cause the protruding fragment end to go back into the wound carrying with it considerable dirt. Such a case serves to illustrate the hazard of a false sense of security concerning contamination in fractures opened from within-out.

On the other hand, there will be many open fractures, usually opened from within-out but sometimes from without-in, in which the surgeon can be sure from the circumstances of the accident and the appearance of the wound and the clothing about the site of injury that no foreign material has been carried into the wound and that soft tissue damage is minimal. Under these circumstances, he may feel that the features discussed above which predispose to wound infection are not present and surgical investigation is not indicated. In such instances he may elect to irrigate the wound thoroughly with sterile saline solution, apply a sterile dressing, reduce the fracture by traction and manipulation and apply immobilization. While such practices cannot be condemned, it should be pointed out that they involve a real risk. In the majority of open fractures some cleansing and débridement of the depths of the wound will be definitely indicated.

Insofar as the fracture is concerned, the same methods of management are applicable in general to open as to closed fractures. In open fractures, however, the question of employing internal fixation at the time of wound excision often assumes paramount importance. As the wound is débrided, the fracture site may be exposed. If the contour of the fracture is such as to permit adequate stabilization by internal fixation, then the decision must be made as to whether that method will be employed. This, too, is a problem which requires expert judgment.

As a practical matter, when the time-lag after injury is not too prolonged, when the wound has been well débrided and when it can be closed by suture without excessive tension, there need be little hesitancy in applying internal fixation to the fracture through the open wound if the internal fixation is indicated otherwise. If, on the other hand, the factors predisposing to infection of the wound are present, internal fixation is probably too hazardous. In doubtful cases it is advisable to employ some method of management of the fracture other than internal fixation and to direct every effort toward obtaining early healing of the wound without infection. If, then, adequate reduction of the fracture has not been maintained, it will be possible to perform a delayed open reduction and internal fixation through a healed intact skin envelope with anticipation of success.

FRACTURES IN CHILDREN

Fractures in children are different. This often-repeated statement is true for several reasons. Incomplete fractures of the greenstick variety are common. Anatomically, the fracture line may cross an epiphyseal plate, or the injury may be a displacement of the epiphysis instead of a true fracture. Fractures in children unite rapidly; the younger the child, the more rapid the healing. For example, a complete fracture of the femoral shaft in a small infant may unite solidly within 10 days (Fig. 20-12).

Of greater significance are certain responses of growing bone which manifest themselves after a fracture during childhood has united. Even if malunion of the fracture has occurred, the normal contour of the bone may be reconstituted by growth according to Wolff's law which states that all changes in the function of a bone are attended by definite alterations in its internal structure. Bone will be laid down where it is needed to restore normal contour, and bone will be absorbed where it disturbs normal contour. This favorable response of growing bone to overcome what otherwise would be malunited fractures means,

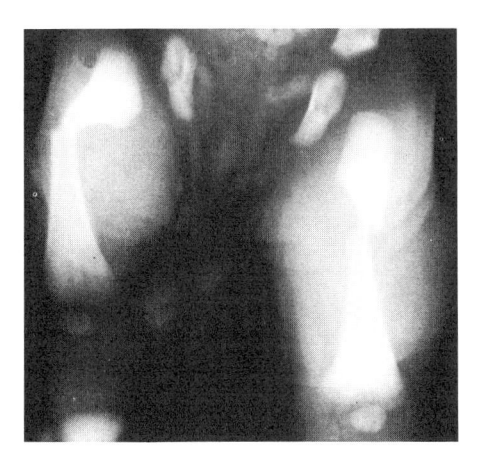

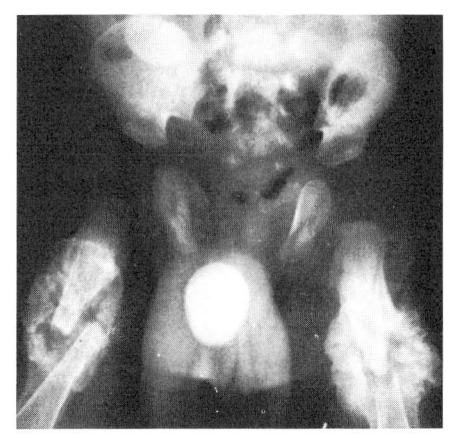

Fig. 20-12. Bilateral fractures of the femoral shafts from birth injury. (*Left*) Roentgenogram taken immediately after birth. (*Right*) Roentgenogram taken 10 days after injury, showing exuberant callus and satisfactory alignment. (From Dr. Robert Cram)

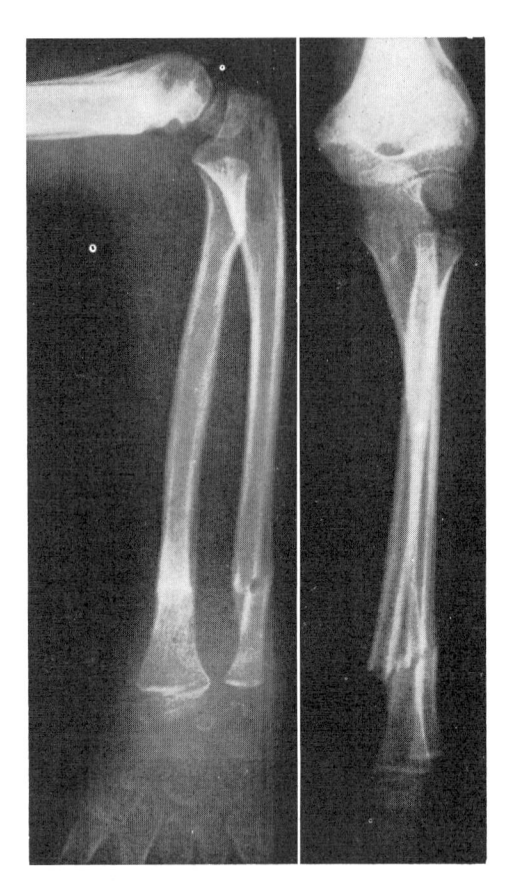

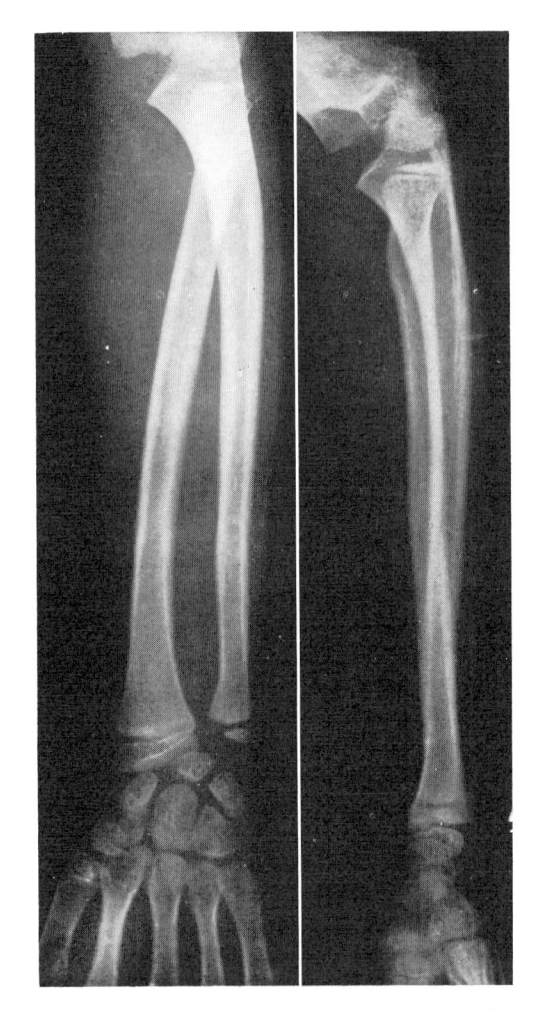

Fig. 20-13. (*Left*) Anteroposterior and lateral roentgenograms showing united fractures of both bones of the forearm in a 5-year-old child with fragments displaced and overriding. (*Right*) Anteroposterior and lateral roentgenograms 18 months later showing no residual evidence of the injury. (Case from Drs. Ward A. McClanahan and Charles K. Wier, Wichita, Kans.)

of course, that although precise reduction of a fracture in a child is desirable, it may not be necessary, and open operation to obtain perfect reduction is, for practical purposes, never justified (Fig. 20-13).

Another unique feature of some fractures in children is a tendency toward a subsequent increased rate of growth of the broken bone. Clinically and experimentally, it has been demonstrated that a displaced fracture of the diaphysis in growing bone will stimulate activity of the epiphyses of that bone, and for a period of time there will be an increased rate of growth. This means, of course, that not only may fractures of the long bones in children be permitted to heal with slight overriding but that such slight overriding is preferable. This is true because the increased rate of growth will enable the fractured bone to catch up in length with its counterpart in the other extremity, whereas if the reduction had been perfect, the increased rate of growth would produce excessive length of the bone which was fractured. However, rotational deformities are not so well corrected by growth processes and this should be taken into account in determining what is a satisfactory reduction of a fracture in a child.

In injuries of the extremities of children, it is often helpful to have roentgenograms of the normal extremity, especially in injuries near joints, because of the frequent difficulty in determining what is normal contour and degree of ossification of the epiphyses for the age of the injured child. Comparison of the roentgenograms of the injured and the uninjured sides may be quite valuable in establishing the presence and the extent of bony or epiphyseal injury.

The statement that open reduction of fractures in children is seldom justified deserves some modification. Open reduction is indicated in certain fractures in children, especially in a group of fractures around the elbow. These include fractures of the medial or the lateral condyle of the humerus with rotation and significant displacement, and fractures of the head and the neck of the radius with severe displacement or severe angulation. Operative intervention is also indicated in irreducible epiphyseal separations such as those at the distal end of the femur and at the distal end of the tibia, although it should be pointed out that operative reduction is not necessary for those injuries when the displacement is minimal.

Birth Fractures

Fractures occurring at birth, usually from the trauma incident to a difficult delivery, are called birth fractures. These usually involve the clavicle, the humerus, or the femur. Those of the clavicle and the humerus require very little treatment. The extremity may be placed in a small sling, a small axillary pad placed between the arm and the chest and the extremity then bandaged to the chest snugly for a week or two. Fractures of the femoral shaft require more attention. They may heal with rotational deformity and 90° anterior angulation if untreated. They are best managed in overhead balanced skin traction (Bryant's traction, p. 533).

Multiple fractures may be seen at birth in osteogenesis imperfecta. Also, congenital pseudarthrosis of the tibia may be observed occasionally. The cause of this condition is not well understood; spontaneous union seldom occurs, and operative treatment at a later date is usually required but even then the results are often poor.

PATHOLOGIC FRACTURES

A pathologic fracture is one involving previously diseased bone and often occurs as a result of little or no trauma. Bone disease predisposing to fracture may be caused by nutritional or hormonal disturbances (hyperparathyroidism, senile osteoporosis) neoplasm, infection, or neurotrophic dystrophies. A fracture may be the earliest manifestation of generalized disease, and physicians treating fractures must be alert to the need for a complete history, physical examination and laboratory investigation. In general, pathologic fractures heal if the same principles of treatment are followed as with nonpathologic fractures.

Although cancer is widely considered as one of our most important medical problems, relatively little attention has been given to fractures caused by metastatic cancer. The incidence of cancer is increasing, and those interested in the surgery of trauma should anticipate treating an increasing number of fractures caused by cancer. Metastatic carcinoma of the breast accounts for the largest percentage of these pathologic fractures. The spine, the femur and the bones of the shoulder girdle are most frequently fractured. Metastases and therefore pathologic fractures distal to the knee and the elbow are uncommon. A hopeless "do-nothing" attitude is unjustified in fractures from metastatic cancer. Vigorous treatment of the fracture relieves pain, reduces hospitalization, simplifies nursing care and permits early ambulation. Open reduction and fixation with an intramedullary nail is often the treatment of choice, especially in fractures of the femoral shaft (Fig. 20-14).

PLASTER OF PARIS

Plaster of Paris* casts or splints serve as the principal means of immobilization in the treatment of fractures and dislocations. As the student will learn with increasing experience, there is a considerable art in the application of a good cast. It must fit snugly enough to immobilize the part and yet not constrict circulation or cause localized pressure. It must be strong enough to avoid breaking, particularly across joints which are the vulnerable areas. Padding beneath the plaster must be

---

* Plaster of Paris is anhydrous calcium sulfate.

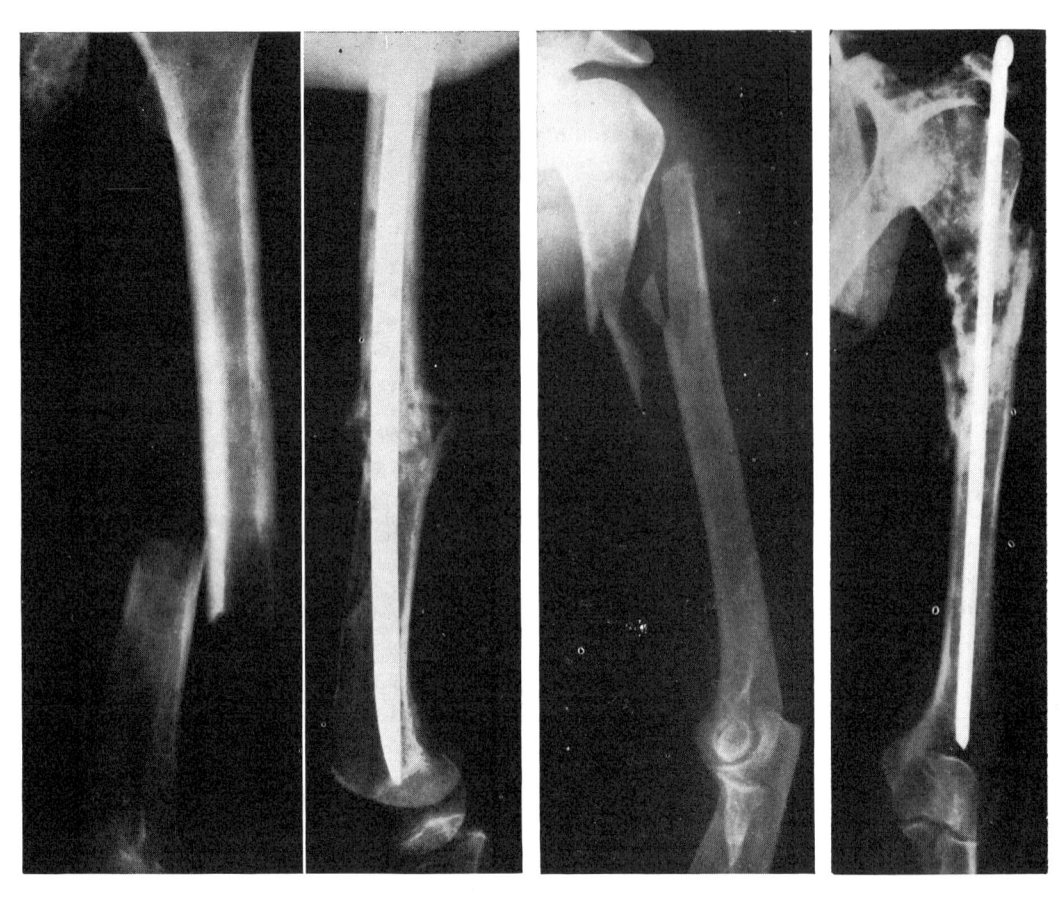

Fig. 20-14. Pathologic fractures of femur and humerus treated by intramedullary nailing. The patient had a radical mastectomy for cancer of the breast in 1949. In 1952 she fractured the left femur through an area of metastatic cancer. Fixation by an intramedullary nail allowed painless weight-bearing within 6 weeks. A year later she fractured the left humerus through another metastatic area. Fixation by an intramedullary nail relieved pain and allowed early motion. She remained comfortable until shortly before her death in 1954. (*Left*) Pathologic fracture of femoral shaft, anteroposterior view. Note metastases in pelvis. (*Center, left*) Four months after open reduction and fixation with intramedullary nail, lateral view. Note callus and evidence of beginning bony union. (*Center, right*) Pathologic fracture of humeral shaft. (*Right*) Three months after open reduction and fixation with an intramedullary nail. Note evidence of union of the fracture despite multiple areas of metastasis in humerus.

smooth and evenly arranged. Point pressure on bony prominences must be avoided both during application of the cast by proper molding and while it is hardening by protection with soft pillows.

Plaster bandages for the application of plaster casts are made by impregnating the meshes of crinoline bandage with plaster of Paris. These bandages must be kept wrapped and not exposed to the air before they are put to use, as the plaster will take up moisture from the air with resulting impairment of its setting qualities.

Plaster casts (or splints) are either padded or nonpadded. A *padded* cast is applied over some material, usually sheet cotton, under which stockinette may or may not be used. The amount of padding varies. For snug-fitting casts, only 2 or 3 thicknesses of sheet cotton should be applied over the extremity. A heavily padded cast may have 6 or 8 thicknesses of sheet cotton; the heavier the padding, however, the less effective the immobilization provided by the cast. A lightly padded plaster cast is used most commonly in the management of fractures. A *nonpadded* or skin-tight cast is, strictly speaking, applied directly to the skin except perhaps for spot padding of bony prominences. Practically, a cast is considered as nonpadded when it is applied over stockinette but without sheet cotton, although bony prominences may be padded with a small portion of sheet cotton or felt.

Various names have been applied to plaster casts according to their location. A *forearm cast* extends from just below the elbow to, as a rule, the proximal transverse crease of the palm. A *long arm* cast extends from the lower level of the anterior axillary fold to the same level on the hand. The elbow is usually immobilized at a right angle. The degree of rotation of the forearm and the position of the wrist in each type vary with the specific fracture under treatment.

A *boot cast* extends from just below the knee to the base of the toes. A *long leg cast* extends from the junction of the upper and the middle thirds of the thigh to the same level. Usually the foot is held at a right angle and in neutral version. In each type of leg cast, a plantar slab of plaster may be made to extend past the toes for their protection. This is at times advantageous and at other times disadvantageous. It protects the toes but prevents active plantar flexion of them.

A *spica cast* incorporates the trunk and an extremity. A *shoulder spica*, therefore, encloses the trunk and the upper extremity; a *hip spica*, the trunk and the lower extremity. A single hip spica covers only one leg; a double hip spica, both legs; and a one-and-one-half spica, one entire leg and only the thigh of the other.

A *body jacket* is a plaster cast applied to the trunk. All extremities remain free.

COMPLICATIONS OF PLASTER CASTS

These complications include constriction of circulation, pressure sores and pressure paralyses.

Constriction of Circulation. This may result because the cast was applied too tightly or because it becomes too tight as a result of swelling of the tissues beneath it, usually at the site of the injury. The tendency toward postoperative swelling may be minimized by elevation of the extremity and early active motion of the digits but, despite these precautions, excessive swelling may occur.

Constriction of circulation must not be allowed to persist. Following the application of every cast to an extremity, continuing observation of the color, temperature and sensation of the toes or the fingers and the patient's ability to move them is mandatory. Some swelling is permissible, but cyanosis and decreasing sensation, range of motion and temperature, together with increasing pain, demand that the cast be split or bivalved and then spread to some degree.

To *split* or *univalve* a cast, it is cut through over its entire length either along the front or the side. To *bivalve* a cast, it is split on each side over its full length into two halves. Whenever a cast is split or bivalved, the underlying sheet cotton should also be cut as it can shrink after being wet with blood and constrict the circulation. A split or bivalved cast must be spread sufficiently to relieve the constriction of the circulation.

Pressure Sores (Decubitus Ulcers). These result from continuing pressure on bony prominences until necrosis of the soft tissue overlying them takes place. While special padding of bony prominences before the cast is applied is some protection, pressure sores may still occur. The most common sites are: in the lower extremity, the back of the heel, the malleoli, the dorsum of the foot, the head of the fibula and the anterior surface of the patella; in the upper extremity, the medial epicondyle of the humerus and the styloid of the ulna. With plaster body jackets or spica casts, the common sites of pressure sores are the sacrum, the anterosuperior iliac spines and the vertebral borders of the scapulae.

Pain at the location of a bony prominence is the warning symptom of an impending pressure sore. A patient with a fracture may be expected to have some pain even after it has been immobilized in a plaster cast. However, if the patient complains of pain, the surgeon and the nurse should make certain that the pain is at a site corresponding to the injury and not over a bony prominence. Too often, when a patient complains of pain, a p.r.n. medication is administered blindly without determining

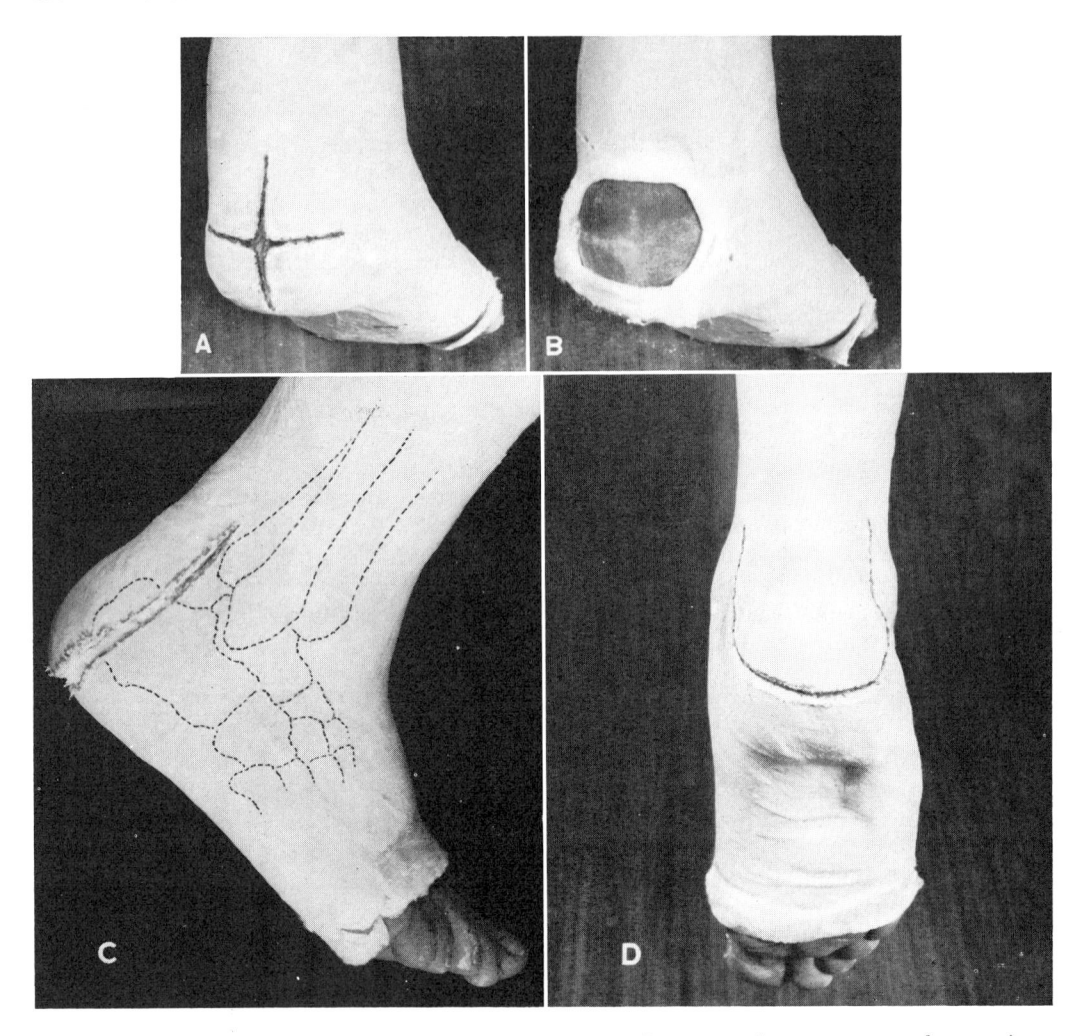

476 Fractures and Dislocations: General Considerations

FIG. 20-15. Methods of cutting plaster casts so as to relieve excessive pressure on the prominence of the heel. A. The cruciate incision over the pressure area. Each quadrant of plaster should be elevated slightly so as to relieve the point pressure in the center. B. The circular window for relief of pressure. This is a somewhat undesirable method as it creates a circular rim against which the heel must rest so that other pressure points may develop. The bulging soft tissue may become edematous and increase the pressure on the circular rim. C. and D. The flap or tongue method for relief of pressure. The long tongue is merely sprung backward. (Hampton, O. P., Jr.: Complications of common fractures. *In:* Hardy, J. D., and Artz, C.: Complications in Surgery. Philadelphia, W. B. Saunders, 1960)

that the pain is at a location which justifies it. This error can easily be avoided by having the patient definitely locate the site of his pain.

Pain over a bony prominence may be relieved and the danger of a pressure sore eliminated by cutting the cast at this point in a crisscross fashion followed by slight elevation of each of the four flaps of plaster (Fig. 20-15). Definitely, this method of relieving the pressure is preferable to the removal of a circular window which allows the skin to bulge through the opening and risks further pressure along the circular margin. Pressure on a bony prominence may also be relieved by cutting the cast over it so as to form a tongue of plaster which is then elevated slightly away from the bony prominence. Pressure sores are preventable complications, and they may be avoided by proper investigation and relief of pressure before necrosis of the skin and other soft tissue occurs.

Pressure Paralyses. These result from prolonged pressure on a nerve trunk, usually at a point where the nerve is rather superficial and overlies bone. Nerve paralyses may occur with little or no evidence of pressure necrosis to the overlying skin.

Paralysis of the peroneal nerve where it encircles the neck of the fibula is the most common nerve palsy in the lower extremity as the result of pressure. The counterpart in the upper extremity is an ulnar paralysis as a result of pressure where the ulnar nerve enters the ulnar notch on the medial condyle of the humerus.

Paralyses from pressure beneath a cast can be avoided by proper padding of the bony prominences and by molding of the plaster while it is setting so as to avoid carefully any pressure which might cause this complication. After the cast has been applied, complaints of pain at a site where a nerve trunk is superficial, accompanied by paresthesias down the course of the nerve as, for example, pain at the head of the fibula and paresthesias down the course of the peroneal nerve, demand that the cast be cut immediately so as to relieve all pressure in this region. As a general rule, pressure paralyses clear up spontaneously, but recovery may be slow. Often the fracture under treatment is firmly united long before the complicating pressure paralysis has disappeared.

REHABILITATION

Rehabilitation of the injured patient with a fracture begins the moment he comes under treatment. Active motion of all joints that do not move the fragments of bone should be carried out frequently. Active contraction of muscle groups which normally move the immobilized joints—for example, the quadriceps group in the thigh—should be carried out many times daily. As soon as the fracture is healed enough so that immobilization is no longer necessary, the contiguous joints should be mobilized. The patient's nutrition and morale must be supported, and he should be encouraged to return to work as soon as this is feasible.

(For Bibliography, see pp. 572 and 573, at end of Chap. 23.)

CHAPTER 21

OSCAR P. HAMPTON, JR., M.D., AND WILLIAM T. FITTS, JR., M.D.

Fractures and Dislocations of the Upper Extremity

Fractures and Dislocations About the Shoulder
Fractures of the Shaft of the Humerus
Fractures and Dislocations About the Elbow
Fractures of the Shafts of the Radius and the Ulna
Fractures and Dislocations About the Wrist

The hand always must be considered carefully in the management of any fracture of the upper extremity. All therapy is designed to safeguard or restore its function even at the cost of some deformity at the site of the fracture. Full length and perfect alignment of the bones of the upper extremity are desirable, but they are not essential in the upper as in the lower extremity. Mobility of the joints should be sufficient to permit the proper placement of the hand for its functions but only if this mobility can be obtained without impairment of the function of the hand. As stated by Mason, "nature has developed in the hand a finely co-ordinated motor and sensory organ which has made possible our present civilization."

FRACTURES AND DISLOCATIONS ABOUT THE SHOULDER

Skeletal injuries about the shoulder may be classified into (1) fractures of the clavicle, (2) fractures of the scapula, (3) fractures of the proximal end of the humerus, (4) dislocations of the shoulder and (5) acromioclavicular dislocations.

With each of these injuries, efforts must be made to avoid edema of the hand and to provide for active exercises of the fingers, measures of great importance in the preservation of hand function. As soon as practicable, pendulum exercises of the shoulder should be initiated in an effort to avoid or minimize restriction of motion in this joint (see Fig. 21-6 D).

FRACTURES OF THE CLAVICLE

The clavicle serves as a strut for the shoulder and holds it upward, outward and backward from the thorax. It is frequently broken, especially in children. The injury usually occurs as a result of a fall on the shoulder or on the outstretched hand. The clavicle usually breaks in the middle third, probably because its two curves join at this point. In a complete fracture of the clavicle with overriding of the fragments, the outer fragment, along with the shoulder, falls downward, forward and inward (Fig. 21-1, *top*); the inner fragment is drawn upward by the sternocleidomastoid muscle. The diagnosis of a fracture of the clavicle is made by clinical examination and an anteroposterior roentgenogram. A lateral roentgenogram of the clavicle is impracticable.

Treatment. All methods of management of fractures of the clavicle aim at holding the shoulder upward, outward and backward until the fracture has united. Actually, there is no completely efficient and comfortable way to do this; accordingly, a multitude of methods have been devised. Practically all employ closed reduction and immobilization by external splinting (Method 1). Open reduction and internal fixation is rarely indicated. A fracture of the clavicle is almost certain to heal solidly regardless of the position of the fragments. However, union usually occurs with some visible deformity which is accentuated by a visible and palpable mass of bony callus. In growing children, remodeling processes usually will eliminate the deformity and excess callus and restore normal size and contour of the bone within 6 months to a year.

Probably the simplest and certainly one of

the most effective ways of obtaining adequate reduction and splinting of a fracture of the clavicle is with a figure-of-8 clavicular strap, such as those furnished by several splint manufacturers (Fig. 21-1, *bottom*). The clavicular strap is easily applied about the shoulders and may be tightened or loosened repeatedly as indicated. With an assistant holding the shoulders in the hyperextended position, the entire strapping may be removed for cleansing of the axilla when indicated and then be reapplied.

Alternative methods of splinting for fractures of the clavicle include a figure-of-8 plaster cast about the shoulders, a clavicular cross or T-splint and even a simple figure-of-8 roller bandage, all of which tend to hold the injured shoulder upward, backward and outward. Each may be used with good result. However, none has been found to be as simple and effective as the standard clavicular strap shown in Figure 21-1.

In children, greenstick fractures of the clavicle are common. No effort should be made to correct the deformity, which is usually one of upward (or superior) angulation. The fracture should be splinted as outlined above or with a sling and swathe bandage and allowed to heal with angulation. The deformity will be corrected rapidly as growth proceeds.

Fractures of the clavicle must be splinted until union has occurred. The time for union varies with many factors, especially the age of the patient. In children of 2 years, for example, the fragments may unite rapidly, i.e., in 2 weeks. In adults, it is advisable to maintain the strapping in place for 5 to 6 weeks although during the last week or two often it may be removed and reapplied by the patient at home.

Whatever the method of splinting selected for adults, stiffness of the shoulder must be prevented by early active exercises. This is not a problem in children. In adults, unless exercise of the shoulder is adequate, a stiff shoulder may produce symptoms long after the clavicle has united.

Fractures of the Scapula

Fractures of the scapula are uncommon. At times direct blows to the body of this bone produce comminuted fractures; blows to the point of the shoulder may result in fractures of the neck of the scapula. In fractures of the neck, the lateral fragment containing the glenoid is often driven medially and impacted firmly into the body.

Treatment. For fractures of the body, complicated treatment is not necessary. If the degree of pain requires some immobilization for its relief, the arm may be bound to the chest wall in a sling and a modified Velpeau bandage for a few days (Fig. 21-2). Then pendulum exercises should be started, followed shortly by active use of the extremity.

For the usual type of impacted fractures of the neck, the same regimen should be followed. Efforts to disimpact the fracture by lateral traction are not worth while. Excellent function of the shoulder may be obtained in these impacted fractures by minimal immobilization and early active exercise.

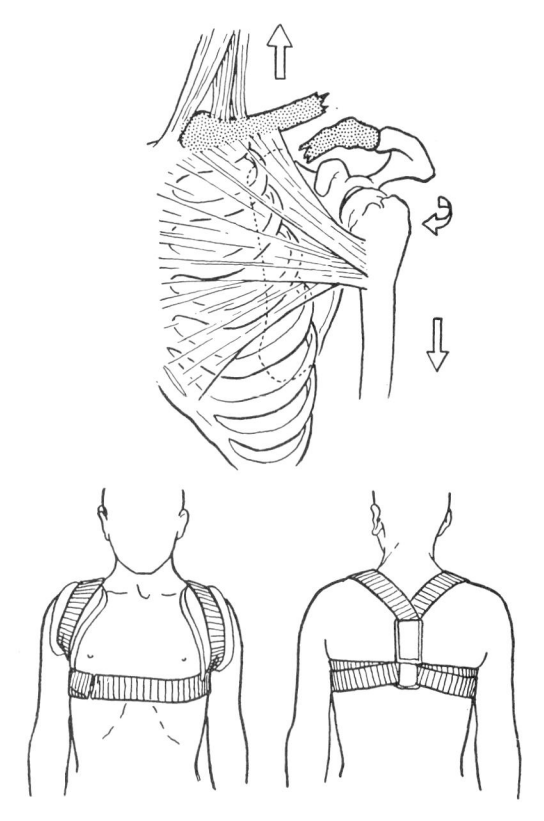

Fig. 21-1. Fracture of the clavicle. (*Top*) Anteroposterior view, showing typical displacement of midclavicle fracture. (*Bottom*) Method of immobilization with a clavicular strap.

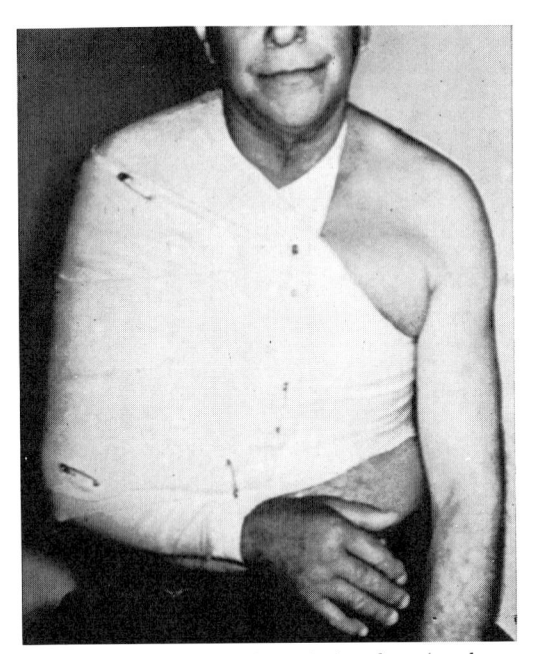

FIG. 21-2. Sling and swathe bandage (modified Velpeau). A sling is first applied in the routine way. Then, 4-inch stockinet, 5 yards long, is split and rolled so as to provide an 8-inch bandage. This is used to bandage the extremity in the sling to the thorax. The stockinet is pinned to the sling at several points.

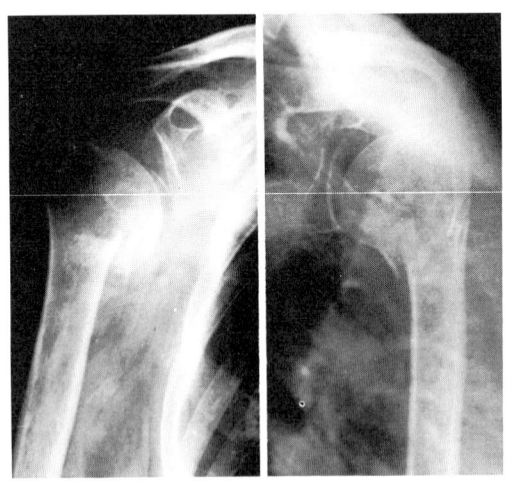

FIG. 21-3. Fracture of the neck of the humerus, adduction type. (*Left*) Anteroposterior view. (*Right*) Lateral view taken through the chest, the only method by which a satisfactory lateral view of the proximal humerus may be obtained.

In those fractures of the neck of the scapula which are not impacted but are badly displaced, lateral skeletal traction using a wire in the olecranon may improve the position of the fragments. This method of therapy keeps the patient recumbent. The surgeon must be sure that the traction offers enough improvement in the position of the fragments to justify the immobilization of both patient and extremity. Too often traction has been employed in such instances without actual improvement in the position of the fragments.

FRACTURES OF THE PROXIMAL PORTION OF THE HUMERUS

Fractures of the proximal portion of the humerus occur usually as the result of an indirect force. They are produced most often by a fall on the outstretched hand or arm in such a way that the head of the humerus is jammed against the glenoid and the overhanging, protecting acromion. The arm may be forced into abduction until either a fracture of the neck of the humerus or a dislocation of the shoulder occurs. A fracture occurring as the arm moves away from the body tends to be an abduction type fracture with medial angulation at the fracture site. On the other hand, if the breaking force is transmitted into the shoulder as the arm moves into an adducted position, an adduction type fracture with lateral angulation results (Fig. 21-3). Both abduction and adduction type fractures may have minimal or severe comminution and either may be impacted.

Fractures of the proximal portion of the humerus, although they may occur at any age, are found principally in the elderly. In the upper extremity fractures about the neck of the humerus are comparable in frequency with fractures about the hip in the lower extremity in the latter decades of life. Injuries in this region in children are more likely to be epiphyseal separations; they are discussed elsewhere (p. 482).

Treatment. From the standpoint of treatment, these fractures fall into 2 large groups: (1) those not requiring reduction and (2) those requiring reduction. Fortunately, the majority of fractures of the upper end of the humerus do not require reduction, as they are impacted fractures of either the anatomic or the surgical neck. Almost without exception, the position of impaction should be accepted and no effort made to disengage and improve the position of the fragments. The functional end results are better and are obtained sooner by accepting the position of impaction, even though the alignment is poor, than by breaking up the impaction in an attempt to improve the position, because the impaction permits very early exercises.

Impacted fractures of the proximal portion of the humerus are managed by Method 5—the no-immobilization method of management. In order to afford the patient some relief from discomfort during the first few days after injury, the arm may be supported in a sling supplemented by a modified Velpeau bandage (Fig. 21-2). Within a few days—at the most a week—the Velpeau bandage is removed, and soon after—never more than 10 to 12 days after injury—the sling is discarded. Pendulum exercises are initiated as soon as the patient will tolerate them, usually less than a week after injury.

With this method of management of impacted fractures of the proximal portion of the humerus, the patient is generally using the arm fairly freely within $2\frac{1}{2}$ to 3 weeks after injury. However, the patient must make continuous efforts to increase the range of motion during the following weeks and months. Obviously, with severely comminuted fractures of the upper end of the humerus and particularly in the aged, some degree of limitation of motion of the glenohumeral joint is to be anticipated. However, limitation of function will be less with the no-immobilization method of management, which permits early passive and active motion, than it would be with a method of management which immobilizes the shoulder for several weeks.

Unimpacted fractures of the proximal portion of the humerus in satisfactory position require no reduction and are managed by a regimen similar to that of an impacted fracture. It is advisable to leave the sling and modified Velpeau bandage in place for some 10 to 12 days after injury, at which time there will be sufficient fixation of the fragments to permit the substitution of a sling and the initiation of active pendulum exercises. Thereafter, management corresponds to that for impacted fractures.

Fractures of the proximal portion of the humerus which are not impacted and in which the fragments are displaced sufficiently to require reduction need a more complicated program. However, before embarking on such a program, the surgeon should be certain that the degree of displacement warrants efforts at improvement. Even though these fractures are near the shoulder joint, anatomic reduction of the fragments is not essential for the return of normal, or almost normal, function. An excellent end result can be obtained with what appears to be poor apposition of the fragments. Further displacement of the fragments from the position into which they are driven at the time of the injury usually does not occur, because the musculotendinous cuff of the shoulder and the tendon of the long head of the biceps muscle serve to retain them in the same relative position.

In displaced fractures of the proximal portion of the humerus, the proximal fragment usually will be drawn into abduction and external rotation by the strong muscles attached to the greater tuberosity, and the distal fragment will be drawn medially by the pull of the pectoralis major. At times a fragment of greater tuberosity will be drawn high into the shoulder by the supraspinatus tendon. Manipulative efforts at reduction of this group of fractures must take into account the cause of these displacements.

In some of these fractures a stable reduction may be obtained by manual traction and closed manipulation (Method 1). Traction on the distal fragment is made with the arm in some abduction against countertraction furnished by the pull of an assistant on a folded sheet looped through the axilla. Traction applied to the region of the elbow makes traction on the long head of the biceps which tends to overcome the abduction and external rotation of the proximal fragment.

If sufficient traction is maintained, the proximal end of the distal fragment usually can be forced outward so as to bring it into apposition with the proximal fragment. If the reduction is stable, apposition of the fragments may be maintained by the sling and the stockinet Velpeau bandage described above. In such instances, about 3 weeks of immobilization is needed to maintain reduction. Then pendulum exercises are initiated, either with the extremity free or with the forearm supported by a sling.

In other displaced fractures some form of continuous traction (Method 2) will be necessary to maintain adequate apposition and alignment of the fragments. This need may be demonstrated immediately after efforts at a manipulative reduction. Following manipulation, a roentgenogram is made with the arm held at the side and the forearm fixed across the abdomen—the position in which a stable fracture would be immobilized. Another roentgenogram is made with the extremity in the same position but with manual traction being maintained at the region of the elbow. By comparison of the 2 roentgenograms it can be determined whether traction affords better apposition and alignment of the fragments.

When traction is necessary, usually it may be adequately obtained and maintained by the use of a properly applied hanging plaster cast. The details of the application of such a cast and the maintenance, for a few days, of traction while the patient is recumbent are presented under fractures of the humeral shaft (see p. 487). The hanging cast, to be effective, requires that the patient be ambulatory. Therefore, when it is used, the patient must be able to walk or sit reasonably erect in a straight chair without resting the elbow. The hanging cast is a traction method—a type of Method 2, Continuous Traction—and not Method 1, Closed Reduction and Immobilization. A "collar and cuff" sling arrangement is an alternative to the hanging cast. The weight of the elbow region provides the traction on the proximal humerus.

The mechanism by which traction may improve reduction of displaced fractures of the proximal portion of the humerus is afforded by the "guy rope" action of the tendon of the long head of the biceps as it passes through the bicipital groove on the proximal fragment and continues downward alongside the distal fragment (see Fig. 21-6 A).

Traction in a hanging cast or collar and cuff sling is continued until sufficient union has been obtained to eliminate all danger of redisplacement and malalignment. During this time it is possible to carry out some degree of pendulum exercises for the shoulder by having the patient lean forward and allow the arm to abduct and rotate. Later, after removal of the cast some 3 weeks after injury, pendulum exercises are carried out.

In selected instances of displaced fractures of the proximal portion of the humerus, in which continuous traction is necessary, such traction may be provided as skeletal traction by means of a Kirschner wire inserted through the olecranon, or as skin traction by means of adhesive tape. Continuous traction may be employed with the arm abducted 90° and resting on the bed and with the forearm suspended toward the ceiling, or with the arm abducted 90° and forward flexed 90° so that the traction is in the direction of the ceiling. In such instances, the forearm is supported by a sling attached to an overhead frame.

Operative reduction (Method 3) is rarely indicated in these injuries, particularly in the elderly age groups. It may be indicated for severely displaced fractures in the young. Open reduction for this injury is usually an extensive operation and should not be selected lightly.

Fractures of the Greater Tuberosity. These fractures are seldom displaced unless they complicate a dislocation of the shoulder. Undisplaced fractures of the greater tuberosity are managed as impacted fractures of the upper end of the humerus and accordingly require very little treatment. Fractures of the greater tuberosity complicating dislocations of the shoulder may be a difficult problem. They are discussed below under dislocations of the shoulder.

FRACTURE-EPIPHYSEAL SEPARATION OF THE
PROXIMAL PORTION OF THE HUMERUS

Fracture-epiphyseal separations at this location usually occur in the second decade of life. Some have minimal displacement and require only immobilization with the arm at the side. In others, there is complete displacement with the shaft usually being drawn inward, upward and forward.

These injuries do not require an accurate reduction. Some angulation and displacement may be accepted with the anticipation of a good functional result and, unless the adolescent is too near maturity, correction of any deformity by growth processes. Efforts at closed reduction should not be too vigorous because of possible damage to the epiphyseal cartilage plate. If closed manipulation does

Fractures and Dislocations About the Shoulder 483

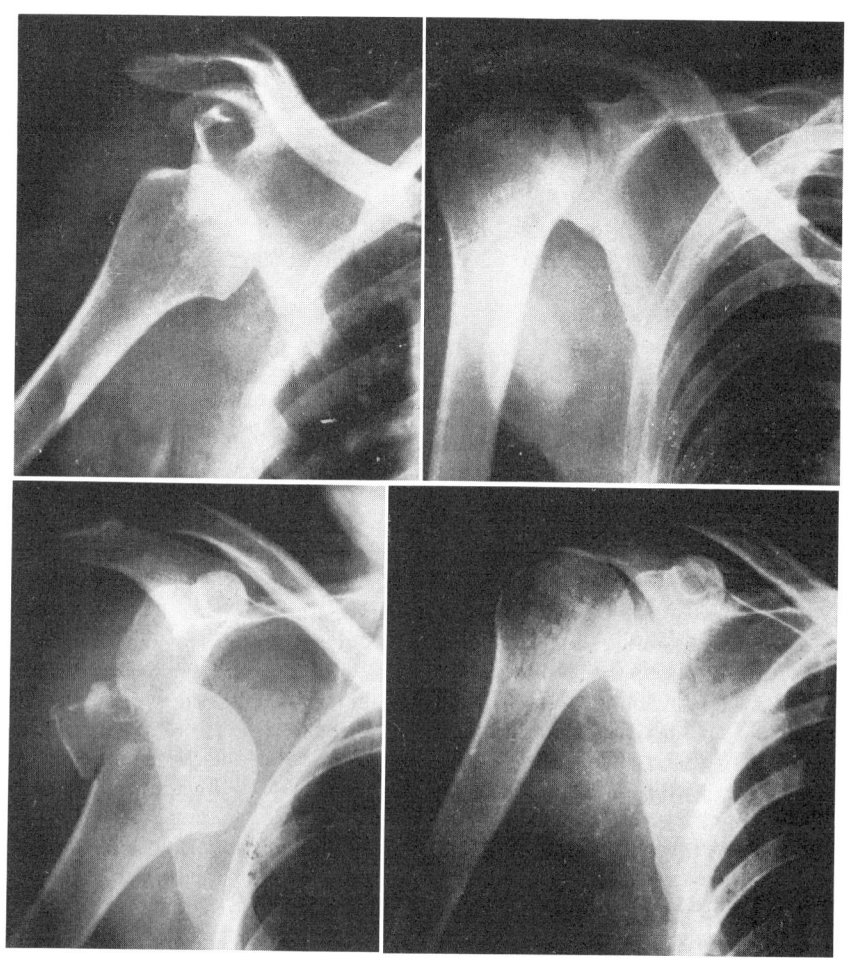

Fig. 21-4. Dislocation of the shoulder. (A, *top, left*) Roentgenogram of subcoracoid dislocation of the shoulder (the common type) without fracture of the tuberosity. (B, *top, right*) Roentgenogram after reduction. (C, *bottom, left*) Roentgenogram of fracture of the greater tuberosity associated with dislocation of the shoulder. (D, *bottom, right*) Postreduction roentgenogram, showing reduction of both fracture and dislocation.

not give a satisfactory reduction, open reduction is required.

Dislocations of the Shoulder

Dislocation of the glenohumeral joint is the most frequent dislocation of a major joint and occurs as a result of forced abduction and external rotation of the arm until the head of the humerus is levered downward out of the glenoid cavity. After the humeral head has torn through the inferior portion of the capsule of the shoulder joint, it may come to rest anteriorly beneath the coracoid process (Fig. 21-4 A) (subcoracoid dislocation, the most frequent position), beneath the glenoid (subglenoid dislocation) or posteriorly behind the glenoid (posterior or subspinous dislocation). The last is rare and is frequently difficult to diagnose. Posterior dislocation of the shoulder should be suspected when routine roentgenograms are not diagnostic of a skeletal injury but pain and restriction of motion indicate a significant injury about the shoulder. In posterior dislocation, the tip of the coracoid process may be prominent. Stereoscopic roentgenograms in the anteroposterior view and conventional vertical views may confirm the diagnosis.

Following anterior dislocation of the humeral head, the arm ordinarily assumes a characteristic position which strongly suggests the diagnosis. The elbow is held forward and is abducted from the side. It cannot be approximated to the side. If the hand can touch the opposite shoulder with the elbow touching the side of the thorax, it may be assumed that an anterior dislocation of the shoulder is not present, unless there is an associated fracture of the humerus. With the humeral head dislocated, the normal contour of the shoulder is lost and is replaced by a shallow hollow. This causes the acromion to be unduly prominent.

While these signs often permit accurate clinical diagnosis, and while occasionally one may be justified in attempting manipulative reduction without roentgenologic confirmation, it is good policy always to obtain a prereduction roentgenogram. This not only confirms the diagnosis but also shows whether or not there is a complicating fracture of the greater tuberosity or other bony injury in this region. Occasionally, it will reveal the distressing complication of a fracture of the neck of the humerus combined with dislocation of the humeral head. This grave injury is discussed below.

Treatment. Manual reduction of the dislocation of the shoulder may be accomplished at times without anesthesia or under sedation provided by morphine. General anesthesia may be employed electively or after reasonable efforts at reduction without anesthesia have been ineffective, provided that conditions for anesthesia are favorable. The relaxation provided by anesthesia usually makes reduction of the dislocation easy and minimizes the hazard of the manipulations causing a fracture of the surgical neck of the humerus or further soft tissue damage.

Technic of Reduction. Dislocations of the shoulder may be reduced in several ways. All methods attempt to return the head of the humerus to a point just inferior to the glenoid by traction and then by gentle rotations to cause it to re-enter the joint through the rent in the capsule. Each method offers advatnages and disadvantages.

In a great many instances reduction may be obtained without anesthesia (perhaps with an injection of morphine) by using the weight of the upper extremity to provide traction (Stimson's method). The patient is placed face down with the injured extremity hanging over the side or the head of the table. A weight of 8 to 12 pounds suspended from the wrist provides traction. This position is comfortable to the patient. Since pain is relieved, spasm of the shoulder muscles subsides. After the extremity has dangled in this position for several minutes, reduction may occur either spontaneously or after the shoulder has been rotated gently a few degrees by the surgeon.

Straight traction without manipulation will reduce the majority of dislocated shoulders. The traction may be made at the wrist with the forearm extended or at the elbow with the forearm flexed. Countertraction is provided by pull on a folded sheet passed through the axilla and resting against the upper lateral chest wall. Traction is made first in the line of the position assumed by the humerus, i.e., slight abduction. While the traction is maintained the arm is brought into slight adduction. If reduction is not obtained immediately, the arm may be rotated inward and outward a few degrees while traction is maintained.

If straight traction does not result in reduction, Kocher's maneuvers may be carried out. These are: (1) traction on the arm in slight abduction with the elbow flexed; (2) as traction is maintained the arm is rotated externally and then adducted; finally, (3) the adducted arm is fully rotated internally so that the hand lies over the opposite shoulder. Kocher's maneuvers must be carried out gently and carefully, with good anesthesia, lest a fracture of the humerus be produced, a tragic complication.

An alternative traction method is known as the Hippocratic maneuver (heel-in-axilla method). In this method the shoeless heel of the surgeon is forced in the axilla, thereby providing countertraction while straight traction is made on the extremity at the wrist with the elbow extended. The pressure of the surgeon's heel against the humeral head is thought to be of some aid in forcing it back into the joint. The method is hazardous and is not recommended. It may injure the axillary vessels and nerves.

Postreduction Management. Authorities

do not agree on postoperative management. Some consider immobilization of the arm and the shoulder of no value, while others insist on immobilization for 5 to 6 weeks. A middle-of-the-road course is 3 to 4 weeks of immobilization with the arm at the side, which may be provided by a sling and modified Velpeau bandage (Fig. 21-2). This is recommended for dislocations of the shoulder in individuals under 40 years of age, the age group in which recurrence of dislocation is the most common. For individuals over 40 years of age, a much shorter period of immobilization, 7 to 14 days, is recommended. Recurrent dislocation in the later decades of life is rare; therefore, all immobilization should be discontinued as soon as comfort of the patient permits, and active pendulum exercises should be initiated as a safeguard against stiffness of the shoulder.

Complications of Dislocations of the Shoulder. These include fractures of the greater tuberosity, fractures of the surgical neck with displacement, damage to the axillary nerve, damage to the axillary vessels and accompanying nerve trunks, and recurrent dislocation of the shoulder.

FRACTURES OF THE GREATER TUBEROSITY OF THE HUMERUS. This not infrequent complication of dislocations of the shoulder occurs in about 20 per cent of cases. In the majority of instances when the glenohumeral dislocation is reduced, the greater tuberosity falls into good position (Fig. 21-4 C, D). In such instances treatment of the dislocation is sufficient treatment for the fracture also. Subsequent displacement of the greater tuberosity need not be feared because the fact that the fragment fell into reduction indicates that the musculotendinous cuff of the shoulder is intact.

In those instances in which the fragment of the greater tuberosity is not replaced when the dislocation of the shoulder is reduced, a more vigorous course of management is indicated. The fragment usually will remain displaced superiorly, and this position indicates that the musculotendinous cuff of the shoulder has been torn. Unless the age and the condition of the patient contraindicate operation, open reduction (Method 3) is indicated. The fragment should be reduced accurately and fixed in position by suture or metallic internal fixation, and then the torn musculotendinous cuff should be repaired. Postoperatively, the course of management is the same as for dislocation of the shoulder without fracture.

FRACTURE-DISLOCATION OF THE SHOULDER. A displaced fracture of the surgical neck with a dislocated humeral head is a highly complicated injury. Efforts at closed reduction are frequently unsuccessful but they may be made carefully. The method of attempted reduction employs traction and countertraction by assistants while the surgeon manipulates the humeral head with his fingers. If reduction can be effected, subsequent therapy follows that described for displaced fractures of the surgical neck. The fracture usually goes into reduction easily if the head can be reduced by closed manipulation.

In the majority of instances, open reduction of the humeral head will be necessary. Actually, the chance of a successful closed reduction is so poor that the effort should be made only after arrangements have been completed to proceed immediately with open reduction, if necessary, under the same anesthesia. Even at operation, reduction is often difficult.

INJURY TO BLOOD VESSELS AND NERVES. Damage to the axillary nerve by the humeral head as it leaves the shoulder joint is a not infrequent complication of dislocation, occurring in about 15 per cent of dislocations. It will manifest itself first by anesthesia in the sensory distribution of the axillary nerve. Later, when it is possible to test the power of the deltoid muscle it will be found that this muscle is paralyzed. Fortunately, the prognosis of this complication is usually good. The nerve is usually bruised but not torn, and spontaneous recovery takes place as a rule. Even if it does not, operative efforts to find and repair the nerve are not considered worthwhile.

Occasionally there is evidence of trauma to the axillary vessels and the large nerve trunks. Usually these are merely bruised and not torn, and any motor or sensory deficit may be expected to disappear spontaneously. Arterial insufficiency persisting after reduction of the dislocation is an indication for immediate arteriogram and probable operative exploration. If anesthesia or paresis has not disappeared within 4 months the problem is neurosurgical.

RECURRENT DISLOCATION OF THE SHOULDER. This distinct clinical entity is, of course, a delayed complication of acute dislocation of the shoulder. The diagnosis is made when the patient finds that he sustains repeated dislocations with minimal trauma which forces the arm into abduction and external rotation. There are several theories concerning the cause of recurrent dislocation. The most prominent, that of Bankhart, holds that the original injury to the labrium glenoidale and the joint capsule commits the patient to the syndrome of recurrent dislocation. He states that the labrium glenoidale and the capsule are so torn away from the anterior inferior rim of the glenoid that repair does not take place and, therefore, redislocation occurs easily. DePalma holds that the trauma to the muscular apparatus, particularly the rotator muscles about the shoulder, results in a loss of tonicity and efficiency which predisposes to recurrent dislocation. Regardless of the underlying cause, recurrent dislocation may be disabling. It is a frequent complication during the first 3 or 4 decades of life and uncommon during the later ones.

When a fracture of the greater tuberosity complicates dislocation of the shoulder, recurrence of dislocation is most unlikely to occur. In other words, the presence of a fracture of the greater tuberosity is excellent evidence that the patient will not develop recurrent dislocation of the shoulder.

The treatment for recurrent dislocation of the shoulder is surgical. Several technics of repair are in general use. For a detailed description of them, the reader must consult more specialized texts.

ACROMIOCLAVICULAR DISLOCATION

Acromioclavicular dislocations or separations result from falls on the point of the shoulder. They may be either complete or incomplete. Complete lesions are described as complete dislocations or separations (Fig. 21-5, *top*). Incomplete lesions are called incomplete dislocations or subluxations.

The stability of the acromioclavicular joint depends upon the strong coracoclavicular and the acromioclavicular ligaments. In patients with complete dislocations, both of these are torn so that the outer end of the clavicle goes upward and backward. In incomplete dislocations or subluxations, the acromioclavicular ligaments are torn to some degree, but the coracoclavicular ligament is not torn, although it may undergo some stretching.

Treatment. Incomplete dislocations or subluxations require very little treatment. It is customary to attempt stabilization of the outer end of the clavicle with adhesive strapping over a felt pad applied just above the outer end of the bone and by a sling applied so as to lift the arm and the shoulder. Such measures are probably of little benefit, although they should be employed until pain about the injured joint has begun to subside. Prolonged immobilization is not necessary. The prognosis for an excellent functional re-

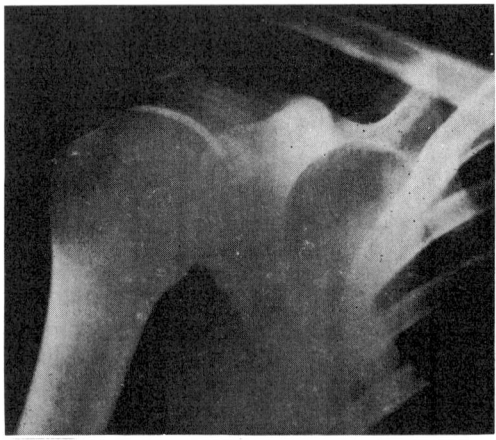

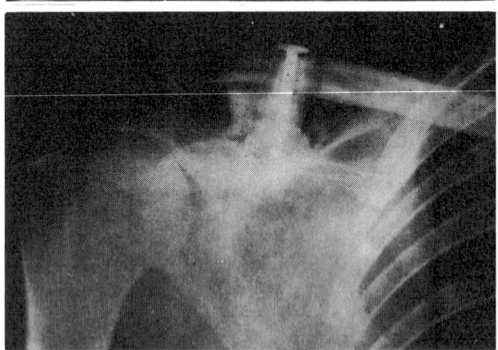

FIG. 21-5. (*Top*) Complete dislocation (or separation) of the acromioclavicular joint. (*Bottom*) Roentgenogram after operative reduction of a complete acromioclavicular separation. A lag screw passing through the clavicle and into the coracoid process stabilizes the reduction.

sult is good, although the outer end of the clavicle may remain somewhat loose and prominent in comparison with the opposite side. These lesions should be undertreated rather than overtreated.

Complete dislocations usually require operative management. Although many cumbersome pieces of apparatus and methods of immobilization have been described for non-operative management of these injuries, none is highly effective, and all are uncomfortable. With open operation, chips of bone and cartilage can be removed from the joint, and tags of torn ligament released and sutured. Some method of internal fixation which stabilizes the reduction must be employed. With operative stabilization, minimal external immobilization, no more than a sling, is necessary, and relatively early pendulum exercises may be initiated. With early operative stabilization of complete dislocations of the acromioclavicular joint, the end result should be a normal or near normal shoulder.

In selected instances of old unreduced dislocations of the acromioclavicular joint, excision of the lateral portion of the clavicle may give a satisfactory final result.

FRACTURES OF THE SHAFT OF THE HUMERUS

The shaft of the humerus extends from a level a short distance above the insertion of the pectoralis major muscle to the supracondylar level. This portion of the humerus has a less abundant blood supply than the regions of the head and neck and the condyles. A unique feature of the anatomy of the arm is the close proximity of the radial nerve as it partially encircles the humeral shaft in the musculospiral groove.

Fractures of the humeral shaft may be transverse, spiral, oblique, or comminuted, depending to some extent on the mechanism of injury. Obviously, these fractures may be caused in many ways, including a direct blow, excessive torsion, or undue leverage on the arm when the shoulder or the elbow is fixed.

Treatment. Despite the many ways these fractures may be caused, the several types which may be sustained, and the anatomic features tending to complicate management, the great majority respond highly satisfactorily to management in a hanging cast. This method, which at first glance appears to be an inadequate application of closed reduction and immobilization (Method 1), actually is a continuous traction method (Method 2) (Fig. 21-6). The hanging cast, applied with the elbow flexed to a right angle and extending from the level of the midhumerus to or including part of the hand, furnishes continuous traction by its weight as it hangs. The continuous traction causes relaxation of the several muscle groups tending to displace the fragments and, with the muscles relaxed, usually causes the fragments to drop into adequate apposition and good alignment. Obviously, the traction is really effective only when the patient is in the erect position. However, it is possible to provide some traction when the patient is recumbent as illustrated in Figure 21-7.

A satisfactory hanging cast usually may be applied without general anesthesia with the patient sitting on a stool or the edge of the table with the extremity held in the position in which it will hang later. The hanging position provides sufficient relief from pain. If general anesthesia is used, the cast should be applied with the arm as close as possible to the hanging position. The cast must not be so heavy that it will distract the fragments. A loop of plaster or wire at the wrist provides for a loop sling suspended around the neck, and another at the elbow provides for traction during periods of recumbency (Fig. 21-7).

During the first 2 or 3 weeks after application of the hanging cast, several check roentgenograms are made at intervals of 4 to 7 days to be certain that satisfactory reduction is being maintained. Anterior or posterior angulation at the fracture site is an indication to shorten or lengthen, respectively, the sling about the neck. Medial or lateral angulation can be corrected at times by moving the loop at the wrist inward or outward or by means of pads of sponge rubber or felt taped to the cast either on the inner side of the proximal end of the cast or at the inner side of the elbow as indicated. Sometimes to correct angulation of fractures at the junction of the middle and the lower thirds it is necessary to change the cast and provide either more pronation or more supination of the forearm and thereby change the direction of muscle pull on

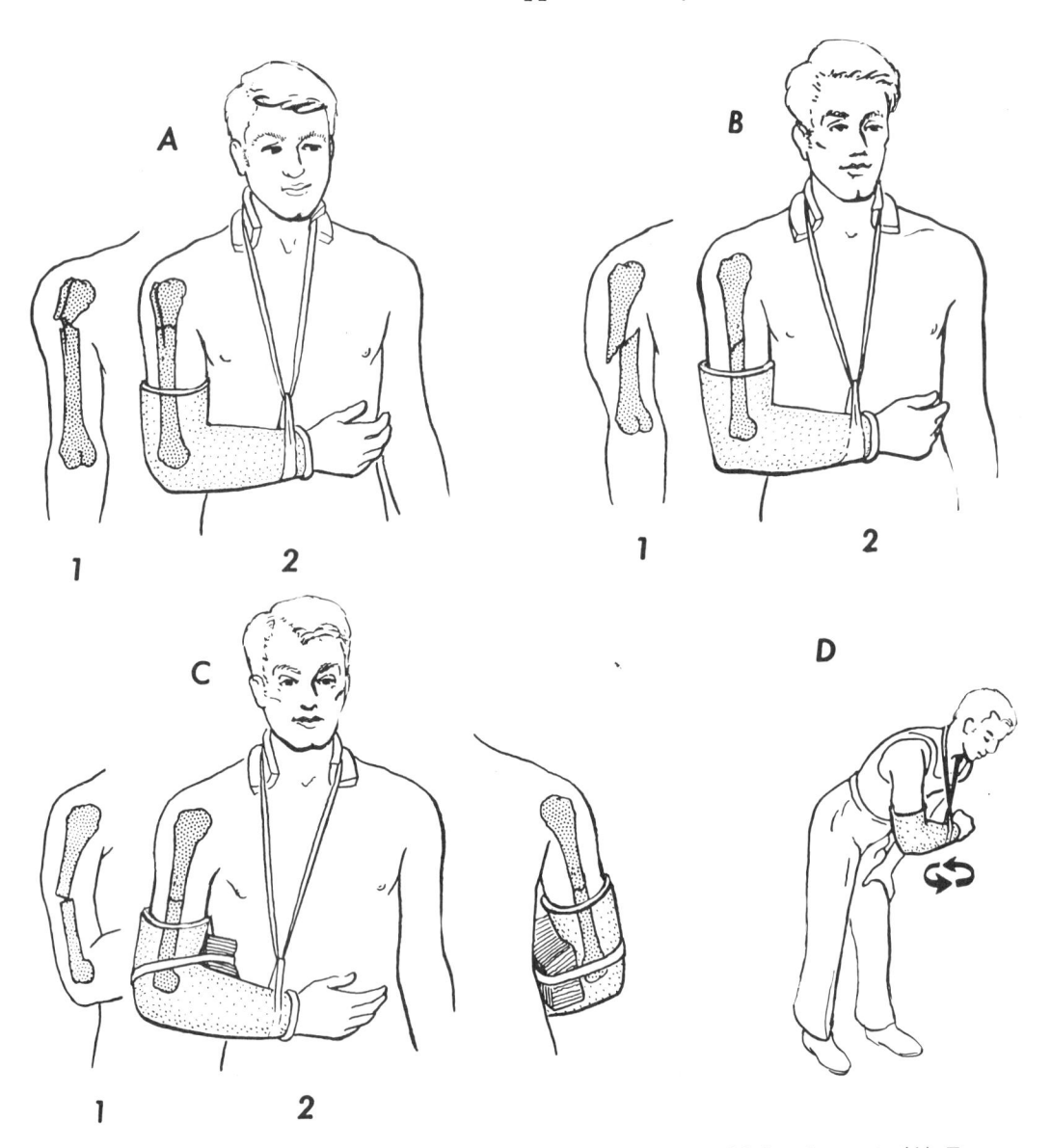

FIG. 21-6. Treatment of fractures of the shaft of the humerus with hanging cast. (A) Fracture of the proximal shaft: (1) abduction of proximal fragment and kinking of long head of biceps; (2) effect of application of hanging cast. (B, 1) Oblique fracture of midshaft with medial displacement and overriding; (B, 2) effect of hanging cast. (C, 1) Transverse fracture of humeral shaft with lateral angulation; (C, 2) after application of hanging cast with pad on medial side of elbow to correct angulation. (D) Circumduction exercises as shown.

the condyles. Occasionally, distraction of the fragments may necessitate substitution of a shoulder spica for the hanging cast.

As a rule, gentle swinging exercises of the shoulder should be instituted within a few days. If the patient leans well forward while the extremity remains suspended by the loop sling, the alignment of the fracture is not disturbed. The fact that these shoulder exercises can be carried out during the period of healing of the fracture is a distinct advantage of the hanging cast method, as other methods men-

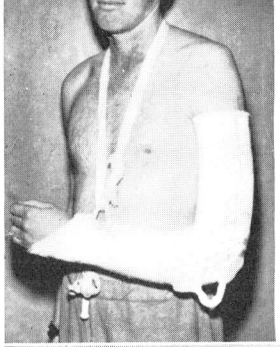

Fig. 21-7. Hanging cast for fracture of the humerus. (*Top, left*) Patient ambulatory. (*Bottom*) Patient recumbent with traction maintained. The cast should not extend as high as shown, but only to about the middle of the arm. (Hampton, O. P.: Wounds of the Extremities in Military Surgery. St. Louis, C. V. Mosby, p. 328)

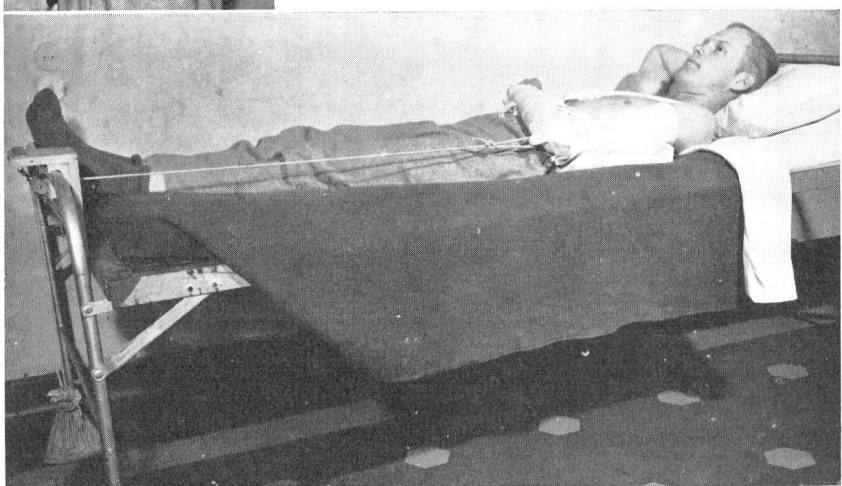

tioned below which do not permit these exercises often are followed by considerable stiffness of the shoulder joint.

Other methods which may be considered for fractures of the humeral shaft include a shoulder spica cast, skeletal or skin traction with the arm abducted from the side and with the forearm suspended from above, and open reduction and internal fixation. About the only indication for a shoulder spica cast is, as mentioned above, when distraction of the fragments results from a hanging cast. Skeletal traction (preferable) or skin traction may be necessary when other injuries or diseases confine the patient to bed.

Open reduction with internal fixation occasionally is indicated when traction methods have not resulted in adequate reduction. This situation may develop when there is interposition of muscle between fragment ends or when the action of certain muscles causing displacement and deformity cannot be overcome. Signs and symptoms of a radial nerve paralysis may indicate early open reduction (see p. 466). Open operation and internal fixation with an intramedullary nail may be the treatment of choice for pathologic fractures of the humeral shaft. Pain is relieved, and x-ray therapy can easily be given to the lesion.

When the hanging cast is used, it is left in place until there is sufficient clinical and x-ray evidence of union to make traction by the weight of the cast no longer necessary. Then a cravat or collar-and-cuff sling may be substituted until union is solid. The usual period for healing of fractures of the humeral shaft varies from 6 to 12 or more weeks after injury. When skeletal or skin traction in recumbency is used, it is continued until other conditions permit the patient to be ambulatory, and then a hanging cast or collar and cuff sling is substituted. When internal fixation is employed, supporting external splinting in some form is usually necessary.

Nerve Injuries. The close proximity of the radial nerve as it winds about the shaft of the humerus in the musculospiral groove makes it particularly susceptible to injury when a fracture of the shaft of the humerus is sustained. In addition, the median and the ulnar nerves are not too far removed from the humeral shaft, and occasionally one of these is injured by a sharp fragment of bone. As in all extremity injuries, at the first examination the surgeon must determine by physical examination whether there is any deficit in the sensory and motor functions of the major peripheral nerve trunks. This is easily done by having the patient carry out the various movements of the fingers and the thumb and also by testing for sensation on the hand. If there are signs of nerve paralysis when the patient is first seen, open reduction may be justified to appraise the extent of damage to the nerve and to make certain that it is free from impingement by the fragments, although the great majority will recover without operative intervention.

It also is important to retest the function of the major peripheral nerves, especially of the radial nerve, throughout treatment of the fracture and especially after the extremity has been placed in a hanging cast or in traction. Signs indicating new nerve damage suggest the possibility of trauma to the nerve during manipulation of the fragments and may indicate an early operation.

FRACTURES AND DISLOCATIONS ABOUT THE ELBOW

Fractures and dislocations about the elbow may be conveniently classified and discussed as (1) fractures of the lower end of the humerus in children, (2) fractures of the lower end of the humerus in adults, (3) fractures of the olecranon, (4) fractures of the head of the radius, (5) Monteggia or "parry" fractures, (6) dislocations of the elbow.

Fractures of the Lower End of the Humerus in Children

These common fractures of childhood may be classified as (1) supracondylar and transcondylar fractures, (2) fractures of the lateral condyle, (3) fractures of the medial condyle, (4) fractures of the medial epicondyle. Of these, the supracondylar and transcondylar fractures are by far the most common and comprise the typical elbow fractures in children.

Roentgenograms of the elbow of a child may be difficult to evaluate because of the many epiphyseal lines and ossifying epiphyses appearing successively as the age of the patient increases. The center of ossification for the capitellum, the first to appear, may be seen in roentgenograms at about 2 years of age. That of the medial epicondyle appears next, at about 5 years of age. The center for the trochlea becomes visible at about the 9th year, and that for the lateral epicondyle at the 12th year. These 4 centers fuse at about the age of 16 to form a single epiphysis which fuses to the shaft at about the age of 18. For the evaluation of roentgenograms of an injured elbow in a child, comparable views of the opposite uninjured elbow for comparison may be an invaluable aid to diagnosis.

One must remember that even though ossification of an epiphysis has not begun and cannot be visualized on roentgenograms, the unossified cartilage can be injured and produce growth disturbances later. What appears to be only a small fragment on the roentgenogram may actually be several times larger because of the nonradiopaque cartilage which surrounds it.

Supracondylar and Transcondylar Fractures. These similar injuries vary only in the exact level of the fracture. The transcondylar level is slightly lower than the supracondylar. From the clinical standpoint, they are customarily considered together and called supracondylar fractures. They usually occur from a fall on the hand with the elbow extended.

Supracondylar fractures are true surgical emergencies. Swelling about the elbow begins promptly and progresses rapidly. Once considerable swelling has developed, manipulative reduction and maintenance of reduction become difficult and perhaps impossible. Massive swelling is likely to result in extensive bleb formation which will handicap proper therapy. Early reduction before excessive swelling has occurred is therefore essential, particularly if the fracture is to be managed by close reduction and immobilization (Method 1).

As soon as the patient is seen and before any attempt at reduction of the fracture is made, the status of the radial pulse and the function of the major peripheral nerve trunks must be determined and recorded. *These valuable prereduction observations must never be omitted.*

TREATMENT. *Management by Closed Reduction and Immobilization (Method 1).*

Supracondylar fractures are preferably reduced by closed manipulation and held reduced in acute flexion (Jones position). Reduction is achieved as illustrated in Figure 21-8. The fundamental maneuvers are strong manual traction with the elbow in extension against equally strong countertraction applied to the arm by an assistant. Once the distal fragment has been unlocked and pulled distally by traction, lateral or posterior displacement, if present, is corrected by direct manual pressure. Then the elbow is flexed acutely. If the fragments have been reduced, acute flexion will maintain the reduction (Fig. 21-9).

Postreduction roentgenograms should be made before the elbow is immobilized. An important criterion of reduction is that in the lateral view the capitellum must extend well forward of the anterior margin of the humeral shaft. Another reduction must be attempted if the roentgenograms show faulty position of the fragments. Slight posterior displacement of the distal fragment may be accepted, but varus (inward) or valgus (outward) deformity resulting from lateral or medial angulation should be overcome if at all possible.

The degree of acute flexion which may be maintained safely is determined by the circulation of the hand. With a swollen elbow, flexion of the forearm may shut off the arterial flow and eliminate the radial pulse. The latter must be felt for at frequent, regular intervals. Only the degree of flexion of the forearm which permits a full radial pulse may be accepted. Moreover, the color of the hand must remain good as evidence that no obstruction of venous return exists. Such obstruction will lead to rapidly increasing swelling which eventually would obstruct the arterial blood flow. (See section on Volkmann's ischemic contracture below.)

The acutely flexed position of the elbow may be held in several ways. Circular adhesive (applied as several half circles) around the arm and the flexed forearm is highly effective. It is unyielding to later swelling, but if

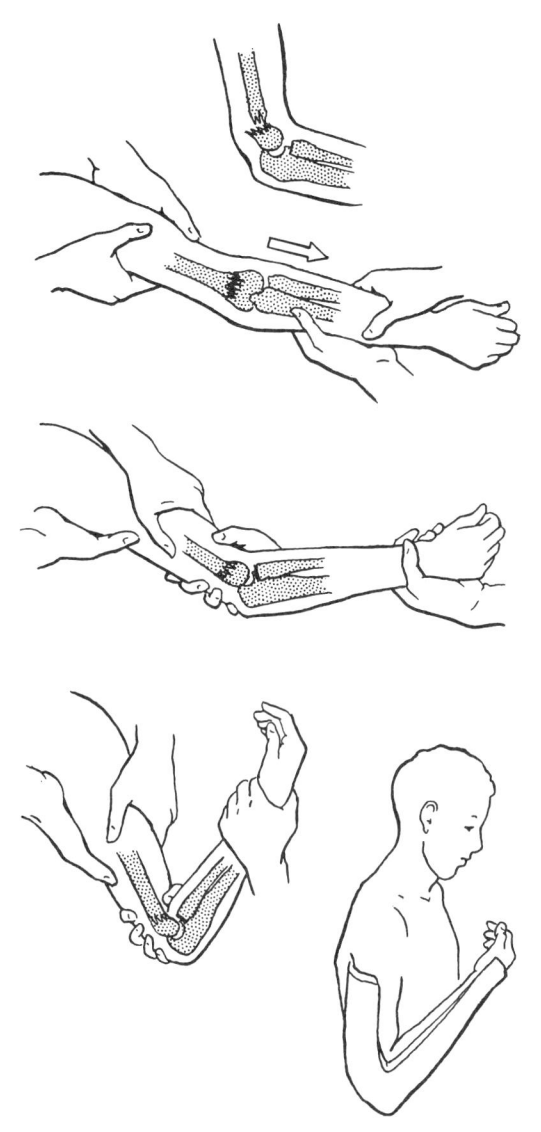

FIG. 21-8. Method of manipulative reduction of supracondylar fracture of the humerus. (See text.)

swelling becomes excessive, the degree of flexion can be diminished easily after cutting across the bands of adhesive. Then more adhesive can be applied easily in the new position without removing that which was applied originally. Instead of adhesive, a posterior molded plaster splint extending from the upper arm to the fingers may be used to hold the elbow in acute flexion. It is somewhat less effective than the adhesive strapping, as it

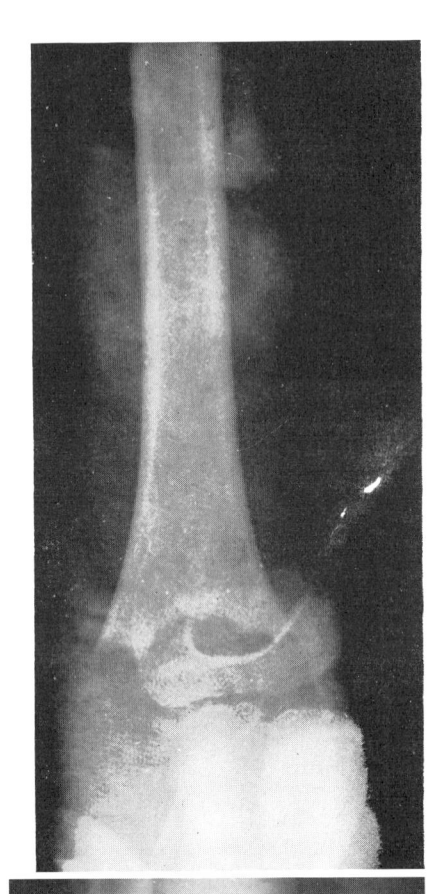

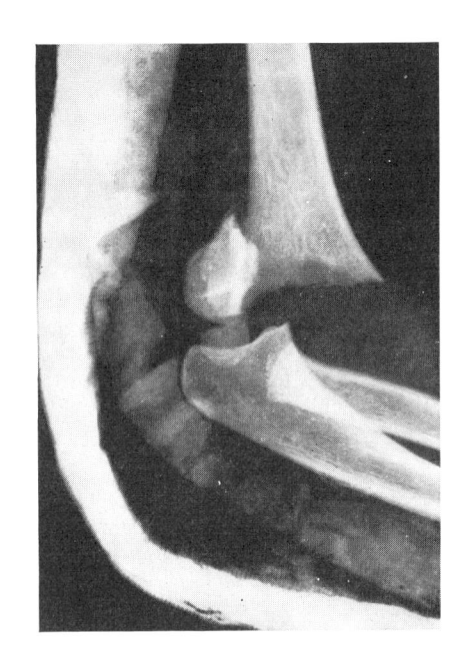

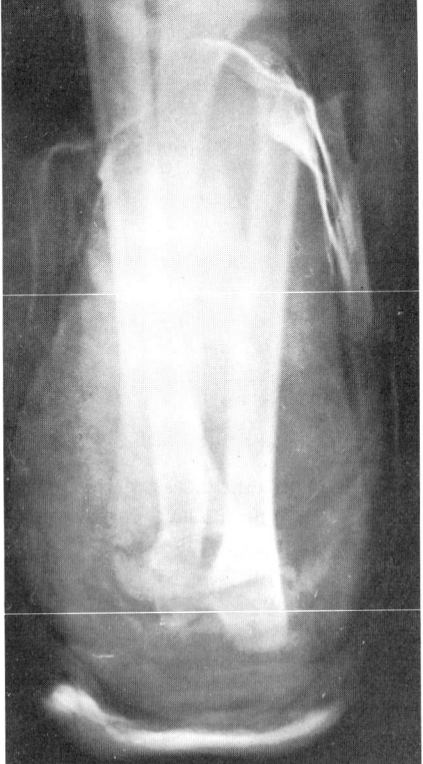

Fig. 21-9. Supracondylar fracture of the humerus. (*Top*) Anteroposterior and lateral roentgenograms before reduction. Note that the elbow is not in acute flexion. (*Bottom*) Postreduction views with elbow held in acute flexion by posterior plaster splint.

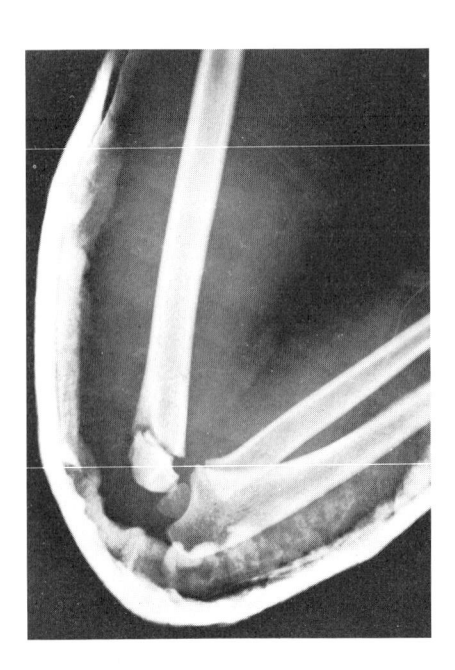

may break and permit the elbow to extend enough to allow displacement of the fragments. However, it does have the advantage that with severe postreduction swelling, some extension of the elbow may be accomplished by slight adjustment of the plaster or may even occur spontaneously as the force of the swelling causes the plaster to give toward extension.

Careful postoperative observation of the circulation is mandatory. If it becomes at all impaired, flexion of the forearm must be decreased until a strong pulse at the wrist is palpable, even if reduction of the fracture is lost. Ideally, the patient should be hospitalized for 2 or 3 days to gain the advantage of continuous and expert observation. Impaired circulation and its sequelae caused by the position of flexion are avoidable.

Volkmann's Ischemic Contracture (see p. 458). This dreaded complication of supracondylar fractures of the humerus in children results from impairment of the arterial flow to the forearm and the hand. The circulation may be obstructed as a result of hematoma and swelling from the injury itself or from flexion of the forearm on the arm to a point that occludes the circulation to the forearm and hand. The possibility of Volkmann's contracture and the importance of maintaining adequate circulation to the forearm and the hand must be kept in mind at all times throughout treatment of these injuries.

Management in Balanced Traction (Method 2). Manipulative reduction and immobilization in acute flexion will not suffice for all supracondylar fractures of the humerus. Some of the patients with this injury will arrive with elbows already so severely swollen that flexion sufficient to maintain a satisfactory manipulative reduction will obliterate the radial pulse. In others, postreduction swelling will impair the circulation and require the release of acute flexion.

When, for any reason, a satisfactory reduction of the fracture cannot be maintained with the elbow in acute flexion, a traction method is indicated. Dunlop's traction is an excellent method for this injury (Figs. 21-10 and 21-11). It is a form of balanced suspension skin traction which usually gives adequate reduction of supracondylar fractures of the humerus even though the forearm is extended to an

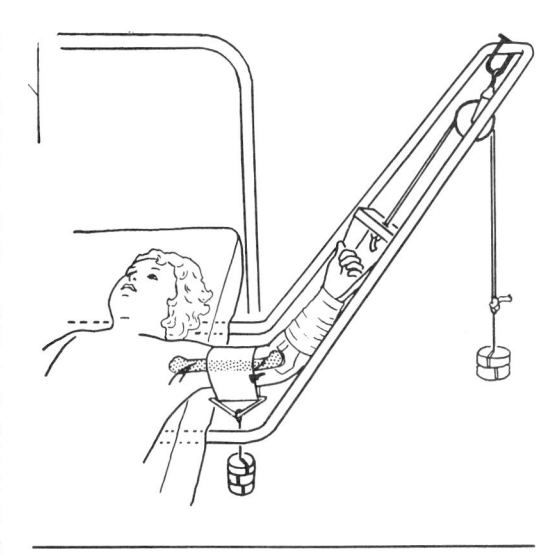

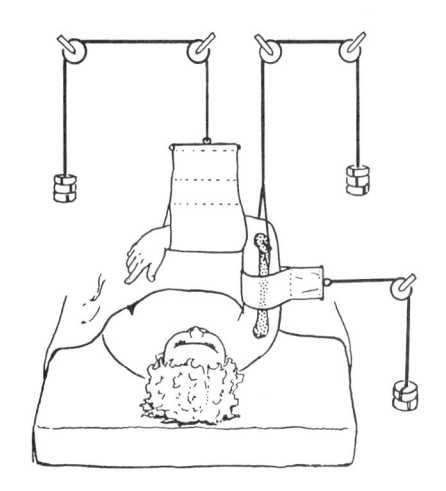

FIG. 21-10. Supracondylar fracture of the humerus. (*Top*) Dunlop's traction. The patient must lie near the edge of the mattress with the injured arm abducted so that it extends from the side of the bed. A loop about the arm which serves to make backward pressure on the proximal fragment may be easily constructed with a piece of felt threaded into stockinet. The skin traction on the forearm is applied in a direction which, with the aid of the weight attached to the loop over the arm, will maintain the elbow at about 135°. The amount of weight required to hold the arm down and that to make sufficient traction on the forearm each will vary from 2 to 4 pounds, depending upon the size of the patient. (*Bottom*) Skeletal traction with Kirschner wire through olecranon.

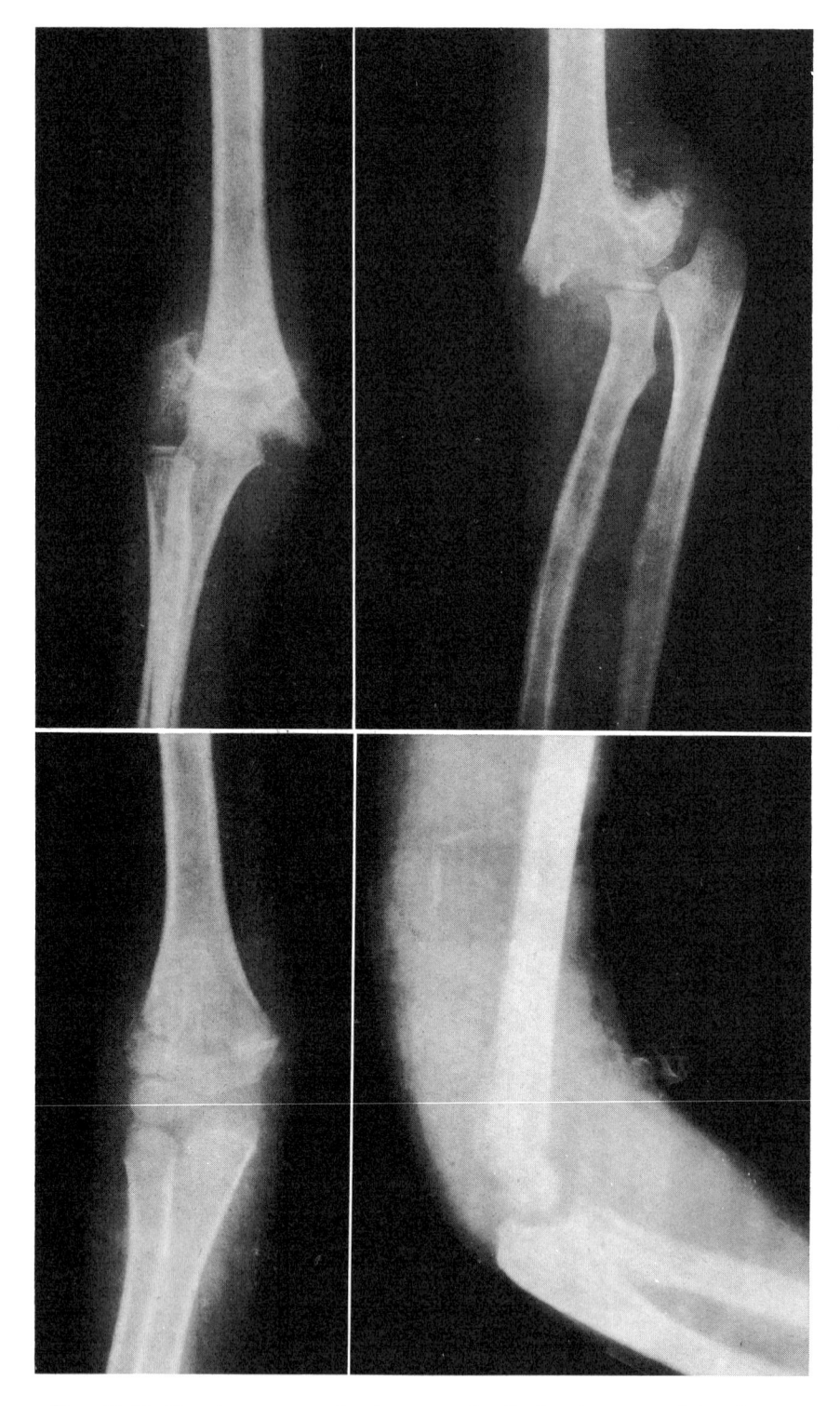

Fig. 21-11. Roentgenograms showing severely displaced supracondylar fracture of a child on admission and the position obtained promptly in Dunlop's traction. (*Top, left and right*) Anteroposterior and lateral views on admission to the hospital (*Bottom, left and right*) Position obtained promptly and maintained until fragments united, with no signs of embarrassment to the circulation of the extremity.

angle about 135°. In this position, circulation is almost never impeded.

The use of skeletal traction directed toward the ceiling with the patient recumbent, using a wire through the olecranon, is an alternative to Dunlop's traction preferred by many surgeons (Fig. 21-10, *bottom*).

Dunlop's or skeletal traction is unlikely to provide as accurate a reduction of the fragments as is usually obtained with a manipulative reduction but, even so, an adequate reduction is usually obtained and maintained, and the hazard of ischemia is avoided. Swelling will usually subside within 1 to 2 weeks, and then the extremity may be immobilized in acute flexion as described above.

Supracondylar fractures of the humerus in children unite rapidly. While displacement of the fragments can recur during the first week, displacement thereafter is most unusual if ordinary precautions are taken. The length of time during which the position of acute flexion must be maintained varies with the age of the patient. In children below the age of 3, acute flexion may be discontinued after 10 to 12 days, and even in children up to the age of 14 the position of acute flexion may be discontinued after 3 weeks. After the retentive apparatus is removed and the position of acute flexion discontinued, it is usually advisable to place the arm in a sling with the elbow at 90° for an additional 7 to 10 days. During this time some active exercises should be carried out. Thereafter full active use of the extremity is allowed. The child should be encouraged to flex the elbow actively to the limit several times daily in order that the range of flexion may be maintained while the ability to extend is being regained.

The ability to extend the elbow completely may return slowly. However, the prognosis for complete or practically complete extension is good. Passive stretching is dangerous and is likely to do more harm than good. Even the carrying of weights to help force extension is inadvisable. Strenuous passive efforts may produce more injury about the joint and may retard or perhaps permanently prevent full extension. Increase in elbow motion may be slow, and the limits of motion which are to be gained may take as long as 2 years.

Fractures of the Lateral Condyle. In fractures of the lateral condyle in children the fragment includes the epiphysis of the capitellum. Any displacement distorts the articular surface of the humerus and, in accordance with the fracture maximum that fractures involving articular surfaces require exact repositioning, this injury requires the most precise reduction. Only in this way can one hope to prevent subsequent growth disturbances with the sequelae of limited elbow function and possible late ulnar nerve paralysis. The latter may occur as long as 20 to 30 years after the original injury from progressive increase in the carrying angle and resulting stretch on the nerve. The carrying angle, usually 10° to 15° of valgus, is formed by the arm and the forearm when the elbow is extended.

The extensor muscles of the forearm attached to the lateral condyle tend to rotate the fragment to a variable extent. With full rotation the articular surface of the condyle may face the fracture surface of the humerus. The fragment must be returned to or near its normal position.

In undisplaced fractures of the lateral condyle immobilization of the elbow in moderately acute flexion for 3 weeks will prevent displacement and is all that is necessary. Aspiration of the hematoma from the joint will minimize pain.

In displaced fractures closed reduction is difficult but is occasionally successful; therefore, an attempt is often worthwhile. The earlier the attempts at reduction the better the chance of success. The surgeon should flex the elbow slightly and then adduct the forearm forcibly to widen the lateral side of the joint. Direct pressure of the thumbs on the fragment is made in an attempt to rotate the fragment backward into place. Fluoroscopic visualization is advantageous. If a satisfactory position cannot be obtained by closed reduction, early open reduction with fixation by sutures or a pin is advisable. Open reduction is usually indicated in displaced fractures of the lateral condyle, an exception to the rule that operative treatment of fractures is seldom indicated in children. Failure to achieve accurate reduction by some method will lead to the complications listed above.

Fractures of the Medial Condyle. Fractures of the medial condyle in children are less common than those of the lateral condyle. The fragment includes the epiphyses for the troch-

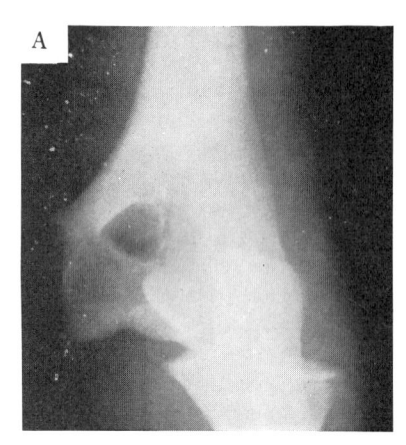

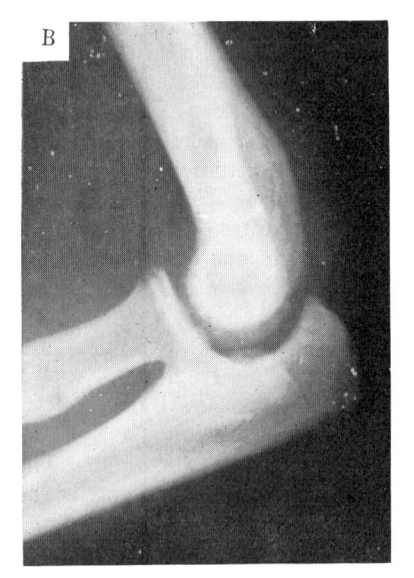

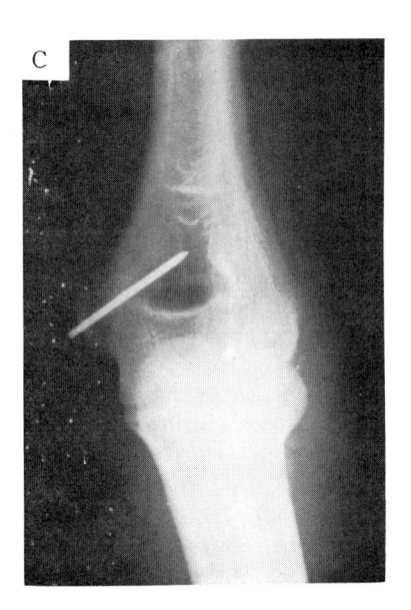

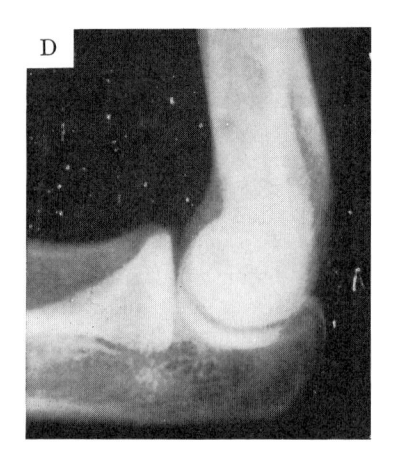

FIG. 21-12. Fracture of the medial epicondyle of the humerus complicating a dislocation of the elbow. (A) Anteroposterior view showing dislocation of the elbow and the displaced fragment of the medial epicondyle. Note the flat appearance of the medial condyle of the humerus and the epicondylar fragment displaced into the elbow joint. (B) Lateral view after reduction of the dislocation. Note that the medial epicondyle remains displaced into the elbow joint, a situation demanding open reduction. (C and D) Anteroposterior and lateral views after union of the medial epicondyle which was reduced at open operation and held by a small pin. The latter was cut short, flush with the bone, and allowed to remain in place permanently. (Hampton, O. P., Jr., and Fitts, W. T., Jr.: Open Reduction of Common Fractures. New York, Grune & Stratton, 1959)

lea and the medial epicondyle. Because the center of ossification for the epiphysis of the trochlea appears late, the size of the fragment is easily underestimated on the roentgenograms.

Management of this injury is comparable to that of fractures of the lateral condyle. For undisplaced fractures, immobilization in moderately acute flexion is sufficient. In displaced fractures, accurate replacement of the condylar fragment is necessary. If efforts at closed reduction are not successful, the fragments must be reduced by open operation and fixed with sutures or pins.

Fractures of the Medial Epicondyle. This injury of childhood and adolescence is really an epiphyseal separation rather than a true fracture. The common tendon of origin of the flexor muscles of the forearm arises in part from the medial epicondyle. When the epiphysis is avulsed, the entire tendon of origin may be torn also. When the tear is severe this muscle group tends to pull the medial epicondyle downward, at times into the joint cavity. This injury may occur at any time before the epiphysis for the medial epicondyle closes at about the age of 17 years. It is produced by a valgus strain at the elbow. It often

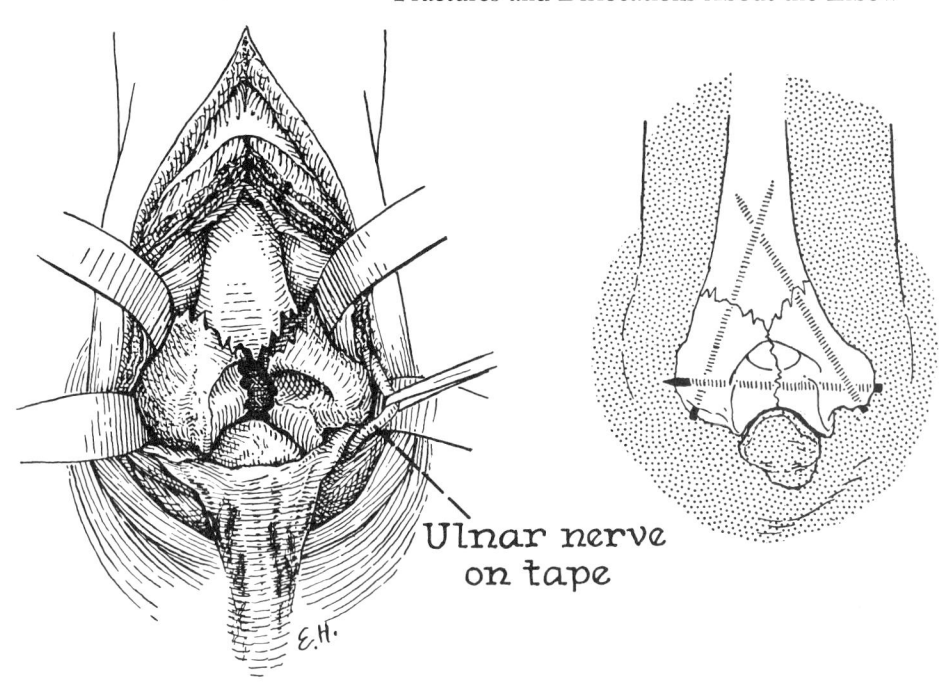

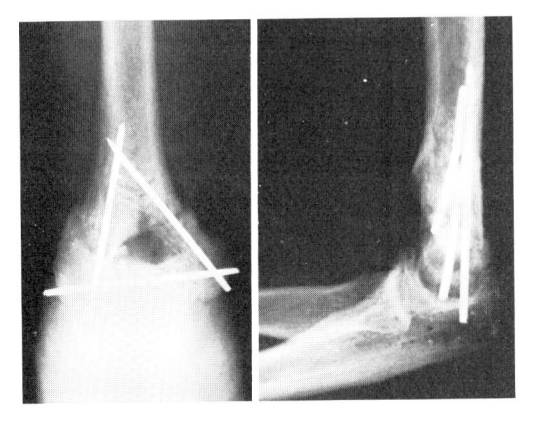

Fig. 21-13. Supracondylar T-fracture of the humerus in adults. (*Top, left*) Drawing to show displaced T-fracture of the lower end of the humerus and depicting the necessity for accurate reduction if the articular surface of the humerus is to be restored. (*Top, right*) Drawing showing internal fixation with multiple threaded pins. (*Bottom, left and right*) Anteroposterior and lateral roentgenograms showing "T" fracture of humeral condyles in an adult following open reduction and internal fixation with multiple threaded pins.

(*Top, left and right* from Hampton, O. P., Jr., and Fitts, W. T., Jr.: Open Reduction of Common Fractures. New York, Grune & Stratton, 1959)

complicates dislocation of the elbow. The ulnar nerve also may be damaged, particularly when the medial epicondyle is greatly displaced.

TREATMENT. With little or no displacement of the medial epicondyle, immobilization of the elbow in moderately acute flexion is sufficient. With considerable displacement as, for example, when the fragment is displaced into the joint, open operation must be performed and the fragment fixed with suture or pin (Fig. 21-12). If the epiphysis is displaced less than 1 cm., only immobilization is necessary, but if the displacement exceeds 1 cm. open operation is indicated. A careful repair of the torn tendon of origin is an important part of this operative procedure.

FRACTURES OF THE LOWER END OF THE HUMERUS IN ADULTS

For purposes of discussion, these injuries may be classified as fractures of the medial or lateral condyle, T-fractures of the distal humerus and fracture of the capitellum. Considerable comminution may accompany any of these types.

Undisplaced fractures in these groups require only immobilization in a plaster cast extending from the upper arm to the proximal palmar crease of the hand with the elbow at a right angle and the forearm, as a rule, in mid-pronation. In displaced fractures of either the medial or the lateral condyle or T-fractures involving both condyles, precise reduction is necessary to restore the articular surface of the lower end of the humerus. In some instances, adequate reduction can be obtained by closed manipulation and maintained by plaster cast immobilization as in undisplaced fractures. In some T-fractures, traction provided by a Kirschner wire through the olecranon or by a hanging cast may suffice to give adequate reduction. In most displaced fractures involving the condyles, including the T-fractures, open reduction with internal fixation is necessary before adequate apposition and alignment of the fragments can be achieved and maintained (Fig. 21-13).

Capitellum. Fractures of the capitellum comprise a unique group peculiar to the elbow. They are usually vertical fractures separating the anterior projecting capitellum from the remainder of the condyle. They are produced by forces transmitted through a fall on the outstretched arm and hand and often are associated with fractures of the head of the radius. The fragment is usually displaced forward and upward anterior to the humerus.

If the fracture of the capitellum is not displaced, only immobilization in a plaster cast is necessary. Large displaced fragments must be replaced, if possible, by closed manipulation, using traction in complete extension combined with direct pressure of the thumbs on the fragment. If reduction cannot be maintained with the elbow in flexion, complete extension may maintain the reduction. The advantage of keeping this difficult fracture reduced by extension outweighs the risks of stiffness from immobilization in extension. If closed manipulation cannot effect reduction, open operation is indicated (Fig. 21-14). Large fragments should be replaced and fixed in position by a pin. Small fragments should be excised.

FRACTURES OF THE OLECRANON

The olecranon is usually broken by a direct fall on the elbow, although it is possible for the injury to result from a fall on the outstretched hand with the elbow slightly flexed, which causes the tense triceps muscle to "snap" the olecranon over the articular surface of the humerus. Fractures of the olecra-

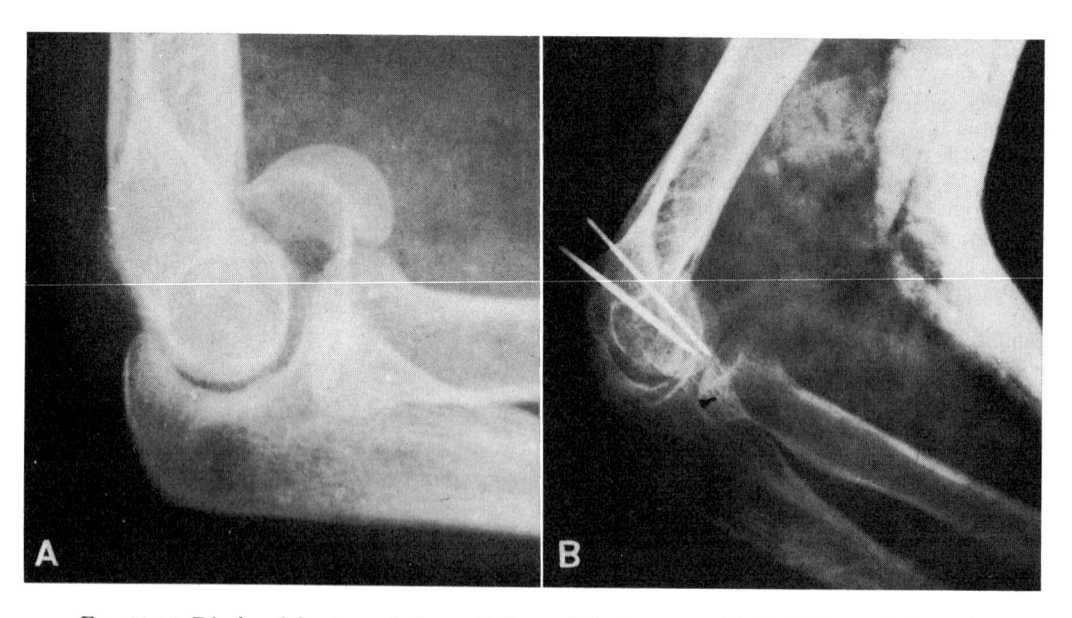

FIG. 21-14. Displaced fracture of the capitellum of the humerus. (*A, Left*) Lateral view, showing large fragment of the capitellum rotated and displaced proximally. (*B, Right*) Lateral view after open reduction and internal fixation with two unthreaded pins inserted from the posterior aspect of the lateral condyle. The pins were cut off just beneath the skin so that they could be removed easily under local anesthesia 4 weeks later.

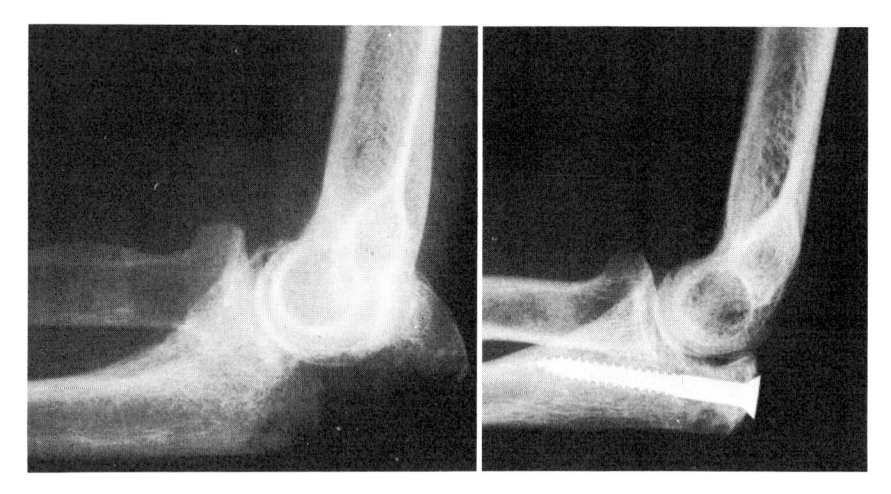

FIG. 21-15. Separated fracture of the olecranon. (*Left*) Roentgenogram taken before reduction. (*Right*) Three months after open reduction and fixation with a lag-type screw. Bony union is complete.

non are comparable with those of the patella in that each bone serves for the attachment of a powerful extensor muscle which also surrounds it. Just as the quadriceps muscle acts on the proximal fragment of the patella, so the powerful triceps muscle causes the proximal fragment of the olecranon to be drawn proximally.

Treatment. The objectives of management are to restore the extensor mechanism at the elbow and to maintain a normal range of motion of this joint. In undisplaced fractures of the olecranon, little active therapy is necessary. Since the fragments are not displaced, the tendinous expansion, including the fascial coverings of the olecranon, have not been torn, and subsequent displacement will not occur. The only treatment necessary is to apply a pressure dressing to the elbow and support the arm in a sling with the elbow at 90° for 3 or 4 weeks (Method 5).

In separated fractures of the olecranon, the best treatment is open reduction and internal fixation by means of a large stainless steel lag type screw, intramedullary pin or loop of strong malleable wire (Method 3) (Fig. 21-15). Some separated fractures of the olecranon may be reduced fairly well by closed manipulation and held in position with the elbow immobilized in extension (Method 1). However, this technic is unlikely to give a cabinetmaker's reduction of the articular surface, is likely to lead to considerable edema of the hand with some permanent restriction of motion of the fingers and may result in permanent loss of flexion of the elbow. For these reasons it is not recommended. Separated fractures of the olecranon are classical indications for the primary use of Method 3, the operative method of management. For severely comminuted fractures of the olecranon the fragments may be excised and the extension mechanism restored by suturing the triceps tendon to the periosteum and the fascia on the proximal part of the ulna.

Fractures of the Head and the Neck of the Radius

Fractures of the head and the neck of the radius usually are caused by a fall on the outstretched hand with the elbow in extension. The resulting force causes the radial head to be jammed against the articular surface of the capitellum. The injury causes limitation of motion of the elbow, pain on pronation and supination of the forearm and tenderness and swelling over the radial head. To determine the extent of damage, roentgenograms in several positions may be necessary, and even then the damage to the cartilage of the radial head and the capitellum often is not demonstrated.

Seemingly trivial fractures of the head and the neck of the radius can result in considerable disability. The head of the radius articulates both with the capitellum of the humerus (within the elbow joint) and with the proximal portion of the ulna at a groove along its radial surface. Malunion of fractures of the head of the radius or excess callus of fractures healed in good position can thus cause limitation of pronation and supination of the forearm as well as limitation of flexion and extension of the elbow. Fractures of the head of the radius, especially those associated with posterior dislocation of the elbow, may be complicated by ossifying hematoma.

Treatment. Fractures of the head and the neck of the radius either require practically no treatment, the "no immobilization" method (Method 5) or they require open operation (Method 3), depending upon the amount of displacement of the fragments. For fissure or

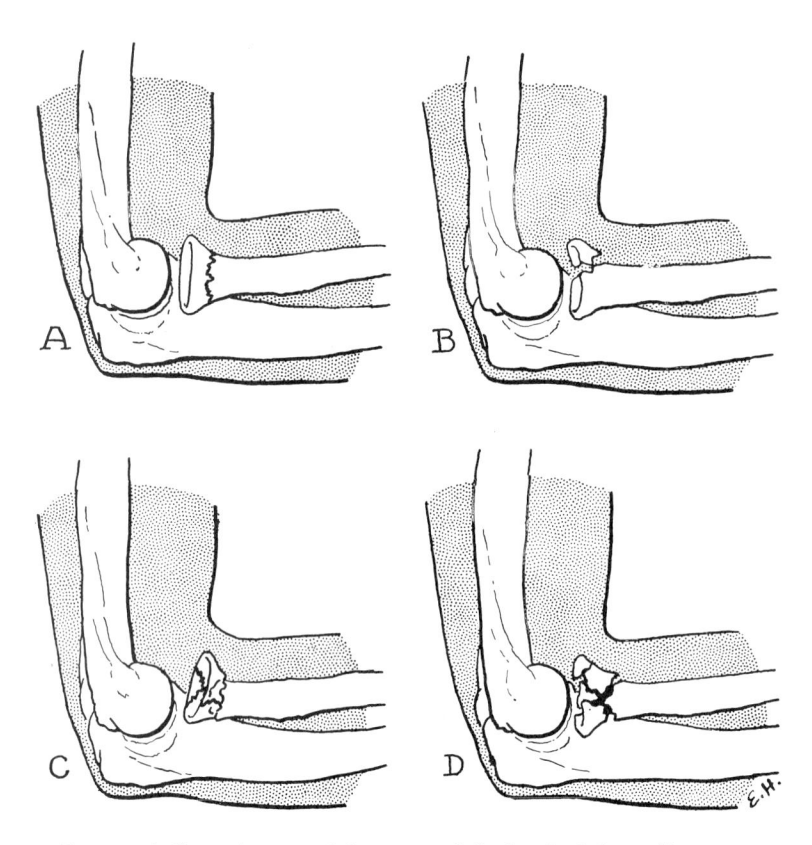

FIG. 21-16. Several types of fractures of the head of the radius.
(A) Undisplaced fracture which should be treated by early active motion of the elbow supplemented by aspiration of the joint.
(B) A small displaced marginal fracture of less than one third of the articular surface for which early operation is indicated. Because this line of fracture is away from the radio-ulnar articulation, merely excision of the small fragment is acceptable.
(C) Comminuted radial head with minimal displacement. Regardless, excision of the radial head is indicated, as much more distortion of the articular surface of the radius is always found at operation than can be seen on the roentgenogram.
(D) Severely comminuted fracture with gross displacement of the fragments. Excision of all of the fragments (the entire radial head) is indicated.
(Hampton, O. P., Jr., and Fitts, W. T., Jr.: Open Reduction of Common Fractures. New York, Grune & Stratton, 1959)

crack fractures of the head and for impacted fractures of the neck with little or no displacement or angulation and for small marginal fractures of the lateral surface displaced away from the joint, the "no immobilization" method is indicated. A sling and sedation will also afford symptomatic relief. Aspiration of the hematoma from the joint decreases pain and allows better motion. Early active motion of the elbow and the forearm is encouraged and, beginning several days after injury, may be aided by hot wet compresses to the elbow region.

For fractures of the head and the neck of the radius with displacement, open operation and excision of the radial head are required. Fractures requiring operation include comminuted fractures involving the articular surface of the head of the radius, marginal fractures of the head with displacement toward the elbow joint, large displaced fractures of the head including more than one third of the articular surface and fractures of the neck with significant angulation (Fig. 21-16). Operation and excision of the radial head should be performed as soon as is practicable, preferably within 1 or 2 days of injury. The entire radial head should be removed, and the neck made smooth. At operation, the injury usually is found to be more extensive than had been anticipated, and often there is evidence of injury to the articular surface of the capitellum. Following excision of the fragments, active motion of the elbow and the forearm is begun within a few days. In adults the disability following removal of the radial head is insignificant compared to that to be expected when such fractures are allowed to heal without operation.

In children excision of the radial head following fracture *is not indicated* because severe growth disturbances would follow. For fractures or epiphyseal separations with severe displacement, open reduction is performed, the epiphysis being replaced and impacted if possible. No foreign material is used for fixation of the fragments unless the reduction is not stable.

Monteggia Fractures

The term "Monteggia fracture" signifies a fracture of the ulna at about the junction of the proximal and the middle thirds and an associated dislocation of the head of the radius. The usual deformity is an angulation of the ulna toward the volar surface of the forearm with a forward dislocation of the radial head (Fig. 21-17, Left). However, a reverse Monteggia fracture can occur, with a dorsal angulation of the ulna and a posterior dislocation of the head of the radius. These injuries result from direct blows on the forearm, and as a consequence they are often open fractures. They are also known as "parry" fractures because the injury is often produced by attempts to parry blows with the forearm.

The dislocation of the head of the radius as an associated injury with a fracture of the shaft of the ulna has been overlooked frequently. This error has resulted because an obvious deformity of the ulna at the fracture site focused attention on this location, and roentgenograms did not include the elbow. It is technically easier, because a patient with this injury holds his elbow flexed, to make roentgenograms showing the bones of the forearm from just below the elbow down to and including the bones of the wrist. Such films

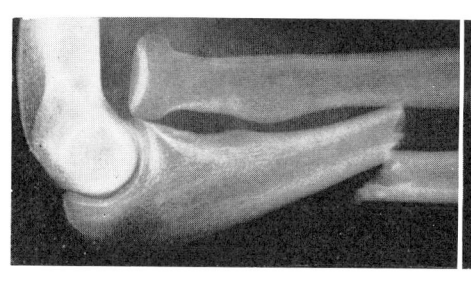

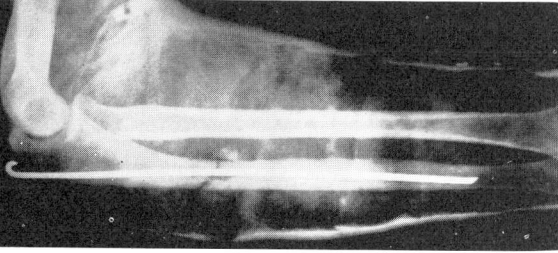

Fig. 21-17. Monteggia fracture. (*Left*) Lateral roentgenogram, showing anterior dislocation of head of radius and fracture of the shaft of the ulna at junction of proximal and middle thirds. (*Right*) Following open reduction of the ulna and fixation with an intramedullary nail. The dislocation of the radial head has been reduced.

show an angulated or overriding fracture of the ulna, but since they do not include the elbow joint, the dislocation of the head of the radius is not visualized. Such an error is disastrous.

The normal radius and ulna bear a constant relationship to each other at the elbow and at the wrist, and if either is intact and in position, it tends to prevent displacement of a fracture of the other. If one bone is broken so that the fragments override or are angulated to any degree, there must be either a fracture or a dislocation of the other. If, therefore, the shaft of the ulna is fractured with overriding or angulation of the fragments so that there is in effect a shortening of the ulna, then the radius is either broken or dislocated at its proximal or distal end. The radius would dislocate at the elbow because its attachments are weakest here. Conversely, if the radius is broken and is overriding or angulated, there must be a fracture of the ulna or a disturbance of its proximal or distal articulation. This would be at the wrist joint because its attachments are weakest here. This guiding principle should serve as a warning to the surgeon when he sees a fracture of the shaft of the ulna which is angulated or overriding. He then may know that there is an associated fracture of the shaft of the radius or a dislocation of the radial head and he must make certain that x-ray films show the elbow joint. As a matter of fact, an excellent principle of radiologic technic is that when the shaft of a bone is broken, enough films should be made to visualize clearly the entire bone and its articulations proximally and distally.

Treatment. Occasionally a Monteggia fracture may be managed by closed reduction and application of a plaster cast (Method 1). In such instances the contour of the fracture of the ulna must be so near transverse that when the fragments are brought into apposition, the reduction will hold, and the full length and alignment of the ulna will be maintained. With such a fracture of the ulna properly reduced, it is then possible for the dislocation of the head of the radius to be replaced by manual pressure over it. The extremity is then immobilized in a long arm cast with the elbow in at least 90° of flexion. Angulation of the ulna and redislocation of the radial head can take place in a cast. Therefore, serial roentgenograms at intervals of 5 or 6 days are necessary for a few weeks in order that such a situation may be detected promptly should it occur.

However, open reduction and internal fixation (Method 3) are indicated in most Monteggia fractures. With an intramedullary pin or a plate with screws, the ulna is stabilized in excellent apposition and alignment. This then usually permits closed reduction of the head of the radius (Fig. 21-17, *Right*). Subsequent immobilization of the extremity in a cast with the elbow at 90° will usually hold the reduction of the radius. If the radial head cannot be reduced adequately following stabilization of the ulna in reduction, the radial head must be reduced by open operation.

DISLOCATION OF THE ELBOW

Dislocations of the elbow usually result from falls on the outstretched hand with the elbow in extension. The forearm is hyperextended until dislocation, usually backward, results. The injury occurs both in children and adults. In adults, associated fractures of the coronoid process of the ulna and of the head of the radius are often present.

Reduction is usually easy with traction on the extended forearm against countertraction by an assistant on the arm. If the dislocation has been medial or lateral, it usually is first manipulated into the posterior position, and then traction is made. When the coronoid process becomes disengaged from behind the lower end of the humerus, flexion of the forearm on the arm will reduce the dislocation.

After reduction of the dislocation the elbow is immobilized at 90° by a cast extending from the upper arm to the proximal palmar crease of the hand. The cast is removed after 10 to 14 days to permit some active motion of the elbow, but full extension is avoided for an additional 2 weeks by the use of a sling as a precaution against redislocation.

FRACTURES OF THE SHAFT OF THE BONES OF THE FOREARM

Fractures of the shaft of the bones of the forearm are common fractures in childhood and not uncommon in adults. Either the ra-

Fractures of the Shaft of the Bones of the Forearm 503

dius or the ulna alone or both bones may be broken at any level.

The forearm presents distinctive anatomic features. It is the only segment of the extremities where one bone rotates around the other (pronation and supination). For proper functioning of the forearm, the interosseous space between the radius and the ulna must be preserved, and the relative length of each bone must be maintained (see p. 500). The radius is the most important at the wrist, and the ulna at the elbow. Each bone of the forearm actually serves to splint the other.

The displacement of fragments following fracture of the shaft of one or both bones of the forearm is the result of the action of muscles which control pronation and supination, and the surgeon must know the anatomy and function of these muscles if he is to manage fractures of the forearm properly. They are the pronator teres, arising from the medial condyle of the humerus and inserting near the mid-point of the radius, the supinator arising from the shaft of the proximal ulna and passing posteriorly about the proximal radius to insert on its anterior surface, the pronator quadratus in the lower forearm passing transversely from the ulna to the radius, and the

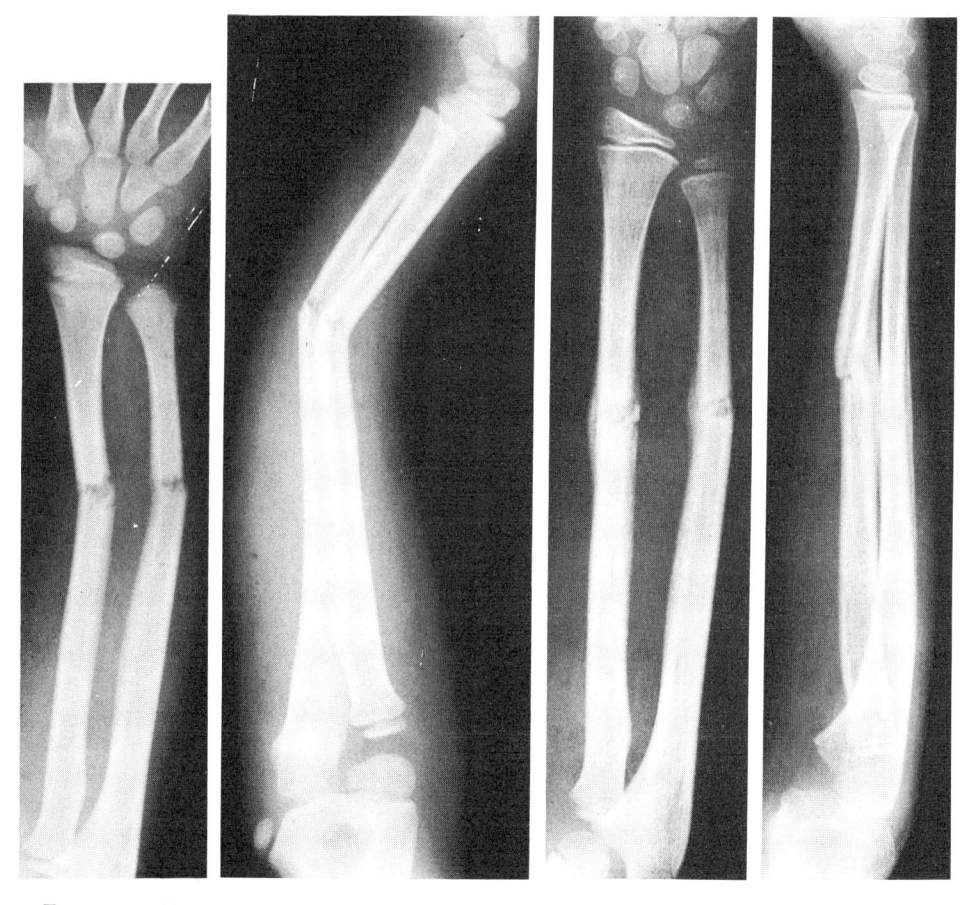

FIG. 21-18. Fractures of shafts of bones of forearm in a child. (*Left*) Roentgenogram of greenstick fractures of radius and ulna, anteroposterior view. (*Center, left*) Lateral view. (*Center, right*) Anteroposterior roentgenogram 1 month after closed reduction. (*Right*) Lateral roentgenogram 1 month after closed reduction. The slight anterior angulation of the radius is undergoing correction according to Wolff's Law.

2 muscles in the arm which act as supinators of the forearm, the biceps muscle inserting into the upper third of the radius, and the brachioradialis, sometimes called the supinator longus, arising from the external supracondyloid ridge of the humerus and inserting on the styloid process of the radius.

Relation of a fracture of the radius to the insertion of the pronator teres is highly significant in the deformity which results and the position in which the forearm must be immobilized to maintain reduction of the fracture. If the fracture of the radius is proximal to the insertion of the pronator teres, the supinating action of muscles described above is unopposed, and the proximal fragment of radius will be held in full supination, and the distal fragment will be held in pronation. To reduce and maintain reduction of such fractures, the forearm must be in full supination. In fractures of the radius below the insertion of the pronator teres, there is both pronator and supinator pull on the proximal fragment and, therefore, in theory at least, it will be held in mid-pronation. This means that such fractures are usually best reduced and immobilized with the forearm in mid-pronation.

Fractures of the Shafts of the Bones of the Forearm in Children

The majority of the fractures of the shaft of the bones of the forearm in children involve both the radius and the ulna. Fractures of the shaft of the radius alone are seen occasionally, but those of the ulna alone are rare and occur only as a result of a direct blow on the ulnar side of the forearm. Fractures of the forearm in children are usually greenstick of one or both bones (Fig. 21-18), although occasionally the fracture of one bone, usually the ulna, will be greenstick and that of the other complete with displacement and overriding. Not infrequently the fractures of both bones are complete and overriding.

For practical purposes, all of these fractures in children are managed by closed reduction and immobilization (Method 1). Open reduction is rarely, if ever, indicated (see Fig. 21-19).

In greenstick fractures, except for those with only minimal angulation, the surgeon should correct the deformity by a combination of traction and pressure against the point of angulation. While displacement of the fragments is to be avoided at all costs, there need be no hesitancy in completing the fracture (indicated by an audible and palpable snap) during the process of restoring alignment. When the fracture is completed and immobilized in good alignment there is no tendency toward recurrence of the deformity; whereas, when the fracture is not completed, angulation may recur in the cast as swelling subsides and the cast becomes loose. Following adequate reduction a long-arm plaster cast is applied from the upper arm to the proximal palmar crease of the hand with the elbow at a right angle and usually with the forearm in midpronation.

Anesthesia for children with greenstick fractures may be a problem. General anesthesia, while desirable from many standpoints, is hazardous unless the child's stomach is empty because of the danger of vomiting and aspiration with its dire consequences. If general anesthesia is used, it is best to wait for 8 or more hours after the last meal for the patient's stomach to empty. Actually, local anesthesia is not impracticable, and our recent experience indicates that it is applicable for the majority of these injuries. Of course, the child often resists and struggles, but, even so, adequate reduction of these fractures is often feasible without the hazards of general anesthesia.

When the fracture of one bone is greenstick and the other is complete and overriding, the problem of reduction is more difficult. For these general anesthesia may be necessary. The deformity of the greenstick fracture is first eliminated to restore full length of that bone and then, by a combination of traction against countertraction, leverage and direct pressure on the displaced fragments of the other bone, this usually can be brought into satisfactory apposition and alignment. Then a plaster cast as described above is applied.

In fractures in which both bones are displaced and overriding, reduction is still more difficult. Under anesthesia, by traction against countertraction, leverage and direct pressure, one bone is guided into reduction. Often the other will fall into reduction simultaneously but, if not, it then must be reduced by the same maneuvers. It is true that often the frac-

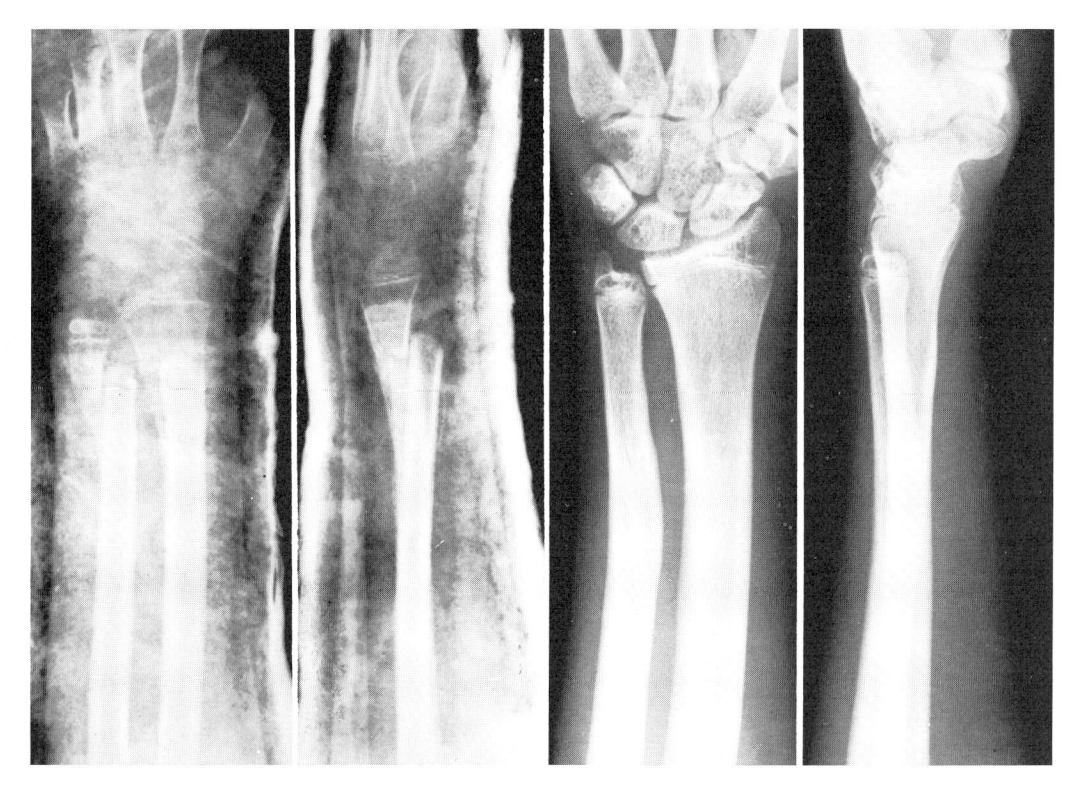

Fig. 21-19. (*Left*) Anteroposterior and lateral roentgenograms showing fractures of both bones of the forearm in a growing child, uniting in poor position. (*Right*) Anteroposterior and lateral roentgenograms taken 4 years later. A perfect anatomic and functional result was obtained. (Drs. Ward A. McClanahan and Charles K. Wier, Wichita, Kansas)

ture first reduced will become displaced again while the other is being forced into position. This may be difficult to prevent, but cognizance of the level of the fracture in relation to the insertion of the pronator teres and the actions of other muscles will aid in reduction, because the manipulations can be made with the forearm held in the right degree of pronation and supination.

While perfect apposition and alignment of the fractures of each bone are desirable, they are not absolutely necessary for a perfect functional result. At times it may be impossible to achieve complete apposition of the fragments of one bone or possibly of both bones. Even though malunion may follow, correction under Wolff's Law and a perfect end result may be anticipated (Fig. 21-19).

The board splint method of Key (Fig. 21-20) which is supplemented by a plaster cast may be highly advantageous in these injuries, not only in preserving the interosseous space but also in furnishing some degree of immobilization following the reduction during application of the plaster cast, thereby serving as a safeguard against redisplacement. The resulting cast appears bulky and cumbersome, but despite this, the board splint-plaster cast method of immobilization is worthwhile in managing these injuries, and it is particularly valuable to the surgeon who must work with relatively inexperienced assistance.

Fractures of the bones of the forearm in children usually require from 4 to 8 weeks of immobilization in the long-arm plaster cast, depending somewhat, of course, on the age of the patient. The younger the patient the more rapid is the rate of union. If the fracture of either or both bones is healing in any angulation, the plaster should remain in place until union is mature.

Refracture is especially common in frac-

Fig. 21-20. Two-board method plus a plaster cast for fractures of the shaft of both bones of the forearm in children. With the forearm supported so that the fragments of each bone of the forearm are in good alignment, a long board *slightly wider* than the forearm itself is applied to the dorsal surface from the elbow to the metacarpophalangeal joints with 3 strips of adhesive tape. Then, a short board of the same width is applied to the volar surface from the elbow to the wrist with 3 additional strips of adhesive tape applied at the same point on the forearm as the first 3. Finally, a long arm plaster cast is applied from well above the elbow to the knuckles. The boards aid in maintaining good alignment of the fragments while the cast is being applied. The compression of the soft parts provided by the boards serves to compress soft parts between the bones and thereby help maintain the interosseous space. Because *the boards are wider than the forearm itself* and are applied individually, circulation is not embarrassed. The 2-board method may be a valuable aid in proper management of fractures of the shaft of both bones of the forearm in children.

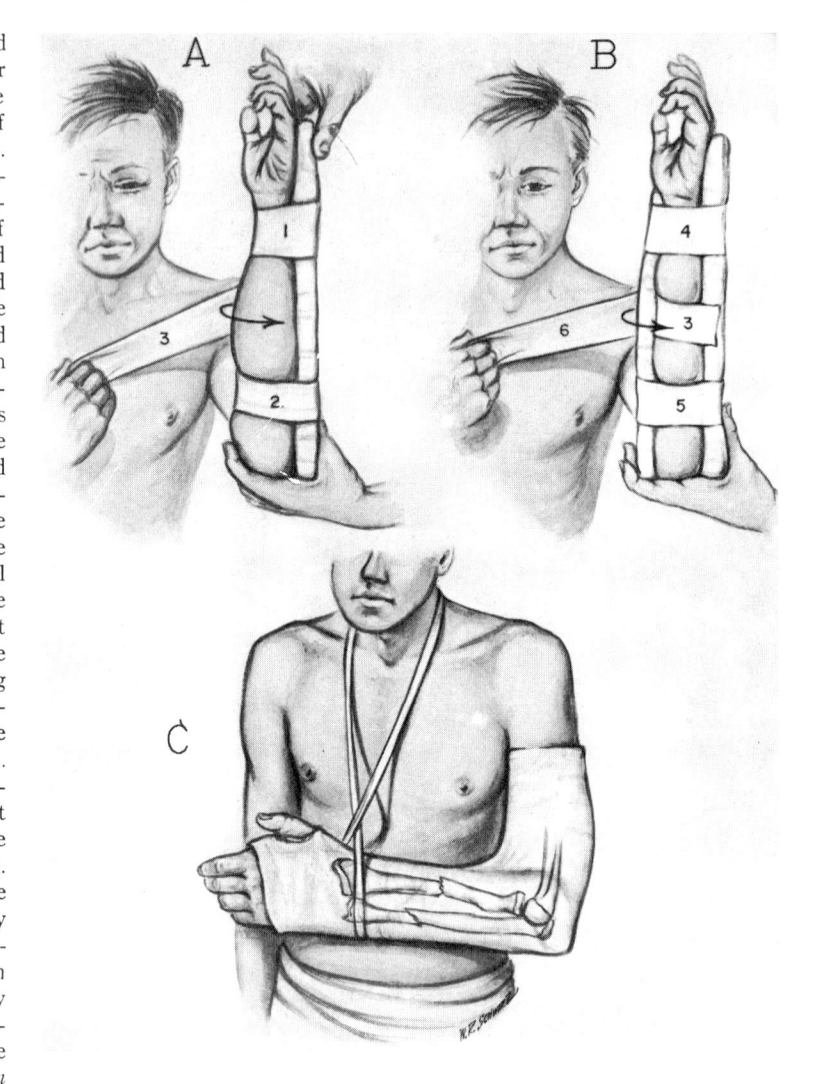

tures of the forearm in children, sometimes occurring years after the original injury, particularly if either bone shows any persisting angulation. For this reason, the parents of the child should be urged to minimize the risk of additional trauma to the part as much as is reasonable and until any angulation has been corrected by growth processes.

FRACTURES OF THE SHAFT OF THE BONES OF THE FOREARM IN ADULTS

Fracture of the Shaft of the Ulna Alone. This injury results from a direct blow on the forearm such as that described above in the production of the Monteggia or "parry" fracture. If the force is sufficient to angulate the fragments of the ulna significantly, the head of the radius must dislocate, producing a Monteggia fracture. It must be kept in mind, as outlined above, that with angulation or overriding of the fragments of the shaft of the ulna, the radius must either be broken or dislocated.

In fractures of the shaft of the ulna without fracture or dislocation of the radius, the fragments usually are not displaced, or if they are displaced, as a rule they are reduced easily by traction and manipulation. Following reduction the extremity is immobilized in a plaster cast extending from the upper arm to the proximal palmar crease of the hand with the elbow at 90° and the forearm in midpronation. Immobilization must be continued until the fracture has united, usually from 8 to 16 weeks, as fractures of the shaft of the ulna may unite slowly. Because of the relatively poor blood supply of the ulna, nonunion of these fractures is not rare.

Fractures of the Shaft of the Radius Alone. Fractures of the shaft of the radius without fractures of the ulna can occur at any level, but they are most common at the junction of the middle and the lower thirds. In fractures at this level, the pronator quadratus muscle in the lower third of the forearm usually pulls the distal fragment of the radius toward the ulna, a displacement which is difficult to overcome by closed reduction. Full radial length must be restored to prevent subluxation of the ulna at the wrist.

If the fracture is transverse, or near transverse, efforts at closed reduction are worthwhile. In some instances an excellent stable reduction will be achieved which can be maintained in a long-arm plaster cast. A plaster cast extending only to the elbow is *not* sufficient immobilization for this injury and must be condemned for any fracture proximal to the level of the Colles' fracture.

In many of these fractures at the junction of the middle and the lower thirds of the radius, the fracture line will be oblique so that a stable closed reduction cannot be achieved. Under these circumstances, open reduction and internal fixation of the fragments of the radius are indicated. Internal fixation may be obtained by an intramedullary pin or by a plate and screws. Because this fracture is an occasional site of nonunion, primary bone grafting supplementing internal fixation is likely to be advantageous.

Fractures of the Shaft of Both Bones. When both the radius and the ulna are broken in the adult, the fragments usually are displaced and overriding. Frequently, one or both fractures are comminuted. These fractures constitute a most difficult problem in management.

Efforts at closed reduction and immobilization may be successful in some instances. If the fractures are transverse so that when the fragments are brought into apposition and alignment the reduction will be stable, then efforts at closed reduction under general anesthesia are worthwhile and will be successful in some instances. Actually, the board splint method supplemented by the long-arm plaster cast described above, under fractures of the shaft of the bones of the forearm in children, may be highly advantageous in these fractures in adults.

However, in fractures of both bones of the forearm in adults, open reduction and internal fixation are often necessary. If there are no important contraindications, operative intervention is often selected primarily by surgeons experienced in the treatment of fractures. It affords accurate reduction of the fragments stabilized in reduction by means of intramedullary pins or plates and screws so that the position will not be lost later during the period of immobilization in a plaster cast (Fig. 21-21). It should be pointed out that nonunion of these fractures is not rare and, therefore, an effort to prevent this complication by supplementary bone grafting at the time of the open reduction and internal fixation is a worthwhile procedure.

Fractures of the bones of the forearm in adults do not unite rapidly, and immobilization must be maintained until the fragments are united—at least 12 weeks and usually longer. It must not be discontinued until there is clinical stability and x-ray evidence of solid bony union of both fractures.

FRACTURES AND DISLOCATIONS ABOUT THE WRIST

Skeletal injuries about the wrist may be grouped for purposes of discussion as: (1) fractures of the distal end of the radius, (2) fractures of the carpus and (3) dislocations of the carpus.

Fractures of the Lower End of the Radius

Fractures of the lower end of the radius are not only the most common fractures of the upper extremity but are also the most common fractures in the body in all age groups except small infants. Each is, to the

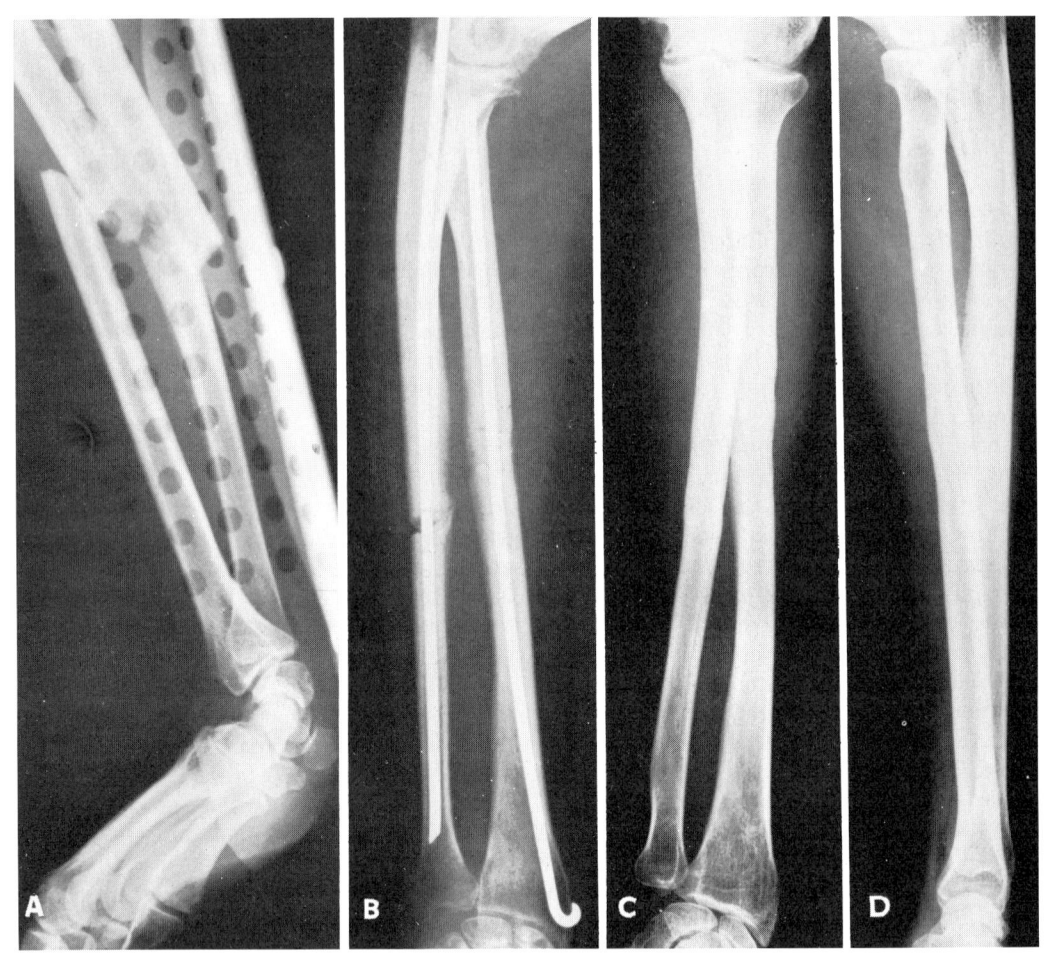

FIG. 21-21. Displaced fractures of the shafts of both bones of the forearm in adults managed by open reduction and internal fixation with intramedullary pins.

(A) Lateral roentgenogram, showing fracture of both bones of the forearm with displacement and overriding.

(B) Anteroposterior roentgenogram of bones of the forearm made immediately postoperative, showing excellent reduction of the fractures and stabilization with intramedullary Rush pins.

(C and D) Anteroposterior and lateral roentgenograms made after union of the fractures and removal of the intramedullary pins. Note that healing of the fractures has been obtained in perfect apposition and alignment.

(Hampton, O. P., Jr., and Fitts, W. T., Jr.: Open Reduction of Common Fractures. New York, Grune & Stratton, 1959)

laity, the typical "fracture of the arm" or "fracture of the wrist." These injuries may have an associated fracture of the styloid or at times of the distal end of the ulna. Even if bony injury of the ulna is not seen on a roentgenogram, the ulnar collateral ligament probably has been damaged. Management of the fracture of the radius suffices for any injury to the distal ulna.

Certain anatomic relationships of the distal ends of the bones of the forearm are important not only in determining the degree of distortion in each of these fractures but also in determining when a satisfactory re-

Fig. 21-22. Colles' fracture. (*Top*) Anteroposterior view: (*left*) showing typical displacement; (*right*) after reduction. (*Bottom*) Lateral view: (*left*) typical displacement; (*right*) after reduction.

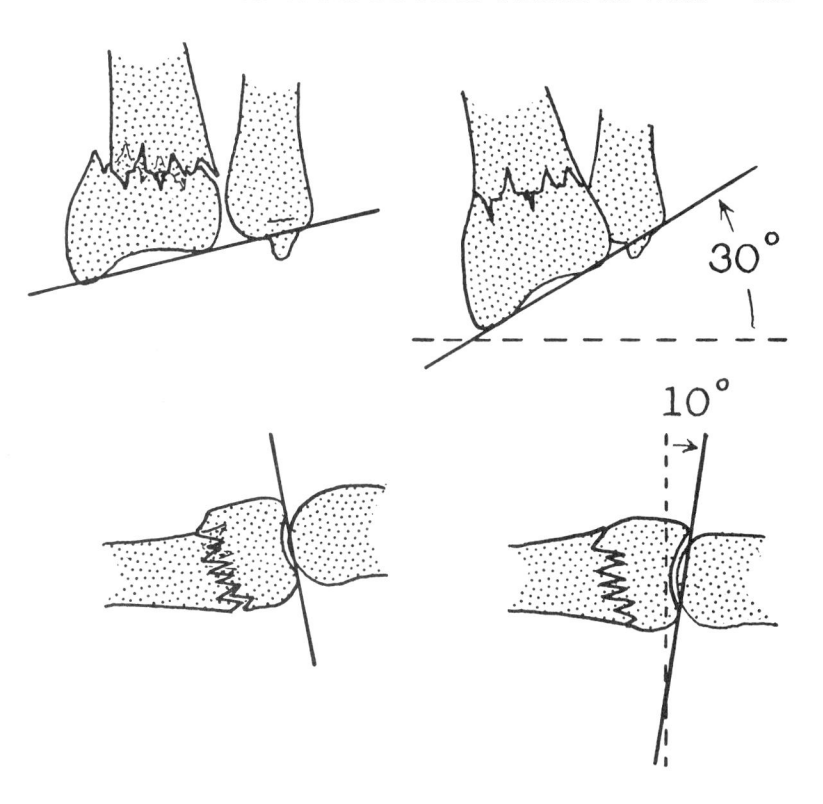

duction has been achieved. Normally, the tip of the styloid process of the radius extends distally about 1 cm. beyond the styloid of the ulna, and the distal articular surface of the radius is inclined toward the ulnar side of the hand at an angle of some 25° to 30°. These relationships, of course, are best observed in the anteroposterior roentgenogram of the wrist. The distal articular surface of the radius also inclines toward the palmar surface of the hand at an angle of some 10° to 15° as seen in the lateral roentgenogram. Unless the inclinations of the distal articular surface of the radius have been restored and full length of the radius has been regained, a fracture of the distal end of the radius has not been completely reduced (see Fig. 21-22).

Fractures of the lower end of the radius may be classified as hyperextension (Colles'), hyperflexion (reversed Colles' or Smith's), marginal (Barton's), and fracture-separation of the radial epiphysis.

Mechanism of Injury. Colles' fracture, Barton's fracture involving the posterior margin of the distal end of the radius, and fracture-separation of the distal radial epiphysis result from falls on the outstretched hand. Reversed Colles' (Smith's fracture) and Barton's fractures involving the anterior margin of the distal end of the radius result from a fall on the back of the hand forcing it into extreme flexion. In each of these fractures all degrees of displacement occur. In Colles' and reversed Colles' fractures, impaction of the distal into the proximal fragment may occur, or there may be severe comminution with lines of fracture entering the articular surface. In marginal fractures (Barton's fracture) displacement is usually not present or is minimal. Fortunately, in fracture-separation of the distal radial epiphysis in children, comminution does not occur.

Management. Closed reduction by manipulation is indicated in all except those that are undisplaced or only slightly displaced. As stated above, the objectives of reduction are the restoration of full radial length and the anatomic relationship of the distal articular surface of the radius. The fundamental maneuvers for closed reduction are strong traction against equally strong countertraction applied at the elbow with the forearm flexed, combined with manipulation of the distal fragment by pressure until it is brought into ex-

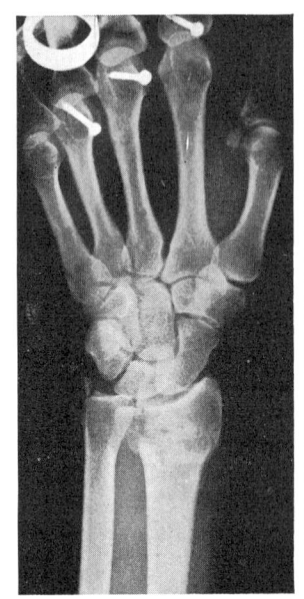

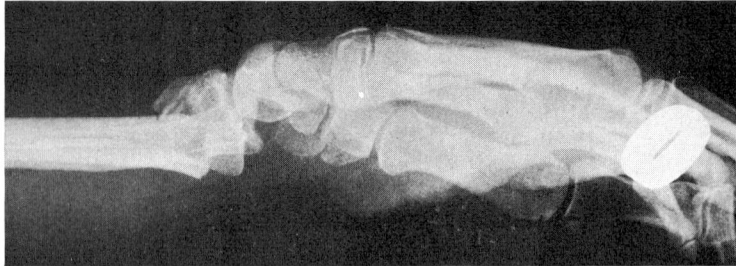

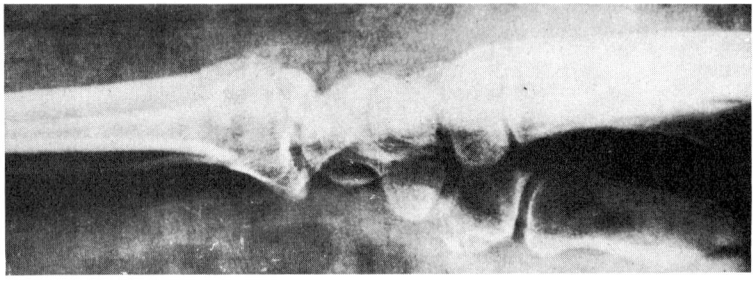

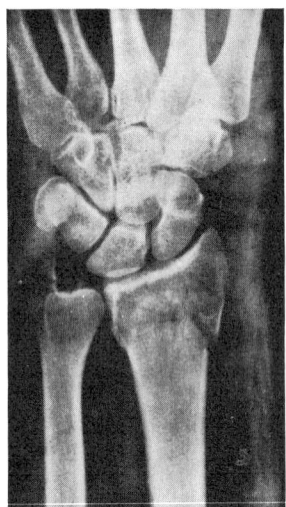

FIG. 21-23. Roentgenograms of Colles' fracture before and after reduction. Note normal inclination of articular surface of radius following reduction. (*Top*) Before reduction. (*Bottom*) After reduction.

cellent apposition and alignment with the proximal fragment.

Anesthesia, either local or general, must almost always be employed. Efforts at closed reduction without anesthesia, particularly in adults, are likely to lead to the acceptance of inadequate reduction because of the painful resistance of the patient. Local anesthesia using about 15 ml. of 1 per cent procaine injected from the dorsum into the hematoma about the fracture of the radius is highly satisfactory in all fractures treated within a few hours after injury. A few milliliters of procaine injected about the distal end of the ulna makes the local anesthesia more effective. Local anesthesia is less likely to be effective in fractures 12 to 24 or more hours after injury because the blood about the fracture site will have clotted, and the procaine diffuses poorly. There is, of course, no objection to the use of general anesthesia if the patient has an empty stomach which minimizes the risk of aspiration of regurgitated gastric contents.

COLLES' (HYPEREXTENSION) FRACTURE. This, the most common fracture of the lower end of the radius, gains the name by which it is commonly known because it was first described in detail by Abraham Colles in 1814. It occurs principally in the middle and the latter decades of life.

In a typical Colles' fracture, all of the relationships of the distal articular surface are distorted (Fig. 21-23). The distal fragment is driven backward and into radial deviation so that the articular surface inclines dorsalward and radially. Radial shortening is present. The distal fragment may be impacted into the proximal fragment with crushing of cancellous bone and it may be severely comminuted. The characteristic displacements result in what is known as a silver-fork deformity because of the analogy of the hump of the dorsum of the wrist to the hump of a silver dinner fork. The radial deviation of the distal fragment results in increased prominence of the distal end of the ulna.

Colles' fractures should be reduced as soon after injury as is surgically feasible. Closed reduction, as outlined above, is based upon a combination of traction and manipulation. In the usual closed reduction, the surgeon grasps the hand of the injured wrist in a handshake manner and applies traction while countertraction is provided by an assistant holding the lower arm just above the elbow with that joint flexed to about 90°. As the surgeon makes strong traction with one hand, he makes pressure against the dorsal surface of the distal fragment with the thumb of the other so as to force it into reduction. The hand is pulled in the direction of some palmar flexion and full ulnar deviation while the forearm is held in pronation. Reduction usually will have been obtained when the normal contour of the wrist has been restored and the tip of the styloid process of the radius extends distal to that of the ulna by about 1 cm.

The principles of traction and manipulation for closed reduction may be applied in another way. Traction may be applied to the hand in a strong steady fashion over a period of several minutes against equally strong countertraction. Strong pull on Chinese finger traps applied to the fingers is an acceptable way of obtaining traction in this method and makes application of plaster easier than when the hand is held by an assistant. After the fragments have become distracted as a result of traction the distal fragment of the radius is molded into reduction.

Following reduction, the wrist is immobilized with the hand in moderate palmar flexion and full ulnar deviation and with the forearm in pronation by either a lightly padded plaster cast or anterior and posterior molded plaster splints. Full palmar flexion, the so-called Cotton-Loder position, is to be avoided. Any advantage to be gained in maintaining a better reduction of a difficult fracture is far overshadowed by the hazard of edema and stiffness of the fingers, which cannot be exercised in this position, and by permanent restriction of motion in the wrist. Either the cast or the splints extend distally only to the proximal transverse palmar crease in the palm and to just behind the metacarpal heads on the back of the hand so that full motion of the fingers is possible. Ordinarily, the plaster is extended proximally to just below the elbow, although in comminuted fractures there is some reason to extend the plaster to the upper arm with the elbow at 90° and the forearm in pronation. Of course, in undisplaced fractures, immobilization is provided with the hand in the neutral position of slight dorsal flexion and ulnar deviation.

Check roentgenograms should be made as soon as the plaster has set (while the anesthesia is still effective) to make certain that adequate reduction has been achieved. If the reduction is not satisfactory, the plaster is removed immediately, and another closed reduction is attempted. While perfect reduction cannot always be obtained, certainly only the best possible reduction should be accepted. Reduction is measured by adequate apposition of the fragments, restoration of radial length and the proper palmar and ulnar inclination of the articular surface of the distal fragment.

The reduction achieved will not always be maintained even in a snug-fitting cast, especially if the distal fragment is badly comminuted. As swelling subsides, the immobilization is less effective, and some redisplacement of fragments may occur. Some telescoping of fragments often occurs, particularly in the aged. Therefore, it is advisable that check roentgenograms be made about the fifth postreduction day and, if all is well then, again about the tenth day. If some slipping of fragments has occurred, another reduction and cast may be indicated, depending upon whether the surgeon believes he not only can obtain but also maintain an improved position.

During postreduction management, objectives are to maintain a full range of motion of the fingers and the shoulder. Edema of the fingers must be minimized as much as possible. Measures to accomplish this include elevation of the hand almost constantly for a few days with strenuous exercises of the fingers. Throughout the period of immobilization, the patient must be encouraged to carry out a forceful full range of motion of the fingers. Similarly, the patient must repeatedly (every hour on the hour) put the

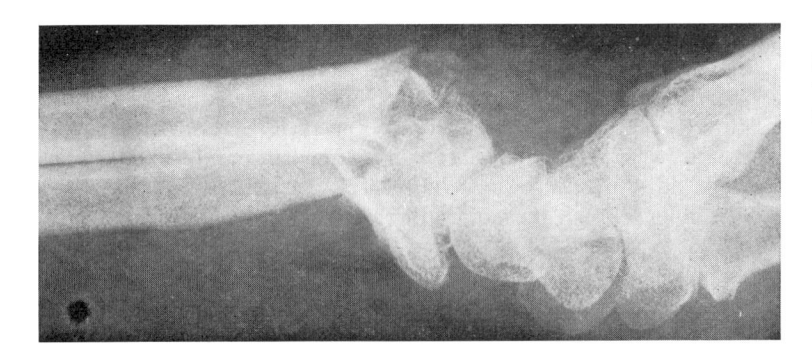

FIG. 21-24. Lateral roentgenogram of reversed Colles' fracture (Smith's fracture).

shoulder through a full range of motion including full overhead reach and full internal and external rotation. Loss of motion in the shoulder joint following fractures of the distal end of the radius is a preventable complication; yet it occurs too often because these exercises of the shoulder have been poorly performed.

Immobilization of the wrist is maintained until union of the fracture has occurred. In adults, about 4 to 6 weeks of immobilization is required. A shorter period is necessary in children. In many patients, particularly in those in the latter decades of life, it is advisable to change casts at the end of 3 weeks in order to bring the hand out of palmar flexion into the neutral position or that of slight dorsal flexion. Obviously, no force should be used in obtaining this corrected position of the hand, as displacement of the distal fragment might occur.

REVERSED COLLES' OR SMITH'S (HYPERFLEXION) FRACTURE (Fig. 21-24). In this fracture, much less common than the Colles', the distal radial fragment is displaced anteriorly, and the articular surface of the radius inclines forward excessively. Some degree of comminution is frequently present. The deformity is usually less pronounced than that of a Colles' fracture.

The principles of manipulative reduction are the same as with a Colles' fracture, except that the hand is brought into hyperextension, and the distal fragment is forced backward with the thumb. Immobilization is provided by a plaster cast or anterior and posterior molded plaster splints holding the hand in full supination and neutral or slight palmar flexion and ulnar deviation. Peculiarly, hyperextension of the hand after the reduction predisposes to volar redisplacement of the distal fragment. The postreduction management is comparable with that outlined for Colles' fractures.

BARTON'S (MARGINAL) FRACTURE. These fractures, which may involve either the anterior or the posterior margin of the distal end of the radius, usually include only a small portion of the articular surface. Displacement, if present at all, is always minimal. Because they involve the articular surface, reduction should be as accurate as possible. By direct pressure on the fragment under local anesthesia it usually can be forced into excellent position.

Immobilization should be provided for about 4 weeks by a plaster cast holding the hand in the neutral or slightly dorsal flexed position. Persistent exercise of the fingers and the shoulder throughout the period of postreduction management are as important as in the other fractures about the lower end of the radius.

FRACTURE-SEPARATION OF THE DISTAL RADIAL EPIPHYSIS. This injury, which occurs generally in children over 10 years of age, is quite comparable with the typical Colles' fracture in adult life. Separation usually occurs between the diaphysis and the epiphyseal cartilage plate so that following adequate reduction there is usually no disturbance of growth.

Reduction can almost always be obtained easily by the maneuvers outlined for Colles' fractures. It is preferable to employ a strong steady traction for several minutes so as to disengage the fragments completely. This permits the epiphysis to be molded into good reduction with a minimum of trauma. Although a perfect reduction is desirable, it is not absolutely necessary, as during subse-

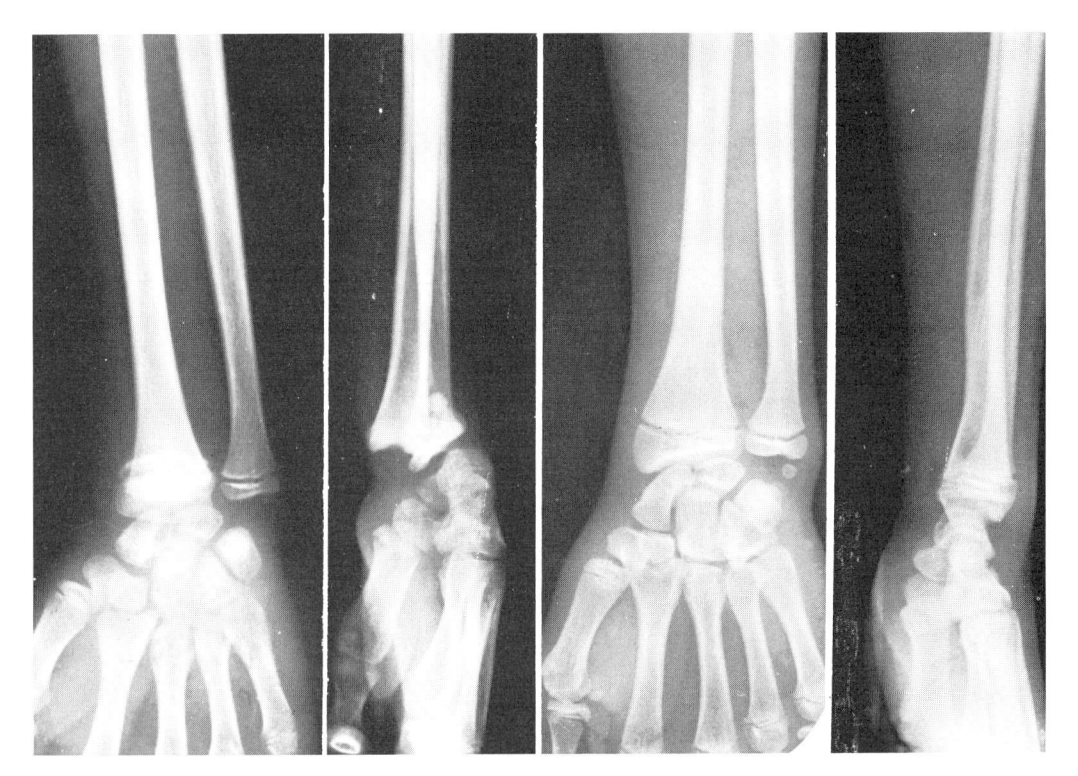

Fig. 21-25. (*Left*) Lateral and anteroposterior roentgenograms of unreduced united fracture, showing epiphyseal separation with severe posterior displacement and anterior angulation. (*Right*) Lateral and anteroposterior roentgenograms taken 2½ years later. Complete correction by growth processes and perfect functional result. (Drs. Ward A. McClanahan and Charles K. Wier, Wichita, Kans.)

quent growth slight malalignment will be corrected (Fig. 21-25).

Immobilization should be provided by a plaster cast holding the hand in slight palmar flexion and ulnar deviation for about 4 or 5 weeks. The end result in these injuries is usually excellent, provided that the epiphyseal cartilage plate was not damaged at the time of injury or during reduction.

Fractures of the Carpus

The most important fracture of the carpal bones is a fracture of the navicular. Fractures involving the other carpal bones are usually mere chips or undisplaced cracks requiring at the most only a few weeks immobilization in a plaster cast with the wrist in the functional position of slight dorsal flexion. Fractures of the navicular, by far the most common fractures of the carpus, deserve special consideration.

Fractures of the Navicular. These injuries, like Colles' fractures, result from falls on the outstretched hand. They occur usually in young adult males whose strong musculature seems to prevent extreme dorsal flexion at the time of injury, thereby causing the navicular (carpal scaphoid) rather than the lower radius to receive the force of impact.

The navicular, the longest of the carpal bones and the only one not cuboidal in shape, has a precarious blood supply. The major blood supply comes from a small artery which usually enters the distal portion of the bone. When a fracture is sustained across the waist or the proximal pole of the navicular, the blood supply of the proximal fragment may be destroyed. The result may be avascular necrosis of that fragment.

The diagnosis of a fracture of the navicular is not always easy. Clinically the patient complains of pain in the wrist, and slight swelling

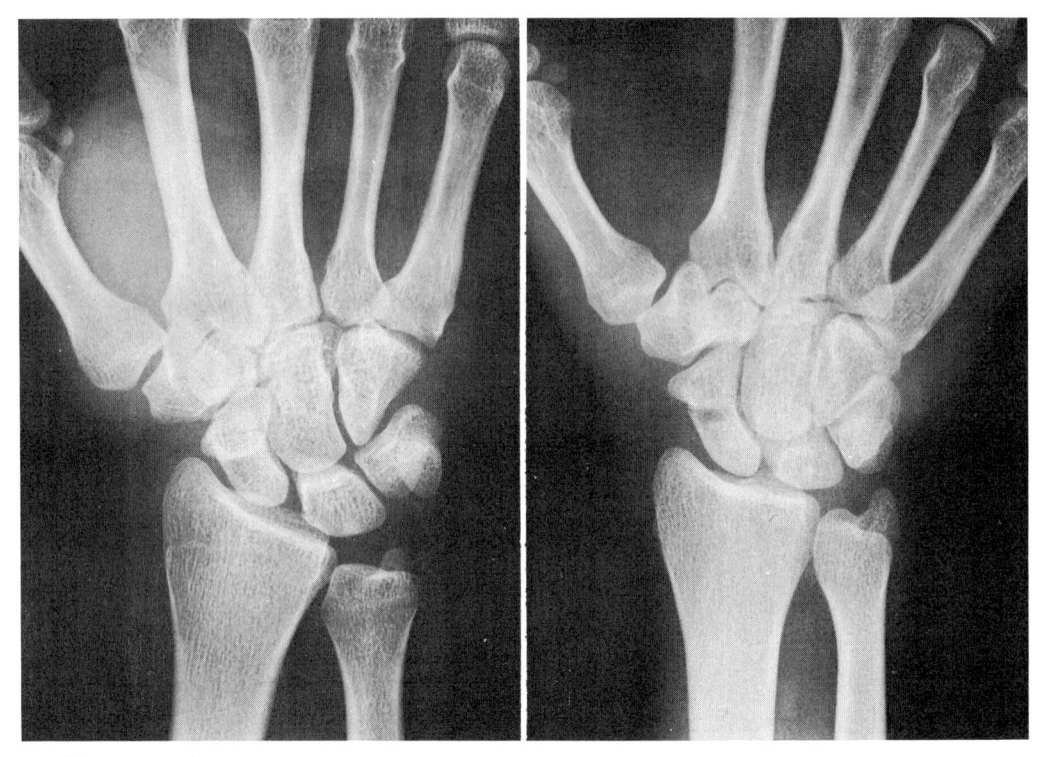

FIG. 21-26. Fracture of the carpal navicular. *(Left)* Roentgenogram in anteroposterior view. Fracture of the navicular is not prominent. *(Right)* Oblique view with hand in ulnar deviation plainly discloses fracture across the waist of navicular.

is present. Tenderness in the anatomic snuffbox is usually severe. With such a clinical picture, an oblique view of the wrist in addition to the routine anteroposterior and lateral views is indicated. Often a fracture of the navicular will be visualized in an oblique view when it has not been disclosed on the routine views (Fig. 21-26). Because of the ever-present possibility of an easily overlooked fracture of the navicular in every injured wrist, 3 views of the region should be routine.

A sprain of the wrist of significance is an exceedingly rare injury. Careful x-ray examination in 3 views usually will disclose a fracture, either of the navicular or of the distal end of the radius. Certainly, a sprain of the wrist which is not completely well in 10 days is likely to be a fracture of the navicular. In some instances, a fracture of the navicular may not be disclosed on x-ray films in all 3 views made soon after injury, and yet repeat films some 10 to 14 days later will show a fracture because the fracture line has become visible as a result of minimal absorption about it. There should be no hesitancy, therefore, in repeating x-ray films after 10 to 14 days if the patient's symptoms have not been completely relieved.

TREATMENT. As a rule, the fragments are in good position, and efforts at reduction are not necessary. If the fragments of a fracture of the navicular are displaced, an associated dislocation of another of the carpal bones is or has been present.

Fortunately the majority of fractures of the navicular will unite if they are immobilized adequately for a long enough period of time. Immobilization is obtained with a plaster cast which extends from just below the elbow to the proximal palmar crease of the palm and to the interphalangeal joint of the thumb with the hand in dorsal flexion and radial deviation. This position of the hand is important, as it tends to approximate the fragments more closely. Immobilization must be provided until the fracture has united, as shown by repeat

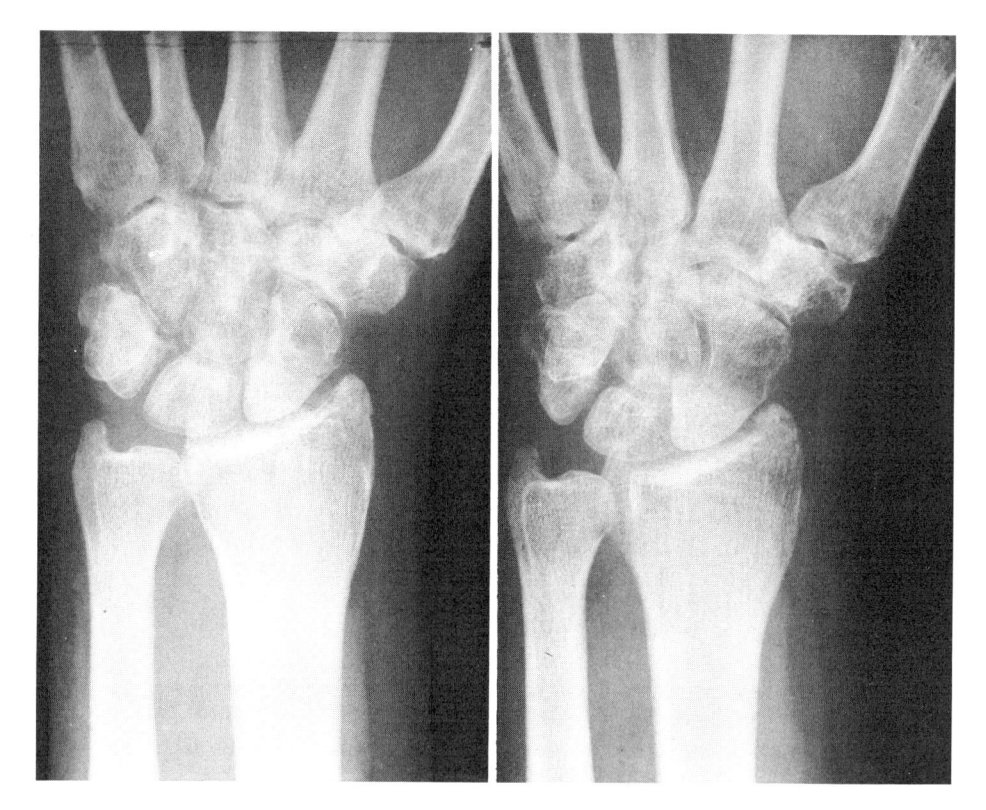

FIG. 21-27. Avascular necrosis of the proximal fragment of a fracture of the carpal navicular. Anteroposterior and oblique views of the wrist, showing a united fracture of the carpal navicular with avascular necrosis of the proximal fragment as indicated by the relative increase in density of this portion of the navicular bone in comparison with the distal fragment and other carpal bones.

roentgenograms. At least 3 months of immobilization is to be expected, and at times from 6 to 9 months or even a year may elapse before the fragments have united. Watson-Jones has emphasized that all navicular fractures will unite if the immobilization is continuous and sufficiently prolonged. Failure of union is the result of delay in providing immobilization or its removal before union has occurred. As a rule the cast should be removed every 6 weeks, new roentgenograms made, and a new cast applied if it is indicated.

The outstanding complication of fractures of the navicular is avascular necrosis of one fragment, usually the proximal fragment (Fig. 21-27). In spite of this, union of the fracture can occur with prolonged immobilization, and the blood supply to the avascular fragment will be re-established so that dead bone will be replaced by living bone by the process of creeping replacement. Immobilization should be continued until the revascularizing process is well established.

With nonunion of the carpal scaphoid, with or without avascular necrosis of the proximal fragment, traumatic arthritis of the wrist joint may develop. This may be an early or a late complication. Once traumatic arthritis has developed, operative fusion of the wrist joint in the position of function is likely to be necessary to provide the patient with a painless, stable wrist.

DISLOCATIONS OF THE CARPUS

Dislocations about the wrist include (1) dislocation of the lunate, (2) perilunar dislocation and (3) midcarpal dislocation. A true dislocation of the wrist joint wherein all of the proximal carpal bones are dislocated out of articulation with the radius does not

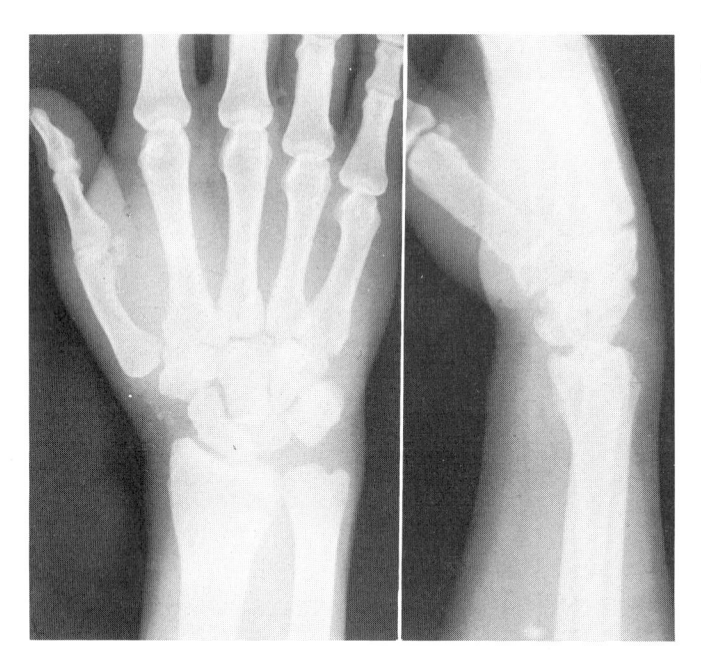

FIG. 21-28. Dislocation of carpal lunate. Anteroposterior and lateral roentgenograms, showing the carpal lunate displaced anteriorly. Note that the injury may be suspected in the anteroposterior view, and the diagnosis is confirmed in the lateral view.

occur for practical purposes except as a complication of fractures of the distal radius.

All of these injuries result from forced hyperextension of the hand such as is sustained from a fall on the outstretched hand or when the hyperextended hand is jammed in attempting to protect oneself from impact against a fall. A miscalculated stiffarm in football could cause these injuries.

While clinically it can be determined from examination that a significant injury has been received to the wrist, exact diagnosis is made by the findings on x-ray examination. The usual anteroposterior and lateral views may be sufficient, but in many instances oblique views will be helpful. Films of the normal uninjured wrist for comparison may be quite advantageous in establishing the exact diagnosis.

Dislocation of the Lunate. In this injury, as the hand is forced into hyperextension the dorsal ligamentous attachments of the lunate are torn, and then the bone is rotated and extruded anteriorly to a point deep to the flexor tendons and the volar carpal ligament. Its only remaining ligamentous attachment is that to the anterior lip of the radius.

In the lateral roentgenogram (Fig. 21-28), the lunate no longer articulates with the radius and is displaced anteriorly. The capitate appears to be in articulation with the radius. In the anteroposterior view, the lunate appears to be elongated and square or rectangular in comparison with its usual round appearance.

Closed reduction under general anesthesia should be attempted as soon as the diagnosis is made. While one assistant provides countertraction, another makes strong traction to open the space for the lunate and hyperextends the hand at the wrist. Pressure is made with the thumbs to replace the lunate, and then the hand is forced quickly into palmar flexion. When the lunate is reduced, the wrist assumes a more normal appearance and can be moved easily through practically a full range of motion. Reduction should be confirmed immediately by x-ray examination before application of the cast. Plaster immobilization with the hand in some palmar flexion is provided for about 3 weeks.

Efforts at closed reduction are not always successful even in fresh injuries. If they are not, either open reduction or excision of the lunate is indicated. Opinions vary as to the most desirable operative procedure. Following open reduction, there is a high incidence of avascular necrosis of the lunate, probably secondary to the further operative destruction of blood supply to the bone. On the other hand, with excision of the bone a weak wrist often follows and may require arthrodesis.

Perilunar Dislocation. In this injury, instead of forward displacement of the lunate as the hand is hyperextended, it remains in normal relationship with the radius, and the remaining carpus with the hand are displaced backward. In some instances, the scaphoid is fractured. If so, the proximal fragment of the scaphoid usually remains behind in the joint with the lunate (Fig. 21-29).

Closed reduction under anesthesia is usually possible by strong traction and manipulation against countertraction. Immobilization by a plaster cast with the hand in slight palmar flexion is provided for 3 to 4 weeks, although, if the carpal scaphoid has been fractured, a much longer period of immobilization is indicated in the position previously described for this fracture.

Perilunar dislocation at the wrist is a serious injury, and some permanent restriction of motion is to be anticipated.

Midcarpal Dislocation. In this injury, as the hand is hyperextended the distal row of carpal bones is dislocated dorsally on the proximal row. Frequently the correct diagnosis has been missed, presumably because the relationship of the carpus was not observed closely on the lateral view. This is a serious injury which can result in severe permanent limitation of function of the hand, particularly if it goes unreduced for any prolonged period of time.

Closed reduction under anesthesia is usually feasible, especially if it is attempted soon

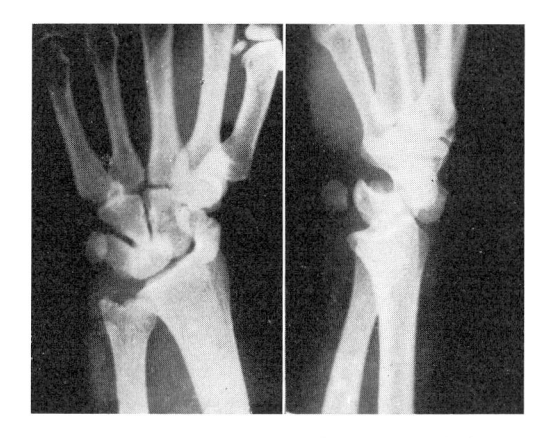

FIG. 21-29. Perilunar dislocation of the carpal bones. Anteroposterior and lateral roentgenograms, showing that the carpal lunate remains in normal articulation with the radius, but all of the other carpal bones have been displaced dorsalward. The proximal articular surface of the capitate now overrides the lunate rather than articulating with its distal surface.

after injury. Reduction is maintained best by immobilization in a plaster cast with the hand in some palmar flexion for a period of 3 or 4 weeks. If efforts at closed reduction are unsuccessful, early open reduction is indicated.

Fractures and dislocations of the bones of the hand are discussed in Chapter 24, Principles of Hand Surgery.

(For Bibliography, see pp. 572 and 573, at end of Chap. 23.)

CHAPTER 22

OSCAR P. HAMPTON, JR., M.D., AND WILLIAM T. FITTS, JR., M.D.

Fractures and Dislocations of the Lower Extremity

Fractures and Dislocations About the Hip
Fractures of the Shaft of the Femur
Fractures of the Distal End of the Femur
Dislocation of the Knee
Internal Derangements of the Knee
Fractures of the Patella
Fractures of the Proximal End of the Tibia
Fractures of the Shafts of the Bones of the Leg
Fractures of the Shaft of the Tibia with an Intact Fibula
Fractures of the Shaft of the Fibula with an Intact Tibia
Fractures and Dislocations of the Ankle
Fractures of the Bones of the Foot
Dislocations of the Foot

The prime objective in treating fractures of the lower extremity is to obtain adequate bony union with full length and normal alignment and without rotational deformity. In addition, full restoration of muscle power and joint motion are highly desirable. In contrast with the upper extremity, stability, and painless weight bearing if possible, even at the expense of mobility, must be obtained in the lower extremity.

Edema is a troublesome accompaniment of almost all injuries of the lower extremities. Its prevention or reduction is often disregarded. In an injury of the lower extremity, elevation, or at least the avoidance of too much dependency, should be carried out from the beginning, provided that the arterial supply to the part is sufficient. Regular exercise of all joints which does not move the bone fragments, including even the small joints of the toes, helps to minimize edema. Following the removal of plaster casts, elastic bandages or elastic stockings should be worn to support the venous circulation. When the patient becomes ambulatory, intermittent elevation will minimize any tendency toward recurring edema.

FRACTURES AND DISLOCATIONS ABOUT THE HIP

Skeletal injuries about the hip may be classified into (1) fractures of the hip (proximal portion of the femur); these are subdivided into fractures of the neck of the femur (intracapsular fractures), and fractures of the trochanteric region of the femur (intertrochanteric, peritrochanteric, subtrochanteric—all extracapsular fractures), (2) dislocations of the hip, and (3) fracture-dislocations of the hip.

FRACTURES OF THE HIP
(PROXIMAL PORTION OF THE FEMUR)

Fractures of the hip fall into two large divisions, depending on whether they involve (1) the intracapsular portion of the neck, or (2) the extracapsular trochanteric region of the femur (Table 22-1). Both groups have much in common. Both occur principally in the elderly. The mean age is in the 70's and almost a third occur in patients 80 or over. About 80 per cent occur in women. Factors which may make women more vulnerable are a natural tendency in the latter decades toward coxa vara deformity and osteoporosis, and a longer life expectancy than men. The hospital mortality rate is high for both types of fractures because of the age of these patients and because the fractures and their treatment demand sharp curtailment of activities in patients who tolerate inactivity poorly. However, these patients do not die from the direct effects of the fracture itself but from complications, such as progression of cardiovascular-renal disease, pneumonia and pulmonary embolism. It may seem paradoxical that the mortality in the group with trochanteric frac-

TABLE 22-1. FRACTURES OF THE HIP

LOCATION	INTRACAPSULAR (NECK)	EXTRACAPSULAR (TROCHANTERIC)
Age	Usually 60 to 75 years	Usually 70 to 85 years
Operative treatment	Internal Fixation (3-flanged nail, collapsing nail-plate or multiple pins) or excision of head and insertion of hip endoprosthesis	Internal Fixation (Nail-plate with screws, such as Jewett, McLaughlin, Neufeld, etc.)
Nonoperative treatment	Ineffective	Continuous traction effective but dangerous and inferior to operative treatment
Nonunion	Common	Very rare
Avascular necrosis of head	Common	Very rare
Mortality before weight-bearing is resumed	15 to 20%	30 to 35%
Expected period for union	4 to 12 months	3 to 4 months

tures is higher than in the group with intracapsular fractures, since fractures of the trochanteric region almost always heal and intracapsular fractures commonly result in nonunion. It is not the nonunion that causes the death of these patients but, as stated above, the complications chiefly related to senility. Trochanteric fractures have a higher mortality rate, probably because they occur, as a rule, in older patients. They also produce more trauma to soft tissues and more blood loss than those of the neck of the femur, and these factors may predispose to thromboembolism.

Mechanism of Injury. Most fractures of the hip occur from a fall. As a rule the patient trips and falls onto the side of the hip. Not infrequently, however, a patient who sustains a fracture of the hip will have the sensation that the hip is broken by a misstep or stumble and that the fall is secondary to the fracture.

Diagnosis. Severe pain in the hip is the outstanding complaint. The patient is unable to arise. The injured lower extremity appears to be shortened and falls into external rotation. This position has been described as "helpless eversion."

The diagnosis always must be confirmed and the type of fracture identified by roentgenograms in two planes. A good lateral roentgenogram of the hip is difficult to make, but it is essential for accurate diagnosis and identification of a fracture of the proximal portion of the femur.

Treatment of Intracapsular Fractures of the Hip. For many years fractures of the neck of the femur as a group have been called the "unsolved fracture." This fracture is unsolved because it ends so often in nonunion or goes on to union only to have the femoral head reveal evidence of avascular necrosis many months or years after union has occurred. Furthermore, even under ideal conditions healing of the fracture takes many months. At one time, these fractures were managed by a concept of "do-nothing," consequently, the great majority ended in nonunion. A great advance was made in 1897 when Royal Whitman advocated a careful manipulative reduction of the hip and immobilization in a plaster hip spica for 3 to 4 months. The next great advance came in 1931 with the introduction of internal fixation by the 3-flanged nail of Smith-Petersen after careful closed reduction. Operative treatment with fixation by one of several types of hip nails remains the treatment of choice. In spite of these advances, the fracture frequently ends in nonunion (15 to 35% in reported series) and still must be considered as unsolved. In recent years, certain of these fractures, usually in the older age groups, have been treated primarily by removal of the femoral head and replacement with a metal hip-joint prosthesis. This form of treatment has gained increasing popularity but it needs further trial and observation before its permanent place in the treatment of fractures of the neck of the femur can be established.

The head and the neck of the femur have an extremely poor blood supply, and it is chiefly for this reason that nonunion is so

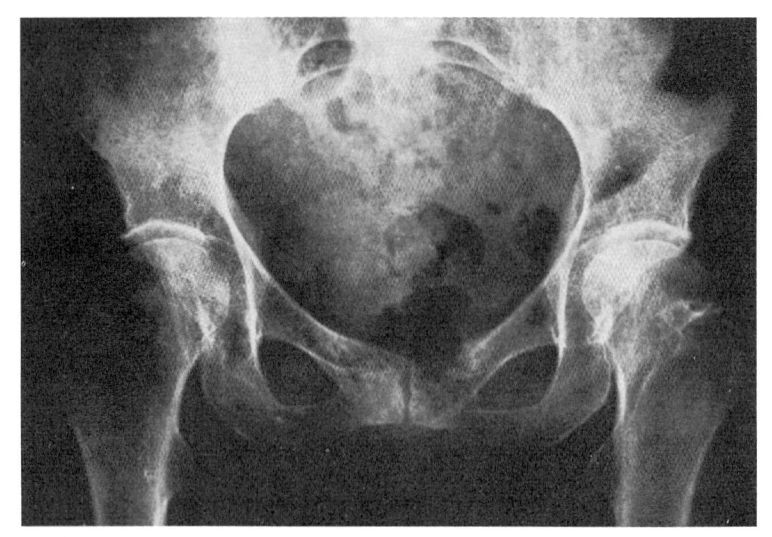

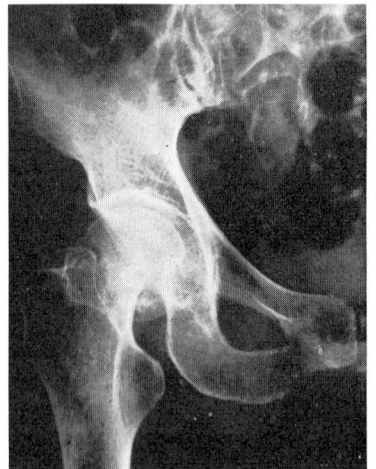

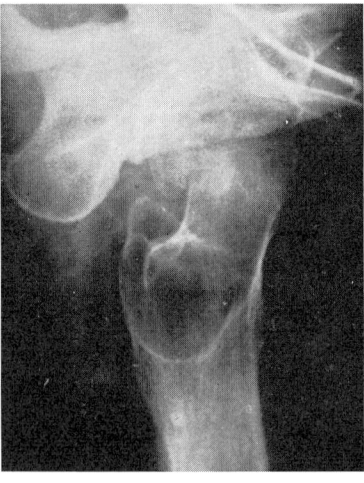

Fig. 22-1. Impacted fractures of the neck of the femur. (*Top*) Roentgenogram showing impaction of the neck of the right femur in abduction. Patient also had sustained an abduction-type impacted fracture of the neck of the left femur 2 years previously which healed with only protection from weight-bearing for 3 months. (*Bottom*) Anteroposterior and lateral roentgenograms of adduction-type impacted fracture of right femur. Since this impaction was unlikely to persist it was managed as an unimpacted fracture by reduction and internal fixation.

common. The head and the neck receive blood from capsular arteries through periosteal and nutrient vessels and to a lesser extent from the small artery in the ligamentum teres. The capsular vessels may be torn by an intracapsular fracture. If so, the artery of the ligamentum teres alone is unlikely to provide a sufficient blood supply for the entire head. Following a fracture of the neck of the femur, aseptic necrosis probably will ensue unless some of the vessels of the capsule remain intact and patent.

Fractures of the neck of the femur may be impacted or unimpacted. The clinical findings and the method of treatment may vary accordingly.

Impacted Fractures of the Neck of the Femur. In some fractures of the femoral neck, the fragments become jammed or impacted together when the fracture is sustained. Under these circumstances, the patient has less pain and may arise from the fallen position and even walk unaided. The foot and the extremity do not fall into helpless eversion. The hip may be moved through a nearly normal range of motion in all directions, particularly if the fragments are firmly impacted. The degree and the position of impaction are determined by roentgenograms in 2 planes. Impacted fractures of the hip are subdivided into abduction or valgus impaction and adduction or varus impaction (Fig. 22-1).

In the abduction impacted fracture of the femoral neck, the fracture line tends to be horizontal, and the head assumes a slight upward or valgus position. In the lateral roentgenogram, the fragments usually are in excellent position. If the fragments are firmly impacted, the fracture is likely to go on to sound bony union with no treatment other than protection from weight-bearing by bed rest for a few weeks, followed by the use of a wheel chair or walker for 3 months. Because occasionally a fracture of this type changes position and becomes disimpacted, internal fixation serves as a safeguard against this hazard. Certainly, if there is any doubt that the fracture is firmly impacted, internal fixation is indicated. Moreover, in those which appear to be firmly impacted, it is reasonable that internal fixation will permit the patient to be out of bed and assume ambulation with a walking aid in a shorter period of time without endangering the position of the fragments.

In the fracture impacted in adduction (Fig. 22-1, *bottom*), the impaction is unlikely to persist. Disimpaction is the rule. These fractures should be managed as unimpacted fractures of the neck of the femur.

Unimpacted Fractures of the Neck of the Femur. The majority of fractures of the neck of the femur are not impacted and require painstaking, accurate reduction of the fragments under anesthesia with the patient, as a rule, on a fracture table. The reduction is followed by internal fixation with a Smith-Petersen three-flanged nail, a nail-plate combination or multiple pins (Method 3) (Fig. 22-2). Most surgeons prefer to perform this operation without exposing the fracture site, the so-called blind nailing. After closed reduction of the fracture confirmed by roentgenograms made in the operating room, the nail is inserted through a lateral incision below the greater trochanter, using additional roentgenograms to confirm the direction of the nail. Occasionally, an accurate reduction of the fragments cannot be obtained by closed reduction. Actually, more and more surgeons are using open reduction in preference to a closed reduction of the fracture in an effort to ensure accurate apposition of the fragments. Unless a good reduction is obtained, nonunion is to be anticipated even though the fragments are transfixed with a nail or pins.

Although patients with fractures of the neck of the femur are usually relatively poor risks, with prompt operation within 4 to 24 hours after admission, skillful anesthesia, adequate blood replacement and antibiotics, the immediate mortality rate should be low. Because of the high incidence of thromboembolic complications in these patients, some advocate the use of anticoagulants prophylactically as a

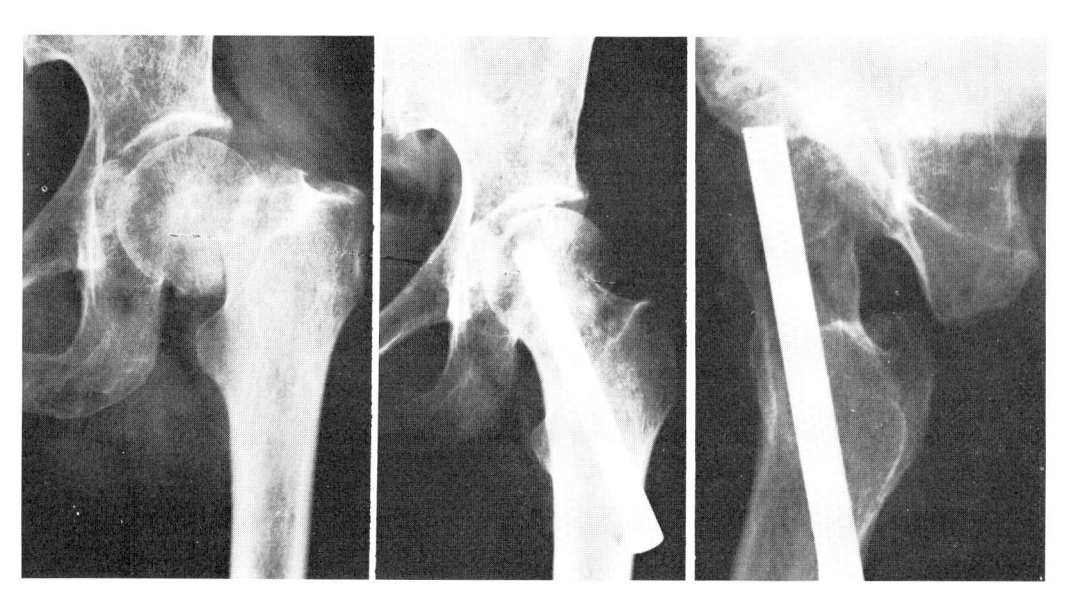

Fig. 22-2. Unimpacted fracture of the neck of the left femur. (*Left*) Roentgenogram before reduction and fixation with a Smith-Petersen 3-flanged nail. Anteroposterior view. (*Center and right*) After internal fixation. (*Center*) Anteroposterior view. (*Right*) Lateral view.

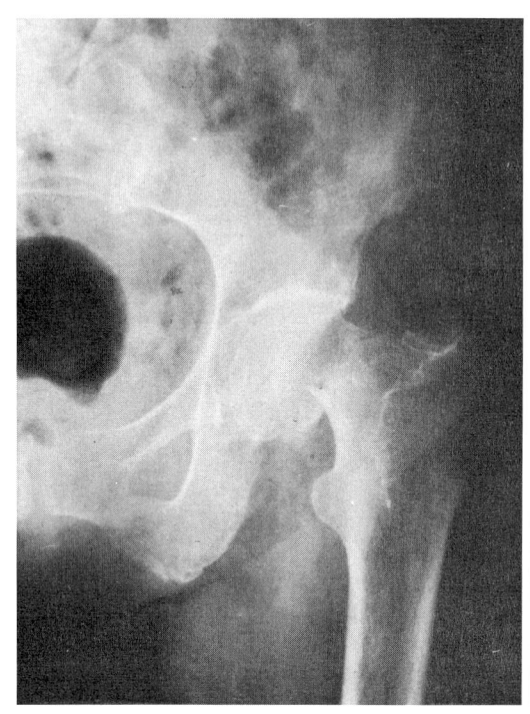

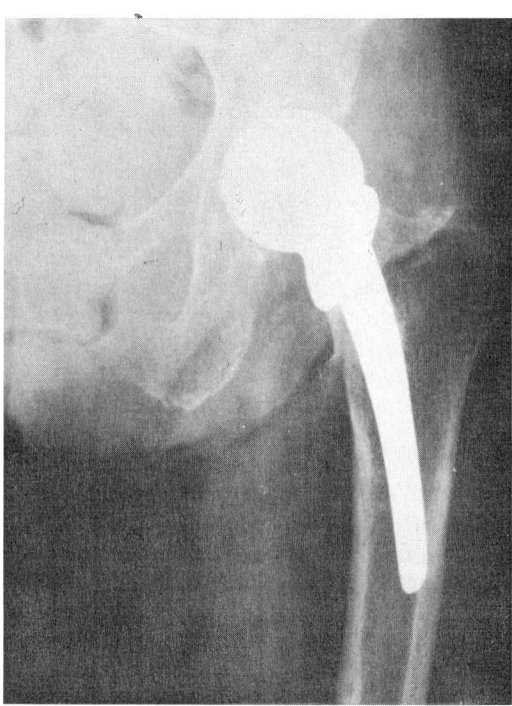

FIG. 22-3. Intracapsular fracture of the neck of the femur treated by replacement with a prosthesis. (*Left*) Anteroposterior view of pelvis showing intracapsular fracture of the neck of the left femur in an 89-year-old woman. (*Right*) Anteroposterior view showing that the femoral head has been removed and replaced by a Fred Thompson hip joint endoprosthesis. Note that with this prosthesis the full length of the femoral neck has been restored. This is important in avoiding postoperative dislocation of the head portion of the prosthesis and in restoring function of the hip. (Hampton, O. P., Jr., and Fitts, W. T., Jr.: Open Reduction of Common Fractures. New York, Grune & Stratton, 1959)

routine measure. Postoperatively, the patient may be turned from side to side and placed in a chair several times a day without endangering the fixation of the fragments. The majority of these patients do not have the strength in the arms to walk with a walker while avoiding weight-bearing on the broken hip. Weight-bearing should not be permitted until there is roentgenographic evidence of union of the fracture. This may require many months.

The operative method of treatment is by far the best for these fractures, not only because it gives the highest percentage of union, but also because it is the best form of treatment for the general condition of the patient. If, for some reason, the operative method is refused or cannot be carried out, the Whitman abduction cast method probably offers the best chances for union of the fracture. However, it does carry a high incidence of complications.

Because of the poor results often obtained with fractures of the neck of the femur (nonunion and avascular necrosis of the head) and the long period of time required to determine the end-result, some surgeons have abandoned internal fixation of these fractures in patients with a short life expectancy, especially when the fracture is subcapital. Instead of reducing and fixing the fracture by internal fixation, the head fragment is excised and replaced with an intramedullary type of metal hip joint prosthesis (Fig. 22-3). Following insertion of a prosthesis, the postoperative management is essentially the same as if the fracture had been reduced and fixed internally, except that weight-bearing may be permitted within a few days or at the most 2 weeks. This com-

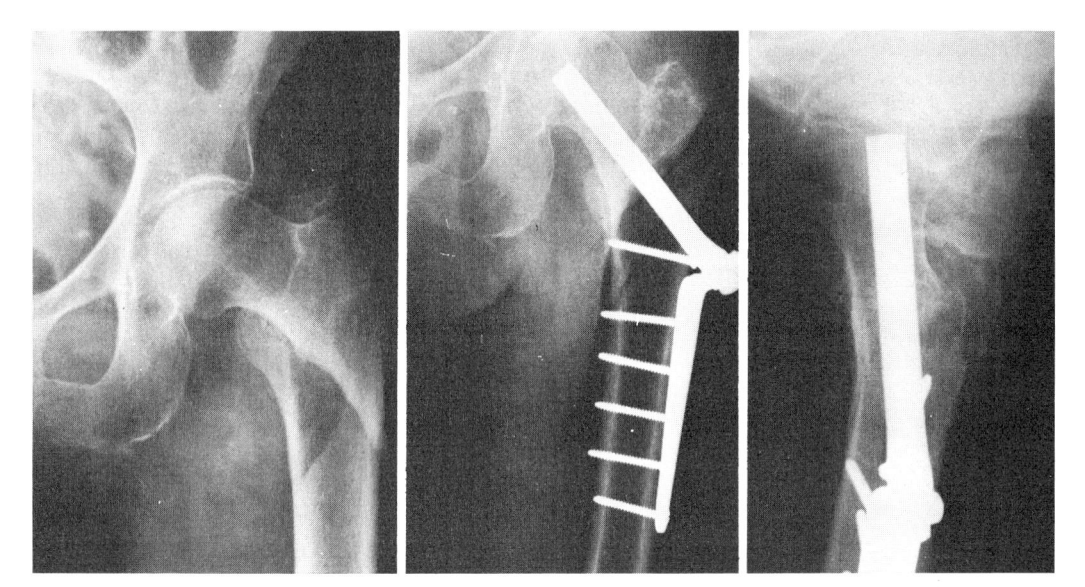

Fig. 22-4. Trochanteric fracture of the femur. Treatment by open reduction and internal fixation. The internal fixation must be of the blade (nail)-plate type, because a nail alone will not fix the fragments adequately. (*Left*) Roentgenogram before operation, anteroposterior view. (*Center*) Roentgenogram after operation and fixation with a Smith-Petersen nail attached to a McLaughlin plate, anteroposterior view. (*Right*) Lateral view.

promise treatment of fractures of the neck of the femur accepts a hip somewhat functionally inferior to one which would be obtained if the fracture united by bone but does offer a slightly inferior hip in a much shorter period of time. It should be anticipated that a cane will be used as an aid to walking and that the patient will experience mild discomfort in the hip, particularly during the first few steps after arising from the sitting position. The final place for this treatment of fractures of the neck of the femur has not as yet been determined, but results to date are most favorable. However, such a radical approach to the problem proves that the treatment of this fracture remains unsolved.

Treatment of Trochanteric Fractures of the Femur. Fractures included in this group are those located between the neck of the femur and a level about 1 inch below the lesser trochanter. The fragments of a trochanteric fracture have an excellent blood supply and for this reason almost always unite if the patient survives and the fragments are held in a reasonably good reduction. The high mortality rate derives from the age of these patients (70 to 85 years as a rule), their poor general condition, and the fact that these fractures, in contrast with those of the neck, result in considerable soft tissue trauma. Considerable blood is lost into the tissues with most trochanteric fractures (it has been estimated at about a liter), and much more blood is lost at operation than at operation for fractures of the neck of the femur.

Trochanteric fractures should be treated by the operative method utilizing a nail-plate type of internal fixation (Method 3) (Fig. 22-4). Union can be obtained with other methods, such as balanced suspension traction (Method 2), but the incidence of complications and the mortality rate are much higher with this method than with open reduction and internal fixation. A patient with this injury treated in traction must be kept constantly in bed on his back. This position predisposes to bed sores, thrombo-embolism, pneumonia, senile dementia, and residual loss of motion in the knee. The operative method permits the patient to be turned in bed frequently and to be out of bed in a chair promptly. The patient has less general discomfort and a much better mental attitude toward the restriction of activities imposed by convalescence. All of this tends to minimize complications. It should be pointed out that the fracture will unite without operative fixation, but that the operative method is indicated because it is best for the patient. Ordinarily weight-bearing must not be allowed until the fracture has united as shown by roentgenograms. Union is more rapid in trochanteric fractures than in fractures of the femur neck and usually occurs in 3 or 4 months.

DISLOCATIONS OF THE HIP

Traumatic dislocations of the hip may be classified as (1) posterior (iliac or sciatic notch) and (2) anterior (obturator or pubic), depending upon where the head leaves the acetabulum and comes to rest. Another form of dislocation, central dislocation of the femoral head through the fracture of the acetabulum, is really a fracture of the pelvis rather than a true dislocation and is discussed under fractures of the pelvis.

Posterior Dislocation of the Hip. Posterior dislocation of the hip occurs most frequently as the result of a strong force applied at the knee when the thigh is flexed and adducted, as when the knee strikes the dashboard after an automobile collision. Dislocation may occur when a heavy weight drops on the low back of a stooping individual, as in a cave-in of dirt or the fall of a roof. A fracture of the posterior wall of the acetabulum frequently accompanies a posterior dislocation of the hip (Fig. 22-5).

DIAGNOSIS. The extremity immediately assumes the position of flexion, adduction and internal rotation at the hip and appears shorter than the opposite side. The position of flexion, adduction and internal rotation is in striking contrast to the position assumed by the extremity with a fracture of the neck of the femur. The position of the extremity and the type of trauma causing it practically establish the diagnosis but it must always be confirmed by an x-ray examination showing the pelvis and both hip joints.

In posterior dislocations, the sciatic nerve may be damaged by the head of the femur or a fragment of the acetabulum. Therefore, before attempts at reduction, a careful motor and sensory examination of the extremity should be made and the results recorded. Otherwise, if the symptoms and signs of damage to the sciatic nerve are found after reduction, it cannot be determined whether they are the result of the injury or the trauma of reduction. Symptoms and signs of injury to the sciatic nerve developing after reduction indicate prompt surgical intervention.

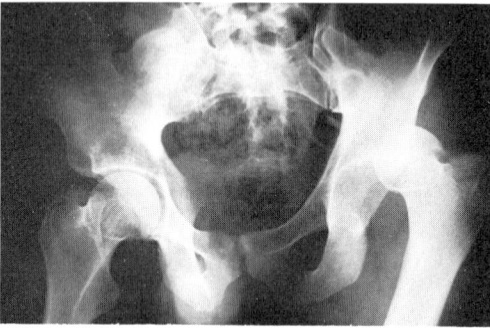

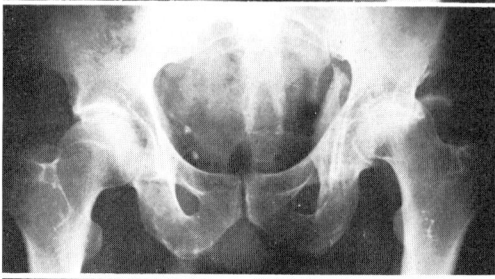

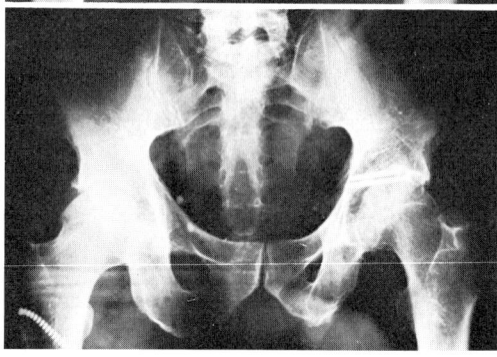

FIG. 22-5. Posterior dislocation of the hip. (*Top*) Roentgenogram of the left hip showing posterior dislocation *without* fracture of posterior wall of acetabulum. (*Center*) Roentgenogram of left hip of another patient showing fracture of posterior wall of acetabulum accompanying posterior dislocation of the hip. Note that the hip is displaced posteriorly but not so far superiorly as in *Top*. (*Bottom*) Roentgenogram following reduction of dislocation, and reduction and internal fixation of acetabular fragment with metal screws.

TREATMENT. Reduction of a dislocation of the hip is a true surgical emergency. Prompt reduction is necessary not only to relieve pain but also to minimize the danger of avascular necrosis, the incidence of which is in direct ratio to the length of time that the femoral head remains dislocated.

Three standard methods exist for reducing a posterior dislocation of the hip. Each method probably offers certain advantages. Reduction at times is most difficult. In some instances one method will fail to give reduction but another will succeed. General or spinal anesthesia, sufficient to give real muscular relaxation, is essential. Ideally suited for the reduction is a one-sided spinal anesthesia with a small dose of the anesthetic agent.

1. Probably the most effective and safest method of reduction is strong traction in the axis of the femur with the hip flexed and slightly adducted, combined with gentle maneuvering of the thigh toward external rotation and mild abduction while an assistant provides countertraction by strong pressure against the pelvis. This, in effect, pulls the femoral head through the rent in the capsule in the reverse direction from that in which it left the joint. Reduction takes place with a satisfying snap or thump. For emphasis, we repeat that traction is made with the hip flexed, not extended.

These maneuvers may be carried out with the patient on a pad on the floor. The surgeon stands over the patient as he reduces the dislocation. An alternative position is provided with the patient on an x-ray table and the surgeon in his stocking feet standing on the table. The latter position offers easy roentgenologic confirmation of the reduction.

2. The time-honored method of Bigelow may be used. In this method, the adducted thigh and leg are fully flexed and then, as traction is applied, the thigh is circumducted lateralward as it is externally rotated and abducted. A disadvantage of this method is that excessive force can cause a fracture of the neck or the shaft of the femur. Moreover, a posterior dislocation may merely be converted into an anterior dislocation.

3. The Stimson method, used too seldom, is really a most atraumatic and effective method. The patient is anesthetized face down with the thighs flexed at the hip over the end of the table and with the legs supported in 90° of flexion at the knee. A heavy weight, up to 20 or 25 pounds, is applied to the affected leg just below the knee, thereby making traction on the thigh. Traction is allowed to persist for several minutes until muscle spasm has been overcome, following which the operator merely rotates the extremity inward and outward. Reduction is sometimes obtained by this method after the two more popular methods described above have failed.

While reduction usually can be achieved with any of the methods just discussed, it is not always easy. Considerable force for traction is often necessary. In the rare instance when closed reduction is unsuccessful, open reduction must be used.

Postreduction Management of Posterior Dislocation of the Hip. Immobilization of the hip in plaster or prolonged traction on the extremity is not necessary. A few pounds of simple skin traction of the Buck's type may be provided for a few days to help overcome spasm of the muscles and thereby to contribute to the comfort of the patient. Redislocation is most unlikely to occur, but as a safeguard against it, the patient may be kept at bed rest without flexion of the thigh at the hip for a period of 3 to 4 weeks. The position of extension prevents pressure of the head of the femur against the rent in the capsule of the joint posteriorly.

Opinions vary as to when weight-bearing may be permitted following dislocation of the hip. One school of thought lays emphasis on the risk of avascular necrosis of the head of the femur and prefers as long as 6 months of crutch-walking without real weight-bearing in order that, if the early signs of this complication have developed, the patient may remain on crutches for a matter of several years anticipating creeping replacement of the dead femoral head. This concept seems to indicate that there will be full creeping replacement of the dead head and the subsequent return of function to the hip will be worth the prolonged period of time on crutches.

A second school recognizes that avascular necrosis of the head of the femur following dislocation may appear at any time after injury, even 4 or 5 years later. Since this is true, an arbitrary period of 6 months on crutches does not seem to be justified. Weight-bearing and full function are permitted approximately 6 weeks after dislocation. This approach to the problem is by far the most practicable and is recommended.

Anterior Dislocation of the Hip. Anterior dislocation of the hip, which is rather rare, may occur when the thigh is forced into extreme abduction and external rotation. The head usually comes to rest in the obturator foramen. The extremity goes into abduction, external rotation and some flexion and appears to be longer than the uninjured limb. While the position of the extremity resembles that assumed when a fracture of the neck of the femur is present, it may be distinguished clinically from that injury because of the mild flexion and the increased rather than decreased length.

TREATMENT. Reduction usually may be achieved by traction in the axis which the femur has assumed, combined with internal rotation and adduction. The Bigelow method for anterior dislocations of the hip also may be used. This, of course, is somewhat the reverse of the maneuver for posterior dislocations of the hip. The thigh and the leg are flexed. Then, as traction is made, the extremity is circumducted toward adduction and brought into internal rotation and extension.

POSTREDUCTION MANAGEMENT. Only a few days of bed rest, avoidance of undue strain toward abduction, external rotation and hyperextension, and about 4 weeks on crutches are necessary. Avascular necrosis of the femoral head is unlikely to develop following anterior dislocation of the hip if reduction is performed within a few hours of injury.

Posterior Dislocation of the Hip With Fracture of the Acetabulum. A fracture of the posterior portion of the acetabulum frequently complicates a posterior dislocation of the hip, the femoral head driving a fragment or fragments ahead of it as it leaves the joint. This combination of injuries frequently results from automobile collisions as a knee of a front-seat occupant strikes the dashboard—hence, it is called the "dashboard dislocation." The fracture of the acetabulum can be diagnosed only by a roentgenogram.

TREATMENT. As the dislocation of the hip is reduced, the fragment or fragments of acetabulum usually fall into position. However, the important consideration in these injuries is the size of the fragments and the potential defect in the acetabular wall rather than whether the fragments go into good position with reduction of the hip. If the fragments are small, they may be ignored even if unreduced and the hip managed as a dislocation without fracture.

On the other hand, when the fragment or fragments are large, even though they are reduced, subsequent displacement and spontaneous redislocation of the hip can easily occur through the defect in the acetabular wall. Therefore, open reduction and internal fixation of large acetabular fragments are indicated to provide a stable posterior acetabulum (Fig. 22-5). Of course, operative reduction and fixation are necessary for unreduced large fragments.

After closed or open reduction of a dislocated hip with a fracture of the acetabulum, external immobilization is not necessary. Flexion of the thigh at the hip is avoided, as this would cause the femoral head to press against the weakened portion of the acetabulum. With the thigh in extension, normal muscle tone holds the femoral head against the intact superior portion of the acetabulum. All that is necessary, therefore, is to keep the patient at bed rest with the thighs in extension for a period of 4 to 6 weeks. So long as the injured hip remains in extension the patient may lie on either side, face down, or on his back.

Posterior Dislocation of the Hip With Chip Fracture of the Femoral Head. Occasionally, a piece of the head of the femur is sheared off as it leaves the acetabulum. This fragment may block reduction of the dislocation or it may fall into the acetabulum and prevent proper seating of the femoral head in the joint. If either situation cannot be overcome by manipulation, then excision of the fragment is necessary. On the other hand, if reduction of the dislocation is achieved without interference by the fragment, usually the latter may be ignored as it is unlikely to interfere with subsequent function of the hip. Early surgical excision is not indicated for 2 reasons: the operation itself may cause further damage to the arterial flow to the femoral head from capsular arteries and increase the chances of avascular necrosis. In addition, the

Fractures of the Shaft of the Femur

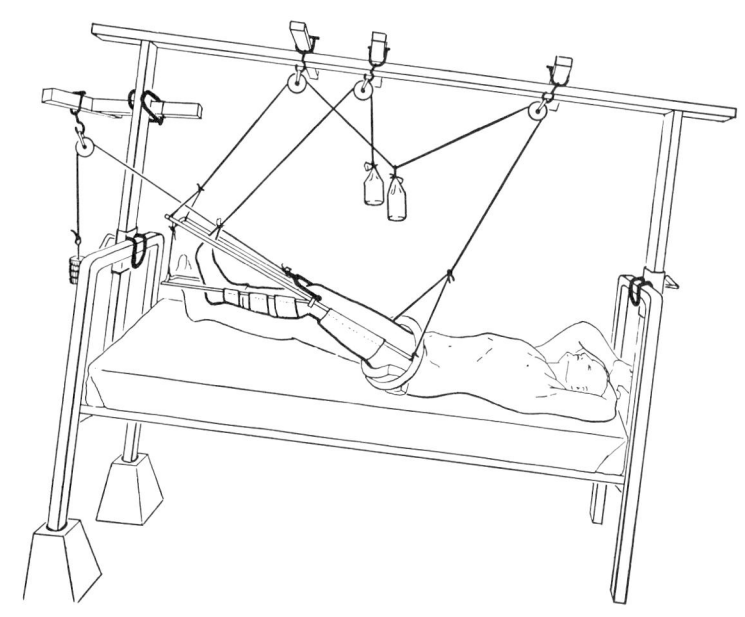

FIG. 22-7. Illustrating use of balanced suspension skeletal traction for treatment of fracture of femoral shaft. The Thomas full ring splint holds the thigh in flexion. The Pierson attachment is attached at the level of the upper border of the patella, with the knee flexed about 15°. The angle of the attachment to the splint should conform to the normal valgus at the knee. The slings for the splint should not overlap, although they must be close to each other. They must support the thigh from the ring of the splint to just proximal to the posterior bulge of the femoral condyles. The slings for the Pierson attachment should support the leg from a point just distal to the posterior bulge of the tibial condyles to the tendo achillis. The foot is supported at 90° by suspension, using stockinet attached over the foot by tincture of benzoin. The ring is placed firmly against the ischial tuberosity. The suspension weights for the splint must not only support the entire splint and the Pierson attachment but also must aid in maintaining the ring against the tuberosity. Elevation of the foot of the bed to increase the countertraction of the weight of the body is essential.

from an overhead frame is the most generally employed method of balanced suspension skeletal traction. The splint must be long enough and wide enough for the extremity to rest comfortably in hammock slings.

A great danger in the use of continuous traction is overpull (distraction) of the fragments. Roentgenograms must be made frequently in the early stages of treatment to detect overpull and other deformities, and to allow the earliest possible reduction in the amount of traction and indicated adjustments of the traction apparatus. The distal fragment and accordingly the leg and the foot must be allowed to remain in sufficient external rotation to conform with the rotation of the proximal fragment.

In our experience, fractures of the upper half of the femoral shaft are treated best with the Kirschner wire through the distal femur, although a wire through the proximal tibia may be satisfactory. An advantage in having the wire above the knee is that knee motion may be instituted earlier. In fractures of the upper third of the shaft, the proximal fragment usually is sharply flexed and abducted and externally rotated. In such instances traction must be made with the thigh flexed, abducted and externally rotated in such a manner as to bring the distal fragment into proper rotation and alignment with the proximal fragment.

Fractures of the lower half of the femoral shaft usually are controlled best with the Kirschner wire inserted through the proximal tibia posterior to the tubercle. It is difficult to control the short distal fragment if the wire is placed through the femur.

The posterior angulation of fractures of the distal end of the femoral shaft, caused by the pull of the gastrocnemii, is difficult to correct. One method is to insert two Kirschner wires: one at the level of the tibial tubercle for longitudinal traction and one just above the condyles for anterior or vertical traction to correct the posterior angulation of the distal

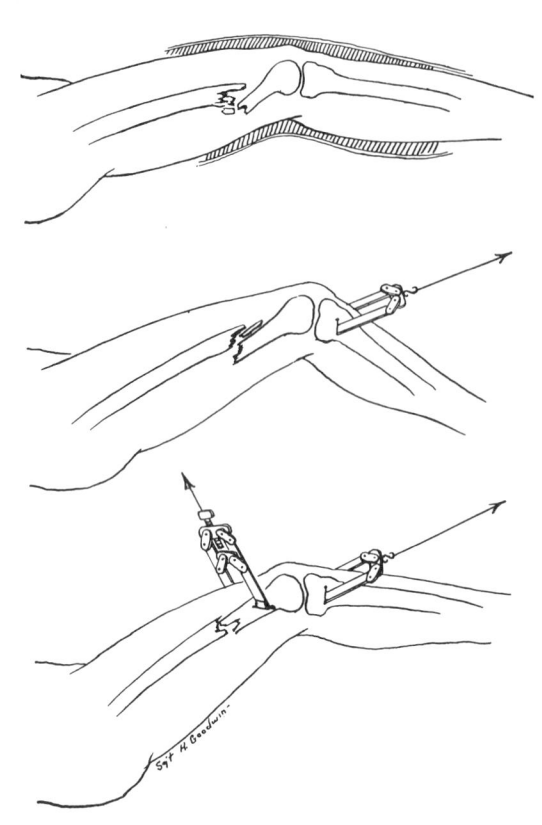

FIG. 22-8. Diagrammatic representation of 2-wire skeletal traction for fracture of femur in distal third. (*Top*) Deformity on admission to hospital. (*Center*) Incomplete reduction in skeletal traction with wire in tibial tubercle. (*Bottom*) Adequate reduction when additional wire is inserted in lower femoral fragment and vertical lift is secured. (Hampton, O. P., Jr.: Wounds of the Extremities in Military Surgery. St. Louis, C. V. Mosby, p. 273)

fragment (Fig. 22-8). Another method is the following: with the Kirschner wire at the level of the tibial tubercle and the hinge of the Pierson attachment at the level of the fracture site instead of at the knee, traction is made parallel with the leg which is kept horizontal with the floor. This is the only situation in which the line of traction is not made parallel with the shaft of the femur. If a satisfactory position cannot be accomplished by traction within 48 to 72 hours, then direct manipulation of the fragments in the traction apparatus should be done with the patient anesthetized, or "two-wire" traction instituted.

Traction should be maintained until bony union has occurred, as shown by clinical and roentgenologic evidence. This may require from 3 to 5 months. Weight-bearing should not be allowed until union is solid. Patients with precarious union preferably should be kept in balanced suspension for an added length of time, during which active and passive knee exercises are instituted, or further immobilization may be provided by a plaster spica. Afterward in instances of relatively precarious union, still in need of some protection, ischial-bearing leg braces should be used until union is mature.

Open Reduction and Internal Fixation (Method 3). The other common method of treating fractures of the femoral shaft is open reduction and internal fixation. Until the introduction of intramedullary nailing for these fractures about 20 years ago, the operative method usually was reserved for those instances in which a satisfactory reduction could not be accomplished with balanced traction. The method of internal fixation then used was a metallic plate with screws (stainless steel or vitallium) which necessitated supplementary immobilization in a plaster hip spica. The incidence of nonunion was high when plates and screws were used and, even if the fracture united, the fact that plaster immobilization was necessary for several months must have contributed to knee stiffness and muscle atrophy. For these reasons internal fixation with plates and screws was not ideal, and intramedullary nailing has largely replaced it. In the last few years the development of the A-O compression plate has led to some resurgence of this method.

Fixation by intramedullary nailing is the preferable method for treatment of fractures of the femoral shaft if the contour of the fracture is such as to permit stabilization by the nail. It is especially applicable for transverse fractures of the middle three fifths of the femur (Fig. 22-9). In addition to an exceedingly high rate of union of the fracture, intramedullary nailing has the great advantage of allowing early weight-bearing with better preservation of joint motion and less muscle atrophy. After a successful medullary nailing a patient with a femoral shaft fracture may be up on crutches with guarded weight-bearing within a few days and resume a

Fractures of the Shaft of the Femur 531

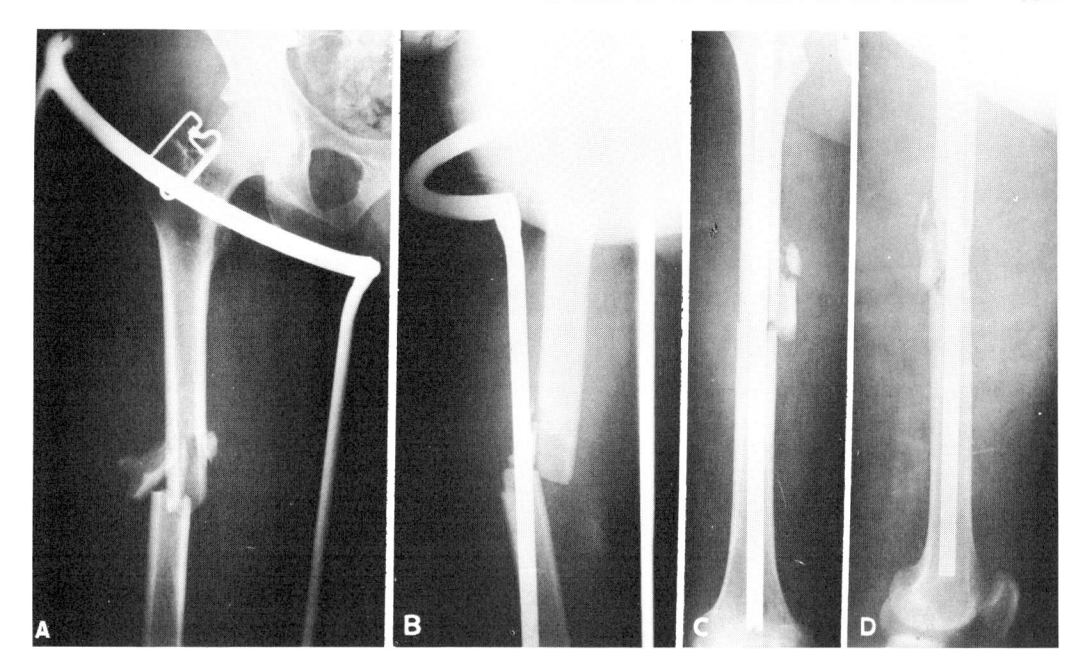

FIG. 22-9. Fracture of the shaft of the femur stabilized in reduction by an intramedullary nail.
(A and B) Anteroposterior and lateral views of a somewhat comminuted fracture of the shaft of the right femur in the upper portion of the middle third immobilized in a half-ring leg splint as emergency splinting.
(C and D) Anteroposterior and lateral views showing the fracture stabilized in excellent reduction with a cloverleaf (Küntscher) intramedullary nail. The fracture went on to solid union in excellent apposition and alignment.
(Hampton, O. P., Jr., and Fitts, W. T., Jr.: Open Reduction of Common Fractures. New York, Grune & Stratton, 1959)

sedentary occupation within a few weeks; whereas, if traction is used, he must spend several months in bed. Intramedullary nailing, in contrast with skeletal traction, permits the patient to be transported about the hospital easily and therefore facilitates the care of other injuries.

Intramedullary nailing of femoral shaft fractures should almost always be done as an open operation. A single nail of adequate diameter is preferred. The Küntscher type of nail is strongly recommended. In certain comminuted or butterfly types of fracture, supplemental wire or plate fixation may be necessary to provide better stabilization of the fracture. (Fig. 22-10. See also Fig. 20-14).

The risk of the nailing operation is that an open operation on bone must be performed with all of its dangers and that technical difficulties may occur in the insertion of the nail. The nail may split, bend, or break. If driven too far distally, the knee joint may be injured. Fat embolism may occur, but serious effects from it are rare. The advantages of a good intramedullary nailing of the femur by far outweigh the disadvantages.

In open fractures of the femur the wounds preferably are débrided, perhaps closed, and allowed to heal while the extremity is held in balanced suspension skeletal traction. After sound wound-healing the advantages of intramedullary nailing may be obtained by operation. Occasionally, for good cause, the open fracture may be stabilized with an intramedullary nail at the time of wound débridement, but this carries a definite risk of catastrophic sepsis.

IN CHILDREN

Fractures of the femoral shaft in children always unite. In addition, children rapidly correct mild or even moderate degrees of angula-

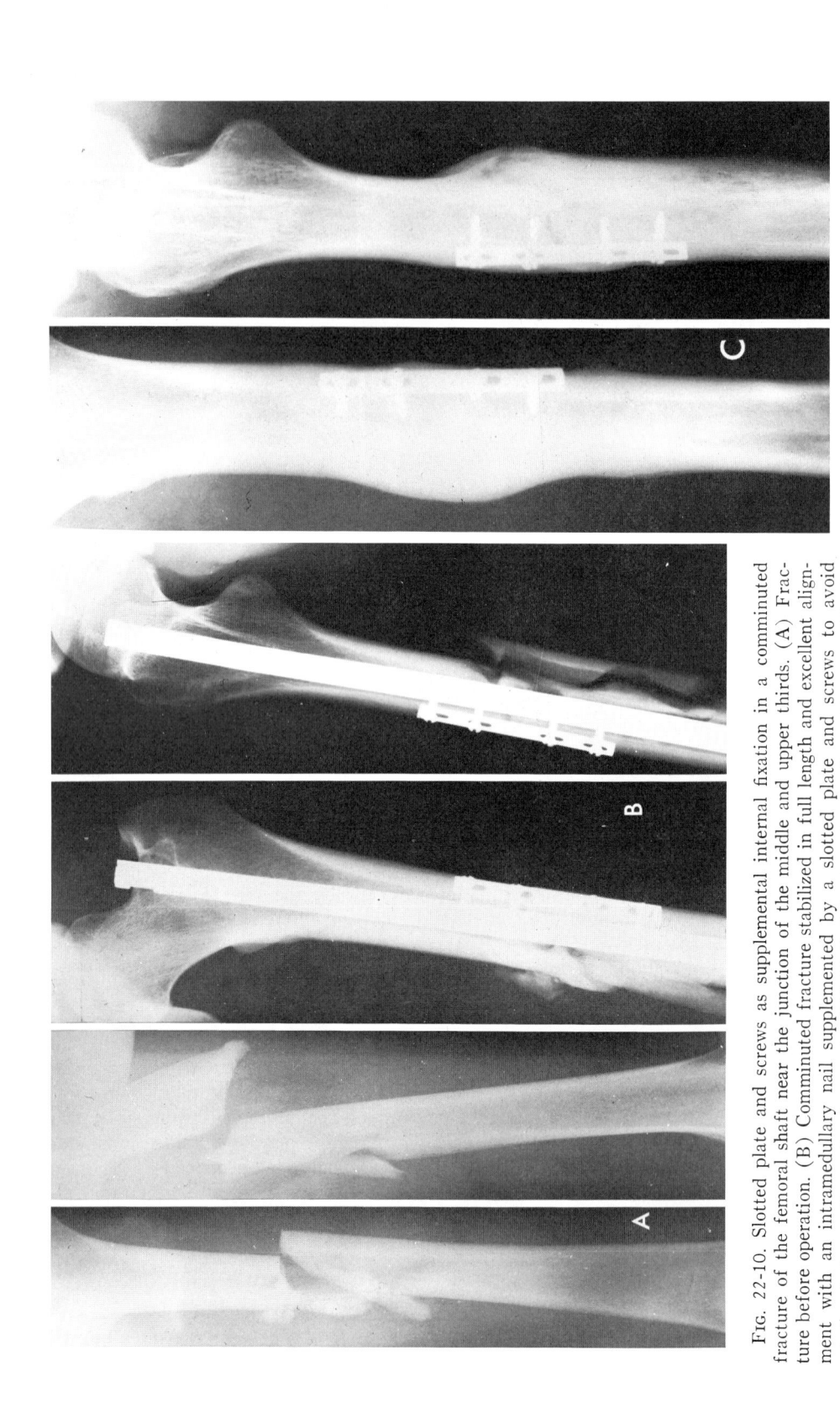

FIG. 22-10. Slotted plate and screws as supplemental internal fixation in a comminuted fracture of the femoral shaft near the junction of the middle and upper thirds. (A) Fracture before operation. (B) Comminuted fracture stabilized in full length and excellent alignment with an intramedullary nail supplemented by a slotted plate and screws to avoid rotation between the major fragments. (C) United fracture in excellent alignment. The intramedullary nail was removed about a year after its insertion. (Hampton, O. P., Jr., and Fitts, W. T., Jr.: Open Reduction of Common Fractures. New York, Grune and Stratton, 1959)

tion and shortening up to 1 inch. Accordingly, reduction does not have to be as precise as in adults.

Traditionally, these fractures in young children have been treated by Bryant's traction (Fig. 22-11), a form of skin traction. In Bryant's traction the hips are flexed 90°, and enough traction is applied on both legs so that the buttocks are lifted just clear of the bed. Depending on the age of the baby, Bryant's traction is usually continued for 2 to 4 weeks, and then if necessary the extremity is immobilized in a plaster hip spica until union is solid—usually another 2 to 3 weeks. Studies by Nicholson showed that Bryant's traction is dangerous above the age of 2 years because this position may cause ischemia of the legs. For children above the age of 2, traction should be skin (as a rule) or skeletal on some splint or inclined plane permitting some flexion of the thigh at the hip, but with the extremity almost horizontal. Traction is on only one leg.

Because children can easily correct some shortening and angulation, plaster immobilization can be used for many of these fractures as long as a reasonable position can be held. Restriction of joint motion and muscle atrophy, which usually follow such immobilization in adults, are not problems in young children.

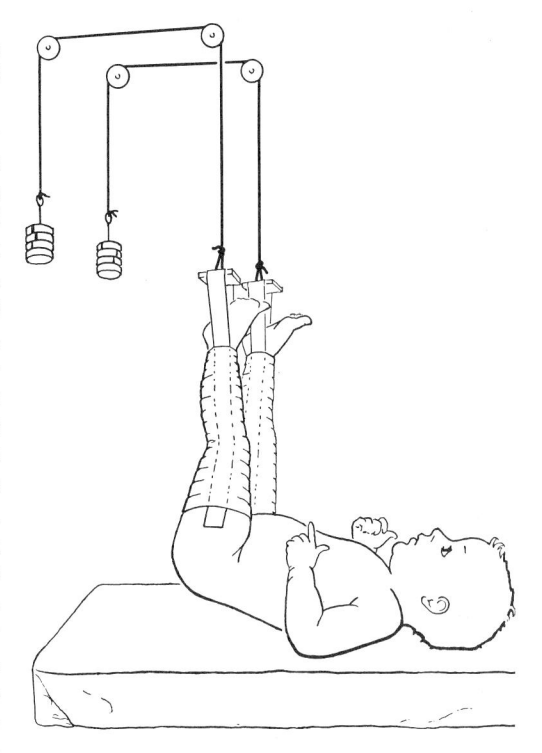

Fig. 22-11. Bryant's traction, a form of balanced suspension skin traction. Bryant's traction may cause ischemia of the feet and the legs (see text).

FRACTURES OF THE DISTAL END OF THE FEMUR

Supracondylar Fracture of the Femur

In almost all fractures of the lower end of the shaft and at the supracondylar level, the distal fragment is angulated posteriorly by the pull of the gastrocnemius, and shortening is usually severe. The sharp edge of the distal fragment as it is pulled posteriorly may injure the popliteal vessels and nerves.

Fractures of the distal femoral shaft and supracondylar fractures with severe posterior displacement may be difficult to reduce by closed methods. The two-wire method described on pages 529 and 530 and illustrated in Fig. 22-8 may be valuable for these injuries. If reduction cannot be obtained by closed methods, satisfactory fixation may be effected at operation as described below under fractures of the condyles.

Fractures of the Condyles

Undisplaced condylar fractures require immobilization in a plaster cast, usually a hip spica, for 6 to 8 weeks. Displaced condylar fractures, however, require an anatomic reduction to minimize the later development of traumatic arthritis. The usual displaced fractures are "T"-fractures, consisting of a transverse fracture just above the condyles with a communicating vertical fracture splitting the condyles apart (Fig. 22-12, A). T-fractures present a difficult problem. They may be managed by open reduction and internal fixation or by balanced skeletal traction suspension with a wire or pin placed below the knee at the level of the tibial tubercle. The latter method is the treatment of choice for severely comminuted fractures.

Treatment by internal fixation usually utilizes a nail–plate combination such as the

534 Fractures and Dislocations of the Lower Extremity

Fig. 22-12. Supracondylar T-fracture of the femur. (A) Drawing of fracture showing disruption of the articular surface and spreading and overriding of the condylar fragments. (B) Drawing showing excellent reduction of the fracture and stabilization with a nail-plate and screws used for internal fixation. (Hampton, O. P., Jr., and Fitts, W. T., Jr.: Open Reduction of Common Fractures. New York, Grune & Stratton, 1959)

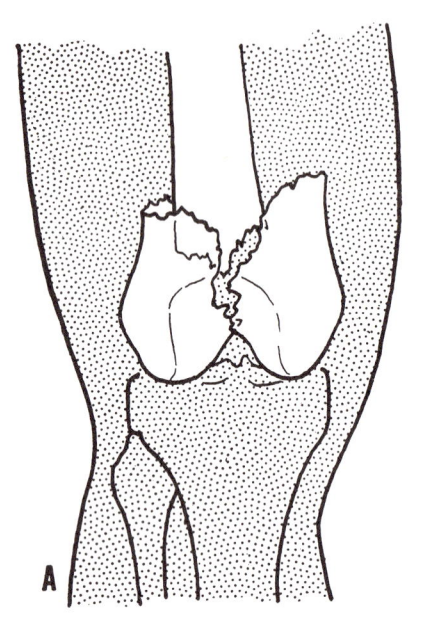

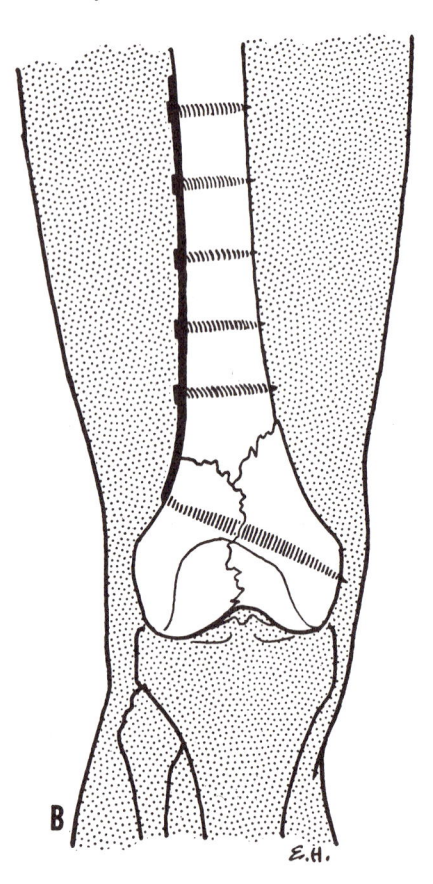

Elliott plate (Fig. 22-12, B). The nail portion transfixes the condyles and holds them together. The plate portion, fixed to the shaft with screws, holds the shaft and condyles in approximation. Postoperative immobilization with a hip spica or, occasionally, a cylinder cast is usually advisable. In some instances 2 crossed intramedullary nails of the Rush type may be satisfactory, but this does not give as good fixation as a nail-plate.

Separation of the Lower Femoral Epiphysis

This is an injury of the 2nd decade of life. In most instances, the displaced epiphysis lies medial and anterior to the shaft. Usually reduction can be effected by closed reduction (Method 1), after which the extremity is immobilized in a single hip spica until union is solid, usually within 6 to 8 weeks. If a satisfactory reduction is not obtained by closed means, open reduction should be done. Fortunately, open reduction is rarely necessary. It is best not to use internal fixation because thereby the epiphysis is further damaged and growth may be disturbed.

DISLOCATION OF THE KNEE

A true dislocation of the knee is a more serious injury by far than the injury which the layman calls a dislocation of the knee. The latter is one of the internal derangements of the knee, usually a torn semilunar cartilage. In a true dislocation of the knee the tibia is completely displaced so that it no longer articulates with the femur. This relatively rare injury is produced by direct violence to the proximal end of the tibia or distal end of the femur while the knee is extended or by forced hyperextension at the knee. For this dislocation to occur, both collateral and both cruciate ligaments must be torn. Probably momentary dislocation with spontaneous reduction occurs occasionally. In such instances, although a dislocation of the knee is not present when the patient is examined, there is marked instability in all directions.

Complications of a complete dislocation of the knee include damage to the popliteal artery and to a major peripheral nerve trunk posterior to the knee, usually the peroneal. The artery may be torn, or its flow of blood obstructed by pressure. This emphasizes the importance of a rapid appraisal of the circulatory status of the leg and the foot when the patient is first seen. Signs of vascular insufficiency demand immediate reduction of the dislocation which, at times, can be done without anesthesia. If after reduction of the dislocation the normal pulsations at the foot do not return, then surgical exploration of the popliteal fossa is indicated with appropriate arterial surgery being carried out, depending on the findings. If there is any doubt about the adequacy of the circulation, an arteriogram should be done.

The peroneal nerve is much more likely to be injured in a dislocation of the knee than is the posterior tibial nerve. The function of each as measured by sensation of the foot and the ability to move the toes and the foot must be tested immediately. This prereduction observation may prove to be advantageous in evaluating the damage to the nerve trunk when a paralysis of the nerve supply to the foot develops after reduction of the dislocation. While the prognosis for eventual recovery is good, it is by no means certain. Even so, immediate exploration for repair of a damaged peripheral nerve trunk is not indicated.

Treatment

Closed reduction of a dislocation of the knee usually can be obtained easily by traction and manipulation. Under ideal circumstances open operation with repair of the collateral and, usually, the cruciate ligaments is indicated and will ensure the best obtainable knee.

Immobilization with the knee flexed 10° in a single hip spica for 4 weeks followed by a snug long leg cast for 4 more weeks may permit sufficient healing of the torn ligaments to give a stable knee and yet permit return of a fairly good range of motion. A hip spica may not be necessary in thin individuals, as a long leg cast may be made to fit snugly; but in all others a hip spica during the first 4 weeks acts as a safeguard against abnormal mobility at the knee which can occur in a long leg cast.

INTERNAL DERANGEMENTS OF THE KNEE

The knee joint, a form of hinge-joint, depends on strong ligaments and the musculature of the thigh for its integrity and stability. The condyles of the femur and the plateau of the tibia are held snugly in contact by these structures in all degrees of flexion and extension of the knee.

An internal derangement of the knee is a mechanical derangement of function of the joint caused by some lesion which eliminates the supporting strength of the major ligaments of the knee or mechanically prevents the constant snug contact and smooth gliding of the plateau of the tibia over the condyles of the femur as the leg is flexed or extended. There are 4 principal internal derangements of the knee:

1. Tears of semilunar cartilages
2. Tears of collateral ligaments
3. Tears of cruciate ligaments
4. Loose osteocartilaginous bodies

All acute closed injuries of the knee without fracture are contusions, sprains (tears of the capsule of some degree, or possibly a tear or contusion of the infrapatellar fat pad) or true internal derangements. The surgeon must differentiate between these as well as is possible by means of the history of injury, the symptoms of the patient and the findings on physical examination. Unless the diagnosis of an internal derangement can definitely be established when the patient is first seen, the injury must be treated as a sprain by means of rest of the joint, compression dressings and possibly aspiration of the accumulated fluid. On the other hand, every acute injury of the knee must not be treated as a simple sprain, as many require specific treatment as outlined below in the discussion of the several internal derangements of the knee.

Tears of Semilunar Cartilages

Tears of the semilunar cartilages result from twisting injuries to the knee. Normally, the semilunar cartilages buffer any rotatory grinding action of the condyles of the femur on the tibia. In some strains, however, one of the cartilages, usually the medial, becomes impinged between the tibia and a condyle of the femur and is torn. The medial cartilage may be torn by an abduction-external rotation strain and the lateral cartilage by an adduction-internal rotation strain. The tear may take the form of a longitudinal split down the long axis of the cartilage (a bucket-handle tear) or a flap may be torn loose at any point along the inner margin. Occasionally, the lateral attachment of the cartilage is avulsed from the tibia. With each type, the torn portion of the cartilage may become caught between a condyle of the femur and the tibia to cause the symptoms of a mechanical derangement.

Diagnosis. In the classical case of a torn medial semilunar cartilage, the patient gives a history of a twisting injury and a painful snapping sensation on the inner side of the knee. Immediately the knee joint is locked* in slight flexion. This usually means a bucket-handle tear with the torn portion of the cartilage displaced into the intercondylar notch of the femur. Pain persists, and considerable effusion develops. Tenderness is fairly well localized over the medial joint line. Roentgenograms are negative, since the semilunar cartilages are not visualized by x-ray examination. This clinical syndrome establishes the diagnosis. However, it occurs in only a small percentage of patients with torn semilunar cartilages.

In the majority of instances, the diagnosis of a torn semilunar cartilage is made on the history of a twisting injury to the knee, perhaps with a snap and subsequent repeated episodes of painful, slipping, catching, near-locking sensations on the inner side of the joint. Tenderness over the cartilage is usually present, and a history of recurring effusions may be obtained. The history also is likely to reveal asymptomatic intervals between these episodes with recurrences brought on by additional twisting injuries of varying severity. Some atrophy of the quadriceps musculature may be discernible. Again x-ray examinations are negative. For diagnostic purposes, a history of repeated actual or impending mechanical derangements well localized to the inner side of the joint is more important than any other symptom or the findings on examination. In a few patients the diagnosis may be justified on only a history of twisting injury, persisting pain and tenderness on the inner side of the knee and a feeling of weakness in the joint, but the diagnosis is made on much sounder grounds if the symptoms of a true mechanical derangement such as locking are present.

The diagnosis of a torn lateral semilunar cartilage is made on comparable clinical symptoms and signs on the lateral side of the joint. This lesion is much less common than a tear of the medial cartilage.

Treatment. Once a semilunar cartilage is torn, it probably never heals. The cartilage has such poor blood supply that any healing efforts are usually ineffective. On the other hand, if, instead of an actual tear of the cartilage, the coronary ligament, which attaches the cartilage to the tibia, is torn so that the entire cartilage is displaced, healing of the torn ligamentous attachment may occur readily if the cartilage is returned to its normal position and held there for a few weeks. With this exception, once a torn cartilage, always a torn cartilage.

Surgical excision of the torn cartilage, or, in selected instances, the torn portion of the cartilage, is the only definitive therapy once the diagnosis has been definitely established. However, surgery may be postponed until a time convenient to the patient, unless the knee remains locked.

Nonoperative treatment includes aspiration of the joint, compression bandages about the knee, the leg and the foot and protection from weight-bearing with crutches until most of the joint reaction has subsided. Actually, nonoperative therapy probably will be employed one or more times in those instances in which the joint is not locked, as the diagnosis cannot be established sufficiently to justify operation without a history of recurring episodes. Occasionally, in first episodes without true locking, a plaster cylinder may be used for 3 or 4 weeks (see page 539 for method of application). The rationale of the plaster cylinder in first episode is based upon the possibility that the entire cartilage has been displaced and, if so, that healing of the coro-

---

* In a locked knee, the leg cannot be extended completely because of a mechanical block. It can be flexed through a good range, although not necessarily a full range.

nary ligament as described above may permanently relieve the patient. With either operative or nonoperative treatment, strenuous quadriceps setting exercises throughout convalescence are highly important in rehabilitation of the patient.

TEARS OF COLLATERAL LIGAMENTS

Tears of the collateral ligaments result from the same type of abduction or adduction strains on the extended knee as those described as the mechanisms of injury for fractures of the tibial condyles (see p. 541). A tear of a collateral ligament on one side and a fracture of the condyle of the tibia on the other side of the knee may result from the same trauma. Tears of the medial collateral ligament are much more common than those of the lateral collateral ligament.

Diagnosis. Tears of the collateral ligaments are acutely painful and are immediately disabling. In all but minor injuries, the patient cannot tolerate weight-bearing. Pain and tenderness are localized over the torn collateral ligament. Hemarthrosis develops rapidly. Within 12 to 24 hours, the skin overlying the torn ligament is likely to become discolored from deep hemorrhage seeping toward the surface.

The diagnosis is confirmed on physical examination. Normally, with the knee extended to 170° or 175° (not hyperextended), abduction and adduction strains elicit little or no lateral movement. With a tear of a collateral ligament, this stabilizing function is impaired or lost so that the extended leg may be abducted (torn medial collateral) or adducted (torn lateral collateral) definitely more than the normal. This is the cardinal sign of a torn collateral ligament of the knee. The degree of abnormal mobility varies with the extent of tear of the ligament.

Treatment. Treatment varies with the extent of the tear which is determined principally by the amount of abnormal lateral mobility. The instability may be masked by the splinting effect of the spasm of the muscles of the thigh produced by the pain of examination as well as the injury itself. Therefore, examination under anesthesia, which relaxes the musculature, may be necessary to demonstrate the full extent of the ligamentous scar.

When the extended leg can be abnormally abducted (or adducted) only 10° or less, probably the injury is essentially a stretching tear rather than a true rupture of the ligament. Under these circumstances, immobilization in a plaster cylinder is indicated (see page 539 for method of application). In these cases the cast should be applied with the knee in 10° to 15° of flexion and with the precaution that the leg is held so as not to place any stretch on the torn ligament. The cast should remain in place for 4 to 6 weeks. During this time, in most instances weight-bearing should be avoided by the use of crutches. When the degree of tear is minimal and when the plaster cylinder remains snug and well fitting, weight-bearing without the use of crutches may be permitted.

When the degree of lateral instability on testing exceeds 10°, primary operative repair, is usually the treatment of choice. In selected instances operative repair may be used for tears of lesser degrees. Operation permits a thorough intra-articular inspection and, if the adjacent semilunar cartilage is torn, it can be removed. The accurate surgical repair of the torn collateral ligament predisposes to the optimal functional result for such a severe injury in the minimum period of time. If for any reason operative treatment is not selected, immobilization for 8 weeks should be provided in a plaster cylinder with the knee flexed 10° to 15°.

TEARS OF CRUCIATE LIGAMENTS

The cruciate ligaments are stretched or torn in injuries which cause excessive movement of the tibia on the femur in the anteroposterior direction. The anterior cruciate ligament, which become taut with the leg in extension and then limits hyperextension, is often torn in twisting-hyperextension injuries. This injury frequently occurs as a result of the extension of a force that ruptures the medial collateral ligament and causes a tear of the medial semilunar cartilage, giving rise to the "unhappy triad" of O'Donaghue: a torn anterior cruciate ligament, ruptured medial collateral ligament and tear of the medial semilunar cartilage. The posterior cruciate ligament, which is taut in flexion and prevents backward displacement of the tibia on the femur, is often torn when the upper portion of the flexed tibia is thrown against a dashboard and as a result is driven backward on the femur.

Diagnosis. The diagnosis of a torn cruciate ligament is made on the basis of physical findings in a patient having all the symptoms of a severe sprain of the knee. Normally, when the knee is in about 90° of flexion, little or no passive movement of the proximal end of the tibia on the femur can be elicited in the anteroposterior direction. When the anterior cruciate ligament is torn, the proximal end of the tibia can be pulled forward excessively (the anterior drawer sign). In addition, excessive hyperextension of the leg may be found. With a torn posterior cruciate ligament, the proximal end of the tibia can be pushed backward on the femur excessively (the posterior drawer sign). Actually, with torn posterior cruciate ligaments, the proximal tibia may remain displaced backward, from which position it can be pulled forward to the normal position. When both cruciate ligaments are torn, the upper tibia can be pushed backward and pulled forward far in excess of the normal. Comparison with the range of passive movement in the anteroposterior direction of the opposite knee is always important in evaluating the findings in a suspected tear of a cruciate ligament. In the acute injury, these tests may be unsatisfactory because of pain; therefore, examination under anesthesia may be advisable.

Treatment. Whether a torn cruciate ligament ever heals spontaneously is subject to question. Many tears of this structure are stretching elongations so that after healing, the ligament remains lax. Complete tears seldom if ever heal so as to restore continuity without operative repair. When the anterior attachment of the anterior cruciate ligament has been avulsed from the anterior tibial spine, it can be held in place by a mattress suture of silk or wire passing through 2 drills holes in the upper tibia (see Fractures of the Tibial Spine, p. 541). Such a repair is frequently a supplemental procedure to operative repair of a torn medial collateral ligament.

If the surgeon suspects a complete tear or an avulsion of a cruciate ligament in an acute knee injury, he is justified in examining the knee with the patient under anesthesia. If his diagnosis is confirmed, operative repair of the torn ligament is usually desirable. After repair the knee is immobilized in a plaster cylinder for about 4 weeks.

In an acute injury, without evidence of a tear sufficient to justify operation, therapy is the same as for a sprain of the knee. If the joint is distended, the fluid is aspirated. If a cruciate ligament has been damaged, the fluid usually contains a considerable amount of blood. A compression dressing is applied, and weight-bearing is restricted or avoided by the use of crutches. This regimen is usually followed until the reaction to injury about the joint has subsided. Occasionally, plaster cylinder immobilization for 4 to 6 weeks is justified. With anterior cruciate lesions, the cast should be applied with the knee in 15° to 20° of flexion. With posterior cruciate tears, the tibia should be held forward and in near complete extension during application of the cast. Strenuous quadriceps-setting exercises during convalescence are important in minimizing residual disability following all tears of the cruciate ligaments.

When a torn cruciate ligament is diagnosed as part of a chronic instability of the knee due to other than a most recent (up to 14 days) injury, about all that can be accomplished is strengthening of the quadriceps, hamstring and calf muscles by an intensive course of exercises. A strong musculature compensates in large measure for loss of the stabilizing effect of a cruciate ligament.

LOOSE OSTEOCARTILAGINOUS BODIES

The exact cause of these is not known. They are generally considered to be secondary to injuries which cause necrosis of a portion of articular cartilage and its subchondral bone. This piece of bone and cartilage is gradually separated from its bed until it falls free into the joint cavity. The most common site of origin of a loose body is the inner or anterolateral surface of the medial condyle of the femur. The condition leading to separation of such a body is called osteochondritis dissecans.

The symptoms of a loose body (joint mouse) in the knee joint are some pain in the knee and recurring slipping, snapping, catching episodes, usually without true locking of the joint. The patient may experience frequent "giving-away" sensations. Recurring effusions are common. The patient actually may palpate a movable particle on either side or the front of the knee.

On examination the surgeon may feel the movable particle. There may be some atrophy of the quadriceps musculature. Otherwise, the physical findings are usually normal.

The diagnosis often is made (or confirmed, if a loose body has been palpable) by the x-ray examination which discloses the loose radiopaque particle varying in size from that of a pea to a large bean. It may lie in the intercondylar notch of the femur or in the knee joint bursa (quadriceps pouch). Occasionally, a loose body may be palpable and not show on x-ray examination. This indicates that the loose body is cartilaginous rather than osteocartilaginous.

Treatment. The indicated therapy is arthrotomy and removal of the loose body or bodies. If this is not done, nonoperative symptomatic therapy is the same as for a sprain of the knee.

FRACTURES OF THE PATELLA

The patella is a large sesamoid bone incorporated in the extensor mechanism of the thigh at the level of the knee. Practically full function of the extremity may be present with the patella removed, yet it does serve several useful purposes. It protects the joint cavity and its contents from injury; it serves as a fulcrum for the extensor mechanism as the flexed leg is extended, thereby permitting better and smoother extensor action; and, cosmetically, it contributes to the contour of the knee.

Fractures of the patella are of real clinical significance only to the extent that the extensor mechanism is divided. An undisplaced or unseparated fracture of the patella on x-ray examination indicates that the surrounding tendon and the retinaculum patellae have not been interrupted. While these injuries are painful and cause some temporary loss of function, essentially the extensor mechanism remains intact, and the power of extension of the leg at the knee is not lost. On the other hand, displacement or separation of the fragments of a broken patella on x-ray examination demonstrates that the soft tissue structures about it have been severed to some extent. In these instances, the extensor mechanism has been interrupted and the power to extend the leg at the knee is lost.

TREATMENT

The objectives of management in fractures of the patella are: the restoration or maintenance of the extensor mechanism of the thigh; a smooth articular surface of the patella; strong musculature of the thigh, particularly the quadriceps muscle group; and maximum range of extension and flexion of the leg at the knee.

WITHOUT SEPARATION OF THE FRAGMENTS

These fractures are accompanied by considerable hemarthrosis, for which aspiration followed by some form of compression dressing is desirable. Immobilization is not necessary if the patient will adequately protect the extremity against a sudden uncontrolled flexion of the leg at the knee which could tear the soft tissues about the patella, resulting in separation of the fragments. Usually, the use of crutches or perhaps only a cane will serve as an adequate safeguard against such a complication. Since early mobility of the knee joint is permitted, this application of the do-nothing method of management (Method 5) predisposes to the maximum return of motion in the knee and minimizes the duration of temporary disability.

When the patient cannot be trusted to protect the knee against additional injury or if he prefers to avoid the use of crutches, the undisplaced fracture of the patella may be protected by a plaster cylinder extending from the upper thigh to a short distance above the ankle with the knee extended to about 175°. The plaster cylinder should be applied over stockinet which is fastened to the skin by tincture of benzoin or some comparable preparation. With the distal end of the stockinet turned back and incorporated in the cast, the cast itself becomes fastened in place and does not tend to drift downward when the patient is ambulatory. With such a plaster cylinder in place, the patient may walk without the aid of crutches. From 4 to 6 weeks of such immobilization is sufficient.

WITH SEPARATION OF THE FRAGMENTS

These fractures present classical indications for primary open reduction (Method 3).

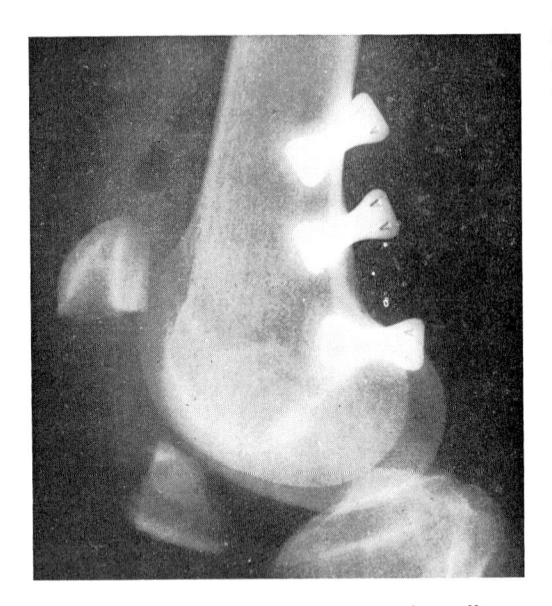

FIG. 22-13. Separated fracture of patella treated by reduction and fixation with a loop of stainless steel wire. (*Top*) Roentgenogram before reduction, lateral view. (*Bottom*) Roentgenograms after reduction, anteroposterior and lateral views.

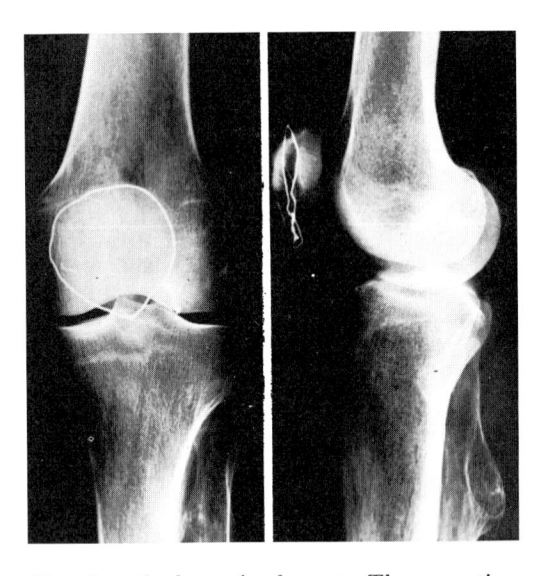

Closed methods are inadequate. The operation is designed to repair the defect in the soft tissue portion of the extensor mechanism and in some instances (see below) accurately approximate the fragments of the patella.

Separated fractures of the patella may be classified as (1) fractures with two major fragments and practically no comminution (2) one major fragment with comminution of the other—usually the distal fragment—and (3) comminuted fractures of the entire patella.

The operative technic varies in these 3 types of displaced fractures of the patella. In fractures with 2 major fragments, a circumferential loop of strong stainless steel wire properly woven in the tendinous tissue, or a mattress suture of wire through parallel transverse drill holes in each fragment may be used to approximate the raw surfaces of bone accurately (Fig. 22-13). In fractures with comminution of the distal or proximal fragment, removal of the comminuted pieces is usually preferable, with approximation of the patella tendon to the raw distal surface of the proximal fragment or of the quadriceps tendon to the raw proximal surface of the remaining distal fragment by a loop, or mattress sutures, of strong wire. In severely comminuted fractures of the entire patella, patellectomy is usually the procedure of choice.

In all of these operative technics, the tears in the extensor mechanism—that is, the expansions of the quadriceps tendon and capsule—must be repaired accurately with interrupted nonabsorbable sutures. When a comminuted fragment of the patella has been removed, often it will be advantageous to imbricate the torn tissues. An accurate repair of the torn tendon and capsule is an integral part of the operative treatment of fractures of the patella.

Postoperative immobilization may or may not be used. If the operative repair has been entirely satisfactory, immobilization is not really necessary, and after soft tissue healing early motion may be instituted. If there is some doubt about the operative repair, a plaster cylinder as described above may be employed for a few weeks.

FRACTURES OF THE PROXIMAL END OF THE TIBIA

Fractures of the proximal end of the tibia may be grouped as fractures of (1) the spine, (2) the lateral condyle (plateau) (3) the medial condyle (plateau) and (4) both condyles (plateaus). In each of these, one or more lines of fracture extend through articular cartilage and enter the knee joint. Objectives of management of each is to achieve as near perfect reduction as possible in order to restore accurately the contour of the articulating surface of the tibia and the stability of the joint.

The diagnosis of these fractures may be suspected by the symptoms and signs at the knee, but only by adequate x-ray studies can it be confirmed and the type of the fracture determined. At times, oblique views supplementing the routine anteroposterior and lateral views will be valuable.

Spine

These are avulsion fractures, as the fragment of bone is pulled away by the anterior cruciate ligament to which it remains attached. They occur in adolescence as an isolated injury. In adults they may be the only significant injury at the knee or they may be part of a comminuted fracture involving one or both condyles of the tibia or complicate an essentially ligamentous internal derangement of the knee (usually a torn medial collateral ligament).

Treatment. When the fragment is not displaced or when a displaced fragment will drop into perfect position upon moderate extension of the knee, a long leg plaster cast is applied. The knee joint is aspirated if hemarthrosis is present. As a rule, in displaced fractures open operation is indicated to fix the fragment in position. This may be accomplished by a mattress suture of catgut, silk or fine wire passing through 2 parallel drill holes beginning over the anterior medial surface of the tibia, emerging through the defect in the articular surface of the tibia and then passing through 2 comparable drill holes in the small bony fragment (Fig. 22-14). In this way, the loop of suture material becomes buried in the substance of the anterior cruciate ligament. Postoperatively, a long leg cast is applied with the knee extended to about 165°. The cast remains in place for 4 to 6 weeks.

Lateral Condyle (Plateau)

These fractures, often called fractures of the lateral plateau, may occur as a result of a force applied to an extended knee from the lateral side such as that provided by the bumper of a moving automobile (the common *bumper fracture*), or from above as might result in a fall from a height when the extremity is somewhat abducted at the hip. These mechanisms force the leg into abduction at

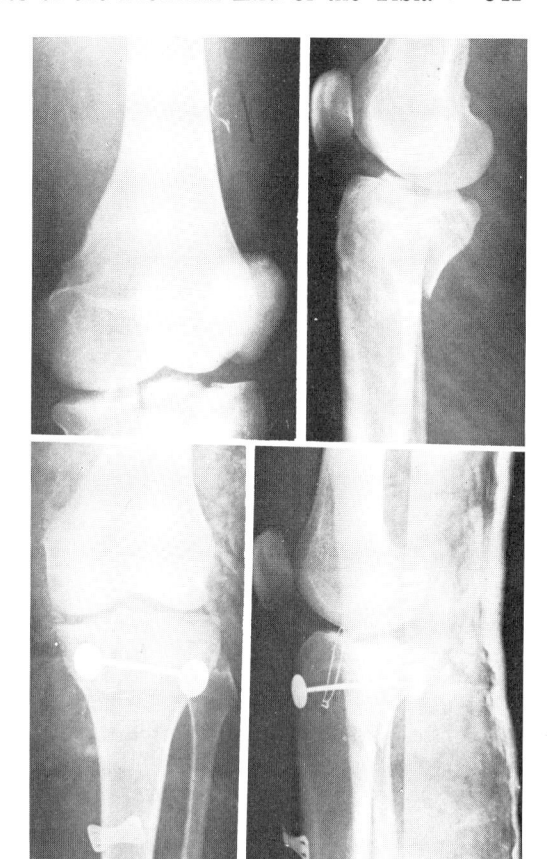

FIG. 22-14. Comminuted fracture of condyles of tibia, including fracture of tibial spine. (*Top*) Anteroposterior-oblique and lateral roentgenograms soon after injury. (*Bottom*) Anteroposterior and lateral roentgenograms after open reduction and internal fixation with tibial bolt. The elevated tibial spine was fixed in position with a loop of wire passed through drill holes.

the knee. The lateral condyle of the femur and the tibia are suddenly compressed against each other. The same mechanisms of injury place a stretching force on the medial collateral ligament (see p. 537). A fracture of the lateral plateau of the tibia or the condyle of the femur or a tear of the medial collateral ligament or some combination of these injuries may result. Also, the lateral semilunar cartilage may be torn by the same force when a fracture of the lateral plateau occurs, or the medial cartilage may be torn when a tear of the medial collateral ligament has resulted.

Fractures of the lateral condyle of the tibia

may consist essentially of one large fragment or they may be severely comminuted. The fragments may remain in good position or be widely displaced. Several fragments of plateau, including portions of the articular cartilage, may be driven downward into the cancellous bone of the condyle.

Treatment. Considerable accumulation of blood in the joint is usually present. This should be removed by aspiration before any form of immobilization is applied.

When the displacement is nil or minimal, a long leg plaster cast usually is provided for 5 or 6 weeks (Method 1). In some instances, when the fragments are so well impacted that further displacement will not occur, a cast may be omitted in favor of a compression dressing for 10 to 14 days. If so, active motion of the joint and quadriceps exercises are immediately instituted. Weight-bearing is avoided, but the patient can be up on crutches. This is an application of Method 5, No Immobilization.

When a large fragment of lateral condyle is displaced laterally or downward, it must be reduced accurately and held reduced until bony union has taken place. Occasionally, reduction can be achieved by lateral compression, for which a carpenter's C-clamp is applicable. After accurate reduction is verified by immediate roentgenograms, a long leg plaster cast, high into the groin, is applied.

However, open reduction of a displaced large condylar fragment is often preferable. The fragment can be reduced accurately under direct visualization and stabilized in excellent position by a bolt passing through it and the medial condyle. While the knee joint is open, any small chips of bone or cartilage and the lateral semilunar cartilage, if torn, are removed. With the fragments firmly fixed in good position, plaster immobilization may be removed after only a few weeks or actually may be omitted altogether so that early active exercises are possible. Open reduction and internal fixation (Method 3) is likely to give the best result obtainable in this type of injury.

In comminuted fractures of the lateral plateau, several fragments are usually depressed downward and spread laterally. Therefore, the articular surface of the plateau is quite distorted. Occasionally, side-to-side compression manually or with a carpenter's C-clamp will give a satisfactory reduction which may be held by a long leg plaster cast. Usually, however, particularly when several fragments including portions of the articular surface are depressed into the substance of the lateral plateau, open reduction is indicated. After the several fragments have been elevated and the articular surface of the plateau reconstituted as best possible, a defect remains in the condyle as a result of the compression of the cancellous bone. This is filled with bone chips removed from the adjacent tibia, the lateral condyle of the femur or the wing of the ilium so as to maintain the elevation of the articular fragments. Usually, supplementary internal fixation is advantageous. At best, a slightly irregular articular surface of the lateral plateau is likely to result. Postoperatively in comminuted fractures, from 6 to 8 weeks of immobilization in a long leg plaster cast is necessary.

In all fractures of the lateral plateau, whether they have been managed by closed reduction and immobilization (Method 1), by open reduction and internal fixation (Method 3), or by no immobilization (Method 5), prolonged protection from weight-bearing is necessary. While ambulation with crutches is permissible, weight-bearing must be avoided until there is solid bony union of the fragments. This usually requires from 3 to 6 months, depending upon the severity of the fracture. Too early weight-bearing while bony union is immature is likely to cause some depression of the lateral plateau with resulting knock-knee, instability and subsequent traumatic arthritis.

Medial Condyle (Plateau)

These fractures, often called fractures of the medial plateau, may occur as a result of a force applied from the medial side to an extended knee, the opposite direction of the force which causes a fracture of the lateral condyle. A fall from a height is unlikely to produce a fracture of the medial condyle, as the extremity is seldom adducted at the hip at the time that the feet strike the ground; moreover, the slight normal valgus of the leg at the knee minimizes the chances of an impact causing a varus strain. The forces which tend to produce a fracture of the medial condyle of the tibia also may cause a tear of the lateral collateral ligament of the knee. Either or both of these may result.

Treatment. Treatment for fractures of the medial condyle of the tibia is entirely analogous to that of fractures of the lateral condyle (see p. 542). The same principles for obtaining reduction of the fracture, for providing immobilization when necessary, and mobilization and exercise as early as possible with prolonged protection from weight-bearing are applicable.

LATERAL AND MEDIAL CONDYLES (T-FRACTURES)

These fractures may occur as a result of a compression force which impacts the plateaus of the tibia and the condyles of the femur together while the knee is extended. They result from falls from a height or in vehicle accidents from the force of an uprising floor board which jams the plateaus of an extended tibia against the condyles of the femur. Each condyle may be essentially a large single fragment or both may be severely comminuted.

Treatment. Aspiration of blood from the knee joint is indicated. The choice of treatment for the fracture depends principally upon the degree of comminution of the fragments.

Occasionally, displacement of the fragments will be so minimal that reduction is not necessary. Mildly displaced fragments can be reduced in some instances by closed manipulation using manual traction applied at the ankle and side-to-side compression at the proximal end of the tibia. In either instance, immobilization is provided by a long leg cast. Much caution is required to make certain that the extremity is held so that neither a knock-knee nor a bowleg strain is made during application of the cast.

When the fragments are significantly displaced, open reduction or continuous traction is usually preferable. At times, a combination of these will give the best result.

When large condylar fragments are spread laterally and medially, they often can be approximated with a tibial bolt so as to restore the articular surface of the tibia (Fig. 22-14). The fixation of the condyles may provide sufficient stability at the fracture site to permit the use of a long leg plaster cast for immobilization. In other instances, continuous skeletal traction using a pin through the distal tibia will be necessary to avoid some telescoping of the shaft between the condyles and resulting shortening.

When the condylar fragments are severely comminuted and displaced, continuous skeletal traction is the preferable method of management. Traction must be maintained until sufficient healing has occurred so that the fragments will not telescope again. This usually requires from 6 to 8 weeks in traction. Then, further immobilization in a cast is usually necessary.

The period of immobilization in these fractures varies. It may be only a few weeks in impacted fractures. In severely comminuted fractures which are displaced, immobilization must be maintained for several months. When union has progressed to a point where redisplacement or angulation will not occur, removal of all immobilization is advisable in order to permit exercise of the knee. As with fractures of either the medial or the lateral plateau, however, weight-bearing must be avoided until bony union is solid and mature.

FRACTURES OF THE SHAFTS OF THE BONES OF THE LEG

Fractures of the shafts of the bones of the leg result both from direct trauma, such as the impact of an automobile bumper, and indirect trauma, such as the rotation or leverage strain incurred when an individual steps into a deep hole while running. One or both bones may be broken, and the fracture of either may be transverse, oblique, spiral, double or even triple, and minimally or severely comminuted. Because the tibia is entirely subcutaneous on its anterior and medial surfaces, open fractures of this bone are common.

Diagnosis of fractures of the shafts of the bones of the leg is usually established easily by the clinical symptoms and signs, especially when the tibia is broken. However, adequate roentgenograms are essential to determine the extent and the contour of the fractures so that the proper method of management can be selected.

A pitfall in diagnosis is the erroneous conclusion that only a fracture of the tibia is present when actually both bones are broken. This is important, not because the fragments of the fibula must be reduced, but because

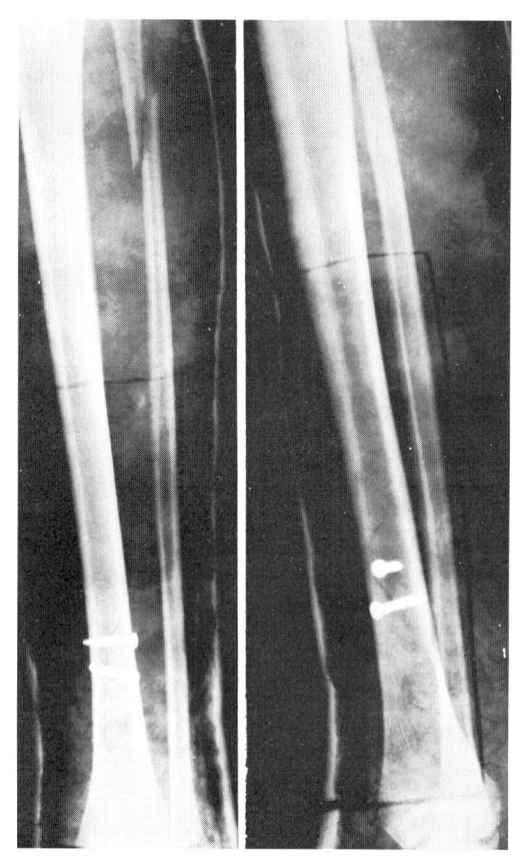

FIG. 22-15. Roentgenograms in 2 planes of spiral-oblique fracture of lower shaft of tibia with associated fracture of proximal fibula. Treatment by open reduction of fracture of tibia and internal fixation with 2 screws. Note the window in the cast made for dressing the wound and removal of the sutures. Replacement of the window minimizes localized edema. (*Left*) Anteroposterior view. (*Right*) Lateral view.

occur. Actually, the fibula may be broken in the unvisualized proximal third, a not uncommon location for such a fracture in association with spiral or oblique fractures of the tibia in the lower third. This combination of injuries is produced by a twisting trauma on the foot and the ankle. It is important that the entire shafts of both the tibia and the fibula be well visualized on roentgenograms before the diagnosis of a fracture of the tibia alone or even of the fibula alone is made (Fig. 22-15).

Fractures of the shafts of both bones of the leg are problem fractures for several reasons. As stated above, many are open fractures so that the hazard of wound infection and prolonged drainage is introduced. Reduction is often not only difficult to obtain but even more difficult to maintain. Circulation to the soft tissues of the leg, particularly on the anteromedial surface in the lower third, is at times so precarious as to make operative intervention too risky. Nonunion of a fracture of the tibia occurs not infrequently, not only because of the reasons just enumerated but chiefly because this bone has meager muscle attachments and blood supply, especially in the lower half.

Treatment

Each of the first 4 methods of management —(1) closed reduction and immobilization, (2) balanced skeletal traction, (3) open reduction and (4) external skeletal fixation (usually by transfixion pins incorporated in plaster)—finds application for certain fractures of the shaft of the tibia. The fact that 1 of 4 different methods may be indicated is further evidence of the complexity of these injuries. Precise surgical judgment is often required for the selection of the best method of management.

The selection of the best method of management is based upon several factors. Of these, the contour of the fracture as revealed by the roentgenograms is probably the most important. Others are the general condition and age of the patient, the quality of the circulation to the foot and the leg, the character of the skin overlying the fracture site, whether the fracture is open or closed, the presence of other injuries, the equipment at hand, and the experience and expertise of the surgeon.

Closed Reduction and Immobilization

when the fibula is broken, its splinting effect on the tibia is lost, a factor which may be significant in the selection of the proper method of management for the tibia. Failure to recognize a fracture of the fibula is most likely to occur with a spiral or oblique fracture of the lower third of the tibia which on roentgenograms of the lower half of the leg is shown in fairly good position with minimal displacement and overriding. If a fracture of the fibula is not visualized, it may be wrongly concluded that the fibula is intact and that further displacement of the fracture of the tibia will not

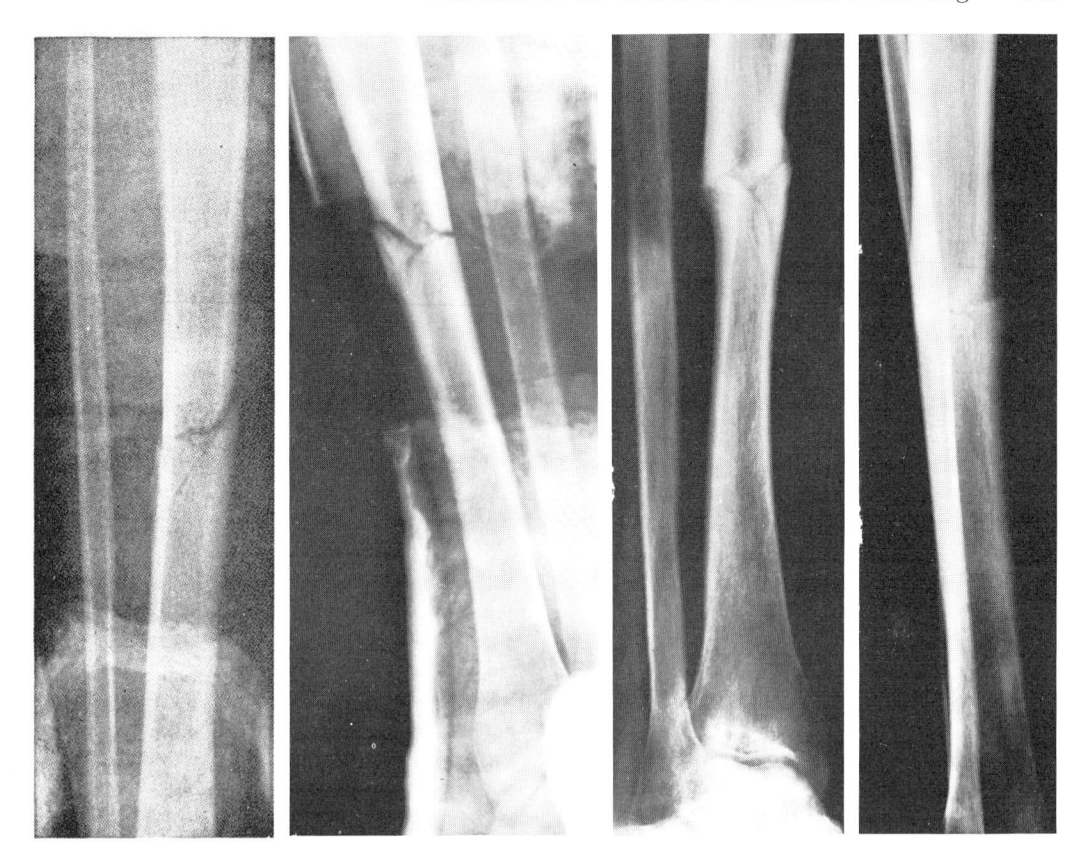

Fig. 22-16. Stable fracture of the tibial shaft. (A and B) Roentgenograms of stable near transverse fracture treated successfully by closed reduction and immobilization in a long leg plaster cast, utilizing the "3-way plaster" technic (see text). Anteroposterior and lateral roentgenograms taken at time of reduction. (C and D) Roentgenograms in 2 planes, showing uniting fractures.

(Method 1). Closed reduction with immobilization in a long leg plaster cast is usually selected for fractures of the shaft of both bones of the leg when a stable reduction of the tibia may be achieved (or is already present in undisplaced fractures) (Fig. 22-16). A reduction is classified as stable when, because the contour of the fracture is transverse or so near transverse, displacement of the fragments is unlikely to recur so long as they are kept in good alignment. A stable reduction is not to be anticipated when the contour of the tibial fracture is oblique, spiral or appreciably comminuted and the fibula is also broken.

Reduction is achieved under general or spinal anesthesia by means of strong traction on the foot and the ankle against equally strong countertraction, usually applied at the knee, together with direct manipulation of the fragments at the fracture site bringing the distal fragment first into apposition and then into alignment with the proximal fragment. The stability of reduction is tested by gently compressing the distal fragment against the proximal fragment while good alignment is maintained. If the reduction is not sufficiently stable to withstand this compression force, it is less likely to be maintained in a plaster cast.

When a satisfactory, stable reduction has been achieved (check roentgenograms at this stage are valuable) a lightly padded, long leg cast is applied. It extends from the upper thigh to the toes and holds the ankle at a right angle, the foot in neutral version, and the knee, as a rule, in 10° to 15° of flexion.

The cast should be well molded, especially about the knee and the foot and the ankle.

The "three-way" plaster technic may facilitate the application of this method. By this technic one segment of plaster is applied from the groin to just above the fracture and another segment from the toes to just below the fracture. The fracture site itself is left uncovered. Then manipulation of the fracture is carried out using the 2 segments covered with plaster (Fig. 22-16). When reduction has been achieved the 2 segments are joined by applying plaster over the fracture site. The advantage of this method is that better control of the proximal and the distal fragments is effected, and one does not incur the risk of redisplacement while the cast is being applied about the knee and the ankle.

Closed reduction and immobilization in a plaster cast can be applied for a large percentage of the fractures of the shaft of both bones of the leg in adults and, for practical purposes, it is indicated for all of these fractures in growing children. It offers many advantages. It is a method with few pitfalls and complications. It entails no risk to life or limb. It makes the patient immediately ambulatory on crutches. It gives a very high percentage of good results, provided that the reduction is maintained in the plaster cast. However, if reduction is unstable, other methods often must be used, even though they are more confining and may entail some risk. When an unstable rather than a stable reduction is to be anticipated from the contour of the fracture, one of the other methods may be selected primarily unless there are contraindications. The choice between these will rest principally on the contour of the fracture, although the other factors mentioned above must also be evaluated carefully.

Continuous Traction (Method 2). This method may be selected for varying reasons. In comminuted fractures precluding a stable reduction by closed or open methods, traction will serve to maintain length and usually adequate apposition and alignment. In oblique or spiral fractures for which open operation might otherwise be preferable but which is contraindicated because of unhealthy skin, the general condition of the patient, inadequate equipment or facilities, or inexperience on the part of the surgeon in the open treatment of fractures, continuous traction affords a highly acceptable method of management.

Skeletal traction using a Kirschner wire or a Steinmann pin through the lower tibia or the os calcis is far preferable to skin traction. The latter is, for practical purposes, ineffective for fractures of both bones of the leg.

Splinting for the skeletal traction may be provided in several ways. Some authorities advise suspension in a Thomas splint with Pierson knee attachment or on a Böhler-Braun frame. More effective splinting, however, is provided by the use of skeletal traction combined with a plaster cast.

Skeletal traction in a cast is provided as follows: after insertion of wire or a pin and attachment of a traction bow, strong manual traction is applied, and the fragments are manipulated until good apposition and alignment are obtained. While the traction is maintained, a long leg padded plaster cast is applied. The padding is usually made rather heavy at the knee in order that the fixation there will not be absolute. The plaster incorporates the pin or wire and traction bow. The foot is immobilized at a right angle, and the knee in only slight flexion. As the plaster is hardening, every effort is made to maintain perfect alignment of the fragments.

Postoperatively, the leg in the cast is placed on one or two pillows, and from 6 to 8 pounds of traction is provided. The patient may be turned to either side so long as the general direction of the traction remains the same. Traction is maintained until sufficient healing has occurred to maintain apposition and length. This usually requires from 5 to 6 weeks. Then, the wire or pin may be removed and a new cast applied for further immobilization. Throughout the period of traction, check roentgenograms in two views are made to ensure that the amount of traction is adequate but not excessive and that good alignment is being maintained.

Open Reduction and Internal Fixation (Method 3). This method may be selected for fractures having a contour permitting a stable internal fixation, provided that the equipment, the facilities and the experience of the surgeon are adequate. Oblique or spiral fractures of the tibia may be fixed with multiple screws (see Fig. 22-15).

Intramedullary nailing of the tibia has been

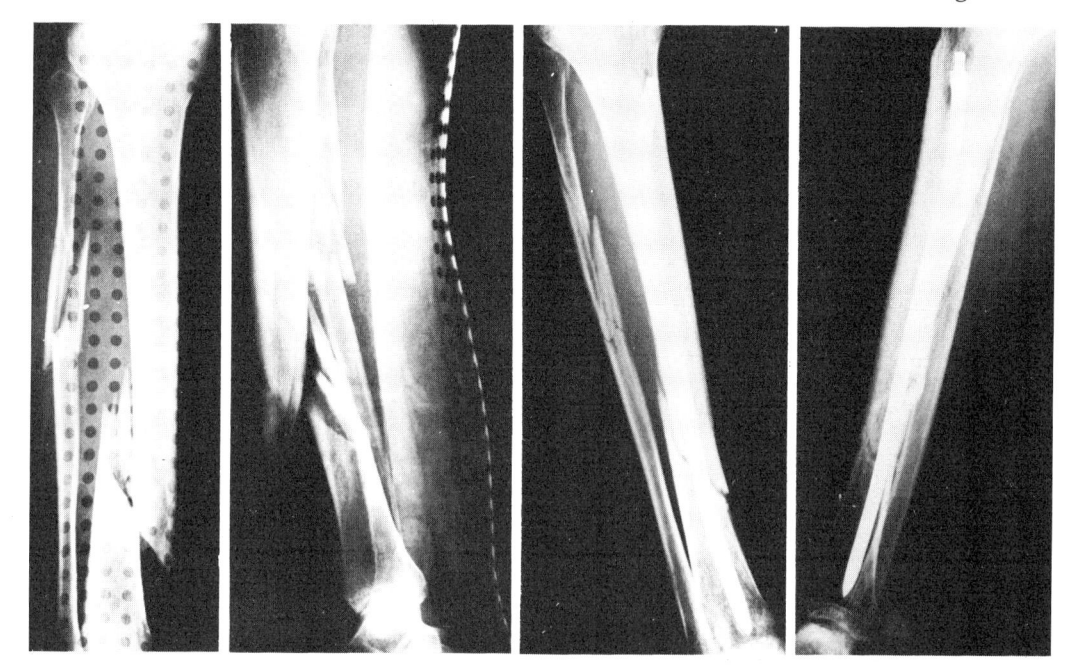

Fig. 22-17. Comminuted open fracture of both bones of leg in lower part of middle third. Treatment by débridement, internal fixation with a Lottes intramedullary nail and primary closure of the wound. (A and B) Roentgenograms in 2 planes with emergency splint in place. (C and D) Several months after operation, showing excellent apposition and alignment and early bony union.

shown to be effective for fractures of the shafts of both bones of the leg (Fig. 22-17). When the contour of the fracture will permit a reasonably stable fixation by an intramedullary nail, it is probably the best type of internal fixation. Fractures with enough comminution to prevent a stable closed reduction can often be stabilized adequately with this technic. Surgeons experienced in the use of intramedullary nails in the tibia can insert them "blindly" in closed fractures, that is, without an incision at the fracture site and thereby avoid any risk of wound complications at that level. Fractures with minimal comminution also may be fixed with a plate, preferably slotted, and held by screws (Fig. 22-18). This method has proved to be inferior to others, and fewer and fewer surgeons are using it.

Supplemental immobilization in a plaster cast is essential following all forms of internal fixation, including intramedullary nailing. With the latter, earlier weight-bearing in a walking cast is feasible, and often this can be initiated a few weeks after operation.

External Skeletal Fixation (Method 4). This method has been used for unstable fractures of both bones of the leg. Its application with true external skeletal fixation apparatus (Roger Anderson or Stader apparatus are examples) is not a recommended procedure. Certainly, this method should be used only by surgeons with extensive experience with it.

An acceptable substitute is provided by a long leg plaster cast incorporating transfixion pins through the upper and the lower major fragments (Fig. 22-19). The pins are inserted, the fracture is held reduced, and the cast is applied. The pins are removed, and a new cast is substituted after enough healing of the fracture has occurred to prevent displacement and overriding of the fragments. The hazards of the method are necrosis and infection about pins and distraction of the fragments with nonunion.

Period of Immobilization. The period of

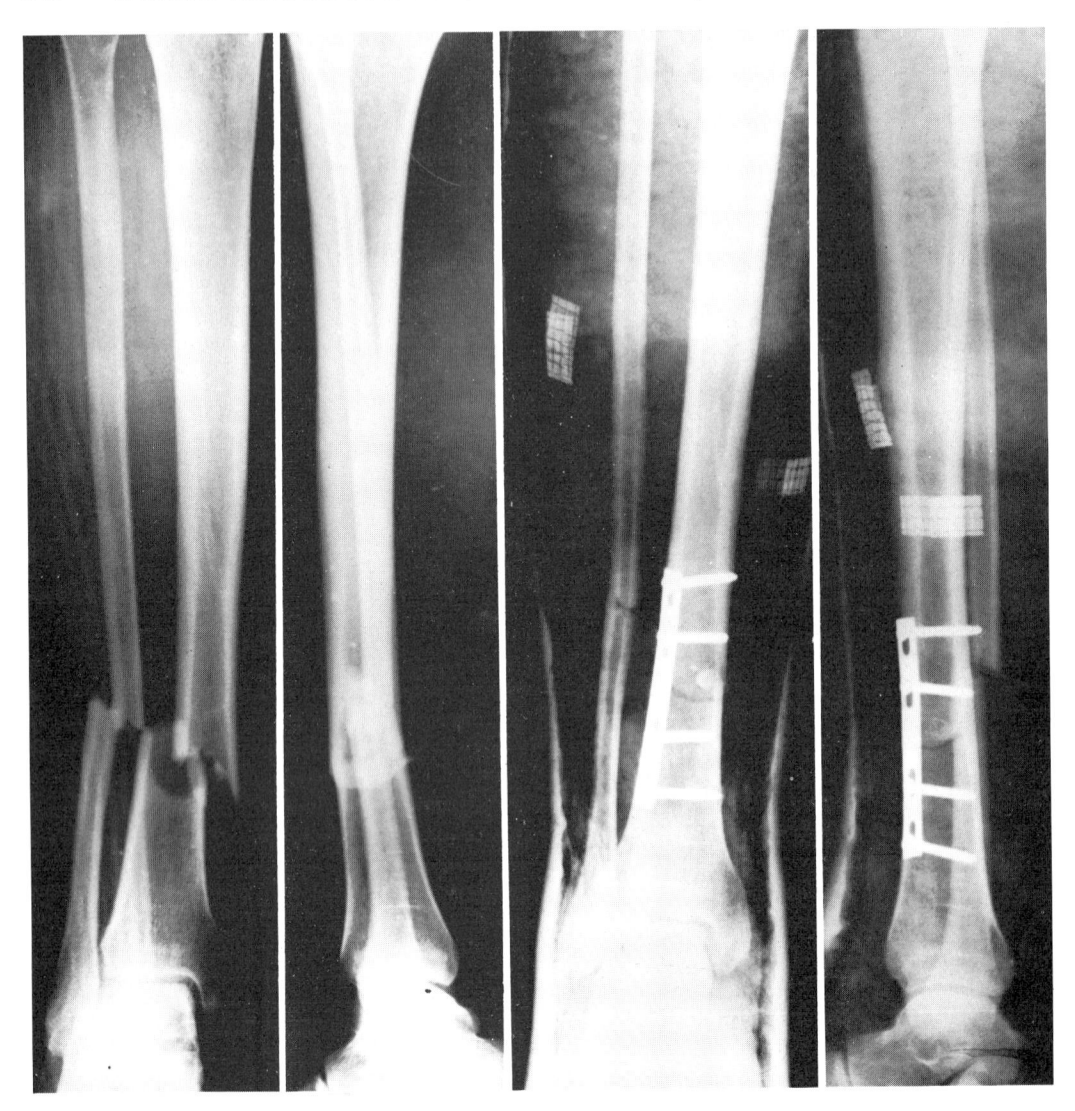

FIG. 22-18. Fractures of both bones of the leg in the distal third. Treatment by open reduction of the tibia and internal fixation with a slotted plate and screws. (A and B) Roentgenograms in 2 planes before operation. (C and D) After operation.

time required for solid healing of fractures of both bones of the leg will vary with the age of the patient, the contour and the location of the fracture of the tibia and the quality of the reduction and immobilization of the fragments. With all methods of management healing is slow and requires many months. While, in general, union is secured faster in closed than in open fractures and when apposition of the fragments is excellent and is maintained, even under these favorable circumstances, a long time may be required for solid union of the fracture of the tibia.

Older textbooks frequently have estimated the period of immobilization and for union of these fractures as from 8 to 12 weeks. This is entirely too short. The average period for adequate union is at least 4 or 5 months. Union does not take place in many for 8 or 10 months. Immobilization must be continued until the fracture of the tibia is solidly united, clinically and as shown on roentgenograms. The immobilization may be discontinued before union of the fracture is complete only in those fractures adequately stabilized by intramedullary nailing and, even with these, a walking plaster cast for several months is less hazardous than early removal of the immobilization.

FRACTURES OF THE SHAFT OF THE TIBIA WITH AN INTACT FIBULA

Fractures of the shaft of the tibia alone usually are not significantly displaced and require only immobilization in a long leg plaster cast (Method 1) with the knee in some 10° to 15° of flexion and the foot at 90° and in neutral version. The splinting effect of the intact fibula may effect a stable reduction of a fracture of the tibia with a contour which otherwise would indicate an unstable situation. Occasionally, however, significant displacement of a fracture of the tibia will occur even with an intact fibula. This often can be overcome and a stable reduction obtained by closed manipulation, following which the cast is applied. Infrequently, usually in spiral fractures in the lower third of the tibia, adequate apposition of the fragments cannot be maintained after closed reduction, so operative reduction and internal fixation (usually with 2 or more screws) are indicated. The perfect reduction obtained at operation avoids the slight shortening of the tibia which would result from overriding of the fragments. Such a shortening would cause permanent disturbance of the ankle joint relationship. Perfect reduction also shortens the healing time by providing excellent contact of the fragments. But even with internal fixation of the fracture, immobilization in a long leg plaster cast is essential.

The period of time required for solid healing of a fracture of the tibia alone, as with fractures of both bones of the leg, will vary with its contour and location and the age of the patient. In children, in whom fractures of the tibia alone are not uncommon, the period of immobilization should be from 3 to 4 weeks in very small children and from 6 to 8 weeks in young teen-agers. In adults a longer period of time is usually required. Certainly, from 8 to 10 weeks of immobilization is the minimum, from 12 to 14 the average, and from 16 to 18 not uncommon. The prognosis for union of a fracture of the tibia alone is excellent, but nonunion may occur, especially in transverse fractures of the shaft of the tibia in the middle or lower thirds.

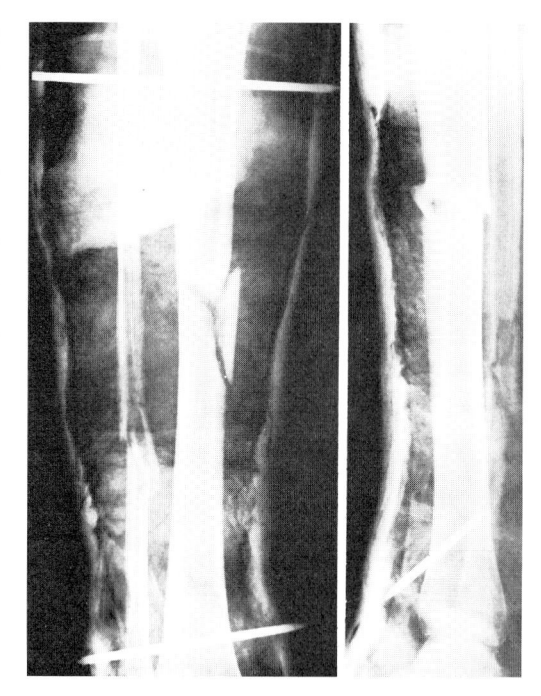

FIG. 22-19. Unstable fracture of both bones of the leg in the midshaft held in good reduction by a transfixion pin above and another below the fracture each incorporated in a long leg plaster cast. (*Left*) Anteroposterior and (*right*) lateral roentgenograms.

FRACTURES OF THE SHAFT OF THE FIBULA WITH AN INTACT TIBIA

Fractures of the shaft of the fibula are not important skeletal injuries. When this fracture accompanies a fracture of the shaft of the tibia, all efforts should be directed toward obtaining and maintaining adequate reduction of the latter, and the fracture of the fibula may be ignored. When the shaft of the fibula alone is broken, the intact tibia splints the fragments and they practically always remain in good position.

Fractures of the shaft of the fibula alone are usually immobilized in a plaster cast in order to minimize pain and maintain the foot in a good functioning position, although healing undoubtedly would occur without immobilization. A plaster cast applied for a fracture

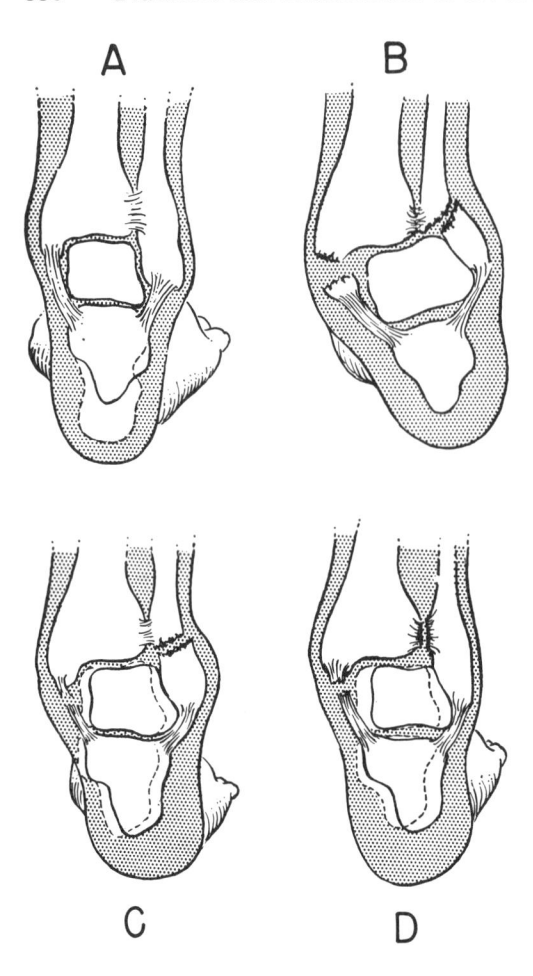

Fig. 22-20. Drawings to show bony and ligamentous support of the ankle mortise.

(A) The normal ankle, showing major ligamentous support of the ankle mortise.

(B) Bimalleolar fracture with lateral displacement of foot. The ligaments are intact.

(C) Fracture of the lateral malleolus and a disrupted deltoid ligament on the medial side of the ankle joint with lateral displacement of the foot. The injuries in (B) and (C) are quite comparable.

(D) Disruption of the deltoid ligament and the ligament supporting the inferior tibial-fibular synchondrosis with lateral displacement of the foot comparable in part to that in (C).

(Hampton, O. P., Jr., and Fitts, W. T., Jr.: Open Reduction of Common Fractures. New York, Grune & Stratton, 1959)

of the shaft of the fibula need not extend above the knee. The plaster need be kept on for only 3 to 4 weeks, although solid union of the fracture may not take place for 6 to 8 weeks.

FRACTURES AND DISLOCATIONS OF THE ANKLE

The ankle joint depends upon ligamentous as well as bony structures for its integrity. The ligaments supporting the inferior tibiofibular synchondrosis contribute materially to the stability of the ankle by maintaining the ankle mortise, the bony framework formed by the malleoli about the talus. The large deltoid ligament on the medial side of the joint and the calcaneofibular and the talofibular ligaments on the lateral side maintain the talus in the mortise and prevent abnormal lateral motion.

In evaluating and managing bony injuries about the ankle joint, it must be determined whether these ligaments have been torn (Fig. 22-20). A torn deltoid ligament, for example, is probably as significant as a fracture of the medial malleolus. Figure 22-20 B shows a bimalleolar fracture with lateral displacement of the malleolar fragments and the foot. Figure 22-20 C shows a fracture of only the lateral malleolus with the same displacement. For this to occur without fracture of the medial malleolus, the deltoid ligament must be torn. The injuries shown in Figures 22-20 B and 22-20 C then are entirely comparable insofar as the integrity of the ankle joint is concerned. Similarly, Figure 22-20 D shows a lateral dislocation of the foot without fracture. For this to occur, there must be disruption of both the deltoid ligament and the ligament supporting the inferior tibiofibular synchondrosis.

In addition to the malleoli and the strong ligaments of the ankle, the surgeon is concerned with the "posterior malleolus" of the tibia in injuries about the ankle. This posterolateral prominence of the tibia contains the posterior portion of the articular surface. It is frequently fractured and displaced away posteriorly or upward from the main body of the tibia. When a fracture of the posterior malleolus is the only injury about the ankle, it remains undisplaced. When it is associated with either a fracture of the medial or the lateral malleolus or of both, or a rupture of a major ligament, the foot and the posterior malleolus often are displaced posteriorly.

Fractures of the ankle result from strong abduction or adduction strains. They may be classified as those of (1) lateral malleolus, (2) medial malleolus, (3) posterior malleolus, (4) bimalleolar (medial and lateral malleoli) and (5) trimalleolar fractures. As outlined above, any of these may be associated with dislocation. A trimalleolar fracture-dislocation of the ankle is not an uncommon injury.

Treatment

Treatment of fractures about the ankle varies with the degree of displacement of the malleolar fragments and the foot. The objectives of management of fractures about the ankle are: (1) to restore the talus to its proper place beneath the tibia; (2) to reduce accurately the fractures of all the malleoli; and (3) to maintain the reduction of the fractures and dislocation until all disrupted bony and ligamentous structures have healed. If any degree of dislocation of the talus or widening of the mortise is allowed to persist, instability, pain, early traumatic arthritis, and considerable disability are likely to follow.

Fractures of the Ankle Without Displacement

These fractures require only plaster cast immobilization (Method 1). Usually, the cast may extend only to just below the knee; but it should extend to the upper thigh if there is any question of subsequent displacement of the fragments in the cast, as in many trimalleolar and bimalleolar fractures. The ankle should be held at 90° and the foot in neutral version. Immobilization in plantar flexion and inversion is to be avoided, as this position predisposes to prolonged disability after the cast is removed. Usually, a walking type cast is advantageous.

Healing of a fracture of the lateral malleolus, even though it has not been displaced, is not rapid, and fracture lines may be visible on roentgenograms for several months. Usually, however, from 6 to 8 weeks of immobilization in a cast will permit sufficient union to make further immobilization unnecessary. A fracture of the medial malleolus in good position unites more rapidly, and 4 weeks of immobilization is usually sufficient. The most rapid healing in fractures about the ankle occurs in those of the posterior malleolus. These fracture lines on roentgenograms have been observed to disappear in $2\frac{1}{2}$ to 3 weeks. Bimalleolar and trimalleolar fractures should be immobilized for 6 to 8 weeks.

Fractures of the Ankle With Displacement

These fractures require precise reduction. Usually closed reduction (Method 1) with immobilization in a plaster cast will suffice, but in many instances open reduction (Method 3) is necessary or advantageous.

Fractures of the Lateral Malleolus With Lateral Dislocation of the Foot (Fig. 22-21). This displacement cannot take place unless the deltoid ligament is torn. This injury usually requires general or spinal anesthesia, although occasionally local anesthesia will suffice. The manipulative maneuvers are manual traction on the foot with pressure on the fragment toward its normal position. These should be carried out with the knee flexed from 45° to 90° to relax the gastrocnemius muscle. Flexion of the knee over the side or the end of the table will provide the necessary flexion. Closed reduction usually is entirely adequate, but a few authorities strongly recommend operative repair of the torn deltoid ligament, which will ensure precise healing of that structure and is a safeguard against recurrence of the lateral displacement of the foot while in the cast. If precise reduction of the dislocation cannot be obtained by manipulation and maintained by a cast, it is likely that torn fibers of the deltoid ligament have become caught between the talus and the medial malleolus. Then operative intervention is mandatory. With removal of the intervening soft tissues, reduction of the dislocation is made easy, and with the deltoid ligament repaired, dislocation will not recur.

In these injuries treated by closed reduction, the plaster cast should extend well above the knee so as to immobilize it and avoid rotation strains at the ankle. These might cause recurrence of the dislocation.

Fractures of the Medial Malleolus. With Displacement of the Malleolus But Without Dislocation of the Ankle. The

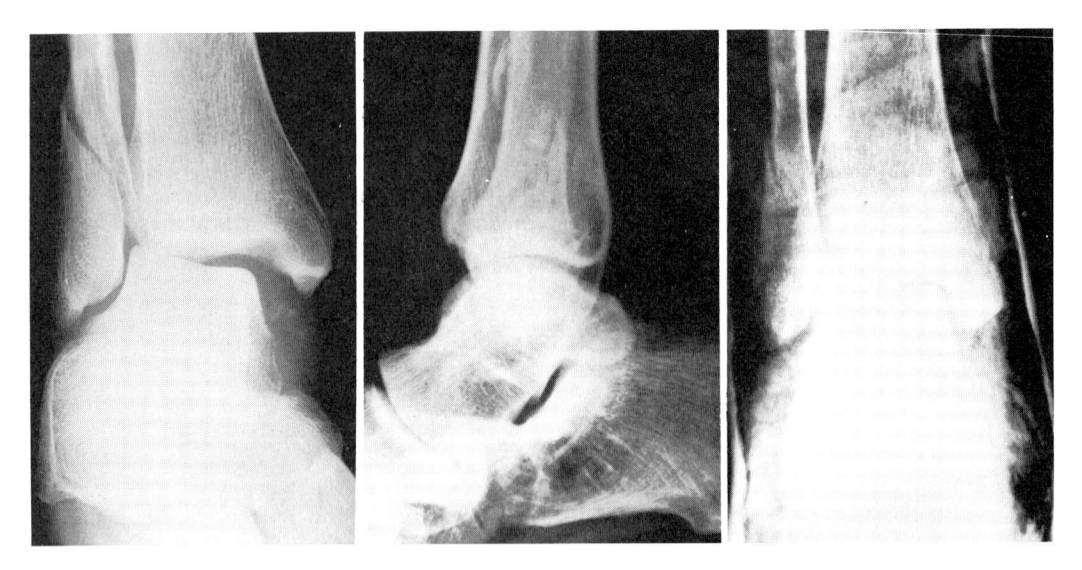

552 Fractures and Dislocations of the Lower Extremity

Fig. 22-21. Fracture of lateral malleolus with lateral dislocation of the foot. Treatment by closed reduction. (*Left and Center*) Anteroposterior and lateral roentgenograms before reduction. For this displacement to occur the deltoid ligament must have been ruptured. (*Right*) After closed reduction and immobilization in a plaster cast, anteroposterior view.

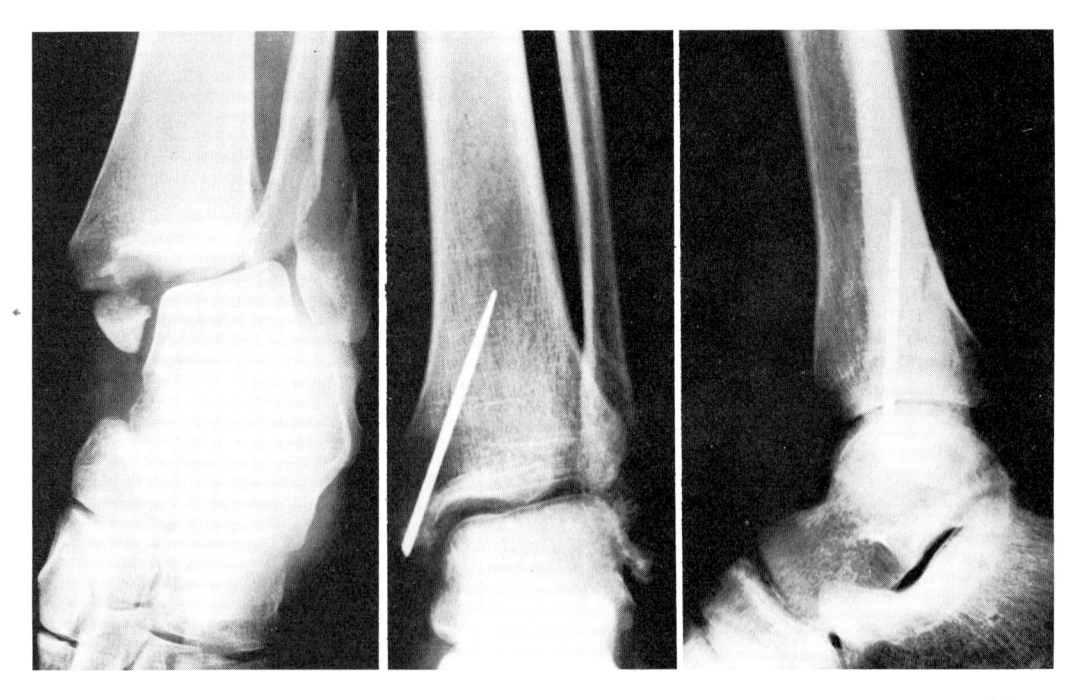

Fig. 22-22. Bimalleolar fracture of the ankle with lateral displacement of the foot, treated by open reduction and internal fixation of medial malleolus. (*Left*) Anteroposterior view before operation. (*Center and Right*) Roentgenograms in 2 planes showing position obtained at operation.

medial malleolus is frequently displaced distally. Usually, under anesthesia, an effort should be made to replace it by full dorsal flexion and perhaps slight inversion of the foot. If the raw edges can be well approximated, immobilization of the leg and the foot in a below-the-knee walking type plaster cast for 4 weeks will permit union of the fragment (Method 1).

In many instances, the raw surface of the medial malleolus cannot be approximated to that of the body of tibia because tags of the periosteum or deltoid ligament have fallen into the fracture site. In such instances, operation is often indicated to permit removal of the soft tissue from the space between the fragments (Method 3). Operative fixation of the medial malleolus usually is obtained by means of a screw or a threaded pin. The internal fixation must be supported by a below-the-knee plaster of Paris cast for at least 4 weeks.

WITH DISPLACEMENT AND LATERAL DISLOCATION OF THE FOOT. As outlined above, this results from disruption of the inferior tibiofibular synchrondrosis. Under these circumstances, manipulative reduction may restore the fibula to its proper place and the medial malleolus into approximation with the tibia, but operative fixation of the malleolus is highly preferable (Method 3). With the malleolus fixed in accurate position, the fibula is pulled back against the tibia, and the ankle mortise is restored. The operative approach is on the medial side of the ankle in this injury, and operation on the outer side of the ankle usually is not necessary. On the other hand, screw fixation of the fibula to the tibia a short distance above the ankle is employed sometimes to aid in maintaining the mortise. If a screw is used, it should be removed before full weight-bearing is allowed.

In this injury a long leg plaster cast for at least 3 weeks, followed by a below-the-knee plaster cast for additional 3 to 5 weeks, is indicated. The use of a walking cast is hazardous, as the force of weight-bearing may tend to cause some spread of the mortise.

Bimalleolar Fracture-Dislocation. These injuries present a combination of the problems outlined above for displaced fractures of either malleolus. Frequently, closed manipulation will provide adequate reduction, which must be maintained in a long leg cast for at least 6 weeks. In many instances manipulation does not provide adequate reduction of the medial malleolus; then operative fixation of the medial malleolus is indicated (Fig. 22-22).

Trimalleolar Fracture-Dislocation of the Ankle. The addition of a fracture of the posterior malleolus to those of the medial and

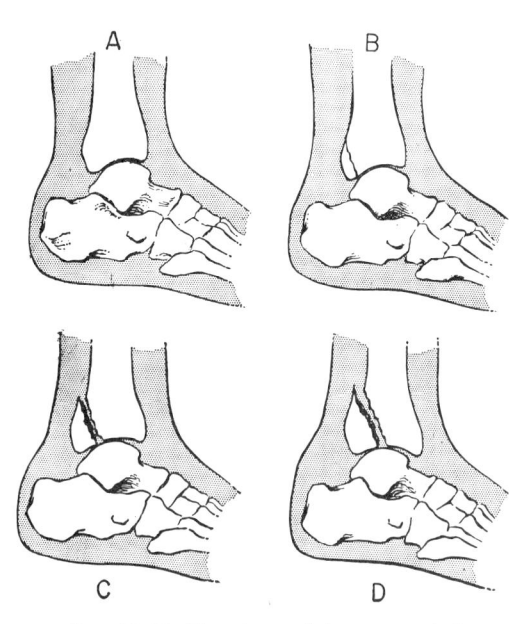

FIG. 22-23. Drawings of fractures of the posterior malleolus.

(A) The uninjured ankle.

(B) The fragment of posterior malleolus makes up only about 10 per cent of the articular surface. Fragments of this size may be ignored even if they are not reduced.

(C) The fragment of posterior malleolus makes up about 25 per cent of the articular surface, and the foot is dislocated posteriorly. Fragments of this size must be reduced and held in perfect reduction. At times this can be achieved by closed reduction; however, many require open reduction and internal fixation.

(D) The fragment of posterior malleolus makes up about 35 per cent of the articular surface. Fragments of this size can seldom, if ever, be held in reduction by closed methods. Primary open reduction and internal fixation are preferable.

(Hampton, O. P., Jr., and Fitts, W. T., Jr.: Open Reduction of Common Fractures. New York, Grune & Stratton, 1959)

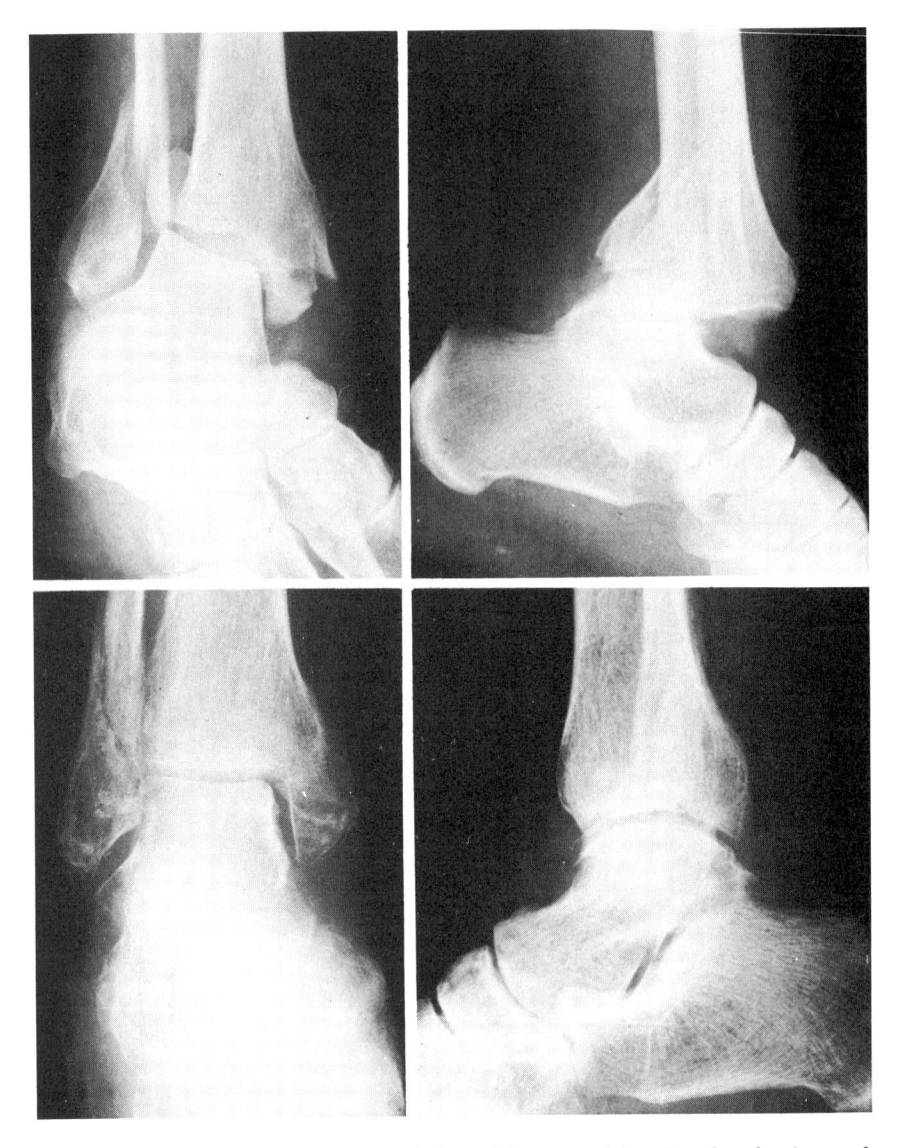

554   Fractures and Dislocations of the Lower Extremity

FIG. 22-24. Trimalleolar fracture of the ankle, treated by closed reduction and long leg plaster cast. (*Top*) Anteroposterior and lateral views before reduction. (*Bottom*) After partial healing of the fractures.

the lateral malleoli with dislocation of the foot creates a more complex problem. If the posterior malleolar fragment is of significant size, accurate reduction of this fragment must be maintained to provide for a smooth articular surface of the tibia (Fig. 22-23). In spite of a perfect closed reduction, displacement of the fragment and redislocation of the foot may occur in a cast.

Actually, the posterior malleolus may determine the preferable method of management. When it includes one third or more of the articular surface of the tibia, closed reduction usually will not be maintained in the cast; therefore, operative fixation of this fragment in reduction is indicated (Method 3). When the posterior malleolus includes less than one third of the articular surface of the tibia, reduction by manipulation may be attempted, and if precise replacement of the posterior malleolus is obtained, a long leg plaster of Paris cast may maintain the reduction

Fig. 22-25. Trimalleolar fracture-dislocation of the ankle after open reduction. Anteroposterior and lateral roentgenograms, showing that a fracture of the medial malleolus and a fracture of the posterior malleolus which contained about one third of the articular surface have been stabilized in excellent reduction so that the danger of redislocation has been eliminated. (Hampton, O. P., Jr., and Fitts, W. T., Jr.: Open Reduction of Common Fractures. New York, Grune & Stratton, 1959)

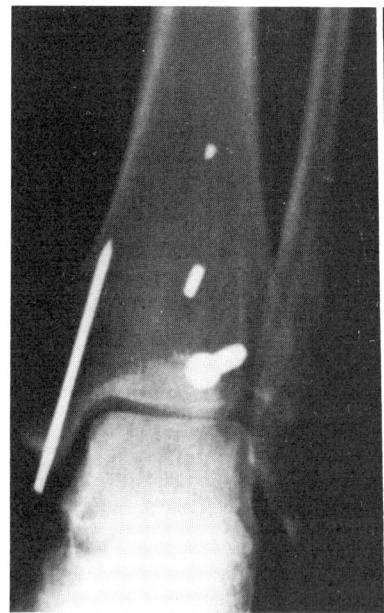

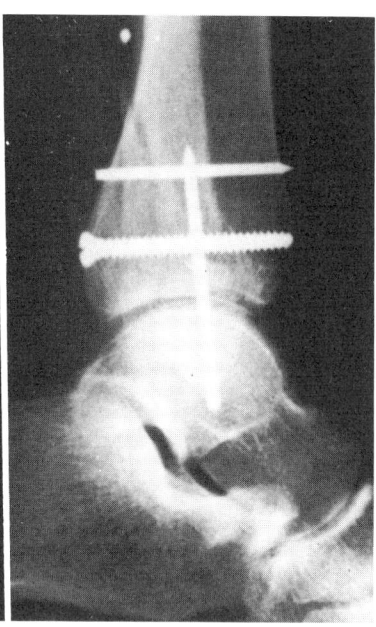

(Fig. 22-24). Check roentgenograms every 4 or 5 days for 3 weeks are essential, since the posterior malleolus may become displaced again, thereby permitting redislocation of the foot. In such instances open reduction is then indicated (Fig. 22-25). If the posterior malleolus occupies only a small portion of the articular surface, perhaps 10 per cent, it requires no special attention. Even though reduction of this small fragment is not complete, there is likely to be little if any effect on future function of the ankle; therefore, operation for replacement of a fragment of this size is not justified.

FRACTURES OF THE BONES OF THE FOOT

Fractures of the bones of the foot may be grouped as fractures of (1) calcaneus, (2) talus, (3) midtarsals (navicular, cuboid and cuneiforms), (4) metatarsals and (5) phalanges of the toes.

FRACTURES OF THE CALCANEUS

These, as a group, are by far the most serious fractures of the bones of the foot. They are very painful injuries. In all but minor fractures temporary disability is prolonged, and considerable permanent disability is to be anticipated in many instances. Disability often exceeds what would be expected from the findings on roentgenograms. Disability results from pain on weight-bearing, loss of inversion and eversion of the foot, and restriction of motion in the ankle joint. Fractures of the calcaneus are indeed serious injuries.

Mechanism of Injury. Fractures of the calcaneus result from falls onto the heels. In military experience, they are also commonly caused by explosion of land mines or the upsurge of the deck of a torpedoed ship. The same force which causes a fracture of the calcaneus is likely to cause a compression fracture of the spine. Therefore, fractures of the calcaneus routinely indicate a thorough clinical examination and, if at all suggested, roentgenograms of the back.

Fractures of the calcaneus are crush fractures. At impact, the calcaneus is crushed between the talus with the superimposed weight of the body and the object onto which the patient fell. Fracture lines may be created in many directions. Characteristic displacements are a downward crushing of the central portion of the calcaneus, including the posterior articular facet into the substance of the bone, lateral and medial spread of cortical fragments, and an upward displacement of a

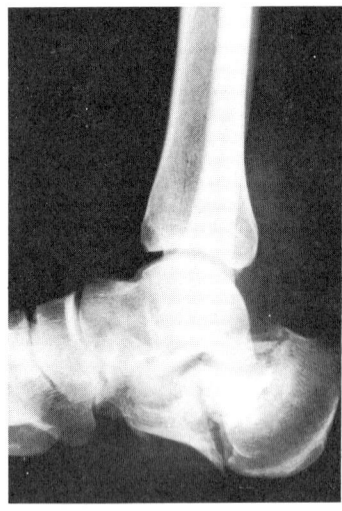

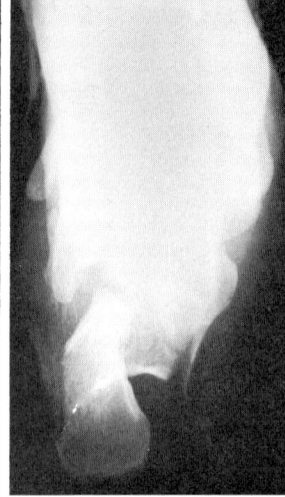

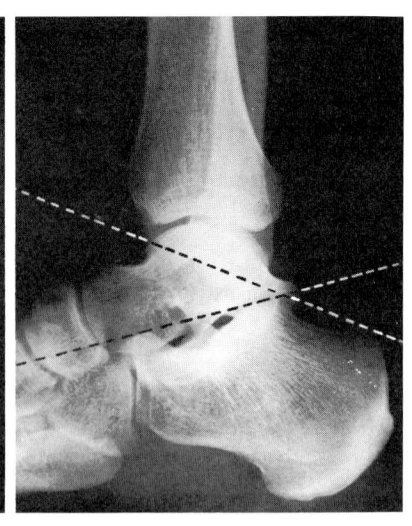

FIG. 22-26. Fracture of the os calcis. (*Left*) Lateral view, showing severe crush fracture with loss of Böhler's angle. (*Center*) Axial view. (*Right*) Normal foot with Böhler's angle demonstrated. This angle is that formed by two lines, one parallel with the superior surface of the tuberosity, and the other joining the anterior and the posterior articular facets. Normally, this angle is about 30°.

large posterior fragment to which the tendo achillis is attached. The tuber angle (Fig. 22-26, *right*) is decreased and may be reversed.

Diagnosis. Fractures of the calcaneus are characterized clinically by severe local swelling and ecchymosis. Swelling may be so severe as to cause massive bleb formation and even spotty necrosis of the skin overlying the bone.

Special roentgenograms are necessary to determine the type and the extent of the bony injury as well as to establish or confirm the diagnosis. In addition to a lateral view of the calcaneus, an anteroposterior or axial view must be made as illustrated in Figure 22-26, *center*. At times, only this special view will demonstrate the fracture. It should be obtained routinely in all suspected fractures of the calcaneus. A lateral view of the uninjured heel should be taken to help in determining the severity of displacement on the injured side (Fig. 22-26, *right*).

Treatment. The principles of treatment of fractures of the calcaneus include: reduction of swelling prior to efforts at reduction of the fracture in most instances (fractures of the calcaneus are a definite exception to the rule of prompt reduction and immobilization); the best possible restoration of the contour of the bone, particularly of its articular surface and the tuber angle; immobilization of the foot and the ankle so long as immobilization is serving a useful purpose; mobilization of the foot and the ankle as soon as feasible in order to minimize any permanent restriction of motion; freedom from weight-bearing until solid bony union has taken place; and prevention of edema as much as possible by elevation and, following removal of plaster, by adequate elastic support. These principles are applied by various means according to the type, the severity and the degree of displacement of the fracture.

Before reduction of the fracture is attempted or immobilization is applied, the severe swelling about the heel and the ankle should be allowed to subside so that the swollen and edematous soft tissues overlying the calcaneus will not be irreparably damaged during the reduction. When the patient is first seen, a large compression dressing is applied immediately to the foot and the ankle. Then the part is sharply elevated if the arterial circulation permits. Depending upon the severity of the fracture, from 5 to 10 days is usually required before swelling has decreased to a point where reduction should be undertaken. If it is attempted too soon, necrosis of the skin overlying the bone may be precipitated.

Fractures of the calcaneus may be grouped as (1) those requiring no reduction, (2) those which can be reduced reasonably well by closed methods, (3) those which will be benefited by open reduction and (4) those in which reduction is impossible.

Several steps are involved in the closed reduction of fractures of the calcaneus. When the fragments appear to be firmly impacted, this impaction must be broken up as a preliminary to reduction. This may be accomplished by strong manipulation of the heel with the hands or by forcibly striking each side of the padded heel with a large wooden or rubber mallet. Upward displacement of the posterior fragment must be overcome by downward traction on it. During this maneuver, the knee should be fully flexed to relax the calf muscles as much as possible. Traction on the heel may be made manually or on a Steinmann pin inserted through or just above the posterior fragment. After the posterior fragment has been pulled downward, traction is made in a posterior direction in an effort to restore the length of the bone. Downward and backward traction on the posterior fragment tends to restore the tuber angle toward normal. Medial and lateral bulging of comminuted fragments is overcome by side-to-side compression with the hands or preferably with a large C-clamp or a special calcaneus redressor made for this purpose. If a pin is used, it is removed after the fracture has been reduced.

Immobilization is provided with a padded plaster cast. In addition to sheet cotton, heavy felt pads are placed on each side of the calcaneus. As the plaster is setting, firm pressure is made with the heels of the hands over the felt pads. The persisting pressure by the cast serves to minimize exuberant callus beneath the malleoli. The ankle is immobilized in about 15° of plantar flexion and the foot in slight inversion, an exception to the rule of immobilizing ankles at 90° and feet in neutral version. In those instances where an upwardly displaced posterior fragment has been pulled downward, the cast must be extended to the mid-thigh with the knee immobilized in some 30° of flexion.

The duration of immobilization varies with the type of fracture, the degree of displacement and what has been achieved by efforts at reduction. In undisplaced fractures, 3 or 4 weeks of immobilization in a below-knee cast will suffice but, thereafter, all weight-bearing is avoided by the use of crutches until bony union is solid. Early removal of the cast permits active exercise of the foot and the ankle and tends to minimize the loss of motion in both the ankle joint and the subtalar joint. Actually, in certain impacted fractures immobilization serves no purpose and should be omitted in favor of early exercise.

When efforts at reduction have achieved little and the fragments remain unreduced, there is no reason to maintain immobilization for an extended period. It is better to remove the cast within a few weeks and initiate active exercises. In this way, permanent restriction of motion, especially in the ankle, will be minimized even though the fracture has not been reduced accurately.

Whenever the patient becomes ambulatory without a cast, elastic bandage support is provided from the base of the toes to just below the knee in an effort to minimize edema. Persisting edema itself tends to restrict motion of the foot and the ankle, and if edema can be prevented by the constant use of elastic support a better end-result will be obtained.

In those fractures consisting principally of a downward displacement of a fragment containing the posterior articular facet with impaction into the substance of the bone, efforts at closed reduction are usually not worthwhile. In these fractures, open reduction is often indicated. The fragment containing the articular surface is elevated into its normal position so as to restore the contour of the articular surface. A small block of bone from the ilium or the upper tibia is used to fill the defect and to maintain elevation of the fragment. In these instances plaster immobilization should be maintained for about 6 weeks.

In severely comminuted fractures in which it is certain that the contour of the bone, particularly the articular surface, cannot be restored by either closed or open methods, it is doubtful whether any effort to reduce them is worthwhile. It may be best to omit immobilization altogether and to start exercise immediately. In this group of cases, primary subtalar arthrodesis may give the best end-

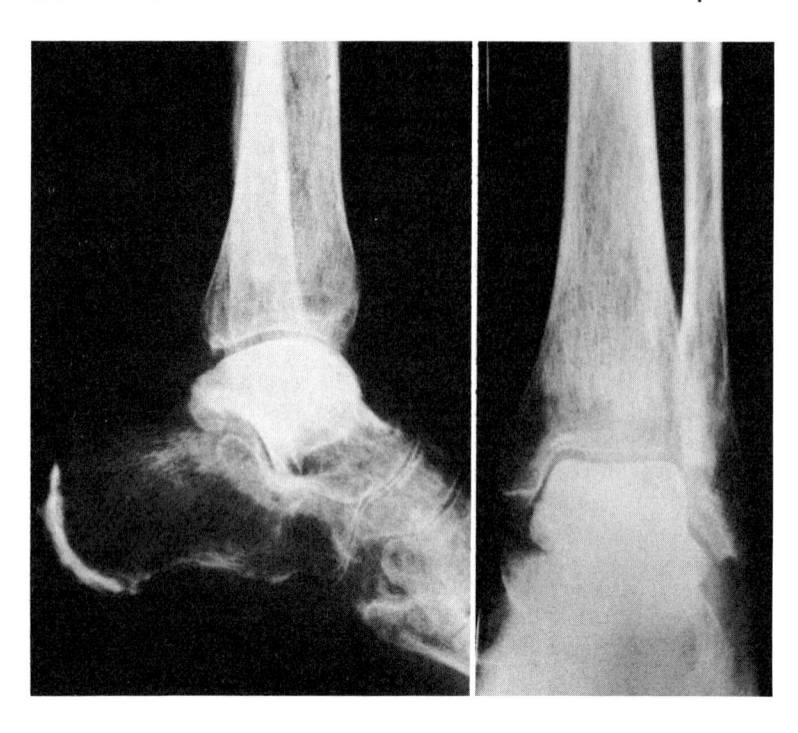

FIG. 22-27. Anteroposterior and lateral roentgenograms of the foot, showing avascular necrosis of the body of the talus, following a fracture through the neck, which had already united.

result. This operation is often indicated in late cases when persisting pain and disability warrant further effort at relief.

FRACTURES OF THE TALUS

These fractures result from injuries which produce excessive dorsiflexion of the foot. The fracture occurs across the neck of the talus when it is forced against the anterior rim of the lower end of the tibia.

Treatment. The fracture may remain undisplaced, but some upward displacement of the distal fragment is common. Accurate reduction is essential if a good result is to be obtained. Often closed reduction can be accomplished under anesthesia by strong plantar flexion of the foot. If, however, the fragments cannot be reduced accurately by closed methods, open reduction and, often, screw fixation is indicated. When the fragments have been reduced accurately, a plaster cast is applied for 5 to 6 weeks. Thereafter, weight-bearing must be protected with crutches until union of the fracture is solid.

A displaced fracture of the neck of the talus may be complicated by a partial or complete dislocation of the body of the bone. Incomplete dislocations or subluxations may be overlooked unless the roentgenograms are studied carefully. A lateral view of the uninjured side may be helpful. Closed manipulation for the fracture may effect reduction of the dislocated body but, if not, open reduction is necessary.

The outstanding complication of a fracture of the neck of the talus is avascular necrosis of the body of the bone (Fig. 22-27). The nutrient arteries for the talus enter through the distal portion of the bone. Therefore, in a fracture of the neck the major blood supply to the body has been destroyed. Avascular necrosis is unlikely to develop in undisplaced fractures but is a distinct possibility when the fracture has been displaced. Dislocations of the body, especially complete or near complete dislocations in which ligamentous attachments to the bone are torn, make avascular necrosis a probability. When this complication ensues, prolonged protection from weight-bearing is necessary until new blood vessels grow into the body and the dead bone is replaced with living bone. This may require from 10 to 12 months or even more. Too early weight-bearing will cause the body of the talus to collapse, and then repair is impossible. Severe traumatic arthritis of the ankle will follow. Early subtalar arthrodesis may hasten the process of revascularization.

Fractures of the Midtarsal Bones (Navicular, Cuboid and Cuneiform)

These fractures are caused by side-to-side crush injuries or by a heavy weight falling on the foot. The skin and other soft tissues of the foot are often badly bruised or torn. After healing of these fractures, considerable disability often remains. This is caused by pain and soreness on twisting strains of the foot and the loss of motion in the midtarsal joints. Prolonged weight-bearing is usually painful.

Displacement of fragments may be corrected in some instances by manual manipulation. In others, open reduction and some form of internal fixation (Method 3) is advantageous. In still others, the midtarsal bones are so crushed that they can be molded only so as to restore the general contour of the foot.

Immobilization is provided by a plaster cast. This should be exceedingly well molded about the foot so as to conform to and support the arches. A walking heel may be added to facilitate ambulation. Weight-bearing in the cast during the period of healing tends to minimize demineralization and atrophy of the bones of the foot. Immobilization is discontinued after 4 to 8 weeks, depending upon the severity of the fracture or fractures.

Fractures of the Metatarsals

These may be considered as fractures of (1) the shafts or the necks of the metatarsals, (2) the base of the fifth metatarsal and (3) march fractures.

Fractures of the Shafts or the Necks of the Metatarsals. These result from compression injuries of the foot. The force may be front to back, side to side or top to bottom. The last includes a heavy object dropping on the foot. These injuries also result from falls onto the balls of the feet.

TREATMENT. Undisplaced fractures may be treated by merely a compression dressing and the use of crutches for 4 to 6 weeks. In many instances a walking cast will be preferable, as it will make the patient ambulatory without crutches and perhaps permit him to return to work. The cast should include a long plantar slab to protect the toes, as a subsequent blow on these might displace the metatarsal fracture. Occasionally the patient may be treated with a metatarsal pad taped to the sole of the foot, after which he is allowed to bear weight.

Fractures with significant displacement should be reduced. Precise reduction of fractures of the first and the fifth metatarsals is especially important so as to restore the weight-bearing heads of these bones to their normal position. Alignment of a fracture of each metatarsal must be restored so that after the fracture is united the head of the broken metatarsal will not project into the sole or the dorsum of the foot and result in painful callus formation.

In transverse or near transverse fractures, reduction can be achieved in many instances by closed manipulation. In oblique or comminuted fractures, continuous traction is often necessary to hold reduction (Method 2). Skeletal traction may be provided by a piece of small Kirschner wire through the tough tissue of the distal phalanx of the toe of the broken metatarsal. Traction is made on the wire by means of a rubber band connected to a loop of heavy wire incorporated in a cast. Skeletal traction may be applied to several toes simultaneously for fractures of several metatarsals. The traction must be maintained for about 4 weeks. In some fractures of metatarsals, open reduction and perhaps internal fixation with an intramedullary pin may be necessary to achieve adequate reduction (Method 3).

Fractures of the Base of the Fifth Metatarsal (Fig. 22-28). These relatively unimportant but common fractures usually result when the foot gives way into inversion as the patient is running or walking rapidly. As a rule they remain undisplaced, although occasionally the small proximal fragment is separated by the pull of the peroneus brevis muscle which attaches to the proximal end of the fifth metatarsal.

TREATMENT. Undisplaced fractures require little active treatment. Many may be treated by strapping with adhesive tape or by an elastic bandage, and immediate weight-bearing can be allowed. A few will require the use of crutches for 10 to 14 days because of pain. Rarely, a walking cast is justified. If there is any significant displacement of the proximal fragment, the cast should be used. The degree of displacement is seldom such as to predispose to nonunion, although the fracture line is often visible for many months.

March Fracture. A march or fatigue fracture results without any known trauma. It is

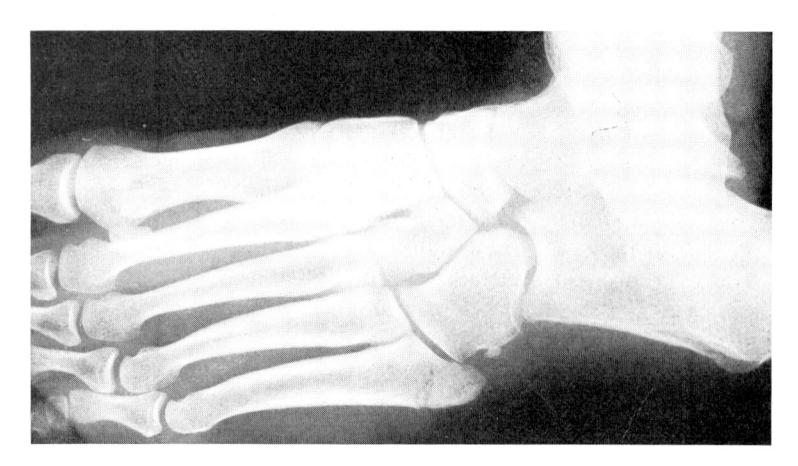

FIG. 22-28. Fracture of base of 5th metatarsal. This fracture should be treated by Method No. 5, no immobilization.

usually seen in unconditioned military personnel who have been subjected to a long and fatiguing march and usually involves the second or the third metatarsal. Pain develops in the metatarsal region of the foot and persists. As a rule, the pain is relatively mild, and since there is no history of injury, x-ray films may not be made. If they are made, a faint line of fracture may be seen. Later, a palpable lump develops in the metatarsal region and this usually leads to roentgenographic examination. The findings on the roentgenogram are those of a healing fracture with some exuberant callus formation. It is important to recognize that a march fracture is present and not to consider the findings as indicative of a bone tumor.

A march fracture may be treated by immobilization in a walking cast for several weeks or, in many instances, by a metatarsal pad in the shoe or a metatarsal bar on the shoe, and restricted activity.

Fractures of the Phalanges of the Toes

These result when some heavy object drops on the toes or when a toe is struck forcibly against an object. Fractures of the fifth toe occur frequently when a barefoot person catches it on a piece of furniture. Except for fractures of the great toe, fractures of the toes are not of great consequence.

Treatment. In undisplaced fractures, including those of the phalanges of the great toe, only protection from additional injury is necessary. Strapping of the injured toe to the adjacent toe or toes with small strips of adhesive tape affords some protection and tends to minimize discomfort. The use of a crutch or cane may make walking more comfortable for the first week or 10 days. With a metatarsal bar applied to the shoe, patients with these injuries often can resume activity long before the fracture is united.

In displaced fractures of the great toe, particularly in those of the proximal phalanx, reduction is necessary. At times this can be achieved by manipulation (Method 1). In some, continuous skeletal traction in a banjo cast, as described for fractures of the metatarsals, is advantageous (Method 2). Open reduction is seldom necessary. These fractures usually unite sufficiently in 3 or 4 weeks to permit the patient to resume weight-bearing without danger of displacement.

In displaced fractures of the small toes, efforts at reduction usually are not indicated. The bones are so small that even with perfect reduction redisplacement occurs easily. However, every effort should be made to restore good alignment, which usually can be maintained by strapping the broken toe to the toe or toes on each side of it.

DISLOCATIONS OF THE FOOT

Dislocations of the foot include (1) peritalar dislocation, (2) tarsometatarsal dislocation and (3) dislocation of the toes.

Peritalar Dislocation

This corresponds to perilunar dislocation at the wrist. The talus remains seated in the ankle joint, but the remainder of the foot is dislocated medially. This means that the articulations between the talus and the calcaneus and between the talus and the navicular are disrupted. The injury may be closed or open.

Prompt reduction is indicated. General anesthesia is usually necessary. Traction and appropriate manipulation usually reduce the dislocation. A plaster cast should be applied to the foot and the leg, holding the ankle at 90° and the foot in neutral version for a period of about 4 weeks (Method 1). The prognosis is rather good for so severe an injury.

TARSOMETATARSAL DISLOCATION

In this injury, usually caused by some force which produces leverage at the mid-foot (as when the forefoot is caught and the body is forced medially or laterally), the metatarsals are torn loose from their articulations with the tarsus. Usually there are multiple chip fractures along these joints. This is a severe injury.

In many instances closed reduction may be successful by traction and manipulation. Then immobilization is provided by a plaster cast, including the leg and the foot (Method 1). When reduction cannot be obtained or maintained by closed methods, operative reduction and usually some form of internal fixation are necessary (Method 3).

DISLOCATION OF THE TOES

Dislocation of a toe without fracture is an unusual injury, but occasionally one of the toes, particularly the great toe, is dislocated at the metatarsophalangeal joint. Reduction by traction and manipulation is usually easy and often may be done without anesthesia.

(For Bibliography, see pp. 572-573, at end of Chap. 23.)

Chapter 23

OSCAR P. HAMPTON, JR., M.D., AND WILLIAM T. FITTS, JR., M.D.

Fractures and Dislocations of the Spine, the Pelvis, the Sternum and the Ribs

Fractures and Dislocations of the Spine
Fractures of the Pelvis
Fractures of the Sternum
Fractures of the Ribs

FRACTURES AND DISLOCATIONS OF THE SPINE

Fractures and dislocations of the spine divide regionally for purposes of discussion into those of the (1) cervical spine, (2) dorsal and lumbar spine and (3) sacrococcygeal spine

Injury to the Spinal Cord

The outstanding complication of fractures and dislocations of the spine is injury to the underlying spinal cord. For practical purposes, there must have been some dislocation of a vertebra for spinal cord injury to occur. A dislocation may show on roentgenograms, usually in association with a compression fracture of the body of a vertebra just below it, or it may have been reduced spontaneously so that only the compression fracture is visualized and the diagnosis of a dislocation made because of the cord injury. In fact, occasionally roentgenograms will show no fracture, and yet the patient will have a complete transverse lesion of the cord. It seems certain, in such instances, that there has been a temporary dislocation of a vertebra with crushing of the cord followed by spontaneous reduction.

Injury to the spinal cord may occur at any level between the first cervical and the second lumbar vertebrae, and below that level the cauda equina may be damaged. Injury to the cord is most commonly found as a complication of injuries to the cervical and upper dorsal spine.

Injury to the spinal cord may produce either complete or incomplete loss of function of the nervous system below the level of the injury. In a complete lesion, motor power, sensation and bladder and rectal sphincter control are lost. In an incomplete lesion, varying degrees of these functions are retained. The seriousness of either a complete or an incomplete lesion of the cord demands an adequate neurologic examination as soon as the patient is seen with a suspected fracture of the spine in order that injury to the cord, if present, may be recognized promptly and every effort made to treat it properly. The ability to move the fingers and the toes fully, and the preservation of normal sensation and normal reflexes show that the function of the nervous system has not been impaired. Such an observation made early may be invaluable from a diagnostic standpoint should signs of injury to the cord develop.

Treatment of a fracture of the spine complicated by some neurologic deficit is designed primarily to relieve pressure of bone on the cord or the cauda equina. Occasionally, pressure on a cord or a cauda equina may be relieved quickly by reduction of the fracture, using hyperextension. However, this maneuver can do more harm than good in some instances. Surgical intervention usually is necessary. The cord is unroofed by partial or complete removal of the lamina (laminectomy) in the area of the injury.

The decision to perform laminectomy requires expert surgical judgment. The procedure is seldom worthwhile in *immediate complete* cord lesions and in itself can lead to a fatal outcome. The operation is indicated in all *incomplete* cord lesions and even in complete lesions which were *not immediate*. Laminectomy is indicated in all lesions of the cauda equina, complete or incomplete—e.g., for all neurologic deficits complicating injuries at or below the second lumbar level.

A Queckenstedt test may help to determine whether the pressure is still present on the cord at the level of the injury. If the Queckenstedt is negative (patent spinal canal), surgical intervention is less likely to lead to improvement. With a positive Queckenstedt (a blocked spinal canal) pressure on the cord remains, and, unless there are other clinical signs that contraindicate it, laminectomy is probably indicated. While the Queckenstedt test may be valuable, good clinical judgment must be relied upon for final decision regarding operative intervention.

FRACTURES AND DISLOCATIONS OF THE CERVICAL SPINE

Compression fractures and dislocations of the bodies of cervical vertebrae are flexion injuries. They usually result from a blow on the head, as from diving into shallow water, an automobile accident, or from a falling object. The extent of injury varies from a fracture of a small fragment of the anterior superior margin of a vertebra or a minimal forward subluxation of a vertebra to a severe compression fracture or a complete forward dislocation. The diagnosis and the extent of injury is determined by adequate roentgenograms.

Compression Fractures. TREATMENT. Minimal compression fractures require only the support of a brace or a Thomas collar for a period of 4 to 6 weeks. More severe compressions require reduction by hyperextension and immobilization usually for 8 to 12 weeks by a plaster cast incorporating the trunk and the head with the latter in hyperextension.

Reduction of a compression fracture may be obtained in several ways. The head may be allowed to lie unsupported in hyperextension over the edge of a table or a mattress. An excellent technic is that provided by 2 mattresses on the bed with the top mattress pulled toward the foot so that the patient's head may hyperextend over the top mattress. Halter traction on the hyperextended head for a few days is another method which may lead to reduction of the compression. A third method is hyperextension of the neck on a fracture table. All modern fracture tables have arrangements for holding the head and the neck in hyperextension during application of a plaster cast to the head, the neck and the trunk. Hyperextension of the neck on a fracture table is the preferable method when the severity of the fracture warrants plaster immobilization, because the other methods of reduction require that the patient be moved to such a table for application of the cast after the fracture has been reduced.

Dislocations of the cervical spine may be (1) incomplete, usually called subluxations, or (2) complete. In a subluxation, the inferior articular facets of a vertebra slide upward and forward on the facets of the vertebra below it, but not far enough for the sliding superior facets to become completely disengaged and to override those below. The body of the superior vertebra moves forward several millimeters on the one below it. In complete dislocations, the superior facets move upward and forward so that all contact with those below is lost and overriding occurs (Fig. 23-1). The body of the superior vertebra is displaced well forward on the one below and may override it. A complete dislocation of a cervical vertebra is often associated with a compression fracture of the vertebra below. In these injuries, a complete transverse lesion of the spinal cord is common.

A subluxation of a cervical vertebra may be overlooked unless a special lateral view of the neck is made with the head flexed. The routine anteroposterior and lateral views are made with the head moderately extended with the patient sitting or recumbent. A subluxation of a cervical vertebra may have been reduced spontaneously so that with the routine position of the head and the neck, the films are negative. In such instances, the subluxation is most likely to recur with the head flexed to the limit of the patient's tolerance. Therefore, if the routine films are negative, it is necessary to obtain a lateral view with full flexion of the neck. In this way, subluxations which have been reduced spontaneously will not go undiagnosed, and proper therapy can be instituted.

TREATMENT. Dislocations of the cervical spine, complete or incomplete, require reduction and immobilization until the damaged capsular and ligamentous structures have

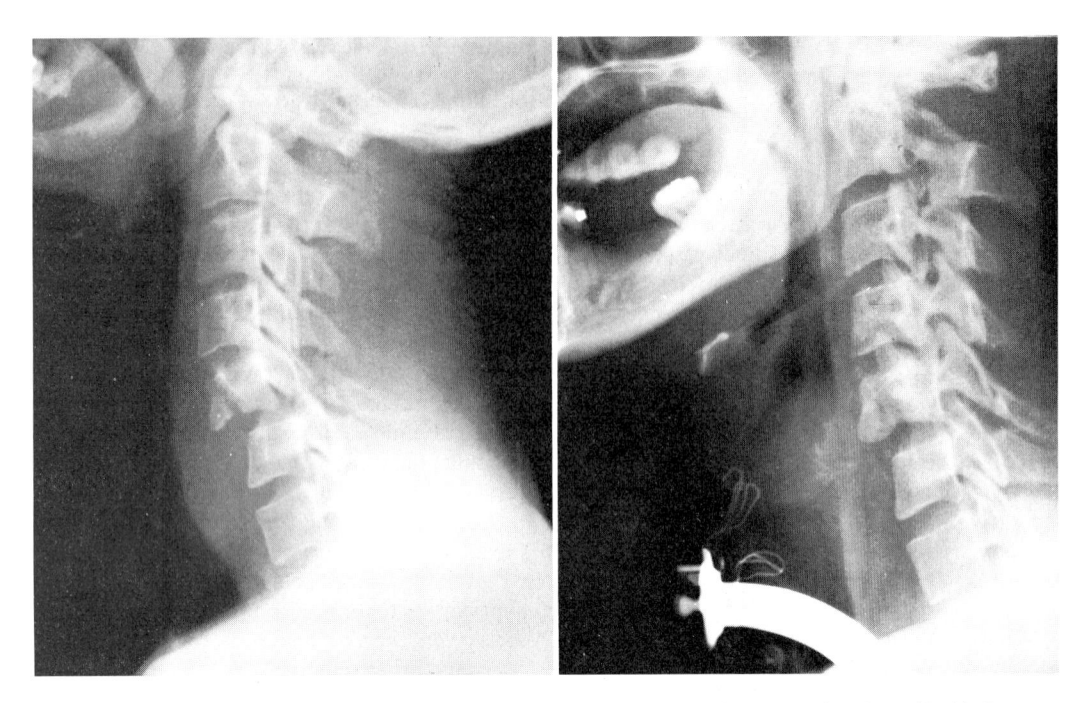

FIG. 23-1. Roentgenograms showing a fracture-dislocation of the cervical spine. (*Left*) Lateral roentgenogram showing a complete anterior dislocation of the 5th cervical vertebra with associated fracture of its body. (*Right*) Lateral roentgenogram showing the dislocation reduced by skeletal traction with Crutchfield tongs. Note the tracheostomy tube, which is often necessary to ensure an adequate airway and to permit aspiration of the tracheobronchial tree.

healed, so that dislocation will not recur. The basic measures by which reduction may be achieved are traction on the head and hyperextension of the neck. The way in which these measures are applied varies with the degree of dislocation.

In incomplete dislocations, the important maneuver is hyperextension of the head so that the facets of the body of the displaced vertebrae will go back into their normal position. Preliminary traction with a canvas head halter will aid in reduction and tend to relieve pain. Hyperextension may be obtained by any of the methods outlined above under Compression Fractures. If immobilization is to be by a plaster cast, obviously the preferable method of obtaining hyperextension is on a standard fracture table.

In complete dislocations, reduction is more of a problem. Traction is of equal and perhaps of greater importance. While head traction may be provided by a canvas head halter, skeletal traction with Crutchfield tongs or some modification of them is highly preferable. Traction at first is made with the head in slight flexion and continued until the facets are no longer overriding and locked. To effect this, as much as 25 to 30 pounds of skeletal traction may be necessary. When the facets are no longer locked, the head is gradually brought into hyperextension as the weights are reduced to about 8 to 10 pounds.

If displacement has been minimal, reduction may be maintained by a hyperextension neck brace which should be worn for 6 to 8 weeks. In more severe yet incomplete dislocations, reduction is preferably maintained by prolonged traction or by a plaster cast incorporating the trunk and the head and holding the head in hyperextension.

In complete dislocations of the cervical spine, the head must be immobilized in hyperextension for a full 3 months. Skeletal traction in some hyperextension may be maintained for a period of about 8 weeks, following which a hyperextension neck brace is worn for an additional 4 weeks. Usually, however, skeletal traction is maintained for only 1 to 3 weeks, following which the trunk and the hyperextended head are immobilized in a plaster cast. Early operative fusion of the involved vertebrae after reduction is often indicated.

FRACTURES AND DISLOCATIONS OF THE DORSAL AND LUMBAR SPINE

Fractures of the dorsal and the lumbar vertebrae may be considered as (1) fractures of the bodies, (2) fractures of transverse processes and (3) fractures of spinous processes. Lamina and articulating processes also may be broken. However, these are usually associated with severe compression fractures or dislocations of vertebrae and need not be considered as separate clinical entities.

Fractures of the Vertebral Bodies (Compression Fractures). Compression fractures of the dorsal and the lumbar vertebral bodies are the typical fractures of the back and comprise some 60 per cent of the bony injuries to the spine. They are produced by hyperflexion or "jackknifing" of the spine as in falling from a height and landing on the buttocks or feet. They often are associated with fractures of the os calcis. A compression fracture may result when an automobile overturns, when an occupant is thrown out of the car following a collision, or when a heavy object falls on the shoulders of an erect or slightly stooped individual. In demineralized spines, as in postmenopausal osteoporosis, a compression fracture may occur merely from lifting strains or other minor trauma.

Compression fractures of bodies of vertebrae are often multiple. In such instances, 1 or at the most 2 vertebrae usually receive the most severe compression.

A compression fracture should be suspected when the patient complains of pain in the back associated with localized tenderness to deep pressure or fist percussion following any trauma which has caused sudden flexion of the back such as those described above. It is confirmed by adequate x-ray visualization in 2 views, the lateral view being the more important. Most compression fractures of the spine occur in the dorsolumbar region and therefore involve the 11th or 12th dorsal or the 1st or 2nd lumbar vertebrae (Fig. 23-2). By coincidence this is the region of the spine where x-ray visualization may be faulty unless the technic is precise.

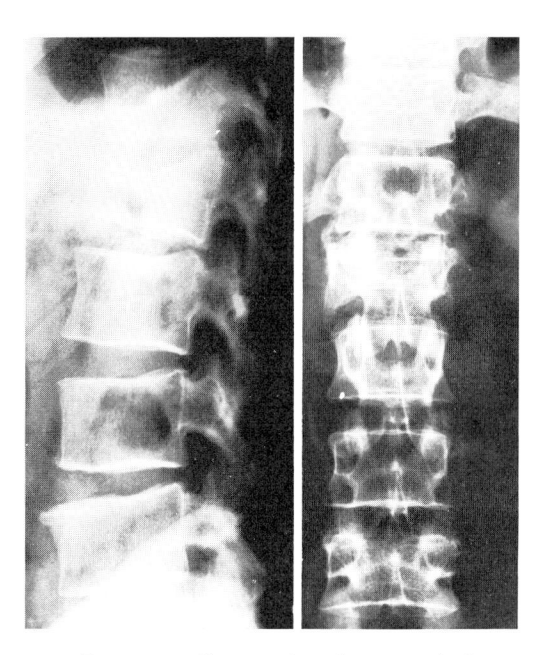

FIG. 23-2. Compression fracture of the lumbar spine. Lateral and anteroposterior views of a severe compression fracture of the 1st lumbar vertebra.

Radiologic technic calls for a different exposure on different films for lateral views of the lumbar spine and the dorsal spine. An error in placement of a film may lead to failure to visualize either the 12th dorsal or 1st lumbar vertebra. The surgeon must be sure that the roentgenograms adequately visualize these vertebrae. Often a detailed view of this region is advisable.

Paralytic or adynamic ileus is usually a problem during the first few days after a compression fracture of the lower dorsal or lumbar spine. Hyperextension for reduction of the fracture, if it is to be used, should be postponed until the ileus has been controlled. It should be managed by the same measures as for adynamic ileus from any cause.

TREATMENT. Until several years ago, the accepted procedure in all these injuries was hyperextension of the spine in an effort to reduce the compression of the vertebral body or bodies, followed by application of a snug plaster jacket. Hyperextension was obtained in several ways. With the patient placed on his back in an adjustable hospital bed so that his head is toward the foot of the bed, the knee rest is gradually elevated so as to provide a fulcrum at the level of the fracture and produce hyperextension of the spine. Watson-Jones introduced the method of placing the patient face down on 2 tables, one of them supporting the lower extremities and the other the head and the neck, so that the trunk dropped into hyperextension between them. Davis used a method which placed the patient face down on a table and then by means of a rope, tied about the ankles passing over an overhead pulley, raised the lower extremities so as to hyperextend the spine fully. All modern fracture tables have methods of hyperextending the spine to its limit of extension with the patient face down or face up.

All of these methods except hyperextension in bed permit application of a plaster jacket. The jacket should extend from the sternal notch to the pubic symphysis anteriorly and should make pressure at 3 points: the upper sternum, the pubic symphysis and the back at the level of the injury. In this way hyperextension of the spine is maintained. The best fitting and therefore the most effective plaster jackets are those applied with the patient in a face-up position. This permits the cast to be made snug-fitting at the 3 pressure points.

While hyperextension and plaster immobilization had not been employed in all compression fractures of the vertebrae by all surgeons, the method had gained wide application. In recent years, however, the method has been used less and less for several reasons. It became recognized that as a spine is hyperextended most of the hyperextension occurs at the lumbosacral joint, and maintenance of this position has predisposed to prolonged low back pain which often was much worse than any residual pain at the site of an unreduced fracture. In many instances prolonged immobilization has led to considerable permanent stiffness throughout the spine. The method is uncomfortable to the patient. Moreover, any improvement in the position of the fracture often has not been maintained in the cast when the patient became ambulatory. Particularly, hyperextension is usually ineffective for compression fractures of the dorsal region above the level of the 9th dorsal vertebra. Certainly hyperextension and plaster immobilization (or immobilization by new hyperextension braces to be described below) need be employed only in selected compression fractures of the lower dorsal and lumbar vertebrae. The following recommendations are guide lines for the management of compression fractures of the dorsal and lumbar vertebrae.

MINIMAL COMPRESSION FRACTURES. These include compressions of about 10 to 15 per cent of the vertical height of the anterior portion of the body and also those chip fractures where the anterosuperior corner of a body is broken away. Effort at reduction of these fractures by hyperextension are seldom indicated regardless of the age of the patient. He should be kept at bed rest on a hard bed until acute reaction to the injury has subsided —that is, until the pain has decreased to the point where he wants to be out of bed. Usually from 2 to 3 weeks is required. If the compression fracture is in the low dorsal or lumbar region, he then is fitted with some kind of back support which may be a broad canvas back belt with strong stays or a full-length back brace. The former will suffice in many instances. The patient is made ambulatory with the support which may be removed when he is in bed.

If the fracture is higher than the 10th dorsal, a full length support (a brace or a full-length corset with shoulder straps and strong stays) becomes necessary if the region of the fracture is to be supported, but actually, for fractures above the 8th or the 9th dorsal, support often may be omitted if the patient is comfortable without it.

MODERATE COMPRESSION FRACTURES. These include compressions of more than 15 per cent but less than 35 per cent of the vertical height of the anterior portion of the body.

In individuals under 35 or 40 years of age, efforts at reduction by hyperextension followed by immobilization are often worthwhile if the fracture is in the last 3 dorsal vertebrae or the lumbar region. The immobilization may be provided in several ways.

As outlined above, the standard method of immobilization for several decades has been the 3-point pressure plaster jacket and this is still acceptable. However, there are several objections to it. Any reduction which is obtained by hyperextension may be lost in the cast which loses its effectiveness in providing continuous 3-point pressure when it becomes loose as a result of the unavoidable atrophy of muscle and fat. The continuous immobility of the spine predisposes to stiffness. Plaster jacket immobilization is uncomfortable and becomes quite disagreeable to the patient as the cast becomes saturated with oil and perspiration from the skin.

The Jewett hyperextension brace (Fig. 23-3) (or an acceptable modification) is a distinct improvement over the plaster jacket. Continuous 3-point pressure can be provided. As atrophy of muscle and fat occurs, the brace is easily tightened to maintain effectiveness. After the first few weeks, the brace may be left off when the patient is in bed, thereby permitting some motion in the joints of the spine, especially in the lumbosacral region, which favors eventual recovery of motion in the back. This limited movement of the spine does not jeopardize the reduction of the compression fracture. A T-shirt under the brace may be changed every few days for cleanliness while the patient is recumbent.

In patients over 35 or 40 years of age, considerable judgment must be used in determining whether the end-result, as measured by a near pain-free useful back, will be obtained by hyperextension and prolonged immobilization or by minimal immobilization and early motion.

Certainly, in older individuals hyperextension which is maintained for any appreciable period of time predisposes to stiffness in the back which, in turn, predisposes to more pain. In this age group the best end-result is likely to be obtained by omitting efforts at reduction of the fracture and by providing just enough immobilization to minimize discomfort and yet permit enough movement in the back at frequent intervals to predispose to a maximum return of motion.

In moderate compression fractures above the level of the 9th dorsal vertebra, efforts at reduction by hyperextension are seldom worthwhile, regardless of the age group of the patient. After a period of bed rest, enough immobilization should be provided to minimize pain, but, as a rule, continuous or prolonged immobilization is not necessary.

SEVERE COMPRESSION FRACTURES. These include compressions of more than 35 to 40 per cent of the vertical height of the anterior portion of the body. This group, fortunately a small percentage of all compression fractures,

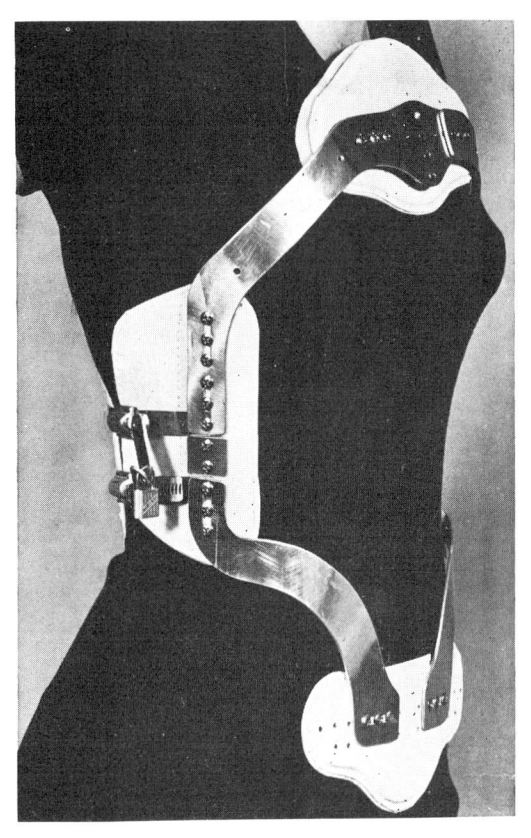

FIG. 23-3. Three-point pressure brace shown from in front (*top*) and behind (*bottom*). By tightening the set screws the pressure pad posteriorly is drawn tighter, and the sternal and the pubic pads are made to press more securely. The brace offers many advantages over a plaster jacket.

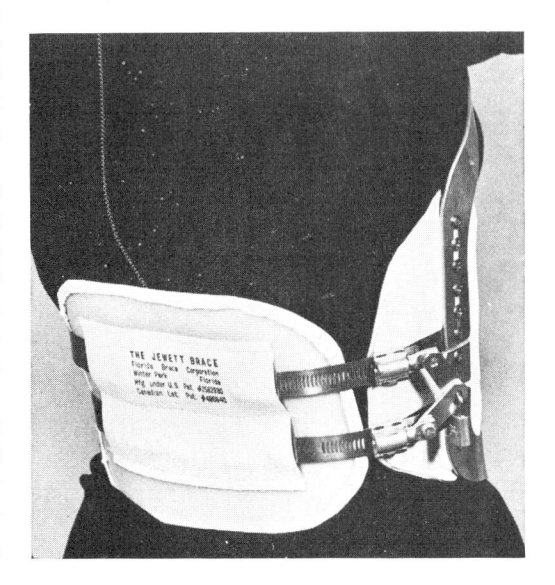

is more likely than the less severe fractures to have associated damage to the spinal cord. Under such circumstances, of course, the fracture itself is of secondary importance, and specific measures to reduce it, as a rule, are indicated only when reduction of the fracture tends to eliminate compression of the spinal cord.

In severe compression fractures involving the last 3 dorsal or the lumbar vertebrae, reduction of the fracture by hyperextension by one of the methods outlined above is indicated except in the aged. Immobilization may be provided by any one of the methods discussed under moderate compression fractures. In individuals under 35 or 40 years of age, loss of reduction should be prevented as much as possible by maintaining 3-point pressure immobilization for at least 3 months and often longer, except when the patient is recumbent in bed. In individuals over 40 years of age, again, considerable judgment must be used in determining whether the advantage offered by prolonged immobilization in maintaining the best position of the fracture outweighs the disadvantages of immobilization in producing a stiff back. In this age group, regardless of the severity of the fracture, continuous immobilization and hyperextension by a plaster jacket for 3 months is hazardous. The Jewett hyperextension brace is preferable to the plaster jacket in this as in all age groups because it can be removed when the patient is recumbent in bed and therefore allows some motion in the spine without jeopardizing the reduction of the fracture.

Fractures of Transverse Processes. These injuries, for practical purposes, occur only in the lumbar region. They generally are avulsion fractures caused by a powerful contracture of the quadratus lumborum muscle which inserts into the 5 transverse processes as well as the 12th rib. The initiating factor in such injuries may be a fall from a height to the back or the side, a heavy blow from the side as when a man is struck by an automobile, or a crushing injury.

The diagnosis is made on the anteroposterior roentgenogram. The fracture may show as a mere crack, or the fragments may be widely separated. In the latter instances, fascia and muscles are torn, and a large hematoma develops. Considerable extracellular fluid may be lost into this severely traumatized area producing shock. A paralytic ileus may follow, as in compression fractures of the vertebral bodies.

TREATMENT. Fractures of transverse processes are treated symptomatically. Following a few days of bed rest on a hard bed, a broad canvas back belt with good stays is fitted to the patient. He may be ambulatory and allowed to resume some activity. For an undisplaced crack in one or two transverse processes, the belt may be needed for only a few weeks. Sometimes a simple adhesive strapping of the back for a week or two will suffice, without the belt. Activity is increased gradually, and practically no residual symptoms should remain after 2 months. When the fragments are widely displaced, however, signifying rather extensive soft tissue injury, the belt may be needed for 5 or 6 weeks. Some residual soreness is to be expected for several months and perhaps permanently as a result of scar formation in the traumatized area. Actually, nonunion of separated fractures of transverse processes is not unusual, but healing by scar re-anchors the fragments.

Fractures of Spinous Processes. This relatively rare injury may result when a spinous process, made prominent and vulnerable because the spine is flexed, is struck "bull's-eye" by some falling object. It also may result in the low cervical or upper dorsal area by strong muscle contracture, as in laborers who are shoveling dirt. For this reason, the injury near the cervico-dorsal junction has been called "clay-shoveler's fracture."

Treatment is usually symptomatic. A Thomas collar for several weeks may benefit those in the lower cervical and upper dorsal area. A lumbosacral corset may help relieve pain for those in the lumbar region. Nonunion may occur. If so, and if pain persists, excision of the small fragment may relieve the symptoms.

FRACTURES OF THE SACROCOCCYGEAL SPINE

Fractures of the Sacrum. These injuries may occur following falls from a height in which the patient lands on the low back or as a result of severe direct blows, as when the patient is struck by an automobile. They usually occur as linear fractures without displacement. Treatment is comparable with that

FIG. 23-4. Fracture of the pelvis. Fracture of superior and inferior rami of left pubis.

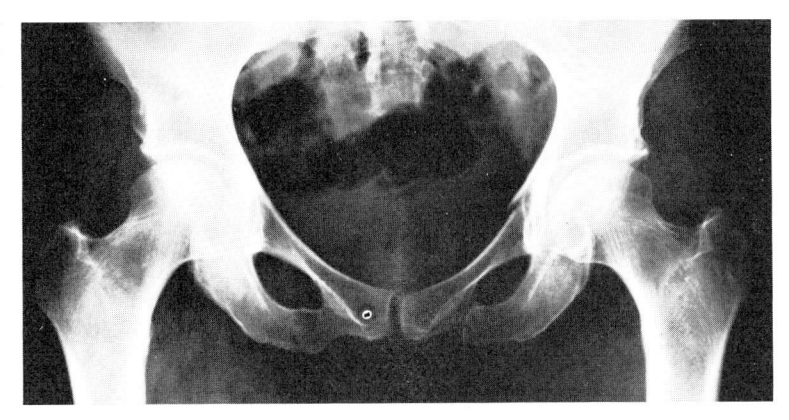

for undisplaced fractures of the pelvis and usually consist of a few weeks of bed rest on a hard bed followed by the support of a good lumbosacral belt.

Fractures of the Coccyx. These result from falls into the sitting position. Usually there is a history that the region of the coccyx struck some protruding object, such as the edge of a step. Although the injury is not serious, it is painful.

If the distal portion of the coccyx is displaced, an effort should be made to achieve reduction by manipulation with one finger in the rectum, for which anesthesia is usually required.

Following reduction, or if the fracture is undisplaced, treatment consists of a rubber ring for sitting, the support of a girdle or a belt about the hips during ambulation, sitting in a tub of hot water several times daily and avoidance of reinjury. Pain on sitting is likely to continue for some time and may persist indefinitely. Under these circumstances, surgical excision of the coccyx may be indicated. At times, however, excision of the coccyx does not relieve the symptoms, particularly in neurotic and hypersensitive individuals. Therefore, the patient must be evaluated carefully before operation is advised.

FRACTURES OF THE PELVIS

Fractures of the pelvis are produced by direct violence, such as falls from a height, automobile accidents and crushing injuries of any kind. The fracture may involve one or both rami of the pubis (Fig. 23-4) or the ischium, or either wing of the ilium. Because of the framework of the pelvis, significant displacement of a fracture usually does not occur. However, with fractures involving both rami and the wing of the ilium on one side, upward and inward displacement of the outer fragment of that innominate bone may occur. With fractures through both rami on each side, as may occur in side-to-side crush injuries, the pelvis may collapse and the fragments override, or with such fractures following front-to-back crush injuries, separation of the fragments and spread of the pelvis may occur.

First consideration with fractures of the pelvis, particularly when the fragments are displaced, concerns not the fractures themselves but the contiguous soft tissues which may have been injured: the bladder, the intestine, or the iliac blood vessels. Unless the patient can void clear urine immediately, catheterization is indicated to determine whether the bladder has been damaged. This investigation is necessary even though the fragments are not displaced, because a full bladder may have been ruptured by the force of the impact. Absence of urine or the finding of bloody urine indicates injury to the bladder; therefore, a cystogram should be made immediately (see Chap. 50, Urology). Repeated examination of the abdomen is indicated to search for signs of injury to an intra-abdominal viscus. The absence of normal peripheral arterial pulsations in either lower extremity would indicate the probability of a torn iliac artery and proper arteriography must be done immediately. The management of these life-endangering complications takes precedence over management of the fractures.

Treatment

Fractures of the pelvis with little or no displacement, which comprise the majority of these injuries, require nothing more than bed rest on a hard bed for a few weeks followed perhaps, by the support of a canvas corset for a few weeks. With a fracture of a single ramus or even of 2 rami on the same side, the patient may easily become ambulatory on crutches in 2 to 3 weeks, but full weight-bearing should be postponed until about 6 weeks after injury. In undisplaced fractures involving rami on both sides, the period of bed rest should be prolonged to 4 to 5 weeks, and crutch-walking postponed until 7 or 8 weeks after injury. The prognosis in these undisplaced fractures of the pelvis is excellent for practically full function. Elderly individuals, in whom these periods of bed rest may be inadvisable, can be safely lifted into a chair after a few days.

In fractures through both rami and the wing of the ilium on the same side with upward and perhaps inward displacement of the lateral fragment of the innominate bone, strong traction, either skin or preferably skeletal, must be applied to the extremity early in the management of the fracture in an effort to pull the displaced fragment back into position. In some instances, efforts at reduction will be more successful if the patient is anesthetized for relaxation; while strong manual traction is being made on the involved extremity, a strong downward and rotary thrust is made manually against the upward displaced wing of the ilium. After reduction, traction must be maintained for several weeks (usually 5 or 6 weeks) to avoid recurrence of the upward displacement.

Those fractures with separation of the fragments and spreading of the lower pelvis require some compressing force. This is most easily accomplished by means of a pelvic sling which serves barely to lift the weight of the pelvis from the mattress and to supply a binding force which tends to mold the fragments back into place. Some caution is necessary to avoid converting a spreading type of fracture into a collapsing type as a result of excessive compression. Bilateral traction on the extremities may aid in obtaining reduction of the fragments and certainly, in the early stages, will contribute to the comfort of the patient.

In bilateral fractures of both rami with overriding and collapse of the pelvis, a pelvic sling is not indicated. Strong bilateral traction with the lower extremities in abduction may effect some improvement in the position of the fragments.

In all these displaced fractures of the pelvis, the period of bed rest must be extended to 6 or 8 weeks, following which the support of a canvas corset should be provided for 1 to 3 months. Immobilization in a plaster cast is seldom worthwhile. When it is used, the cast must incorporate the trunk and one or both thighs.

Fractures Associated with Dislocations of the Hip

Fracture of Margin of Acetabulum. (This lesion is discussed on p. 526.)

Central Fracture-Dislocation of the Hip Joint (Fracture of the Floor of the Acetabulum). A blow in the line of the shaft of the femur, especially when the thigh is abducted, or a fall onto the greater trochanter may drive the head of the femur through the floor of the acetabulum and into the pelvis, pushing fragments of the acetabulum ahead of it (Fig. 23-5). The dislocated femoral head frequently can be reduced by skeletal traction. At times the acetabular fragments fall into good position but frequently they are not pulled back into place by traction so that the acetabulum remains distorted. Even so, open reduction of the acetabular floor is an extensive and dan-

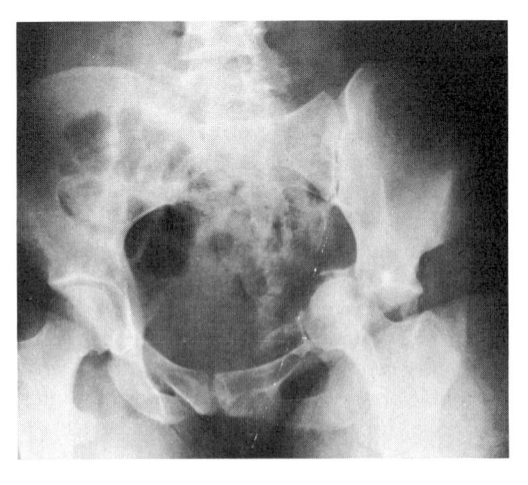

Fig. 23-5. Central dislocation of the hip.

gerous procedure and should seldom be attempted in these circumstances, especially since a satisfactory functional result is often obtained even though the acetabular fragments are not reduced accurately. The explanation for this is probably that the weight-bearing part of the acetabulum is chiefly the superior undisplaced aspect rather than the central, displaced portion. Occasionally, an early operation with the implantation of a large vitallium cup of the type designed for a cup arthroplasty may be indicated. If traumatic arthritis develops later, arthrodesis or arthroplasty may be performed.

FRACTURES OF THE STERNUM

Fractures of the sternum occur usually as the result of an automobile collision in which the driver is thrown forward so that his sternum strikes the steering wheel. Rarely, they occur in association with compression fractures of the dorsal spine following severe sudden jackknifing compression injuries, such as when a very heavy weight falls across the shoulders of a stooped individual.

The fragments, if displaced at all, may overlap slightly. The diagnosis is based upon pain, tenderness, discoloration and at times a palpable offset at the fracture site confirmed by visualization of the fracture on roentgenograms. The routine lateral view of the dorsal spine usually shows the sternum in the lateral projection.

TREATMENT

Efforts at reduction are seldom indicated as no impairment of function results even when the fragments unite in slight overriding. The patient is treated symptomatically, but the presence of a fracture of the sternum should serve as a warning for careful observation of the patient for signs and symptoms of intrathoracic injury. If reduction seems to be indicated, it may be attempted by strong hyperextension of the dorsal spine, or open operation may be employed.

FRACTURES OF THE RIBS

Fractures of the ribs result from direct trauma or compressions of the thoracic cage. The fractures cause pain, usually aggravated by respiration, localized tenderness, sometimes crepitus and perhaps subcutaneous emphysema. The diagnosis is confirmed by roentgenograms, but fractures of the ribs are at times difficult to demonstrate on roentgenograms, especially in the first 1 to 2 weeks after injury.

Although fractures of the ribs cause considerable pain, they are of little consequence in themselves. Even if untreated they will unite with no residual impairment of function. Their principal importance comes from the injury to the pleura and the lung and the impairment of pulmonary function which may accompany them. At the time of injury the pleura and the lung may be torn, resulting in pneumothorax or hemothorax or traumatic pneumonitis. These problems are discussed in Chapter 45, Lung.

Even without damage to the underlying pleura and lung, fractures of the ribs may result in altered pulmonary function. The pain which they produce may decrease respiratory excursion and prevent coughing. Under these circumstances tracheobronchial secretions are not coughed up. As they collect in the tracheobronchial tree, aeration of the lung fields is minimized, and a predisposition to pneumonia and atelectasis is created. These considerations are exceedingly important in treating a patient with fractures of the ribs. An especially serious type of double fracture of several adjoining ribs results in a flail chest (see Chap. 45, Lung).

TREATMENT

The pain of fractures of 1 or 2 ribs may be alleviated by a "rib belt," adhesive strapping (adhesive straps should extend either about the entire chest or cover the involved side with extension onto the uninjured side; enough strips should be used to cover the chest wall from the level of the nipple downward to the belt line) or a wide elastic bandage applied around the lower thorax in circular fashion. A disadvantage of adhesive is that many patients are sensitive to it and develop painful blisters that may cause more disability than the broken ribs. For this reason the skin must always be protected. While these time-honored methods may be employed for fractures of the ribs in selected instances, it should be kept in mind that each adds further restriction to the respiratory excursion and therefore may further impair the effectiveness of respiration, even though they do provide the patient with some relief of pain.

A more rational effective and safe approach to the treatment for fractures of the ribs is provided by posterior intercostal nerve block. Five cc. of 1 or 2 per cent procaine is injected in the region of the intercostal nerves on the inferior surfaces of each of the ribs involved (usually including 1 or 2 ribs above and below those obviously fractured) posterior to the fracture sites and usually at the posterior prominence of the rib some 2 inches from the mid-line of the spine. An adequate intercostal block relieves all pain of respiration, permits strong coughing to empty the tracheobronchial tree of its secretions and allows full inspiration so as to aerate the lung fields fully. Obviously, this procedure tends to restore the normal pulmonary function in contrast with strapping about the thoracic cage. It is surprising how often the patient remains pain-free long after the effects of the procaine have worn off. In many instances, however, the posterior intercostal nerve block should be repeated several times at intervals of 8 to 24 hours.

A combination of intercostal nerve block followed by strapping may be employed. The block serves to restore reasonably normal pulmonary function, leaving the tracheobronchial tree free of secretions and the lungs well aerated. Then, a rib belt or adhesive strapping will afford the patient some prolonged relief and any impairment of pulmonary function resulting from the compression will be minimal and probably insignificant.

The treatment of flail chest presents special problems and is discussed in Chapter 45, Lung.

BIBLIOGRAPHY

Chapters 20-23

Bankart, A. S. B.: The pathology and treatment of recurrent dislocation of the shoulder joint. Brit. J. Surg., 26:23, 1938.

Blount, W. P.: Fractures in Children. Baltimore, Williams & Wilkins, 1955.

Boyes, J. H.: Bunnell's Surgery of the Hand. ed. 4. Philadelphia, J. B. Lippincott, 1964.

Cave, E. F. (ed.): Fractures and Other Injuries. Chicago Year Book Pub., 1958.

Committee on Trauma, Am. Coll. Surgeons: The Management of Fractures and Soft Tissue Injuries. ed. 2. Philadelphia, W. B. Saunders, 1965.

Compere, E. L., Banks, S. W., and Compere, C. L.: Pictorial Handbook of Fracture Treatment. ed. 5. Chicago, Year Book Pub., 1963.

Crenshaw, A. H. (ed.): Campbell's Operative Orthopedics. ed. 4. St. Louis, C. V. Mosby, 1963.

Darrach, W.: Treatment of fractures. Ann. Surg., 124:607-616, 1946.

DePalma, A. F.: Surgery of the Shoulder. Philadelphia, J. B. Lippincott, 1950.

Dunlop, J.: Transcondylar fractures of the humerus in childhood. J. Bone & Joint Surg., 21:59, 1939.

Eggers, G. W. N.: The Internal Fixation of Fractures of the Shafts of Long Bones (Monographs on Surgery. Baltimore, Williams & Wilkins, 1952.

Essex-Lopresti, P.: Results of reduction in fractures of the calcaneum. J. Bone & Joint Surg., 33-B: 284, 1951.

Fitts, W. T., Jr., Lehr, H. B., Bither, R. L., and Spelman, J. W.: An analysis of 950 fatal injuries. Surgery, 56:663-668, 1964.

Fitts, W. T., Jr., Roberts, B., Grippe, W. J., Muir, M. W., and Allam, M. W.: The treatment of fractures complicated by contiguous burns. Surg., Gynec., Obstet., 97:551-564, 1953.

Fitts, W. T., Jr., Roberts, B., and Ravdin, I. S.: Fractures in metastatic carcinoma. Am. J. Surg., 85:282, 1953.

Friedenberg, Z. B.: Recent advances in bone physiology. Internat. Abstr. Surg., 98:313-320, 1954.

Friedenberg, Z. B., and French, G. O.: The effects of known compression forces on fracture healing. Surg., Gynec., Obstet., 94:743, 1952.

Hampton, O. P., Jr.: Fundamentals of surgery in contaminated and infected wounds. J.A.M.A., 154: 1326-1328, 1954.

———: The prevention of gas gangrene and tetanus. Indust. Med., 23:309, 1954.

———: Wounds of the Extremities in Military Surgery. St. Louis, C. V. Mosby, 1951.

Hampton, O. P., Jr., and Fitts, W. T., Jr.: Open Reduction of Common Fractures. New York, Grune and Stratton, 1959.

Hampton, O. P., Jr., and Holt, E. P., Jr.: The present status of intramedullary nailing of the tibia. Am. J. Surg., 93:597, 1957.

Hanlon, C. R., and Estes, W. L., Jr.: Fractures in childhood. Am. J. Surg., 87:313-323, 1954.

Key, J. A., and Conwell, H. E.: The Management of Fractures, Dislocations and Sprains. ed. 5. St. Louis, C. V. Mosby, 1951.

McLaughlin, H. L.: The Principles of Fracture Treatment. Committee on Trauma of the American College of Surgeons, 1954.

McLaughlin, H. L. (ed.): Trauma. Philadelphia, W. B. Saunders, 1959.

Magnuson, P. B., and Stack, J. K.: Fractures. ed. 5. Philadelphia, J. B. Lippincott, 1949.

Müller, M. E., Allgöwer, M., and Willenegger, H.: Technique of Internal Fixation of Fractures. New York, Spring-Verlag, 1965.

Murray, C. R.: The timing of the fracture-healing process; its influence on the choice and application of treatment methods. J. Bone & Joint Surg., 23:598, 1941.

Nicholson, J. T., and Heath, R. D.: Bryant's traction; a provocative cause of circulatory complications. J.A.M.A., 157:415-418, 1955.

O'Donoghue, Don H.: Treatment of Injuries to Athletes. Philadelphia, W. B. Saunders, 1962.

Palmer, I.: The mechanism and treatment of fractures of calcaneus; open reduction with the use of cancellous grafts. J. Bone & Joint Surg., 30-A:2, 1948.

Peltier, L. F.: A few remarks on fat embolism. J. Trauma, 8:812-820, 1968.

Ralston, E. L.: Handbook of Fractures. St. Louis, C. V. Mosby, 1967.

Rogers, W. A.: The treatment of fracture-dislocation of the cervical spine. J. Bone & Joint Surg., 24:245, 1942.

Rush, L. V.: Atlas of Rush pin techniques. Mississippi Doctor (Book Section), March 1954.

Saltzman, E. W., Harris, W. H., and DiSantis, R. W.: Anticoagulation for prevention of thromboembolism following fractures of the hip. New Eng. J. Med., 275:122-130, 1966.

Shires, G. T. (ed.): Care of the Trauma Patient. New York, McGraw-Hill, 1966.

Stewart, M. J., and Milford, L. W.: Fracture-dislocation of the hip. An end-result study. J. Bone & Joint Surg., 36-A:315, 1959.

Trueta, J.: The Housing Problem of the Osteoblast. J. Trauma, 1:5, 1961.

Wade, P. A.: Fractures in children. Am. J. Surg., 107:531-536, 1964.

Watson-Jones, R.: Fractures and Joint Injuries. ed. 4. Baltimore, Williams & Wilkins, 1955.

CHAPTER 24

ERLE E. PEACOCK, JR., M.D.

Principles of Hand Surgery

Introduction
Soft Tissue Injuries Exclusive of Nerves and Tendons
Soft Tissue Infections
Nerves
Tendons
Bones and Joints
Compound Wounds
Secondary Reconstruction of the Hand
Joints
Disease and Congenital Deformity
Tumors
Rehabilitation and Disability

INTRODUCTION

In 1855 Sir Charles Bell wrote:

The human hand is so beautifully formed and has so fine a sensibility, that sensibility governs its motion so correctly, every effort of the will is answered so instantly, as if the hand itself were the seat of that will; its actions are so powerful, so free, and yet so delicate, that it seems to possess a quality instinct in itself, and there is no thought of its complexity as an instrument or of the relations which make it subservient to the mind; we use it as we draw our breath, unconsciously, and have lost all recollection of the feeble and ill dictated efforts of its first exercise, by which it has been perfected. . . .

The surgeon's search for the biophysical, biochemical, and mechanical foundations for the hand function so eloquently described by Bell is one of the most recent and interesting chapters in medical achievement. Not until World War II was the hand considered susceptible of reconstruction following architectural disruption. The progress in hand surgery which has occurred in so brief a period is magnificent.

Yet 25 years after the achievements of military surgeons were directed to civilian problems, a significant portion of the terrible economic and human disability resulting from injury to the upper extremity is still attributable directly to mistakes in diagnosis and judgment rendered after a potentially reconstructable defect comes under medical care. Permanent disability seldom is the result of nothing being available for an injured hand; it is more often the result of a physician not being aware of the natural course of specialized healing and the havoc that contracture, fibrous protein synthesis, and the peculiar remodeling of deep scar can cause in the hand when allowed to progress in an uncontrolled manner. The major threat to successful restoration of function following a hand injury, therefore, must be defined as the failure of the first physician who treats the patient to recognize the sinister threat of total disability which hovers over even a cut no larger than the point of a sharp knife. There is hardly any other area in the body where failure to consider the disastrous potential of secondary complications in a simple wound takes such a toll in permanent disability.

SOFT TISSUE INJURIES EXCLUSIVE OF NERVES AND TENDONS

The most important principle in the care of any wound of the hand is to obtain as quickly as possible a healed wound without complications. Secondary closure of hand wounds is permissible only when frank infection is present. Contaminated wounds should be treated by careful and accurate débridement under the best conditions, followed by immediate closure of the wound. The reason for this is that secondary healing of a wound is invariably accompanied by edema and some degree of immobilization of the small joints. In addition, wound contraction, which also restricts small joint function, will occur. Uncomplicated primary healing is the only certain way to prevent prolonged immobilization, edema, contracture, and small joint stiffness.

Lacerations should be treated by copious irrigation, accurate excision of devitalized tissue, with careful preservation of nerves and tendons, and closure with fine sutures. Deep sutures should not be used in the palm, because the reactive palmar fascia often develops extensive deep scar around permanent sutures, producing painful nodules. Subcuticular sutures in dorsal skin do not create foreign body reaction and will decrease the width of a cutaneous scar in most instances. Injuries resulting in loss of skin in the hand are of special significance, because there is no extra skin in the hand of a young person. Small avulsions often can be closed by flexing or extending a joint in the vicinity of the wound, but permanent reduction in range of motion of the joint is the price that must be paid for this maneuver. Skin does not regenerate, and no more skin is normally present in the hand than is needed to allow all of the small joint to be put through a complete range of motion simultaneously. Except in old people, therefore, skin loss should be treated by skin replacement as soon as careful débridement has converted a contaminated wound into a surgically clean one. In older people, redundant skin usually can be mobilized and a free graft may not be needed. In wounds in which a movable structure such as tendon or a nonvascular structure such as denuded bone or joint space is not present, replacement is most simply accomplished by a free split thickness skin graft. When movable or avascular structures comprise a portion of the wound surface, however, a pedicle flap may be required. This can be accomplished by local rotation of tissue, following which the donor site is resurfaced by a free split thickness skin graft or by a distant flap such as an abdominal or pectoral pedicle flap. Pedicle flaps (particularly distant flaps) are time consuming and expensive; they should be used only as a last resort to preserve deep tissue that will not support a free graft.

Avulsion. A frequent injury characterized

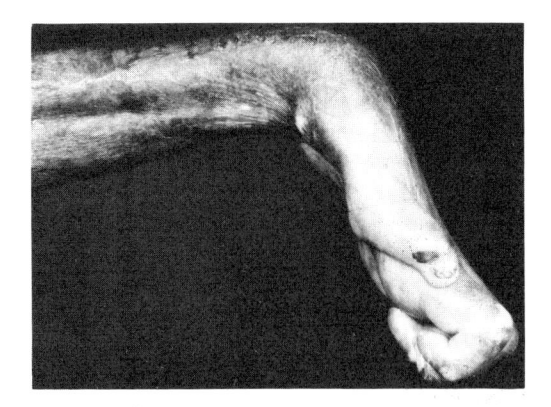

Fig. 24-1. Severely contracted hand. The result of uncontrolled healing and prolonged immobilization.

by avulsion of tissue is amputation of all or some part of a digit. When bone is not exposed in a fingertip amputation, a split thickness skin graft can be used to close the wound. The amputated tip of a digit can provide an excellent full thickness skin graft to resurface the proximal wound. When bone is exposed, particularly in the prime digits (thumb or index), experienced surgeons may choose to preserve length of the digit by performing a complex shift of local tissue or performing a small skin flap from another digit (cross finger flap). The occasional hand surgeon should not attempt complex coverage of this type in an amputation stump, however, because the danger of producing an objectionable donor site scar or the risk of immobilizing the hand for two to three weeks is considerable. In the small, ring, or long finger and in all digits when an inexperienced surgeon is caring for the injury, the simplest possible closure should be done. This usually means sacrifice of a few millimeters of bone so that soft tissue flaps can be mobilized and brought together without tension to produce a wound that will heal without complications. Sacrifice of a few millimeters of length is a small price to pay for insurance against the complications of immobilization and more complex tissue transfers. Although scattered reports of replantation of amputated fingers have appeared, vascular anastomosis in the digits is not feasible except under unusual circumstances and by highly trained individuals. Replantation of a digit should not be considered at this time except

576   Principles of Hand Surgery

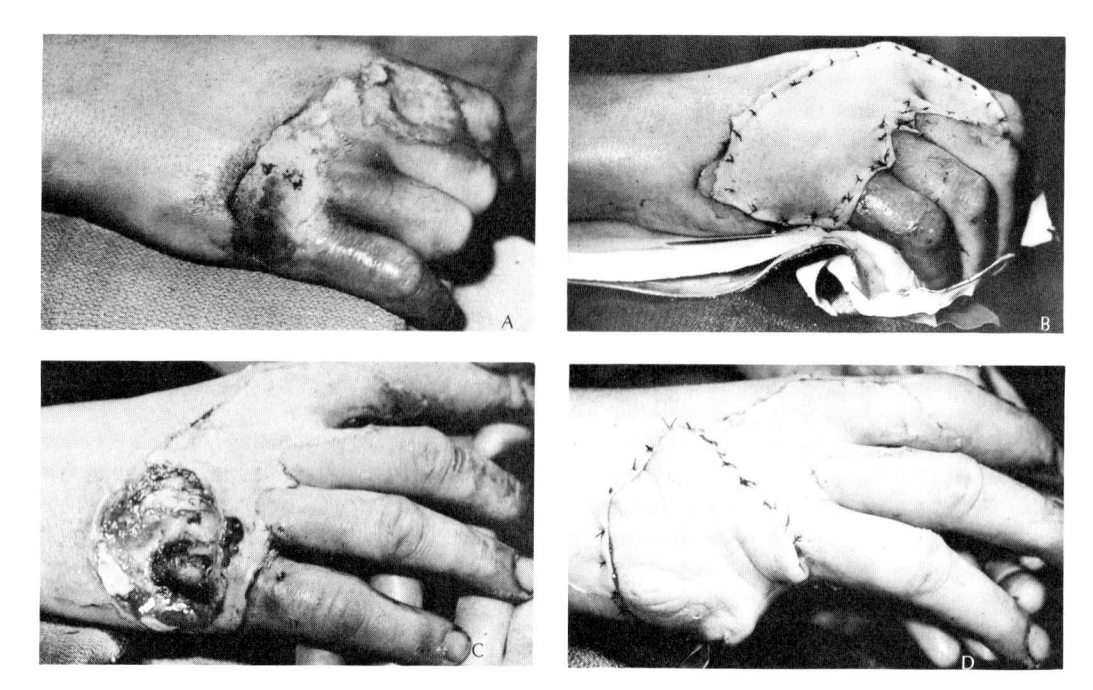

Fig. 24-2. A. An electrical burn of the dorsum of the hand. B. Excision of burn followed by immediate resurfacing with a split thickness skin graft. C. Failure of the ulnar side of the graft to take because of unrecognized deep necrosis. D. Conversion of the small finger into a local pedicle flap to produce a healed wound before extensive contraction and fibrous protein synthesis occurred.

under very unusual circumstances and by specially trained surgeons.

Circumferential avulsion of skin from a digit is usually the result of sudden force on a ring. Although a circumferentially denuded finger can be resurfaced by a free split thickness skin graft, only a trace of normal function usually results, and subsequent amputation often is requested. A free skin graft is all that should be attempted following ring

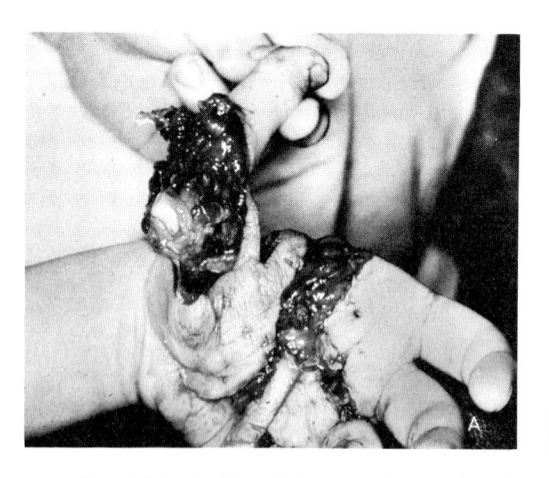

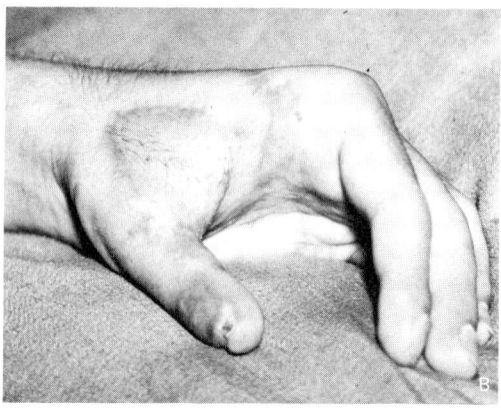

Fig. 24-3. A. Blast injury of the hand with near total amputation of the thumb. B. Salvage of the thumb by thorough débridement of the wound and application of a primary abdominal pedicle flap.

avulsion injuries; distant flaps do not produce any better coverage, and these procedures are much more dangerous to the rest of the hand than is a free graft.

First and second degree burns of the hand are best treated conservatively until re-epithelization occurs; motion should be preserved during healing. Third degree burns should be excised and resurfaced with free split thickness skin grafts as soon as possible. The combination of deep second degree burns and third degree burns presents the greatest problem for surgeons. If motion is preserved and infection prevented, healing of the entire area without loss of function can be accomplished by the use of topical antibiotics, attentive wound care, and skillful physiotherapy. Because secondary grafts may be required to correct contractures which develop during prolonged healing, early excision of mixtures of partially damaged and full thickness damaged skin is a better plan, in the judgment of some surgeons. A difference of opinion exists, however, and in all probability either course can be utilized successfully if complications do not occur. Successful management of the burned hand is measured in preservation of joint function; any therapy that produces a healed wound without loss of small joint function is an excellent one. Any course of treatment that leaves the hand with stiff interphalangeal joints is less than adequate.

Electrical burns are especially serious because the extent of damage usually cannot be appreciated for several days. The objective of early excision of damaged tissue, followed by replacement with the new skin as quickly as possible, although more difficult to achieve than after a thermal burn, is still sound.

Short-wave radiation effect in skin of the hand is most often encountered following x-ray therapy of eczema or hemangiomas. Radiation dermatitis from improper use of a fluoroscope is more rare now than 25 years ago. Skin which has typical radiation effect should be replaced before open ulcers or epidermoid carcinoma appears. If short-wave-damaged skin is not replaced relatively early, ulceration, pain, and finally change to epidermoid carcinoma will necessitate radical and sometimes mutilating surgery.

SOFT TISSUE INFECTIONS

Subcutaneous infection in the hand is often, although not always, the result of a known penetrating injury. Pain and tenderness are more intense in the hand than in many areas because of rigidly limited spaces which prevent diffuse swelling. Edema and erythema may not be as prominent in the hand as in other areas of the body because the retinacular structures separate the hand and fingers into rather rigid compartments; infections at first are limited by fibrous membranes and produce characteristic diagnostic signs for each compartment.

Felons. The most distal compartment is the volar pulp surrounding the distal phalanx. Multiple fibrous septi convert the distal pulp into a multilocular container. Infections developing in this area are sharply limited to the distal phalangeal section of the digit, and are called felons. The characteristic signs and symptoms of a felon include history of a penetrating injury in some cases (but not in others) and throbbing pain relieved partially by elevation (patients often state that they can count their own pulse by the throbbing pain). Physical signs include a tense and shiny skin, erythema, and exquisite tenderness to superficial pressure on the end of the finger. Fever and leukocytosis are serious signs that the infection may not be limited to the pulp space. If adequate surgical drainage, including division of a large number of the fibrous septi, through a midlateral incision is not accomplished early, the intraspace pressure will exceed the arterial blood pressure and septic necrosis with osteomyelitis of the distal phalanx will occur. A felon is a serious emergency which must be treated aggressively by an experienced surgeon as soon as possible.

Paronychia. Dorsal infections around the nailbed are called paronychia. A common term for paronychia is "a run around." Signs of infection soon follow the course of the cuticle in a semi-circular outline. Early surgical drainage is mandatory for, if adequate drainage is not established, removal of the nail may be necessary to prevent a subungual abscess.

Tenosynovitis. The most serious deep infection of the finger is infection of the flexor tendon sheath; this entity is called tenosynovitis. All of the signs and symptoms of infection in the soft tissues are present throughout the finger but, in addition, an important sign is present indicating that the tendon sheath also is involved. This sign is elicited by gently holding the proximal finger so that motion cannot occur in the proximal interphalangeal joint and then, with the other hand, briskly extending the distal interphalangeal joint passively. If the infection involves only the soft tissues external to the tendon sheath, discomfort greater than that produced by direct pressure from holding the finger is not produced. If tenosynovitis is present, the patient will experience severe, lancinating pain when the distal interphalangeal joint is extended. The diagnosis is seldom in doubt if the test is performed skillfully. Accurate diagnosis is extremely important when tenosynovitis is considered, because this condition is a dangerous infection which not only ruins the involved finger but spreads quickly throughout the sheath mechanism to involve other areas of the hand. An entire hand may be converted into an immovable fibrous claw by the severe scarring and joint fixation which follows healing in the wake of tenosynovitis. Conversely, the operation to drain the flexor tendon sheath and prevent such a complication will create a tenosynovitis if a subcutaneous cellulitis is mistakenly diagnosed as tenosynovitis. Accurate diagnosis, therefore is critical in the proper management of digital soft tissue infections.

Infections in the Palmar Spaces. The various palmar spaces (thenar, hypothenar, or midpalmar) also are distinctly outlined by fascial membranes, and deep infection is restricted for some time by these structures. Infections in the palmar spaces are accompanied by edema, which is usually more severe on the dorsum of the hand than on the volar surface where the tough palmar fascia lies between a collection of pus and the surface. Accurate localization of the abscess by history, physical findings, and unerring anatomic knowledge, followed by adequate surgical drainage performed so that resulting scar tissue will not restrict hand function, is essential if permanent disability is to be prevented.

Management of Pyogenic Infections. The most important principle in management of pyogenic infections of the hand is that the seriousness of even a dermal cellulitis is so great that experienced surgical consultation and, possibly, hospitalization are needed early to prevent permanent disability or even death. The complex fibrous retinacular system in the hand which gives rise to the term "closed space infections" must be understood both anatomically and biologically before treatment is instituted. Finally, the healing process with its inevitable production of unyielding fibrous protein is so devastating to hand function that time is of the essence both for diagnosis and experienced surgical therapy.

Tuberculous infections usually involve skin, tendon sheath, bone and joints. Although no evidence of the disease may be readily apparent in other organs, involvement of the hand usually is caused by hematological dissemination. The frequency of this condition in cattle handlers suggests that bovine tuberculosis is prevalent. Drug-resistant mutants are common, and combination therapy with streptomycin, isoniazid, and PAS is usually required. Radical excision of involved tissues with protection of nerves and normal tendons, combined with adequate antibiotic therapy, will cure approximately 75 per cent of patients.

NERVES

Diagnosis of a sensory defect is difficult only when patients are inebriated or too young to be cooperative. In these patients a crude sweat test can be performed which, if positive, is of diagnostic significance. The test is performed, if possible, in a warm room. The area supplied by a sensory nerve which may be divided is sponged with ether until it is completely dry. If the skin is then examined carefully with the aid of magnification from a low power lens such as the $+8$ lens on an ophthalmoscope, tiny droplets of sweat can be seen to appear if the nerve is intact. Unmistakable appearance of cutaneous sweating is strong evidence that peripheral sensory innervation is intact. Absence of sweating is strong suggestive evidence that a peripheral nerve has been interrupted, particularly if surrounding skin supplied by another nerve sweats normally.

For inexperienced examiners, examination of intrinsic muscle function can be considerably more difficult than sensory evaluation.

There are two reasons why this is true. One is that variation in the nerve supply to intrinsic muscles of the hand is surprisingly common. The other is that substitution patterns are possible in many hands. The unwary examiner can be tricked more often than is commonly appreciated into believing that motor function is normal. For instance, opposition of the thumb is often recommended as a test for median nerve function. But there is a 60-40 variation in the nerve supply to the long head of the short flexor muscle in the thenar group, and this muscle alone can oppose the thumb. A more reliable motor test for suspected median nerve palsy is circumduction of the thumb through a 360° arc. A 360° sweep of the thumb is impossible if all of the thenar muscles are not functioning. Abduction and adduction of the fingers is frequently used as a test of ulnar nerve function; mixed innervation of the intrinsics and lumbricals, as well as substitution of some of the long tendons, can be responsible for an erroneous estimation of intrinsic function. Froment's sign (maintaining a perfect circle with the index finger and thumb during hard pinch) is a reliable sign of ulnar nerve integrity; the first dorsal interosseus and the adductor muscles are more constantly supplied by the ulnar nerve than are the lumbricals or intrinsics. One side of the circle invariably will collapse during hard pinch without normal contraction of these muscles.

Wrist drop and inability to extend the fingers at the metacarpophalangeal joint are reliable signs of radial nerve palsy.

Repair of Peripheral Nerves

The question of whether repair of a divided peripheral nerve should be made immediately or delayed until after soft tissue healing and scar maturation is complete cannot be answered at this time. The theoretical advantages of delaying a nerve anastomosis include allowing Wallerian degeneration to occur so that advancing axons will have open channels in the distal nerve and being certain of the extent of proximal nerve damage so that a traumatized proximal end incapable of regeneration will not be anastomosed to the distal nerve. Advantages of primary repair include the obvious elimination of a second operation and the relatively rapid innervation of muscles before degeneration of motor end plates occurs.

About all that can be said now is that excellent results have been otained from both primary and secondary repairs when performed by experienced surgeons. When damage to nerve and surrounding tissue has been considerable (as in a crushing injury) or where danger of infection is increased (as in heavily contaminated wounds) or when a high velocity missile has caused the damage, so that the extent of proximal damage cannot be determined, secondary anastomosis is clearly indicated. In a clean laceration, primary repair may be indicated. So much of the fundamental biology of axoplasm and Schwann cell reaction to injury is unknown for human nerves that only the most general recommendations can be made at this time.

The result of nerve anastomosis in the sensory digital nerves is excellent. Digital nerves are small pure sensory nerves, and failure to recover excellent sensation after anastomosis is good evidence that something went awry locally, and that the anastomosis should be repeated. Results following repair of the median nerve are much better than results following repair of the ulnar nerve at the wrist level. The median nerve is approximately 90 per cent sensory, and the motor fasciculus often can be identified and properly oriented at the time of primary repair. Recovery of sensation is not as good following suture of the median nerve at the wrist as it is following repair of digital nerves in the palm or fingers. Protective sensation (ability to detect when an affected area is being touched but not able to discriminate accurately) is usual. Motor return is not predictable, although excellent return of function in paralyzed thenar muscles is observed with gratifying frequency. Return of sensation following anastomosis of the ulnar nerve is less predictable than following repair of either the median or digital nerves. Return of significant motor function following anastomosis of the proximal ulnar nerve is not usual unless the motor branch alone was divided and repaired. The ulnar nerve is an evenly mixed motor and sensory nerve without discrete localization of fibers; thus regenerating axons have a considerably smaller chance of finding the correct distal channel following repair than they do in some other nerves.

Regeneration of axons following repair of a peripheral nerve occurs at an average rate of approximately one millimeter a day. Progress in regeneration can be estimated fairly accurately by the use of Tinel's sign, which is obtained by tapping the course of the nerve distal to an anastomosis until a point is reached where tapping no longer elicits a tingling sensation in the skin supplied by that nerve. Persistence of a positive Tinel's sign at the site of the anastomosis and palpation of an oval smooth mass in the scar tissue are good evidence of formation of a neuroma. A neuroma usually means that, for some local reason, distal regeneration of axons did not occur. A second attempt at reconstruction of the nerve is usually indicated.

Pain syndromes such as causalgia and hyperesthesia can be differentiated from the hypersensitivity of a neuroma by history and examination. These perplexing syndromes—often severely disabling and usually difficult to treat—are more often associated with partial injury to a nerve than with complete division of a nerve. The longer such syndromes persist, the more difficult they are to treat. Experienced consultation should be obtained as soon as an unusual pain pattern becomes fixed.

Finally, many factors are involved in recovering hand function following repair of a peripheral nerve. In addition to regrowth of axons in the distal segment, the ability to use the eyes to substitute for peripheral sensory reception, an increase in sensitivity of surrounding intact peripheral receptors, and an integration of other receptors such as kinesioreceptors are but a few of the possible ways in which hand function may be improved. It is often difficult to be certain how much the regeneration of axons contributes to the overall return of function in the hand; critical appraisal of hand function by a person thoroughly acquainted with anatomic variations and substitution patterns is needed to properly evaluate the true effectiveness of many complex procedures such as free nerve grafts, pedicle nerve grafts, etc.

TENDONS

Diagnosis of divided tendons is usually obvious, although it may be several weeks before division of some tendons such as a single flexor sublimis or wrist flexor becomes apparent if surrounding tendons are functioning normally. Division of tendons with relatively large amplitudes of motion, such as the digital flexors, is more difficult to repair than is division of tendons with relatively small amplitudes, such as finger extensors or intrinsic tendons.

One of the most complex and, at times, difficult problems in restorative surgery is to re-establish mechanical continuity between two tendon ends by the formation of a fibrous scar while sustaining movement of the entire tendon scar complex so that distal function is possible. In a sense, precisely what must happen between tendon ends (synthesis and assembly of a rigid nonelastic scar) must not happen around the tendon if motion and transmission of force are to be accomplished. Biologically, this means that the early amorphous gel of cells, new collagen, and ground substance, which diffuses throughout the wound, must differentiate into a scar of one type between the tendon ends and differentiate into a scar with entirely different physical characteristics around the tendon. Because there is only one wound (including tendon, surrounding tissue and overlying skin) and consequently only one scar, what is really being asked is that secondary remodeling of the early scar proceed along lines so that collagen between the tendon ends will be assembled in closely packed longitudinally oriented patterns resembling normal tendon, while surrounding the tendon a different portion of the same scar will remodel to produce a loosely disorganized network which by physical weave and internal arrangement will have physical qualities similar to those of loose areolar tissue.

Although many of the factors that govern synthesis, assembly, and remodeling of new connective tissue are unknown, most of those that are known are not controllable by surgeons; surgical judgment and technic in tendon repair are based upon the factors which can be controlled at this time to influence collagen synthesis and remodeling. Examples of judgments and technics that have been found to influence physical characteristics of scar tissue following healing of a tendon laceration are time of repair (immediate versus delayed), suture of divided tendons or replacement of an entire tendon by a free graft, immobilization and type of remobilization, and preparation of the tissues through which a repaired tendon ultimately must glide. Other factors such as selection of suture material, configuration of sutures within the wound, position during immobilization, use of drugs, etc. do not appear now to be based on sound biochemical and biophysical knowledge of healing and scar remodeling; consequently, they do not influence the end result as much as has been supposed.

FLEXOR TENDONS

The only real emergency involving laceration of tendons is division of the finger flexors in the proximal wrist. In the proximal wrist there are no restraining structures, such as lumbrical muscles and vincula, to prevent complete contraction of the muscle and retraction of the proximal tendon ends. Consequently, it is always difficult to locate proximal tendon ends immediately after they are lacerated in this area, and prospects for locating and repairing them after proximal fibrosis and atrophy of the muscle belly has occurred are not good. Digital flexor tendons, therefore, should be anastomosed in the wrist as soon after injury as possible. It is preferable not to attempt anastomosis of all of the sublimis and all of the profundus tendons at the same time. The difference in amplitude of motion between the sublimis and profundus tendons is considerable, and a common scar in the wrist assures that profundus excursion will be reduced to that of the sublimis group. Because profundus function alone usually gives adequate finger flexion for most activities, the reduction in operating time, reduction in suture materials inserted, and reduction in tissue reaction and subsequent scar tissue formation present a compelling argument for repairing only four digitorum profundus tendons and the flexor pollicis longus when all twelve flexor tendons have been divided in the wrist. Wrist flexion is adequate following restoration of the profundus tendons without repairing the three wrist flexors.

Elsewhere in the hand, repair of flexor tendons can be performed with as good, and in many instances even better, results as a secondary procedure. This does not mean that an experienced surgeon working under ideal conditions cannot repair primarily, or even graft primarily, tendons in almost every area in the hand or fingers with superb functional results. It does mean that factors that affect significantly the synthesis and remodeling of scar tissue are often less controllable during primary repair of a wound than after soft tissue healing has occurred. Therefore, if there is any doubt about conditions of the wound, preparation and experience of the surgeon, available facilities, etc., the overlying skin could be closed primarily without any attempt to repair a divided tendon. Secondary restoration following this type of primary surgical care is always *as good as* and in some areas even better than repair by primary anastomosis. This is particularly true in special areas such as the restricted confines of the digital theca or where tendons pass through each other or through an area where unmovable structures such as bone also have been damaged and will become part of a single scar. Under favorable circumstances, modern surgical technics have made it possible to restore predictably normal finger flexion following injury of flexor tendons proximal to the digital sheath in the palm and distal to the insertion of the sublimis tendon in the middle phalanx. Restoration of flexion sufficient to do more than touch the palm with the fingertip is unusual (although possible) following division of both flexor tendons within the digital sheath.

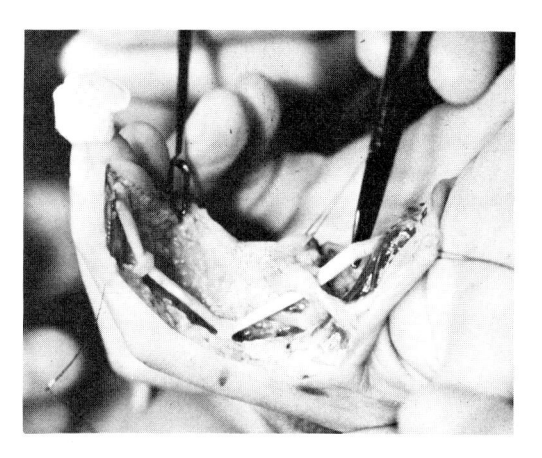

FIG. 24-4. Palmaris longus used as a free tendon graft to replace the flexor sublimis and profundus tendons. Note two pulleys salvaged from digital theca to prevent bowstringing of tendon.

EXTENSOR TENDONS

Because the extensor tendons have a relatively short amplitude of motion (less than one centimeter to extend completely the metacarpophalangeal joint), and because these tendons pass through large expanses of movable loose areolar tissue in contrast to the tight restricted passages of the immovable digital sheaths, scar tissue involving extensor tendons does not restrict function as often or as severely as the scar surrounding a repaired flexor tendon. As a result, primary repairs almost always can and usually should be performed if the wound is one that can be closed safely. A notable exception is a wound that includes a fracture or denuded bone. Involvement of an extensor tendon in scar that is attached to an immovable structure such as bone means not only that active extension of the involved digit will be restricted but that passive flexion of the distal joint also will be limited by a checkrein or tenodesis effect. Secondary repair or rerouting of the repaired tendon to avoid fixation to an immovable structure is necessary to restore extension and permit a full range of passive flexion. It should be remembered that extensor tendons can be divided in some areas without loss of active extension of the digit; in these instances, repair of the tendon should not be attempted, for there is nothing to be gained by doing so, and much can be lost if the repaired tendon becomes adherent to an immovable structure and restricts flexion. The extensor tendons are often multiple in number and attach to each other at varying levels and in varying patterns so that laceration of a single tendon in the metacarpal area may not deprive a digit of its only source of extension.

INTRINSIC TENDONS

Intrinsic tendons are not often divided, but when they are, it is easy to overlook them, particularly in the area of the neck of a metacarpal. Repair in restoring intrinsic function is successful when the diagnosis of a divided intrinsic tendon is made at the time of the original injury and immediate repair is carried out. Secondary repairs usually must be made in the form of a tendon transfer, and the results are not comparable to those obtained with immediate recognition and repair of a lacerated intrinsic tendon. Thenar and hypothenar disabilities are not difficult to diagnose, as the level of the injury combined with absent or abnormal intrinsic function leaves little doubt as to what has occurred. Intrinsic tendon lacerations in the metacarpal area usually cause deviations of digits, particularly ulnar deviations, which may be missed during care of the initial wound unless power of abduction and adduction is tested.

BOUTONNIERE DEFORMITY

Disruption or attenuation of the central portion of the extensor mechanism over the dorsum of the proximal interphalangeal joint allows the lateral bands to subluxate below the axis of rotation of that joint. In this position, intrinsic power is directed straight to the distal interphalangeal joint. With the lateral bands in this position, the intrinsic muscles produce unopposed flexion of the proximal interphalangeal joint and overpowering forces of extension of the distal phalanx. The result is a finger which reposes in flexion at the proximal interphalangeal joint and cannot be actively extended. The deformity, called a boutonnière (button hole) deformity, can be repaired only by surgical relocation of the lateral bands of the intrinsic mechanism to a position dorsal to the axis of rotation of the proximal interphalangeal joint.

MALLET FINGER

Division or forcible avulsion of the insertion of the extensor mechanism from its terminal insertion in the base of the distal phalanx produces unopposed flexion of the distal interphalangeal joint. This deformity is called mallet finger or baseball finger because of the frequency with which a blow on the tip of the finger produces dehiscence or avulsion of the terminal slip. Splinting the distal interphalangeal joint in hyperextension for four weeks usually results in reattachment (particularly when a fragment of bone is dislodged with the tendon) of the tendon to the point of insertion. Splinting must be started early and maintained rigidly to be successful; otherwise, operative repair is needed to restore distal interphalangeal extension.

HEALING

Approximately three weeks is required for tendons to heal and for the scar to become

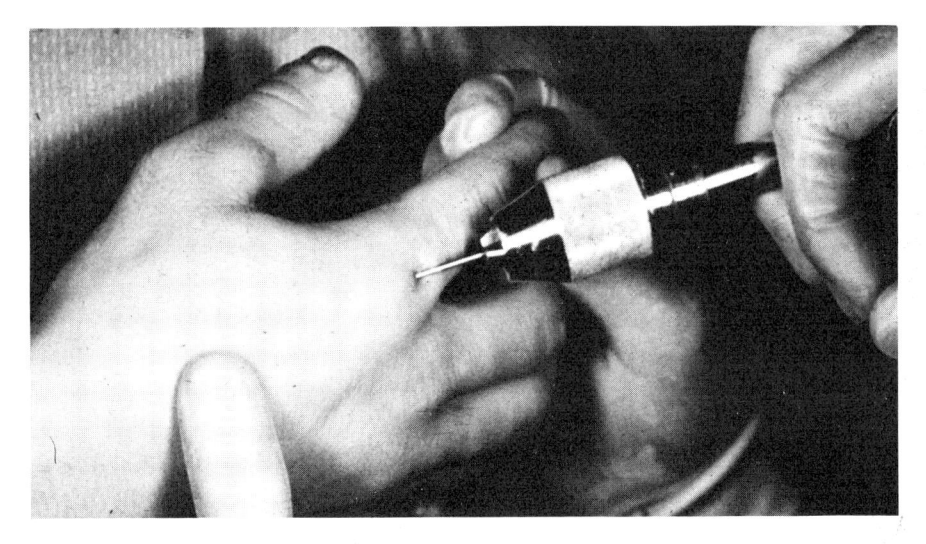

FIG. 24-5. Insertion of a longitudinal Kirschner wire to stabilize a transverse fracture of the index metacarpal.

mature enough to permit active and passive motion. During the immobilization period it is extremely important that joints not be kept in extreme positions of flexion or extension, particularly in older people. Permanent joint fixation is a frequent complication of tendon repair. So disabling that it should be kept in mind continually, it can be prevented by not placing small joints in extreme positions and by removing restraining dressings periodically to put joints through a careful passive range of motion when possible.

BONES AND JOINTS

An old principle in the treatment of fractures of the extremities—immobilize a joint below and a joint above the fracture—is seldom applicable to fractures of the hand. As in all other injuries of the hand, the devastating complications of loss of motion in small joints must be prevented, not treated. After World War II, the term "position of function," which refers to the position of the hand when the joints are in an approximately neutral position such as when an object the size and shape of a tennis ball is being grasped, became popular. The connotation that immobilization was permissible, provided all joints were in this position, was a step in the right direction, as it did much to destroy the popular use of straight board splints or banjo traction from the tip of a finger to an outrigger which immobilized in extension every joint. In the final analysis, however, universal hand splints and the position of function only assured that when a joint became stiff it would be in a neutral position. At the moment a great deal of effort is being expended to go another step and develop more strongly the concept of preservation of motion by not immobilizing any small joints if possible. Such a concept can be very productive in reducing permanent disability due to joint stiffness from immobilization.

Immobilization of fractures without immobilizing joints is accomplished usually by either open or closed reduction of a fracture and by stabilizing the fractures with local intramedullary pins. Phalangeal fractures, metacarpal fractures, and special fractures such as a Bennett's fracture (a fracture dislocation of the base of the first metacarpal) usually can be reduced and immobilized with local pins so that motion in all of the joints remains normal. A possible exception, of course, is a fracture involving a joint surface. Operative reduction and skeletal traction may be required in these fractures. When traction is required, however, it is important to utilize skeletal fixation as close to the fracture as possible so that only the affected joint will

584   Principles of Hand Surgery

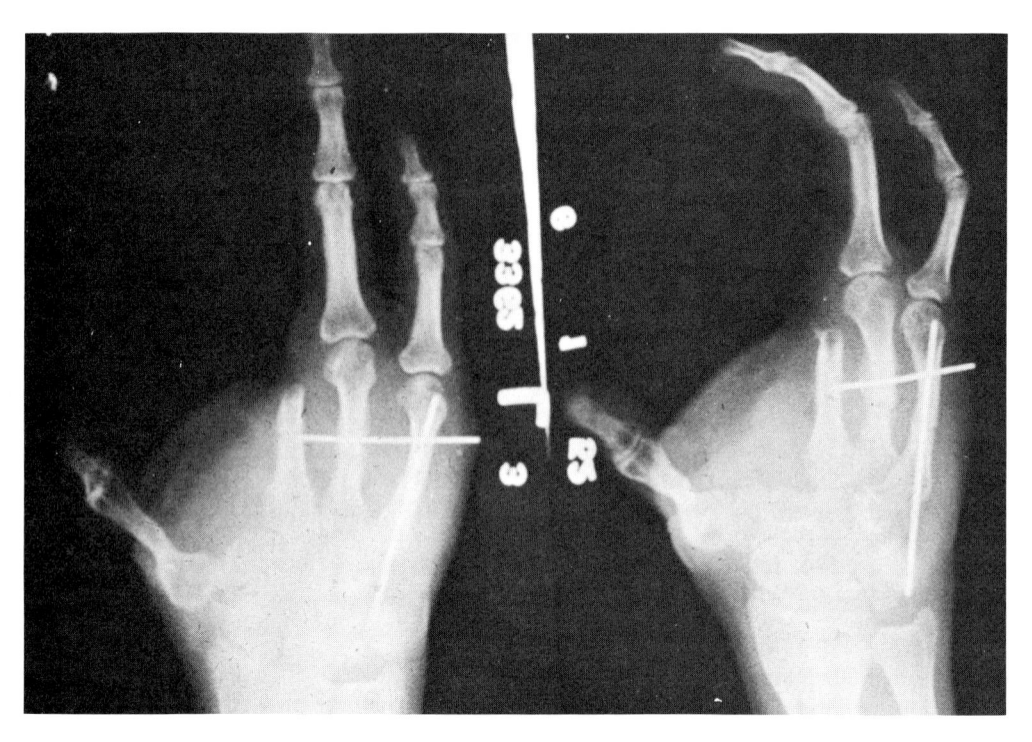

Fig. 24-6. Utilization of Kirschner wires in two planes to stabilize multiple fractures of the metacarpals.

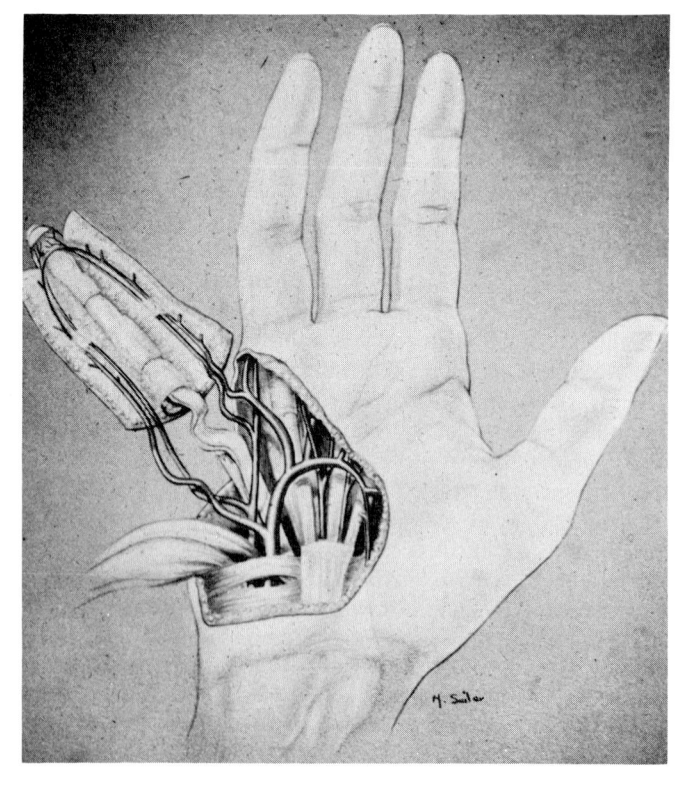

Fig. 24-7. Artist's conception of the exploded finger, demonstrating dual radial-oriented blood supply to potential source of spare parts.

be immobilized while all joints distal to the affected joint will be movable.

Wounds of joints should be treated by careful débridement, repair of ligaments and joint capsule, and restoration of adequate soft tissue covering by whatever means is necessary to provide full thickness skin without tension and with adequate blood supply. A period of seven to ten days of complete immobilization to permit soft tissue healing, followed by incomplete immobilization for an additional two weeks, usually is required to regain any function. During the two weeks of incomplete immobilization, an external splint should be removed at least every two days while the reconstructed joint is put through a careful passive range of motion within the limits imposed by inflammation and pain.

COMPOUND WOUNDS

Most wounds of the hand involve more than one tissue, and some perforating wounds may destroy simultaneously skin, nerve, tendon, bone, and joints. The proper order of surgical procedures can be pivotal in the success of attempted restoration. With the exception of tendon injuries at the wrist level, a good rule is that the only objective that has to be accomplished during primary care of the wound is reconstruction of soft tissue by the simplest possible method. A split thickness skin graft used to resurface a complex wound will prevent infection and edema and will assure that joint stiffness does not occur. Even if such a graft has to be replaced later by a distant pedicle flap, successful closure by a temporary graft is mandatory if later restorative procedures are going to be possible.

The usual order of reconstruction is to restore adequate soft tissue and then to restore sensation. This is followed by reconstruction of the bony architecture and mobilization of joints. Replacement of tendons by free grafts or tendon transfers obviously must be delayed until a solid skeletal framework has been provided and flexible joints have been obtained. Neither bone nor tendon surgery is predictably successful in an anesthetic or inadequately covered extremity. Thus, definitive skin coverage and restoration of sensation are important prerequisites to bone, joint, and tendon replacement.

A penetrating gunshot wound of the palm that lacerates extensor or flexor tendons, cuts a neurovascular bundle, and splinters the center third of a metacarpal might be treated in the following way: The large stellate wound of exit on the dorsum of the hand could be grafted with a split thickness skin graft after thorough débridement. Two months later the split thickness skin graft could be excised and the defect resurfaced with an abdominal pedicle flap. Six weeks later the common volar digital nerve in the palm could be repaired. Approximately three months later, the flap on the dorsum of the hand could be partially elevated and an iliac bone graft inserted to reconstruct the missing portion of a metacarpal; a capsulotomy and collateral ligament excision to restore motion in the distal metacarpal phalangeal joint might or might not be required. Approximately three months later, adequate coverage, sensation, stability, and joint motion having been obtained, an extensor or flexor tendon graft could be inserted to complete the restoration. Although this amount of surgery in the hand may be justified, a single finger so badly damaged probably should be deleted. A general rule is that if any three of the five major tissues (skin, nerve, tendon, bone, joint) of a digit have to be replaced, amputation should be considered.

SECONDARY RECONSTRUCTION OF THE HAND

After the initial wound has healed and soft tissue scars have become soft and mature, the reconstructive surgeon turns his thoughts to rebuilding the hand through a series of reconstructive procedures. The condition of the proximal interphalangeal joints often is the critical limiting factor in what can be accomplished. A hand that reaches the stage of secondary reconstructive surgery with supple joints usually can be reconstructed to near pre-injury status, but a hand that has developed serious loss of interphalangeal joint range of motion has very limited potential, regardless of the skill of the surgeon.

Skin and Subcutaneous Tissue

Replacement of badly scarred skin, addition of new skin when coverage is inadequate, and

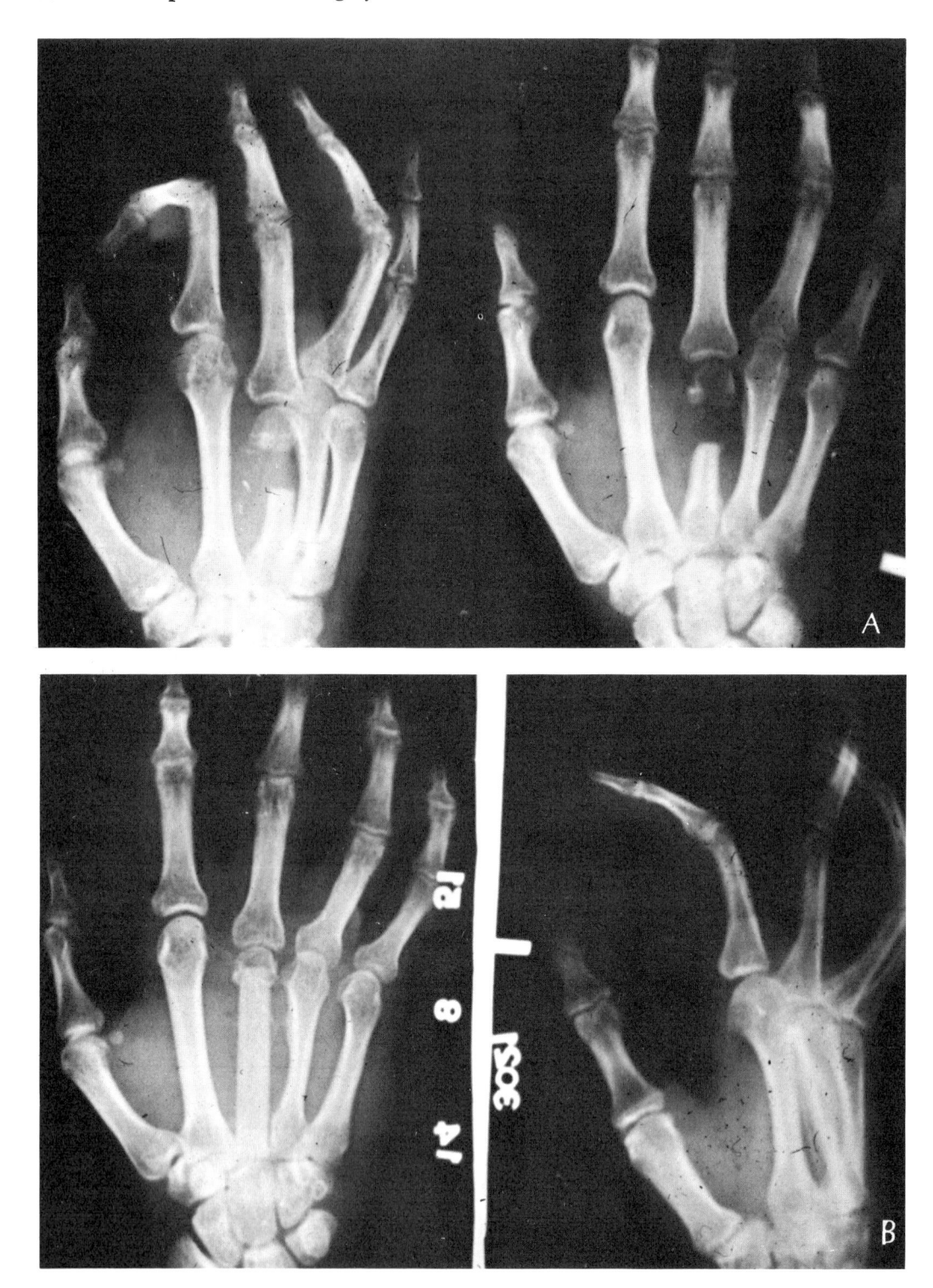

Fig. 24-8. A. Loss of substance of the long metacarpal from a gunshot wound. Note recession of long finger into palm. B. Replacement of metacarpal bone with a full length bone graft from the tibia.

grafting of composite tissue when there is deficient subcutaneous tissue must be accomplished first. Abdominal and pectoral pedicle flaps, local digital flaps, and island pedicle flaps are the main technics used to provide definitive cover. Distant (abdominal or pectoral) flaps are not as desirable as a local flap because skin from the abdomen or chest is too hairy, too thick, and too anesthetic even after some sensation is regained to replace satisfactorily the thin, highly specialized skin of the hand and fingers. Thus, distant flaps should be reserved for those patients in whom the remaining fingers are too good to be sacrificed and converted into a local pedicle flap.

A full thickness defect in the hand can be superbly resurfaced by converting a damaged finger into a local skin flap containing adequate subcutaneous tissue. Such a flap has perfect texture, specialized elasticity, and good color, and often tactile sensation is intact, wholly or partially. When a finger flap is too short to reach a distant soft tissue defect, it can be converted into an island pedicle by dissecting away all of the soft tissue from the neurovascular bundle supplying the finger. The skin and subcutaneous tissue is left attached to the hand only by relatively long neurovascular bundles. After the dissection is complete, the flap can be threaded subcutaneously to almost any position in the hand or wrist. Occasionally a small neurovascular island pedicle flap is removed from the inside of a central finger and transplanted to the tip of the thumb or index finger to provide sensation when nerve repair is impossible. An example would be taking an island pedicle from the ulnar side of the ring finger where sensation is not critical and transferring it to the tip of the thumb where sensation is badly needed in a patient with an irreparable injury to the median nerve.

NERVES

The most reliable procedure for restoring peripheral sensation is to anastomose the proximal and distal ends of a severed nerve. As much as an 8-cm. defect in the median nerve and a 12-cm. defect in the ulnar nerve can be overcome by transplanting the proximal nerve to a superficial position in the forearm and flexing the elbow, wrist, and fingers as much as possible. Regenerating nerves should be immobilized with the extremity in a flexed position for three weeks, following which the arm and wrist should be extended gradually so that the nerve and surrounding soft tissue can be gradually stretched.

Defects in nerves too great to be overcome by transplanting the nerves can be bridged by a free nerve graft. In the case of digital nerves, a free graft results in about 50 per cent as much return of sensation as can be obtained by a single, direct anastomosis. Axons have to cross twice as many anastomotic sites in a nerve graft as in a single anastomosis. A digital nerve from an amputation stump or a free graft of the sural nerve can be utilized. Free nerve grafts of larger diameter, such as using the ulnar nerve to graft the median nerve, are usually unsuccessful. Although good data are not available on the changes in large nerves following transplantation, the failure of these grafts to function is presumably the result of a graft being too large to survive by diffusion of gases and nutrients after transplantation. The central area of the nerve appears to become necrotic, and fibrosis occurs. Some success has been reported by utilizing two or three small nerve grafts (cable grafts) to bridge a defect in a large nerve, but, at present, the best method of overcoming a large defect when both median and ulnar nerves have been destroyed is by transfer of a nerve by the pedicle method. Based on the reasoning that blood supply in a nerve is longitudinal as well as segmental, the ulnar nerve can be sutured to the end of the median nerve without disturbing the segmental circulation at the first operation. Three months later, after the ulnar nerve graft has acquired some longitudinal circulation from the proximal median nerve, and the proximal axons from the median nerve have penetrated the graft, the ulnar nerve can be dissected out of its bed; the entire median and ulnar nerve complex can be pulled into a defect in the wrist and sutured to the distal median nerve in the hand. Return of sensation following such a procedure is appreciable, but fundamental data on the amount and rate of axonal regeneration following such rearrangement of the blood supply are lacking.

Distal nerve transfers by which an intact

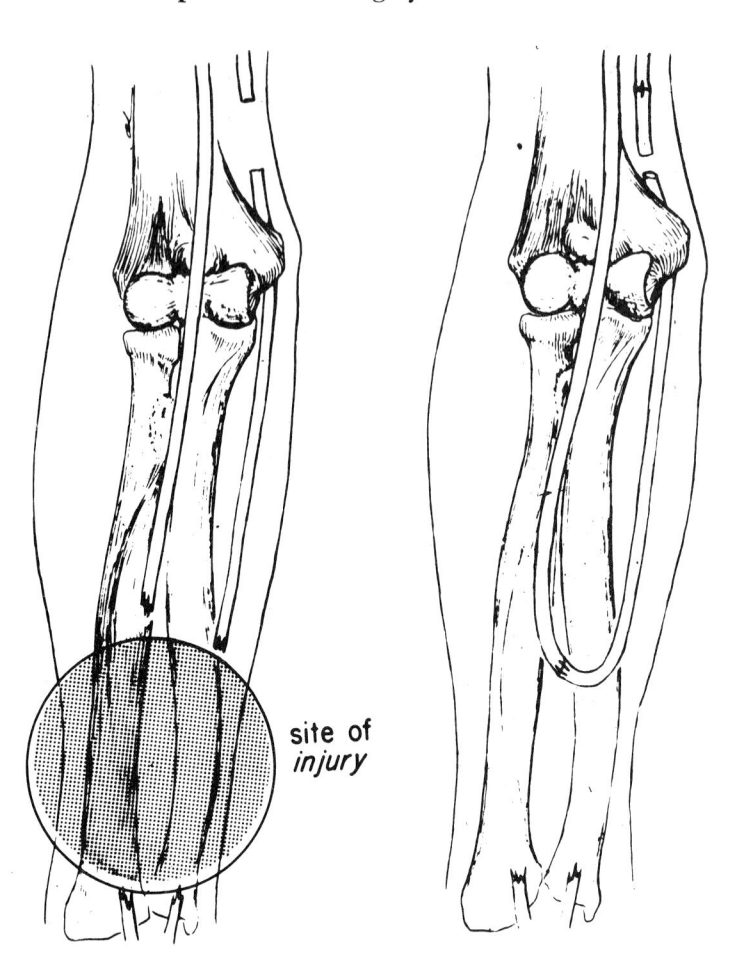

FIG. 24-9. Diagram of a first stage of a pedicle nerve transplant in which the ulnar nerve is sutured to the median nerve and then rotated into the lower forearm and wrist defect.

ulnar proper volar digital nerve on the medial side of the small finger is divided in the finger and transferred to an unrepairable distal nerve in the index finger or thumb can switch relatively unimportant sensation to a critically important area. However, the price of anesthesia in the donor area following such a procedure is just as great as when an island flap is transferred for the same purpose. Because the quality of sensation regained after suture of a nerve is never as good as normal sensation, the island pedicle method usually is to be preferred.

The use of irradiated and lyophilized free nerve grafts has been reported in animals and human beings but, at this time, the laboratory data are difficult to interpret and the clinical data which would suggest that very much has been accomplished by this approach are far from convincing.

TENDONS

Tendons are usually reconstructed by free tendon grafts. Such grafts can extend as far as from the wrist and distal forearm to the tip of a finger on either the volar or extensor surfaces. When the long flexor tendons have to be replaced, great technical skill is required to restore a useful range of motion. Moreover, condition of the tissue has to be optimal, and patients should be carefully selected. Adequate soft tissue, at least one functioning digital nerve, adequate passive joint motion, and a highly motivated patient are essential to obtain satisfactory results. A recent innovation which has enlarged the effective application of flexor tendon grafting has been the utilization of a composite tissue allograft of the entire flexor mechanism from a recently deceased cadaver. Such a graft consists of both flexor tendons, surrounded by an intact digital sheath. Healing following insertion of such a graft occurs only between the recipient digital bed and the outside of the transplanted digital sheath. The highly specialized surface between tendons and internal surface of the sheath is not involved in the fibrous tissue reaction of the healing process. It is possible to put such a graft in a severely scarred finger that would be unsuitable for a conventional autograft.

Balance of motor power in the hand can be restored following paralysis of an important muscle or muscle group by transferring the tendons of a normally functioning muscle to the point of insertion of the paralyzed one. For instance, one of the three wrist flexors can be converted into a wrist extensor without significantly reducing power of wrist flexion. A wrist extensor can be transferred to all of the finger intrinsic muscle insertions to overcome the claw deformity of an intrinsic palsy. To be considered as a possible transfer, a muscle must have normal strength, be independently innervated, have a course reasonably close to a straight line in its new location, and be retrainable. It is desirable to transfer a muscle which normally functions synchronously with the muscle which it is to replace. Such a transfer would be a wrist extensor to a metacarpophalangeal joint flexor. Almost any muscle in the forearm and hand can be retrained to perform a new function in a highly motivated, alert patient.

BONE

Metacarpals are reconstructed by free bone grafts from the ilium or tibia. Iliac grafts of cancellous bone become vascularized more dependably than cortical grafts. When intricate bone carpentry is needed to introduce a graft into a complicated defect, however, cortical bone from the tibia is preferable; small dowels and interlocking surfaces cannot be cut accurately from soft cancellous bone.

An operation known as metacarpal transfer

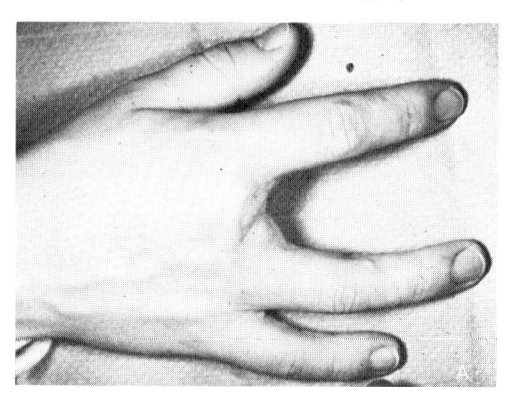

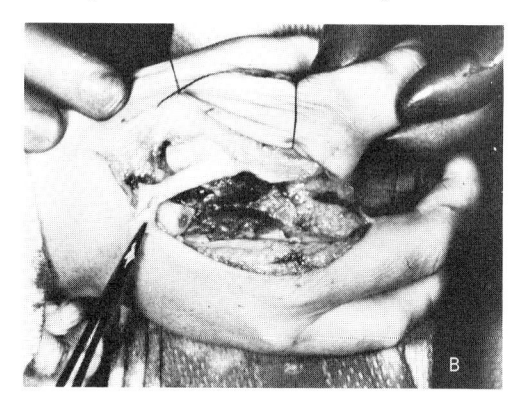

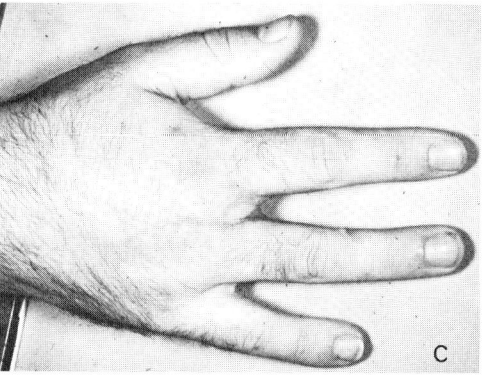

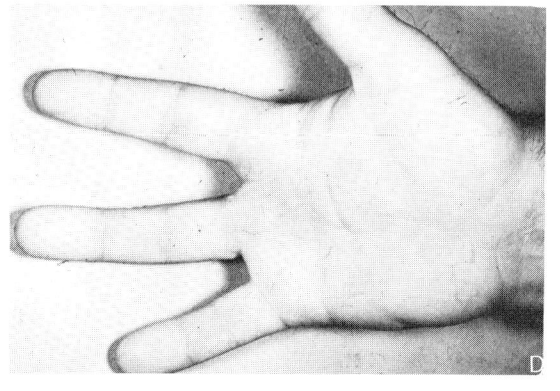

FIG. 24-10. A. Amputation of the long digit creating an asymmetrical appearance and a space in the middle of the hand. B. Excision of the long metacarpal and osteotomy of the base of the index metacarpal. C. Dorsal appearance of hand after metacarpal transfer of index finger. D. Volar appearance of the hand after metacarpal transfer of index finger.

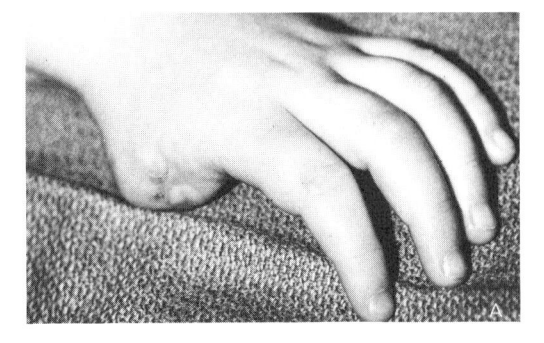

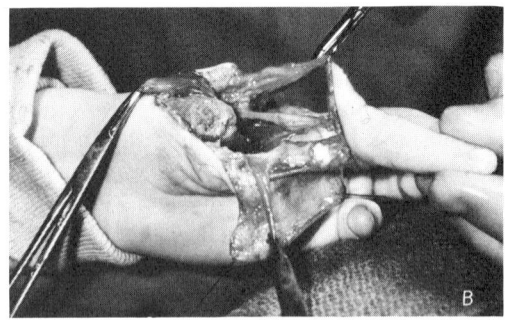

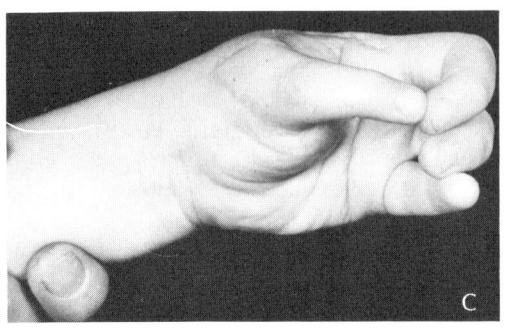

FIG. 24-11. A. Amputation of the thumb through the base of the first metacarpal in a 4-year-old child. B. Mobilization of the index finger following excision of the metacarpal and proximal third of the proximal phalanx. C. Pollicized index finger being utilized for prehensile function.

produces a dramatic change in both the appearance and function of a hand that has lost a central (ring or long) digit. In this operation, the base of the marginal ray (index or small) is transected in the proximal metacarpal area. The metacarpal proximal to the stump or amputated digit is excised and, after appropriate relocation of the dorsal intrinsic muscles, the marginal ray is transplanted to the base of the amputated metacarpal. By so doing, the hand is converted into a symmetrical three-fingered hand without a central gap or amputation stump to mark the site of amputation. Appearance is dramatically improved and function is increased by eliminating a space through which small objects escape. Contrary to some opinions, the strength of the hand is not significantly reduced by this procedure, and it should be considered whenever amputation is necessary.

Reconstruction of the thumb has been one of the most interesting and rewarding chapters of restorative hand surgery. Presently the island pedicle method has been accepted as the best method of transferring a digit into a prehensile position. If a digit has been damaged in a proximal area (metacarpophalangeal joint or proximal phalanx), that digit usually should be selected for transfer because a transplanted digit needs to be shortened one phalanx and one joint in the proximal region. When all of the digits are normal, for technical reasons the index finger usually is selected. The metacarpal and proximal portion of the proximal phalanx are discarded, and the distal portion of the finger is converted into an island pedicle flap of proper length which remains attached to the hand by two neurovascular bundles and the flexor and extensor tendons. The base of the first metacarpal—or occasionally the greater multangular bone—is prepared to receive the transfer, which will be fixed to it by intramedullary pins. Thus, in one operation, an index finger can be converted into a thumb that appears and performs surprisingly close to a normal thumb. Loss of the thumb on the dominant hand is generally recognized as producing a 60 per cent permanent disability. Thus, even the financial advantages of successful reconstruction of prehensile function by this method are obvious.

In the subtotal amputation of the thumb (disarticulation at the metacarpophalangeal joint) an adequately functioning thumb can be developed by merely deepening the cleft between the first and second metacarpals. This procedure is often referred to as pollicization of the metacarpal. Cosmetically, the operation

Secondary Reconstruction of the Hand

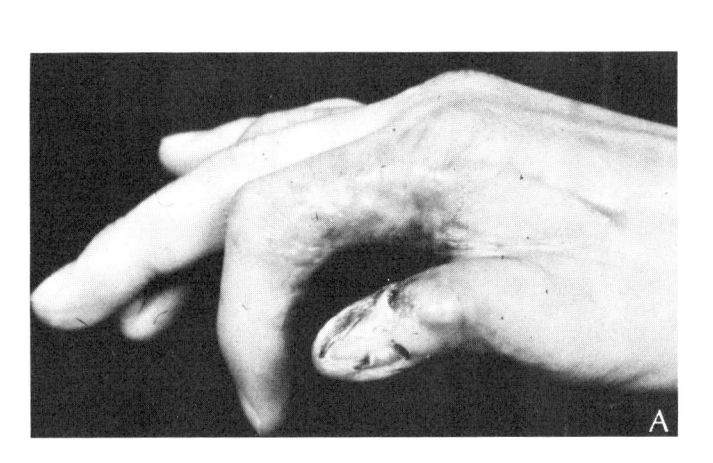

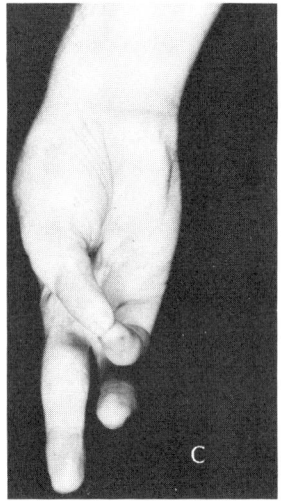

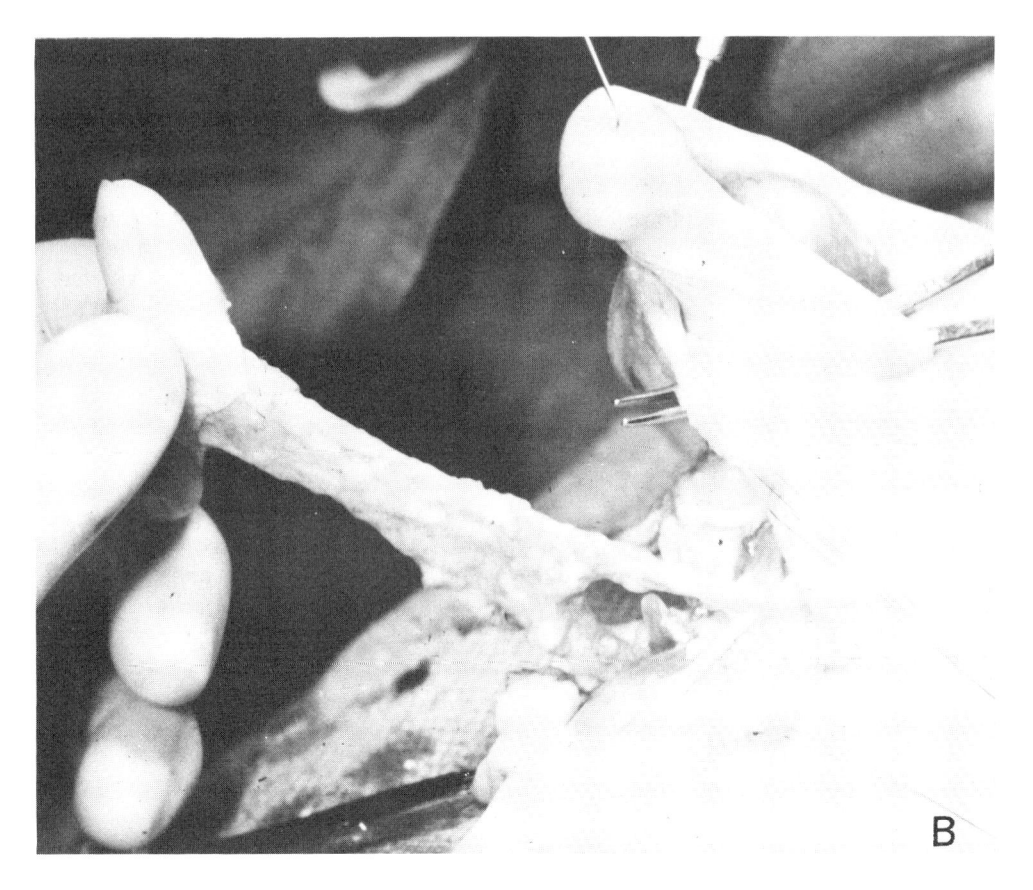

FIG. 24-12. A. Example of a common injury in which the distal end of the thumb and the proximal portion of the index finger are damaged. B. Utilization of the good parts of both damaged digits. The distal end of the index finger is being transplanted as an island pedicle to the proximal portion of the thumb. C. Thumb as reconstructed, using the distal end of the index finger and the proximal portion of the thumb.

is not as satisfactory as a digit transfer; functionally, it is adequate. Reconstruction of the thumb with a distant flap and free bone graft rarely is indicated; reconstruction of the thumb by transfer of a toe is not acceptable by modern standards.

JOINTS

Stiff metacarpophalangeal joints can be mobilized by excising collateral ligaments and the dorsal capsule, provided that surrounding intrinsic muscles are functioning normally. If a major nerve palsy has caused paralysis of intrinsic muscles, the collateral ligaments are the last remaining structure providing lateral stability; excision of the ligaments under these conditions results in disastrous lateral dislocation of the joints and instability.

Despite a few scattered reports of successful operations on the interphalangeal joints, surgical procedures designed to restore mobility in these delicate structures have met with failure. Replacement by allografts and replacement by artificial joints are being attempted with unpredictable results. A successful method of restoring interphalangeal joint motion by revising or replacing this intricate structure has not been developed. Interphalangeal joint stiffness remains, therefore, one of the major frontiers in further development of reconstructive hand surgery.

DISEASE AND CONGENITAL DEFORMITY

RHEUMATOID ARTHRITIS

Rheumatoid arthritis is a systemic disease of unknown etiology which affects synovial membranes, articular surfaces, ligaments, and tendons in the hand. The synovial reaction is a villous proliferation which appears to undermine and, at places, actually invades the cartilage on the articular surface of joints until all of the cartilage is destroyed and the end of the bone becomes remodeled. A similar thickening and proliferation of the synovial tissue surrounding tendons occurs to the extent that rupture of long tendons, particularly where they change direction over bony prominences on the dorsum of the hand and wrist, occurs. Ligaments and tendons at their points of attachment to bone appear to be particularly vulnerable to deterioration of the tendon by the rheumatoid process. Flexor tendons often pull away from their distal insertions, and collateral ligaments become detached at their origin and insertion. Deterioration of dense connective tissue throughout the hand strongly suggests abnormal collagenolytic activity, and direct measurements to support this clinical impression have recently been made. It is possible that part of the deterioration of ligaments and tendons is caused by simple mechanical pressure and interference of blood supply secondary to proliferating synovial reaction.

Gross deformities of the hand include characteristic enlargement of the joints. Usually the disease is more manifest in either the metacarpophalangeal joints or the proximal interphalangeal joints, although occasionally both groups of joints are equally involved. Attenuation of the extensor mechanism over the metacarpophalangeal joints allows the long extensor tendons to become dislocated from their normal position on top of the joint to a lateral position between the metacarpals. In this position the tendons are so close to the axis of rotation of the joints that they exert almost no effect on extension of the proximal phalanges. Destruction of the metacarpal heads and attenuation of the collateral ligaments accompany volar dislocations of the proximal phalanges. Simultaneously, the fingers become laterally deviated in an ulnar direction. The exact reason why the fingers shift to an ulnar position is not clear, but it is probably a combination of several factors related to the normal orientation and configuration of tendons and articular surfaces.

Spasm in the intrinsic muscles also is a part of the rheumatoid process, and the development of an intrinsic plus deformity (metacarpophalangeal joint flexion and IP joint hyperextension) frequently occurs. This manifestation of rheumatoid arthritis may be very severe; combined with attenuation or detachment of the terminal insertion of the extension mechanism into the base of the distal phalanx it produces a clinical picture known as swan neck deformity. In a classical swan neck deformity, the extensor hood stands out over the dorsum of the proximal phalanx and proximal interphalangeal joint, the proximal interpha-

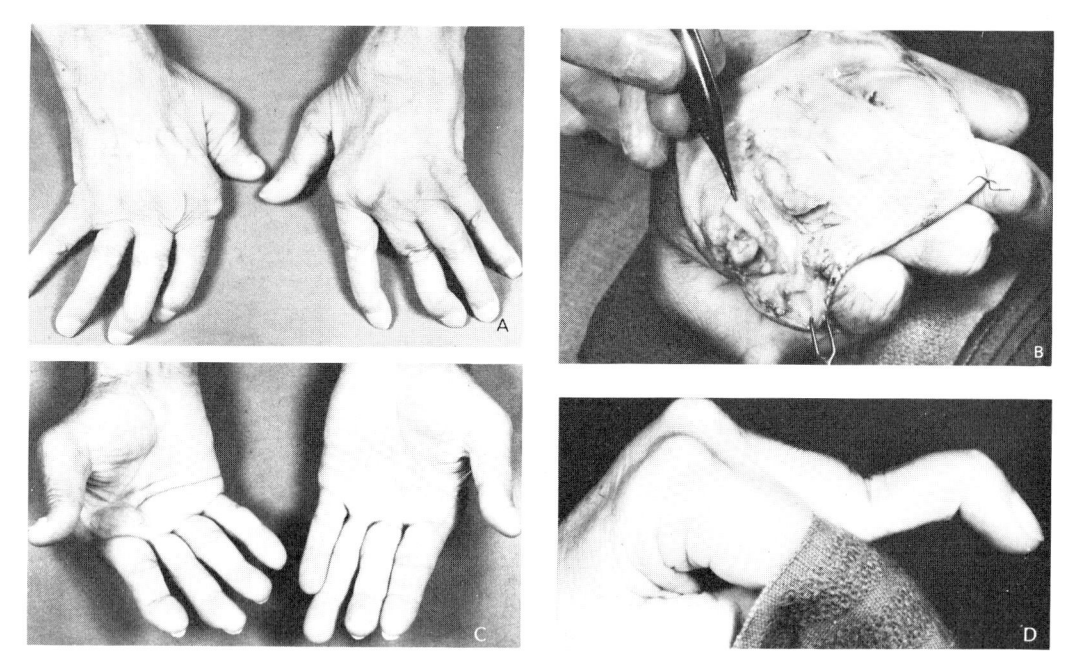

FIG. 24-13. A. Typical advanced rheumatoid arthritis. Note severe ulnar deviation of fingers and complete dislocation of metacarpophalangeal joints. B. Operative exposure of hand with severe rheumatoid arthritis. Note dislocation of the extensor tendons into the valley between the metacarpal heads and complete dislocation of the metacarpophalangeal joints. The metacarpal head of the index metacarpal is exposed, although it is hardly recognizable because of severe erosion. C. Volar appearance of both hands of a patient with rheumatoid arthritis. The right hand has not been operated upon; the left hand has been operated upon. Note correction of alignment of digits. D. Severe "swan neck" deformity of long finger in a patient with rheumatoid arthritis.

langeal joint goes into a dorsal recurvatum or hyperextension deformity, and the distal interphalangeal joint goes into acute flexion. Again, the exact mechanism by which this frequently encountered deformity is produced is unknown, but it probably is the end result of both destruction within the joint and abnormal stress on long and short tendons secondary to proximal muscle and tendon involvement.

A stage in the involvement of tendon sheaths can produce symptoms which are called snapping finger or trigger finger. Patients experience a catching or locking sensation when the tendon passes through the proximal sheath in the distal palm. This is due to an enlargement of the tendons in this area, a thickening of the tendon sheath, or both. Trigger finger can be congenital (frequently involving the thumbs bilaterally in infants). Another frequently encountered area of tendon sheath involvement is where the abductor pollicis longus and extensor pollicis brevis tendons pass over the styloid process of the radius. A painful tenosynovitis sharply located at this area and markedly exaggerated by ulnar deviation of the wrist is called deQuervain's stenosing tenosynovitis. Both trigger finger and deQuervain's disease are seen as an isolated condition of the hand; occasionally, however, they occur as a manifestation of rheumatoid arthritis.

A syndrome of pain following distribution of the sensory branches of the median nerve, followed by anesthesia in the same area and thenar weakness or paralysis, is often referred to as carpal tunnel syndrome. Compression of the median nerve is found beneath the unyielding volar carpal ligament, and recovery is usually prompt following division of the ligament. The cause is not always apparent, although compression is due to proliferating tenosynovitis more often than is realized. The syndrome, quite common in patients with rheumatoid arthritis, is also found in patients with no evidence of proliferating tenosynovitis or rheumatoid arthritis.

The most prominent symptom of rheumatoid arthritis in the hand is pain in the affected joints. Swelling and tenderness are prominent signs. All of the joints including the wrist may be involved or only a group of joints, such as the metacarpophalangeal joints, may be diseased. Occasionally only a single joint may be all that is involved, and the diagnosis may be difficult during early stages.

Surgical treatment of rheumatoid arthritis constitutes one of the latest accomplishments in surgery of the hand. The objectives are to remove as much diseased synovial tissue from joints and around tendons as possible and to restore normal anatomic relations where it is feasible to do so. Excision of synovial tissue (synovectomy) relieves pain in that area and prevents further deformity from occurring. The operation, therefore, has both therapeutic and preventive aspects. In addition, it can be helpful in establishing a diagnosis when isolated joint involvement has produced a perplexing diagnostic problem. It is becoming apparent that synovectomy can hardly be performed too early when evidence of severe synovial reaction is present. Synovectomy does not damage a joint, and the beneficial effects of relief of pain, prevention of further deformity, and obtaining a tissue diagnosis should not be denied a patient because preoperative diagnosis is uncertain. As far as we know now, synovectomy can prevent most of the mutilating deformities produced by untreated rheumatoid arthritis in the hand, and the effect provided by removing diseased synovial tissue is permanent in that joint. Recurrence of rheumatoid arthritis in joints which have had synovectomy is rare; recurrences seem to be the result of incomplete synovectomy rather than a recurrence of the disease.

Function and appearance of a hand with rheumatoid arthritis can often be improved by restorative procedures such as arthroplasty, fusion, tendon replacement, and readjustment of the intrinsic mechanism. Trigger finger, deQuervain's disease, and carpal tunnel syndrome are easily repaired by merely incising the proper sheath or restricting ligament. Joint replacement by artificial hinges has been tried extensively and is still undergoing study. A satisfactory artificial interphalangeal joint has not yet been designed, however; thus, preventive synovectomy is the most reliable procedure the surgeon has at this time for preventing deformity in the wrist and metacarpophalangeal joints.

Dupuytren's Contracture

The name of Baron Guillaume Dupuytren has become associated with an enigmatic contracture of the palmar aponeurosis which most often affects the ulnar side of the hand in elderly men. This condition affects approximately 1 per cent of Caucasians and is found very infrequently in Negroes or in Orientals. It affects men six times more frequently than women. The disease may occur as early as the second decade of life, although it characteristically appears first during the fourth or fifth decade. It is often bilateral, and in 5 per cent of patients it is associated with Peyronies' syndrome (induration and fibrosis of the corpora cavernosa). There is a tendency to develop transient arthritis in the small joints of most patients.

The disease usually starts as either a subcutaneous nodule or a small dimple at the base of the ring or small finger. There is a variable rate of progression to severe involvement of the skin and development of longitudinal bands which may produce a flexion contracture of the proximal interphalangeal and metacarpophalangeal joints. The disease in some patients never progresses beyond the small dimple or single nodule stage, while in others the longitudinal bands and contractures of the digits develop very early. The condition usually is painless, but a few patients complain of mild tenderness on deep palpation of a nodule. Nodules and bands can occur anywhere in the hand where palmar fascia extends, including the first web and thumb.

On gross examination there is not a clear demarcation between the thin inelastic dermis and the hypertrophic bands of dense connective tissue; furthermore, involved areas may be separated by normal appearing fascia. Microscopic examination reveals relatively more cells during the early nodular stage than later, when heavy collagenous bundles predominate. Staining technics which show iron deposited in the tissues have raised the question of

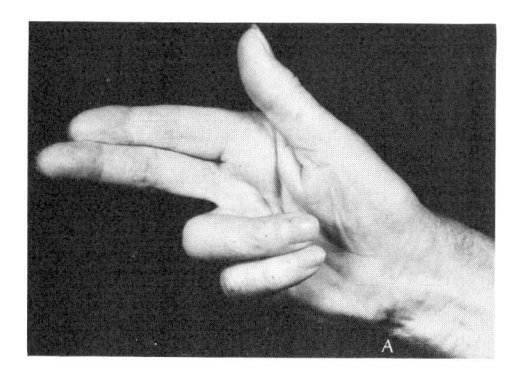

FIG. 24-14. A. Typical appearance of a hand with moderately severe Dupuytren's contracture involving the small and ring fingers. B. Longitudinal band of hypertrophied palmar fascia in a patient with Dupuytren's contracture involving primarily the ring finger. C. Operative exposure of hypertrophied band of palmar fascia producing flexion contraction of the metacarpophalangeal joint of the ring finger.

whether microscopic hemorrhages secondary to trauma are a cause of Dupuytren's disease.

Although cortisone injections, subcutaneous tenotomy, dynamic splinting, radiation, ultrasound, and Vitamin E have been recommended in the past to treat Dupuytren's disease, accurate surgical excision of the involved fascia is the only predictable and reliable treatment at this time. Properly performed, excision of the palmar fascia alleviates the disease in that area. Other areas of palmar fascia subsequently may become involved. It is not necessary to operate on all patients with Dupuytren's contracture: only those in whom the hypertrophic fascia is symptomatic or in whom skin deterioration and joint contracture are progressive should be treated by surgery. As a rule, only the involved fascia should be excised; prophylactic excision of uninvolved fascia increases the possibility of delayed healing and joint stiffness. Occasionally severe arthritis follows excision of the palmar fascia; the likelihood of this condition arising seems to be related, among other things, to the extent of the operative procedure.

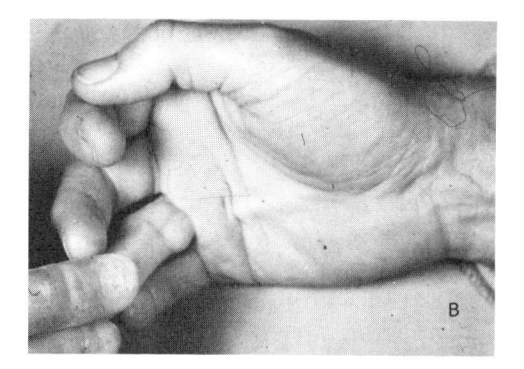

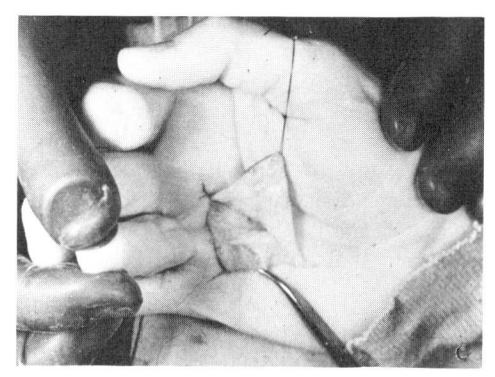

TUMORS

A section on tumors of the hand can only be a compendium of the experience of a number of surgeons. Most tumors are relatively rare, and no single surgeon has had personal experience with a large enough number of tumors to describe them authoritatively. It can be stated, however, that tumors that occur in skin, nerves, ligaments, bones, and joints elsewhere in the body also occur in the hand although relatively infrequently. For the most part, the same general principles which apply to diagnosis and treatment of these tumors elsewhere apply to their diagnosis and treatment in the hand. Slight variations may be encountered, such as the extremely capricious nature of subungual melanomas and synovial sarcomas, but most tissues behave and respond to treatment when located in the hand much the same as in the rest of the body.

There are a few benign tumors that occur more commonly in the hand than in the rest of the body. An example is a cystic tumor—usually located at the wrist—called a ganglion. A ganglion, or ganglion cyst as it is frequently called, has a predilection for young females. Characteristically it is a cystic structure composed of a tough fibrous capsule and a mucoid highly viscous center. The cyst is usually attached to a ligamentous structure by a pedicle which may be long and have a devious course between the flexor or extensor tendons. Smaller cysts may be found in the vicinity of origin of the main pedicle, which suggests that a ganglion may be the result of mucoid degeneration of dense connective tissue.

Treatment of a ganglion is by surgical excision. They may disappear for a few weeks following trauma sufficient to rupture the capsule, but recurrence is inevitable if they are not excised. Surgical removal should be attempted only in the operating room under general or regional block anesthesia and tourniquet hemostasis.

A tumor that ranks second in frequency to a ganglion is a giant cell tumor of the tendon sheath. These tumors are round, subcutaneous nodules which usually are painless and may attain large size. On pathologic examination they contain fibrous stroma, foam cells, capillaries, various connective tissue cells, and multinucleated giant cells in varying numbers. The very cellular tumors are occasionally misdiagnosed as malignant sarcomas. The capsule is fragile and may not contain the tumor completely in some areas. The tumor is benign, however, and even though it may have to be dissected from around nerves and tendons, cure is usually possible. Recurrence of a giant cell tumor of tendon sheath does not mean malignancy, and repeated excision should be performed until the tumor is completely eradicated.

REHABILITATION AND DISABILITY

Surgical technic is only a part of the total picture of rehabilitation of a badly damaged hand. Surgery of the hand is primarily surgery of fibrous tissue, and fibrous tissue healing is subject to considerably more variation and requires more time to be complete than does healing in nonfibrous tissue. Though much is known about synthesis of collagen, the breakdown of collagen and remodeling of old and new collagenous structures are important aspects of rehabilitation about which we know very little. Remodeling of scar tissue may require a long time: no fundamental is more important in reconstructive hand surgery than to allow sufficient time for inflammation to subside, excess collagen to be reabsorbed, and softening of surface scars to occur. Delicate secondary reconstructive surgery cannot be performed through hard, hyperemic, immature scar tissue. The changes that occur in such scars are not well understood, although many of the problems encountered in trying to operate through them may be due to what is thought to be accelerated healing in a secondary wound (primary wound reopened). In all probability, however, the apparent rapid healing of a secondary wound is no more than a demonstration of the continued healing of a primary wound; the clinical significance of this observation is considerable, however, and every experienced surgeon knows that going back into a healing wound in the hand too quickly may be followed by excessive tissue reaction and excessive scar production. When difficulty in dissecting nerves and tendons from scar is anticipated, all procedures that are designed to increase active motion should be delayed until the surface scar is soft and pliable, and perceptible changes in the deep tissues have occurred.

In this regard, physical agents such as heat, cold, ultrasound, stretching, massage, etc. have been thought for some time to exert a beneficial effect on scar maturation. In addition, such physical agents seem to be helpful in mobilizing stiff joints and reducing discomfort.

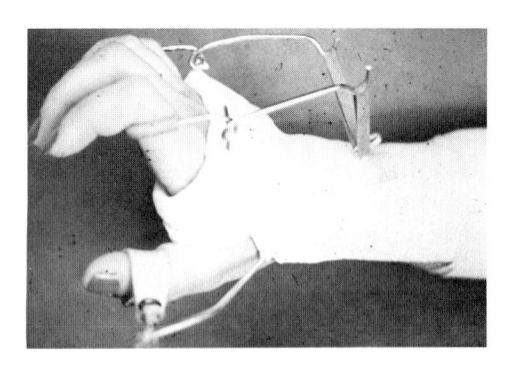

FIG. 24-15. Dynamic splint made of brass welding rod and plaster. Such splints are designed individually for each patient. Rubber bands substitute for paralyzed radial nerve innervated muscles.

Unfortunately, an overzealous approach to the use of physical agents on connective tissues may be responsible for failure to achieve desired results. We do not have data that can tell us whether the application of physical agents to scar tissue in the hand is uniformly beneficial or not. Recent measurements strongly suggest that hot and cold applications are valuable from the standpoint of producing analgesia during or after physical manipulations. That temperature variations within physiologic limits change significantly the physical properties of collagenous tissue, however, has not been shown.

Occupational therapy can be of great help in rehabilitation of the hand, provided that the program is one that has as its objective the return of the patient to gainful employment and personal independence. Antiquated technics, often featuring craft skills such as basketweaving, etc., are useful only if they are carefully designed and prescribed to activate a specific joint or increase power in a specific muscle. Such exercises can actually be detrimental in rehabilitation of a whole person, however. A male patient accustomed to heavy labor is not often totally rehabilitated unless his occupational therapy program includes use of tools and progression to work of a type which he desires to perform.

Perhaps nothing is more important in rehabilitation of the hand than motivation. It must be remembered that even amputation of upper extremity does not totally disable highly motivated individuals. Patients who are willing to be totally disabled by injury of a finger or even the whole hand frequently are difficult to rehabilitate by surgery alone. So much is dependent upon the will to succeed in activation of a surgically repaired extremity that absence of this important ingredient can be the cause of functional failure after a perfectly performed operation. A great deal of time, effort, and money can be expended to no avail if surgical feats are attempted just because they are technically possible. Performing such operations indiscriminately on all patients who, on first examination, appear to have surgical indications for restorative surgery can be the cause of unpredictable and often disappointing results. There is literally always something else that can be done for a severe composite tissue wound of the hand—even if it is no more than revising a surface scar. At the moment, however, technical expertise is more easily achieved than the ability to select patients and determine the correct answers to the critical question of whether it is worthwhile to perform surgery. In some individuals a badly damaged finger can make its greatest contribution to the hand as a source of spare parts to reconstruct another area; in another patient, a similarly damaged finger might be worthy of prolonged reconstructive surgery and rehabilitative efforts. In addition to the technical possibilities which modern reconstructive surgery offers, age, sex, occupation, intelligence, hobbies, social background, and ambition are but a few of the important criteria which must be considered for each patient. Above all, the surgeon must realize that all hands are not salvageable and that at times the greatest contribution an experienced hand surgeon can provide is to make a decision and inform the patient and sponsoring agency that further treatment is not going to change the final disability enough to make expensive hospitalization worthwhile. To be able to select the patients for reconstructive surgery who will be benefited by modern surgical skill and to estimate accurately what the potential in a damaged hand is likely to be may be much more difficult than mastering the technic of performing a flexor tendon graft. Great technical skill in manipulating the intricate structures of the hand, combined with a broad appreciation of the hand as a portion of a complex human being, can make it possible, however, to provide some of the most widely needed and gratifying services in the practice of medicine.

BIBLIOGRAPHY

Boyes, J. H.: Flexor-tendon grafts in the fingers and thumb: an evaluation of end results. J. Bone Joint Surg., 32A:489, 1950.

Bunnell, S.: Ischemic contracture, local, in the hand. J. Bone Joint Surg., 35A:101, 1953.

———: Surgery of the Hand. ed. 3. Philadelphia, J. B. Lippincott, 1956.

Curtis, R. M.: Capsulectomy of the interphalangeal joints of the fingers. J. Bone Joint Surg., 36A: 1219, 1954.

Dupuytren, G.: De la retraction des doigts par suite d'une affection de l'apponevrose palmaire, description de la maladie, operation chirurgicale qui convient dans de cas. J. Univ. med. chir. Par., 5:

352, 1831-1832. (Eng. translation in Lancet, 2:222, 1834. Reprinted in Med. Classics, 4:86, 1939.)
Entin, M. A.: Reconstruction of congenital abnormalities of the upper extremities. J. Bone Joint Surg., 41A:681, 1959.
Flatt, A. E.: The Care of the Rheumatoid Hand. St. Louis, C. V. Mosby, 1963.
Flynn, J. E.: Hand Surgery. Baltimore, Williams & Wilkins, 1966.
———: Subcutaneous beryllium granuloma of the hand. Ann. Surg., 137:265, 1953.
Fowler, S. B.: Mobilization of metacarpophalangeal joint, arthroplasty and capsulotomy. J. Bone Joint Surg., 29:193, 1947.
Goldner, J. L.: Volkmann's contracture. J. Bone Joint Surg., 37A:621, 1955.
Graham, W. C.: Transplantation of joints to replace diseased or damaged articulations in the hands. Am. J. Surg., 88:136, 1954.
Harris, C., Jr., and Riordan, D. C.: Intrinsic contracture in the hand and its surgical treatment. J. Bone Joint Surg., 36A:10, 1954.
Howard, L. A., Jr.: Surgical treatment of rheumatic tenosynovitis. Am. J. Surg., 89:1163, 1955.
Larsen, R. D., and Posch, J. L.: Dupuytren's contracture with special reference to pathology. J. Bone Joint Surg., 40A:773, 1958.
Lewis, G. K.: Electrical burns of the upper extremities. J. Bone Joint Surg., 40A:27, 1958.
Littler J. W.: Extensor habitus. J. Bone Joint Surg., 42A:913, 1960.
———: Neurovascular pedicle method of digital transposition for reconstruction of thumb. Plast. Reconstr. Surg., 12:303, 1953.
———: Principles of reconstructive surgery of the hand. Am. J. Surg., 92:88, 1956.

———: The physiology and dynamic function of the hand. S. Clin. N. Am., 40:259, 1960.
———: The severed flexor tendon. S. Clin. N. Am., 39:435, 1959.
McCormack, R. M.: Primary reconstruction in acute hand injuries. S. Clin. N. Am., 40:337, 1960.
Moncrief, J. A., Switzer, W. E., and Rose, L. E.: Primary excision and grafting in the treatment of third degree burns of the dorsum of the hand. Plast. Reconstr. Surg., 33:305, 1964.
Peacock, E. E., Jr.: Biological principles in the healing of long tendons. S. Clin. N. Am., 45:461, 1965.
———: Management of conditions of the hand requiring immobilization. S. Clin. N. Am., 33:1297, 1953.
———: Preservation of interphalangeal joint function: a basis for the early care of injured hands. Southern Med. J., 56:56, 1962.
Peacock, E. E., Jr., and Hartrampf, C. R.: The repair of flexor tendons in the hand. Internat. Abstr. Surg., 113:411, 1961.
Peacock, E. E., Jr., and Madden, J. W.: Human composite flexor tendon allografts. Ann. Surg., 166:624, 1967.
Pulvertaft, R. G.: Tendon grafts for flexor tendon injuries in fingers and thumb. A study of technique and results. J. Bone Joint Surg., 38B:175, 1956.
Rank, B. K., and Wakefield. A. R.: Surgery of Repair as Applied to Hand Injuries. ed. 2. Baltimore, Williams & Wilkins, 1960.
Riordan, D. C.: Congenital absence of the radius. J. Bone Joint Surg., 37A:1129, 1955.
Verdan, C. E.: Primary repair of flexor tendons. J. Bone Joint Surg., 42A:647, 1960.
———:Repair of Tendons. *In* Flynn, J. E., (ed.): Hand Surgery. Baltimore, Williams & Wilkins, 1966.

CHAPTER 25

JOHN M. HOWARD, M.D. AND ROBERT B. BROWN, M.D.,
  Vice Admiral, M.C., U.S.N.

Military Surgery

Function of a Combat Medical Service
Organization of a Combat Medical Service
Wounding Agents
Wound Ballistics
Problems Related to the Management of Combat Wounds Caused by Specific Ordnance
The Battle Wound
Resuscitation and Evacuation
Regional Surgery: Principles of Surgery
Specific Complications
Principles of Management of Atomic Casualties
Submarine Medicine
Chemical Warfare
Arctic Medicine

FUNCTION OF A COMBAT MEDICAL SERVICE

To understand military surgery one must appreciate the basic concept that the first principle of the military force is to win the battle. The functions of the medical services are secondary to this basic military principle.

The field medical service is designed with a twofold mission: (1) to help win the war; (2) to give the greatest support to the greatest number of casualties.

Obviously, the function of helping to win the war is important. Over the centuries, soldiers in the front line have developed great faith in the medical corpsmen and battalion aid surgeons, believing that in the event of their being wounded, medical assistance would reach them immediately, regardless of the danger to the medical personnel. By educating troops as to the value of the protective helmet or the armored vest, casualties can be prevented. Following thousands of cold injuries in North Korea, further casualties were prevented by the provision of better clothing and the education of the troops as to their proper use. Sanitation and immunization are other examples of means of conserving troop strength. Finally, casualties with minimal injuries must be given appropriate treatment in the forward area and returned to combat duty.

The heritage of civilian medicine is that every conceivable support must be given the individual patient. This is based on the assumption that unlimited resources are available. Under combat conditions, this basic assumption may become untenable. Depending upon combat activities, the flow of casualties may vary from day to day between a dozen and a thousand. When the number of casualties impose an overwhelming load on a medical unit, complete immediate care cannot be given each casualty. Under such conditions, the medical officers must decide who is to have immediate care and who can await delayed care. This function is designated "triage," the French word meaning "sorting, picking, choosing." Obviously, triage may necessitate compromises in the treatment of individual patients, but compromises that are designed to provide the greatest number of men with the best care.

ORGANIZATION OF A COMBAT MEDICAL SERVICE

Because of its nature as a supporting unit of a combat army, the medical service in a combat area must be organized so as to be mobile. The units in the front lines must be able to move under their own manpower at any time; a unit 10 miles behind the front lines must be able to move in a few hours; a unit 100 miles behind the lines must be able to move within approximately 24 hours. This prerequisite of mobility is basic in the organization. Thus, a forward unit which must be capable of moving its personnel and equip-

```
                                    Battle Field
                                         │
   ┌─────────────────────────────────────┼─────────────────────────────────────┐
Battalion Aid Station          Battalion Aid Station              Battalion Aid Station
                               located in forward combat
                               area. Designed to offer im-
                               mediate life-saving and limb-
                               saving measures: splinting,
                               control of hemorrhage, thora-
                               centesis, tracheostomy, blood-
                               volume replacement, initiation
                               of antimicrobial therapy

Divisional Clearing Station    Divisional Clearing Station       Divisional Clearing Station
                               One in each brigade area (8
                               to 20 Km. behind front);
                               one in division near area (15
                               to 30 Km. behind front). De-
                               signed to provide further re-
                               suscitation short of major
                               surgery

          Divisional Clearing
          Station                                              Surgical Hospital
                                                               Mobile 60-bed hospital. Re-
                                                               ceives highly perishable or
                                                               "nontransportable" casualties
                                                               requiring intensive resuscita-
                                                               tion and immediate major
                                                               operation

Evacuation Hospital
Semimobile 400-bed hospital,
50 to 70 Km. behind front.
Receives all classes of pa-
tients. Provides definite care
and return to duty, or initial
care and preparation for evacu-
ation to fixed hospitals in the
rear.

                    Fixed Hospitals Far to the Rear or in the Zone of the
                                             Interior
                    (Large hospitals, nonmobile, designed to complete medical
                    care)
```

In the Vietnam-type war, the battalion aid station is often over-flown by helicopters which carry patients from frontal areas to medical facilities in the rear.

ment, without assistance and within an hour, cannot be elaborate nor can it contain at any time many critically ill, and thus immobilized, casualties. To a lessening extent, this characteristic pattern is true of medical facilities at increasing distances behind the front lines. Based on this need, the policy of evacuation was evolved. Since a forward unit cannot be large or elaborate, casualties must be evacuated toward the rear, being held at forward units only as their condition necessitates treatment or does not permit transportation.

The organization of a medical service in a combat theater varies, being adaptable to combat activity, but the diagram on page 600 is the basic pattern as revised during the Vietnam conflict. Actually in Vietnam, the majority of casualties have bypassed the forward units, being carried by helicopter directly from the battle field to the mobile hospital.

The above organization necessitates that patients pass from one doctor to another without continuity of physician-patient relationship.

WOUNDING AGENTS

Military weapons are of 3 basic patterns:

1. **Small Arms.** Machine guns, submachine guns ("burp guns"), rifles and pistols. These weapons vary in range, velocity and rapidity of firing but all of them fire a preformed mis-

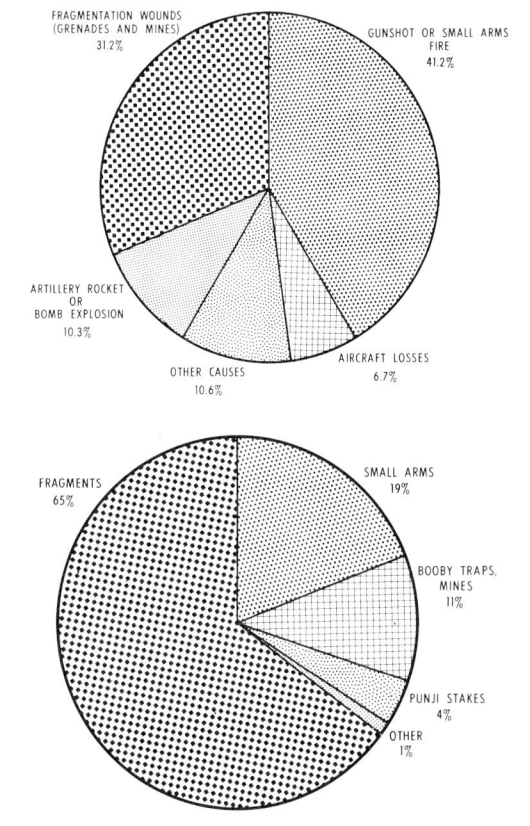

(*Top*) Chart 1. U. S. Forces killed in action or died of wounds in Vietnam, 1961-1968, by cause. (OSD Report, Sept. 5, 1968)

(*Bottom*) Chart 2. U. S. Army, nonfatal wounds in Vietnam, Jan. 1965–July 1968, by cause. (OTSGAMSA Report, Sept. 9, 1968)

sile which is not designed for fragmentation.

2. **Fragmentation Shells.** These larger missiles, consisting of mortar shells, artillery shells, conventional bombs, grenades, rockets, booby traps and mines, are designed to explode into thousands of fragments.

3. **Atomic and Thermonuclear Weapons.** These weapons are designed to produce blast, thermal and irradiation damage. In addition to the direct destructive effect of the blast, the target is fragmented, producing millions of secondary missiles.

The relative number of casualties produced by the first 2 types of weapons has been:

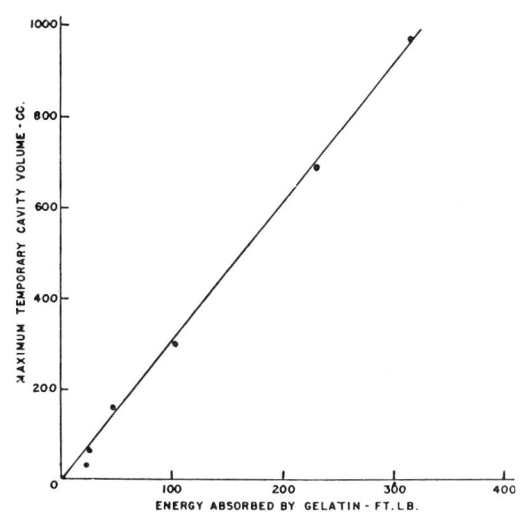

FIG. 25-1. Plot of energy absorbed in producing a "wound" in a gelatin body model (horizontal scale) versus maximum size of the temporary wound cavity (vertical scale). (Herget, C. M.: Wound ballistics. *In* Bowers, W. F. (ed.): Surgery of Trauma. Philadelphia, J. B. Lippincott, 1953)

Burns accounted for approximately 1 per cent in each instance.

In World War II, approximately 23 per cent of men hit by small arms fire died, and approximately 18 per cent of men hit by fragmentation missiles died.[3] Thus, because of the much higher incidence of injury, fragmentation missiles have been the chief cause of death.

WOUND BALLISTICS

Wound ballistics[37] is the science of the motions and the effects of projectiles, or other missiles, in the body upon and after impact.

Studies of wound ballistics have added materially to the knowledge of the nature of combat wounds. For the first time wounds can be described in terms of the amount of energy transmitted from the missile to the

WOUNDING AGENT	WORLD WAR II[3]	KOREAN CONFLICT[33]	VIETNAM CONFLICT*
Small arms	27%	23%	19%
Fragmentation missiles	72%	76%	65%

* Nonfatal wounds only. Other injuries included booby traps and mines 11% and punji stakes 4%.

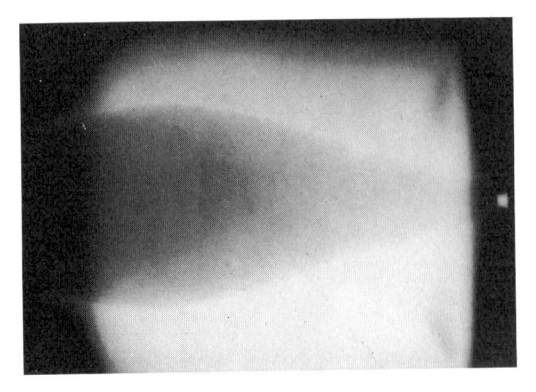

Fig. 25-2. Microsecond roentgenogram showing an early stage in the production of a temporary "wound" cavity in a gelatin body model by a 10-grain fragment which hit with a velocity of about 5,400 ft./sec. and is shown leaving the model. The maximal size of this "wound" cavity was much larger. (Herget, C. M.: Wound ballistics. *In* Bowers, W. F. (ed.): Surgery of Trauma. Philadelphia, J. B. Lippincott, 1953)

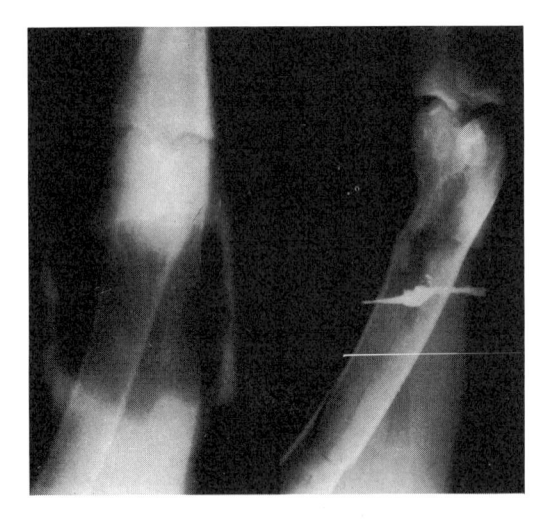

Fig. 25-3. On the left is a microsecond exposure roentgenogram showing the maximal size of a temporary wound cavity in an animal's limb. By comparison (*right*), a subsequent roentgenogram following the injection of a radiopaque fluid demonstrates the small size of the permanent wound tract. Note that the fracture is quite remote from the permanent wound tract. (Herget, C. M.: Wound ballistics. *In* Bowers, W. F. (ed.): Surgery of Trauma. Philadelphia, J. B. Lippincott, 1953)

body rather than simply in terms of centimeters of tissue destroyed. By using bullets of known weight, investigators have measured the velocity of the missile as it struck the experimental animal and as it left the animal. Thus, the energy lost by the missile and transmitted to the animal could be calculated. These physical measurements of wounds permit description or classification on the basis of energy transmitted (Fig. 25-1). Thus, mechanical injuries can be compared quantitatively with each other, with electrical or irradiation injuries, or with the clinical course of the experimental subject.

As a high-velocity missile strikes the body, the resistance offered by the tissue results in the transmission of energy to the tissues. Thus, every cell in the pathway of the bullet becomes a secondary missile traveling at right angles to the primary missile. As a result of these secondary missiles, the scope or size of the wound is increased greatly. Serial roentgenograms, taken with exposures of only a microsecond, demonstrate the transient development of a cavity that is far greater in size than that of the wounding agent (Fig. 25-2). The cavitation does not persist and would not be suspected by examination of the final gross anatomic defect (Fig. 25-3). During such studies, defects in large blood vessels, nerves, and even fractures, have been produced by the secondary force, even though the structures were not touched by the bullet. This concept of energy transmission as a measure of the magnitude of a wound can be correlated roughly with clinical experiences. A penetrating soft tissue wound is associated with a minimal absorption of kinetic energy. A bullet that encounters the resistance of bone and transmits enough energy to produce a compound fracture is a wound of greater magnitude. Finally, a traumatic amputation of an extremity, evulsing soft tissues and bone, requires a still greater force.

Wound	Number of Casualties	Mortality
Soft tissue penetration[35]	280	0
Compound fracture	82	1.2%
Traumatic amputation	32	9.7%

The correlation between this rough index of the magnitude of the wound and the resultant mortality in military surgery is not unexpected.

These basic studies of ballistics have confirmed and extended 2 well-recognized clinical observations: (1) that the wounds of entrance and exit do not depict the degree of damage to underlying structures; and (2) that the edges of the wound do not delineate the lateral extent of injury. This concept of lateral injury is the basis for the surgical principle of débridement.

PROBLEMS RELATED TO THE MANAGEMENT OF COMBAT WOUNDS CAUSED BY SPECIFIC ORDNANCE

The type of casualty seen at the various hospitals accurately reflects the tenor of the conflict. Major offensive deployments, whether allied or enemy, yield high proportions of bullet wounds and high velocity fragment (artillery) wounds. Search and destroy type missions, on the other hand, produce the highest proportion of mine and booby trap injuries.

Not only is this of general interest, but it also plays an important role in patient care, particularly in regard to times required for triage and surgery. For example, mine and booby trap injuries will not only take significantly longer to prepare for surgery, but the actual surgical procedures will be more time consuming as well.

However, more important than the differences in patient handling times are the specific differences of the wounds, even though over 90 per cent of the wounds are lumped into the missile-caused category. Each kind of ordnance results in characteristic wounds and problems. The following are some general observations on this topic.

Wounds Caused by Mines and Booby Traps

Although this is considered as a specific category of wounds, the etiologic agents are anything but specific. They are grouped together because of the nature of contamination, as well as the fact that the explosive force is, in most cases, from below upward. The category includes all explosive ordnance which is buried. Although usually detonated by the patient or a comrade, the device may be activated by a vehicle or remotely, by the enemy.

Unless the explosive device consists wholly of a specific weapon (e.g., an M-26 grenade), the observed or recovered fragments are of little value in determining the weapon involved.

Frequently the device is little more than a box filled with explosive and metal scraps, the latter having been picked up from bomb craters, etc. The resultant wounds vary widely in size, distribution and destructive power.

The casualties resulting from these devices do, however, have one thing in common—the explosive forces that resulted in the injuries came from below upward. Not only are the fragments from the weapon itself propelled in this direction (primary missiles), but also bits of sand, wood, dirt, gravel, rock, pieces of boot and, indeed, even pieces of other injured people (secondary missiles). As often as not, these secondary fragments cause as much or more damage than the weapon itself.

Contamination is the grossest imaginable. Frequently handsful of sand or dirt are blown upward, dissecting between tissue planes, to be found 12 to 18 inches proximal to the wound of entrance. This is particularly true of the adductor region of the thigh and the posterior leg.

The force of the blast itself is often sufficient to strip the periostium from the entire tibia and at the same time filet out all major muscle groups of the leg. However, this may not be evident prior to operation, as the tissues often will have fallen back into nearly normal relationships. As a result, the initial examination (both physical and radiographic) may reveal a relatively clean amputation at the ankle but operative exploration will reveal the necessity for a high, below knee amputation.

Initial surgical management of these casualties involves the usual surgical principle of débridement of all nonviable tissue, copious irrigation and adequate drainage, and, in addition, requires that the following be kept in mind:

1. Recovery of all but the most minute of the fragments is essential. The body could undoubtedly tolerate many of these metallic foreign bodies but the depths of the tract cannot be thoroughly cleansed unless they

are totally examined. This requires exploration of the area deep to the fragment, which will often reveal a piece of cloth or boot driven in ahead of the fragment.

2. Any wound that perforates the dermis must be opened. If, due to the superficial nature of the wound, the surgeon elects not to formally débride the skin then the wound must be at least opened more widely. More often than not, "slitting open" the wound will reveal the rock or piece of gravel that caused it and would cause the subsequent infection.

3. When dirt has been blown up into tissue planes, first remove the largest amounts of dirt or sand (handful) then irrigate, then sharply débride the dirty exposed tract. If the tract is débrided initially, removal of the bolus of mud from the depths at the close of the procedure will recontaminate the tract and it will require débridement.

4. As the débridement and irrigation of each wound is completed, the wound should be drained prior to going on to another area. When many wounds are involved, unless this procedure is followed, areas needing drains will be missed or forgotten if all wounds are drained at the conclusion of the procedure.

5. Primary closure of these wounds, as is true with virtually all combat wounds, is mentioned only to be condemned.

Wounds Caused by Grenades

From the standpoint of wound-causing capabilities, there are two general types of hand grenades currently in use in Vietnam. The first is the small fragment type, manufactured by the United States but used with equal effectiveness by both sides. The larger fragment grenades have less well defined origins and are used primarily by the enemy.

When hand grenades are actually thrown, they account for less than 15 per cent of the total battle casualties. However, grenades are more frequently used as booby traps or as detonating devices for mines and thus account for many more injuries.

Of the small fragment grenades, the only one in general use is the M-26. The fragments measure $2 \times 3 \times 7$ mm. The wounds are multiple, and, although the skin perforations are small and reasonably clean because of the high velocity, the destruction occurring to deeper tissues is considerable. Fractures are most often of the "punch-out" or perforating type, but one fragment is capable of severely comminuting a tibia.

The wounds, while destructive, are generally clean. Pieces of clothing are usually not pushed in ahead of the fragment, as the fragment tears rather than punches out. However, even though clean, the wounds often require extensive débridement, owing to the massive tissue destruction.

If the patient is on the periphery of the wounding radius, damage to deeper structures may be minimal but each skin wound *must* be opened if not completely débrided. The fragments can usually be left embedded in deeper tissues possessing a good blood supply.

The grenades yielding large ($1.5 \times 1.5 \times 0.5$ cm.) fragments are generally of enemy origin and are, at best, crudely made. Their fragmentation pattern is inconsistent and it is not uncommon to recover three or four connected fragments that have failed to break apart on detonation. The fragments from these weapons travel at a lesser velocity but this seeming disadvantage in effectiveness is more than compensated for by the facts that (1) they come in contact with (and thus contaminate) more tissue and (2) they punch out fragments of clothing and push them ahead into deeper tissues.

Thus, it is essential that large fragments be removed. Removal is prerequisite to retrieving the fragmented clothing deep to the metallic fragment. The wound tracts also require thorough débridement because of their greater degree of contamination.

Wounds Caused by Artillery (Rockets, Mortars, Etc.)

The fragment size and shape varies greatly in this category of weapons. Fragments as large as a saucer have been recovered from patients but this is the exception rather than the rule.

Often this ordnance will explode in the air or upon impact, thereby yielding fewer secondary fragments from dirt, rocks, etc. Upper extremity, trunk and head wounds are more common with artillery than with mines and booby traps.

The position of the patient at the time of explosion is of more than academic interest in this category. If the patient is sitting at the time of an explosion occurring in front of him, he may have intra-abdominal fragments that entered through his thighs. Thus, appropriate diagnostic measures (e.g., x-rays) can be carried out only with a knowledge of the mechanism and position of injury.

The larger artillery fragments are also capable of driving clothing in ahead of them and should be dealt with as with the large grenade fragments.

Gunshot Wounds

Gunshot wounds are frequently the cleanest and most easily handled of all battle casualties. There are, however, problems involving gunshot wounds that are rarely seen in casualties from other ordnance.

"Refragmentation" is commonly seen in this group of casualties. What appears to be an exit wound may only be the exit of the copper jacket of the round or even a piece of bone (a secondary fragment). The major portion of the round may still be in the patient, but unless it is in an area where it is likely to cause mechanical problems, the round may usually be left in unless it can be easily recovered. Heroic efforts to "recover the bullet" are usually ill-advised. Clothing is rarely carried into the wound ahead of the bullet.

Frequently, the only "débridement" required of the tract is thorough irrigation. However, a through-and-through wound of a major joint (e.g., knee) will still require a formal arthrotomy and sharp débridement.

It must be remembered that with gunshot wounds (as well as with any high velocity missiles), tissue destruction is not limited to the tract per se. The tract is enveloped in a cylindrical zone of variable diameter and degree of tissue destruction caused by the energy expended by the missile passing through the tissues. Therefore, before the surgeon elects not to formally débride the tract, he should examine it thoroughly. It must also be remembered that the path of the missile (bullet) may have but a cursory relationship to a straight line drawn between entrance and exit wounds. The varying densities of the tissues through which the missile passes all have the capability of changing the trajectory of the missile.

Punji Stakes

The use of sharpened bamboo stakes, metal spear-like devices, etc., has recently decreased with the increased sophistication of enemy weaponry. Pits in which the stakes are placed are often mined to detonate when the stakes are touched, resulting in mine injuries rather than impalement.

When the isolated punji stake injury is seen, it is best handled by cutting off the barb and pulling the device back through the wound. The wound is then treated like any grossly contaminated, through-and-through wound.

Flechettes. Recently a new type of ordnance has been used—the "beehive" round. Projectiles of this type can be fired from a variety of weapons ranging from a 12-gauge shotgun to a 154 mm. gun.

The projectiles are loaded with small metallic darts appearing not unlike a shingle nail with a four-finned tail instead of a flattened head.

Because of the finned configuration and pointed nose, the wound of entrance appears as a four-pointed star, which is usually self-sealing and will be missed in a normal physical examination.

Unless bone or major neurovascular structures are encountered, the tract will be equally obscure if not completely untraceable. The diagnostic problem is further complicated by the relative translucency of the "dart" rendering it invisible with low-resolution x-ray equipment, particularly if overshadowed by bone.

Thus, the physician must be aware of the existence of such a weapon to maintain the high degree of suspicion necessary to diagnose these wounds.

Treatment varies with wound location. If in anatomically benign areas (the buttock, calf, etc.), the flechette can probably be left with impunity after minimally débriding the wound of entrance. They cannot, however, be allowed to remain in joints, nor can the tracts remain unexplored so long as the possibility exists that a major structure might have been violated.

THE BATTLE WOUND

The passage of a bullet through the body requires only a fraction of a second, and the

COMBAT STRESS
Urinary Excretion of Adrenal Steroids

Stress: On Front Line 40 days. Under heavy mortar fire throughout this day of study.

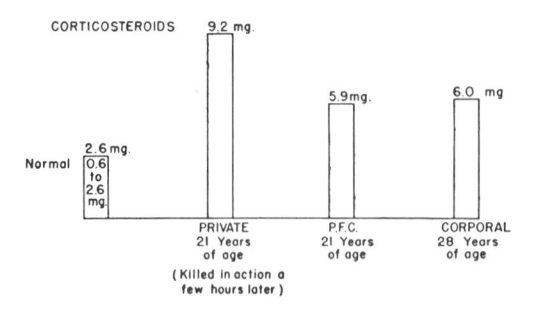

FIG. 25-4. Demonstrating simultaneously the stress response of 3 soldiers who were sharing the same combat bunker.

combat soldier has sustained an injury. But lives, like wars, seldom are lost instantaneously. There is a struggle—an injury and a response—a continuing injury and a continuing response. Death may occur moments or weeks thereafter.

The missile has inflicted its damage and then the wound itself exerts a deleterious effect on the body—as deleterious an effect, perhaps, as cancer. The injury is not a wound of the moment; it is a dynamic injury, progressive or regressive until death or healing results. Thus, it is a continuing injury, not just of the missile pathway, but of the entire body, which persists not for the moment but for days or weeks. Every system, every organ and, presumably, every cell in the body responds to this injury. Like the wound, this response continues for days or weeks. In general, it appears to be proportional to the magnitude of the injury.

Because of the stress of combat, the response in part may precede the physical trauma. During 48 hours of an intensive artillery barrage by the enemy on the Eastern Korean Front in the spring of 1952, volunteers of an infantry division were studied by means of 24-hour urine collections and analyses of adrenal steroids. The 1st day the incoming artillery fire was intense. The 2nd day the fire was less intensive but remained heavy; one of the subjects was killed, several others had their bunkers destroyed. The 3rd day was quiet with rain so heavy that the collecting vessels for urine overflowed, and the specimens were lost. The 4th day was quiet.

The stress of such men is intense. Studies of the corticosteroid excretion of these men revealed a stress response comparable with that following major trauma.[20]

The 1st day every man demonstrated the stress response. The second day the stress response had subsided in some, not in others. The 4th day the stress response had subsided in every man (Table 25-1; Figs. 25-4, 25-5).

A wound is inflicted, and a compensatory response occurs. This response may be lifesaving. The response is fully activated by the time the casualty undergoes operative treatment. Anesthesia blocks, in part, this response and, therefore, for the moment furthers the injury.

COMBAT STRESS
Urinary Excretion of Adrenal Steroids

Subject: Master Sergeant, 34 years of age
Stress: On Front Line 40 days. Under heavy artillery fire during first day of the study

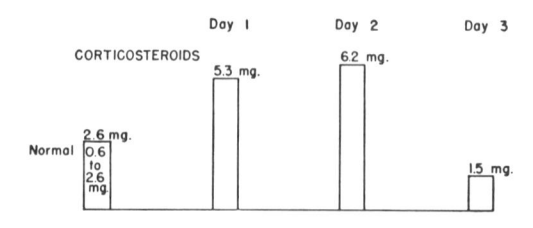

FIG. 25-5. Serial studies of individual soldiers revealed the continuation of the stress response throughout the 48-hour combat period.

TABLE 25-1. COMBAT STRESS—ALL MEN ON FRONT LINE 40 DAYS. A STUDY OF 15 SOLDIERS

DAY	ACTIVITY	AVERAGE CORTICOSTEROID EXCRETION* (mg. per 24 hr.)
1st Day	Heavy artillery fire	6.3 mg.
2nd Day	Fewer incoming shells	3.7 mg.
3rd Day	Rain—quiet	—
4th Day	Quiet day	1.5 mg.

* Normal range 0.6 to 2.6 mg.

What is the nature of the injury from which a soldier may die?

Transmission of Energy

The basic nature of the injury has been described as the transfer of energy from the missile to the tissue. For the first time the magnitude of injury is being measured not in centimeters of tissue destroyed but in the amount of energy transmitted.

How does the passage of a missile exert its deleterious effect? Perhaps there is a transmission of energy to every cell of the body with a resulting deleterious effect, but at present at least the following 4 components of the battle injury are recognized. Any one of the components may predominate and result in a fatality, but the summation of injuries produces a distinct, continuing, deleterious effect.

1. Mechanical Defects

Defects such as an open chest, tracheal obstruction, cardiac tamponade, increased intracranial pressure or a perforated bowel carry an immediate threat to life that needs no elucidation here.

2. Destruction of Tissue

Destruction of tissue produces injury in 2 ways: (1) the acute injury—the loss of function of a vital organ; (2) the subacute injury—the production of necrotic tissue.

Only by seeing those killed in action can one appreciate the magnitude of a battle wound. A vital organ, such as the brain, can be destroyed, and death is inevitable. The destruction of such a vital organ is one of the two chief reasons why approximately 20 per cent of all men injured in battle die before reaching medical facilities. This figure has not been reduced appreciably during the 20th century. By contrast, the mortality rate of those casualties dying after reaching medical facilities has dropped steadily, reaching an all-time low of approximately 2 to 3 per cent in Korea and Vietnam. These 2 categories are referred to in military statistics as "Killed in Action" and "Died of Wounds," respectively. Efforts to reduce the number of men killed in action have centered in the use of the protective helmet and the armored vest. Both have proved to be valuable in helping to offset the increasing destructiveness of modern weapons.

Studies in Korea indicated that 68 per cent of missiles striking the vests were stopped. This does not imply that 68 per cent of casualties were prevented, since many casualties (and vests) were struck by multiple missiles. It does indicate, however, a degree of protection against fragmentation missiles. Most small arms missiles penetrated the armored vest.[16]

The second syndrome, centering in the subacute injury of necrotic tissue, is of historical importance in military surgery. One needs only to turn back to the medical history of the American Civil War[25] to appreciate the progress made in this field. The Surgeon General's report of the Civil War included 283 patients with wounds of the extremities who developed gangrene secondarily. The resultant mortality was 56 per cent.

The wound is dynamic. It is continuing to insult the body, and the body is continuing to respond. Dead tissue, contaminated with virulent bacteria, accentuates the injury, since this part of the wound is isolated from the blood stream. Serum collections and hematomas, like necrotic tissue, are isolated from the active circulation, and so behave like dead tissue in offering a springboard for infection. The fundamental principle of wound surgery is débridement—the removal of debris—so as to bring the defense mechanism, the blood supply, to the frontier of the continuing assault, the open wound.

If life is maintained, the dead tissue will be removed. Either the surgeon takes a few minutes to accomplish it with knife and scissors (débridement) or the body responds and takes 2 to 3 weeks to remove the dead tissue as a slough or metabolic débridement.

The shaggy, shredded tissue lining the missile pathway is identified easily as nonviable tissue, which must be removed. That immediately adjacent to the pathway may be obviously nonviable. But inevitably, as the surgeon débrides away from the pathway into the area of the indirect trauma, tissues become less obviously viable or nonviable.

The color of the muscle, the presence of bleeding on the cut surface, the contraction of the muscle bundles when pinched, may all suggest viability; yet often the surgeon simply cannot delineate, on the day of injury, the extent of devitalized tissue. It is for this paramount reason that the procedure of delayed closure of war wounds still is justified today. Thus, the basic principle of wound surgery is to excise the dead and foreign tissue and thus bring the blood supply to the wound frontier. Delayed closure is not a principle, only a means of ensuring the basic principle of débridement by providing drainage and the opportunity to reinspect the wound at a later time when any nonviable tissue has become obvious.

Split thickness skin grafting has been used extensively as a method of secondary closure, especially where a large skin defect could be otherwise closed only by rotating flaps or tubular grafts. It is most useful in obtaining rapid coverage of a wound where secondary repair of an underlying nerve or tendon will be necessary.

3. Blood Loss

Blood is lost, and thus the body's defense is injured seriously—its supply chain and communication system are disrupted. Death may result, as no part of the body is self-sufficient, each part being dependent upon the circulation for support. Thus, blood loss and systemic ischemia promote injury to the entire individual, so that the entire patient, not just the tissues of the open wound, is fighting for survival. Literally speaking, the wound then is the entire individual.

Three aspects of the problem are pertinent: control of bleeding; correction of blood-volume deficiency; and repair of damage from prolonged ischemia.

Control of bleeding is essential, and yet it constitutes one of the real challenges of surgery today. Usually, control of external bleeding is relatively simple, but control of intra-abdominal bleeding from major vessels or a large wound of the liver may prove to be difficult and sometimes impossible. When anesthesia is superimposed on deep or impending shock in an effort to control hemorrhage, death may result. This is the crucial problem today in the control of hemorrhage once the patient has reached the hospital.

The correction of blood-volume deficit in combat casualties in Korea and Vietnam reached a peak in efficiency. Never before in the history of military surgery was blood used so freely and so effectively. The concept of hopelessly severe injury does not exist except in an occasional patient with massive destruction of the brain. Instead, patients with massive traumatic amputations or massive intra-abdominal injuries are tackled with the concept of expectant salvage as blood was begun within seconds of arrival through 2 to 4 portals. Crossmatch is unnecessary, due to the universal donor program of low titer Type O blood, and time and again patients have received from 15 to 20 pints of blood without crossmatch and without transfusion reaction (Table 25-2). Transfusion has been much more effective, of course, if hemorrhage could be controlled first. In lieu of whole blood or sterile plasma, plasma-volume expanders were introduced and used extensively in the front lines, for nature provides a relatively greater reserve in red cell mass than in blood volume. Large infusions of Ringer's lactate are being evaluated in Vietnam.

The effect of prolonged ischemia, the third problem, is a matter of keeping the patient alive until he can repair the damage.

Postanesthetic, postoperative hypotension usually reflects a marked persistent blood-volume deficiency, although the body tolerates a deficiency of considerable magnitude at this time much better than it does immediately after injury.[32] Additional transfusion usually is the treatment of choice.

Post-traumatic renal insufficiency has carried a mortality of 80 to 90 per cent. Because of the gravity of the prognosis, a Renal Failure Center was established at an Evacuation Hospital in Korea to receive all casualties of the United Nations' troops in Korea with this complication. Slow, steady progress resulted in lowering the mortality to approximately 50 per cent.[40] Progress in Vietnam continues.

TABLE 25-2. EXPERIENCES IN KOREA IN THE ADMINISTRATION OF TYPE O BLOOD, WITHOUT CROSSMATCH[18]

PINTS OF TYPE O BANKED BLOOD	HEMOLYTIC TRANSFUSION REACTIONS	INCIDENCE
10,000	3	0.03%

Policy:
High titer—Type O patients.
Low titer—All other patients.

4. Bacterial Contamination

The open wound is a contaminated one. Studies by the Surgical Research Team in Korea re-emphasized several factors. The extremity wound, at the time of primary débridement, contains pathogenic aerobic and anaerobic organisms. In a study of 154 battle wounds, a single bit of tissue from each wound revealed clostridia in 47 per cent, pathogenic clostridia in 27 per cent. In addition, 84 per cent of the cultures yielded aerobic organisms.[22] In a more detailed study of a smaller group of wounds, clostridia were found at the time of primary débridement in 82 per cent.[39] Blood cultures, taken from the most severely injured at the time of hospitalization, approximately 3.5 hours after injury, occasionally but infrequently revealed the presence of virulent organisms.[23] So, these wounds represent a break in the body's defense against bacteria and contain the virulent organisms necessary to produce life-endangering infections.

In order to minimize the continuing nature of the injury, débridement is necessary. This can be performed only by blocking, in part, the lifesaving response as one introduces the fifth element of injury, anesthesia. The responses of the patient, particularly of the autonomic nervous system, are mobilized fully. Anesthesia depresses this response and so temporarily furthers the injury. This may be a critical moment, to be minimized only by correcting part of the injury, mechanical defects and *blood-volume deficiency* prior to adding the anesthetic insult. To add anesthesia to the earlier insults prior to correcting the blood-volume deficit may be necessary sometimes, but it is comparable with shooting the bullet-ridden casualty one time more.

Finally, the day of combat injury is a day of continuing injury: combat stress, extremes of temperature, combat injury, painful litter rides, continued bleeding, repeated bacterial contamination, transfusion with cold blood, anesthesia, operation and fear of death. This is continuing trauma inflicted from without the wound. Korea saw this period of injury greatly shortened. The helicopter shortened the pre-hospitalization period in Korea to from 1.0 to 2.5 hours, the average time lag in the severely injured, combining helicopter and ambulance evacuees, being 3.5 hours. In Vietnam, the evacuation time has been further shortened, usually ranging between 30 and 90 minutes.

Because of continuing improvements in treatment, the mangling combat wound has continued its historic loss in its ability to kill and deform. The mortality rate of those wounded in action has continued to drop: World War II, 4.5 per cent; Korea, 2.4 per cent; Vietnam, 1.7 per cent.[34] Wounds of certain anatomic areas have shown marked decreases in mortality, especially those influenced by infection (Table 25-3).

RESUSCITATION AND EVACUATION

Principles of Resuscitation and Evacuation

Resuscitation includes emergency therapy designed to stop the injury and to correct its previous damage. The wound continues to exert its deleterious effect. The body con-

TABLE 25-3. COMPARATIVE STATISTICS FOR MORTALITY RATES WORLD WAR II* (1942-45) AND KOREA† (1952-53)

Site of Injury	World War II Number of Casualties	World War II Mortality	Korean Conflict Number of Casualties	Korean Conflict Mortality
Abdomen	1,185	21%	402	12.6%
Colon	1,106	23%	140	9.3%
Jejunum and ileum	1,168	14%	134	3.0%
Stomach	416	29%	45	0 %
Liver	829	10%	102	9.0%
Spleen	341	12%	54	0 %

* Second Auxiliary Surgical Group.
† Surgical Research Team in Korea.

610   Military Surgery

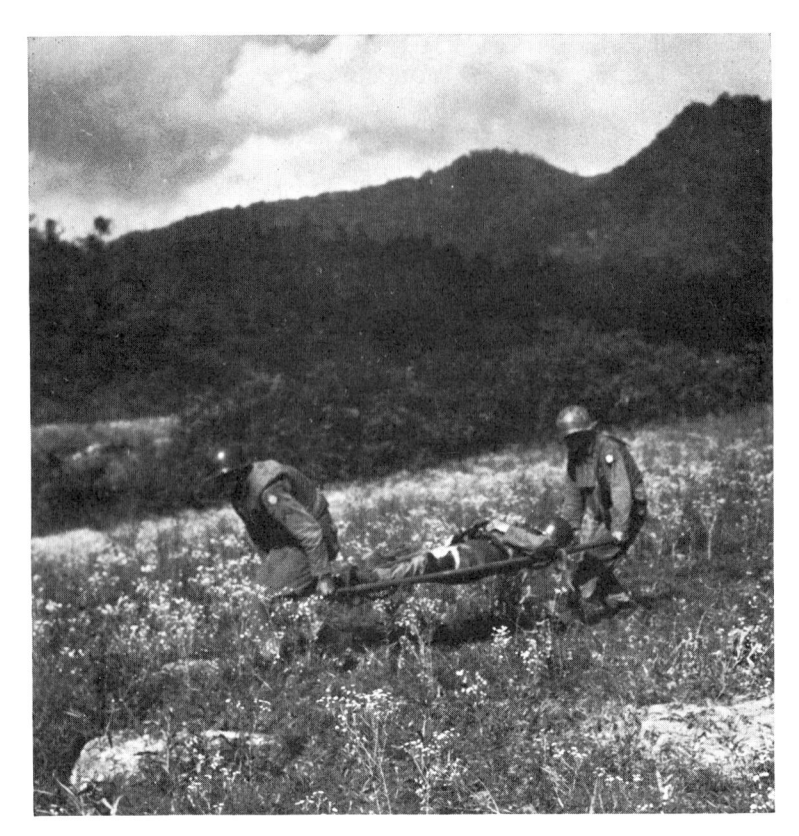

FIG. 25-6. (*Top*) Bringing a casualty off the front lines to the battalion aid station. The casualty will remain on the litter until he reaches the operating room at the forward surgical hospital. (*Bottom*) A marine receives first aid after being injured in a landing craft. (Official U. S. Navy photograph)

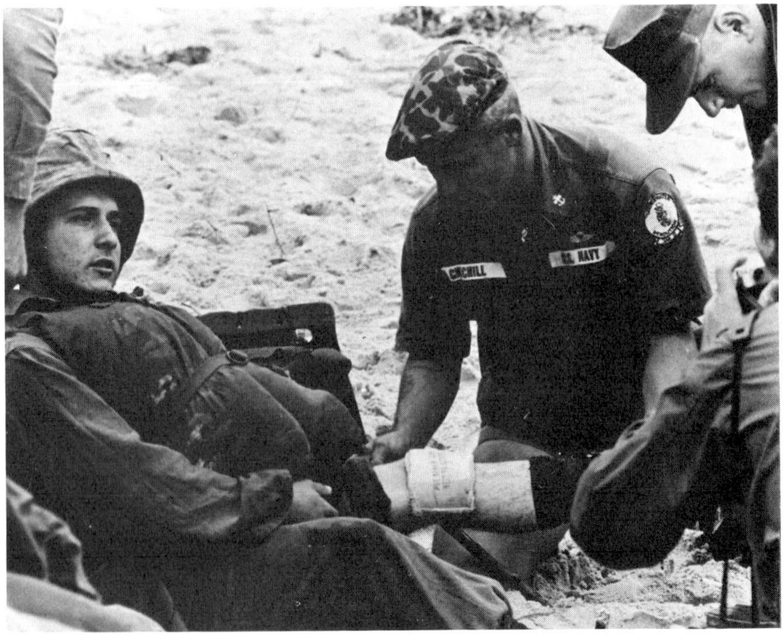

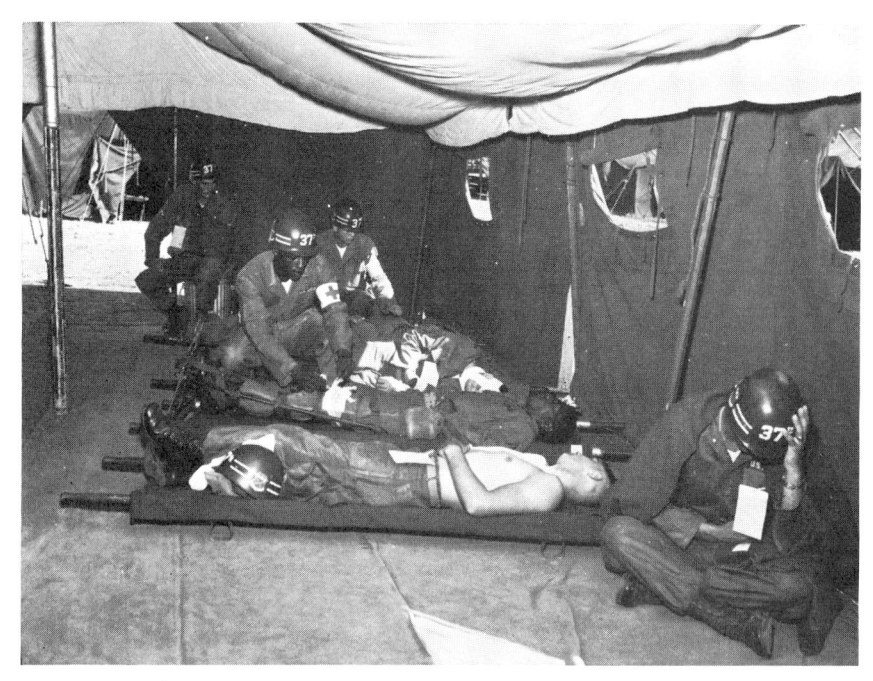

Fig. 25-7. (*Top*) Inside a battalion aid station. These simulated conditions lack the protective elements of sandbags and trenches. (Lt. Col. H. H. Ziperman, MC., U.S.A.) (*Bottom*) The receiving area of the U. S. Naval Hospital in Da Nang. (Official U. S. Navy photograph)

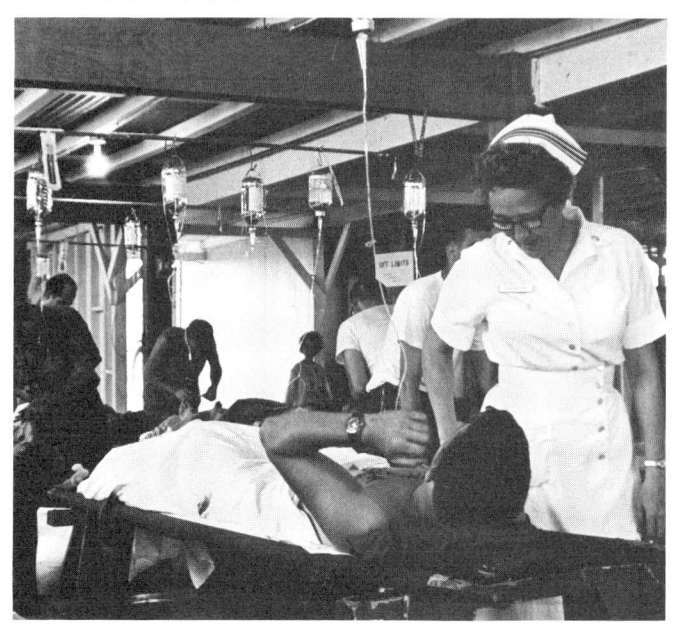

tinues to respond. Treatment also must be continuous. Within such a concept, it is difficult to define the point at which resuscitation ends. From the practical point of view, resuscitation includes first aid, correction of mechanical defects, control of hemorrhage, correction of blood-volume deficit, definitive surgery, including excision of the wound and continued supportive measures until the body, and especially the circulatory system, becomes stabilized. Most casualties who die are lost within the first 48 hours. It is during this

612 Military Surgery

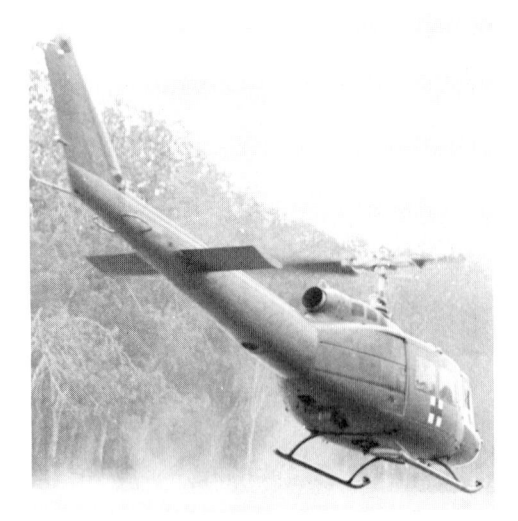

FIG. 25-8. A helicopter comes in for a landing in Vietnam to pick up casualties wounded nearby. (U. S. Army photograph)

period, and particularly during the first 24 hours, that resuscitation includes almost the total therapy.

Resuscitation is begun by the medical corpsmen or sometimes by a fellow combat soldier who first sees the casualty. The first responsibility is to stop the progression of the injury. In the front line, this consists of stopping hemorrhage by the application of a tourniquet if bleeding is profuse. The casualty either walks or is placed on a litter (Fig. 25-6) and traditionally has been carried the necessary distance, usually a few hundred yards, to the battalion aid station (Fig. 25-7). Here, usually, he has been seen first by a medical officer. The wounds are inspected, are covered with sterile dressings, and hemostasis is obtained by tourniquets, pressure dressings or, occasionally, by the clamping and the ligation of vessels. The most important responsibility of the battalion surgeon is to stop hemorrhage and correct any major blood-volume deficiency so as to make the soldier better able to withstand transportation to a forward hospital. The battalion aid stations often have to move and often are under artillery, mortar or small arms fire. As a result, they must be simple and improvised for protection. Only the most fundamental treatment can be carried out. Blood banks are impractical, due to the lack of electricity at this level. As a result, concentrated albumin and plasma volume expanders are maintained and used. Although these substances are not as beneficial as whole blood, they may be a life-saving compromise in the absence of blood. Coincident with the correction of blood-volume deficiency, mechanical defects are corrected. Sucking chest wounds are closed with occlusive dressings, and fractures are splinted. Occasionally, tracheotomy, thoracentesis or pericardiocentesis may be necessary. When the press of casualties permits, tetanus toxoid and antibiotics are administered at this time. When necessary, morphine is administered for the control of pain.

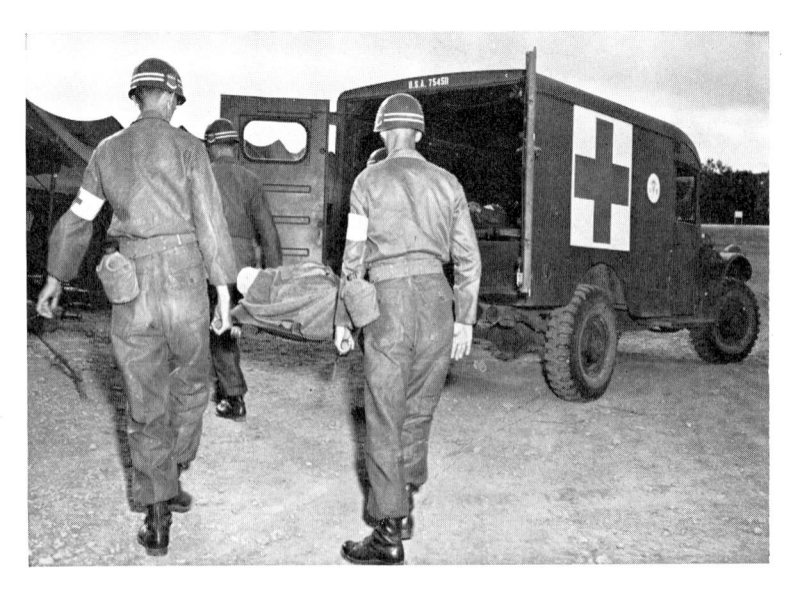

FIG. 25-9. This compact ambulance carries 4 patients on litters—2 tiers with 2 litters on each tier. (Lt. Col. H. H. Ziperman, MC., U.S.A.)

Fig. 25-10. A Mobile Army Surgical Hospital (Field Hospital) located within 10 miles of the front lines. This unit, containing 60 beds, consists of tents and sufficient equipment and personnel to perform definitive surgery. Helicopters land in the foreground; ambulances drive to the hospital entrance.

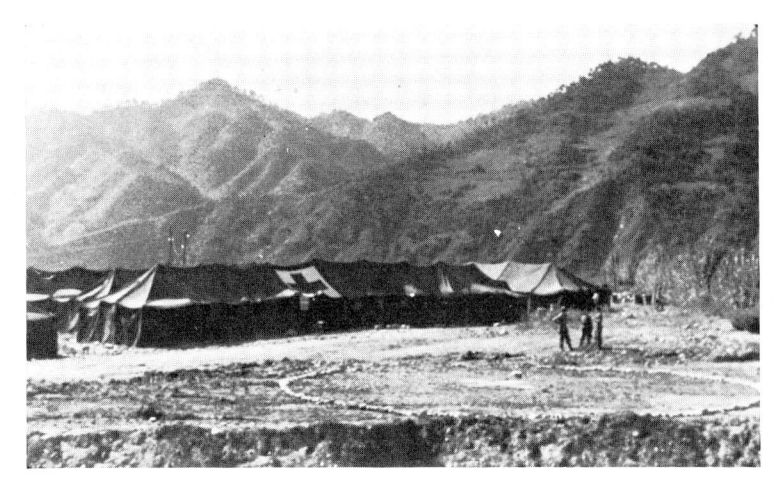

If the medical corpsman has not previously started the patient's record, it is begun at this level. The time of injury, the nature of the wounding agent, the description of the wound, vital signs and therapy are recorded.

In Korea, the most critically injured were evacuated by helicopter (Fig. 25-8) directly to the forward hospital, but most casualties (and all casualties at night) are evacuated by ambulance (Fig, 25-9). From the battalion aid station, the casualty was formerly carried approximately 1,000 yards to the company collecting station and then to the clearing station several miles to the rear. The clearing station serves fundamentally as a triage or routing center, although resuscitation is continued when necessary. It derives its name from the organizational fact that a casualty who is evacuated to the rear of the clearing station leaves the control of the infantry division, the control passing to a higher headquarters. At the clearing station, a casualty may be examined and returned to duty (a function also served by the battalion aid station), may be held for observation, may be transported to an adjacent forward surgical hospital for emergency surgery (Fig. 25-10), or may be transferred to an evacuation hospital far to the rear for delayed care (Figs. 25-11 and 25-12). These decisions depend not only on the casualty's condition but also on the combat activity and the number and the needs of the fellow casualties.

Helicopter evacuation, begun in Korea and perfected in Vietnam, has unquestionably saved thousands of lives by permitting sophisticated treatment early after wounding before exsanguination, irreversible shock, interference with the airway and other fatal complications have developed and progressed to advanced stages. Helicopters often deliver patients who cannot be saved due to the gravity and multiplicity of their wounds and, in previous wars, would have died on the field of battle. These deaths, formerly were classified as "killed in action." They are now counted as "died of wounds" and serve to complicate comparative statistics.

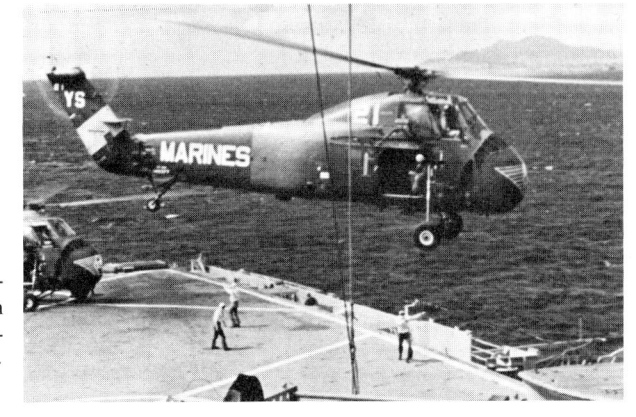

Fig. 25-11. A marine helicopter carrying injured servicemen is guided down to the landing pad of a U. S. Navy Hospital Ship off the coast of Vietnam. (Official United States Navy photograph)

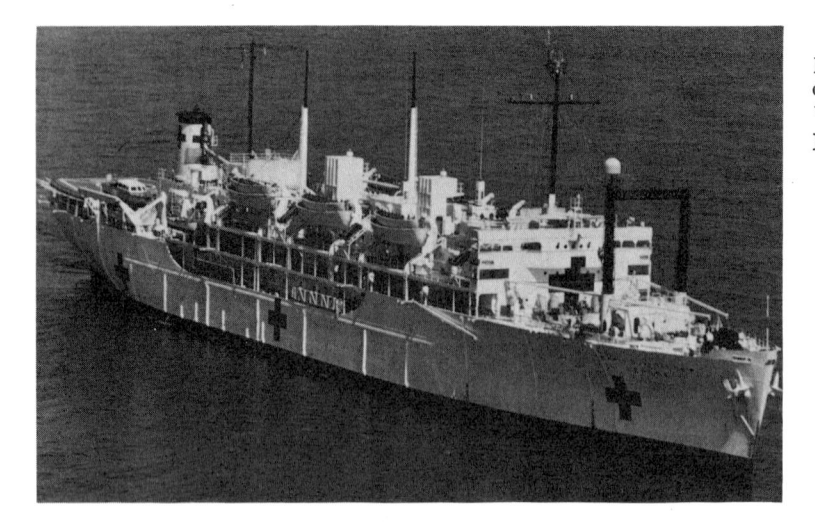

FIG. 25-12. The Hospital Ship *U.S.S. Repose* off the coast of South Vietnam. (Official U. S. Navy photograph)

High speed Air Force jet ambulance planes have produced great changes in the total care of combat casualties. In those cases where complex or long range surgical care is indicated, the patients may be evacuated to "base hospitals" in the war theater or in the United States. This principle does not apply to those having physiologic imbalance, pulmonary problems, infection not completely controlled, potential problems (such as being in the early stages after vascular surgery), etc.

When the load of casualties exceeds the resources of the medical personnel, priorities for evacuation and definitive surgery must be established. These priorities represent a compromise based on the guiding principles of (1) promoting the greatest good of the greatest number and (2) the age-old surgical principle that life takes precedence over limb, function over anatomic deformity.

This function of triage, or sorting, of casualties requires mature surgical judgment, for occasionally many lives may depend upon proper immediate decisions as to the disposition of large numbers of casualties.

Priorities in the Surgical Management of Traumatic Casualties

Top Priority. Mechanical correction of defects that immediately endanger life.
  Relief of respiratory obstruction
  Control of external hemorrhage
  Relief of intracranial pressure
  Closure of sucking chest wound or relief of tension pneumothorax.
  Control of internal hemorrhage
  Relief of cardiac tamponade
  Shock, coma or evisceration, which places any casualty in this group as regards priority of medical attention.

Second Priority. Correction of defect that ultimately endangers life.
  Relief of progressive spinal cord pressure
  Definitive repair of perforations of gastrointestinal tract or biliary-pancreatic tract
  Débridement of cerebral wounds
  Exploration of wounds of mediastinum
  Surgical amputations following traumatic amputation (to control bleeding and prevent sepsis)

Third Priority. Correction of defect that immediately endangers limb or organ: Repair of major arterial wound.

Fourth Priority. Correction of defect that ultimately endangers limb or organ:
  Exploration of ocular injuries
  Immobilization of compound fractures and reduction of dislocated joints

Fifth Priority:
  Débridement of soft tissues
  Realignment of fractures

Sixth Priority:
  Closure of soft tissue wounds
  Repair of peripheral nerves

CLINICAL EXPERIENCES IN RESUSCITATION

Military surgery has provided a few groups with the clinical opportunity of participating actively in the resuscitation of several thousand casualties. Valuable observations have resulted. The following discussion is based on such experiences in World War II and in the Korean and Vietnamese Wars.

All major combat injuries are associated with significant losses of blood. To this loss the body responds by vasoconstriction and by increased cardiac activity. As the magnitude of blood loss increases, the clinical picture may change gradually as the body becomes unable to compensate for the loss. The basic concept is that all degrees of hemorrhage may be associated with these injuries. There is no magic point at which hypotension occurs or at which transfusion is required. "Shock" is not an end-point; instead, as the basic process of hemorrhage continues, vasoconstriction and increased cardiac activity cannot maintain a normal blood pressure. Hypotension results. A casualty may lose 1,000 ml. of blood and maintain a normal blood pressure. After he loses another 100 ml. he may be hypotensive and be described as "in shock." Actually, very little difference exists in his status in the two circumstances. With the loss of 1,000 ml. of blood he was in incipient shock. Hypotension might then follow evacuation, movement on a litter, change of position or the administration of morphine. Profound hypotension would follow the induction of anesthesia. It is absolutely essential to good surgery that this deficit be recognized, even though the blood pressure is normal. In the normotensive patients, the deficit can be estimated only by the other vital signs, the blood loss on the dressings and the magnitude of the wound. It is more difficult to estimate in the patient with intra-abdominal injuries. Because these patients are young and previously healthy, it is safer, when in doubt, to transfuse the compensated casualty with from 500 to 1,000 ml. of blood preoperatively.

The rapid loss of from 1,200 to 1,500 ml. (2 to 25% of the blood volume) is associated characteristically with a modest drop in systolic blood pressure from the normotensive level to a range of from 90 to 110.[4, 13] If the bleeding can be stopped, the patient's pressure responds immediately to transfusion.

Not infrequently, casualties arrive at a forward surgical hospital with a systolic blood pressure below 50 mm. Hg—even imperceptible. Such patients require immediate intensive transfusion. Transfusions must be started through 2, 3 or even 4 portals, large bore needles or Rochester type plastic catheters being used. Under supervision, pressure is used to increase the rate of transfusion.

In the massively injured casualty, a therapeutic error encountered occasionally is to transfuse distally to a severed vein. Thus, if a laceration of the inferior vena cava is a possibility, the surgeon must not depend entirely upon transfusion portals in the lower extremities.

In Korea and Vietnam, where the evacuation time has been short, the concept of hopelessly severe injury has not existed except in the presence of mangling injuries of the brain. Preoperative irreversible shock is not recognizable, for, without exception, the blood pressure can be returned to normal in the preoperative period if bleeding can be controlled. Continued hypotension means continued bleeding or inadequate transfusion.

Since the restoration of a normal blood pressure is a rough indication of the correction of the blood-volume deficit in the young subject, ideally this has been a prerequisite to anesthesia and operation. So long as the pressure was rising toward normal, transfusion was continued, and anesthesia was postponed. The more difficult decisions arose when intra-abdominal bleeding continued during the period of transfusion. So long as the blood pressure continues to rise, vigorous transfusion should be continued and operation delayed. Should the bleeding be so profuse that the blood pressure fails to respond or stabilize at a subnormal level, operative control of the hemorrhage is the only recourse. The surgeon and the anesthetist must realize, however, that to block such a patient's compensatory mechanism with anesthesia carries the grave risk of immediate death. This problem of continued massive intra-abdominal hemorrhage has not been solved. Its solution probably will depend upon finding means of controlling hemorrhage without the use of general or spinal anesthesia. Hemostasis may be attained under local anesthesia when a single vessel has been injured, but it becomes more difficult when multiple missiles have produced many points of injury.

Operative correction of the wound, being necessary to stop the continuing injury, is a part of resuscitation. In itself, it is an added injury with added blood loss. Transfusion must be continued. In an analysis of a large military experience,[2] it was found that approximately 40 per cent of the blood was transfused preoperatively, 40 per cent during operation and 20 per cent during the first 24 hours after operation. Throughout this period, the seriously injured casualty was unstable and required active support—continuing resuscitation.

Studies in Vietnam have emphasized the value of monitoring arterial blood oxygen tension and pH. A failure of adequate pulmonary perfusion, following non-thoracic trauma, has often been noted to result in a low arterial oxygen tension. Similarly, inadequate perfusion of skeletal muscles has been found to lead to an increased blood level of lactic acid and a falling pH—metabolic acidosis.

The use of central venous pressure (CVP) measurements as an aid in transfusion therapy has been widely evaluated.[15] The CVP is an important adjunct in the evaluation and management of the patient in shock. It is the function of four measurable and independent forces: the volume and flow of blood in the central veins; the distensibility and contractibility of the right chambers of the heart during filling of the heart; venomoter activity in the central veins, and intrathoracic pressure. The response of this measurement during resuscitation depends as well on the type of fluid infused and the rate of infusion. In the presence of hemorrhagic shock the CVP becomes extremely helpful in monitoring fluid replacement. In this respect, the trend of the CVP and especially the response to therapy are often more important than any isolated CVP reading. However, a CVP reading above 15 to 20 cm. H_2O indicates that the infusion of additional fluid would be hazardous.

Patients with wounds of the central nervous system form a separate resuscitative group. These patients seldom lose large volumes of blood, yet they may be markedly hypotensive. Large transfusions are seldom useful, for the basic deficiency is not in the blood volume but apparently in the autonomic nervous system.

Experience has demonstrated several other points of clinical importance. The casualty seldom complains of severe pain. Unless severe pain exists, morphine often does more harm than good. Patients with intracranial injuries should not receive morphine, as the additional depression makes accurate evaluation difficult. The drug should be avoided also in patients with severe intrathoracic injuries, for the pharmacologic repression of respiration adds to the already embarrassed respiratory function. Finally, the drug should be administered with discretion in the presence of impending or incipient shock, as hypotension may result, presumably from the depression of the nervous system. As pointed out by Beecher, one of the rather frequent errors made formerly was the overdosage to patients in deep shock. In such patients, a single subcutaneous or intramuscular injection had little effect, as the circulation was so inadequate that the drug was not absorbed. When pain persisted, a second injection was given. Following transfusion and improvement in the peripheral circulation, increased absorption sometimes resulted in the signs of overdosage. When the drug is to be given to patients in shock, the intravenous route is preferable.

Unlike the civilian patient undergoing elective surgery, the battle casualty very often has a full stomach, with the inherent danger of vomiting and aspiration on the induction of anesthesia. In estimating this hazard, the critical period is not the duration between the last meal and operation but the time lapse between the last meal and injury, for gastric emptying is diminished greatly after injury. In fact, under the stress of active combat, gastric motility may be reduced greatly prior to injury. In such circumstances, food may be found occasionally in the stomach from 12 to 24 hours after eating. As a result of this stasis, the patient should be forced to vomit, or a gastric tube should be inserted and the stomach emptied prior to anesthesia when a full stomach is suspected.

The administration of antibiotics at the earliest feasible time is part of resuscitation. Penicillin with either streptomycin or chloramphenicol is being used widely in Vietnam. Like morphine, the antibiotics are absorbed slowly while the patient is in shock.[33] In the face of peripheral vascular collapse, the intravenous route of administration probably is to be preferred. The efficacy of prophylactic antibiotic therapy in combat casualties has yet to be thoroughly investigated. Although facilities for undertaking culture and sensitivity studies are frequently available, rapid patient turnover precludes their use in a controlled study situation. However, even though antibiotic therapy is, and should be, considered a step in initial resuscitation, the physician must guard against the sense of complacency that often accompanies high antibiotic blood levels in his patients. Antibiotics, regardless of type or time and route of administration, are no substitute for strict adherence to the well established surgical principles of adequate débridement, copious irrigation and *delayed* primary closure of wounds. At the same time, it must be remembered that the physician involved in the initial care of battle casualties will encounter specific infections such as pneumonitis, urinary tract infection and, not uncommonly, septicemia. Septicemia may be more commonly encountered in a combat zone than in a civilian environment due to massive, open wounds which, if not contaminated on admission, easily become contaminated with the pathogens of nosocomial infection. These patients must be treated aggressively and specifically.

As in all phases of surgery, the maintenance of good records is essential. This is emphasized here, for it is neglected frequently in the combat theater. The press of mass casualties occasionally makes the keeping of good records impossible. This compromise must not become standard practice or be acceptable when the flow of casualties is slow. Vital signs, therapy and response to therapy should be recorded in an orderly, continuous manner. Urinary output, measured on an hourly basis when feasible, is a vital sign of considerable importance in the critically injured man. It cannot be overemphasized that the compromises and the short cuts acceptable and advisable in the treatment of mass casualties must be recognized clearly as compromises, to be practiced when necessary but unacceptable when the casualty load is light. Combat medical records often reflect the need for this emphasis.

REGIONAL SURGERY: PRINCIPLES OF SURGERY

The distribution of total wounds over the body corresponds roughly with surface areas. The distribution of total wounds, however, is not representative of the problems in military surgery, for the professional requirements on

TABLE 25-4. REGIONAL DISTRIBUTION OF WOUNDS[17]

LOCATION OF WOUNDS	"WOUNDED IN ACTION"*	"KILLED IN ACTION"†	"DIED OF WOUNDS"‡
Head	14%	42%	25.5%
Neck	3%	4%	3 %
Thorax	19%	36%	24 %
Abdomen	11%	9%	22 %
Upper extremities	25%	6%	20.5%
Lower extremities	27%		
Genitalia	1%	—	—
Buttocks	—	3%	5 %
Total	100%	100%	100 %
Multiple wounds	53%		

* Includes all fatal and nonfatal battle casualties.
† Battlefield deaths.
‡ Died after reaching medical units.

the one hand and the resultant mortality on the other hand follow a far different distribution (Table 25-4).

WOUNDS OF THE BRAIN

As shown in Table 25-4, approximately 14 per cent of all combat wounds occur in the head. Many of these involve the brain. Because of the resistance offered by the skull, most of the injuries are penetrating rather than perforating, the ratio being approximately 15:1.[17]

Many fatal wounds of the brain result from negligence in not wearing the protective steel helmet.

Most of the intracranial injuries are open injuries from penetrating missiles. These open wounds tend to decompress themselves, so that the rapid onset of increased intracranial pressure is unusual. As a result, operation may be less urgent than in many closed head injuries in which intracranial pressure may increase more rapidly. Because of the autodecompression, these patients tolerate transportation fairly well.

Blood loss from an intracranial wound is seldom of major proportion—a fact that adds to the relative stability and transportability of the preoperative patient.

At the battalion aid station, the primary concern centers in the problem of the care of the unconscious patient. First, attention should be directed toward maintaining an adequate airway, a tracheotomy often being required. The immediate insertion of a nasal or oral endotracheal tube may often be preferable, permitting the tracheostomy to be done under less hectic circumstances. Second, bleeding from scalp wounds or associated injuries should be controlled and replacement therapy instituted as needed. Then a neurologic examination should be *done* and *recorded*. A sterile dressing should be applied to minimize further contamination.

Transportation of the unconscious patient entails several real hazards. The most important is the mechanical obstruction of the airway by the tongue, by blood clots, by faulty positioning or by *vomiting* and *aspiration*. This hazard is minimized by performing tracheotomy prior to transportation when a reasonable doubt exists and by positioning the patient on his side with his head, shoulders and pelvis tilted ventrally. In such a position saliva, blood and vomitus may escape aspiration. Morphine and Demerol should be avoided, as pain seldom is a factor, and mental and respiratory depression is contraindicated. Helicopter transportation is highly desirable.

Because of the need for specialized care and because of the relative shortage of neurosurgeons, neurosurgical centers were established in the Combat Zone in World War II and in Korea. In Vietnam most fixed hospitals and hospital ships provide neurosurgical care. Definitive surgery is performed, usually within a few hours of injury. Operation consists essentially of débridement. Bone fragments, devitalized brain tissue, foreign bodies and hematomas are removed meticulously by excision and irrigation. Hemostasis is obtained accurately, and the wound is closed primarily, because of the fear of secondary infection. Because of the rich blood supply in the scalp and the brain, secondary necrosis and residual infection are infrequent. Meticulous early surgery and consistent use of antibiotics have made secondary abscesses rare and secondary meningitis almost unknown. In Vietnam, neurosurgeons have emphasized the value of x-rays of the skull in at least 2 planes both pre- and postoperatively in order to localize bone and metal fragments, as well as initially determining penetration of the cranial vault.

Postoperatively, anticonvulsant medication should be used almost routinely.

Spinal Cord Injuries

Therapy in these patients is designed (1) to minimize the effects of the local wound and (2)—often of more importance—to rehabilitate the paraplegic patient.

These patients have been handled in neurosurgical centers in the Combat Zone, as have the patients with wounds of the brain. Transportation to such centers is done best by helicopter, as was demonstrated in Korea. The patient may be placed in either a prone or a supine position for transportation, but every care must be taken not to increase the spinal cord injury by flexing or extending the vertebral column, thereby permitting bone fragments further to lacerate the cord.

Early laminectomy is indicated in almost every penetrating wound of the spinal canal and the spinal cord.[6] The aim of early intervention is to relieve pressure by bone fragments, hematoma or foreign bodies on the spinal cord, the cauda equina or the spinal nerve roots; to débride and close the wound primarily, and to determine the anatomic extent of injury. Laminectomy usually can be performed under local anesthesia. Only by direct visualization can anatomic transection be distinguished from physiologic transection.

The postoperative care of these patients determines the extent to which they can be rehabilitated. The surgeon who treats only an occasional paraplegic patient and adopts a fatalistic outlook may not realize the degree of success that has been developed in military centers in rehabilitating these men to useful creative positions.

There are several essential points in rehabilitation. At the very onset, and preferably beginning before operation, the neurologic defect, its possible or definite permanence, and the aims and the possibilities of rehabilitation should be discussed frankly with the patient, because his proper motivation is essential to recovery.

Transection of the spinal cord interrupts central control of the urinary bladder. A secondary center in the conus medullaris, governing the bladder through the sacral reflex arc, subsequently may assume control of bladder function. It is the aim of the surgeon to bring this secondary center into control and produce a reflex neurogenic bladder.[6] (See Chap. 52, Urology.)

To achieve this goal it is essential from the very first day to prevent overdistention of the bladder by the use of an indwelling Foley catheter. A suprapubic cystostomy should generally be avoided. Urinary tract infections also must be prevented. At a very early date, tidal drainage, as described by Munro,[26, 27] must be instituted. A successfully functioning bladder will result in most, but not all, patients.

Additional effort is necessary to prevent overdistention of the incontinent colon, decubitus ulcers and malnutrition. Physiotherapy should be instituted within the first week. Finally, leg braces, continued skilled assistance and encouragement will result in subsequent ambulation of many of these patients.

Wounds of the Face and the Neck

Initial treatment will determine whether these casualties live or die. With proper early care, almost all should survive.

These injuries are characterized by profuse hemorrhage and by a tendency to produce respiratory obstruction. Wounds of the scalp, the cheek, the tongue or the floor of the mouth may result in a surprising loss of blood, even though no single large vessel has been lacerated. Finally, the battalion surgeon may gain a false impression that a wound, such as the avulsion of the lower jaw, is of hopelessly severe magnitude. Final results justify no such fatalism.

The battalion surgeon first must ensure an adequate airway; next, control hemorrhage; and, finally, assess and record the neurologic status, since the incidence of associated injuries to the brain and the cervical spinal cord is high. In evaluating the factor of respiratory obstruction, the surgeon must consider the fact that the casualty is about to enter the chain of evacuation, during part of which time he will not be under direct medical observation. If he is in doubt as to the presence or the potential development of respiratory obstruction, tracheotomy should be done by the physician initially treating the patient. As a generalization it should be performed for wounds of the trachea and the pharynx and for large wounds of the floor of the mouth and the lower jaw. In addition, if the patient is unconscious, tracheotomy should be performed if the presence of intra-oral or pharyngeal bleeding predisposes to aspiration. Blood clots, foreign bodies, broken teeth and dentures should be removed from the mouth and throat and the tongue brought forward with a finger or forceps. A suture through the tongue or a towel clip may be required to maintain the tongue in a forward position. Anterior traction of the mandible may be required when the normal anterior fixation of the tongue is lost following anterior fractures of the mandible.

Because of the fear of respiratory complications, morphine should be avoided, thereby protecting the cough reflex and its resulting defense against aspiration of blood.

When endotracheal suction is required, it can be obtained by connecting a rubber catheter to a bulb syringe.

At the forward surgical hospital, the airway, hemostasis and neurologic status should be rechecked first. Any appreciable blood-volume deficiency should be corrected, and the stomach should be emptied by vomiting or by gastric tube prior to anesthesia. Loose teeth should be removed before or at the beginning of operation. Roentgenograms of the bones of the face and the skull should be obtained prior to operation.

Except in the patient with neurologic damage, primary repair should be attempted.

In the face and the neck, more than in any other part of the body, except perhaps the hand, loss of tissue or excessive scarring leads to serious functioning impairment as well as to disfigurement. The principles of treatment are the same as for wounds elsewhere. However, the rich vascular supply to the face and the neck limits the extent of lateral necrosis around a wound and minimizes infection. As a result of the excellent blood supply, it is possible to obtain good wound healing after minimal but meticulous débridement and primary closure. There are many exceptions when this is not possible, but the goal of therapy is to close the wound as soon as possible and thereby limit fibrosis and deformity. In general, every effort is made to conserve tissue, and, when feasible, primary closure offers the best cosmetic result.

When primary closure is not possible because of infection due to delay in reaching the hospital, secondary suture should be performed within the shortest feasible time. When primary suture is impractical because of the magnitude of the wound, the principle of early closure still holds, the wound being closed with a split thickness skin graft.

From the combat zone, these casualties are evacuated to the Zone of the Interior, where plastic centers, developed by the medical services, have contributed materially to the total knowledge of reparative surgery. The subsequent reconstructive surgery does not differ in principle from that of civilian practice. Obviously, the medical service has not discharged its full responsibility to such a combat casualty until the best possible functional and cosmetic result has been obtained.

Wounds of the Eye

Injuries of the eye constitute from 2 to 3 per cent of combat injuries. The initial management frequently determines the severity of late complications. Tiny particles elsewhere in the body cause little difficulty, often hardly requiring medical attention, but, in the eye, penetration of a tiny particle may destroy the usefulness of the organ.

Superficial foreign bodies may be removed after the topical application of ½ per cent Pontocaine.

Major penetrating injuries of the eye should be treated by an ophthalmologist. In order to prevent movement of the injured eye, with the possibility of secondary retinal detachment, both eyes should be bandaged. Antibiotic solutions should be applied topically, for bloodborne antibiotics penetrate the tissues of the eye poorly from the blood stream, and infection may mean the loss of vision. Mydriatics should not be used.

A principle of definitive surgery is to repair primarily any eye in which there has not been too great a loss of intra-ocular contents. Enucleation is not an emergency operation. One report from Korea indicated that 70 per cent of wounds of the eye were repaired.[10] Conservative management is especially important in bilateral injuries.

The general medical officer seldom is prepared to evaluate these injuries. Evacuation, if necessary, should be carried out to permit specialized attention by an ophthalmologist.

Wounds of the Chest

Wounds of the chest constitute 19 per cent of all combat injuries. In one large series,[41] 70 per cent were penetrating in type, 28 per cent were perforating, and 2 per cent were due to crushing injuries. The incidence of thoracic wounds in Vietnam has fallen to approximately 8 per cent, but such wounds still account for approximately 20 per cent of all deaths.

Of all combat soldiers receiving wounds of the chest, many die from cardiac or major vascular injuries before reaching medical assistance. This constitutes 36 per cent of the total number "killed in action." Thereafter, only about 7 per cent of the group reaching the forward hospital are lost, but this constitutes a major problem, representing almost one fourth of the total hospital deaths. Body armor, as developed in Korea, and used extensively in Vietnam, covers the thorax as a vest and, by stopping many of the missiles, reduced the incidence of thoracic wounds after the vest was introduced.

The surgical management of most thoracic injuries differs from that of injuries to other parts of the body. The aims of management of intrathoracic injuries are (1) to correct the mechanical defects, (2) to replace the blood loss and (3) to prevent infection. These principles are not unlike those applied to other parts of the body, but the means of application differ.

The mechanical defects—pneumothorax, hemothorax, an open sucking thoracic wound, tension pneumothorax and hemopericardium—exert an immediate deleterious effect, and they should be corrected at the earliest possible time, often forward of the surgical hospital. Operative control of hemorrhage seldom is necessary. Almost inevitably, bleeding from the pulmonary parenchyma will stop spontaneously. Usually, this tendency to self-limited bleeding is attributed to the low arterial pressure in the pulmonary system and its high thromboplastin titer. Only an occasional injury due to laceration of a large hilar vessel, an intercostal or internal mammary artery, or a subclavian vein or artery will continue to bleed and require operative hemostasis. Blood loss frequently is of major proportions, however, and vigorous transfusion may be necessary.

TABLE 25-5. WOUNDS OF THE CHEST

WOUNDS	WORLD WAR II Number of Casualties	Mortality	KOREAN CONFLICT Number of Casualties	Mortality
Thoracic wounds				
Immediate results				
Forward Surgical Hospital	2,000[11]	10%	33[32]	6 %
Late results				
Army General Hospital	—	—	2,305	0.6%
Thoraco-abdominal wounds				
Immediate results				
Forward Surgical Hospital	903*	27%	29[19]	10 %
Late results				
Army General Hospital	—	—	506[38]	0.8%

* Second Auxiliary Surgical Group.

Efforts to prevent infection center in the prevention of atelectasis, the aspiration of blood and exudate from the pleural space, and the liberal use of antibiotics.

Débridement of the lung seldom is practiced. Occasionally, foreign bodies, such as bits of clothing or large metallic fragments, may have to be removed, but exploration rarely is advisable on the day of injury. Relatively few of these patients will ever require thoracotomy.

The practice of not débriding pulmonary wounds rests upon both a theoretic and a clinical basis. The elasticity of the lung permits the tissue to expand as the missile cavity forms, without secondary tearing. In contradistinction to hepatic wounds, stellate fractures of the parenchyma do not occur. Instead, the lung stretches with resultant minimal destruction of the parenchyma. Thereafter, the rich blood supply minimizes the extent of devitalization and infection and promotes healing. Clinical experience has demonstrated a lower mortality and a smoother clinical course since the more conservative management has been instituted (Table 25-5).

When the casualty with a penetrating thoracic wound is first seen, the open wound in the chest wall should be closed. This can be achieved temporarily with several thicknesses of petrolatum gauze reinforced with a thick dressing and adhesive tape. Such a casualty retains a pneumothorax, but the sucking aspect of air moving in and out of the pleural space with each respiratory cycle is stopped. This has the advantage of overcoming the rhythmic shift of the mediastinum with each respiratory movement. After closing the wound in this way, the air and the blood in the pleural space can be aspirated, so that, temporarily at least, the positive (atmospheric) intrapleural pressure is relieved and the normal pressure relationships are restored. This not only permits re-expansion and function of the collapsed lung but restores the function of the thoracic pump mechanism in aiding the return of venous blood to the right side of the heart. Simultaneously, it may be necessary to begin transfusion of blood or of available blood substitutes. When respiratory obstruction is suspected tracheotomy is mandatory.

Vietnam has witnessed a decline in the use of thoracentesis and an increased use of a large bore (40 French) intrapleural plastic tube with a flutter type valve (Heimlich). Such valves have been especially useful during transportation.

Because the pneumothorax and intrapleural bleeding tend to recur, these casualties should not be delayed unduly in the evacuation chain. Experience in World War II suggested a significant increase in mortality as the time lag before definitive care increased.

As soon as the patient's condition warrants movement, roentgenograms of the chests should be made. These should be made with the patient sitting upright, both anteroposterior and lateral views being taken. The films demonstrate not only the degree of collapse of the lung and the degree of hemothorax and pneumothorax but also the nature and the location of retained missiles. The latter information may be of some assistance in estimating the pathway of the missile and possible damage to mediastinal or abdominal structures.

Repeated aspiration of the pleural space and continued transfusion often are necessary. It is essential that the expansion of the lung be maintained. If, after several thoracenteses, air and blood continue to collect, it is often advisable under local anesthesia to insert a fenestrated catheter into the pleural space and connect it to a bottle with an underwater seal. Respiratory movements then will expel the air and the fluid into the bottle. The catheter should not be inserted through the initial wound. The soft tissue wound of the chest wall should be débrided and closed primarily.

Occasionally, continued bleeding will require immediate thoracotomy. Such patients who bleed into shock in spite of transfusion, and repeatedly and rapidly refill their pleural space with blood, usually have a wound of a major systemic vessel (e.g., intercostal, internal mammary, subclavian artery or subclavian vein, or a large mediastinal vessel). Operative hemostasis may be lifesaving. Thoracotomy has been used more frequently in Vietnam, approximately 10 per cent of patients with thoracic injuries being subjected to it. Pulmonary resection (usually lobectomy) has been employed for treatment of hilar damage to a bronchus or vessel or for massive lobar destruction.

All patients with thoracic injuries should receive antibiotics parenterally in an effort to minimize pleural infection. Tracheal aspiration via the nasopharyngeal route is of assistance in preventing or overcoming atelectasis with its resultant parenchymal infection. Procaine block of intercostal nerves often is an adjunct to therapy in the relief of pain, especially when the injury includes rib fractures. This also has the advantage of assisting the patient in coughing.

Preferably the patients should remain at the forward surgical hospital for several days to permit stabilization of their condition, as casualties with residual deficiency in pulmonary function do not tolerate well the high altitude of air evacuation.

Follow-up studies[41] of 1,395 casualties from Korea demonstrated that 80 per cent recovered completely after only thoracenteses, antibiotics and blood. Within a few weeks 68 per cent were returned to duty. The remainder were returned to the Zone of the Interior (U.S.A.) largely because of associated injuries to other parts of the body. Of the patients with residual hemothorax 2 weeks after injury, one fourth became infected and required surgical drainage or decortication.

Decortication was deemed to be necessary in approximately 10 per cent of the total group, and it was performed optimally within 3 to 5 weeks after injury. The operation was elected because of decreased pulmonary function or infection associated with large, clotted or organized, hemothoraces. Residual infection was the indication in three fourths of the patients.

Delayed thoracotomy was performed in 12 per cent of the casualties for removal of large foreign bodies, usually shell fragments. This indication has not been established clearly, but it rests on the belief that the incidence of infection and erosion of vessels is high when a large metallic foreign body remains.

Mediastinal Injuries

Five per cent or less of thoracic wounds will include mediastinal injuries. They are infrequently seen by combat surgeons because they are so often associated with lethal injuries to the heart or great vessels. Injuries to the mediastinal trachea or bronchi may be suspected by the presence of mediastinal emphysema on the roentgenogram or occasionally by the presence of subcutaneous emphysema. Injuries to the esophagus can be suspected by the location and the pathway of the missile. An esophagogram, using Lipiodol, Diodrast or Urokon as a contrast medium, may demonstrate a perforation. In the absence of fluoroscopy, additional evidence of esophageal perforation may be obtained by having the patient swallow a few cubic centimeters of dilute methylene blue prior to thoracentesis. The dye then may be demonstrated in the pleural fluid. Evidence of tracheal, bronchial or esophageal perforation in the mediastinum is an indication for immediate repair. These injuries are quite infrequent, but they must always be considered.

Cardiac Injuries

In contradistinction to civilian surgery, in which many cardiac wounds are due to stab injuries, most military casualties with cardiac injuries due to bullets or shell fragments die before reaching the hospital. Of those who reach the hospital alive, most will have small wounds with self-limiting hemorrhage. Immediate exploration and suture seldom are justified. This procedure should be reserved for the occasional patients with more massive hemorrhage. Most patients will have a small leak into the pericardial sac. If the pericardial laceration remains patent, the blood may pass into the pleural cavity, and the cardiac component of the injury may not be suspected. The more classic injury is that in which the pericardial wound closes or that in which the wound involves a part of the heart not covered by pleura. Blood then is retained in the pericardial sac. As the hemopericardium develops, the increasing pressure in the pericardial cavity results in cardiac tamponade. Pressure on the heart, especially the auricles, prevents adequate filling, the result being a decreased cardiac output. Clinically, the diagnosis can be made by the low systolic and pulse pressures, the faint heart sounds, distention of neck vessels and elevated central venous pressure.

The overall condition of the patient is the major determinant in the course of treatment that should be employed. If pericardiocentesis is unsuccessful in relieving symptoms, immediate thoracotomy is indicated. If the initial aspiration was successful and the signs of cardiac tamponade reoccur, then surgical exploration is indicated. Thoraco-abdominal incisions are rarely employed. If both laporatory and thoracotomy are required, separate incisions are indicated. In all cases with penetration of both the abdominal and the thoracic cavities by the same missile, the diaphragm should be repaired. In most instances this can be accomplished during the abdominal procedure. Occasionally a separate small thoracotomy incision is required for repair of the right diaphragm not possible from below. Wounds of the right diaphragm into the "bare area" of the liver are rarely associated with herniation of the abdominal viscera into the chest early or late. Rather than subjecting the patient to the additional surgery necessary to "take down" the liver to expose and repair the diaphragmatic wound, treatment of the liver injury and adequate draining is sufficient in such cases.

Cardiopulmonary by-pass with pump oxygenator has been seldom employed in combat injuries. Conservative approach in dealing with foreign bodies of the heart is recommended.

THORACO-ABDOMINAL INJURIES

Frequently, missiles penetrate the chest and reach the abdomen. These patients have thoracic wounds that usually are handled nonoperatively and abdominal wounds that require laparotomy. The mortality of thoraco-abdominal wounds in World War II (Table 23-5) approximated that of abdominal wounds in contradistinction to that of thoracic wounds.

The thoracic component of the injury is treated as in other thoracic injuries. Care must be taken during anesthesia for laparotomy that the injured lung does not again undergo collapse and remain unrecognized. If catheter drainage of the pleural cavity is to be performed, sometimes it is well to insert the catheter at the beginning of operation or before laparotomy to assist in maintaining or restoring normal intrapleural pressures as the diaphragmatic wound is manipulated.

Unless thoracotomy is indicated for the specific wound of the chest, peritoneal exploration usually should be performed by the abdominal approach.

Most thoraco-abdominal injuries involve the liver. Less frequently, the spleen, the colon, the stomach and the kidney will be injured. Treatment includes closure of the diaphragm and proper management of the wounds of the abdominal viscera. Occasionally, exposure of small wounds of the diaphragm covered by the dome of the right lobe of the liver is so traumatic as hardly to justify the procedure.

In World War II, the mortality of thoraco-abdominal wounds of the left side of the body was greater than that of wounds of the right side. This presumably was due to the increased frequency of injuries to hollow viscera on the left side. Because of improvements in the treatment of infections, this difference apparently disappeared or was reversed in the Korean conflict.[5]

Pulmonary Complications of Nonthoracic Trauma

Pulmonary complications following nonthoracic war wounds include retained secretions with atelectasis, aspiration pneumonia, bacterial pneumonia, embolism of thrombus or fat to the lungs, oxygen toxicity, and pulmonary edema without congestive heart failure. The latter is a syndrome which has attracted great interest during the Vietnam war. It has been the subject of much clinical and laboratory research by the U. S. Navy.*

Patients who develop pulmonary edema typically have sustained massive soft tissue wounds with a large blood loss and profound hypovolemic shock. They have required multiple transfusions and large volumes of electrolyte solutions during resuscitation. When extensive wound débridement and multiple other surgical procedures are completed, they are discovered, within a variable period of time ranging from minutes to days, to be in severe respiratory distress. Central venous pressure is often normal or low. In laboratory preparations, left atrial pressure has also been found to be low. Blood gas analysis early reveals a widening of the alveolar-arterial gradient for PO_2 due to increased venous admixture or right-to-left shunting through the lungs. Later changes are a fall in the arterial pO_2 to less than 80 mm Hg. despite oxygen therapy, a lowered pCO_2, and an O_2 saturation of less than 90 per cent. When these changes become manifest, the clinical picture deteriorates rapidly, with almost total dependence on a respirator and increasing resistance to ventilation (reduced pulmonary compliance). The mortality exceeds 50 per cent. At autopsy, the lungs are heavy and congested. From the cut surface there is ooze of bloody, bubbly fluid. Microscopically, there is intense capillary congestion, and the alveoli are filled with edema fluid, red blood cells, and pigment-laden macrophages. Hyaline membranes and scattered foci of bronchopneumonia have also been noted.

The etiologies of this syndrome remain unclear. There is sufficient evidence that the excessive administration of intravenous fluids may play a role to recommend that during resuscitation of the severely wounded patient the rate and volume of fluid therapy be curtailed as soon as there is adequate peripheral circulation, as indicated by examination of the extremities and the urine output. Restoration of a "normal blood pressure" is not always necessary or desirable.

Adequate treatment of this syndrome demands the use of a volume-cycled respirator and the availability of blood gas analysis. To avoid oxygen toxicity in the lungs, the pO_2 of the inspired air must be monitored and kept as low as is consistent with a minimum of 90 per cent saturation of the arterial blood with oxygen. The use of diuretics, corticosteroids, and continuous positive pressure ventilation is being evaluated.

Wounds of the Abdomen

Physiologically, patients with abdominal injuries respond somewhat differently from those with wounds of the extremities. This appears to be due only in part to the increased prominence of the element of infection associated with intraperitoneal injuries. Patients with massive intraperitoneal injuries are not unlike the burned patient; they appear to lose plasma in large amounts into the peritoneal cavity. The hematocrit may remain stable or increase after injury and for a day or two after operation and transfusion. On the contrary, patients with massive wounds of the extremities tend to develop a falling hematocrit after injury, a trend that may persist in spite of massive transfusions. Casualties with moderate wounds of the extremities occasionally develop a hypertensive response, a finding seldom observed in patients with abdominal injuries (see Chap. 7, Shock). Patients with muscle destruction often excrete large amounts of creatine; presumably this is due to the destruction of muscle, since patients with abdominal injuries excrete much less. Paralytic ileus is much more marked in the presence of abdominal injuries. Furthermore, measurements of hepatic and renal function indicate greater impairment following abdominal injury. The incidence of demonstrable bacteremia appears to be about the same for the two groups. Finally, abdominal injuries result in a stormier clinical course and a higher mortality rate.

---

* Mills, Mitchell: The pulmonary complications of nonthoracic trauma, the clinical syndrome. U. S. Navy. J. Trauma, 8:651, Sept. 1968.

Although remarkable progress has been made in the treatment of abdominal injuries, these wounds remain one of the major problems in military surgery. In earlier wars penetrating wounds of the abdomen were treated nonoperatively. The surgeons of World War I began to wonder if laparotomy would not be a preferable form of treatment. During World War II, laparotomy was performed on all casualties with intra-abdominal injuries except the very occasional patient who was in so critical a condition that the surgeon felt that the additional operative trauma per se would be fatal. The mortality rate in World War II, as reported by the 2nd Auxiliary Surgical Group, was 23.5 per cent. The latter phases of the Korean conflict saw this mortality reduced by half, a mortality of 12 per cent being reported by the Surgical Research Team in Korea during 1953.

Many abdominal injuries are of massive extent involving multiple organs. The mortality rate is directly proportional to the number of organs injured, as indicated in Table 25-6.

A second factor that influences the mortality is the time lag before surgery. From the statistics of World War II, Beebe and De Bakey calculated an increase in mortality of approximately 0.5 per cent for every hour's delay before operation.

The reduction in mortality in Korea and Vietnam is attributable to the more liberal use of whole blood, the routine use of penicillin, the frequent use of wide spectrum antibiotics and the availability for helicopter evacuation for the more critically injured.

The goal in resuscitation and evacuation is to get the casualty into the operating room as soon as feasible.

Management at the Forward Surgical Hospital

Because hemorrhage is intra-abdominal and thus hidden, the inexperienced surgeon can be misled into underestimating the extent of blood loss in these patients. In such circumstances, anesthesia and laparotomy convert the patient from a state of impending shock to one of profound hypotension. As a result of this widespread experience, the maxim was developed of transfusing the patient with abdominal injuries "a pint or so more than he seems to need."

Preoperative evaluation and preparation include the insertion of an indwelling gastric tube and a urinary catheter, with attention to whether stomach or bladder contains blood. When injury to the rectum is suspected, the rectum should be checked for blood by digital and proctoscopic examination prior to operation.

Roentgenograms should be taken routinely. The demonstration of unexpected positions of missiles, multiple foreign bodies or vertebral fractures is occasionally of real assistance to the surgeon. Its aid in the evaluation of the individual patient cannot be predicted, but the experienced surgeon will utilize this adjunct to evaluation in most patients.

Principles of Abdominal Operations

Incisions. Almost always, vertical incisions are used for laparotomy in military surgery. The mid-line abdominal incision is the one of choice because of rapidity in opening and closing and of its adequate exposure of all areas of the abdomen. A systemic search of the abdominal cavity is imperative. Where indicated the lesser sac opened, the duodenum kocherized, the peritoneal reflections about the cecum and colon taken down if there is the slightest possibility of injury in these areas. All hematomas must be explored. Hepatic laceration should be repaired early to prevent excessive blood loss and to allow for as long a period of observation as possible prior to closure of the incision. Copious irrigation of the abdominal cavity with tepid physiologic saline solution to complete the peritoneal toilet is recommended.

TABLE 25-6. COMPARISON OF MORTALITY RATES FOR ABDOMINAL WOUNDS BY NUMBER OF ORGANS INJURED*

NUMBER OF ORGANS INJURED	WORLD WAR II No. of Casualties	WORLD WAR II Mortality Rate	KOREAN CONFLICT No. of Casualties	KOREAN CONFLICT Mortality Rate
0	98	5%	36	3%
1	496	10%	181	7%
3	132	42%	45	27%
5	13	92%	16	16%

* Casualties operated upon within approximately 7 hours after injury.

Thorough evaluation of mesenteric blood supply is mandatory prior to closing the abdomen. Single loop vessel injuries may be ligated. However, multiple vessel drainage and large areas of hematoma may be associated with deficient blood supply to a portion of the bowel, requiring resection and anastomosis at a viable level.

Hepatic Wounds. These are among the most frequent and sometimes the most dangerous of intra-abdominal injuries. The surgical problem, primarily, is that of hemostasis and, secondarily, that of preventing infection and bile leakage. In World War II and in Korea, the mortality remained from 9 to 10 per cent among patients whose only injury was of the liver.

The consistency of the liver is such that a high velocity missile produces extensive lateral damage resulting in stellate fractures that bleed profusely. Attempts to suture the wound sometimes increase bleeding, so that no single method of obtaining hemostasis is uniformly satisfactory. Hemostatic methods include ligature, suture, absorbable hemostatic agents, such as Gelfoam and, when absolutely necessary, massive packs of nonabsorbable gauze. Belause of inability to control bleeding, débridement is often practical. As a result, secondary necrosis and secondary hemorrhage occur occasionally. The latter also may follow the removal of large hemostatic packs.

Control of hemorrhage during débridement or resection can be facilitated by hepatic inflow occlusion, which can be safely performed on the normothermic patient for 15 minutes and up to one hour under hypothermia. This allows for individual ligation of the biliary vessels and ducts. The line of resection should be the edge of the devitalized tissue. Total hepatic lobectomy is necessary only in the severest injuries.

T-tube decompression of the biliary system is recommended in all cases requiring partial hepatectomy and lobectomy (liver wounds of a serious nature) to prevent bile leakage. An additional benefit of T-tube decompression is its use postoperatively for cholangiography to determine presence, position and size of abscesses and biliary fistulae.

All wounds of liver must have adequate drainage through generous incisions in the posterolateral abdominal wall to allow for dependent drainage. Sump drainage is recommended in the early postoperative period (recommended for wound in either upper quadrant).

Butyl cyanocrylate as a sprayed-on hemostatic agent for the cut surface of the liver is under investigation.

The most common complicating factor in liver injuries has been the development of abscesses; the majority appear to be infected hematomas.

Gallbladder. Almost always, injuries of the gallbladder are complicated by injury to the overlying liver. Cholecystectomy usually is followed by an uneventful course. Injuries to the extrahepatic bile ducts are seen infrequently, and usually they are associated with massive wounds and fatal hemorrhage because characteristically the wound traverses the hilum of the liver. Isolated injuries of the common duct should be repaired over a T-tube inserted through a separate opening in the duct.

Spleen. Injuries of the spleen are frequent and usually are accompanied by penetration of the adjacent abdominal organs and the overlying diaphragm and lung. Although splenectomy offers adequate therapy and few casualties of uncomplicated splenic trauma died in Korea, approximately 1 out of 6 casualties with splenic trauma died from associated injuries, accentuated doubtlessly by preoperative hemorrhage.

Stomach. Gastric injuries present few problems except that wounds of its posterior surface may be overlooked. Primary suture is followed by good wound healing due to the excellent blood supply of the stomach. Secondary leakage is almost unknown. The 29 per cent mortality in World War II for wounds that involved only the stomach was reduced to almost zero in Korea.[20]

Duodenum. Duodenal injuries are far more serious than gastric injuries. The retroperitoneal position of the duodenal is such that inevitably several other organs are injured. Bleeding often is profuse. Secondary necrosis of the suture line with the development of a duodenal fistula is not an uncommon complication. As a result, the mortality for all wounds involving the duodenum was over 50 per cent in World War II and approximately 40 per cent in Korea.

Resection and anastomosis is proving safer in Vietnam than is simple closure of the duodenal wound. The greatest hazard, however, remains the possibility of overlooking a wound of the duodenum unless the surgeon examines the duodenum in all injuries in this area.

Jejunum and Ileum. Injury to the small bowel is the most frequent of abdominal injuries. Often the injuries are massive, involving from 10 to 20 perforations of the bowel and its mesentery. If multiple injuries are found closely approximated, localized resection with end-to-end anastomosis may be necessary. As a generalization, however, simple suture is adequate. The rich blood supply of the small bowel makes formal débridement of the wound edges unnecessary; healing usually is uncomplicated. When innumerable perforations are found, the experienced surgeon always counts his suture lines to be certain that an even number is found, for almost inevitably an odd count implies that a hidden point of entrance or exit has been overlooked. Injuries limited to the small bowel have a negligible mortality (Korea); yet wounds of the small bowel compounded by injury of other organs still resulted in the loss of 1 of every 8 casualties.

Colon. Injuries to the colon, approximately as frequent as those of the small bowel, have led to more numerous complications.

RIGHT COLON. Wounds of the cecum and ascending colon are essentially the same as small bowel injuries and can be treated in a similar manner.

A. Small penetrating wounds, 1 cm. or less, may be débrided and closed primarily after careful examination of the retroperitoneal space. No cecostomy may be necessary.

B. Large or multiple wounds not involving the mesentery or associated with severe contiguous organ injuries or gross fecal contamination may be treated by resection and ilioascending colostomy.

C. Large or multiple wound with severe associated injury of continguous organs or gross fecal contamination are best treated by resection of the involved bowel and a matured ileostomy and distal mucous fistula.

D. Exteriorization of the cecum or ascending colon may occasionally be necessary.

Associated iliac fossae wounds must be adequately débrided to include the underlying fracture of the pelvis.

TRANSVERSE AND LEFT COLON INJURIES. All wounds of these sections of the bowel must be treated in either of two ways:

A. The wound must be repaired and the bowel returned to the peritoneal cavity with a proximal diverting colostomy, *or*

B. The traumatized area of the colon must be exteriorized.

Perforation of the Rectum. Wounds of the rectum are characterized by inaccessibility, difficulty of diagnosis, frequent damage to other structures and the hazard of pelvic and ascending retroperitoneal cellulitis. Due to the solid nature of the stool, perforations may be temporarily occluded and overlooked at the time of exploratory surgery. This possibility must be kept in mind and a very thorough search made in all known or suspected cases. Colostomy (not cecostomy) is mandatory, as is free posterior drainage. This is best provided by incision of the fascia propria exposing the rectal, sacral, and lateral paramedian spaces. Attempts to drain the retroperitoneal space by utilizing the missile wound of the buttock have been disastrous. In establishing posterior drainage it may be desirable to increase the exposure by removal of the coccyx, by disarticulation from the sacrum by sharp dissection and erasure of exposed articulating cartilage. Incomplete amputation with bone forceps should not be done.

Pancreas. Like duodenal injuries, injuries to the pancreas usually include injuries to several other organs. Injuries to large or small pancreatic ducts are inevitable. Since the ducts cannot be repaired adequately, drainage is essential to prevent collections of pancreatic juice. Although most fistulas result from injuries to major ducts in the head of the pancreas, almost inevitably they will close spontaneously if given a prolonged period of time.

Urinary Tract. Approximately 3 out of 4 wounds of the kidney are associated with injuries to other organs; therefore, the management of renal injuries usually is carried out through the laparotomy wound used for the repair of the associated injuries.

The renal injury may be suspected by the presence of hematuria, which should be checked preoperatively, as occasionally the retroperitoneal position of the kidneys may obscure renal injuries. A preoperative intravenous urogram should be considered if urinary involvement is suspected.

Like the liver and the spleen, the kidney often fractures from the lateral force of a missile. Bleeding may be very profuse, and it is the chief cause of death.

Small penetrating wounds may simply be drained to prevent possible urinary extravasation and to demonstrate any secondary bleeding. Not infrequently, larger wounds require nephrectomy. The advisability of partial nephrectomy for injuries to one pole of the kidney is unsettled; many surgeons believe that the high incidence of late complications make a conservative approach inadvisable, provided that the other kidney is present and uninjured. Small tears of the capsule or injuries to the renal pelvis may be repaired. In the future, it should prove to be feasible to repair injuries to the renal artery, but to date these injuries have required nephrectomy.

Injuries to the ureter are extremely rare. They should be treated by primary suture with drainage and proximal diversion of the urinary stream by pyelostomy or nephrostomy.

Wounds of the bladder are not rare; they occur most often when the bladder is distended with urine. Such wounds should be treated by primary repair and by decompression of the bladder by suprapubic cystostomy or by indwelling urethral catheter.

One of the more difficult injuries to treat is that of the posterior urethra. These injuries may be due to perforation by missiles or to the shearing force associated with pelvic fractures. Considerable progress has been made in the primary repair of these injuries, but it is probably too early to generalize as to the applicability of the procedure. The alternative is the insertion of an indwelling urethral catheter as a splint and the decompression of the bladder by the catheter or by a suprapubic cystostomy. With perineal wounds, the advisability of creating a diverting colostomy should be considered.

Associated Pelvic Fractures. Pelvic fractures ordinarily occur from missile fragments or gunshot wounds entering through the upper thigh and buttocks, penetrating the bony pelvic wall and entering the pelvic cavity. They frequently continue and exit through the opposite perimeter of the body. Care of these wounds is a combined General Surgical, Urologic and Orthopedic Surgical problem. The wound of the buttock and hip should be handled as any other seen in war and not handled as a fracture per se: that is, approach to the hip joint should be performed in order to reach the depths of the wound and complete a thorough débridement of bone, muscle, pelvic wall and iliac muscle wherever it is involved. Loose pelvic bone fragments should be removed. The penetrating wound of the pelvic wall should be enlarged with a rongeur. The bladder will be managed as a penetrating bladder wound, frequently requiring a suprapubic cystostomy. Ureteral injuries must be managed with catheters and the urinary stream may be diverted through a nephrostomy tube. The colon wounds are treated with standard technics and a diverting colostomy is usually mandatory. When urinary and fecal contamination and diversion have thus been accomplished, the wound of the hip and the pelvis will heal as any other well débrided war wound will heal. It can then be closed secondarily at 7 to 10 days if clinically clean. Drainage of the deep pelvis may be accomplished by posterior coccygectomy.

Wounds of the Extremities

In a study of the regional distribution of wounds among soldiers wounded in action in Korea, the Wound Ballistics Research unit found that over half of the wounds were of the extremities. Thus, although most men killed in action have injuries to the head or the trunk, most of the surgery done is for wounds of the extremities.

Soft Tissue Injuries

The principles of management of soft tissue wounds have been discussed under the heading, "The Battle Wound." These wounds are contaminated and may become infected if they are left untreated. Small wounds may require only incision, inspection as to the extent of damage, irrigation to remove loose debris and drainage by leaving the wound open. Larger wounds require extensive débridement (Fig. 25-13, *top* and *bottom*).

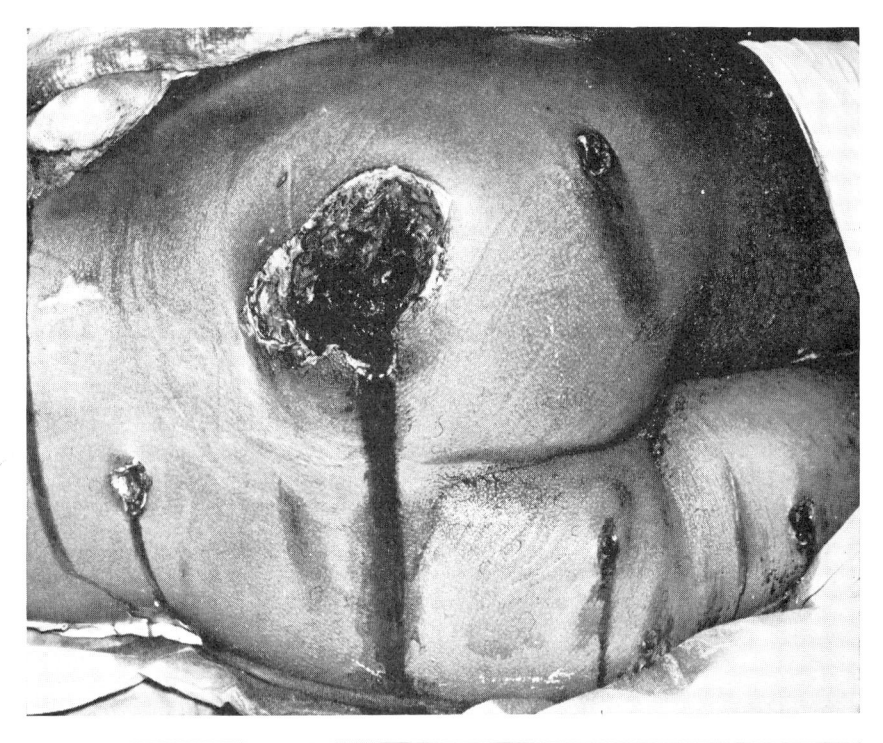

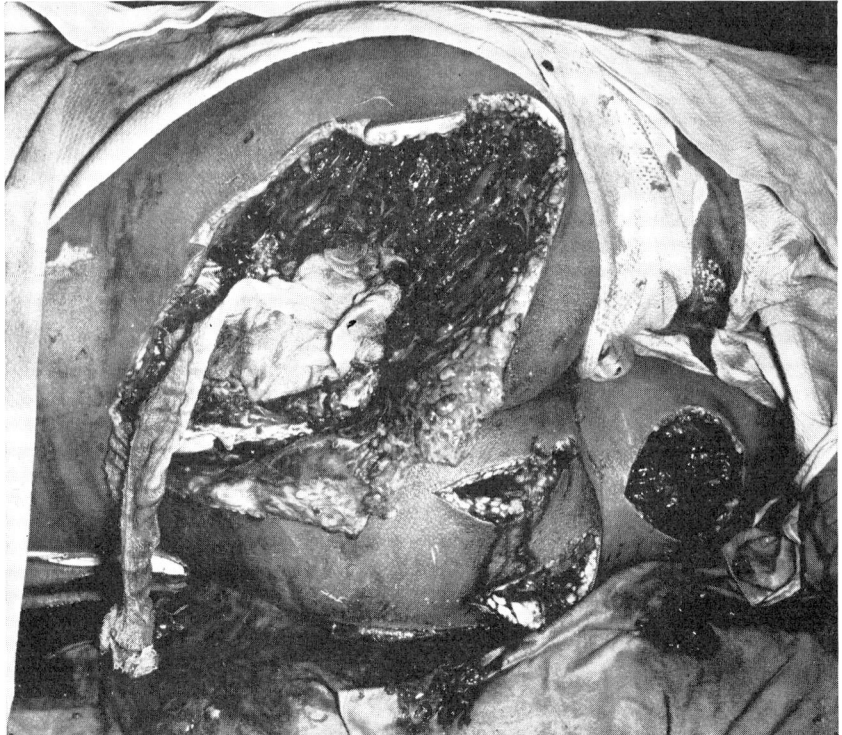

Fig. 25-13. (*Top*) Demonstrating the external appearance of penetrating shell fragment wounds of various sizes. (*Bottom*) Débridement includes adequate exposure and excision in order to prevent wound necrosis and infection. (Lt. Stephen Dittman, U. S. Army)

Almost all of these wounds are contaminated with virulent bacteria, many containing pathogenic clostridia. A group of battle casualties were studied by Strawitz and his associates in Korea by serial biopsies of the open wound over a period of the first week after injury.[39] At the end of débridement, culture of the remaining viable muscle revealed the presence of residual clostridia. Repeated biopsy cultures at 2-day intervals revealed the disappearance of the clostridia, provided that the wound was free of necrotic tissue. If débridement had been inadequate, virulent clostridia remained in the wound. During the first 2 to 3 days after injury, histologic study (Vickery) of the open wound demonstrated an exudate and surface necrosis. About the 4th to the 6th day, granulation tissue and fibroblastic proliferation became evident, and the exudate and the necrosis diminished. This sequence of events is the basis for selecting the 4th to the 6th day as the time for secondary closure of the soft tissue wounds. The absence of residual necrotic tissue or spreading infection is evident then; healing has begun, and it will continue and be expedited by secondary closure.

Arterial Injuries

Few casualties with injuries to the aorta survive to reach medical assistance. An occasional patient with injuries of a large intraabdominal artery, such as an iliac, reaches the forward surgical hospital alive, but he may die before or during operative hemostasis. The use of tourniquets and pressure dressings always has permitted most casualties with injuries of the extremities to reach the forward hospital. Until the Korean conflict, definitive treatment consisted of ligation of the severed artery. Under such a regimen, the area of the wound either had a collateral circulation sufficient to permit viability of the distal extremity or gangrene resulted.

The vascular pattern is similar in the upper and the lower extremities. A main arterial trunk gives off a deep branch to the arm and the thigh. The main artery divides at the knee or the elbow to form 2 smaller trunks. Thus, injury of the main trunk at the axilla or the groin, proximal to the origin of the deep branch, is associated with a poor collateral circulation and a graver risk of gangrene. Distal to the profunda branches, injury to brachial or femoral artery is associated with collateral circulation through the intact profunda. Distal to the elbow or the knee, ligation of 1 of the 2 arterial branches usually is not attended by gangrene. One of the most critical areas, however, is that of the popliteal artery. Here collateral circulation is poor, and, with the destruction of part of the collaterals by the wound and by the surgical incision, ligation is often disastrous.

In the American Civil War, 75 per cent of the casualties with injuries of the popliteal artery died because of the resulting gangrene, which probably had clostridial infection superimposed. In World War II, the incidence of gangrene and amputation following ligation of the popliteal artery was 73 per cent. In the Korean conflict, primary repair of the severed arteries was developed. As a result, the amputation rate following injury to the popliteal artery fell to 18 per cent. When feasible, the arterial wound was débrided and resutured directly. Such débridement should take cognizance of the fact that the damage on the inner walls of a large artery may extend from 2 to 3 mm. beyond the limits of that apparent on the outside. When the defect is too long to permit of primary suture, autogenous vein grafts (saphenous or cephalic veins) should be inserted. Neither sympathectomy nor anticoagulants appear to be necessary. The overall results in Korea were excellent, as demonstrated in Table 25-7. Even better results are emerging from Vietnam. Arterial injuries associated with an unstable fracture, especially the femur and humerus, are treated by a venous replacement graft to preclude tension on the suture line. Soft tissue is interposed between the fracture and the arterial repair to avoid impingement on the graft. Adequate stabilization is afforded by a circular cast, monovalved rather than bivalved. Only in rare instances is intramedullary fixation required or justified to protect the arterial repair.

Concomitant fasciotomy of the leg compartments is frequently required in arterial injuries when there has been an undue time lapse between injury and repair, when total venous interruption has occurred in the severely ischemic limb with beginning edema and when there has been significant soft tis-

TABLE 25-7. MANAGEMENT OF ACUTE ARTERIAL INJURIES. AMPUTATION RATE

ARTERY INJURED	LIGATION WORLD WAR II[8]		REPAIR KOREAN CONFLICT[20]	
	Number	% Amputated	Number	% Amputated
Axillary	74	43%	4	0%
Brachial	—	—	25	0%
Above profounds	97	56%	—	—
Below profounds	209	26%	—	—
Common femoral	106	81%	9	0%
Superficial femoral	177	55%	12	8%
Popliteal	502	73%	17	18%

sue injury of the extremity. In the postoperative period any signs of compartment compression require immediate and generous fasciotomy.

The débridement of all devitalized tissues is extremely important in wounds with vascular injuries. Infection accounts for practically all of the failures of vascular repairs. Primary repair of wounds of large veins is now often preferable to ligation.

Peripheral Nerve Injuries

All patients with combat wounds of the extremities should be examined specifically prior to débridement for evidence of peripheral nerve injury. It is equally important that the findings be recorded, for the patient with peripheral nerve injuries has embarked on a prolonged course of evacuation, surgical treatment and rehabilitation by many surgeons, each of whom will find the record of inestimable value in determining treatment and prognosis. Management at the forward surgical hospital consists primarily of treatment of associated injuries, débridement, repair of arterial injuries and treatment of compound fractures. In addition, the record is of considerable assistance in the subsequent management of the patient if the extent of anatomic injury to the nerve can be ascertained; that is, whether the nerve is contused, severed or lacerated incompletely. In combat injuries caused by high velocity missiles, immediate peripheral nerve repair is contraindicated. This question was explored extensively in World War II; the casualties were followed for several years afterward, and no new evidence accrued to change this concept.[42]

Immediately following débridement, an active program of physiotherapy is begun. Unless necessitated by associated fractures, splinting is reserved for radial or sciatic nerve injuries. Such splints are not used continuously; they are removed intermittently to permit physiotherapy.

Definitive nerve suture is postponed for from 1 to 3 months, and the patients are transferred to specialty centers in the Zone of the Interior (U.S.A.). Within a month, the secondary degeneration of the nerve ends has occurred, allowing the extent of damage to be ascertained accurately. Meanwhile, the soft tissue wound has healed, and the danger of infection has lessened. If the wound has healed and if physiotherapy has protected joint motility, nerves known to have been divided should be repaired within 3 months after injury, and always within 6 months. These time limitations are based on the extensive follow-up studies from World War II.[42] Exploration appears to be advisable if, after 3 months, nerves injured in continuity or lacking a description of injury demonstrate no return of function. If tests of function reveal normally progressive regeneration, exploration should be postponed.

Regardless of the type of injury, the prognosis as to the extent of functional recovery must be guarded until progressive recovery is demonstrated.

Compound Fractures

The characteristics of compound fractures in combat surgery are their frequency, the massive destruction of bone and soft tissues that often is present (Fig. 25-14), the associated life-endangering injuries to other parts of the body and the repeated need for transportation of the casualty.

At the battalion aid station, a sterile dress-

632   Military Surgery

ing should be applied and immobilization begun. Various splints usually are available for the different parts of the body, but the battalion surgeon often finds himself forced to improvise to meet inevitable shortages of supplies or unpredicted combinations of injuries. His aim is to prevent further damage and to minimize pain by immobilization. If splints are not available, the fractured leg may be bound to the uninjured leg. The fractured

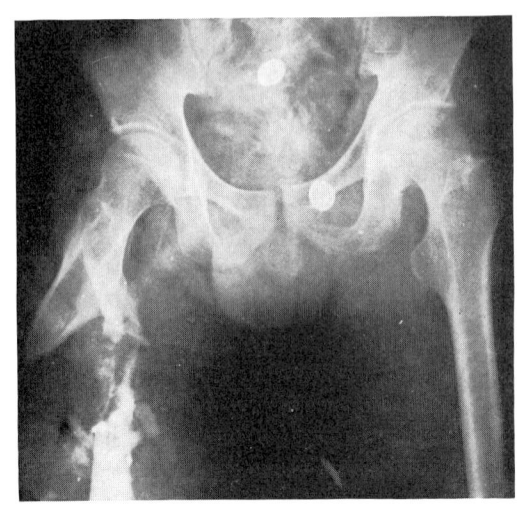

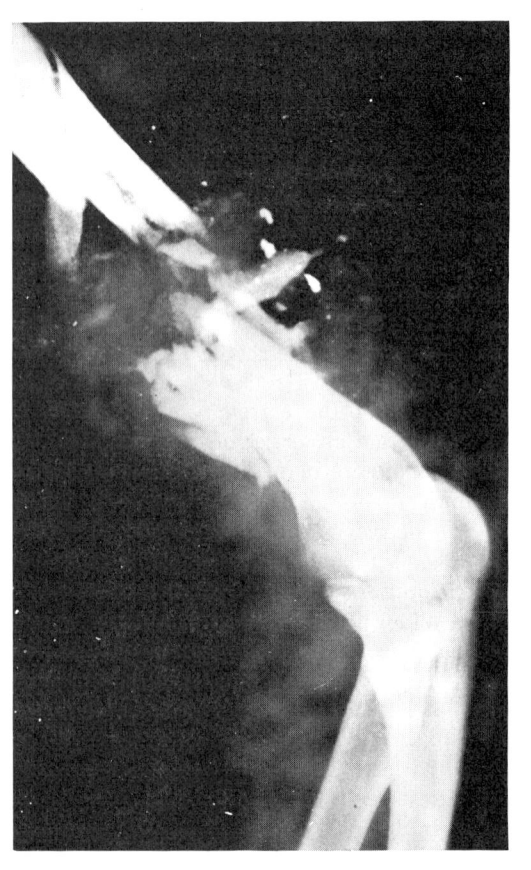

FIG. 25-14. Demonstrating the massive destruction of bone and soft tissues in compound fractures. (Lt. Stephen Dittman, U. S. Army) (*Continued on facing page*)

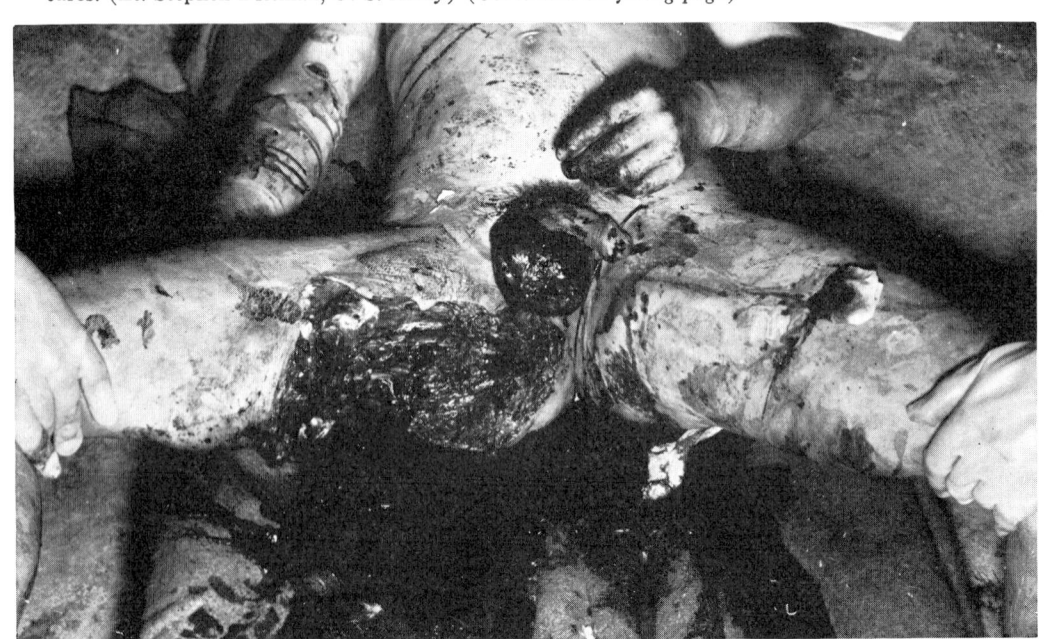

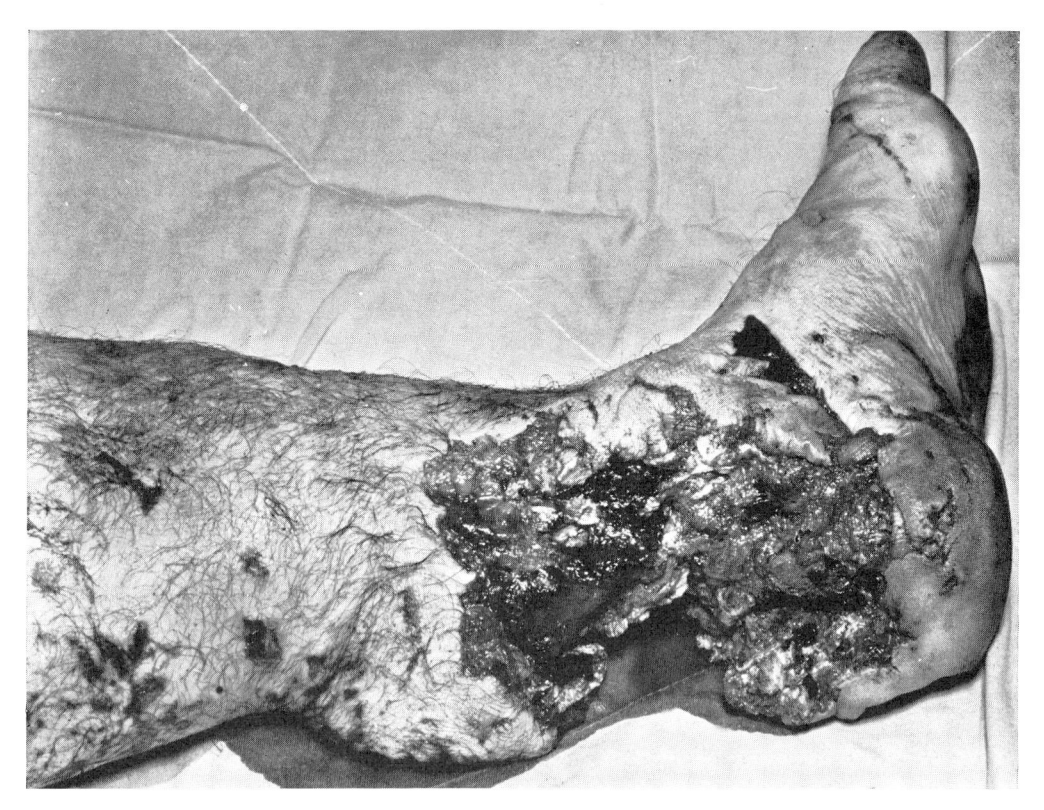

FIGURE 25-14 (*Continued*)

arm can be bound to the chest wall. Rifles or tent poles may become improvised splints.

At the forward surgical hospital, roentgenograms must be obtained prior to surgery, as the extent of bony injury from a high velocity missile cannot be predicted.

The aim of initial surgery is to prevent infection, for osteomyelitis results in a tremendous handicap to healing of a shattered bone. Débridement must be meticulous. Dead muscle and shredded fascia must be excised. Bone fragments attached to periosteum should be left in situ. Accessible shell fragments and all bits of clothing should be removed. Following hemostasis the wound should be irrigated copiously with sterile saline. Then the wound is left open.

A sterile dressing is applied, and the extremity is immobilized in a plaster cast. Immediately afterward, the cast and the underlying padding should be split longitudinally and spread to permit decompression. The injured extremity will swell, and, unless decompression is ensured, ischemia and gangrene may result. Experience has demonstrated the absolute need for this precaution in military surgery.

A line drawing of the site and the extent of the injury should be inscribed on the cast to assist personnel in the subsequent chain of evacuation.

The soft tissue wound is closed secondarily as soon as feasible after the first 4 to 5 days. Thereafter the needs of continued treatment are similar to those encountered in civilian practice.

Wounds of Joints

All penetrating or perforating wounds of joints should have examination by biplanar x-rays, followed by a formal arthrotomy to accomplish débridement. If the joint location permits, the visualization and débridement will be far more thorough under tourniquet ischemia. Copious irrigation of the joint fol-

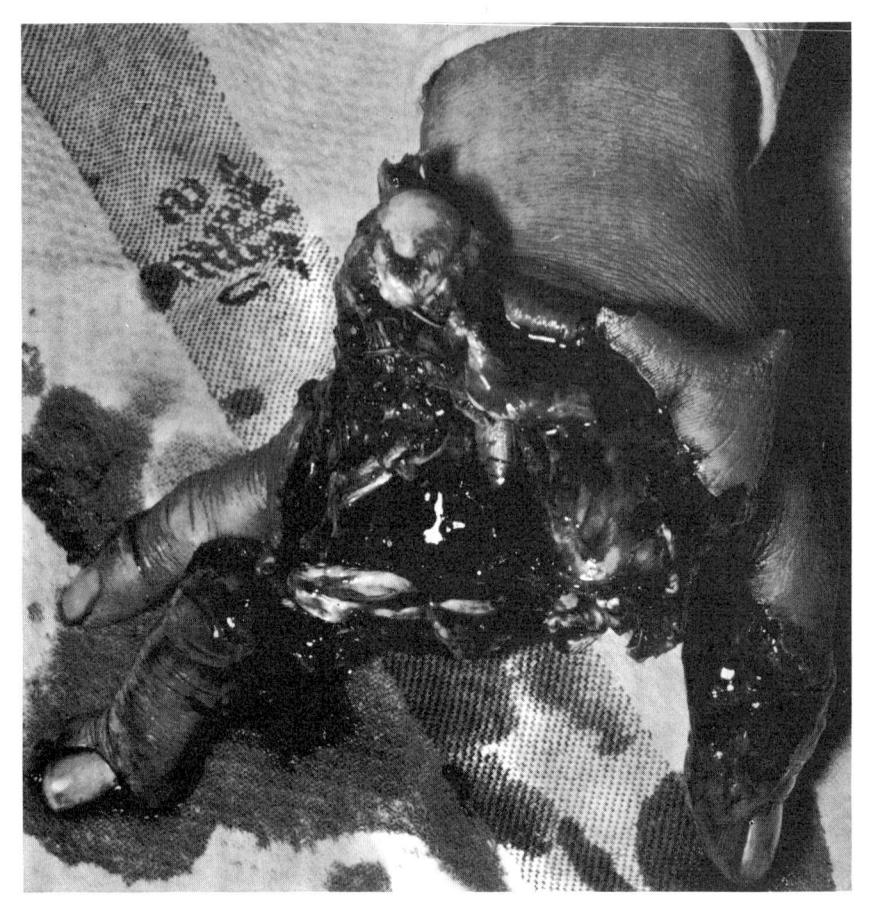

FIG. 25-15. A mangled wound of the hand. Initial conservation of tissue and subsequent reconstruction resulted in a useful hand. (*Continued on facing page*)

lowing débridement of all deep devitalized tissue should be performed. An interrupted, loose approximation of the synovial joint lining should be performed. Skin closure should not be performed. No drains should be inserted. The wound should then be encased in a plaster cylinder which is bivalved over the surgical dressing. Prophylactic antibiotics should be routine. The patient with such a wound can then be evacuated in a few days to have delayed primary closure performed at some other hospital.

Wounds of the Hand

Wounds of the hand are handled as are other wounds of the extremities, except that débridement of skin and tendons can be very conservative. Copious saline irrigation is indicated, bone fragments with soft tissue attachments are not removed. Kirschner wires may be used at time of initial surgery in special conditions where stabilization of dislocations and fractures are required. Severed nerves and tendons are not repaired initially. The hand is dressed with a fine mesh gauze lining for the wound, covered with fluff gauze with the fingers and wrist in the functional position. This dressing is supported by a light plaster splint and the hand is maintained in elevation to prevent edema.

It must be stressed that because of its unique anatomy and irreplaceable role in the productive life of an individual, intelligent conservatism must be practiced in the care of hand injuries and all viable, healthy tissue must be preserved (Fig. 25-15).

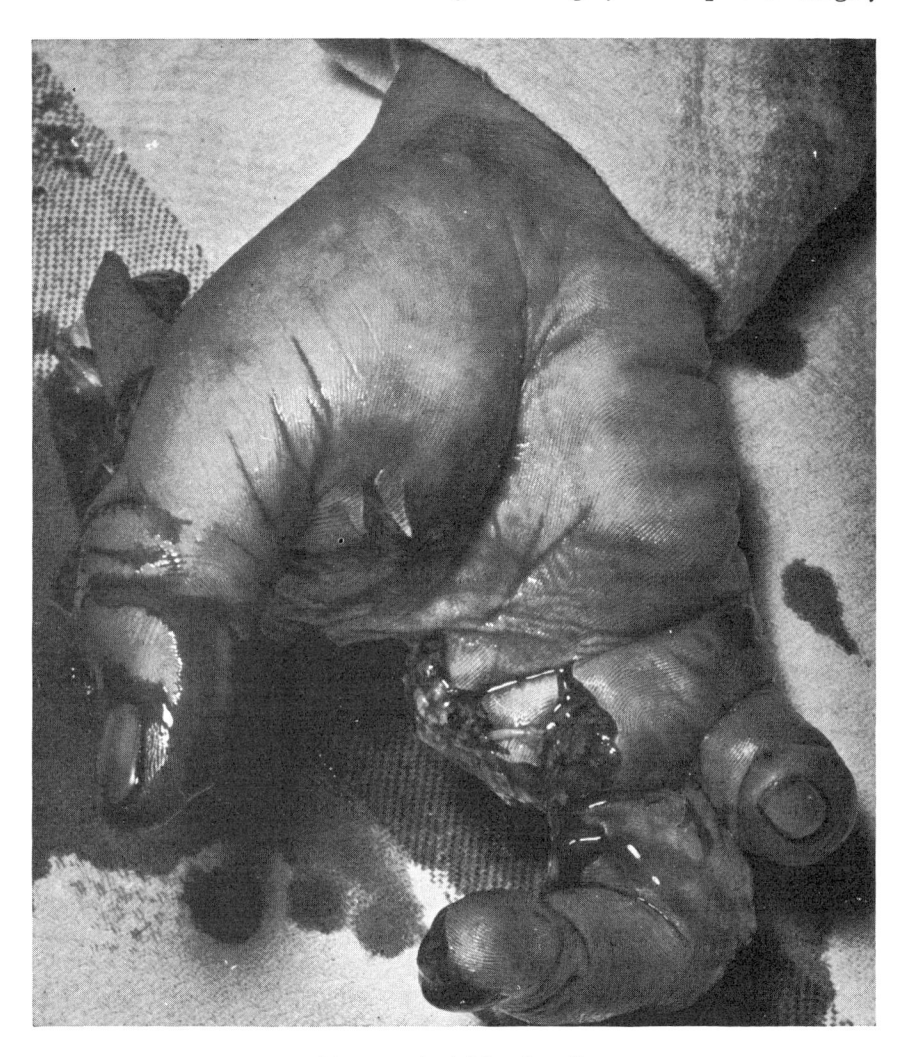

FIGURE 25-15 (*Continued*)

Wounds of the Foot

In many mine explosion wounds, severe injuries of the foot are seen with multiple embedded small fragments and debris. Such a wound cannot be adequately débrided unless the sole of the foot is approached. Consequently, civilian rules for avoiding plantar incisions must be temporarily put aside in favor of adequate débridement. Extension of the plantar incision should be planned to obtain complete fascial decompression and débridement of the small muscles of the foot on both plantar and dorsal surfaces. Usually incisions on both surfaces will be required for adequate débridement. Early and continuous elevation of the involved extremity is essential in these injuries.

Traumatic Amputations

The many blasting mine injuries seen in Vietnam are causing multiple injuries throughout the extremity. Open circular amputation at the most distal level of good circumferential skin frequently results in unnecessary sacrifice of lengths. For this reason, the modified type of amputation has been used in the mutilated type of extremity seen with land mine injuries. First the entire extremity is completely and thoroughly débrided. When only viable skin, muscle and bone remain,

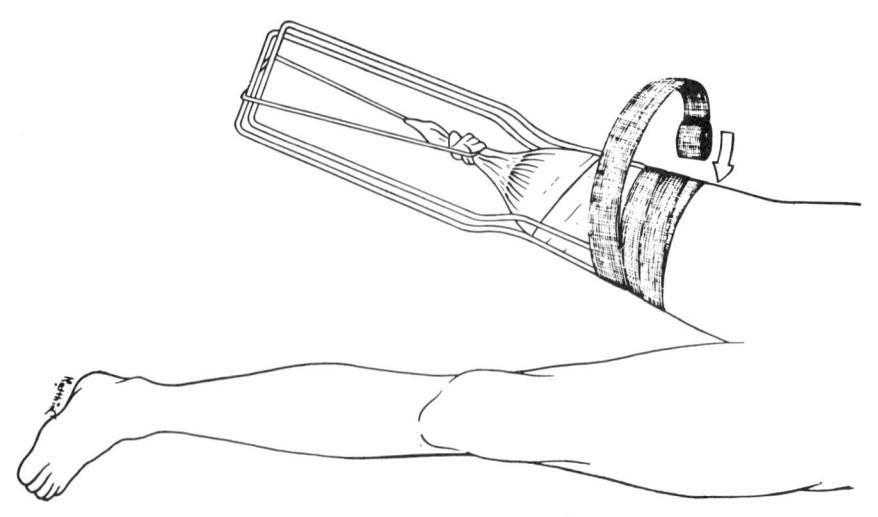

FIG. 25-16. Skin traction for amputees. The wire frame is incorporated in a plaster cast, thus permitting continuous skin traction during evacuation.

the site of election for amputation is determined by the most distal level of a major viable skin flap, provided that the muscle is viable over the bone at this level. Circumferential skin traction cannot always be applied to this type of a stump and for this reason modified skin traction and anchoring suture procedures are necessary. It is important to consider this type of an amputation as a major open war wound and at the end of 3 to 7 days it can be partially closed with skin graft and the modified skin flaps, or sutured in the most desirable position without tension. The objective in this type of an amputation is to achieve a clean healed wound as quickly as possible. Revision of this amputation should be done at rear echelon hospitals as an elective rather than an emergency procedure after the swelling and infection have subsided. In practice, the majority of these modified type of amputations following mutilating extremity injuries are closed by modified skin flaps, plus split thickness skin grafts.

The cost of rehabilitation and the pension of a soldier with an amputation of a leg has been estimated by the Veterans Administration as $100,000.

Transportation of Amputees. The open circular amputation in stockinette skin traction can be evacuated with traction remaining on the skin by the means of a self-contained outrigger bar formed by the wire ladder splint. In this manner, the patient can be placed in air-evacuation channels and will not suffer loss of skin length while in transit.

WHITE PHOSPHORUS BURNS

Burns are a common injury in the combat zone and are handled in a manner similar to burns in civilian practice. However, white phosphorus burns are unique to warfare and require treatment different from that used in thermal burns.

Elemental white phosphorus can be incorporated into several different types of weapons, artillery shells, mortar rounds, grenades, bombs, etc. In addition to the effects of the explosion and metallic fragments of the weapons casing, fragments of phosphorus are driven into the body where, if the phosphorus is exposed to air, it continues to smolder and burn the local tissues. Phosphorous and phosphoric acids which result from oxidization of the elemental phosphorus in the wound are absorbed, as is elemental phosphorus which is extremely toxic and may result in severe hepatic damage (50 mg. is a lethal dose).

The immediate treatment of white phosphorus injuries is to exclude the phosphorus from contact with air. Any type of wet compress will suffice. Definitive treatment consists of careful débridement of the wound to remove all phosphorus particles. Copious physiologic saline irrigations are an important adjunct to the débridement. Historically, Copper sulfate solution, 0.5 to 5 per cent, has been recommended in the treatment of white phosphorus burns. A protective coating of black cupric phosphate forms on the surface of phosphorus particles, which makes easier their identification and removal. However, the use of copper sufate solution is attended with some danger. Systemic absorption will occur with the use of strong solutions or with prolonged contact in the wound and may cause a hemolytic diathesis. The mechanism of this hemolysis is obscure. Studies reported by Mital *et al.* suggest a possible relationship between erythrocytic glutathione and glutathione stability to acute copper sulfate poisoning. On this basis, individuals with glucose-6-phosphate dehydrogenase deficient red cells (approximately 10% of Negro population and some of Mediterranean or Near East origin) would be particularly prone to develop hemolysis if copper sulfate were used to treat phosphorus burns. Therefore, it should be used in dilute solutions only and applied just for a few minutes to blacken the phosphorus particles.

SPECIFIC COMPLICATIONS

Tetanus

Basic immunization, including a booster injection prior to entering the combat theater and followed by an emergency booster after injury, offers an effective prophylaxis against tetanus. The incubation period for tetanus is approximately 7 days; the antibody response to the booster requires only 4 to 5 days.

Edsall[9] collected only 15 cases of tetanus among the 2,500,000 wounded men in the U. S. Armed Forces during World War II. Only 6 had received the full scheduled immunization. All soldiers should be immunized and should receive a booster injection of the toxoid as soon as feasible after injury. Thus this complication of injury can be prevented.

In considering the possible mass casualties of atomic warfare, the problem must be reconsidered, for atomic casualties might include civilian (often nonimmunized) casualties. In World War I, the incidence of tetanus among the armies of the world varied from 2 to 8 per 1,000 wounded, falling to about 1 per 1,000 when wound surgery and tetanus antiserum became routine (Table 25-8).

Deaths from tetanus among the German soldiers were estimated at 12,000. The problem of mass civilian casualties was described best by Glenn[12] in World War II. Among the untreated, malnourished civilian casualties of the siege of Manila (1945), the incidence of tetanus was about 40 per 1,000. Tetanus wards were established, and, of 473 patients treated, 82 per cent died.

Gas Gangrene

Whereas tetanus can be prevented by prophylactic immunization, gas gangrene can be prevented by active surgical treatment. When the problem is applied to the situation of mass

TABLE 25-8. Incidence of Tetanus in Military Campaigns

War	Years	Number of Casualties	Incidence of Tetanus (per 1,000 Casualties)
American Civil War	1861–65	246,172	2.07
Franco-German War	1870–71	—	8.0
World War I			
British troops			
Before antiserum	1914–15	—	8.0 ⎫ 1.47
After antiserum	1915–18	—	1.0 ⎭
World War I			
German troops	1914–18	4,000,000	3.8
World War II			
American troops	1941–45	2,500,000	0.006
World War II			
Manila civilians	1945	—	40.0*

* Estimated.

casualties, as from an atomic disaster, gas gangrene becomes a greater problem, for its prevention rests primarily on early adequate surgery.

As a generalization, almost all large battle wounds contain pathogenic clostridia that are capable of producing gas gangrene. However, gas gangrene develops only in necrotic tissue, and almost invariably it is preceded by proximal interruption of the main artery to the extremity. Altemeier described the average incubation period of gas gangrene (*Clostridium perfringens*) as 24 hours, and Trueta found in the Spanish Civil War that an untreated patient who survived 48 hours or longer without signs of anaerobic infection probably would escape gas gangrene. Once the infection has developed in experimental animals, penicillin prolongs life, but it does not affect the mortality if the wound is not treated.[1] Hyperbaric oxygen has proved to be a valuable adjunct to the treatment of clostridial infection and has removed the necessity for limb amputation in some cases. Hospital ships and some larger hospitals ashore are equipped with chambers that can be used for this purpose. Cases with clostridial infections should be transferred to these activities as early as possible.

TABLE 25-9. GAS GANGRENE IN WORLD WAR I[1]

TYPE OF INJURY	NUMBER OF CASUALTIES	INCIDENCE OF GAS GANGRENE	MORTALITY
Soft tissue	128,265	1.1%	48.5%
Compound fractures	25,272	5.2%	44.6%

These facts explain the progress in military surgery in controlling gas gangrene, and they highlight the problem anew in terms of the management of possible atomic casualties.

In the latter half of the Korean conflict, gas gangrene almost disappeared. Among 4,900 consecutive casualties, 4 developed gas gangrene, and all 4 survived. This remarkable success was not due to lack of wound contamination; it was due to early consistent débridement, the repair of injured arteries and, perhaps, in part to the routine use of antibiotics. Antiserum was not used. In all 4 instances above, arterial injury had been followed by an unsuccessful surgical repair.

This represents quite a difference from the earlier experiences (Tables 25-9, 25-10) in World Wars I and II. Coupal[7] reported an incidence of gas gangrene of 1.1 per cent of soft tissue wounds and 5.2 per cent of compound fractures among American troops in World War I. Pettit[31] wrote of the more seriously injured of the Saint-Mihiel and Argonne-Meuse operations in World War I when a hospital received 4,377 casualties over a 2-month period, the time lag often being as long as 48 hours. These conditions as to time lag are pertinent to the problem of mass casualties. Pettit wrote that, of the 4,377 patients, 221, or 5 per cent, developed gas gangrene. This presumably represents approximately 10 per cent of the casualties with wounds of the extremities. The mortality of such infections was 27.6 per cent.

POST-TRAUMATIC RENAL INSUFFICIENCY

Among the massively injured casualties, post-traumatic renal insufficiency is a major problem. Although its incidence approximated

TABLE 25-10. CLOSTRIDIAL MYOSITIS (GAS GANGRENE)

	WORLD WAR I[31] EVACUATION HOSP. NO. 8 Sept. 20, 1918–Nov. 13, 1918	WORLD WAR II[28] Hospital, India	KOREAN CONFLICT[19] 46th Surgical Hosp. Jan., 1952–June, 1953
Number of casualties	4,377	4,600	4,900
Number developing clostridial myositis	221	32*	4
Percentage developing clostridial myositis	5.0%	0.7%	0.08%
Case fatality rate	27.6%	31.3%	0 %

* An additional 37 patients developed serious clostridial wound infections, making a total incidence of serious infection by *Clostridium perfringens* of 1.5%.

smaller atomic bombs used in World Wa offer the only base line in experience. principles of care of mass casualties are parently the same after the explosion of weapon of this type.

A small atomic bomb similar to those ploded over Japan might be equivalen 20,000 tons of TNT; therefore, the b might be called a "20 KT" or a "20 kilo bomb. Other bombs are designated meg (million tons) in capacity.

The detonation of an atomic bomb is lowed immediately by a heat wave that about a second. Initially, the heat prod has been estimated to be in the million degrees centigrade. In spite of this tremen radiant energy, its destructive power is c pated rapidly as the distance from the center (point on ground directly beneath explosion) increases. Heat in excess of 8 ories per square inch will char clothing skin; heat of 2 to 3 calories per square will produce first-degree burns. Ordinary c ing offers protection against the flash beyond a distance of from 3,500 to 4,500 (20 KT bomb); within this range, both c ing and skin are burned, so that unshelt people would receive third-degree burns. to a range of 12,000 feet from the epice unprotected people may receive first-de and second-degree burns.

Other effects of the radiant energy inc a temporary blindness, usually lasting a minutes, due to staring at the fireball.

Whereas the initial flash will produce n primary burns, many other thermal inj will result from secondary burns—bur clothing, houses, gas lines, overturned st disrupted electrical lines, etc.

The experience of Hiroshima and Naga indicates that approximately 35 per cer the casualties requiring medical care w suffer from uncomplicated thermal burns, that an additional group would have the burns complicating mechanical injuries. incidence of burns would have been lowe Japan had a warning period permitted people to take cover.

Approximately 50 to 60 per cent of casualties suffered from mechanical inj secondary to the blast. Immediately after explosion there is a tremendous surge o creased pressure. This blast wave is relat

2. **Frostbite.** This lesion is probably the most acute cold injury encountered in man. It results from exposure for a few minutes to several hours to temperatures of extreme "dry cold" ($+20°$ F. to $-100°$ F.). Frostbite is very similar to a thermal burn of the skin and has been classified into two degrees of severity.

First degree: early blanching of the skin at onset with a characteristic tingling sensation followed by numbness. In very mild cases, if rewarmed at this point, no further injury may be noted; or redness of the area may develop, followed by scale desquamation.

Second degree: blister formation appears in 12 to 36 hours, followed by sheet desquamation.

When palpated, frostbite skin is cold, but soft and resilient, and moves freely over bony prominences. Should any treatment be considered necessary, it is the same as for a first or second degree burn.

3. **Immersion or (Cold) Trench Foot.** This injury results from longer exposures (several days or weeks) to milder temperatures (slightly above or below freezing) accompanied by conditions where the feet are exposed to moisture (from excess sweat accumulation in the boot or from standing in water and mud). It is most likely that the excess moisture plays the largest part in this injury, as a similar condition occurs in South East Asia, where the troops are exposed to a hot humid environment and spend much of their time in swamps and rice paddies. This condition is referred to as "Rice Paddy Foot."

The injury can be divided into two stages. In the ischemic state, the foot is cold, swollen, cyanotic or mottled. Walking is difficult, and the skin may be anesthetic due to nerve injury.

Following the first stage is a period of hyperemia which can last from days to weeks. The feet are red, swollen, and hot, with deep pain and superficial burn. In some cases the pain can be so severe as to require narcotics for relief. Untreated cases can result in wet gangrene with extensive loss of tissue.

4. **Frozen Injury.** Freezing of a tissue takes place when intracellular ice crystals form. An extremity may be considered frozen when tissues deeper than the skin are affected. It is always preceded by frostbite and occurs most often in the feet, ears and nose, and occasionally in the hands. The skin appears waxy with a yellowish color, sometimes translucent in nature, and is stiff and firm to palpation. It will not move normally over bony structures. Once the patient is brought into shelter, the skin overlying frozen tissues collects moisture droplets from the atmosphere. Depending on the severity of the injury, blisters will appear over the frozen area in one day to a week, with hyperemic discoloration appearing from about the second to the fifth day. The end stage is the development of dry gangrene with autogenous amputation of destroyed tissue. In less severe cases the recovered extremity may have residual hyperesthesia, paresthesia, and extreme sensitivity to even moderate cold. The generally accepted treatment today is rapid rewarming in a water bath or whirlpool with the water temperature about 104 to 110° F.

Surgical intervention should be delayed for several months, as the superficial line of demarcation is not indicative of deep tissue loss. Many extremities can now be saved which were lost in the past by premature amputation.

5. **Generalized Hypothermia.** This condition results from the general loss of body heat to the extent that the core temperature may be lowered to a lethal degree. The symptoms are extreme fatigue, muscle weakness, joint stiffness, and overpowering sleepiness. A feeling of warmth and comfort has often been reported. Unconsciousness and death may follow. The treatment of choice is total body rewarming by the use of blankets and hot water bottles, immersion in a hot bath, or by diathermy. Two conditions are considered serious complications during the period of rewarming. The patient may develop a generalized vasodilation with a resultant hypotensive episode. The second and most dangerous is the development of cardiac fibrillation.

The military problem with cold injuries is not primarily treatment; it is prevention. Prophylactic measures consist, in part, of ascertaining weather predictions and avoiding, when possible, undue exposure. When exposure is necessary, heat loss can be minimized by proper clothing, based on the principle of insulation by air spaces. Constricting clothes prevent air insulation, and moisture increases heat conduction. Because of the deleterious effect of moisture, many injuries have been prevented by the simple expedient of changing socks every day—something that under com-

bat conditions can be achieved
tinued educational program for
sulated rubber boots have been
have proved to be effective pr
provided that the troops obse
foot hygiene. No clothing can
effective in conserving heat if
immobilization are prolonged u
fore, the prevention of cold inju
the responsibility of commandin
is of the medical officer. Howev
officer must be responsible for
command and troops the dar
preventive measures involved.

IMMERSION FOOT

In contrast to the experiences
war, the problem in Vietnam is
water or tropical immersion foc
when the feet are exposed to co
ing in warm water for prolong
time (several days to over a we
keratin layer of the sole absor
ating the distinctive triad of w
painful feet. Quite often, the sy
companied by a macerated derm
sides and dorsal aspects of the
onto the ankles, where the pro
is not thickened (boot distri
acute injury responds rapidly
the patient is usually fully reco
few days. In contrast to the im
where the water temperature is
ing (25°-60° F.) there are
sequelae in tropical immersion f
be anticipated, persons with
soles (e.g., congenital hyperkera
sities) more readily develop
than persons with normal feet
formulated silicone ointment ha
to be effective in reducing the
severity of this condition.

In *cold-water* immersion fo
represent variations of the sam
like thermal burns, represent ir
ing degrees—superficial, dermal
section on Cold Injuries). Trea
specific. Unfortunately, the lesso
to be learned afresh in each war
amputation is unnecessary. Cons

* Carson, T. E.: Dermatology, U.
Hospital, Danang, Republic of Vi
communication).

a few seconds the small bombs over Hiroshima and Nagasaki produced the following casualties:

	Hiroshima	Nagasaki
Killed and Missing	70,000	36,000
Injured	70,000	40,000

Faced with responsibilities of such magnitude, the medical profession must plan, in generalities, its approach to therapy.

It is quite obvious that the hydrogen bomb has a much greater range of devastation. Perhaps very small atomic weapons may be utilized. In either instance, the principles remain unchanged.

On the basis of extensive military experiences and limited experience in civilian disasters, principles of management of mass casualties can be outlined tentatively. These principles should include the following items, divided under several general headings:

GENERAL PRINCIPLE

1. The plan of treatment must be designed to accomplish the greatest good for the greatest number of people. The saving of a life takes precedence over the saving of a limb. However, it is conceivable that the return to military duty might, under conditions of total warfare, take precedence over either.

TRAUMA

2. Within the first 24 hours, most fatalities occurring after patients reach medical installations are due to hemorrhage, mechanical defects or thermal burns.

3. Traumatic wounds are contaminated wounds containing pathogenic aerobic and anaerobic organisms.

4. Primarily, the prevention of infection is dependent upon the adequacy of débridement. Antibiotics will not prevent infection in the presence of necrotic tissue. When débridement is not feasible because of the press of casualties, incision and drainage may be advantageous. Soft tissue wounds should not be closed under these conditions.

5. Gas gangrene develops primarily in patients with arterial injuries. It has an incubation period of from 24 to 48 hours. In the presence of gangrene tissue, it cannot be prevented by antibiotics. Its prevention requires surgical removal of the mass of nonviable tissue.

SHOCK

6. Nature has supplied man with a relatively greater reserve in red cell mass than in plasma volume. A young man who loses rapidly 50 per cent of his whole blood is almost dead. The use of plasma or plasma volume expanders, while not restoring his red cell mass, restores his circulating volume and assists him materially to compensate for his injury. Plasma or plasma volume expanders can be used as a compromise to replace blood loss in amounts of 1,000 to 2,000 cc. In greater amounts, units of whole blood and plasma substitutes may be administered alternately so as to extend the supply of blood.

7. When the supply of available blood is limited, it can be used most efficiently in patients in whom hemorrhage has been controlled. Therefore, a limited quantity of blood will save more patients with injuries of the extremities than with intra-abdominal hemorrhage.

BURNS

8. Burn wounds are contaminated, and, since immediate débridement is not feasible technically, immediate surgery has little to offer the patient with uncomplicated burns in mass casualty situations.

9. Since the burn wound is already contaminated, sterile dressings are not essential to the management of these patients.

10. The cause of early death in patients with thermal injuries is blood-volume deficiency. This deficiency is primarily in the plasma component. Whole blood is not absolutely essential in the immediate treatment of thermal injuries. Plasma or plasma volume expanders will suffice. Sodium chloride and sodium bicarbonate, given orally in isotonic solution, lowers substantially the mortality rate in the first 2 days.

11. Patients with burns of from 5 to 15 per cent of their body surface will survive if given oral fluids. Most patients with burns of from 60 to 100 per cent of their body surface will die in spite of intensive therapy. In the presence of mass casualties, first priority in the treatment of thermal injuries should be those

casualties with burns of from 20 to 40 per cent.

Head Wounds

12. In the absence of increased intracranial pressure, patients with wounds of the brain tolerate transportation to fixed hospitals without greatly increasing the mortality.

Thoracic Wounds

13. Intrathoracic injuries, while seldom requiring formal thoracotomy, apparently result in a marked increase in mortality if treatment of the mechanical pulmonary defects and blood-volume deficiency is delayed. As a result, these injuries deserve a fairly high priority.

Abdominal Wounds

14. Patients with perforating wounds of the bowel appear to deteriorate rather rapidly with the passage of time. They, too, deserve a fairly high priority.

Sedation

15. Under conditions in which survival may depend upon one's ability to care for one's self, morphine or other sedatives may immobilize an individual to his ultimate detriment.

Fluid Administration

16. Limitations in personnel and supplies will make the routine use of intravenous fluids impractical. All patients should be given water or, better, a hypotonic saline solution orally, except those who are unconscious, in profound shock, have gastrointestinal perforations or are about to undergo anesthesia. Although the absorption of water is retarded after injury, thirst and fluid requirements often can be controlled by drinking.

Evacuation

17. Evacuation of patients to hospitals in neighboring cities must be controlled in such a way that no single hospital is overcrowded while other hospitals are not utilized.

Radiation Injuries

18. Although experience is limited, radiation injuries appear to produce delayed manifestations and deserve little consideration during the immediate postdisaster period. Fatalities during the first few days result principally from thermal and mechanical injuries.

SUBMARINE MEDICINE

Atmosphere Control. On board the nuclear-powered submarine, the doctor is required to be not only physician and surgeon, but also an expert in atmosphere control. Since the nuclear submarine is a system closed from the earth's atmosphere, oxygen must be provided and waste products eliminated. Oxygen is generated by first distilling seawater to an essentially ion-free state and then, by the process of electrolysis, producing oxygen for breathing.

Until recently, the primary problem of submarine medical officers has been the control of carbon dioxide levels in the atmosphere of the submerged ship. However, this has now been controlled adequately, even under conditions of prolonged submergence (several months) in the nuclear-powered submarines. A continuing problem is the wide variety of contaminants in the air of the closed environment: tobacco smoke, hydrocarbons from lighter fluid, solvents, polishes, decomposition products of lubricants, and even by-products of the process used to "scrub" carbon dioxide and other contaminants from the atmosphere. The nuclear submarine, nevertheless, continues to demonstrate the ability to control its atmosphere in a highly satisfactory manner. Contaminants are eliminated either by electrostatic precipitation of the ions and aerosols in high voltage units installed in the ship's ventilation system, or through the carbon monoxide-hydrogen burning units by conversion to carbon dioxide and water. Odors and certain hydrocarbons are removed by an activated charcoal filter. As an adjunct to atmosphere control, submarines maintain a list of strictly prohibited items and all new items on-board are screened for toxic or contaminant properties.

Nuclear Medicine. The practice of nuclear medicine in submarines includes the identification, monitoring, and recording of radiation levels and exposures that are encountered in our nuclear ships. Radiation hazards are minimal and are well controlled aboard the nuclear powered vessels of the U. S. Navy.

Surgery at Sea. Surgical intervention in an incommunicado ship, submerged far at sea, is a calculated risk. Although a few cases of heroic surgery are well chronicled, there is no basis for condoning any major surgical procedure when an acceptable alternative exists. In addition to the impediments of physical isolation, environment and restricted communication, surgery is further hampered by lack of equipment and suitable means of anesthesia. Even though all submarines are outfitted with at least basic surgical supplies and instruments, the diversity of materials, equipment, and trained personnel essential in today's sophisticated operating room are not to be found on board the submarines.

Anesthesia presents a principal barrier to a surgical undertaking on the submarine. The use of any gas, of course, is precluded. Anesthesia is restricted to local, regional or spinal block.

Patients who obviously cannot be retained for treatment are evacuated. This decision is often difficult if circumstances necessitate radio silence. In such instances, submarine-doctor-corpsman teams have successfully applied nonoperative treatment to conditions ordinarily considered surgical.

CHEMICAL WARFARE*

The medical problems of chemical warfare include the prevention of injury or the resuscitation after injury by several types of agents, which include the following.

Lethal Agents

Anticholinesterases. Loosely referred to as "nerve gases," these chemicals block the action of acetylcholinesterase and therefore lead to muscarinic and nicotinic signs and symptoms. Treatment includes artificial respiration, the administration of atropine in large doses and the administration of one of several oximes.

Vesicants. Sulfur mustards, nitrogen mustards and certain arsenical compounds produce chemical burns of the skin and the eyes. Healing may be prolonged, but otherwise the surgical problem may be considered to be analogous to the treatment of thermal burns of comparable extent and severity.

Lung Irritants. The vesicants attack the respiratory tract when inhaled, producing severe tracheobronchitis and pneumonitis. Certain compounds, such as phosgene, have relatively little effect on the proximal tracheobronchial tree but produce pulmonary edema by damaging the alveolar membrane. Treatment is supportive (antibiotics, oxygen) and is disappointingly ineffective.

Incapacitating Agents

A wide variety of pharmacologic effects may be utilized to produce temporary, nonlethal impairment of purposeful activity. Such effects include paralysis, rigidity, tremors, convulsions, postural hypotension, physiologic blindness and other physical effects, or hallucinations, delusions, delirium, depersonalization and other psychological effects. Treatment will depend on careful diagnosis and the postulation of logical pharmacological counteraction.

ARCTIC MEDICINE†

Military commitments today include the deployment of troops to all climates. In arctic combat, man is the limiting factor; his success will depend upon his state of fitness, training, initiative and adaptability. A temperature of $-30°$ F. is probably the lower limit for efficient, prolonged outdoor operations. At $-40°$ F., even animal activity is markedly reduced. At $-60°$ F., many kinds of outdoor activities become exceedingly difficult but by no means impossible.

The limitation of the soldier's ability to operate in a cold environment depends ultimately on his ability to maintain positive heat balance. This depends in turn on the severity of the environmental exposure, his heat production and his heat conservation, including insulation and clothing.

There are few, if any, specific evidences of general physiologic acclimatization in man. From a practical standpoint, such changes are in any case small compared with the importance of factors such as accustomization, experience, training and fitness. On the other hand, there may be some clear-cut evidence of local acclimatization to cold, such as the maintenance of high skin temperature and blood flow of the face and the hands during cold exposure in cold-acclimatized individuals.

* Col. Douglas Lindsey, M. C.

† Dr. Kaare Rodahl.

The present military arctic uniform, providing somewhat less than 4 clo units, would offer adequate protection during moderate or light work at −40° F. when there is protection from the wind. During prolonged periods of exposure more severe than this, the soldier has to rely on physical exercise to augment heat production in order to maintain thermal balance. Therefore, a high level of physical fitness is essential in cold-weather operation, and simple, heated shelters should be provided whenever possible for troops who are resting. Casualties must be protected immediately.

The caloric requirements of troops in the Arctic are only slightly higher than those of soldiers stationed in temperate climates, the difference being due mainly to the hobbling effect of the Arctic winter clothing and the greater energy expenditure required by movement through snow, etc. The percentage of calories furnished by protein, fat and carbohydrate in the diet of American troops living in Alaska is not significantly different from that reported for United States troops eating a garrison ration in temperate or tropical climates. There is no increased metabolism in the clothed man exposed to the Arctic environment under normal conditions of environmental protection. Nor is there any increase in thyroid activity under these conditions.

To a great extent, the success of the Arctic soldier will depend on his ability to adapt himself psychologically to the cold environment, to overcome his fear of the cold and to realize that snow is a very excellent protector against cold. Nevertheless, he must be aware of hazards such as hypothermia and frostbite. A severe degree of hypothermia may occur, especially in soldiers who are forced to remain inactive in extreme cold—for instance, while under fire in a foxhole. The recommended treatment is rapid rewarming. First-degree frostbite is a minor matter, commonly experienced by all who live or work in a cold environment. The treatment is simply to warm the frozen skin by applying heat.

REFERENCES

1. Altemeier, W. A., and Furste, W. L.: The problem of gas gangrene. *In:* Advances in Military Medicine. vol. 1. Boston, Little, Brown & Co., 1948.
2. Artz, C. P., Howard, J. M., Sako, Y., Bronwell, A. W., and Prentice, T. C.: Clinical experiences in the early management of the most severely injured battle casualties Ann. Surg., 141:285-296, 1955.
3. Beebe, G. W., and DeBakey, M. E.: Battle Casualties. Springfield, Ill., Charles C Thomas, 1952.
4. Board for the Study of the Severely Wounded: The Physiological Effects of Wounds. Washington, D.C., U. S. Government Printing Office, 1952.
5. Bronwell, A. S., Artz, C. P., and Sako, Y.: Abdominal and thoraco-abdominal wounds. *In:* Recent Advances in Medicine and Surgery, Based on Professional Medical Experiences in Japan and Korea, 1950-1953. vol. 1. Medical Science Publication No. 4, Washington, D.C., Army Medical Service Graduate School, 1954.
6. Campbell, E., and Meirowsky, A.: Penetrating wounds of the spinal cord. *In:* Bowers, W. F. (ed.): Surgery of Trauma. Philadelphia, J. B. Lippincott, 1953.
7. Coupal, J. F.: Pathology of gas gangrene following war wounds. *In:* The Medical Department of the United States Army in the World War. vol. 12. section 2. U. S. Government Printing Office, 1929.
8. De Bakey, M. E., and Simeone, F. A.: Battle injuries of the arteries in World War II: an analysis of 2,471 cases. Ann. Surg., 123:534-579, 1946.
9. Edsall, G.: Immunization of adults against diphtheria and tetanus. Am. J. Pub. Health, 42:393-400, 1952.
10. Edwards, J. E.: Practical considerations in the treatment of eye casualties. *In:* Recent Advances in Medicine and Surgery, Based on Professional Medical Experiences in Japan and Korea, 1950-1953. vol. 1. Medical Science Publication No. 4, Washington, D.C., Army Medical Service Graduate School, 1954.
11. Forsee, J. H.: Thoracic wounds. *In:* Bowers, W. F. (ed.): Surgery of Trauma. Philadelphia, J. B. Lippincott, 1953.
12. Glenn, F.: Tetanus—a preventable disease. Including an experience with civilian casualties in the battle for Manila (1945). Ann. Surg., 124:1030-1040, 1946.
13. Grant, R. T., and Reeve, E. B.: Observations on the General Effects of Injury in Man. With Special Reference to Wound Shock. Medical Research Council Special Report No. 277, London, 1951.
14. Hampton, D.: Wounds of joints. *In:* Bowers,. W. E. (ed.): Surgery of Trauma. Philadelphia, J. B. Lippincott, 1953.
15. Hardaway, Robert, *et al.*: Intensive study and treatment of shock in man. J.A.M.A., 199:779, 1967.
16. Holmes, R. H.: Wound ballistics and body armor. J.A.M.A., 150:73-78, 1952.
17. Holmes, R. H., Enos, W. F., Jr., and Beyer, J. C.: Medical aspects of body armor in Korea. *In:* Recent Advances in Medicine and Surgery, Based

on Professional Medical Experiences in Japan and Korea, 1950-1953. vol. 1. Medical Science Publication No. 4, Washington, D.C., Army Medical Service Graduate School, 1954.
18. Howard, J. M.: The battle wound. Mil. Med., 117:247-256, 1955.
19. Howard, J. M., and Inui, F. K.: Clostridial myositis—gas gangrene. Observations of battle casualties in Korea. Surgery, 36:1115-1118, 1954.
20. Howard, J. M., Olney, J. M., Frawley, J. P., Peterson, R. E., Smith, L. H., Davis, J. H., Guerra, S., and Dibrell, W. H.: Studies of adrenal function in combat and wounded soldiers. A study in the Korean Theatre. Ann. Surg., 141:314-320, 1955.
21. Inui, F. K., Shannon, J., and Howard, J. M.: Arterial injuries in the Korean War: experiences with 111 consecutive injuries. Surgery, 37:850-857, 1955.
22. Lindberg, R. B., Wetzler, T. F., Marshall, J. D., Newton, R., Strawitz, J. G., and Howard, J. M.: The bacterial flora of battle wounds at the time of primary débridement. Ann. Surg., 141:369-374, 1955.
23. Lindberg, R. B., Wetzler, T. F., Newton, A., Howard, J. M., Davis, J. H., Strawitz, J. G., and Wynn, J. H.: The bacterial flora of the blood stream in the Korean battle casualty. Ann. Surg., 141:366-368, 1955.
24. Matson, D. D.: The Treatment of Craniocerebral Injuries Due to Missiles. Springfield, Ill., Charles C Thomas, 1948.
25. Medical and Surgical History of the War of the Rebellion. Third Surgical Volume. Washington, D.C., Government Printing Office, 1883.
26. Munro, D.: The rehabilitation of patients totally paralyzed below the waist, wlth special reference to making them ambulatory and capable of earning their living. 3. Tidal drainage, cystometry and bladder training. New Eng. J. Med. 236:223-235, 1947.
27. Munro, D., and Hahn, J.: Tidal drainage of the urinary bladder: a preliminary report of this method of treatment as applied to "cord bladders" with a description of the apparatus. New Eng. J. Med., 212:229-239, 1935.
28. North, J. P.: Clostridial wound infections and gas gangrene. Surgery, 21:364-372, 1947.
29. Office of the Surgeon General of the Army /MSA. Report of 9 Sept. 1968.
30. Orr, K. D.: Developments in prevention and treatment of cold injury. In: Recent Advances in Medicine and Surgery, Based on Professional Medical Experiences in Japan and Korea, 1950-1953. vol. 2. Washington, D.C., Army Medical Service Graduate School, 1954.
31. Pettit, R. T.: Infections of wounds of war J.A.M.A., 73:494, 1919.
32. Prentice, T. C., Olney, J. M., Artz, C. P., and Howard, J. M.: Studies of blood volume and transfusion therapy in the Korean battle casualty. Surg., Gynec., Obstet., 99:542-554, 1954.
33. Pulaski, E. J.: War wounds. New Eng. J. Med., 249:890-897 and 932-938, 1953.
34. Report of Casualties. Released by OSD Sept. 5, 1968.
35. Sako, Y., Artz, C. P., Howard, J. M., Bronwell, A. W., and Inui, F. K.: A study of evacuation, resuscitation and mortality in a forward surgical hospital. Surgery, 37:602-611, 1955.
36. Sborov, V. M., Giges, B., and Mann, J. D.: Incidence of hepatitis following use of pooled plasma. A follow-up study in 587 Korean casualties. Arch. Int. Med., 92:678-683, 1953.
37. Silliphant, W. M.: Wound ballistics. Mil. Med., 117:238-246, 1955.
38. Smith, L. H., Jr., et al.: Post-traumatic renal insufficiency in military casualties. II. Management; use of an artificial kidney; prognosis. Am. J. Med., 18:187-198, 1955.
39. Strawitz, J. G., Wetzler, T. F., Marshall, J. D., Lindberg, R. B., Howard J. M., and Artz, C. P.: The bacterial flora of healing wounds. Surgery, 37:400-408, 1955.
40. Teschan, P. E., et al.: Post-traumatic renal insufficiency in military casualties. 1 and 2. Am. J. Med., 18:172-198, 1955.
41. Valle, A. R.: An analysis of 2,811 chest casualties of the Korean conflict. In: Recent Advances in Medicine and Surgery, Based on Professional Medical Experiences in Japan and Korea, 1950-1953. vol. 1. Medical Science Publication No. 4, Washington, D.C., Army Medical Service Graduate School, 1954.
42. Woodhall, B., and Nulsen, F.: Peripheral nerve wounds. In: Bowers, W. F. (ed.): Surgery of Trauma. Philadelphia, J. B. Lippincott, 1953.

CHAPTER 26

CARL A. MOYER, M.D., AND JONATHAN E. RHOADS, M.D.

Skin and Subcutaneous Tissues

Introduction
Benign Tumors of the Skin
Malignant Tumors of the Skin

INTRODUCTION

The skin, as the dermatologists point out, is the largest organ of the body. It is a highly complex system of tissues capable of many and unexplained reactions. It is subject to immediate contact with the environment and hence to many types of trauma—mechanical, thermal, chemical or that due to ionizing radiation. It is a major defense against microorganisms but may become invaded by them. Likewise, it is a common site for tumors, both benign and malignant in type. Some of the skin elements extend into the subcutaneous tissue, and the subcutaneous fat and connective tissue layer is the site of an additional group of diseases, as well as being in a position to be involved early by many of the diseases of the skin.

It is not intended in this chapter to present a systematic review of the many conditions arising in the skin and the subcutaneous tissue because a majority of these are treated in other chapters. Cross references will be provided for a discussion of most of the injuries and infections of the skin, and brief statements of the more common tumors of the skin and their management will be presented:

Abrasions and lacerations (see Chaps. 2, 24, 25 and 47)

Avulsions of the skin (see Chaps. 24, and 25)

Burns of the skin, see Chaps. 17 on burns and 18 (on radiation injury)

The common infections of the skin and the subcutaneous tissues are discussed in Chapters 4 and 24.

Acne. Only a few afflictions of the sebaceous glands have surgical significance. *Acne conglobata* and *acne aggregata seu conglobata* are chronic inflammatory diseases of the sebaceous glands of males after puberty. They are characterized by scores of comedones, and their pitted scars spread over all of the body excepting the palms and the soles. Acne conglobata is separable from acne aggregata by virtue of the association of abscesses, cutaneocutaneous fistulas, and sinuses with the former. Acne conglobata is especially troublesome when located over the lower sacrum, the buttocks and the perineum. When it is widespread it produces chronic illness and septic wasting. The diagnosis is made by biopsy. Excision of the whole of the skin containing the abscesses, the fistulas and the sinuses and the immediate coverage of the denudation with split-thickness autografts is the only way known of ridding the person of acne conglobata.

Deep within the perineal segment of acne conglobata pictured in Figure 26-1, a squamous cell carcinoma was found. This case does not constitute evidence of a causal relationship between acne conglobata and cutaneous squamous carcinoma but it does tell us to suspect their co-existence and to look for cancers within the lesion of acne conglobata.

Acne rosacea ("brandy nose, drunkard's face") in its advanced form, rhinophyma, peculiarly affects the nose and the forehead, producing great facial disfigurement. The nose becomes bulbous and splayed, and all of its earlier contours are buried by nodules and ridges of hyperplastic epidermis containing acnelike pustules. A person having this disease may be the butt of malicious gossip, especially should he be a theologian, a doctor, or a lawyer. Its synonyms such as "brandy nose," "brandy face" and "rosy drop" are indicative of public misconceptions regarding the alcoholic origin of this disease. Actually, it afflicts

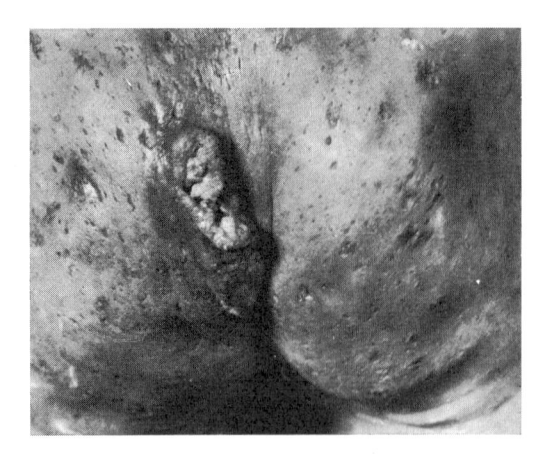

FIG. 26-1. Acne conglobata covering the sacral, the gluteal and the perianal regions of a man with a squamous carcinoma of the skin of the left buttock. All of the skin covering the buttocks and the perineum was excised with the carcinoma, and the cutaneous defect was covered immediately with split grafts that functioned successfully. (F.B., 52-5033)

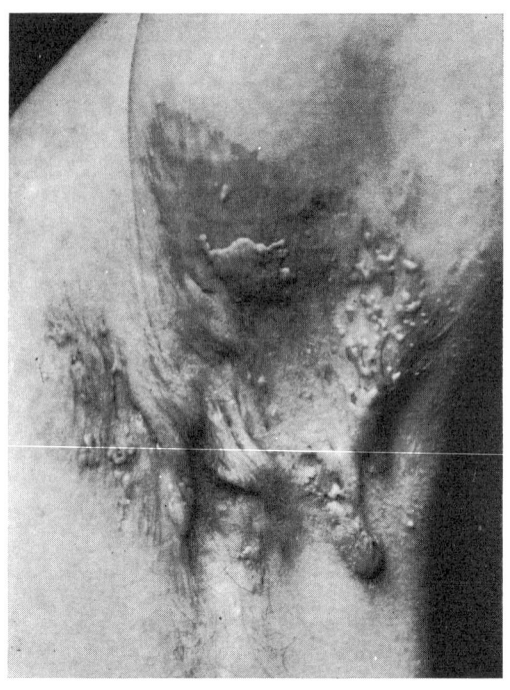

FIG. 26-2. Hidradenitis suppurativa of the right axilla. The skin of the entire axilla was excised and replaced immediately with split grafts. This cured the disease without cicatrix. (A.G., 52-4428)

both imbibers and abstainers just as the rain falls upon both the just and the unjust. The diagnosis is made readily by inspection and biopsy. The treatment is simply shaving off the hyperplastic epidermis. One experienced with the procedure should do it because one must have sufficient experience so as to know when to stop shaving the skin from the bulbous member.

Diseases of the Sweat Glands. The diseases of the sweat glands with which the surgeon needs be concerned are hyperhidrosis, hidradenitis suppurativa, and tumors of the sweat glands. *Hyperhidrosis* is rarely a primary affliction but it is often associated with a number of diseases. The "dripping paw or hand" appears to be of congenital or familial origin. It often becomes intolerable to nonmanual workers and is a menace to mechanics and other manual laborers. Actually, it is a bar to some trades such as tool- and die-making, watch-making and repair and other skilled trades in which *dry hands* are required. Anxiety states and palmar hyperhidrosis are associated very frequently. Hyperhidrosis often is one of the symptoms of such ills as Sudeck's atrophy, Raynaud's phenomenon, chronic pernio, livedo reticularis, chronic immersion foot or trench foot, and chronic dermatophytosis. A proper sympathectomy stops hyperhidrosis, whatever may be its cause.

Hidradenitis suppurativa (Fig. 26-2) is a chronic cicatrizing suppuration of apocrine sweat glands. Either staphylococci or streptococci, or both types of organisms, are isolatable from the suppurating lesions. It tends to spread steadily, ultimately involving the whole of the region in which it began. The axilla, the pubic, the perianal and the mammary regions are the corporal areas affected by the disease. Rarely, large subcutaneous abscesses complicate it. No antibiotic cures or even controls the disease for any appreciable length of time. The excision of all of the skin containing the infected glands, followed by its replacement with split grafts, cures the disease.

The tumors of sweat glands are biologic oddities: mixed tumor of the skin is practically never malignant and is especially prone to occur on the face and the palms and the soles; the turban tumor is benign and often attains great surface extent, completely covering the scalp or large areas of the back or the arms; the syringomas are benign yellow, soft small nodules that appear in the skin of the eyelids, the thighs and the trunks of girls at puberty. The hidradenoma is benign and occurs most frequently in the skin of the labium majus and the perianal region. The sweat gland carcinoma is malignant. The vulva, the scrotum and the axilla are its principal loci. They are reddish-purple, smooth, polypoid tumefactions. The sweat gland carcinomas should be widely excised because they are prone to persistent and recurrent growth. The diagnosis of all sweat gland tumors requires biopsy.

Cutaneous blastomycosis is often mistaken for cutaneous cancer. It begins as a small papule, enlarges slowly, ulcerates and heals centrally as the papulopustular lesions spread circumferentially (Fig. 26-3). The diagnosis is best made from a biopsy. Treatment consists of surgical excision of the lesion if the area can be encompassed readily and if systemic blastomycosis does not exist. Local and systemic therapy with amphotericin is the method of choice (Abernathy, R. S., 1966).* The prognosis is very good if the disease is localized.

Cutaneous tuberculosis has many forms. All of the forms are chronic, indolent, relatively painless papular or papulo-ulcerative lesions. The ulcerative forms are called scrofulous dermatitis or scrofuloderma, and the variants are descriptively designated as gummosa (deep ulcers), papular (superficial ulcers), pustular (mimicking furunculosis), verrucous (wartlike), papulonecrotica (papules and nodules which undergo necrosis). Shallowly ulcerative tuberculosis of the skin about body orifices—the mouth, vagina and anus—is called T. cutis orificialis or T. ulcerosa. Tuberculosis cutis indurativa is a chronic, deep, indurative and ulcerative tuberculosis of the skin of girls that is recurrent. The early lesion is a bluish plaque. Tuberculosis paronychia is an indolent, chronic painless lesion of the fingers. Diagnosis is made by biopsy and culture.

---

*Abernathy, R. S.: Amphotericin therapy of North American blastomycosis. Antimicrob. Agents Chemother., 6:208, 1966.

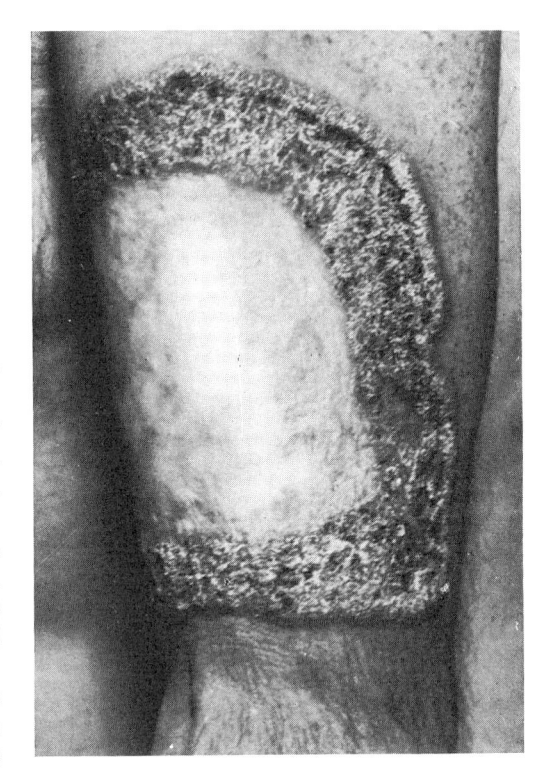

FIG. 26-3. Blastomycosis of the skin with central healing and scarring.

Treatment is medical with streptomycin, para-aminobenzoic acid and isoniazid, singly or in appropriate combinations.

Molluscum contagiosum is a viral disease of the pox group occurring mainly on the face, the arms and the genital regions.

It appears singly or in groups of small, discrete, firm, gray-white hemispherical nodules having umbilicated central areas. It is often mistaken for basal cell carcinoma.

The diagnosis is made by biopsy.

Surgical removal of the lesions is curative. Oxytetracycline has been reported to effect regression of the lesions.

Granuloma annulare is a lesion of unknown etiology, consisting of hard red nodules which gradually enlarge to form a red ring or plaque in skin, often on the extremities. It may be confused with early cutaneous blastomycosis and cutaneous neoplastic metastases. Biopsy is needed to make the diagnosis. The lesion resolves rapidly when treated with ointments containing glucogenic adrenocortical steroids.

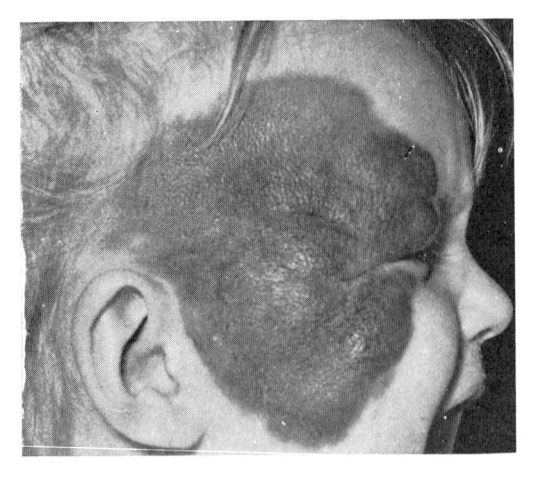

Fig. 26-4. (*Top*) Large hairy benign nevus in a child. This type of lesion is not prone to malignancy. (*Right*) Large blue benign nevus of the lower extremity. Note the intact covering epithelium. This type of nevus is not prone to malignancy.

cised in administering it. Large doses of vitamin A (50,000 units daily) for weeks or months have been regarded as helpful. The subverrucous injection of 1 per cent procaine has also been followed by their disappearance in some instances. Surgical excision is sometimes necessary, but recurrence is not rare, and it should be remembered that plantar skin is specialized, and grafted skin tends to break down in this area under the stress of weight-bearing. Therefore, the amount of plantar skin which can be sacrificed with impunity is small. Furthermore, healing on the foot is slow, and use militates against primary healing so that a considerable period of rest (2 or more weeks)

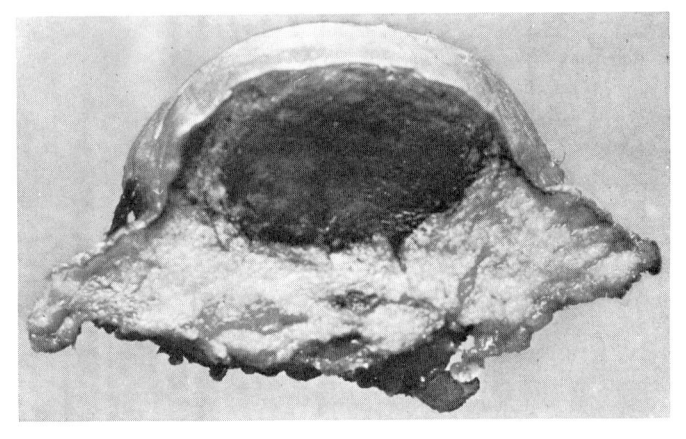

BENIGN TUMORS OF THE SKIN

Warts (Verrucae)

One of the commonest tumors of the skin is the ordinary wart (verruca vulgaris). It has been demonstrated that this lesion is due to a virus, and it is not uncommon to see groups of warts appear close together. They are especially common on the hands. Often they will persist for months or years and then may disappear inexplicably. Excision is sometimes followed by recurrence but is usually successful in chronic lesions. Small doses of irradiation often lead to regression. Another method which has been successful at times is the injection of vaccinia virus beneath the lesion. This should not be done in a person who has not been vaccinated recently, lest a "take" occur in an unfavorable area.

Plantar warts often cause marked disability. Sometimes small doses of x-ray therapy have been helpful, but great care must be exercised is often advisable if excision is carried out. Deep curettement under local anesthesia and cautery of the bleeding dermal base with lunar caustic (solid $AgNO_3$) or electrocautery once or twice will cure practically all plantar warts.

Venereal Warts (Condyloma Lata and Condyloma Acuminata) (see Chap. 40)

The Mole or Nevus

Although the term "mole" is used rather indiscriminately for any elevated thickening of the skin, it usually refers to the nevus, which is a small tumor of the skin, ordinarily benign but capable of appearing in a malignant form, the melanoma. The nevus may occur in both a pigmented and nonpigmented form. It may present hair growth or absence of hair growth. The areas may be small and elevated or even pedunculated, or they may be flat. They may be as small as 1 or 2 mm. in diameter, or they may extend over an area of many centimeters (Fig. 26-4).

FIG. 26-5. Pigmented mole (compound type). Note "nevus cells" in dermis and at dermal epidermal junction.

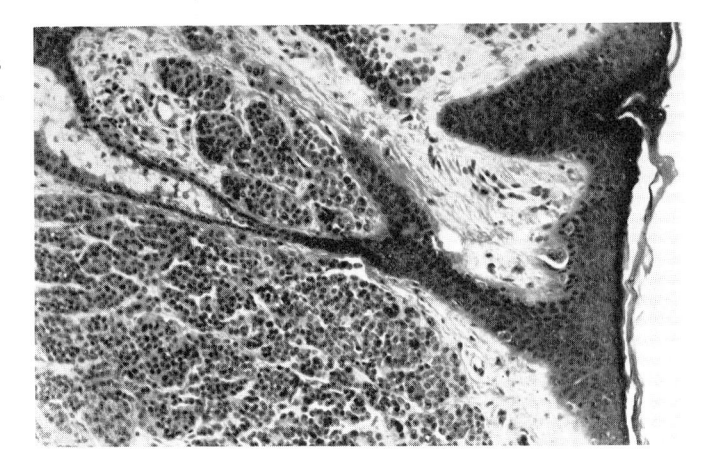

A typical one is about 1.5 cm. in diameter, somewhat raised from the surface of the surrounding skin, soft and pliable, brown to black in color, and subject to considerable bleeding on light trauma due to the fact that the cornified layer is very thin and that many of these lesions are rather vascular. In the past, many of these have been removed by electrocoagulation. This method is not advised because it affords no chance for histologic examination of the tissue, and there is always a real possibility that destruction of the lesion will be incomplete. These lesions are characterized by the presence of mole cells (see Fig. 26-5), and the color is determined by the amount of pigment or melanin which the particular lesion produces.

(For malignant melanomas see section on Malignant Tumors of the Skin.)

Vascular Tumors or Angiomas

These are sometimes hemangiomas and sometimes lymphangiomas, and sometimes there are a mixture of the two. The "capillary" hemangiomas are red areas of the skin, with or without thickening, and these comprise the commonest form of birthmark. In the newborn these lesions sometimes show a tendency to decrease in size or to go away during the first year (Fig. 26-6). Many physicians prefer to wait 6 to 12 months before instituting definitive therapy unless the tumor is very large or becomes ulcerated and/or infected.

In infancy they are sometimes treated with x-rays in the hope of blanching them, but in view of the hazards of radiation in infancy which have been demonstrated in the cervical and the mediastinal areas (see Chap. 28), it is preferable to remove them surgically when they ulcerate or grow rapidly, or to neglect them if they are not seriously disfiguring. They have also been attacked by cryotherapy (freezing), but it is doubtful whether this form of destruction has material advantages over

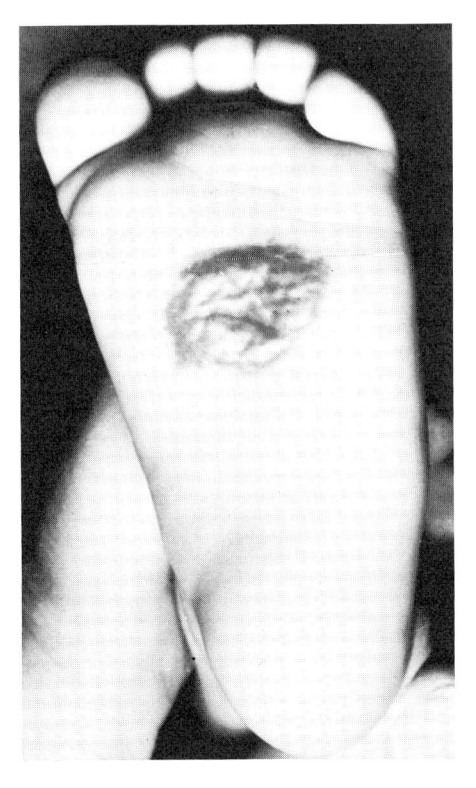

FIG. 26-6. Capillary hemangioma in an unusual location, on the plantar surface of the foot in a child.

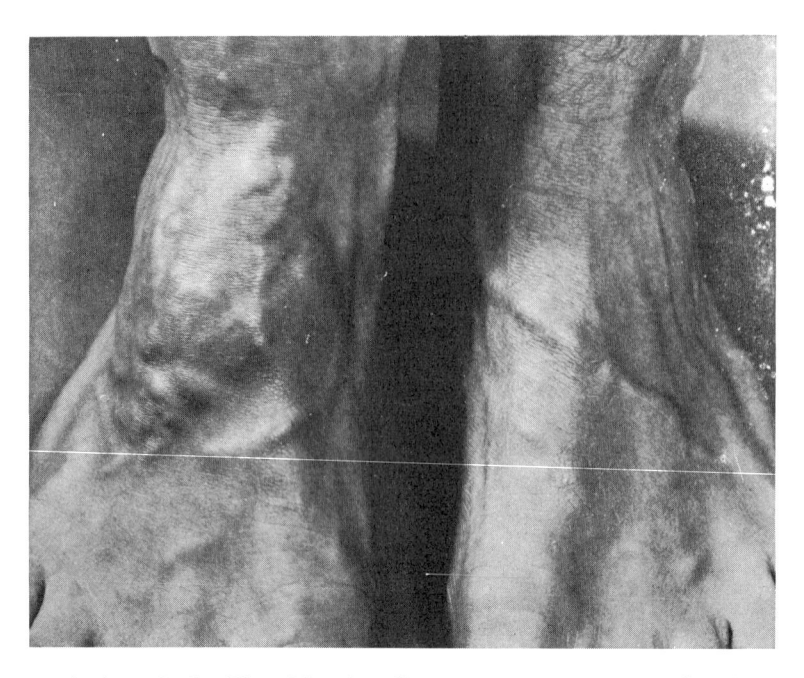

654 Skin and Subcutaneous Tissues

FIG. 26-7. Cavernous hemangioma of the dorsal surface of the ankle without overgrowth of the part.

surgical methods. The risk of malignancy in these lesions is small, and a great many people carry them throughout their lives without difficulty. Small ones are very common and are present on close inspection of the body surface of a large percentage of individuals. The indications for removal are usually three: (1) cosmetic reasons; (2) confusion with moles in an area of the body which may be subject to irritation; and (3) suspicion of hemangio-endothelioma which can occur in a malignant form.

Cavernous Hemangioma. Deeper angiomas containing large vascular lakes are often called cavernous hemangiomas (Fig. 26-7). If they are large and extend deeply into muscles or between the structures of the hands and the feet, their removal may be a difficult or impossible task. Hemorrhage from them may be formidable.

A peculiar variant of the cavernous hemangioma is the diffuse dermal, subcutaneous, and intermuscular and intramuscular angioma attended by a remarkable overgrowth of the part of the body wherein it is located (Fig. 26-8). It most often involves the lower ex-

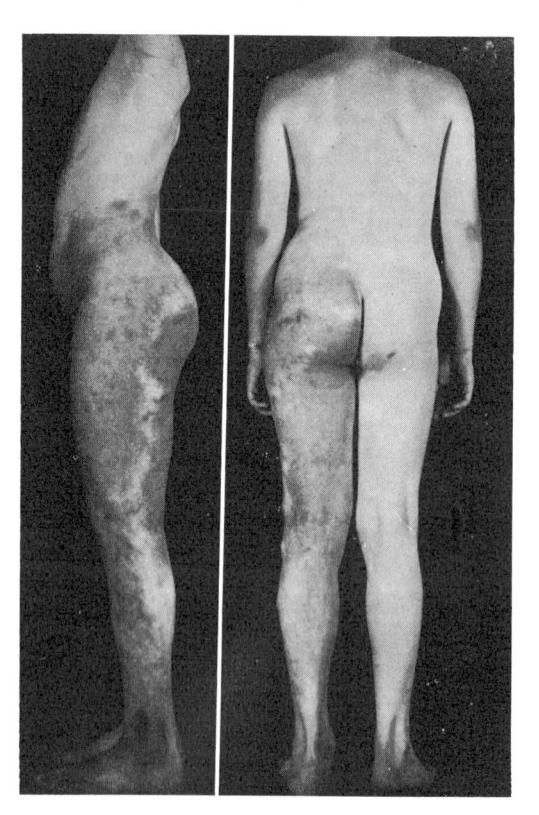

FIG. 26-8. Boy of 11 years with an extensive cutaneous hemangioma of the left leg, thigh and lower torso. There are extensive venous varicosities, overgrowth of the left femur, tibia, fibula, and bones of the foot, and an ulcer overlying the outer aspect of the left ankle.

Fig. 26-9. Superficial lymphangioma of the lower eyelid.

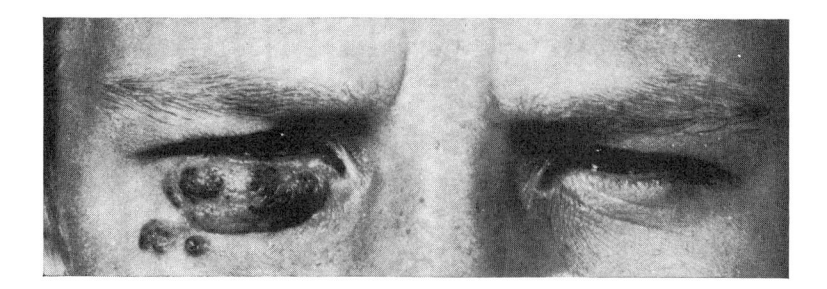

tremity, producing excessively rapid growth of the bones of the leg distal to the upper visible limits of the lesion. Extensive varicose veins and stasis ulceration appear very early. As time passes, grossly detectable arteriovenous communications with audible continuous bruits and systemic signs such as polycythemia and cardiac enlargement appear.

Treatment of the varicose veins is often attempted because they are so large. As a rule they cannot be eradicated completely by any suitable means.

The ligation of major arteries to the extremity effects only temporary benefit. Only excision of the lesion or amputation of the part will cure it. X-ray therapy is useless.

Lymphangiomas. There are 3 main varieties: lymphangioma simplex, lymphangioma cutis circumscriptum and lymphangioma cysticum. They are all benign tumors.

LYMPHANGIOMA SIMPLEX is a grayish pink, soft cutaneous nodule and often is associated with lymphangiectatic macroglossia. The tongue associated with lymphangioma simplex weeps lymph continuously from eroded dilated lymphatics that protrude above the mucosal surface and are covered by very thin epithelium. These lymphatic protrusions give the tongue, anterior to the circumvallate papillae, the appearance of being covered with hair.

Surgical excision of part of the tongue is requisite for the prevention of macrocheilia and chronic ulceration of the tongue.

Excision of the lymphangioma simplex is indicated solely for the improvement of appearance and effecting certainty of diagnosis.

LYMPHANGIOMA CUTIS CIRCUMSCRIPTA appear as soft warts. They may be removed for appearance's sake.

LYMPHANGIOMA CYSTICUM (Fig. 26-10) is a soft cystic tumor covered with normal skin appearing predominantly in the neck, the mediastinum and the axilla. When limited to the neck it is called *hygroma colli* or cystic hygroma. Nine tenths of these tumors appear before the age of 2. Usually their growth period is limited, and they disappear from sight during late childhood. However, they may become infected and occasionally become so large as to interfere with deglutition and breathing. Drainage of infected tumors should be performed whenever a frank abscess occurs or antibiotics are ineffective.

Excision is indicated whenever they inter-

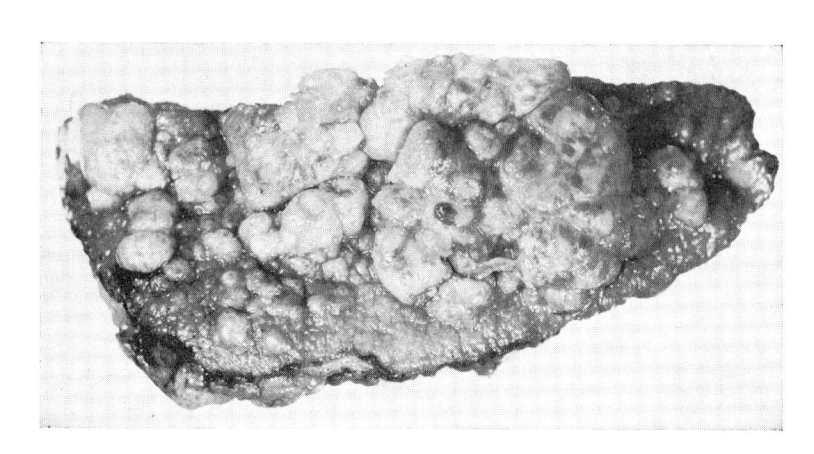

Fig. 26-10. Large complex cystic lymphangioma of the skin.

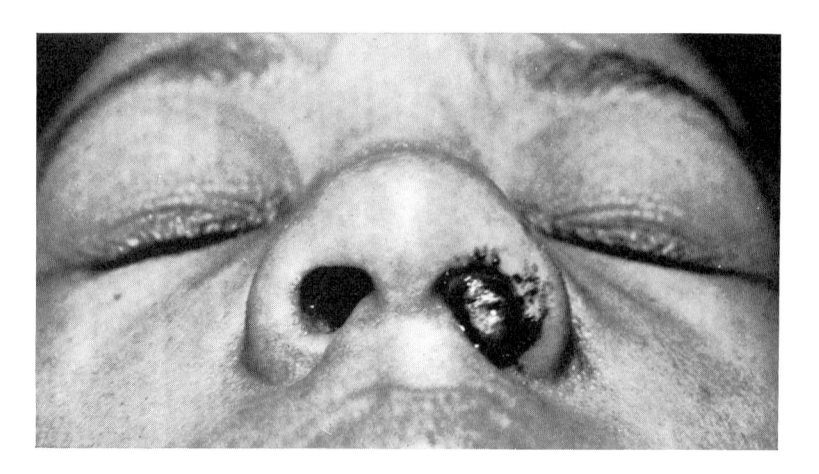

FIG. 26-11. Juvenile fibroma protruding from the nares.

fere with breathing or swallowing. Preparations for the transfusion of blood should be made before undertaking their extirpation. The operation is difficult, and blood loss is relatively large in many instances.

Juvenile nasopharyngeal angiofibroma (fibroid of adolescence) is a highly vascular nasopharyngeal lesion largely peculiar to adolescent boys. It is a smooth fibrous tumor which bleeds profusely when traumatized and at times may fill the nasal cavity (Fig. 26-11). When large they may erode contiguous bones and thereby be mistaken for sarcoma.

Biopsy is requisite for diagnosis. Because they have no malignant propensity and most of them regress spontaneously during the second decade of life, excision need not be performed unless recurrent exsanguinating epistaxis occurs or they are otherwise symptomatically very troublesome.

The excision of a juvenile nasopharyngeal angiofibroma is often a disquietingly, and at times, a dangerously hemorrhagic affair. For this reason preparations for the transfusion of much blood should be made before the excision.

Glomus Tumor (see Chap. 24)

Lipomas

A very common subcutaneous tumor is the lipoma. It is composed mainly of fat and is sometimes difficult to distinguish from normal subcutaneous tissue. It is characterized by a thin, fibrous capsule and varying amounts of fibrous tissue, forming trabeculae which run through it. The trabeculae frequently extend somewhat beyond it, with the result that lateral pressure upon the subcutaneous mass may produce a slightly dimpled or cobblestone appearance of the skin overlying the lesion.

By definition, a lipoma is a benign, fatty tumor, whereas the malignant forms are called liposarcomas. Fortunately, the benign variety greatly predominates, and liposarcomas, while not rare, are infrequent. Whether they represent malignant degeneration of a lipoma or a separate cell species from the beginning is uncertain.

The benign lipomas are especially frequent over the back and the shoulders and the interscapular area of the back. If a linear incision is made down to the fibrous capsule, many of them shell out quite easily. Others have firmer attachments to the surrounding tissues. Their removal often leaves a considerable dead space which may tend to collect serum, with the result that primary healing is not always obtained. Such tumors may range from a very small size to a very large size. Treatment consists of excision. Some physicians advise doing nothing when these lesions are asymptomatic and apparently not growing. However, they may be confused with small sweat gland carcinomas, occasionally with sebaceous cysts, occasionally with neurilemmomas, granular cell myoblastomas and a few rare lesions such as malignant neurilemmomas, rhabdomyosarcomas, et cetera. For these reasons the authors are inclined to recommend their removal unless important contraindications are present.

Fat Necrosis. Localized traumatic fat necrosis is a benign lesion which is often grossly indistinguishable from an infiltrating neoplasm. Its sites of predilection are the breasts, the buttocks and areas subject to hypodermic injections. Characteristically, it appears some time after the injury or injection as a well-defined though nondiscrete unencapsulated mass. It is often cystic. The skin overlying it is more or less fixed to it.

Excepting when located over points subject to pressure it is practically symptomless. By virtue of the impossibility of distinguishing fat necrosis within the breast from mammary cancer without a microscopic examination, its diagnosis should not be assumed excepting after biopsy.

Excision is curative.

Weber-Christian disease or idiopathic panniculitis is a peculiar lesion of fat involving the skin immediately over it. When located upon the legs, as it often is, usually it is mistaken initially for stasis dermatitis, acute thrombophlebitis, or cellulitis. A similar condition occasionally may afflict the omentum and the mesentery.

In the early phase, it is a painful, irregular, sharply circumscribed, thick plaque covered by reddened, tender, slightly edematous, immobile skin. As the lesion resolves the involved subcutaneous panniculus practically disappears, leaving a crater lined by abnormally thin skin.

Biopsy is requisite for diagnosis. The removal of medications and salt containing iodine and the administration of cortisone, prednisone, or prednisolone usually effect a remarkably rapid resolution of the process. Should treatment with steroids fail, excision of the involved skin and fat and the immediate coverage of the defect with a thick partial-thickness autograft of skin shortens the period of disability.

Xanthoma

A subcutaneous or intracutaneous deposit of a yellowish character not infrequently appears on the eyelid. These are called xanthomata and are due to a deposit of cholesterol in the tissues. They sometimes, but not always, signify hypercholesterolemia and sometimes, but not always, indicate a tendency toward atherosclerosis. Occasionally, they will disappear in individuals who are successful in lowering their blood cholesterol concentrations by taking a very low fat diet. Usually, surgical treatment is not indicated.

Myxoma

These tumors are of mesenchymal origin and are associated with a relatively large production of ground substance. They occur both in benign and malignant form and may arise in the subcutaneous tissues involving the skin

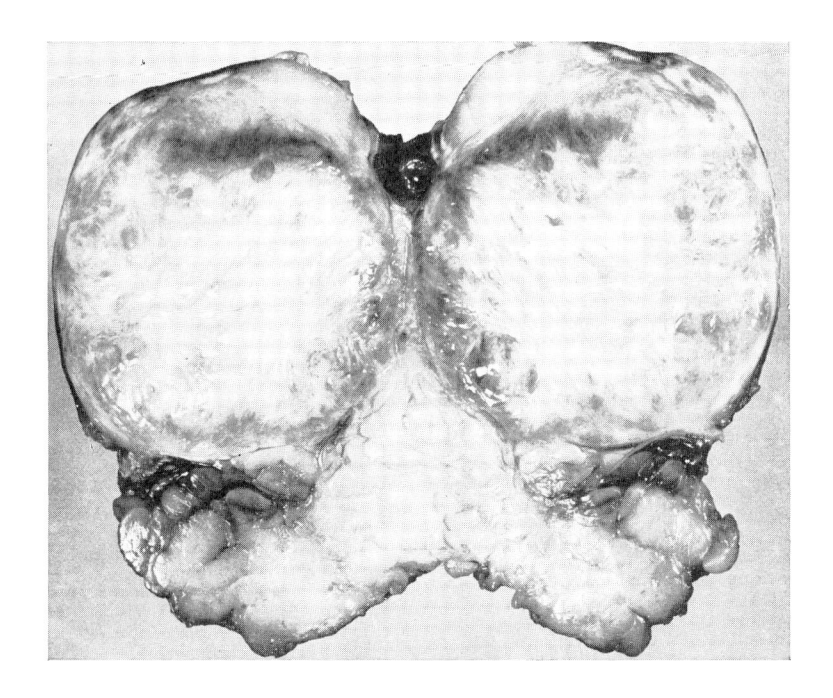

Fig. 26-12. Classic example of a desmoid tumor of the abdominal wall. Note fibrous tissue replacement of muscle.

658   Skin and Subcutaneous Tissues

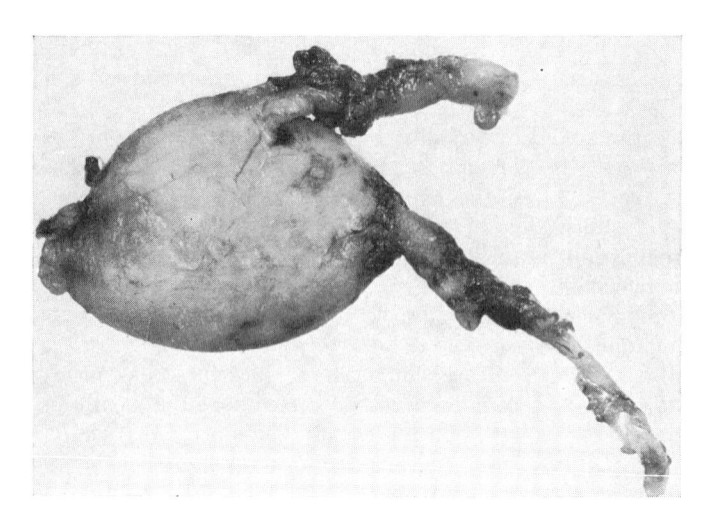

FIG. 26-13. A well-delimited neurilemmoma with nerve filaments expanding over its surface. This type of neurogenous tumor does not often become malignant.

or in the deeper tissues. Diagnosis is usually made microscopically subsequent to excision or biopsy. Treatment is excision where possible.

DESMOID TUMOR

The desmoid tumor is found in various areas such as the abdominal wall, usually in muscle. It consists of firm, fibrous tissue. Excision is apt to be carried out in order to establish the diagnosis, though it is not clear that the course might not be benign if it were not removed. However, occasionally the desmoid is locally invasive, and when located within the pelvis or about the hip or the axilla it may produce severe pain by virtue of its growth into large nerves. When this is threatened, the tumor must be extirpated (Fig. 26-12). A hemipelvectomy may even be needed in exceptional cases of pelvic desmoids when recurrent.

NEURILEMMOMA

Neurilemmoma is a tumor arising from the sheath cells of Schwann and formerly was

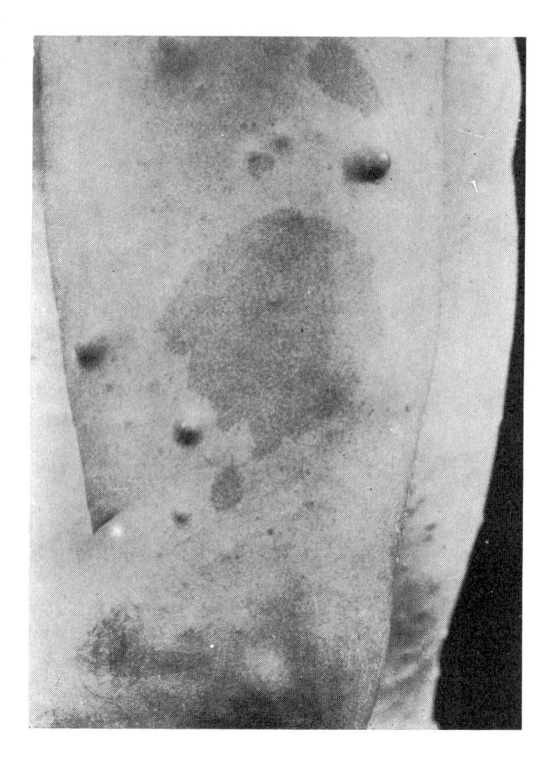

FIG. 26-14. Neurofibromatosis (von Recklinghausen's disease) with multiple fibromata and café-au-lait spots. The tumors are soft.

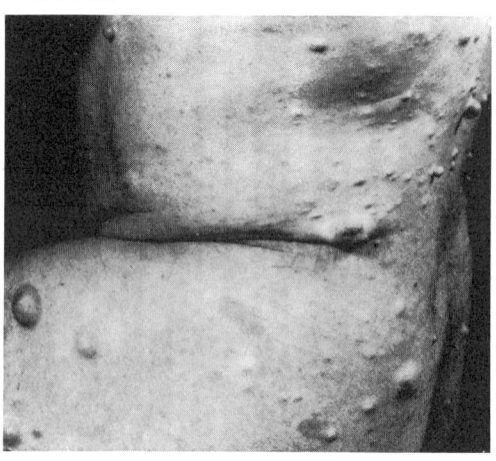

called a schwannoma. These tumors arise along nerve trunks but are not infrequent on the extremities, as well as within the interior of the body. Furthermore, they frequently arise from relatively small nerves. Characteristically, they do not produce much pain, so that the diagnosis should not be excluded because pain is lacking (Fig. 26-13).

Treatment is excision. A small proportion of these tumors show malignant changes. The author (J.E.R.) encountered one malignant neurilemmoma in the lower part of the back which recurred locally and metastasized to the lung on the opposite side of the body with a fatal issue, despite seemingly liberal resection of the original lesion and the surrounding tissue.

NEUROFIBROMA

These are subcutaneous masses of neurofibromatous tissue, usually multiple. They are soft and usually may be easily depressed into the subcutaneous tissue with a little pressure upon them. When pressed upon by a thin object such as a sharpened pencil, they deform only beneath the point of pressure, permitting the tip of the pencil to be depressed 5 to 10 mm. without deforming the contour of the mass. This has been termed pressure umbilication and differentiates cutaneous neurofibroma from fibroma, lipoma, and sebaceous cysts. In the multiple form, this condition is known as von Recklinghausen's disease. The masses sometimes cause protrusions of the skin which form hanging grapelike masses of tissue. These tend slowly to grow in the course of life and may become quite troublesome in the later years. These tumors are widely distributed within the body as well as in the skin. When located within osseously confined spaces they produce difficulty such as deafness and signs of cerebellopontine angle tumor when growing from the 7th or the 8th cranial nerves in the internal auditory canal and into the posterior fossa; they cause paralyses when growing from spinal nerve roots into the spinal canal and exophthalmos when arising from nerves within the orbit. Persons with neurofibromatosis are prone to develop certain other tumors, namely, meningioma; gliomas, including glioma of the optic nerve, especially in children; pheochromocytoma, (rarely) fibromas of colon (Chap. 39); and other diseases, such as localized gigantism, fibrous dysplasia, subperiosteal bone cysts, scoliosis and pseudoarthrosis. In addition, with von Recklinghausen's disease sarcomatous degeneration of one or more of the neurofibromas occurs in 5 to 10 per cent of cases. There is no effective treatment other than excision of particular tumors that are giving symptoms. (See Chap. 47, Carcinoma of the Lung.)

GRANULAR CELL MYOBLASTOMA

This tumor may present as a nodule under the skin or mucous membrane, particularly in the tongue. Histologically, it is composed of nests of large cells with small round nuclei and cytoplasm stippled with eosinophilic granules. The origin of these cells has not been definitely determined, although many sources have been suggested, such as striated muscle, nervous tissue, endothelial cells and fibroblasts. Most observers lean toward the former myogenic origin. A distinctive feature of this tumor is the characteristic pseudoepithelial hyperplasia overlying the lesion which may simulate squamous cell carcinoma. Many observers believe that this lesion represents the lowest grade of muscle tumors in which there may be a transition to the highly malignant rhabdomyosarcoma (Murphy, et al.*). Allen† feels that this transition cannot be substantiated and prefers to regard the tumor as a distinct and benign entity with its histogenesis still unsolved. Simple excision is the treatment.

Calcifying Epithelioma of Malherke. This peculiar tumor seemingly arises from skin appendage precursor cells. It is a benign tumor appearing most often on the face and the upper extremities and often occurs in children.

The lesion is a hard, rounded, well-demarcated nodule located in the deep dermis or the subcutaneous fat and frequently contains calcium, and rarely bone.

It is treated by excision.

Keratoacanthoma (Molluscum Sebaceum, Self-healing Epidermoid Carcinoma) (Fig. 26-15). This is a benign, usually self-limited, cutaneous, tumorous affliction that is readily confused clinically and occasionally confused

---

* Murphy, G. H., Dockerty, M. B., and Broders, A. C.: Myoblastoma, Am. J. Path. 25:1157-1181, 1949.

† Allen, A. C.: The Skin: A Clinicopathological Treatise, St. Louis, Mosby, 1954.

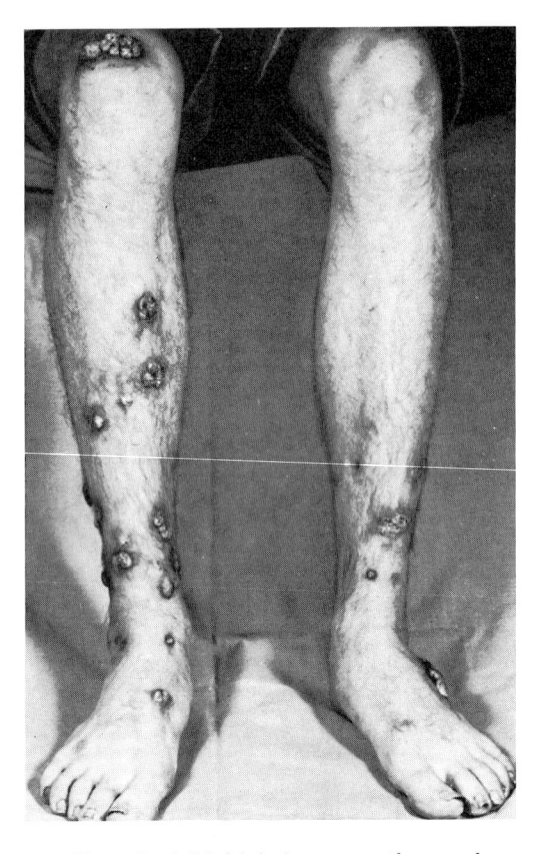

FIG. 26-15. Multiple keratoacanthoma of the skin. These lesions may be mistaken for epidermoid carcinoma, clinically and microscopically.

microscopically with epidermoid carcinoma.

The tumors tend to come and go singly or in crops over many years. Because a well-documented case of malignant transformation is lacking and the disease tends to be self-limited, excision of the lesions need not be practiced after the diagnosis is made.

Dermatofibrosarcoma Protuberans. This rare tumor arises within the connective tissue of the dermis (Fig. 26-16). It is a malignant tumor in that it is locally invasive, though it practically never metastasizes. It first appears as slowly growing, reddish, firm nodules which in time coalesce to form large multinodular masses that may ulcerate. It is usually curable by simple local excision without resection of contiguous lymphatic vessels or nodes. It may recur locally if excised inadequately. Distant metastases practically never occur.

Subepidermal Nodular Fibrosis (Sclerosing Hemangioma, Dermatofibroma Lenticulare, Histiocytoma). Subepidermal nodular fibrosis (Fig. 26-17) is a benign tumor of dermal origin occurring chiefly on the extremities and possibly incited by trauma. It usually appears as a small, nonpainful and nontender nodule or depressed area within the skin. The overlying epidermis is frequently pigmented. Often it is mistaken microscopically for fibrosarcoma or malignant melanoma.

Keloid (Fig. 26-18). When devoid of its cutaneous covering a keloid is practically indistinguishable cellularly from a desmoid. It is a fibrous tissue tumor that appears after

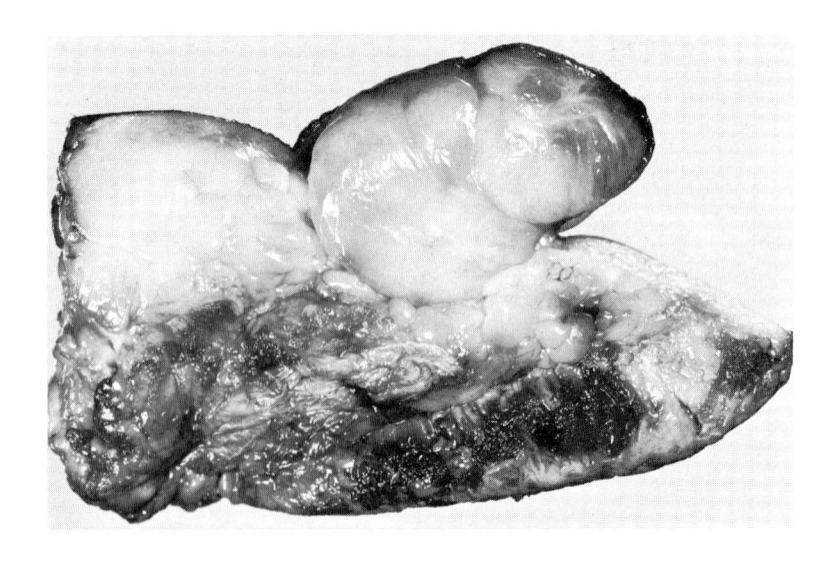

FIG. 26-16. Gross photograph of dermatofibrosarcoma protuberans with its typically multinodulated surface.

FIG. 26-17. Subepidermal nodular fibrosis (sclerosing hemangioma) of the dorsal surface of the leg in a young adult. This lesion was bright yellow in color on cross section.

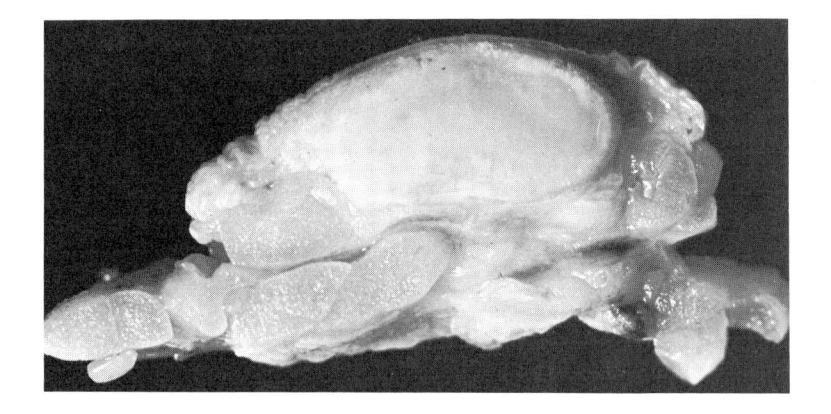

traumatic or incisional disruption and healing of the skin. Attenuated epidermis practically devoid of lymphatics is closely attached to the tumor. Other than unsightliness and susceptibility to injury, it has no clinical significance.

Subtotal excision with incision through the outermost limits of the tumor and meticulous suture of the skin to secure primary union usually will secure a significant reduction of the mass. Excision of the entire tumor with incision through the normal skin around the tumor is followed frequently by another keloid as large or larger than the first. The author's experience (C.A.M.) with subtotal and total excision leads him to prefer the subtotal.

Dermoid Cysts, Sebaceous Cysts and Inclusion Cysts

According to Ackerman, dermoid cysts, sebaceous cysts and epidermal inclusion cysts are almost always diagnosed as sebaceous cysts but are readily susceptible to differentiation. The dermoid cyst occurs in the embryonic cleavage lines and is rare. It is benign and is lined by stratified squamous epithelium and may contain hair. True sebaceous cysts are lined by sebaceous cells which are an integral part of the living wall. The epidermal inclusion cysts, which Ackerman rates as the commonest, he believes to be related to traumatic displacement of epidermis into the deeper layers of the skin where sebum is produced and collects within the keratinized cyst wall.

These last two forms are retention cysts arising from sebaceous glands about the hair follicles. They may grow to a surprisingly large size. The author (J.E.R.) has removed one from the posterior axillary fold which was approximately 6 inches in diameter. They are subject to infection and abscess formation. Malignant degeneration as such occurs very rarely. Some of the instances of carcinoma supposedly arising with a sebaceous cyst represent cystic degenerations within squamous cell carcinoma; others, partially necrotic squamous cell carcinomas metastatic in superficial lymph nodes.

Treatment is excision, with care to remove the entire lining of the sac and the skin pore

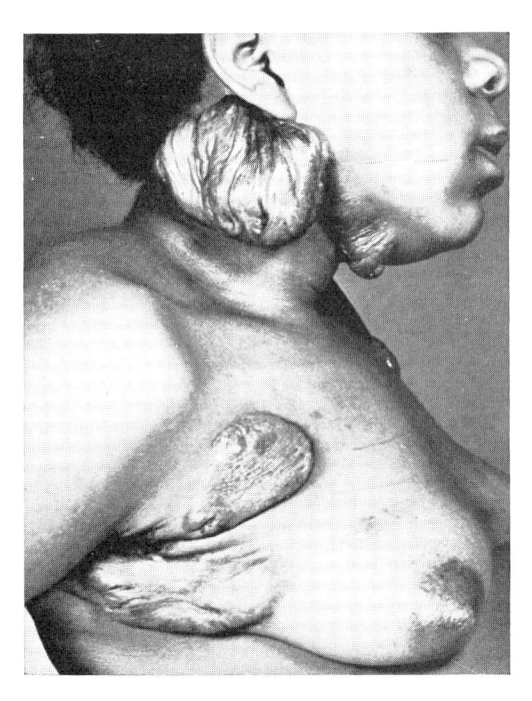

FIG. 26-18. Multiple large deforming keloids.

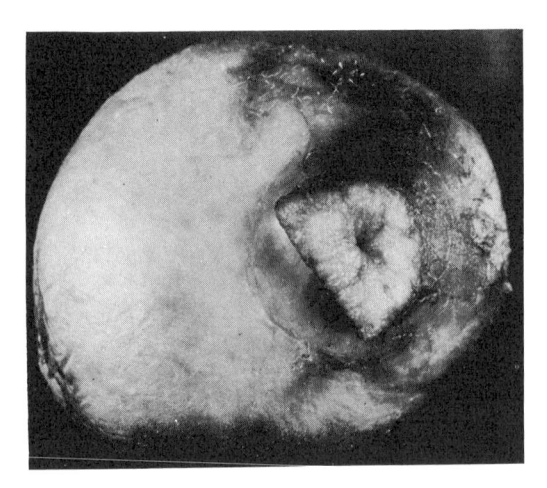

FIG. 26-19. Gross photograph of a slightly magnified epidermal inclusion cyst. Note the characteristic dimple in the piece of skin attached to the tumor.

with which it is connected. If they are infected, preliminary incision and drainage is often preferable, followed by excision a few weeks later after the acute inflammation has subsided. On the scalp they are called wens and are frequently multiple. Inclusion cysts occur sometimes in the region of wounds due to small amounts of epithelium being carried into the depth of a wound or a needle tract; sometimes one appears in the webs between the fingers, where it apparently has been carried in through some previous injury, or occasionally in other locations of the body (Fig. 26-19). Dermoid cysts are not common in the skin or the subcutaneous tissue. They are characterized by the presence of tissues originating from more than one of the early embryonic layers ectoderm, mesoderm and entoderm.

PILONIDAL CYSTS

A common inclusion cyst of the body is the pilonidal cyst, thought by some authors to be due to the inclusion of epithelial remnants in the sacral region possibly early in the course of fetal life.

Treatment is excision, which in the case of the *pilonidal cyst* presents a rather special problem. These cysts always present at or very close to the midline between the buttocks. They are posterior to the rectum and seldom connect with it, though occasionally they may be confused with perirectal abscesses. Characteristically, close inspection reveals a pore with one or more hair shafts sticking out through it. These cysts, like sebaceous cysts, commonly become infected, and when acute inflammation supervenes it is best to open them with a midline incision which affords drainage and to defer any attempt to extirpate them until after the acute inflammation has subsided.

Three methods of treatment are then available. One is excision, leaving the wound open to heal by secondary intention. The other is excision with primary suture. By either method of treatment, completeness of excision is a prerequisite for success. If any of the epithelial elements are allowed to remain, recurrence is almost inevitable and frequently prompt. The first method (permitting healing by secondary intention) is more certain of success but usually requires 3 months or more for complete healing. The second method (primary suture) is often employed. It requires technical competence and should not be attempted if the excision must be so wide that the resulting closure requires much tension. Primary union may be obtained in upward of three quarters of the cases with a 10- to 14-day period of disability, followed by some protection of the area. If the wound does not heal primarily, the sutures may be removed and the wound opened widely which, in effect, constitutes the first method.

The third method consists in excision of the cyst and suture of the skin edges down to the sacral fascia leaving a narrow strip (about 5 mm. wide) of the fascia exposed for a distance of 3 to 5 cm. This is more certain than the primary closure and takes a shorter time for healing than the first. Except for the primary attack on uninfected favorable cases in which primary closure is preferred the third method is most frequently the method of choice.

Another method proposed is that of marsupialization in which the posterior wall of the cyst is left in place, and the skin edges are sutured to its edge. This seems less sound than the third method, and one of us has had 4 consecutive unsatisfactory results with it in chronically infected cases. Therefore, we do not recommend it in spite of the fact that there are some favorable reports in the literature.

Fig. 26-20. Gout, involving the joints of both hands. Tophi.

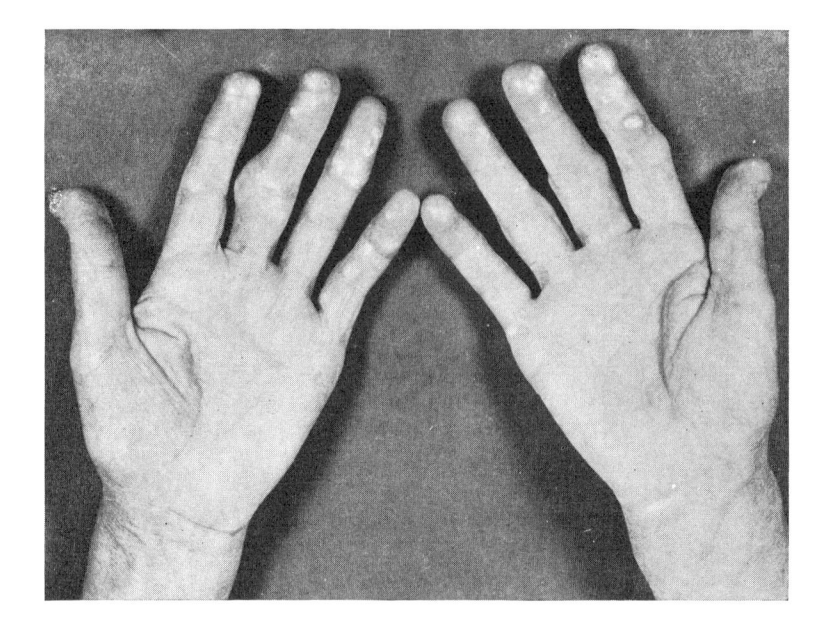

Malignancy in pilonidal cysts is rare, but Weinstein, Roberts and Reynolds report a collected series of 11 cases (J.A.M.A. 170: 1394-1395, 1959). Pilonidal sinuses must be differentiated from a low-lying congenital dermal sinus occurring especially in children.

Congenital Dermal Sinus

The congenital dermal sinus may open through the skin overlying the midline of the sacrum. It is associated with a defect in the vertebra beneath it that is readily demonstrable radiographically. It needs to be treated by resection, but the surgeon who removes it must be prepared to remove it from the cauda equina and not merely remove the superficial portion.

Hematoma

A hematoma is a swelling produced by extravasation of blood. Such extravasations are apt to be associated with a considerable amount of ecchymosis within a few days following the injury, but subsequently a fibrous capsule may form around the main collection of blood, and this may persist for months or years unless it is evacuated. Such encapsulated hematomas in contact with bones of the head tend to erode the bone. Also, there is a tendency toward calcification in such lesions if they are permitted to endure for long periods of time.

In the abdominal wall, an occasional cause of hematoma is rupture of the *deep epigastric vessels*. In this case bleeding may be severe enough to result in shock. Also, it not infrequently produces sufficient irritation of the parietal peritoneum to give the symptoms of an acute abdominal catastrophe.

A rupture of the rectus abdominis muscle occasionally occurs as the result of severe coughing or straining. The torn end of the muscle contracts, producing a thickening that may present as a tumor. Other band-shaped muscles which are torn or severed may also form tumorlike masses where the unattached muscle contracts and thickens.

Tophi

These manifestations of gout consist in deposits of uric acid crystals. They are especially common about the ears, fingers and toes and, while they constitute tumors, they are not to be thought of as neoplasms (Fig. 26-20).

Foreign Bodies

Occasionally, a subcutaneous tumor will prove to be the site of an old splinter or other foreign body. It should be remembered that common forms of glass are not very radiopaque, and one cannot be confident of detecting them by radiography, though examination is worthwhile and is sometimes positive. Wooden splinters are usually not radiopaque.

The mass is formed not only by the foreign body itself but also by the surrounding inflammatory reaction or fibrosis. The patient does not always recall the injury.

MALIGNANT TUMORS OF THE SKIN

Carcinoma of the Skin

This lesion occurs in 2 forms: a *squamous cell carcinoma*, generally called an epithelioma, and a *basal cell carcinoma*. Both are slow to metastasize, the basal cell being somewhat less likely to metastasize than the squamous cell type. When metastasis occurs, it is apt to be to regional lymph nodes. The most frequent cutaneous sites of origin of epidermoid carcinoma are the ears, the temples, the dorsum of the hand and the mucous membrane of the lips, while the predominant sites of the basal cell carcinoma are the skin of the nose, the hair-bearing skin of the lips, the eyelids and the chin. All of these sites are on parts of the body directly exposed to air and sunlight. Epidermoid carcinoma is also the predominant cutaneous neoplasm arising in irradiated skin (x-rays, etc.) and old scars that are thick and avascular and may have healed and broken down repeatedly (Marjolin's ulcer); basal cell carcinoma arises only rarely in these loci.

Epitheliomas of the skin and the mucous membranes frequently represent a malignant transition from various "precancerous lesions" such as kraurosis vulvae, xeroderma pigmentosum, senile keratosis, and keratoses caused by irradiation, arsenicals or exposure to tar.

Treatment is liberal excision, or deep x-ray therapy except for neoplasms arising in previously irradiated skin. Irradiation therapy is sometimes preferable in areas such as the eyelids, where the sacrifice of tissues is especially undesirable. Five-year cure rates as high as 95 per cent are claimed for skin carcinoma. However, if the lesions are not recognized early and dealt with accordingly, they can get beyond the range of curability and produce a high degree of destruction with great pain, sloughing, offensive odor, disability and slow death. Therefore, they always should be treated thoroughly and wholeheartedly at the outset.

Bowen's Disease

Bowen's disease as a pathologic entity is noninvasive epidermoid carcinoma. Clinically it presents with superficial, salmon-pink lines with slightly elevated margins. Common sites are the posterior surface of the chest and the face. Treatment is usually surgical excision. Radiation is also generally effective.

Kaposi's disease or multiple idiopathic

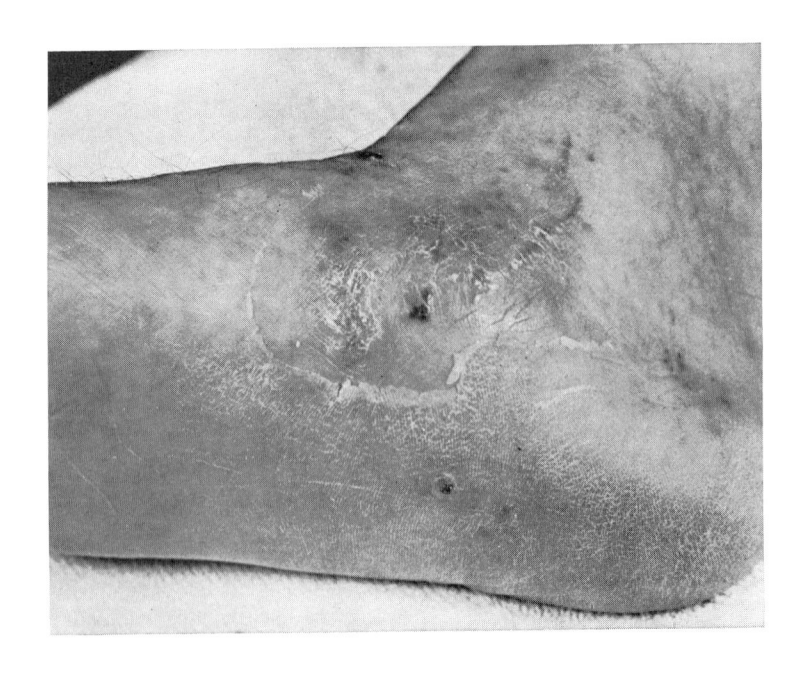

Fig. 26-21. Multiple black nodules of Kaposi's sarcoma involving the foot. Such lesions mimic melanocarcinoma.

hemorrhagic sarcoma (Fig. 26-21) is possibly of reticuloendothelial origin. It occurs most frequently on the lower extremities. It is a slowly progressive malignant tumor. However, it may develop foci within viscera. It metastasizes late in its course to lymph nodes and distant organs and may be mistaken for malignant melanoma, especially when it appears on the lower extremities.

Multiple hemorrhagic sarcoma usually appears as discrete or grouped maculopapular to nodular, red-brown lesions of usually less than 1 cm. in diameter. It occurs predominantly in males and usually is associated with edema of the lower extremities.

Irradiational therapy is useful. Although the prognosis is poor insofar as control of the growth of the tumor is concerned, the afflicted person may live for many years by virtue of the tumor's slow natural growth.

Malignant Melanoma

The malignant melanoma (Fig. 26-22) is one of the most deadly of all tumors and is certainly the most deadly of the skin tumors. It metastasizes early, both through the lymphatics and often through the blood stream. Metastases to internal organs, including the stomach, are common. Those arising within the upper part of the body, excepting those within the scalp, are more often curable than those arising in the lower extremity. The smaller the lesion is, when it is widely excised, the better the prognosis is. It used to be regarded as almost uniformly fatal. In recent years many 5-year survivals have been achieved through radical surgery and removal of regional lymph nodes and lymphatics. It is one of the few tumors that, when widespread within the skin of an extremity, may often be temporarily controlled by the localized perfusion of the extremity with cancerocidal agents.

The feeling that chronic irritation predisposes to malignant degeneration of a junctional nevus into a malignant melanoma is based on observations of various tumors in various parts of the body subject to irritation. Incomplete removal which may result from electrocoagulation is also thought of as a procedure which may increase the risk of malignant degeneration, although this has not been proved.

Diagnosis of this lesion requires a high index

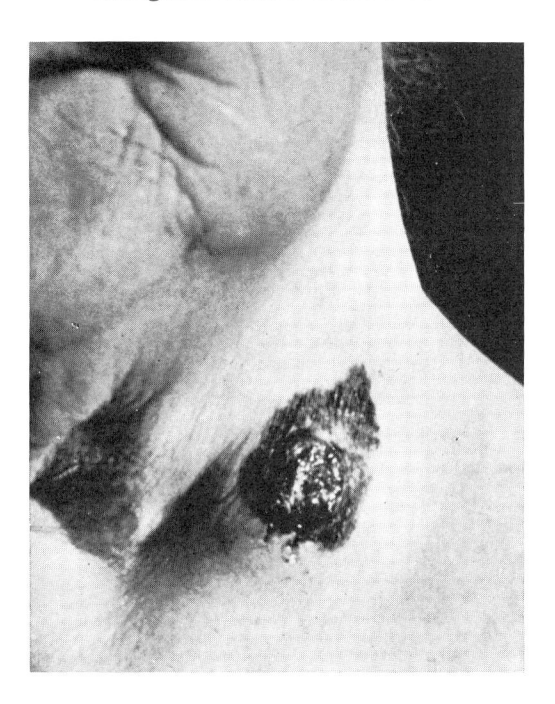

FIG. 26-22. Malignant melanoma.

of suspicion. Juvenile moles (pre-puberty) are almost invariably benign. The junction mole as opposed to the intradermal or common mole is considered as premalignant. Suspicious signs include: a slate blue to black color (but it may be amelanotic), change in pigmentation, appearance after puberty, an increase in size, the presence of a pigmented ring around the primary lesion, and the location of lesions on plantar or palmar surfaces where they are subject to excessive irritation. Preferred treatment is always excision biopsy rather than punch biopsy or electrodesiccation.

In excising moles, it should be remembered that the mole cells often extend to a considerable depth in the subcutaneous tissue, and that they not infrequently extend laterally, well beyond the visible confines of the lesion. In general, such lesions should be excised with a margin of skin equal to at least one half of the diameter of large lesions and equal to the diameter of small lesions of 1.0 cm. or less all around it, and excision should be carried down to the fascia over the muscle in most instances. Where such a procedure is likely to have especially unfortunate cosmetic or functional results, it is sometimes wise to remove the lesion with a narrower margin for histologic study of the tissue. Then additional tissue is removed only if necessary. In removing these lesions, it is well to orient the specimen by inserting a black silk suture through one corner of the normal skin margin, so that if an extension of mole cells is demonstrated beyond the limits of the excision, the surgeon will know at what point to remove additional tissue.

Before undertaking a radical removal of lymphatics and other tissues for a malignant melanoma, one should exclude distant metastases insofar as possible by chest roentgenogram, thorough examination of the body surface and a scan of the liver with an appropriate radioactive isotope. However, as long as there are no signs of distant metastases to parts of the body other than the skin, the excision of satellite lesions, appearing after the excision of the primary, should be performed even though it may require the denudation and the skin grafting of a large part of a leg, an arm, the neck or the thigh and the removal of appropriate deep lymph node chains and vessels such as the iliac and the deep cervical. This attitude is permissible because of the unpredictability of the growth characteristics of a particular melanoma.

The removal of grossly unremarkable regional lymph nodes as a prophylactic measure is favored provided that there is no evidence of remote metastasis that would be left behind and provided that the group of nodes to which the lesion would be expected to metastasize is reasonably well defined. The latter is apt to be true for melanomas on the extremities or those near a groin or an axilla and for some of those on the head and the neck. It is often difficult when they occur at the surface of the torso well away from axillae and groins.

The advantage of this step has not been measured accurately nor has the advantage or disadvantage of removing the intervening skin and subcutaneous tissue between the primary lesion and the nodes, nor the advantage or the disadvantage between immediate excision and waiting 3 weeks or more to permit malignant cells in the lymphatics to arrive in the nodes.

Lymphangiograms made by the injection of opaque colloidal material through skin lymphatics and then making roentgenograms sometimes contribute to the diagnosis of metastasis in lymph nodes.

The advantages of prophylactic removal of nodes in which there is no evidence of metastasis are not clear enough to subject poor-risk patients to procedures which would be highly hazardous for them.

LIPOSARCOMA

This is the malignant variety of fatty tumor arising from mesoderm. It has much the same potentialities as a fibrosarcoma and in many instances it does not metastasize until late. However, it is a very persistent tumor, and attempts at eradication frequently fail, so that local recurrence is not infrequent, even when the surgeon feels that a liberal excision has been done.

Both lipomas and liposarcomas often extend deeper than the subcutaneous tissues, sometimes lying between muscle bundles, and sometimes lying partly within the muscular tissue and partly in the subcutaneous area. They also occur within a body cavity and presumably may arise wherever fat is present. Very wide and deep excision is necessary to cure liposarcoma. Hemiplevectomy and scapulohumeral disarticulation are often necessary to cure such a tumor originating in the upper thigh or the shoulder, respectively.

FIBROSARCOMA

These lesions may arise anywhere, and when they appear in the subcutaneous tissues or in the more superficial muscles, they are frequently slow-growing tumors capable of being eradicated by a wide resection. All too frequently, they recur. Whether this is due to failure to carry out a wide enough excision, to the secondary implants created at the time of operation, or to multicentric origin is not entirely clear. Ordinarily, amputation is not recommended for these tumors but it may have to be considered in some cases when an extremity is extensively involved and when no evidence can be obtained of metastasis beyond the confines of the limb.

LYMPHOMA

The *lymphomas* will sometimes affect the skin and the subcutaneous tissues by the invasion of these structures by collections of tumor cells. This is apt to be a late manifestation of lymphosarcoma or Hodgkin's disease.

METASTATIC TUMORS

Malignant tumors of many varieties may metastasize to the skin. This is frequently a late manifestation and in most instances a contraindication to therapeutic surgery. Exceptions are the excision of satellite nodules near the site of a primary tumor, e.g., breast carcinoma or malignant melanoma where surgical removal is often palliative and occasionally, though not frequently, curative.

ACANTHOSIS NIGRICANS

Acanthosis nigricans is a cutaneous change associated in perhaps half of the cases with an internal cancer. It occurs especially in the axilla or in skin folds but may be generalized. The change consists in an increased pigmentation of the skin with a roughening of its surface. It requires no treatment itself but is an indication for a thorough search for internal cancers which may require treatment.

CHAPTER 27

J. GARROTT ALLEN, M.D.

Breast

Embryology
Anatomy
Inflammatory Diseases
Benign Tumors
Cancer: Pathology, Diagnosis, Treatment and Prognosis
Attempts To Improve Survival Results
The Male Breast
Prognostic Considerations

The female breast is an organ subject to many disorders. Although the majority of these relate to benign lesions, the fact that the breast is one of the two most frequent primary sites of cancer in women underscores the importance of determining promptly the nature of any breast lesion detected. Moreover, because of its physiologic change in menstruation, pregnancy, lactation and postmenopausal atrophy, the breast is subject to many alterations in gross and microscopic structure during life. These changes are to be distinguished from the disease encountered. The vestigial breast in the male is largely exempt from important pathologic disease, although not entirely.

The detection and the definition of breast lesions are not accomplished as readily as might be expected for an organ on the body's surface. In many instances, reliance on biopsy procedures for final diagnosis is the only possible means for establishing an accurate diagnosis.

EMBRYOLOGY

The mammary gland is both ectodermal and mesodermal in origin. It is an analogue of the sweat gland and arises along the milk line or ridge which extends from the neck perpendicularly through the midclavicular line to the thigh. Usually, 7 papilla make their appearance embryologically along each line, but only one remains at birth, located in the 5th interspace in the midclavicular line. Occasionally, one or more of these rudimentary structures persist as supernumerary nipples; they may secrete small quantities of milk during normal lactation. Infrequently they have been the site of cancer.

ANATOMY

The anatomy of the breast important to surgical pathology centers about its glandular and ductal structure. The ducts proceed in retrograde fashion from the nipple. As they radiate peripherally, they subdivide into primary, secondary and tertiary ducts, the last receiving the milk secretions during lactation.

The glandular tissue is firm in texture, convex anteriorly and concave posteriorly, thicker in the center than at the periphery. The superior part of each breast extends nearly to the axillary fold, deviating slightly laterally. This uppermost lateral part is known as the tail of Spence and is easily cut across and portions left behind when performing a simple mastectomy.

The gland is subdivided into lobes; and these, in turn, into lobules enmeshed in areolar tissue interspersed with fat. Between the lobules course numerous fibrous strands known as Cooper's ligaments. These ligaments support the breast, running vertically from the deep fascia through the breast to the skin.

The epithelium of the female breast varies according to its physiologic state. Normally, the alveoli are small and usually filled with masses of glandular cells. During pregnancy these cells undergo rapid proliferation. Near term, fatty degeneration occurs, and fat globules are excreted in the first milk as colostrum corpuscles. The colostrum is rich in antibodies.

Fibrous tissue surrounds the entire breast and invests all structure of the gland.

The Lymphatics of the Breast and Their Relation to Operation. There are few, if any, organs within the body where knowledge of the lymphatic circulation and its drainage is more important to the surgeon than that of the breast. In recent years, the excellent studies of the surgeon, Handley (1955), have greatly increased our information on this subject and that which follows is largely a summary of his writings.

There appears little reason to believe that the lymphatic vessels of the skin over the breast are different from those in the skin elsewhere. Normally, this skin is comprised of four lymphatic plexuses, the small lymph channels from the dermal papillae, the subpapillary intradermal plexus into which the lymph vessels from the dermal papillae drain, the intermediate plexus deep in the dermis and the deep plexus coursing over the surface of the deep fascia.

The breast lies between the deep dermal plexus and the deep fascial plexus. Communications between these two plexuses exist, permitting cancer cells to metastasize in either or both directions.

Handley believes that the subareolar plexus of Sappey is less important than was described previously and concludes that it drains away from the areolar tissue. Grant, Tabah and Adair (1953) came to the opposite conclusion from their studies.

The lymphatic nodal system of the axilla is fed by numerous lymph channels arising about the neck, the arm and the pectoral girdle, in addition to those from the breast. The lateralmost nodes in the axilla drain primarily the arm and are not frequently involved in metastatic disease of the breast unless higher lymphatic channels to the axilla have been blocked. The subscapular nodes course along the anterior surface of the latissimus dorsi, the teres major and the subscapularis muscles in close proximity to the subscapular blood vessels. These should be identified and removed along with the corresponding blood vessels and fascia of these muscles, particularly for inferior-lying and lateral-lying breast lesions.

The pectoral nodes follow the course of the lateral thoracic blood vessels close to the margin of the pectoralis minor. They drain principally the upper and outer quadrants of the breast, terminating in the same central nodes of the axilla as do the subscapular channels. Between the pectoralis major and minor is a small group of nodes which ascend along the course of the acromiothoracic artery, draining both the inner and the outer upper quadrants of the breast to empty into the apical nodes of the axilla.

The central lymph nodes of the axilla are numerous. Fortunately, they are mostly situated below the axillary vein between the lateral thoracic and subscapular vessels. Often they are imbedded in axillary fat. These are the nodes usually detected clinically when enlarged. They receive lymph drainage from the pectoral, the subscapular and the lateral groups and in turn drain more centrally to the apical nodes.

The apical or subclavicular nodes lie between the lateral margin of the first rib and the mesial border of the pectoralis minor muscle. They tend to lie behind the axillary vein and the clavicle. These are probably the last nodal barriers of any significance, draining the pectoral girdle and the breast before the lymph enters the subclavian or internal jugular veins. These apical nodes are biopsied (also the second node of the internal mammary chain) by Haagensen (1959) as a preliminary step in determination of operability.

The internal mammary chain of lymph nodes, although recognized and described nearly 200 years ago, has received little attention surgically until recent times. Their efferent channels arise from the anterior pericardial nodal system, ascending in close proximity to the internal mammary artery and vein on the posterior surfaces of the upper 6 costal cartilages. They receive drainage from the adjacent chest wall, including the parietal pleura and the pectoral muscles. They may enter directly into one of the neighboring large veins beneath the clavicle or converge upon another lymphatic channel near the apex of the axilla. There is little evidence of cross communication with the contralateral internal mammary chain, which again is suggestive evidence that a carcinoma appearing in the contralateral side is more likely a second primary tumor than a secondary one.

As these nodes receive much of the lymphatic drainage from the mesial aspect of the breast, lesions lying within this area tend to metastasize to this system. Such metastases in the patient have been overlooked. The reawakening of an interest in this drainage system is explained by the surgeon's efforts to improve his 5-year survival rates following radical mastectomy. However, because of difficulties encountered in resecting this channel, some surgeons prefer to biopsy the nodes in the 2nd and the 3rd interspaces adjacent to the internal mammary blood vessels and, finding the nodes positive in either of these areas, prefer less radical procedures. Others consider such findings a challenge for more radical surgery (Urban). However, both the biopsy and the resections of the internal chain procedures are still in the experimental stage.

Handley has demonstrated the lymph drainage from the lower portion of the breast, particularly its mesial side, may enter the fascial lymphatics of the abdominal wall and from these to the liver via lymph channels of the round ligament. Fortunately, tumors in the lowest portion of the breast are comparatively rare, but when present one should consider removing the central portion of the anterior rectus sheath and the round ligament, in addition to the usual radical mastectomy procedure.

Although the lymphatic circulation as described above does segregate itself into groups draining more prominently one area of the breast, the skin or the fascia than another, nonetheless they intercommunicate fairly freely. In consequence, there is no one route that metastases may be expected to follow simply because the tumor lies predominantly in a particular region of the breast. However, a surgeon's approach to a radical mastectomy should be governed in part at least by the location of the tumor and its likely course of drainage, spending perhaps more time in certain areas than others. Therefore, in all radical mastectomies, the central, the subscapular, the pectoral and the apical nodes of the axillary system should be removed en bloc.

The cutaneous nerve supply of the breast is segmental and arises from T-2 to T-6. The first interspace is usually supplied by the nerves to the subclavius. Two nerves are important in performing radical mastectomy or other operations on the anterolateral chest wall.

The long thoracic nerve or the external respiratory nerve of Bell supplies the serratus anterior muscles. It arises from the roots of the 5th, the 6th and the 7th cervical nerves to descend behind the brachial plexus and the axillary vessels to reach the serratus. It may be sacrificed if necessary but usually should be avoided in the course of operation. The other nerve is the thoracodorsal, arising from the posterior cord of the brachial plexus after deriving its fibers also from the 5th, the 6th and the 7th cervical nerves. It passes behind the medial cord and the axillary vessels to touch lightly on the upper lateral chest wall before entering the anterior border of the latissimus dorsi. Its division or injury results in paralysis of a major portion of this muscle.

The nipple of the breast is perforated with a number of small ductal openings which drain various segments of the breast. Occasionally, these become important clinically because a bloody discharge may arise from a particular duct. The circular pigmented area surrounding the nipple is known as the areola, which contains from 12 to 15 elevations arranged in circular fashion. These mark the site of Montgomery's glands, which resemble sebaceous glands. During pregnancy these glands actively secrete sebum and at times become the site of low-grade and persistent infections.

INFLAMMATORY DISEASES

Acute Pyogenic Mastitis and Breast Abscess

This disease is usually an infection caused by the staphylococcus, but other pyogenic organisms, particularly the streptococcus, may also infect the breast. Although acute mastitis may occur in the adult female breast at any time, it is observed most frequently during lactation and in late pregnancy. It usually starts from abrasions about the nipple or the areolar tissue. By retrograde extension of a superficial infection along the ducts or the lymphatics, it becomes deep-seated in breast tissue, forming an abscess. The local signs of heat, redness, tenderness and pain usually are associated with those of fever, malaise and occasionally a chill. Diagnosis can be difficult.

Its treatment should include the use of a suitable antibiotic, heat and analegesics until localization and suppuration warrant surgical drainage. Should the infection occur during lactation, breast-feeding is discontinued immediately, and stilbestrol is given to induce involution and cessation of lactation. When symptoms persist several days without detectable localization, aspiration of suspicious deep areas of the breast may reveal the site of abscess which can then be incised and drained. Deep-lying abscesses may require counterdrainage if drainage is to be adequate. A persistent draining sinus may form in a few patients and require excision later.

Tuberculous Mastitis

This disease is rarely seen these days and is usually of the bovine type. It is primary in about 60 per cent of cases and secondary to systemic tuberculosis in the rest. The male breast is seldom affected. Occasionally, human tuberculous chondritis may spread to the breast with sinus formation, giving rise to tuberculous mastitis. Infrequently, it is associated with or arises from other nonpulmonary sites of bovine tuberculosis. Improved public health measures, especially pasteurization of milk, have reduced effectively the attack rate of tuberculous mastitis (Wilson and MacGregor, 1963).

A tuberculous abscess usually opens spontaneously and drains chronically. Its treatment is the surgical excision of the sinus and the abscess wall, followed by primary closure. A course of PAS with isoniazid or streptomycin for a number of months is usually advisable, and the usual family and public health preventive measures should be observed.

Idiopathic Mammary Phlebitis (Mondor's Syndrome)

A form of thrombophlebitis, usually idiopathic, may occur in one or more superficial branches of the axillary vein, of the upper arm and of the upper anterior chest wall (Mondor's syndrome, 1939). It is referred to here only because an occasional case may occur in a female patient in whom there is or has been breast cancer or in one who has fibrocystic disease. Classically, when the breast is placed under tension, cordlike structures representing thrombosed veins may be felt. Under these circumstances, its occurrence may be alarming if the cause is not recognized; in reality, this form of phlebitis is self-limiting, inconsequential and requires no therapy other than to avoid aggravation by manipulation or surgical intervention. In more acute cases, the adjacent breast tissue may become inflamed secondarily, but rarely has latent fat necrosis been observed. A similar form of idiopathic thrombophlebitis occurring in the axillary vein was described by Matas (1934); Mondor's syndrome appears to be only a variant of Matas's syndrome which is a variant of the more frequent forms of thrombophlebitis occurring in other locations and is called idiopathic thrombophlebitis. The process in the breast usually clears in 3 to 6 weeks and seldom recurs (Hogan, 1964).

Fat Necrosis

Fat necrosis may occur from a blow to the breast or from a breast abscess. It is an occasional sequela of a breast biopsy and is observed more frequently under these conditions in obese women. The necrotic area becomes soft and fluctuant; if aspirated, the fatty globules in the fluid resemble that in broth. Later on, scarring may dimple the overlying skin, become adherent to the fascia, form a hard mass and, upon the cut section, grossly resemble carcinoma (Fig. 27-1).

BENIGN TUMORS

Fibroadenoma

Fibroadenoma is seen most frequently between the ages of 15 and 35, with a maximum incidence rate at approximately age 25. Only about 10 per cent of cases occur in the postmenopausal state. It is by far the most commonly encountered benign tumor in women under the age of 30 and almost the only tumor found under the age of 20. Usually, the lesion is a solitary one, although several may exist independently within the same breast or in both breasts. The lesion ordinarily ranges from 2 to 5 cm. in diameter, averaging closer to 2 than to 5. The lesion is usually mild to moderately painful but may be quite tender to the touch. It is firm, discrete and freely movable.

Pathologically, fibroadenomas may arise

from the intraductal tissue (intracanicular fibroadenoma) or from that lying between the lobules (interductal fibroadenoma). They may undergo myxomatous degeneration, and some are thought to be the source of origin for cystadenoma phyllodes (see p. 683). The treatment is their surgical excision.

Intraductal Papilloma

This benign tumor of epithelial origin arises within the ducts, usually close to the nipple. It is usually solitary in contrast with the multiple papillary folds observed in chronic cystic mastitis. There is no indication that it will become malignant; rather, most intraductal carcinomas are considered to be of that nature from the beginning. In 283 women with proved intraductal papilloma, Hendrick (1957) did not observe the subsequent development of cancer among the 92 per cent of patients he was able to trace 5 to 15 years. The significance and the treatment of lesions, benign or malignant, which give rise to bleeding from the nipple are discussed on page 684 and will not be elaborated upon here. Contrast mammography may be helpful in locating the papilloma.

Lipoma

Lipoma of the breast is encountered occasionally and is easily recognized by its soft rubbery consistency, its mobility and usual "cluster of grapes" contour when lying near the surface. Other benign tumors affecting the breast are those seen in the skin and the subcutaneous tissue elsewhere and need not come under discussion here (see Chap. 26, Skin and Subcutaneous Tissue).

Ectasia of the Breast

Ectasia of the breast is a dilatation of the mammary ducts and is a benign disease. It occurs usually in middle-aged women and can be indistinguishable from carcinoma of the breast (Asch and Frey, 1962). The disease is usually bilateral; it may be associated with nipple discharge and tends to present as a painless tumor mass. Not infrequently, signs of local inflammation are caused by irritation from the inspissated intraductal material which may erode through the ducts into the surrounding tissue, occasionally causing a sterile abscess. Later, this abscess is followed by the development of a firm fibrocystic mass. The clinical picture at this stage may be one of retraction of the overlying skin and nipple and of adherence of the lesion to the pectoral fascia, much as may occur after the scarring process of pyogenic abscess or from fat necrosis of the breast. Moreover, calcific debris may be scattered throughout the lesion and may be interpreted falsely as positive for cancer on mammographic examination (see p. 688). Unless microscopic examination of biopsy tissue is first performed, the mistaking of ectasia for carcinoma of the breast can occasionally cause surgeons to perform radical mastectomy for this disease because upon gross examination the texture resembles that of carcinoma.

Chronic Cystic Mastitis

This disease is also known as cystic hyperplasia, fibrocystic disease, Schimmelbusch's disease, chronic interstitial mastitis, adenosis and others.

The cause of this disease is unknown, though its symptoms tend to increase at the time of ovulation, during menstruation, and to subside during pregnancy and after menopause.

Pathology. The symptoms tend to be chronic and cystic but not always. While they may be associated with inflammatory-like reactions (subacute and chronic), these reactions are not those of the usual types of inflammation. In some patients, fibrosis of the periductal tissue predominates; in others, dilatation of the ducts with or without hyperplasia of their epithelial lining and the formation of papillary folds projecting into the lumen are among some of the changes noted. During the active stages of the disease, old hemorrhage, cholesterol and round cell periductal infiltration are commonly observed. Chronic cystic mastitis thus appears to be a syndrome that may assume one or more of several histologic patterns, to be bilateral but not necessarily to be of the same extent in each breast. It is reported to be asymptomatically present in about 50 per cent of autopsies performed on patients with clinically "normal" breasts (Frantz et al., 1951). Clinically, this syndrome is observed most commonly between the ages of 25 and 45, but in some patients it may be clinically evident throughout life. The association of exacerbations and remissions in relation to altered hormonal activity leads many to consider this syndrome as due to hyperestrogenism, although conclusive evidence is lacking. Its persistence after menopause in some patients has been attributed to the adrenal origin of estrogens (Tellem, et al., 1965).

Symptoms are chiefly those of painful and tender lump or lumps in the breasts. Often the entire breast is painful. Pain is usually intermittent, or at least not constantly present to the same degree of intensity. It tends to be accentuated during menstruation. In other patients, pain is most prominent at the time of ovulation. Spontaneous nipple discharge occurs in at least 10 per cent of cases and is greenish yellow to brown in color but may be bloody. Pressure applied to the subareolar area and the nipple may elicit a slight secretion not previously known to the patient. When the discharge is bloody, usually it is associated with an intraductal papilloma and infrequently complicated by the presence of an intraductal carcinoma. Papanicolaou (1954) and others have examined these secretions for carcinomatous cells, making the diagnosis in 20 per cent of all cases by this technic, but cellular distortion by the secretions limits seriously the usefulness of this procedure in screening for breast cancer.

The possibility that chronic cystic mastitis is a precursor of cancer has been the subject of much study, the results of which are discussed below.

Physical findings of chronic cystic mastitis are those of a tender, firm, nodular breast, shotty to palpation. The edge of the breast tissue is frequently quite prominent when normally it is often difficult to make out. The greatest diagnostic problem that these patients present is the differentiation of this disease from cancer. It is not sound to imply that the finding of a cyst, whether of the blue-dome variety or of the more commonly encountered greenish-yellow type, provides strong evidence against the diagnosis of carcinoma. It simply means that chronic cystic mastitis likely exists; the diagnosis of carcinoma or its exclusion must stand on its own merits, and if it is overlooked, it will come to light—often too late.

Clinical significance of chronic cystic mastitis can be even more uncertain than its cause and the meanings of its variations in histopathology. The basic issue centers about its relationship to breast cancer. If, as Frantz, et al. claim, about half the female population over the age of 30 have histologic evidence of this syndrome, and if as Warren (1940) reported, the incidence of breast cancer is 11.7 times greater in women between the ages of 30 and 50 who have chronic cystic mastitis than among those without this condition, it would appear that more than 85 per cent of patients who develop cancer of the breast in this age group have also some degree of chronic cystic mastitis. Nonetheless, it may still be that whatever causes chronic cystic mastitis might also be capable of producing breast cancer independently; therefore, breast cancer may not necessarily be the sequel to chronic cystic mastitis. Warren also found that the coexistence of breast cancer in women after the age of 50 suffering from chronic cystic mastitis was 2.5 times greater than among those of similar ages without chronic cystic mastitis. In other studies, Haagensen (1956) found the incidence of breast cancer to be about 4 times greater among patients showing evidence of chronic cystic mastitis than among those without. The significance, if any, of this association is not easily determined, because there is considerable variation of opinion among pathologists as to what constitutes the histopathologic evidence of chronic cystic mastitis. However, until much more is known about chronic cystic mastitis as well as about the fundamental biologic disturbances causing cancer, one must be aware that these relationships exist clinically but recognize that their nature is not understood.

Another side of this vexing situation is that in patients with proved chronic cystic mastitis, a cancerous lump may appear and be accorded less attention than it deserves simply because of the numerous other lumps that may coexist. It is often a very difficult matter to decide how much to rely upon repeated manual examinations of the breast once the initial lumps have been biopsied and found to be compatible with the diagnosis of chronic cystic mastitis. Simple mastectomy for benign disease without evidence of cancer seems to be too radical a procedure in most patients, and it is too small an operation for most patients with breast cancer. One should not hesitate to advise surgical biopsy in patients with chronic cystic mastitis when uncertainty arises, despite one or more previous biopsies. Occasionally, simple mastectomy provides the only reasonable solution.

At times, a large solitary cyst is the primary evidence of chronic cystic mastitis. These usually transilluminate and may be aspirated, but cytologic examination of the desquamated cells in the aspirate is seldom helpful. These cysts may or may not recur. Carcinoma may occur in the walls of such cysts in about 1 to 3 per cent of cases; thus it is necessary to caution these patients to continue under surveillance.

Mastodynia (*painful breasts*) usually is associated with chronic cystic disease of the breast. It may occur also without any demonstrable lesion and occasionally is associated with heavy and pendulous breasts. One or both breasts may be painful. In acute unilateral mastodynia, breast abscess or hemorrhage into a cyst should be considered; if present, it should be drained or excised. Occasionally, a solitary fibroadenoma is found to account for unilateral mastodynia and should be removed; fibroadenomas occur most frequently in patients under 35 years of age.

Frequently, mild sedation, analgesics and reassurance are useful. If a mass is present, nothing is as reassuring to both patient and doctor as is the exclusion of cancer by biopsy evidence. Rarely, the surgeon may feel forced to perform a simple mastectomy to relieve the patient of her pain; but because emotional disorders often are associated with mastodynia and because pain in the area may persist after operation, he will do well to avoid mastectomy for mastodynia if possible, unless there is strong evidence of the presence of a fibroma.

Treatment. No very happy form of treatment of chronic cystic mastitis exists. Mild sedatives and aspirin may give temporary relief. The use of estrogens and of androgens has been recommended by some, but the author has not found this form of therapy to be very useful. In most patients, operation, other than for purposes of biopsy, is not likely to be indicated. In some, the pain experienced is disabling and may require partial or subtotal mastectomy, even bilaterally. It is usually better to make a lateral incision at the periphery of the breast, removing as much tissue as necessary, than to perform a simple mastectomy, removing the nipple. Patients with chronic cystic mastitis should be taught to practice breast examination by themselves and to report to a physician at regular intervals.

CANCER

It is from human breast cancer that we have learned most of what we know about the nature of cancer in patients, the interrelationship of this cancer to the hormonal activity of the individual, and have developed the rationale for several methods of treatment. Perhaps more important, we are beginning to learn how to analyze results of treatment to determine if treatment is more effective than none at all. In this connection, it is distressing that what we have learned about statistics and epidemiology has come so late in our long experience with this disease. Thus, problems that could have been settled 50 or 60 years ago still go begging for answers because the appropriate statistical methods are so recent in origin and in application.

Gradually, there is emerging a view, among both physicians and the laity, that the earlier the diagnosis, the less likely it is that the tumor has metastasized, and that when treatment is delayed, the tumor tends to be larger and the effectiveness of any form of treatment is reduced quite significantly. However, there is a cynicism about the curability of cancer in any stage that leads some physicians to believe that early diagnosis is of little significance. Fortunately, an abundance of evidence contradicts this contention. But it is discouraging that among the lower socioeconomic group of patients, there has been little tendency for their cancers to be diagnosed and treated earlier, in contrast with private patients. However, the problem is not this simple, as Breslow (1963) has pointed out rather sharply in an analysis of the differences in cancer survival rates in the State of California, when patients are treated surgically for breast cancer by private physicians as opposed to those treated by resident staffs in charity teaching hospitals. These differences in survival are evident even when the comparison is strictly limited to groups where the disease has progressed to the same extent at the time of treatment. Breslow therefore states: "It is clear, however, that persons in lower social classes experience a double penalty; they are generally diagnosed at a later stage of the disease and, even when the disease is localized at the time of diagnosis, they do not survive as well as private patients with localized disease." He carefully points out that half of the private patients were seen and treated for breast cancer prior to the age of 55; whereas at this same age only 25 per cent of the total with carcinoma of the breast in the charity series had been diagnosed and treated. In other words, 71 per cent of the patients in the latter series were over age 55 when they were diagnosed and treated for this disease. Therefore, it is possible that some or most of the differences observed in survival rates can be attributed to increased rates at which death occurs from other causes as the population ages. Stated otherwise, the primary cause of death may not be cancer in a substantial number of the older group, even though they may have cancer at the time of death. There is also a notable increased susceptibility to breast cancer in women in higher socioeconomic circumstances.

Every cancer has its beginning and, though some grow more rapidly than others, if the disease is discovered early and treated adequately while it is localized, it is curable in the fullest sense of this term. When it has extended beyond the confines of surgical resection, it is not. The shades of gray are those in which there are regional metastases, but even here better results are usually achieved by surgical resection of the primary lesion along with its regional nodes, and possibly by the additional use of other forms of therapy, including irradiation.

Breslow's data (1963) indicate the distribution of breast cancer according to age and show little difference in incidence for any one age group between females and males with breast cancer (Table 27-1).

Family history of breast cancer tends to increase the risk rate. Daughters of mothers who had breast cancer tend to have an increased incidence of this disease (Oliver, 1958). To a lesser extent this is also observed among sisters of patients who develop cancer of the breast but whose mothers did not have breast cancer. The numbers of cases in the several reports on this aspect of breast cancer

TABLE 27-1

Age	No. of Cases of Breast Cancer Female	Male	Per Cent Breast Cancer of All Cancer Sites Female	Male
Under 15	1	—	0.2	
15–24	24	—	3.5	
25–34	502	2	17.1	<1
35–44	2,254	11	30.4	<1
45–54	3.110	14	27.5	<1
55–64	3,125	31	23.3	<1
65–74	2,777	46	21.0	<1
75 and over	1,565	29	19.0	<1
	13,392	133	23.1	<1

From California Tumor Registry report, 1963.

are not large enough to bear much statistical reliability, but the results of all are in the same direction. In Oliver's studies he found that breast cancer had occurred with a little greater frequency in the mothers of patients with cancer than in the mothers of the noncancerous group which served as controls. The pertinent data are shown in Tables 27-2, 27-3 and 27-4 taken from Oliver; their limitations, though obvious, do not deny that family history for breast cancer is one of the factors to be considered in this disease. The major question is: "How much?"

INCIDENCE

Age. The most significant single fact that affects the incidence of cancer of the breast in women is the age of the patient. For example, the incidence rate among women 15 through 34 is 1.9 cases per 100,000; whereas in women 75 and older, it is 139.9 cases per 100,000, or 73 times greater (Table 27-5). Not only is the attack rate for breast cancer per 100,000 greatly increased in the older age patient, but also affecting the total numbers in any age group is the fact that there has been a great shift in the age of our population in recent decades. For example, the number of females in the United States under the age of 15 in 1900 was 13,200,000 compared with 6,900,000 who were at that time 45 years of age or older. By 1960, there were 27,576,000 females under the age of 15, and 27,627,000 who were age 45 or older—a startling change in age ratios in 60 years.

TABLE 27-2. OCCURRENCE OF CANCER IN SISTERS OF PATIENTS WITH BREAST CANCER AND IN NONCANCER CONTROL GROUP

| GROUP | No. IN GROUP | HISTORY OF SISTERS ||||
		No Family History of Cancer	Breast Cancer Only Positive	Breast and Other Sites Positive	Nonbreast Sites Positive
Breast cancer patients	312	29.4%	6.1%	26.2%	38.3%
Control group	134	41.0%	8.9%	12.7%	37.3%

From Oliver, 1958.

TABLE 27-3. OCCURRENCE OF BREAST CANCER AMONG SISTERS OF PRIMARY PATIENTS WITH CANCER OF BREAST HAVING MOTHERS WITH OR WITHOUT BREAST CANCER

| MOTHERS | | SISTERS* OF PRIMARY PATIENTS |||
	No. in Groups	No. in Groups	No. Developing Breast Cancer	Per Cent Developing Breast Cancer
With breast cancer	19	41	6	14.6
Without breast cancer	259	576	16	2.8
Totals	278	617	22	

* All sisters were 20 years or older at time of study.

TABLE 27-4. CANCER IN MOTHERS OF BREAST CANCER PATIENTS AND IN CONTROL NONCANCER GROUP

| GROUP | No. IN GROUP | BREAST CANCER IN MOTHERS || CANCER IN OTHER SITES IN MOTHERS ||
		No. Found	Per Cent	No. Found	Per Cent
Breast cancer patients	312	19	6.10	34	16.0
Noncancer controls	134	3	2.24	8	6.0

Tables 3 and 4 from Oliver, 1958.

Breast cancer in the State of California accounted for 23 per cent of all cancer in white females compared with 18 per cent of all cancer in Negro females. Undoubtedly, this difference is in part a function of the greater life expectancy of white females, which is 74.4 years, compared with 66.8 years for Negro females (Table 27-6). Of the white women living to their expected age of 74, a little less than 6 per cent will have developed cancer of the breast. The incidence of breast cancer is significantly less among the Chinese and Japanese.

These racial differences in incidence of breast cancer are said to exist, but how much of this is due to differences in efficiencies of reporting among countries and how much represents actual racial differences, whether genetic or environmental, are questions yet to be answered. Illustrating this problem is the adjusted death rate of 3.8 per 100,000 from female breast cancer in Japan compared with 26.6 in the United States, 12.1 in Finland and 18.2 in Sweden. The children of nationals, once living in another country, tend to assume the rate of their new country (Breslow, 1963).

While the high death rates for breast cancer correlate with those countries where birth rates are low, there is also a remarkable correlation with the amount of fat consumed per capita (Table 27-7). The higher the amount of fat consumed, the higher the death rate from breast cancer, with exceptions, of course. The significance of these data is interesting, but not clear.

Wynder et al. (1960) reviewed the problem of breast cancer in relation to marital status, age at marriage, nursing habits and numbers

Table 27-5. Comparison of Breast Cancer Mortality With That of the 5 Leading Cancer Sites in Females (United States, 1960)

Age Groups	15–34			35–54			55–74			75 & Over		
No. in Groups & Per Cent of Female Population	23,800,000 (37%)			22,800,000 (36%)			14,000,000 (22%)			3,200,000 (5%)		
	Deaths			Deaths			Deaths			Deaths		
	Site*	Number Reported	No. per 100,000	Site*	Number Reported	No. per 100,000	Site*	Number Reported	No. per 100,000	Site*	Number Reported	No. per 100,000
	Uterus	520	2.2	BREAST	7,827	34.3	BREAST	10,983	78.4	Colon & Rectum	7,174	224.2
	BREAST	462	1.9	Uterus	4,503	19.7	Colon & Rectum	10,439	74.5	BREAST	4,477	139.9
	Leukemia	397	1.6	Colon & Rectum	2,837	12.4	Uterus	6,940	49.5	Stomach	3,044	95.1
	Hodgkins	272	1.2	Ovary	2,428	10.6	Ovary	4,313	30.8	Uterus	2,445	76.4
	Brain	258	1.1	Lung	1,344	5.9	Stomach	3,731	26.6	Pancreas	1,854	57.9
TOTALS		1,911	8.0		18,939	83.0		36,406	260.0		18,994	593.5

* Listed in order of frequency of disease. (Computed from "1964 Cancer Facts and Figures," American Cancer Society. Source: Vital Statistics of the United States, 1960.)

Table 27-6. Life Expectancy in Years of Females in the U.S.

	White				Nonwhite*			
	1850	1900	1950	1964	1850	1900	1950	1964
	40.5	51.08	72.03	74.6		35.04	62.7	67.2

* Of the nonwhite, 92 per cent are Negro. Source: U. S. Bureau of the Census.

TABLE 27-7. DEATH RATE PER 100,000 FEMALES (LIVING) FROM BREAST CANCER, AND CONSUMPTION OF FATS AND OILS

COUNTRY	FAT CONSUMPTION (Kg. per person/year)	DEATH RATE*
Japan	2.6	3.8
Mexico	9.9	3.8
Greece	17.3	4.5
Columbia	5.5	5.6
Spain	14.0	6.5
Yugoslavia	9.5	6.9
Chile	7.7	7.1
Venezuela	7.8	8.0
Portugal	15.0	11.0
Finland	17.7	12.1
Italy	13.1	13.6
France	12.9	14.4
Austria	17.1	14.9
Germany	22.9	15.5
Norway	24.7	17.1
Sweden	21.1	18.2
Ireland	19.3	18.9
Belgium	21.6	19.8
Switzerland	17.2	21.5
New Zealand	19.2	21.6
United Kingdom	21.9	23.0
Netherlands	25.1	23.4
Denmark	25.0	24.0

* Compiled from WHO Report, 1967.

of children, and concluded as others had that the incidence rate of breast cancer may be a little higher in the unmarried, in the childless married female, and in those who did not nurse their children.

Hormones, especially steroids, which appear to be carcinogens in the murine species, give no evidence yet of having increased the incidence rate of breast cancer in women. The occasional beneficial influence of steroids upon primary and metastatic cancer of the breast is well known and this, too, is not clearly understood. Symmers (1968) however, has reported cancer of the breast in two transsexual individuals after surgery and hormonal interference with their primary and secondary characteristics. Both patients had primary metastasizing adenocarcinoma and in both the tumor was noticed about five years after the surgery procedures intended to effect a change of sex from male to female. Estrogens had been administered by inunction into the skin of the breasts by subcutaneous implantation and oral administrations. Contraceptive pills may change the breast, but more time is necessary to evaluate their carcinogenic potential.

An unexpected increase in breast cancer among women exposed to the Hiroshima and Nagasaki bombing radiation has been observed by the Atomic Bomb Casualty Commission (Wanebo et al., 1968). A comparable observation was made by McKenzie in 1965 in women with pulmonary tuberculosis who had been frequently examined by fluoroscopy. Provisional conclusions are that women exposed to 90 rads or more, as was the case in most of these patients, develop breast cancer at 2 to 4 times the expected rate, and that in the irradiated group, the disease begins earlier in life.

Breast Cancer in Pregnancy and Lactation. The incidence of cancer of the breast in pregnant and lactating women is said to be less than in the total child-bearing age group. However, if true, the reason may not relate to pregnancy and lactation at all, because the

TABLE 27-8. COMPARISON OF INCIDENCE OF BREAST CANCER AND BIRTH RATE BY AGE GROUPS (1962)

	15 & under	15–24	25–34	35–44	45–54	55–64	65–74
Patients with breast cancer	0.05%	0.2%	3.7%	16.8%	23.2%	23.2%	20.7%
Live births	0.05%	49.3%	40.3%	10.3%	0.05%		

incidence of breast cancer rises sharply in the age groups where the incidence of pregnancy declines (Table 27-8). Steiner (1954) found that only 5 (1.6%) of the 315 cases of breast cancer he encountered occurred below the age of 30 and only 25 (8.0%) of the total were under 40 years of age. Finn (1952) reported 46 cases of carcinoma of the breast among 62,561 pregnancies. Harrington (1937) reported 92 patients among 4,638 patients with carcinoma of the breast who were either lactating or pregnant when their carcinoma was discovered. McWhirter (1955) encountered carcinoma in this group 26 times among his series of 1,882 patients. Rosemond (1963) reported 56 cases of breast cancer among 7,381 pregnant patients treated during the preceding 10 years, and Devitt et al. (1964) observed 43 among 1,600.

In general, the prognosis is poor when cancer of the breast is first detected in pregnancy or lactation. Several factors may contribute. First, the outlook for cancer of any type is usually less favorable in pregnant patients. Second, physiologic breast engorgement tends to mask early detection of the tumor. The associated mammary hyperemia may favor an early spread by the vascular route. Finally, there is the unsettled effect of hormonal change with the pronounced elevation of estrogen levels encountered in pregnancy and lactation; most consider this hormonal effect to be adverse.

Lest one consider surgery contraindicated in patients whose breast lesions are first detected during pregnancy or lactation, the reader's attention is directed to a 25 per cent 5-year survival at Memorial Hospital, New York (Adair, 1952), and a 35 per cent 5-year survival reported by McWhirter (1955). Erwald (1967) concludes that the same treatment should be given during pregnancy as when the patient is not pregnant. In the absence of metastases, there is no reason to interrupt the pregnancy since it is not established that the prognosis is improved by this measure. If metastases are found, the prognosis is extremely poor, but not hopeless. There is no evidence that subsequent pregnancy worsens the prognosis in a woman previously treated for breast cancer if metastases are not already present. Thus the views of White and White (1956) that coincident pregnancy and lactation should not serve as categorical reasons for inoperability of breast cancer seem to be sound.

Bilateral carcinoma of the breast is an infrequent occurrence among the female population. However, the patient who has had a cancer in one breast has twice the chance of developing cancer in the remaining breast within the next 5 years than has the average white woman in the general population of developing an initial cancer in either breast in a lifetime. It is possible that bilateral breast cancer may represent a cross metastasis, but for a variety of reasons it appears more likely that in most cases it represents a primary cancer in each breast. The multicentric origin of cancer in the same breast is common enough, and it appears that factors which predispose to the development of cancer in one breast quite likely are capable of affecting the other adversely.

The incidence rate for cancer of the breast is also increased in patients with chronic cystic mastitis as discussed on page 673.

Aberrant or ectopic breast tissue is reported to be present in 1 to 5 per cent of the female population. The most frequent location is in the upper outer quadrant, although mammary ectopia may occur anywhere along the "milk line." Cancer arising in such tissue has been reported. That which is most frequently considered to be cancer in ectopic tissue is in the upper outer margin of the breast (tail of Spence) which fairly frequently may be classified erroneously as ectopic tissue because the upper margin of the breast rises higher on the pectoral fold more frequently than is generally appreciated. The interesting experimental work in which a high rate of occurrence of mammary cancer has been produced in the murine species, especially that produced by hybridization followed by the administration of steroid hormones, appears to bear little relationship to the occurrence of breast cancer in women, as stated. While these controlled studies have provided a very useful experimental tool, particularly in relation to therapy, there is no evidence yet that exogenous steroids produce breast cancer in the human population though it may be anticipated.

PATHOLOGY

The clinical grading of breast cancer has resulted in several classifications in which the general purpose is to categorize patients with this disease as to (1) whether the disease clinically appears localized to the breast, (2) whether it has extended so as to involve axillary nodes but without evidence of generalized spread, and (3) whether distant metastases are evident. At times the latter may be the case even when the primary lesion and axillary metastases are not detected clinically. Although such clinical classifications are useful and in a general way correlate with the effectiveness of treatment and the prognosis, if the primary lesion is small and may be missed, if the axillary metastatic nodes have not enlarged sufficiently to be palpable, or if the patient is obese and therefore at times the axillary nodes may be obscured, even though they are rather large, erroneous classifications on a clinical basis may result.

Several microscopic classifications of breast cancer exist, and each depends on one or more of the following factors: (1) the extent to which breast cancer is observed histologically —i.e., limited to the breast, or to the breast and the axillary nodes, or to the breast, the axillary and the mediastinal nodes, etc.; (2) the degree of anaplasia that the tumor exhibits in these areas; and (3) its tendency to invade venules and lymphatics and its tendency to invade the basement membrane and surrounding fibrous tissue, whether or not there is a lymphocytic response at the periphery of the tumor. Collectively, these are among the more important indicators of what the tumor is doing, and they hint as to whether or not it is highly invasive, whether it is being partially contained by resistance on the part of the host, or whether its biologic activity is somewhere between. For these reasons the older morphologic classifications of scirrhous, adenomatous or medullary cancer are of little value. The necessity for a simplified and more uniformly acceptable pathologic classification for breast cancer is especially obvious if one is to compare the results obtained from two particular forms of treatment. Unfortunately, even among pathologists, the same terms do not necessarily connote pathologic similarity of breast cancer. For example, some consider colloid cancer of the breast to be so benign that it should not be considered in computing end-results, whereas others find it to be a highly malignant lesion (Bonser et al., 1961). Obviously, all do not agree on what is and what is not colloid cancer of the breast. Unless one is assured that the same classification and grading are used for all patients, comparison of survival data on the basis of descriptive pathology is not practical on a national scale. Therefore, it is extremely difficult to compare the results from one series with those of another unless the same author reviews both series, and this is seldom possible.

Precancerous Lesions. Stewart (1950) expresses the view that the change of a lesion from a benign status to one of malignancy probably takes place before it is detectable under the microscope; he finds the term "premalignant" less and less appropriate as the years go by. Occasionally, it is applicable, but the question is "where and when." In this connection, most will agree with the suggestions of Stewart that "the most frequent precancerous lesion of the breast is a cancer in the opposite breast"—in fact, that "the female breast is a precancerous organ." Cancer may and does occur in any postpubertal breast, whether "normal," the hyperplastic breast of pregnancy and lactation, the atrophic breast or in conjunction with chronic cystic mastitis. There are no barriers or inhibiting factors that cancer will respect in the breast.

In situ lobular carcinoma is a preinvasive form of breast cancer which, if inadequately treated, will frequently progress to infiltrative cancer. A follow-up study of patients with in situ lobular carcinoma (McDivitt et al., 1967), treated in most instances by local excision, reveals the subsequent cumulative risk of infiltration to be: 8 per cent after 5 years, 15 per cent after 10 years, 27 per cent after 15 years, and 35 per cent after 20 years. After 23 years, the cumulative risk is thought to exceed 50 per cent. In addition, the cumulative risk of cancer developing in the breast contralateral to that in which in situ lobular carcinoma was found was 10 per cent after 10 years, 15 per cent after 15 years, and 25 per cent after 20 years. The cumulative risk of contralateral breast cancer after 22 years appears to exceed 30 per cent. These data argue for performing a simple prophylactic mastectomy of the "normal" breast in patients whose cancer in the opposite breast has been removed.

Paget's Disease of the Nipple. This entity was described by Sir James Paget in 1874, only 2 years before his description of Paget's disease of the bone. It is characterized by an erythematous eruption of the nipple and/or the areolar tissue. A sensation of itching or burning about the nipple is often the first symptom. It is to be distinguished only from bilateral eruptions about the nipple which generally connote some allergic or local irritant factor. Bilateral Paget's disease rarely occurs.

Paget's disease of the nipple is diagnostic of carcinoma within the breast. Usually, it is carcinoma of the intraductal type, although other types of carcinoma occasionally also produce the skin eruptions. The cutaneous eruption probably represents an extension of carcinoma cells into the skin from the underlying ducts, and most evidence is suggestive that the initial lesion arises within the ducts and often some distance from the nipple. The lesion is also to be distinguished from tuberculosis or syphilis, either of which may present at times gross appearances which raise the question of Paget's disease, but usually the differentiation is not a difficult one. There is no structural distinction relative to the changes in the ducts that would distinguish this clinical entity from ductal carcinoma unaccompanied by skin eruption. Often the nipple is enlarged, inflamed and granular in appearance, although late in the disease it may be destroyed.

The microscopic examination of the skin discloses the classic Paget cells which are large, round or "pavement stone" in appearance. Edema and some inflammatory response may also be noted. The Paget cells are present most abundantly in the malpighian layer of the skin but may extend to its surface.

In many instances, no tumor mass can be felt in the breast, but should Paget cells be present in the skin, without exception a carcinoma exists within the breast. A radical mastectomy is indicated and without delay. At times axillary metastases are already evident in spite of the failure to feel the tumor. Careful sectioning of the breast will disclose the presence of a ductal carcinoma, often minute but infiltrative. Usually extensive adenosis or intraductal epithelial proliferation, with piling up of cells, is noted. If there are any changes in the opposite breast, a biopsy usually is indicated, as ductal carcinomas account for most bilateral independent carcinomas of the breast, in the author's experience. The prognosis is generally fair, provided that the physician recognizes the connotation of Paget's disease and does not wait for a palpable lump in the breast to appear.

Paget's disease may also occur in the skin elsewhere, and thus is not limited to the breast (Holleran and Schmutzer, 1965).

Carcinoma of Mammary Ducts. Noninfiltrating ductal tumors or papillary carcinoma may display all gradients between benign and malignant disease. The features of adenosis and the piling-up of ductal epithelium usually are observed microscopically; the lumen of the duct is correspondingly reduced or obliterated. Usually, the cells are well differentiated, and mitotic figures are not abundantly noted. Carcinomas in this category may not extend beyond the basement layer, in which case the lesion is not invasive cancer. Indeed, the diagnosis of cancer is often most difficult to make with certainty. On the other hand, if there is any one "benign" lesion likely to assume malignant characteristics at a later date, it is this one. Breast amputation under these conditions may be advisable as a cancer often develops later, which suggests that this lesion when first seen was cancerous. Intraductal hyperplasia, with the piling up of epithelium, is frequently found in the contralateral breast. Should this be the case, a simple mastectomy should be seriously considered and, if acceptable, should be performed on the opposite breast as soon as practical. In some instances, multiple foci of ductal carcinoma are found in the breast once the entire tissue becomes available for microscopic examination.

Intraductal carcinoma, if diagnosed early and treated by radical mastectomy, carries perhaps the best prognosis of any breast carcinoma. On the other hand, when operation is delayed until more positive evidence of carcinoma is available, prognosis is likely to be poor indeed.

Carcinoma with fibrosis is among the more commonly encountered histologic varieties. Grossly, these lesions usually are not well circumscribed because they tend to radiate toward the periphery of the breast. They are unusually hard, and the cut surface discloses the striated appearance of tumor intermingled with fibrous tissue which cuts with a hard and gritty feeling. Microscopically, the pattern varies extensively between one of an orderly arrangement with the cells lying in columnar fashion between heavy strands of fibrous tissue and one of such extensive fibrous proliferation that the carcinoma cells are not always readily found.

Carcinoma with Lymphoid Infiltration (Circumscribed). In contrast to the fibrous qualities of scirrhous carcinoma, these are generally bulky tumors which cut with little resistance and tend to be circumscribed, although not encapsulated. The surface after cutting is pearly gray in color, often containing hemorrhagic and necrotic areas. Unlike scirrhous carcinoma which tends to be adherent to adjacent normal breast tissue, subcutaneous fat, skin or fascia, the medullary carcinoma is comparatively free from attachment and seems to metastasize later than the scirrhous tumors.

This carcinoma usually is composed of large rounded cells with basophilic staining cytoplasm and large vesicular nuclei. The lymphocytic response at the periphery and indeed in some of the central areas of the tumor has been interpreted by some as a manifestation of "immune" response on the part of the host. This phenomenon often implies a better prognosis than is observed in the more infiltrative fibrous or scirrhous types of carcinomas.

Infiltrative lobular carcinomas are poorly demarcated grossly; they are tough and firm and frequently display the striations characteristic of scirrhous cancers. From microscopic examination, it may not be readily evident that this form of infiltrating carcinoma is one arising within the lobules of the breast; nor is its infiltrating nature always apparent. Once infiltration has occurred, "threadlike strands of tumor" are dispersed fairly loosely throughout the adjacent fibrous tissue.

Intraductal infiltrating carcinoma tends to metastasize early. Stewart points out that its metastases often may simulate lymphosarcoma. The author has observed several cases wherein the final diagnosis from a biopsy of the axillary node in the absence of a palpable breast tumor could not be distinguished from a lymphosarcoma histologically until permanent sections were available.

Relatively Rare Cancers. Among these are the so-called "sweat gland" carcinomas, the intracystic carcinoma, the adenoid cystic carcinoma, the squamous cell carcinoma, the spindle cell carcinoma, the carcinoma with osseous and cartilaginous metaplasia, and fibrosarcoma and angiosarcoma.

The *"sweat gland" carcinoma* involves the ducts with transitions ranging from typical apocrine epithelium to the hyperplasia of the intraductal carcinoma. It may or may not infiltrate as a cellular structure having the same cell type as apocrine epithelium. There is not sufficient evidence to justify the sweat gland as the site of origin for this tumor to the exclusion of the lobular epithelium as its origin. The fact that the breast is a sweat gland in embryonic origin has confused the picture of this tumor. In general, these cancers tend to grow slowly and to metastasize comparatively late.

The *intracystic carcinomas* are rare, possibly because the epithelium of most cysts is destroyed or lost as it enlarges. This tumor often arises within a residual portion of the epithelium in a fairly large cyst. Such cysts may be aspirated, obtaining as much as 30 to 50 ml. or more of yellow cholesterol-bearing fluid occasionally tinged with blood. As the incidence of carcinoma in such cysts is probably less than 1 per cent, the practice of aspiration continues. In the occasional patient, however, a small carcinoma may be found within the wall of the cyst; if overlooked, it can metastasize with fatal consequence. Occasionally, the staining of the fluid aspirated by the Papanicolaou technic discloses suspicious cells, but more often these cells are either crenated and destroyed or so distorted as to defy diagnosis by this cytologic technic.

The *adenocystic carcinomas* are extremely rare and probably need to be mentioned only because of their ability to metastasize in spite of their generally very slow-growing nature. Stewart states they are indistinguishable histologically from adenoid cystic carcinoma of the salivary glands as well as from those arising in the mucous glands of the tracheobronchus.

Squamous cell carcinoma connotes a tumor arising within the breast itself and not one from the overlying skin as the term might imply. In reality, it is an infiltrating ductal carcinoma with squamous metaplasia. However, its histologic structure is predominantly that of the squamous cell carcinoma with keratohyaline granules, intracellular bridges and epithelial pillars with transitional changes from ductal carcinoma also being detectable.

The *spindle cell carcinoma* is comprised microscopically of areas simulating sarcomatous tumors arising within the connective tissue. It may be difficult to distinguish from the malignant form of "cystosarcoma" phyllodes. Spindle cell carcinoma is rarely encountered. Stewart adroitly sums up the best methods for avoiding the controversy as to whether such tumors are carcinoma or sarcoma by acknowledging that "some doubt as to the ultimate accuracy of the diagnosis" may exist. However, these tumors metastasize to the regional lymph nodes unlike the usual expected behavior in sarcoma which, as a general rule, tends to metastasize via the blood stream. "As a general rule, applicable to neoplasms as a whole, it may be stated that it is much more common for an epithelial tumor to show pseudosarcomatous areas than for a connective tissue tumor to show pseudoepithelial areas" (Stewart, 1950).

Mammary carcinoma with osseous and cartilaginous metaplasia provides many unusual microscopic manifestations of metaplasia. Such aberrations may be limited to the tumor or arise in certain parts of the areas it infiltrates. In some parts osseous and cartilaginous tissue may predominate to the exclusion of most other histologic characteristics. The predominance of cartilage over osseous material or its reverse is an individual variant. It is most unlikely that these tumors represent either osteogenic or chondrosarcomas, but rather they are extreme examples of metaplasia occurring in epithelial tumors.

Cystosarcoma phyllodes generally attains enormous size and may actually burst. It usually behaves as a benign tumor, but occasionally a malignant variant is found. Its spectacular size and its infrequent occurrence undoubtedly is cause why this tumor is reported with the highest frequency of all rare tumors of the breast. It usually arises from a fibroadenoma of the intracanalicular type.

The malignant variant involves the connective tissue rather than the epithelium in most patients. Blood stream invasion, more characteristic of sarcoma than carcinoma, is the probable reason that when metastases occur from this tumor, generally they are discovered first in the lung or in some distant area instead of the regional lymphatics. More frequently than not, the tumor is benign. The choice of treatment is radical as opposed to simple mastectomy, as portions of the tumor may show malignant change not discernible from biopsy samplings.

Sarcomas arising from the fat, blood vessels, including the lymphatics, are exceedingly rare, as are fibrosarcomas, leiomyosarcomas and osteogenic sarcomas in the breast.

Metastatic Breast Cancer

Breast cancer may metastasize to any and all organs, and it may do so before the primary lesion is detected. Not infrequently a distant metastasis is the only presenting finding. As with any metastatic carcinoma, its microscopic structure may assume such unusual patterns of growth as to give no indication of its site of origin.

Occasionally, nodes are detected in the axilla or the supraclavicular region on the contralateral side when these same areas are apparently normal above the breast in which carcinoma is suspected. In some, perhaps in most cases, these are harbingers of bilateral carcinoma.

Metastasis to bone is a prominent feature of advanced breast cancer. The lumbar vertebrae, the pelvis and the proximal femoral areas are the bones most commonly involved, but no bone is exempt. Occasionally, occult metastatic carcinoma is first detected upon the examination of a marrow smear, searching for the cause of an "unexplained" anemia.

Curiously, the adrenal glands are common organ sites of metastatic breast cancer, although metastases to the lungs, the brain and the liver are encountered more frequently. Tumor extension to the parietal pleura from the chest wall is observed fairly regularly in advanced stages of breast malignancy. The lungs and the liver, when affected, usually receive tumor by lymphatic or hematogenous routes. The abdominal cavity may be affected similarly with the appearance of ascites and the occurrence of intestinal obstruction.

Direct spread of tumor through the intracutaneous lymphatics may occur over a fairly wide area of the chest wall (carcinoma *en cuirasse*). It is possible that skin metastases arrive at the distant areas by the same route. Metastatic carcinoma to the brain is frequently from the breast, but tumors of the thyroid and the lung are more likely to involve the brain. The route and the nature of metastases for any particular breast cancer, and perhaps for all cancer, are highly variable, and factors influencing the route and extent are not understood. An important question to answer is whether secondary and tertiary metastases may occur from a primary metastasis, as this information would be of considerable assistance in determining the value of removing metastasis at the time the primary cancer is excised.

CLINICAL PATTERN OF CARCINOMA OF THE BREAST

The course of untreated breast cancer invariably is fatal if intercurrent causes of death do not supervene in the natural course of the disease. Death is rarely due to the localized lesion; almost always death is from metastatic involvement of a vital organ or organs or from general debility too nonspecific to assign to any one organ alone.

History. There is no one factor or set of factors to be found in the past or family history which can be assigned an important role in the clinical history, except for a previously recognized carcinoma in the opposite breast. True, certain degrees of positive statistical correlation may exist in relation to a lump in the breast, but none is specific. Then too, a lump in the breast of an older patient is much more likely to be cancerous than in a woman under 25 years of age. Such minor variants as menstrual or gynecologic disorders, celibacy, failure to nurse or to be able to nurse, familial background of cancer, and socioeconomic position are of interest to note but are of statistical importance only to groups of patients, and can be of interest retrospectively only in the individual patient when an unexpected lump is discovered incidentally.

Trauma as an antecedent history of breast cancer is often spontaneously conjured up from the distant past by the patient seeking to explain why she should become victim of an established breast cancer. Moritz (1954) attributes the patient's persistent attitude in desiring to involve trauma to "claim value," especially that of compensation. But it is also possible that this attitude of the patient persists from the fact that after trauma to the breast, she may massage her breast and by this unintended "self-examination" find for the first time a breast mass. This she may choose to watch silently by herself. Often several months elapse before she seeks medical advice. Should a cancer be found at that time, she may assume that the "bruise" had undergone spontaneous malignant transformation. And who can say it has not? We just don't know.

Nipple discharge, particularly a bloody discharge, alarms many patients. Its most likely cause is a benign intraductal papilloma. Occasionally an intraductal carcinoma causes a bloody discharge. Fitts and Horn (1951) report nipple discharge to have been the only sign of an otherwise occult carcinoma in some patients.

Discharges that are yellow or dark green in color generally connote benign "cystic" disease of the breast. Study of this fluid may prove to be useful in the early diagnosis of cancer in some patients. Papanicolaou examined the fluid obtained by gentle massage and was able to detect cancer cells. Of 560 patients entering the Strong Prevention Clinic for an asymptomatic check-up, he was able to express breast secretions in 19.3 per cent. By the use of an improved breast pump, secretions were obtained in 50 per cent of patients who had cancer of the breast.

Breast pain as a dominant complaint usually arises from one of several causes, most of which are not malignant in nature. It is more important when unilateral. Bilateral breast pain (mastodynia) is observed fairly frequently prior to or during the early phases of menstruation and usually represents physiologic engorgement of the breast attending menstruation. It also occurs in pregnancy, particularly during the early part of the first trimester and in the last stages of the third trimester. Bilateral pain is often a severe complaint in women with heavy pendulous breasts; often pain of this origin radiates down the inner surfaces of the arms. Bilateral pain is also a frequent complaint of patients with chronic "cystic mastitis," but, as this disease may be more severe in one breast than the other, or limited to one breast, the complaint may refer to one side only. The duration of pain in this disease is often long and one of slowly growing worse until after the menopause. Complete remissions are not uncommon, but generally some recurrence at or just prior to menstruation is noted.

Pain of recent origin and localized to one breast is an important complaint. It is found in 15 to 25 per cent of patients with carcinoma with or without a lump or a mass in the breast noted by the patient. It is more suggestive of the presence of cancer in the postmenopausal period than in the premenopausal era. Reassurance of the patient as being free of cancer simply because her breast is painful is not warranted under these conditions.

In patients under 30 years of age, a painful and tender discrete hard lump is most commonly a fibroadenoma. An acute or chronic abscess of the breast may simulate a fibroadenoma in some ways but usually can be excluded readily on other grounds. Occasionally, fibroangiomata, a breast scar, or fibrosis secondary to fat necrosis may also be painful.

The sudden onset of pain often indicates hemorrhage into a pre-existing cyst; a hemorrhagic cyst is rare but when present is strong supporting evidence that it may contain a carcinoma. Acute distention of a benign cyst from the rapid accumulation of fluid may suddenly produce pain. Both of these lesions are usually very tender.

Thus the recent onset of breast pain is an important complaint and one to be evaluated and its cause determined. Its presence does not exclude cancer.

Lumps. The finding of a lump is a most common complaint in patients with breast cancer. Usually, the patient has noted a mass or lump in her breast while bathing, massaging after painful injury, or while practicing self-examination. Lumps found during self-examination are usually painless, though at times slight pain is the factor initiating self-examination. The physician is occasionally surprised by the frequency with which the patient may find very small masses in spite of obese breasts. It is equally surprising how large some masses may become without the patient's apparent knowledge. Often, cancers of the latter variety are discoid or flat, occurring in an obese female. Occasionally, however, they are rounded or oblong and actually affect the contour of the breast to a degree that seems impossible to escape the patient's attention. Perhaps, it really has not; fear of the truth can prove to be fatal.

Examination of the Breast. The normal texture of the breast varies considerably in accordance with the age of the patient, whether or not previous pregnancies have occurred, the strength of the suspensory (Cooper's) ligaments of the breast, atrophy or lobular separation which often give the impression of a granular or shotty nodularity. Previous disease such as chronic cystic mastitis, breast abscess or fat necrosis may distort the breast as well as the normal direction that the nipple should point. None of these variations is in itself necessarily significant but may create difficulties in detecting the presence of a lesion and in suspecting its nature.

Both breasts should be equal in size, the nipples pointing in isometric directions and protruding to a comparable extent. Any particular area more prominent than others should arouse suspicion. The nipples and the areolar tissue should be inspected closely for evidence of scaling, desquamation, retraction or asymmetric tilting. Skin retraction is searched for and usually is detected best with the patient in the normal sitting position, placing both outstretched arms above the head. Skin retraction implies skin invasion or involvement of Cooper's ligaments and more often than not tumor spread to the regional lymphatics as well (Fig. 27-1). The

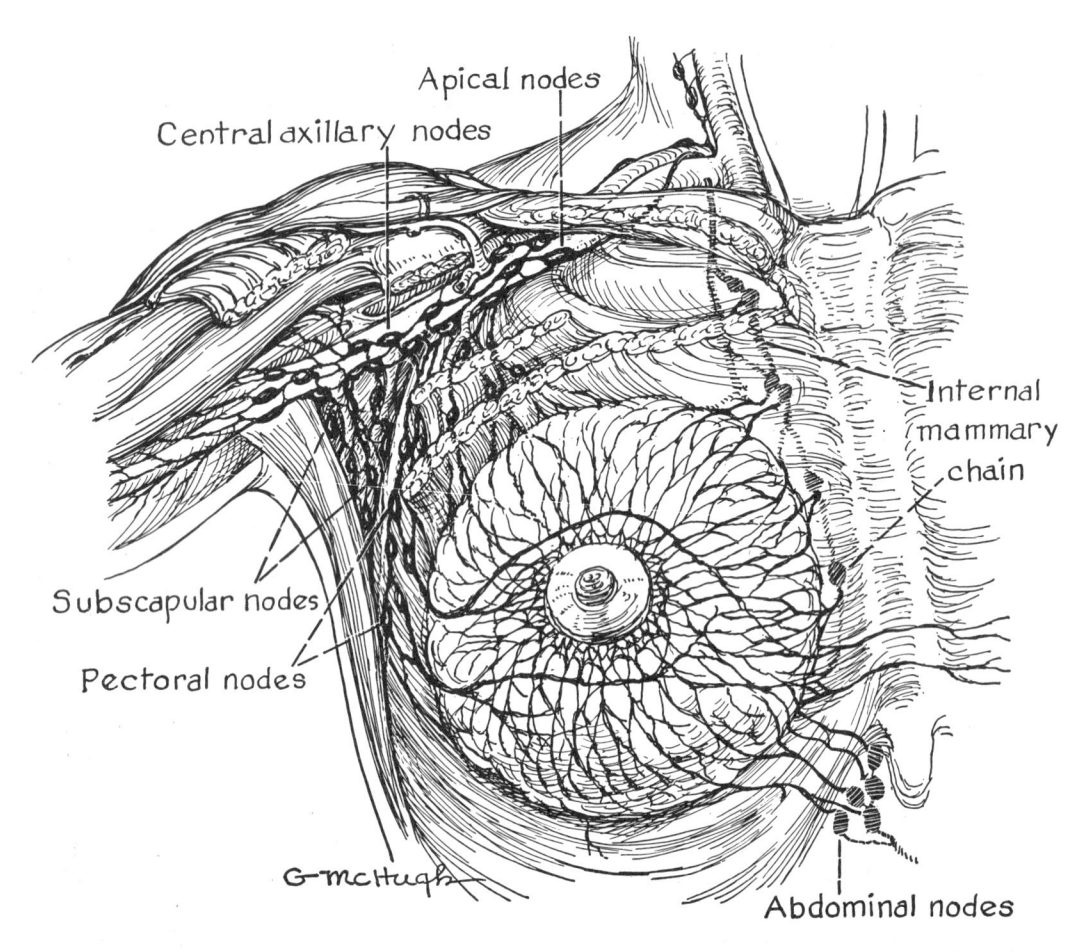

FIG. 27-1. Principal channels of the lymph drainage from the breast are illustrated. It is evident that carcinoma of the breast may spread in any direction, although metastases are more likely to follow the course of the dominant channels for the area of the breast in which the tumor arises. When nodes are involved, in about two thirds of the operable cases, the spread is to axillary lymph nodes; in the remaining third the internal mammary chain is involved. When axillary nodes are involved, the tendency to drain to substernal nodes may be increased.

same applies to the orange-peel or "pigskin" appearance of the skin, often referred to as *peau d'orange*. This appearance is created by intracutaneous lymphostasis, causing intradermal pores to be widely separated, and is usually associated with intracutaneous metastatic nodules locally or even at some distances from the primary site. Compared with the minor skin retraction, *peau d'orange* usually carries a much less favorable prognosis, although in neither instance is the prognosis good. Both are late signs (Chiu-Chen Wang, 1967).

Carcinoma *en cuirasse* is the classic example of widespread intracutaneous dissemination of cancer through its lymphatics, with brawny induration being more prominent than *peau d'orange*. Often the entire breast, the shoulder and the upper abdomen may be involved. Discoid or rounded nodularity is present. When the skin is red and appears to be inflamed, the term "inflammatory carcinoma" is often used to describe it. The prognosis in such patients is especially poor, usually hopeless.

Inflammation and dimpling of the skin in the presence of an underlying mass does not always indicate an advanced cancer at all. In

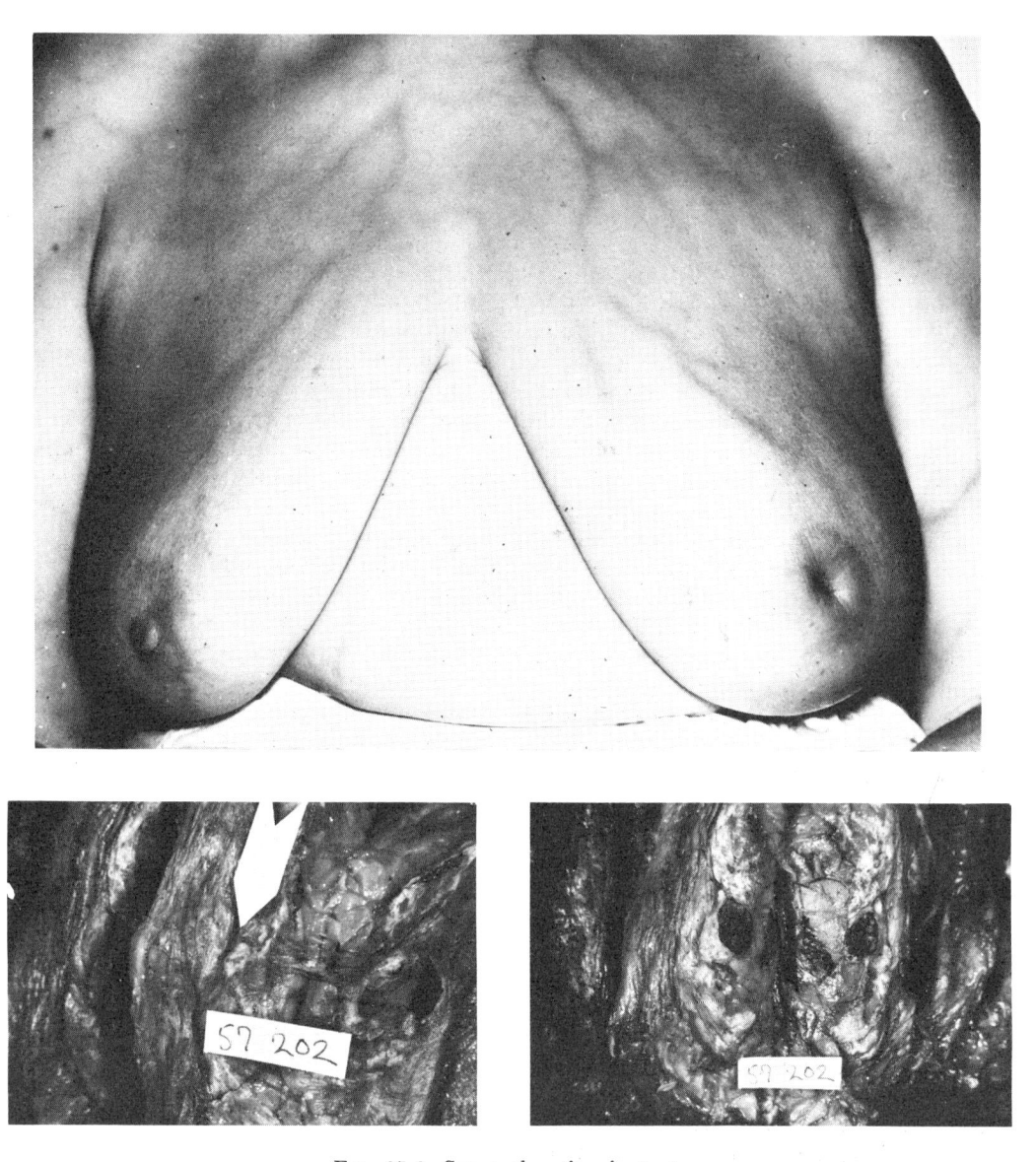

Fig. 27-2. See explanation in text.

Fig. 27-2, is an infrared photograph of the breast of a 63-year-old female who developed inflammatory changes in the skin similar to those seen in inflammatory cancer and in addition, a six weeks' history of retraction of the nipple. The photograph shows some increase of venous vascularity and all physical findings except for the absence of metastases, suggested the diagnosis of an inflammatory cancer. There is no effective treatment for this lesion; nonetheless, we attempted a radical mastectomy, avoiding biopsy since the diagnosis was so obvious clinically, and at the time the prevailing opinion was to remove the breast with a minimum of manipulation. This procedure was carried out after suitable consultation, including another surgeon and a radiologist. Great care was taken to manipulate the breast the least possible and successful radical mastectomy was carried out. To our chagrin, the diagnosis was a lipoma with hemorrhage into its center as also shown in Fig. 27-2. This case serves to emphasize once again that there are few if any contra-indications to a biopsy that are as bad as an unnecessary extensive surgical operation.

Upon palpation, usually one lump may prove to be more prominent than others if carcinoma is present. It is often referred to as the *dominant lump* because of one or more of the following features: it is usually firm to hard, often nontender and may be fixed to adjacent tissue. The lump may be adherent to the skin, producing dimpling or it may be adherent to the fatty tissue, or to the fascia and not affect the skin, depending upon the depth of its origin and whether it introduces traction of Cooper's ligaments. Advanced local carcinoma may be fixed to all four of the structures; an early cancer may be fixed to the skin should its site of origin be close to the dermal structures. Occasionally, the tumor is relatively soft and extends over a wide area and does not arouse much suspicion. Unnecessary manipulation once the diagnosis is suspected is to be avoided as this may disseminate tumor cells.

Examination of the axilla is carried out best with the forearm of the patient resting upon the examiner's arm or with one hand supporting the elbow of the patient. With his other hand, the axilla is examined gently, beginning at its base along the margin of the pectoralis major. The fingers are introduced gently into the truncated portion of the axilla, depressing the skin and the underlying subcutaneous tissue gently against the thoracic cage, trying to reach the apex. Any suspicious nodule encountered is rolled gently under the finger against the thoracic cage. Its size, consistency and freedom of mobility are noted. Obviously, perfectly innocent lymph nodes are palpable and usually they may be palpable to a similar degree in the contralateral axilla. Failure to detect nodes in the axilla is no assurance that nodal involvement does not exist, because only the larger and more laterally situated ones can usually be reached. Some lymph nodes may be replaced completely by carcinoma and still remain fairly soft and freely movable. Others may be small, shotty and create little suspicion when extensively involved. Hence, in examination of the axilla, errors are fairly common, even among the most experienced clinicians.

The supraclavicular areas along the lower neck on both sides should be examined gently but firmly, searching especially for nodes lying just below the posterior margin of the mesial third of the clavicle and along the jugular vein and carotid artery.

Examination of the opposite breast where the other breast has cancer will often reveal masses which may or may not be cancerous. From 3 to 9 per cent of patients with carcinoma of one breast may be expected to have or to develop tumor in the opposite breast, simultaneously or within a year or two. Occasionally, carcinoma of the breast is multicentric in one breast so that more than one "dominant lump" may be found. When there are other signs raising suspicions as to the presence of a malignant lesion in one breast, the presence of a similar lesion, perhaps without fixation, should not delude the examiner into the belief that he is dealing with widespread benign disease, such as chronic cystic mastitis. Search is made for metastases in the abdomen, especially the liver. Roentgenograms of the chest, the skull, the vertebral column and the pelvis may be helpful.

MAMMOGRAPHY

In 1953 Gershon-Cohen *et al.* reported some success with the use of roentgenographic technics to detect breast lesions, now known as mammography. As experience accumulated and methods improved, the merits of this procedure became established, especially as a means for the detection of breast cancer not previously suspected. It is useful also as a means for determining the status of both breasts before operating on a patient with a primary cancer, unilateral as far as can be ascertained clinically without the aid of a mammogram.

In the hands of experts, the diagnostic accuracy of mammographs is remarkably good when the technical quality of the films is satisfactory (Gershon-Cohen *et al.*, 1961). Egan (1962), without the aid of clinical information, was able to interpret correctly from mammograms alone the diagnosis of breast cancer in 501 (96.7%) of 518 proved carcinomas and to recognize 351 (91.6%) of the 383 lesions that proved benign. In addition, he detected 58 carcinomas that were present and not clinically suspected among the combined total of 2,522 mammograms, an incidence of about 2 per cent of occult carcinoma. Egan's results have been reviewed carefully by Robbins (1962), who wrote: "There is no practical importance of Egan mammography to cancer control, unless there exists in the local community the ability to reproduce these results." It seems probable that mammography will be generally adopted as the technics are mastered by others, though thus far progress has been slow. It is probable that 80 to 90 per cent of breast cancer determined by surgical biopsy can also be suspected from mammography (Witten, 1964). Therefore, the latter technic is quite useful as an additional screening device but is not intended to replace surgical biopsy once a lesion has been detected (see p. 678).

Egan, whose more recent results were published in 1964, believes that mammography is indicated (1) when signs and symptoms of breast disease are present; (2) as a means of observing the opposite breast after mastectomy (see also Missakian et al., 1965); (3) in patients with a strong family history of breast cancer; (4) in pendulous or lumpy breasts; (5) in patients with cancerophobia; and (6) in women with cancer when the primary site is undetermined.

Funderburk et al. (1964), injecting a 50 per cent solution of diatrizoate sodium into the duct from which bloody discharge had emerged and followed by mammography, located the intraductal papilloma in each of the 34 patients examined.

An initial screening examination of 20,211 women of ages 40 to 60 for carcinoma of the breast was carried out as part of a periodic screening study conducted by the Health Insurance Plan of Greater New York. Mammography was performed and a group of control patients was assigned. Strax et al. (1967) found that screening has resulted in substantial detection of cancer; mammary cancer is detectable through screening an average of 21 months sooner than usual. A higher proportion of cancers, or 65 per cent, has been detected in the screened group in an early stage, as shown by the absence of axillary node involvement, than in the control group, where the rate was 41 per cent. Both mammography and clinical examination contribute to the early detection of cancer in mass screening.

Barnes and Gershon-Cohen (1963) have been exploring the use of "clinical thermography" in a variety of diseases, including breast cancer—thermomammography. The principle involved depends on temperature differentials produced by disease, including cancer, and the making of infrared photoscans to detect abnormal variations in the body's natural infrared radiations. However, Hitchcock et al. (1968) and others have found thermography too nonspecific to be useful in mass screening for occult breast cancer, although Samuel et al. (1969) seem to find it beneficial.

Breast Biopsy

Indications for Biopsy or for Repeated Observations. The examiner's findings are not always evaluated easily. He may experience even more difficulty in articulating the reasons for his recommended course of action, even to himself.

The consideration which most reliably favors a benign lesion is the patient's age. If the physician is not completely satisfied that the lesion is benign, it should be biopsied without delay. If the diagnosis of cancer of the breast is to be made early, the only attitude that the surgeon can assume is early biopsy of any lesion, even if it is only remotely suspicious. Unfortunately, this course of action will force him to perform biopsy on a considerably larger number of patients whose ultimate diagnosis will prove to be benign than on those who will prove to have breast cancer. However, he cannot afford a course of delayed action in suspected cases. Waiting for fixation, skin retraction or *peau d'orange* is to be avoided assiduously, as these are the usual late manifestations of the disease.

Admittedly, the problem facing the family doctor is a different one. He may not encounter a patient with breast cancer more than once in several years, as there are more than 200,000 practicing physicians in the country, but there are about 68,000 new cases of breast cancer annually encountered. The family physician, however, often has the advantage of his previous examinations, as well as the opportunity afforded by an established rapport with the patient, which is so essential to a program of repeated examinations at frequent intervals. The surgeon, on the other hand, sees a different segment of patient population. His patients often are those who are screened by the family doctor. This factor serves to concentrate the population of positive or very suspicious breast masses in the office of the surgeon, who therefore needs to recommend biopsy more frequently.

If the surgeon is not entirely satisfied that the lesion under suspicion is benign, he has no recourse other than to advise *biopsy*, especially in females 25 years of age or older. The sooner this is carried out, the better. Delay of one week is often necessary for the patient to arrange for the care of her family. Should the patient be refractory to the suggestion of biopsy and refuse consultation after careful explanation, additional reappointments should be made in the hope that her confidence may be gained and biopsy performed. For those patients whose lesions are not suspicious the following schedule is a reasonable one: return in 3 weeks after the initial detection of the lesion, return again in 6 weeks, then 3 months, and thereafter at 4-month intervals for at least 3 to 5 years. These examinations should be made between menstrual periods. Additional safety is gained by instructing the patient thoroughly in self-examination to be carried out between her visits to the doctor's office.

Technics of Biopsy. Three types of procedures are practiced fairly commonly, but only one is recommended for most patients; that is excision biopsy. *Needle biopsy* is a poor substitute for a surgical biopsy and usually should not be performed unless the tumor mass is fluctuant, transilluminates readily, or the patient is under 25 years of age or refuses surgical biopsy. Often the pathologist is placed at a disadvantage with such specimens and may not be able to provide information as definitive as he could otherwise.

Incision biopsy is to be avoided in most patients unless the tumor mass is so large that its removal amounts essentially to a simple mastectomy. When performed, a small incision is made parallel with and equidistant from the elliptical incision planned if radical mastectomy proves to be necessary. A wedge of tissue is removed, noting whether it grates when stroked with the scalpel blade. The incision should not extend to the pectoral fascia nor into areas to be exposed later in the course of surgical removal of the breast. Once the tissue is removed, its bed should be closed carefully and the skin reapproximated with closely placed stitches sealing the skin from any possible seepage from beneath.

While closing the biopsy wound, the frozen section is performed. In more than 90 per cent of the cases, the diagnosis can be established accurately this way. If the pathologist is unable to reach a definite decision by this technic, no further operation should be performed until the permanent sections can be reviewed a few days later; otherwise, the breast should be removed as soon as the frozen section information is decisively positive. In the interest of avoiding tumor implants, the biopsy instruments are discarded, the surgeon and his assistants don another pair of gloves, the wound is "re-prepped" and redraped before starting the radical mastectomy. The mastectomy incision should be wide of the biopsy wound not only at the surface but also in the depths of the wound and should never enter into the biopsy wound at any point—tumor asepsis.

Excision biopsy is the procedure of choice and most commonly performed. The tumor is removed, giving it a fairly wide berth, so that noncancerous breast tissue surrounds the excised tumor. This avoids tumor implantation. The wound is closed carefully, and if the biopsy is positive for cancer, then radical mastectomy is performed.

Contralateral Breast Biopsy. Because of the possibility of concurrent or delayed occurrence of carcinoma in the contralateral breast, some authors consider that it is generally wise to biopsy that breast at the same time that the suspected breast is biopsied, and thereby to determine if there are ductal changes or other abnormalities present. Often no masses are felt in the "normal" breast, but this does not imply that serious changes have not occurred; hence, it is occasionally rewarding to sample its tissue for present and future reference.

Two points of caution should be mentioned. Surgical biopsy should not be performed in the office or under local anesthesia. Breast biopsy is a procedure to be carried out under general anesthesia and with the patient's permission and thorough understanding that a radical mastectomy is a distinct possibility at that time, depending upon the biopsy findings.

Anatomic Staging of Breast Cancer

A variety of attempts to classify clinically the stages of breast cancer have been devised. Most of these serve a useful purpose, but none is without its limitations. The Columbia classification by Haagensen and Foote (1943) was the first to prove a useful guide in determining operability of patients with breast cancer. More recently, the International Classification of Breast Cancer advocated a clinical staging based on the T (primary), N (nodes), and M (metastases) system (Table 27-9). At first glance, it is accurate, but detailed, cumbersome, and difficult to remember. However, once read, the broad principles are fully appreciated and are based upon Haagensen's criteria of operability and inoperability. The Columbia Clinical Staging System, developed by Haagensen himself and lettered A, B, C, D, is essentially similar to the International Classification's stages I, II, III, and IV. Characteristically, stage I (or A) is an early breast cancer, localized to the breast without axillary nodes; stage II (or B) is a similar early cancer with palpable and involved axillary nodes; stage III (or C) is characterized by a locally advanced cancer showing skin infiltration, ulceration, fixation, or edema; and stage IV (or D) has evidence of distant metastases.

Treatment of Breast Cancer

Radical Mastectomy. As this operation is designed to remove the breast and the entire axillary contents *en bloc*, leaving no known tumor behind, the choice of the initial incision should be tailored to the needs of the particular patient. Various types of incisions have been developed to serve these purposes (Fig. 27-3). For the most part, the surgeon employs only one as the incision of his preference. The author prefers the Deaver incision, a modification of the Meyer type. Should the lesion lie on either the lateral or the mesial side of the central portion of the breast, a modification of the Steward or the Orr incision may be preferred.

The tumor is ellipsed by the incision of choice, allowing at least 1½ to 2 inches of normal skin to be taken on all sides of the tumor. The subcutaneous tissue is undermined generously, leaving an estimated ¼ to ⅜ inch of subcutaneous tissue on the underside of the skin flap. The author prefers to leave this amount of subcutaneous fat in nontumor-bearing areas to avoid direct adherence of skin to the chest wall after the wound heals. This small amount of subcutaneous fat allows a small degree of gliding motion of the undermined skin edges which seems to be more comfortable to the patient later on. If the amount of skin ellipsed in the course of operation creates too large an area to be closed by approximating the undermined mesial and lateral flaps without undue tension, the remain-

TABLE 27-9. Abridged TNM* System of Classification of Carcinoma of the Breast†

Symbol	Description
T_1	Less than 2 cm. No skin fixation
T_2	2 to 5 cm. Skin tethered or dimpled No pectoral fixation
T_3	5 to 10 cm. Skin infiltrated or ulcerated Pectoral fixation
T_4	More than 10 cm. Skin involvement not beyond breast Chest wall fixation
N_0	No nodes
N_1	Axillary nodes movable Not significant Significant
N_2	Axillary nodes fixed
N_3	Supraclavicular nodes Edema of arm
M_0	No metastases
M	Metastases including skin involvement beyond breast and contralateral nodes

Four Clinical Stages Designated by TNM Symbols

Stage I	$T_1 N_0 M_0$
	$T_2 N_0 M_0$
Stage II	$T_1 N_1 M_0$
	$T_2 N_1 M_0$
Stage III	$T_1 N_2$ or $N_3 M_0$
	$T_2 N_2$ or $N_3 M_0$
	$T_3 N_0, N_1, N_2,$ or $N_3 M_0$
	$T_4 N_0, N_1, N_2,$ or $N_3 M_0$
Stage IV	Any combination of T and N symbols including M

* T = tumor; N = nodes; M = metastases.
† From Copeland, M. D.: American Joint Committee on Cancer Staging and End Results Reporting: Objectives and progress. Cancer, 18:1637, 1965.

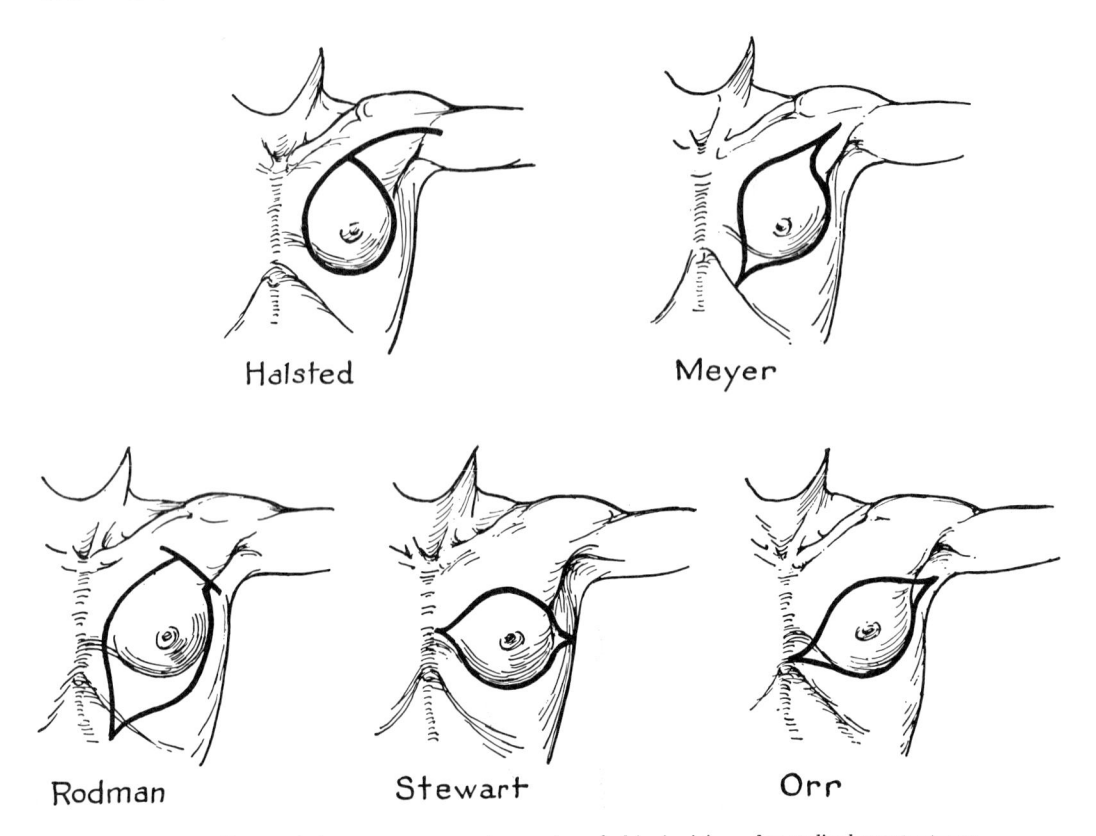

FIG. 27-3. Some of the more commonly employed skin incisions for radical mastectomy.

ing defect is closed with a split-thickness skin graft at the end of the operation (Fig. 27-4 B).

The superior aspect of the elevated skin flap is retracted to expose the tendinous attachment of the pectoralis major, which is then divided. One may leave the clavicular portion of the pectoralis major if the tumor does not lie in the upper quadrants of the breast. Usually, a little better exposure of the apical portion of the axilla is obtained by its removal. The pectoralis minor now comes into view, and its tendinous process is divided as it inserts into the coracoid process of the scapula. If the insertions of these 2 muscles are cut sufficiently close to the bone, little or no bleeding occurs from the residual ends. Together, these 2 muscles are retracted gently downward and mesially, exposing the axillary fat, the brachial plexus, the axillary artery and vein, and the lymphatics of the area. Then the fascia enveloping the neurovascular bundle of the axilla is incised on its uppermost margin, and the incision is carried laterally from the apex to the base of the axilla. This permits dissection of the fascia and the overlying fatty tissue to be carried out from above downward over the entire anterior surface of the neurovascular bundle to its lowermost margin, at which point the subscapular artery and vein and the lateral thoracic vessels come into view (Fig. 27-4, B, C and D).

The axillary artery and veins, like the lymphatics, are of surgical importance and deserving of special attention in radical mastectomy. For convenience, the axillary artery and vein are arbitrarily considered in three portions (Fig. 27-4). The *mesial* portion is a direct continuation of the subclavian artery and runs from the outer margin of the first rib over its superior surface to the mesial border of the pectoralis minor. One small artery, the superior artery, is encountered in this segment as it passes to the second intercostal space. In this area also is the apical group of lymph nodes. This artery is divided and ligated. The second or *middle* portion of the

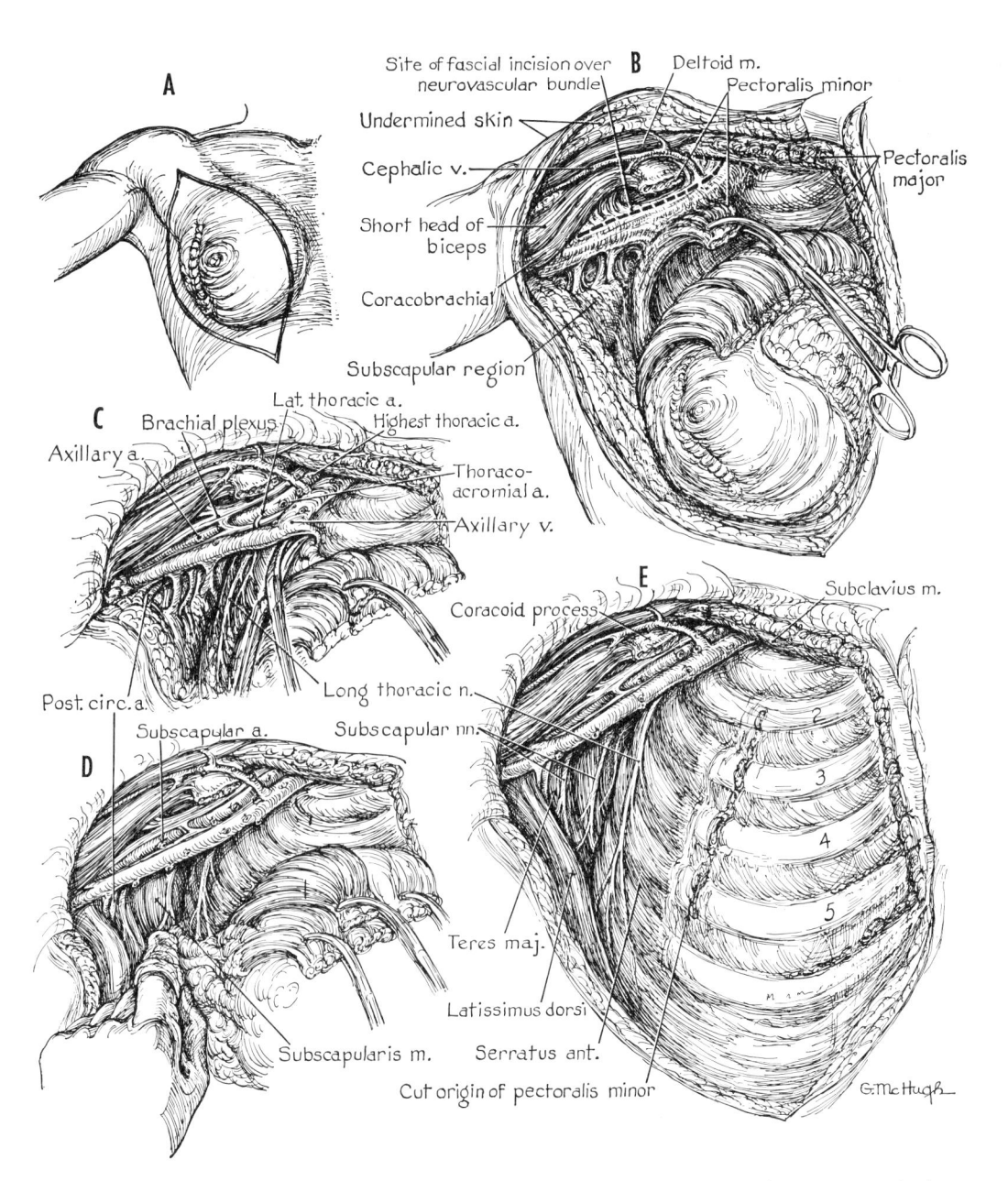

FIG. 27-4. Illustrations of operative principles in radical mastectomy (see text, p. 691). (A) Skin incision after excision biopsy. (B) Reflections of pectoralis major and minor after dividing at their respective insertions. Axillary contents are exposed. (C) Central and superior portions of axillary neurovascular bundle are cleaned of fat, fascia and lymph nodes. (D) Subscapular dissection of lymph nodes and fat. (E) Residual incision; note the perivascular fat and lymphatics along the long thoracic and thoracodorsal nerves have been resected. Resection of internal mammary lymph channels is not yet an established procedure and hence is not shown.

axillary artery and vein lies behind the pectoralis minor. The thoraco-acromial and the lateral thoracic arteries and veins lie in this segment. The thoraco-acromial vessels constitute the axillary blood supply to the pectoralis major and to a lesser extent that of the minor. The lateral thoracic vessel descends perpendicularly for about 2 cm. along the long thoracic nerve of Bell and is one of the surgical landmarks of this nerve. This vessel supplies the anterior serratus, the intercostals and the mammary gland. Lymphatic channels ascending from the upper and more centrally located portions of the breast often are encountered in close proximity to these two vessels. They are carefully resected in mastectomy. The third or *lateral* portion of the axillary vessels emerges from behind the lateral margin of the pectoralis minor and extends laterally to the surgical neck of the humerus. Three arterial branches are derived from this portion of the axillary artery; the largest is the subscapular and then the anterior and posterior circumflex humeral vessels which mark the distal end of the lateral segment of the axillary vessels. Paralleling these vessels are the ascending lymphatic circulation and nodes draining the corresponding areas. The circumflex vessels usually are the only ones of the 6 axillary vessels herein described which the author does not routinely divide and resect in the course of *en bloc* axillary dissection. The subscapular vessels along with the subscapular lymphatics and the underlying subscapular fascia are carefully resected in all cases.

The cephalic vein carries the venous return from most of the subcutaneous and cutaneous areas of the lateral portion of the arm. Entering the axilla, it lies in the deltopectoral groove passing along the upper margin of the pectoralis major in the axilla, serving as a surgical landmark to identify the cleavage plane between these muscles. Its mesial extremity pierces the costocoracoid membrane covering the subclavius muscle and then enters the first portion of the axillary vein just mesial to the pectoralis minor. This vein is usually preserved in mastectomy, for it may prove to be a useful channel for collateral venous return if tumor-bearing nodes are adherent to the second or the third portions of the axillary vein and necessitate its resection.

The 5 branches of the axillary vessels are clamped separately and ligated close to their parent vessels, thereby permitting the posterior aspect of the neurovascular bundle to be cleaned of its fascia and fatty contents (Fig. 27-4 E).

Once again the surgeon turns his attention to the area of the axilla, dissecting away the fascia of the anterior serratus muscle from the center laterally. Care is taken to avoid injury to the long thoracic nerve and the more laterally placed thoracodorsal nerve which respectively supply the anterior serratus and the latissimus dorsi muscles. Then the subscapular dissection, beginning with the division of the subscapular artery and vein from the axillary artery and vein, is carried out from above and downward by undermining the underlying fascia for a distance of at least 1 to $1\frac{1}{2}$ inches on either side of these vessels. The axillary vein should be spared, but if tumor is attached to it, a segment of this vein can be removed safely—with little increased danger of arm edema—so long as the cephalic vein is spared, and infection does not occur.

At this point, it is usually more convenient to clamp the sites of origin of the pectoralis major along its mesial border as it arises from the lateral half of the anterior portion of the sternum and the anterior surfaces of the first 7 or 8 costal cartilages. Its nerve supply, the lateral and the mesial thoracic nerves, are divided. The breast and the pectoralis major and minor are now elevated and rotated laterally until the origin of the pectoralis minor is encountered, arising from the 2nd to the 5th ribs anteriorly. The few slips of muscle encountered beneath are clamped separately and ligated against the bared thoracic cage before being divided.

Finally, the inferior portion of the pectoralis major and its fascia (continuous with the rectus sheath below) are clamped and divided adjacent to the chest wall. All tissue lateral to the pectoralis major and extending to the anterolateral margin of the latissimus dorsalis is removed *en bloc*, avoiding, if possible, injury to the long thoracic and the thoracodorsal nerves.

This effects complete removal of the breast with the axillary and lateral contents attached intact. Then final inspection of the axilla follows to make certain that the dissection has been carried above and behind the neurovascular bundle of the axilla, that the retroclavicular area has been cleaned of its normal contents and the brachial plexus with the axillary artery and veins have been cleaned carefully of small bits of fat and adventitia which may contain nodes. A soft rubber drain of the Penrose type is introduced through a laterally placed stab wound in the axilla, carried posteriorly to the neurovascular bundle and allowed to lie in the denuded subscapular space. Suction may be attached later.

Next, the wound is closed, suturing the subcutaneous tissue to the chest wall whenever possible to obliterate dead space insofar as possible. If a skin graft is required to effect closure without tension, it is cut and applied at this time. The studies of Conway and Neuman (1949) suggest that the routine grafting does not reduce the incidence of cutaneous metastasis appearing later as frequently as originally believed by Halsted.

The operative mortality should be no greater than that from the administration of anesthesia. Early morbidity may occur largely as the result of one of two problems. If the axillary dissection has been carried too far down into the arm, lymphedema may result because of interference with the return of its lymphatic supply which enters the lateralmost group of the axillary nodes. Only rarely does arm edema result from venous obstruction. The second complication, more easily avoidable, is skin necrosis; this complication is nearly always caused by attempting to close the skin under too much tension rather than to use a skin graft under these circumstances. Skin grafting to avoid tension is time and effort well spent. The likelihood of skin necrosis when infection occurs is great. Making the skin flaps too thin is also a cause of postoperative necrosis. It is better to apply split-thickness grafts initially than to utilize skin flaps too thin.

Simple Mastectomy. If a simple mastectomy is to cure breast cancer in which the axillary nodes are involved with tumor, one must assume that such metastases do not continue to grow after the breast is removed and that from such nodes secondary or more distant spread does not occur. However, there is no evidence to support either of these contentions. Thus, a simple mastectomy is not an operation designed for the surgical cure of cancer of the breast except when the cancer is limited to the tissues of the breast removed. It may be employed palliatively in the removal of an ulcerated carcinoma and when distant metastases are already recognized. In some patients with intraductal adenosis in one breast and cancer in the other, a simple mastectomy of the noncancerous breast is usually in order as a prophylactic measure. In a few patients with extensive abscesses of the breast, granulomatous disease of the breast, especially tuberculosis and certain of the mycotic infections, simple mastectomy may be the most effective form of therapy; in other words, it is used curatively for some benign lesions. The same holds true for the rarely encountered patient with crippling mastodynia, but only as a last resort.

Many surgeons performing a simple mastectomy do not appreciate the extent to which the superior and the lateral portions of breast tissue may reach. Consequently, occasionally the tail of Spence (the upper outermost breast tissue) may be cut across and left behind. Stated otherwise, a *complete* simple mastectomy is difficult to perform and may not be accomplished unless one is keenly aware of these anatomic extensions of the breast tissue. If the breast tissue is not all removed, cancer may develop in that which remains.

Postoperative Radiation. Many methods for the application of postoperative radiation have been used in the past, and a review of this material reveals discouraging results in many instances. In general, however, the reports of poor response center about series of patients who received comparatively small doses of radiation therapy, 2,000 r or less tumor dose. When more intense radiation has been employed, tumor dosage of 5,500 to 6,000 r, more encouraging results have been obtained. The latter dosage ranges are more safely administered over a time interval of 8 to 12 weeks (McWhirter, 1955). This somewhat longer timespread usually avoids desquamation and the "wet epidermis," as well as other serious sequelae. However, latent pulmonary fibrosis with severe permanent disability is observed occasionally when this quantity of irradiation is used, and in the first few months to a year or more, acute transient pneumonitis may also accur. The tangential radiation to the chest wall largely spares the underlying lung. Postoperative radiation should begin as soon as the wound is healed.

Most surgeons employing postoperative radiation limit its use to those patients whose axillary nodes were shown to be positive for tumor metastasis. In several series, about half the patients whose axillae were apparently free from metastatic disease also received this course of therapy. Concerning this group, the decision to radiate postoperatively was based largely on the histologic nature of the tumor and its degree of invasiveness. In others this decision represented personal choice on the part of the surgeon, who recognizes that the failure to demonstrate tumor in the axilla does not necessarily imply that none was present or left behind.

X-ray therapy delivered to painful and localized metastases, particularly those in bone, may give a surprising amount of relief for a few months, and in rare instances for even years. This should be considered as a palliative measure before attempting more radical forms of palliative treatment.

Preoperative radiation has been advocated many times. Interest in this type of radiation ebbs and flows. For the most part, the dosage acceptable to the surgeon has been too slight to be considered beneficial. Larger dosages hamper subsequent surgical resection; therefore, this technic is not used extensively. Prevailing opinion is one of discouragement toward preoperative radiation; this is the dominant conclusion of most surgeons and radiotherapists at this time.

Lymphedema of the upper extremity is one of the unpleasant after-effects of radical mastectomy. It may result from resection of the axilla being carried too far laterally, from postoperative wound infection with obliteration of the lymphatic and/or venous return, or from tumor invading the lateral lymph channels and nodes, from phlebitis, from excision of too long a segment of the axillary vein or from reaction to radiation therapy. In some patients, careful dissection of the axilla and avoidance of wound infection eliminates or greatly reduces the extent of such swelling. The progressive increase of edema suggests local axillary recurrence occluding the residual lymph channels and/or the axillary vein. When edema is severe, the arm becomes less and less useful to the patient and may be so painful that narcotics are required or surgical transection of the posterior roots of the brachial plexus is needed. Neither of these forms of treatment is pleasant to contemplate. Infection, acute sunburns or trauma are to be avoided if possible as they may result in further edema.

Postoperative radiation may produce transient edema when it did not exist previously but does not constitute a contraindication to extensive radiation unless pronounced edema exists prior to treatment.

Sleeping with the arm elevated and carrying it in a sling during waking hours may afford some relief, but generally the amount of improvement is not an impressive one.

Postoperatively, limited exercises should be encouraged, beginning as early as the first postoperative day, to avoid restriction of motion of the arm and the shoulder on the affected side. At the beginning this may require considerable encouragement, especially among timid patients. It is therefore important that any pressure dressing applied at the conclusion of operation be placed about the shoulder girdle and the chest wall so as not to restrict early shoulder and arm motion.

Extending the arm above the head with the elbow flexed across the top of the head, touching the ear on the opposite side, and using the hand of the affected arm to comb the hair are early exercises to perform after operation. The patient should be encouraged to abduct her arm and swing it in a circular fashion. With the arm abducted and the patient standing within reach of the wall, she should be encouraged to move her fingers stepwise up the wall as high as possible. If a certain amount of subcutaneous fat can be safely left under the skin flaps, motions of this kind are usually accomplished more easily.

Operability and Curability

The term "operability" does not connote curability, but operability does imply more than a surgical exercise. (1) The operation must do no harm. (2) The operation should provide a good chance that the patient will receive substantial palliative relief despite the recognized possibility that it may not prolong life. For example, the removal of an ulcerated carcinoma of the breast may abolish only the stench of necrotic tumor and its soiling of clothing; but the relief from these troubles will allow the patient to regain her social acceptability and lessens her burden to some extent. (3) Operability may accomplish an extension of her expected survival period, although any increase in survival time is of little merit unless it is accompanied by relief from or the avoidance of distressing symptoms.

Some of the criteria for operability are obvious and undebatable; hepatic metastases or spread of the tumor to the brain are not likely to respond to any form of therapy. Pulmonary and osseous metastases may respond very well for a while to one or more of the endocrine attacks upon the disease (see p. 704). Certain of the local findings often considered indicative of inoperability in the past may also need to be revised in view of the substantial relief afforded some patients by adrenalectomy and allied procedures. True, these patients may not survive a great deal longer, but if such ancillary procedures are effective, their residual life is a much happier one. Take the case of a young mother with carcinoma; an operative procedure may enable her to run her home effectively and to teach her children much longer without necessarily increasing her survival period. How can one evaluate these benefits if the only yardstick for measuring results is that of the "5-year" survival?

Haagensen and Stout (1943) set up certain criteria for operability of carcinoma of the breast, based upon the 5-year survival rates obtained from 1,040 patients operated upon at the Presbyterian Hospital in New York during the years 1915 through 1934. Their purpose in reviewing the experience at that hospital was to establish criteria wherein it could be concluded that patients with these findings could be classified as *categorically inoperable*. They believed that any one of the following criteria was cause to consider a patient with carcinoma as "categorically inoperable":

1. When the carcinoma is one which developed during pregnancy or lactation
2. When extensive edema of the skin over the breast is present
3. When satellite nodules are present in the skin over the breast
4. When intercostal or parasternal tumor nodules are present
5. When there is edema of the arm
6. When proved supraclavicular metastases are present
7. When the carcinoma is the inflammatory type
8. When distant metastases are demonstrated
9. When any two, or more, of the following signs of locally advanced carcinoma are present:
   a. Ulceration of the skin
   b. Edema of the skin of limited extent (less than one third of the skin over the breast involved)
   c. Fixation of the tumor to the chest wall
   d. Axillary lymph nodes measuring 2.5 cm. or more, in transverse diameter, and proved by biopsy to contain metastases
   e. Fixation of axillary lymph nodes to the skin or the deep structures of the axilla, and proved by biopsy to contain metastases

Unfortunately, these criteria make no distinction between operability and curability. These two terms may have entirely different meanings and in some patients operability may have little bearing upon curability; yet an operation may be very worthwhile from the patient's point of view. Certainly one could not assemble a group of criteria in which the 5-year survival could be lower. On the other hand, certain important exceptions exist and have been reported. Perhaps this classification should be modified to serve as a guide to operability rather than as a firm rule connoting "categorical inoperability."

Finally, Haagensen and Stout conclude from the study of their patients that the duration of the postoperative period among those listed in the category of inoperability was actually shortened because of the operative procedure performed. This conclusion may be an erroneous one, for it was based on the fact that their patients did not survive as long after treatment as those of Daland's untreated group (1927). In reality, the survival period for both groups seems to be the same if the survival time is computed on the same basis, i.e., the date of apparent onset of disease which, for the era covered by their survey, was generally 10 to 12 months earlier than the time at which treatment was begun (Nathanson and Welch, 1936).

A patient may be alive and well 3 years after operation; recurrences may manifest themselves at that time and the patient be dead 6 months thereafter. She was operable but not curable. On the other hand, the result of her operation may represent a better one than the patient who is considered categorically inoperable but survives 3½ years, with the last 3 of these years being spent in misery. Hence, in the field of carcinoma of the breast, the surgeon must evaluate each patient on an individual basis and plan his course of action accordingly. The results he obtains also must be individually evaluated, considering not only the duration of survival but also the degree of relief or lack of it that the patient may have experienced.

Results of Primary Treatment

Most of the debates about results of treatment of operable breast cancer could be avoided if both sides were in possession of all the facts. A very important consideration is pointed out in the California Tumor Registry report (1963), which is that the charity or county hospital results were decidedly poorer than those of private hospitals. Also, the latter are for the most part teaching hospitals—some university affiliated, some not. It is because the California Tumor Registry is the largest in the United States that some of these data are used and because, for the hospitals concerned, follow-up averaged 95 per cent for all cancers studied, including breast cancer. The results are not easily explained, but they seem to bear upon the clinical results of treatment reported in this state and probably elsewhere.

Shown in Table 27-10 are the basic data pertinent to this survey, which included 13,392 patients with breast cancer, in whom the stage and the age were known in 12,867. Of the total, 10,660 were treated in 25 private hospitals, and 2,699 were treated in 12 county and state institutions. Five of every 6 were private patients, and a greater per cent of

TABLE 27-10. Per Cent Distribution by Age. Female Breast Cancer Cases by Stage of Disease and Type of Hospital, 1942-56

	ALL STAGES		LOCALIZED		WITH SPREAD	
AGE	County	Private	County	Private	County	Private
Total, Age Known	100.0	100.0	100.0	100.0	100.0	100.0
	(2,699)	(10,660)	(620)	(4,530)	(1,846)	(5,871)
Under 45	12.4	22.9	11.0	23.8	13.4	22.5
45–54	13.6	25.7	11.0	25.1	14.8	26.4
55–64	18.5	24.7	13.5	23.6	20.6	25.6
65–74	29.0	18.7	32.1	19.0	28.6	18.3
75 and over	26.6	8.0	32.4	8.5	22.6	7.2
Median Age	*66.9*	*55.5*	*69.5*	*55.5*	*65.4*	*55.4*

From California Tumor Registry: Cancer registration and survival in California, State of California Department of Public Health, Berkeley, 1963.

TABLE 27-11. Per Cent Distribution by Course of Treatment. Breast Cancer Cases, Various Registries

REGISTRY	TIME PERIOD	TOTAL NUMBER	PER CENT			
			Total	Surgery	Surgery and Radiation	Other or None Reported
					Radiation	
California	1942–56	13,525	100	63	6	19	12
Connecticut	1947–51	2,916	100	75	3	17	5
Massachusetts	1956–57	410	100	52	13	16	18
New Zealand	1948–55	3,690	100	33	11	50	6
Saskatchewan	1946–58	2,274	100	31	12	43	14

TABLE 27-12. PER CENT DISTRIBUTION BY FIRST COURSE OF TREATMENT. FEMALE BREAST CANCER CASES BY TIME PERIOD AND STAGE OF DISEASE, 1942-56

TREATMENT	TOTAL	1942-46	1947-51	1952-56
	ALL STAGES			
TOTAL	100.0	100.0	100.0	100.0
	(13,392)	(2,935)	(4,534)	(5,923)
Surgery	63.5	61.0	62.7	65.4
Radiation	5.9	8.4	6.3	4.4
Surgery and radiation	18.6	16.1	17.2	21.0
Other or none reported	11.9	14.5	13.8	9.2
	LOCALIZED			
TOTAL	100.0	100.0	100.0	100.0
	(5,159)	(972)	(1,734)	(2,453)
Surgery	82.6	78.8	82.7	83.9
Radiation	1.9	3.8	1.9	1.1
Surgery and radiation	10.8	11.5	9.2	11.5
Other or none reported	4.8	5.9	6.2	3.5
	WITH SPREAD			
TOTAL	100.0	100.0	100.0	100.0
	(7,739)	(1,810)	(2,627)	(3,302)
Surgery	52.4	52.5	51.8	52.9
Radiation	8.4	10.9	8.5	6.8
Surgery and radiation	24.5	19.0	23.1	28.6
Other or none reported	14.7	17.6	16.6	11.7

TABLE 27-13. PER CENT DISTRIBUTION BY FIRST COURSE OF TREATMENT. BREAST CANCER CASES BY STAGE OF DISEASE CALIFORNIA REGISTRY AND CONNECTICUT REGISTRY, 1947-51

TREATMENT	ALL STAGES	LOCALIZED	WITH SPREAD
	California Registry		
TOTAL	100.0	100.0	100.0
	(4,578)	(1,752)	(2,652)
Surgery	62.6	82.6	51.7
Radiation	6.3	1.9	8.6
Surgery and radiation	17.2	9.2	23.0
Other or none reported	13.9	6.3	16.8
	Connecticut Registry		
TOTAL	100.0	100.0	100.0
	(2,916)	(1,273)	(1,514)
Surgery	75.0	87.5	66.1
Radiation	3.2	0.8	4.4
Surgery and radiation	16.6	9.9	22.2
Other or none reported	5.2	1.8	7.3

Tables 27-11, 27-12, and 27-13 from California Tumor Registry: Cancer registration and survival in California, State of California Department of Public Health, Berkeley, 1963.

TABLE 27-14. RELATIVE SURVIVAL RATES FEMALE BREAST CANCER CASES BY TYPE OF HOSPITAL ALL STAGES AND LOCALIZED, 1942-56

STAGE OF DISEASE AND HOSPITAL	YEARS AFTER DIAGNOSIS (Relative Rate—Per Cent)				
	1	3	5	10	15
All Stages					
County	66.3	45.8	34.7	22.8	21.9
Private	90.3	72.8	61.5	46.0	37.5
Localized					
County	90.8	79.3	67.4	52.8	—
Private	98.3	90.8	83.1	68.3	58.2

Note: Dash (—) indicates that rate has a standard error of 10.0 per cent or higher.

TABLE 27-15. COMPARISON OF 5-YEAR SURVIVAL. PERCENTAGES FOR SURGICALLY TREATED PATIENTS WITH LOCALIZED BREAST CANCER BY AGE GROUPS AND TYPE OF HOSPITAL

TYPE OF HOSPITAL	PERIOD	PER CENT SURVIVAL
Age group 45–54		
County	1950–54	71.7
	1955–59	73.2
Private	1950–54	81.4
	1955–59	85.1
Age group 55–64		
County	1950–54	69.9
	1955–59	65.6
Private	1950–54	80.2
	1955–59	81.2

the private patients were younger when first seen than were the county hospital patients. Likewise, the per cent of private patients whose lesions were clinically localized when first seen was substantially higher under the age of 65; thereafter, the per cent of localized lesions was higher for the county group.

The kinds of "first" treatment are shown in Table 27-11, which compares with similar data from 4 other registers. In Table 27-12 are data from the California Registry which show the general trend to be toward increased use of surgical treatment. This increasing use of surgical treatment for localized and advanced breast cancer is also shown in Table 27-13, which compares the California Registry experience with that of Connecticut.

In general, the breast cancer patients treated in county hospitals in California had a much lower survival rate than that experienced by patients in private hospitals (Table 27-14). The fact that county patients are first seen and treated at later stages of their disease than private patients seems to be an unsatisfactory explanation for the differences observed, because the same differences still exist when surgically treated patients in similar age groups with only localized lesions are considered (Table 27-15).

One is left with only one other possible explanation, which is that the life expectancy among lower socioeconomic groups (county hospital patients) is substantially lower than among those more fortunate. Several reports suggest this to be true but, upon examination of these life tables, this difference in life expectancy is accounted for by higher mortality rates in the younger age brackets of the lower socioeconomic groups, and it is shown that the life expectancy at the ages of 35 through 65 for both groups is sufficiently similar that the observed over-all life expectancy differences do not appear to apply. Whatever the reason may be, Breslow's statement that patients in the lower social classes do not survive as well as those in more fortunate circumstances is probably correct, and this fact very seriously affects previously published data which have failed to define the socioeconomic status of the patients involved. Were similar data from other states available, probably they would show the same differences in the results of surgical treatment of breast cancer between private and county hospital patients. Unfortunately, most of our earlier data on the results of surgical treatment of cancer of the breast are derived from the larger series encountered in county hospitals, where indeed it does appear true that little improvement in 5-year survival has occurred during the last 60 years.

On the other hand, in private hospital series, such as that of the Mayo Clinic, a steady improvement in the end-results of radical mastectomy among patients with axillary metastasis has been shown over several decades (Table 27-16). There has also been a steady decline in the percentage of patients

TABLE 27-16. FIVE-YEAR SURVIVAL IN PRIVATE PATIENTS IN DIFFERENT PERIODS

PERIOD OF TIME	TOTAL NO. OF PATIENTS OPERATED ON	PER CENT OF TOTAL WITH METASTASIS	PER CENT 5-YEAR SURVIVAL AFTER MASTECTOMY		
			Entire Group	Without Metastasis	With Metastasis
1910–24	2,363	66.6	40.1	70	25.6
1925–34	2,032	66.4	49.5	78–82	34.6
1935–44	2,480	57.0	58.6	78–82	41.5
1945–49	1,358	51.2	61.0	78–82	43.0
1950–54	1,416	47.6	65.1	78–82	46.4

Compiled from data by Berkson et al. (1957).

who had axillary metastases at the time of operation. Inasmuch as operative technics and the criteria for operability did not change over the period of the study, it is suggested that an increasing number of patients with axillary metastasis had less advanced disease at the time of operation and also that fewer had disease that had advanced beyond the axilla. In contrast, rather steady, unimproved 5-year survival rates for indigent patients was observed in a study of this group of patients at the Johns Hopkins Hospital (Lewison, 1963).

There is a good basis for the conclusion that radical or superradical (Urban, 1959) mastectomy is superior to simple mastectomy. There are substantial data to indicate that the earlier the patient with this disease is operated upon the better the results are likely to be, regardless of which operation is used. We, therefore, cannot expect better results from the same operation for the same disease, unless we can bring the patient to her operation at an earlier date, thus improving her opportunity for achieving a better result. Beyond this is the important unexplained difference in results between comparable age groups operated on in county and in private hospitals. Logically and objectively, if cancer has not spread, simple mastectomy should be as beneficial as radical mastectomy; if cancer has extended to the lymph nodes, it may well have spread more generally, and thus the radical operation may fail to "cure," as often as simple mastectomy fails. Most surgeons are reluctant to accept this possibility because they believe, correctly or not, that in some patients axillary metastases may be all that have occurred; hence, in their removal with radical mastectomy, metastases from metastases are prevented. Although what is the best form of primary operative treatment may not be settled as yet, it is clear that even in the face of long and revered tradition, we must accept the need for a new and fresh approach to the entire subject. It is equally clear that we cannot discard radical mastectomy as the method of choice until a substitute form of treatment is found that gives decisively better results in the hands of all concerned. And it has not. A recent survey of 5-year survival after radical mastectomy is shown in Table 27-17.

It is possible that advances in biostatistical

TABLE 27-17. FIVE-YEAR SURVIVAL AFTER RADICAL MASTECTOMY

SOURCE OF DATA	NO. OF PATIENTS	FOLLOW-UP %	FIVE-YEAR SURVIVAL		
			OVERALL %	− AXIL	+ AXIL
Conn State Survey	8,396		57.2	70.0	41.1
Mayo Clinic	7,325	98.4	51.2	78.3	32.5
Memorial Hosp NYC	3,494	97.8	54.4	77.5	39.4
Haagensen	495	96.2	47.2	71.0	34.8
Middletown, USA	271	100.0	55.0	73.0	31.0
Johns Hopkins Hosp	204	94.5	44.1	64.0	31.7
FGH* Series	121	96.9	62.8	76.1	54.6

* Fitzsimmons General Hospital, After Muir and White: Carcinoma of the Breast. Arch. Surg., 95:170, 1967.

TABLE 27-18. HISTORICAL LANDMARKS IN CLINICAL BIOMETRY IN RELATION TO ACHIEVEMENT IN CLINICAL SURGERY WITH EMPHASIS UPON TREATMENT OF BREAST CANCER

YEAR	STATISTICAL METHOD*	YEAR	RELATED SURGICAL PROGRESS
1835	Pierre Charles Alexandre Louis: Devised "Numerical Method."	1653	Johann Schultes (Scultetus): His "Simplified Simple Mastectomy" published.
1846	Adolphe Quetelet: Devised "Theory of Probability and Normal Curve."	1846	William Thomas Green Morton: Introduced ether at the Massachusetts General Hospital.
1869	Francis Galton: Devised correlation coefficients in relation to "Natural Inheritance."	1867	Joseph Lister: Discovered antisepsis.
1900	Karl Pearson: Devised Chi square test for significance.	1889	William Stewart Halsted: Devised radical mastectomy for cancer.
1908	William Gosset: Devised technics for testing of small samples of large populations.	1908–13	Ruben Ottenberg: Introduced crossmatching procedures for blood transfusion.
1935	Ronald Fisher: Design of experiments with statistical considerations.	1936	Ira T. Nathanson and Claude E. Welch: Published first clinical paper in which survivals in patients with breast cancer were considered in relation to normal life expectancy; i.e., concept of adjusted mortality.
1945	Bradford Hill: Design of clinical trials before attempting statistical evaluation of results.	1945	Charles B. Huggins and William W. Scott: First adrenalectomy for hormonal dependent tumors (prostate).
		1952	Urban, J. A.: The *en bloc* extended radical mastectomy for cancer.
		1955	McWhirter, R.: First definitive work on simple mastectomy and radiotherapy for breast cancer.

* After Shimkin.

methods will eventually solve some of the problems discussed above. Unfortunately, however, as indicated in Table 27-18, developments essential to safe surgery preceded developments in the biostatistical methods suitable for application to these problems. As a result, there is some confusion, and even contradiction, in the data published, such as in reports of 5-year survival in relation to simple versus radical mastectomy. It is clear that conclusions drawn from a retrospective study in which modern statistical methods were used to evaluate data that were inadequately prepared for that purpose cannot always be valid. Unfortunately too, the statistical approach to the effectiveness of early diagnosis, to improved technics of treatment, accurate follow-up and to evaluation of end-results have not often given evidence that the biometrician was aware that these are among the answers sorely needed in evaluating breast cancer. Until we design a program in conjunction with highly competent biometricians with full knowledge of the limitations of the history, the physical examination, of the lack of uniformity in methods used by surgeons in performing a radical or a simple mastectomy, of the wide variations in the extent to which removed tissue is studied, its lymph nodes counted, sectioned and reviewed by the pathologist, more questions remain to ask than have been answered. If valid comparisons of different treatment are to be made, certainly all series should resemble each other as nearly as possible in all respects except for the method of treatment itself. As yet this has not been accomplished.

SURVIVAL IN UNTREATED BREAST CANCER

It is fundamental that the course of the untreated patient should be established before it can be assumed that any benefit has been derived from the treatment applied. In this connection, it should be borne in mind that in the untreated series survival times are computed from apparent date of onset of the disease until death, whereas in the treated series these computations are based on date of onset of treatment until death and omit the period of time which may have elapsed before treatment was instituted.

Greenwood (1926) collected data from several British hospitals relative to the eventual outcome of 651 patients who were known to have cancer of the breast which for one reason or another were untreated. This was when life expectancy ranged from 44 years of age to 60, compared with today's 74 years. Fifty per cent of Greenwood's patients were dead within 6 months after onset of symptoms. Another 25 per cent had died by the 46th month. The remaining 25 per cent died over the next 10-year period. The mean survival time was 38 months. Shimkin (1951) arranged the mean survival time of Greenwood's patients according to the age of the patient when each developed cancer. These are tabulated in Table 27-19.

Daland (1927) reported the mean survival time for 100 untreated patients with cancer of the breast seen in 2 Boston hospitals. The mean survival time for his group was also 38 months, with a similar spread in time of the percentage of patients surviving at any particular month. Later, Nathanson and Welch (1936) reported almost identical data once again. Tabulated in Table 27-20 are the percentages of untreated patients surviving each year after the onset of symptoms.

TABLE 27-19. SURVIVAL IN UNTREATED BREAST CARCINOMA RELATIVE TO AGE

AGE RANGE	NO. OF PATIENTS	MEAN SURVIVAL TIME IN MONTHS
25–34	40	35
35–44	105	42
45–54	159	37
55–64	152	38
65–74	130	41
75 and older	37	36

The average percentage of patients surviving in each of the 3 groups of untreated patients is 19 per cent, being 18, 19 and 20 per cent respectively and remarkably similar. Stated otherwise, 80 per cent of patients with untreated breast cancer will be dead in 5 years after apparent onset of the disease.

ATTEMPTS TO IMPROVE SURVIVAL RESULTS

Of all the known methods for increasing the survival and cure rates for carcinoma of the breast, those technics that assist in the establishment of early diagnosis are likely to be the most successful, provided that the establishment of the diagnosis is followed immediately by adequate treatment. The cooperative patient can be the greatest factor in assisting in the early diagnosis. She should be taught the art of periodic self-examination as well as the value of an examination by a competent physician at least once a year. Despite the use of both technics, some tumors will not be detected, and a few of those which are found early will be of such a nature that blood stream or lymphatic channel invasion will not enable a surgical "cure."

The so-called "super" radical operations in selected patients continues under investigation. Many lesions situated in the mesial quadrants of the breast, particularly those in the upper mesial quadrant, tend to metastasize

TABLE 27-20. PER CENT OF UNTREATED PATIENTS WITH CARCINOMA OF THE BREAST ALIVE EACH YEAR AFTER ONSET OF SYMPTOMS

1 yr.	2 yrs.	3 yrs.	4 yrs.	5 yrs.	6 yrs.	7 yrs.	8 yrs.	10 yrs.	15 yrs.
75%	58%	40%	25%	18%	15%	10%	7%	4%	0%

Nathanson and Welch, 1936

to the internal mammary chain. The extended radical operation has been largely concerned with the removal of this chain in addition to the axillary system. Three approaches to these parasternal nodes have been employed: splitting the sternum to expose the internal mammary chain, *en bloc* excision of the parasternal chest wall from the 2nd through the 5th ribs inclusive, followed by a grafting procedure, and the division of the costal cartilages of these same ribs to expose the chain. The last procedure carries the least risk insofar as increasing mortality and morbidity rates are concerned but in none are these prohibitive. To date, results obtained are insufficient to allow an adequate appraisal of the inclusion of this chain along with those of the axilla. Certainly more experience is required before such a radical procedure can be advised as routine for even selected series of patients. Its final evaluation must be made on the basis of comparing the end results with those of the standard radical procedure.

Some idea as to the location of the primary tumor site and the frequency of nodal metastases to various regions may be evident from the observations of Handley and Thackeray (1954) which are presented in Table 27-21.

In Urban's series (1959) of 300 cases in which surgical excision of the parasternal chest wall was carried out, the site of the primary tumor lay in the mesial quadrants 3 times more often than in the outer quadrants among the 82 cases who proved to have positive nodal involvement along the internal mammary chain. In 100 cases of breast cancer in which there were metastases to the internal

TABLE 27-21

	LOCATION OF THE BREAST LESION	
	INNER QUADRANTS	OUTER QUADRANTS
When all nodes were negative	16 cases	33 cases
When only the axillary nodes were positive	12 cases	40 cases
When only the internal mammary nodes were positive	6 cases	2 cases
When both groups were positive	27 cases	14 cases

TABLE 27-22. NODE FINDINGS IN 300 CASES

	LATERAL PER CENT	MEDIAL PER CENT	TOTAL PER CENT
Number	61–20	239–80	300–100
All nodes clear	16–26	117–48	133–44.3
Internal mammary nodes +	2–3	21–9	23– 7.7
Axillary nodes +	21–34	40–17	61–20.3
Both int. mammary and axillary nodes +	22–36	61–26	83–27.7

If axillary nodes are positive, then internal mammary nodes are positive in:
58% Over-all group
61% Medial half
51% Lateral half
If axillary nodes are negative, then internal mammary nodes are positive in:
15% Over-all group
15.2% Medial half
11% Lateral half
(After Urban)

mammary nodes, the most frequent involvement appeared in the 2nd interspace, and then in decreasing order, in the 3rd, the 1st, the 4th and the 5th interspaces. In Table 27-22 are the nodal findings reported for Urban's 300 cases.

The mortality for this series was less than 1 per cent. The 5-year survival of 100 patients with primary operable breast cancer treated by this method was 67 per cent, and the 5-year survival rate clinically free of disease was 61 per cent. These are excellent results, and continued evaluation of the technic is imperative.

PALLIATIVE FORMS OF TREATMENT FOR METASTATIC CANCER

The procedures under discussion here relate primarily to hormonal control, including the administration of sex or corticoid hormones, oophorectomy, adrenalectomy and hypophysectomy. The effectiveness of these forms of therapy is based on the concept that many breast cancers are in part hormonal-dependent. Precise knowledge is lacking.

The extent of palliation accomplished varies considerably, and which patient will respond to which form of therapy is unpredictable. In some patients the results are so striking as to permit a bedridden patient to return to work for several years entirely free of symptoms. Eventually, the disease escapes hormonal control, and the patient dies. Thus there is to be considered not only the possible duration of benefit from this form of therapy but, more important, the fact that frequently considerable or complete relief is obtained for months to several years. Fortunately, when benefit no longer is maintained, death usually follows rapidly—often within a few days or weeks, avoiding prolonged and painful final stages of the disease. The percentage of useful and happy life is increased considerably, although the increase of mean duration of survival is not as long as is desired.

Estrogen Therapy. Although these substances are carcinogenic in certain species and strains, they are capable of inducing tumor regression in the human female with breast cancer and metastases. Haddow et al. (1944) were the first to report beneficial results with this form of therapy. In some patients, the results have been striking for a while, usually doubling the mean survival time for similar cases receiving no estrogen. This effect is not limited to any particular product; a patient who fails to respond to one estrogenic substance is unlikely to respond to another. Most reports indicate that the results are better for the postmenopausal group than for those of younger age, though many who fail to respond to estrogens may respond to androgens.

Landau et al. (1962) observed improvement in 9 of 15 patients, including one male, with advanced breast cancer by treatment with a combination of 50 mg. of progesterone and 5 mg. of estradiol benzoate administered intramuscularly. Seven of the 9 who improved for a while had previously responded either to ablative or supplemental endocrine therapy. Freckman et al. (1964) observed objective clinical improvement for a minimum of 6 months in one third of the patients given prednisolone in combination with an alkylating agent, the latter given intrapleurally when necessary in addition to its daily systemic administration. Additional data published in Cancer Chemotherapy Reports (Gardner et al., 1962), reflect some of the general problems and results encountered in a cooperative study which included not only the administration of various hormones but also of anti-cancer chemotherapeutic agents.

Androgen Therapy. Although several workers noted some degree of tumor regression as early as 1939 with the administration of testosterone, it was the report of Adair and Herrmann in 1946 which awakened a keen investigative and clinical interest in this subject. Methyltestosterone administered orally in large doses seems to be nearly as effective as intramuscular testosterone propionate, although long-acting depotestosterone affords more certainty of response. In this author's experience, this form of therapy has produced a higher percentage of good results, often lasting longer than the effects of oophorectomy, x-ray castration or estrogen administration. One patient who developed pathologic fractures of several bones, including the hip, experienced complete remission for $4\frac{1}{2}$ years without other forms of therapy. This is the exception and not the rule; usually, improvement lasts only a few months. Peters (1956), in her experience, comes to the opposite conclusion—that estrogens are more often effective than are androgens.

Goldenberg (1964) summarized the results of the Cooperative Breast Cancer Group which observed objective remission in one fifth of 521 women after administration of testosterone propionate, 100 mg. in sesame oil administered intramuscularly 3 times a week. The highest rate of remissions occurred in breast, skin and lymph nodes (31.5%), whereas those for osseous and visceral lesions were about equal (18%).

As the recent literature is replete with experiences favoring one or the other group of sex hormones, even among the same age group, one is left with the conclusion that both are helpful to many patients. If estrogens fail to give relief, androgens should be tried, and vice versa. As yet there appears to be no rational basis for a decision as to which to employ other than clinical trial in the individual patient, and possibly age.

The unpleasant side-effects of testosterone, such as masculinization, salt retention with edema and an increased libido are largely overcome by the use of certain synthetic analogues.

Oophorectomy. As early as 1896, Beatson demonstrated the beneficial response from oophorectomy in a 33-year-old patient with recurrence of cancer in the surgical scar. She responded well, though temporarily, to oophorectomy. As this antedated the recognition of hormones, Beatson's report was subject to

TABLE 27-23. ENDOCRINE MODIFICATION IN ADVANCED MAMMARY CANCER: PERCENTAGE OF IMPROVEMENT

AUTHORS	TOTAL CASES	OBJECTIVE IMPROVEMENT NUMBER	PER CENT	REMARKS
Ovariectomy				
Thomson, 1902	80	18	22	16 Premenopausal and 2 postmenopausal
Lett, 1905	75	22	29	Premenopausal
	24	1	0	Postmenopausal
Adair et al., 1945	31	4	12	Premenopausal
Sicard, 1947	5	5	0	Premenopausal
	1	1	0	Postmenopausal
Dargent, 1949	10	2	20	
Ovarian Irradiation				
Ahlbom, 1930	16	0	0	
Dresser, 1936	30	9	30	Premenopausal
Taylor, 1939	50	20	40	
Adair et al., 1945	304	47	15	Premenopausal
Douglas, 1952	175	36	20	2 Postmenopausal improved
Testosterone				
Adair and Herrmann, 1946	11	4	36	Premenopausal
Cutler and Schlemenson, 1948	19	8	42	
Adair et al., 1949	48	9	19	Bone metastasis
	54	8	15	Extraskeletal metastasis
A.M.A. Council on Pharmacy and Chemistry, 1949	82	15	18	Bone metastasis
	77	15	20	Extraskeletal metastasis
Segaloff, 1952	48	13	27	
Douglas, 1952	30	8	36	
Estrogen				
Haddow et al., 1944	40	16	40	
Ellis et al., 1944	100	14	14	Age less than 60 yrs.
	68	27	39	Age over 60 yrs.
Adair et al., 1949	35	8	23	
A.M.A. Council on Pharmacy and Chemistry, 1949	144	36	25	Postmenopausal
Douglas, 1952	322	98	30	Majority postmenopausal

From Huggins and the National Cancer Institute

severe criticism, and the idea did not take hold. Nonetheless, periodically others tried the procedure and found benefit in about 20 per cent of patients with such metastases.

Ablation of ovarian function by x-radiation in patients with carcinoma of the breast was suggested by Courmelles in 1905 but was little pursued until 1930 and thereafter. The results of these experiences have been summarized by Huggins in Table 27-23. Castration appears to be beneficial even when the urinary secretion of estrogen is low, although the best response seems to occur among premenopausal women and those with excessive estrogen excretion. Bony metastases appear to respond better and more frequently than those in soft tissue. Prophylactic castration has been advocated, but there is more agreement in its theory than observed when practiced. Kennedy (1964) found no difference in survival times in patients who underwent castration before metastases than when castrated after metastases appeared. He did find that, within limits, the later in the advanced stages of the disease oophorectomy was performed, the more likely it was to be beneficial.

Bilateral adrenalectomy was first accomplished successfully by Huggins and Scott in 1945 as a means of palliative relief for advanced carcinoma of the prostate. These observers found the urinary excretion of 17-ketosteroids to be essentially abolished following the combination of orchiectomy and adrenalectomy (see Chap. 29, Part 2). Huggins and Bergenstal (1951) reported that adrenalectomy alone was beneficial in many patients with metastatic breast cancer when maintained on corticoids.

After bilateral adrenalectomy, the patient's general condition improves rapidly if she is to improve at all. She becomes animated, possibly from cortisone or possibly from relief of pain, her appetite improves, and she looks happily to the future. Osseous lesions appear to heal, and so do some pathologic fractures. Fluid may disappear from the chest, the local tumor and even some of the cutaneous metastases may diminish or may disappear entirely. She literally may arise from her death bed, walk and resume a full and active normal life, sometimes for several months to several years.

Of course, adrenalectomy is no cure, but the excellence of palliation, if for only 6 months, seems to warrant the use of this procedure in many patients. The subjective improvement noted tends to outstrip the objective changes; however, this is better than the reverse.

Methods for the selection of patients in whom there is a chance of improvement after adrenalectomy have been studied seriously. Probably there is no absolute single criterion, but there are certain "straws in the wind" which are helpful (Table 27-24).

Hypophysectomy was first performed by Perrault for the treatment of metastatic breast cancer in 1951, and Luft, Olivecrona and Sjögren (1952) at about the same time. The reasoning behind this procedure was that the ablation of the pituitary removed the trophic hormones and hence theoretically could diminish more effectively hormonal activity and production in the target organs.

Rasmussen et al. (1953) have accomplished the same end by the implantation of yttrium[90] beads in the pituitary gland (see Fig. 29-10). Illingworth and colleagues (1956) implanted radon seeds into the pituitary for the same purpose. The early results of both groups continue to be encouraging.

Most impressive results from hypophysectomy have been reported by Pearson and Ray (1959). These authors reported on 109 patients with advanced carcinoma followed for at least 17 months. About 50 per cent of the patients obtained objective remissions, and 35 per cent had remissions of 6 months or longer. The average remission was over 15 months, and the average survival was over 21 months. The question still remains whether hypophysectomy is superior to adrenalectomy or combined adrenalectomy and oophorectomy. At the present time, hypophysectomy seems to be a worthwhile procedure in the palliative treatment of patients with metastatic breast cancer when adequate facilities are available to carry out this technic.

TABLE 27-24. CHANCES OF BENEFIT FROM ADRENALECTOMY

AGE OF PATIENT	FAIRLY GOOD 40 TO 65 YRS.	LIKELY TO BE POOR UNDER 40 AND OVER 65
Duration of breast carcinoma	3–5 yrs.	Less than 2 yrs. and longer than 6
Type of Carcinoma		
1. "Carcinoma en cuirasse"	+++	
2. "Adenocarcinoma"	++	
3. "Ductal carcinoma"	+	
4. Highly anaplastic	0	
Location of metastases		
1. Bone	+++	
2. Skin	++	
3. Lung	++	
4. Liver	0	
Increased estrogen excretion	++	
Calcium balance	Not yet sufficient data to evaluate	

Key: 0 Essentially no change
 + Slight chance for improvement
 ++ Moderate chance for improvement
 +++ Good chance for improvement

Atkins *et al.* (1966) undertook a prospective study to determine the timing of adrenalectomy or hypophysectomy. Of the 191 patients included, all now have been followed up on for at least a year. One group was treated conventionally, i.e., initial treatment of hormones or radiotherapy or both, and then adrenalectomy or hypophysectomy only if and when that treatment failed. The other group was treated immediately with adrenalectomy or hypophysectomy. The survival and remission rates between the 2 groups were not significantly different and there was no advantage in carrying out adrenalectomy or hypophysectomy at the first sign of recurrence. The response from hormone treatment gave no guide to the subsequent result of adrenalectomy or hypophysectomy.

Chemotherapy. The various chemotherapeutic agents that have been tried have not as yet produced results of palliative benefit equal to those of endocrine alterations (see Chap. 10, Neoplastic Disease).

Operative procedures that alter the hormonal balances and achieve palliation in patients with metastatic breast cancer, in a sense, represent a chemotherapeutic approach. Hypophysectomy is as effective as adrenalectomy, but it carries a greater mortality and morbidity in most hands.

The administration of sex hormones to patients with breast cancer can produce a number of unpleasant side effects, and give only minor relief of symptoms. Minor alterations in the chemical structure of the steroid compounds has produced certain compounds that are more acceptable to the patient, but not necessarily more effective. Combinations of steroid therapy with 5-fluorouracil (Moore *et al.*, 1967), appears to produce the most effective palliative therapy to date.

Because of the increasing use of surgical adjuvant chemotherapeutic agents in the treatment of breast cancer without true assessment of their worth or hazard, 36 institutions entered into phase 2 of the Surgical Adjuvant Breast Project (Cohn *et al.*, 1968). This project has supplied data on 1,328 patients. The results disclose that 45 per cent of all patients receiving a placebo had one or more local or systemic complications to impair normal surgical convalescence, suggesting that the morbidity from this procedure may not be as negligible as generally believed. Leukopenia occurred in 2 per cent of patients receiving fluorouracil and in only 15 per cent of those patients receiving triethylenethiophosphoramide.

Neither chemotherapeutic group differed from the placebo group regarding the number of patients in each that required blood transfusions during their hospital stay. The use of fluorouracil was associated with a statistically significant increase in local and systemic complications over that occurring in the placebo group. They did not occur subsequent to triethylenethiophosphoramide therapy. The fluorouracil proved much more toxic than the triethylenethiophosphoramide therapy. There were 16 postoperative deaths—8 in each group. All were thought to be associated with the effects of the drug. The experience of this group was very discouraging in two ways: first, there was a high incidence of local, systemic and hematologic complications associated with the use of fluorouracil; and second, the anti-tumor effect was not demonstrated to the satisfaction of the group in most patients.

Nadler and Moore (1968) came to the opposite conclusion, namely, that the repeated treatment or maintenance therapy with fluorouracil was beneficial, and in their opinion, individualized schedules of treatment combined with other forms of therapy offered some hope for patients with advanced breast cancer. Thus far no single approach has uniformly met with a high degree of success, although spectacular improvement is occasionally seen and definite improvement observed in 35 to 40 per cent of patients treated.

Hypercalcemia in metastatic breast cancer has been reported with increasing frequency, once it was recognized that, in the late stages of breast cancer, the occasional drowsiness and stupor were frequently associated with a remarkable elevation of serum calcium levels. Usually, under these circumstances, serum phosphate is reduced. Similar observations with regard to other tumors led Albright (1941) to suggest that some tumors may produce parathyroid hormone. The problem may not be that simple; but, if not, certainly many of the responses observed are analogous. Gardner *et al.* (1962) reported that urinary calcium excretion in women with metastatic breast cancer, with or without bony metastasis, was not a reliable index of progression or regression of metastases. They believe that the rise in calcium and phosphate levels probably is due to osteolysis at sites distant from the tumors and that androgens decrease these levels and probably reduce osteolysis without significantly altering renal clearance or tubular resorption. Some attribute this form of hypercalcemia to the use of hormones in the treatment of breast cancer, but it may occur without hormone therapy. This phenomenon is interesting but not yet well understood.

Phosphate and citrate infusions have proved useful in reducing the elevated serum calcium levels in patients with hypercalcemia due to metastatic breast cancer (Kahil et al., 1967). These are temporary measures, but they may prove of considerable value until adrenalectomy can be performed.

Pain in metastatic breast cancer may become so severe and unrelenting that some form of interruption of pain-conducting fibers is indicated if other palliative measures fail. Methods to accomplish the relief of pain are considered in the chapters on anesthesia and neurologic surgery.

SUMMARY OF PALLIATIVE ENDOCRINE INTERFERENCE WITH ADVANCED BREAST CANCER. The benefits of the appropriate utilization of endocrine therapy in relieving the patient's symptoms are well stated in an editorial in the *New England Journal of Medicine*: "The doctor who regards the complex endocrinology of carcinoma of the breast as 'just a confusing fog' had best do some reading and studying so that he can find a few landmarks in the fog." Perhaps this overstates the facts but not the principles.

The surgeon today has a much better chance than 5 years ago to relieve his patients with advanced carcinoma of the breast and to prolong their lives. Hormonal therapy, endocrine ablation and better technics of radiotherapy all are useful tools. The fullest possibility of each alone or in combination is not yet known, but surely substantial progress has been made.

THE MALE BREAST

GYNECOMASTIA—"PHYSIOLOGIC" HYPERTROPHY

In the course of sexual maturity, enlargement of one or both breasts often occurs in the male, usually between the ages of 12 to 15 years. Enlargement is encountered so frequently that it might well be considered a variant lying within the normal range. These little subareolar buttons of tissue disappear before the age of 20, and their entire duration of existence is usually only a matter of a few months to a year or two.

The term gynecomastia generally has been applied to those patients in whom the breast enlargement at puberty does not subside. More often this type is unilateral and to be differentiated from fibroadenoma, lipoma and dermoid cysts.

Although the breast may be slightly painful and moderately tender, the two reasons for seeking medical advice are that the lesion creates embarrassment and that the parents of the boy are often concerned about the hypertrophied breast representing a malignancy or at least a premalignant lesion.

The etiology is related to the hormonal changes occurring with puberty. These are aptly described by some pediatricians as "the hormonal confusion of adolescence." In some patients, especially with bilateral gynecomastia first appearing after ages 18 to 20, more important aberrations in endocrinology should be considered, particularly the estrogen-producing tumors. Of these, teratoma of the testis is perhaps the most commonly encountered; certain of the hormonally active adrenal tumors, benign or malignant, also should be considered. Enlargement of the male breast is also noted in many patients in the advanced stages of liver disease and is explained on the basis of impaired or faulty metabolism of the sex hormones due to the derangement of liver function. Testicular atrophy, from orchitis or trauma, may be followed by the appearance of bilateral hyperplasia of the breasts in the male. These days, bilateral hyperplasia is commonly seen in the adult male, as many men with carcinoma of the prostate are receiving stilbestrol as part of their treatment. Often the breast in this group of patients is painful and tender.

Treatment depends on the cause of gynecomastia. In patients receiving stilbestrol for prostatic cancer, toleration of the associated gynecomastia is the lesser of the two evils. When due to an estrogen-producing tumor, breast enlargement subsides when the tumor is removed. In the adolescent, reassurance with observation is the only rational course in most instances. Occasionally, persistence of pubertal gynecomastia may require excision, largely because of the psychological and social disturbances it may create. However, the surgical cosmetic result must be better than that created by gynecomastia and involves removal of the hypertrophied gland, but with preservation of the nipple. Finally, removal of the enlarged breast is essential should breast carcinoma be suspected.

Carcinoma of the Male Breast

Malignant disease of the male breast is rarely encountered. Most reported series disclose that cancer incidence of the female breast is at least 100 times greater than that of the male. The average age of males with this disease is slightly higher than that found for women.

In patients with Klinefelter's syndrome, which occurs in males and is associated with gynecomastia, cancer of the breast occurs with the same frequency that it does in the normal female population (Jackson et al., 1965). In other words, in patients with this syndrome, cancer of the breast occurs about 100 times more frequently than among normal males.

The symptoms are variable; pain and tenderness and bloody discharge from the nipple are among the more common ones. Most frequently, the complaint is that of a painless lump. The occasional patient does not present himself until the skin over the lesion becomes ulcerated.

Examination of the breast will disclose the lump readily. It is much more commonly fixed to the nipple and the skin than is carcinoma of the female breast. Nipple retraction or distortion likewise is more frequently evident, as the amount of normal breast tissue is small and usually lies directly beneath the areolar tissue. Involvement of the axillary nodes in resected specimens seems to occur in a higher percentage of breast malignancies of the male than in the female, but these nodes may go undetected on physical examination, particularly if the pectoralis musculature is well developed.

The pathologic findings encountered in malignant tumors of the male breast are similar to those of the female breast. The rare occurrence of this tumor prevents a reliable evaluation as to the frequency of the various types.

Treatment is radical mastectomy unless distant metastases already can be demonstrated. A skin graft is nearly always necessary to close the defect. In the event that distant metastases are established, simple mastectomy should be performed to avoid likely ulceration later on.

Hormonal therapy and adrenalectomy should be considered, but experience is too limited to evaluate either at present. In one patient, aged 73, osteolytic metastases became osteoclastic with relief of pain for 15 months under stilbestrol therapy. In another 34-year-old male at the University of Chicago Clinics, pulmonary and bony metastases receded surprisingly well for more than 48 months after bilateral orchiectomy was performed.

The prognosis in general is poor, being less favorable than for carcinoma of the female breast.

However, Edelman (1967) observed carcinoma of the male breast in 21 patients during a 13-year period. The patients reported are all Caucasian and the age range is from 39 to 72 years. Histologically the tumors were similar to those found in females. A total of 12 of the 19 patients followed are currently alive, with a 5-year survival rate of 63 per cent and an absolute 5-year survival rate of 43 per cent.

PROGNOSTIC CONSIDERATIONS

Of the several methods for the pathologic grading of breast cancers, none seems to reflect so well the future course of the individual patient as does the actual size of the tumor, measured in the freshly resected specimen. Cancer has a small beginning; it must grow to invade the surrounding structures, especially the lymphatics and the blood vessels. This takes time, longer in some than in others, and upon these inherent relationships or growth characteristics depends the outcome. The smaller the tumor and the more fibroplasia and lymphocytic response it provokes, the less anaplastic it is likely to be, and the slower its rate of metastasis is apt to be. Age of the patient appears to have less relationship to survival, at least after 35, than was presumed earlier. In spite of the controversy as to the preference of operation, it still appears best to perform the standard radical mastectomy when there is no evidence of distant metastases. That axillary metastases, left behind in the simple mastectomy but which may be removed with the carefully performed radical operation, do not give rise to other metastases is a concept difficult to accept.

With 50 per cent of all private patients with cancer of the breast being seen before the age of 55 and only 25 per cent of charity cases seen by this age, nearly twice as many charity patients have evidence of metastasis when first seen compared with the private group. The most obvious improvement in the treatment of breast cancer has occurred among private patients, who are being treated earlier with each decade; in this respect the educational efforts of such agencies as the American Cancer Society have been most worthwhile. It is hoped that the same can be accomplished in the lower socioeconomic groups.

It is probably wise to consider that cancer is never "cured" but that when patients can be treated early enough, many survive to their full life expectancy. But also, and especially for breast cancer, the operation is only one phase of treatment. Additional forms of palliative treatment may be necessary, each at the most judicious time. If ever the surgeon needs to assume the role of the family doctor or to continue to work with the family doctor, it is in the life-time management of patients with cancer of the breast.

REFERENCES

Adair, F. E.: Report of symposium at the sectional meeting of the American College of Surgeons, Feb. 11, 1952.
Adair, F. E., and Herrmann, J. B.: The use of testosterone propionate in the treatment of advanced carcinoma of the breast. Ann. Surg., 123:1023, 1946.
Albright, F.: Case records of the Massachusetts General Hospital (Case No. 27461). New Eng. J. Med., 225:789, 1941.
Asch, T., and Frey, C.: Radiographic appearance of mammary-duct ectasia with calcification. New Eng. J. Med., 266:86, 1962.
Atkins, H., Falconer, M. A., Hayward, J. L., MacLean, K. S., and Schurr, P. H.: The timing of adrenalectomy and of hypophysectomy in the treatment of advanced breast cancer. Lancet, 1:827, 1966.
Barnes, R. B., and Gershon-Cohen, J.: Clinical thermography. J.A.M.A., 185:949, 1963.

Beatson, G. T.: On treatment of inoperable carcinoma of the mammae: suggestions for a new method of treatment, with an illustrative case. Lancet, 2:104, and 162, 1896.
Berkson, J., Harrington, S. W., Clagett, O. T., Kirklin, J. W., Dockerty, M. B., and McDonald, J. R.: Mortality and survival in surgically treated cancer of the breast. Proc. Mayo Clin., 32:645, 1957.
Bittner, John J.: Experimental aspects of mammary cancer in mice. In: Breast Cancer and Its Diagnosis and Treatment. Baltimore, Williams & Wilkins, 1955.
Bonser, G. M., Dossett, J. A., and Jull, J. W.: Human and Experimental Breast Cancer. Springfield, Ill., Charles C Thomas, 1961, p. 368.
Breslow, L.: See California Tumor Registry.
Bryant, M. F., Lampe, I., and Coller, F. A.: Cancer of the breast. Surgery, 36:863, 1954.
California Tumor Registry: Cancer registration and survival in California. State of California, Department of Public Health, Berkeley, 1963.
Cohn, I., Jr., Slack, N. H., and Fisher, B.: Complications and toxic manifestations of surgical adjuvant chemotherapy for breast cancer. S. G. & O., 127:1201, 1968.
Conway, H., and Neuman, C. G.: Evaluation of skin grafting in the technique of radical mastectomy in relation to local recurrence of carcinoma. Surg. Gynec., Obstet., 88:45, 1949.
Cooperative Breast Cancer Group: Testosterone propionate therapy in breast cancer. J.A.M.A., 188:1069, 1964.
Courmelles, de F.: Quoted by Huggins (1954).
Daland, E. M.: Untreated cancer of the breast. Surg. Gynec., Obstet., 44:264, 1927.
Devitt, J. E., Beattie, W. G., and Stoddart, T. G. Carcinoma of the breast and pregnancy. Canad. J. Surg., 7:124, 1964.
Edelman, S.: Carcinoma of the male breast. J. Mount Sinai Hosp., 34:578, 1967.
Egan, R. L.: Mammography, an aid to diagnosis of breast carcinoma. J.A.M.A., 182:839, 1962.
———: Mammography in the evaluation of breast lesions. Hosp. Med., 1:2, 1964.
Erwald, Rolf: Mammary carcinoma and pregnancy. Acta obstet. gynec. scand., 46:316, 1967.
Finn, W. F.: Pregnancy complicated by cancer. Bull. Margaret Hague Maternity Hosp., 5:2, 1952.
Fitts, W. T., and Horn, R. C.: Occult carcinoma of the breast. J.A.M.A., 147:1429, 1951.
Frantz, V. K., Pickren, J. W., Melcher, G. W., and Auchincloss, H., Jr.: Incidence of chronic cystic disease in so-called normal breasts. Cancer, 4:762, 1951.
Freckman, H. A., Fry, H. L., Mendez, F. L., and Maurer, E. R.: Chlorambucil-prednisolone therapy for disseminated breast carcinoma. J.A.M.A., 189:23, 1964.
Funderburk, W. W., Syphax, B., and Smith, C. W.: Contrast mammography in breast discharge. Surg. Gynec., Obstet., 119:276, 1964.
Gardner, B., Gordan, G. S., Loken, H. F., and Thomas, A. N.: Calcium and phosphate metab-

olism in disseminated breast cancer: effects of site, progression or regression, and hormonal control. Cancer Chemotherapy Reports, No. 16, p. 299, Feb. 1962.

Gershon-Cohen, J.: Technical improvements in breast roentgenography. Am. J. Roent., Radium Therapy and Nuclear Med., 84:224, 1960.

Gershon-Cohen, J., Hermel, M. B., and Berger, S. M.: Detection of breast cancer by periodic x-ray examinations; a 5 year survey. J.A.M.A., 176: 1114, 1961.

Gershon-Cohen, J., Ingleby, H., and Hermel, M. B.: Roentgenographic diagnosis of calcification in carcinoma of the breast. J.A.M.A., 152:676, 1953.

Goldenberg, I. S.: (See Cooperative Breast Cancer Group.)

Grant, R. N., Tabah, E. J., and Adair, F. E.: The surgical significance of the subareolar lymph plexus in cancer of the breast. Surg., 33:71, 1953.

Greenwood, M.: A report on the natural duration of cancer. Ministry of Health Reports on Public Health and Medical Subjects, No. 33, London, Her Majesty's Stat. Off., 1926.

Haagensen, C. D.: Diseases of the Breast. Philadelphia. W. B. Saunders, 1956.

Haagensen, C. D., and Obeid, S. J.: Biopsy of the apex of the axilla in carcinoma of the breast. Ann. Surg., 149:149, 1959.

Haagensen, C. D., and Stout, A. P.: Carcinoma of the breast: II. Criteria of operability. Ann. Surg., 118:859, 1943.

Haddow, A., Watkinson, J. M., and Paterson, E.: Influence of synthetic oestrogens upon advanced malignant disease. Brit. Med. J., 2:393, 1944.

Handley, R. S.: The anatomy of the breast. *In*: Breast Cancer and Its Diagnosis and Treatment. p. 8. Baltimore, Williams & Wilkins, 1955.

Handley, R. S., and Tackeray, A. C.: Invasion of internal mammary lymph nodes in cancer of the breast. Brit. Med. J., 1:61-64, 1954.

Harrington, S. W.: Carcinoma of the breast—results of surgical treatment when cancer occurred in the course of pregnancy or lactation and when pregnancy occurred subsequent to operation (1910-33). Ann. Surg., 106:690, 1937.

———: Results of surgical treatment of unilateral carcinoma of the breast in women. J.A.M.A., 148:1007, 1952.

Hendrick, J. W.: Intraductal papilloma of the breast. Surg., Gynec., Obstet., 105:215, 1957.

Hitchcock, C. R., Hickok, D. F., Soucheray, J., Moulton, T., and Baker, R.: Thermography in mass screening for occult breast cancer. J.A.M.A., 204:419, 1968.

Hogan, G. F.: Mondor's Disease, Arch. Int. Med., 113:881, 1964.

Holleran, W. M., and Schmutzer, K. J.: Paget's disease of the groin. J.A.M.A., 193:193, 1965.

Huggins, C. B.: Endocrine methods of treatment of cancer of the breast. J. Nat. Cancer Inst., 15:1, 1954.

Huggins, C., and Bergenstal, D. M.: Surgery of the adrenals. J.A.M.A., 147:101, 1951.

Huggins, C., and Scott, W. W.: Bilateral adrenalectomy in prostatic cancer: clinical features and urinary excretion of 17-keto-steroids and estrogen. Ann. Surg., 122:1031, 1945.

Illingworth, C. F. W., Forrest, A. P. M., and Brown, D. A. P.: A simple method of implanting radon seeds into the pituitary gland in treatment of advanced breast cancer. Surg. Forum, 6:406, 1956.

Jackson, A. W., Muldal, S., Ockey, C. H., and O'Connor, P. J.: Carcinoma of male breast in association with the Klinefelter syndrome. Brit. Med. J. 1: 223, 1965.

Kahil, M., Orman, B., Gyorkey, F., and Brown, H.: Hypercalcemia. J.A.M.A., 201:721, 1967.

Kennedy, B. J.: The role of castration in breast cancer. Arch. Surg., 88:743, 1964.

Landau, R. L., Ehrlich, E. N., and Huggins, C.: Estradiol benzoate and progesterone in advanced human-breast cancer. J.A.M.A., 182:632, 1962.

Lewison, E. F.: Breast Cancer and Its Diagnosis and Treatment. Baltimore, Williams & Wilkins, 1955.

———: An appraisal of long-term results in surgical treatment of breast cancer. J.A.M.A., 186:975, 1963.

Luft, R., Olivecrona, H., and Sjögren, B.: Hypofysektomi pa människa. Nord. med., 47:351, 1952.

Matas, R.: On the so-called primary thrombosis of the axillary vein caused by strain. Am. J. Surg., 24:642, 1934.

McDivitt, R. W., and Hutter, R. V.: In situ lobular carcinoma. J.A.M.A., 201:96, 1967.

McDivitt, R. W., and Stewart, F. W.: Breast carcinoma in children. J.A.M.A., 195:388, 1966.

McKenzie, I.: Breast cancer following multiple fluoroscopies. Brit. J. Cancer, 19:1, 1965.

McWhirter, R.: Simple mastectomy and radiotherapy of breast cancer. Brit. J. Radiol., New Series, 28:128, 1955.

Missakian, M. M., Witten, D. M., and Harrison, E. G., Jr.: Mammography after mastectomy. J.A.M.A., 191:1045, 1965.

Mondor, H.: Tronculite sous-cutanée subaiguë de la paroi thoracique antéro-latérale. Mém. Acad. chir., 65:1271, 1939.

Moore, F. D., Woodrow, S. I., Aliapoulios, M. A., and Wilson, R. E.: Carcinoma of the breast (Concluded). New Eng. J. Med., 277:460, 1967.

Moritz, A. R.: The Pathology of Trauma. ed. 2. Philadelphia, Lea & Febiger, 1954.

Nadler, S. H., and Moore, G. E.: A clinical study of fluorouracil. Surg. Gynec. Obstet., 127:1210, 1968.

Nathanson, I. T., and Welch, C. E.: Life expectancy and incidence of malignant disease: I. Carcinoma of the breast. Am J. Cancer, 28:40-53, 1936.

New England J. Med.: Carcinoma of the breast—endocrinology and statistics. Editorial. 254:961, 1956.

Oliver, C. P.: Studies on human cancer families. Ann. N. Y. Acad. Sci., 71:1198, 1958.

Papanicolaou, G. M.: The value of exfoliative cytology in the early diagnosis and control of neoplastic disease of the breast. CA (Bull. Cancer Progress), 4:191, 1954.

Pearson, O. H., and Ray, B. S.: Results of hypophysectomy in treatment of metastatic mammary carcinoma. Cancer, 12:85, 1959.

Perrault, J.: Discussion. Bull. Soc. méd. hôp. Paris, 68:209, 1952.

Peters, M. V.: The influence of hormonal therapy on metastatic mammary cancer. Surg., Gynec., Obstet., 102:545, 1956.

Ramirez, G., and Ansfield, F. J.: Carcinoma of the breast in children. Arch. Surg., 96:222, 1968.

Rasmussen, R., Harper, P. V., and Kennedy, T.: The use of a beta ray point source for destruction of the hypophysis. Surg. Forum, 4:681, 1953.

Robbins, L. C.: Purposes of the mammography reproducibility study. Cancer Bull., 14:102, 1962.

Rosemond, G. P.: Breast cancer during pregnancy. Clin. Obstet. Gynec., 6:994, 1963.

Rubin, P.: Carcinoma of the breast. J.A.M.A., 199:142, 1967.

Samuel, E., and Young, G. B.: Early detection of cancer. Lancet, 1:149, 1969.

Shimkin, M. B.: Duration of life in untreated cancer. Cancer, 4:1-8, 1951.

Simmons, C. C., Daland, E. M., and Wallace, R. H.: Delay in the treatment of cancer. New Eng. J. Med. 208:1097, 1933.

Steiner, P. E.: Cancer: Race and Geography. Baltimore, Williams & Wilkins, 1954.

Stewart, F. W.: Tumors of the Breast. Washington, D. C., Armed Forces Inst. Path., 1950.

Strax, P., Venet, L., Shapiro, S., and Gross, S: Mammography and clinical examination in mass screening for cancer of the breast. Cancer, 20:2184, 1967.

Symmers, W. St. C.: Carcinoma of breast in transsexual individuals after surgical and hormonal interference with the primary and secondary sex characteristics. Brit. Med. J., 2:83, 1968.

Tellem, M., Shane, J. J., and Imbriglia, J. E.: Breast cancer in the postmenopausal years. Surg., Gynec., Obstet., 120:17, 1965.

Urban, J. A.: Extended radical mastectomy. *In*: Breast Cancer and Its Diagnosis and Treatment. p. 295. Baltimore, Williams & Wilkins, 1955.

———: Radical mastectomy in continuity with en bloc resection of the internal mammary lymph-node chain: a new procedure for primary operable cancer of the breast. Cancer, 5:992-1008, 1952.

———: Clinical experience and results of excision of the internal mammary lymph node chain in primary operable breast cancer. Cancer, 12:14, 1959.

Wanebo, C. K., Johnson, K. G., Sato, K., and Thorslund, T. W.: Breast cancer after exposure to the atomic bombings of Hiroshima and Nagasaki. New Eng. J. Med., 279:667, 1968.

Wang, Chiu-Chen: Carcinoma of the breast; associated problems: IV. Management of inflammatory carcinoma of the breast. J.A.M.A., 201:533, 1967.

Warren, S.: The relation of chronic mastitis to carcinoma of the breast. Surg., Gynec., Obstet., 71:257, 1940.

White, T. T., and White, W. C.: Breast cancer and pregnancy. Ann. Surg. 144:384-393, 1956.

Wilson, T. S., and MacGregor, J. W.: The diagnosis and treatment of tuberculosis of the breast. Canad. Med. A. J., 89:1118, 1963.

Witten, D. M.: Mammography: advantages and limitations. Postgrad. Med., 36:242, 1964.

Wynder, E. L., Bross, I. J., and Hirayama, T.: A study of the epidemiology of cancer of the breast. Cancer, 13:559, 1960.

CHAPTER 28

OLIVER COPE, M.D.

Thyroid, Thymus and Parathyroids

The Thyroid Gland
  Pathogenesis of Goiter
  Hyperthyroidism
  Nodular Goiter
  Thyroiditis
  The Normal Gland
  Suggestions About the Investigation of the Patient
  Pointers on Surgical Technic
The Thymus Gland
  Surgical Anatomy
  Pathologic Physiology
  Status Thymicolymphaticus

The Thymus Gland (Cont.)
  As a Seat of Tumor
  As an Instigator of Myasthenia Gravis
The Parathyroid Glands
  Introduction
  History
  Hypoparathyroidism
  Hyperparathyroidism
    Pathophysiology
    Anatomic Pathology
    Diagnosis
    Treatment

The Thyroid Gland

The surgery of goiter has been an integral part of the development of modern surgery. The peculiar anatomic and physiologic difficulties have stubbornly challenged the surgeon. Their conquest has contributed much to the technic of surgery, and the effect of the surgical removal much to the understanding of the physiology of the gland. A colorful phase of this surgical history is to be found in Halsted's *Story of Goiter* (1924).

In the latter part of the 19th century and the first portion of the 20th, surgery emerged as the only successful treatment of the various types of goiter. The final third of the 20th century finds much of the therapy of goiter in transition from surgical methods to medical.

First, the establishment that lack of iodine was the cause of endemic goiter provided an opportunity for preventive medicine (Marine and Kimball, 1917). The introduction of iodized salt has steadily reduced the incidence of endemic goiter throughout the world, and the need for operative care in this condition is vanishing.

Next, two effective medical therapies have appeared since 1941 for the control of hyperthyroidism. The earlier use of external irradiation and iodine have been only sporadically or incompletely effective. Radioactive iodine was the first adequate medical therapy. Its use started in 1941 (Hertz and Roberts, 1946). The second was the antithyroid drugs initiated by Astwood (1943). However, surgery is occasionally advisable in younger patients and in those whose goiter is suspected of containing a neoplasm.

In sporadic nonhyperfunctioning goiter, surgery still has a role. In spite of much new knowledge regarding the pathogenesis of such goiters and the common success of medical therapy, neoplasia, benign and malignant, are problems and surgery their treatment.

The study of the effects of the antithyroid drugs has occasioned new concepts of the pathogenesis of goiter. These concepts are described initially as an introduction to the subsequent section on hyperthyroidism and nontoxic goiter.

The chapter includes short accounts of thyroiditis and of attempts to alleviate heart disease by reduction of the activity of the normal gland. It is completed by remarks on the examination of patients with goiter, and pointers on surgical technic.

PATHOGENESIS OF GOITER

Hyperplasia was recognized as a part of most goiters and has been considered by some to be the primary etiologic stimulus of tumor formation. Experiments with iodine by Marine (1912) and its clinical introduction by Plummer (1923) in the treatment of hyperthyroidism gave rise to the concept of iodine involution as a cause of tumors. Recent experiments using the blocking agents or antithyroid drugs have recapitulated the gamut of human goiters to a striking degree and have led to a possible consolidation of our ideas regarding the pathogenesis. The newer knowledge can be construed to reinforce the concept that hyperplasia is an essential of all goiter. If reasonable, the concept is to be used to guide the therapy of goiter. The following three processes are to be considered.*

Hyperplasia: The Primary Process

Primary hyperplasia of the thyroid gland has been classically described both clinically and experimentally. There are 4 aspects recognizable by clinician, surgeon and pathologist.

1. The epithelial cells of the follicles are increased in number. The mitotic figures are visible on microscopic section, and there are papillary infoldings due to crowding of the cells. The process is diffuse throughout the gland, all areas taking part. Clinically, the thyroid gland increases in size.

2. The secretory activity is increased. Microscopically, this is seen as resorption of the colloid of the follicles. Clinically and experimentally, there is an increased turnover of radioactive iodine. The cells of the follicles change from cuboidal to columnar form, and there are large secretory droplets.

3. The blood flow through the gland is increased. The examiner recognizes this as a bruit and sometimes a thrill in the gland. The surgeon sees it as enlarged, engorged major vessels and unusual prominence of the minor vessels.

4. Hyperplasia of the lymphoid follicles takes place both in the thyroid gland and in the lymph nodes surrounding the thyroid. This is still an incidental finding, the meaning of which is not clear.

These 4 changes appear to be due to an increased secretion of the thyrotropic hormone of the anterior pituitary. On clinical grounds this is believed to be true because sometimes the same findings are encountered in patients with acromegaly. The identical changes have been produced in several experimental animals and more recently in man by thyrotropic hormone of the anterior pituitary. An iodine-deficient diet is accompanied by the same changes. The thyroid-blocking agents or antithyroid drugs also produce them, but here a direct effect of the antithyroid drugs upon the thyroid gland cannot be excluded absolutely. The effect of iodine deficiency and of these drugs can be canceled by the simultaneous administration of desiccated thyroid or one of the synthetic thyroid hormones thyroxin or tri-iodothyronine.

Iodine Involution

The 4 manifestations of primary hyperplasia of thyroid gland can be reversed by iodine. This action of iodine has been termed "involution." Although it has been postulated that part of this involuting effect may be due to a direct inhibiting effect of the iodine upon the anterior pituitary gland, it is more probably due to a local effect on the thyroid itself. In patients with the spontaneous hyperplasia of acute hyperthyroidism, as a rule the involution does not return the gland to normal. In experimental animals the involuting effect varies with the dosage of the anterior pituitary extract. The involution is only moderate when the stimulus in intense.

Iodine has no visible effect upon the normal gland, either clinically or experimentally. Therefore, a demonstration of the involuting effect depends upon the existence of a pre-existing hyperplasia. The involution represents restraint rather than stimulation.

The involution may be accompanied by some disturbance in the architecture of the gland (Reinhoff, 1926). This disturbance has been mistaken for the beginning of early nodule formation. It is more likely, on the basis of recent evidence, that the storage of iodine within the follicles and the consequent expansion of the thyroid tissue, together with

---

* During the first half of this century, observation of the life history of endemic goiter and of the goiter associated with acute hyperthyroidism led to a number of theories regarding the pathogenesis of goiter.

the loss of vascularity, may bring about an exaggeration of the normal lobulations of the thyroid, resulting in apparent nodule formation. Historically, iodine involution has provided the oldest explanation of nodule formation, and now it is probably of little importance. Nodules are more likely due to continued hyperplasia.

Continued Hyperplasia

The life history of endemic goiter first gave rise to the concept that continued hyperplasia was the reason for tumor formation. The initial process of formation of goiters in people living in an iodine-deficient area was hyperplasia. With continued iodine deficiency, a variety of nodules appeared, scattered here and there in the hyperplastic tissue. All sorts of tumors formed, including adenomas, cysts and, in later life, carcinomas.

The entire sequence of hyperplasia and a variety of tumors, including malignant ones, has been recapitulated in experimental animals given the antithyroid drugs (Bielschowsky, 1945; Griesbach et al., 1945; Money and Rawson, 1950; Morris et al., 1951; Paschkis et al., 1948). Rats and mice have been fed thiouracil or other antithyroid drugs over a period of from many months to 2 years. The drug promptly initiates an intense hyperplasia. If the drug is continued, in 3 to 4 months tumors begin to appear. Their occurrence may be expedited by the simultaneous administration of a carcinogen (Bielschowsky et al., 1949). Some adenomas are composed of embryoniclike cells, some of fetal cells, and others are typical papillary tumors. More differentiated follicular adenomas may occur, with central necrosis and healing by fibrosis. In later months, cysts of inactive cuboidal epithelium appear immediately adjacent to the continued hyperplastic tissue. The apparent inactivity has given rise to the concept of cellular exhaustion (Money and Rawson, 1950). Comparable cysts have been encountered in the pancreas of dogs and cats injected with large doses of a suitable anterior pituitary extract (Richardson and Young, 1938). Eventually, after 18 months to 2 years of continued stimulation, malignant tumors appear. The simultaneous use of the carcinogens does not seem to make these appear any earlier. The humors metastasize and eventually grow to a size sufficient to kill the animal. They can be transplanted to other animals (Bielschowsky et al., 1949).

In the pathogenesis of goiter, 3 other factors are to be considered: the endocrine phases of normal life, diet and the nervous system. Puberty and pregnancy are associated with an enlargement and increased activity of the thyroid gland. Diffuse goiter and thyroid nodules are apt to appear as abnormal accompaniments of both these phases of endocrine change. The menstrual cycle and the menopause may normally be associated with slight changes in thyroid stimulation and activity. Though the menstrual cycle has not been incriminated, at the time of the menopause a pre-existing goiter is commonly prone to renewed or intensified growth. These relationships to ovarian function are believed to be the reason why goiter is so much more frequent in women than in men.

Certain foods contain thiocyanates and other goitrogenic substances (Astwood et al., 1949). Such foods have been suggested as possible causes of sporadic goiter, but beyond the occurrence of goiter in a number of monks of a monastery whose diet had been limited to cabbage for 2 or 3 years, such an origin has not been substantiated.

Because of the occurrence of the hyperplastic goiter of hyperthyroidism in patients subjected to undue emotional stress, the central nervous system has been suggested as the stimulator of the anterior pituitary's thyrotropic secretion, thus making it the primary cause of thyroid enlargement. Experimental proof of the pathways of such a stimulation has been offered by Harris (1958).

HYPERTHYROIDISM

Hyperthyroidism occurs both as an acute disease and as a secondary complication of a pre-existing goiter. Acute hyperthyroidism is the most dramatic disease of the thyroid gland. It is generally known as exophthalmic goiter because of its frequent association with a characteristic form of exophthalmos. The disease was first recognized by Parry (1825), a physician of Bath, England. It was described more fully by Graves of Ireland (1835) and 5 years later by von Basedow of Germany (1840). In English-speaking countries it is commonly known as Graves's disease and on the continent of Europe as Basedow's disease.

Pathogenesis. Exophthalmic goiter is generally acute in onset because the enlargement of the thyroid, the initial symptoms from hypersecretion, and the appearance of the eye signs have a date of onset known by patient, family and friends. The disease is 4 times as common in women as in men, and it characteristically occurs during the phase of active ovarian life. It occasionally occurs in childhood before puberty, when the sex incidence is approximately equal. It also occurs, but less commonly, in both men and women after the age of 50. In the older group the exophthalmos is often absent.

Clinical evidence indicates that the acute form of hyperthyroidism is a psychosomatic disease (Lidz and Whitehorn, 1949). The people from childhood to older age who succumb to this disease are emotionally anxious. Shortly before or at the time of onset of the hyperthyroidism a history of an additional emotional insult is almost always found. There is nothing specific known about the character or the type of emotional insult. The insults are the kind frequently encountered in other individuals who do not succumb to any psychosomatic disorder or may be afflicted by another type of organic disease. Therefore, it is probable that some predisposition exists. The disease has been encountered occasionally in several members of the same family, and it has been postulated, therefore, that there is a genetic factor (Boas and Ober, 1946). At least the stimulus seems to fall upon fertile ground.*

An intact anterior pituitary gland and an excess of its thyrotropic hormone are probably essential to the development of hyperthyroidism. Clinically, several arguments point to this. Sometimes exophthalmic goiter is encountered in patients in the initial phase of acromegaly. Reports of its occurrence in patients without intact pituitary tissue are open to question. Sometimes the disease can be arrested by x-ray irradiation of the anterior pituitary, much as Cushing's disease of the adrenal cortex is sometimes relieved by pituitary irradiation (Pope and Raker, 1955; Thompson and Thompson, 1944). The disease is prone to blossom in women at times when the anterior pituitary is undergoing abrupt changes in function—namely, during or at the termination of pregnancy and at the menopause. The cells of the anterior pituitary of patients dying with hyperthyroidism are consistent with increased anterior pituitary function (Russfield, 1955). Experimentally, a comparable hyperplasia and increased activity of the thyroid gland are produced by TSH, LATS† and antithyroid drugs. Hypophysectomy, or the administration of thyroid, prevents the effect of the antithyroid drugs but not of the hormones. Thus, the concept emerges that emotional stress acting upon the hypothalamus of a susceptible person increases the secretion of the Thyrotrophic Releasing Factor (TRF) which, in turn, increases the TSH of the pituitary and finally stimulates the thyroid to grow and oversecrete. The thyroid gland is the end organ of abnormal function, not the origin of the disease.

Signs and Symptoms. The prominent, characteristic eye signs of exophthalmic goiter have a dual origin. The exophthalmos is independent of the thyroid level and stems apparently from a pituitary secretion closely related to the thyrotropic hormone, while the stare and the lid lag depend upon the excess of thyroid (Dobyns, 1950). Usually the eye signs develop coincidentally with the goiter and hyperthyroidism. Sometimes, however, the eye signs antedate by weeks or months the development of the goiter. Occasionally one eye may be involved first and the other eye only many months later or not at all. The eye

---

* Objection has been raised to the psychosomatic concept of Graves's disease on the very ground that emotional conflicts are common and Graves's disease relatively rare. The occurrence of Graves's disease may be likened to that of lobar pneumonia. A large portion of our population in winter harbors the pneumococcus in the upper respiratory tract; only an occasional person develops lobar pneumonia, and only when the balance between virulence of the organism and immunity of the host provides the right conditions. Pneumococcus lobar pneumonia never occurs in the absence of the pneumococcus. Does acute hyperthyroidism ever afflict emotionally adjusted people living in a stable environment? The author has not seen such a case.

† LATS, a Long Acting Thyroid Stimulating hormone, has recently been identified in the blood plasma and in lymphocytes of human beings and experimental animals in a variety of conditions. Its possible role in the pathogenesis of Graves's disease is not as yet agreed upon.

signs may be absent even after prolonged enlargement and hypersecretion of the thyroid. Finally, the exophthalmos may become worse if treatment of the thyroid reduces the function to below the normal level (Means, 1948).

The eye signs usually come into abeyance with therapy of the hyperthyroidism. The stare and the lid lag are the first to disappear. The recession of the eyeballs may be slow. Occasionally, the exophthalmos is increased after therapy, and the eyes may be endangered by the forward displacement of the eyeballs—so-called progressive exophthalmos. Hypothyroidism is to be avoided. Surgical decompression of the orbital cavities may be necessary to save the eyes.

Hyperthyroidism developing in a patient with a pre-existing goiter generally is termed "toxic nodular goiter." In contrast with exophthalmic goiter, it occurs principally in patients of the older age group, both sexes being involved, but with a continued preponderance in the female. It often develops insidiously and is characteristically slow in onset. The degree of hyperthyroidism usually is less severe. In those patients in whom the activity of the goiter has been studied and found to be normal prior to the development of hyperthyroidism, there usually has been a slow increase in size of the goiter coincident with the onset of hyperthyroidism.

The intimate pathology of the nodular goiter often fails to show any hyperplasia. Because of the increase in size prior to the recognition of the hyperthyroidism, it is felt that accretion in size gives rise to the hyperthyroidism rather than increase in activity of any part. In many women, the onset of renewed growth of the goiter and the development of the hyperthyroidism follow closely on the menopause, an argument that the anterior pituitary is an essential etiologic link in this type of goiter as well.

Differential Diagnosis. Much has been written differentiating the 2 types of hyperthyroidism, but basically the two are probably the same disease. The extremes are not alike, but there are transitional forms where one melts into the other. For example, long-standing acute hyperthyroidism without exophthalmos cannot be differentiated from toxic nodular goiter because nodules develop gradually in any hyperthyroidism of long standing. The intensity differs, and this may be related to the difference in age. The acute disease arises in flamboyant form; in the secondary nodular type the etiologic stimulus appears to be less virulent. In acute hyperthyroidism cardiac signs are less prominent because the patients are younger and more elastic; the nervousness and the irritability of the excessive thyroid hormone dominate the clinical picture. In the older age group, a modicum of hyperthyroidism quickly uses up the cardiac reserve, and signs of cardiac insufficiency are prominent. The absence of exophthalmos in the nodular type may well be due to loss of sensitivity of the orbital tissues with advancing age. The eye signs are absent in older people with no previous goiter and acute hyperthyroidism.

Treatment. SURGERY. Surgery was the first successful therapy of hyperthyroidism. In its initial years the therapy was faltering, largely because of the vascularity of the gland and the precarious cardiac and physiologic status of the hyperthyroid patient. Therefore, external irradiation by x-rays was tried and was successful in about one third of the patients. The discovery that iodine, with its involution of the hyperplasia, induced a partial remission of the hyperthyroidism (Plummer, 1923) opened the surgical era of therapy. The iodine-induced remission made it possible for the operation to be carried out when the patient was less toxic, and the success of operation rose precipitously. From 1923 to 1941, refinements such as staged operations, attention to nutrition and the regaining of strength during remission under iodine brought mortality and complications to the level of other major surgical procedures.

The introduction of the thiouracil compounds by Astwood (1943) enabled the surgeon to do even better. The metabolic rate could now be brought to normal, the nutrition of the patient restored, and the operation carried out without urgency on an essentially normal person. It became possible to operate under controlled conditions without fear of any mortality or complications such as hemorrhage, recurrent nerve palsy, or parathyroid insufficiency. Surgery, therefore, remains today as one of the 3 successful therapies of hyperthyroidism. Less often used in acute hyperthyroidism, it is still to be considered in some patients with nodular goiters and secondary hyperthyroidism. The slightly higher frequency of a concomitant malignant lesion in such goiters and the size of the goiter with the complication of pressure unrelieved by medical therapy make surgery preferable.

RADIOACTIVE IODINE was introduced in 1941 by Hertz (1946) in the therapy of hyperthyroidism. In principle, it is like surgery; instead of surgical extirpation of the larger part of the goiter, it eliminates the excess thyroid tissue by radiation necrosis. With experience, the right amount of radiation can be landed in the thyroid cells, and the desired necrosis accomplished (Chapman and Maloofa, 1955). Sometimes repeated doses are needed. It is as controlled a procedure as the surgical extirpation, but it takes more time to accomplish the desired result. Surgery brings an abrupt ending to the hyperthyroidism; radiation necrosis may take from 4 to 6 months or even longer. Initially, it is equally sure, and far easier for the patient. However, there are disadvantages. After 10 to 15 years one third have developed clinical hypothyroidism needing thyroid therapy. Some have become myxedematous, making their restitution therapy more difficult. Since such progressive hypothyroidism is rare following surgery, it appears that there are later effects after irradiation.

Another drawback to its use has been found in children. Tumors with malignant potential have been seen in the thyroid of patients whose hyperthyroidism was treated 15 or more years previously when they were children. Comparable tumors have not been encountered in patients treated when they were adults.

The final disadvantage, still an unproved, theoretical one, is the possible genetically deleterious effect upon the gonads of the initial therapeutic doses. Many feel that the therapy should be withheld from patients still in the child-bearing ages.

ANTITHYROID DRUGS. The second successful medical therapy is the use of the antithyroid drugs, introduced by Astwood. These drugs eliminate hyperthyroidism by blocking chemically the elaboration of iodine into the thyroid hormone. There are 3 forms of drugs, each apparently acting at a different chemical phase—the thiocyanates, the thiouracils and perchlorate. Propylthiouracil, Tapazole and potassium perchlorate are the drugs used most commonly. If a sufficient dosage of the drug is given, thyroid activity can be reduced to normal in all patients and can be so maintained with suitable adjustment of dosage. An excessive dose produces hypothyroidism.

The use of antithyroid drugs has been disappointing as definitive therapy for hyperthyroidism. If the metabolic rate is maintained at the normal level for only a few months and the drug then omitted, the hyperthyroidism returns in a large percentage of patients. If the drug is administered for a 2-year period, somewhat more than half of the patients have no recurrence. The disease process, being self-limited, apparently has run its course.* Of those who have a recrudescence of hyperthyroidism, a subsequent prolonged period of drug therapy may be followed by a permanent remission in another half. Such prolonged therapy means close care of the patient and is a nuisance to patient and physician; therefore, some of the clinics which at first advocated the use of the antithyroid drugs as the definitive therapy have abandoned it in favor of radioactive iodine.

PSYCHOSOMATIC CONSIDERATIONS. Evidence is accumulating that attention to the psychosomatic aspect of acute hyperthyroidism may lead to greater success with the prolonged drug therapy. If attention is paid to the emotional origin of the disease and irritating influences eliminated during the course of the drug therapy, it is more likely to be followed by a successful remission. Thus, the drug therapy has the additional advantage of calling to the physician's attention those very aspects of the patient's life which have been troublesome. Whether the emotional stress is etiologic or not becomes academic, for the combined use of drug and psychosomatic therapy brings to the patient relief that is more nearly complete. Such psychosomatic therapy also can be linked to the surgical and the radiation methods.

* In 1926, Friedrich von Mueller, Professor of Medicine in Munich, advocated sending patients with exophthalmic goiter to the Tyrol Mountains for a minimum of 2 years. He stressed the need for a 2-year stay. The reason for the success of his therapy is now clear. The deficiency of iodine in these mountains deprived the thyroid gland of iodine as effectively as the use of the antithyroid drugs.

NODULAR GOITER

Nodular goiter includes a heterogeneous group of clinical entities, from small to large goiters, from single nodules to multiple, and from benign to malignant. The causes are obscure. Some case histories reveal only the ravages merely of living, of bearing babies, or working hard and living long. Many people go to their graves not knowing that they had a lump in their thyroid. Though many lumps are innocent and many vanish under thyrotoxin therapy, lumps *are* tumors, and tumors are still the concern of the surgeon.

Nodular goiter is a descriptive term. In some communities, "adenomatous goiter" is preferred. The use of "adenomatous" implies that the nodules in the goiter are adenomas, that is, benign neoplasms. Since there is often doubt regarding the true nature of the nodules, the use of the descriptive word is to be preferred. The term "adenoma" should be reserved for those nodules in which there is substantial evidence that the growth is both anatomically and physiologically independent of the remainder of the gland.

Classification

A number of classifications of nodular goiter have been proposed. The differences between the classifications depend upon differences of opinion regarding the nature of the origin and the character of the nodules. The following classification is in use in the Thyroid Clinic of the Massachusetts General Hospital. In relation to tumors it follows most closely that of Warren and Meissner (1953).

Diffuse nodular goiter means that the disease process involves to some extent the entire thyroid apparatus, that the entire thyroid is enlarged, and that at least one or more areas are nodular. Endemic goiter and sporadic goiter encountered in nonendemic, noniodine deficient areas are such goiters. The goiter of a patient with burned-out Graves's disease is also such a goiter. Secondary hyperthyroidism occurs in these goiters when growth is renewed, for example, after the menopause.

The nodules are of a variety of types, varying from exaggerated lobulations without clear-cut capsules through cysts to localized adenomas and occasionally carcinomas. They are comparable to the isolated tumors described later (see Adenomas and Carcinomas), and they are the variety of tumors mimicked in the experimental animals exposed to prolonged thiouracil therapy described above under Pathogenesis of Goiter.

A single goiter may have nodules of one or more types. Two or three types are common. When several are present they have been called pudding-stone goiters. Approximately 4 per cent of such goiters coming to operation at the Mayo Clinic and at the Massachusetts General Hospital harbor a carcinoma as one of the nodules (Beahrs *et al.*, 1951; Cope *et al.*, 1949). The incidence of cancer in diffuse nodular goiter in the population at large must be considerably smaller. Sokol has estimated that 40,000 of each 1 million of North American population harbor thyroid lumps 1 cm. or greater. Of these 40,000, only 25 are cancerous in any one year.

Localized goiter is the term applied to those goiters in which the enlargement and the nodularity are limited to one area of the gland, the remainder of the gland being essentially normal. By definition, the nodules of these goiters are more likely to be adenomatous, since they fulfill the definition of autonomous growth.

The nodule of the diffuse or localized nodular goiter may be any one of the following:

Exaggerated Lobulation. In the embryologic development of the normal thyroid, the lateral lobe is rarely fused into a smooth mass. The surface is frequently indented by two or three or more sulci. A hyperplastic process increases the depth of such sulci, the adjacent tissue bulging out to form a rounded nodule. Separately encapsulated pieces of thyroid, which occur in at least 10 per cent of normal people, also enlarge under a stimulus and push forward, mimicking an adenoma. On cut section these exaggerated lobulations have no capsule separating them from the body of the lobe. Desiccated thyroid is effective therapy when the nodular goiter is limited to this lobular phase of development. The medication suppresses the anterior pituitary's thyrotropic action, and the goiter shrivels. Such therapy is not effective in eliminating true neoplasms described below, for they have developed an autonomy and an integrity independent of the thyrotropic stimulation.

Cysts filled with colloid and lined by low

cuboidal epithelium are not infrequent. The probability that such cysts represent exhaustion phenomena has been described already. They grow slowly and are to be differentiated from papillary cystadenomas.

Adenomas. PAPILLARY CYSTADENOMAS are uncommon. They usually have a thick, well-demarcated capsule. The tumors may vary from largely cystic to essentially solid, in which case they may be called a papillary adenoma. There is no absolute line that can be drawn between papillary adenoma and papillary carcinoma described below. A locally benign-appearing papillary adenoma may have been accompanied by metastases to the regional lymph nodes.

EMBRYONAL ADENOMA denotes a localized, encapsulated tumor consisting of cords of cells similar to the cells of the thyroid in the embryonic stage of development. These are considered by some to be potentially malignant.

FETAL ADENOMA is a circumscribed, encapsulated tumor consisting of cells arranged in a rudimentary follicular configuration, with little or no colloid in the follicles. The cells resemble those of fetal thyroid, being somewhat more differentiated than the embryonal but less so than those of the follicular adenoma. The fetal adenoma is also considered by some as potentially malignant, though most surgical pathologists classify them as benign.

HÜRTHLE ADENOMA is a rare tumor with cells having a special staining reaction. The cells are arranged usually in the fetal or embryonic manner, the tumor probably being a variant of the relatively undifferentiated adenoma. Occasionally, it gives rise to distant metastases, particularly to bone, and therefore is potentially malignant. Probably less than 10 per cent of such adenomas are actually malignant.

FOLLICULAR ADENOMA is the most common of all adenomas and is a frequent lesion of the thyroid. Always encapsulated, it may grow to considerable size. When it reaches the size of a lemon, it usually is necrotic in the center with evidence of healing by fibrosis. Hemorrhage sometimes occurs into such adenomas. The cells form well-differentiated follicles with varying amounts of colloid secretion. Occasionally, such an adenoma gives rise to a blood-borne metastasis, usually to bone, even though the local lesion appears to be benign. Blood vessel invasion may be found if diligently searched for. Rarely do these adenomas spread their cells in the lymphatics. When a locally benign adenoma has given rise to distant metastases, perforce it must be called a carcinoma. The German pathologists have tried to combine both features by the awkward term of "benign metastasizing struma or adenoma." Since the follicular adenoma is a common tumor, and bone metastasis from such a tumor is rare, it is obvious that the vast majority of such adenomas are benign, in keeping with their local appearance. The benign form are the tumors most commonly found incidentally in the thyroid at autopsy in the majority of people over 65 dying from any cause (Schlesinger et al., 1938).

All of these benign lumps are encountered more frequently in the female than in the male, and probably more often in women who have had one or more pregnancies. Their incidence increases with each decade in both sexes. Some are subject to physiologic influence. Their rate of growth may be slowed occasionally by thyroid medication, and frequently the rate is accelerated by pregnancy. Thyroid medication has not been proved to dissolve any of the adenomas. Therefore, the only known effective therapy is surgery, and it is indicated if the diagnosis is in doubt or the growth is rapid.

Carcinomas. The carcinomas are of 3 general types: the papillary carcinomas, the adenocarcinomas and the undifferentiated. In contrast with the benign adenomas of the thyroid, which are common lesions in the population, the carcinomas are rare. Thus, they constitute a very small proportion of the nodules of the thyroid.

The carcinomas probably start *de novo*, as do the adenomas. The engrafting of a carcinoma on a part of a follicular or other benign adenoma has been described, but it is probably a rare occurrence. Only twice has the author encountered findings consistent with such a development. Mixed types of carcinomas are encountered not infrequently, the biologic behavior of the tumor following both types. It is believed that sometimes metastases deviate from the primary type.

PAPILLARY CARCINOMA is the most prevalent malignant lesion, representing approximately 60 per cent of the carcinomas. Biologically, no other tumor in the body is quite like these papillary lesions. They occur in all decades of life, as frequently in the later teens and twenties as in any other decade. They are no more malignant in the child or the adolescent than in any other age group. In other words, they do not follow the classic age distribution of malignancy. They have a sluggish growth, and this in spite of a wildly growing appearance of many on microscopic section. They are slow to invade surrounding tissues. Even if they have invaded the cartilage of the larynx, for example, extirpation is easy and curative. They spread early through the lymphatics to the lymph nodes, and here the cells may stay for years without metastasizing through the blood stream. The cells grow luxuriantly in the lymph nodes so that the lymph node metastasis frequently outgrows the primary lesion. Only when the lymph node capsule is overdistended does the papillary growth spread into the neighboring tissue. The life span from initial lesion to lymph nodes to neighborhood spread may extend over several years.

A number of the papillary carcinomas have an occasional well-developed follicle containing colloid. Because of such follicles pathologists call them "papillary adenocarcinoma," a term describing their microscopic appearance rather than their biologic behavior. Occasionally, and almost always in the older patient, the follicular areas are adenocarcinoma, the tumor being of mixed types.

The papillary carcinoma is the type of malignancy encountered in an occasional patient with Graves's disease or nodular goiter of long standing. The clinical occurrence in Graves's disease indicates that long-continued hyperplasia is a dominant stimulus giving rise to the tumor. Usually the patients are above the age of 40 and have had long-standing Graves's disease. The youngest patient in the Massachusetts General Hospital series with hyperthyroidism complicated with papillary carcinoma was a girl of 15 who had had Graves's disease certainly since the age of 8 and probably since the age of 4.*

ADENOCARCINOMAS. The adenocarcinomas are more like carcinomas of other organs such as the stomach or the breast. They have the typical age distribution and, except for the well differentiated, are locally invasive. Lymph node metastases are less prominent than are blood-borne; bones and lungs are particularly fertile ground for seeding. If the cells of the metastasis are well differentiated to begin with or become biologically so by total thyroidectomy, significant therapeutic restraint may be obtained with radioactive iodine. This form of radiation is most useful in the well-differentiated tumor described in the previous section under Follicular Adenoma. Their metastases may be held in abeyance for a number of years, although no radiation cure has been reported as yet. The metastases grow so slowly with or without radiation that, if single and accessible, surgical excision should be considered as the most desirable therapy.

UNDIFFERENTIATED CARCINOMAS. These are a highly malignant group. Usually they are subclassified according to their cell type and include the small cell, the giant cell and the epidermoid. When first recognized, ordinarily they have spread beyond the limits of surgical extirpation; they have a bad prognosis. The cells are biologically undifferentiated and do not concentrate any radioactive iodine. Therefore, external radiation is the sole therapy available beyond the effort at surgical extirpation. They follow the usual age distribution of malignancies.

Lymphoma has been reported arising in the lymph follicles of the thyroid. This tumor is difficult—sometimes impossible—to differentiate microscopically from the undifferentiated small cell carcinoma and from sarcoma of the thyroid. Malignant tumors of other organs metastasize occasionally to the thyroid, producing a goiter as the patient's first symptom and sign. Hypernephroma, myeloma and carcinomas of the gastrointestinal tract are such tumors.

THYROIDITIS

Included under the term "thyroiditis" are a small group of poorly understood goiters. An occasional streptococcus abscess forms in the thyroid gland following an acute throat infection. In rare cases, a tuberculous abscess is encountered. The origin of these is clear enough.

---

* In younger patients in whom a papillary carcinoma has been found as the only lesion in the thyroid, there have been an early history of rediation therapy and an antedating stress. It is hard to escape the conclusion that both are involved in the trigger mechanism.

They are abscesses like those in any organ, the bacteria being blood-borne.

ACUTE THYROIDITIS

Acute thyroiditis is an acute inflammation that behaves like a virus infection. Sometimes patients with this condition are encountered in waves, as if there were a mild epidemic. The thyroid becomes acutely tender and swollen in a few hours, to subside a week or 10 days later. Usually there is a moderate fever. The acute attack is characteristically recurrent once or twice after intervals of a month or two. Efforts to culture a virus have thus far failed. There is no residuum and no proven treatment, although many have been claimed. Often the inflammation is localized to one lobe of the gland; the alternate lobe may be affected in the subsequent attack.

CHRONIC THYROIDITIS

Three types of chronic goiter enlargement are included under chronic thyroiditis: nonspecific lymphoid, Hashimoto's and Riedel's. Each has its characteristic cell picture. The lymphoid type is a probably nonspecific accompaniment of long-standing diffuse goiter. Hashimoto's thyroiditis is a specific process associated with destruction of the thyroid follicles. The goiter is spongy and bulging and often grows over a period of many months, with increasing compression of the trachea and the esophagus. Its etiology is debatable, an autoimmune reaction being the current popular concept. The only established therapy is surgical decompression if the size of the goiter warrants intervention. The isthmus and the anterior portion of the lateral lobes are removed, providing mobility for the remaining tissue. The process usually burns itself out and may leave the patient with an inadequate amount of secreting thyroid tissue and a consequent hypothyroidism. Thyroid therapy is indicated.

Riedel's struma is characteristically hard and has been termed *ligneous thyroiditis*. The gland is fibrosed, contracts and may constrict the trachea. Surgical decompression also may be indicated. Some think that this process is the end result of the Hashimoto type, but against this concept is the fact that Hashimoto's thyroiditis is common, and Riedel's struma is rare.

THE NORMAL GLAND

Surgical resection of the normal thyroid gland has been practiced in patients with decompensated heart disease. Benefit was only occasional—occurring in some of the patients with angina. Later, the same program was advocated, using radioactive iodine to ablate the thyroid (Blumgart et al., 1957). Limited use by cardiologists suggests a limited benefit. Success, presumably, depends on the wisdom used in selecting the patients. The failure of most hearts to improve under the diminished load of hypothyroidism may be due to the effect of the hypothyroidism on the action of the heart muscle.

SUGGESTIONS ABOUT THE INVESTIGATION OF THE PATIENT

Comprehensive investigation of the patient suspected of thyroid disease includes taking the history, and making the physical, the behavior and the laboratory examinations. The

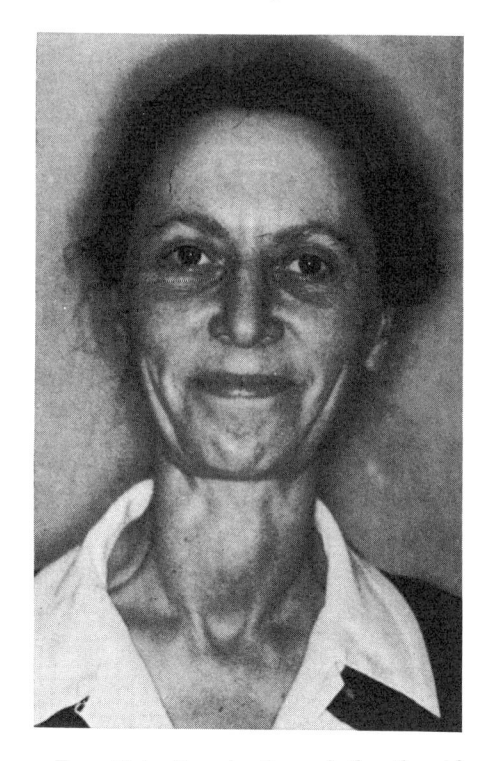

FIG. 28-1. Examination of the thyroid gland. Inspect as the first step. Watch as the patient swallows. Asymmetries and mediastinal extensions are readily picked up.

diagnosis usually can be established with surprising confidence by the history and a knowledgeable physical examination; the laboratory examination is needed only for confirmation. The behavior examination contributes, for the most part, to therapy.

The principles of diagnosing hyperthyroidism are well established. The elevated metabolic rate of the tissues, even when only of mild degree, increases the circulatory load and the irritability of the entire nervous system—peripheral, autonomic and central. In more extreme forms it undermines strength and disturbs organ function. In anyone with such symptoms or with a goiter, hyperthyroidism is to be considered. Confirmation of the clinical impression is secured through determination of the basal metabolic rate, the radioactive iodine tracer and the thyroid molecule in the blood serum.

A painstaking physical examination of the thyroid itself is most telling in relation to tumors. The basic principle of the examination is that a neoplasm is a localized disease and that a goiter, if it contains one, must give evidence of a localized change, one area out of line with the rest. Confusion between the diffuse process of hyperplasia and the localized neoplasia occurs when the original thyroid is unusually asymmetric or irregular. Such a gland enlarged by hyperplasia exhibits the asymmetry or the irregularity in exaggerated form. The right thyroid lobe is most often confusing in this regard. The normal right lobe

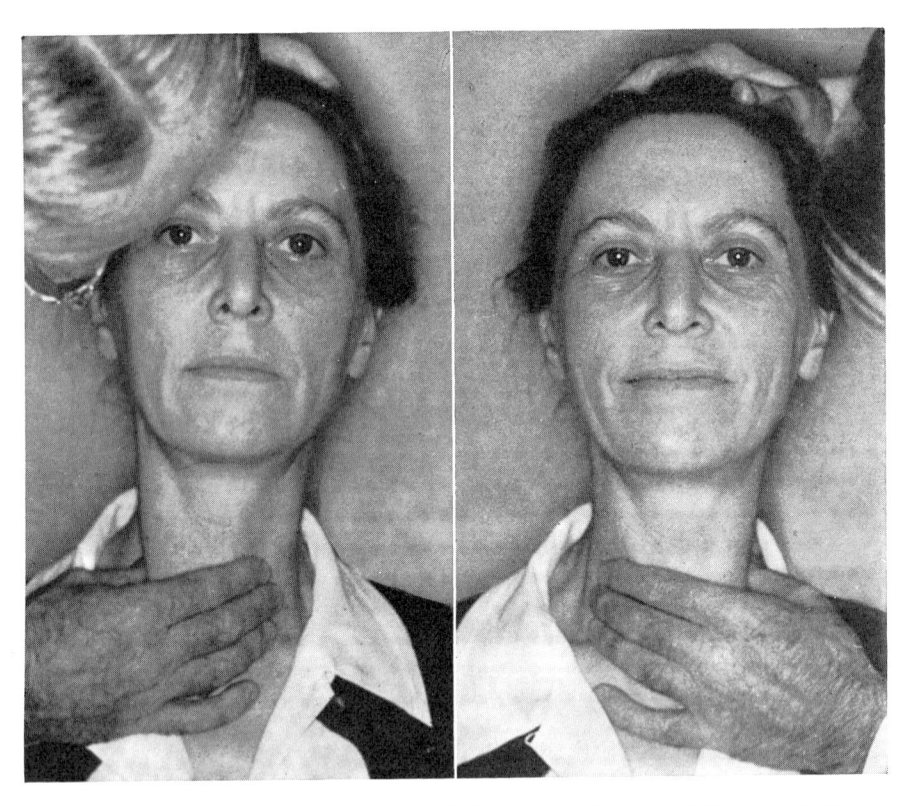

Fig. 28-2. Palpate as the second step, and always from in front of the patient. Examine one side at a time, use the thumb to displace the goiter toward the examining fingers. Steady the patient's head with the nonexamining hand, relaxing the sternocleidomastoid muscle by slight rotation of the head. A small goiter may be felt by insinuating the fingers between the thyroid and the muscle; a large one must be felt through the muscle.

averages 25 per cent heavier than the left. In a diffuse goiter the right lobe is expectedly larger than the left. The difference in size does not necessarily indicate a neoplasm in the right lobe. On the other hand, a left lobe larger than the right should arouse suspicion of neoplasia in the left.

Refinements of the local examination include checking for mobility of a nodule within the thyroid substance, smoothness of the capsule, tenderness and hardness. If a lump is stuck, rough, hard and not tender, malignancy should be suspected. Care must be taken not to render a lump tender by overpalpation.

Lymph nodes are to be sought. Normal nodes are rarely large or firm enough to be felt. The easiest place to pick up initial enlargement is in the Delphian and the pretracheal groups (Cope, 1948). The Delphian node lies in the midline just above the thyroid isthmus. It can be identified against the firm background of the cricoid cartilage. Always there is one node in this position and often two. The pretracheal nodes lie below the isthmus and can be felt against the trachea. Their position is not so constant and they are harder to find. Nodes of the jugular chains have to be palpated against the soft background of the jugular veins. They have to be larger to be felt. When the Delphian or the pretracheal nodes are palpable, then the thyroid disease is to be differentiated between thyroiditis and malignancy.

Many physicians examine the thyroid from behind the patient, using both hands. This approach has two disadvantages. First, the fingers are disadvantageously placed for palpation of the deeper parts of the gland. Only the anterior surface can be well felt. Stand to the side, slightly in front. Examine the right thyroid lobe with the left hand. The bulb of the fingers can feel the front and also slide around to the side and posteriorly. Place the right or nonexamining hand on the patient's head. Rotate the head slightly toward the examiner, thus relaxing the right sternocleidomastoid muscle. The fingers of the left hand can now be pushed in medial to the sternocleidomastoid to closer contact with the lateral and the posterior surfaces of the lobe. The thumb of the examining hand is placed against the left or contralateral lobe. Pressure pushes

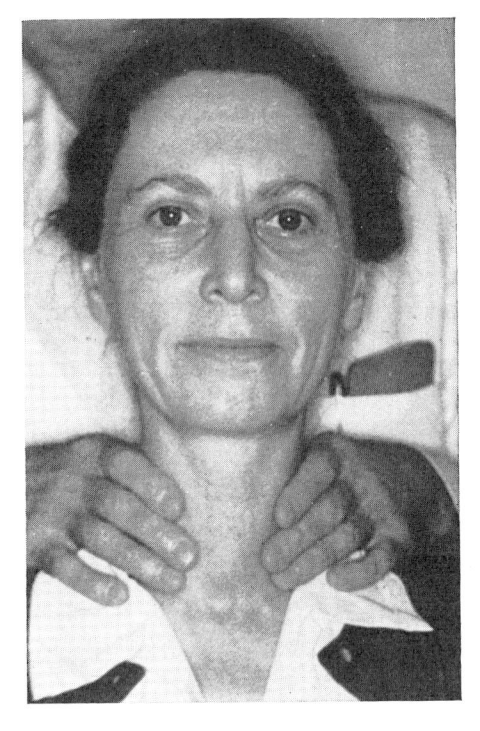

FIG. 28-3. The blind approach from behind, both hands at once. Only the front of the goiter is readily palpated from this position, and the patient's expression cannot be watched. Tenderness and anxiety are missed.

the right lobe out where it can be felt better. The left thyroid lobe is to be examined in comparable fashion by standing to the right side of the patient, using the right hand on the thyroid and the left hand on the patient's head.

The second reason that the position somewhat in front of the patient is to be preferred is that the patient's expression can be watched. Tenderness and the presence of anxiety are picked up readily. In examining from behind these two important points may be entirely overlooked. Besides, it is more comforting to the patient to be able to watch the physician's face. The hidden position behind does not consider the patient's concern. Too often physicians examining the thyroid from behind look off into the ceiling dreamily, inattentive of the patient, as if they were playing the piano.

Much of the emotional pattern can be learned by observing the patient during the taking of the history and the making of the physical examination. This is the behavior examination. During the talk the reaction of the patient rather than the specific answer to a question may be informative. The way the patient hesitates or talks voluntarily should be noted. The patient's attitude or reluctance during the physical examination may be revealing. These reactions should be looked for particularly at the first interview. Later, when the patient is accustomed to the physician, there is less to be noted.

What is observed of the patient's behavior is more than mental status, that final designation of the customary physicial examination. It appraises his equanimity as well as his anxieties, including his fear of the disease. It contains matters relating to the genesis, if the disease is considered to be psychosomatic. It also yields the clue to much of the management of the patient. It tells the sore points of the patient with hyperthyroidism that are to be rectified if possible during the course of the therapy of the thyroid. It tells the amount of anxiety about a possible cancer, which is to be taken into account in advising the removal of a tumor. Its thorough consideration and use will end in making the patient happier.

POINTERS ON SURGICAL TECHNIC

The technical approaches to thyroid operations may be classified as either dashing or deliberate. Which is chosen is a matter somewhat of training and somewhat of temperament of the surgeon. In the days before means were available to control the hyperthyroidism, the surgeon was forced to operate when the goiter was vascular, the nutrition poor, the anesthetic uncertain, and the procedure perilous. Time was precious, and the surgeon hurried, thinking that he would lose less blood. He contented himself with a subtotal resection, leaving a thick wad of gland to protect parathyroids and recurrent nerves. These were the horse-and-buggy days when the surgeon knew little of what he did.

The use of the antithyroid drugs and iodine in those patients with hyperthyroidism, attention to nutrition, and collaboration with a competent anesthesiologist provide all the time needed to carry out exactly the operation desired. Parathyroids can be identified and laid aside safely if they lie in the path of the dissection; so also with the recurrent nerves. Now, total excision of a lateral lobe can be accomplished with the same avoidance of complications or protection of the patient formerly sought by partial removal of the lobe. It is now possible to follow the precepts of Halsted, but it still takes curbing or self-discipline on the part of the surgeon inclined to be vigorous.

Hemorrhage, a dreaded complication of thyroidectomy, can be eliminated by deliberate care. The vessels in the thyroid bed along the trachea, the esophagus and the larynx deserve the most attention. Tie every vessel, lay all knots down squarely. Do not cut the ends too short; otherwise the knots will untie when the larynx goes up and down with swallowing after operation.

Drains in a thyroid wound are a relic of the dashing days. If care is taken with the size of the bites and the hemostasis, there is no need to drain. Infection will not be introduced, and the scar will heal much better. If the bites behind the snaps are big, and oozing here and there is not controlled, do not try to get away without a drain.

Parathyroid tetany and laryngeal nerve palsy can be avoided by forethought, training and attention at operation. There are two ways of not falling down a mountain. One is never to go near a mountain, and the other is to walk carefully when climbing. The surgeons of a generation ago got around these complications by avoiding the areas where parathyroids and nerves lurk. Satisfactory surgery today demands that the surgeon approach these danger spots, but he must recognize them and deal with them. To do this he must prepare himself. Parathyroids are hard to identify. Dissections at the postmortem table provide excellent schooling. There also the surgeon can learn the vagaries of the inferior laryngeal nerves, including the nonrecurrent anomaly on the right side. He will also learn of the variations of the normal thyroid gland. It is gratifying to note how normal these tissues appear on fresh postmortem material. The effort will be well repaid in technical competence at the operating table.

The Thymus Gland

At the turn of the century the thymus gland was considered to be an organ important only to fetal development, becoming vestigial early in postuterine life. If it persisted in the child, it was a dangerous thing. Since Laquer and Weigert (1901) described a thymic tumor in a patient dying with myasthenia gravis, it has slowly become accepted that the gland survives with a function, is sometimes the seat of tumor and the instigator of mischief. Recent experimental evidence points to an important role in the development of both the lymphatic system and antibodies. Composed of epithelial and lymphoid cells, a comprehensive account of its function is still to be written.

SURGICAL ANATOMY

The thymus gland develops embryologically from the 3rd branchial clefts (Norris, 1938). Each lateral component descends during fetal life behind the lateral lobe of the thyroid gland to rest in the anterior mediastinum. Each component usually leaves a thin tongue behind in the neck, stretching downward from the lower pole of the thyroid, broadening out as they pass the left innominate vein. The two components fuse in front of the ascending aorta, forming the body of the thymus. Sometimes driblets are left behind the thyroid lobe, well above the tongue of each component. The left tongue is normally a little longer, reaching higher in the neck. The left side of the body of the thymus is a little larger than the right. Sometimes the fusion in the mid-line is only partial, since there is a long or a complete cleft in the mid-line. Usually the thymus passes in front of the left innominate vein, sometimes behind, and occasionally it splits, with the vein running through the middle. In its final resting place each component lies against the pleura laterally, stretching down in front of the lung root and medially along the ascending aorta down over the upper pericardium. The gland receives its arterial supply locally. The larger part of venous return is directly to the left innominate vein.

The bulk of the thymus is composed of lymphoid follicles and fat. Here and there, scattered in the lymphoid tissue, are so-called Hassall's corpuscles, characteristic whorls, presumably of epidermoid origin (Norris, 1938).

The lower pair of parathyroid glands also develop embryologically from the 3rd branchial clefts and descend along with the thymus in the neck to their usual position behind the lower pole of the thyroid lobes (Norris, 1937). Not infrequently, during their descent they are carried down beyond the thyroid with the thymus. In 10 per cent of normal people one or more of this pair is contained within the thymic capsule, usually in the upper tongue. In resecting the thymus or in looking for a parathyroid tumor, this frequent relationship is to be remembered.

PATHOLOGIC PHYSIOLOGY

The full physiologic role or roles of the thymus gland is still to be unfolded. A specific substance with a curarelike action has been sought but not found. Because of the lymphoid tissue, a relation to immune body production is not surprising. One substantial fact known about the thymus is that it enlarges when lymphoid tissue generally is hyperplastic and shares in the atrophy when lymphoid tissue atrophies (Dougherty, 1952). Thus, it is hyperplastic in patients with Graves's disease when lymphoid tissue generally is hyperplastic.* It waxes with the lymphoid hyperplasia of Addison's disease or experimental adrenal insufficiency and wanes with the lymphoid atrophy following cortisone or ACTH. It has not been proved how much of these changes are due to the adrenal hormone secreted in response to the anterior pituitary stimulation or how much directly to the anterior pituitary itself. The thymus atrophies following experimental hypophysectomy.

STATUS THYMICOLYMPHATICUS

Infants, children and adolescents dying suddenly in accidents or during operation sometimes were found at autopsy to have had a

---

* European clinicians speculated concerning the relation of the thymic hyperplasia in Basedow's disease to the myasthenia. As early as 1911 von Garré and Sauerbruch resected the thymus but without definitive relief of the myasthenia (Sauerbruch, 1925).

swollen thymus gland and generalized lymphadenopathy. So firmly was it believed that the sudden death was due to the thymic hypertrophy that as late as the middle 1920's many hospitals routinely x-rayed the chests of children below the age of 10 before undertaking an operation of any sort. If evidence of an enlarged thymus was found, it was treated with a small dose of x-rays before the operation. This dose of irradiation usually was followed by shriveling of the thymus. Although so-called status thymicolymphaticus never has been resolved to the satisfaction of everybody, it is no longer the practice to take chest roentgenograms and to carry out irradiation of the thymus. The sudden deaths are generally held to have been due to some cause other than the enlarged thymus.

AS A SEAT OF TUMOR

Thymus tissue is the not infrequent source of benign and malignant tumors arising in the anterior mediastinum. Primary tumors include both lymphomas and epithelial neoplasms. Teratomas also are encountered. The tumors are often silent until they have reached considerable size, sometimes beyond surgical extirpation. The thymus is a rare site for a metastasis to settle from malignancy in another organ.

Although the early growth of malignant tumors of the thymus may be silent, when they have reached a relatively massive proportion, symptoms and signs of myasthenia gravis not infrequently appear as a harbinger of early death. In an occasional thymoma agammaglobulinemia is an accompaniment.

In general, whenever a tumor in the region of the thymus is diagnosed, immediate surgical exploration is indicated, since early eradication is considered at present to be the only possible chance for cure. Irradiation is palliative only.

AS AN INSTIGATOR OF MYASTHENIA GRAVIS

On the basis that thymic enlargement is the cause of myasthenia gravis, 3 different therapeutic approaches have been used in attacking the thymus—x-ray irradiation, surgical extirpation and ACTH. Although hundreds of patients with myasthenia gravis have been treated by one or a combination of these methods, it must be admitted that success is sporadic and unpredictable, and that the relationship between the thymus and the myasthenia is poorly understood.

Pierchalla (1921) reported that irradiation of the thymus improved patients with myasthenia gravis. Two years later Mella (1923) recorded 2 patients similarly benefited. The therapy attracted little attention and soon was abandoned. In 1936, Blalock excised a thymic tumor from a man with myasthenia gravis (Blalock et al., 1939). The patient improved, and the surgical era was initiated. In subsequent patients whose thymus was resected at the Johns Hopkins Hospital the good effect was obtained only sometimes, and enthusiasm for this approach has waned (Blalock, 1944).

Thymectomy has been carried out in several centers. The claims of benefit from operation are criticized by those who have observed the life history of the disease in many patients without operation. Spontaneous remissions are common, and particularly in those patients in whom the disease has been of short duration. It is argued that many successful cases might have recovered without operation. The experience with Case 1 is a case in point.

Case 1. A married woman of 42, mother of 3, complaining of lower abdominal pain, was found to have a simple cyst of an ovary and erosion of the uterine cervix. An ovariectomy and hysterectomy were performed under ether anesthesia. Upon regaining consciousness the patient noted diplopia. This persisted, generalized weakness appeared, and 5 days after operation the diagnosis of myasthenia gravis was established with Prostigmin. In 1 month the disease had increased to moderate severity; the patient was incapacitated in spite of frequent Prostigmin tablets. Thymectomy was considered.

The patient had noticed occasional transient diplopia in the previous 5 years. The husband reported that the episodes were always at times when the patient was under stress. Recently she had been increasingly worried over the illness of the oldest daughter. It became obvious that much could be done to help the patient with her emotional problems. Therefore, thymectomy was delayed, and a series of interviews was undertaken by an interested physician.

By the 10th month after the pelvic operation, the patient had gained some understanding of her problems and a return of confidence in her doctors. Her daughter was also in better health. All signs of the myasthenia gravis disappeared. She has remained well for the ensuing 10 years.

At the Massachusetts General Hospital 180 patients have undergone thymectomy for myasthenia gravis since 1939. Appraisal of the benefit of operation is difficult, since it involves the opinion of what would have happened if operation had not been performed. The author has the following general impression: ⅓ of the patients were significantly improved; a few of them were completely relieved; ⅓ were somewhat improved; and in ⅓ the severity of the disease was not influenced by thymectomy. This distribution suggests that the operation has only the effect of a placebo.

Keynes and Schwab agree that the most favorable group are the younger women with disease of short duration. The disease is less likely to be influenced favorably when in men, in older patients or when a thymoma is present. There are exceptions to each of these groups among the author's cases. For example, a 40-year-old man with a malignant thymoma and severe myasthenia was relieved by resection of the thymoma. A year later with regrowth of the tumor from an implant the myasthenia rapidly recurred, and the patient died in crisis.

What one advises about thymectomy in an individual patient depends upon one's concept of the disease. It is like an endocrine disease in that it is found most commonly in women and in the childbearing, active ovarian phase of life. Like acute hyperthyroidism and Cushing's disease, it appears to be a psychosomatic disease. Its onset is frequently coincidental with psychological trauma and emotional upset. It also bears a curious relationship to pregnancy and ovarian function. Pregnancy may induce a complete remission. The origin may be associated with resection of an ovary.

Thymectomy is indicated in any patient with myasthenia gravis with evidence of a tumor of the thymus. The tumor in itself demands the exploration. It is also to be carried out in any patient, man or woman, who is gettting worse and in whom all other efforts fail. Adjustment to the problems of life are to be attended to in all patients.

In patients with a severe degree of myasthenia gravis, operation is hazardous. Everything that can be done to improve the myasthenia before undertaking the operation is wise. Roentgen-ray therapy to the thymus is such a measure. For some years it was the author's rule to irradiate all patients, waiting at least 3 weeks before operating; but there has been no consistent correlation between those improving with irradiation and those from thymectomy, throwing further doubt on the role of the thymus.

The Parathyroid Glands

INTRODUCTION

Disease of the parathyroid glands is a latecomer to the endocrine field. Not until 1925 was a primary disease established. For the 45 years from the time of their discovery until 1925, their sole interest for the surgeon was as danger spots, areas to be avoided when operating upon the thyroid gland. Since 1925, gradually it has dawned that disease of these glands is not uncommon, and their relation to the metabolism of calcium and phosphorus has made them a subject of wide interest to physiologist and biochemist, as well as the clinician. In spite of the wide interest in these glands there is still little but speculation regarding the etiology of the disease, and only a glimpse of understanding in regard to the counterbalancing, reciprocating physiologic forces.

HISTORY

The parathyroid glands were first discovered in the rhinoceros by Owen (1853), the British zoologist, and subsequently independently discovered in the rabbit, by the Swedish anatomist, Sandström (1880). They were anatomic curiosities until the French physiologist Gley (1891) later proved that their removal led to tetany, disclosing the etiology of the tetany that sometimes followed thyroidectomy. The relation of the calcium level of the blood to this tetany was demonstrated experimentally by MacCallum and Voegtlin (1908). These discoveries established the effect of the removal of the normal glands.

Discovery of disease of the parathyroid glands came about more slowly. Overactivity of the glands was the first disease described.

The story of how overfunction became recognized is important because it led at first to an overemphasis on the associated bone disease. Knowledge first came from the European pathologists. Von Recklinghausen (1891) described the generalized disease of bone which now bears his name. Askanazy (1903) found a parathyroid tumor at autopsy in a patient who had died of this disease. In the next few years other examples of this association were described. In the meantime, Erdheim (1907, 1914) in a clinical and experimental study showed that the parathyroid glands were slightly enlarged or hyperplastic in conditions such as rickets, osteomalacia and even pregnancy. These enlargements, he felt, represented a compensatory hyperplasia in response to the changes in the bones. Because of Erdheim's influence, it was assumed by most pathologists that the parathyroid tumors encountered clinically were secondary to the bone disease. Another pathologist, suggested that the reverse might be true—that the parathyroid tumor might be the cause of the bone changes (Schlagenhaufer, 1915). Not until 10 years later did a surgeon test this concept (Mandl, 1926). After failing to benefit a patient with von Recklinghausen's disease of bone by engrafting parathyroid tissue, he explored the patient's neck, removing a parathyroid tumor. The patient's bones improved, and parathyroid enlargement as the cause of the bone changes was established. Hyperparathyroidism and von Recklinghausen's disease of bone were considered as synonymous.

On the west side of the Atlantic, knowledge of disease of the parathyroids grew from the physiologic rather than pathologic point of view. This difference had far-reaching consequences, since it led eventually to a broader recognition of the disease. The first step was the successful extraction of the hormone from the parathyroid glands of animals. Hanson (1924) and Collip (1925) independently succeeded in obtaining a potent extract. Collip showed that when the extract was injected into dogs in sufficient quantity the serum calcium rose, even doubled in concentration, with thickening of the blood and the death of the animal. The serum phosphorus level was reduced, and he observed calcium pouring out in the urine. The same effects on blood levels of calcium and phosphorus and of calcium excretion were found by Aub in patients with lead poisoning (Hunter and Aub, 1927). He employed Collip's extract to hasten the elimination of lead from the bone. Thus, the effect of an excess of parathyroid hormone upon calcium and phosphorus metabolism was established in the experimental animal and in man.

The next step came when DuBois found the same metabolic abnormalities in a patient with a widespread bone disease (Hannon et al., 1930). He postulated overactivity of the parathyroid glands as the cause and sent the patient to Aub for further study (Bauer et al., 1930). The changes in blood levels of calcium and phosphorus and the outpouring of both through the kidney were confirmed. In April, 1926, 8 months after Mandl's operation in Vienna, surgical exploration of the parathyroid glands was undertaken at the Massachusetts General Hospital. Unfortunately, the Americans were unaware of the discoveries of the German pathologists and of Mandl, and the surgeon had little idea of what he should look for. No abnormal parathyroid gland was found. It was not until 6 years later that the parathyroid tumor was found in this patient (Churchill and Cope, 1934).

Blocked at the beginning by lack of knowledge of pathology, the physiologic point of view has led eventually to a more comprehensive view of the nature of hyperparathyroidism. Albright, a student of both Aub and Erdheim, first realized that the renal stones frequently found in patients with hyperparathyroidism were a complication of the metabolic disorder. The excess of calcium in the urine, he reasoned, must lead to the precipitation of calcium and the production of stones. Calcium metabolism was investigated in patients entering the hospital with renal stones. Soon the diagnosis of hyperparathyroidism was made in such patients; as more were encountered, evidence of bone disease was frequently absent (Albright et al., 1934). It was realized for the first time that bone disease was not an essential part of hyperparathyroidism. Both the bone changes and the renal stones presumably were complications of the disordered metabolism, not primary effects.

When, for the first time, such a patient, with kidney stones and no bone disease, was operated on in 1932, a new era in regard to hyperparathyroidism was begun. Since then other clinical forms of the disease have been recognized. Instead of being rare, as at first supposed, it is now known to be common.

HYPOPARATHYROIDISM

Hypoparathyroidism is of two types—the idiopathic, and the iatrogenic. The spontaneous disease is extremely rare. The first case was diagnosed by Aub and Bauer in 1927. The symptoms are those of chronic unremitting tetany of low calcium origin. Marble stones have been postulated as an accompaniment. Cataract is common. Oversecretion of thyrocalcitonin is possible but unproven.

The disease is easily confused with pseudohypoparathyroidism, a bizarre condition with frequent convulsions and characteristic physical changes, including a moon face and stubby fingers and toes. This condition has been described by Albright who believed that it was due to immunity to the parathyroid hormone (Albright et al., 1942). The parathyroid glands are normal grossly and microscopically. Here, also, oversecretion of Thyrocalcitonin has recently been implicated. It is probably a genetic or microsomal disease.

Hypoparathyroidism complicating thyroidectomy is due either to damage to the parathyroid glands or to their resection. If the glands have merely been bruised by operative trauma, the function will return, and the tetany will be of short duration. If 3 glands have been removed and the 4th one remain *in situ* undamaged, the tetany will also be of short duration. Only if the remaining gland has been damaged or its life endangered by interference with its blood supply will the tetany endure. If parathyroid tissue remains intact, the hypoparathyroidism will be reduced gradually as the remnant undergoes hyperplasia. If there was insufficient tissue for adequate regeneration, the hypoparathyroidism may be permanent.

The tetany of hypoparathyroidism should be treated by a high calcium and low phosphorus intake. In the severe acute phase the calcium is to be given intravenously in order to preclude laryngeal spasm. Calcium chloride, because it is highly ionized, is most promptly available for the relief of tetany; calcium gluconate, more slowly. Calcium gluconate may be given intramuscularly.

If the tetany is mild, oral intake will be adequate. The calcium salt most readily available by mouth is the gluconate. Calcium lactate is absorbed slowly. It is believed that the addition of vitamin D to the diet is useful to increase the absorption of calcium from the intestinal tract. AT 10* is a variant of high vitamin D therapy. Overdose of either vitamin D or AT 10 may result in hypercalcemia and loss of calcium in the urine, with renal calcification and damage.

HYPERPARATHYROIDISM

Although hyperparathyroidism exists as a disease without complications, from a practical point of view it is diagnosed usually by one of its complications. The recognized complications, in order of their frequency, are calcification in the urinary tract, decalcification of the bones, peptic ulceration of duodenum or stomach, pancreatitis, fatigue and pseudogout (see Table 28-1). Rarely is the

TABLE 28-1. CLUES TO DIAGNOSIS OF HYPERPARATHYROIDISM IN THE FIRST 398 CASES AT M.G.H.

1. Bone Disease	88 Cases
2. Renal Stones	224
3. Peptic Ulcer	35
4. Pancreatitis	12
5. Fatigue	12
6. Hypertension	6
7. Mental Disturbance	3
8. Central Nervous System Signs	7
9. No symptoms	2
10. Multiple Endocrine	4
11. Lump in Neck	2
12. Pseudogout	3

diagnosis made by the presence of a tumor in the neck; this is because the parathyroid glands are so small that tumors of them are not large enough to be recognized by patient or examiner. The diagnosis is made only by keeping hyperparathyroidism in mind when caring for patients with renal and bone disease, peptic ulceration and pancreatitis. Before describing each form of the disease fully, it is essential to understand the pathophysiology.

* Dihydrotachysterol.

PATHOPHYSIOLOGY

Parathormone, the secretion of the parathyroid glands, dominates calcium metabolism and strongly influences aspects of phosphorus metabolism. These actions have been found to be opposed in large measure, but not wholly, by thyrocalcitonin, the secretion of the thyroid gland. Because of their mutually opposing forces, the actions of these two hormones will be considered together. The best evidence indicates that the hormones affect the integrity of bone, the sensitivity of nerves and the excretory function of both kidney and large bowel. The following are the generally accepted actions:

The calcium level of blood plasma and extracellular fluid is regulated predominantly by the parathyroid hormone. A decreasing function lowers the calcium level, and an excessive function induces a rise. Thyrocalcitonin exerts the opposite effect, but less strongly.

The calcium in the plasma and the extracellular fluid can be isolated into 2 fractions—the protein-bound and the free or ionized. It is about equally divided in the plasma, but, because of its low protein concentration, the spinal fluid normally contains about half as much as the plasma. The hormones presumably influence the concentration of the ionized fraction only. In diseases associated with an elevated plasma protein (e.g., myeloma) the calcium of the plasma is elevated. Conversely, the plasma concentration is low in patients with hypoproteinemia. In diagnosing hyperparathyroidism it is always wise to measure the concentration of the serum protein simultaneously with that of the calcium.

It is believed that it is the ionized fraction that affects the sensitivity of nerves and muscles. A low level is associated with hyperactivity or tetany, and a high level with a reduced sensitivity, producing fatigue and lassitude. The Q-T interval of the electrocardiogram is lengthened when the calcium is low and shortened when elevated.

The inorganic phosphate level of the blood plasma and the extracellular fluid is lowered by both hormones. If renal damage is present, the level may be normal or elevated in the presence of continued parathyroid hyperfunction.

Calcium excretion is raised by hyperfunction of the parathyroids. In the absence of renal impairment the increased excretion is through the kidney. The elimination from the bowel may be slightly decreased compared with the expected normal. It is the increased excretion of calcium through the kidney that may lead to supersaturation of the urine and deposition of calcium somewhere in the urinary tract. The deposition may start in the renal tubule, the kidney pelvis, the ureter, the bladder or the prostate. If oxalates are present, the stones may be of calcium oxalate. Most commonly they are of calcium phosphate, since there is always an excess of phosphate in the urine.

If the pathologic calcification is extensive in the renal tubules, impairment of renal function ensues. The urine has a fixed, low specific gravity, and the excretion of calcium may be reduced to the normal level or even less than normal. In the face of continued hyperparathyroidism the bowel takes over the excessive excretion of calcium. Therefore, in a patient whose blood level of calcium indicates hyperparathyroidism but whose renal excretion is within normal limits, the fecal calcium should be measured if the urine specific gravity is continuously low.

Phosphorus excretion is increased by hyperparathyroidism. Excretion is through the kidneys, except when damage has occurred; then phosphorus is retained. With such retention, the level of phosphorus rises to normal or even above normal.

The action of the parathyroid hormone on bone has long been a question and is still unsettled. The European pathologists felt that the primary action of the hormone was in decalcifying bone with a resulting rise in the blood level. The presence of patients with hyperparathyroidism without demonstrable bone disease suggested that the effect upon bone might be secondary, since the primary force is a disturbance of the fluid equilibrium of calcium and phosphorus. Studies by Krane, using radioactive calcium, indicate a more rapid than normal turnover of calcium in bone in some but not all patients with hyperparathyroidism. A turnover more rapid than normal also occurs in hyperthyroidism. Thyrocalcitonin, in contrast, fixes calcium in bone.

The excessive loss of calcium through the kidney is paid for either from the skeleton or from the food intake. If the amount of calcium in the food is adequate to meet the extra loss, the skeleton remains normally calcified. If the intake is less than the excretion, the calcium comes from the bones, and the bones slowly become depleted.

The alkaline phosphatase activity of the blood serum is not directly affected by the parathyroid hormone. In patients with hyperparathyroidism and no bone disease, the activity is within normal limits. Only when there is bony depletion with active regeneration is the phosphatase elevated. The activity is proportionate to the osteogenesis and is a good indicator of the amount of calcium that the skeleton will absorb immediately following operation. Patients with a high activity (10 Bodansky units or more) are to be warned that after operation they will be prone to the tetany of the recalcification period. Such patients need large amounts of calcium postoperatively.

Thyrocalcitonin probably exerts a reciprocating mechanism to the parathormone. To what extent this action takes place in hyperparathyroidism is not as yet understood.

No clue has been found regarding the etiology of hyperparathyroidism. A secondary form is known to be the sequel of chronic renal disease (Castleman and Mallory, 1937), but a history of pre-existing renal disease is seldom disclosed in patients with hyperparathyroidism of the primary type.

ANATOMIC PATHOLOGY

Demonstrable anatomic changes of hyperparathyroidism are confined to the parathyroid glands, the bones, and certain tissues which become pathologically calcified.

The Parathyroids

Proof of the presence of hyperparathyroidism depends upon finding a clearly defined abnormality in one or more of the parathyroid glands. Hyperplasias involving all of the glands and neoplasias involving one or more have been found (Castleman, 1952; Castleman and Mallory, 1935). Neoplasias are the more common (see Table 28-2).

Neoplasia. Hypersecreting neoplasms of the parathyroid glands may be either benign or malignant. The benign form, an adenoma, is found in nearly 90 per cent of patients with

TABLE 28-2. HYPERPARATHYROIDISM—M.G.H. SERIES 400 CASES—1930-1968

Neoplasia	
Single Adenoma	312 Cases
Double Adenoma	13
Carcinoma	17
Primary Hyperplasia	
Clear Cell	16
Chief Cell	42

hyperparathyroidism. Usually only one gland is affected. Occasionally two adenomas have been found, one in each of two glands.

The cell type is variable, the chief cell being the commonest variety. Usually adenomas are of a single cell type. The clear cells have not constituted an entire adenoma, although they may appear here and there in either a chief cell or an oxyphil cell adenoma.

CARCINOMA is a form found occasionally. It was encountered in 17 of 400 cases. Since 4 of these patients were referred after establishment of the diagnosis of carcinoma, it is probable that the incidence is not over 3 per cent. The growths are sluggish, the cells well differentiated. All of the primary tumors have been large. They have been locally invasive. They spread by both the lymphatics and the blood stream. After local eradication of the tumor, a metastasis may carry on hyperfunction. A single metastasis in the liver has been found in at least two patients at autopsy (Albertini et al., 1953; Cope et al., 1953). The capsule of the tumor may be broken at the time of the initial resection. In such cases the incidence of seeding throughout the wound has been high and there has been repeated local recurrence.

In an occasional case the malignant process may be a degeneration of a hyperplasia. A carcinoma was found growing in one area of hyperplastic gland, invading the benign portion of the enlargement.

Hyperplasia. The hyperplasias associated with hyperparathyroidism are both primary and secondary. The primary hyperplasias are the more important clinically and are of two cell types: chief cell and clear cell. Of the primary type, clear cell hyperplasia was recognized initially and was at first thought to be the more common (Castleman and Mallory, 1935).

Hyperplasia of the parathyroid glands is the type of hyperplasia comparable with that of the thyroid in Graves's disease. In contrast with disease of the thyroid, it is found less often than the neoplastic form, accounting for between 10 and 25 per cent of all the patients. Only the clear cell hyperplasias can be recognized on frozen section because, the cells are huge, being distended with fluid. The cells are usually concentrically arranged with basally oriented nuclei. At first sight, the concentric grouping suggests follicles of thyroid without any colloid in the center. Also, the huge clear cells have been mistaken for those of renal cell carcinoma.

Clear cell hyperplasias are usually recognizable grossly. They are a darker chocolate brown than other tumors; they have an irregular surface, frequently with pseudopod projections. The upper pair is nearly always larger than the lower (Castleman and Cope, 1951).

Chief cell hyperplasia, as a cause of primary hyperparathyroidism, is a comparative newcomer to the field of parathyroid pathology (Owen, 1953). It was not recognized until the 142nd case at the Massachusetts General Hospital. Each of the enlargements resembles a benign adenoma. However, all of the glands are so characteristically involved in the process that it is difficult to assume that each constitutes a separate adenoma. In one of the 42 patients of this type there were 5 such enlargements, the first case with 5 enlarged parathyroids on record. In this case, four were found at the first operation. Resection of three and ⅔ of the fourth failed to relieve the hyperparathyroidism. Search of the mediastinum at a second operation disclosed a fifth within the thymic capsule. It weighed 1.9 Gm., as much as the previous four together. Its resection was followed by a prompt drop of the calcium level to below normal with reversion of the calcium balance (Case 172).

The 42 patients with chief cell hyperplasia were of various clinical groups. Some had osteoporosis and several had renal complications. The parathyroid enlargements were much bigger than the relatively mild chief cell hyperplasia found secondary to renal disease or in vitamin D deficiency. Six patients had associated endocrine abnormalities: an older man a pituitary enlargement; his daughter a pancreatic islet-cell adenoma; another woman bore her only child in the middle of a many-year period of amenorrhea.

Secondary chief cell hyperplasia is found in patients with long-standing chronic nephritis and occasionally in a patient with rickets and osteomalacia (Castleman and Mallory, 1937). The parathyroid enlargement is much less than in the previous group. The enlargements are bulbous and vascular and usually not more than 4 to 5 times the size of the normal gland.

THE BONES

The resorption of calcium from the bones under an excessive action of the parathyroid hormone results in 2 general types of anatomic change: simple decalcification and the classic disease of von Recklinghausen. In the first, the decalcification is diffuse, all bones sharing to some degree. It may be mild and presumably is present more often than is recognized because of the difficulty of diagnosis, so considerable is the variation in density of normal bones. Occasionally, the decalcification is sufficient to lead to pathologic fractures. The vertebral bodies of the thorax and the lumbar region not infrequently crumple, giving the fishbone type of vertebral body. At times, the bones of the feet also give way under the weight of the body.

The classic type of bone disease described by von Recklinghausen, *osteodystrophia fibrosa* or *osteitis fibrosa cystica generalisata*, is so characteristic that there is no mistaking it by roentgenogram or often by physical examination. In addition to a generalized demineralization, cysts and brown tumors are diffusely distributed throughout the skeleton. The cysts apparently start in the marrow and swell, with cortical necrosis and pathologic fracture. The brown tumors probably start in the bone trabeculae. The microscopic picture of the trabeculae is diagnostic. In an orderly arrangement on one side there is active bone resorption with large numbers of osteoclasts, and here and there one finds osteoclastomata. On the opposite side there is active bone regeneration.

The brown tumors appear to be adenomas of the giant cell osteoclasts. There may be a hundred or more distributed throughout the skeleton. They often attain considerable size. In one patient, there were 2 the size of grapefruit, one on either side of the pelvis.

The tumors are distinguishable microscopically from the single giant cell tumors occasionally found in adolescence. Although the latter may be malignant, no case of malignancy developing in the giant cell tumors of hyperparathyroidism has been recorded. This is peculiar, because the cellular activity is often intense.

Following correction of the hyperparathyroidism, the brown tumors resolve quickly. First, they lose their vascularity with disappearance of the majority of the giant cells in a week. By 2 weeks, there are numerous islands of calcification. By 2 years, all evidence of the former tumor may have been eradicated by bone growth and re-formation of the normal bony contours. The vacuoles of the cysts, in contrast, do not recalcify, but the cortex surrounding the original cystic area is thickened.

The marrow is characteristically fibrosed. An anemia is usually present when the bone disease is advanced; it may be related to the fibrous displacement of the cellular marrow although it occurs in patients without the bone disease. The anemia disappears spontaneously following correction of the glandular overactivity.

Pathologic Calcification

During the active phase of hyperparathyroidism, pathologic calcification occurs in a number of organs and diseases. The most common is the kidney. It is believed to be due to supersaturation of the urine with calcium, but the deposition of calcium occurs not only within the lumen of the tubule but also in the surrounding tubular cells. There are calcium-containing casts in the tubules. Stones are formed throughout the urinary tract.

Small, stonelike bodies form in the prostate, the pancreas and the salivary glands.

Pathologic calcification also occurs in a number of other tissues, the gastric mucosa and the pancreas. There is deposition of calcium in the conjunctivae and the cornea of the eye (Cogan et al., 1948; Walsh and Howard, 1947). These deposits are in contrast with the cataracts which form in hypoparathyroidism. Thick calcification of the capsule of the parathyroid adenoma itself has been encountered in 2 instances (Churchill and Cope, 1934).

DIAGNOSIS

It is rarely possible to make a diagnosis of hyperparathyroidism before the onset of one of its complications. Although an excess of the hormone upsets the calcium equilibrium and affects the nervous system, the symptoms produced are so common or so easily mistaken for other conditions that the diagnosis is rarely made on these alone. With the hormone overactivity and elevated calcium level, neuromuscular tension is decreased. Patients commonly feel fatigued. Their muscles and joints are relaxed. Their feet flop along, and they trip more easily. They are subject to backaches, presumably being unable to hold themselves erect. They may notice some mental perturbation, perhaps irritation, or failure to concentrate. All these symptoms are so common among the population that they are hardly characteristic. Yet, the diagnosis has been made when these were the sole symptoms. The following case is illuminating.

Case 107. A man, aged 45, was seen first by Dr. Resnick of Stamford, Conn., in November, 1949. Dr. Resnick made a diagnosis of hyperparathyroidism in the following manner.

A resident of suburban New York, the patient had a desk job in the Navy in Washington, D. C. during World War II. He felt lackadaisical, without his usual energy. He ascribed this to the uprooting of his wartime job. With the cessation of hostilities, he returned to his old life. He continued to feel out of sorts and was checked over by his physician in New York. All tests were negative. A prominent right thyroid lobe was felt, and a right thyroidectomy was carried out in 1946. No nodule was found. The right lobe was larger than the left; therefore, part was resected. For 3 months following operation he felt better, then lapsed back into his previous state. He described his feelings as nothing in particular, simply no energy. Before World War II, when he returned home from work he repaired screen doors, did odd jobs about the house, and frequently played tennis. Now when he returned home all he wanted to do was sit and do nothing.

Discouraged, in 1949 he changed doctors. Dr. Resnick too found nothing on physical examination, but his laboratory routine included the Sulkowitch test for calcium content of the urine The test was 3+, a definitely elevated concentration. Dr. Resnick asked the patient to return, and the check test was the same. He then obtained a fasting blood for calcium and phosphorus levels. The day following, in the late afternoon, the laboratory reported 12.0 mg. and 2.5 mg. per 100 ml., respectively. He intended to recall the patient for a check blood analysis.

That very night the patient was awakened by severe left flank colic and called Dr. Resnick who told the patient that he had a left ureteral calculus and to go directly to the hospital.

A stone passed spontaneously. The blood calcium and phosphorus levels were persistently altered. The patient was referred to the Massachusetts General Hospital for parathyroid exploration. On December 20, 1949, a single benign adenoma was excised. The patient's phosphorus and calcium metabolisms returned promptly to normal. In 3 months the patient had noticed a return of well-being and has remained well during the ensuing years.

Examination of the slides of the thyroid tissues resected in 1946 revealed normal thyroid gland. Presumably the usual preponderance of the right thyroid lobe, perhaps exaggerated in this patient, had been mistaken on physical examination and at operation as representing an abnormality.

Polydipsia and polyuria are occasionally present. In four of the Massachusetts General Hospital patients, a diagnosis of diabetes insipidus had been entertained. Apparently these symptoms are occasioned by the increased excretion of calcium and the need for water. They are more suggestive than those due to muscular relaxation.

For practical purposes, the presence of a complication is needed to call attention to the diagnosis. The deposition of calcium in the renal tract is the commonest source of symptoms. In all patients with renal stones, or calcification in the region of the kidneys and prostate, hyperparathyroidism is to be considered. In the population served by the Massachusetts General Hospital, hyperparathyroidism constitutes approximately 5 to 8 per cent of all renal tract stones. Confirmation of the diagnosis depends upon careful chemical analysis and metabolic study. Many of the patients with renal stones have mild or borderline degrees of the disease. Therefore, the blood levels are borderline and need to be repeated at intervals, perhaps of weeks. It must be borne in mind that many endocrine diseases fluctuate in intensity with exacerbations and remissions. Of cases diagnosed at the Massachusetts General Hospital and by Keating at the Mayo Clinic a large number were brought to light by painstaking effort on the part of the internist, with repeated observation of the patients (Cope, 1942; Keating and Cook, 1945). In addition to the blood levels, the calcium excretion must be measured on a controlled diet. In view of the usual absence of bone disease, particularly in the mild cases, the phosphatase level of the blood is normal and is of no help diagnostically. Serum protein is always to be measured for correction of the calcium level if the protein concentration is low.

Chemical analysis of the stone is also helpful if a stone is available. Calcium phosphate is the commonest; calcium oxalate stones constitute approximately 10 per cent. The absence of calcium is against hyperparathyroidism.

The presence of decalcification is also helpful. Hyperthyroidism and Cushing's disease must be excluded, since they too decalcify the skeleton. Cushing's disease also causes renal stone. However, the thyroid and adrenal diseases do not disturb the blood levels of either calcium or phosphorus.

The classic form of bone disease can be diagnosed by roentgenogram alone. In the typical advanced case, chemical confirmation really is not needed. The bone disease is distributed throughout the skeleton and more or less evenly. Fibrous dysplasia of the bone, which in any one bone may give a picture mimicking exactly hyperparathyroidism, is distributed irregularly throughout the skeleton, following the distribution of peripheral nerves. Roentgenograms of sufficient areas of the skeleton must be taken in all patients to make sure that the disease is not a localized one. No other endocrine disease gives the picture of diffuse calcification with cysts and brown tumors.

Diffuse osteoporosis without cysts and brown tumors has a much wider differential diagnosis. It can be associated with hyperparathyroidism and Cushing's disease, and is found in older patients, particularly women past the menopause. Of these endocrine conditions, hyperparathyroidism is the only one affecting the blood levels of calcium and phosphorus. Acromegaly affects the skeleton, producing some diffuse osteoporosis with a negative calcium balance. However, it does not simulate the classic bone disease of hyperparathyroidism. The overgrowth of the extremities of bone, and the widening of the jaw should not be mistaken for the resorption and the fracture of the terminal phalanges of the fingers and the loss of lamina dura and vacuolization of the jaws seen in hyperparathyroidism.

Patients with peptic ulcers of the duodenum and the stomach (Rogers and Keating, 1947), and likewise patients with acute pancreatitis (Cope et al., 1957), should be screened for hyperparathyroidism. The most difficult differential diagnosis lies in patients with peptic ulceration and renal calcification who have received a high calcium and alkali intake. The renal damage is much like that encountered with primary hyperparathyroidism and secondary renal damage with a normal or elevated phosphorus level of the blood. Differential diagnosis lies in evaluation of the calcium level of the blood and the fecal calcium excretion. In hyperparathyroidism both are elevated.

TREATMENT

Medical and irradiation therapies of hyperparathyroidism have not proved to be successful. A high calcium diet has spared the skeleton but has ruined the kidneys. No antiparathyroid drug has emerged, and the high incidence of neoplasia in parathyroid disease, in contrast with that of the thyroid, lessens the advisability of such a therapy, were it available.

Irradiation too has failed. The tumors perhaps are radioresistant, but also their variable position and number make it hard to focus sufficient irradiation upon the offending glands.

The treatment of hyperparathyroidism is still surgical. It must be precise to meet the challenge of the diagnostician. The problems involve the nature, the number, the site and the size of the tumors.

It is essential to recognize the nature of the offending glands. The surgeon must keep in mind 7 types of glands. Prompt recognition of the pathologic type expedites the exploration and the judgment concerning resection.

First comes the normal gland; it must not be resected. It varies considerably in size and shape. The gland is soft and conforms to its surroundings. It is like a flat pancake when on the surface of the thyroid but, caught in a sulcus, it may be triangular or bulbous. It varies normally in color according to age. In children and older people it is browner because it contains less fat. With adolescence and early adult life, there is a larger proportion of fat to epithelial tissue, and the glands are yellower. Maximum fatty infiltration is found in people 30 to 35 years of age.

Second is the atrophic parathyroid. When the disease is of long standing and due to a single adenoma, the other 3 parathyroids, although not diseased, are not really normal. They are atrophic and therefore yellower than the normal gland. The may be hard to see in the fatty tissue and recognizable only by their form and vascular pattern rather than by their color. They too are not to be damaged or resected. An atrophic parathyroid, when recognized at the first gland found indicates that an adenoma must be present in one or two of the others.

Next are the pathologic glands. Their types have been described under Anatomic Pathology. Surgically, the following aspects are to be kept in mind. The adenoma is the commonest. Grossly, it is smooth, vascular, reddish brown and contains no fat. If the adenoma is only 1 or 2 mm. in diameter, there may be a rim of normal tissue surrounding it or a piece at one pole. Two adenomas are found in 10 per cent of the patients having the adenoma type. The importance of size will be described below.

The clear cell hypertrophy and hyperplasia is identified by its darker chocolate color and by the irregularity of its surface and pseudopod projection. It is essential in the pathologic type to identify all 4 glands. Generally, it is wise not to remove any one until all 4 have been found. Three of the enlargements should be resected, and a small piece of the 4th left with its blood supply intact. A 40 to 100 mg. remnant has sufficed in 14 of the patients of the Massachusetts General Hospital series. It is sound practice to use the most accessible enlargement for the subtotal resection so that if too large a remnant is left and there is residual hyperparathyroidism, it can be uncovered readily at a secondary operation.

Realization that the hypertrophied upper gland usually is considerably larger than the lower should facilitate the search for a missing enlargement. If the upper has not been found

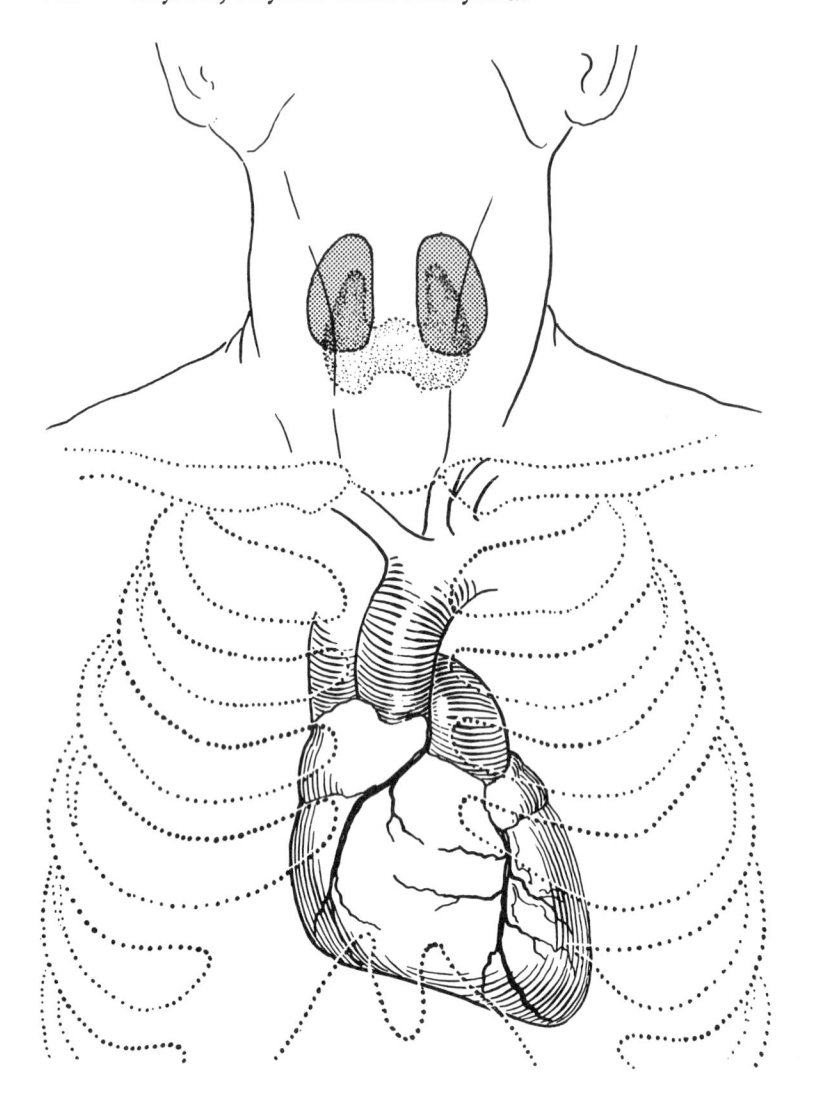

Fig. 28-4. Surgical anatomy, upper parathyroid, lateral and anterior views. The shading shows the extent of possible positions of the normal upper parathyroids due to differences in development during fetal life. The limited area facilitates the surgical identification of these parathyroids. (Cope, O.: Ann. Surg. 114:706)

in the usual position, it will have been displaced downward and posteriorly. If the lower is the missing gland, the neck having been searched, it will lie in the anterior mediastinum.

The chief cell hyperplasias resemble the adenomas. The clue that the patient has this type of the disease lies in finding 2 enlargements when the first 2 parathyroids have been identified. Then the search should be continued until an undiseased gland is found or until all 4 hyperplastic glands have been uncovered. The same principle as that used for the hypertrophied glands applies to the subtotal resection.

In order to establish the diagnosis of hyperparathyroidism, sometimes it is wise to explore the parathyroids in patients in whom the character of the disease is not clear. Trouble in differential diagnosis frequently lies between patients having minimal primary hyperparathyroidism with severe renal impairment and patients with primary nephritis with sceondary hyperparathyroidism. In the latter condition, the parathyroid enlargements, the secondary chief cell hyperplasias, are only 4 to 5 times as large as the normal gland, much smaller than the primary chief cell hyperplasias. The importance of size is well documented.

FIGURE 28-4
(*Continued*)

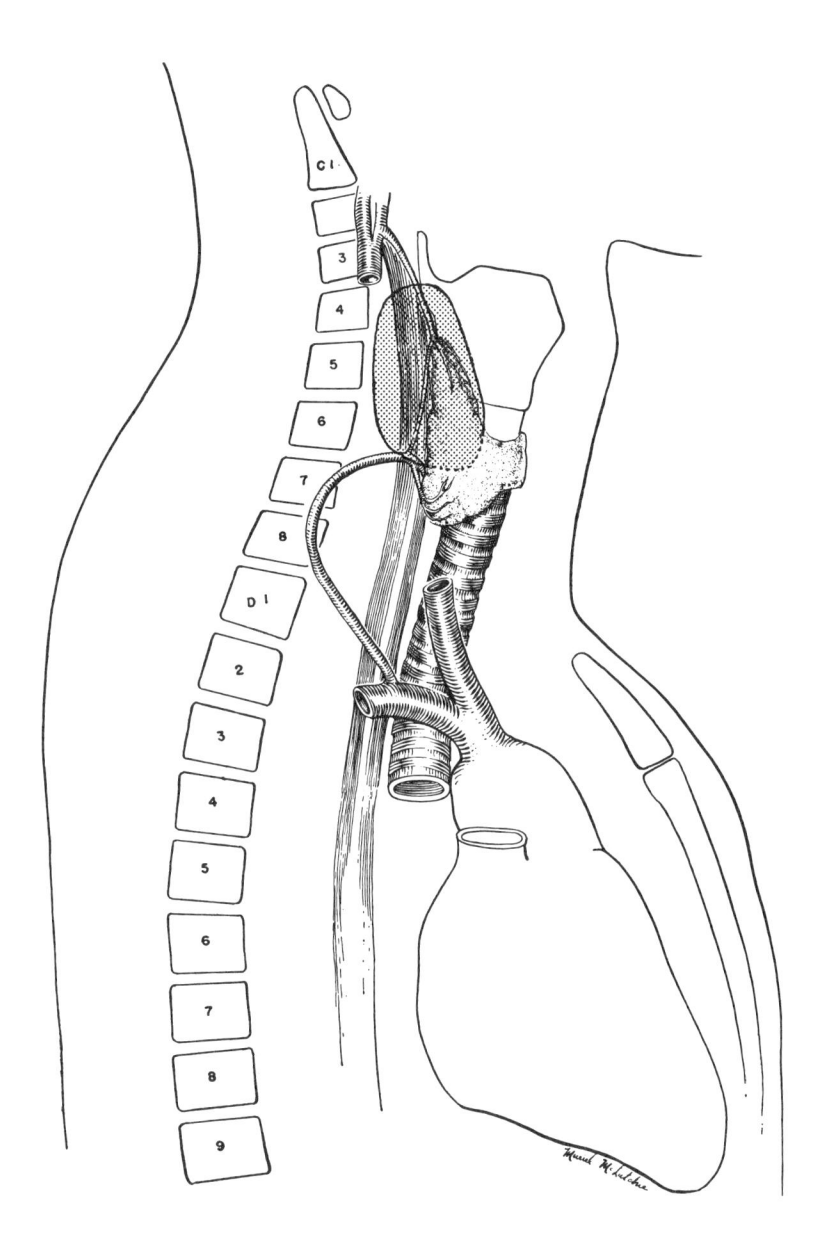

The surgeon should be suspicious of carcinoma if a single tumor is unexpectedly large for the degree of the disease and also if it is stuck. All the carcinomas encountered at the Massachusetts General Hospital have been encased by a fibrous chronic inflammatory reaction. This reaction has not been encountered surrounding a benign adenoma or hyperplasia and therefore is characteristic.

The normal parathyroid glands may be distributed over a wide area of the neck and the mediastinum, and when enlarged they may be shoved to a new position. The upper pair usually have the more confined distribution; therefore, they are the easier pair to isolate. Embryologically, the upper pair arise from the 4th branchial cleft along with the thyroid anlage (Norris, 1937). They descend during embryonic life, together with the thyroid, to their final position in the neck. These upper glands are generally in close association with the lateral thyroid lobes.

Thyroid, Thymus and Parathyroids

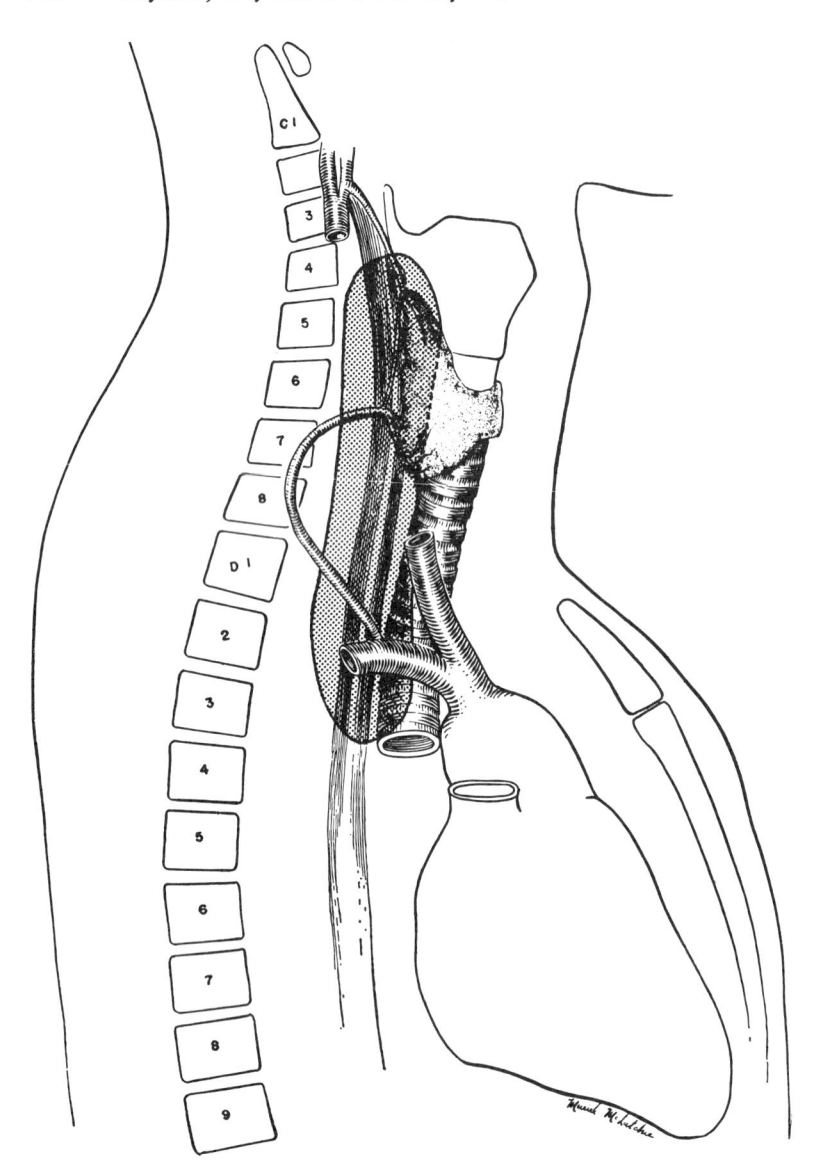

FIG. 28-5. Surgical anatomy. Lateral view of enlarged upper parathyroid (IV). The area of embryologic occurrence is extended by downward displacement of enlarged glands. (Cope, O.: Ann. Surg. 114: 706)

When enlarged, the gland may be displaced from its final embryologic position. The parathyroid gland is attached solely by its vascular pedicle. It does not have a fibrous attachment to the trachea and the cricoid cartilage comparable with that by which the thyroid gland is held firmly in place. As it enlarges and bulges out, it is pushed by the motion of the thyroid on swallowing and also sucked down by the negative intrathoracic pressure. It drags its vascular pedicle with it. Sometimes the upper gland is caught on the recurrent nerve or on a branch of the inferior thyroid artery. When it does move past the inferior thyroid artery, generally it is drawn posteriorly into the posterior superior mediastinum. The upper gland is to be found anywhere from above the upper pole of the thyroid, the length of the thyroid lobe, and down into the posterior superior mediastinum.

The lower pair of parathyroids normally have a wider distribution. They arise from the 3rd branchial cleft along with the thymus and descend with the thymus. Usually they stop off somewhere behind the thyroid gland or at the lower pole of the thyroid, the thymus continuing its descent. Sometimes they pass

Fig. 28-6. Surgical anatomy, lower parathyroid, lateral and anterior views. The shading shows the extent of possible positions of the normal lower parathyroids due to differences in development during fetal life. The extensive area accounts for the surgical difficulty frequently encountered in identifying these glands. The glands may lie anterior or posterior to the left innominate vein. (Cope, O.: Ann. Surg. 114:706)
(*Fig. 28-6 continued on p. 742*)

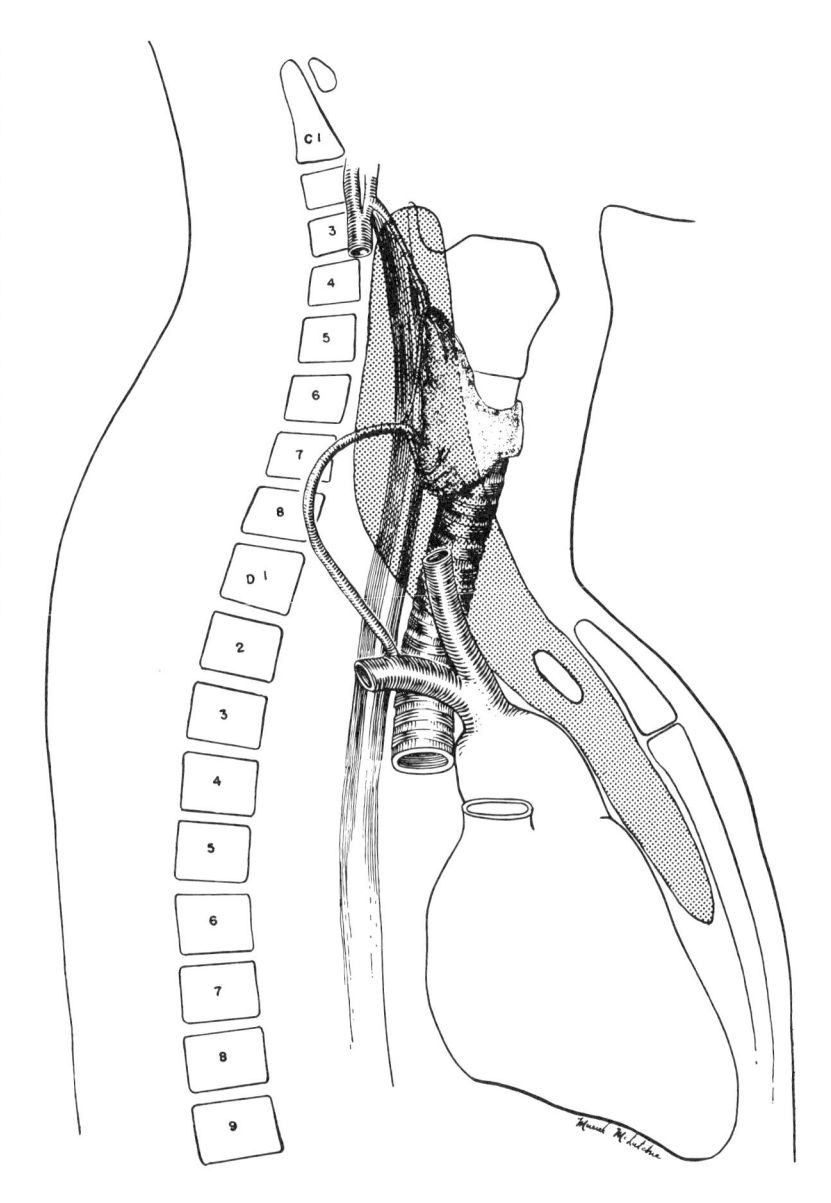

farther down with the thymus into the anterior superior mediastinum. In 10 per cent of normal persons, one or more of the lower parathyroids is in the anterior mediastinum, and frequently one or more is within the thymic capsule, usually near the upper end of the tongue of thymus which stretches up from the body toward the neck.

The lower gland when enlarged also may be displaced by swallowing and suction into the chest. Because of its more anterior position at the level of the lower pole of the thyroid, it may be displaced into the anterior mediastinum. It lies usually in front of the innominate vein, but like the thymus it also may lie posterior to the innominate vein. Because of their close association with the thymus, Norris has suggested that this pair should be called the *parathymus gland*. The lower pair of parathyroids has a considerably wider distribution and are found anywhere from the upper pole of the thyroid into the anterior mediastinum to a point as low as the pericardium.

742   Thyroid, Thymus and Parathyroids

Figure 28-6 (*Continued*)

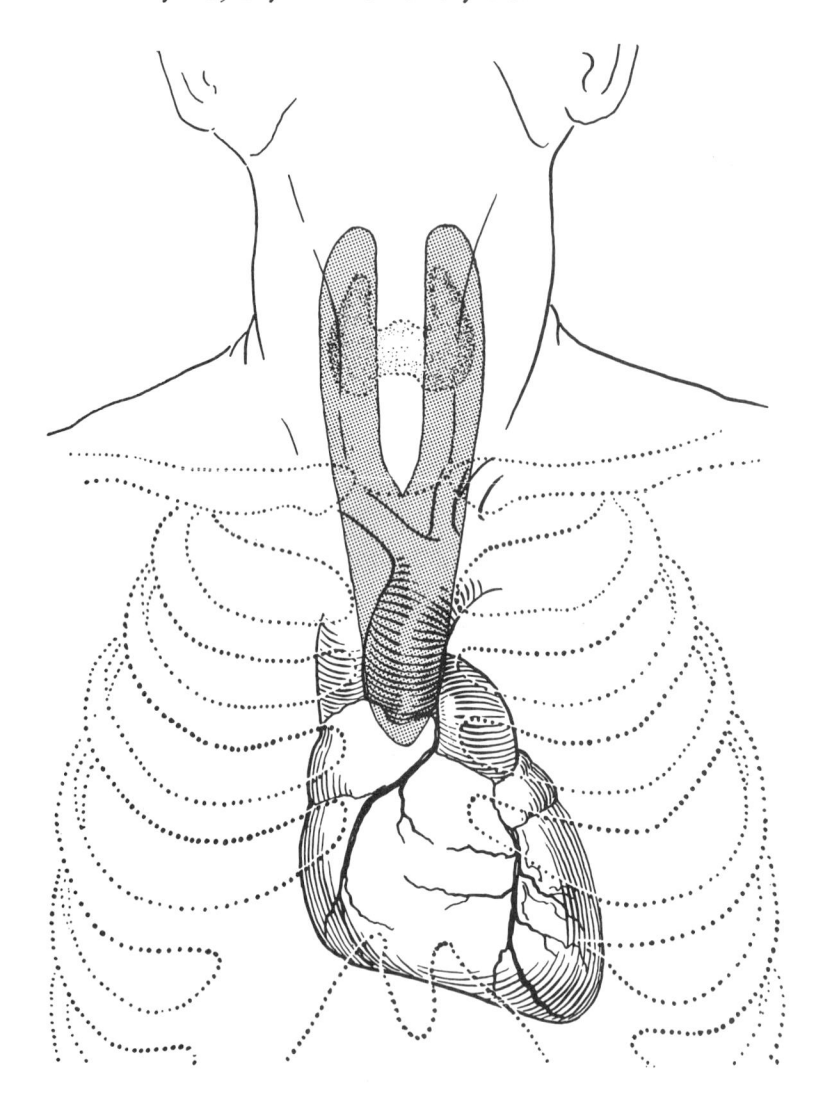

The size of the tumor often directs surgical management. It has been referred to already in relation to carcinoma and secondary chief cell hyperplasia. It is perhaps most significant in relation to the adenoma type. Here, the size of the adenoma is roughly proportionate to the intensity of the disease. In the patients with the classic type of bone disease with a calcium level of 14 mg. or higher, and due to a single adenoma, the adenoma is recognized readily, since it will be at least 2 cm. in diameter and may be considerably larger. In the patients with mild disease, particularly those with the renal stones and no bone disease, the adenoma may be small, no larger than the normal gland itself. The volume of the hyperplasias also varies somewhat with the intensity of the disease, although the total volume of tissue in the primary hyperplasias is greater for the degree of the disease than in those due to an adenoma. If a patient has a moderate or severe degree of the disease and the adenoma found in a small one, search should be continued until all 4 glands have been identified in order to exclude the presence of a second adenoma. Because of the large variation in size from case to case, if an adenoma has been found on the first side of the neck explored, generally it is wise to identify the other gland on that side before ter-

FIG. 28-7. Surgical anatomy. Lateral view of enlarged parathyroids (III) displaced from their original position in the neck. Glands having had embryologic position posterior to thyroid after enlargement may be displaced into the posterior mediastinum; those having had embryologic position caudal to thyroid in a more anterior plane may be displaced into the anterior superior mediastinum. (Cope, O.: Ann. Surg. 114:706)

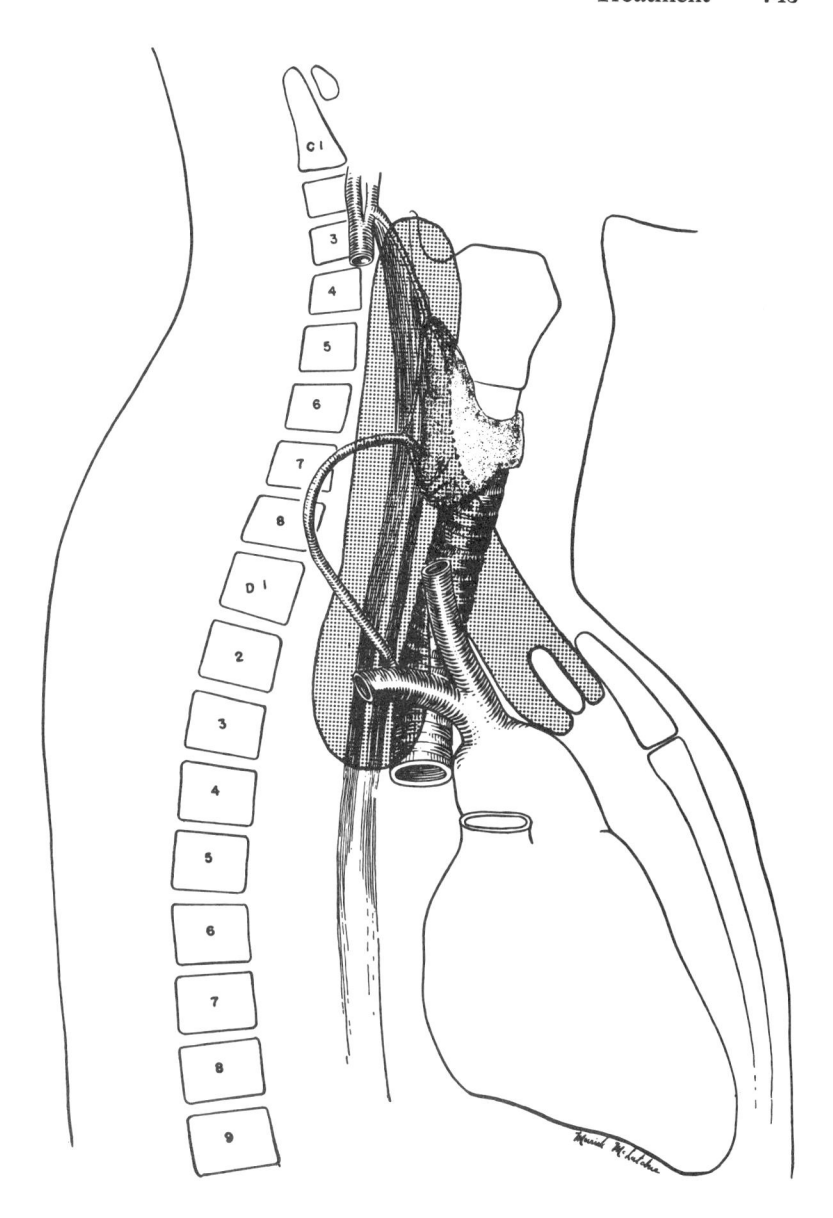

minating the operation to make certain that it does not contain a second adenoma.

The number of parathyroids for practical surgical purposes is assumed to be four. However, supernumerary glands are not rare. In a careful series of dissections at the postmortem table, C. A. Wang has identified 5 glands in five and 6 glands in two of 50 cases. In 5 patients it has been necessary to invoke the presence of a 5th gland to settle satisfactorily the hyperparathyroidism (see Case 172 under Anatomic Pathology). The surgeon never should be content that he has excluded disease if he has found only 3 normal-appearing glands.

The first exploration is the golden opportunity to identify parathyroid tissue. Scarring always makes re-exploration more difficult.

It is obvious that the surgeon must be tutored in what parathyroids look like before embarking on a parathyroid exploration. Many cases technically are easy, but a minority are difficult, and in a number of patients the surgeon has had to retreat and let

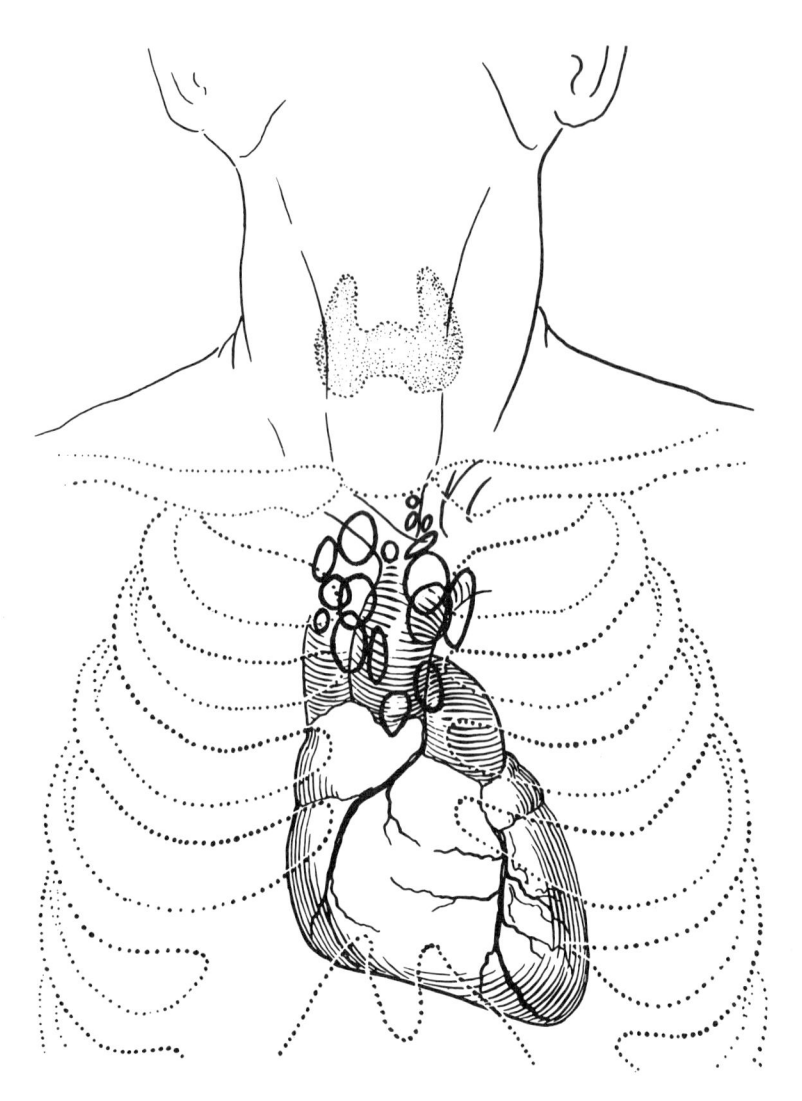

Fig. 28-8. Surgical anatomy. The position and the size of parathyroid adenomata recovered from the anterior mediastinum in 17 patients.

somebody else try again. The postmortem room is a place in which the surgeon can tutor himself. The parathyroid glands of people recently dead are remarkably like the living, and their lurking places become familiar to the surgeon who goes after them.

The tutored surgeon approaches the exploration with care and restraint. His hemostasis is painstaking, because only a little blood may so discolor the areolar and fatty tissues that he may overlook an undiseased gland or small tumor.

A swallow of barium sometimes reveals a nick on one side of the esophagus if a large enough mass is pressing against it. If no such evidence is available to indicate where an enlargement may be, where does the surgeon start? In the neck, obviously, but on which side? The number of tumors has been equal on the two sides in the Massachusetts General Hospital series and as many in the upper as in the lower gland. In choosing the side to start on, it has seemed wise to palpate the thyroid regions after the skin and the platysmal flaps have been elevated. Due allowance is to be made for the normally larger right thyroid lobes (see Case 107 under Diagnosis).

Sometimes the parathyroid exploration should be divided into 2 stages. This is the case if the search in the neck has been prolonged by scarring of a previous operation or if the offending gland is judged to be in the anterior mediastinum. It is not possible to see very far into the anterior mediastinum from a collar thyroid incision in the neck, and blind dissection is not likely to turn out the desired gland.

REFERENCES

THYROID

Astwood, E. B.: Treatment of hyperthyroidism with thiourea and thiouracil. J.A.M.A., 122:78, 1943.

Astwood, E. B., Greer, M. A., and Ettlinger, M. G.: The antithyroid factor of yellow turnip. Science, 107:631, 1949.

Basedow, von, C. A.: Exophthalmos durch Hypertrophie des Zellgewebes in der Augenhöhle. Wschr. ges. Heilk., 6:197, 1840.

Beahrs, O. H., Pemberton, J. de j., and Black, B. M.: Nodular goiter and malignant lesions of thyroid gland. J. Clin. Endocrinol., 11:1157, 1951.

Bielschowsky, F.: Experimental nodular goitre. Brit. J. Exp. Path., 26:270, 1945.

Bielschowsky, F., Griesbach, W. E., Hall, W. H., Kennedy, T. H., and Purves, H. D.: Studies on experimental goitre: transplantability of experimental thyroid tumours of rat. Brit. J. Cancer, 3:541, 1949.

Blumgart, H. L., Freedberg, A. S., and Kurland, G. S.: The treatment of incapacitated euthyroid cardiac patients by producing hypothyroidism with radioactive iodine. New Engl. J. Med., 245:83, 1951.

Boas, N. F., and Ober, W. B.: Hereditary exophthalmic goitre—report of 11 cases in one family. J. Clin. Endocrinol., 6:575, 1946.

Chapman, E. M., and Maloof, F.: The use of radioactive iodine in the diagnosis and treatment of hyperthyroidism: 10 years' experience. Medicine, 34:261, 1955.

Cope, O.: Diseases of the thyroid gland. New Eng. J. Med., 246:368, 408, 451, 1952.

———: The surgery of the thyroid. In: Means, J. H.: The Thyroid and Its Diseases. ed. 2. pp. 507-509. Philadelphia, J. B. Lippincott, 1948.

Cope, O., and Barnes, B. A.: Nodular goiter: the 18 year experience in the treatment of 400 cases with desiccated thyroid. Manuscript in preparation.

Cope, O., Dobyns, B. M., Hamlin, E., Jr., and Hopkirk, J.: What thyroid nodules are to be feared. J. Clin. Endocrinol., 9:1012, 1949.

Cope, O., and Raker, J. W.: Cushing's disease: the surgical experience in the care of 46 cases. New Eng. J. Med., 253:119, 165, 1955.

Dobyns, B. M.: Present concepts of pathologic physiology of exophthalmos. J. Clin. Endocrinol., 10:1202, 1950.

Graves, R. J.: Clinical lectures. London M. & S. J. (Part II), 7:516, 1835.

Griesbach, W. E., Kennedy, T. H., and Purves, H. D.: Studies on experimental goitre: thyroid adenomata in rats on Brassica seed diet. Brit. J. Exp. Path., 26:18, 1945.

Halsted, W. S.: Surgical Papers, The Operative Story of Goitre: The Author's Operation. vol. 2. p. 257. Baltimore, Johns Hopkins Press, 1924.

Harris, G. W., and Woods, J. W.: The effect of electrical stimulation of the hypothalamus or pituitary gland on thyroid activity. J. Physiol., 143:246, 1958.

Hertz, S., and Roberts, A.: Radioactive iodine in the study of thyroid physiology; VII. The use of radioactive iodine therapy in hyperthyroidism. J.A.M.A., 131:81, 1946.

Lidz, T., and Whitehorn, J. C.: Psychiatric problems in thyroid clinic. J.A.M.A., 139:698, 1949.

Marine, D.: The anatomic and physiologic effects of iodine on the thyroid gland of exophthalmic goiter. J.A.M.A., 59:325, 1912.

Marine, D., and Kimball, O. P.: The prevention of simple goiter in man. J. Lab. Clin. Med., 3:40, 1917.

Means, J. H.: The Thyroid and Its Diseases. ed. 2. pp. 415-423. Philadelphia, J. B. Lippincott, 1948.

Money, W. L., and Rawson, R. W.: Experimental production of thyroid tumors in rat exposed to prolonged treatment with thiouracil. Cancer, 3:321, 1950.

Morris, H. P., Dalton, A. J., and Green, C. D.: Malignant thyroid tumors occurring in mouse after prolonged hormonal imbalance during ingestion of thiouracil. J. Clin. Endocrinol., 11:1281, 1951.

Parry, C. H.: Collections from the Unpublished Papers of the Late Caleb Hilliel Parry. vol. 2. p. 111. London, 1825.

Paschkis, K. E., Cantarow, A., and Stasney, J.: Influence of thiouracil on carcinoma induced by 2-acetaminofluorene. Cancer Res., 8:257, 1948.

Plummer, H. S.: Results of administering iodine to patients having exophthalmic goiter. J.A.M.A., 80:1955, 1923.

Richardson, K. C., and Young, F. G.: Histology of diabetes induced in dogs by injection of anterior-pituitary extracts. Lancet, 1:1098, 1938.

Rienhoff, W. F., Jr.: Involutional or regressive changes in the thyroid gland in cases of exophthalmic goiter and their relation to the origin of the so-called adenomas. Arch. Surg., 13:391, 1926.

Russfield, A. B.: Histology of the human hypophysis in thyroid disease—hypothyroidism, hyperthyroidism and cancer. J. Clin. Endocrinol., 15:1393, 1955.

Schlesinger, M., Gargill, S. L., and I. H.: Studies in nodular goiter; I. Incidence of thyroid nodules in routine necropsies in a non goitrous region. J.A.M.A., 110-1638, 1938.

Thompson, W. O., and Thompson, P. K.: Treatment of toxic goiter by irradiation of pituitary. J. Clin. Invest., 23:951, 1944.

Warren, S., and Meissner, W. A.: Tumors of the thyroid gland. In: Atlas of Tumor Pathology. Washington, D. C., Armed Forces Institute of Pathology, 1953.

Thymus

Blalock, A.: Thymectomy in the treatment of myasthenia gravis; report of 20 cases. J. Thoracic Surg., 13:316, 1944.

Blalock, A., Mason, M. F., Morgan, H. J., and Riven, S. S.: Myasthenia gravis and tumors of the thymic region. Ann. Surg., 110:544, 1939.

Dougherty, T. F.: Effect of hormones on lymphatic tissue. Physiol. Rev., 32:379, 1952.

Eaton, L. M., and Clagett, O. T.: Thymectomy in the treatment of myasthenia gravis; results in 72 cases compared with 142 control cases. J.A.M.A., 142:963, 1950.

Keynes, G.: The results of thymectomy in myasthenia gravis. Brit. M. J., 2:611, 1949.

Laquer, and Weigert: Beiträge zur Lehre von der erb'schen Krankheit. Neurol. Centralbl., 20:594, 1901.

Mella, H.: Irradiation of the thymus in myasthenia gravis. Med. Clin. N. Am., 7:939, 1923.

Norris, E. H.: The morphogenesis and histogenesis of the thymus gland in man: in which the origin of the Hassall's corpuscles of the human thymus is discovered. Contrib. Embryol., no. 166, pp. 191-207, May 31, 1938.

———: The parathyroid glands and the lateral thyroid in man: their morphogenesis, topographic anatomy and prenatal growth. Contrib. Embryol., no. 159, pp. 249-294, January 30, 1937.

Pierchalla, L.: Über die Röntgenbehandlung der hyperplastischen Thymus bei Myasthenia pseudoparalytica. Therap. Halbmonatsch, 16:504, 1921.

Sauerbruch, F.: Chirurgie der Brustorgane; Die Chirurgie des Thymus. vol. 2. pp. 512-514. Berlin, Springer, 1925.

Schwab, R. S., and Viets, H. R.: Thymectomy in myasthenia gravis (Scientific Exhibit). Interim Session of the A.M.A., Boston, Mass., Nov. 29–Dec. 2, 1955.

Soffer, I. J., Gabrilove, J. L., Laqueur, H. P., Volterra, M., Jacobs, M. D., and Sussman, M. L.: The effects of anterior pituitary adrenocorticotropic hormone (ACTH) in myasthenia gravis with tumor of the thymus. J. Mount Sinai Hosp., 15:73, 1948.

Torda, C., and Wolff, H. G.: Effects of adrenocorticotrophic hormone on neuromuscular function in patients with myasthenia gravis. Proc. Soc. Exp. Biol. Med., 71:432, 1949.

Parathyroid Glands

Albertini, von, A., Koller, F., and Gaiser, H.: Functioning parathyroid tumor with liver metastasis. Acta endocrinol., 12:289, 1953.

Albright, F., Baird, P. C., Cope, O., and Bloomberg, E.: Studies on the physiology of the parathyroid glands; IV. Renal complications of hyperparathyroidism. Am. J. M. Sci., 187:49, 1934.

Albright, F., Burnett, C. H., Smith, P. H., and Parson, W.: Pseudohypoparathyroidism—an example of Seabright's bantam syndrome. Endocrinology, 30:922, 1942.

Askanazy, M.: Über Ostitis Deformans ohne ostoides Gewebe. Arb. Geb. path., Anat. Inst. Tübingen (Leipzig), 4:398, 1903.

Bauer, W., Albright, F., and Aub, J. C.: A case of osteitis fibrosa cystica (osteomalacia?) with evidence of hyperactivity of the parathyroid bodies: metabolic study II. J. Clin. Invest., 8:229, 1930.

Castleman, B.: Tumors of the parathyroid glands. In: Atlas of Tumor pathology. p. 74. Washington, D. C., Armed Forces Inst. Path., 1952.

Castleman, B., and Cope, O.: Primary parathyroid hypertrophy and hyperplasia: a review of 11 cases at the Masschusetts General Hospital. Bull. Hosp. Joint Dis., 12:368, 1951.

Castleman, B., and Mallory, T. B.: Parathyroid hyperplasia in chronic renal insufficiency. Am. J. Path., 13:553, 1937.

———: The pathology of the parathyroid gland in hyperparathyroidism: a study of 25 cases. Am. J. Path., 11:1, 1935.

Churchill, E. D., and Cope, O.: Parathyroid tumors associated with hyperparathyroidism: 11 cases treated by operation. Surg., Gynec. Obstet., 58:255, 1934.

Cogan, D. G., Albright, F., and Bartter, F. C.: Hypercalcemia and band keratopathy: report of 19 cases. Arch. Ophth., 40:624, 1948.

Collip, J. B.: The extraction of a parathyroid hormone which will prevent or control parathyroid tetany and which regulates the level of blood calcium. J. Biol. Chem., 63:395, 1925.

Cope, O: Hyperparathyroidism: 67 cases in 10 years. J. Missouri M. A., 39:273, 1942.

———: Surgery of hyperparathyroidism: the occurrence of parathyroids in the anterior mediastinum and the division of the operation into 2 stages. Ann. Surg., 114:706, 1941.

Cope, O., Culver, P. J., Mixter, C. J., Jr., and Nardi, G. L.: Pancreatitis, a diagnostic clue to hyperparathyroidism. Ann. Surg., 148:857, 1957.

Cope, O., Keynes, W. M., Roth, S. I., and Castleman, B.: Primary chief-cell hyperplasia of the parathyroid glands: a new entity in the surgery of hyperparathyroidism. Ann. Surg., 148:375, 1958.

Cope, O., Nardi, G. L., and Castleman, B.: Carcinoma of the parathyroid glands: 4 cases among 148 patients with hyperparathyroidism. Ann. Surg., 138:661, 1953.

Erdheim, J.: Über Epithelkörperbefunde bei Osteomalacie. Sitzungsb. Akad. Wissensch. Math. naturw. Cl., 116:311, 1907.

———: Rachitis und Epithelkörperchen. Aus der Kaiserlich-Königlichen Hof- und Staatsdruckerei, Vienna, 1914.

Gley, E.: Sur les fonctions du corps thyroïde. Compt. rend. Soc. biol., 43:551, 567, 583, 841 and 843, 1891.

Hannon, R. R., Shorr, E., McClellan, W. S., and DuBois, E. F.: A case of osteitis fibrosa cystica (osteomalacia?) with evidence of hyperactivity of the parathyroid bodies: metabolic study. I. J. Clin. Invest., 8:215, 1930.

Hanson, A. M.: The hydrochloric x sicca: a parathyroid preparation for intramuscular injection. Mil. Surgeon, 54:218, 1924.

References

Hunter, D., and Aub, J. C.: Lead studies: XV. The effect of the parathyroid hormone on the excretion of lead and of calcium in patients suffering from lead poisoning. Quart. J. Med., 20:123, 1927.

Keating, F. R., Jr., and Cook, E. N.: The recognition of primary hyperparathyroidism—an analysis of 24 cases. J.A.M.A., 129:994, 1945.

Krane, S.: Unpublished data.

MacCallum, W. G., and Voegtlin, C.: On the relation of the parathyroid to calcium metabolism and the nature of tetany. Bull. Johns Hopkins Hosp., 19:91, 1908.

Mandl, F.: Klinisches and Experimentelles zur Frage der lokalisierten and generalisierten Ostitis Fibrosa (unter besonderer Berücksichtigung der Therapy der letzteren). Arch. klin. Chir., 143:245, 1926.

Norris, E. H.: The parathyroid glands and the lateral thyroid in man: their morphogenesis, topographic anatomy and prenatal growth. Contrib. Embryol., no. 159, pp. 249-294, January 30, 1937.

Owen, R.: Richard Owen and the Discovery of the Parathyroid Glands in Science, Medicine and History: Essays on the Evolution of Scientific Thought and Medical Practice. E. A. Underwood, Editor, London, Oxford University Press, 1953, 2:217.

Recklinghausen, von, F. D.: Die Fibröse oder deformirende Ostitis, die Osteomalacie und die osteoplastische Carcinose in ihren gegenseitigen Beziehungen. Festschrift f. Rudolf Virchow, Berlin, 1891.

Rogers, H. M., and Keating, F. R., Jr.: Primary hypertrophy and hyperplasia of the parathyroid glands as a cause of hyperparathyroidism. Am. J. Med., 3:384, 1947.

Sainton, P., and Millot, J. L.: Malignant degeneration of eosinophil adenoma of the parathyroids in the cause of von Recklinghausen's disease. Ann. anat. path., 10:813, 1933.

Sandström, I.: On a new gland in man and several mammals (glandulae parathyreoideae). Upsala läkaref, förh., 15:441, 1879-80.

Schlagenhaufer: Zwei Falle von Parathyreoideatumoren. Wien. klin. Wchnschr., 28(2):1362, 1915.

Walsh, F. B., and Howard, J. E.: Conjunctival and corneal lesions in hypercalcemia. J. Clin. Endocrinol., 7:655, 1947.

CHAPTER 29, SECTION 1

DAVID Y. COOPER, M.D.

Physiology of the Pituitary and Adrenal Glands

Introduction
Physiology and Biochemistry—Pituitary
Response in Surgical Stress
Diagnosis of Adrenal and Pituitary Insufficiency
Pathologic Changes Caused by Excess of Adrenal Steroids or ACTH

INTRODUCTION

The hormones secreted by the pituitary and adrenal, as a class of compounds, have three major functions—integrative, regulative, and morphologic. Integrative action is possible because the hormones are carried by the blood stream to their sites of action, enabling the body to function as a unit in response to stimuli. The regulative actions of hormones are related to the homeokinetic reactions of carbohydrate, salt and water balance, thus maintaining a constant internal body environment. Certain of the hormones, the tropic hormones, are of importance in controlling the rate and type of growth of the body (Brown and Barker, 1962). The key to the role of the pituitary adrenal system in surgical stress is "sufficient function," since excessive adrenal and pituitary activity gives no added protection to the individual, whereas insufficient function leads to circulatory collapse and death. In order to give the surgeon a better insight in assessing pituitary adrenal function in surgical patients, the following topics will be discussed.

1. Biochemistry and Physiology of the Pituitary and Adrenal
2. Response in Surgical Stress
3. Detection of Pituitary Adrenal Adequate Function
4. Pathologic Changes caused by an Excess of Adrenal Steroids or ACTH

PHYSIOLOGY AND BIOCHEMISTRY

Pituitary

Morphology

The pituitary is a small organ, with normal dimensions of 10 × 13 × 6 mm. and weighing

TABLE 29-1. DIVISION OF PITUITARY GLAND*

Adenohypophysis (Lobus glandularis)		Pars distalis Anterior lobe Pars tuberalis Pars intermedia Posterior lobe Processus infundibuli
Neurohypophysis	(Lobus neurosis) (neural lobe) Infundibulum (neural stalk)	Pediculus infundibularis (stem) Bulbus infundibularis (bulb) Lobum infundibularis (rim) or Median eminence of the tuber cinereum

* Terminology recommended by the International Commission on Anatomical Nomenclature.

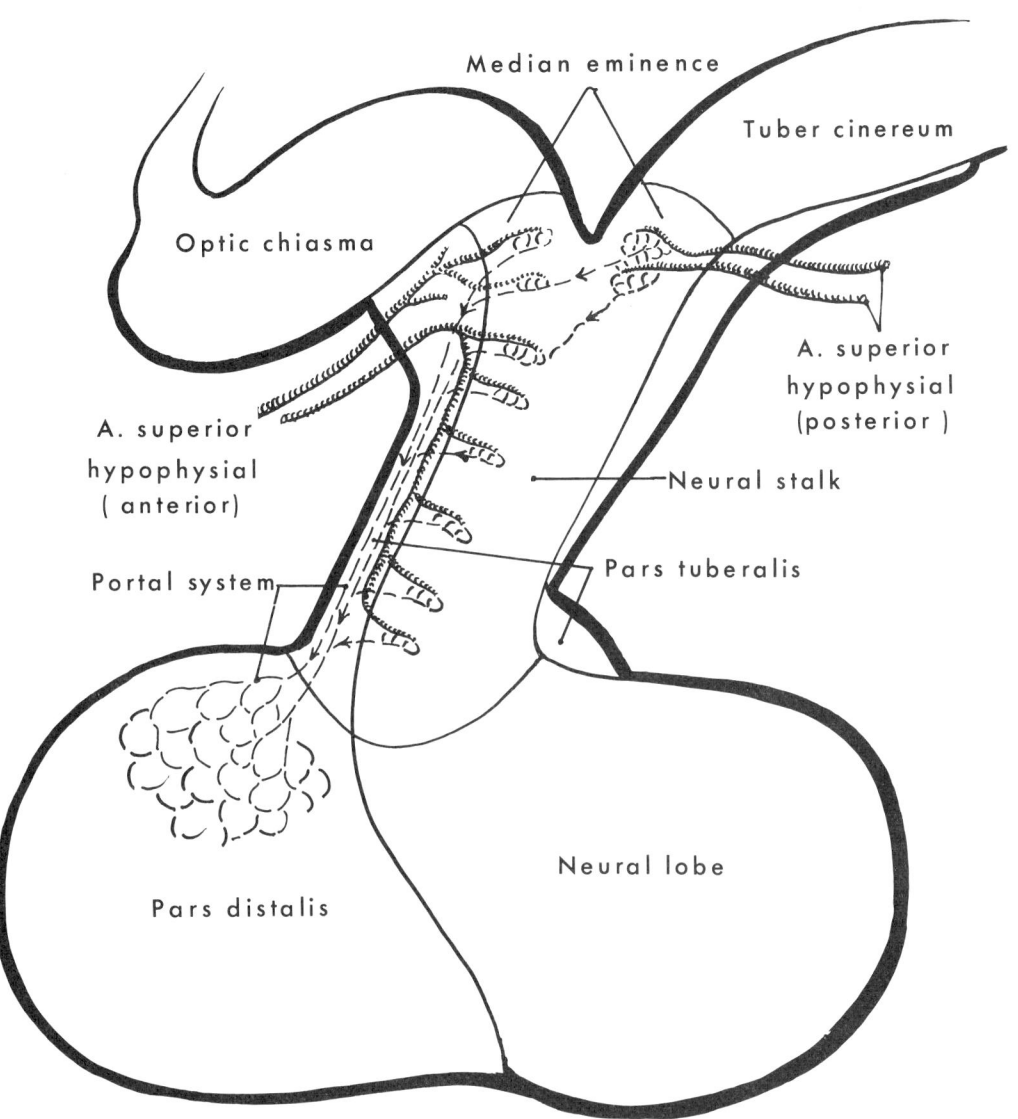

FIG. 29-1. Diagram showing anatomic relationships of the anterior pituitary, posterior pituitary and hypothalamus.

about 0.5 Gm. This complex structure lies in a bony wall cavity, the sella turcica, in the sphenoid bone at the base of the skull. The anterior lobe constitutes 15 per cent of the weight. The terminology recommended by the International Commission for the different parts of the pituitary is given in Table 29-1.

Microscopic Anatomy

The pituitary gland is composed of at least three, and possibly five, distinct cell types.

1. *Basophils*—round oval cells with ovoid nuclei and clearly defined boundaries with intensely Schiff-positive granules.

2. *Acidophils*—round ovoid cells with round ovoid nuclei and distinct boundaries; Schiff-negative, but stain bright orange with orange G counterstain.

3. *Chromophils*—cells smaller than basophils or acidophils, with ovoid nuclei and denser chromatin, indistinct cell boundaries and granular cell boundaries.

4. *Amphophils*—pleomorphic, irregular in shape, with predominantly indistinct boundaries containing some orange granules. Most of the granules are weakly Schiff-positive.

5. *Hypertrophic Amphophils*—clearly derived from the amphophils by degranulation, diminution of the cytoplasm, and enlargement of the nucleolus.

The pituitary cells are not distributed uniformly throughout the pituitary gland. Acidophils are concentrated at the stalk in the infundibular region, while the basophil cells are found in the anterior and inferior margins of the gland.

The specific secretory activities of the individual cell types described is not clearly known. Present information with regard to the secretory activity of the various cell types is summarized in Table 29-2. Data seem to indicate that the acidophilic cells are associated with the production of growth hormone (somatotropin), while thyrotropin, gonadotropin, follicle stimulating hormone and corticotropin are formed by the basophilic cells. Little evidence is available in regard to which of the cells form prolactin.

Pituitary Hormones

Six hormones have been isolated from the anterior lobe of the pituitary (Table 29-2). Four of these—the lactogenic (luteotropic) hormone, the interstitial cell stimulating hormone (ICSH), the adrenocorticotropic (ACTH) hormone, and the growth hormones—have been obtained in pure forms. Follicle stimulating hormone (FSH) and thyrotropic (TSH) hormone, although highly purified, are not considered homogeneous at present. These six hormones can be classified on the basis of general activity:

1. The gonadotropins: follicle stimulating hormones, interstitial cell stimulating hormone and luteotropic or lactogenic hormone;

2. The so-called metabolic hormones; adrenocorticotropic hormone (ACTH), thyrotropic hormone and growth hormone. These hormones may also be divided into two chemical groups: simple proteins (ACTH, LTH, and STH), and glycoproteins (TSH, FSH and ICSH). Other substances with hormonal activity, ascribed to the pituitary, are the exophthalmus-producing substance, which has been found related to TSH, and the fat-mobilizing substance (peptides of 10,000 to 20,000 molecular weight). The latter mobilize fatty acids from adipose tissue and may play an important role in fat metabolism. The hypoglycemic factor and the various pituitary "releasing factors" are not yet as well characterized.

Somatotropin (Growth Hormone; GH, STH). Removal of the anterior lobe of the pituitary in laboratory animals or man markedly retards but does not completely suppress skeletal growth. From pituitary extracts a variety of growth hormone preparations have been made that support growth in hypophysectomized animals. Repeated injection of GH into normal rats that have reached a plateau of growth development results in the production of giant animals. (This apparently does not occur in man.) Hypophysectomized animals are more sensitive to growth hormone than are normal animals and, therefore, they are more useful for assay of the hormone. Specifically affected by the hormone is the growth of epiphyseal cartilage of the long bones of hypophysectomized animals. This phenomenon also is the basis of an assay for this hormone.

Tumor growth, wound healing, growth of hair and teeth, and regeneration of liver can occur in the absence of growth hormone. At present the physiologic role of growth hormone is extremely difficult to evaluate.

Li and Evans (1948) summarized the effects of growth hormone on protein metabolism as follows: The growth hormone causes: (1) nitrogen retention, (2) lowering of blood amino acids, (3) an increase in protein content and a decrease in fat content of the carcass of the animal, (4) an increase in alkaline phosphatase and inorganic phosphorus, (5) enlargement of the liver and thymus, and (6) a slight increase in the ribonucleic acid content of the liver. Growth hormone does not seem to have a direct effect on fatty acid synthesis or oxidation yet it may influence cholesterol biosynthesis. Administration of growth hormone to fasted subjects elevates plasma concentration of unesterified fatty acids. In fed animals the fatty acid release is not as large. Growth hormone effects on carbohydrate metabolism are an insulinlike hypoglycemic effect and an anti-insulin diabetogenic effect; these are not yet understood.

TABLE 29-2. PITUITARY HORMONES

HORMONE	SYNONYMS	CELL SOURCE	PREPARATIVE SOURCE	MOL. WT.	AUTHORITY
Growth hormone (GH)	Somatotropin Somatotropic	Anterior lobe eosinophils center	whale simian human	39,900 25,400 21,500	Li (1963) Li (1963) Li (1963)
Thyroid stimulating hormone (TSH)	Thyrotropin Thyreotropic hormone Thyrotropic hormone	Anterior lobe	human	26,000 30,000	Bates & Condliff (1960)
Prolactin	Luteotropin Lactogenic hormone Mammotropic hormone Luteotropic hormone	Largely basophils of anterior pit.	sheep	24,000	Li (1963)
Follicle stimulating hormone (FSH)	Follicle stimulator Thylakintrin	Largely basophils of anterior pit.	pig human (urinary)	29,000 30,000	Steelman (in Albert, 1961) Steelman and Segaloff 1963
Interstitial cell stimulating hormone (ICSH)	Follicle Luteotropin Lactogenic hormone Mammotropin Luteotropic hormone Galactin	Largely basophils of anterior pit.	sheep	30,000	Steelman (in Albert, 1961)
Adrenocorticotropic hormone (ACTH)	Corticotropic hormone Adrenotropin Corticotropin Adrenotropic hormone	Largely basophils of anterior pit.	human	4,567	Li (1963)
Melanocyte stimulating hormone (MSH)	Melanotropin Chromotropic hormone Intermedia	Intermediate lobe	α beef β pig	1,823 2,734	Dixon (1964)
Vasopressin	Pitressin Vasopressor principle Anti diuretic principle	Post. pituitary	synthetic beef hog	~1000	du Vigneaud (1953) Dixon (1964)
Oxytocin	Pitocin Oxytoxic hormone	Post. pituitary	synthetic beef hog	~1000	du Vigneaud (1953)

Thyrotropin (Thyrotropic Hormone; Thyroid Stimulating Hormone; TSH). Administration of thyrotropin reverses thyroid atrophy and relieves the suppression of thyroid secretion observed after removal of the anterior hypophysis. TSH has been studied extensively; however, its structure is not yet known. It has a molecular weight in the range of 26,000 to 30,000 and contains a high content of cystine. Glucoseamine, galactosamine, mannose and fucose may be the carbohydrate components of the hormone.

TSH effects on the thyroid gland are multiple. The primary effect is probably to cause the thyroid to discharge its stored hormone into the circulation. As thyroid iodine values fall, acinar cell height, thyroid weight and the ability of the thyroid to concentrate iodine increase. Which of these responses are primary and which are secondary is not known. Administration of excess exogenous thyroid hormone suppresses the secretion of TSH. Administration of excessive TSH to the laboratory animal or man, or hypersecretion of TSH by the anterior hypophysis, produces a state of hyperthyroidism. Thyroid secretory activity does not fail completely in the absence of hypophyseal TSH. Thyroidectomy as well as goitrogenic drugs such as thiourea and thiouracil markedly increase TSH secretion.

Prolactin; Lactogenic Hormone; Luteotropic Hormone (Luteotropin). Prolactin maintains the functional state of the corpus luteum, stimulates proliferation of the crop gland in birds and exercises a galactopoietic effect in mammals. This hormone was one of the first of the pituitary hormones to be purified and crystallized. It has a molecular weight of 24,000 to 26,000 in the different species from which it is prepared. It may play a role in a number of the phases of lactation but its principal action is initiation of lactation. After complete morphologic development of the mammary gland, prolactin plays an important role in stimulating progesterone formation by formed corpora lutea. Prolactin elicits a variety of other metabolic and behavioral responses in different species studied, indicating it may have a broader role in controlling metabolic function.

Follicle Stimulating Hormones (FSH) and Interstitial Cell Stimulating (ICSH) Hormones. Removal of the pituitary gland before maturity causes a cessation of sexual development. In mature animals hypophysectomy produces atrophy of the testes in males and degeneration and atrophy in the ovaries of females. The effect of hypophysectomy during pregnancy has different effects in different animals. Abortion is induced by hypophysectomy in dogs, cats and rabbits, whereas in rats, mice and guinea pigs, if the hypophysectomy is done in the second half of gestation, a prolonged gestation period may result.

The multiple nature of these hormones has been shown by Fevold, Hisaw and Leonard (1944) who separate pituitary extracts into a follicle-stimulating fraction (FSH) and a luteinizing-hormone fraction (LH). The follicle-stimulating fraction was shown to produce spermatogenic activity in testes and the luteinizing fraction to cause Leydig cell development and function, with the production of the male hormone testosterone. The latter fraction, generally called interstitial cell stimulating hormone, is the same as luteinizing hormone. At the present time it is possible to replace all gonadotropic function by FSH, ICSH and luteotropic hormone. Purified preparations of FSH have been made but the structure is not yet known. One of the better preparations has a molecular weight of around 29,000.

Highly purified ICSH has been prepared (Mol.wt., human 26,000; sheep 30,000). Both α and β forms of ICSH have been isolated. Prolonged administration of estrogenic or androgenic steroids produces ovarian or testicular atrophy by suppressing excretion of FSH or ICSH.

Corticotropin (Adrenocorticotropic Hormone; ACTH). Loss of function of the anterior pituitary results in atrophy of all three layers of the adrenal cortex and marked reduction of the secretion of all adrenocortical steroids. However, a low level of adrenocortical secretory activity remains. There is no atrophy of the adrenal medulla, and secretion of the medullary hormones likewise is not influenced by loss of anterior pituitary function. It was found that injection of anterior pituitary extracts resulted in hyperplasia of all three layers of the adrenal cortex. Further work resulted in purification of corticotropin, a straight chain polypeptide consisting of 39 amino acids with a molecular weight of about 4,500. Fig. 29-2 summarizes the structural similarities of

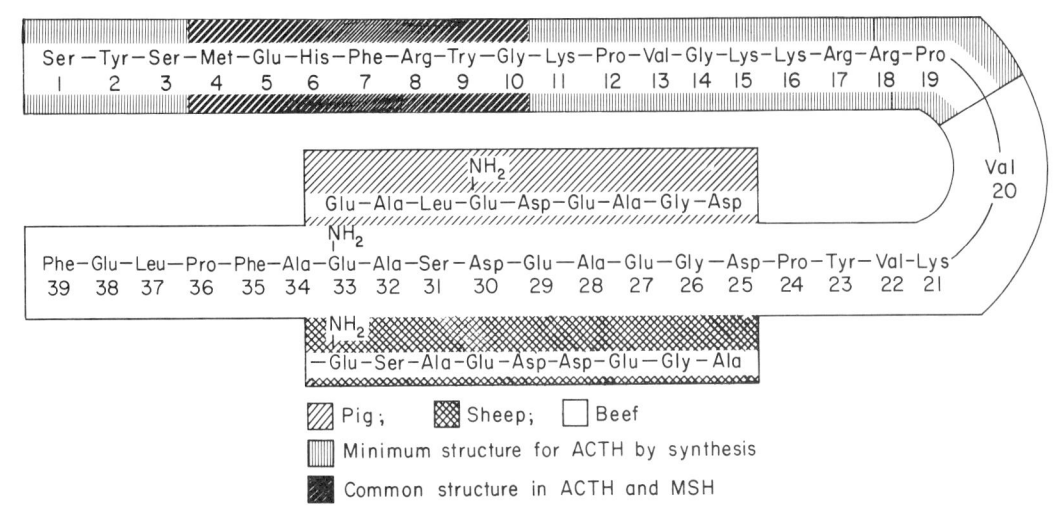

```
Ser—Tyr—Ser—Met—Glu—His—Phe—Arg—Try—Gly—Lys—Pro—Val—Gly—Lys—Lys—Arg—Arg—Pro
 1   2   3   4   5   6   7   8   9   10  11  12  13  14  15  16  17  18  19

                            NH₂
                Glu—Ala—Leu—Glu—Asp—Glu—Ala—Gly—Asp                                   Val
                       NH₂                                                             20
Phe—Glu—Leu—Pro—Phe—Ala—Glu—Ala—Ser—Asp—Glu—Ala—Glu—Gly—Asp—Pro—Tyr—Val—Lys
 39  38  37  36  35  34  33  32  31  30  29  28  27  26  25  24  23  22  21

                            NH₂
                  —Glu—Ser—Ala—Glu—Asp—Asp—Glu—Gly—Ala
```

Pig;   Sheep;   Beef
Minimum structure for ACTH by synthesis
Common structure in ACTH and MSH

Fig. 29-2. Molecular structure of ACTH of pig, sheep, and beef cattle.

ACTH prepared from pig, sheep, and beef pituitaries respectively. The main difference in the ACTH from the various species occurs in the amino acid sequences of positions 25 to 33. The mechanism by which ACTH acts on the adrenals is not clear. A specific action of ACTH is the stimulation of the conversion of cholesterol to pregnenolone. Some extra-adrenal actions of ACTH have been demonstrated: (1) production of ketonuria in fed, fasted, and fasted-adrenalectomized animals; (2) liberation of free fatty acids from adipose tissue (this effect appears to require adrenocortical steroids); (3) production of hypoglycemia and improved glucose tolerance, an increase in adipose tissue glycogen and some effects on muscle glycogen, and (4) apparently, a decrease in urea formation from infused amino acids.

Melanocyte Stimulating Hormone. This hormone is primarily produced in the intermediate lobe of the pituitary; however, it is found in lower concentrations in other parts of the hypophysis in different species of animals. Both α and β melanocyte stimulating hormone have been purified and the amino acid sequence determined. αMSH is made up of 13 amino acids and has the same structure regardless of animal source. βMSH contains 18 to 23 amino acids and varies from species to species. The thirteen amino acids of the αMSH are the first 13 amino acids of ACTH. The amino acid sequences of representative MSH structures are shown in Figure 29-2. MSH produces the skin darkening in frogs and other amphibians that is important for camouflage. The function of MSH in humans is not clear. Human skin is darkened by MSH but the differences in color of Negroes, Caucasians and Albinos appear to be related more to genetic factors than to MSH function. Synthetic MSH darkens human skin. Although ACTH is structurally similar to MSH, it has only slight effects on the skin color.

Hormones of the Posterior Lobe; Neurophyseal Hormones. Substances formed in the posterior lobe of the pituitary cause contraction of the mammalian uterus, diuresis and antidiuresis in mammals, as well as pressor and other effects such as milk let-down, changes in membrane permeability, etc. Du Vigneaud (1953) and his colleagues have isolated some of the "active principles" and have defined their chemical nature as oligopeptides (Fig. 29-2A). At present four octapeptides, oxytocin, vasopressin, vasotocin and isotocin, are thought to be the natural neurohypophyseal hormones. Of these the first two have been observed in mammals.

Injection of vasopressin produces a sharp rise in blood pressure due to constriction of peripheral vessels and a slowing of the heart, frequently resulting from constriction of the coronary arteries.

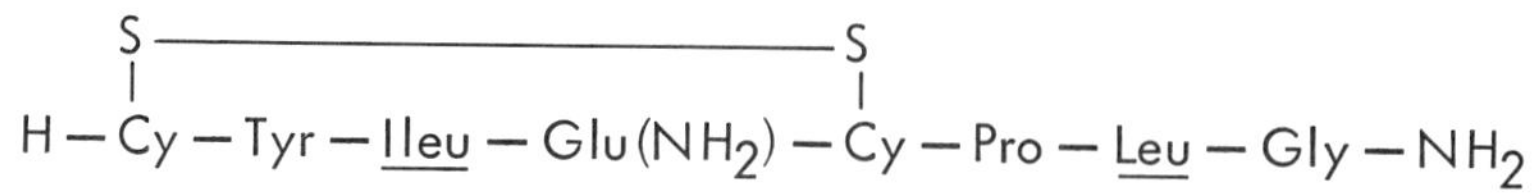

$$\text{H}-\underset{|}{\overset{\text{S}\relbar\joinrel\relbar\joinrel\relbar\joinrel\relbar\joinrel\relbar\joinrel\relbar\joinrel\relbar\joinrel\relbar\joinrel\relbar\joinrel\relbar\joinrel\relbar}{\text{Cy}}}-\text{Tyr}-\underline{\text{Ileu}}-\text{Glu}(\text{NH}_2)-\underset{|}{\overset{\text{S}}{\text{Cy}}}-\text{Pro}-\underline{\text{Leu}}-\text{Gly}-\text{NH}_2$$

Oxytocin

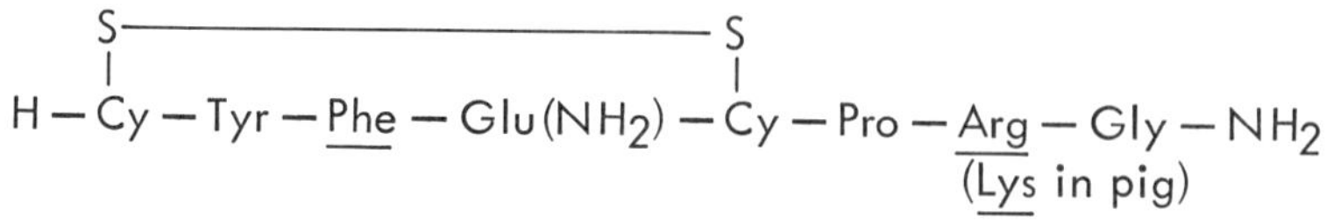

$$\text{H}-\underset{|}{\overset{\text{S}\relbar\joinrel\relbar\joinrel\relbar\joinrel\relbar\joinrel\relbar\joinrel\relbar\joinrel\relbar\joinrel\relbar\joinrel\relbar\joinrel\relbar\joinrel\relbar}{\text{Cy}}}-\text{Tyr}-\underline{\text{Phe}}-\text{Glu}(\text{NH}_2)-\underset{|}{\overset{\text{S}}{\text{Cy}}}-\text{Pro}-\underline{\text{Arg}}-\text{Gly}-\text{NH}_2$$
$$(\underline{\text{Lys}}\text{ in pig})$$

Vasopressin

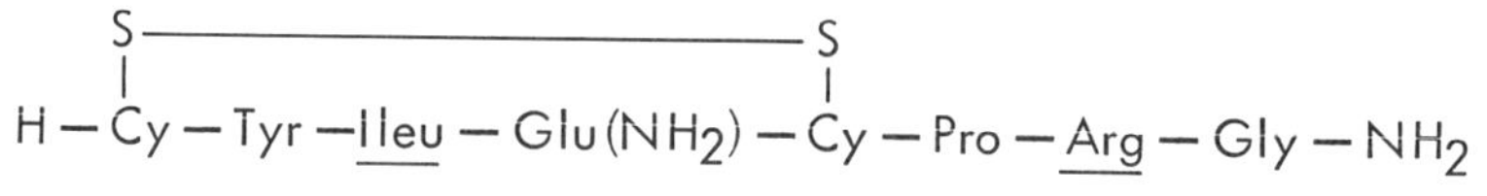

$$\text{H}-\underset{|}{\overset{\text{S}\relbar\joinrel\relbar\joinrel\relbar\joinrel\relbar\joinrel\relbar\joinrel\relbar\joinrel\relbar\joinrel\relbar\joinrel\relbar\joinrel\relbar\joinrel\relbar}{\text{Cy}}}-\text{Tyr}-\underline{\text{Ileu}}-\text{Glu}(\text{NH}_2)-\underset{|}{\overset{\text{S}}{\text{Cy}}}-\text{Pro}-\underline{\text{Arg}}-\text{Gly}-\text{NH}_2$$

Vasotocin

$$\text{H}-\underset{|}{\overset{\text{S}\relbar\joinrel\relbar\joinrel\relbar\joinrel\relbar\joinrel\relbar\joinrel\relbar\joinrel\relbar\joinrel\relbar\joinrel\relbar\joinrel\relbar\joinrel\relbar}{\text{Cy}}}-\text{Tyr}-\underline{\text{ileu}}-\text{Ser}-\text{Asp}(\text{NH}_2)-\underset{|}{\overset{\text{S}}{\text{Cy}}}-\text{Pro}-\underline{\text{Ileu}}-\text{Gly}-\text{NH}_2$$

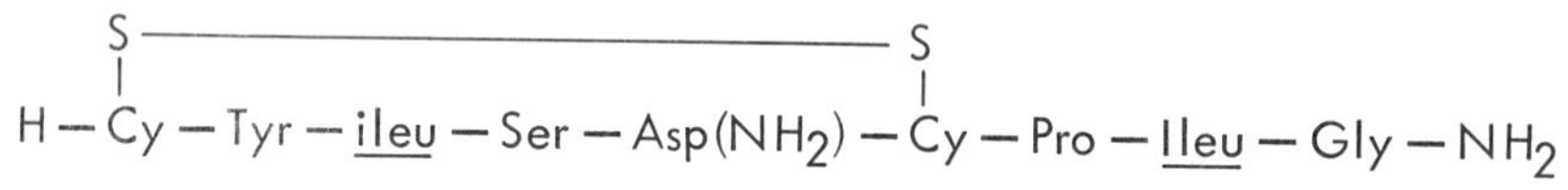

Isotocin

FIG. 29-2A. The amino acid sequence of natural neurohypophyseal hormones.

Oxytocin causes marked constriction of smooth muscle, particularly the uterus and certain portions of the gastrointestinal tract. Since the gravid uterus near term is particularly susceptible to oxytocin, this substance is used frequently in initiating labor. Stimulation of contraction of smooth muscle strips serves as a convenient assay for this hormone.

Posterior lobe extracts, as well as vasopressin, have a profound effect on water balance. Diabetes insipidus, a condition characterized by excessively dilute urine excretion, results when posterior lobe function is lost. Injection of the purest pressor preparations has shown this hormone to have antidiuretic effects when the urine is dilute, as in diabetes insipidus; and to have diuretic effects when injected into animals with normal pituitary function.

THE ADRENAL GLANDS

The adrenal gland is composed of a cortex and a medulla. Steroid hormones are secreted by the cortical tissue; the medullary hormones are amines. The cortex is derived from mesoderm in close association with the developing gonads. The medulla is ectodermal since it is differentiated from the neural crest along with the sympathetic ganglia. Medullary cells are modified ganglion cells and remain in intimate contact with preganglionic fibers of the sympathetic nervous system. It follows, therefore, that medullary secretions are largely under nervous control. In contrast, the cortex has few nerve terminals. Its control is largely humoral, by hormones from the anterior pituitary.

Anatomy

The anatomic relationship of the adrenal gland to the kidneys, renal blood vessels, vena cava and aorta are given in Fig. 29-3. The adrenals are supplied with arterial blood from many small arteries that arise from the inferior phrenic artery superiorly, the adrenal branches of the aorta medially and the renal artery inferiorly. Frequently, additional vessels arise from the ovarian or spermatic artery on the left side and from the intercostals bilaterally. These small vessels join to form sinusoids that are devoid of any endothelial phagocytic

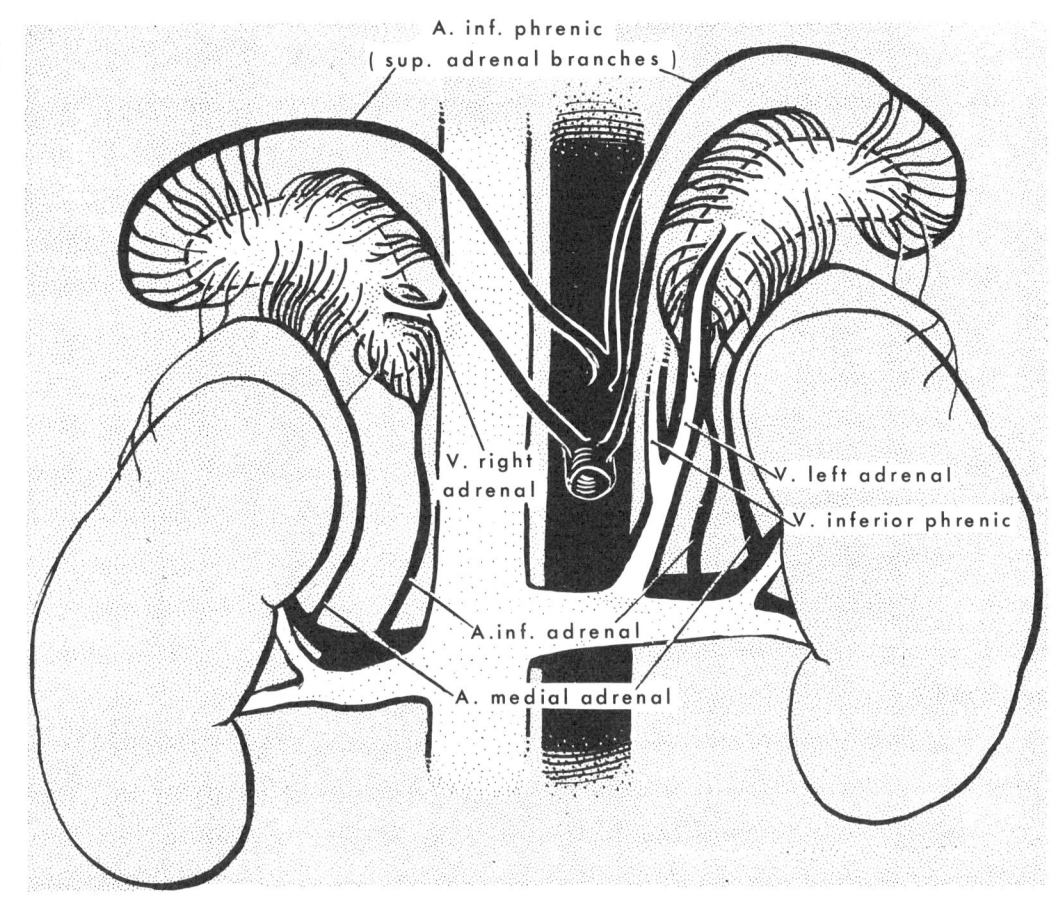

FIG. 29-3. Diagram of the anatomy of the arterial blood supply and venous drainage of the human adrenal glands.

cells. These sinusoids run through the substance of the adrenal cortex and end in large venous lacunae in the medulla. The blood is collected from these lacunae in a large single venous trunk with a thick media (the adrenal vein) as well as other small unnamed veins.

This hemodynamic arrangement explains why blood infections such as tuberculosis destroy the gland more completely, whereas spontaneous atrophy generally affects the innermost layers which are poorly oxygenated and largely spares the glomerulosa which has a richer oxygen supply.

The short right adrenal vein drains medially into the vena cava; the left is often joined by the inferior phrenic vein prior to its entry into the left renal vein.

Histology

Histologically the cells of the adrenal cortex are arranged into three vaguely defined layers:
1. The zona glomerulosa;
2. The zona fasciculata;
3. The zona reticularis.

The zona glomerulosa is the thin layer lying immediately below the capsule and is composed of irregular groups of cells. The zona fasciculata is the widest zone and is composed of radially arranged cords of polyhedral cells. The innermost layer, the zona reticularis, is composed of netlike cords of cells bordering on the adrenal medulla. The zona glomerulosa appears to be little affected by ACTH and produces steroids that function in the regulation of electrolytes. The inner layers produce glu-

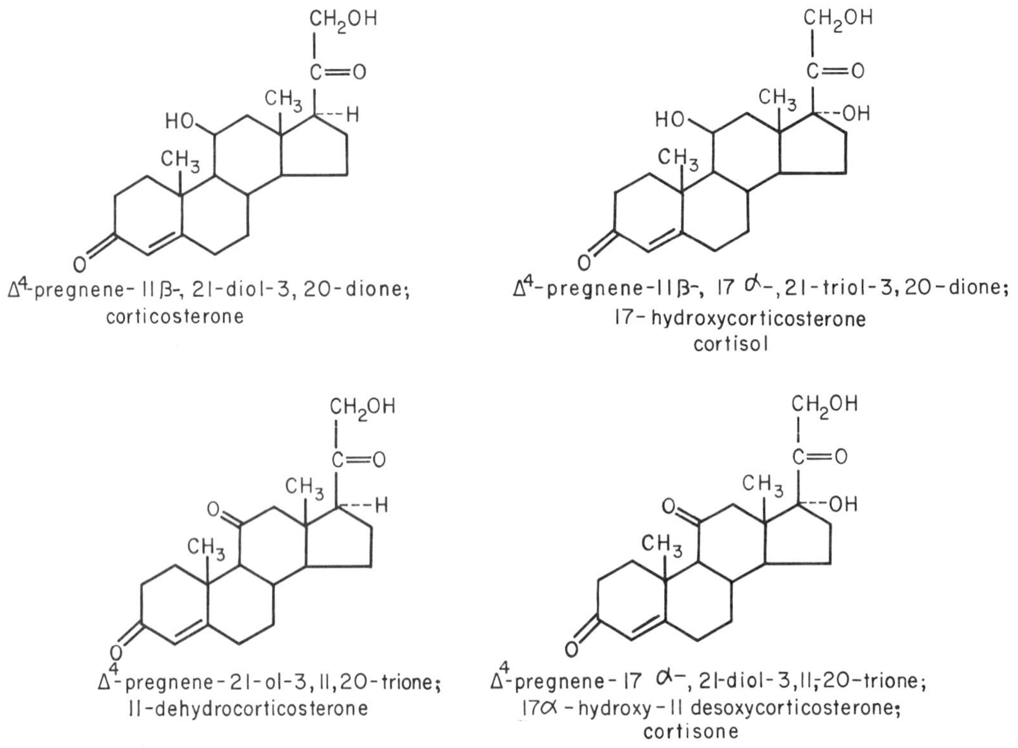

Physiology of the Pituitary and Adrenal Glands

FIG. 29-4. Structure of some steroids of clinical interest.

Δ⁴-pregnene-11β-, 21-diol-3, 20-dione; corticosterone

Δ⁴-pregnene-11β-, 17α-, 21-triol-3, 20-dione; 17-hydroxycorticosterone cortisol

Δ⁴-pregnene-21-ol-3, 11, 20-trione; 11-dehydrocorticosterone

Δ⁴-pregnene-17α-, 21-diol-3, 11, 20-trione; 17α-hydroxy-11 desoxycorticosterone; cortisone

cocorticoids, 17-ketosteroids, progestins and estrogens and are dependent upon corticotropin for growth and secretory stimulation.

Histology of the Medulla. The medulla is composed of masses and strands of cells separated by sinusoidal vessels. Most medullary cells contain fine granules which stain with chromium salts, hence they are called "chromaffin cells." These granules are also stained green with ferric chloride. The adrenal medullary cells are generally regarded as modified postganglionic neurons. The nerve centers involved in controlling medullary secretion are located in the posterior hypothalamus. These centers relay their impulses to the adrenal medulla through the splanchnic nerve.

Adrenocortical Hormones

Since 1930, and as the result of work of many laboratories (Dorfman and Ungar, 1965) 40 or more steroids have been isolated from adrenal cortical tissue or cortical extracts. Most of the steroids isolated from the adrenal cortex possess 21 carbon atoms and 3 or more oxygen atoms. Nineteen-carbon atom steroids are also formed by the adrenal cortex. Of the 40 numerous steroids isolated from adrenal tissue, only three steroids have been demonstrated in human blood—corticosterone, 17-hydroxycorticosterone and aldosterone.

The structure and names of steroids of clinical and physiological interest are given in Figure 29-4.

Relationship of Structure and Physiological Activity. The four key chemical structures that are related to physiologic activity are:

1. The α, β unsaturated ketone group C-3.
2. The ketone oxygen at C-20 adjacent to the primary hydroxyl at C-21.
3. The space orientation of the side chain at C-17.
4. An alcoholic or ketonic oxygen at C-11.

All steroids do not have these four groups. Variation of one or more of these functional groups bestows the biologic variability on the

Physiology and Biochemistry

different steroids. All active adrenal steroids have the α, β unsaturated bond associated with the ketone at C-3. Reduction of either the ketone or the double bond between C-4 and 5 results in loss of activity.

The α ketol side chain is essential to all activity except maintenance of life. Diminished activity is seen with lengthening the α ketolic side chain and by spatial isomers of the C-17 side chain. Reduction of the C-20 ketone or addition of a tertiary hydroxyl at C-17 results also in reduced activity (Fig. 29-5).

Physiologic Activity of Corticoids. Removal of cortical function results in death of the animal, as a result of numerous biochemical disturbances. Since the adrenal gland is only a part of a balanced endocrine system controlled by a neuro-endocrine system, it is hard to assign specific roles to the individual corticoids. It is definite, however, that adrenal hormones are related to:
Fluid and electrolyte balance
Renal function
Carbohydrate and protein metabolism

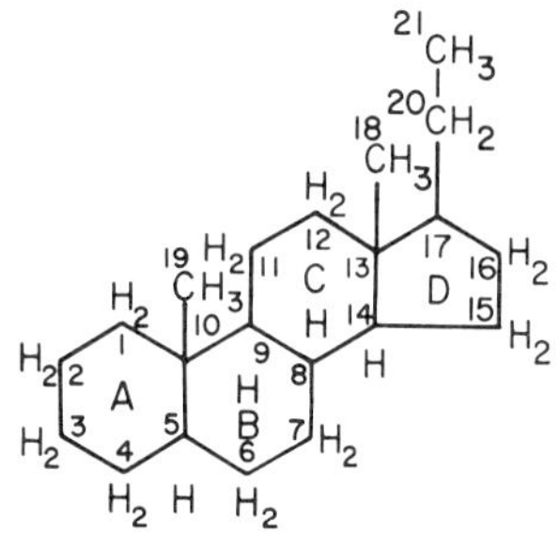

allopregnane

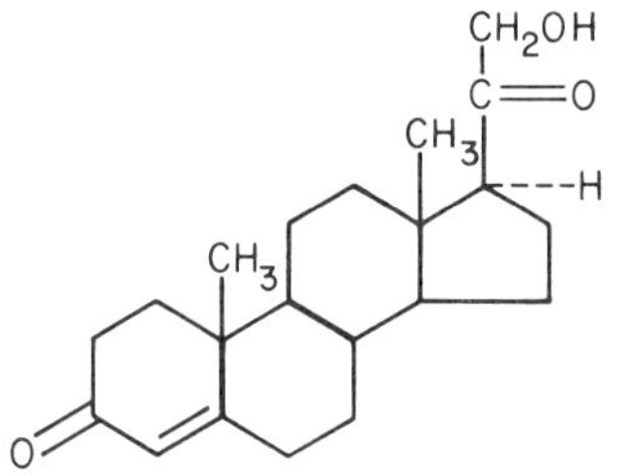

Δ⁴-pregnene-21-ol-3, 20-dione;
11-desoxycorticosterone
(DOC)

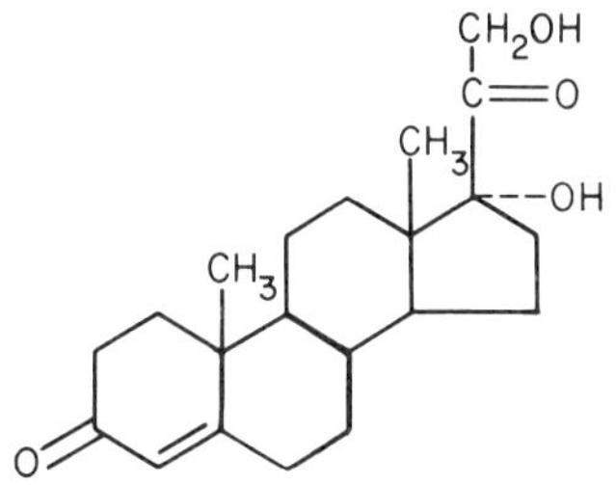

Δ⁴-pregnene-17α-, 21-diol-3,20-dione;
17α-hydroxy-11 desoxycorticosterone,
11-deoxycortisol

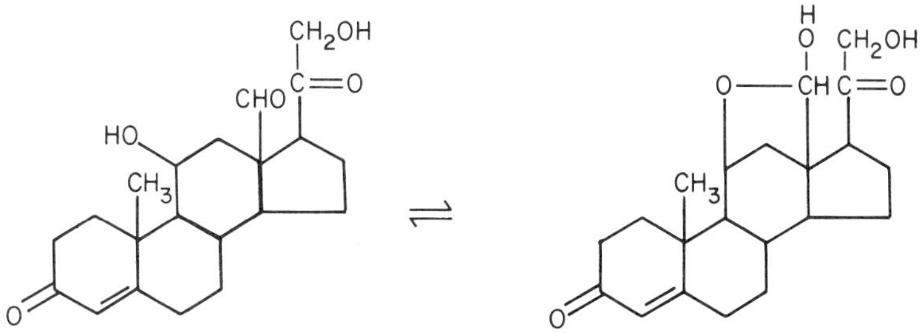

(aldehyde) ⇌ aldosterone (hemiacetal)

Figure 29-5

Growth of young animals
Resistance to stress
Control of blood pressure
Muscle activity

FLUID AND ELECTROLYTE BALANCE. Aldosterone and 11-desoxycorticosterone exert their influence primarily on fluid electrolyte balance.

It has long been known that in Addison's disease or after experimental adrenalectomy a condition develops characterized by the following changes:

Excessive loss of sodium and water
Retention of potassium
Decreased serum sodium
Increased serum potassium
Metabolic acidosis
Decreased plasma and extracellular fluid volume

The Addisonian can be maintained on high sodium, low potassium diets with added sodium bicarbonate. Treatment with 11-desoxycorticosterone or aldosterone will correct the electrolyte disturbance. Cortisone and hydrocortisone are required also for complete restoration of normal adrenal function.

Although aldosterone is known to be of major importance in the control of water and electrolyte balance, its exact mechanism of action is not yet clear.

CARBOHYDRATE METABOLISM. Cortisone and hydrocortisone aid in control of the level of blood sugar. Adrenalectomy produces hypoglycemia and a decrease in liver and muscle glycogen. Many of the effects of glucocorticoids appear related to the decreased gluconeogenesis observed after adrenalectomy.

PROTEIN METABOLISM. Glucocorticoids stimulate gluconeogensis from the metabolism of proteins. Administration of large doses of glucocorticoids produces changes characteristic of protein breakdown such as inhibition of growth, negative nitrogen balance and muscle wasting. These glucocorticoid effects of high steroid concentrations can be harmful in wound healing and recovery of patients in the postoperative period.

FAT METABOLISM. Observed effects of corticoids on fat metabolism are believed to be secondary to the influence of corticoids on protein and carbohydrate metabolism.

MUSCLE FUNCTION. Muscle weakness—a primary symptom in adrenal insufficiency—is reversed by cortisone or hydrocortisone in physiologic doses. Large doses may cause muscle wasting. Corticoids have effects on bone, the central nervous system, the gastrointestinal tract, blood cells and mesenchymal cells. The action of corticoids on these systems is observed only after the administration of large or pharmacologic doses of steroid.

Other Adrenal Steroids isolated from adrenal tissue include two estrogenic C-17 steroids, estrone and equilenin; nine C-19 steroids similar to androgens; and progesterone, pregnenolone and 5β hydroxyallopregnen-20-one.

The relationship of these steroids to normal sex function is not understood. In adrenal tumors and adrenal hyperplasia the various sex hormones can be produced in excessive amounts and, depending on the substance produced, result in feminization or masculinization.

Lymphoid tissue has a marked sensitivity to administration of cortisol, cortisone and other synthetic steroid analogs. Likewise formation of neoplastic lymphoid tissue is inhibited by administration of cortical steroids. Eosinophils are reduced after corticoid therapy—this phenomenon is used to assess the effectiveness of ACTH therapy.

Proliferation of fibroblasts is inhibited by corticoid administration, as is collagen formation. It is this action that makes corticoids of value in the treatment of inflammation.

Catabolism. Many studies on the catabolism of adrenocortical steroids and administered anabolic steroids, involving the isolation and identification of steroid excretory products in the urine, have been carried out. The metabolic pathways of formation of these urinary excretory products are given in detail by several authors (Dorfman and Ungar, 1965). The main reactions are (a) the reduction of both the C-3 ketone and the double bond between carbon atoms 4 and 5, and (b) the removal of the carbon atom side chain to produce C-17 steroids.

Many steroids are conjugated with glucuronic acid at the C-3 hydroxyl group. This conjugation with a water-soluble sugar renders the steroids more water soluble and allows them to be more readily excreted in the urine.

Hormones of the Adrenal Medulla

Epinephrine, also called adrenaline or adrenin, and norepinephrine (noradrenalin) are the two hormones excreted by the adrenal

TABLE 29-3. ADRENERGIC RESPONSE OF EPINEPHRINE AND NOREPINEPHRINE

EFFECT	NOREPINEPHRINE	EPINEPHRINE
Vascular	+	0
Constriction of veins and arteries		
Dilatation of arteries	0	+
Cardiac		
Increase of heart rate	0	+
Increase in atrial contractility and conduction rate	0	+
Increase in conduction velocity of A.V. node	0	+
Increase in ventricular contractility, automaticity and conductive velocity	0	+
Pulmonary		
Dilatation of bronchial musculature	0	+
Metabolic		
Increase fasting blood glucose and free fatty acid levels following formation of cyclic Amp.	±	+

medulla. Both of these hormones (but primarily norepinephrine) are also found in postganglionic nerve fibers. In the medulla the ratio of epinephrine excreted to norepinephrine is 5 to 1. Within the physiologic range epinephrine acts as an over-all vasodilator. It increases blood pressure by increasing cardiac output. Norepinephrine increases blood pressure by an over-all vasoconstrictor effect. There is no change or a slight decrease in cardiac output. The norepinephrine effect on liver breakdown of glycogen to glucose is much smaller than that of epinephrine.

In addition to the circulatory effects, epinephrine rapidly raises blood glucose and lactic acid content in blood. Secretion of epinephrine, therefore, is important in the reaction to acute emergencies.

Four mechanisms of inactivation of catecholamines are known. Probably the most important mechanism is the reuptake of catecholamines by the storage granules which are located at the nerve endings. Two enzymatic inactivation mechanisms appear to be of less importance. Catechol-o-methyl transferase (COMT) is responsible for the initial inactivation of physiologic amounts of circulating catecholamines. Monoamine oxidase (MAO) apparently has little function in inactivating circulating catecholamines. Monoamine oxidase is thought to be of importance for the rapid inactivation of catecholamines as they are released from the storage granules into the cytoplasm by the nerve endings. Excretion of catecholamines unchanged into the urine is a minor route of biologic inactivation of catecholamines.

Chemical Tests for Catecholamines

Blood catecholamines are difficult to measure and these determinations are usually done

TABLE 29-4. NORMAL RANGE OF CATECHOLAMINE AND METABOLITE CONCENTRATION

Urine	
Catecholamine*	
Norepinephrine	10-70 µg./24 hrs.
Epinephrine	0-20 µg./24 hrs.
Normetanephrine and Metanephrine	< 1.3 mg./24 hrs.
Vanilmandelic acid	1.8-9.0 mg./24 hrs.
Dopamine	< 20 µg./24 hrs.
Blood	
Catecholamines	< 1 µg./liter
Adrenal Medulla	
Norepinephrine	0.04-0.16 mg./Gm.
Epinephrine	0.22-0.84 mg./Gm.

* Urinary total catecholamines in pheochromocytoma > 300 µg./day.

Urine collections should be made over a 24-hour period and should contain 15 ml. of 6N HCl. To simplify interpretation, certain drugs and foodstuffs that might interfere with the test should be withdrawn at least 48 hours before collection of the urine specimen. Drugs such as exogenous catecholamines, highly fluorescent compounds (e.g., tetracyclines), and antihypertensive agents such as α-methyldopa interfere with catecholamine determination but not with VMA and metanephrine determinations.

Monoamine oxidase inhibitors cause misleading increase in urinary metanephrine and a decrease in VMA secretion.

Several VMA screening tests detect other phenolic substances, and, therefore, patients should be given no coffee, vanilla and certain vegetables and fruits prior to the test.

TABLE 29-5. SUMMARY OF CONTROL MECHANISMS OF HORMONE SECRETION*

CONTROL MECHANISM	SYSTEM CONTROLLED		DESCRIPTION OF CONTROL MECHANISM
Simple endocrine control	Insulin → blood sugar Glucogen → blood sugar Parathyroid hormone → plasma calcium thyrocalcitonin → plasma calcium Aldosterone → plasma sodium (to some extent)	(diagram: E.G. and Cell with arrows X→, h, X'—, inhibitor)	Hormone (h) released from endocrine gland (E.G.) (→) acts on target (cell) to release a substance which by negative feedback (- - →) inhibits E.G. production of h. X and X' are factors acting independently of the feedback loop and influencing the endocrine gland or cell.
Endocrine control by release of a hormone precursor (hormogen) from one organ and activation of the hormone by enzyme released from a second organ	Angiotensinogen → angiotensin → aldosterone	(diagram: EOA (releases enzyme), EOB (releases hormonogen), Enzyme + Hormone → EG → cell; Inhibits; X→, X'→)	Hormone precursor (hormonogen) released by EOB is activated by enzyme released by EOA to produce hormone (h) which acts as tropic hormone on peripheral cells.
Endocrine control by hypothalamus → endocrine gland → target cell mechanism	Posterior pituitary → vasopressin → kidney and plasma H$_2$O (neural control between hypothalamus and E.G.) Adrenal medulla → epinephrine (neural control between hypothalamus and E.G.) Anterior pituitary → growth hormone	(diagram: CNS → Hypothalamus → (N) or (h) → (EG) → h → cell; X→, X'→, X"→)	Neurogenic signal from CNS stimulates hypothalamus to give a neural (N) or a hormonal (h) signal to endocrine gland (E.G.) which acts on cell by secretion of specific hormone (h); (——→) represents inhibition by secretion from cell. X, X', X" are additional factors which modulate respectively the activity of the hypothalamus endocrine gland or cell

TABLE 29-5. SUMMARY OF CONTROL MECHANISMS OF HORMONE SECRETIONS (*Continued*)

CONTROL MECHANISM	SYSTEM CONTROLLED	DESCRIPTION OF CONTROL MECHANISM
Endocrine control by hypothalamus → anterior pituitary → endocrine gland → target cell mechanism	Hypothalamic control of thyroxine, cortisol. Gonadal hormones are similar but additional positive feedback loops serve to coordinate sequential release of the pituitary and sex hormones.	CNS acts on hypothalamus by neural mechanism. Hypothalamus produces hormone (h_1), which activates anterior pituitary (AP) to release h_2, which stimulates EG to produce h_3, which exerts negative feedback control mainly on hypothalamus. There is some evidence that some h_3 feedback control (⎯⎯→) is exerted on anterior pituitary. X, X', X'' are factors regulating respectively and independently activities of hypothalamic anterior pituitary, endocrine gland and cell.

$$X \longrightarrow \text{Hypothalamus} \overset{\text{CNS}}{\longleftarrow}$$
$$\quad\quad\quad\quad (h_1) \downarrow$$
$$X' \longrightarrow \text{AP}$$
$$\quad\quad\quad\quad (h_2) \downarrow$$
$$X'' \longrightarrow \text{EG}$$
$$\quad\quad\quad\quad (h_3) \downarrow$$
$$X''' \longrightarrow \text{cell}$$

*Summarized from Rasmussen, H. S. (1968)

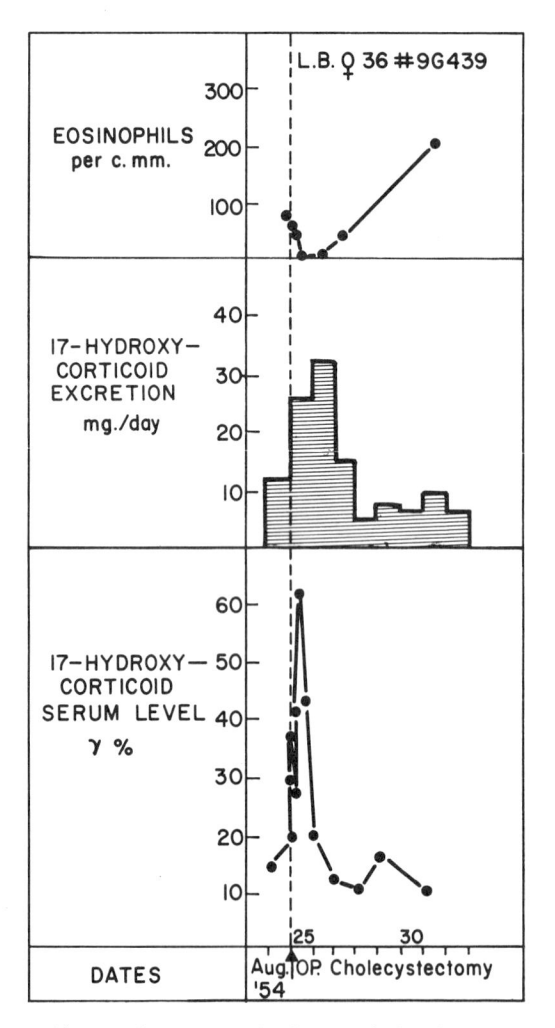

FIG. 29-6. Pituitary-adrenal response to an uncomplicated surgical procedure and anesthesia. Patient LB, age 36, underwent a cholecystectomy for removal of gallstones. Anesthesia was induced with ether and maintained for about one hour until the incision was made. Note that the corticoid concentration rose in response to ether induction (first spike in curve beginning at arrow). The cholecystectomy produced a further rise.

By the next morning the corticosteroid concentrations were back down to essentially the normal range. Had sepsis or other complications developed, the steroid level would have remained elevated or risen to a high value.

Note also that the blood steroid level showed little change in the immediate postoperative period. The eosinophil count remained low for 2 to 3 days.

The urinary excretion of 17-hydroxy corticosteroids was measured by the method of Reddy, Jenkins and Thorn. This is a measure of the total of 17-hydroxy corticosteroids in the urine. Most of this urinary steroid is in the conjugated form and the greater part is reduced to the tetrahydro derivative before conjugation.

Note that the peak of urinary secretion comes the day after operation, indicating that the downslope of the free blood steroid after operation is in part due to conjugation, hydrogenation, inactivation and excretion of steroid, as well as to its decreased output from the adrenal. This steroid excretion pattern is characteristic of noncomplicated surgery with little tissue injury. (Redrawn from Moore, F. D., Metabolic Care of the Surgical Patient. p. 81, Philadelphia, W. B. Saunders, 1959)

in research laboratories. The clinician, however, can gain useful information from quantitative tests measuring urinary excretion of catecholamines and their metabolites, metanephrine, normetanephrine and vanilmandelic acid (VMA). The normal range of catecholamine concentrations in urine, blood and adrenal medulla and that for urinary VMA and normetanephrine are listed in Table 29-4.

Endocrine Control Mechanisms

The various mechanisms that control the hormone secretion of the various endocrine glands are summarized in Table 29-5. The mechanisms outlined in this table are those described by Rasmussen (1968).

RESPONSE IN SURGICAL STRESS

Pituitary-Adrenocortical Changes After Surgery

Increased excretion of adrenal corticoids has been recognized as a normal response to stress (Moore, 1959) ever since the original work of Braune and Cope. These investigators demonstrated significant increase in urinary 17-ketosteroids after trauma and burns. With the development of better methods for measuring plasma and urinary steroids, it has been demonstrated that 17-hydroxycorticoids are increased after all surgical trauma also.

The increase in 17-hydroxycorticoids corresponds to the fall in eosinophils. In the first four days after trauma, increased steroid excretion correlates well with increased total urinary nitrogen excretion; after this period, there is no further correspondence. By the use of thin-layer and paper chromatographic methods, all steroid changes in the postoperative period can now be isolated and identified. The results of such studies have not changed the basic concept of adenocortical function in the postoperative period.

Aldosterone Increases in Response to Dehydration, Salt Loss and Hemorrhage. Aldosterone assays are now available in most medical centers, however, owing to the difficulty of the assay these studies are generally done only in special cases.

The adrenocortical response to mild surgical trauma—e.g., in a cholecystectomy—lasts only about 24 hours (Fig. 29-6), whereas in a case with multiple complications, the response lasts throughout the periods of the stress associated with the complications (Fig. 29-7).

Since the mechanism by which adrenal steroids exert their action in the various tissues is not known, the function of the postoperative steroid increases also remains unknown.

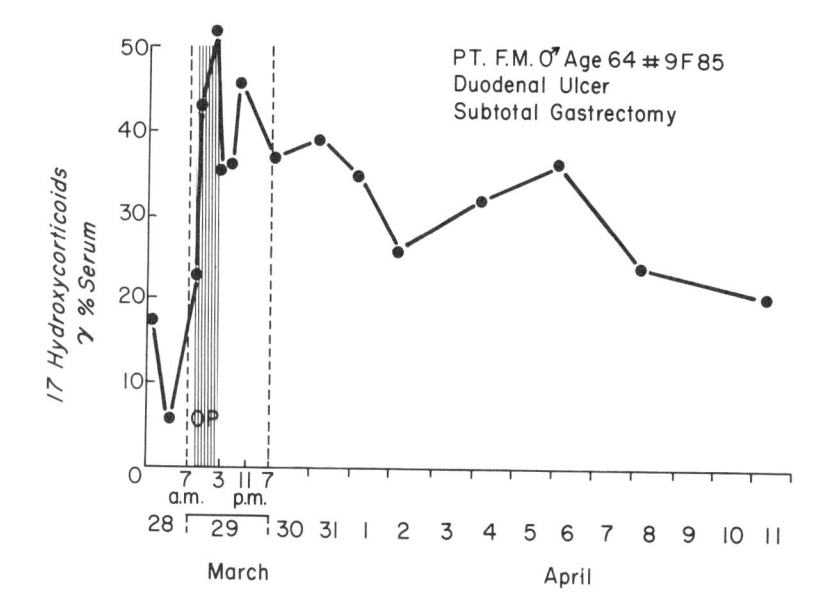

FIG. 29-7. Corticosteroid concentrations in blood of a patient who had undergone a subtotal gastrectomy for duodenal ulcer, with complications in the postoperative course.

The patient had severe pain in the right upper quadrant with spasm and tenderness 4 days after operation. In the four days after operation he was afebrile, but after the onset of pain on the fourth day he ran a low grade fever until approximately the eighth postoperative day. Neither symptoms nor physical signs were severe enough to demand re-exploration. It was presumed that he had a small area of peritonitis in the subhepatic region, which was handled without drainage. The blood steroid curve increased in response to the operation and after the onset of the right upper quadrant pain on the fourth day. After the eighth postoperative day the steroid level decreased slowly; 14 days after operation it had not returned to normal. The eosinophil count remained depressed throughout this time, indicating an increase in pituitary secretion of ACTH in response to the stress of the postoperative complication.

The patient's final convalescence was uneventful. (Redrawn from Moore, F. D.: Metabolic Care of the Surgical Patient. p. 91, Philadelphia, W. B. Saunders, 1959)

DIAGNOSIS OF ADRENAL AND PITUITARY INSUFFICIENCY
(Soffer, Dorfman, and Gabrilove, 1961)

In an acute adrenal crisis, the presence of dehydration and shock with a low serum sodium, elevated serum potassium and increased urinary excretion of sodium, together with darkly pigmented skin, is enough to establish the diagnosis of acute adrenal insufficiency. Improvement of symptoms after administration of adrenal steroids confirms the diagnosis.

Diagnosis of adrenal insufficiency in the absence of a crisis is more subtle and depends upon the clinical picture and laboratory evidence of impaired adrenocortical function. The following laboratory findings are useful for this purpose:

1. A reduction in the plasma levels of 17-hydroxycorticosteroids, and their failure to rise following intravenous or intramuscular injection of corticotropin.

2. A lack of increase in the urinary excretion of the neutral 17-ketosteroids and 17-hydroxycorticoids following an 8-hour intravenous infusion of 25 I.U. of corticotropin on two successive days, or after injection of 25 I.U. of corticotropin every 6 hours for 48 hours.

3. Lack of an adequate 5-hour urine volume response following the oral administration of a water load, and improvement in the response, after the water loading, by administration of a glucogenic steroid.

4. An increase in salivary Na/K ratio above 2.0.

5. The salt deprivation test, with resultant clinical and laboratory evidence of acute adrenal insufficiency.

6. A reduction of less than 50 per cent in the peripheral eosinophil count 4 hours after intramuscular injection of 25 I.U. of corticotropin.

7. A decrease in 24-hour excretion of the neutral 17-ketosteroids and 17-hydroxycorticoids.

8. A reduction of the serum sodium and elevation of serum potassium levels.

9. The roentgen demonstration of calcium in the region of both adrenals, in the presence of a suggestive clinical picture.

10. Hypoglycemia and an increase in blood urea nitrogen.

PATHOLOGIC CHANGES CAUSED BY EXCESS OF ADRENAL STEROIDS OR ACTH

Treatment with adrenocortical steroids and potent synthetic derivatives of naturally occurring steroids (Soffer, 1961; Curii, 1962; Applezweig, 1962) may produce physiologic and morphologic abnormalities both in man and in laboratory animals. Likewise, administration of excessive doses of ACTH activates the adrenal cortex to produce dangerous amounts of steroids. Side effects resulting from high steroid level are hypertension, edema and congestive heart failure. Hyperglycemia and glycosuria may occur in individuals predisposed to diabetes. Convulsive episodes have been observed in patients on prolonged ACTH. Mental changes also have been observed.

Gastric and duodenal ulcers are not uncommon complications of corticotropin and steroid therapy. Some patients on prolonged steroid therapy develop osteoporosis and pathologic fractures. Wound healing may be delayed when patients are maintained on high doses of corticoids. Adrenal function may be impaired after prolonged steroid therapy, owing to the inhibition of ACTH secretion by the pituitary as a result of high corticoid levels.

REFERENCES

Albert, A. (ed.). Human Pituitary Gonadotropins—A Workshop Conference. Springfield, Ill., Charles C Thomas, 1961.

Applezweig, N.: Steroid Drugs. New York, McGraw-Hill, 1962.

Bates, R. W., and Condliff, P. G.: Recent Prog. Hormone Res., 16:309, 1960.

Brown, J. H. U., and Barker, S. B.: Basic Endocrinology. Philadelphia, F. Davis, 1962.

Curii, A. R., Symington, T., and Grant, J. K.: The Human Adrenal Cortex. Baltimore, The Williams and Wilkins Co., 1962.

Dixon, H. B. F.: *In*: The Hormones, Pincus, G., Thuman, K. U., and Astwood, E. B. (eds.): vol. 5. New York, Academic Press, 1964.

Dorfman, R. A., and Ungar, F.: Metabolism of Steroids. New York, Academic Press, 1965.

du Vigneaud, Ressler, C., and Tripput, S. J. Biol. Chem., 205:949, 1953.

Fevald, H. L.: *In*: The Chemistry and Physiology of Hormones. Washington, D. C., American Association for the Advance of Science, 1944.

Li, C. H.: *In*: Von Euler, U. S., and Heller, H. (eds.). Comparative Endocrinology. New York, Academic Press, 1963.

Li, C. H., and Evans, H. M.: Recent Prog. Hormone Res., 3:3, 1948.

Moore, F. D.: Metabolic Care of the Surgical Patient. Philadelphia, W. B. Saunders, 1959.

Rasmussen, H.: *In*: Robert H. Williams (ed.): Textbook of Endocrinology. Philadelphia, W. B. Saunders, 1968.

Soffer, L. J., Dorfman, R. I., and Gabrilove, J. L.: The Human Adrenal Gland. Philadelphia, Lea & Febiger, 1961.

CHAPTER 29, SECTION 2

J. GARROTT ALLEN, M.D.

Pituitary and Adrenal Glands
Their Interrelationships, Hyperplasia, Endocrine-producing Adenomas and Carcinomas

Pituitary Gland
  The Anterior Lobe
  Hypophysectomy, Its Complications and the "Posterior" Lobe Hormones
  Controlled Radiative Destruction of Pituitary
Adrenal Gland
  General Considerations
  Adrenal Cortex
  Adrenal Medulla

Pituitary function and its interrelationships with those of other endocrine organs and its broad influence upon many metabolic functions of the body place this organ in a category of unusual interest. In recent years, its interaction and interdependence upon adrenal cortical functions have caught the imaginations of many. The developments in the fields of pituitary-adrenal relationships have occurred so rapidly that it is still impossible to discuss the general subject with any degree of finality at this time. This point of view and caution are emphasized by Cooper and by Moore in their respective writings in this book.

PITUITARY GLAND

THE ANTERIOR LOBE

The anterior lobe of the pituitary is known to produce at least 6 different hormones. With the exception of ACTH, TSH, and growth hormone, the rest have not been sufficiently purified to permit their repeated injection in man without risk of sensitization. Thus far, these hormones appear to be proteins or polypeptides. The question as to whether the corresponding hormones of the anterior pituitary derived from different species are chemically and biologically identical remains unsettled. Species differences are known to exist for the growth hormones. The hormones of the pituitary and adrenal glands have been identified in Section 1 of Chapter 29.

Those conditions resulting from excessive hormone production may call for surgical consideration directed toward partial or total hypophysectomy. Of particular concern at present are excesses in production of ACTH and the growth hormone. With the exception of growth hormone, the other 5 tropic hormones appear to direct their action toward specific organs. However, there is an increasing evidence that some systemic responses, as well as those of the "target" organs, may occur with some of the other hormones also.

Human Growth Hormone (HGH)

This hormone probably is produced by the eosinophilic cells of the anterior pituitary, but other pituitary components also may take an active part in its elaboration, directly or indirectly. Growth or somatic hormone appears to regulate growth of the skin and of bone and cartilage. Visceral growth and, to a lesser extent, growth of the vascular system also are affected. Growth hormone has little effect upon growth of the brain.

Growth hormone favors a positive nitrogen balance, characteristic of growth and other anabolic states. However, in order that a positive nitrogen balance may be obtained with growth hormone, insulin appears to be essential and may act in a cofactor role. Carbohydrate metabolism is also profoundly affected by growth hormone. In the absence of the hypophysis, extreme sensitivity to insulin develops, and the individual is unable to maintain his glycogen stores during the fasting state; he is unable to develop severe diabetes mellitus after pancreatectomy, as pointed out 40 years ago by Houssay. Growth hormone appears to be synonymous with the diabetogenic hormone or to be closely allied with it; its influence upon carbohydrate metabolism appears to be independent of that governed by the adrenal cortex (see below).

Growth hormone causes an increase in size of many tissues without accelerating the rate of maturation or promoting sexual development. It appears to function without apparent aid from other pituitary hormones. In the absence of thyroid hormone, growth hormone is less effective. It acts to enhance anabolism of protein more than of fat; with it, positive nitrogen balance has been achieved in man on a calorically inadequate diet, and blood urea is decreased. A rise in serum fatty acids occurs with very small doses, and larger doses produce diabetes which may become permanent. Hypophysectomy in man has been successfully used in the treatment of diabetic retinopathy (Pearson et al., 1964). Phosphorus and calcium are retained and calcium absorption is enhanced (see Table 29-6).

Species specificity has retarded progress in this field because the risks of reactions in man from the administration of growth hormones from other species present a formidable problem, though, of greater importance, its effectiveness is so diminished as to be clinically useless. Simian growth hormone may be effective but has not been used for a long enough period of time. At present, the only reliable source of clinically useful material is from man himself. At this time, enough human growth hormone (HGH) to meet the needs of 1 patient for 1 year requires 50 to 100 human pituitary glands.

Its action is unique in that no single target tissue or organ seems to exist; most, if not all, tissues seem to be affected by its presence or absence. Clearly, too, its effect is not only upon growth, for its production does not cease when growth ceases, and its concentration in plasma and, indeed, in the pituitary itself remains relatively constant throughout life. Growth ceases but the hormone lingers on. Virtually unique among hormones, no feedback mechanism to dampen its production

TABLE 29-6. EFFECTS OF HUMAN GROWTH HORMONE REPORTED TO OCCUR IN MAN*

EFFECT	
Growth promotion	Increase in fat mobilization:
Anabolic by balance study:	Increase in plasma free fatty acids
Nitrogen storage	Ketogenic effect
Phosphorus storage	Effects on carbohydrate metabolism:
Potassium storage	
Sodium storage (not regularly)	Diminution in insulin sensitivity
Calcium absorption increased	No change or decrease in glucose tolerance
Decrease in blood urea nitrogen	Transient fall in blood sugar
Slow increase in serum phosphorous & alkaline phosphatase	Increase in urinary citrate
Increase in calcium in urine	Enlargement of chloride space
Increase in serum "sulfation factor"	Increase in renal clearance of inulin, creatinine, PAH & Tm_{PAH}

* Raben, M. S.: Growth hormone. I. Physiologic aspects. New Eng. J. Med., 266:31, 1962.

rate has been described thus far. It appears to circulate with a half-life of about 30 minutes.

Although HGH has proved to be clinically useful in a variety of conditions, it is still to be considered as an experimental tool—first, because its advantages and disadvantages need to be defined, along with dosage requirements, and second, until another source for growth hormone can be found (preferably synthetic), its availability precludes extensive clinical use. Its uses in surgery would seem to be many, and one of these may be to reverse catabolic states in cachectic diseases—cancer, trauma, infection, and in protracted postoperative care —all yet to be established.

Acromegaly and Gigantism. These syndromes are generally the result of an adenoma of the pituitary, usually of its eosinophilic tissue. In some patients, eosinophilic hyperplasia without adenoma may be responsible. In still others, more than one cell type and more than this hormone alone may be involved in the primary disease so that the clinical picture may become mixed and less well-defined.

Much of the information remaining in ques-

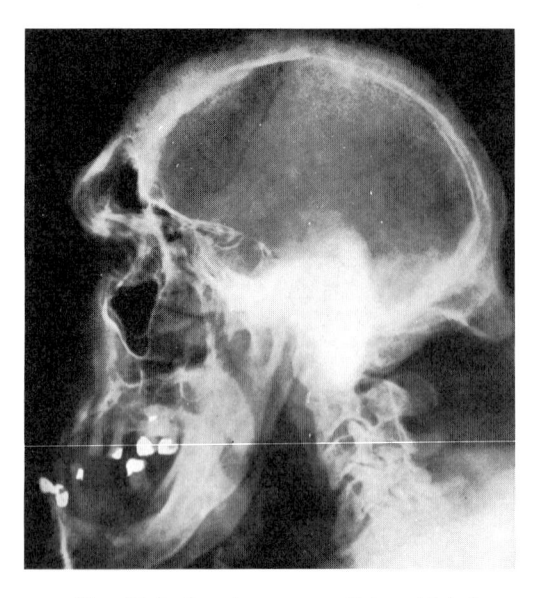

FIG. 29-8. Roentgenogram (14 × 17 in.) of skull in acromegaly. Note (1) enlarged sella, 32 × 25 mm.; (2) huge paranasal sinuses; (3) prognathism; (4) increased thickness but not increased density of tables of skull; (5) exostosis of occiput.

tion would be clarified were there suitable methods for assay or analysis of growth hormone, though recently much progress has been made in this area. Such technics would help especially in determining how often the disease totally destroys the pituitary and leaves the patient ultimately with moderate to severe hypopituitarism; whether in such patients there is cyclic function with periods of "rest"; or whether the disease continues to progress slowly with growth hormone continuing to be elaborated in excess of normal.

The enlarging pituitary eventually exerts its pressure upon the sella turcica. Several changes in this bony structure may then be demonstrated roentgenologically. By no means, however, is the absence of these findings to be considered as excluding pituitary disease when there are other sound grounds to suspect its presence. However, as the pituitary enlarges, the sella generally does also. Usually its floor is depressed, and its cavity is ballooned out. Its dorsum may be displaced somewhat posteriorly and in time may be eroded and destroyed along with the clinoid processes. When this state of affairs obtains and is demonstrated roentgenographically, it is diagnostic of abnormal pituitary enlargement, regardless of cause. On the other hand, fairly wide ranges of variations in the size of the normal sella occur—8 to 12 mm. in depth and 9 to 16 mm. in length, respectively, are the usual extremes of normality as measured on the skull roentgenogram. Figure 29-8 is a roentgenogram of an acromegalic patient with a pituitary tumor in which the sella measures 32 mm. in length and 25 mm. in depth. This film also demonstrates the huge excavations of the paranasal sinuses, the increase in length and breadth of the mandible with blunting of its angle and thickening of the orbital ridge, so characteristic of acromegaly.

Among the somatic changes occurring in acromegaly and/or gigantism are the following:

Changes in bony structure. Those that occur from growth hormone-producing tumors are modified considerably by the age of the patient at the time the onset of its excessive secretion begins. If the onset occurs prior to ossification of the epiphyseal plates of the long bones, the rate of growth is accelerated and the duration of growth prior to epiphyseal closures usually is prolonged by several years beyond that of the normal. Until epiphyseal ossification takes place, the excessive rates of growth are fairly uniform. Thereafter, growth continues in isolated skeletal areas, particularly the mandible, the maxilla, the orbital ridges, the bones of the hands and the feet, with thickening of the long bones and of the vertebrae (Fig. 29-9). Later, the characteristics of acromegaly may be superimposed upon those of gigantism, should the patient with gigantism live long enough. When excessive elaboration of growth hormone does not occur until after full and normal growth has been attained with epiphyseal closures effected, only acromegaly occurs. More often the latter is observed; such patients often survive beyond 50 years of age.

With the continued growth of the mandible, prognathism becomes a prominent feature of acromegaly. The teeth protrude beyond the incisors of the maxilla, and the mandibular overgrowth causes a separation of its teeth. The bones of the hands and the feet are usually enlarged in pronounced acromegaly and are associated with tufting of the terminal phalanges. However, part of the enlargement or "spading" of the digits is due to thickening of the skin, subcutaneous and periarticular tissue.

Although the rate of osteogenesis is accelerated, so also is that of bony resorption. The end result is that the enlarged bones contain less calcium per gram of tissue rather than more. Calcium absorption and excretion are both enhanced, with the net result that they largely cancel out; citrate in the urine is increased. Blood volume expands and is associated with an increase in the total quantity of exchangeable sodium.

The epiphyseal plates, if still active, continue to promote longitudinal growth. Ossification of cartilages is normally favored by sexual maturity because of the increased production of sex hormones and gonadal activity at this time. In excessive production of growth hormone, however, gonadal activity and the sex hormones are reduced; hence, the delayed ossification may be explained on the basis of the hypogonadism, permitting further growth than might otherwise occur.

Enlargement or growth of the cartilaginous structures of the ears, the nose and the larynx add further to the grotesque features that these patients eventually display. Aside from disfiguring enlargement of the ears and the nose, caused by the cartilaginous overgrowth, the voice is deepened, often rasping in character, due to an overgrowth of the cartilaginous structures of the larynx. The growth of the costal cartilages in excessive, causing an abnormal enlargement of the bony thorax which, along with the usual dorsal kyphosis and elongated extremities, imparts the gorillalike features that many of these patients display.

Skin Changes. Enlargement of the soft parts of hands, feet, face, nose and lips often is nearly as disfiguring as are the skeletal changes. The skin thickens, and hypertrichosis is commonly noted. The total mass of sweat glands is said to be increased. Connective tissue is excessive within the skin, as well as in the subcutaneous and submucosal areas. The brow and the face often take on the "bulldog" appearance. The fibrous proliferation about the joints contributes to the arthritic complaints that many of these patients express. The ligamentous attachments (Sharpey's fibers) like-

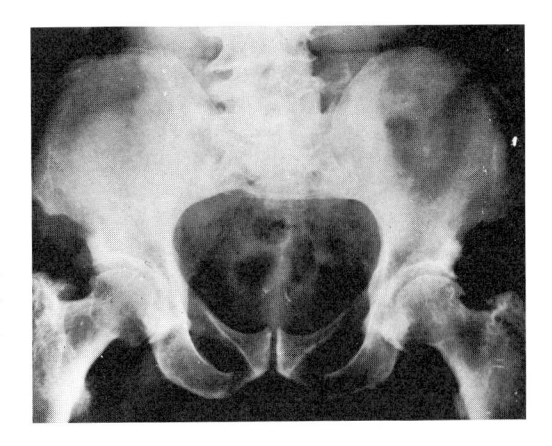

FIG. 29-9. This picture demonstrates the increased width of the bony pelvis, the 17-inch roentgenogram being scarcely large enough to contain both ilial wings. Note ossifications at sites of attachments of abductor muscle to greater trochanters, the increase in width of L-5, and the osteoarthritis of lower spine and hip sockets.

wise increase, favoring immobility; actually they may become encased or ossified at their sites of attachment to bone as the bones increase in diameter, particularly the spine (Fig. 29-9).

Organ Hypertrophy. This is the rule in advanced acromegaly, with or without gigantism. The tongue enlarges, becoming broader and thicker, and the papillae hypertrophy. The heart may exceed by several times its normal weight. The weight of the liver may be increased by more than 100 per cent of its normal limits. Similar increases are frequently noted in lungs, adrenals, pancreas, intestine, thymus and kidneys. However, the brain does not increase in weight, although the perineural tissue of the peripheral nerves often proliferate, contributing to the paresthesia and the numbness often encountered. Enlargement of the ganglia also usually occurs. It is suspected that some of the neurologic complaints are due to vascular insufficiency and tension upon the nerves in gigantism, caused by the stretch effect of unusual longitudinal growth. Personality changes may occur.

Physiologic disturbances created by the enlargement of organs are related primarily to the heart, the skeletal muscle and possibly to the unusual stretch of arteries and nerves when gigantism is present. Fragmentation of the individual muscle fibers of the heart and hypertension (probably not related) are fairly common findings. Diabetes mellitus is detectable in 15 to 20 per cent of patients, presumably from the demonstrated degeneration of islet cell tissue from the diabetogenic effect of growth hormone. It may be insulin-resistant. Early, sexual drive may be increased; later, impotence often occurs.

Many patients display an increase in basal metabolic rate; findings of plus 20 to 30 or more are not uncommon. Exophthalmos also may occur along with other features of hyperthyroidism, including tachycardia and goiter. These occur with sufficient frequency to present a confusing diagnostic picture at times. Presumably the thyroid changes result from coexisting excessive secretion of thyrotropic hormone (TSH).

In some patients with acromegaly, muscular strength even in fairly advanced stages of the disease may remain excellent for many years. For example, the roentgenographic illustrations of acromegaly in Figures 29-8 and 29-9 are those made of a professional wrestler who continued several engagements a week for many years after severe skeletal and cutaneous manifestations of his disease first appeared. He abandoned his wrestling career only 2 years prior to death at the age of 50. In others, however, muscular strength, while pronounced and perhaps greater than that of the normal in the early stages of the disease, is eventually superseded by weakness, the explanation of which is wanting.

CLINICAL FINDINGS AND DIAGNOSIS. If uncomplicated and other concurrent abnormalities such as hyperthyroidism or myxedema (latent) are not marked, skeletal and cutaneous changes together usually make the diagnosis of acromegaly obvious. Confirmation of this clinical picture by roentgenographic demonstration of erosion of the posterior sella, with ballooning of the sella and destruction of the clinoid processes, establish the diagnosis beyond question.

In patients in whom such changes are less severe or those who are seen early in the stages of their disease, the diagnosis may not be established so easily. Often the first complaints are those of paresthetic hyperesthesia, pains about the joints associated with headaches, and impotence. These are the complaints so often associated with functional disorders or other ill-defined entities that acromegaly may not be considered. Moreover, the sella may appear perfectly normal in spite of the presence of an adenoma; the sella enlarges only as the tumor increases in size. In other patients with similarly mild complaints, the sella may be enlarged beyond average size but still remain within the normal range, causing one to suspect acromegaly, when in reality some other disorder may be at fault, especially hyperthyroidism or functional complaints.

Visual fields may be distorted in time if the tumor ruptures the diaphragm above the sella and exerts pressure upon the optic chiasm. Classically, loss of color vision precedes loss of the ability to recognize shape and form. Bitemporal hemianopsia, when present, is usually a latent development and eventually total blindness may occur in a few of these patients. Visual field disturbances are found in about 20 per cent of patients. Choking of the optic disks is seldom encountered, presumably because the tumor is slow-growing and is small by comparison with other intracranial tumors. The adenoma may become cystic.

Laboratory aids may become more specific than in the past, but the several "new leads" that have occurred have not been extensively tested. Technics for the measurement of growth hormone have been substantially improved but, for routine clinical use, are only now being evaluated. The increase in metabolic rate and the diabetic type of glucose tolerance curve, occasionally with frank, frequently insulin-resistant, diabetes, are valuable diagnostic aids when in the presence of physical findings and x-ray observations compatible with acromegaly.

TREATMENT of acromegaly with or without gigantism centers about the ablation of pituitary function. This has been pursued historically along 3 lines: hypophysectomy, external x-radiation, and more recently local radiation (Harper et al., 1964).

Hypophysectomy as performed by Cushing was incomplete. This occurred not only for technical reasons, but because it now appears that total hypophysectomy in man creates an addisonian state requiring exogenous cortisone or ACTH to sustain life. As the clinical usefulness of these substances was not explored until a decade after Cushing's death, hypophysectomy probably was doomed to fail in his time, irrespective of the development status of surgical technic.

Recent experience with hypophysectomy suggests that once again its usage may be explored. However, most of the good results reported are in patients with normal glands in whom its removal is employed as a palliative measure in the management of breast carcinoma. Removal of pituitary tumors presents more difficulty and is not performed so readily.

X-radiation therapy to the pituitary has proved to be partially effective in the treatment of acromegaly and gigantism in many patients. Fortunately, brain tissue and the optic nerves are fairly resistant to radiation. Dosages of 3,000 r carefully administered over a period of 3 to 4 weeks are generally employed.

Local Irradiation Implants. More recently, stereotaxic placement of yttrium-90 beads throughout the pituitary has been employed, especially by Evans and Rasmussen, with Harper (see Chap. 9, "The Principles of Isotope Technics in Surgery"). Radon seeds have been similarly employed by Illingworth and colleagues. The dosages of such radiation are designed so as to ablate completely all pituitary tissue without damage to the neighboring hypothalamus and optic nerves. The ultimate place of this combined form of radiation and surgery remains to be determined (Fig. 29-10).

The urgency of diagnosis, particularly in the presence of gigantism among the young, cannot be stressed too strongly. This disorder, even more than that of untreated acromegaly, is likely to lead to serious social maladjustment, with the creation of difficulty and intense psychological problems in the shortened life span. Death usually occurs before the age of 30 in serious gigantism. These are a lonely lot of patients—almost outcasts. Therefore, the treatment to be undertaken should be effective and carried out as soon as the diagnosis can be made.

Pituitary Dwarfism. In the absence or the severely diminished production of growth hormone, dwarfism results. As this is of no surgical consequence, here it is referred to only briefly because it appears to be the counterpart of gigantism. Patients with this condition

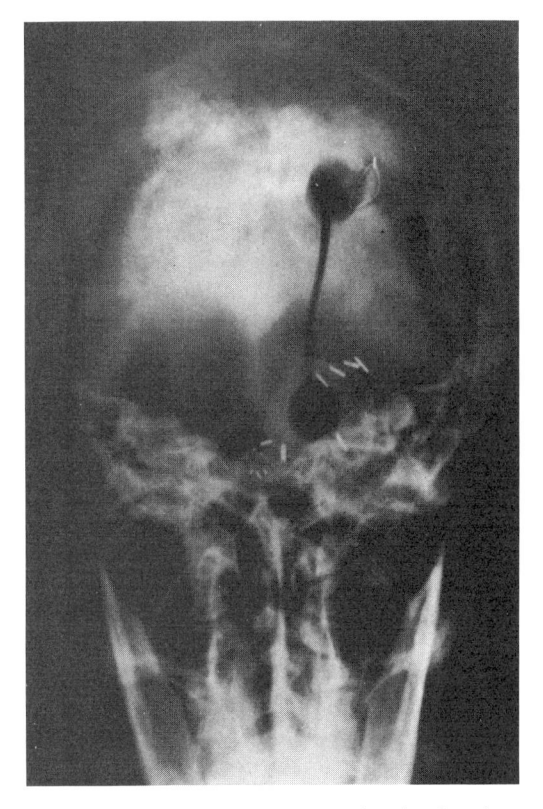

FIG. 29-10. Six yttrium-90 beads placed in the pituitary are shown in (*above*) the A-P and (*below*) the lateral roentgenograms of the skull. Large opacities are silver clips.

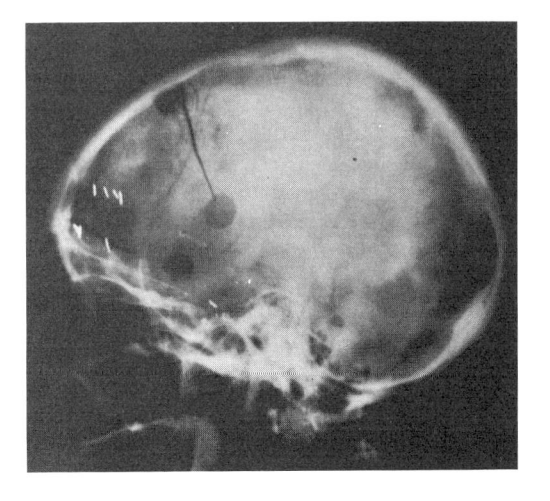

usually respond well to HGH; the problem is early diagnosis so that maximal response may be achieved (Rosenbloom, 1966).

If the growth functions of the pituitary

tissue are interfered with in infancy or childhood, growth is retarded uniformly. The time of epiphyseal closure usually is delayed in dwarfism as well as in gigantism. Usually, but not always, other endocrine activities dependent upon the pituitary tropic hormones are also present.

Adult Hypopituitarism. When this occurs, growth having already been attained, the problem involves several deficiencies: HGH, thyrotropic, adrenotropic and gonadotropic hormones. Except for HGH because it has no known specific target gland, the administration of thyroid extract, ACTH, and either estrogen in females or androgens in males results in reasonably good responses.

Cushing's Syndrome (Pituitary Basophilism). Basophilic pituitary tumors cause abnormal amounts of ACTH to be secreted, which stimulates the production of cortisol by the adrenal cortex. The symptoms observed are often indistinguishable from those of adrenocortical tumors. Normally, the increased production of cortisol would suppress the pituitary's release of ACTH, but when the increased ACTH is from a basophilic adenoma, this regulatory mechanism does not prevail. Thus adrenal cortical hyperactivity continues, with the result that the symptoms are those of an adrenal cortical tumor and, therefore, this syndrome is detailed under the adrenal gland (p. 778). Most of the cases Cushing described proved to be from primary adrenal cortical tumors and not from basophilic adenomas, as these appear to account for only a small number of cases with the Cushing syndrome. When basophilic adenoma is the cause, treatment is hypophysectomy or ablation of the gland by other means.

Chromophobe adenomas of the pituitary, which tend to enlarge and to destroy the sella more frequently than basophilic adenomas, also tend more often to compress the optic chiasm and to produce the usual visual disturbances of tumors in this area. Before the pituitary is entirely destroyed by a chromophobe adenoma, it may stimulate massive secretion of ACTH so that a Cushing picture appears from the adrenal cortisol produced, to be followed years later by hyperpigmentation of the skin, in a pseudo-addisonian picture, due to the pituitary destruction which allowed the adrenal cortex to vegetate and atrophy. A rapid suppression test for Cushing's Syndrome, using dexamethasone, has been described by Tucci et al., 1967.

Finally, the Cushing pattern may result from excessive function or hyperactivity of the pituitary. Its etiology is not understood, and it appears not to decrease its function because of the excess of circulating cortisol.

Ray et al. (1968) have subjected patients with diabetic retinopathy to pituitary ablation. In his study, 37 (78.7%) were benefited. After the early experience with hypophysectomy in 18 unselected patients resulting in four postoperative deaths, a more rigid selection on the basis of age and cardiovascular and renal function resulted in avoiding postoperative mortality in the next 38 patients. Hypophysectomy appears to be a desirable method of treatment in the carefully selected diabetic patient who is threatened with blindness. With the early encouraging results of hypophysectomy in patients with diabetic retinopathy reported by Luft et al. in 1955, this operation appears justified in selected patients.

Hypophysectomy, Its Complications and the "Posterior" Lobe Hormones

Cushing (1906) first operated successfully upon the pituitary and developed the field. The early experiences were frequently associated with injuries to the optic chiasm and to the neurohypophysis. The procedure soon was largely abandoned and was cause for the surgeon to compromise his operative attempts, settling for incomplete hypophysectomy with multiple operations if needed rather than the total removal of the gland.

Hemorrhage. Uncontrolled hemorrhage and diabetes insipidus were serious problems and not infrequently fatal complications of surgical hypophysectomy which beset Cushing and continue to plague the neurosurgeon of today. The control of hemorrhage in such deep wells as required in many neurosurgical operations caused Cushing early to focus his attention sharply upon the problems of neurosurgical hemostasis. He introduced the use of bits of muscle fragments obtained from the exposed temporalis muscle, recognizing its thromboplastic action; he may have been informed of this potential by the physiologist, William H. Howell, Professor of Physiology at Hopkins at the time Cushing began his experimental and clinical neurosurgery in that institution. Howell was studying problems in blood coagulation. Bone wax to plug the bleeding of cut bone edges was introduced by Victor Horsley but was used infrequently by Cushing. At Cushing's instigation, Ernest Grey (1915) explored the use of fibrin clots placed at the bleeding site, but this technic proved to be of little value. The silver clip applied to bleeding points or to vessels before transection was developed by Cushing in 1910 with his first report on its use being made in 1911. (Note x-ray appearance in Fig. 29-10.)

In 1926 Cushing explored the hemostatic effect of high-frequency current in cerebral surgery but not upon the hypophysis. This technic had been employed as early as 1911 in urologic surgery. Working with W. T. Bovie (1928), Cushing first employed electrocoagulation in neurosurgery on October 1, 1926. The patient suffered from a highly vascular "myeloma." Although nearly all methods currently in use for the control of intracranial hemorrhage were either developed or first employed in this field by Cushing, many hemostatic problems remain to be solved. Hypotensive anesthesia has been used in recent years and has proved to be helpful, but there is as yet no perfect answer.

Antidiuretic Hormone and Diabetes Insipidus. The second disquieting complication of hypophyseal surgery is the complication of diabetes insipidus, first described by Claude Bernard. Originally, this operative complication was attributed to injury to the posterior pituitary. Later it was realized that injury to the pituitary stalk, the hypothalamus or the supra-optic nuclei likewise could induce this disorder. With hypophysectomy being reintroduced in recent years, many of the earlier interpretations appear to need reconsideration. Re-examination of the newer evidence is necessary, for it becomes increasingly evident that the original simple explanations of a few years ago do not satisfy all observations being encountered in patients today.

Many surgeons believe that total hypophysectomy performed by clipping the stalk as near the gland as possible is least likely to produce diabetes insipidus. However, no one procedure appears to avoid this complication completely, nor can any one procedure be relied upon to induce the disorder consistently.

Fortunately, the magnitude of this complication often lessens to some extent over that immediately observed after hypophysectomy.

The physiologic disorder believed to be responsible for diabetes insipidus is the interference with the production or release of an antidiuretic hormone (ADH) known also as *vasopressin*. This hormone appears to be under the nervous control of the posterior neurohypophysis. The identity of the chemical structure of the antidiuretic hormone is of added interest because it marks for the first time that a polypeptide hormone was identified chemically and synthesized. This feat was accomplished by du Vigneaud in 1953, for which he became the Nobel laureate in 1955. He also identified and synthesized a second hormonal polypeptide believed to be associated with the function of the posterior pituitary—*oxytocin*.

The physiologic action of the antidiuretic hormone (vasopressin or ADH) appears to be directed specifically toward resorption of water from the distal renal tubules. It promotes water absorption in some manner without much apparent influence upon electrolyte resorption. Thus it enables the body to conserve essentially osmotically free water. Should excess salt need to be disposed of in the urine, this may be accomplished without the serious losses of water which otherwise might occur were salt and water resorption not under separate means of control.

As the name "vasopressin" implies, the antidiuretic hormone also affects arteriolar tension as well as cardiac function. This action favors an increase in arterial blood pressure and diminishes renal blood flow.

In diabetes insipidus, ADH is of indispensable aid; it is administered best, at present, as a crude extract by nasal insufflation, 40 mg., several times daily. Pure ADH may be administered in oil, each dose generally lasting several days. Because of its current expense, this product is not yet widely used.

ADH increases intestinal tone and promotes peristalsis and may be of some therapeutic value in the treatment of adynamic ileus.

Oxytocin appears to be concerned primarily with uterine contraction in late pregnancy. The oxytocin content of the neurohypophysis is said to be diminished during lactation, when this hormone is believed to be elaborated to assist the periductal myoepithelium of the mammary ducts in expressing milk (Richardson, 1949). Oxytocin appears to depress vasomotor responses of the heart and the arteriolar vessels, lowering blood pressure. To this extent, its action seems to oppose mildly the vasopressor effects of ADH.

Again it seems essential to caution the student about the changing status in regard to knowledge about the pituitary gland—and, for that matter, endocrines in general. Recent evidence tends to demonstrate that many of the views held earlier as fact may not be true. At least many of the well-accepted interpretations of a few years need to be re-examined, as a number of the pituitary functions now appear to be much too complex to support unitarian points of view.

Controlled Radiative Destruction of Pituitary

The method of trans-sphenoidal radiative destruction of the pituitary, described by Harper et al. (1964), appears likely to replace surgical hypophysectomy. Their method, involving the use of a 54-mc. sealed source of ^{90}Sr-^{90}Y in a 19-gauge needle under stereotaxic vision fluoroscopy and with an image intensifier, appears to be generally applicable and to be relatively free from complications. Under appropriate circumstances, it may be used in many, if not in most, patients requiring hypophysectomy. Morbidity is minimal and hospitalization is greatly reduced.

ADRENAL GLAND

General Considerations

Anatomic and Surgical Considerations. The adrenal glands lie on the upper mesial aspect of the pole of each kidney which they cover as a cap. Normally, each gland weighs between 1 and 1.5 Gm.

Small accessory adrenal tissue occasionally is said to be found in the connective tissue adjacent to the adrenal itself; such an occurrence is rare.

The adrenal cortex is derived from celomic epithelium and hence is of mesodermal origin; the medulla is of ectodermal derivation, arising from the neural crests. Microscopic examination shows the cortex to consist of glandular epithelium enmeshed loosely in a fine stroma of connective tissue. The cortical architectural structure suggests 3 areas or zones stratified one upon another. The *zona glomerulosa* has its cells arranged in rounded clusters and is situated just beneath the thin external fibrous capsule. The cells are fairly large, polyhedral in shape and contain many granules. Just beneath the zona glomerulosa is the *zona fasciculata* with its cells arranged in columnar fashion, radiating toward the glomerulosa. Their cytoplasm also contains granular and much lipoid material. Most mesially situated is the *zona reticularis*. Its distal contact is with the fascicularis and mesially with the adrenal medulla. The cells of the reticularis often contain pigment granules in their cytoplasm which are not seen in those of the glomerulosa of the fasciculata.

The possible loci of origin of the various adrenal cortical hormones as to the cell-type or zone in the adrenal gland remain unsettled. Reports by Conn and Louis (1956) and by Carr et al. (1964) provide reasonably good but not conclusive evidence that in Cushing states the predominant cytologic activity is in the *zona fasciculata*; in hyperactive androgenic states the *zona reticularis* appears to be hyperactive; and in primary aldosteronism, hyperplasia of the *zona glomerulosa* occurs.

The demonstration by Cooper and his associates (1960) that medullary tissues and, to some extent, the catechol amines themselves enhance the production of the steroids of the cortex supplies a logical explanation of the intimate anatomic relationship of the medulla and the cortex of the adrenal. These effects were demonstrated by incubating fresh tissue slices of human and of bovine adrenals.

The adrenal arteries usually arise from the aorta, the inferior phrenics and/or the renal arteries. The lymphatic circulation terminates for the most part within the lumbar nodes.

The adrenal veins pass centripetally to form the left and the right adrenal veins, respectively. Generally, the vein from the left adrenal enters either the left renal or the vena cava; that on the right more frequently enters the vena cava directly. More than one vein leaving each gland is frequently found. Their walls are thin and easily torn; when this happens at operation, severe retrograde bleeding occurs from the vena cava and/or from the renal veins. Unless the surgical field has excellent exposure, control of this type of hemorrhage may be both difficult and dangerous, especially if one attempts blindly the placement of hemostats in the puddle of blood which continues to flood the field at a rate which is usually more rapid than can be cleared. The vena cava or renal veins also may be torn in attempting hemostasis, inviting not only more extensive hemorrhage but air embolism as well. Unless small sutures can be easily placed under direct vision, packing may be the safer hemostatic procedure to employ. The pack must not occlude the flow of blood in the vena cava, as this may create the acute vena cava syndrome with shock from the intravascular pooling of blood in the distal veins. Should shock appear an hour or so after packing, when there is insufficient evidence of continuing extensive blood loss, and be associated with distention of the veins of the legs as well as cyanosis of the distal extremities, the patient should be returned to the operating room, the wound reopened and the pack gently loosened until improvement in color of the distal extremities occurs. Transfusions under these conditions should be administered through the antecubital veins of the arms and not in the saphenous veins because of the diminished distal venous return. The acute vena cava syndrome, however, is a complication which generally can be easily avoided by careful dissection carried out under direct vision with good exposure.

In the performance of adrenalectomy, many surgeons prefer to apply silver clips (Cushing), cutting between the distal and the proximal clips. As these veins are small and not easily recognized as such, the author places 2 clips on any periadrenal thread of tissue which conceivably might be mistaken in identity as a nerve or a bit of fibrous tissue. As might be expected, many of the clips are placed upon the nerve plexus entering the adrenal as well as on the veins. These nerves are numerous and are derived principally from the celiac and the renal plexuses and probably also from the phrenic and the vagal nerves.

Adrenal Cortex

Physiologic and Pharmacologic Actions of Corticoid Hormones. The cortical hormones have in common with the sex hormones the steroid nucleus. Many such compounds have been isolated from cortical extracts, and of these some are known to possess sufficient biologic activity to sustain life and good health after bilateral adrenalectomy as well as to treat successfully the patient with Addison's disease. Over a period of years, Kendall and associates and others have methodically isolated and identified the chemical composition of many of these compounds prior to much knowledge as to their biologic activity or therapeutic importance. A number of these compounds probably are parent substances from which the active hormones are biosynthesized. It is also possible that a few may have been created artificially in the course of chemical extraction procedures.

The gland seems to elaborate and to dispense these hormones so rapidly in meeting the body's normal needs that little storage is undertaken by the gland itself. Thus the adrenal cortex is a relatively poor commercial source of these compounds.

As Ingle points out, the original concepts as to the biologic functions of cortical hormones were oversimplified. It was early suggested that those hormones bearing oxygen at the 11 position of the steroid nucleus, such as cortisone, hydrocortisone and corticosterone, regulated gluconeogenesis of carbohydrate derived from proteins. Those lacking in oxygen at position 11 were believed to be concerned essentially with the metabolism of water and electrolytes. It is now known that the cortical hormones may affect nearly all of the body's tissues and functions, but until these mechanisms are better understood, it serves no useful purpose to classify them at this time. Some of the known metabolic functions that they influence will be discussed with the realization that these, too, are complex, and incompletely understood, and that many may be either interdependent or interrelated.

Cortisone and hydrocortisone (cortisol) probably have the greatest influence of all natural cortical hormones upon metabolic functions under partial or complete adrenal control (Table 29-7).

Protein Metabolism. The patient with Addison's disease or the animal subjected to adrenalectomy without replacement therapy encounters difficulty in mobilizing and metabolizing endogenous protein. As the normal

TABLE 29-7. FOUR GENERAL CLASSES OF
ADRENAL CORTICAL HORMONES

Glucocorticoids
 11-hydroxycorticoids
 11-17 hydroxycorticoids
Adrenal Androgens
 17-ketosteroids
 Testosterone (small amount)
Estrogens
Mineral Corticoids
 Aldosterone
 Desoxycorticosterone Acetate

human or mammal derives a certain amount of glucose from protein metabolism (gluconeogenesis), the addisonian patient and the adrenalectomized animal are prone to develop hypoglycemia. In the case of exogenous protein, as Ingle has pointed out, there is a much less demonstrable defect of metabolism. When the adrenal-insufficient patient or animal is fed protein and allowed a normal caloric intake, nitrogen is excreted in normal amounts, and the hypoglycemic tendency is reduced materially. However, the decreased potassium excretion in the addisonian is not affected unless cortical replacement is employed. The ease of fatigue upon exercise has been demonstrated most dramatically by Ingle in adrenalectomized rats without corticoid supportive therapy.

When excessive amounts of cortisone and/or hydrocortisone are present, whether from excessive cortical activity or administration, the nitrogen excretion is increased materially. This is a response about which much is known, but the information available is not sufficient to establish whether it results from an accelerated rate of catabolism or a diminished rate of anabolism or both.

CARBOHYDRATE METABOLISM and its dependence upon cortical function in the adrenalectomized rat in the fasting state was first demonstrated by Cori and Cori in 1927. They showed that neither the normal blood sugar nor the stores of liver glycogen could be maintained under these conditions. This phenomenon occurs in many species, including man. Diabetes mellitus may be ameliorated by adrenalectomy but may be produced by hypercorticism when diabetes did not previously exist.

Two factors appear to play a role in the diminished ability of the addisonian patient or the adrenalectomized animal to maintain the normal level of blood glucose. One is the retarded rate of gluconeogenesis from protein. The other is the apparent acceleration in the rate of glucose utilization after adrenalectomy in the fasting state. Presumably, the latter phenomenon is due to an antagonism between certain of the cortical hormones and insulin but further study is needed for elucidation.

In hypercorticism, the effect upon carbohydrate metabolism is reversed. Glycosuria, decreased glucose tolerance, frank diabetes and an increased insulin tolerance characteristically occur. Again, it should be remembered that in addition to an increased insulin tolerance (Thorn et al., 1940) more carbohydrate is also made available from the accelerated rate of gluconeogenesis from protein when excesses of cortisone and hydrocortisone occur.

FAT METABOLISM is disturbed in that a diminished transport of fat to the liver as well as a reduction in the total lipid content in this organ occurs. Ketonuria and ketonemia are observed with less frequency and to a lesser extent than in the normal; this is not yet explained. In the addisonian, the respiratory quotient is reported to be increased, and to be diminished in hypercorticism. The cause of abnormal distribution of fat in the Cushing's state is unknown.

WATER AND ELECTROLYTE METABOLISM are among the more dramatic and acute disorders created by either the hypocortical or the hypercortical state. There are many internal factors and mechanisms which can alter water and electrolyte balance; those of hormonal origin are as important as any (see Chap. 5, Fluid and Electrolytes). Whereas the types of these disorders in the hypocortical and the hypercortical states are well known, the exact mechanisms by which they occur are not.

So far as the mineral electrolytes are concerned, sodium and potassium are among those subject to the most apparent and most important changes noted (see p. 783, Aldosteronism). In hypocorticism, sodium excretion in the urine is increased; in hypercortical states, sodium tends to be retained. These changes reflect differences in tubular rates of absorption due to corticoid activity.

The first progress in the treatment of the addisonian patient resulted from the recognition that such patients required large quantities of salt (Harrop et al., 1933; Loeb, 1933). The synthetic desoxycorticosterone acetate (DOCA) was introduced as a therapeutic agent at that time. Its administration favored sodium retention in the normal patient as well as in the addisonian. The brilliant researches of Luetscher et al. in 1948 (Luetscher, 1964) and of Simpson et al. (1954) and the chemical identification of the naturally occurring, potent, salt-retaining hormone, aldosterone, may lead to the explanation of many of the unknowns in mineral and water balance. Aldosterone, milligram per milligram, exerts more than 20 times the effect upon sodium retention exerted by DOCA.

It is probable that the excessive loss of sodium in the addisonian patient accounts for many of the well-established features of this disease: hypovolemia, reduction in extracellular water, the increase in hematocrit reading and in plasma protein concentration and blood viscosity, all of which render these patients very susceptible to the development of hypovolemic shock.

In hypercorticism, sodium is retained abnormally and along with this are the excesses in extracellular water with edema. Soon after the hypercortical state occurs, sodium equilibrium is established at a slightly higher level than normal, but in some it remains unchanged and at the normal level. The hyponatremia of the hypocortical state is usually much more alarming and serious than is the sodium retention in hypercortical activity. Certainly, the latter is not to be considered lightly, especially in the elderly patient or in those with pre-existing or concurrent cardiovascular, renal or hepatic disease.

The urinary excretion of potassium and its concentrations in the body fluids are also influenced considerably by the state of adrenal cortical function. In the addisonian or untreated adrenalectomized patient, potassium retention is the rule. Many believed earlier that death in these patients was due primarily to potassium intoxication. Undoubtedly in some patients this was true, but as many other important and vital changes also occur in adrenal insufficiency, and these associated disorders, each in themselves or in combination, can be lethal.

In hypocorticism, the potassium concentrations of serum, extracellular and intracellular water are increased. As the concentration of potassium in heart muscle increases, changes in the electrocardiogram occur which are believed to be characteristic of impending potassium intoxication. ECG tracings are often useful aids in the management of the hypocortical and the hypercortical states. However, these findings are not entirely reliable.

The mechanisms involved in the altered potassium metabolism from abnormalities in cortical activity are probably more intricate than those that affect sodium. In addition to considerations of disordered tubular absorption and internal fluid shifts, there are also the disturbances in protein metabolism. Normal concentrations of potassium are usually essential to normal protein metabolism; the reverse also is true and probably of equal importance. To what extent the abnormalities in protein metabolism are responsible for the altered potassium responses in adrenal cortical disorders is not established. Favoring the altered metabolism of protein is the reported observation that aldosterone, which has no known influence upon protein metabolism, appears to exert less influence upon potassium excretion than upon sodium retention (Luetscher and Johnson, 1954; Swingle et al., 1954).

The changes in water metabolism caused by some adrenal cortical hormones are in part due to the electrolyte shifts, especially sodium. In part they may also result from the ill-defined changes in tubular resorption assigned to the cortical hormones. In the addisonian patient there is a diminished diuretic response to water (Keppler water test). If large quantities of water are administered, water intoxication may occur. This abnormality appears to be more amenable to the administration of the 11, 17-oxysteroids than to the 11-deoxysteroids or to aldosterone. There is also considerable evidence to suggest that the antidiuretic hormone of the neurohypophysis and some of the adrenocortical steroids are antagonistic.

The general ranges of adrenal cortical hormones produced in normal man are shown in Table 29-8.

Diseases of the Adrenal Cortex. CUSHING'S DISEASE (HYPERCORTICISM). Harvey Cushing recorded in 1912 his first observations of the disease that now bears his name. This

TABLE 29-8. ADRENAL STEROID SECRETION IN MAN (COMPOUNDS ISOLATED FROM ADRENAL VEIN BLOOD OF NORMAL SUBJECTS)

GROUP	COMPOUND	MEAN 24-HOUR SECRETION IN ADULTS
Glucocorticoids	Cortisol	15–30 mg.
	Corticosterone	2–5 mg.
Mineralocorticoids	Aldosterone	50–150 μg.
	11-Desoxycorticosterone	Normally only traces
	Dehydroepiandrosterone	15–30 mg.
Androgens	$\Delta4$,Androstenedione	0–10
	11-β Hydroxyandrostenedione	0–10
Progestins	Progesterone	0.4–0.8 mg.
Estrogens	Estradiol	Trace

patient was a young woman who suffered from headache, pain in the back, obesity about the face, the neck and the trunk but not of the extremities, and from hirsutism and hypertension. The dorsal kyphosis and "buffalo hump" obesity that she displayed, with hirsutism, florid complexion, ease of bruising and purple striae of the lower trunk, along with diabetes mellitus, were to characterize this syndrome which he did not encounter again until 1932. Cushing's first patient, he believed, suffered from a pituitary disorder; his second patient, a male, received pituitary radiation and improved promptly.

Clinical Course and Diagnosis of Cushing's Syndrome. As others entered this field of study, additional clinical and metabolic disturbances were noted. The round "moon facies" was noted frequently. Weakness was commonly encountered. Hypertension was detected in about 75 per cent of cases. Osteoporosis was an important finding and to this was attributed the skeletal pain, the backache and the dorsal kyphosis often experienced by many of these patients. Negative calcium balance is the rule, and about 25 per cent develop renal stones, presumably due to the excessive quantities of calcium appearing in the urine.

Diabetes mellitus or a diminished glucose tolerance curve was encountered less commonly in Cushing's cases than the known physiology of hypercorticism might suggest. The syndrome occurs about 3 times more often in females than in males.

Perhaps the most characteristic and constant finding revealed by careful physical examination is the loss of muscular mass. This can be overlooked in the presence of the unusual obesity. It seems reasonable to explain the patient's muscular weakness on the basis of this finding alone, although other factors also may be involved.

The skin is thin, especially the corium, and sometimes is described as having a marblelike appearance. The wasting of fascial and fibrous connective tissue probably accounts for the striae of the skin so often noted over the areas of the abdomen where the skin may be stretched from obesity. These striae are usually "purple" in color and are attributed to the thinning of skin, allowing the color of blood contained in the underlying vessels to be transmitted more readily than in the striae of pregnancy or other types of obesity wherein the skin thickness is normal. Cope (1955) states that these vessels are often enlarged, lacking in resiliency and strength; the latter may account for the ease of bruising often noted.

Associated with wasting of the skin, is wasting of most, if not all, organs, including occasionally also the brain.

The frequency of occurrence of the various complaints that Cope's patients present is tabulated in Table 29-9.

Prior to our understanding or interpretation of these findings, Albright and Bloomberg (1941) attempted the use of testosterone as a means of re-establishing positive nitrogen balance with some reported success. The rationale of this approach was based upon the gonadal atrophy that these patients display and the demonstration by Kenyon in 1937 of the anabolic effect of testosterone with the increase in nitrogen balance when this hormone was given to the eunuchoid patient. In a few of Albright's cases, the negative calcium balance was restored to one of equilibrium or to

TABLE 29-9. COMPLAINTS OF THE 46 PATIENTS*

SYMPTOM	PRESENTING COMPLAINT No. of Cases	AS ADDITIONAL SYMPTOM No. of Cases	TOTAL OCCURRENCE No. of Cases
Fatigue and weakness	16	19	35
Weight gain and obesity	6	28	34
Changed appearance	2	31	33
Amenorrhea or irregularity	3	26	29
Bruising		18	18
Nervousness, depression, irritability	4	11	15
Back pain and bone pain	5	9	14
Hirsutism	3	10	13
Headache	1	9	10
Ankle and hand edema	1	8	9
Decreased libido (females); impotence (males)		8	8
Paresthesias	1	3	4
Lower voice		4	4
Blurred vision	1	2	3
Poor wound healing and leg ulcers	1	2	3
Cessation of growth	1		1
Difficulty in walking	1		1
General aching and malaise	1		1

* Cope, Oliver, and Raker, J. W.: Cushing's disease, the surgical experience in the care of 46 cases. New Eng. J. Med., 253:119, 1955.

a slightly positive balance; in only one was there suggestion that remission of the disease occurred.

The electrolyte disturbances tend to be a hypokalemic alkalosis with an elevated content of serum carbon dioxide. Lowered serum sodium is encountered infrequently. Despite the negative calcium balance and its increased rate of excretion, the values of serum calcium, phosphorus, phosphatase activities and chloride are usually found to be within normal range.

Specific laboratory diagnostic findings, including roentgenographic observations, exist but are not always detectable. Arterial hypertension is detectable in approximately three fourths of these patients. Although its cause is not understood, it usually returns fairly promptly to normal after adrenalectomy.

Glycosuria and/or frank diabetes are by no means a constant finding. Blood sugar was normal more often than not in Cope's series.

The urinary 17-ketosteroid excretions are also variable. They are generally elevated in malignant cortical tumors but less constantly so in the benign ones. When the disease appears to be due to adrenal hyperplasia, the ketosteroids are usually increased in the urine. Studies made to identify the more specific chemical nature of the increased steroid secretion indicate that those steroids bearing the oxygen atom in the 11 position are increased more frequently than others.

Urinary ketosteroids as usually measured in urine represent the "total neutral" 17-ketosteroids. It may be useful to summarize the usual ranges under different conditions wherein no original adrenal pathology has existed. Slightly different values may be obtained by different methods of urine extraction. The following 24-hour values are usually obtained:

Young adult males	10 to 15 mg.
Aged adult males	3 to 8 mg.
Adult females	5 to 15 mg.
Newborn infant, 1st week of life	2.5 mg.
Children under 10	0 to 1 mg.
Children 12 to 16	2 to 5 mg.
Late pregnancy	15 to 20 mg.
Castrated males	7 to 24 mg.
Castrated females	10 to 15 mg.
Postmenopausal females	10 to 15 mg.
Castration and adrenalectomy	2 to 4 mg. on cortical extracts

Additional fractionation and separation into the ketonic and nonketonic fractions is possible; about 10 to 15 per cent or slightly more of the total is nonketonic normally. The larger ketonic fraction portion is comprised of alpha and beta fractions. The beta fraction comprises about 5 per cent normally but may be increased to 50 per cent or more in patients with adrenal cortical tumors with hypercortical secretory activity, in cortical hyperplasia and in patients with the adrenogenital syndrome (see p. 781). Abnormally low values are usually found in patients with hypopituitarism (Simmonds' disease), hypophyseal infantilism, Addison's disease, myxedema and occasionally in anorexia nervosa.

The increased calcium and nitrogen excretions in Cushing's disease, with the resultant negative balances they entail, have been alluded to above. Potassium excretion also is increased and probably relates to the general wasting of body protein; Albright reported its restoration to normal in some patients given testosterone as their only form of treatment. The fact that neither sodium balance nor the sodium "space" appears to be distinctly abnormal in this disease generally eliminates consideration of Addison's disease from the differential diagnosis. However, there are other clinical features that are more decisive in the elimination of Addison's disease than muscular weakness, for example—hypertension and obesity in the "Cushing" patient.

Thyroid function as revealed by the basal metabolic state is generally somewhat hypoactive; protein-bound iodine measurements are usually within normal range.

Origin of the Endocrine Disorder and the Pathology of Cushing's Disease. Cushing's original concept was that the primary pathology lay within the anterior lobe of the pituitary and was concerned chiefly with adenomatous formation of the basophilic cells. Soon the term "basophilism" was employed as descriptive of the presumed pathology for this syndrome, for it connoted the site which he believed to harbor the primary disturbance as well as the cell type. His report in 1932 was so convincing that when others observed patients with the same phenomenon but with normal pituitary histology at autopsy, faith was shaken as to the validity of Cushing's concept and interpretations. Most patients failed to respond to pituitary radiation. As a number of these patients came to autopsy, a new phase of its historical development began to unravel. Many died of primary adrenocortical tumors, benign or malignant—more often the latter. In a smaller group, cortical hyperplasia, usually bilateral, was observed.

Final proof as to the nature of the hormonal disturbances did not come about until 1948 when ACTH and cortisone were first employed clinically. These agents, particularly ACTH, seemed to duplicate almost completely the Cushing picture. Although excessive and prolonged cortisone therapy produced many of these manifestations, acne, the moderate degree of virilism and the florid complexion were less striking and seemingly less frequently encountered than with ACTH administration. However, the question as to whether or not these are the only hormonal disturbances of the adrenal cortex in Cushing's disease remains an unsettled one. The demonstration of primary pituitary disorders in this disease is infrequent; in fact, the paucity of such pathologic material has been cause for some to conclude that the pituitary is seldom the site of the primary disturbance. With bilateral adrenalectomy or the removal of a unilateral tumor being so effective a form of treatment, these patients survive and return to normal life. Hence it may be many years before enough autopsy material is available from pituitary examinations to establish how often the origin of the disease lies within the pituitary. In most patients, the primary pathology appears to arise within the adrenal cortex.

Treatment. As the hypersecretory activity of cortical adenomas or tumors usually is not suppressed by the administration of cortisone or ACTH, complete unilateral adrenalectomy is performed with removal of the cortical adenoma or carcinoma if possible. Although multiple adenomas are found occasionally, they are usually located within the same gland; these adenomas or tumors may occur bilaterally, and bilateral adrenalectomy may be advisable.

When one adrenal is the cause of the Cushing syndrome, the activity of the contralateral one is always depressed; its cortex atrophies. Hence, unless such patients are maintained on cortisone after unilateral adrenalectomy, addisonian crisis is likely to develop postoperatively. In the postoperative period, ACTH therapy is administered to awaken cortical function in the remaining adrenal; cortisone therapy is reduced cautiously while ACTH is administered until finally both can be discontinued—generally within 8 to 10 days.

Subtotal adrenalectomy for bilateral adrenal hyperplasia would seem to be the ideal treatment of Cushing's syndrome of this origin. It is the treatment generally preferred and most commonly employed. It is not always possible to resect the proper amount of adrenal tissue to control completely the course of the disease. On the other hand, subtotal adrenalectomy is preferable to total removal of both glands despite the fact that replacement therapy in the bilaterally adrenalectomized patient poses a less serious problem than was anticipated earlier. Should more adrenal tissue need to be removed, this can be done at a later date.

Prognosis. Except for huge adrenal tumors and the technical difficulty that they may pose in removal, surgical mortality in adrenalectomy for this disease should be less than 5 per cent. Total cure is effected when the cortical tumor is benign or due to hyperplasia. Should cortical carcinoma be the cause, the prognosis is generally poor. These tumors tend to metastasize early, frequently to the liver, the lungs, the brain and bone. In this respect they appear to follow metastatic pathways to the organs of predilection which are similar to those characteristic for hypernephroma.

Testosterone is the steroid of testicular origin. It is many times as potent as androsterone in promoting comb growth of the cock and seminal vesicular activation in the castrate rat. In the castrate human male or female, however, androsterone and dehydro-iso-androsterone continue to appear, but the quantity is less than normal. When adrenalectomy is added to castration, the 17-ketosteroids essentially disappear from the urine unless corticoids are administered. It was upon this observation that adrenalectomy in combination with orchiectomy was explored by Huggins in the palliative management of the partially dependent tumors of the breast or the prostate (see Chap. 27, Breast).

There is a close quantitative correlation between urinary androgens and the biologic activity that the patient displays clinically. Their excretion is diminished in castrates and is increased in hypercorticism, interstitial tumors of the testes or the ovary, in pregnancy and in acromegaly or gigantism of pituitary origin.

ADRENOGENITAL SYNDROMES. The most significant masculinizing hormone is testosterone, and its major site of origin is the testes. Its androgenic activity is 40 to 60 times that of any of the 17-ketosteroids. Normally, only a small proportion of testosterone is produced by the adrenal cortex and a small amount by the ovary. In both sexes, the adrenal cortex normally produces, in much larger quantities, a number of other masculinizing compounds, principally the 17-ketosteroids, dehydroepiandrosterone, etiocholanolone, androsterone, and 11-oxy derivatives thereof, which are excreted as sulfates and glucuronides. Though all these compounds are weakly androgenic, they account for most of the masculinizing qualities observed in the adrenogenital syndromes because of the large quantities produced. When excessive amounts of adrenal androgens are released, because of hyperplasia of the cortex, functioning cortical adenomas or cortical adenocarcinomas, alterations in secondary sex characteristics and in somatic development due to their anabolic effects occur. The clinical patterns of these effects depend upon the sex and the stage of growth and development of the patient at the time abnormal increases in adrenal androgens first occur, and obviously they are much more conspicuous in the female than in the male.

The adrenogenital syndromes develop because somewhere along the line of biologic synthesis by the adrenal cortex, one or more pathways leading from pregnenolone to the elaboration of cortisol are inhibited or blocked, whereas those concerned with androgen production are not. Thus the adrenal fails to produce sufficient cortisol to regulate the production of ACTH by the pituitary gland. The resulting excesses of ACTH stimulate some, if not all, of the pathways for synthesis of adrenal androgen. Now that these pathways are better understood, it is quite obvious that some, but not all, forms of the adrenogenital syndromes, when due to a blockade in the formation of cortisol, should respond to the administration of hydrocortisone—and some do, as evidenced by the return of the 17-keto-

782   Pituitary and Adrenal Glands

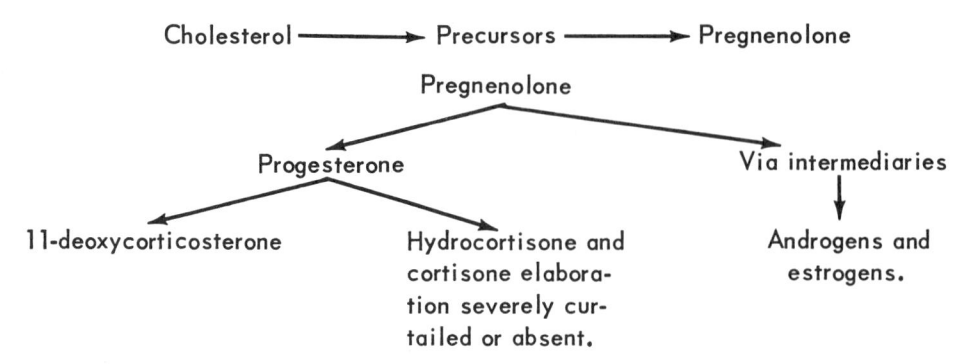

```
Cholesterol ──────▶ Precursors ──────▶ Pregnenolone
                      Pregnenolone
          ◀──────────────┴──────────────▶
    Progesterone                    Via intermediaries
   ◀────┴────▶                              ↓
11-deoxycorticosterone   Hydrocortisone and     Androgens and
                         cortisone elabora-      estrogens.
                         tion severely cur-
                         tailed or absent.
```

FIG. 29-11. Simplified schematic illustration of the several causes of adrenogenital syndromes.

steroid secretion to normal and the complete disappearance of symptoms. However, when the excess production of androgens is due to biologic activity of an adenoma or an adenocarcinoma, the excess production of androgens usually is no longer under the control of ACTH as the tumor itself does not appear to respond.

The scheme of the more important chemical pathways shown in Figure 29-11 may be useful to an understanding of the principles of the adrenogenital syndromes; many details are omitted.

Prenatal Block in Steroid Synthesis. The most interesting and perhaps informative aspects of the adrenogenital syndromes are those usually classified as occurring prenatally and from a blockade of one or more enzymes involved in the synthesis of adrenal cortical steroids from cholesterol. These include the androgens, the glucocorticoids and the mineral corticoids, and small amounts of testosterone and estrogen of adrenal origin. These latter two hormones, however, are not discussed here. Somewhat schematically, these steroids are briefly detailed as follows:

1. TOTAL BLOCK OF ALL STEROID PRODUCTION (LIPOID HYPERPLASIA). Patient is addisonian and, because intra-uterine müllerian ductal system remains unchanged in the genotype male, he develops female external genitalia and is born as a male pseudohermaphrodite. Rare. There is no production of corticosteroids, aldosterone, androgens, or testosterone or estrogen.

2. SELECTIVE BLOCK OF ADRENAL STEROIDS
A. *Block of 17-Ketosteroid Synthesis.* In the absence of androgens, the genotype male is born as a pseudohermaphrodite with female external genitalia. Genotype female is sexually normal.

B. *Block of Cortisol Synthesis.* Patient will not survive unless his addisonian state is recognized and treated. In the absence of cortisol, or if cortisol synthesis is subnormal, ACTH production is stimulated continuously, which stimulates adrenal androgen production, creating prenatal adrenal virilism. The genotype male develops macrogenitosomia and other evidence of virilism. The genotype female develops masculinization of external genitalia and hair distribution and is a pseudohermaphrodite female (see salt-retaining syndrome, below).

C. *Block of Mineral Corticoids*
a. SALT-LOSING SYNDROMES. Block at pregnenolone level and thus all steroids except androgens are absent.

(1) In the absence of aldosterone, salt is lost, profound hyponatremia develops, with early death when the defect is that which prevents transformation of pregnenolone to progesterone.

(2) More commonly, the defect is at the level of progesterone so that the formation of aldosterone and cortisol is inhibited or retarded. In about two thirds of cases the block is partial, with subnormal production of aldosterone and cortisol. The patient is therefore either a total or a partial addisonian, and the absence or deficiency of cortisol results in the excessive production of ACTH. Hence, all the complications of the excess of adrenal androgens this creates are found in these patients (because of the limited cortisol), i.e., pseudohermaphroditism in genotype females, and in

genotype males, macrogenitosomia and masculinization.

b. SALT-RETAINING SYNDROME (Hypertensive Syndrome). This is due to a block that prevents the synthesis of cortisol and of aldosterone. The usual excessive production of the 17-ketosteroids continues, and the male genotype develops macrogenitosomia and the female genotype develops pseudohermaphroditism. The block in aldosterone occurs at the level of its precursor, 11-deoxycorticosterone, which has potent properties of sodium retention but, unlike aldosterone, is not under the control of plasma sodium concentration.

Postnatal Adrenogenital Syndromes. In this group there is an increased production of 17-ketosteroids which is most often caused by an adrenocortical adenocarcinoma. Depending upon sex, the penis or the clitoris is enlarged in response to the excessive adrenal production of androgens, but neither the testes nor the ovaries mature. The excess of adrenal androgens suppresses the release of gonadotropins and this appears to account for the failure of the gonads to mature and is the point of differentiation between patients with the adrenogenital syndrome and those with precocious puberty, wherein a tumor in the region of the hypothalmus stimulates the production of gonadotropins as well as adrenal androgens so that in such children sperm are found in the ejaculate and the female child appears to ovulate.

In the adrenogenital syndrome in the child, hair is excessive and of masculine distribution. The anabolic effect of androgens is also evident because there is an increase of total muscle mass with a minimal amount of adipose fat; not infrequently these children create a physical impression of herculean strength. Nitrogen balance is strongly positive, and bone growth is facilitated.

Adrenogenital Syndrome in the Adult. An increase of 17-ketosteroids also may occur in the adult from a cortical hyperplasia or from adenomas or carcinomas of the adrenal. The effect is best described in the female adult, whose body habitus resembles that of the male, with loss of normal feminine adipose tissue and the development of heavier musculature. She develops hirsutism of the body and the face and the male distribution of pubic hair. There is atrophy of the breasts and the uterus and an enlargement of the clitoris. Menstruation usually ceases, as does ovulation. There is deepening of the voice.

All of these masculine changes are reversible if the tumor can be removed or if hydrocortisone is administered to suppress ACTH production and its stimulating effect upon 17-ketosteroid synthesis.

The same condition may occur in the adult male, and when it does, it tends to be less apparent because it simply accentuates his masculine characteristics and may therefore go unnoticed for longer periods of time. The individual usually becomes sterile because of hypospermia or aspermia resulting from the suppression of gonadotropins by the excess of adrenal androgens.

The particular cause of the adrenogenital syndrome in children and in adults is partially elucidated by the quantity of urinary ketosteroids excreted daily. The ranges usually are these:

Cortical hyperplasia ... moderately elevated—
15-20 mg.

Cortical adenoma or
carcinoma .... pronounced elevations
—30-150 mg.

Normal values ...... 4-12 mg.

Virilism and Adrenal Hyperplasia. Hyperplasia of the adrenal cortex may occur with or without acceleration of growth or bone maturation. It is apparently a mild condition when it occurs without manifestation of an acceleration of bone growth (Aceto et al., 1960). More commonly, it occurs in late childhood, but it may occur as early as 21 months of age. Cortisol by mouth appears the treatment of choice, as it tends to block the pituitary stimulus of the adrenal gland.

Aldosteronism. Aldosterone is a corticoid with a potent influence upon sodium retention. Its identification clarifies one of the important mysteries regarding adrenal function. Although deoxycorticosterone acetate (DOCA) has a moderate influence upon sodium retention and has been useful to a limited extent in the treatment of Addison's disease, it is a synthetic compound and not a hormone normally produced by the adrenal cortex. It has been clear that some factor was needed to explain satisfactorily the incompleteness of corticoid replacement therapy after bilateral adrenalectomy, if salt and water were to be normal. Aldosterone secretion is stimulated by sodium depletion and suppressed when sodium is retained. Excessive amounts of aldosterone have been reported in the urine in nephrotic edema, congestive failure, decompensated cirrhotics, and in eclampsia (Luetscher and Johnson, 1954).

PRIMARY ALDOSTERONISM. Conn (1963) infers this to be a disease entity due primarily to the excessive production of aldosterone. Cortical tumors are the principal causes and appear to arise from cells in the *zona fasciculata* (Luetscher, 1964; Priestley et al., 1968). This syndrome also differs from secondary aldosteronism in that edema does not develop. The electrolyte disorder is comparable, if not identical, with that of the disease known as "potassium-losing nephritis." Increasing numbers of cases are being reported of aldosterone-producing cortical tumors; a few are bilateral.

The clinical pattern of primary aldosteronism varies with the degree that aldosterone is produced. Full-blown, it includes muscle weakness and fatigue, polyuria, headache, polydipsia, paresthesia, visual disturbances, intermittent paralysis, and tetany. Indications for exploration are hypertension without other cause, hypokalemic alkalosis with potassium loss in the urine, and increased excretion of aldosterone. The essential negative findings when uncomplicated are normal 17-hydroxycorticosteroid excretion, normal serum sodium, and normal renal angiograms. The diagnosis is easily made, if thought of.

Most of the more than 300 cases of primary aldosteronism that have accumulated since Conn (1956) reported the first case have occurred in persons between the ages of 30 and 50 years, though it has been found in children and in the elderly. It occurs about 2.5 times more frequently in females than in males. In the vast majority of cases the cause is an adenoma in one cortex of the adrenal. The clinical pattern of primary aldosteronism and its biochemical aberrations are shown in Tables 29-10 and 29-11. An etiologic classification of co-existing hypertension and hypokalemia has been proposed by Conn (1963) and is shown in Tables 29-12.

Treatment of primary aldosteronism is limited to surgical exploration of both adrenals

TABLE 29-10. SYMPTOMS AND SIGNS IN PRIMARY ALDOSTERONISM (TUMOR)*

A. Renal
  1. Polydipsia†
  2. Polyuria†
  3. Nocturia†
B. Muscular
  1. Weakness, usually episodic†
  2. Flaccid paralysis, occasional
  3. Tetany, manifest or latent (paresthesias)
C. Hypertensive
  1. B.P. elevation—mild to very severe (270/160)†
  2. Headache—a major symptom†
  3. Retinopathy—minimal in relation to B.P. elevation
  4. Cardiomegaly—minimal in relation to B.P. elevation
D. Important negative findings
  1. Peripheral edema—absent or minimal
  2. Grade IV retinopathy—absent

* Conn, J. W.: J.A.M.A., 183:871, 1963.
† Most common

TABLE 29-11. BIOCHEMICAL AND FUNCTIONAL ALTERATIONS OBSERVED IN PRIMARY ALDOSTERONISM (TUMOR)*

A. Blood
  1. Hypokalemia†
  2. Hypernatremia
  3. Hypochloremia
  4. Hypomagnesemia
  5. Alkalosis†
B. Urine
  1. Increased aldosterone excretion and/or secretion†
  2. Normal 17-KS and 17-OHCS†
  3. Decreased concentrating ability
     (a) Water restriction
     (b) Vasopressin resistance
  4. Decreased ability to acidify
     (a) Neutral or alkaline urine
     (b) Decreased H+ and increased NH_4^+
  5. Decreased renal conservation of K+
C. Na, K and body fluids
  1. Increased body exchangeable Na†
  2. Decreased body exchangeable K†
  3. Low sweat Na concentration†
  4. Low Na/K of saliva
  5. Increased plasma volume (decreased hematocrit reading)
D. EKG—Changes compatible with hypokalemia

* Conn, J. W.: J.A.M.A., 183:871, 1963.
† Most common.

TABLE 29-12. ETIOLOGICAL CLASSIFICATION OF CO-EXISTING HYPERTENSION AND HYPOKALEMIA*

A. Primary aldosteronism (tumor)
B. Congenital aldosteronism (bilateral hyperplasia)
C. Diuretic therapy in hypertensive patients
D. Accelerated ("malignant") hypertension (Renal ischemia, unilateral or bilateral)
E. Potassium-wasting renal disease
   1. Fanconi syndrome
   2. Renal tubular acidosis
   3. Advanced chronic nephritis
   4. Chronic pyelonephritis
F. Conditions associated with large production of hydrocortisone
   1. Cushing's syndrome
      a. Adrenal hyperplasia or tumor
      b. Corticotropin-producing pituitary tumor
   2. Neoplasm producing corticotropinlike compounds (Lung, thymus, pancreas, gallbladder)
G. Miscellaneous
   1. A few benign hypertensives with *all* the characteristics of primary aldosteronism but no tumor
   2. Aberrant aldosteronoma
   3. Factitious (pseudo-primary aldosteronism)
      a. Chronic ingestion of licorice (4 cases) (subnormal aldosterone excretion and secretion)

* Conn, J. W.: J.A.M.A., 183:871, 1963.

with removal of the adenoma. The symptoms then disappear, the normal electrolyte pattern returns, and after a few weeks normal blood pressure is re-established. If no adenoma is found, adrenalectomy should be considered, provided that sound evidence of primary aldosteronism exists and biopsy suggests hyperplasia.

SECONDARY ALDOSTERONISM is a condition in which edema exists. It is found principally in diseased states in which there is sodium loss by mechanisms not herein under discussion, though a variety of clinical conditions are involved. Only occasionally does such a patient present a surgical problem. Secondary aldosteronism in relation to angiotensin is discussed by Davis (1964). Some confusion may occasionally arise in diagnosis because in potassium-wasting renal disease there is acidosis with *hypo*natremia, in contrast with the *hyper*natremia found in primary aldosteronism.

The first effective antagonist of aldosterone for clinical use was spironolactone (Aldactone). Another derivative of the same basic compound now available is Aldactone-A, claimed to be 4 times more effective than Aldactone. These agents, by inhibiting aldosterone, favor sodium secretion and may be of some benefit in secondary aldosteronism, but also are used when sodium overload has occurred in the course of intravenous therapy.

Corticoid Therapy in Surgical Patients. As corticoid therapy is employed in a variety of medical disorders, in due course some of these patients may require operation, either for the disease under cortisone treatment (ulcerative colitis) or for independent disorders. In either case, certain adjustments in cortisone dosages appear to be necessary in the immediate preoperative and postoperative periods.

Early studies implicated cortisone therapy as an agent that disposed toward poor healing in surgical wounds. Certainly there are some patients whose wounds do not appear to heal well when they have received large doses of cortisone for weeks to months. In doses of 50 to 100 mg. of cortisone per day, however, there is little evidence of impaired wound healing when the total period of therapy is less than 2 weeks in duration for the average patient.

The claim has been made by Grey *et al.* (1951) that cortisone and/or ACTH therapy produces peptic ulcer. This view seems to have gained support by the accumulated experience of others, though the means by which an ulcer is produced is still in question.

Because ACTH and cortisone increase the appetite for food, Cole (1953) and others have administered cortisone for a few days to postoperative patients who are able to eat and are in need of food, but without appetite. Daily dosages beginning with 300 mg. of cortisone, tapered down each day, are generally used to this end, but for no longer than 5 to 6 days. Although the corticoids have a catabolic effect at these dosage levels, the benefit of the increased caloric intake appears to offset this disadvantage. Often the patient may consume in excess of 4,000 calories daily. After the

TABLE 29-13. RELATIVE ANTI-INFLAMMATORY POTENCIES OF SOME THERAPEUTIC CORTICOIDS

COMPOUND	RELATIVE POTENCY COMPARED WITH CORTISOL*	RELATIVE SODIUM-RETAINING ACTIVITY
Cortisol Hydrocortisone	1	++
Cortisone Acetate	0.8	++
Prednisolone (1–2 dehydrocortisol)	4	+
Prednisone (1–2 Dehydrocortisone)	3.5	+
Triamcinolone (9 α-fluoro-16-α hydroxyprednisolone)	5	0
6-Methylprednisolone (6-α-methyl-prednisolone)	5	0
Haldranolone (6 α-fluoro-16-α-methyl-prednisolone)	10	0
Betamethasone (9 α-fluoro-16-β-methyl-prednisolone)	25	0
Dexamethasone (9 α-fluoro-16-α-methyl-prednisolone)	25	0
9 α-fluorohydrocortisone	15	+++++

* When used orally as anti-inflammatory agent.

drug has been discontinued, the patient usually continues to display an active interest in his diet and appears to recover more rapidly than otherwise. However, this is not a practice widely employed or one to be used indiscriminately.

Corticoid and Salt Management of the Adrenalectomized Patient. It is remarkable how easily the bilateral adrenalectomized patient can be managed; the problem appears to be more simple than that of many diabetics. Thus, the ability to maintain such patients in good health poses no contraindication to adrenalectomy, should the operation be necessary. Just as the diabetic must be advised about his insulin dosage, so must the adrenalectomized patient be instructed and advised about his corticoid and salt therapy and seen at regular intervals to guide his course.

In Table 29-13 are shown the comparative anti-inflammatory potencies for some of the therapeutic corticoids.

ADRENAL MEDULLA

Knowledge of the function of the adrenergic nervous system has increased considerably during this century. It has become clear that there are two fundamentally different types of adrenergic receptors, each of which can combine in ways not yet entirely known (Epstein and Braunwald, 1966). First, we have drugs available that can stimulate these receptors that simulate nerves of the sympathetic system. Secondly, there are drugs that block the alpha-adrenergic receptors that have been available for many years. More recently, pharmacologic agents capable of blocking beta-adrenergic receptors have become available. The mechanisms of action presently known for the beta receptors are complex and they have not yet been employed extensively in the pharmacologic treatment of patients. The value of blocking these beta receptors appears to lie mainly in the management of disorders affecting the cardiovascular system, especially the heart.

Chromaffin tissue, wherever found, is so named because it is stained yellow or brown with chromium salts. This tissue is associated with the ganglia of the sympathetic nervous system, of which the adrenal medulla embryologically is a part. The size of the autonomic system is proportionately much larger in fetal life than after birth, when it is reduced remarkably, except for a few areas. The remaining structures in adult life are the paraganglionic areas which connect with the principal sympathetic trunks, i.e., the celiac, renal, adrenal, aortic and hypogastric plexuses and the carotid body. The adrenal medulla is the largest single site of chromaffin tissues.

It is not surprising that factors that affect the autonomics may also affect the adrenal medulla and vice versa. The major hormone elaborated by the medulla is epinephrine, the first natural hormone to be isolated in crystalline form. Its biologic activity was recognized by Abel in 1897. Epinephrine and norepinephrine were synthesized by Stolz in 1904. More that 45 years elapsed before norepinephrine was to be employed clinically. Norepinephrine is a neurohumor as well as a hormone. Epinephrine is only a hormone. Both hormones are normally found in medullary tissue, epinephrine being predominant. Circulating levels of both epinephrine and norepinephrine vary markedly, with bursts being released in response to various physiological stimuli (e.g., hypotension and hypoglycemia), as well as to psychological stimuli (e.g., fear and anger). These bursts are readily cleared from the circulation by various tissues, many of which can extract over half of the catecholamine which perfuses them in a single passage, either by enzymatic degradation or inert binding.

Tissue catecholamine is stored in two pools —one that turns over rapidly and is released by tyramine and sympathetic nerve stimulation, the other "storage" pool which turns over slowly and is relatively refractile to tyramine.

Norepinephrine is felt to be the neuro-transmitter at most post-ganglionic sympathetic endings in the autonomic nervous system. It is usually present in larger quantities than epinephrine in pheochromocytoma. Both adrenergic hormones are stable in blood, although they are destroyed rapidly *in vivo*, probably by either conjugation or oxidation or both. Most, if not all, tissues appear to be capable of inactivating them (Wurtman, 1965).

It has long been known that the adrenal medulla is not essential for life. However, this is no justification for the conclusion that its 2 vasopressor hormones are unessential, for they are produced generously by other pheochromaffin tissues as well as by the adrenal medulla; therefore, removal of the adrenal medulla does not abolish all of their sources of production.

Pharmacologic Action of Epinephrine and Norepinephrine. The action of these hormones mimics direct stimulation of the adrenergic nerves, though response appears to be upon effector cells of specific organs. Many of the actions ascribed to epinephrine are also common to norepinephrine, but there are also major differences, many of which can be attributed to their disparate alpha- and beta-receptor activity. These differences play an important role in the ultimate decision as to which is the most suitable preparation for use in the particular surgical patient. Among the important sites of actions of these agents are the heart, the arterioles and the kidney. A rise in pulse rate and an elevation of arterial blood pressure occur. Pulmonary circulation and bronchial musculature are also quite responsive. The metabolic response is an increase in blood glucose and lactate and an increase in circulating free fatty acids. Glycolysis may be sufficiently stimulated to overcome insulin shock and may produce frank diabetes in some patients with tumors producing these hormones over prolonged periods of time.

Cardiac response is an increase in rate and stroke volume. The heart beat is more forceful and may be very distressing symptomatically to some patients during the systolic thrust. The minute volume output of the heart is greatly increased over normal. Ventricular irritability is exaggerated; extrasystoles and fibrillation may occur. The effect upon ventricular irritability is the chief reason why these agents should not be used in "cardiac arrest," hypoxia, hypercapnia, hypothermia, in hyperthyroidism or in conjunction with cyclopropane anesthesia, all of which may also create an increased irritability of the ventricles. To superimpose the irritant properties of these drugs under conditions wherein an increase in ventricular irritability already exists may lead to fatal ventricular fibrillation.

Vascular effects are largely limited to the small arterial vessels, especially the arterioles. Vasoconstriction is the rule if one limits consideration to the skin and the splanchnic bed. However, vasodilation is the general response of the arteriolar vessels in the myocardium and the skeletal muscles.

Arterial blood pressure is elevated promptly. Within limits, this response is usually in proportion to the quantity of epinephrine or norepinephrine administered. Some state that the diastolic pressure is reduced in man, but this is not in accord with the observations of many, including the author. More often than not, the diastolic pressure is also elevated; so is the mean arterial pressure. When the vasopressor effect of epinephrine "wears off," transient hypotension may occur as a rebound phenomenon.

Renal blood flow is usually reduced by more than 50 per cent and is accompanied by an increase in peripheral arteriolar resistance. Glomerular filtration and tubular resorption are not consistently altered, although excretion of sodium and chloride is said to be decreased.

Pulmonary arterial pressure is elevated, but it is not certain that this effect is due to vasoconstriction alone. Bronchial musculature is relaxed by epinephrine; hence, the usefulness of this agent in the relief of bronchial spasm of asthma.

The metabolic response is through stimulation of adenyl cyclase which in turn has two major effects: (1) activation of phosphorylase of liver and skeletal muscle producing, via glycolysis, an increased blood glucose and blood lactate respectively, the latter in turn being converted by the liver back to glycogen; and (2) stimulation of lipase in adipose tissue producing hydrolysis of triglycerides and increased circulating free fatty acids. Epinephrine has been employed upon occasion in the treatment of hypoglycemia when exogenous sources of glucose were not available.

Intestinal tone is diminished, but the sphincters of the pylorus and the ileocecal areas contract. Gastric secretion is inhibited.

Contraction of the Spleen. In man the volume of blood contained in the spleen is small, but in the dog and the rabbit, when the spleen contracts, considerable quantities of blood are expressed into the circulation. In these species, the effect is that of an autologous transfusion; in man this seems to be of little consequence.

Blood and plasma volumes are unchanged. The distinctions between epinephrine and norepinephrine are largely those related to specific functions of cardiovascular response. These are summarized in Table 29-14.

Should norepinephrine be administered for many hours or for a day or two as a continuous intravenous drip, vasoconstriction along the venous subcutaneous channel of the extremity may be so intense as to cause cutaneous and fat necrosis on either side of the vessel for a distance of several centimeters. From a practical point of view it is best that a transfusion of blood or plasma be administered into a vein of another extremity while norepinephrine is given *only* by a venous cannula, lest the rate of flow of the blood transfusion be sharply curtailed, or norepinephrine leak into the tissues and cause necrosis.

LIMITATIONS AND CONTRAINDICATIONS OF EPINEPHRINE AND NOREPINEPHRINE IN HYPOVOLEMIC SHOCK. With epinephrine, its rebound hypotensive effect, its tendency to cause ventricular fibrillation, and other side reactions virtually eliminate this drug from serious con-

TABLE 29-14. COMPARISON OF THE EFFECTS OF INTRAVENOUS INFUSION OF EPINEPHRINE AND NOREPINEPHRINE IN MAN*

INDEX	EPINEPHRINE	NOREPINEPHRINE
Cardiac		
Heart rate	+	—**
Stroke volume	++	++
Cardiac output	+++	0, —
Arrhythmias	++++	++++
Coronary blood flow	++	+++
Blood Pressure		
Systolic arterial	+++	+++
Mean arterial	+	++
Diastolic arterial	+, 0, —	++
Mean pulmonary	++	++
Peripheral Circulation		
Total peripheral resistance	—	++
Cerebral blood flow	+	0, —
Muscle blood flow	++	0, —
Cutaneous blood flow	— —	+, 0, —
Renal blood flow	—	—
Splanchnic blood flow	++	0, +
Metabolic Effects		
Oxygen consumption	++	0, +
Blood sugar	+++	0, +
Blood lactic acid	+++	0, +
Eosinopenic response	+	0
Central Nervous System		
Respiration	+	+
Subjective sensations	+	0, +

(After Goldenberg, Aranow, Smith, and Faber, Dec., 1950. A.M.A. Archives of Internal Medicine.)
* 0.1 to 0.4 microgram per kilogram per minute.
+ = Increase.
0 = No change.
— = Decrease.
** After atropine, +.

sideration in most cases of hemorrhagic, burn or traumatic shock. The author has not used this agent for the treatment of shock for many years because 50 years ago it was shown by Phemister and by Blalock that the underlying cause of hypovolemic shock was failure of transport, now called perfusion, and vasoconstrictor drugs restrict perfusion to a remarkable degree.

Norepinephrine, while seemingly capable of "raising the dead" in some instances, should rarely be used in hypovolemic shock unless blood and/or plasma are immediately at hand and can be administered rapidly to expand blood volume. The peripheral collapse in hypovolemia results from the diminished circulating blood volume—not from lack of peripheral resistance. In reality, physiologic peripheral vasoconstriction is already almost maximal and no longer capable of sustaining the arterial pressure without blood replacement. Although admittedly exogenous, norepinephrine administered under these circumstances can induce the smaller arteries and arterioles, and possibly the veins also, to squeeze down a bit further in the agonal state; this is not a practice to follow. The agent that is needed in hemorrhagic shock is that which has been lost—blood (even commercial blood: see Chap. 8)—and very quickly!

On the other hand, occasionally after prolonged and complicated surgery or following extensive trauma, loss of peripheral tone does occur and norepinephrine may be indicated. Although almost always such patients require and may have received adequate blood replacement, further transfusion in volumes greater than needed can easily lead to cardiac failure and pulmonary edema, especially in patients with marginal cardiac reserve. These are the few patients in whom the use of an intravenous drip of norepinephrine is strongly indicated, and its administration may be life-saving. To recognize when the continued use of blood or plasma may be harmful in shock and when the powerful vasoconstrictor, norepinephrine, should be employed, may tax the judgment of the most experienced observer. Generally after a few hours (often less), norepinephrine administration may be slowed or discontinued. However, one should wait several hours longer before removing the cannula from the vein, in case norepinephrine therapy should need to be resumed.

Norepinephrine administration has proved to be more useful in the treatment of the vasoplegic shock of toxemia—septic or chemical. Here the primary circulatory problem is usually one of loss of peripheral tone, although plasma loss may also occur. A vasoconstrictor as the definitive treatment in the hypovolemic shock of hemorrhage, burns or dehydration is contraindicated.

A specific effect of epinephrine and of norepinephrine is the stimulation of the thyroid to release protein-bound iodine, including triiodothyronine, into the blood stream. This was demonstrated in the dog by Ackerman and Arons (1956).

Pheochromocytoma (Adrenal Medullary Hyperfunction). This tumor produces another series of spectacular disorders in hormonal physiology. There may be a familial tendency for these to occur, as Tisherman *et al.* (1962), Kingdon *et al.*, (1966), and several others suggest. The symptoms and signs are those which result from the excessive epinephrine and norepinephrine that these tumors produce. The tumor is of pheochromoblastic tissue and most often located within the adrenal medulla; hence, the origin of its name. They may also arise occasionally from the urinary bladder and the chromaffin tissue of the paraganglia. (Van Buskirk *et al.*, 1966). They are comparatively rare.

CLINICAL PATTERN. In pheochromocytoma the course of the patient results from excessive production of epinephrine and norepinephrine, usually more norepinephrine than epinephrine. Both agents may be found in the urine. The patient may experience paroxysms or bursts of extreme hypertension, due to sudden releases into the circulation of large amounts of these powerful drugs. These attacks may last for minutes to several hours. Anxiety, throbbing headache, palpitation, blurring of vision, nausea and vomiting, perspiration, dilation of pupils, and prostration are among the patient's complaints. Hyperglycemia is often present, and hypercalcemia may occur in some. Generally, such bursts of adrenergic activity are associated with body motion, such as flexion or hyperextension of the spine, or a tight belt or girdle which causes mild pressure on the adrenal area. The systolic pressure may exceed that which can be measured by the usual sphygmomanometer. Death from a cerebrovascular accident, cardiac arrest from ventricular fibrillation, or pulmonary edema may occur; occasionally, a shocklike state develops with high fever as the terminal pattern.

In about half of the patients encountered, however, a base line hypertension is present and is not readily distinguished from essential hypertension. Some clue is to be found in the elevated basal metabolic rate and the diabetic state which frequently are also present. It is thought that the patients in this group are those in whom hypersecretion of the longer-acting norepinephrine, rather than of epinephrine occurs.

DIAGNOSIS. In considering pheochromocytoma, one may try to produce an attack or paroxysm deliberately by palpating the adrenal areas or by asking the patient to perform such activities as he knows to precipitate an attack; however, this procedure is not without risk. Routine laboratory work is of little value other than in a negative way. An elevated basal metabolic rate is often found which is not usually accompanied by the expected avidity for thyroid uptake of iodine[131] or the usual expected altered relationships between the free and the bound serum iodine. Should the tumor be large, it may be detected by intravenous pyelography or the retroperitoneal insufflation of air.

Other lines of evidence for or against the diagnosis of pheochromocytoma may be uncovered through the application of certain pharmacologic tests. One may try to provoke a paroxysm by the administration of several types of drugs which incite the adrenergic hormones. Among them are histamine phosphate and methylcholine hydrochloride. Normally, these drugs produce slight hypotension and flushing. A rise in blood pressure, greater than that noted when the cold pressor test is applied, usually occurs in patients with pheochromocytoma. Neither test is free of the fairly frequent occurrence of false negative or false positive responses.

More useful diagnostically, as well as in the management of the paroxysms, are the so-called adrenergic "blocking agents." They should not be used excepting under resting conditions; preferably the patient should re-

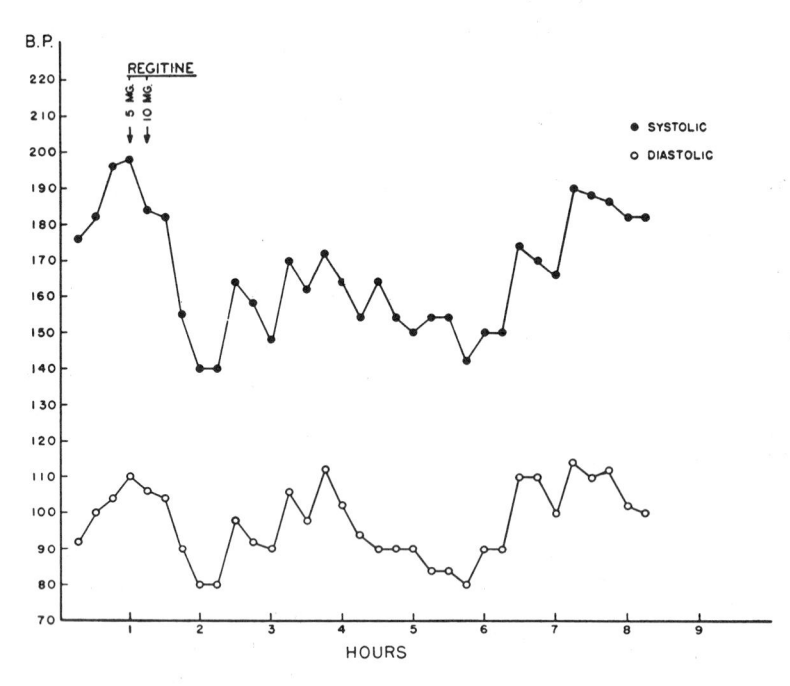

FIG. 29-12. A positive Regitine response in a patient in whom subsequently a pheochromocytoma was removed. (Chart from Dr. Dwight E. Clark)

main in bed for at least 24 hours to secure adequate blood pressure readings under basal conditions. Of these, benzodioxane and Regitine are especially helpful. The former is chemically related to epinephrine. While it retains certain of the pharmacologic actions of epinephrine, it also loses some. Instead of inducing hypertension, it produces hypotension in a remarkably high percentage of patients with pheochromocytoma. Benzodioxane, in dosages of 10 mg. square meter of body surface, is administered intravenously over a period of about 2 minutes. At this rate and dosage, a fall in arterial pressure of up to 50 mm. Hg or greater usually occurs when pheochromocytoma is present. False positive responses are rarely encountered. This same dosage similarly administered to the normal subject usually induces a slight rise in pressure.

Regitine (phentolamine) reacts similarly but with less side effects; 5 mg. of this compound given intravenously produces a lowering in blood pressure, should pheochromocytoma be present. Regitine is preferred to benzodioxane, although both are occasionally used (Fig. 29-12).

PATHOLOGY. Although the incidence of pheochromocytoma is rare, in about 15 per cent of patients with this disease multiple tumors are found. A like number is found to lie outside of the adrenal glands, as paragangliomas of the retroperitoneal or retropleural areas along the sympathetic chains, and at the periaortic plexus at its bifurcation and in the carotid body. The vast majority of these tumors are benign; only a few are malignant.

Usually these tumors are well encapsulated, highly vascular and relatively small. Hemorrhages and cystic degeneration are fairly common; the cut surface is usually brown in color.

SURGICAL TREATMENT. When the diagnosis

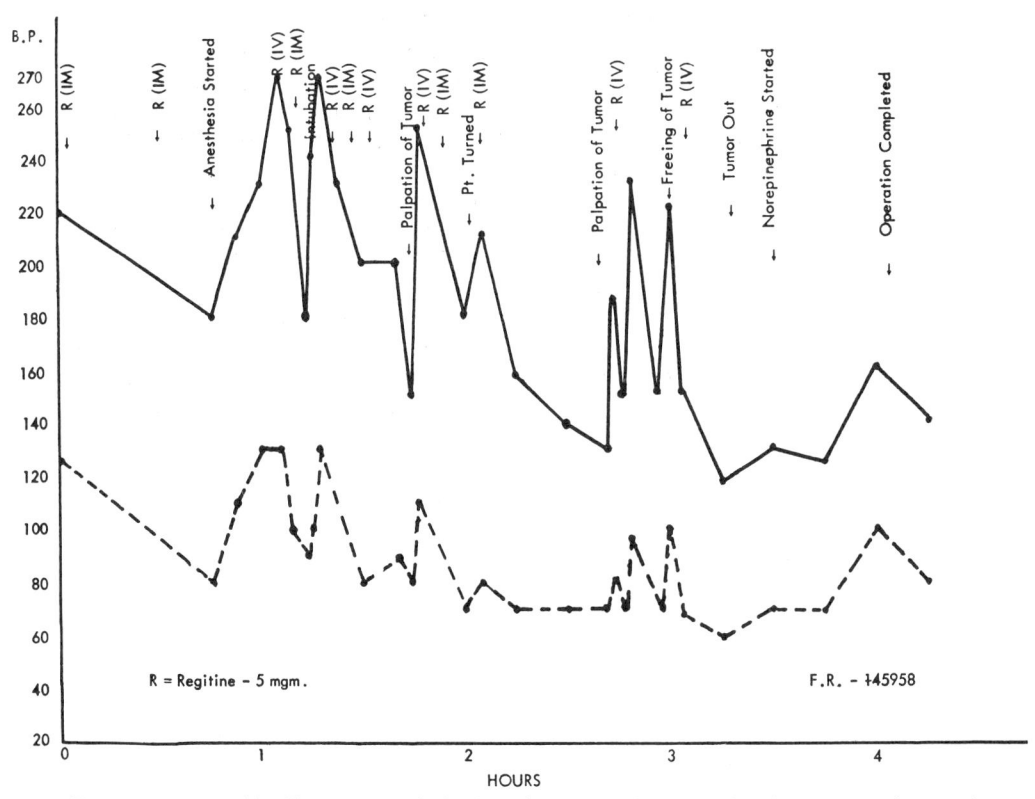

FIG. 29-13. Graphic illustration of the blood pressure increases in the course of operative manipulation of pheochromocytoma. Note response to Regitine and that after tumor was removed, norepinephrine was administered. (Chart from Dr. Dwight E. Clark)

seems to be reasonably well established or carries a sufficiently high index of suspicion, surgical exploration of the adrenal glands and the paraganglionic tissue is indicated. In fact, it is mandatory in most patients, as no other effective treatment exists.

From 1927, when C. H. Mayo removed successfully the first of these tumors, until the advent of the "blocking agents," surgical exploration was extremely hazardous. There were no means available to control the releases of epinephrine and/or norepinephrine induced by surgical manipulation of the adrenals essential to their surgical exploration and removal. Fatal cardiac arrest or cerebrovascular accident from the hypertensive bursts were often caused by surgical exploration and proved to be discouraging to many surgeons. Still others attempted to ligate the adrenal veins and the usually numerous collaterals to and from the tumor, prior to palpating for the tumor. Often this could not be accomplished successfully and usually entailed prolonged anesthesia under the most unfavorable of circumstances.

With the introduction of the blocking agents, carefully and continuously administered and regulated according to need throughout the operation, the risk of operation is greatly reduced. Should the surgeon's manipulations cause a burst of epinephrine to enter the circulation, the elevation of arterial pressure is controlled promptly and readily. An example of this type of control of blood pressure change during the operative phase in a patient with pheochromocytoma during operation is demonstrated in Figure 29-13.

Opinions differ among surgeons as to the operative approach to be employed. Many prefer a transverse abdominal incision in order that both adrenals may be explored, as well as the paraganglionic area. Others prefer the extraperitoneal flank approach, each adrenal being explored separately. These tumors may be situated bilaterally, though they are usually within the same gland. When possible, ligation of their blood supply should be carried out before the tumor is removed.

A precipitous fall in blood pressure often occurs as soon as the tumor is removed. This response presumably is a rebound one and due to release of the arteriolar vasospasm formerly caused by the excess of adrenergic hormones.

A solution of norepinephrine should be prepared in advance and the catheter for its administration already inserted into an appropriate extremity vein. Should the sudden onset of hypotension occur, control of rebound hypotension and the prevention of other untoward effects are easily accomplished. Usually after a few hours, the drip of norepinephrine can be slowed and discontinued when the patient's pressure and circulatory dynamics stabilize. In some, administration of norepinephrine may need to be continued for a day or two. The risk of a skin slough is real. Regitine may be given subcutaneously in small amounts to avoid slough.

The surgical results, as well as the low mortality experience since the advent of the blocking agents and norepinephrine, have encouraged physicians to search more diligently for the presence of this syndrome among their patients with hypertension, especially those with hypermetabolism without hyperthyroidism.

Nonfunctioning Medullary Tumors of the Adrenals. The sympathogonioma, the ganglioneuroma and the neuroblastoma are nonhormonal tumors which may also arise from paraganglionic tissue, including the adrenal medulla. The first is rare and usually malignant, with early metastasis being the rule. The ganglioneuroma is essentially benign; it is well encapsulated and slow-growing, often producing few, if any, symptoms. The neuroblastoma, on the other hand, is highly malignant; it is a fairly commonly encountered tumor in the retroperitoneal area in children. As none of the 3 is a hormone-producing tumor, their symptoms and detection depend upon pressure displacements and metastasis.

Treatment is surgical removal when possible, followed by intensive radiation therapy and actinomycin D; most are fairly resistant to radiation alone. The 2 malignant ones are amenable to chemotherapy after surgery.

REFERENCES

Abel, J. J., and Crawford, A. C.: On the blood-pressure raising constituent of the suprarenal capsule. Bull. Johns Hopkins Hosp., 8:151, 1897.

Aceto, T., MacGillivray, H. H., Caprano, V. J., Munschauer, R. W., and Raiti, S.: Congenital virilizing adrenal hyperplasia without acceleration of growth or bone maturation. J.A.M.A., 198:1341, 1966.

Ackerman, N. B., and Arons, W. L.: Effect of epinephrine and nor-epinephrine on the thyroidal release of thyroid hormones in dogs. J. Clin. Endocrinol., 16:926, 1956.

Albright, F., Parson, W., and Bloomberg, E.: Cushing's syndrome interpreted as hyperadrenocorticism leading to hypergluconeogenesis: results of treatment with testosterone propionate. J. Clin. Endocrinol., 1:375, 1941.

Bovie, W. T.: Electro-surgery as an aid to the removal of intracranial tumors; with a preliminary note on a new surgical-current generator. Surg., Gynec. Obstet., 47:751, 1928.

Carr, H. E., Jr., Curtis, G. W., and Thorn, G. W.: A clinical-biochemical-histologic correlation in hyperadrenocorticism caused by acquired hyperplasia. Am. J. Surg., 107:123, 1964.

Cole, W. H., Gross, W. J., and Montgomery, M. M.: The use of ACTH and cortisone in surgery. Ann. Surg., 137:718, 1953.

Conn, J. W.: Aldosteronism in man. Some clinical and climatological aspects, Part I and II. J.A.M.A., 183:775 and 871, 1963.

Conn, J. W., and Louis, L. H.: Primary aldosteronism; a new clinical entity. Ann. Int. Med., 44:1, 1956.

Cooper, D. Y., Rosenthal, O., Foroff, O., and Blakemore, W. S.: Action of noradrenalin and ascorbate on hydroxylation of progesterone by bovine adrenocortical homogenates. S. Forum, 11:127, 1960.

Cope, O., and Raker, J. W.: Cushing's disease: the surgical experience in the care of 46 cases. New Eng. J. Med., 253:119, 1955.

Cori, C. F., and Cori, G. T.: The fate of sugar in the animal body. VII. The carbohydrate metabolism of adrenalectomized rats and mice. J. Biol. 74:473, 1927.

Cushing, H.: The basophil adenoma of the pituitary body and their clinical manifestations (pituitary basophilism). Bull. Johns Hopkins Hosp., 50:137, 1932.

————: The control of bleeding in operations for brain tumors, with the description of silver clips for the occlusion of vessels inaccessible to the ligature. Ann. Surg., 54:1, 1911.

————: Sexual infantilism with optic atrophy in cases of tumor affecting the hypophysis cerebri. J. Nerv. Ment. Dis., 33:704, 1906.

Davis, J. O.: Aldosterone and angiotensin. J.A.M.A., 188:1062, 1964.

du Vigneaud, V., Lawler, H. C., and Popenoe, E. A.: Enzymatic cleavage of glycinamide from vasopressin and a proposed structure for this pressor-antidiuretic hormone of the posterior pituitary. J. Am. Chem. Soc., 75:4880, 1953.

Epstein, S. E., and Braunwald, E.: Beta-adrenergic receptor blocking drugs. N. Eng. J. Med., 275:1175, 1966.

Evans, J.: Personal communication. 1956.

Grey, Ernest: Fibrin as a hemostatic agent in cerebral surgery. Surg., Gynec. Obstet., 21:452, 1915.

Grey, S. Benson, J. A., Reifenstein, R. W., and Spiro, H. H.: Chronic stress and peptic ulcer: I. Effect of corticotropin (ACTH) and cortisone on gastric secretion. J.A.M.A., 147:1489, 1951.

Harper, P. V., Strandjord, N., Paloyan, E., Moseley, R. D., Warner, N. E., and Lathrop, K. A.: Destruction of the hypophysis with a Sr^{90}-Y^{90} needle. Ann. Surg., 160:743, 1964.

Harrop, G. A., Weinstein, A., Soffer, J. L., and Trescher, J. H.: Diagnosis and treatment of Addison's disease. J.A.M.A., 100:1850, 1933.

Houssay, B. A., and Biasotti, A.: Hypophysis, carbohydrate metabolism and diabetes. Endocrinology, 15:511, 1931.

Illingworth, C. F. W., Forrest, A. P. M., and Brown, D. A. Peebles: A simple method of implanting radon seeds into the pituitary gland in treatment of advanced breast cancer. S. Forum, 6:406, 1956.

Kenyon, A. T., et al.: Urinary excretion of androgenic and estrogenic substances in certain endocrine states: studies in hypogonadism, gynecomastia and virilism. J. Clin. Invest., 16:705-717, 1937.

Kingdon, H. S., Cohen, L. S., Roberts, W. C., and Braunwald, E.: Familial occurrence of primary pulmonary hypertension. Arch. Intern. Med., 118:422, 1966.

Loeb, R. F.: Effect of sodium chloride in treatment of patient with Addison's disease. Proc. Soc. Exp. Biol. Med., 30:808, 1933.

Luetscher, J. A.: Aldosteronism. Disease-a-Month. May, 1964.

Luetscher, J. A., and Johnson, B. B.: Observations on the sodium-retaining corticoid (aldosterone) in the urine of children and adults in relation to sodium balance and edema. J. Clin. Invest., 23:1441, 1954.

Luft, R., Olivecrona, H., Ikkos, D., Kornerup, T., and Ljunggren, H.: Hypophysectomy in Man: Further experiences in severe diabetes mellitus. Brit. Med. J., 2:752, 1955.

Pearson, O. H., Ray, B. S., McLean, J. M., Peretz, W. L., Greenberg, E., and Pazianos, A.: The treatment of diabetic retinopathy. J.A.M.A., 188:117, 1964.

Priestley, J. R., Ferris, D. O., Remine, W. H., and Woolner, L. B.: Primary Aldosteronism: Surgical management and pathologic findings. Mayo Clin. Proc., 43:761, 1968.

Raben, M. S.: Growth hormone. I. Physiologic aspects. New Eng. J. Med., 266:31, 1962.

Rasmussen, T., Harper, P. V., and Kennedy, T.: The use of a beta ray point source for destruction of the hypophysis. S. Forum, 4:681, 1953.

Ray, B. S., Pazianos, A. G., Greenberg, E., Peretz, W. L., and McLean, J. M.: Pituitary ablation for diabetic retinopathy. J.A.M.A., 203:101, 1968.

Richardson, K. C.: Contractile tissue in the mammary gland, with special reference to the myoepithelium in the goat. Proc. Roy. Soc., London, ser.B., 136:30, 1949.

Rosenbloom, A. L.: Growth hormone replacement therapy. J.A.M.A., 198:364, 1966.

Simpson, S. A., Tait, J. F., Wettstein, A., Nehr, R., von Euw, J., Schindler, O., and Reichstein, T.: Konstitution des Aldosterons, des neuen Mineralocorticoid. Experientia, 10:132, 1954.

Stolz, F.: Ueber Adrenalin und Alkylaminoacetobenzcatechin. Ber. deutsch. chem. Ges., 37:4149, 1904.

Swingle, W. W., Maxwell, R., Ben, M., Baker, C., LeBrie, S. J., and Eisler, M.: Effect of aldosterone and desoxycorticosterone on adrenalectomized dogs. Proc. Soc. Exp. Biol. Med., 86:147, 1954.

Thorn, G. W., Emerson, K., Jr., Koepf, G. F., Lewis, R. A., and Olsen, E. F.: Carbohydrate metabolism in Addison's disease. J. Clin. Invest., 19:813, 1940.

Tisherman, S. E., Gregg, F. J., and Danowski, T. S.: Familial pheochromocytoma. J.A.M.A., 182:152, 1962.

Tucci, J. R., Jagger, P. I., Lauler, D. P., and Thorn, G. W.: Rapid dexamethasone suppression test for Cushing's syndrome. J.A.M.A., 199:379, 1967.

Van Buskirk, K. E., O'Shaughnessy, E. J., Hano, J., and Finder, R. J.: Pheochromocytoma of the bladder. J.A.M.A., 196:293, 1966.

Wurtman, R. J.: Catecholamines. N. Eng. J. Med., 273:746, 1965.

CHAPTER 30

K. ALVIN MERENDINO, M.D.

Esophagus

Anatomy and Physiology
Foreign Bodies
Benign Stricture
Spontaneous Rupture of the Esophagus
Esophageal Diverticula
Reflux Esophagitis (Peptic Esophagitis)
Cardiospasm
Tumors of the Esophagus

ANATOMY AND PHYSIOLOGY

The esophagus is a muscular tube approximately 25 cm. long, extending from the pharynx to the stomach. It begins in the neck at the inferior border of the cricoid cartilage at the level of the 6th cervical vertebra and descends in front of the vertebral column through the posterior mediastinum, passes through the diaphragm and upon entering the abdomen ends at the cardiac orifice of the stomach at the level of the 11th thoracic vertebra. It is narrowest at its beginning and a few centimeters proximal to the point where it passes through the diaphragm. In addition, while not narrowed, it may be compressed anteroposteriorly in two additional areas, viz., at the level of the aortic arch and the left main bronchus (Fig. 30-1).

The esophagus consists of 4 coats: an outer fibrous, a muscular, a submucous and an inner mucous coat. The muscular coat consists of 2 layers, an outer longitudinal and an inner layer which is in part circular, elliptical and spiral. The upper fourth of the esophagus is made up of striated or skeletal muscle, a continuation from the constrictor pharyngei, which in the second fourth is gradually supplanted by smooth muscle. The lower half of the esophagus possesses only smooth muscle with few exceptions; racemose glands of the mucous type are lodged in the submucous tissue, and each opens upon the surface by an excretory duct. The inner layer consists of stratified squamous epithelium.[12]

The cervical esophagus receives its blood supply mainly from the inferior thyroid artery. Esophageal arteries may arise from the ascending pharyngeal and the common carotid arteries. In approximately 13 per cent of cases, the esophageal arteries to the cervical esophagus originate from sources other than the inferior thyroid artery. The blood supply to the thoracic portion of the esophagus is mainly from the thoracic aorta, with the major supply being derived from the bronchial arteries; most frequently, there are 3 bronchial arteries: 2 on the left and 1 on the right. In addition, the thoracic portion of the esophagus receives blood supply from the right intercostals in 20 per cent of cases. Exceptional origins of esophageal arteries occur rarely from the internal mammary, the costocervical trunk and the subclavian artery. These vessels tend to course longitudinally and to anastomose with vessels which supply the abdominal portion of the esophagus coming up from below. The arterial supply to the abdominal portion of the esophagus is mainly from the left gastric and the left inferior phrenic arteries. These arteries extend upward through the esophageal hiatus of the diaphragm. In approximately 10 per cent of cases, esophageal arteries originate from an accessory left hepatic and splenic arteries and from the celiac axis.[35] The venous drainage tends to follow the arterial supply. Consequently, it is apparent that the thoracic esophagus between the jugular notch and the aortic arch is the most avascular segment. It is for this reason that if the esophagus must be transected in this area, thus depriving the organ of any arterial supply from the bronchial arteries, the anastomosis should be done at the apex of the chest. Thereby, the surgeon can take advantage of the blood supply to

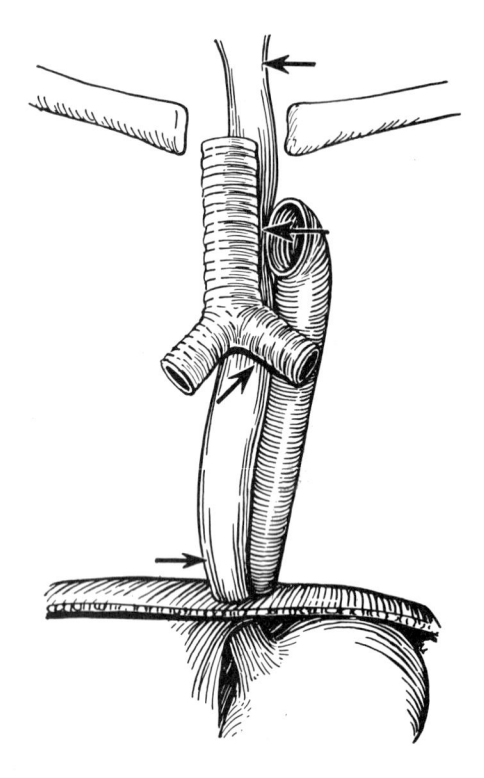

FIG. 30-1. The anatomic relationships of the intrathoracic esophagus indicating its relative inaccessibility and proximity to vital structures. Two normal sites of apparent narrowing of the esophagus exist at the beginning of the esophagus immediately below the cricopharyngei at the cricoid cartilage level and immediately above the diaphragm. This latter is variable from individual to individual and likewise variable in location. In addition, the esophagus is compressed by the aortic arch and also between the left main bronchus and the descending aorta.

the proximal segment from the inferior thyroid arteries.

The nerves are derived from the vagi and from the sympathetic trunks. These form a plexus in which are groups of ganglion cells: one between the 2 muscular layers, and a second in the submucous tissue.

The function of the esophagus is concerned with the conduction of food and liquid from the pharynx to the stomach during the third stage of deglutition. X-ray studies including cinefluorography have contributed greatly to our understanding of the actual behavior of the esophagus in man. The mechanism by which food reaches the stomach varies with the consistency of the food and the position of the patient. Three forms of esophageal contractions are noted: primary and secondary peristaltic waves and apparent purposeless tertiary contractions. The primary peristaltic wave is initiated by the act of swallowing and is largely responsible for the progression of the bolus along the esophagus. In the standing position the passage of the bolus is assisted by gravity. A liquid bolus drops quickly through a relaxed esophagus and collects above the contracted cardiac sphincter. Here it awaits the arrival of the primary peristaltic wave. With the approach of this wave the sphincter relaxes, and the contents are passed into the stomach. If the patient drinks rapidly, the entire length of the esophagus and the cardiac sphincter may remain relaxed, so that the fluid drops abruptly from the mouth into the stomach without interference. Apparently, the relaxation of the esophageal muscle is caused by waves of inhibition which precede the waves of contraction. The waves of contraction, which would be initiated by rapid swallows of liquid, find the esophagus in a phase of inhibition and, therefore, do not occur. If the bolus is firmer in consistency and dry, the wave of contraction is the primary factor in its transport. With the patient horizontal or in Trendelenburg's position, the force of gravity is eliminated, leaving the peristaltic waves as the sole propelling force. The wave initiated by the contraction of the pharyngeal muscles continues in an unbroken pattern down the esophagus. This is referred to as the primary peristaltic wave. The "law of the intestine," viz., contraction behind the bolus with relaxation ahead, applies here also. The speed of the wave of contraction is more rapid in the upper than in the lower portion of the esophagus. This difference is attributed to the nature of the muscular coat. Striated muscle is more rapidly contractile than is smooth muscle.

In some patients, particularly those having either a physiologic or an organic obstruction of the lower esophagus, another form of peristaltic wave is sometimes observed. This wave is termed the secondary peristaltic wave. It is thought by some to be set up by sensory stimulation of the walls. These waves are rarely seen during x-ray examination. When observed, they arise in the region of the aortic arch. Here a segment of the esophagus undergoes spontaneous contraction and forces barium toward the mouth and toward the stomach. The secondary wave, once initiated, progresses as does the primary wave described earlier. Barium that flows toward the mouth may enter the pharynx where its presence may cause the patient's swallow to initiate another primary wave. The inhibitory phase of the primary wave may overtake and inhibit the secondary before it reaches the diaphragm. Primary peristaltic waves sometimes cease at the level of the aortic arch, and secondary waves begin at this point, continuing down the esophagus. This may be due in part to the apparent break in peristalsis resulting from changes in the musculature at that level. Tertiary waves are minute indentations which are observed throughout the esophagus, particularly in its lower portion. These waves simulate the segmental contractions observed in the intestine. These contractions frequently are seen in patients with cardiospasm and, particularly in older individuals without any diseases of the esophagus. Their true significance is unknown.[37]

The harmony of sequence as food passes from the pharynx along the upper esophagus depends upon an extrinsic nervous mechanism and not upon a simple conduction of contractions from one portion of the wall to the next. The exact innervation and nervous control of the act in man is not definitely known. From animal experimentation it is presumed that the motor impulses come through the vagi and that the sensory impulses pass over the 5th, the 9th and the 10th (vagus) cranial nerves. Clinical evidence for the dependence of peristalsis on extrinsic innervation can be observed in patients with large carcinomas of the esophagus. In these cases, when a primary wave progresses down to the tumor, it ceases but continues down the esophagus distal to the tumor an instant later. The coordinating mechanism lies in the medulla; apparently, the nucleus ambiguus supplies the striated and the dorsal nucleus the unstriated muscle. In the lower portion of the esophagus, the wave apparently is independent of the extrinsic nerves. This difference is attributed to the presence of smooth muscle.

The function of the esophagus is to convey material from the pharynx to the stomach and sometimes vice versa.[16] Between swallows and regurgitation, mechanisms at either end of the tube prevent easy access of air from above and gastric contents from below. These barriers are easily inhibited or forced under various circumstances. At the esophagogastric junction esophageal mucosa is immediately adjacent to gastric mucosa. Because of the sensitivity of esophageal mucosa to acid-peptic damage, considerable interest has been evidenced concerning the mechanism here which normally prevents the regurgitation of gastric juice into the lower esophagus. While there is some anatomic support that a sphincter is present, the muscular arrangement is unlike other areas of the enteric tract where true sphincters exist.[20] Some believe that a valvelike mechanism exists because of the oblique entrance of the esophagus with the stomach. This obliquity may be accentuated by the slinglike arrangement of the diaphragm and the oblique muscular fibers of the esophagus itself. Others stress the importance of a rosette of gastric mucosal folds which act as a valve mechanism.

Recently, radiography and intra-esophageal pressure studies simultaneously carried out have revealed unequivocal evidence of the presence of a sphincteric mechanism at or near the level of the diaphragm. This is manifested by a zone of high pressure 2 to 4 cm. in length with maximum pressures of 5 to 10 cm. on either side of the effective diaphragmatic hiatus. While the resting pressure of this area varies with respiration and expiration, it is higher than either gastric or esophageal pressures during certain phases of respiration. In addition, swallowing is followed by a fall in pressure before the arrival of the peristaltic wave. Therefore, the evidence seems to indicate clearly the tonic contraction characteristic of a sphincter and reflex relaxation with swallowing.[3, 9]

FOREIGN BODIES

Incidence

The incidence of esophageal foreign bodies is approximately equal in children and adults. Carelessness is responsible for the majority of instances in children. Most cases occur in unattended children who have easy access to pins, coins, buttons, etc. Under the age of 2, children instinctively put everything in their mouths; those between 2 and 5 years will do likewise unless under careful observation. In adults, foreign body ingestion is almost always accidental; however, some psychotic patients swallow objects intentionally. Artificial dentures are the underlying cause of many of these accidents in adults. The hard palate is rendered insensitive by the dental plate, and the swallowed object is under the reflex action of the constrictor muscles before it is detected. The presence of pathologic conditions of the esophagus (e.g., stricture) is sometimes responsible for the impaction of foreign bodies which ordinarily would create no difficulty.

The most common foreign bodies are fish, chicken and meat bones, metals, including safety pins, buttons, and a miscellaneous category which covers a remarkable variety of items. The commercial practice of chopping chicken rather than disjointing it, is another contributing factor. This custom, while time saving, creates many dangerous bone splinters which otherwise would not be present. The majority of bones will be impacted in the cervical esophagus. However, if this area is passed, they may be located anywhere in the esophagus and, particularly, at the sites of natural narrowing of the esophagus.

Diagnosis

The history of a swallowed foreign body is easy to obtain from an adult but is often missed in children. If the initial symptoms of gagging, choking or coughing are not observed, a foreign body may not be suspected until obstructive symptoms, mediastinitis or an unexplained grave illness occurs.[4, 6] While vomiting is common, often dysphagia or the overflow of oral secretion into the trachea are the first symptoms noted. Children often hold their heads to one side and keep their necks stiffened.

Adults are usually immediately aware of the accident by the discomfort produced and often can locate the level at which the foreign body is lodged. Persistent pain and tenderness over the point of lodgment in the neck, the accumulation of saliva in the hypopharynx and evidence of oropharyngeal trauma may be the only important physical signs. A sticking sensation, particularly with fish bones, is not uncommon. On occasion, cervical crepitus may be present.

When the foreign body cannot be seen by examination of the hypopharynx, anteroposterior and lateral cervical x-ray studies are in order. The lateral view is the more important.[11] Opaque foreign bodies create no difficulty. The diagnosis can be made readily by x-rays in about 75 per cent of patients. While more difficult, with care and overexposure of film, certain types of fish bones may be seen. If complications are present, widening of the cervical area between vertebrae and esophagus, and/or air may be noted.

If after routine x-ray studies no final conclusion can be drawn, a swallow of opaque material should be given. Barium is best, unless perforation is suspected; then water-miscible iodinated contrast material such as Hypaque should be used. A filling defect or an obstruction to flow may be evident. The material may be divided into two streams and go around the obstruction. Radiotranslucency is the one common quality of foreign bodies that go undetected for periods from weeks to years. The plastic materials are characteristically difficult in this regard.

X-ray studies always should precede esophagoscopy; however, on occasion endoscopy may be necessary as a diagnostic and therapeutic endeavor.

Complications

Foreign bodies may be complicated by periesophagitis, with or without abscess, mediastinitis or actual perforation. In long-standing cases, stricture and proximal diverticula may develop. The latter tend to recede in size after removal of the foreign body.

Treatment

Speedy removal of the foreign body is the best treatment. Esophagoscopy should be done as an emergency when damaging objects are at fault. The procedure may be delayed a day or two with smooth objects, such as coins, when they are asymptomatic, as many of these pass safely out of the esophagus. If the foreign body is not arrested or impacted in the esophagus, or is accidentally pushed into the stomach at esophagoscopy, these objects, even open safety pins, frequently will pass through the intestinal tract without difficulty. Occasionally, external incision is necessary.

BENIGN STRICTURE

Localized

Benign strictures are relatively common. They may occur after gunshot wounds, lacerations of the throat or foreign-body ingestions. Strictures may follow operations for tracheoesophageal fistula, diverticulectomy and any operation in which an esophagogastrostomy has been performed (see reflux esophagitis).

The major symptom is dysphagia of varying degree. X-ray studies are important. Esophagoscopy and biopsy are essential for a histologic diagnosis.

Treatment ordinarily consists of simple periodic dilatation by bougies over a previously swallowed thread. However, in selected cases more extensive procedures are indicated. If localized, excision of the area with end-to-end esophageal anastomosis can be performed. Unfortunately, recurrent stenosis may occur. Other measures consist of esophageal substitution for localized areas by means of a jejunal segment or a bypass of the block by means of a jejunal segment en-Roux-Y as shown in Figure 30-5. Yudin's use of the jejunum as a bypass conduit deserves special mention.[42] However, jejunal bypass or interposition presently is used only for lower esophageal strictures in situations where the esophagojejunal anastomosis can be readily effected below the aortic arch. In all other situations for bypassing high localized or extensive esophageal strictures, the right transverse or left colon is used for interposition between the esophagus and the stomach. An end of the colon is delivered into the neck retrosternally for anastomosis to the cervical esophagus. The distal esophagus is closed and left in situ. Excision with esophagogastrostomy also has been utilized. Reflux esophagitis may follow this procedure.

Extensive

The largest group of benign strictures is comprised of patients who have swallowed strong alkalis, acids, or phenols, either accidentally or with suicidal intent. These lesions may be extensive with component areas of injury in the oropharynx and the stomach. The treatment is especially important.

Management of the Acute Burn. The history usually reveals the nature of the material that has been ingested. Weak antidotes, such as vinegar after alkalis, alumina gel or soda after acids, and milk or egg white after phenols, rather than strong agents are advised. Close observation for possible laryngeal edema is important in children. Occasionally, tracheotomy within the first 24 hours may be necessary. In adults the possibility of a chemical mediastinitis or perforation of the stomach due to the ingestion of a large amount of caustics must be considered. Fluids and nourishment must be administered intravenously if the patient is unable to swallow liquids. Gastrostomy should be considered early if there is a complete inability to swallow fluids or saliva. Formerly, the esophagus was placed at complete rest with no further treatment. During recent years, however, active treatment is advised within 24 hours after the caustic is ingested to prevent stricture. Because of the possibility of generalized and localized (perforation) complications secondary to steroid therapy and lack of any evidence that they prevent stricture, the use of steroids is not advocated.

The treatment consists of passing well-lubricated, mercury-filled bougies. The bougies are allowed to pass through the esophagus into the stomach by their own weight. Generally, 3 bougies are passed each day, beginning with a No. 16 French and increasing the size as one determines what the lumen will accept. Usually, the 1st day No. 16 or 18 French bougies are passed. The size is increased gradually until No. 30 to No. 40 French mercury-filled bougies are accepted readily by the esophagus. The size depends upon the age of the patient. Usually, an infant 1 year of age can accept a No. 30 bougie fairly easily, while in adults the sizes are carried up to as high as No. 40 or No. 50 French. When the maximum size has been reached, treatment is reduced from daily dilatations to dilatations every 3rd or 4th day. After the 1st month, bouginage is continued at intervals of 1 week, then once every 2 weeks, and finally once a month. In the absence of stricture formation, dilatations can be performed at greater intervals. Occasional dilatations should be done during the remainder of the patient's life at intervals of 1 or 2 years to prevent the possibility of a tight stricture at a later date. A chronic stricture may develop weeks, months or even years after the initial burn. *It is extremely important to stress the fact that once the esophagus has been burned, stricture formation may develop at any time in the life of the patient. Under no circumstances should treatment be discontinued when normal deglutition returns.*[15]

Management of Chronic Strictures. Simple dilatations may be satisfactory for most chronic strictures. These dilatations are accomplished with olive-tipped bougies passed over a previously swallowed thread. In cases of multiple tight strictures, the patient should be treated by an early gastrostomy followed by retrograde or peroral dilatation. If a No. 6, 8, or 10 bougie can be advanced through the esophagus either from below or from above, the bougie can be grasped at the opposite end, either in the stomach or in the mouth, and brought to the outside. Then a string is attached to it and drawn through the esophagus. Thus, with a string in the lumen, periodic dilatations can be carried out rapidly over a relatively short period of time. When adequate stabilization in luminal size has been established, dilatations may be carried out in the usual peroral manner.

In certain cases, more extensive procedures may be in order. These operations are similar to those discussed under localized strictures.

SPONTANEOUS RUPTURE OF THE ESOPHAGUS

INCIDENCE

The syndrome of spontaneous rupture of the esophagus presumably occurs unassociated with esophageal disease, foreign body, manipulation of the esophagus or any external force. However, many reported cases have shown evidence of pre-existing esophageal disease, viz., esophagitis. Usually such disease has been asymptomatic prior to perforation. Suffice it to say, spontaneous rupture can occur in the presence of a normal or an abnormal esophagus. This catastrophe is seen predominantly in males in the ratio of 8:1, mainly between the age of 35 and 55 years. Although this condition has been recognized for over 200 years, successful treatment has occurred largely in the last few years.

ETIOLOGY

Esophageal rupture nearly always occurs in the terminal 3 or 4 inches of the esophagus. Experimentally, this area represents the weakest portion. In the human cadaver an average pressure of 7 lbs. per square inch is necessary to rupture the adult esophagus. Approximately 4 times as much pressure is required to rupture the esophagus of a child below 12 years of age. The rapidity of the rise in intraluminal pressure rather than the total pressure may be an important factor in perforation. Certain anatomic explanations have been made concerning the propensity of the lower esophageal wall to rupture. It has been stressed that the esophageal muscles at the lower end are tapered and extremely thin; these muscles are relatively weaker than the muscles of the stomach, and segmental defects are found occasionally in the circular muscle layer.

Whether the esophagus is normal or abnormal, the fact that rupture usually occurs in that portion of the esophagus, which experimentally and anatomically has proved to be the weakest, leads one to believe that internal force plays an important role as a causative factor. Because vomiting is observed frequently in spontaneous rupture, some believe that vomiting precipitates rupture by the sudden increase in intraluminal esophageal pressure. Consequently, the term postemetic rupture has been suggested.[33] However, vomiting is not always present until after rupture has occurred, suggesting in certain cases that the vomiting may be the result of rupture and not its cause. Actually, some patients never vomit.

PATHOLOGY

In 90 per cent of the patients with spontaneous rupture of the esophagus, the tear occurs on the posterolateral wall of the left side in the lowermost 8 cm. of the esophagus. It is usually vertical. When the stomach wall is involved also, severe bleeding may occur. However, perforation of the middle third of the esophagus and complete disruption of the lower esophagus have been described. These situations are extremely rare. In "true" spontaneous rupture no disease process, either gross or microscopic, is demonstrable at the site of tear. Esophagitis of varying degree has also been observed. It is difficult to be certain whether these changes are the result or the cause of the rupture.

Diagnosis

The attack often is preceded by a large meal or an alcoholic bout. The acute onset is usually marked by a sudden severe pain. It may be preceded, followed, or unassociated with vomiting. The pain may be substernal, epigastric, or abdominal, and it is severe. The pain characteristically is unrelieved by ordinary doses of morphine. From minutes to hours, the epigastric or abdominal pain becomes substernal, occasionally radiating around into the back and between the scapula. Pleural pain may occur on either side.

The triad of rapid respiration, with or without cyanosis, abdominal rigidity and subcutaneous emphysema has been emphasized as being diagnostic.[2]

X-ray examination may reveal a hydrothorax and, occasionally, mediastinal air. Under fluoroscopic examination, a swallow of water-miscible iodinated contrast material such as Hypaque (not barium) often will delineate the perforation or reveal a para-esophageal pocket with a direct communication into the pleural cavity.

Thoracentesis may yield turbid or blood-stained fluid. It should be examined for food particles and hydrochloric acid, using Toepfer's solution as an indicator. Methylene blue may be given by mouth, and, if immediately recovered in the chest aspirate, the presence of a fistulous communication is proved beyond doubt.

It is apparent that this clinical picture could be confused with many different disease entities, viz., ruptured peptic ulcer, acute pancreatitis, coronary thrombosis, dissecting aneurysm, pulmonary embolism and spontaneous pneumothorax. However, if the patient relates the usual history, exhibits the diagnostic triad, has fluid in the chest and lacks free air under the diaphragm, most of the other conditions can be ruled out quickly. Most diagnostic failures are due to the fact that the examiner is unaware of the symptoms of spontaneous esophageal rupture or simply fails to consider it a possibility.

Treatment

This condition is a surgical emergency. Treatment may be divided into conservative and radical management or, better, by surgical drainage of the pleural cavity versus thoracotomy with direct surgical repair of the site of rupture.

If the diagnosis is established early the patient should be operated upon as soon as possible.[17] Shock is almost always present and is attributable to fluid sequestration in the areas affected, which rapidly become very edematous, and to blood loss, pain and anoxic hypoxia (see Chap. 7, Shock). With proper attention to these factors, operation may be carried out. A left thoracotomy is performed, and the pleural cavity is cleansed. The opening in the mediastinal pleura is readily apparent. The pleura should be opened widely above this area in order to decompress the mediastinum into the pleural cavity. The esophageal rent is identified immediately, and the defect is closed in layers, with nonabsorbable sutures, utilizing finally the mediastinal pleura locally. A plastic nasogastric tube is passed through this area beyond the perforation into the stomach. The chest always should be drained anteriorly and posteriorly in order to ensure proper drainage and complete pulmonary expansion. Ordinarily, the nasal tube is left in place for approximately 1 week. Healing is sometimes retarded. Therefore, a prolonged period is required before peroral feeding is safe. Postoperative complications are empyema, mediastinitis and break-down of repair, with formation of an esophageal pleural fistula.

Conservative therapy may be reserved for those patients who have been seen 24 to 48 hours or longer after the onset of rupture. If the patient has survived this period, closed thoracotomy drainage may suffice, combined with nasogastric suction and prolonged parenteral feeding. Furthermore, exploration at this time may reveal edematous and friable tissue at the rupture site. Attempted closure at this stage may be harmful. If the patient survives with conservative management, residual fistulae and empyema usually require subsequent thoracotomy.

ESOPHAGEAL DIVERTICULA

Two varieties of diverticula occur in the esophagus: (1) pulsion and (2) traction types. These descriptive terms indicate the mechanism of formation. A pulsion diverticulum is thought to develop because of a force from within the esophagus pushing outward. Pulsion diverticula frequently develop in areas of muscular weakness existing naturally or acquired. Consequently, they are mainly false diverticula in that the sac usually is made up of mucosa and submucosal elements and is deficient in regard to the muscular layer. On the other hand, traction diverticulum develops on the basis of a force pulling on the esophageal wall from without. Therefore, all layers of the esophagus are involved, and a true diverticulum occurs.

Pulsion Types

Pulsion diverticula may occur anywhere in the esophagus. However, the most common site is at the pharyngo-esophageal junction; the second most common site is just above the diaphragm. These lesions are encountered in older patients for the most part.

Pharyngo-esophageal Diverticulum (Fig. 30-2). The propensity of diverticula to occur at the junction of the pharynx with the esophagus presumably is due to the relationship of the inferior constrictor muscle and the obliquely passing fibers of the cricopharyngei as they descend on the posterior wall of the esophagus to become longitudinal. Posteriorly at the junction of these muscular layers there is a relative weakness of the surrounding muscular coat of the digestive tube, probably more marked in some individuals than in others. The neuromuscular coordination, which brings about propulsion of food from the pharynx into the esophagus, acts normally when with contraction of the constrictors the cricopharyngei relax to permit the propelled food to pass into the esophagus. When there is incoordination in this neuromuscular effort, the pressure from the constrictors above, combined with the obstruction below created by the unrelaxed cricopharyngei, may result in a posterior bulge, known as the pharyngeal dimple. Recurring pressure on this point eventually creates a sac.[14, 19]

DIAGNOSIS. Usually no symptoms are observed in the initial stages of pharyngo-esophageal diverticulum. In the intermediate stages there may be few if any symptoms. However, when symptoms are present, there may be minor difficulty in swallowing, although most complaints are referrable to a regurgitation of undigested food particles into the mouth with saliva when assuming the horizontal position, or with "gurgling" and unexpected belching. This latter symptom may be embarrassing to the patient; if severe, the patient frequently eats away from the company of other people. In the final stages of the development of a diverticulum, these symptoms become more marked, and dysphagia becomes prominent. In time the patient may become severely malnourished.

On physical examination, the diagnosis occasionally can be made with the patient's mouth open and pressure exerted by the examining fingers at the base of the neck immediately above the clavicles. With backward pressure against the cervical muscles, gas and fluid may be compressed so that a belch can be heard very audibly, not only by the patient, but by any other individuals in the room.

The final diagnosis is made by x-ray studies following a barium swallow. On a straight anteroposterior view, an esophageal "web" in

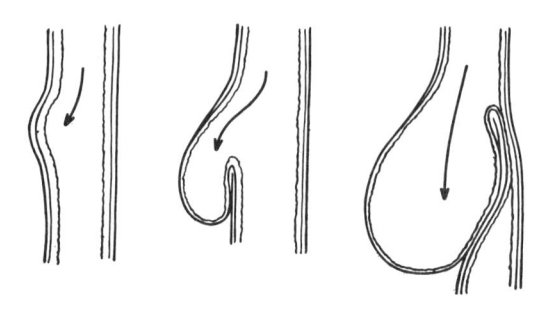

FIG. 30-2. Early, intermediate and late phases in the development of pharyngo-esophageal diverticulum. When fully developed, the diverticulum is in a completely dependent position, and its orifice appears on esophagoscopy to be the continuation of the esophagus. At the same time, compression of the esophagus by the sac containing food and fluid compromises the distal esophageal orifice. It can be understood that the blind passage of a nasal tube or esophagoscopy, unless expertly performed, may result in perforation of the diverticulum.

this area may give an x-ray picture similar to a diverticulum directed posteriorly. Therefore, to avoid this error, an oblique film should be taken which differentiates the two (Fig. 30-3).

Esophagoscopy is contraindicated in the ordinary case because of the danger of perforation of the diverticulum, with mediastinitis. For the same reason, any attempt to pass blindly a nasal tube into the stomach should be avoided. In the presence of severe starvation, if a feeding vent is considered to be important, a nasal tube often may be guided into the stomach under direct vision by means of the esophagoscope.

TREATMENT. This disease is a progressive one. Surgery offers the only means of cure. However, surgical therapy is reserved for symptomatic patients. When symptoms are present, the diverticulum is at least in the intermediate stage. It appears best to advise surgery at this stage prior to the development of the final stages when surgical therapy is more difficult.

The surgical approach is dependent upon the side to which the diverticulum presents. In any event, the incision right or left is identical. Usually the operation is carried out by a vertical incision extending along the anterior border of the sternocleidomastoid muscle. A transverse cervical incision is preferred by some. The omohyoid muscle is severed, and the thyroid gland and the strap muscles are retracted medially and the sternocleidomastoid laterally. It is necessary to retract laterally also the common carotid artery and the internal jugular vein. Care must be taken to avoid undue trauma to these vessels and inadvertent obstruction of the cerebral circulation. Usually, without great difficulty, the sac can be demonstrated protruding lateral to the esophagus and dissected free of its loose attachment. If any difficulty is encountered in identifying the sac, it may be packed with gauze through the mouth, transilluminated with an esophagoscope, or if local anesthesia is being used it can be distended by having the patient drink water. As the neck of the sac is approached, the wall of the diverticulum may be attached intimately to the esophagus proper. This part of the procedure is clean, unless there has been severe infection in the diverticulum or a previous rupture has occurred.

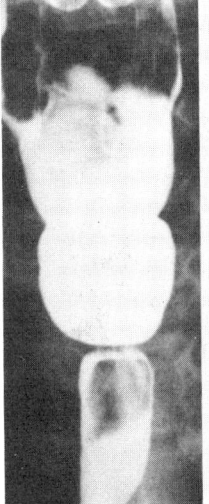

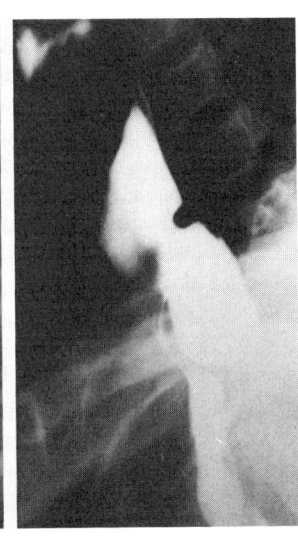

FIG. 30-3. (*Left*) Anteroposterior view of patient with a pharyngo-esophageal diverticulum. In this view this situation could be confused with a congenital esophageal web or the Plummer-Vinson syndrome. (*Right*) Lateral or oblique views are necessary for proper diagnosis. Here the diverticulum is clearly profiled with a spillover of barium into the distal esophagus.

If a nasal tube is desired in the stomach for early postoperative decompression and, perhaps, later for feeding purposes, it should be passed at this stage. With the sac elevated and by direct palpation of the esophagus, the nasal tube is passed from above with ease. The neck of the sac should be amputated flush with the esophageal wall. Care must be exercised to assure removal of all the sac and at the same time to avoid esophageal narrowing at this site. The presence of a nasal tube in the esophagus will help to avoid these dangers.

The neck of the sac may be closed by running or interrupted sutures of the mucosal and the submucosal layers with interrupted nonabsorbable sutures in the muscular layer. Some have advocated transverse closure of the neck and longitudinal closure of the esophageal musculature. A sterile gauze pack may be placed in the defect created by the diverticulum if large and a portion removed daily until all has been removed by the fourth postoperative day. This irritation causes an obliterative reaction which tends to seal off the fascia planes of the neck which communicate with the mediastinum. A Penrose drain may be inserted down to the site of esophageal closure and be led out by a separate stab wound in the inferior portion of the neck.

Others advocate a 2-stage procedure. In the first stage, the diverticulum is elevated and sutured to the strap muscles covering the thyroid so that the sac, rather than being dependent, drains by gravity into the esophagus. At a second stage, usually performed from 7 to 12 days later, the sac is amputated, and the repair is done in the usual manner. The 2-stage method was thought to protect the patient from a descending mediastinitis but has been used very little since antibiotics became available.

In a small number of cases, an esophagocutaneous fistula will develop. However, these close spontaneously. In good hands, the operative mortality should be in the neighborhood of 1 to 2 per cent and the recurrence rate extremely small.

Epiphrenic or Supradiaphragmatic Diverticulum. Such diverticula are uncommon. In general, the symptoms, the x-ray findings, the stages of development and the indications for operation are similar in all respects to a pharyngo-esophageal diverticulum (Fig. 30-4). The major differences relate to the level of the lesion and the fact that some cases are associated with lower esophageal spasm or fibrosis immediately distal to the diverticulum. The mechanism of formation may be related to these obstructive factors and localized muscular weakness. In general, the same surgical principles apply to the treatment of these lesions as with the pharyngo-esophageal diverticulum. The procedure of choice is 1-stage transthoracic removal of the lesion. However, at the time of surgery one must be satisfied that no other obstructive mechanism exists below the diverticulum which might affect the result. If present, attention must be directed to this lesion as well.

Traction Types

Traction diverticula are likewise uncommon. They are seen characteristically about the tracheobronchial bifurcation. In contrast with the globular shape of the pulsion type, the traction diverticulum is cone-shaped. The apex of the cone usually is pointing directly to the inflammatory attachment of cicatrized bronchial lymph nodes. The esophageal opening is open-mouthed and dependent. Therefore, such diverticula empty readily, are usually small, and ordinarily produce no symptoms. They are frequently an incidental x-ray finding. No treatment is needed.

REFLUX ESOPHAGITIS (PEPTIC ESOPHAGITIS)

This clinical entity is characterized by the chemical irritation of the lower esophagus and is believed to be secondary to the regurgitation of acid-peptic gastric chyme. While an alkaline-tryptic esophagitis occasionally occurs following reconstructive surgery for total gastrectomy, the most common and troublesome type of reflux esophagitis is of acid-peptic origin.

Etiology

Considerable controversy exists concerning the exact mechanism at the junction of the esophagus and the cardia of the stomach which

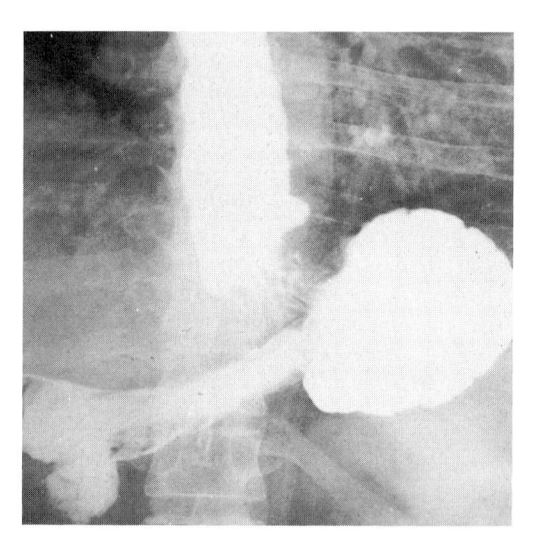

Fig. 30-4. Patient with free reflux of barium from the stomach up the esophagus during the Mueller maneuver (chalasia). A small epiphrenic diverticulum is demonstrated. While some have stressed that an obstructive mechanism usually exists distal to this type of diverticulum, its presence in this patient indicates that other mechanisms also are responsible for the development of epiphrenic diverticula.

normally prevents the regurgitation of gastric chyme into the lower esophagus. Some believe that a sphincter is present in the area, others deny its presence and offer various explanations for the valvelike competence observed. However, it is generally agreed that some protective mechanism exists, otherwise peptic lesions probably would be more common in the esophagus than in the stomach and the duodenum.

When this mechanism is incompetent for any reason, reflux esophagitis develops. This entity has been observed in association with congenitally short esophagus, sliding esophageal hiatus hernia, repeated vomiting, prolonged use of indwelling nasogastric tubes, and following surgical procedures which destroy this mechanism either by incision or excision of this area with restoration of gastrointestinal continuity by esophagogastrostomy. In addition, reflux esophagitis is observed in individuals with normal anatomic relationships in this region unassociated with any other apparent lesion.

PATHOLOGY

Peptic esophagitis usually is limited to the lower esophagus and, particularly, immediately above the cardiac orifice. The esophageal mucosa is the most sensitive of the entire gastrointestinal tract to acid-peptic digestion. The irritation produced by contact with acid-peptic juice results in varying degrees of injury.

In its early stages, a granular erythema with edema is manifest. As the disease progresses superficial ulcerations develop and may eventuate in large ulcers which penetrate into the mediastinum or the pleural cavity. With periodic ulceration alternating with periods of healing, stricture may develop with or without the formation of proximal pulsion diverticula. On microscopic examination there may be epithelial necrosis and hyperplasia with marked polymorphonuclear infiltration and hypertrophy of the muscularis above the stricture. With advanced stages local fibrotic changes become prominent.

DIAGNOSIS

Lower substernal discomfort on swallowing, associated with heartburn, regurgitation and hemorrhage, may be presenting symptoms. Dysphagia may progress until liquid foods only can be swallowed. Physical signs are absent, although in later stages inanition may be manifest.

X-ray studies may be diagnostic. The findings will be dependent upon the stage of the disease. Early in the course of the disease there may be fine irregularity without clear delineation of the mucosal pattern. At times, spasm of the lower esophageal segment occurs also. In advanced cases, lower esophageal stenosis is prominent. The transition from the proximal esophagus which may be dilated to the strictured area usually is gradual and symmetrical. There may be esophageal ulcer or other associated disease, e.g., short esophagus, hiatal hernia, etc. At times, reflux esophagitis in its final stages may be difficult to differentiate from cardiospasm and carcinoma.[41]

Esophagoscopy with biopsy is indicated in all cases in order to establish the correct histologic diagnosis.

TREATMENT

Medical treatment is similar in many respects to the treatment of the ordinary patient with peptic ulcer of the stomach or the duodenum. This consists of small frequent feedings of a bland, nonirritating diet, antacids at intervals of 1 or 2 hours during active phases and less frequently during quiescence. Some advise a conventional Sippy diet. Anticholinergic drugs are of considerable help. In severely symptomatic cases, therapy must be continued in modified form throughout the night as well as during the daytime.

In addition, to minimize reflux, patients should be advised to avoid intra-abdominal pressure by garment compression, and to sleep with the head and the chest elevated at least 8 inches, stooping by bending the knees and the hips and not by spinal flexion.

Where symptoms of esophagitis are associated with a sliding hiatus hernia in an obese individual, weight reduction is important. With reduction in weight, the hernia sometimes reduces itself, with amelioration of symptoms. However, if this combined with other medical measures is of no avail, surgical repair of the hernia is indicated. With the restoration of normal anatomic relationships, the symptoms of esophagitis usually disappear.

806   Esophagus

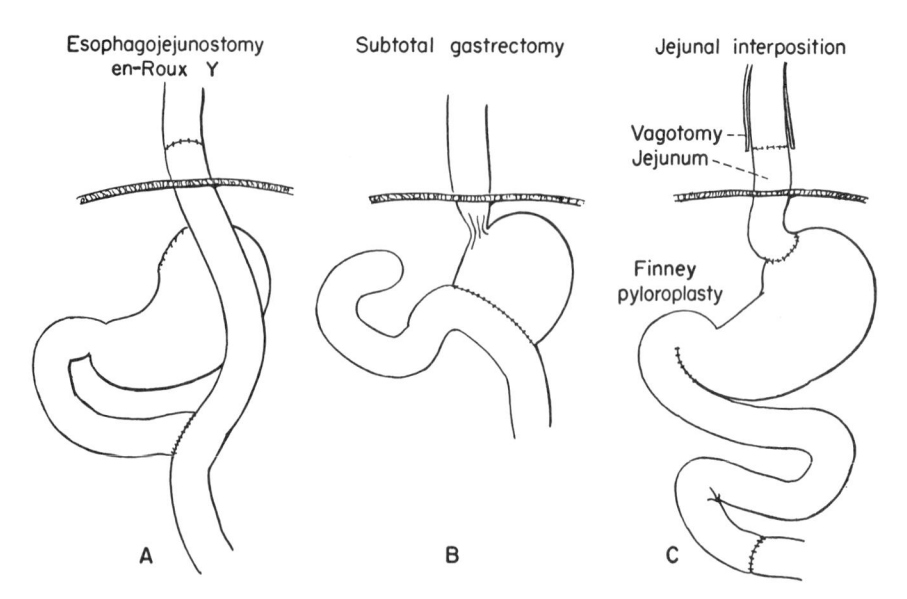

FIG. 30-5. These procedures may be considered acceptable surgical measures in the therapy of reflux esophagitis. (A) An esophagojejunostomy en-Roux Y with the stomach out of circuit has been done. Thus, there no longer exists the possibility of contact of gastric chyme with the esophageal mucosa. (B) A subtotal gastrectomy has been performed in order to reduce acid-peptic secretion, thereby protecting the esophagus. The stenotic segment is left in situ. (C) An interposed jejunal segment which behaves as a substitute sphincteric mechanism has been utilized. This is accompanied by a bilateral vagotomy and a pyloroplasty (see text).

When stricture formation is present, bouginage in the usual fashion over a swallowed string may be necessary. Such dilatations must be carried out at intervals for the remainder of the life of the patient. It should be pointed out that dilatation of the stricture, while allowing food to pass more readily into the stomach, also may allow extension of the lesions by permitting easier regurgitation of gastric juice to more proximal levels. Consequently, bouginage is a complement to and not a substitute for medical measures.

Major surgical procedures for esophagitis and its complications without an associated correctable lesion have left much to be desired. In order to be successful, such procedures must be directed not only to the relief of obstruction but also to the reduction of gastric secretion. Therefore, operations concerned with excision of the strictured area with re-establishment of continuity by esophagogastrostomy are followed not infrequently by recurrent esophagitis. If this procedure is combined with vagotomy and a Finney pyloroplasty or gastrojejunostomy, the chances of success may be improved. Experimentally, it has been suggested that the reflux of gastric contents following esophagogastrostomy may be prevented by implanting the esophagus into a submuscular tunnel in the gastric wall.[31]

Another physiologic approach involves the use of the conventional subtotal gastric resection identical with that performed for peptic ulcer of the stomach or the duodenum.[40] The stricture is left in situ and treated by bouginage. In some patients, dilatations may be discontinued without recurrent stenosis (Fig. 30-5). In order to prevent the contact of gastric secretion with the sensitive esophageal mucosa, excision of the stricture with esophagojejunostomy en-Roux Y with the stomach out of circuit has been used successfully.[1] More recently, it has been proposed that the surgical need is a new sphincter mechanism. A jejunal segment interposed between the esophagus and the stomach with excision of

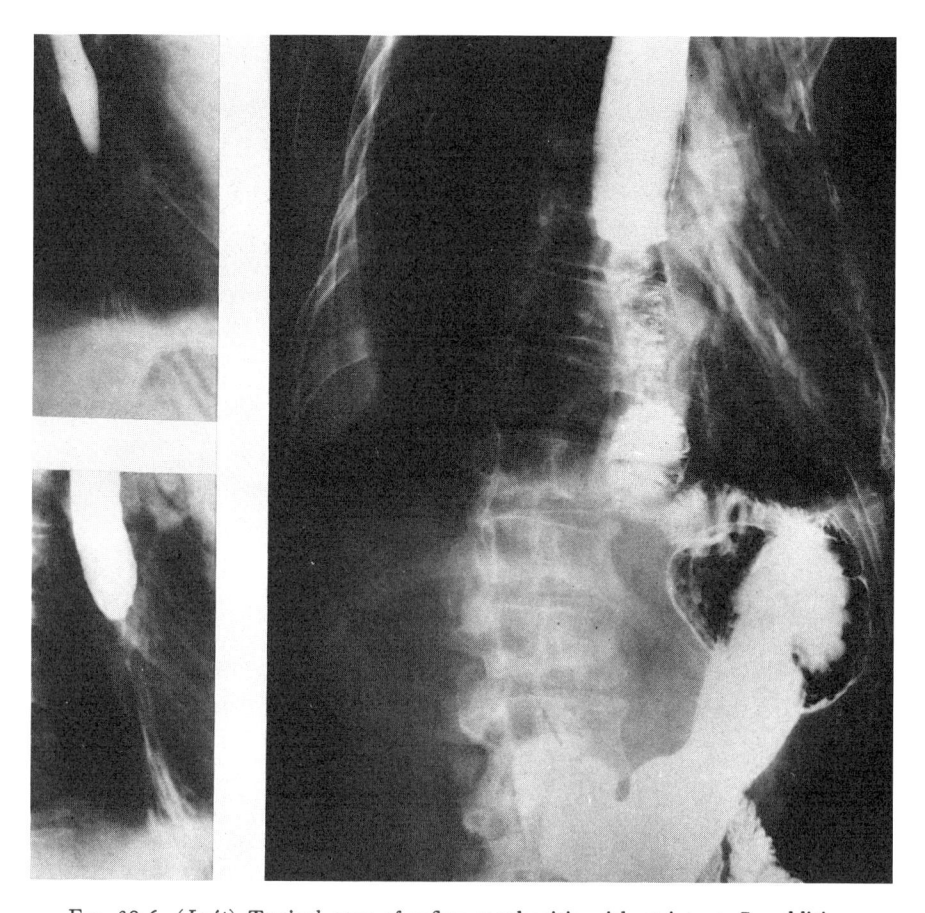

Fig. 30-6. (*Left*) Typical case of reflux esophagitis with stricture. In addition, a hiatus hernia is seen with gastric mucosal folds extending up to the stenotic area. Several years previously while this patient was hospitalized for pulmonary tuberculosis it was noted that he had a hiatus hernia. (*Right*) A jejunal segment has been interposed between the esophagus and the cardia of the stomach with vagotomy and pyloroplasty following resection of the stricture. An old left thoracoplasty can be noted as well as a healed empyema of the right pleural cavity. This patient is now asymptomatic.

the stenosed area combined with vagotomy and a Finney-type pyloroplasty has been found to be satisfactory[23, 38] (Fig. 30-6).

The colon has been used as a substitute for the esophagus in certain benign disorders, including stricture due to reflux. Some are attracted to its use because the blood supply is less tenuous than that of the jejunum. However, the peristaltic pattern of the colon makes it behave more as a conduit and reservoir, rather than as a substitute sphincter, when compared to the jejunum. The complications of stenosis at the anastomosis[22] and the occurrence of peptic ulcer in the colon when used as an esophageal substitute[28] make its use here less attractive.

CARDIOSPASM

Synonyms: Achalasia, mega-esophagus, phrenospasm, esophagospasm.

This disease is a specific clinical entity with definite but not completely understood anatomic abnormalities. It is characterized by spasm of the lower esophagus and the cardia, delayed passage and retention of food with dilatation of the proximal esophagus. The etiology is unknown. One theory suggesting au-

808   Esophagus

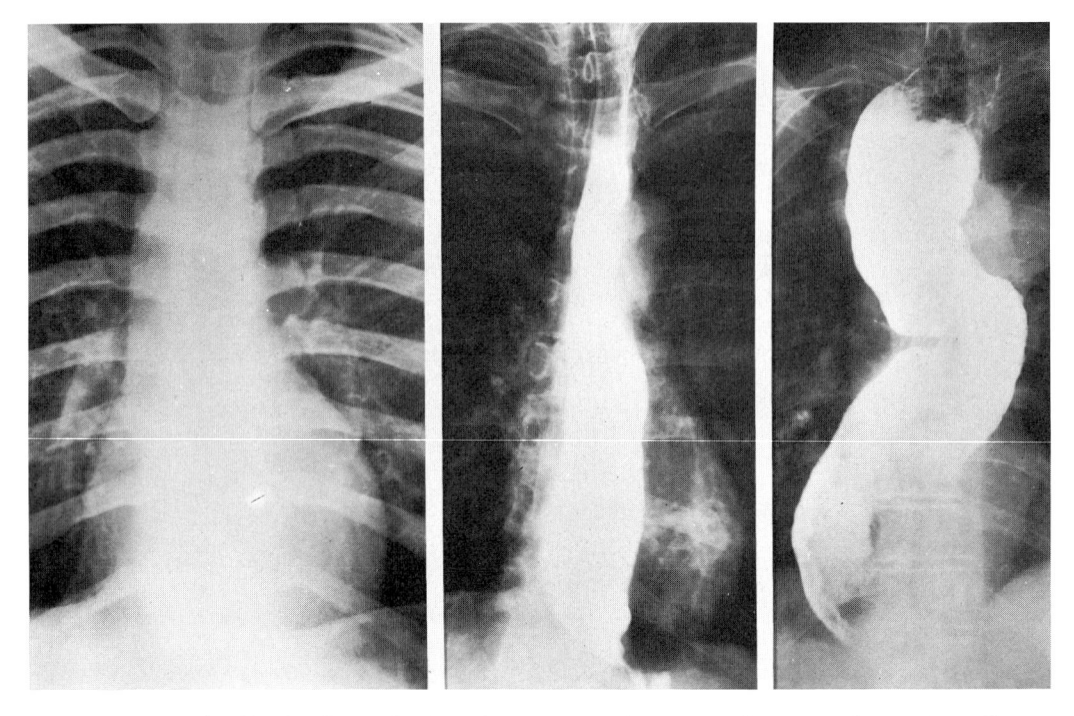

FIG. 30-7. (*Left*) The diagnosis of cardiospasm may be suggested on an ordinary chest film. The outline of the dilated esophagus can be seen behind the heart shadow. (*Center*) A relatively early case of cardiospasm. (*Right*) S or sigmoid contour of the esophagus typical of the late stages of this disease.

tonomic imbalance seems to be the most acceptable. This imbalance may be due to degenerative changes either in the vagus or the sympathetic (Auerbach's plexus) nerves. Mega-esophagus is one of the manifestations of Chagas' disease and is caused by the trypanosome T. cruzi. This organism elaborates chemicals which destroy terminal ganglion cells within the walls of the esophagus, colon and ureter. Because no organic lesion can be found distal to the dilated esophagus, one must consider this disease to be due to a disordered neuromuscular mechanism. A strong psychosomatic overlay is noted in most patients.

DIAGNOSIS

Cases of cardiospasm divide themselves into 2 groups: (1) those starting early in life, in children even below the age of 5, and (2) those starting commonly after middle age. Males predominate in the ratio of 3:2. The characteristic symptoms are dysphagia, epigastric or substernal pain and regurgitation. This disease is the most frequent cause of dysphagia in the female and is second only to carcinoma as a cause in the male. The pain usually occurs immediately upon the ingestion and the swallowing of food and liquids and may be referred upward to the throat. Dysphagia and pain may occur long before the patient has difficulty with regurgitation. In the early stages of regurgitation it is prompt and partial and accompanied by a marked weight loss. As the tone of the esophagus decreases and esophageal dilatation ensues, regurgitation may be delayed for hours, and the emesis may contain material ingested many hours before.[13]

X-ray examination reveals the characteristic findings of spasm of the lower esophagus with dilatation above. The contour of the esophagus may be fusiform, flask-shaped or the S or "sigmoid" type, depending upon the stage of the disease (Fig. 30-7). Many cases are discovered accidentally during routine roentgenography with advanced changes in the esophagus while symptoms are slight, if present at all.

COMPLICATIONS

There exists no tendency toward natural cure, and, if neglected, the disease progresses steadily to a fatal termination over a prolonged period of time. The complications are concerned mainly with pulmonary aspiration and malnutrition. In the later stages of the disease a hugely distended esophagus may be present. Because of lower esophageal spasm, the esophagus fails to empty and consequently becomes a storage bin for food and saliva. At times, and particularly during sleep, overflow may occur into the posterior pharynx, with tracheal aspiration. This results in recurring pneumonitis and lung abscess.

TREATMENT

There are neither drugs nor other medical means of ameliorating the patient's symptoms or the course of the disease.

Minor Surgical Procedures. BOUGINAGE is the most conservative method for the alleviation of the obstruction due to cardiospasm.[39] All dilatations should be carried out over a previously swallowed heavy silk thread. By the passage of a size No. 60 French bougie through the area of spasm, complete temporary relief of all symptoms occurs in approximately 10 per cent of patients. About half of these remain well for prolonged periods. When bougies are used, repeated periodic dilatations are necessary. However, bouginage may be dangerous, particularly in the large S-shaped esophagus, in spite of taking the precaution of attempting dilatation over a prepassed guide thread. Mercury-weighted dilators also have been used. In the late stages of the disease, the esophagus is frequently edematous and friable.

Hydrostatic Dilatation. Either as the primary therapy or if bouginage is unsuccessful, hydrostatic dilatation of the lower esophagus and the cardia may be attempted. Such dilatation should be done only after a No. 60 French bougie has been passed. It is reported that 70 per cent of the patients treated in this fashion will be asymptomatic. Some patients will require subsequent treatment by the hydrostatic method. In experienced hands, hydrostatic dilatation appears to be dependent upon the uncontrolled rupture of the muscular coat in the area of cardiospasm. Among surgeons there is growing support for the management of cases refractory to or unsatisfactory for bouginage by direct surgical means, thereby avoiding hydrostatic methods.

Major Surgical Procedures. It is apparent that a group of patients remains in which the above-mentioned methods are unsuccessful. Currently, major surgical procedures are reserved mainly for this group. Most surgical procedures involve destruction of the cardiac sphincteric area by either incision or excision of this area or an attempt to bypass the area of narrowing.

While it is agreed that cardiospasm is unrelated to acid-peptic disease, the destruction of the cardiac sphincter allows gastric secretion to reflux into the lower esophagus. Because the esophageal mucosa is extremely sensitive to acid-peptic digestion, the patient frequently traded his original disease, viz., cardiospasm, for the more serious entity—reflux esophagitis. Consequently, certain procedures previously advocated for cardiospasm are performed less and less frequently. A list of these operations is included for historical purposes only.

Mikulicz (1904). Gastrostomy with retrograde manual or instrumental dilatation.

Wendel (1910). Longitudinal incision through all layers of the cardiospasm with cardioplasty by transverse closure.

Heyrovsky (1913). Side-to-side anastomosis of the distal portion of the dilated esophagus with the dome or fundus of the stomach.

Gröndahl (1916). Longitudinal incision through all layers of the lower esophagus and the upper stomach with reconstruction similar to a Finney-type pyloroplasty.

Other operations concerned with reconstruction of the esophageal hiatus and on the autonomic nervous system also have been attempted without success and have been abandoned.

Presently, the following operations are thought to possess some merit in the surgical treatment of cardiospasm recalcitrant to more conservative measures:

The Heller operation (1913) originally included longitudinal incision, both anteriorly

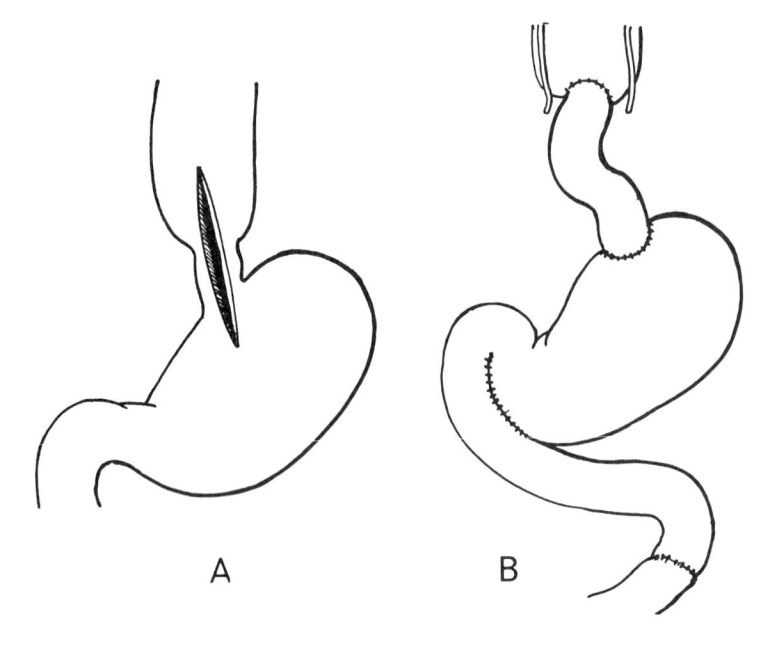

FIG. 30-8. These schematic drawings indicate procedures that might be considered acceptable in the therapy of surgical cardiospasm. (A) Zaaiger-Heller anterior cardiomyotomy is considered to be of value. Because the complications of the modified Heller operation when they occur are related to acid-peptic reflux with esophagitis, some have suggested the addition of bilateral vagotomy and pyloroplasty in order to decrease gastric acidity and volume and to allow a larger gastric efferent outlet. (B) The interposition operation, utilizing a jejunal segment as a substitute sphincter with vagotomy and pyloroplasty (Merendino). This procedure has been carried out in a few patients with success; however, it is not recommended as the primary operation.

and posteriorly, through the muscular layers of the area of cardiospasm, thus allowing the submucosa of the area to bulge outward. In current practice, only an anterior incision is utilized (Zaaiger-Heller). This operation is similar in concept to the *Fredet-Ramstedt operation* for congenital hypertrophic pyloric stenosis. *The Zaaiger-Heller operation* was discarded many years ago presumably because of unsatisfactory results. However, some proponents of this procedure have reported numerous successes. For the latter reason together with the discouraging results with other operations, the Zaaiger-Heller operation has been revived. It is a simple procedure and probably should be attempted if conservative measures are unsuccessful (Fig. 30-8).

Merendino (1955)[23] suggested that the true surgical need in cardiospasm is a new sphincter. He has excised the area of spasm with restoration of gastrointestinal continuity by means of a segment of jejunum interposed between the proximal esophagus and the cardia of the stomach. This procedure is accompanied by a bilateral vagotomy and a Finney pyloroplasty. The clinical results to date in a few patients have been excellent.

TUMORS OF ESOPHAGUS

Tumors of the esophagus are primarily malignant. Carcinoma is the most important tumor of this organ.

CARCINOMA

The average age of the patient with carcinoma of the esophagus is 63 years. The majority of patients fall into the 5th and the 6th decades of life. The next important decade is the 7th, and a poor fourth is the 8th. Males predominate in the ratio of 10:1.

Pathology. Macroscopically, two varieties exist. The most common type produces stenosis (90%) and, eventually, occludes the esophageal lumen. Nonstenosing tumors (0 to 20%) do not occlude the lumen, even in the terminal stages of the illness. Typically, carcinoma of the esophagus is of a squamous cell type. Primary adenocarcinoma of the esophagus accounts for less than 5 per cent of all cases. In the lower esophagus where an adenocarcinoma is contiguous with gastric mucosa, it is frequently impossible to determine whether such a tumor is primary in the esophagus or the stomach.

Carcinoma of the esophagus tends to spread locally by direct infiltration and widely by the lymphatics in the wall of the esophagus and about contiguous nerves, as well as by metastasizing to regional nodes and distantly. Because of the intimate relationship of the esophagus to other important structures passing through the posterior mediastinum, direct extension of the tumor may result in the development of fistulae between the trachea, the bronchi, the pleura, or the aorta. Perforation locally may occur without the development of a fistula. The site of regional metastases is dependent upon the location of the lesion. Carcinomas of the lower third of the esophagus tend to metastasize to the para-esophageal nodes at the diaphragmatic level, to the nodes about the left gastric artery and the celiac axis. Lesions of the middle third tend to involve the para-esophageal nodes locally and the hilar lymph glands at the tracheal bifurcation and downward as well. Carcinomas of the upper third of the intrathoracic esophagus involve superior mediastinal and cervical nodes, tending to follow the venous drainage of this area.

Because of its surgical significance, considerable attention has been directed to the incidence of localized esophageal carcinoma without nodal involvement at the time of autopsy of persons dying of esophageal carcinoma. In large series of cases, the incidence of localized carcinoma without nodal involvement varies from 19 to 48 per cent. On the other hand, in one series of 50 cases, all had involvement, either regionally or distantly at time of death.

The anatomic location of the tumor conditions not only the probable site of regional metastases but also the magnitude of the operative procedures which might be necessary. When only squamous carcinoma of the esophagus is included for study, thereby excluding adenocarcinomas of questionable primary site, the mid-portion of the esophagus is the most frequent site for carcinoma of the esophagus. When one includes those adenocarcinomas thought to be primary in the esophagus, the lower esophagus becomes the most frequent area for carcinoma.

Diagnosis. Ordinarily, the history is invaluable in directing the attention of the physician to the esophagus. 90 per cent of the patients complain of dysphagia at the time of their initial visit, 63 per cent complain of pain, usually associated with swallowing, and 30 per cent complain of vomiting or regurgitation of food immediately ingested or of the regurgitation of salivary juice. Pain may be described as dull, burning, pressure, sharp, or anginal. It may be restrosternal, in the chest, the epigastrium, subcostal, in the back, or in the cervical area. Hematemesis rarely may be the presenting complaint. Rarely, aural pain aggravated by swallowing may be present. This symptom is ascribed to the reflex irritation of the tympanic branch of the 5th and the 9th cranial nerves or the auricular branch of the 10th.

A typical history usually reveals progressive dysphagia, together with voluntary restriction of solid foods to the point where only liquids are taken. Occasionally, early dysphagia is followed by a free interval, subsequent to which a recurrence of the difficulty makes its appearance. Consequently, transient dysphagia has the same implication as does permanent progressive dysphagia. With non-stenosing carcinomas, dysphagia may be absent, even at the time of death.

Many common digestive complaints have been said to represent early symptoms of esophageal carcinoma; none is specific. Although dysphagia is a relatively late symptom, nonetheless, from the practical viewpoint it is the earliest symptom which directs attention to the esophagus. Dysphagia, whether transient or permanent, when combined with the rejection of solid food or a voluntary liquid diet, should suggest the diagnosis of carcinoma in the patient over 45 years. Obviously, some benign conditions can produce this symptom complex; nevertheless, carcinoma of the esophagus should be suspected, and every diagnostic measure explored until carcinoma is proved or excluded.

The correct diagnosis can be made by the roentgenologist in about 75 per cent of the patients. The roentgenograms should suggest the possibility of esophageal carcinoma in almost all cases. Esophagoscopy with biopsy is the final step in making the definitive histologic diagnosis.

Starvation and dehydration are extremely common in patients with carcinoma of the esophagus. These complications are related to dysphagia, which produces either a lack of desire or the inability to swallow. Many patients, with starvation only, die because they are thought to exhibit terminal stages of the disease with widespread metastases. In the absence of any evidence that distant metastases are in fact present, severe weight loss must not be construed as evidence of inoperability.

Prognosis. After the appearance of dysphagia, with few exceptions, untreated carcinoma of the esophagus appears to be a rapidly fatal disease. The patient with carcinoma of the esophagus has an average life expectancy varying from 7 to 12 months from the onset of symptomatology until death. These time relationships pertain to untreated patients or patients given palliative therapy only. Palliative procedures exert no significant prolongation of life, although their value in certain instances is unquestioned.

In the average patient the time from the onset of symptoms until the diagnosis is established varies between 4 to 6 months. Consequently, about half of the patient's survival time is dissipated in making the diagnosis. Unfortunately, undue delay is created by the physician as well as by the patient.[24]

"Carcinosarcoma" is a term used to designate a neoplasm with both carcinomatous and sarcomatous histologic elements. It is a rare lesion—only 28 acceptably documented cases have been found in the world's literature. Because these tumors, in contrast with the common epidermoid carcinoma, have a striking tendency to be polypoid, nonulcerated, only superficially invasive, and metastasize late in the course of the disease, it is possible that the prognosis with surgery should be hopefully more optimistic.[26, 36]

Treatment. Intrathoracic carcinoma of the esophagus poses a serious problem for the surgeon and the elderly patient. Because of the age of the average patient with esophageal carcinoma and the presence of other stigmata associated with normal aging, one must make a meaningful evaluation of the patient's ability to tolerate the rigors of major surgery. The location of the lesion will dictate the magnitude of the operation necessary and should be an important consideration in the final decision. In view of the fact that the hope for cure is presently relatively small, one should not indiscriminately subject all patients to major surgery, even though there is no clinical evidence of tumor spread beyond the local lesion. Obviously, the general condition of the patient may contraindicate a direct surgical attack. For this group of patients and those with evidence of distant metastases, only palliative measures are available. In all other patients an exploratory thoracotomy is indicated.

For purposes of discussion, the treatment of carcinoma of the esophagus will be considered under the headings of palliative and curative methods.

PALLIATIVE METHODS
1. Bouginage
2. Intubation (metal or plastic)
3. Gastrostomy
4. Plastic prosthetic substitution with excision of the lesion
5. Bypass procedures using the jejunum or colon
6. X-ray therapy

Periodic bouginage or dilatation is one of the better means of palliation. Most intubation tubes are of metals or plastics. They are usually funnel-shaped. The flange rests upon the proximal tumor mass with the stem extending through the lesion. This allows a passageway for the ingestion of food by mouth. Fixation of the tube is used by some. The Celestin plastic tube has several advantages in this regard. A midline supraumbilical incision is necessary. With the aid of the esophagoscope, the narrow lead of the prosthesis is passed through the tumor into the stomach. This is retrieved by the surgeon who, by exerting gentle traction, completes the impaction of the flanged proximal end into the tumor.[7] Neither a thoracotomy nor an esophageal incision is needed, thus minimizing morbidity and mortality. On occasion all such tubes may become obstructed with food and require special care. This problem may be accentuated in the elderly patient who for various reasons may not masticate solid food well. Gastrostomy establishes a feeding vent below the obstruction, thus bypassing the esophageal lesion. Gastrostomy in the starved individual is accompanied by some mortality, does not greatly prolong life and, in general, is unsatisfactory to the patient in that he is unable to eat by mouth. Recently, the use of a plastic prosthesis has been advocated with and without excision of the lesion.[5] The risk is great, and the value of this procedure is questionable.

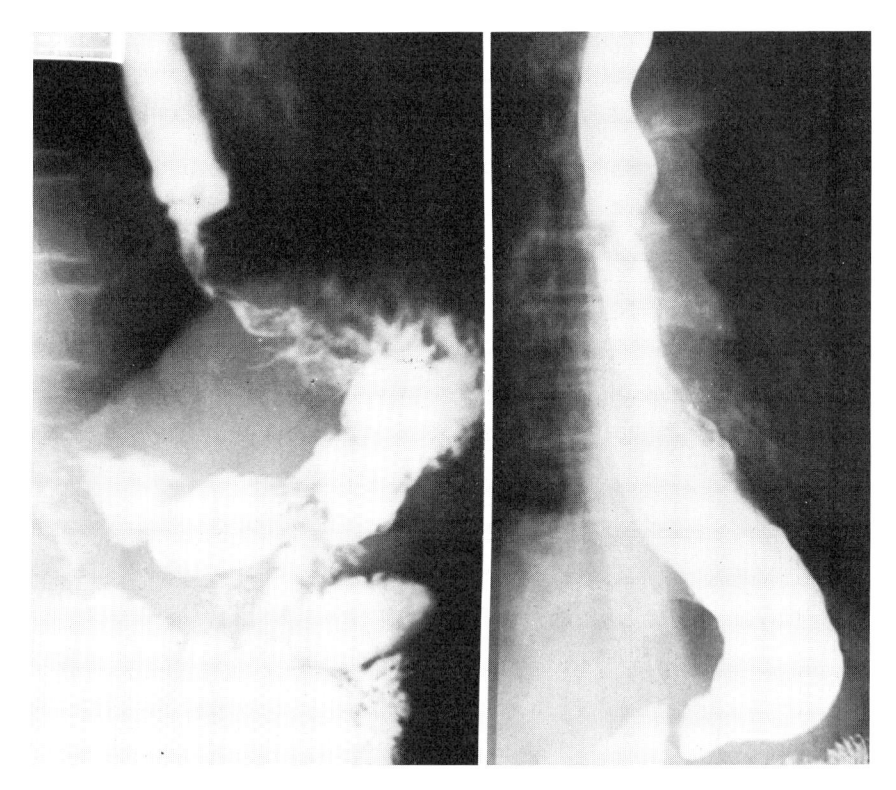

FIG. 30-9. (*Left*) Typical carcinoma of the lower third of the esophagus. (*Right*) Resection of almost the entire lower two thirds of the esophagus, combined with an upper gastrectomy, has been carried out. Restoration of intestinal continuity has been effected by esophagogastrostomy immediately below the aortic arch. The indentation of the esophagus by the aorta is seen readily.

The jejunum has been used to bypass the obstruction. The esophagojejunostomy has been effected in the neck, and a jejunojejunostomy en-Roux Y has been performed in the abdomen with the stomach out of circuit. This intestinal segment may be placed subcutaneous or via the anterior mediastinum.[32] The surgeon then has the option at a second stage of attempting excision of the lesion if the situation looks favorable. For the most part, however, this has been used as a palliative method.

X-ray therapy as a means of treating carcinoma of the esophagus has been utilized for decades. Discarded in the past, it has been revived as a means of palliation. X-ray therapy is capable of sterilizing squamous cell carcinoma on the surface of the body. Unfortunately, the esophagus is disadvantageously placed in juxtaposition to other important structures. Consequently, to destroy the tumor one runs a simultaneous risk of destroying adjacent tissues, for x-rays are relatively unselective with regard to the tissues affected. The revival of this method of therapy is based upon the development of higher voltage machines and the concept of rotational therapy. By rotation of the patient a more nearly accurate and uniform dosage of x-ray with a higher cancerocidal potentiality may be delivered with less damage to the skin and other organs situated radially to this lesion. In addition, the renewed interest has come about because of the morbidity, the mortality and the small cure yield of radical surgery. While carcinomas of the cervical esophagus have been cured by x-ray therapy on rare occasions, this method must be considered mainly as palliative. It has been the experience that if the tumor has spread to regional nodes, a cure by means of x-ray therapy is impossible .

CURATIVE METHODS. Radical surgical procedures involve the wide excision en masse of

814 Esophagus

the esophageal lesion, together with the nodal areas to which the lesion tends to spread.

Radical surgical excision with restoration of gastrointestinal continuity.

Esophagogastrectomy with esophagogastrostomy.[10, 34]

Carcinomas of the lower esophagus ordinarily are approached through the bed of the left 7th rib. Because of the propensity of esophageal lesions to spread in the submucosa, the esophagus should be transected just distal to the aortic arch (Fig. 30-9). Distally, the upper one third to one fourth of the stomach should be removed, including the left gastric artery at its origin from the celiac axis. Restoration of gastrointestinal continuity is made by esophagogastrostomy. Because the vagi must be sacrificed, a pyloroplasty should be performed also.

For lesions of the midthoracic esophagus, a 2-incision approach is gaining favor among surgeons; one incision involves a mid-line supra-umbilical approach. This allows easy access for freeing the attachments of the stomach, leaving intact the right gastric and the right gastroepiploic arteries. By severance of the duodenal attachment to the posterior peritoneum, the duodenum and the pancreas may be mobilized sufficiently for deliverance of the stomach high in the chest. The second inci-

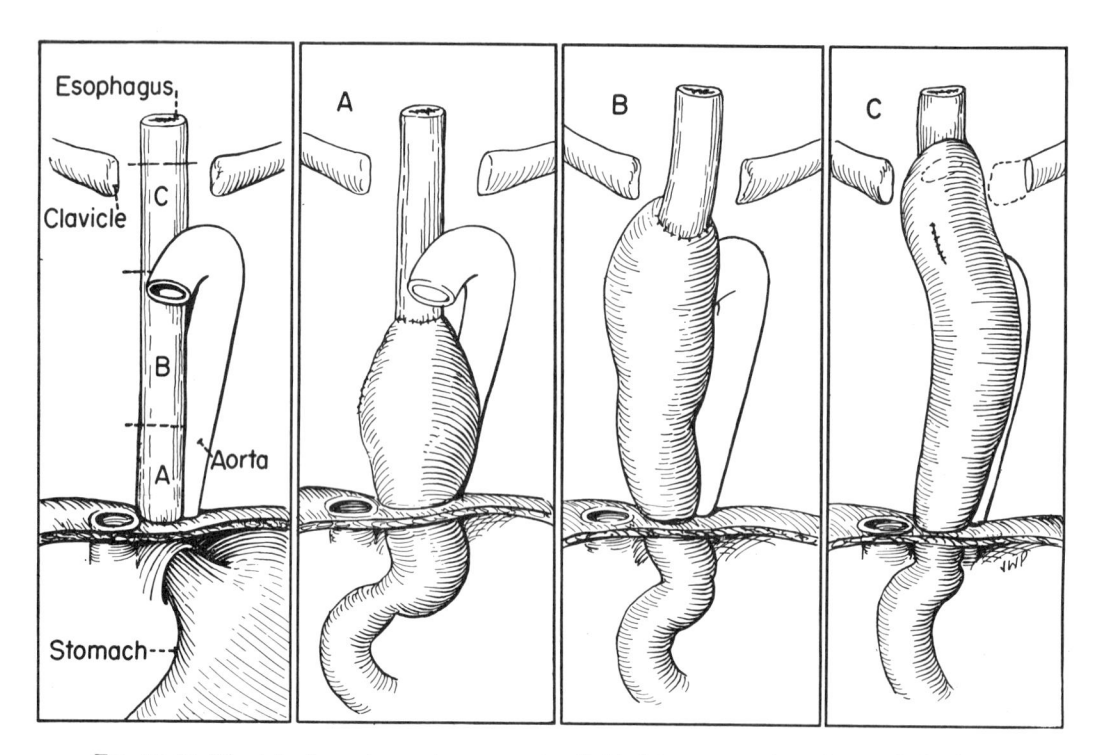

FIG. 30-10. The intrathoracic esophagus can be divided into approximately equal thirds. The location of the esophageal carcinoma conditions the surgical approach and the procedure to be done. (A) Lesions of the lower third may be approached by a left thoracotomy with a transdiaphragmatic component. In order to enhance the chances of cure, most of the lower two thirds of the esophagus should be excised. This also is combined with upper gastrectomy. (B) Lesions of the middle third should be treated by separate abdominal and right thoracic incisions. The esophagogastric anastomosis is made at the apex of the thorax. (C) Few lesions in this area have been handled successfully. Separate abdominal, right thoracic and cervical incisions are necessary. Removal of the medial clavicular head aids in exposure.

If during surgery it becomes apparent that the operation is only palliative and/or the patient a poor risk, many surgeons presently prefer to terminate the operation. Rather than subject the patient to the high risk of a definitive resection, they depend upon lesser surgical procedures or x-ray therapy for palliation.

sion is a right-sided thoracic one. This incision may be made anteriorly through the 4th or the 5th intercostal space with severance of the costal cartilages or by a posterolateral thoracic incision with removal of the 4th or the 5th rib. With the anterior thoracic approach, the patient's position need not be changed; the posterolateral approach is more direct and gives wider exposure, but the patient's position must be changed. There are advantages and disadvantages inherent in either method. After excision of the primary lesion, the freed stomach is displaced into the chest, and the esophagogastrostomy is made at the apex of the chest.

For lesions above the aortic arch, one may combine the abdominal incision, a separate right thoracic incision, and a separate cervical incision for the deliverance of the stomach into the cervical area. This maneuver is facilitated by resection of the medial portions of the left clavicle and the left first rib (Fig. 30-10). Because of the high mortality rate with lesions in the upper third of the thoracic esophagus, most surgeons now feel that carcinomas in this location should not be resected and should be treated by x-ray therapy. Others feel that only carcinoma of the lower third of the esophagus is primarily a surgical disease, and that carcinoma of the esophagus at all other levels should be treated by x-ray therapy.[27]

Obviously, the proper approach to esophageal carcinoma still remains unclear. There is growing favor for substernal transverse and left colonic interposition between the cervical esophagus and the stomach for either palliation or cure. In the former situation the distal cervical esophagus is closed, and the entire organ is left in situ. If no evidence of distant spread is noted at abdominal exploration, the colonic interposition can be done as a first stage to subsequent total esophagectomy preceded or followed by x-ray therapy.

Because of the manner in which esophageal carcinoma spreads in continuity and by lymphatics, some feel that total esophagectomy should be carried out regardless of the site of the primary lesion in the esophagus. Consequently, colonic interposition would be necessary in all cases in which operative attack of the carcinoma was contemplated. There is no evidence presently available which indicates that an improved cure rate follows total esophagectomy. In general, most surgeons still utilize esophagogastrectomy with esophagogastrostomy at the aortic arch for lesions of the lower third of the esophagus.

For carcinoma of the cervical esophagus without evident lymph nodal involvement on examination or at the time of exploration, resection of the area with reconstruction by means of a full-thickness skin tube manufactured from cervical skin is considered as the procedure of choice. This operation must be staged. A split-thickness skin graft over a tantalum splint has been used to bridge the gap.[8] Free autografts of sigmoid colon utilizing the subclavian artery and vein for anastomosis to the colonic artery and vein have been used for replacement of the cervical esophagus after resection for carcinoma and stricture. These are preliminary experiences but encouraging.[30] In the absence of nodal cervical metastases where direct extension to the larynx may be present, a laryngectomy with a distal tracheotomy may be necessary. Such lesions are frequently complicated by early cervical metastases. In this situation, x-ray therapy offers the best means of palliation.

Results. While radical surgical measures have been termed curative, unfortunately the results to date indicate that such measures are mainly palliative. In general, approximately 60 to 70 per cent of the cases seen by the surgeon are operable. This implies that some cases already have been screened prior to the request for surgical consultation. Of those explored, approximately 85 per cent of patients with lesions of the lower esophagus and 70 per cent with midesophageal lesions are resectable. The mortality for lower esophageal lesions varies between 12 and 21 per cent, while the mortality with anastomoses above the aortic arch varies between 25 and 30 per cent. The number of cases involving the upper third of the thoracic esophagus in the superior mediastinal area who have been treated surgically is inadequate for the establishment of a definite mortality rate.

It is apparent, even at the time of intervention, that most operations for carcinoma of the esophagus are palliative. For the entire esophagus and cardia, the 5-year cure rate following resection, in certain major series which are roughly comparable, has varied between 10 and 15 per cent. The 5-year cure rate following resection for carcinoma of the lower esophagus and cardia has been approximately 16 per cent, whether the growth is epidermoid or adenocarcinoma.[21]

In summary, of 100 cases coming to a hospital many will evidence distant spread of tumor when first seen. With additional screening, others for medical reasons will be unsuitable candidates for major surgery. Of those considered operable some will be unresectable. Of those surviving resection, some will be cured. Only about 7 per cent of the total number of cases seen result in 5-year cures. While this is a discouraging picture, the curability of esophageal carcinoma closely parallels the curability of carcinoma of the stomach and carcinoma of the lung. However, in order to gain this yield the patient must be subjected to a higher risk of morbidity and mortality than in the case of gastric and pulmonary lesions.

BENIGN TUMORS

Benign tumors of the esophagus are rare. In one autopsy series of approximately 7,500 consecutive cases only 44 benign tumors of the esophagus were found.[25] None were symptomatic. Approximately 60 such tumors have been treated surgically. The lower third of the esophagus is the most common location for such lesions. Histologically, leiomyoma is the most frequent benign tumor found in the esophagus. In addition, other histologic types, such as myoma, fibromyoma, papilloma, neurofibroma, endothelioma, lipoma, and bronchogenic and esophageal cysts have been described. While a great variety have been reported on a histologic basis, macroscopically all fall into one or the other of two main groups.[18]

Classification

MUCOSAL OR INTRALUMINAL. These tumors arise in the submucosa, grow into the lumen and stretch the esophageal mucosa before them as they grow, being at first sessile, later becoming pedunculated. They nearly always arise at the upper end of the esophagus. These tumors are commonly fibromyxomyomata or fibrolipomata. Some tumors have been described as cystic. It is probable that cystic changes are noted in tumors which have undergone extensive degeneration. They are of all sizes and, if large, become sausage-shaped, conforming to the contour of the esophageal lumen. They rarely become malignant, but may do so.

EXTRAMUCOSAL OR INTRAMURAL. This group is more common than the first. These tumors originate from the smooth muscle, the connective tissue, the nerve sheath elements and the cysts developing from bronchial or esophageal cell rests. Unlike the intraluminal group, they are usually sessile but rarely may become pedunculated. Occasionally, leiomyomata will become malignant, or they may have been malignant from the beginning. Next to leiomyomata, cysts of esophageal and bronchial origin are the second most common benign esophageal tumors. Embryologically, esophageal and bronchial cysts have a gross relationship, and histologically the lining mucosa shares common characteristics, which makes differentiation difficult. Since the embryologic esophagus has ciliated epithelium, cysts of either origin may have a respiratory-like mucosal lining. The single distinguishing characteristic microscopically is that whereas bronchogenic cysts may contain cartilage, true esophageal cysts do not.

Diagnosis. Usually, benign esophageal tumors are asymptomatic. If there is some obstruction, dysphagia may be present. One should consider the diagnosis of a benign lesion if dysphagia has been present for several years. Dysphagia may be intermittent and slowly progressive. Some patients may complain of substernal distress, tightness or fullness, or pain in the chest. In addition, with intraluminal types, regurgitation of the tumor sometimes occurs after violent expulsion efforts, such as vomiting or coughing. If the neoplasm is regurgitated into the larynx, choking and coughing may ensue. Death due to suffocation has been reported.

Significant physical findings are usually absent. The diagnosis rests on fluoroscopic and contrast roentgenographic examination of the esophagus (Fig. 30-11). The demonstration of a smooth, dome-shaped cap of barium adjacent to a rounded protrusion into the lumen of the esophagus suggests a benign intramural tumor. Esophagoscopy should be done and serves chiefly as a means of evaluating the esophageal mucosa overlying the tumor. Biopsy is usually of no value since, with the exception of tumors located near the cardia which may ulcerate, the overlying mucosa is intact. Biopsy through the intact mucosa is dangerous and may jeopardize easy enucleation by introducing infection into the tumor bed.

Treatment. For pedunculated intraluminal tumors, particularly of the upper esophagus, removal may be accomplished by means of a long snare, with or without diathermy. Should the pedunculated tumor be very large, an external incision may be necessary.

With the exception of the relatively uncommon intramural lesion of the cervical esophagus, the transpleural approach to these tumors is preferred. In most instances, the simple enucleation is uniformly successful in true cysts. Less frequently, the tumor may be firmly attached to the mucous membrane. In such situations, the tumor-bearing mucosa should be excised, with closure of the defect.[29] More extensive lesions may require resection of the esophagus and reconstruction. Once the diagnosis of tumor is established, a definite histologic diagnosis seems to be imperative in view of the danger of possible malignancy.

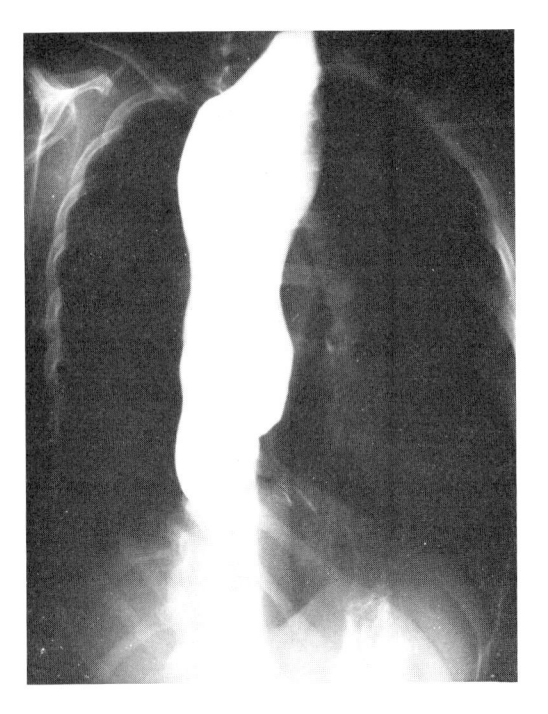

FIG. 30-11. An esophagogram of a 21-year-old female with a history of recurrent pneumonitis, and without dysphagia. The smooth indentations of the lower esophagus suggested a benign intramural esophageal lesion. The preoperative diagnosis—and the correct one—was leiomyoma, and was made on the basis that that is the most common benign lesion of the esophagus. This large benign tumor—11 x 9 x 4 cm.—could not be enucleated and required extensive resection of the esophagus and the stomach, with reconstruction. The esophageal dilatation (misdiagnosed cardiospasm) suggests long-standing obstruction, and it is of interest that this patient denied having any dysphagia. Although they are benign histologically, leiomyoma recurrences are not infrequent.

REFERENCES

1. Allison, P. R.: Peptic ulcer of the esophagus. J. Thoracic Surg., 15:308-317, 1946.
2. Anderson, R. L.: Rupture of the esophagus. J. Thoracic Surg., 24:369-383, 1952.
3. Atkinson, M., Edwards, D. A. W., Honour, A. J., and Rowlands, E. N.: Comparison of cardia and pyloric sphincters. A manometric study. Lancet, 2:918-922, 1957.
4. Barrett, J. H.: Foreign bodies in the air and food passages; observations in 108 private patients. A.M.A. Arch. Otolaryng., 54:651-665, 1951.
5. Berman, E. F.: Carcinoma of the esophagus: a new concept in therapy. Surgery, 35:822-835, 1954.
6. Boyd, G.: Oesophageal foreign bodies, Canad. M.A.J., 64:102-107, 1951.
7. Celestin, L. R.: Permanent intubation in inoperable cancer of the esophagus and cardia. A new tube. Ann. Roy. Coll. Surg. Eng., 25:165-170, 1959.
8. Edgerton, M. T.: One-stage reconstruction of cervical esophagus or trachea. Surgery, 31:239-250, 1952.
9. Fyke, F. E., Jr., Code, D. F., and Schlegel, J. F.: The gastroesophageal sphincter in healthy human beings. Gastroenterologia, 86:135-150, 1956.
10. Garlock, J. H.: Surgical treatment of carcinoma of the esophagus. Arch. Surg., 41:1184-1214, 1940.
11. Goldman, J. L.: Fish bones in the esophagus. Ann. Otol., 60:957-973, 1951.
12. Goss, C. M.: Gray's Anatomy, ed. 28. Philadelphia, Lea & Febiger, 1966.
13. Gray, H. K., and Sharpe, W. S.: Benign lesions at the lower end of the esophagus. Am. J. Surg., 54:252-261, 1941.
14. Harrington, S. W.: The surgical treatment of pulsion diverticula of the thoracic esophagus. Ann. Surg., 129:606-618, 1949.

15. Holinger, P. H., and Johnson, K. C.: Benign strictures of the esophagus. S. Clin. N. Am., 31:135-152, 1951.
16. Ingelfinger, F. J.: Esophageal motility. Physiol. Rev., 38:533-584, 1958.
17. Kinsella, T. J., Morse, R. W., and Hertzog, A. J.: Spontaneous rupture of the esophagus. J. Thoracic Surg., 17:613-631, 1948.
18. Korkis, F. B.: Benign tumours of the oesophagus. J. Laryng., 65:638-645, 1951.
19. Lahey, F. H.: Esophageal diverticula. Arch. Surg., 41:1118-1140, 1940.
20. Lerche, W.: The Esophagus and Pharynx in Action. Springfield, Ill., Charles C Thomas, 1950.
21. Logan, A.: The surgical treatment of carcinoma of the esophagus and cardia. J. Thorac. Cardiov. Surg., 46:150-161, 1963.
22. Malcolm, J. A.: Occurrence of peptic ulcer in colon used for esophageal replacement. J. Thorac. Cardiov. Surg., 55:763-772, 1968.
23. Merendino, K. A., and Dillard, D. H.: The concept of sphincter substitution by an interposed jejunal segment for anatomic and physiological abnormalities at the esophagogastric junction; with special reference to reflux esophagitis, cardiospasm, and esophageal varices. Ann. Surg., 142:486-506, 1955.
24. Merendino, K. A., and Mark, V. H.: An analysis of 100 cases of squamous-cell carcinoma of the esophagus: Part I. With special reference to the delay periods and delay factors in diagnosis and therapy, contrasting state and city and county institutions. Cancer, 5:52-61, 1952; Part II. With special reference to its theoretical curability. Surg., Gynec., Obstet., 94:110-114, 1952.
25. Moersch, H. J., and Harrington, S. W.: Benign tumors of the esophagus. Ann. Otol., 53: 800-817, 1954.
26. Moore, T. C., Battersby, J. S., Vallios, F., and Loehr, W. M.: Carcinosarcoma of the esophagus. J. Thorac. Cardiov. Surg., 45:281-288, 1963.
27. Morrison, D. R.: The treatment of carcinoma of the esophagus. Surgery, 46:516-520, 1959.
28. Mullen, D. C., Young, W. G., Jr., and Sealy, W. C.: Results of twenty years experience with esophageal replacement for benign disorders. Ann. Surg., 5:481-488, 1968.
29. Myers, R. T., and Bradshaw, H. H.: Benign intramural tumors and cysts of the esophagus. J. Thoracic Surg., 21:470-482, 1951.
30. Nakayama, K., Yamamoto, K., Tamiya, T., Makino, H., Odaka, M., Ohwada, M., Tokahashi, H.: Experience with free autografts of the bowel with a new venous anastomosis apparatus. Surgery, 55:796-802, 1964.
31. Redo, S. F., Barnes, W. A., and Ortiz della Sierra, A.: Esophagogastrostomy without reflux utilizing a submuscular tunnel in the stomach. Ann. Surg., 151:37-46, 1960.
32. Robertson, R., and Sarjeant, T. R.: Reconstruction of the esophagus. J. Thoracic Surg., 20:689-701, 1950.
33. Samson, P. C.: Postemetic rupture of the esophagus. Surg., Gynec., Obstet., 93:221-229, 1948.
34. Sweet, R. H.: Carcinoma of the midthoracic esophagus: its treatment by radical resection and high intrathoracic esophagogastric anastomosis. Ann. Surg., 124:653-666, 1946.
35. Swigart, L. L., Siekert, R. G., Hambley, W. C., and Anson, B. J.: The esophageal arteries: anatomic study of 150 specimens. Surg., Gynec., Obstet., 90:234-243, 1950.
36. Talbert, J. L., and Cantrell, J. R.: Clinical and pathologic characteristics of carcinosarcoma of the esophagus. J. Thorac. Cardiov. Surg., 45: 1-12, 1963.
37. Templeton, F. E.: X-ray Examination of the Stomach. Chicago, Univ. Chicago Press, 1944.
38. Thomas, G. I., and Merendino, K. A.: Jejunal interposition operation—analysis of thirty-three clinical cases. J.A.M.A., 168:1759-1766, 1958.
39. Vinson, P. P.: Diagnosis and treatment of cardiospasm. Postgrad. Med., 3:13-18, 1948.
40. Wangensteen, O. H., and Leven, N. L.: Gastric resection for esophagitis and stricture of acid-peptic origin. Surg., Gynec., Obstet., 88:560-570, 1949.
41. Winkelstein, A., Wolf, B. S., Som, M. L., and Marshak, L. H.: Peptic esophagitis with duodenal or gastric ulcer. J.A.M.A., 154:885-889, 1954.
42. Yudin, S. S.: The surgical construction of eighty cases of artificial esophagus. Surg., Gynec., Obstet., 78:561-583, 1944.

CHAPTER 31

HENRY N. HARKINS, M.D. AND LLOYD M. NYHUS, M.D.

Stomach and Duodenum

> Some have made the stomach a mill; some would have it to be a stewing-pot; and some a wort-trough: yet all the while, one would have thought that it must have been very evident, that the stomach was neither a mill, nor a stewing-pot, nor a wort-trough, nor any thing but a stomach.—WILLIAM HUNTER (1718-1783).

Introduction
Peptic Ulcer
Carcinoma of the Stomach
Hypertrophic Pyloric Stenosis
Operative Procedures on the Stomach
Late Complications of Gastric Surgery: The Postgastrectomy Syndrome
Miscellaneous Surgical Diseases of the Stomach and Duodenum

INTRODUCTION

The stomach and the duodenum have important functions and at the same time are the frequent site of serious diseases. In few organs that are diseased so frequently can the majority of affections be attributed to only 3 pathologic conditions. These 3 are peptic ulcer, gastric carcinoma and hypertrophic pyloric stenosis—an inflammatory, a neoplastic and a congenital condition, respectively. Together these 3 conditions are a major cause of morbidity (about 17,000,000 persons in the United States alone are affected during their lifetime) and of mortality (34,000 deaths per year or 2,400,000 of those persons now alive in the United States alone). All other affections of the stomach and the duodenum, while important, are so dwarfed in relative significance by the 3 major conditions cited above that they are listed separately at the end of this chapter so as not to interfere with the main discussion. Before proceeding with the description of the individual diseases of the stomach and the duodenum, a brief basic background description will be given.

EMBRYOLOGY

The stomach appears as a spindle-shaped dilatation of the foregut during the 4th week of embryonic life. There are at this stage both dorsal and ventral mesenteries, the latter extending only as far as the umbilicus. A rotation occurs because the dorsal and the cardiac portions of the stomach grow more rapidly than the ventral and the pyloric portions. The result of this uneven growth is that the dorsal-cardiac portions turn to the left and the ventral-pyloric portions to the right. The dorsal portion thus becomes the greater curvature with the dorsal mesentery forming part of the lesser sac and the greater omentum. The ventral portion becomes the lesser curvature with the ventral mesentery forming the lesser omentum and the falciform ligament. The vagus nerves go along with the rotation of the stomach, the left becoming anterior and the right posterior (rule to remember: "LARP").

ANATOMY

The stomach lies between the cardiac and the pyloric sphincters and includes the fundus, the corpus and the antrum (see Fig. 31-1). The lower part of the antrum is loosely termed the "pyloric" or "prepyloric" region. The lesser and the greater curvatures are of some surgical significance, the former being the site of most benign gastric ulcers, while most ulcers on the latter are malignant. The lesser curva-

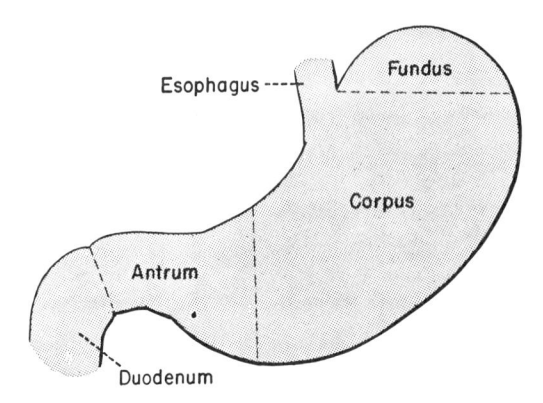

FIG. 31-1. The anatomic divisions of the stomach.

ture is also referred to as the *Magenstrasse* or gastric pathway; it is the shortest route through the stomach, being the course traveled by ingested liquids. The term *Magenstrasse* was introduced by Waldeyer (1908) and popularized by Bauer (1923).

The arteries to the stomach are plentiful. This excellent blood supply has the advantage that healing is prompt after operation (cf. esophagus and colon, which are the opposite in this respect), but, at the same time, the disadvantage that bleeding is difficult to control. Bentley and Barlow (1952) demonstrated that while in the rest of the stomach the mucosal arteries come from a rich submucosal plexus, along the lesser curvature they arise directly from long slender branches of the right and the left gastric arteries which pierce the muscularis directly. This apparently more precarious arrangement of the vascular supply may explain the predisposition of the *Magenstrasse* to develop gastric ulcer. The presence of arteriovenous anastomoses in the stomach was demonstrated by Barclay (1947), Barlow, Bentley and Walder (1951) and was confirmed by Sherman and Newman (1954). Glass spheres of maximum diameters of 100 to 180 μ were passed through the gastric circulation of living dogs by the latter authors.

The veins and the lymphatics tend to follow the arteries (Fig. 31-2).

The gastric secretion-stimulating nerves comprise the parasympathetic gastric branches of the left anterior and the right posterior vagal trunks. It should be pointed out that the left trunk has additional "hepatic" branches (coursing to the right in the gastrohepatic omentum and going to the liver, the biliary tract and the pylorus). Also, the right trunk has an additional celiac branch (coursing posteriorly and to the right in the same mesenteric fold which contains the left gastric artery and the coronary veins, and going to the pancreas, the entire small bowel and the right half of the colon). The apparent sympathetic fibers have been established as the pathways for the perception of visceral pain. The stomach and the duodenum receive most of their sympathetic innervation from the seventh and eighth thoracic spinal segments. Pain of peptic ulcer is therefore most commonly perceived in the seventh and eighth thoracic dermatomes (the epigastrium). Since the

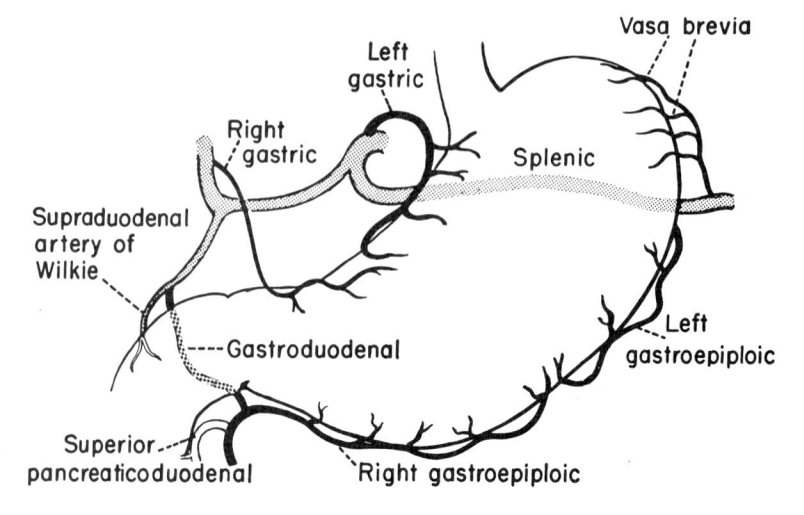

FIG. 31-2. The arterial blood vessel supply to the stomach.

fifth or sixth or ninth and tenth thoracic dermatomes may occasionally contribute fibers to the stomach and the duodenum, pain may be noted in patients with peptic ulcer in the lower thorax or about the umbilicus.

HISTOLOGY

The most important cells in the stomach are the parietal (oxyntic) cells which are especially plentiful in the corpus. There are essentially *no* parietal cells in the antrum. The parietal cells secrete HCl; the chief cells secrete pepsin. It has been shown that there is a relationship between the size of the parietal cell mass and acid output (Bruce, Card, Marks and Sircus, 1959; Card and Marks, 1960). In the proximal duodenum there is a special layer of cells, the so-called Brunner's glands, which secrete mucin that may protect the duodenum against peptic digestion. It is of interest that Moffat and Anderson (1955) reported an adenoma of a Brunner's gland. Such tumors are said to comprise 10 per cent of benign duodenal tumors.

PHYSIOLOGY

The physiology of the stomach and the duodenum is of great importance in studying and understanding the different affections of this region, not only peptic ulcer but the others as well. The following factors will be considered separately: (1) gastric acid secretion, (2) neutralization, (3) gastric pepsin and mucin secretion, (4) altered resistance of gastric and duodenal mucosa, (5) variations in mucosal resistance at different levels in the intestinal tract, and (6) gastric motility.

Gastric Acid Secretion. The secretion of hydrochloric acid is of especial importance clinically. The rule may be given: *No acid, no ulcer*. Acid activates the enzyme pepsin which works best at a pH below 4.0.

Acid secretion may be expressed in clinical units (numbers of ml. N/10 NaOH to neutralize 100 ml. gastric juice using Töpfer's

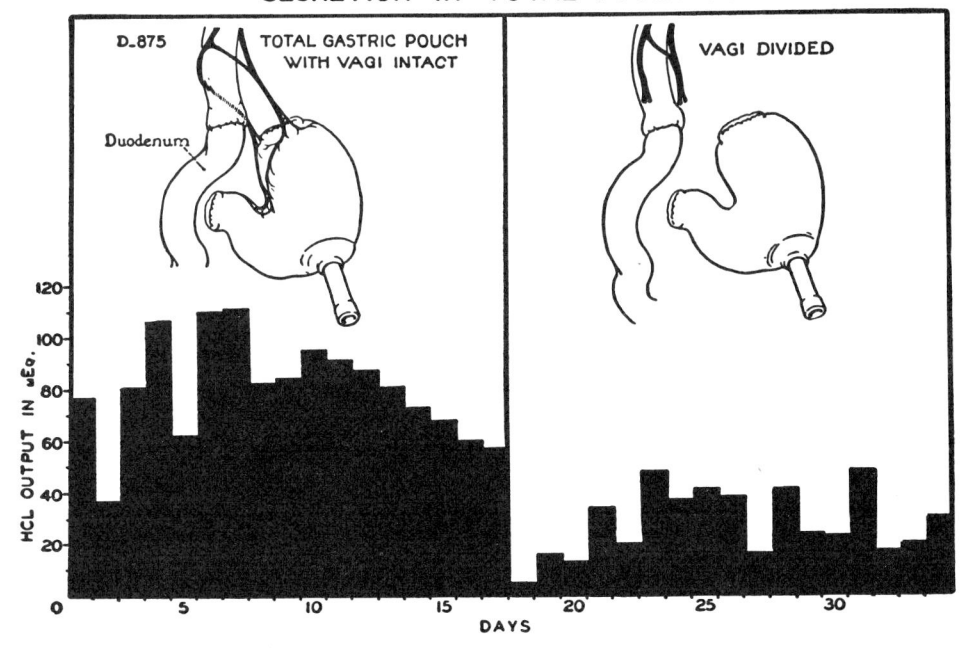

FIG. 31-3. The effect of vagotomy on gastric secretion in the total pouch dog. At the left the control 24-hour secretion of free HCl in mEq. from the total gastric pouch is shown over a 17-day period. At the right the same is shown after vagotomy, demonstrating the marked decrease. (Dragstedt, L., *et al.*: Ann. Surg., 132:626)

822 Stomach and Duodenum

reagent as indicator) or in volume of secretion in liters. We prefer to express it as the product of these 2 factors, or the number of clinical units of free hydrochloric acid × the volume of secretion in liters = mEq. of free hydrochloric acid, usually using an overnight (12 hours) specimen.

Acid secretion is *stimulated* by the following factors:

CEPHALIC (NERVOUS OR PSYCHIC) PHASE by action of the vagi. This usually acts early in the course of a meal, occurring even at the sight or the smell of food. Hypoglycemia sufficient either to reduce the blood sugar level to below 50 mg. per cent or to produce definite symptoms of hypoglycemia acts upon the vagal centers, producing an increased secretion of gastric acid. This action is the basis of the so-called insulin or Hollander test for vagal function. If the test shows no increase in free hydrochloric acid secretion after administration of sufficient insulin to fulfill the requirements listed above, vagotomy has been complete. Because of the importance of the vagal factor in gastric secretion, representative experimental studies upon which our modern concept are based will be listed below:

1. Vagotomy eliminates the secretory response of the stomach to sham feeding (Pavlov, 1910).

2. Sectioning of the vagi to an isolated total stomach pouch or to a Pavlov pouch* causes a marked reduction in acid secretion from that pouch (Dragstedt, Woodward, Storer, Oberhelman and Smith, 1950) (Fig. 31-3).

3. Sectioning of the vagus nerves to the stomach in the Shay rat preparation (if the pylorus is ligated in the fasting rat, an aver-

* Pavlov pouch = a partial stomach pouch with the nervous connections still intact.

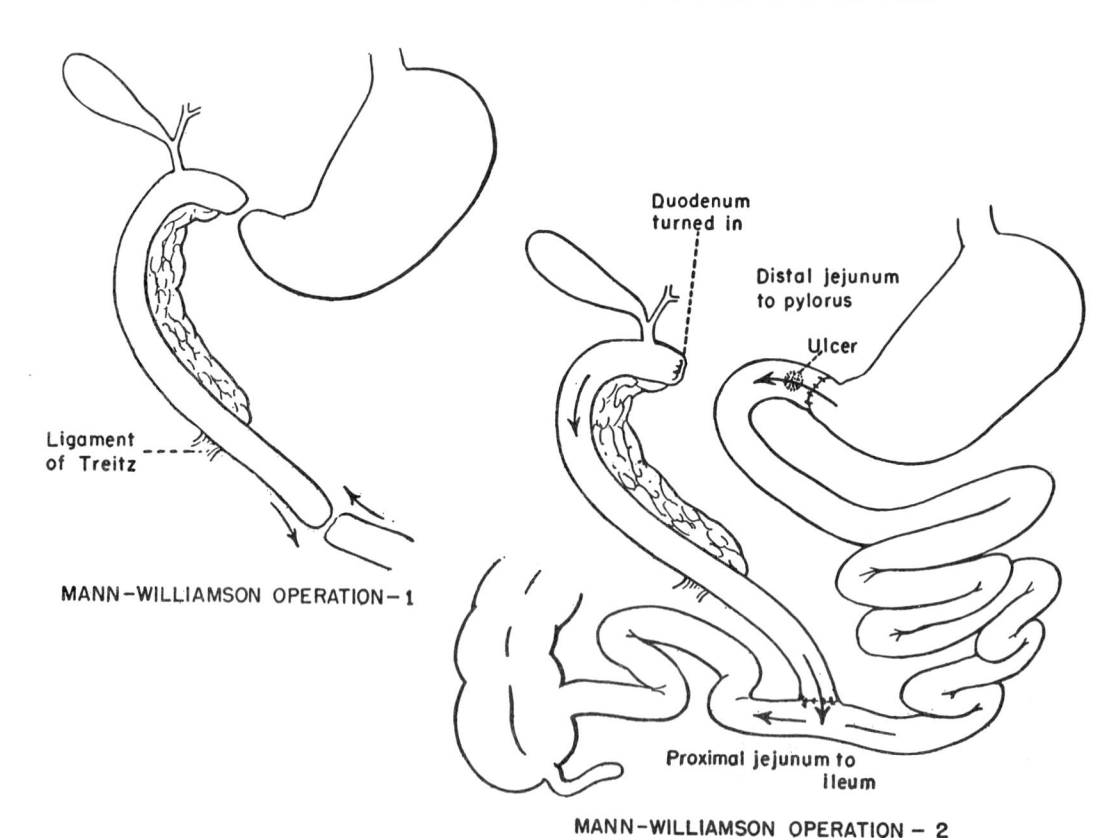

FIG. 31-4. The Mann-Williamson preparation for the production of experimental ulcer. On the left the lines of division of the bowel are shown. On the right, the reconstituted intestinal tract is demonstrated. The diversion of the neutralizing biliary and pancreatic juices away from the gastrojejunal anastomosis leads to ulceration at the point shown.

age of 22 gastric ulcers per rat develop within 24 hours) prevents the formation of gastric ulcers (Harkins, 1947).

4. Sectioning of the vagus nerves to the stomach in the Mann-Williamson preparation markedly lowers the incidence of marginal ulcer formation (Harkins and Hooker, 1947) (Fig. 31-4).

5. Sectioning of the vagus nerves to the stomach pouch in the Sauvage pouch preparation decreases the incidence of stomal peptic ulceration in the connecting jejunal loop (Sauvage, Schmitz, Storer, Kanar, Smith and Harkins, 1953).

6. To show that the action of the vagi is not a simple one, it was demonstrated that cutting the vagi to the *main stomach* causes an *increase* in the acid output of a Heidenhain pouch,* possibly because of secondary stimulation of the hormonal phase (Storer, Schmitz, Sauvage, Kanar, Diessner, and Harkins, 1952).

ANTRAL (GASTRIC OR HORMONAL) PHASE by stimulation of the antrum to produce gastrin which travels by the blood stream acting as a hormone to stimulate the parietal cells of the corpus and the fundus to secrete, in turn, more gastric acid. There is some evidence that the cephalic phase exerts its full effect in the presence of an intact antrum and vice versa, indicating some interdependence of the two stimulating mechanisms. The hormone gastrin is an internal secretion of the antral mucous membrane which contains no parietal cells, and

* Heidenhain pouch = a partial stomach pouch with no vagal fibers leading to it.

acts on the rest of the stomach which secretes no gastrin.

Representative points demonstrating the importance of the antrum are as follows:

1. Edkins of England in 1906 was the first to show that an extract of antral mucosa contains a gastric secretagogue. It is now well accepted that this secretogogue (gastrin) is a low molecular weight polypeptide containing at most 17 amino acids (Gregory and Tracy, 1959, 1964).

2. The hard-learned clinical fact that if the excluded antrum is left in place after a partial gastric resection, marginal ulcer is more apt to occur (see below).

3. The fundamental observations of Dragstedt, Woodward, Storer, Oberhelman and Smith (1950) relative to transplantation or removal of the antrum. As shown in Figures 31-5 and 31-6, when the antrum is in contact with intestinal contents, it stimulates the secretion of hydrochloric acid from Pavlov or total stomach pouches in dogs. When it is isolated, excised, or transplanted subcutaneously, it does not act in this stimulatory manner.

4. Foods and other chemicals placed in the isolated antrum of dogs stimulate acid production of Heidenhain pouches (Oberhelman, Woodward, Zubiran and Dragstedt, 1952).

5. Physical stimuli, including distention, to the antrum attached to the colon of dogs, cause an increase in Heidenhain pouch acid secretion (Dragstedt, Oberhelman, Evans and Rigler, 1954).

6. Antrectomy in the Sauvage pouch prepa-

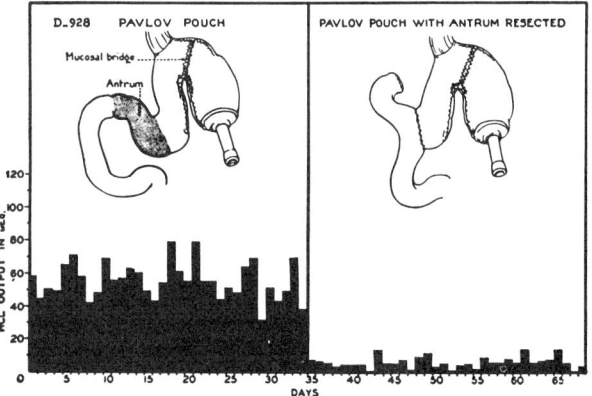

FIG. 31-5. The effect of antral resection on Pavlov pouch secretion of free HCl in the dog. (Dragstedt, L., et al.: Ann. Surg., 132:629)

COMPARATIVE EFFECT OF ANTRUM TRANSPLANTATION INTO COLON AND DUODENUM

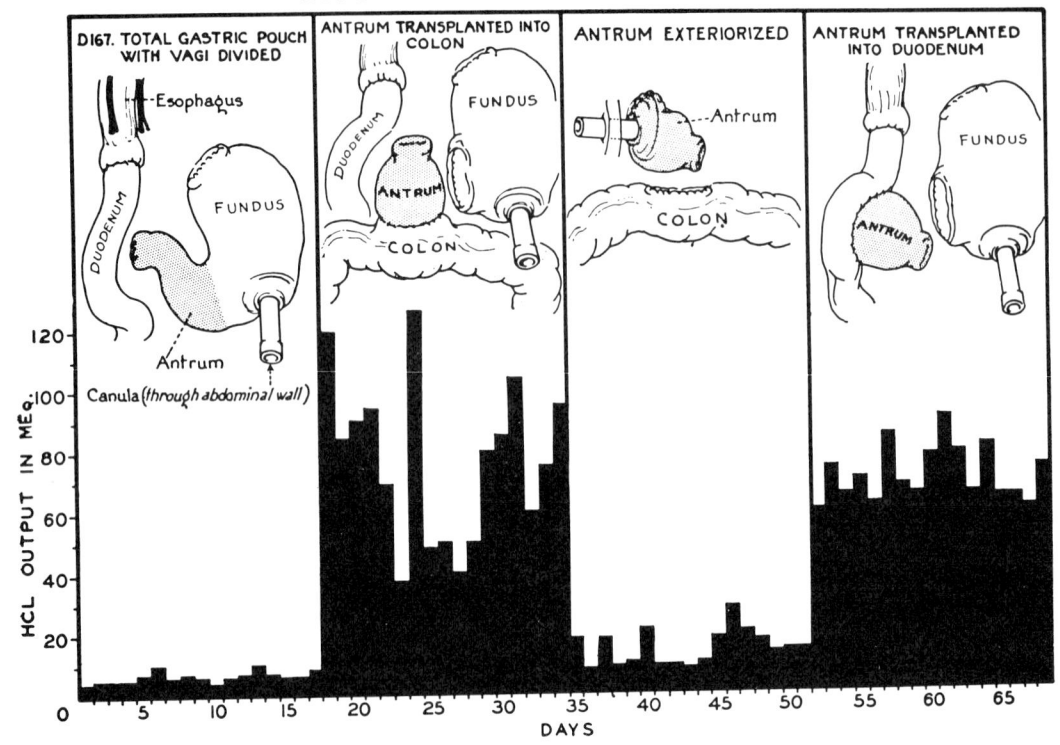

FIG. 31-6. The effects of the antrum in different situations on gastric pouch secretion in the dog. *Phase 1:* Antrum in contact with acid but not with intestinal contents—very low secretory rate. *Phase 2:* Antrum in contact with intestinal contents but not with acid—very high secretory rate. *Phase 3:* Antrum in contact with neither acid nor intestinal contents—quite low secretory rate. *Phase 4:* As Phase 2, except antrum is attached to duodenum instead of to colon. (Dragstedt, L., et al.: Ann. Surg., 134:333)

ration is a more potent factor than vagotomy in reducing the incidence of marginal ulcer in the connecting jejunal loop (Sauvage, Schmitz, Storer, Kanar, Smith and Harkins, 1953).

7. *Effect of portasystemic shunting on gastric secretion:* That gastrin or other acid-stimulating substances which reach the parietal cells via the blood stream may normally be partly destroyed or inactivated while passing through the liver was postulated by Clarke, Ozeran, Hart, Cruze and Crevling (1958). Experiments indicated that portacaval shunts caused an increase in Heidenhain pouch production. The exact role of liver damage following shunt procedures, gastric secretogogues and other factors as background for this type gastric hypersecretion remains unclear (Silen et al., 1963; Orloff and Windsor, 1966).

8. *Criteria for retention of the antrum.* Many gastric operations performed for duodenal ulcer retain the antrum (e.g., gastrojejunostomy). On the basis of many studies, including some listed previously in this chapter, Chapman, Nyhus and Harkins (1959) established 3 criteria for retention of the antrum. These are as follows. The antrum must:

A. Be vagally denervated
B. Remain in the acid stream
C. Have antral stasis prevented.

Experience has shown that if all 3, or even 2, of these rules are disobeyed (e.g., by gastrojejunostomy) a very high incidence (in this case, 35%) of secondary stomal ulcer results. It is a pity that these rules were not worked out on animals before thousands of patients the world over were given unsuitable operations. The reader can think of some now abandoned antrum-retaining operations for duodenal ulcer and see how many of the 3 criteria were left unfulfilled by each.

Only 3 antrum-retaining operations fulfill 2 or more of the 3 criteria. These are the Dragstedt operation (vagotomy and gastrojejunostomy) (p. 854), the Weinberg operation (vagotomy and pyloroplasty) (p. 854) and the Wangensteen segmental resection with pyloroplasty (p. 853).

INTESTINAL PHASE. A hormone similar to but less powerful than gastrin may be secreted by the intestinal mucous membrane when in contact with food. This hormone is not believed to be enterogastrone, an inhibitory hormone.

Just as vagotomy of the main stomach increases Heidenhain pouch acid production, probably due to greater output of gastrin from the antrum (see p. 823), so Kelly, Nyhus and Harkins (1964) have shown that vagotomy of the small intestine does the same, possibly for a similar reason relating to the output of a gastrinlike hormone from the small intestine.

PITUITARY-ADRENAL PHASE. Stimulation of the posterior hypothalamus may act on the stomach by way of the adrenal cortex as an intermediary. Villarreal, Ganong and Gray (1955) similarly found that in the dog ACTH stimulates gastric acid secretion after a latent period of 3 to 4 hours and despite antrectomy or vagotomy, but that its action is blocked by bilateral adrenalectomy.

PANCREATIC PHASE. The pancreas plays a double role in the etiology of peptic ulcer. The first depends upon the fact that exclusion of the external secretion of the organ increases the tendency to ulceration of the duodenum. This observation is the main basis of the Mann-Williamson preparation to produce experimental ulcer.

Elman and Hartmann (1931) found that complete diversion of the pancreatic secretion away from the duodenum resulted in duodenal ulcer in all of the 6 dogs they studied. Dragstedt (1942) reported that external drainage of the pancreatic secretions produced peptic ulcer in 100 per cent of dogs, but that in 300 pancreatectomies the incidence of ulcer was only 1.3 per cent, indicating a curious difference. Poth, Manhoff and DeLoach (1948) further helped to establish the role of the pancreas in the production of peptic ulcer.

The importance of the internal secretions of the pancreas in gastric secretion is more complex. The administration of insulin is the basis of the well-known Hollander test for completeness of vagotomy. In addition, Preshaw (1966) has demonstrated a relationship between gastrin and pancreatic secretion.

Another important observation is that patients with hyperfunctioning islet cell tumors seldom develop peptic ulcer. The report of Janowitz and Crohn (1951) represents one of the few in the literature of coexistent peptic ulcer and hyperfunctioning islet cell tumor. Furthermore, in their case, removal of the islet cell tumor, while restoring the blood sugar values to normal, did not affect the clinical course of the ulcer.

These basic studies on the role of the pancreas indicate that its external secretion may prevent marginal ulcers, and its internal secretions may be a factor in (1) stress ulcers of both the Curling and the Cushing types, and (2) intractable ulcer (q.v.).

Acid secretion is *inhibited* by the following factors:

1. *Nervous Factor.* The action of the sympathetic fibers may either affect the stomach directly, or hold the vagal stimuli in check (Cushing, 1932; Gregory and Tracy, 1960). Holle (1968) has demonstrated an acid control mechanism effective when the vagal supply to the antrum remains intact.

2. *"Antral Acid-Inhibition."* It is believed that when excess acid strikes the antrum, this acts as a signal to the parietal cells to slow down in the production of acid. It is of interest that one organ, the antrum, can be active in both stimulating and inhibiting the production of acid.

A. Oberhelman, Woodward, Zubiran and Dragstedt (1952) demonstrated that in the dog the flow of acid gastric juice through an antral pouch attached to the colon markedly diminishes the secretory stimulating effect of the antral pouch.

B. State, Katz, Kaplan, Herman, Morgenstern and Knight (1955) demonstrated that after wedge resection the incidence of histamine-induced ulcers in dogs is significantly less when the antrum is preserved and anastomosed to the residual gastric pouch than when it is excised and continuity restored by Billroth I or II anastomosis.

C. Brackney, Campbell and Wangensteen (1954) performed a modification of the Sauvage pouch experiment, except that in one variant the antrum was in contact with the acid secretions of the stomach. The incidence of ulcer was much less than when the antrum was not bathed by acid.

D. Shapira, Morgenstern and State (1960) studied antral inhibitions with twin antrum pouches.

3. *"Antral Inhibitory Hormone."* The presence of an antral inhibitory hormone produced by the antrum was postulated by Harrison, Lakey and Hyde (1956), and Thompson *et al.* Studies of Jordan and Sand (1957); Woodward, Trumbull, Schapiro and Towne (1958) and of Dragstedt, Kohatzu, Gwaltney, Nagano and Greenlee (1959) tend to cast doubt on this hypothesis. However, the extraction of an inhibitor substance from human gastric juice has been reported by Smith, DuVal, Joel and Wolf (1959) and Smith, DuVal, Joel, Hanska and Wolf (1960).

4. *"Duodenal Acid-Inhibition."* This is a postulated mechanism similar to antral inhibition except that the excess acid acts upon the duodenum rather than on the antrum to cause a supposed hormonal warning which passes to the stomach which, in turn, cuts down on the production of acid. Enterogastrone, a possible inhibitory hormone produced by the duodenum, may be the factor in duodenal inhibition. Evidence for duodenal inhibition is as follows:

A. Sokolov (1904) reported that the instillation of 0.5 per cent HCl into the duodenum inhibits gastric secretion.

B. Day and Webster (1935) and Griffiths (1936) confirmed this observation. Pincus, Thomas and Rehfuss (1942) reported that acid inhibition resulted only if the pH in the duodenum was 2.5 or lower. The extent of inhibition was dependent upon the level of pH produced.

C. Dragstedt, Oberhelman and Smith (1951) and later Harkins, Schmitz, Nyhus, Kanar, Zech and Griffith (1954) performed subtotal gastric resections in dogs after attaching the antrum to the colon. In half the animals the continuity was restored by gastroduodenal and in half by gastrojejunal

TABLE 31-1. EFFECT OF TYPE OF ANASTOMOSIS ON INCIDENCE OF EXPERIMENTAL ULCER PRODUCED BY ANTRAL TRANSPLANT TO COLON (COMBINED RESULTS OF DRAGSTEDT ET AL., 1951, AND HARKINS ET AL., 1954)

TYPE OF ANASTOMOSIS	NO. OF DOGS	NO. WITH ULCER	% WITH ULCER
Billroth I	18	4	22
Billroth II	17	14	82

anastomosis. In the former, 22 per cent of the dogs developed stomal ulcer (as shown in Table 31-1) while in the latter, 82 per cent developed ulcer. In other, and almost similar experiments, Harkins *et al.* (1954) used histamine-in-beeswax as the stimulus to excess gastric secretion. With this preparation, 25 per cent of the animals developed ulcer after gastroduodenal anastomosis and 100 per cent after gastrojejunal anastomosis. These experiments can be used to argue either for a greater resistance of the duodenum, as compared with the jejunum, or for duodenal acid-inhibition, or for both.

D. The experiments of Brackney, Thal, and Wangensteen (1955), Sircus (1958) and Jones and Harkins (1959) clearly indicate the presence of duodenal acid-inhibition: Resection of the duodenum and transplantation of the bile and pancreatic ducts into the jejunum, or transplantation of the duodenum lower into the intestinal tract—both resulted in a definite increase in Heidenhain pouch secretion in dogs.

5. *Enterogastrone.* This chalone is prepared from the first 6 to 8 feet of fresh hog intestine. The colorless product is easily soluble in water, and 25 mg. will suppress histamine-induced gastric secretion in the total pouch dog. Greengard, Atkinson, Grossman and Ivy (1946) reported that only 25 per cent of 8 Mann-Williamson dogs injected with purified enterogastrone daily for 1 year developed ulcer, whereas 100 per cent of 10 such dogs given hog muscle extract injections as controls developed ulcer. Preliminary clinical trial by these authors is suggestive of benefit, but the drug is not commonly accepted as being of clinical benefit at present.

Interrelations Between the Phases of

Gastric Secretion. Experimental studies (Oberhelman, Rigler and Dragstedt, 1957; Woodward, Robertson, Fried and Shapiro, 1957; Thein and Schofield, 1959; Chapman, Nyhus and Harkins, 1960; Nyhus, Chapman, DeVito and Harkins, 1960; Harkins, Chapman and Nyhus, 1963; Nyhus, Condon and Harkins, 1963) indicate that vagal action probably releases gastrin. These interrelationships may explain the confusing reports concerning antral inhibition and antral inhibitory hormones. Other studies (Gillespie et al., 1960) indicate that gastrin, besides its acid-stimulatory property, is able to influence the "reactivity" of the parietal cells to other stimuli, including vagal action. Apparent acid inhibition may be nothing other than removal of this facilitatory influence. Also, Gillespie (1959) showed that acidification of the antrum is capable of reducing the response of the parietal cells to histamine. A study on the final common pathway of gastric secretion is that of Peters and Womack (1958).

Based on these studies, as well as on that of Stavney, Kato, Savage, Harkins and Nyhus (1964) relating to parietal cell reactivity, it can be proposed that instead of the conventional 3 phases of gastric secretion (cephalic, antral and intestinal), there are 4 phases, as follows:

1. The *cephalic phase* of acid secretion—direct stimulation of the parietal cells via the vagus nerves.

2. The *vagal-antral phase* of acid secretion—release of gastrin from the antrum in response to vagal stimulation.

3. The *gastric (local antral) phase* of acid secretion—stimulation of the parietal cells by gastrin released as a result of direct stimulation of the antrum.

4. The *intestinal phase* of acid secretion—parietal cell stimulation resulting from a release of "hormones" by intestinal mucosa.

Neutralization. Since acid causes peptic ulcer, attempts at treatment within the stomach, both medical (Sippy powders) and surgical (gastrojejunostomy) have been partly based on an attempt to neutralize the acid. Both attempts have resulted in partial failure. Alkaline powders are followed by a "rebound phenomenon" and gastrojejunostomy has been followed by a high incidence (34%, Lewisohn, 1925) of marginal ulceration. In the duodenum, however, the normal alkaline bile and pancreatic juice play an important neutralizing role. (See pp. 822 and 828 relative to [1] the Mann-Williamson preparation which is based upon deflecting these secretions away from the pylorus and [2] studies on the decrease in acid-buffering capacity of the intestine proportionate to the distance from the ampulla of Vater.)

Gastric Pepsin and Mucin Secretion. Although these two substances have different purposes, the one to act as the enzyme of protein digestion in the stomach, the other to lubricate the organ and to protect its wall from the digestive action of the more active constituents of the gastric juice, the two will be considered together here.

PEPSIN is believed to come from the body chief cells of the gastric glands. Unlike hydrochloric acid, its secretion is believed to be essentially continuous, although, of course, it cannot act in the absence of acid. Alterations in pepsin production after different surgical operations have been studied by Farmer, Burke and Smithwick (1954). Book, Chinn and Beams (1952) reported that in patients with duodenal ulcer there is no reduction in the secretion of pepsin per unit of volume of secretion following vagotomy, unlike the finding for free hydrochloric acid which is reduced following vagotomy. However, since vagotomy reduces the total volume of secretion, the total amount of pepsin secreted in 12 hours is reduced.

MUCIN. The surface epithelial cells, the neck chief cells of the glands of the corpus, and the cardiac and the pyloric glands all secrete mucus. Mersheimer, Glass, Speer, Winfield and Boyd (1952) reported that in patients, mucin secretion, similar to hydrochloric acid, no longer responds to insulin hypoglycemia after vagotomy. Following partial gastric resection, on the other hand, the acid response to insulin was largely lost, while the mucous response was maintained at its preoperative level.

Altered Resistance of Gastric and Duodenal Mucosa. This factor has been brought forward repeatedly as an explanation for certain types of peptic ulcer. Overaction of the sympathetic fibers may not only decrease acid secretion but also by producing local ischemia may produce a lowered resistance to peptic

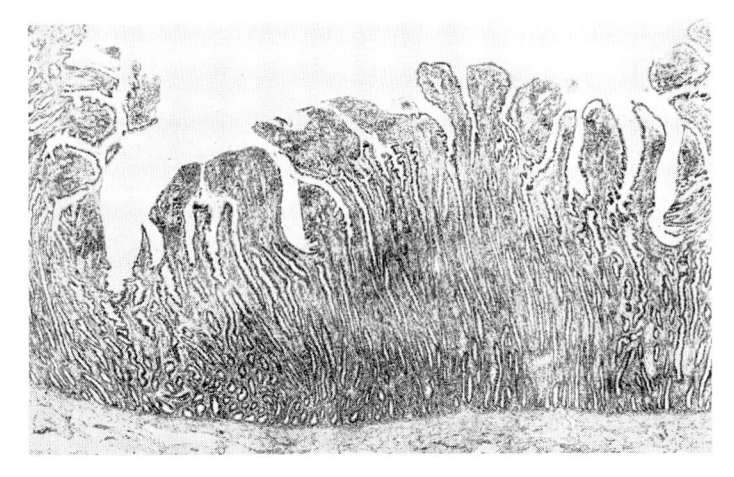

FIG. 31-7. (*Top*) Normal jejunum of man (8 cm. distal to ligament of Treitz) without Brunner's glands. (*Bottom*) Normal duodenum of man (3 cm. distal to pylorus) with solid mass of these glands (layer BC) lying below the muscularis mucosae. (Griffith, C., and Harkins, H.: Ann. Surg., 143:161)

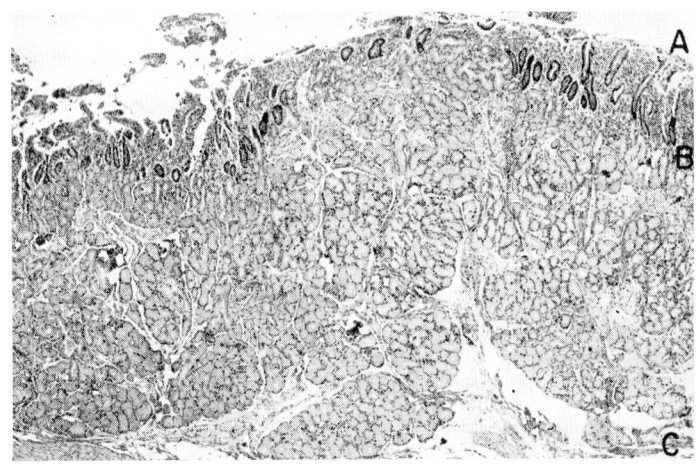

digestion. A decrease in the mucin secretion of the gastric mucosa may cause a comparable decrease in its resistance. Friesen (1950) reported that hemoconcentration, with "its resultant mucosal congestion," is a factor in the causation of gastroduodenal ulceration following burns. Lillehei, Roth and Wangensteen (1952) extended this hypothesis to demonstrate "that a number of stress-provoking agencies in experimental animals fail to influence gastric secretion or even depress gastric acidity; but nevertheless, they exert a powerful ulcer abetting effect by reducing the resistance of the gastroduodenal mucosa to autodigestion." Menguy and Masters (1963) demonstrated the decrease in mucus production and an altered composition following cortisone administration. They proposed a steroid-induced lowering of the threshold of susceptibility to peptic ulceration by interference with the rate of renewal of the mucous barrier. (See also section on Acute Ulcer, p. 830.)

Variations in Mucosal Resistance at Different Levels in the Intestinal Tract. In the duodenum of man, Brunner's glands extend as a dense sheet immediately below the muscularis mucosae from the pylorus to or beyond the ampulla of Vater (Fig. 31-7), but never beyond the ligament of Treitz. These cells are capable of secreting an abundant alkaline mucus which may be a leading factor in the protection of the normal duodenum, as shown by Griffith and Harkins (1956). It is of interest that the distribution of Brunner's glands in man and the pig is almost identical, whereas these glands are almost absent in the dog, upon which animal so much experimental work relating to ulcer has been done.

In the dog, below the level of the upper duodenum where the only Brunner's glands are present, Kiriluk and Merendino (1954) have shown that there is little variation in inherent sensitivity between the lower duodenum, the jejunum and the ileum.

At the same time, the esophagus, which is lined with squamous epithelium, is *much* less resistant than any portion of the intestinal tract from cardia to pectinate line.

Gastric Motility. Alterations in gastric motility are known to be a factor in hunger and also may be responsible for some of the pain of peptic ulcer. Section of the vagi decreases gastric motility—does not decrease tone as is popularly believed—as well as gastric secretion. Rowe, Grimson and Flowe (1953) devised a gastrometric balloon test for the completeness of vagal section which they stated is more reliable than the insulin test of Hollander.

Pharmacology

The possible compound effect of neutralizing drugs has been cited above. The important role of the antisecretory drugs (atropine, methantheline bromide, etc.) will not be elaborated upon here. Other drugs are also useful, and the pharmacologic aspects of gastric secretion are important. The introduction of histamine-in-beeswax as a method of experimental study of peptic ulcer by Code and Varco (1940) has been of great importance.

Bacteriology

In the presence of normal acidity the stomach is the least contaminated portion of the main intestinal tract. When acid is reduced after operation, or in many patients with carcinoma of the stomach, bacterial contamination increases. After vagotomy, not only the lowered acidity but also the decreased motility with resultant stasis tends to increase bacterial contamination of the stomach.

Pathology

The typical chronic peptic ulcer is surrounded by thickened, scarred gastric or duodenal wall. Acute ulcers are punched out, and there is little fibrous tissue between them and the surrounding intestinal wall. Two rules are of some practical significance: (1) Gastric ulcers are quite apt to be malignant; duodenal ulcers almost never so. (2) Perforated duodenal ulcers are *usually* anterior and do not bleed; bleeding duodenal ulcers are *usually* posterior and do not perforate (they penetrate into the pancreas and erode the gastroduodenal artery).

PEPTIC ULCER

Peptic ulcer is a medical and surgical problem of great significance. It is accompanied by a considerable morbidity and, because of its complications, is a major cause of death. By definition, peptic ulceration involves the autopeptic digestion of the patient's own tissues. This is rendered possible by either an excess acidity—which enables the pepsin secreted by the chief cells to act at its optimum pH—or by the reduced resistance of the tissues in question.

Peptic ulcer occurs in a number of special types according to etiology and location. Each of these headings with its various subheadings will be considered, after which a separate account of duodenal ulcer, the most common and most important of all the peptic ulcers, will follow.

Special Types of Peptic Ulcer According to Etiology

In this section, 5 special types of peptic ulcer will be considered, each with a special etiology according to present concepts. These include: (1) gastric ulcer, (2) duodenal ulcer, (3) Cushing's acute ulcer, (4) Curling's acute ulcer and (5) intractable ulcer.

Gastric Ulcer. Such ulcers are undoubtedly peptic but have several differentiating features from duodenal ulcers. They tend to occur in older individuals. They may be associated with chronic atrophic gastritis, whereas there is no such atrophic gastritis in cases of duodenal ulcer. There is a different geographic distribution, gastric ulcer being more common on the continent of Europe and duodenal ulcer being more common in Great Britain and America, especially in the latter. Persons who eat rough foods are probably more susceptible to gastric ulcer, whereas persons living under conditions of emotional tension may be more liable to develop duodenal ulcers. The 12-hour night secretion of free hydrochloric acid is normal (average 18.6 mEq.) or on the average less (12 mEq.), as opposed to the elevated value in duodenal ulcer patients (average 63 mEq.) (Dragstedt, Oberhelman, Evans and

Rigler, 1954). These authors and Dragstedt (1954) attributed gastric ulcers to an overproduction of gastrin by the antrum, possibly due to stasis.

Another factor pertaining to the etiology of gastric ulcer relates to why the majority of such ulcers occur along the lesser curvature, the *Magenstrasse*. Dragstedt (1955) pointed out that the lesser curvature is relatively fixed, and the mucous membrane is relatively smooth and has less rugae than the remainder of the corpus. Other factors to consider are the different anatomic arrangement of the end-arteries and the drinking of liquids which may wash the mucus off the lesser curvature, since they pass directly along it.

Additional differences are based on responses to treatment. After a minimal gastric resection, e.g., 40 to 50 per cent, including the entire antrum, however, for gastric ulcer, stomal ulcer seldom develops. Duodenal ulcer, on the other hand, responds well to vagotomy plus a drainage procedure and frequently (about 12% or more) is followed by a stomal ulcer when a 40 to 50 per cent gastrectomy is performed.

Duodenal Ulcer. Such an ulcer seems to be due to an increased cephalic phase of gastric secretion, possibly due to the tensions and strain of modern life. It responds well to either vagotomy-drainage procedure or to vagotomy-antrectomy.

Acute Ulcer (Curling's Ulcer, Stress Ulcer, Posterior Hypothalamus-Stimulated Ulcer). In 1842, Curling described acute ulcers of the stomach or the duodenum following burns. More recently such ulcers have been noted following various types of trauma. Fletcher and Harkins (1954) reported 42 such cases at the King County Hospital, Seattle, during the 7-year period 1946-1953. The 42 cases occurred in 4,102 autopsies, an incidence of almost exactly 1 per cent. Of the ulcers 20 were gastric, 14 duodenal, 6 both gastric and duodenal, 1 gastrojejunal and 1 esophageal. The ulcer was not the cause of death in all of these cases, but in at least 15 cases there was perforation, massive hemorrhage, or both. Only 1 of the 42 cases occurred following a burn. Bogardus and Gustafson (1956) reported a somewhat similar series wherein 28 cases (4.9%) of 566 consecutive autopsies revealed a coincident duodenal ulcer. Not all of these ulcers were acute, but a number of them were.

Other workers have approached this problem from the aspect of mechanism. Gray, Benson, Reifenstein and Spiro (1951) postulated that in stress the cells of the anterior hypothalamus secrete a humoral substance which stimulates the pituitary gland to release corticotropin which in turn acts on the adrenals to liberate cortisone. Zubiran, Kark, Montalbetti, Morel and Dragstedt (1952) showed that cortisone stimulation of gastric secretion occurs even when the antrum is removed and the vagi are sectioned, thus indicating a direct action on the parietal cells. Dragstedt (1953) utilized this evidence along with the recognized relief of duodenal ulcer by vagotomy to indicate that chronic duodenal ulcer, unlike the stress or acute ulcer under consideration here, cannot be due to this mechanism. Risholm (1956) postulated that "acute portal hypertension" may be a factor in these acute stress ulcers.

The particular type of Curling's ulcer following burns was reviewed by Moncrief, Switzer and Teplitz (1964). When hemorrhage occurs, surgical intervention is mandatory.

Acute Ulcer (Cushing's Ulcer, Anterior Hypothalamus-Stimulated Ulcer). Such ulcers may be due to acute or chronic involvement of the central nervous system, especially the anterior hypothalamus, and were first described by Rokitansky in 1846 and by Cushing in 1932. Such ulcers also may be related to gastromalacia (see p. 863). They are especially apt to occur in acute bulbar poliomyelitis; Schaberg, Hildes and Alcock (1954) reported that in 480 cases of acute bulbar poliomyelitis, there were 34 instances (7%) of upper gastrointestinal tract hemorrhage, of which 23 cases (5%) resulted in death. In addition, 2 patients died of perforation of the duodenum. Cabieses and Lecca (1955) reported 10 cases of acute gastrointestinal hemorrhage following neurosurgical operations. Rupture of the esophagus was observed in 19 of 1,590 autopsies during a 4-year period by Maciver, Smith, Tomlinson and Whitby (1956). Seventeen of the 19 (89%) were associated with lesions of the central nervous system. While these authors favored a mechanical tear as the most com-

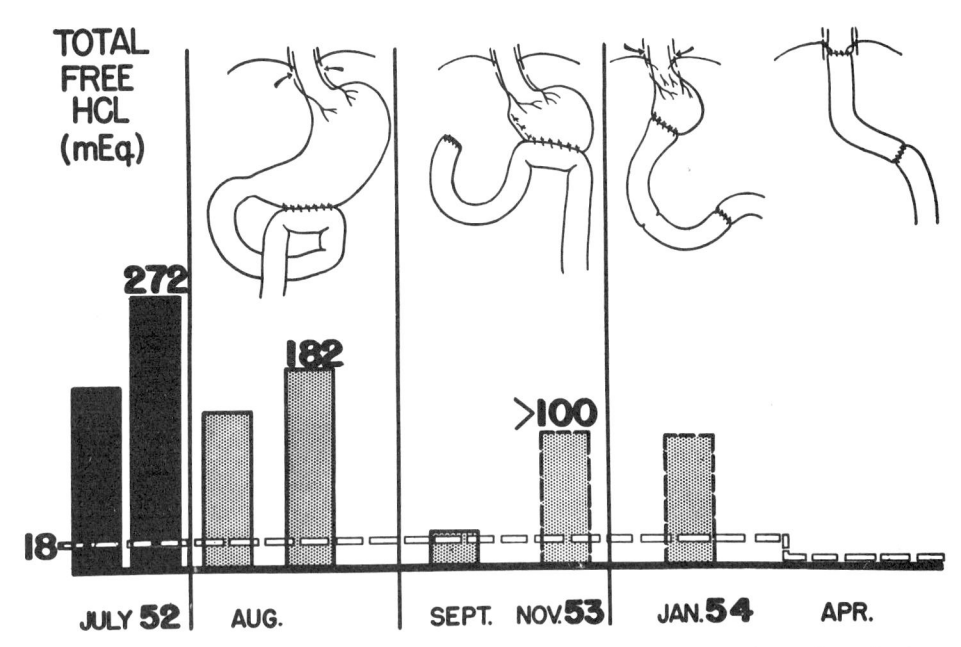

FIG. 31-8. Total mEq. of free HCl found in repeated 12-hour nocturnal gastric aspirations of patients with intractable ulcer (36-year-old married white female), showing the effects of a succession of operative procedures utilized to reduce the hyperacidity. The normal value is indicated by the broken horizontal line. (Zollinger, R., and Ellison, E.: Ann. Surg., 142:712)

mon explanation, erosion could not always be ruled out.

The relationship between these 2 types of acute ulcer was portrayed graphically by Shay (1954).

Intractable Ulcer (Ulcer Diathesis, Zollinger-Ellison Ulcer). For a long time it has been observed by those doing a considerable amount of gastric surgery that an occasional patient—possibly 1 in 100 or 200—will have repeated recurrences despite supposedly adequate medical and surgical therapy. A typical history might run as follows: perforated duodenal ulcer, simple closure; intractable duodenal ulcer, gastrojejunostomy; marginal ulcer, subtotal gastrectomy; second marginal ulcer, vagotomy plus reresection; third marginal ulcer, thoracic revagotomy; finally total gastrectomy. These cases, although rare, present a serious situation.

In 1952, Strøm reported a case of peptic ulcer with "insuloma." In his patient no preoperative studies were made before the removal of the 8-Gm. tumor. The tumor contained "atypical beta-cells." Strøm postulated the possible relationship of the tumor to a possible increase in gastric secretion.

Observations of Zollinger and Ellison (1955), Ellison (1955, 1956) and Dragstedt (1961), Amberg, Ellison, Wilson and Zboralske (1964), Bryant, Moore and Carney (1964), Zollinger and Grant (1964), and Ellison and Wilson (1964) reporting their own cases and collecting other cases and suggestive reports from the literature, furnished the solution to this problem. In their first classic paper the Columbus, Ohio authors reported 2 personal cases plus 7 collected cases (Fig. 31-8).

Zollinger and Ellison concluded: "A clinical entity consisting of hypersecretion, hyperacidity, and atypical peptic ulceration associated with non-insulin-producing islet cell tumors of the pancreas is suggested." The therapeutic implications are twofold and clear: (1) examine the pancreas routinely in cases of peptic ulcer; and (2) in cases of intractable ulcer or ulcer in atypical locations (e.g., third portion of duodenum or jejunum) make a meticulous search of the pancreas. Some of the basic studies upon which these observations are based are discussed in the section on gastric physiology (see p. 825, Pancreatic Phase of Gastric Secretion).

It is of interest in this connection that 4 cases of ulcer, 2 coincident with parathyroid tumor and 2 with hyperplasia, have been reported (Rogers, Keating, Morlock and Barker, 1947; Robinson, Black, Sprague and Tillisch, 1951; Albright and Kerr, 1952). Polyglandular involvement by multiple adenomata has been surveyed by Ellison and Wilson (1964) and a consistent rate of 20 per cent was found. Zollinger and Moore (1968) recommend that hyperparathyroidism or other endocrine hyperfunction should be ruled out in any patient suspected of having an ulcerogenic tumor.

Special Types of Peptic Ulcer According to Location

No matter where it occurs, peptic ulcer is due to the acid-peptic autodigestion of the lining of some portion of the alimentary tract. There are 7 special types of peptic ulcer according to the various locations in the alimentary tract in which they may occur, as follows:

1. **Ulcer from Ectopic Islands of Gastric Mucosa in the Upper Esophagus.** This type of ulcer is essentially hypothetical and, to the author's knowledge, has not been reported in the literature. However, it is mentioned for completeness and to emphasize the contrast with Type 2, discussed below.

In the esophagus ectopic gastric mucosa occurs most frequently in the postcricoid region of the upper esophagus. Islands of such mucosa ranging in size from microscopic dimensions to 1 or 2 cm. in diameter were found in 70 per cent of autopsied cases (Schridde, 1904). Barrett summarized this by stating: "I cannot believe that the tiny volume of acid diluted by pints of saliva, would be likely to harm the lower reaches of the gullet."

2. **Ulcer From Heterotopic Sheets of Gastric Mucosa in the Lower Esophagus (Peptic Ulcer of Gastric Mucosa-Lined Esophagus, Barrett's Ulcer).** Unlike the theoretically possible, but never yet described, ulcers postulated in the first type, these ulcers, while rare, represent a distinct and important entity, especially in older people. They occur in heterotopic gastric mucosa in the lower esophagus which is continuous with the gastric mucosa of the stomach. Jackson (1929) reported gastric mucosa in 7 of his 21 personal cases of peptic ulcer of the lower esophagus.

Barrett (1950, 1954) believed that such a portion of the esophagus is part of the stomach, while Allison and Johnstone (1953) preferred to call this condition "esophagus lined with gastric mucous membrane" because the outer walls are typical of the esophagus. Whether the presence of the gastric mucosal sheet is always congenital and a part of the syndrome of congenitally short esophagus (see Chap. 30, Esophagus) or whether it may result from an eccentric healing of a marginal squamous membrane ulcer (the gastric side healing more readily so that the gastric mucous membrane gradually "climbs" into the esophagus) is not yet settled. Also, it is not settled whether the Barrett's ulcers within this gastric mucosa-lined segments or possible peptic esophagitis in the squamous mucous membrane above it, if present, are caused by secretion of acid from the segment in question or due to reflux from the stomach proper below. The absence of oxyntic cells in the gastric mucosa-lined segment would tend to support the latter view, as would also the fact that most of the patients with gastric mucosa-lined esophagus do not get into trouble until later life, when a sliding hiatal hernia and consequent reflux occur. In all of Allison and Johnstone's cases of Barrett's ulcer a sliding hernia was present. Thus we have a paradox wherein a condition which presumably is congenital affects patients almost entirely in later life.

Barrett's ulcer behaves like an ulcer of the abdominal stomach. It may bleed profusely; it may perforate; it rarely causes stenosis, and then only if it is circumferential. If it is localized to one segment of the circumference, it may heal on medical treatment, unlike peptic esophagitis (see below) which seldom regresses once a rigid tube is present. Perforation of Barrett's ulcers may occur into the mediastinum or the pleural cavity. When stenosis is present with Barrett's ulcer, it is usually a marginal stenosis in the squamous mucous membrane-lined esophagus immediately above.

Treatment of Barrett's ulcer is complicated and includes that of the almost always associated sliding hiatal hernia below, and of the squamous mucous membrane-lined esophagus above. The most radical treatments include: (1) complete excision of the affected segments with jejunal interposition between normal esophagus above and stomach below (see Chap. 30, Esophagus) and (2) complete excision with esophagojejunal anastomosis by-passing the stomach. Less radical procedures include: (3) complete excision with esophagogastric anastomosis (this may lead to secondary marginal reflux esophagitis) and (4) local excision of a strictured or ulcerated segment, preserving the cardia and anastomosing the normal squamous mucous membrane-lined esophagus above to the stump of gastric mucous membrane-lined esophagus below. Morris (1955) performed this last procedure in 2 cases with success. It should be accompanied by repair of the hiatal hernia if possible to prevent recurrence. The success of this operation may depend on the possibly greater resistance of the gastric mucosa-lined esophageal segment than of the squamous mucosa-lined esophagus to peptic digestion (see p. 828, immunity of different segments of the gastrointestinal tract).

All of these procedures should be coupled with a drainage procedure to the stomach, preferably of the Finney pyloroplasty type. Treatment of patients with perforation or massive hemorrhage is urgent and in some instances of the former may involve drainage of the mediastinum or the pleura only as a temporary procedure pending more definitive treatment when the patient is in better condition.

3. Reflux (Peptic) Esophagitis (Esophagitis and Peptic Ulceration of Squamous Mucous-Membrane-Lined Esophagus). This condition was first described by Winkelstein (1935) and frequently has been elaborated upon since (see Chap. 30, Esophagus). It is the most common nonspecific inflammatory condition of the esophagus. There are several varieties (see below) of the condition, but they have certain features in common. This condition is secondary to regurgitation of gastric contents, and competence of the cardia is lost. Ulcerations are not as characteristic of the syndrome as is the esophagitis. Ulcerations tend to be superficial and serpiginous (Jones, 1955). There is a nonpenetrating ulceration with thin yellow surface slough, slow blood loss from the surface, and progressive fibrosis and stenosis. The submucous fibrosis which is present leads to stenosis and stricture formation which is much more severe than with Barrett's ulcer. Perforation, on the other hand, almost never occurs, and bleeding, while frequent, is usually not massive. However, De Vito, Listerud, Nyhus, Merendino and Harkins (1959) have reported 3 cases with massive hemorrhage. The response to medical treatment is poor, but bouginage is useful so long as the main cause of obstruction is spasm and a rigid tube does not exist. In the latter instance, surgical treatment is required.

Esophagitis occurs in three quarters of the cases of sliding hiatal hernia but may exist in the absence of such hernias. Reflux is usually present but is not always demonstrable. The small superficial ulcerations which may be present are seldom seen in roentgen examination.

Bombeck, Aoki, and Nyhus (1967) have suggested that hiatal hernia and acid-peptic reflux esophagitis are two separate entities, the former due to attenuation of the phrenoesophageal ligaments which normally tether the stomach in the abdominal cavity and the latter due to lower esophageal sphincter failure. Successful repair of a hernia must be considered separately from successful alleviation of reflux. Any procedure that maintains hernial reduction while allowing reflux to continue is a failure. The converse is of little consequence, provided that the recurrent hernia does not reach sufficient size to cause symptoms as a space-occupying lesion.

Carver and Sealy (1954) pointed out that in their series of 130 cases of peptic esophagitis, the following 3 factors were causative: (1) hiatus hernia, 76 per cent; (2) surgical excision or destruction of the cardiac sphincter, 13 per cent; and (3) persistent vomiting, 11 per cent. The important symptoms in descending order of frequency included dysphagia, substernal pain, regurgitation, weakness and anemia, and hemorrhage and hematemesis. Related to these factors in causation, reflux esophagitis may be divided into the following 4 types:

TYPE 1. Cases which follow intubation or

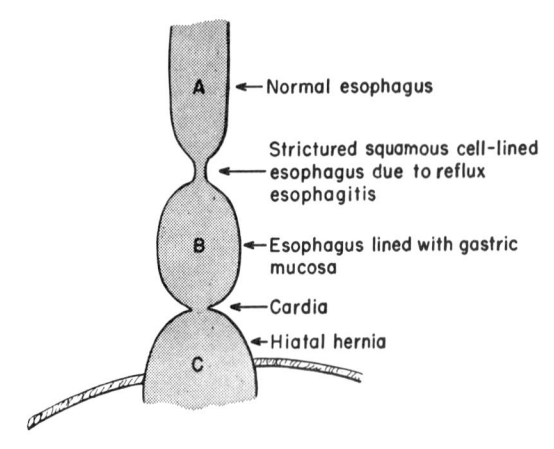

FIG. 31-9. Diagram of triple barium shadow above diaphragm indicative of heterotopic sheet of gastric mucosa at lower end of esophagus. (A) Normal esophagus. (B) Gastric-mucosa-lined esophagus. (C) Hiatal hernia.

persistent vomiting or are associated with duodenal ulcer. Such cases are apt to be severe and acute. Hiatal hernia is often absent.

TYPE 2. The usual milder variety associated with sliding hiatal hernia. In such instances, at least in the early stages, roentgen signs of esophagitis are lacking. When stenosis does occur it is present immediately above the cardia.

TYPE 3. Marginal ulceration occurring in the squamous mucous-membrane-lined esophagus immediately above a segment lined with gastric mucosa. Bosher and Taylor (1951) reported such a case (without a hiatal hernia), but Allison and Johnstone (1953) and Morris (1955) have elaborated their reports into an elucidation of a definite and interesting syndrome in which the reflux esophagitis and associated stenosis, unlike that in Type 2, are usually high in the chest and are associated with hiatal hernia. Wolf, Marshak, Som and Winkelstein (1955) discussed a special type of this syndrome in which the segment of gastric mucosa-lined esophagus is short, discrete ulceration is more apt to occur in the area of esophagitis above it (possibly because it is nearer the source of reflux), the associated hiatal hernia is more triangular in shape than usual, the condition may occur in childhood, and the prognosis is especially poor.

Allison and Johnstone (1953) collected all the cases of esophageal stenosis seen in their clinic and found that 115 patients had stenosis from squamous ulcer of the esophagus and 10 from gastric (Barrett's) ulcer of the esophagus. Of the 115 patients with squamous ulcer and stenosis there was definite evidence in 11 of a segment of esophagus lined with gastric mucosa between the stenosis and the hernia. Thus, in these 125 cases, 21 had gastric mucosa in the esophagus, 10 had Barrett's ulcer of that mucosa (roughly half), and the relative changes of a peptic stenosis being squamous or gastric were about 10 to 1.

When the combined condition of esophagus lined with gastric mucosa and (squamous) peptic esophagitis at its upper end exists, a very interesting picture is present (Fig. 31-9). The stricture marks the lower limit of squamous epithelium. The esophagus below this, lined by gastric mucosa is normal or a little dilated. The position of the cardia can be identified as the place where the lumen widens out again to form the sac of the herniated stomach. As Allison and Johnstone pointed out, this gives a triple segmentation of barium in the chest, from above downward: (1) normal esophagus, (2) esophagus lined by gastric mucosa and (3) sliding hiatal hernia. The first is separated from the second by the stricture, and the second from the third by the cardia. As these authors stated, "When this picture occurs it can be concluded that the intermediate tubular stricture is esophagus lined by gastric mucous membrane." To complicate the situation further, sometimes typical Barrett ulcers are present in this intermediate tubular stricture below.

TYPE 4. Marginal ulceration following operations in which the cardiac sphincter has been sacrificed. This is a common clinical occurrence and has been studied experimentally by Hoag, Kiriluk and Merendino (1954). Esophagogastrectomy in dogs, with or without vagotomy, led to a high percentage of fatal esophageal ulceration, as did the Gröndahl esophagocardioplasty and the long Heller extramucous esophagocardiomyotomy procedures.

Treatment of reflux esophagitis varies according to the type and the stage of the disease but involves bouginage and/or repair of the associated hiatal hernia when the main obstruction is spastic, and surgical excision when it is present because of a rigid tubelike obstruction. If manometric studies prove the absence of the lower esophageal sphincter, a valvuloplasty of the Nissen (1964) or Thal (1965) type may be considered. Surgical repair, as discussed previously under the consideration of Barrett's ulcer, should include that of an associated hiatal hernia in some cases and, since in cases with resection preservation of the cardiac sphincter usually is not possible, esophagogastrostomy with jejunal interposition is the ideal procedure in advanced cases.*

4. **Gastric Ulcer.** As stated previously, gastric ulcer may be of different origin than duodenal ulcer. The acute gastric ulcer or erosion may heal on medical management, but the typical chronic gastric ulcer is very apt to recur. Wangensteen (1953) reported that 11 of 12 gastric ulcers thought to have healed on roentgen examination were found to be still present at subsequent operation. Swynnerton and Tanner (1953) concluded that the healing of gastric ulcer by medical treatment was followed by recurrence in 75 per cent of the patients, while in the surgically treated patients, 80 per cent had very successful results, 10 per cent satisfactory results, and only 10 per cent poor results. Tanner (1951), in discussing the special indications of gastric resection for gastric ulcer, stated:

"Gastric ulcer is a disease of wear and tear and will not be cured medically until wrinkles will be." The repeated and chronic healing of a chronic gastric ulcer can cause considerable shortening of the lesser curvature (Tanner, 1951). Dolphin, Smith and Waugh (1953) reported that multiple ulcers are present in 21.9 per cent of stomachs removed with benign gastric ulcer and in only 5.6 per cent of the specimens removed with malignant gastric ulcer, a ratio of 4:1.

The symptoms of gastric ulcer are quite similar to those of duodenal ulcer. There is a little less tendency to periodicity, the pain is sometimes a little more on the left side, and the patients are usually about 8 years older at the time of onset. Sometimes an older patient with gastric ulcer will present a history of a duodenal ulcer in his youth, now healed. This substitution of one ulcer for another is based on the lowered acidity yet increased susceptibility of the gastric mucous membrane due to a degenerative gastritis (Tanner, 1951). Johnson (1956) observed coincident gastric and duodenal ulcer in 10 per cent of his patients with peptic ulcer. In 130 cases of combined ulcer, the following facts were observed: (1) in 93 per cent the duodenal ulcer appeared first, and (2) in 64 per cent there was associated pyloric stenosis and retention, possibly indicating an antral hyperstimulation as postulated by Dragstedt (1954).

Other differences are that gastric ulcer seldom leads to stomal ulcer following gastric resection (not once in 700 gastric resections for gastric ulcer—Tanner, 1952), and that the differentiation between gastric ulcer and gastric carcinoma is difficult. This last point deserves special emphasis on two scores.

The question as to whether gastric ulcer becomes carcinomatous, or gastric carcinomas ulcerate is still not settled. Notkin (1955) reported 2 resected cases in which the pathologic findings strongly suggested the possibility of subsequent malignant degeneration in a previously benign ulcer. However, the author ascribes to the views of Palmer (1950) and others who stated that for all practical purposes gastric ulcers do not turn into carcinoma, but that carcinomas regularly ulcerate.

The differentiation between gastric ulcer and gastric carcinoma brings in an application of Hippocrates' dictum, because, in such instances, truly "experience is fallacious and judgment difficult." In general, about 10 per cent or more of gastric lesions thought to be ulcer turn out to have carcinoma at operation (Table 31-2).

Jones and Doll (1953) reported that 11 per cent of their patients with simple closure of a perforated gastric ulcer were dead of carci-

---

* The student may wonder why so much space is given to the elucidation of this complicated subject of peptic ulcer of the esophagus and reflux esophagitis which may involve such major surgical procedures. This is done for the following reasons: (1) These conditions are far more common than is generally realized. (2) Their recognition by medical men, as well as by surgeons, is important. (3) Prompt simple treatment may eliminate the necessity for more radical therapy later.

TABLE 31-2. PER CENT OF PREOPERATIVELY DIAGNOSED GASTRIC ULCERS WHICH TURN OUT TO BE MALIGNANT AT OPERATION

AUTHOR	TOTAL CASES	PER CENT MALIGNANT
Allen and Welch (1941)	277	14.0
Allen and Welch (1953)	295	10.8
Walters (1942)	...	10.0
Ransom (1947)	246	10.1
Marshall (1953)	411	15.8

noma of the stomach after an average follow-up period of 6.3 years.

Differentiation on the basis of roentgen examination, gastroscopy, gastrocamera and determination of acidity are all helpful but seldom definitive in borderline cases. Cytologic studies are promising and are useful when performed by one experienced in this technic.

Cytologic studies of the stomach involve specimens that are obtained by mechanical means (brush technic, etc.) or by aspiration after the instillation of mucolytic agents. This latter technic is less traumatic, and good results have been reported by Traut, Rosenthal, Harrison, Farber and Grimes (1953) and Rubin and Benditt (1955). The latter authors found that papain lavage is simple and rapid but does not regularly yield well-preserved cells. Chymotrypsin (a freshly prepared solution of 7 μg. of crystallized d-chymotrypsin in 500 ml. of 0.1 M acetate buffer) is instilled into the stomach with a Levin tube and removed in 10 minutes. The stained sediment shows well-preserved cells, and the test was positive in 19 of 20 patients who proved to have cancer. Brandborg et al. (1967) presented their results of chymotrypsin lavage in 1,247 patients. The correct diagnosis of benignancy was made in 1,001 of 1,006 patients. The correct diagnosis was made by cytology in 223 of 241 with malignancy.

While the decision is difficult as to whether or not a gastric ulcer is malignant, the results of surgical treatment in such cases are encouraging. Ranson (1947) and also Lampert, Waugh and Dockerty (1950) reported that resection in such instances resulted in a 41 per cent 5-year survival rate, which is almost twice that of preoperatively diagnosed carcinoma of the stomach. Olsson and Endresen (1956) also compared the results in a series of 25 "ulcer cancers," i.e., those thought to be ulcer before pathologic examination, with 176 ordinary gastric cancers, both series including only cases with no metastases. The 3-year survival figures were 64 per cent and 42 per cent, respectively.

Amberg and Rigler (1956) approached this subject in a different way by comparing a series of 39 cases of gastric cancer, selected because the roentgen diagnosis was made after an earlier negative one, thus indicating relatively early or small lesions, with a control group of 866 cases. In the special series the incidence of cases without positive nodes was 46 per cent as compared with the 15 per cent in the control group.

The decision as to whether to operate for gastric ulcer is based on the known high recurrence rate after medical therapy and the danger of unrecognized carcinoma. Some advise gastric resection for all gastric ulcers. As will be shown below, this has some logical basis. In the large clinics, from 37 to 95 per cent of gastric ulcers are treated by resection. The present author believes the higher figure is more nearly correct but that under certain circumstances routine resection is not advisable. Acute ulcers may be followed medically if *prompt* improvement occurs within 3 weeks, corroborated by roentgen studies. The aid of a competent internist and an expert cytologist is also of help. (See section on Carcinoma of the Stomach, p. 844.)

An analysis of the problem of whether or not to do routine gastric resection for gastric ulcer is taken from Moore and Harkins (1954) and is as follows:

If we consider 2 hypothetical series, each composed of 100 clinically benign gastric ulcers, and if we treat 1 series using subtotal gastric resection and the other using only medical measures, the outcome can be predicted with reasonable assurance based on available statistics. In each series it will be assumed that 10 patients will have carcinomatous ulcers. Other assumptions will be considered when the outcome of each separate series is discussed.

In the surgical series, all of the 100 patients will be benefited except the following; 6 of the 10 patients with carcinoma will die despite operation, 2 of the total series will be expected to die from operation, and 9 patients will develop disabling postgastrectomy symptoms. (Whereas some other patients will develop nondisabling postgastrectomy symptoms, we are assuming that these will be balanced out by the group of 6 carcinomatous ulcer patients which, even though counted as mortalities, will receive definite palliation.) Thus, a total of 17 of the 100 patients treated surgically will not be benefited (including 8 deaths) and 83 will be.

In the medical series, all of the 10 carcinoma patients will die; 20 of the remainder will have difficulty with medical management in the form of intractability, hemorrhage, perforation, or obstruction, and approximately 2 of these 20 will die of such complications. Thus, a total of 30 of the 100 patients treated medically will not be benefited (including 12 deaths), and 70 will be. Such is the case for subtotal resection for gastric ulcer.

This type of reasoning by probability would tend to support the use of routine gastric resection for gastric ulcer; however, individualization of each patient has certain advantages that cannot be denied.

The technical aspects of the surgical treatment of gastric ulcer involve the following: (1) Resection should include the ulcer but need not be more radical than is necessary for this technical requirement. However, it should always include the antrum. (2) Because of the normal duodenal stump, after resection gastroduodenal anastomosis is preferable. (3) In cases where carcinoma is suspected, gastrotomy and observation and biopsy of the ulcer from within the stomach may be of help in deciding on the extent of resection. Care must be taken not to scatter the cells from the biopsy wound. (4) In similar cases, the omentum should be removed with the stomach, and an attempt to include the lymph-node-bearing mesentery should be made.

Gastric ulcer high on the lesser curvature ("juxta-esophageal gastric ulcer") presents 2 special problems. (1) There is the relatively high chance of malignancy in such ulcers. Figure 31-10 shows data from Plenk and Lin (1954) which indicate that a preponderance of such ulcers, including those in the fundus, is malignant. Marshall (1953) also reported that in his series of 411 gastric ulcers, despite the fact that only 15.8 per cent were malignant, this was *one* part of the stomach where the malignant tumors outnumbered the benign 6:4. Since these figures include the fundus,

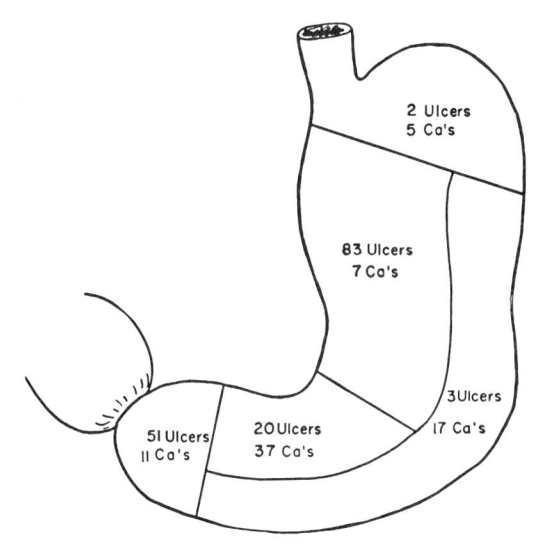

FIG. 31-10. Distribution of benign and malignant gastric lesions in Utah series. (Plenk, H., and Lin, R.: Am. Surgeon, 20:351)

they may not apply strictly to the high lesser curvature, but the danger of malignant lesions in this region is to be borne in mind. The second point concerning these ulcers is that they are technically difficult to remove. For this reason some (Editorial, J.A.M.A., 1954) advise a longer than usual trial with medical management. However, before such a policy is adopted, the other factor, namely, the increased hazard of malignancy, must also be considered.

Treatment of gastric ulcer high on the lesser curvature involves the following: Subtotal distal gastric resection, including the ulcer, should be the intended procedure. If certain technical steps listed below are utilized, this can be attained more often. Total gastrectomy is not desirable, while the Kelling-Madlener operation (distal resection leaving the ulcer in place) is a compromise. The left gastric artery should be doubly ligated and divided as well as the associated vagus nerve (the latter for purposes of mobilization, not to affect the cephalic phase). If at any time during the operation it becomes obvious that a high-lying ulcer is malignant, a carcinoma-type of operation is done which is usually a proximal subtotal resection—seldom a total—and involves removal of the lower end of the esophagus above and a pyloroplasty below.

Since most high gastric ulcers are slightly on the posterior surface, Tanner (1952) advised rotation of the stomach in such cases, bringing the lesser curvature forward and to the left so that the ulcer is now where the lesser curvature was. After resection, the closure of the lesser curve and the anastomosis are made in this rotated position. In removing a high gastric ulcer it is also best to do the operation by the open method without clamps, cutting the stomach above the ulcer with scissors. During closure of the lesser curve after resection, the surgeon should check the cardia frequently from within to be sure that it is not impinged upon too much.

Other points of importance in the treatment of gastric ulcer are as follows: (1) Massive hemorrhage from gastric ulcer is more dangerous than from duodenal ulcer. Therefore, if the diagnosis is known, an earlier operation is indicated in such instances. (2) Perforation of a gastric ulcer is more dangerous than of a duodenal ulcer. Also, the danger of carcinoma makes a definitive resection operation more strongly indicated.

The operation of vagotomy and drainage procedure for benign gastric ulcer has not proved effective to date. The experience of Stemmer et al. (1968) of a 36 per cent recurrence rate following this modality of treatment seems representative of the result of others.

5. Duodenal Ulcer. Since duodenal ulcer, the most common and most important of all peptic ulcers, will receive further elucidation in an entirely separate section below, only a few points of its relationship to the other types of peptic ulcer will be listed here. Duodenal ulcer is believed to be caused by an exaggerated cephalic phase of gastric secretion. Therefore, it can be approached both from the standpoint of eliminating this phase (vagotomy) or of cutting down on the source of acid from the parietal cells (gastric resection). Duodenal ulcer has a very high incidence of recurrence, and operations for duodenal ulcer are the main cause of stomal ulcer. Thus, from this standpoint, any surgical treatment to be successful must be thorough and radical. At the same time the danger of unrecognized malignancy is almost nil in duodenal ulcer, so that from this standpoint surgical therapy need not remove the omentum or lymph-gland-bearing mesentery.

6. Stomal Ulcer (Marginal Ulcer). Stomal ulceration is the most serious late complication of gastric surgery. Its one favorable feature is that with an additional major operative procedure it can be remedied, whereas some less severe complications tend more to persist despite therapy. The usual stomal ulcer is in the jejunum following a gastrojejunostomy (incidence 34%, Lewisohn, 1925) or a Billroth II gastric resection (incidence 2 to 6% or more). The ulcer may be at the actual stoma (stomal or gastrojejunal ulcer) or on the adjacent or opposite wall of the jejunum, in which case it is termed a jejunal ulcer. If it has broken into the adjacent colon, the more serious gastrojejunal-colic fistula results.

Whenever a surgeon performs a gastrojejunostomy he identifies the upper jejunum to be used for the anastomosis by its proximity to the ligament of Treitz. He always fears that he will mistake the ileocolic fold for the ligament of Treitz and perform an inadvertent gastro-ileostomy (Thomford, Bachulis and Brashear, 1968). This serious surgical error is evidenced by loss of weight, passage of recently eaten material in the stools, and general cachexia. Treatment is always surgical and involves takedown of the gastro-ileostomy with performance of a gastrojejunostomy in the proper place, or if the stomach has not been resected, an ulcer is present, and the patient is in reasonably good condition, performance of a gastric resection with correct anastomosis. The far rarer inadvertent gastro-colostomy is an unforgivable technical error and is never performed by a trained surgeon (Landry, 1951).

Stomal or marginal ulceration also occurs in the duodenum, or more often at the stoma itself, following the Billroth I type of gastric resection. The incidence of such ulceration for the same extent of resection is probably at least as low as for the Billroth II resection. Ulceration on the gastric side of the anastomosis was found to be much more common after Billroth I than Billroth II resections by Ordahl, Ross and Baker (1955) and by Goligher, Moir and Wrigley (1956). Other observers have not found these ulcers on the gastric side of the anastomosis except in rare instances. The results in our own patients have been summarized by Kanar et al. (1956).

Marginal ulcerations following esophagogastrostomy have been considered already. Stomal ulceration is more liable to occur under the following circumstances:

1. Original operation for duodenal rather than for gastric ulcer.
2. Original operation for perforated ulcer.
3. Inadequate resection (less than 70% if done without vagotomy).
4. Incomplete vagotomy if the intended original procedure was a hemigastrectomy plus vagotomy.
5. Excluded remnant of antrum (for the acid-potentiating capacities of such a stump, originally advocated by Devine, 1925, 1928, see Kelly, Cross and Wangensteen, 1954, Nyhus, 1960, Thompson and Peskin, 1961).
6. Too long (> 15 cm.) jejunal loop.

One interesting point is that it takes a stomal ulcer much longer to show up after gastrojejunostomy than after gastric resection. Walters, Chance and Berkson (1955a) reported the mean interval in 186 cases of the former until subsequent surgical repair was 11.2 years, while in 115 cases of the latter it was 3.7 years. (These intervals were 8.0 and 3.9 years, respectively, Edwards, Herrington, Cate and Lipscomb, 1956.) Thompson (1956) reported that 75 per cent of marginal ulcers following gastrectomy occurred within 5 years as opposed to only 20 per cent of those following gastroenterostomy. Similarly, only 7 per cent of those following gastrectomy occurred after 10 years as opposed to 66 per cent following gastroenterostomy. In the Walters, et al. (1955b) series 91 per cent of patients were men. Gastrojejunocolic fistula was present in 20 of their 301 cases (6.5%) and 16 of these (80%) followed an original gastrojejunostomy.

Complications of stomal ulcer include intractable pain, obstruction, hemorrhage and perforation, as with the original ulcer. However, the treatment is surgical in a much higher percentage of cases than with primary duodenal ulcer. In fact, operative management should be used unless there are definite reasons to the contrary in any case of stomal ulcer which has been diagnosed positively and persists after a few weeks of medical treatment.

If the original operation was a gastrojejunostomy, the preferred surgical treatment is an adequate gastric resection after takedown of the anastomosis. If the original operation was a gastric resection of known adequacy, transthoracic vagotomy, or abdominal vagotomy with reresection should be tried. As shown in Table 31-3, the results are much poorer if vagotomy is not used in such cases. On the other hand, the data of Walters, Chance and Berkson (1955) also demonstrate that the use of gastric resection or reresection reduces the chance of subsequent hemorrhage after operation for stomal ulcer as opposed to procedures in which vagotomy alone is used, the percentages being 3.4 as contrasted with 10.4 per cent.

If the stomal ulcer follows a previous gastrojejunostomy plus vagotomy, an insulin test to determine the completeness of the vagotomy is indicated. In all of 13 such cases, Everson and Allen (1954) found the test to indicate incomplete vagotomy. In such instances, another attempt at vagotomy, or a vagotomy plus resection should be utilized.

Schirmer and Bowers (1955) give an excellent review of secondary surgical indica-

TABLE 31-3. RESULT IN 301 CASES OF GASTROJEJUNAL ULCER TREATED SURGICALLY*

SECONDARY OPERATION	GASTROJEJUNOSTOMY			GASTRIC RESECTION		
	Total Cases (186)	% Mortality	% Good Results	Total Cases (115)	% Mortality	% Good Results
Vagotomy alone	29	0	⎫	88	1.1	70.5
Vagotomy with resection (or reresection)	3	0	⎬ 77.8	14	14.3	100.0
Vagotomy with other operations	9	0	⎭	..	..	..
Resection (or reresection)	145	0.7	86.5	13	15.3	57.1

* From Walters, Chance and Berkson: Surg., Gynec., Obstet., 100:1-10, 1955b.

tions for stomal ulcer following inadequate surgery. In all cases in which the original resection was of unknown adequacy, abdominal exploration should be made with a check as to length of loop, possible presence of an excluded antral stump, and adequacy of the extent of resection. Depending on the findings, a decision as to election of abdominal vagotomy, reresection, adjustment of the loop length (preferably less than 4 in. from the ligament of Treitz), or removal of an antral stump should be made. In such cases the pancreas should be examined for the presence of tumor.

7. **Peptic Ulcer of Meckel's Diverticulum.** Heterotopic gastric mucosa occurs in 54 per cent of Meckel's diverticula (Gross, 1953). This congenital anomaly, in turn, is present in 1.4 per cent of autopsies (Harkins, 1933). The gastric mucosa may involve part or the entire diverticulum and may be grossly similar to that in the stomach with rugae. The usual ulcer develops in the diverticular or ileal epithelium adjacent to the gastric mucosa, and hence is similar to a marginal ulcer. Most cases of peptic ulcer occur before the 6th year, involving boys 3:1. Pain and dyspepsia do not occur, but hemorrhage does occur frequently, and perforation rarely.

In 149 Meckel's diverticula which Gross removed, 50 (33%) were the site of ulcer and hemorrhage. This latter figure did not include 18 other cases with inflammation with or without perforation, in some of which the diverticulum contained gastric mucosa. In a series of 25 consecutive cases of symptom-producing Meckel's diverticulum, Berman, Schneider and Potts (1954) found 14 with bleeding, 2 with perforation, and 2 with both bleeding and perforation. Of 4 other cases gastric mucosa was present in 2. The hemorrhage may be severe and recurrent. It is followed by melena, but we have never seen hematemesis. While this gastric mucosa is probably not under vagal control, it undoubtedly responds to gastrin, and the secretion is especially dangerous because the acid-buffering capacity of the ileal contents is much less than that of the upper jejunum or duodenum. Diagnosis usually is made only by exploration. Removal of the Meckel's diverticulum whenever found on laparotomy is advised, both therapeutically and prophylactically, and should include a portion of the base since gastric cells are at the neck, not at the apex.

DUODENAL ULCER; INDICATIONS FOR OPERATION

Duodenal ulcer is not only an important factor in morbidity, but also in mortality. According to the U. S. 1953 Vital Statistics (Dunn, 1955), there were 4,511 deaths from ulcer of the duodenum. In the records of 2,837 of these, there was no mention of perforation while in 1,674 there was a mention of perforation. In 1,036 additional deaths, gastrojejunal ulcer, duodenitis, etc., were cited which might have been related to duodenal ulcer.

Estimate of all deaths from peptic ulcer in 1965 was 12,500 (Blumenthal, 1967). Since duodenal ulcer is the most common form of peptic ulcer, the trend toward an increased death rate from this cause becomes apparent. An increase of more than 10 per cent in the death rate due to ulcer has been noted (Klebba, 1966). It affects particularly males between the ages of 20 and 50, but individuals of both sexes and all ages are susceptible. Persons with blood-group O are more prone to duodenal ulcer (Aird, Bentall, Mehigan and Roberts, 1954; Wright, Grant and Jennings, 1955). The symptoms include postprandial pain, usually coming on more than an hour after meals and often temporarily relieved by food, milk, or alkali, and with a definite periodicity and remissions and recurrences. Physical signs are usually absent in uncomplicated cases, but often the patient will point to the epigastrium with one finger to indicate the location of pain. Roentgen examination of the upper gastrointestinal tract is very important in the diagnosis. Gastroscopic studies may show mild hyperplastic gastritis. Gastric analysis usually reveals an elevated level of free hydrochloric acid. The more nearly accurate 12-hour night secretion study indicates both an elevated acidity and volume of juice, so that the mEq. of free hydrochloric acid excreted in 12 hours (clinical units × volume in liters = mEq.) is usually higher than the average normal value of 18, being in the range of 60 on the average. Most duodenal ulcers are in the first portion of the duodenum, but postbulbar ulcers are more common than is generally recognized (Clark, 1956).

Uropepsin, or the inactive proenzyme pepsinogen, is normally found in human urine. In a study of 72 patients with a history of definite duodenal ulcer, Nyhus (1957) found a tendency to increased excretion of uropepsin in the urine.

Most (about 75% or more) duodenal ulcer patients should be treated medically. During the first attack without complications, medical management almost always should be given a trial. Patients who do not respond to medical management and those who develop complications should be treated surgically. There are thus 4 indications for the surgical management of duodenal ulcer which will be considered separately below:

Obstruction. True organic obstruction at the pylorus or below it is rare, but a combination of stenosis due to scar with edema is common. Kozoll and Meyer (1964) found obstruction to occur exactly half as often as either perforation or massive hemorrhage in their series of 5,900 duodenal ulcers. If the history is of short duration, medical management almost always should be tried. On the other hand if the obstruction is of long standing, operation is indicated. The surgeon has a choice of operations in the following order of preference: (1) hemigastrectomy plus vagotomy with gastroduodenal (or gastrojejunal) anastomosis; (2) vagotomy plus drainage procedure; (3) subtotal (75%) gastrectomy with gastroduodenal (or gastrojejunal) anastomosis; (4) gastrojejunostomy, in aged or seriously ill patients, and (5) some of the newer experimental operations, such as the wedge resections. (See section on Operative Procedures on the Stomach found on page 852.)

Perforation. The perforation of a peptic ulcer is a surgical emergency. The standard treatment is simple suture closure of the perforation, covered by an attached omental tag to act as a plug. Including this method, there are 3 methods of treatment, each with special indications: (1) simple suture closure of the perforation (Byrd and Carlson, 1956), (2) primary subtotal gastric resection (Moore, Harkins and Merendino, 1954; and Jordan and De Bakey, 1961) and (3) conservative or medical treatment by suction (Seeley and Campbell, 1956). In the United States, in 1953, there were 3,440 deaths from perforated peptic ulcer, 1,766 from perforated duodenal ulcer and 1,674, or almost as many, from the much rarer, but more dangerous perforated gastric ulcer.

A study of our own material at the King County Hospital, Seattle, and that of the Central Middlesex Hospital, London, leads us to the following conclusions and method of managing these cases based on these conclusions:

Certain patients will be too sick for operation, either because of associated disease or advanced peritonitis and shock. In these instances, we use the third method mentioned above, paying especial attention to seeing that the gastric suction tube is working at all times. Supportive treatment, including blood transfusions, is also given.

It appears that patients with perforated peptic ulcer requiring surgical intervention can be divided into 3 roughly equal groups on the basis of future possible difficulties, history of their disease, and the pathologic findings at operation:

GROUP 1. Patients who will have no further difficulty with ulcer symptoms following simple closure of a peptic perforation (patients with perforation of a stress ulcer).

GROUP 2. Patients who satisfy the criteria for definitive surgical therapy, i.e., primary gastric resection, vagotomy and pyloroplasty, or vagotomy and antrectomy. These criteria will be given later. Simple closure in these patients is followed by recurrent symptoms requiring further surgery.

GROUP 3. Patients who may have mild or moderate recurrent ulcer symptoms following simple closure of a perforation but do not satisfy the criteria for resectability at the time of exploration.

It is evident that two thirds of the patients with peptic ulcer perforations should be treated by simple closure of the perforation even though some of the patients in Group 3 may require subsequent surgical treatment. The patients falling into Group 2 should be treated by a definitive operation, provided that these factors of safety are observed: (1) satisfactory general condition of the patient; (2) adequate operating facilities are available; (3) the operation is performed by a competent surgeon experienced in gastric surgery; (4) proper facilities for satisfactory postoperative care are present; (5) consideration of the patient's physiologic rather than chronologic age; (6) sex of the patient. Female patients should have more of the preceding factors in their favor than males.

The criteria for placing the patients in Group 2 are as follows:

1. History of ulcer symptoms for over 1 year
2. Presence of a previously diagnosed peptic ulceration
3. Failure of adequate medical treatment or unreliability of patient's cooperation in following such treatment (alcoholics)
4. History of a previous perforation
5. Perforation of a large callused peptic ulcer
6. Presence of multiple peptic ulcers
7. Perforation with concomitant or previous hemorrhage
8. Perforation which is less than 12 hours in duration
9. Perforated gastric ulcer—fear of later gastric carcinoma
10. Perforated gastric carcinoma with ulceration
11. Perforation of an ulcer associated with a fixed pyloric obstruction

A definitive operative procedure for peptic perforation is technically easier to perform than an elective procedure for a chronic penetrating type of ulceration because the perforation is usually anterior. The morbidity and the mortality for definitive treatment in properly selected patients are better than the mortality and morbidity of simple closure of peptic perforation (Burdette and Rasmussen, 1968). In addition, one third of the patients with perforation will be saved the morbidity and the mortality of additional operative procedures if the criteria of selectivity for a definitive operation are observed.

Currently, in those cases in which a definitive ulcerocurative resection seems to be indicated, we utilize vagotomy combined with antrectomy or Heineke-Mikulicz pyloroplasty.

Massive Hemorrhage. Massive hemorrhage is defined as hemorrhage with a resultant hematocrit of 28 or less corresponding to a blood volume loss of 30 per cent and usually with fainting or shock. It is interesting that mortality is sometimes higher when the *admission* hematocrit is only slightly depressed. This is probably because there has not been time in rapid bleeding for the dilutional effect to have lowered the hematocrit (Cammock, Hallett, Nyhus and Harkins, 1963).

It is of interest that the onset of bleeding often impels the patient to go to the bathroom, and often he faints there. Massive hemorrhage is the most frequent cause of death from peptic ulcer, causing 46 per cent of ulcer deaths (Wangensteen, 1954). The patient with massive hemorrhage should be seen by the surgeon from the beginning of the attack.

Bleeding duodenal ulcers, unlike perforated ulcers, are usually posterior, have penetrated into the pancreas and often erode the gastroduodenal artery. The duodenum and the stomach become filled with clots, and the jejunum and remainder of the intestine below have a bluish appearance at operation due to the contained blood.

Two important questions must be answered: (1) Is the bleedng from an ulcer? (2) Is it continuing? With regard to the first question, it is indeed fortunate when a patient enters the hospital during his bleeding attack with a well-verified history backed by roentgen diagnosis of old duodenal ulcer. Not all cases present this advantage. Carcinoma of the stomach, bleeding from esophageal varices, and other causes of upper gastrointestinal hemorrhage should be ruled out. Bleeding gastric ulcers and esophageal varices tend to have more hematemesis than melena; bleeding duodenal ulcer is the opposite. Palpation of an enlarged spleen may indicate varices, but most cases of varices do not have a palpable spleen. A barium swallow is in order to arrive at a diagnosis, although it is usually not advisable to wash out clots in the stomach. On the basis of probability, upper gastrointestinal hemorrhage is due to duodenal ulcer (80% of all cases).

Arteriography may become increasingly useful in the diagnosis of the exact site of gastrointestinal bleeding. (Baum *et al.*, 1965; Ternberg and Koehler, 1968; Reuter and Bookstein, 1968. See also Nusbaum, Baum, Blakemore and Finkelstein, 1965.)

With regard to the other question, a useful positive sign is continued hematemesis after admission to the hospital. Blood volume studies, if available, should be utilized and are far more helpful than blood counts alone, or pulse and blood pressure changes alone (Stewart, Sanderson and Wiles, 1952). A positive head-up "tilt test" may be of value (Wechsler, Roth and Bockus, 1956). A falling blood volume despite adequate blood replacement indicates continued hemorrhage. Gastroscopic examination just before operation may be helpful (Tanner, 1951).

Additional factors which *tend* to influence the decision in favor of operation include the following: generalized arteriosclerosis, age over 50 years or especially over 60 years, history of previous massive hemorrhage, history of long-standing ulcer or many previous mild hemorrhages, and a history of previous perforation. If the bleeding is from a gastric ulcer or from a "stress" ulcer, it is less apt to stop without operation.

Medical management should be tried in almost all cases of bleeding peptic ulcer. The essential feature of medical management is also the best preoperative preparation, namely, adequate blood replacement. If bleeding continues, operation should be performed *before* the patient's condition deteriorates further. A useful adjunct to medical treatment is gastric cooling (Wangensteen, Salmon, Griffen, Paterson and Fattah, 1959; and Nicoloff, Griffen, Salmon, Peter and Wangensteen, 1962). This method does not cure the ulcer, but it may stop the hemorrhage.

Allen and Oberhelman (1955) have classified surgical intervention into 4 categories:

GROUP 1. INTERVAL SURGERY carried out after the patient has fully recovered from his hemorrhagic episode.

GROUP 2. EMERGENCY SURGERY when blood transfusion fails to keep up with blood loss and shock occurs or persists.

GROUP 3. URGENT SURGERY where shock is corrected but bleeding slowly continues. These patients cannot be weaned from their bottle of blood.

GROUP 4. ELECTIVE INTERVENTION because of the likelihood of a recurrent bout of bleeding during the same episode.

Surgical therapy requires that the patient come to the operating room in as good condition as possible, particularly so far as blood replenishment is concerned. As Allen and Oberhelman (1955) emphasized, the error in these cases is almost always in giving too little blood. Because of the clots in the stomach, gastric suction may be deficient, and if general anesthesia is used a cuff around the tracheal catheter is advisable to prevent aspiration of gastric contents. A recent trend is toward a vagotomy plus pyloroplasty with a figure-of-eight suture of the bleeding point, using a nonabsorbable suture (Foster, Hickok, and Dunphy, 1965).

The operation of choice is vagotomy and pyloroplasty with transfixion of the bleeding point. However, occasionally, subtotal gastrectomy with removal of the ulcer will be indicated. When the latter procedure is elected, the duodenum should be divided below the ulcer if possible, and if an artery is seen with pulsatile bleeding in the ulcer bed in the head of the pancreas, it should be oversewn. Palliative operations, such as gastrojejunostomy, ligation of the major arteries supplying the stomach, or even subtotal gastrectomy leaving the ulcer in place and without suturing the bleeding point, are not advised.

The stomach stump should be anastomosed by the open method so that all clots can be removed and a careful search made for additional ulcers.

If no ulcer is found, and if the portal vein pressure is normal, and if the bleeding is obviously from the upper gastrointestinal tract, and if a thorough abdominal exploration has been done, a so-called "blind" gastric resection is indicated. Use of a wide gastrotomy may reduce the indications for "blind" resections.

Intractability Despite or Incompatibility With Medical Treatment. Either of these situations is an indication for operative treatment. Incompatibility with medical treatment involves those patients whose lack of intelligence, lack of stick-to-itiveness, alcoholism, or job requirements make adequate medical therapy impossible. After a thorough trial, sometimes including psychiatric assistance, the operations of choice are the same as those listed above under "Obstruction."

The mortality of operations for duodenal ulcer varies with the indications, being higher with massive hemorrhage or with perforation treated after 8 hours. Generally speaking, it is 1 to 3 per cent for gastric resection and 0.5 per cent for vagotomy plus drainage procedure. Acute complications are those of the operation in question and include blowout of the duodenal stump (in resection with gastrojejunostomy), wound infection, pneumonia, etc. Chronic complications are listed in the previous section. About 65 per cent have an excellent result, 27 per cent a satisfactory result (mild dumping but no pain, etc.), and 8 per cent have a poor result (operative mortality, stomal ulcer, severe dumping, etc.).

The concept of gastric freezing to treat duodenal ulcer was introduced by Wangensteen (1962). This technic has not proved to be effective and must be considered completely in the realm of an experimental approach. Gastric cooling for massive hemorrhage (see p. 843) is a different matter, and the author does believe that it sometimes has merit as a medical adjunct for this complication.

CARCINOMA OF THE STOMACH

Carcinoma of the stomach is a leading cause of death in this country today. The death rate from this cause is decreasing in this country for unknown cause but is still high. Approximately 24,000 patients die of cancer of the stomach in the United States each year; in other words, of those persons now alive in this country, 1,700,000 will die from this disease.

Etiology

The cause of cancer of the stomach is essentially unknown. Studies indicate that the idea of Konjetzny (1913) that chronic gastritis is a precursor of cancer (which idea was discredited by Guiss and Stewart, 1943) may be important. Morson (1955) studied the occurrence, distribution and relation of "intestinal metaplasia" of gastric mucosa, a form of chronic atrophic gastritis, to gastric carcinoma. Intestinal metaplasia is a condition in which the stomach glands take on the appearance of colonic glands with goblet cells (which stain red with mucicarmine), and Paneth cells (which are low columnar cells with basal nuclei and cytoplasm packed with coarse granules that stain brightly with eosin). Such intestinalization was present in at least a portion of the stomach in patients operated upon for duodenal or gastric ulcer or carcinoma in 78.2 per cent of stomachs. Its presence was most common in carcinoma, least common in duodenal ulcer, while gastric ulcer took an intermediate position. In all cases it was most common near the pylorus (antrum), but in gastric ulcer and carcinoma this preponderance of location was not so marked (Table 31-4).

TABLE 31-4. INCIDENCE OF INTESTINAL METAPLASIA IN DIFFERENT SITES IN THE STOMACH IN SURGICAL SPECIMENS*

Site	D.U. (%)	G.U. (%)	Carcinoma (%)
Antrum	59.6	71.4	87.1
Lesser curve	15.4	57.1	79.5
Greater curve	9.6	39.3	66.7

* From Morson, B. C.: Brit. J. Cancer, 11:369, September, 1955.

Morson also related the "signet ring" cells in colloid carcinomas to the goblet cells seen in intestinal metaplasia. He also pointed out that most gastric carcinomas originate in areas where intestinal metaplasia also is most common. In pernicious anemia, on the other hand, as shown by Schell, Dockerty and Comfort (1954), carcinoma is especially apt to occur in the cardiac and fundic portions of the stomach, and in pernicious anemia this is the site of predilection for intestinalization of the mucosa. Morson concluded his discussion by showing examples of gastric carcinoma which appeared to arise from epithelium of the intestinal type and by stating, "Evidence has been considered which suggests that about 30 per cent of gastric carcinomas arise from areas of intestinal metaplasia in the gastric mucosa."

Pathology

The pathology of carcinoma of the stomach includes a variety of primary tumor forms which can be divided roughly, in ascending order of malignancy, into polypoid, ulcerating and infiltrating varieties, of about equal frequency. Microscopically, they can be divided, also in ascending order of malignancy, into adenocarcinoma, colloid carcinoma, carcinoma simplex and undifferentiated carcinoma.

Local Spread and Invasion of Contiguous Organs. Such spread is apt to be far more extensive than can be detected with the naked eye or the palpating finger at the operating table. In the stomach wall it is most extensive and at the same time least conspicuous in the submucosal and subserosal layers, but it also occurs in the intramuscular layer. As shown by Zinninger (1954), spread into the duodenum is chiefly by the muscular and subserosal layers, while spread to the esophagus is chiefly by the submucosal route. In 101 cases, spread to the duodenum occurred in 43 per cent (Coller, Kay and McIntyre, 1941, reported a figure of 26.4% for duodenal spread). In only 3 of 43 cases (7%) was such spread for more than 3 cm. In 9 of the 101 cases (9%) there was extension to the esophagus; in only 1 case was the spread for more than 3 cm. In no instance did a carcinoma of the cardia extend into the duodenum or a carcinoma of the prepyloric or the antral regions extend into the esophagus. Fundic lesions, however, spread both to the duodenum (28%) and to the esophagus (8%). Therefore, the rule of removing at least 3 cm. of duodenum in low-lying carcinomas and 3 cm. of esophagus in high-lying carcinomas would seem to be in order.

In many instances sufficient stomach is not removed. Berne and Freedman (1951) reported an incidence of "recurrence" in the gastric stump in 78.6 per cent and in 10.7 per cent in the duodenal stump in autopsies. Coller, Kay and McIntyre (1941) reported that in 24.5 per cent of operative specimens the carcinoma had extended to the upper limit of the resection. McNeer, Sunderland, McInnes, VandenBerg and Lawrence (1951) reported recurrence in the gastric remnant in 50 per cent of 92 patients. Helsingen and Hillestad (1956) reported the interesting finding of development of carcinoma in the gastric stump after 11 of 229 gastrectomies for histologically verified peptic ulcer (4.8%). A breakdown of this incidence indicated 10.5 per cent of the 95 gastric ulcer cases and only 0.8 per cent in the 125 duodenal ulcer cases. (In the 9 cases with combined gastric and duodenal ulcer there was no development of carcinoma.)

Even when total gastrectomy is performed, there is a tendency to leave carcinoma behind at the ends of the resection. Ransom (1956) reported that in 38 histologically studied total gastrectomy specimens, the operations being all performed for carcinoma, there was cancerous involvement of one or both ends of the specimen in 26 (68%). Since in 19 of the cases the proximal end was involved, this would argue for resecting the lower esophagus more often in such cases.

Spread by way of the blood stream to lungs, brain, etc., does occur but is rare. Spread by way of the peritoneal cavity also occurs (the involvement of the greater omentum, of the bottom of the pelvis—"Blumer's shelf"—and the Krukenberg tumor of the ovary from colloid carcinoma of the stomach are examples).

Lymphatic Spread. This is extremely common. In the classic study of Coller, Kay and McIntyre (1941), evidence of metastases was present microscopically in 75.5 per cent of cases (plus 12.5% additional in which only a palliative operation was done, total 88%). The 4 zones of lymph node involvement are shown in Figure 31-11. The most commonly involved are Zones I and III. Of the sessile neoplasms, 95.4 per cent had metastasized in comparison with only 60 per cent of the polypoid carcinomas. The authors concluded: "Whether palpable lymph nodes are present or not, the 4 zones of lymphatic metastases should be included within the resection to increase the likelihood of cure."

Metastases to the hilum of the spleen are frequent. Eker's series (1951) contained 46 stomachs with the attached spleen. The high over-all (21.7%) incidence of metastases is shown in Table 31-5. It is true that these cases were selected, since in only those cases in which it was thought necessary was the spleen removed. However, 16 of the 46 carcinomas were in the lower part of the stomach, including 8 on the lesser curve. Fly, Dockerty

TABLE 31-5. INCIDENCE OF METASTASES TO THE HILUM OF THE SPLEEN IN 46 CASES OF GASTRIC RESECTION FOR CARCINOMA*

Gross Type of Tumor	Metastases to Hilum of Spleen Number	Per Cent
Polypoid (21 cases)	1	4.8
Ulcerating (6 cases)	0	0.0
Infiltrating (19 cases)	9	47.4
Total (46 cases)	10	21.7

* From Eker, R.: Acta chir. scandinav., 101:123, March 22, 1951.

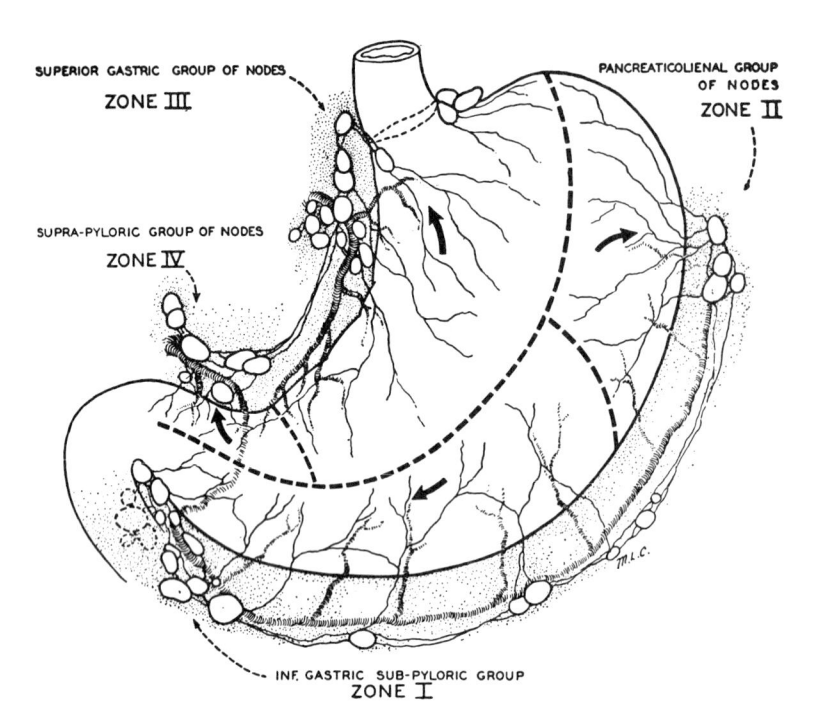

FIG. 31-11. Diagrammatic representation of zonal lymphatic metastases of carcinoma of the stomach. (Coller, F., Kay, E., and McIntyre, R.: Arch. Surg., 43:751)

and Waugh (1956) found the splenic hilar nodes involved in 36.3 per cent of 102 resected stomach specimens. Furthermore, in the group of 20 carcinomas involving the distal half of the stomach, the percentage of splenic hilar involvement was almost as great, namely 30 per cent. Because the spleen is an "expendable" organ and also easily removed, it should be included en bloc with the stomach in resections for carcinoma.

Eker also reported that the frequency of histologically verified metastases in all locations was 70 per cent in his 100 subtotal resections and 82.9 in his 70 total resection specimens. Incomplete removal of nodes in Zone III seemed to be apparent in the subtotal resections as compared with the total resections.

Arhelger, Lober and Wangensteen (1955), during "second look" operations for gastric cancer, obtained positive findings in 11 of 26 patients in the hepatic pedicle and retropancreaticoduodenal areas (Zones IV and I, respectively). On the basis of these observations, a more nearly complete dissection of these areas was done in 24 patients. In 11 of the latter patients positive nodes were found in Zone IV and in 4 patients in Zone I. These authors concluded, "It is apparent that the lymph node dissection in present-day operations for cancer of the stomach is incomplete. An extension of the operation to include dissection of the hepatic pedicle and retropancreaticoduodenal area is recommended."

Classification. The importance of classification of carcinoma of the stomach is of especial significance from the standpoint of prognosis. Most classifications consider only the local lesion, while that of Hoerr (1954) takes into account both the element of metastases and of invasion, as follows:

Metastases. The extent of metastases is estimated preoperatively (as for example for osseous or pulmonary metastases) and at the time of operation. Capital letters (A, B and C) are used to denote 3 stages in descending order of favorableness.

STAGE A. No metastases.

STAGE B. Regional metastases to lymph nodes that usually are resectable.

STAGE C. Distant metastases, connoting incurability.

Invasion. Invasion and local extension are determined at the time of laparotomy and are classified according to the degree to which the primary growth has penetrated the walls of the stomach. Three stages of invasion are recognized by Roman numerals (I, II and

Fig. 31-12. Three stages of carcinoma of the stomach according to extent of metastasis. A fourth stage, C-NX, is listed as a variant of stage C. (Hoerr, S.: Surg., Gynec. Obstet. 99:282)

Stage A. No metastases, grossly or microscopically.

Stage B. Regional metastases, usually resectable. Must be verified histologically since involved nodes may appear normal grossly, and enlarged nodes may represent only chronic inflammation. These metastases will be resectable unless fixed to aorta or in gastrohepatic ligament.

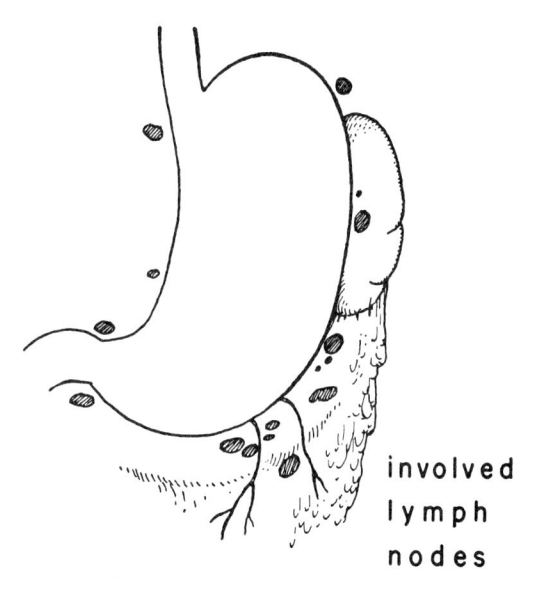

Stage C. Distant metastases. Included are metastases to supraclavicular nodes, peritoneum, liver, lung, or bone. Usually will be verified histologically. At the present time they mean incurability.

Stage C-NX. Distant metastases. No operation. Distant metastases without surgical exploration of the stomach. A special case of stage C, such as might occur in a patient who has cancer in a biopsied supraclavicular lymph node, x-ray evidence of a gastric neoplasm, but no abdominal operation. "NX" is "no exploration" for grouping of invasion.

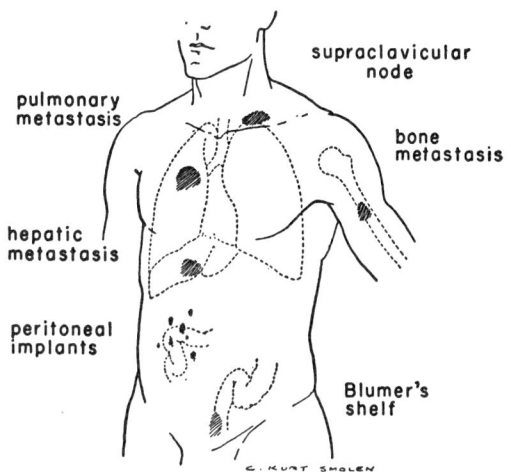

III), once more in descending order of favorableness.

STAGE I. The growth is superficial and is confined to mucosa and muscularis.

STAGE II. All gastric layers are involved, including the serosa, but there is no extragastric extension.

STAGE III. The tumor has extended in continuity to neighboring structures, such as mesocolon, colon, liver, or pancreas.

In Stages I and II the primary lesion is resectable, but in Stage III only if the involved neighboring structures also are resectable.

Hoerr summarized the application of this classification by pointing out that at the time of operation the situation may be expressed by a combination of the two symbols: *metastases* represented by a letter A, B, or C, and *invasion* by a numeral I, II, or III. For example, superficial cancer with no clinical or pathologic evidence of metastases would be grouped as A-I, the most favorable type. On the other hand, the most serious would be C-III, with metastases to the liver and invasion of neighboring structures. (Hopeless carcinoma, e.g., with proved supraclavicular lymph node metastases and a gastric filling defect, but *no* laparotomy would be designated as Stage C-NX.) A pictorial represen-

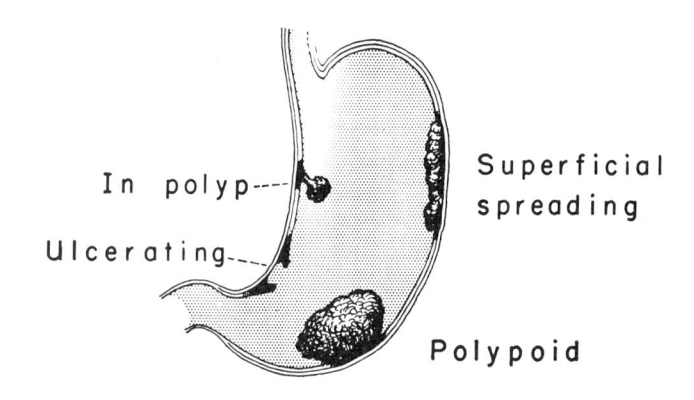

FIG. 31-13. Three stages of carcinoma of the stomach according to extent of invasion. (Hoerr, S.: Surg., Gynec., Obstet., 99:283)

Stage I. Superficial cancer. Growth confined to mucosa and muscularis, irrespective of extent within the stomach. All are resectable.

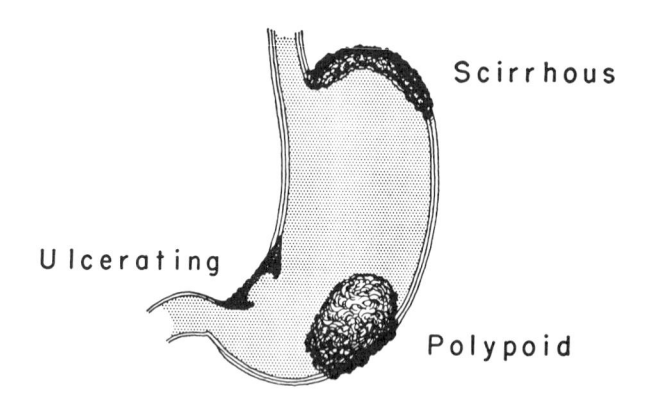

Stage II. All gastric layers. Penetration to serosa but not involving extrinsic structures. Growths may extend into duodenum or esophagus if there is no external invasion. All are resectable.

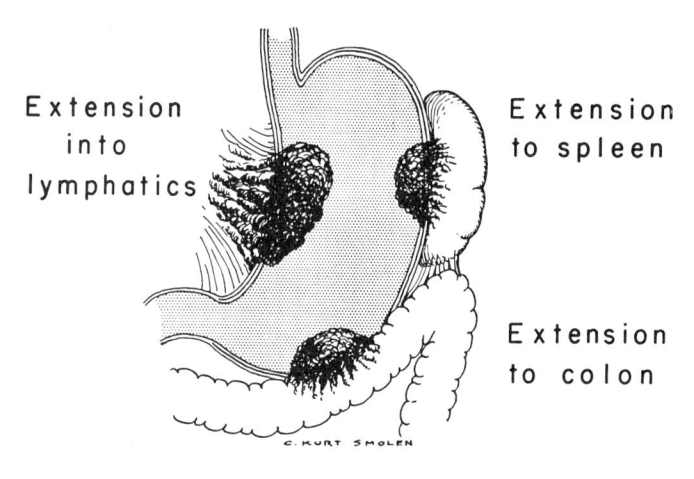

Stage III. Extragastric invasion. Direct invasion of neighboring structures. These structures may be omentum, mesocolon, colon, pancreas, liver, spleen, diaphragm, aorta, adjacent lymphatics, or lymph nodes, or any combination of these. Resectability depends upon the structures that are invaded.

tation of the six individual stages is shown in Figures 31-12 and 31-13.

In a series of 100 patients with 1- to 4-year follow-up in 100 per cent of the cases. Hoerr summarized the mortality. He found a progressive and marked decrease in the percentage of patients still alive as they were listed according to the different stages from A to C and from I to III.

DIAGNOSIS

The important program of diagnosis of cancer of the stomach has been handicapped by certain mistaken attitudes relating to prognosis. As will be seen in the section on "Prognosis" (p. 850), the situation is not as bleak as some would persuade us to think. Jenson, Shahon and Wangensteen (1960) have shown that annual examinations of asymptomatic patients in a cancer detection center turn up a relatively large number of cases of carcinoma of the stomach. Unfortunately, in their experience, only 43 per cent of such discovered cases were without positive lymph nodes at the time of discovery.

The very important subject of the differential diagnosis between gastric ulcer and carcinoma has been covered in the section on ulcer. In summary, and extending the criteria of McGlone and Robertson (1953), malignancy is suggested by any of the following:

1. Roentgen evidence of malignancy, as determined by competent roentgenologic investigation
2. Gastroscopic evidence of malignancy
3. Cytologic evidence of malignant cells in the gastric aspirate
4. The presence of histamine-proved achlorhydria
5. Location of lesion
   A. Greater curvature
   B. Prepyloric portion of lesser curvature
   C. Fundus
6. Failure of a lesion in any part of the stomach to heal within 3 weeks. (Not all agree even to giving medical treatment a trial, Edwards, 1950, stating, "Such a therapeutic test should be completely eliminated from practice.")

There are no typical symptoms of gastric cancer. Epigastric pain, loss of weight, anorexia, tiredness, or even a protracted siege of "flu" (Wangensteen, 1951) may herald the onset of this most serious of all cancers. The physical examination is of limited value, because once a mass is palpable, cure is extremely unlikely. Among the simple laboratory tests, the determination of achlorhydria in the gastric contents, of normochromic or hypochromic anemia, and of occult blood in the stools is helpful.

Males are affected about 3 times as often as females, and the average age of the patients is about 63 years, but neither of these two is of help in the diagnosis in an individual patient.

Boyce (1953) deplored the fact that a comparison of a recent series of cases of carcinoma of the stomach with other series he reported in 1933 and 1941 indicated that while the surgeon was doing his share of improvement by greatly lowering the operative mortality, the patients were still seeking treatment late. He advised more vigor in the prosecution of the diagnostic routine and a prompter and far more general resort to exploratory laparotomy in doubtful cases. He also stated: "An alarming tendency was noted in this most recent analysis, i.e., the invocation of psychosomatic medicine to explain symptoms and signs caused by gastric cancer."

Treatment

The only curative treatment of cancer of the stomach known at present is complete surgical excision of the tumor and its metastases. Roentgen therapy is of no curative value and of little, if any, palliative benefit. There was a trend in favor of more radical operations, going in two different but parallel directions. The first was a trend toward more frequent total gastrectomy (Lahey, 1950; Lahey and Marshall, 1950; McNeer, Sunderland, McInnes, VandenBerg and Lawrence, 1951). This approach has lost favor because of a failure to significantly improve survival. The second is toward a more radical subtotal gastrectomy, avoiding total gastrectomy in most pyloric or antral lesions, but including a more radical removal of lymph-node-bearing areas or portions of contiguous organs, especially the spleen, which are involved (Boyden, 1953; Fretheim, 1955; Arhelger, Lober and Wangensteen, 1955; and Hoerr, 1961).

The operations for gastric cancer can be listed as follows:

1. Radical subtotal distal gastrectomy (for lesions of the distal stomach).
2. Radical subtotal proximal gastrectomy (for lesions of the upper stomach). The lower portion of the esophagus also is removed along with the spleen. A combined thoraco-abdominal incision is used.
3. Total gastrectomy (for lesions of the body, or extensive lesions of the lower or upper stomach). An abdominal approach is possible, but a thoraco-abdominal one is preferable. As indicated, this procedure is used less frequently today than it was a decade ago.
   A. With esophagojejunostomy by anastomosis to a jejunal loop coupled with enteroenterostomy
   B. With esophagojejunostomy Roux-en-Y

CANCER OF THE STOMACH
ANALYSIS OF 5-YEAR LOSSES

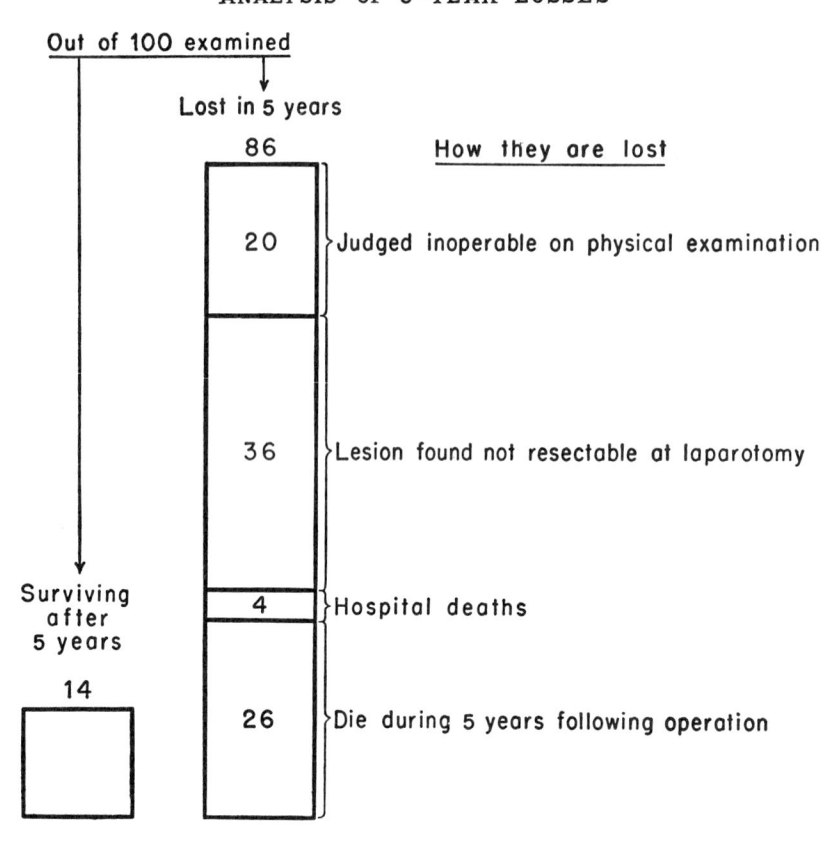

Out of 100 examined → Lost in 5 years: 86

How they are lost:
- 20 — Judged inoperable on physical examination
- 36 — Lesion found not resectable at laparotomy
- 4 — Hospital deaths
- 26 — Die during 5 years following operation

Surviving after 5 years: 14

FIG. 31-14. Analysis of 5-year losses from cancer of the stomach. (Berkson, J., Walters, W., Gray, H., and Priestley, J.: Proc. Mayo Clin., 27: 150)

    C. With esophagoduodenostomy:
        a. Direct anastomosis
        b. With ileocolic segment as pouch (Hunnicut, 1952)
        c. Jejunal segment as pouch (Hunt, 1955)
    4. Palliative operations: gastrojejunostomy, gastrostomy, etc. (often of value).

PROGNOSIS

While the prognosis of carcinoma of the stomach could be improved markedly, the outlook is far from hopeless. It is true, as Berkson, Walters, Gray, and Priestley (1952) reported, of 100 patients examined with carcinoma of the stomach, that only 14 will be alive at the end of 5 years (Fig. 31-14). However, if one takes 100 patients who survive gastric resection for carcinoma of the stomach and in whom no metastases are found, 48.5 will be alive in 5 years. Ferguson and Nusbaum (1964) even report a 61.6 figure in this respect. The differences in survival between resection, palliative operation and exploration only are shown in Figure 31-15, and the effect of metastases in Figure 31-16. In these charts the entire survival curve is included for as long a period as the follow-up of a sufficient number of patients allowed. The actuarial method of calculation of the curves was used.

Other authors have reported somewhat similar figures. Landelius (1948) found 31 per cent of 62 resected patients who survived operation were still alive in 5 years. In 343 resections for cure with survival after operation, Ransom (1953) found 28 per cent still alive at the end of 5 years (26 per cent if the 31 palliative resections are included). In 91 with negative nodes there were 49.5 per cent still alive at the end of 5 years and in 184 with positive nodes, only 15.8 per cent (nodes not recorded in 68). Shahon, Horowitz and Kelly (1956) found 57.1 per cent 5-year sur-

FIG. 31-15. Survival rates in successive years after operation (resection, palliative operation, or exploration only) for cancer of the stomach. (Berkson, J., Walters, W., Gray, H., and Priestley, J.: Proc. Mayo Clin., 27:143)

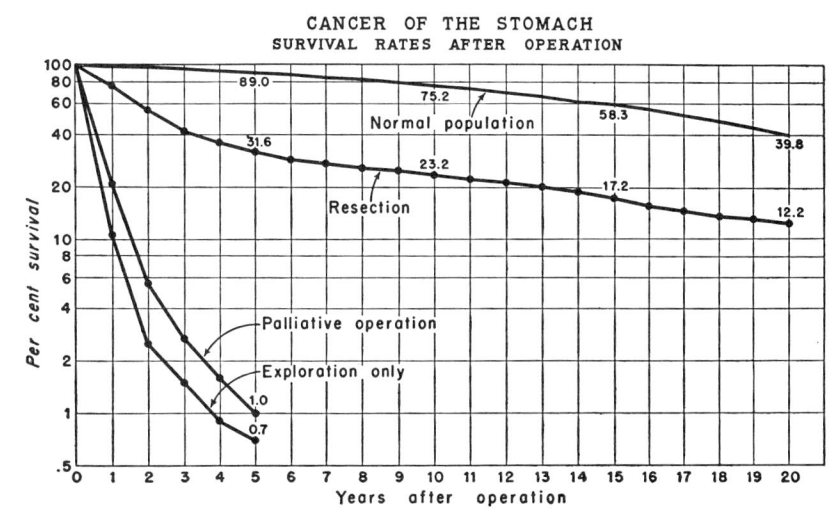

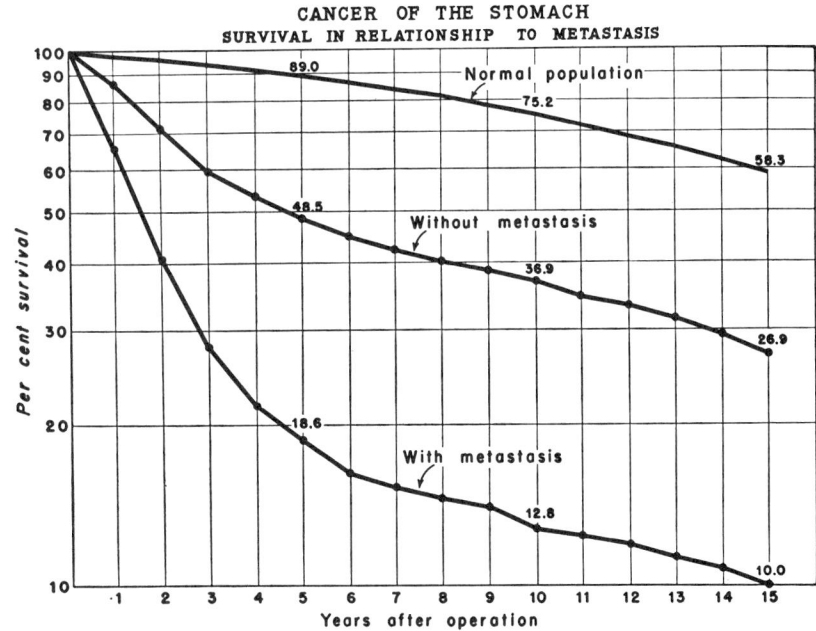

FIG. 31-16. Survival rates in successive years after gastric resection for cancer of the stomach, according to absence (middle line) or presence (lower line) of metastases. (Berkson, J., Walters, W., Gray, H., and Priestley, J.: Proc. Mayo Clin., 27: 144)

vivals in cases without nodes and 14.5 per cent in those with nodes. Beal and Hill (1956), after 133 definitive subtotal resections, reported similar figures of 48.6 and 15.9 per cent (33.1% in the entire group). The figures of Brown, Cain and Dockerty (1961) indicate an even more hopeful outlook.

Muto et al. (1968) noted an improvement in the survival rate in recent years, i.e. from 22.6 per cent in the period 1941 to 1945 to 34.9 per cent from 1956 to 1960. These trends in the end results of the surgical treatment of gastric cancer were well correlated with the relative frequency of the mucosal or submucosal carcinomas in the resected specimens. They attributed this improvement in results to earlier diagnosis and surgical treatment of the disease.

HYPERTROPHIC PYLORIC STENOSIS

This condition, while one of the 3 most important lesions of the stomach and the duodenum, will not be discussed here (see Chap. 50 where the story of hypertrophic pyloric stenosis and its treatment by the very effective Fredet-Ramstedt operation will be given in detail).

OPERATIVE PROCEDURES ON THE STOMACH

In the following compilation, only those surgical procedures which are currently in use will be discussed. Operations such as gastropexy are not listed here because it is believed that these procedures are obsolete. Some other rare or optional operations also are not listed.

When any operation is performed on the stomach or the duodenum, a careful preoperative and postoperative regimen must be followed as described in Chapter 5. Special attention must be directed toward getting the stomach as empty as possible before operation. Aspiration and irrigation with the large tube may be necessary in cases of pyloric obstruction. In most cases the patient comes to the operating room with a Levin tube in the stomach. Such a tube is left in the stomach a varying period after operation, usually less than 5 days, and the present tendency is to use the tube for a shorter period postoperatively than formerly, except after vagotomy.

DRAINAGE PROCEDURES

These are utilized either alone or with vagotomy to drain the stomach.

Pyloromyotomy (Fredet-Ramstedt). This operation is used not only in cases of hypertrophic pyloric stenosis for which it is almost specific but also in conjunction with certain upper and wedge gastric resections (see Chap. 50, Pediatric Surgery).

Heineke-Mikulicz. This is used as a drainage procedure in conjunction with vagotomy or wedge resection. It involves a longitudinal incision through the pylorus which is then closed transversely, usually with one layer of interrupted sutures. Its plastic principle gives added diameter to the lumen (Fig. 31-17).

Finney Pyloroplasty. This involves a more extensive longitudinal incision than with the Heineke-Mikulicz. Then this is closed separately for the lower and the upper leaves of the incision in an inverted-U fashion. It has the same uses as the Heineke-Mikulicz but is used when one desires a bigger opening.

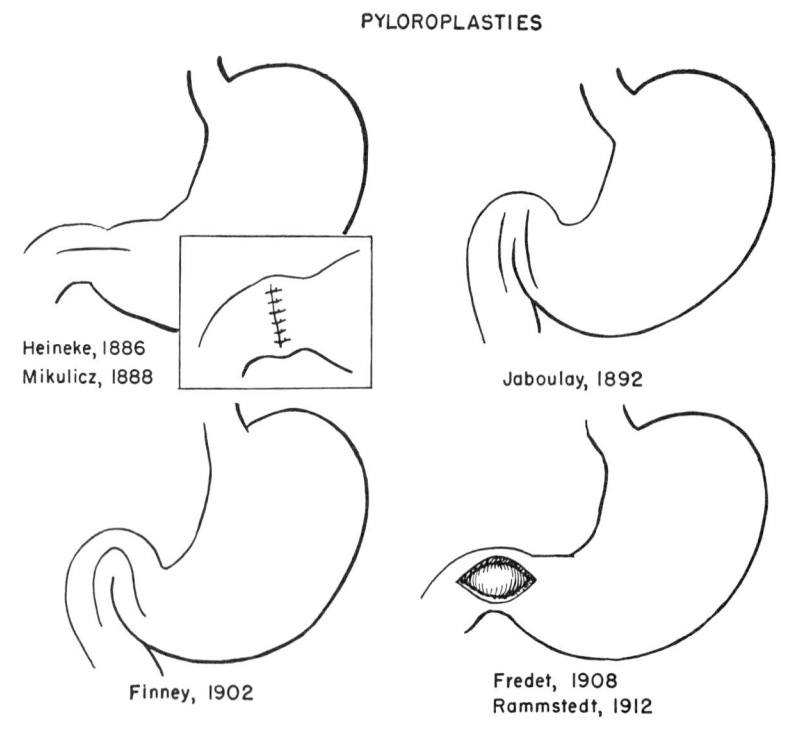

Fig. 31-17. Different types of pyloroplasty procedures. The Heineke-Mikulicz involves the principle of longitudinal incision with transverse closure to enlarge the lumen. The Jaboulay involves an anastomosis of 2 longitudinal incisions. The Finney involves a closure of an inverted U-incision. Finally, the Fredet-Ramstedt involves a longitudinal incision of muscularis down to but not through the mucosa; after separation of the muscle layer the mucosa should pouch out to a level even with the adjoining serosa. (Redrawn from Waugh, J., and Hood, R.: Quart. Rev. Surg., 10: 205)

Gastrojejunostomy. This procedure anastomoses the jejunum, preferably within 4 inches of the ligament of Treitz, to the stomach. The loop of jejunum can be brought up either anteriorly or posteriorly with relation to the colon. Some surgeons do not realize that an anterior anastomosis can be performed with a loop shorter than 4 inches, but if the transverse colon is pulled to the right and the loop brought up toward the left side, this can be done easily in most cases.

Gastric Resections

Billroth I (Gastroduodenostomy Anastomosis After the Resection). This operation has the advantage of restoring normal continuity. It is especially applicable to the treatment of gastric ulcers or perforated duodenal ulcers (which are usually anterior). With adequate mobilization of the duodenum and preparation of the duodenal stump surgeon with experience in doing this operation can perform it in almost all instances where subtotal resection is indicated and without sacrificing the extent of resection (Harkins and Nyhus, 1956).

1. The Finney-von Haberer variety of this operation anastomoses the end of the cut stomach to the side rather than to the end of the duodenum.

2. Another variant is "gastrectomy with replacement" (Henley, 1952) in which a jejunal loop connects the end of the stomach to the end of the duodenum, obviating tension on the anastomosis.

(*Application:* Gastric or duodenal ulcer or carcinoma of the lower stomach. See Fig. 31-18.)

Billroth II (Gastrojejunostomy Anastomosis After the Resection). There are several varieties of this operation, depending upon whether the jejunal loop is brought up anterior or posterior to the colon, and whether the entire stomach opening is anastomosed to the jejunum (Polya) or only its lower half (Hofmeister or Schoemaker), after closure of the duodenal stump (Fig. 31-19) in either instance.

(*Application:* Duodenal, or gastric ulcer, or carcinoma of the lower stomach. See Figs. 31-20A and 31-20B.)

Segmental Resection With Pyloroplasty. This procedure has the advantage that it leaves the antrum in place and removes more

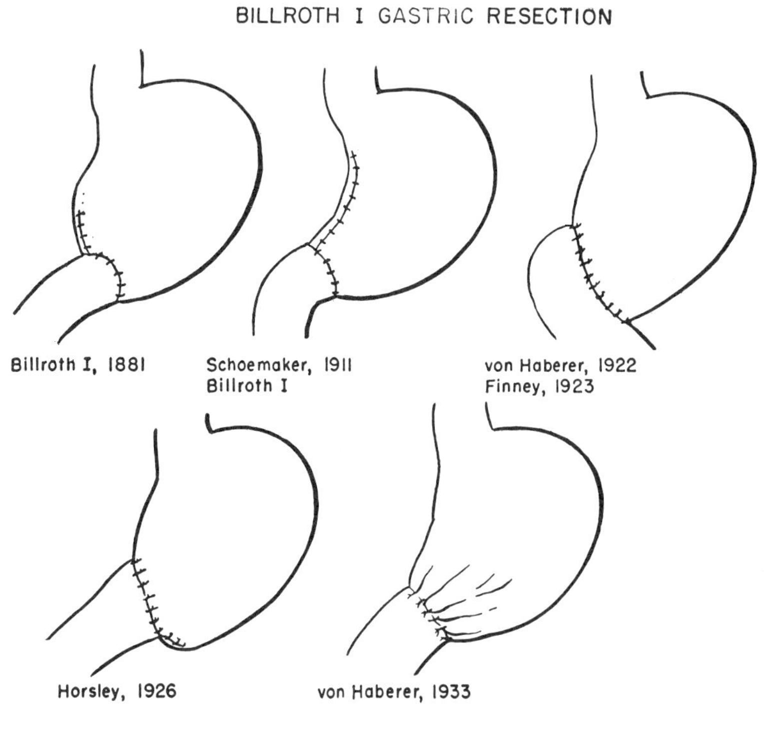

BILLROTH I GASTRIC RESECTION

Billroth I, 1881

Schoemaker, 1911
Billroth I

von Haberer, 1922
Finney, 1923

Horsley, 1926

von Haberer, 1933

Fig. 31-18. Different types of gastroduodenostomy following subtotal gastric resection (Billroth I).

DUODENAL STUMP CLOSURE

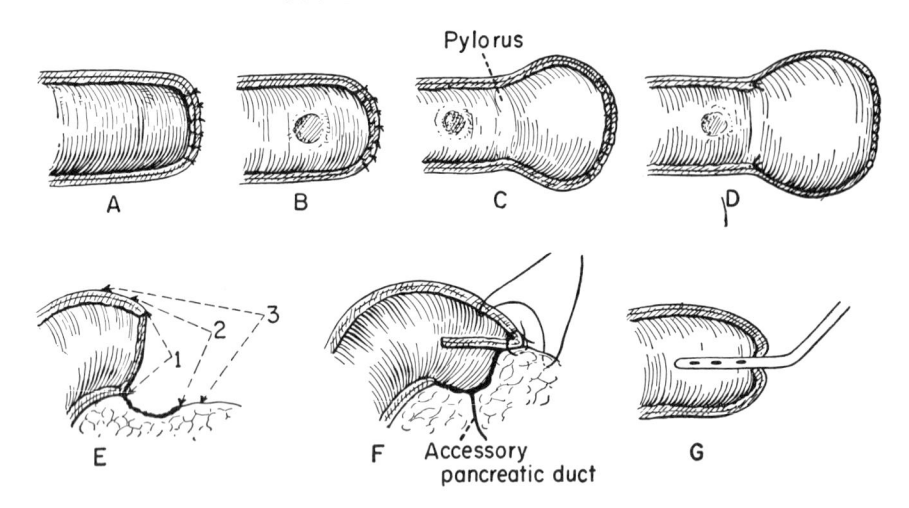

FIG. 31-19. Different methods of duodenal stump closure. (A) Routine closure distal to the removed ulcer. (B) A similar closure proximal to the ulcer which is left in situ. (C) The Devine exclusion of the distal stomach with the antral mucosa in place. (D) The Bancroft-Plenk exclusion with the antral mucosa excised. (E) The Nissen-I with the anterior duodenal flap sutured as follows: (1) Inner layer to distal edge of ulcer in situ in the bed of the pancreas. (2) The inner serosal sutures to the proximal edge of the ulcer bed. (3) The outer serosal sutures to the capsule of the pancreas. (F) The Nissen-II for ulcers which not only are left in situ but also may contain the opening of the duct of Santorini. The anterior edge of the duodenal stump is sutured in 2 layers to the proximal edge of the ulcer. (G) Closure over a tube which is brought out through a stab wound in the abdominal wall. (Modified from Dr. John A. Duncan)

parietal cells, at the same time leaving a larger stomach. It has been popularized by Wangensteen (1952) and reported on by MacLean, Hamilton and Murphy (1953). Because of the vagal interruption to the distal segment, a Heineke-Mikulicz pyloroplasty is necessary for drainage.

Proximal (Upper) Gastrectomy. This operation, a type of esophagogastrectomy, involves an end-to-end anastomosis between the lower esophagus and the remaining lower stomach. Usually it must be supplemented by a pyloroplasty (Tanner, 1954, 1955).

(*Application:* Tumor of the upper stomach. Not suitable for high-lying ulcer because of the danger of peptic esophagitis.)

Total Gastrectomy. A thoraco-abdominal approach is advised (Tanner, 1951).

(*Application:* Carcinoma of body or fundus of stomach.)

VAGOTOMY

Vagotomy, introduced by Dragstedt and Owens (1943), is used for duodenal ulcer, not for gastric ulcer. It also requires a drainage procedure or a coincident resection.

1. *With drainage procedure* (gastrojejunostomy), Dragstedt, 1945; Holt and Robinson, 1955; Hoerr, 1955; Heineke-Mikulicz pyloroplasty, Weinberg, 1953, 1964

2. *With hemigastrectomy* (45 to 50 per cent, removing all the antrum)

    A. Billroth II anastomosis (Farmer, Howe, Porell and Smithwick, 1951; Stock, Hui and Tinckler, 1956, and others)

    B. Billroth I anastomosis (Harkins, Schmitz, Harper, Sauvage, Moore, Storer and Kanar, 1953; Zollinger and Williams, 1956; Harkins, Jesseph, Stevenson and Nyhus, 1960; Herrington, Classen and Edwards, 1961; and Harkins and Nyhus, 1962)

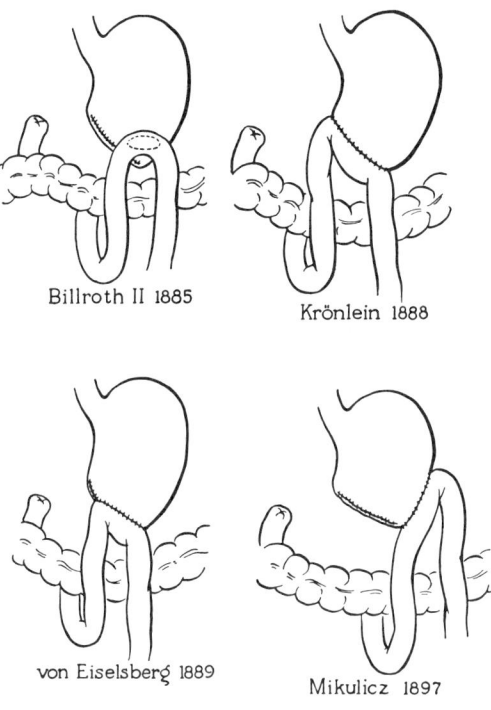

FIG. 31-20A. Different types of gastrojejunostomy following subtotal gastric resection (Billroth II). (Waugh, J., and Hood, R.: Quart. Rev. Surg., 10:212)

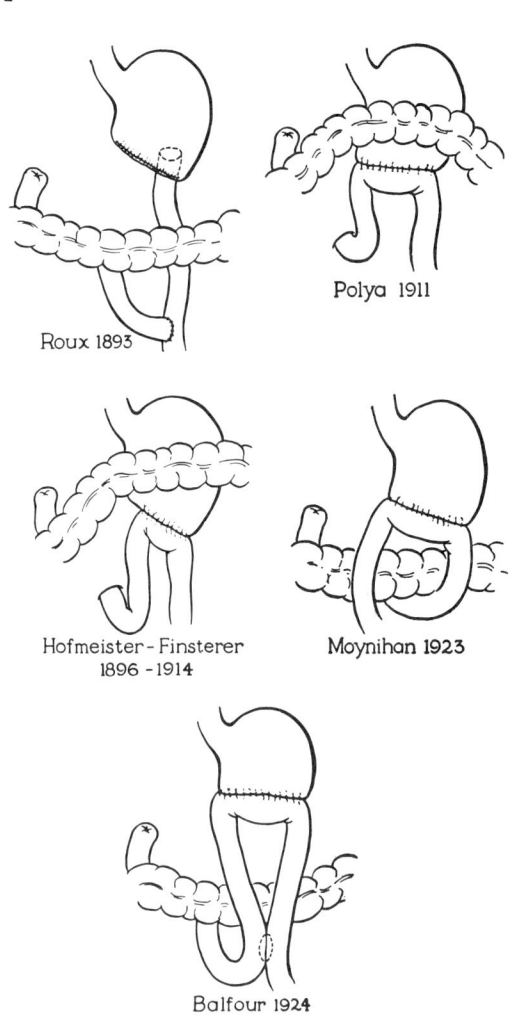

FIG. 31-20B. Billroth II gastrectomies (*Cont.*) (Waugh, J., and Hood, R.: Quart. Rev. Surg., 10:213)

3. *Selective gastric vagotomy.* With either drainage procedure or hemigastrectomy (Griffith and Harkins, 1957; Griffith, 1960; Burge, 1960). This technic spares the celiac and the hepatic branches of the vagi, sectioning only those to the stomach, and purportedly eliminates diarrhea and other complications that sometimes follow total abdominal vagotomy. Historically, the technic of selective vagotomy was introduced by Jackson of Ann Arbor and by Franksson of Stockholm independently in 1947. These surgeons did not combine the operation with a drainage procedure, and it remained for Griffith and Burge to reintroduce the technic in its modern combined form a decade later.

The author's own experience with this procedure plus studies of the literature lend interest to his studies (Harkins, Stavney, Griffith, Savage, Kato and Nyhus, 1963; Harkins, Stavney, Griffith, Savage and Nyhus, 1964; Burge, Hutchison, Longland, McLennan, Miln, Rudick and Tompkin, 1964; Ruckley, 1964; and Rudick and Hutchison, 1964; Scheinin and Inberg, 1967). However, because these investigations are still in progress, the author will not advocate the method at this time in a definitive fashion in a textbook. Suffice it to say that to vagotomize almost the entire abdominal contents—as is done by standard truncal vagotomy—seems to be as illogical as to amputate an entire leg for the cure of an ingrown toenail. Furthermore, the oft-cited objection to the selective technic, that it would be less effective in accomplishing its primary aim, namely to vagotomize the stomach, is not correct. If anything, the selective technic vagotomizes the stomach more effectively than does truncal vagotomy (Sawyers *et al.*, 1968).

Miscellaneous Operations

Gastrostomy. These are more applicable for feeding below an obstruction in an attempt to maintain or get the patient in better shape than they are for palliation of a malignant process (Connar and Sealy, 1956).

Tube (Temporary) Gastrostomy (Stamm). Such a gastrostomy of the Stamm type involves introduction of a catheter into a hole in the stomach around which the wall is closed with 3 overlapping purse-string sutures. The catheter is brought out through the omentum and then through a stab wound in the abdominal wall (Farris and Smith, 1956). Use such a catheter as a temporary measure in place of nasogastric suction after many major operations.

Gastric-Wall-Lined (Permanent) Gastrostomy (Spivack). While there are several varieties of permanent gastrostomy, the author prefers the Spivack variety which has a mucous-membrane-lined valve to prevent leakage. Another type of gastric mucous-membrane-lined gastrostomy is that of Glassman (1939) as modified by Gibbon, Nealon and Greco (1956). Another permanent type of gastrostomy, an interposed jejunal loop (Nyhus, Stevenson, Jones, DeVito and Harkins, 1958) is useful.

Simple Closure of a Perforated Peptic Ulcer. About 3 sutures are placed across the defect, without inversion and then are tied loosely over the tip of an attached omental tag.

LATE COMPLICATIONS OF GASTRIC SURGERY: THE POSTGASTRECTOMY SYNDROME

Mortality is the most serious complication of all surgery. Fortunately, for most of the common gastric operations it is relatively low (gastrojejunostomy, 0.5%; subtotal gastric resection for ulcer, 1 to 3%; subtotal gastric resection for carcinoma, 3 to 7%; total gastrectomy, 5 to 12%, and vagotomy with pyloroplasty, 0.5%).

In those patients who recover from a technically correct gastric operation, a number of late effects are observed in a varying proportion of patients. Sometimes these are lumped together as the "postgastrectomy syndrome"; sometimes this term is used to include only "dumping," and sometimes it is used to include all but recurrence. In the following discussion, the 5 main late complications of gastric surgery will be considered.

Stomal Ulcer

Such a complication is often called a recurrence. This involves a matter of definition since a stomal ulcer after a Billroth II gastric resection for duodenal ulcer is situated many inches away from the original ulcer and, from this standpoint, is hardly a recurrence. This type of complication has been considered previously under special types of ulcer according to location and will not be discussed further here.

"Dumping Syndrome"

Dumping may be defined as the occurrence of sweating, unpleasant warmth, subjective flushing, nausea, palpitation, or explosive diarrhea, with onset during or within 15 minutes after eating and lasting up to 45 minutes and partially or completely relieved by lying down. Parenthetically, it may be observed now, in connection with the discussion which will follow, that most if not all of these symptoms are similar to those of mild hypovolemic shock. These symptoms are more common following gastric resection, particularly when the resection has been radical in extent, but they occur following any gastric procedure. Since most of the symptoms are subjective, the incidence of dumping has been reported variously as ranging from 0 to 100 per cent following the same procedure, partly depending on the thoroughness of the follow-up studies. After gastric resection, 4 per cent severe or moderate dumping and an additional 15 per cent slight dumping are reasonable average incidences.

Many theories have been postulated to explain the dumping syndrome since its first description by Hertz (1913) and its first designation by the term "dumping" by Andrews (1920). Among these are the following:

Theory 1. Secondary hypoglycemia following initial hyperglycemia due to rapid passage of food into, and absorption by the jejunum (Gilbert and Dunlop, 1947)

Theory 2. Nervous reflex from rapid overdistention of the jejunum (Hertz, 1913)

Theory 3. Loss of supporting structures holding the gastric remnant in place (Butler and Capper, 1951)

Theory 4. Alimentary hyperglycemic shock (Glaessner, 1940)

Theory 5. Reflex pooling of blood in the splanchnic vascular bed due to rapid entrance of food into the intestine, with secondary decrease in cerebral blood flow (Hoffmann, 1939)

Theory 6. Hypopotassemia (Smith, 1951; Kleiman and Grant, 1954)

Theory 7. Allergy to partially digested food (Zeldis and Klinger, 1952)

Theory 8. Hypovolemic shock due to osmotic inflow into the jejunum of plasma constituents (Roberts, Randall and Farr, 1953)

Theory 9. In 1957, Hinshaw, Joergenson, Davis and Stafford made the interesting observation that there is an *increase* in peripheral blood flow coincident with the onset of symptoms of dumping. (If hypovolemic shock were the only cause, there should be a *decrease* in blood flow.) Later, Hinshaw, Joergenson and Stafford introduced a "dumping test" involving the administration of 150 ml. of 50 per cent glucose rapidly by stomach tube to the sitting patient. Dumping symptoms accompanied by plasma volume fall and increased peripheral blood flow occurred in "positive" tests.

Johnson, Sloop, Jesseph and Harkins (1962) and Jesseph and Harkins (1963) corroborated the association of symptoms with increased peripheral blood flow by digital plethysmography in patients and paw plethysmography in dogs (see Fig. 31-21). These authors also postulated that a serotoninlike substance may be released from the intestinal wall when dumping occurs; therefore, they treated some dumping patients with an antiserotonin agent (cyproheptadine) with generally favorable results.

Theory 1 represents a satisfactory explanation of the late hypoglycemic dumping syndrome (see below) but does not explain the early dumping syndrome now under discussion, in which the symptoms may be at their maximum in the presence of hyperglycemia. Several of the theories agree in postulating that the rapid entrance of food into the jejunum is the initiating factor. Until recently Theory 2, the mechanical distention

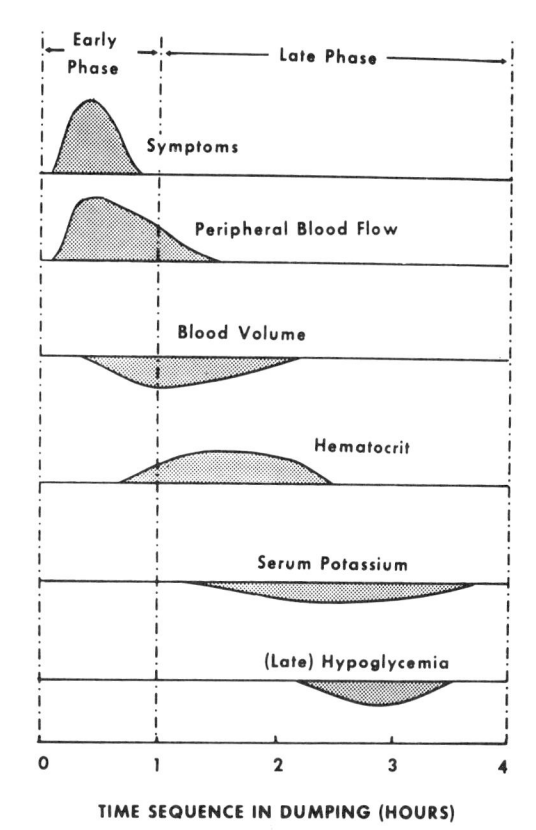

Fig. 31-21. The early symptomatic phase of dumping, beginning almost immediately after meals, is concomitant with the early increase in peripheral blood flow. The later occurring blood volume, glucose and electrolyte changes are consequences of intestinal hyperosmolarity, and not causes of the earlier symptoms. (Johnson, L. P., Sloop, R. D., Jesseph, J. E., and Harkins, H. N.: Serotonin antagonists in experimental and clinical "dumping." Ann. Surg., 156:538)

theory, was the most popular. At present, Theory 8, the shock theory (Fig. 31-22), possesses merit. As seen in Figure 31-23, there is a marked drop in plasma volume coincident with the administration of hypertonic solution sufficient to produce symptoms of dumping. However, Theory 9 seems to be most useful to us at present even though we accept Theory 8 in addition (Fig. 31-24).

Many of the early vasomotor symptoms of this syndrome have been ascribed to the vasoactive polypeptide bradykinin. Macdonald, Webster and Drapanas (1969) found a sig-

858 Stomach and Duodenum

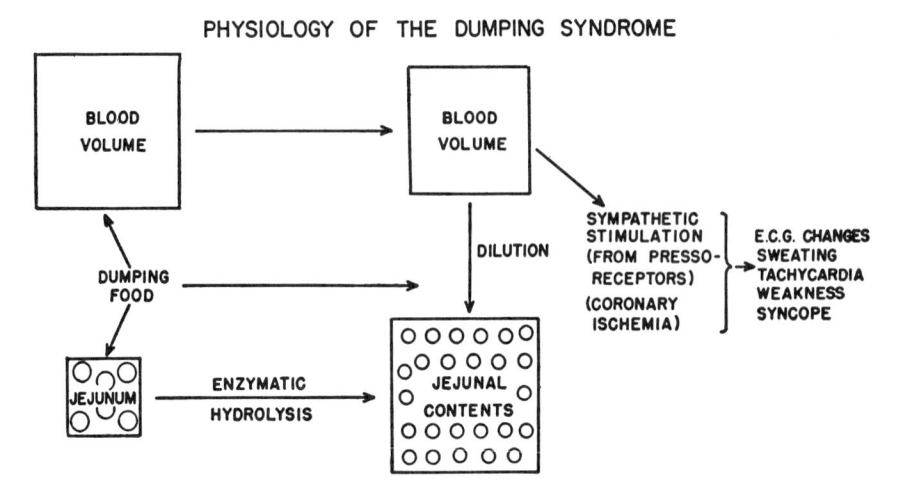

FIG. 31-22. The postprandial-hypovolemia concept of the dumping syndrome. (Walker, J., Roberts, K., Medwid, A., and Randall, H.: Arch. Surg., 71:546)

nificant increase in plasma bradykinin levels in both portal and arterial blood following challenge of intraduodenal hypertonic glucose in the dog. An excellent temporal correlation existed between the onset of dumping and these alterations.

Fisher, Taylor and Cannon (1955), advocates of Theory 2, devised a test for dumping involving the onset of symptoms after drinking of 150 cc. of 50 per cent glucose in water, while seated. In 53 postoperative patients, the incidence of clinical dumping was 36 per cent, and the incidence of test dumping 34 per cent. After either vagotomy and pyloroplasty or the Billroth I resection, the incidence of test dumping was 29 per cent, and after the Billroth II it was 48 per cent.

The treatment of the dumping syndrome is largely medical. Many patients lose their symptoms after several months. Others learn to eat less at one time. In severe cases a "conversion operation" (Billroth II to Bill-

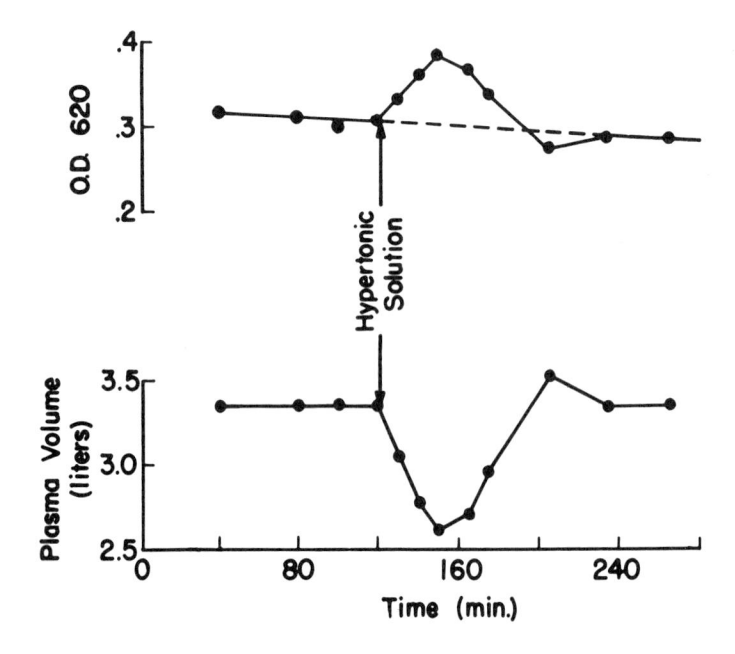

FIG. 31-23. Changes in plasma concentration of the dye (upper half) and in plasma volume (lower half) following the administration of hypertonic solutions to a gastrectomized patient. (Roberts, K., Randall, H., and Farr, H.: S. Forum, 4:302)

FIG. 31-24. Pathophysiology of the dumping syndrome. (From Dr. Gerald W. Peskin)

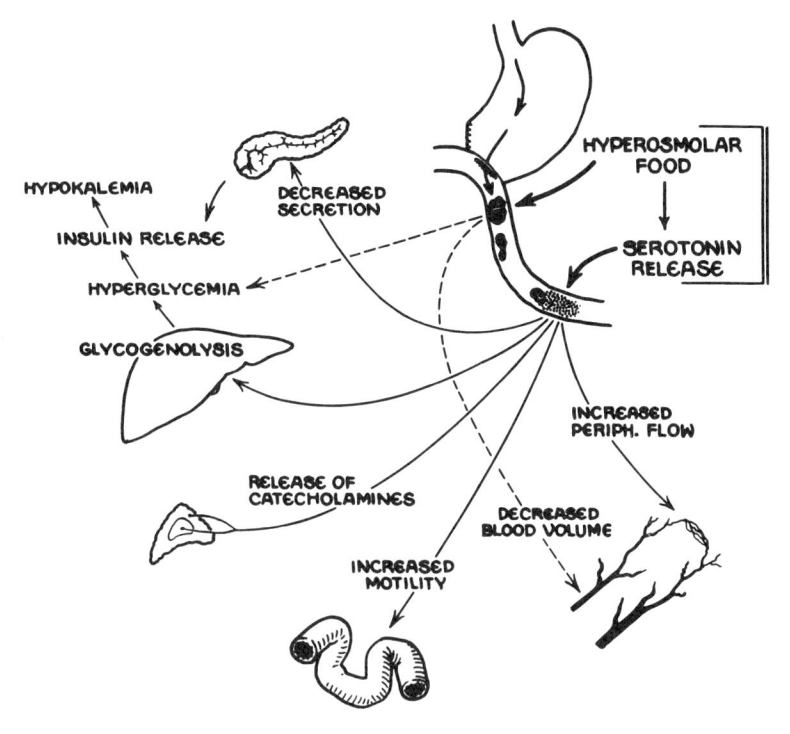

roth I) can be tried, or an attempt can be made to narrow the anastomotic stoma (Woodward, Desser and Gasster, 1955; Zollinger and Williams, 1956), or a 15 cm. jejunal loop —a vagotomy must be added as well—as advocated by Henley (1959) and by Hedenstedt and Heijenskjöld (1961) can be inserted between the lower end of the previously resected stomach and the duodenum.

LATE HYPOGLYCEMIC DUMPING SYNDROME

This syndrome is believed to be due to a secondary hypoglycemic phase occurring 2 to 3 hours after the initial hyperglycemic phase. The treatment involves the use of proteins, avoidance of carbohydrates, and the use of other measures to prevent the initial hyperglycemia. In such patients the syndrome involves an abnormal glucose tolerance curve, but in cases with recurrent ulcer as well, the pancreas should be examined for the presence of islet cell tumors.

POSTGASTRECTOMY ANEMIA

Owren (1952) emphasized that poor absorption of iron following subtotal gastrectomy is related to the rapid emptying of the gastric remnant. Postgastrectomy anemia has been reported in from 0 to 39 per cent of men and from 17 to 82 per cent of women. The fact that menstruating women normally lose comparatively more iron from the body stores than other individuals explains why they comprise such a large proportion of postgastrectomy anemias. Fortunately, this anemia is usually amenable to oral or intravenous iron therapy and causes very little disability to the patient. Because sufficient intrinsic antianemic factor is produced in the residual stomach pouch following subtotal gastrectomy, it is rare to observe a macrocytic anemia in such cases.

The interrelationship between the various types of postgastrectomy syndrome was shown by Wallensten (1955). He found a definite correlation between postcibal symptoms, including dumping, and the existence of anemia and especially of sideropenia. Furthermore, intravenous iron therapy relieved the postcibal symptoms in many of the postoperative patients with sideropenia.

WEIGHT LOSS

A postoperative weight loss, or inability to gain weight in those already underweight, is a frequent complication. In this respect the

TABLE 31-6. FECAL FAT AND NITROGEN LOSSES IN DOGS FOLLOWING VARIOUS TYPES OF GASTRECTOMY*

OPERATION	LOSS IN FECES, PER CENT	
	Fat	Nitrogen
Billroth II	27.7	24.4
Billroth I	10.6	19.3
Segmental	6.4	12.6
Control	4.9	14.9

* Everson, T. C.: Surgery, 36:525-537, 1954.

Billroth I type of anastomosis seems to have an advantage over the Billroth II. In the former, from 8 to 42 per cent of patients are reported as losing weight, and in the latter from 16 to 75 per cent.

Experimental studies indicate that almost any kind of gastric operation decreases fat and protein absorption, but that, in general, this impairment is less with the Billroth I than with the Billroth II. Everson (1954) compared these two procedures along with segmental gastrectomy as shown in Table 31-6. It is seen that the Billroth I was distinctly superior to the II regarding both fat and nitrogen loss but was inferior to the segmental resection. The work of MacLean, Perry, Kelly, Mosser, Mannick and Wangensteen (1954) who performed metabolic studies on patients after various types of gastric resections was referred to in the section on Operative Procedures on the Stomach (see p. 852).

TABLE 31-7. FECAL FAT AND NITROGEN LOSSES IN DOGS FOLLOWING VARIOUS GASTRIC OPERATIONS*

OPERATION	LOSS IN FECES, PER CENT	
	Fat	Nitrogen
1. ⅔ Polya gastrectomy	17.1	26.2
2. Vagotomy, transthoracic	5.0	21.7
3. Vagotomy plus gastroenterostomy	16.2	13.8
4. Gastroenterostomy	5.6	8.4
5. ⅔ Polya gastrectomy + vagotomy	32.1	31.5
Control	5.0	13.6

* From Javid, H.: Surgery, 38:641-651, 1955.

Javid (1955) also performed metabolic studies on 5 series of dogs as shown in Table 31-7.

The treatment of excessive weight loss following gastric operations is partly prophylactic, as shown by Zollinger and Ellison (1954) who advised avoiding extensive resections in patients who have had difficulty in maintaining weight before operation. From the therapeutic standpoint the treatment is largely medical but includes surgical measures to overcome underlying stomal ulcer, etc. If weight loss persists, a conversion, without additional resection, from a Billroth II to a Billroth I may be tried.

The increased tendency to tuberculosis following gastrectomy may well be a secondary phenomenon due to the malnutrition which frequently occurs following gastrectomy (Waugh, 1956). Stammers (1955) and Boman (1956) pointed out the importance of this complication.

MISCELLANEOUS SURGICAL DISEASES OF THE STOMACH AND THE DUODENUM

A number of miscellaneous affections of the stomach and duodenum, including benign tumors and malignant tumors of the stomach other than carcinoma, are listed below alphabetically with brief discussions.

STOMACH

Benign Tumors of the Stomach. The comprehensive review by Palmer (1951) on this subject is outstanding. The relative incidence of reported cases of such tumors collected from the literature is shown in Table 31-8.

This table does not represent the true incidence, if the smallest tumors are to be considered but does signify the relative incidence of those intramural tumors large enough to be reported. Certain tumors such as neuromas, leiomyomas, fibromas, "gastritis cystica," etc., may be very frequent and are often multiple. If all sizes of tumor are included, the leiomyoma probably is the most frequent intramural or nonepithelial tumor of the stomach (q.v.). If both epithelial and nonepithelial tumors of the stomach are considered, the polypoid adenoma is probably the most common benign gastric tumor (Woodruff, 1961).

TABLE 31-8. RELATIVE INCIDENCE OF BENIGN INTRAMURAL TUMORS OF THE STOMACH AS COLLECTED FROM THE WORLD LITERATURE*

TYPE OF BENIGN INTRAMURAL TUMOR OF THE STOMACH	NO. OF REPORTED CASES	PER CENT
1. Aberrant pancreatic tumors	215	13
2. Vascular tumors	93	6
A. Gastric angioma	59	
B. Gastric endothelioma	34	
3. Fatty tumors (lipoma, 95)	103	6
4. Neurogenic tumors	263	16
5. Leiomyomas	610	37
6. Fibromas	289	17
7. Cystic tumors	87	5
Total	1660	100

* From Palmer, E. D.: Medicine, 30:81-181, 1951.

Bezoars and Concretions. Such foreign bodies are similar to the hair balls occurring in long-haired domestic animals. In human beings, certain types of foreign bodies are more common in children or in the mentally deranged, while others occur more generally. A brief classification is as follows:

1. INDIVIDUAL OBJECTS (single or multiple): coins, bobby pins, etc. Most of these will pass into the jejunum if given sufficient time.
2. BEZOARS: Concretions resulting from the repeated ingestion of swallowed material which is unable to pass the pylorus:
   A. *Trichobezoars:* hair balls (more common in female children)
   B. *Phytobezoars:* vegetable fibers (persimmons—"diospyrobezoars,") dried apricots, etc. (more common in male adults)

The diagnosis is based chiefly on the history and roentgen confirmation. Symptoms ranging from poor appetite to those of complications such as obstruction, hemorrhage, or perforation may be present. In the 14 cases of diospyrobezoar reported by O'Leary (1953), most were associated with gastric ulcer, 5 with bleeding, 4 with penetration, and 1 with perforation. In some instances, however, no symptoms may be present, even though the foreign body be large enough to indicate potential danger. Morey, Means and Hirsley (1955) reported a diospyrobezoar removed 8 years after a subtotal gastrectomy.

Treatment of patients with single objects in the stomach includes: close observation, with immediate operation for complications; bulky diet, mineral oil, and removal by gastrotomy if the object does not pass within 96 hours (a longer trial may be given if the object has no sharp edges or points). Multiple foreign bodies and bezoars almost always require laparotomy, gastrotomy and removal. If marked chronic ulceration is present, gastric resection occasionally may be necessary. The method of nonoperative treatment of bezoars results in a mortality of about 60 per cent (De Bakey and Ochsner, 1938-39) as opposed to 6 per cent in the operative cases.

Dreiling and Marshak (1956) pointed out that while ingestion of indigestible foreign bodies is always to be avoided, it is particularly hazardous in patients who already have duodenal obstruction from peptic ulcer. These authors reported 2 cases with chronic duodenal obstruction resulting from the impaction of ingested fruit pits in an area of duodenal stenosis resulting from chronic peptic ulcer.

Boerhaave Syndrome (see "Mallory-Weiss Syndrome"). Literally speaking, the designation "Mallory-Weiss syndrome" refers to massive painless hematemesis from longitudinal lacerations which traverse the gastroesophageal junction. Such lacerations extend into the submucosa but by definition do not rupture through the entire thickness of the wall. The true esophageal rupture syndrome, on the other hand, was described by Boerhaave (1668-1738) in 1724. The Boerhaave syndrome is more serious, leads to mediastinitis, or more rarely peritonitis, and the patient needs urgent thoracotomy to lower the currently reported 65 per cent mortality. Bruno, Grier and Ober (1963) cited 3 cases of Boerhaave's syndrome from their own experience.

Congenital Malformations. Unless the relatively common congenital hypertrophic pyloric stenosis is included, it can be said that congenital malformations of the stomach occur less frequently than in any other part of the intestinal tract. This is of interest in view of the fact that the stomach stands high in the list of organs with acquired abnormalities. Another condition that should not be included with the stomach is congenital diaphragmatic hernia containing the organ. Rare abnormalities include atresia at the cardia or the pylorus, congenital hourglass stomach, and aberrant pancreatic tissue near the pylorus.

Dilatation, Acute, of the Stomach. This condition usually occurs as a postoperative or post-traumatic complication, especially after abdominal operations and when peritonitis is present. It may be present even though the patient vomits frequently (generally in small amounts) and in such instances is similar to the urinary bladder retention present despite repeated small urinations. The upper abdomen is tympanitic and distended. Careful observation as to which part of the abdomen is distended is important, as some cases have been treated with a rectal tube or with enemas. The dangers of acute dilatation are: (1) aspiration of vomitus into the lungs (see "Mendelson's Syndrome"), (2) disruption of operative suture lines and (3) occasionally rupture of the stomach. Continuous or repeated aspirations of the stomach, maintenance of fluid balance, and prevention of aspiration pneumonia by avoidance of narcosis are important in the treatment. In one postoperative patient following partial gastric resection for carcinoma of the stomach, the author saw a measured 5,200 ml. (approximately half air and half liquid) aspirated from the stomach during a 1 hour period 5 days after operation.

Diverticulum of the Stomach. In a series of 1,750 gastroscopic examinations, Tanner (1952) found 5 gastric diverticula, 4 being in the upper stomach. Treatment is medical unless the diverticulum is very large, retains barium more than 24 to 48 hours, or causes symptoms. Inversion is a satisfactory treatment unless the diverticulum is near the cardiac orifice, in which instance it may produce obstruction if inverted. In these cases, as well as in some others, it should be excised. Hillemand, Patel and Lataste (1955) have written a good review of this subject.

Eosinophilic Granuloma of the Stomach. This condition, described by Booher and Grant (1951), includes a granulomatous infiltration of the wall of the stomach and occasionally of the jejunum and the ileum. The patient may have an eosinophilia suggesting an allergic basis, possibly with sensitivity to certain foods. An eosinophilia was present in 2 of the more extensive cases collected by Booher and Grant and in 1 of the 2 reported by McCune, Gusack and Newman (1955), being 34 per cent in the latter. Also the condition may be due either to the traumatic introduction of food particles into the gastric wall or to the necrotizing effect upon the patient's own gastric wall tissues of gastric juice which has extravasated. At present this is not a surgical condition.

Booher and Grant pointed out that the most common manifestation of the disease, on the basis of the 10 cases they collected, is the formation of a poorly circumscribed submucosal nodule which tends to become pedunculated and polypoid and occurs most frequently in the pyloric antrum. In their own case such a tumor intermittently prolapsed through the pylorus.

McCune, Gusack and Newman also reported a case of generalized eosinophilic gastroduodenitis with an eosinophil percentage of 59 per cent.

Gastritis, Acute. Behrend, Katz and Robertson (1954) divided acute gastritis into 5 types: (1) simple (due to alcohol, irritating foods, drugs, or allergens), (2) corrosive (due to strong caustics, acids, or other chemicals), (3) infectious (associated with influenza, pneumonia, scarlet fever, etc.), (4) phlegmonous (due to suppurative infection by streptococci or the colon bacillus), and (5) necrotizing (due to infection by necrotizing bacteria, such as fusiform bacilli and spirochetes, but without occlusion of the major arterial supply to the stomach). Treatment of the simple variety involves avoidance of the causative agent, antacids, bland diet and parasympatholytic drugs. Treatment of the infectious variety includes that of the causative disease, and antacids, diet and drugs as in the simple type. Corrosive, phlegmonous and necrotizing gastritis will be considered separately.

Gastritis, Atrophic. Atrophic gastritis occurs in older people and represents a lessened capacity to secrete acid. Young individuals with high gastric acids and duodenal ulcer, on reaching an older age, may have less acid and develop a gastric ulcer. The relationship between chronic atrophic gastritis and carcinoma of the stomach was studied by Konjetzny (1934, 1938), who believed that the relationship is a close one and that the gastritis is a precancerous lesion with 85 per cent of gastric carcinomas developing on the basis of pre-existing "gastritis hyperplastica atrophicans." Guiss and Stewart (1943) opposed this theory, but more recent studies have revived it (see p. 844).

Gastritis, Chronic. A chronic condition possibly representing acute hypertrophic gastritis in a late stage. Postoperative gastritis is a variety of chronic gastritis and follows most stomach operations. Chronic gastritis is said to occur in 6 per cent of the general population.

Gastritis, Corrosive. In some instances ingested caustic agents may produce a sufficiently localized lesion that recovery occurs, yet scarring with atrophy and achlorhydria results. If pyloric obstruction is present, gastrojejunostomy or partial gastric resection may be advisable.

Gastritis, Emphysematous. A variant of phlegmonous gastritis (Han, Collins and Petrany, 1965).

Gastritis, Hypertrophic. This condition is said to occur in 2 to 17 per cent of gastroscopic examinations and to comprise 18 to 57 per cent of cases of chronic gastritis. It does not occur in children and in adolescents, the majority of the cases being in the 4th to the 6th decades. The cause of the condition is not known. According to Fieber (1955), the cardinal symptoms are pain (74%), weight loss (60%), vomiting (42%), and hemorrhage (20%). The average duration of these symptoms is 2 years. The term "hypertrophic gastritis," as used by Fieber, in reality combines the 2 types of Menetrier, *polyadenomes polypeux*, a hyperplastic variety, and *polyadenomes en nappe*, a hypertrophic variety. The classification of the hypertrophic gastritides and polyps is still uncertain.

Gastritis, Necrotizing. This lesion is one of the 5 types of acute gastritis and usually is due to infection with fusiform bacilli and spirochetes from severe mouth infections. The necrosis results from the infection, despite the fact that the major arterial vessels to the stomach are not occluded. In the case reported by Behrend, Katz and Robertson (1954) death resulted despite antibiotic therapy and drainage of the peritoneal cavity.

Gastritis, Phlegmonous (Gastric Phlegmon). This rare lesion may be diffuse or localized. It includes a suppurative involvement, usually by streptococci, of the submucosa with the occasional occurrence of fibrin and pus on the outside of the stomach. Males are afflicted 3 times as often as females, and over 80 per cent of patients are between 30 and 60 years of age. Most patients are seen on charity wards, and many are excessive users of alcohol. The condition is somewhat related to acute necrotizing gastritis but does not involve the mucosa. Sachs and Angrist (1945) compared phlegmonous gastritis with phlegmonous cholecystitis. Three of their 4 cases had no break in the mucosa of the stomach in the form of an ulcer, a neoplasm or an operative wound. They concluded that phlegmonous gastritis is a "manifestation of sepsis with localization in the stomach wall rather than a lesion following local invasion from the lumen." Complications include localized and subdiaphragmatic abscess and the results of general pyemia. Treatment involves drainage of secondary abscesses, maintenance of nutrition by jejunostomy feedings and adequate vitamin C intake (Cutler and Harrison, 1940), and antibiotics.

Gastritis, Postoperative. Palmer (1953) reported that many instances of postoperative gastritis represent a continuation of a preoperative process; however, 22 of 45 postoperative patients, all with normal preoperative gastric mucosa, showed postoperative gastritis. Such gastritis, once it had developed, tended to remain static. It occurred following various types of gastric operations.

Gastromalacia. This condition has been defined as an acute, erosive phenomenon, manifested by a gelatinous softening of a poorly defined area of stomach wall, with little or no inflammatory response (King and Reganis, 1953). There may be multiple small mucosal ulcerations, or large areas of dissolution of the entire stomach wall. The condition is related to Cushing's ulcer and may be due to an interference with the central autonomic control mechanism (see section on Cushing's ulcer). Bell, Thomas and Skillicorn (1956) reported the first instance of recovery after repair of a 5-inch-long gastric perforation in a case of gastromalacia. The association with poliomyelitis in this patient is of interest, and these authors pointed out that in their hospital in 1953 there were 8 bulbospinal deaths from poliomyelitis. Five of these 8 had antemortem perforations of the upper gastrointestinal tract (1 esophagus, 3 stomach, and 1 of the duodenum). Treatment will succeed only if applied promptly because of the large size of the perforations and large amount of leakage into the peritoneal cavity within a short time. If the perforation is low in the stomach, gastric resection may be done, but in Bell, Thomas, and Skillicorn's case, the necrotic area on the anterior wall was débrided longitudinally and closed longitudinally.

Glomus Tumor of the Stomach. These tumors, related to the hemangiopericytomas, are rare benign tumors similar to glomus tumors found elsewhere. Allen and Dahlin (1954) reported 2 such tumors.

Leiomyoma of the Stomach. This tumor probably is not only a very common benign tumor but also the most common subepithelial tumor of the stomach. Meissner (1944) found an incidence of 46 per cent in 50 necropsies. Many of these subepithelial tumors are small, and they rarely grow to a size that proves to be of clinical significance. As pointed out by Appleby (1950), those large enough to produce symptoms usually produce ulceration and hemorrhage, the latter sometimes sudden and severe. Many are discovered inadvertently on roentgen examination. Treatment includes removal, even when symptoms are absent, because the exact nature of the tumor is uncertain until examined microscopically. If frozen sections reveal benign tissue, localized removal is permissible; if not, the treatment is as for leiomyosarcoma.

Leiomyoma of the duodenum is much rarer, but Campbell and Young (1954) collected 30 cases, including 2 of their own.

Lymphoid Tumors of the Stomach. Such tumors comprise about two thirds of all sarcomas of the stomach (q.v.) and are, next to carcinoma, the most common gastric malignancy. In turn, about half the lymphoid tumors are true lymphosarcomas, the remainder being Hodgkin's disease, reticulum cell sarcoma and malignant lymphoma. In the present discussion, the lymphoid tumors are grouped together under the general term of lymphosarcoma. Approximately 2 per cent of malignant tumors of the stomach are in the group of lymphosarcomas. The average age is about the same as for carcinoma, and there is a preponderance of males of from 2:1 to 6:1. Since these tumors do not involve the gastric mucosa as much as does carcinoma, hemorrhage and secondary anemia are less common.

The life expectancy of patients with lymphosarcoma of the stomach is appreciably greater than for those with carcinoma. Surgical excision involving either subtotal or total gastrectomy, possibly combined with roentgen therapy, offers the best chance for prolonged survival. Snoddy (1952) recommended that roentgen therapy be used only when lymph nodes are involved and only postoperatively. He re-emphasized 2 important points: "Certainly some cases of lymphosarcoma of the stomach represent a solitary lesion which can be cured if adequately removed. Lymph node involvement reduces the chances of cure, but does not preclude the possibility of a 5-year survival." (See also Welborn, 1965.)

Mallory-Weiss Syndrome. This condition was first reported by Mallory and Weiss in 1929. It results from a tear across the gastroesophageal junction, often caused by vomiting or similar stress. The tear is by definition only through the submucosa, and a perforation is not present (see "Boerhaave syndrome"). Massive painless hematemesis is the presenting syndrome. This syndrome is undoubtedly more common than formerly realized (Dobbins, 1963).

Mendelson's Syndrome. This syndrome is not strictly a gastric condition per se, but most certainly it is a potential danger in operations on the stomach. The syndrome, as originally described by Mendelson (1946), involved an acid pneumonitis due to vomiting of acid gastric juice during obstetric anesthesia. As currently used, the term denotes such aspiration of acid vomitus during any anesthesia or from the complications of peptic ulcer from which such aspiration is especially apt to occur; *viz.* pyloric obstruction and massive hemorrhage. Mendelson's original report included studies on the instillation of fluid into the lungs of rabbits. One-tenth normal HCl or unneutralized liquid gastric juice produced the specific serous pneumonitis syndrome, while normal saline solution or neutralized liquid gastric juice was relatively innocuous. Since the acid output in duodenal ulcer is especially high, the surgeon dealing with this condition should be cognizant of Mendelson's syndrome.

Perforation, Traumatic, of the Stomach. Such perforation of the stomach, in the absence of other severe injury, is relatively rare. It can occur from overdistention (beer drinkers), accidental perforation from a gastroscope, and from stab and gunshot wounds. Perforation of the stomach should be considered not only in cases of upper abdominal but also in instances of lower thoracic trauma. The symptoms and signs include those of perforation of peptic ulcer, plus those of associated hemorrhage and other injury. Treatment by simple suture is usually adequate, although partial resection may be necessary.

Rupture of the stomach in the newborn infant is a special condition which, while rare, deserves more attention so that prompter treatment may be instituted. Vargas, Levin and Santulli (1955) collected 55 cases and added 11 of their own. In 30 cases in the over-all series, surgical repair had been attempted with 11 survivals (37%). No patients survived without operation. Gastric ulcer, muscle defects, sepsis and trauma were factors in the etiology. Prompt surgical repair offers the only hope for survival. Neonatal rupture of the stomach is possibly more common than is generally realized (Arrants, Brogdon and Jurkiewiecz, 1965).

Polyadenoma en Nappe (*Polyadénomes en Nappe* of Menetrier, 1888, giant hypertrophic gastritis, localized hypertrophic gastritis). This condition, first described by Menetrier (1888) and later clarified by Berne and Gibson (1949), is a rare but interesting condition. It is most likely a form of diffuse gastric neoplasm which may be an indication for subtotal or even total gastrectomy.

Polyps of the Stomach (*Polyadénomes Polypeux* of Menetrier, 1888; gastric polyps). Polyps may be associated with similar lesions elsewhere in the intestinal tract or even in the urinary bladder. They are usually single but may be multiple and may undergo malignant change. Unlike polyps of the colon, there does not seem to be a hereditary factor, although they may be congenital or inflammatory. The incidence varies from 0.3 to 0.8 per cent in autopsy examinations and 1.6 per cent in gastroscopic examinations (Yarnis, Marshak and Friedman, 1952). Bleeding is a significant symptom. Achlorhydria and atrophic gastritis are quite common. Coincident hypertrophic gastritis is seldom present.

Treatment should include resection of the polyps with the underlying wall, at least down to the muscle, if the polyps are not too numerous. In localized cases of diffuse polyposis subtotal gastrectomy should be performed. Instances of diffuse polyposis which involve the entire stomach present a serious problem. There are no current conclusive data, such as there are for multiple polyposis of the colon, to help the surgeon reach the important decision as to whether or not he should do a total gastrectomy. Consequently, this serious decision must be reached separately in each individual case. If polyps are left behind, careful postoperative observations, including gastroscopy at frequent intervals, are mandatory.

Prolapse of Gastric Mucosa Through the Pylorus. Such prolapse was first described by Schmieden (1911). While it is agreed that severe degrees of prolapse will produce symptoms, there is some argument as to whether minor degrees of prolapse are of clinical significance. Peptic ulcer, polyps, and malignant change in polypoid gastric mucosa must be differentiated. Feldman, Morrison and Myers (1952) in a thorough review of the subject reported that the incidence of the condition is 1.8 per cent of patients subjected to upper gastrointestinal roentgen studies. However, they concluded that "prolapse of the gastric mucosa is ordinarily a medical problem and in only the severe intractable cases and those with complications is surgery indicated." Medical treatment includes bland diet and particularly antispasmodics. If obstruction, hematemesis, severe pain or other complications exist, operation is indicated and includes gastrotomy, followed by removal of the prolapsed mucosa, or gastrojejunostomy, or often preferably gastric resection.

Peutz-Jeghers Syndrome. This condition includes the presence of pigmented spots on the lips with polyps of the intestinal tract, including the stomach. The first descriptions were by Peutz (1921) in Holland and by Jeghers (1944) in this country.

Sarcoidosis. Gastric sarcoidosis is rare. In most of the reported cases this condition is a part of the generalized disease. Pearce and Ehrlich (1955) pointed out that the gastric lesions of sarcoidosis may ulcerate secondarily (as in carcinoma), necessitating gastric resection for the complication of the ulcer.

Sarcoma of the Stomach. Such tumors, while rare, are more common than is generally realized. There are 2 chief classes of sarcoma: the leiomyosarcomas (see Rosenberg, 1964) (possibly related to the benign leiomyomas) comprising about 1 per cent of all gastric malignancies, and the lymphomas (mainly lymphoid tumors including lymphosarcoma [q.v.]) but also including some cases of Hodgkin's disease, comprising about 2 per cent of gastric malignancies. Eker and Efskind (1956) reported 21 personal cases of another rare malignant gastric tumor, namely, hemangio-endothelioma (1.2% of their resected malignant tumors). Thus, the total incidence of the sarcomas is about 3 per cent (Marshall, 1955). Usually, the diagnosis is not made before operation.

Treatment includes gastric resection. Postoperative roentgen treatment is not advised for leiomyosarcoma but is to be considered for lymphoma (q.v.). Marshall and Meissner (1950) reported that the over-all 5-year arrest rate in 41 cases of sarcoma of the stomach was 44 per cent as opposed to 27 per cent for carcinoma of the stomach. In the leiomyosarcoma group alone, the 5-year arrest rate is even better, 67 per cent.

Syphilis of the Stomach. This tertiary lesion, while never common, is becoming rarer. Males are affected about twice as frequently as females. Patients with gastric syphilis are apt to be 20 to 40 years of age. The onset of symptoms occurs on an average of 10 years after the primary lesion. The symptoms include epigastric pain, fullness and heaviness. The pain resembles that of peptic ulcer except that it lacks the periodicity and the relief by food of the latter. Pyloric obstruction, vomiting and emaciation may be present. The most common pathologic lesion is a broad, plaquelike, spongy thickening of the gastric wall, sometimes with superficial ulceration of the mucosa. The *sine qua non* of gastric syphilis is the importance of differentiating it from gastric cancer *before* definitive operation. The occurrence in a young age group, a positive serology, and the atypical nature of the lesion, with the patient's emaciation being out of proportion to the anemia, and the size of the lesion to the general condition of the patient, all tend to indicate the presence of syphilis. A therapeutic test of antisyphilitic therapy may be helpful in those cases in which obstruction is not present.

Treatment includes a trial at medical therapy and the treatment of obstruction. Since syphilitic proliferative lesions tend to heal by cicatrization, gastroenterostomy is often necessary. Occasionally, gastric resection is required.

Tuberculosis of the Stomach. This rare condition usually is associated with advanced generalized tuberculosis of the intestinal tract in the presence of open pulmonary tuberculosis. Ulceration, usually on the posterior wall of the stomach near the pylorus, occasionally may reveal visible tubercles. Ulcers of the duodenum may lead to stenosis. Achlorhydria, palpable tumor and gastrointestinal hemorrhage are common. Differential diagnosis, particularly on the basis of the roentgenographic studies, should rule out ulcer or carcinoma. Treatment includes a high protein diet, PAS, streptomycin, isoniazid and occasionally, if obstruction exists or the differentiation from carcinoma cannot be made, gastrojejunostomy or partial gastrectomy.

Volvulus of the Stomach. This condition, first described by Berti in 1866, probably is more frequent than is generally recognized. In all cases of upper abdominal symptoms, particularly when acute, and when a definite diagnosis cannot be made, volvulus should be considered, especially if the Borchardt-Lenormont triad of symptoms is present. This triad includes: (1) strong efforts to vomit without result, circumscribed epigastric pain, and impossibility of passing a stomach tube. Because of the excellent blood supply of the stomach, rotation up to 180° usually is tolerated without strangulation, often for prolonged periods of time, but more severe cases require urgent surgical reduction. The von Haberer (1912) classification of gastric volvulus is as follows:

TYPE A. MESENTERO-AXIAL. Rotation of the stomach from right to left or left to right about the long axis of the gastrohepatic omentum. In the series of Gottlieb and associates, all 3 cases of this type were idiopathic and also infracolic.

TYPE B. ORGANO-AXIAL. Rotation of the stomach upward around the long axis of the stomach, i.e., around the coronal plane. This is usually supracolic but rarely may be infracolic. In the series of 20 cases, reported by Gottlieb, Lefferts and Beranbaum (1954), 17 were of this type; and of these, 16 were supracolic. The organo-axial can be further divided into idiopathic and secondary, there being 6 and 11 cases, respectively, in the series cited. Among the causative factors in secondary organo-axial volvulus were eventration of the diaphragm (3), parahiatal hernia (3), ulcer or adhesions (3), diverticulitis coli (1), and carcinoma of the pancreas (1). (See Fig. 31-25.)

Because of the relationship of the colon, roentgen studies should include examination of this organ. Differentiation from "cascade stomach," a spastic deformity, is based on the following points: (1) one fluid level in cascade stomach, 2 in volvulus; (2) the greater curvature is uppermost only in volvulus; (3) only in volvulus does the greater curvature form a convex curve continuous with the duodenum; and (4) in volvulus the cardia is apt to have a low position due to the rotation, whereas in cascade stomach it is in its normal position.

In general, the more common organo-axial type of volvulus of the stomach is seen in connection with parahiatal diaphragmatic hernia (see Chap. 42, Hernia), the so-called "upside-down stomach" being popularly associated with such a hernia. Treatment of chronic volvulus with symptoms includes removal of the causative factor and repositioning of the stomach. If symptoms are not present, the decision will rest upon the size and the type of volvulus present. If acute symptoms are present, immediate operation is mandatory as advocated by Sawyer, Hammer and Fenton (1956).

Wounds of the Stomach. (See perforation, traumatic.)

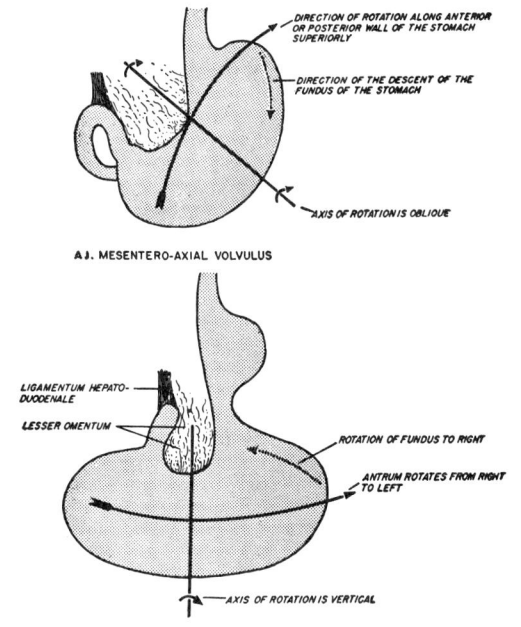

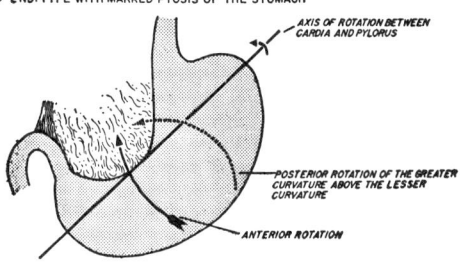

Fig. 31-25. Different types of volvulus of the stomach according to the von Haberer classification. (A-1) Mesentero-axial volvulus with stomach in usual position. (A-2) Mesentero-axial volvulus with marked ptosis of the stomach. (B) Organo-axial volvulus with either anterior or posterior rotation of the greater curvature above the lesser curvature. (Gottlieb, C., Lefferts, D., and Beranbaum, S.: Am. J. Roentgenol., 72:611)

DUODENUM

Arteriomesenteric Duodenal Compression Syndrome. First described by Rokitansky in 1849, this condition was elucidated clinically by Wilkie in 1921, then by Barling (1923), and finally clarified by Jones, Carter, Smith and Joergenson in 1960. The symptoms usually are considered due to obstruction of the third portion of the duodenum where it passes around the superior mesenteric vessels. Because of the large volume of secretion of gastric juice, bile and pancreatic juice, vomiting is profuse and, unlike cases of pyloric obstruction, always contains bile. The head-down prone position may give relief, but if vomiting persists, a short-circuiting duodenojejunostomy should be performed as advised by Jones, Carter, Smith and Joergenson (1960). Annular pancreas may produce a similar duodenal obstruction with indications for relief by duodenojejunostomy (Brant and Hamlin, 1960).

Carcinoma of the Duodenum. Primary carcinoma of this organ is rare (about 0.04% of all autopsies). The condition was first described by Hamburger (1746). In 1932, Mateer and Hartman correlated the clinical and pathologic findings. The distribution of duodenal carcinoma is as follows: suprapapillary, 23 per cent; peripapillary, 59 per cent, and infrapapillary, 18 per cent. Brenner and Brown (1955) pointed out that while the older literature included ampullary carcinoma with duodenal carcinoma, they believe that the two are separate entities as regards mucosal origin (biliary versus duodenal) and clinical picture. Symptoms of duodenal carcinoma are those of high intestinal obstruction, hemorrhage, biliary obstruction and peptic ulcer-type symptoms. Roentgen examination reveals deformity or obstruction, but usually it is only at operation that the final diagnosis can be made. Metastases are frequent, and the results of operation are poor, resulting in only about 5 per cent 5-year arrests in those cases treated by resection. Burgerman, Baggenstoss and Cain (1956) recently reported 31 cases of primary malignant neoplasms of the duodenum, excluding those of the papilla of Vater. Barclay and Kent (1956) reported 8 similar cases. Sarcoma of the duodenum, while rare, is almost as frequent as carcinoma. Benign tumors of the duodenum are also rare and include polyps, lipomas and heterotopic pancreas.

Cyst (Enterogenous) of the Duodenum. Enterogenous cysts of the duodenum are rare, 22 cases having been collected from the literature by Polson and Isaac (1953). Most of these cysts are believed to arise from a diverticulum with a constricted opening or from congenital abnormalities. Obstruction of the duodenum is a common symptom and requires excision.

Diverticula of the Duodenum. Two important points of discussion exist concerning such diverticula, namely, as to their true incidence and as to the proportion of them that should be treated surgically. Ackermann (1943) stated that the true incidence is far higher than the reported one, and that roentgenographic studies reveal only a small proportion of such abnormalities. Now it is recognized that primary duodenal diverticula of the pulsion type, as distinguished from diverticula secondary to traction of scarring, are found in 1 to 2 per cent of roentgenographic surveys and in 10 to 14 per cent of careful duodenal dissections. The true diverticula must be differentiated from the false or traction or scar diverticula of the upper duodenum, which most often evidence themselves by the clover-leaf deformity associated with duodenal ulcer.

True diverticula usually occur in the second portion of the duodenum, often are in the posterior wall in close association with the pancreas and the ampulla of Vater, and may produce diverticulitis. Blegen, Swanberg and Cox (1952) reported a case in which the common duct emptied into the diverticulum, which also was associated with a peptic ulcer, necessitating partial gastric resection with removal of the first and the second portions of the duodenum and reimplantation of the common duct.

If a diverticulum is asymptomatic, usually it should be left alone, although the rule of Zinninger (1953) may be applicable. This author stated that in addition to the rare cases of duodenal diverticula which cause symptoms, "in those instances in which the diverticulum is large and retains barium for 24 hours or longer and in which no other cause for the patient's symptoms can be demonstrated, operation for removal of the diverticulum is indicated." Invagination of this diverticulum into the duodenal lumen as advocated by Ferguson and Cameron (1947) may be advisable in some cases. If resection is elected, extreme care must be taken not to injure the closely associated biliary and pancreatic ducts and the duodenal blood supply.

In a series of 525 patients with a clinical diagnosis of duodenal diverticulum, 30 underwent surgical exploration of the upper abdomen as reported by Waugh and Johnston (1955). In only 8 of the explorations was the presence of the diverticula the basic reason for operation. Diverticulectomy was performed in 17 of these patients, and inversion of the diverticula in 2. Fewer than half of the surgically treated patients with adequate follow-up data were found to have relief of their symptoms. These authors concluded that, "Operative intervention is indicated in less than 1 to 2 per cent of the cases of duodenal diverticula noted on roentgenograms."

Duodenitis. Judd (1921) pointed out that in some patients thought to have a duodenal ulcer there is only a congestion and stippling of the serosal surface, a narrowing of the duodenum without scarring, or minute ersions of the mucosa or any of these 3 signs in combination. Such cases are thought to be chronic duodenitis, but an acute variety also has been described. The author does not dispute the existence of acute or chronic duodenitis but does believe that the majority actually represent various stages of the healing of a duodenal ulcer. In the past, most gastric resections have been performed by closing the duodenum over a clamp so that many surgeons do not see into the duodenum during this operation. When the open method of duodenal closure, or anastomosis, is used direct vision demonstrates small ulcer scars that otherwise might be missed.

Fistulas of the duodenum are divided into the external and the internal varieties:

(1) *External duodenal fistulas.* These again may be subdivided into 2 types: (A) the end type, in which there is leakage of *duodenal* contents from the duodenal stump following the different varieties of Billroth II gastric resections, and (B) the lateral type, in which there is no interruption of continuity of the duodenum, occurring usually after duodenotomy for exposure of the ampulla of Vater or other similar operations. Craighead and St. Raymond (1954) reported a 66 per cent mortality in the end type and only 40 per cent in the lateral type. Other authors have reported that the end type is less dangerous, probably because the peristalsis goes the other way in most of them. The average onset of the 2 types in Craighead and St. Raymond's series was 8 and 5 days respectively, after operation. The lateral type of fistula can be closed by suturing a loop of jejunum over the defect by the method of Jones and Joergenson (1963), and Jones et al., 1964.

The end type of fistula should be treated prophylactically by utilizing a proper closure of the duodenal stump (see Fig. 31-19). As soon as a "blowout" is suspected, if an external fistula is not already present, the abdomen should be opened to permit reclosure of the stump, or secondary catheter drainage of the duodenum, or drainage of the perforation site. The first of these 3 measures is not often feasible; hence one of the latter 2 usually must be adopted. In all cases of external duodenal fistula, whether end or lateral, the following measures should be adopted to keep the patient in as good general condition as possible. These measures include: (A) adequate fluids, electrolytes (including potassium), blood, protein and vitamins, (B) sump drainage and (C) jejunostomy feedings through a tube inserted either orally or abdominally. The fistula usually closes spontaneously in 3 weeks if the patient survives the 1st week and if there is no obstruction distal to the perforation.

2. Internal duodenal fistula. Such a fistula most commonly results from ulceration of a single large gallstone from the gallbladder into the duodenum. Cowley and Harkins (1943) reported that only 3 (12%) of the 25 cases of perforation of the gallbladder seen at the Henry Ford Hospital involved formation of a fistula into the bowel and, in turn, only 1 of these was into the duodenum. Such a fistula into the bowel is termed Class I perforation of the gallbladder according to the classification of Niemeier (1934). In such instances, of course, if the gallstone has not already passed the rectum, it may herald its presence by being impacted at the ileocecal valve with production of the classical syndrome of gallstone ileus (see Chap. 32, Biliary Tract).

Duodenal ulcer occasionally may ulcerate into the biliary tract—usually the gallbladder —or into the colon, producing an internal fistula.

Treatment includes cholecystectomy, if this organ is involved, with closure of the fistula and removal of the gallstone if still present.

Regional Enteritis Involving the Duodenum. The rare cephalad involvement of the small intestine by this disease has recently been emphasized. Segal and Serbin (1956) reported a case of their own and referred to 18 additional cases in the literature. Berk (1956) reported 3 cases. Treatment is more difficult than lower down in the small intestine because of the difficulties involved in either sidetracking or resection.

Traumatic Perforation of the Duodenum. A special type of perforation, and the most common perforation of the duodenum, is that of the *retroperitoneal duodenum*. Such a perforation usually is the result of closed trauma—although it can result from penetrating wounds—and occurs at any point which is well fixed; i.e., the retroperitoneal duodenum, the jejunum where it crosses the spinal column just distal to the ligament of Treitz, and the lower ileum where it crosses the spine near its fixation to the cecum. Such fixed regions of the bowel are especially susceptible to transection or perforation because the organ cannot move in relation to the pressure exerted by the traumatic force. Such force may result from a steering wheel of an automobile. Diagnosis may be difficult because: (1) intestinal perforation may not have been considered in the list of possibilities; and (2) certain regions especially prone to perforate (retroperitoneal portion of the duodenum, Cottrell, 1954, and proximal jejunum) are in "blind" areas not readily visualized on exploration. (See also: Fistula, duodenal.) The diagnostic importance of retroperitoneal gas bubbles in the roentgenograms was emphasized by Rothchild and Hinshaw (1956). Treatment is surgical and is urgent.

Wilkie's Syndrome (see Arteriomesenteric Duodenal Compression Syndrome).

REFERENCES

Ackermann, W.: Diverticula and variations of the duodenum. Ann. Surg., 117:403-413, 1943.

Aird, I., Bentall, H. H., Mehigan, J. A., and Roberts, J. A. F.: The blood groups in relation to peptic ulceration and carcinoma of colon, rectum, breast, and bronchus: an association between the ABO groups and peptic ulceration. Brit. M.J., 2:315-321, 1954.

Albright, H. L., and Kerr, R. C.: Primary hyperplasia of parathyroid glands: report of a case with coincident duodenal ulcer. J.A.M.A., 148:1218-1221, 1952.

Allen, J. G., and Oberhelman, H. A.: The problem of the bleeding peptic ulcer. Surgery, 37:1019-1028, 1955.

Allen, R. A., and Dahlin, D. C.: Glomus tumor of the stomach. Proc. Mayo Clin., 29:429-436, 1954.

Allison, P. R.: Reflux esophagitis, sliding hiatal hernia, and the anatomy of repair. Surg., Gynec., Obstet., 92:419-431, 1951.

Allison, P. R., and Johnstone, A. S.: The oesophagus lined with gastric mucous membrane. Thorax, 8:87-101, 1953.

Amberg, J. R., Ellison, E. H., Wilson, S. D., and Zboralske, F. F.: Roentgenographic observations in the Zollinger-Ellison syndrome. J.A.M.A., 190:185-187, 1964.

Amberg, J. R., and Rigler, L. G.: Results of surgery in carcinoma of the stomach discovered by periodic roentgen examination. Surgery, 39:760-775, 1956.

Andrews, E. W.: "Dumping stomach" and other results of gastrojejunostomy: operative cure by disconnecting old stoma. S. Clin. Chicago, 4:883-892, 1920.

Appleby, L. H.: The outlook for patients with leiomyomas of the stomach. J. Int. Coll. Surg., 14:512-516, 1950.

Arhelger, S. W., Lober, P. H., and Wangensteen, O. H.: Dissection of the hepatic pedicle and retropancreaticoduodenal areas for cancer of stomach. Surgery, 38:675-678, 1955.

Arrants, J. E., Brogdon, B. G., and Jurkiewicz, M. J.: Neonatal gastric perforation. Am. Surg., 31:96-101, 1965.

Barclay, A. E.: Micro-arteriography. Brit. J. Radiol., 20:394-404, 1947.

Barclay, T. H. C., and Kent, H. P.: Primary carcinoma of the duodenum. Gastroenterology, 30:432-446, 1956.

Barling, S.: Chronic duodenal ileus. Brit. J. Surg., 10:501-508, 1923.

Barlow, T. E., Bentley, F. H., and Walder, D. N.: Arteries, veins, and arteriovenous anastomoses in the human stomach. Surg., Gynec., Obstet., 93:657-671, 1951.

Barrett, N. R.: Chronic peptic ulcer of the oesophagus and "oesophagitis." Brit. J. Surg., 38:175-182, 1950.

———: Hiatus hernia: a review of some controversial points. Brit. J. Surg., 42:231-244, 1954.

Bauer, K. H.: Über das Wesen der Magenstrasse. Arch. klin. Chir., 124:565-629, 1923.

Baum, S., Nusbaum, M., Blakemore, W. S., and Finkelstein, A. K.: The preoperative radiographic demonstration of intra-abdominal bleeding from undetermined sites by percutaneous selective celiac and superior mesenteric arteriography. Surgery, 58:797-805, 1965.

Beal, J. M., and Hill, M. R., Jr.: An evaluation of the surgical treatment of carcinoma of the stomach. Surg., Gynec., Obstet., 102:271-278, 1956.

Behrend, A., Katz, A. B., and Robertson, J. W.: Acute necrotizing gastritis. Arch. Surg., 69:18-24, 1954.

Bell, L. G., Thomas, E. E., Jr., and Skillicorn, S. A.: Gastromalacia: a review and report of one case with recovery. Ann. Surg., 143:106-111, 1956.

Bentley, F. H., and Barlow, T. E.: Stomach: vascular supply of in relation to gastric ulcer. *In* Surgical Procress, 1952. London, Butterworth, 1953.

Beranbaum, S. L., Gottlieb, C., and Lefferts, D.: Gastric volvulus. III. Secondary gastric volvulus. Am. J. Roentgenol., 72:625-638, 1954.

Berk, M.: Regional enteritis involving the duodenum. Gastroenterology, 30:508-516, 1956.

Berkson, J., Walters, W., Gray, H. K., and Priestley, J. T.: Mortality and survival in cancer of the stomach: a statistical summary of the experience of the Mayo Clinic. Proc. Mayo Clin., 27:137-151, 1952.

Berman, E. J., Schneider, A., and Potts, W. J.:

Importance of gastric mucosa in Meckel's diverticulum. J.A.M.A., 156:6-7, 1954.
Berne, C. J., and Freedman, M. A.: Local recurrence following subtotal gastrectomy for carcinoma. Am. J. Surg., 82:5-7, 1951.
Berne, C. J., and Gibson, W. R.: Giant hypertrophic gastritis. West. J. Surg., 57:388-391, 1949.
Berti (1866): Cited by Gottlieb, Lefferts, and Beranbaum (see reference below), 1954.
Blegen, H. M., Swanberg, A. V., and Cox, W. B.: Entrance of common bile duct into duodenal diverticulum: report of a case corrected by surgery. J.A.M.A., 148:195-197, 1952.
Blumenthal, I. S.: Social cost of peptic ulcer. Paper presented at Conference on Digestive Disease as a National Problem, Bethesda, Md., February 5-7, 1967.
Boerhaave, H.: Atrocis, nec descripti pruis, morbi historia: Secundum medicae artis leges conscripta, Lugduni Batavoum, Boutestiana, 1724 (cited in Editorial: The Boerhaave syndrome. J.A.M.A., 187:57, 1964).
Bogardus, G. M., and Gustafson, I. J.: Gastroduodenal ulceration complicating other diseases. Surgery, 39:222-229, 1956.
Boman, K.: Tuberculosis occurring after gastrectomy. Acta chir. scandinav., 110:451-457, 1956.
Bombeck, C. T., Aoki, T., and Nyhus, L. M.: Anatomic etiology and operative treatment of peptic esophagitis. An experimental study. Ann. Surg., 165:752-764, 1967.
Booher, R. J., and Grant, R. N.: Eosinophilic granuloma of the stomach and small intestine. Surgery, 30:388-397, 1951.
Book, D. T., Chinn, A. B., and Beams, A. J.: Studies on pepsin secretion. II. Effect of vagal resection for duodenal ulcer. Gastroenterology, 20:458-463, 1952.
Bosher, L. H., Jr., and Taylor, F. H.: Heterotopic gastric mucosa in the esophagus with ulcer and stricture formation. J. Thoracic Surg., 21:306-312, 1951.
Boyce, F. F.: Carcinoma of stomach; comparison of 3 series of surgical cases in large general hospital. J.A.M.A., 151:15-20, 1953.
Boyden, A. M.: Radical gastrectomy for benign gastric ulcer. Surg., Gynec., Obstet., 97:1-8, 1953.
Brackney, E. L., Campbell, G. S., and Wangensteen, O. H.: Role of antral exclusion in development of peptic stomal ulcer. Proc. Soc. Exp. Biol. Med., 86:273-277, 1954.
Brackney, E. L., Thal, A. P., and Wangensteen, O. H.: Role of duodenum in the control of gastric secretion. Proc. Soc. Exp. Biol. Med., 88:302-306, 1955.
Brandborg, L. L., MacDonald, W. C., Rubin, C. E., and Gottlieb, S.: Cytological diagnosis of gastric cancer by chymotrypsin lavage. Recent Advances in Gastroenterology, 1:300-307, 1967.
Brant, J., and Hamlin, H. H.: Annular pancreas, report of case with unusual presenting symptoms and cure. J.A.M.A., 173:1586-1588, 1960.
Brenner, R. L., and Brown, C. H.: Primary carcinoma of the duodenum. Gastroenterology, 29:189-198, 1955.

Brown, P. M., Cain, J. C., and Dockerty, M. B.: Clinically "benign" gastric ulcerations found to be malignant at operation. Surg., Gynec., Obstet., 112:82-88, 1961.
Bruce, J., Card, W. I., Marks, I. N., and Sircus, W.: The rationale of selective surgery in the treatment of duodenal ulcer. J. Roy. Coll. Surg. Edinburgh, 4:85-104, 1959.
Bruno, M. S., Grier, W. R. N., and Ober, W. B.: Spontaneous laceration and rupture of esophagus and stomach: Mallory-Weiss syndrome, Boerhaave syndrome, and their variants. Arch. Intern. Med., 112:574-583, 1963.
Bryant, L. R., Moore, T. C., and Carney, E. K.: Islet cell adenomas of the duodenum with recurrent peptic ulceration (Zollinger-Ellison). Ann. Surg., 160:104-107, 1964.
Burdette, W. J., and Rasmussen, B.: Perforated peptic ulcer. Surgery, 63:576-585, 1968.
Burge, H. W.: Vagal nerve section in chronic duodenal ulceration. Ann. Roy. Coll. Surg. Eng., 26:231-244, 1960.
Burge, H., Hutchison, J. S. F., Longland, C. J., McLennan, I., Miln, D. C., Rudick, J., and Tompkin, A. M. B.: Selective nerve section in the prevention of post-vagotomy diarrhoea. Lancet, 1:577-579, 1964.
Burgeman, A., Baggenstoss, A. H., and Cain, J. C.: Primary malignant neoplasms of the duodenum, excluding the papilla of Vater. Gastroenterology, 30:421-431, 1956.
Butler, T. J., and Capper, W. M.: Experimental study of 79 cases showing early post-gastrectomy syndrome. Brit. M.J., 1:1177-1181, 1951.
Byrd, B. F., and Carlson, R. I.: Simple closure of peptic ulcer: a review of end results. Ann. Surg., 143:708-713, 1956.
Cabieses, F., and Lecca, G. G.: Acute gastrointestinal hemorrhage in neurosurgical patients. Gastroenterology, 29:300-307, 1955.
Cammock, E. E., Hallett, W. Y., Nyhus, L. M., and Harkins, H. N.: Diagnosis and therapy in gastrointestinal hemorrhage. Arch. Surg., 86:608-614, 1963.
Campbell, R. E., and Young, J. M.: Leiomyoma of the duodenum. Am. J. Surg., 88:618-622, 1954.
Card, W. I., and Marks, I. N.: The relationship between the acid output of the stomach following "maximal" histamine stimulation and the parietal cell mass. Clin. Sci., 19:147-163, 1960.
Carver, G. M., Jr., and Sealy, W. C.: Peptic esophagitis. Arch. Surg., 68:286-295, 1954.
Chapman, N. D., Nyhus, L. M., and Harkins, H. N.: The antrum: its role in the surgery of duodenal ulcer. Scientific Exhibit, 45th Clinical Congress Am. Coll. Surgeons, Atlantic City, N.J., Sept. 28-Oct. 2, 1959.
———: The mechanism of vagus influence on the hormonal phase of gastric acid secretion. Surgery, 47:722-724, 1960.
Clark, C. W.: Peptic ulcer of the second part of the duodenum. Ann. Surg., 143:276-279, 1956.
Clarke, J. S., Ozeran, R. S., Hart, J. C., Cruze, K., and Crevling, V.: Peptic ulcer following portacaval shunt. Ann. Surg., 148:551-566, 1958.

Code, C. F., and Varco, R. L.: Chronic histamine action. Proc. Soc. Exp. Biol. Med., 44:475-477, 1940.

Coller, F. A., Kay, E. B., and McIntyre, R. S.: Regional lymphatic metastases of carcinoma of the stomach. Arch. Surg., 43:748-761, 1941.

Connar, R. C., and Sealy, W. C.: Gastrostomy and its complications. Ann. Surg., 143:245-250, 1956.

Cottrell, J. C.: Nonperforative trauma to abdomen. Arch. Surg., 68:241-251, 1954.

Cowley, L. L., and Harkins, H. N.: Perforation of the gallbladder: a study of 25 consecutive cases. Surg., Gynec., Obstet., 77:661-668, 1943.

Craighead, C. C., and St. Raymond, A. H.: Duodenal fistula: with special reference to choledochoduodenal fistula complicating duodenal ulcer. Am. J. Surg., 87:523-533, 1954.

Cushing, H.: Peptic ulcers and the interbrain. Surg., Gynec., Obstet., 55:1-34, 1932.

Cutler, E. C., and Harrison, J. H.: Phlegmonous gastritis. Surg., Gynec., Obstet., 70:234-240, 1940.

Day, J. J., and Webster, D. R.: The autoregulation of the gastric secretion. Am. J. Digest. Dis. 2:527-531, 1935.

De Bakey, M., and Ochsner, A.: Bezoars and concretions. Surgery, 4:934-963, 1938; 5:132-160, 1939.

Devine, H. B.: Basic principles and supreme difficulties in gastric surgery. Surg., Gynec., Obstet., 40:1-16, 1925.

———: Gastric exclusion. Surg., Gynec., Obstet., 47:239-243, 1928.

DeVito, R. V., Listerud, M. B., Nyhus, L. M., Merendino, K. A., and Harkins, H. N.: Hemorrhage as a complication of reflux esophagitis. Am. J. Surg., 98:657-663, 1959.

Dobbins, W. O.: Mallory-Weiss syndrome: a commonly overlooked cause of upper gastrointestinal bleeding; report of three cases and review of the literature. Gastroenterology, 44:689-695, 1963.

Dolphin, J. A., Smith, L. A., and Waugh, J. M.: Multiple gastric ulcers: their occurrence in benign and malignant lesions. Gastroenterology, 25:202-205, 1953.

Dragstedt, L. R.: Pathogenesis of gastroduodenal ulcer. Arch. Surg., 44:438-451, 1942.

———: Vagotomy for gastroduodenal ulcer. Ann. Surg., 122:973-989, 1945.

———: Gastric vagotomy in the treatment of peptic ulcer. Postgrad. Med., 10:482-490, 1951.

———: The role of the nervous system in the pathogenesis of duodenal ulcer. Surgery, 34:902-903, 1953.

———: The etiology of gastric and duodenal ulcers. Postgrad. Med., 15:99-103, 1954.

———: Sites of peptic ulceration. Arch. Surg., 70:326-327, 1955.

Dragstedt, L. R., Kohatzu, S., Gwaltney, J., Nagano, K., and Greenlee, H.: Further studies on the question of an inhibitory hormone from the gastric antrum. Arch. Surg., 79:10-21, 1959.

Dragstedt, L. R., Oberhelman, H. A., Jr., Evans, S. O., and Rigler, S. P.: Antrum hyperfunction and gastric ulcer. Ann. Surg., 140:396-404, 1954.

Dragstedt, L. R., Oberhelman, H. A., Jr., and Smith, C. A.: Experimental hyperfunction of the gastric antrum with ulcer formation. Ann. Surg., 134:332-341, 1951.

Dragstedt, L. R., and Owens, F. M., Jr.: Supradiaphragmatic section of vagus nerves in treatment of duodenal ulcer. Proc. Soc. Exp. Biol. Med., 53:152-154, 1943.

Dragstedt, L. R., Woodward, E. R., Storer, E. H., Oberhelman, H. A., Jr., and Smith C. A.: Quantitative studies on the mechanism of gastric secretion in health and disease. Ann. Surg., 132:626-640, 1950.

Dreiling, D. A., and Marshak, R. H.: Chronic duodenal obstruction from ingested fruit pits in patients with duodenal ulcer: report of 2 cases, Arch. Surg., 72:411-414, 1956.

Dunn, H. L.: Vital statistics of the United States, 1953, vol. 2, Washington, U.S. Government Printing Office, 1955.

Editorial: The treatment of gastric ulcer. J.A.M.A., 154:766-767, 1954.

Edkins, J. S.: The chemical mechanism of gastric secretion. J. Physiol., 34:133-144, 1906.

Edwards, H. C.: Carcinoma of the stomach. Brit. M.J., 1:973-990, 1950.

Edwards, L. W., Herrington, J. L., Cate, W. R., Jr., and Lipscomb, A. B.: Gastrojejunal ulcer: Problems in surgical management. Ann. Surg., 143:235-244, 1956.

Eker, R.: Carcinomas of the stomach: investigation of the lymphatic spread from gastric carcinomas after total and partial gastrectomy. Acta chir. scandinav., 101:112-126, 1951.

Eker, R., and Efskind, J.: Rare types of malignant gastric tumors. I. Hemangioendotheliomas. Acta path. microbiol. scandinav., 38:14-26, 1956.

Ellison, E. H.: Personal communication, October 30, 1955.

———: Personal communication, June 15, 1956.

———: Ulcerogenic tumor of the pancreas. Surgery, 40:147-170, 1956.

Ellison, E. H., and Wilson, S. D.: Zollinger-Ellison syndrome: Re-appraisal and evaluation of 260 registered cases. Ann. Surg., 160:512-530, 1964.

Elman, R., and Hartmann, A. F.: Spontaneous peptic ulcers of duodenum after continued loss of total pancreatic juice. Arch. Surg., 23:1030-1040, 1931.

Everson, T. C.: Experimental comparison of protein and fat assimilation after Billroth II, Billroth I, and segmental types of subtotal gastrectomy. Surgery, 36:525-537, 1954.

Everson, T. C., and Allen, M. J.: Gastrojejunal ulceration. Arch. Surg., 69:140, 1954.

Farmer, D. A., Burke, P. M., and Smithwick, R. H.: Observations upon peptic activity of the gastric contents in normal individuals and in patients with peptic ulceration. Surg. Forum, 4:316-325, 1954.

Farmer, D. A., Howe, C. W., Porell, W. J., and Smithwick, R. H.: The effect of various surgical procedures upon the acidity of the gastric contents of ulcer patients. Ann. Surg., 134:319-331, 1951.

Farris, J. M., and Smith, G. K.: An evaluation of

temporary gastrostomy as a substitute for nasogastric suction. Ann. Surg., 144:475-486, 1956.

Feldman, M., Morrison, S., and Myers, P.: The clinical evaluation of prolapse of the gastric mucosa into the duodenum. Gastroenterology, 22:80-102, 1952.

Ferguson, L. K., and Cameron, C. S., Jr.: Diverticula of the stomach and duodenum: treatment by invagination and suture. Surg., Gynec., Obstet., 84:292-300, 1947.

Ferguson, L. K., and Nusbaum, M.: Survival after surgical treatment of carcinoma of the stomach. CA, 114:116-118, 1964.

Fieber, S. S.: Hypertrophic gastritis: report of 2 cases and analysis of 50 pathologically verified cases from the literature. Gastroenterology, 28:39-60, 1955.

Fisher, J. A., Taylor, W., and Cannon, J. A.: The dumping syndrome: correlations between its experimental production and clinical incidence. Surg., Gynec., Obstet., 100:559-565, 1955.

Fletcher, D. G., and Harkins, H. N.: Acute peptic ulcer as a complication of major surgery, stress or trauma. Surgery, 36:212-226, 1954.

Fly, O. A., Jr., Dockerty, M. B., and Waugh, J. M.: Metastasis to the regional nodes of the splenic hilus from carcinoma of the stomach. Surg., Gynec., Obstet., 102:279-286, 1956.

Foster, J. H., Hickok, D. F., and Dunphy, J. E.: Changing concepts in the surgical treatment of massive gastroduodenal hemorrhage. Ann. Surg., 161:968-976, 1965.

Franksson, C.: Paper given at Meeting of Svensk kirurgisk Förening. Stockholm, Sweden, October 24, 1947.

Fretheim, B.: Gastric carcinoma treated with abdominothoracic total gastrectomy. Arch. Surg., 71:24-32, 1955.

Friesen, S. R.: The genesis of gastroduodenal ulcer following burns; an experimental study. Surgery, 28:123-158, 1950.

Gibbon, J. H., Jr., Nealon, T. F., and Greco, V. F.: A modification of Glassman's gastrostomy with results in 18 patients. Ann. Surg., 143:838-844, 1956.

Gilbert, J. A. L., and Dunlop, D. M.: Hypoglycemia following partial gastrectomy. Brit. M.J., 2:330-332, 1947.

Gillespie, I. E.: Influence of antral pH on gastric acid secretion in man. Gastroenterology, 37:164-168, 1959.

Gillespie, I. E., Clark, D. H., Kay, A. W., and Tankel, H. I.: Effect of antrectomy, vagotomy with gastrojejunostomy and antrectomy with vagotomy on the spontaneous and maximal gastric acid output in man. Gastroenterology, 38:361-367, 1960.

Glaessner, C. L.: Hyperglycemic shock. Rev. Gastroenterol., 7:528-533, 1940

Glassman, J. A.: A new aseptic double-valved tubogastrostomy. Surg., Gynec., Obstet., 68:789-791, 1939.

Goligher, J. C., Moir, P. J., and Wrigley, J. H.: The Billroth-I and Polya operations for duodenal ulcer: a comparison. Lancet, 1:220-222, 1956.

Gottlieb, C., Lefferts, D., and Beranbaum, S. L.: Gastric volvulus: Part I. Am. J. Roentgenol., 72:609-615, 1954.

Gray, S. J., Benson, J. A., Jr., Reifenstein, R. W., and Spiro, H. M.: Chronic stress and peptic ulcer. I. Effect of corticotropin (ACTH) and cortisone on gastric secretion. J.A.M.A., 147:1529-1538, 1951.

Greengard, H., Atkinson, A. J., Grossman, M. I.. and Ivy, A. C.: The effectiveness of parenterally administered "enterogastrone" in the prophylaxis of recurrences of experimental and clinical peptic ulcer: with a summary of 58 cases. Gastroenterology, 7:625-649, 1946.

Gregory, R. A., and Tracy, H. J.: The preparation and properties of gastrin. J. Physiol., 149:70-71 P, 1959.

———: Secretory responses of denervated gastric pouches. Am. J. Digest. Dis., 5:308-323, 1960.

———: The constitution and properties of two gastrins extracted from hog antral mucosa. Part I. The isolation of two gastrins from hog antral mucosa. Part II. The properties of two gastrins isolated from hog antral mucosa. (By W. H. Taylor): A note on the nature of the gastrin-like stimulant present in Zollinger-Ellison tumors. Gut, 5:103-117, 1964.

Griffith, C. A.: Gastric vagotomy vs. total vagotomy. Arch. Surg., 81:781-788, 1960.

Griffith, C. A., and Harkins, H. N.: The role of Brunner's glands in the intrinsic resistance of the duodenum to acid-peptic digestion. Ann. Surg., 143:160-172, 1956.

———: Partial gastric vagotomy: an experimental study. Gastroenterology, 32:96-102, 1957.

Griffiths, W. J.: The duodenum and the automatic control of gastric acidity. J. Physiol., 87:34-40, 1936.

Gross, R. E.: The Surgery of Infancy and Childhood: Its Principles and Techniques. Philadelphia, W. B. Saunders, 1953.

Guiss, L. W., and Stewart, F. W.: Chronic atrophic gastritis and cancer of the stomach. Arch. Surg., 46:823-843, 1943.

Haberer, von, H.: Volvulus des Magens bei Carcinoma. Deutsche Z. Chir., 115:497-532, 1912.

Hamburger, G. E. (1746): Cited by Brenner and Brown (see reference above), (1955).

Han, S. Y., Collins, L. C., and Petrany, Z.: Emphysematous gastritis. J.A.M.A., 192:914-916, 1965.

Harkins, H. N.: Intussusception due to invaginated Meckel's diverticulum: report of 2 cases with a study of 160 cases collected from the literature. Ann. Surg., 98:1070-1095, 1933.

———: The prevention of pyloric ligation-induced ulcers of the gastric lumen of rats by trans-abdominal vagotomy: a preliminary report. Bull. Johns Hopkins Hosp., 80:174-176, 1947.

Harkins, H. N., Chapman, N. D., and Nyhus, L. M.: Studies on the vagal release of gastrin and its mechanism. Bull. Soc. Int. Chir., 22:48-52, 1963.

Harkins, H. N., and Fletcher, T. L.: The present status of the gastric secretion stimulating hormone gastrin. Bull. Soc. Int. Chir., 22:435-439, 1963.

Harkins, H. N., and Hooker, D. H.: Vagotomy for peptic ulcer. Surgery, 22:239-245, 1947.

Harkins, H. N., Jesseph, J. E., Stevenson, J. K., and Nyhus, L. M.: The "combined" operation for peptic ulcer. Arch. Surg., 80:743-752, 1960.

Harkins, H. N., and Nyhus, L. M.: A comparison of the Billroth I and Billroth II procedures: clinical and experimental studies. Bull. Soc. Int. Chir., 15:111-118, 1956.

———: Surgery of the Stomach and Duodenum. Ed. 2. Boston, Little, Brown & Co., 1969.

Harkins, H. N., Schmitz, E. J., Harper, H. P., Sauvage, L. R., Moore, H. G., Jr., Storer, E. H., and Kanar, E. A.: A combined physiologic operation for peptic ulcer: (partial distal gastrectomy, vagotomy and gastroduodenostomy): a preliminary report. West. J. Surg., 61:316-319, 1953.

Harkins, H. N., Schmitz, E. J., Nyhus, L. M., Kanar, E. A., Zech, R. K., and Griffith, C. A.: The Billroth I gastric resection: experimental studies and clinical observations on 291 cases. Ann. Surg., 140:405-427, 1954.

Harkins, H. N., Stavney, L. S., Griffith, C. A., Savage, L. E., Kato, T., and Nyhus, L. M.: Selective gastric vagotomy. Ann. Surg., 158:448-480, 1963.

Harkins, H. N., Stavney, L. S., Griffith, C. A., Savage, L. E., and Nyhus, L. M.: Scientific exhibit: selective gastric vagotomy. Postgrad. Med., 35:289-298, 1964.

Harrison, R. C., Lakey, W. H., and Hyde, H. A.: The production of an acid inhibitor by the gastric antrum. Ann. Surg., 144:441-449, 1956.

Hedenstedt, S., and Heijenskjöld, F.: Secondary jejunal transposition for severe dumping following Billroth I partial gastrecomy. Acta chir. scandinav., 121:262-273, 1961.

Helsingen, N., and Hillestad, L.: Cancer development in the gastric stump after partial gastrectomy for ulcer. Ann. Surg., 143:173-179, 1956.

Henley, F. A.: Gastrectomy with replacement—a preliminary communication; with an introduction by Rupert Vaughan Hudson. Brit. J. Surg., 40:118-128, 1952.

———: The surgical correction of the post-gastrectomy syndromes. Presented at the 18th Congress of Int. Soc. Surgeons, Munich, Sept., 1959.

Herrington, J. L., Jr., Classen, K. L., and Edwards, L. W.: Experiences with a Billroth I reconstruction following vagotomy and antrectomy for duodenal ulcer. Ann. Surg., 153:578-580, 1961.

Hertz, A. F.: The cause and treatment of certain unfavorable after-effects of gastro-enterostomy. Ann. Surg., 58:466-472, 1913.

Hillemand, P., Patel, J., and Lataste, J.: A propos des diverticules gastriques. Presse méd., 63:1808-1810, 1955.

Hinshaw, D. B., Joergenson, E. J., Davis, H. A., and Stafford, C. E.: Peripheral blood flow and blood volume studies in the dumping syndrome. Arch. Surg., 74:686-693, 1957.

Hinshaw, D. B., Joergenson, E. J., and Stafford, C. E.: Preoperative "dumping studies" in peptic ulcer patients. Arch. Surg., 80:738-742, 1960.

Hoag, E. W., Kiriluk, L. B., and Merendino, K. A.: Experiences with upper gastrectomy, its relationship to esophagitis with special reference to the esophagogastric junction and diaphragm. Am. J. Surg., 88:44-45, 1954.

Hoerr, S. O.: A surgeon's classification of carcinoma of the stomach; preliminary report. Surg., Gynec., Obstet., 99:281-286, 1954.

———: Evaluation of vagotomy with gastroenterostomy performed for chronic duodenal ulcer. Surgery, 38:149-157, 1955.

———: Carcinoma of the stomach. Am. J. Surg., 101:284-291, 1961.

Hoffmann, V.: Klinische Krankheitsbilder nach Magenoperationen. I. Die nicht regulierte Sturzentleerung; II. Die nutritive Gastrojejunitis. München. med. Wschr., 86:332-335, 1939.

Hollander, F.: The insulin test for the presence of intact nerve fibers after vagal operations for peptic ulcer. Gastroenterology, 7:607-614, 1946.

Holle, F.: Spezielle Magenchirurgie. Berlin, Springer-Verlag, 1968.

Holt, R. L., and Robinson, A. F.: The treatment of duodenal ulcer by vagotomy and gastrojejunostomy. Brit. J. Surg., 42:494-502, 1955.

Hunnicut, A. J.: Replacing stomach after total gastroectomy with right ileocolon. Arch. Surg., 65:1-11, 1952.

Hunt, C. J.: Subtotal versus total gastrectomy for gastric malignancy: with a discussion of the various technics advocated in the operation of total gastrectomy. West. J. Surg., 63:337-343, 1955.

Irvine, W. T., Duthie, H. L., Ritchie, H. D., and Waton, N. G.: The liver's role in histamine absorption from the alimentary tract. Lancet, 1:1064-1068, 1959.

Irvine, W. T., Duthie, H. L., and Waton, N. G.: Urinary output of free histamine after a meat meal. Lancet, 1:1061-1063, 1959.

Jackson, C.: Peptic ulcer of the esophagus. J.A.M.A., 92:369-372, 1929.

Jackson, R. G.: Anatomic study of vagus nerves, and a technic of transabdominal gastric vagus resection. Univ. Hosp. Bull., Ann Arbor, 13:31-35, 1947.

Janowitz, H. D., and Crohn, B. B.: Hyperinsulinism and duodenal ulcer: a rare combination. Gastroenterology, 17:578-580, 1951.

Javid, H.: Nutrition in gastric surgery with particular reference to nitrogen and fat assimilation. Surgery, 38:641-651, 1955.

Jeghers, H.: Medical progress: pigmentation of the skin. New Eng. J. Med., 231:88-100, 1944.

Jenson, C. B., Shahon, D. B., and Wangensteen, O. H.: Evaluation of annual examinations in the detection of cancer. J.A.M.A., 174:1783-1788, 1960.

Jesseph, J. E., and Harkins, H. N.: Chemical and vascular factors in the dumping syndrome. Bull. Soc. Int. Chir., 22:446-450, 1963.

Johnson, H. D.: Associated gastric and duodenal ulcers, Surg., Gynec., Obstet., 102:287-292, 1956.

Johnson, L. P., Sloop, R. D., Jesseph, J. E., and Harkins, H. N.: Serotonin antagonists in experimental and clinical "dumping." Ann. Surg., 156:537-549, 1962.

Jones, F. A.: Discussion of paper by Wolf, Marshak, Som, and Winkelstein (see reference below), 1955.

———: Hematemesis and melena: with special reference to causation and to the factors influencing the mortality from bleeding peptic ulcers. Gastroenterology, 30:166-190, 1956.

Jones, F. A., and Doll, R.: Treatment and prognosis of acute perforated peptic ulcer. Brit. M.J., 1:122-127, 1953.

Jones, S. A., Carter, R., Smith, L. L., and Joergenson, E. J.: Arteriomesenteric duodenal compression. Am. J. Surg., 100:262-277, 1960.

Jones, S. A., and Joergenson, E. J.: Closure of duodenal wall defects. Surgery, 53:438-442, 1963.

Jones, S. A., Gregory, G., Smith, L. L., Saito, S., and Joergenson E. J.: Surgical management of the difficult and perforated duodenal stump. Am. J. Surg., 108:257-263, 1964.

Jones, T. W., and Harkins, H. N.: The mechanism of inhibition of gastric acid secretion by the duodenum. Gastroenterology, 37:81-86, 1959.

Jordan, G. L., Jr., and DeBakey, M. E.: The current management of acute gastroduodenal perforation: an analysis of 400 surgically treated cases, including 277 treated by immediate subtotal gastrectomy. Am. J. Surg., 101:317-324, 1961.

Jordan, P. H., Jr., and Sand, B. F.: A study of the gastric antrum as an inhibitor of gastric juice production. Surgery, 42:40-49, 1957.

Judd, E. S.: Pathologic conditions of the duodenum. Lancet, 41:215-220, 1921.

Kanar, E. A., Nyhus, L. M., Olson, H. H., Schmitz, E. J., Scott, O. B., Stevenson, J. K., Jesseph, J. E., Sauvage, L. R., Finley, J. W., and Harkins, H. N.: The Billroth I subtotal gastric resection: a follow-up report on 493 cases. Arch. Surg., 72:991-1002, 1956.

Kelly, K. A., Nyhus, L. M., and Harkins, H. N.: The vagal nerve and the intestinal phase of gastric secretion. Gastroenterology, 46:163-166, 1964.

Kelly, W. D., Cross, F. S., and Wangensteen, O. H.: The importance of the spatial relationship of the gastric antrum in the development of gastrojejunal ulcer in the dog, S. Forum, 4:339-345, 1954.

Kiriluk, L. B., and Merendino, K. A.: An experimental study of the buffering capacity of the contents of the upper small bowel. Surgery, 35:532-537, 1954.

———: The comparative sensitivity of the mucosa of the various segments of the alimentary tract in the dog to acid-peptic action. Surgery, 35:547-566, 1954.

Klebba, A. J.: Mortality trends in the United States 1954-1963. National Center for Health Statistics, Report Series 20, No. 2, 1966.

Kleiman, A., and Grant, A. R.: The role of K+ in the pathogenesis and treatment of the postgastrectomy dumping syndrome. S. Forum, 4:296-301, 1954.

Konjetzny, G. E.: Ueber die Beziehungen der chronischen Gastritis mit ihren Folgeerscheinungen und des chronischen Magenulcus zur Entwicklung des Magenkrebses. Beitr. klin. Chir., 85:455-519, 1913.

———: Chronische Gastritis und Magenkrebs. Mschr. Krebsbekämpfung. pp. 65-78, 1934.

———: Eine besondere Form der chronischen hypertrophischen Gastritis unter dem klinischen und röntgenologischen Bilde des Carcinoms. Chirurg., 10:260-268, 1938.

Kozoll, D. D., and Meyer, K. A.: Obstructing gastroduodenal ulcers: general factors influencing incidence and mortality. Arch. Surg., 88:793-799, 1964.

Lahey, F. H.: Total gastrectomy for all patients with operable cancer of the stomach. Surg., Gynec., Obstet., 90:246-248, 1950.

Lahey, F. H., and Marshall, S. F.: Should total gastrectomy be employed in early carcinoma of the stomach? Ann. Surg., 132:540-565, 1950.

Lampert, E. G., Waugh, J. M., and Dockerty, M. B.: The incidence of malignancy in gastric ulcers believed preoperatively to be benign. Surg., Gynec., Obstet., 91:673-679, 1950.

Landelius, E.: Results of partial and total gastrectomy in cancer of the stomach. Acta chir. scandinav., 96:441-460, 1948.

Landry, R. M.: Gastroileostomy and gastrocolostomy. Surgery, 30:528-533, 1951,

Lefferts, D., Beranbaum, S. L., and Gottlieb, C.: Gastric volvulus. Part II. Idiopathic gastric volvulus. Am. J. Roentgenol., 72:616-626, 1954.

Lewisohn, R.: The frequency of gastrojejunal ulcers. Surg., Gynec., Obstet., 40:70-76, 1925.

Lillehei, C. W., Roth, F. E., and Wangensteen, O. H.: The role of stress in the etiology of peptic ulcer: experimental and clinical observations. S. Forum, 2:43-48, 1952.

McCune, W. S., Gusack, M., and Newman, W.: Eosinophilic gastroduodenitis with pyloric obstruction. Ann. Surg., 142:510-518, 1955.

McGlone, F. B., and Robertson, D. W.: Diagnostic accuracy in gastric ulcer. Gastroenterology, 25:603-613, 1953.

McNeer, G., Sunderland, D. A., McInnes, G., VandenBerg, H., Jr., and Lawrence, W.: A more thorough operation for gastric cancer. Cancer, 4:957-967, 1951.

Macdonald, J. M., Webster, M., and Drapanas, T.: Serotonin and bradykinin in the dumping syndrome. Am. J. Surg., 117:204, 1969.

Maciver, I. N., Smith, B. J., Tomlinson, B. E., and Whitby, J. D.: Rupture of the oesophagus associated with lesions of the central nervous system. Brit. J. Surg., 43:505-512, 1956.

MacLean, L. D., Hamilton, W., and Murphy, T. O.: An evaluation of segmental gastric resection for the treatment of peptic ulcer Surgery, 34:227-237, 1953.

MacLean, L. D., Perry, J. F., Kelly, W. D., Mosser, D. G., Mannick, A., and Wangensteen, O. H.: Nutrition following subtotal gastrectomy of 4 types (Billroth I and II, segmental and tubular resections). Surgery, 35:705-718, 1954.

Mallory, G. K., and Weiss, S.: Hemorrhages from lacerations of the cardiac orifice of the stomach due to vomiting. Am. J. Med. Sci., 178:506-515, 1929.

Marshall, S. F.: The relation of gastric ulcer to

carcinoma of the stomach. Ann Surg., 137:891-903, 1953.
———: Gastric tumors other than carcinoma, S. Clin. N. Am., 35:693-702, 1955.
Marshall, S. F., and Meissner, W. A.: Sarcoma of the stomach. Ann. Surg., 131:824-837, 1950.
Mateer, J. G., and Hartman, F. W.: Primary carcinoma of the duodenum: clinical and pathologic aspects, with differential diagnosis. J.A.M.A., 99:1853-1859, 1932.
Meissner, W. A.: Leiomyoma of the stomach. Arch. Path., 38:207-209, 1944.
Mendelson, C. L.: Aspiration of stomach contents into the lungs during obstetric anesthesia. Am. J. Obstet., Gynec., 52:191-205, 1946.
Menetrier, P.: Des polyadénomes gastriques et de leurs rapports avec le cancer de l'estomac. Arch. Physiol. Norm. Path., 1:32-55, 236-262, 1888. Cited by Yarnis, Marshak, and Friedman (see reference below), 1952.
Menguy, R., and Masters, Y. F.: Effect of cortisone on mucoprotein secretion by gastric antrum of dogs: Pathogenesis of steroid ulcer. Surgery, 54:19-28, 1963.
Mersheimer, W. L., Glass, G. B. J., Speer, F. D., Winfield, J. M., and Boyd, L. J.: Gastric mucin —a chemical and histologic study following bilateral vagectomy, gastric resection and the combined procedure. Tr. Am. S. A., 70:331-342, 1952.
Meyer, K. A., and Steigman, F.: The surgical treatment of corrosive gastritis. Surg., Gynec., Obstet., 76:306-310, 1944.
Moffat, F., and Anderson, W.: Adenoma of Brunner's gland. Brit. J. Surg., 43:106-107, 1955.
Moncrief, J. A., Switzer, W. E., and Teplitz, C.: Curling's ulcer. J. Trauma, 4:481-494, 1964.
Moore, H. G., Jr., and Harkins, H. N.: The Billroth I Gastric Resection: With Particular Reference to the Surgery of Peptic Ulcer. Boston, Little, Brown & Co., 1954.
Moore, H. G., Jr., Harkins, H. N., and Merendino, K. A.: The treatment of perforated peptic ulcer by primary gastric resection. Surg., Gynec., Obstet., (Internat. Abstr. Surg.) 98:105-123, 1954.
Morey, D. A. J., Means, R. L., and Hirsley, E. L.: Diospyrobezoar in the postgastrectomy stomach. Arch. Surg., 71:946-948, 1955.
Morris, K. N.: Gastric mucosa within the oesophagus Aus. New Zeal. J. Surg., 25:24-30, 1955.
Morson, B. C.: Intestinal metaplasia of the gastric mucosa. Brit. J. Cancer, 9:365-376, 1955.
———: Carcinoma arising from areas of intestinal metaplasia in the gastric mucosa. Brit. J. Cancer, 9:377-385, 1955.
Moyer, C. A.: Personal communication, July 12, 1964.
Muto, M., Maki, T., Majima, S., and Yamaguchi, I.: Improvement in the end-results of surgical treatment of gastric cancer. Surgery, 63:229-235, 1968.
Nicoloff, D. M., Griffen, W. O., Salmon, P. A., Peter, E. T., and Wangensteen, O. H: Local gastric hypothermia in the management of massive gastrointestinal hemorrhage. Surg., Gynec., Obstet., 114:495-503, 1962.

Niemeier, O. W.: Acute free perforation of the gallbladder. Ann. Surg., 99:922-924, 1934.
Nissen, R.: The treatment of hiatal hernia and esophageal reflux by fundoplication. In Nyhus, L. M., and Harkins, H. N., (eds.). Hernia. p. 488. Philadelphia, J. B. Lippincott, 1964.
Notkin, L. J.: Carcinoma occurring on the basis of pre-existing gastric ulcer. Canad. M.A.J., 72:288-296, 1955.
Nusbaum, M., Baum, S., Blakemore, W. S., and Finkelstein, A. K.: Demonstration of intraabdominal bleeding by selective arteriography: Visualization of celiac and superior mesenteric arteries. J.A.M.A., 191:389-390, 1965.
Nyhus, L. M.: Uropepsin excretion: its relation to duodenal ulcer disease in diagnosis and therapy. Surgery, 41:406-415, 1957.
———: The role of the antrum in the surgical treatment of peptic ulcer. Gastroenterology, 38:21-25, 1960.
Nyhus, L. M., Chapman, N. D., DeVito, R. V., and Harkins, H. N.: The control of gastrin release: an experimental study illustrating a new concept. Gastroenterology, 39:582-589, 1960.
Nyhus, L. M., Condon, R. E., and Harkins, H. N.: The evolution of surgery for duodenal ulcer during the mid-twentieth century. J. Roy. Coll. Surg., Edinburgh, 8:91-104, 1963.
Nyhus, L. M., Stevenson, J. K., Jones, T. W., DeVito, R. V., and Harkins, H. N.: Jejunal gastrostomy. Bull. Soc. Int. Chir., 17:254-259, 1958.
Oberhelman, H. A., Jr., Nelsen, T. S., Johnson, A. N., Jr., and Dragstedt, L. R., II: Ulcerogenic tumors of the duodenum. Ann. Surg., 153:214-227, 1961.
Oberhelman, H. A., Jr., Rigler, S. P., and Dragstedt, L. R.: Significance of innervation in the function of the gastric antrum. Am. J. Physiol., 190:391-395, 1957.
Oberhelman, H. A., Jr., Woodward, E. R., Zubiran, J. M., and Dragstedt, L. R.: Physiology of the gastric antrum. Am. J. Physiol., 169:738-748, 1952.
O'Leary, C. M.: Diospyrobezoar: a review of 14 cases with an analysis of 46 collected cases from the literature. Arch. Surg., 66:857-868, 1953.
Olsson, O., and Endresen, R.: Ulcer cancer of the stomach. Acta chir. scandinav., 111:16-21, 1956.
Ordahl, N. B., Ross, F. P., and Baker, D. V., Jr.: The failure of partial gastrectomy with gastroduodenostomy in the treatment of duodenal ulcer. Surgery, 38:158-168, 1955.
Orloff, M. J., and Windsor, C. W. O.: Effect of portacaval shunt on gastric acid secretion in dogs with liver disease, portal hypertension and massive ascites. Ann. Surg., 164:69-80, 1966.
Owren, P. A.: The pathogenesis and treatment of iron deficiency anemia after partial gastrectomy. Acta chir. scandinav., 104:206-214, 1952.
Palmer, E. D.: Benign intramural tumors of the stomach: a review with special reference to gross pathology. Medicine, 30:81-181, 1951.
———: Further observations on postoperative gastritis: histopathologic aspects with a note on jejunitis. Gastroenterology, 25:405-415, 1953.
Palmer, W. L.: Certain aspects of benign and malig-

nant gastric ulcer. Bull. N. Y. Acad. Med., 26: 527-537, 1950.
Pavlov, I. P.: The Work of the Digestive Glands. p. 54. London, Griffin, 1910.
Pearce, J., and Ehrlich, A.: Gastric sarcoidosis. Ann. Surg., 141:115-119, 1955.
Peters, R. M., and Womack, N. A.: Hemodynamics of gastric secretion. Ann. Surg., 148:537-550, 1958.
Peutz, J. L. A.: Very remarkable case of familial polyposis of mucous membrane of intestinal tract and nasopharynx accompanied by peculiar pigmentation of skin and mucous membrane. Ned. mschr. Geneesk., 10:134, 1921. (Cited by Weber, R. A.: Ann. Surg., 140:901-905, 1954.)
Pincus, I. J., Thomas, J. E., and Rehfuss, M. E.: A study of gastric secretion as influenced by changes in duodenal acidity. Proc. Soc. Exp. Biol. Med., 51:367-368, 1942.
Plenk, H. P., and Lin, R. K.: Gastric ulcer and gastric carcinoma: a correlative study. Am. Surg., 20:348-354, 1954.
Polson, R. A., and Isaac, J. E.: Enterogenous cyst of the duodenum. Gastroenterology, 25:431-434, 1953.
Poth, E. J., Manhoff, L. J., Jr., and DeLoach, A. W.: The relation of pancreatic secretion to peptic ulcer formation: effect of pancreatectomy, ligation of pancreatic ducts, and diabetes on the production of histamine-induced ulcers in dogs. Surgery, 24: 62-69, 1948.
Preshaw, R. M.: Stimulation of pancreatic secretion by gastrin extracts. In Grossman, M. I. (ed.): Gastrin. Los Angeles, University of California Press, 1966.
Ransom, H. K.: Subtotal gastrectomy for gastric ulcer: a study of end results. Ann. Surg., 126: 633-652, 1947.
———: Cancer of the stomach. Surg., Gynec., Obstet., 96:275-287, 1953.
———: Cancer of the stomach: report on cases treated by total gastrectomy. Gastroenterology, 30: 191-207, 1956.
Reuter, S. R., and Bookstein, J. J.: Angiographic localization of gastrointestinal bleeding. Gastroenterology, 54:876-883, 1968.
Risholm, L.: Acute upper alimentary tract ulceration and haemorrhage following surgery or traumatic lesions. Acta chir. scand., 110:275-283, 1956.
Roberts, K. E., Randall, H. T., and Farr, H. W.: Acute alterations in blood volume, plasma electrolytes, and electrocardiogram produced by oral administration of hypertonic solutions to gastrectomized patients. S. Forum, 4:301-306, 1953.
Robinson, A. W., Black, B. M., Sprague, R. G., and Tillisch, J. H.: Hyperparathyroidism due to diffuse primary hyperplasia and hypertrophy of the parathyroid glands: report of a case. Proc. Mayo Clin., 26:441-446, 1951.
Rogers, H. M., Keating, F. R., Morlock, C. G., and Barker, N. W.: Primary hypertrophy and hyperplasia of the parathyroid glands associated with duodenal ulcer. Arch. Int. Med., 79:307-321, 1947.
Rokitansky, C. (1846): Cited by Cushing (see reference above), 1932.
———: (1849): Lehrbuch der pathologischen Anatomie (3rd ed.). Vol. 3. Wien, Braumüller, 1855-1861. (Cited by Barling, 1923).
Rosenberg, J. C.: Gastroduodenal leiomyosarcomas: A report of the clinical roentgenologic, and pathologic features of three surgical cases. Am. J. Digest. Dis., 9:213-220, 1964.
Rothchild, T. P. E., and Hinshaw, A. H.: Retroperitoneal rupture of the duodenum caused by blunt trauma; with a case report. Ann. Surg., 143:269-275, 1956.
Rowe, C. R., Jr., Grimson, K. S., and Flowe, B. H.: Comparison of insulin and gastrometric tests for completeness of vagotomy. S. Forum, 3:1-5, 1953.
Rubin, C. E., and Benditt, E. P.: A simplified technique using chymotrypsin lavage for the cytological diagnosis of gastric cancer. Cancer, 8:1137-1141, 1955.
Ruckley, C. V.: A study of the variations of the abdominal vagi. Brit. J. Surg., 51:569-573, 1964.
Rudick, J., and Hutchison, J. S. F.: Effects of vagal-nerve section on the biliary system. Lancet, 1:579-581, 1964.
Sachs, L. J., and Angrist, A.: Phlegmonous gastritis as a manifestation of sepsis. Ann. Int. Med., 22: 563-584, 1945.
Sauvage, L. R., Schmitz, E. J., Storer, E. H., Kanar, E. A., Smith, F. R., and Harkins, H. N.: The relation between the physiologic stimulatory mechanisms of gastric secretion and the incidence of peptic ulceration: an experimental study employing a new preparation. Surg., Gynec., Obstet., 96: 127-142, 1953.
Sawyer, K. C., Hammer, R. W., and Fenton, W. C.: Gastric volvulus as a cause of obstruction. Arch. Surg., 72:764-772, 1956.
Sawyers, J. L., Scott, H. W., Jr., Edwards, W. H., Shull, H. J., and Law, D. H., IV.: Comparative studies of the clinical effects of truncal and selective gastric vagotomy. Am. J. Surg., 115:165-172, 1968.
Schaberg, A., Hildes, J. A., and Alcock, A. J. W.: Upper gastrointestinal lesions in acute bulbar poliomyelitis. Gastroenterology, 27:838-848, 1954.
Scheinin, T. M., and Inberg, M. V.: Clinical experiences with selective vagotomy. Acta chir. scand., 133:533-537, 1967.
Schell, R. F., Dockerty, M. B., and Comfort, M. W.: Carcinoma of the stomach associated with pernicious anemia: a clinical and pathologic study. Surg., Gynec., Obstet., 98:710-720, 1954.
Schirmer, J. F., and Bowers, W. F.: Operation for duodenal ulcer after inadequate surgery. Arch. Surg., 71:80-90, 1955.
Schmieden, V.: Die Differentialdiagnose zwischen Magengeschwür und Magenkrebs; die pathologische Anatomie dieser Erkrankungen in Beziehung zu ihrer Darstellung im Röntgenbilde. Arch. klin. Chir., 96:253-344, 1911.
Schridde, H.: Über Magenschleimhaut-Inseln vom Bau der Cardialdrüsenzone und Fundusdrüsenregion und den unteren, oesophagealen Cardialdrüsen gleichende Drüsen im obersten Oesophagusabschnitt. Virchows Arch. path., Anat., 175: 1-16, 1904.
Seeley, S. F., and Campbell, D.: Nonoperative

treatment of perforated peptic ulcer: a further report. Surg., Gynec., Obstet. (Int. Abstr. Surg.), 102:435-446, 1956.

Segal, G., and Serbin, R.: Regional enteritis involving the duodenum. Gastroenterology, 30:503-507, 1956.

Shahon, D. B., Horowitz, S., and Kelly, W. D.: Cancer of the stomach: an analysis of 1152 cases. Surgery, 39:204-221, 1956.

Shapira, D., Morgenstern, L., and State, D.: Critical examination of the "acid-inhibition" phenomenon in dogs with twin antrum pouches. S. Forum, 10: 143, 1960.

Shay, H.: Stress and gastric secretion, Gastroenterology, 26:316-319, 1954.

Sherman, J. L., and Newman, S.: Functioning arteriovenous anastomoses in the stomach and duodenum. Am. J. Physiol., 179:279-281, 1954.

Silen, W., Hein, M. F., Albo, R. J., and Harper, H. A.: Influence of liver upon canine gastric secretion. Surgery, 54:29-36, 1963.

Sircus, W.: Studies on the mechanisms in the duodenum inhibiting gastric secretion. Quart. J. Exp. Physiol., 43:114-133, 1958.

Smith, W. H.: Potassium lack in the postgastrectomy dumping syndrome. Lancet, 2:745-749, 1951.

Smith, W. O., DuVal, M. K., Joel, W., Hanska, W. L., and Wolf, S.: Gastric atrophy in dogs induced by administration of normal human gastric juice. Gastroenterology, 39:55-61, 1960.

Smith, W. O., DuVal, M. K., Joel, W., and Wolf, S.: The experimental production of atrophic gastritis using a preparation of human gastric juice. Surgery, 46:76-82, 1959.

Snoddy, W. T.: Primary lymphosarcoma of the stomach. Gastroenterology, 20:537-553, 1952.

Sokolov, A. P. (1904): Cited by Brackney, Thal, and Wangensteen (see reference above), 1955.

Stammers, F. A. R.: The complications of partial gastrectomy. Ann. Roy. Coll. Surg. Eng., 17:373-385, 1955.

State, D., Katz, A., Kaplan, R. S., Herman, B., Morgenstern, L., and Knight, I. A.: The role of the pyloric antrum in experimentally induced peptic ulceration in dogs. Surgery, 38:143-148, 1955.

Stavney, L. S., Kato, T., Savage, L. E., Harkins, H. N., and Nyhus, L. M.: Parietal cell reactivity. Surg., Gynec., Obstet., 118:1269-1272, 1964.

Stemmer, E. A., Zahn, R. L., Hom, L. W., and Connolly, J. E.: Vagotomy and drainage procedures for gastric ulcer. Arch. Surg., 96:586-592, 1968.

Stewart, J. D., Sanderson, G. M., and Wiles, C. E., Jr.: Blood replacement and gastric resection for massively bleeding peptic ulcer. Ann. Surg., 136:742-748, 1952.

Stock, F. E., Hui, K. K. L., and Tinckler, L. F.: Vagotomy and pylorectomy in the treatment of duodenal ulceration. Surg., Gynec., Obstet., 102: 358-368, 1956.

Storer, E. H., Schmitz, E. J., Sauvage, L. R., Kanar, E. A., Diessner, C. H., and Harkins, H. N.: Gastric secretion in Heidenhain pouches following section of vagus nerves to main stomach. Proc. Soc. Exp. Biol. Med., 80:325-327, 1952.

Strøm, R.: A case of peptic ulcer and insuloma. Acta chir. scand., 104:252-260, 1952.

Swynnerton, B. F., and Tanner, N. C.: Chronic gastric ulcer: a comparison between a gastroscopically controlled series treated medically and a series treated by surgery. Brit. M. J., 2:841-847, 1953.

Tanner, N. C.: The indications for surgery in peptic ulcer. Edinburgh M.J., 58:261-278, 1951.

———: Non-malignant affections of the upper stomach. Ann. Roy. Coll. Surg. Eng., 10:45-60, 1952.

———: Surgery of peptic ulceration and its complications. Postgrad. M.J., 30:448-465, 523-531, 577-592, 1954.

———: The treatment of carcinoma of the stomach. Ann. Roy. Coll. Surg. Eng., 17:102-113, 1955.

———: Cited by Allen and Oberhelman (see reference above), 1955.

Ternberg, J. L., and Kochler, R. R.: The use of arteriography in the diagnosis of the origin of acute gastrointestinal hemorrhage in children. Surgery, 63:686-689, 1968.

Thal, A. P., Hatafuku, T., and Kurtzman, R. A.: A new method for reconstruction of the esophagogastric junction. Surg., Gynec., Obstet., 120:1225-1231, 1965.

Thein, M. P., and Schofield, B.: Release of gastrin from the pyloric antrum following vagal stimulation by sham feeding in dogs. J. Physiol., 148: 291-305, 1959.

Thomford, N. R., Bachulis, B. L., and Brashear, R. E.: Stenosis of an inadvertent gastroileostomy with severe metabolic alkalosis. Ann. Surg., 167: 595-597, 1968.

Thompson, J. C., Daves, I. A., Davidson, W. D., and Miller, J. H.: Studies on the humoral control of gastric secretion in dogs with autogenous and homotransplanted antral and fundic pouches. Surgery, 58:84-109, 1965.

Thompson, J. C., and Peskin, G. W.: The gastric antrum in the operative treatment of duodenal ulcer. Surg., Gynec., Obstet. (Intern. Abst. Surg.), 112:205-227, 1961.

Thompson, J. E.: Stomal ulceration after gastric surgery. Ann. Surg., 143:697-707, 1956.

Traut, H. F., Rosenthal, M., Harrison, J. T., Farber, S. M., and Grimes, O. F.: Evaluation of mucolytic agents in gastric cytologic studies. S. Forum, 3: 28-33, 1953.

Vargas, L. L., Levin, S. M., and Santulli, T. V.: Rupture of the stomach in the newborn infant. Surg., Gynec., Obstet., 101:417-424, 1955.

Villarreal, R., Ganong, W. F., and Gray, S. J.: Effect of adrenocorticotrophic hormone upon the gastric secretion of hydrochloric acid, pepsin and electrolytes in the dog. Am. J. Physiol., 183:485-492, 1955.

Waldeyer, W. (1908): Cited by Bauer (see reference above), 1923.

Walker, J. M., Roberts, K. E., Medwid, A., and Randall, H. T.: The significance of the dumping syndrome. Arch. Surg., 71:543-550, 1955.

Wallensten, S.: The relation between sideropenia and anemia and the occurrence of postcibal symptoms following partial gastrectomy for peptic ulcer. Surgery, 38:289-297, 1955.

Walters, W., Chance, D. P., and Berkson, J.: The surgical treatment of gastrojejunal ulceration. Arch. Surg., 70:826-832, 1955a.

———: Comparison of vagotomy and gastric resection for gastrojejunal ulceration: follow-up study of 301 cases. Surg., Gynec., Obstet., 100: 1-10, 1955 (b).

Wangensteen, O. H.: Cancer of the Esophagus and the Stomach. New York, Am. Cancer Soc., 1951.

———: Segmental gastric resection for peptic ulcer. J.A.M.A., 149:18-23, 1952.

———: Evolution and evaluation of an acceptable operation for peptic ulcer. Rev. Gastroenterol., 20:611-626, 1953.

———: The surgical treatment of peptic ulcer. J. Iowa M. Soc., 44:356-373, 1954.

———: Gastric cooling. *In* Harkins, H. N., and Nyhus, L. M., Surgery of the Stomach and Duodenum. (ed.). Boston, Little, Brown & Co., 1962.

Wangensteen, O. H., Salmon, P. A., Griffen, W. O., Jr., Paterson, J. R. S., and Fattah, F.: Studies of local gastric cooling as related to peptic ulcer. Ann. Surg., 150:346-360, 1959.

Waugh, J. M.: Quart. Rev. Surg., 13:18. 1956.

Waugh, J. M., and Hood, R. T., Jr.: Gastric operations: an historic review. Quart. Rev. Surg., 10: 201-214, 1953; 11:1-18, 1954.

Waugh, J. M., and Johnston, E. V.: Primary diverticula of the duodenum. Ann. Surg., 141:193-200, 1955.

Wechsler, R. L., Roth, J. L. A., and Bockus, H. L.: The use of serial blood volumes and head-up tilts as important indicators of therapy in patients with bleeding from the gastrointestinal tract. Gastroenterology, 30:221-231, 1956.

Weinberg, J. A.: Personal communication, April 4, 1953.

———: Pyloroplasty and vagotomy for duodenal ulcer. *In* Current Problems in Surgery. Chicago, Year Book Publishers, April, 1964.

Welborn, J. K.: Lymphoma of the stomach. Arch. Surg., 90:480-487, 1965.

Welch, C. E., and Allen, A. W.: **Gastric ulcer:** a study of the Massachusetts General Hospital cases during the ten-year period 1938-1947. New Eng. J. Med., 240:276-283, 1949.

Wilkie, D. P. D.: Chronic duodenal ileus. Brit. J. Surg., 9:204-214, 1921.

Winkelstein, A.: Peptic esophagitis: a new clinical entity. J.A.M.A., 104:906-909, 1935.

Wolf, B. S., Marshak, R. H., Som, M. L., and Winkelstein, A.: Peptic esophagitis, peptic ulcer of the esophagus and marginal esophagogastric ulceration. Gastroenterology, 29:744-766, 1955.

Woodruff, J. F.: Personal communication, March 29, 1961.

Woodward, E. R., Desser, P. L., and Gasster, M.: Surgical treatment of the postgastrectomy dumping syndrome. West. J. Surg., 63:567-573, 1955.

Woodward, E. R., Robertson, C., Fried, W., and Schapiro, H.: Further studies on the isolated gastric antrum. Gastroenterology, 32:868-877, 1957.

Woodward, E. R., Trumbull, W. E., Schapiro, H., and Towne, L.: Does the gastric antrum elaborate an antisecretory hormone? Am. J. Digest. Dis., 3:204-213, 1958.

Wright, J. T., Grant, A., and Jennings, D.: A duodenal-ulcer family. Lancet, 2:1314-1318, 1955.

Yarnis, H., Marshak, R. H., and Friedman, A. I.: Gastric polyps. J.A.M.A., 148:1088-1094, 1952.

Zeldis, A. M., and Klinger, J. R.: Sindrome postgastrectomia. Rev. méd. Valparaiso, 4:311, 1951. *In* Surg., Gynec., Obstet., (Int. Abstr. Surg.), 94: 546, 1952.

Zinninger, M. M.: Diverticula of the duodenum: indications for and technique of surgical treatment. Arch. Surg., 66:846-856, 1953.

———: Extension of gastric cancer in the intramural lymphatics and its relation to gastrectomy. Am. Surg., 20:920-927, 1954.

Zollinger, R. M., and Ellison, E. H.: Nutrition after gastric operations. J.A.M.A., 154:811-814, 1954.

———: Primary peptic ulcerations of the jejunum associated with islet cell tumors of the pancreas. Ann. Surg., 142:709-728, 1955.

Zollinger, R. M., and Grant, G. N.: Ulcerogenic tumor of the pancreas. J.A.M.A., 190:181-184, 1964.

Zollinger, R. M., and Moore, F. T.: Zollinger-Ellison Syndrome comes of age. J.A.M.A., 204: 361-365, 1968.

Zollinger, R. M., and Williams, R. D.: Considerations in surgical treatment for duodenal ulcer. J.A.M.A., 160:367-373, 1956.

Zubiran, J. M., Kark, A. E., Montalbetti, A. J., Morel, C. J. L., and Dragstedt, L. R.: Peptic ulcer and the adrenal stress syndrome. Arch. Surg., 65:809-815, 1952.

CHAPTER 32

JONATHAN E. RHOADS, M.D.

Liver, Gallbladder and Bile Passages

Anatomic Considerations
Physiologic Considerations
Tumors of the Gallbladder and the Extrahepatic Bile Ducts
Hemobilia
Acute Cholecystitis
Perforation of the Gallbladder with Abscess, Peritonitis or Biliary Fistula
Chronic Calculous Cholecystitis and Chronic Noncalculous Cholecystitis
Diagnosis of Common Duct Stone and Other Indications for Choledochostomy
The Jaundiced Patient
The Prognostic Significance of Obstructive Jaundice
Preparation of the Jaundiced Patient for Operation
Standard Operative Procedures on the Gallbladder and the Extrahepatic Biliary Passages
Pathologic Conditions of the Liver Parenchyma with Notes Regarding Surgical Therapy

INTRODUCTION

Surgery of the biliary tract includes the problems of the gallbladder and the extrahepatic biliary ducts as well as those of the liver itself. The gallbladder and the ducts will be considered first in this chapter. The surgeon should know the anatomic relationships between the gallbladder, the cystic duct, the common hepatic duct, the common bile duct, the portal vein, the hepatic artery and its branches, including the cystic artery, as they normally occur. He will require also an appreciation of the variability of these structures and their interrelationships and should bear in mind at least the more dangerous of the common anomalies which are illustrated in Figure 32-1.

Many of the surgical catastrophes which have occurred during endeavors to benefit the patient with biliary tract symptoms have resulted from ignorance of or failure to recognize such anomalies.

He will also need to know the signs and symptoms of acute cholecystitis, the indications for immediate and delayed operation, and the basis on which a decision is made as to whether to do a cholecystectomy or merely to drain the gallbladder (cholecystostomy).

In the nonacute cases, he must learn the even more difficult problem of assessing the various signs and symptoms of cholelithiasis with chronic cholecystitis. Here, he needs to gain a practical knowledge of the uses of cholecystography and biliary drainage and of other laboratory aids in diagnosis. It is also of major importance for him to understand the accepted indications for opening and exploring the common bile duct (choledochostomy).

The jaundiced patient presents a complex problem in diagnosis which often calls for elaborate clinical and laboratory study and also requires as much knowledge as is available of liver physiology in order to assess the risks of operation and to prepare the patient as thoroughly as possible in order to diminish these risks. Biliary tract patients and especially those with common duct obstruction may be subject to certain special complications more or less peculiar to this field, such as the hemorrhagic tendency of obstructive jaundice (hypoprothrombinemia), liver shock, "pancreatic asthenia" and the hepatorenal syndrome.

The portion of this chapter devoted to the pathologic processes of the gallbladder and the extrahepatic bile ducts will be focused on these particular subjects. The surgery of the liver itself will be considered briefly, utilizing the material on liver physiology referred to in connection with obstructive jaundice.

It should be noted that there are two specific hazards to the surgeon and members of his team who handle diseased gallbladders on the one hand and jaundiced patients on the other. The first is that of contracting typhoid fever, especially from adults who were alive before the decline in the incidence of this disease which occurred about 1910. The second is the danger of serum hepatitis in patients with jaundice. This disease may be contracted through any break in the skin.

The surgery of portal cirrhosis is considered in Chapter 35.

ANATOMIC CONSIDERATIONS

The common hepatic duct is formed by the union of the ducts draining the right and the left lobes of the liver. It runs from the transverse fissure of the liver inferiorly and posteriorly, lying in the right border of the lesser omentum. Here, it follows a course to the right of and anterior to the portal vein and also to the right of the hepatic artery. The duct is approximately 4 cm. long and is joined by the cystic duct to form the common bile duct.

The cystic duct runs a course of approximately 3.5 cm. from the neck of the gallbladder inferiorly, to the left, and posteriorly to enter the lesser omentum between the portal vein and the hepatic artery and finally to join the hepatic duct at an acute angle.

The common bile duct passes downward in the right border of the lesser omentum with the same relationships as the common hepatic duct. From here it passes behind the superior portion of the duodenum, entering the duodenum obliquely in its descending portion, and in over 50 per cent joining the main pancreatic duct to form the terminal portion known as the ampulla of Vater. The entrance from the ampulla to the duodenum is surrounded by a portion of the sphincter of Oddi which also surrounds the terminal pancreatic and the common bile ducts. Frequently, the common bile duct and the duct of Wirsung join to form a common channel for a significant distance before emptying into the duodenum. According to Howard and Jones (1947), this amounted to 0.5 cm. or more in 17 per cent of cadavers, but they demonstrated reflux into the pancreatic duct of fluid injected into the common duct in 54 per cent of 150 cadavers.

The gallbladder is a pear-shaped sac, about 10 cm. in length, nestled against the inferior portion of the liver between the right and the quadrate lobes and covered with a layer of peritoneum which is reflected from Glisson's capsule. The gallbladder may be divided into 3 parts: the fundus, or superficial portion; the body; and the neck, or infundibulum, which joins the cystic duct. If the infundibulum has an abnormal sacculation, often it is referred to as Hartmann's pouch. Such a pouch may be adherent to surrounding structures, seriously obscuring important anatomic relationships at the time of dissection. The main arterial supply of the gallbladder is the cystic artery, which arises from the hepatic artery or more commonly from the right branch of the hepatic artery. This may cross in front of, behind, or at some distance from the common duct to join the cystic duct or infundibulum and thus supply the gallbladder. (See Chap. 33, Pancreas.)

Embryologically, the liver, the bile ducts and the gallbladder arise as a diverticulum from that portion of the gut which later becomes the second part of the duodenum. This diverticulum is lined by entoderm and grows upward and forward into a mesodermal mass called the *septum transversum*. Two solid buds of cells then arise from it to form the right and the left lobes of the liver by growing into columns and cylinders called *hepatic cylinders*. They branch into a very fine network which invades the vitelline and the umbilical veins to form a series of tiny vessels called *sinusoids*. These capillarylike vessels ramify throughout the cellular network and finally develop into the venous capillaries of the liver. This growth and ramification continues until ultimately the mass of the liver is formed.

As this occurs, it gradually divides the ventral mesogastrium into 2 parts: the falciform and the coronary ligaments developing from the anterior part, and the lesser omentum from the posterior. By the 3rd month of embryonic life, the liver, having differentiated from the septum transversum, has grown downward and almost filled the abdominal cavity. The left lobe later degenerates somewhat and maintains a smaller size than the right lobe. Thereafter, the relative development of the liver is slower, but it maintains a relatively larger size during later fetal life and infancy than it does in the adult. At times, all or part of the extrahepatic biliary system fails to develop, which usually

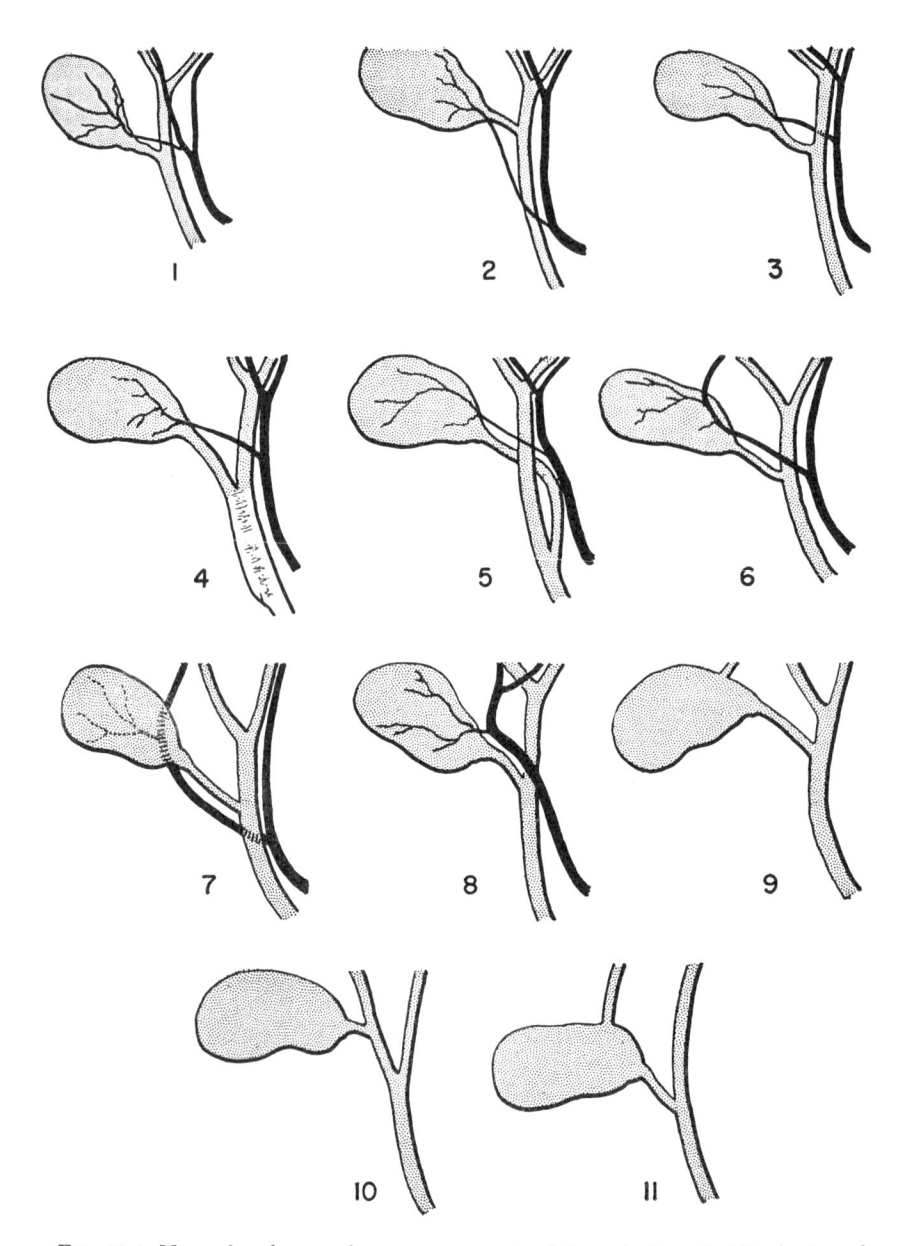

Fig. 32-1. Normal and anomalous arrangements of the extrahepatic bile ducts and their adjoining arteries.

1. Normal arrangement.
2. Caudad origin of cystic artery (frequent variation).
3. Placement of the cystic artery posterior to the common hepatic duct.
4. Long cystic duct attached to the common hepatic duct for some distance prior to the confluence to form the common bile duct.
5. Long cystic duct passing behind the common hepatic duct and joining it medially at a lower level.
6. Normal ductal system with anomalous right hepatic artery reaching the gallbladder wall where it gives off the cystic artery and then turns into the liver. In this anomaly, which is not rare, the right hepatic artery is often ligated either with the cystic duct or as a separate structure erroneously identified as the cystic artery.
7. Anomalous right hepatic artery in a posterior position presenting the same dangers as in No. 6.

(*Continued on facing page*)

results in biliary atresia or agenesis. (See Chap. 48, Pediatric Surgery, for this and other congenital anomalies of infants.) A study of the phylogeny of the liver has revealed an order with no gross extrahepatic ducts in the adult—the cyclostomata, which includes the lampreys and hagfishes.

PHYSIOLOGIC CONSIDERATIONS

The physiology of the liver parenchyma is so complex that a description of what is known about it could readily fill several volumes. The liver has certain excretory functions. Beyond this, it is the central organ of intermediary metabolism. Despite its complex function, its cellular composition seems to be remarkably simple. In addition to its supporting stroma, capsule and 3 sets of blood vessels (portal vein, hepatic artery and hepatic vein systems), it has its excretory ductal system surrounded in the bile canaliculi only by the parenchymal liver cells which are the principal functional unit of the liver. The other cells of note are the reticuloendothelial cells situated in the vascular channels. These are not peculiar to the liver, but the liver is the site of the largest aggregation of them.

The liver also possesses an extensive and important lymphatic system. Among the substances which the liver excretes are the following: water, sodium, chloride, bicarbonate, calcium, bile pigments (bilirubin; biliverdin), bile salts (sodium taurocholate; sodium glycocholate), cholesterol, certain dyes (e.g., bromsulphalein, when this is injected into the circulation; tetraiodophenolphthalein, whether injected intravenously or absorbed from the gastrointestinal tract); and alkaline phosphatase of intestinal origin.

When injured by disease or poisons the liver's excretion of bile salts declines first—probably because of interference with their formation. When excretion is impaired by obstruction of the ductal system, bilirubin and alkaline phosphatase levels both mount in the blood. The itching which is so characteristic of obstructive jaundice has been attributed to the retention of bile salts. The disappearance of bromsulphalein from the blood stream is retarded when this drug is given in test doses.

The liver is largely responsible for the reduction of amino acids to urea and glucose. It is an important site of the conversion of glucose to glycogen, the storage of glycogen, and of the conversion of glycogen to glucose. It is one of the sites in which fat is converted to fatty acids and glycerol, and vice versa. It is a site of formation of uric acid. It is the principal site of formation of albumen.

It is vital for at least two major components of the coagulation mechanism, as it is the principal site of formation of fibrinogen and of prothrombin. It is the site of conjugation of benzoic acid with glycine, which is the basis for the hippuric acid conjugation test of liver function. It is the site of hydrolysis of certain sugars, and this is the basis of the galactose tolerance test of liver function.

It is the organ that removes certain steroids from the blood, preventing an excess. Thus, when the liver is damaged by cirrhosis, estro-

---

FIG. 32-1 (*Continued*)

8. A very dangerous anomaly of the entire hepatic artery which follows the cystic duct to the gallbladder before turning into the liver. Accidental ligation of the entire hepatic artery was almost always fatal before the development of penicillin and chlortetracycline and is still hazardous.

9. Anomalous bile duct entering gallbladder through its bed in the liver. Cholecystectomy in such instances is usually followed by profuse drainage of bile and is likely to result in fatal bile peritonitis unless external drainage is afforded.

10. Anomalous insertion of cystic duct into right hepatic duct. The section of the right hepatic duct caudad to its junction with the cystic duct can easily be mistaken for the cystic duct and ligated, thus occluding the drainage of the right lobe of the liver into the intestine.

11. Anomalous arrangement of the right hepatic duct in which it enters the gallbladder so that all of the bile from the right lobe of the liver must drain through the cystic duct.

gens accumulate in the blood of male subjects to a degree which often causes mammary hypertrophy. Hydrocortisone is continuously metabolized in the normal liver with reduction to biologically inactive compounds and conjugation with glucuronic acid. The effective half life of this compound is of the order of 80 minutes. In the presence of liver damage the rate of inactivation is retarded, with the result that administration of normal dosages of hydrocortisone may produce symptoms suggestive of Cushing's disease in such patients.

It is an important site of destruction of various drugs—notably morphine and several barbituric acid derivatives, so that serial doses of these agents in usual amounts may result in an accumulation to toxic levels in subjects with damaged livers.

As physiologic investigation continues, more and more activities have been found to be attributable to the liver. The foregoing is by no means a complete list of known actions of hepatic cells, and there is a strong probability that additional hepatic activity will be revealed in the future.

New insight has been gained into the method by which the liver metabolizes certain drugs e.g., codeine and acetanilide. This story is an excellent example of serendipity. Cooper, Estabrook and Rosenthal (1963; Estabrook, et al., 1963) were studying the synthesis of corticoids by the adrenal cortex in vitro. They identified an enzyme in adrenal cortical microsomes capable of converting 17-OH progesterone to cortexolone by hydroxylation of the 21 carbon in the presence of triphosphopyridine nucleotide. Study of the enzyme showed that its effect was inhibited by carbon monoxide in a reversible manner. Reversal was effected by light—maximally by light of 450 millimicrons wavelength—the same wavelength which was maximally absorbed by the enzyme when treated with CO.

It was found that a similar enzyme had been described in liver microsomes by Klingenberg (1958) and Garfinkel (1958), but no function was assigned. Further study indicated the similarity and possible identity of these enzymes—one from the liver and one from adrenocortical sources—and showed the capacity of the enzyme for hydroxylation of acetanilide and demethylation of codeine. It is believed that certain carcinogens may be similarly detoxified or activated. The question of whether sufficient carbon monoxide is given off from a cigarette to interfere with the enzyme and its ability to detoxify carcinogens has been studied. As of the date of writing no data which when considered quantitatively could substantiate this interesting theory has been reported. The enzyme—referred to as the 450 millimicrons CO combining pigment (P-450)—has been concentrated and at least partially purified and its role in the metabolism of certain drugs demonstrated.

A role for the liver in the regulation of renal function has recently been suggested by Berkowitz, Miller, and Itskovitz (1968). These workers believe that the normal physiologic action of the renin-angiotensin system, previously unassigned, is to function as a controlling mechanism over the intrarenal distribution of blood flow, resulting in marked alterations in renal functional parameters. Utilizing an isolated, blood-perfused kidney system, they demonstrated that, with prolonged perfusion, renal function deteriorates concomitantly with a drop in the renin substrate level in the perfusate. At this point, infusions of renin substrate, alone—the necessary precursor for intrarenal angiotensin formation—results in significant improvement in glomerular filtration rate, renal vascular resistance, and the excretion of sodium and water. Since renin substrate is produced by the liver, in the alpha-2 globulin fraction, these findings may provide a partial explanation of the renal sequelae of advanced liver disease, the so-called *hepatorenal syndrome*, which has been shown to be a renin substrate-deficient state (Berkowitz, Miller and Itskovitz, 1968).

The reticuloendothelial cells are important in removing particulate matter, such as carbon particles (as when India ink is injected intravenously experimentally), bacteria, et cetera, from the blood stream. Thus, they have an important function in resistance to infection. They are specifically involved with the conversion of hemoglobin derived from old erythrocytes to bilirubin which is carried in the plasma conjugated with albumin to the hepatic parenchymal cells, where it is separated from albumin and excreted in the bile conjugated with glucuronides. They are the site of accumulation of heparin which may be released by peptone shock. It was formerly thought that this occurred following exposure of the whole body to ionizing radiation and accounted for some of the hemorrhagic tendency found in radiation victims. It is now believed that this is not a major factor in this clinical picture (Hewitt, 1953; DiLuzio, 1957).

This brief list is sufficient to show that an individual whose liver has been severely damaged by acute poisoning, such as chloroform, by acute infection, such as hepatitis, or by chronic damage as in various types of cirrhosis, is liable to many physiologic derangements. Especially important among these are hypoalbuminemia, hypoprothrombinemia, intermittent hypoglycemia—which at times has been falsely attributed to hyperinsulinism, and failure to detoxify drugs at the expected rate, with consequent overdosage. It is clear that the liver is an essential organ and cannot be sacrificed.

At the same time it must be borne in mind constantly that the liver has a large margin of reserve function, so that in some experimental animals four fifths of it can be sacrificed with survival. Hepatic lymph is peculiar; it contains almost as high a concentration of serum albumen as does plasma.

Bile in a quantity of 350 to 1,000 ml. per day is secreted by the liver. With the sphincter of Oddi closed, pressure relationships exist whereby most of this bile flows to the gallbladder. Hepatic bile consists mainly of water, cholesterol, bile pigments, inorganic salts and salts of bile acids. In the gallbladder, water with chlorides and bicarbonates is absorbed, increasing the relative concentration of bile pigments and bile salts. The concentrate is stored in the gallbladder until it is expelled.

When gastric chyme comes into contact with the duodenal mucosa, a hormone, *cholecystokinin*, is released which causes the gallbladder to contract and the sphincter of Oddi to relax, thus making bile available for digestion.

In pathologic states, such as cholecystitis, the gallbladder very often loses progressively its capacity to concentrate bile salts and bile pigment. Figure 32-2, taken from the paper of Riegel, Ravdin, Johnston and Morrison (1936), demonstrates this graphically.

In the presence of jaundice or of liver damage without jaundice, the composition of hepatic bile will be altered also (compare section on The Jaundiced Patient).

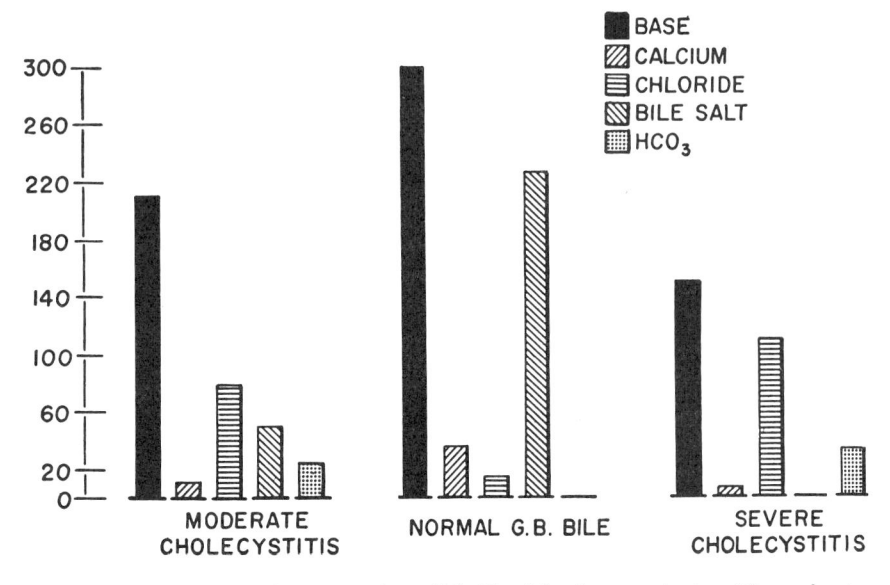

FIG. 32-2. Chemical differences in gallbladder bile from patients with moderate cholecystitis, patients with normal gallbladders, and patients with severe cholecystitis. Note particularly the profound diminution in bile salt concentration in the bile from diseased gallbladders. (Riegel, C., Ravdin, I., Johnston, C., and Morrison, P.: Surg., Gynec., Obstet., 62:933, 1936)

TUMORS OF THE GALLBLADDER AND THE EXTRAHEPATIC BILE DUCTS

Benign papillomas occasionally occur in the gallbladder. At times the roentgenologist can suggest the diagnosis on the basis of fixation of an isolated shadow seen on a cholecystogram. The malignant potential of such lesions is not accurately known. Their removal by cholecystectomy is recommended because of the possibility of malignant degeneration, the possibility that they may cause symptoms—perhaps by acting like a ball valve—and the considerable doubt that surrounds their diagnosis by roentgenography. A shadow suggestive of such a papilloma may turn out to be due to stone or, conceivably, to carcinoma.

Carcinoma is the only primary malignant tumor occurring in the gallbladder with any frequency. It was found in 1.41 per cent of a series of 3,842 gallbladders removed at the Hospital of the University of Pennsylvania. The survival rate of patients who develop carcinoma of the gallbladder is pitifully low—under 5 per cent in most series. Those few who do survive are apt to be among cases in which the malignancy was an unexpected pathologic finding.

Since 73 per cent of gallbladder carcinomas are associated with stones, it has been suggested that all gallbladders containing stones should be removed for cancer prophylaxis. Certain authors have reported a 5 per cent incidence of carcinoma of the gallbladder among stone-bearing gallbladders. We do not believe that such a figure is representative but would analyze the problem as follows:

1. The incidence of gallstones increases in autopsy material with each decade of life.
2. The average age of death from gallbladder carcinoma is between 50 and 60 years.
3. The incidence of gallstones in this decade (50 to 60) is 21 per cent.
4. Autopsy studies reveal that the incidence of gallstones in the presence of gallbladder carcinoma is 73 per cent, and the over-all incidence of gallbladder carcinoma in long series of autopsies is only 0.39 per cent.

Therefore, if 73 per cent of the carcinomas occur in the 21 per cent of patients who have stones, the incidence of gallbladder carcinoma among stone-bearers is 1.42 per cent—not far different from the figure of 1.41 per cent actually found in our clinic at operation. Thus, it appears that the incidence of carcinoma is about as high among the asymptomatic stone-bearers as among those who come to operation.

The average expectation that a person aged 59 will live 5 years is 89 per cent (Life Insurance Fact Book, 1959). Those who have gallbladder carcinoma can expect to live 5 years in only about 3 per cent of instances. Therefore, the salvage from gallbladder carcinoma death would be the incidence, $1.42\% \times (89\% - 3\%) = 1.22\%$ per 100 stone-bearers cholecystectomized before developing carcinoma. If the operative mortality can be held down to 0.5 per cent, one can theoretically justify removing the gallbladders of all stone-bearers at about age 50. However, the margin is rather narrow and, if due to mischance the mortality should rise to 2.0 per cent, one would lose more patients than he saved by such a policy. (Campbell, 1941; Cooper, W. A., 1937; Illingworth, 1935; Jankelson, 1937; Kirshbaum, 1941; Roberts, 1957; Robertson, 1944; Sainburg, 1948; Sawyer, 1956; and Swinton, 1948).

The tumors of the common hepatic and common bile ducts are similar to those of the gallbladder. Benign papillomas occur but are rare. Carcinomas may produce early jaundice leading to operation and diagnosis. Those arising in the intrapancreatic portion of the common duct and the papilla of Vater may sometimes be saved and are discussed with the pancreaticoduodenal carcinomas in Chapter 33. Those arising cephalad to the level of the duodenum have been uniformly fatal in the author's experience. Palliative relief of jaundice can sometimes be achieved by shunts of one type or another.

In a few instances, carcinoma of the gallbladder discovered at operation has been treated by right hepatic lobectomy as well as cholecystectomy and removal of lymph nodes about the common bile duct. This high risk procedure is not yet sufficiently well evolved to permit a recommendation but, at present, it seems doubtful if it will help to solve the problem of gallbladder carcinoma.

HEMOBILIA

Bleeding from the biliary tract into the duodenum may occur and occasionally becomes life-threatening. While hypoprothrombinemia may be a contributory factor, the term hemobilia is not usually applied to hypothrombinemia which may be equated to the earlier term "hemorrhagic tendency of obstructive jaundice."

The latter is a general tendency, even though it may be manifest from the biliary tract after operations on it.

Hemobilia is a term introduced by Philip Sandblom (1948) to describe a group of cases which presented with gastrointestinal hemorrhage but in which it was found that the bleeding was coming from the biliary tract and entering the duodenum by way of the common duct. The causes of this phenomenon include tumors (rare) and traumatic wounds of the liver, those due both to penetration from the body surface and to blunt trauma. Such hemorrhage may be delayed. Some of the former are iatrogenic and have resulted from attempts at needle biopsy or direct injection of contrast media into the ductal system for radiography.

ACUTE CHOLECYSTITIS

Acute cholecystitis is a condition characterized by hyperemia, edema and polymorphonuclear cell infiltration and, in many instances, patchy or extensive necrosis of the mucosa of the gallbladder. Although the gallbladder is essentially a diverticulum of the main bile duct, an inflammatory process may not affect the other ducts in ways that are apparent. On the other hand, there is evidence in many cases that the inflammatory process does affect the biliary tract more widely. This is manifested by mild rises in serum bilirubin, typically of 1.0 to 2.0 mg. per 100 ml. While stones usually are found in patients with acute cholecystitis, this is not always the case. Berk (1940, 1946) found calculi obstructing the neck of the gallbladder in 92 per cent of such cases. Acute cholecystitis can be produced experimentally in the goat by ligating the common channel formed by the common bile duct and the pancreatic duct, thus causing a retrograde flow of pancreatic juice into the gallbladder and stasis of bile (Bisgard, 1940). Thus, it is postulated that pancreatic ferments may contribute to an occasional case of acute cholecystitis in human patients.

Experimentally, Gatch (1946) produced acute cholecystitis by injecting bile salts into the portal veins of dogs, increasing the concentration in the bile. The experimental production of cholecystitis seemingly has little relation to the clinical condition. Though infection often plays an important role in acute cholecystitis, this appears to be secondary to other factors such as stones. In addition to *Salmonella typhosa*, which characteristically gains access to the gallbladder and may persist there for many years, common bacteria found in this organ include *Escherichia coli*, other organisms of the coliform group, *Pseudomonas aeruginosa*, common pyogens, such as the streptococcus and the staphylococcus, and various representatives of the clostridium group.

Signs and Symptoms

The signs and symptoms of acute cholecystitis are usually rapid rather than sudden in onset. Fever and leukocytosis are well marked. Vomiting may be serious, leading to dehydration. Slight hyperbilirubinemia may be present. Local symptoms are striking; usually there is persistent pain in the right upper quadrant or the epigastrium. If the pain radiates to the back, in the region of the angle of the scapula or in the interscapular area, the diagnosis is strengthened. The pain is associated with tenderness commonly maximal just below the right costal margin, and deep breathing often aggravates the pain. Rebound tenderness is often demonstrable and may be referred to the gallbladder area. Moderate to marked muscle spasm, generally more or less localized to the right upper quadrant, is the rule. Peristalsis diminishes somewhat; however, the sounds seldom cease for more than a minute or 2 unless the gallbladder ruptures. A mass, usually the gallbladder, may be palpated in a third or more of the cases. Muscle spasm often prevents palpation; therefore, the gallbladder may become palpable for the first time after the attack has begun to subside or after anesthesia is induced.

While gallbladder pain is typically lateralized to the right, it may be bilateral or occasionally predominantly on the left side. The mechanism of this is not clear, but it is a fact to be reckoned with in diagnosis, as left-sided reference does not rule out the presence of an acute cholecystitis.

DIAGNOSIS

The diagnosis may be easy but at times can be confused with ruptured ulcer or necrotizing pancreatitis, which is often more severe, or with edematous pancreatitis, which frequently may coexist with cholecystitis.

Other conditions that may give rise to similar symptoms are acute appendicitis, coronary insufficiency with angina pectoris or coronary thrombosis, chronic passive congestion affecting the liver, pneumonia, pleurisy, renal colic, intestinal obstruction, tabetic crisis, lead colic, herpes zoster, phlegmonous gastritis, and gonococcal peritonitis with adhesions forming between the diaphragm and the liver (Curtis—Fitz-Hugh Syndrome). The diagnosis usually is confirmed at the operation if the symptoms do not improve fairly promptly, and by roentgenogram if improvement supervenes. Before operation an electrocardiogram and x-ray examination of the chest and the abdomen are frequently indicated.

After making the diagnosis, the decisions (1) when to operate and (2) whether to do a cholecystostomy (drainage of the gallbladder) or a cholecystectomy (removal of the gallbladder) have to be reached. If symptoms do not abate, complications may ensue, such as gangrene and perforation leading to internal biliary fistulas connecting with bowel or the common duct, pericholecystic abscess, or even spreading peritonitis, pylephlebitis (inflammation in the portal venous system), cholangitis, pancreatitis, hepatitis or septicemia. In the acute case, edema and hyperemia are often so severe as to interfere seriously with safe dissection and exposure of the common duct and the cystic ducts. To insist on carrying out cholecystectomy under these circumstances is to risk injury to the main ductal system or the hepatic artery. Therefore, the safe surgeon sometimes will perform only a cholecystostomy when operating during the acute phase. Most of these patients will require a second operation later for removal of the gallbladder. Donald and Fitts' follow-up study (1949) indicates that it is wise to recommend elective cholecystectomy within several months in almost all patients having cholecystostomy. In general, three months is a suitable interval between a cholecystostomy and the subsequent cholecystectomy. Rarely, another acute attack will supervene within this period, but early reoperation is usually handicapped by the postoperative reaction to the first procedure.

PERFORATION OF THE GALLBLADDER WITH ABSCESS, PERITONITIS, OR BILIARY FISTULA

Rupture of the gallbladder is less frequent than rupture of the appendix. Nevertheless, it constitutes a grave hazard in acute cholecystitis, especially in elderly patients, and it is this danger that forces operation in a considerable number of poor-risk patients at times when they are acutely ill.

Rupture of the gallbladder is of 3 types: (1) it may rupture slowly into a previously prepared abscessed pocket—rupture with localized abscess; (2) it may rupture suddenly into the general peritoneal cavity—rupture into free peritoneal cavity; or (3) it may rupture slowly into an adjoining viscus attached by adhesions, especially the duodenum, the stomach or the colon—rupture with biliary fistula.

After rupture into the free peritoneal cavity, bile leakage through the cystic duct into the open gallbladder may lead to bile peritonitis. This is the only one of the 3 types of rupture of the gallbladder which causes bile peritonitis which, if untreated by early drainage, is apt to result in a fatal issue. Bile peritonitis is harmful not only because of infection but also because of the irritant action of the bile. This irritant action leads to shock due to plasma leakage from the peritoneal surfaces (see Chap. 7, Shock) and also to fat necrosis due either to damage to the pancreas or to reflux of pancreatic enzymes (see Chap. 33, Pancreas).

The third type of rupture of the gallbladder (rupture with biliary fistula) may lead to the interesting syndrome of gallstone ileus (see Chap. 38, Intestinal Obstruction) if a large gallbladder stone passes through the fistula into the upper intestinal tract and then becomes impacted in the narrow lower ileum or elsewhere in the gut.

In modern hospital experience 2 per cent of the patients operated upon for disease of the biliary tract have rupture of the gallbladder, while the incidence rises to 10 per cent in cases of acute cholecystitis. The mortality rate among the patients with all types of gallbladder perforation averages about 20 per cent. The mortality for the type of perforation with localized abscess is usually less than this overall figure. On the other hand, perforation with biliary fistula has a relatively low immediate mortality, but when the mortality of operations for cure of the fistula is included, the total mortality for cases with biliary fistula rises toward that for free perforation. For additional data on the incidence and the mortality of gallbladder rupture, the reader is referred to the work of the following authors and their collaborators: Stevenson (1957); Fletcher (1951); Pines (1954); Cowley (1943); Massie (1957); McCubbrey (1960); Becker (1957); and Morse (1957).

DIAGNOSIS

Typically, the attack of free perforation is similar to other attacks of acute gallbladder disease, but instead of subsiding, the acute symptoms spread—usually after 24 hours—and the local and systemic signs of peritonitis supervene. Unfortunately, the complication is prone to occur in elderly and debilitated persons and often is not attended by the amount of fever and/or leukocytosis which would be expected in a typical case of peritonitis. For this reason, persons over the age of 65 or persons who are weak and debilitated at any age should, in general, be operated on for an acute gallbladder attack if it persists over 24 hours without clear evidence that it is subsiding.

Unfortunately, not all cases of gallbladder perforation are preceded by sufficiently characteristic symptoms to lead to the diagnosis. In fact, some patients who develop fistulae into the intestine may seek medical advice only after the stone has passed down the intestine and caused an obstruction.

The diagnosis of biliary fistula can often be made preoperatively by a combination of the patient's history and the finding of gas or barium in the biliary tract on x-ray examination. Ingestion of a carbonated beverage may be helpful in demonstrating this phenomenon.

PATHOLOGY

The gallbladder may have only a single point of necrosis, which gives way or becomes gangrenous with escape of bacteria through it, or the entire organ may rarely become gangrenous as though its blood supply had become compromised by distention or by thrombosis. As is usual when stones are present, bacteria are apt to be present, so that one is generally dealing with a bacterial as well as with a chemical peritonitis when the gallbladder ruptures.

TREATMENT

The objectives of the immediate treatment of free perforation are removal of necrotic material and stones and adequate drainage to the outside of the body. Thus, a cholecystostomy plus the placing of drains in the subhepatic space and, if the peritonitis is extensive, in the subdiaphragmatic space and the pelvis is usual. If the gallbladder wall is gangrenous, the gangrenous part should be removed even if this requires a cholecystectomy. However, one need not be concerned with completing the cholecystectomy to within 5.0 mm. of the common duct but can stop it as soon as viable tissue is reached and drain the cystic duct or the infundibulum, as the case may be. These patients are actually or potentially very ill, and the procedure should be aimed solely at saving life with virtually no concern about the question of whether or not a subsequent operation may be required.

The treatment of perforation with localized abscess is little different from that of acute cholecystitis in a seriously ill patient except that an additional drain to the site of the abscess is generally required.

The treatment of perforation with biliary fistula is usually an elective procedure and, unless there is accompanying gallstone ileus, the patients are not acutely ill, although they may be seriously debilitated. However, the technical aspects of dealing not only with the diseased gallbladder but also with closure of the fistula into the intestine—all in scar tissue—may make this a formidable operation. Furthermore, the fistula may be kept open by obstruction at the ampulla of Vater by a common duct stone—the bile draining through the fistula into the intestinal tract, so that the patient is not jaundiced. In such cases, when the fistula is closed, the common duct should be carefully palpated for the presence of stones and, if stones are present, they should be removed. It is essential to establish the patency of the common duct either by actual exploration or by operative cholangiography or both when closing a fistula between the biliary tract and the intestinal tract.

Postoperative treatment is of great importance in the free perforation, as in any case of peritonitis. It consists in a regimen which includes gastrointestinal rest produced by giving nothing by mouth and by nasogastric suction; by support of blood volume with lactated Ringer's solution and transfusions of blood; and by antibiotics—at first selected by guess and then chosen on the basis of bacterial sensitivity studies. Nutritional support is given by parenteral routes. It includes water, sodium, potassium, chloride, glucose and, if the course is long, other nutritive substances. With timely intervention and vigorous but judicious support, a great majority of such patients can be saved.

CHRONIC CALCULOUS CHOLECYSTITIS AND CHRONIC NONCALCULOUS CHOLECYSTITIS

As in the case of acute cholecystitis, chronic cholecystitis can occur without stones. Unfortunately, surgical experience in treating noncalculous chronic cholecystitis has been exceedingly unsatisfactory. According to most authors, the majority of such patients have residual postoperative digestive complaints, frequently of greater magnitude than those for which the operation was carried out. From the surgical standpoint, therefore, the objective in studying patients suspected of having chronic cholecystitis is to establish the presence or the absence of cholelithiasis with reasonable certainty. The association of cholelithiasis with symptoms of discomfort after eating generally are considered as an indication for operation unless outweighed by contraindications, such as severe renal disease, etc.

There are 3 principal avenues through which a diagnosis of cholelithiasis is approached. First, there is the history and the physical examination. Most typically, the patient is a woman in middle life and inclined toward obesity who has intermittent attacks of severe pain in the right upper quadrant of the abdomen or the epigastrium, most often coming on in the evening or at night following a heavy meal. Often it is associated with radiation of the pain to the back in the region of the angle of the right scapula or the angles of both scapulae, at about the level of the 8th dorsal segment and with nausea and vomiting. Often the patients have such severe pains that they call their physicians during attacks and are given morphine or other narcotics hypodermically. Many of them have been pregnant, and frequently the initial symptoms start during or immediately after a pregnancy. In addition to the severe attacks, such individuals often have postprandial fullness and distress in the epigastrium, accentuated by fatty foods and sometimes by cabbage or other closely related vegetables. Belching and sour eructations are common. Always it is important to inquire for a history of jaundice or of the appearance of especially dark urine, or of light-gray or putty-colored stools. Such symptoms, especially if they are of brief duation and intermittent, are highly suggestive of common duct obstruction due to stones. If the bouts of jaundice are ushered in by a fever and a chill, one has the classical picture of common duct obstruction due to stones described by Charcot (Charcot's intermittent hepatic fever).

Even without symptoms of common duct obstruction, if the patient has severe acute bouts of epigastric or right upper quadrant pain radiating to the right scapula with upper quadrant tenderness and a palpable mass, one can feel relatively certain that the patient has cholelithiasis. In fact, the existence of the above triad—typical pain, tenderness and mass—is indicative of the presence of gallstones 9 times out of 10. Babcock (1937) has stated that 94 per cent of patients with the typical clinical history have gallstones.

In the great majority of instances, however, the history is far less typical. It may consist only of some postprandial distress and upper abdominal discomfort. Under such circumstances, it is necessary to rely heavily on laboratory methods in order to reach a definitive diagnosis of cholelithiasis. Roentgenographic technics undoubtedly constitute the most valuable of these methods. A simple scout film of the abdomen will reveal gallstones in only about 10 to 15 per cent of patients having them. The amount of calcium necessary for a stone to show varies markedly with the distribution of the calcium in the stone. If it is evenly diffused through the substance of the stone, it may take much more calcium to render the stone sufficiently opaque to be demonstrable on an x-ray film than if the calcium is deposited in a particular layer or lamina of the stone so that it forms ring-shaped shadows (Fig. 32-3).

Because such a small percentage of gallstones are radiopaque, as contrasted with the urinary tract, where upward of 90 per cent may be demonstrated on a scout film, Graham, Cole and Copher (1925) devised a method of successfully demonstrating many of the nonopaque stones by the oral or intravenous administration of tetraiodophenolphthalein. This dye, absorbed into the blood stream, is excreted by the liver and is concentrated in the gallbladder. Thus, the functional gallbladder may be visualized roentgenographically, usually about 12 to 18 hours after ingestion of the dye. Nonopaque stones then stand out as negative shadows. The use of this dye intravenously was abandoned in many clinics because of occasional severe reactions, sometimes leading to death.

Other preparations, such as Priodax (iodoalphionic acid; beta-(4-hydroxy-3,5-diiodophenyl)-alpha-phenylpropionic acid), Telepaque (iopanoic acid; 3-(3-amino-2,4,6-triiodophenyl)-2-ethyl propionic acid) and Cholografin (meglumine iodipamide; [3,3'-(adipoyldiimido)bis - (2,4,6 - triiodo - benzoic acid)] (Frommhold, 1953), have been introduced and appear to have some advantages over the original material, although they are effective for the same reasons. Cholografin is the first material to be excreted in sufficient concentration in hepatic bile to make possible more or less routine films of the common bile duct. This is obviously a real advance, although it is to be hoped that still futher gains may be possible in this field. It is of considerable importance that a flat film be done as a routine before the dye appears, as a stone of density equal to that of the dye may blend in with the dye if only a cholecystogram is done.

Practical points to remember in connection with cholecystograms are: (1) that films should be taken in various degrees of obliquity in order to throw the shadow of the gallblad-

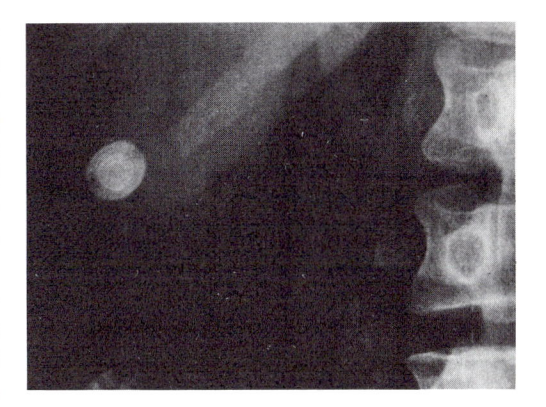

FIG. 32-3. Laminated gallstone.

der away from the colon which, when containing a pocket of gas, may suggest a gallstone if superimposed on the gallbladder shadow; (2) that some of the dyes induce vomiting or diarrhea. Therefore, if the gallbladder fails to visualize, it is important to inquire whether the patient did vomit or whether he had diarrhea after taking the tablets. It is important, of course, to be sure that the patient did take the tablets, and finally it is often best to give the patient additional tablets and to make a second attempt at demonstrating the gallbladder if the first attempt fails to do so. Repetition of the original recommended dose is appropriate. The doubling of the second dose was a common practice until renal toxicity was encountered with Priodax (Malt, Olsen and Good, 1963). Tincture of paregoric in adult doses of 4 to 8 cc. may be very helpful in preventing or diminishing the diarrhea.

The results of such tests may clearly demonstrate gallstones (Fig. 32-4) or they may show that the gallbladder does not visualize, or that it visualizes very weakly. A well-visualized gallbladder that shows no stones, taken in conjunction with a flat film which showed no opaque stones, is fairly strong evidence against cholelithiasis in the gallbladder. Rarely, a stone may be small enough to be overlooked on the cholecystogram and yet large enough to block the cystic duct. If the gallbladder is not visualized in either of 2 cholecystograms for which an appropriate dye was given in recommended doses and retained within the gastrointestinal tract satisfactorily, it is reasonable to suppose that cholelithiasis and gallbladder disease exist. This may be

892   Liver, Gallbladder and Bile Passages

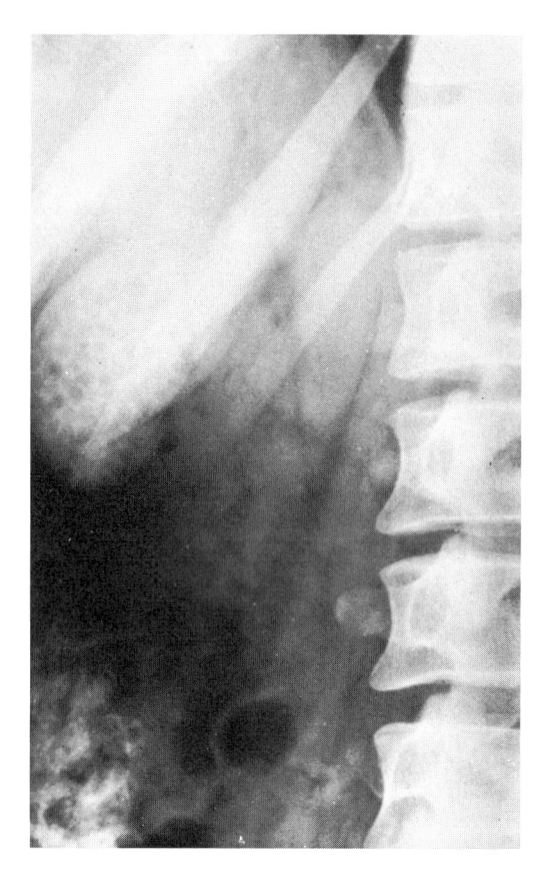

FIG. 32-4. Typical cholecystogram, showing 71 stones (nonopaque).

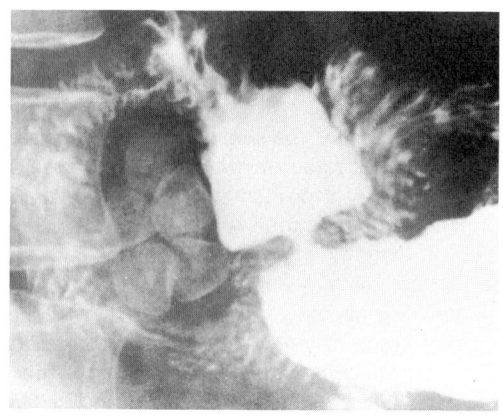

FIG. 32-5. Oblique film, showing radiopaque gallstones in gallbladder projected over duodenal loop. Duodenum is opacified with barium.

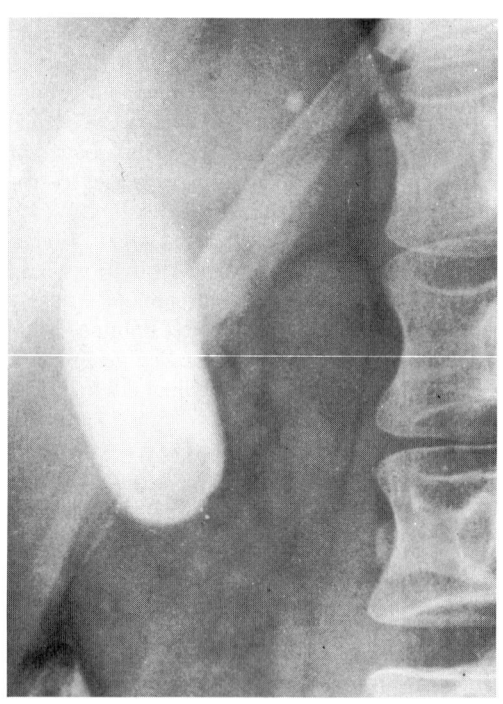

FIG. 32-6. Cholecystogram, showing solitary large stone in fundus of the gallbladder.

due to an actual cystic duct obstruction, or it may be due to loss of the chemical functions of the gallbladder (see section on Physiology).

In many instances, the decision to operate rests on failure to visualize the gallbladder in the cholecystogram plus a suggestive but not classic history of gallbladder symptoms.

The direct demonstration of stones in patients with cholelithiasis is raised to the range of 55 or 60 per cent by means of the cholecystogram. In most of the remaining individuals who harbor stones, the gallbladder will fail repeatedly to concentrate the dye sufficiently for visualization. In other words, repeated failure of the gallbladder to visualize is good evidence that it contains stones (present in more than 85%).

It is important in assessing gallbladder function to recognize that severely impaired liver function may be a cause of the failure of the gallbladder to visualize. Thus, in patients with jaundice, no weight can be given to failure of the gallbladder to visualize, and usually the decision for or against operation is arrived at best without recourse to a cholecystogram.

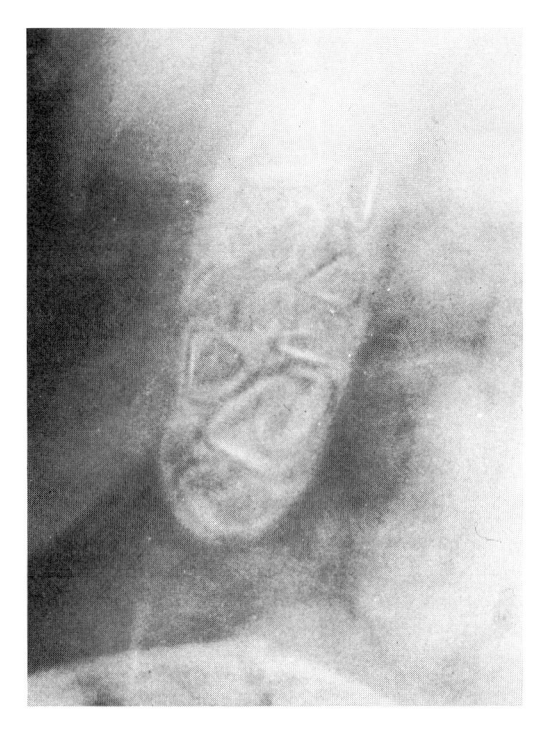

FIG. 32-7. Multifaceted stones in the gallbladder, showing peripheral calcification.

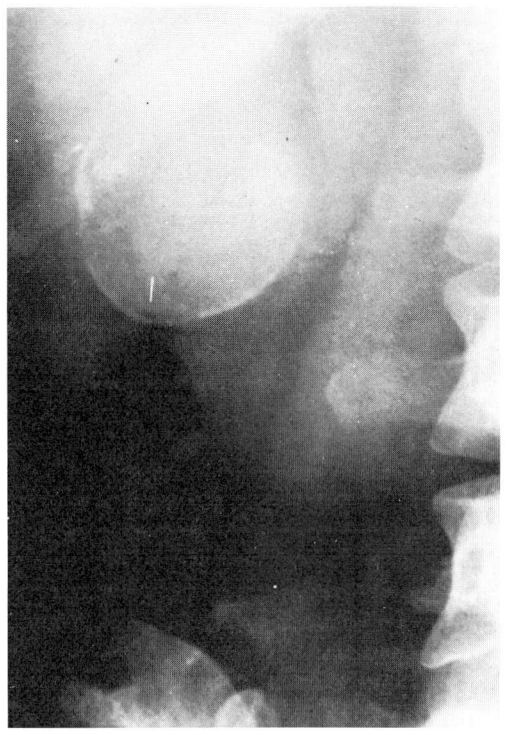

FIG. 32-8. Calcification in the wall of the gallbladder. A marble-sized stone was impacted in the cystic duct at the time of operation.

Additional examples of roentgenologic studies of the biliary tract are shown in Figures 32-5 to 32-20.

The third method of diagnosis is biliary drainage. For this purpose, a rubber tube 3 or 4 ft. long and about 16 mm. in circumference is passed through the patient's nose, pharynx and esophagus into the stomach and from there is advanced so that the tip lies beyond the pylorus. Suitable tubes for this purpose have all of their openings close to the distal end of the tube, so that once this has passed the pylorus, aspiration will not withdraw material from the stomach simultaneously with that from the duodenum. In order to get the tube past the pylorus, the patient is placed on his right side, and sometimes a metal weight is used on the end of the tube. The position of the end of the tube must be checked, either by fluoroscopy or by aspiration of the tube and testing the samples aspirated with litmus paper —an alkaline reaction indicating that the tube has passed beyond the stomach. With the tube in this position, duodenal contents are aspirated, and this is designated as "A-bile." Then the gallbladder is stimulated to contract by the administration of either olive oil or concentrated magnesium sulfate. Most workers feel that the oil is unsatisfactory because it interferes with the microscopic examination of subsequent samples. In normal individuals, stimulation of the gallbladder is followed by the recovery of dark black-brown concentrated bile. This is the sample (B-bile) most likely to give evidences of cholelithiasis. The presence of amorphous aggregates of calcium bilirubinate and of the flat platelike crystals of cholesterol are indicative of cholelithiasis. These are illustrated in Figure 32-21. If both are present in fresh biliary drainage samples, the incidence of cholelithiasis, according to Bockus, Shay, Willard and Pessel (1931), is 90 per cent. Such findings, taken in conjunction with symptoms suggestive of biliary tract disease, are commonly used as an indication for operation when the roentgenogram is doubtful or difficult to interpret. Frequently, a

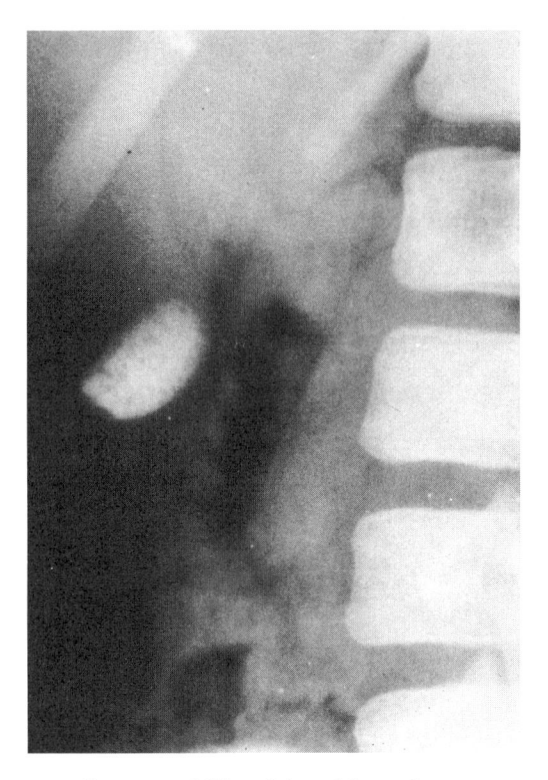

FIG. 32-9. Milk calcium bile and stones in 8-year-old patient with congenital hemolytic anemia. (Stones palpated during splenectomy.)

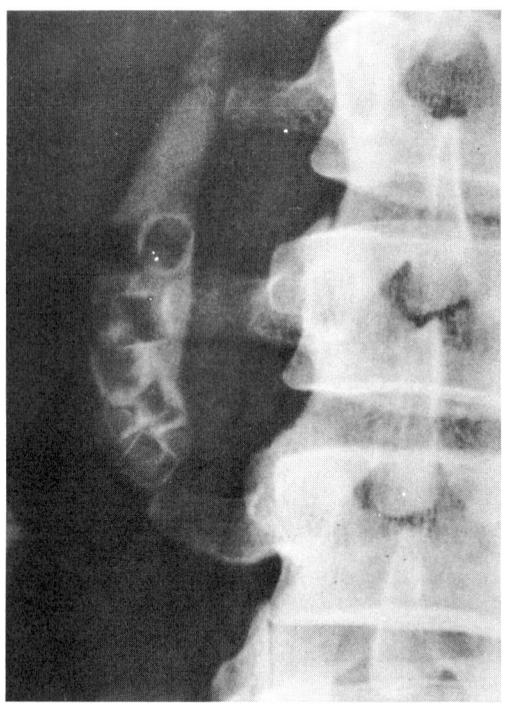

FIG. 32-10. Cholecystogram, showing faceted stones in a gallbladder that shows some function.

third sample of bile is collected following stimulation of the gallbladder and aspiration of the B-bile; this is spoken of as C-bile and is thought to represent hepatic bile as it comes from the liver. The results of biliary drainage studies have been strikingly related to the experience and the interest of the individual making the examination. Under most circumstances, negative findings should not be given much weight.

Therefore, it is readily seen that diagnosis of patients with chronic calculous cholecystitis may be difficult and that the diagnostic criteria on which we rely are not completely accurate. If an operation is undertaken on these criteria and the gallbladder appears entirely normal at operation, it is difficult for the surgeon to know what to do, or for the medical consultant to advise him. It has been the author's experience that if the gallbladder shows evidence of fibrosis, adhesions or thickening of the wall, generally it is best to remove it, for in most such instances small granular stones have been found in the region of the cystic duct. However, if the gallbladder really appears normal in every respect, at times he has preferred to do an exploratory cholecystostomy, and if no stones can be recovered by stone forceps and scoop and if no cholesterosis is present, the gallbladder has not been removed but has been drained to the outside with a catheter or a plain rubber tube for about 2 weeks.

Cholesterosis, the deposit of cholesterol in the gallbladder wall, may be visible only from the mucosal side when it appears as a network of fine straw-colored lines. If the mucosa is hyperemic, the appearance is reminiscent of the surface of a strawberry (strawberry gallbladder). Such gallbladders should be removed when encountered at operation, even though no stone is found in the lumen. Whenever the gallbladder is opened and not removed, it should be drained.

Despite the many impressive series of cholecystectomies that have been done without drainage, the editors feel strongly that when-

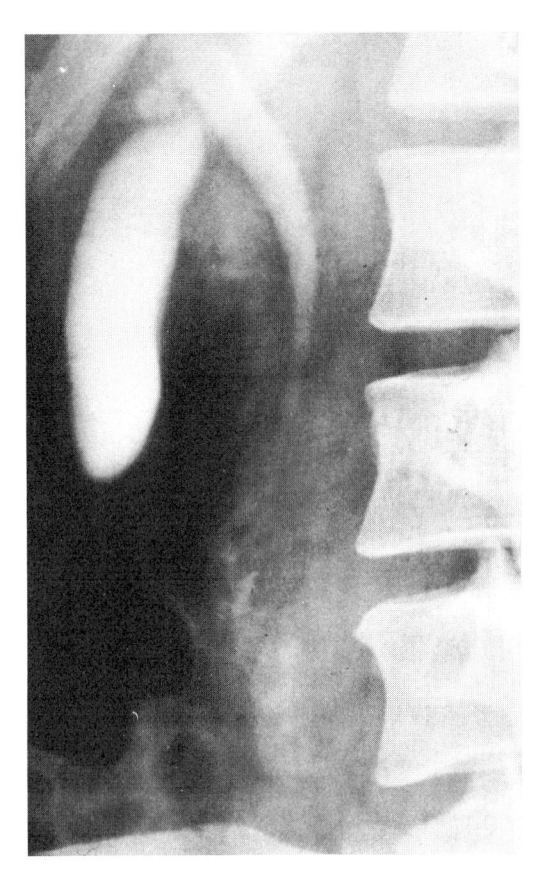

FIG. 32-11. Demonstration of the common bile duct and the cystic duct during a routine cholecystogram.

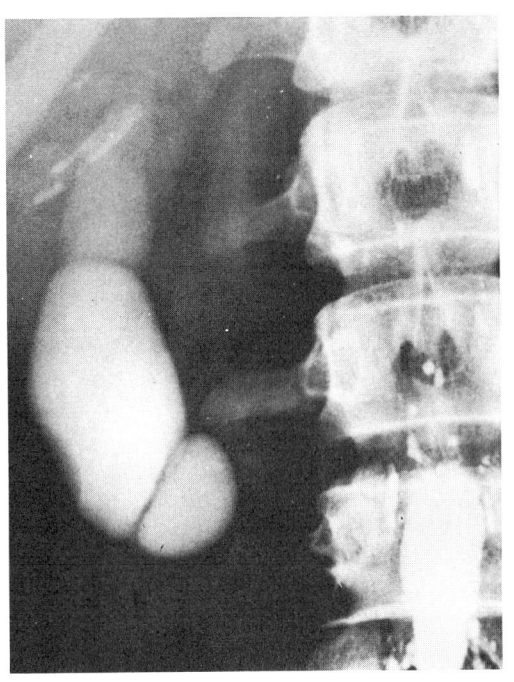

FIG. 32-13. Cholecystogram, showing functioning gallbladder with phrygian cap. (Note also contrast material in spinal canal introduced previously for myelography.)

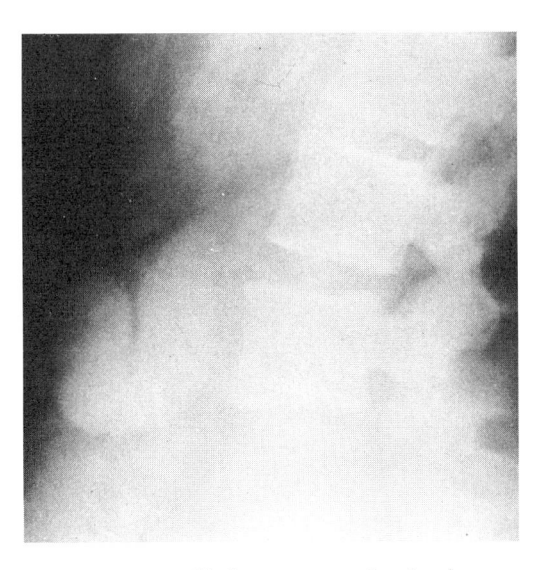

FIG. 32-12. Cholecystogram, showing long S-shaped gallbladder, a normal variant.

ever the biliary tract is entered, drains should be employed. (See section on Biliary Tract Operations.)

DIAGNOSIS OF COMMON DUCT STONE AND OTHER INDICATIONS FOR CHOLEDOCHOSTOMY

In a patient with cholelithiasis, jaundice is prima facie evidence of a stone in the common duct and, if there are indications for any elective biliary tract operation in such a case, choledochostomy is almost always indicated. The history of previous jaundice in a patient presenting other indications for operation on the biliary tract is accepted by most surgeons as an indication for choledochostomy. Palpation of a stone in the common duct at the time of operation is likewise an indication, and palpation should be carried out not only at the beginning of the procedure but also after the common duct is mobilized as fully as the surgeon feels is justified. The existence of a dilated common duct is generally accepted as an

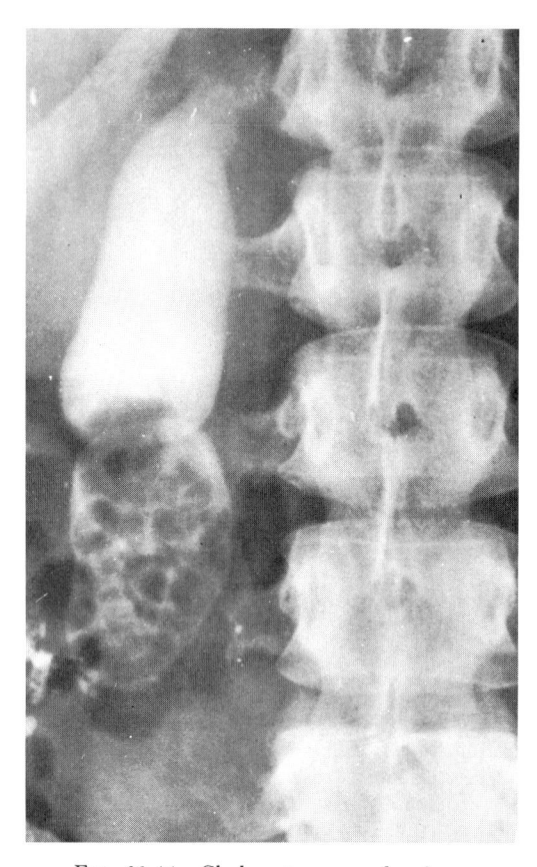

FIG. 32-14. Cholecystogram, showing a gallbladder with an hourglass constriction and stones appearing in the distal half only.

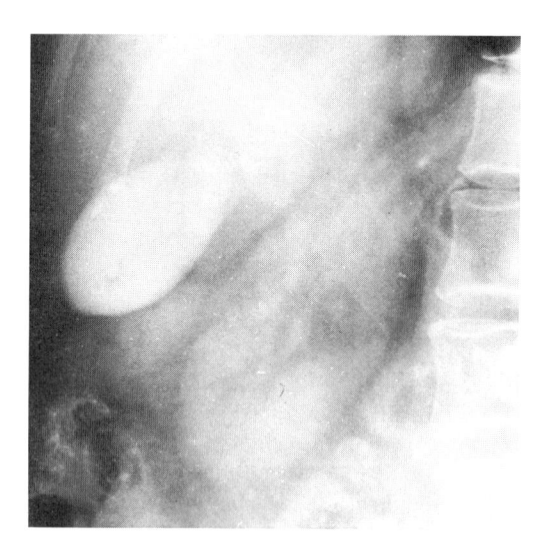

FIG. 32-15. Cholecystogram, showing stellate area of radiolucency due to a gas pocket within a stone.

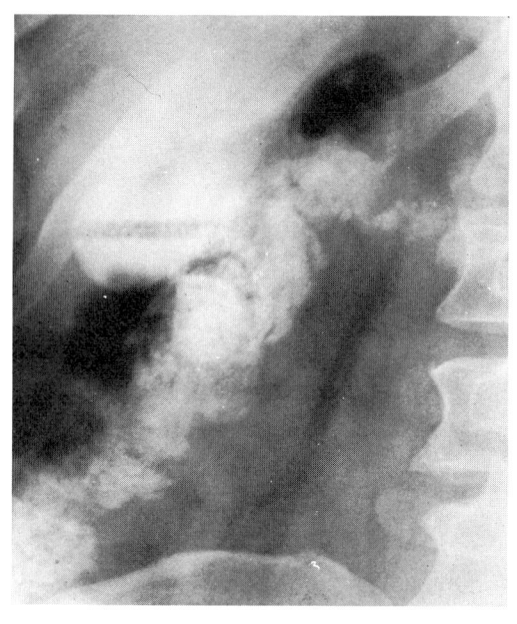

FIG. 32-16. Layering of nonopaque gallstones as seen on a cholecystogram. Film made with patient erect.

indication to explore it and to carry out a choledochostomy. Some allowance should be made for the physiologic dilatation that occurs if a cholecystectomy has been done many months previously. The existence of small

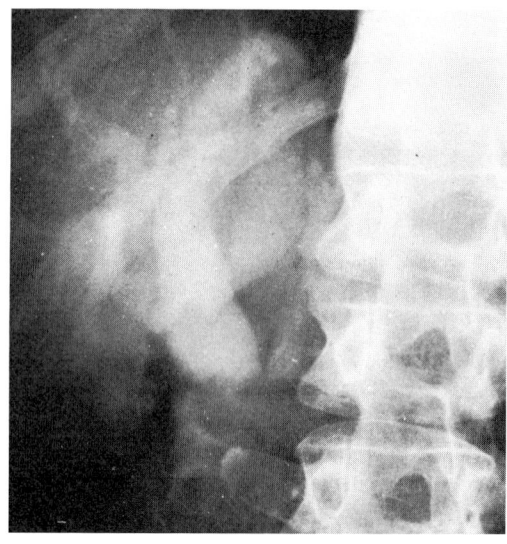

FIG. 32-17. Cholografin study, showing dilated common duct with stones (confirmed at operation).

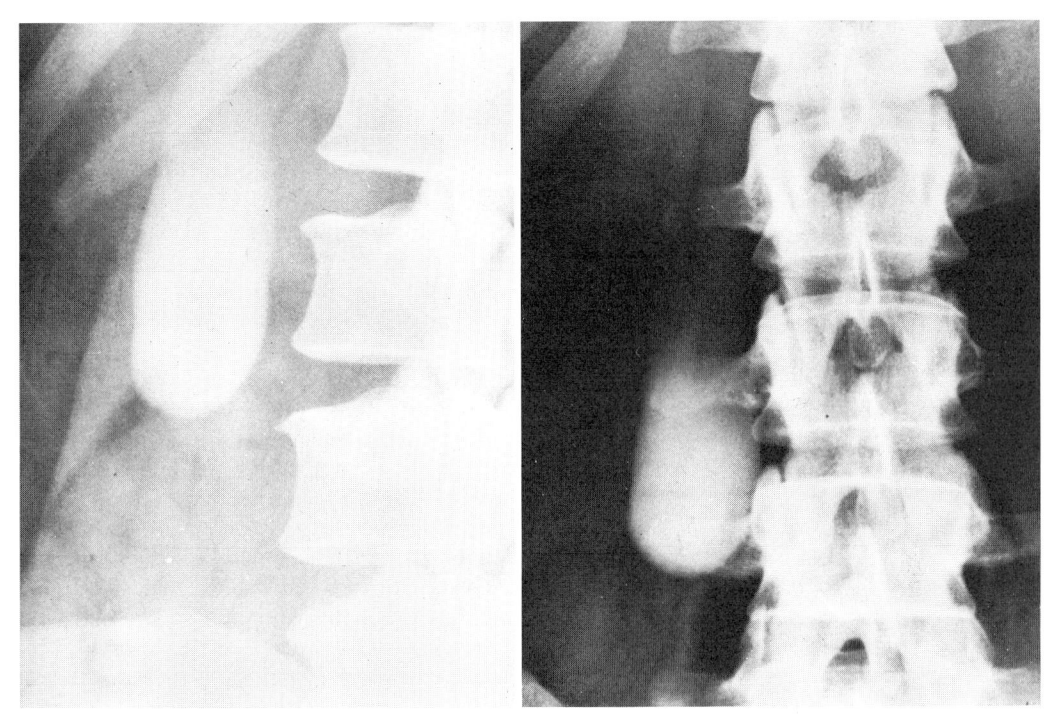

Fig. 32-18. Cholecystogram, of S. R. (*Left*) Film made with patient lying down. Functioning gallbladder. No stone shadow seen. (*Right*) Film made with patient erect. Note line of stones which have formed a radiolucent layer at the junction of the distal and the middle thirds of the gallbladder.

stones in the gallbladder with a cystic duct which appears large enough to transmit them is accepted by many surgeons as an indication for exploration of the common duct.

A conservative policy, and one which is followed in the great majority of clinics, is always to drain the common bile duct with a T-tube if it is opened. In clinics in which operative cholangiography is carried out, a defect in the cholangiogram may well prove to be the indi-

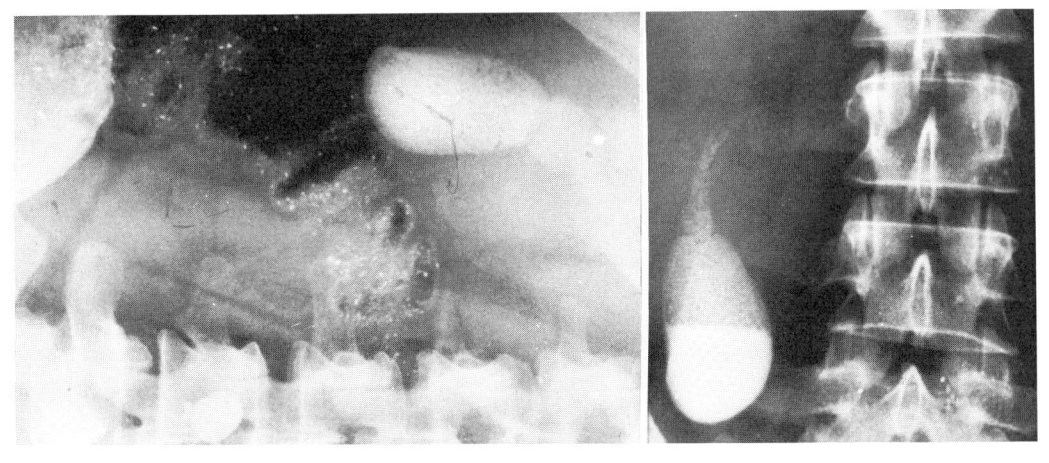

Fig. 32-19. Multiple stones with layering of the contrast medium. (*Left*) Horizontal position. (*Right*) Erect position. Direction of x-rays was horizontal in both films.

898 Liver, Gallbladder and Bile Passages

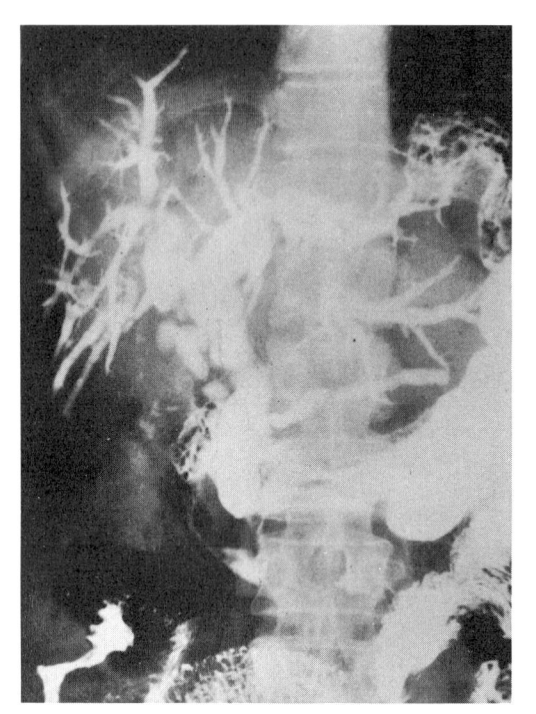

FIG. 32-20. The biliary tree filled with barium sulfate in a patient with a duodenobiliary fistula after administration of a water barium meal.

cation for opening the duct. Great care should be taken in carrying out such cholangiograms to avoid the introduction of air bubbles which may cast a shadow similar to that produced by a calculus on the x-ray film. Injection

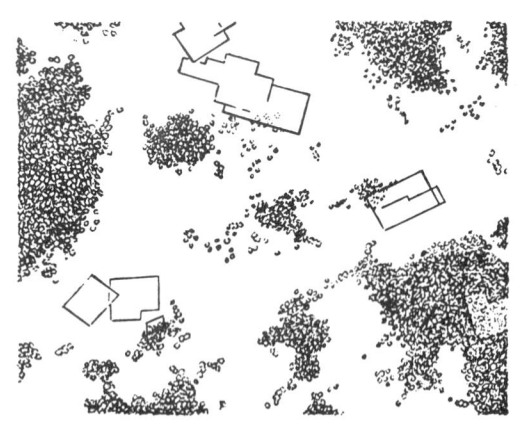

FIG. 32-21. Showing platelike crystals of cholesterol and masses of calcium bilirubinate sediment as they characteristically appear in specimens obtained by biliary drainage from patients with cholelithiasis.

through the cystic duct may be helpful (see Fig. 32-29).

The proper role of operative cholangiography is by no means agreed upon. The author has made wide use of this technic, usually injecting the dye through the cystic duct. He uses the findings when positive as additional indications for opening the common duct. He does not use a negative operative cholangiogram as a basis for omitting choledochostomy and common duct exploration when other clear indications are present.

He also uses cholangiography performed through a T-tube in the common duct at times to check the completeness of the common duct evacuation, particularly when multiple stones were present. Proceeding in this way, it is only infrequently that common duct stones are found which would otherwise have been missed. However, this additional precaution adds only about 15 minutes to the operative procedure, so that there is little reason to withhold it whenever there is even a slight suspicion of common duct calculus. When the common duct is below average in size and none of the indications for choledochotomy mentioned above is present, the procedure is often omitted. Acute pancreatitis as a sequela of this procedure has been reported by Zech (1949) and others, and recently discussed by Bergkvist (1957-58). The injection of Diodrast (iodopyracet) should be made gently and not in a way that is likely to build up excessive pressure in the ductal system.

Other indications for exploring the common duct may be found in the existence of anomalies, the existence of strictures not tight enough to produce jaundice, etc. (See also section on The Jaundiced Patient and section on Biliary Tract Operations.)

In jaundiced patients whose livers do not secrete cholografin in sufficient concentration for adequate visualization of the common duct direct injection of contrast media into an intrahepatic duct by a needle introduced from the skin surface has been proposed (Evans, 1964). course, the chances of success in entering the ductal system are increased by the dilation of the ducts characteristic of obstructive jaundice and are determined by aspiration of bile. The dangers are three: (1) leakage of bile into the peritoneal cavity, (2) bleeding into the peritoneal cavity and (3) hemobilia or bleeding into the biliary ducts. At present the method is restricted by the more conservative surgeons to situations in which the patient is ready for surgery, and the operation is carried out immediately after the needle puncture unless obstruction can be ruled out by the examination and continued observation of the patient rules out extravasation of blood or bile into the peritoneal cavity.

THE JAUNDICED PATIENT

Jaundice is the yellow color of skin, sclerae and mucous membranes due to an increase in bilirubin in the plasma. This increase may be due to obstruction of the ducts which carry the bile from the liver to the duodenum (obstructive jaundice), to disease of the cells which execrete bilirubin (hepatocellular jaundice) or to an overproduction of bilirubin due to increased breakdown of erythrocytes (hemolytic jaundice).

Jaundice is to be differentiated from other yellow colorations of the skin. The most important of these are the lemon-yellow color of individuals with profound anemia in whom the color of the fat shows through the skin more than usual and carotenemia due to ingestion of excessive amounts of carotene, either as carrots or as vitamin A precursor in drug form. The gray color of argyria sometimes has given rise to confusion, especially with long-standing or declining icterus.

Frequently, obstructive jaundice is relieved by operation, whereas hepatocellular jaundice is apt to be made worse by anesthesia and operation. Thus, the differentiation between the two is often crucial to the survival of the patient. Hemolytic jaundice does not usually call for operation but may do so if the increased production and excretion of bile has led to the formation of gallstones, or if the hemolysis is largely occurring in the spleen, in which case splenectomy may be helpful (see Chap. 34).

Obstructive Jaundice

The most common cause of obstructive jaundice during adult life is a stone in the common duct. A second common cause is carcinoma of the head of the pancreas (see Chap. 33). Metastatic carcinoma involving the liver is a third and fairly frequent cause, though usually it is one of the terminal events in malignant disease.

Other neoplasms which may cause obstructive jaundice are primary carcinoma of the liver, carcinoma of the gallbladder, carcinoma of the bile duct and carcinoma of the papilla of Vater. Rarely, jaundice may be caused by a benign polyp in the bile duct.

The author has seen obstructive jaundice resulting from abscesses pressing against the duct from the right side, from chronic pancreatitis, from penetrating ulcer of the duodenum, from primary carcinoma of the duodenum, from enlarged lymph nodes pressing against the duct, from congenital (or spontaneous) stricture of the common duct in a man of 18, from so-called chronic hypertrophic biliary cirrhosis, and iatrogenic jaundice from various injuries to the duct—transection, excision of part of the wall, occlusion with sutures during cholecystectomy, occlusion during gastrectomy and after accidental clamping of the duct. Parasites, such as *Ascaris lumbricoides* or *Schistosoma japonicum,* have caused common duct obstruction. While this occurs very rarely in the United States, common duct obstruction due to parasites is by no means uncommon in certain geographic areas in which infestation with the parasites is more frequent. During the neonatal period the common causes of obstructive jaundice are ductal atresia, ductal agenesis and choledochal cysts.

Principal interest in the differential diagnosis of obstructive jaundice is focused on cholelithiasis versus carcinoma of the head of the pancreas. The French surgeon Courvoisier* enunciated the law that bears his name: "When the common bile duct is obstructed by a stone, dilatation is rare; when the duct is obstructed in some other way, dilatation is common." A palpably distended gallbladder indicates carcinoma of the head of the pancreas, whereas in cholelithiasis the gallbladder is usually too shrunken and fibrotic to become palpably distended. Unfortunately, the exceptions to the law are so common as to permit only the most modest emphasis of it.

Jaundice is likely to be accompanied by pain when due to stone, and that accompanying car-

---

* While Courvoisier is identified with French surgery, he was born in Basel and for a period was Professor of Surgery at the University of Basel (Nissen, 1959).

TABLE 32-1. CHARACTERISTIC FINDINGS IN LIVER FUNCTION IN THREE TYPES OF JAUNDICE

	OBSTRUCTIVE	HEPATOCELLULAR	HEMOLYTIC
Bilirubin—total	+	+	+
1-minute reading	+	±	±
Cephalin cholesterol flocculation	±	+	±
Thymol flocculation	±	+	±
BSP retention	+	+	N
Alkaline phosphatase	+	N	N
Urine urobilinogen	0, if complete	±	+
Prothrombin response to vitamin K*#	>75% of N	<75% of N	

N = Normal   + = Increased   ± = Sometimes Increased   0 = None.

* = Response within 24 hours to 20 mg. of Synkayvite in afebrile patients whose initial prothrombin levels are below 75% of normal.

\# = Allen, J. G. (1940, 1943).

cinoma of the head of the pancreas is apt to be relatively painless at the time of onset ("silent jaundice"). Unfortunately, there are exceptions in both directions. However, painless jaundice is not very frequent with stones but does occur. On the other hand, pain is by no means rare in carcinoma of the head of the pancreas, even by the time the jaundice is noted (see Chap. 33).

Laboratory aids in differentiating between the 3 basic types of jaundice are summarized in Table 32-1.

Most important in the differentiation of hemolytic jaundice is the dark color of the stools. In severe anemia (< 6 Gm./100 ml.) patients with hemolytic jaundice may not show these findings. Of outstanding value in differentiating obstruction from hepatocellular jaundice has been the alkaline phosphatase level in the serum. However, none of the tests has been infallible, and the experiments of Mann (1926) indicate that large fractions of the liver can be resected without significant reductions in various of the function tests.

The levels of 2 enzymes in the serum are of some value in differentiating hepatocellular jaundice (Pryse-Davies and Wilkinson, 1958). The S.G.O.T. (serum glutamic oxaloacetic transaminase) and the S.G.P.T. (serum glutamic pyruvic transaminase) are apt to rise sharply in hepatocellular jaundice. They also rise in some other forms of cell deaths—for instance, in myocardial infarction.

Differential diagnosis is, of course, most important when it involves the decision to operate. Thus, the diagnosis of hepatitis versus obstruction is tremendously important. However, if hepatitis can be excluded and the jaundice is clearly obstructive, it is often not essential to know whether stone or carcinoma is the cause, as both usually need to be explored surgically if only to relieve the jaundice.

If no satisfactory differentiation is reached by laboratory methods and the patient does not improve on supportive therapy within a reasonable time (usually about 3 weeks), laparotomy should be done. Some clinicians resort to needle biopsy of the liver, provided that the prothrombin concentration is above 75 per cent of normal. Occasional serious hemorrhages have occurred, either into the peritoneal cavity or into the bile ducts, producing hemobilia. However, the principal objection to the procedure is the likelihood of missing significant areas by blind sampling and the difficulties encountered by the pathologist in interpreting the scanty material obtained.

Patients with hemolytic jaundice have a high incidence of gallstones, typically of the pure bilirubin type (jackstones).

THE PROGNOSTIC SIGNIFICANCE OF OBSTRUCTIVE JAUNDICE

Obstructive jaundice is a serious symptom. Cholelithiasis associated with jaundice is accompanied by a higher mortality than cholelithiasis alone. If it is due to carcinoma, the ultimate outlook is probably more than 99 per cent unfavorable. In the author's experience, all of the metastatic cases have gone on to die; all of the primary carcinomas of the liver have gone on to die; all except one of the primary carcinomas of the gallbladder have gone on to die within 5 years, and all of the carcinomas of the bile ducts have gone on to die, except for a rare few involving the papilla of Vater or the adjacent area of the duct who have survived several years and may possibly turn out in the final analysis to be cured. In a recent compilation from the literature, there were over 100 instances in which patients with

Whipple resections of the duodenum and the head of the pancreas for malignant disease have survived for 5 years or more. (See Chap. 33.)

As mentioned above, cholelithiasis with jaundice is accompanied by a much higher mortality than is cholelithiasis confined to the gallbladder. One can point to various series of cholecystectomies in which the operative mortality (death in the hospital within 30 days) was less than 1 per cent for cholecystectomy. Yet, the same clinics commonly report a mortality rate of 4 to 8 per cent for individuals with obstructive jaundice. This mortality represents a decided improvement from that of a few decades ago when it frequently ranged around 15 per cent or higher.

The cause of the higher death rate is explained partly by certain special complications to which the jaundiced patient is subject. These are: the hemorrhagic tendency in obstructive jaundice, "pancreatic asthenia," "liver shock" and "hepatorenal syndrome." In the past the most important of these has been the hemorrhagic tendency. About 20 per cent of patients undergoing major operations for relief of jaundice used to have hemorrhagic episodes in the postoperative period as reported by Ravdin *et al.* (1939) and Ulin (1943).

This problem was solved by 2 discoveries: (1) the discovery of vitamin K, the coagulation vitamin, by Dam in 1935; (2) the discovery by A. J. Quick that prothrombin deficiency is the basic coagulation defect in obstructive jaundice. E. D. Warner and his associates (1938) demonstrated that hypoprothrombinemia in patients actually could be relieved in many instances by the oral administration of vitamin K with bile salts, to facilitate its absorption. In order to avoid this complication, it is customary to give vitamin K_1 or one of the synthetic preparations with similar action, such as menadione, preoperatively until the prothrombin level has returned to normal or has been brought up as close to normal as possible. It is important to continue therapy into the postoperative period until the wound is healed. Late hemorrhagic episodes have been reported 3 or 4 weeks after operation when vitamin K is stopped before wound healing has occurred. Experience rapidly showed that about 18 per cent of patients with obstructive jaundice and hypoprothrombinemia failed to respond to vitamin K therapy, and an additional 12 per cent or so responded only partially. Failure of the prothrombin level to respond adequately to vitamin K is seen more frequently in patients with jaundice due to malignancy or in people with very long-standing liver damage or infectious hepatitis than in other jaundiced patients.

Many bits of evidence combined to demonstrate that vitamin K is effective only in the presence of a functioning liver. Impairment of function can be produced by chloroform or the liver can be removed surgically in animals, after which the prothrombin falls progressively and at a much more rapid rate than fibrinogen, the level of which in the blood is also dependent on the liver (Warren and Rhoads, 1939).

Further study of the coagulation mechanism indicates that the prothrombin, as measured by the Quick test, is not a single factor but is composed of at least 2 factors—one of which diminishes on storage of blood in a blood bank (accelerator globulin), whereas another is diminished by Dicumarol (pure prothrombin). Both are diminished by chloroform anesthesia. When the prothrombin level does not respond to vitamin K, it is possible to give the patient some prothrombin through transfusion of fresh blood. Frequently, stored blood also can have a beneficial effect, if the deficiency as determined by the 1-stage method of Quick happens to be in the component which is not much affected by storage (prothrombin).

Vitamin K_1 prepared as an emulsion for intravenous use and given intravenously in doses of 15 to 100 mg. or more will often produce a brief rise not obtained by ordinary doses. This is specifically indicated in Dicumarol poisoning or in patients under the influence of Dicumarol who must have emergency operations. It can be tried in other situations.

The second of these complications, pancreatic asthenia (a term introduced by Whipple, 1923), is now believed to result from prolonged bile drainage. The symptoms are anorexia and progressive weakness. A sodium and chloride deficiency may be part of the picture, but simple replacement of sodium and chlorides has failed practically always to bring about marked improvement. Refeeding of bile, however, in amounts of 150 ml. a day or more, usually will restore appetite and improve the patient greatly within 2 or 3 days. Because of the bitter taste, it is often necessary to refeed the bile through a nasogastric tube introduced into the stomach. Sometimes hardy patients can drink it mixed with pineapple juice, tomato juice or some other flavoring.

Liver shock is a picture that can be reproduced experimentally in the dog by ligation of the hepatic artery close to the hilum of the liver. It has been seen occasionally in patients who had injury or thrombosis of the hepatic artery. Such injuries can occur easily during cholecystectomy in those instances in which the hepatic artery runs up along the cystic duct, giving off the cystic artery opposite the infundibulum of the gallbladder and then turning back into the liver. Here the main hepatic artery or the right hepatic may be ligated instead of the cystic artery.

Markowitz (1949) showed that dogs receiving penicillin frequently do not develop liver shock after ligation of the hepatic artery. Fitts and his associates (1950) confirmed this observation and found also that chlortetracycline would protect similarly; however, streptomycin did not.

The present concept is that death results from an overgrowth of anaerobes which are resident in the liver. Appropriate antibiotics may suppress the growth of these organisms until such time as the liver has established an adequate collateral arterial circulation.

As a result of the improvements that have occurred in the understanding of the pathology of jaundice, it is now possible to operate on simple cases of jaundice produced by common duct stones with a large probability of success.

The fourth of the complications listed, hepatorenal syndrome, is described sometimes as including a chronic phase. The acute phase is, in effect, liver shock. The chronic phase corresponds to liver failure with cholemia, frequently with evidence of renal irritation, so-called bile nephrosis and with coma (see section on Physiology, p. 884). Studies by McDermott et al. (1954) indicate that hepatic coma is associated sometimes with a rise in the blood ammonia level. This change is observed routinely in Eck-fistula dogs fed on a meat diet. In the normal animal, ammonia concentrations in the portal vein are considerably higher than in the systemic circulation, and the ammonia is removed by the normal liver as the blood flows through it. In the experimental animal, a critical level is often reached at which the rise in blood ammonia is accompanied by coma (so-called meat intoxication). The level varies for different individuals but, according to McDermott, is fairly constant for any one animal. Therefore, it appears unwise to feed much protein to a jaundiced patient if coma is impending. McDermott and his associates have advised that, in patients with advanced cirrhosis of the liver, blood escaping from esophageal varices be aspirated from the stomach to reduce ammonia formation in the intestine. That the intestine is the actual site of the formation of free ammonia was reported by Folin (1912). Apparently, it is due to the activity of microorganisms, and patients in hepatic coma have at times been brought out of coma by the administration of broad-spectrum antibiotics into the gastrointestinal tract (Stormont, 1958).

PREPARATION OF THE JAUNDICED PATIENT FOR OPERATION

After the appropriate diagnostic studies are completed or, where possible, while they are being carried out, certain steps should be taken to be sure that the patient with jaundice is in as good condition as possible for operation. Menadione (vitamin K) should be given in doses of 5.0 mg. 2 to 4 times a day. In the event that this does not bring the prothrombin back to normal, vitamin K_1 emulsion may be given intravenously. Most surgeons prefer to give vitamin K to all patients with jaundice who are to undergo operation, even though the prothrombin happens not to be particularly depressed in advance of operation.

It also appears advisable to place the patient on a diet containing as close to 3,000 calories per day as he can be persuaded to take, and to supply about 70 per cent of these calories as carbohydrate, not less than 20 per cent as protein, and a relatively small portion as fat. There is some evidence that it may be suitable to go as high as 20 per cent of the calories from fat which, in general, permits a more palatable diet. When it is necessary to sacrifice one objective for another in planning the diet, the total caloric intake is probably

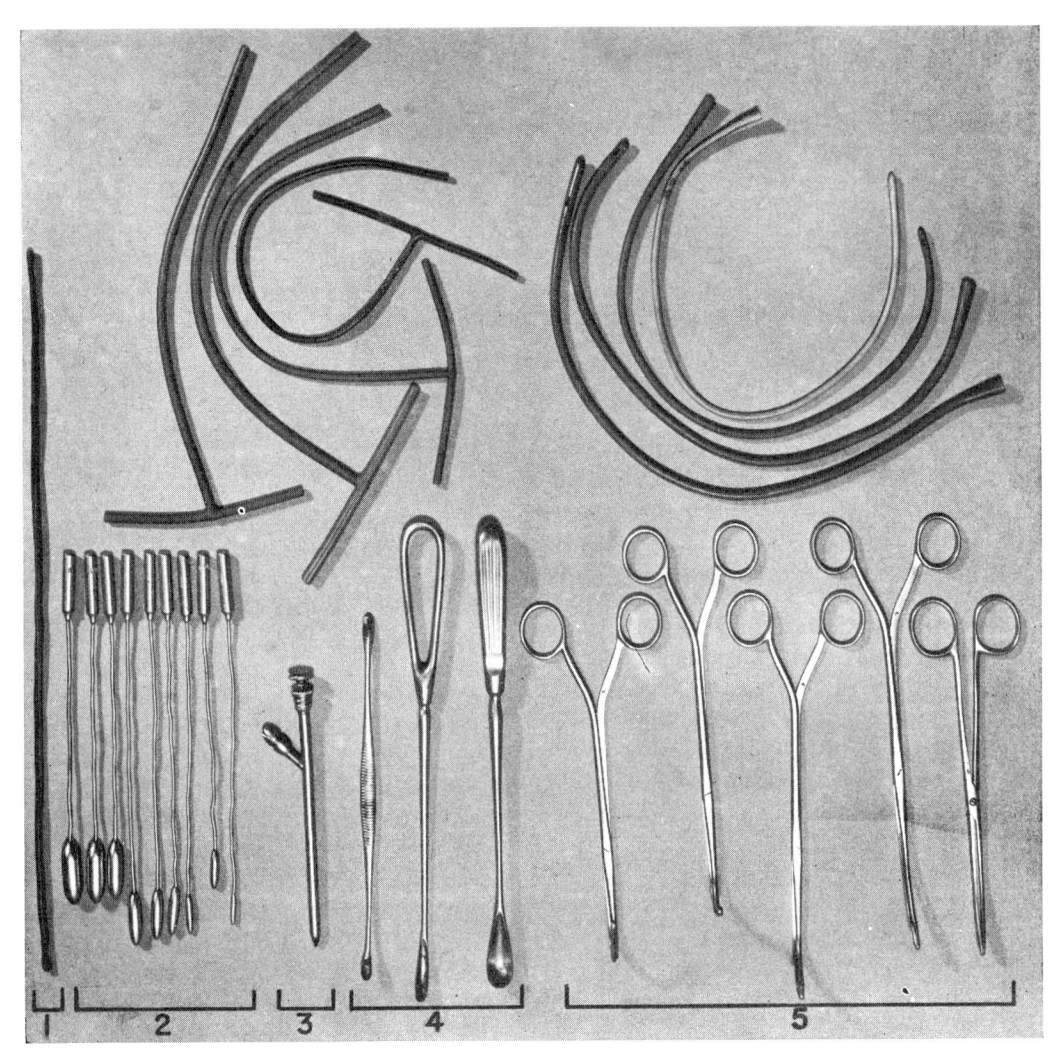

FIG. 32-22. Instruments commonly used in biliary tract surgery. (*Top, left*) Rubber T-tubes of various sizes. (*Top, right*) Straight rubber catheters of various sizes. (*Bottom, left to right*) (1) Malleable common duct probe. (2) Graduated common duct dilators (Bakes). (3) Trochar aspirator point for entering the distended gallbladder. Suction tubing fits on side arm and sharp point is withdrawn by drawing back plunger after the trochar has entered the gallbladder. (4) Three types of stone scoops. (5) Five stone forceps of varying degrees of curvature.

the most important, and the relatively high protein intake next most important.

The studies of Ravdin *et al.* (1943) suggest that when such a diet is actually ingested by patients for 5 to 7 days before operation, it is rare that one finds the high fat content of liver biopsy specimens which are encountered frequently in patients not prepared in this manner. It is believed that patients are better risks for anesthesia and operation as the result of such dietary preparation.

Occasionally, the progression of symptoms, particularly of pain and tenderness in the upper abdomen, make it inadvisable to take the time required for such careful dietary preparation. Under these circumstances it is usually advisable to carry out the minimum procedure which will relieve the patient of his acute symptomatology.

Other aspects of the preoperative preparation of a patient with biliary tract disease are similar to the steps used in preparing other patients for major abdominal operations and are set forth in Chapter 15.

STANDARD OPERATIVE PROCEDURES ON THE GALLBLADDER AND THE EXTRAHEPATIC BILIARY PASSAGES

In the following paragraphs certain operations performed on the biliary tract for indications already discussed are described briefly. These include cholecystostomy, cholecystectomy, choledochostomy, duodenotomy with transduodenal exploration of the common duct, sphincterotomy, cholecystojejunostomy, choledochojejunostomy and choledochoduodenostomy and, finally, pancreaticoduodenectomy. The surgeon who opens the peritoneal cavity to perform biliary tract surgery should be capable of doing any combination of these procedures when indicated and therefore should have all of them available in his armamentarium. It is sometimes difficult, if not impossible, to differentiate before operation exactly which patients will need which of these procedures (see Fig. 32-22, which shows instruments commonly used in biliary tract surgery).

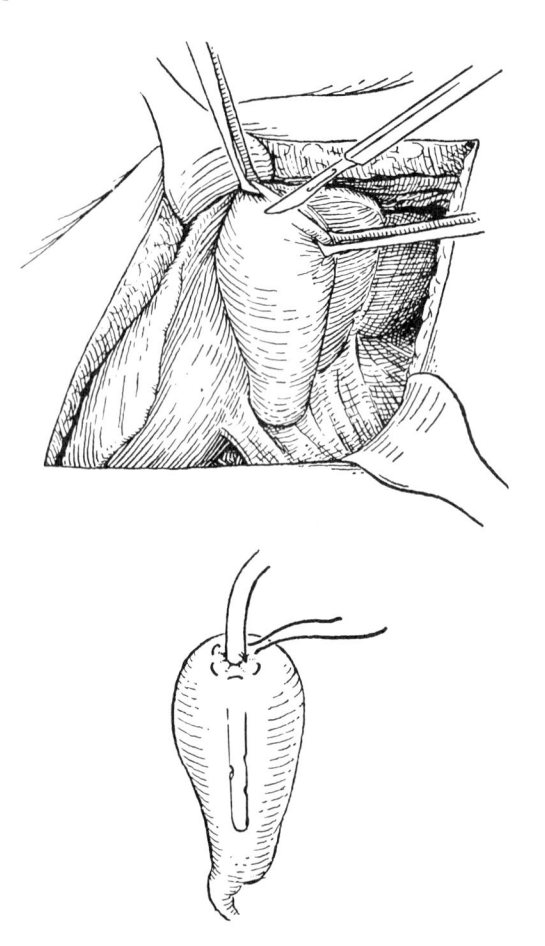

FIG. 32-24. Surgical exposure of the gallbladder for cholecystostomy, showing insertion of tube after evacuation of the organ by suction, stone forceps and scoops. The trochar aspirator tip shown in Figure 32-22 (3) is often used when the gallbladder is tense to diminish leakage of bile. Then the opening is enlarged as necessary with the scalpel.

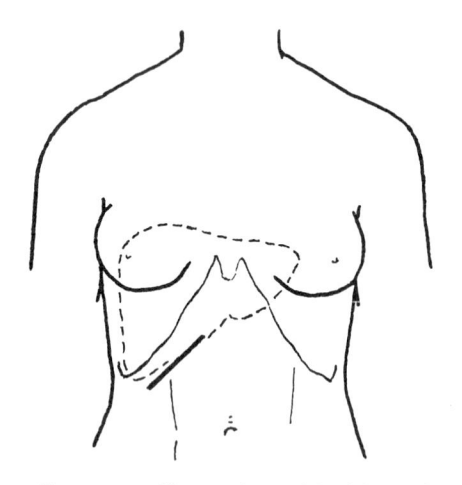

FIG. 32-23. Short subcostal incision suitable for cholecystostomy. Local, regional, or general anesthesia may be used.

CHOLECYSTOSTOMY

The gallbladder is opened, usually through its fundus (see Figs. 32-23 and 32-24); an effort is made to remove all stones. Then a rubber tube, fenestrated near the end, is introduced into its lumen, and the gallbladder is closed tightly around it with purse-string and accessory sutures of catgut. The end of the tube leads outside the body wall where it is connected to a drainage bottle. The subhepatic space usually is drained to the outside with a "cigarette" or other soft drain.

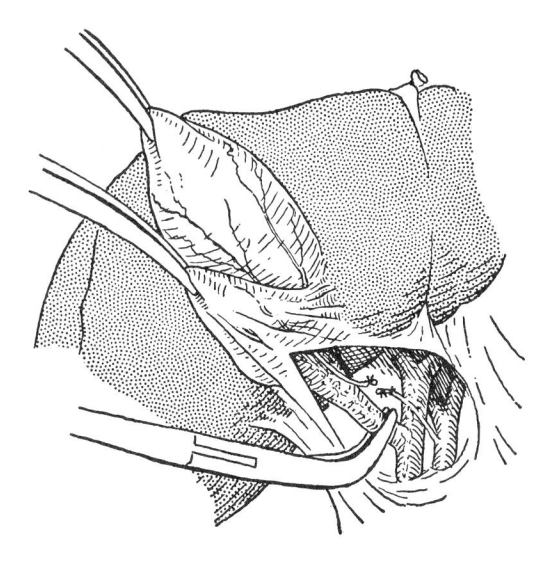

FIG. 32-25. Retrograde cholecystectomy, showing the application of a Shallcross clamp to the cystic duct after division and double ligation of the cystic artery.

The procedure can be done with local infiltration anesthesia, using 0.5 to 1.0 per cent procaine hydrochloride solution and is admirably adapted as a minimal procedure to prevent rupture of the gallbladder in very elderly or debilitated persons.

Cholecystectomy

It is believed that the first cholecystectomy was performed by Langenbuch and reported by him (1882). The first such operation to be reported in the United States is believed to be that performed by Ohage (1886, 1887).

The gallbladder is removed, beginning either at the fundus or at the infundibulum (see Figs. 32-25 and 32-26). The great dangers are injury to the main bile ducts, injury to the hepatic artery or the right hepatic artery, and postoperative hemorrhage. Anatomic variations in the arrangements of the various structures account for a considerable proportion of the accidents which occur. While the possibilities of injury are as many as the anatomic variations which have been described (see Fig. 32-1), the main dangers are:

1. Clamping of the bile duct in a blind effort to control hemorrhage from the cystic artery or some other vessel at the hilum of the liver. Even though the clamp is removed,

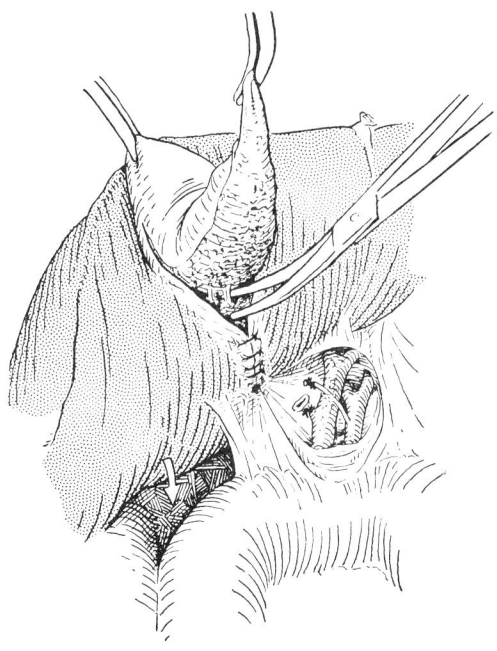

FIG. 32-26. A later stage in the retrograde removal of the gallbladder, showing the 2 ligatures on the stump of the cystic duct placed close to but not quite flush with the wall of the common duct. Note the interrupted sutures used in closing the liver bed. Arrow points to Morison's pouch. After removal of the gallbladder has been completed, the author employs a rubber tube drain in Morison's pouch and a Penrose drain which overlies the site from which the gallbladder has been removed. These drains may be exteriorized through the lateral end of the incision when the subcostal approach is used, or a separate stab wound may be made to accommodate them. Subsequently, they are removed in stages, usually in 3 to 7 days.

there is reason to believe that stricture may form in the crushed area. This is avoided best if, at the outset of dissection, the foramen of Winslow is identified, so that unexpected hemorrhage can be controlled by placing a finger through the foramen behind the hepatic artery and the portal vein, and then compressing these vessels digitally.

2. Tenting of the common duct upward by traction on the cystic duct with application of the cystic duct clamp across all or a part of the main bile duct (see Fig. 32-27).

3. Laceration or actual division of the com-

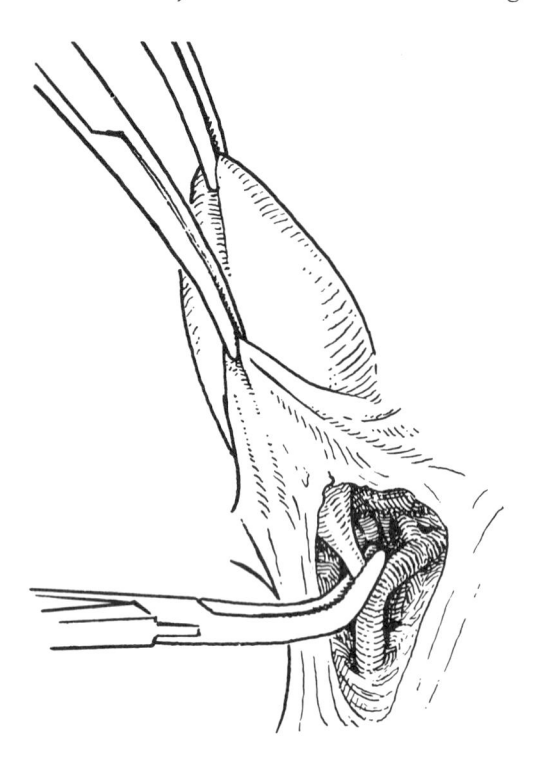

FIG. 32-27. Shows tenting of common duct due to traction on cystic duct with application of clamp on cystic duct in such a manner as to encroach on the common duct. This error in technic is a frequent cause of stricture of the common duct.

mon duct or of the right hepatic duct which may join the cystic duct or even the gallbladder before uniting with the left hepatic duct. The complications (2 and 3) are preventable by complete identification of the cystic duct, the common duct and the common hepatic duct before ligation and division of the cystic duct.

4. Injury and subsequent ligation of the common hepatic artery or the right hepatic artery. First, one should identify the course of the hepatic artery by palpation. At operation, whenever that which appears to be the cystic artery looks unusually large, it is wise to dissect it up on to the gallbladder and make sure that it does not turn back into the liver before ligating or clamping or dividing it. These two steps help to avoid liver shock. The reliability of antibiotics in protecting against liver shock after these injuries is uncertain but, when injury occurs or is suspected, they certainly should be used in large doses (300,000 units of penicillin every 3 hours, and 250 mg. of chlortetracycline every 12 hours, by vein or 1 Gm. twice daily by mouth). If the structures at the infundibulum and the common duct region cannot be exposed easily, it is safer to begin the dissection at the fundus, gradually separating the gallbladder from the liver. This requires more time for hemostasis because the cystic artery is not secured until near the end of the dissection. The gallbladder bed is drained with a soft drain, and the kidney fossa (Morison's pouch) is drained in a similar manner.

The author's present technic is to locate the cystic artery after palpating the hepatic artery and its right branch. Once satisfied that the artery supporting the gallbladder is of appropriate caliber as compared with a right hepatic artery, he divides and ligates the cystic artery just distal to the cystic lymph node.

With this secured, dissection of the gallbladder is begun at the fundus. With the arterial supply ligated it is usually easy to keep the field dry and to dissect the cystic duct free to its junction with the common bile duct. Usually, one or more arterial twigs supply the cystic duct and must be ligated individually.

This technic gives maximal opportunity to see, to recognize and to deal with anomalies of the ductal system. In 1964, it permitted recognition and prevention of ligation of a third hepatic duct draining about 15 per cent of the right lobe of the liver which joined with the cystic duct before confluence with the common hepatic duct to form the choledochus.

Choledochostomy

Choledochostomy is employed not only to remove stones from the common duct but also to explore the common duct for possible stricture or tumor (see Fig. 32-28). After freeing the anterior surface of the common bile duct of fat for a short distance, it is finally identified by aspiration of bile through a fine 22-gauge needle. Then the duct is held forward by two traction sutures placed in its anterior wall for the purpose. It is opened longitudinally between the sutures for a distance of about 8 mm. This permits exploration of the lumen with probes and stone forceps; the introduction of dilators to stretch the sphincter of Oddi; and of catheters to irrigate the duct

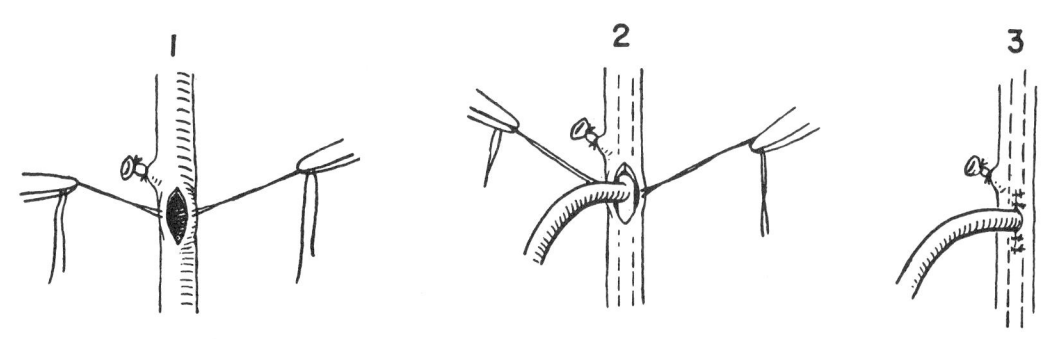

Fig. 32-28. Shows an opening in the anterior wall of the common duct slightly caudad to the cystic duct. The opening is made in the long axis of the common bile duct between 2 sutures which are used to support the anterior wall of the duct, thus preventing the likelihood of injury to the posterior wall. Through this opening, the duct is explored with appropriate probes, scoops and stone forceps. Frequently, it is irrigated with a straight rubber catheter. The sphincter of Oddi in the lower end of the duct usually grips the Bâkes dilators, so that the operator can tell when the duodenum is entered. By passing dilators of successively larger sizes, the sphincter may be gently dilated sufficiently to accommodate a small rubber catheter. Irrigation of this catheter determines quite accurately when the sphincter has been passed in doubtful cases. If the openings in the side of the catheter remain in the common duct, the irrigating fluid regurgitates; whereas if these openings have passed the sphincter into the duodenum, the fluid does not regurgitate.

When the operator is satisfied that the common duct is empty and communicates freely with the duodenum below and the hepatic duct above, a rubber T-tube is introduced. This provides drainage to the outside for bile which otherwise might leak into the peritoneal cavity. It also forms a splint which is helpful in preventing narrowing of the common bile duct by the absorbable sutures used to close the choledochotomy. After 12 days or longer, the stem of the tube is enclosed in a fibrous tract, and, after having done a T-tube cholangiogram, the T-tube can be removed by simple traction from the outside with the expectation that the common duct will seal off spontaneously and that bile will not drain into the general peritoneal cavity.

and to pass through the sphincter in order to demonstrate its patency (sterile saline solution injected through such a catheter will regurgitate through the opening of the common duct until the eyes of the catheter have passed the sphincter, then the fluid will be retained in the duodenum). Other instruments, such as choledochoscopes and choledochophones (Kirby, 1950), have been designed to aid in the exploration of the common bile duct.

Standard practice is never to close the duct without a drain tube. The almost universally accepted type of drain is the T-tube, the cross bar of the T lying in the common duct and the stem extending out to the exterior of the body. The opening in the duct is closed with 2 or 3 fine sutures of swaged catgut about the stem of the tube. Care should be taken to take small bites so that the duct is not narrowed appreciably as the result of the suture. Such a tube is useful both at the operating table and subsequently, to introduce radiopaque material into the common duct and to obtain cholangiograms (Fig. 32-30). This should be done at the time of operation if the requisite x-ray equipment is available in the operating room and always should be done before removal of the T-tube. After about 12 days, the tube may be removed by simple traction, provided that the sutures have absorbed sufficiently. The wound in the duct then heals by itself, and there is little, if any, tendency toward stricture formation.

Although some have advocated complete closure of the duct after choledochostomy, this procedure is not recommended here.

Duodenotomy With Transduodenal Exploration of the Common Duct

Mobilization of the duodenum by cutting the avascular peritoneal attachments to the right (Kocher, 1903) not only renders duodenotomy more feasible but also permits palpation of the ampullary region to be carried out

908 Liver, Gallbladder and Bile Passages

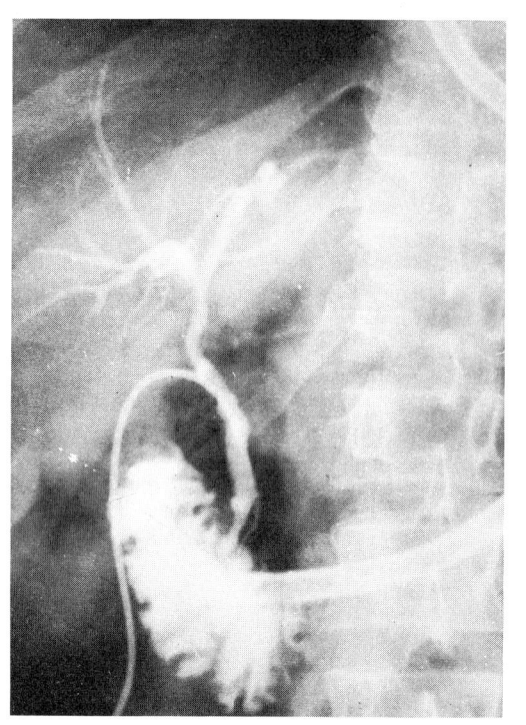

FIG. 32-29. Normal cholangiogram made at operation by use of a catheter introduced through the cystic duct. The large tube entering the duodenum from the patient's left is a gastric suction tube introduced through the nasopharynx, which has slipped through the pylorus.

more definitively (see Fig. 32-31). Duodenotomy (see Chap. 34) is performed best by a short longitudinal or diagonal incision in the duodenum at a level determined by the location of the tip of a common duct probe inserted from above. After exposing the ampulla, a probe can be inserted from below. With the combined action of the 2 probes plus palpation, stones may be recovered which were not found with the use of probes from above alone. If the duodenal incision is longitudinal (i.e., parallel to the long axis of the duodenum), the incision should be closed transversely according to the Heineke-Mikulicz principle to avoid narrowing of the duodenal lumen.

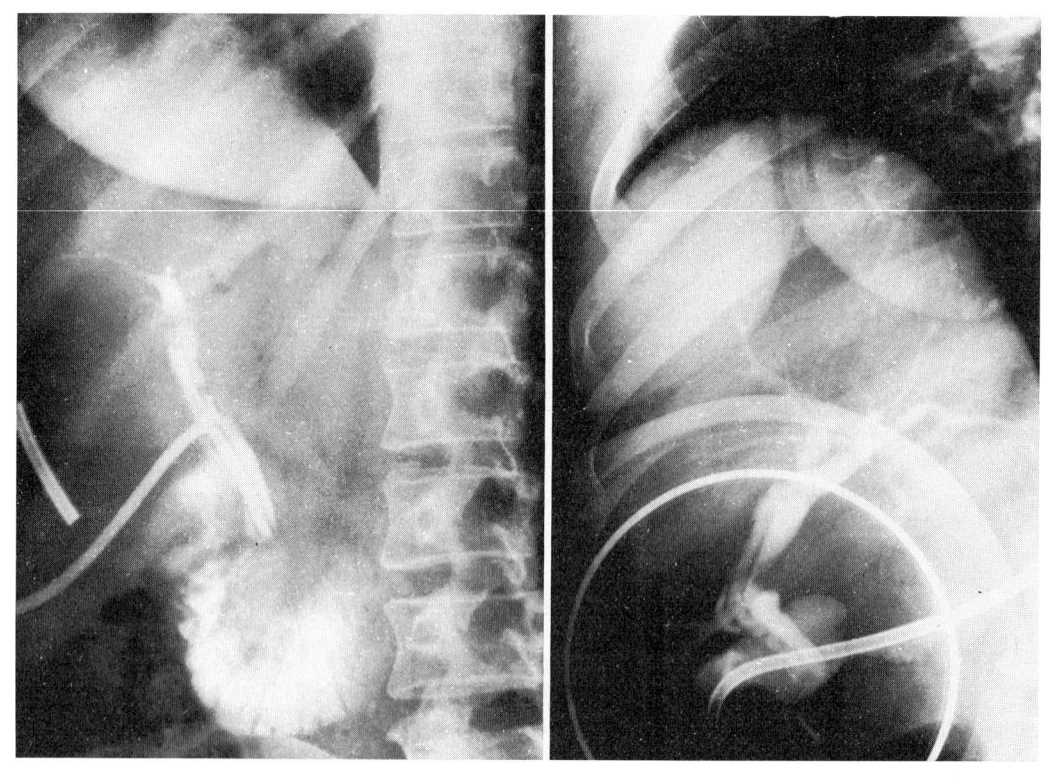

FIG. 32-30. The use of an inflated balloon in the duodenum to aid in filling the hepatic radicles during a postoperative cholangiogram. (*Left*) Attempt without the balloon. (*Right*) Attempt with the balloon.

SPHINCTEROTOMY

In certain very rare instances, an impacted stone can be dislodged only after sphincterotomy. Other indications for this procedure are discussed in Chapter 33, Pancreas.

CHOLECYSTOJEJUNOSTOMY

This procedure is used to sidetrack the common duct when the latter is obstructed and direct removal of the obstruction seems to be unwise for one reason or another. A 2-layer anastomosis is done between the inferior surface of the fundus of the gallbladder, and a loop of jejunum which is drawn up anteriorly in front of the transverse colon. The anastomosis should be placed as high as possible in the small bowel but not so high as to result in any tension. As demonstrated by Fitts (1948) and others, the sphincter of Oddi mechanism is very important in preventing retrograde cholangitis from the bowel. None of the anastomoses of the extrahepatic biliary system to the intestinal tract have been entirely free of this complication in all cases.

Allen, A. W. (1945) and Cole (1951) independently have recommended defunctionalizing the loop of jejunum which is to be used for the anastomosis (see Chap. 33). This is done by means of the Roux-Y principle and probably is helpful to some extent in reducing the incidence of cholangitis. There is experimental evidence to show that the defunctionalized loop should be at least 30 cm. long. The idea of taking tucks in one side or the other of the bowel to produce so-called valves has been advanced, but it is doubtful if it confers much advantage.

Now it is generally accepted that cholecystogastrostomy is a less satisfactory procedure, and this is seldom practiced.

CHOLEDOCHODUODENOSTOMY

This procedure is seldom well adapted to relieve local obstructions due to tumor in the head of the pancreas or in nearby structures. It has been strongly advocated by Madden for patients with a strong tendency to form stones in the bile ducts. He believes that most instances of cholangitis following choledochoduodenostomy are due to failure to make a large enough opening (Madden, 1965).

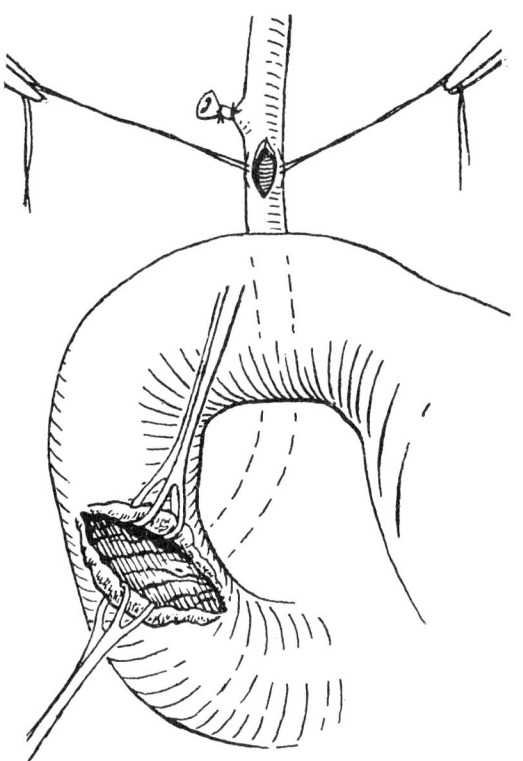

FIG. 32-31. Shows transduodenal exploration of the papilla of Vater. The author prefers a diagonal incision in the anterolateral wall of the duodenum which may be closed from side to side without danger of constricting the duodenum. Choledochotomy always is made in the supraduodenal position. The lateral attachments of the duodenum are also incised so that the duodenum may be mobilized and delivered into the wound. This also permits the operator's fingers to palpate posteriorly over the pancreas traversed by the common duct. Closure of the duodenal wound must be thorough. The author uses an inverting Connell suture of catgut as the first layer, followed by two layers of interrupted nonabsorable sutures. In addition, a tag of omentum is held in place by other interrupted sutures so as to cover the suture line in the duodenum. A T-tube is placed in the choledochotomy. A sump drain is often used in Morison's pouch.

CHOLEDOCHOJEJUNOSTOMY

A defunctionalized loop of jejunum may be brought up and anastomosed either to the side of the common duct or the common duct may be transected and anastomosed end-to-end or end-to-side to a jejunal loop. This is a necessary part of a local resection for removal of the distal end of the common duct, the head of the pancreas, and the duodenum. The length of the loop should be not less than 30 cm.

PANCREATICODUODENECTOMY

In a small number of patients, usually those with surgical jaundice due to carcinoma of the region of the head of the pancreas or the ampulla of Vater, radical resection by the method of Whipple must be resorted to (see Chap. 33).

GENERAL PRINCIPLES FOR SECONDARY OPERATIONS ON THE BILIARY TRACT

Secondary operations are not infrequent in biliary tract surgery. These extend in magnitude and difficulty from cholecystectomy following cholecystostomy to very difficult procedures for recurrent stricture of the common duct. Adhesions form with great regularity in the region of the gallbladder and the subhepatic space as the result of previous operation and/or inflammation. The safe exposure of the parts of the biliary tract without injury to them or to other organs can be a very perplexing problem—especially to the novice.

There is one rule which has been of inestimable help to many surgeons: Find the anterior caudad edge of the liver and then keep the plane of dissection directly against Glisson's capsule as you separate the adherent organs from the undersurface of the liver. This plan is supplemented by periodic palpation for the hepatic artery, remembering that it is often not palpable if the blood pressure is as low as 80 mm. of mercury. Once the hepatic artery is located, it may be useful to locate the common duct by aspiration through a fine (22-24 gauge) needle, remembering that if complete obstruction of the common duct is present, only "white" bile looking like water or lymph may be found.

PATHOLOGIC CONDITIONS OF THE LIVER PARENCHYMA WITH NOTES REGARDING SURGICAL THERAPY

The problems of portal hypertension are discussed in Chapter 34 in connection with shunt operations. Portal hypertension may result from either intrahepatic obstruction to the portal flow or extrahepatic obstruction. Whereas the common cause of the latter is thrombosis, the common cause of the intrahepatic obstruction is cirrhosis.

Cirrhosis may be described as a progressive involvement of the liver with fibrous tissue, presumably resulting from progressive and repeated liver damage with replacement with scar tissue. The histologic picture is frequently one of both fibrosis and regeneration. In the Laennec's form, the fibrosis results in diffuse scarring, with the lobulations of medium size. As judged by the irregularities in the surface of the liver, the trabeculae become prominent at distances of the order of perhaps ¼ inch apart. In Hanot's cirrhosis, the trabeculation is finer, whereas in biliary cirrhosis the trabeculation is coarser. The latter form of the disease is apt to follow chronic or recurrent obstruction of the bile ducts and is more frequently associated with jaundice in its earlier stages than the other forms.

Whereas obstruction resulting in hematemesis from rupture or ulceration of dilated esophangeal veins usually is treated by vascular shunts or direct attack on the affected portion of the esophagus, cirrhosis resulting in ascites primarily is less susceptible to surgical treatment. Nevertheless, portal systemic shunts of the side-to-side type have at times been helpful (see chapter on portal cirrhosis or hypertension). Many procedures have been recommended to increase anastomoses between the portal circulation and the systemic circulation. One of these is the Talma-Morison procedure in which the parietal peritoneum is scarified and the omentum sutured to it. The variations of this include forming pockets in various layers of the abdominal wall into which the omentum or another organ, such as the spleen, is fitted.

Another group of procedures involves removal of segments of the peritoneum or making apertures to allow the ascitic fluid to penetrate the peritoneum into other layers of the abdominal wall, especially the subcutaneous layer in the hope that it will be absorbed there. In still other procedures efforts have been made to anastomose the stump of the saphenous vein to the abdominal cavity in the hope that fluid actually will be pumped back into the vascular system. Another method is to anastomose the pelvis of one kidney to the abdominal cavity so that the fluid may make an exit via the urinary tract.

None of these procedures can be recommended with much enthusiasm. If any is to be undertaken, perhaps the removal of large segments of parietal peritoneum offers the most to recommend it. Such ascites usually represent a fairly advanced form of cirrhosis, and the average life expectancy is not long, although individuals sometimes exceed the average by a number of years. Treatment of this condition should be primarily medical along the lines thas are recommended in the section on the preparation of the jaundiced patient but continued for many months. Such dietotherapy may be quite helpful. Most authors believe it important to avoid all alcohol.

A number of other processes involve the liver, such as actinomycosis, tuberculosis and syphilis. All of these conditions are now rare, and the reader is referred to special articles such as that by Ravdin (1941).

Cysts of the Liver

There are 2 principal types of liver cysts: congenital cysts which may contain either bile or mucus, and hydatid cysts due to echinococcus disease. Both are rare in this country. The echinococcus cysts should be removed intact if possible. In the event of rupture, there is danger of an allergic reaction to the antigen in the cysts, and there is also great likelihood that daughter cysts will become engrafted in other viscera and grow, producing a series of secondary symptoms. The congenital cysts may require no treatment or, if they become infected, may require drainage as in the case of a liver abscess. Where feasible, excision is perhaps the best treatment for those that become symptomatic, but this is not always possible for those that are close to the large blood vessels. Partial excision, cauterization of the remaining lining and packing may be successful.

Echinococcus Cysts

Echinococcus cysts are still common among pastoral peoples who live with their dogs. The *Taenia echinococcus* or dog tapeworm uses the intestinal tract of the dog as a primary breeding ground and then may be ingested by man, penetrate the wall of his alimentary canal and lodge in various organs, of which the most common are the lung and the liver. Here the cysts are characterized by large fibrous envelopes (the false cyst) containing a soft lining or membrane (the true cyst). The latter contains fluid in which may float the scolices, which are the organs by which the future tapeworm will attach itself to the alimentary tract of a future canine host. Many of these will be embedded in or at least attached to the true cyst wall. In additon, the true cyst will often contain daughter cysts or smaller compartments made up of the same kind of walls as the true cysts.

Two species of this parasite have been described—*Echinoccocus granulosus* which uses man, cattle, sheep, horses and hogs as its intermediate host and the dog, the wolf, the coyote and other Canidae as its definitive host, and *Echinococcus multilocularis* which invades the microtine rodents as intermediate host and the dog and the fox as definitive hosts. The latter has been found in Eurasia, Alaska and the Kurile Islands. The lesions it produces are destructive because of their invasive character. It should be noted that the canine host must eat the uncooked tissues of the intermediate host in order to complete the life cycle of these parasites—a fact probably accounting for the rarity of the lesions among owners of pet dogs.

Current practice in Iran, where echinococcus disease is frequent, is to aspirate the cyst through a hollow needle and then carefully to open the false cyst and dissect out the collapsed true cyst. The object is to remove the true cyst wall intact. After this is completed, the false cyst wall may be excised, or, if this is not feasible, it may be closed about drains. Cahill (1964) suggests aspiration of the cyst and injection of 10 per cent formalin, followed by a 20-minute wait before further manipulation and excision in order to reduce the chance of spread. The toxicity of formalin itself would have to be kept in mind.

Wounds of the Liver

Wounds of the liver are important because this is the most frequently injured of the solid viscera within the abdomen. Hemorrhage is apt to be profuse and not infrequently is attended by a slow pulse until late in the development of shock. Suture should be undertaken promptly, using a large blunt needle and coarse suture material tied over omentum or some absorbable hemostatic agent, such as gelatin foam. The abdomen always should be drained as the wounds frequently leak bile and not infrequently give rise to subhepatic or subphrenic abscesses. Merendino (1963) has recommended that the ductal system be drained routinely in all cases of liver laceration. Often large amounts of blood must be transfused to save the lives of patients with large liver wounds, as these commonly bleed very rapidly.

Particularly after blunt crushing injuries a portion of the liver may be so lacerated that it is impossible or impractical to repair it. Such portions are better removed, since this permits more accurate hemostasis. Even large amounts of the liver may be sacrificed. An amount equivalent to the left and caudate lobes is sufficient, if normal, to permit survival and the body can regenerate liver in accordance with its needs from such remnants.

In the case of penetrating wounds of the liver some surgeons have recommended laying the liver open by incision along the tract to assure hemostasis. This may be necessary if hemorrhage is not controlled by simpler means such as absorbable packing and suture of the wound of entrance. It is necessary to examine the common duct for evidence of bleeding and, if the duct is filled with clot, to open the duct, remove the clot and see if there is active bleeding by this route.

With penetrating injuries, the vessels to the liver also may be injured, and here the chance of saving the patient's life is slight unless the patient is seen early, and intervention is prompt. The vascular channels should be restored by suture. Should it be necessary to tie off the hepatic artery or a major branch of the hepatic artery, penicillin or chlortetracycline are recommended to reduce the chances of liver shock.

The earlier literature contains much about ptosis of the liver and corset liver, but neither of these conditions requires treatment frequently enough to justify emphasis in a book of this length. The reader is referred to Ravdin (1941).

Hepatic Biopsy

A biopsy of 0.5 or 1.0 Gm. of liver can be taken conveniently from the anterior edge of the liver, preferably an inch or more away from the gallbladder. Hemostasis can be obtained by swaged catgut sutures if they are tied judiciously and not so tight as to cut through the liver tissue. It is believed that this is a safer procedure than the use of needle biopsy. A needle biopsy is ordinarily done: (1) without visualization of the point at which the needle enters the liver; (2) without visualization of any organs or tissues which may be present between the skin and the liver at the site selected; and (3) without visualization of the amount of bleeding which follows the puncture; nevertheless, needle biopsy sometimes avoids laparotomy; if avoided in persons with low prothrombin levels, it has been carried out at a risk of less than 1 per cent (Zamcheck, 1953).

Partial Hepatectomy

Relatively large segments of the liver have been removed in man. Many times, most of the left lobe has been sacrificed, and various substantial proportions of the right lobe. At times, the entire right lobe has been sacrificed with survival. The indications for these procedures are not encountered very frequently because most of the malignancies of the liver are either metastatic from another site or are multicentric or diffuse in their growth. Therefore, it is seldom that a case presents in which there seems to be a worthwhile chance of eradicating a tumor by a partial hepatectomy. Multiple abscesses in a given localized part of the liver, echinococcus cysts, severe injury to the liver, and so forth, occasionally may provide a sufficient indication for a partial hepatectomy.

Technically, the problem is mainly one of hemostasis. Clamping of the entire blood supply of the liver at its hilum is interdicted because this results in a pooling of blood in the portal bed which may be fatal. It also interrupts the blood supply to the liver for a period which is undesirable. The use of the electric knife and the electric cautery, the use of coarse catgut swaged on larger curved needles and absorbable sponge such as foam gelatin are valuable technical aids. Sutures must be placed deep and tied loosely. If they are tied over Gelfoam or omentum, they cut the tissue less.

If the dissection is begun at the hilum, the divisions of the hepatic artery and the portal vein going to the various parts of the liver may be identified. It is then best to ligate those branches going to the portion to be excised, e.g., the right lobe. With this done, blunt dissection through the liver with the handle of a scalpel will expose the larger communicating vessels in time to doubly clamp, divide and ligate them. The most hazardous part of the procedure is apt to be that which concerns the hepatic veins. These should be identified before they are entered. Vascular sutures may be required to close the junctions of these veins with the inferior vena cava.

Drainage of Hepatic Abscesses

Liver abscesses may be drained transperitoneally through an incision below the costal margin. They may be drained transpleurally, but if this is to be done it is wise to utilize a 2-stage procedure which permits a 5-day period for the pleura to seal off in the costophrenic angle before one traverses the pleural cavity. Usually a resection of the 9th and the 10th ribs is carried out at the posterior axillary line. Packing is introduced against the pleura; and after 5 days, if the pleural surfaces appear to be glued together, an incision is made through the parietal pleura and then through the parietal pleura on the diaphragm, and thence through the diaphragm into the subdiaphragmatic space and on into the liver as necessary. To avoid possible air embolism, it is well to have the patient in a slight head-up position when the liver is transected.

Ordinarily, an aspirating needle of large gauge is utilized to locate the abscess, and frequently a cautery is used to form a larger tract along the needle into the abscess cavity. Then such a tract can accommodate rubber drain tubes. Care must be taken with this plan not to go too close to major vessels, such as the inferior vena cava or the main hepatic veins.

The lung itself does not present a problem with this approach, as it lies higher at rest, and the packing and the splinting of the diaphragm prevent its downward excursion after the first stage.

Another route by which abscesses of the liver can be drained is the so-called extraperitoneal route proposed by Ochsner (1938). The 12th rib is resected, its bed is incised, care being taken not to enter the pleura above. One then dissects bluntly under the diaphragm, more or less at the top of the perirenal fat. This permits a plane to be developed between the reflected peritoneal surface and the muscle fibers of the diaphragm. This allows one to expose from the outside a clear area near the dome of the liver where there is no peritoneal covering. Sometimes, the abscess will present there. In other instances, it may be necessary to explore for it with an aspirating needle. This method has found considerable application where amebic abscesses are frequent. Greater experience with chemotherapy of amebic abscesses has reduced the frequency with which this operation must be done. However, it is still necessary occasionally for amebic abscesses which become secondarily infected and it may be useful in the approach to subdiaphragmatic collections of infected material occurring after operations of various kinds in the abdomen.

Where there are multiple small abscesses in the liver, effective surgical drainage seldom can be accomplished, and in general one must pin his hopes on chemotherapy which will sometimes effect recovery. (See also Chap. 37, on drainage of subdiaphragmatic abscesses.)

REFERENCES

Allen, A. W.: A method of re-establishing continuity between the bile ducts and the gastrointestinal tract. Ann. Surg., 121:412, 1945.

Allen, J. G.: The diagnostic value of prothrombin response to vitamin K therapy as a means of differentiating between intrahepatic and obstructive jaundice; collective review, Int. Abstr. Surg., 76:401, 1943.

Allen, J. G., and Julian, O. C.: Response of plasma prothrombin to vitamin K substitute therapy in cases of hepatic disease. Arch. Surg., 41:1363, 1940.

Becker, W. F.: Perforation of the gallbladder. Surg., Gynec., Obstet., 105:636, 1957.

Bergkvist, A., and Seldinger, S. I.: Pancreatic reflux in operative cholangiography in relation to pre- and postoperative pancreatic affection. Acta chir. scand., 114:191, 1957-1958.

Berk, J. E.: Chapter C *In* Bockus: Gastroenterology. vol. 3. Philadelphia, Saunders, 1946.

———: Management of acute cholecystitis. Am. J. Digest. Dis., 7:325, 1940.

Berkowitz, H. D., Miller, L. D., and Itskovitz, H. D.: Liver disease, renal function, and the renin-angiotensin system. Surg. Forum, 19:391, October 1969.

Bisgard, J. D., and Baker, C. P.: Studies relating to the pathogenesis of cholecystitis, cholelithiasis and acute pancreatitis. Ann. Surg., 112:1006, 1940.

Bockus, H. L., Shay, H., Willard, J. H., and Pessel, J. F.: Comparison of biliary drainage and cholecystography in gallstone diagnosis. J.A.M.A., 96:311, 1931.

Cahill, K.: Tropical Diseases in Temperate Climates. pp. 28-29. Philadelphia, J. B. Lippincott, 1964.

Campbell, D. A.: A clinical study of carcinoma of the gallbladder. Ann. Surg., 113:1068, 1941.

Cole, W. H., Reynolds, J. T., and Ireneus, C., Jr.: Strictures of the common duct. Ann. Surg., 128:332, 1948.

———: Strictures of the common duct. Ann. Surg., 133:684, 1951.

Cooper, D. Y., Estabrook, R. W., and Rosenthal, O.: Stoichiometry of C-21 hydroxylation of steroids by adrenocortical microsomes. J. Biol. Chem., 238:1320, 1963.

Cooper, W. A.: Carcinoma of the gallbladder. Arch. Surg., 35:431, 1937.

Cowley, L. L., and Harkins, H. N.: Perforation of the gallbladder; a study of twenty-five consecutive cases. Surg., Gynec., Obstet., 77:661, 1943.

DiLuzio, N. R., Simon, K. A., and Upton, A. C.: Effects of x-rays and trypan blue on reticuloendothelial cells. Arch. Path., 64:649, 1957.

Donald, J. D., and Fitts, W. T., Jr.: Cholecystostomy: a study of patients 10 to 16 years later. Am. J. Surg., 78:596, 1949.

Estabrook, R. W., Cooper, D. Y., Rosenthal, O.: Reversible carbon monoxide inhibition of the steroid C-21 hydroxylase system of the adrenal cortex. Biochem., 338:741-755, 1963.

Evans, J. A.: Specialized roentgen diagnostic techniques in the investigation of abdominal disease. Radiology, 82:579, 1964.

Fitts, W. T., Jr.: Personal communication. 1948.

Fitts, W. T., Jr., Scott, R., and Mackie, J. A.: Antibiotics in the prevention of death following ligation of the hepatic artery in dogs. Surgery, 128:458, 1950.

Fletcher, A. G., Jr., and Ravdin, I. S.: Perforation of the gallbladder. Am. J. Surg., 81:178, 1951.

Folin, O., and Denis, W.: The origin and significance of the ammonia in the portal blood. J. Biol. Chem., 11:161, 1912.

Frommhold, W.: Ein neuartiges Kontrastmittel für die intravenöse Cholezystographie. Fortschr. Geb. Röntgenstrahlen, 79:283, 1953.

Garfinkel, D.: Studies on pig liver microsomes. I. Enzymic and pigment composition of different microsomal fractions. Arch. Biochem., 77:493, 1958.

Gatch, W. D., Battersby, J. S., and Wakim, K. G.: The nature and treatment of cholecystitis. J.A.M.A., 132:119, 1946.

Graham, E. A., Cole, W. H., and Copher, G. H.: Cholecystography: The use of sodium tetraiodophenolphthalein. J.A.M.A., 84:1175, 1925.

Hewitt, J. E., Hayes, T. L., Gofman, J. W., Jones, H. B., and Pierce, F. T.: Effects of total body irradiation upon lipoprotein metabolism. Am. J. Physiol. 172:579, 1953.

Howard, J. M., and Jones, R.: The anatomy of the pancreatic duct. Am. J. Med. Sci., 214:617, 1947.

Illingworth, C. F. W.: Carcinoma of the gallbladder. Brit. J. Surg., 23:4, 1935.

Jankelson, I. R.: Clinical aspects of primary carcinoma of the gallbladder. New Eng. J. Med., 217:85, 1937.

Kirby, C. K.: Instrument for detection of stones in the bile ducts. Am. J. Surg., 80:133, 1950.

Kirshbaum, J. D., and Kozoll, D. D.: Carcinoma of the gallbladder and extrahepatic bile ducts. Surg., Gynec., Obstet., 73:740, 1941.

Klingenberg, M.: Pigments of rat liver microsomes. Arch. Biochem., 75:376, 1958.

Kocher, T.: Textbook of Operative Surgery. London, Black, 1903.

Lagenbuch, C.: Ein Fall von Exstirpation der Gallenblase wegen chronischer Cholelithiasis; Heilung. Berlin klin. Wschr., 19:725, 1882.

A case of extirpation of the gallbladder for cholelithiasis by C. Langenbuch (Trans. by S. Brandeis). Louisville M. News, 15:161, 1883.

Life Insurance Fact Book 1959. New York, Institute of Life Insurance, p. 126.

McCubbrey, D., and Thieme, E. T.: Perforation of the gallbladder. Arch. Surg., 80:204, 1960.

McDermott, W. V., Jr., Adams, R. D., and Ridell, A. G.: Ammonia metabolism in man. Ann. Surg., 140:539, 1954.

Madden, J. L., Gruwez, J. A., Tam, P. Y.: Obstructive (surgical) jaundice: An analysis of 140 consecutive cases and a consideration of choledochoduodenostomy in its treatment. Am. J. Surg., 109:89, 1965.

Malt, R. A., Ollsen, H. G., and Goode, W. J., Jr.: Renal tubular necrosis after oral cholecystography. Arch. Surg., 87:743-747, 1963.

Mann, F. C., and Bollman, J. L.: Liver function tests. Arch. Path., 1:681, 1926.

Markowitz, J., Rappaport, A., and Scott, A. C.: Prevention of liver necrosis following ligation of the hepatic artery. Proc. Soc. Exp. Biol. Med., 70:305, 1949.

Massie, J. R., Coxe, J. W., III, Parker, C., and Dietrick, R.: Gallbladder perforations in acute cholecystitis. Ann. Surg., 145:825, 1957.

Merendino, A. K., Dillard, D. N., and Cammock, E. E.: Concept of surgical biliary decompression in the management of liver trauma. Surg., Gynec., Obstet., 117:285-293, 1963.

Morse, L., Krynski, B., and Wright, A. R.: Acute perforation of the gallbladder. Am. J. Surg., 94:772, 1957.

Nissen, R.: Personal communication, May 14, 1959.

Ochsner, A., De Bakey, M., and Murray, S.: Pyogenic abscess of liver: II. An analysis of 47 cases with a review of the literature. Am. J. Surg., 40:292, 1938.

Ohage, J.: Report of case at meeting of County Medical Society, Sept. 27, 1886. Northwestern Lancet, 6:55, 1886.

———: The surgical treatment of diseases of the gallbladder. Med. News Phila., 50:202, 233, 1887.

Pines, B., and Rabinovitch, J.: Perforation of the gallbladder and acute cholecystitis. Ann. Surg., 140:170, 1954.

Pryse-Davies, J., and Wilkinson, J. H.: Diagnostic value of serum-transaminase activity in hepatic and gastrointestinal diseases. Lancet, 1:249, 1958.

Ravdin, I. S.: Surgery of diseases of the liver. In Bancroft, F. W. (ed.): Operative Surgery. New York, Appleton-Century-Crofts, 1941.

Ravdin, I. S., Rhoads, J. E., Frazier, W., and Ulin, A. W.: The effect of recent advances in biliary physiology on the mortality following operations for common duct obstructions. Surgery, 3:804, 1939.

Ravdin, I. S., Thorogood, E., Riegel, C., Peters, C., and Rhoads, J. E.: The prevention of liver damage. J.A.M.A., 121:322, 1943.

Riegel, C. R., Ravdin, I. S., Johnston, C. G., and Morrison, P. J.: Studies of gallbladder function: XIII. The composition of the gallbladder bile and calculi in gallbladder disease. Surg., Gynec., Obstet., 62:933, 1936.

Roberts, B., and Dex, W. J.: Primary carcinoma of the gallbladder. *In* Proceedings of the Third National Cancer Conference. p. 802. Philadelphia, J. B. Lippincott, 1957.

Robertson, H. E., and Dochat, G. R.: Pregnancy and gallstones; collective review. Int. Abstr. Surg., 78:193, 1944.

Sainburg, F. P., and Garlock, G. H.: Carcinoma of the gallbladder; report of seventy-five cases. Surgery, 23:201, 1948.

Sandblom, P.: Hemmorrhage into the biliary tract following trauma: "traumatic hemobilia." Surgery, 24:571-586, 1948.

Sawyer, C. D., and Minnis, J. F., Jr.: Primary carcinoma of the gallbladder. Am. J. Surg., 91:99, 1956.

Stevenson, J. K., and Harkins, H. N.: Acute perforations of the gastrointestinal tract. West. J. Surg., 65(5):286, 1957.

Stormont, J. M., Mackie, J. E., and Davidson, C. S.: Observations on antibiotics in the treatment of hepatic coma and on factors contributing to prognosis. New Eng. J. Med., 259:1145, 1958.

Swinton, N. W., and Becker, W. F.: Tumors of the gallbladder. S. Clin. N. Am., 28:669, 1948.

Ulin, A. W.: Therapeutic trends and operative mortality in cases of obstructive jaundice. Arch. Surg., 46:504, 1943.

Warner, E. D., Brinkhous, K. M., and Smith, H. P.: Bleeding tendency of obstructive jaundice: prothrombin deficiency and dietary factors. Proc. Soc. Exp. Biol. Med., 37:628, 1938.

Warren, R., and Rhoads, J. E.: Hepatic origin of the plasma-prothrombin-observations after total hepatectomy in the dog. Am. J. Med. Sci., 198:193, 1939.

Whipple, A. O.: Pancreatic asthenia as a post-operative complication in patients with lesions of the pancreas. Ann. Surg., 78:176, 1923.

Zamcheck, N., and Sidman, R. L.: Needle biopsy of the liver. I. Its use in clinical and investigative medicine. New Eng. J. Med., 249:1020, 1953.

Zamcheck, N., and Klausenstock, O.: Liver biopsy (concluded). II. The risk of needle biopsy. New Eng. J. Med., 249:1062, 1953.

Zech, R. L.: Acute pancreatitis following cholangiography. West. J. Surg., 57:295, 1949.

CHAPTER 33

JONATHAN E. RHOADS, M.D.

Pancreas

Anatomy
Physiology
Acute Pancreatitis
Postoperative Pancreatitis
Chronic Pancreatitis and Chronic Relapsing Pancreatitis
Unusual Associations of Acute Pancreatitis With Other Conditions
Trauma
Islet Cell Tumors
Pancreaticoduodenal Cancers
Cysts
Benign Solid Tumors
Pancreatic Heterotopia
Metabolic Effects of Total Pancreatectomy

ANATOMY

The pancreas, variously called by such eponyms as the "hermit organ" and the "abdominal salivary gland," is a yellowish, elongated, retroperitoneal gland situated at about the level of the 2nd lumbar vertebra on the posterior wall of the upper abdomen (Fig. 33-1). It is a transverse L-shaped organ about 15 cm. long, 2 to 3 cm. thick and approximately 65 to 125 Gm. in weight, consisting of a head, a neck, a body and a tail. The head nestles in the concavity of the duodenum with which it is intimately associated. The neck overlies the superior mesenteric vessels and the origin of the portal vein. The body and the tail extend upward and laterally to reach the hilum of the spleen. The uncinate process, an inferior extension of the head, is in apposition with the third portion of the duodenum and lies posterior to the mesenteric vessels. Thus, the pancreas is wrapped around the superior mesenteric artery and vein on 3 sides: anteriorly, to the right and posteriorly.

The arterial supply is derived from 3 principal sources. The *superior pancreaticoduodenal artery* arises from the hepatic artery via the gastroduodenal artery and supplies the duodenum and the pancreas in part. It anastomoses with the *inferior pancreaticoduodenal artery*, which usually arises from the superior mesenteric artery, and the two vessels form an arcade between the duodenum and the pancreas and supply principally the duodenum and the uncinate process, the head and the neck of the pancreas. The splenic artery, a branch of the celiac axis, courses along the posterosuperior border of the pancreas en route to the spleen. It is the principal source of supply to the body and the tail of the gland.

Numerous variations of the vascular supply may occur to plague the surgeon. Ligation of certain anomalous vessels may result in such catastrophies as necrosis of the liver or the transverse colon. If attention is paid to the pulsation in the hepatic artery at the hilum of the liver and the pulsations in the middle colic artery and its major branches before dividing, ligating, or crushing any major blood vessel, such injuries will be rare. The principal veins correspond to the arteries except that the superior pancreaticoduodenal vein sometimes empties into the terminal portion of the splenic vein.

There are 3 principal groups of lymph nodes closely associated with the pancreas. These comprise the subpyloric group, the pancreaticolienal nodes and the group in proximity to the uncinate process and the superior mesenteric vessels at that level. Lymphatics accompany the major vessels and may terminate in the pancreatic nodes; they anastomose freely with lymphatics which terminate in the nodes about the stomach and the aorta. Branches of the sympathetic and the parasympathetic nerves accompany the vessels, terminating as fine filaments about the acini.

Duct System

The duct of Wirsung, coursing throughout the length of the pancreas, is the main pancreatic duct. In the head of the pancreas it becomes closely associated with the terminal portion of the common bile duct and, in the majority of cases, the 2 ducts terminate jointly at the papilla of Vater on the concave side of the second part of the duodenum (about 7 cm. from the pylorus). The ampulla of Vater is a channel lined by epithelium and formed by the confluence of the common bile duct and the main pancreatic duct. The sphincter of Oddi encompasses the ducts just proximal to their terminus on the papilla.

Since 1901 when Opie first presented his common channel theory of the etiology of acute pancreatitis (Opie, 1903) interest has centered in the termination patterns of the 2 ducts. In 29 per cent of cases (Rienhoff and Pickrell, 1945) the 2 ducts enter the duodenum through separate openings on a common papilla. However, in the majority of cases the 2 ducts communicate to form a single short channel before entering the duodenum. Various classifications have been employed using as a criterion the depth of the ampulla. In from 54 per cent (Howard and Jones, 1947) to 66 per cent (Cameron and Noble, 1924) of cadavers it was found that a stone impacted distally could divert the flow of bile into the pancreatic duct or alternatively the flow of pancreatic juice into the biliary tract. Millbourn (1949), using cholangiographic technics in postmortem specimens, found a common channel in 91.5 per cent.

The duct of Santorini, the accessory pancreatic duct, is present in the majority of glands and drains a portion of the head of the pancreas. It opens separately, without a sphincter, into the duodenum proximal to the papilla of Vater. The 2 pancreatic ducts were found to communicate in 36 per cent (Howard and Jones) and in 89 per cent (Rienhoff and Pickrell) of cases.

HISTOLOGY

The pancreas has no true capsule but is enveloped by loose connective tissue from which septa extend to divide the gland into lobules. It is covered on the anterior surface by the posterior parietal peritoneum. Both the exocrine and the endocrine secretory cells are derived from the finer ductules, although the latter lose their connection with the duct system. The exocrine gland cells form the main

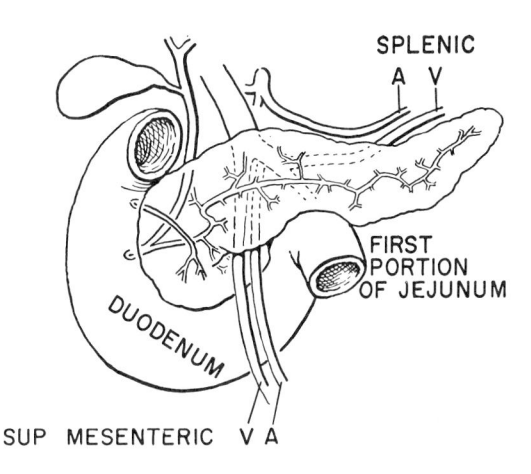

FIG. 33-1. Anatomy of the pancreas and its relation to surrounding structures.

mass of the organ and form acini whose component secreting cells are characterized by basal nuclei and zymogen granules. Spheroidal aggregations of light-staining cells, the islets of Langerhans, are found scattered throughout the gland but are more numerous in the tail. The islets number from 200,000 to 2,000,000.

ANNULAR PANCREAS

Pancreatic tissue surrounding the second portion of the duodenum is termed annular pancreas. It represents a developmental defect and is occasionally symptomatic, causing the picture of high intestinal obstruction, especially in children, due to the formation of a constriction. It is usually best treated by anastomosis of the jejunum to the duodenum proximal to the point of narrowing. (See Chap. 50, Pediatric Surgery.)

PANCREATIC HETEROTOPIA

Another developmental abnormality is the occurrence of pancreatic tissue along various parts of the alimentary tract not connected with the main organ. These too are occasionally symptomatic.

PHYSIOLOGY

The pancreas is a dual gland, having both an exocrine and an endocrine function.

Pancreas

The Pancreas as an Exocrine Gland

Pancreatic juice, the daily production of which is about 1,500 to 2,000 milliliters, is a clear, limpid fluid with an alkaline pH. It contains trypsinogen, chymotrypsinogen, amylase, pancreatic lipase (steapsin) and maltase. Pancreatic juice also contains a carboxypolypeptidase capable of digesting certain peptides.

Trypsinogen is activated (converted to trypsin) by the action of enterokinase, an enzyme found in the succus entericus and also by the action of trypsin itself. *Activated trypsin* splits proteoses, peptones and polypeptides to simple peptides in an alkaline medium. It is more potent than pepsin. *Chymotrypsinogen* is activated by trypsin and has a similar action but is a weaker proteolytic agent. *Amylase* converts long-chain carbohydrates such as starch and glycogen to dextrins and sugars. *Pancreatic lipase* splits fats into glycerin and fatty acids. *Bile salts* increase the efficiency of this process by helping to emulsify the fats.

The author is indebted to his associate Dr. Howard Reber for the following description of pancreatic exocrine physiology.

Pancreatic Exocrine Physiology

Pancreatic secretion is a clear limpid fluid with an alkaline pH; the daily output of the human pancreas approximates 1.5 liters. The rate and composition of the secretion is influenced by humoral and neural mechanisms. When acid chyme comes into contact with the mucosa of the duodenum, a hormone, *secretin*, is released into the bloodstream and stimulates the pancreas to secrete a large volume of watery fluid that is rich in bicarbonate and poor in enzymes. The presence of various foods in the duodenum causes the release of another hormone, *pancreozymin*, that causes the output of a juice rich in enzymes, but does not greatly influence total volume or bicarbonate concentration in the juice. The gastric mucosal hormone, *gastrin*, has effects similar to pancreozymin. Vagal stimulation also causes the release of an enzyme-rich juice; it is unclear at present whether this effect is mediated through the release of gastrin or by direct action on the pancreas (Gregory and Tracy, 1964). These vagal effects can be inhibited by atropine or vagotomy. There is some recent evidence that the sulfa drugs and some antibiotics (colistin, kanamycin, erythromycin) are excreted in pancreatic juice (Dainko *et al.*, 1963).

Organic Constituents. The protein fraction of pancreatic juice is comprised almost entirely of enzymes: these include trypsinogen and chymotrypsinogen (inactive precursors of trypsin and chymotrypsin, the classical endopeptidases), and procarboxypeptidase (precursor of carboxypeptidase, an exopeptidase); also several ribonucleases, as well as elastase, amylase, and lipase (Neurath, 1963).

Trypsinogen is activated to trypsin by the action of enterokinase, an enzyme found in the succus entericus, and by trypsin itself. Chymotrypsinogen is activated by trypsin. Amylase converts long chain carbohydrates such as starch and glycogen to dextrins and sugars. Lipase splits fats (triglycerides) into monoglycerides and fatty acids. All these enzymes are secreted by the acinar cells, whose zymogen granules contain the inactive precursors (Palade *et al.*, 1963).

Inorganic Constituents. Pancreatic juice contains greater or lesser amounts of all the major ions. Of the cations, sodium and potassium are present in the juice in roughly the same concentrations as they appear in plasma, and do not vary with the flow rate. Calcium, which plays an important role in the activation of trypsinogen (Desnuelle *et al.*, 1963), is present in lower concentration than in plasma. The

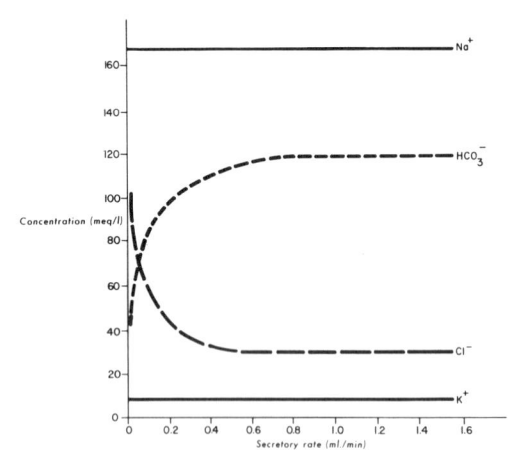

FIG. 33-2. Relation between the rate of secretion and the concentrations of electrolytes in dog pancreatic juice. (From Bro-Rasmussen *et al.*, 1956)

anions behave more interestingly; the anionic composition is a function of flow rate. Bicarbonate concentration, which ranges from 25 to 150 mEq/L, varies directly with the rate of flow, while chloride varies inversely with the bicarbonate concentration, so that the sum of the two anions remains constant (Janowitz and Dreiling, 1963). (Fig. 33-2.)

This relationship between rate of flow and bicarbonate holds true in the healthy pancreas no matter what the stimulus to fluid secretion may be, exogenously administered secretin or secretin endogenously released from the duodenum. However, this apparently invariant relationship may be altered by drugs, hormones, or disease in two directions: (1) the secretion of juice at high rates of flow with lowered bicarbonate concentration (in chronic inflammation in man) and (2) the preservation of high bicarbonate concentrations at low rates of secretion (following the carbonic anhydrase inhibitor, acetazolamide, or anticholinergic drugs) (Dreiling and Janowitz, 1959).

The exact cell of origin of the water and bicarbonate remains unknown. Since secretory rate does not influence the output of enzymes, nor visibly alter the appearance of the zymogen granules in the acinar cells, the ductular epithelium is most widely held to be the site of elaboration of the alkali. This belief is strengthened by the finding that carbonic anhydrase can be demonstrated histochemically in the ductular system only, and not in the acinar cell (Becker, 1963).

Many theories have been advanced to explain the interesting relationship between secretory rate and bicarbonate concentration. Most investigators hold the theory put forth by Dreiling and Janowitz (1963), that the pancreatic fluid as it flows through the smaller ducts of the collecting system is acted upon by the cells which comprise the ductular wall. However, recent work by Reber and Wolf (1968) employing micropuncture technics has shown no difference in bicarbonate or chloride concentration along the smaller ducts. These differences may be resolved by more recent evidence that the main duct of the rabbit pancreas is able to reabsorb bicarbonate, and that the rate of fall of bicarbonate concentration is inversely proportional to flow rate through the duct. Whether the reabsorption is active or passive, or under the influence of neurons or hormones is not yet known.*

Pure pancreatic juice does not digest living tissue such as skin. Erosion of the skin about abdominal fistulas implies that the pancreatic juice has become activated. Aluminum paste and building cement powder (bentonite) have found favor in minimizing the skin excoriation. However, constant wound suction still remains the single most effective method of reducing skin damage from activated pancreatic enzymes.

THE PANCREAS AS AN ENDOCRINE GLAND

Insulin, a product of the beta cells of the islets of Langerhans, is the hormone which plays a vital role in carbohydrate, fat and protein metabolism. Without it men soon die. Its exact mechanism of action has not yet been completely elucidated.

Cells of the islets of Langerhans have also been shown to produce a blood-sugar-raising principle (glucagon).

Because it was found that completely depancreatized dogs maintained on insulin still died in a few months and at postmortem demonstrated fatty infiltration of the liver, it was postulated that the pancreas elaborated yet another hormone. Dragstedt (1936) prepared an extract of the pancreas, which he called "lipocaic," that prevented fatty infiltration and permitted prolonged survival of depancreatized dogs maintained with insulin. The dose was about 1 Gm. daily. Lecithin, choline and methionine had been found to possess similar properties.

Rhoads *et al.* (1951) studied the effect of a lipotropic extract, produced by the method of Bosshardt, Ciereszko and Barnes (1951), on depancreatized dogs. They found that it was effective in preventing fatty infiltration of the liver, and the observations suggested that the material acted as an enzyme, since it was less effective in dogs that ate poorly (insufficient methionine?).

Haanes and Gyorgy (1951) found that Bosshardt's extract contained a powerful proteolytic enzyme (probably trypsin), the action of which was masked by an excess of an inhibitor. Duodenal juice (from a depancreatized dog) destroyed the effect of this inhibitor,

* Reber and Wolf, 1969.

leaving the proteolytic enzyme free to liberate methionine from casein.

In certain depancreatized patients Nardi (1952, 1954) and his collaborators have found that no replacement therapy except insulin has been necessary. Marked differences apparently occur between species and probably between individuals so that replacement therapy is provided after total pancreatectomy until detailed studies show that digestion is reasonably complete without it.

NON-BETA CELL TUMORS

The cells of the islands of Langerhans have been classified histologically as alpha cells, beta cells and other types. The beta cells are the site of formation of insulin. Non-beta cells are believed to produce glucagon (a glycogenolytic substance). Certain non-beta cell tumors produce gastrin or a similar material (*See* Zollinger-Ellison syndrome, Chapter 31).

ACUTE PANCREATITIS

Acute pancreatitis is an inflammation of the pancreas affecting all or, more rarely, a part of the gland. It may be evidenced only by edema and leukocytic infiltration, or by these signs and evidence of necrosis in the gland and necrosis of fat in the vicinity of the pancreas or even at a distance in the peritoneal cavity due to the escape of enzymes. In severe cases fat necrosis also has been observed in the thoracic cavity. Severe pancreatitis may be associated with hemorrhage into the gland or even hemorrhage from the gland into the peritoneal cavity (hemorrhagic pancreatitis) or by actual necrosis of macroscopic portions of the gland with sloughing (necrotizing pancreatitis). In the past, a considerable effort has been made to distinguish edematous pancreatitis from hemorrhagic and necrotizing pancreatitis. The mortality of those cases showing only edema is slight, whereas the mortality in the hemorrhagic and necrotizing forms has exceeded 50 per cent in some series. However, available evidence suggests that these are 2 stages of the same disease rather than separate entities. Some patients who have been operated on in the edematous stage have recovered from that attack only to experience subsequent development of the hemorrhagic necrotizing form from which they died. Surely differentiation of the two at the time of a hospital admission is uncertain unless operation or autopsy is subsequently performed. Men are afflicted by the severe forms of the disease more frequently than women.

In a series of cases reported from the Hospital of the University of Pennsylvania, the range and average for temperature, pulse rate, respirations and leukocyte count on admission were almost identical for those cases in which edematous pancreatitis was found at laparotomy and for those cases in which necrotizing pancreatitis was found at laparotomy. Probably it is possible to pick out as hemorrhagic or necrotizing a few of the very severe cases on the clinical picture, but for the large majority differentiation can be made only on the basis of the course of the disease and the pathologic findings at operation or at autopsy.

The development of practical methods for the determination of the serum amylase and lipase have revolutionized the diagnosis of pancreatitis within certain limitations to be discussed below. However, it is not claimed that the studies of these enzymes at the time of admission to a hospital will effectively distinguish the edematous form of the disease from the hemorrhagic or necrotizing forms, as very high values frequently occur in edematous pancreatitis as well as with the more severe types of the disease.

CLINICAL PICTURE

The milder forms of pancreatitis are associated with pain in the epigastrium, frequently radiating to the back near the angles of the scapulae; this radiation may be to the left side of the back, to the right side of the back or to both sides. Vomiting may or may not occur. The chief differential problems in diagnosis at this stage are acute cholecystitis, peptic ulcer with a slow leak or a leak that is sealed off, or a penetrating ulcer that has given rise to inflammation without frank perforation. From this picture one sees various degrees of severity up to and including the patient who has had a rapid onset of severe abdominal pain, with prostration, marked tachycardia, high fever and a gray, shocklike appearance. Such patients often become distended early from adynamic ileus and not infrequently vomit profusely. The vomitus is sometimes fecal in character. Associated with these symptoms will usually be found very marked abdominal tenderness, rebound tenderness, diminution or absence of peristaltic sounds on auscultation of the abdomen, and marked muscle spasm and rigidity. Here the differential diagnosis includes ruptured peptic ulcer, renal colic, acute phlegmonous gastritis and possibly perforation of the gallbladder, mesenteric occlusion, volvulus, dissecting aneurysm of the abdominal aorta or myocardial infarction.

The most useful confirmatory studies from the laboratory are the serum amylase and the serum lipase. The amylase is of greater value in the first 48 hours of the disease, whereas the lipase remains elevated for a longer period, usually 5 to 7 days. Unfortunately, the elevation of the serum amylase is not absolutely pathognomonic for primary pancreatitis. Elevations occur frequently in patients in whom an ulcer penetrates against the pancreas, setting up a local inflammatory process. Elevations have also been noted in a miscellaneous group of patients undergoing operation, especially operations in the region of the pancreas, and in patients with acute cholecystitis. The editors of this volume have seen marked elevations of amylase in high intestinal obstruction, volvulus of the small intestine, mesenteric vascular occlusion, trauma to upper lumbar and lower thoracic space (laminectomy), and acute renal insufficiency. The significance of this is that when one wishes to treat pancreatitis without operation, one would like to have a test which would remain unaffected by other diseases entering into the differential diagnosis which do require operation. Hence, in the present state of our knowledge, it is still frequently necessary to operate on patients suspected of having an acute pancreatitis because the picture is sufficiently compatible with that of a perforated peptic ulcer, a very acute cholecystitis with rupture, or mesenteric occlusion.

Determination of serum amylase by the method of Somogyi (1938) requires approximately 1½ hours, whereas determination of lipase by most of the standard methods requires from 4 to 24 hours. Therefore, for emergency use the amylase test has been of greater value. The normal level runs up to about 200 Somogyi units; in the presence of acute pancreatitis, this value usually is exceeded by more than 100 units and not infrequently mounts as high as 1,000 units or more. Institutions caring for patients with acute abdominal disease should provide for the performance of this test on emergency admissions on a 24-hour-a-day, 7-day-a-week basis.

The concentration of serum calcium often falls from 36 to 48 hours after the beginning of an attack of severe pancreatitis. Levels as low as 7 mg./100 ml. have been seen. This is not known to occur in any other acute abdominal condition except occasionally in a leaking duodenal stump, a perforated peptic ulcer, or ulcerative colitis with ileostomy. The fall in serum calcium is commonly attributed to the binding of calcium with fatty acids to form insoluble calcium soaps in areas of fat necrosis. Symptoms and signs of hypocalcemia are described in Chapter 28 (Parathyroid).

Etiology

Acute pancreatitis can be reproduced experimentally in the dog by injecting bile into the main pancreatic duct under pressure. Opie (1910) originally postulated that some instances of the disease in man might be due to the entrance of bile into the pancreatic duct as the result of a stone lodged in the papilla of Vater. This presupposes a common channel of sufficient length to permit the bile to move into the pancreatic duct behind the stone. According to the studies of Jones and Howard (1947), there was a common channel of at least 0.5 cm. in 54 per cent in a series of 100 individuals examined at necropsy whom they had opportunity to study. It also presupposes a higher pressure in the biliary tract than in the pancreatic ductal system. However, experimental evidence does not support this presupposition with uniformity.

Also, it has been suggested that pancreatitis arises by virtue of bacterial infection coursing toward the pancreas from the gallbladder and the hilum of the liver through the lymphatics. Others have postulated that the infection is an ascending one through the ductal system into the pancreas from the duodenum. There are authenticated cases in which an acute pancreatitis has followed trauma. While this may be penetrating in type, it also has followed blunt trauma to the abdomen without a break in the skin. Another small group of cases has occurred after operation, particularly operations on the biliary tract or the stomach where, of course, there may be some disturbance or even trauma to the pancreas. A further occasional cause of pancreatitis is apparently the mumps virus, which attacks primarily the salivary glands but may attack the gonads and the pancreas also.

The frequency with which severe acute necrotizing and hemorrhagic pancreatitis occurs among alcoholics is so much higher relative to its frequency among the nondrinkers that alcoholic debauchery may be considered as a predisposing factor.

Mallet-Guy (1944) and others of the French workers have produced pancreatitis in the experimental animal by electrical stimulation of autonomic nerves leading to the pancreas.

Treatment

The treatment of acute pancreatitis has gone through cycles, between operative and nonoperative treatment. In the severe forms of the disease attempts at drainage of the pancreas have been attended by mortality rates as high as 70 per cent (Babcock, 1930). The present consensus is that wherever the diagnosis can be established safely, operation should not be done during the acute stage, though if the process goes on to the formation of abscesses or collections of necrotic material in the pancreas, usually these will require free drainage, perhaps in the 2nd or the 3rd or subsequent weeks after the onset of the attack.

If early operation is done, as is not infrequently necessary in order to exclude the possibility of other serious intra-abdominal conditions, and if at the time of operation acute pancreatitis is found it is our practice to do a simple cholecystostomy in order to permit an easy route for bile to escape in the event that the common channel is occluded at its termination either by stone or spasm, and to lay drains down to the pancreas without injuring its substance in any way. Then the wound is closed, all unnecessary surgical manipulation being scrupulously avoided. Waterman and colleagues (1967) have dissented from the consensus of the last few decades and favor early operation and sump drainage of the peripancreatic spaces. They report a mortality rate of 10 per cent in 10 cases.

Nonoperative treatment includes antibiotics, which have had a profound effect on the course of acute pancreatitis. Penicillin is administered in divided doses totaling 1,000,000 units a day; one of the polyvalent antibiotics parenterally and possibly chlortetracycline by mouth or through a stomach tube may be given. According to the experiments of Fine and his collaborators on the dog, chlortetracycline by mouth was especially beneficial in the reduction of the mortality rate in experimental pancreatitis (Persky et al., 1951). It also depends on the application of standard methods of treating peritonitis, hypotension and hypovolemia, including suction drainage of the stomach, water and electrolytes in sufficient amounts to maintain the internal environment of the body normal with respect to sodium, potassium, chloride and pH, and transfusions of blood or plasma sufficient to maintain blood volume and hemoglobin and protein concentrations near the normal range. If the serum calcium is reduced, calcium gluconate should be given intravenously in doses up to 1 Gm. every 2 to 4 hours until it is restored to the normal range.

The role of paravertebral injections of local anesthetic agents deserves especial mention. This method of treatment in pancreatitis was advocated vigorously by Mims Gage (1948) in New Orleans. From 10 to 20 cc. of 1 per cent procaine is introduced on each side of the spine just below the level of the 12th rib along the anterolateral surface of the vertebral body. Often the procedure is followed by a striking relief of pain, even in patients whose pain has not been relieved by 15 to 30 mg. of morphine sulfate. Gage (1948) believed that the procaine relieves vascular spasm and exerts a therapeutic as well as a symptomatic effect. The method was very widely practiced, although perhaps more on an empiric basis than anything else. It is now used chiefly for relief of pain. In our own clinic, it is customary to give 1 or 2 procaine injections on each side during the first 24 hours and to repeat them once a day for 2 or 3 days if pain persists.

The combined use of gastroduodenal suction and atropine constitutes a very important part of the treatment of acute pancreatitis by virtue of the fact that atropine prevents vagal stimulation of the pancreas, and the gastroduodenal suction removes the stimulus for the elaboration of secretin, the principal humoral stimulant.

A pancreatic enzyme inhibitor, developed and marketed under the name "Trasylol," is prepared from bovine parotid gland and has the property of inhibiting trypsin and chymotrypsin. It is prepared in suitable form for intravenous administration and has been applied in clinical as well as experimental pancreatitis. Reports, while favorable, are impressionistic and as yet do not afford a convincing basis for establishing its value in clinical pancreatitis.

It has also been used by Inouye and Vars in experimental animals to protect enterally administered insulin from digestion until significant amounts of the insulin could be absorbed. While the authors were able to maintain a depancreatized dog in this way for several weeks, the method is uneconomic because many times as much insulin was required as is needed by the subcutaneous route (Moss, 1960).

PROGNOSIS

If one takes all patients diagnosed as having acute pancreatitis with the support of an elevated serum amylase, mortality is relatively low; Howard (Rhoads et al., 1949) reported 3 per cent. On the other hand, if one restricts the series to those cases known to have hemorrhagic or necrotizing pancreatitis on the basis of laparotomy, mortality rates are much higher, usually 20 per cent and up. A review of the statistics from the Hospital of the University of Pennsylvania by Kirby and Senior yielded the following data (Table 33-1). Severe acute pancreatitis remains a serious disease despite all forms of present-day therapy, including antibiotics. Mortality rates are likely to reflect more the zealousness of an institution in establishing the diagnosis in a large number of mild or borderline cases than any other one factor. It should be remembered that before the development of the amylase test, only the severe forms were recognized.

Early deaths from pancreatitis indeed appear to be much rarer than was the case before the advent of the antibiotics and other concomitant advances. In those days it was common for pancreatitis to be fatal in the first few days—sometimes in the first 24 hours. With the exception of a single case in our recent experience, all of the patients have lived for over a week, and most of the fatal cases have survived from 2 to 6 weeks. In these individuals a suppurative autolyzing process is set up in the pancreas, which it seems impossible to control by drainage or even by the removal of some of the necrotic tissue after an appropriate interval of some weeks. Activated pancreatic ferments apparently continue to be released, and the terminal event is frequently hemorrhage from a large artery, the wall of which is digested away. This may be the hepatic artery or some other major branch of the celiac axis or the superior mesenteric artery. Necrosis involves not only the pancreas but seems to extend some distance into the retroperitoneal fat. It is difficult to define what the factors of resistance may be to this process, but some individuals clearly have greater powers of localizing the process than do others.

Experience with acute pancreatitis in Moscow was reported by Bystrov (1959) in a series of 810 cases. Of these, 60 patients or 7.4 per cent of the series were classified as having hemorrhagic necrosis of the pancreas. Twenty-three patients, including all of the 8 not operated upon, died, so that the per cent of mortality was 38.

It is evident that recovery from one attack of pancreatitis does not guarantee that the individual will not suffer a subsequent attack. In a series of 47 cases of acute pancreatitis followed by Howard (Howard and Ravdin, 1948), 5 were found to have had subsequent attacks of pancreatitis, 2 of them fatal. Cholelithiasis is present in about 75 per cent of the

TABLE 33-1. ACUTE PANCREATITIS*
Hospital of the University of Pennsylvania
Mortality Before and After 1946 (Per cent)

	EDEMATOUS	NECROTIZING	TOTAL	POSTOPERATIVE
1922–46	11.9	76.2	28.8	...
1946–53	4.6	33.3	13.8	57.1

* Rhoads, J. E., Senior, J. R., Kirby, C. K., and Rhoads, D. V. Surgery of the Pancreas. Presented at the 66th annual meeting of the Mid-South Postgraduate Medical Assembly, Memphis, Tenn., Feb. 8-11, 1955.

patients in most series of cases of fatal acute pancreatitis. In most clinics it is routine to investigate the gallbladder by cholecystography after the acute attack has passed and to remove those in which there is evidence of cholelithiasis. We believe this to be good practice.

Eleven series of acute pancreatitis cases in which the diagnosis was determinate were collected by Howard and comprised a total of 591 patients; 300 (50.7%) of these had cholelithiasis.

Howard gives the recurrence rate of pancreatitis in the presence of cholelithiasis at 53 per cent (average follow-up period 36 months) and compares this with a figure of 3 per cent among 160 cases who had undergone cholecystectomy and had been followed for from 1 to 7 years.

The use of dyes for visualizing the gallbladder after pancreatitis raises certain questions. When the dye originally advocated by Graham and Cole (1924), tetraiodophenolphthalein, was employed in the presence of jaundice, several instances of acute pancreatitis were reported. Dick and Wallace (1928) found that if the dye were given to an animal and the contents of the gallbladder aspirated at a time when the dye was concentrated there, this material seemed to be especially toxic when injected into the pancreatic duct. However, Howard (1948) was unable to confirm this finding with iodoalphionic acid. So far iodipamide has not been incriminated, but we have not studied it from this standpoint experimentally. A case of acute pancreatitis occurring immediately following an operative cholangiogram occurred in 1954 and was reported by Hershey and Hillman (1955).

Acute pancreatitis apparently due to parasitic infestation has been reported from Hanoi by Tong That Tung and his associates (1960). Among 103 patients, there was one in whom the parasite was actually found in the pancreatic duct. In 19 patients ascarides were found in the bile duct without stones; in 17 patients ascarides and stones were found; and in the remaining patients (67) only "ascaridic" stones were found containing eggs of Ascaris, pieces of dead worms, or both.

These cases require operation, and the authors report that acute, severe "ascaridic cholecystic-pancreatitis" treated expectantly is accompanied by a mortality rate approaching 100 per cent. Operation usually included clearing the common bile duct, except in the sickest patients in whom cholecystostomy was used as a first stage.

The editors know of no matching experience in the United States with which to compare this unusual report.

POSTOPERATIVE PANCREATITIS

Acute postoperative pancreatitis has been reported not only after surgical procedures in close proximity to the pancreas such as gastric resection, biliary tract surgery and splenectomy, but also following cholangiography, transurethral resection, thyroidectomy, appendectomy, cesarean section, dorsolumbar laminectomy and colon resection. Hotchkiss et al. (1954) reviewed the literature of postoperative pancreatitis and studied the effects of intra-abdominal and extra-abdominal operations on the serum lipase and amylase. Possible etiologic factors concerned in the mechanism of postoperative pancreatitis may be as follows:

1. Mechanical injury to the parenchyma of the pancreas
2. Injury to pancreatic vessels
3. Injuries to the pancreatic ducts, especially the duct of Santorini
4. Obstruction of the pancreatic ducts associated with an actively secreting gland
5. Spasm of the muscles about the ampulla, producing a common channel permitting a reflux of bile into the pancreatic ducts
6. An increase in the viscosity of pancreatic secretion induced by dehydration, atropine and ether during operation and by pancreatic manipulation (Dunphy, Brooks and Achroyd, 1953)
7. Postoperative infection in the region of the pancreas
8. Overzealous palpation of the pancreas at operation

Hotchkiss found that there is a moderate depression of serum amylase and a moderate and consistent depression of serum lipase in most postoperative patients. Elevations of serum amylase without significant elevations in serum lipase were found in some cases after both the intra-abdominal operations and extra-abdominal operations, especially after operations upon or near the pancreas. None of the patients he studied had clinical signs of pancreatitis, and the author concluded that such a diagnosis is hazardous on the basis of elevated serum amylase alone.

The author has seen several cases of postoperative pancreatitis of a severe degree (with hemorrhage and massive necrosis)—one following a common duct exploration which seemed to be uneventful at the time of operation. The mortality has been extremely high, 57 per cent in the author's experience, 50 to 80 per cent as stated by Howard and Jordan (1960). The very high mortality may be colored by difficulty in making the diagnosis except in the severe cases.

CHRONIC PANCREATITIS AND CHRONIC RELAPSING PANCREATITIS

Chronic Pancreatitis

This term is reserved largely for fibrosis in the pancreas without acute symptoms, whereas chronic relapsing pancreatitis is marked by remittent symptoms with significant pain.

These two conditions are almost certainly different forms of the same process. Chronic pancreatitis may be relatively "silent" with vague digestive disturbances. Occasionally, it causes sufficient constriction of the lower end of the common bile duct to produce jaundice. It then is almost indistinguishable from carcinoma of the head of the pancreas. Biopsy of the head of the pancreas is difficult and uncertain and is sometimes followed by severe reactions. Because it and the frozen section examination are unreliable, sometimes these patients are subjected to pancreaticoduodenectomy. This is an unnecessarily extensive procedure, because these patients usually do very well with a simple sidetracking procedure such as a cholecystojejunostomy. Therefore, the more radical procedure should not be done unless it is believed that malignancy is present and resectable.

The decision to resect is a difficult one. There must be a tumor in the pancreas so situated as to explain the symptoms. Involvement of the entire gland is suggestive of chronic pancreatitis rather than malignancy. If there are enlarged lymph nodes adjacent to the pancreas, often one can be removed for frozen section. The finding of malignant cells would militate against resection. Age and debility may be deciding factors against resection. The existence of fat necrosis suggests inflammation but does not absolutely rule out neoplasm.

The experience cited by Rhoads, Zintel and Helwig (1960) suggests that 7 per cent of hard pancreatic swellings accompanied by jaundice probably were due to chronic inflammation rather than carcinoma.

Chronic Relapsing Pancreatitis

Whereas the diagnosis of chronic pancreatitis must most often be made at operation, that of chronic relapsing pancreatitis can be made preoperatively with a fair degree of accuracy.

A typical case is the following. A middle-aged man, a regular consumer of alcohol, began having epigastric pain of a dull aching character extending through to the back at about the 8th dorsal segment but not sharply localized. It tended to be accentuated by eating, and he noted anorexia but no vomiting. He lost 15 pounds in weight over a period of 6 months. The pain would flare up acutely for 1 to 3 days at a time. At such a period he would run a low-grade temperature, 99 to 101° F. He usually had mild tenderness in the epigastrium, and during exacerbations this became more marked but was not associated with much muscle spasm or rebound tenderness. Gradually, he had come to use codeine with increasing frequency.

Roentgenograms of the abdomen were first interpreted as showing only calcified mesenteric lymph nodes. Then the patient was referred to a psychiatrist with the impression that the symptoms might be psychosomatic.

Later x-ray studies showed calcification in the region of the pancreas (Fig. 33-3). A sugar tolerance curve was diabetic in type, and postprandial blood sugars were high. Finally, a tube was passed into the duodenum, and specimens were collected before and after stimulation of the pancreas by secretin. The specimens were analyzed for enzyme concentration, and marked reductions were found in fat, starch and protein-splitting activity. A diagnosis of chronic relapsing pancreatitis was made and confirmed at operation.

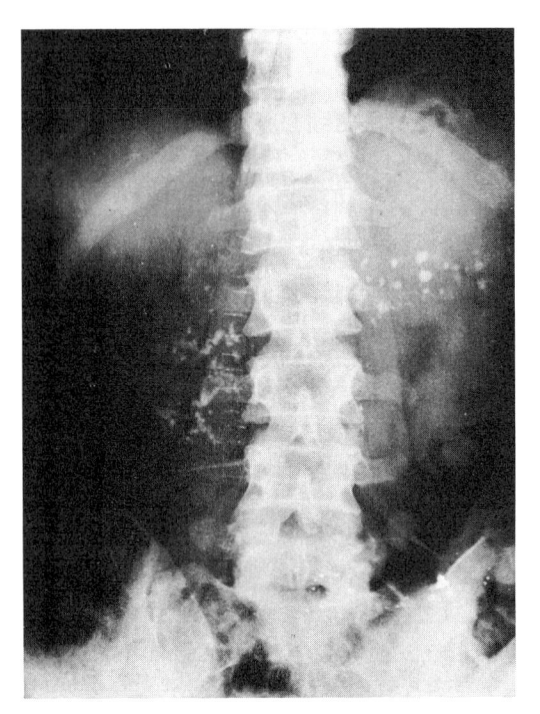

FIG. 33-3. Roentgenogram showing calcification in pancreas in chronic relapsing pancreatitis.

Some patients develop marked diffuse calcification which delineates the whole gland. In others this may not be found. Some patients develop discrete calculi in the pancreatic ducts. Formerly, attempts were made to remove such stones, but at present the balance of evidence seems to be that they are usually a part of the picture of chronic relapsing pancreatitis and should be treated as such. Simple removal of the calculi rarely afforded lasting relief. Large solitary calculi constitute most of the exceptions.

Likewise, diabetes is not necessarily present, but as the disease progresses the sugar tolerance curve may go up, and eventually frank diabetes may appear.

The enzyme studies of duodenal content after secretion stimulation (lipase, amylase, trypsin) are at times very helpful but are very time-consuming.

Another finding which may be helpful is a rise in blood amylase and/or lipase early in the exacerbations. Late in the course of the disease, however, the pancreas may act as though it were "burned out," so that the absence of such rises does not exclude the diagnosis. In fact, low amylase values may be suggestive of chronic pancreatitis.

Except in very fully developed cases, the diagnosis requires confirmation at laparotomy. Grossly, the pancreas feels firm to hard and usually a bit enlarged. The surrounding tissues are edematous, fibrotic or rubbery, as the case may be, and generally show evidence of inflammation in adjacent tissues. If biopsy is done, it shows increased fibrosis and round cell infiltration. There may or may not be dilatation of the ducts, calcification, or polymorphonuclear cell infiltration. Occasionally, a cystlike area will mark the site of a subsiding abscess or focus of necrosis. Both the acinar cells and the islet cells are replaced in varying degrees by fibrous tissue.

While the chronic relapsing pancreatitis is not frequent, its chronicity makes it a pressing problem whenever it is encountered. One of the difficult features of this disease is the frequency with which patients seeking relief from its symptoms become addicted to narcotics.

Therapy is still at the stage where the number of the methods of treatment advocated indicates that none is ideal. The following are among those reported:

1. **Total Pancreatectomy.** This eradicates the disease process but leaves the patient diabetic and handicaps his digestion. Operative mortality has been high. Unexpected coma following the ingestion of alcohol has resulted in the death of a number of those individuals who have survived the operation.

2. **Sphincterotomy** (Doubilet and Mulholland, 1949; 1951). Good results have been claimed following division of the sphincter of Oddi, but it is not clear that the process is due to obstruction at the sphincter. Most follow-up reports have been short. Relief from symptoms has not been uniform by any means.

3. **Ligation of the Ducts** (Rienhoff). The objective here is to complete the process of fibrosis as observed in the dogs used by Banting and Best in the discovery of insulin. Little experience has been reported with this method as yet.

4. A. **Anastomosis** of the duct of Wirsung to the jejunum (Cattell, 1947).

B. **Amputation** of the tail of the pancreas and anastomosis of the duct to a defunctionalized loop of jejunum.

C. Side-to-side anastomosis between the duct of Wirsung and a jejunal loop (filleting operation of Puestow and Gillesby, 1958).

These again are procedures to improve drainage of the ductal system.

5. **Vagotomy, Sympathectomy, Splanchnicectomy** (Rienhoff and Baker, 1947). The objective here is to relieve symptoms by interruption of the sensory nerve fibers. It appears that vagotomy is not necessary for this.

6. **Lumbodorsal Sympathectomy and Splanchnicectomy.** The studies of Ray (1949) indicate that the afferent nerve impulses from the pancreas travel over the sympathetic system. They can be interrupted by bilateral removal of the sympathetic chain from D11 to L2 inclusive and resection of the greater, the lesser and the least splanchnic nerves bilaterally.

Next to sphincterotomy, this procedure is probably the one most often employed and gives good relief of symptoms in about 50 per cent of instances. It has certain disadvantages. It leaves the pancreas in situ, and there was evidence in some of Ray's cases that flare-ups of the inflammatory process continue. It also interrupts the sensory pathways from the gallbladder, the duodenum and part of the stomach so that intercurrent disease in these organs may develop quite far without the usual warning symptoms. Eventually, however, inflammation arising from any of these sources will reach areas such as the parietal peritoneum where sensory innervation is intact and symptoms will supervene. Finally, the procedure is apt to require 3 operations: (1) laparotomy to establish the diagnosis and to exclude other pathologic changes; (2) a right lumbodorsal sympathectomy; (3) a left lumbodorsal sympathectomy. Some cases have been relieved after the second step, but usually only temporarily.

Ralph Bowers (1956) reported good results in 16 of a series of 17 patients with chronic relapsing pancreatitis by anastomosis of a defunctionalized loop of jejunum to the common bile duct.

Some changes in outlook have developed about chronic relapsing pancreatitis.

Howard divides these cases into 3 groups: the first associated with cholelithiasis, the second with chronic alcoholism, and the third with neither. The first group has responded well to corrective biliary tract surgery—usually the removal of the gallbladder and the removal of stones from the bile ducts by choledochostomy.

Owens and Howard (1958) have focused attention on the correlation between pancreatic calcification and the chronic use of alcohol. In 32 consecutive cases of pancreatic calcification observed by them, a well-documented history of chronic relapsing pancreatitis and alcoholism was established in 29. The other 3 also had a record of chronic alcoholism.

The authors' current approach is the following: (1) If cholelithiasis is found, correct it surgically. (2) At the first operation intubate the duct of Wirsung after duodenotomy and sphincterotomy and do a pancreatogram on the operating table, using a contrast material such as Hypaque injected at physiologic pressures. (3) If the duct is obstructed, try amputation of the distal portion if this is all accessible, or if there is obstruction to the right of the superior mesenteric vessels, drain the distal duct of Wirsung into a loop of jejunum (preferably defunctionalized by the Roux en Y technic). (4) If the involvement of the pancreas is generalized, one decides between the symptomatic approach (sympathectomy and splanchnicectomy) and a Whipple resection, depending on the severity of the process.

If a Whipple resection is decided upon, the suggestion of Longmire and associates (1956) that a segment of the tail be conserved to prevent or at least ameliorate the diabetes is a good one. If subsequent symptoms demanded its removal, this could be done later.

In the calcific form of the disease alcoholism must be strongly suspected. Total abstinence should be tried. Unfortunately, subsequent attacks are frequent, and it is often impossible to know absolutely whether these are due to a relapse in the alcoholism or to a relapse in the disease in the absence of alcohol. Whichever is the explanation, it is rare that the disease having progressed to the calcific stage becomes asymptomatic for long.

UNUSUAL ASSOCIATIONS OF ACUTE PANCREATITIS WITH OTHER CONDITIONS

Attention is called to 10 case reports of patients who developed acute pancreatitis in association with or immediately after surgical removal of a parathyroid tumor. Two cases have followed thyroidectomy, and perhaps a dozen cases have been associated with familial hyperlipemia, a condition in which the serum neutral fats are unusually high. See Howard and Jordan (1960).

TRAUMA

Injuries to the pancreas result most commonly from operations upon the pancreas or structures in close proximity to it, such as the biliary tract, the duodenum, the stomach and the spleen. In operations in this area, pancreatic parenchyma, ducts or vessels may be injured, with resultant hemorrhage, escape of pancreatic ferments and necrosis. Obviously, prevention is the most important part of treatment.

Penetrating (gunshot and stab wounds), nonpenetrating (automobile accidents, falls and contact sports), abdominal and, less commonly, flank trauma may cause pancreatic injury. Penetrating pancreatic trauma usually is associated with damage to contiguous structures and nearly always requires exploratory laparotomy. If the gland is found to be injured, silk sutures are employed to stop hemorrhage, but accurate suture of lacerated parenchyma is rarely feasible. Adequate drainage with sump or Penrose drains is mandatory. Continuous suction is instituted to prevent wound digestion from the pancreatic juice, in case it is activated.

Nonpenetrating abdominal or flank trauma need not necessarily be so severe as to cause extensive pancreatic injury. Injury of the smaller pancreatic ducts with escape of pancreatic juice may result in extensive pancreatic necrosis and severe hemorrhage from autodigestion of contused parenchyma. The most common clinical picture is that of pancreatitis which may be associated with surgical shock by virtue of blood loss or with adynamic ileus as a result of widespread peritoneal irritation.

Treatment is similar to that of acute pancreatitis. Laparotomy will almost always be necessary to evaluate the extent of the damage and to establish the diagnosis.

The principal sequelae of pancreatic trauma are pancreatic abscess, pancreatic fistulas and the formation of pseudocysts (Fig. 33-4). The first two are treated with antibiotics and surgical drainage followed usually by continuous aspiration of the drainage tract; treatment of the last is discussed in the section on pancreatic cysts.

External pancreatic fistulas should be treated conservatively, with continuous suction, in the hope that the fistula will close. If the amount of drainage has not decreased significantly in several weeks, further treatment is indicated. The treatment of choice is excision of the tract down to and including the segment of the pancreas from which it arises plus excision of all pancreatic tissue distal to this point. If this is impossible, implantation of the tract into the gastrointestinal tract, preferably jejunum, may be performed.

As long as fluid balance can be maintained

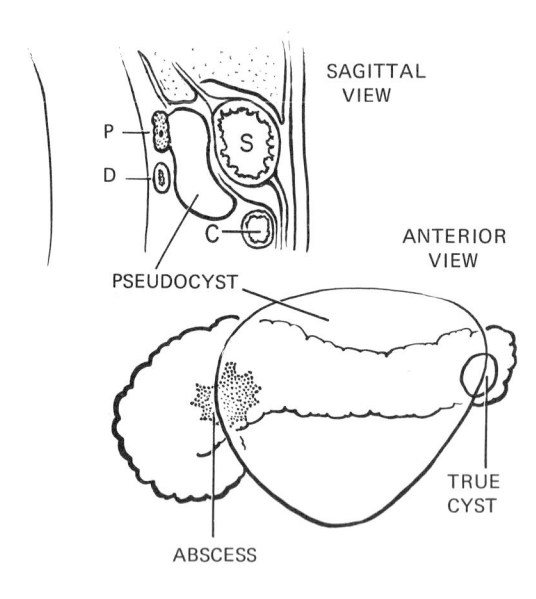

Fig. 33-4. Diagrammatic representation showing difference between true cysts, pseudocysts and abscess of the pancreas. P-pancreas; D-duodenum; S-stomach. C-transverse colon.

it is best to be quite patient, as many of these fistulas will close spontaneously even after several months.

ISLET CELL TUMORS

Tumors of the islet cells of the pancreas were first described by Nichols, a pathologist, in 1902. However, it was not until 1927, after the discovery of insulin by Banting and Best (1927) and the elaboration of the concept of hyperinsulinism by Harris (1924), that Wilder et al. (1927) first established the unquestioned correlation between clinical hyperinsulinism and a malignant islet cell tumor which was found at operation. Roscoe Graham (1929) recorded the first surgical cure of organic hyperinsulinism in 1929 with the excision of an islet cell adenoma. The tumors may be benign or malignant, functional or nonfunctional. The majority of these circumscribed, vascular, reddish-gray tumors are about 1 to 2 cm. in diameter, although some have been reported up to 15 cm. They occur in the head, the body and the tail of the pancreas, with a somewhat higher incidence in the tail. Microscopically, the tumor cells closely resemble normal islet cells.

Howard, Moss and Rhoads (1950) collected 388 cases and added 10 from the Hospital of the University of Pennsylvania. They found that 78.6 per cent were benign adenomas, 12.1 per cent were microscopically malignant but clinically benign, that is, there was no evidence of recurrence or metastasis, although histologically these tumors demonstrated anaplasia, blood vessel invasion or lack of well-defined encapsulation; and 9.3 per cent (37 cases) were carcinomas of which 22 were hyperfunctioning tumors. Of the 361 localized tumors, 200 were operated upon for hyperinsulinism, and 161 were found at autopsy. The incidence of multiple tumors was 12.6 per cent. Ectopic pancreatic tissue was found to be the site of islet cell tumors in 9 patients, 8 of whom presented clinical evidence of hyperinsulinism. This collected series has been extended to 1959 (Moss and Rhoads, 1960).

Symptoms

Nonfunctioning islet cell tumors are rarely diagnosed during life unless quite large or malignant. Functioning tumors manifest themselves by the symptoms of hyperinsulinism. These patients have periodic attacks of hypoglycemia which may present as weakness, anxiety, "nervousness," sweating, palpitation and syncope, convulsions and coma. Often they are admitted to the neurologic or neurosurgical service of a hospital. Misdiagnoses as functional hypoglycemia, epilepsy, encephalitis, psychoneuroses, alcoholic intoxication and brain tumor are not uncommon.

During an attack, the blood sugar frequently drops to 30 mg. per cent or lower, causing increased nervous excitability of central nervous system origin which in its severe form is manifested by epileptiform convulsions, followed by depression of the central nervous system which may be severe enough to cause coma. Prolonged episodes of hypoglycemia or repeated attacks may cause irreversible nerve cell damage leading to mental deterioration and death, particularly in infants.

Diagnosis

The criteria for diagnosis of a functioning islet cell tumor are as follows:

1. Signs and symptoms of insulin shock, frequently induced by the fasting state or during exercise
2. Repeated fasting blood sugar concentrations below 50 mg. per cent
3. Relief of symptoms by glucose administration
4. Lack of relief by low-carbohydrate, high-protein diet to exclude functional hypoglycemia as far as possible

The first 3 of the above criteria constitute Whipple's triad.

The principal differential diagnostic problem is functional hypoglycemia which is largely ruled out by the above criteria. Conn (1955) believes that functional hypoglycemia is responsible for 70 per cent of cases with hypoglycemic manifestations. It is due to an exaggerated insulin response to an elevation of the blood sugar such as occurs with meals, especially carbohydrate foods, and excitement (adrenalin response) (Fig. 33-5). Tests based on the effect of insulin on blood sugar levels and the effect of epinephrine on blood sugar levels are no longer widely used in the diagnosis of organic hyperinsulinism.

Rare causes of hypoglycemia are due to the following: (1) biliary cirrhosis of the liver

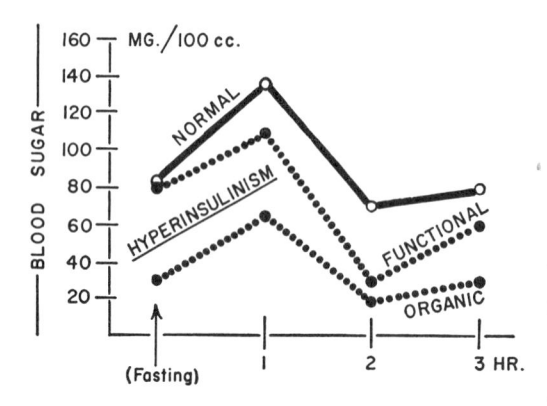

FIG. 33-5. Glucose tolerance curves differentiating functional from organic hyperinsulinism.

with decreased storage of glycogen, (2) von Gierke's disease and (3) functional hypoglycemia after gastric operations.

TREATMENT

Carefully planned laparotomy with simple enucleation of the adenoma if found is the treatment of choice. Excision of surrounding normal pancreatic tissue is unnecessary, as there is no evidence that the adenoma is a premalignant lesion. A very careful examination of the entire pancreas must be carried out, even though one or more adenomas are easily found, because multiple tumors occur in about 12 per cent of these patients.

If no localized adenoma is found in an individual having all the criteria requisite to a diagnosis of organic hyperinsulinism, a resection of all but a small section of the head of the pancreas is advocated by many surgeons. Occasionally, small adenomas are thus removed blindly (see below). The operative mortality should be below 5 per cent in experienced hands. Alloxan has been demonstrated to be ineffective and dangerous in the treatment of these tumors (Brunschwig and Allen, 1944).

RESULTS

The results of surgical therapy have been remarkably good. In the 398 cases collected by Howard, Moss and Rhoads (1950), operative removal consisted of exploration and enucleation in 153 patients, and exploration and partial resection in 48 patients. The mortality was about 9 per cent, and end results were reported as good in 87.3 per cent of the survivors.

In 118 patients no tumor could be located at the time of exploration. Of these, 37 eventually were found to have an islet cell tumor, 12 having the adenoma removed at a subsequent operation, and 12 having it resected blindly during subtotal pancreatectomy. Adenomas were found in 13 cases at autopsy. In 81 patients the tumor never was found. Of these, 56 had a partial pancreatectomy with an operative mortality of 7.1 per cent and a satisfactory therapeutic result was obtained in 46.4 per cent. Only 1 of the 37 patients with carcinoma was alive when last reported.

PANCREATICODUODENAL CANCERS

Cancers of the lower end of the common duct, the papilla of Vater, the pancreas and the duodenum were termed pancreaticoduodenal cancers by Child (1949). Whipple emphasized that patients with these tumors have much in common in the insidious onset of symptoms and in their common confusion with digestive and biliary disturbances. Consequently, they frequently receive nonoperative symptomatic therapy for prolonged periods of time. The relative incidence of these tumors is shown in Table 33-2.

Warren and his associates (1967) reported their experience with pancreatoduodenectomy for periampullary carcinoma as shown in Table 33-3.

CARCINOMA OF THE AMPULLA OF VATER

There are 2 principal types of ampullary carcinoma, the papillary and the ulcerating carcinomas. Microscopically, both are adeno-

TABLE 33-2. TYPES OF PANCREATICODUODENAL CANCER
(1931-1950 Massachusetts General Hospital)
(McDermott and Bartlett, 1953)

CANCER	NO. OF CASES 1931–1940	NO. OF CASES 1941–1950
Head of pancreas	112	136
Ampulla of Vater	9	24
Common bile duct	10	17
Duodenum	1	6
Totals	132	183

TABLE 33-3*

CANCER	OPERATIVE MORTALITY (PER CENT)	FIVE YEAR SURVIVAL RATE (PER CENT)
Head of pancreas	11.4	12.5
Ampullary	10.8	29.8
Distal bile duct	19.2	35.7
Duodenum	21.6	41.2
Totals	13.5% (of 253 cases)	24.1% (of 170 cases)

* Warren, K. W., et al.: Surg. Clin. N. Am., 47: 689, 1967.

carcinomas. The former rises from the ampulla itself and by its growth, edema and invasion tends to cause early obstruction of the terminal common bile duct and in some instances also of the pancreatic duct. The ulcerating variety arises from the epithelium of the papilla and invades the ampulla and the ducts secondarily. Cattell and Warren (1953) stated that the gallbladder is distended in 90 per cent of these cases.

Spread of ampullary carcinoma occurs by direct extension and by lymphatic and vascular dissemination. The liver is the most common site of visceral metastasis. Carcinoma of the ampulla of Vater offers the best prognosis with radical surgery, perhaps because it tends to cause biliary tract obstruction early in the course of the disease and because the more common type, the papillary variety, tends to remain localized for a longer period than most other tumors in this area. The tumor tends to bleed and slough and thus may mimic the intermittent jaundice caused by a common duct stone. Whereas all types of pancreaticoduodenal carcinomas may give rise to occult blood in the stool, this symptom in a patient with jaundice should direct attention particularly to the possibility of ampullary carcinoma.

Carcinoma of the Duodenum

This rare adenocarcinoma is difficult to diagnose in an operable state unless it occurs near or in contact with the papilla of Vater, in which case the signs and symptoms resemble those of ampullary carcinoma.

The results of a study of the incidence of carcinoma of the duodenum are shown in Table 33-4.

Carcinoma of the Common Duct

This infiltrating, stenosing type of carcinoma has less tendency to bleed and slough than has the tumor of the papilla of Vater. Such tumors produce symptoms usually indistinguishable from those of carcinoma of the head of the pancreas, unless the duct is affected above the junction of the cystic duct when the gallbladder usually would not be dilated. The prognosis in these tumors has been very poor, especially if they occur cephalad to the duodenum.

Carcinoma of the Pancreas

This tumor presents itself as a hard, irregular mass in the pancreas. In over two thirds of the cases it is located in the head of the gland. Differential diagnosis with chronic inflammation is often difficult, as is the determination of the extent of the tumor, because of associated inflammation and fibrosis sometimes secondary to ductal obstruction.

Miller, Baggenstoss and Comfort (1951) reported that 81.6 per cent of their series of carcinoma of the pancreas arose from ductal epithelium. A smaller number arise from acinar epithelium. The vast majority are adenocarcinomas; a few are squamous cell carcinomas. Pancreatic carcinoma also may arise from the islet tissue (see above).

The spread of these tumors occurs by direct invasion of the contiguous structures and by metastasis via the abundant lymphatic and vascular systems. Cattell and Warren (1953) refer to 77 of 108 cases of carcinoma of the pancreas found to be inoperable because of

TABLE 33-4. INCIDENCE OF CARCINOMA OF DUODENUM
Review of World Literature
(Deaver and Ravdin, 1920)

1. Carcinomas of duodenum—0.033% of hospital autopsies
2. Inch for inch the duodenum is much more liable to undergo carcinomatous change than the jejunum or ileum
3. Relative frequency at various sites of duodenal carcinoma
    1st portion 22.15%
    2nd portion 65.82%
    3rd portion 12.02%

metastasis or invasion of major vessels. Peripheral venous thrombosis not uncommonly accompanies carcinoma of the pancreas, especially of the body. Therefore, a search for signs of a neoplasm of the pancreas always should be made in persons with peripheral venous thromboses.

Pancreaticoduodenal cancer is found most frequently after age 55. Men are affected twice as often as women. The duration of symptoms before medical consultation is most commonly from 3 to 5 months. Only about 25 to 30 per cent are resectable by the time the patient is hospitalized. The disease runs a rapid course.

Symptoms and Signs of Pancreaticoduodenal Cancers

While the earliest symptoms are local pain, anorexia and weight loss, jaundice has attracted the most attention. Jaundice frequently may be the first sign, especially in ampullary or common duct cancers. Contrary to earlier opinion, painless jaundice is not a regular finding in pancreatic carcinoma, nor is a palpable gallbladder with intense jaundice found in most patients with operable cancer.

When the common bile duct is obstructed by a stone, dilatation of the gallbladder is rare (Courvoisier's Law). When the duct is obstructed in some other way, dilatation is frequent. This is valid in the majority of cases of carcinoma of pancreaticoduodenal origin, although its converse that a nonpalpable gallbladder with jaundice signifies choledocholithiasis is by no means always correct, as the gallbladder is not felt in some of the cases of carcinoma. The law is based on the finding that stones in the common duct generally are preceded by inflammation in the gallbladder with resultant fibrosis and shrinkage of the organ and its inability to dilate when the pressure in the biliary tract rises due to blockage.

Pain is one of the most common symptoms and is more frequent as the presenting complaint than is jaundice. The reverse is true for ampullary carcinoma where jaundice often without pain is the cardinal complaint. The pain may be paroxysmal or steady and deep in the epigastrium. Very frequently it radiates through to the back. On occasion it radiates to the right or even to the left upper quadrants or may be girdling in character. Biliary tract or peptic ulcer pain may be mimicked. Da Costa (1858) noted relief of the pain by leaning forward. It may be aggravated by the dorsal recumbent position. As the disease progresses the pain may become excruciating.

Therefore serious consideration should be given to cordotomy if pain, anorexia and weight loss persist and cannot be relieved satisfactorily by careful study and treatment. Only about 75 per cent of the patients are icteric. Painless jaundice was present in 25 per cent of the Lahey Clinic series. If unrelieved, the biliary obstruction may cause intractable pruritus and will result in severe hepatic damage. In spite of the fact that jaundice is often not an early symptom, Cliffton (1952) noted that in 75 patients it was the only symptom or sign actually bringing them for definitive treatment in an operable state.

Weight loss is probably the most common serious symptom and occurs early. It is often as much as 20 pounds by the time the patient is hospitalized.

Anorexia and weakness, nearly always present, are early symptoms, though nonspecific.

Constipation is frequent, although not helpful in diagnosis. Diarrhea is less common and tends to occur when the pancreatic duct is obstructed. However, typically foul, bulky stools are quite uncommon, and at times patients may have complete duct obstruction without any obvious changes in the stools. Nausea and vomiting are frequent. Occasionally, chills and fever may occur with neoplastic biliary obstruction, but more often they are associated with stones. Ascites and unexplained migratory phlebitis, particularly of the lower extremities, may occur. The appearance of mild diabetes has been noted occasionally.

Physical Findings

There may be no physical findings, especially in the early operable cases (Table 33-5).

Jaundice is common, as noted above. Its absence does not rule out early carcinoma of the head and, of course, is not to be expected early in carcinoma of the body and the tail of the pancreas.

An enlarged palpable liver is fairly common, appearing in 75 per cent of the cases according to Berk (1941).

Palpable gallbladder with jaundice is fre-

TABLE 33-5. DIFFERENTIAL DIAGNOSIS OF COMMON DUCT OBSTRUCTION

	OBSTRUCTION DUE TO STONE	OBSTRUCTION DUE TO CARCINOMA OF HEAD OF PANCREAS
Symptoms		
Pain	+++ Colicky	± early +++ Aching later
Jaundice	++++ Often intermittent. Rapid onset	++++ Insidious onset. Persistent and progressive
Weight loss	++	++++
Fatigue	++	++++
Anorexia	+++	+++
Nausea, vomiting	++++	++
Chills, fever	+++	±
Physical Findings		
Jaundice	++++	++++
Hepatomegaly	++	+++
Palpable gallbladder	Rare	+++
Migratory phlebitis	Rare	Occasional
Laboratory Findings		
Bile pigment in stools	Usually present intermittently	Usually absent constantly
Occult blood in stools	0	±
Excess fat and undigested meat fibers in stool	0	+++
Hyperbilirubinemia	++++	++++
Serum alkaline phosphatase and cholesterol	Elevated	Elevated
Liver function tests indicating the presence of hepatocellular injury	±	±
Pancreatic enzymes in duodenal contents	Normal	Often decreased
Anemia	±	+
Hyperglycemia and glycosuria	0	±
Glucose tolerance test (oral)	Normal	±
Plasma anti-thrombin titer	0	Occasionally elevated

quently but not uniformly present. However, at operation the biliary tract and/or the pancreatic ducts are dilated in the majority of cases. As emphasized by Cattell and Warren (1953), resection is not carried out unless common duct dilatation can be demonstrated, since, in many cases, it is necessary to proceed without a histologic diagnosis because of the unreliability of biopsy of this area.

A palpable epigastric tumor is rare and must be regarded as of poor prognosis.

PANCREATIC BIOPSY

Frequently at operation an area of pancreas is found which is either thicker or firmer than one expects. A histologic diagnosis would be helpful. However, there are two cogent reasons for not undertaking pancreatic biopsies lightly. The first is that many of the lesions are in the head of the gland and one does not know where the common bile duct or the pancreatic ducts lie precisely. The result is that the biopsy obtained must be limited and therefore inconclusive if negative. The second danger is that sometimes incision into the pancreas is followed by acute pancreatitis or a pancreatic fistula. Therefore, pancreatic biopsies are to be avoided and should be undertaken only for well-considered reasons. In pancreaticoduodenal carcinomas sometimes a satisfactory biopsy may be obtained from inside the duodenum after duodenotomy. Ackerman and his associates (1959) have achieved considerable success in the diagnosis of specimens by frozen section of material obtained at laparotomy, often by needle biopsy.

LABORATORY DATA

A mild to moderate anemia is usually present. Elevated levels of serum bilirubin, alkaline phosphatase and cholesterol are present in pancreaticoduodenal carcinomas as they are in most instances of biliary tract obstruction. Liver function tests will indicate the presence of obstructive rather than hepatocellular jaundice in the earlier cases. However, in prolonged obstruction varying degrees of parenchymal damage may coexist. The prothrombin determination and its response to parenteral vitamin K is a valuable test (Ravdin, I. S., 1939). Serum amylase and lipase may be elevated, but usually the values are not significant. Stool examination for neutral fats and undigested meat fibers may show excessive amounts of both.

Aspiration of the duodenal contents with a double lumen tube as emphasized by Bauman (1939) and stressed by Whipple (1952) may be a valuable test for diagnosis and for differential diagnosis between choledocholithiasis and various types of pancreaticoduodenal tumors obstructing the pancreatic ducts near the duodenum (Fig. 33-6). Tumors of the body of the pancreas do not result, as a rule, in low enzyme levels in material aspirated from the duodenum.

The value of these studies depends on the expertness and the thoroughness with which they are carried out.

ROENTGENOGRAPHIC FINDINGS

An upper gastrointestinal series may show, at times, enlargement of the duodenal loop or displacement, distortion or actual invason of contiguous organs (Figs. 33-7 and 33-8). The inverted-3 sign of Frostberg (1938) is suggestive but rare. The films are most often negative; in fact, Cattell and Warren (1953) state that: "We have come to regard negative studies as one of the important indications of the presence of pancreatic disease in those patients who have dyspepsia, fatigue and progressive weight loss."

A method of visualizing the pancreas by radiographic means suitable for preoperative use has long been sought. If operation is done, duodenotomy, intubation and injection of the duct of Wirsung will often throw light on the pathology.

Radioactive selenomethionine has proved to be of some use in outlining at least the larger lesions of the pancreas by means of "scanning." It is known that methionine moves into the pancreas in fairly high concentration. Selenium may be substituted for sulfur in the "methionine" and there is an appropriate radioactive isotope of selenium which emits gamma rays and with a suitable collimator may be well localized in the body. At present the method is of limited value, but it gives

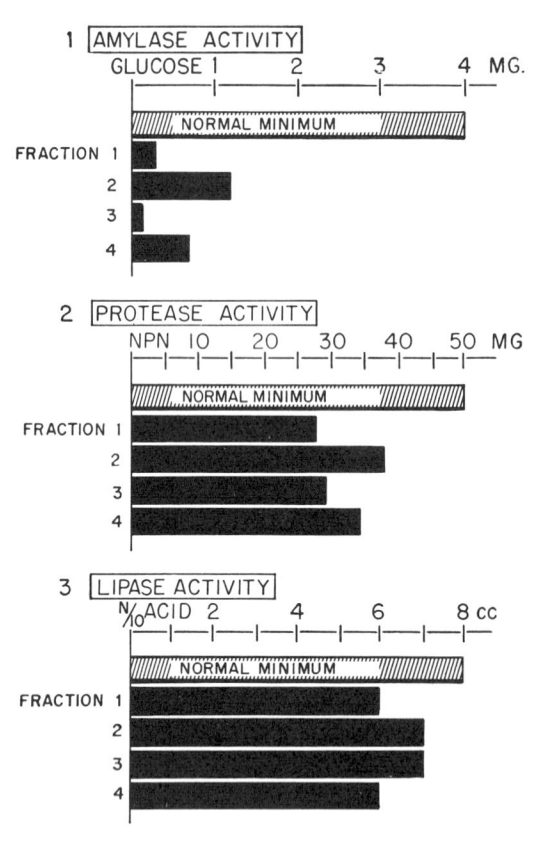

FIG. 33-6. Pancreatic function tests (from Bauman). Pancreatic enzyme determinations in a case of carcinoma of the head of the pancreas as compared with the normal minimums when no pancreatic disease is present.

Pancreaticoduodenal Cancers 935

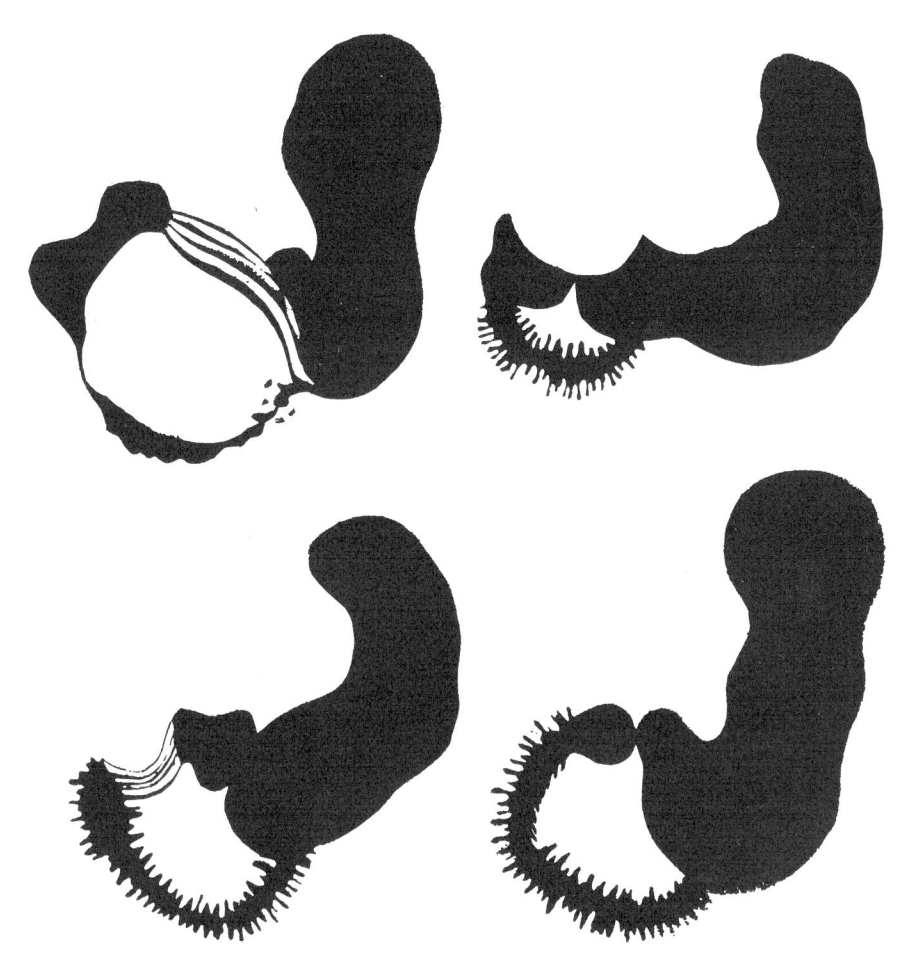

FIG. 33-7. Various x-ray changes sometimes produced by pancreaticoduodenal carcinoma. (*Top, left*) Diagrammatic representation of gastrointestinal series, showing widening of duodenal loop due to pancreaticoduodenal carcinoma. (*Top, right*) Diagrammatic representation of gastrointestinal series showing compression by dilated gallbladder on upper border of duodenum and pyloric antrum due to pancreaticoduodenal carcinoma. (*Bottom, left*) Diagrammatic representation of gastrointestinal series, showing postbulbar impression due to pressure of the obstructed biliary tract due to pancreaticoduodenal carcinoma. (*Bottom, right*) Diagrammatic representation of gastrointestinal series showing distortion of mucosal folds on medial side of second portion of duodenum due to pancreaticoduodenal carcinoma. (From Dr. Philip J. Hodes)

promise of more adequate methods to be achieved along similar lines.

None of the rises in the serum levels of the several enzymes commonly measured in the blood is currently regarded as pathognomonic for carcinoma of the pancreas.

SUMMARY

The diagnosis of pancreaticoduodenal cancer is made most often if the possibility is kept in mind. A middle-aged patient who presents himself with persistent abdominal pain, anorexia and unexplained weight loss and in whom physical examination and an upper gastrointestinal series are negative should suggest immediately the possibility of carcinoma of the pancreas, even in the absence of jaundice. However, jaundice remains the symptom which most often leads to the diagnosis.

936   Pancreas

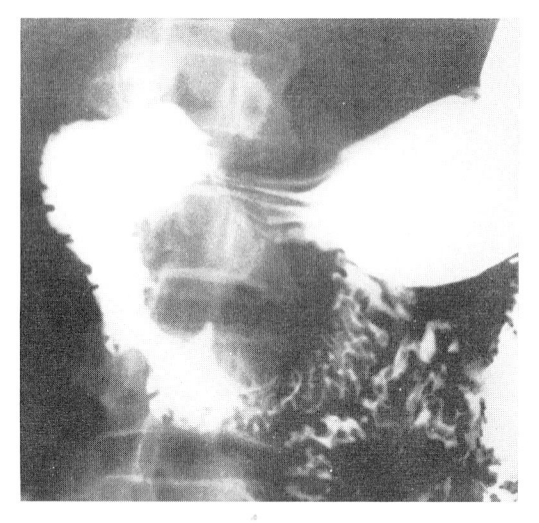

FIG. 33-8. The inverted 3-sign of Frostberg which is indicative (though not pathognomonic) of carcinoma of the pancreas when it occurs.

Treatment

The treatment of pancreaticoduodenal cancers by resection has been and remains relatively unsatisfactory. Prior to 1935, curative procedures had been given up. Then, Dr. Allen O. Whipple (1935) reported a radical resection in 2 stages. He and other surgeons soon modified this to a 1-stage procedure (Trimble, 1941). Only about 25 per cent of the lesions are resectable, and for the majority of individuals, the procedure has turned out to be palliative. Preoperative preparation includes parenteral vitamin K therapy to restore the prothrombin activity, a high protein, high carbohydrate diet and blood transfusions. A glucose tolerance test should be performed preoperatively, since diabetes mellitus is present in 10 per cent of cases.

Essentially 2 general types of operations are available:

1. Strictly palliative procedures for inoperable carcinoma
   A. Cholecystojejunostomy
   B. Cholecystojejunostomy with enteroenterostomy (Fig. 33-10, *right*)
   C. Pancreatojejunostomy
   D. Ligation of the gastroduodenal and inferior pancreaticoduodenal arteries
   E. Gastrojejunostomy
   (See also Cattell and Warren (1953).)

The majority of such patients are dead within 12 months after palliative operations.

2. Possibly curative procedures
   A. Pancreaticoduodenal resection is the procedure most commonly employed. Essentially, this consists of the block resection of the head of the pancreas, the duodenum, the pylorus, the distal stomach, and the lower end of the common duct. Then the remainder of the stomach is anastomosed to the jejunum. The common duct and the pancreatic duct also are anastomosed to the jejunum proximal to the gastrojejunostomy. Failure to place the gastric anastomosis distally has led to fatal peptic ulceration of the jejunum. Some surgeons do not anastomose the pancreatic ducts but simply ligate them. The absence of the external secretion can be compensated by the oral administration of animal pancreatic enzymes when necessary; indeed, some patients without external secretion have apparently normal stools and regain their weight without such therapy. However, anastomosis is generally considered desirable because it is thought to reduce the incidence of fistulas and to preserve a part of the exocrine function of the gland (see Fig. 33-11).

Anastomosis of the cut end of the pancreas to the posterior wall of the stomach has been recommended by Millbourn (1958) and by

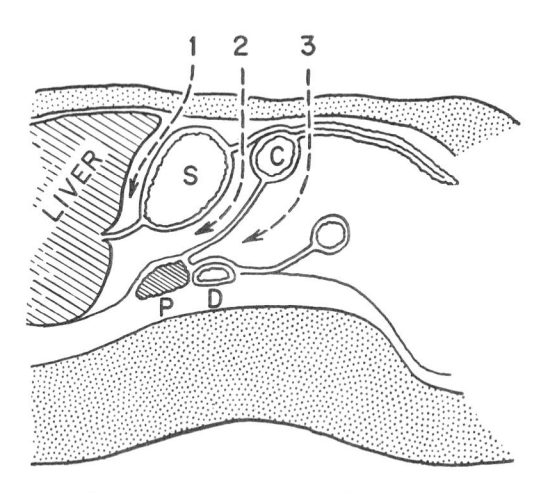

FIG. 33-9. Approaches to the body of the pancreas: (1) Through the gastrohepatic omentum. (2) Through the gastrocolic omentum. (3) From below through the transverse mesocolon. D—duodenum; P—pancreas; S—stomach.

Fig. 33-10. Two palliative procedures for inoperable carcinoma of the pancreas: (*Left*) Loop cholecystojejunostomy. (*Right*) Cholecystojejunostomy en Y.

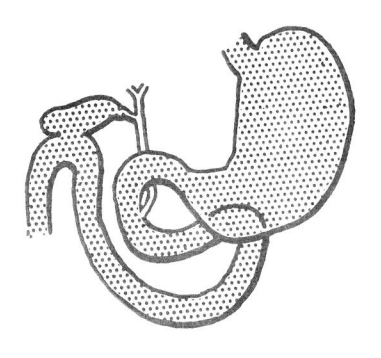

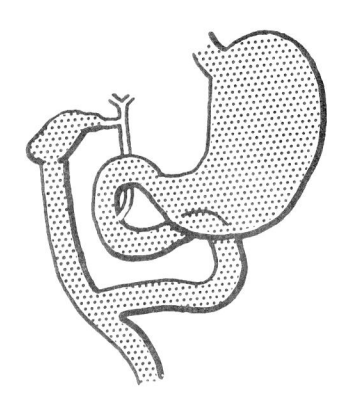

Park, Mackie and Rhoads (1967). The objective has been lower operative mortality. The advantages are:

   a. The proximity of the 2 structures

   b. The thickness and strength of the gastric wall

   c. The fact that pancreatic enzymes are not strongly proteolytic at an acid pH

   d. The specific activator of trypsinogen and chymotrypsinogen has been identified in succus entericus.

It is believed that the enzymes are not destroyed in the stomach but persist to function in the small intestine as they are carried down with food and other secretions. Measurements of changes in stomach content due to secretion and to histamine, with respect to pH and bicarbonate, have been made several months after operation. These indicate that the anastomoses are functional. A patent duct of Wirsung also was seen through the flexible gastroscope in one of these patients.* Table 33-6 summarizes mortality experience with this procedure.

Though the mortality of pancreatoduodenectomy has been reported in the literature as about 30 per cent, now it is under 10 per cent in several of the leading surgical clinics. Howard (1968) reported a personal series of pancreatoduodenotomies numbering 41 cases, with no operative mortality.

B. Total pancreatectomy is similar to the preceding operation except that all pancreatic tissue and the spleen are removed—the spleen because of the arrangement of the blood supply. The splenic vein and artery course within or immediately contiguous to the pancreas.

The author feels that for the present at least these two operations should be reserved for patients without evidence of distant metastasis or involvement of the major vessels. However, Brunschwig (1952) reported 3 five-year survivals in patients who had lymph node involvement at the time of pancreaticoduodenal resection. Furthermore, Child and others (1952) investigating resection of the portal

* (Norman Cohen, M.D. Personal communication, 1968)

Fig. 33-11. Restoration of pancreatic, biliary and gastrointestinal continuity after radical pancreaticoduodenal resection. (*Left*) Poor method. (*Center*) Fair method. (*Right*) Satisfactory method.

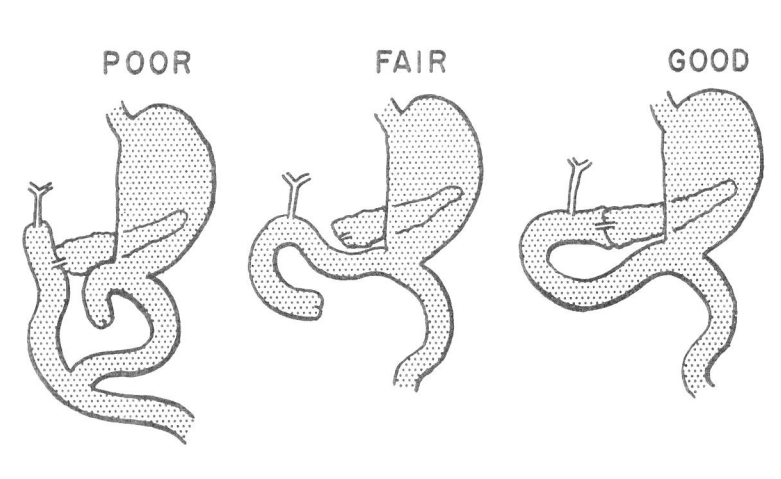

POOR   FAIR   GOOD

vein have reported success in experimental animals and in a limited number of patients.

POSTOPERATIVE COMPLICATIONS

Pancreatic fistula, hemorrhage, biliary fistula, peritonitis, diabetes mellitus, obstruction of the gastrojejunostomy, and necrotizing pancreatitis in the pancreatic remnant have all been encountered. Hemorrhage resulting from autodigestion of vessels by escape of activated pancreatic juice has been the most serious in the author's experience.

(See also section on Metabolic Effects of Total Pancreatectomy.)

RESULTS OF TREATMENT OF PANCREATICODUODENAL CANCER

The reported results of radical pancreatic surgery were very poor at the time of the first edition of this text. There has been some improvement reported since. McDermott and Bartlett (1953) compared all cases treated at the Massachusetts General Hospital in the decade 1931 to 1940 (132 cases), when only palliative procedures were done, with all cases in the decade 1941 to 1950 (183 cases), when 35 per cent of the tumors were resected by pancreatoduodenectomy with a 34 per cent mortality. The average duration of life after pancreatoduodenectomy was 11 months. The average survival of resected and palliative cases between 1941 and 1950 was 6.2 months for carcinoma of the pancreas compared with 7.7 months in the preceding decade when only palliative procedures were done.

For carcinoma of the ampulla the survivals were 21 months in the first decade and only 18.5 months in the second decade. Of the 183 cases, there were only 2 five-year survivals among the 65 per cent resected. None of the cases with carcinoma of the pancreas survived 5 years.

Logan and Kleinsasser (1951), in their review of the literature, collected 123 cases of pancreaticoduodenal cancer for which pancreatoduodenectomy was performed between 1942 and 1949 (35 for ampullary carcinoma, 62 for carcinoma of the pancreas, and 23 for other cancers). In the 35 resections for ampullary carcinoma, the operative mortality was 23 per cent, the average survival was 23 months, and 8 of 28 patients were alive at the end of 5 years. In the 62 resections for carcinoma of the pancreas, mortality was 31 per cent, an average survival 13 months, and only 1 patient of 30 was alive after 5 years. In the 23 resections for all other cancers requiring pancreatoduodenectomy, mortality was only 4.5 per cent, average survival was 20 months, and 1 of 15 patients was alive in 5 years.

Orr (1952) was able to collect from the literature 17 patients who lived for 5 or more years after pancreatoduodenectomy for cancer. Only 3 of these patients had carcinoma of the pancreas. Most of the remaining had ampullary carcinoma.

Cattell and Warren (1953) reported 5 of 32 patients (16%) living after 5 years.

Dennis and Varco (1956) reported 13 5-year survivors of radical pancreatoduodenal resection. Eight of these patients had primary lesions in the head of the pancreas.

Kaufman and Wilson (1955) reviewed the American literature and reported 36 5-year survivors following pancreatoduodenectomy, 8 of them having had carcinoma of the head of the pancreas and 21 ampullary carcinoma.

Muir (1955) made inquiries in Great Britain and found 4 unpublished cases which had survived 5 years after pancreatoduodenectomy. He also reported 2 5-year survivors who had carcinoma of the head of the pancreas.

A further series of radical operations for pancreaticoduodenal carcinoma was reported by Rhoads, Zintel and Helwig (1957; 1960), and several more reports have appeared, including one from the Lahey Clinic in two parts (Cattell, Warren and Au, 1959; Warren and Cattell, 1959), reporting 41 5-year survivors (Table 33-6).

More than 100 5-year survivors of carcinoma in the pancreaticoduodenal region have been reported. Practically all of these tumors invade pancreatic tissue to some extent. Those deemed to be primary in the head of the pancreas are decidedly less favorable than those arising at the papilla of Vater.

In conclusion, it now appears that, if the pancreaticoduodenal carcinomas are considered collectively, about 25 per cent of the cases are resectable, and about 25 per cent of those resected survive 5 years or longer. In the series from the Hospital of the University of Pennsylvania, the average survival was 30.5 months for the resected cases, 11 months for those undergoing palliative shunts,

TABLE 33-6. ONE HUNDRED 5-YEAR SURVIVALS OF CARCINOMA OF THE PANCREATICODUODENAL REGION AFTER OPERATIONS OF THE WHIPPLE TYPE

AUTHOR AND YEAR	HEAD OF PANCREAS	BILE DUCT	DUO-DENUM	PAPILLA OF VATER	NOT STATED	Total
Orr (1952)	3	..	..	11	2	16
Muir (1954–55)	1	..	..	1	..	2
Dennis & Varco (1956)	8	..	1	3	1	13
Smith (1956)	1	..	2	3	..	6
Rhoads, Zintel & Helwig (1957)	..	3	1	2	..	6
Ross (1957)	1	..	..	..	..	1
Waugh & Giberson (1957)	3	..	2	5	..	10
Porter (1958)	..	..	1	3	..	4
Warren & Cattell (1959)	7	3	7	24	..	41
Rhoads, Zintel & Helwig (1960)	..	..	..	1	..	1
Total	24	6	14	53	3	100

and 2.5 months for those who were merely explored. This, of course, reflects the fact that the most favorable cases were apt to be chosen for resection. Nevertheless, resection would seem to offer some hope of cure for the more favorable cases. The report of Monge, Judd and Gage (1964) indicates an 18 per cent 5-year survival after Whipple operations performed for carcinoma of the head of the pancreas, 39 per cent for papilla of Vater, 28 per cent for duodenum and 11 per cent when operation was done for those in the bile duct.

If merely a shunt for bile is decided upon, experience dictates that a gastroenterostomy be constructed also, as duodenal obstruction frequently follows bile obstruction by a short interval.

CYSTS

Cysts of the pancreas are uncommon but not rare. There are many etiologic varieties. Of the many classifications that have been proposed, a modification of that of Mahorner and Mattson (1931) appears to be most useful.
1. Cysts resulting from defective development
    A. Fibrocystic disease
    B. Cysts associated with polycystic disease of other viscera
    C. Simple cysts
    D. Dermoid cysts
2. Cysts resulting from disruption of pancreatic tissue, either traumatic or inflammatory
    A. Pseudocysts
    B. Hemorrhagic cysts
3. Retention cysts
4. Neoplastic cysts
    A. Cystadenoma
    B. Cystadenocarcinoma
    C. Teratoma
5. Cysts resulting from parasites: echinococcus cysts

Two main types of non-neoplastic cysts are encountered—the true cysts which have an epithelial lining, and the false or pseudocysts which do not. Of the neoplastic cysts, the cystadenoma is the most common, although only 53 of these had been reported in the literature up until 1954. Of a total of 46 pancreatic cysts of all types treated at the Lahey Clinic, 30 were pseudocysts.

PSEUDOCYSTS

Pseudocysts of the pancreas are the result of fluid accumulations in or about the pancreas which apparently do not undergo resorption. The exact mechanism of formation is not known; presumably, disruption of pancreatic tissue with hemorrhage and escape of pancreatic juice in addition to local exudation accounts for the accumulation of fluid. A proliferation of connective tissue forms a fibrous wall which may include parts of the pancreas or neighboring organs and tissues. Either trauma to the pancreas or acute and chronic pancreatitis may be the cause of disruption of the parenchymal tissue. The trauma is usually a severe blow to the epigastrium or

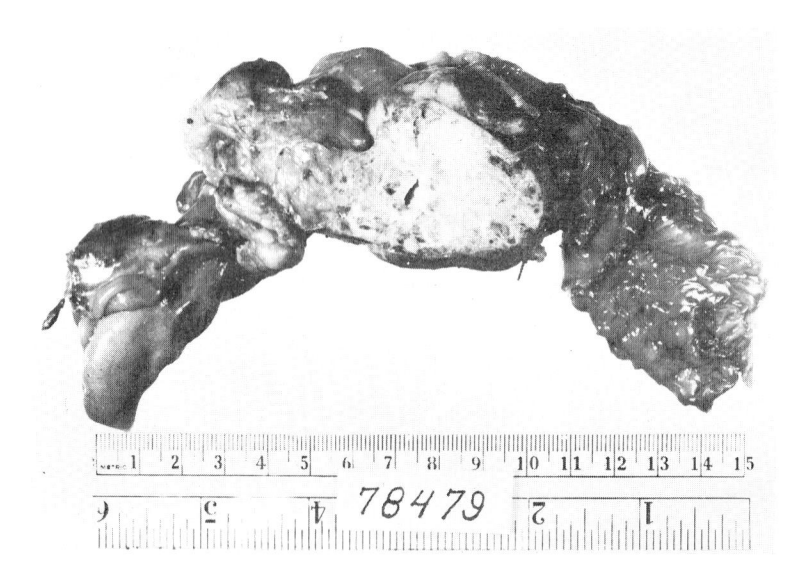

FIG. 33-12. Benign cystadenoma. Gross appearance of a sectioned lesion in relation to the duodenum.

the midabdomen, and the latent period before the cyst becomes evident may vary from a few days to a few years but usually it is a few months. Fallis and Plain (1939) believe that pseudocysts occur as a sequel of acute pancreatitis in about 10 per cent of cases. The author's experience would not place the figure nearly so high.

The pseudocyst has no epithelial lining and usually has only a single cavity. The contained fluid is usually cloudy, and pancreatic enzyme activity may be demonstrable. It, as do most pancreatic cysts, presents most commonly in the lesser peritoneal cavity, displacing the stomach forward and up and the transverse mesocolon downward. Anteriorly, it is covered by the gastrocolic omentum.

CYSTADENOMAS

Cystadenomas are rare (Figs. 33-12 and 33-13). Generally, they are considered to be true neoplasms arising from the parenchymal cells. These coarsely lobulated, multicystic tumor masses are found most commonly in the tail of the pancreas. They usually vary in size from 2 to 8 cm. and though larger tumors have been reported, they are generally smaller than non-neoplastic cysts. The tumors have a definite semitranslucent capsule, and Brunschwig has likened them to a cluster of grapes. They feel cystic and when sectioned appear spongelike or honeycombed. The fluid contained in them is clear, yellow or brown and varies in viscosity. Microscopically, the cystic spaces are lined with cuboidal or flattened epithelium, and there may be papillary projections of epithelium into the spaces. Though these tumors are usually well encapsulated and grow by expansion, infiltration of surrounding tissue also may occur.

Mozan (1951) collected 49 histologically verified cystadenomas from the literature. The ratio of females to males was 7 to 1. He found that a palpable tumor mass in the epigastrium was usually the first recognizable sign of the lesion. Zintel, Enterline and Rhoads (1954) reported 4 cases of cystadenoma of which 3 were papillary. All patients had long survivals without metastases, and the authors reiterate that malignancy should not be diagnosed on the basis of papillary projection alone. However, though malignant degeneration is rare, these tumors may occur in a malignant form.

SIGNS AND SYMPTOMS OF PANCREATIC CYSTS

Though the symptoms and signs of pancreatic cysts are dependent somewhat upon etiology, size, location and duration, they are quite similar and are usually insidious unless associated with trauma or inflammation (pancreatitis).

Epigastric pain, which may radiate to the back or flanks, occasionally associated with sharp, darting pains in the abdomen, is the most prominent symptom. It is usually dull and intermittent but may be severe.

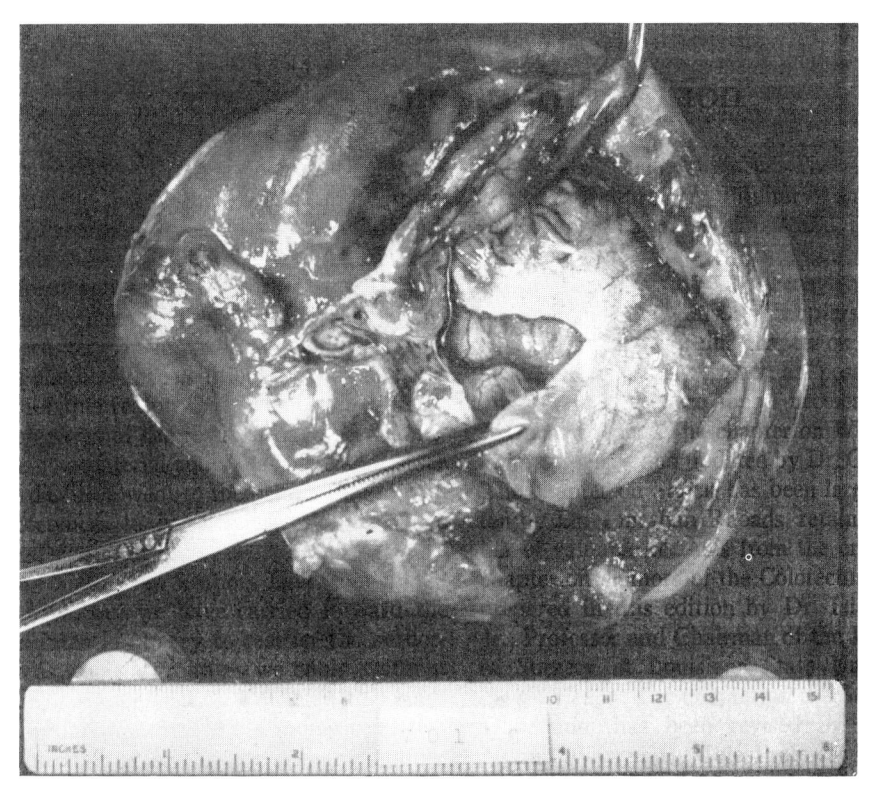

FIG. 33-13. Gross appearance of a large cystadenoma of the pancreas.

Dyspepsia and anorexia are common, and icterus rare. When jaundice exists it may be due to pressure upon the common duct or to concomitant biliary tract disease.

Weight loss and fatigue are common symptoms. Constipation and a sense of fullness in the abdomen may be present. Chills and fever and glycosuria are uncommon. Steatorrhea is rare.

A palpable abdominal mass, usually epigastric, is present in 90 per cent of cases, according to Cattell and Warren. Often the mass is not tender to moderate pressure and may be mobile.

Laboratory findings are seldom very helpful in diagnosis.

ROENTGENOGRAPHIC EXAMINATION

A gastrointestinal series is usually negative but may reveal displacement and compression of contiguous organs if the cyst is large. In rare instances, calcification in the cyst wall may be visible. The administration of radioactive seleno-methionine followed by scanning may reveal some of these lesions as "cold areas."

DIFFERENTIAL DIAGNOSIS

Pancreatic cysts are to be differentiated from other pancreatic tumors and from tumors, cysts or enlargements of surrounding organs. These include retroperitoneal tumors and lymph node enlargement, splenomegaly, renal and hepatic masses, hydrops of the gallbladder, cysts of the omentum and the mesentery, tumors of the stomach and aneurysms.

TREATMENT

The treatment of choice of pancreatic cysts is complete excision if compatible with the extent and the size of the cyst and the condition of the patient. This may necessitate amputation of a portion of the tail and the body of the pancreas. Even pancreatoduodenectomy has been done when the lesion involves the head of the pancreas or if differentiation from carcinoma is uncertain (see discussion of pancreatic biopsy above). It is doubtful, however, if pancreatoduodenectomy is justified in the absence of malignancy. Ordinarily the true cysts can be excised. Some true cysts and most pseudocysts involve surrounding organs or tissues so extensively that excision is impossible.

Because of this and because marsupialization with external drainage may be followed by prolonged drainage (many years) or by recurrence of a collection if the external tract is not kept open, internal drainage has gained in popularity. This is usually to the stomach for pseudocysts occupying the lesser peritoneal cavity but a loop of the jejunum—usually defunctionalized by the Roux en Y technic—may also be used. While these methods should not be used when complete excision is safe, they have worked surprisingly well. Howard and Jordan present a collected series of 572 pseudocysts: 63 were excised with 3.2 per cent recurrence, 274 were drained externally with 17.2 per cent recurrence, and 235 were drained internally with 2.6 per cent recurrence. Of the last group cystoduodenostomy was done 20 times with 1 recurrence, cystogastrostomy 121 times with 3 recurrences, cystojejunostomy (simple loop) 27 times with 1 recurrence, cystojejunostomy (proximal jejunojejunostomy) 8 times without recurrence and cystojejunostomy (Roux en Y) 59 times with 1 recurrence. Operative mortality in the same series was 8.7 per cent when excision was done and 4.5 per cent both for external drainage and internal drainage. Although follow-up studies were not complete, reoperation was estimated at 5.5 per cent when external drainage was practiced.

BENIGN SOLID TUMORS

Excluding islet cell tumors, solid benign tumors of the pancreas are very rare. In addition to solid adenomas, which may represent an early stage in the development of cystadenomas, lipomas, fibromas, myxomas and chondromas may occur in the pancreas. Hemangiomas of the pancreas also have been reported.

Signs and symptoms, when present, namely, dyspepsia and epigastric distress or pain, resemble those of cysts of the pancreas. The tumors may reach sufficient size to become palpable. Small benign tumors are asymptomatic unless compression of the ductal system occurs.

Treatment is surgical excision. The prognosis is good provided that the benign nature of the lesion is recognized before the surgeon subjects the patient to a high-risk procedure under the impression that the lesion is malignant.

PANCREATIC HETEROTOPIA

Aberrant or ectopic pancreatic tissue, subject to all the pathologic changes of the pancreas itself, has become of increasing clinical significance. Barbosa, Dockerty and Waugh (1946) of the Mayo Clinic reported 41 histologically proved surgical cases, of which 61 per cent were of clinical significance. Such ectopic tissue was found about once in every 500 upper abdominal operations, the highest percentage of the total (70%) being in the duodenum, the stomach and the jejunum. However, occurrences in the biliary tract, ileum, diverticuli of the small bowel including Meckel's diverticulum, spleen, liver, omentum, mesentery and mediastinum (teratoma) have been reported.

Symptoms produced resemble those of peptic ulcer, duodenal obstruction, biliary tract disease, intussusception, or indefinite gastrointestinal complaints. Pathologically, edema, ulceration, hemorrhage, fat necrosis and inflammation may be observed. It is believed that malignant change is more likely to occur than in normal pancreas. Since most of these lesions are not recognized preoperatively and the findings may be misinterpreted at operation, frozen section examination is very helpful.

The treatment of choice is local excision whether the lesions are symptomatic or are found incidentally at laparotomy.

Howard et al. (1950) summarized 9 cases of ectopic islet cell tumors, 8 of which produced hypoglycemia. Autopsy incidence of pancreatic heterotopia in the literature as collected by Barbosa (1946) ranged from 0.6 per cent to 5.6 per cent.

METABOLIC EFFECTS OF TOTAL PANCREATECTOMY

Thirty-three total pancreatectomies were collected from the literature by Cattell and

Warren (1953). These were performed for carcinoma, sarcoma, chronic pancreatitis, and for hyperinsulinism, where no adenoma was found. The mortality was 36.4 per cent. A number of metabolic studies have been reported, a careful one being that of Nardi (1954).

INSULIN REQUIREMENT

The insulin requirement is relatively low, usually 40 units daily or less. The patient with pre-existing diabetes may have his insulin requirement slightly increased, unaltered or decreased following pancreatectomy. Thorogood and Zimmerman (1945) found that pancreatectomy reduced the insulin requirements of alloxan-diabetic animals and postulated the presence of a diabetogenic factor in the pancreas. However, Mirsky et al. (1951) have shown that fasting depancreatized dogs, previously rendered alloxan-diabetic, have an aggravation of the diabetic state.

The apparent mildness of diabetes following pancreatectomy is explained by Mirsky et al. by the absence of external secretion, since these authors found that pancreatectomy produces a decrease in absorption of proteins and carbohydrates from the gastrointestinal tract.

Lukens (1955) also believed that pancreatectomy produces the severest form of diabetes. However, Nardi's patient required only 10 units each of protamine zinc and crystalline insulin for adequate control of the diabetes. The usual experience has placed the requirement in the range of 30 to 40 units per day.

FATTY LIVERS

In contradistinction to dogs, fatty infiltration of the liver seldom has been reported in man. Brunschwig (Ricketts, Brunschwig and Knowlton, 1946) reported one instance in a patient with diabetes prior to surgery. However, most patients have been protected by choline, methionine or pancreatic extracts.

PHOSPHOLIPID METABOLISM

Barker et al. (1950), working with pancreatectomized dogs, found a reduced ability of the animals to incorporate radioactive phosphorus into phospholipid and postulated that the post-pancreatectomy fatty livers may be related to this. However, Nardi repeated the experiment in his patient and found no such abnormality.

STOOLS

Whipple (1946) reported 2 patients who showed no fecal disturbances after total pancreaticoduodenectomy. Nevertheless, some patients have bulky, soft, diarrheic stools. The nutritional status of Nardi's patient was better without pancreatin than with it. Thus, it appears that such supplements are not always necessary although very helpful in a majority of cases.

SERUM ENZYMES

Normal or low normal levels of serum amylase and lipase have been found in nearly all reported cases.

Despite the interesting studies reported, the author is impressed with the moderate and relatively constant insulin requirement of depancreatized patients, including one who survived 9 years and gained weight and remained active to the age of 71.

In the present state of knowledge a methionine supplement of 5 to 6 Gm. per day is recommended to prevent fatty infiltration of the liver.

FIBROCYSTIC DEGENERATION OF THE PANCREAS

This congenital malformation is discussed in Chapter 48, under "Meconium Ileus."

REFERENCES

Ackerman, L. V., and Ramirez, G. A.: The indications for and limitations of frozen section diagnosis; A review of 1269 consecutive frozen section diagnoses. Brit. J. Surg., 46:336, 1959.

Babcock, W. W.: Principles and Practice of Surgery. p. 1331. Philadelphia, Lea & Febiger, 1930.

Banting, F. G., and Best, C. H.: Internal secretion of pancreas. J. Lab. Clin. Med., 7:251-266, 1922.

Barbosa, J. J. DeC., Dockerty, M. B., and Waugh, J. M.: Pancreatic heterotopia. Surg., Gynec. Obstet., 82:527-542, 1946.

Barker, W. F., Rogers, K. E., and Moore, F. D.: Effect of pancreatectomy on phospholipid synthesis in dogs. Arch. Surg., 61:1151-1162, 1950.

Bauman, L.: The Diagnosis of Pancreatic Disease. Philadelphia, J. B. Lippincott, 1949.

Becker, V.: Histochemistry of the exocrine pancreas. In: de Reuck, A. V. S., and Cameron, M. P. (eds.): The Exocrine Pancreas—Normal and Abnormal Functions. pp. 56-62. Boston, Little, Brown and Co., 1963.

Berk, J. E.: Diagnosis of carcinoma of pancreas. Arch. Int. Med., 68:525-559, 1941.

Bosshardt, D. K., Ciereszko, L. S., and Barnes, R. H.: Preparation of a pancreas derivative having lipotropic activity. Am. J. Physiol., 166:433-435, 1951.

Bowers, R. F.: Discussion of a paper by Longmire, W. P., Jr., Jordan, P. H., Jr., and Briggs, J. D.: Experience with pancreatic resection for chronic relapsing pancreatitis. Tr. Am. S. A., vol. LXXIV, 1956.

Bro-Rasmussen, F., Killman, S-A., and Thaysen, J. H.: Acta physiol. scand., 37:97, 1956.

Brunschwig, A.: Pancreatoduodenectomy: "curative" operation for malignant neoplasms in pancreatoduodenal region; report of three over-five-year survivors. Ann. Surg., 136:610-624, 1952.

Brunschwig, A., and Allen, J. G.: Specific injurious action of alloxan upon pancreatic islet cells and convoluted tubules of kidney: comparative study in rabbit, dog, and man; attempted chemotherapy of insulin-producing islet cell carcinoma in man. Cancer Res., 4:45-54, 1944.

Bystrov, N. V.: Clinical forms of acute pancreatitis, their diagnosis and treatment. Khirurgiia, 35:7, 1959.

Cameron, A. L., and Noble, H. F.: Reflux of bile up the duct of Wirsung caused by an impacted biliary calculus. J.A.M.A., 82:1410-1414, 1924.

Cattell, R. B.: Anastomosis of duct of Wirsung; its use in palliative operations for cancer of head of pancreas. Surg. Clin. N. Am., 27:636-643, 1947.

Cattell, R. B., and Warren, K. W.: Surgery of the Pancreas. p. 374. Philadelphia, W. B. Saunders, 1953.

Cattell, R. B., Warren, R. W., and Au, F. T. C.: Periampullary carcinomas, diagnosis and surgical treatment. Surg. Clin. N. Am., 39:781, 1959.

Child, C. G., III: Advances in management of pancreaticoduodenal cancer. In: Andrus, W. D. (ed.): Advances in Surgery. vol. 2. pp. 495-561. New York, Interscience, 1949.

Child, C. G., Holswade, G. R., McClure, R. D., Jr., Gore, A. L., and O'Neill, E. A.: Pancreatoduodenectomy with resection of the portal vein in the Macaca mulatta monkey and man. Surg., Gynec. Obstet., 94:31-45, 1952.

Cliffton, E. E.: Carcinoma of pancreas: symptoms, signs, and results of treatment in 122 cases. Arch. Surg., 65:290-306, 1952.

Conn, J. W., and Seltzer, H. S.: Spontaneous hypoglycemia. Am. J. Med., 19:460-478, 1955.

DaCosta, J. M.: Cancer of the pancreas. N. Am. Med-chir. Rev., 2:883-909, 1858.

Dainko, E. A., Paul, H. A., Gabel, A., and Beattie, E. J.: Pancreatic secretion of antibacterial agents through a new pancreatic fistula in the dog. Arch. Surg., 86:1050, 1963.

Deaver, J. B., and Ravdin, I. S.: Carcinoma of the duodenum. Am. J. Med. Sci., 159:469-477, 1920.

Dennis, C., and Varco, R. L.: Survival for more than five years after pancreatoduodenectomy for cancers of the ampulla and pancreatic head. Surgery, 39:92, 1956.

Desnuelle, P., Reboud, J. P., and Ben Abdeljlil, A.: Influence of the composition of the diet on the enzyme content of rat pancreas. In: de Reuck, A. V. S., and Cameron, M. P. (eds.): The Exocrine Pancreas. pp. 90-107. Boston, Little, Brown and Co., 1963.

Dick, B. M., and Wallace, V. H. G.: Cholecystography: toxic effects of the dyes. Brit. J. Surg., 15:360-369, 1928.

Doubilet, H., and Mulholland, J. H.: Results of sphincterotomy in pancreatitis. J. Mt. Sinai Hosp., 17:458, 1951.

———: The surgical treatment of pancreatitis. Surg. Clin. N. Am., 29:339-359, 1949.

Dragstedt, L. R., Van Prohaska, J., and Harms, H. P.: Observations on a substance in pancreas which permits survival and prevents liver damage in depancreatized dogs. Am. J. Physiol., 117:175-181, 1936.

Dreiling, D. A., and Janowitz, H. D.: The secretion of electrolytes by the human pancreas. The effect of Diamox, ACTH, and disease. Am. J. Digest. Dis., 4:137-144, 1959.

Dunphy, J. E., Brooks, J. R., and Achroyd, F.: Acute postoperative pancreatitis. New Eng. J. Med., 248:445-451, 1953.

Fallis, L. S., and Plain, G.: Acute pancreatitis; report of 26 cases. Surgery, 15:358-373, 1939.

Frostberg, N.: Characteristic duodenal deformity in cases of different kinds of perivaterial enlargement of the pancreas. Acta radiol., 19:164-173, 1938.

Gage, M.: Treatment of acute pancreatitis with report of cases. Surgery, 23:723-724, 1948.

Graham, E. A., and Cole, W. H.: Roentgenologic examination of gallbladder. J.A.M.A., 82:613-614, 1924.

Graham, R.: Quoted by Howland, G., Campbell, W. R., Maltby, E. J., and Robinson, W. L.: Dysinsulinism: convulsions and coma due to islet cell tumor of the pancreas, with operation and cure. J.A.M.A., 93:674-679, 1929.

Gregory, R. A., and Tracy, H. J.: The constitution and properties of two gastrins extracted from hog antral mucosa. Gut, 5:103, 1964.

Haanes, M. L., and Gyorgy, P.: In vitro action of a new lipotropic fraction in the pancreas. Am. J. Physiol., 166:441-450, 1951.

Harris, S.: Hyperinsulinism and dysinsulinism. J.A.M.A., 83:729-733, 1924.

Hershey, J. E., and Hillman, F. J.: Fatal pancreatic necrosis following choledochotomy and cholangiography. Arch. Surg., 71:885-889, 1955.

Hotchkiss, D., Jr., Fitts, W. T., Jr., and Rosenthal, O.: The effect of abdominal operations upon the serum amylase and serum lipase. Surg. Forum, 1954. V, 490-495.

Howard, J. M.: Experimental studies on the toxicity of beta-(4-hydroxy-3,5-diiodophenyl)-alpha-phenyl-propionic acid (Priodax). Am. J. Roentgenol., 59:408-415, 1948.

———: Pancreatico-duodenectomy. Forty-one consecutive Whipple resections without an operative mortality. Ann. Surg. 168:629-640, 1968.

Howard, J. M., and Jones, R., Jr.: Anatomy of pancreatic ducts; etiology of acute pancreatitis. Am. J. Med. Sci., 214:617-622, 1947.

Howard, J. M., and Jordan, G. L.: Surgical Diseases

of the Pancreas. Philadelphia, J. B. Lippincott, 1960.
Howard, J. M., Moss, N. H., and Rhoads, J. E.: Hyperinsulinism and islet cell tumors of the pancreas. Internat. Abstr. Surg. (Surg., Gynec. Obstet.), 90:417-455, 1950.
Howard, J. M., and Ravdin, I. S.: Acute pancreatitis: a study of 80 patients. Am. Pract., 2:385-395, 1948.
Inouye, W. Y., and Vars, H. M.: Intestinal absorption of insulin in dogs. Surg. Forum, 13:316-317, 1962.
Janowitz, H. D., and Dreiling, D. A.: The pancreatic secretion of fluid and electrolytes. *In*: de Reuck, A. V. S., and Cameron, M. P. (eds.): The Exocrine Pancreas. pp. 115-133. Boston, Little, Brown and Co., 1963.
Kaufman, L. W., and Wilson, G. S.: Carcinoma of the head of the pancreas and periampullary region. Am. J. Med. Sci., 230:200-212, 1955.
Logan, P. B., and Kleinsasser, L. J.: Surgery of the pancreas: results of pancreaticoduodenal resections reported in the literature. Internat. Abstr. Surg. (Surg., Gynec. Obstet.), 93:521-543, 1951.
Longmire, W. P., Jr., Jordan, P. H., Jr., and Briggs, J. D.: Experience with resection of the pancreas in the treatment of chronic relapsing pancreatitis. Ann. Surg., 144:681, 1956.
Lukens, F. D. W.: Experimental diabetes and its relation to diabetes mellitus. Am. J. Med., 19:790-797, 1955.
McDermott, W. V., Jr., and Bartlett, M. K.: Pancreaticoduodenal cancer. New Eng. J. Med., 248:927-931, 1953.
Mahorner, H. R., and Mattson, H.: The etiology and pathology of cysts of the pancreas. Arch. Surg., 22:1018-1033, 1931.
Mallet-Guy, P., Jeanjean, R., and Feroldi, J.: Provocation expérimentale de pancréatites aiguës par excitation électrique du splanchnique gauche. Lyon chir., 39:437-447, 1944.
Millbourn, E.: Excretory ducts of pancreas in man, with special reference to their relations to each other, to common bile duct and to duodenum. Acta anat., 9:1-34, 1950.
———: Pancreatico-gastrostomy in pancreatico-duodenal resection for carcinoma of the head of pancreas or the papilla of Vater. Acta chir. scand., 116:12, 1958.
Miller, J. R., Baggenstoss, A. H., and Comfort, M. W.: Carcinoma of the pancreas: effect of histologic type and grade of malignancy on its behavior. Cancer, 4:233-241, 1951.
Mirsky, I. A., Futterman, P., Wachman, J., and Perisutti, G.: The influence of pancreatectomy on the metabolic state of alloxandiabetic dog. Endocrinology, 49:73-81, 1951.
Monge, J. J., Judd, E. S., and Gage, R. P.: Radical pancreatoduodenectomy: Twenty-two years experience with the complications, mortality rate, and survival rate. Ann. Surg., 160:711-719, 1964.
Moss, N. H., and Rhoads, J. E.: Hyperinsulinism and islet cell tumors of the pancreas. *In*: Howard, J. M., and Jordan, G. L. (eds.): Surgical diseases of the pancreas. Philadelphia, J. B. Lippincott, 1960.
Moyer, C. A.: Personal communication.

Mozan, A. A.: Cystadenoma of the pancreas. Am. J. Surg., 81:204-214, 1951.
Muir, E. G.: Resection for carcinoma of the head of the pancreas; two five-year survivals. Brit. J. Surg., 42:489-490, 1954-55.
Nardi, G. L.: Metabolic studies following total pancreatectomy for retroperitoneal leiomyosarcoma. New Eng. J. Med., 247:548-550, 1952.
———: Phospholipid synthesis in patients with pancreatic disease. Arch. Surg., 69:726-731, 1954.
Neurath, H.: Considerations of the occurrence, structure and function of the proteolytic enzymes of the pancreas. *In*: de Reuck, A. V. S., and Cameron, M. P. (eds.): The Exocrine Pancreas. pp. 67-86. Boston, Little, Brown and Co., 1963.
Opie, E. L.: The anatomy of the pancreas. Bull. Johns Hopkins Hosp., 14:229-232, 1903.
———: Diseases of the Pancreas. ed. 2. p. 291. Philadelphia, J. B. Lippincott, 1910.
Orr, T. G.: Some observations on the treatment of carcinoma of the pancreas. Surgery, 32:933-947, 1952.
Owens, J. L., and Howard, J. M.: Pancreatic calcification: a late sequel in the natural history of chronic alcoholism and alcoholic pancreatitis. Ann. Surg., 147:326, 1958.
Palade, G. E., Siekevitz, P., and Caro, L. G.: Structure, chemistry and function of the pancreatic exocrine cell. *In*: de Reuck, A. V. S., and Cameron, M. P. (eds.): The Exocrine Pancreas. pp. 23-49. Boston, Little, Brown and Co., 1963.
Park, C. D., Mackie, J. A., and Rhoads, J. E.: Pancreatogastrostomy. Am. J. Surg., 113:85, 1967.
Persky, L., Schweinburg, F. B., Jacob, S., and Fine, J.: Aureomycin in experimental acute pancreatitis of dogs. Surgery, 30:652, 1951.
Porter, M. R.: Carcinoma of the pancreaticoduodenal area, operability and choice of procedure. Ann. Surg., 148:711, 1958.
Puestow, C. B., and Gillesby, W. J.: Retrograde surgical drainage of pancreas for chronic relapsing pancreatitis. Arch. Surg., 76:898, 1958.
Ravdin, I. S.: Some recent advances in surgical therapeusis. Ann. Surg., 109:321-333, 1939.
Ray, B. S., and Console, A. D.: Relief of pain in chronic (calcareous) pancreatitis by sympathectomy. Surg., Gynec. Obstet., 89:1-8, 1949.
Reber, H. A., and Wolf, C. J.: Micropuncture study of pancreatic electrolyte secretion. Am. J. Physiol., 215:34-40, 1968.
Reber, H. A., Wolf, C. J., and Lee, S. P.: The role of the main duct in pancreatic electrolyte secretion. Surg. Forum, 20:1969.
Rhoads, J. E., Howard, J. M., and Moss, N. H.: Clinical experiences with surgical lesions of the pancreas. Surg. Clin. N. Am., 29:1801-1816, 1949.
Rhoads, J. E., Liboro, O., Fox, S., Gyorgy, P., and Machella, T. E.: In vivo action of a new lipotropic fraction of the pancreas. Am. J. Physiol., 166:436-440, 1951.
Rhoads, J. E., Zintel, H. A., and Helwig, J., Jr.: Results of operations of the Whipple type in pancreaticoduodenal carcinoma. Ann. Surg., 146:661, 1957.
———: An evaluation of palliative and curative op-

erations in the treatment of pancreatoduodenal carcinomas. Acta Un. int. Cancr., 16:1397-1401, 1960.

Ricketts, H. T., Brunschwig, A., and Knowlton, K.: Effects of total pancreatectomy in a patient with diabetes. Am. J. Med., 1:229-245, 1946.

Rienhoff, W. F., Jr., and Baker, B. M.: Pancreatolithiasis and chronic pancreatitis; preliminary report of case of apparently successful treatment by transthoracic sympathectomy and vagotomy. J.A.M.A., 134:20-21, 1947.

Rienhoff, W. F., Jr., and Pickrell, K. L.: Pancreatitis; anatomic study of pancreatic and extrahepatic biliary systems. Arch. Surg., 51:205-219, 1945.

Ross, D. E.: Cancer of the pancreas with two case reports of five-year survivals. Am. J. Surg., 93:990, 1957.

Smith, R.: Long-term survival after pancreatectomy for cancer. Brit. J. Surg., 44:294, 1956.

Somogyi, M.: Micromethods for estimation of diastase. J. Biol. Chem., 125:399-414, 1938.

Thorogood, E., and Zimmerman, B.: The effects of pancreatectomy on glycosuria and ketosis in dogs made diabetic by alloxan. Endocrinology, 37:191-200, 1945.

Tong That Tung, Nguyen Duong Quang and Hoang Kim Tinh: The diagnosis and treatment of acute pancreatitis caused by parasites. Vestn. Khir. Grekov., 84:3, 1960.

Trimble, I. R., Parsons, J. W., and Sherman, C. P.: A one stage operation for the cure of carcinoma of the ampulla of Vater and of the head of the pancreas. Surg., Gynec. Obstet., 73:711, 1941.

Warren, K. W., and Cattell, R. B.: Pancreatic surgery (concluded). New Eng. J. Med., 261:387, 1959.

Warren, K. W., Veidenheimer, M. C., and Pratt, H. S.: Surg. Clin. N. Am., 47:639-645, 1967.

Waterman, N. G., et al.: The treatment of acute hemorrhagic pancreatitis by sump drainage. Surg., Gynec. Obstet., 126:963, 1968.

Waugh, J. M., and Giberson, R. G.: Radical resection of the head of the pancreas and of the duodenum for malignant lesions. Surg. Clin. N. Am., 965, August, 1957.

Whipple, A. O., Parsons, W. B., and Mullins, C. R.: Treatment of carcinoma of the ampulla of Vater. Ann. Surg., 102:763, 1935.

Whipple, A. O.: Radical surgery for certain cases of pancreatic fibrosis associated with calcareous deposits. Ann. Surg., 124:991-1008, 1946.

————: The radical surgery of pancreaticoduodenal cancer. In: Carter, B. N.: Monographs on Surgery. pp. 1-19. Baltimore, Williams & Wilkins, 1952.

Wilder, R. M., Allan, F. N., Power, M. H., and Robertson, H. E.: Carcinoma of the islands of the pancreas; hyperinsulinism and hypoglycemia. J.A.M.A., 89:348-355, 1927.

Zintel, H. A., Enterline, H. T., and Rhoads, J. E.: Benign cystadenoma of pancreas. Surgery, 35:612-620, 1954.

CHAPTER 34

J. GARROTT ALLEN, M.D.

Spleen

Historical Note
Anatomy
Physiology
Splenic Function, Hyperfunction and Dysfunction
Auto-immune Diseases Benefited by Splenectomy
Diseases of the Spleen
Inherited Diseases Benefited by Splenectomy
Splenic Tumors
Technic of Splenectomy
Splenic Transplantation in Classical Hemophilia A

The spleen is of surgical importance because many of its diseases, whether primary or secondary, respond to splenectomy. On the other hand, the role of most surgeons in performing splenectomy for its nontraumatic diseases has been a passive one more often than not. At times they may rely too heavily upon the judgment of the hematologist or the pathologist for the detailed examination of the blood marrow, and the splenic pulp essential to the diagnosis, not acquainting themselves with the reliability of the diagnosis.

HISTORICAL NOTE

Although the spleen has often been referred to as an "organ of mystery," a review of some of the early writings on the subject discloses no unusual deficiency in knowledge or lack of thought on the part of physicians. Among the writings of the laity, however, the spleen has been assigned bizarre, apocryphal, and imaginary functions. Perhaps this accounts for some of the luster in folklore and fiction surrounding functions of the spleen.

Aristotle recognized the spleen as belonging to the hepatic and portal circulations, but he erroneously believed it to be the "second liver." Galen, who added much sparkle to early medical history but little to medical knowledge, believed "yellow bile" to be disposed of by the liver and "black bile" to be attracted to the spleen. Aretaeus of Cappadocia (Adams, 1856) may have been influenced by Galen's writings. He, Aretaeus, thought that the spleen "strained black blood," believing the spleen to be porous, and recognized that it often was enlarged. It is interesting to speculate why he found that the spleen was "often enlarged" among the Greeks and the Romans of 2,000 years ago; to what extent did parasitic diseases and perhaps Mediterranean anemia contribute to his conclusion?

Marcello Malpighi was the first to study the spleen by means of the microscope. In 1659, he described its capsule, the contractile nature of its trabeculae and its lymph follicles, later to bear his name. He proved that the spleen is essentially an organ of the vascular system, especially of the splanchnic bed.

Florian Matthis is said to have performed the first splenectomy in dogs in the late 16th century. This feat was repeated a few years later by Paul Barbette (1629-1699) in dogs but was not achieved in man until 2 centuries later.

An interesting sidelight relating to the history of surgery of the spleen is that found in the condemnation of John Blundell (see Chap. 8, Blood Transfusion). He was a bold surgeon for his day, and his exploits in blood transfusion in 1818 were soon to be followed by his performing "radical" intra-abdominal operations which proved to be the source of severe criticism resulting in his disrepute. The *Lancet* expressed the fear in 1825 that his next activity might well be the surgical removal of the spleen. Thirty-two years later (1857), Gustav Simon (1824-1876) did perform the first human splenectomy, and later Spencer Wells exploited the operation to advantage.

As the physiologic, pathologic and clinical consequences of splenic diseases developed, the developments assumed many aspects of interest and importance. Some of these will be mentioned briefly in the appropriate sections which follow.

ANATOMY

The spleen arises embryologically from the dorsal mesogastrium just above the tail of the pancreas. When fully developed, it lies in contact with the lateral and the posterior margins of the diaphragm to which its superior pole is suspended by the phrenicolienal ligament. All of its ligaments are in reality reflections of the parietal peritoneum upon the splenic surface as visceral peritoneum. Its posterior border abuts the abdominal wall in the regions of the 11th rib, where it is held by a continuation of the phrenicolienal ligament which attaches along the posterior parietal peritoneal wall. This ligament departs from the abdominal wall, the tail of the pancreas, the splenic vessels, and the splenic flexure of the colon at its superior-posterior margin, to encapsulate the spleen as visceral peritoneum. The inferior and posterolateral portions of the spleen are covered with peritoneum derived from that over the area of the kidney, forming the lienorenal ligament.

Thus, except for the posterior line of parietal reflections of peritoneum over the spleen, more than 90 per cent of its surface faces into the peritoneal cavity and is covered with serosa. In some patients its ligamentous attachments are fairly long so that the spleen may be somewhat mobile and subject to torsion. In others these peritoneal reflections are short, holding the spleen firmly in place. Should the spleen enlarge, it must do so in the anterior and inferior direction. Its posterior ligamentous attachments are stretched, and it may acquire more mobility. This increase in mobility often facilitates splenectomy, and for this reason the enlarged spleen at times is more easily removed surgically than the one normal in size.

The spleen is also held by the gastrolienal ligament which is a reflection of anterior and posterior visceral peritoneum of the stomach as they come together along the lateral uppermost part of the greater curvature. This omental ligament attaches to the splenic hilum. Between its leaves run several short arteries and veins from the distal portion of the left gastroepiploic vessels which supply the gastric fundus. Thus on its mesial surface the spleen receives both parietal and visceral ligamentous attachments. The major splenic vessels enter via the posterior visceral peritoneal reflection; the short gastrics enter through its anteromesial gastric attachments.

The color of the normal spleen is dark purple. Its normal weight in the adult is from 200 to 225 Gm., and it cannot be felt. In infancy the normal spleen weighs more in proportion to body weight; its greater weight in infancy is attributed to its hematopoietic activity at that time, especially in the formation of lymphocytes—the dominant leukocytic cell in this age group. The organ is normally palpable in most infants under the age of 2 years. The amount of blood contained within the normal human spleen is not great. Motulsky et al. (1958) found the normal spleen to contain from 1 to 2 per cent of the total circulating red cell mass. In normal man there is neither splenic sequestration of red cells of any significance nor a noncirculating reserve of red cells (Ebert and Stead, 1941). These latter observations are in contrast with findings in the dog. Reeve and his associates (1953) indicated that in the dog up to one third of the red cell mass could be sequestered temporarily in the spleen during barbiturate narcosis. These observations emphasize the important species differences in the function of this organ.

The splenic artery is usually the first and largest branch of the celiac artery. It is remarkably tortuous, the most tortuous artery normally within the abdomen. As it departs from its source, it passes horizontally to the left just above the superior margin of the pancreas in the retroperitoneum of the lesser omental bursa. Along its lateral half, the artery usually parallels the course of the splenic vein, which lies slightly below and anterior to the artery. Within 1 to 3 cm. of the spleen, the artery divides into 2 or 3 major branches before entering the splenic hilum. Venous drainage leaves the spleen through several branches which quickly converge to form the splenic vein.

The lymphatic drainage of the spleen is certainly grossly inconspicuous. The lymph channels converge upon the hilum from within the spleen and then drain into the nodes in the region of the tail of the pancreas; the author seldom has encountered them.

Accessory spleens, ranging from a few hundred milligrams to several grams in weight, are found in about 12 to 15 per cent of patients at operation, whether or not splenic disease is present. Usually they lie near the hilum, in the adjacent omentum, or to the left side of the esophageal hiatus. They are important in certain of the hypersplenic diseases; in some patients with these disorders, failure to respond to splenectomy is attributed to accessory splenic tissue left behind (see below). Accessory spleens are often multiple, 2 to 10 or more.

The splenic capsule is comprised of serosa and a subserosal fibro-elastic coat. The serosa is its visceral peritoneum derived from the peritoneal reflections described above. The fibro-elastic coat is easily torn at operation. This coat surrounds the spleen and on its internal surfaces interlaces its way toward the center, forming the trabecular network that Malpighi described. This is the basic internal structural architecture of the spleen in which is enmeshed the splenic pulp and its internal vascular system. The trabecular network with its fibro-elastic tissue converges upon the major splenic vessels.

PHYSIOLOGY

Although the spleen is not essential to normal childhood development or to adult life, it does partake in certain functions shared also by the "reticuloendothelial system," and at times may share some of those of the marrow, especially in fetal life and early infancy. In certain diseases that encroach upon the marrow space in adults, the spleen, as well as the liver, may resume its embryonal functions of hematopoiesis; in fact, under these circumstances, they may be the major portion of the blood-forming tissue. Hence, splenectomy under these circumstances can prove to be disastrous.

When the normal spleen is removed from man for acute trauma or to facilitate another surgical procedure, transient thrombocytosis and leukocytosis lasting several weeks is the rule. Platelet and leukocyte counts several times normal may occur. Several report definite but less conspicuous increases of the circulating red cells also. These observations usually are interpreted as implicating the spleen as an organ involved in the normal destruction of the formed elements of blood.

Jacobson and co-workers (1951) showed that shielding the spleen during fatal doses of total body radiation protected the animal from the lethal effects of the irradiation. Cole et al. (1952) showed that intravenous infusions of spleen cell homogenates also conferred protection from lethal irradiation. For a time the protective effect of the administered spleen cells was thought to be due to a humoral factor. However, Barnes and Loutit (1956) showed that the protective effect of spleen cells could be achieved only with living cells and was not due to a humoral or chemical agent. Lorenz et al. (1951) showed that bone marrow infusions would also protect against irradiation injury. It appears that the benefit of shielding the spleen is a general phenomenon, since shielding other portions of the hematopoietic tissue from lethal doses of total body radiation will produce the same protective effect. The protective effect of shielding hematopoietic tissue is related to the fact that the shielded tissue will quickly recover its normal function. The protective effect of the injected spleen or marrow cells is related to the fact that the injected cells live and multiply within the recipient and assume the functions of the destroyed hematopoietic tissue.

The spleen is intimately related to the production of antibodies, but its presence is not essential to this end. Other organs are also involved.

When the spleen alone is exposed to x-rays, Hektoen, as observed in 1916, found that the capacity for the body to elaborate antibodies during the next few weeks is diminished. Friedell and others (1947) observed an even greater depressed antibody production capacity after total body radiation in rabbits. The transient depression in antibody production following depressed antibody response of the spleen after splenic x-radiation in man has been used as a partial treatment in the past for various forms of hypersplenism in which the formation of auto-antibodies is believed to be their cause.

Rowley (1950) has studied antibody response in patients splenectomized for a variety of conditions, including trauma and surgical extirpation of normal spleens necessary to other surgery. His studies disclosed the same results regardless of whether splenectomy had been performed a few weeks to several years before. Compared with the capacity of his normal human subjects to produce antibodies to a standard antigen, the ability of the splenectomized individual to produce high titers of antibodies was diminished. Steiner (1956) has extended this type of study experimentally and demonstrated the enormous capacity of splenic tissue to form antibodies in tissue culture. Thus the relation of the spleen to antibody formation seems to be unquestioned, but the problem as to the susceptibility of infection in man is not. The end result clinically is of no obvious importance in later life, if serious infection is the indication measured.

The splenic pulp is comprised of reticular cells and splenocytes in which are enmeshed lymphocytes, granulocytes, erythrocytes and platelets. It is this structure that appears to be responsible for most of its physiologic functions. Lymphoid follicles (malpighian corpuscles) are numerous and located throughout the normal spleen. They are believed to be one of the sites of lymphocyte and monocyte production in adult life. In fetal life and early infancy, the spleen is also the site of normal hematopoiesis, an atavistic function observed in certain diseases, as mentioned above.

SPLENIC FUNCTION, HYPERFUNCTION AND DYSFUNCTION

The term hypersplenism was popularized by Eppinger (1922) to describe those syndromes—anemia, leukopenia and thrombocytopenia—where they could be relieved or cured by splenectomy. However, we know very little about the normal functions of the spleen, and for more than 50 years we have assumed that the hematopoietic disorders that respond to splenectomy somehow represent an increase of normal function. Presumably, splenism is that state that characterizes the splenic or normal person, and the state of hyposplenism exists when the spleen is removed and no splenic tissue is left behind. When all three of the formed elements of blood are deficient in the same patient and these deficiencies are relieved by splenectomy, the term panhypersplenism is used.

But these terms are not yet well defined, nor are the abnormalities of splenic function which they describe. In prenatal life the normal spleen is the site of myelopoiesis, including erythropoiesis. Ordinarily, these functions disappear at birth or shortly thereafter but may be reactivated when the marrow becomes fibrotic, sclerosed or is largely replaced by metastatic cancer. In the first few years of life, the spleen apparently contributes materially to the production of lymphocytes, and it is thought that splenectomy performed in the infant or the young child may render him more susceptible to bacterial infection than does splenectomy in the adult. There are large and small lymphocytes; the small lymphocytes are thought to be associated with hypersensitivity reactions.

The concept that the spleen is the slaughterhouse for the aging cellular population of blood may be true in part, but the same rate of cellular destruction continues after the normal spleen has been removed. When splenectomy has been performed because of rupture or for surgical convenience in other operative procedures, the levels of circulating platelets, leukocytes and erythrocytes may be increased temporarily but soon resume their normal values. It may be that the normal spleen assists in the regulation of the levels at which the formed elements of blood are normally maintained; but this role, while possibly contributory, is not essential.

Neonatal Thrombocytopenia

Isoimmune Purpura. There are several kinds of platelet antibodies which occur in human serum. One of these antibodies identifies an antigen (or antigens) shared by the granulocytes, lymphocytes and other tissues. It is not naturally occurring, but arises following stimulation by transfusion and or pregnancy. This antigen (or antigens) may induce symptomatic thrombocytopenia occurring in the neonatal period. It can be a potentially serious disorder resulting in death in approximately 14 per cent of reported cases (Morris, 1954). In about 20 per cent of the reported cases of neonatal thrombocytopenia, there is no history of maternal hematologic disease. Sensitive technics based on complement fixation have been developed for detecting and characterizing antiplatelet isoantibodies (Shulman et al., 1961).

The ideal therapy regimen for such patients is early exchange transfusions with the use of blood from a normal platelet[A1] negative donor. In this way a hemostatic level of circulating compatible platelets would be established at the same time that platelet antibodies are being removed. The immunologic sequence of this disease is analogous to that of erythroblastosis foetalis or the erythrocytes (Adner et al., 1969), and requires much the same treatment—exchange transfusions.

Autoimmune Neonatal. Autoimmune thrombocytopenia produces a low platelet count in the patient and, if she is pregnant, she may transmit her antibodies to the platelets of the fetus and cause it to develop severe thrombocytopenic purpura *in utero* (Allen et al., 1947).

The thrombocytopenia of autoimmune disease is acquired and not somatic. In the case of a pregnant woman who develops autoimmune antibodies to her own platelets, and consequently, thrombocytopenic purpura, because her antibodies are transmitted across the placental membrane, the infant also develops thrombocytopenia. However, in neonatal thrombocytopenia from this cause, exchange transfusions are not necessary because once the baby is delivered and detached from its source of antibodies, they are soon exhausted and the baby makes a spontaneous recovery (Bogardus et al., 1949).

The mechanism by which autoimmune antibodies develop against the platelets, is not well understood. The term itself is an unfortunate one, for it implies automation without sequence of causes. The autoimmune mechanisms responsible for this hematologic complication are often self-limited and the clinical course may wax and wane for periods of time ranging from weeks to years. In children and young adults, thrombocytopenia is frequently associated with common infections. The same may also be true when patients are taking certain drugs. If these associations are recognized, the drugs discontinued and the infection appropriately treated, petechial hemorrhage may disappear and the platelet count return to normal.

After splenectomy there is often cited an increase of risk of infection (Eraklis et al., 1967). It is alleged that, because the spleen plays a role in antibody response, the reticuloendothelial system does not compensate fully after splenectomy. Patients whose courses are most commonly associated with post splenectomy fever are those who have reticulo-endothelial disease or inborn errors of metabolism: Cooley's anemia, Wescott-Aldrich syndrome, diffuse cancer, histiocytosis and lipidosis, Niemann-Pick disease, or Gaucher's disease. Allergic purpura may also occur with any infection.

The rate of antibody production of a particular bacterial antigen or hemolysin may be depressed after removal of the normal spleen, but this depression in the adult patient does not appear to make him more vulnerable to endemic infections.

Can the spleen suppress hematopoiesis either in health or disease? Possibly, but evidence is not convincing, and much of these data could be explained equally well by the fact that after splenectomy there is an adjustment of the functions governing the levels of formed elements in the blood and that a few days to a few weeks may be necessary for this transition to occur.

Are there antibodies to formed elements of blood that by "coating" their surfaces, or through other mechanisms, predispose them to more rapid removal from the circulation as they traverse the splenic bed? This appears to be a reasonable explanation as to why, in acute autohemolytic disease with an indirect Coomb's reaction and so-called splenic anemia, removal of the spleen effects relief if not a cure. Antibodies against the formed elements are illustrated best by two observations in connection with platelets. The first is that a young woman with idiopathic thrombocytopenic purpura (ITP) in the course of her pregnancy will give birth to an infant who, for a few days to several weeks after birth, may exhibit mild to moderate evidence of this disease (Bogardus et al., 1949). Apparently, the platelet-sensitizing antibodies cross the placental membrane to enter the fetal circulation, causing the infant's spleen to destroy its own passively sensitized platelets. After birth there is no longer this passive transfer of antibodies, and recovery of the infant is spontaneous. A more elaborate series of observations are those of Harrington et al. (1951), who noted that plasma transfused from a patient with ITP produced the disease transiently in the recipient. He further observed that these platelet antibodies persisted in the patient whose spleen had been removed some time previously with symptomatic cure. Thus it appears that in this syndrome, ITP, the auto-antibodies which sensitize the platelets continue to do so in the absence of the spleen, and that the spleen is apparently normal except that in receiving sensitized platelets, it disposes of them promptly either by lysis or by phagocytosis.

Platelets are rich in acid phosphatase, which Oski et al. (1963) found reflected in an elevated acid phosphatase plasma in patients with active idiopathic thrombocytopenic purpura. It was also elevated to some extent in 13 of 15 patients with chronic ITP in contrast with values below normal found in all patients whose platelet deficiency was due to marrow failure. However, Cohen and Gardner (1961) reported that, if such patients require large doses of corticoid steroids for prolonged periods of time, remissions may occur, but a form of thrombocytopenia may then develop which is secondary to the high doses of corticosteroids administered. If the administration of corticosteroids is necessary to sustain remissions of thrombocytopenia, splenectomy may be advisable within a few months to obviate some of the complications that may arise from the prolonged use of high doses of corticosteroids.

We owe much to Evans (1951), who recognized the similarities of idiopathic thrombocytopenic purpura (ITP) and acquired hemolytic anemia. He was able to demonstrate platelet agglutinations and suggested that the disease was an auto-immune process, as did Coombs et al. (1956). Dameshek (1960) suggested that ITP and acute hemolytic anemia may be the first manifestations of systemic lupus erythematosus—an interesting suggestion that is not yet established.

ITP, as well as hemolytic anemia, may occur under circumstances in which the increased rate of platelet or erythrocyte destruction or removal is more transient and possibly caused by different mechanisms. For example, thrombocytopenia, anemia, leukopenia and even neutropenia may develop in any patient whose spleen is enlarged and, as the spleen returns to normal or is removed, the levels of these formed elements return to normal. This suggests that the spleen itself is primarily responsible for suppression of the levels of one or more of these elements. Presumably the abnormal spleen may in some manner sensitize the patient's platelets or erythrocytes or leukocytes so as to accelerate their rates of removal by the spleen, or, as some have suggested, the enlarged spleen, without a concurrent increase of blood flow per gram of tissue, allows the formed elements to remain exposed for a longer period of time to the normal mechanisms for removal or destruction of these elements with the result that the opportunity for their destruction is greatly enhanced (Motulsky, 1958). However, this latter theory does not explain why antibodies to erythrocytes are formed and can be demonstrated by a positive Coomb's reaction, nor why the Coomb's test becomes negative after the spleen is removed. Prevailing evidence suggests that in splenic anemia, with or without neutropenia or thrombocytopenia, a circulating autoimmune mechanism is initiated from within the spleen itself.

The platelets have been implicated in the formation of atheromatous plaques and it is thought by some (Abrahamsen, 1968) that one of the explanations for the appearance of atheromatous plaques at the bifurcations of the arteries is the adhesiveness of the platelets to the arterial walls just distal to the arterial bifurcations. If true this would help explain why the location of such plaques appear earliest at such levels.

There is thought to be a reduced atherosclerotic process distal to these arterial bifurcations in von Willebrand's disease. This is attributed to the diminished adhesiveness of platelets, and a diminished factor XII deficiency. While factor XII deficiency gives rise to hemorrhagic disease due to a platelet deficit, it is not well established that people with such a disease have less atherosclerosis. Their life expectancy is less than normal.

Negus et al. (1969) studied platelet adhesiveness in 36 patients undergoing surgical operations. They found no significant change in platelet adhesiveness between those patients who developed deep-vein thrombosis and those who did not.

What then can we say of splenic function in those diseases of the blood in which splenectomy effects improvement or cure? We cannot generalize too much, but the few facts described above may be summarized as follows:

1. Abnormal blood cells, whether because of coating with antibodies, or because of abnormality in shape, or because of age, are removed or destroyed by the spleen at greatly accelerated rates.

2. Auto-antibodies or autosensitization of platelets in ITP appears to be an auto-immunologic process that continues to be active after splenectomy, though in the absence of the spleen, the platelet count usually remains normal. The spleen in this disease is probably otherwise normal and removes platelets at an excessive rate only because of the abnormality of the platelets themselves and not because of any particular abnormal function of the spleen. Therefore, cure of the disease by splenectomy is symptomatic rather than organic.

3. In enlarged spleens, whether from chronic passive congestion, portal hypertension, splenic tumors or cysts, or other forms of splenic disease, frequently there is an accelerated rate of destruction of platelets, of erythrocytes and leukocytes, which usually subsides when the size of the spleen returns to normal, when its internal pathology is arrested, or when splenectomy is performed. In these patients, the Coomb's test is positive and reverts to normal after splenectomy or when spontaneous remission of the splenic disorder occurs.

4. There is evidence to suggest that, if blood flow is not commensurately increased in splenomegaly, the duration of time that the formed elements are exposed to the splenic circulation is sufficiently increased so as to be a contributing, if not important, factor in the increased rate of destruction of platelets, erythrocytes or leukocytes.

AUTO-IMMUNE DISEASES BENEFITED BY SPLENECTOMY

In this group of disorders, the benefit of splenectomy is upon the associated hematologic complications. The auto-immune mechanisms may persist after splenectomy but, in the absence of the spleen, the sensitized formed elements usually are no longer destroyed at an accelerated rate.

In theory the hematologic complications of auto-immune disease may respond to one of two therapeutic approaches. First, often the auto-immune phenomenon can be suppressed by the use of glucocorticoids to a point where the accelerated rate of destruction of the formed elements of blood does not occur. Second is splenectomy which may abolish the site of accelerated cellular destruction but may have little or no effect upon the underlying auto-immune disease.

If, as some claim, the flow of blood through the bed of the enlarged spleen is retarded, presumably the removal of blood elements would proceed at a normal rate but, because of this greater exposure time, the usual number of cells or platelets would be removed from the circulation without necessarily entailing the action of an auto-immune mechanism. In these latter conditions, splenectomy exerts its benefit much as in the case of congenital spherocytic anemia.

The auto-immune mechanisms responsible for these hematologic complications are often self-limited, or the clinical course may wax and wane for periods of time ranging from weeks to years. Most of the cases that subside and do not recur are those in which a disease develops before puberty, and frequently in the wake of an infection, particularly of the upper respiratory system, or in association with allergic disease. However, at this young age are also observed some of the most severe cases, particularly of thrombocytopenic purpura and of acquired hemolytic anemia. Usually these patients respond to the administration of glucocorticoids, though occasionally a splenectomy may be necessary.

Idiopathic Thrombocytopenic Purpura (ITP) as a clinical entity was first described by Werlhof in 1735 and is centered about the following brief case history.

An adult girl, robust, without manifest cause, was attacked recently, towards the period of her menses, with sudden severe hemorrhage from the nose, with bright but foul blood escaping together with a blood vomiting of a very thick extremely black blood. Immediately there appeared about the neck and on the arms, spots partly black,

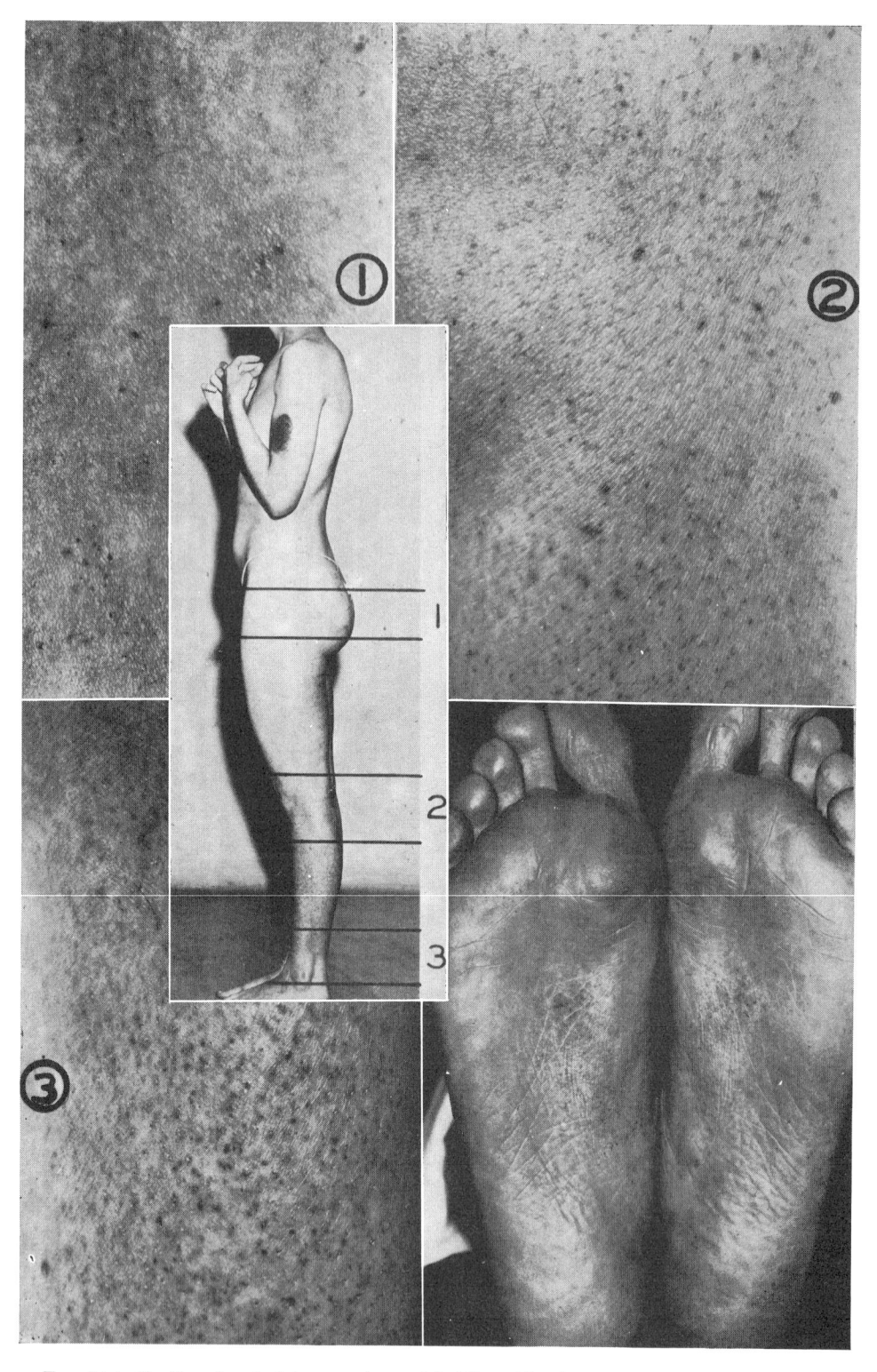

Fig. 34-1. Profile of ambulatory patient with idiopathic thrombocytopenic purpura. Note hematoma on arm which followed a hypodermic injection. Pictures 1, 2, and 3 are enlargements of correspondingly numbered skin segments and show an increase in numbers of petechiae in more dependent parts of the body. Note that petechiae on soles of feet are largely limited to nonweight-bearing portions of skin.

partly violaceous or purple, such as are often seen in malignant smallpox. . . .

She recovered spontaneously.

As blood platelets were not recognized for another 100 years, the above case can only be presumed to have been one of thrombocytopenia. Not until 1883 did Brohm describe the first case of purpura ascribed to a demonstrated thrombocytopenia.

CLINICAL PATTERN of the Werlhof syndrome is one of petechial hemorrhage, more numerously distributed over the more dependent portions of the body (Fig. 34-1). The increased venous pressure from gravity causes the number of petechial hemorrhagic points to increase. This phenomenon is simulated artificially by the so-called Rumpel-Leede or tourniquet test and in recent years has been demonstrated by the application of suction cups applied to the skin.

The petechial areas tend to become confluent, forming intracutaneous ecchymotic areas. At autopsy, the organs of motion usually display more evidence of hemorrhage than those which are inactive. Ease of bruising is one of the prominent features noted (Fig. 34-1). Nonetheless, should the platelet count be seriously depressed, spontaneous extravasations can occur with fatal consequence in organs which display no motion and are not likely traumatized. The most common cause of death in these patients is spontaneously occurring intracranial hemorrhage; this complication may appear while the patient is lying in bed. Abnormal bleeding may be found in all organs and tissues in severe thrombocytopenia. The seriousness in symptoms varies generally in accordance with the degree of platelet depression. Massive gastrointestinal hemorrhage, melena, hematuria, epistaxis and intracranial hemorrhage may occur together, or in various combinations. In mild cases, hematuria or a "skin rash" over the lower legs may be the patient's only complaint. Each of these symptoms upon occasion has been the first manifestation of hemorrhage to be encountered. Often the physician confronted with complaints of abnormal bleeding may center his attention so closely upon the organ source of bleeding that he overlooks the necessity for a careful examination searching for the clotting abnormalities in general.

In many patients with Werlhof's disease, spontaneous remission occurs, especially in the group under 12 years of age. True Werlhof thrombocytopenia is seldom seen after the age of 30. It is encountered 4 to 5 times more commonly in females and is likely to have its onset at the time of menstruation. Curiously, in this connection, estrogen administration in the dog, followed about 10 days later by its sudden withdrawal, usually is followed promptly by thrombocytopenia and an abnormal bleeding state resembling that in man.

DIAGNOSIS is not especially difficult. Certain features are essential: (1) the demonstration of thrombocytopenia; (2) the demonstration of normal or hyperplastic marrow aspirates which are much more meaningful and accurately interpreted if fixed and permanent sections are made, as described by Block (1947), than when examined by direct smear. The results following splenectomy for this disease are in large measure a function of the correctness of diagnosis.

Classically, the marrow shows an abundance of megakaryocytes but few platelets. The erythroid elements are also normal or hyperplastic, determined by the presence and the extent of hemorrhage. It is important to establish that there is no other dysplasia of the marrow; hypoplasia of the marrow is usually a contraindication of splenectomy.

The clotting time usually is described as being normal in this disease. From a practical point of view, this is true, as most who perform clotting times fail to obtain any increase. With the use of skilled technic, including the entrance into the vein with only one puncture, placing the blood gently in the series of glass test tubes which need not be lined by silicone or similar anti-wetting agents, the clotting time is found almost always to be prolonged. It is not generally realized that all errors in measuring the clotting time of blood in vitro hasten coagulation. The values of 3 to 8 minutes, usually reported as normal, represent the summation effect of multiple errors, for a carefully performed clotting time of the Lee-White technic will yield normal values of 30 to 40 minutes in uncoated glassware. In Figure 34-2 are shown the differences in whole blood clotting time after heparin when the only difference is one in excellence of venipuncture.

One other simple laboratory test also is

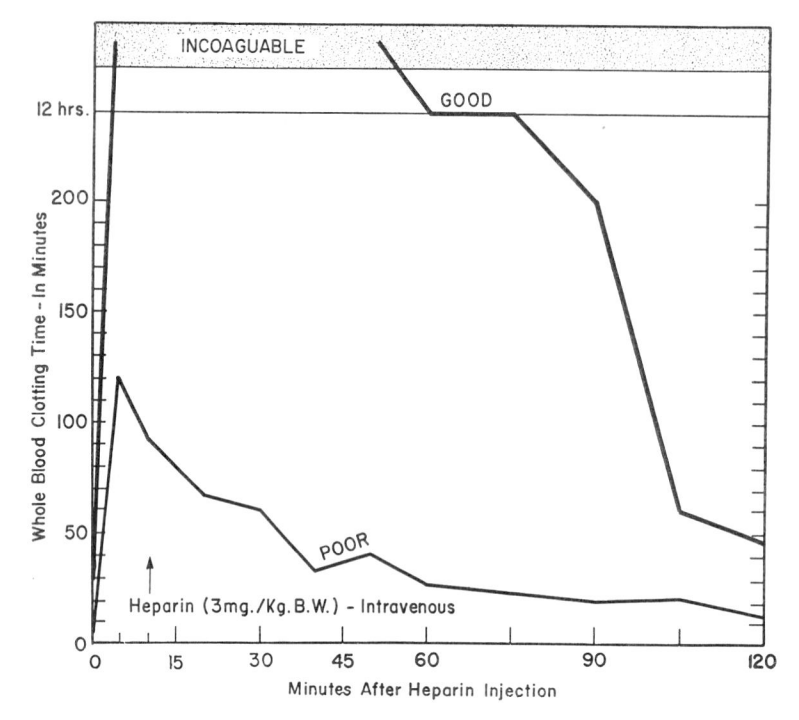

FIG. 34-2. Effect of good and poor venipuncture technics upon the Lee-White whole blood clotting time. Punctures for samples were made at the same time but from opposite extremity veins. Faulty venipunctures are prominent causes for the usually short clotting times reported.

positive; clot retraction (syneresis) is usually impaired or lacking. Platelets appear to be essential to the occurrence of this phenomenon.

There are no findings upon physical examination which will disclose the nature of thrombocytopenic purpura except for the indirect supporting evidence of one negative finding. In the true Werlhof picture, the spleen classically is not enlarged and therefore not palpable. Should the spleen be palpable, the diagnosis is very frequently one of secondary dysfunction of the spleen, which may also respond well to splenectomy, or it is one of a blood dyscrasia which is usually unresponsive to operation because of the inability to produce platelets. At times after splenectomy temporary improvement may occur among patients with hypersplenism and blood dyscrasias, either because of some reduction of their hypersplenic component or because other elements of the reticuloendothelial system take over.

Two other major categories of disease exist which can induce thrombocytopenia without splenomegaly and from which recovery is spontaneous if the patient survives. Splenectomy is not beneficial and often harmful in either instance and therefore to be avoided assiduously. These are the allergic purpuras usually seen in conjunction with infection or the administration of certain drugs, or following exposure to certain noxious agents, including ionizing radiation.

The pathogenesis of this disease is discussed on page 958, though it is not well understood. The platelets are obviously involved, for not only is their normal concentration sharply diminished, but as the platelet count returns toward normal, whether spontaneously, from the administration of glucocorticoids, from platelet transfusions, or in response to splenectomy, purpuric bleeding promptly ceases. At times, the bleeding tendency ceases before there is evidence of an impressive rise in the platelet count, which suggests the possibility that the platelet deficiency may also have in part a qualitative component.

Platelets arise from the fragmentation of megakaryocytes by a process that Wright described and illustrated in 1906. The megakaryocytes respond to ITP by an accelerated rate of production of platelets; they appear in the marrow larger than normal and stain lighter than the more mature forms of megakaryocytes normally present. The role of circulating platelets is not fully understood, though they are essential to the prevention of spontaneous and abnormal bleeding, as first shown by Bizzozero in 1882, by means not yet defined. Among their physiologic properties is adhesiveness, which enables them to stick to traumatized areas of endothelium. They bear a negative electrical charge, as does the intimal surface; the charge of the latter is reversed in injury, and presumably this is an important factor, causing platelets to migrate quickly to such areas where they adhere. Many then undergo lysis, liberating enzymes which greatly accelerate the rate of thrombin formation; hence, the deposition of fibrin follows almost immediately. This process was observed accurately in great detail by Howell and Holt in 1918.

In this connection, the observations of Soldant and Best (1940) are interesting; they observed that platelet adhesiveness could be completely prevented by heparin—possibly because heparin bears a strongly negative charge in contrast to the positive charge of platelets. There is an exponential relationship between the concentration of platelets and that of heparin (Fig. 8-4, p. 180). The clotting time of thrombocytopenic blood is extremely sensitive to heparin. Similarly, in patients whose platelet counts rise above normal, more than the usual amount of heparin is required to control thrombophlebitis.

TREATMENT. Kaznelson (1916) of Prague persuaded Professor Schloffer to perform splenectomy on a 36-year-old female patient with thrombocytopenic purpura and splenomegaly in 1916. His suggestion was based on the possibility that the spleen was destroying platelets at an excessive rate. This concept he carried over from the established benefits of splenectomy in familial hemolytic anemia. An excellent result was obtained. That a medical student could persuade a professor of surgery to try something of this nature is remarkable in itself!

Three courses are open to the physician today in the management of Werlhof's disease. Should the disease be mild, watchful waiting with or without the administration of cortisone or ACTH is reasonable. These agents are employed because of their depressing effects on antibody formation, in this instance the auto-antibody of Evans. Good results are often obtained in milder forms of the disease on this conservative therapy, especially in children. As the disease tends to diminish in recurrence rate after the age of 20, the remissions successfully induced in many young patients tend to be permanent as the child grows older.

In severe cases, serious consideration must be given to the possibility that a beneficial effect from cortisone or ACTH may not be obtained soon enough to avoid intracranial hemorrhage. Some deaths under these conditions have been reported with this form of therapy. Splenectomy should be performed in some of these patients, as the beneficial response it induces is often almost immediate. Abnormal bleeding frequently ceases soon after the splenic pedicle is ligated, although the rise in platelet count may be delayed several days to several weeks. Cortisone therapy as an adjunct to splenectomy may be useful.

Platelet transfusions have been alluded to in Chapter 8, Blood Transfusion, and they can be exceedingly helpful, but, due to the enormous quantities of blood required, their usage often is delayed until the day of operation or employed only when the response to splenectomy is slow and bleeding continues. In the latter situation, they may tide the patient over until he makes a satisfactory response of his own.

Results of splenectomy for idiopathic thrombocytopenic purpura are contingent upon the accuracy of diagnosis and removal of accessory splenic tissue. Not all accessory spleens appear to be capable of inducing a continuation or a recurrence of ITP but, when failures do develop or when the disease recurs, the presence of accessory spleens or of splenosis should be suspected. Miller and Hagedorn (1951) reported 32 of 47 patients living and well after 5 years, although 4 had episodes of expistaxis and hematemesis too slight to cause the patient concern. These authors reported only 1 hospital death; 3 others died later. In one, the cause of death was Albers-Schönberg disease; in another the cause was chronic myeloid leukemia; and in the third, the cause of death was unknown. Thus, in at least 2 of the 3 late deaths, the initial diagnosis was incorrect, leaving 1 hospital death from continuing hemorrhage in true Werlhof's disease that failed to respond to splenectomy, and 1 late death where the patient died of unknown cause 18 months after splenectomy.

Cole *et al.* (1949) reported no operative

mortality among 26 patients with the Werlhof syndrome. Platelet response in 2 was slow at first but did return to normal later; 1 died of tuberculosis; 2 had good symptomatic relief but poor hematologic results.

Walter and Chaffin (1955) reported their experience with idiopathic thrombocytopenic purpura in infants and children conservatively managed for the most part. Of 41 patients in this age group, 31 responded to conservative management, and 5 died; 2 of these 5 deaths occurred on the day of admission, another died of pneumonia, nephritis and hemorrhage; 2 died of hemorrhage 1 and 2 months after coming under their care, and both of these deaths occurred prior to the cortisone-ACTH era. Splenectomy was performed in only 5, all of whom were cured; however, 2 of these patients continued with low platelet counts. The results of Walter and Chaffin from conservative treatment are similar to those of others and those of the author.

Accessory Spleens. Accessory spleens overlooked and therefore left behind are believed to be responsible for failure of improvement in many of these patients. To Curtis (1946) belongs the credit for alerting the surgeon to this possible hazard, although Morrison *et al.* called attention to this possibility in 1928. Curtis reported accessory spleens to be present in 56 of 176 patients subject to splenectomy, or an incidence of 31.8 per cent. Others report a somewhat lower incidence. The location of accessory spleens is usually in the following regions: the hilus, the pedicle, the omentum, the retroperitoneum, the splenic ligaments (gastric and colic) and the small bowel mesentery. The last three locations are rare sites of accessory spleens. A number of patients with recurrences of the disease after splenectomy are reported to be relieved completely by removal of accessory spleens found at re-exploration. Thus it is important to search for accessory spleens at the time of splenectomy.

Secondary Thrombocytopenic Purpura With Splenomegaly. This condition as referred to here is hemocytologically similar to those connoted as primary, except for the fact that the spleen per se is pathologic, often secondary to another disease. Platelet autoantibodies in the plasma of some of these patients, too, have been identified (Harrington *et al.*, 1953). The principal differences between primary and secondary thrombocytopenic purpura of the hypersplenic variety then are the enlarged spleen in the latter and that its enlargement results from a variety of causes. In many instances, the cause of the enlarged spleen is either its involvement in a more generalized disease or any one of the various forms of portal hypertension. Among the diseases in which secondary hypersplenism has occurred are the following: cysts and tumors of the spleen, acquired hemolytic anemia, tuberculosis or histoplasmosis, leishmaniasis and echinococcal disease of the spleen, malaria and filariasis, the various leukemias and Hodgkin's disease, a number of the "storage" diseases of which Gaucher's disease is a common example, portal hypertension and chronic passive congestion, occasionally congenital hemolytic anemia, sickle cell anemia in early stages, Felty's syndrome and, in fact, almost any disease should it affect the spleen, including lymphoma.

Splenectomy is the treatment of choice if the purpuric manifestations are severe, although we recognize that many of these diseases cannot be cured medically. Therefore, splenectomy in this group is largely one of palliation, although in some instances curative. Hence, the palliation anticipated must be weighed against that of life expectancy if the problems of abnormal bleeding are relieved.

Of those causes of splenomegaly for which splenectomy more commonly provides a prolonged survival are Gaucher's disease, Banti's syndrome and some of the acquired splenic anemias. In some of the cases of splenomegaly where the primary disease is eventually fatal, relief from the associated thrombocytopenic purpura may be required to permit survival. An occasional patient may survive indefinitely; therefore, withholding splenectomy should not be done lightly or discouraged simply because of the poor prognosis implied by the primary diagnosis. Moreover, the diagnosis may be in error or at least carry less serious import than was believed at the time of hemorrhage. Death from untreated purpuric hemorrhage may be a more likely outcome than death from the primary disease. A case in point is that which follows.

A 22-month-old male infant was admitted with the diagnosis of Letterer-Siwe disease (reticulo-

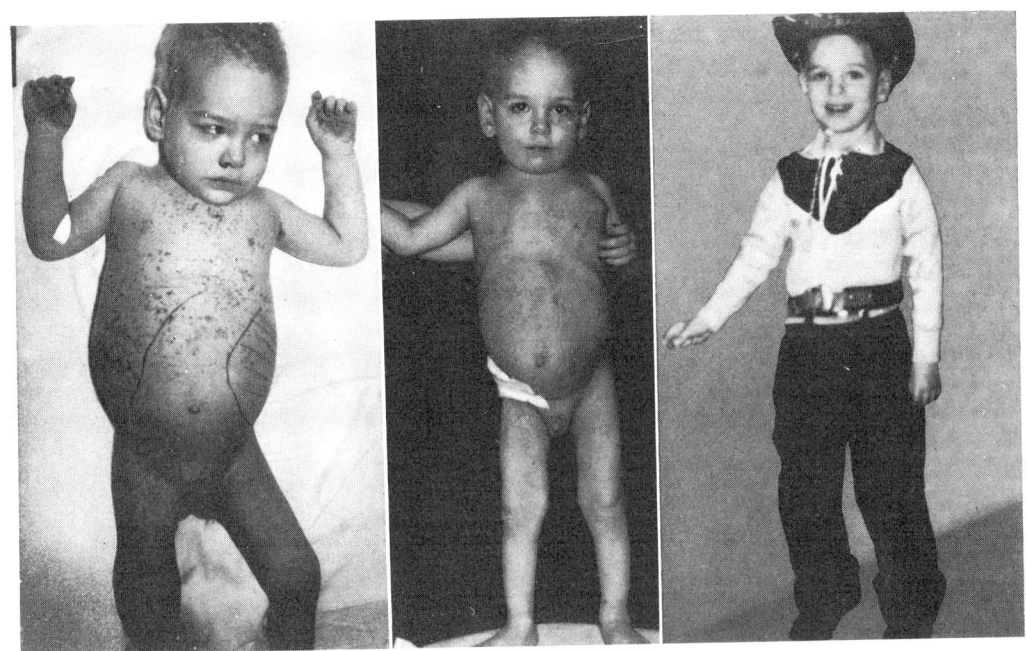

FIG. 34-3. Letterer-Siwe's disease and thrombocytopenic purpura. The photograph on left was taken 2 weeks prior to serious deterioration. The picture in center was on the 16th postoperative day. The photo on right was taken 4 years later when no evidence of disease remains. (53-78-00 U. of C.)

endotheliosis) involving the left scapula, the right ilium, the left femur and the skull. Radiophosphorus was administered, and local radiation was superimposed. The enlarged spleen was not altered. Petechial hemorrhages, present on admission, progressively worsened, and bleeding from the mouth and the alimentary tract appeared. ACTH and cortisone were to no avail. Pneumonia developed, and the child was placed in an oxygen tent. Anemia rapidly progressed in spite of transfusions. Severe neutropenia appeared, and the platelet count was less than 10,000 per cu. mm. Marrow studies revealed hyperplasia but with the characteristic "reticuloendothelial cells" also being present.

The infant was transported from his oxygen tent to the operating room where splenectomy was performed. His general condition began to improve at once; his temperature promptly began to fall toward normal levels. Bleeding ceased, and the platelet count 12 hours later was 31,000 and gradually reached 200,000 by the 6th day. He was discharged on the 43rd postoperative day (Fig. 34-3).

Surprisingly, the bony lesion began to disappear, and 24 months later none remained. The child, at 16 years of age, appeared to be well and free of disease. As Letterer-Siwe's disease is so frequently fatal, there may be reason to question the diagnosis, which conceivably may have been eosinophilic granuloma; if so, the cellular pattern was unusual.

In any case, however, to have concluded that the infant should have been spared splenectomy, in favor of the assumed fatal course that his diagnosis implied, almost certainly would have been in error. There are, of course, many clinical situations in which less heroic procedures are indicated. In this child, a conservative course would have been a fatal mistake. The proper decision in many patients in such categories is not easily made upon a rational basis.

DISEASES OF THE SPLEEN

Plasma Iron Clearance in Plasma and Marrow and Its Significance in Splenic Disorders

Iron normally circulates within the plasma as a complex beta globulin. The total quan-

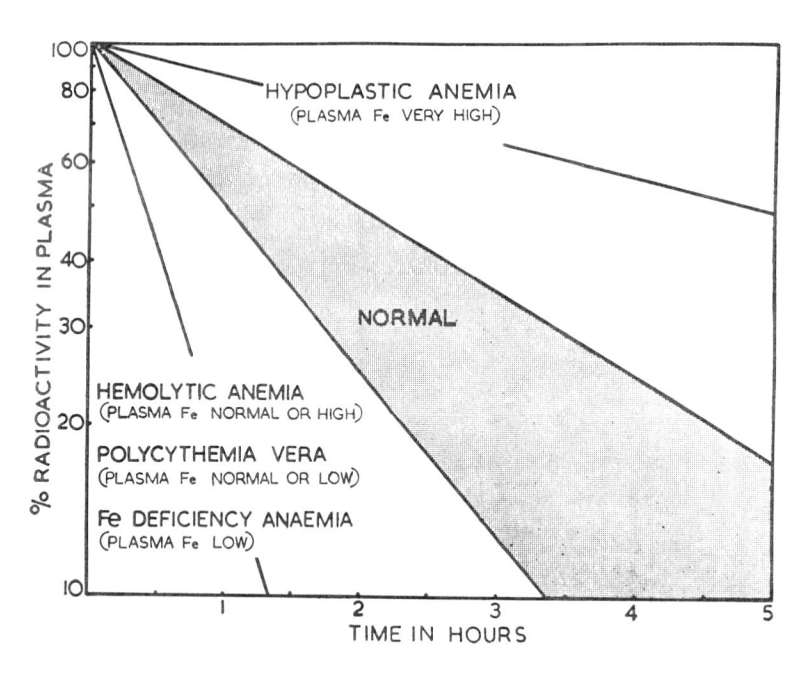

FIG. 34-4. The usual patterns of radioiron clearance from the plasma in normal subjects and in patients with various blood disorders. (Bothwell, T. H., Callender, S., Mallett, R., and Witts, L. J.: Brit. J. Haemat. 2:1)

tity of iron within the plasma normally is only about 0.1 per cent of the entire amount of the body; plasma iron is important, for it represents the only means of transport of iron from one part of the body to another.

In recent years a number of investigators have employed radioiron (^{59}Fe) as a means of studying the turnover rates of iron in normal and pathologic hematopoietic states. Although there is evidence that the status of the iron stores within the body may influence to some extent the rate at which iron is incorporated into new hemoglobin, usually iron liberated by hemolysis is re-utilized promptly in the formation of new hemoglobin (Figs. 34-4 and 34-5).

For the most part, those conditions that favor an increased rate of hematopoiesis disclose a high rate of plasma iron turnover. In those in which hematopoiesis is reduced in

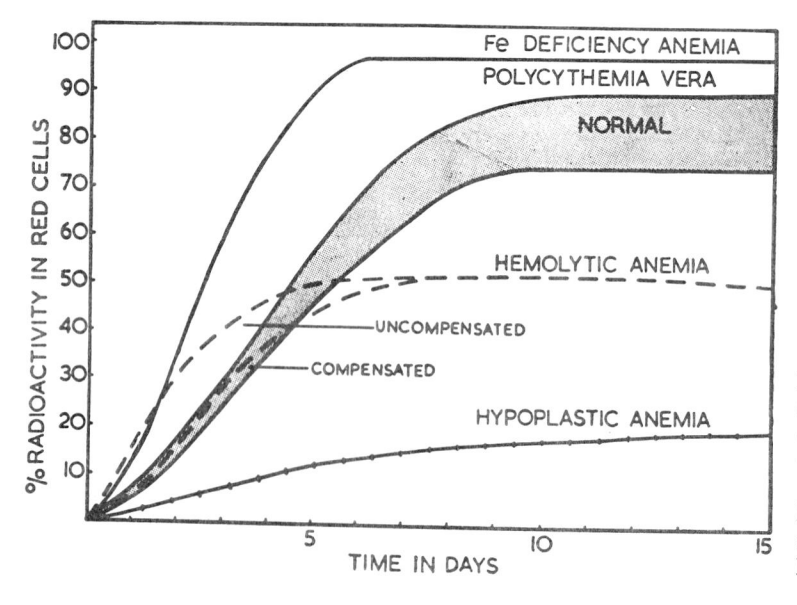

FIG. 34-5. The usual patterns of red-cell utilization in normal subjects and in patients with various blood disorders. (Bothwell, T. H., Callender, S., Mallett, B., and Witts, L. J.: Brit. J. Haemat. 2:1)

activity, the turnover rates of plasma iron are retarded correspondingly. Thus, there is a rapid clearance of radioiron from plasma in iron-deficiency anemias, hemolytic anemias and polycythemia vera, indicating true hyperplastic states of the marrow in these conditions. However, it should be pointed out that many studies of iron metabolism are currently under way and that a thorough understanding of this mechanism is not yet at hand.

RUPTURE

Rupture of the spleen is a serious surgical emergency because of blood loss and hypovolemic shock. Trauma is the most common cause; rarely, the spleen may enlarge rapidly in disease and rupture spontaneously, or it may do so because of torsion when its ligamentous attachments are long—the so-called "wandering spleen" (Dowidar, 1948). In some patients with splenomegaly, the spleen may undergo torsion, or its weight may shear it from its artery and/or vein with fatal hemorrhage if not recognized promptly and treated surgically. Splenosis may follow.

Traumatic rupture of the spleen was a rare entity until mankind became victim to high speed transportation. It is occasionally seen in patients who have back injuries and who may be encased in a plaster cast. It should be the diagnosis most frequently thought of when acute hypotension develops a few days after blunt abdominal trauma.

Acute Traumatic Rupture From Nonpenetrating Injuries. Rupture of the spleen caused by nonpenetrating trauma usually tears its capsule or shears the spleen from its vascular attachments. The spleen is the most commonly injured organ in closed abdominal trauma. Usually, the history of trauma is one of an acute blow to the left lower chest or to the upper left abdomen. An injury that causes fractures of rib segments in the lower left chest should, in particular, arouse suspicion that the spleen may have been ruptured. Whitesell (1960) reported that 90 per cent of his patients with ruptured spleen were hospitalized for symptoms within 6 hours of injury. In 10 per cent symptoms were absent or not sufficiently marked for them to seek hospitalization until 1 to 6 days after the injury. Pain in the left upper quadrant was the dominant complaint in three fourths of his series. Of these it was steady or increased in severity in 83 per cent and, among this group, pain that radiated to the left shoulder was present in 40 per cent of the cases. Shock was present on admission in 30 per cent of cases, and in only 25 per cent was the PCV less than 34 per cent.

The clinical pattern is fairly consistent. The symptom most frequently encountered is generalized abdominal pain. In about one third of the cases, pain is limited or predominantly located in the left upper quadrant. Pain radiating to the left shoulder is present less often than might be expected (15% of cases).

Abdominal rigidity and hypovolemic shock are present in about 75 per cent of patients with ruptured spleen when first seen. Dullness to percussion in the flank and the "doughy abdomen" are usually observed if sought for. Nausea and vomiting are frequently complained of. The association of other injuries is to be expected in many instances. Lacerations of the liver and the kidneys as alternate or co-existing diagnoses also must be considered and sought for at the time of exploration. Occasionally, the bowel or the stomach may be torn.

Delayed Traumatic Rupture. Not all spleens rupture at the time of injury. In some patients, the rupture may not occur until 48 hours or longer after injury. Baudet (1907) suggested that the term "delayed rupture" be applied as a means for emphasizing the latent possibilities of splenic rupture following injury. The incidence of traumatic rupture of the normal spleen in which the onset of symptoms is delayed ranges from 5 to 40 per cent of reported cases, averaging about 15 per cent. Although the onset of hemorrhage is delayed, possibly several days to a week, when it does occur the same serious set of consequences as those of acute rupture results. The criteria for this diagnosis were defined by McIndoe in 1932 and further elaborated upon by Zabinski and Harkins in 1943.

Delay in rupture of the spleen after injury lies in the fact that there is no immediate complete tear in the capsule. Rather, there is an intracapsular or subcapsular tear into which blood continues to seep, enlarging the tear until the capsule is finally ruptured. At this point, blood flows freely into the abdomen. In others, a subcapsular tear or contusion of the pulp gives rise to a splenic hematoma which continues to distend the spleen until this is able to rupture the capsule. In some patients the capsular tear is slight and may be "self-sealing" in a short time, only to reopen or to be torn further by the enlarging subcapsular hematoma. In a few, the bleeding ceases, and later the hematoma may form a false cyst of the spleen and calcify or resorb. Such favorable responses are uncommon.

The syndrome of delayed splenic rupture is hazardous because in the interval of time between trauma and the onset of rupture, the patient often is symptom-free. Many of these patients have been treated for their initial injuries and sent home before the first indication of splenic rupture is evident (Lorimer, 1964).

Treatment of rupture of the spleen is splenectomy as soon as the diagnosis is made and the patient can be prepared for operation. Often the rate of blood loss is faster than that which can be replaced; under these circumstances one is forced to operate, removing the spleen, so that he may secure hemostasis while continuing blood replacement. Once the spleen is out and hemostasis effected, blood transfusion should be continued until the patient's circulation is stable—shock-free. Search for tears in the liver, the kidneys, the stomach, the bowel and the urinary bladder is important.

As the splenic bed in the traumatized patient may later be the site of abscess formation, the author prefers to employ a broad-spectrum antibiotic prophylactically in some cases, and in most cases to drain the splenic bed.

Needle biopsy of the spleen, a useful diagnostic procedure, occasionally has been followed by unrelenting bleeding from the site of needle puncture. In some instances, the capsule has been torn. Occasionally, splenectomy has been necessary to control this complication. Spleen biopsy should not be undertaken lightly, but fear of this consequence is seldom warranted if the information expected is important and can be obtained in no other way. In the author's experience needle biopsy of the spleen carries a little greater risk of serious hemorrhage than does needle biopsy of the liver. In most patients neither of these procedures should be undertaken when serious platelet or prothrombin deficiency is present.

Operative tears of the normal spleen occasionally occur incidental to other upper abdominal operations, particularly gastric resection, vagotomy, and surgery performed on the splenic flexure. Seldom are the major vessels torn. Usually, unrealized tension upon the gastrolienal ligament in gastrectomy or vagotomy tears the capsule or, less frequently, the vasa brevia. The capsule of the lower pole may be torn in dissecting free the splenic flexure of the colon; again, this usually is encountered without realization.

Its treatment is splenectomy at the time, unless the tear is minor and bleeding ceases promptly. Sutures may be employed successfully if applied carefully, and splenectomy may not always be necessary.

Splenosis is a clinical entity resulting from the autotransplantation of splenic tissue. It was first related to rupture of the spleen by von Küttner in 1910, who regarded these auto-implants as accessory spleens. Fifty or more implants have been found in some patients afflicted with this disorder, in contrast with 1 to 10 accessory spleens (Buchbinder and Lipkoff, 1939; Cotlar and Cerise, 1959). Blood supply enters the capsule of such implants rather than through the hilum as in the normal or accessory spleens. Some report that splenosis does not follow rupture of the diseased spleen (Cotlar and Cerise), although Stobie (1947) reported a case of recurrence of congenital hemolytic anemia in a patient in whom the enlarged spleen was ruptured at the time of splenectomy. Experimental implantation of splenic tissue is easily accomplished; even homologous splenic tissue will survive for a while (see Chap. 18, Radiation Injury).

Splenosis produces symptoms not unlike those of endometriosis; in either case complaints are referable to their location and may simulate almost any acute abdominal condition. If the tissue cannot be totally removed, recurrence of symptoms is frequent.

Cysts

Cysts of the spleen may be classified as true cysts, false cysts and those caused by parasites. True cysts are thought to represent an embryonal defect or rest. They are lined with flattened epithelium which may be cuboidal or squamous in nature. False cysts are thought to be the end-result of intrasplenic hemorrhage. The wall consists of flattened epithelium and trabeculated or fibrous tissue. Occasionally, these cysts are multiple. Many true or false cysts give little or no distress and are found only at autopsy. Others become large and burdensome and may be associated with signs of hypersplenism, in which case splenectomy may be in order.

Echinococcus cysts may occur in the spleen, although they are found more often in the liver and elsewhere. The parasites may be alive; hence, splenic puncture and its tear at operation are to be avoided. The diagnosis may be suspected in patients with masses palpable in the splenic area, especially among those who have lived in regions where the disease is endemic. Eosinophilia of varying degree is usually found. Roentgenographic examination of the upper abdomen frequently discloses the rather large cyst whose wall is usually calcified. Intradermal injection of the echinococcal antigen usually gives a positive reaction.

Treatment is splenectomy when this is possible. Occasionally, the spleen is totally destroyed, and only the cyst remains. At times the cyst can be excised without the risk of spilling its contents into the abdominal cavity which may give rise to other cysts later on. Should splenectomy or excision of the cyst *in toto* be impossible, the wall of the cyst nearest the portion of the abdominal wall is marsupialized by suture. From 48 to 72 hours later, the cyst is opened, and its contents are carefully evacuated. Its wall is sponged gently with formalin, and a gauze pack is placed in the cavity, to be removed slowly over a few days. Usually, it is necessary to reapply a clean pack, removing it also in piecemeal fashion over a period of several days. When the cavity is nearly collapsed, a cigarette drain is applied to its base and removed slowly while the entire cavity fills in from the bottom. This is the same form of treatment often employed in the drainage of echinococcus cysts of the liver.

Infections of the Spleen

Infections of the spleen are comparatively rare in the total consideration of its diseases. They may be bacterial, parasitic, or viral in origin. The spleen may enlarge in the course of systemic infections without necessarily harboring the specific agent. The splenomegalic reaction must be distinguished from those in which the spleen is a host organ to infection.

Bacterial infections involving the spleen may give rise to abscess formation requiring splenectomy or drainage. Usually, splenic abscesses are secondary to pyemia with some other focus serving as the point of origin. In a few instances, splenic abscess may result from nearby bacterial infections in the upper abdomen, of which perforated peptic ulcer is an example. Septic thrombi of arterial or venous origin may produce a splenic abscess. Splenic hematomas may become infected at times and result in abscess formation. Among the organisms more commonly encountered as pathogens are the staphylococcus, the pneumococcus, the salmonella and the coliform groups.

Abscess. The splenic abscesses induced by septic emboli or infarcts are largely confined within the spleen and may not be recognized readily. Should they not respond to antibiotic therapy or go unnoticed, the abscess cavity often continues to enlarge, and in time the capsule may be perforated with the formation of a subphrenic abscess, presenting its usual complications, including empyema of the left chest and bronchopleural fistula. Septic thrombi may form in the splenic vein as a result of splenic abscess. The clots may embolize via the portal vein to form intrahepatic abscesses. In a few, rupture of the abscess occurs into the free peritoneal cavity, giving rise to peritonitis. Often the spleen is totally destroyed by the abscess, and its vessels are completely thrombosed. Once necrotic tissue develops, the abscess continues until drained. In about one third of cases, fragments of splenic tissue will be discharged through surgical wound as "sequestra."

Clinical features of splenic abscess are as variable as is the nature of the antecedent history of infection responsible. Should a septic infarct be the origin and sufficient occlusion of the circulation occur to create perisplenitis, pain referred along the left phrenic nerve may be a complaint. In others, pain in the region of the spleen may be the only complaint and is perhaps the one most commonly encountered. A febrile course is the rule. The left diaphragm is usually elevated and is immobile as determined by respiratory excursions upon percussion or fluoroscopic examination. Its continuing presence unrecognized may lead to weight loss and the debility and the septic course common to any chronic but serious infection. Frequently, there is a palpable tender mass in the left hypochondrium; this may be spleen or the omentum.

Treatment depends upon the stage of abscess development at the time the diagnosis is first suspected. A heavy course of antibiotic therapy is indicated in any event, using a broad-spectrum agent such as a tetracycline. Splenic abscesses may subside without splenectomy or surgical drainage when antibiotics are used. Splenectomy is still the treatment of choice in many patients, draining the splenic bed through a stab wound. The spleen may be so adherent to adjacent structures that the surgeon may be forced to drain the abscess through a lateral incision, leaving the spleen in place. In such cases the wall of the abscess should be sutured to the peritoneum at the point intended for drainage; in the case of abscesses of the upper pole, the left transpleural approach may be advisable. Drainage of the spleen involves the same principle as entailed in the surgical drainage of suprahepatic or intrahepatic abscesses (see Chap. 35, Mesentery, Splanchnic Circulation and Mesenteric Thrombosis). Drainage is likely to persist for weeks to months, unless all sequestra of necrotic splenic pulp are expelled early. Once healed, delayed splenectomy is rarely indicated.

TUBERCULOSIS of the spleen occasionally requires splenectomy to correct the secondary manifestations of the hypersplenic states which may also develop. Otherwise, the patient should be treated for his systemic disease, realizing that the spleen, too, will heal in due course if medical therapy is successful. Calcifications form within the spleen, often giving the appearance of buckshot, each of the larger miliary tubercules becoming calcified. The same is the end result for histoplasmosis involving the spleen, which may be found roentgenographically. This fungus disease may also induce thrombocytopenic purpura when it involves the spleen, as may sarcoid. If healing occurs, miliary calcifications of the spleen are often observed on roentgenography of the upper left abdomen. The response of the thrombocytopenic purpura to splenectomy is excellent and may be lifesaving; the patient should not be deprived of the benefits afforded by splenectomy simply because of the systemic nature of tuberculosis, histoplasmosis or sarcoid (see p. 958).

Parasitic infections involving the spleen are comparatively rare in the northern half of the United States. Principally concerned are malaria and leishmaniasis (kala-azar) encountered overseas and echinococcal disease; the last is discussed under "Cysts of the Spleen."

MALARIA occasionally induces extreme enlargement of the spleen. When this occurs rapidly, the spleen may rupture spontaneously, requiring emergency splenectomy. If medical management of the acute phase is successful, the splenomegaly subsides, usually without further difficulty. When the disease has been chronic and untreated, the enlargement of the spleen also can be huge; its weight may be so great as to shear it from its ligamentous moorings, and in doing so tear the major splenic vessels at its hilum. Emergency extirpation of the spleen is necessary, with ligation of the severed vessels; such an event is likely to be fatal unless the accident occurs in the hospital and is recognized early. It is for this reason that elective splenectomy should be strongly considered when the spleen becomes huge, regardless of cause, unless life expectancy is obviously very short.

LEISHMANIA INFANTUM OR DONOVANI are parasitic diseases affecting the spleen, often causing huge splenomegaly similar to that seen in chronic malarial infections. Neither of these diseases is encountered frequently in this country. The diagnosis is made on biopsy tissue obtained by splenic puncture; portions of the biopsy material should be cultured. Antimony therapy or the more recently developed ethylstibamine (Neostibosan) is usually effective. But if the spleen remains very large splenectomy may be necessary.

Among other rarely encountered parasitic infections which on occasion have been the origin of huge splenomegaly are *Toxoplasma pyrogenes* and *Cryptococcus farciminosus*. The spirochetal infections—syphilis, yaws and Weil's disease—usually respond to medical therapy; splenectomy is rarely required unless an associated uncontrolled hypersplenic disorder appears.

Felty's Syndrome. This syndrome of febrile polyarthritis is characterized by splenomegaly, lymphadenopathy, anemia, thrombocytopenia, cutaneous pigmentation, and leukopenia of the neutropenic variety. It has been known by many names; among these are Chauffard-Still's disease and von Jackson's syndrome. Felty's report in 1924 was the first in the English language, and so in this country it bears his name, although Still's description antedates Felty's report by 28 years (1896). Felty's syndrome is a clinical rather than a pathologic entity.

THE CLINICAL PATTERN is one of chronic arthritis affecting few or many of the joints. Weakness and abdominal pain are frequent complaints. Brownish pigmentation of the skin may be noted, and lymphadenopathy is fairly general. Usually, these nodes are not matted together, thus assisting in the distinction of Felty's syndrome from that of lymphoma or Hodgkin's disease. However, the nodes are generally fixed to the adjacent tissue and often tender to palpation. Gastric achlorhydria or diminished secretion is a common finding, but usually normal responses are elicited to Gastramine or histamine. Anemia is present, usually mild to moderate, and normochromic in character. The marrow is not usually abnormal to any particular degree, nor does it possess any distinct characteristics.

Some have reported the occasional finding of *Streptococcus viridans* on blood culture or cultures of biopsied nodes. Fever is usually present; more often it is low-grade rather than serious. The consensus today is that this disease is a form of rheumatoid arthritis.

TREATMENT is medical which, for the want of a better understanding as to its pathogenesis, is largely symptomatic. Corticoids and salicylates are commonly used.

Splenectomy has been performed in a number of these patients for the associated blood disorders with reported improvement. Its rationale is that hypersplenic disorders may account for granulocytopenia and/or thrombocytopenia. The response to splenectomy is variable; an early good response often is not sustained. However, Flatow *et al.* (1966) reported 3 patients with aplastic anemia who had received a number of platelet transfusions for several years until they apparently developed an immunity to the platelet levels and this kind of transfusion had to be abandoned. Splenectomy was then performed without complication on all 3 patients when they became refractory to platelet transfusions and was followed by an improved post-transfusion survival rate of platelets.

INHERITED DISEASES BENEFITED BY SPLENECTOMY

Congenital Spherocytic Anemia. This is a hereditary disease whose basic disorder is attributed to the spherocytic shape of the patient's erythrocytes instead of their usual discoid character. The disease is inherited as a mendelian dominant characteristic and, as occurs under similar circumstances, does not imply that all progeny of a parent so afflicted will display this disorder. The abnormality is not sex-linked.

HISTORICAL CONSIDERATIONS. This disease was first described by Murchison in 1885; its familial nature was pointed out later by Minkowski (1886). Chauffard (1914) reported in 1907 the increased fragility of erythrocytes to trauma in this disease which he attributed to the spherocytoidal properties of the cells. Thereafter osmotic fragility was reported and studied by several observers, especially Dawson (1931). However, it has been Haden's study in 1934 which serves as the basis for most of the present-day saline dilution tests employed. Splenectomy as its treatment was first employed by Spencer Wells in 1887.

CLINICAL PATTERN is one of mild icterus, with or without anemia, a slowly enlarging spleen, with the eventual formation of bilirubinate gallstones in many patients. Icterus may be present at birth or may not appear until later in life. There is a positive correlation between the degree of anemia, the serum level of bilirubin, and the incidence of gallstones. The disease tends to be one of remission and exacerbation, although the sallow color of the skin tends to remain. Once severe anemia and intense icterus develop, there is little likelihood of spontaneous remission. Chronic leg ulcers are observed in this disease, as is true in a number of other chronic hemolytic states.

The most striking and unusual feature of this disease is the hemolytic crisis which may occur at any time in life. While these are characterized by severe abdominal pain, nausea and vomiting, fever, palpitation, dyspnea, and often the acute onset of profound anemia, serum bilirubin is not increased above its pre-existing levels; in fact, Owren (1948) reports a decline in serum bilirubin, urobilinuria, and reticulocytosis, with the onset of acute aplasia of the marrow during crises. These findings led him to conclude that the cause of the crisis is one of acute suppression of erythropoiesis rather than that of a suddenly increased rate of red cell destruction. Leukopenia and thrombocytopenia also are usually present during these episodes.

Of interest is the observation reported by Marson et al. (1950) that crises may occur in several members of the family at the same time, suggesting a common trigger mechanism. Presumably such "epidemics" could result from the exposure to a common toxin or some other pathogen to which the family is exposed simultaneously. Owren's postulations as to the pathogenesis of these crises have subsequently proved to be true in some instances, although it seems that there are also occasions when a rapid increase in the rate of hemolysis may occur.

The question as to whether the reticulocyte response of the marrow in patients with spherocytic anemia is a normal one to hemorrhage or hemolysis, either before or after splenectomy, should be studied and settled if possible, though during crises in spherocytic anemia the hemolytic feature is clearly accelerated. It may be that whatever causes the accelerated rate of hemolysis is also capable of suppressing marrow activity temporarily, or that the byproducts of hemolysis retard the rate of hematopoiesis. There is no evidence that if the spleen is removed during the crisis the claimed marrow depression recovers with accelerated promptness.

The presence of pigmented gallstones is reported in 40 to 70 per cent of cases. The range of such an incidence is undoubtedly influenced by the nature of medical practice, especially the frequency of or time lapse before splenectomy is performed. This varies from one community to another. After stones have formed, these patients are subject to attacks of biliary colic to the same degree as patients with cholelithiasis from other causes. The formation of gallstones requires time; it is likely that the incidence of cholelithiasis will be higher among patients in communities where the prevailing clinical practice is to withhold splenectomy until late in the course of the disease. Such stones in themselves are indications for operation in many patients.

Several infrequently encountered skeletal abnormalities have been described in association with the disease, including the "tower" skull, the one observed most commonly. Growth impairment and endocrine disorders occur in a few children if the disease is severe.

Roentgenographic changes of the skull and the long bones may disclose the striation changes of the former and evidence of increased marrow mass in the long bones. As these are the same findings of any severe anemia associated with hyperactive marrow patterns, they are confirmatory and not diagnostic. Spherocytosis, the increased red cell fragility and the familial history of the disease superimposed upon the above establish the origin of the hemolytic anemia as familial or spherocytic anemia. Whereas the usual life span of the circulating normal red cell is in the neighborhood of 3 to 4 months, studies employing tracer or other technics suggest that the life span of erythrocytes in familial hemolytic anemia is reduced markedly, from a few days to a few weeks.

PATHOLOGY of familial hemolytic anemia is most interesting, although again neither its exact nature nor its entire mechanism is understood. The most logical and usual explanation of the augmented erythropoiesis is its stimulation by the increased rate of red cell destruction. Presumably the stimulus here is a nonspecific one and does not differ from the erythroid stimulation induced by blood loss from other causes, such as hemorrhage or hemolysis, except that in this disease its chronicity (years rather than days, weeks or months) may pose certain special problems in relation to hemosiderin deposits and the greater frequency of gallstone formation. Hemosiderosis is seen classically in the spleen, in or near its smaller blood vessels, occasionally forming deposits in the adventitia and the elastic coats of smaller arteries; sometimes the latter deposits are referred to as Gandy-Gamma nodules (Wells, 1931). Hemosiderin deposits are also found frequently in most other body tissues, particularly in the Kupffer cells of the liver, the lymph nodes, the marrow and in the loops of Henle of the kidney. Fatty degeneration of the heart with brown atrophy is noted occasionally.

The marrow may be exceedingly hyperactive in severe cases. Cut sections of the vertebrae, the ribs and the long bones showing the beefy red character of marrow hyperplasia are strikingly impressive. Normoblasts are more numerous than megaloblasts, and mitotic figures are seen commonly. Leukopoiesis is less pronounced, but the number of mitoses may be increased in the myeloblastic elements, too. Extramedullary marrow activity may occur in severe cases, especially in infants and children.

For a time, hematopoiesis seems to be capable of matching the increased rate of red cell destruction, but as the disease progresses, marrow exhaustion may occur. Cellular hyperplasia becomes less and less efficient in erythrocytic replacement. The number of megaloblasts at this stage may exceed that of the dominant cell type, the erythroblast, found earlier in the disease.

As for the *circulating* blood, the most notable feature is microcytic anemia and the characteristic spherocyte. This abnormal shape of the circulating red cells is the primary disorder usually believed to account for the clinicopathologic aspects of the disease. To the increased fragility of spherocytic red cells after mechanical agitation has been attributed most if not all of the abnormalities associated with this disease. Although the fragility of these cells may be due in part to defects in stroma and possibly in the cellular membrane, most have entertained the possibility that the spheroidal shape itself posed certain mechanical problems in addition to the increased fragility. There has been no convincing evidence that there is a circulating antibody to account for hemolysis; this is of some assistance in the differential diagnosis of other hemolytic disorders associated with the splenomegaly.

Whipple *et al.* (1954) presented observations which suggest that spherocytes may experience more difficulty traversing the splenic circulation than normal cells. Perfusing the normal spleens with mixtures of spherocytic and normal erythrocytes disclosed that a distinctly higher percentage of normal cells finally reached the venous side of its circulation. Microscopic sections of the spleen disclosed upon examination that the spherocytes were predominant among the cells retained. It is possible that the erythrocytic engorgement of the spleen in this disease is due in part to the impairment in cell transit across the splenic pulp. It is not known whether the capillaries of other organs pose similar problems; possibly they do. It would seem reasonable that cells that are more fragile than normal might well be broken up more rapidly, particularly if they encountered more trauma in passing through the capillary vessels. As pointed out in Chapter 8, Blood Transfusion, the rate of destruction of red cells transfused to a normal recipient is increased exponentially in accordance with the age of the cells.

Testing for the increase in *red cell fragility* when exposed to diminishing concentrations of saline solution is not as easy as might be expected. Many suggest refrigeration storage of the blood sample overnight before testing for altered osmotic fragility.

DIAGNOSIS is usually fairly easy to establish, especially when hemolytic anemia, spherocytes and their increased osmotic fragility are demonstrated in multiple members of the same family who are mildly icteric and display splenomegaly. The accuracy of the diagnosis depends upon the certainty that spherocytosis and an increased osmotic fragility exist, plus the hyperplastic marrow. Measurements of fecal urobilinogen excretion or plasma iron "clearance" disclose an increase in both. These tests provide specific evidence of hemolysis, but they do not disclose its cause. Family history in the presence of the other classic findings establishes the diagnosis beyond much question. However, family history is not essential to the diagnosis nor is it always present, for occasionally the patient is the first member of his family to develop the mendelian mutant necessary for this disease. In this respect the situation is similar to the familial aspects of congenital hemophilia.

The deer mouse (*Peromyscus maniculatus*) is described in which spherocytosis occurs with the formation of gallstones (Fitzpatrick *et al.*, 1963). In this rodent, there appears to be a separation of hereditary factors predisposing to the formation of gallstones that, while related to spherocytosis, is not necessarily dependent upon it. There are no available data in man to suggest that the formation of gallstones in this disease is not dependent primarily upon spherocytosis and continuing hemolysis.

TREATMENT. Spencer Wells, cited by Dawson in 1931, appears to have performed the first successful splenectomy for this disease in 1887 in a 27-year-old female with "bouts" of jaundice since the age of 9. The operation was performed 3 years before the disease was first described by Minkowski. The spleen weighed "11 lbs. 4 oz." Jaundice disappeared, and the patient survived at least 40 more years. Her only son developed jaundice, splenomegaly and gallstones at about the age of 14; he was operated upon for obstructive jaundice as well as for his hemolytic spherocytic anemia. By this time, the disease was known and the diagnosis clearly established in the boy.

Of all the nontraumatic indications for splenectomy, this is the one disease in which this operation has the perfect record in effecting a permanent cure, if accessory spleens or splenic tissue left behind does not give rise to splenosis later on. Conservative treatment is nonspecific and relies upon spontaneous remission. The few surgical failures reported are likely the result of diagnostic error.

Because of the prompt improvement after splenectomy, most hematologists believe that the operation may be carried out at the time of a crisis if required. In general, however, it is better to avoid crises, performing splenectomy prior to their onset if possible or during a quiescent interval. Blood transfusions during operation possibly should be withheld until after the spleen's blood supply is ligated, as transfusion reactions are encountered more commonly in hemolytic anemias and are also more difficult to avoid.

Splenectomy should be performed in most young people with icterus in whom the diagnosis is established. Should the disease not be detected or give symptoms only late in life, splenectomy may be deferred, if other circumstances suggest that the risk of splenectomy is greater than that of pursuing an expectant course. There is no medical management that will prevent the crises, the formation of gallstones, leg ulcers, etc.

The finding of gallstones alone is usually an indication for cholecystectomy in most patients under the age of 60 in whom contraindications do not exist (see Chap. 32, Biliary Tract). Gallstones in the presence of familial hemolytic anemia greatly strengthen the operative indication for either disease. Most surgeons believe that cholecystectomy and splenectomy can and should be carried out through the same incision at the same time if the patient is in good condition.

PROGNOSIS is excellent if splenectomy is performed. Once the diagnosis of familial spherocytic anemia is made, splenectomy is often justified, particularly in patients from 5 to 15 years of age, irrespective of symptoms. Expectant treatment, when anemia, icterus and gallstones are present, has nothing to offer. The operative mortality is much less than that of the untreated disease. Although icterus may be remitting in early life, over the years it tends to increase and to be associated with other complications.

The lessening of spherocytosis or its complete disappearance after splenectomy is reported occasionally. This has caused some to question the accepted concept that a primary constitutional defect is responsible for spherocytosis. It is probable that some error in the original or subsequent diagnosis accounts for these few reports.

Krueger and Burgert (1966) presented data pertaining to 100 consecutive pediatrics patients with congenital spherocytosis. There was little difference in the course of the disease among the 57 boys and 43 girls. The most common complaint was anemia, although only 64 patients had normal hemoglobin values postoperatively.

In four fifths of the patients, the spleen could be felt, and the serum bilirubin was mildly elevated in 49 of the 86 upon whom this test was performed. Spherocytes were found in the 100 patients and reticulocytosis appeared in 82 of the 92 patients tested. At operation the spleen was generally 2 to 4 times its normal size. They encountered no problems with infection postoperatively, an experience different from that of Diamond *et al*. (1965).

From the Mayo Clinic experience Krueger and Burgert concluded that splenectomy was justified in the child beginning at the age of 2 when anemia, splenomegaly, or icterus was present.

Congenital Nonspherocytic Anemia is a rare clinical entity that is inherited similar to spherocytic anemia but differs in that spherocytes are not found, that osmotic fragility is not present, and that splenectomy is without benefit. It is mentioned here only for the last reason.

Gaucher's Disease is another hereditary disease that occurs in "horizontal spread" rather than in the more usual vertical distribution (Groen, 1948). It is observed in the brothers and the sisters or the cousins of the same generation, whereas only occasionally is a case found among their parents or grandparents. Usually the children of these patients are healthy. Groen (1964) presents the interesting hypothesis that the first mutant in the family develops no evidence of the metabolic disturbance or does so late in life. The defect, he writes, is transferred to the 2nd and even the 3rd generation in increasing severity, "penetrance," until 50 per cent of a particular generation is affected; half of the next generation is affected so severely as to be fatal in utero or early infancy, the other 50 per cent being unaffected but through them the cycle is perpetuated.

It occurs most frequently among the Ashkenazi Jews and is nonsexlinked, but apparently it is rarely if ever found among the Sephardi and Oriental Jews. Groen writes: "Most geneticists nowadays conceive a mutation as a fixed metabolic or structural entity, but there is no reason why the fact (in Gaucher's disease) should not teach us to modify this standpoint." The basic metabolic defect in this disease is unknown, though metabolism of cerebrosides is among the abnormalities recognized; they contain glucose instead of galactose.

Splenectomy may be indicated in the middle-aged or older patients only if the weight of the spleen threatens torsion or tearing from its vascular pedicle, or if the enlarged spleen produces hemolytic anemia or thrombocytopenia. If splenectomy is planned, the possibility exists that the marrow may not be able to respond properly.

Sickle Cell Anemia. This interesting hereditary disease, for which splenectomy occasionally is performed, was first recognized by James B. Herrick (1910). It is predominantly a disease of Negroes and characterized by hemolytic anemia with the hyperplasia of the marrow of any hemolytic disease. The clinical pattern is that of chronic leg ulcers, attacks of acute abdominal pain, osteoarthritis, abnormal bleeding with remission and exacerbations frequently encountered. The seriousness of the disease and its manifestations are variable. Should complaints appear in early childhood or early adult life, the eventual outlook is likely to be poor. Few in this group survive beyond the age of 30.

Among the causes of death are cardiac failure, often with cor pulmonale, thrombosis, hemorrhage, intercurrent infection, or shock in association with abdominal crises attributed to vascular stasis. The spleen is usually enlarged in children but almost never palpable in adults, as it tends to fibrose and shrink below its normal size.

Sickle cell trait is to be distinguished from sickle cell anemia. The finding of the trait is seldom of consequence. The diagnosis of symptomatic sickle cell anemia is aided by the fact that studies indicate that the disease is limited to those in whom both parents bear the sickle trait. Most patients with the disease die within the first 2 decades of life.

The sickle shape is demonstrated best at 37° C. in an atmosphere devoid of oxygen, with the pH of the blood slightly reduced. A drop of blood mixed with a 2 per cent solution of sodium metabisulfite and examined 15 minutes after placing a cover slip over the slide usually shows that sickling is present. Kitchen et al. (1964) found sickle cells to be the normal characteristic of hemoglobin in the Florida white-tailed deer, which apparently causes no disease.

The cause of sickle cell anemia is an abnormal hemoglobin (HbS) found in the red cells of patients with this disease (Pauling et al., 1949). Hemoglobin S is less soluble than normal hemoglobin (HbA) and forms a gel more easily than other varieties of hemoglobin. When hemoglobin S is subjected to low oxygen tensions, its solubility is reduced even more, and in such low oxygen tensions it assumes a sicklelike shape. These sickled cells are easily destroyed; they also increase the viscosity of the blood and somehow propagate the painful and destructive infarctions which are characteristic of the disease.

A curious association is the fact that most

cases of osteomyelitis due to Salmonella infection occur in patients who have sicklemia or the sickle cell trait (Brit. Med. J., 1957).

Sicklemia and the acute abdominal symptoms it may cause have occasionally led the physician erroneously to recommend abdominal exploration. This disease is among the differential diagnoses to be considered in patients with acute abdominal complaints, especially young Negroes. When acute abdominal pain with fever and leukocytosis occurs, the diagnosis of a surgical condition within the abdomen is difficult if not impossible to exclude in some of these patients. However, the increased nucleated red cells, sicklemia and anemia are very helpful. Wilson et al. (1950) tabulate the following "surgical features" of this disease:

1. Acute abdominal symptoms, more often simulating colic, intussusception, or other forms of acute mechanical ileus
2. Jaundice
3. Bone and joint pains
4. Occasionally, bony lesions representing osteomyelitis due to *B. salmonella* are found by roentgenography.
5. Leg ulcers
6. Priapism
7. Hematuria may be associated with the clinical picture of renal colic.
8. Cerebral accidents

Satisfactory treatment does not exist. Splenectomy ordinarily is not indicated, unless one or more of the hypersplenic manifestations develop secondarily, in which case, as Egdahl et al. (1963) recommend, splenectomy may be useful but only for those secondary auto-immune blood disorders.

Many believe that the shape of the cells imposes difficulties upon its traversing the capillary bed throughout the body and not just that of the spleen. The tortuous vessels of the eye grounds leading to visual disturbances provide a direct opportunity to note this effect. It is also proposed that cardiomegaly with its cor pulmonale is another manifestation of the same phenomenon of vascular stasis.

The surgeon needs to bear in mind that often the abdominal crises may simulate the picture of the acute abdomen except that peristaltic activity usually persists. If he overlooks this disorder, he may perform a needless abdominal exploration, particularly on the Negro patient. However, sickle cell anemia does not immunize against acute appendicitis or other concurrent surgical conditions.

Thalassemia (Cooley's Anemia). This disease also has been reason for splenectomy in a few instances. Operation is performed primarily for relief of the distress from splenomegaly; it has no apparent benefit upon the disease per se. Lichtman et al. (1953) provided some evidence that the spleen may play a hemolytic role in this disease after a year or two of age and that splenectomy may then lessen the frequency of transfusion requirements.

Smith et al. (1962) observed that young patients splenectomized for thalassemia major showed "a predisposition to overwhelming infection" with 7 severe infections among 33 splenectomized patients of whom 5 died. In contrast, in 23 nonsplenectomized patients suffering from this disease, there were 3 cases of infection with no deaths. However, in the 33 subjected to splenectomy their primary disease was more severe; therefore, this difference may not be as meaningful as the figures suggest.

Acquired Autohemolytic Anemia. The term "splenic anemia" was introduced to describe cases of anemia attributed to splenomegaly. Since this term was first introduced about a century ago, any anemia associated with splenomegaly from any cause has often been referred to as being of splenic origin. With the recognition of auto-antibodies and their probable relation to increased red cell destruction, the term "splenic anemia" today is usually restricted to patients with autoantibodies and splenomegaly. In this group, the hemolytic process is curable by splenectomy. Unfortunately, knowledge is not advanced to the point wherein the presence of a hemolytic component can be expected simply because the spleen is enlarged in association with certain anemic states, although most cases of splenomegaly demonstrate a hemolytic component at one time or another.

The clinical picture is one of mild to moderate anemia, developing usually over a period of several years. Severe anemia is the exception but does occur. Icterus is seldom evident and when present is usually slight. These patients often live for many years with few or no symptoms related to the pathogenesis of the splenomegaly save for the distress of an enlarged or heavy spleen, and anemia.

The anemia encountered is usually hypochromic and normocytic. If repeated bouts of hemorrhage are superimposed, as in portal hypertension with bleeding varices, the hypochromic anemia may be severe. Hyperplastic marrow activity is usually found. If the marrow is hypoplastic, splenectomy is contraindicated.

Once the marrow and peripheral blood studies have been concluded, splenic puncture should be considered in doubtful cases, lest the spleen prove to be an important source of extramedullary erythropoiesis. Should this be so, splenectomy is strongly contraindicated.

Plasma iron clearance rate may be an important diagnostic aid in hemolytic anemias. The technics employed in such patients appear to be promising as an accessory means for establishing the diagnosis of hemolysis, but it does not delineate this from other forms of hemolytic anemia with hyperactivity of the marrow (Figs. 34-4 and 34-5, p. 960).

Auto-antibodies are demonstrated most reliably by the "diagnostic Coombs' test" (see Chap. 8, Blood Transfusion). Should this test be negative in the presence of splenomegaly and anemia, other causes of anemia should be considered more seriously. Whether the increased red-cell destruction is caused by a normally functioning but greatly enlarged spleen—that is, whether it is a quantitative rather than a qualitative abnormality—is not known.

A curiosity is that there is no evidence that these patients suffer from an increased tendency for gallstones to form, even though many have suffered for years from their hemolytic disease.

There are other causes of hemolytic anemia besides auto-immune mechanisms. At times other lytic processes are involved, and among them are those caused by the action of certain lipids and fatty acids, as well as by those of cholesterol, certain proteins, and protein-bound phospholipids, including certain snake venoms. When acquired hemolytic anemia is due to one of these causes, splenectomy and the administration of glucocorticoids are of little value. Usually, the Coombs' test is negative for this group (J.A.M.A., 1962).

Splenectomy is the treatment of choice and indeed of necessity when severe anemia of this origin is demonstrated. However, it should be restricted to those patients in whom normal or hyperplastic marrow activity and a positive diagnostic Coombs' test can be demonstrated. As many of these patients survive for years or appear to live a normal life-span, splenectomy is not required unless anemia becomes profound. The following case (Carpenter and Allen, 1941) illustrates the prolonged story and complications in a female patient observed for a number of years, beginning in February, 1940:

At that time she was treated for an unexplained anemia and nonthrombocytopenic purpura. Other than severe anemia ranging between 3 and 6 Gm. per cent of hemoglobin, no other blood or marrow abnormalities were noted. Her bleeding time, clotting time and prothrombin time were normal, although her Rumpel-Leed test was positive. Clot retraction was normal. She was 30 years of age when seen here in 1940.

Her history of abnormal bleeding dated back to the onset of menstruation and even in childhood as her parents forbade spanking because of her tendency to "bruise easily." Each menstrual flow had been excessive since adolescence, generally lasting for 1 to 2 weeks. In consequence, her severe anemia had been known and present for 15 years. An attempt to correct her hemoglobin concentration by repeated blood transfusion and iron therapy were met with little success. After transfusion of sufficient blood to elevate the hemoglobin concentration to 10 Gm. per cent, she complained of the symptoms of plethora and stated that she was more comfortable with her anemia, to which she had become accustomed. The platelet count remained normal during the periods of her observation from 1940 until 1947, at which time mild thrombocytopenia developed, and for the first time the spleen became palpable that year. Over a 12-month period the platelet count gradually fell to levels of 40,000 per cu. mm., and characteristic petechial hemorrhage appeared. On July 6, 1948, splenectomy was performed without incident. The platelet count promptly returned to normal, and for the first time her menstrual periods assumed a normal character. Her hemoglobin concentration slowly increased to its normal values at 15 to 16 Gm. per cent. Once this normal hemoglobin concentration was achieved, the patient again complained of the symptoms of plethora, and these complaints remained present and very unpleasant for her for 18 months following splenectomy. Thereafter she began to feel better and for the last 16 years she has been well.

Comment: The nature of the initial purpura in this patient is not understood, nor is it known why the thrombocytopenic component should have finally appeared after more than 30 years of nonthrombocytopenic purpura. Perhaps she had two separate bleeding states, although after splenectomy no further bleeding has occurred in 8 years. Of special interest are the pronounced adjustments that she had made to her near-lifelong severe hypochromic anemia as well as the difficulties that she encountered once her anemia was corrected by the avoidance of further blood loss after splenectomy was performed.

Splenic Neutropenia and Panhypersplenism. Splenic neutropenia may also occur in conjunction with splenomegaly. It is much more frequently a part of thrombocytic or of hemolytic disease than an isolated form of hypersplenic disease. The more commonly encountered forms of neutropenia are those from drug reactions, especially the amidopyrine series, or from other hemocytologic toxins which also cause aplastic anemia. In others, neutropenia may be a manifestation of one of the malignant blood dyscrasias. In some individuals, moderate neutropenia (1,000 to 2,500 total leukocyte count per cu. mm. of blood) may exist without much difficulty being encountered other than the more frequent occurrence of upper respiratory infections. In time, some of the patients with splenic neutropenia may develop an aplastic anemia or a leukemia.

In profound neutropenia (250 to 800 leukocytes per cu. mm. of blood) from any cause (hypersplenism, leukemia, or aplastic anemia) the clinical pattern is one of infection, cutaneous ulceration, poor wound healing, and mucosal desquamation of the alimentary tract. These are the same symptoms frequently noted in total body exposure to ionizing radiation in the near-lethal range. One is more impressed by the role of the leukocytes in the control or the prevention of infection when they are absent than by the usual and normal leukocytosis accompanying primary infections. Such was the case in the following patient

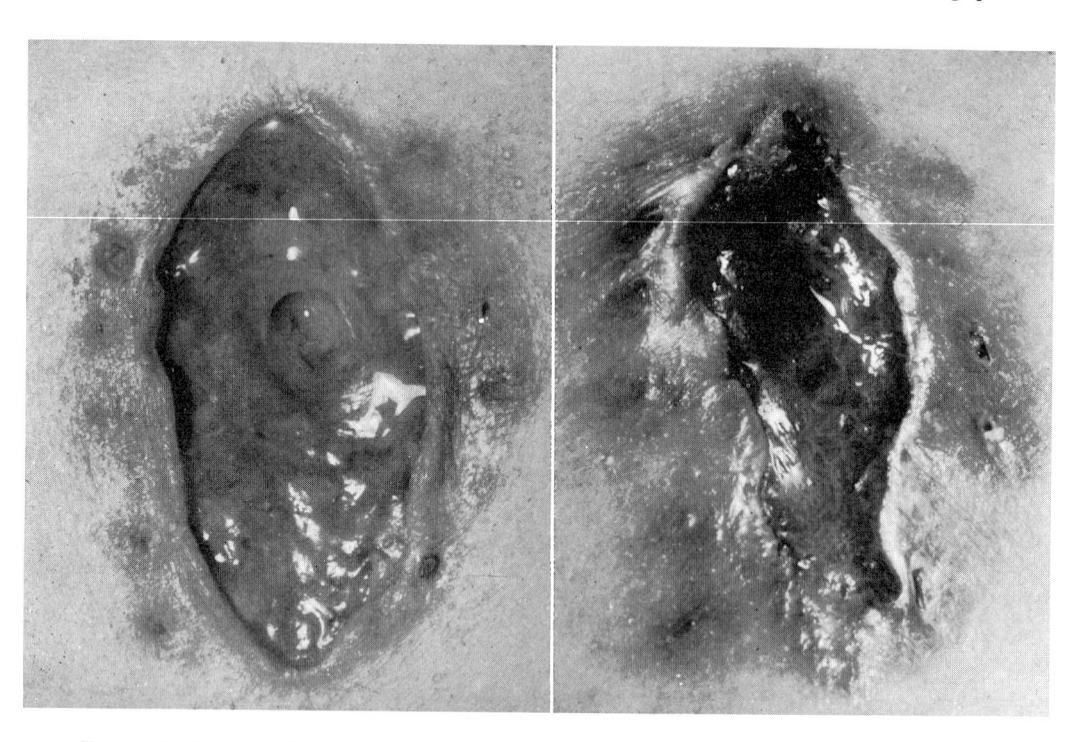

Fig. 34-6. Surgical biopsy of sternal marrow in patient with hypersplenism, predominantly of the neutropenic type. Picture on left shows grayish color of granulating wound after it separated. No pus is seen. Photo on right was taken 5 days after splenectomy and shows wound healthy and beginning to heal. Leukocyte response promptly followed operation.

who suffered from pancytopenia or panhypersplenism in whom the dominating picture was that resulting from her profound neutropenia.

The patient (40-65-32), a 50-year-old female, was admitted to the hospital on April 20, 1947. Her chief complaints were weakness of 10 weeks' duration and daily fever ranging between 100° and 103° F. for the last 4 weeks. The remainder of her history was negative, and there was no history of exposure to drugs or known toxins. The lungs were clear, the heart and blood pressure normal, but the spleen was palpable, enlarged and firm. Laboratory findings revealed a hemoglobin concentration of 8 Gm. per cent, the leukocyte count was 1,050 with 7 per cent neutrophils, and the platelet count was 139,000. The urine was negative. A surgical biopsy of the sternal marrow was performed the day following admission. Although the incision was closed, it became infected, failed to heal, and broke down (Fig. 34-6). This open wound produced no detectable pus, presumably because there were so few neutrophils. During the first week of hospitalization, the patient's course was rapidly downhill. Her temperature increased from 102° to 105° F. Bronchial pneumonia developed, and the patient was placed in an oxygen tent. Her anemia and neutropenia became more pronounced. The diagnosis of primary splenic neutropenia and splenic anemia were made. Splenectomy was performed on the 9th day. Her improvement was remarkably rapid, and within 48 hours her fever disappeared, and the pneumonitis began to clear. The day of operation, her leukocyte count was 1,250; 18 hours after splenectomy the total white blood count was 10,000 with 44 per cent neutrophils. There was a sharp increase in the lymphocytes as well. The surgical biopsy incision promptly changed its color from a grayish red to a bright red and was nearly healed by the 17th day, when the patient was discharged. When last seen 3 years later, she was in excellent health.

Comment: The patient's general condition was desperate by the time splenectomy was performed. The operation was undertaken at this time only because a fatal outcome was expected unless splenectomy relieved rapidly the course she displayed.

Summary of Indications and Contraindications for Splenectomy

Indications. Splenectomy is the only effective treatment currently available in the following disorders:
1. Rupture or torsion of the spleen
2. Splenic abscess
3. "Wandering" spleen
4. Cysts and tumors of the spleen
5. Aneurysm of the splenic artery
6. Spherocytic hemolytic anemia
7. Severe forms of auto-immune diseases
   A. Primary or secondary thrombocytopenic purpura
   B. Acquired autohemolytic anemia
   C. "Splenic" neutropenia
   D. Panhypersplenism
8. In the performance of certain operations as a technical necessity
9. In Banti's syndrome (splenic vein block only), otherwise as a necessity in splenorenal shunts
10. In certain general diseased states when hypersplenic manifestations dominate the picture and threaten the life of the patient who otherwise might live in comfort many years with his disease. Gaucher's disease is an example (also case example, p. 971).

Contraindications. The spleen should not be removed when it is an important organ of erythropoiesis as in secondary myeloid metaplasia, in hypoplastic and malignant disorders of the marrow, or in most infections amenable to medications.

1. Secondary myeloid metaplasia. Examples include
   A. Sclerosing osteitis
   B. Extensive marrow replacement by fibrous tissue or metastatic tumor
2. Aplastic or hypoplastic anemia
3. The "leukemoid" states, with few exceptions
4. In portal hypertension unless the surgeon is prepared to perform a splenorenal anastomosis or is satisfied than an anastomosis cannot be carried out satisfactorily by him or someone more experienced.

SPLENIC TUMORS

Malignant tumors of the spleen unassociated with blood dyscrasia are extremely rare. A few patients suffering from primary sarcoma of the spleen have been reported. Fibroma, myoma, leiomyosarcoma and angiomatous tumors may occur. For the most part, however, any splenic enlargement is much more likely to be secondary to infection, cyst formation, lymphoma, Hodgkin's disease, portal hypertension, or chronic congestive failure than tumor. The positive diagnosis is made by needle biopsy or from the removed specimen.

Metastatic tumors to the spleen are also rare by comparison with metastases found in other organs. This may be due in part to the scanty lymphatic supply to the spleen. However, experimentally implanted tissues grow as well in the spleen as in other organs, implying that the infrequent occurrence of tumor metastasis is not likely due to any particular noxious influence that the spleen may have on tumor cells. Apparently, the infrequency of metastasis to this organ is simply one of failure of significant quantities of tumor cells to arrive there, or to remain long enough to be seeded.

TECHNIC OF SPLENECTOMY

The experienced surgeon does not often find this to be a difficult operation, although numerous adhesions may be encountered, and extensive collateral veins may give rise to troublesome bleeding in some patients. Almost all technical difficulties can be attributed to one of two technical faults or both: inadequate surgical exposure and failure to secure adequate hemostasis. The best and surest means for securing hemostasis is the benefit afforded by adequate exposure.

Two other points in technic contribute to or are primarily responsible for the majority of the postoperative complications of splenectomy. One is surgical injury to the tail of the pancreas which often abuts or is included in the hilus of the spleen. The other is the inclusion in a hemostat or ligature of a small portion of the greater curvature of the stomach in the course of ligating the vasa brevia. As the greater curvature may have some temporary impairment of blood supply along the splenic margin after ligation of the gastroepiploic and short gastric vessels (vasa brevia), gastric perforation with subphrenic abscess or peritonitis may occur. Both injury to the pancreas and the stomach are avoided best by gaining adequate surgical exposure before attempting splenectomy (Fig. 34-7).

A long left paramedian incision is made, beginning at the upper left portion of the xiphoid cartilage and extending below to at least half way between the umbilicus and the pubic symphysis, slanting to the left, and terminating over the midportion of the lower rectus muscle. The additional exposure provided by a "T" with the vertical arm to the left and extending horizontally for several inches is seldom necessary but nonetheless should be taken advantage of in difficult cases, especially when the spleen is huge. Some prefer the transthoracic approach.

Once the abdominal exposure is obtained, the gastrocolic omentum is carefully dissected away from the anterior surface of the colon, beginning slightly to the right of the center of the transverse colon and proceeding gently to the left until the splenocolic ligament is divided and the entire left portion of the transverse colon is freed of its omental and splenic attachment.

At this point the following optional procedure may be carried out: The greater curvature of the stomach with its freed omentum is gently retracted upward and mesially, exposing the lesser peritoneal sac. This usually brings the tortuous splenic artery into view 5 to 10 cm. away from the splenic hilus as the artery courses above the pancreas in the retroperitoneum, from the celiac axis to the spleen. Usually a ligature can be easily slipped under the artery at this point and tied securely and cut after gaining access to it by incising a small area of its overlying peritoneum. However, the artery is not yet to be divided. Care is taken to avoid injury to the body of the pancreas and the splenic vein lying just below and often in direct contact with the artery. The ligature serves to reduce any loss of blood that may be entailed should the spleen be torn later in the course of its removal.

The next step is the cutting with scissors of the lateral peritoneal reflection along the posterior margin of the spleen. Gentle retraction is applied along the left costal margin and directed upward and laterally. This assists in securing the exposure necessary to extend the cut along the posterior peritoneum to the upper pole of the spleen and to its mesial aspect, thereby dividing the phrenicolienal ligament, which is the upper suspensory ligament of the spleen. Any adhesions between the lateral and/or the superior surfaces of the spleen and the diaphragm encountered in this maneuver are carefully clamped if necessary and cut more closely to the diaphragm than the spleen.

Then the "cupped" hand is introduced

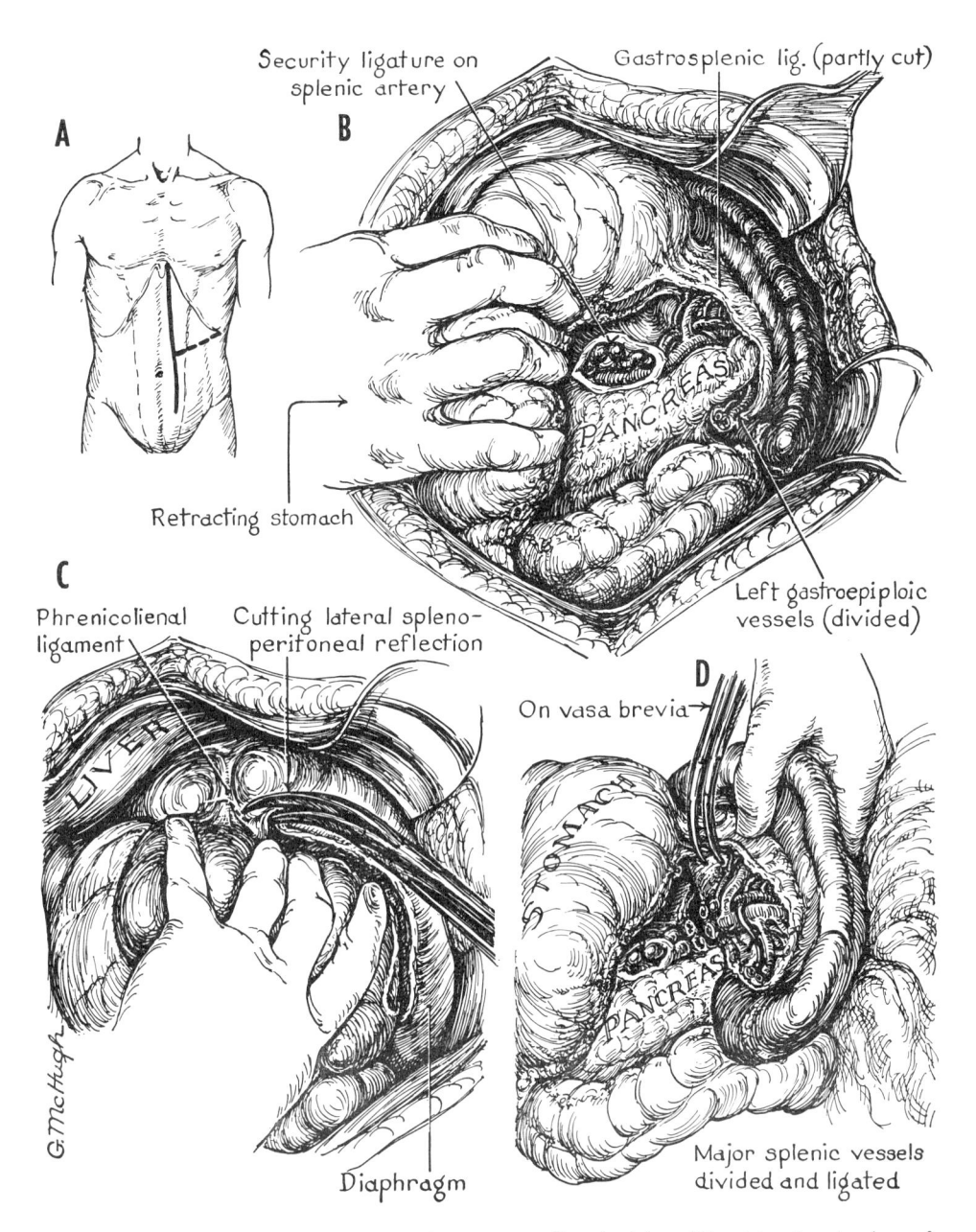

FIG. 34-7. Drawing A illustrates a long paramedian incision. The lateral extension of the incision is optional. (B) Security ligature placed about splenic artery after entering lesser peritoneal cavity. Lienocolic ligament has been divided to prevent tearing of splenic capsule. (C) Spleen is gently rotated mesially, exposing its retroperitoneal attachments; the lateral leaf is divided, extending upward to include the phrenicolienal ligament. Should the vasa brevia be readily accessible at this time, they, too, are clamped and ligated, being careful not to include any portion of adjacent wall of gastric fundus. (D) Cupped hand is introduced through the posterior lateral cut margin, and the fingers are advanced gently through the divided lateral margin into the retroperitoneum of the lesser peritoneal cavity, freeing the spleen with its pedicle and the distal third of the pancreas, permitting the spleen to be advanced safely to a forward position. With one hand supporting the mobilized spleen in its new position, the gastrolienal omentum is divided, exposing the splenic artery and vein at hilum. These vessels are divided and ligated separately. Finally, the vasa brevia are divided if not already cut.

through the incised lateral splenoperitoneal reflection, entering the retroperitoneum. The fingers gently dissect mesially beneath the spleen, the tail of the pancreas and the splenic vessels. This allows the spleen and its pedicle to be rotated forward and advanced to the anterior portion of the abdominal cavity. Several laparotomy pads are carefully placed in the splenic bed to support the spleen in its new forward position; this has the additional effect of hastening coagulation should there be a seepage of blood from the denuded retroperitoneum.

The pedicle is now easily exposed by the careful dissection of the retroperitoneum as it is reflected from the pedicle onto the mesial surface of the spleen covering anteriorly the splenic vessels. Then each branch of the splenic artery and vein is clamped separately, divided and ligated as encountered. With this accomplished (without injury to the tail of the pancreas), the surgeon rotates the upper pole forward a little more if need be, exposing the vasa brevia. The peritoneum along the anterior surface is cut *close* to the spleen. With these vessels thus exposed, each is clamped separately with small hemostats close to the spleen, divided and ligated under direct vision. Care is taken to avoid enclosure or encroachment upon the stomach at any point.

The spleen is now entirely free and is lifted from the abdomen. Then the greater curvature is inspected for hemorrhage, the packs are removed, and the denuded splenic bed is inspected for bleeding, as is the underside of the diaphragm. A final check is made for the presence of any accessory splenic tissue which may have been left behind. The distal portion of the lienocolic ligament is sutured to a location similar to its original site, and the abdomen is closed without drainage unless the tail of the pancreas was injured or splenectomy was performed for an abscess.

Mortality for splenectomy is less than 3 per cent when the patients are presented to the surgeon before they are seriously ill or moribund. If not, mortality rates of 10 to 30 per cent may be expected; stated more accurately, 70 to 90 per cent of these moribund patients may be salvaged by splenectomy, especially those with splenic rupture or hypersplenism.

Anesthesia. The choice of the anesthetic agent and its method of administration deserve special consideration in patients with hypersplenic thrombocytopenic purpura. In some patients, liver or other systemic diseases pose special problems to be considered.

Intubation, spinal anesthesia or intercostal "blocks" are to be avoided lest the trauma entailed cause extensive local hemorrhage in the face of the generalized tendency toward abnormal bleeding. The use of cyclopropane is thought by some to augment bleeding, a point not convincingly settled at this time. Third is the need for good relaxation which is essential to adequate exposure. Augmenting the general anesthetic agent with the very careful use of drugs with curarelike action is most helpful, but the anesthesiologist must bear in mind that in these patients intubation offers unusual risk; hence, the use of such agents is compromised if not contraindicated in the purpuric patient. Due consideration also must be given to the liver which is diseased in many, especially those with portal hypertension (see Chap. 36, Portal Hypertension).

Blood transfusion in hypersplenic disorders and congenital hemolytic anemia should be withheld if possible until the splenic artery has been ligated or, better, until the spleen has been removed. Blood should be "type-to-type" and Coombs' negative. Although these reactions are seldom serious if the patient is not critically ill, they may become so under these circumstances. If platelet transfusions are to be employed, they, too, should not be given until after the spleen is out; this author does not rely upon platelet transfusions but does not object to their usage, if available, especially should bleeding continue after splenectomy.

Nonhemolytic complications after splenectomy are principally thrombosis and infection. Thrombosis of the splenic vein with extension into the portal vein was encountered more commonly in the days before splenorenal or portacaval shunting procedures. Two factors peculiar to splenectomy favor thrombosis. First is the thrombocytosis which often follows a few days after removal of the spleen. Platelet counts 3 to 5 times the normal value may occur. The second and likely the more important one is splenectomy performed for portal hypertension when the increased venous pressure is not relieved. This leads to venous stasis which always favors intravascular thrombosis. Thrombocytosis and stasis together provide such fertile soil for coagulation that it is amazing that this complication is not encountered more frequently. Pancreatitis also may occur and may contribute to splenic and portal vein thrombosis.

Subphrenic abscess may occur occasionally, and its prevention by drainage of the subphrenic space via a stab wound in the flank always should be considered before closing the abdomen. This possibility is obviously needed should splenectomy be performed for an abscess of the spleen. Drainage should be considered if the tail of the pancreas has been injured. If there remains some doubt, the author prefers to drain.

SPLENIC TRANSPLANTATION IN CLASSICAL HEMOPHILIA A

The spleen has been thought to be a site of formation for antihemophilic globulin (AHG). Thus far no convincing evidence has been put forward in support of this thesis. The evidence is much better that AHG is formed within the liver and that hepatic transplants might be a solution. However, this too is a very drastic form of treatment, since hemophilia can be controlled by the appropriate dosage of cryoprecipitated AHG administered periodically. To continue experimental transplants of spleens and liver for the treatment of this disease in man seems ill-conceived, especially since it is possible to perform such studies on hemophiliac dogs (Brinkhous *et al.*, 1951). Not only is the threat of hemophilia a factor, but so also is the probability of uncontrolled rejection of the spleen when the immunosuppressive agents will suppress the platelets sufficiently to have hemorrhage from thrombocytopenia alone. Surgery is not that far ahead of science. On the other hand, there is reasonably acceptable evidence that cultures of hepatic cells are capable of elaborating AHG. Marchioro *et al.* (1969) found the concentration of factor VIII (AHG) and partial thromboplastin times became normal and remained normal for 140 days after orthotopic transplantation of a normal liver to a hemophiliac dog. Transplantation of a normal spleen into a hemophiliac animal did not result in a significant change of factor VIII although there was evidence that the splenic graft remained viable for at least 47 days.

The problem with most of these experiments has been that AHG titer may vary spontaneously rather widely, and therefore that operations are occasionally tolerated surprisingly well. The same may hold true for experimental animals. The solution for hemophiliac bleeding, or for urgent operations in hemophiliacs, is the transfusion of adequate quantities of cryoprecipitated AHG (Pool and Shannon, 1965). (See Chapter 8.)

REFERENCES

Abrahamsen, A. F.: Platelet survival studies in man. Scandinavian J. Haematology, Supplement No. 3, Copenhagen, 1968.

Adams, F.: The Extant Works of Aretaeus the Cappadocian. London, 1856.

Adner, M. M., Fisch, G. R., Starobin, S. G., Aster, R. H.: Use of "Compatible" platelet transfusions in treatment of congenital isoimmune thrombocytopenic purpura. N. Eng. J. Med., 280:274, 1969.

Allen, J. G., Bogardus, G., Jacobson, L. O., and Spurr, C. L.: Some observations on bleeding tendency in thrombocytopenic purpura. Ann. Int. Med., 27:382, 1947.

Aristotle: Quoted by Mettler, C. C.: History of Medicine. p. 358. New York, Blakiston Div. of McGraw-Hill, 1947.

Barbette: Cited by Mettler, C. C.: History of Medicine. p. 2. New York, Blakiston, 1947.

Barnes, D. W. H., and Loutit, J. F.: The immunological and histological responses following spleen treatment in irradiated mice. *In:* Progress in Radiobiology. Oliver and Boyd, London, 1956. p. 291.

Baudet, R.: Rupptures de la rate. Med. prat., 3:565 and 581, 1907.

Bizzozeri, J.: Ueber einen neuen Formbestandtheil des Blutes und die Rolle bei der Thrombose und der Blutgerinnung. Virchows Arch. path. Anat., 90:261, 1882.

Block, M. H.: Personal communication. 1947.

Bogardus, G., Allen, J. G., Jacobson, L. O., and Spurr, C. L.: Role of splenectomy in thrombopenic purpura. Arch. Surg., 58:16, 1949.

Bothwell, T. H., Callender, S., Mallett, B., and Witts, L. J.: The study of erythropoiesis using tracer quantities of radioactive iron. Brit. J. Haemat., 2:1, 1956.

Brinkhous, K. M., Graham, J. B., Penick, G. D., and Langdell, R. D.: Studies on canine hemophilia. *In:* J. E. Flynn (ed.): Transactions of Fourth Conference on Blood Clotting and Allied Problems. Jan. 22-23, 1951. Josiah Macy, Jr. Foundation, New York, 1951.

British Medical Journal: Sickle cells and salmonellae. No. 5060, p. 1537, Dec. 28, 1957.

Brohm: Cited by Quick, A. J.: The Hemorrhagic Diseases and the Physiology of Hemostasis. p. 130. Springfield, Ill., Charles C Thomas, 1942.

Buchbinder, J. H., and Lipkoff, C. J.: Splenosis: multiple peritoneal splenic implants following abdominal injury. Surgery, 6:927, 1939.

Carpenter, G., and Allen, J. G.: A defect in clot formation observed in three cases of chronic agnogenic hemorrhagic disease. Am. J. Med. Sci., 202:655, 1941.

Chauffard, A.: Pathogénie de l'ictere hémolytique congenital. Ann. méd., 1:3, 1914.

Cohen, P., and Gardner, F. H.: The thrombocytopenic effect of sustained high-dosage prednisone therapy in thrombocytopenic purpura. New Eng. J. Med., 265:611, 1961.

Cole, L. J.. Fisher, M. C., Ellis, M. E., and Bond, V. P.: Protection of mice against x-irradiation by spleen homogenates administered after exposure. Proc. Soc. Exp. Biol. Med., 80:112, 1952.

Cole, W. H., Walter, L., and Limarzi, L. R.: Indications and results of splenectomy. Ann. Surg., 129:702, 1949.

Coombs, R. R. A., Marks, J., and Bedford, D.: Specific mixed agglutination: mixed erythrocyte-platelet anti-globulin reaction for the detection of platelet antibodies. Brit. J. Haemat., 2:84, 1956.

Cotlar, A. M., and Cerise, E. J.: Splenosis: autotransplantation of splenic tissue following injury to spleen. Report of two cases and review of literature. Ann. Surg., 149:402, 1959.

Curtis, G. M., and Movitz, D.: The significance of the accessory spleen. J. Lab. Clin. Med., 31:464, 1946.

Dameshek, W.: Controversy in idiopathic thrombocytopenic purpura. J.A.M.A., 173:1025, 1960.

Dawson (Lord of Penn): Hemolytic icterus (The Hume Lecture No. 1), Brit. Med. J., 1:921, 1931.

Diamond, L. K., Eraklis, A. J., and Kevy, S. V.: The hazard of overwhelming infection post splenectomy. (Abstr.) J. Pediat., 67:1022, 1965.

Dowidar, M. L.: Wandering spleen. Ann. Surg., 129:408, 1948.

Ebert, R. V., and Stead, E. A., Jr.: Demonstration that in normal man no reserves of blood are mobilized by exercise, epinephrine and hemorrhage. Am. J. Med. Sci., 201:655, 1941.

Egdahl, R. H., Martin, W. W., and Hilkovitz, G.: Splenectomy for hypersplenism in sickle cell anemia. J.A.M.A., 186:745, 1963.

Eppinger, H.: Das retikulo endothelial System. Klin. Wchnschr., 35:1078, 1922.

Eraklis, A. J., Kevy, S. V., Diamond, L. K., and Gross, R. E.: Infection risk after splenectomy. N. Eng. J. Med., 276:1225, 1967.

Evans, R. S.: Primary thrombocytopenic purpura and acquired hemolytic anemia: Evidence for common etiology. Ann. Int. Med., 87:48, 1951.

Evans, R. S., and Duane, R. T.: Acquired hemolytic anemia. Blood, 4:1196, 1949.

Felty, A. R.: Chronic arthritis in the adult associated with splenomegaly and leukopenia; a report of 5 cases of an unusual clinical syndrome. Bull. Johns Hopkins Hosp., 35:16, 1924.

Fitzpatrick, W. K., Jr., Burdette, W. J., and Huestis, R. R.: Cholelithiasis and spherocytosis in *Peromyscus*. Arch. Surg., 86:897, 1963.

Flatow, F. A., and Freireich, E. J.: Effect of splenectomy on the response to platelet transfusion in three patients with aplastic anemia. N. Eng. J. Med., 274:242, 1966.

Friedell, H., Sanderson, M., Kirschon, A., Milhan, M., and Allen, J. G.: A study of hemolysin titrations in sensitized irradiated rabbits. *In:* Quart, Rep. Biological & Medical Res. Div., No. 4078, pp. 78-93, Chicago, Argonne National Laboratory, 1947.

Galen: Cited by Walsh, J.: Galen's writings and influences inspiring them. III. Ann. M. Hist. [n.s.], 7:428, 1935.

Groen, J. J.: The hereditary mechanisms of Gaucher's disease. Blood, 3:1238, 1948.

———: Gaucher's disease: Hereditary transmission and racial distribution. Arch. Int. Med., 113:543, 1964.

Haden, R. L.: The mechanism of the increased fragility of the erythrocytes in congenital hemolytic jaundice. Am. J. Med. Sci., 188:441, 1934.

Harkins, H. N.: Personal communication, 1956.

Harrington, W. J., Minnich, V., Hollingsworth, J. W., and Moore, C. V.: Demonstration of a thrombocytopenic factor in the purpura. J. Lab. Clin. Med., 38:1, 1951.

Harrington, W. J., Sprague, C. C., Minnich, V., Moore, C. V., Aulvin, R. C., and Dubach, R.: Immunologic mechanism in idiopathic and neonatal thrombocytopenic purpura. Ann. Int. Med., 38:433, 1953.

Hektoen, L.: Further studies on the effects of roentgen rays on antibody production. J. Infect. Dis., 22:28, 1916.

Herrick, J. B.: Peculiar elongated and sickle-shaped red corpuscles in a case of severe anemia. Arch. Int. Med., 6:517, 1910.

Howell, W. H., and Holt, E.: Two new factors in blood coagulation—heparin and pro-antithrombin. Am. J. Physiol., 47:328, 1918.

Jacobson, L. O.: Evidence for humoral factors concerned in recovery from radiation injury: A review. Cancer Res., 12:315, 1952.

Jacobson, L. O., Simmons, E. L., Marks, E. K., and Gaston, E. O.: Further studies on recovery from irradiation. J. Lab. Clin. Med., 37:683, 1951.

J.A.M.A.: (editorial): Tissue abnormalities in hemolytic anemias. 179:721, 1962.

Kaznelson, P.: Verschwiden der hämorrhagischen Diathese bei einem Fälle von essentieller Thrombopenie (Frank) nach Milzextirpation; splenogene thrombolytische Purpura. Wien. klin. Wschr., 29:1451, 1454, 1916.

Kitchen, H., Putnam, F. W., and Taylor, W. J.: Hemoglobin polymorphism: Its relation to sickling of erythrocytes in white-tailed deer. Science, 144:1237, 1964.

Knopp, L. M., and Harkins, H. N.: Traumatic rupture of the normal spleen. Surgery, 35:493, 1954.

Krueger, H. C., and Burgert, E. O., Jr.: Hereditary

spherocytosis in 100 children. Mayo Clin. Proc., 41:821, 1966.

Küttner: Discussion at Medical Section of the Silesian Society for Patriotic Culture in Breslau. Berlin. klin. Wschr., 47:1520, 1910.

Lichtman, H. C., Watson, R. J., Feldman, F., Ginsberg, V., and Robinson, J.: Studies of thalassemia. J. Clin. Invest., 32:1229, 1953.

Lorenz, E., Uphoff, D., Reid, T. R., and Shelton, E.: Modification of irradiation injury in mice and guinea pigs by bone marrow injection. J. Nat. Cancer Inst., 12:197, 1951.

Lorimer, W. S., Jr.: Occult rupture of the spleen. Arch. Surg., 89:434, 1964.

Malpighi, Marcello: De Pulmonibus Observations Anatomicae. *In* a letter to Borelli, tr. by Foster: Lane Lectures on History of Physiology. London, Cambridge, 1901.

Marchioro, T. L., Hougie, C., Ragde, H., Epstein, R. B., and Thomas, E. D.: Hemophilia: role of organ homografts. Science, 163:188, 1969.

Marson, F. G., Meynell, M. J., and Tabbush, H.: Familial crisis in acholuric jaundice. Brit. Med. J., 2:760, 1950.

Matthis, Florian: Opera omnia medica et chirurgica. Leyden, 1672. Quoted by Mettler, C. C.: History of Medicine. p. 862, New York, Blakiston Div. of McGraw-Hill, 1947.

McIndoe, A. H.: Delayed hemorrhage following traumatic rupture of the spleen. Brit. J. Surg., 20:249, 1932.

Miller, E. M., and Hagedorn, A. B.: Results of splenectomy: a follow-up of 140 consecutive cases. Ann. Surg., 134:815, 1951.

Minkowski, O., and Naunyn, B.: Über den Icterus durch Polycholie und die Vorgänge in der Leber bei demselben. Arch. exper. Path. Pharmakol., 21:1, 1886.

Morris, M. B.: Thrombocytopenic purpura in the newborn. Arch. Dis. Child., 29:75, 1954.

Morrison, W., Lederer, M., and Fradkin, W. Z.: Accessory spleens: their significance in essential thrombocytopenia purpura haemorrhagica. Am. J. Med. Sci., 176:672, 1928.

Motulsky, A. G., Casserd, F., Giblett, E. R., Brown, G. O., Jr., and Finch, C. A.: Anemia and the spleen. New Eng. J. Med., 259-1164, 1958.

Murchison, C.: Clinical Lectures on Diseases of the Liver, Jaundice, etc., edited by Lander. Brunton, London, 1885.

Negus, D., Pinto, D. J., and Brown, N.: Platelet adhesiveness in postoperative deep-vein thrombosis. Lancet, 1:220, 1969.

Norman, J. C., Covelli, V. H., and Sise, H. S.: Transplantation of spleen–enduring AHF synthesis in canine hemophilia. Fed. Proc., 27:373, 1968.

Oski, F. A., Naiman, J. L., and Diamond, L. K.: Use of the plasma acid phosphatase value in the differentiation of thrombocytopenic states. New Eng. J. Med., 268:1423, 1963.

Owren, P. A.: Congenital hemolytic jaundice: The pathogenesis of the hemolytic crisis. Blood, 3:231, 1948.

Parsons, L., and Thompson, J. E.: Traumatic rupture of the spleen from nonpenetrating injuries. Ann. Surg., 147:214-223, 1958.

Pauling, L., Itano, H. A., Singer, S. J., and Wells, I. C.: Sickle cell anemia, a molecular disease. Science, 110:543, 1949.

Reeve, E. B., Gregersen, M. I., Allen, T. H., and Sear, H.: Distribution of cells and plasma in normal and splenectomized dog and its influence on blood volume estimates with P^{32} and T-1824. Am. J. Physiol., 175:195, 1953.

Rowley, D. A.: The formation of circulating antibodies in the splenectomized human being followin intravenous infusion of heterologous erythrocytes. J. Immunol., 65:515, 1950.

Shulman, N. R., Aster, R. H., Leitner, A., and Hiller, M. C.: Immunoreactions involving platelets. V. Post-transfusion purpura due to a complement-fixing antibody against a genetically controlled platelet antigen. A proposed mechanism for thrombocytopenia and its relevance in "autoimmunity." J. Clin. Invest., 40:1597, 1961.

Simon, Gustav: Die Extirpation der Milz am Menschen, Giessen, 1857.

Smith, C. H., Erlandson, M. E., Stern, G., and Hilgartner, M. W.: Postsplenectomy infection in Cooley's anemia. New Eng. J. Med., 266:737, 1962.

Soldant, D. Y., and Best, C. H.: Time-relation of heparin action on blood clotting and platelet agglutination. Lancet, 1:1042, 1940.

Steiner, D. F.: The formation of antibodies *in vitro*. Recipient of Borden Student Award, University of Chicago School of Medicine, 1956.

Stobie, G. H.: Recurrence of congenital hemolytic anemia due to splenosis. Canad. M. A. J., 56:374, 1947.

Walter, L. E., and Chaffin, L.: Splenectomy in infants and children. Ann. Surg., 142:798, 1955.

Wells, Spencer: (Quoted by Lord Dawson of Penn), Hemolytic icterus (The Hume Lecture No. 2), Brit. Med. J., 1:963, 1931.

Werlhof, Paul Gottlieb: Opera medica. p. 748. Paris, Wichmann, 1775.

Whipple, A. O., Parpart, A. K., and Chang, J. J.: A study of the circulation of the blood in the spleen of the living mouse. Ann. Surg., 140:261, 1954.

Whitesell, F. B.: A clinical and surgical anatomic study of rupture of the spleen due to blunt trauma. Surg., Gynec. Obstet., 110:750, 1960.

Wilson, Harwell, Patterson, R. H., and Diggs, L. W.: Sickle cell anemia: a surgical problem. Ann. Surg., 131:641, 1950.

Wright, J. H.: The origin and nature of blood plates. Boston M. & S.J., 154:643, 1906.

Zabinski, E. J., and Harkins, H. N.: Delayed splenic rupture: A clinical syndrome following trauma. Arch. Surg., 46:186, 1943.

Chapter 35

J. GARROTT ALLEN, M.D.

Mesentery, Splanchnic Circulation and Mesenteric Thrombosis

Anatomic Considerations of the Mesentery and the Splanchnic Circulation
Diseases of the Mesentery
Mesenteric Thrombosis

From the beginning of the modern era of intestinal surgery, surgeons have been acutely aware of the importance of relationships of the arterial and the venous blood supply to and from the small and the large bowel and of the considerable extent to which these relationships are determining factors in limiting any bowel resection undertaken. In recent years the venous drainage of the alimentary tract has received additional attention in connection with the surgical developments in the treatment of portal hypertension. In yet another direction, surgery of the alimentary tract has been extended in the treatment of malignant disease wherein the origin and the course of the lymphatic circulation also play an important role in the extent of bowel resection required. Finally, any discussion of the abdominal portion of the intestinal tract must consider the mesentery, *in part* or *in toto*, not only because the blood and the lymphatic circulations to and from the bowel traverse the mesentery, but also because certain anomalies of the mesentery are responsible occasionally for acute surgical diseases. Hence, it is useful to consider the splanchnic circulation and the mesentery somewhat independent of the alimentary tract.

ANATOMIC CONSIDERATIONS OF THE MESENTERY AND THE SPLANCHNIC CIRCULATION

The Mesentery and the Omentum

The jejunoileum is attached to the anterior margin of its mesentery throughout its entire length and is confined principally within the midabdomen. Its restriction to this position in the peritoneal cavity is determined largely by length of the mesentery, its "encapsulation" by the omentum and the transverse mesocolon, and by the "picture frame" peripheral position of the abdominal colon within whose confines the small bowel tends to remain.

The superior boundary of the midabdomen is the undersurface of the transverse mesocolon. This mesocolon serves as a cupola and drapes the small bowel, suspended superiorly, and continues anteriorly below the transverse colon, fusing with the greater omentum. These 2 structures essentially eliminate the possibility that the small bowel may wander into the upper abdomen; thus, there is little chance that the subcolic small bowel (not including the duodenum) will become directly adherent to stomach, duodenum, gallbladder, liver or spleen in acute inflammatory lesions affecting these organs (Fig. 35-1). The pancreas, which lies in the upper abdomen with its inferior margin located just above the margin of the superior leaf of the transverse mesocolon at its posterior attachment, is an occasional exception, in that inflammation of the pancreas may involve the small bowel secondarily. In acute pancreatitis, the adjacent mesocolon may become sufficiently inflamed to produce an inflammatory response in the loops of neighboring small bowel, causing them to become adherent to the underside of the mesocolon and perhaps to give rise to small bowel obstruction.

The mesentery of the small bowel is essentially a reflection of the parietal peritoneum from the posterior abdominal wall onto the mesenteric vessels and the surface of the bowel. The parietal peritoneum becomes visceral peritoneum when it leaves the abdominal wall to encase the mesenteric vessels as

Anatomic Considerations of the Mesentery and the Splanchnic Circulation

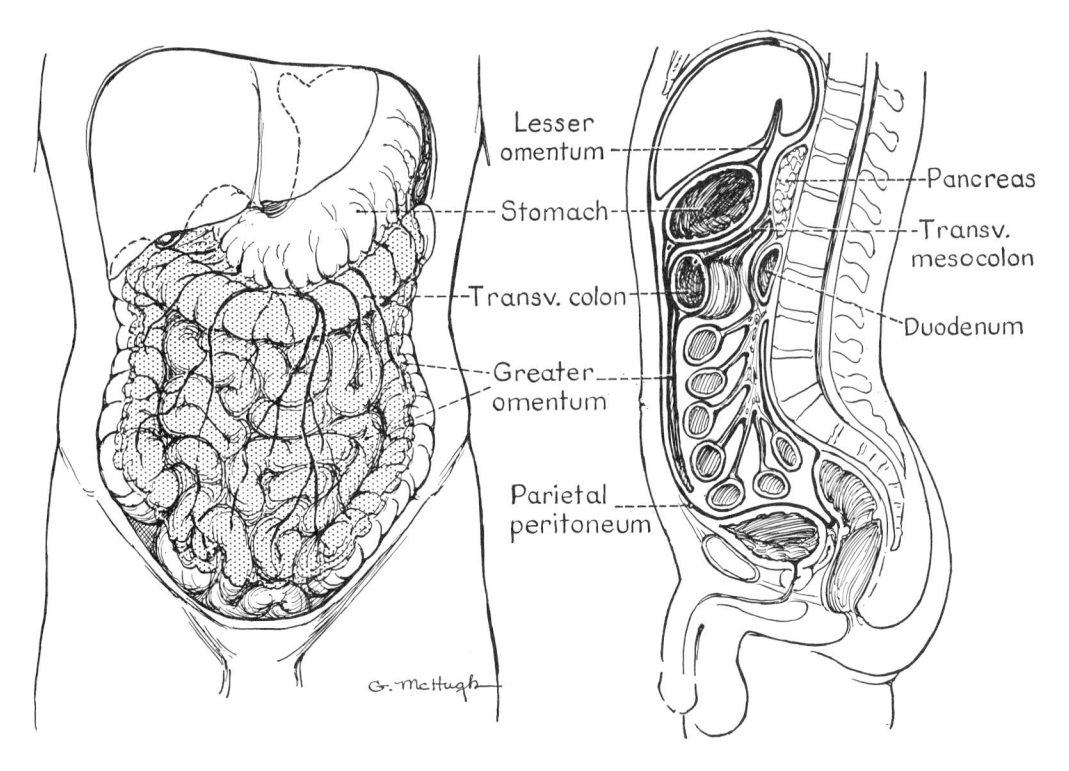

Fig. 35-1. Illustrates the effective manner by which the transverse mesocolon, in conjunction with the greater omentum, normally confines the small bowel to the midabdomen.

they travel from the aorta to the intestinal tract. The free mesentery of the small bowel begins at the ligament of Treitz, located at the level of the body of the 3rd lumbar vertebra. From this ligament to the ileocecal valve the entire small bowel is suspended from its mesentery, which allows motion in any direction, bounded only by the limits of the mesenteric length. The root, or origin, of the small bowel mesentery at the posterior abdominal wall descends obliquely to the right, terminating in the iliac fossa near the right sacral joint. In doing so, it passes about 1.5 cm. to the right of the retroperitoneal course of the right ureter and the common iliac vessels on this side (Fig. 35-2).

The mesentery of the ascending and descending colon differs from that of the small bowel in that the lateral leaves of peritoneum adjacent to the ascending and the descending portions of the colon usually are short or functionally nonexistent. Usually the lateral portions of the posterior parietal peritoneum pass directly from the abdominal wall over the ascending and the descending colon, respectively, in its course toward the midline and the root of the mesentery of the small bowel. When the parietal peritoneum reaches the centrally located mesenteric vessels, where it forms the peritoneum of the small bowel mesentery, it continues over the entire jejunoileum as visceral peritoneum. Occasionally, a freely moving mesentery is formed for the ascending and descending colon so that these structures may become as mobile as the small bowel. When this anomaly exists, these portions of the colon are subject to torsion, with resulting intestinal obstruction and ischemic necrosis if not relieved promptly.

We now recognize that occlusive arterial disease may impair circulation of the celiac and the superior mesenteric arteries and produce the syndrome known as intestinal angina.

The mesentery of the transverse colon is fully developed in contrast with those of the ascending and the descending colon. This mesentery is known as the transverse mesocolon. The transverse colon is adherent ante-

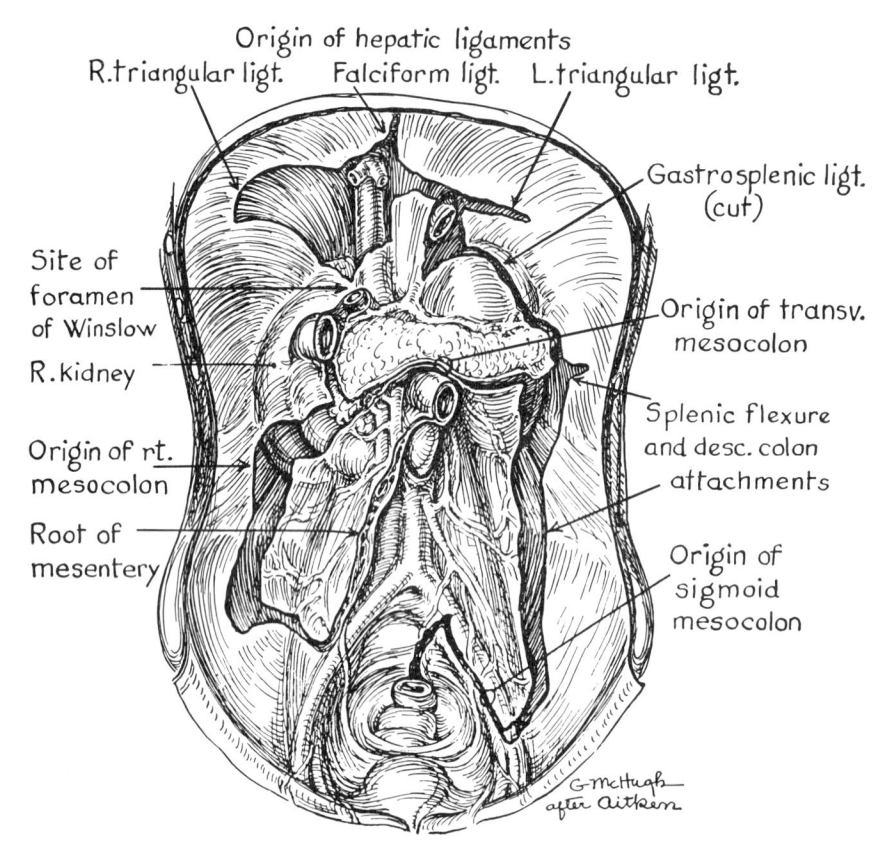

FIG. 35-2. The abdominal viscera and their mesenteric suspensions have been excised, including suspensory or triangular ligaments of the diaphragm and the posterior abdominal wall. Shown are the portions of the abdominal wall and the diaphragm not covered by parietal peritoneum as they are the sites of origin of the visceral peritoneum. (Drawn from Aitken)

riorly to the undersurface of the greater omentum, which suspends this part of the colon superiorly from the greater curvature of the stomach, in addition to its posterior suspension by the transverse mesocolon from the abdominal wall. Suspension of the transverse colon in two directions accounts for the rare occurrence of torsion of this part of the colon compared with that of its lateral portions, when unattached to the retroperitoneum.

The mesentery of the sigmoidal colon usually is well developed, and in this respect is like that of the small bowel, except for location. Normally, the sigmoidal mesentery begins at the end of the descending colon in the left iliac fossa, and from this point of origin its posterior margin runs diagonally upward and mesially along the left iliac vessels nearly to the bifurcation of the aorta, where it turns downward sharply into the sacral fossa and terminates in the pelvis, as the sigmoid-rectum leaves the peritoneal cavity to become the rectum (Fig. 35-2). If the sigmoidal mesentery is stretched and relaxed, as it tends to be with advancing age, volvulus or torsion may occur.

The normal colon, then, is covered with visceral peritoneum, except for those portions lying in direct contact with the posterior abdominal wall, where no mesentery exists (Fig. 35-2). Occasionally, the cecum also has little or no mesentery; its posterior portion has a broad area of direct contact with the iliac fossa, and this area of the posterior cecum is free of peritoneum. On the other hand, the dependent cecum may have a fairly well-developed mesentery, which may be further relaxed, especially in the aged and malnourished patient, causing it to be more mobile pancreas. This artery passes between the leaves of transverse mesocolon, dividing into a right and a left branch, whose primary arcades in turn anastomose with those of the right and the left colic arteries (see Fig. 35-5, A-D).

The distal colon, which includes the splenic flexure from its proximal side, the descending colon and the sigmoidal colon, and the upper rectum, receives its blood from the *inferior mesenteric* artery originating from the aorta opposite the 3rd lumbar vertebra. The principal branches of the inferior mesenteric artery are the *left colic* artery, which supplies the distal transverse colon, beginning near its splenic flexure, and most of the descending colon. The *sigmoidal* artery and its branches run obliquely to the sigmoidal colon in its mesentery; they anastomose with the primary arcades of the left colic artery above and the primary and the secondary arcades of the superior hemorrhoidal artery below. The *superior hemorrhoidal* artery is the terminal continuation of the inferior mesenteric and descends almost vertically in the sigmoidal mesentery to form usually 2 systems of arcades in its course before entering the wall of the lower sigmoid and the rectum. The superior hemorrhoidal artery also communicates with the *middle* and the *inferior hemorrhoidal* arteries, which are the near-terminal branches of the internal iliac artery, giving the rectum a dual source of arterial blood. However, the superior hemorrhoidal artery is the more important source of arterial blood to the rectum (Fig. 35-6).

Colon Resection and Arterial Supply

Knowledge of the arterial blood supply to the large bowel and the rectum is essential to the performance of safe operative procedures upon these structures. In resecting malignant lesions involving the cecum or the ascending colon, not only must the surgeon take into consideration the extent of the operation needed to remove potential sites of tumor spread within the mesentery and the segmental periaortic nodes, but also he must be certain that the remaining bowel has an uncompromised blood supply (see Figs. 35-4 and 5).

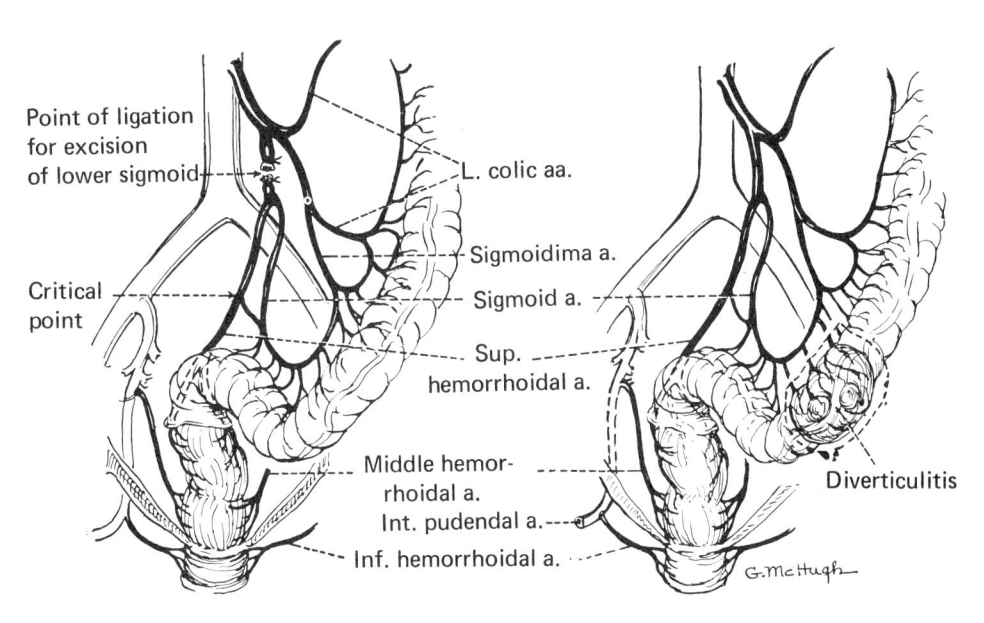

FIG. 35-7. On the left is designated the point of ligation of the superior hemorrhoidal artery for resection of the lower sigmoid for benign disease. Note that if the ligature were placed at the critical point shown, it would be necessary to resect not only the sigmoid but also the rectum as well.

It is for this reason that the extent of the bowel resection beyond the tumor site may sometimes be greater than that required to circumvent the tumor and its likely area of lymphatic spread.

Resection of the right colon necessitates the inclusion of about 6 in. of the terminal ileum, the appendix, the cecum, the ascending colon, and the hepatic flexure to a point at which there can be no doubt that the remaining portion of the transverse colon can be well sustained by the blood flow of the middle colic artery. The extent of the resection is determined by position and adequacy of the blood flow from the middle colic artery. Resections of lesions involving the transverse colon require division of the middle colic artery at its point of origin from the superior mesenteric artery. Removal of the entire transverse colon is required in order that the remaining portions of the hepatic and the splenic flexures receive sufficient blood from the right and the left colic arteries, respectively (see Fig. 35-5, A-D).

Resection of the descending colon, the sigmoid and the rectum may be necessary should the removal of the inferior mesenteric artery and its mesenteric wedge be essential to elimination of probable sites of tumor spread.

Noncancerous lesions, such as diverticulitis and polyps, may be removed by local bowel resection, only such segments being excised as required to eradicate the local area of bowel involved. In these diseases some conservation of colon may be possible, but usually the saving of a few inches of colon is an unimportant consideration, provided that previous bowel resection has not been performed and further resection at a later date does not seem to be a likely possibility. Excepting these circumstances, it may be easier to resect the bowel segment required after ligation of its arterial supply an inch or two from its point of origin from the superior or the inferior mesenteric artery than to attempt a less anatomic resection designed to conserve only small portions of colon (Fig. 35-7).

The Small Vessel Circulation of the Mucosa and the Submucosa of the Intestinal Tract

One of the characteristics of many capillary circulations appears to be the coexistence of arteriolar venular anastomosis capable of shunting or bypassing a segment or a major portion of the capillary bed when the latter's function is not needed (Boyd, 1953). This intermittent shunting is to be suspected in most organs which have a phasic function and whose active phase depends in part upon blood flow. The alimentary tract is an example of such a system of organs whose principal functions are predominantly phasic in character.

The suggestion of arteriolar-venular shunts to bypass a capillary circulation is not new. Renewed interest in this phenomenon can be credited to the studies of Spanner in 1931. In a series of observations, Spanner demonstrated beyond reasonable doubt the existence of such shunts within the villi and the mucosa of the stomach and the bowel. Confirmation of Spanner's studies has been reported by Barlow (1953), Walder (1953), and Grayson (1953); all studies to date, whether of anatomic, physiologic or pharmacologic nature, seem to come to the same conclusion, namely, that shunts exist within the villi and the mucosa of the stomach and the intestine. They appear to shunt blood away from the villous mucosa during the fasting state, and are said to be under nervous rather than humoral control.

Evidence thus far demonstrates considerable lability of the intraluminal circulation of the alimentary tract, a lability comparable with that exhibited by the capillary bed of the skin. The control of the circulation of the bowel and the skin is largely autonomic in nature; that of the striated muscle appears to be free of nervous control, responding chiefly to altered concentrations of serum metabolites, particularly those bearing upon CO_2 and pH values of the blood itself.

Venous Drainage, the Portal Circulation

The venous return from the splanchnic viscera has assumed a role of surgical importance and of anatomic and physiologic consequence, due to the developments in the operative treatment of portal hypertension.

The venous drainage of the small bowel and the colon is through a confluence of veins that terminate ultimately in the portal vein, which drains into the liver. The portal tributaries correspond in nomenclature and location to those of the arterial supply of corresponding segments of the small bowel, the colon and the rectum. The primary arteries to the intra-abdominal alimentary organs, including the liver and the spleen, arise directly from the aorta as 3 separate vessels (celiac axis, superior mesenteric artery and inferior mesenteric artery) and at 3 distinct aortic levels. The venous return differs in that all of it culminates in the large solitary portal vein.

The portal circulation differs from the systemic venous circulation in at least 4 respects:

1. The normal venous pressure of the portal vein usually is 12 to 15 cm. of water compared with the normal pressure values of the inferior vena cava which fluctuate between a positive pressure of 1 to 3 cm. of water during the expiratory phase of respiration and a negative pressure of 1 to 3 cm. during inspiration.

2. When venous blood from the gastrointestinal tract finally is collected into the single common channel, it must circulate through the sinusoidal or capillary circulatory bed of the liver before reaching the inferior vena cava via the hepatic veins. In this respect, the venous return from the splanchnic bed resembles the arteriovenous system between the right and the left sides of the heart, save for the fact that portal blood manages to pass through the liver by virtue of the much lower venous pressure at its point of exit through the hepatic veins compared with that of the portal vein.

3. The portal system, like the vena cava, has no valves, although valves are abundantly present in the veins of the extremities leading to the vena cava.

4. The venous drainage of the alimentary tract, along with that of the splanchnic lymphatic circulation return, is the only known source for the normal transport of ingested food products aside from the lacteals.

The portal circulation also receives venous return from the spleen. As the spleen has no known function related to alimentation, there is no very obvious physiologic explanation for its anatomic location within the splanchnic circulation (see Fig. 35-6).

The portal system begins with the capillary circulation within villus folds of the intestinal mucosa. After these coalesce to form the venules and the veins in the submucous layer, eventually they emerge alternatingly from the bowel wall about 1 cm. or so apart in a fashion corresponding to the small arteries entering the bowel. From here they pass directly into their respective mesenteric segments to converge upon a system of venous arcades corresponding in location and number to those of the mesenteric arteries. From these anastomotic arcades, blood enters the major branches of the superior or the inferior mesenteric vein and eventually into the portal vein. Usually the venous and the arterial channels in the corresponding areas of the gut and the mesentery run parallel and in close proximity.

The inferior mesenteric vein usually drains the distal portion of the transverse colon, its splenic flexure, the descending and sigmoidal colon, and the upper half of the rectum. The most distal portion of the inferior mesenteric vein is its superior hemorrhoidal branch, which begins at the superior margin of the venous plexus surrounding the midportion of the rectum. The lower portions of this plexus drain through the middle and the inferior hemorrhoidal veins into the "headwaters" of the internal iliacs, hence into the systemic rather than into the portal circulation (see Fig. 35-6).

The confluence of the superior hemorrhoidal, the sigmoidal and the left colic veins forms the inferior mesenteric vein, which then ascends along the psoas muscle beneath the parietal peritoneum, passing under the ligament of Treitz at its left margin to disappear beneath the body of the pancreas, where usually it joins the splenic vein as the latter passes in its mesial direction to unite with the larger superior mesenteric vein in the formation of the portal vein. From this junction the portal vein emerges and continues in an upward direction, leaning slightly to the right until it reaches its termination, the right and left branches at the porta hepatis, before entering the capillary and the sinusoidal network of the liver.

The superior mesenteric vein receives the venous return from the middle, the right and the ileocolic veins and drains the colon proximal to its splenic flexure. These veins are joined by 12 to 15 major tributaries from the small bowel; they account for all venous return of this portion of the colon and all of the small bowel short of a few centimeters distal to the ligament of Treitz. The superior mesenteric vein runs within the mesentery of the small bowel at the left of the superior mesenteric artery. As the two pass over the duodenum and the uncinate process of the pancreas, the artery is directed more posteriorly, allowing the vein to cross anterior to the artery. The vein deviates slightly to the right to ascend in the gastrohepatic ligament as the portal vein. Under the pancreas the superior mesenteric vein usually receives several pancreatic veins, some of which are major branches of the superior and the inferior pancreatoduodenal veins, and usually the gastroepiploic veins, which drain the greater omentum and the greater curvature of the stomach.

The coronary vein, which drains most of the blood from the lower esophagus, the fundus and the lesser curvature of the stomach, normally is of no unusual consequence in the course of surgical operations performed on patients without portal hypertension. However, should portal hypertension exist, it is largely the small branches of the coronary vein that become varicosities in the esophagus and the upper stomach, due to the increased portal pressure transmitted to them. To a lesser extent, the gastroepiploics and the short gastric veins also may contribute to esophageal and gastric varices (see Fig. 36-4).

The portal vein, from 6 to 9 cm. in length, passes in the posterior edge of the gastrohepatic omentum after emerging from behind the superior margin of the mesial portion of the head of the pancreas. Usually the common duct lies along the anterior right surface of the portal vein; to the posterior left of the vein is the hepatic artery. These relationships and positions are fairly constant, though not always so. Less constant anatomic relationships are found among some of the major tributaries to the portal vein, especially the gastroepiploics and the coronary veins, which may enter the portal vein directly or at the junction of the superior mesenteric with the splenic vein.

DISEASES OF THE MESENTERY

Cysts of the mesentery are congenital, caused by the presence of aberrant embryonic lymph tissue which, because of the absence of drainage, becomes distended with serous or chylous fluid. The walls are thin and are lined with epithelium and, hence, these are true cysts. They are slow to grow and cause vague to more pronounced distress in the abdomen and occasionally in the back. A mass may be palpable and, depending upon its location, may displace loops of small bowel to either side. Occasionally, the cyst may cause symptoms of obstruction, and rarely they may also become secondarily infected. Treatment is usually achieved easily by enucleation.

Lipogranuloma of the mesentery may occur, particularly in the mesentery of the small bowel. It is characterized as a mild localized area or areas of necrosis of mesenteric or omental fat, producing a mass, but its primary cause is not known (Weeks ct al., 1963). The question may be raised that this is a form of mesenteric panniculitis (see below).

Panniculitis of the mesentery is a systemic form of panniculitis that may also occur in the abdomen where it may cause chronic and fairly severe abdominal pain not unlike that of chronic pancreatitis in many patients (Ogden et al., 1960). The pathologic findings are similar to those found in Weber-Christian disease and, in the mesentery, consist of loss of normal nodularity of fat, scattered areas of reddish-brown to yellow patches resembling fat necrosis, and abundant macrophages filled with "foamy" cytoplasm with focal collections of lymphocytes but no giant cells. The clinical course of the patient is one of relapsing pain and fever, malaise and recurrent episodes of abdominal pain with intermittent nausea. Laparotomy is occasionally necessary for diagnostic purposes but, unless intestinal obstruction secondary to adhesions is present, no specific treatment is indicated, once the diagnosis is made.

Torsion of the omentum occasionally may occur with resulting infarction of the omentum. It is caused most commonly by a distal portion becoming attached by herniation or inflammation and allowing the intermediate portion to twist. Treatment is resection.

Tumors that arise primarily in the mesentery and the omentum may be liposarcomatous, angiosarcomatous, lymphosarcomatous and fibrosarcomatous. Treatment differs from similar lesions elsewhere only if intestinal obstruction or fistula develops.

MESENTERIC THROMBOSIS

Arterial Thrombosis

Embolic occlusion of the superior mesenteric artery may be treated successfully by embolectomy. Most persons with this disease are cardiac patients with fibrillation, and the embolus usually represents the dislodgment of a mural thrombus, though a plaque or a thrombus dislodged from the aorta may also produce this disease. Depending upon the status of the circulation of the small bowel and that of its collateral channels through the celiac axis and the inferior mesenteric artery, as well as the size of the embolus and its location, the embolic result may range from simple ischemia to extensive infarction. Two places the embolus may frequently lodge in the superior mesenteric artery are just proximal to, and just distal to, the egress of the midcolic artery.

There is no clinical pattern that is diagnostic of this entity, but the suddenness of onset of abdominal pain and pain in the lumbar area, and its rapid progression, particularly when it occurs in a cardiac patient with mitral disease or fibrillation, should alert one to the possibility that an embolus to the superior mesenteric artery has occurred. Exploration should be undertaken without delay if embolectomy is to be successful and hopefully without bowel resection. Vomiting and diarrhea often accompany the onset of pain, but it is not colicky in nature unless intussusception also occurs (Harkins, 1936; Hardy, 1960). At first peristalsis may be hyperactive and, as ischemia threatens to advance to infarction, peristaltic activity diminishes and disappears. Distention is not a usual finding. In the first few hours, x-ray films disclose little or no gas in the small bowel; later, scattered pockets of gas may be evident.

Mesenteric arterial embolization in children is a rare complication of the dislodgment of a clot during operations on the heart and has also been observed following cardiac catheterization. The tendency is to consider arterial occlusion as a complication of the older age group, as this disorder in children has been recognized only recently (DeMuth, 1962).

Treatment is early operative intervention with surgical excision of the nonviable segment of bowel, which is the only treatment that will prevent death when the bowel is deprived of its arterial supply. In those patients in whom occlusion is either incomplete or located in vascular segments which collateral circulation can sustain, resection is not necessary and is perhaps contraindicated, as the intact cyanotic bowel may recover. If such bowel is resected, the healing of the anastomosis may be impaired, and it may leak a few days later. In cases of questionable viability, the bowel segment may be exteriorized and covered with a protective sterile dressing for a day or two to observe its course (Wangensteen, 1955).

Black bowel does not always indicate dead bowel; the petechial subserosal hemorrhages of contused bowel may hemolyze, become confluent, and the hematin pigments turn black. In several patients in whom the hemorrhagic bowel segment (usually the colon) was jet black but its peristaltic activity persisted, the author exteriorized the loops involved. A day or two later the color returned entirely to normal, and the bowel was obviously viable. The loops were returned to the abdomen, and the patients recovered. Black bowel is observed in the occlusion of a vein of the mesentery more often than it is in the occlusion of an artery.

With increasing awareness of the entity of superior mesenteric artery occlusion, more cases can be treated successfully by thrombectomy, endarterectomy and/or resection of the involved bowel (Glotzer and Shaw, 1959; Shaw and Maynard, 1958; Stewart *et al.*, 1960). Subsequent to the patient's recovery from arterial embolic occlusion, the author prefers to maintain the older patients on Dicumarol or a suitable derivative indefinitely if the potential sources of emboli from the heart or the aorta persist.

Superior mesenteric artery syndrome (intestinal angina) is another form of ischemia of the splanchnic arterial blood supply to the small bowel (Shaw and Maynard, 1958). Pain after eating, the result of a relative increase in the metabolic demands of the small bowel during digestion that are not associated with the usual augmentation of arterial splanchnic flow, may become so severe that the patient prefers not to eat rather than to suffer the consequence. Nearly always the blood supply from at least 2 of the 3 splanchnic arteries (the celiac, the superior mesenteric and the

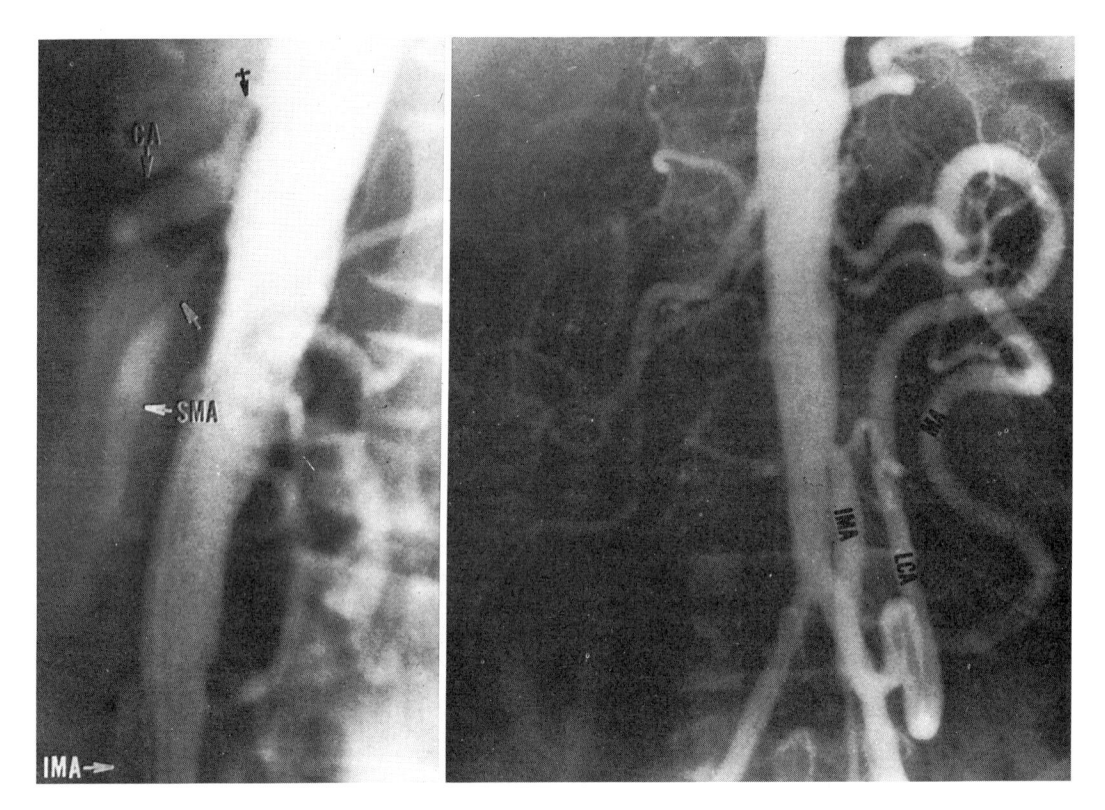

FIG. 35-8. (*Left*) Lateral view of abdominal aortogram showing marked arteriosclerotic narrowing of the celiac and superior mesenteric arteries. (*Right*) Abdominal aortogram in same patient showing marked elongation and dilatation of the marginal artery of Drummond. The collateral circulation provided by this artery was such that the small bowel circulation was adequate and the patient asymptomatic. CA—celiac artery. SMA—superior mesenteric artery. IMA—inferior mesenteric artery. LCA—left colic artery; MA—dilated marginal artery.

inferior mesenteric) must be compromised severely by atherosclerotic plaques before symptoms of angina develop. Often the marginal artery of Drummond is enlarged as shown by arteriography (Fig. 35-8). Such dilatation and elongation of the marginal artery of Drummond is diagnostic of obliterative disease of the superior mesenteric artery, as Connolly (1964) has indicated. Also, this enlargement is indicative of the necessity for protecting the inferior mesenteric artery, which may be the major source of arterial blood for the small bowel in such patients. As Connolly points out, patients with marked dilatation and elongation of Drummond's artery, despite the slow occlusion of the superior mesenteric artery, are frequently asymptomatic, and thrombo-endarterectomy or the use of a bypass graft may not be necessary (Zuidema *et al.*, 1964).

Rob (1966) points out that abdominal symptoms due to partial or total occlusion of visceral arteries are likely to increase as our population ages. It is better to operate at the stage of stenosis in order to prevent the sometimes disastrous effect of a complete arterial occlusion.

Dick *et al.* (1967) properly emphasized the importance of angiography in the investigation of obscure abdominal pain which may occasionally arise from partial occlusion of one or more of the mesenteric vessels, including the celiac axis, especially if weight loss, diarrhea, intestinal malabsorption, and intestinal angina following meals are present.

Originally it was thought that at least two

of the three major arteries to the bowel had to be occluded or markedly stenosed before symptoms were produced. Cases had been reported in which symptoms were due to occlusion of only one of the three arteries (Terpstra, 1966). Moreover, the disease may occur in relatively young individuals and may be related to partial compression of the celiac axis by the median arcuate ligament of the diaphragm. Lysis of this ligament has been performed in some of these patients and has been followed by complete relief; the follow-up, however, has been too brief, in this author's opinion, to demonstrate permanent relief by this procedure, and psychosomatic disorders have not been completely excluded. It is also true that pronounced stenosis of the celiac artery may be observed and yet no abdominal symptoms result (Drapanas, 1966).

Generally the therapeutic approach is to expose the arteries involved, to perform a thromboendarterectomy if this is feasible and, if not, to resect and use a prosthesis or a patch graft. It appears that the results have been striking where the diagnosis has been properly established, psychosomatic complaints properly evaluated, and the stenosing or occluded vessels reopened.

Mesenteric arteriolar ischemia, without necessarily threatened arterial occlusion, may occur as the result of widespread atherosclerosis of the smaller, more peripherally located branches of the mesenteric arteries (Gooding and Couch, 1962). Multiple areas of small bowel necroses, ranging from punctate ones to those several centimeters in length, are found occasionally. Malabsorption is a symptom more prominent than pain in this disease, at least until necrosis of the bowel occurs. Adler *et al.* (1962) report this form of arteritis with infarction of the bowel as a complication of rheumatoid arthritis in 2 patients, one of whom had received cortisone and the other (aged 30) had not. Both required bowel resection and were alive 2 years later, maintained on cortisone and anticoagulants. Microscopic sections of the smaller mesenteric arteries disclosed extensive atherosclerosis and inflammation. Treatment for infarction of the bowel is always surgical, though if the thrombosis of the smaller arterioles is very extensive, the results may be disappointing.

Traumatic destruction of the superior mesenteric artery poses many immediate problems, including those of multiple injuries, some of which are clean but others may be contaminated. Treatment is urgent, and restoration of the circulating blood volume may have to proceed simultaneously with an operation for repair of the artery if possible. Meyer (1962) reported an interesting case history of the destruction of the superior mesenteric artery, the result of a war wound in a 19-year-old male. The small bowel, 18 inches beyond the ligament of Treitz, was resected because of necrosis, as was the large bowel to the midportion of the transverse colon. End-to-end continuity was re-established between the upper jejunum and the distal half of the transverse colon. For 18 years, the patient has done remarkably well, considering the extent of the resection. He has maintained his weight at 125 pounds, compared wtih his pre-injury value of 145 pounds, and has experienced bouts of loose watery stools, intermittent clinical manifestation of vitamin deficiencies, and chronic macrocytic anemia. For 14 years, the author has had a similar case with the same extent of bowel resection in a 207-pound male who had embolic occlusion for 48 hours. The patient has done equally well, is now 68 years of age and weighs 210 pounds.

Acute occlusion of the inferior mesenteric artery as a complication of translumbar aortography has been reported by Guilfoil (1963), and a similarly acute syndrome may occur in some patients following resection of an abdominal aortic aneurysm. The accidents from aortography are in most instances the result of intramural, rather than of the intended intraluminal, injection of the contrast media, and in at least 8 of the 11 reported cases, the contrast media outlined perivascularly the blood supply to the descending colon. Necrosis of the descending colon and the sigmoid followed. Ordinarily, the inferior mesenteric artery can be ligated at any point without necrosis of the left colon because the anastomotic arterial supply via the inferior hypogastric and the superior mesenteric arteries is a substantial one and quite sufficient to eliminate the contributions of the inferior mesenteric artery. The most common cause of threatened or occluded patency of the inferior mesenteric artery is atherosclerosis; arterial emboli are usually larger than the lumen of this vessel. The ordinarily adequate collateral arterial sources are also apt to be severely compromised. Treatment is surgical exploration and resection of the distal third of the transverse to the lower sigmoid in accordance with what is found.

Angiomata and phlebectasia may occur in the mucosa of the intestinal tract; in this location, they are disorders of the terminal branches of the arterial or venous portions of the splanchnic circulation. At times they may bleed and, because they are small, they may be difficult to locate and remove. When found, treatment is surgical removal (Calem and Jimenez, 1963).

Aneurysms (mycotic or dissecting) may produce sufficient pain to encourage surgical exploration before bowel necrosis occurs. In some of these patients, the aneurysm may have occluded the vessel slowly and therefore usually can be ligated or excised, as adequate collateral circulation will have been established. In others, the situation may be less favorable, and in a few patients rupture of the aorta or the superior mesenteric aneurysm results in death promptly from hemorrhage or from bowel necrosis caused by dissection of the arterial wall by blood, compressing the lumen of the mesenterics.

Extent of Bowel Resection Compatible With Life. Most resections of the magnitude of the two described above are incompatible with life for more than a few months to a year in spite of careful management. Experience has shown that some patients with as much as three fourths of the small bowel resected survive to lead a normal existence after a few months (Bierman *et al.*, 1950). Usually such extensive resections are tolerated better by adults than by children. As discussed above, a number of successful resections of major portions of the small bowel, often with resection of the right colon, have been reported in recent years. Most of these patients suffer severe diarrhea for a few weeks but may appear to be able to compensate for bowel loss after a few months. Thereafter, they may have 1 to 3 liquid bowel movements a day and maintain or gain weight. On the other hand, some patients do not respond, and eventually after many months they die, in spite of vigorous medical management.

PORTAL VEIN THROMBOSIS

Factors favoring thrombosis of the vessels of the splanchnic (portal) circulation are similar to those predisposing to thrombosis in vessels elsewhere.

Stasis in unrelieved portal hypertension is a common cause of portal thrombosis. It is exemplified by the reported occurrence of thrombosis of the splenic and the portal veins after splenectomy is performed for portal hypertension of any type. A patient with the Budd-Chiari type of portal hypertension, measuring 65 cm. of water, explored by the author and with no possible site for a shunting procedure found, died on the 4th postoperative day of acute portal vein thrombosis. Presumably, the trauma of venous exposure plus stasis to hepatic vein outflow prepared the ground for the sequence of events that followed operation.

Inflammatory diseases of the bowel, such as diverticulitis, appendicitis, and secondarily infected carcinoma of the bowel, are the sources of septic mesenteric thrombophlebitis usually encountered. Such thrombi are extensive and may involve the entire portal system; or they may fragment, giving rise to septic emboli that lodge within the liver, causing intrahepatic abscess formation. Dehydration with hemoconcentration, or pronounced polycythemia with its elevated platelet levels, is occasionally associated with either thrombosis or embolic disorders in the splanchnic vesssels. The thrombotic tendency of Buerger's disease also affects the mesenteric vessels occasionally and can cause mesenteric thrombosis.

Acute venous occlusion of the portal or the superior mesenteric vein is followed promptly by hyperemia, edema and subserosal petechial hemorrhages of the infarcted segment of bowel and its mesentery. In massive venous occlusion, death from hypovolemic shock occurs usually in less than 24 hours and is believed to be due to the continuing arterial blood flow into the splanchnic bed without adequate venous drainage or return. The bowel and the mesenteric surfaces are found "weeping" serosanguineous fluid; and the patient, aside from having abdominal pain, usually has bloody diarrhea, presumably due to venous engorgement of the intestinal mucosa. Should the patient survive long enough, thrombosis of the mesenteric artery is the likely sequela.

Acute occlusion of the mesenteric arteries produces bowel necrosis without the hypovolemic disturbances seen in extensive venous thrombosis. Bloody diarrhea is less common, although abdominal pain is usually present. Death from the gangrenous bowel and its peritonitis is the usual outcome if the bowel is not resected. Of these 2 types of vascular occlusion, arterial embolic occlusion is more likely to be amenable to successful surgical treatment than is venous thrombosis.

REFERENCES

Adler, R. H., Norcross, B. M., and Lockie, L. M.: Arteritis and infarction of the intestine in rheumatoid arthritis. J.A.M.A., 180:922, 1962.

Barlow, T. E.: Vascular patterns in the alimentary canal. In Visceral Circulation (Ciba Foundation Symposium). Boston, Little, Brown & Co., 1953.

———: Variations in the blood-supply of the upper jejunum. Brit. J. Surg., 43:473, 1956.

Bierman, L. G., Ulevitch, H., Haft, H. H., and Lemish, S.: Metabolic studies of an unusual case survival following resection of all but 18 inches of small bowel. Ann. Surg., 132:64, 1950.

Boyd, J. D.: General survey of visceral vascular structures. In Visceral Circulation (Ciba Foundation Symposium). Boston, Little, Brown & Co., 1953.

Calem, W. S., and Jimenez, F. A.: Vascular malformations of intestine. Arch. Surg., 86:571, 1963.

Connolly, J. E., Abrams, H. L., and Kieraldo, J. H.: Observations on the diagnosis and treatment of obliterative disease of the visceral branches of the abdominal aorta. Arch. Surg., 90:596, 1965.

DeMuth, W. E.: Mesenteric vascular occlusion in children. J.A.M.A., 179:130, 1962.

Dick, A. P., Graff, R., Gregg, McC., Peters, N., and Sarner, M.: Arteriographic study of mesenteric arterial diseases. Gut, 8:206, 1967.

Drapanas, T., and Bron, K. M.: Editorial: Stenosis of the celiac artery. Ann. Surg., 164:1085, 1966.

Drummond, Hamilton: Some points relating to the surgical anatomy of the arterial supply of the large intestine. Proc. Roy. Soc. Med., London, 7:185, 1914.

Glotzer, D. L., and Shaw, R. S.: Massive bowel infarction: an autopsy study assessing the potentialities of reconstructive vascular surgery. New Eng. J. Med., 260:162, 1959.

Gooding, R. A., and Couch, R. D.: Mesenteric ischemia without vascular occlusion. Arch. Surg., 85:186, 1962.

Grayson, J.: Observations on the blood flow in the human intestine. In Visceral Circulation (Ciba Foundation Symposium). Boston, Little, Brown & Co., 1953.

Guilfoil, P. H.: Inferior-mesenteric-artery syndrome after translumbar aortography. New Eng. J. Med., 269:12, 1963.

Hardy, J. D.: Surgery of the aorta and its branches. Am. Pract. Digest Treat., 11:317, 1960.

Harkins, H. N.: Mesenteric vascular occlusion of arterial and venous origin. Arch. Path., 22:637, 1936.

Laufman, H., Nora, P. F., and Mittelpunkt, A. I.: Mesenteric blood vessels: Advances in surgery and physiology. Arch. Surg., 88:1021, 1964.

Meyer, H. W.: Sixteen-year survival following extensive resection of small and large intestine for thrombosis of the superior mesenteric artery. Surgery, 51:755, 1962.

Michels, N. A.: Newer anatomy of liver-variant blood supply and the collateral circulation. J.A.M.A., 172:125, 1960.

Ogden, W. W., II, Bradburn, D. M., and Rives, J. D.: Panniculitis of the mesentery. Ann. Surg., 151:659, 1960.

Rob, C.: Surgical diseases of the celiac and mesenteric arteries. Arch. Surg., 93:21, 1966.

Shaw, R. S., and Maynard, E. P.: Acute and chronic thrombosis of the mesenteric arteries associated with malabsorption: A report of two cases treated successfully by thromboendarterectomy. New Eng. J. Med., 258:874, 1958.

Spanner, R.: The artero-venous anastomoses in the intestine. Anat. Anz., Supp., pp. 24-26, 1931.

Stewart, G. D., Sweetman, W. R., Westphal, K., and Wise, R. A.: Superior mesenteric artery embolectomy. Ann. Surg., 151:274, 1960.

Terpstra, J. L.: Intestinal angina secondary to compression of the celiac axis. Arch. Chir. Neerl., 18: 245, 1966.

Walder, D.: Some observations on the blood flow of the human stomach. In Visceral Circulation Ciba Foundation Symposium, Boston, Little, Brown & Co., 1953.

Wangensteen, O. H.: Intestinal Obstructions. ed. 3. pp. 789-790. Springfield, Ill., Charles C Thomas, 1955.

Weeks, L. E., Block, M. A., Hathaway, J. C., Jr., and Rinaldo, J. A.: Lipogranuloma of mesentery producing abdominal mass. Arch. Surg., 86:615, 1963.

Zuidema, G. D.: Surgical management of superior mesenteric arterial emboli. Arch. Surg., 82:267, 1961.

Zuidema, G. D., Reed, D., Turcotte, J. G., and Fry, W. J.: Superior mesenteric artery embolectomy. Ann. Surg., 159:548, 1964.

CHAPTER 36

J. GARROTT ALLEN, M.D.

Portal Hypertension and Ascites

Portal hypertension is a complex syndrome that may or may not be associated with ascites or with liver disease. Similarly, ascites need not be associated with primary or secondary liver disease.

If portal hypertension persists, esophageal varices usually develop. The problem with portal hypertension is that by the time such varices bleed, the patient often has also developed other very severe metabolic disturbances of the liver that are not amenable to treatment. Hence surgical correction of the bleeding varices in patients with advanced liver disease may be life-saving at the moment, but within a year or two death may supervene from liver failure.

In the United States, cirrhosis of the liver is largely associated with alcoholism. Approximately 90 per cent of patients dying with cirrhosis die from Laennec's or alcoholics' cirrhosis. In 1965 there were approximately 22,200 deaths attributed to this disease alone and its complications.* If untreated, one third die of hemorrhage.

Many of the surgical aspects of portal hypertension were reviewed in detail by Child (1964).

DEFINITION AND DIAGNOSIS

Portal hypertension is a syndrome characterized by esophagogastric varices and splenomegaly, caused by the increase in portal pressure, and often accompanied by hepatomegaly and ascites. The varices may bleed with exsanguinary vigor, and frequently this is the first manifestation of the existence of portal hypertension. In some patients the splenomegaly may create serious problems in secondary hypersplenism (see p. 958). Because there usually is serious impairment of liver function, hepatic coma and death from liver failure may occur. The ascites, as well as the liver disease and the hemorrhaging varix, can contribute to severe nutritional and metabolic disorders, which often are lethal.

Portal hypertension is associated most frequently with hepatic cirrhosis. As a clinical entity, portal hypertension is fairly easy to diagnose, although the primary nature of its pathology is not necessarily clear or well defined. Usually, the diagnosis may be suspected, or should be considered, in any patient suffering from upper gastrointestinal hemorrhage; the history or the finding of liver disease should increase the index of suspicion that "silent" portal hypertension may exist in these patients, and that a bleeding varix is the source of blood loss. Bleeding varices account for the points of origin of acute upper gastrointestinal hemorrhage in 15 to 25 per cent of all patients over the age of 30. Accuracy of diagnosis is very helpful in the bleeding patient preoperatively, but it may not be possible to carry out the necessary tests because the patient is frequently too ill and the necessity to secure hemostasis so urgent that the diagnosis may have to be established at operation or later.

In children and young adults with massive gastrointestinal hemorrhage, the likelihood that the bleeding point is from a varix is much greater than in the older age group. One factor which seems to be responsible for this difference is that peptic ulcer accounts for about 80 per cent of all massive bleeding from the upper gastrointestinal tract in adults, and that peptic ulcer is a comparatively rare disease among children and adults under 20 years of age. Another factor is that some of the causes of portal hypertension, hence the bleeding varix, either are congenital or are acquired in early life. Many of these young patients do not live to adult life or much beyond.

---

* *Alcoholism,* U. S. Dept. of Health, Education & Welfare, Sept. 23, 1965.

ANATOMIC CAUSES OF PORTAL HYPERTENSION

Most patients with portal hypertension also suffer from liver disease, although in about 10 per cent of cases portal hypertension is caused by occlusion of the portal or of the splenic vein external to the liver. The site of venous constriction or occlusion creating portal hypertension is rarely, with the exception of cardiac failure, located in the hepatic veins or above them in the inferior vena cava. Therefore, the customary sites lend themselves to an anatomic classification of the causes of portal hypertension, which are suprahepatic, intrahepatic and subhepatic. Nearly 80 per cent of all cases of portal hypertension in this country are intrahepatic. The treatment depends on the cause, which may be determined by one or more forms of roentgenographic visualization of the portal system, and by needle biopsy of the liver supplementing studies on its functional capacity.

Intrahepatic Portal Hypertension. The most commonly encountered cause in the United States is Laënnec's cirrhosis, though there is an increasing number of patients with so-called postnecrotic cirrhosis, which also may give rise to portal hypertension with esophageal-gastric bleeding from varices. Among the causes of postnecrotic hepatitis are the various hepatotoxins and viral hepatitis, but the pathologic findings are so similar that a distinction on this basis alone is usually not possible. Prominent among the causes of cirrhosis with portal hypertension and bleeding in the tropics is *Schistosoma mansoni* or *Schistosoma japonicum* infection. Ova from these parasites lodge in the portal triads or in the intrahepatic radicles where they give rise to the formation of granuloma with enlargement of the liver; esophageal varices and hemorrhage are frequent complications of this form of cirrhosis and portal hypertension. If the patient is well nourished, hepatic failure is uncommon in this disease, though bleeding from varices is a prominent complication and, unless treated, may be fatal. Another group of causes of cirrhosis giving rise to portal hypertension and bleeding varices are the various forms of biliary or obstructive cirrhosis, whether congenital or acquired. Some are idiopathic or cryptogenic.

These same forms of cirrhosis also may exist in children, but certain additional types of liver disease not often seen in adult life also must be considered. Among these are hepatic agenesis or atrophy, including the so-called Cruveilhier-Baumgarten syndrome. Hepatic atrophy in this syndrome is attributed to a congenital communication between the portal and the systemic circulations through the patent umbilical vein. The reduced flow of portal blood through the liver is believed to cause atrophy or agenesis of the liver. An explanation that is equally or more plausible would seem to be the failure of the umbilical vein to undergo its usual postnatal fibrosis because of the existence of intrahepatic portal hypertension at the time of birth, presumably from hepatic agenesis or cirrhosis acquired *in utero*. Both of these conditions do occur and should favor the development of collateral venous circulation *in utero* at a time in life when the umbilical vein is still patent and in direct communication with the portal vein. Should agenesis or atrophy of the liver occur *in utero*, it may be anticipated that the channel most likely to shunt the portal circulation to the systemic circulation would be the umbilical vein, and in doing so it would form extensive communications with the systemic veins in the anterior abdominal wall. In a few adult patients with portal hypertension, the recanalization of the umbilical vein and its ability to form collaterals with those of the abdominal wall also seem to occur.

The interesting and diagnostic clinical feature in the Cruveilhier-Baumgarten syndrome is the venous hum and thrill usually detectable in the veins of the abdominal wall near the umbilicus.

Subhepatic portal vein obstruction is encountered more commonly in children and young adults than in older people. Usually, it is referred to as Banti's syndrome. If portal vein occlusion alone is responsible for portal hypertension, the liver appears to be perfectly normal. In rare instances, only the splenic vein may be thrombosed, leaving the superior mesenteric and the portal veins intact and normally patent. It is in this small group of patients that splenectomy has proved to be curative at times. The importance of splenoportography to ascertain the patency of the splenic and the portal veins is apparent.

The cause of portal vein occlusion in the young probably is inflammation, although no specific etiologic agent can be implicated. Much of the gross pathology observed at operation or autopsy suggests the basic disturbance to be one of a chronic phlebitis, with progressive obliteration of the major veins of the portal system. Cavernous segments of the portal vein or its major radicals are seen frequently. In many areas of the peripheral portal system, the veins appear to be relatively normal and uninvolved.

In most young patients with subhepatic portal hypertension, numerous enlarged and chronically inflamed lymph nodes are found along the course of the portal vein or adjacent to it, particularly in the upper abdomen at the junction of the superior mesenteric and the splenic veins, and in the retroperitoneum of this area. The peritoneum in these same regions usually is chronically inflamed.

Certainly, the causes of these inflammatory changes are not known; indeed, one cannot be certain that the phlebitis, the periphlebitis and the venous occlusion are the primary cause of this type of subhepatic portal hypertension or the sequelae of another. One may postulate a low-grade phlebitis arising shortly after birth from a postnatal omphalitis which extends from the umbilical vein into the portal as one possibility; another is that of a phlebitic process beginning in the portal system in childhood and secondary to some other intra-abdominal disease, such as mesenteric adenitis, regional enteritis or ulcerative colitis. At best these are highly speculative suggestions as to the otherwise unexplained origin of portal hypertension in early life.

Suprahepatic portal hypertension may result from chronic passive congestion whether due to right heart failure, constrictive pericarditis, or compression of the inferior vena cava above the hepatic veins. Regardless of which of these suprahepatic mechanisms is involved, the effect is the classic picture of cardiac cirrhosis. Varices may occur with the portal hypertension from right heart failure or pulmonary hypertension but, if the primary cardiac or pulmonary disease is amenable to medical therapy, disappearance of the varices results, and, if not responsive to medical treatment, the patient usually dies of his primary disease before his varices bleed.

Obstruction of the hepatic veins may occur from thrombosis or compression by tumor above the liver. The condition known as the Budd-Chiari syndrome is caused by idiopathic thrombosis with obliteration of the hepatic veins. It is characterized by the prompt appearance of extensive ascites and huge esophageal varices. The resulting increases in portal pressure are among the highest readings encountered in portal hypertension from any cause, in contrast with the relatively mild portal hypertension secondary to cardiac or pulmonary disease. The microscopic appearance of the liver in the Budd-Chiari syndrome is very similar to that of cardiac cirrhosis, though some extension of the thrombosis may be found in some of the central veins of the liver lobules, as well as in the portal vein. There is seldom an opportunity to employ a portal caval shunt for the relief of this type of portal hypertension, and death usually occurs within a few weeks after the symptomatic onset of the disease.

The cause of cirrhosis usually determines the benefit of surgical correction of portal hypertension. Portal hypertension may persist long after the cirrhotic process has become inactive. In these patients, shunting procedures are very worthwhile because, with progressive liver disease not a problem, the correction of portal hypertension avoids death from bleeding esophagogastric varices. On the other hand, little may be accomplished by the surgical relief of portal hypertension in the ligation of bleeding esophageal varices in patients with advanced alcoholic cirrhosis because their drinking patterns often continue. In addition, it appears that in some patients the cirrhotic process in Laënnec's disease seems to continue irrespective of abstinence from alcohol and the practice of improved dietary habits. Thus, our methods for the correction of portal hypertension and bleeding are more effective than are our methods of treatment of cirrhosis and alcoholism.

Many of the patients, by the time they have developed extensive cirrhosis with either bleeding varices or ascites or both, have also developed other complications due to impending liver failure and portal hypertension. Among these are umbilical hernia, due to extensive abdominal distention; cancer of the breast, presumably because of an accumulation of steroids in the blood that would normally be esterified within the liver; diabetes, which is thought to be due to an impairment of glycogen storage within the liver and, at times, complicated by chronic pancreatitis associated with alcoholism; and polyarthralgia, which most characteristically affects the shoulders.

There are only two reasons that surgery is applied to patients with portal hypertension from cirrhosis: first, to prevent or to treat hemorrhage; second, to treat the complication of ascites when it occurs, if unmanageable medically. There is no reason to expect that either of these operations will alter the course of the liver disease itself, for they do not. There are, however, many kinds of cirrhoses and many causes for them. Knowledge is so insufficient in this field that most clinicians recognize only three kinds of cirrhosis: alcoholic, postnecrotic and cryptogenic. However, any disease that may affect the liver can result in latent fibrosis and cirrhosis. In this country and in certain European countries, it is alcoholic cirrhosis that is the most difficult to treat because no one has yet solved the problem of the treatment of alcoholism (Table 36-1).

Unfortunately, most of those writing on the subject do not classify their cases of cirrhosis according to etiology. Until the importance of the pathology of the underlying liver disease is recognized, the internist and the surgeon will continue to be confused as to whether surgery is advantageous or not.

There seems little question that bleeding episodes can be stopped by an appropriate shunt, but if the liver substance continues to

TABLE 36-1. PER CENT DISTRIBUTION OF 2 PRINCIPAL CAUSES OF CIRRHOSIS AND PORTAL HYPERTENSION

	ALCOHOLIC	CRYPTOGENIC
London*	25	75
Boston†	83	17
New York‡	71	29

* Sherlock, S. 1968.
† Garceau et al., 1964.
‡ Panke et al., 1968.

TABLE 36-2. THE BENEFIT OF PROPHYLACTIC AND THERAPEUTIC SHUNTING IN PATIENTS WITH VARICES AND CIRRHOSIS*

OCCURRENCE OF HEMORRHAGE (per cent of cases)

	WITH SHUNTING		
	THERAPEUTIC	PROPHYLACTIC	UNTREATED
Splenorenal	19.0%	—	26%
Portacaval	2.8%	1.5%	

* Data from Grace, N. D., Muench, H., and Chalmers, T. C.: The present status of shunts for portal hypertension in cirrhosis. Gastroenterol., 50:684, 1966.

deteriorate, the patient will die of hepatic failure. However, in cases such as cirrhosis associated with ulcerative colitis, schistosomiasis, and, in many instances, so-called post hepatitis cirrhosis, prevention of hemorrhage may indeed extend substantially the life of the patient.

The experience of Grace et al. (1966) with therapeutic and prophylactic shunts for the control of hemorrhage is shown in Table 36-2. The mystery, however, is how many of these patients would ordinarily die from a hemorrhagic episode if untreated. It is this part of the analysis of any series which remains unknown. Can it be that when a patient begins to hemorrhage he is operated upon and therefore is transferred to the surgery category?

Distribution of Esophagogastric Varices and Their Tendency to Bleed. Portal vein pressure ordinarily is expressed as centimeters of water and is measured by the insertion of a needle into one of the tributaries of the portal vein or better, into the vein itself, at the time of operation. It may be measured as splenic pulp pressure by introduction of a needle percutaneously without significant risk of bleeding, or it can be measured as wedge pressure by a percutaneously placed intravenous catheter threaded through the cephalic vein under fluoroscopic control into the hepatic vein. Normal pressures range between 10 to 20 cm. of water; in portal hypertension with extensive esophageal varices, the pressure is often between 30 and 50 cm. of water. These are useful measurements, and the errors are nearly always on the low side, usually because the pressures are measured with the patient under sedation or anesthesia, both of which may reduce portal venous pressure as well as systemic arterial pressure.

The demonstrated presence of esophageal varices implies portal hypertension, though for technical reasons measurements of portal venous pressure may not always disclose an elevated reading at the time of measurement. The rare occurrence of an arteriovenous fistula involving the portal vein is the only other known cause of an elevated portal venous pressure.

The distribution of major radicles of the portal vein may vary extensively. These variations seem to account for the several different "normal patterns" that are described in textbooks of gross anatomy. More nearly accurate anatomic descriptions have become available only as the surgical control of portal hypertension has developed; many of these variations are summarized clearly by Child (1964).

The usual sites of bleeding are the varices at the lower end of the esophagus, which are the distal tributaries of the coronary (left gastric) vein. This vein normally drains the lesser curvature and fundus of the stomach and the lower two thirds of the esophagus. These also anastomose with the splenic vein via the vasa brevia of the stomach and the gastroepiploic vessels so that control of back pressure is not obtained by ligation of the coronary vein. While varices may be equally prominent in the upper stomach, the gastric mucosa overlying gastric varices appears to be more substantial than the overlying squamous epithelium of the esophagus; presumably, this is the reason gastric varices are less likely to bleed than esophageal varices.

Five collateral venous channels, in addition to those between the coronary and the esophageal veins, may be drawn upon to assist in the natural decompression of portal hypertension. Seldom if ever are they effective, and for the most part we are concerned with their presence because of the increased vascularity and hemorrhage encountered at operation. They are these: (1) the esophageal anastomoses between the coronary or left gastric vein and the azygos system; (2) hemorrhoidal communications from inferior mesenteric vein and middle and inferior hemorrhoidal veins to the hypogastric system; (3) channels between the retroperitonealized portions of the duodenum, the pancreas, the ascending and the descending colon (veins of Retzius), and the perirenal and the lumbar veins; (4) channels between pancreatic and splenic veins and the renal veins; and (5) the accessory portal veins (veins of Sappey) which include the deep cystic vein, the vaso vasorum of the hepatic artery and of the inferior vena cava, veins in the triangular ligament and the surface of the liver which, as they become engorged, collateralize via the umbilicus with the superior hypogastric veins and account for the caput medusae. Of these 5 pathways, the veins of Retzius and those of Sappey are usually the most significant, aside from the collaterals between the coronary and the esophageal veins which, of course, are the largest and account for the esophagogastric varices.

What initiates bleeding in esophageal varices is not known. Baronofsky (1949) suggested that regurgitation of gastric juice into the esophagus in the patient with varices was a frequent occurrence and produced a chemical esophagitis that provoked superficial erosion over the varices and exposed the distended esophageal veins to acid-peptic digestion. Orloff et al. (1963), in a biopsy study of patients at the time of surgical treatment of bleeding esophageal varices, found no histologic evidence of peptic esophagitis in 19 of 20 consecutive patients whose bleeding varices were caused by portal hypertension from Laënnec's cirrhosis. It may be that bleeding occurs because of the increased venous pressure alone. The varices do not disappear after successful portacaval shunting; they only collapse when the shunt successfully reduces the portal pressure. Also, there is no evidence to suggest that esophageal varices predispose to regurgitant peptic esophagitis.

PATHOGENESIS OF ASCITES IN PORTAL HYPERTENSION

Ascites, except for modest fluid accumulations found at operation, usually is not detectable by clinical examination in patients with subhepatic portal hypertension if the liver is otherwise normal and other causes do not exist. Usually, subhepatic portal occlusion in middle or late life is from tumor invasion or its compression of the larger radicles of the portal system. Tumors of the kidney (the hypernephroma in particular), carcinoma of the stomach, the pancreas and the common bile duct, metastatic tumors, abdominal lymphomas, or tumors of the stomach and the duodenum are many of those conditions producing portal hypertension without cirrhosis of the liver. Tumor obstruction of the portal vein, even when complete, usually results in only mild increases in portal venous pressure and, infrequently, in the formation of a few small varices. Under these conditions, the bleeding varix is seldom encountered, and death from the malignancy usually supervenes. On the other hand, migratory phlebitis of the portal system may occur in the adult and, as in children, result in severe portal hypertension and varices which may bleed.

Many studies tend to confirm the importance of diminished sodium excretion in the urine, in sweat, saliva and in the stool in the formation of ascites in cirrhosis. The reason is largely because of an inappropriate increase in aldosterone, due on one hand to a 10- to 15-fold increase of its production by the adrenal cortex and, in the case of cirrhosis, to a great delay in its metabolism by the liver. The retention of sodium leads to an increase in extracellular water (see p. 1005).

It appears that the decrease in aldosterone is much more pronounced with the side-to-side anastomosis than with an end-to-side. This return of aldosterone to normal values is accompanied also by a return of serum sodium to normal values.

While many of these patients may be successfully handled by the appropriate use of diuretics and the limitation of salt intake, the ones in the New York series had had substantial medical trials under hospital control preoperatively for 3 months to 10 years, with a mean of 12.6 months. Their series of 63 patients was carried out through the years 1961 to 1967. In the summer of 1968 60 per cent were known to be alive. In more than 90 per cent of the patients in this series, prevention of variceal hemorrhage and amelioration of resistant ascites were also achieved.

The cause of ascites is obviously more complex than the mechanism described, because the stimulus for this form of secondary aldosteronism does not begin until other causes favoring edema or ascites have developed— i.e., increased venous pressure or diminished concentration of serum albumin, probably both. The plasma volume is then sacrificed extravagantly at the expense of the formation of edema and ascitic fluid. The reduction in renal blood flow stimulates the release of renin from the juxtaglomerular apparatus leading to increased circulating levels of angiotensin II (Davis, 1964) which stimulate hypersecretory rates of aldosterone production.

It is not clear why hypertension does not develop in the cirrhotic patient from the increase in angiotensin levels when the same increase would ordinarily produce hypertension in the patient with primary aldosteronism. Potassium-wasting disease is a prominent feature in primary aldosteronism (adrenal tumor), although it is inconspicuous or absent in the cirrhotic patient as long as his sodium excretion is low, but wasting may develop if diuretics are administered (Luetscher, 1964) or if repeated paracenteses are performed.

The formation of ascites is obviously complex and is probably the result of several factors, including those detailed above, especially the influences of the increased hydrostatic pressure and reduced colloid osmotic pressure from hypoalbuminemia and possibly others. In most patients with portal hypertension from tumor, ascites is caused by local peritoneal reaction from tumor implants which may also secrete mucin or extracellular water.

Increased hydrostatic pressure within the sinusoidal circulation of the liver, whether from superhepatic obstruction to the venous outflow of the liver or from intrahepatic obstruction, undoubtedly initiates and perpetuates the formation of ascites. An additional factor contributing to the formation of ascites is the reduced colloidal osmotic pressure in the circulation when serum albumin is reduced in liver disease. These facts suggest the possibility that the increased hydrostatic pressure may result in an increase in the rate of formation of hepatic lymph and its flow rate. Under these conditions, the concentration of protein in the lymph may approach that of the proteins of plasma. In effect, the accumulation of ascitic fluid in cirrhotics with portal hypertension resembles more an active exudative process than a passive transudate.

In a series of experimental studies, Drapanas et al. (1960) demonstrated that after partial constriction of the hepatic veins not only was there a sharp increase in the collateral venous circulation as chronic ascites developed but also an increase in the lymphatic channels in the region of the hilum of the liver, which were prominently distended and tortuous. This group observed beads of lymph accumulating on the surface of the liver much the same as on the surface of the intestine after partial occlusion of its venous drainage. An analysis of the protein content in lymph and ascitic fluid in this form of subacute ascites is as follows:

PROTEIN CONCENTRATIONS IN GRAMS PER CENT IN ASCITIC FLUID IN DOG 31

	TOTAL PROTEIN	ALBUMIN	GLOBULIN
Plasma	6.9	1.7	5.2
Lymph	6.0	1.6	4.4
Ascitic fluid	4.8	1.4	3.4

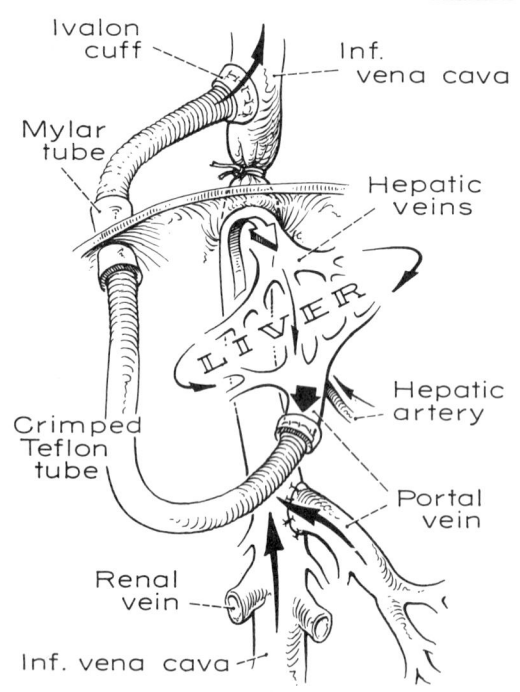

FIG. 36-1. Operative procedure used to reverse flow of blood through liver. (David, C., Bollman, J. L., Grindlay, J. H., and Hallenbeck, G. A.: An experimental study of the effectiveness of the portal vein as a hepatic outflow tract. Surg., Gynec., Obstet., 117:67, 1963)

Flow measurements disclosed that for the normal animal the total hepatic blood flow (venous and arterial) was about 40 ml. per minute per kilo of body weight; one third of this was arterial, and two thirds was venous in origin. Curiously, these flow rates were not altered by the partial occlusion that they employed to produce ascites. However, these authors reported that the total hepatic blood flow was diminished in a patient with portal hypertension and that, after a successful portal caval shunt, the rate of blood flow in the hepatic artery was doubled.

David, Bollman et al. (1963) confirmed the experimental observations of Drapanas and also provided experimental data in support of McDermott's clinical experience. It will be recalled that with substantial constriction of the hepatic veins in the dog, ascites routinely develops. The preparation of David and Bollman was first to ligate in the dog the inferior vena cava just above the point of entrance of the hepatic veins; therefore, they obstructed both the portal and the systemic venous return below this point. Then a long vascular prosthesis was introduced into the proximal end of the portal vein and carried through the diaphragm above the liver and anastomosed with the inferior vena cava just *above* the point of its previous ligation. By this procedure the portal circulation and the total systemic venous blood below the diaphragm were shunted retrogradely through the liver and, with the aid of the bypass, into the inferior vena cava above the point of ligation. The splanchnic venous return was also included in this diversion because the distal end of the divided portal vein was anastomosed as the usual end-to-side portal caval shunt (Fig. 36-1). Ascites did not develop in any of the animals unless the vascular anastomoses were occluded later by thrombosis. An interesting additional point in their observations was that these animals developed none of the symptoms of meat intoxication associated with the formation of Eck fistula. It is also interesting that the complete reversal of flow did not in itself create obstructive symptoms, that the metabolic function of the liver did not appear grossly disturbed in this preparation, and that in adding the venous flow from the inferior vena cava, which is approximately twice that of the portal vein, the total retrograde circulation was approximately 3 times that of the normal portal flow.

Lymph flow in the thoracic duct in cirrhotic patients appears to be implicated in the formation of ascites and in the presence of portal hypertension. For example, in patients with Laënnec's cirrhosis but with normal subclavian venous pressure, the thoracic duct may be greatly distended with lymph under 30 to 70 cm. of water pressure, and flow rate is greatly increased. After cannulation of the duct with relief of pressure, the ascites disappeared, the liver diminished in size, and portal pressure was reduced (Dumont and Mulholland, 1962). When the cannula was removed, ascites returned, the liver enlarged, and portal pressure increased. The significance of these observations remains to be seen.

THE NATURAL HISTORY OF PATIENTS WITH ESOPHAGO-GASTRIC VARICES

Survival studies among patients with portal hypertension and varices are essential to establish the contribution of surgery to the relief of the bleeding varix. Some data are available,* but more are needed to arrive at definite conclusions, particularly as to any merits that prophylactic surgical decompression in portal hypertension may have, because surgical intervention at the time of a bleeding episode is difficult and carries a substantially higher mortality than when carried out as an interval or elective procedure. Obviously, important considerations are the underlying cause of cirrhosis, whether the process continues to be active or stationary, and what the capacity is of the liver to perform its essential metabolic functions. The report of Resnick, Chalmers and the Boston Inter-Hospital Liver Group (1969) is of interest because it is concerned with studies in an ongoing or prospective, rather than retrospective, group of cirrhotic patients. In an earlier study of 471 patients, 390 (83%) suffered from alcoholism which presumably was the cause of their cirrhosis and varices. The cause in the other 17 per cent is not given. The clinical features of the total group are shown in Table 36-3.

At the time of the Boston report, 253 of the 471 under study had died of the causes

Annotations. Lancet, 1:1076, 1968.

TABLE 36-3. CLINICAL FEATURES IN 471 PATIENTS WITH ESOPHAGEAL VARICES

FEATURE	No. OF CASES	PERCENTAGE
Ascites	383	81
Jaundice	367	78
Coma or precoma	285	61
Triad of ascites, jaundice & coma	217	46
Spider angiomas	330	70
Palpable spleen	240	51
Significant hemorrhage	238	51
Peptic ulcer	71	15
Diabetes mellitus	25	5

TABLE 36-4. MODES OF DEATH IN UNTREATED PATIENTS

CAUSE OF DEATH	No. OF CASES	PERCENTAGE
Hemorrhage	86	34
Hepatic failure	82	32
Renal shutdown when all else seemed stable	27	11
Infection	22	9
Indeterminate & other	36	14
Totals	253	100

listed in Table 36-4. Although unequivocal varices were present in all, death from hemorrhage accounted for only one third of all deaths; another third died in hepatic failure without hemorrhage; and another third died of conditions often associated with hepatic failure but without objective evidence of hemorrhage.

In spite of better treatment available, "the survival is only 30 to 40 per cent at one year, a rate quite comparable to that for acute lymphocytic leukemia." Of the 253 deaths reported, 180 (71%) died during the first 6 months of observation; another 19 patients died the second 6 months; and 26 more died during the second 12 months. The fact is obvious that many of the patients in this group were acutely ill with advanced liver disease at the time they entered the study, that the vast majority suffered from far-advanced Laënnec's cirrhosis, and, as the Boston group points out, the return to alcoholism was high among patients discharged from the hospital. This study, while very useful, does not answer the question of how much longer patients with cirrhosis and varices will survive if bleeding from varices is prevented or treated successfully by portacaval shunts to correct portal hypertension, or if in addition the function of the liver in some manner could be improved. Presumably, shunts performed successfully could prevent about one third of deaths occurring in patients with alcoholic cirrhosis if their liver disease were not progressive. However, the Boston data (Garceau et al., 1964) and the earlier studies of Ratnoff and Patek (1942) suggest that death from esophageal hemorrhage may be a late or nearly preterminal event in the seemingly unrelenting clinical course of advanced Laënnec's cirrhosis. The question that cannot be answered yet is what is the recovery power of the liver when associated with alcoholism if the patient never again drinks alcohol. Sherlock (1968) expresses a more encouraging viewpoint than most in the United States for this group of alcoholic patients.

The story is quite different for survival when bleeding from the esophageal varices is due to extrahepatic portal block. Although the incidence of hemorrhage from varices is much higher in this group of patients, presumably because hepatic function is normal, survival rates are greatly increased. Similarly, the risk of mortality from repeated hemorrhages from esophageal varices is considerably less in patients with extrahepatic portal block than when the varices are due to cirrhosis. Similar data have been reported by Patton (1963).

It seems probable that, in addition to the significance of impaired nutrition in the genesis of Laënnec's cirrhosis, there are both direct and indirect metabolic actions of alcohol upon the liver, which Isselbacher and Greenberg (1964) reported.

DIAGNOSIS

The diagnosis of portal hypertension always must include a search for liver disease and an evaluation of hepatic function, secondary hypersplenism, a careful evaluation of renal function and of the patient's general health. As most effective operative procedures for the relief of portal hypertension are rather formidable in magnitude, all reasonable possibilities for evaluating the patient's general condition and hepatic function should be explored prior to the decision as to the treatment to be followed.

When liver disease is present, the symptoms may be anorexia, weakness, fatigability and impotence, and there is often a history of alcoholism or other antecedent factors (hepatitis, hepatotoxins, biliary surgical procedures, etc.). The findings may include the appearance of "spider" nevi on the chest and arms, eyelid retraction and lid lag, palmar erythema and liver flap, muscle wasting, loss of axillary and pubic hair, gynecomastia, testicular atrophy, distention of inferior and superior epigastric veins, the caput medusae, ascites, jaundice, ecchymosis if secondary hypersplenism is present, enlarged liver and enlarged spleen.

Of these findings, distention of the abdominal veins, the caput medusae and the palpable spleen, with or without ecchymoses, are the principal findings of uncomplicated or subhepatic portal block.

THE ONSET OF THE CLINICAL HISTORY

The onset of the clinical history of portal hypertension in the otherwise asymptomatic patient often has for its outstanding feature a massive bout of hematemesis. Patients who bleed from gastric or duodenal ulcer also may bleed massively (see Chap. 31, Stomach and Duodenum); but in the case of the bleeding duodenal ulcer the quantity of blood vomited is likely to be less than when bleeding is from either the esophageal varix or the gastric ulcer, even though the total quantity of blood lost is the same or greater. Usually this clinical pattern is explained on the basis that much or most of the blood lost from the bleeding duodenal ulcer tends to continue downward in the small bowel rather than to back up and enter the stomach. Blood from the bleeding varix or a gastric ulceration tends to accumulate within the stomach and to cause rapid distention which induces massive hematemesis.

In most patients, especially those suffering from symptoms of heart or liver disease, diagnostic evidence of portal hypertension is obtained by searching for signs of portal hypertension in the course of the general work-up. Not infrequently, patients with portal hypertension present themselves to the doctor because of unexplained weight gain in spite of a drawn facies or because of a recent increase in girth, obvious ascites, or the recent detection of mild to moderate icterus. A few will have noted an enlarged liver and/or spleen, which may or may not cause distress, but such findings alarm the patient and prompt him to seek his physician's advice.

Preceding episodes of viral hepatitis, "toxic" hepatitis, or cirrhosis can be elicited among a few patients with portal hypertension. Of some interest in this connection are the histories of 8 patients operated on by the author for portal hypertension that developed several years after the onset of nonspecific ulcerative colitis. Four of these received multiple transfusions of blood in previous years; the others did not. It is possible that the cirrhotic and portal hypertensive states in these patients represented latent manifesations of serum hepatitis, or that the virus of infectious hepatitis can and did enter the portal circulation more readily in ulcerative colitis patients than in the normal individual, or that the hepatitis and the cirrhosis were primarily a problem of malnutrition or of "auto-immune disease" and possibly an associated increased susceptibility to virus hepatitis, or that during the active stage of the disease, the colon allowed the absorption of other substances capable of producing cirrhosis.

The Physical Examination

The physical examination, when the portal hypertension is of the *suprahepatic* variety, almost always discloses 3 important corollaries. These are hepatomegaly, splenomegaly and massive ascites.

Ascites presents a special problem in diagnosis and treatment, as well as in establishing its etiology both clinically and experimentally. The association of ascites with suprahepatic portal hypertension is present so reliably that its absence, when other evidence of portal hypertension is present (hepatomegaly, splenomegaly and demonstrable esophageal varices), is usually sufficient evidence to question or to eliminate the Budd-Chiari syndrome from consideration.

Although Burchell *et al.* (1968) have reported an impressive series of results for the treatment of cirrhosis ascites in 63 patients using the side-to-side shunt, it is to be pointed out that the medical treatment of ascites is perhaps the one therapeutic advance in cirrhosis that has been developed within the past 8 to 10 years. More effective diuretics have been developed and the use of low sodium diet has proved effective in many patients.

Patients with portal hypertension of *intrahepatic* origin nearly always have splenomegaly, but they may or may not have ascites. Extensive ascites is a more common accompaniment of advanced portal cirrhosis than when the liver disease is from other causes or is less severe, though ascites may be encountered in all types and stages of liver disease. Extensive ascites is rare indeed in patients with subhepatic portal vein obstruction; the presence of moderate to large accumulations of ascitic fluid in patients with portal hypertension and without evidence of heart or renal disease, or of malnutrition, should direct attention first to the liver as its cause, second to the Budd-Chiari syndrome, and third, if at all, to subhepatic portal vein occlusion as the cause of the portal hypertension.

Peripheral edema is not likely to be present in patients with a moderate degree of hepatic cirrhosis if they do not also have ascites or hypoproteinemia. In general, the cirrhosis is associated with sodium retention, hypoalbuminemia and possibly to some extent an increased intra-abdominal pressure upon the inferior vena cava from ascites. This combination can easily induce edema. Edema may involve the sacral area and the back, as well as the lower extremities, in patients who are bedridden.

Splenomegaly is present nearly always in portal hypertension, whether or not liver enlargement is present. However, before the enlarged spleen may be palpable, it usually must be enlarged from 2 to 3 times its normal size, except in infants. If it remains posterior as it enlarges, it may not be felt in spite of its increased size. In the abdomen distended with ascitic fluid, even very large spleens may not be palpable until the fluid is removed. Assessment of splenic size by percussion is subject to many errors and has little merit when evaluated in the face of operative or autopsy findings. Some have sought to determine the size of the liver or the spleen by the use of pneumoperitoneum, wherein air contrast about these organs outlines them upon roentgenographic films. Information provided by such ancillary procedures is seldom of great importance, either to the diagnosis or to the treatment to be followed.

Icterus may or may not be present in patients with long-standing portal hypertension from chronic liver disease. When present and of intrahepatic origin, it is a sign of need for caution. Usually, icterus infers the presence of an active or a subacute form of hepatitis or cholangitis; otherwise, it infers extensive replacement of liver cells by fibrous tissue. In either instance the patient's prognosis is likely to be poor unless obstructed by stones.

Cutaneous and subcutaneous venous collaterals may be evident in many patients with portal hypertension from any cause, especially in those who are thin and malnourished. As the circulating blood volume usually is reduced to 75 per cent or less its normal value during periods of active formation of ascitic fluid, the systemic veins, including the collaterals, may not seem to be as distended as they did before ascites began to appear. The extent of collateral vein development can be demonstrated easily by means of infrared photography. The presence or the absence of internal hemorrhoids from the increased pressure transmitted to them through the superior hemorrhoidal vein seldom is cause for some consideration of the existence of portal hypertension should other findings be absent. Patients with portal hypertension frequently also have hemorrhoids, but hemorrhoids are encountered so commonly that their presence without other evidence is little reason to suspect portal hypertension.

ROENTGENOLOGIC DIAGNOSTIC AIDS

The presence of portal hypertension is inferred diagnostically by the fluoroscopic demonstration of esophageal and/or gastric varices. During early phases of portal hypertension, esophageal varices may not be evident; thus a negative fluoroscopic result does not always exclude the possibility of portal hypertension. A series of films taken over a period of several months to a year or two often demonstrate clearly an increase in size and number of varices if the disease progresses and the patient is unrelieved of his portal hypertension. Varices disappear after successful shunting procedures, though in reality, probably they remain but become inconspicuous once their intraluminal pressure is relieved (Fig. 36-2).

It is important to search for the presence of gastric varices at the time of fluoroscopy. Varices in this location can bleed as briskly as those in the esophagus. One of the reasons for failure of esophageal tamponade to control the bleeding of portal hypertension is the bleeding gastric varices beyond the reach of the balloon employed (see below). The oversewing of varices in the esophagus when hemorrhage continues from those of the stomach has accounted for some of the failures in this form of surgical treatment.

A second use of diagnostic roentgenography in patients with portal hypertension is the preoperative demonstration of the location of the venous obstruction in the portal system (Fig.

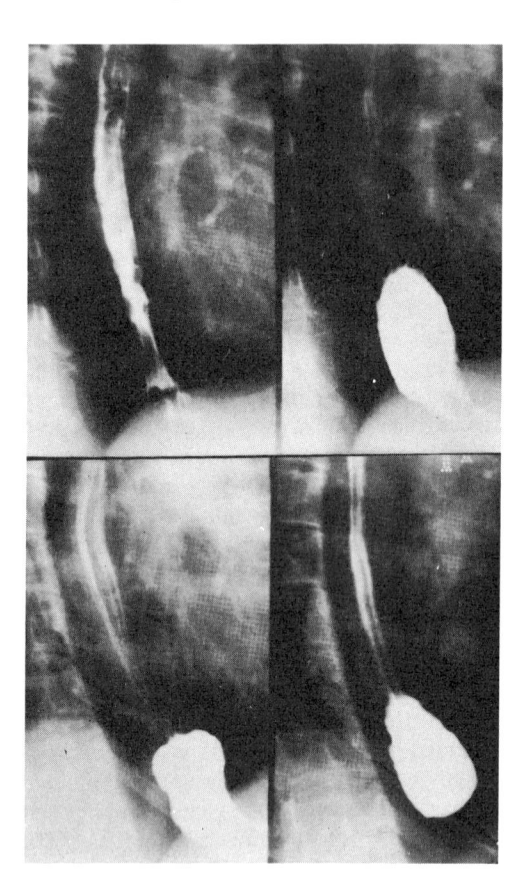

FIG. 36-2. Compares the preoperative demonstration of moderate esophageal varices with their total absence 4 years following splenorenal anastomosis for portal hypertension. This patient died in the eighth post-shunt year.

FIG. 36-3. Demonstrates by splenoportography a communication between the portal vein and the vena cava. Note also that the portal vein appears partially obstructed at its point of entrance into the liver (Cruveilhier-Baumgarten syndrome).

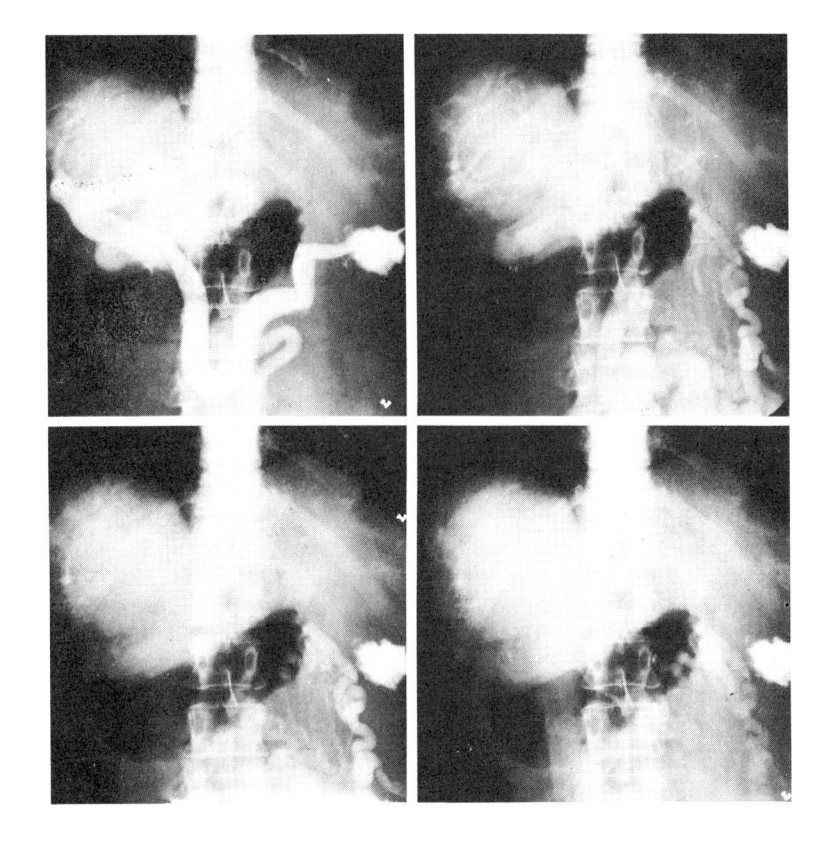

36-3). This procedure is known as splenoportography. It has proved to be a valuable diagnostic aid and of great practical help to the surgeon, as it may provide advance information as to the location of portal obstruction of the subhepatic type. This is a procedure that is performed easily in the operating room just before surgical decompression of the portal system is to be carried out. Prior to the splenoportogram, a splenic pulp pressure determination may be made which may confirm the clinical impression of portal hypertension (Rousselot et al., 1960). Occasionally, the percutaneous catheterization of an intrahepatic venous radicle is used to outline the portal system when splenectomy previously has been performed (Bierman et al., 1955).

Esophagoscopy may be used to detect the presence of esophageal varices and the bleeding site. While many favor and use this procedure, some are fearful that such an examination may induce bleeding, if the varix should be traumatized. In selected cases and in competent hands, esophagoscopy may be a procedure of diagnostic merit when other technics fail. Some have attempted to measure portal pressure by the insertion of a needle attached to a manometer, introduced through the esophagoscope into a varix. Such attempts to measure portal pressure may be dangerous and also may yield variable results.

GENERAL EVALUATION OF PATIENTS WITH PORTAL HYPERTENSION

Operations of any type performed on patients with liver disease carry certain risks related to the extent of impairment of hepatic function. The complications arising from the operation and anesthesia employed are principally hepatic and renal failure (see below) and, less often, bile nephrosis which is known also as hepatorenal syndrome. It appears that renal failure in hepatic disease is more a function of extracellular accumulations of fluid, as ascites and edema, at the expense of intravascular volume (Gornel et al., 1962). Renal failure of this type is characterized by the rapid onset of a reduced glomerular filtration rate and the formation of small volumes of concentrated urine. If these conclusions are correct, it may be that paracentesis for the relief of ascites may, as it re-forms, play a role in the production of renal failure.

Hepatic failure in patients with severe liver disease may be precipitated by an operation as minor as hemorrhoidectomy, by infection, or by exertion. Usually, in such patients more than three fourths of the hepatic parenchyma has been replaced by fibrous tissue, or an acute loss of function has occurred secondary to actue hepatitis, whether of bacterial, viral, or chemical origin.

Recovery of hepatic function from acute hepatitis may be complete in many patients. In some, subacute hepatitis is believed to persist with exacerbations and remissions over periods of months to years, leading eventually to cirrhosis, ascites, hemorrhage, coma, and death.

Recovery of hepatic structure from cirrhosis of any type, as determined by histologic study, seldom occurs unless its cause can be relieved early before fibrotic changes take place. Relief of chronic obstruction of the extrahepatic biliary tract at times will allow a remarkable degree of functional improvement, and improvement in any cirrhotic condition is more likely to be functional than anatomic. Similarly, recovery from cardiac cirrhosis may be essentially complete if cardiac failure can be cured by either medical or surgical means. Although improvement in the histologic patterns of the liver is discernible in many patients whose biliary or cardiac cirrhosis is relieved, varying degrees of permanent fibrous change usually remain. The extent and eventual consequence of the liver damage is often difficult to evaluate.

TESTS OF LIVER FUNCTION

The functions of the liver are numerous and diverse, and no one test will disclose reliably the total functional capacity of this organ. Therefore, the best that can be hoped for at present is an estimation based upon data obtained from several tests each of which attempts to appraise a different kind of hepatic function.

If a battery of tests are to be used, certain criteria should be considered in the selection of those that may be most practical: (1) they should be simple, easily performed and with reproducible accuracy in the average hospital laboratory; (2) the function each measures should be one performed only by the liver; and (3) when an impairment in function is detected, it should have a high degree of correlation with the extent of organic hepatic disease present. Negative results from such tests need not exclude the presence of organic liver disease, but they should be of such nature as to indicate little chance of early hepatic failure. Thus, in selecting patients with liver disease for operation, the surgeon is searching for indications that suggest strongly the presence or the absence of seriously impaired hepatic function rather than for evidences of minor deviations from normal. For the most part the surgeon is already aware of some degree of hepatic dysfunction, but he needs additional information in order to appraise the ability of the liver and the patient to withstand the operation and the anesthesia that he plans.

A number of commonly used tests of hepatic function and the capacities that they appear to measure are listed in Table 36-5. Only a few of these are useful in solving the problems presented to the surgeon by patients with known liver disease. The author prefers the use of the serum bilirubin concentration and the Bromsulphalein test as tests of the excretory function of the liver; the serum albumin and the prothrombin time as general indicators of the liver's ability to synthesize protein; and the free cholesterol and cholesterol ester ratio as a crude index of lipid metabolism within the liver. If all 3 of these functions appear to be good in patients with hepatic disease, the prognosis is likely to be favorable, and usually such patients withstand surgical operations well.

Among these groups of tests, and in the absence of ascites, the serum albumin level is probably the most important in assessing hepatic functional capacity. In certain patients a positive Bromsulphalein excretion test in the absence of icterus may be the most important indication of impaired hepatic function that we have, but in most patients a positive BSP test is not as reliable an indication of serious hepatic impairment as is the reduced serum albumin concentration, with a reversal of the

TABLE 36-5. TESTS OF HEPATIC FUNCTION USED COMMONLY IN PATIENTS WITH LIVER DISEASE WITH SPECIAL ATTENTION TO SURGICAL PATIENTS

TEST	ORIGINATOR	VALUE TO SURGEON
Excretory Tests:		
Bromsulphalein	Rosenthal & White, 1924	Excellent in detection of liver disease in absence of icterus (moderate to severe liver disease)
Bilirubin excretion	von Bergmann, 1927	Offers no advantages over BSP and is more difficult to perform
Detoxication Tests:		
Hippuric acid synthesis	Quick, 1932	Good but of limited value and too complex for simplicity. Positive in other diseases
Cholesterol and cholesterol ester ratio	Feigel, 1918	Excellent when positive but positive in diabetes and thyrotoxicosis also (advanced liver disease)
Galactose tolerance	Bauer, 1906	Excellent when positive (advanced liver disease)
"Flocculation" Tests:		
Takata-Ara	Takata-Ara, 1925	Of little value
Cephalin	Hanger, 1939	Of little value
Colloidal gold	Gray, 1940	Of little value
Thymol turbidity	Maclagan, 1944	Of little value
Prothrombin Assays and Response of vitamin K:	Allen & Julian, 1940	Good when observing course of hepatic disease. Excellent when positive as differential test of jaundice (obstructive versus nonobstructive)
Serum Protein Concentration:		
Albumin	Many observers	Excellent for advanced disease in absence of starvation or albuminuria
Globulin	Many observers	Excellent for advanced liver disease
Serum alkaline phosphatase	Many observers	Elevated in both intrahepatic and extrahepatic jaundice; levels tend to be higher in obstructive jaundice
Glutamic Oxaloacetic transaminase Glutamic pyruvic transaminase	Many observers	Elevated in acute liver injury and in myocardial infarction. These better reflect course of injury than locate what has been injured

albumin and globulin ratio, assuming that neither malnutrition nor albuminuria is present.

The various flocculation tests, as well as those measuring enzymatic activity, including the transaminase and phosphatase groups, provide useful means for following the clinical course of hepatic function; if all show improvement, this usually reflects clinical improvement and vice versa. But these groups are not as useful as the serum albumin and bilirubin concentrations in attempting to appraise liver function when a decision needs to be made soon after the patient is seen. The surgeon under these conditions is in search of evidence that liver function is disturbed so severely that operation should not be performed. These two tests are most useful in this respect.

As in most clinical situations, the information that they provide must be reviewed and interpreted in light of the data gleaned from the taking of a careful history, the physical examination, the routine blood and urine analysis, and other special tests.

The Bromsulphalein test is performed by

the intravenous injection of 5 mg. of this material per Kg. of body weight (Mateer et al., 1943). Normally, all of this dye will be excreted by the liver in bile within less than 45 minutes. The detection of its presence in excess of 10 per cent in the serum after 30 minutes indicates impaired hepatic excretion, as this is its major means of rapid escape. Usually the greater the percentage of dye retention, the more pronounced the disturbance in excretory hepatic function, and usually the more extensively diseased the liver if extrahepatic biliary obstruction is not present.

The BSP test serves no useful purpose if the serum bilirubin is elevated. Icterus is evidence enough that excretory function is impaired, provided that acute hemolysis has not occurred recently. Moreover, the elevated serum bilirubin level obscures the BSP color and invalidates the use of the latter.

The serum albumin level normally is about 4.5 Gm. per cent. A reduction in its concentration may come about from diseases other than of hepatic origin, but these are so conspicuous that they are not likely to be overlooked or to confuse the general picture; they are principally the various forms of starvation and the abnormal losses of albumin secondary to other conditions such as burns, cutaneous ulcers and the nephroses.

Some patients with ascites and liver disease may have a hypoalbuminemia only because of the loss of albumin in ascitic fluid, especially if they are tapped frequently; or they may be unable to synthesize albumin at a rate sufficient to sustain the normal serum concentration irrespective of ascites. When ascites is present, hypoalbuminemia is not so dependable an indication of the status of hepatic reserve, but it is reassuring indeed when the serum albumin level is normal in the presence of ascites.

Prothrombin activity may or may not be altered seriously in extensive liver disease (Allen, 1944). Usually, the more depressed the prothrombin activity and its unresponsiveness to vitamin K administration, the more severe the liver damage. Exceptions, however, are encountered with sufficient frequency to disqualify the level of prothrombin activity as a superior indicator of hepatic function. However, over a period of time a rise or a fall in prothrombin activity correlates fairly well with regression or advancement of hepatic disease.

The use of the prothrombin time as an index of hepatic function in patients with known liver disease is not to be confused with its employment to measure the response to vitamin K administration as a means of distinguishing between obstructive and intrahepatic jaundice.

The prothrombin level has a third connotation; it is a good indicator as to the likelihood of abnormal bleeding at the time of operation or needle biopsy of the liver from hypoprothrombinemia. Most observers agree that the prothrombin activity as measured by the Quick 1-stage technic should be in excess of 50 per cent of its normal value before operative procedures are undertaken.

Cholesterol ester formation appears to be a function performed only by the liver. Normally, from 25 to 40 per cent of the total serum cholesterol is so conjugated. Usually this function continues to be performed at a rate sufficient to maintain the normal ratio between free and esterified cholesterol; only in severe liver disease or hepatic failure does the percentage of esterified cholesterol begin to fall. It is a sound presumption that serious impairment of hepatic function may be present when less than 10 per cent of the total cholesterol is esterified, particularly if the total serum cholesterol level is not elevated materially.

As the drop in the percentage of cholesterol esters usually is a late occurrence in liver disease, normal values are not necessarily harbingers of good fortune.

EVALUATION BY HISTOLOGY EXAMINATION (LIVER BIOPSY)

The nature of the pathologic process responsible for the altered hepatic function can be established only by histologic examination of liver tissue. Until the development of the Silverman needle technic (Iverson and Roholm, 1939), biopsy material could be made available only at the time of operation or autopsy. The needle-biopsy technic has largely overcome the need for surgical exploration as the means for establishing the diagnosis and the nature of liver disease. It is a procedure to be performed whenever the nature and the extent of liver disease are important in the choice of treatment. From the sample tissue obtained, it is usually possible to distinguish between intrahepatic and extrahepatic biliary obstruction to determine the presence or the absence of hepatitis and, less frequently but occasionally, the detection of metastatic tumor within the liver. However, the biopsy material may not shed much information on the liver's functional capacity; hence the need to test liver function continues and is to be considered as an important separate series of studies to be carried out, even though the final diagnosis of hepatic disease is based on histologic evidence.

Bleeding from the needle site of liver puncture seldom is a serious problem, although some bleeding usually occurs in most instances. Most clinicians believe that the prothrombin time should be in excess of 50 per cent of normal if needle biopsy is to be performed. In the face of serious hypoprothrombinemia and/or thrombocytopenia, needle biopsy usually should be avoided; the value of the information obtained from needle biopsy in selected patients should outweigh the risk of bleeding, despite the fact that the bleeding encountered in a few patients may require surgical hemostasis.

COMPLICATIONS

Hepatic Coma

Hepatic coma and hepatic encephalopathy are associated with changes in protein and amino acid and ammonia metabolism. The alterations within the brain are unclear. As early as 1893 Hahn, Massen, Nenki and Pavlov described a form of hepatic encephalopathy related to an increased intake of nitrogenous food in Eck-fistula dogs. Monguio and Kraus (McDermott *et al.*, 1955) detected elevated levels of blood ammonias in these circumstances and concluded that this type of encephalopathy was the result of ammonium intoxication. Several clinical studies 30 years ago related ammonium intoxication to hepatic coma in patients with cirrhosis of the liver. Bollman and Mann (McDermott *et al.*, 1955) demonstrated a rise in the concentration of ammonia in the peripheral blood after hepatectomy, again implicating the liver as the organ of ammonia detoxification.

Krebs (1935) showed ammonia to be used in the synthesis of urea by the liver cells, and Foster *et al.* (1939) demonstrated that ammonium nitrogen was converted rapidly to amide nitrogen, probably as the amide group of glutamine through an interaction of ammonia with glutamic acid. This reaction probably is the normal mechanism for preventing excessive accumulations of blood ammonia. These are the basic papers leading to our current understanding of ammonium intoxication and encephalopathy and their relationship to glutamic acid metabolism.

Based on Krebs observations that brain slices were able to synthesize glutamine from glutamic acid and ammonia at a fairly rapid rate in the presence of glucose, Sapirstein (McDermott *et al.*, 1955) demonstrated that convulsions in rabbits caused by the intravenous injection of ammonium chloride could be prevented if glutamic acid were given first. McDermott *et al.* (1955) reported ammonium intoxication in patients with liver disease and portacaval shunts. In 1954 McDermott *et al.* instituted a series of studies demonstrating a critical elevation of blood ammonia in the peripheral blood to be a constant finding in Eck-fistula animals with "meat intoxication." This Boston group and others claimed that the administration of L-glutamine acid (25 Gm. daily intravenously or orally) was an effective means of lowering the blood-ammonia concentration in patients with hepatic coma; apparently a number of their patients responded with the prompt disappearance of their neurologic symptoms. The glutamine formed from glutamic acid binds the circulating blood ammonia, and the end product, glutamine, appears to be excreted promptly in the urine.

This method of management of hepatic coma may be particularly useful when recovery depends primarily on survival of ammonia encephalopathy. It does not appear to alter the course of liver disease. As other causes of coma exist in the terminal phase of hepatic disease, the relief of hepatic coma achieved by the administration of arginine glutamate intravenously depends on the importance of the etiologic role of ammonium intoxication in the production of the encephalopathy in the particular patient (Council on Drugs, 1964).

Ammonia is a by-product of protein digestion in the bowel, and it is converted to urea by the liver. Ammonium encephalopathy may occur simply because, in patients with advanced cirrhosis, this process is sufficiently impaired to allow the accumulation of ammonium ion in the systemic circulation, a tendency that may be greatly enhanced after performing a portacaval shunt, especially in such patients. However, methionine may produce hepatic coma without elevating blood ammonia, and high ammonia levels are not always followed by hepatic coma. Hyponatremia and hypokalemia, among other disturbances, may contribute to hepatic coma, as may certain of the diuretics.

Formation of ammonia in the bowel occurs primarily in the colon from enzymatic action of bacteria. This action may be diminished by the oral administration of appropriate antibiotics, by restriction of ingested protein, by early control of gastrointestinal bleeding and by purgation. McDermott et al., (1962) reported improvement in some cases of intractable hepatic encephalopathy by ileoproctostomy with by-pass of the colon. This procedure continues to be useful where other methods fail (Hume et al., 1966).

The normal peripheral blood-ammonia concentration is about 50 μg per cent. Symptoms of intoxication begin to appear between levels of 150 and 250 μg. Most patients are comatose when the level exceeds 250 μg per cent, and it may rise to 450 or 500 μg before death, especially after hemorrhage into the alimentary tract (McDermott et al., 1954).

The neuropsychiatric abnormalities and electroencephalographic changes are frequent in patients with portacaval shunts. Indeed this is the one objection to side-to-side portacaval shunt. Polli et al. (1969) report the prophylactic value of administering neomycin and a low protein diet to prevent such disturbances. Such a regimen reduces the amount of ammonia generated in the intestinal tract. By this measure, they were able to minimize the occurrence of mental disturbances and at no time did their patients demonstrate hepatic encephalopathy. They observed also an increase in cerebral blood flow under this form of treatment, and in most cases the cerebral metabolic rate was slightly higher than normal, with a greater increase in the metabolic rate of glucose utilization. In 20 cirrhotic patients with chronic hepatic coma or encephalopathy, they observed a striking decrease in cerebral blood flow and in cerebral metabolism. In the shunted patient, these increased values were observed from one to two years after their operation—as long as their studies had been conducted. They concluded that the presumptive mechanism of the cerebral metabolic disorder is a partial glycolysis blockade by deamination of α-ketoglutarate to form glutamic acid and glutamine.

Peptic Ulcer

Peptic ulcer, usually duodenal, occurs in 8 to 10 per cent of patients with cirrhosis; therefore, in the cirrhotic patient with known portal hypertension, the possibility of coexisting ulcer as the source of bleeding should be considered. Clarke et al. (1959) have shown that, following portacaval transposition or shunts in dogs, the secretion of gastric juice and its acidity are markedly elevated. This effect appears the result of a humoral factor, because it is observed in the isolated fundic gastric pouch (Heidenhain), which continues to hypersecrete despite vagotomy and antrectomy. Thus, the response is histaminelike, and it may be that an increase in blood histamine does occur with portacaval transposition in dogs. Clarke believes that the responsible agent probably arises in the small bowel or colon and bypasses the liver in shunted patients, or is not destroyed in the cirrhotic patient.

It is not clear that such a mechanism is responsible for the increased incidence of duodenal ulcer observed in cirrhosis in man or for the apparent increase in the *de novo* appearance of duodenal ulcer after portacaval shunts in patients. A basic difference exists in that in Clarke's observations the dog's liver was normal, whereas the few observations in man have been made on patients with portal hypertension due to cirrhosis.

INDICATIONS FOR OPERATION AND SELECTION OF PATIENTS

Evaluation of surgical risk in patients who have liver disease but require surgical operation for other causes is the same as for patients requiring surgical decompression or hemostatic operations for intrahepatic or suprahepatic portal hypertension.

The 2 principal features of portal hypertension amenable to surgical therapy are the bleeding varix and the relief of portal hypertension itself. The major point of concern is the surgical decompression of the portal system: (1) When should it be performed? (2) And what does it offer in long-term gains to the patient? These questions beg 2 more: (1) What percentage of patients with esophagogastric varices will experience bleeding before death? (2) Is there any evidence that restoring the normal portal pressure reduces the extent of residual liver damage or retards or reverses its course? Neither can be answered with much assurance at this time.

Usually those patients with subhepatic portal hypertension are free of liver disease (see p. 997). However, tests of liver function, as well as needle biopsy of the liver, usually are also essential to the correct interpretation of the pathogenesis and the general location of portal obstruction and the state of hepatic reserve. In addition, the information provided by a splenoportogram can be very helpful, often enabling the surgeon to accomplish his shunt more rapidly and with less dissection. These studies are basic to case selection in the surgical treatment of portal hypertension and to the choice of operative procedure.

The clinical classification presented herein is modified from that employed by Linton (1948). In each instance portal hypertension with demonstrated esophagogastric varices is presumed, with or without a previous episode of bleeding. One may prefer Child's classification, shown in Table 36-3.

Excellent surgical risks are those patients with subhepatic portal hypertension and no evidence of cirrhosis or hepatitis. Varices with or without a previous history of bleeding are their only evidence of portal hypertension. Secondary hypersplenism may or may not be present. The one disappointing surgical feature in this group of patients that is of fairly common occurrence is splenic and/or portal vein thrombosis with cavernous recanalization, leaving little or no opportunity for shunting the portal circulation. Operative mortality is minimal, and, so far as is known now, long-term survival is compatible with normal life expectancy if an adequate shunting procedure can be performed and maintained. Most agree that the diameter of the shunt should be more than 1.0 cm.

Good surgical risks are those patients with mild to moderate liver disease, without jaundice, fever or ascites and in whom the serum albumin level is above 3.5 Gm. per cent. These are patients in whom cirrhosis is minimal to moderate and not complicated by hepatitis or cholangitis. A shunting procedure usually can be performed with less than 10 per cent mortality and with good reason to anticipate a 5-year or longer survival without difficulty.

Moderate surgical risks are those patients whose tests of hepatic function are not altered severely. The serum albumin remains above 3.0 Gm. per cent; these patients may have 15 to 25 per cent bromsulphalein retention but no icterus, or elevation of serum bilirubin, histologic evidence of active hepatitis, fever or leukocytosis. With these limitations the presence or the absence of ascites is not too important; in fact, the maintenance of the serum-albumin level above 3.0 Gm. per cent when ascites is present is fairly good evidence that hepatic function is better than reflected by the serum-albumin level. Shunting procedures usually can be carried out in this group of patients with less than 15 per cent operative mortality and with an expectation that 4 out of 5 surviving will live a normal life for a number of years without ascites or hemorrhage.

Poor surgical risks are those patients with icterus, ascites, muscle wasting, and cirrhosis of long standing and increasing in severity, in whom the serum albumin is less than 3.0 Gm. per cent with a reversal of the A/G ratio, often with fever and leukocytosis. An analysis of the course of such patients discloses that it is within this group that posthemorrhagic hepatic coma is most likely to develop, that ascites is not relieved by shunting operations, and liver disease is most likely to progress, with death from hepatic failure only months to a year or two away despite any form of treatment. A successful shunting operation may avoid subsequent hemorrhage, but generally it has little if any other influence upon the clinical causes of liver disease. Yet, within this group there are a few patients who may benefit from a shunting procedure with relief from ascites, avoidance of hemorrhage and survival for periods longer than 5 years. These are the patients whose general condition improves under conservative management over a period of time. Usually, they are those whose hepatic function is impaired temporarily and disproportionately and whose liver disease is, by comparison, less severe than suggested by either clinical or laboratory findings. Some are patients with an exacerbation or superimposed bout of hepatitis. If operation can be delayed until the patient's general condition improves, then he may be operated upon as a moderate-risk patient and possibly with a good prognosis.

Causes of Death in Patients With Bleeding Varices. There is little disagreement among surgeons that surgery should not be performed for the relief of portal hypertension when the patient is bleeding actively. This opinion has crystallized out of the bad experience of the past decade in surgical attempts at hemostasis or portal diversion carried out during active episodes of bleeding. In spite of the successful control of hemorrhage and hemorrhagic shock, two complications have not been avoided often or treated successfully in these circumstances. They are hepatic coma and aspiration pneumonitis.

Hepatic coma, already discussed, may arise from the digestion of blood remaining within the alimentary tract.

Aspiration bronchopneumonitis in the absence of hepatic failure is the major cause of death in patients with massive upper gastrointestinal bleeding, short of exsanguination itself (Allen and Head, 1956). The bleeding varix or, for that matter, the bleeding gastric ulcer usually fills the stomach with blood fairly promptly, and about the time the stomach is distended sufficiently to induce vomiting the sensorium is dulled by the hypoxia of hypovolemic shock from blood loss. The patient feels faint and often becomes unconscious before he has a massive bout of hematemesis. Thus the stage is set for aspiration of some of the gastric contents into the tracheobronchial tree. The gastric aspirate is highly irritating and induces edema of the bronchial mucosa shortly after contact; generally this continues as a bronchopneumonia. The presence of blood in the gastric aspirate may neutralize partially the acidity of gastric juice, but this potential benefit is overcome by the numerous small clots of blood lodged in the periphery of the bronchial tree and the excellent culture media that they provide for prompt bacterial growth. The mortality rate from these misfortunes is high.

MANAGEMENT OF THE PATIENT WITH THE BLEEDING VARIX

The patient with the bleeding varix presenting himself for the first time is an unresolved risk in that his hepatic function cannot be assessed rapidly or accurately under such conditions. Conservative management with esophagogastric tamponade is strongly indicated. Later a shunting procedure may be useful.

Esophagogastric Tamponade

Because of the high mortality rate in patients with cirrhosis and portal hypertension whose varix bleeds—75 per cent in the Sengstaken-Blakemore (1950) series—nonoperative measures to control hemorrhage have been explored vigorously. To date the most successful is the employment of a balloon tamponade devised by these 2 investigators. This is a triple lumen tube: one arm of it serves to inflate a sausage-shaped balloon to compress against the esophageal wall; the 2nd arm leads to a globular-shaped balloon which, when inflated, remains in the stomach; the third leads to the distal tip of the tube, serves to aspirate the stomach and enables the surgeon to wash it free of clots. To be effective in the arrest of hemorrhage, both balloons are inflated to a pressure of 25 to 30 mm. of mercury under fluoroscopic control. When they are in proper position, traction is placed on the tube entering the patient's nasal passage or mouth. This in turn exerts its greatest point of pressure at the esophagogastric junction, occluding the veins in this area and often controlling bleeding. The tube leading into the stomach is irrigated at hourly intervals to be certain that bleeding does not recur. Within 48 to 96 hours the inflation pressures and traction are released. If further bleeding does not occur within 24 hours, the tube is removed. This is a very useful form of treatment, and it should be carefully tried in all patients bleeding from the varices of portal hypertension. Bennett *et al.* in 1952 and Conn in 1958 have clearly presented an intrinsic danger in the use of these tubes. Sudden rupture of one of the balloons while in position within the esophagus can lead to a calamitous situation; the counterweight utilized for traction may pull the remaining intact balloon suddenly into the oropharynx with asphyxiation of the patient.

Conn and Simpson in 1967 reported the complications of esophageal tamponade in 40 consecutive patients. It was effective in 55 per cent of the patients. Major complications occurred in 14 patients or 35 per cent and resulted in death in 9 of the patients or 42 per cent. They recommend prophylactic tracheostomy or endotracheal intubation prior to the use of the balloon tubes if these complications are to be prevented.

Injection of Varices With Sclerosing Solutions. Transesophageal injection of the esophageal varices with sclerosing solutions was introduced in 1930 by Crafoord and Frenckner. The results were occasionally good, but usually only temporary, multiple repeated injections being required. This procedure still should be tried if bleeding is not controlled with tamponade and the patient's general condition does not permit of more elaborate surgery when seen.

USE OF DRUGS TO DECREASE PORTAL HYPERTENSION

Intravenous pituitrin or pitressin, because it reduces portal pressure, among other actions, has been used in the treatment of bleeding varices. It is probable that the bleeding varix reduces portal hypertension more effectively than does pitressin in sublethal doses, and that in many patients with portal hypertension bleeding ceases for the hypotensive reasons of shock rather than because of pitressin. Nor is there evidence that pitressin exerts a direct influence on blood coagulation. In a disease in which this natural or endogenous hormone is already excessive, along with aldosteronism, the potentially adverse effects of its administration seem to have received little attention. The administration of this drug as a trial in the place of the prompt introduction of esophagogastric tamponade can, at times, delay more effective treatment.

PORTAL SHUNTS

Direct Shunting of Portal Blood Around the Liver. This procedure was performed first by von Eck in 1877, a side-to-side anastomosis being made between the portal vein and the vena cava. After the anastomosis was completed, the portal vein adjacent to the porta hepatis was ligated so that all portal blood circumvented the liver. Although this has been a useful physiologic preparation, the operation was used in patients only rarely prior to 1945 and then, with few exceptions, usually to anastomose smaller branches of the portal bed with the vena cava.

Whipple attacked the problem of portal hypertension directly, beginning about 1943. He anastomosed the splenic vein to the left renal vein. Since that time various modifications of his procedure were introduced with the successful decompression of portal hypertension in suitable patients. Among the more prominent modifications are the end-to-side or the side-to-side portacaval anastomosis. The end-to-side anastomosis is the easier to perform technically and is the least likely to thrombose; its disadvantage may be largely theoretical. It diverts all portal flow away from the liver, and in doing so may present a greater threat of ammonium intoxication. The lateral portacaval or the splenorenal anastomosis has in its favor the theoretical advantage that not all portal blood bypasses the liver. Most surgeons prefer the side-to-side portacaval because of the ease with which it can be accomplished. When ascites is present, there is a marked difference of opinion as to the most efficacious method, i.e., end-to-end or side-to-side (Welch *et al.*, 1959; Madden, 1959). Berstein *et al.* (1968) find no basis for physiologic choice of end-to-side and side-to-side portacaval anastomosis in portal hypertension except when ascites is present. A side-to-side is then preferable—portacaval or splenorenal.

Burchell *et al.* (1968), as well as others (Berstein *et al.* 1968), report the effectiveness of a side-to-side portacaval shunt for ascites caused by cirrhosis is considerably more effective in relieving the ascites than is an end-to-side shunt.

In the Burchell series, the patients in whom they performed a side-to-side anastomosis were

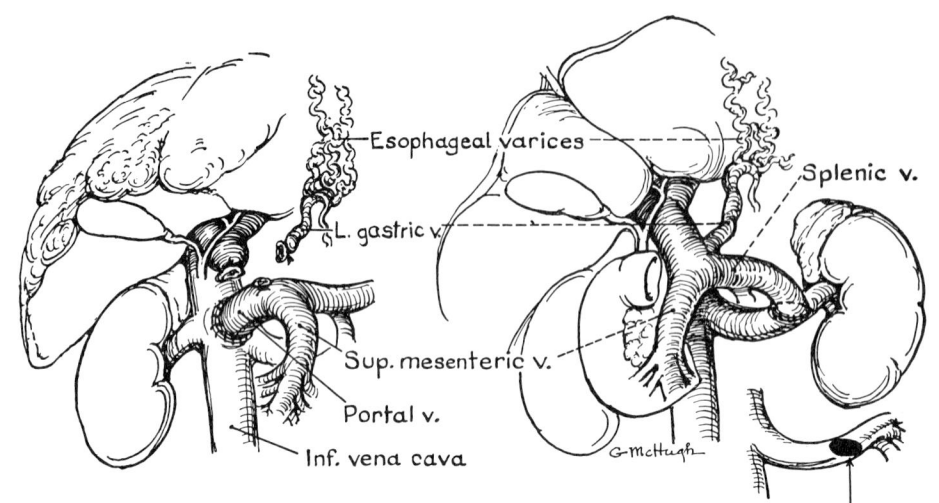

FIG. 36-4. (*Left*) Shows a portacaval end-to-side anastomosis wherein the coronary vein is divided and ligated in this particular instance in the treatment of portal hypertension. (*Right*) Illustrates the technics of end-to-side splenorenal anastomosis. Note the oval window made in the renal vein to ensure its continued patency.

clinically more severely ill than were their earlier patients in whom they performed an end-to-end shunt. Yet the mortality and morbidity rates from the side-to-side group were substantially lower and the patients in general fared better than those in the earlier series.

Turcotte *et al.* (1969) observed better results in patients with ascites when side-to-side anastomosis had been performed, but, just as Burchell *et al.* (1968) pointed out, the incidence of hepatitic encephalopathy occasionally presented a serious problem.

Shunting the superior or the inferior mesenteric veins may be all that can be accomplished in patients whose portal and/or splenic vein is thrombosed. These are less satisfactory procedures, as usually they do not divert sufficient blood to decompress the portal pressure adequately. Merendino and Dillard (1955) suggested the use of an interposed jejunal segment between the esophagus and the stomach to prevent regurgitation of acid onto the varix. Habif (1959) has reported excellent results with this technic.

Portal pressure increases in the range of 25 to 65 mm. are usually found in portal hypertension. Most observers believe that portal pressure should be reduced below 20 mm. of water, preferably below 15, if recurrence of bleeding is to be avoided.

Results of Portacaval Shunting for the Control of Variceal Hemorrhage. More recent data suggest a substantial advantage to portacaval shunting both as a means of extending life and as a means of controlling hemorrhage. The key to these improvements over the Boston series lies in the better selection of patients for operation as used by the New York and Ann Arbor groups. Panke *et al.* (1958) reported the operative mortality in relation to operative risk in 210 patients with elective end-to-side shunts (Table 36-6). Their survival rate by years is shown in Figure 36-5. Burchell *et al.* show a lower mortality rate in 63 patients upon whom an elective side-to-side shunt was performed for ascites (see Fig. 36-6).

TABLE 36-6. CAUSES OF LONG-TERM MORTALITY: 55 OPERATIVE SURVIVORS OF 63 ELECTIVE SIDE-TO-SIDE SHUNTS

Liver failure (hepatoma-1)	12
Exsanguinating ulcer hemorrhage	1
Serum hepatitis	1
Epistaxis with aspiration	1
Brain abscesses with septicemia	1
Bizarre neurologic syndrome	1
Partial followup; considered dead from date of last followup	4
Total	21

FIG. 36-5. Long-term survival rate (189 operative survivors of 210 elective end-to-side shunts). The percentages apply only to the number of patients available for each year, as indicated within the bar of the graph. (Panke, W. F., Rousselot, L. M., and Burchell, A. R.: Ann. Surg., 168:957, 1968)

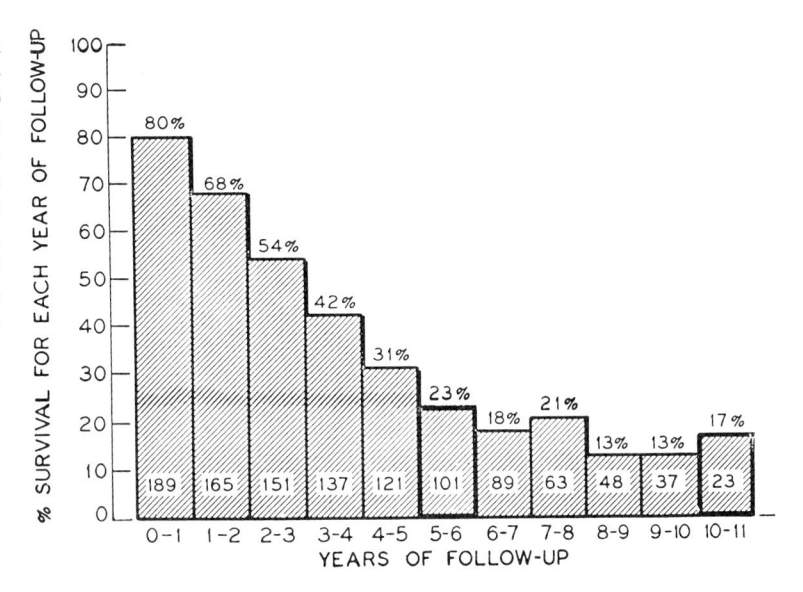

TABLE 36-7. LATE CAUSES OF DEATH AFTER SHUNTING FOR PORTAL HYPERTENSION

	NEW YORK (273)	ANN ARBOR (102)
Liver	53	17
Ulcer disease	13	6
Pneumonia	8	—
Serum hepatitis	4	—
Aspiration	1	—
Cardiovascular	3	5
Recurrent variceal hemorrhage	3	—
Infection	1	—
Bizarre neurological syndrome	1	—
Others	17	9
Total Dead	105	35

In Table 36-7 are shown the late causes of death in the two New York series and the Ann Arbor series.

The end results for any surgical procedure for portal hypertension can be improved only by better patient selection and by the development of effective medical methods for the treatment of cirrhosis itself. Until such time that medical treatment can be improved, portacaval shunts will continue to have a place in the treatment of hemorrhage from esophageal varices.

There has been substantial experience with this technic for the control of hemorrhage and many surgeons prefer to perform a shunting procedure as soon as the patient can be prepared. Earlier caution seems unwarranted.

Elective portacaval shunt, when it can be carried out from 1 to 3 weeks after cessation of a bleeding episode, is the procedure preferred if the patient's bleeding can be controlled by tamponade or ceases spontaneously.

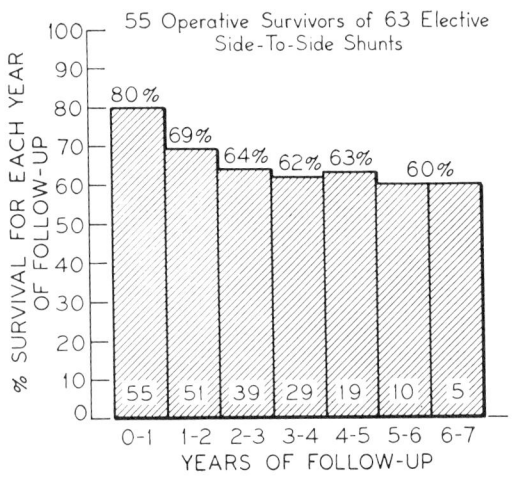

FIG. 36-6. Long term survival rate (55 operative survivors of 63 elective side-to-side shunts). The percentages apply only to the number of patients available for each year of follow-up; not to the entire 55 patients. The number of patients available for each year is indicated within the bar of the graph. (Burchell et al.: Ann. Surg., 168:655, 1968)

The lapse of time allows the patient's circulation to become stabilized and possibly his metabolic state and hepatic function to improve. It also provides an opportunity to evaluate the patient's general condition; to assess the nature of his liver function and ascertain the cause of his cirrhosis; and to evaluate the status of the portal circulation and the site of the block, when it is subhepatic.

There are three technical advantages of a portacaval anastomosis without splenectomy: (1) if bleeding recurs, splenoportography may be repeated to determine the patency of the anastomosis; (2) if patency of the splenic vein exists, a splenorenal shunt can be added as a second operation; and (3) results are better.

The disadvantage of an end-to-side portacaval anastomosis is that direct decompression of the liver is not possible because the proximal end of the divided portal vein is ligated. The side-to-side portacaval shunt would appear to obviate this disadvantage. Retrograde flow may not always be achieved by the side-to-side procedure because this flow would have to compete with the higher pressure of the distal flow.

The experience of most surgeons at the present time is that side-to-side portacaval anastomosis is a better procedure to decompress the liver as well as to prevent ascites.

Other Procedures. *Omentopexy* was introduced by Drummond and Morison, Talma, and others about 1900. It was their hope that suturing the omentum to the abdominal wall would promote vascular adhesions and thereby shunt some of the portal blood to the systemic circuit through such collaterals. Its failure is now understood in that the volume of blood such adhesions may carry is much too small to be effective in reducing portal hypertension. An expansion of this concept is the supradiaphragmatic transposition of the spleen into the left thorax to encourage collateral circulation. This procedure may be performed at the time of a thoracoabdominal exposure of the esophagus for the direct suture of varices (Hoffman and Freedlander, 1960).

Splenectomy crept into the treatment of portal hypertension originally because it afforded a means of relief of the discomfort produced by the enlarged spleen. Any benefits to portal hypertension soon were recognized as being limited to patients without cirrhosis. It was not realized until much later that the patients whose course splenectomy relieved were those few patients whose portal obstruction was limited primarily to the splenic vein. The concept of segmental portal occlusion was largely an outgrowth of the work of Whipple and Blakemore; this concept has done much to explain the heretofore random results obtained from splenectomy in portal hypertension.

The relief from the secondary hypersplenism that is often associated with enlargement of the spleen (see Chap. 34, Spleen) is reason enough for removal of the spleen in portal hypertension. However, this procedure should not be carried out in this disease unless the surgeon is certain that he can perform either a splenorenal or a portacaval anastomosis at that time. He may not do this later.

Surgical Hemostasis. Treatment of bleeding varices, otherwise uncontrolled, has been explored by many, and occasionally it is the only successful therapy that can be employed. In general, it is not the primary surgical treatment of choice; nonetheless, in a few patients it may be the only treatment possible. In 1926, Flerow attempted to devascularize in part the blood-flow to and from the lower esophagus and the upper stomach by ligating the left gastric artery and vein, the short gastrics and the inferior mesenteric vein. These procedures have failed to prevent hemorrhage.

Suture of the bleeding varix by the transthoracic approach, exposing and opening the lower esophagus and the upper stomach, has been advocated by Linton (1949, 1953), Crile (1960) and Cohn and Mathewson (1957). This procedure has given good temporary relief in bleeding patients whose hemorrhage is uncontrolled by tamponade. Its disadvantage is the transthoracic approach required. When performed during the active bleeding state, the patient's condition usually is poor, and already he may have developed aspiration pneumonitis to compromise his air exchange.

Esophagogastrectomy, Subtotal Gastrectomy and Gastric Bisection. In 1947 Phemister and Humphreys reported on esophagogastrectomy as a means of controlling bleeding varices. This procedure is reserved for patients whose portal and splenic veins are not suited for shunting operations. The results reported have been good. The development of collaterals later on with return of hemorrhage is anticipated but has been an infrequent event. Subtotal gastrectomy, dividing all venous connections between the fundus, the spleen, the pancreas, the triangular ligament and the esophagus, seems to have advantages over esophagogastrectomy, gastric bisection and possibly also over suturing the varices.

Tanner (1954) and later the author (1956) introduced gastric bisection, wherein the left gastric artery and vein are ligated and divided, splenectomy is performed, and the stomach is sectioned completely at the level of its proximal fourth and simply re-anastomosed. Occasionally, a sleeve of the distal segment of stomach is resected to avoid necrosis, in the event that the blood supply to this portion appears to be impaired after bisection. This eliminates successfully all venous bridges between the major portal tributaries and the collaterals of the lower esophagus and the upper stomach. It has the advantage that it can be performed through an abdominal incision, if need be, without entering the chest. As neither this procedure nor the Phemister resection can be performed without a vagotomy, a gastroenterostomy or pyloroplasty should be carried out at the time of section or bisection. The resulting hypoacidity should favor the healing of any peptic esophagitis.

Hepatic Artery Ligation. Ligation of the hepatic artery proximal to the gastroepiploic artery, thereby allowing some collateral arterial flow to enter the distal hepatic artery via the gastroduodenal artery, is a method devised in 1951 by Rienhoff for the treatment of portal hypertension and bleeding varices. Its merits rest on the 1907 report of F. C. Herrick, who believed that he demonstrated the development of abnormal arteriolar connections with the small portal radicles in cirrhosis; thus it is concluded that to reduce the arterial blood flow would lower portal pressure. The merits of both the concept and the therapeutic results claimed remain in controversy; some who have tried this operation report death from hepatic necrosis. The procedure is not advocated at this time.

SUMMARY

The bulk of experience and reported data indicate that in good- to moderate-risk patients with portal hypertension and cirrhosis who have bled from a varix, the side-to-side shunt appears as the most effective means for the control of hemorrhage and the prevention of subsequent bleeding. Most patients who have a good arterial supply to the liver appear to do better in the postoperative period insofar as hepatic function is concerned. It also appears that benefits are substantial and persisting after shunts that are properly performed, if the liver disease does not advance. These patients generally fall into the good- to moderate-risk class. In the poor-risk patients, operative mortality of 40 to 50 per cent is not uncommon. It is doubtful the shunt holds any promise other than to permit the patient to die of another cause.

The problems of hepatic coma require constant surveillance and treatment if they are not to dominate the postoperative period. Needed most is some means of improving the function of the liver, especially in patients with alcoholic cirrhosis.

REFERENCES

Allen, J. G.: The clinical value of the functional tests of the liver; a review with a special study of the plasma prothrombin. Gastroenterology, 3:6, 1944.

Allen, J. G., and Head, L. R.: The diagnosis of portal hypertension with notes on treatment. Surg. Clin. N. Amer., 36:119-130, 1956.

Annotations: Natural History of Cirrhosis. Lancet, 1:1076, 1968.

Baronofsky, I. D.: Portal hypertension with special reference to the acid-peptic factor in the causation of hemorrhage and extensive gastric resection in its treatment. Surg., 25:135, 1949.

Bennett, H. D., Baker, L., and Baker, L. A.: Complications in use of esophageal compression balloons (Sengstaken tube). Arch. Int. Med., 90: 196-200, 1952.

Bernstein, J. E., Nutting, R. O., and Orloff, M. J.: Comparison of the effects of end-to-side and side-to-side portacaval shunts on liver function in dogs. Surg. Forum, 19:328, 1968.

Bierman, H. R., Kelly, K. H., White, L. P., Coblentz, A., and Fisher, A.: Transhepatic venous catheterization and venography. J.A.M.A., 158: 1331, 1955.

Britton, R. C., and Shirey, E. K.: Cineportography and dynamics of portal flow following shunt procedures. Arch. Surg., 84:25, 1962.

Burchell, A. R., Rousselot, L. M., and Panke, W. F.: A seven-year experience with side-to-side portacaval shunt for cirrhotic ascites. Ann. Surg., 168: 655, 1968.

Child, C. G.: The Liver and Portal Hypertension. Philadelphia, W. B. Saunders, 1964.

Clarke, J. S., McKissock, P. K., and Cruze, K.: Studies on the site of origin of the agent causing hypersecretion in dogs with portacaval shunt. Surg., 46:48, 1959.

Cohn, R., and Mathewson, C., Jr.: Observations on patients during the surgical treatment of acute massive hemorrhage from esophageal varices secondary to cirrhosis of the liver. Surgery, 41:94-99, 1957.

Conn, H. O.: Hazards attending the use of esophageal tamponade. New Eng. J. Med., 259:701-707, 1958.

Conn, H. O., and Simpson, J. A.: Excessive mortality associated with balloon tamponade of bleeding varices: A critical reappraisal. J.A.M.A., 202:135, 1967.

Council on Drugs: An ammonia detoxicant, arginine glutamate. J.A.M.A., 187:359, 1964.

Crafoord, C., and Frenckner, P.: New surgical treatment of varicose veins of the esophagus. Acta otolaryng., 27:422-429, 1939.

Crile, G., Jr.: Transesophageal ligation of bleeding esophageal varices. Arch. Surg., 61:654-660, 1950.

Cruveilhier, J.: Traité d'anatomie descriptive. Paris, Bechet, 1834-6; ed. 2, Paris, Labe, 1943-5; ed. 4, Paris, Asselin, 1862-71.

David, C., Bollman, J. L., Grindlay, J. H., and Hallenbeck, G. A.: Experimental study of the effectiveness of the portal vein as a hepatic outflow tract. Surg. Gynec. Obstet., 117:67, 1963.

Drapanas, T., Schenk, W. G., Jr., Pollack, E. L., and Stewart, J. D.: Hepatic hemodynamics in experimental ascites. Ann. Surg., 152:705, 1960.

Drummond, D., and Morison, R.: A case of ascites due to cirrhosis of the liver, cured by operation. Brit. Med. J., 2:728, 1896.

Dumont, A. E., and Mulholland, J. H.: Alterations in thoracic duct lymph flow in hepatic cirrhosis: Significance in portal hypertension. Ann. Surg., 156:668, 1962.

Eck, von (See Von Eck).

Flerow: Quoted by Child, C. G.: The Hepatic Circulation and Portal Hypertension. p. 225. Philadelphia, W. B. Saunders, 1954.

Foster, G. L., Schoenheimer, R., and Rittenberg, D.: Studies in protein metabolism. V. the utilization of ammonia for amino acid and creatine formation. J. Biol. Chem., 127:319, 1939.

Garceau, A. J., Chalmers, T. C., and the Boston Inter-hospital Liver Group: The natural history of cirrhosis. I. Survival with esophageal varices. New Eng. J. Med., 268:459, 1963.

Garceau, A. J., Donaldson, R. M., Jr., O'Hara, E. T., Callow, A. D., Muench, H., Chalmers, T. C., and the Boston Inter-Hospital Liver Group: A controlled trial of prophylactic portacaval-shunt surgery. N. Eng. J. Med., 270-496, 1964.

Gornel, D. L., et al.: Acute changes in renal excretion of water and solute in patients with Laënnec's cirrhosis, induced by administration of pressor amine, metaraminol. J. Clin. Invest., 41: 594, 1962.

Habif, D. V.: Treatment of esophageal varices by partial esophagogastrectomy and interposed jejunal segment. Surgery, 46:212-237, 1959.

Herrick, F. C.: An experimental study into the cause of the increases of portal pressure in portal cirrhosis. J. Exp. Med., 9:93-104, 1907.

Hoffman, H. L., and Freedlander, S. O.: Supradiaphragmatic transposition of the spleen for portal hypertension. Arch. Surg., 80:452, 1960.

Hume, H. A., Erb, W. H., Stevens, L. W., and Hallahan, J. D.: Treatment of hepatic encephalopathy by surgical exclusion of the colon. J.A.M.A., 196:593, 1966.

Isselbacher, K. J., and Greenberg, N. J.: Metabolic effects of alcohol on the liver. New Eng. J. Med., 270:351, 1964.

Iverson, P., and Roholm, K.: On aspiration biopsy, of the liver, with remarks on its diagnostic significance. Acta med. scandinav., 102:1, 1939.

Krebs, H. A.: Metabolism of amino acids. IV. Synthesis of glutamine from glutamic acid and ammonia, and enzymic hydrolysis of glutamine in animal tissues. Biochem. J., 29:1951-69, 1935.

Linton, R. R.: Portacaval shunts in the treatment of portal hypertension. New Eng. J. Med., 238:723-727, 1948.

————: Surgical treatment of bleeding esophageal varices by portal systemic venous shunt. Ann. Int. Med., 31:794-804, 1959.

Linton, R. R., and Warren, R.: The emergency treatment of massive bleeding from esophageal varices by transesophageal suture of these vessels at the time of acute hemorrhage. Surgery, 33: 243-255, 1953.

Luetscher, J. A.: Aldosteronism. Disease-a-Month, May, 1964.

McDermott, W. V., Jr., and Adams, R. D.: Episodic stupor associated with Eck fistula in humans with particular reference to metabolism of ammonia. J. Clin. Invest., 33:1, 1954.

McDermott, W. V., Jr., Adams, R. D., and Riddell, A. G.: Ammonia metabolism in man. Ann. Surg., 140:539-556, 1954.

McDermott, W. V., Jr., Victor, M., and Point, W. W.: Exclusion of the colon in the treatment of hepatic encephalopathy. New Eng. J. Med., 267: 850, 1962.

McDermott, W. V., Jr., Wareham, J., and Riddell, A. G.: Treatment of hepatic coma with L-glutamic acid. New Eng. J. Med., 263:1093, 1955.

Madden, J. L.: Discussion, paper of Welch, C. S., Welch, H. F., and Carter, J. H.: The treatment of ascites by side to side portacaval shunt. Ann. Surg., 150:442-444, 1959.

Mateer, J. G., Baltz, J. I., Marion, D. F., and MacMillan, J. M.: Liver function tests. J.A.M.A., 121:723, 1943.

Merendino, K. A., and Dillard, D. H.: The concept of sphincter substitution by an interposed jejunal segment for anatomic and physiologic abnormalities at the esophagogastric junction: with special reference to reflux esophagitis, cardiospasm and esophageal varices. Ann. Surg., 142:486-508, 1955.

Merendino, K. A., and Volwiler, W.: Medical and

surgical aspects of portal hypertension. Northwest Med., 52:724, 1953.

Michels, N. A.: Newer anatomy of liver-variant blood supply and collateral circulation. J.A.M.A., 172: 125, 1960.

Orloff, M. J., and Thomas, H. S.: Pathogenesis of esophageal varix rupture: Study based on gross and microscopic examination of esophagus at time of bleeding. Arch. Surg., 87:301, 1963.

Panke, W. F., Rousselot, L. M., and Burchell, A. R.: A sixteen-year experience with end-to-side portacaval shunt for varical hemorrhage. Ann. Surg., 168:957, 1968.

Patton, T. B.: Surgical treatment of portal hypertension: A 15-year follow up. Ann. Surg., 157: 859, 1963.

Phemister, D. B., and Humphreys, E. M.: Gastroesophageal resection and total gastrectomy in the treatment of bleeding varicose veins in Banti's syndrome. Ann. Surg., 126:397-410, 1947.

Polli, E., Bianchi Porro, G., and Maiolo, A. T.: Cerebral metabolism after portacaval shunt. Lancet, 1:153, 1969.

Ratnoff, A. D., and Patek, A. J., Jr.: Natural history of Laënnec's cirrhosis of liver: Analysis of 486 cases. Medicine, 21:207, 1942.

Resnick, R. H., Chalmers, T. C., et al., and the Boston Inter-hospital Liver Group: A controlled study of the prophylactic portacaval shunt: a final report. Ann. Int. Med., 70: 675, 1969.

Rienhoff, W. F., Jr.: Ligation of the hepatic and splenic arteries in the treatment of portal hypertension with a report of 6 cases: preliminary report. Bull. Johns Hopkins Hosp., 88:365-375, 1951.

Sherlock, S.: Diseases of the liver and biliary system. Philadelphia, F. A. Davis, 1968.

Talma, S.: Chirurgische Offnung neuer Seitenbahnen für das Blut der Vena Porta. Klin. Wschr., 35: 833, 1898.

Tanner, N. C.: Hemorrhage as a surgical emergency. Proc. Roy. Soc. Med., 43:147, 1950, and personal communication, 1954.

Turcotte, J. G., Wallin, V. W., Jr., and Child, C. G.: End to side versus side to side portacaval shunts in patients with hepatic cirrhosis. Am. J. Surg., 117:108, 1969.

Von Eck, N. V.: Ligature of portal vein. Voyemo-Med. J., 130:1, 1877.

Wantz, G. E., and Payne, M. A.: The emergency portacaval shunt. Surg. Gynec. Obstet., 109:549-554, 1959.

Welch, C. S., Welch, H. F., and Carter, J. H.: The treatment of ascites by side to side portacaval shunt. Ann. Surg., 150:428-444, 1959.

Whipple, A. O.: The problem of portal hypertension in relation to hepatosplenopathies. Ann. Surg., 122:449-475, 1945.

CHAPTER 37

J. GARROTT ALLEN, M.D.

Appendicitis, Peritonitis, and Intra-abdominal Abscesses

Introduction
Nonperforative Acute Appendicitis
Perforative Acute Appendicitis
Appendicitis in Pregnancy
Recurrent Appendicitis
Removal of the Normal Appendix in the Course of Other Intra-abdominal Operations
Complications of Acute Appendicitis
Mortality From Appendicitis
Tumors of the Appendix
Abdominal Pain
Differential Diagnosis of Appendicitis
The Peritoneum
Subdivisions of the Abdominal Cavity
Acute Peritonitis
Chronic Peritonitis
Intra-abdominal Abscesses

Section 1. Appendicitis and the Acute Abdomen

INTRODUCTION

Acute appendicitis is the acute inflammatory condition that taught us most of what we know of the diagnosis and the treatment of all intraperitoneal inflammatory diseases. It was the first disease in which the importance of early diagnosis and of prompt surgical intervention was emphasized as essential to reduction in mortality from a specific disease entity. It was also the first of the surgical diseases in which the signs and the symptoms of early diagnosis were widely publicized among the laity, leading to a lowering of mortality rates. It is the disease that, when complicated by perforation and abscess, taught surgeons how best to treat the peritonitis and the abscesses resulting from perforation of other inflammatory lesions of the stomach, the small bowel and the colon.

For reasons not clear, the numbers of cases of appendicitis in the United States have been decreasing fairly steadily for at least a decade. Table 37-1 presents familiar data that are representative of most urban and rural hospitals.

The mortality rate from acute appendicitis is nearly zero when the patient is operated on before perforation has occurred but varies from 0.5 per cent to 6.0 per cent and higher when the appendix is ruptured. As the incidence of the disease has decreased, so also has mortality; the reduced mortality percentages are probably functions of earlier operation and of antibiotics. In general, the higher mortality rates are reported, as Egdahl (1964) has shown, in hospitals whose patient populations are comprised of the indigent. In his report, the patients who died after appendectomy were symptomatically ill with appendicitis 1 to 14 days before seeking hospital treatment, the mean being 5½ days.

TABLE 37-1. DECREASING INCIDENCE OF ACUTE APPENDICITIS

METROPOLITAN HOSPITALS									
All Admissions		All Surgical Cases		Primary Appendicitis		Acute Appendicitis		Nonacute Appendicitis	
1941	1956	1941	1956	1941	1956	1941	1956	1941	1956
211,138	383,841	106,794	204,405	7,388	3,920	3,869	2,878	2,295	1,042
A GROUP OF RURAL AND SUBURBAN HOSPITALS									
50,887	99,848	23,352	39,228	2,974	1,752				

Castleton, K. B., Puestow, C. B., and Sauer, D.: Is appendicitis decreasing? Arch. Surg., 78:794, 1959.

Although appendicitis is seen most frequently in patients between the ages of 10 and 20, it is probably still the most frequent inflammatory surgical condition arising in the right lower quadrant in any decade of life (Table 37-2 and Ross et al., 1962).

In some areas of the world, acute appendicitis is said to be unusual or rare; certain areas of Asia and Africa have been cited as examples. Newbold (1962) stated that in the 15 years he had been engaged in practice in Ruanda, Africa, performing annually approximately 200 major abdominal procedures, he had encountered only 1 case of acute appendicitis. The explanation usually given is one pertaining to dietary habits of more primitive peoples, though the precise reason is not known. As a history of constipation is fairly frequent in patients with acute appendicitis in this country, the lack of it in countries whose inhabitants eat more fruits and vegetables may contribute to, if not account for, the reported differences in attack rates. However, these reports do not take into account the high infant mortality rates or the poor quality of medical records in such areas. In consequence, these claims (low incidence of acute appendicitis and its explanation on dietary and bowel habits) cannot be accepted readily without greater assurance as to the validity of the original data. For example, Kelley (1968) observed that 98 per cent of the patients operated upon for acute appendicitis at the Dhahran Health Center between 1952 and 1968 were Saudi Arab nations and Muslims of the neighboring areas. He concludes that the alleged low incidence of appendicitis among people not highly civilized, living under unsanitary conditions and eating a diet high in roughage, is a myth.

Barnes et al. (1962) reviewed the classification of cases in which appendectomy was

TABLE 37-2. APPENDICITIS IN A COMMUNITY HOSPITAL: 1946–60

MORTALITY		
Diagnosis	Number	Deaths
Acute appendicitis	1,351	12
Normal appendix	971	0

CASE DISTRIBUTION															
	1946	−47	−48	−49	−50	−51	−52	−53	−54	−55	−56	−57	−58	−59	−60
Normal	159	199	141	100	74	60	50	30	29	21	25	20	28	19	16
Acute	110	126	111	92	117	115	67	86	94	81	82	73	56	61	80

AGE DISTRIBUTION								
	0–9	10–19	20–29	30–39	40–49	50–59	60–69	70+
Normal	108	368	251	153	61	19	8	3
Acute	220	428	284	169	107	69	49	26

Ross, F. P., Zarem, H. A., and Morgan, A. P.: Appendicitis in a community hospital. Arch. Surg., 85:1036, 1962.

Table 37-3. Classification of 7,810 Cases in Appendectomy Study
1937–1959, Massachusetts General Hospital

		Deaths		Survivors		Total
				Drainage of Incision or Secondary Closure	Primary Closure	
Group	Gross Pathology	No.	%	No.	No.	No.
A	Normal appendix	4	0.2	12	1,962	1,978
B	Inflamed appendix, not gangrenous	5	0.1	136	3,990	4,131
C	Gangrenous appendix, not perforated	4	0.6	85	555	644
D	Perforated appendix with or without small abscess formation	29	3.6	457	320	806
E	Appendiceal abscess *not* treated initially by appendectomy	33	13.1	142*	76†	251
	Totals	75				7,810

* These cases had initial incision and drainage of appendiceal abscess followed, in 82 per cent of the cases, by interval appendectomy.

† These cases had initial period of nonoperative management for appendiceal abscess. Subsequently, they had interval appendectomy or right colon surgery for treatment of sepsis of appendiceal origin. (Barnes et al., 1962)

performed between the years 1937 and 1959 at the Massachusetts General Hospital. These are shown in Table 37-3. In that institution, the cases of acute appendicitis were seen no earlier in the evolution of their disease in 1959 than in 1937, whereas in some other areas, the patients appear to seek medical assistance earlier.

Historical Note

In 1759 Mestivier reported one of the first cases of acute appendicitis. This report is believed to be the first valid description of this disease, although Heister and Fernel may have been discussing appendicitis in their writings in 1581 and 1711 respectively. John Parkinson in a case report published in 1812 is credited with the first description of a death from peritonitis following perforation of the appendix. Nearly 50 years earlier, de Lamotte described autopsy findings wherein he attributed death to intestinal obstruction secondary to recurring attacks of appendicitis in which its lumen was occluded by "cherrylike" stones. Melier in 1827 pointed out that perforating appendicitis was a frequent cause of peritonitis and death in the young adult, but the value of his observations and those of others were to be negated by the erroneous conclusions of the more influential Dupuytren who attributed the disease process to the cecum rather than the appendix. Dupuytren persuaded Husson and Dance to accept his views, and they were expressing his views in their report of 1827. Dupuytren subsequently made known his own feelings in his lectures on clinical surgery in 1833.

It is not clear to this author that the indictment of Dupuytren in this connection should be as severe as generally quoted. True, Goldbeck wrote his thesis at Heidelberg, expressing and adopting the French views in 1830; he coined the term perityphlitis, attributing the disease to peri-inflammatory disease of the cecum (typhlon) in spite of the fact that his report contained also a recognized case of perforative appendicitis from fecal concretions and was associated with peritonitis. Burne in 1837 recognized the fallacy of the French conclusions and made a strong appeal that their views be modified.

Boyce credits Voltz in 1846 as reporting 38 cases of "intra-abdominal inflammation followed by perforation of the appendix as the result of fecal concretion." He is said to doubt that perforation of the appendix ever occurred in the absence of concretions except in tuberculosis and typhoid fever; he believed that perityphlitis is secondary to perforation of the cecum. Voltz distinguished between nonperforative and perforative appendicitis and subdivided the latter into those forming localized abscess and those which were not localized but progressed to generalized peritonitis. Boyce also states that Leudet concluded in 1859 that

Perforation of the ileocecal appendix is in itself more common than all other perforations of any part of the intestine whatever; it at least equals in frequency all perforations of the digestive tract taken collectively.

On the surface, these appear as convincing proof that acute appendicitis was generally recognized prior to 1886; but this was not true. This author examined several medical and surgical texts published between the years 1875 and 1885 and found no mention of appendicitis or that perityphlitis, typhlitis or paratyphlitis was considered as the result of appendicitis. As late as 1884, J. Graham Brown of Edinburgh, writing in *Birmingham's Medical Library,* discussed carefully the patient's attitude in acute peritonitis from "typhilitis," stating that "A patient with acute peritonitis lies with knees drawn up"; but nowhere is there reference in his writing to the fact that perforation of the inflamed appendix was a cause of this condition. That same year, 1884, Krönlein apparently first recognized a case of peritonitis as due to perforating appendicitis and performed the first planned appendectomy for this disease but the patient died (Kelly and Hurdon, 1905).

Hall of New York recorded in June of 1886 the first appendectomy performed in the United States. His preoperative diagnosis—strangulated hernia—was in error. Thomas G. Morton of Philadelphia, according to Kelly and Hurdon, appears to have performed the first successful appendectomy wherein the preoperative diagnosis was perforative appendicitis; the operation was performed for this disease; and the patient recovered. A concretion the size of a "cherry stone" was found near the appendix, both the concretion and the appendix lying in an abscessed cavity. Concretions, pins and other foreign bodies usually were reported to lie within the appendix or the abscess cavity in most of the early cases reported—from Mestivier's patient whose appendix contained a pin to the patient of Morton alluded to above.

The recognition of appendicitis as a clinical and pathologic entity, for which the surgical therapy was essential to recovery, was largely the result of the efforts of two men: Reginald Fitz, Professor of Pathologic Anatomy at Harvard, and Charles McBurney (1889, 1894), a surgeon at St. Luke's Hospital in New York City. Fitz reported before the first meeting of the American Association of Physicians, held in Washington, D.C., on Friday, June 18, 1886, the general problem of perforative appendicitis and its sequelae—peritonitis and abscess formation. He discarded the terms of typhlitis, perityphlitis and paratyphlitis calling attention "to the importance of the fact that in the vast majority of cases, the primary disease was an inflammation of the cecal appendix." He presented 257 cases of perforative appendicitis diagnosed anatomically and recognized that the one treatment which could be expected to give good results was an appendectomy performed early in the course of the disease. The Fitz report was convincing and was not allowed to lie dormant; he persisted in repeating his views and presented his data in an accurate and understandable manner. No one can doubt the importance of his contributions.

McBurney's contributions consisted in the formulating in an orderly and accurate arrangement the clinical features of early appendicitis, making possible the diagnosis prior to rupture. He contributed to the operative considerations of appendectomy and insisted upon early appendectomy. The principles set forth by this surgeon continue as the basis for our therapeutic practices of today. A review of more historical details was made for this disease by Meade in 1964.

ANATOMY OF THE APPENDIX

The vermiform appendix is the remnant of the apex of the cecum. The 3 longitudinal muscular bands (taenia coli) of the cecum arise at the base of the appendix and traverse the colon throughout its intra-abdominal length. Occasionally, the appendix is not easily located; if present it always will be found by following the taeniae downward to their point of origin at the apex of the cecum which conforms to the point of origin of the appendix. The appendix varies in length from 1 to 10 inches. It has its own mesentery, triangular

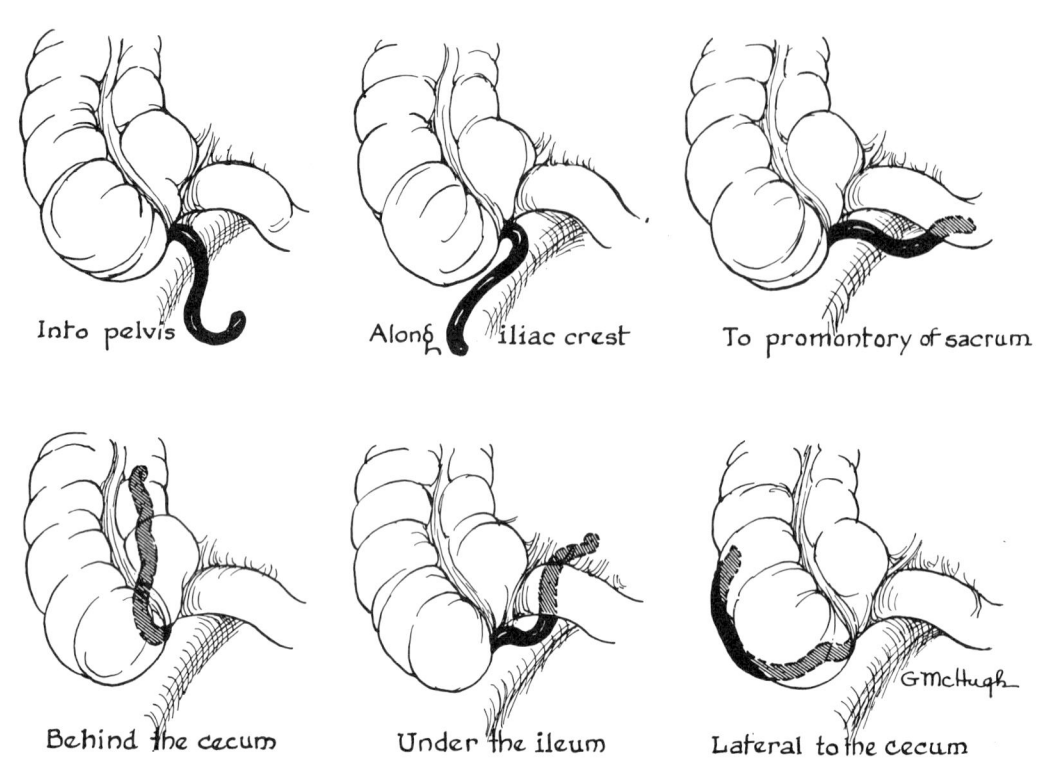

Into pelvis | Along iliac crest | To promontory of sacrum

Behind the cecum | Under the ileum | Lateral to the cecum

FIG. 37-1. The position of the appendix varies considerably; the more commonly encountered locations are illustrated. This factor of variation in its position can be important to the location of pain in general and of tenderness in particular.

in shape, in which course its blood and lymphatic vessels. The arterial blood supply is the appendicular artery, a branch of the terminal portion of the ileocolic artery.

The position of the appendix in relation to the caput of the cecum and the terminal ileum varies considerably. Some of these variations account for minor but important differences in the location of pain and tenderness which accompany an attack of appendicitis. The more commonly encountered positions of the course and the tip of the appendix in the abdomen are listed below in the order of the frequency generally found. These are also illustrated in Figure 37-1.

Positions in Which the Appendix Is More Commonly Found:

1. The right side of the false pelvis
2. The right iliac fossa beside the right iliac vessels
3. Mesially toward the sacral promontory
4. Posterior to the cecum, usually referred to as the retrocecal position
5. At the inferior angle of the ileocecal junction
6. Mesial or lateral to the cecum
7. Along the anterior surface of the cecum (infrequent)
8. The left side if situs inversus is present
9. (Rarely) totally absent (Elias et al., 1967)

The histology of the appendix is important to the cause of appendicitis in some patients, especially in the young (see below). The mucosa resembles that of the colon. In the submucosa are situated numerous lymph follicles which gradually atrophy with age. The muscular and serosal coats are also similar to those of the colon.

PATHOGENESIS OF ACUTE APPENDICITIS

The most frequent cause (about 90%) of acute appendicitis is occlusion of the lumen of the appendix. The cause is usually a fecal impaction or concretion and rarely a foreign body such as a seed. These concretions (fecaliths) may be solitary or multiple and may be located in the lumen at any point from appendiceal-cecal junction to its distal tip.

Locally, the concretion may produce ulceration of the mucosa with inflammatory response which, if allowed to continue, usually induces necrosis, gangrene and perforation. Occasionally, concretions are found in the appendix incidentally; thus, not all concretions produce appendicitis. Some of these may be calcified and identifiable by roentgenographic examination. At a later date, they may no longer be visible; presumably, in such cases, the fecalith has been expelled uneventfully into the cecum. Others may remain inactive indefinitely. Still others may lie dormant, sometimes for months to years, only to give rise to acute appendicitis at a later date. A case in point is that of a 62-year-old male who was on periodic medical management for the treatment of duodenal ulcer over a 20-year period. The roentgenogram in Figure 37-2 shows the presence of an appendiceal concretion present for at least 1 year prior to an attack of acute gangrenous appendicitis. Chemical analysis of the opaque concretion removed at appendectomy proved that it was largely barium sulfate. Presumably this resulted from one of the several barium meals administered in following the course of his duodenal ulcer. The last barium meal had been administered 12 months prior to the onset of acute appendicitis; the appendiceal concretion had been observed 18 months prior to that examination, or 30 months prior to his attack of appendicitis and appendectomy.

Obstructive appendicitis may result from causes other than appendiceal concretions, fecaliths or foreign bodies. In children or young adults, the abundant lymphoid tissue in the submucosa of the appendix may undergo acute hyperplasia along with the lymphoid tissue elsewhere in response to systemic infections, especially those of the upper respiratory tract. The lymphoid hyperplasia may obstruct the appendiceal lumen temporarily, giving rise to appendicitis. In a large university student population, the incidence of acute appendicitis increases at times of epidemics of respiratory diseases, possibly for this reason. In the older age patients, acute appendicitis may be a manifestation of carcinoma of the cecum or of the appendix itself, obliter-

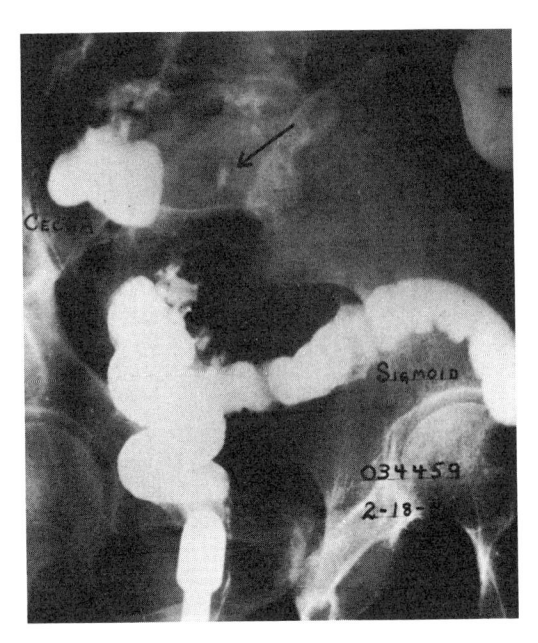

FIG. 37-2. Photograph of an opacity in the region of the appendix which had been interpreted as a probable appendiceal fecalith in a 62-year-old male. Thirty months later appendectomy was performed for perforative appendicitis. The fecalith proved to be barium sulfate. The lumen was completely occluded by this barium concretion at the time of appendectomy, illustrating that some concretions within the appendix may remain dormant for long periods of time, but eventually some may produce trouble.

ating or obstructing the appendiceal lumen. A carcinoma of the cecum should be searched for at the time of appendectomy if peritonitis is not present. A month or 6 weeks later the patient should be examined fluoroscopically and the stools examined at this time for the presence of occult blood. Bierman (1968) presents preliminary evidence which he concludes indicates that the appendix tends to suppress the occurrence of neoplastic disease. Thirty-five per cent of patients who had cancer had had a previous appendectomy, whereas only 24 per cent of 679 patients without cancer had had an appendectomy. One cannot be certain from his report of the meaning of his data, if indeed they mean anything.

As the individual ages, the appendix tends to atrophy; often this atrophy is not uniform, leaving certain areas in which the lumen is partially or totally obliterated and more distal ones in which the lumen remains. If the obliterated lumen involves only the proximal end of the appendix, the more distal portion remains patent and subject to subsequent infection. This is not an infrequently encountered setting responsible for acute appendicitis among older patients. Intestinal parasites, especially pinworms, may infest the appendiceal lumen, giving rise to acute appendicitis. Regional ileitis or ileo-ulcerative colitis at times also obstructs the proximal lumen and may cause appendicitis.

When regional enteritis is encountered at laparotomy, the prevailing opinion is that incidental appendectomy should be performed at the time unless the cecum is also involved (Marx, 1964). When the cecum and the appendix are involved in regional enteritis, appendectomy is usually not warranted because of the frequent occurrence of external fistula from the appendiceal stump.

About 10 per cent of cases have no demonstrable or obvious cause to explain the attack. The author has seen one case in which a small arterial embolus to the appendicular artery caused gangrenous appendicitis in a 69-year-old male. In this patient, the onset of pain began in the right lower quadrant; there was no epigastric distress.

The pathologic sequelae of acute appendicitis which occur within the first few days to few weeks after the attack are primarily peritonitis and abscess formation and septic thrombi of the portal tributaries which may in turn give rise to abscesses in the liver. Latent complications (months to years) are almost always related to adhesions. The small bowel is either enmeshed in these adhesions from the beginning or a segment of bowel insinuates itself between adhesive bands, causing obstruction or volvulus. In either case, "closed loop" obstruction and ischemic necrosis of the bowel wall may occur.

NONPERFORATIVE ACUTE APPENDICITIS

There are several forms of appendicitis that should be distinguished. These include mild appendicitis, edematous and suppurative appendicitis, gangrenous appendicitis and perforative appendicitis.

CLINICAL ASPECTS OF ACUTE NONPERFORATIVE APPENDICITIS

Onset of Pain and Tenderness. The symptoms of nonperforative appendicitis were first described by Charles McBurney of New York in 1889. He observed the early onset to be usually that of mild general abdominal pain beginning in the epigastrium; usually this is associated with acute loss of appetite and occasionally with nausea and vomiting. After a few hours, the pain localizes or "settles" in the right lower quadrant. Then the early and more generalized abdominal pain or distress may subside. A history of recent constipation is the rule, but the occasional patient may have experienced some diarrhea or no change in bowel habits.

Fever in nonperforative appendicitis, as McBurney pointed out, is slight, generally 99° to 100° F. The pulse rate is usually normal. The patient sometimes prefers to lie with flexion of the right thigh. Occasionally, reflex hyperesthesia is present along the cutaneous area supplied by the distribution of the right 10th, 11th and 12th intercostal nerves in the lower right side of the abdomen.

The point of greatest early *tenderness* usually is located in the region referred to as *McBurney's point*. This point he described as being "located exactly between an inch and a half and two inches from the anterior spinous process of the ilium on a straight line drawn from that process in the umbilicus." As experience accumulated, so exact a location is not always possible, nor is the point of maximum tenderness always so specific. This tenderness is a function of the position in which the appendix lies. In malrotation of the colon, the tenderness in acute appendicitis may not be in the right lower quadrant at all should the cecum lie elsewhere in the abdomen. If the inflamed tip of the appendix lies deeply in the pelvis, the point of greatest tenderness may be high on the right side elicited only by rectal examination. Occasionally, the cecum is felt to be distended with gas.

The quality of the tenderness varies considerably. If the inflamed appendix lies anteriorly and in contact with the abdominal wall, tenderness is maximal. If the appendix is retrocecal, tenderness may be slight. If the tip lies deep in the pelvis, little or no tenderness may be elicited by abdominal examination. *The diagnosis may be missed unless rectal and pelvic examinations are made.*

Rebound tenderness, that is, pain referred to the region of the appendix when the examining hand releases its pressure suddenly from the abdomen, is commonly seen in appendicitis. In nonperforative appendicitis, the rebound tenderness is localized to the appendiceal area. Contralateral abdominal pressure with sudden release also may cause rebound pain in the right lower quadrant. This is highly suggestive of inflammatory disease confined to the region of the appendix but is noted less often than when the sudden release is from pressure applied directly over the cecum.

Muscle spasm of the right lower abdomen often is seen early. At first, this is a voluntary type of splinting which can be overcome by gentle pressure, particularly if the patient's attention is distracted. Muscle spasm tends to become involuntary or reflex as the disease progresses, especially if perforation occurs and peritonitis develops. However, as Cope states, the appendix may be on the verge of perforation without the slightest evidence of rigidity being demonstrable. Thus, the absence of voluntary rigidity is not an all-important consideration.

The use of the stethoscope to determine whether or not bowel sounds are present is of the greatest importance in establishing the presence or the absence of generalized peritonitis. With peritonitis bowel sounds are often infrequent and may be absent. The stethoscope can be a very important instrument in the examination of the acute abdomen; in some instances, the information obtained may be decisive.

Laboratory Aids. An elevation of the leukocyte count is commonly found within a few hours after the onset of the first symptoms of appendicitis. As the disease progresses, the count continues to rise; minor changes may be due to error or to diurnal variation; and such changes do not constitute good reason either to wait or to intervene. Initially, a count of 10,000 to 12,000 per mm. of blood is found; at this level, the leukocyte count is not very helpful or necessarily reliable. When it reaches 14,000 or higher, it assumes a role of major importance, especially when accompanied by other symptoms and signs suggestive of appendicitis. In debilitated or critically ill patients, as well as in the aged and diabetic, the leukocyte count may not be elevated or is increased only slightly, even in acute perforative appendicitis. However, a blood smear in most instances shows an increase in the number of neutrophilic granulocytes even when the total leukocyte count is not elevated. Valuable as the leukocyte count has proved to be, failure to find an elevated white count in the face of other dominant clinical findings of appendicitis should not discourage or delay appendectomy. A blood smear should be done in connection with the diagnostic work-up for acute appendicitis for other reasons also. On occasion, it has been the first evidence for the presence of some blood dyscrasia or infectious disease. Such a finding indicates the need for further study but does not preclude the diagnosis of acute appendicitis or the need for appendectomy.

The sedimentation rate also may be elevated but is not diagnostic and is not usually employed by this author in most patients suspected of having appendicitis. A greatly accelerated sedimentation rate within a few hours after onset of symptoms should make one search for other causes or explanations, especially pelvic inflammatory disease or some associated disease characterized by macroglobulinemia.

Examination of the clean voided urine is essential. The finding of glycosuria, albumin, or casts suggest the presence of other important co-existent disease which may modify the program of fluid therapy and possibly the choice of anesthesia. Large quantities of red or white blood cells in the urine suggest that the symptoms attributed to acute appendicitis may be the result of urologic disease such as pyelitis, cystitis, renal tract tumor, renal calculi and renal tuberculosis. However, the presence of 10 to 30 erythrocytes per highpowered field in the uncentrifuged urine is an occasional finding in acute appendicitis should the inflamed appendix lie alongside the course of the ureter or be in contact with the urinary bladder. Bacilluria in fresh catheterized urine usually is not found in acute appendicitis; when present, it is cause to suspect renal tract infection as the basis of the patient's complaints.

A plane roentgenographic film of the abdomen occasionally may be desirable. The diagnosis of a radiopaque fecalith in the region of the appendix when other manifestations of appendicitis are present strongly supports the presumptive diagnosis of appendicitis. Also, a chest roentgenogram may be useful, as pain in the right lower abdomen may be referred along the 9th, 10th, 11th or 12th nerves irritated by disease such as pneumonia located in the lower right chest giving rise to pleurisy. The author does not employ either of these roentgen procedures routinely except for chest roentgenograms in young children but has utilized either or both roentgenographic procedures in puzzling cases, especially in the aged patient.

Diagnosis of Nonperforative Acute Appendicitis

The clinical features of early acute appendicitis are by no means as constant as may be implied above. But the trend is usually there, and in most cases the diagnosis is made fairly easily. In the first place, the fact that acute appendicitis is the most commonly encountered inflammatory disease in the right lower abdomen of all age groups is reassuring. Acute pain and tenderness within this region always should alert the suspicion of the surgeon to the possibility of this diagnosis. Although there may be evidence to implicate other sources for the origin of symptoms, such as a slow leak from a perforated duodenal ulcer, an inflamed gallbladder or pelvic inflammatory disease, often the possibility of acute appendicitis cannot be excluded readily.

When acute appendicitis is present, usually more than one complaint or finding is observed. Some of these findings are more important than others; given a patient whose history is of short duration with abdominal tenderness over the region of the appendix, or with rectal tenderness elicited on the right side by digital examination, this alone is sufficient evidence to make the diagnosis of appendicitis, barring indications of disease elsewhere. However, pain and/or tenderness may not always be pronounced or severe in acute appendicitis, especially should the appendix lie retrocecally or deep in the pelvis.

In the author's experience, the following are the findings most commonly observed in acute appendicitis; they are listed in the order of their importance to this diagnosis.

1. Point tenderness over the region of the appendix, whether from abdominal or rectal examination, in patients with a short history of epigastric or periumbilical distress and pain which localizes in the right lower abdomen a few hours later
2. The above findings with a slight fever (99° to 100.6° F.)
3. Co-existing moderate leukocytosis (12,000 to 18,000) or a pronounced increase in the percentage of neutrophils in the blood smear should the total white count not be elevated
4. Normal urinary sediment
5. Absence of disease elsewhere

If any error is more common than others in making the diagnosis of acute nonperforative appendicitis, it is the tendency to be too precise as to the nature of the pathology present. It is more important to arrive at the conclusion that an acute surgical condition exists in the right lower abdomen and to explore promptly for its cause and surgically to correct it than to risk perforative appendicitis while waiting for better interpretation of symptoms. Some diagnostic errors cannot be avoided, but the percentage will not be high when the patient is examined thoughtfully and carefully. In doubtful cases, wherein the patient has little systemic or localized findings, repeated examinations by the same individual at intervals of 1 to 4 hours is a most useful practice, often saving the patient from needless operation on one hand and needless perforation on the other.

Certain alterations in pain and tenderness are thought to have special connotations; at times they may relate to the onset of gangrenous appendicitis, the occurrence of perforation of the appendix and to recovery from an attack.

Once the diagnosis of acute appendicitis is made, treatment is prompt appendectomy if not contraindicated for reasons of the patient's general condition. Some patients will recover spontaneously from an attack, but the incidence of recurrent attacks a few weeks to months later is dangerously high, and recurrence may be under less favorable circumstances than the initial attack. One third of the 257 fatal cases comprising Fitz's original report (1886) died from a recurrent attack. Others have reported this same impressively consistent trend. If, in any case of subsiding appendicitis, the decision is to wait and the attack subsides without complication, then the appendectomy should be performed within 8 weeks.

The Significance of the Relief of Pain and Tenderness

Acute Gangrenous Appendicitis. In this type of appendicitis, pain may abate temporarily and, in some cases, even disappear for a few hours. Tenderness, likewise, may be less pronounced. This may give the false impression that the pathologic process is improving. However, fever and leukocytosis are likely to persist or to increase during this same short period of time.

Perforation of the Appendix. Should the distended and inflamed appendix undergo perforation, there may also be a sudden relief of pain for a short time, even though the remainder of the appendix is viable. Tenderness also may abate temporarily after perforation. However, fever and leukocytosis are likely to increase after perforation, in spite of a brief period of relief of symptoms. The relief of pain and tenderness following perforation or gangrene is not frequent in this author's experience; usually, pain and tenderness become more pronounced—not less so.

Spontaneous Recovery From Acute Appendicitis. The relief of pain and tenderness is also associated with a recession of an attack of acute appendicitis. In such cases, fever and leukocytosis also diminish and may return to normal within a few days. Relief of symptomatic complaints in subsiding appendicitis is likely to be at a slower rate than when associated with the onset of gangrenous or perforative appendicitis.

Treatment of Nonperforative Appendicitis

The treatment of acute appendicitis is appendectomy. This should be carried out as soon as the diagnosis is made. Any serious fluid or electrolyte imbalance that might exist can be corrected while the operating room is being readied and during the operation itself. The administration parenterally of one of the broad-spectrum antibiotics or one of their combinations before and during the operation, especially if peritonitis exists, reduces the danger of life-threatening wound infections and sepsis (see p. 1039). If the patient has eaten within 8 hours, a stomach tube is passed, and the gastric contents are aspirated prior to the induction of anesthesia (see Chap. 14, Operative Surgical Care).

Anesthesia. The choice of the anesthetic agent is conditioned by the age and the general state of the patient, as well as the one that the anesthetist feels most competent to administer. Before the incision is made, the surgeon should again palpate the abdomen in the region of the appendix because an occasional mass that otherwise would not be detectable may be felt when the patient is relaxed by anesthesia.

Incision. The muscle-splitting incision was designed originally for the purpose of performing an appendectomy and for the lateral drainage of abscess so commonly present. Also, as McArthur (1894) pointed out, this incision reduces the incidence of postoperative hernia. It remains to this day the incision of choice and is the one which all 4 editors of *Surgery: Principles and Practice* recommend for most patients.

The technic of this incision is as follows: The skin is incised parallel with its nerve supply. The author prefers to place the incision beginning just mesial to the anterior superior spine of the ilium. It is carried in a slightly curved line, crossing the lateral margin of the right rectus muscle for a distance of about ¾ in. The mesial end of the cut lies about ½ in. lower on the abdominal wall than does the lateral end. The entire length of the skin incision is 4 to 6 in.

The midportion of the edges of the skin with its subcutaneous fat is elevated above and below for a distance of about 2 in. in each direction. Retractors are placed at the centers of each skin flap, and the assistant pulls gently in both directions so as to expose the underlying tendinous portion of the external oblique.

Then these fibers are incised for a distance of 4 to 6 in. in the descending direction in which they run, passing about 1 in. mesial to the anterior superior spine.

The fascial incision should be placed so that

one third of its length lies above a projected line from the anterior superior spine to the umbilicus and two thirds of its length lie below this imaginary line.

The internal oblique is now exposed and incised in the parallel horizontal direction at a level corresponding to that of the skin incision. At times it may be necessary to incise the fascia at the lateral margins of the rectus muscle to permit better mesial exposure. The transversalis fascia is similarly incised or separated with scissors.

The peritoneum is now incised obliquely but only for a short distance, beginning about 1 in. mesial to the anterior superior spine. The author prefers to stretch the incised peritoneum with the retractors rather than to incise the full length of the available area, as this makes its upper and lower ends more easily seen when ready for closure after appendectomy. The end result of these 4 incisions is a "gridiron" effect, a term by which this incision occasionally is known.

The "gridiron" incision has certain advantages: There is little blood loss. The nerves to the musculature of the abdominal wall are spared. It affords ready access for the drainage of an appendiceal abscess if this be present. Should adhesions form, they are likely to be lateral and of little consequence. Finally, the healed wound, because of its crosshatch nature, is stronger than any other type. Those objecting to its use do so on the basis that the exposure is limited in patients where pathology lies elsewhere, particularly in the left tube or ovary. Because the incision can be expanded or extended readily, this criticism seems to be unwarranted. Others believe it to be impracticable should the primary disease be that of a perforated gallbladder or duodenal ulcer. To this the author agrees, but such cases are rare and when they are encountered, it is simple to close this incision and to make another in a more appropriate area. The appendix is first removed, however.

Of historical interest is the question of to whom should go the credit for the introduction of the muscle-splitting incision for acute appendicitis. Undoubtedly, the first publication on this subject was McBurney's which appeared in the July issue of the *Annals of Surgery* in 1894. He had employed this technic in 4 cases, the first being operated upon December 18, 1893. Also, in 1894, the independent report of McArthur appeared in the November issue of the *Chicago Medical Recorder*, at which time he described the use of this incision in 59 cases. From the published discussion it appears clear that McArthur had employed this incision for at least 18 months prior to its use by McBurney and certainly in many more cases. McArthur's report had been submitted to the secretary of the Chicago Medical Society in the spring of 1894 but could not be read before that society until after the summer's vacation. While the students and the admirers of each of these men have debated the question of to whom priority should be given, it is to the credit of both of these great surgeons that this was never a point of concern to them.

Usually, the appendix is located easily after the peritoneum is incised unless it is retrocecal or adherent to pelvic structures or the sacral promontory. The caput of the cecum is lifted gently out of the wound along with a short portion of the terminal ileum. If the tip of the appendix comes out easily, its arteries and veins are divided and ligated; the appendix then remains attached only to the cecum. Should the tip of the appendix be bound down too tightly to permit its gentle deliverance into the wound, or if it is too friable or necrotic to permit flexion without rupture, the base of the appendix is clamped and severed from the cecum first. Then the clamped base is lifted gently and separated from its mesentery, from its base to its tip. Every vessel is ligated individually after being clamped adjacent to the appendix.

The management of the appendiceal stump is a point of considerable variance in practice. In general, there are 3 methods of closure that can be employed. Some prefer to crush momentarily the base of the appendix at its junction with the cecum and to ligate the short stump at this site, and do no more. Others prefer not to crush the base of the appendix; rather, they incise the appendix at its point of junction with the cecum and then close this opening with interrupted fine catgut sutures. Still others prefer to ligate the base of the appendix and to bury the short ligated stump by means of a purse-string suture placed in the cecum. The author prefers the last technic, using No. 000 plain catgut to ligate the base of the appendix and No. 000 medium chromic catgut as the cecal purse-string suture. In theory, should an abscess form at the site of the buried appendix, it might rupture more easily into the cecum than into the peritoneal cavity as the plain catgut ligature should digest much more rapidly than the chromic purse-string ligature.

The placement of a drain into the region of the amputated appendix to be led to the outside through a laterally placed stab wound depends largely on whether there was rupture of the appendix or spillage of pus from an abscess encountered during appendectomy. In either of the latter instances, the author employs a small soft rubber drain of the Penrose type which is led to the outside through a laterally placed stab wound. Also, a small slip of a drain is placed in the subcutaneous tissue and brought out through the lower end of the skin incision. Clean cases are not drained.

Closure of the wound is then effected, gently approximating each layer separately. The one layer likely to be missed is the transversus muscle. This is found readily by turning back the edges of the internal oblique muscle. These two layers may be approximated as one.

Unless other factors contravene, ambulation is possible the day of operation. Oral feeding usually can begin the next day, with liquid to soft to regular diet progressing over a period of 3 to 4 days. At the end of this period of time the patient may be ready for discharge.

Mortality in Nonperforative Acute Appendicitis

Death of patients with nonperforative acute appendicitis is nearly always from other causes: anesthesia, pulmonary embolism, cardiovascular accidents and bronchopneumonia. These are largely unpreventable deaths. Thus death from the operative procedure—appendectomy—is indeed rare, less than 0.3 per cent when the operation is performed prior to perforation, even when deaths from all other causes are included. The story is quite different for perforative appendicitis.

PERFORATIVE ACUTE APPENDICITIS

Once perforation has occurred, the essentially nonexistent operative mortality and morbidity of nonperforative appendicitis no longer obtain. Peritonitis and intra-abdominal abscesses are serious sequelae to be reckoned with; pylephlebitis and miliary abscesses in the liver are another set of complications to be expected in some patients; bowel obstruction, fecal fistula and malnutrition are still other serious consequences which may appear. The folly of surgical delay or of expectant management of acute appendicitis is so obvious as to point up sharply that any practice other than appendectomy prior to perforation has nothing to recommend it and indeed much to condemn it.

Clinical Aspects and Course

Prior to the time of perforation, the symptomatology from acute appendicitis which will rupture if left unattended cannot be distinguished from that of one that will not perforate. However, after perforation the symptoms change. Rupture of the appendix seldom or never occurs without symptoms preceding the perforation by hours or even days.

Why then does perforative appendicitis continue to occur? There can be only two possible explanations: either acute appendicitis is not recognized by the patient or his physician; or the patient is in a sufficiently isolated area that he cannot or does not seek medical counsel.

Much has been accomplished by public education; undoubtedly, it has brought many patients to the surgeon earlier than they might come otherwise. At the same time, there are certain patients who, when seen by their physician, exhibit mimimal complaints in the face of advanced suppurative acute appendicitis; these are most often elderly people, young children, or infants.

For some reason appendicitis in the child, the aged and the diabetic is likely to progress more rapidly to the stage of perforation than is usually observed in adults. Perhaps the fairly frequent gastrointestinal upsets in children from dietary indiscretion or other causes lead parents to conclude that this is only another upset stomach or "bellyache." While all agree that these may cause unnecessary delays in children, the fact remains that the time interval from onset of symptoms to perforation in the child is, by comparison with the same course in adults, often relatively short. For this reason most surgeons do operate for suspected appendicitis earlier in children when the complaints are suggestive of the diagnosis but not as fully confirmatory as may be desired in the adult.

The importance of perforation in acute appendicitis in children is attested to by Boles et al. (1959). These authors found that 30 per cent of the children in their series of 837 cases had perforation. Furthermore, in preschool children, this increased to 66 per cent. Also, the complication rate in the patients with perforation was seven times that of those with simple acute appendicitis. Similar findings are reported by Jackson (1963), who found the appendix ruptured in 154 of 303 children 12 years old or younger. In only 1 of 36 children operated on after 48 hours of hospitalization was the appendix not ruptured. Maddox et al. (1964) reported a 20 per cent incidence of peritonitis with or without perforation among 405 children at the time they were operated on for acute appendicitis. There were no deaths. They found no difference in the incidence of complicated appendicitis in infants from that observed in children.

Acute appendicitis in the aged patient is also likely to have reached the stage of perforation before the physician is aware that rupture may have taken place already. This situation may be attributed to several factors. The threshold of pain in the aged person usually is increased, partly from tolerance by habit and partly from some loss of cerebral sensory interpretation. His febrile response develops more slowly, and his leukocyte count may rise surprisingly slowly; in some there may be little or no rise. Atrophy of the abdominal musculature with advancing age and the accompanying loss of tone tends to minimize muscle spasm.

Although the debris and the feces contained within the lumen of the appendix at the time of perforation escape and cause local peritonitis, large quantities of feces are seldom found when the abdomen is opened. It is doubtful that a continuous flow of feces from the cecum occurs very often in spontaneous perforative appendicitis, because the site of perforation is usually distal to that of the appendiceal obstruction. Nonetheless, the discharge of pus and feces contained in the obstructed appendix at the time of perforation serves as an excellent source for a continuing and spreading infection—peritonitis.

Tenderness in the abdomen immediately after perforation usually increases, often becoming steady and severe. If peritonitis spreads or becomes generalized, abdominal tenderness becomes more diffuse. If, on the other hand, perforation occurs into the omentum or between agglutinated loops of small bowel, it may remain restricted largely to the right lower abdomen. Thus, the fingerpoint tenderness of nonperforative appendicitis usually is no longer observed once perforation occurs. It is the diffuse character of the tenderness, even though it still may be limited to the right lower abdomen, that largely distinguishes clinically spreading or generalized from local peritonitis, and all three from nonperforative appendicitis.

Rebound tenderness continues after perforation, but its localization is no longer as sharp as that of nonperforative appendicitis; rather, it is likely to conform to the extent of the area involved in peritonitis at the time that the examination is made, extending or receding in accordance with the progress or the recession of peritonitis.

Palpation of the abdomen in perforative appendicitis generally reveals rather intense and extensive spasm of the muscles of the abdominal wall, roughly corresponding to the area of the peritoneum involved in active inflammation. In the author's experience the "boardlike" rigidity, so often characterizing peritonitis of the perforated duodenal ulcer with its highly irritating contents, is not often observed early in peritonitis of bacterial origin, including that of perforative appendicitis. This, too, is not of strong differential diagnostic significance but rather is an observation which, with other considerations, may add or subtract a little from the over-all clinical picture in favor of one diagnosis over another (see Chap. 37, Section 2, Peritonitis).

If peritonitis is spreading or generalized, the gentle palpation of the abdomen may reveal a certain degree of "doughiness" of the skin and the subcutaneous tissue. This sign is generally fairly distinct when present, but some degree of experience and skill is required to detect its presence; it is nondiagnostic. The experience of most surgeons, the author included, is that the doughy abdomen is observed more commonly after intra-abdominal hemorrhage than in chemical or bacterial peritonitis.

The auscultatory findings of peritonitis are largely those of the adynamic ileus in that portion of the peritoneum involved. Bowel sounds are at first hypoactive and, as the disease progresses, they may be entirely absent. Seldom, if ever, are bowel sounds hyperactive unless a portion of the bowel is uninflamed and, proximal to this, mechanical obstruction exists. In most patients with less than a generalized peritonitis, peristalsis ceases; this may be due in part to the reflex adynamic ileus, similar to that observed in the early postoperative stages following intra-abdominal operations and anesthesia; it is also from the local effects of peritonitis.

Laboratory Aids. Some of these are of considerable value in establishing the general condition of the patient with peritonitis but they are of little specific diagnostic consequence. The loss of plasmalike fluid into the peritoneal cavity and the subperitoneal spaces is likely to result in hemoconcentration relative to the preperitonitis values of the hemoglobin and the hematocrit reading; the degree of hemoconcentration is influenced also by the loss of fluids from gastric intubation, an essential part of the treatment of both adynamic and mechanical ileus (see Chap. 37, Section 2, Peritonitis).

The leukocyte count generally rises fairly sharply in perforative appendicitis; it soars above that usually observed in the earlier preperforation stages of acute appendicitis. The infrequently encountered exceptions in the aged, diabetic, or debilitated patients should be mentioned once again. The sedimentation rate usually is increased considerably over that noted in nonperforative acute appendicitis, even when corrected for any preexisting anemia and taking into account that the hemoconcentration of peritonitis is likely to yield normal or increased red cell volume also.

Roentgenographic examination of the abdomen in perforative appendicitis may disclose one of two features or both; neither is diagnostic. The first is the pattern suggestive of adynamic ileus, and the other is the disclosure of an intra-abdominal abscess. Save for the clinical history and physical findings upon which the diagnosis of perforative appendicitis depends, x-ray findings are largely confirmatory. In the author's opinion roentgenographic studies are of greater value in following the progress of the patient, particularly with reference to subsequent abscess formation in areas distal to the site of the appendix. Such examinations may be useful in connection with the initial diagnosis if certain other acute intra-abdominal conditions need to be evaluated and if possible to be excluded by this technic. This author never has seen a case of perforative acute appendicitis in which free intraperitoneal air has been demonstrated. Although this possibility does exist, the obstructive nature of perforative appendicitis seldom allows the free retrograde flow of feces or gas from the cecum.

DIAGNOSIS OF PERFORATIVE APPENDICITIS

The diagnosis of perforative appendicitis is largely the differential diagnosis of local, spreading or generalized peritonitis. Clinically, the events antecedent to perforation and peritonitis are most important to the knowledge of the origin of peritonitis.

The physical findings are largely those relating to peritonitis if the patient is seen for the first time after perforation has occurred. Two features of the examination may be useful to the diagnosis of perforative appendicitis: (1) the localization of the finding of peritonitis largely to the right lower abdomen; (2) the detection of a tender mass within the abdomen or the right pelvis, suggesting an abscess or agglutination of omentum or small bowel to the appendix. Finally, some consolation and possible confirmation are derived from the fact that appendicitis, more than any other inflammatory disorder, accounts for peritonitis limited to the right lower abdomen. Should peritonitis be full-blown and generalized when the patient is first seen, one may have only this statistical possibility in favor of acute appendicitis to aid in formulating his impression of its origin. Should a mass be detectable in the right lower abdomen, the diagnosis of perforative appendicitis is nearly certain in younger people. The possibility of a perforating carcinoma of the cecum with abscess must be considered in older patients; the presence of occult blood in the stool favors the diagnosis of carcinoma. (See also Regional Enteritis and Ulcerative Colitis, Chap. 39.)

Thus, 3 features favor the diagnosis of perforative appendicitis as the cause of peritonitis and form a reasonable basis for this presumptive diagnosis:

1. A history compatible with acute appendicitis prior to the onset of peritonitis
2. A mass palpable in the right lower abdomen or high on the right side of the pelvis as determined by rectal examination. This diagnosis is reinforced by the failure to find occult blood in the stool.
3. The statistical probability of appendicitis in the absence of other disease, especially of peptic ulcer, cholecystitis and diverticulitis.

TREATMENT OF PERFORATIVE APPENDICITIS

Certain clinical facts should be made clear about abscess formation in acute perforative appendicitis as they bear upon the time at which appendectomy can be performed to the best advantage. One has been discussed already. By no means are all masses felt in the right lower quadrant in cases with appendicitis due to abscesses. Many of these are masses of omentum and/or small bowel agglutinated to an inflamed but not perforated appendix. Such masses often are misinterpreted as abscesses, and expectant treatment is pursued; the appendix may perforate, a fate which could have been avoided had appendectomy been carried out sooner. Should the patient not be seen until the 4th to the 6th day and found to appear toxic with a fever of 103° to 105° F., such masses are very likely to be abscesses; this author believes these, too, should be operated on at once in many instances. Drainage through a laterally placed McBurney incision is the operation of choice and usually can be done with little risk. The appendix should be sought for and removed at this same time, provided that its identification does not require the surgeon to explore beyond the confines of the abscess cavity. If no abscess has formed and if local or spreading peritonitis is found and the perforated appendix lies in the free peritoneal cavity, it must be found and removed. The earlier opening of the appendiceal abscesses with appendectomy under these circumstances is a more recent practice made possible primarily by the advent of chemotherapeutic and antibiotic agents.

In experienced hands, this change in attitude toward the treatment of appendiceal abscesses or spreading peritonitis has much to recommend it. In the past, some of these abscesses have ruptured into the peritoneal cavity. Others have dissected into the pelvic area or upward to the regions of the duodenum or have formed fistulae. Spreading peritonitis often has extended rather than receded on conservative management. The relief of fever and intoxication is in itself a desirable accomplishment if early drainage and/or appendectomy can be performed safely. Finally, it is possible but not proved that a reduction in incidence of intrahepatic abscess from migratory septic thrombi arising in the venous radicals of the appendiceal veins may result from draining the abscess with earlier surgical intervention. Pulmonary emboli, septic or sterile, arising from the iliac, the pelvic, or the more distal veins of the extremities, are also to be considered, as these account for a not inconsiderable number of deaths in perforative appendicitis and other inflammatory diseases arising within the lower abdomen, especially in adults.

Appendectomy for perforative appendicitis has been a subject of much discussion by surgeons since Day One (June 18, 1886). Until the past 4 decades, the dominant school was that popularized by A. J. Ochsner: namely, bed rest, opium "around the clock" and nothing by mouth. This was known as the "expectant treatment," awaiting a well-defined abscess to form and to drain it within 10 days of the initial onset of the attack. J. B. Murphy and others held the opposite view for most cases, referring despairingly to the Ochsner method as the "expectans mortans" regimen.

Those who advocated the expectant method were not without fairly sound grounds, at least for many patients seen in their time. They held that the silent abdomen was important to avoiding rupture of the abscess; to this end they stopped feedings, the use of purgatives and enemas, and endorsed the use of opium to quiet bowel activity. They also maintained that time favored the development of an immune response, believing that in due course antibodies to the offending organisms would form. This latter view may be more substantial in theory than in fact, as its importance is not yet settled. To this end, Murphy maintained that the abscess wall and the immune response were very minor considerations compared with leaving the source of the infection within the abdomen, namely, the necrotic appendix.

Today early appendectomy is recognized as the best thing to do for perforative appendicitis. Most of the older arguments favoring delay are not germane to current practice. The surgeon now has additional supportive measures not available in the days of Ochsner or of Murphy. These are, in the order of their development: intravenous fluid therapy, prompt intragastric intubation and the use of safe blood and plasma transfusion.

Fowler's (1900) positioning of the patient with peritonitis to favor the gravitational flow of pus into the pelvis still may be used, but it should be avoided in the presence of impending or actual shock. This author does not employ Fowler's position as frequently as before the days of antibiotic therapy because it favors stasis and embolism, theoretically at least.

Gradients of Conservative and Operative Intervention in Patients with Perforative Appendicitis First Seen After 48 Hours. It is better to decide for each patient the advantages and the disadvantages of operative management of perforative acute appendicitis, realizing that appendectomy must be performed in each case but that timing is the important consideration. This approach perhaps is the most useful and widely practiced method of treating cases of suspected perforative appendicitis at this time. It employs the sound principle of case selection, applying initially to each patient one treatment or the other or their combination once a careful clinical appraisal is made of his particular problem. Such an appraisal should include the possibility that the case is one in which nonperforative appendicitis exists surrounded by a mass of omentum or small bowel and that abscess formation or spreading peritonitis has not yet occurred or will not occur. It also takes into account the possibility that the mass is really an abscess, that a spreading or full-blown generalized peritonitis is already present, and that these latter two complications do not necessarily imply that early drainage and appendectomy will be more harmful than beneficial in all instances. To individualize each case, considering each of these points separately at the time the patient is first seen, is useful, but it must be recognized that an accurate clinical appraisal which will correlate with the actual state of the pathologic process at any one time is difficult. Yet this approach can be employed to good advantage, provided that thoughtful consideration is given to each patient. This may require several visits and examinations of some patients at hourly intervals, before a basis for sound judgment can be reached to determine the therapy best suited for the patient. For some patients the merits of the conservative approach over that of prompt appendectomy are quite obvious, even when they are seen as late as a week after the onset of symptoms.

Favoring prompt appendectomy in suspected perforative appendicitis is the good general condition of the patient and the absence of serious complications. In the author's opinion the suspicion of an abscess and/or the presence of a local or spreading peritonitis are less important considerations, provided that the abscess and the appendix are to be approached from a laterally placed McBurney incision without entering the free peritoneal cavity. The purpose of appendectomy in these cases is the removal of this necrotic organ which, if left in place, continues as the nidus for the growth of pathogenic bacteria and especially of the highly dangerous anaerobes. This more bold attitude assumes that appendectomy and lateral drainage will at least maintain the *status quo* and can be done without entering the free peritoneal cavity save in those cases in which no abscess has been formed. It is also predicated upon the vigorous use of appropriate antibiotic drugs preceding, during and after the operation, the use of blood, plasma and saline to combat shock and sodium depletion, the use of gastric intubation, and the near-constant vigilance on the part of the physician, resetting his therapeutic "compass" as the patient's course indicates.

Coran and Wheeler (1966) observed 28 consecutive cases of acute appendicitis in patients between the ages of 60 and 91. While the clinical picture was similar, it was generally less striking than observed in younger adults. In 17 of the 21 patients operated upon more than 24 hours after onset of symptoms, perforation had occurred. It had also occurred in 1 of 6 patients operated upon earlier than 24 hours. The mortality rate was 7 per cent.

Most surgeons adopted the plan of prompt appendectomy in perforative appendicitis in children many years ago because they found that the expectant treatment did not seem to favor localization (abscess formation) of the infection to the extent that it did in adults.

The mortality of appendicitis continues to decline, again owing to a wider adoption of the practice of early appendectomy. Marcucci et al. (1967) reported 1399 cases of appendicitis occurring between 1961 and 1966 for which operation was performed with no mortality. Pathologic diagnosis of appendicitis was confirmed. The only complications were delayed adhesions with intestinal obstruction, wound abscesses and one wound dehiscence. This totaled less than 1 per cent of the cases.

Favoring delayed surgery in perforative appendicitis are 2 factors: (1) incontrovertible evidence of recession of the peritonitis; and (2) evidence that more than one abscess has formed (subdiaphragmatic, intrahepatic, subhepatic or intermesenteric). Primary concern usually centers about the drainage of these satellite abscesses after a vigorous use of antibiotic drugs having broad-spectrum influence on the usual organisms found in perforative appendicitis (see Chap. 37, Section 2, Peritonitis, and Chap. 4, Surgical Infections).

If the patient recovers from his attack of perforative appendicitis without removal of the appendix, how long should appendectomy be delayed? Barring the persistence of other sequelae, the appendix should be removed within 2 months, because another attack of appendicitis is likely in the relatively near future, and it may be more severe than the initial one. A case in point was a patient observed by Harkins (1956) wherein the patient experienced 3 separate attacks of perforative appendicitis within less than 4 months. Interval appendectomy as soon as symptoms subsided was advocated by Fitz in his original paper. A number of the fatalities that he reported in 1886 resulted from 2nd or 3rd attacks, some coming on within a matter of weeks after the initial one.

APPENDICITIS IN PREGNANCY

Acute appendicitis in pregnancy requires special and separate consideration because in these cases a special hazard exists, as pointed out first by McArthur in 1895. Once an appendiceal abscess forms during the last 2 trimesters of pregnancy, it usually has for its mesial or posteromesial wall the adjacent enlarged uterus. Should abortion or labor occur, shrinkage of the uterus may tear the mesial wall of an appendiceal abscess, allowing free flow of pus throughout the abdomen.

Conservative management of nonperforative appendicitis in pregnancy is likely to be more disastrous than in the population at large. The tendency of the patient to abort or miscarry is slight indeed when appendectomy is performed for acute appendicitis during pregnancy prior to perforation. There is no justification for delay. The removal of a normal appendix in a mistaken diagnosis under these circumstances cannot be condemned, because the risk of a nonoperative error when appendicitis exists is likely to be of much greater consequence.

Priddle and Hesseltine (1951) reported a series of 51 cases of appendicitis subjected to appendectomy in Chicago Lying-in Hospital between 1930 and 1950, and they found that acute appendicitis occurred in 0.07 per cent of all expectant mothers seen at that hospital during that 20-year period. The cases encountered were distributed essentially equally for each trimester. Five more occurred during early postpartum. All but 6 of the 51 patients were under 30 years of age. Only 2 in this series had premature labor. Progesterone was used in none of the 51 patients. One maternal death occurred, which was in 1931. This case is typical of many others reported for neglected appendicitis in pregnancy. The patient, a 32-year-old gravida VI, para V, was 5 months pregnant when seen for the first time. Her history was one of 4 days of nausea, vomiting, abdominal pain and tenderness. She was admitted promptly when first seen and, after rehydration, she was explored immediately for perforative appendicitis. An abscess was found behind the cecum; it contained about 60 ml. of pus arising from retrocecal perforative appendicitis. Drains were placed, and the appendix was removed. Hemolytic streptococci were cultured from this pus. Her recovery was slow, and she was discharged on the 25th day. Two days later she went into premature labor, delivering a 980-Gm. fetus which promptly died. On the 3rd postpartum day, a painful swelling appeared in the region of the previous drain site; this was reopened, and large quantities of pus escaped. Two weeks later a pelvic abscess was drained of 400 ml. of pus; this recurred and resulted in death from sepsis on the 41st postpartum day.

The treatment of suspected appendicitis during pregnancy is appendectomy. The author performed appendectomy in 2 patients in early normal labor in the above hospital; in another patient whose symptoms did not occur until late in the 2nd stage of labor, appendectomy was delayed 4 hours until after delivery was completed.

There is little fear of wound disruption should the patient go into labor soon after appendectomy. The McBurney incision should be used, as this gives the strongest wound. The skin incision usually is placed higher and more laterally than in other cases, and the incision of the internal oblique may need to be longer than is customarily applied to achieve adequate exposure.

RECURRENT APPENDICITIS

This type of appendicitis was first described by Fitz in 1886. A patient recovered or recovering from one attack experiences another. It is for this reason that the appendix always should be removed within 2 months after perforation, should it not have been removed at the time of the initial attack of perforative appendicitis.

REMOVAL OF THE NORMAL APPENDIX IN THE COURSE OF OTHER INTRA-ABDOMINAL OPERATIONS

Opinion is not unanimous as to the wisdom of removing the normal appendix in the course of other intra-abdominal operations. This procedure is to be considered not only as an elective one but also as one which is prophylactic in nature. In favor of appendectomy under these conditions is the prevention of appendicitis at a later day; few surgeons can practice surgery for many years without encountering appendicitis among his own patients on whom he had operated previously for some other intra-abdominal conditions.

This author favors removal of the normal appendix in the course of another operation, provided that appendectomy can be performed through the incision already in use, especially if the patient's general health and operative condition are good, and that if in the surgeon's judgment appendectomy can be performed without threat, including wound contamination. It seems to be logical that appendectomy under these conditions is likely to carry less risk than that of the second anesthetic needed should acute appendicitis occur later. From time to time incidental appendectomy has been recommended as an acceptable procedure to perform in the course of repair of a right inguinal hernia. More recently, Eiseman et al. (1962) and Keeley and Schairer (1962) presented evidence that appendectomy may be performed without an increase in infection in the course of hernia repair, but their cases were not followed long enough to learn if appendectomy under these conditions increased the recurrence rate for the hernia. The basic problem in repair of a hernia is just that—repair. Appendectomy may be performed along with repair of the hernia if it is certain that no risk is entailed.

Occasionally, the presenting symptoms of regional enteritis are those of appendicitis. At operation, if the surgeon observes the classic picture of regional enteritis, should incidental appendectomy be performed? Marx (1964) observed no difficulty when appendectomy was performed on persons with Crohn's disease if the cecum was not edematous or inflamed. However, the removal of the appendix in the face of regional enteritis involving both the terminal ileum and the cecum has been followed by enterocutaneous fistulae arising from the appendiceal stump (Barber et al., 1962). Nonetheless, an incidental appendectomy should be performed when operating for Crohn's disease if the cecum is not involved, in order to exclude appendicitis from the differential diagnosis of possible future abdominal pains.

COMPLICATIONS OF ACUTE APPENDICITIS

The nature and the incidence of the common complications of acute appendicitis are largely conditioned by the character of an attack of appendicitis itself. Complications from appendectomy for *nonperforative* acute appendicitis are rare; of those which have been encountered during the postoperative period, infection in the subcutaneous tissue or an abscess in the region where the appendix lay are the principal ones. Pylephlebitis with miliary abscess formation in the liver, pulmonary embolism and fecal fistula are seldom seen in simple appendicitis. Most complications from appendectomy for nonperforative appendicitis are from anesthesia, poor hemostasis, failure to observe the principles of aseptic surgical technic and sponges left inadvertently in the wound. Latent complications are largely referable to small bowel obstruction from adhesions; obstruction usually makes its first appearance years later but may occur at any time during the remainder of the patient's life.

The complications of *perforative* appendicitis, in comparison with those of the nonperforative form of the disease, are encountered much more frequently. Most of the complications of perforative appendicitis are inseparable from and synonymous with bacterial peritonitis and/or abscess formation. (See Chap. 37, Section 2, Peritonitis and Intra-abdominal Abscesses.)

Peritonitis from Perforative Appendicitis

The onset of perforative appendicitis is generally also the onset of peritonitis. The extent to which peritonitis develops varies immensely; it may progress to involve the entire abdominal cavity or may be largely contained within the right lower quadrant, forming peri-appendiceal or residual abscesses and occasional cecal fistulae. The incidence and the extent of peritonitis from perforated appendicitis varies among hospitals. This is partly because of the type of patient encountered (charity or private) and in part from the lack of uniformity of well-defined or similar terminology when reporting this complication. As bacterial peritonitis may result from many intra-abdominal sites and causes, this subject and its sequelae are discussed more extensively below.

Abscess Formation From Appendicitis

Intra-abdominal abscesses from appendicitis are of 3 types: (1) those localized to the appendiceal area, (2) those situated more distally, as in the subphrenic spaces or pelvis, and (3) those located within other organs, especially the liver, and resulting from pylephlebitis and other pyemias. In addition, subcutaneous or superficial abscesses may occur in the incision. None of these is peculiar to appendicitis, as they may come from any other cause of intra-abdominal infection. However, they are reported more frequently in acute perforative appendicitis, as this is the most commonly encountered cause of bacterial peritonitis.

The incidence of true abscess within the abdomen after appendicitis as well as after ruptured peptic ulcer is difficult to calculate because many surgeons still employ conservative management of some cases of perforative appendicitis, and consequently the actual frequencies of masses of omentum and periappendiceal abscess are not known. Boyce (1949) reports a mortality rate of 13.2 per cent from periappendiceal abscess at the Charity Hospital in New Orleans and believes that abscess formation is a fortunate outcome of perforative appendicitis only insofar as this is a lower mortality than that experienced with spreading peritonitis. Pericecal abscess is largely limited to the perforative form of appendicitis, but it also occurs from contamination during operation in patients with nonperforative appendicitis.

Pylephlebitis (Portal Pyemia) in Appendicitis

This is perhaps the most serious complication of appendicitis, but it is very rare. Pylephlebitis is portal pyemia—that is to say, a septicemia with abscesses in the liver. It is usually associated with septic thrombosis within the portal venous system. Evidently, the abscesses within the liver arise from septic thrombi, or from emboli from the portal venous thromboses. Although the abscesses are usually many and the disease mortal, in some cases the abscesses are few and, if drained or removed by resecting the part of the liver containing them, recovery may be effected.

The clinical picture is one of recurrent chill, fever, mild icterus and enlargement of the liver, following perforative appendicitis. The blood culture is often positive. A scintigram of the liver is very valuable in making the diagnosis and in determining the locations of the hepatic abscesses. Scintigrams of the liver should be made before attempting exploration of the liver for abscess because it is the only way that deeply situated ones can be detected with any degree of certainty.

Drainage or resection of the abscess or abscesses is the treatment. Wide spectrum antibiotics, should the blood culture be positive, can be selected to fit the sensitivities of the organisms and are valuable in treatment. However, it is doubtful that they alone can cure a pyogenic hepatic abscess in the absence of its spontaneous drainage into a large bile duct or of adequate surgical drainage.

Adynamic Ileus and Mechanical Obstruction in Perforative Appendicitis

Adynamic ileus often accompanies spreading or generalized peritonitis from appendicitis and may continue for a week or longer. Gastric or intestinal intubation with continuing suction until bowel tone returns and the patient expels flatus and has a bowel movement is usually effective treatment. However, operative decompression of the dilated intestine may be necessary when intubation (gastric or intestinal) fails to relieve the abdominal distention. (See Chap. 39, Intestinal Obstruction.)

Mechanical obstruction as a complication is observed much less frequently in the early weeks of recovery from perforative appendicitis and is usually a sequel of the increasing adhesions about an abscess or fecal fistula. However, this complication is more likely to occur several months or years later and is seen more often when right paramedian incisions have been used. Appendectomy for nonperforative appendicitis through the lateral McBurney's incision rarely produces adhesions of consequence due only to the operation.

Wound Infection, Fecal Fistula and Malnutrition After Appendectomy

These comprise a complex series of events which may occur in perforative appendicitis with or without abscess formation. These also may be complicated by other types of intraperitoneal infection. Abscess may cause fecal fistula, or fecal fistula may cause abscess. Malnutrition may result from either or both, as well as from other persisting serious complications of appendicitis. The enterocutaneous fecal fistula is the least harmful of this group of complications and is more often the result of necrosis of the adjacent cecal wall from periappendicitis or periappendiceal abscess than from blowout of the ligated or impacted appendiceal stump. Foreign bodies, especially sponges left at operation, should be searched for whenever bowel fistula persists.

MORTALITY FROM APPENDICITIS

Incidence of Peritonitis From All Causes and From Appendicitis in Particular

The mortality in appendicitis is largely from spreading or generalized peritonitis. The remarkable reduction in mortality from acute appendicitis is attributed primarily to 2 factors: (1) more patients being operated on earlier, before perforation, and (2) the improved therapeutic measures for the management of peritonitis. Earlier operation has done more to reduce mortality than have the advances made in the management of peritonitis; nonetheless, the improvement in the management of the latter is by no means inconspicuous or of little consequence.

Peritonitis from perforative appendicitis, although still a serious problem, carries a much lower morbidity and mortality rate than it did at the turn of the century. Ochsner et al. reviewed this subject in 1930 and reported variations in the incidence of peritonitis from 7 to 78 per cent for perforative appendicitis. The Commission on Acute Appendicitis Mortality in Pennsylvania (Bower, 1940), reported 68 per cent of all cases of spreading peritonitis as due to perforative appendicitis. Some years later only 9 per cent of cases of perforative appendicitis developed spreading peritonitis (Commission on Acute Appendicitis Mortality). In the Charity Hospital of New Orleans, spreading peritonitis from perforative appendicitis has declined remarkably (Boyce, 1949). Cannon (1955) observed and reported the same phenomenon at the University of Chicago (Fig. 37-3).

Death From Peritonitis

Cannon (1955) has shown that death from peritonitis of any origin has been reduced. The ratio fell from 32 cases of fatal peritonitis per 500 unselected autopsies in 1927 to

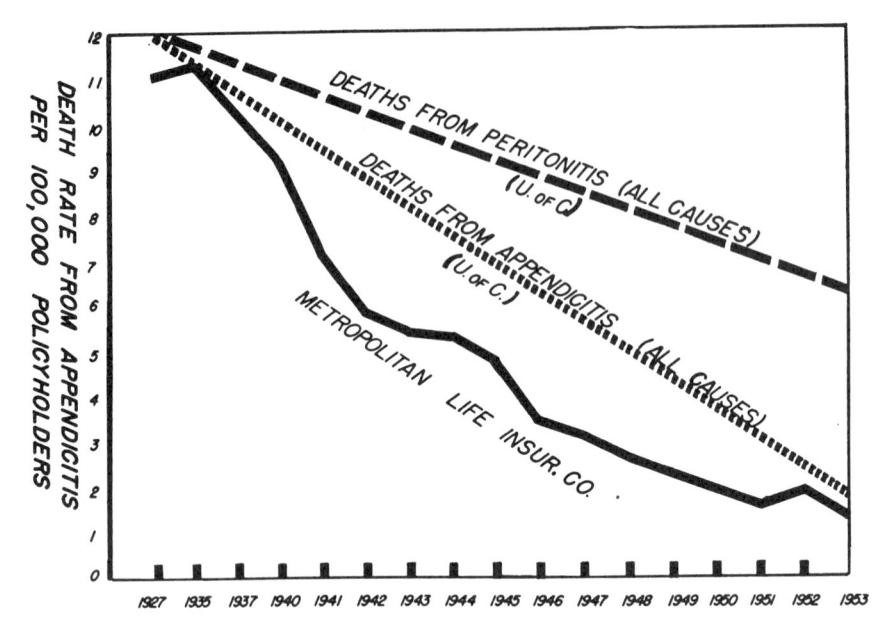

FIG. 37-3. Mortality trends in peritonitis from all causes, graphically compared with that of peritonitis from acute appendicitis. Decline in mortality rate for appendicitis percentages is about 4 times that of peritonitis from all causes over corresponding years. (Data compiled by Paul R. Cannon, University of Chicago, in 1955, and by the Metropolitan Life Insurance Company in 1953)

16 cases per 500 autopsies in 1951. This decline of 50 per cent in mortality rate has been steady, and at no point has it shown a sharp drop.

During the same period, improved fluid management, gastric intubation, increased use of blood and plasma and finally the sulfonamides and the antibiotics became widely used in the therapy of peritonitis. At the same time, public education had its effect too, causing more patients to seek help earlier.

Death From Appendicitis

Appendicitis was frequently fatal 50 years ago. Now the mortality is very low among causes of death. At the University of Chicago Clinics, death occurred 17 times from peritonitis of appendicitis among 2,556 autopsies performed consecutively from 1927 to 1941, but only twice in 2,436 autopsies performed from 1941 to 1952 (Cannon, 1955). This is a reduction 4 times as great as the reduction in deaths occurring from bacterial peritonitis from any and all causes during the same period. The trend of these data is remarkably similar to those compiled by the Metropolitan Life Insurance Company wherein death from appendicitis in 1937 was 11.3 per 100,000 policyholders, and 1.3 in 1953. A still broader sampling disclosed that there were 21,000 deaths from appendicitis in the United States in 1931; by 1946 there were only 6,000, representing a saving of 15,000 lives per year.

This reduction in mortality rate among persons having appendicitis was accomplished largely by education—education of both laity and the profession alike. A higher index of suspicion for this disease and a broad understanding of its consequences if untreated have led to earlier and earlier appendectomy, reducing the number of patients coming to operation after peritonitis has developed. It is likely to continue to play an important role in the future if further substantial reduction in mortality is to be achieved. Much credit should be accorded to such men as John B. Deaver (1855-1931) of Philadelphia, Mont Reid (1889-1943) of Cincinnati, and John Bower (1885-1960), formerly chairman of the Commission on Acute Appendicitis Mortality of the Pennsylvania State Medical Association, for preaching early diagnosis and treatment in appendicitis.

TUMORS OF THE APPENDIX

Mucocele is a rare disorder, in which the lumen of the appendix is obstructed, and the distal portion becomes distended with mucus. The distention may be very great, with the diameter exceeding 2 inches and the length 6 to 12 inches. Rupture and the resulting spillage of mucus into the peritoneal cavity are usually followed by widespread foreign-body reaction unless the appendix is retrocecal. Many consider that cells from the appendiceal mucosa are disseminated throughout the peritoneal cavity where they secrete mucus and cause adhesions, creating intestinal obstruction, a condition known as pseudomyxoma peritonei. This is a condition originally described in association with mucus-secreting carcinomas of the ovary, later with pseudomucinous adenomatous carcinoma of the appendix and even the colon and the stomach. Among 229 cases thought to be mucocele by Hilsabeck et al. (1951), 29 were cancers arising from the appendix. It seems more reasonable that the syndrome pseudomyxoma peritonei is from the cellular distribution of myxomatous cancers within the peritoneal cavity than from the seeding of normal mucosal cells when a simple mucocele of the appendix perforates. Perforative appendicitis occurs frequently enough that one should expect to find some of these epithelial cells surviving and giving rise to peritoneal implants, which they do not.

Carcinoid. This tumor has many characteristics of other argentaffin tumors. It may be benign or malignant, but in the appendix it is rarely malignant in contrast to those found in the small bowel, the colon and the rectum. Although it may cause appendicitis or may be found in the appendix at the time of operation for another disease, it is rarely diagnosed preoperatively. Previously unrecognized carcinoid of the appendix is found at autopsy in 0.1 per cent of the cases (Farringer and Tarasidis, 1964).

Carcinoma of the appendix occurs with about the same frequency as does carcinoid. This statement is based on the fact that both carcinoma and carcinoid of the appendix occur more frequently than is usually appreciated. The channels through which carcinomas of the appendix and of the cecum metastasize are essentially the same, only with carcinoma of the appendix rupture into the peritoneal cavity commonly occurs (Callaghan and Del Beccaro, 1962). The symptoms of carcinoma and carcinoid in the appendix simulate those of appendicitis because they may obstruct the lumen, following which actual appendicitis may develop.

Lymphoma and reticulo-cell sarcoma have also been reported and carry about the same prognosis as when found elsewhere in the alimentary tract.

ABDOMINAL PAIN

Clinical Considerations

Acute appendicitis can be mimicked fairly successfully at times by certain other acute intra-abdominal diseases. Although there are many causes of pain and tenderness in the right lower quadrant of the abdomen with slight fever and moderate leukocytosis, acute appendicitis always should receive first consideration. Therefore, a working knowledge of the origin of abdominal pain is essential to the understanding of the nature of the patient's complaint.

The small monograph by Sir Zachary Cope (1968) on the acute abdomen, now in its 13th edition, is one of the few classics in medicine that should be read by every medical student. Its brevity and clarity permit this. Also in 1968, Shepherd published a much larger volume on the same subject which serves better as a reference book than as a text. It, too, is well written.

Nature, Pathways and Clinical Interpretation of Peritoneal Pain

As abdominal pain is a subjective complaint and not readily analyzed objectively, any analysis of its nature, nervous pathways and interpretation is complicated by such vagaries as "threshold of complaint," the individual's capacity to make known the character of his pain, and the ability of the observer to record, as well as re-interpret, the patient's communications. Nonetheless, much is known about abdominal pain, the types of stimuli that provoke it, the difference between parietal and visceral peritoneal pain, and the disorders most likely to produce many of the patient's complaints. Obviously, interpretation of abdominal pain is as much an art as a science and not easily acquired save by experience.

Capps (1932) initiated an important clinical study of parietal and visceral pain. His findings, along with the later ones of Lewis (1942), serve as the basis upon which most of our present-day knowledge is based. Capps's views as to the importance of abdominal pain are largely held today. He wrote: "Pain (peritoneal) is perhaps the most important evidence upon which we base our interpretation and diagnosis of abdominal disease."

Parietal Pain. The stimuli that provoke pain from the parietal peritoneum more nearly correspond to those causing pain when applied to the skin. They include contact with sharp or cutting instruments, pain of pressure, thermal pain, and pain from irritants, either chemical or bacterial in nature.

Visceral Pain. The only stimulus that appears to be capable of provoking pain from the visceral peritoneum of the alimentary tract is distention. Cutting, pinching or cautery applied to this visceral peritoneum produces no pain.

The nature of the peripheral sensory nerve endings is not well known. However, it appears that these sensory origins are located in the peritoneum itself as well as in its adjacent subserosal tissue, particularly that of the parietal peritoneum. There is some reason to conclude that the sensory nerve terminals of the visceral peritoneum may arise largely from the subserosa and the muscularis of the alimentary tract rather than the visceral peritoneum itself.

Sensory Nerve Pathways. PARIETAL. These pathways of the parietal peritoneum are somatic in distribution. The peritoneum of the abdominal wall is supplied by sensory nerves which correspond to the overlying skin. Both enter the posterior roots of the thoracic sensory nerves from T-7 to T-12 inclusive. The diaphragm likewise is supplied by somatic nerves which enter principally C-4 and to some extent C-3 and C-5. Any appropriate painful stimulus to the parietal peritoneum is referred along to the corresponding cutaneous nerve(s); hence, diaphragmatic pain is characteristically referred to the shoulder cap cutaneous distribution of C-3, C-4 and C-5. Pain from the abdominal peritoneum is referred to the corresponding cutaneous segment(s) of T-7 to T-12. In general, these cutaneous points of pain reference correspond fairly precisely to the site of parietal peritoneal irritation. Thus, pain from acute appendicitis usually is localized to the 10th or the 11th thoracic cutaneous nerve distribution on the right. Pain from the gallbladder usually is in the region of the 8th nerve distribution and follows its course to the back. The pain of acute salpingitis is usually bilateral and of 11th nerve distribution, and so on.

VISCERAL. Pain pathways from the visceral peritoneum of the alimentary tract are believed to be transmitted along somatic pathways and, in the course of reaching the dorsal root of the spinal nerves, they find their way along the course of the autonomic nervous system. This intermingling of the afferent somatic sensory nerves and the efferent autonomic fibers usually is cited as the explanation for pain experienced when the central ends of the divided splanchnic nerves are stimulated. Lewis (1942) maintains that the painful response from stimulation of the central and of the autonomic fibers is not reason for

regarding the pain nerves of the sympathetic system as distinct from those supplying the deep-lying somatic structures . . . the fact that those (pain fibers) from the somatic structures at first use the channel of the spinal nerves and that those from the visceral structures at first use the channel of the autonomic system before entering the posterior roots is really immaterial.

This may be an oversimplification which will be elucidated later when more information becomes available. Lewis cites Barrington as observing that the pain of ureteral colic has the segmental distribution of somatic pain corresponding to the particular level at which the stone is lodged, provided that the stone remains above the bladder. Pain from the visceral peritoneum of the alimentary tract cannot be localized as precisely by the patient as the pain of parietal peritoneum irritation. For example, the pain (visceral) of distention in small intestinal obstruction usually is more diffuse, being localized to the anterior and the lateral portions of the abdomen. Similarly, distention of a colostomy by the finger causes the patient to experience cramplike pain of the abdomen which often is associated with pain in the back. However, this lack of preciseness is no reason to question the somatic origin of visceral pain; rather, it indicates certain possible differences in quality between parietal and visceral peritoneal pain.

Pain arising from stimulation of the parietal peritoneum often is associated with spasm of the overlying abdominal musculature. Should the stimulus and the pain be of mild intensity, guarding or muscle spasm is not great and generally can be overcome by gentle pressure of the examining hand; this is known as "voluntary muscle spasm." Should the painful stimulus be more intense, such as occurs when the highly irritating acid gastric juices escape into the peritoneal cavity from a perforation of a duodenal ulcer, muscle spasm is likely to be maximum, and the "boardlike" rigidity of the abdominal wall it produces is not overcome by the physician's examining hand and, for this reason, is commonly referred to as "involuntary muscle spasm." This difference between voluntary and involuntary spasm of the muscles of the abdominal wall appears to be largely a quantitative one.

The skin surface location by the patient of his abdominal pain, when of visceral origin, is in general as follows: pain of gastric or duodenal origin is experienced above the region of the umbilicus. That of the small bowel and the appendix is often periumbilical; and that of the colon usually is localized below the umbilicus.

Certain experimental observations made by Lewis and Kellgren (1939) are interpreted by these workers as indicating the somatic nature of visceral pain. They claim to have produced many types of pain by the injection of hypertonic saline into the regions of various interspinous ligaments. When injected into the proper interspinous ligament, they report that their subjects were unable to distinguish between the pain induced by saline and that experienced by the abdominal disorder producing the pain for which the patient was seen. For example, the injection into the first lumbar interspinous ligament caused pain resembling that of "renal colic." Injection of the saline solution into the 9th thoracic interspinous ligament caused pain in the back and over the distribution of the 9th intercostal nerve. An analysis of data from more patients similarly studied might be useful in providing more information as well as providing means for interpretation of the patient's localization of his pain.

The location of the patient's pain in general is of much greater practical value when it arises from the parietal peritoneum than from the visceral peritoneum. However, even for visceral pain, the physician may obtain information by a careful analysis of the patient's complaints, especially the location of his pain, which can play an important role in the differential diagnosis of the acute abdomen.

Operative Pain and Splanchnic Block. Unless the patient is maintained in the 3rd plane of a general anesthesia or under a fairly high spinal anesthetic, the peritoneal stimuli attending the operation result in an involuntary spasm of the muscles of the abdominal walls and may interfere with both surgical exposure and surgical closure of the abdominal cavity. Two very useful additions in the technics and the principles of anesthesia have been devised to assist the surgeon when his procedure requires the maximum of muscular relaxation. The first is the transabdominal procaine block of the celiac ganglia which usually abolishes the transmission of stimuli induced by retraction or tugging upon the mesentery. It is often helpful to supplement this by infiltration of the parietal peritoneum about the wound edges. The second and more widely used technic is the temporary paralysis of somatic motor nerves at the myoneural junctions by the use of drugs having a curarelike action. These drugs are effective regardless of the persistence of perceptive painful stimuli and make possible a lighter plane of general anesthesia. As muscular relaxants they are useful indeed, but they also paralyze temporarily the action of all striated muscles, including those of respiration.

DIFFERENTIAL DIAGNOSIS OF APPENDICITIS

Ruptured Graafian Follicle. This lesion may produce a picture like that of appendicitis. It is sudden in onset, usually producing mild abdominal distress localized to the lower abdomen and often to the right side. Acute loss of appetite, nausea and occasional vomiting may occur. Fingerpoint tenderness is absent or not well defined. If much blood escapes, the patient may experience phrenic pain referred to the left shoulder with distribution over the 3rd, the 4th and the 5th cervical nerves when lying down, as blood may migrate to the under surfaces of the diaphragm. The most important diagnostic clue is to be found in the history; the sudden onset of pain occurring in the midterm of the intermenstrual period. Hence, this syndrome is known as *mittelschmerz*. Anemia may be present, but leukocytosis and fever are mild or nonexistent in the first day or two.

Ectopic Pregnancy. Generally, this is associated with some irregularity of the recent menstrual cycle. This condition may produce pain simulating in part that of appendicitis. Maximum tenderness is lower than McBurney's point. A right tubo-ovarian mass may be felt on pelvic examination. If rupture has occurred, shoulder pain may be complained of, and shock may appear soon if operation is delayed. The abdominal wall develops the doughy consistency characteristic of intra-abdominal blood, and peristaltic activity may be reduced or absent. Fever, if present, is slight, although leukocytosis and anemia may be observed.

Twisted Ovarian Cyst or Tumor. This lesion produces sudden and sharp lower abdominal pain and vomiting. In a few cases reference of pain may be to the medial aspect of the thigh. As with the ruptured ectopic pregnancy, the acuteness and the seriousness of the signs and symptoms make unnecessary a discussion of details, because soon the necessity for prompt exploration of the lower abdomen is obvious.

Acute Salpingitis. This condition is by no means always easily distinguishable from acute appendicitis. Pain is usually hypogastric in location. Tenderness is low and often bilateral. Motion of the cervix is usually very painful, and often bilateral tender pelvic masses can be felt. From the purulent discharge it may be possible to demonstrate the intracellular gonococcus by stained smear. Fever and leukocytosis are usually greater than for early appendicitis, and the sedimentation rate is substantially increased early over that seen in nonperforative appendicitis (Girardet and Enquist, 1963). Occasionally, appendectomy is necessarily resorted to simply because acute appendicitis cannot be excluded satisfactorily by any other means. And it may co-exist!

Mesenteric Adenitis. This occurs more commonly in children and young adults. This syndrome is characterized by generalized abdominal pain which may be more pronounced in the right lower quadrant. It usually accompanies or follows a respiratory infection and may or may not be associated with fever and leukocytosis. If this disease resembles too closely the symptoms of acute appendicitis, the diagnosis of the latter always should be made and appendectomy performed.

Regional Enteritis. This type of inflammation also may resemble appendicitis and indeed, may give rise to the latter by obstructing the lumen of the appendix. Its symptom complex in the acute and first attack so often resembles appendicitis that most patients whom the author has seen with regional enteritis have had appendectomy at the time of a previous attack of similar nature. In some patients the "sausage roll" swelling of the terminal ileum may be felt, but even though regional enteritis may be suspected, concurrent appendicitis is often difficult, if not impossible, to exclude.

Ureteral Stone. This condition occasionally simulates appendicitis, particularly if lodged in the right ureter, and produces pain without colic. Reference of pain in the scrotum and the penis is often complained of. Hematuria, no fever and the absence of leukocytosis strongly suggest the presence of a ureteral stone. However, more often than not ureteral stone is associated with fever and leukocytosis. Cystoscopy and pyelograms usually produce the indisputable evidence necessary to eliminate the need for further concern about the appendix, barring the coexistence of both diseases.

Perforated Peptic Ulcer. Such an ulcer may simulate an attack of acute appendicitis, especially if the perforation is small and the leakage of gastroduodenal juices is at a slow rate. Pain in the epigastrium with nausea and occasional vomiting may mark its onset. As the fluid tends to flow down into the right iliac fossa, pain and tenderness in the right lower quadrant become prominent findings and may resemble acute appendicitis. Often the diagnosis is confused with perforative appendicitis, especially if rigidity of the abdominal wall is present and bowel sounds are absent. Leukocytosis and slight fever may be present early and tend to rise later on.

The differential points are chiefly the history of peptic ulcer. The fact that pain, tenderness and muscular rigidity are more pronounced than are seen in early appendicitis is helpful; the presence of air under the diaphragm on roentgenographic examination is usually diagnostic but it may also be observed in small perforations (see Chap. 31, Stomach and Duodenum).

On the other hand, a history of peptic ulcer, even of perforated ulcer, does not weigh too heavily against the diagnosis of acute appendicitis. It is the impression of this author that the incidence of the latter disease among ulcer patients on medical management is greater than that among similar age groups in the population at large. The author has seen one patient, in whom there was a history of 3 perforations of duodenal ulcer, who presented himself with a sudden attack of severe epigastric pain of 3-hours' duration and in whom the diagnosis of another perforation seemed to be much more likely than that of acute appendicitis. At operation, perforated appendicitis proved to be the correct diagnosis. The incidence of acute appendicitis and of duodenal ulcer is greater in men than in women. Fortunately, both conditions require early surgical exploration, at which time the correct diagnosis can be established.

Acute Cholecystitis. Occasionally, acute cholecystitis can and does simulate acute appendicitis. The pain onset is usually epigastric, which slowly localizes slightly to the right. Colic may or may not be present, and often the pain is referred to the right flank and/or the right subscapular area. Acute loss of appetite, nausea, and vomiting are more prominent features than are generally seen in appendicitis, as is the associated fever and leukocytosis. If muscular rigidity is not pronounced, occasionally a distended gallbladder or a mass of surrounding omentum can be felt. However, in some cases the gallbladder lies lower than usual, and the distinction between acute cholecystitis and appendicitis is made more difficult. In doubtful cases early exploration is indicated.

Acute Pancreatitis. This is another condition to be considered, as it too may give rise to right lower abdominal pain in some patients (see Chap. 33, Pancreas).

Pleuritis of the Right Lower Chest or of the Right Diaphragm. The pleuritis of the right lower chest or of the right diaphragm may be difficult to distinguish from appendicitis, especially in children. Loss of appetite, nausea and vomiting are infrequently present, although leukocytosis and fever are commonly present. Voluntary spasm of the abdominal muscles and hyperesthesia are commonly present and to an extent greater than might be expected early in the course of appendicitis. Bowel sounds are nearly always present. A roentgenogram of the chest may or may not disclose evidence of pleuritis or pneumonitis. The most important single sign in the author's experience is that achieved by splinting of the lower chest by hand compression over the right lower chest cage and having the patient breathe deeply. This usually relieves the pleuritic pain. If it does not, then the procedure is repeated, applying manual splinting to the abdomen below the thoracic cage. Thus thoracic motion is accentuated, and as a rule pleuritic pain is accentuated upon deep inspiration.

Intussusception. (See Chap. 50, Pediatric Surgery.)

Intestinal Obstruction. (See Chap. 38, Intestinal Obstruction.)

In Table 37-4 are listed the sites of origins of pain, the location of reference of pain, and the character of pain frequently observed in many of these acute intra-abdominal emergencies.

Many other conditions must be considered which at times can resemble acute appendicitis. These are encountered less frequently and also confused less frequently with acute appendicitis. Among these are: spinal cord and vertebral diseases, tabes dorsalis, sickle cell anemia, porphyria (including lead poison-

TABLE 37-4. PAIN IN ACUTE INTRA-ABDOMINAL EMERGENCIES

SITE OR ORIGIN OF PAIN	LOCALIZATION OR REFERENCE OF PAIN	CHARACTER OF PAIN
Subphrenic abscess, or irritation from blood, bile, or other irritating fluids in this area	Shoulder cap and at times also to the hypochondrium and the upper and the middle portions of the abdominal wall of the affected side.	Made worse by deep inspiration and generally is diminished by splinting of the abdomen by manual pressure.
Perisplenitis, abscess, infarct, or tear of spleen	Similar to that of left subphrenic abscess.	Made worse by inspiration.
Gallbladder disease:		
1. Acute distention	Subscapular pain, 8th nerve.	Fairly continuous unless distention is intermittent.
2. Acute inflammation	Over the region of the gallbladder and generally along the course of T-8 sensory distribution.	Continuous.
3. Cystic or common duct stone	Right hypochondrium and right subscapular area.	Generally continuous, occasionally intermittent and often recurring.
Penetrating duodenal ulcer	Anteriorly, over region of duodenum and generally to back in area of penetration.	Continuous. Made worse by sligh amount of hydrochloric acid through Levin tube. Generally relieved by gastric drainage and milk or alkaline therapy.
Appendicitis:		
1. Early	Usually mild and in periumbilical or midepigastric area.	Usually mild and ill-defined, tends to recede.
2. Within a few hours	Right lower abdomen and generally conforming fairly well to location of appendix.	Well localized and continuous. Mild to moderate in severity.
3. With local or spreading peritonitis	More extensive and less sharply defined.	Generally more severe and diffuse.
Salpingitis or impending rupture of ectopic tubular pregnancy	Low in abdomen and lateralized to area involved and does not tend to disappear when the patient is placed in Trendelenburg position.	Dull to sharp and constant.
Ruptured graafian follicle	Mild to moderate. Generally located to lower abdomen. If much blood escapes, subphrenic pain in recumbent position may be experienced. Onset sudden.	Usually mild and somewhat ill-defined. Constant and may be of sudden onset, occurring in the midintermenstrual cycle.
Ruptured ectopic pregnancy	First lateralized in lower abdomen, tends to become more diffuse and may give rise to subphrenic pain if in recumbent position.	Sudden, moderate to severe, continuous. May be bilateral.
Twisted ovarian cyst	Low in abdomen and may radiate also to upper mesial side of thigh.	Sudden in onset and usually intense. Continuous.

TABLE 37-4. PAIN IN ACUTE INTRA-ABDOMINAL EMERGENCIES (*Cont.*)

SITE OR ORIGIN OF PAIN	LOCALIZATION OR REFERENCE OF PAIN	CHARACTER OF PAIN
Sigmoidal diverticulitis	Generally left-sided or bilateral and located low in abdomen.	Mild but progressing in intensity.
Acute intestinal obstruction (mechanical ileus)	Pain at first may be diffuse and later tends to localize over region of obstruction.	Early or sudden in onset. In the early stages is generally cramp-like, severe and intermittent; this remains, but as bowel becomes inflamed, a local persistence of pain appears in region of the inflamed bowel.
Mesenteric thrombosis	Onset may be sudden; first is generalized and a little later may be associated with dull pain in upper lumbar area. As bowel becomes inflamed it may produce localization at site of necrotic bowel.	Is mild to moderate. Is continuous and often ill-defined.

ing), rheumatic fever, hepatic or subhepatic abscesses, herpes zoster, periarteritis nodosa with extraperitoneal hematoma, rupture of the abdominal musculature, intra-abdominal hernia, mesenteric thrombosis, torsion of the omentum or of an appendices epiploicae, coronary thrombosis, and last but not least is acute retention of urine in children.

If the diagnosis of appendicitis remains in doubt, take the appendix out.

Section 2. Peritonitis and Intra-abdominal Abscesses

THE PERITONEUM

Structure and Surface Area

The peritoneum is a glistening, serous lining, enveloping all of the abdominal viscera and their mesenteries (the visceral peritoneum), as well as the peripheral confines of the abdominal cavity (the parietal peritoneum). The visceral peritoneum is attached loosely to its underlying structures by the subserosal areolar tissue, while the parietal peritoneum overlies the transversalis fascia and in places is rather firmly attached to it. The peritoneal surface consists of a single layer of flattened mesothelium moistened by a small quantity of serous fluid, which permits the viscera to glide about in the abdominal cavity.

The surface area of the peritoneum is approximately equal to that of the skin. Consequently, it is one of the largest absorptive, transudative and exudative surfaces of the body.

SUBDIVISIONS OF THE ABDOMINAL CAVITY

The anatomic subdivisions of the abdominal cavity are only 2: the greater and the lesser peritoneal sacs. They communicate through the foramen of Winslow, the epiploic foramen.

The Lesser Peritoneal Cavity or Omental Bursa. The boundaries of the lesser cavity are: anteriorly, the posterior wall of the stomach; inferiorly and left laterally, the superior surface of the transverse mesocolon; and posteriorly, the peritoneum over the pancreas and the diaphragmatic peritoneum above the pancreas. Its right lateral limit is the mesial border of the gastrohepatic ligament which envelops the hepatic artery, the portal vein and the common duct. Because the gastrohepatic ligament is reflected onto the posterior surface of the stomach but not onto the posterior abdominal wall, a foraminal connection is left connecting the greater and the lesser peritoneal cavities. This opening between the greater and the lesser omental cavities is the foramen of Winslow.

The Greater Peritoneal Cavity. It contains most of the abdominal viscera. Each organ or vessel contained in or traversing this cavity is covered with peritoneum on its surface facing into the abdominal cavity. Where such organs as the liver, the kidney and pancreas lie against the abdominal musculature the visceral peritoneum of these organs passes onto the abdominal wall where it continues as the parietal peritoneum. Organs having portions of their surfaces not covered with peritoneum and other portions which are covered are said to be retroperitoneal.

That part of the greater peritoneal cavity which lies below the brim of the true pelvis is considered to be a somewhat separate division of the greater omental cavity because it contains most of the urogenital organs.

ACUTE PERITONITIS

Peritonitis is an inflammatory reaction of the peritoneum, to bacterial, chemical, thermal, irradiation and physical injuries and to foreign bodies. The inflammatory response evoked is qualitatively similar to that induced by similar agents in other tissues. Because of the vast surface area of the peritoneum, generalized bacterial or chemical peritonitis is attended by the rapid movement of large quantities of extracellular fluid, plasma proteins, and white blood cells into the peritoneal cavity and into the soft areolar tissues beneath the visceral and parietal peritoneum. This intraperitoneal and subperitoneal sequestration of extracellular fluid is attended by a decrease in the plasma volume and consequently by an oligemia that contributes a great deal to the shock that at times results in early death. Related to the speed of absorption through its large surface area is the speed with which septic toxemia accompanies acute generalized peritonitis—a generalized peritonitis being somewhat analogous to a fulminant subcutaneous cellulitis covering almost the entire skin surface.

The magnitudes of water and mineral losses in generalized peritonitis and the reasons why they may result in early death, irrespective of toxemia, are evident from the following: 0.5 mm. swelling of the peritoneal surfaces would require the sequestration of 5,000 ml. of extracellular fluid, or approximately one third that normally present in a 70-Kg. lean individual. This is minimal because edema may involve the abdominal musculature as well.

CLASSIFICATION OF PERITONITIS

Although any classification of peritonitis is to some extent arbitrary, it can be effected on the bases of: temporal relationships, extent of the peritoneal surface involved, the nature and the sources of the pathogens responsible, and whether peritonitis is primary or secondary in origin.

The most frequent as well as the most dangerous form is *acute peritonitis*. This may cause death within a few hours or a day or two.

Acute peritonitis may be confined to a relatively small part of the abdominal cavity. This is *localized peritonitis*. At times it may spread quickly or gradually during a day or two and is then called *spreading peritonitis*. When the entire peritoneal cavity is involved it is called *generalized peritonitis*. Peritonitis may exist for a time as local peritonitis and then may spread and evolve in 12 to 48 hours through the spreading stage to a full-blown generalized peritonitis. These developments can occur so rapidly that the local and intermediate stages are difficult or impossible to identify.

Bacteria and Chemicals and Their Relationships. Both usually provoke extensive inflammation of the peritoneal cavity, causing extensive outpouring of fluid and, generally, an adynamic ileus. With perforation of a peptic ulcer into the peritoneal cavity large quantities of chemically irritating fluids pour into the peritoneal cavity within a matter of minutes. In such cases if the leak is not stopped, and if removal of the inflammatory chemicals is not effected, shock may ensue rapidly. Death from shock (Altemeier and Cole, 1958) may occur in such cases before infection and septicemia assume serious or irreparable proportions. Noon et al. (1967) evaluated the advantages of irrigation of the peritoneal cavity with an antibiotic in normal saline against irrigating with normal saline alone. Among 404 patients undergoing the operation for either traumatic or spontaneous perforation of the gastrointestinal tract, half were given antibiotics plus saline and half were given saline alone. The antibiotics used were bacitracin and kanamycin. The incidence of wound infection after each operation was studied, and it was found that infection occurred twice as frequently with saline alone as in the group with antibiotic irrigation.

In many cases of secondary peritonitis, the inflammation is localized for a time; this is especially true with appendicitis, salpingitis, and cholecystitis. The initial localized phase of peritonitis is associated with the inflammation of and about the sick organ; the peritonitis becomes a spreading one, often progressing to a generalized one, after the appendix or the gallbladder perforates or the tubal abscess ruptures. The time that elapses between the beginning of the localized peritonitis and the time it begins to spread is decidedly variable, being only a few hours in some cases of appendicitis, and weeks with tubal abscesses. In these cases, septicemia is more likely to cause death than is hypovolemia, although both are involved in any case.

The substances that most often produce chemical peritonitis are gastric juice, bile, pancreatic juice and urine. With the exception of a sterile urine, all of these fluids very often, if not almost always, contain, or become contaminated with, intestinal bacteria; consequently, in almost all cases of chemical peritonitis, a bacterial peritonitis soon becomes imposed upon the chemical one unless the leak of the irritating chemicals is stopped very soon after it starts.

Primary and Secondary Peritonitis. Primary peritonitis, while rare, is most frequently due to pneumococci, hemolytic streptococci or gonococci and is often associated with recognizable infections due to these organisms elsewhere. Primary peritonitis is largely limited to children, young women and persons with ascites. The symptoms and signs are essentially identical with those of secondary acute bacterial or chemical peritonitis.

Primary acute chemical peritonitis occasionally occurs with certain systemic diseases, such as polyserositis and uremia.

Secondary bacterial peritonitis usually results from perforation of the alimentary tract, penetrating abdominal wounds, or from septic pelvic inflammatory disease. The distinction between primary and secondary bacterial peritonitis is often very difficult to make. Consequently, it is frequently impossible to avoid surgical exploration in some cases of primary bacterial peritonitis. Whenever the circumstances are such that one cannot make a distinction, the chance of overlooking an early case of secondary bacterial perforative peritonitis is too great, and the consequences of a mistake are too grave, to warrant an expectant course hoping that the passage of time will permit a sure differentiation of whether the peritonitis is primary or not.

Idiopathic retroperitoneal fibrosis is a rare disease occurring more commonly in males (Kerr et al., 1968), and is characterized by the formation of a dense plaque of fibrous tissue in the retroperitoneum. Usually there is some evidence of a moderate degree of hydronephrosis and a mesial deviation of the ureters. Its cause is unknown, and freeing up the ureter seems the most effective treatment. It may be viral in origin.

THE BACTERIOLOGY OF ACUTE PERITONITIS

A wide variety of organisms, many of which are not usually regarded as pathogenic, have been found within the peritoneal cavity in this disease. Table 37-5 summarizes the kinds of bacteria most often found in peritonitis and the antibiotic agents usually effective against these bacteria. Table 37-6 shows the in-vitro sensitivities of these organisms to the principal antibiotics. Table 37-7 lists the concentrations of various antibiotics effective for *Staphylococcus aureus*.

DIAGNOSIS OF PERITONITIS

The history, the physical examination of the chest and the abdomen, the differential white blood count, the hematocrit, simple roentgenographic examinations of the abdomen, and aspiration of fluid from the peritoneal cavity are the bases for diagnosing the various forms of peritonitis.

Pain. The pain suffered with peritonitis is varied. With a chemical peritonitis secondary to rupture of an ulcer of the stomach or the duodenum, pain usually comes suddenly, often without an antecedent illness; it is usually a severe, burning and at times even an excruciating cutting agony; it spreads rapidly and within minutes or in an hour or two occupies the entire abdomen; it is aggravated by every sort of movement and immediately or very

TABLE 37-5. BACTERIA COMMONLY ASSOCIATED WITH PERITONITIS

ORGANISMS	ANTIBIOTICS OF CHOICE
Escherichia coli	Streptomycin, chloramphenicol, neomycin
Aerobacter aerogenes	Streptomycin, chloramphenicol, neomycin
Klebsiella aerogenes	Streptomycin, chloramphenicol, neomycin
Streptococcus pyogenes	Penicillin, erythromycin, tetracycline
Staphylococcus aureus	Penicillin, erythromycin, tetracycline
Diplococcus pneumoniae	Penicillin, erythromycin, tetracycline
Proteus vulgaris	Streptomycin, chloramphenicol, neomycin
Pseudomonas aeruginosa	Neomycin, streptomycin, tetracycline, colimycin
Neisseria gonorrhoeae	Penicillin, erythromycin, tetracycline
Streptococcus faecalis	Chloramphenicol, tetracycline, vancomycin
Clostridia perfringens	Penicillin, tetracycline, chloramphenicol, vancomycin

TABLE 37-6. ANTIBIOTIC SENSITIVITY OF SOME PATHOGENS IMPORTANT IN PERITONITIS

NORMAL MINIMUM INHIBITORY CONCENTRATIONS (μg./ml.)

	Peni-cillin	Eryth-romycin	Tetra-cycline	Chlor-am-pheni-col	Neo-mycin	Strep-tomy-cin	Vanco-mycin	Novo-biocin	Baci-tracin	Poly-myxin	Olean-domy-cin	Spira-mycin	Coli-mycin
Escherichia coli	20->100	32	1	8	1	2				0.25			5
Aerobacter aerogenes	250		2	8	0.5	2				0.25			2
Streptococcus pyogenes	0.006	0.03	0.25	2	>128	32	0.5	2	0.25		0.25	0.25	>500
Staphylococcus aureus	0.012	0.12	0.12	8	1	2	1	0.12	2		0.5		250
Diplococcus pneumoniae	0.006	0.03	0.25	2	128	64	0.5	1	10		0.25		50
Proteus vulgaris	5-100		40->80	10	1	2	>500	4					500
Pseudomonas aeruginosa			20	200	1	2	>100	2	5	1	2	1	0.5
Neisseria gonorrhoeae	0.003	0.06	1	1	10	5	32+	2	5				
Streptococcus faecalis	5.0	6	5		50	50	2	50		500			1000
Klebsiella aerogenes	250		2	8	0.5	2				0.25			
Clostridia perfringens	0.12	2	0.03-0.25	4			1	32	4		16	64	

After Garrod, L. P., and Scowen, E. F.: The Principles of Therapeutic Use of Antibiotics. Brit. Med. Bul, Vol. 16, 1960.

TABLE 37-7. CONCENTRATIONS (μg./ml.)
REQUIRED FOR HEMOLYTIC
STAPHYLOCOCCUS AUREUS

	μg./ml.
Bacitracin	5.0
Carbomycin	1.5
Chlortetracycline	1.0
Erythromycin	0.4
Neomycin B*	1.0
Kanamycin	3.9
Leucomycin	0.5
Novobiocin	0.8
Ristocetin	5.0
Spiramycin	3.5
Thiostrepton*	0.1
Oleandomycin	1.6
Vancomycin	1.8

* For reduction of bacterial flora of the gastrointestinal tract before surgery.

soon incapacitates the sufferer. The pain of peritonitis secondary to appendiceal or cholecystic rupture usually follows pain different in character from that of peritonitis. At times, with appendicitis this first type of colicky pain suddenly decreases or even disappears, signaling rupture of the appendix. Then the gradually increasing burning ache of secondary bacterial peritonitis begins, first in the region of the site of the organ that perforates and from there may spread over the entire abdomen. The pain of secondary bacterial peritonitis is rarely excruciating.

The pain of acute primary peritonitis is preceded frequently by an acute febrile illness such as pneumonia, erysipelas, a streptococcal pharyngitis in children, or acute gonorrhea, a septic abortion, or a puerperal sepsis in women. The pain is usually described by the ill person as a terrible soreness of the entire abdomen, though often excepting the epigastrium. Abdominal pain is usually absent in chronic tuberculous peritonitis and the primary chemical peritonitis of uremia.

Tenderness. Abdominal tenderness tends to vary in severity with the pain. It is quick in onset and severe with acute secondary chemical peritonitis, begins locally and spreads with acute secondary bacterial peritonitis, is diffuse from the beginning with primary bacterial peritonitis and is seldom present in chronic bacterial and uremic chemical (nonbacterial) peritonitis.

Muscle Spasm. Reflex spasm of the abdominal musculature is characteristic of all forms of acute peritonitis. With local peritonitis only the parts of the muscle supplied by the neural segments affected by the inflammation of the parietal peritoneum are in spasm, but with a general peritonitis all of the abdominal musculature is affected. One must be able to distinguish reflex from "voluntary" muscle spasm. The latter is stimulated whenever pressure is applied over any part of the abdomen overlying abscesses, closed loop intestinal obstructions, or acutely swollen lymph nodes and is not a sign of peritonitis. In order to distinguish between voluntary and reflex muscle spasm, the search for spasm should be made by gentle pressure applied steadily while the patient takes 4 to 5 breaths. If tenseness of the abdomen does not decrease and does not vary with breathing, waxing during expiration and waning during inspiration, the spasm is likely to be reflex; if the spasm waxes and wanes and decreases in intensity, it is probably voluntary.

Reflex muscle spasm comes immediately and is often so intense that the abdomen is rigid or "boardlike" with rupture of duodenal and gastric ulcers but is usually less intense with acute bacterial peritonitis and acute pancreatitis.

Ileus. With all forms of acute generalized peritonitis, peristalsis soon becomes feeble and infrequent, and, unless gastric intubation is done quickly, the intestine may fill rapidly with gas and fluid. Ileus associated with generalized peritonitis is in part reflex in origin. However, bacterial toxemia also plays a role because adynamic ileus is prone to attend any sepsis, such as lobar pneumonia or septicemia. These diseases and others associated with severe electrolyte imbalances also may cause ileus as a sequelae; particularly prominent in this respect is serum potassium deficiency.

Occasionally, localized peritonitis partially obstructs loops of bowel, and the patient may experience diarrhea rather than ileus.

Changes in Blood. Leukocytosis too is a variable accompaniment of peritonitis. An acute generalized peritonitis, such as that following rupture of the cecum, is associated at times with a polymorphonuclear leukopenia—not leukocytosis; with tuberculous peritonitis, the white blood cell count is often within normal range, and it is unpredictable in uremia. However, excepting tuberculous peritonitis and uremic peritonitis, a shift to the left of the neutrophils (shift to young form) is the usual finding in acute peritonitis.

A rising hematocrit value regularly attends acute generalized chemical peritonitis. However, a falling, rather than a rising, hematocrit may accompany severe acute bacterial peritonitis. In the case of a falling hematocrit, the patient soon develops jaundice, presumably because hemolytic bacterial toxins absorbed from the peritoneal cavity lyse the red blood cells very rapidly. Frequently, the serum transaminase level rises under these conditions.

Temperature. With all forms of bacterial peritonitis, even tuberculous, some fever is the rule. However, the body temperature may be normal or subnormal during the first 3 to 6 hours after the perforation of gastric or duodenal ulcers. When hypothermia occurs with bacterial peritonitis, it is a sign of nearness to death; when it occurs during the first few hours of an acute chemical peritonitis, it is a sign of sodium deficit.

Pulse and Respiration. Tachycardia accompanies all forms of peritonitis. Tachypnea and restriction of abdominal respiratory movements are characteristic of all forms of acute chemical and bacterial generalized peritonitis but are observed also in pneumonitis.

Roentgenograms of the abdomen and the intestine are often very helpful in the differential diagnosis of peritonitis. Plane films of the abdomen taken after the patient has been sitting upright for 5 minutes often show an extragastric air level or air-fluid level beneath the diaphragm whenever peritonitis is secondary to the perforation of the intraabdominal gastrointestinal tract. Because most of the very rapidly developing generalized secondary peritonitis arises from perforation of the stomach or the duodenum, the oral giving of 50 to 100 ml. of a water-miscible iodinated radiopaque fluid is a fairly safe, quick and rather accurate way of determining roentgenographically if perforation of gastric or duodenal ulcers is the cause of the generalized peritonitis, especially when there are indications that a primary bacterial, rather than a secondary chemical, peritonitis may exist. Barium should never be used for this purpose because, should it escape into the peritoneal cavity with gastrointestinal fluids, a disabling and life-endangering adhesive peritonitis may be produced.

Perforations may seal, at least for a while; therefore, failure to demonstrate passage of an aqueous solution of radiopaque material into the peritoneal cavity does not necessarily exclude the presence of a perforation of a peptic ulcer. Rarely, perforation of the appendix is associated with intraperitoneal free-air which may be due to gas-producing bacteria within the peritoneal cavity, rather than to leakage of intestinal air. Some gas-producing organisms may be the cause of primary peritonitis and also produce intraperitoneal air without perforation. In more than 90 per cent of the demonstrated cases of gas in the free peritoneal cavity, the cause is perforation of the alimentary tract, most often secondary to peptic ulcer.

Peritoneal Aspiration. For a number of years the aspiration of fluid from the peritoneal cavity has been practiced sporadically for the purpose of ascertaining the cause of an acute generalized peritonitis. Many have found peritoneal aspirations to be of considerable diagnostic help both when hemorrhage is present and when there is a visceral perforation. It is generally done as a 4-quadrant tap. It is less useful in localized intra-abdominal inflammatory diseases (Baker et al., 1967).

Differential Diagnosis. LOBAR PNEUMONIA. The differentiation of peritonitis from conditions which have a number of the same features that peritonitis has is usually rather easy, provided that the physician is alert. During the acute pleuritic phase, lobar pneumonia in the lower lobes of the lungs is often associated with continuous abdominal pain, abdominal distention and hyperesthesia but not with genuine reflex muscular spasm over the abdomen; peristaltic activity may be reduced, but it is not absent. However, the lower lobar pneumonic consolidation (x-ray and physical signs), the pleuritis and the chill with which the illness began serve to differentiate a lobar pneumonia with abdominal signs from peritonitis. But also the physical signs are more helpful because in pleurisy, if the examiner splints the chest with his hands, the patient can take a deep breath with ease. If the pain is peritoneal in origin, splinting the lower chest accentuates motion of the abdominal muscles and thus accentuates pain. The reverse is true when the abdomen is splinted; respiration is less painful when the disease is peritonitis, and pain is accentuated when the disease is in the chest.

SPIDER BITE. The boardlike abdominal rigidity and severe abdominal pain caused by the bite of *Latrodectus mactans* (the black widow) are also easily distinguished from peritonitis. There is no fever or leukocytosis, and the muscles of the back, the legs and the neck may also be in spasm after the spider bite, but not with acute peritonitis. Bee stings on the abdomen, especially those by wasps, may also elicit generalized abdominal rigidity and may more commonly be fatal than the bite of the black widow spider.

ABDOMINAL CRISES. More difficult is the differentiation of the abdominal crises that occur with such conditions as sickle cell anemia, anaphylactoid purpura, acute porphyria, lead poisoning, spherocytic anemia, tertiary syphilis and Hodgkin's disease. However, with all of these, the abdominal spasm, tenderness and pain wax and wane rather rapidly, shift from one place to the other, and are not associated with the type of fever or the leukocytoses that peritonitis is; also, peristaltic activity is present and in some patients may be increased. It is most important, when making the diagnosis, to think of these nonsurgical conditions to avoid unnecessary operations.

From the practical point of view, the only important differentiation is the one between primary and secondary peritonitis. At times one cannot differentiate with certainty primary from secondary without recourse to diagnostic celiotomy. When in doubt, it is better to perform a laparotomy in error for primary peritonitis than to let a person die of secondary peritonitis without attempting to stop the leak.

TREATMENT OF PERITONITIS

The treatment of peritonitis may be divided into support and specific measures.

The supportive treatment consists of:

1. Preventing aspiration pneumonitis and distention with proper intestinal intubation and drainage (see Chap. 38).

2. The alleviation of pain with the analgesics, morphine or Demerol.

3. Restitution of the extracellular fluid volume deficit produced by intra-abdominal exudation, the sequestration of edema fluid beneath the parietal peritoneum and in the intestinal wall, and the collection of fluid within the adynamic intestine. Because the body fluid aberrations with peritonitis are so similar to those of bad burns and intestinal obstruction, the principles of fluid therapy applicable to burns and intestinal obstruction are applicable also to peritonitis (Chaps. 17 and 38).

4. In cases of peritonitis complicated by rapid hemolysis, septic shock or anemia, the transfusion of blood is a very important supportive measure.

5. Feed the person parenterally something safe, such as glucose.

The specific therapeutic measures are: for *spreading* or *generalized secondary peritonitis* —stop the leak, remove the exudate and the intra-abdominal debris, drain surgically, and give antibiotics parenterally; and for *primary peritonitis*—give the appropriate antibiotics. Stopping the leak that has produced the secondary peritonitis may require appendectomy for appendiceal rupture, resection of ileum for Meckel's diverticular perforation, colostomy for perforation of the neoplastically obstructed colon, resection of the colon with perforated ulcerative colitis, continuous gastroduodenal drainage, omental or suture closure for perforated duodenal and gastric ulcers, and closure and external drainage for the torn bladder.

In all cases of spreading secondary peritonitis and of generalized peritonitis, the sooner the leak is stopped, the better is the person's chance of recovering (see Chap. 12).

The principles of antibiotic therapy of established infections in Chapter 4 are immediately applicable to the use of antibiotics for peritonitis. Because of the heterogeneity of the bacteria associated with secondary peritonitis, large doses of tetracycline (250 mg.-500 mg. every 6 hours) should be used intravenously until the organisms in a particular case have been identified and their sensitivities to the various antibiotics ascertained. Then the principles of Chapter 4 can be followed readily.

The treatment of septic shock is partially discussed in Chapter 7. Buffered saline solutions, plasma, blood, large amounts of appropriate antibiotics, oxygen therapy and possibly the judicious use of a vasopressor agent such as norepinephrine constitute the basic materials for treating septic shock (Altemeier and Cole, 1958). The case for large doses of cortisol and the use of vasodilators is an unsettled one at this time.

Hypothermia, though sporadically used for the treatment of septic shock, has not been proved to be effective by itself.

SOME SPECIAL FORMS OF PERITONITIS

Because of the peculiarities of peritonitis that are relatable somewhat to a particular etiology, some individual attention needs to be given to these special forms.

Bile peritonitis is a relatively rare cause of acute peritonitis. Some of the chemical constituents of bile are irritating and may induce rapid exudation into the peritoneal cavity. Consequently, shock tends to occur soon.

Extensive bile peritonitis is not frequently seen from perforation of the gallbladder. When this viscus ruptures, the cystic duct is usually obstructed by impacted gallstones. Thus, the spillage is limited in amount, unless the release of intracystic pressure attending rupture of the gallbladder dislodges the impacted stone.

McCarthy and Picazo (1968) found that bile peritonitis is more severe when complicated by bacterial contamination. Jaundice is frequently present and the serum levels of conjugated bilirubin increase. The rise of alkaline phosphatase occurs later.

Bile peritonitis is more commonly secondary to operation upon the biliary tract, and penetrating injuries or traumatic avulsions of the gallbladder than to perforation of the diseased gallbladder. Several types of surgical accidents account for most intraperitoneal extravasations of bile. During cholecystectomy an unrecognized small accessory hepatic or cystic duct may be cut and not ligated. Necrosis or "blowout" of the cystic duct stump or a dislodgment of its ligature may occur a few days after the operation, especially should the flow of bile into the duodenum be partially or totally obstructed by a stone lodged in the ampulla of Vater. Postoperative bile leakage may also occur from simple aspiration of the common ducts through a needle. When such a procedure is used for cholangiography, catheter drainage of the duct should be employed. Unrecognized operative injury to the common duct and spontaneous localized necrosis of this structure are additional causes of bile peritonitis.

Pancreatic peritonitis in its early stage is usually a sterile inflammatory process and is attributable to the effects of enzymatic activity and the cleavage products of pancreatic lipase and tryptase upon the peritoneal surfaces and the subserosal fat. (See Chap. 33, Pancreas.)

Blood "Peritonitis" (Hemoperitoneum). Blood within the peritoneal cavity may arise from any vascular or visceral injury, even those so slight as peritoneal lacerations due to mild muscular effort (Deol et al., 1967). More commonly, however, it is associated with severe trauma or spontaneous rupture of the abdominal aorta and its mesenteric vessels, or the spleen. It is diagnosed best by a four-quadrant tap (see Chap. 34, Spleen).

Blood in the peritoneum may produce a mild peritoneal inflammatory response which may not be detectable for a day or two. Common nontraumatic sources of intraperitoneal hemorrhage are ruptured graafian follicles or cysts and tubal pregnancies. Aside from the early appearance of mild distress in the lower abdomen in the former, the characteristic complaint is one of pain in one or both shoulder regions when lying down. The rate of blood loss in ruptured ectopic pregnancy may be rapid indeed. The blood loss may be fatal unless surgical intervention is prompt and blood replacement is adequate.

Urine peritonitis is usually at first sterile. Later, especially with rupture of the dome of the bladder, signs of peritonitis may be strangely lacking even though the bladder has been ruptured for 2 or 3 days and there are 6 or more liters of uriniferous ascites. In such cases, the urine is sterile, and presumably it is not so acid or hypertonic as to produce inflammation. After all, a sterile urine with a pH of about 7 and a specific gravity of 1.012 to 1.018 is a rather physiologic saline solution containing urea which is practically nonirritating to many tissues. Ruptures of the vesical urethra or the bladder are the usual frequent causes of urine peritonitis (see Chap. 52, Urology).

CHRONIC PERITONITIS

Chronic bacterial peritonitis is exemplified almost exclusively by tuberculous peritonitis.

FIG. 37-4. The adherence and the appearance of the omentum and the bowel in a 30-year-old man with tuberculous peritonitis.

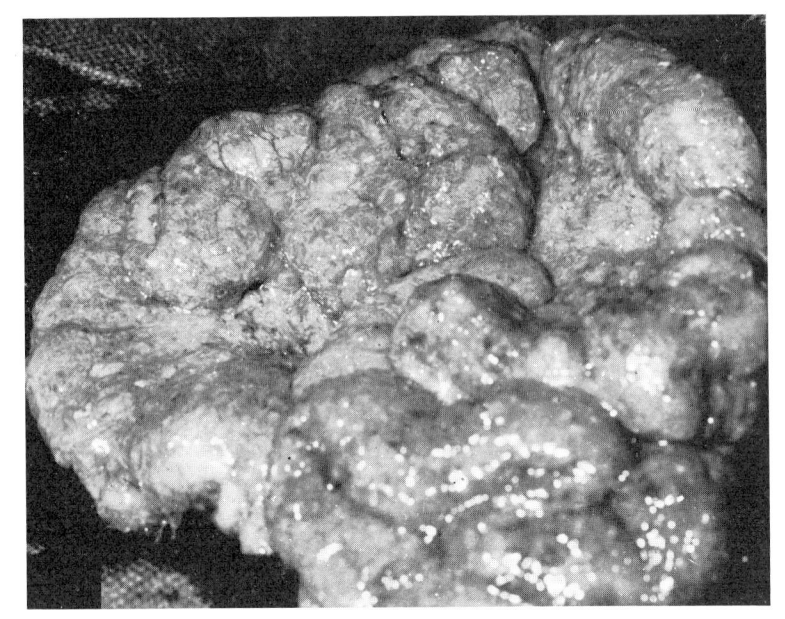

This granulomatous disease usually involves the entire peritoneum (Fig. 37-4). When it complicates acute miliary tuberculosis, the visceral and parietal peritoneal surfaces are often covered in their entirety by miliary tubercles and with fronds of fibrin. In these cases the peritoneal fluid is fibrinous and frequently scanty.

When tuberculous peritonitis is associated with nonmiliary tuberculosis it assumes a somewhat different form. The peritoneal tubercles are larger and occasionally fibrotic; adhesions are numerous and occasionally cause intestinal obstruction. Fluid accumulations are large, low in protein content and contain little or no fibrin.

The prognosis of tuberculous peritonitis is good since the advent of certain of the antitubercular drugs, but the fibrotic form is often complicated by intestinal obstruction, and consequently, its ultimate outcome is seldom certain.

Chronic chemical peritonitis is perhaps best illustrated by the talc and starch granulomata resulting from dusting of surgical gloves with these materials. The disease smolders along for many years and may require many operations for release of intestinal adhesions causing obstruction. Barium sulfate perforating the bowel or entering the peritoneal cavity via an unsuspected perforation also causes a chronic inflammatory reaction similar to that produced by talc in the peritoneum. This can largely be avoided if the barium is removed promptly from the abdomen.

Meconium peritonitis occurs from the intra-abdominal perforation of the gut in utero or in the neonatal period. This is a sterile chemical peritonitis if it develops in utero (see Chap. 50, Pediatric Surgery).

Idiopathic chronic peritonitis is observed occasionally in patients with long-standing ascites. It is not clear that the thickened serosa with its granular surface is the cause or the result of accumulations of ascitic fluid. This condition is observed more frequently in children or young adults in whom ascites and portal hypertension are the result of portal vein thrombosis than in adults with cirrhosis and ascites.

Chylous ascites and peritonitis are accompanied by a nonspecific inflammatory reaction to chylous lymph within the abdominal cavity. Most frequently, spontaneous chylous ascites is caused by the blockage of the flow of chyle in the region of the cisterna chyli by lymphomas and malignant tumors of the pancreas, the retroperitoneal connective tissue (sarcomas) and the kidney. However, chylous ascites may also be idiopathic and persist for many years with the patient otherwise remaining in good health, having only a swollen fluid-containing abdomen to plague him. Nitrogen mustard or radioactive colloidal gold have been used to treat chylous ascites of neoplastic origin with reported success. A low-fat diet limits the ascites in the idiopathic form.

COMPLICATIONS OF PERITONITIS

The most frequent complications or sequelae of peritonitis are intra-abdominal inflammatory masses, abscesses, adhesions with mechanical intestinal obstruction, and enterocutaneous fistulas. Rarer sequelae are septicemia, septic thrombosis of pelvic and mesenteric veins, intrahepatic abscesses, empyema, and enterovaginal and enterovesical fistulae.

Inflammatory Masses. Intra-abdominal inflammatory masses should be distinguished from intra-abdominal abscesses when possible because the former often disappear without surgical intervention while the latter usually require drainage. Intra-abdominal inflammatory masses are made of fibrin-adherent edematous inflamed loops of intestine and parts of the omentum and do not contain pus. This inflammatory conglomeration of tissue is tender and readily felt through the abdominal wall or the rectum, depending upon its location. It is also attended by leukocytosis and some fever. The only way the inflammatory mass can be distinguished from an abscess without recourse to a diagnostic celiotomy is to examine repeatedly the mass and the patient, noting what is happening to the size of the mass and the overlying tenderness, and taking cognizance of the course of the illness. If within 24 to 48 hours the mass decreases in size, if the tenderness subsides, and if there is steady recovery from the general illness, the tender intra-abdominal tumor is an inflammatory mass, and nothing need be done about it. Should the lump increase in size, the tenderness not subside, and the patient remain septic, it is probably an abscess and should be drained.

Adhesions and intestinal obstruction are discussed in Chapter 38. All that need be said here is: the long intestinal tube is a fairly effective way of treating adhesive mechanical intestinal obstruction should it occur within the first week or two after the peritonitis began. But celiotomy is usually the better treatment for adhesive mechanical intestinal obstruction that may occur later.

Pylephlebitis is discussed in Chapter 37, Sect. 1, and hepatic abscesses in Chapter 32.

INTRA-ABDOMINAL ABSCESSES

These are the most frequent complications of peritonitis. They are classified mainly on the basis of their anatomic locations: subphrenic, mid-abdominal and pelvic.

SUBPHRENIC ABSCESSES

The subphrenic space is that portion of the abdominal cavity bounded by the diaphragm above and the transverse colon and the mesocolon below. Barnard's (1908) description of the subphrenic spaces quoted for so many years is not anatomically correct. The subphrenic space is divided by the liver into the suprahepatic and the infrahepatic compartments. The falciform ligament further divides the space into the right and the left divisions. The triangular ligaments and the coronary ligament do not suspend the liver from its superior diaphragmatic surface but are actually dorsal mesenteries attaching the liver to the transversalis fascia overlying the base of the right crus and the posterior third of the right dome of the diaphragm. Consequently, on the right there is only one large space above the liver—the right suprahepatic space. The so-called posterior suprahepatic abscesses really occupy the posterolateral part of the suprahepatic space lying anterior and lateral to the coronary and the right triangular ligaments. Below the right lobe of the liver there is only one space, the right infrahepatic space; its most posterior recess is known as the pouch of Morison. On the left side of the abdomen the space above the left lobe of the liver is the left suprahepatic space. Because of the small size of the left lobe of the liver, this space freely communicates anteriorly and laterally with the space below the liver and anterior and superior to the stomach and the spleen, and for this reason it is considered to be only a single space, the left anterior infrahepatic. The lesser peritoneal sac constitutes the left posterior infrahepatic space. Abscesses within these spaces rarely occupy more than a part of a particular space. Consequently, an abscess may be located either anteriorly or posteriorly, medially, centrally or laterally, in any of the spaces described above excepting the omental bursa; abscesses in it usually occupy it in entirety. Approximately two thirds of all the subphrenic abscesses are located on the right side, the suprahepatic spaces being occupied by them more frequently than the infrahepatic spaces. Approximately one sixth of the abscesses affect more than one of these spaces simultaneously, and about 6 per cent of them are so large as to be bilateral.

Diagnosis of Subphrenic Abscess. Subphrenic abscesses are often conspicuous by the lack of local signs of inflammation. After all, they are usually buried far away from the abdominal wall, the structures about them contain few somatic sensory nerves, and the ribs keep us from feeling them. Therefore, the old saying, "When there must be pus somewhere, but it is seemingly nowhere, there is pus under the diaphragm" is often appropriate. Pain and tenderness over the upper abdomen or the lower chest is most often inconspicuous; however, subphrenic or suprahepatic abscesses are frequently attended at one time or another by a pleuritic pain that may be referred to the shoulder. Widening and bulging of the intercostal spaces and edema of the skin are seen only rarely and then only late. Often about the only signs of a subphrenic abscess are: a spiking temperature, an occasional chill (10 to 15% of patients), tachycardia, anorexia, malaise, diminished or absent diaphragmatic motion on the affected side, leukocytosis with a shift to the left, anemia, and a pleural effusion. Most of these signs may be suppressed by antibiotics, and when they are, the subphrenic abscess may burst catastrophically into the free peritoneal or pleural cavities before the diagnosis is made.

RADIOLOGIC EXAMINATION is most important for the diagnosis and the localization of subphrenic abscesses. Demonstration of an air fluid level separable from the gastrointestinal tract is to be seen in approximately 25 per cent of the cases and is diagnostic. Elevation and loss of mobility of the affected diaphragm occur in approximately two thirds of the cases. A sterile pleural effusion on the affected side is present in 90 per cent. Occasionally, the stomach when distended with barium or carbonated beverage is found to be displaced, and with a barium enema the hepatic or the splenic flexures may be found out of place and distorted. Occasionally, a pneumoperitoneum (750 to 1,000 cc.) may be used to demonstrate obliteration of the normal spaces between the liver and the adjacent structures. Diagnostic aspirations are somewhat hazardous because of the danger of contaminating the pleural space with them. In addition, they are unreliable because the abscess is readily missed by the needle. Once an abscess is localized, it should be drained (Carter and Brewer, 1964). The main consequences of an undrained subphrenic abscess, besides septicemia and death, are related to rupture of the abscess into the abdomen, producing a usually fatal generalized peritonitis, or into the thorax, followed by empyema, pyopneumothorax, or bronchopleural fistula.

Treatment of Suprahepatic Abscesses. Ever since the introduction of the posterior extraperitoneal approach by Nather and Ochsner (1923), and the anterior extraperitoneal approach of Clairmont and Meyer (1926), the mortality from suprahepatic abscesses has been reduced to approximately half that associated with the previously used transperitoneal and transpleural routes. Suprahepatic abscesses may be drained under local or light general anesthesia.

Abscesses located posteriorly are usually drained by subperiosteal resection of the 12th rib on the affected side. Melinkoff found in cadavers that the pleura extended below the 12th rib in 62 per cent but never extended below the level of spinous process of the 1st lumbar vertebra. Therefore, after resection of the appropriate 12th rib, a transverse incision, not one paralleling the bed of the rib, is made at the level of the spinous process of L-1, thereby permitting assured entrance into the retroperitoneum below the diaphragm. With the index finger, the transversalis fascia is stripped from the diaphragm upward until the abscess is felt, perforated, and drained (Fig. 37-5).

For the drainage of abscesses located anteriorly, subcostal incisions located approximately 1 inch below the costal margin and extending from the middle of the rectus abdominus laterally and downward for 3 inches paralleling the costal margin are very satisfac-

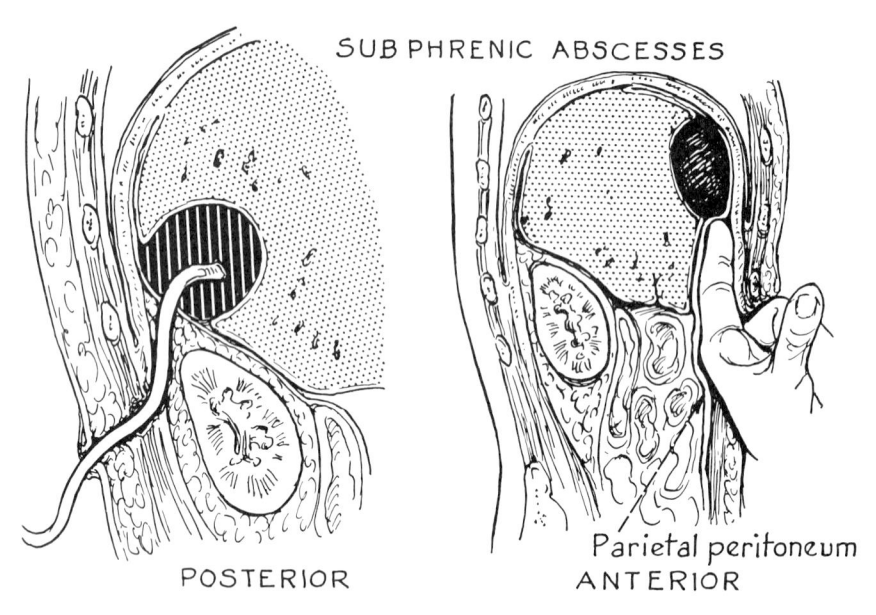

FIG. 37-5. Technics for surgical drainage of subphrenic abscesses. (After Clairmont, Ochsner and De Bakey)

tory. The incision is carried down to but not through the transversalis fascia, and then with blunt dissection with a finger the transversalis fascia is separated from the diaphragm, taking care to keep out of the peritoneal cavity until the abscess cavity is located and drained (Fig. 37-5). In a few instances when the location of the abscess is uncertain, particularly in subhepatic abscesses, it may be necessary to open the free abdominal cavity first in order to identify the limits of the abscess. Then this incision is closed, and another is made so as to drain the abscess without traversing the free peritoneal cavity. Recently, the transpleural approach has been resurrected for the drainage of posteriorly located suprahepatic abscesses. The 9th or 10th rib is resected in the posterior axillary line. The pleura is displaced superiorly when possible; when this is impossible, it is separated from the posterior chest wall, pushed against the diaphragm, and carefully sutured to the diaphragm all about the selected site for the diaphragmatic incision in order to seal off the pleural cavity before incising into the abscess. This is now a safer method than it used to be, presumably because of the use of antibiotics.

Treatment of subhepatic abscess in a few instances may involve locating the abscess by exposing first the free peritoneal cavity away from the suspected site of the abscess. A counter incision is then made directly into the abscess without entering the peritoneal cavity, where the visceral and parietal surfaces adhere. Caution is necessary lest the exploratory intraperitoneal incision become contaminated; if possible, the skin area to be incised should be marked and the exploratory incision closed before attempting stab-wound drainage directly into the abscess cavity through the marked skin surface. More often, subhepatic abscesses can be entered directly from the overlying abdominal skin. Usually the site of location can be established by nonsurgical means and the drainage incision properly placed to ensure against transperitoneal drainage or contamination.

Mid-abdominal Abscesses

Abscesses in the mid-abdomen may be located anywhere between the transverse mesocolon superiorly and the rim of the true pelvis inferiorly. The right colic gutter is the most usual site, the left gutter the next, and between the folds of the small intestinal mesentery the rarest.

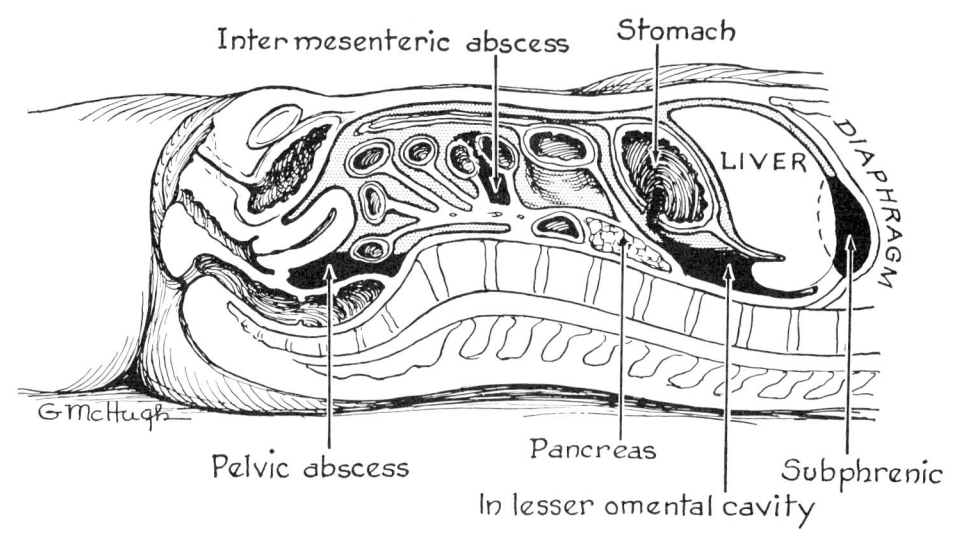

FIG. 37-6. Illustration of the dependent areas of the peritoneal cavity when the patient is in the supine position. These are the same areas in which intra-abdominal abscesses are encountered most frequently.

Abscesses in the mid-abdomen most often follow perforative appendicitis, diverticulitis and carcinoma of the colon, ulcerative colitis, traumatic perforations of large and small intestines, regional enteritis, and the leaving of sponges in the abdomen during laparotomy. Occasionally, perforations of the biliary tract or of a peptic ulcer are followed by a mid-abdominal abscess located in the region of the cecum. The diagnosis of abscesses lying in the gutters of the mid-abdomen is usually relatively easy. A septic fever and a tender growing mass in the abdomen that is easily felt, excepting in very obese persons, are the only signs requisite for diagnosis.

The diagnosis of intermesenteric abscesses lying between folds of the jejuno-ileal mesentery or below it (see Fig. 37-6) is much more difficult because abscesses thus located are usually small and multiple and do not come in contact with the anterior abdominal wall. Continued sepsis and partial mechanical obstruction of the small intestine are practically the only signs of intermesenteric abscesses unless they become so large as to be felt through the anterior abdominal wall.

Because of the paucity of signs that abscesses produce when located between folds of the mesentery, their existence must always be suspected when sepsis continues after the acute phase of peritonitis has passed and localizing signs of abscess cannot be found anywhere else. Especially in case of failure to find subphrenic abscess, when it is operatively searched for, the mid-abdomen should be explored for intermesenteric abscesses.

The treatment of mid-abdominal abscesses is drainage, using incisions that will permit a retroperitoneal or a direct approach into the abscess without traversing any open part of the peritoneal cavity. This is often possible with abscesses located in the colic gutters. It is usually impossible with abscesses located between folds of mesentery. The latter must be drained by the complete evacuation of their pus and the separation of the mesenteric folds one from the other.

At times the free peritoneal cavity must be opened first to delineate the boundaries of an abscess. When this is done, the exploratory wound is closed, and another is made to drain the pus from the abscess without permitting its entry into the peritoneal cavity.

All foreign bodies and dead organs such as the appendix or the gallbladder should be lifted out from the abscess should this be possible without breaking through the abscess wall or opening into the intestine that almost always makes up a part of the wall of the abscess.

Pelvic Abscesses

Pelvic abscesses most often follow pelvic inflammatory disease in women, perforative appendicitis, and diverticulitis of the colon. Pus draining into the pelvis from perforation of the upper or mid-abdomen may also lead to abscesses within the pelvis. It is said that should any patient with peritonitis be kept in Fowler's position (semirecumbent), the abscess that may form is more likely to do so in the pelvis, making it easy to diagnose and drain. The symptoms of pelvic abscess include pain and tenderness in the lower abdomen, fever, frequency of urination, and dysuria.

Often the only symptom of a pelvic abscess in either sex is fever and a general feeling of being sick. The "silent pelvic abscess" may usually be found by performing a digital examination of the rectum every day after all appendectomies and during and after any acute peritonitis.

Pelvic abscesses are tender masses that are readily palpated through the anterior rectal wall because they push this part of the rectum posteriorly and downward. The anterior rectal mucosa becomes thick and edematous, and the rectal sphincter becomes lax. One must be careful to distinguish between a pelvic inflammatory mass and a pelvic abscess. About two thirds of the tender pelvic masses felt through the rectum after peritonitis from perforation of a duodenal ulcer disappear spontaneously. Should an attempt be made to drain such a pelvic inflammatory mass (not an abscess) through the rectum or the vagina all that may be accomplished is the creation of an anterorectal or enterovaginal fistula. In general, the inflammatory mass does not bulge into the rectum, while the abscess does; the inflammatory mass has indefinitely palpable limits, while the abscess is discrete and hemispherical; the inflammatory mass becomes smaller and less discrete over a day or two, while the abscess grows steadily larger; and the inflammatory mass is associated with an improving patient, while the abscess is associated with a continuing or worsening illness.

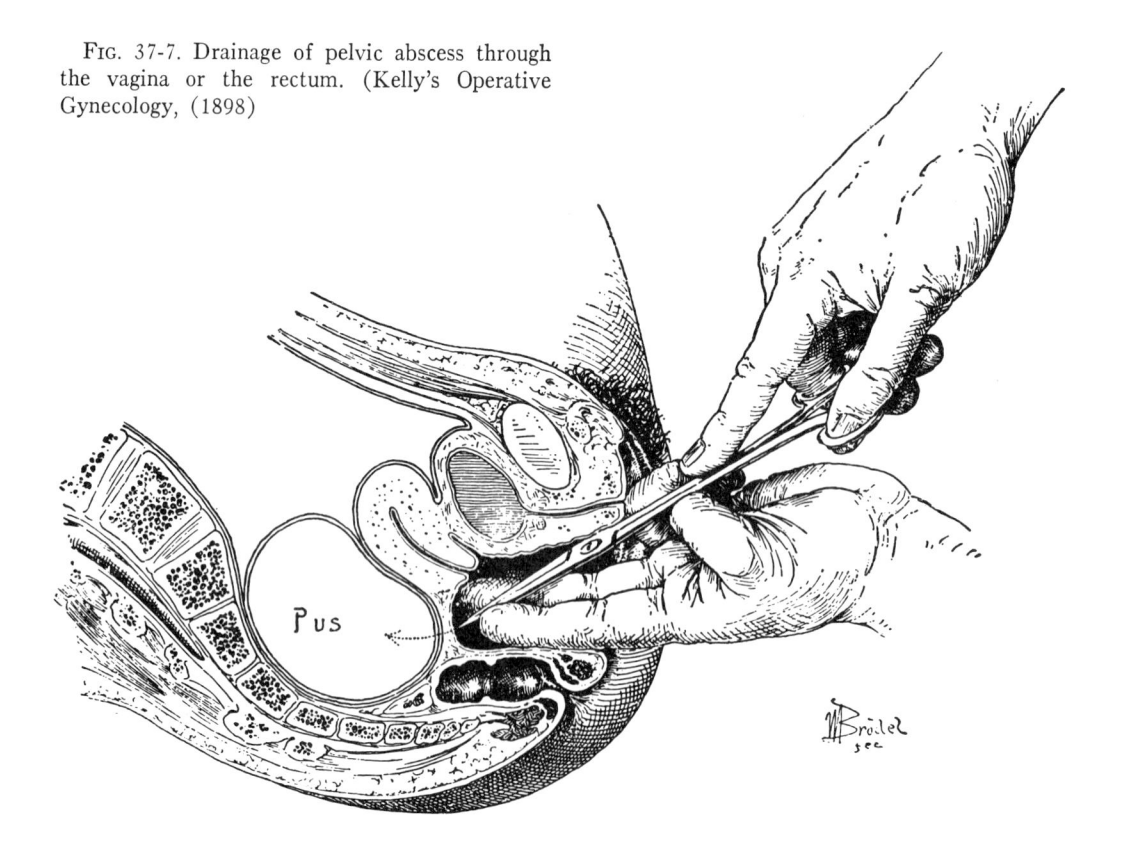

FIG. 37-7. Drainage of pelvic abscess through the vagina or the rectum. (Kelly's Operative Gynecology, (1898)

The treatment of a pelvic abscess is drainage into the rectum or the vagina (Fig. 37-7). Needle aspiration, once such an abscess is felt by rectal or pelvic examination, usually can be performed with reasonable safety. A 16-gauge, 4-inch needle is inserted through the posterior wall of the vaginal vault, or through the anterior wall of the rectum entering directly into the previously palpated abscess. Once pus is obtained, the site of needle puncture is enlarged by spreading with a hemostat or a pair of scissors inserted directed into the abscess cavity (Fig. 37-7). A soft but noncollapsible piece of rubber tubing is left in the abscess cavity and led to the outside. A piece of heavy silk is firmly secured to the tubing and appropriately attached to the adjacent external skin.

In all cases of spontaneous intra-abdominal abscess further studies should be made to determine its cause as soon as the patient's condition permits. Removal of the appendix should be carried out within 6 to 8 weeks after drainage of an appendiceal abscess. Carcinoma or other serious disorders which may require more surgery should be sought for and treated as required.

Occasionally, pelvic abscesses communicate with abscesses in the mid-abdomen; in these cases combined rectal or vaginal and abdominal drainage is often needed.

In all drainages of abdominal abscesses, wherever they may be, continuous drainage must be maintained until the cavity of the abscess has disappeared. The principles of drainage are discussed in Chapter 2 (Wound Healing).

The persistence of an abdominal enterocutaneous fistula after the drainage of an intra-abdominal mass or abscess complicating peritonitis is almost always relatable to one or more of six factors: (1) the persistence of an abscess between the abdominal wall and the intestine, (2) partial obstruction of the intestine distal to the fistula's enteral orifice, (3) a foreign body within the peritoneal cavity, (4) a chronic granuloma within the intestine such as actinomycosis or tuberculosis, (5) a neoplasm of the bowel about the enteral orifice of the fistula, and (6) the juncture of skin with mucous membrane within the fistula. The injection of water-miscible radiopaque contrast media through a catheter into the fistula during fluoroscopy and subsequent filming of the region is the simplest means of ascertaining whether one or more of the first three causes are operative. Biopsy and proper culturing of scrapings from the depths of the fistula serve to examine whether causes 4 or 5 may exist, and close inspection of the fistula, which is usually very short, in cases of cutaneous mucosal juncture, serves to examine possibility 6. The treatment of chronic enterocutaneous fistulas rests upon removing the cause: e.g., wide direct drainage for residual abscesses, resections of the intestine and lysis of adhesions for distal obstruction, proper antibiotic therapy for actinomycosis and tuberculosis, resection for neoplasm, and separation of intestinal mucosa from the skin for cutaneous-mucosal juncture.

REFERENCES

Appendicitis

Baker, W. N. W., Mackie, D. B., and Newcombe, J. F.: Abdominal wall, peritoneum, hernia. Brit. M. J., 3:146, 1967.

Barber, K. W., Jr., Waugh, J. M., Beahrs, O. H., and Sauer, W. G.: Indications for and the results of the surgical treatment of regional enteritis. Ann. Surg., 156:472, 1962.

Barnes, B. A., Behringer, G. E., Wheelock, F. C., and Wilkins, E. W.: Treatment of appendicitis at the Massachusetts General Hospital (1937-1959). J.A.M.A., 180:122, 1962.

Bierman, H. R.: Human appendix and neoplasia. Cancer, 21:109, 1968.

Boles, E. T., Ireton, R. J., and Clatworthy, H. W., Jr.: Acute appendicitis in children. Arch. Surg., 79:447, 1959.

Bower, J. O.: Report on the first statewide survey of acute appendicitis from statewide hospital records of 1937. Penn. Med. J., 43:1145, 1940.

Boyce, F. F.: Acute Appendicitis and Its Complications. New York, Oxford University Press, 1949.

Burne, J.: M. Chir. Tr., 20:219, 1837. Quoted by Fitz, 1886.

Callaghan, P. J., and Del Beccaro, E. J.: Adenocarcinoma of the appendix. J.A.M.A., 180:333, 1962.

Cannon, P. R.: The changing pathologic picture of infection since the introduction of chemotherapy and antibiotics. Bull. N. Y. Acad. Med., 31:87, 1955.

Capps, J. A.: Pain in the Pleura, Pericardium and Peritoneum. New York, Macmillan, 1932.

Castleton, K. B., Puestow, C. B., and Sauer, D.: Is appendicitis decreasing in frequency? Arch. Surg., 78:794, 1959.

Commission on Acute Appendicitis Mortality: Report

of the third state-wide survey of acute appendicitis mortality. Penn. Med. J., 55:449, 1952.

Cope, Z.: The Early Diagnosis of the Acute Abdomen. Ed. 13, London, Oxford University Press, 1968.

Coran, A. G., and Wheeler, H. B.: Early perforation in appendicitis after age 60. J.A.M.A., 197:745, 1966.

de Lamotte, J.: Observations made at the opening of a body of a person dead of tympanites. J. med., chir. pharm., 22:65. Quoted by Major, R. H.: Classic Descriptions of Disease. p. 617, Springfield, Ill., Charles C Thomas, 1932.

Dupuytren, B. G.: Leçons orales. Clin. chir., 3:330, 1833. Quoted by Fitz, 1886.

Egdahl, R. H.: Current mortality in appendicitis. Am. J. Surg., 107:757, 1964.

Eiseman, B., Robinson, R. M., and Brown, J. H.: Simultaneous appendectomy and herniorrhaphy without prophylactic antibiotic therapy. Surg., 51:578, 1962.

Elias, E. G., and Hults, R.: Congenital absence of vermiform appendix. Arch. Surg., 95:257, 1967.

Farringer, J. L., Jr., and Tarasidis, G.: Carcinoid tumors of the appendix. Arch. Surg., 88:354, 1964.

Fitz, R. H.: Perforating inflammation of the vermiform appendix; with special reference to its early diagnosis and treatment. Tr. A. Am. Physicians, 1:107, 1886.

Fowler, G. R.: Diffuse septic peritonitis, with special reference to a new method of treatment, namely, the elevated head and trunk posture, to facilitate drainage into the pelvis, with a report of 9 consecutively treated cases of recovery. Med. Rec., 57:617, 1900.

Girardet, R., and Enquist, I. F.: Differential diagnosis between appendicitis and acute pelvic inflammatory disease. Surg., Gynec., Obstet., 116:212, 1963.

Goldbeck: Über eigenth. entz. Geschw, i.d. rechten Huftbeingegend. 1830. Quoted by Fitz, 1886.

Harkins, H. N.: Personal communication. 1956.

———: Unpublished data, 1956.

Hilsabeck, J. R., Judd, E. S., Jr., and Woolner, L. B.: Carcinoma of the vermiform appendix. Surg. Clin. N. Amer. 31:995, 1951.

Husson, and Dance: Répertoire gen. d'anat., etc., 4:154, 1827. Quoted by Fitz, 1886.

Jackson, R. H.: Parents, family doctors, and acute appendicitis in childhood. Brit. Med. J., 2:277, 1963.

Keeley, J. L., and Schairer, A. E.: Incidental appendectomy during repair of groin hernias. Surgery, 52:421, 1962.

Kelley, E. P.: Letter to editor. J.A.M.A., 206:647, 1968.

Kelly, H. A., and Hurdon, E.: The Vermiform Appendix and Its Diseases. Philadelphia, W. B. Saunders, 1905.

Kerr, W. S. Jr., Suby, H. I., Vickery, A., and Fraley, E.: Idiopathic retroperitoneal fibrosis; Clinical experiences with 15 cases, 1956-67. J. Urol., 99:575, 1968.

Lewis, T.: Pain. New York, Macmillan, 1942.

Lewis, T., and Kellgren, J. H.: Observation relating to referred pain, visceromotor reflexes and other related phenomenon. Clin. Sci., 4:47, 1939.

Maddox, J. R., Jr., Johnson, W. W., and Sergeant, C. K.: Appendectomies in a children's hospital: A five-year survey. Arch. Surg., 89:223, 1964.

Marcucci, A., and Monosi, V.: Observations on 1,399 instances of acute appendicitis. Osped. Ital. Chir., 17:443, 1967.

Marx, F. W., Jr.: Incidental appendectomy with regional enteritis. Arch. Surg., 88:546, 1964.

McArthur, L. L.: Choice of incisions of abdominal wall; especially for appendicitis. Chicago Med. Rec., 7:289 and 330, 1894.

———: Gestation complicated by appendiceal abscess. Am. J. Obstet., 31:181, 228, 1895.

McBurney, C.: Experience with early operative interference in cases of diseases of the vermiform appendix. N. Y. Med. J., 50:676, 1889.

———: The incision made in the abdominal wall in cases of appendicitis, with a description of a new method of operating. Ann. Surg., 20:38, 1894.

Meade, R. H.: The evolution of surgery for appendicitis. Surgery, 55:741, 1964.

Melier, F.: Mémoire et observation sur quelques maladies de l'appendice caecale. J. gén. méd. chir. pharm., 100:317, 1827.

Mestivier, M.: On a tumor situated near the umbilical region on the right side, produced by a large pin found in the vermiform appendix of the cecum. J. med., chir. et pharm. tom., 1:441, 1759. Quoted by Major, R. H.: Classic Descriptions of Disease. p. 617. Springfield, Ill., Charles C Thomas, 1932.

Newbold, R. S.: Personal communication to the author (1962).

Noon, G. P., Beall, A. C. Jr., Jordan, G. L. Jr., Riggs, S., and De Bakey, M. E.: Clinical evaluation of peritoneal irrigation with antibiotic solution. Surgery, 62:73, 1967.

Ochsner, A. J.: The cause of diffuse peritonitis complicating appendicitis and its prevention. Chairman's address, delivered before Section on Surgery and Anatomy. 55th Annual Meeting, A.M.A., June 4-7, 1901.

Ochsner, Alton, Gage, M. I., and Garside, E.: The intra-abdominal postoperative complications of appendicitis. Ann. Surg., 91:544, 1930.

Parkinson, J.: Case of diseased appendix vermiformis. Med. Chir. Tr., 3:57, 1812.

Priddle, H. D., and Hesseltine, H. C.: Acute appendicitis in the obstetric patient. Am. J. Obstet. Gynec., 62:150, 1951.

Reid, M. R.: The mortality of appendicitis—a national disgrace. South. Surgeon, 8:404, 1938.

Ross, F. P., Zarem, H. A., and Morgan, A. P.: Appendicitis in a community hospital. Arch. Surg., 85:1036, 1962.

Shepherd, J. A.: Surgery of the acute abdomen. Baltimore, Williams & Wilkins, 1968.

Peritonitis and Intra-abdominal Abscesses

Altemeier, W. A., and Cole, W. R.: Nature and treatment of septic shock. Arch. Surg., 77:498-507, 1958.

Carter, R., and Brewer, L. A., III: Subphrenic abscess: a thoracoabdominal clinical complex. Am. J. Surg., 108:165, 1964.
Clairmont, P., and Meyer, M.: Erfahrungen über die Behandlung der Appendicitis. Acta chir. scandinav., 60:55, 1926.
Deol, J. S., and Updegrove, J. H.: Peritoneal laceration due to muscular effort: an unusual cause of hemoperitoneum. J.A.M.A., 199:500, 1967.
McCarthy, J. D., and Picazo, J. G.: Bile peritonitis: diagnosis and course. Am. J. Surg., 116:664, 1968.
Ochsner, Alton, and De Bakey, Michael: Amoebic hepatitis and hepatic abscess. Surgery, 13:635, 1943.
Other reading material on the subject of peritonitis is to be found in the bibliography of Section 1, Appendicitis and the Acute Abdomen.

CHAPTER 38

J. GARROTT ALLEN, M.D.

Anatomy and Physiology of the Small Bowel and Colon, and Intestinal Obstruction

Anatomy
Physiology
Diagnosis of Intestinal Obstruction
Clinical Features
Treatment

ANATOMY

The jejuno-ileum or the "small bowel" extends from the ligament of Treitz to the ileocecal valve and is about 20 feet in length. About 40 per cent of its proximal length is considered to be jejunum and the distal 60 per cent as ileum. It is all covered by serosa except for its point of mesenteric attachment. There is no discernible gross anatomic feature which allows an accurate or exact separation of the jejunum from the ileum. The jejunum is usually of a little larger diameter and its muscular coats are a little thicker than those of the ileum, and most of the lymphoid tissue known as Peyer's patches is found in the distal half of the ileum. The entire jejuno-ileum is attached to the anterior border of the mesentery in which course its blood vessels and lymph channels. Situated about 3 to 4 feet from the ileocolic junction and on the antimesenteric border of the ileum, occasionally there is to be found a fingerlike projection, Meckel's diverticulum (see Chap. 50, Pediatric Surgery), and it may cause intestinal obstruction at any time in life (Seagram *et al.*, 1968).

Intra-abdominal Colon. The colon is about 5 feet in length and, except during infancy, is about twice the diameter of the small bowel. Its musculature differs from that of the small bowel in that the longitudinal muscle fibers are collected together in 3 bands, the *taeniae coli*. Each taenia is located equidistantly; one of them lies along the site of the embryologic attachment of the mesentery of the colon. The circular fibers of smooth muscle of the colon also are more or less collected together at intervals of 1 or 2 cm. and account for the haustra that give the colon its sacculated appearance. An important contributory factor is that the taeniae are shorter than other muscular coats of the colon, tending to encourage the saccular pleating observed, which is more pronounced in the proximal than the distal half of the colon.

The rectum averages 12 cm. in length and is below the peritoneal reflection. It usually begins near the level of the 3rd sacral vertebra posteriorly and terminates as the top 2 cm. of the "anorectum" (see Chap. 41). The anus, or anal canal, itself is also about 2 cm. in length, making the entire anorectum about 4 cm. (1.75 in.) long. The anorectum has a common difference from the upper rectum in that the nonstriated circular muscle is much thicker for this 4 cm. of length than in the rectum above. This thickened portion of the circular muscle is the internal anal sphincter. The dividing line between the rectal and the anal portions of the anorectum is the circular line of shelflike pockets known as the valves, or crypts of Morgagni, which are related to the pectinate line.

The anatomy of the cecum and the appendix has been discussed in Chapter 37. The mesenteric relationships and the vasculature of the small and the large intestine have been presented in Chapter 35.

Electron microscopy of the mucosa of the alimentary tract, as elsewhere, has only recently been attempted (Trier et al., 1963), and though such studies may be of great assistance as experience is acquired, discussion at this time is premature.

Lymph Drainage. The lymphatic circulation from the small bowel, the colon, the rectum and the anus must be known by the surgeon in planning operations on malignant tumors arising from these organs. The lymphatic spread of tumors arising within these portions of the alimentary tract tends to be through the regional lymph channels and nodes draining the particular bowel segment involved. Consequently, the *en bloc* removal of the regional lymphatics and lymph nodes affords the patient his best chance for cure.

To a large extent, the lymph channels of the small bowel, the abdominal colon and the rectum correspond in location and distribution to those of the blood vessels of the same organs (see Figs. 35-5 and 35-6, Chap. 35). However, when the lymphatics reach the root of the mesentery, this relationship no longer strictly obtains.

Lymphatics of the anus usually drain anteriorly, uniting with those from the scrotum or the labia majora and terminating in the superficial inguinal nodes, but occasionally they also may drain upward to join the lymphatics of the anal canal and the rectum, and thus to the thoracic duct and to the retroperitoneum.

Lymphatics of the anal canal drain the lower rectal mucosa and usually follow the course of the middle and the inferior hemorrhoidal blood vessels, to the hypogastric (internal iliac) nodes. These particular lymph channels are fairly diffuse and may course along the superior surface of the levator ani muscles, reaching the sacral nodes prior to entering the hypogastric lymph glands.

The lymphatics of the rectum and the colon are described in Chapter 41.

Lymphatics of the jejunum and the ileum serve as conduits for chyle. These lymphatics pass through or around the preaortic nodes of the superior mesenteric region before entering the cisterna chyli which is the central point of collection of all three preaortic nodal clusters (celiac, superior and inferior mesenteric). Thus it receives lymph from all of the intra-abdominal organs, and occasionally from the rectum and the anus.

The cisterna chyli is an irregular, somewhat conical, saccular structure located on the anterior surface of the 2nd lumbar vertebra to the right side of and behind the aorta. From its cephalic end arises the *thoracic duct* which passes into the posterior mediastinum along the anterior surface of the thoracic vertebra between the right side of the aorta and the mesial side of the azygos vein. At the level of the top of the 5th thoracic vertebra, the duct crosses to the left, where it continues its upward course, to empty into the left jugular or the subclavian veins or their point of juncture. Through this duct tumor cells from the alimentary tract may reach the systemic venous blood without passing through the liver. Virchow recognized that occasionally tumors (from the stomach especially) may reach lymph nodes in the left supraclavicular area via the thoracic duct route. Such nodes are often referred to as "Virchow's nodes," but they are more often spoken of than found.

Between the leaves of the mesentery of the small intestine and the intra-abdominal portions of the colon are large numbers of mesenteric lymph nodes. These are the nodes that are frequently the earliest sites for metastases from tumors of the bowel. The mesenteric nodes are frequently very prominent and enlarged in regional enteritis and ulcerative colitis.

PHYSIOLOGY

Intestinal Motility (Including Peristalsis)

Four types of intestinal motion occur: peristalsis, segmental contractions, pendular movements and an undulating motion of the intestinal villi. Electrical activity in relation to muscular contractility is under study in several laboratories in this country and abroad. These studies should increase our understanding of peristalsis and aid in our appreciation of its stimulating and inhibiting factors.

Peristaltic motions propel the bolus of food in the aboral direction; the segmenting and pendular contractions do not. Peristalsis is a contraction wave of the circular muscle that progresses in the aboral direction a few centimeters per second for distances of 5 to 30 cm. before stopping. Although the role of the long muscle coat in peristalsis is not known, some shrinkage in the length of the contracted segment of bowel appears to occur which may represent the contraction of the longitudinal muscles. The distance traveled and the vigorousness of the peristaltic contraction are usually greatest in the upper jejunum. The contractions of the lower ileum are less vigorous.

The bolus of food is propelled forward and spread out by each peristaltic motion. It then remains stationary until another propelling wave of contraction comes along.

From time to time, a much more vigorous type of peristalsis occurs. These movements are known as *"peristaltic rushes"* and they swiftly sweep all that lies before them for distances of 20 to 50 cm. or farther within a second or two before they die out.

Mechanical distention of the lumen appears to be the main stimulus to peristalsis. In the normal person, food is propelled most rapidly through the upper jejunum. Lower in the small bowel, peristaltic activity is less active, and the transit time is longer. The distance traveled by each peristaltic wave is less in the ileum than in the jejunum. Moreover, there is evidence that competitive antiperistaltic waves (damming back of intestinal contents) may occur normally in the lower ileum and oppose those traveling in the aboral direction. Throughout the small bowel, the process of food transit becomes a "two steps forward—one step backward" sort of affair, though this motion is more noticeable in the duodenum and in the lower ileum.

Segmental Contractions. These have no capacity to propel food. Cannon described them as groups of simultaneous contractions, occurring at intervals, spaced fairly regularly throughout the small bowel. They occur more frequently than peristaltic waves, usually 6 to 15 a minute.

The segmenting movements appear to disseminate the bolus of food, in addition to turning the bolus over, thereby exposing fresh portions to the intestinal mucosa and facilitating absorption. These contractions also speed the flow of lymph through the lacteals. Some of these contractions may continue to occur in an adynamic ileus.

Pendular or oscillating motions are also annular contractions. They travel up and down a small segment of bowel for short distances. Because they may travel in both the oral and the aboral directions, their motion suggests the swinging of a pendulum, hence their name. They, too, knead and churn the food, spreading it forward and backward for short distances within the lumen of the small bowel.

Pendular motions are less obvious in man than peristaltic or segmenting contractions. Their function, when present, is very similar if not identical with those of the segmenting contractions.

The undulating motion of the intestinal villi may be most important in facilitating food absorption. Such motions constantly change the food environment at the absorptive surfaces, bringing into contact with each villus new fluid constituents. Each villus has its own capillary and lymph vessel and its own smooth muscle fibers. Contractions of the latter seem to account for the swaying or undulating motion of the villi.

Nervous control of intestinal peristalsis is under the influence of 2 sets of nerve plexuses; one is extrinsic and the other is intrinsic. At least pendular motion is capable of functioning independently of the functional integrity of either plexus; therefore, like the heart, it is myogenically activated.

The motor functions of the extrinsic nerves are as follows: stimulation of the parasympathetics—the vagus nerves—increases the tonus and the motor activity of the bowel. Tonus is decreased and motility temporarily inhibited by stimulation of the sympathetics—the splanchnic nerves.

Experimentally, the stimulation of the sympathetics is believed to reduce intestinal tone and to stimulate contraction of sphincters; increase of parasympathetic activity is said to have the reverse effect. In man, vagotomy retards temporarily gastric motility but has little if any demonstrable influence upon intestinal activity. The removal of the celiac ganglia, together with the cutting of the preganglionic fibers, may be followed by an intractable diarrhea in the dog but not always in man.

The intrinsic nerves are comprised of Auerbach's and Meissner's plexuses—the myenteric plexuses. Auerbach's plexus lies between the longitudinal and the circular coats of the bowel. This plexus contains numerous ganglion cells whose absence is the primary defect in Hirschsprung's disease of the colon (see Chap. 50, Pediatric Surgery). The myenteric plexus may be destroyed in Chagas' disease which is caused by *Trypanosoma cruzi*. This infection has a predilection for the reticuloendothelial system, the myocardium, the meninges and the myenteric plexuses of the alimentary tract, as well as other motor centers. The alimentary manifestations are those of a functional obstruction like Hirschsprung's disease, except more frequently motility of the esophagus, the duodenum and upper jejunum are affected.

The ganglia in Auerbach's plexus are believed by some to be the terminal connections of the vagus nerves and other parasympathetic nerves to the intestines; conclusive evidence is lacking. Meissner's plexus lies in the submucosa and, compared with Auerbach's, contains relatively few ganglion cells. This plexus is said to be largely sympathetic in function; stimulation inhibits action of the smooth muscle.

Megacolon may also occur in childhood and adolescence in which the myenteric plexus is normal. In any child with this finding, psychogenic causes are often considered, especially poor early toilet training. It has been speculated that since the hindgut has a definite embryologic innervation, idiopathic megacolon, as this condition is known, might be due to an alteration in the activity or release of cholinesterase or acetylcholine. Roy (1968) describes marked improvement in 5 adolescents by resection of the hindgut, implying the disease may not be psychogenic.

Finally, it should be stated again that the churning and mixing motions (largely segmenting and pendular motions) of the intestine continue in the absence of either extrinsic or intrinsic nervous control and are not affected when strips of smooth muscle are suspended in solutions of cocaine or other ganglionic blocking agents. Therefore, this type of movement is considered to be myogenic and to be independent of nervous control, though not necessarily unresponsive to neural influences.

LeVeen *et al*. (1967) have pointed out that the irritant action of castor oil, which depends upon its soluble sodium soaps and the free fatty acid, ricinoleic acid, can be prevented by the administration of a calcium salt, which is chelated by the fatty acid, forming insoluble soap. Hence the irritant action of free ricinoleic acid or its soluble sodium soap is largely avoided.

Defecation. As peristaltic activity gradually propels food through the small bowel and the colon, the feces distend the rectum. As the intraluminal pressure in the rectum rises to 40 to 50 mm. of mercury, the reflex of defecation is set in motion. This reflex is characterized by strong peristaltic contractions of all the smooth muscular coats of the descending and the sigmoid colons. Both longitudinal and circular contractions take place. Contraction of the longitudinal musculature (the taeniae coli) shortens the colon. These two contractions are associated with the simultaneous relaxation of the anal sphincters, and feces are expelled.

Additional forces are applied by certain of the striated muscles which seem to act automatically but are under voluntary control. The simultaneous contraction of the musculature of the abdominal wall exerts considerable increase in the intra-abdominal pressure when the diaphragm is held in the fixed position of deep inspiration.

Voluntary control of defecation is largely effected by relaxation of the musculature of the abdominal wall and the diaphragm, while maintaining the tonus of the external anal sphincter. The latter is supplied by the 4th sacral and the internal pudendal nerves. If these nerves are cut, voluntary sphincter control is lost.

Intestinal Absorption

The absorptive surface of the small bowel in man is estimated to exceed 10 square meters or about 8 times the area of the skin of an average adult. The large surface of the bowel mucosa is made possible by its innumerable villus folds.

There is no disagreement as to the intestine's ability to absorb water, alcohol, glucose, some polypeptides, amino acids and fat, but the mechanisms by which these various substances are absorbed are not well understood. Until such time that more precise information is available, perhaps it is best in a text such as this to state that foodstuffs are absorbed primarily in the small bowel and that the function of the colon is largely restricted to the absorption of water. The colon will also absorb certain aqueous solutions, in limited amounts, such as isotonic or hypotonic solutions of glucose and saline; consequently, these substances may be administered by proctolysis if given slowly. Water absorption in the colon takes place mainly in the cecum and the right half of the colon. The descending colon, the sigmoid and the rectum are largely reservoirs for feces.

INTESTINAL SECRETIONS

Intestinal juice or succus entericus is comprised of water, electrolytes, glucose and urea essentially in isotonic concentrations.

In a normal man, enormous quantities of water pass into and out of the intestinal tract during a day. Approximately 8,000 to 10,000 ml. enter the alimentary tract in the course of 24 hours, while normally less than 200 ml. of water is excreted in feces. In other words, more than 96 per cent is reabsorbed, a ratio of water salvage close to that of the normal kidney in its recovery of the glomerular filtrate.

Diarrhea and intestinal fistulae result in excessive losses of water and electrolytes from the alimentary tract and for this reason alone may be rapidly fatal unless water and salts are given rapidly and properly. The tragic but dramatic stories of John Snow and others about epidemics of cholera of more than a century ago tell of progression of symptoms from onset to death in less than 24 hours. Snow recognized the lethal effect of uncontrollable purgation with its loss of water and salt and proposed their replacement as the most effective form of treatment.

Consider for a moment the result of losing most of the intestinal secretions (shown in Table 38-1). It can be readily appreciated that the entire loss of any one of the secretory fluids which normally enters the alimentary tract could be rapidly fatal if uncorrected. Death was a common sequel to duodenal, pancreatic or biliary fistulae as recently as 30 years ago. Elucidation of the quantitative and qualitative aspects of water and mineral metabolism has enabled us to treat these abnormalities effectively. Assuming a case of midilial obstruction, with the patient losing about 2,500 ml. of gastrointestinal contents, his approximate electrolyte replacements for these gastrointestinal losses would be as follows:

TABLE 38-1. RATES OF TURNOVER OF WATER BY VARIOUS ORGANS IN A 70-KILO HUMAN INDIVIDUAL IN CUBIC CENTIMETERS PER 24 HOURS

ORGANS	MINIMUM	LIBERAL
Salivary glands	500	1,500
Stomach	1,000	2,400
Intestinal wall	700	3,000
Pancreas	700	1,000
Liver (bile)	100	400
Lymph	700	1,500
Total recovered by body	3,700	9,800

(Adoph, after Wangensteen, O. H.: Intestinal Obstructions. ed. 3. Springfield, Ill., Charles C Thomas)

AVERAGE CONCENTRATION OF SODIUM, POTASSIUM AND CHLORIDE IN THE GASTROINTESTINAL TRACT SECRETIONS REMOVED BY INDWELLING TUBES, MILLIEQUIVALENTS PER LITER

	SODIUM	POTASSIUM	CHLORIDE
Through Gastric Tube Salivary Gastric	59	9.3	89.0
Through Small Bowel Tube Bowel Wall Bile Pancreas	104.9	5.1	98.9
Through Miller-Abbott Suction Ileum	116.7	16.2	105.8
Through Ileostomy	129.5	20.6	109.7
Through Cecostomy	79.6		48.2

(Randall, H. T.: Surg. Clin. North Am., 32:2, 457, 1952)

Estimated Loss

Sodium	290 mEq.
Chloride	266 mEq.
Potassium	12-25 mEq.
Bicarbonate	50 mEq.

These losses, aside from insensible and urinary losses, could be replaced by approximately 2.5 liters per day of lactated Ringer's solution. These estimates should be substantiated by daily records of the volume lost, and by measuring the serum electrolyte concentrations as necessary. (See Chap. 5, Fluids and Electrolytes.)

Mucus is an important constituent of intestinal secretions. It is a protein-polysaccharide complex whose function appears to be the maintenance of a "nonwettable" bowel surface, especially in the colon. Mucus is secreted in response to mechanical and nervous stimulation and does not appear to be under hormonal control, though it may be affected by such agents as pilocarpine, atropine and adrenergic agents.

The volume of intestinal juice is modified by a number of stimuli: mechanical, nervous, humoral, osmotic and chemical. Secretin increases its secretion, as does the intravenous injection of saline solutions and sympathetic denervation.

Origins of Intestinal Gases

The normal intestinal tract contains only small amounts of gas within the stomach and the colon. The small bowel of normal persons, excepting infants, is largely free of gas. Normally, about 300 to 500 ml. of flatus is expelled in the course of the day.

Much of the intestinal gas enters the gut through the esophagus during swallowing, deep breathing and coughing. However, some of it is formed in the intestine by chemical and bacterial action, namely, methane and carbon dioxide. Actually, about 7½ liters of carbon dioxide is elaborated in 24 hours by the interaction of hydrochloric acid of gastric juice upon the bicarbonates of biliary and pancreatic secretions, but because CO_2 is absorbed readily, this gas is usually an unimportant cause of intestinal distention.

The enzymatic degradation of certain foods potentially may yield surprisingly large quantities of gas. Schwartz (1909), for example, calculated that 30 liters of carbon dioxide, methane and hydrogen could come from the digestion of 100 Gm. of cellulose. Since no mammalian enzymes can attack the cellobiose bond of cellulose and since bacterial hydrolysis of cellulose in man is not a prominent activity, this figure of Schwartz may be more theoretical than actual.

Portis (1953) described the composition of intestinal gases with particular diets (Table 38-2).

Normally, gases are absorbed from the intestinal tract at rates that are directly proportional to their diffusibility, the latter property being related to the function of the partial pressures of the particular gas in the tissues and the intestine and in the plasma and in the air breathed. For example, under normal circumstances, the partial pressure of carbon dioxide is highest in tissues, intermediate in the plasma and very low in the air breathed. Consequently, there is a net diffusion of CO_2 from tissues to plasma to air. However, with nitrogen the partial pressures of this gas are the same in tissue, in plasma and in air; consequently, the net diffusion of nitrogen is zero as long as air is breathed.

TABLE 38-2.

	MILK DIET %	MEAT DIET %	LEGUMES %	NORMAL DIET %
CO_2	16.8	13.6	34.0	10.3
CH_4	0.9	37.4	44.6	0.7
H_2	43.9	3.0	2.3	29.6
N_2	38.4	46.0	19.1	59.4

Malabsorption and the Blind-Loop Syndromes

We are learning more about intestinal absorption in man from the nature of and the basic disturbances associated with the malabsorption syndromes than perhaps from studies upon the normal. Most, if not all, causes of malabsorption are associated with chronic diarrhea, weight loss, and one or more manifestations of deficiencies of specific nutritive factors. These deficiencies may be due to excessively rapid transit time with inadequate time for absorption, to lack of cofactors necessary to absorption, to competition from intestinal bacteria for certain factors, to losses or absences of digestive enzymes including those of some bacteria that may be essential to absorption, to diminished surface areas, or to the diminished ability of the normal areas of the intestine that are essential to absorption of a particular nutrient factor.

Some of the arterial vascular anomalies resulting in ischemia to the small bowel are also causes for impaired absorption and may produce the malabsorption syndromes (see Chap. 35).

Impairment of fat absorption occurs from exclusion of bile and/or pancreatic juice from the intestinal lumen and tends to produce deficiencies in the absorption of essential fats, fatty acids and fat-soluble vitamins; vitamin K deficiency is the most conspicuous in surgical patients, though vitamin A, D and E deficiencies are occasionally encountered clinically. Calcium depletion may also occur because, with the increased fat in the stool when bile or pancreatic secretions are absent, insoluble calcium soaps are formed. A similar nutritional disorder, with poor fat absorption, occurs in celiac disease which in many patients is largely controlled by the elimination of gluten from the diet—wheat, rye, oats, barley and buckwheat and their products. Remarkable improvement in general health occurs, frequently with a regression of the microscopic abnormalities observed in the intestinal epithelium in this syndrome, simply by excluding all gluten-containing food. Although in these syndromes, absorption of fat and of fat-soluble vitamins is the most conspicuous deficiency, alterations in protein, carbohydrate and mineral metabolism are not uncommon.

The blind-loop syndrome is a term used to describe a host of events that may complicate certain operations on the gastrointestinal tract, in which one of the associated deficiencies is that of vitamin B_{12}. Chronic diarrhea and weight loss are the most obvious early complaints.

Vitamin B_{12} is one of the more interesting food factors because in nature it is nearly always bound to a protein or polypeptide, which for the most part is of the glycoprotein type, whether in plasma, milk, Castle's intrinsic factor in gastric secretions, or in bacterial ribosomes. Orally ingested vitamin B_{12} was formerly designated as the extrinsic factor essential—with the intrinsic factor—to prevent or treat pernicious anemia. Vitamin B_{12} ingested orally is not absorbed in the absence of intrinsic factor, and hence there is the possibility that pernicious anemia may develop after total gastrectomy.

Calcium is also essential for the absorption of the vitamin B_{12}–intrinsic factor complex. In the malabsorption syndromes there is an excessive amount of undigested fat which may be due to (1) disturbances in secretion of bile or pancreatic juices, (2) mucosal disorders such as celiac disease, or (3) the short-circuiting of small bowel either because of an operation or because of internal fistulae. The resulting calcium deficiency favors inadequate absorption of vitamin B_{12} and consequently megaloblastic anemia and polyneuritis are fairly common under these conditions.

It appears that the primary source of vitamin B_{12} is its natural synthesis by certain bacteria and that vitamin B_{12} is an essential nutrient factor for the replication of certain organisms. Other bacteria are unable to create vitamin B_{12} and, if they need it, they acquire it as in a parasitic relationship. As will be noted later, in the blind-loop syndrome the stasis which occurs favors bacterial fermentation and, in the process, some organisms may digest the complex of intrinsic factor-B_{12}-calcium and thus make the absorption of vitamin B_{12} an impossibility.

The site of absorption of vitamin B_{12} is the lower ileum (Drapanas et al., 1963). Vitamin B_{12} deficiency develops when extensive portions of the lower ileum are resected or when its mucosal surface is extensively diseased. It also develops when this organ is bypassed intentionally as in the treatment of regional enteritis, or is unintentionally bypassed when gastroenterocolic and similar internal fistulae develop as a complication of an operation or of a disease. These are syndromes in which the transit time of food is accelerated, impeding absorption of vitamin B_{12}. In addition, the diarrhea observed in gastroenterocolic fistula and ileal bypass is in part due to fermentation of ileal contents by bacteria, some of which also may have the capacity to destroy the intrinsic factor-B_{12}-calcium complex essential to absorption of vitamin B_{12} in the ileum, or to compete successfully for vitamin B_{12} in microbial metabolism. The latter is especially impressive when diarrhea with vitamin B_{12} deficiency occurs after a side-to-side enteroenterostomy or enterocolostomy has been performed for any purpose, or after an end-to-side anastomosis in which there is a nonfunctioning segment of bowel, as little as 5 cm. in length, to act as a reservoir for intestinal fermentation. Because of the technical advantages and safety, it has been common practice to perform side-to-side or end-to-side entero-enterostomy or enterocolostomy in patients with intestinal obstruction. The reason an end-to-end anastomosis is usually not feasible or safe under these conditions is that the diameter of the proximal bowel is much larger than that of the collapsed distal portion. But it is necessary to be aware that the blind-loop syndrome may develop. If it does, it is a simple matter either to revise the anastomosis with end-to-end continuity or to resect the blind loop. Either procedure is usually curative, both of the vitamin B_{12} deficiency and of the chronic diarrhea, if other causes for the latter do not remain. The diarrhea in the blind-loop syndrome is not caused by the vitamin B_{12} deficiency but by the bacterial fermentation which is the common denominator in this syndrome and in the vitamin B_{12} deficiency as well. Vitamin B_{12} is, by weight, the most potent of the food factors essential to human life. Therapeutically it is among the most effective and most rapid to act when needed.

To summarize, inadequate mucosal absorption of B_{12} may occur from several causes of surgical interest: (1) lack of intrinsic factor because of total gastric resection, (2) lack of vitamin B_{12} or excessive competition of bacteria in intestinal fermentation, (3) altered binding of bacterial material with excess of alimentary fat and decrease in available calcium, (4) decreased transit time, (5) ablated ileal mucosal surfaces, and (6) to this, the fact that vitamin B_{12} is lost in bile which, if not resorbed or replaced, rapidly depletes the body stores when a bile fistula exists. The major consequence of vitamin B_{12} deficiency in man appears to be impairment of desoxybiotide synthesis and the methyl group of methionine.

INTENTIONAL "SHORT-CIRCUITING" AND THE MALABSORPTION SYNDROME

This is a procedure designed to assist the obese patient in losing weight without the inconvenience of self-discipline or the treatment of the more important underlying reasons that seem to compel him to eat in excess of his metabolic demands. It is a sort of "have-your-cake-and-eat-it-too" malabsorption syndrome. The procedure performed is the surgical diversion of the mid or high jejunal contents into the colon. The patient usually loses weight along with vitamin B_{12}, calcium, iron, protein, carbohydrates, fat-soluble vitamins, fats and cholesterol, among other things (Lewis et al., 1962). What this operation lacks in physiologic wisdom it makes up for in pathologic interest to some physicians, and in social incapacitation and personal inconvenience to some patients (Wood and Chremos, 1963). DeMuth and Rottenstein (1964) reported a case of fatal calcium deficiency in a 38-year-old patient after this procedure. Report of other deficiencies characteristic of the malabsorption syndrome may be expected. The advisability of its use was open to considerable question in this author's opinion, in 1964—and more so now.

Vitamin C deficiency also may occur in the "blind-loop" syndrome because of bacterial competition, rapid transit time and disordered mucosal function. There is some suggestion that vitamin B_{12} is necessary to prevent the oxidation of ascorbic acid, because as plasma vitamin B_{12} levels are restored to normal, those of vitamin C tend to rise.

Folic acid deficiency may develop in patients with sprue and possibly also in other malabsorption states. The use of folic acid, because of the usefulness of this agent in the enhancement of the megaloblastic response to vitamin B_{12}, is probably a worthwhile additional measure. Moreover, it is possible that some of the impairment of intestinal absorption observed when anti-folic-acid compounds are administered may be caused in minor degree by folic acid deficiency on a nutritional basis.

Iron deficiency also develops as part of the malabsorption syndrome and may be quite severe when it is associated with mucosal lesions. Vitamin B_{12} plasma levels may in part depend upon normoferremia (Cox et al., 1958). There also is the suggestion that hypoferremia may adversely affect the metabolism of intestinal mucosa; stated otherwise, the parenteral administration of 1 to 2 Gm. of iron may improve intestinal absorption in malabsorption syndromes. Parenteral iron is advisable because of the poor tolerances of iron when fed orally in such patients.

Fluid and electrolyte losses, because of the

chronic diarrhea of malabsorption syndromes, though less exotic as considerations, can nonetheless be life-threatening. Increased intakes of water, sodium and potassium may be necessary. Often it is the electrolyte losses that account for listlessness, fatigability, abdominal distention and anorexia which facilitate, and conceivably may initiate, the development of the malabsorption syndromes. The studies of Cooke (1957) disclose the magnitudes of the daily losses of sodium and potassium in relation to the volume of stool excreted.

Magnesium deficiency has received little attention as part of the malabsorption syndrome. Magnesium is principally absorbed in the upper intestine, and depletion of this ion has been observed most commonly in protracted drainage of upper intestinal juices unless magnesium is among the ions included in fluid replacement. Such depletion is also observed in some alcoholic patients. Usually the symptoms of magnesium deficiency are mental confusion, transient multifocal seizures, neuromuscular excitability, hyperreflexia, tremor, a positive Chvostek sign with a negative Trousseau, and sinus tachycardia (Gerst et al., 1964). Thus it resembles in some ways the symptoms of hypocalcemia. Treatment is the slow intravenous administration of 2 to 4 Gm. of hydrated magnesium sulfate in 500 to 1,000 ml. of isotonic saline, or, more safely, the same amount may be administered intramuscularly as a 50 per cent aqueous solution.

Conjugated bilirubin products apparently are not reabsorbed from the intestine in rat or man, whereas the unconjugated portions of bilirubin are (Lester and Schmid, 1963). Since nearly all bilirubin in man is excreted as a conjugate of glucuronic acid, there is little recirculation of bilirubin. A congenital syndrome exists in which bilirubin is not conjugated (Crigler-Majjar syndrome) with hyperbilirubinemia being the result.

The functions of bile salts in the alimentary tract (to be distinguished from bilirubin) are to assist in the emulsification of fats in the intestine and to dissolve fatty acids and water-insoluble soaps. In man, bile salts are the derivatives of 4 bile acids: cholic acid, deoxycholic acid, chenodeoxycholic acid and lithocholic acid, which are excreted as conjugates of glycine and taurine. When bile is absent from the alimentary tract, the excesses of fats tend to coat food particles, which impairs their enzymatic digestion.

The blind-loop syndrome may be corrected temporarily by the administration of broad-spectrum antibiotics.

Whipple's disease (1907) is an absorption defect of the small bowel that has been considered to be a lipodystrophy, although recent evidence suggests that the primary defect may be in carbohydrate, rather than lipid, metabolism. It may be a systemic disease instead of one that simply involves the intestinal mucosa and mesenteric lymph nodes as originally believed. It has no known surgical importance, but it needs to be distinguished from those causes of malabsorption which are amenable to operative treatment (Fisher, 1962).

DIAGNOSIS OF INTESTINAL OBSTRUCTION

General Considerations

It is estimated that approximately 8,000 deaths occur each year from intestinal obstruction. The mortality rates reported vary from 5 to 20 per cent, which would imply that more than 160,000 cases of intestinal obstruction occur annually. An analysis of the fatal cases discloses that death is usually the result of the sequelae of intestinal obstruction, e.g., perforation, peritonitis, fluid and electrolyte loss, shock and aspiration pneumonitis. These are sequelae which for the most part are avoidable if treatment can be implemented early.

The mortality rate from acute intestinal obstruction over the past 50 years has diminished sharply due to earlier diagnosis, preoperative decompression as established by Wangensteen, fluid and electrolyte replacement, blood and plasma administration, antibiotic therapy, earlier surgical intervention and improvements to operative technics.

Definitions. *Ileus* is a word derived from the Greek and literally means "to twist." However, ileus is a synonym now for intestinal obstruction from any cause.

There are two rather distinct forms of ileus: the mechanical and the adynamic or paralytic. They may be functionally subclassified as shown in Table 38-3.

TABLE 38-3. INTESTINAL OBSTRUCTION (ILEUS)

TYPE	SUBTYPE		PREDOMINANT CAUSES
Mechanical Ileus	Without direct interference to intestinal flow of blood	(a) Intraluminal:	Bezoars, gallstones, foreign bodies, polyps, atresia, diaphragms
		(b) Mural:	Inflammatory, irradiational and neoplastic strictures, hemorrhage into wall of bowel (Dicumarol, hemophilia, crushing trauma)
		(c) Extraintestinal:	Annular pancreas, intra-abdominal congenital bands, perienterostomy strictures, incomplete dehiscence of laparotomies, nonstrangulating hernias, simple adhesional obstructions
	With direct interference to intestinal flow of blood	(a) Extraintestinal:	Strangulated hernias, intraperitoneal adhesions with closed loop obstructions
		(b) Mural:	Intussusception
		(c) Mesenteric:	Volvulus
Adynamic or Paralytic	Without direct interference to intestinal flow of blood	(a) Metabolic:	Potassium deficiency, severe sodium deficiency, diabetic ketosis
		(b) Reflex:	Handling of the intestine; injuries to the thoracic and the lumbar spine; obstructions of ureters, cystic duct, common duct or appendix; acute distention of the bladder; chemical and bacterial peritonitis
		(c) Septic:	Bacteremia, septicemia, lobar pneumonia, acute pyelitis, meningitis, bacterial peritonitis
	With direct interference to intestinal flow of blood	(a) Mesenteric arterial occlusive:	Emboli, thrombi and ligatures
		(b) Venous occlusive:	Thrombi and ligatures

Mechanical intestinal obstruction is a structural occlusion of the intestine. There are 3 categories of obstructing mechanisms: (1) the closure of the intestinal lumen by occlusion from such things within it as polypoid tumors, congenital diaphragms, foreign bodies, gallstones, bezoars, or impacted feces; (2) the closure of the intestinal lumen by intramural abnormalities such as congenital atresia and duplications, intussusception, stenosing inflammations of the intestine (segmental enteritis, regional ileitis), strictures from primary cancer or metastases to the intestinal serosa, and occasionally from intramural hemorrhage; and (3) the closure of the lumen by extrinsic abnormalities, such as hernial rings, adhesive bands and volvulus. Some of the mechanisms of mechanical intestinal obstruction are shown in Figures 38-1 to 38-5.

Nearly 80 per cent of all mechanical intestinal obstructions fall in the third causal category. Groin, umbilical, incisional and internal hernias alone account for about a third; hernias and the adhesive bands collectively account for about 70 per cent of all causes of mechanical intestinal obstructions (Table 38-4). Thomas (1968) found that obstruction of a small bowel was more frequently caused by femoral hernias than by all other external hernias combined.

Anatomy and Physiology of the Small Bowel and Colon, and Intestinal Obstruction

TABLE 38-4. CLASSIFICATION OF INTESTINAL OBSTRUCTION AND THE APPROXIMATE PERCENTAGES OF EACH TYPE USUALLY ENCOUNTERED AMONG ADULT PATIENTS IN A LARGE GENERAL HOSPITAL

SMALL BOWEL AND COLON	APPROXIMATE PERCENTAGE OF ALL CAUSES
Mechanical obstruction	
A. Simple obstruction	40 (of total)
a. Adhesive bands	25
b. Tumors and foreign bodies	15
B. Strangulated obstruction	45 (of total)
a. External strangulated hernia	25
b. Adhesive bands	20
C. Special types of strangulation obstruction*	15 (of total)
a. Volvulus	7
b. Intussusception	5
c. Mesenteric thrombosis or embolism	3
	100

* It is essential that early operative intervention be carried out for relief of strangulation before necrosis occurs.

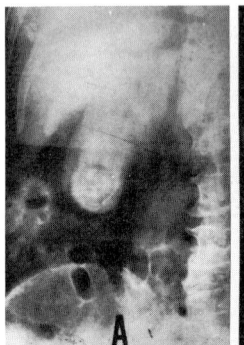

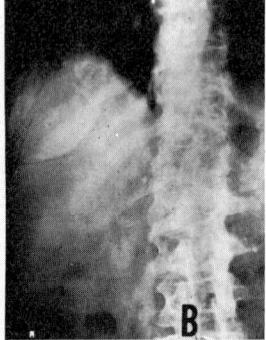

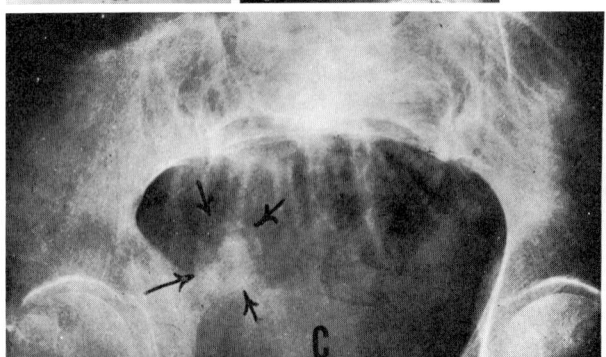

SYMPTOMS AND SIGNS OF INTESTINAL OBSTRUCTION

The symptoms and signs of intestinal obstruction are rather variable. Their variability depends a great deal upon the type of obstruction, its location within the intestine and when it occurs; for example: (1) cramping pains occur regularly with mechanical intestinal obstruction in which intestinal blood flow is not interfered with, while constant pain characterizes a strangulated obstruction; (2) abdominal distention is often great with simple mechanical obstruction and adynamic ileus but is small early in the course of closed-loop obstructions, excepting sigmoid volvulus; (3) vomiting regularly and soon accompanies obstruction of the proximal jejunum, and inconstantly and tardily attends mechanical obstruction of the sigmoid colon; and (4) simple mechanical obstruction of the small intestine during the first week after an abdominal

FIG. 38-1. Simple obturator obstruction caused by a gallstone in the ileum. Roentgenographic records depict the events in a 74-year-old woman with a large solitary gallstone which led to "gallstone ileus." (A) Shows the calcified gallstone in the gallbladder in May, 1946. (B) A roentgenogram 3 months later when she first experienced persistent right upper quadrant pain of 3 days' duration, associated with increasing upper abdominal tenderness, mounting fever and leukocytosis. Note that calcified gallstone is not seen on this film. (C) A roentgenogram of the lower abdomen taken 4 days after B, showing small bowel distention and the calcified gallstone. This stone was removed from the terminal ileum. (D) Photograph of the calculus removed during operation.

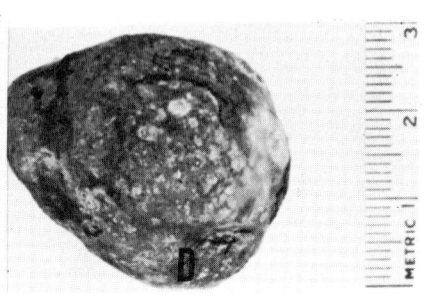

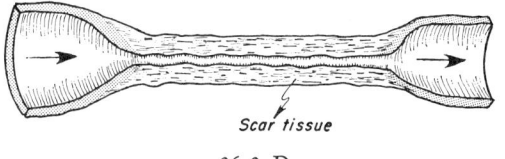

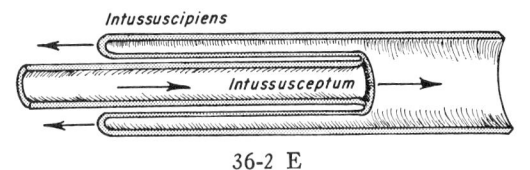

FIG. 38-2. Varieties of mechanical intestinal obstruction. Intraluminal obstruction due to: (A) polyp; (B) gallstone; and (C) cancer. Mural obstruction due to (D) scar tissue, and (E) intussusception.

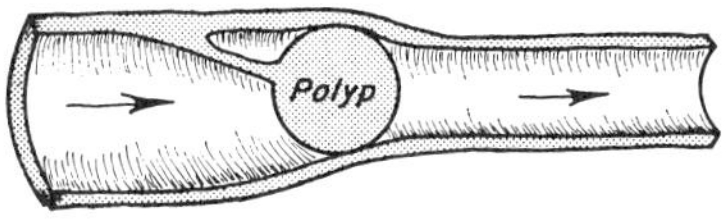

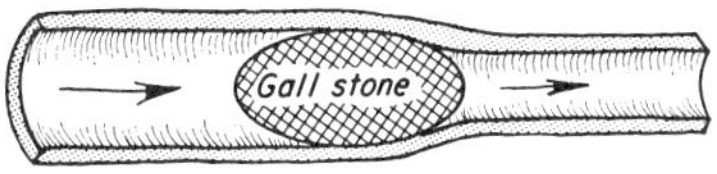

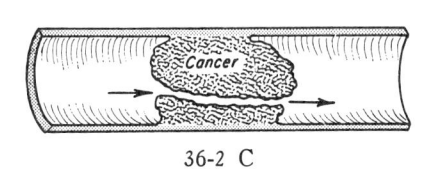

operation is often relatively painless and crampless but is rarely so later. The diagnosis of intestinal obstruction can be difficult at times.

The history is important. Questions relative to a previous condition which could produce intra-abdominal adhesions should be searched for, and the answers should be evaluated critically. A history of an intra-abdominal operation or abscess, a bout of peritonitis or pelvic inflammatory disease, regional enteritis or diverticulitis can readily provide the necessary intra-abdominal adhesions to account for acute mechanical obstruction.

Postoperative adhesions, especially following mid-abdominal or lower abdominal operations, and pelvic peritonitis or inflammatory disease, are the most commonly encountered elements in the past history that give rise to acute mechanical obstruction. In the absence of an abdominal operative scar or external hernia, and with no history of nonoperative peritonitis or pelvic inflammatory disease, attention is directed toward tumor, volvulus,

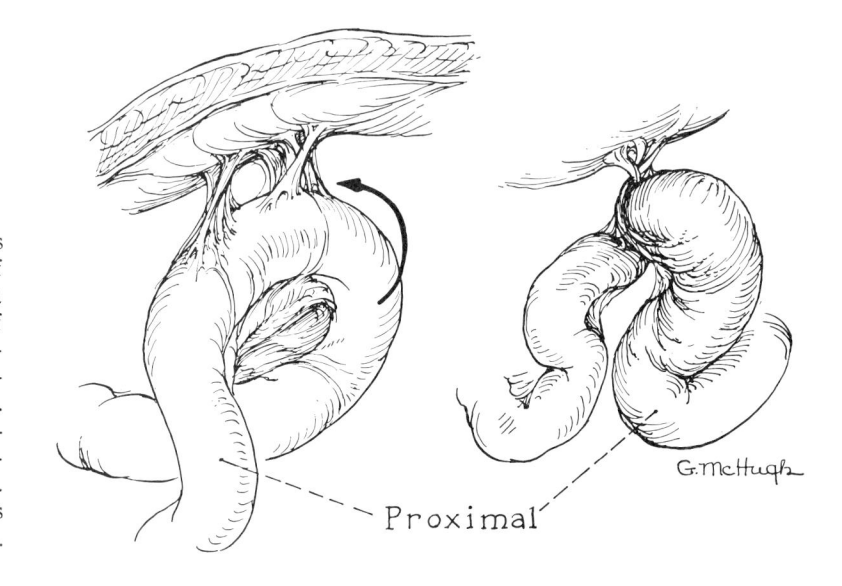

FIG. 38-3. Volvulus with obstruction of small bowel due to a twist of a loop of small bowel about adhesions on its antimesenteric border. Note distended proximal loop and collapsed distal loop. Other mechanisms may produce volvulus.

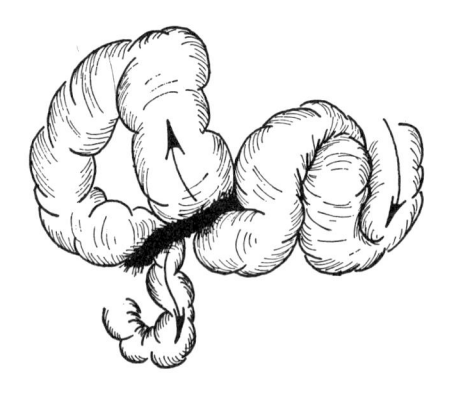

FIG. 38-4. Strangulated closed-loop obstruction with a loop of bowel under an adhesive band. As the loop of bowel that passed beneath the band distends, strangulation occurs.

intussusception, fecal impaction, mesenteric thrombosis or embolism, or foreign body in declining order of frequency as causes of intestinal obstruction in the adult.

Actually the problem of diagnosis may be approached best by discussing the variances of the symptoms and signs of ileus.

Pain With Intestinal Obstruction. Intestinal colic characterizes the pain of simple mechanical ileus (mechanical obstruction without interference with intestinal blood flow). Intestinal colic is pain that comes and goes away coincident with the coming and the going away of intestinal peristalsis. The person having intestinal colic will often say that the pain comes while gurgling is heard and felt within the abdomen. Ascertainment of the coincidence of the pain with peristalsis is the only way of being certain that an abdominal pain that comes and goes is intestinal colic. Ureteral colic comes and goes too, but the colics of ureteral obstructive pain are not associated with intestinal peristalsis but are disassociated with it. At times, to establish the coincidence of abdominal pain with intestinal peristalsis requires 15 or more minutes of continuous auscultation of the abdomen.

As the obstructed intestine becomes distended with fluid and gas, the colic and the peristalsis decrease in intensity and may even disappear. As this happens, a steady abdominal pain takes its place. This disappearance of intestinal peristalsis in simple mechanical obstruction is ascribed to its decompensation. Presumably, the obstructed intestine becomes too distended to contract. The steady pain associated with decompensation of the intestine is usually not severe. Peculiarly, simple mechanical ileus occurring during the immediate postoperative period may not be accompanied by intestinal colic. Severe steady or increasing abdominal pain that soon supersedes intestinal colic usually signifies that strangulation of the obstructed intestine has taken place. With volvulus the pain may be so excruciating that the sick person may lose his self-control.

During the height of paralytic or adynamic ileus, abdominal pain is diffuse and steady and is rarely severe. However, during the recovery phase of adynamic ileus, typical intestinal colic occurs—"gas pains" they are called. The steady pain of adynamic ileus, caused by occlusions of the mesenteric vessels by thrombi or emboli, grows steadily worse until shock occurs, and then it abates. In fact, whenever shock complicates any type of intestinal obstruction, the pain partially or wholly subsides, as is also true of somatic pain in hypovolemic shock.

Meteorism. Some abdominal distention usually follows all types of intestinal obstruction. However, the amount of distention is highly variable. It is often very great with adynamic ileus, with simple mechanical obstructions of the ileum and the left colon, volvulus of the sigmoid colon, and Hirschsprung's disease. It is often almost nonexistent with simple mechanical obstructions in the proximal jejunum, with closed-loop obstructions of the small bowel and with

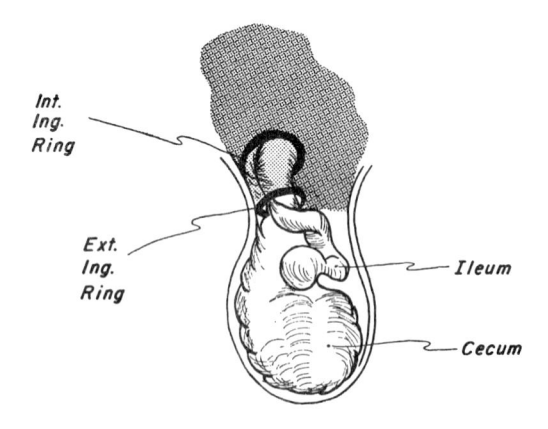

FIG. 38-5. Strangulated mechanical intestinal obstruction of a sliding hernia of the cecum and terminal ileum.

mesenteric arterial obstructive ileus, particularly early.

Nausea and vomiting usually accompany most forms of intestinal obstruction sooner or later. When the obstruction is located within the proximal intestine, such as in the duodenum or the upper jejunum, nausea and vomiting occur almost immediately or soon after the intestine is obstructed. In addition, the vomiting often completely relieves the intestinal colic temporarily when the obstruction is located in the proximal small intestine, just as it relieves the pain of pyloric obstruction, probably because distention may be partially relieved. In general, the more distal in the intestine the obstruction is located, the longer the time will be between the beginning of ileus and the onset of vomiting. Actually, complete obstruction of the sigmoid colon may be unattended by vomiting for days, and sometimes vomiting may not occur at all.

CHARACTER OF VOMITUS. Before roentgenography was developed, the character of the vomitus was considered to be important diagnostically and prognostically. Today all that need be said about the significance of the character of vomitus with ileus is: feculent vomitus signifies that the bacteria normally largely restricted to the colon and the distal ileum are now growing freely throughout the small intestine. For this to take place the intestine usually needs to have been obstructed for 1 or more days and widely distended with fluid and gas. Prognostically, feculent vomitus tends to be a dire omen.

Obstipation is a universal accompaniment of complete intestinal obstructions. To be sure, individuals may pass feces or gas either spontaneously or following an enema after the small intestine or the proximal colon has become completely obstructed, but this act only represents the passage of the gas and the excrement located distal to the obstruction. Consequently, the passage of feces or flatus after the intestinal colic has begun does not mean that complete mechanical small intestinal obstruction does not exist. The old test of the trial enema is worthless and often misleading.

Diarrhea. The frequent passage of liquid feces is often a sign of partial mechanical intestinal obstruction, because secretions are increased by the resultant distention and because of stasis, with fermentation and liquefaction of formed fecal material. Persistent diarrhea through ileostomies and colostomies is almost a certain sign of partial intestinal obstruction proximal to or at the site of the enteral stomata. Rectal fecal impactions are heralded by diarrhea. Partially obstructing neoplasms of the colon are often accompanied by alternate periods of diarrhea and obstipation.

Temperature With Intestinal Obstruction. Fever with mechanical intestinal obstruction is predominantly a sign that: (1) the blood flow to the closed part of the intestine is obstructed and that part of the intestine is dead or dying (the obstruction is strangulated); (2) that the intestine is perforated; or (3) that the obstruction is related to, or associated with, an infection within the intestinal wall and about it such as with diverticulitis or deeply ulcerating neoplasms. Very rarely is fever with intestinal obstruction caused by hypernatremia and water deficit.

Hypothermia occasionally occurs with intestinal obstruction. When it does, it almost always means that the person has been severely depleted of sodium and is hyponatremic.

Concentration of Cellular Elements in the Blood. Just as fever is usually a sign of strangulation, so is leukocytosis. However, a slight degree of leukocytosis may be attributable to dehydration alone. Dehydrational leukocytosis is not usually associated with increased numbers of immature forms of polymorphonuclear leukocytes. Consequently, a differential count of the leukocytes is very important in patients with intestinal obstruction. Polymorphonuclear leukopenia will occasionally occur with such forms of intestinal obstruction as strangulating obstructions, volvulus and mesenteric vascular occlusions, with almost all the polymorphonuclear cells in the blood being immature.

The hematocrit reading is often somewhat increased in all forms of intestinal obstruction because of dehydration.* However, rapidly

---

* Dehydration refers to loss of water. It has been shown that one can add or remove water from blood and not change the hematocrit, based upon the fact that water is not only extracellular but intracellular. To change the hematocrit, a loss of colloid or saline is necessary. Water alone will equilibrate its increments or decrements between the intracellular and extracellular compartments proportionately, while colloid and saline remain for the most part extracellular and therefore affect the hematocrit.

rising and very high hematocrits are indicative of volvulus, mesenteric venous occlusion, or of strangulation obstruction with peritonitis; all of these conditions promote the rapid loss of plasma from the blood, and therefore the concentration of red blood cells rapidly rises. This is one of the reasons why a person with intestinal obstruction and a very high or rapidly rising hematocrit value is so often precariously ill.

Localized Abdominal Tenderness. Tenderness that is restricted to a limited part of the abdomen of patients with mechanical ileus means strangulation of the mechanically obstructed intestine. Should this tenderness overlie a palpable mass, a strangulated, closed-loop intestinal obstruction almost certainly exists. Should the tenderness overlie a mass and the abdominal musculature over it be reflexly rigid, the obstructed intestine is most likely dead or perforated or both.

Serum Amylase and Serum Lactic Dehydrogenase. For reasons that are as yet poorly understood, the concentration of serum amylase rises very rapidly in some patients with only obstructed intestines and especially so when the larger arteries and veins to a long piece of intestine are occluded. No evidence of pancreatitis can be found in such patients when operated upon or subjected to necropsy. Serum amylase values higher than 3,600 Somogyi units have been found with small intestinal volvulus, strangulation of long segments of jejunum beneath adhesive bands and in internal hernias, and mesenteric arterial thromboembolic occlusions.

Lactic dehydrogenase, an enzyme contained in moderately large amounts within the normal intestine and its mucosa, has been found in amounts more than three times the normal in the sera of 8 to 11 human beings with *infarction of the intestine* (volvulus, strangulated closed-loops and mesenteric arterial and venous occlusions). The serum lactic dehydrogenase concentrations were normal in: 4 cases of peritonitis without intestinal infarcts, 2 infarcted herniated pieces of omentum, 18 cases of intestinal obstruction without death of intestine, and 5 cases of pancreatitis (serum amylases above 1,000 S. U. in 4 of them) (Calman et al., 1958). The levels of these enzymes obviously should not be given the same significance as many of the clinical observations and findings described.

DIFFERENTIAL DIAGNOSIS

The differential diagnosis of intestinal obstruction is two-phased. One phase is concerned with the differentiation of intestinal obstruction from other conditions that mimic it, and the other pertains to the differentiation of the types of ileus one from the other.

The main conditions that may simulate intestinal obstructions are: (1) acute bacterial and toxic enteritis, (2) the various abdominal visceral crises, such as arise from tabetic intestinal and renal sources, the abdominal crises associated with porphyria, the hemolytic anemias, with Henoch's and the Schönlein-Henoch purpuras, (3) renal colic, (4) acute pancreatitis, (5) acute cholecystitis, (6) pseudocyesis, and (7) the acute meteorisms that are suffered by persons having intractable asthma or disabling pulmonary emphysema or fibrosis. The conclusion that mechanical intestinal obstruction exists may not be easily reached, and the chance of making diagnostic errors is good unless medical conditions that may simulate the clinical patterns of intestinal obstruction are also considered.

Acute Bacterial Enteritis. The initial pains of acute bacterial enteritis (such as dysentery and toxic enteritis, including lead and arsenic poisoning) are typical intestinal colics; the pains are synchronous with hyperperistalsis. Initially, these attacks are accompanied by obstipation for lengths of time varying from a few minutes to hours. During the obstipational period of dysentery and toxic enteritis, even the abdominal roentgenographic appearance may mimic mechanical obstruction of the small intestine. About the only thing which may serve to make one aware of the possibility of toxic enteritis during the obstipational period is the severity of the general illness that develops so soon after the beginning of the colic. Anyone who has been afflicted with acute toxic enteritis needs no instruction; and no amount of instruction will convince the uninitiated how welcome death is momentarily to the patient at this point in his illness.

Abdominal Crises. The differential characteristics of the various abdominal crises are beyond the scope of this text. The diagnoses of renal colic, pancreatitis, and cholecystitis are discussed in Chapters 52, 33 and 32, respectively. The differentiation of acute hemorrhagic pancreatitis from volvulus and from large closed-loop and mesenteric arterial occlusive intestinal obstruction is particularly difficult because adynamic ileus, fever, tachycardia, leukocytosis and shock attend both hemorrhagic pancreatitis and these forms of ileus, and so does hyperamylasemia. Celiotomy may be the only way to differentiate with certainty acute hemorrhagic pancreatitis from volvulus, strangulating intestinal obstructions and mesenteric vascular occlusion.

Pseudocyesis or spurious pregnancy is an organic manifestation of hysteria that will often lead the unwary into performing laparotomies for what they take to be intestinal obstruction. The abdomen appears to be distended, but true meteorism does not exist. With pseudocyesis, breathing is fast, shallow and almost completely thoracic. The thoracic cage is chronically held in the inspiratory position even at the end of expiration. Fluoroscopically, the diaphragm is held in the inspiratory position, and it moves little with breathing. The lateral abdominal musculature is rigid, and the central part of the abdominal wall is pushed forward. With all this, the sufferer complains of continuous or "crampy" pains in the abdomen, and of breathlessness—a pattern similar to a number of emotional ones that are not necessarily restricted to the female or to specious pregnancy. The abdominal walls of these patients are frequently "battle scarred," occasionally bearing as many as 10 to 15 scars of laparotomies. The diagnosis of pseudocyesis is easy: the ostensible abdominal distention disappears upon having the patient rebreathe into a tight-fitting quart-sized paper bag for 3 or 4 minutes, or upon having her breathe from a closed breathing system containing 5 per cent carbon dioxide in oxygen. True meteorism is unaffected by these maneuvers.

Meteorism. Acute periods of meteorism accompanied by intestinal colic occasionally bedevil the severely emphysematous and the so-called chronic pulmonary cripple. The differentiation of this meteorism from that of intestinal obstruction is usually easy. Obstipation does not accompany the abdominal distention and cramps. On the contrary, excessive amounts of flatus are passed, and the entire intestine, including the colon and the rectum, contains gas.

Types of Ileus. Concerning the differentiation of the types of ileus one from the other, the most important thing is the differentiation of ileus without mechanical interference to the flow of blood to the obstructed intestine from ileus that is associated with mechanical interference to the flow of blood to the obstructed intestine. A delay in the operative correction of an ileus such as a volvulus, a strangulated obstruction, or that which accompanies mesenteric vascular occlusion may lead to death of the obstructed intestine and to the death of the patient from overwhelming peritoneal sepsis and shock. For these reasons, often one cannot safely await the analytical reports of the serum amylase or lactic dehydrogenase; the decision as to the state of blood flow to the obstructed intestine should and must be reached whenever possible upon the bases of other evidences that can be gathered more quickly. These have already been discussed or are listed in Table 38-5. In other words, ileus accompanied by occlusion of blood flow to the obstructed intestine is an immediate surgical emergency, and one cannot afford to delay making a decision for want of erudite chemical evidence. Frequent repeated examinations of the abdomen for localized tenderness, a mass, and changing character of peristalsis, the pulse, the temperature and the leukocytes constitute the main ways of determining whether or not an ileus has an intestinal vascular occlusive component. Often the signs of intestinal vascular occlusion will be few and meager during the initial hours of a strangulated ileus, although the blood vessels to the intestine are then already partially choked and may become completely occluded at any moment. Consequently, one should not assume that an ileus which at first ostensibly has no evidences for vascular occlusion actually does not have or will not develop one. Therefore, a person with an ileus that lacks signs of intestinal vascular impairment must be examined at intervals not longer than 1 or 2 hours apart until the obstruction is removed.

Roentgenographic Examination. A relatively simple roentgenographic examination of the abdomen is very valuable for the differential diagnosis of ileus.

Stereoscopic filming of the abdomen with

TABLE 38-5

		Type of Obstruction Cause	Character of Pain	Abdominal Distention	Peristaltic Sounds
Without Interference With Intestinal Blood Flow	Mechanical	Bezoars, gallstones, foreign bodies	Severe sudden colics that often suddenly stop for days at a time	Variable	Hyperactive during pains
		Strictures inflammatory or neoplastic	Colics that are rarely severe and tend to increase over days or weeks	Usually great unless obstruction is high in gut	Variable if colic is severe, hyperperistalsis is great; if pain is weak, peristalsis is weak
		Hernias and adhesions	Severe colics that usually come suddenly	Variable	Hyperactive during colics
	Adynamic	K deficit, severe Na deficit, peritonitis, sepsis, handling of bowel	Diffuse soreness or discomfort	Usually great if ileus persists for more than a day	Few in number faint and tinkling
With Interference With Intestinal Blood Flow	Mechanical	Strangulation of hernias and intestine beneath adhesions	Continuous pain that is usually preceded or accompanied by colics	Variable	Few or absent usually
		Volvulus	Steady and severe until shock occurs, then it subsides		
	Adynamic	Mesenteric thrombotic or embolic occlusion		Usually small	

the patient in the *supine* position is the basis of all abdominal roentgenologic diagnosis. Examination should not be done with the patient prone because of the alteration of normal location of abdominal viscera due to external pressure against the abdominal wall in this position.

Prior to obtaining the supine abdominal film, it is important that no cleansing enema be administered. Not only may such an enema be painful and dangerous to the patient, but, in addition, it almost certainly will produce confusing collections of air and fluid on the abdominal x-ray examination.

Despite the popularity of the erect film of the abdomen, it seldom proves to be a significant diagnostic aid. Certainly gas-fluid levels within the bowel ("stepladder pattern") can be seen by this method, but no reliable information concerning location of or degree of intestinal distention can be obtained by this procedure. Such gas-fluid levels are not pathognomonic of mechanical ileus as is widely believed but may be seen also in cases of adynamic ileus, regional enteritis, ulcerative colitis, sprue, or even in patients with normal abdomens following cleansing enemas. Nor does the finding of such a gas-fluid level ensure that it is intraluminal in position; such a finding is frequent, for instance, in subdiaphragmatic abscess in which the fluid is pus in the peritoneal cavity, and bacteriogenic gas caught under the diaphragm forms the level.

If the simple radiologic procedures outlined above indicate that there is a lesion of the colon, obstructive or otherwise, without evidence of perforations, then barium enema may be performed safely and is frequently diagnostic of not only the site but also the nature of the lesion. In cases of obstructive lesions of the colon, the oral administration of barium sulfate suspension is contraindicated because of the tendency of this material to convert a partially obstructing lesion to a complete acute obstruction. This occurs because colonic water absorption tends to inspissate barium sulfate suspensions. These factors lead to technical difficulties in bowel preparation and at laparotomy.

However, if it is certain that the area of obstruction is in the small bowel, no such difficulties attend the oral administration of contrast medium, and frequently the site and the nature of the obstructive lesion in the small

Table 38-5 (Continued)

Tempera-ture	Pulse Rate	W.B.C.	Hemato-crit	Serum Amylase	Serum Lactic Dehydro-genase	X-Ray Signs	Obstipation
							Intermittent
Normal unless complicated by severe dehydration or infection	Normal unless complicated by severe dehydration or infection	Normal differential. Count normal unless complicated by severe dehydration or infection	Rise that is proportionate to the apparent dehydration	Normal	Normal	Intra-intestinal fluid and gas above the obstruction and very little or none below the obstruction	Often alternating diarrhea and obstipation
							Complete
						Intra-intestinal fluid and gas throughout the intestine	Variable, often incomplete
Fever	Tachycardia	Leukocytosis and shift to left (young cells) / Occasionally leukopenia	Rise that is disproportionately greater than the apparent dehydration	Occasionally elevated / Often much elevated (up to 4,000 S. U.)	Usually much elevated	Intra-intestinal fluid and gas above the obstruction / Often little gas in bowel but fluid distention may be enormous (sigmoid volvulus) / Little gas or fluid in the intestine	Complete after evacuation of the intestine below the obstruction

bowel can be demonstrated by this method. Barium sulfate suspensions may be administered by mouth in such patients or, better, may be injected through a long intestinal tube of the Miller-Abbott type. In the latter instance, the progress of the tube is observed until the distention is relieved and the point of obstruction is reached. Then the introduction of the barium suspension directly through the tube is observed fluoroscopically and by appropriate filming at the time of fluoroscopy. The water-miscible contrast media, long used for pyelography, have been employed successfully to examine rather quickly and definitively the small intestines of people with ileus. One need not worry about giving these materials orally to patients with colonic lesions; they cannot convert a partial into a complete colonic obstruction as barium sulfate may do.

Simple stereoscopic filming of the abdomen will often permit the discovery of intestinal obstructing foreign bodies that otherwise may escape detection.

Foreign Bodies

Most foreign bodies that are ingested will pass through the gastrointestinal tract without incident (Barnes, 1964). Occasionally, a large or peculiarly shaped ingested object will fail to pass, and surgical removal will be necessary (Teimourian et al., 1964). If the foreign body is opaque to x-rays, usually its location and progression can be determined. Plastic, glass and other radiolucent foreign bodies afford more difficulty, and their presence may be determined only if they produce complications. The findings of a perforated viscus may be produced by such an object, or the clinical and radiologic picture of intestinal obstruction may result (Fig. 38-6).

The location, the level and the degree of obstruction in large or small bowel usually can be determined from radiologic examination. Except for direct inspection at laparotomy, supine abdominal x-ray examination is the most dependable means of determining the location and the degree of distention of the small bowel. If dilated gas-filled loops of small bowel are present, a diagnosis of ileus may be made with reasonable confidence.

In a typical case of low small bowel obstruction, diagnosis is usually easy, but with increased experience one tends to be less certain of the location of obstruction when it is

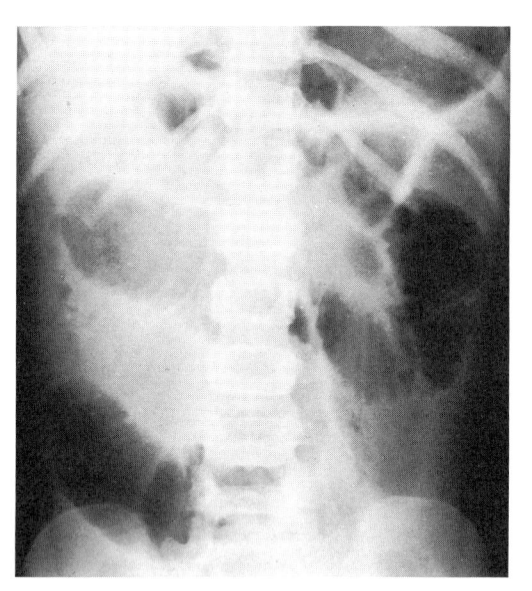

FIG. 38-6. (*Left and right*) Dilated gas-filled loops of small bowel indicate the presence of intestinal obstruction. Mechanical ileus in this case was due to a nonopaque foreign body (trichobezoar).

in the small bowel. The presence of distended loops of jejunum and ileum arranged transversely in the central portion of the abdomen with little or no gas in the colon strongly suggests mechanical obstruction (Fig. 38-7).

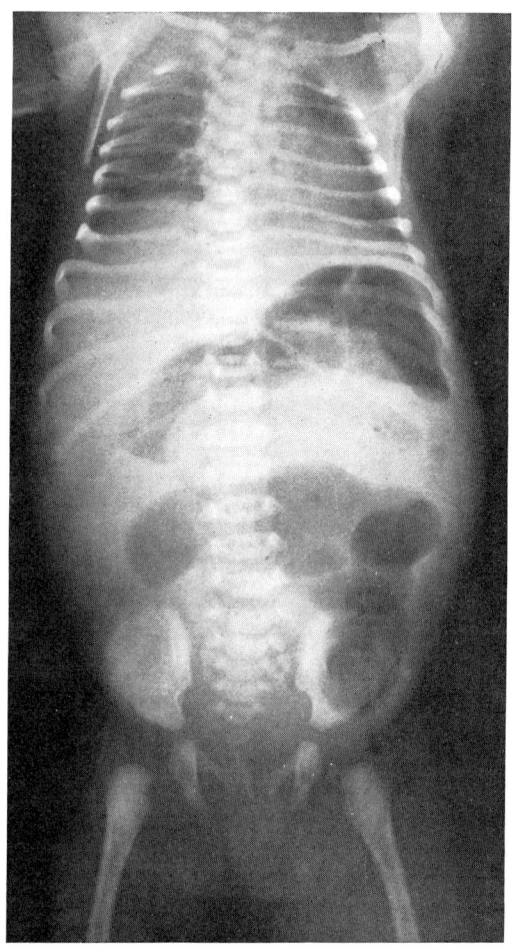

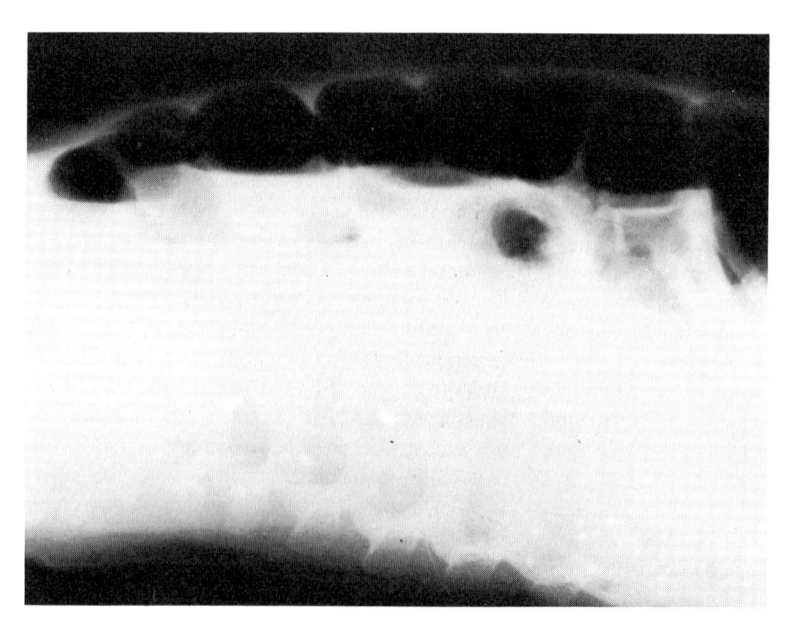

FIG. 38-7. Classic roentgen appearance of mechanical ileus. Note that the "translateral" view (*left*) made with the patient supine and with the radiation horizontal demonstrates the distended loops. However, it gives no useful information as to extent or the location of these loops; as a matter of fact, it fails even to make possible the differentiation of large and small bowel.

Diagnosis of Intestinal Obstruction 1085

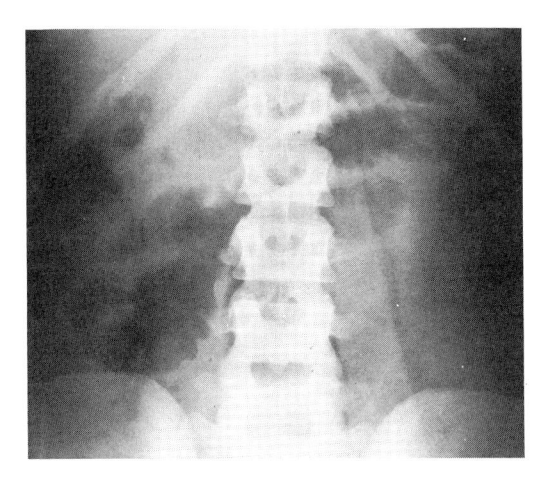

FIG. 38-8. Closed loop obstruction with large "pseudotumor" in the left lower abdominal quadrant.

Small bowel is identified by the presence of the plicae circulares forming their characteristic pattern of circular transverse ridges in the distended lumen and by the usual central abdominal position that distended small bowel

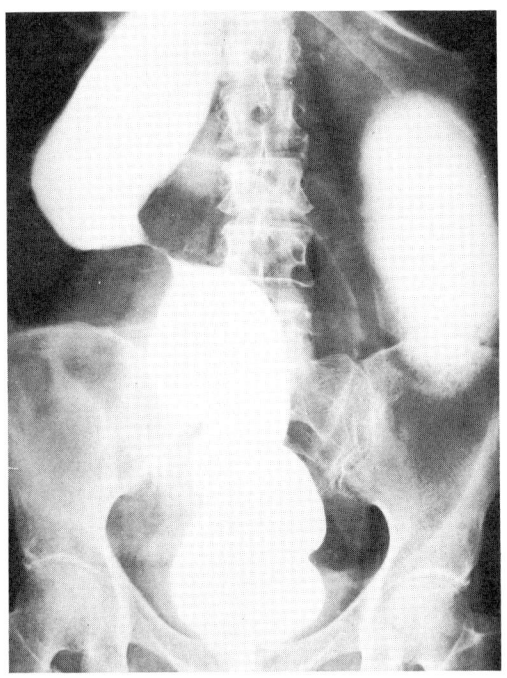

FIG. 38-10. Typical appearance of barium enema in case of sigmoid volvulus of Figure 36-9 (bird-beak or ace of spades deformity).

assumes. Distended colon does not have this appearance; the haustra do not cross the entire distended lumen.

In closed-loop obstruction, the distended fluid-filled loop of small bowel forms an abdominal mass which displaces other abdominal viscera (Fig. 38-8). The closed loop contains fluid and no significant amount of gas. The closed loop becomes edematous and fluid-filled due largely to embarrassment of venous return. Prompt radiologic recognition of the presence of a closed-loop obstruction may lead to surgical intervention prior to permanent vascular damage and gangrene.

Volvulus of the sigmoid colon is the most frequent form of torsion of the colon and produces a quite characteristic roentgen appearance (Fig. 38-9). There is a grossly dilated loop of bowel which has no plicae circulares (valvulae conniventes, Kerckring's folds) but it may have haustral indentations. The bowel walls lead to the two distinct points of obstruction. Barium enema demonstrates the

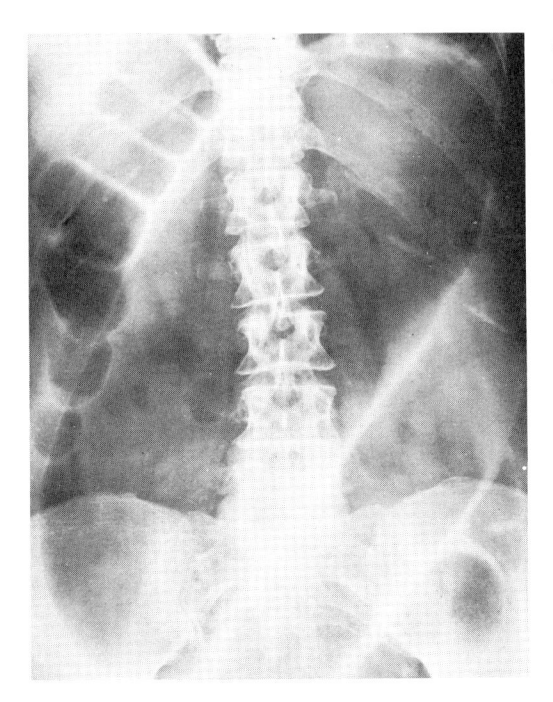

FIG. 38-9. Volvulus of the sigmoid colon.

abruptly tapering (bird-beak deformity) of the

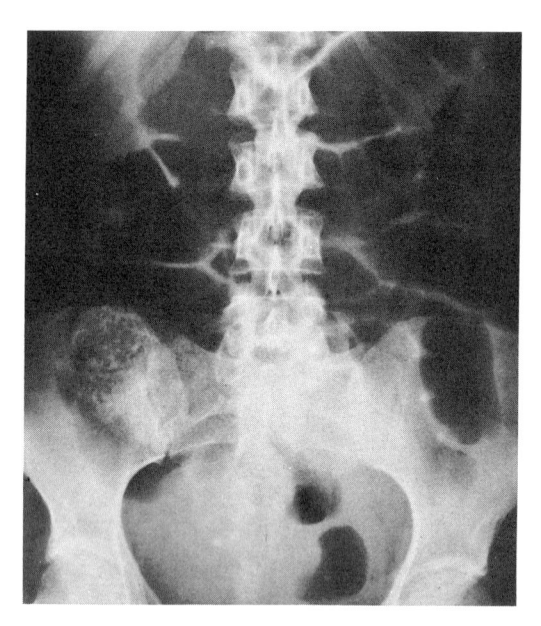

FIG. 38-11. Peritonitis with adynamic ileus.

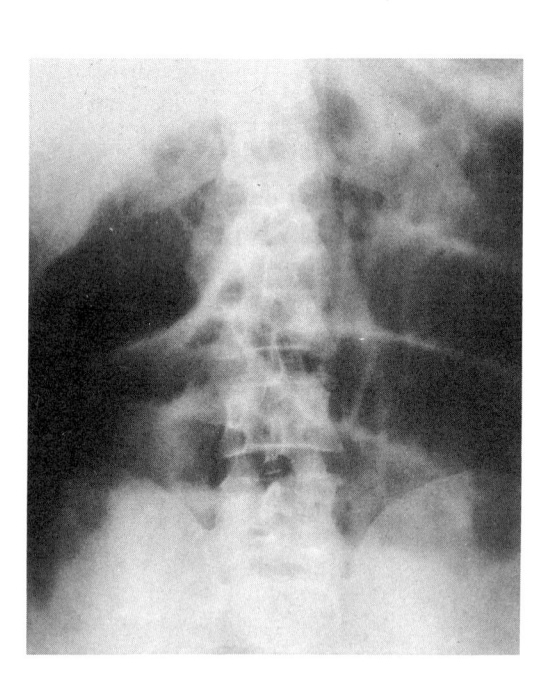

FIG. 38-12. Distended small bowel and right colon leading to the erroneous conclusion that there was mechanical colon obstruction with incompetent ileocecal valve. Adynamic ileus was the true situation.

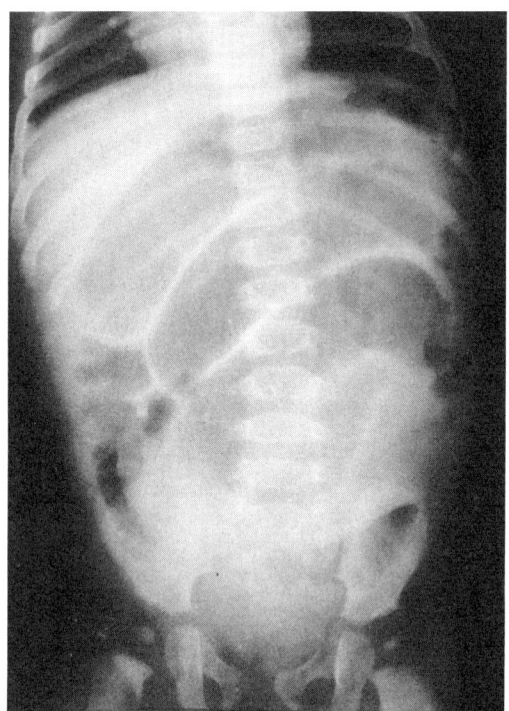

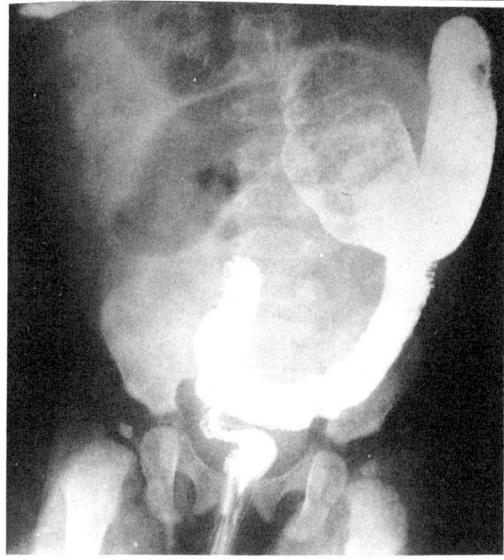

FIG. 38-13. The etiology of mechanical ileus is demonstrated by barium enema. In this case the intussusception was not reduced by this diagnostic procedure.

colon distal to the volvulus (Fig. 38-10). This finding is diagnostic of torsion.

The presence of distended loops of large and small bowel is said to be typical of ady-

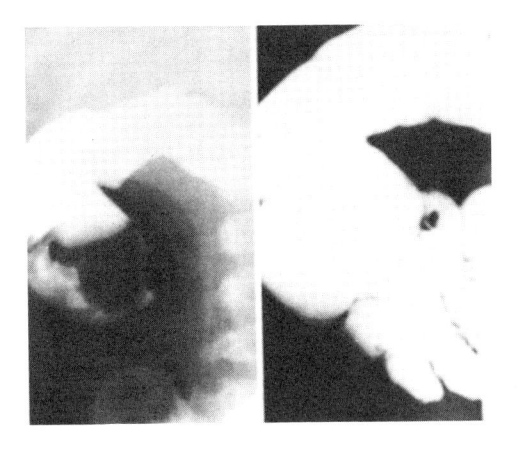

FIG. 38-14. (*Left*) The diagnosis of intussusception is made. (*Right*) The invagination is corrected during the procedure.

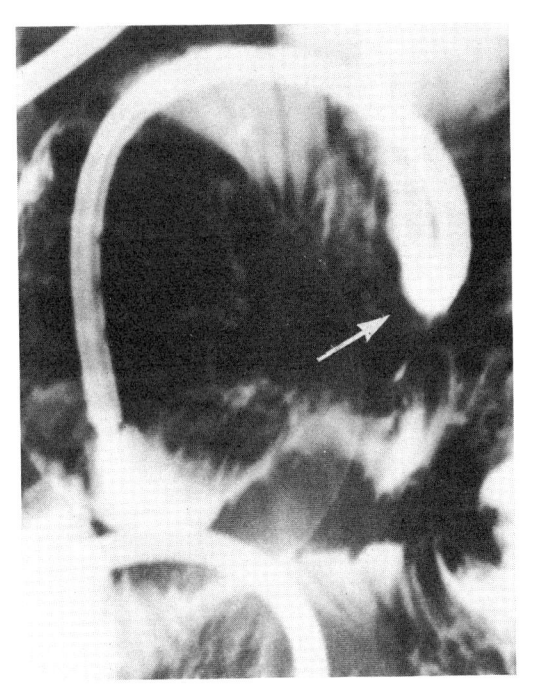

FIG. 38-15. The small bowel distention and its deflation by means of a Miller-Abbott tube may be seen. Barium administered after decompression when the tube ceased advancing demonstrates the point of obstruction that was caused by an adhesive band.

namic ileus (Fig. 38-11). However, in obstructive lesions of the colon, distention of the large bowel proximal to (and occasionally even outlining) the point of obstruction is found frequently. If the ileocecal valve is incompetent, there is also small bowel distention in such cases, and roentgen differentiation between adynamic and mechanical ileus becomes difficult or impossible. Only the clear outlining of the obstructing lesion may lead to the diagnosis; even this may be misleading, as cases of adynamic ileus with a spurious obstruction in the colon are commonplace (Fig. 38-12). A barium enema is necessary at times to ascertain colonic patency in cases such as this.

The most reliable method of differentiating mechanical and adynamic ileus is by auscultation of the abdomen. Fortunately, this method is accurate early. The absence of bowel sounds in functional neuromuscular disturbances is characteristic, whereas increase in borborygmi at the height of colic is a characteristic of mechanical intestinal obstruction.

Diagnosis of ileocolic or colocolic intussusceptions as the etiology of mechanical intestinal obstruction is best done by barium enema (Figs. 38-13 and 38-14).

Administration of barium sulfate suspension through a double lumen tube after it has reached the point of obstruction will demonstrate the point and the nature of the obstructing lesion (Fig. 38-15). The presence of normal mucosal folds in the constricted area is suggestive of an extrinsic obstruction, such as one caused by adhesions; occasionally, a small bowel tumor is demonstrated by this method.

Bowel obstruction due to the presence of a large gallstone which has perforated the gallbladder and the duodenum and entered the small bowel lumen through the resultant fistula is one of the types of intestinal obstruction in which the etiology is frequently apparent on the supine abdominal film (Thomas *et al.*, 1962). The presence of air in the biliary tree is pathognomonic of the fistulous connection, and this finding coupled with that of bowel obstruction is sufficient to make the diagnosis (Fig. 38-16). In about one fourth of such patients, the gallstone contains sufficient calcium so that it can be identified radiographically.

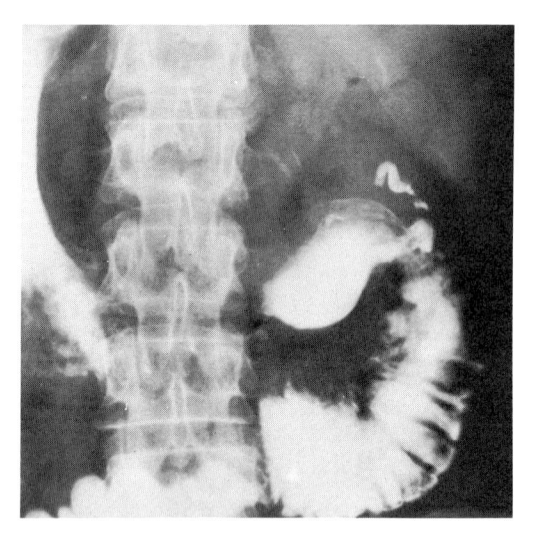

FIG. 38-16. Gallstone ileus. Air and some barium in the biliary tree are noted. A large radiolucent gallstone was found at the ligament of Treitz. The dilated duodenum is seen, and the point of obstruction is sharply outlined by orally administered barium. (Also see Fig. 38-1.)

CLINICAL FEATURES

The treatment of ileus needs to fit its cause and the physiologic disturbances that are found. The physiologic deformations that attend ileus are mainly hydrational, circulatory and respiratory.

The hydrational disturbance that more or less is present in all forms of ileus is extracellular fluid volume deficit. Within minutes after intestinal obstruction begins, interstitial fluid begins to collect within the lumen and the walls of the obstructed intestine; whether this fluid is subsequently vomited or not does not matter; interstitial fluid sequestered within the lumen and the walls of the intestine is as certainly lost from about the nonintestinal tissue cells and the red blood cells as if it were lost through vomiting or diarrhea. The amount of interstitial fluid that may collect within the lumen of a mechanically or adynamically obstructed small intestine within 12 hours is occasionally fantastically large, sometimes constituting one half of the entire corporal interstitial fluid. With mechanical obstructions of the terminal ileum and with toxic adynamic ileus among adults the small intestine frequently attains a diameter up to 4 cm. Should such a dilated small intestine be filled only with interstitial fluid, from 7 to 9 liters would be needed to fill it.

As the intestine distends, its volume increases as the square of the radius. Within the ranges of distention that may be observed with intestinal obstructions, the intraluminal capacities are approximately those tabulated in Table 38-6.

Fortunately, the content of the distended intestine is rarely only interstitial fluid; usually half or more of it consists of gas. However, interstitial fluid often constitutes practically the total amount of the content of the obstructed intestine in cases of volvulus, mesenteric vascular occlusion and strangulated

TABLE 38-6

	DIAMETER OF INTESTINE	VOLUME PER METER LENGTH OF INTESTINE		VOLUME IN ENTIRE LENGTH OF UNIFORMLY DISTENDED BOWEL	
	cm.	mls.	pints	mls.	pints
Small intestine normal length —7 meters	2	300	.75	2,000	4.6
	3	700	1.5	4,900	10.9
	4	1,250	2.75	8,750	19.4
	5	2,000	4.4	13,700	30.4
	6	2,800	6.2	19,600	43.5
	7	3,850	8.5	26,950	59.5
Colon length— 1.5 meters	10	7,800	17.2	11,700	26
	11	9,500	21	14,250	31.6
	12	11,300	25.1	16,900	37.5
	13	13,200	29.3	19,800	43.9
	14	15,400	34.2	23,100	51.3

closed-loop obstruction. In such cases as well as others in which fluid makes up a significant part of the distended intestine's contents, severe extracellular fluid deficit and even dehydrational shock are to be expected.

Acidosis is a rare accompaniment of ileus, except with diabetes and infancy, and usually requires for its treatment only insulin and glucose for the diabetic and glucose for the infant.

Potassium deficiency with hypokalemia is one of the primary causes of adynamic ileus and frequently complicates simple mechanical intestinal obstruction secondarily when the obstruction has been partial and accompanied by diarrhea or repetitive vomiting. Potassium deficiency infrequently complicates acute simple mechanical or strangulating intestinal obstruction.

Because of the rarity of severe acidosis or potassium deficit with acute mechanical ileus, the repair solutions best fitted to the treatment of the interstitial fluid volume deficit of mechanical ileus are glucose containing Hartmann's solution (lactated Ringer's solution), or slightly hypotonic (¾ strength) Locke's solution (bicarbonate Ringer's solution) (see Chap. 5). Occasionally, the amount of repair solution needed may be very large. Some idea of the amount needed may be gained from the assessment of the amount of the vomitus, the degree of fluid distention of the intestine measured on roentgenograms, and measurement of the volume of fluid removed from the intestine by nasogastric intubation or operative decompression. No glucose in water need be given during the restitution of the dehydration of ileus so long as the patient requires 2.5 to 3.0 liters or more of Hartmann's solution or of dilute Locke's solution containing glucose daily.

Whenever potassium deficiency occurs with or causes ileus it should be treated with appropriate solutions of potassium salts in glucose (see Chap. 5).

Occasionally, severe hypo-osmolarity (hyponatremia) complicates ileus; when it does from 500 to 1,000 ml. of 3 per cent sodium chloride solution may be used with the other repair solutions. The hypertonic sodium chloride is especially indicated should physical signs of water intoxication exist.

The respiratory derangements that accompany intestinal obstructions are relatable to meteorism. With an adynamic ileus in which the entire length of the small intestine is dilated to 5 cm. and the colon to 10 cm. (not unusual with toxic adynamic ileus) the intra-abdominal visceral volume has been increased by about 20 liters, or more than 5 gallons. Such intestinal distention cannot be accommodated within the abdomen without pushing the diaphragm far up into the thoracic cavity and thereby choking the person from below. At times intestinal meteorism may so impede breathing as to threaten life immediately. The only sure way of treating acute life-threatening respiratory insufficiency related to acute meteorism of ileus is operative decompression of the intestine.

The general circulatory disturbances of ileus without organic interference with blood flow to the obstructed intestine are largely relatable to the dehydration and the meteorism, and upon proceeding far enough become manifest as peripheral circulatory failure. Adequate treatment of the dehydration and the meteorism correct these circulatory disorders. However, whenever organic obstruction of intestinal blood vessels occurs, additional circulatory disturbances take place that are relatable to the movement of bacteria and bacterial products into the peritoneal cavity and then through the peritoneum into the general circulation. Many bacterial toxins weaken heart muscle, injure capillary walls and affect vasomotion and attack nerve cells. Couple these with dehydrational oligemia and dehydrational cellular metabolic disturbances, and a very profound and often therapeutically unresponsive form of shock, called septic shock, occurs.

The treatment of the intestinal obstruction itself is individual and is outlined in Table 38-7.

Complications of Ileus

Aspiration pneumonitis, disruption of the continuity of the intestine and pulmonary embolism are the main complications of ileus.

Aspiration pneumonitis is to be feared with all kinds of ileus. Vomiting, while the person is weak or drugged by soporifics or analgesics, is especially prone to lead to pneumonic aspiration of the vomitus. The aspiration of a large amount asphyxiates and kills within minutes,

TABLE 38-7. SPECIFIC TREATMENT OF MECHANICAL ILEUS

TYPES	SPECIFIC CAUSE	TREATMENT	CHAPTER REFERENCE THIS TEXT
I. Intraluminal	Bezoars, gallstones, foreign bodies	Push obstructing object back into a part of the proximal dilated intestine *that is not inflamed* and remove it through a short longitudinal antimesenteric incision that is closed transversely	This chapter
	Polyps	Local removal, or local resection of bowel	40
	Diaphragms	Local excision, or diverting enteroenterostomy	50
	Atresia	Resection of proximal bulbous end and enteroenterostomy	50
	Malignant neoplasms	Small intestine and right colon—wide primary resections and anastomosis; left colon—decompressive colostomy followed by wide resection	30, 31, 40 and 41
II. Intramural and Mural	Inflammatory strictures	Resect or bypass with an appropriate enteroenterostomy	18, 40 and 50
	Neoplastic strictures	As for intraluminal obstructing neoplasms, or bypass enteroenterostomy if there are numerous peritoneal metastases	
	Intussusception	Reduce in infants by methods described in Chapter 50	50
		Resect without attempting to reduce in older children or adults because among older children and adults *malignant neoplasms* constitute *the lead point of the lesion* in from 30 to 50 per cent of cases	This chapter
III. Extra-intestinal and Mesenteric	Annular pancreas	Duodenojejunostomy	50
	Congenital and postinflammatory adhesions	Excise band adhesions, do not merely transect them	50
	Volvulus of sigmoid colon	Decompress through sigmoidoscope with a rectal tube if possible; otherwise surgically decompress after exteriorizing	This chapter
	Volvulus of small intestine	Reduce operatively	50
	Hernias of all types	Reduce operatively and repair	42
	Ileostomy or colostomy strictures	Excise stricture and effect a meticulous coaptation of mucous membrane to the skin with sutures	2 and 39
IV. Adynamic	*K deficit	Potassium salts	
	Na deficit	Sodium salts	
	Diabetic ketosis	Insulin	5
	*Reflex	Gastric and/or intestinal intubation	
	*Septic	Drain abscesses, remove gangrenous parts, antibiotics	3 and 4
	Vascular occlusive	Embolectomy, endarterectomy, bypass grafting, resection of dead intestine	44

* In cases of adynamic ileus of these types in which meteorism threatens life because of respiratory embarrassment, operative decompression of the intestine is the best treatment.

while the aspiration of lesser amounts leads to a gangrenous type of pneumonitis that kills within days. Prompt irrigation of the tracheobronchial tree may be life saving. Prevention of aspiration rests upon keeping the stomach empty! This can be done only by the proper placement of and attention to the continuous functioning of an inlying gastric tube. Occasionally, a gastrostomy is needed to ensure emptiness of the stomach should the patient be comatose, very weak, or so uncooperative as to remove the nasogastric tube repeatedly.

Should the gastric tube be connected to a mechanical suction pump, the tube leading from the gastric tube to the pump should always be vented with a No. 20 or 22 hypodermic needle. If this is not done, the mucosa of the stomach is often sucked into the holes of the gastric tube, the stomach fills with liquid, and vomiting and aspiration occur even though the tube is properly placed. Straight gravity drainage of the gastric tube directly into a plastic bag that is simply fastened to the patient's gown or the mattress cover is a very simple and effective way to keep the stomach empty provided that there are no vertical U-loops in the tubing connecting the gastric tube with the plastic receptacle. Should there be such a loop, it acts as a hydraulic obstructive valve because the fluid part of the gastric drainage collects in the loop, and the gas part of the gastric drainage collects behind it and precedes it. When this happens nothing will leave the stomach through the tube until the pressure in the stomach reaches a level which is higher than the weight of the column of water in one side of the U-loop. If the vertical height of a loop, half filled with a liquid that has air in front of and behind it, is 13 cm., the pressure in the stomach must rise above 13 cm. of water (10 mm. Hg) before any gas or fluid will leave the stomach through the tube. When U-loops are kept out of the tubes, simple drainage works very satisfactorily.

Irrigation of the gastric tube, using a syringe and a saline solution once an hour, is very important. It is the only way that one is able to ensure emptiness of the stomach. Saline should always be used to irrigate inlying gastric and intestinal tubes. Should water be used to flush the tubes and wash the stomach, sodium and potassium salts pass into the water from the gastric and the intestinal mucosa very rapidly and are washed out of the body.

Disruption of the continuity of the wall of an obstructed intestine is a catastrophe. The postoperative mortality rate for intestinal obstruction without peritonitis is now less than 7 per cent, while the postoperative mortality rate is about 30 per cent for intestinal obstruction when complicated by peritonitis, arising from dissolution of the continuity of the obstructed intestine.

There are a number of ways that intestinal continuity may be broken functionally: (1) localized pressure necrosis of the wall immediately under hernial rings or adhesive bands, (2) avascular necrosis from pressure occlusion or thrombo-embolic occlusions of large intestinal arteries by twisting, intussusception, hernial or adhesive bands, mesenterc arterial thrombosis or embolism, and (3) localized avascular necrosis arising from distentional occlusion of intramural intestinal arterioles, capillaries, or veins.

The first mechanism of necrosis is relatively rare but is especially important as a cause of rupture of the intestine caught in a Richter's hernia or under a fixed adhesion (see Chap. 42).

The second mechanism is the most frequent cause of intestinal disruption. The third is not rare and pertains especially to the colon.

In the past, occasional disruptions of the wall of the obstructed colon were thought to be directly attributable to simple physical rupture by the pressure built up between the ileocecal valve and the obstructing lesion. The normal small intestine of man bursts when subjected to intraluminal pressures of 120 to 230 mm. Hg, and the colon when pressured to 90 mm. Hg (Gatch et al., 1927). The ileocecal valve is forced open by intracolonic pressures of 40 to 55 mm. Hg. Obviously, the ileocecal valve will be breached before the normal colon bursts from pressure alone; if this were not true, bursting of the colon would be an important hazard of roentgenographic examination of the colon with the barium enema which, as practiced today, regularly is attended by retrograde filling of a part of the terminal ileum.

However, acute complete left-sided colonic obstruction is very dangerous because localized colonic rupture affecting usually the cecum or the ascending colon is so prone to complicate it. Van Zwalenberg (1907) discovered that upon increasing the intraluminal pressure within exteriorized human appendices (exteriorized to decompress obstructed colons through appendicostomy) circulatory arrest would occur within the wall of the distended appendix. Others (Dragstedt et al., 1929; Noer and Derr, 1949; Oppenheimer and Mann, 1943) have demonstrated that intestinal capillary stasis occurs with intraluminal pressures of 30 to 50 mm. Hg, venular occlusion with pressures of 50 and 60, and intramural arterial occlusion with pressures higher than 90 mm. Hg.

Obviously, localized avascular necrosis of the colon may follow its being subjected to intraluminal pressures that have actually been measured in obstructed human colons, namely, 10 to 40 mm. Hg (Wangensteen, 1955).

Whatever the mechanism may be, cecal rupture does complicate complete colonic obstruction; consequently, operative decompression of the completely obstructed colon is a surgical emergency.

Peritonitis may complicate strangulated closed-loop obstruction without actual physical dissolution or rupture of the intestine (Medins and Laufman, 1958).

Ordinarily, the intestinal wall is remarkably capable of preventing diffusion of its intraluminal contents into the peritoneal cavity and vice versa. However, when the bowel is severely distended or even distended moderately for protracted periods of time, many substances are then capable of diffusing into the peritoneal cavity. Bacteria, hemoglobin and pigments of hemoglobin may be detected in the peritoneal fluid. Colloidal dyes which normally would not diffuse into the peritoneal cavity may stain the serosal surface of the distended bowel and color the intra-abdominal fluid. Nemir et al. (1953) and many before them have studied the effects of the intravenous injection of peritoneal exudates obtained in the presence of strangulated obstruction. Often these exudates have been fatal to recipient animals. This type of observation has been the principal anchor for the toxic theory of mortality from intestinal obstruction.

TREATMENT

INDICATIONS FOR INTUBATION IN INTESTINAL OBSTRUCTION

Short Tubes. Besides being useful for the prevention of pneumonic aspiration, the short or gastric tube is employed most frequently during the early postoperative period of any operation performed upon the abdomen which is likely to produce temporary inhibition of peristaltic activity. The tube may be used for 1 to 3 days, by which time peristalsis usually has returned. The short-tube intubation is often the most effective type of intubation in the prevention of further distention in paralytic ileus from peritonitis. It is also employed occasionally as a supplement to long-tube intubation to prevent accumulation of swallowed air in the stomach when the long tube lies far down the ileum.

The chief drawback to the use of short-tube or gastric suction in attempting decompression of intestinal obstruction is its failure to remove appreciable amounts of gas or fluid distal to the pylorus. This criticism is not as serious as might appear, for the usefulness of long-tube intubation in the relief of mechanical intestinal obstruction is fairly limited due to the fact that more than 80 per cent of mechanical obstruction occurs within the small bowel where short tubes are fairly effective in avoiding distention.

Long Tubes. Intestinal intubation with a tube of the Miller-Abbott (1934) type may be indicated in some patients with simple small bowel obstruction, particularly incomplete obstruction. Occasionally, the release of distention in such patients will permit the bowel to disengage itself from its point of obstruction. It may slip out from under an adhesive band, or retract from a hernial sac if not incarcerated or volvulated. However, long-tube intubation has its greatest usefulness in patients with recurring bouts of small bowel obstruction during and for a short time after acute peritonitis from any cause and in cases of multiple neoplastic metastases to the wall of the intestine. It is also occasionally useful in the late stages of paralytic ileus from peritonitis when relief of distention occasionally hastens the return of peristaltic activity (Smith, 1956).

In most patients with intestinal mechanical

obstruction, even when not associated with obstruction of blood flow to the intestine, an operation is the best treatment. Procrastination usually does not avoid necessity for operation and carries with it the threat of unrecognized bowel necrosis occurring during the interval of intubation as well as problems in fluid and electrolyte balance.

Decompression of the colon by long tubes is practically impossible; the fecal matter within an obstructed colon cannot be drawn through the tube. Consequently, the passage of a long tube in cases of colonic obstruction with the hope of decompressing the colon and preventing its disruption only wastes time. A proximal colostomy works and prevents colonic rupture.

Any sign of restricted blood flow to obstructed intestine contraindicates any attempt at passage of a long intestinal tube; one cannot afford to waste this time doing something that cannot take the intestine out of vascular jeopardy (Cantor, 1949; Paine, 1934).

Surgical Intervention and Procedures for the Relief of Mechanical Obstruction of Small Bowel and Colon

Before these operations are undertaken for simple mechanical ileus, it is presumed that the deficits of fluids and electrolytes have been at least partially corrected, that blood has been administered as indicated, and that other disorders have been appropriately considered and treated insofar as possible. All of these things need to be accomplished within a matter of hours with simple mechanical intestinal obstruction. In case of ileus with signs that the blood flow to the intestine is impaired, and with complete colon obstruction with a greatly distended cecum, there can be no time wasted. In such cases the operating room is the place, and the period of the operation itself is the time to treat the dehydration and the shock. This can be done more readily during the operation because then the causes of the dehydration and the shock are removed, and the fluids given are consequently more effective than they are when given while the causes are still operative. Delay in release of an incarcerated and strangulated loop of bowel is the most important secondary factor contributing to bowel necrosis and hence to the mortality rate.

The aims of surgical intervention in acute mechanical obstruction are:
1. Release of obstruction
2. Resection of nonviable bowel
3. Re-establishment of intestinal continuity or at least of a segment sufficient in length to avoid excessive losses of water and electrolytes and to provide for adequate absorption and nutrition in the days or years ahead.

How these aims may best be accomplished will vary from one patient to another, but the most important determining factor related to treatment is the site of obstruction. The operative procedure of choice for large bowel obstruction can be the most harmful one which may be performed on the obstructed small bowel and vice versa.

Choice of Anesthesia. The safest anesthesia for operative correction of ileus is one that permits the anesthetist to maintain full control over breathing and to keep gastric fluid out of the trachea and the lungs. A cuffed intratracheal tube is the instrument which permits him to do both things. Whether the basal anesthetic be spinal, local, or inhalation, the intratracheal tube should be used. This can now be done by skilled anesthetists on fully conscious persons (see Chap. 13, Anesthesia).

Relief of Simple Obstruction. Except for the performance of operative decompression for asphyxiating meteorism of adynamic ileus and for colostomy, the incision must be long enough to permit removal of the entire small intestine from the abdomen if need be. The site of the most distal obstruction can be located most readily by first finding collapsed bowel and following it upward. One should never assume that a mechanical obstruction of the intestine has been relieved until the entire small intestine has been examined by sight and feel. Whenever the small intestine is significantly dilated with gas and fluid, it should be decompressed surgically before any attempt is made to replace it within the abdomen. A person able to breathe with meteorism before being operated upon may be readily choked by it after the operation when he is weaker and the incision hurts with each breath. Great care must be taken during the replacement of intestine into the abdomen so that the jejunum lies within the left upper abdominal quadrant, the terminal ileum in the pelvis, and that the base of the mesentery runs straight from the ligament of Treitz to the cecum to be sure that a volvulus has not been created during the replacement of the intestine.

DIVISION OF ADHESIONS. In many patients with simple obstruction of the small bowel, removal of adhesions is all that is required. Often the excision of one adhesive band is sufficient. However, the remainder of the peritoneal cavity should be inspected carefully for the presence of other adhesions likely to give rise to obstruction. Care should be taken to avoid denuding the serosal surface of bowel insofar as possible.

Reduction of Strangulated Hernia. Reduction by external pressure applied over the hernia should not be attempted if obstruction is more than 6 hours in duration, or if fever and leukocytosis are present. It is better that these patients be subjected to operation, exposing the hernial sac and opening the sac to inspect the bowel for viability before replacing it in the abdomen. If viable, the bowel is manipulated gently under direct vision, returned to the abdomen, and the hernia is repaired (see Chap. 42, Hernia). In some patients, the hernial ring may need to be enlarged by incision to allow re-entry of the bowel into the abdomen without trauma or taxis. Traction or taxis on the afferent or the efferent loops from within the abdominal cavity is to be avoided as the occluded loop may be torn with surprisingly little tension.

Occasionally, an awkward situation arises in which an incarcerated hernia with bowel obstruction of a few hours' duration cannot be reduced prior to operation but does reduce spontaneously under anesthesia in the operating room prior to operation. Then the question arises: can it be assumed that the bowel is viable and that the hernia can be repaired without inspection of the bowel to determine its viability? The answer is usually no. One may enlarge the hernial ring surgically so that the visceral contents can be inspected adequately. Once the decision is made to operate and gentle attempts at pre-anesthetic reductions have failed, further manipulation should be avoided until the obstructed loop is exposed surgically and inspected to determine its viability while remaining *in situ*.

Removal of Foreign Bodies, Bezoars and Gallstones. Occasionally, a large gallstone obstructing the intestine may be so friable that it breaks up when a little firm pressure is applied to it. Should this happen, that is all one needs do. In general, whenever one can do so readily without risiking puncture of the bowel, all obstructing intraluminal foreign bodies should be pushed up into the proximal dilated noninflamed bowel before making the intestinal incision to remove it. Making the incision through the inflamed intestine overlying the lodged body invites an intestinal fistula. The incision should be made through uninflamed bowel, linearly and antimesenterically, and closed transversely so not to obstruct the bowel by the closure.

Loop Colostomy for Relief of Distention. Decompression by colostomy of the proximal colon in simple complete colon obstruction is the safest and most satisfactory means yet devised. It affords prompt relief of distention with minimal risk of soilage or bacterial contamination.

The location of the colostomy along the course of the colon should receive special consideration. Two factors are concerned in arriving at the proper incision: (1) The colostomy must be proximal to the point of obstruction. (2) In locating and devising the type of colostomy, one needs to bear in mind the types of colostomy appliances available for subsequent usage, especially if the colostomy is to be permanent.

In general, there are 3 sites where a colostomy may be located on the anterior abdominal wall: over the descending colon (Fig. 38-17), over the transverse colon (Fig. 38-18) and over the cecum (Fig. 38-19). Each decompresses the colon proximal to the site of obstruction without leaving a long distal obstructed segment. As more than 75 per cent of obstructing lesions in the colon and the rectum are distal to the descending colon, the transverse colostomy is the one most often employed as well as the one most easily performed. Barium enema to locate the site of colon obstruction is a most helpful procedure in patients with large bowel obstruction and should be performed in all cases before the colostomy unless contraindicated by signs of perforation.

To perform a transverse colostomy, a vertical incision is made in the mid-line or, better,

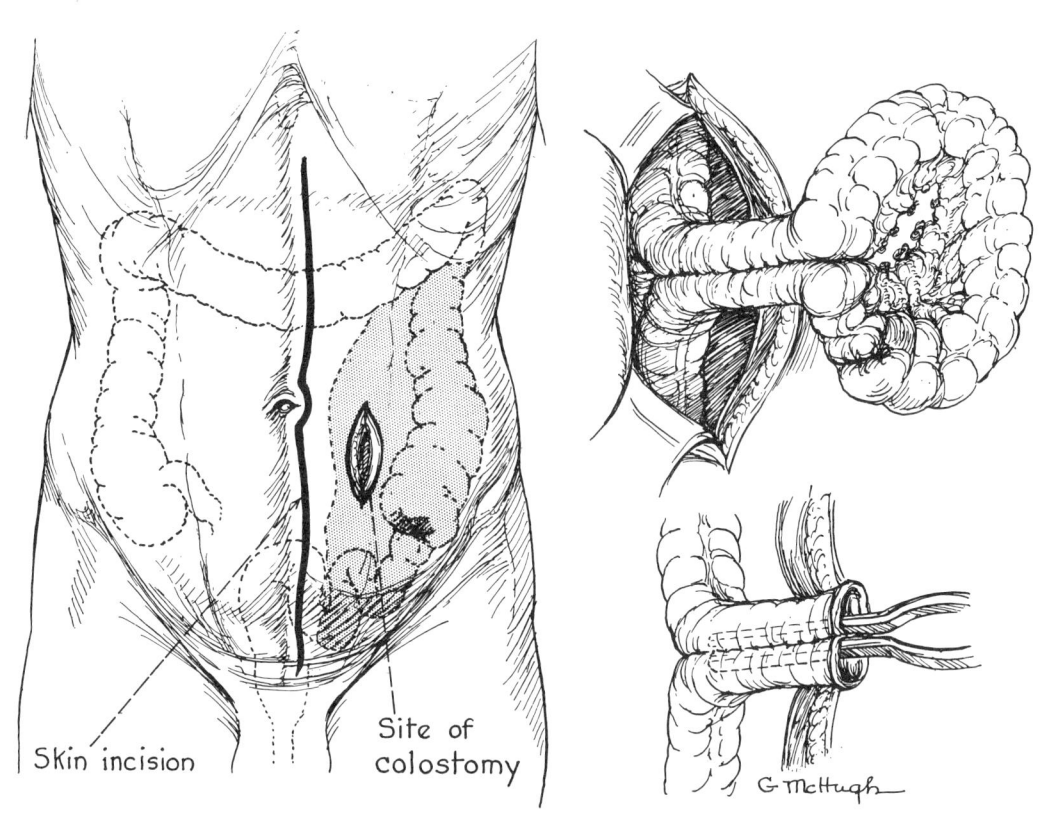

Fig. 38-17. A colostomy of the descending colon is performed. Mikulicz type of exteriorization of the sigmoid colon for diverticulitis or necrotic bowel from volvulus of sigmoid. The mesenteric borders of afferent and efferent segments are sutured together to prevent a loop of small bowel from slipping in between and becoming obstructed. The site for colostomy is indicated. A few days later a crushing clamp is applied, necrosing the bowel between the afferent and the efferent limbs, hoping that a spontaneous fistula will develop between them and that normal fecal current will be re-established. If successful, the colostomy often will undergo spontaneous closure.

a right paramedian one, usually above the umbilicus. If distention is massive and its cause is established as tumor or diverticulitis without threat of strangulation, a large incision should be avoided, as it will allow distended loops of small bowel to escape to the outside and complicate wound closure. However, the incision should be large enough to permit the introduction of the hand to palpate the site of obstruction. It is often possible to establish that the distally situated tumor is locally operable or not operable, and to establish the presence of nodules within the liver, presumably from metastatic tumor, by passing the hand over the various hepatic surfaces. If it can be satisfactorily established that the tumor is inoperable due to local extension or hepatic metastases, the patient is spared a second operation. However, it must be realized that blind palpation is a poor substitute for palpation with inspection and biopsy, particularly biopsy of hepatic nodules. Sclerosing hemangioma or lymphangioma, concretions or stones within the liver, hamartoma and fibroma are among the many benign lesions that may erroneously imply hepatic metastases, hence inoperability. Massive hepatic metastases are usually easy to recognize by palpation with a high degree of reliability, but small nodules on or just under the surface of the liver are often most deceiving.

Similar errors are common to palpation of

colostomy is performed for relief of distention. The careful dissection essential to curative operations for carcinoma of the colon cannot often be carried out satisfactorily in the presence of distended loops of bowel. Moreover, even though the tumor may seem to be resectable at the time colostomy is being performed for relief of obstruction, the patient cannot be spared the need for a second operation to close the colostomy, as primary anastomosis cannot be performed safely with the colon distended.

In cases of even obstructing carcinoma of the cecum or the ascending colon without very great dilatation of the small intestine, wide and adequate resection usually can be carried out initially to advantage. In these patients the proximal bowel may be decompressed by trocar drainage at the operating table (see

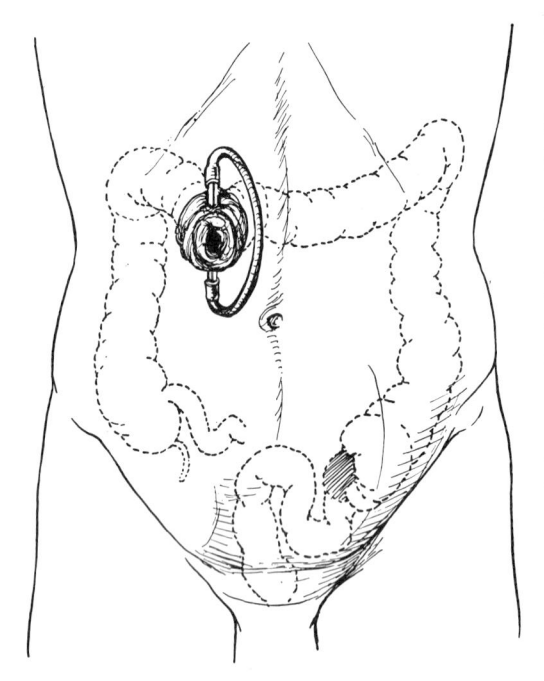

FIG. 38-18. Transverse colostomy through a right paramedian incision about 2 inches above the umbilicus. A glass rod is carried under the transverse colon and is used as a temporary support to hold the loop of colon outside the abdomen. This location of colostomy is best suited to patients whose obstructions are in the splenic flexure and distally.

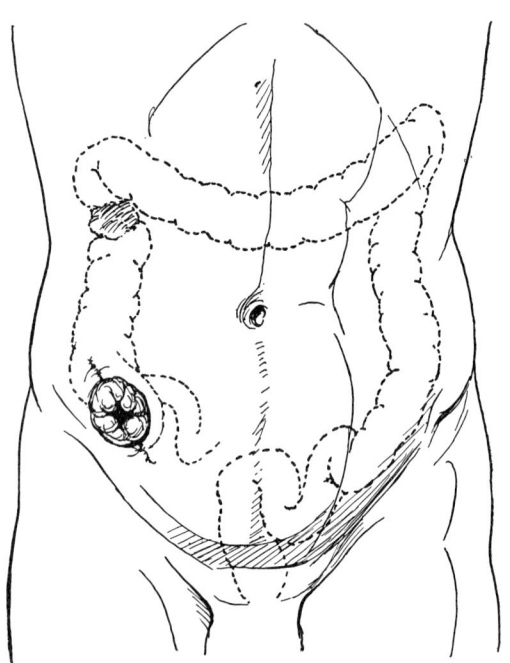

FIG. 38-19. Cecostomy drainage for decompression of the colon with lesion lying at hepatic flexure. Cecostomy here is a temporary one, and bowel resection is planned within 2 to 3 weeks. Location of the cecostomy site is too low in this illustration for a colostomy appliance, but in this instance it is purposefully placed low, as incision for the second operation will be largely above the present cecostomy.

bowel tumors. Much of the apparent fixation may represent local cellulitis secondary to infection of the bowel tumors rather than local tumor extension. Despite the drawbacks and the limitations of palpation, a fair number of inoperable cases can be established at the time of colostomy, saving the patient a useless second operation (see Carcinoma of the Colon).

A loop colostomy of the descending colon may have several disadvantages when used as a means of decompression. It should be avoided if possible, in favor of a transverse colostomy. Colostomy at the lower site at times interferes seriously with a curative operative procedure that is planned for several weeks later, whether the obstructing lesion is inflammatory or neoplastic.

No attempt should be made to resect carcinoma of the transverse or descending or sigmoid segments of the colon at the time that below). Then the necessary bowel is resected, and a careful anastomosis is performed between the terminal ileum and the transverse colon. In such patients, carcinoma of the cecum or the ascending colon may be transplanted locally by attempting cecostomy or ileostomy close to the tumor.

The location of the colostomy wound on the abdominal wall should be well away from the anterosuperior spines of the ilium, preferably about halfway along a line between the spine of the ilium and the umbilicus if a descending colostomy or cecostomy is to be performed. This precaution allows the colostomy appliance to fit snugly against skin and avoids resting upon the iliac spine, causing pressure necrosis of the skin or leakage with soiling of clothing later on. This error is illustrated in Figure 38-19.

The transverse colostomy is better suited to the majority of appliances if placed 2 to 3 inches above rather than below the umbilicus. In this location, the colostomy is cared for more easily and is less likely to be displaced, especially in patients with protuberant abdomens. Moreover, there is less chance that diastasis or colostomy hernia will occur in the upper abdomen, as the forces of gravity are less than in the lower abdomen; also the posterior rectus sheath is present in the epigastrium but not in the lower abdomen.

In most cases with loop colostomy and distention, the colostomy should be opened as soon as the abdominal incision is closed and its proximal and distal segments aspirated. A closed colostomy has no decompressing value and may distend upon the surface of the abdomen, dragging more colon to the outside.

TROCAR DECOMPRESSION of the distended small bowel is often desirable at the time of operation. This can be performed safely by carefully packing off a segment of bowel and placing a purse-string suture, encircling the site intended for the introduction of the trocar into the enteric lumen. As soon as the trocar (with its suction tube vigorously active) perforates into the intestinal lumen, the purse-string suture is immediately drawn tight about the shaft of the trocar to avoid leakage. The sharp trocar tip is then pulled back and the outer tube (sheath of the trocar) is gently directed upward, pleating the bowel onto the shaft. Then it is directed distally, and the procedure is repeated. As the metal tube is removed, the purse-string is closed, sealing the enterostomy site, which is then reinforced with 2 or 3 interrupted serosal sutures.

Trocar decompression has the following advantages: it provides better surgical exposure and avoids a large spill within the abdomen should the distended bowel wall accidentally be perforated while handling. With the bowel collapse, wound closure is greatly facilitated. The possibility for a postoperative leak at the suture line occurring because of continual distention is hereby largely avoided. It has the physiologic advantage that the collapsed bowel affords more rapid recovery of normal bowel activity. Trocar drainage introduces no important hazards if carefully performed, and at times its usage can avoid unnecessary delay in attempting long-tube intubation as its alternative.

Should a long tube with an inflatable balloon on its tip have passed successfully beyond the ligament of Treitz, the balloon tip can be threaded down the small bowel without much difficulty. Suction applied at the head end of the tube collapses the bowel and, of course, avoids the necessity for trocar drainage. Such tubes are very difficult to manipulate distally at operation unless they have already traversed the duodenum.

Relief of Strangulated Obstruction With Bowel Necrosis

DETERMINING BOWEL VIABILITY. This is the all-important question to be answered in strangulation obstruction. The circulation of the strangulated bowel may be impaired but recovers when obstruction is released; it may be impaired and fail to recover when released, or the bowel segment may be obviously dead when first inspected.

Although a number of valid clinical observations have been employed to determine the viability of the strangulated loop, the only practical ones are those which are decisive. There is no room for doubt. The following 3 points are likely to be valid under most circumstances in determining the viability of the segment in question.

1. Restoration of color promptly (1 to 15 minutes) when strangulation is released
2. Return of pulsation in small arteries on the surface of the bowel
3. Return of peristaltic activity and the

peristaltic contraction following stimulation (pinching, etc.)

Should doubt remain, "There is no better rule than this: ... resect"; this statement by Wangensteen summarizes all that needs to be said.

SURGICAL MANAGEMENT OF DEAD AND DISTENDED BOWEL

Colon. Exteriorization of the dead segment of colon and its excision after the abdominal wound has been closed about living colon proximal and distal to the dead part are the safest operative procedures that can be carried out where a necrotic segment of the transverse, descending, or sigmoid colon is encountered, especially if there is co-existent distention. The blood supply to the colon, being less dependable than that of the small bowel, is even less dependable when the colon is obstructed, distended or its wall edematous. Hence, primary colocolic anastomoses are to be avoided under these circumstances, because the suture line may leak a few days later. A necrotic ascending colon is treated as is necrotic small intestine. It is excised, and an ileocolic anastomosis performed.

The exteriorization of necrotic distal colon is performed as follows: mesentery at the proximal and the distal ends of the segment involved is divided, and the segment of dead bowel is lifted gently to the exterior surface of the abdomen along with about 4 or 5 cm. of the adjoining viable bowel at either end (Fig. 38-17). This technic is known as the Mikulicz exteriorization procedure or the Mikulicz-Brun-Mayo resection. Many modifications exist, but the principles embodied are the same as those described by Mikulicz. The segment of necrotic bowel is not resected or decompressed until after the abdomen is closed, thereby avoiding operative spillage or soilage within the peritoneal cavity.

The disadvantages of the Mikulicz type of resection are inconsequential when dealing with obstruction and/or a dead segment of colon. Essentially only one disadvantage exists: a second operation is required to close the colostomy that the Mikulicz procedure creates.

Small Bowel. Primary resection and anastomosis in high intestinal obstruction with a nonviable segment of the small bowel is the only practical procedure in most patients. External drainage of the mid-ileum or the jejunum nearly always creates more trouble than it solves. The volumes of fluids and electrolytes lost through most high intestinal enterostomies are no less that those of high intestinal obstruction itself. Malnutrition also continues.

Primary resection and intra-abdominal anastomosis of the obstructed dead segment of small bowel fortunately do not carry the risk entailed in similar resection of the obstructed colon. While primary resection and anastomosis of the dead distal colon is condemned, this is the only feasible and safe operation possible in small bowel obstruction with necrosis. Ordinarily, an end-to-end anastomosis of the small bowel fortunately does not carry the risk most frequently employed after resection of an unobstructed segment of small bowel. However, when obstruction exists, the proximal segment may be so distended, its wall so edematous, and the diameter of its proximal lumen so large that to join it to the collapsed distal one would be unsafe.

Therefore, the proximal and the distal transected ends are carefully sutured closed, the ends enfolded and reinforced with serosal stitches, and a lateral (side-to-side) anastomosis performed to re-establish intestinal continuity. This type of anastomosis is easily carried out, and the lateral opening in the distended proximal segment can be cut to the same size as the lateral opening in the collapsed distal segment. With rubber-shod intestinal clamps applied to both the proximal and the distal segments at the proposed anastomotic site, the operative field is carefully walled-off with laparotomy pads, and a lateral anastomosis (isoperistaltic) is carried to completion without risk of spillage of intestinal contents and with only minimal surface soilage.

Trocar decompression of the small bowel prior to closure of the abdomen should be carried out whenever anastomoses of small intestine are done and the proximal intestine is distended if long-tube intubation has not been successful.

TREATMENT OF INTUSSUSCEPTION IN ADULTS

This is different from the treatment of intussusception in infants (see Chap. 50). In infants, reduction by hydrostatic pressure or manually should be attempted if the bowel is not dead or the intussusception is not too longstanding. Intussusception in adults, excepting for very short ones with a Meckel's diverticulum as the lead point, should not be reduced but should be resected because malignant intestinal tumors make up a significant portion, about 30 per cent, of the lead points of the intussusceptions in older children and adults, and one runs too much risk of breaking the tumor and spreading it if reduction of the intussusception is attempted. After all, in adult intussusception the bowel must almost always be opened to remove the lead point even if it is benign, and this is as dangerous, if not more dangerous, than a resection with anastomosis between normal bowel parts because incision through bowel that was in the intussusception and is inflamed and edematous if not ulcerated is less likely to heal well.

MECHANISMS AND TREATMENT OF PRIMARY VOLVULUS IN ADULTS

The frequency with which volvulus or torsion of the small and large intestine is reported to occur varies widely. These discrepancies are in part artificial (differences in semantics) and in part real. For example, if one considers rotation of a loop of small bowel about the axis of an adhesion, an ileostomy or colostomy stoma, etc., then volvulus is a very frequent cause of acute small bowel obstruction in adults. If the term is restricted to those which are primary in origin in that torsion is due to the congenital failure of fixation of the duodenum and/or of the colon, then torsion of the intestines in the adult is indeed a rare occurrence (see Chap. 50, Pediatric Surgery).

Using the latter definition, primary torsion or volvulus is much more frequently encountered in the cecum or sigmoid colon than in the small bowel, though still not a commonly encountered cause of acute intestinal obstruction among the populations of western Europe and the United States.

When primary volvulus occurs, obstruction is usually sudden, and always of the closed-loop variety if obstruction is complete. Ischemia or total vascular occlusion is often present from the onset.

Primary Volvulus of the Colon. This nearly always occurs in the cecum or the sigmoidal segments. Volvulus of the transverse colon is exceedingly rare, probably because this segment of colon is suspended posteriorly from the mesocolon and superiorly by the gastrocolic omentum (see Fig. 35-1).

Volvulus of the Cecum. This is a form of torsion which nearly always involves also the terminal ileum just proximal to the cecum and the adjacent ascending colon at its distal end. This disorder accounts for about 1 per cent of all causes of acute intestinal obstruction (Byrne et al., 1952). The predisposing factor is the inadequate fixation of the ascending colon by the posterior parietes. Instead, it is usually partially or totally mobile upon a mesentery. Volvulus of the cecum is much more commonly encountered in malnourished patients whose mesenteries are very thin.

The severity of symptoms depends upon the extent to which torsion is possible. Minor degrees of mobility are not likely to provide the soil for a volvulus that can obstruct completely; more often partial obstruction occurs, giving rise to right lower abdominal crampy pains whose origin is not likely to be recognized unless surgical intervention is required.

Wolfer et al. (1942) maintained that in addition to the unduly mobile ascending colon, the terminal ileum must be less mobile than usual if volvulus of the cecum and the ascending colon was to occur. They believed that the point of hyperfixation of the ileum is essential and that it serves as the axis about which the cecum and the ascending colon may rotate.

Other factors have been described as providing a higher degree of mobility to the ascending colon and the cecum. Among these are malrotation or incomplete rotation of the midgut embryologically, or its counterpart—too much rotation with an exaggerated degree of descension, allowing excesses of the cecum and part of the ascending colon to lie free within the right pelvis.

To some extent, dietary habits are thought to play an inciting role in volvulus of the mobile cecum and the sigmoid, too. Large amounts of diet roughage have been suggested to explain the higher frequency of volvulus of the cecum claimed for populations of the eastern European countries. In Russia, Turkey, India and Africa, volvulus of the cecum is reported to be one of the commonest causes of acute obstruction in adults (Figiel and

Figiel, 1953), and also malnutrition is very common. According to Donhauser and Atwell (1949), the cecum and the ascending colon are sufficiently mobile in about 20 per cent of the population to permit pathologic rotation. If this be the case, it would seem plausible that the incidence of torsion might be higher among those individuals in whom the cecum becomes heavily weighted with feces, thereby favoring rotation in response to gravity or exertion. Clinical experience possibly tends to support this thesis.

DIAGNOSIS presents the problem of deciding upon the specific cause of acute intestinal obstruction. The nature of onset and the clinical findings are not distinctive, but the roentgenographic findings may be fairly diagnostic. Figiel and Figiel (1953) describe the ectopic position of the cecum which is simulated by only a few clinical entities. Partial torsion should be suspected when the cecum is severely distended and displaced. Volvulus of the cecum without displacement is not likely to be distinguished from incomplete obstruction from other cause, such as carcinoma of the ascending colon, without the aid of contrast studies (barium enema). A large intra-abdominal abscess containing gas and lying in the right mid and lower abdomen constitutes the most difficult radiologic distinction usually encountered, but the longer history and the septic state associated with infection generally tip the scale in favor of abscess. In volvulus the barium enema shows the contrast medium cut off at the hepatic flexure and having the appearance of the apex of the "ace of spades" with no alterations of mucosal pattern. The cecum tends to wander toward the left upper quadrant as distention progresses, for the cecum and the ascending colon swing mesially from their distal point of twist and fixation which is usually near the hepatic flexure.

TREATMENT is operative and is carried out as promptly as the diagnosis is suspected. More commonly, the nature of the distention is not discovered until the time of operative intervention for the relief of acute intestinal obstruction. This may be sufficiently late that viability of the bowel is threatened, if the bowel is not actually gangrenous.

Most surgeons believe that it is best to perform an exteriorization procedure of the Mikulicz type (Fig. 38-17), resecting the cecum after the abdomen is closed, leaving the patient with a temporary ileostomy, to be closed as a transverse ileocolostomy a few weeks later. In some patients, right hemicolectomy with a primary anastomosis may be performed safely.

When the cecum is fully viable, a cecocoloplicopexy may be performed. "Cecocoloplicopexy" (incising the lateral parietal peritoneum and suturing its cut edge to the cecum and the ascending colon) is a method devised to anchor these structures to the posterior parietes to avoid subsequent torsion. Although this technic has been employed successfully in the management of the detorsed cecum, it carries the risk of needle or suture perforation in view of the acutely distended and ischemic bowel. This hazard coupled with occasional failure to maintain anchorage of the cecum and ascending colon in position favors resection over cecocoloplicopexy; i.e., resection performed at the time of volvulus.

However, coloplicopexy for abnormal mobility of the cecum or sigmoid is at times a procedure to be elected when the conditions of abnormal mobility are discovered in the course of other abdominal operations, preferably if distention presents no problem.

Volvulus of the sigmoid in the adult is encountered most often after the age of 50. Occasionally, it is a complication of megacolon or sigmoidal obstruction from carcinoma. In a few it is the result of adhesions suspending the sigmoid from the abdominal wall. In the latter instance, the rotational axis is about the adhesive bands; in the case of the long mesentery the volvulus is about the mesenteric axis and the sigmoidal vessels.

Usually the twist is in the counterclockwise direction with the upper loop coming to lie in front of the distal segment. This creates a very efficient check-valve at the proximal end, allowing gas and liquid feces to enter the closed loop but none to leave. Gas and feces continue to accumulate. There is no cause of bowel obstruction which produces larger coils of distended bowel loops than volvulus of the sigmoid. The heavier the loop becomes, the more tightly closed is the distal site of occlusion. The distal end, too, has a check-valve action but not when entered from below. Therefore it may be possible to introduce very gently a proctoscope or long rectal tube through the lower check-valve to enter the "omega" loop, achieving explosive decompression, often with total relief. (See Figs. 38-9 and 38-10.)

CLINICAL PATTERNS may be those of chronic constipation associated with bouts of colicky pain, distention and obstipation. Occasionally, the condition is self-relieved by the expulsion of huge quantities of air and liquid stool. As the disease progresses, there is less likelihood of spontaneous remission. The obstruction usually develops over a period of several days to a week or longer in older patients. Often by the time they present themselves, distention is pronounced, the abdomen tympanitic, and respiratory embarrassment is obvious. Bloody exudates accumulate within the bowel lumen and may lead to hypovolemic shock. Bowel necrosis is the sequela, followed by perforation.

Less commonly encountered is the sudden onset of symptoms which usually occurs in younger patients, especially those with megacolon. After the sudden onset, the course usually progresses more rapidly than that noted above for older patients. Peripheral circulatory collapse from dehydration is frequent, and necrosis of the bowel with rupture or perforation tends to occur soon.

DIAGNOSIS of a sigmoid volvulus should be suspected in any patient with pronounced abdominal distention.

TREATMENT. As mentioned above, the simplest procedure to attempt is decompression by proctoscopy. If this is successful, surgery need not be performed, although peripheral collapse may occur a few hours later unless the extracellular fluid volume deficit is sufficiently treated. In order to determine the approximate amount of Hartmann's solution needed to treat the dehydration, the amount of fluid that flows out through the sigmoidoscope and the rectal tube, or that removed from the loop by trocar drainage must be measured. An amount of Hartmann's solution equal to this, plus a liter more to allow for the edema of the colon, should be given intravenously. At times this may amount to 5 to 8 liters (see Table 38-6). Antibiotics may be given for several days. Surprisingly, recurrence of sigmoidal volvulus after decompression in this manner is not a certainty; only about 1 out of 4 or 5 patients ever have trouble again.

Operative management is designed for detorsion. But before this can proceed safely, it is better to perform trocar decompression, being very careful to avoid splitting the colon and causing extensive fecal contamination. Once bowel distention is relieved, the volvulus may be untwisted. At this point, the decision is whether to perform a Mikulicz exteriorization of the sigmoid colon, ligating its vessels, or whether to return the bowel to the abdomen, and perform a decompressing transverse colostomy in the course of closure of the abdomen. The bowel should be left *in situ* only when its circulation is not impaired.

INTRAPERITONEAL ANTIBIOTICS

The intraperitoneal instillation of antibiotics after celiotomy for the relief of simple mechanical intestinal obstruction is not indicated. The "prophylactic administration" of antibiotics when overt contamination of the peritoneal cavity has *not* taken place accomplishes nothing. Should necrotic bowel have to be resected, or spillage of intestinal contents into the peritoneum have occurred, antibiotics should be given parenterally as for peritonitis (see Chap. 37) and an antibiotic may be placed in the peritoneal cavity. However, if an antibiotic is put into the peritoneal cavity, no antibiotic having a curarelike action (such as neomycin) should be used. Fatal respiratory failure may be induced. Penicillin is usually safe.

REFERENCES

Barnes, W. A.: Management of foreign bodies in the alimentary tract. Am. J. Surg., 107:422, 1964.

Byrne, J. J., Swift, C. C., and Farrell, G. E.: Volvulus of the cecum. Arch. Surg., 64:378, 1952.

Calman, C., Hershey, F. B., and Skaggs, J. O.: Serum lactic dehydrogenase in the diagnosis of the acute surgical abdomen. Surgery, 44:43-52, 1958.

Cannon, W. B.: The Mechanical Factors of Digestion. London, Longmans, 1911.

Cantor, M. O.: Intestinal Intubation. Springfield, Ill., Charles C Thomas, 1949.

Cooke, W. T.: Water and electrolyte upsets in steatorrhea syndrome. J. Mount Sinai Hosp., New York, 24:221, 1957.

Cox, E. V., Gaddie, R., Matthews, D., Cooke, W. T., and Meynell, M. J.: An interrelationship between ascorbic acid and cyanocobalamin. Clin. Sci. 17: 681, 1948.

DeMuth, W. E., Jr., and Rottenstein, H. S.: Death associated with hypocalcemia after small-bowel short circuiting. New Eng. J. Med., 270:1239, 1964.

Donhauser, J. L., and Atwell, S.: Volvulus of the

cecum with a review of 100 cases in the literature and a report of 6 new cases. Arch. Surg., 58:129, 1949.

Dragstedt, L. R., Lang, V. F., and Millet, R. F.: The relative effects of distention on different portions of the intestine. Arch. Surg., 18:2257, 1929.

Drapanas, T., Williams, J. S., McDonald, J. C., Heyden, W., Bow, T., and Spencer, R. P.: Role of the ilium in the absorption of vitamin B_{12} and intrinsic factor (NF). J.A.M.A., 184:337, 1963.

Figiel, L. S., and Figiel, S. J.: Volvulus of the cecum and ascending colon. Radiology, 61:495, 1953.

Fine, J., Banks, B. M., Sears, J. B., and Hermanson, L.: Treatment of gaseous distention of intestine by inhalation of 95 per cent oxygen: description of apparatus for clinical administration of high oxygen mixtures. Ann Surg., 103:375, 1936.

Fisher, E. R.: Whipple's disease; Pathogenic considerations. J.A.M.A., 181:396, 1962.

Gatch, W. D., Trusler, H. M., and Ayres, K. D.: Effects of gaseous distention on obstructed bowel: incarceration of intestine by gas traps. Arch. Surg., 14:1215, 1927.

Gerst, P. H., Porter, M. R., and Fishman, R. A.: Symptomatic magnesium deficiency in surgical patients. Ann. Surg., 159:402, 1964.

Lester, R., and Schmid, R.: Intestinal absorption of bile pigments. II. Bilirubin absorption in man. New Eng. J. Med., 269:178, 1963.

LeVeen, H. H., Borek, B., Axelrod, D. R., and Johnson, A.: Cause and treatment of diarrhea following resection of the small bowel. Surg., Gynec., Obstet., 124:766, 1967.

Lewis, L. A., Turnbull, R. B., Jr., and Page, I. H.: "Short-circuiting" of the small intestine. J.A.M.A., 182:77, 1962.

Medins, G., and Laufman, H.: Hypothermia in mesenteric arterial and venous occlusions. Ann. Surg., 148:747-754, 1958.

Melzer, Von H., and Kollert, W.: Ein Beitrag zur Klinik und Therapie der Chagas-Krankheit. Deutsche med. Wsch., 8:368, 1963.

Miller, T. G., and Abbott, W. S.: Intestinal intubation: a practical technique. Am. J. Med. Sci., 187:595, 1934.

Nemir, P., Hawthorne, H. R., Cohn, I., and Drabkin, D. L.: Cause of death in strangulation obstruction: II. Lethal action of the peritoneal fluid. Ann. Surg., 130:874, 1949.

Noer, R. J., and Derr, J. W.: Effect of distention on intestinal revascularization. Arch. Surg., 59:542, 1949.

Oppenheimer, M. J., and Mann, F. C.: Intestinal capillary circulation during distention. Surgery, 13:548, 1943.

Paine, J. R.: The history of the invention and development of the stomach and duodenal tubes. Ann. Int. Med., 8:752, 1934.

Portis, S. A.: Diseases of the Digestive System. ed. 3. p. 176. Philadelphia, Lea & Febiger, 1953.

Randall, H. T.: Water and electrolyte balance in surgery. Surg. Clin. N. Am., 32:445, 1952.

Roy, A. D.: Resection of hindgut for idiopathic megacolon in adolescence. Brit. J. Surg., 55:106, 1968.

Schwartz, E.: Ueber Flatulenz. Med. Klin., 5:1339, 1909.

Seagram, C. G. F., Lough, R. E., Stephens, C. A., and Wentworth, P.: Meckel's diverticulum. Canad. J. Surg., 11:369, 1968.

Smith, G. A.: Long intestinal tubes for operative decompression and postoperative ileus. J.A.M.A., 160:266, 1956.

Teimourian, B., Cigtay, A. S., and Smyth, N. P. D.: Management of ingested foreign bodies in the psychotic patient. Arch. Surg., 88:915, 1964.

Thomas, D.: Acute small bowel obstruction. Aust. N. Zeal. J. Surg., 37:302, 1968.

Thomas, H. S., Cherry, J. K., and Averbook, B. D.: Gallstone ileus. J.A.M.A., 179:625, 1962

Trier, J. S., Phelps, P. C., and Rubin, C. E.: Electron microscopy of mucosa of small intestine J.A.M.A., 183:768, 1963.

Wangensteen, O. H.: Intestinal Obstructions. ed. 3. Springfield, Ill., Charles C Thomas, 1955.

Whipple, G. H.: Hitherto undescribed disease characterized anatomically by deposits of fats and fatty acids in intestinal and mesenteric lymph nodes. Bull. Johns Hopkins Hosp., 18:382, 1907.

Wolfer, J. A., Beaton, L. E., and Anson, B. J.: Volvulus of the cecum: Anatomic factors in its etiology; report of a case. Surg., Gynec., Obstet., 78:882, 1942.

Wood, L. C., and Chremos, A. N.: Treating obesity by "short-circuiting" the small intestine. J.A.M.A., 186:63, 1963.

van Zwalenburg, C.: Strangulation resulting from strangulation of hollow viscera; its bearing upon appendicitis, strangulated hernia and gallbladder disease. Ann. Surg., 46:780, 1907.

CHAPTER 39

J. GARROTT ALLEN, M.D.

Small Bowel and Colon

Congenital Disorders of the Intestinal Tract Afflicting Adult Patients
Trauma of the Small Bowel and the Colon
Inflammatory Diseases of the Small Bowel and the Colon
Tumors of the Small Bowel
Pseudomembranous Enterocolitis

The anatomy and the physiology of the small bowel, the colon and the peritoneal cavity have been discussed in preceding chapters and are not under discussion here:

Chapter 35—Peritoneum and splanchnic circulation of blood

Chapter 37—Anatomy of appendix and cecum and the differential diagnosis of the acute abdomen.

Chapter 37—The peritoneum's response to peritonitis

Chapter 38—Lymphatic circulation of small bowel and colon, physiology of peristalsis, intestinal secretions and absorption, intestinal air and gases, intestinal intubation, abnormal fluid and electrolyte losses and their replacements in small and large bowel obstruction

CONGENITAL DISORDERS OF THE INTESTINAL TRACT AFFLICTING ADULT PATIENTS

Most congenital anomalies of the bowel manifest their presence shortly after birth, especially the obturator obstructions (imperforate anus, atresias of small or large bowel) (see Chap. 50, Pediatric Surgery). Most others are likely to give symptoms within the first 2 years of life. Duplications of portions of the alimentary canal and other anomalies generally produce symptoms before the age of 10. Thus, the only congenital anomalies giving rise to symptoms in adults as frequently as they do in infants and children are the Meckel's diverticulum and the abnormally mobile cecum and sigmoid which may create volvulus, usually for acquired rather than for congenital reasons.

The mucosa of the small intestine depends for its normal appearance upon an adequate intake of Vitamin B_{12} (cyanocobalamine) (Foroozan and Trier, 1967). In deficiency of B_{12} there is a diminished number of mitoses in crypts, a shortening of villi, a megaloblastosis of the epithelial cells, and an increase in cellular elements of the lamina propria. In relation to other food essentials, the requirements of B_{12} in micrograms are the least of all, and, microgram for microgram, it exerts its effect at the same level as the miniscule dosage of botulism toxin. Despite the small amount of B_{12} required in the normal diet, patients on antibiotics for such conditions as diverticulitis and chronic intestinal disease (i.e., chronic ulcerative colitis, Crohn's disease and the blind loop syndrome) may develop B_{12} deficiency remarkably rapidly. No mention is made here of pernicious anemia for which B_{12} is also required.

MECKEL'S DIVERTICULUM

Incidence. Meckel's diverticulum is found in 1 to 2 per cent of all patients coming to autopsy, being present 3 times more often in males than in females. About half of the diverticuli which become symptomatic do so before the age of 2.

Historical Considerations. This diverticulum is a developmental remnant of the vitelline duct. Normally, the duct atrophies; failure to do so may leave only a residual fibrous cord which extends from the lower ileum to the umbilicus. The duct may remain patent with an umbilical sinus or a fecal fistula presenting, or more commonly the proximal portion remains patent on the antimesenteric margin of the ileum (95% of cases) where the ductal remnant constitutes a pouch. This lesion was named for Johann Friedrich Meckel, the younger (1781-1833) whose several works on comparative anatomy made Germany the center for this discipline in the early 19th century and earned him recognition as the German Cuvier.

Johann Friedrich Meckel, the elder (1724-74) of Wetzlar, was graduated at Göttingen in 1748 with a noteworthy inaugural dissertation on the 5th nerve (Meckel's ganglion) and became the first teacher of obstetrics in Berlin. His son, Philipp Friedrich Theodor Meckel (1756-1803) was graduated at Strassburg in 1777 with an important dissertation on the internal ear. He was Professor of Anatomy and Surgery in Halle in 1779 and was also a favorite obstetrician in the Russian Court. His son, in turn, Johann Friedrich Meckel (1781-1833), called the younger, was born in Halle, was an eminent pathologist and the greatest comparative anatomist in Germany before Johannes Müller. It was he who discovered Meckel's diverticulum of the intestine.

Unlike another great and almost contemporary family in anatomy, the three Monros of Edinburgh—*primus, secundus* and *tertius*—the flame of genius burned brightest with the third generation of the Meckels, rather than dimmest as with the Monros.

According to Maingot (1955), Lavater first mentioned the existence of such a diverticulum in 1671; Ruynch illustrated its presence in 1701; and Littre in 1742 described its presence in a hernial sac, but to Meckel belongs the credit for recognizing its embryologic and anatomic significance about 150 years after Lavater's discovery. Zenker (1861) described the occasional presence of ectopic pancreas in its wall; Salzer (1904) reported the occasional finding of gastric mucosa lining the diverticulum; Schaetz (1925) described local peptic ulceration as accounting for the hemorrhagic complications the diverticulum occasionally presents.

Complications. A number of other complications may arise from the presence of Meckel's diverticulum. To a large extent these depend upon the structural nature of the remnant. Should a cord attachment persist between the ileum and the umbilicus, the ileum may rotate on this axis (antimesenteric), causing volvulus and closed loop obstruction. Also, a loop of small bowel may slip innocently behind the cord, causing acute intestinal obstruction. This type of Meckel's diverticulum cannot intussuscept in the usual manner as the intussuscipiens is held in traction by the cord, tending constantly to disengage any but a retrograde type of intussusception. If the diverticulum is free to intussuscept or to twist upon its own axis, it can produce strangulation volvulus and obstruct its own lumen, causing gangrenous Meckel's diverticulitis. If its neck is small or its lumen is obstructed by concretions or a foreign body, preventing drainage, obstruction diverticulitis, gangrenous perforation and peritonitis may follow in the same manner as acute obstructive appendicitis (see "Appendicitis and the Acute Abdomen").

If its wall contains gastric mucosa, peptic ulcer may develop within the diverticulum or in the wall of the ileum, usually a little distal to the ostium of the diverticulum. Acute rectal bleeding, without pain, is the usual complaint when bleeding is from an ulcer of this sort. The ulcer may perforate, especially one lying within the diverticulum. Colonic or duodenal heterotopia may also comprise part or all of the lining of the diverticulum; each may appear singularly or in combination and are asymptomatic.

For so small an anomaly, this diverticulum has been the site of origin of a variety of tumors, benign and malignant. Among them are lipomas, fibromas, angiofibromas, fibrosarcomas, argentaffinomas, lymphosarcomas and carcinomas. However, the total number of tumors encountered is exceedingly small.

Diagnosis. The diagnosis of the diverticulum obviously is a speculative one. The physician must envisage the numerous pathologic entities which can arise from Meckel's diverticulum but realize that these are also common to many other alimentary disorders. The diagnosis may be suspected and it may be difficult to prove short of operation. Usually, one or more of the following complaints are among the indications for operation:

Intestinal hemorrhage: if cramplike pain persists, one may suspect intussusception and Meckel's diverticulum with intussusception as one of many possible causes.

Hemorrhage without pain is frequently present and suggests peptic ulceration.

Intestinal obstruction from volvulus, bands, intussusception but only when the diagnosis of intestinal obstruction is tenable, Meckel's diverticulum being one of the less common causes of obstruction in adults.

Acute Meckel's diverticulitis resembles appendicitis in particular and other right lower abdominal inflammatory lesions in general.

The umbilical sinus or ileal-umbilical fecal fistula are rare conditions but are more usually recognized as due to the presence of Meckel's diverticulum.

Therefore, the indications for operations are the same as those for surgical intervention in seeking to establish the cause and to institute treatment for intestinal bleeding, acute obstruction or acute intra-abdominal inflammatory disease with or without abscess or peritonitis. About two thirds of all symptomatic Meckel's diverticula are those causing intestinal obstruction or those which bleed, the two sharing about equally in frequency.

The remaining third of complications caused by Meckel's diverticula are largely concerned with acute diverticulitis, perforation and tumors. In excess of 70 per cent of all patients with Meckel's diverticulum have no symptoms, its presence being established at the operating table incidentally or at autopsy.

Treatment of the complications of Meckel's diverticulum is early operation. If the diverticulum has undergone torsion or intussusception, they are relieved as described. If the bowel segment is nonviable, the segment is resected and appropriately anastomosed. If the bowel is viable and the diverticulum is necrotic, the latter is resected. A clamp is placed across its base at a 45° angle to the axis of the bowel lumen, cutting away the diverticulum and suturing with 2 layers of interrupted fine silk without infolding. Some prefer to resect a wedge of the antimesenteric edge of the ileum, which also permits closure without encroachment upon the lumen and has the advantage of resecting a segment of adjacent bowel whose blood supply may have been partially impaired.

A Meckel's diverticulum, found incidentally in the course of another operation, is usually resected unless the nature of the primary operation is one which will contraindicate any additional or elective surgery at the time. Especially those diverticula which are long and have a narrowed proximal lumen should be resected if they can be removed without risk. Similarly, those with attachments to the umbilicus should be removed to avoid volvulus.

OTHER CONDITIONS

Other conditions exist and give rise to symptoms in the adult which may be considered "quasi-congenital" in origin, because factors in addition to congenital disorders undoubtedly contribute to the onset of their complications in adult life.

These are (1) the superior mesenteric artery syndrome, (2) volvulus of the cecum, (3) volvulus of the sigmoid colon, and (4) intestinal obstruction due to internal hernia. The superior mesenteric artery syndrome results in partial obstruction of the third portion of the duodenum as the artery crosses its anterior surface, compressing and partially occluding the duodenal lumen (see Chaps. 31 and 35). Volvulus of the cecum or of the sigmoid colon is made possible by weight loss and an unusually mobile cecum or ascending colon. Internal hernias are the result of strangulation of intestine in abnormal peritoneal folds that result from failure of normal fusion of the peritoneum. The sites at which internal intestinal incarcerations may occur are (1) diaphragmatic hernia, (2) hernia of the foramen of Winslow, (3) hernias of the paraduodenal fossae, (4) congenital hole in the mesentery, (5) hernia into the intersigmoid fossa, and (6) pericecal hernias (see Chap. 38, Intestinal Obstruction).

A variety of reduplications of the alimentary tract may not give rise to symptoms until adult life when a "blind" reduplication, gradually having accumulated secretions, may compress the portion of the adjacent alimentary tract, causing partial obstruction or intussusception. Similarly, embryonal cysts of the mesentery may not cause symptoms until adult life.

The Peutz-Jeghers syndrome of familial polyposis (almost always noncancerous) consists of deposits of melanin about the mouth, the lips and the buccal mucosa, less often around the nose and the eyes, the fingers and the toes. Polyps, mostly in the small bowel, may cause intussusception. They may bleed, and melena and fatigue from anemia are frequent symptoms. Such polyps are considered polypoid hamartomas. Another familial disease is that known as Gardner's syndrome, which consists of multiple polyposis associated with osteomas and certain soft-tissue tumors; here, the chance of a polyp turning into a cancer is sufficiently great that prophylactic measures may be advisable, as they are for familial multiple polyposis of the colon. Whipple's disease and celiac disease both appear to result from genetic aberrations, though their natures are not understood, nor are they amenable to surgical therapy. There are suggestions that several other genetic abnormalities exist, but the evidence is insufficient to judge or evaluate them. Genetic factors in intestinal polyps are discussed by McKusick (1962).

TRAUMA OF THE SMALL BOWEL AND THE COLON

Traumatic injuries suffered by the small bowel and the colon usually are classified as nonpenetrating injuries to the abdomen, penetrating wounds from without, and perforations of the bowel arising from within the lumen.

Nonpenetrating Injuries

The classification of injuries sustained by any part of the body necessarily is arbitrary, and a particular injury may fall into more than one category. The very nature of the trauma sustained is one of chance; so, too, is the pattern of the injury sustained.

Classification. Nonpenetrating or blunt injuries to the abdomen usually fall into 3 categories: crushing injuries where the bowel is squeezed against unyielding structures such as bone. At times it may be pinched or "exploded." Tearing injuries are usually the result of a tangential blow or one wherein the body is displaced more rapidly than the mobile intestine. Acute compression injuries may burst the bowel or shear it from its mesenteric attachment. Of course, any one of these types of trauma may produce symptoms which are characteristic of another.

Much of our knowledge on nonpenetrating abdominal wounds has been derived from military activities, although in recent decades the high-speed modes of travel provide an equally or even larger experience among the civilian population (see Chap. 25, Military Surgery).

Seat belt injuries can be serious, but fortunately their occurrence in auto accidents is rare (LeMire et al., 1967).

The pathology of traumatic lesions to the bowel produced by nonpenetrating injuries includes complete or partial tearing, rupture of the bowel, subserosal hematoma and infection following tearing of mucosa and/or the muscular coats. The bowel may be severed from its mesenteric vessels, and rents of the mesentery, the mesocolon, the gastrocolic or the greater omentum are not uncommon.

Tearing and rupture of the bowel, pathologically and clinically, can be the same entity. Only the physical forces producing them tend to differ. Tears more frequently are the result of indirect violence. For example, the individual may fall, landing on his feet or buttocks, tearing the intestine from portions of its mesenteric attachments. Intraperitoneal hemorrhage with shocks occurs early. Should the bowel subsequently necrose, perforation with peritonitis is inevitable.

Delayed rupture of the bowel may occur several days later, often after the patient has been discharged from the hospital; this situation is reminiscent of delayed rupture of the spleen. Such instances are rare and usually are caused by an infected subserosal hematoma which perforates or devitalizes the adjacent bowel by interference with its blood supply. Not infrequently, more than one contusion or tear in the bowel is present. At times delayed perforations are minute compared with the several centimeters of tears or the complete division of bowel that is usually seen early.

The location of the perforation may be anywhere along the circumference of the bowel. The tear may be on the retroperitoneal surface facing into the mesentery, commonly giving rise to hematoma and abscess formation which later may burst into the free peritoneal cavity. This type of injury is likely to devitalize the adjacent segment of bowel as it frequently injures the mesenteric vessels as they enter and leave the bowel.

Most tears resulting from indirect violence occur near the points of bowel fixation. Neighboring portions of bowel will shift positions quickly, but in "rolling with the punch" a tear may occur in close proximity to a portion which is fixed. Injuries of this type are found in the upper jejunum near the ligament of Treitz or in the distal ileum. Occasionally the proximal or distal ends of the sigmoid colon are torn in a similar manner.

The mesentery of the small bowel, the transverse mesocolon, the gastrocolic omentum and the greater omentum are torn or detached in about 30 or 40 per cent of injuries sustained by the intestine. The direction of the mesenteric tear bears upon the hazard involved. Vertical tears are less likely to sever the mesenteric blood vessels.

Clinical pattern of nonpenetrating injuries sustained by the small bowel and the colon: With rare exceptions, the most frequent early clinical finding is that associated with hypovolemic shock. The loss of blood from the torn surfaces of the bowel or one of the mesenteric vessels, the irritant action of intestinal juices and the rapid outpouring of peritoneal exudates, and the fact that other injuries also are often sustained provide adequate explanations for the pallor, the clammy and moist extremities, the thready and rapid pulse, and the hypotension commonly observed. As blood accumulates within the abdomen, pain and tenderness increase if the patient is conscious. Rigidity of the abdominal musculature with shifting dullness in the flanks and the presence of a boggy mass felt in the cul-de-sac are all indications of internal hemorrhage.

Pain and muscle spasm are usually present when the patient is first seen. Both tend to increase steadily unless the patient is treated promptly. At first pain may be localized, but it rapidly becomes diffuse. Occasionally, the patient complains of pain referred to the shoulder cap distribution of the phrenic nerve, due to subdiaphragmatic irritation from blood or intestinal contents.

Nausea and vomiting are frequent complaints from any acute and painful injury, whether to the abdomen or elsewhere. However, when vomiting continues an hour or 2 later, it is suggestive evidence of bowel perforation.

Muscular rigidity may be deceptive, as it can arise from associated compression fractures of the vertebrae or broken ribs and from hemorrhage into the abdominal wall.

Abdominal distention may develop very promptly, or not for a day or two. Early, the distention is in part the result of air swallowing associated with apprehension and the dyspnea caused by hemorrhage or splinting of the chest or the abdomen to avoid pain. Subsequently, distention usually results from the air which normally is swallowed but not expelled because of paralytic ileus from peritonitis or injury to the spinal cord.

Subcutaneous crepitation may occur from the escape of free intestinal air dissecting over the abdominal wall. It is found in a few patients having ruptured the bowel along its mesenteric attachments, particularly ruptures of the second and the third portions of the duodenum and the ascending and the descending colons. Intestinal emphysema can occur from air or gas dissecting under the serosa when the mucosal and the muscular layers are torn but the serosa remains intact.

X-ray examination of the abdomen is useful primarily for the detection of free air in the peritoneal cavity. Failure to see air is not acceptable evidence that rupture or perforation has not transpired.

Diagnosis of injury to the intestinal tract is not readily obvious in most patients soon after injury. However, it always should be suspected and the patient observed for more definite signs; these are early peritonitis and hypovolemic shock. It is most important that the diagnosis be made within the first few hours to avoid the hazards of generalized peritonitis or fatal hemorrhage. The use of the "4-quadrant tap" to detect free blood or intraperitoneal bowel contents that may have entered the free cavity should be considered.

One of the distressing features of a rupture of any viscus within the abdomen is that it may follow any seemingly inconsequential injury. A sneeze, a cough, or a very trivial blow to the abdomen has been at times the only history of trauma that can be elicited.

Mortality. The urgency of early diagnosis and early treatment is reflected in the mortality rates of the many reports. Mortality rate increases exponentially with the duration of time after injury and perforation prior to treatment. Lockwood reported in 1934 mortality rates as low as 15 per cent when patients were subjected to operation within 2 to 4 hours after the injury. A year later, Counsellor and McCormack reported mortality of 60 per cent among all patients injured, but Maingot in 1955 stated that the mortality rate from a tear of the bowel is not higher than 10 per cent if operation is carried out within the first 6 hours. Needless to say, the mortality rate is also a function of the presence or the absence of other injuries, but for the most part the high mortality rate from ruptured bowel continues to be attributable to delayed diagnosis, inadequate replacement of blood, and delay in surgical treatment and age of patient (Roof, Morris and DeBakey, 1960; Biggs et al., 1963).

Treatment. Surgical intervention is indicated in any patient in whom a tear or rupture of the intestinal tract or intraperitoneal hemorrhage is suspected. Nasogastric suction is instituted immediately. Favoring early exploration are shock, intra-abdominal pain with referred pain to the shoulder cap, persistent vomiting, increasing abdominal tenderness, fever, leukocytosis, and intraperitoneal air.

A matter of priority in the treatment of other injuries should be considered. For example, the co-existence of hemopericardium and/or pneumothorax must be corrected first if the patient is to survive his abdominal operation.

The correction of hypovolemic shock is mandatory. Unless the patient is bleeding actively at a brisk rate, shock can be corrected within a matter of an hour or less by the rapid infusion of blood during the period in which the operating room is being set up to receive the patient. Unless contraindicated, a general anesthetic, with supplemental oxygen, has much to recommend its use. The vasodilatation of splanchnic circulation from spinal anesthesia can be troublesome. Antibiotics should be administered prior to operation.

A long paramedian incision is made in order to explore the entire abdominal cavity, making possible satisfactory examination of the stomach, duodenum, liver, kidneys, spleen, pancreas and rectum, as well as careful examination of the entire small bowel and colon. The exploration should be carried out expeditiously but without haste. Unless pulmonary, cardiac, or central nervous system damage has occurred, these patients withstand prolonged surgery remarkably well, provided that adequate blood replacement is continued throughout the entire period of the operation and usually for a few hours at a slower rate while the patient is in the recovery room.

When the abdomen is opened, hemostasis should receive first attention. Continued hemorrhage not only implies continued blood loss and shock, but the dry, clean abdomen is essential if a careful search for perforations and tears is to be made. The stomach, the duodenum, the small bowel and the colon are examined thoroughly throughout for evidences of contusion, subserosal tears, or perforations. One need not fear that shock will be induced by exploring the bowel several times, provided that sufficient blood has been and is being administered. If inadequate transfusion is employed, the manipulation of any abdominal viscera, having a vagotonic action, superimposes vasodilatation upon existing hypovolemia, a bad state of affairs!

The types of lacerations and tears found within the bowel vary considerably and repair may tax the ingenuity of the surgeon. Although the perforation may be only 2 or 3 mm. in diameter, it is advisable to excise the wedge of small bowel extending 1 to 2 cm. beyond the site of perforation. This procedure removes traumatized tissue at the edges of the perforation which otherwise might subsequently become necrotic. One must bear in mind always that more than one perforation may have occurred or that the perforation can be on the mesenteric border and hidden. Consequently, the mesentery, as well as the bowel, should be explored.

When the mesentery artery or one of its branches has been severed, the segment of bowel it supplied should be inspected carefully as to viability. If any question remains, the segment should be resected.

Nonpenetrating wounds of the abdomen produce injury to the small bowel much more frequently than to the colon (Albers, Smith and Carter, 1956). When perforation of the colon is found, the loop involved should be either exteriorized (see Fig. 17, in Chap. 38, Intestinal Obstruction) or resected with a proximal colostomy being performed.

EXTERNAL PENETRATING INJURIES

Penetrating wounds of the abdomen may present serious diagnostic problems to the surgeon in his appraisal as to whether or not the bowel has been perforated. He must recognize the well-established fact that he often may need to explore the abdomen if he is to detect penetrating perforations early. Usually he has no choice. Wounds with ice picks, hat pins, razors and knives in particular are difficult to evaluate. The presence of more than incisional pain and especially the presence of tenderness within the abdomen are very suggestive of bowel perforation and peritoneal soilage, demanding early surgical exploration. It is better to explore such a patient early, finding no perforation, than to delay 10 or 12 hours while a spreading peritonitis develops. When penetrating wounds are present, laparotomy carries little risk.

Abdominal wounds inflicted by bullets and high-velocity missiles vary in extent, according to the velocity, the size and the shape of the penetrating fragment. The abdominal wound may bleed very slightly and yet several loops of bowel may have been penetrated. The introduction of a probe into such wounds to determine whether or not the probe will pass into the peritoneal cavity provides positive information only. More often than not, the probe cannot be passed freely along the path of the penetrating missile, despite the fact that the missile entered the peritoneal cavity.

A roentgenogram is valuable in 2 respects: (1) it may disclose the presence of pneumoperitoneum and be diagnostic of perforation, and (2) it may disclose the site of the missile. Except for the presence of pneumoperitoneum, the early x-ray findings are likely to be uninformative as to bowel perforation.

Gunshot Wounds

Gunshot wounds of the abdomen and the bowel encountered in the military experience during World War II, the Korean War, and Viet Nam have been discussed in Chapter 25, Military Surgery. The best results were obtained when the simplest technical procedures were employed. For wounds of the colon, exteriorization of the injured segment was singularly the best immediate form of therapy. Wounds of the rectum were managed most effectively by closure and the performance of a proximal colostomy, supplemented with the generous use of antibiotics and blood. The average time lapse was about 11 hours from time of injury to operation, according to Chunn's experience (1947), and the mortality rate was 36 per cent in his series. The cause of death was attributed to infection when death from co-existing head and thoracic wounds was excluded; 80 per cent of deaths were attributed to peritonitis.

The mortality rate was highest for wounds of the cecum and the ascending colon and diminished when perforations were situated more distally. The lowest mortality was in injuries to the rectum. These differences have been attributed to the more liquid nature of feces in the proximal colon which allowed greater soilage of the peritoneal cavity.

Better results were achieved during the Korean campaign due to more rapid evacuation and to the more liberal usage of antibiotics, the increased availability of agents with a broader spectrum of antibacterial action, and to administration of more generous quantities of blood and, of course, to the recent experiences and lessons learned from World War II. Experience in Viet Nam shows improvement over Korea, due probably to even better methods of evacuation of the injured.

Compressed Air Injuries

Pneumatic or compressed air injuries of the colon constitute a serious but rare surgical emergency occurring largely in industries employing high-pressure air guns. The usual story is that a prankster fellow worker places the nozzle of the air gun against the anus of the victim who is stooping or perched on a ladder. Occasionally, a worker falls on an air-gun nozzle or is cleaning his clothing with compressed air while wearing them, forgetting or being untutored in the hazard of the air gun. The sudden burst of air ruptures the colon completely or incompletely. Abdominal pain quickly follows. Pneumoperitoneum may or may not be present.

Rupture of the colon is believed to be due more commonly to the quick distention of the lumen more often than to the air volume introduced. However, the pressures encountered from such injuries are many times those encountered in the most severe forms of intestinal obstruction.

While numerous areas of colon may rupture from air gun injuries, there is usually only one which actually perforates (Burt, 1931). Most perforations are located in the sigmoid. The size of the rupture varies from a just discernible split, to a longitudinal laceration running the entire length of the colon (Waugh and Leonard, 1951). Swenson and Harkins (1944) and others describe the lesions as characteristically lying on the antimesenteric border. Burt (1931) found in his studies on cadavers that rupture most frequently took place longitudinally, along the teniae; however, transverse rupture was not a rare occurrence. Waugh and Leonard (1951) state that the longitudinal rupture is fundamentally a series of adjoining transverse ruptures.

Treatment is prompt surgical exploration. In some patients extreme meteorism may exist; immediate trocar decompression of the abdomen may be lifesaving and is a preliminary maneuver essential to the release of associated respiratory embarrassment prior to the administration of anesthesia.

Penetrating Injuries of the Bowel From Within

Swallowed objects, capable of penetrating the wall of the gut, seldom succeed in doing so. Henderson and Gaston (1938) reported only 1 per cent of perforations occurring among 800 patients treated for ingested foreign bodies in the Boston City Hospital. Usually ingested small bones are completely digested within the stomach, although bones of similar size often will pass unchanged when the patient is achlorhydric (Faber, 1938). It is remarkable how many foreign bodies, open safety pins, glass and sharp metal objects pass without difficulty. Undoubtedly many pins perforate the bowel but continue to pass, and healing takes place without leakage.

Perforations more often occur from small objects entering the appendix or a Meckel's diverticulum where they become trapped and may perforate (Bunch, Burnside and Brannon, 1942). Such objects may produce an abscess or peritonitis. Once the foreign body enters the peritoneal cavity, it may migrate to form an abscess some distance away, or become fixed in a position because of the foreign body reaction it may induce without abscess formation.

Treatment is usually expectant. If the foreign body is radiopaque, its progression may be checked by serial roentgenograms or fluoroscopy. Should pain, tenderness, fever and/or leukocytosis occur, surgical exploration is advised. The feeding of a bulky diet to "coat the foreign body" is a dubious procedure. Such a program implies that the foreign body is hung up in the alimentary tract and that bread, cotton or other materials will overtake the foreign body, encase it and aid in its passage. This seldom happens; in some patients the ingested material has surrounded the foreign body and produced obturator obstruction. Catharsis is contraindicated. A regular diet seems to be best (Siddons, 1939).

Proctoscopic injuries or perforations of the bowel from the use of dilators to overcome strictures of the rectosigmoid are hazards to be borne in mind when these procedures are employed. If such an accident occurs, laparotomy should be performed with repair of the perforation and a temporary transverse loop colostomy created at the same time.

Summary of Management of Bowel Trauma

If the management of bowel trauma including gunshot wounds and pneumatic injuries of the abdomen and bowel can be reduced to principles in treatment, the following might be included:

1. Adequate blood replacement: preoperative, operative and postoperative.

2. Institution of gastric suction and catheter drainage of urinary bladder immediately.

3. Assume that the bowel and/or the mesentery have been injured when the bullet(s) or knives, etc., have pierced the abdominal wall or are found by x-ray examination to have lodged within the abdomen: explore within 2 to 4 hours of injury if possible. It is seldom wise to wait for evidence of peritonitis before operating.

4. Secure hemostasis of mesenteric or other vessels before attempting repair of perforations.

5. Ligation of several vessels and correction of shock usually will improve the color of viable bowel and more distinctly delineate between viable and nonviable bowel. Examine carefully all other abdominal organs for perforations and lacerations, including those in the lesser peritoneal cavity.

6. Examine carefully the entire abdominal alimentary tract for contusion, subserosal hemorrhage and perforations. A missile penetration of the bowel almost always will have

a point of exit as well. If none is obvious, enlarge the point of entrance with scissors and examine the mucosa. Search for the point of exit along the mesenteric attachment or the retroperitoneum, duodenum, cecum, ascending and descending segments of colon in particular.

7. Resect any segment of small bowel whose circulatory status is in question.

8. Primary, 2-layer repair of the lacerated colon is indicated if injury is not extensive. When the colon is badly damaged, perform a segmental resection with 2-layer end-to-end anastomosis. Exteriorization should be used in situations where long segments of colon have been destroyed, making repair unduly hazardous or difficult. If the low sigmoid or rectum has been injured, a defunctionalizing proximal colostomy should be performed; the importance of doing a proximal colostomy when in doubt can hardly be overstated.

9. Trim back edges of perforated bowel before suturing the injured area closed, especially should subserosal hematomata exist. This avoids necrosis of the area a few days later.

10. Evacuate and drain all retroperitoneal hematomata through appropriately placed stab wounds.

11. Remove all intraperitoneal collections of intestinal contents by suction, followed by the gentle absorption of the areas involved with warm saline-moistened sponges or laparotomy pads. Irrigation with Ringer's solution may be helpful in some patients.

12. Inspect urinary bladder.

13. Close abdomen but continue the administration of blood and plasma slowly until circulatory status is stable.

14. Dilate rectum if colostomy has not been performed.

15. Administer larger than usual dosages of antibiotics during first 4 postoperative days.

16. Continue nasogastric suction until bowel sounds are heard and flatus is expelled.

17. Observe for latent abscess formation and drain when appropriate (see Chap. 37, Appendicitis, Peritonitis and Intra-abdominal Abscesses).

INFLAMMATORY DISEASES OF THE SMALL BOWEL AND THE COLON

Inflammatory diseases of the intestinal tract are fairly numerous, but idiopathic diverticulitis, ulcerative colitis and regional enteritis are by far the most commonly encountered ones likely to require surgical intervention. Other diseases which on rare occasion require surgical attention are tuberculosis, amebiasis, blastomycosis or actinomycosis, and drug-induced small bowel lesions. The surgeon must bear in mind that bacillary dysentery, food poisoning and pseudomembranous enterocolitis are entities which may confront him in the differential diagnosis of the "acute abdomen" and which call for surgical intervention only if perforation or abscess formation develops as a complication.

Drug-Induced Small Bowel Lesions

Nonspecific ulceration, followed by stenosis, of the small bowel has been reported by several investigators and is believed to be due to the administration of enteric-coated preparations of thiazide-potassium chloride. Apparently, when thiazide-potassium salts are administered without enteric coating, this does not occur. In some, this condition may lead to intestinal obstruction and require operative repair. Presumably, the tablet comes to rest at one site and then dissolves with the full concentration of the potassium salt discharged on a small area of mucosa, producing local edema and ulceration, which may go on to stenosis and obstruction. As Boley *et al.* (1965) and others have shown, it is the potassium salt in these tablets that is responsible for the ulcerations.

Amebiasis

Amebiasis is encountered as a surgical problem for 4 reasons: (1) the erroneous interpretation of intrahepatic or other intraabdominal or pulmonary abscesses; uncomplicated amebic abscesses are preferably treated primarily with amebicidal drugs; (2) when the nature of such abscesses is recognized, they may require surgical drainage should they become secondarily infected with bacteria, usually one of the coliform group; they may also require surgical drainage when they fail to respond to antiamebal drugs; (3) perforation of the colon, usually the cecum; (4) obstruction from amebic granuloma, a rare complication in this disease.

Amebiasis is a systemic disease which is said to mimic as many clinical syndromes as undulant fever, syphilis and tuberculosis combined. It is world-wide in distribution; chronic carriers frequently are nearly asymptomatic. But the surgeon is usually concerned only with its consideration in his differential diagnosis of patients with hepatic or intra-abdominal abscesses of unexplained origin, and in establishing the diagnosis of idiopathic ulcerative colitis or regional enterocolitis.

Amebiasis occurs 5 to 8 times more frequently in men than in women. The pathogen is the *Endamoeba histolytica*, a protozoan usually transmitted from person to person in contaminated food and water supplies. Once within the alimentary tract, the trophozoite resides in the cecum where it attaches itself to the mucosa and begins to invade by virtue of its mobility, aided by the cytolytic enzymes it produces (Frye, 1956). More often, only the mucosa is penetrated; the muscular coats seem better able to withstand the cytolytic action. Once beneath the mucosa, the colony tends to undermine and destroy the submucosa. The result is the small mucosal perforation with a large undermined area, the so-called "flask-shaped" abscess. These abscesses may become confluent with others nearby. For some time the mucosa between the surface perforations remains normal, and only the pinhead-sized ulcerations with their grayish-yellow exudates are seen. If the disease continues to progress, the mucosa is devitalized. It sloughs, leaving the "buffalo-hide" appearance occasionally noted upon proctoscopic examination or at autopsy. It is present more commonly in the cecum.

Lesions are found more frequently in the cecum, the rectum and in the region of haustral valves. Sawitz (1943) attributes the predilection for these regions to the assumption that the fecal current moves more slowly in these areas, affording more leisure for invasion by the protozoan.

Occasionally, the muscularis and the serosa are penetrated, giving rise to amebic peritonitis or to a perityphlic abscess. Nearly always such abscesses are also infected with bacteria of enteric origin.

Toxic megacolon developing during the course of fulminating ulcerative colitis was described in 1950 by Marshak and Lester. Five years later Lumb *et al.* reported 7 cases of "ulcerative colitis with dilatation of the colon."

In 1959 Roth and his associates coined the term "toxic megacolon." This expression was used to describe extreme dilatation of a segment of the colon or of the entire diseased colon that occurred during a fulminating phase of nonspecific ulcerative colitis.

The clinical pattern and complaints of intestinal amebiasis are protean, ranging from constipation to bloody diarrhea. Often malaise, fatigue, constipation and fever are the only complaints, so unless one initiates a self-stimulated search for the organism in the stool, he is not likely to make the diagnosis. In others, bloody diarrhea (occult blood is nearly always present) immediately arouses suspicion.

Representative flecks of feces or mucus are removed with an applicator and examined for the organism, using the direct film method of D'Antoni (1942) or preferably the zinc sulfate centrifugal flotation technic of Faust (1952). In the final analysis, the diagnosis is a laboratory one, depending upon the demonstration of *Endamoeba histolytica* in the stool, body fluids or tissues. As other nonpathogenic ameba may be found within the colon or the feces, e.g., *Endamoeba coli*, these are to be distinguished and not confused as pathognomonic of amebiasis. These nonpathogenic amebae often coexist with *Endamoeba histolytica*.

Occasionally, amebic granulomata, the "ameboma," occur within the small bowel, but more often in the cecum. Definite tumor formation may be observed by palpation and by roentgenogram. Ameboma is the result of massive granulomatous reaction within the cecum and occasionally is confused with carcinoma, stricture or abscess. Unless intestinal obstruction supervenes, the treatment of choice is the use of amebicidal drugs in conjunction with a low-residue diet. Operative intervention should employ only Mikulicz's exteriorization resection with ileostomy, for primary anastomoses in amebiasis of the colon are notorious for subsequent leakage.

Extra-intestinal amebic lesions occur most frequently in the liver and the lung. The amebae are transported from the primary intestinal ulcers to the liver via the portal venous system, resulting in amebic hepatitis and amebic hepatic abscesses. Amebic lesions in the lung may be embolic in origin but are usually secondary to direct extension of subcapsular liver abscesses by rupture through the diaphragm. Although free rupture into the pleural or the pericardial cavities does occur, more often the lung becomes adherent to the inflamed diaphragm, and rupture is direct into the lower lobe (Takaro and Bond, 1958).

Treatment of amebic hepatic abscesses is somewhat debated among authorities in this field. Most prefer a trial of one of the amebicidal drugs, particularly chloroquine or emetine, aspirating the abscess periodically as indicated by the clinical findings. Under this regimen the abscess may subside and disappear permanently. However, in many cases which improve markedly on drug therapy, complete recovery may be delayed until the abscesses are drained. If an amebic abscess becomes secondarily infected, extraperitoneal drainage should be employed (see Chap. 37, Appendicitis, Peritonitis, and Intra-abdominal Abscesses). Transperitoneal or transpleural routes for drainage should be avoided.

Reports of De Bakey and Ochsner (1951) and of Ochsner and De Bakey (1943) extending over a period of 16 years clearly indicate the value of drainage of hepatic abscesses due to amebiasis. The abscess may be aspirated beforehand to determine its nature. The New Orleans group states that the "pus" is typically sterile and that in the stages of early focal necrosis, the protozoa can be demonstrated readily. Later on, however, amebae in such aspirates are difficult to detect.

De Bakey and Ochsner experienced a mortality of 42.9 per cent when amebic abscesses of the liver were present against 6.8 per cent when they were absent. Secondary infection of the amebic abscess was a grave consequence, where the mortality rate of 40 per cent prevailed in contrast with 5.5 per cent when the abscess was sterile. More recent experiences are not available.

Should perforation of the bowel occur, nothing but bold surgical exteriorization of the involved segment will prove to be effective. Operative mortality is high, but with conservative management mortality approaches 100 per cent.

INTESTINAL TUBERCULOSIS

Tuberculosis of the intestinal tract is most frequently secondary to systemic tuberculosis. It may occur in the small bowel or the colon. Usually secondary intestinal tuberculosis is seen in the late stages of pulmonary tuberculosis, although it can occur when the pulmonary is healing. Most physicians consider secondary tuberculosis of the intestinal tract to be the result of the continuous swallowing of sputum containing the bacillus. Once secondary tuberculosis of the intestinal tract with ulceration of its mucosa becomes established, healing is extremely difficult to obtain unless the primary pulmonary disease can be arrested. Continued exposure of the intestinal tract to sputum containing the bacillus favors continuation of alimentary tract tuberculosis.

Primary tuberculosis of the intestinal tract rarely occurs in this country and seldom is observed in conjunction with tuberculosis of other organs. The primary form is probably bovine in origin, whereas the secondary variety is due to the human form of the tuberculous bacillus.

In a study by Rubin (1931), 2 out of 3 patients dying of pulmonary tuberculosis had intestinal tuberculosis. Secondary intestinal tuberculosis is an uncommon finding today when pulmonary disease is not advanced.

Pathology. The pathologic change in secondary intestinal tuberculosis is usually mucosal ulceration. That of primary tuberculosis is more likely to be hypertrophic, a fact which seems to explain why many patients with regional enteritis, a hypertrophic disease of the small bowel in which noncaseating tubercles are found, formerly were considered to have an aberrant form of hypertrophic or primary intestinal tuberculosis.

In the ulcerative form of tuberculosis, the mucosa may become necrotic and desquamate, producing an ulcer. In others, the mucosa remains intact, and the lymph nodes are the only site in which infection can be detected. Although the disease may be located from the stomach to the anus, the terminal ileum is the most frequently involved portion of the alimentary tract, possibly because of its higher content of lymphoid tissue (Peyer's patches) and the affinity of the tubercle bacillus for lymphoid tissue. Peyer's patches are gray and translucent early in the disease but later become swollen, caseous and yellow. The overlying serosa is normal or chronically inflamed.

Healing usually occurs if the systemic disease can be controlled.

Clinical Course and Diagnosis. The disease when present is so frequently a complication of the terminal stages of systemic tuberculosis that secondary intestinal tuberculosis is more often diagnosed at autopsy than during life. Diarrhea with blood and pus in the stool may be observed. However, massive intestinal bleeding is unusual.

Intestinal tuberculosis in patients with pulmonary tuberculosis is to be suspected when the pulmonary disease is healing but the patient suddenly becomes febrile and his condition changes from one of improvement to one of deterioration, an unexplainable course of events on the basis of pulmonary findings. Abdominal pain is the principal symptom aside from diarrhea. If the mucosa is ulcerated and the adjacent peritoneum is irritated, tenderness is also found. Tuberculous peritonitis (the "wet" variety) may follow, but the latter is often seen in the absence of intestinal tuberculosis (Chap. 38, Intestinal Obstruction).

The patient continues to run a downhill course with bizarre manifestations, especially his daily temperature records. Usually, his previous temperature had its maximum point of elevation in the late afternoon, but now he may exhibit his highest fever for the day before noon.

Barium studies may disclose filling defects, particularly in the lower ileum. This finding may suggest intestinal tuberculosis when the disease is known to exist elsewhere. Ileal stasis may be noted when oral barium is administered and is a finding considered suggestive of tuberculosis in this region.

The differential diagnosis centers chiefly about the distinction between other granulomatous diseases such as sarcoidosis, amebiasis, regional enteritis, lymphoma and nonspecific ulcerative ileocolitis.

The prognosis is dependent upon the ability to control pulmonary tuberculosis. If the latter can be arrested, the prognosis for secondary intestinal tuberculosis is good. On the other hand, when intestinal tuberculosis complicates advancing pulmonary tuberculosis, the prognosis is poor indeed.

The treatment is primarily medical and conservative. It consists first of all in controlling the pulmonary disease. A bland diet high in caloric value and containing supplemental vitamins usually is administered. Surgery is rarely indicated unless perforation, intestinal obstruction, abscess or fistulation occurs.

The hypertrophic form of the disease is more likely to produce partial intestinal obstruction and occasionally complete occlusion of the bowel. As this disease is seldom recognized preoperatively, most commonly the lesions are resected without suspecting its nature. This disease, like that of the secondary type, is most commonly present in the ileocecal region.

The hypertrophic form still persists fairly commonly in England and upon the continent of Europe and in other parts of the world where pasteurization of milk is seldom practiced. Its persistence in England and Europe is interesting, for despite the fact that the most effective measure for elimination of bovine tuberculosis had its origin in France, pasteurization as a routine prophylactic measure there, and in many European countries, was slow to be used widely. The only patients whom the author has encountered with hypertrophic primary tuberculosis were seen on shipboard in 2 members of the British crew. Curiously, the 2 British surgeons performing the emergency operations for relief of obstruction in these patients also had been operated upon a few years previously for the same disease.

Fistula-in-ano may develop from intestinal tuberculosis, although this, too, has largely disappeared as a cause of perirectal fistulae in this country. However, all patients with fistula-in-ano should be investigated to exclude tuberculosis as its cause. A normal chest film coupled with a history of drinking pasteurized milk is generally sufficient to exclude tuberculosis as the cause of perirectal fistula in most patients in this country, but smears of pus and tissue examination should be carried out in suspicious cases.

REGIONAL ENTERITIS

In 1932, Crohn, Ginzberg and Oppenheimer resolved a group of nonspecific inflammatory tumors of the small bowel into a single pathologic entity to which they gave the name "regional ileitis." In retrospect, many granulomatous lesions of the small bowel previously attributed to hyperplastic tuberculosis and other granulomatous diseases probably were this entity instead.

For the most part, the disease is found in the terminal ileum; hence the name "terminal" ileitis was used earlier. As multiple diseased areas were soon described affecting different levels of the small bowel, and at times the colon, too, the names "regional" or "segmental" enteritis seemed to be more appropriate. In many quarters the entity is known as Crohn's disease, as it perhaps should be known, since "Crohn's disease" connotes a very specific intestinal granulomatous disease.

Regional enteritis and nonspecific ulcerative colitis have certain features in common, but there is no evidence that these two pathologic states are the same pathologic process. They coexist in about 2 to 5 per cent of all patients. In neither entity is the cause known. Both diseases affect more commonly the young and the middle-aged groups, and neither disease occurs more frequently in one sex than the other. Both have a higher attack rate in the same families than in the population at large. There is some evidence of a strong familial linkage in occurrence rate (Aronson, 1967). Regional enteritis may occur in one member of the family and ulcerative colitis in another. In both diseases personality changes occur, but the patient with ulcerative colitis usually suffers more. However, the pathologic findings are quite different (Lockhart-Mummery and Morson, 1960, and Laipply, 1957).

Etiology of regional enteritis is unknown. No virus or bacterial agent has been recognized as causing the disease. That it is a form of an "auto-immune" phenomenon has been suggested but without evidence, perhaps because we really do not understand what an auto-immune disease consists of.

Pathology. The segment of small bowel involved most frequently is the terminal portion of the ileum, usually extending for a distance of a few inches to several feet. In about 15 per cent of patients, the lesions may be found elsewhere, either as single segments in continuity or as multiple segments with normal regions in between. Rarely is an isolated segment found in the colon; more often lesions in the colon are located in the region of the ileocecal valve and the cecum and are involved in continuity or by extension with that of the terminal ileum. Regional enteritis is primarily a disease of the small bowel. Ulcerative colitis is primarily a disease of the colon.

The diagnosis of regional enteritis at the operating table can be readily suspected from the gross appearance of the bowel alone, although actinomycosis, tuberculosis, sarcoidosis and intestinal lymphoma, including Hodgkin's disease, occasionally have similar gross and roentgenographic appearances. In a few instances, the diagnosis of regional enteritis is possible only when the adhesions are freed and the bowel can be inspected and microscopic examination of tissue is possible.

The involved segment of bowel is inflamed; often its color is livid. Fibrinous exudation is commonly present on the serosal surfaces of the diseased segment and its mesentery during the acute stages. The circumference of the bowel is enlarged, its wall thickened, often causing encroachment upon its lumen so that partial obstruction is a fairly frequent finding. Uninvolved proximal small bowel may be dilated or normal, depending upon the presence or the absence of obstruction. The thickened diseased portions resemble a "rubber garden hose," an analogy commonly used in the gross description of the diseased segments.

Fistulous communications between loops of adjacent small bowel and/or the colon, the bladder, and the vagina are commonly encountered. Abscess pockets between the leaves of mesentery of nearby segments are present not infrequently. Abscesses may be located in the lateral gutters of the posterior abdomen or in the pelvis.

The mesentery is classic in its appearance in this disease. Its serosa is often slightly fibrotic so that its high gloss may be lost. More distinctive, however, is its thickness. At times, the thickness of the mesentery is equal to the diameter of the small bowel that it sustains. The mesenteric lymph glands are always prominent and enlarged in the segment of the involved mesentery. These nodes may reach 2 to 4 cm. in diameter. Should operation be performed early in the stage of the disease, the lymph nodes may not be as enlarged as later on. But they may appear more prominent, as the mesentery is not likely to be as edematous or as thickened as in the subacute or chronic stages of active disease.

The extent of adhesions is a matter of time and continued activity of the disease. Adhesions are usually more prominent when abscess and fistula are present. As a rule, adhesions are short and are found principally between adjacent loops of bowel and parietal peritoneum, agglutinating the gut into a mass which may be felt while palpating the abdomen. Adhesions may be scanty or absent, or they may be prolific. In some patients inspection of the gut at the time of operation discloses a large mass of adhesions, so extensive that the individual loops of bowel are not identifiable. Loops of bowel are encased in fibrous tissue. However, the diagnosis should be suspected, as there are not many other pathologic conditions that produce similar changes within the abdomen.

The mucosa is swollen; its transverse folds are edematous; and small ulcerations are noted fairly frequently along the mesenteric border where they may become confluent, forming linear ulcerations, oval in shape, which may be several centimeters long or run the entire length of the involved segment. Secondary infection often extends into the mesentery or into adherent adjacent loops of bowel, the bladder or the visceral peritoneum. Fistula or satellite abscesses tend to form at these sites.

Microscopically, two features dominate the picture. One is the appearance of multiple granulomatous areas which are characterized by large multinucleated giant cells not dissimilar from those seen in tuberculosis, except that caseation does not occur. Occasionally, these are centered about small foreign bodies which have the appearance of food particles, possibly cellulose, or other material which may have entered from the diseased mucosa.

The second prominent microscopic feature is sclerosing lymphangitis which appears to obstruct the lymphatics and the lacteals. Warren and Sommers (1954) describe the process as being focal with widely dilated lacteals and lymphatics in between. The end result is "elephantiasis" of the bowel segment and mesentery. Indeed, the primary disturbance may well be the obliteration of the lymph and lacteal channels of the mesentery with engorgement of the lymph nodes, lymphedema of the mesentery and finally lymphedema of the bowel itself leading to mucosal ulceration. Reichert and Mathes (1936) recognized the close relationship between the pathologic changes seen in regional enteritis and the changes following experimental chronic mesenteric lymphedema. They felt that the more extensive stenosis and mucosal ulceration found in clinical regional enteritis as compared with their experimental preparations might be due to the presence of a persistent low-grade bacterial infection in the clinical disease. Can regional enteritis be the end result of "mesenteric adenitis" with mesenteric lymphangitis and lactealitis? Further study will be necessary to establish its basic disturbance.

Clinical Pattern and Course. Regional enteritis is a chronic disease characterized by remissions and exacerbations and sometimes spontaneous "cures." The disease is found most frequently in young adults, the average age of onset of symptoms being about 25. However, it may have its symptomatic onset at any age, although 75 per cent of patients acquire the disease before the age of 35. The attack rate is essentially the same for both sexes.

In general the symptoms, signs and clinical course are functions of the rapidity at which the disease progresses, the segment(s) and the lengths of bowel involved, and the complications that develop.

ACUTE SYMPTOMS often simulate an attack of smoldering or subacute appendicitis and more frequently are observed in patients under 25 years of age. Nausea, vomiting, and pain in the right lower quadrant with tenderness and muscular rigidity often are observed. Fever and leukocytosis are generally parts of the total picture in all forms of the disease, although they tend to be more pronounced in the acute stages or when abscesses are present or perforation occurs. Appendicitis is the disease usually suspected, and frequently appendectomy is performed in patients of this group. The fundamental disease may not be detected at the time, as the appendix is often inflamed, and after it has been removed, the surgeon may not choose to explore for the presence of other disease. At times, acute appendicitis is coexistent but usually its inflammatory reaction is secondary to regional enteritis

If the appendix is normal and regional ileitis is found to be the cause of the patient's symptoms, appendectomy is generally advisable if the appendix is not involved. This is done so that, when subsequent bouts of abdominal pain occur, the possibility of recurrent acute appendicitis as a cause no longer exists. There are those who contend that the innocent appendix, when found under these circumstances, should be left untouched because of the possibility that the appendiceal stump may leak and an external fistula develop. Van Patter et al. (1954) reported fistulation in about 25 per cent of cases in which appendectomy was performed. More recently, van Heerden et al. (1967), also of the Mayo Clinic, reported appendectomy without fistulation in patients with Crohn's disease, and endorse prophylactic appendectomy, as do most surgeons today.

ENTERIC SYMPTOMS with chronic diarrhea, pain in the abdomen and the back, weight loss, malaise, fever, moderate leukocytosis and anemia are usually present. These are the symptoms and the symptom complexes most often observed. Gross blood in the stool may occur but is infrequent; occult blood is common. Tenderness of the abdomen is less severe than in the acute group, and a sausage-shaped mass may be felt in the abdomen, located in the right lower quadrant in about 85 per cent of patients in whom it is detected. As the disease progresses, diarrhea and pain become more troublesome. When the pain becomes crampy in nature, impending obstruction should be suspected. The personality changes are similar to those encountered in patients with idiopathic ulcerative colitis.

OBSTRUCTIVE SYMPTOMS in this disease seldom occur in the absence of a previous history of diarrhea, mild to moderate abdominal distress, or pain. Obstruction may be partial or complete. Operative intervention should not be delayed.

ABSCESS AND FISTULATION are late manifestations of the disease, although in unrelenting acute forms these complications may appear within a few months after onset of initial symptoms. They are often associated with signs of partial intestinal obstruction; less frequently they are independent of obstruction but seldom are present without a previous and fairly prolonged history of diarrhea, malaise, weight loss, increasing abdominal pain with tenderness, fever and leukocytosis. This group comprises about 30 per cent of all patients seen with regional enteritis.

Pain is the complaint most consistently given. Diarrhea is present in about 75 per cent of patients, and a palpable mass can be made out in the abdomen in many patients examined.

Roentgenographic findings, when demonstrable, strongly support the diagnosis of regional enteritis but are not specific, as other granulomatous and malignant lesions of the small bowel may produce similar findings. Barium enema filling the terminal ileum may disclose the "string sign" of Kantor (1934) and can be demonstrated in many patients if the wall of terminal ileum is swollen and has encroached upon the lumen, allowing only a thin thread of barium to pass into the ileum on barium enema examination. This thin thread of the barium shadow may be several inches in length (Fig. 39-1). It is usually a late manifestation of the disease and often likely to be associated with symptoms of partial intestinal obstruction.

The significance of the genetic and environmental factors in the incidence of nonspecific inflammatory disease of the bowel continues to stimulate great interest. Studies of multiple occurrences in family units have been published (Mendeloff et al., 1966). Theories as to such occurrences, ranging from a common immunologic defect within a family to an environmental factor such as early weaning, have been proposed.

Finding multiple cases of granulomatous enteritis within a family unit is probably more than a casual coincidence. The reported prevalence of regional enteritis in England varies from 9 per 100,000 to 14 per 100,000. Figures obtained in the United States are slightly higher (Almy and Sherlock, 1966).

Other x-ray findings are "feathering" of the plica circulares with some separation of the mucosal pattern due to edema. Later the mucosal pattern is largely destroyed. These findings are helpful in detecting the presence of disease in the jejunum and the upper ileum when the diagnosis is rarely established for the terminal ileum. The lesions of the proximal small bowel are detected when the small bowel is filmed serially after the administration of oral suspensions of barium. Oral barium should not be administered when symptoms of intestinal obstruction are present.

Diagnosis and the differentiation of regional enteritis from other diseases of the small bowel is largely a presumptive one, to be confirmed by microscopic examination of the re-

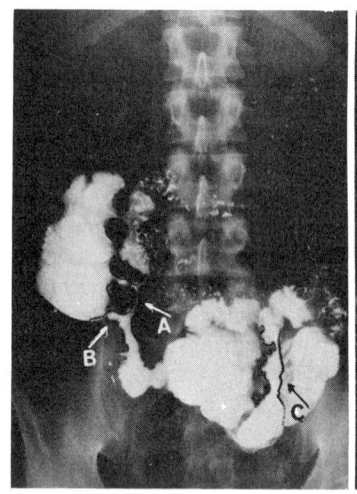

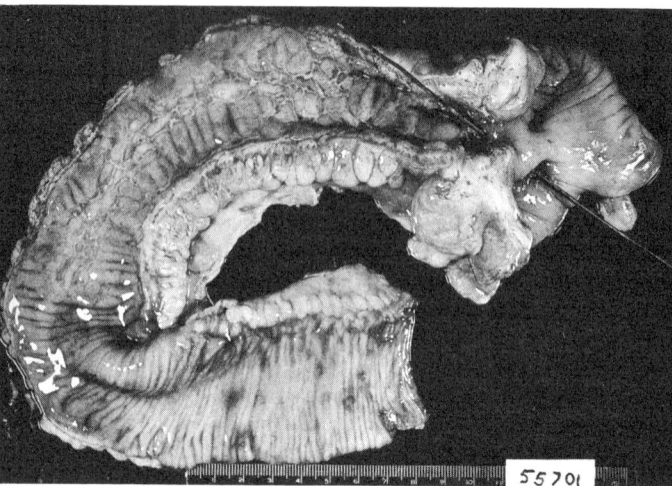

FIG. 39-1. Barium enema of a 34-year-old male with regional ileitis, showing narrowed segments of ileum at points A and C. Point A resembles a "string." Point B is a fistulous communication between the lower ileum and the cecum. Also shown is the resected specimen with the probe passing through this fistulous tract. Note the edema and the "trough" of confluent ulcerations of the mucosal folds along the mesenteric border. Thickening of the bowel wall is clearly indicated; the edematous mesentery is not shown.

sected specimen. Nonetheless, the presumptive diagnostic evidence in favor of Crohn's disease is usually strong despite the fact that at times lymphoma, tuberculosis and mycotic infections may produce local hypertrophic lesions that may simulate regional enteritis. Two features of regional enteritis usually not well mimicked when the specimen is viewed at the operating table are the hypertrophic mesenteric lymph nodes and the thickened mesentery. The history, the physical findings and the positive x-ray findings of the bowel with negative chest films are very helpful. However, the extensive hypertrophy of the wall of the small bowel in primary intestinal tuberculosis usually is not suspected until the resected specimen is examined histologically. If in doubt at the operating table, biopsy of an enlarged lymph node usually will disclose tubercles with caseation in tuberculosis but not in regional enteritis.

Amebiasis is largely a diagnostic problem when the stools are negative for parasites in patients with amebic granuloma of the ileocecal area. In patients with amebic granuloma, "ameboma," the diagnosis may be established only when the resected specimen is examined histologically. Amebiasis much more often affects the cecum and the ascending colon; regional enteritis affects primarily the small bowel. The cecum and the proximal portion of the ascending colon are usually involved in regional enteritis, secondary to this disease in the terminal ileum.

Carcinoma is exceedingly rare in the small bowel but commonly found in the cecum and the ascending colon. This seldom presents a serious diagnostic problem in regional enteritis, especially if the terminal ileum can be visualized with barium. Ulcerative colitis extending into the ileum may be very difficult to distinguish from regional enteritis extending into the cecum and the ascending colon.

Treatment of the complications of regional enteritis is primarily surgical at the present time. Symptomatic regional enteritis may improve under medical therapy, which includes corticoids and ACTH therapy.

Once abscess, stricture or fistulation occurs, nothing short of surgical intervention affords any benefit. Crohn (1953) sums it up in the following manner:

A specific conservative or medical approach does not exist; the long, slowly downward course cannot be interfered with or changed by any method now known . . . sulfonamides occasionally produce good results. Penicillin is useless, and Aureomycin may cause diarrhea and vomiting. . . . Streptomycin, given orally or parenterally, and chloramphenicol, given orally, frequently produce strikingly favorable results, but follow-up studies are too limited to warrant definite opinions as to their ultimate value. . . .

Even with the newer antibiotics, the situation medically has not improved very much.

In adults with ulcerative colitis, the indications for operation include such major complications as exsanguinating hemorrhage and fulminating disease with toxic megacolon; colonic obstruction; colonic carcinoma; and "intractability"—best defined as disease that is so severe and resistant that the patient cannot follow a normal pattern of living. What are the indications for operation in children with colitis? Do these differ essentially from those generally accepted in treating colitis in adults?

Tumen *et al.* (1968) state that the indications for surgery in children with ulcerative colitis are often the same as in adults with the disease. Thus, four of the 18 patients reviewed were operated upon for such emergencies as toxic megacolon, massive hemorrhage, or colonic perforation, and five were operated upon because of intractable disease. This review emphasizes, however, two features of ulcerative colitis in children that have particular significance and that must be considered to be related specifically to the problem of the surgical treatment of colitis in young patients. Four patients were operated upon because the bowel disease had caused stunting of growth and infantilism. Removal of the colon was followed by gain in weight, attainment of normal growth, and in the two patients who had passed the age of normal puberty without sexual development, subsequent normal pubescence. There are probably multiple reasons why ulcerative colitis in childhood may interfere with growth and development. These include malnutrition, blood and protein loss, chronic infection, and the effect of all of these on pituitary and adrenal function. Long-continued steroid therapy and emotional factors may also have some influence. Whatever the mechanism, the dire effects of active ulcerative colitis in young and preadolescent children must be recognized. A child with colitis must be observed carefully for any evidence of retardation of growth or lack of normal development. Inadequate growth must be considered an indication for operation. Operation, even though colectomy is required, must be accepted at an age when removal of the diseased bowel will still permit normal growth and development to be achieved. To delay operation unduly adds immeasurably to the risk of permanent stunting and infantilism.

The form that surgical therapy should take is slowly becoming better defined, and there is better, though not complete, agreement as to which particular operation should be applied to the particular clinical forms of the disease.

The indications for surgical intervention are:

1. Medical failure
2. Abscess with or without fistula
3. Stricture with partial or complete obstruction
4. Massive hemorrhage (rare)

If resection is carried out, the enlarged lymph nodes and edematous mesentery present certain technical and pathologic considerations and problems, for which there is no very conclusive answer. The author, inclined toward the theory that primary obstruction of the mesenteric lymphatics and lacteals may be the basic disturbance responsible for the changes in the ileum or the jejunum in regional enteritis, attempts to resect the enlarged lymph nodes and edematous mesentery of the segment of bowel involved unless this procedure should entail resection of too large a bowel segment. In early cases, however, such resections along anatomic lines are readily feasible. The results are usually good when this type of resection is possible.

Resection of bowel always demands the removal of 10 to 20 inches of grossly normal bowel on either side of the lesion if one is to remove all microscopic evidence of disease. This concept may be useful in the opposite direction, too, for if the amount of bowel which needs to be resected to eliminate diseased mesentery is too great, a bypass procedure may be necessary.

Ileocolostomy with exclusion is an operation which has regained some popularity within the past decade. It has been recommended as the primary operation when the terminal ileum is the only segment diseased. By this method, the terminal ileum is divided about 12 to 18 inches above the diseased segment. The distal portion of the divided segment is closed. The proximal end of the ileum is anastomosed to the ascending or right portion of the transverse colon. Thus all feces are diverted around the diseased terminal ileum. The chief advantage claimed for this procedure is that it carries a lower mortality rate. To date, the recurrence rate is said to remain about the same as that following resection. However, this bypass procedure is successful only if an adequate amount of normal small bowel proximal to the diseased portion is included. Subsequent exploratory laparotomy discloses in many instances regression of the disease with scarring, and in some patients evidence of gross disease disappears. However, the same course of events is noted when an ileotransverse colostomy is performed without further exclusion of the diseased bowel (Heaton, Ravdin, Blades and Whelan, 1964).

Not all accept the bypass and exclusion operation as the preferred method of surgical treatment (Colcock and Vansant, 1960). Moreover, among those who elect to perform this procedure, the indications for its use also vary considerably. In general, the bypass-exclusion procedure is preferred when more than one area of the jejuno-ileum is involved and the major disease is affecting the terminal ileum. The bypass procedure is not well suited for other diseased areas of the small bowel. Some believe it to be the procedure of choice for early disease; others prefer to restrict its use for more advanced stages. A complication reported in the use of extensive bypass procedures or extensive resections of the small bowel for regional enteritis, as well as for other conditions, has been the occasional development of hypocalcemia (DeMuth and Rottenstein, 1964). In addition, among other abnormalities that may develop are generalized malnutrition, disturbances in electrolytes, and especially vitamin B_{12} deficiency in the blind-loop syndrome (see Chap. 38).

This author prefers to limit the use of bypass procedures to patients with previous resections above the terminal ileum who now have recurrences involving the terminal ileum, or to those who have other segments of the bowel involved but in whom the dominant disease is found in the distal ileum. The results with resection are good if the mesenteric involvement also can be removed completely without resecting more than 4 to 8 feet of small bowel.

Some British surgeons (Aylett, 1960; Hughes, 1963) report good results by restoring continuity of the bowel, resecting the abdominal colon, and then anastomosing the ileum to the rectum. The good results they report are unusual to most American surgeons whose results have been so poor with this procedure that it has generally been abandoned in favor of abdominal colectomy with excision of the rectum and performance of ileostomy (Waugh et al., 1964).

It is to be admitted that no one operation has gained universal acceptance. The diversity of procedures currently employed reflects the problems clinically encountered and the continued failures in about 15 per cent of cases regardless of which operation is performed. The most likely cause of recurrence is the inability or the failure to remove all of the disease originally present, including mesentery.

Primary regional enteritis of the colon is being reported with increasing frequency. It appears to be the same pathologic entity as Crohn's disease of the small bowel. In the colon it may or may not be associated with involvement of the small bowel, and vice versa. Among 151 patients operated upon for primary ulcerated disease of the colon, Hawk et al. (1967) reported 87 cases to be Crohn's disease. The appearance of the colon is similar in every way to the appearance of the involved small bowel with Crohn's disease. The colon is thickened, its surface tends to be covered with mesenteric fat, its wall is edematous and its mucosa is ulcerated, with irregular islands of uninvolved mucosa between serpiginous ulcerations. The surgical treatment of Crohn's disease of the colon is colectomy with ileostomy when medical treatment fails. There are other causes of granulomatous colitis, of which Crohn's disease is one—sarcoid, eosinophilic granuloma and other infrequent disorders.

NONSPECIFIC ULCERATIVE COLITIS

Nonspecific ulcerative colitis may be acute and fulminant, subacute, chronic, relapsing and recurring in nature. As its cause is unknown and its courses at times spontaneously remitting, methods of treatment often have been controversial. After examination of the patient and consideration of his course, appropriate treatment is often self-evident when contemplated in light of the pathologic process and the clinical facts at hand.

Etiology. As the name implies, the cause of nonspecific idiopathic ulcerative colitis is not established. There are many agents that may cause an ulcerative colon, such as amebiasis, bacillary dysentery, tuberculosis and mercuric poisoning, but these are not of concern here.

From time to time, various suggestions have been made as to its pathogenesis. Among them are bacterial and virus infections, toxins, allergens, enzymatic disorders, collagen disturbances, and emotional or psychiatric disturbances. Some evidence can be marshalled in defense of each claim but in no instance is it sufficient to warrant the conclusion that a specific pathogen is uniformly responsible for the disease or, for that matter, solely responsible for the disease in any one patient.

A most impressive clinical feature is the emotional instability of most patients with this disorder. So striking is the psychological overlay that some have expressed the belief that such disturbances alone accounted for its pathogenesis. There is, however, no evidence to support this contention and much information to suggest that the psychological disorders are secondary. There is some evidence that pre-existing emotional disorders may precipitate the *initial* attack; however, there is strong evidence that emotional or physical stress often precipitates *subsequent* ones (Lepore, 1965). The precipitating role of emotional distress in acute relapse, once the disease has been established, is illustrated by the following case abstract:

A 32-year-old salesman was admitted in March, 1939. His history was that of fairly mild ulcerative colitis of 7 months' duration. The diagnosis was arrived at by exclusion; the barium enema and the proctoscopic examination findings were compatible with mildly severe chronic ulcerative colitis. With bed rest, sedation, dietary adjustments and reassurance, symptoms remitted.

For 2 months following hospital discharge he remained symptom-free. On the 66th day, his twin brother developed acute perforative appendicitis and died 2 days later. Our patient suffered an immediate fulminant relapse from which he died 72 hours later.

Until an etiologic agent is established, the possibility exists that nonspecific ulcerative colitis is a clinical syndrome which may result from a variety of causes and that no one specific therapeutic agent may prove to be uniformly effective.

Pathology. The systemic and local manifestations of nonspecific ulcerative colitis are sufficiently variable that it is not surprising the pathologic findings also should vary considerably.

FULMINANT NONSPECIFIC ULCERATIVE COLITIS with death occurring within a few days to a few weeks discloses the colon to be grossly dark and seminecrotic. Its serosal surface ranges from dusky red in color to purple or black. Fibrinous exudate is scanty. Free serosanguineous fluid is often present within the peritoneal cavity, but unless perforation has occurred, the exudate is not very purulent nor especially fibrinous. Numerous enteric bacteria often can be cultured from the fluid. The mesentery is moderately edematous, but there is remarkably little enlargement of its lymph nodes in contrast to regional enteritis.

The colon is usually shortened by one third or less of its usual length, particularly if the fulminant course is superimposed upon the chronic disease. Usually the entire colon and the rectum are involved in the fulminant form of the disease. The mucosal surface is seminecrotic if not desquamated. The ileocecal valve and the terminal 2 to 6 inches of ileum may show similar changes.

Microscopically, there may be little or no mucosal surface remaining. That which may be found frequently contains numerous small abscesses within the crypts of the glandular epithelium. The muscular and serosal layers are infiltrated with polymorphonuclear leukocytes. Numerous thrombi are found throughout the intramural vessels of the colon. Acute vasculitis is widespread in the walls of the colon and the rectum. Focal necrosis is common and often confluent. Perforation and multiple areas with small pericolonic abscesses may be found. However, extension of thrombi beyond the marginal mesenteric vessels into the larger portal radicals is seldom observed.

Ulcerative colitis in children tends to follow a slightly different course than in adults (Michener *et al.*, 1964). The extracolonic symptoms tend to appear before symptoms of

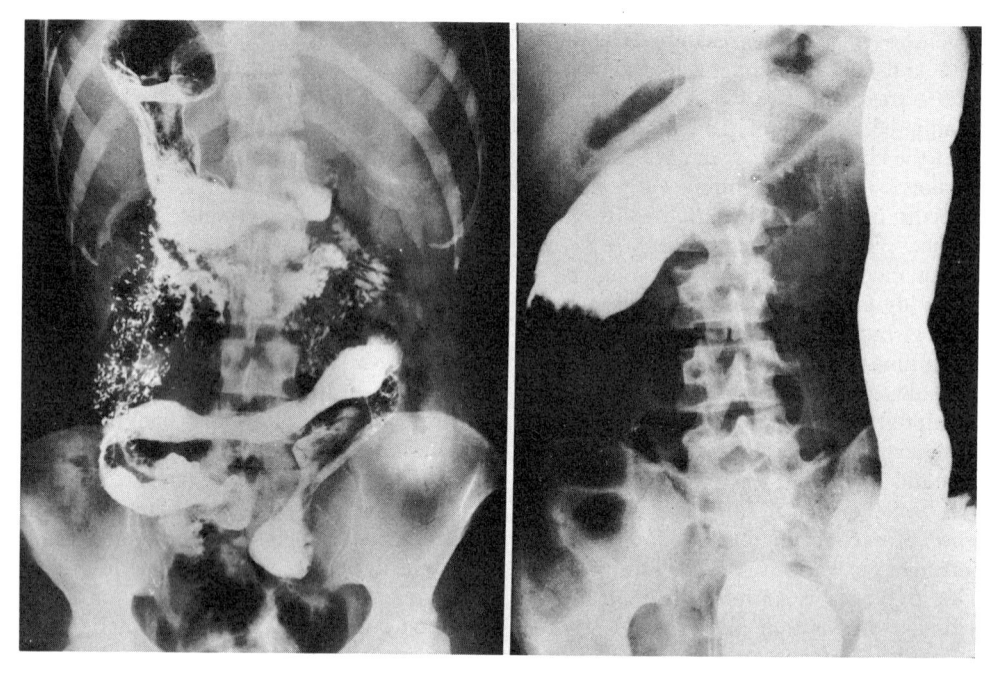

FIG. 39-2. Roentgenograms of the colons of 2 patients with chronic nonspecific ulcerative colitis. (*Left*) The shrunken colon; the ascending and the descending colon segments lie more mesially than they usually do and are contracted, drawing the transverse colon into the lower abdomen. (*Right*) Shows less shortening, but note the loss of haustral markings throughout and the stricture at the hepatic flexure which proved to be inflammatory when the resected specimen was examined. Preoperative decision as to malignant or benign nature of the stricture was not possible on the basis of the barium studies alone.

diarrhea and blood loss. Medical treatment is less likely to be effective, and in this group the complications are often worse. Growth is retarded, sexual maturity is usually delayed, and cancer of the colon is a more frequent complication in the later life of those who develop ulcerative colitis in their youth.

CHRONIC NONSPECIFIC ULCERATIVE COLITIS displays a less uniform pathologic appearance. It most frequently affects the rectum, least often the cecum. In order of frequency are the rectum, the rectosigmoid, the rectosigmoid-descending colon, etc. Occasionally, the disease is segmental, or at least some portions of the colon are more extensively diseased than others. In most patients with advanced disease the entire colon is involved.

Grossly, the colon is shortened considerably, often less than half of its normal length. The splenic flexure no longer rises high into the splenic fossa, the sigmoid redundancy is lost, the cecum, the ascending and the transverse colonic segments are short, all of which tend to give the x-ray appearance on barium enema examination of a "sickle-shaped" structure. The lateral portions of the colon are usually drawn to a more mesial position than its usual "picture-frame" location (Fig. 39-2). The haustral markings are lost, providing the "lead-pipe" characteristics seen on the barium contrast films (Fig. 39-3).

The serosal surface has lost much of its sheen; it is dull and grayish pink in color. Its surface is usually free of fibrinous exudate, save for areas of impending perforation. The wall of the colon is thickened, perhaps twice as thick as normal, but this is still an unremarkable finding compared with the thickening of the small bowel or the colonic segments in regional enteritis.

Several small perforations on the mesenteric margins with abscess formation in the mesentery are frequent findings in the advanced stages, particularly in the sigmoid-rectum

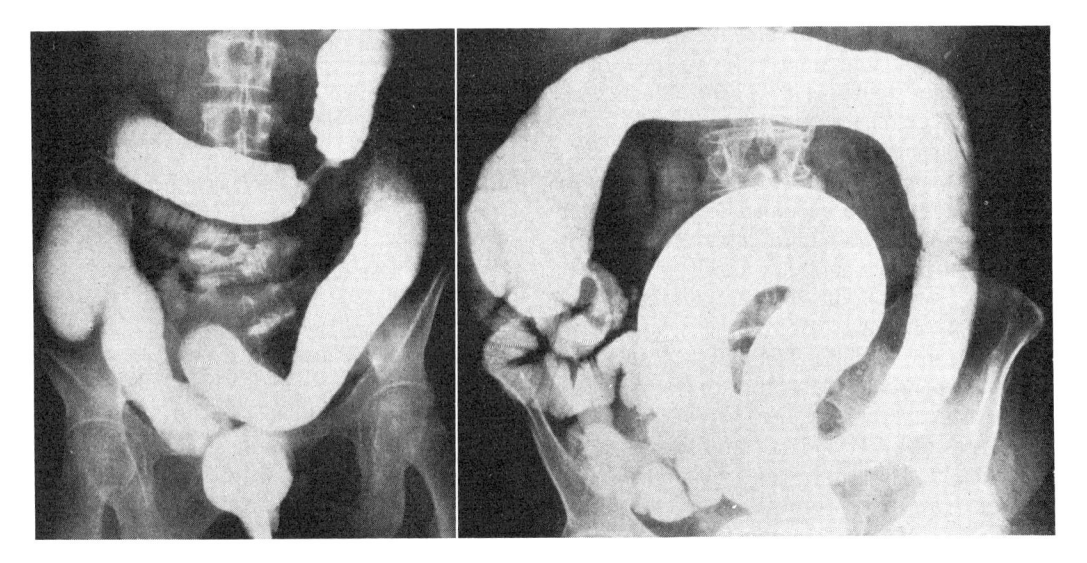

FIG. 39-3. (*Left*) Shows the "lead-pipe" appearance of the colon silhouette in nonspecific chronic ulcerative colitis. In addition, note the stricture in the left portion of the transverse colon which proved to be carcinoma. (*Right*) Also has a "lead-pipe" appearance, but this patient did not have ulcerative colitis. Instead, she suffered from chronic constipation and had taken mineral oil daily for 25 years; mineral oil, chronically administered, is known to produce this change in some patients.

where they tend to dissect downward, often forming perianal, rectovesical or rectovaginal fistulae. Abscess formation is also a frequent finding at the sites of stricture formation, the latter being a fairly common complication in the chronic state and one of the stellar indications for operation.

The mucosal surface in chronic ulcerative colitis shows a variety of changes. Ulcerations tend to run in the longitudinal axis of the colon and to be more prominent along the teniae coli with lateral cross extensions, similar to a spider web. The remaining mucosa is edematous with the ulcerated edges overhanging the denuded and undermined surfaces, often giving the appearance of multiple polyps —pseudopolyps. The strictures encountered may nearly occlude the lumen.

Carcinoma is encountered in 2 to 5 per cent of all cases with chronic ulcerative colitis and in 10 to 15 per cent of cases which develop in childhood and are severe but do not receive surgical treatment. The longer the duration of the disease the higher the percentage of carcinoma. The threat of carcinoma does not reach such proportions that prophylactic colectomy should be considered for this reason alone. Its frequency rate is 6 to 8 times greater than in the general population, it tends to occur in the more proximal portions of the colon, and the prognosis appears to be worse when carcinoma occurs in a colon with ulcerative colitis than in a normal colon (Welch and Hedberg, 1965). Cancer, as a complication of Crohn's disease of the colon, by contrast, is rarely seen.

Microscopically, the colonic mucosa is infiltrated with inflammatory cells. Its surface, where mucosa remains, is superficially ulcerated as well. Therefore, the crypts are shallow, though often plugged with detritus and leukocytes, giving rise to myriads of small, almost miliary abscesses. Submucosal layers are edematous and fibroplasia is usually evident. Muscular hyperplasia is often described, but it is difficult to determine whether this is true hyperplasia or a functional thickening due to the longitudinal shortening of the colon. Except where abscess or perforation is present, the seromuscular coats show surprisingly little pathologic reaction for so extensive a disease that is present in the mucosa.

Clinical Course. *Fulminant or colitis gravis* form may occur as the first attack or it may be superimposed as an exacerbation upon the chronic form. Bowel movements are frequent, 15 to 30 a day, and almost always show blood with pus and mucus also. Fever, anemia and exhaustion are characteristic.

The anus and the lower rectum can be very painful; fissures often are observed. The entire colonic area of the abdomen becomes tender, and moderate distention may be present. Cramps are frequent and usually associated with an attitude of gloom, irritability and despair.

Weight loss is rapid. The hollow cheeks and the sunken eyeballs resemble those of severe shock or dehydration. These are due to excessive losses of water and salt and to loss of fat and protein. The hands, the arms and the legs show a remarkable loss of muscular substance. The bony thorax, the anterosuperior spines of the ilium, the spinous processes of the vertebrae and the bony sacrum are all prominently visible; pressure necrosis of skin and subcutaneous tissue is difficult to avoid over these weight-bearing areas when in bed.

Peristalsis is hyperactive.

Anemia is prominent, requiring frequent transfusions, often several a day, to keep ahead of blood loss and peripheral circulatory collapse. Crossmatching becomes increasingly difficult because of the frequent occurrence of "cold agglutinins" (see Chap. 8, Blood Transfusion). Leukocytosis is pronounced, often in excess of 25,000 cells per cu. mm. of blood. Leucoantigens may develop.

Fever mounts higher and higher, frequently ranging between 104° and 106° F. in the fulminant state.

The patient becomes increasingly toxic and confused and lapses into coma if he fails to respond. Death then may occur from 24 to 36 hours later from irreversible shock, peritonitis, exhaustion or toxemia—singularly, in combination, or collectively.

Chronic nonspecific ulcerative colitis as well as the fulminant variety are largely diseases of the young and the middle-aged adults. The age and sex distribution of 100 illustrative patients studied by Kirsner and Palmer (1948) is shown in Table 39-1 and is fairly representative of the experience of others in 1968.

The duration of the disease in their patients at the time they were first seen ranged from a few months to more than 15 years. The mor-

TABLE 39-1.

	AGE AND SEX		
Decade	Male	Female	Total
1–9	3		3
10–19	7	17	24
20–29	17	21	38
30–39	12	9	21
40–49	7	4	11
50–+	2	1	3
Total	48	52	100

(Kirsner, J. B., Palmer, W. L., Maimon, S. N., and Ricketts, W. E.: J.A.M.A., 137:922, 1948.)

tality rate was highest within the first 2 years of illness and became progressively lower as chronicity increased. The course characteristically was one of remissions and exacerbations with only 6 whom these authors were willing to consider as possible "cures."

The severity of clinical symptoms tended to parallel the degree to which the colon was involved. This relation was no means a constant one. Nor did the severity of the roentgenographic findings correlate more than in a general way with the severity of the clinical manifestations, although the presence of stricture was more commonly associated with the more serious complications: continued hemorrhage, diarrhea, distention, cramps, abscess and fistulation.

Relapses in the Kirsner-Palmer series of patients could be associated with emotional disturbances in 34 per cent, respiratory infections in 29 per cent and physical fatigue in 14 per cent. It is to be emphasized that relapses are commonly associated with trials of everyday life. This association is not evidence that such stresses play a fundamental etiologic role (see Etiology). As these same stimuli often cause diarrhea among the normal population, it was believed that their effects should be more pronounced among those with inflammatory disease of the colon, a postulate which, indeed, is difficult to deny.

Despite the serious pathologic changes of the bowel, many of these patients had little disability, and some remained in good health for longer than a decade. Disability in this disease is relative, largely a matter of the patient's tolerance for inconvenience, and it is therefore hard to evaluate. Fourteen per cent died

—9 per cent while on medical management and 5 per cent after operation.

The complications were and are numerous and varied in this particular series as well as in all others similarly studied. Nineteen per cent developed stricture; 17 per cent developed abscess and fistula; in 16 per cent polyps occurred; 12 per cent had severe bleeding from the bowel; 8 per cent had arthritic manifestations; perforation with peritonitis occurred in 6 per cent; and carcinoma in 2 percent. Infections of various types were frequent, and thrombophlebitis occasionally noted. About half of the patients developed pronounced hypochromic anemia; and in the more debilitated, hypoproteinemia was usually present with occasional reversal of the albumin-globulin ratio. Vitamin deficiencies occurred unless combated actively in most who were chronically ill for prolonged periods. Many patients developed more than one complication.

The initial roentgenographic findings in 24 of 89 patients were normal. The entire colon was abnormal in 30 patients; the rectosigmoid involvement alone was found in only 11. Involvement from the rectum to the splenic flexure occurred in 12 with another 8 having involvement from the rectum to the hepatic flexure (see Table 39-2).

This experience is rather typical for any group of carefully managed patients with this disease carried on conservative or medical therapy. Perhaps the complications of abscess, perforation, peritonitis and carcinoma are higher than this series indicates, as some patients with these complications were admitted directly to the surgical services and hence not included in the Kirsner-Palmer series.

The author has encountered 8 patients with chronic nonspecific ulcerative colitis who developed cirrhosis and portal hypertension later on. These were successfully treated by portacaval shunts. Possibly the hepatitis and the cirrhosis were secondary to ulcerative colitis, recognizing the ease with which the virus particles of hepatitis might enter the portal circulation, from the ulcerative surface of the colon or that the cirrhosis could have been in part nutritional in origin or perhaps a combination of both (see Chaps. 35 and 36), but other reasons for this association may exist.

The personality of the patient with nonspecific ulcerative colitis deserves special mention and understanding upon the part of the physician and the surgeon alike, if cooperation of the patient is to be elicited in the therapeutic program that they wish the patient to follow. To conclude that the personality is more than a complex combination of neuroses accumulating in the course of a most distressing illness does not seem to be warranted from the data at hand. Infantilism, dependency and emotional instability are characteristic, but these seem to be manifest expressions of persistent cramps and painful diarrhea rather than descriptive of psychological disturbances.

Once relieved of their disease, many of the overt personality disorders disappear, although not without leaving their marks. In the meantime, persistent patience on the part of the physician is as rewarding as most other forms of conservative therapy. An excellent review is that of Zetzel (1964) who comes to these same general conclusions. Medical treatment should not be persisted in unless rewarding results are being achieved.

Diagnosis. The diagnosis of nonspecific ulcerative colitis is one of exclusion: exclusion of amebiasis, bacillary dysentery, tuberculosis, polyposis, diverticulitis, carcinoma and specific causes of ulcerative colitis. Stool culture and repeated examinations for the presence of parasites within the bowel exclude

TABLE 39-2.

Extent of Roentgenographic Involvement	Less Than 1 Yr.	1–9 Yrs.	10–20 Yrs.	Total
Normal	10	12	2	24
Rectosigmoid only	3	7	1	11
Rectum to splenic flexure	6	5	1	12
Rectum to hepatic flexure	2	6		8
Entire colon	10	16	4	30
Segmental	1	2	1	4
Total	32	48	9	89

(Kirsner, J B., Palmer, W. L., Maimon, S. N., and Ricketts, W. E.: J.A.M.A., 137:922)

most infections other than tuberculosis and ameboma.

Proctoscopic examination is perhaps the most direct diagnostic technic when the results of other tests are known. The diffusely granular, friable, superficially ulcerated and bleeding mucosa are diagnostic findings in the absence of other specific causes of inflammation.

The barium enema examination discloses the so-called "lead-pipe" character of the bowel wall with the absence of haustral markings in the involved segment. Frequently, the major or entire colon is shortened. However, the lead-pipe appearance may occur from other causes, particularly the chronic use of mineral oil (Fig. 39-3), wherein the patient's complaint is constipation rather than diarrhea. However, it is to be noted in Figure 39-3 that, while the haustral markings are lost, the colon is not shortened. The loss of mucosal detail is an early finding in ulcerative colitis but not necessarily diagnostic of the disease. Roentgenographic lesions limited to the cecum and the ascending colon should raise suspicion of tumor, amebiasis or tuberculosis in addition to ulcerative colitis. The last has a predilection for more distal portions of the colon and seldom is seen as an isolated disease entity involving only the cecum and the ascending colon. In about 15 to 25 per cent of the patients, the terminal ileum is also involved in ulcerative colitis and may be demonstrated by edematous folds and often with destroyed mucosal patterns in the ileum.

The repeated use of the barium enema and proctoscopic examination over the years is the best protection that can be afforded the patient against delayed detection of carcinoma in chronic ulcerative colitis. Unfortunately, carcinoma developing in the colon with ulcerative colitis carries a poor prognosis. Cytology may be helpful.

The differential diagnosis, aside from amebiasis, tuberculosis, polyposis, diverticulitis, etc., should consider also nonspecific proctitis and lymphopathia venereum. Both of these latter diseases are detected proctoscopically, and the history of bubo with a strongly positive Frei test weighs heavily in favor of the diagnosis of lymphopathia venereum. Nonspecific proctitis may be a form of nonspecific ulcerative colitis and is best treated medically on a regimen similar to that used for mild ulcerative colitis.

Treatment. Divergence of opinion exists as to the best means for treating the patient with nonspecific ulcerative colitis, although the lines drawn are more rational than a decade ago. Operation after a short period of conservative management is no longer frequently practiced today. However, to persist in medical management when the patient's condition continues to fail is equally unsound.

The chief problem centers about the indications for surgical intervention. Considerable variations exist as to the threshold levels of resistance or capitulation on the part of the physician to permit the operative management of his patient. Perhaps the one point about which there is most confusion relates to the emotional disorders of the patient. The disease in the colon may be brought under control medically, but the patient's emotional disorders may continue to be incapacitating. Freed of his colon, many of his emotional ills may disappear, but is this an indication for colectomy? Most believe not.

Patients with mild disease do well on conservative therapy about 85 per cent of the time, although recurrences are the rule. These, too, tend to be mild. About 50 per cent of those with moderately severe disease will respond to conservative management, including corticoids and ACTH, although several months are often necessary to achieve results.

Continued efforts are rewarding unless an early recurrence supervenes. Should this occur, it is well to take stock of what has been accomplished. Hospital costs and loss of gainful employment deserve serious attention, too. The treatment employed should provide not only relief of symptoms but rehabilitation and restoration to gainful employment and a useful life when possible.

Several clinical factors tend to forecast the likelihood for recovery on conservative management: the older the patient at the time of onset of the disease, the better his prognosis is likely to be. Most deaths occur within 2 years after onset and most often before the age of 30; the moderately severe disease in the younger patient may not respond well to conservative treatment. When the disease is limited to the left colon, the prognosis is a more favorable one; the longer the segment of proximal uninvolved colon, the better the outlook is likely to be. The lack of disease in the right colon, the absence of stricture, fistulation and pseudopolyposis are favorable signs, indicating that a good response to conservative treatment may be obtained.

The term toxic megacolon is an unfortunate one. It is thought to apply to a patient with a distended colon from idiopathic ulcerative colitis and is usually associated with impending perforation or an abscess formation because of perforation. It is perhaps better to realize that there are many causes of megacolon, some of which are associated with toxic manifestations not due to idiopathic chronic ulcerative colitis. But there are some patients with a very severe degree of idiopathic ulcerative colitis who have megacolon and symptoms of toxicity. It is in this last classification that the term toxic megacolon is more precisely used.

The indications for surgical therapy are reviewed by Dukes and Lockhart-Mummery (1957). Most physicians and surgeons would agree that surgery is indicated for:

1. Acute fulminating disease with uncontrollable hemorrhage, toxic megacolon, or a continued downhill course despite aggressive medical management.

2. Complications of acute or chronic disease, such as stricture with partial or complete obstruction, perforation of the colon, peritonitis, abscess formation, fistula formation.

3. Medical failure; that is, chronic invalidism or the continued presence or progression of chronic bleeding, arthritis, dermatitis, etc.

4. Carcinoma, proved or suspected. The onset of carcinoma in ulcerative colitis patients is at an average age of 42 years after an average duration of disease of 14 years.

The type of operation performed is no longer held in much dispute. *Total abdominal colectomy and ileostomy* as a 1-stage procedure is the operation of choice for the management of the above indications. Compromise and procrastination add to the complications and have been responsible for many of the poor results and much of the mortality rate. In most patients the 1-stage colectomy is feasible and safe. The rectum may be removed at the same time; this is desirable for 3 reasons: (1) it spares the patient a second operation; (2) no residual disease exists; and (3) the improvement obtained will often make it difficult to persuade the patient that removal of the rectum is necessary at a later date.

Diversionary ileostomy performed to "place the colon at rest" seldom accomplishes anything in advanced disease. For example, in those patients with abdominal colectomy, an intact rectum nearly always continues to show active disease upon proctoscopic examination. Patients who might benefit with temporary ileostomy are those in whom the disease is mild and will improve on conservative management alone. To perform only ileostomy in fulminant nonspecific ulcerative colitis does not rid the abdomen of seminecrotic bowel, and the results are indeed poor. There are few survivals among patients upon whom this was attempted as a last resort procedure. If any operation is to be performed in this moribund group of patients, it should be colectomy. The patient who will withstand ileostomy will also generally withstand at least a total abdominal colectomy.

ACUTE FULMINANT NONSPECIFIC ULCERATIVE COLITIS. Most patients with the malignant form of colitis, colitis gravis, should be subjected to total abdominal colectomy as soon as this course is evident. The clinical problem involved is largely defining when this condition exists. In another sense, the question revolves about what constitutes a medical failure in acute ulcerative colitis. There is no better answer than this: any patient whose stools continue to increase in frequency with larger quantities of blood being lost, whose fever continues to mount, whose abdomen becomes increasingly tender and whose general status continues to go down hill despite vigorous conservative management, should be subjected to colectomy. Once the decision is made to operate, the procedure should be carried out as soon as the operating room can be made ready. Tomorrow may be too late.

As these patients are critically ill, often moribund, it is difficult for the surgeon to muster sufficient courage to perform colectomy; he would rather settle for the diversionary ileostomy under local anesthesia. However, there is no disease within the abdomen other than hemorrhage and panhypersplenism where a patient so near to death will respond as promptly as these patients do once the colon is removed. Each should be given a chance, but the fair chance depends upon

1128 Small Bowel and Colon

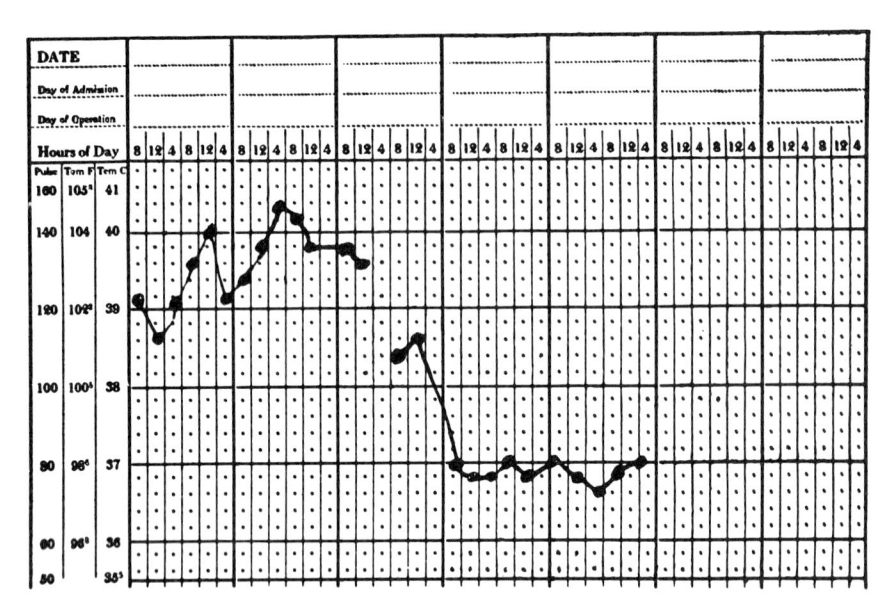

FIG. 39-4. Graphic chart shows the return of temperature to normal the day following total abdominal colectomy. The rectum was removed at the same time.

nothing less than complete abdominal colectomy. Diversionary ileostomy has no place here. The author has employed this approach without mortality in all fulminant cases operated upon since 1950. The abdominal rectum may be divided, closed and tucked beneath the pelvic peritoneum if desired, with extraperitoneal stab-wound drainage established, or it may be removed at the same time.

The response of a patient with the fulminant disease to 1-stage colectomy is shown in Figure 39-4. The high temperature and tachycardia promptly drop and are often near normal within 12 to 24 hours. Toxemia disappears within the same period. Within 2 to 4 days, the patient is able to eat, and complete recovery usually follows rapidly.

Corticoids are administered preoperatively if the patient is not already receiving them. If he is on corticoids or ACTH, as usually is the case, his daily dosage is doubled during the day of operation. Half of the increase is given within 2 hours prior to operation, and the remainder is distributed equally throughout the rest of the day, being added to the base-line dosage levels used prior to operation. These are administered over the next 4 doses given at 6-hour intervals. During the second 24-hour period, the increased increments of corticoids are usually cut in half so that each 6-hour dose now is only 25 per cent greater than the preoperative one. On the second postoperative day, the dosage is reduced to its preoperative level and thereafter is reduced judiciously each 2 or 3 days until discontinued between the 8th and the 10th postoperative days.

The *technical features* of ileostomy construction are important, since the future uncomplicated function of the ileostomy depends on attention to small details. We utilize the technic of Brooke (1954) as modified by Durham (1957).

The location of the ileostomy should be on the right side of the anterior abdominal wall at least 1½ inches away from both the umbilicus and the anterior spine of the ilium. Otherwise, a skin-tight ileostomy seal cannot be maintained. For this reason, the abdominal skin incision for abdominal colectomy should be in the mid-line or slightly to the left and deviating around the left of the umbilicus (Fig. 39-5). It is well to remember that the patient will wear a belt to support his ileostomy appliance so that the stoma should not be placed in or near the waistline; otherwise, the belt will tend to pull the appliance out of position.

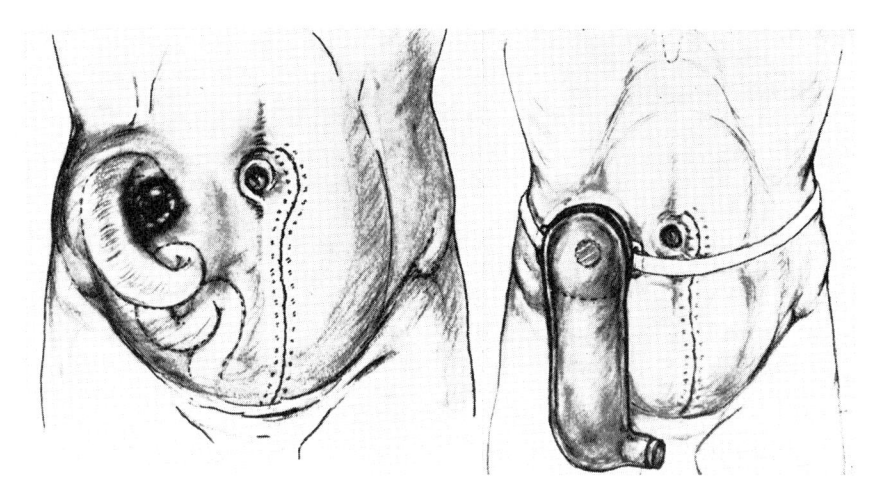

FIG. 39-5. The 2 drawings illustrate the construction of an ileostomy. Note (*left*) that the ileum adjacent to the inner aspects of the abdominal wall can twist and cause obstruction unless this portion of the ileal mesentery is sutured to the parietal peritoneum so that volvulus is prevented. (*Right*) Illustrates the application of a watertight or "skin-seal" ileostomy bag. Note that the location of the ileostomy is such that this appliance does not rest on the anterior superior iliac spine or encroach upon the umbilicus. The operative incision is placed slightly to the left of the mid-line to avoid interference with the ileostomy appliance and its seal.

After selecting the ileostomy site, a circular excision of skin, subcutaneous fat and anterior fascia is made; the muscle fibers are separated, and the posterior fascia incised. If the fascial edges are at all tight, portions are excised so as to obviate the possibility of any stricture. Then the end of the small bowel is brought through this wound and turned back upon itself, forming a double-layered ileostomy stoma with no exposed serosal surface. This prevents the serositis, inflammation, stricture and ileostomy dysfunction which were so common with the older technics. The free edge of bowel mucosa is immediately sutured to the skin margins.

The serosal surface of the mesentery should be sutured to the parietal peritoneum about the ileostomy site internally and along the posterior and lateral surfaces of the right abdominal wall. No sutures should be placed in the bowel segment as it traverses the abdominal wall lest a fistula develop. As an alternative, the extraperitoneal tunnel technic of Goligher (1958) may be used. This internal anchoring of the mesentery to the parietes is said to eliminate the possibility of three postoperative complications of ileostomy: internal hernia, rotational volvulus of the terminal ileum, and prolapse of the ileum through the ileostomy.

Early postoperative management of ileostomy. Immediate application of a temporary water-sealed ileostomy appliance or the use of catheter drainage of the terminal ileum is essential to preventing excoriation of the skin which delays the application of a permanent appliance. More important, skin excoriation promotes low-grade infection of the exteriorized ileum which contributes to stenosis of the ileostomy stoma and the partial obstruction that stenosis may cause.

A No. 26 fenestrated soft latex catheter introduced into the ileostomy for a distance of 5 to 6 inches will often drain away ileal juices for a few days, leaving the skin dry. A ligature snugging or tying the tube to the *tip* of ileal stoma to prevent leakage may be used *only* if it is realized that the distal segment will slough and may result in a skin-flush stoma if an inadequate length of ileum is exteriorized. The final stoma should protrude from $\frac{1}{2}$ to 1 inch from the abdominal wall.

The catheter should be removed on or before the 5th postoperative day after which time plastic ileostomy bags are sealed to the skin and a week or two later a permanent appliance may be worn. Care must be exercised that the portion of the appliance adjacent to the ileostomy does not cause excoriation or pressure necrosis of the ileum, as this will create a small external fistula and cause leakage.

Gentle dilatation of the ileostomy should be performed with the index finger, at least 4 times a week for 5 to 6 weeks.

Before discharge, the patient should demonstrate to the surgeon his ability to apply the sealed bag without injury to the ileostomy and to dilate the stoma satisfactorily. His diet should be bland, avoiding fruit juices and roughages for several months, by which time the ileal contents should be semisolid, if not as formed stools.

A well-performed colectomy and ileostomy is a great satisfaction to the patient with chronic ulcerative colitis. He is free to leave his home to resume normal activity, to raise his family and to be self-supporting. Bacon (1960) has reported a personal service of 468 patients with both acute fulminant and chronic forms of ulcerative colitis who underwent colectomy. The long term survival and rehabilitation rate in this series was 98 per cent at 5 years and 90.5 per cent at 10 years postoperatively.

DIVERTICULITIS AND DIVERTICULOSIS

Diverticular disease includes both diverticulosis and diverticulitis. Diverticulosis eventually affects two thirds of patients who live to be 85 years of age. Diverticula are present in one fifth of all persons over 40 years of age who have barium enema examinations of the colon. Diverticulitis occurs as a complication in 15 per cent of patients who have diverticulosis (Ryan, 1958). As the name implies, this is an inflammatory disease of one or more diverticula occurring in the colon. More than 80 per cent of patients with diverticulosis have their disease situated within the distal descending and sigmoidal segments of the colon. Next in frequency is the cecum, and in some patients the entire colon is involved.

Etiology of diverticulitis is nearly always obstruction at the neck of the diverticula or the impaction of desiccated feces within the pouch which eventually is cause for stercoraceous ulcerations and inflammation of adjacent tissue. These facts do not explain the origin of the basic disturbance—the diverticula. They may be acquired, although certain anatomic features, congenital if you choose to call them, may account for their development in some individuals and not in others.

The diverticulum represents a herniation of colonic mucosa through the muscular layers. This herniation may occur between muscle coats. The muscular layers may be pushed ahead of the mucosal pouch and thinly dispersed over its surface. Diverticula rarely are found in the rectum or along the taeniae coli. Generally, they are located on the mesenteric border or beneath the appendices epiploicae. However, some diverticula appear in regions of the bowel not commonly covered with appendices.

For the most part, however, diverticula appear to arise in areas penetrated by the small vessels entering and leaving the colon. Many pathologists and anatomists attribute the location of diverticula to these regions as related to etiology. It should be easier for the mucosal outcroppings or herniations to proceed along the paths made by these vessels than to make new ones. In some cases the diverticulum dissects between two muscular planes and is therefore incomplete, but nonetheless troublesome.

The diverticulum tends to become larger and its wall thinned out, becoming "teardrop" in shape. The diverticulum does not perforate because of distention unless it becomes inflamed. It is surprising how frequently most or all diverticula empty readily despite the attenuation of the muscular coats. They seem to fill readily when enemas of barium sulfate suspension are administered and to empty fairly promptly soon after the enema is expelled.

Diverticulosis may be found in children and young adults but much less frequently than in older patients. It is observed more commonly in fat individuals with poor muscular tone and in those who have a history of mild or moderate constipation over a number of years. Some of these clinical features are encountered frequently in patients with hiatus hernia and cholelithiasis. In fact, the concurrence of hiatus hernia, cholelithiasis and diverticulosis is fairly common and sometimes is referred to as Saint's triad.

Pathology. Inflammation of diverticula, resulting in diverticulitis, may be acute, subacute, chronic or recurring.

The length of the colon involved is usually 4 to 10 inches. Inflammation of one diverticulum causes sufficient edema to occlude the openings of those adjacent to it. These diverticula, now closed, often become secondarily infected. The length of the bowel segment involved may be fairly extensive if diverticula are extensive. Frequently, the disease may only stop its progression when there are no more diverticula above or below to be occluded by edema or the distance between them is greater than can be bridged by the inflammatory reaction. In some patients with diverticulosis of the entire colon, the disease commences in the sigmoid and extends in retrograde fashion to involve most if not all of the colon. One of the author's patients required resection from the hepatic flexure to the rectum, and in another abdominal colectomy was necessary; however, such occurrences are rare.

Slight bleeding, though often occult, is frequent, occurring in about one fourth of patients with diverticular disease. As the location of a diverticulum is usually alongside a blood vessel, it is not unexpected that ulceration caused by fecal impaction of the diverticulum may erode into blood vessels. The concept has often been expressed in past years that "if the sigmoidal lesion bleeds, it is carcinoma."

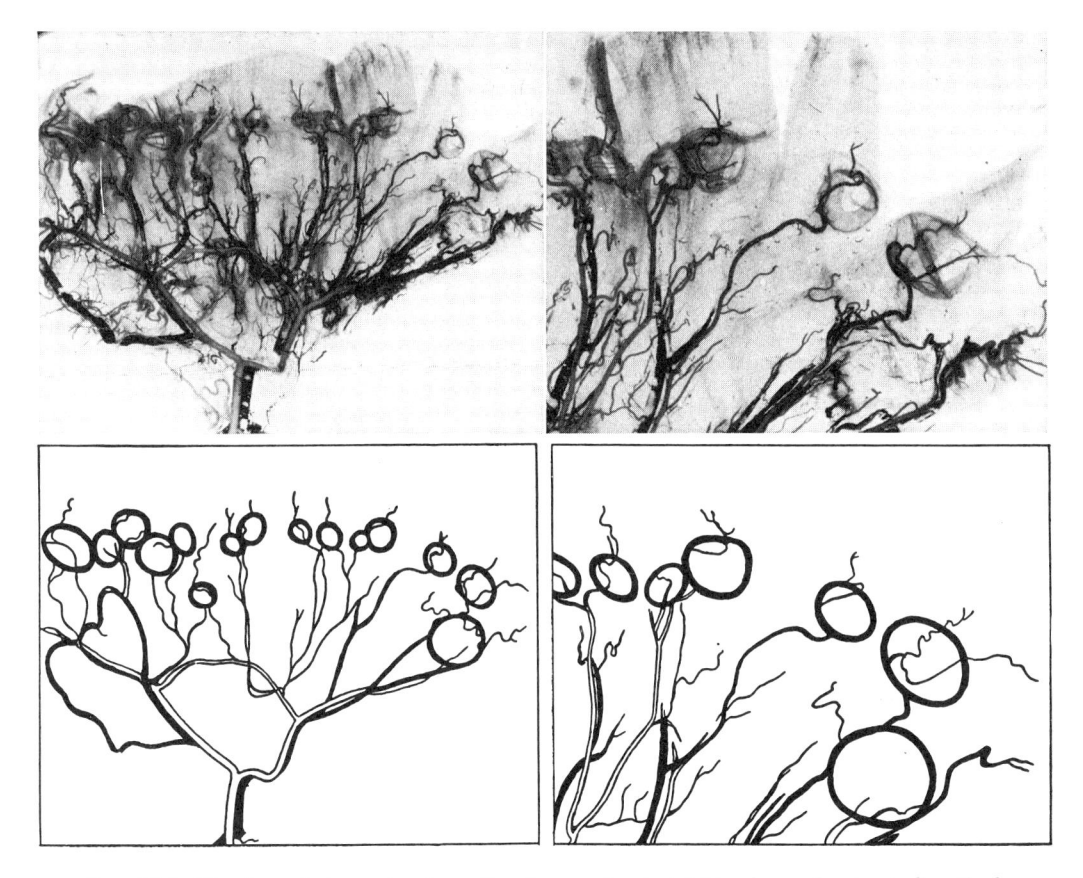

FIG. 39-6. The two photographs show the abnormal arterial blood vessels about diverticula in a resected specimen of colonic wall in which liquid latex was injected to outline the vessels. The specimens were then cleared by the Spalteholtz technic. The arteries are light and the veins are dark. The two drawings below are shown to clarify the nature of the vascular abnormalities. Each corresponds to the photograph immediately above. (Noer, R. J.: Ann. Surg., 141:674)

This point of view is contested by Noer (1955) who believes it to be an erroneous one. Noer's studies disclosed some rather unusual features of the vessels in the regions of diverticula, which he believes to favor bleeding (Fig. 39-6). Studies by Ponka, Brush and Fox (1960) substantiate the opinion that bleeding is not a useful criterion in differentiating diverticulitis from carcinoma of the colon, and the subject has been reviewed by Laufman et al. (1962).

Although serious hemorrhage is a less frequent complication, it does occur in 12 per cent of patients with known diverticula disease (Harkins, 1960). At times, hemorrhage from a diverticulum may nearly exsanguinate the patient and dictate very aggressive treatment (Ulin, Sokolic and Thompson, 1959).

The inflammatory changes in diverticulitis are often extensive locally. Whether or not perforation occurs, pericolitis is usually pronounced, the wall of the colon becomes edematous, and partial or complete obstruction not infrequently occurs. Perhaps the most impressive feature of the disease, noted at the operating table, is the extent of the edema of the mesocolon, the adjacent pelvic structures and loops of small bowel. Certainly, the extent of the gross pathology is usually greater than expected on the basis of preoperative studies. An abdominal mass may be palpated or felt on digital examination of the rectum or the vagina.

Abscess formations within the mesentery, between loops of small bowel or the adherent bladder, are not uncommon and occasionally contain several hundred milliliters of pus.

Fistulous communications between the colon and the small bowel, the bladder or the skin (usually perianal) are not as commonly encountered as in regional enteritis but are by no means rare complications. Pylephlebitis of the sigmoidal veins with miliary or larger abscesses forming in the liver is an infrequent complication, but when jaundice appears in a patient with diverticulitis, this is an easy association to recognize. Adhesions form and are among the more common nonsurgical causes of small bowel obstruction in patients who have had no previous surgery.

Less than 1 per cent of cases have carcinoma as a co-existing feature. The major diagnostic hazard is the failure to recognize that carcinoma may be a "sleeper." There is no evidence that diverticulitis induces carcinoma; the coincidence appears to be explainable on predilection of both diseases for the sigmoid segment of colon.

Clinical Pattern and Course. The symptoms of diverticulitis and the nature of complications are dependent upon the segment of the colon involved, the length of the segment affected, the presence or the absence of intestinal obstruction, perforation, abscess formation with or without fistulation, and bleeding.

Pain is the most common complaint and is located most often low in the abdomen. As the sigmoid is often redundant and may lie across the lower abdomen, bilateral lower abdominal pain is often complained of. Pain is usually constant and not very intense unless perforation or pericolitis occurs with irritation of the adjacent parietal peritoneum. The patient may state that pain is worse with defecation or if jolted when riding in an automobile. He is restless and decidedly uncomfortable in most instances.

When the lesion lies in the low sigmoid, he may complain of a sense of rectal fullness unrelieved by defecation, especially if an abscess is developing. The stools are frequently loose and may be small in caliber.

Chills and fever may be noted. A chill with high fever raises the alarming question of migratory pylephlebitis of the sigmoidal veins with possibly early intrahepatic abscess formation. On the other hand, these symptoms may be the result of abscess formation with or without cystitis and urinary tract infection, or they may imply perforation. Low-grade fever is commonly encountered in the active stages of the disease.

Bilateral lower abdominal tenderness is commonly present when the disease is active; of course, tenderness may be elsewhere if diverticulitis is in a part of the colon other than the sigmoid. Abdominal tenderness is maximum over the point of inflammation, except for perforation, abscess and pericolitis. Tenderness usually is not exquisite, although it may be pronounced.

Hemorrhage and its cause have been discussed under Pathology.

Leukocytosis is generally present, and its degree is roughly commensurate with the extent and the activity of infection.

The clinical course is one of remissions and exacerbations. Often the intervals between attacks are years rather than months apart, a point which favors conservative management. At the same time, the attacks are weeks in duration rather than days; occasionally they linger for several months. They may not clear up short of operative excision of the segment involved (see Treatment).

Proctoscopic examination is of value primarily because usually the scope will not pass readily into the narrowed sigmoid. If it does, the proctoscopist recognizes the fact that he has entered a narrowed segment whose mucosa is intact without polyps or carcinoma, and that such a finding is indirect evidence of diverticulitis. Few, if any, other inflammatory lesions of the colon mimic diverticulitis upon proctoscopic examinaton. Bleeding mucosa is infrequent, and ulcerations are rare. Pus may be noted upon occasion. The openings of diverticula are almost never observed in diverticulitis because edema of the mucosa generally occludes their lumina.

Barium enema should not be administered in the presence of crampy pains, as partial obstruction may be present. Iodinated oil may be used, as this will not obstruct a partially occluded lumen, but this is a technic inferior to barium sulfate examination. Pain without cramps does not contraindicate barium administration.

The features of the barium enema examination which suggest diverticulitis are: First, the mucosal pattern is normal in the narrowed segments. Second, both the proximal and the distal segments of the involved loop are funnel-shaped, indicating the more gradual narrowing of the bowel lumen in contrast to the abrupt constriction seen in carcinoma. Third and most helpful, of course, is the demonstration of diverticula of the colon adjacent to the diseased segment. As the ostia of diverticula in the inflamed narrowed segment of bowel are occluded or narrowed, they seldom visualize (Fig. 39-7).

A mass may be felt in the left lower abdomen. Aiding in the abdominal palpation is the fact that the general muscular tonus is poor in many of these patients. With gentle palpation the mass can be detected in many patients.

Digital examination of the rectum may disclose bogginess of the cul-de-sac and often a

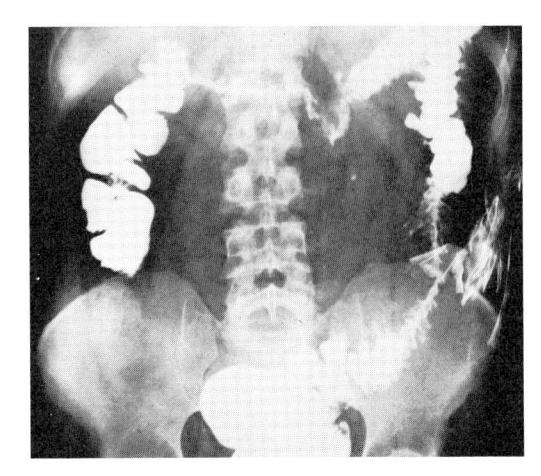

FIG. 39-7. Roentgenogram of colon in patient with diverticulosis and diverticulitis. Note the tapered narrowing of the upper and the lower ends of the constricted descending and transverse colonic segments. Diverticula are noted near the splenic flexure which were not extensively diseased, which barium could enter and leave. Absence of diverticula in diseased portions is due to closure of their ostia in the inflamed regions.

sense of a mass above the reach of the finger when the patient bears down at the time of bimanual palpation.

The diagnosis is largely one of exclusion plus the important positive findings disclosed by the barium enema. The location and the bilaterality of pain in the lower abdomen, the palpable mass, fever and leukocytosis, the absence of positive findings by proctoscopic examination, all favor the diagnosis. But it is to be remembered that carcinoma in this same segment and diverticulitis may coexist, and the tumor be obscured.

Treatment. MEDICAL OR CONSERVATIVE TREATMENT is the one most often employed unless perforation, fistulation, intestinal obstruction or serious hemorrhage prevail. Conservative management consists largely of mineral oil, a bland diet, bedrest, heat to the abdomen, sulfasuxidine or sulfathalidine, streptomycin, and/or one of the tetracycline compounds administered parenterally during the acute phases. The disease subsides in most patients, although recurrences later on may be unpleasant and require a repetition of the same therapeutic program. Avoidance of constipation or diarrhea are important prophylactic measures to be carried out throughout the rest of the patient's life.

Surgical Treatment. The results of conservative management are sufficiently good and recurrences sufficiently infrequent that it is not easy for the surgeon to protest vigorously in most cases, should one wish to advocate resection instead. However, Babcock (1941), Bartlett and McDermott (1953), Judd and Mears (1955) and Rosser (1945) have expressed the view that surgical intervention has more to offer than is generally realized. This position is tenable largely because of the advent of intestinal sulfonamides and antibiotics, and a better understanding of the problems of bowel preparation with improvement in methods to accomplish this purpose. A more aggressive attitude in favor of earlier surgical intervention is desirable in many of the patients eventually referred for surgical therapy. In the past, they have been patients with difficult complications which resulted in a higher mortality rate than occurs today.

Indications for surgical intervention in diverticulitis continue to be largely those of the pre-antibiotic era. They are:

1. Partial or complete obstruction
2. Abscess
3. Perforation
4. Fistulation
5. Severe hemorrhage
6. Carcinoma

Many surgeons are broadening the indications for operative treatment to include patients who fail to respond to medical management during an acute attack or have repeated attacks of diverticulitis (McCune *et al.,* 1957; Schlicke and Logan, 1959; Boyden and Neilson, 1960; Brown and Toomey, 1960, and Smithwick, 1960).

The types of operation performed depend upon the nature of the complication requiring surgical intervention.

For partial or complete intestinal obstruction, the goal of the immediate operation is decompression. One of two procedures may be employed. A transverse colostomy is all that is required in most patients in whom the disease is distal to this point. It is a very useful temporary procedure and, of course, simple to perform. The second is the Mikulicz resection wherein the involved segment of colon is freed by cutting the lateral peritoneal reflection of the colon as required. The colon segment is dissected free and reflected mesially, being careful to avoid the ureter which may be adherent to its undersurface. Then the involved segment is exteriorized, being brought to the outside through a stab-wound incision.

It is advantageous when possible to resect the area involved, for in many patients there is no significant local improvement following a diversionary colostomy, leaving the inflamed bowel in place. However, the risks entailed in freeing up the diseased bowel need to be considered for the individual case, and this usually can be assessed only at the operating table when the extent of the lesion is known.

Any abscesses encountered should be drained. Generally, such abscesses are fairly chronic, having been present for several weeks or months. For reasons not well understood, the peritoneum seems to gain some degree of immunity under these circumstances, and generalized peritonitis is not likely to follow. Pus should be thoroughly aspirated, the cavity sponged dry, a soft latex drain placed in the cavity and led to the outside, preferably through an extraperitoneal stab-wound incision. As many abscesses are situated low in the pelvis or the cul-de-sac, a drain may be inserted into the upper rectum or the vagina and led externally through the anus or the vagina, where it is sutured to the skin to avoid premature removal. Cultures are taken of the pus, and a broad-spectrum antibiotic likely to be effective in the treatment of bacteria of enteric origin is administered parenterally in large doses for several days, changing to another should the culture data so indicate.

The patient must be observed and examined for evidence of new abscesses or recurrences of old ones during his recovery period. Blood and plasma are used as indicated to prevent and combat shock. Short-tube intubation is employed to avoid distention from swallowed air until peristaltic activity returns.

Perforation requires immediate surgical intervention. The need to support the patient promptly by the administration of plasma and blood in the prevention or treatment of shock is often as essential as the operation itself. One of two operative procedures is indicated when perforation occurs. Exteriorization of the perforated segment of bowel is the procedure of choice but is not always feasible to perform; however, exteriorization should not be abandoned without serious try. Second is the closure of the perforation, resorting to a proximal colostomy. With either technic, the peritoneum and its recesses are cleared of feces and pus, extraperitoneal stab-wound drainage is instituted, and large doses of antibiotics are administered. Continued support of the patient with blood and plasma transfusions may be necessary for many hours after operation to counteract shock. Short-tube intubation is also continued until return of bowel function has occurred.

Fistulation requires exteriorization of the segment of bowel serving as a source of the fistula. Abscesses are frequently encountered along the way and are to be treated as described above.

When hemorrhage is the indication for surgical intervention in diverticulitis, the surgical problem is hemostasis. Essentially, only one method of surgical therapy exists—Mikulicz resection of that segment of bowel which is the source of bleeding.

TUMORS OF THE SMALL BOWEL

Compared with inflammatory lesions of the small bowel, tumors are remarkably rare, particularly malignant tumors. Tumors of the duodenum have been discussed elsewhere (see Chap. 31, Stomach and Duodenum). Those comprising this discussion are only those of the jejuno-ileum.

Benign Tumors. Most tumors of the small bowel are benign, as indicated in Table 39-3 by Shandalow (1955).

River, Silverstein and Tope (1956) have presented a most comprehensive review of benign small bowel tumors, compiling and classifying all of these tumors reported in the world literature (Table 39-4).

The incidence of benign tumors of the small bowel depends upon the character of reports consulted and the polysemantics of descriptive pathology. Small bowel tumors account for about 10 per cent of all benign tumors of the gastrointestinal tract. There is no striking difference in occurrence between sexes. As most of these tumors are small and asymptomatic,

TABLE 39-3. RATIO OF BENIGN AND MALIGNANT TUMORS OF THE SMALL INTESTINE

SOURCE	CASE No.	BENIGN %	BENIGN No.	MALIGNANT %	MALIGNANT No.
Morison	17	77	13	23	4
Dundon	62	77	44	29	18
Raiford	88	57.8	51	42.2	37
Eckel	19	37	7	63	12
Shandalow	25	88	22	12	3

Morison, J. E.: Tumors of the small intestine. Brit. J. Surg., 29:139, 1941.

Dundon, C. C.: Primary tumors of the small intestine. Am. J. Roentgenol., 59:492, 1948.

Raiford, T. S.: Tumors of the small intestine. Arch. Surg., 25:122, 321, 1932.

Eckel, J. H.: Primary tumors of the jejunum and ileum. Surgery, 23:467, 1948.

Shandalow (this series).

Adenomas were the most frequently found, followed by myomas and leiomyomas.

(This table from Shandalow, S. L.: Arch. Surg., 71:761, 1955)

the numbers found at autopsy greatly exceed those encountered in surgical specimens; about 15 are incidental findings at autopsy for every one resected surgically. Even so, the occur-

TABLE 39-4. TYPES AND NUMBERS OF TUMORS STUDIED; 20 CASES PREVIOUSLY UNREPORTED FROM COOK COUNTY HOSPITAL ARE INCLUDED

Adenomas	227
Polyps	170
Polyposis (adenomatosis) with melanin pigmentation (Peutz-Jeghers and Gardner's syndromes)	59
Lipomas	219
Myomas	179
Fibromas	163
Angiomas and hemangiomas	127
Neurogenic tumors	90
Fibromyomas	81
Fibromyxomas and myxofibromas	26
Lymphangiomas	18
Fibroadenomas	15
Myofibromas	12
Myxomas	8
Reticulofibromatosis	1
Teratoma	1
Hemangiopericytoma	1
Osteoma	1
Osteofibroma	1
Total	1,399

River, L., Silverstein, J., and Tope, J. W.: Surg., Gynec., Obstet. (Internat. Abstr. Surg.), 102:1, 1956.

rence at autopsy is no greater than 0.02 per cent; that of surgical specimens is about 0.002 per cent.

The association of generalized polyposis of the intestine, particularly involving the jejunoileum, and melanin spots of the buccal mucosa and the lips (Peutz-Jeghers syndrome) has been recognized (Dormandy, 1957; Staley and Schwarz, 1957). Gardner's syndrome appears to be a variant of the Peutz-Jeghers picture.

Despite their rare occurrence, they should be discussed briefly, as small bowel tumors are among the causes of occult abdominal pain, melena and intermittent intestinal obstruction. Failure to consider benign small bowel tumors in diagnosis accounts in part for the near 20 per cent mortality associated with operative treatment; many of these patients are seen late when intussusception, necrosis, perforation and hemorrhage have taken their toll.

The pathology tumors found at operation in the survey by River *et al.* (1956) is reported as follows: The majority of benign tumors are located in the ileum—606 of 1,399; 272 were found in the jejunum, 198 were found in the duodenum, and 323 were multiply located.

Clinical pattern and diagnosis are evident in less than 10 per cent of all benign tumors because most are asymptomatic. Obstruction was present in 877 patients, absent in 359 and unstated in 163 of the reports surveyed by River *et al.* Intussusception was the most common cause of obstruction, occurring in 627, and frequently was self-reducing. Occasionally, there is more than one clinical episode of intussusception, as many of these tumors are multiple.

Intestinal bleeding was present in 426 or 30 per cent of those included in River's review and ranged in severity from serious hemorrhage to occult blood. Adenomas, polyps, polyposis, myomas, neurogenic tumors and angiomas accounted for most of the bleeding, in the order of descending frequency.

Small bowel tumor is much more often suspected than proved preoperatively. The cramplike pain of intestinal obstruction which remits and recurs days, weeks or months later is suggestive of recurring intussusception of the small bowel due to Meckel's diverticulum or tumor. Bleeding from the rectum when the esophagus, stomach, colon, rectum and anus are negative to endoscopic and barium contrast studies leaves the small bowel the site of suspicion. Small bowel fluoroscopy is not often helpful, as many of these tumors are small, and their presence is difficult to detect. Such studies should be carried out nonetheless.

One of the most useful diagnostic technics when small bowel tumors are suspected is the use of long-tube intubation, sampling the aspirate for the presence of gross or occult blood. As soon as blood is found, barium may be introduced through the tube and the particular segment studied fluoroscopically. If this fails, the patient is explored, and the segment, a few feet on either side of the end of the tube, is thoroughly inspected and palpated. If this also fails to reveal the bleeding point, the bowel is opened 6 to 12 inches above the end of the indwelling tube, and a sterile sigmoidoscope is passed into the lumen. The mucosa is carefully explored as far as possible in both directions.

The surgeon should not be satisfied upon the finding of one tumor, as multiple ones are not infrequent. If necessary, one should not hesitate to open the bowel in 3 or 4 areas to permit inspection of the entire small bowel with the sigmoidoscope.

Treatment of benign tumors is local resection; generally a wedge resection is sufficient, although resection of a loop of small bowel may be necessary in about 20 per cent of cases. Frozen sections of such tumors are advisable and may avoid the need for a second operation.

Pneumatosis Cystoides Intestinorum. This is a rare and generally symptomless curiosity in which gas-containing cysts lined by endothelium are found in the subserosa and the submucosa, usually of the distal ileum, rarely of the duodenum, the rectum or the appendix. The origin of the gas cysts is unknown. They may spontaneously regress or slowly enlarge and ultimately project into the peritoneal cavity or into the bowel lumen. They may be mistaken for polyps.

Malignant tumors of the small bowel, excluding carcinoid tumors, account for 0.5 to 3.0 per cent of all malignancies of the gastrointestinal tract. The incidence may be slightly higher in the duodenum and the ileum than in the jejunum. Conflicting statements exist as to whether sarcoma or carcinoma is the more commonly encountered tumor.

Pathology of cancers discloses no outstanding differences between those of the small bowel and those of the colon. They may be polypoid, or annular and constricting. Obstruction and anemia are the usual symptoms and findings. Wide resection is indicated. The prognosis is not as favorable as for carcinoma of the large bowel, possibly because of the more extensive lymphatic and lacteal channels in the small bowel. Malignant tumors, like the benign ones of the small bowel, tend to be multiple.

The sarcomas principally encountered are leiomyosarcoma, neurofibrosarcoma, fibrosarcoma, angiosarcoma and lymphosarcoma. The prognosis of sarcoma of the small bowel, like that of carcinoma, is poor, although lymphosarcoma is less rapidly fatal than other intestinal sarcomas.

Symptoms produced and diagnostic procedures to be employed are the same as those of benign small bowel tumors.

Carcinoids. Carcinoid tumors of the small bowel deserve special mention, as there is much confusion as to their pathologic significance and clinical consequence. As is the case with any rarely encountered tumor, the incidence varies according to the surgeon's experiences. Carcinoids may be malignant or benign. Although the author has encountered more carcinoids of the small bowel than carcinoma in this same structure, the reverse is the general experience reported.

These tumors stain with chromic acid and therefore are of argentaffin origin. When malignant, they may or may not metastasize early; of those encountered, many had metastasized at the time of operation, or metastasis became evident within a few months or a year or two later. The carcinoid syndrome occurs in about one fourth of patients with these tumors (see discussion in Chap. 40, Tumors of the Colorectum). The carcinoid syndrome represents a spectrum of signs and symptoms in association with elevated levels of tryptophan metabolites and one or several biologically active peptides. Each of these substances may be responsible for certain of the symptoms, or the symptoms may be due to a preponderance of one of these substances, an abnormal metabolic pathway, or a complex interaction among several of them. Once thought to be explained solely on the basis of serotonin release, the carcinoid syndrome has proved to be a complex disorder involving multiple biologically active substances, and the complete solution to this problem has not yet been found.

These tumors are not infrequently multiple, and hemorrhage has been the complaint most commonly encountered. Some bleed with surprisingly large amounts of blood being lost within a few days, considering their small size; this seems to be explained on occasion when large dilated vessels are found within the tumor on microscopic examination.

PSEUDOMEMBRANOUS ENTEROCOLITIS

Pseudomembranous enterocolitis, a disease entity first described within recent years, occasionally occurs as a postoperative complication of bowel surgery and may be fatal. Originally, this disorder was attributed to an overgrowth of the *Micrococcus pyogenes*, one of the staphylococcal family. It was presumed to grow excessively because of the diminished or near absence of other normal bacterial inhabitants of the colon when intestinal antibiotics were administered orally. More recently the disease has been recognized in patients receiving no antibiotics or chemotherapeutic agents; hence the initial concept as to the cause for the overgrowth by this organism may not be true.

This disturbance is characterized by gaseous distention of both the large and the small bowel, diarrhea, fever, leukocytosis, peripheral collapse and death. At autopsy, the bowel is distended, often hemorrhagic; the lumen of the colon is frequently filled with blood. The peritoneal cavity usually contains large quantities of exudate. The amount of blood and plasma lost contribute materially to peripheral vascular collapse. Most consider peripheral collapse in this disease to be the result of the enterotoxin elaborated by the Micrococcus (Prohaska, Long and Nelsen, 1956).

Microscopic examination of the diseased bowel shows intense inflammatory changes involving all of its layers, with pronounced edema and partial or complete destruction of the mucosa.

REFERENCES

Albers, J. H., Smith, L. L., and Carter, R.: Perforation of the cecum. Ann. Surg., 143:251, 1956.

Almy, T. P., and Sherlock, P.: Genetic aspects of ulcerative colitis and regional enteritis. Gastroenterol., 51:757, 1966.

Aronson, A. R., and Ruoff, M.: Regional enteritis—occurrence in a father and both siblings. J.A.M.A., 201:267, 1967.

Aylett, S. O.: Diffuse ulcerative colitis and its treatment by ileo-rectal anastomosis. Ann. Roy. Coll. Surg. Eng., 27:260, 1960.

Babcock, W. W.: Diverticulitis. Rev. Gastroenterol., 8:77, 1941.

Bacon, H. E., Bralow, S. P., and Berkley, J. L.: Rehabilitation and long-term survival after colectomy for ulcerative colitis. J.A.M.A., 172:324, 1960.

Bartlett, M. K., and McDermott, W. V.: Surgical treatment of diverticulitis of the colon. New Eng. J. Med., 248:497, 1953.

Biggs, T. M., Beall, A. C., Jr., Gordon, W. B., Morris, G. C., Jr., and DeBakey, M. E.: Surgical management of civilian colon injuries. J. Trauma, 3:484, 1963.

Boley, S. J., Schultz, L., Krieger, H., Schwartz, S., Elguezabal, A., and Allen, A. C.: Experimental evaluation of thiazides and potassium as a cause of small-bowel ulcer. J.A.M.A., 192:763, 1965.

Boyden, A. M., and Nielson, R. O.: Reappraisal of the surgical treatment of diverticulitis of the sigmoid colon. Am. J. Surg., 100:206, 1960.

Brooke, B. N.: Ulcerative Colitis and its Surgical Treatment. Edinburgh, Livingstone, 1954.

Brown, D. B., and Toomey, W. F.: Diverticular disease of the colon. Brit. J. Surg., 47:485, 1960.

Bunch, G. H., Burnside, A. F., and Brannon, L. J.: Intestinal perforation from ingested fishbone. Am. J. Surg., 55:1, 1942.

Burt, C. A. V.: Pneumatic rupture of the intestinal canal; with experimental data showing the mechanism of perforation and the pressure required. Arch. Surg., 22:875, 1931.

Cahill, K. M.: Tropical Diseases in Temperate Climates. Chap. 10. Amebiasis. pp. 92-104, Philadelphia, J. B. Lippincott, 1964.

Chunn, C. F.: Wounds of the colon and rectum. J. Florida Med. A., 34:260, 1947.

Cohn, I., Jr.: Antibiotics for colon surgery. Gastroenterology, 35: 583, 1958.

Cohn, I., Jr., and Rives, J. D.: Protection of colon anastomosis with antibiotics. Ann. Surg., 144:738, 1956.

Colcock, B. P., and Vansant, J. H.: Surgical treatment of regional enteritis. New Eng. J. Med., 262: 435, 1960.

Counsellor, V. S., and McCormack, C. J.: Subcutaneous perforations of the jejunum. Am. J. Surg., 102:365, 1935.

Crohn, B. B.: Regional ileitis. In: Portis, S. A.: Diseases of the Digestive System. ed. 3. p. 738. Philadelphia, Lea & Febiger, 1953.

Crohn, B. B., Ginzberg, L., and Oppenheimer, G. D.: Regional ileitis, a pathological and clinical entity. J.A.M.A., 99:1323, 1932.

D'Antoni, J. S.: Amebiasis: recent concepts of its prevalence, symptomatology, diagnosis and treatment. Int. Clin., 1:101, 1942.

De Bakey, M., and Ochsner, A.: Hepatic amebiasis: a 20-year experience and analysis of 263 cases. Surg. Gynec. Obstet. (Int. Abstr. Surg.), 92:209, 1951.

DeMuth, W. E., and Rottenstein, H. S.: Death associated with hypocalcemia after small-bowel short circuiting. New Eng. J. Med., 270:1239, 1964.

Dormandy, T. L.: Gastrointestinal polyposis with mucocutaneous pigmentation (Peutz-Jeghers Syndrome). New Eng. J. Med., 256:1093, 1141, 1957.

Dukes, C. E., and Lockhart-Mummery, H. E.: Practical points in the pathology and surgical treatment of ulcerative colitis. A critical review. Brit. J. Surg., 45:25, 1957.

Durham, M. W.: Simplified technique for ileostomy construction. Surg., 41:984, 1957.

Faber, Knud: Quoted in Henderson, F. F., and Gaston, E. A.: Ingested foreign body in the intestinal tract. Arch. Surg., 36:66, 1938.

Faust, E. C.: Modern criteria for the laboratory diagnosis of amebiasis. Am. J. Trop. Med., 1:140, 1952.

Foroozan, P., and Trier, J. S.: Mucosa of the small intestine in pernicious anemia. New Eng. J. Med., 277:553, 1967.

Frye, W. W.: The pathogenesis and therapy of human amebiasis. Am. J. Gastroenterol., 25:315, 1956.

Goligher, J. C.: Extraperitoneal colostomy or ileostomy. Brit. J. Surg., 46:97, 1958.

Harkins, H. N.: Discussion in Howard, M. A.: The management of bleeding diverticula of the colon. Am. J. Surg., 100:217, 1960.

Hawk, W. A., Turnbull, Jr., R. B., and Farmer, R. G.: Regional enteritis of the colon. J.A.M.A., 201:738, 1967.

Heaton, L. D., Ravdin, I. S., Blades, B., and Whelan, T. J.: President Eisenhower's operation for regional enteritis: A footnote to history. Ann. Surg., 159:661, 1964.

Henderson, F. F., and Gaston, E. A.: Ingested foreign body in the intestinal tract. Arch. Surg., 36:66, 1938.

Hughes, E. S. R.: Right-sided colitis. Gut, 4:316, 1963.

Judd, E. S., Jr., and Mears, T. W.: Diverticulitis: progress toward wider application of single-stage resection. Arch. Surg., 70:818, 1955.

Kantor, J. L.: Regional (terminal) ileitis: its roentgen diagnosis. J.A.M.A., 103:2016, 1934.

Kirsner, J. B., Palmer, W. L., Maimon, S. N., and Ricketts, W. E.: Clinical course of chronic nonspecific ulcerative colitis. J.A.M.A., 137:922, 1948.

Laipply, T. C.: Pathological anatomy of regional enteritis. J.A.M.A., 165:2052, 1957.

Laufman, H., Silberman, W. W., and Poticha, S. M.: Surgical management of diverticulitis. Surg., Gynec. Obstet., 115:409, 1962.

LeMire, J. R., Earley, D., and Hawley, C.: Intraabdominal injuries caused by automobile seat belts. J.A.M.A., 201:735, 1967.

Lepore, M. J.: The importance of emotional disturbances in chronic ulcerative colitis. J.A.M.A., 191:819, 1965.

Lockhart-Mummery, H. E., and Morson, B. C.: Crohn's disease (regional enteritis) of the large intestine and its distinction from ulcerative colitis. Gut, 1:87, 1960.

Lockwood, A. L.: Traumatic lesions of the abdomen. Int. J. Med. Surg., 47:35, 1934.

Lumb, G., Protheroe, R. H. B., and Ramsay, G. S.: Ulcerative colitis with dilatation of colon. Brit. J. Surg., 43:182, 1955.

McCune, W. S., Iovine, V. M., and Miller, D.: Resection and primary anastomosis in diverticulitis of the colon. Ann. Surg., 145:683, 1957.

McKusick, V. A.: Genetic factors in intestinal polyposis. J.A.M.A., 182:271, 1962.

Maingot, R.: Abdominal Operations. ed. 3. New York, Appleton, 1955.

Marshak, R. H., and Lester, C. J.: Megacolon, complication of ulcerative colitis. Gastroenterol. 16:768, 1950.

Mendeloff, A. I., Monk, M., Siegel, C., and Lilienfeld, A.: Some epidemiological features of ulcerative colitis and regional enteritis: A preliminary report. Gastroenterol. 51:748, 1966.

Michener, W. M., Brown, C. H., and Turnbull, R. B., Jr.: Ulcerative colitis in children. I. Diagnosis. II. Medical and surgical therapy. Am. J. Dis. Child., 108:230, 1964.

Noer, R. J.: Hemorrhage as a complication of diverticulitis. Ann. Surg., 141:674, 1955.

Ochsner, A., and DeBakey, M.: Amebic hepatitis and hepatic abscess. Surg., 13:635, 1943.

Ponka, J. L., Brush, B. E., and Fox, J. D.: Differential diagnosis of carcinoma of the sigmoid and diverticulitis. J.A.M.A., 172:515, 1960.

Poth, E. J.: The role of intestinal antisepsis in the preoperative preparation of the colon. Surgery, 47:1018, 1960.

Prohaska, J. V., Long, E. T., and Nelsen, T. S.: Pseudomembranous enterocolitis. Arch. Surg., 72:977, 1956.

Reichert, F. L., and Mathes, M. E.: Experimental lymphedema of the intestinal tract and its relation to regional cicatrizing enteritis. Ann. Surg., 104:601, 1936.

River, L., Silverstein, J., and Tope, J. W.: Benign neoplasms of the small intestine; a critical comprehensive review with reports of 20 new cases. Surg., Gynec. Obstet. (Int. Abstr. Surg.), 102:1, 1956.

Roof, W. R., Morris, G. C., Jr., and DeBakey, M. E.: Management of perforating injuries to the colon in civilian practice. Am. J. Surg., 99:641, 1960.

Rosser, C.: Diverticulitis; indications for resection. South. Med. J., 38:161, 1945.

Roth, J. L. A., Valdes-Dupena, Skin, G. A., and Bockus, H. L.: Toxic megacolon in ulcerative colitis. Gastroenterol. 37:239, 1959.

Rubin, E. H.: Laryngeal intestinal tuberculosis. Am. J. Med. Sci., 191:663, 1931.

Ryan, P.: Emergency resection and anastomosis for perforated sigmoid diverticulitis. Brit. J. Surg., 45:611, 1958.

Sawitz, W. G.: The diagnosis of amebiasis. Clinics, 2:828, 1943.

Schlicke, C. P., and Logan, A. H.: Surgical treatment of diverticulitis of the colon. J.A.M.A., 169:1019, 1959.

Shandalow, S. L.: Benign tumors of the small intestine. Arch. Surg., 71:761, 1955.

Siddons, A. M. H.: The fate of swallowed foreign bodies. J.A.M.A., 113:17, 1577, 1939.

Smithwick, R. H.: Surgical treatment of diverticulitis of the sigmoid. Am. J. Surg., 99:192, 1960.

Staley, C. J., and Schwarz, H., II: Gastrointestinal polyposis and pigmentation of the oral mucosa (Peutz-Jeghers Syndrome). Int. Abstr. Surg., 105:1, 1957.

Swenson, S. A., and Harkins, H. N.: Rupture of the rectosigmoid by compressed air. Am. J. Surg., 63:141, 1944.

Takaro, T. M., and Bond, W. M.: Pleuropulmonary, pericardial and cerebral complications of amebiasis. Inst. Abstr. Surg., 107:209, 1958.

Trinkle, J. K., Fisher, L. J., Ketcham, A. S., and Berlin, N. I.: The metabolic effects of preoperative intestinal preparation. Surg., Gynec. Obstet., 118:739, 1964.

Tumen, H. J., Valdes Dapena, A., and Haddad, H.: The indication for surgical intervention in ulcerative colitis in children. Am. J. Dis. Child., 116:641, 1968.

Ulin, A. W., Sokolic, I. H., and Thompson, C.: Massive hemorrhage from diverticulitis of the colon. Ann. Int. Med., 50:1395, 1959.

van Heerden, J. A., Sigler, R. M., and Lynn, H. B.: Regional enteritis in children: Surgical aspects. Mayo Clin. Proc., 42:100, 1967.

van Patter, W. N.: Regional enteritis. Gastroenterology, 26:347, 1954.

Warren, S., and Sommers, S. C.: Pathology of regional enteritis and ulcerative colitis. J.A.M.A., 154:190, 1954.

Waugh, J. M., Peck, D. A., Beahrs, O. H., and Sauer, W. G.: Surgical management of chronic ulcerative colitis. Arch. Surg., 88:556, 1964.

Waugh, R. L., and Leonard, F. C.: Rupture of the colon due to compressed air, with particular reference to the character of the lesion. Mil. Surgeon, 108:294, 1951.

Welch, C. E., and Hedberg, S. E.: Colonic cancer in ulcerative colitis and idiopathic colonic cancer. J.A.M.A., 191:815, 1965.

Wruble, L. D., Duckworth, J. K., Duke, D. D., and Rothschild, J. A.: Toxic dilatation of the colon in a case of amebiasis. New Eng. J. Med., 275:926, 1966.

Zetzel, L.: Treatment of ulcerative colitis. New Eng. J. Med., 271:891, 1964.

CHAPTER 40

ISIDORE COHN, JR., M.D.

Tumors of the Colorectum

Benign Tumors: Polyps
Benign Tumors: Rarer Lesions
Premalignant Lesions of the Colon
Malignant Tumors: Adenocarcinoma
Malignant Tumors: Rarer Lesions

The colon and rectum are common sites for tumors, many of which are malignant. Colonic lesions may present with the dramatic suddenness of an intestinal obstruction, or may be silent until they have spread beyond the area where cure is possible. Because of the frequency with which colonic lesions occur, knowledge of their major characteristics and therapy is of considerable importance to all physicians, regardless of whether their primary interest is surgical or medical.

The majority of lesions of the colon tend to be polyps or carcinomas. Some polypoid lesions may be carcinomas. There are other rarer tumors, but these two groups dominate the field so completely that the bulk of this discussion will revolve around these two types. Important lesions in the "gray areas" between these two pathologic variants are discussed as Premalignant Lesions. Malignant lesions of the colon are often discussed in terms of whether they are right sided or left sided lesions, because these two types of lesions differ in so many ways as to be almost two separate entities. This kind of distinction is pointed out later in the chapter.

Some polyps and adenocarcinomas also may be found in the rectum. These lesions will be discussed in the appropriate places in this chapter.

The distal rectum and the anus will be considered separately in Chapter 41. Because of its embryologic origin, the anus may be the seat of squamous cell carcinoma, which is a different problem from those discussed in the present chapter.

BENIGN TUMORS: POLYPS

Polyps of the colon and the rectum (colorectal polyps) present certain general features. They may be pedunculated or sessile; they often present no symptoms; they tend to bleed; their presence may be associated with a mucous discharge; they may serve as the initiating point for an intussusception (but not as often as in the small bowel); they produce direct intestinal obstruction less often than do similar polyps in the small bowel (probably because of the greater diameter of the colon); they may be diagnosed with difficulty by roentgen studies or digital anal examination and with ease (in the lower 10 in., 25 cm., of the bowel) with a sigmoidoscope. Colorectal polyps may be very small, but they are extremely important.

Polyps of the colon and the rectum can be divided into 5 main clinical types. Two types are discussed in this section: polypoid adenoma and juvenile polyposis. The three other types are more properly discussed in the subsequent section on Premalignant Lesions: familial polyposis and Gardner's syndrome, villous tumors, and the pseudopolyposis of ulcerative colitis.

Polypoid Adenoma

(*Synonyms:* Pedunculated polyp, lobulated adenoma, adenomatous polyp.)

Polypoid adenomas are the most commonly occurring tumors of the colon and rectum. These lesions are important because of the frequency with which they are found, the symptoms they may produce, and their possible, though unproved, association with carcinoma of the colon.

Incidence. Reported frequencies of occurrence of adenomatous polyps have varied widely. Statistics depend on whether autopsy or clinical material has been used, and upon the diligence of the investigator and/or his definition of adenomatous polyp. Clinical studies have been based mainly on routine sigmoidoscopic studies of asymptomatic individuals performed at cancer detection centers or gastroenterological clinics. In the combined series of 55,816 patients collected by Rider et al. (1954) the incidence was 5.1 per cent. Their own incidence was 5.4 per cent in 7,487 patients. The incidence rises with age in both clinical and autopsy series. Males are affected more commonly, in a ratio of 3.5 to 2. In clinical reports 65 to 90 per cent of polyps are diagnosed by proctoscopy (and are thus located in the distal 25 cm. of the large bowel). The remainder have been scattered throughout the colon.

Autopsy studies have almost always given a higher incidence, varying in the extreme from Helwig's 9.5 per cent (1947) to Atwater and Bargen's 69 per cent (1945; the colon was examined with a hand lens). Of greater significance is the altered distribution of polyps observed in autopsy material. Thus in Arminski and McLean's recent study of 1,000 colons (1964), the distribution of polyps was as follows:

Right colon	39.3%
Left colon	41.9%
Rectum	18.8%
(Distal 25 cm.	30.9%)

Blatt (1961) reports similar figures.

Symptoms are not common in patients harboring colorectal polyps. Indeed Rider et al. reported that symptoms were as common in their patients *without* polyps as in those *with* polyps. When symptoms are present they may be due to other causes. In a study by

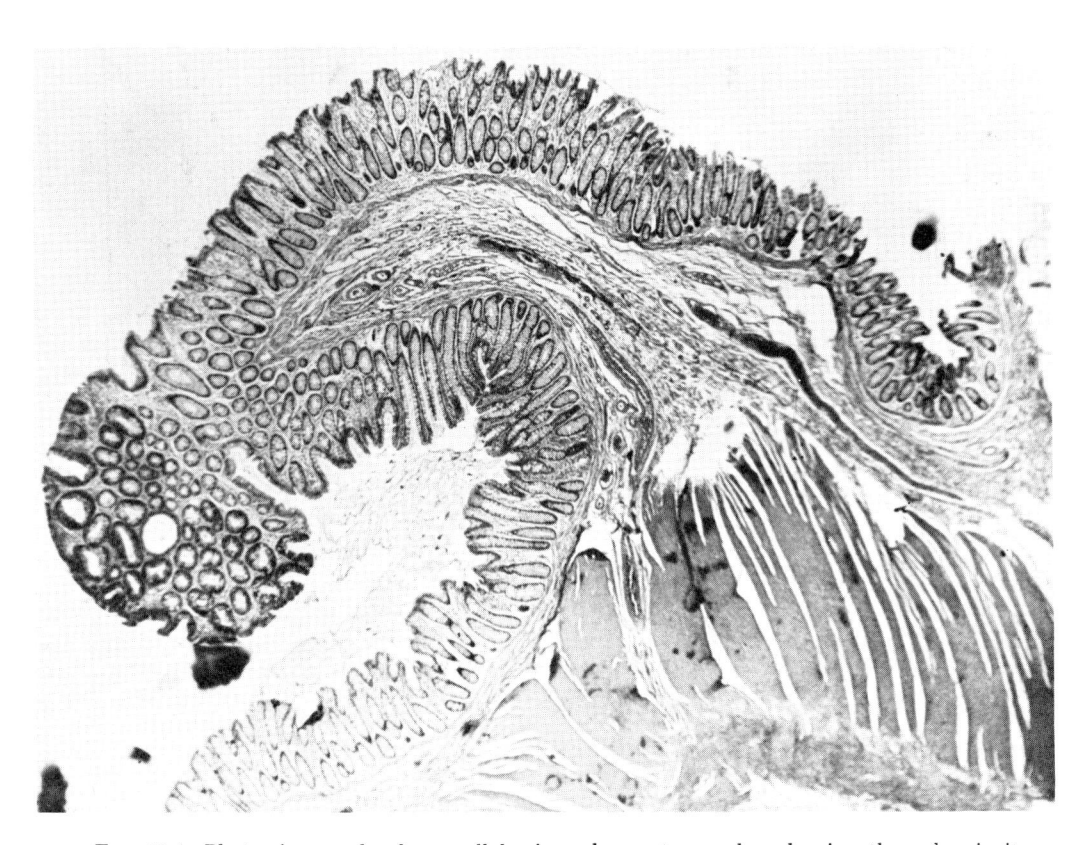

FIG. 40-1. Photomicrograph of a small benign adenomatous polyp showing the polyp in its early stages of development with the connective tissue stroma of the pedicle of the polyp, and the adenomatous character of the covering epithelium and tip of the stalk.

Bockus et al. (1961) of symptomatic patients with polyps, the only symptoms of consequence were bleeding in 47 per cent, disturbed bowel function in 26 per cent, and abdominal pain in 23 per cent.

Pathology. Adenomatous polyps are usually small, the majority being less than 1 cm. in diameter. Lesions larger than 4 cm. are exceedingly rare. The earlier lesions appear grossly as small elevations in the mucosa. Larger tumors are granular or mottled, somewhat darker than the surrounding mucosa, often sitting atop a stalk much like a soft mushroom. The stalk may be short or very long. Occasionally a polyp on a short stalk may be mistaken for a sessile growth.

Histologically the glandular epithelium exhibits an orderliness approaching that of normal colon. There is lengthening of mucosal tubules with cystic dilatation. The number of goblet cells is decreased. The polyp is supported by a central vascular stroma, often containing an increased number of mononuclear leukocytes (Fig. 40-1).

Relationship to Carcinoma. Until very recently the concept was accepted almost universally that adenomatous polyps were premalignant and preceded cancer. In 1958, Spratt, Ackerman and Moyer challenged that concept and thereby began a lively controversy which still rages. The subject is of sufficient importance that both sides of the argument will be given.

The conclusion that adenomatous polyps give rise to carcinoma rests upon 5 observations (Turrell and Haller, 1964): (1) similar location of cancer and adenoma; (2) age succession from adenoma to cancer; (3) higher incidence of adenomas in patients with cancer of the colon; (4) high incidence of cancer among patients with familial polyposis, and (5) microscopic areas of transition from adenoma to adenocarcinoma.

SIMILAR LOCATION. Clinical reports of the frequency of polyps and of carcinoma show a striking similarity of location. Such a congruence of location, however, is not seen when autopsy material is used. To quote Spratt, Ackerman and Moyer: "The frequency distributions of adenomatous polyps and cancers in the colon are not homogeneous (not congruent). Adenomatous polyps are more evenly distributed throughout the colon than cancers are. . . ."

AGE SUCCESSION. It has been reported that there is an age difference between patients with adenomas and those with cancers. The inference has been that the difference represents the time it takes for an adenoma to turn into cancer. The more recent studies of Bockus et al. (1961) and Enterline et al. (1962) give an average age of 55 years for both groups of patients. Neither noted any significant difference in the ages of patients with adenoma or cancer.

HIGHER INCIDENCE OF ADENOMAS IN PATIENTS WITH CANCER. It is observed commonly that adenomas are found in association with carcinomas. A satellite adenoma was noted in 30 to 76 per cent of cases in variously reported series. However, Spratt, Ackerman and Moyer have pointed out that the individual adenomatous polyps associated with colonic cancers are not randomly distributed above and below the cancers as they should be if colonic cancers predominantly arose from adenomatous polyps.

FAMILIAL POLYPOSIS. This clearly premalignant disease has been cited as strong evidence for the close association between adenomas and cancer. The adenomas of familial polyposis are histologically indistinguishable from singly occurring adenomas. However, the association of the two lesions may well be explained by a genetic susceptibility both for adenomas and for carcinoma.

HISTOLOGIC EVIDENCE FOR MALIGNANT CHANGE. Much of the evidence for the association of cancer and benign polyps has rested on histologic evidence. Unfortunately, a great deal of confusion has existed with respect to definition of terms. A celebrated case in point is the paper by Castleman and Krickstein (1962). These authors reviewed a series of 60 "carcinomatous polyps" previously reported from their own institution. They stated that the diagnosis had been in error and gave the following revised list of diagnoses:

Adenomatous polyp—no cancer	33
Adenomatous polyp with cancer	1
Papillary adenomas	4
Papillary adenomas with carcinoma	5
Polypoid adenocarcinoma, no polyp tissue	14

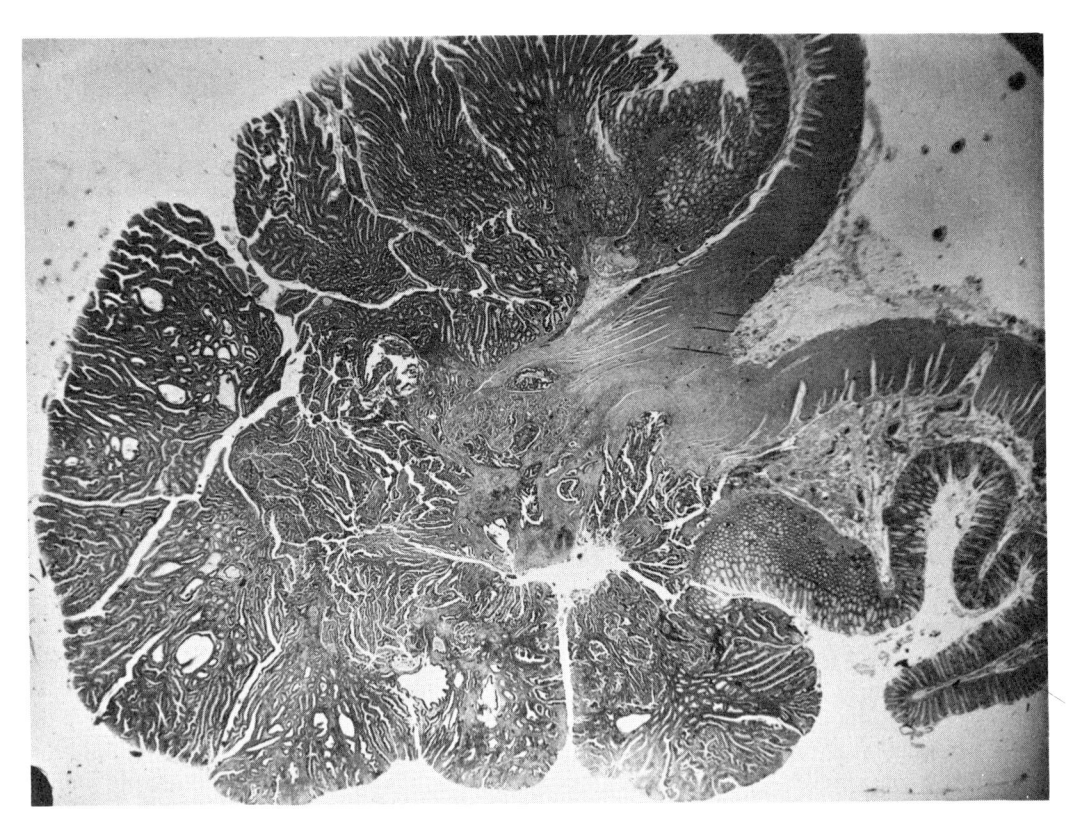

FIG. 40-2. Polyp with malignant changes in the polyp. Note changes in the mucosal character of the polyp on the upper margins and also note invasion of the stalk by carcinomatous tissue. Comparison with Figure 40-3 shows the significant differences between the microscopic appearance of juvenile polyp and true carcinoma.

These authors maintain that focal atypicality (carcinoma in situ) had been incorrectly diagnosed as carcinoma. They pointed out that none of their cases with such changes had metastases. A similar observation has been made by Enterline *et al.* and by others. Proper understanding of the biologic potential of a polyp with carcinoma in situ on the tip is the crux of the problem of what to do with adenomatous polyps. A lesion is *biologically* benign and will be cured if the polyp and its stalk are excised, so long as invasion of the stalk of an adenomatous polyp has not occurred, even though the polyp itself may meet the cytologic criteria of malignancy. Unfortunately for the surgeon it is not always possible during the operation, even with frozen section, to obtain complete assurance that the stalk is free from invasion. A difference in approach to these lesions has resulted from this uncertainty. Some surgeons prefer to take no chances and advocate wedge resection for all polypoid lesions. Others believe that the lesser mortality of simple polypectomy through a colotomy incision justifies this approach for benign-appearing lesions (Fig. 40-2).

Older studies, which claimed a histologic association between adenomatous polyps and cancer, are rendered suspect by their failure to clearly separate villous tumors from adenomas. As will be discussed later in this chapter, almost all pathologists concede that villous tumors are premalignant lesions. Although case reports of metastases from cancer developing in adenomatous polyps occasionally appear, they are less often encountered than one would expect if the development of frank malignancy from polyps were a common occurrence.

The question of the malignant potential of

adenomatous polyps is not settled. The current beliefs may be summarized as follows:

(1) It is possible that occasionally metastasizing cancers arise in previously benign polyps;

(2) Only a tiny fraction of polyps become cancers;

(3) A majority of cancers arise *de novo*.

Diagnosis. The diagnosis of benign polyps rests primarily on the educated finger and especially on proctosigmoidoscopy. Since most of these lesions are asymptomatic, they are often discovered during the course of routine screening studies. The value of such studies can hardly be overestimated. Like the vaginal smear, the routine proctoscopic examination is an important method of early cancer detection. Few screening examinations are so productive. Enquist's series (1957) is instructive: Of 7,608 patients examined in his clinic 11.5 per cent were found to have one or more polyps. There were 12 frank adenocarcinomas, 3 carcinoid tumors, 3 villous adenomas and 3 polyps with "non invasive malignant change." More important, the finding of polyps in the rectum of a patient increased the chance of finding pathologic lesions more proximal in the colon in the same patient. If a polyp was seen in the rectum, a patient had a 4.5 per cent chance of having a polyp discovered more proximally and 0.34 per cent chance of having a frank carcinoma.

The polyp-bearing patient has a 41 per cent chance of developing another polyp within 4 to 11 years (Kirsner *et al.*, 1960) and his risk of developing carcinoma of the colon is higher than that of the general population. Thus the routine proctoscopy is useful in the early diagnosis of cancer, and also serves to identify those individuals with a relatively high risk of developing cancer of the colon at some time in the future.

Other diagnostic studies helpful in identifying polypoid lesions are barium enema, barium enema with air contrast, foam enema, cytology, and studies of stool specimens. These will be discussed further in the section on colorectal cancer.

Coloscopy. This technic requires a laparotomy and may be used in patients undergoing operative polypectomy. With mobilization of the colon flexures, the entire colon may be examined by introducing a sterile sigmoidoscope through two colotomy incisions. The technic has an increased morbidity from infection and it should be used only in selected patients but not as a routine. A variation of this method, the so-called ano-transabdominal technic, permits examination and polypectomy as high as the splenic flexure without a colotomy incision. In this technic an assistant introduces the proctoscope from below while the surgeon guides it through the left colon.

Therapy. Polypoid adenomas should be removed—first, because their biologic potential is not completely understood and, second, because the differentiation between a polypoid cancer and a polypoid adenoma can be made only with a biopsy. For lesions below 15-20 cm. this can be easily accomplished, with negligible risk, through a sigmoidoscope. Excision may be made with the biopsy forceps or snare, and the base of the polyp electrocauterized. All lesions should be submitted for histologic study. Larger or sessile lesions may require preliminary biopsy and more extensive therapy.

The management of polypoid lesions beyond the reach of the sigmoidoscope requires more circumspection. One must be careful not to substitute an operative death for a potential death due to disease. Careful evaluation of all factors is important, but, unfortunately, there is no nonoperative method to determine with certainty the histologic and biologic nature of a polypoid mass seen on barium enema.

Symptomatic polypoid masses and large or sessile masses should be removed surgically unless there is a serious medical contraindication. Most surgeons would advise removal of *any* polypoid lesion in good risk patients. Most would agree on careful observation of asymptomatic, small, stalked lesions in elderly *poor risk* patients. In asymptomatic patients, the size of the lesion is a guideline accepted by some but not all surgeons. Spratt, Ackerman and Moyer have shown that only 0.6 per cent of lesions less than 1 cm. in diameter will contain invasive cancer. They recommend following those patients with small (less than 1 cm.) asymptomatic lesions.

Surgical therapy for polypoid lesions of the proximal colon may include colotomy with polypectomy, wedge resection, or subtotal resection. Each of these methods has its advocates. Colotomy and polypectomy is the simplest procedure. Careful localization of the lesion preoperatively is necessary but, in spite of this, a long stalk and the softness of the lesion may make it difficult for the surgeon to find. Palpation of the bowel, transillumination and coloscopy are aids to localization. For a typical benign appearing polypoid adenoma, excision of the lesion with the base of the stalk through a colotomy incision is all that is necessary. Cure will result even with microscopic carcinoma-in-situ, if the stalk is free of invasion.

Some authorities feel that *all* lesions should be treated by wedge resection or subtotal colectomy. Resection carries with it an increased mortality—0.5 per cent for colotomy, 3.8 per cent for resection (Spratt and Ackerman, 1960). We employ wedge resection only for sessile or bulky lesions or for lesions with suspicious areas of induration on palpation.

A careful search for other polypoid lesions should be made by palpation and/or coloscopy at the time of operation.

All patients who have polyps should have periodic proctoscopic examinations at yearly intervals. As stated previously, these patients have an increased risk of cancer of the colon,

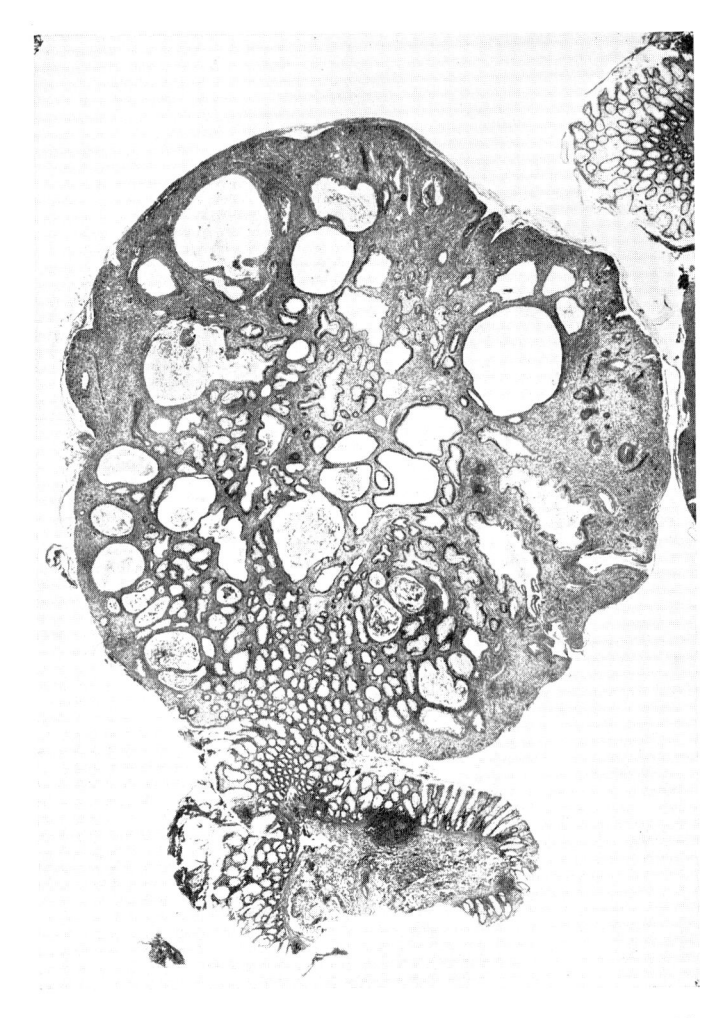

FIG. 40-3. Photomicrograph of retention polyp from a child. This shows uniformity of glandular epithelium and retention of mucus in some distended glands (Spratt, J. S., Jr., Ackerman, L. V., and Moyer, C. A.: Ann. Surg., 148:683).

and a 40 per cent chance of developing another polyp.

JUVENILE POLYPS

(*Synonym:* Retention polyp)

The most common colorectal tumor in children is the juvenile polyp. Although they are frequently confused with neoplastic adenomatous polyps, they are more like warts than adenomas. Despite their name, juvenile polyps are also seen in young adults (Roth and Helwig, 1963). The average age of patients is 4.1 years and the peak incidence is at ages 2 to 6. Males are affected more commonly than females.

The most prominent symptom of juvenile polyps is rectal bleeding and has occurred in 80 to 99 per cent of reported series. The bleeding is usually mild, and exsanguinating hemorrhage is seldom observed. Protrusion of the tumor through the anus is seen in 20 to 30 per cent of cases (Mallam and Thomson, 1959). Occasionally, juvenile polyps are the lead points of intussusception. Some patients will report passage of tissue through the rectum. Pain is seldom encountered.

The polyps are most commonly located in the rectum (69%) and sigmoid colon (9%), and are multiple in 14 per cent of patients. They may be sessile or pedunculated. The surface is red, smooth and glistening. The cut surface of the tumor usually has grossly visible cysts filled with gray-white mucus. There is a prominent stroma with abundant vascular tissue and polymorphonuclear leukocytes. The epithelium is usually ulcerated and a thick layer of granulation tissue is present. Dilated glands containing retained mucus are common (Fig. 40-3).

Treatment. Excision biopsy is proper for polyps within the reach of the proctoscope. If multiple polyps are present in a child, one polyp should be biopsied. If one is a juvenile polyp, all are likely to be juvenile polyps and the rest may be observed. These polyps have no malignant potential and may disappear spontaneously. Lesions of the proximal colon which bleed continuously may require excision through a colotomy, but most surgeons agree that extensive operative procedures should not be employed to remove asymptomatic juvenile polyps (Smilow, Pryor and Swinton, 1966).

BENIGN TUMORS: RARER LESIONS

Leiomyoma. Such tumors are grossly similar to those which appear elsewhere in the intestinal tract and are essentially submucosal. Only rarely do they produce symptoms. Very rarely they are malignant.

Fibroma. Neurofibromas in patients with von Recklinghausen's disease have been reported.

Lipoma. With the exception of adenomas, lipomas are the most common benign tumors of the large intestine. They may be sessile or pedunculated and are usually located in the submucosa of the bowel wall. Most occur in the right colon. They occur at an average age of 60. Males and females are affected equally. Pain has been the most common symptom, but rectal bleeding is encountered in half the patients. Twenty per cent of patients present with intussusception. An intramural filling defect can usually be demonstrated by barium enema and the correct diagnosis is occasionally made on the basis of roentgenographic characteristics. Lipomas should be removed surgically. Usually they can be identified at operation as lipomas by their very soft consistency. If the diagnosis is certain, enucleation is sufficient treatment. Segmental resection is appropriate in cases where doubt exists as to the nature of the lesion (Haller and Roberts, 1964).

Carcinoid. Carcinoid tumors of the cecum and proximal colon are rare. Carcinoids arising in this portion of the gastrointestinal tract are usually quite malignant and have the highest rate of metastasis of any of the carcinoid tumors (67%). The symptoms are similar to those of carcinoma except that bleeding is unusual. Right lower quadrant pain, obstruction, or a right lower quadrant mass are usually found. Patients with hepatic metastases may exhibit the carcinoid syndrome. Carcinoids of the proximal colon are treated as any colonic malignancy (see below).

Rectal carcinoids are more common than carcinoids of the proximal colon. They are frequently silent lesions. Most are found in the course of routine rectal examination or sigmoidoscopy and are located 5 to 8 cm. from the anus. They appear as pale-yellow submucosal nodules covered by an intact epithelium. Carcinoid tumors of the rectum often resist impregnation by silver stain and may appear deceptively benign. The most reliable histologic criterion of malignancy is evidence of local extension into and beyond the muscular coat of the bowel. Peskin and Orloff (1959) found that lesions less than 2 cm. in diameter had only a 7 per cent incidence of muscular invasion. On the other hand, 90 per cent of lesions over 2 cm. showed evidence of invasion and lymph node metastasis. On this basis they have recommended local therapy for the smaller lesions and more radical therapy for larger lesions.

Carcinoids should be excised totally. Small submucosal nodules may be treated by full thickness excision. Large tumors greater than 1.5 cm. in size or lesions which have invaded the bowel wall should be treated as carcinomas. The prognosis is poor if muscle invasion has occurred.

The *carcinoid syndrome* of cutaneous flushing, asthma, intermittent diarrhea, skin rash and collagen deposits on the endocardium results from metastatic carcinoid tumor in the liver. This interesting syndrome is due in part to the excess production of serotonin by the tumor. Serotonin affects bronchial, intestinal and vascular smooth muscle and produces pulmonary vasoconstriction, bronchoconstriction and increased intestinal peristalsis which leads to diarrhea. Serotonin also promotes connective tissue proliferation, possibly explaining the fibrotic heart lesions.

The usual association of the syndrome with hepatic metastases may be due to direct release of serotonin into the general circulation, by-passing the large amount of hepatic monoamine oxidase which inactivates serotonin. The rarity of cardiac lesions in the left side of the heart except in instances of bronchial carcinoid or right-to-left intracardiac shunts has been explained by inactivation of serotonin by pulmonary monoamine oxidase.

Carcinoid tumors are most common in the small intestine and appendix although metastases from appendiceal carcinoids are rare. A few tumors occur in the stomach, duodenum and rectum. Rectal tumors rarely produce the carcinoid syndrome. Carcinoids spread by local invasion through the bowel wall and are often asymptomatic until metastasis to the liver has occurred. Some patients even have liver metastasis without symptoms. Metastatic lesions may be very slow growing—a 5 year survival of 21 per cent for patients with metastatic carcinoid has been reported.

Carcinoid heart disease usually develops late in the disease. Only right sided lesions occur unless there is a right-to-left shunt. A fibrous tissue, free of elastic fibers, is deposited on valves, endocardium and intima, causing thickening, adherence and valvular stenosis or insufficiency. Heart failure is the usual cause of death in patients with carcinoid syndrome. Operative correction of carcinoid heart disease has been unsuccessful.

Local symptoms in patients with the carcinoid syndrome are usually indistinguishable from those of other intestinal neoplasms. Obstruction may be the earliest sign of the tumor. Gastric carcinoids may present with hemorrhage, duodenal carcinoid with symptoms of pyloric obstruction. Patients with appendiceal carcinoid may have symptoms of acute appendicitis. Rectal carcinoids are often locally asymptomatic or may produce rectal bleeding. Symptoms of pellagra may appear, as a result of the diversion of dietary niacin to the production of excessive serotonin.

The presence of episodic flushing and diarrhea in association with a palpable liver should raise the suspicion of carcinoid tumor. The flushing may be provoked by catecholamines, and there is evidence that other vasoactive substances such as bradykinin may be involved in the production of flushing. The determination of urinary 5-hydroxy 3-indoleacetic acid, an inactive serotonin metabolite, is a simple screening test. Certain drugs may provoke false positive tests, and ingestion of bananas should be avoided, since they are high in serotonin content.

TREATMENT of patients with the carcinoid syndrome has employed both pharmacologic and surgical approaches. Serotonin antagonists, notably cyproheptadine and methysergide maleate, have been used in the symptomatic treatment of patients with carcinoid syndrome. Unfortunately, results have been variable and unpredictable. A tendency to become refractory to the drugs has been noted, and significant side effects have appeared.

Cytotoxic agents have been used with limited success to control tumor growth. Nitrogen mustard, cyclophosphamide, thioTEPA and 5-fluorouracil have been reported to have therapeutic benefit. Phenylalanine mustard and vinblastine sulfate have been ineffective.

General supportive therapy should include supplementary niacin, other vitamins and adequate diet. Avoidance of foods that trigger attacks should be counseled. Lomotil and codeine have been useful in controlling diarrhea. Chlorpromazine may be of value in controlling the vasomotor symptoms.

Local therapy includes resection of involved intestine together with the mesentery. Carcinoids are frequently multiple in origin. Palliative procedures to correct obstruction, fistula or bleeding are useful, since long term survival is common even in the presence of metastases.

Excision of hepatic metastases to control the symptoms due to excessive serotonin has been successful in several patients. Second operations for removal of hepatic tumors have even been performed. Photoscan localization of hepatic tumor masses is a useful preoperative diagnostic test.

Patients with the carcinoid syndrome present an increased operative risk. Severe hypotension and flushing may occur with the induction of anesthesia. Cardiac failure may occur also.

The reviews of Dollinger and Gardner (1966) and of Sanders and Axtell (1964) are particularly useful.

Hemangioma. Such a tumor involves the colon, or more rarely the rectum, and presents several distinguishing features.

Rectal bleeding is common. By roentgenographic examination, phleboliths may be seen, and the tumor usually extends over a longer segment of bowel than does carcinoma, often with no obstruction to the retrograde flow of barium. If the tumor does not extend up into the sigmoid loop, ligation of the inferior mesenteric artery may effect improvement, but resection of large tumors may be preferable.

Endometriosis. This lesion may produce obstruction in the absence of mucosal involvement. Up to two thirds of women with pelvic endometriosis may have involvement of the lower rectal wall. Growths higher on the colon may be present in 20 per cent of patients with endometriosis (Gray, 1966). When bowel symptoms are marked, or when obstruction is present, surgical procedures directed toward the bowel are obviously necessary. If the bowel involvement is only a minor part of an extensive endometriosis, then hormone or hormone-ablative therapy may be sufficient. Occasionally the differential diagnosis between endometriosis and cancer of the colon may be difficult, if not impossible, and, under these circumstances, the therapy should be directed at removing any focus of potential cancer.

Benign Lymphoma. Holtz and Schmidt (1958) found 24 cases of lymphoid polyps in 20 years at the University of Michigan. This condition is not rare, over 300 cases having been reported in the literature. McGraw and Bonenfant (1960) confirm the benign nature of these tumors.

Granuloma. Granulomas, amebic or nonspecific, are of interest chiefly because they may simulate carcinoma.

Peutz-Jegher's Syndrome. (See Chap. 39.) Although small bowel polyps are characteristic in this syndrome, large bowel tumors occur in about one third of the patients. Grossly the tumors resemble adenomatous polyps but microscopically they are characterized by smooth muscle components not found in adenomas. These are actually hamartomas and are not prone to malignant change.

Other benign tumors include:
Congenital Cyst;
Xanthoma;
Melanoma.

PREMALIGNANT LESIONS OF THE COLON

FAMILIAL POLYPOSIS OF THE COLON

(*Synonyms:* Hereditary multiple polyposis, diffuse polyposis, polypoid adenomatosis, multiple adenomatosis.)

This disease is perhaps the most clearly premalignant condition known in clinical medicine. It was first accurately described by Virchow in 1863. The familial nature of the disease was noted by Cripps in 1882. The studies of Lockhart-Mummery and of Dukes clarified the genetic features and established the predisposition to carcinoma.

The disease is characterized by an excessive proliferation of the glandular epithelium of the colon and rectum, leading to the development of myriads of sessile and polypoid tumors. The distribution and numbers of polyps are variable but they tend to be most numerous in the distal colon and rectum. The smaller lesions consist of scattered patches of epithelial hyperplasia. The larger lesions have the histologic structure of adenomata.

Familial polyposis is a hereditary disease transmitted as a Mendelian dominant. Males and females are affected equally. Since one half the children of a patient with polyposis have the gene and the condition has an 80 per cent penetrance, 40 per cent of the offspring of an affected parent exhibit the disease (Raynham and Louw, 1966). Virtually all afflicted patients will develop carcinoma of the colon in time. Fifty per cent of patients harbor an infiltrating colonic carcinoma by age 30 (Mayo, deWeerd and Jackman, 1951), and Dukes (1952) noted 41.6 years as the average age of death from cancer of the colon. The occasional occurrence of multiple polyposis in patients without a family history is thought to be due to mutation. It is not yet known whether these individuals will transmit the disease.

Patients are not born with polyps but tend to develop them at some time during their childhood, usually about the time of puberty. The condition has been described in a child of 4 months and there is one verified case in which the polyps did not appear until age 39. The initial symptoms are mild, consisting of looseness and frequency of stools which may progress to frank diarrhea. Excess mucus and rectal bleeding may occur. The presence of pain or other severe symptoms in these patients is ominous and usually indicates that cancer is present.

Rectal examination and sigmoidoscopy are usually sufficient to establish the diagnosis. The digital examination may show multiple small masses or there may be a sensation of mucosal granularity. The appearance of multiple small sessile and pedunculated tumors separated by normal mucosa is quite characteristic. Almost the only lesion which could be confused with familial polyposis at sigmoidoscopy is the pseudopolyposis of ulcerative colitis. Biopsy of a typical lesion and of any suspicious lesion should be performed. A barium enema helps to establish the extent of the disease and to rule out a more proximal carcinoma.

Treatment must be radical, since virtually 100 per cent of affected patients will develop carcinoma. Symptomatic patients already have a 50 per cent risk of harboring a frank carcinoma. All adults, symptomatic or not, should have colectomy. Children who have symptoms probably should have a colectomy but definitive therapy may be deferred until age 14 or 15 in asymptomatic children with polyposis.

Two methods of therapy have been advocated: Total proctocolectomy with establishment of an abdominal ileostomy, and subtotal colectomy with ileorectal anastomosis preceded by fulguration of remaining polyps in the rectal stump.

Total colectomy is necessary in the presence of carcinomatous changes in the rectum. Even in patients without a frank carcinoma this procedure has the advantage of obviating the risk of carcinoma developing at a later date. It has the disadvantage of disturbing normal bowel function and requiring a permanent ileostomy, a not inconsiderable inconvenience, particularly in young patients. It is occasionally difficult to persuade some asymptomatic patients with polyposis to undergo total colectomy.

Subtotal colectomy with ileorectal anastomosis has been advocated as a compromise procedure (Dukes, 1952; Lockhart-Mummery, Dukes and Bussey, 1956; Everson and Allen, 1954). Usually prior to the operation the rectum is cleared of all polyps by fulguration through a sigmoidoscope. Subtotal colectomy with ileorectal anastomosis about 12 to 15 cm. from the anus is then carried out. Repeated postoperative sigmoidoscopy must be performed at 3- to 6-month intervals to destroy new polyps as they develop. The procedure permits anal continence and relatively normal bowel function (2-3 stools per day). In addition, in some cases, the rectal polyps have been noted to regress following establishment of the ileorectal anastomosis. However, faithful, regular follow-up for the rest of the patient's life is absolutely mandatory and in practice this has been difficult to achieve in all patients. In addition, even in adequately followed patients the risk of carcinoma developing in the rectal stump has been at least 3 to 5 per cent.

Total colectomy is recommended for most patients when the diagnosis of familial polyposis has been established. We do not feel that carcinoma of the rectal stump can be adequately prevented even if all the visible rectal polyps can be removed.

Adequate treatment of any patient with multiple polyposis should include thorough investigation of all members of the family. Sigmoidoscopic examination of each member should be carried out as soon as possible and at periodic intervals. A method of predicting which individuals of an affected family carry the polyposis gene has not been developed and sigmoidoscopy remains the only reliable means of identifying the patients. All patients over the age of 15 who have developed polyps should undergo colectomy. If by the age of 40 no polyps have appeared, it is unlikely that polyposis will develop.

Gardner's Syndrome

The association of soft tissue tumors, bone tumors and multiple colonic polyposis is known as Gardner's syndrome. It was first recognized as a familial syndrome inherited as a Mendelian dominant by Gardner and Stephens in 1950. Most authorities separate this syndrome from familial multiple polyposis (Jones and Cornell, 1966).

The symptoms vary but are generally attributable to the polyposis. The soft and hard tissue tumors appear early in life but, except for cosmetic problems, cause little difficulty. The onset of bowel symptoms usually occurs in late adolescence. Diarrhea, mucorrhea, and rectal bleeding are most common. Symptoms have usually been present for several years before medical advice is sought.

The osseous tumors are benign osteomas ranging from simple cortical thickening to protuberant bony masses. The mandible is most commonly involved but almost any portion of the skeletal system may be affected. Soft tissue tumors may be the first external manifestation of the disease. The types of tumors associated include epidermoid inclusion cysts, desmoid tumors, lipomas, leiomyomas, retroperitoneal fibrous tissue tumors and neurofibromas.

The polyposis of Gardner's syndrome seems to be indistinguishable from that of familial multiple polyposis. The risk of cancer is similar. The polyposis of Gardner's syndrome is no less dangerous than that of classic familial polyposis, and the treatment should be the same (Thomas et al., 1968).

Villous Tumors

(*Synonyms:* Villous adenoma, villous papilloma, papillary adenoma, papilloma, true papilloma.)

These lesions are dangerous and might well be classified with the malignant tumors later in this chapter. The tumors may be defined as sessile, poorly demarcated polyps consisting of villi which project above the level of the surrounding intestinal mucosa. The villi are made up of fingerlike projections of loose supporting vascular stroma covered by a single layer of columnar epithelial cells. Grossly, they are often large bulky tumors. The tumor has a very characteristic soft, velvety feel by which the educated finger may make a tentative diagnosis. The softness of the tumor is treacherous and tumors may be missed on routine digital or sigmoidoscopic examination. When seen at proctosigmoidoscopy, the tumor is grayish-pink to port wine in color. Delicate fronds of villi may be seen projecting from the tumor. They are quite friable, and bleeding is common.

Villous tumors are relatively rare, making up 2 to 5 per cent of all colorectal polyps. They occur in males and females with equal frequency.

The average age of patients with villous adenomas has been reported to be 63 years (Wheat and Ackerman, 1958; Sunderland and Binkley, 1948). The highest incidence occurs in the 7th decade. Villous tumors occur in an older age group than either benign adenomas (54.5 years) or rectosigmoid carcinoma (55.1 years).

The most common symptom of villous tumors is rectal bleeding, which occurs in 60 to 70 per cent of cases. Diarrhea or excretion of mucus is seen in over half of the cases. Protrusion of the tumor occurs in 10 per cent. Less frequent symptoms include constipation, weight loss, tenesmus and anal pain. A few patients have no symptoms. The duration of symptoms has ranged from 2 days to 15 years, with an average of 2.5 years (Wheat and Ackerman).

Villous adenomas occur predominantly in the distal large bowel. Seventy per cent have been palpable by digital examination and 79 per cent are found in the rectosigmoid area within reach of the sigmoidoscope (Fig. 40-4).

The rest of the tumors are found scattered along the rest of the proximal colon. Goldfarb reported that the right colon was involved in 7.8 per cent of the cases at Barnes Hospital. Villous tumors range in size from a small 0.5 cm. in diameter to a huge 20 cm., but the majority are between 4 and 6 cm. in transverse diameter. A very broad base is common: in Bacon, Lowell and Trimpi's series (1954), 39 per cent of the tumors were completely circumferential. Involvement of more than half of the rectum is relatively common.

A tentative diagnosis of villous tumor may be made by the characteristic consistency and gross appearance. Roentgenologic features which suggest the diagnosis are a large size, with lack of infiltration of the adjacent bowel wall and a lacy reticulated surface pattern.

Careful biopsy of these lesions is imperative in the diagnostic evaluation of villous adenomas because of their dangerous propensity to harbor a cancer. An invasive carcinoma within a villous adenoma is not readily visible and may be buried within the depths of the tumor. The finding of a firm or ulcerated area in a given tumor is ominous, and such areas should be included in the biopsy. In the final analysis, assurance of benignancy cannot be made unless the pathologist examines the entire tumor minutely with serial sections. All villous adenomas should be treated with deep suspicion. The incidence of invasive carcinoma within villous adenomas ranges from 30 to 70 per cent in variously reported series.

Treatment should be radical. Snaring, cautery, piecemeal excision and radiation have no place in the treatment of this lesion. Invasive carcinoma is found so frequently that we recommend a proper "cancer operation" for all villous tumors. This means a Miles resection for tumors of the distal rectum and a radical wedge resection for tumors high enough to spare the rectum.

"Adequate local excision" has been recommended by some authorities for small, apparently benign tumors which are located in the distal rectum (where a Miles resection would be necessary for cancer). Adequate local excision means removal of the entire villous adenoma in one piece, including the stalk and a margin of tissue on *all* sides including depth. This may be done through a posterior approach or, on occasion, through the anus. In addition to their very clearly established malignant potential, villous adenomas have a high incidence of recurrence when inadequately excised. In Sunderland and Binkley's series (1948), 17 of 48 patients treated by cautery, or cautery and radiation had invasive cancer or recurrence.

To reiterate: Villous adenomas should be treated as cancer, by radical resection. With adequate therapy, the prognosis following adequate excision of villous adenomas is excellent if invasive carcinoma is not present in the resected specimen. Periodic sigmoidoscopic examinations should be performed to ensure against recurrence.

Hypersecreting Villous Tumors. An occasional patient with a villous adenoma presents with an unusual syndrome characterized by loss of large quantities of clear, thin mucoid fluid from the rectum. This may result in the rapid development of severe dehydration, oliguria, and circulatory collapse. The syndrome was first described by McKittrick and Wheelock in 1954. All patients with this syndrome have been found to have large bulky villous tumors located in the rectum or rectosigmoid area. The average age of patients has been 66 and symptoms have been present for an average of 5.8 years.

The syndrome is interesting and important. Death may result from inadequate fluid and

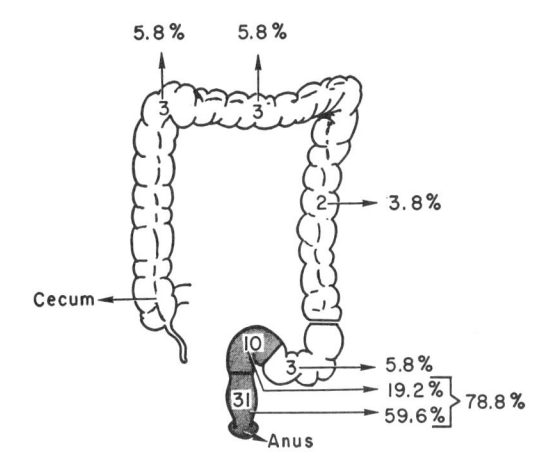

Fig. 40-4. Distribution of villous tumors of the large intestine (Wheat, M. W., Jr., and Ackerman, L. V.: Ann. Surg., 147: 476)

electrolyte replacement. Mucous diarrhea usually has been present in these patients for years but they may present with sudden circulatory collapse. The rectal discharge of mucus tends to become continuous, with daily fluid losses ranging from 375 to 3,400 ml. The volume is almost invariably underestimated unless it is carefully measured. The fluid secreted by the tumor contains Na^+ and Cl^- in concentrations similar to serum but the concentration of K^+ may be as high as 80 mEq./L. Virtually all patients present with prerenal azotemia, with blood urea nitrogen levels of 100 mg. per cent or greater. Hyponatremia, hypochloremia, hypokalemia and dehydration may be marked. The electrolyte disturbances may be accompanied by shock, neuromuscular symptoms and ECG changes. Serum proteins and calcium usually are normal.

Treatment is urgent and requires prompt fluid and electrolyte replacement. Potassium deficits are particularly hard to correct and more than 120 mEq. of K^+ per day may be required. Careful recording of rectal losses should be instituted. Definitive treatment involves removal of the villous tumor as soon as the patient is in suitable operative condition. Proximal colostomy alone will not prevent the massive fluid loss and therefore is inadequate therapy (Eisenberg et al., 1964; Shnitka et al., 1961).

ULCERATIVE COLITIS AND PSEUDOPOLYPOSIS

Pseudopolyposis is a complication of severe ulcerative colitis. These lesions are inflammatory and not neoplastic. Three types are encountered: (1) polypoid edematous mucosal tags; (2) polyps of granulation tissue; (3) polyps of connective tissue covered by glandular epithelium. In the series of de Dombal et al. (1966) pseudopolyps occurred in 12.5 per cent of patients with ulcerative colitis. The "polyps" may occur in any portion of the colon but rectal involvement occurs in only 40 per cent. Recognition of the importance and interrelationship of cancer, ulcerative colitis, and pseudopolyposis is relatively recent. Some clarification of previous confusion is apparent in Hinton's statement:

It was once thought that pseudo-polypi represented pre-cancerous change. It is now generally accepted that they have no causal relationship with cancer. Pseudo-polypi occur in association with severe disease, and this in turn usually involves the whole of the colon. Patients with total colitis are the ones liable to develop cancer. But cancer can also occur in colitics who do not have pseudo-polypi: in the St. Mark's series these were the majority.*

Some agreement can be found in the reports of individuals in several different disciplines (Morson, 1966; Hinton, 1966; Bargen, 1962; Goldgraber and Kirsner, 1964; Slaney and Brooke, 1959).

Some of the salient features of cancer in ulcerative colitis are:

1. Cancer develops up to eight times more frequently in patients with ulcerative colitis than it does in the population at large.

2. Cancer develops 20 years earlier in patients with ulcerative colitis than in the population at large.

3. Cancer is most likely to develop in people whose ulcerative colitis began in childhood. Morson states that "The incidence of cancer in colitis beginning before the age of 25 years is twice as great as those with symptoms beginning after this age."

4. The incidence of cancer increases with the duration of the symptoms and with the degree of involvement of the colon. It becomes of major proportions after ulcerative colitis has been present for ten or more years. The risk is so high in patients with total involvement of the colon that many surgeons now recommend total colectomy in any patient with symptoms or x-ray changes of ulcerative colitis which persists more than ten years.

5. Previous ileostomy and diversion of the fecal stream do not protect the remaining colon from the development of carcinoma.

6. The diagnosis of cancer of the colon in a patient with ulcerative colitis is particularly difficult because there may be no change in symptoms when the cancer begins, or even when it grows to significant proportions.

7. The cancers in ulcerative colitis have a different distribution in the colon from those cancers developing in the population at large (Fig. 40-5).

8. Cancers in ulcerative colitis are more likely to be multiple, possibly related to the

* Hinton, J. M.: Risk of malignant change in ulcerative colitis. Gut, 7:427-432, 1966.

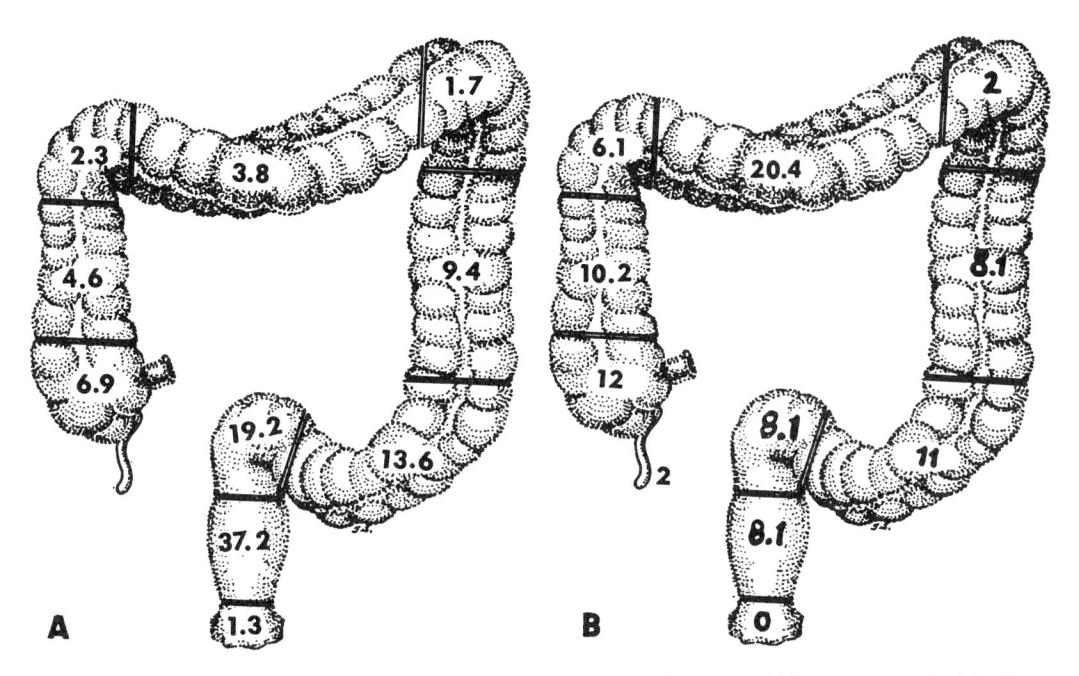

FIG. 40-5. Location of 478 "ordinary" cancers of the colorectum (A) as compared with 49 cancers in 33 patients with ulcerative colitis(B). (Goldgraber and Kirsner, Cancer 17:661)

more diffuse involvement of the entire large bowel which is usually present.

9. The prognosis is generally considered to be quite poor. Figures as low as 18 per cent for 5-year survivals have been reported. The poor prognosis is probably a result of the difficulty in diagnosis, the inflammatory condition of the bowel, which aids the spread of the malignancy, the multiple sites of origin and other factors not well understood.

Treatment should be total colectomy, including rectum and anus, with establishment of permanent ileostomy.

Total colectomy can be accomplished in the male patient with ulcerative colitis with little or no sacrifice of sexual function, in contrast to the common loss of sexual function when an abdominoperineal resection is performed for cancer. Thus the younger patient with ulcerative colitis—prior to the development of cancer—need not have this fear of the operative procedure. Since the operation is being performed for benign disease, it is possible to carry the resection close to the bowel wall, in contrast to the need to remove surrounding tissues and lymphatics when the operation is performed for frank malignancy. We advise the removal of the entire colon in any patient who has had symptomatic ulcerative colitis for ten years, because of the prohibitive danger of leaving the colon in under these conditions. The operation can be done electively with minimal risk.

MALIGNANT TUMORS

Adenocarcinoma

The importance of colorectal cancer is attested by the following facts:

First, it ranks first or second in incidence and estimated deaths in the United States (Fig. 40-6). It is estimated there will be 73,000 new cases of cancer of the colon and rectum in the United States in 1968, as compared with 65,000 new cases of cancer of the breast, the nearest second. (Both of these are exclusive of cancer of the skin, which will have 105,000 cases, but almost no associated deaths.) Anticipated deaths from the leading cancer causes are as follows: lung—55,000; colon and rectum—45,000; breast—28,000;

1154 Tumors of the Colorectum

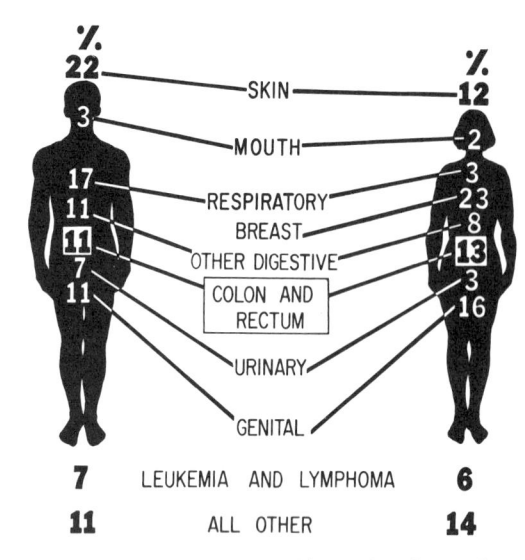

FIG. 40-6. Cancer incidence by site and sex as predicted for 1968. (Data from 1968 Cancer Facts and Figures, American Cancer Society)

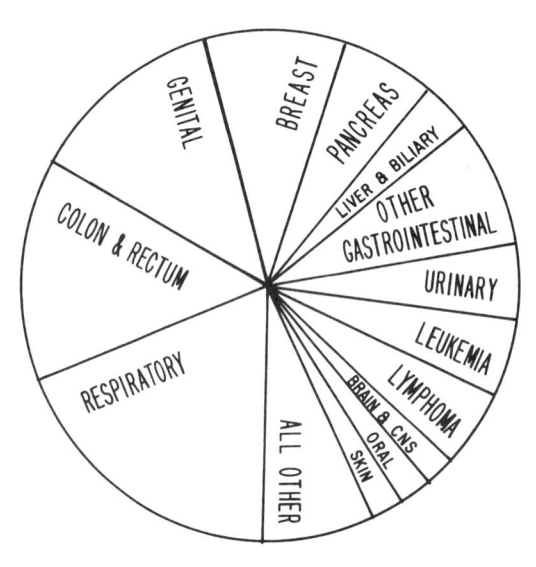

FIG. 40-7. Estimated cancer deaths by site, predicted for 1968. (Data from 1968 Cancer Facts and Figures, American Cancer Society)

stomach, prostate and lymphomas—17,000 each; uterus—14,000 (Fig. 40-7).* Age adjusted cancer death rates show a slight decrease for 1963-65 as compared with 1953-55

* 1968 Cancer Facts and Figures, American Cancer Society.

for colon and rectal cancer. Shimkin and Cutler indicated that 1.3 per cent of men and 1 per cent of women develop carcinoma of the rectum some time during their lives.

Second, this mortality can be significantly reduced by the use of relatively simple procedures which should be available to every physician: digital rectal examination and sigmoidoscopic examination of all patients. The vast majority of colonic lesions are within reach of these two methods of examination. A vigorous antipolyp campaign may aid this attempt at cancer eradication by its early detection of malignant lesions and/or by the removal of any and all polyps that might otherwise become malignant. Figure 40-8 shows this distribution in our series and Table 40-1 shows a comparable distribution for a larger, collected series.

Third, the five year survival rate following definitive operation for cancer of the colon and rectum is quite high (see section on Prognosis) and is better than that for stomach, lung, or pancreas.

Most of the material that follows, dealing with specific clinical experience, is based on a study at Charity Hospital in New Orleans of 1,687 histologically confirmed cases of cancer of the colon, rectum, and anus, and most of these data are confirmed in publications from other institutions where similarly large groups of patients have been analyzed (Colcock, 1964; Galante, Dunphy and Fletcher, 1967; Garlock *et al.*, 1962; Gilbertsen, 1963; Glenn and McSherry, 1966; Grinnell, 1953; Hughes, 1963; Liechty *et al.*,

TABLE 40-1. LOCATION OF CANCERS OF THE COLON

LOCATION	INCIDENCE (IN PERCENT)
Cecum	8
Ascending	5
Hepatic flexure	2
Transverse	5
Splenic flexure	3
Descending	4
Sigmoid	21
Rectosigmoid and rectum	50
Anus	2

Data derived from summation of 13,380 cases of colon cancer from 9 separate reports.

1968; McSwain, Sadler and Main, 1962; Postlethwait, Adamson and Hart, 1958; Welch and Burke, 1962).

Age. Colorectal carcinoma is usually a disease of older persons (Fig. 40-9).

Symptoms and Physical Signs. The colon may be divided into right and left halves on the basis of a number of different features. If the division is made at the distal transverse colon, there are differences with respect to embryologic origin, blood supply, function, fecal content, type of lesion to be found, clinical syndrome produced (Table 40-2), diagnostic considerations, and type of therapy to be employed.

In essence, the right colon is derived from and has the same blood supply as the mid gut. Its arterial supply comes from the superior mesenteric artery via the right colic and middle colic arteries. The contents are mainly liquid and a major function of the right colon is water absorption.

The left colon is derived from the hind gut, and has its blood supply from the inferior mesenteric artery via the left colic, the sigmoid, and the superior hemorrhoidal arteries. The contents are more solid, and the major functions are storage and excretion.

The venous supply parallels that of the arterial supply, and all empty ultimately into the portal vein so that all blood from the colon drains directly to the liver. The lymphatics follow the main vascular pathways. Knowledge of each of these is essential to any plan of surgical removal of cancer of any part of the colon.

The colon is not essential to life, and any part or all of it may be removed without shortening the life span, though some disruption of normal routines may be produced.

TABLE 40-2. QUALITATIVE DIFFERENCES IN SYMPTOMS AND SIGNS OF RIGHT AND LEFT COLORECTAL CARCINOMA

	RIGHT	LEFT
Occult blood in stools	+	−
Bright blood in stools	−	+
Anemia	+	−
Obstructive signs	−	+
Gallbladderlike symptoms	+	−
"Sentinel polyps"	+	+
"Sentinel hemorrhoids"	−	+
Small caliber of stools	−	+

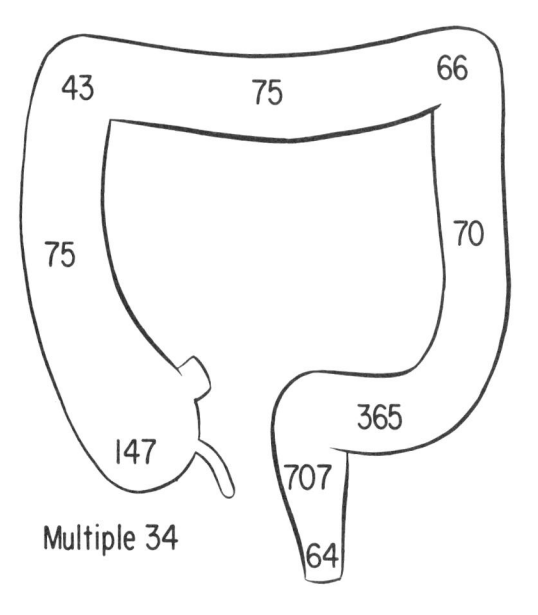

FIG. 40-8. Distribution of colonic cancer in 1,687 histologically verified cases at Charity Hospital in New Orleans. (Floyd, C. E., Stirling, C. T., and Cohn, I., Jr.: Ann. Surg., 163:831)

The malignant lesion in the right colon is typically a bulky, fungating, ulcerating carcinoma that projects into the lumen of the bowel and, although it rarely causes obstruction, is commonly the cause of unexplained bleeding from its large surface area. The bleeding goes unnoticed by the patient because it is mixed in with the rest of the stool. Anemia, weakness, and a mass in the right lower quadrant are the common clinical manifestations of right-sided lesions.

The typical lesion of the left colon is an annular napkin ring tumor which encircles the bowel and is likely to cause obstruction. A change in bowel habit, obstructive symptoms, and gross blood in the stool are common symptoms for lesions on the left side. The change in bowel habit may be the onset of constipation, obstipation, diarrhea, or alternating periods of constipation and diarrhea. The development of small-caliber "pencil" stools is a particularly important sign. Obstructive symptoms are related to the circumferential nature of the tumor and the solid

TABLE 40-3. INCIDENCE IN PER CENT OF SYMPTOMS IN CANCER OF THE COLON

AUTHORS	FLOYD, STIRLING AND COHN	GLENN AND MCSHERRY	MCSWAIN, SADLER AND MAIN			POSTLETHWAIT, ADAMSON AND HART		
Number of cases	1,687	1,026	708			1,023		
Location of lesion	Entire colon	Distal bowel	Cecum (61)	Ascending to rectosigmoid (359)	Rectum and Anus (288)	Right colon (171)	Left colon (306)	Rectum and rectosigmoid (546)
Pain	70	—	90	78	52	74	65	26
Change in bowel habits	59	64	32	78	84	35	52	77
Weight loss	54	29	75	60	60	—	—	—
Bloody/tarry stools	54	57	—	—	—	37	54	81
Palpable mass	44	—	50	—	—	19	6	0.7
Anemia	35	—	—	—	—	35	4	0
Partial/complete obstruction	27	—	38	42	—	7	6	5
Occult blood in stool	21	—	—	—	—	—	—	—

nature of the feces. Obstruction may be mild in onset or, by contrast, acute symptoms may be the first of which the patient is aware. The role acute obstruction plays in altering prognosis and therapy is indicated in the section on Prognosis.

The importance of change in bowel habits, blood in the stools, pain and anemia cannot be overemphasized. The frequency of various signs and symptoms is shown in Table 40-3. Perhaps the most important thing to remember is that *any change in bowel habits in an individual over 40 is an observation that deserves further study.*

Physical signs relate most closely to findings on rectal examination and sigmoidoscopy. The relative importance of these studies and of barium enemas is indicated in Table 40-4, and

TABLE 40-4. POSITIVE DIAGNOSTIC STUDIES IN 1,687 PATIENTS WITH CANCER OF THE COLON*

X-ray	1,131
Proctoscopy or sigmoidoscopy	803
Rectal examination	748

* Floyd, Stirling and Cohn: Ann. Surg., 163:829, 1966.

this experience is echoed by all who have dealt with cancer of the colon. Any lesion which is felt or seen should be biopsied immediately and decision as to therapy based upon histologic examination of the specimen. Any patient can be sigmoidoscoped on his first visit to the physician's office. Preparative cleansing enemas obviously permit better visualization of the colonic mucosa but are not essential. The presence of an abdominal mass is usually suggestive of late disease, as is the presence of liver enlargement, but neither of these alone should be a contraindication to further study and/or treatment. Hemorrhoids must not be accepted as the complete explanation for patients' symptoms, as this fatal error has led too many patients and physicians to delay further study until curative procedures were no longer possible.

Obstruction. Cancer of the colon, rectum and anus has been implicated as the cause of approximately 75 per cent of large bowel obstructions. The survival rate for patients with malignant obstructing lesions of the colon re-

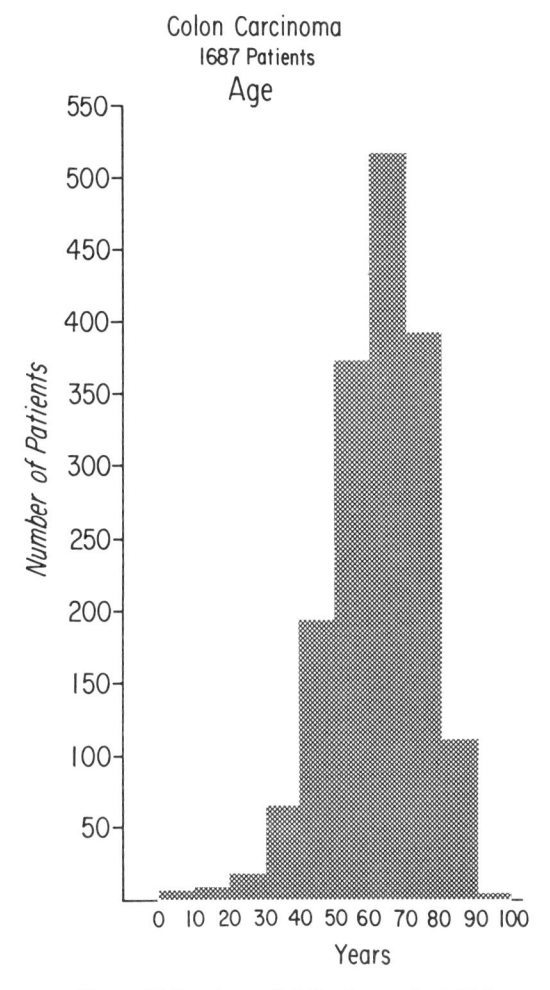

FIG. 40-9. Age distribution of 1,687 patients with cancer of the colon (Floyd, C. E., Stirling, C. T., and Cohn, I., Jr.: Ann. Surg., 163:830)

mains in the distressingly low range of 10 to 33 per cent despite the many advances in colon surgery. The experience at Charity Hospital in New Orleans with 512 patients with colonic obstruction due to carcinoma and an additional 1,467 reported cases is shown in Figure 40-10.

Obstruction of the large bowel occurs more frequently in the left colon. Acute complete obstruction in the sigmoid may be explained on the basis of a narrowed lumen, solid feces, the predominance of annular lesions and the high incidence of lesions in this area. However, if one compares the *ratio* of obstructing

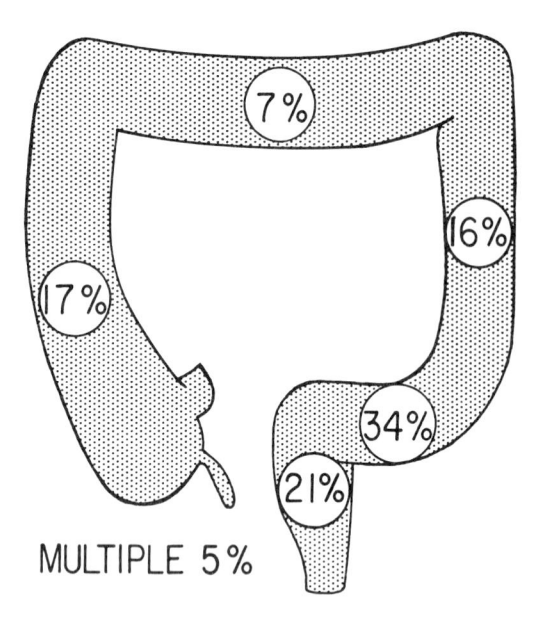

FIG. 40-10. Distribution of malignant lesions in the colon in patients with obstruction resulting from their lesions. (Modified from Floyd, C. E., and Cohn, I., Jr.: Ann. Surg., 165:722)

to total lesions in any one location, it is noted that there are other areas in the colon where the proportion of lesions causing obstruction is higher than in the sigmoid. The higher incidence in other areas has been overlooked because of the greater number of lesions in the sigmoid.

The significant and deleterious influence of obstruction on survival is discussed in the section on Prognosis.

TREATMENT. When the obstructing lesion is on the right side, the patient should be subjected to a one-stage decompression, resection, and primary anastomosis, even when this must be done as an emergency procedure. On the right side of the colon a primary resection permits one to remove the diseased bowel, and restore continuity by anastomosing small bowel to large bowel and have an anastomosis over which only liquid contents will pass. Because the contents of the bowel are liquid, the size of the bowel lumen is large and the blood supply of the bowel is good, this would seem to be an acceptable procedure.

Within recent years there has been interest in a similar approach to lesions on the left side (Windsberg, 1959; Herrington et al., 1967). In the left colon, conditions are quite different and the dangers of primary resection are considerably magnified. This approach has had little backing in past surgical experience. Primary resection of obstructing left colon lesions requires the emptying of a dirty, distended, friable large bowel, contamination of the entire field no matter how careful one's technic, the performance of an anastomosis of distended thin-walled bowel with a poor blood supply, and the risk of an anastomosis which will immediately be traversed by solid feces with all the attendant danger to a fresh suture line. Until further experience is obtained in the hands of a number of careful observers, it cannot be recommended for widespread use.

The preferred management of obstructing lesions on the left side is a proximal decompressing colostomy, with later, staged resection of the malignant lesion and closure of the colostomy. These are poor-risk patients, and even the colostomy must be performed with care when significant distention and dehydration are present.

The colostomy should be placed in an area which will permit subsequent definitive resection of the left colon. In order to allow sufficient length of distal colon for anastomosis, decompressive colostomy for left sided lesions usually is accomplished by exteriorizing a loop of the right transverse colon.

Perforation. The simultaneous occurrence of cancer and perforation of the colon represent a dual threat to life. Of the two threats to life, perforation, with its attendant fecal peritonitis, presents the more immediate cause for alarm, and is the one that dictates urgent care of such patients. Surgical care of perforation and the resultant peritonitis or abscess must take precedence over that of the cancer. The gravity of the combination of perforation and cancer and the poor long-term survival rates, combined with the apparently better results of a more radical approach, suggest that immediate resection should be considered more often (Crowder and Cohn, 1967). Perhaps Madden (1965) is correct when he says: "In perforations of the colon caused by cancer, primary resection is considered mandatory because of the frequent and rapid peritoneal spread of the tumor cells." Standard present day practice, however, still calls for preliminary proximal colostomy followed by staged resection for perforated lesions of the left colon.

X-Ray Studies. Barium enema studies are so important they need to be stressed. Barium enema preferably should be done after sigmoidoscopic examination so that neither will interfere with the other. Every effort should be made to have the colon as clean as possible. If a polyp is visualized, any surgical procedure should be delayed until a confirmatory barium enema can be obtained.

An air-contrast study is of particular importance in the visualization of small and polypoid lesions. If a lesion is identified on two separate barium enema examinations by a competent radiologist, then it is encumbent on the surgeon to find the lesion at the time of operation.

Angiographic technics can be utilized to specifically localize the site of bleeding, or to outline the location and vascular characteristics of a tumor (Kanter and Fleming, 1967). Lymphangiography may determine the presence and extent of lymph node metastases from lesions in the lower bowel (Nusbaum et al., 1967).

Laboratory Examinations. The specific procedures which relate to lesions in the colon include (1) biopsy for lesions which can be visualized, (2) hemoglobin determination, and (3) cytologic studies where the pathologist is specifically interested in this type of evaluation (Overholt and Pollard, 1967). Silicone foam enemas (Cook and Margulis, 1963), which originally looked promising for diagnosis of lesions above the reach of the sigmoidoscope, have not been as effective as had been hoped. Improvements in the formulation of the silicone foam may improve its usefulness. The complete evaluation of the patient, including laboratory studies, is discussed elsewhere.

Differential diagnosis includes the ruling out of diverticulitis (more apt to have leukocytosis), lymphopathia venereum (Frei test), tuberculosis (usually pulmonary tuberculosis is present), endometriosis (does not involve the mucosa, and the symptoms usually are made worse at the time of the menstrual periods), appendicitis, simple ulcer of the colon, and of course, benign polyps. In all instances of low-lying lesions, biopsy is the surest and really the only way to make the diagnosis. There are many benign conditions which can be confused with carcinoma.

The important differential diagnosis between diverticulitis and carcinoma of the colon was studied by Colcock and Sass (1954). These authors pointed out that the roentgenograms would differentiate most cases, but that the history is important as well. On the basis of 50 consecutive cases of each condition, nausea and vomiting, colicky pain, chills and fever, and rectal tenderness were all more common in diverticulitis. Constipation and blood per rectum were more common in carcinoma. Massive hemorrhage may occur, not only with diverticulitis but also with diverticulosis of the colon. Abscess and fistula formation were more common in diverticulitis. However, it should be mentioned in emphasizing the difficulties of this differential diagnosis that all of these listed differential features occurred in both conditions except for rectal tenderness which, while present in only 8 cases (16%) of the patients with diverticulitis, did not occur in any of those with carcinoma.

However, the differentiation between diverticulitis and carcinoma does not solve all the problems. Ponka, Fox and Brush (1959) pointed out that 75 (21%) of their cases of carcinoma of the colon had coexistent diverticulosis and diverticulitis.

Pathologic Variants. In addition to the usual adenocarcinoma of the colon, there are squamous cell, adenocanthomatous, mucoepidermoid, small cell, and physaliferous types.

Preparation of the Patient for Colon Surgery. Since surgery of the large bowel is major surgery, and since the complication rate for this type surgery is known to be high, it is important that all possible preoperative measures be employed to put the patient in optimum condition for the surgical procedure. The following should be considered a *minimum* for any prospective large bowel operation:

1. Blood count—to detect any anemia and the presence of any inflammatory disease.

2. Chest x-ray—as part of any preoperative work-up, and to detect presence of any metastases.

3. Sigmoidoscopy—as part of routine for any patient with colon disease.

4. Barium enema—even when a lesion has already been seen sigmoidoscopically, to de-

tect the presence of other lesions in the large bowel.

5. Intravenous pyelogram—particularly for lesions on the left side, to detect any displacement of ureters, in connection with sigmoid or rectosigmoid surgery.

6. Electrolyte studies in patients with any element of obstruction.

7. Liver function studies, x-rays of the pelvis and lumbosacral spine, serum proteins, alkaline phosphatase, liver scan, and clotting studies may be indicated under special circumstances.

Specific preparation of the patient for the operative procedure should include cleansing of the bowel for all elective colon surgery, unless inflammatory large bowel disease is present. Our routine is as follows:

1. Preparation should be conducted in the hospital for 72 hours.

2. Low residue diet for this period, preferably clear liquids.

3. A cathartic the first day.

4. Enemas for each day during the period, the last one to be administered the night before operation, *not* the morning of operation, to be sure the operative field is not flooded with liquid bowel contents.

5. Enema returns should be seen by the responsible surgeon to be sure the bowel is clean. This is particularly important in operations performed for polyps which may be extremely difficult to find in a dirty colon.

6. Intestinal antisepsis for 72 hours, with any of the drugs listed in Table 40-5. Our own

TABLE 40-5. DRUGS RECOMMENDED FOR INTESTINAL ANTISEPSIS

Amphotericin-neomycin
Bacitracin-neomycin
Kanamycin
Nystatin-neomycin
Polymyxin B-neomycin
Sulfathalidine-neomycin
Thiostrepton-neomycin

(Cohn, I., Jr.: Intestinal Antisepsis. Springfield, Ill., Charles C Thomas, 1969.)

choice is kanamycin as follows: 1 gm. every hour for four hours, then four times a day for total of 72 hours.

In addition to mechanical cleansing of the bowel, the patient being prepared for large bowel surgery should have a nasogastric tube in place prior to surgery, and, if the operation is to be a long one, or is to involve the distal bowel, an indwelling catheter should be placed in the bladder. We do not routinely place catheters in the ureters when an abdominoperineal is contemplated, but some surgeons use this additional safeguard, and all should know how helpful it can be in a difficult case.

Blood volume should be restored to as nearly normal as possible in the preoperative period, and adequate supplies of blood should be available during the operative procedure.

Treatment. The treatment of cancer of the colon and rectum is surgical excision. Colonic cancers should be removed as soon after diagnosis as possible. If the patient is obstructed, consideration must be given to relief of the obstruction prior to a definitive resection of the lesion. The management of patients with obstructive lesions has been discussed previously.

If the patient has metastases that cannot be removed, resection should still be attempted if it is possible to remove the primary lesion, even though a curative resection cannot be performed. The justification for resection under these circumstances is that the primary lesion is removed, the possibility of obstruction is eliminated, the chances of bleeding are minimized, and the opportunities for perforation, fistulization, infection, and the continuing discharge of foul-smelling material is diminished. The major fear of infection and hemorrhage are the determining factors here, in contrast to the management of malignant lesions in other parts of the body. Even the presence of known metastases in the liver should not be a deterrent to resection of the primary lesion. Some would even attempt curative resection with removal of a solitary liver metastasis as part of the primary procedure. Direct extension to other organs also should not be a deterrent to removal of the primary.

Interest in roentgen therapy has been revived, mainly as a result of the efforts of the group at Memorial Hospital. The most recent reports from this group (Stearns, Berg and Deddish, 1961; Quan, 1966) suggest that there is some benefit from preoperative x-ray therapy to lesions in the rectum, but the evidence is no longer as convincing as it was in the earlier studies. Truly randomized studies are currently underway at Memorial Hospital and elsewhere (Galante, Dunphy and Fletcher), and the long-term results of these studies will be awaited with interest. Cady's excellent review (1968) of the overall problem of preoperative radiation should be read by anyone interested in the subject.

Electrocoagulation or surgical diathermy was originally proposed by Strauss et al. (1935) as a means of palliation in the poor-risk patient. More recently Strauss et al. (1965) and Madden and Kandalaft (1967) have revived interest in this method of therapy, even for the good-risk patient, but this proposal needs additional evaluation by other surgeons before it can be recommended generally.

Perfusion with various cancer-chemotherapeutic agents has not been too successful in most hands.

THE SECOND LOOK. The second look was originally proposed by Wangensteen et al. as a deliberate re-exploration at 6-month intervals of patients with intra-abdominal cancer as a means of eradicating any disease left behind during the first operative procedure. The most recent report by Gilbertsen and Wangensteen (1962) is not sufficiently optimistic to warrant frequent use of the technic, and the lack of enthusiasm for this approach is apparent from the almost total absence of reports from other centers. When there is some justification for another operation—e.g., the development of gallstones in a patient who has previously had intra-abdominal cancer—then it should be utilized to search for recurrent or residual cancer, but the primary planned second look cannot be widely recommended.

DEFINITIVE RESECTION involves a consideration of 6 factors in the spread of the tumor, as follows: (1) the local tumor and its intramural spread; (2) the lymphatic metastases; (3) the venous spread; (4) the implantation of tumor cells from within the bowel lumen in the lines of anastomosis; (5) spread by direct extension to contiguous organs, and (6) transperitoneal spread.

Intramural Spread. The extent of such spread is important, and the surgeon should consider an adequate margin at all times. Studies include those of Dunphy and Broderick (1951), and of Lofgren, Waugh and Dockerty (1957).

Lymphatic Metastases. The classic studies of Gilchrist and David (1938) on lymphatic spread from lesions of the rectum are a landmark in the study of this problem, and should be reviewed by anyone interested in the subject. From a detailed study of all the nodes detectable in cleared specimens, they were able to reach the following conclusions: (1) The size of the tumor is of little value in determining the presence or absence of lymph node metastases. (2) Low-lying tumors may have very high metastases. (3) Retrograde metastases downward may occur when the upward lymph channels are blocked by metastases. (4) Tumors at the level of the levator ani muscle have a double lymphatic drainage, the more common being upward along the superior hemorrhoidal artery, the other being laterally along the superior surface of the levator ani muscle, indicating the necessity of resecting these muscles. (5) Squamous cell carcinoma may involve two lymphatic systems, upward along the course of the superior hemorrhoidal artery and laterally to the inguinal lymph nodes, indicating the necessity for a different operative approach to these lesions (See next chapter). (6) About 68 per cent of all operative specimens will be found to have involved lymph nodes if the specimens are studied by clearing technics. (7) Palpation is not a reliable method of detecting the presence of lymph nodes or their involvement. (8) The Miles operation is an ideal operation for rectal lesions because it removes all the areas discussed.

Ault (1953) has divided the lymphatic spread of rectal lesions on the basis of their relation to the middle valve of Houston. The demonstration of lymphatic spread only to the abdominal pathway as contrasted with the spread by both abdominal and pelvic routes for lesions below the middle valve is convincing.

The presence of lymph node metastases in general reduces 5-year survival by approximately one half the figure usually accepted for lesions without such involvement (See section on Prognosis).

Venous Spread. Spread occurs by the venous route more commonly than is popularly

1162   Tumors of the Colorectum

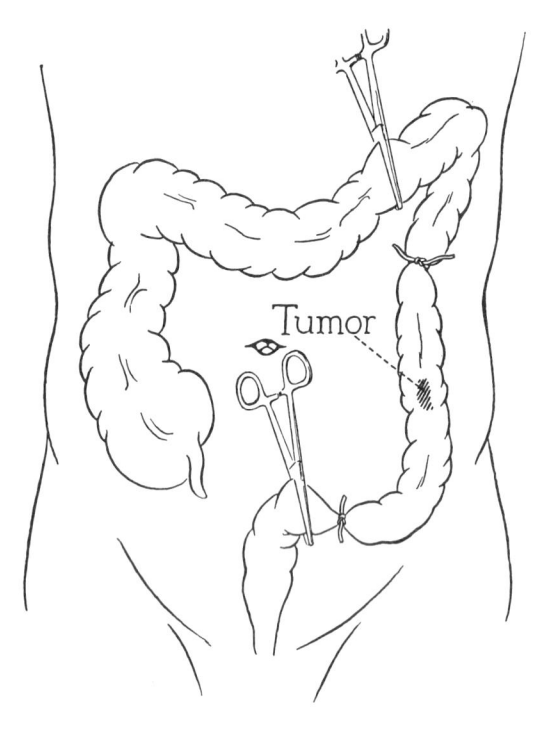

FIG. 40-11. First step in effort to prevent recurrence in colonic carcinoma from implantation of intraluminal tumor cells in suture lines: ligation of bowel on each side of tumor. (Cole, W. H.: Arch. Surg., 65: 267)

realized, and Cole and associates (1965) believe it is the most important route. Dionne (1965) found good evidence for blood-borne metastases in one third of the cases of cancer of the rectum. Fisher and Turnbull (1955) found tumor cells in the blood of the major mesenteric venous channels in patients being operated on for colorectal cancer. From this has grown a voluminous literature on the identification of tumor cells in the circulation, but the relationship of these specific tumor cells to the development of metastatic implants is not yet clear.

Clinically, early ligation of the venous supply to the colon prior to its mobilization is a direct outgrowth of these observations. This is a reversal of previous methods when ligation of the blood supply was almost the last step in resection. An even more recent modification has been the development of the "no-touch isolation" procedure in which "the cancer-bearing segment was not manipulated or handled in any manner until after the lymphovascular pedicles were divided and ligated and the colon was divided at the elected sites for resection" (Turnbull et al., 1967). The evidence indicates a better 5-year survival rate for some patients handled in this rather than the more conventional manner. Greater use of this technic seems almost certain for the immediate future, followed by a more careful evaluation of the results in other institutions.

Implantation of Tumor Cells From Within the Bowel Lumen in the Lines of Anastomosis. Between 1948 and 1951 three different groups of workers (Cole, 1951; Goligher, Dukes and Bussey, 1951; Lloyd-Davies, 1948) independently noted a high incidence of tumor recurrence in the suture line (10-14%) following resection of the colon for carcinoma. The first good experimental study of this problem was published in 1954 (Vink). Summary of our own work, Table 40-6, shows which agents and technics are effective in controlling tumor spread when studied in the rabbit, using the Brown-Pearce tumor as the experimental model.

A number of different clinical approaches to the control of this newly recognized form of tumor spread have been proposed. English

TABLE 40-6. INFLUENCE ON TUMOR IMPLANTATION*

No Effect	Effective		
	Suture Line	Peritoneal Cavity	Both
Clorpactin XCB irrigation	Iodized suture	Irradiation	Closed anastomosis
DMSO		Low molecular weight	
Iodine irrigation		dextran	
Nitrogen mustard		Mechanical control	
Saline irrigation			

* Based on data from Cohn, I., Jr.: Surg., Gynec., Obstet., 124:501, 1967.

surgeons have favored chemical irrigation of the ends of the bowel to prevent tumor implantation, but their use of bichloride of mercury has not been favorably received in the United States. Cole's suggestion of isolating the segment of bowel containing the cancer so as to prevent any spillage of tumor cells has been considered by many to be one of the major recent advances in surgery of gastrointestinal cancer (Fig. 40-11). Rousselot *et al.* (1968) advocate intraluminal chemotherapeutic agents for the control of spread, but his treated series is still too small to warrant any far-reaching conclusions. Other major reviews of the subject may be found in the works of Keynes (1961), and Cole and his associates (Cole *et al.*, 1961; Cole *et al.*, 1965).

Both clinical and experimental data now indicate that implantation following spillage of tumor cells during operations on the gastrointestinal tract is an important feature of cancer spread, and one that must be considered in all future advances in surgery of colon cancer.

Spread by Direct Extension to Contiguous Organs. In males spread to the prostate or from the prostate to the rectum may make the decision difficult at the time of operation as to exactly where the tumor arose. Involvement of the small bowel is a simpler matter, since the tumor has almost always arisen in the colorectum. Such spread is not a reason for defeatism, and the results of pelvic exenteration in such cases are often surprisingly good (Butcher and Spjut, 1959).

Transperitoneal Spread. Such spread usually means inoperability, except occasionally to relieve or forestall obstruction. In the case of one prominent American, such spread was found in a hernial sac during an incidental hernioplasty.

SELECTION OF OPERATION FOR TUMORS AT

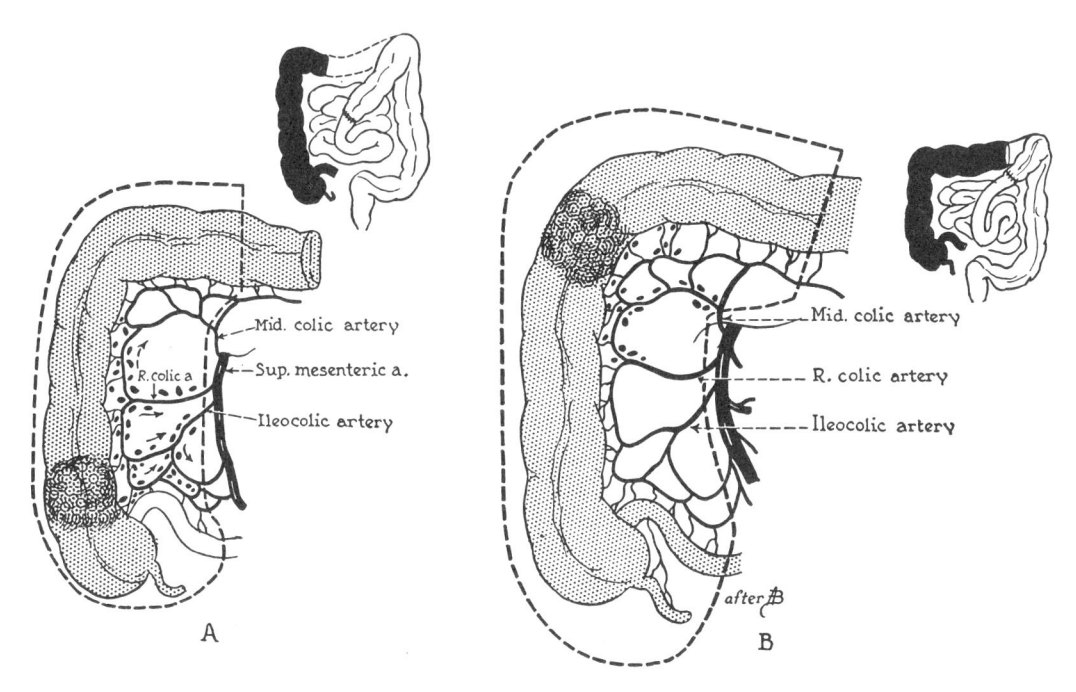

FIG. 40-12. (A) Carcinoma of the cecum. Lymphatic spread is along the ileocolic group of lymph nodes. Extent of resection, indicated by dotted line, includes tumor and potentially involved regional lymph nodes. In our opinion, the lowest branch of the superior mesenteric artery (A) should be ligated proximal to its first branching and not distally as shown. Inset shows site of ileocolic anastomosis. (B) Carcinoma of hepatic flexure. Lymphatic spread is along the right and the middle colic arteries. Line of resection includes tumor, omentum and regional lymph nodes. Inset shows the continuity of the bowel re-established by an anastomosis of the ileum to the splenic flexure. (Rosi, P. A.: Surg. Clin. N. Am., 34:225)

1164 Tumors of the Colorectum

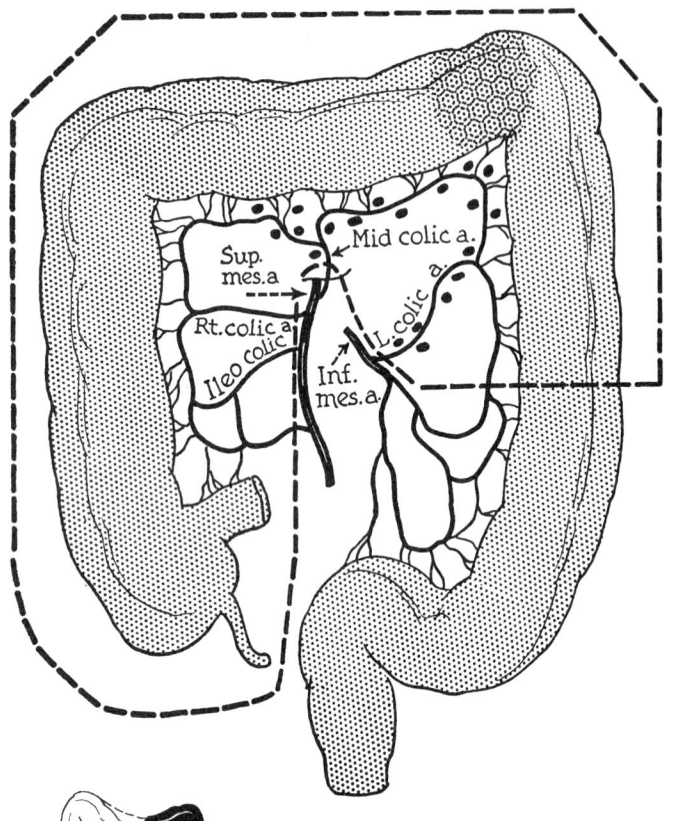

FIG. 40-13. Carcinoma of the splenic flexure. Lymphatic spread is to the nodes that lie on the middle colic and the left colic arterial arcade. Line of resection includes ascending (not all surgeons would remove this, since the nodes along the right colic and the ileocolic arteries are seldom involved), transverse and descending colon and all the lymph nodes along the middle colic and the left colic arteries. Inset shows anastomosis between the ileum and the sigmoid. (Rosi, P. A.: Surg. Clin. N. Am., 34:226)

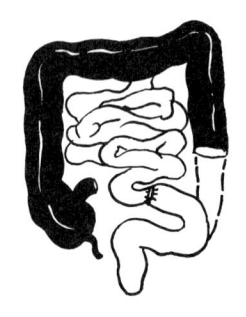

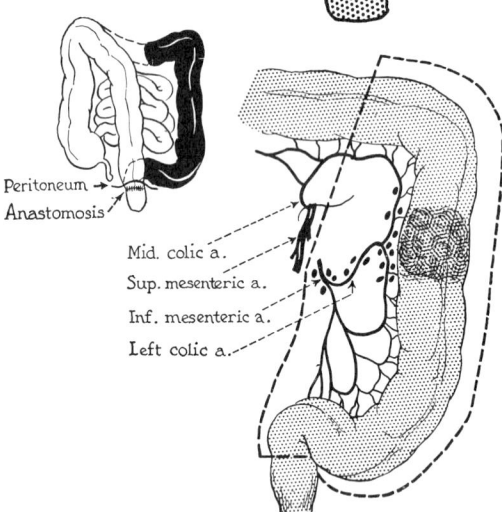

FIG. 40-14. Carcinoma of the descending colon and sigmoid. Lymphatic spread is to the regional lymph nodes and the inferior mesenteric and the periaortic group of nodes. Line of resection includes the tumor and the entire mesentery of the left colon. Inset shows continuity of the bowel reestablished by transverse colon-rectal anastomosis. (Rosi, P. A.: Surg. Clin. N. Am., 34:226)

DIFFERENT SITES IN THE COLORECTUM. An adequate cancer operation should remove the tumor, as much of the organ in which it arises as is necessary or practical, and all the appropriate vascular and lymphatic pathways. This is as true for colonic cancers as for any other type cancer. In removing carcinomas in some parts of the colon, adequate lymphatic dissection entails simultaneous vascular dissection that may require sacrifice of additional colon. Knowledge of the lymphatic and vascular anatomy is essential to a clear understanding of the principles of colonic resection.

Excellent plans for dealing with tumors in various parts of the large bowel are shown in Figures 40-12 to 40-16, based on the work of Rosi.

The older surgical literature repeatedly stresses the importance of the marginal artery of Drummond and of Sudek's critical point in terms of whether a proposed colonic resection would lead to viable or nonviable segments of bowel. Recently there has been less concern with either of these anatomic features,

Fig. 40-15. Carcinoma of the rectosigmoid. Lymphatic spread is upward toward the inferior mesenteric group of nodes, but retrograde spread into the nodes of the mesorectum may occur. Line of resection includes the tumor, the inferior mesenteric and the periaortic nodes and from 12 to 15 cm. of bowel and mesentery below the tumor. The tumor shown in this figure is so low that only surgeons with considerable experience can safely remove it by anterior resection. Inset shows descending colon-rectal anastomosis. (Rosi, P. A.: Surg. Clin. N. Am., 34:229)

provided that proper attention is devoted to other elements during the resection of the bowel. A comprehensive anatomic review of the vasculature of the colon is presented by Michels, Siddharth, Kornblith, and Parke (1963).

The final test of viability of any stump of rectum or colon should be the continuation of normal bowel wall color after several minutes observation, *plus* the presence of arterial bleeding from the cut edge of the stump.

There is controversy in regard to the level at which the vascular pedicle should be ligated when resecting lesions of the left colon. Ault (1958) probably presents the best arguments and best illustrations for ligation of the inferior mesenteric artery flush with the aorta and the inferior mesenteric vein where it crosses the left renal vein. He also argues that the method of handling the entire approach to cancer of the colon should be changed in favor of primary isolation of the vascular-lymphatic pedicle followed by clamping the colon on both sides of the lesion as a means of controlling all known routes of tumor spread. This is much the same approach that Turnbull calls the "no-touch isolation technic." However, at the time of its original presentation, Ault's proposal stimulated debate mainly on the question of the advisability of such a high ligation of the inferior mesenteric vessels. Grinnell's (1965) conflicting evidence concludes that none of the patients who already have metastases at this high a level would be helped by this extended form of resection because they already have metastases to other areas.

Our own impression is that the high ligation of the vessels should be practiced when it can be done, until such time as there are larger series of cases to confirm or deny the value of additional operative time and risk. However, there is not sufficient justification for carrying the operative procedure to these limits in the poor-risk patient, the obese patient, or in any patient in whom the additional operative time would increase the operative risk.

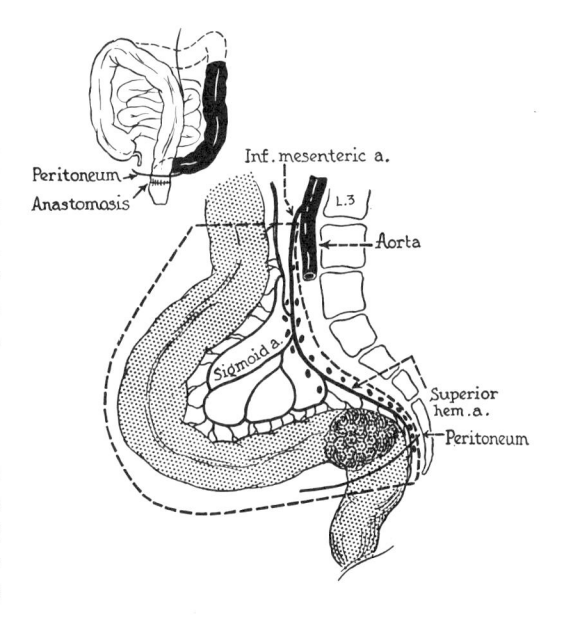

ABDOMINO-PERINEAL RESECTION. The description in 1908 by Ernest Miles of the abdomino-perineal approach to tumors of the rectum is a landmark in the history of surgery of the colon. It is notable for what it says and for the brevity with which it is said, the entire article encompassing only one and a half pages in *The Lancet*. Since the appearance of the original article, only minor modifications in the operative approach and principles have been developed, and thus it seems worthwhile to quote from portions of the original:

Removal of the rectum by a combined abdominal and perineal operation was first performed by Czerny in 1884. Since that time several other surgeons have employed the method with certain modifications. . . . The technique of these operators seems to have failed in one important respect—namely the complete eradication of the *zone of upward spread* of cancer from the rectum,

1166   Tumors of the Colorectum

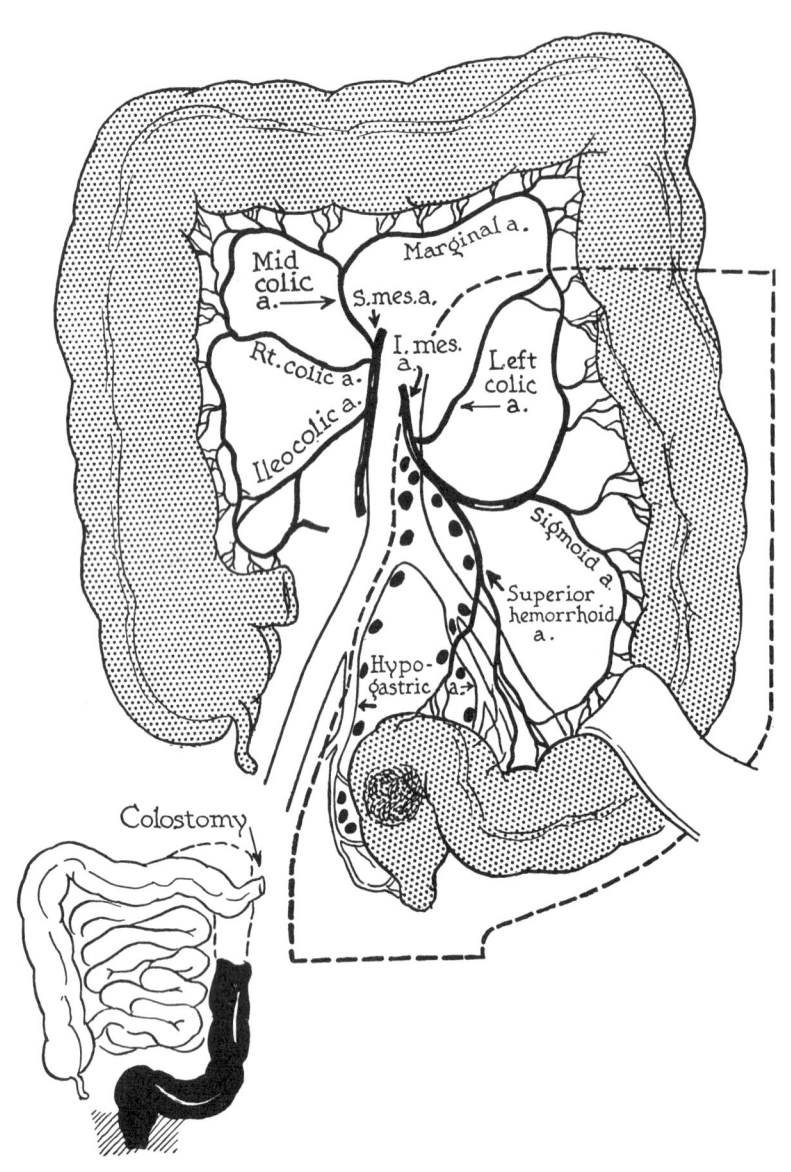

FIG. 40-16. Carcinoma of the lower rectum. Lymphatic spread is upward toward the inferior mesenteric group of nodes and laterally along the middle hemorrhoidal, the hypogastric and the iliac groups of nodes. Line of resection includes the tumor, the mesentery of the left colon, and nodes along the middle hemorrhoidal, the hypogastric and the iliac arteries and the perianal muscles and the skin. Inset shows completed abdominoperineal resection with colostomy in the region of the splenic flexure. Whereas the colostomy comes from the splenic flexure, in our opinion it should be placed more centrally on the abdomen. (Rosi, P. A.: Surg. Clin. N. Am., 34:229)

whereby the chance of recurrence of the disease, above the field of operation, can be diminished if not entirely obviated.

. . . I found that, even after the most complete and extensive (perineal) removal possible, . . . recurrence took place within periods ranging from six months to three years in 54 instances (of 57).

. . . Recurrence appeared in situations that were beyond the scope of a removal from the perineum. Post-mortem examination showed that these situations were (a) the pelvic peritoneum, (b) the pelvic mesocolon, and (c) the lymph nodes situated over the bifurcation of the left common iliac artery.

The study of the spread of cancer from the rectum has led me to formulate certain essentials in the technique of the operation . . . (1) that an abdominal anus is a necessity; (2) that the whole of the pelvic colon with the exception of the part from which the colostomy is made, must be removed because its blood supply is contained in the zone of upward spread; (3) that the whole of the pelvic mesocolon below the point where it crosses the common iliac artery together with a strip of peritoneum at least an inch wide on either side of it, must be cleared away; (4) that the group of lymph nodes situated over the bifurcation of the common iliac artery are in all instances to be removed; and lastly, (5) that the perineal portion of the operation should be carried out as widely as possible so that the lateral and downward zones of spread may be effectively extirpated.*

The Miles operation is the standard against which any new proposal is measured in terms of long-term results, morbidity, mortality, and patient satisfaction. From time to time there have been attempts to displace the Miles procedure with various operative procedures that did not require a permanent abdominal colostomy. Babcock (1947) summarized his experience with a pull-through operation which was a modification of the Hochenegg procedure, and claimed to have morbidity, mortality, and survival figures on a par with that of the Miles procedure. Best and Rasmussen (1956) also recommended a sphincter-saving procedure for which they claim results superior to that of an abdomino-perineal resection.

The major controversy in regard to the treatment of lesions of the rectum at the present time is related to whether to do an anterior resection or an abdomino-perineal resection. Excellent articles by proponents of each side seem to provide indisputable evidence for the validity of their viewpoint. The wide variation in viewpoint only serves to point up the importance of an open mind. The high incidence of tumor recurrence at or near the suture line has been one of the cogent arguments against the use of an anterior resection, particularly for low-lying lesions where an adequate margin cannot be obtained. Advocates of the anterior resection include Muir (1958); Mayo and Cullen (1960); and Vandertoll and Beahrs (1965). In a critical review of both the literature and their own clinical experience in the field, Dunphy and Broderick concluded that the anterior resection should

... be employed only: (1) to extend the scope of resection for lesions of the lower sigmoid colon, (2) to avoid colostomy in the presence of distant metastases provided that the local disease can be completely extirpated, and (3) to restore continuity of the bowel in carefully selected cases of cancer of the upper rectum and lower pelvic colon in which the pelvic fascia is not invaded, there are no obvious lymph node metastases, and there is a minimal "operative margin" of 10 cm. below the tumor.†

* Miles, W. E.: Lancet, 2:1812-1813, 1908.
† Dunphy, J. E., and Broderick, E. G.: Surgery, 30:106-115, 1951.

This is a sound approach with which the present author agrees. Almost everyone now agrees that, for tumors located in the distal rectum, the abdomino-perineal resection is the operation that more nearly fits the ideals of cancer surgery, but most also agree that there are definite instances when the anterior resection must be given proper consideration. For lesions above the perineal reflection most surgeons would perform an anterior resection. For lesions located between 8 and 15 cm. some surgeons would perform an anterior resection if technically feasible, but the present author prefers an abdomino-perineal. For lesions closer to the anus than 8 cm. the Miles resection is the operation of choice.

A *colostomy* or an *ileostomy* needs special care. The technics for making any gastrointestinal stoma are well outlined by Turnbull and Weakley (1967), but there are certain precautions in addition to the technical details that should be part of the basic knowledge of any physician who cares for these patients. In the immediate postoperative period the stoma should be inspected frequently, and certainly at intervals no further apart than every 12 hours for the first 48 to 72 hours. During this time the color, amount of edema, and presence of any retraction or prolapse should be noted. Any unusual bleeding should be noted. In the case of an ileostomy, the amount and type of discharge should be observed, and an ileostomy bag should have been applied at once to prevent any skin excoriation. A bag is not necessary for a colostomy and early fecal discharge is not expected. If the patient has had an abdomino-perineal resection, the perineal wound should be examined each time the colostomy is observed, to note the amount of bleeding. Urinary output also should be monitored particularly carefully in any such patient because of the danger of hypotension during or after the operative procedure and the danger to the ureters during the dissection.

Complications. Urinary complications and sexual malfunction are among those complications which follow these operations which extend into the true pelvis.

The complications of colorectal surgery are not inconsiderable. Nearly 100 per cent of the patients have temporary difficulties with voiding, some have serious delay in recovery

TABLE 40-7. THE INFLUENCE OF EXTENT OF DISEASE ON SURVIVAL IN CANCER OF THE COLON. BASED ON 14,865 REPORTED CASES*

	No. CASES EVAL.	5 YEAR SURVIVAL	No. CASES EVAL.	10 YEAR SURVIVAL
I. Absolute Survival Rates	14,865	34.0%	1,187	30.1%
II. Determinate Survival Rates	12,525	39.8%	888	35.7%
Stages				
Stage I	838	80.3%	141	68.8%
Disease strictly confined to bowel wall. No evidence of metastases.				
Stage II	1,202	70.6%	220	55.9%
Extension into the pericolonic tissues but not involving other organs. No evidence of metastases.				
Stage III	1,934	31.9%	297	21.5%
Regional lymph node metastases.				
Stage IV	577	1.2%	0	
Extension into other organs or with distant metastases.				

* Modified from James, A. G.: Cancer Prognosis Manual. New York, Am. Cancer Soc., 1967.

in this respect, some never recover entirely. Many men have need for a later prostatectomy. Almost all patients with abdomino-perineal resection for carcinoma have some postoperative sexual difficulty, either with erection or ejaculation or both, in contradistinction to a similar resection for ulcerative colitis, or congenital polyposis for which the dissection is close to the rectum. In operation for carcinoma with adequate pelvic resection there is no adequate way of preventing such a complication and younger male patients should be warned concerning it before operation. Other complications include late wound infections in the properitoneal fat, necrosis of the colostomy stump if proper attention is not paid to the blood supply of the colon loop, and leakage at the site of the anastomosis, particularly when colon is joined to colon or to rectum.

Prognosis and Results. The results of therapy for cancer of the colon depend on a number of factors, which include: location of the tumor, its extent, presence of positive lymph nodes, the operation performed, environmental factors, geographic distribution, and probably a long list of other factors about which not enough is yet known. Good discussions of this problem may be found in the following references (See Bibliography): Dukes and Bussey; Colcock; Galante, Dunphy and Fletcher; Garlock et al.; Gilbertsen; Glenn and McSherry; Goligher; Grinnell (1953); Hughes; Liechty et al.; McSwain, Sadler and Main; Postlethwait, Adamson and Hart; Welch and Burke; Wynder and Shigematsu.

The importance of metastases to lymph nodes is immediately apparent from even a cursory look at the figures from the Cancer Prognosis Manual, in which the results of various reported series have been tabulated to give the final figures on over 14,000 cases (Table 40-7). These figures show that both the 5-year and the 10-year survival figures are decreased to less than half when lymph node metastases are present.

From our own experience (Floyd, Stirling and Cohn, 1966) where a sufficiently large group of patients was studied to permit various types of analyses, and where *all* patients were considered, it is possible to provide interesting survival data. Regardless of what type therapy is employed, the drop-off during the first year is marked, and only 43 per cent of all patients were alive one year after the diagnosis was made. The subsequent decline was precipitous. The differences between survival of patients subjected to "curative" procedures, "palliative" procedures, or simple

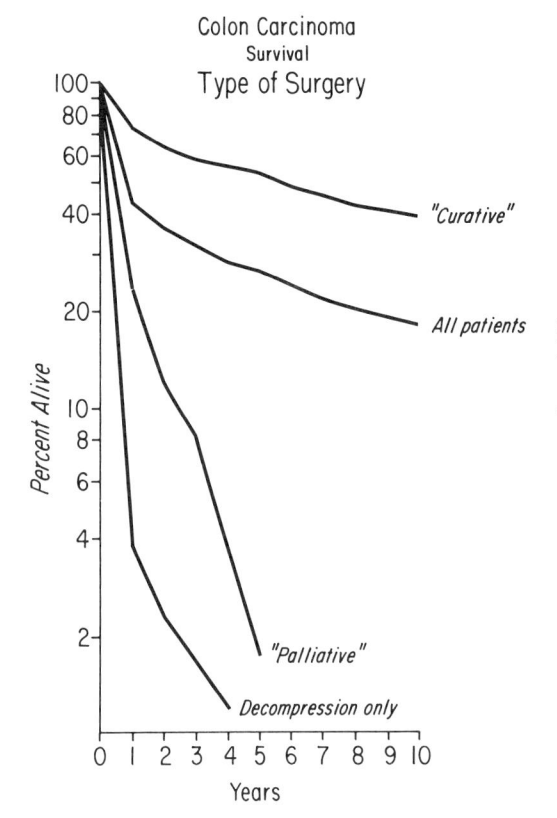

FIG. 40-17. Survival after diagnosis of cancer of the colon, rectum and anus computed by life-table method for 1,687 patients reviewed at Charity Hospital. The curves are based upon all patients and the various surgical procedures are those listed by the surgeon at the time of operation. Curves for "palliative" and decompressive procedures are discontinued because there were too few survivors to make meaningful calculations. (Floyd, C. E., Stirling, C. T., and Cohn, I., Jr.: Ann. Surg., 163:835)

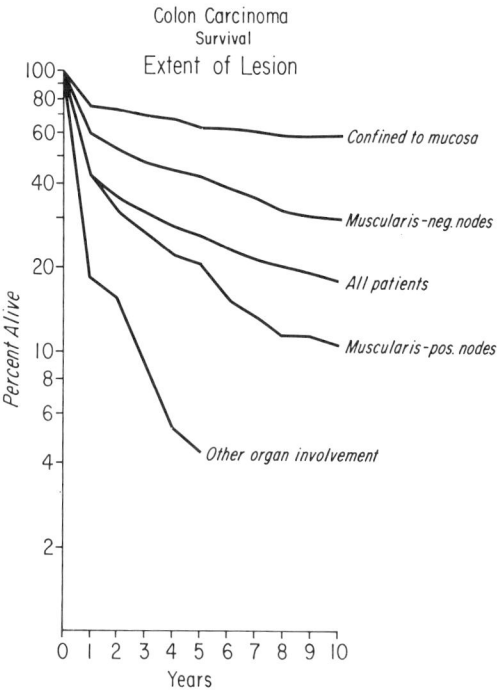

FIG. 40-18. Survival curves based upon the microscopic extent of the lesion, computed by the same technic as in Figure 40-17, and from the same data. There were too few survivors after 5 years in the group with other organ involvement to permit calculation of data. (Floyd, C. E., Stirling, C. T., and Cohn, I., Jr.: Ann. Surg., 163: 835)

decompressive procedures is so striking as to be one of the major observations of this particular study (Fig. 40-17).

A different type evaluation, but equally instructive, can be obtained by studying survival based upon the extent of the lesion histologically (Fig. 40-18). It is obvious that the survival decreases as the lesion extends. The negligible decline in survival from the 5th to the 10th year for those whose lesion was confined to the mucosa suggests that the term "cure" may have application after 5 years for these patients. These studies confirm other observations that the 5-year and 10-year survival figures for cancer of the colon are better than those for most other common types of cancer, and this is an area in which proper education of the public and of the medical profession can do much to improve our overall results in cancer therapy.

The impact of obstruction on survival can be seen from the fact that the 53 per cent 5-year survival rate for patients subjected to curative procedures was reduced to 17 per cent when obstruction was present. However, extensive disease alone is not responsible for the poor prognosis in patients with obstructing lesions, since a number of patients who did not survive the 5-year period had negative lymph nodes. Patients with obstruction on the left side had the best 5-year survival, and those

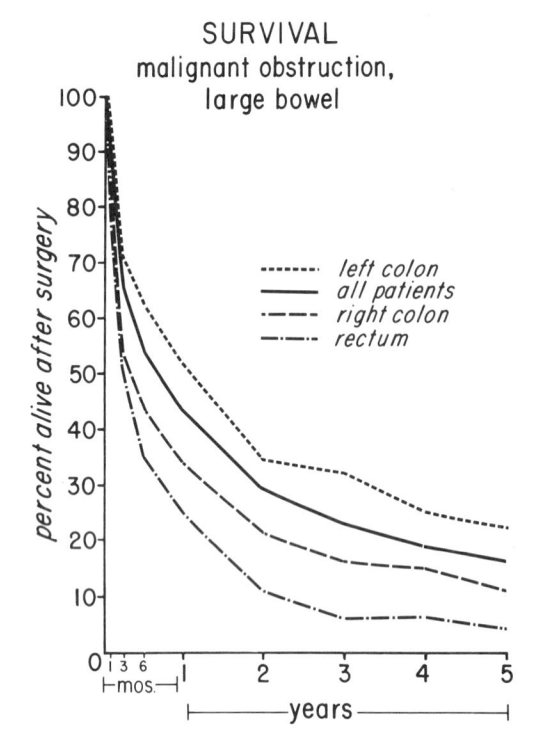

FIG. 40-19. Survival curves based upon location of lesions for patients with malignant lesions causing obstruction of the large bowel. (Modified from Floyd, C. E., and Cohn, I., Jr.: Ann. Surg., 165:729)

with obstruction in the rectum had the poorest results (Fig. 40-19). The improved survival rate of patients with left colon lesions may be related to the earlier detection of the lesion as a result of earlier obstruction. By comparison, the poor survival of patients with rectal lesions may be related to the late appearance of obstructive symptoms, the lack of serosal covering, and the additional avenues of spread of rectal lesions.

The relatively good results obtained in cancer of the colon when the disease is properly treated at an early stage indicate this is one form of cancer that will respond to appropriate therapy. If the patients can be educated to come to the physician early and if the physicians can be educated to think of the disease and to do the simple things necessary to establish a diagnosis, the long-term results should begin to show significant improvement.

MALIGNANT TUMORS: RARER LESIONS

Among malignant tumors, adenocarcinoma is so preponderantly of major importance among the lesions of the colon and the rectum that other lesions will only be listed. These include: (1) fibrosarcoma, (2) leiomyosarcoma, (3) lymphosarcoma, (4) leukemic infiltration, (5) malignant carcinoid metastasizing to distant organs, (6) malignant melanoma, (7) squamous cell carcinoma of the colon, (8) hemangiopericytoma, and (9) secondary tumors.

BIBLIOGRAPHY

American Cancer Society, Inc.: 1968 Cancer Facts and Figures. New York, American Cancer Society, 1967.
Arminski, T. C., and McLean, D. W.: Incidence and distribution of adenomatous polyps of the colon and rectum based on 1,000 autopsy examinations. Dis. Colon Rectum, 7:249-261, 1964.
Atwater, J. S., and Bargen, J. A.: The pathogenesis of intestinal polyps. Gastroenterology, 4:395-408, 1945.
Ault, G. W.: Carcinoma of the rectum: factors responsible for recurrent or residual disease. Am. Surg., 19:1035-1044, 1953.
———: A technique for cancer isolation and extended dissection for cancer of the distal colon and rectum. Surg., Gynec., Obstet., 106:467-477, 1958.
Babcock, W. W.: Radical single stage extirpation for cancer of the large bowel, with retained functional anus. Surg., Gynec., Obstet., 85:1-7, 1947.
Bacon, H. E., Lowell, E. J., Jr., and Trimpi, H. D.: Villous papillomas of the colon and rectum: a study of 28 cases with end results of treatment over a 5-year period. Surgery, 35:77-87, 1954.
Bargen, J. A.: The nature of the carcinoma associated with ulcerative colitis. Dis. Colon Rectum, 5:356-360, 1962.
Best, R. R., and Rasmussen, J. A.: Sphincter-preserving operations for cancer of the rectum. Arch. Surg., 72:948-956, 1956.
Blatt, L. J.: Polyps of the colon and rectum: Incidence and distribution. Dis. Colon Rectum, 4:277-282, 1961.
Bockus, H. L., Tachdjian, V., Ferguson, L. K., Mouhran, Y., and Chamberlain, C.: Adenomatous polyp of colon and rectum; Its relation to carcinoma. Gastroenterology, 41:225-232, 1961.
Butcher, H. R., Jr., and Spjut, H. J.: An evaluation of pelvic exenteration for advanced carcinoma of the lower colon. Cancer, 12:681-687, 1959.
Cady, B.: Preoperative radiation. Surg., Gynec., Obstet., 126:851-865; 1091-1105, 1968.
Castleman, B., and Krickstein, H. I.: Do adenomatous polyps of the colon become malignant?, New Eng. J. Med., 267:469-475, 1962.

Cohn, I., Jr.: Implantation in cancer of the colon. Surg., Gynec., Obstet., 124:501-508, 1967.
———: Intestinal Antisepsis. Springfield, Ill., Charles C Thomas, 1969.
Colcock, B. P.: Early diagnosis in carcinoma of the right colon. Dis. Colon Rectum, 7:482-485, 1964.
Colcock, B. P., and Sass, R. E.: Diverticulitis and carcinoma of the colon: differential diagnosis. Surg., Gynec., Obstet., 99:627-633, 1954.
Cole, W. H.: Measures to combat the menace of cancer. Am. Surg., 17:660-663, 1951.
———: Recurrence in carcinoma of the colon and proximal rectum following resection for carcinoma. Arch. Surg., 65:264-270, 1952.
Cole, W. H., McDonald, G. O., Roberts, S. S., and Southwick, H. W.: Dissemination of Cancer. Prevention and Therapy. New York, Appleton-Century-Crofts, 1961.
Cole, W. H., Packard, D., and Southwick, H. W.: Carcinoma of the colon with special reference to prevention of recurrence. J.A.M.A., 155:1549-1553, 1954.
Cole, W. H., Roberts, S. S., Webb, R. S., Jr., Strehl, F. W., and Oates, G. D.: Dissemination of cancer with special emphasis on vascular spread and implantation. Ann. Surg., 161:753-770, 1965.
Cook, G. B., and Margulis, A. R.: Detecting small sessile colon cancers with silicone foam. J.A.M.A., 183:66-68, 1963.
Crowder, V. H., Jr., and Cohn, I., Jr.: Perforation in cancer of the colon and rectum. Dis. Colon Rectum, 10:415-420, 1967.
deDombal, F. T., Watts, J. McK., Watkinson, G., and Goligher, J. C.: Local complications of ulcerative colitis: Stricture, pseudopolyposis, and carcinoma of colon and rectum. Brit. Med. J., 1:1442-1447, 1966.
Dionne, L.: The pattern of blood-borne metastasis from carcinoma of rectum. Cancer, 18:775-781, 1965.
Dollinger, M. R., and Gardner, B.: Newer aspects of the carcinoid spectrum. Surg., Gynec., Obstet., 122:1335-1347, 1966.
Drummond, H.: Some points relating to the surgical anatomy of the arterial supply of the large intestine. Proc. Roy. Soc. Med. (Surgical Section, Subsection of Proctology), 7:185-193, 1914.
Dukes, C. E.: Familial intestinal polyposis. Ann. Roy. Coll. Surg. Eng., 10:293-304, 1952.
Dukes, C. E., and Bussey, H. J. R.: The spread of rectal cancer and its effects on prognosis. Brit. J. Cancer, 12:309-320, 1958.
Dunphy, J. E., and Broderick, E. G.: A critique of anterior resection in the treatment of cancer of the rectum and pelvic colon. Surgery, 30:106-115, 1951.
Eisenberg, H. L., Kolb, L. H., Yam, L. T., and Godt, R.: Villous adenoma of the rectum associated with electrolyte disturbance. Ann. Surg., 159:604-610, 1964.
Enquist, I. F.: The incidence and significance of polyps of the colon and rectum. Surgery, 42:681-688, 1957.
Enterline, H. T., Evans, G. W., Mercado-Lugo, R., Miller, L., and Fitts, W. T., Jr.: Malignant potential of adenomas of colon and rectum. J.A.M.A., 179:322-330, 1962.
Everson, T. C., and Allen, M. J.: Subtotal colectomy with ileosigmoidostomy and fulguration of polyps in retained colon: evaluation as method of treatment of polyposis (adenomatosis) of colon. Arch. Surg., 69:806-817, 1954.
Fisher, E. R., and Turnbull, R. B., Jr.: The cytologic demonstration and significance of tumor cells in the mesenteric venous blood in patients with colorectal carcinoma. Surg., Gynec., Obstet., 100:102-108, 1955.
Floyd, C. E., and Cohn, I., Jr.: Obstruction in cancer of the colon. Ann. Surg., 165:721-731, 1967.
Floyd, C. E., Stirling, C. T., and Cohn, I., Jr.: Cancer of the colon, rectum and anus: Review of 1,687 cases. Ann. Surg., 163:829-837, 1966.
Galante, M., Dunphy, J. E., and Fletcher, W. S.: Cancer of the colon. Ann. Surg., 165:732-744, 1967.
Gardner, E. J., and Stephens, F. E.: Cancer of the lower digestive tract in one family group. Am. J. Hum. Genet., 2:41-48, 1950.
Garlock, J. H.: Lerman, B., Klein, S. H., Lyons, A. S., and Kirschner, P. A.: Twenty-five years' experience with surgical therapy of cancer of the colon and rectum: an analysis of 1,887 cases. Dis. Colon Rectum, 5:247-263, 1962.
Gilbertsen, V. A.: Results of treatment of bowel cancer. Ann. Surg., 157:198-203, 1963.
Gilbertsen, V. A., and Wangensteen, O. H.: A summary of thirteen years' experience with the second look program. Surg., Gynec., Obstet., 114:438-442, 1962.
Gilchrist, R. K., and David, V. C.: Lymphatic spread of carcinoma of the rectum. Ann. Surg., 108:621-642, 1938.
Glenn, F., and McSherry, C. K.: Carcinoma of the distal large bowel: 32-year review of 1,026 cases. Ann. Surg., 163:838-849, 1966.
Goldfarb, W. B.: Villous adenomas of the right colon, Cancer 17:264-271, 1964.
Goldgraber, M. B., and Kirsner, J. B.: Carcinoma of the colon in ulcerative colitis. Cancer, 17:657-665, 1964.
Goligher, J. C.: Surgery of the Anus, Rectum and Colon. Springfield, Ill., Charles C Thomas, 1967.
Goligher, J. C., Dukes, C. E., and Bussey, H. J. R.: Local recurrences after sphincter-saving excision for carcinoma of the rectum and rectosigmoid. Brit. J. Surg., 39:199-211, 1951.
Gray, L. A.: The management of endometriosis involving the bowel. In: Fuchs, F., and Green, T. H., Jr. (eds.). Clincial Obstetrics and Gynecology. pp. 309-330. New York, Harper & Row, 1966.
Grinnell, R. S.: Results in the treatment of carcinoma of the colon and rectum. An analysis of 2,341 cases over a 35 year period with 5 year survival results in 1,667 patients. Surg., Gynec., Obstet., 96:31-42, 1953.
———: Results of ligation of inferior mesenteric artery at the aorta in resections of carcinoma of the descending and sigmoid colon and rectum. Surg., Gynec., Obstet., 120:1031-1036, 1965.
Grinnell, R. S., and Lane, N.: Benign and malig-

nant adenomatous polyps and papillary adenomas of the colon and rectum. An analysis of 1856 tumors in 1335 patients. Surg., Gynec., Obstet., 106:519-538, 1958.

Haller, J. D., and Roberts, T. W.: Lipomas of the colon: A clinicopathologic study of 20 cases. Surgery, 55:773-781, 1964.

Helwig, E. B.: The evolution of adenomas of the large intestine and their relation to carcinoma. Surg., Gynec., Obstet., 84:36-49, 1947.

————: Adenomas and the pathogenesis of cancer of the colon and rectum. Dis. Colon Rectum 2:5-17, 1959.

Herrington, J. L., Jr., Lawler, M., Thomas, T. V., and Graves, H. A., Jr.: Colon resection with primary anastomosis performed as an emergency and as a non-planned operation. Ann. Surg., 165:709-720, 1967.

Hinton, J. M.: Risk of malignant change in ulcerative colitis. Gut, 7:427-432, 1966.

Holtz, F., and Schmidt, L. A., III: Lymphoid polyps (benign lymphoma) of the rectum and anus. Surg., Gynec., Obstet. 106:639-642, 1958.

Hughes, E. S. R.: Results of treatment of carcinoma of colon and rectum. Brit. Med. J., 2:9-12, 1963.

James, A. G.: Cancer Prognosis Manual. pp. 53-54. New York, American Cancer Society, 1967.

Jones, E. L., and Cornell, W. P.: Gardner's syndrome. Review of the literature and report on a family. Arch. Surg., 92:287-300, 1966.

Kanter, I. E., and Fleming, R. J.: Recent advances in abdominal aortography. Angiology, 18:334-348, 1967.

Keynes, W. M.: Implantation from the bowel lumen in cancer of the large intestine. Ann. Surg., 153:357-364, 1961.

Kirsner, J. B., Rider, J. A., Moeller, H. C., Palmer, W. L., and Gold, S. S.: Polyps of the colon and rectum; Statistical analysis of a long term follow-up study. Gastroenterology, 39:178-182, 1960.

Liechty, R. D., Ziffren, S. E., Miller, F. E., Collidge, D., and DenBesten, L.: Adenocarcinoma of the colon and rectum: Review of 2,261 cases over a 20-year period. Dis. Colon Rectum, 11:201-208, 1968.

Lloyd-Davies, O. V.: Discussion on radical excision of carcinoma of the rectum with conservation of the sphincter. Proc. Roy. Soc. Med., 41:822-827, 1948.

Lockhart-Mummery, J. P.: The causation and treatment of multiple adenomatosis of the colon. Ann. Surg., 99:178-184, 1934.

Lockhart-Mummery, H. E., Dukes, C. E., and Bussey, H. J. R.: The surgical treatment of familial polyposis of the colon. Brit. J. Surg., 43:476-481, 1956.

Lofgren, E. P., Waugh, J. M., and Dockerty, M. B.: Local recurrence of carcinoma after anterior resection of the rectum and the sigmoid. Relationship with the length of normal mucosa excised distal to the lesion. Arch. Surg., 74:825-838, 1957.

McGraw, J. Y., and Bonenfant, J. L.: Anorectal lymphomas. Canad. J. Surg., 3:225-228, 1960.

McKittrick, L. S., and Wheelock, F. C., Jr.: Carcinoma of the Colon. Springfield, Ill., Charles C Thomas, 1954.

McSwain, B., Sadler, R. N., and Main, F. B.: Carcinoma of the colon, rectum and anus. Ann. Surg., 155:782-793, 1962.

Madden, J. L.: Primary resection and anastomosis in the treatment of perforated lesions of the colon. Am. Surg., 31:781-786, 1965.

Madden, J. L., and Kandalaft, S.: Electrocoagulation. A primary and preferred method of treatment for cancer of the rectum. Ann. Surg., 166:413-419, 1967.

Mallam, A. S., and Thomson, S. A.: Polyps of the rectum and colon in children. A ten year review at the Hospital for Sick Children, Toronto. Canad. J. Surg., 3:17-24, 1959.

Mayo, C. W., and Cullen, P. K., Jr.: An evaluation of the one stage, low anterior resection. Surg., Gynec., Obstet., 111:82-86, 1960.

Mayo, C. W., DeWeerd, J. H., and Jackman, R. J.: Diffuse familial polyposis of the colon. Surg., Gynec., Obstet., 93:87-96, 1951.

Michels, N. A., Siddharth, P., Kornblith, P. L., and Parke, W. W.: The variant blood supply to the small and large intestines: Its import in regional resections. J. Int. Coll. Surg., 39:127-170, 1963.

Miles, W. E.: A method of performing abdominoperineal excision for carcinoma of the rectum and of the terminal portion of the pelvic colon. Lancet, 2:1812-1813, 1908.

Morson, B. C.: Cancer in ulcerative colitis. Gut, 7:425-426, 1966.

Muir, E. G.: Carcinoma of the rectum and anterior resection. Aust. New Zeal. J. Surg., 27:174-182, 1958.

Noer, R. J.: Hemorrhage as a complication of diverticulitis. Ann. Surg., 141:674, 1955.

Noer, R. J., Hamilton, J. E., Williams, D. J., and Broughton, D. S.: Rectal hemorrhage: Moderate and severe. Ann. Surg., 155:794-805, 1962.

Nusbaum, M., Baum, S., Rajatapiti, B., and Blakemore, W. S.: Intestinal lymphangiography in vivo. J. Cardiov. Surg., 8:62-68, 1967.

Overholt, B. F., and Pollard, H. M.: Cancer of the colon and rectum. Current procedures for detection and diagnosis. Cancer, 20:445-450, 1967.

Peskin, G. W., and Orloff, M. J.: A clinical study of 25 patients with carcinoid tumors of the rectum. Surg., Gynec., Obstet., 109:673-682, 1959.

Ponka, J. L., Fox, J. D., and Brush, B. E.: Co-existing carcinoma and diverticula of the colon. Arch. Surg., 79:373-384, 1959.

Postlethwait, R. W., Adamson, J. E., and Hart, D.: Carcinoma of the colon and rectum. Surg., Gynec., Obstet., 106:257-270, 1958.

Quan, S. H. Q.: Preoperative radiation for carcinoma of rectum. New York J. Med., 66:2243-2247, 1966.

Raynham, W. H., and Louw, J. H.: Familial polyposis of the colon, S. Afr. Med. J., 40:857-865, 1966.

Rider, J. A., Kirsner, J. B., Moeller, H. C., and Palmer, W. L.: Polyps of the colon and rectum: their incidence and relationship to carcinoma. Am. J. Med., 16:555-564, 1954.

————: Polyps of the colon and rectum, a four-year to nine-year follow-up study of five hundred thirty-seven patients. J.A.M.A., 170:633-638, 1959.

Rosi, P. A.: Selection of operations for carcinomas of the colon. Surg. Clin. N. Am., 34:221-230, 1954.

Roth, S. I., and Helwig, E. B.: Juvenile polyps of the colon and rectum. Cancer, 16:468-479, 1963.

Rousselot, L. M., Cole, D. R., Grossi, C. E., Conte, A. J., Gonzalez, E. M., and Pasternack, B. S.: A five year progress report on the effectiveness of intraluminal chemotherapy (5-fluorouracil) adjuvant to surgery for colorectal cancer. Am. J. Surg., 115:140-147, 1968.

Sanders, R. J., and Axtell, H. K.: Carcinoids of the gastrointestinal tract. Surg., Gynec., Obstet., 119:369-380, 1964.

Shimkin, M. B., and Cutler, S. J.: End results in cancer of the rectum. Dis. Colon Rectum, 7:502-505, 1964.

Shnitka, T. K., Friedman, M. H. W., Kidd, E. G., and MacKenzie, W. C.: Villous tumors of the rectum and colon characterized by severe fluid and electrolyte loss. Surg., Gynec., Obstet., 112:609-621, 1961.

Slaney, G., and Brooke, B. N.: Cancer in ulcerative colitis. Lancet, 2:694-698, 1959.

Smilow, P. C., Pryor, C. A., Jr., and Swinton, N. W.: Juvenile polyposis coli. A report of three patients in three generations of one family. Dis. Colon Rectum, 9:248-254, 1966.

Spratt, J. S., Jr., and Ackerman, L. V.: Pathologic significance of polyps of the rectum and colon. Dis. Colon Rectum, 3:330-335, 1960.

Spratt, J. S., Jr., Ackerman, L. V., and Moyer, C. A.: Relationship of polyps of the colon to colonic cancer. Ann. Surg., 148:682-698, 1958.

Stearns, M. W., Jr., Berg, J. W., and Deddish, M. R.: Preoperative irradiation of cancer of the rectum. Dis. Colon Rectum, 4:403-408, 1961.

Stearns, M. W., Jr., Deddish, M. R., and Quan, S. H. Q.: Preoperative irradiation for cancer of the rectum and rectosigmoid: Preliminary review of recent experience (1957-1962). Dis. Colon Rectum, 11:281-284, 1968.

Strauss, A. A., Appel, M., Saphir, O., and Rabinovitz, A. J.: Immunologic resistance to carcinoma produced by electrocoagulation. Surg., Gynec., Obstet., 121:989-996, 1965.

Strauss, A. A., Strauss, S. F., Crawford, R. A., and Strauss, H. A.: Surgical diathermy of carcinoma of rectum: Its clinical end results. J.A.M.A., 104:1480-1484, 1935.

Sunderland, D. A., and Binkley, G. E.: Papillary adenomas of the large intestine: a clinical and morphological study of 48 cases. Cancer, 1:183-207, 1948.

Thomas, K. E., Watne, A. L., Johnson, J. G., Roth, E., and Zimmermann, B.: Natural history of Gardner's syndrome. Am. J. Surg., 115:218-226, 1968.

Turell, R., and Haller, J. D.: A re-evaluation of the malignant potential of colorectal adenomas. Surg., Gynec., Obstet., 119:867-887, 1964.

Turnbull, R. B., Jr., Kyle, K., Watson, F. R., and Spratt, J.: Cancer of the colon: The influence of the *no-touch isolation* technic on survival rates. Ann. Surg., 166:420-427, 1967.

Turnbull, R. B., Jr., and Weakley, F. L.: Atlas of Intestinal Stomas. C. V. Mosby, St. Louis, 1967.

Vandertoll, D. J., and Beahrs, O. H.: Carcinoma of rectum and low sigmoid. Evaluation of anterior resection of 1,766 favorable lesions. Arch. Surg., 90:793-798, 1965.

Vink, M.: Local recurrence of cancer in the large bowel: The role of implantation metastases and bowel disinfection. Brit. J. Surg., 41:431-433, 1954.

Wangensteen, O. H., Lewis, F. J., Arhelger, S. W., Muller, J. J., and MacLean, L. D.: An interim report upon the "second look" procedure for cancer of the stomach, colon, and rectum and for "limited intraperitoneal carcinosis." Surg., Gynec., Obstet., 99:257-267, 1954.

Welch, C. E., and Burke, J. F.: Carcinoma of the colon and rectum. New Eng. J. Med., 266:211-219, 1962.

Wheat, M. W., Jr., and Ackerman, L. V.: Villous adenomas of the large intestine. Ann. Surg., 147:476-487, 1958.

Windsberg, E.: Intestinal obstruction of the distal colon due to malignancy: single-stage decompression and resection. Surgery, 46:305-318, 1959.

Wood, D. A.: Tumors of the Intestine. Washington, D. C., Armed Forces Institute of Pathology, 1967.

Wynder, E. L., and Shigematsu, T.: Environmental factors of cancer of the colon and rectum. Cancer, 20:1520-1561, 1967.

CHAPTER 41

HENRY N. HARKINS, M.D.

Anorectum

Definition
General Considerations
Anatomy
Diagnosis
Clinical Conditions

DEFINITION

The anorectum is the distal 1½ inches (4 cm.) of the intestinal tract. The upper ¾ inch (2 cm.) of the anorectum is the distal end of the rectum while the lower ¾ inch (2 cm.) comprises the anus itself. As seen in Figure 41-2, the rectal portion of the anorectum is bounded above by the anorectal ring and below by the pectinate line. The anal portion of the anorectum is bounded above by the pectinate margin and below by the anal verge.

The anorectum is not the anus *and* the rectum. It includes all of the anus, but only the distal ¾ inch (2 cm.) of the rectum. To avoid confusion, and yet to discuss the portion of the intestinal canal which functions as a unit, even though it is composed of 2 separate organs, we have used the term anorectum.

GENERAL CONSIDERATIONS

Even though the anorectum or distal portion of the intestinal tract is relatively short, it is, like the mouth, very important. Pathologic conditions in the anorectum are frequent, painful, sometimes dangerous (carcinoma) and often difficult to cure.

One feature of the anorectum is that an understanding of its diseases largely involves a knowledge of *anatomy*. Unlike the parathyroids or the adrenals, for example, where the problems are chiefly physiologic or chemical, in the anorectum pathologic conditions—and their correction—have a primarily anatomic basis. The principle that different basic sciences have a different extent of application in different parts of the body is well illustrated by these contrasting conditions.

Probably the second most important feature in the anorectum is infection; it involves a knowledge of *bacteriology*. With a few exceptions involving specific infections such as syphilis (chancre and condylomata lata), tuberculosis, etc., most of the infections of the anorectum are nonspecific and have an anatomic basis of causation. Usually when an anatomic correction has been made, the nonspecific infection will be cured. Among the specific infections, lymphopathia venereum leads to stricture involving the lower rectum as well as the anus. Nonvenereal warts, condylomata acuminata, should be treated by anal hygiene, including the use of a dusting powder to keep the area dry, and 25 per cent podophyllin in tincture of benzoin applied directly to the lesions, avoiding contact of the drug with uninvolved skin. Another type of infection is that by *Schistosoma mansoni* (liver fluke). The large shift of population to the United States from Puerto Rico, where the parasite is endemic, has brought the disease to the attention of proctologists. A precise method of diagnosis (Warner, 1957) involves sigmoidoscopy with biopsy of small specimens of rectal mucosa for identification of the eggs.

The anorectum has a close relationship with surrounding structures, and particularly with the remainder of the intestinal canal above. The physician who treats the anorectum, whether he be general surgeon, proctologist, or general practitioner, must be cognizant of these relationships and must not direct his attention only to the obvious lesions at hand. An example of the danger of such a narrow approach is the report that at one large clinic

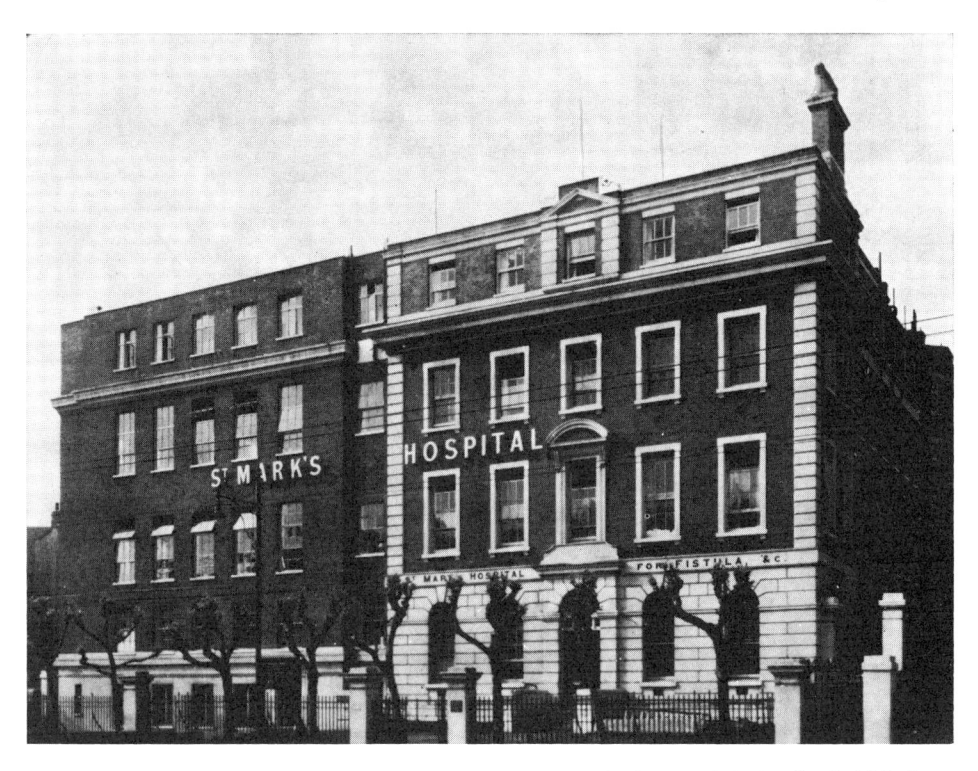

FIG. 41-1. Picture of St. Mark's Hospital For Fistula & C., London, England. This hospital has played a greater role in the development of anorectal and colorectal surgery than any other institution in the world. It was built in 1835; Charles Dickens was a subscriber. (From Mr. C. Naunton Morgan, F.R.C.S.)

over 20 per cent of the patients submitted to radical excision of the rectum for carcinoma had had a simple hemorrhoidectomy elsewhere within 3 months, invariably without a sigmoidoscopic examination.

ANATOMY

The anorectum is collapsed when empty so that it is an anteroposterior slit. Two clearly palpable landmarks are felt by the examining finger, the anorectal ring at the upper end of the anorectum and the interhemorrhoidal groove at the junction of the middle and the upper thirds of the anus proper.

The anatomy of the rectum has been worked out both by anatomists and by surgeons. Many of the surgeons who have contributed to this field were or are at St. Mark's Hospital, London, an institution devoted entirely to diseases of the anus and the rectum (see Fig. 41-1). Ernest Miles, Lockhart-Mummery, Cuthbert Dukes, Gabriel, Milligan, Morgan, and many of the other world leaders in this field are or have been on the staff of St. Mark's Hospital. The classic anatomic studies of this region, done by Milligan and Morgan, have been accepted by proctologists throughout the world, even though in some instances they may have differed from the writings of the anatomists. Figure 41-2 presents a recent concept of the anatomy of the anorectum. Figure 41-3 depicts the classic Milligan-Morgan diagram on the left as contrasted with the newer concept based upon the observations of other surgeons, including Eisenhammer (1951, 1953, 1965), Goligher, Leacock and Brossy (1955), also of St. Mark's, Parks (1955, 1956), Morgan and Thompson (1956), Hughes (1956, 1964a), Fowler (1957), and Walls (1958). These later observations are more in accord with those of the anatomists and, it is believed, with the patient. The rest of this chapter will be based

MUCOSA
A. Columnar
B. Cuboidal
C. Modified squamous
D. Skin

1. Lateral hemorrhoidal groove
2. Interhemorrhoidal groove
3. Pectinate line
4. Crypts of Morgagni

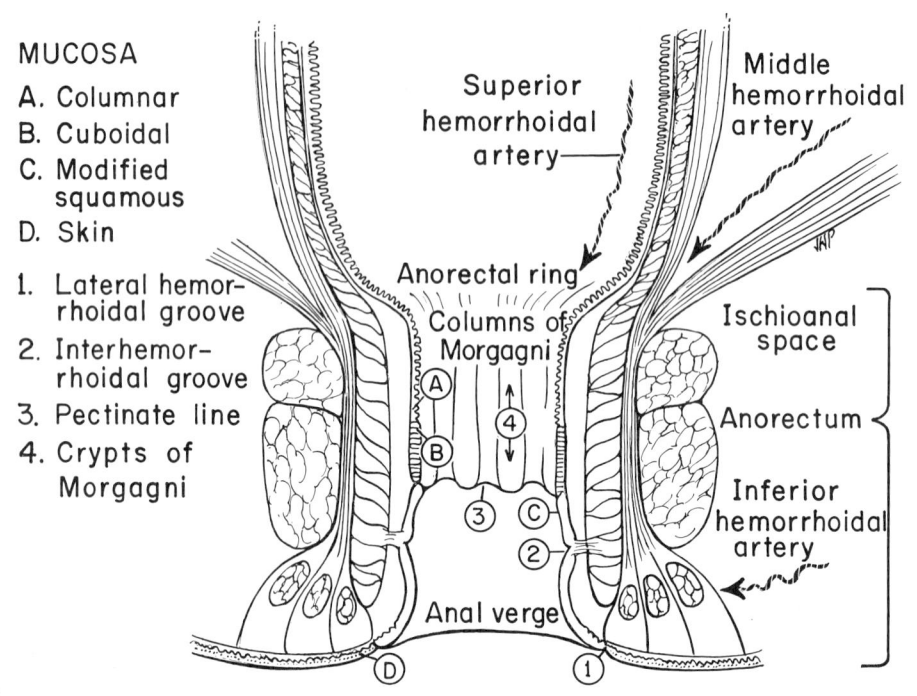

FIG. 41-2. Master drawing of anorectum and lower rectum showing epithelium, muscles, arteries and landmarks. The anorectum itself is the portion of the intestinal canal between the anorectal ring above and the anal verge below.

on the newer ideas of anatomy, especially those of Parks.

MEMBRANES

The rectal mucous membrane is composed of columnar epithelium (pale pink as is the membrane above). The mucous membrane of the rectal portion of the anorectum is covered by a columnar-cuboidal epithelium (red, due to the underlying vessels of the superior hemorrhoidal plexus) according to the classical description. Goligher, Leacock and Brossy (1955), however, found the mucous membrane between the pectinate line and the anorectal ring to be multilayered.

Going from the skin to the rectum, the epithelial lining may be divided into 4 zones. Lateral to the most median attachment of the conjoined terminating fibers of the levator ani and longitudinal muscles (Fig. 41-3), at a point which Parks (1956) terms the squamous border, there is true skin. Medial to this there are 3 additional zones, and the entire arrangement is as follows:

Zone 1. *True skin*, with sweat glands and hair follicles.
Dividing margin: squamous border (lateral hemorrhoidal groove, anal verge).

Zone 2. *Stratified squamous epithelium* with only occasional sweat glands and hair follicles (1.0-1.5 cm.).
Dividing margin: line of anal crypts (interhemorrhoidal groove, mucocutaneous line, point of attachment of mucosal suspensory ligament—see Fig. 41-3).

Zone 3. *Stratified columnar epithelium* (middle zone): mucus secreting and moist (0.25-1.0 cm.).
Dividing margin: pectinate or dentate line.

Zone 4. *Columnar glandular rectal epithelium*, above the pectinate line.

Zones 2 and 3, combined, are known as the pecten (Stroud, 1896). Zones 1, 2 and usually 3 are sensitive; Zone 4 is supplied by visceral nerves and is insensitive. Zone 1 has the normal color of the patient's skin elsewhere or is slightly darker. Zones 2 and 3 are slightly bluish.

Anatomy

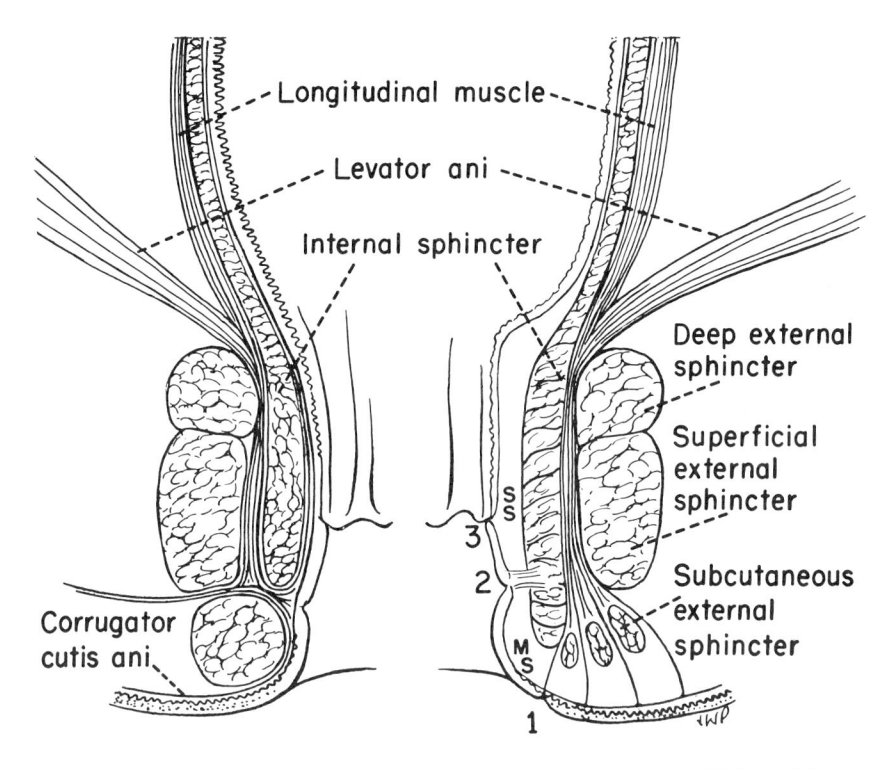

FIG. 41-3. Muscles and fascial septa of anorectum. The classical Milligan-Morgan concept is shown on the reader's left, the *newer* concept of Parks and others on the right. (1—lateral hemorrhoidal groove, 2—attachment of mucosal suspensory ligament, or interhemorrhoidal groove, 3—pectinate line, MS—marginal space, and SS—submucous space.)

The skin is adherent to the underlying structure at the squamous border. The mucous membrane is similarly adherent at the mucocutaneous line. Between these two points of attachment the subepithelial space is termed the "marginal space" (in which are the external hemorrhoidal vessels); lateral to the squamous border it is the "ischiorectal space," while above the mucocutaneous line is the "submucous space" (in which are the internal hemorrhoidal vessels).

The pectinate line is made prominent by the

FIG. 41-4. Relationships of the *visible* "interhemorrhoidal" groove (a) and the palpable "intersphincteric" groove (b). (From E. S. R. Hughes, Melbourne, Australia)

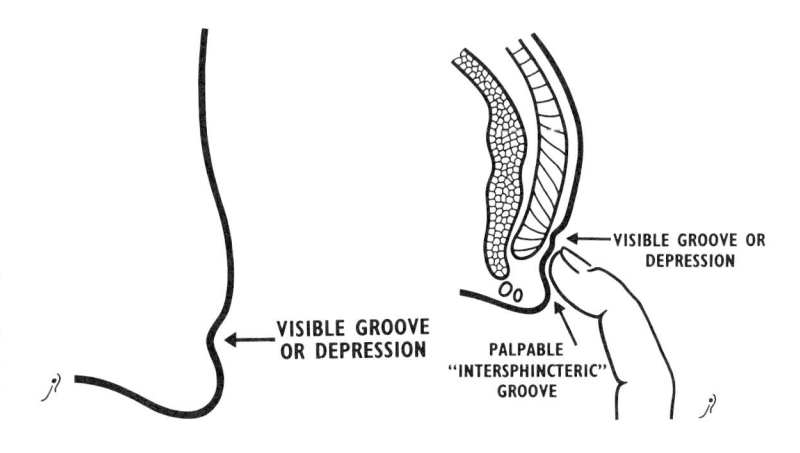

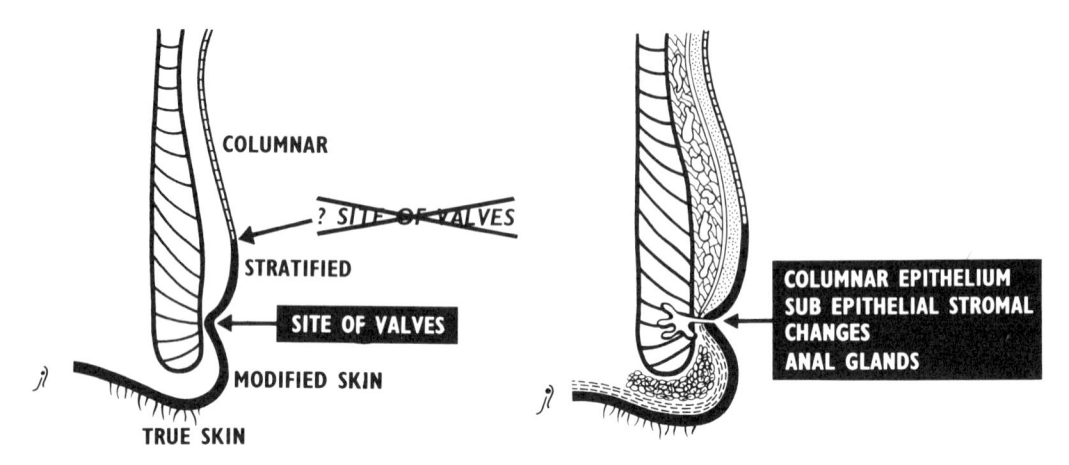

FIG. 41-5. The site of the valves is *not* at the line of transition from stratified epithelium (a) (below) to columnar epithelium (above), but *is* at the visible groove (b). (From E. S. R. Hughes, Melbourne, Australia)

presence of small epithelial processes, the anal papillae, on the free margins of the anal valves of Ball. These papillae represent the remnants of the proctodeal membrane which in early embryonic life separated the proctodeum from the postallantoic gut. The sinuses of Morgagni are small depressions or pockets which occur above each anal valve. These sinuses are deeper posteriorly than elsewhere and may be subject to infection through lodging of foreign material in them. The infection of the sinuses and of the anal glands at their bases is known as cryptitis and may be the starting point for other infections of the anorectum (abscess, fistula and possibly fissure). The anal glands may be several millimeters long and may extend down to the interhemorrhoidal groove or into the circular muscles. Hypertrophy of the papillae usually is associated with cryptitis and is known as papillitis.

The relationships of the *visible* "interhemorrhoidal" groove and the palpable "intersphincteric" groove are shown in Figure 41-4. Similarly, the site of the anal glands at the visible interhemorrhoidal groove is shown in Figure 41-5 and in a synthesis of these concepts, as shown in Figure 41-6.

Nerve Supply

Only the external sphincter and the levator ani muscles are under voluntary control, and there is sensitivity to pain just above the anal valves only (Duthie and Gairns, 1960).

Blood Supply

The superior hemorrhoidal artery sends branches which course down the rectum beneath the mucosa and are collected in 6 to 8 vertical folds or columns of Morgagni in the rectal portion of the anorectum (Fig. 41-2). The middle hemorrhoidal artery comes to the rectum at the inferior angle of the pelvirectal space. The inferior hemorrhoidal arteries approach the anus through the perianal space.

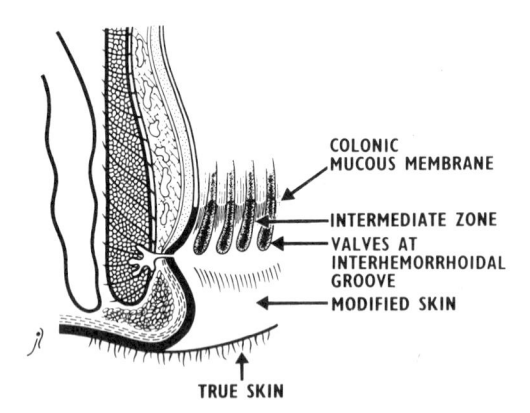

FIG. 41-6. A synthetic depiction of the sites of mucous membrane transition (above); the valves at the interhemorrhoidal groove, and the true skin (below). (From E. S. R. Hughes, Melbourne, Australia)

These vessels anastomose freely, except at the interhemorrhoidal groove, and the corresponding veins form an extensive plexus about the anorectum with many of the vessels lying just beneath the mucosa. Because of the effects of gravity upon venous congestion, the horizontal position relieves pain in most anorectal conditions.

MUSCLES (FIG. 41-3)

The external sphincter and the levator ani, being voluntary striated muscles, are red, while the internal sphincter and the longitudinal sphincter, being involuntary nonstriated muscles, are paler.

Longitudinal Sphincter. The 3 taeniae coli of the colon become spread out over the wall of the rectum. The muscle is strongest and thickest on the anterior and the posterior surfaces and laterally is thinner. The longitudinal muscle, involving nonstriated fibers, is continued down in this way to the rectal portion of the anorectum where it envelops the internal sphincter and ends by passing through the subcutaneous portion of the external sphincter, dividing it into many segments, and inserting in the anal skin (Wilde, 1949). The *corrugator cutis ani* muscle is a continuation downward and outward from the cutaneous insertion of the longitudinal muscle. Extending upward and inside the canal from the cutaneous insertion of the longitudinal muscle (lateral hemorrhoidal groove) is the *musculus submucosae ani* (Fine and Lawes, 1940, Gorsch, 1955). These longitudinal fibers lie between the internal hemorrhoidal plexus (toward the lumen) and the circular internal sphincter (away from the lumen). They are the counterpart of the *muscularis mucosae* elsewhere in the intestinal tract. The "pecten band," so well described by Miles, is the lower portion of the internal sphincter.

External Sphincter. Santorini in 1715 first described the external sphincter as being composed of 3 parts. These 3 parts are now termed the deep, the superficial and the subcutaneous portions of the external sphincter. They are usually fused together more in the patient than the diagrams would indicate. Their respective locations are shown in Figure 41-3.

FIG. 41-7. Demonstration of the sling-like action of the puborectalis (one of the 3 components of the levator ani) muscle. (A) Lateral view of puborectalis sling (posterior to left, anterior to right). (B) Diagrammatic representation of similar situation with regard to right crus of diaphragm, forming a sling for the esophagogastric junction (Allison). (C) Lateral view shows that the finger palpating the posterior rectal wall meets resistance of puborectalis. (D) Lateral view shows that finger palpating anterior rectal wall meets no resistance at level of puborectalis.

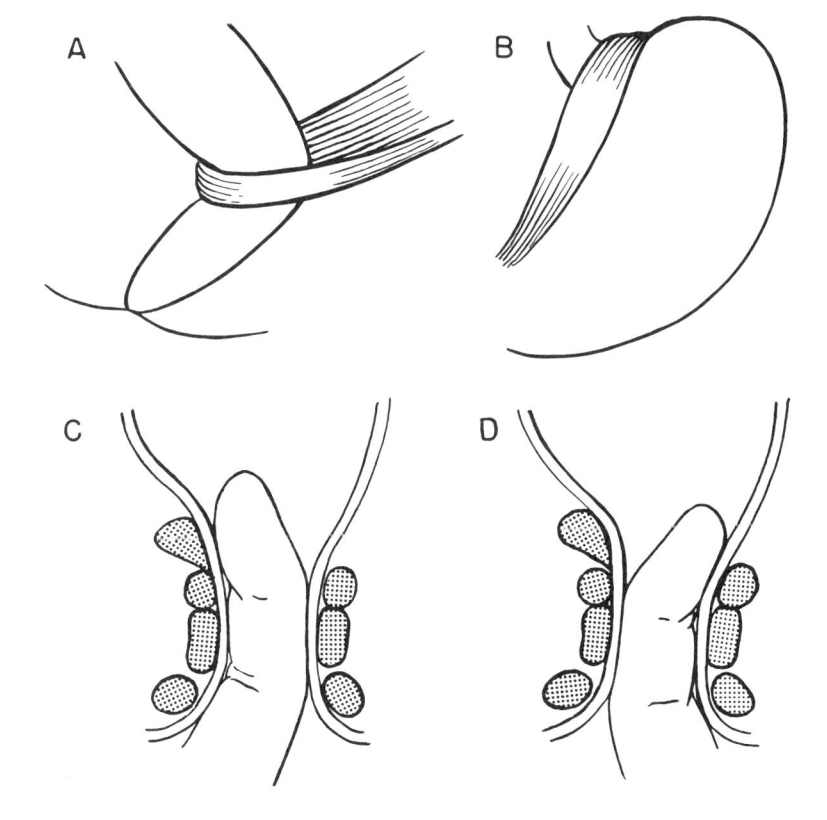

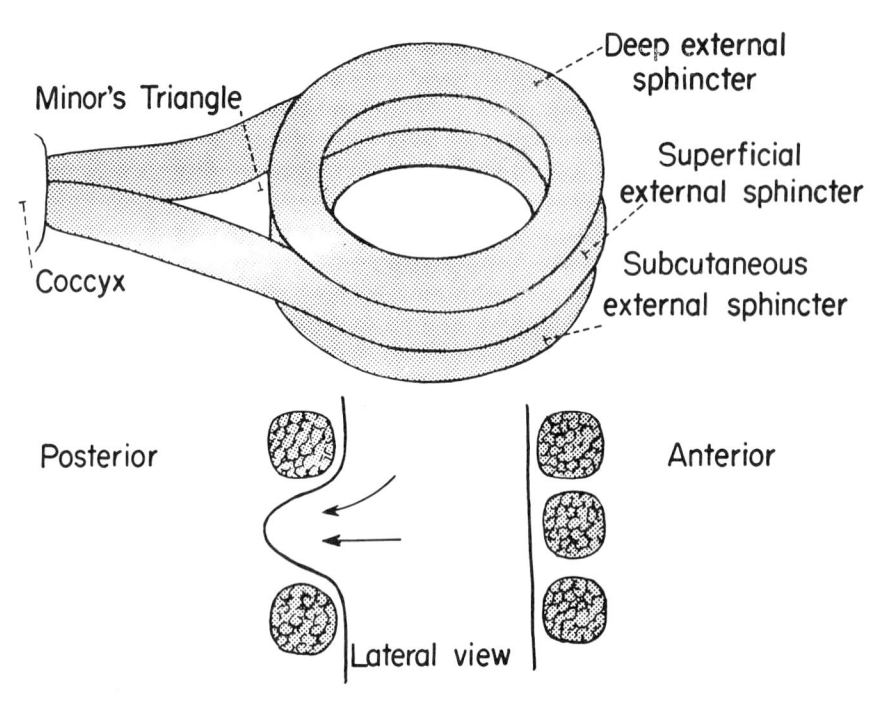

FIG. 41-8. Diagrammatic representation of Minor's triangle. The upper drawing is a lateral view showing the same defect as that caused by the attachment of the superficial portion of the external anal sphincter. The lower drawing is a lateral view showing the same defect as that caused by the presence of Minor's triangle.

The subcutaneous portion has been likened by Gabriel to an umbrella ring. It is about ¼ inch in cross section and lies immediately beneath the skin lateral to the anal margin and to the lateral hemorrhoidal groove.

The muscle "seen" in the bed of a hemorrhoidectomy wound was formerly believed to be the subcutaneous portion of the external sphincter. Work by Eisenhammer (1951, 1953), Goligher, Leacock and Brossy (1955), Parks (1956), and others, indicates that this is actually the lower end of the internal sphincter. Biopsy of this muscle was performed by Vetto, Harkins, McMahon and White (1956), and in 18 of 20 patients microscopic study revealed nonstriated muscle, confirming the Eisenhammer-Goligher-Parks hypothesis. The paper by Swinton and Mumma (1956) is the first in the American literature, to the author's knowledge, taking cognizance of these new anatomic concepts.

Associated Muscles. These include the levator ani, including the puborectalis, as well as all of the muscles of the pelvis and the perineal floor.

Anal Muscular Defects. Certain normal muscular defects are important in the surgical anatomy of the anorectum. These are as follows:

PUBORECTALIS "SLING." The puborectalis, which has been called the best-developed muscle in the pelvic diaphragm, acts like a sling around the upper portion of the anorectum, as shown in Figure 41-7. It is of interest that this slinglike action has been compared with that of the oblique muscles of the stomach around the cardia of the stomach. The result of the arrangement of the puborectalis as depicted is that the anal canal is shorter anteriorly than posteriorly, 1¼ in. (3 cm.) as opposed to 1½ in. (4 cm.).

MINOR'S TRIANGLE. Of the 3 portions of the external sphincter, two (the deep and the subcutaneous) are essentially circular, while the superficial is the only one of the three that attaches to the coccyx. The angular defect produced by this insertion is known as Minor's triangle (Fig. 41-8). It may have considerable clinical importance because of a lack of support of the anal wall at this level posteriorly. The downward passage of feces may cause trauma because of this irregularity of the wall and may be a factor in the causation of anal fissure, which is most common in the midline posteriorly. The relative protuberance of the subcutaneous external sphincter below Minor's triangle is known as Blaisdell's bar. Eisenhammer (1951, 1953) has contested the importance of Blaisdell's bar in the genesis and the perpetuation of fistula and has stated that the only "bar" at fault is the internal sphincter.

DIAGNOSIS

In various conditions occurring in different parts of the body the diagnosis is made by the history and the physical examination, supported by laboratory studies. The inexperienced doctor is apt to fall into two errors of concept in this regard, wrongly assuming: (1) that the history is always the most important of these 3 methods and (2) that their relative importance is the same, irrespective of the lesion. Granting that the history is generally the basic diagnostic tool and that laboratory studies play in general only a supportive and corroborative role, the relative usefulness of these 3 methods varies markedly with the lesion. In cases of epilepsy or peptic ulcer the history is most important; in instances of parathyroid tumor or islet cell tumor of the pancreas laboratory studies have a special applicability; but in diseases of the anorectum, the physical examination is the *sine qua non*.

After a preliminary history, examination of the anorectum involves *inspection* of the anal orifice and the surrounding skin. Following this, a *digital examination* should be done. Since fissures usually occur in the mid-line posteriorly and since, with the exception of the thrombosed external hemorrhoids, they are the most sensitive anorectal lesion, in cases where fissure is suspected the examining finger should hug the anterior wall on introduction into the anal canal to minimize pain. The digital examination should be thorough and systematic. In postoperative cases, fecal impaction should be searched for, and a history of frequent stools may be misleading and delay disimpaction (Dresen and Kratzer, 1959).

Following the digital examination, a *proctosigmoidoscopic examination* should be performed. A sigmoidoscope is one of the first instruments that a surgeon or a general practitioner should purchase upon entering practice. The importance of the sigmoidoscope in anorectal examination is exceeded only by the palpating finger and direct inspection. An anoscope is a useful adjunct.

For a proctosigmoidoscopic examination (Jackman, 1958, and Turell, 1959, give detailed instructions), the patient should come with the rectum well cleansed and prepared. Adequate preparation includes: (1) a light or liquid supper the night before, (2) castor oil, 1½ ounces (50 cc.) the night before, (3) two enemas in the morning and (4) tea and toast for breakfast preceding the examination. Despite these measures, preparation may be incomplete, and it is advantageous to have suction available in the proctoscopy room. In old and debilitated patients it may be advisable to adopt a less rigorous preparation, and it may be preferable to avoid some of the head-down positions for examination to be listed below. The position, whether it be the knee-chest-left shoulder down position, the Sims' or left lateral position, the lithotomy position, or the prone jackknife position, is relatively immaterial so long as the surgeon is familiar with it. Any firm table is adequate for the first two positions, while special tables are necessary for the latter two. The examination should be done, if possible, to the full length (25 cm.) of the instrument, and the history sheet should have a special form, possibly a rubber stamp diagram such as is used at St. Mark's Hospital, London, for recording of the findings.

CLINICAL CONDITIONS

In the brief summary of surgery of the anorectum given in this chapter, an outline of 10 surgical conditions of this region will be given. Certain other lesions, such as lymphopathia venereum, ulcerative colitis, proctitis, viral verrucae (Young, 1957), polyps and adenocarcinoma, are considered to be more in the province of the colon or the rectum

TABLE 41-1. SOMMERSCHILD, KNUTRUD AND
FRETHEIM CLASSIFICATION OF
ANAL ATRESIA (1964)

Grade I. *Low atresia* (anal type)
　　　　The bowel ends *below* the pelvic floor, possibly with a fistula to:
　　　　(1) The anus (microscopic anus)
　　　　(2) The perineum
　　　　(3) The vestibule of the vagina
Grade II. *High atresia* (rectal or anorectal type)
　　　　The bowel ends *above* the pelvic floor, possibly with a fistula to:
　　　　(1) The urethra
　　　　(2) The bladder
　　　　(3) The vagina
　　　　(4) The uterus *or*
　　　　(5) A cloaca

proper and are discussed in Chapters 39 and 40.

IMPERFORATE ANUS

Imperforate anus may occur in both sexes and may be classified in various ways. In this country the classification of Ladd and Gross is usually adopted. More recent classifications are those of Partridge and Gough (1961) and Sommerschild, Knutrud and Fretheim (1964). The latter is given in Table 41-1.

This subject is more completely dealt with in Dr. Ravitch's Chapter 50, Pediatric Surgery, and will not be definitively discussed here. Two points, however, will be emphasized since they represent modern developments important to the planning of surgical management which are not in all the other texts.

First is the importance of frequent fistulas into the bladder, the vagina, the urethra, etc. This has been pinpointed by Stephens (1953a), Bill and Johnson (1958), Brayton and Norris (1958), Scott, Swenson and Fisher (1960), Swinton and Palmer (1960), and Sauvage and Bill (1965).

Second is the importance of the puborectalis sling in the repair of high atresia. Stephens (1953b, 1959) first showed that many repairs bring down the rectum *posterior* to this sling rather than *anterior* to it as is the normal situation. This is partly because the sling itself, having no rectum to "hug," is more anterior than normal, and also because the anal opening may not have migrated properly (Bill, 1958).

At any rate, for a proper functional result, the rectum must be enclosed by the sling. To do this properly requires that colostomy be performed and that the definitive operation be accomplished several months after birth, rather than immediately as by older technics. This important principle has been re-emphasized by Lynn and Arcari (1962), Swain and Tucker (1962), Kiesewetter and Turner (1963), Sauvage and Bill (1965), and Harkins (1965).

Classic texts on anatomy express divergent views concerning the relation between the urethra and the rectum, often in the same text. They may show the two in immediate approximation or quite widely separated. Obviously, both of these concepts cannot be correct at the same time. Since it is important in doing a sacroperineal pull-through to bring the rectal stump through the muscles, especially the puborectalis sling so as to obtain anal continence, the anatomic texts must furnish more precise information than is provided by this wide difference of opinion. The rectum should be brought down in the midline just in front of the puborectalis sling (*not* through or behind the fibers) and just posterior to the prostate or the vagina, as shown so well by Sauvage and Bill (1964).

(For a more complete discussion of this condition, see Chap. 50, Pediatric Surgery.)

The somewhat related but different condition of *duplication of the rectum* is also to be considered (Stockman, Young and Sholes, 1960; Kraft, 1962).

PROLAPSE

Prolapse of the rectum can be classified into 3 types as shown below:

CLASSIFICATION OF PROLAPSE OF THE RECTUM
(Modified from Altemeier, Hoxworth and Giuseffi, 1955)

Type I. Mucosal Prolapse (Partial Protrusion of the Rectum, False Prolapse). This type occurs especially at the extremes of life and in the debilitated. Constipation, straining at stool, and reading on the toilet are etiologic factors. Treatment involves correction of these factors, but with avoidance of cathartics and diarrhea. In children the buttocks may be strapped together for a few days. The straight vertical rectal canal of children may be a factor in the etiology. This type of prolapse is seldom longer than 4 to 6 cm. and is usually shorter. Since the protrusion involves only the mucosa it is thin to palpation.

Type II. Intussuscepted Prolapse (Incomplete Prolapse). This type involves a prolapse of all layers of the rectum. It usually starts at a point above the anorectal ring, having as a point of origin one of the valves of Houston or the pelvic rectal junction. Both areas correspond to the junction of a higher, comparatively mobile portion of the rectum with a lower, more fixed portion. In early cases there may be a groove around the prolapsed bowel between it and the skin extending up to the point of invagination. If the groove is deeper than 3 cm., the lesion is more apt to be a true intussusception rather than a prolapse. In advanced cases of intussuscepted prolapse the anus becomes everted as well as the rectum, and the groove is no longer present.

Type III. Sliding Prolapse (Complete or Massive Prolapse, Pelvirectal Sliding Hernia). Such a lesion represents a herniation of the pelvic peritoneum or cul-de-sac through a defect in its underlying endo-abdominal fascia and the pelvic diaphragm. As the hernia progresses and slides downward, the cul-de-sac invaginates the anterior wall of the rectum to produce an intussusception. The anal sphincter becomes progressively relaxed with continued protrusion. Such prolapses are larger than the other types. The anterior wall is thicker than the posterior (due to contained sac and even small bowel) and may be tympanitic. As a result of this asymmetry the rectal opening faces posteriorly, while in Types I and II the opening of the bowel is centrally located. Type III is rare in children. In adults it is not restricted to the older age group as in Type I.

Those who have worked at St. Mark's Hospital—Goligher (1964) and Hughes (1964b), as well as Moyer (1964) and others—divide prolapse of the rectum into only 2 types—mucosal and complete. The intermediate type is considered to be an early stage of the complete.

Differential diagnosis includes such conditions as prolapsing internal hemorrhoids or an intussuscepting tumor of the upper rectum or sigmoid.

Treatment of Type I or Type II is relatively simple and involves sleeve excision of the mass with mucosa-to-mucosa approximation. Perisphincteric wiring (Thiersch operation) has been revised for Type II by Burke and Jackman (1959). The correction of true prolapse, Type III, on the other hand, is a difficult problem which has led to devising a number of operative approaches (Nigro and Walker, 1957). These involve the abdominal approach (Moschcowitz, 1912; Graham, 1942; Orr, 1947; Frykman, 1955; Tendler, 1956; Goligher, 1958, 1961, 1964; MacKenzie and Davis, 1958; Baden and Mikkelsen, 1959; Shann, 1959; Rhoads, 1960; Palmer, 1961; Wells, 1961; and Ripstein and Lanter, 1963), the combined abdominal and perineal approach (Dunphy, 1948), and the perineal approach (Miles, 1933, 1955; Altemeier, Hoxworth and Giuseffi, 1955; Inberg, 1958; Hughes and Gleadell, 1962; Hughes, 1964b; and Altemeier, Culbertson and Alexander, 1964). The original Moschcowitz operation pulled up the pelvic colon and closed the pelvic structures in front of it with a pursestring suture, but did not suture the levators themselves in front of the rectum. The Roscoe Graham (1942) modification of the Moschcowitz operation (see also Rhoads, 1964) pays special attention to suturing the levators in front of the rectum.

The perineal approach was utilized in 49 cases of Type III prolapse with good results in all but 1 case and presents some advantages.

This technic involves a 1-stage operation with less risk to the patient, since it utilizes the perineal approach. An incision is made about the circumference of the protruding mass 3 mm. proximal to the pectinate line. This incision is carried through the first of the 2 layers of bowel, the cut layer then being stripped distally from the underlying or inner loop. The hernial sac is located anteriorly and dissected free superiorly as far as possible. Then the sac is opened, and the peritoneal cavity is explored. The sliding character of the hernia now becomes apparent because the posterior peritoneal layer of the sac is the serosa of the rectum. The redundant loop of rectum and sigmoid with its attached mesentery is marked for the site of resection with a silk stitch. This point is selected so as to permit ready anastomosis to the anus previously cut across 3 mm. proximal to the pectinate line at the first step.

The peritoneal cavity is closed with a Y-shaped suture, the levator ani muscles are approximated in front of the rectum with interrupted sutures, the bowel is divided at the point previously marked and is anastomosed in one layer to the anus. In the event no hernial sac or levator defect is found, it can be assumed that the prolapse is Type I. If a levator defect is found without a hernial sac, the prolapse is Type II. Resection of the elongated rectum with anastomosis is performed as for Type III, with or without repair of the levators as indicated in the case at hand.

(Since Type III, or sliding prolapse, is also a type of pelvic hernia, see Chap. 42, Hernia, section on Perineal Hernia.)

STRICTURE

Stricture of the anus may follow trauma, infection (Kark, Epstein and Chapman, 1959) or poorly performed hemorrhoidectomies, particularly of the Whitehead type (Anderson, Pontius and Witkowski, 1955). The best method of treatment, aside from prevention, is an S-shaped incision (S-plasty), swinging the skin flaps into the tightened anal ring (Ferguson, 1959). Such operations involve the Z-plasty principle (see Chap. 49).

INCONTINENCE

Anal incontinence is due to overenthusiastic muscle-cutting operations for anal fistula, to trauma and to neurologic conditions. Karlan, McPherson and Watman (1959) have studied factors affecting fecal incontinence in the dog. The 4 chief methods of surgical treatment in patients are as follows:

Treatment of Anal Incontinence
1. Lawson-Tait operation (like a Heineke-Mikulicz)
2. Blaisdell operation (1957)
   a. Advance muscle flaps
   b. Close as Lawson-Tait
3. Lockhart-Mummery operation (superficial external sphincter pleating)
4. Thiersch's operation (circumferential wire suture)

PRURITUS ANI

This condition is common, annoying to the patient, and difficult to treat. Possibly more than with some other anorectal lesions the

CLASSIFICATION OF PRURITUS ANI

(Modified from Fromer, 1955)

The percentage figures represent relative incidences of the different groups of patients as seen at the Lahey Clinic.

Type 1. Anorectal (25%). (Best treated by surgical care of the underlying condition)

   a. Fissures
   b. Fistulas
   c. Draining sinuses
   d. Ulcers
   e. Mucosal prolapse
   f. Papillitis
   g. Cryptitis
   h. Skin tags
   i. Hemorrhoids
   j. Neoplasms

Type 2. Dermatologic (20%). (Best treated locally by medical means)

   a. Psoriasis
   b. Seborrheic dermatitis
   c. Bacterial dermatitis
   d. Mycotic dermatitis
   e. Lichen sclerosus
   f. Syphilis
   g. Contact dermatitis

Type 3. Medical (10%). (Best treated generally to overcome or remove the underlying condition)

   a. Jaundice
   b. Diabetes
   c. Lymphoblastomatosis
   d. Antibiotic irritation
   e. Allergy (foods, deodorants, hygienic pads, etc.)
   f. Parasites (especially pinworms)

Type 4. Idiopathic (45%). (Treatment difficult, see text) patient as a whole must be considered. Psychic factors, general medical conditions, such as jaundice, spread from vaginal lesions including Trichomonas, and spread of pinworms from the rectum above, are all to be considered. Furthermore, an underlying anorectal cause *per se* is often a factor, and cryptitis (with involvement of the associated anal glands), fistula, hemorrhoids, hypertrophied anal skin tags, etc., should be taken care of adequately before the diagnosis of idiopathic or primary pruritus ani is made. In secondary pruritus ani the condition is a symptom rather than a disease. Ruiz-Moreno lists 71 causes of pruritus ani (1964).

A classification of pruritus ani, modified from Fromer (1955), is given on page 1184. The percentage figures listed after each group of patients indicate the relative frequency of such patients at the Lahey Clinic.

Another classification, listed in Table 41-2, is that of Turell (1955) which, while less useful for general purposes than the Fromer classification, serves as a guide for hydrocortisone therapy.

If the pruritus continues despite a careful and thorough diagnostic study to determine causative factors with the carrying out of indicated therapeutic measures, the condition can be classified as idiopathic (essential or primary) pruritus ani. Before reaching this conclusion a dermatologic and/or a psychiatric consultation may be advisable.

In cases of idiopathic pruritus ani, as well as in some cases of secondary pruritus, 4 types of therapy should be considered. The first of these is adoption of a regimen of anal hygiene. This does no harm and may be sufficient to cure most cases of pruritus ani. Directions for anal hygiene are as follows and may be given to the patient in the form of a mimeographed schedule:

Anal Hygiene. After defecation immediately cleanse the perianal skin with wet absorbent cotton or, if possible, take a shower, or a partial bath or a partial shower, avoiding strong soaps. Basis soap or some other superfatted soap is nonirritating to most people. The lubricating action of the soap helps to reduce the hemorrhoids. Do not use toilet tissue. Dry well with cotton and powder well with cornstarch or nonaromatic powder. Cleansing with wet cotton and dusting with powder must be repeated about 4 times daily, depending on the amount of moisture and the degree of itching. Always keep the skin around the anus clean and dry. Carry cotton and talcum in separate envelopes on the person in a pocket or a handbag. Before retiring repeat the "low" enema and cleanse, dry and powder the anal region. Once a week, after retiring, daub a small amount of bland ointment or mentholphenol paste into the perianal skin. The latter may cause mild burning for several minutes. Osborne and Stoll (1959) also emphasize the importance of local hygiene in the treatment of pruritus ani. In our opinion, especially as a prophylactic measure in early cases, local hygiene, usually without enemas, is the cornerstone of all treatment for this condition.

Sedatives. Phenobarbital gr. 1 ss (90 mg.) at bedtime and gr. ¼ (15 mg.) t.i.d. may be useful in quieting the nervous patient who still has to work. For patients confined to bed, larger daytime doses may be allowed. An ice bag applied to the itching area may be helpful.

Hydrocortisone Ointment. This method of treatment is very helpful for certain types of pruritus ani. Turell (1955, 1957) reported that

TABLE 41-2. GROUPING OF CASES OF PRURITUS ANI ACCORDING TO RESPONSE TO HYDROCORTISONE OINTMENT THERAPY (Turell, 1955)

GROUP	NO. OF CASES TREATED	RESPONSE
1. Intractable (with moderate lichenification), of less than 3 years' duration	36	Good
2. Intractable (with advanced lichenification) of over 3 years' duration	5	Good
3. Acute exacerbations	2	Trace
4. Refractory, without cutaneous changes	15	None
5. Secondary to diarrhea	12	Trace
6. Secondary to antibiotic therapy	14	Trace
7. Severe, accompanying fistula, fissure, or hemorrhoids	16	Trace
8. Severe, caused by pediculosis, enterobiasis or leukemia	6	None

it is particularly effective in the treatment of patients with intractable anal pruritus (Group 1, Table 41-2) but completely ineffective for patients of Groups 4 or 8. Hydrocortisone acetate, prednisolone, or free sterol in 1 per cent or 2.5 per cent ointment base is applied locally by the patient in the night and the morning, or more often in severe cases. When associated infection is present, oxytetracycline or neomycin and mycostatin may be added to the ointment. While this treatment is almost specific in many instances, its chief danger is that it will be used indiscriminately without utilizing proper diagnostic methods. If the pruritus is due to pinworms, hydrocortisone ointment therapy, even if it helps the itching, will be of symptomatic value only; if the pruritus is due to discharges from undiagnosed carcinoma of the rectum, the ointment, by its symptomatic benefit, may actually delay definitive treatment of the carcinoma until metastases have occurred.

Operative Management. In the most severe and intractable cases of pruritus ani when diagnostic measures have failed to reveal a causative factor and when all conservative measures (anal hygiene, sedatives, and hydrocortisone ointment) have been tried, operative management, beyond that necessary to remove causative fistulas, etc., may be indicated. In many instances, such treatment is necessary more to heal the skin which has been damaged by incessant scratching than for the itching itself. Included in the category of treatments to be considered are tattooing with cinnabar; subcutaneous injections of procaine, long-acting anesthetics, or even alcohol; presacral neurectomy (Smith, Malkiewicz, and Massenberg, 1955); undermining of skin flaps; or even excision of skin flaps with skin grafting. The multiplicity of such procedures reflects the unreliability of all of them. Fortunately, these radical measures are becoming less and less necessary as conservative treatment is improved.

FISSURE

An anal fissure is essentially a very sensitive crack in the mucous membrane of the anal canal. Most fissures occur in the midline posteriorly at or above the interhemorrhoidal groove (attachment of mucosal ligament to the anal wall). The next most common site is in the midline anteriorly. Goodsall's fissure site rule (1900) states that anterior fissure occurs in 1 per cent of male patients with fissure and in 8 per cent of female patients with fissure; hence, since fissure as a whole is twice as common in women as in men, there is a 1:16 ratio between the sexes for anterior fissure.

In chronic fissure one sees the circular muscle (formerly thought to be the subcutaneous portion of the external sphincter but now considered to be the lower portion of the internal sphincter). An anal fissure develops an "anal skin tag" at its lower end. This is not an anal papilla from the pectinate line but is edematous skin. It can be likened to a terminal moraine in the realm of geology, the stools corresponding to the glaciers. Tearing down of the associated anal valve may be a cause of fissure.

Treatment. The treatment of fissure involves 2 different types of therapy, depending on the stage of the disease:

Best in acute fissure ↑ 1. Medical treatment
2. Surgical treatment ↓ Best in chronic fissure

MEDICAL TREATMENT includes the avoidance of constipation and of rough foods or those containing seeds, the use of a regimen of anal hygiene, as for pruritus ani, mineral oil by mouth, soothing suppositories and externally applied ointments, and occasionally the injection of long-lasting anesthetics under the bed of the fissure. Supposedly, such injections will relax the sphincters, allow bowel movements to pass without trauma, and in turn permit healing. Because of the danger of infection and necrosis, injections are not advised.

SURGICAL TREATMENT includes either dilatation or excision. Dilatation puts the sphincters at rest for several days, usually allowing a subacute fissure time to heal. Since this method requires an anesthetic, local, regional, or general, one usually excises the fissure at the same time as one performs a dilatation. In chronic fissures, Gabriel stated that, "I have come to the conclusion that cure cannot be given for certain except by operation." Recur-

TABLE 41-3. INCIDENCE OF POSTOPERATIVE SYMPTOMS AFTER OPERATIONS FOR HEMORRHOIDS, FISTULA AND FISSURE*

| SYMPTOM | PERCENTAGE WITH SYMPTOM ||||
	NORMAL CONTROLS	AFTER HEMORRHOIDECTOMY	AFTER ORTHODOX OPERATION FOR ANAL FISTULA	AFTER INTERNAL SPHINCTEROTOMY
Inadvertent flatus	10	9	16	24
Occasional unexpected leakage of feces	3	6	12	11
"Soiling"	2	17	24	28
One or more of these 3 symptoms	10		36	43

* Based on Leeds University figures, papers of Bennett, et al., 1962-1963, loc. cit.

rence does occur occasionally following surgical treatment, but the results following this type of management are generally good, despite the fact that its use is reserved for the most severe fissures.

Two features of fissurectomy are also important: (1) one should remove a triangle of skin for drainage during the healing process external to and including the anal skin tag (sentinel pile). (2) The "pecten band," which actually is the lower portion of the internal sphincter, may be divided in the bed of the fissure (total internal sphincterotomy was advised by Eisenhammer [1951] and by Brossy [1956]), or an 0.8-mm. square section of it may be excised.

Due largely to the influence of Eisenhammer (1951, 1959), partial internal sphincterotomy is now our preferred operation for intractable anal fissure. Bennett and Goligher (1962) speak of cure resulting from the procedure as follows: "We doubt if it is surpassed in this respect by any other treatment for this condition." The one objection to the operation is that there is some interference with anal function. "Soiling" of the underclothes is the commonest complication, occurring in 30 per cent of cases and showing no tendency to improve with time. On the other hand, incontinence for flatus or feces occurred in 34 and 15 per cent of cases, respectively, but tended to definitely improve with time, the percentages being 13 and 9 per cent, respectively, after 3 years. To be entirely fair to the Eisenhammer internal sphincterotomy operation for anal fissure, these complications also follow hemorrhoidectomy (*without* sphincterotomy) and "orthodox" operations for fissure and even occur in normal persons. Table 41-3 presents a synthesis of data from Bennett (1962), Bennett and Goligher (1962), and Bennett, Friedman and Goligher (1963). Bennett and Duthie (1964) have studied the results of internal sphincterotomy in 16 patients relating to anal pressures recorded with open-type catheters through a Statham strain gauge. A definite decrease as compared with normals was observed.

In view of the tabulated experience we believe that most of the internal sphincter should be left intact in the primary treatment of most fissures. If they then fail to heal or if they recur, a greater risk of these troublesome symptoms may probably be incurred in exchange for a better chance for lasting cure.

In place of this standard operation, Pope (1959) advises an anorectoplastic procedure.

ABSCESS ("THE FORERUNNER OF FISTULA")

As shown in Figure 41-9, abscesses occur with varying frequency in the different spaces near the anus. There is a 5 to 1 preponderance in males. The origin of abscesses is considered to be an infection, often originating in anal glands or crypts, which penetrates into the perirectal spaces. Perirectal abscesses are associated with malaise, fever, pain and swelling until they either rupture externally or internally into the anorectum, or are incised and drained. Because of the thickness of the skin of the buttocks, fluctuation is not felt early. Similar conditions exist around the mouth at the opposite end of the intestinal tract, or on the palm of the hand; a contrasting situation

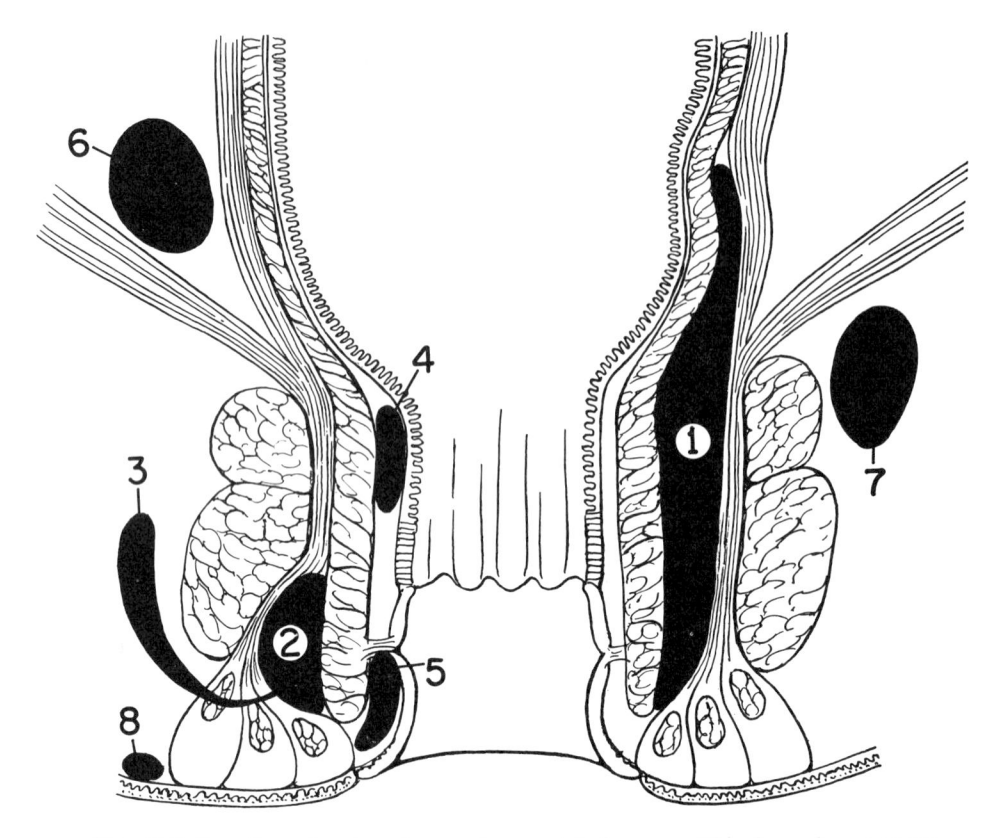

Fig. 41-9. Location of various types of anorectal abscesses. This figure incorporates the concepts of Eisenhammer (1958). The eight types are designated by numbers in the above figure as follows:
1. High intermuscular fistulous abscess
2. Low intermuscular fistulous abscess
3. Intermuscular ischiorectal fistulous abscess (horseshoe abscess)
4. High submucous nonfistulous abscess
5. Low mucocutaneous fistulous abscess
6. Pelvirectal abscess, nonanorectal
7. Ischiorectal fistulous abscess
8. Subcutaneous fistulous abscess

exists on the dorsum of the hand where incision seldom should be done unless definite signs of fluctuation are present. Gabriel (1963) stated in this regard: "The great majority of anorectal abscesses should be incised and given proper drainage at the earliest possible moment, and this policy has acquired additional importance following Eisenhammer's published work which stresses the common occurrence of the intermuscular abscess lying deep to the internal sphincter, which work is referred to below."

The submucous space extends downward only as far as the interhemorrhoidal groove. It contains the internal hemorrhoidal plexus. The perianal (marginal) space is inferior and lateral to the interhemorrhoidal groove. More laterally, infections superficial to the corrugator cutis muscle usually heal spontaneously, while those beneath it generally result in low-level anal fistula.

According to Nesselrod there are 5 deep spaces:
  2 ischioanal (one on each side)
  2 pelvirectal (anterior and posterior)
  1 retrorectal

Papers by Eisenhammer (1953, 1958, 1959, 1961, 1965) of Johannesburg, South Africa,

TABLE 41-4. EISENHAMMER CLASSIFICATION OF ANORECTAL ABSCESS

It is to be noted that the pelvirectal abscess, not being a primary anorectal condition, is not included in the percentage incidences. Note that 95 per cent of the fistulas are intermuscular according to this classification.

Group	Type	Etiology	Incidence
A. Internal	1. High intermuscular	Deep cryptoglandular infection	10%
	2. Low intermuscular	Deep cryptoglandular infection	81%
	3. High submucous	Shallow cryptoglandular infection, infected hematomas, direct trauma	2%
	4. Low mucocutaneous	Shallow cryptoglandular infection, infected hematomas, direct trauma	
B. External	5. Pelvirectal	Pelviabdominal infection	..
	6. Ischiorectal	Primary lymphatic or blood borne infection	2%
	7. Subcutaneous	Local tegumentary infection	1%
C. Interno-external	8. Intermuscular ischiorectal fistulous abscess (horseshoe type)	Secondary break-through of low intermuscular abscess into both the subcutaneous space and the outer portion of the ischiorectal fossa	4%
		Total	100%

have emphasized a new concept in the origin, the development, the classification and consequently the treatment of anorectal abscesses. This concept is that many abscesses are of an "intermuscular" variety, lying between the internal and the external sphincters (Fig. 41-9). Such abscesses result, according to Eisenhammer, from infection of anal glands which end deep to the internal sphincter in the intermuscular space. This space may be similar to the "anal intermuscular interstice" so well described by Shropshear (1960). The classification of anorectal abscess, with etiologic factors in each instance, is given in Table 41-4.

The high intermuscular abscess, situated deep to the internal sphincter and occupying the intermuscular space, is universally described and diagrammatically represented as the "submucous abscess" (Fig. 41-9). A true submucous abscess, a very superficial lesion, resolves spontaneously before operation is required. Eisenhammer (1958) states: "The failure to recognize the intermuscular space abscess is responsible for much of the present-day unsatisfactory treatment of the anorectal fistulous abscess." When fully developed, with a subcutaneous projection, the high intermuscular space abscess, instead of being mistaken for the simpler submucous abscess is confused with the more serious deep postanal or ischioanal abscess. This mistake results in formidable incorrect surgery, whereas the correct diagnosis requires only the simple surgical procedure of total internal sphincterotomy over the central axis of the abscess in order to bring about a cure (Eisenhammer, 1958, 1959). This author also refers to the intermuscular space as the "breeding ground of the more complicated fistulas" and "the key to the surgery of this complex subject." Table 41-4 also shows that the total per cent of abscesses which are of cryptoglandular origin amounts to at least 95 per cent. Similarly, at least 90 per cent of fistulas occur in the posterior quadrant because this is where most of the glands are.

The pelvirectal and retrorectal spaces have only visceral sensation; hence, they are not so painful and they produce only vague symptoms. The ischioanal space abscesses are painful (as well, of course, as the perianal ones) Batson's rule is also of importance in differentiating: the ischioanal space has a capacity of only 2 or 3 ounces; on the other hand, the pelvirectal space can enlarge considerably by floating up the peritoneum. Hence, if over 2 to 3 ounces is obtained by incision and drainage, the lesion is not an ischioanal abscess. Pelvirectal abscesses may be confused with true pelvic abscesses.

Eisenhammer (1960, 1961) described two special varieties of the anterior anorectal intermuscular fistulous abscesses, namely the "anovulvar high" and the "anoscrotal low" varieties. Since these are so frequently misinterpreted, a separate account of each is in order.

1. **Acute Anovulvar High Intermuscular Fistulous Abscess.** In the female, the acute high anterior anorectal intermuscular fistulous abscess lies to the side of the rectovaginal septum and bulges posteriorly into the deep aspect of the lower vulva above the anorectal line. It is distinctly palpable digitally and is about the size of a walnut. It has the misleading features of a primary vulval abscess. There are two diagnostic features: (A) the acute pain is of distinctly anorectal distribution, and (B) there is edema at the anal verge. There are no superficial inflammatory changes of the vulva as in an acute Bartholin abscess in which the pain is vulval. This type anterior abscess is relatively rare.

2. **The Anoscrotal Low Intermuscular Fistulous Abscess.** In the male, the anterior low acute anorectal intermuscular fistulous abscess points, in the majority of cases, to the right of the median perineal raphe at the base of the scrotum. In the ensuing recurring inflammatory attacks, the infection spreads higher up the scrotum until it is grossly involved in the chronic suppurative process and now appears to be the primary site. In the advanced scrotal involvement, the testes may be pushed up by the cicatrized scrotum. The diagnosis is made from the fact that there are no signs of epididymo-orchitis, and the testicle remains free and mobile. More important signs are telltale healed scars nearer the anal verge. The chief diagnostic sign is a well-developed cord representing the chronic granulomatous fistulous tract which is distinctly palpable from the base of the scrotum to the anal verge. This lesion forms about 5 per cent of the lower intermuscular fistulous abscess group and is, in nearly all cases, on the right side.

Antibiotics have a limited application in the treatment of these abscesses. Their use should not delay necessary operation, as they seldom, if ever, eliminate the requirement for it. The use of antibiotics for the definitive treatment of anorectal abscess "should be condemned; it is the best way in the world to get a bigger and better abscess" (Ferguson, 1965). Drainage usually involves a radial or cruciate incision over the abscess, sometimes with complete unroofing of the overlying skin. Drainage is maintained for a few days with either a Penrose drain or a gauze pack. Even though abscesses are the "forerunner of fistula," there is little that one can do at the time of treating the abscess to prevent the development of a fistula although McElwain (1959) has used primary fistulotomy in the treatment of 100 consecutive anorectal abscesses of all types. The advocates of anorectoplasty also treat abscesses definitively in one stage in selected instances. The patient should be warned of this probable eventuality and be examined periodically until either the danger is over or the time for treating the fistula has come.

Fistula

A fistula-in-ano involves the two openings of the sinus tract left behind by an abscess. Because of inadequate drainage due to scarring, first one opening and then the other may clog up. If too long a period of time is allowed to elapse, both openings may close off, the abscess may become reactivated, and a new site of spontaneous rupture may occur. This process, if repeated several times, results in the so-called "pepper pot anus." Formerly, 10 per cent of fistulas were tuberculous; at present, the true percentage is undoubtedly lower (2 to 3%, Dunphy and Pikula, 1955). Martin (1957), basing his observations on experience with 29 cases, mostly at a tuberculosis sanatorium, outlines rules for adjunctive chemotherapy. He also points out that in 112 cases with tuberculosis, viable and virulent tubercle bacilli were present in the lower portion of the rectum in 30 per cent, indicating how tuberculous fistula may originate. Differential diagnosis of fistula, tuberculous or otherwise, should include furunculosis, pilonidal sinuses and perineal sinuses, hidradenitis, sacrococcygeal cysts (Jackman, 1965), and teratomas, the latter particularly in the female.

Most fistulas originate from abscesses or other infection related to an anal gland. An infected internal or external thrombosed hemorrhoid may occasionally lead to a simple type fistula of the submucous or the subcutaneous types, respectively. Of the abdominal causes, primary Crohn's disease of the colon and the rectum (more frequent than formerly believed —Cornes and Stecher, 1961) should be considered. If there is an ulcerative process complicated by fistula, this combination is much more apt to occur in Crohn's disease than in ulcerative colitis (Morson and Lockhart-Mummery, 1959; Cornes and Stecher, 1961). In such cases any biopsied material should be searched for noncaseating tubercles with Langhan's-type giant cells which would suggest a diagnosis of unsuspected Crohn's disease of the large intestine. It is possible that some of the "tuberculous" fistulae diagnosed in the past were actually of this origin. At the same time, a fistula from Crohn's disease or ulcerative colitis is usually a perfectly typical pyogenic fistula without microscopic earmarks of the predisposing disease.

Fistulas occur mainly in adults. Males predominate 3:1 as would be expected, since antecedent abscesses are the cause ("Invariably results from abscess"—Gabriel, 1963). In truth, fistulas can lead "anywhere," and the process of tracing out their full course is often difficult but important, since unless the tract is found *in toto*, cure cannot be expected.

The rule propounded by Goodsall (1900) is a very practical one in understanding anal fistula: Fistulas with posterior external openings have their internal openings in the midline posteriorly; fistulas with anterior external openings have their internal openings radially opposite thereto (Fig. 41-10). Eisenhammer (1965) re-emphasizes a forgotten point of Goodsall's rule, namely that if the external opening is more than 1 inch from the midline, whether posterior or anterior, it originates from an internal opening in the midline posteriorly. Most fistulas, like most fissures, and possibly for the same reasons, have posterior openings.

Delineation of the course of fistulas may be made with probes, with injection of a peroxide-dye mixture (the writer uses 1% peroxide and methylene blue) and with the use of Lipiodol, bismuth paste, or other radiopaque injections followed by x-ray examination.

Treatment is essentially surgical. The surgeon, fortified with the armor of knowledge of the exact course of the fistula, still stands

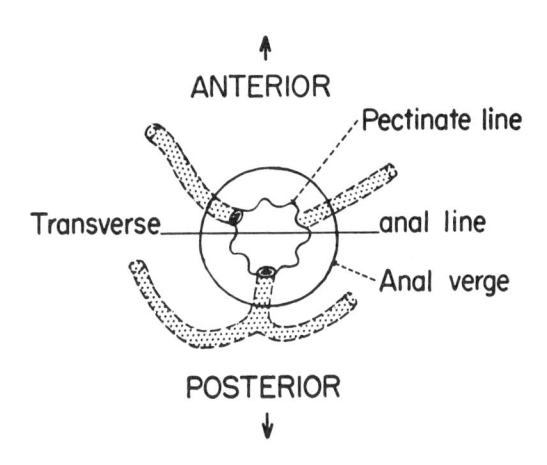

Fig. 41-10. Goodsall's rule: Fistulas with posterior external openings have their internal openings in the midline posteriorly; fistulas with anterior external openings have their internal openings radially opposite thereto.

between the Scylla of inadequate surgery and resultant recurrence and the Charybdis of complete excision and cure of the fistula, but with such extensive sphincter division that fecal incontinence results. Fortunately, in the most common types of fistula this is not a problem, and the entire fistula can be laid open and excised quite safely. If a fistula is soft it should merely be laid open; if it has a hard core it should be excised. It is quite safe to cut the subcutaneous and the superficial portions of the external sphincter; it is moderately unsafe to cut everything as high as the anorectal ring. (In this connection it is fortunate that some very high fistulas can be treated with thorough exposure and drainage without cutting the anorectal ring even by a 2-stage operation.) Between these extremes, the lower portion of the internal sphincter and the deep portion of the external sphincter can be cut when absolutely necessary in cases of high level anal fistulas by experienced surgeons using certain precautions. The incision should be perpendicular to the muscle and sometimes should be done in 2 stages, inserting a seton at the time of the first operation, although setons are used less often than formerly. The seton is left in place beneath the muscle to be cut at the second stage about 7 days later, the fistulous tract having been excised at the first stage. Use of the seton permits the muscle to become fixed so that its cut ends will not separate too widely. Swerdlow (1958) advocates a 2-stage technic in most lateral fistulas.

Ischiorectal abscess and fistula in cases of ulcerative colitis present a special problem. Before an extensive fistula is to be excised, ileostomy should be done; until the ileostomy is functioning it is only safe to drain.

Concepts concerning fistula should take cognizance of the newer ideas regarding abscess, particularly the intermuscular variety described by Eisenhammer. As Eisenhammer (1958, 1961, 1964) pointed out, about 97 per cent of abscesses are of the intermuscular variety (Fig. 41-9). The resultant fistulas are related to these abscesses, particularly the common "low intermuscular fistulous abscess." Parks (1961) has also shown that many of the operations in the past may have been unnecessarily radical in sacrificing external sphincter muscles. This is due to blind cutting of muscle in an effort to cure which at the same time leaves behind a portion of the abscess with its internal connections. If the abscess is completely unroofed *internally*, the *external* tract need only be cored out externally with no sacrifice of external sphincter muscles and with the avoidance of large, deforming external wounds. This internal operation also excises the related infected anal gland area which has been shown by Parks (1961) to be responsible for at least 90 per cent of fistula-in-ano. The chief difference between this operation and the formerly used "core-out" procedures for high-level fistula is that the new technic combines "core-out" with an intra-anal operation designed to eradicate the source of infection. The older procedures either did not always cure or, if they assured cure, often led to fecal incontinence.

When excising the fistulous tract it is advisable to remove a generous bit of tissue from 1 to 3 mm. in thickness at the site of the internal opening so as to assure extirpation of the adjacent anal glands which so often are the origin of the fistula. Such tissue should be sent for biopsy. Wide saucerization of the wound, especially at the external end, is not necessary with the Eisenhammer-Parks type of operation. Thus, if the entire lesion is removed in one piece it is like a long dumbbell with the fistulous tract connecting the excised skin margin at one end and the less widely removed portion of mucosa at the other. Packs should be used only for hemostasis and should never be left in longer than 4 days (Stelzner, Dietl and Hahne, 1956) or not be used at all (Parks, 1961). Immediate splitthickness skin grafting of the fistula defect, utilizing a stent, as advocated by Hughes (1957a,b), may save considerable time in healing. In a limited experience with this technic, the author has been impressed by how well these grafts take. Anorectoplasty, bringing down a mucosal flap to cover the internal opening, may simplify the treatment of these patients and may obviate the cutting of muscles. This has been utilized by McMahon (1956) and Rhoads (1960). Any treatment of fistulas must also take cognizance of Eisenhammer's newer ideas (1958) on "Abscess" (p. 1188-1189).

Hemorrhoids

A hemorrhoid is a vascular enlargement of either the internal or the external venous hemorrhoidal plexus or of both. The internal plexus is situated in the submucous space above the interhemorrhoidal groove, while the external plexus lies in the marginal space between the interhemorroidal groove above and the lateral hemorrhoidal groove below. The interhemorrhoidal groove is quite visible on a prolapsed combined internal-external type of hemorrhoid (Fig. 41-11). When the hemorrhoids enlarge, the whole mass tends to prolapse and to carry with it the mucosal ligament and interhemorrhoidal groove to a more superficial position, as shown on the right of Figure 41-11.

Hemorrhoids represent one of the most common ailments to afflict mankind. Fortunately, the treatment is relatively simple and safe, and the results are good when operation has been performed properly. From the anatomic standpoint it should be noted that there are 3 primary hemorrhoidal masses (piles): a left lateral and 2 right ones—anterior and posterior. These are also designated as being at 3, 7 and 11 o'clock, the mid-line anterior being high noon. It is interesting for the student to consider other places in the body where asymmetry exists (cerebral lobes, heart, lungs, en-

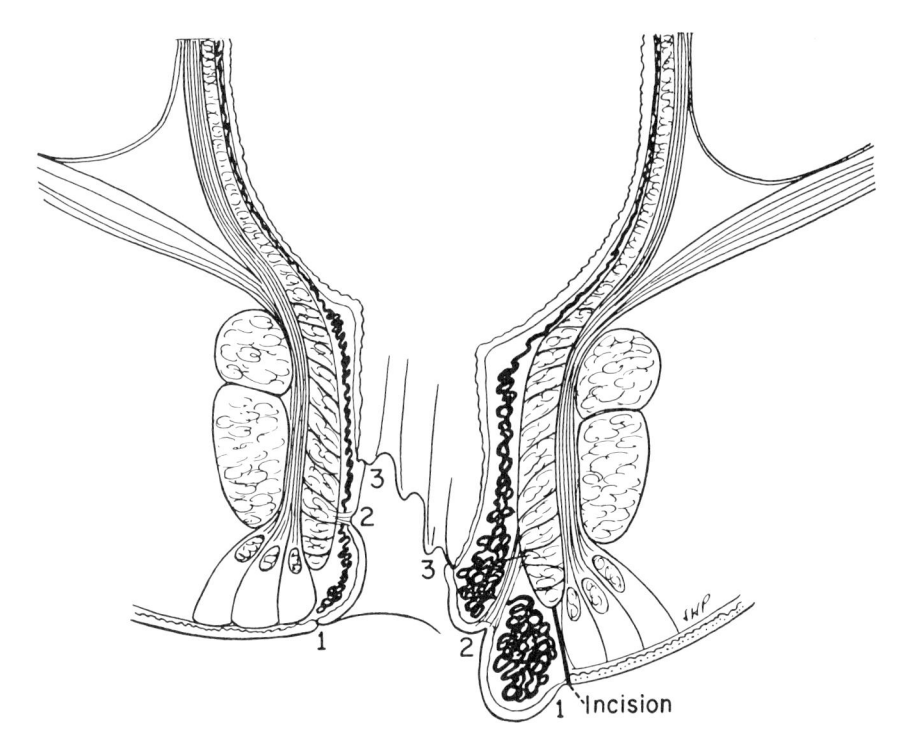

Fig. 41-11. Hemorrhoids. The portion of the drawing on the left shows the normal hemorrhoidal plexuses with the internal plexus above the external plexus below the interhemorrhoidal groove (Point 2 on the diagram). The portion of the drawing on the right shows how advanced prolapsed internal-external hemorrhoids still maintain their relationship to the interhemorrhoidal groove. The solid black line depicts the line of first incision for either the St. Mark's Hospital operation or for submucosal hemorrhoidectomy. The surgeon should avoid cutting into the internal sphincter muscle. Point 1 is the lateral hemorrhoidal groove; Point 3 is the dentate line.

trance of ovarian veins into renal vein and vena cava, etc.).

Internal hemorrhoids are insensitive, except at their lower portions and when prolapsed or infected, while external ones are very sensitive. The appearance of both may be considerably altered as a result of thrombosis, infection, ulceration, sloughing, or, in their later stages, by the processes of repair.

Predisposing factors include the erect posture of all mankind, constipation, long straining at the toilet, pregnancy, and a general hereditary venous weakness or pressure factor as evidenced by the frequent concomitant presence of hemorrhoids and varicose veins. Hemorrhoids are rarely present in portal hypertension (according to the author's view; some believe they are more frequent) but may occur in patients with neoplasms of the rectum and the sigmoid. Hemangiomata of the anus are a rare cause of hemorrhoids, excepting in children.

Parks (1956) presented a reasonable theory of the etiology of hemorrhoids. He postulated that the descending fecal scybalous mass forces the blood in the superior hemorrhoidal vessels downward, much as an interne will "milk" a blood transfusion rubber tube. Normally the blood may escape through vascular connections penetrating the internal sphincter, but in the presence of sphincter spasm, this is interfered with. Escape of the blood into the external hemorrhoidal plexus is meager, due to the mucosal ligament which separates the two plexuses. All this time, arterial blood continues to enter the venous plexus from above, until the venous pressure equals the arterial. The result is an internal hemorrhoid which bleeds easily.

Once a large internal hemorrhoid occurs, partial prolapse stretches the mucosal ligament. The external plexus now begins to fill due to free communication between the two plexuses, i.e., between the submucous and the marginal spaces, and a combined internal-external pile results, according to Park's view. At this stage when a bowel movement occurs, the pressure within the internal hemorrhoidal plexus can be dissipated by a flow of blood to the external hemorrhoidal plexus, and bleeding is less apt to result. Other factors rendering chronic prolapsed hemorrhoids less apt to bleed than some early hemorrhoids are squamous metaplasia of the overlying rectal mucosa due to the prolapse, and recurrent minor thrombosis and resultant fibrosis.

Differential Diagnosis. Before considering the treatment of hemorrhoids, one point deserves special emphasis. Hemorrhoids may occur coincidentally with, be confused with (because both give rectal bleeding and possibly pain) and even may be caused by carcinoma of the rectum or the rectosigmoid.

Hemorrhoids represent a distinct entity, but the number of hemorrhoidectomies performed when unrecognized coincident cancer of the rectum exists is not a tribute to the hemorrhoidectomist in question (see also p. 1157). Moore (1961) stated: "It is tragic that many patients with rectal cancer are still being first treated for hemorrhoids, some even with hemorrhoidectomy, before the malignancy is found." Thus, diagnosis, with universal proctosigmoidoscopic examination is requisite in all cases of hemorrhoids.

No patient ever should be operated upon for hemorrhoids (except for acute thrombosis of an external hemorrhoid and then he should be urged to return for subsequent study) without a complete anal and rectosigmoidoscopic examination. Any surgeon treating a large number of patients with carcinoma of the lower bowel has seen repeated instances in which advanced cases are admitted with a history of recent hemorrhoidectomy elsewhere.

Acute involvement of hemorrhoids may affect either the internal or the external plexuses. Prolapse of internal hemorrhoids is usually a chronic process associated with laxity of the anal musculature. In certain instances an internal hemorrhoid may be "strangulated," and reduction into the anal canal is in order. Most usually, however, advanced internal hemorrhoids become infected, ulcerated, thrombosed and permanently prolapsed. An erroneous diagnosis of strangulation is often made. In such instances reposition is not possible, the hemorrhoids being completely irreducible, and the preferred treatment is conservative, involving moist dressings, bed rest, heat and sitz baths. Operative treatment, or even attempts at forcible "replacement," in the presence of acutely infected internal hemorrhoids, may lead not only to spread of local infection but also to liver and lung abscesses due to the double (portal and systemic) venous drainage of the hemorrhoidal masses.

Acutely thrombosed *external* hemorrhoids (sometimes called "perianal hematoma"), on the other hand, if infection is not marked, may be safely treated as follows: under local infiltration anesthesia, a radial ellipse of overlying skin over the hemorrhoid (Anderson, 1959; Turell, 1960) plus a small wedge of skin lateral to it is removed. The clot may be plucked out intact, or split, and the two halves are removed (Inberg, 1955). All visible clots are picked out of the vein with forceps, and with the finger in the rectum the remainder of the clot may be gently milked out. Because the thrombosis extends back to the nearest branches, serious bleeding is seldom a problem, and this operation truly is one of the most succcessful in all of surgical practice. However, it is usually unwise to perform simple excision of thrombosed external hemorrhoids situated in the mid-line anteriorly or posteriorly because of the danger of resultant fissure.

Treatment. The treatment of chronic internal hemorrhoids is essentially surgical. Historically, the "complete hemorrhoidectomy" of Whitehead (1882) removing a circumferential cuff of hemorrhoid-bearing mucosa is of interest. In fairness to this surgeon it should be pointed out (Starr, 1957) that not all of his hemorrhoidal operations were radical. Whitehead stated: "Whenever it is possible with strict regard to removing every evidence of hemorrhoidal growth, I invariably leave longitudinal strips of mucous membrane continuous with the skin." Injections are not recommended, because of the danger of infection, necrosis and occasional resultant stricture.

Surgical methods include: (1) *The St. Mark's (Morgan and Milligan) method* (*vide infra*); see also Söderlund, (1962). (2) *The clamp and cautery method.* The author of this chapter was taught this technic but does not advise it. It is an old method, but still has its advocates (Cormie and McNair, 1959). A co-editor of this book (C.A.M.) believes that it is a "relic of barbarism and should have been cast into oblivion with the rack and the iron-woman." (3) *The Parks submucosal hemorrhoidectomy*, Parks (1956), *vide infra*. This method is also used by Shackelford (1958), Rainer (1959), and Silen and Brown (1960); and in modified form by Bartlett (1959); Vajrabukka (1965), and Moran (1964). (4) *The office ligation method* (Barron, 1962). (5) *Radical anorectoplastic hemorrhoidectomies* have been introduced, such as the technics of Lewis (1955), McMahon (1956) and others, which are modifications of Whitehead's second operation (1887) but utilize the principles of anorectoplasty. These radical methods have the disadvantage that they lead to a high incidence of stricture unless used by experts in this field. They are not advocated for general use.

The operation to be outlined here is the St. Mark's Hospital technic, a conservative one which involves the removal, after ligation, of the 3 primary internal hemorrhoids with the associated external hemorrhoid and with preservation of a bridge of mucosa of at least 8 to 10 mm. between each line of excision. In general, it is preferable to remove too little rather than too much.

Technical details of the St. Mark's Hospital hemorrhoidectomy are as follows:

Preoperative preparation of the lower bowel is similar to that for sigmoidoscopy. Using either general or low spinal anesthesia, the patient is placed in the lithotomy position. The anal canal and the lower rectum are cleansed with pieces of moist cotton wool introduced with the index finger.

Using a pair of nontoothed dissecting forceps, one of the anal skin tags is drawn downward and outward to expose the lower end of the internal hemorrhoid. When the dark-red mucosa covering the hemorrhoid is seen, this is grasped with an artery forceps, and the same thing is repeated with each of the 3 primary internal hemorrhoids. Morgan (1955) described the next important steps as follows:

When traction is now made on the artery forceps, pink rectal mucosa is delivered, and upon it, longitudinal ridges will be noted running downwards, one to each hemorrhoid—these are the *pedicles* of the piles. Each artery forceps is removed in turn from the pile mass and placed on each pile pedicle, which is then drawn downwards until there is a ridge of *pink* mucous membrane seen between each hemorrhoid. These ridges form a complete triangle of pink mucous membrane with a hemorrhoid at each corner. It is important to demonstrate this triangle of pink mucous membrane, which has been called, by Milligan, the *"triangle of exposure,"* since until this is produced, the hemorrhoids are not fully delivered (Fig. 41-12 A).

The left lateral hemorrhoid is dealt with first, the right posterior one second, and the right anterior one last, so that bleeding from this anterior one will not obscure dissection of the others.

The technic of ligature of each of the hemorrhoids is essentially the same and is as follows:

A second hemostat is placed on the skin overlying the external hemorrhoid corresponding to the internal one to be removed. With a pair of scissors the skin is cut in a V-shape up to the pectinate line on each side of the external hemorrhoid (Fig. 41-12 B). This dissection is carried upward, exposing the lower border of the pale internal sphincter (Fig. 41-12 C). Occasionally, the relaxed subcutaneous portion of the external sphincter is seen at the lateral angle of the wound and is recognized by being redder than the internal sphincter. The internal hemorrhoid is ligated with a transfixion suture of No. 1 catgut on a round needle at the level of the lower border of the internal sphincter and on the mucosal side at the level of the triangle of exposure (Figs. 41-11 and 41-12 D). The skin should not be included in the ligature.

A complete bridge of skin and mucous membrane at least 8 to 10 mm. wide should be left between each of the 3 incisions. After ligation of all 3 hemorrhoids, they are excised, leaving an adequate stump below the point of ligature. If it has been necessary to remove

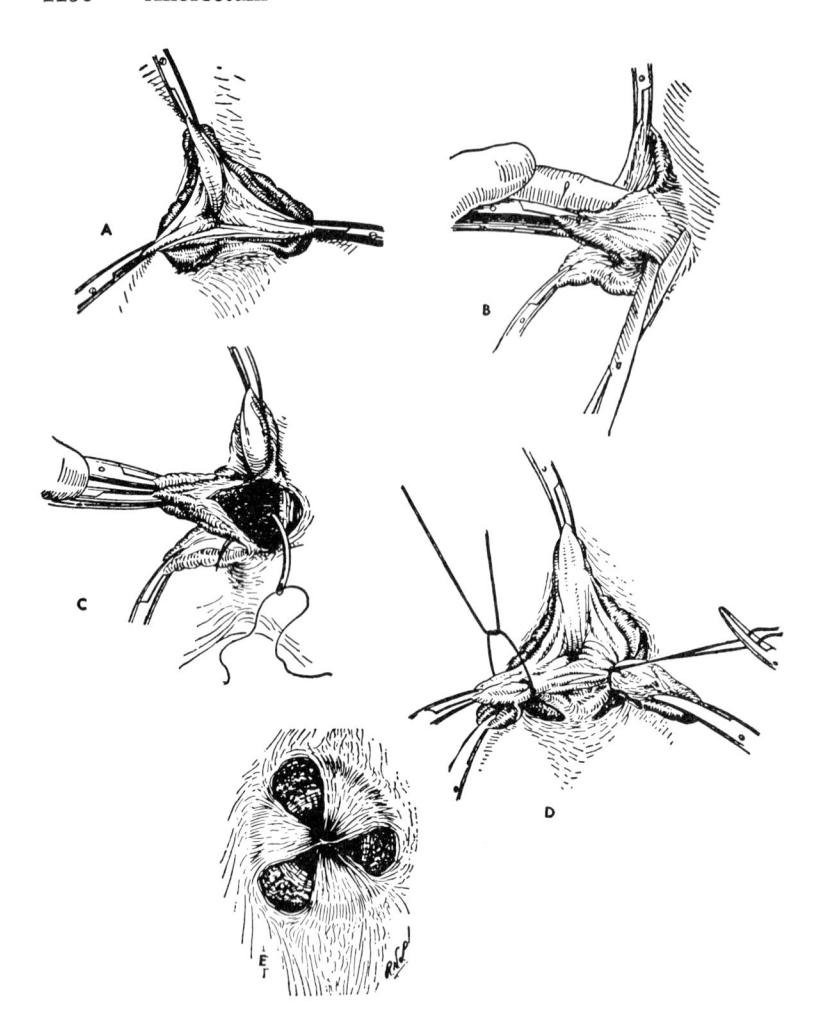

FIG. 41-12. The St. Mark's Hospital operation for hemorrhoids. (A) The triangle of exposure. (B) Commencement of dissection with initial incisions. (C) Dissection completed with the lower end of the internal sphincter (white) and the ligamentous fibers passing to the dissected hemorrhoid exposed. (D) The left lateral hemorrhoid has already been ligated, and the right posterior hemorrhoid is in the process of being ligated. (E) The 3 flat perianal wounds with complete skin bridges in between. (Morgan, C. N.: Hemorrhoids *in* Turner, G. G., and Rogers, L. C.: Modern Operative Surgery, London, Cassel)

skin in the anterior or the posterior mid-line of the anal canal, the lower 8 mm. of the internal sphincter should be divided at this point. Generally, except in cases with associated fissure, the hemorrhoid removal should not cross the mid-line anteriorly or posteriorly.

The skin edges are trimmed, and external hemorrhoidal masses protruding from beneath them are avulsed (Fig. 41-12 E). Ligatures are avoided here if at all possible. A proctoscope is inserted to see if the pedicles are bleeding, and after its removal a Penrose drain is inserted. No gauze is inserted into the anal canal, but saline gauze strips are placed on each side between the buttocks. The drain is removed in 24 hours, while the gauze dressings are removed by irrigation in 48 hours and changed at least daily thereafter for the first week, after which they are discontinued except for wearing a pad to protect the clothing. The second evening after the operation the patient is given 15 ml. of mineral oil. The next morning, 48 hours after operation, the patient is given an enema of 5 ounces (150 ml.) of olive oil.

A finger is passed very gently into the rectum on the 7th day and twice weekly thereafter until the skin wounds heal, which usually takes from 3 to 6 weeks.

Postoperative bleeding following hemorrhoidectomy is of two main types. The first is early, major, or arterial hemorrhage occurring the day of the operation and requiring a prompt trip to the operating room to find the bleeding point. The second is delayed, usually minor, or venous, occurring about the 7th to the 9th day after operation and is possibly due to sloughing of tissues, or separation of a ligature. Usually, conservative measures in the patient's bed are sufficient. Sometimes the delayed type of bleeding may be exigent. The following method of control of postoperative anorectal bleeding has been advocated by Marshall (1955). A lubricated No. 16 French urethral catheter with a 30-ml. balloon is inserted 10 cm. into the rectum, the balloon is distended, gentle traction is exerted upon the catheter, it is taped to the buttocks and usually is withdrawn in 24 to 36 hours. This method has the advantage that it does not require a second trip to the operating room or additional anesthesia. Thorlakson (1963) utilized gelatin foam packs to control postoperative bleeding.

The author has utilized the "submucosal hemorrhoidectomy" of Parks (1956) with good results, but it is still early to recommend this method in preference to ligature and excision, as described above, since we have used the Parks method in only 22 cases. The Parks technic involves infiltration of the skin and the mucous membrane overlying the hemorrhoids with a 1:400,000 solution of epinephrine in normal saline. The skin ellipse overlying the external hemorrhoid is excised in the usual manner, but the mucous membrane is cut longitudinally over each hemorrhoid. The artificial edema produced by the injection permits the surgeon to dissect up two mucosal flaps over each hemorrhoid and to ligate and excise each hemorrhoid without excision of any mucosa and without including any mucosa in the ligature. The method presents advantages in being radical as far as the hemorrhoidal varices are concerned but conservative as far as the mucous membrane is concerned. Thus the operation is not apt to produce pain or to lead to stricture or recurrence. It is not suitable for early hemorrhoids because of the friability of the mucosa in such instances.

The postoperative management of these cases includes the following 10 points:

1. Mineral oil—30 ml./day for 1 week
2. Dioctyl sodium sulfosuccinate (Doxinate, Colace, Aerosol O.T.), either 1 teaspoonful of liquid (1% solution) in fruit juice b.i.d. or 1 capsule (60 mg.) daily for 3 weeks
3. Ice bag over dressing for pain
4. No sulfonamides
5. No antibiotics
6. No drain or pack
7. Sitz baths beginning in 24 hours
8. Inspect wound with applicator
9. Dilatation: none except by bowel movements first week, little finger second week, and index finger third week
10. If postoperative bleeding of severe degree occurs, an attempt should be made to control it by the method of Marshall (1958), using a balloon catheter, or the technic of Blaisdell (1958), which aims at avoiding sloughing of tissue.

The essential problems of all treatment of hemorrhoids are to avoid resultant pain, stricture and recurrence. Pain is especially to be feared in the early postoperative period, and most particularly at the time of the often dreaded first bowel movement. Dickson Wright, speaking in his inimitable descriptive fashion stated (1964): "I make it a custom never to visit the patient at the time of the first defecation which may be like the passing of a red hot cannon ball wrapped in the skin of a hedgehog."

Goligher (1964) compared the immediate and the long-term results in a study of the St. Mark, the Parks and the clamp and cautery methods as to pain, healing and recurrence. The differences were not significant. The history of hemorrhoidectomy is discussed by Parks (1955).

Carcinoma of the Anus

Such carcinomas are usually epidermoid carcinomas, although basal cell and melanotic carcinomas may occur. Differential diagnosis should include viral warts (Young, 1964).

Basal cell carcinomas are rare, but Wittoesch, Woolner and Jackman (1957) reported 28 cases of basaloid tumors, 10 of which they called true basal cell carcinomas. Bunstock (1958) collected 47 cases from the literature, including the 10 of Wittoesch *et al*. Lemeh (1964) collected 59 cases and emphasized that these cancers affect elderly men, metastases are frequent, and that if the sphincters are involved, a Miles-like operation is indicated. Lone, Berg and Stearns (1960) reviewed 110 cases of primary invasive anal cancer seen at Memorial Hospital over an 18-year period. Of these, 21 (19%) were purely basaloid, and another 21 were basaloid plus either epidermoid or squamous. It is of interest that the basaloid tumors had a 5-year survival rate of

57 per cent, whereas the mixed or nonbasaloid groups had a 26 per cent survival. The use of preoperative radiation in these cases is not yet established.

Anorectal malignant melanoma is also rare (Probstein, 1957; Pack and Martins, 1960), but Hume and Marshall (1957) stated that over 100 have been reported in the literature while Quan, White and Deddish (1959) reported 21 (0.5% of all malignant tumors of the anorectal region) from the Memorial Center, New York City. Anorectal melanoma represents about 1 per cent of all malignant melanoma.

Epidermoid carcinomas arise from the true anus, in other words from the portion of the anorectum external to the pectinate line. The lesion is relatively rare, and only about 3 per cent of cases of cancer of the rectosigmoid, the rectum and the anus arise from the anus. While adenocarcinoma of the rectum is twice as common in men as in women, there is little or no sex predisposition with carcinoma of the anus. Buckwalter and Jurayj (1957) believed that chronic infection plays an important etiologic role. Patients with carcinoma of the anus are, on the average, about 4 years older than those with adenocarcinoma of the rectum (61 as opposed to 57 years). The lesion is especially apt to involve the anterior quadrant of the anorectum. In females this has a clinical application in that the posterior vaginal wall frequently has to be removed.

Turell (1962) emphasized the role of fistula, hidradenitis suppurativa, etc., as an etiologic factor in the causation of squamous cell cancer in this region just like the similar effects of chronic irritation elsewhere in the body. The prophylactic implications of this as to eradication of these chronic inflammatory conditions are clear.

The routes of spread of the tumor have a relation to selection of treatment. Local extension may involve the skin, the perianal and the ischioanal spaces, and the levator ani muscles. Extension to the prostate, the vagina (except in anterior lesions, see previous paragraph), the cervix and the bladder is rare except late in the course of the disease.

Blood-borne metastases are rare when compared with those from rectosigmoid carcinomas, being respectively 4 and 11 per cent to the liver, and 0 and 8 per cent to the lungs, the spine and the brain (Grinnell, 1955). This may explain why radical surgery may give better results in the treatment of anorectal (squamous cell) carcinoma than in rectosigmoid carcinoma.

Metastases by way of the lymphatics are common. Because of the position of carcinoma of the anus it metastasizes by lymphatic spread, both to the inguinal glands and upward to the pelvic glands. Upward metastatic involvement of either the perirectal or the mesocolic lymph nodes by way of the superior hemorrhoidal artery to the inferior mesenteric vessels occurs almost as frequently as in carcinoma of the rectum (33 as opposed to 42%; Grinnell, 1955). Involvement of the inguinal nodes can occur by 2 routes: an external and an internal one. The external route is via the anal plexus through the perineal lymphatics up over the upper thigh, emptying into the superficial groin nodes. The internal route is via the middle hemorrhoidal plexus to the hypogastric and the obturator nodes, then to the external iliac nodes and finally to the inguinal nodes.

The standard treatment of carcinoma of the anus is combined abdominoperineal resection of the rectum associated with the following 7 procedures: (1) ligation of the superior hemorrhoidal vessels just below the left colic, (2) wide removal of the peritoneum, (3) wide perianal skin incision, (4) complete removal of the ischioanal fossa contents, (5) division of the levator muscles close to their origin, (6) abdominopelvic node dissection which includes removal of the tissue about the aorta and its bifurcation, the vena cava, the iliacs (common, external and internal), and the obturator and the presacral spaces, and (7) inguinal node dissection if these nodes are involved. This is essentially the method of treatment advocated by Stearns (1955, 1958) and by Grinnell (1955) and used at the Memorial and the Presbyterian Hospitals respectively, in New York. Sawyers, Herrington and Main (1963), reporting from the Vanderbilt University Hospital, are also in essential agreement with this program. The usefulness of preoperative radiation in carcinoma of the anus is suggested but as yet not established.

Variations from this standard treatment should be assessed carefully before being adopted. Roentgen therapy alone is not recommended, and in combination with surgery has not been used in most big centers. Less radical surgery than a combined abdominoperineal resection should not be used for high lesions but is still used at the Memorial Hospital for small and superficial lesions very low in the anal canal. Such low lesions are sometimes treated by wide local excision.

While all surgeons agree that involved inguinal nodes are an indication for *therapeutic* groin dissection, either at the time of the posterior operation or within a few weeks thereafter, there is a difference of opinion as to whether a bilateral *prophylactic* groin dissection is to be advocated. Stearns studied the patients with epidermoid carcinoma of the anus treated at the Memorial Hospital during the 11-year period 1942 to 1952, inclusive. In 53 of these patients there were no recognizable inguinal metastases at the time the primary lesion was treated. Forty of these failed to develop metastases, while 13 (25%) did. Further breakdown of the 13 indicated that in only 3 could a prophylactic groin dissection have been of possible value. Thus, 53 bilateral groin dissections with their attendant morbidity, including possible leg edema, etc., would have had to be performed to salvage at the most 3 patients or 6 per cent. Further analysis of large series of patients will be necessary to settle the question as to the advisability of prophylactic groin dissection in this condition. However, one point is clear, namely, that if a prophylactic groin dissection is not done the patient should be examined periodically for the subsequent development of involved groin lymph nodes. The Memorial Hospital schedule for such check-ups is as follows: examination at monthly or bimonthly intervals the first 2 years (the time interval during which 85% of the nodes which are to become positive do so), at intervals of 3 or 4 months from then to 5 years, and at yearly intervals thereafter. Furthermore, it was found that the results following groin dissection on such delayed metastases were actually much better than in cases in which the groin nodes were involved initially, possibly because in the delayed cases the tumor is less active biologically.

Hohm and Jackman (1964), of the Mayo Clinic, after studying a series of 85 cases, concluded that the location of the squamous cell carcinoma with respect to the pectinate line is of importance. For those cases above, or involving, the line, they recommend a Miles-type of operation; for those below they advise a conservative resection or other indicated conservative treatment from below.

The results of radical surgery for epidermoid carcinoma of the rectum are obtainable only from the few large series reported. Stearns reported an over-all 5-year survival rate of 30 per cent (50% in patients without groin metastases and 12.5% in those with groin metastases—all of the latter representing patients in whom the groin metastases occurred after removal of the primary lesion). Grinnell reported an over-all 5-year survival rate of 39 per cent, but in those with curative surgery it was 55 per cent. These figures are quite comparable with those obtained after abdominoperineal resection for carcinoma of the rectum or the rectosigmoid.

Villous tumor of the rectum is rare, usually sessile, occurs in adults, may cover a wide area of the rectum and extend down to but not below the pectinate line of the anorectum. Its 3 chief points of interest are (1) its microscopic nature with numerous stalklike or frondlike thin villous processes which appear to be quite fragile, (2) its frequent tendency to malignant change, possibly in one third, or more, of cases, and (3) its tendency when large to secrete so much mucus that shocklike syndromes may result. (For a more extensive discussion of *colorectal* villous tumors, see Chap. 40, pages 1150-1152.)

BIBLIOGRAPHY

Altemeier, W. A., Culbertson, W. R., and Alexander, J. W.: One-stage perineal repair of rectal prolapse. Arch. Surg., 89:6-15, 1964.

Altemeier, W. A., Hoxworth, P. I., and Giuseffi, J.: Further experiences with the treatment of prolapse of the rectum. S. Clin. N. Am., 35:1437-1447, 1955.

Anderson, R. E.: The humble thrombosed hemorrhoid. Northwest Med., 58:114-1120, 1959.

Anderson, R. E., Pontius, G. V., and Witkowski, L. J.: Complications following surgery for benign anorectal lesions. J.A.M.A., 159:9-17, 1955.

Baden, H., and Mikkelsen, O.: The results of rectopexy in complete prolapse of the rectum in adults. Acta chir. scand., 116:230-234, 1959.

Barron, J.: Personal communication. 1962.

Bartlett, W.: Freedom from pain after hemorrhoidectomy. Arch. Surg., 78:916-922, 1959.

Bennett, R. C.: A review of the results of orthodox

treatment for anal fistulae. Proc. Roy. Soc. Med., 55:756-757, 1962.
Bennett, R. C., and Duthie, H. L.: The functional importance of the internal anal sphincter. Brit. J. Surg., 51:355-357, 1964.
Bennett, R. C., Friedman, M. H. W., and Goligher, J. C.: Late result of haemorrhoidectomy by ligature and excision. Brit. Med. J., 2:216-219, 1963.
Bennett, R. C., and Goligher, J. C.: Results of internal sphincterotomy for anal fissure. Brit. Med. J., 2:1500-1503, 1962.
Berg, J. W., Lone, F., and Stearns, M. W., Jr.: Mucoepidermoid anal cancer. Cancer, 13:914-916, 1960.
Bill, A. H., Jr.: Pathology and surgical treatment of "imperforate anus." J.A.M.A., 166:1429-1432, 1958.
Bill, A. H., Jr., and Johnson, R. J.: Failure of migration of the rectal opening as the cause for most cases of imperforate anus. Surg., Gynec., Obstet., 106:643-651, 1958.
Birnbaum, W., and Sproul, G.: The treatment of postoperative fecal incontinence. S. Clin. N. Am., 35:1487-1495, 1955.
Blaisdell, P. C.: Repair of the incontinent sphincter
———: Prevention of massive hemorrhage secondary
ani. Am. Surg., 94:573-576, 1957.
to hemorrhoidectomy. Surg., Gynec., Obstet., 106: 485-488, 1958.
Brayton, D., and Norris, W. J.: Further experiences with the treatment of imperforate anus. Surg., Gynec., Obstet., 107:719-726, 1958.
Brossy, J. J.: Anatomy and surgery of anal fissure, Ann. Surg., 144:991-998, 1956.
Buckwalter, J. A., and Jurayj, M. N.: Relationship of chronic anorectal disease to carcinoma. Arch. Surg., 75:352-361, 1957.
Bunstock, W. H.: Basal cell carcinoma of the anus. Am. J. Surg., 95:822-825, 1958.
Burke, R. M., and Jackman, R. J.: A modified Thiersch operation in treatment of complete rectal prolapse. Dis. Colon Rectum, 2:555-561, 1959.
Cormie, J., and McNair, T. J.: The results of haemorrhoidectomy. Scot. Med. J., 4:571-574, 1959.
Cornes, J. S., and Stecher, M.: Primary Crohn's disease of the colon and rectum. Gut, 2:189-201, 1961.
Crumpacker, E. L., and Baker, J. P.: Proctosigmoidoscopy in periodic health examinations. J.A.M.A., 10:1033-1035, 1961.
Dickson Wright, A.: Surgical treatment of hemorrhoids. Panel presentation before Joint Meeting of American Proctologic Society and the Section on Proctology of the Royal Society of Medicine. Philadelphia, May 11, 1964.
Dresen, K-A., and Kratzer, G. L.: Fecal impaction in modern practice. J.A.M.A., 170:644-647, 1959.
Dunphy, J. E.: A combined perineal and abdominal operation for the repair of rectal prolapse. Surg., Gynec., Obstet., 86:493-498, 1948.
Dunphy, J. E., and Pikula, J.: Fact and fancy about fistula-in-ano. S. Clin. N. Am., 35:1469-1477, 1955.
Duthie, H. L., and Gairns, F. W.: Sensory nerve-endings and sensation in the anal region of man. Brit. J. Surg., 47:585-595, 1960.

Eisenhammer, S.: The surgical correction of chronic internal anal (sphincteric), contracture. S. Afr. Med. J., 25:486-489, 1951.
———: The internal anal sphincter: its surgical importance. S. Afr. Med. J., 27:266-270, 1953.
———: The internal anal sphincter and the anorectal abscess. Surg., Gynec., Obstet., 103:501-506, 1956.
———: A new approach to the anorectal fistulous abscess based on the high intermuscular lesion. Surg., Gynec., Obstet., 106:595-599, 1958.
———: The evaluation of the internal anal sphincterotomy operation with special reference to anal fissure. Surg., Gynec., Obstet., 109:583-590, 1959.
———: Personal communication. August, 1960.
———: The anoscrotal and anovulval fistulous abscess. Surg., Gynec., Obstet., 113:519-520, 1961.
———: The long-tract anteroposterior intermuscular fistula. Dis. Colon Rectum, 7:438-440, 1964.
Ferguson, J. A.: Repair of "Whitehead deformity" of the anus. Surg., Gynec., Obstet., 108:115-116, 1959.
Ferguson, L.: The role of antibiotics in the treatment of anorectal abscesses and fistulas. Dis. Colon Rectum, 1965 (in press).
Fine, J., and Lawes, C. H. W.: On the muscle-fibers of the anal submucosa, with special reference to the pecten band. Brit. J. Surg., 27:723-727, 1940.
Fowler, R.: Landmarks and legends of the anal canal. Aust. N. Zeal. J. Surg., 27:2-18, 1957.
Fromer, J. L.: Dermatologic concepts and management of pruritus ani. Am. J. Surg., 90:805-815, 1955.
Frykman, H. M.: Abdominal proctopexy and primary sigmoid resection for rectal procidentia. Am. J. Surg., 90:780-789, 1955.
Gabriel, William B.: The Principles and Practice of Rectal Surgery. ed. 4. London, Lewis, 1948.
Goligher, J. C.: The treatment of complete prolapse of the rectum by the Roscoe Graham operation. Brit. J. Surg., 45:323-333, 1958.
———: Prolapse of the rectum. Postgrad. Med. J., 40:125-129, 1964.
———: In Nyhus, L. M., and Harkins, H. N.: Hernia. Chap. 46. Philadelphia, J. B. Lippincott, 1964.
———: Healing after hemorrhoidectomy. Dis. Colon Rectum, 7:441-443, 1964.
Goligher, J. C., Leacock, A. G., and Brossy, J. J.: The surgical anatomy of the anal canal. Brit. J. Surg., 43:51-61, 1955.
Gorsch, R. V.: Proctologic Anatomy. ed. 2. Baltimore, Williams & Wilkins, 1955.
Graham, R. R.: The operative repair of massive rectal prolapse. Ann. Surg., 115:1007-1014, 1942.
Granet, Emil: Manual of Proctology. Chicago, Year Book Pub., 1954.
Grinnell, R. S.: Squamous cell carcinoma of the anus. S. Clin. N. Am., 35:1289-1294, 1955.
Harkins, H. N.: Correlation of the new knowledge of surgical anatomy of the colorectum and anorectum. Dis. Colon Rectum., 8:154-157, 1965.
Hohm, W. H., and Jackman, R. J.: Anorectal squamous-cell carcinoma: Conservative or radical treatment? J.A.M.A., 188:241-244, 1964.

Hughes, E. S. R.: Anal fissure. Brit. Med. J., 2:803-804, 1953a.
———: Ano-rectal suppuration. Aust. N. Zeal. J. Surg., 23:41-47, 1953b.
———: Fistula-in-ano. Med. J. Aust., 1:198-200, 1953c.
———: Surgical anatomy of the anal canal. Aust. N. Zeal. J. Surg., 26:48-55, 1956.
———: The classification of anorectal fistula. Aust. N. Zeal. J. Surg., 26:273-280, 1957a.
———: Treatment of ischiorectal anal fistula. Aust. N. Zeal. J. Surg., 26:281-288, 1957b.
———: Ulcerative colitis. Personal communication. May 5, 1964a.
———: Prolapse of the rectum. Personal communication. May 4, 1964b.
Hughes, E. S. R., and Gleadell, L. W.: Abdominoperineal repair of complete prolapse of the rectum. Proc. Roy. Soc. Med., 55:1077, 1962.
Hume, A. H., and Marshall, S. F.: Anorectal malignant melanoma. Lahey Clin. Bull., 10:174-177, 1957.
Inberg, K. R.: Perianal haematoma. Acta chir. scand., 109:203-205, 1955.
———: Complete rectal prolapse. Acta chir. scand., 114:310-318, 1958.
Jackman, R. J.: Technique of proctoscopy. J.A.M.A., 166:1510-1513, 1958.
———: Perianal sinuses: Unusual cases. Am. J. Surg. Dis. Colon Rectum 8:115-118, 1965.
Kark, A. E., Epstein, A. E., and Chapman, D. S.: Nonmalignant anorectal strictures. Surg., Gynec., Obstet., 109:333-343, 1959.
Karlan, M., McPherson, R. C., and Watman, R. N.: An experimental evaluation of fecal continence—sphincter and reservoir—in the dog. Surg., Gynec., Obstet., 108:469-475, 1959.
Kiesewetter, W. B., and Turner, C. R.: Continence after surgery for imperforate anus: A critical analysis and preliminary experience with the sacroperineal pull-through. Ann. Surg., 158:498-512, 1963.
Kraft, R. O.: Duplication anomalies of the rectum. Ann. Surg., 155:230-232, 1962.
Leifer, W.: Pruritus ani, S. Clin. N. Am., 35:1479-1482, 1955.
Lemeh, C. N.: Basal cell carcinoma of the anus: Review of the literature and report of a case. Ann. Surg., 30:213-220, 1964.
Lewis, A. E.: Anorectoplasty for hemorrhoidal surgery. Am. J. Surg., 90:767-772, 1955.
Lieberman, W.: Spasm of the external sphincter ani muscle. Am. J. Proct., 1960.
Lone, F., Berg, J. W., and Stearns, M. W., Jr.: Basaloid tumors of the anus. Cancer, 13:907-913, 1960.
Lynn, H. B., and Arcari, F. A.: Anal atresia: Results of surgical treatment. Surgery, 51:691-693, 1962.
MacKenzie, R. J., and Davis, D. A.: Prolapse of the rectum in infants and children. West. J. Surg., 66:323-325, 1958.
Marshall, G. R.: A method for control of anorectal hemorrhage. J. Int. Coll. Surg., 24:97-99, 1955.

———: Control of anorectal hemorrhage with balloon catheter. Northwest Med., 57:334, 1958.
Martin, C. L.: Tuberculous fistula-in-ano: Diagnostic criteria and current therapy. J. Int. Coll. Surg., 27:649-655, 1957.
McElwain, J. W.: Primary fistulotomy in the treatment of anorectal abscesses. Surgery, 45:945-948, 1959.
McMahon, W. A.: Personal communication. May 9, 1956.
Miles, W. E. (1904): Cited by Altemeier, Hoxworth, and Giuseffi (see reference above), 1955.
———: Recto-sigmoidoscopy as a method of treatment for procidentia recti. Proc. Roy. Soc. Med., 26:1445-1452, 1933.
Milligan, E. T. C.: Rectum-haemorrhoids. In British Surgical Practice. vol. 7. London, Butterworth & Co., 1948.
Milligan, E. T. C., and Morgan, C. N.: Surgical anatomy of the anal canal with special reference to anorectal fistulae. Lancet, 2:1150-1156, 1213-1217, 1934.
Milligan, E. T. C., Morgan, C. N., Jones, L. E., and Officer, R.: Surgical anatomy of the anal canal, and the operative treatment of hemorrhoids. Lancet, 2:1119-1124, 1937.
Milligan, E. T. C., Morgan, C. N., Lloyd-Davies, O. V., and Thompson, H. R.: Fistula in ano. In British Surgical Practice. vol. 4. London, Butterworth & Co., 1948.
Minkari, T.: Rectosigmoidal rupture caused by effort during defecation and acute evisceration of several loops of the small intestine through the anus. Ann. Surg., 154:967-971, 1961.
Moore, G. E.: CA, 11:149, 1961.
Moran, T. F.: Advantages of minimal excision of normal skin in anorectal surgery. Am. J. Surg. Dis. Colon Rectum, 7:445-447, 1964.
Morgan, C. N.: Hemorrhoids and their surgical treatment: A description of the St. Mark's Hospital operation for hemorrhoids. S. Clin. N. Am., 35:1457-1464, 1955.
———: Hemorrhoids. In Turner, G. G., and Rogers, L. C.: Modern Operative Surgery. London, Cassel & Co., 1955.
Morgan, C. N., and Hughes, E. S. R.: The anal canal and rectum. Aust. N. Zeal. J. Surg., 21:161-172, 1952.
Morgan, C. N., and Thompson, H. R.: Surgical anatomy of the anal canal with special reference to the surgical importance of the internal sphincter and conjoint longitudinal muscle. Ann. Roy. Coll. Surg. Eng., 19:88-114, 1956.
Morson, B. C., and Lockhart-Mummery, H. E.: Anal lesions in Crohn's disease. Lancet, 2:1122-1123, 1959.
Moschcowitz, A. V.: The pathogenesis anatomy, and cure of prolapse of the rectum. Surg., Gynec., Obstet., 15:7-21, 1912.
Moyer, C. A.: Personal communication. July, 1964.
Nigro, N. D., and Walker, G. L.: An evaluation of the mechanism and treatment of complete rectal prolapse. Am. J. Med. Sci., 234:213-226, 1957.
Orr, T. G.: A suspension operation for prolapse of the rectum. Ann. Surg., 126:833-840, 1947.

Osborne, E. D., and Stoll, H. L.: Pruritus ani et vulvae. J.A.M.A., 169:108-111, 1959.
Pack, G. T., and Martins, F. G: Treatment of anorectal malignant melanoma. Dis. Colon Rectum, 3:15-24, 1960.
Palmer, J. A.: The management of massive rectal prolapse. Surg., Gynec., Obstet., 112:502-506, 1961.
Parks, A. G.: A note on the anatomy of the anal canal. Proc. Roy. Soc. Med., 47:997-998, 1954.
———: De haemorrhois. Guy's Hosp. Rep., 104:135-156, 1955.
———: The surgical treatment of haemorrhoids. Brit. J. Surg., 43:337-351, 1956.
———: Pathogenesis and treatment of fistula-in-ano. Brit. Med. J., 1:463-469, 1961.
Partridge, J. P., and Gough, M. H.: Congenital abnormalities of the anus and rectum. Brit. J. Surg., 49:37-53, 1961.
Pope, C. E.: An anorectal plastic operation for fissure and stenosis and its surgical principles. Surg., Gynec., Obstet., 108:249-252, 1959.
Probstein, J. G.: Malignant melanoma of the anorectum. Arch. Surg., 75:253-255, 1957.
Quan, S. H., White, J. E., and Deddish, M. R.: Maligant melanoma of the anorectum. Dis. Colon Rectum, 2:275-283, 1959.
Rainer, W. G.: Discussion of paper by Bartlett (see reference above), 1959.
Rhoads, J. E.: Personal communication. July 16, 1960.
———: Personal communication. July 29, 1964.
Ripstein, C. B., and Lanter, B.: Etiology and surgical therapy of massive prolapse of the rectum. Ann. Surg., 157:259-264, 1963.
Ruiz-Moreno, F.: Anal pruritus. Scientific Exhibit at Meeting of American Proctologic Society and the Section of Proctology of the Royal Society of Medicine. Philadelphia, May, 1964.
Sauvage, L. R., and Bill, A.: Imperforate anus repair utilizing a buttock-reflecting incision. Surgery, 57:448-453, 1965.
Sawyers, J. L., Herrington, J. L., Jr., and Main, F. B.: Surgical considerations in the treatment of epidermoid carcinoma of the anus. Ann. Surg., 157:817-824, 1963.
Scott, J. E. S., Swenson, O., and Fisher, J. H.: Some comments on the surgical treatment of imperforate anus. Long term results and postoperative management. Am. J. Surg., 99:137-143, 1960.
Shackelford, R. T.: Personal communication. November, 1958.
Shann, H.: The complete prolapse of procidentia of the rectum, an unsolved surgical problem. Int. Abst. Surg., 109:521-534, 1959.
Shropshear, G.: Surgical anatomic aspects of the anorectal sphincter mechanism and its clinical significance. J. Int. Coll. Surg., 33:267-287, 1960.
Silen, W., and Brown, W. B.: Submucosal hemorrhoidectomy. Am. Surg., 26:123-128, 1960.
Smith, C., Malkiewicz, G. M., and Massenberg, G. Y., Jr.: The autonomic nervous system in pruritus ani: perianal skin temperatures after sympathetic block in control subjects. Am. J. Surg., 90:790-794, 1955.

Söderlund, S.: Results of haemorrhoidectomy according to Milligan: A follow-up study of 100 patients. Acta chir. scand., 124:444-453, 1962.
Sommerschild, H., Knutrud, O., and Fretheim, B.: Anorectal anomalies. Acta chir. scand., 127:536-542, 1964.
Starr, K. W.: The heritage of Walter Whitehead. Surg., Gynec., Obstet., 104:751, 1957.
Stearns, M. W., Jr.: Epidermoid carcinoma of the anal region: inguinal metastases. Am. J. Surg., 90:727-733, 1955.
———: Epidermoid carcinoma of the anal region. Surg., Gynec., Obstet., 106:92-96, 1958.
Stelzner, F., Dietl, H., and Hahne, H.: Results of radical operations in 143 anal fistulas (evaluation of one-step sphincteral division in one-stage and in multi-stage operations). Chirurg., 27:158-162, 1956, Abstr. J.A.M.A., 161:1189, 1956.
Stephens, F. D.: Congenital imperforate rectum, recto-urethral and recto vaginal fistulae. Aust. N. Zeal. J. Surg., 22:161, 1953a.
———: Imperforate rectum: A new surgical technique. Med. J. Aust., 2:202, 1953b.
———: Imperforate anus. Med. J. Aust., 2:803, 1959.
Stockman, J. M., Young, V. T., and Sholes, D. M.: Duplication of the rectum. Dis. Colon Rectum, 3:223-229, 1960.
Stroud, B. B.: On the anatomy of the anus. Ann. Surg., 24:1-15, 1896.
Swain, V. A. J., and Tucker, S. M.: The results of operation in 46 cases of malformation of the anus and rectum. Gut, 3:245-251, 1962.
Swerdlow, H.: Fistulotomy and fistulectomy for fistulas about the anus and rectum. Am. J. Surg., 95:818-821, 1958.
Swinton, N. W., and Mumma, J. F.: The treatment of hemorrhoids. S. Clin. N. Am., 36:761-772, 1956.
Swinton, N. W., and Palmer, T.: The management of rectal prolapse and procidentia. Am. J. Surg., 99:144-151, 1960.
Tendler, M. S.: Massive prolapse of the rectum. Arch. Surg., 72:667-672, 1956.
Thorlakson, R. H.: Pain and bleeding after anorectal operations with special reference to anal dressings. Surg., Gynec., Obstet., 117:56-60, 1963.
Turell, R.: Hydrocortisone therapy in control of anogenital pruritus. J.A.M.A., 158:173-175, 1955.
———: Modern treatment of pruritus ani. Surg., Gynec., Obstet., 104:233-237, 1957.
———: Colonic and anorectal function and disease. Surg., Gynec., Obstet., 107:417-448, 1958.
———: Sigmoidoscopy and biopsy. Surgery, 45:880-882, 1959.
———: Hemorrhoids: advances and retreats. Am. J. Surg., 99:154-167, 1960.
———: Epidermoid squamous cell cancer of the perianus and anal canal. Surg. Clin. N. Am., 42:1235-1241, 1962.
Vajrabukka, C.: Submucous hemorrhoidectomy. Dis. Colon Rectum (in press) 1965.
Vetto, R. M., Harkins, H. N., McMahon, W. A., and White, T. T.: Unpublished data, 1956.
Walls, E. W.: Observations on the microscopic anatomy of the human anal canal. Brit. J. Surg., 45:504-512, 1958.

Warner, B. W.: Diagnosis of schistosomiasis by sigmoidoscopy and rectal mucosal biopsy. J.A.M.A., 163:1322-1325, 1957.

Wells, C.: Personal communication. Sept. 1, 1961.

Whitehead, W.: The surgical treatment of haemorrhoids. Brit. Med. J., 1:148-150, 1882.

Wilde, F. R.: The anal intermuscular septum. Brit. J. Surg., 36:279-285, 1949.

Wittoesch, J. H., Woolner, L. B., and Jackman, R. J.: Basal cell epithelioma and basaloid lesions of the anus. Surg., Gynec., Obstet., 104:75-80, 1957.

Young, H. M.: Viral verrucae in the anorectum. Surgery, 41:292-305, 1957.

―――: Viral warts in the anorectum possibly precluding rectal cancer. Surgery, 55:367-380, 1964.

Books

There are numerous special monographs on anorectal surgery. Among these some of the best are as follows:

Bacon, H. E.: Cancer of the Colon, Rectum and Anal Canal. Philadelphia, J. B. Lippincott, 1964.

Gabriel, W. B.: The Principles and Practice of Rectal Surgery. ed. 5. London, H. K. Lewis, 1963.

Goligher, J. C.: Surgery of the Anus, Rectum and Colon. Springfield, Ill., Charles C Thomas, 1961

Hughes, E. S. R.: Surgery of the Anus, Anal Canal and Rectum. Edinburgh E. & S. Livingstone, 1957.

Turell, R.: Diseases of the Colon and Anorectum. Philadelphia, W. B. Saunders, 1959.

CHAPTER 42

HENRY N. HARKINS, M.D.

Hernia

> There is, perhaps, no operation which has had so much of vital interest to both physician and surgeon as herniotomy, and there is no operation which, by the profession at large, would be more appreciated than a perfectly safe and sure cure for rupture.—Halsted, 1892.

> In the entire history of surgery no subject has been so controversial as the repair of groin hernias.—McVay, 1954.

Introduction
Historical Considerations
Definition, Diagnosis, Incidence and Prognosis
The Hernia Problem Today
Subsidiary Problems in the Field of Hernia
Aids to Repair
Rarer Hernias: Treatment and Glossary of Terms

INTRODUCTION

The subject of hernia is an important one in surgery today, and probably will be so for some time to come. The number of persons now alive who either have had or will develop hernia runs into the millions. Thus, hernia is a practical subject. Its repair is largely a structural one, and is based on a sound correction of the existing anatomic defects. At the same time, many of the advances in the fundamental knowledge of wound healing have and will come from a study of their almost controlled and repetitive application in the treatment of countless patients afflicted with the deformity of hernia.

One factor which is responsible today for part of the poor results following the repair of hernia is that operations for hernia are often considered to be minor or easy. On the contrary, it is difficult to learn the anatomy of the inguinofemoral region, repairs are not easy, and it is necessary to utilize great judgment in selecting the proper procedure for the particular patient being treated and to develop a facile technic in performing the operation. Only too often in training programs these operations are done by the younger and more inexperienced assistant residents. Ideas concerning the repair of hernias are passed on from one resident generation to another, often with no direct supervision by or infusion of new ideas from the chief of the service who is interested in more "major" procedures. In practice, surgeons who have learned their craft by other means than training do herniorrhaphies when they would not venture into more "major" fields. The philosophy that "anyone" can get good results with the repair of hernia makes even some trained surgeons careless. While experienced surgeons have fewer immediate complications involving such things as inadvertent division of the vas deferens, puncture of femoral vein by sutures, wound infection, etc., the matter of recurrence is the chief one at stake. For example, in good hands repair of direct hernia is followed by about a 7 per cent recurrence, while in less well-trained hands it may be 30 per cent (or higher). To the 70 out of 100 patients who may get a satisfactory result whether they go to an expert or a novice (or to the 7% who would get a recurrence anyway), the matter is not important; but to the 23 patients who do have a recurrence only because they have gone to a less capable surgeon, the matter is vitally significant.

HISTORICAL CONSIDERATIONS

The treatment of hernia has gone through an evolution similar to that in other fields of surgery. The careful anatomic repair of today had to wait for the development of anesthesia and antisepsis. Before the introduction of these two advances, operation was both hurried, because of pain, and dangerous, because of frequent sepsis, permitting operation only in the larger hernias which demanded treatment and in which it was often impossible to ascertain the anatomic relationships. Mass ligatures, and even the cautery, were widely used. One clinic visitor observed even as great a surgeon as Dupuytren (1777-1835) cut into the bowel with the original skin incision during the performance of 2 consecutive herniotomies.

In a delightful tract, Ravitch (1969) recalled the great Boston controversy concerning permanent cure of reducible hernia or rupture. The following appeared in the Dec. 18, 1851 issue of the *Boston Evening Transcript:*

IMPORTANT TO THE MEDICAL PROFESSION. Drs. Geo. Hayward, J. Mason Warren and S. Parkman, acting as a Committee of the American Medical Association, request their professional brethren throughout the Union to send them, before 1st March next, any practical information they may have on the possibility of "a radical cure of reducible hernia." This important branch of surgery is to be considered at the next annual meeting of the Association to be held in Richmond, Va.

It was an unusual way to obtain follow-up information, unique to the times but, as it turned out, not very useful.

In the last decade of the last century there was an especially rapid advance in the knowledge of hernia, particularly in so far as surgical treatment was concerned. The stage was set for careful dissections without the previous handicaps of haste and fear of infection, and able observers in a number of countries made distinct and almost simultaneous contributions. The classic reports of Bassini (1888), Halsted (1889, 1903), Lucas-Championnière (1892), Andrews (1895), Lotheissen (1898), Ferguson (1899) and McArthur (1901) appeared during this period. Essentially, these observers devised different varieties of layer closure of the defects remaining after sac ligation, and most of today's repairs, of groin hernias at least, are based upon the technics of 60 years ago. The details of repair introduced by some of these men will be discussed in the section on groin hernia later in this chapter. The historical development of herniorrhaphy has beeen reviewed by Carlson (1956), Brown and Galletti (1960), Galletti and Brown (1960), Lytle (1954), Koontz (1963) and Olch and Harkins (1964).

DEFINITION, DIAGNOSIS, INCIDENCE AND PROGNOSIS

Definition

A hernia is an abnormal protrusion of an organ or a portion of it through the containing wall of its cavity, beyond its normal confines. The usual meaning of the term is restricted to the abdominal cavity, so that such things as muscle hernia of the leg, hernia of the lung, etc., are not usually considered and will not be in this chapter.

Diagnosis

The diagnosis of a hernia is made primarily on the basis of the physical examination, not on the history. However, there are exceptions to this rule. If the patient, or the patient's mother in the case of a child, states that a hernia is present, the physician should not dismiss the patient with a negative diagnosis on the basis of a single examination. If repeated examination is negative, the patient should be urged to return at a time when the hernia is present. Furthermore, a patient wearing a truss may have negative findings at the first examination. In such instance he should be requested to leave the truss off for several days, or until the hernia becomes manifest, and then return for a second examination.

A dragging sensation, sometimes with pain at the onset, is the one feature in the history common to many groin hernias, but, as stated above, the diagnosis is based primarily on the physical examination. A hernia usually is most painful at the onset, while the gradual spreading of tissues in the later stages only gives a vague discomfort.

The physical examination involves 4 steps. The first 3 require that the examiner be seated on a low stool before the patient, who is standing with the area from above the groin to the knees exposed. Furthermore, the patient should be masked or should be required to hold a towel in front of his mouth when coughing to prevent the spread of germs, particularly *Mycobacterium tuberculosis*. The patient is encouraged to cough while the examiner (1) observes the groin region for appearance of a swelling; (2) palpates it to feel for an impulse and later for a swelling which gives a gurgling sensation on being reduced; and (3) palpates through the invaginated neck of the scrotum with a single examining finger for an impulse or reducible swelling. The 4th step involves repetition of the examination with the patient lying down.

The "thumb test" (Moyer, 1955) is an added means of examination. With the hernia reduced, the flat of the thumb is held firmly over the site of the internal ring (just above a point halfway between the anterior superior iliac spine and the symphysis pubis), and the patient is encouraged to cough. If the hernia is indirect, the thumb will retain it; if the hernia is direct, the thumb cannot hold it in, and it will protrude medial to the point being pressed upon.

In infants, the "water-silk" sign (see Gross, 1953) may be helpful. The middle finger is placed over the inguinal canal and moved back and forth from below and laterally to above and medially. An increased thickness can be felt if an inguinal hernia is present, and there is a sensation of silken surfaces sliding over each other.

Zieman (1940) emphasized the importance of the second step in the physical diagnosis of hernia, as listed above. In brief, his method consists of standing behind and to the side of the erect patient and using the right hand for examination of the right side and the left hand for the left. The 1st, the 2nd and the 3rd fingers of the hand are placed over the region of Hesselbach's triangle, the external ring and the femoral region, respectively, with the fingers pointing downward and medially. When the patient coughs or strains, a peculiar gurgling, sliding or slipping motion occurs under one finger. If under the index finger, the hernia is more apt to be direct; if under the other 2, indirect or femoral hernia. If a bulge is present before coughing, it is reduced before applying the test.

Other methods also are used to decide the difficult question as to whether the hernia is indirect or direct inguinal, or femoral. An oblique impulse, a hernia that goes all the way down into the scrotum, or palpation of a rounded edge of the fascial defect medially indicates a possible indirect inguinal hernia. A more vertical or outward impulse, a hernia that protrudes diffusely anteriorly and medially and does not go all the way down into the scrotum, and a straight vertical edge of the medial fascial defect indicate a possible direct inguinal hernia. Preoperative palpation of the pulse in the superficial inferior epigastric artery through the abdominal wall so as to determine whether the hernial impulse is lateral or medial to it, hence indirect or direct, is not possible in the experience of the author.

The decision as to whether the hernia is inguinal or femoral is arrived at on accurate palpation of the lower edge of the external oblique aponeurosis. If the bulge comes out above, it is inguinal; if below, it is femoral. At the same time the examiner should remember that femoral hernias first descend, then protrude, anteriorly; then they may even curl upward slightly. The common error is to overlook a femoral hernia; it is much more common to label a femoral hernia as an inguinal one than the reverse. The author's rule epitomizes this as follows: "If in doubt, it is a femoral hernia."

In the differential diagnosis from other conditions, the following must be considered: (1) inguinal adenitis (to one side of the empty inguinal canal); (2) ectopic testis (characteristic shape to mass combined with absence of testis in scrotum on that side); (3) hydrocele of the cord (usually moves when cord is tightened by scrotal traction, may be transilluminated, examining finger may get above mass with the finding of absent cough impulse); (4) psoas abscess (dull to percussion, associated with change in the spine); (5) femoral adenitis (lacks the impulse of a femoral hernia); and (6) saphenous varix (compressible, has an impulse on percussion of saphenous vein below —Schwartz's sign—and a thrill or a transitory impulse as a result of pressure from above during coughing).

INCIDENCE AND PROGNOSIS

It is difficult to arrive at the incidence of the various types of hernia, since different hospitals treat different types of material and,

TABLE 42-1. INCIDENCE OF HERNIA

	PERCENTAGE
Indirect inguinal	56
Direct inguinal	22
Femoral	6
Ventral and incisional	10
Umbilical	3
Esophageal hiatus	1
Others	2
Total	100

furthermore, different hernias, due to diagnostic difficulties, etc., are treated in different proportions in relationship to their occurrence in the untreated population. However, for practical purposes, the following outline serves as a basis of departure. These figures are reached by combining percentages given in various texts plus personal observations, taking into special consideration the belief that direct hernia, if properly tested for and searched for at operation, is much more common than is generally realized. These figures are given in Table 42-1.

As Elman (1952) pointed out in an editorial, it is a surprise to learn that in the 1948 United States mortality tables, hernia (exclusive of intestinal obstruction) is listed as responsible for 5,000 deaths, a figure which exceeded the death rate for acute appendicitis in that year. Moreover, this mortality remained nearly constant for 2 decades, a period during which the mortality from acute appendicitis was cut sharply—to about one third. Elman urged more frequent practice of herniorrhaphy before the onset of the complications of strangulation and obstruction, which are responsible for the high death rate cited above.

Elman pointed out further that the United States Public Health Service estimated that there were 800,000 individuals in this country with unrepaired hernias—a figure that correlates well with the annual sale of trusses, which is said to exceed 1 million a year. He concluded his observations by stating: "The hernia problem is a simple one which can be solved by using adequate surgery earlier and more frequently."

Hagan and Rhoads (1953) discussed the prognosis following 1,082 groin herniorrhaphies on 957 patients in 1,022 operations at the University of Pennsylvania Hospital from 1945 to 1948 (Table 42-2). The operative mortality rate was 0.3 per cent. The distribution of these cases gives an indication of the relative incidence of the more common types of groin hernia in hospital practice, as follows: 86 per cent of the total hernias occurred in males, while 84 per cent of the femoral hernias occurred in females. It is significant that in conformity with most other reports, while femoral hernia is *relatively* more common in females, its *absolute* frequency in females is less than indirect inguinal hernia (41% femoral, as opposed to 52% indirect inguinal, the most common among all groin hernias in women).

TABLE 42-2. RELATIVE INCIDENCE OF
GROIN HERNIAS
(HAGAN AND RHOADS, 1953)

	PERCENTAGE
Indirect inguinal	66.1
Direct and direct-indirect	20.2
Recurrent inguinal	6.9
Femoral	6.8
Total	100.0

TABLE 42-3. RECURRENCE RATES IN INGUINAL HERNIA RELATIVE TO TIME
ELAPSED SINCE PRIMARY REPAIR

AUTHOR	NO. OF CASES	To 1 yr.	RECURRENCES PERCENTAGE To 2 yr.	To 5 yr.
Fallis (1937)	200	37	48	68
Clear (1951)	114	17	28	62
Zawacki and Thieme (1951)	105	51		75
Borgström (1951)	88	55	71	87
Hagan and Rhoads (1953)	75		55	75

Hagan and Rhoads reported 4.6 per cent of hernias in women as being direct or pantaloon in type. This is considerably more than has occurred on the author's service (1 in approximately 1,000, or 0.1%). However, the figure of 4.6 per cent represents only 0.4 per cent of the direct hernias in both sexes and only 0.9 per cent of the entire series of 1,082 groin hernias. For the student who may not see a large number of hernias, the rule taught the author by Andrews (1933), that "There is no such thing as a direct hernia in a woman," may be valuable as a teaching point to emphasize that such hernias are indeed very rare.

Recurrences were noted by Hagan and Rhoads as late as 39 years after the original operation: 55 per cent of the recurrences were evident within 2 years and an additional 20 per cent during the following 3 years. Thus, 25 per cent occurred after 5 years following operation. Fallis (1937) reported similar figures: 48 per cent recurrences within 2 years, an additional 20 per cent within the following 3 years and 32 per cent after 5 years following operation. Recurrence rates relative to the time since repair in various reported series are shown in Table 42-3. The entire subject of recurrence of groin hernias has been analyzed by Ryan (1953) on the basis of his experience with 369 recurrent cases.

The recurrence rate relative to age in Hagan and Rhoads' series is of interest. The over-all recurrence rate at the end of 2 years was 5.4 per cent. There were no recurrences in children under 10 years of age. The recurrence rate rose by decades from 10 to 60 years with percentages of 2.3 rising progressively to 12.2 per cent. After 60, the recurrence rate again dropped to 3.7 per cent, probably because of less physical activity in patients over that age. The sex differences in recurrence rate also were interesting, being 6.1 per cent for males and 1.1 per cent for females.

Guy, Werelius and Bell (1955) give an overall summary of the probable recurrence rates now occurring in the United States, as shown in Table 42-4.

The incidence of recurrences in different parts of the inguinal floor was studied by Zawacki and Thieme (1951), as shown in Table 42-5.

These authors pointed out that 75 per cent of recurrences were due to failure either to close the internal ring properly or to take a firm stitch at the pubic spine. In general, it can be said that most recurrences are direct, except when the sac has been left behind or the internal ring has not been tightened properly.

TABLE 42-4. RECURRENCES AFTER HERNIORRHAPHY

	PERCENTAGE RECURRENCE
Indirect inguinal hernia:	
Children and females	1 to 4
Adult males	5 to 10
Direct inguinal hernia	15 to 30
Recurrent inguinal hernia	15 to 40
Ventral and incisional hernias	20 to 30

THE HERNIA PROBLEM TODAY

The hernia problem today is essentially surgical. Its major facets are two: (1) the problem of incarceration (irreducibility) and strangulation; and (2) technical factors in the repair of the 4 most common types of hernia (groin, ventral incisional, umbilical and esophageal hiatus hernias) with the prevention of recurrence.

These 2 major groups of problems, which concern the medical student, will be considered here. Then at the end of the chapter the following items which concern the specialist will also be covered: (1) subsidiary problems in the field of hernia, (2) a consideration of certain "aids" to repair which are not applicable routinely but are useful methods in the arma-

TABLE 42-5. ANATOMIC LOCALIZATION OF 105 RECURRENCES FOLLOWING INGUINAL HERNIORRHAPHY

TYPE OF RECURRENCE	PERCENTAGE OF TOTAL CASES	
At internal ring:		
Small at ring	18	
Above and lateral	12	
Typical indirect hernia	20	50
At pubic tubercle		22
Direct hernia		22
Miscellaneous		6
Total		100

mentarium of any surgeon, and (3) a glossary of terms, including a discussion of some of the rarer, but important, types of hernia for which a few details of therapy will be given.

The Problem of Incarceration (Irreducibility), Obstruction and Strangulation

In cases of incarcerated (irreducible) hernia (see glossary at end of chapter), it is often difficult to tell whether such a hernia is strangulated or soon will be, and, from a practical viewpoint, it would seem advisable to look upon all incarcerated hernias as potentially strangulated and to treat them as emergencies along with the truly strangulated hernias. This same argument also applies to obstructed hernias to an even greater degree. The line of differentiation between incarceration (syn.: irreducibility) and obstruction on the one hand and strangulation on the other is often tenuous and may change from hour to hour, particularly in the case of a hernia that has become incarcerated only recently. The safest procedure would be early operation for all, and emergency operation for incarceration, and always, of course, for strangulation.

Strangulation, implying obstruction of the flow of blood to the contents of a hernia, is an important catastrophe. It is one of the two most common causes of death from intestinal obstruction (the other being adhesive bands), and it kills about 5,000 persons in the United States every year. In 1946, strangulation was responsible for 3,985 deaths in England and Wales in a total population of 43 million. Smith, Moore and Perry (1955) reported that 44 per cent of all strangulating bowel obstructions at the University of Minnesota were due to external hernia with strangulation. A prophylactic means of reducing this mortality would be to treat reducible hernias surgically. Therapeutically, 2 means are available: (1) the physician always should look at and feel the hernial rings in any patient with intestinal obstruction or abdominal symptoms which might presage intestinal obstruction; (2) one should recognize the early signs of obstruction in any patient who has a hernia. These include general and abdominal symptoms (see Chap. 38) or local symptoms and signs, including pain in the region of the hernia, tenderness over an irreducible or an incarcerated hernia, recent development of irreducibility, and discoloration of the tissues over the hernia.

Certain hernias—for the most part those with small rigid rings—are more apt to become strangulated than others. Femoral hernias, umbilical hernias in adults and indirect inguinal hernias are apt to strangulate in that order, while direct inguinal hernias are less apt to do so. Hagan and Rhoads (1953) observed that of 19 strangulated hernias, 12 were indirect inguinal, 6 were femoral, 1 was recurrent inguinal and none was direct inguinal. Dennis and Enguist (1964) point out that incisional and epigastric hernias are also very apt to strangulate and that in their experience such strangulation has a high mortality (44 and 100%, respectively).

The treatment of a strangulated hernia involves several general principles in addition to that of anatomic repair of the hernia:

1. The operation is an urgent emergency.
2. The general condition of the patient may be precarious, and supportive measures (blood, etc.) should be given if at all indicated.
3. Infection is apt to occur, particularly if intestinal resection becomes necessary, and antibiotics may be indicated.
4. The questionable loop of bowel must not be allowed to escape into the general peritoneal cavity until the *all-important decision* as to its viability has been made. Querna (1955) pointed out that reduction of hernia en masse, even in the absence of strangulation, may be dangerous and lead to later intestinal obstruction. When strangulation is present, such reduction en masse, in which the hernia remains in its peritoneal coat—hence is not really reduced at all—is particularly hazardous. Persistent tenderness may give an indication as to the diagnosis. Such reduction usually occurs in inguinal hernias, but 1 of Querna's 3 cases was femoral. Furthermore, even when the strangulated loop of bowel is apparently viable and is not resected, late stenosis of the intestine may result. Cherncy (1958) reported such a case and reviewed 82 others cited in the literature.
5. It must be recognized that the operative wound, following repair of a strangulated hernia, is especially liable to become infected. For this reason, steel-wire sutures are to be considered in the closure.

If intestinal resection proves to be neces-

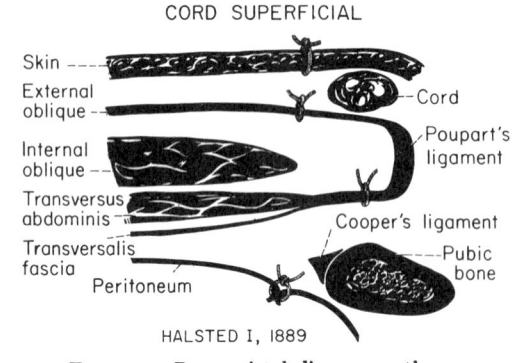

FIG. 42-1. Parasagittal diagrammatic representation of groin hernia repair with *cord superficial to the external oblique anastomosis*. It should be pointed out that in Halsted's original description, a separate layer-by-layer suture was not used. This figure denotes how a Halsted I would be done by such a technic today. Note that in Figures 42-2 through 42-4 the layer that is usually called the "conjoined tendon" but really is—or at least *should* be—the fused transversus abdominis aponeurosis, or "arch," and transversalis fascia, is sutured to the shelving edge of Poupart's ligament. Actually, the "conjoined tendon," or fusion of internal oblique aponeurosis and transversus abdominis aponeurosis, has been found in cadavers in only 3 per cent of dissections. Also, the depiction in Figures 42-1 through 42-5 could apply to either direct or indirect inguinal hernia. (Nyhus, L. M., and Harkins, H. N.: Hernia. Philadelphia, J. B. Lippincott, 1964)

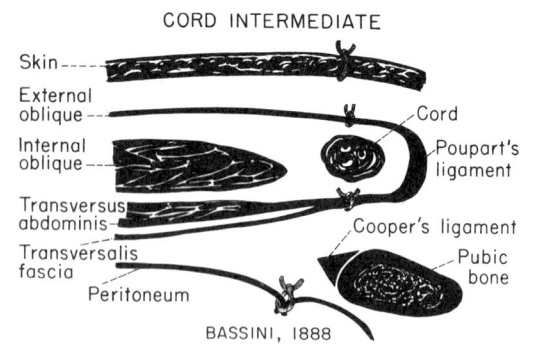

FIG. 42-2. Parasagittal diagrammatic representation of groin hernia repair with *cord in intermediate position between external oblique aponeurosis and fused transversus abdominis aponeurosis and transversalis fascia*. (See note to Fig. 42-1.) (Nyhus, L. M., and Harkins, H. N.: Hernia. Philadelphia, J. B. Lippincott, 1964)

sary, it should be done with as little contamination of the wound as possible. In seriously ill or moribund patients, all the means of dealing with a complicated situation available to a thoroughly trained abdominal surgeon may be necessary. It is estimated that 20 per cent of strangulated external hernias require bowel resection. Despite all safeguards, the operation is difficult, it requires a careful decision as to viability of the bowel, the mortality is high relative to that for other hernias (about 25% or more), and, if the patient survives, the recurrence rate is higher than that for corresponding nonstrangulated hernias.

In the special instance of treatment of femoral hernia with gangrenous bowel, the method of Dennis and Varco, 1947 (elaborated upon by Enquist and Dennis, 1955) represents a distinct advance when gangrene is present and resection is required. The entire sac and contents are resected intact in order to avoid bacterial contamination of tissues to be used for repair. This is accomplished by freeing the sac and its contents above without releasing the neck. The peritoneum is opened parallel with the oblique skin incision, involved omentum is cut and ligated close to the neck, and the mesentery of the small intestine entering the sac is divided from the proximal to the distal side of the incarcerated intestinal loop. Each limb of bowel is clamped by 2 Ochsner clamps, and the intestine is divided between them with the cautery. Next, the inguinal ligament is divided near its attachment to the pubis and split laterally, enough of the heavy aponeurotic tissue being left in front of the neck of the sac to prevent it from relaxing and releasing the contaminated contents. Then the entire sac is freed by dissection down to the remains of the ring, which is cut under direct vision, and the complete contaminated mass is removed without soiling the field. Then Cooper's ligament repair is performed.

THE PROBLEM OF THE 4 MOST COMMON TYPES OF HERNIA

This problem will be considered for each of these general types with a consideration of diagnosis, indications for operation and methods of procedure to prevent recurrence.

GROIN HERNIAS

Indirect Inguinal Hernia

This is the most common type of hernia in both sexes and at all ages. Millions of persons now alive in this country have had or will develop an indirect inguinal hernia. The operative treatment of this condition is one of the most important subjects in surgery today. This type of hernia stands in an intermediate position in its tendency to strangulate between direct hernia (rare strangulation) and femoral hernia (frequent strangulation).

Important anatomic studies within the past 10 years have clarified the structural arrangement of the fascial layers in the groin. Emphasis on ligaments which previously received scant notice, such as Cooper's ligament (ligamentum pubicum superius) and the iliopubic tract (intermediate iliopubic ligament), has altered surgical concepts. Outstanding anatomic studies are those of McVay and Anson (1942), Clark and Hashimoto (1946), Donald (1948), Anson, Morgan and McVay (1949), Burton (1952, 1953) and Griffith (1959).

The surgical treatment of inguinal hernia can be simplified by considering it from 3 standpoints: (1) a clarification of the exact nature of some of the historically significant operations for groin hernia; (2) a consideration of 4 grades of hernia, increasing in severity, each of which requires a different surgical operation, also increasing in complexity; and (3) a step-by-step outline of the radical operation for hernia required for the severest indirect inguinal hernia, not all of the steps being necessary in the repair of the simpler grades of hernia.

Clarification of Certain of the Historically Significant Operations for Groin Hernia. Because of the common misuse of eponymic terminology as related to certain of the classic operations, the diagrammatic representations of these are shown in Figures 42-1 to 42-5. Koontz (1949) has helped in the elucidation of the origin of these operations. It is noted that these technics are classified as to whether the cord is superficial, intermediate or deep in the first 4 diagrams, all of which portray various Poupart's ligament re-

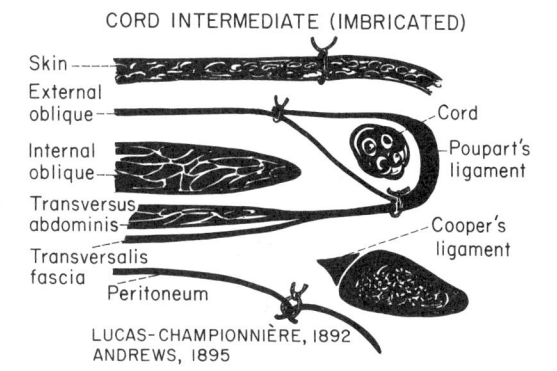

FIG. 42-3. Parasagittal diagrammatic representation of groin hernia repair with *cord in intermediate position with imbrication between layers of external oblique aponeurosis.* (See note to Fig. 42-1.) (Nyhus, L. M., and Harkins, H. N.: Hernia. Philadelphia, J. B. Lippincott, 1964)

pairs, while the 5th shows the Cooper's ligament repair. It is of interest that just as in gastric surgery there is renewed interest in the Billroth I gastric resection, so in the surgery of hernia the swing is definitely toward the Halsted I herniorrhaphy among those surgeons who use a Poupart's ligament type of repair (Fig. 42-1).

Grades of Groin Hernia Repair. Groin hernias can be divided according to severity into 4 grades. The type of operation required

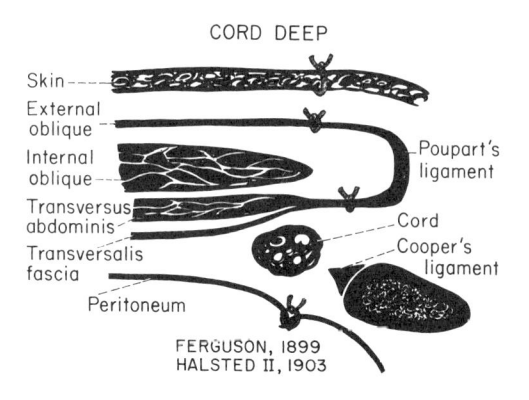

FIG. 42-4. Parasagittal diagrammatic representation of groin hernia repair with *cord deep to fused transversus abdominis aponeurosis and transversalis fascia.* (See note to Fig. 42-1.) (Nyhus, L. M., and Harkins, H. N.: Hernia. Philadelphia, J. B. Lippincott, 1964)

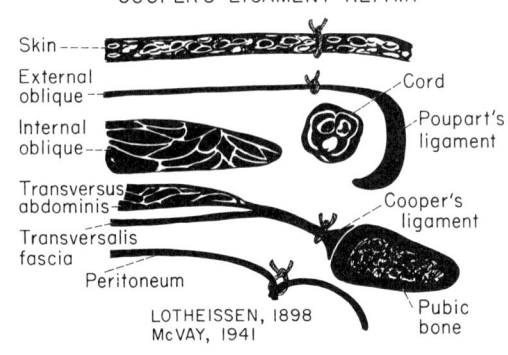

FIG. 42-5. Parasagittal diagrammatic representation of groin hernia repair with *cord in intermediate position and fused transversus abdominis aponeurosis and transversalis fascia sutured to Cooper's ligament.* (Nyhus, L. M., and Harkins, H. N.: Hernia. Philadelphia, J. B. Lippincott, 1964)

TABLE 42-6. GRADES OF HERNIA REPAIR

Grade 1. Infant repair. Indication: infants. Repair: high ligation of sac.

Grade 2. Simple repair. Indications: older children, young and healthy adults with indirect inguinal hernia. Repair: high ligation of sac. Tighten internal ring.

Grade 3. Intermediate repair. Indications: adults with indirect inguinal hernia plus slight weakness of Hesselbach's triangle. Repair: high ligation of sac. Tighten internal ring. Close Hesselbach's triangle, suturing transversalis fascia to iliopubic tract.

Grade 4. Radical repair. Indications: older adults with poor musculature; recurrent, direct or femoral hernias. Repair: high ligation of sac. Tighten internal ring. Close Hesselbach's triangle, suturing conjoined tendon to Cooper's ligament.

in each grade is shown in Table 42-6. This grading of the severity of hernia is similar to that introduced by Ogilvie (1937) and Harkins (1952), except that the 3rd grade of these 2 previous classifications has been expanded into a 3rd and a 4th grade. Some surgeons omit the 2nd grade (McVay, 1947). It is seen that, in general, each successive grade adds an additional step to the procedure but also keeps the steps of the lower grade. The borderline between the grades is not always sharp, and treatment in borderline cases must be individualized.

Grade 1. Infant Type of Hernia (Repair: High Ligation of Sac). Two current concepts should be emphasized: (1) in infants, as Potts, Riker and Lewis (1950) showed, there is an urgent indication for surgical repair; and (2) such a repair primarily should consist of sac ligation. When the author received his training, he was taught to avoid operation in infants under 2 years of age, except in face of the most urgent circumstances, because it was then believed that the repair would be easier after that age, that the danger of strangulation was slight, and that many of the hernias would be cured spontaneously. At present, less credence is given to these 3 beliefs, and early operation is urged. As Fisher (1951) pointed out, even if most infantile hernias do disappear spontaneously, many of them will reappear in later life. He stated: "Children should be operated at any age they present themselves—this, of course, providing there are no complicating conditions."

Heifetz (1953) also emphasized that inguinal sacs do not tend to obliterate themselves after birth.

The operation described by Potts *et al.* (Figs. 42-6 and 42-7) embraces the following features:

1. Short transverse skin incision
2. Opening the external oblique aponeurosis in the direction of its fibers, but in the routine case *"the external ring is not opened"*
3. Exposure, separation, division and high ligation of the sac without disturbing the cord
4. Simple closure of the external oblique aponeurosis and of the skin over the undisturbed cord

According to Potts:

The treatment of the typical inguinal hernia in infants and children is surgical removal of the sac without elevating the structures of the cord and without any plastic repair of the muscles or fascia of the inguinal region.

Packard and McLauthlin (1953) and Clatworthy and Thompson (1954) advocated essentially the same type of repair, based on an experience with 332 and 940 cases operated upon at the Denver and the Cincinnati Children's Hospitals, respectively. The Denver authors stated:

Recurrence is so rare that when it does occur, it suggests a technical error. Apparently the simple

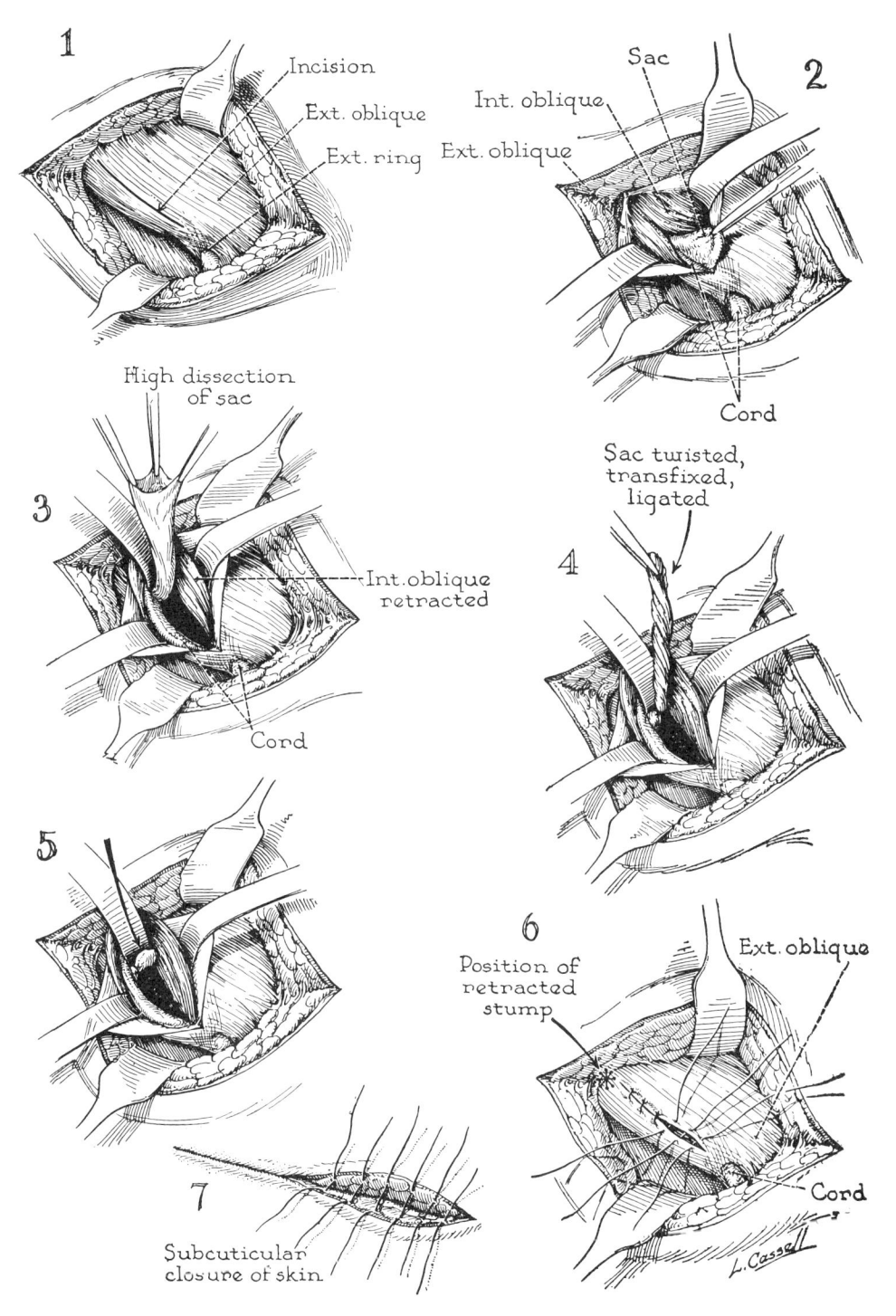

Fig. 42-6. Technic of repair of infantile hernia. (1) Opening the external oblique aponeurosis—*not* down to external ring. (2) Finding sac. (3) High dissection of sac. (4) Twisting, transfixion and ligation of sac. (5) Retraction of stump of sac. (6) Closure of external oblique aponeurosis. (7) Superficial wound closure. (Potts, W. J., Riker, W. L., and Lewis, J. E.: Ann. Surg., 132:571)

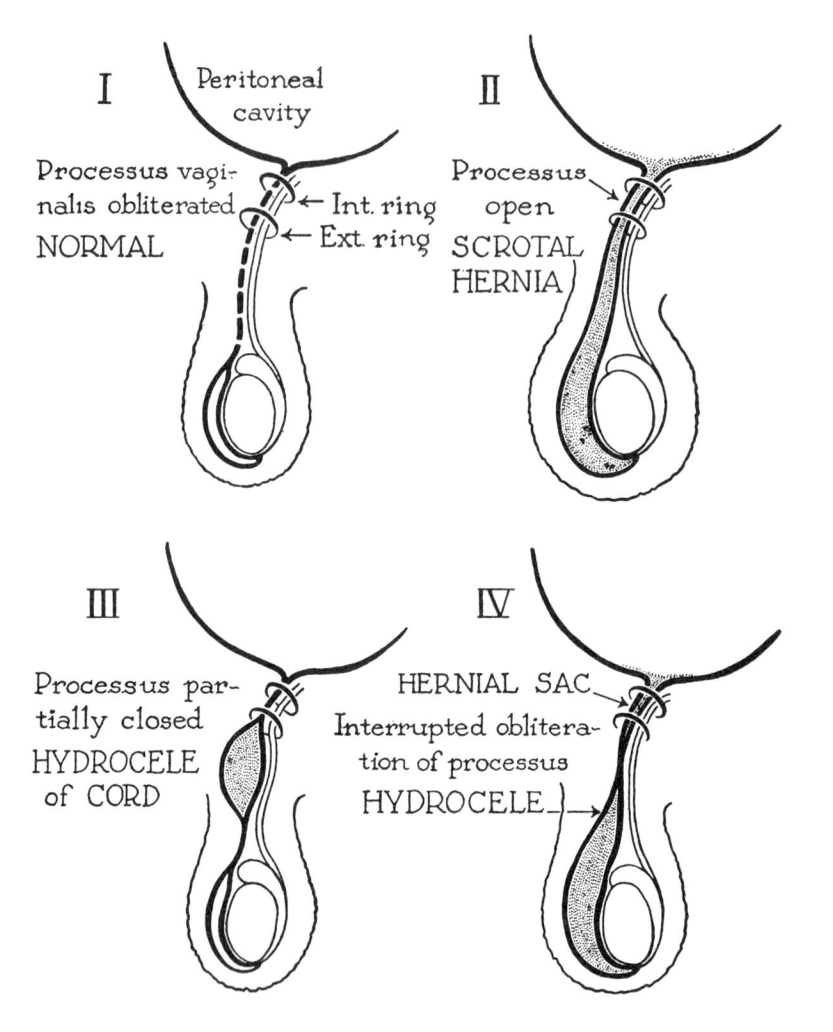

I NORMAL — Processus vaginalis obliterated; Peritoneal cavity; Int. ring; Ext. ring

II SCROTAL HERNIA — Processus open

III HYDROCELE of CORD — Processus partially closed

IV HYDROCELE — HERNIAL SAC; Interrupted obliteration of processus

Fig. 42-7. The pathology of hernia, hydrocele of the cord and hydrocele in the male child. (Potts, W. J., Riker, W. L., and Lewis, J. E.: Ann. Surg. 132:573)

removal of the sac is as effective as any other method. Some tightening of the ring in large hernias may possibly be indicated, but it is hard to see how the approximation of the internal oblique to the inguinal ligament over the cord (Ferguson method) can be of any help; and transplantation of the cord by the Bassini method seems absolutely contraindicated.

McVay (1947), in speaking of small indirect hernias, stated this another way:

> Any additional imbricating, plicating, or other sutures are not only superfluous but may damage the posterior inguinal wall so as to cause a direct or femoral recurrence.

Grade 2. Simple Type of Hernia (Repair: High Ligation of Sac Plus Plastic Closure of the Internal Ring). This grade of repair is used in older children and in young adults or in middle-aged individuals with primary indirect inguinal hernia and with good muscular and fascial structures. It is the repair most suitable for the majority of military personnel. It emphasizes the closure of the neck of the sac by high suture ligation—which may be said to be the essential foundation of the repair of all hernias—but adds a few additional steps because the structures are older and the hernia is more complex than in infants.

The surgical procedure delineates the following features:

1. Transverse skin incision
2. Opening the external oblique aponeurosis in the direction of its fibers and usually by opening the external ring
3. Exposure, separation, division and high ligation of the sac
4. Separation of the cord near the internal

ring so as to delineate the margins of the latter

5. Plastic closure of the internal ring (MacGregor maneuver)
6. Closure of the external oblique aponeurosis, Scarpa's fascia, and skin over the minimally disturbed cord

Technical details of some of these steps will be given below in the discussion of the radical type of repair.

The essential added feature in the simple type of repair is the careful plastic closure of the internal ring to guard against recurrence at this point, the frequency of which has been pointed out, among others, by Levy, Wren and Friedman (1951).

Grade 3. Intermediate Type of Hernia (Repair: High Ligation of Sac Plus Plastic Closure of the Internal Ring Plus Closure of Hesselbach's Triangle, Suturing Transversalis Fascia to Iliopubic Tract). This type of hernia is that encountered in young adults with large indirect inguinal hernias, or older persons with small hernias or especially strong inguinal floors. Most military inductees with inguinal hernias present Grade 3 (or Grade 2) indications for repair. The first 5 steps in the procedure are similar to those in Grade 2. Step 6 involves a row of interrupted fine silk sutures between the transversalis fascia above (at the upper edge of the slight bulge in the inguinal floor) and the iliopubic tract below. Step 7 then involves a closure of the external oblique aponeurosis, Scarpa's fascia, and skin over the cord; Harkins (1964a); McVay and Savage (1964).

Grade 4. Advanced Type of Hernia (Radical Repair: High Ligation of Sac Plus Plastic Closure of the Internal Ring Plus Closure of Hesselbach's Triangle, Suturing Conjoined Tendon to Cooper's Ligament) (Fig. 42-8). This grade of repair is indicated: (1) in recurrent hernias; (2) in femoral hernias; (3) in direct hernias; and (4) in indirect hernias in older individuals or in those with weak musculature or fascial structures (Harkins, 1943, 1949; McVay and Anson, 1949).

The radical repair advised involves high ligation of the sac and plastic closure of the internal ring, as discussed above in connection with the simpler grades of repair. The additional essential feature is the closure of Hesselbach's triangle by suturing the conjoined tendon to Cooper's ligament. A relaxing incision in the anterior rectus sheath facilitates this maneuver.

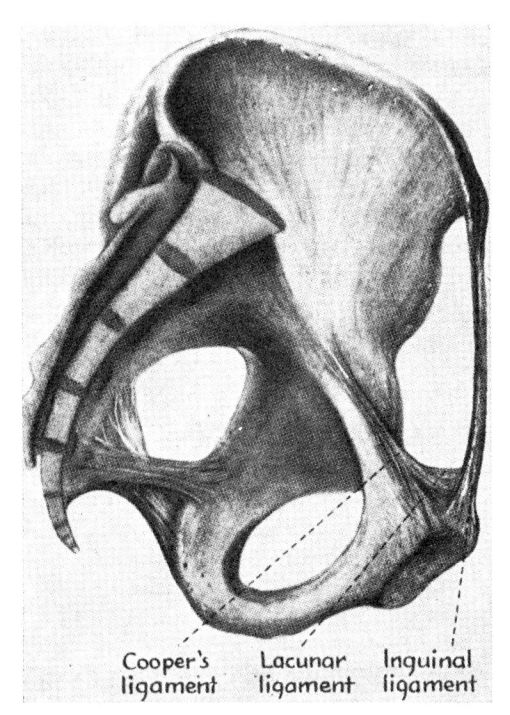

FIG. 42-8. Cooper's ligament. View of the left half of the pelvis with attached ligaments. The relationships between the firmly anchored Cooper's ligament and the loose inguinal ligament are clearly shown. (Harkins, H. N.: Surg. Clin. N. Am., 23:1281)

Within the past few years the author has adopted the "preperitoneal" approach for the majority of groin hernias (Nyhus, Condon and Harkins, 1960; see also p. 1222). While we recognize that this method has advantages, at the same time we do not feel that it is ready for recommendation for general adoption in a standard text. Through this approach, the suture of transversalis fascia to Cooper's ligament can be accomplished—and with better visualization, we believe—as is recommended below in the account of the classic Cooper's ligament repair:

Ten Steps in Radical Groin Hernia Repair (Cooper's Ligament, Lotheissen-McVay Technic). The technical details may be divided into 19 steps, but in individual cases the available armamentarium should include use of such ancillary suture materials as steel wire and fascia lata strips and such accessory patches as tantalum mesh, cutis grafts and buried whole skin grafts. The author has utilized these adjuncts, with the exception of whole skin, in selected cases, but their use is seldom necessary.

Step 1. Exposure of the Cord and Opening the Indirect Sac. The skin incision is made in one of the skin folds, ending about 2 cm. above the pubic spine medially. The semitransverse skin incision has several advantages. It avoids part of the hairy area over the pubis and is less prone to infection. In addition, because it follows the lines of skin cleavage, the cosmetic result is better. The external oblique aponeurosis and the external ring are exposed, and the external oblique aponeurosis is split in the direction of its fibers even with the upper border of the ring to allow for an adequate lower flap. This splitting with the scalpel should be begun 3 cm. from the ring to avoid the nerves when they are adherent to the ring. Then the split is extended laterally and upward with scissors and then downward in the direction of the external ring after the iliohypogastric nerve, which is often adherent to the undersurface of the external oblique aponeurosis at this level, has been peeled away carefully. When cutting occurs accidentally, it is usually near the external ring, and it may be prevented by approaching the latter from the lateral side. The cord and the surrounding structures are separated from the lower leaf of the external oblique aponeurosis and Poupart's ligament, then from the region of the pubic spine and the conjoined tendon, so that finally the cord is freed entirely except at both ends. The cremaster muscle is split longitudinally anteriorly and posteriorly, and 2-inch segments are removed from the internal ring outward, including the internal spermatic fascia and the external spermatic vessels, which are doubly ligated. The cord is thus narrowed so that the internal ring can be closed more tightly as emphasized by Koontz (1956). The vas deferens and the internal spermatic vessels, including the veins, are carefully preserved. The indirect sac, which is always present even in normal persons, is located upward and medially from the internal ring and is opened in all instances, whether the hernia is indirect or direct. In many instances of direct inguinal hernia or femoral hernia the indirect sac is normal in size, but it always can be found above and medial to the cord. In cases of complete indirect in-

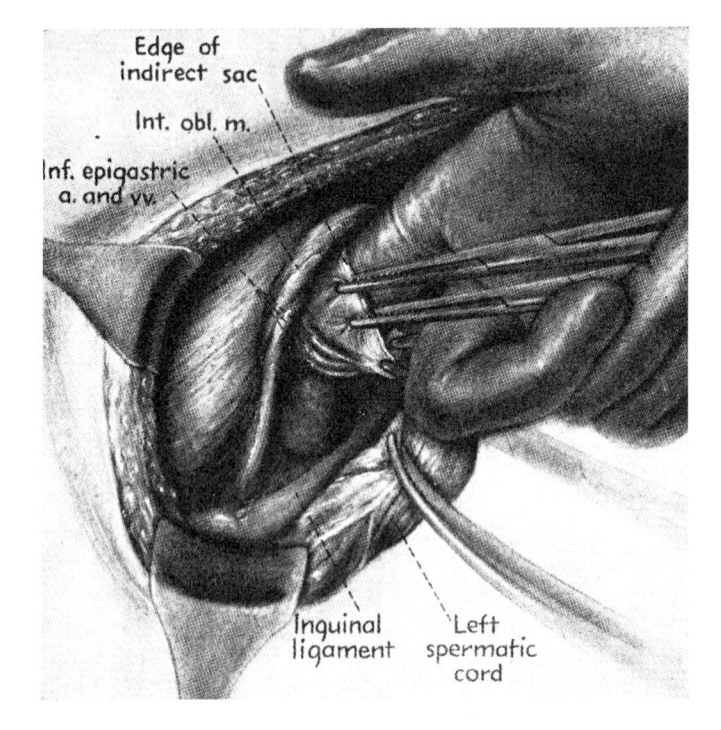

FIG. 42-9. Hoguet's maneuver. The indirect sac is opened, and any femoral or direct (as shown above) sac is transposed so as to become a part of the indirect sac. In this figure, the tip of the examining finger is in a small direct sac. (Harkins, H. N.: Surg. Clin. N. Am., 23:1284)

guinal hernia of the congenital type or in patients in whom the hernial sac is long, the latter is cut across near the internal ring and separated from the cord. The proximal end is closed by an internal purse-string suture, as outlined later, while the distal end is left in place.

Step 2. Exploration of Hesselbach's Triangle and of the Femoral Ring. Once the indirect sac is opened, it is a simple matter to insert the gloved finger to feel Hesselbach's triangle for a direct weakness or obvious direct hernia and to feel the femoral ring. It is indeed surprising how few surgeons will take the extra 30 seconds needed to perform this exploration, and many femoral and direct hernias that "recur" are overlooked because this maneuver was not performed. Exploration of the femoral ring and Hesselbach's triangle with the fingertip should be an essential feature of the repair of all groin hernias.

Step 3. Hoguet's Maneuver—Transposition of Direct and/or Femoral Sacs into the Indirect Sac (Fig. 42-9). If a direct sac is present, it should be transposed lateral to the inferior epigastric vessels by the technic of Hoguet (1920), which has since been popularized by Fallis (1938). Thus, the direct and the indirect sacs are converted into one. This step may be described in Hoguet's own words as follows:

By traction outward on the indirect sac, all of the peritoneum of the direct sac may be pulled external to the vessels and the two sacs converted into one. An indirect sac can always be found in these cases, although it may be very small.

The same procedure can be used to convert a femoral sac into an indirect sac, as practiced by McClure and Fallis (1939). This maneuver is extremely useful. In general, no matter how large a direct sac is, it is not opened but is merely transposed. In the case of large direct sacs the transversalis fascia can be infolded with numerous interrupted silk sutures. One advantage of not opening a direct sac is the fact that the danger of opening the bladder is largely obviated. In some instances all 3 sacs can be converted into a single indirect sac, which in turn can always be dealt with as described in Step 4.

Step 4. Internal Purse-string Closure of Indirect Sac (Fig. 42-10). The indirect sac,

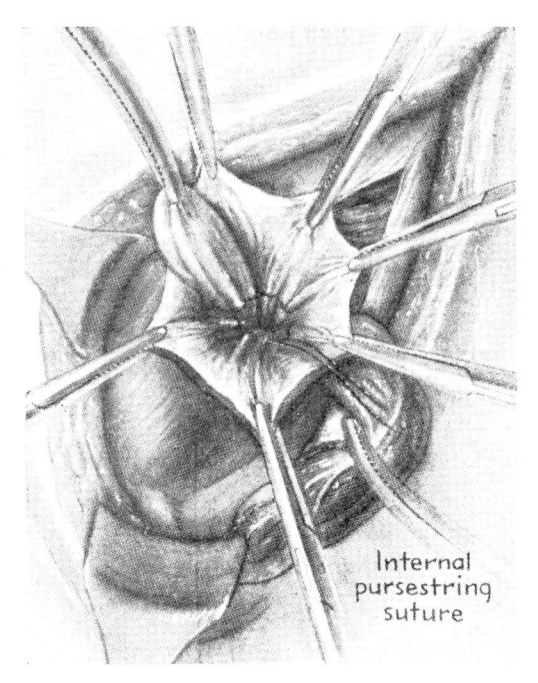

FIG. 42-10. Internal purse-string suture. The indirect sac is closed by an internal purse-string suture which obliterates all of its folds. The redundant indirect sac is usually replaced inside the internal ring, but, if large, it may be excised. The forceps in the upper left-hand portion of the figure grasp the transposed and inverted direct sac. (Harkins, H. N.: Surg. Clin. N. Am., 23:1286)

whether it is simple or enlarged by the added conversion of direct and femoral sacs, is then closed with an internal purse-string suture of medium or heavy silk. Many stitches are taken with a round noncutting needle so as to include all crevices. Such a closure is done as high as possible to prevent indirect recurrences, although the sac is not attached beneath the abdominal wall, as is done by Collins (1942).

Step 5. Tightening of the Internal Ring—MacGregor's Maneuver (Fig. 42-11). When the free ends of the purse string are cut and the peritoneum snaps back, the defect in the transversalis fascia at the internal ring is seen to be large, and in many instances it will admit even 3 or 4 fingers. The fascia is grasped with Allis clamps at numerous points round the internal ring above and medially as far as the

1218 Hernia

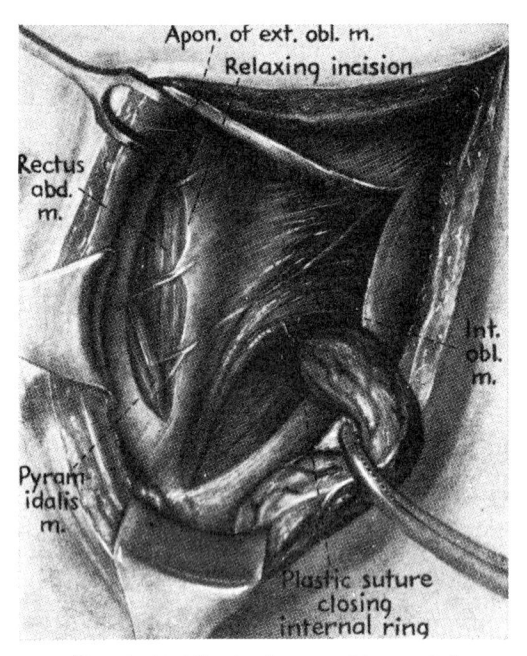

FIG. 42-11. Plastic closure of internal ring and relaxation of internal oblique muscle. The internal ring has been closed by a plastic stitch in the transversalis fascia, while the internal oblique has been relaxed close to its junction with the external oblique aponeurosis to form the linea alba. An attempt is made to spare the nerves and accompanying vessels. (Harkins, H. N.: Surg. Clin. N. Am., 23:1287)

inferior epigastric vessels, but not entirely around the circumference lateral to the cord, and the defect is closed vertically with interrupted silk sutures. The reason for narrowing the cord structures is now manifest, and the internal ring is narrowed so that it barely admits the tip of a little finger. This is a most important step; essentially it involves suturing the transversalis fascia, Hesselbach's ligament and the iliopubic tract to tighten the internal ring. Incomplete closure of the internal ring is a common cause of recurrence. Occasionally the conjoined tendon may be included in the sutures, but the shelving edge of Poupart's ligament should not be included, since the normal and desirable retractile sphincterlike action of the internal ring demonstrated by MacGregor (1929, 1930, 1945, 1949) would be interfered with. Occasionally the lateral sutures to close the internal ring are not placed until Step 7 is completed, so that when they are inserted there will be a continuous closure from the pubic spine to internal ring, eliminating the open space that otherwise might result. Marshall (1960) has re-emphasized recently the importance of this step.

Step 6. Relaxation of the Internal Oblique Muscle. The inner layer of the anterior rectus fascia usually is split for a distance of about 7 cm. from a point 2 cm. above the pubic spine upward and laterally, as described by Rienhoff (1940). The external oblique aponeurosis is lifted up by the assistant, and the internal oblique aponeurosis is cut just lateral to the junction of the two where they form the linea alba. The rectus and the pyramidalis muscles are exposed. The iliohypogastric nerve and the adjoining nerves and vessels that enter the rectus muscle through the internal oblique aponeurosis at this point can be avoided easily. This relaxation allows the internal oblique and the attached transversalis fascia to be pulled down for the subsequent repair without tension. This step is called the "Tanner slide" in Great Britain (Tanner, 1942) and more recently has been readvocated by Doran (1955).

Step 7. Sutures into Cooper's Ligament (Fig. 42-12). The "red" muscle of the internal oblique is disregarded and elevated with a small retractor, and the conjoined tendon is located with a gauze (Küttner) dissector. If the transversalis fascia plus the transversus muscle appear strong enough, they alone are used for the upper leaf of the repair. If they are not adequate, one must go higher and include the internal oblique aponeurosis. In no instance should "red" muscle be used. The transversalis fascia plus transversus muscle, and often the conjoined tendon, therefore, form the *upper leaf* of the repair, while Cooper's ligament is the *lower leaf.* As stated previously, Cooper's ligament is an extremely tough thickening of the periosteal structures on the anterosuperior surface of the anterior ramus of the pubis. Cooper's ligament is visualized by cutting the transversalis fascia from the pubic spine lateral to and occasionally including the inferior epigastric vessels (which are doubly ligated and divided on one side). This incision in the transversalis fascia is just anterior and superior to the iliopubic tract.

The left index finger now is placed on the

anterior ramus of the pubis near the spine and moved laterally along the crest until the femoral vessels are reached. This is usually about 4 cm. lateral to the spine of the pubis. Since the finger is held in close contact with the bone, the vessels being kept lateral, and the 1st stitch is placed medial to the finger, there is little danger of damaging the vessels. Thus, the 1st stitch is usually from 3 to 5 cm. lateral to the pubic spine. Therefore, since the upper leaf is to be taken with the suture first, the needle goes through the transversalis fascia a corresponding distance of 3 to 5 cm. from the pubic spine and then through the thick Cooper's ligament on the upper border of the pubic ramus. Then the stitch is tied, and the intervening gap between this point and the pubic spine is closed with 3 or 4 similar sutures. The most medial sutures usually go through Gimbernat's (lacunar) ligament, as well as Cooper's. Often it is important that the most lateral suture be placed first, as otherwise it is more difficult to protect the vein. The sutures into Cooper's ligament are of double heavy 00 silk and are applied with a small (No. 6) round curved Mayo needle or a Davis tonsil needle, held with a Bland or a Jones needle holder. The double strands are made into a double (or triple) knot, and the individual strands are separated and tied in pairs (this is called "braiding"). The braiding technic has been found useful in other operations when one is especially anxious that a double suture should not become untied and yet the making of the knot is difficult because of the depth of the wound. The relatively large amount of silk seldom has caused trouble. In certain cases, because of the prominence of Rosenmüller's gland (a lymph gland lying over Cooper's ligament about 2 cm. medial to the femoral vessels) or because of the large size of the vein, the sutures must be placed with special care. Babcock (1927) advised one medial Cooper's ligament suture in conjunction with his operation for direct hernia.

The space between the most lateral stitch in Cooper's ligament and the plastic suture on the internal ring often seems to be a possible weak spot to those doing the operations for the first time. Actually this is not so, because the arched internal oblique muscle will tend to close this defect on contraction. Any attempt to tighten it by suturing the internal oblique or conjoined tendon to Poupart's ligament, as is done by Baritell (1944) and others, would seem to defeat the purpose of the operation. Such a suture interferes with the sphincterlike action of the internal ring and tends to pull the transversalis fascia away from Cooper's ligament. Furthermore, the gap can be closed by an additional layer of fine interrupted silk sutures tacking down the superior edge of the lower flap of transversalis (just superior to the iliopubic tract where it was incised to expose Cooper's ligament), including the iliopubic tract and the superficial portion of the medial femoral sheath, to the outer surface of the conjoined tendon and continuing this suture line laterally to join with the line of closure of the internal ring (Griffith, 1959). The methods of McVay (1954) and of Burton (1954, 1956) to close the weak spot are also to be considered.

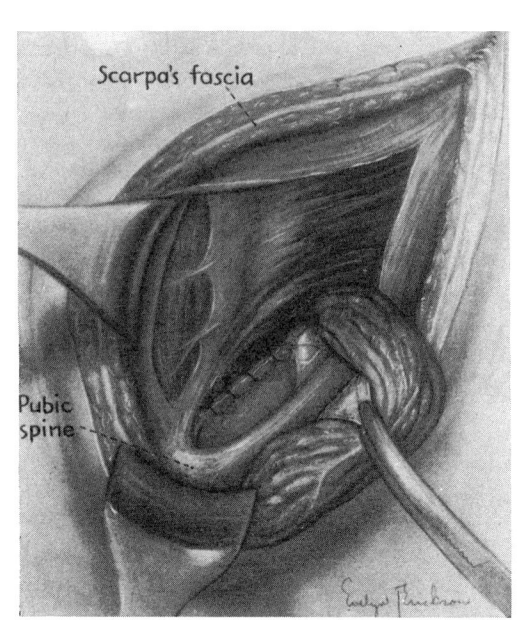

FIG. 42-12. Stitches attaching conjoined tendon and Cooper's ligament in place. (Harkins, H. N., and Schug, R. H.: Arch. Surg., 55:702)

Step 8. Closure of the External Oblique Aponeurosis (Fig. 42-13). The external oblique aponeurosis is closed over the cord in most patients. Occasionally, in severe recurrent hernias the cord is brought out sub-

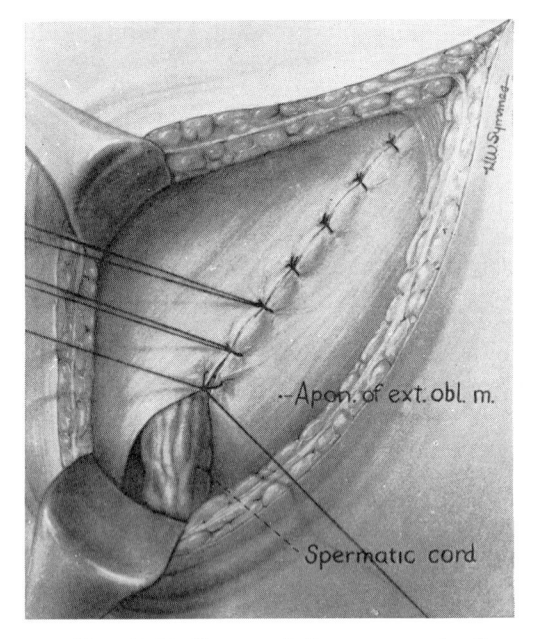

FIG. 42-13. Closure of the aponeurosis of the external oblique over the cord. Then Scarpa's fascia (well shown in this illustration) and the skin are also closed with interrupted sutures over the cord. (Harkins, H. N., and Schug, R. H.: Arch. Surg., 55:703)

cutaneously (Halsted I position), but in the past few years this has been done less and less. In both procedures the external oblique is closed with interrupted fine or medium silk sutures, little if any imbrication being used.

Step 9. Closure of Scarpa's Fascia. Closure of Scarpa's fascia with small bites of the suture seems more sound anatomically and leaves less silk than does suture of the fat with large bites taken at random. This closure is especially important with a Halsted I type of repair, as it gives the already superficial cord additional protection. By preference the sutures are placed so that the knot will be down.

Step 10. Closure of the Skin. Interrupted sutures of silk are advisable for this step. The proper closure of the medial fourth of the wound inside the hairline is of especial importance.

Direct Inguinal Hernia

A direct inguinal hernia is more common than is popularly believed; it is often a bulge more than a long sac; it protrudes anteriorly rather than primarily downward; it will not descend entirely into the scrotum; it affects older patients more often than does indirect inguinal hernia; for practical purposes, it never occurs in a woman; it does not strangulate as often as an indirect inguinal hernia, but more often it contains bladder (patients with bladder hernia may have to urinate twice on arising in the morning, even in the absence of prostatic obstruction); and, finally, its surgical repair is followed by a much higher recurrence rate. The results of such repair were so bad 20 years ago (about 50% recurrence in some series, and 30% even in 1949—Wangensteen) that Andrews and Bissell (Surg., Gynec., Obstet. *58*: 753,-761, 1934) entitled their paper: "Direct Hernia: A Record of Surgical Failures." In older patients with small direct hernias, operation is not as essential as it is in the case of inguinal and femoral hernias.

Direct inguinal hernia occurs through a weakness in Hesselbach's triangle. It represents a weakness in the inguinal floor, i.e., in the transversalis fascia. Lateral direct hernias protrude laterally to the obliterated hypogastric artery (in the lateral triangle) and medial ones medial to the artery (in the medial triangle). Medial direct hernias (Ginzburg and Freund, 1954) are more apt to be funicular in shape, whereas the lateral hernias are usually domelike.

Three technics seem to be suitable for the repair of direct inguinal hernia. These are the Halsted I procedure (especially advocated by Fallis, 1938, and by Palumbo and Mighell, 1954), the Cooper's ligament repair (McVay, 1941; Harkins, Szilagyi, Brush and Williams, 1942; and Harkins and Schug, 1947), and the Nyhus operation by the preperitoneal approach (Nyhus, Condon and Harkins, 1960) (see also p. 1222).

Since the defect in direct hernia is in Hesselbach's triangle, this area should be buttressed. The author uses only the Cooper's ligament method, but occasionally supplements it in difficult cases with imbrication of the external oblique aponeurosis beneath the cord. Such a supplemented operation could be termed a "Halsted I-McVay," or a McVay repair putting the cord in the Halsted I (superficial) position.

The technic of the Cooper's ligament repair for direct hernia is essentially as outlined in the section on indirect inguinal hernia. Usually the direct sac is not opened, but is transposed to the indirect opening by the Hoguet maneuver. Avoiding opening the sac cuts down on the incidence of trauma to the bladder.

Femoral Hernia

This type of hernia is relatively more common in the female but still not as common in absolute figures in that sex as are indirect inguinal hernias. While femoral hernias are essentially a condition of adult life, they do occur in childhood, as Owen, Kirklin and Du Shane (1954) have pointed out. There is one important difference in the treatment of inguinal hernias as opposed to femoral hernias in early childhood; whereas the former should be treated in the simplest way possible (sac ligation only), contrariwise true radical repair of femoral hernia is indicated irrespective of age.

Femoral hernias are most important from 2 standpoints: (1) often they are overlooked, even at operation; and (2) they tend to strangulate.

As to the first point, the author has operated upon 3 women for femoral hernia in whom his operation was the 4th, the 5th and the 7th operation for hernia, respectively. While it is difficult to prove, it is likely that the total of 13 previous operations on these unfortunate patients was all for inguinal hernia—probably nonexistent—and that the cause of their troubles (and even of their swellings) was femoral hernia from the beginning. It is of interest that when reporting 8 cases of "ectopic recurrence" of femoral hernia after inguinal hernia repair, Easton (1933) did not even mention the possibility that they might have been overlooked at the first operation. The importance of exploration of the femoral region from within the peritoneal cavity with the gloved finger at the time of any operation for hernia has been emphasized in the discussion of inguinal hernia above. Whereas the differentiation between direct and indirect inguinal hernia, at least preoperatively, is somewhat academic, that between inguinal and femoral hernia is always of practical importance.

Regarding the second point, Monro (1950a) stated: "Strangulation of a femoral hernia is in my experience the commonest strangulation."

The subject of strangulation has been considered in the general section on strangulation above. Femoral hernias are especially liable to strangulate because of the rigid edges of the opening. The diagnosis of strangulated femoral hernia may be very easy with the patient pointing to the lesion, or very difficult. A tense, tender lump which has lost its expansile impulse on coughing should be present. Tenseness is always present, but the occasional complete absence of tenderness may throw the physician off guard. Furthermore, tenderness alone may be due to acute femoral lymphadenitis, and the corresponding foot should be examined. General signs are also late in development, particularly in the case of Richter's hernia (see page 1247). Taxis is entirely out of place in an incarcerated or strangulated femoral hernia. In approximately 80 per cent of strangulated femoral hernia, bowel resection is not necessary at least at the time of operation. Because the remaining 20 per cent will die without prompt surgical treatment, immediate operation is mandatory. In fact, because of the frequency of strangulation in femoral hernias (10 to 25% in *hospital* statistics, the incidence for persons with femoral hernia who do not enter hospitals is undoubtedly lower), all femoral hernias should be operated upon at once after diagnosis, irrespective of season or accompanying minor ailments. Intestinal decompression is advisable after operation in strangulated cases until bowel sounds return.

The treatment of femoral hernia per se is in a state of flux. Three methods are vying with one another for standard adoption, and all 3 have their supporters. These 3 methods are as follows:

1. The lower approach, from the thigh, below Poupart's ligament.
2. The upper, or inguinal, approach
3. The abdominal extraperitoneal approach through a mid-line, or paramedian, incision

1. **The Lower Approach** (Bassini, 1893; Monro, 1964). This is the simplest and the most direct operation, and it permits one to see the sac without disturbing the inguinal region. Disadvantages of this approach include inability to treat associated inguinal hernia at

the same time, inability to close the femoral weakness high up at its beginning, and, last but not least, inability to deal adequately with strangulated bowel from below. The lower approach has considerable disadvantages in cases in which resection is necessary. Monro (1950b) indicated that the recurrence rate (including inguinal hernia on the same side) is about 10 per cent. Waugh and Hausfeld (1942) reported on the use of a femoral approach with sac removal without attempting to close the femoral canal (Socin-A. J. Ochsner technic). Waugh and Hausfeld used the the method in 12 cases of simple femoral hernia with good results. They did not advise the technic in complicated or strangulated cases. Birt (1947) advised the femoral route for nonstrangulated hernias and the inguinal route for strangulated femoral hernias. Butters (1948) also was an advocate of the lower approach. It is of interest that Butters' experience with 120 repairs by the lower approach with 3.3 per cent recurrences plus 7 per cent inguinal recurrences (total = 10%) seemed favorable to him, yet it is the basis for Monro's critical opinion stated above.

The technic involves a low oblique incision, freeing and opening the sac, careful observation of the contents for viability, reduction of normal contents, high ligation of the sac, and closure of the femoral ring and fossa ovalis by suturing Poupart's ligament to the tenuous pectineus fascia. The saphenous vein usually is doubly ligated and divided.

Three technical points deserve comment. The first involves the fact that femoral hernias are covered with much fat, each layer of which may be confused with omentum. True omental fat appears more granular than other fat, and in addition, when the sac is opened, fluid (hernial water, the Bruchwasser of the Germans) escapes. The second is that, while omentum may be ligated and amputated, one should remember that omentum descends from colon and therefore one should avoid clamping the latter. The third point is that while in 75 per cent of cases the obturator artery arises from the internal iliac, in 25 per cent it arises from the external iliac, swinging above the femoral vein to descend to the obturator foramen. A femoral hernia may push it to one side or other of the femoral ring, where it may be injured during the repair.

2. **The Inguinal Approach.** This was introduced by Annandale (1876), but modernized by Lotheissen (1898), who in a classic paper first advocated suture of the conjoined tendon to Cooper's ligament. Another type of inguinal approach involves suturing Poupart's ligament to Cooper's ligament (Ruggi, 1892; Moschcowitz, 1907), while other surgeons suture both to Cooper's ligament. The Lotheissen-McVay method seems preferable and has the advantages of treating any coincident direct inguinal weakness at the same time and of not suturing together 2 such rigid structures as Poupart's and Cooper's ligaments. The inguinal approach gives a good visualization of strangulated bowel. If the hernia is irreducible, the following means of handling the situation are available: (1) expose, and possibly open, the sac by retracting the lower skin flap; (2) cut Gimbernat's (lacunar) ligament medially; and (3) cut Poupart's ligament loose from the pubic spine (Hey Groves maneuver, 1923) to give more room in all directions. (The ligament is resutured in place at the end of the operation.) Hagan and Rhoads (1953) pointed out that the Lotheissen-McVay repair of femoral hernia may not be necessary, even though adequate, since they had no femoral recurrences in 74 femoral hernias repaired as follows: 62 by the femoral route, 2 each by the Halsted I and the Bassini procedure, and only 8 by the Lotheissen-McVay repair.

Technical steps include a somewhat low inguinal incision followed by a typical Lotheissen-McVay operation (McVay, 1964), transposing the femoral sac into the indirect one by the Hoguet maneuver in simple cases. In the more difficult instances, the additional tricks mentioned above may have to be utilized. Resection may be necessary. An all-important rule is that *bowel loops in a femoral sac never should be permitted to escape into the general peritoneal cavity before first being scrutinized carefully for viability.*

3. **The Preperitoneal Approach.** On the Services of Dr. Harkins the preperitoneal approach has been used for the treatment of all groin hernias. The results were satisfactory in most of the thousand cases that were operated upon in this manner. It is still in the developmental stage and not all agree to its value.

The anatomic basis of the method is well

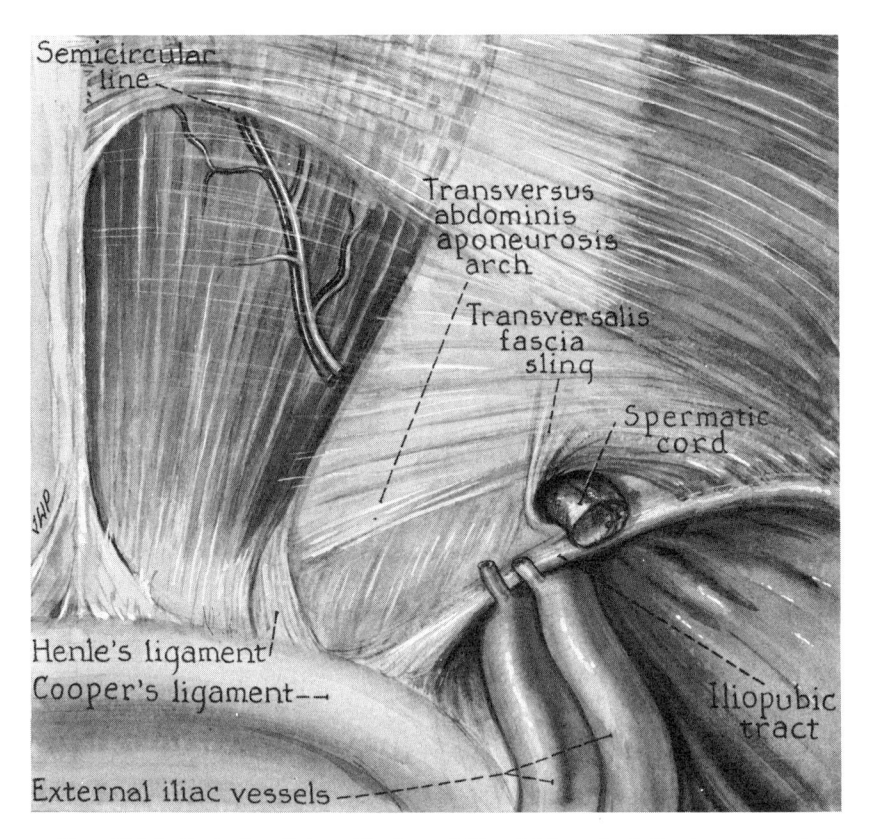

FIG. 42-14. Posterior (internal) view of the right groin following removal of the peritoneum, preperitoneal fat and lymphatics and the iliacus fascia. The spermatic cord has been transected just internal to the deep inguinal ring. The structures of the transversus abdominis lamina are well shown. The inferior epigastric vein is more frequently a double channel where it lies upon the rectus abdominis, and its junction with the external iliac vein is often a little more proximal.

This drawing is also a good illustration of the difficulties of medical illustration in the groin region; the problems are similar to those faced by the cartographer in attempting to depict a curved surface on a flat plane. In order to present a drawing with no discontinuities, increasing distortion and exaggeration must be introduced as one proceeds from the central focus to the margins of the picture. The geographic exaggerations of a world map drawn on Mercator's projection are analogous to those of this figure. (Nyhus, L. M., and Harkins, H. N.: Hernia. Philadelphia, J. B. Lippincott, 1964)

portrayed by Condon (1964). Historically, it is based on contributions by Cheatle (1920, 1921), Henry (1936, 1964), McEvedy (1950), Mikkelsen and Berne (1954), Rogers (1959) and Nyhus (1964a,b).

Nyhus has synthesized the procedure into a modern technic which we denote as the Nyhus operation. It includes not only the *approach* but a *technic* utilizing certain concepts of *anatomy* which have seldom been recognized by surgeons. The technic is briefly as follows, all by the preperitoneal approach:

(a) *For indirect inguinal hernia:* Suture the arms of the internal ring transversalis fascia crura lateral to the cord (Fig. 42-14).

(b) *For direct inguinal hernia:* Suture the transversus abdominis arch to the iliopubic tract (Fig. 42-15).

(c) *For femoral hernia:* Suture the iliopubic tract to Cooper's ligament (Fig. 42-15).

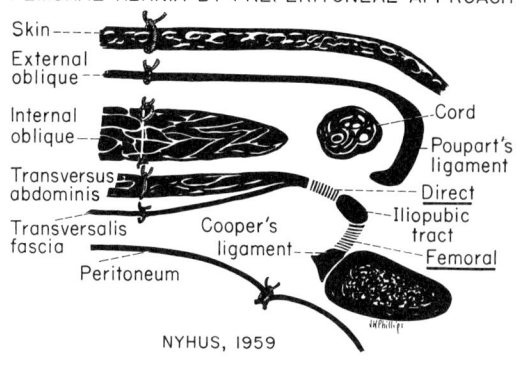

FIG. 42-15. Parasagittal diagrammatic representation of groin hernia repair (in this instance direct *or* femoral hernia) *utilizing a preperitoneal approach for an iliopubic tract repair.* Note: The abdominal wall closure in layers subsequent to repair of the hernia through the preperitoneal approach is shown. As in Figs. 42-1 through 42-5, the peritoneal sac has been closed after high ligation—in this instance a *true* high ligation. If the hernia is *direct*, the fused transversus abdominis aponeurosis and transversalis fascia are sutured to the iliopubic tract. If the hernia is *femoral*, the iliopubic tract is sutured to Cooper's ligament. The difference between this type of repair and the Lotheissen-McVay repair shown in Fig. 42-5 is that, by the anterior approach, the iliopubic tract is not readily visualized and hence cannot be used, as it can by the preperitoneal approach, so as to actually shorten the distance that must be bridged in the repair. (Nyhus, L. M., and Harkins, H. N.: Hernia. Philadelphia, J. B. Lippincott, 1964)

TABLE 42-7. FACTORS LEADING TO RECURRENCE FOLLOWING THE REPAIR OF INGUINAL HERNIA (MACKENZIE, 1955)

Failure to:
1. Ligate the sac high enough in indirect inguinal hernia
2. Constitute the internal ring adequately
3. Close the fascial defect adequately in direct hernia
4. Rule out associated direct or femoral hernia
5. Recognize and repair sliding hernia adequately
6. Avoid tension by relaxing incisions
7. Place sutures properly and utilize adequate technic
8. Control sepsis
9. Utilize hemostasis, particularly in the cord structures

The LaRoque (LaRoque, 1919, 1922; Williams, 1947, 1964; and Phetteplace, 1955) abdominal or intraperitoneal approach presents some, but in my opinion not all, of the advantages of the preperitoneal approach.

Recurrent Groin Hernia

The subject of the prevention of recurrence has been dealt with under the headings of individual hernias (see Table 42-7). The present discussion emphasizes the therapeutic approach to recurrences already present. Such treatment involves a radical herniorrhaphy utilizing certain of the "Aids to Repair" considered in the section relating to them below. If the patient is old, cord division may be considered. A careful Cooper's ligament (Lotheissen-McVay) repair utilizing nonabsorbable sutures is adequate in most instances. Fascia lata sutures (Swenson and Harkins, 1943b), cutis grafts (Swenson and Harkins, 1943a; Harkins, 1945) or tantalum-mesh patches, and suturing the external oblique aponeurosis beneath the cord (Halsted I position), in addition to the underlying Cooper's ligament repair, should all be considered. Thorough exploration to rule out previously overlooked femoral hernia is mandatory. Hagan and Rhoads (1953) found that in a series of 75 recurrent inguinal hernias, there were 21 per cent recurrences after secondary repair. This high figure may be significant when it is noted that in only 4 of the 75 cases was a Lotheissen-McVay repair performed. The problem is a difficult one, and a single Cooper's ligament operation for recurrent hernia may take from 90 to 120 minutes, but with care a secondary recurrence rate of less than 5 per cent can be obtained. The placing of wire-stitch markers on the edges of the layers to be approximated, as introduced by Doran and Lonsdale (1949), and extended by Olson, Kanar and Harkins (1954), enables one to determine if there is recurrence by roentgenologic means in some cases. The edges pull apart, and the markers become separated.

VENTRAL INCISION HERNIAS

The occurrence of such hernia testifies to the lack of perfection in the closure of abdominal wounds. The incidence of incisional hernia varies from 0.5 to 8.0 per cent, depending on a number of factors, many of which are covered elsewhere in this book. No one incision, type of suture material, manner of closure or individual surgeon is immune from occasional wound disruption. However, careful attention to the general preoperative care of the patient, to the use of the correct incision for the particular patient, to the insertion of nonabsorbable sutures which do not "miss" the fascia and do not constrict the blood supply to the flaps being sutured, and to the maintenance of nutrition in the postoperative state—all these will help to prevent wound disruptions and ventral incisional hernias.

The surgical care of these hernias is difficult and simple at the same time. The scarred skin is removed by an elliptical incision. The fascial margins of the ring, which usually is smaller than would appear from the outside before operation, are freed, and the peritoneal cavity is opened, preferably at a point at which there are no adhesions. The sac is trimmed away, taking into consideration the fact that one does not wish to leave weak tissue behind, but at the same time one does not wish to sacrifice good tissue.

A decision as to the direction of closure must now be reached. Whereas, other things being equal, one would wish to close a ventral hernia transversely (i.e., by bringing an upper flap down and a lower flap up), most herniated incisions are vertical, leaving the surgeon with no other choice than to close the gap vertically. If the closure is to be horizontal, the flaps should be tested to see if they can be imbricated. If so, fat should be cleared from the undersurface of the upper flap and from the outer surface of the lower flap for a distance equal to that to be imbricated. The surgeon should approach each incisional hernia with the aim of at least getting the edges together. With proper care usually they can be imbricated a little, even in the largest hernias.

The flaps now are sutured with a first row of mattress sutures at the edge of the lower flap to upper flap at the distance from the edge corresponding to the imbrication. The second row of mattress sutures approximates the lower edge of the upper flap down over and to the outer surface of the lower flap. If a vertical closure is necessary, the same thing is done by overlapping one lateral flap over the other. If imbrication is not possible, the edges should be sutured together. If the edges cannot be brought together, the surgeon should consider carefully whether the fault is his or the anatomic situation is insurmountable. In 10 years the author did not find a ventral hernia the edges of which could not be brought together.

Next, the superficial wound is closed, often with large mattress sutures, to obliterate the dead space. A drain is inserted in the wound for 48 hours.

Additional technical points are as follows:

It is usually impossible to make a separate peritoneal closure. A common error is to mistake the anterior edge of a daughter sac for the inner fascial flap to be used for closure. The most common error is to give up too easily in trying to see if the true flap edges can be approximated. It is especially difficult to close epigastric incisional hernias because of the unyielding nature of the near-by costal margins. The surgeon will need a knowledge of all the methods listed below under "Aids to Repair" in dealing with a difficult ventral incisional hernia.

UMBILICAL HERNIAS

This type of hernia is most common in infancy and in young children. Small umbilical hernias in infants often may be treated by adhesive strapping, as many of them will close spontaneously as the patients grow. This is especially true of those umbilical hernias which are hemispheric in shape. As Gross (1953) pointed out, the two requirements are relaxation of lateral tension and the emptying of the sac. These requirements are not met by strapping a metal coin over the protruding navel or by spring trusses or rubber belts with protruding attachments. Adhesive strapping must be applied carefully if it is to be successful. Even then it is difficult to be sure if the good results are not those of a natural cure. Strapping is accomplished by cutting two pieces of 2-in. adhesive, one with a hole and the other with a tongue so that they can be interlaced.

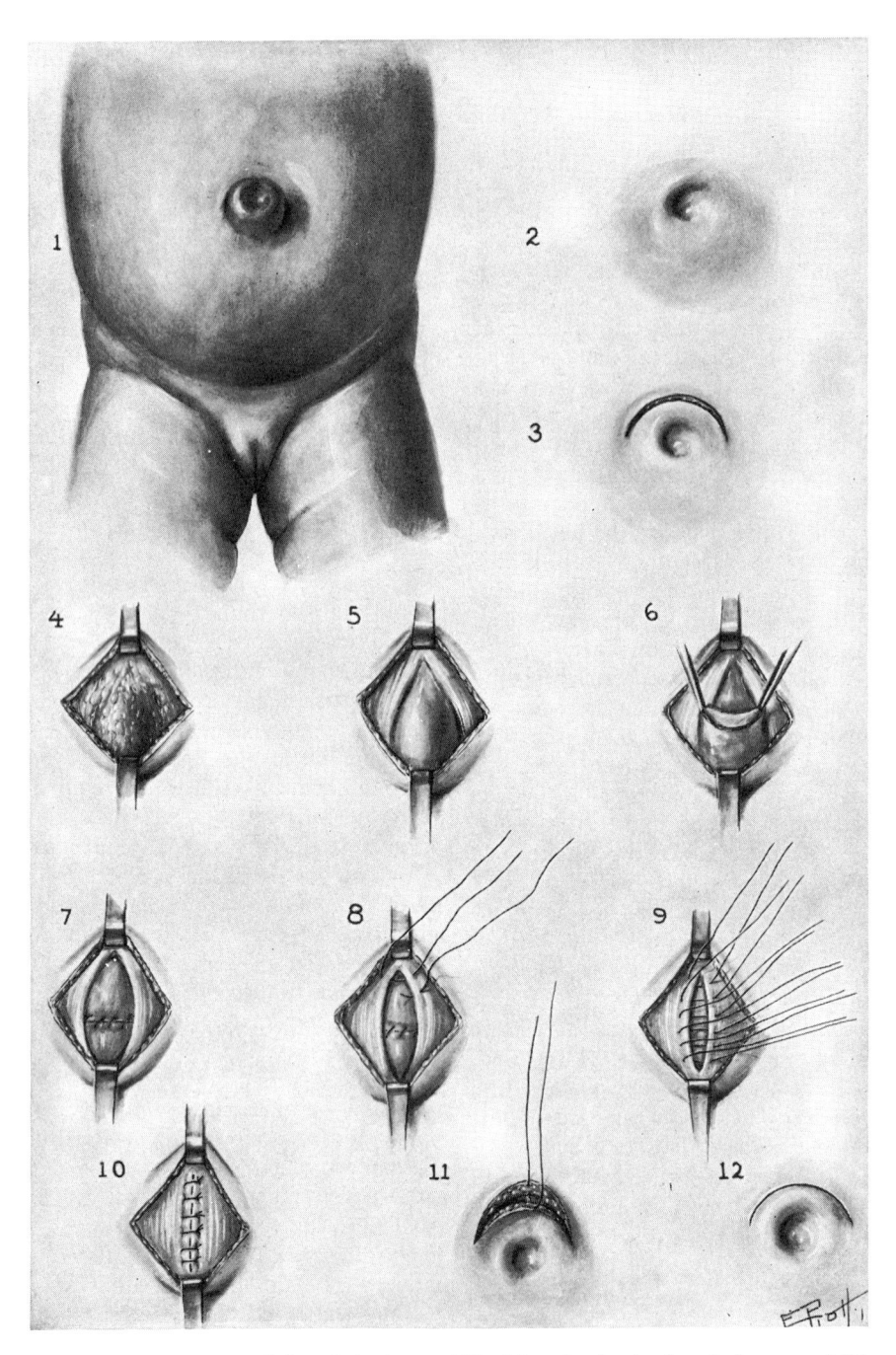

FIG. 42-16. Recommended technic for umbilical herniorrhaphy in a baby or a child. (1) Showing the navel swelling. (2) When relaxed under anesthesia, the navel becomes depressed. (3) Position of the curved incision in skin just above the navel. (4) Skin flaps freed from underlying tissues and retracted. (5) Rectus sheaths cleared of overlying fat. Hernial sac cleared. (6) Hernial sac cut away from undersurface of navel skin. (7) Peritoneum (hernial sac) closed. (8) Stitches (of silk) being taken in the edges of the rectus sheaths. (9) Rectus sheath stitches in place. (10) Rectus fasciae brought together in midline. (11) Subcuticular stitches (of 6-0 Deknatel silk) just beneath the corium. Skin edges brought together by the subcuticular stitches. (12) No cutaneous sutures are necessary. (Gross, R. E.: Surgery of Infancy and Childhood. Philadelphia, W. B. Saunders, 1953)

They are applied with tension after previously preparing the abdominal skin with tincture of benzoin. Such support is renewed every week or two and is maintained for several months. Strapping is of little value in the treatment of conical or "elephant-trunk" umbilical hernias. Few of this type can be controlled adequately by strapping. Strapping should be abandoned if it is unsuccessful after 6 months' trial or if the child is over 1 year of age. Surgery may be indicated more urgently in females for the same size hernia because of the future possibility of strain upon the opening by pregnancy. On the other hand, McVay (1954) stated that in his experience the serious complication of strangulation was most common in the elderly debilitated male. After the first year of life, umbilical hernias larger than 8 mm. in diameter (2.0 cm. in younger infants) should be repaired surgically. The repair in children involves the following steps. (Fig. 42-16):

1. A semilunar "frowning" skin incision above and sparing the umbilicus
2. Freeing the sac with transverse closure of it
3. Longitudinal closure of the fascia with interrupted fine (4-0) silk sutures. When the recti muscles are immediately adjacent to the umbilical hernia ring, the anterior and the posterior rectus sheaths can be closed longitudinally and separately in layers (Brown, 1960).
4. Interrupted subcuticular (6-0) silk closure of the wound.

In adults, an umbilical hernia with symptoms, or with incarceration, or larger than 1 cm. should be treated surgically. In the surgical repair in adults, the following steps are suggested:

1. Separate and ligate the sac.
2. Incise the anterior rectus sheath transversely on each side for about 1 cm. in small hernias and up to 3 cm. in large hernias.
3. Retract the rectus muscle and incise the posterior sheath in a similar manner.
4. Imbricate the upper flap over the lower ("vest over pants") with 2 layers of mattress sutures of nonabsorbable material. In any imbrication procedure it is important that the 2 layers in contact be as fat free as possible. Farris (1964) does not advocate imbrication.
5. If possible, preserve the umbilicus; if not, in younger patients fashion an artificial umbilicus with skin tucked down to the deeper tissues.

ESOPHAGEAL HIATAL DIAPHRAGMATIC HERNIA

General Considerations

These hernias are the most common type of herniation through the diaphragm. They are also the type that most commonly require surgical treatment. Harrington (1955), whose outstanding work has helped to develop this field and whose experience based on 489 repairs of these hernias is the basis for his statements, lists a number of factors which make these hernias of general interest, as follows: their indefinite causation; their relatively frequent occurrence; the variation of the relationship between the defective esophageal hiatus and the esophagus resulting in involvement of different structures and in different types of esophageal hiatal hernias; their progressive development; their varied and complex symptoms which often simulate those of other organic disease (this, coupled with the not infrequent presence of unassociated and coincidental conditions, such as malignant disease, of the esophagus or the stomach, cholecystic disease, angina pectoris, and duodenal ulcer, which may be confused with the hernia, make appropriate its designation as the "masquerader of the upper abdomen"); the complications such as incarceration of the viscera involved in the hernia; the occurrence of incompetency of the sphincteric mechanism at the cardia which permits a retrograde flow of acid-peptic secretions into the esophagus with resultant occurrence of esophagitis, ulceration of the esophagus and the cardia, and, in some instances, stricture of the esophagus; and, finally, spasm of the esophagus which may be secondary to the herniation, or may be a primary condition causing the hernia.

Saint's triad (hiatal hernia, gallstones and diverticulosis coli) is of great interest from the diagnostic standpoint. This syndrome, first described by Muller (1948) and elaborated upon by Palmer (1951), denotes that about 10 to 15 per cent of patients with hiatal hernia will have *both* the other two conditions at the same time. Furthermore, if such patients have either of the other two conditions, they are extremely likely to have both. In most cases, symptoms which are present are attributed to the gall-

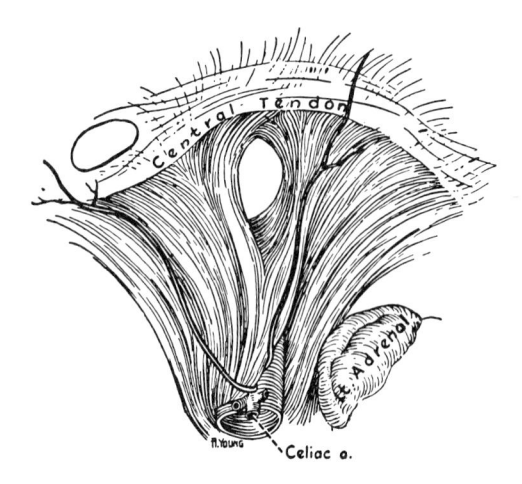

FIG. 42-17. The usual mode of formation of the esophageal hiatus as seen from below. The aorta is posterior, and the opening represents the hiatus. The right crus forms the hiatus. (Carey, J. M., and Hollinshead, W. H.: Surg., Gynec. Obstet., 100:198)

bladder pathology. It is significant that the symptomatic relief from the cholecystectomy is usually slight, whereas that from the repairs of the hiatal hernia is usually good. Saint's triad may explain the course of events in at least some of the patients with the "postcholecystectomy syndrome."

Anatomic Considerations

The esophageal hiatus permits the traversing of the diaphragm by the esophagus, both vagi and the connections between the left gastric artery and the coronary vein below and the corresponding thoracic esophageal blood vessels above. These structures actually penetrate the phreno-esophageal ligament (see below). So far as the action of the hiatus on the esophagus is concerned, in conjunction with the cardiac sphincter, the esophagus maintains the flow of food in one direction, downward, and, when this sphincter mechanism is impaired, the patient becomes subject to the evils of bidirectional flow with its possible complications listed above. The action of the diaphragm and the attached fascia is termed the *extrinsic mechanism* in maintaining competency; the cardiac sphincter is termed the *intrinsic mechanism*. Lendrum (1937), Allison (1951) and others believed that the extrinsic mechanism was most important, while Lam (1954), Braasch and Ellis (1956), Dillard (1964) and others credit the intrinsic sphincters with significance. In addition, the oblique entry of the esophagus into the stomach acts as a valve (Nauta, 1955, 1956).

As to the hiatus itself, Carey and Hollinshead (1955) considered the anatomy from the standpoint of 3 layers, going from outside inward: (1) muscle, (2) fascia, and (3) peritoneum.

1. **Muscular Relations of the Hiatus.** The crura of the diaphragm, right and left, arise by stout tendinous bands from the anterolateral surfaces of the first 3 or 4 lumbar vertebrae and their intervening fibrocartilages. The 2 crura are separated immediately anterior to the spine by the upper end of the abdominal aorta and its first main anterior branches (celiac axis and superior mesenteric artery). In 25 human dissections by Carey and Hollinshead, the right crus was found to be larger than the left in 24. In most instances, the superficial (viewed from the abdomen, hence caudad) portion of the right crus forms the right margin of the esophageal hiatus (Fig. 42-17) and the deep (craniad) portion the left margin. This confirms the observation of Low (1907), that the right crus usually sends fibers on both sides of the esophagus (Fig. 42-18). From their positions bordering the esophagus, medial fibers of the right crus continue anterior to the hiatus to complete the muscular collar, while lateral ones insert in a fan-shaped manner into the central tendon of the diaphragm. The anterior muscular collar

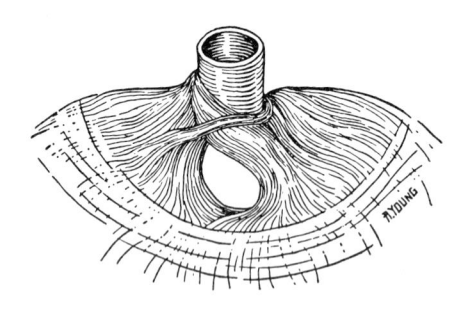

FIG. 42-18. The same as in Figure 42-17 from above and anteriorly. The accessory bundle of Low from the left crus passes forward to the right. (Carey, J. M., and Hollinshead, W. H.: Surg., Gynec. Obstet., 100:198)

separating the esophagus from the diaphragm is less than 1.5 cm. in almost all instances. The role of the right crus in forming a sling for the esophagogastric junction is similar to that of the puborectalis around the anorectal junction.

The left crus usually passes forward to abut against, but not to contribute to, the muscular collar of the diaphragm. The left crus then passes to the central tendon of the diaphragm.

On the basis of 204 fresh cadaver dissections, the variations in the muscular anatomy of the esophageal hiatus were divided into 11 types (Listerud and Harkins, 1958, 1959). The most common, Type I, is that referred to in the previous paragraph (49% of total series). The next most common, Type II (31%), has a divided left crus, the right portion of which *does* contribute to the right margin of the hiatus. The important facts for the student to remember are: First, while in the most common type, and in the rare Type VIII (0.5%), only the right crus contributes to the hiatal margins, in the other 9 types (comprising slightly over 50.5% of the series), the left crus also contributes. Second, in operating in this region, the surgeon should be aware of these anatomic variations. Allison (1951) summarizes his view of the hiatus as follows:

Examination of the esophageal hiatus shows it to be a split in the muscle fibers of the right crus lightly reinforced by fibers from the left. In front the esophagus is supported by a sling of muscle fibers continuous on each side with the perpendicular fibers of the crus and decussating with one another to form a stoutly reinforced raphe, but behind there is less support, for it is here that the crus splits to form the hiatus. If the opening is enlarged the pressure felt in front and at the sides may cause some atrophy of muscle fibers, but it can do little more because it is acting "across the grain." The pressure at the back, however, is felt "along the grain" and splits the fibers to increase the size of the opening. This . . . forms the key to the problem of surgical repair.

2. **Fascial Relations of the Hiatus.** There are 2 fascial layers involved in the esophageal hiatus: (1) the strong diaphragmatic reflection of the endo-abdominal fascia below, and (2) the weak diaphragmatic reflection of the endothoracic fascia above. The fascial lining of the abdominal parietes (endo-abdominal

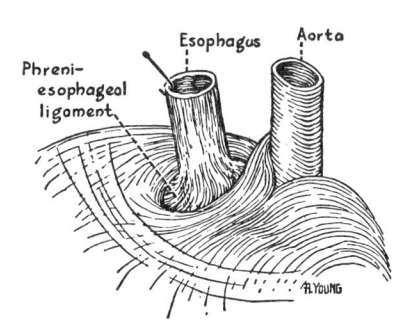

FIG. 42-19. Phreno-esophageal ligament as seen from above. (Carey, J. M., and Hollinshead, W. H.: Surg., Gynec. Obstet., 100:198)

fascia) commonly is given the local name of the muscle under which it lies (much as certain rivers used to be known locally by the name of the town through which they flowed). Thus, in the inguinal region, a portion of the endo-abdominal fascia is designated the *transversalis fascia* (see p. 1218), where it lies beneath the transversus muscle, and in the region of the esophageal hiatus a portion is designated the *diaphragmatic fascia* on the inferior surface of the diaphragm. As the diaphragmatic fascia approaches the hiatus it overlies the crura, then passing the margins of the esophageal hiatus it ascends through the hiatus and out of the abdomen to be attached about the entire circumference of the lower end of the thoracic esophagus about 2 to 3 cm. above the cardia (Fig. 42-19). The portion involved in this attachment is known as the phreno-esophageal ligament (Laimer's ligament, 1883). It is a relatively strong fascia which normally holds the structures in their proper relationships and is stretched in cases of hernia. Another way of putting it is to state that the ligament is the normal antagonist of the longitudinal musculature of the esophagus and prevents the stomach from herniating into the chest upon esophageal contraction. Thus, while the muscular ring of the normal esophageal hiatus approximates the lower end of the esophagus, it is not directly attached to it. The phreno-esophageal ligament serves this function. Many of the hiatal hernias of elderly people result from incompetence of the hiatus due to atrophy of this protective and normally elastic membrane. This is especially true when the hiatus itself is already abnormally large and the ligament has to carry the burden of holding back increased intra-abdominal pressures from coughing, etc.

The diaphragmatic portion of the endothoracic fascia, especially where it reflects onto the esophagus is, in marked contrast with the endo-abdominal layer (true phreno-esophageal ligament), a weak and tenuous layers of loose connective tissue underlying the pleura.

3. **Peritoneal Relations of the Hiatus.** The peritoneal layer which closely invests the major portion of the stomach becomes quite loose anteriorly 2 to 3 cm. from the cardia. It becomes separated from the wall of the stomach before passing anteriorly to become firmly attached to the diaphragm by a variable amount of loose areolar tissue.

The laxity of the peritoneum at this point is the reason why the surgeon can invaginate his fingers for a short distance through the normal hiatus when doing an abdominal exploration. Surgeons are urged to do this exploratory maneuver, when the abdomen is open and when no contraindications are present, to accomplish 2 purposes: (1) to detect abnormally large hiatal openings; and (2) to acquaint themselves with the size of the normal opening—usually "2 fingers, 3 cm." (Two fingers admitted to a depth of 3 cm. The author has included this maneuver as a part of his routine abdominal exploration since 1942.) Harrington (1955) stated that while there was considerable variation in the size of the hiatus, which is palpated as a part of a routine abdominal exploration,

a hiatus that will admit 1 or 2 fingers may be considered normal if there is no infolding of the peritoneum into the mediastinum but, in all cases in which the hiatus admits 3 fingers, the possibility of a hernia should be considered. Each of these patients should have a roentgenogram of the stomach. Even though hernia may not be demonstrated by a subsequent roentgenogram, it should be considered as a potentiality and the patient, if obese, should reduce and have periodic physical examinations.

There is some discussion as to whether the enlarged esophageal hiatal opening, which is usually elliptical in shape, has its long axis mainly in an anteroposterior direction (vertically) or in a transverse direction (horizontally). Many published pictures of operative procedures indicate that it is transverse. The

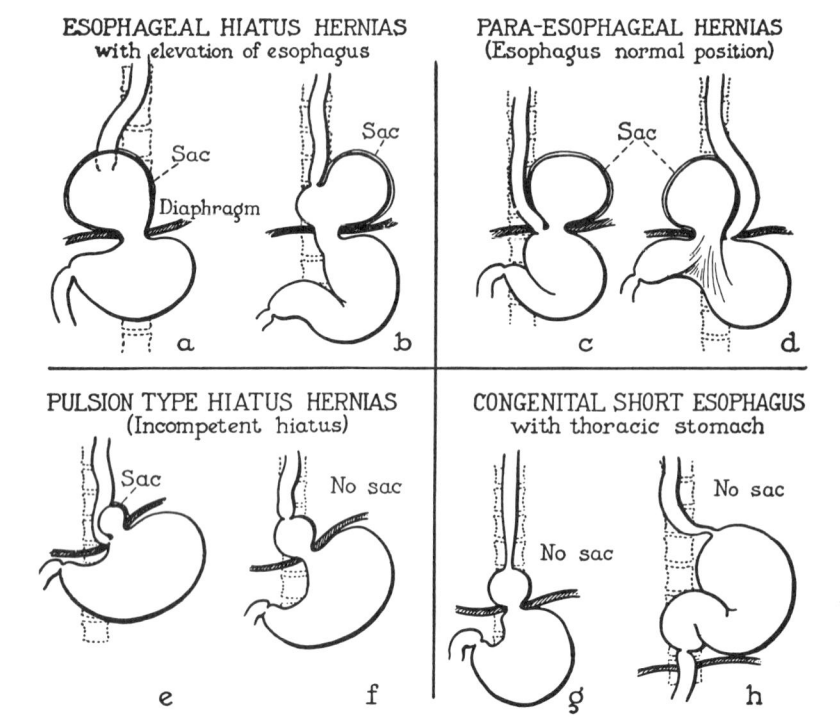

FIG. 42-20. Harrington's classification of herniation through the esophageal hiatus. (Harrington, S. W.: Surg., Gynec. Obstet., 100:279)

author is in accord with Lam and Kenney (1954), who stated that it is essentially vertical.

Classification

Harrington's (1955) classification of esophageal hiatal diaphragmatic hernia is as follows (Fig. 42-20). In the instance of the more common types, as seen at surgery, the percentage incidence is listed:

Esophageal Hernia With Elevation and Displacement of the Esophagus. The esophagus is of normal length but does not extend to the diaphragm (many so-called "short esophagus" cases are probably of this type). There is a true sac. This is the most common type (67%) in Harrington's series, and the incidence of recurrence was higher than with other types. Almost always the sac is anterior and incompletely embraces the portion of the stomach that has slid up posterior to the sac. Usually the herniation is of the stomach, and it may be large and into either or both sides of the thoracic cavity (Fig. 42-21). This type is also called a "sliding" hiatal hernia. It almost never leads to strangulation but is a definite causative factor of esophagitis.

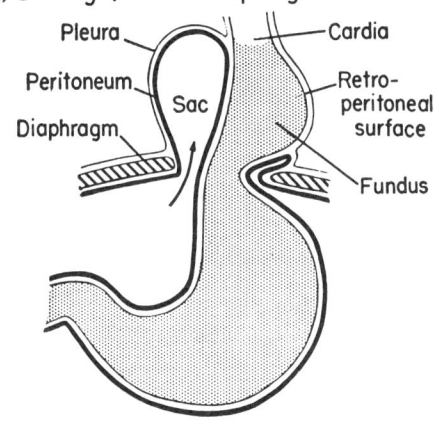

Para-esophageal Hernia. The esophagus is of normal length but is not displaced and remains attached to, and is not elevated above, the diaphragm. There is a true sac that lies anterior to the stomach (as shown in Fig. 42-22). This is the second most common type (15%) in Harrington's series, but, unlike Group 1, the most satisfactory results are obtained from surgical treatment in these cases, because correction of the hernia requires only repair of an abnormal and enlarged hiatus after replacement of the herniated viscera. These hernias usually are of the stomach, although other intestinal loops also may herniate, and, while they may be of any size, more often they are small or of moderate size. The herniation into the posterior mediastinum may extend into either or both sides of the thoracic cavity. This type constitutes the true "upside-down" stomach. Almost always there is a small remnant of the hiatus between the esophagus and the sac, although the main crural fibers may be found displaced by the sac.

Short Esophagus. These have no sac.

Congenital Type. In such instances the esophagus is not long enough to permit the

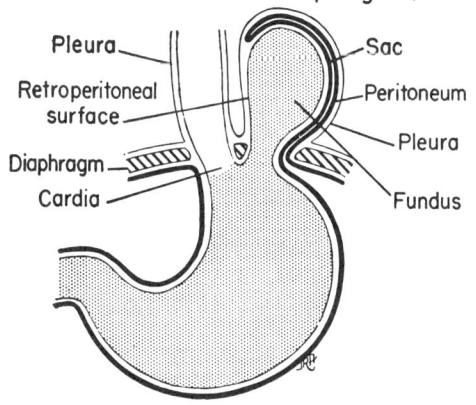

FIG. 42-21. (*Top*) Diagram illustrating the anatomic relations of the sliding type of herniation through the esophageal hiatus of the diaphragm. The drawing is made as a sagittal section through the area involved to show the relation of the herniated portion of the stomach to the hernia sac. (*Bottom*) Diagram illustrating the anatomic relations of the parahiatal type of diaphragmatic hernia. (Sweet, R. H.: Ann. Surg., 135:2, 5)

stomach to reach its normal position below the diaphragm, with the result that the organ is held suspended above the diaphragm in the posterior mediastinum. This type is not a true hernia, since the stomach never has been below the diaphragm. Harrington, who reported this as being present in 5 per cent of his operative cases, stated: "I believe the condition could be described better as congenitally short

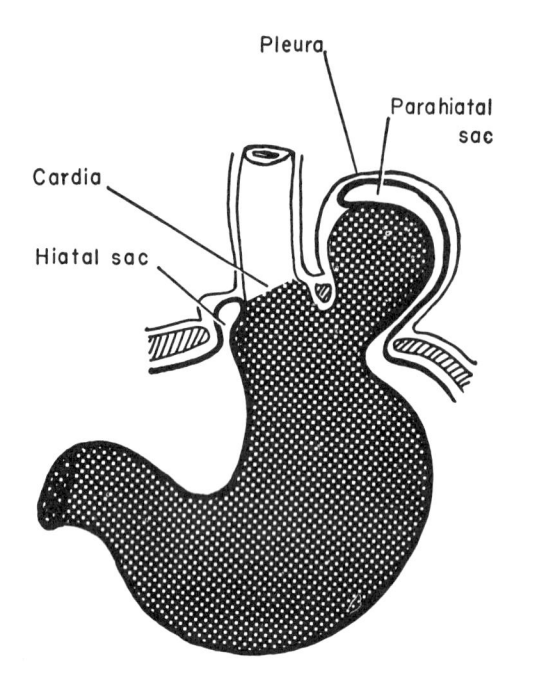

FIG. 42-22. Diagram illustrating the anatomic relations of the type of diaphragmatic hernia at the esophageal hiatus which consists of a combination of both sliding hiatal and parahiatal varieties. The term *composite* is suggested to designate this double arrangement. (Sweet, R. H.: Ann. Surg., 135:5)

esophagus with partially thoracic stomach than as an esophageal hiatal hernia."

Other writers put the incidence of this condition as lower than 5 per cent, while Lam (1954) stated that for practical purposes there was no such thing as a congenitally short esophagus. The editors of this textbook agree with Lam in this regard. The condition involves a mucosal factor as shown by Barrett (1950) and Morris (1955), i.e., the growth of the gastric mucosa up the esophagus. Therefore, the problem is one of esophageal surgery rather than of diaphragmatic surgery (see Chap. 30, Esophagus). Preoperative esophagoscopy, sometimes immediately before operation, is often helpful in cases of hiatal hernia if esophagitis is suspected. In general, it can be said that the relative roles and relationships between esophagitis and hiatal hernia are still unsettled. Moyer (1955) advocated a Finney pyloroplasty in conjunction with hernial repair when there was associated esophagitis. Peptic esophagitis, being a type of peptic ulcer, is also considered in Chapter 31, Stomach and Duodenum.

Acquired Type. As a result of ulceration or, occasionally, malignancy of the esophagus, the cardia of the stomach may be pulled above the diaphragm. No true hernia exists, and any stricture that may be present is a result of the primary condition rather than of the elevation of the stomach. Treatment is either by dilatation or resection and is also directed to the primary condition.

Pulsion Type of Hernia. Harrington adds a 4th type, which in turn is divided into (1) a small para-esophageal type of hernia with a sac and (2) incompetent hiatus without sac. The exact place which this group will occupy in the classification of hiatal hernia will be determined by future observations.

Incidence. Esophageal hiatal diaphragmatic hernia is noted most commonly in adult life, particularly in obese females over 50, but it may be found at any age, or in males, or in persons of normal weight. This type is less commonly found at birth than certain other types of congenital diaphragmatic hernia. Nelson (1953) reported 4 cases of hiatal hernia seen at the Sydney Children's Hospital. It is difficult to arrive at a figure for its overall incidence at all ages, but in the larger hospitals it may represent 1 per cent of the hernias treated surgically.

Predisposing Factors. These include: (1) age changes due to decreased elasticity of connective tissue, atony of the diaphragmatic muscles and loss of fat (or excessive fat) around the structures in the hiatus; and (2) changes due to increased subdiaphragmatic pressure caused by coughing, vomiting, constipation with flatulence, pregnancy, ascites and abdominal tumors.

Symptoms. The chief feature of the symptoms of early esophageal hiatal diaphragmatic hernia is the vagueness of their nature. Pain is substernal, precordial or epigastric. It may be exaggerated by lying down; thus, it may occur at night. It may be relieved by getting up in the morning or by sleeping in a semi-erect position at night; also by belching, swallowing and induced vomiting. Pain resulting from postural changes, particularly forward bending, is significant. Helpful diagnostic information also is supplied by a history of postural heartburn, probably due to regurgitation of acid liquid or of food, chiefly on forward bending or lying down; it may disturb sleep and is helped by assuming an erect or semierect position. Vomiting is rare, but eructation is not, and hiatal hernia should be suspected when there is aerophagia.

Additional symptoms include dysphagia, regurgitation, heartburn, hiccough, vomiting, hematemesis, anemia, palpitation, tachycardia, difficulty in breathing and cough. Differential diagnosis should consider heart disease, especially angina pectoris, gallbladder disease, gastroduodenal ulcer, and other lesions of the esophagus, some of which may be associated with hernia, including peptic ulcer, cardiospasm, diverticula and tumors. The importance of differential diagnosis from coronary insufficiency was emphasized by Kohli and Pearson (1953).

Diagnosis. Except that most patients are over 40 years of age and are obese, physical examination is of little value. The history of symptoms referable to hiatal hernia may be of some help, but confirmation is made with roentgen examination. Such a study should be performed in a number of positions, including the prone, the supine and sometimes the head-down position. If a hiatal hernia is suspected, it is important to inform the roentgenologist about it, since the lesion may be missed easily on a routine upper gastrointestinal examination. Pressure on the stomach region, as by bending forward during fluoroscopic examination, may force the stomach to herniate upward. Hillemand and Watteblede (1953) emphasized the importance of observation of the position of the cardia on fluoroscopic examination to determine if it was thoracic (sliding hernia) or abdominal (para-esophageal hernia). For study of the gastro-esophageal reflux, the patient swallows a few mouthfuls of water to clear the esophagus of barium. Then, in the decubitus position, retrograde flow into the esophagus is looked for. O'Connor and Ritvo (1955) pointed out that while the diagnosis of hiatal hernia by roentgen examination after the administration of opaque contrast material is a well-established procedure, it is not generally recognized that plain films of the upper abdomen may lead to a positive or a suggestive diagnosis. Observation of soft tissue densities, with or without air inclusion, is the essential feature in this method. Esophagoscopic examination also is indicated frequently.

Berry, Holbrook, Langdon and Mathewson (1955) introduced an important new procedure in the differential diagnosis of hiatal hernias. They produced pneumoperitoneum in 15 patients with diaphragmatic hernia of the hiatal type. This caused a reduction in the hernia and concomitant cessation of certain of the symptoms that previously had been difficult to attribute only to the hernia. They concluded that this might "be a useful technic for selecting patients who will benefit from surgical intervention."

Complications. These include ulceration, hemorrhage, incarceration and, very rarely, strangulation and rupture. Anemia frequently is present, probably because of chronic hemorrhage. Ritchey and Winsauer (1947) found anemia in 27 per cent of their series of 41 hiatal hernia patients. While as a general rule hemorrhage in cases of peptic esophagitis with or without associated hiatal hernia is of the chronic slow type (see Chap. 31), in exceptional instances sudden massive hemorrhage does occur (De Vito, Listerud, Nyhus, Merendino and Harkins, 1959). In the 39 cases of strangulated diaphragmatic hernia collected by Carter and Giuseffi (1948), all but 4 with the etiology stated were traumatic, and these 4 were congenital; in other words, in no instance in their collected series did strangulation occur in a hiatal hernia. The incidence of complications as reported by Stensrud (1954) in his 42 cases was 26 per cent (11 patients). These included stricture in 6, hematemesis or melena in 4, and incarceration in 1 patient.

Surgical Treatment

Indications. When an opening that normally admits 2 fingers for 3 cm. is found on routine abdominal exploration in a patient with no symptoms attributable to the esophageal hiatus, operation is not required. A patient with a large fist-sized or larger herniation, and with symptoms most likely attributable to it, needs repair. Those cases with indications varying in intensity between these extremes pose a difficult problem. Lam (1954) pointed out that the "incidental" finding of a hiatal hernia on "routine" upper gastrointestinal examination might not be as incidental as might be thought, as otherwise why did these patients have the examination performed in the first place? Most certainly, patients with a combination of severe symptoms, complications and large hernias require operative care. Obese patients should be requested to reduce. Evarts Graham (1954) summarized his opinion concerning the operative indications in hiatal hernia by saying:

Too many roentgenologists and physicians are accustomed to think that repair is not indicated unless the symptoms are extreme. The operative risk is extremely small. Unquestionably, many more hernias should be operated on.

The author agrees that symptomatic hiatal hernias should be repaired surgically in the absence of definite contraindications. Blades and Hall (1956) summarized their conclusions in this regard as follows: "(1) The incidental finding of a hiatal hernia without symptoms does not justify surgical treatment at the present time. In the future this attitude may change. (2) All symptomatic hiatal hernias should be treated surgically unless the patient's condition precludes operation." Harrington (1956) stated: "At the Mayo Clinic we have operated on about 16 to 18 per cent of the hiatal hernias that have been recognized roentgenologically."

Operative Technic. Aside from the decision as to whether to repair a sliding hiatus hernia by the thoracic or the abdominal route, the surgical world is faced with the problem of adopting 1 of 3 popular technics. These are as follows:

(1) CRURORAPHIA: Suture of the crura of the hiatus, usually behind the esophagus, combined with closure of the phreno-esophageal ligament and repositioning of the stomach into the abdominal cavity. This is less popular than it was five years ago (Allison, 1951; Sweet, 1952; Lam, 1954; Harrington, 1955, 1964; Tanner, 1955b; Madden, 1956; Beardsley, 1956, 1964; Hayward, 1964, and many others). If associated peptic esophagitis is present, cruroraphia is usually combined with vagotomy and pyloroplasty (Herrington, Edwards and Sawyers [1963], truncal vagotomy; Berne [1964] selective gastric vagotomy).

(2) GASTROPEXIA ANTERIOR GENICULATA (lesser curvature gastropexy): Suture of the lesser curvature of the stomach to the anterior abdominal wall so as to hold the stomach down in the peritoneal cavity (Boerema and Germs, 1955; Nissen, 1956; Boerema, 1964; and Ziperman, 1964).

(3) CARDIOFUNDOPLASTY (fundoplication): Suture of the gastric fundus around the abdominal esophagus (Nissen, 1964; with selective gastric vagotomy and Heineke-Mikulicz pyloroplasty, Berne; 1964; and with envelopment of only half the circumference of the esophagus—esophagofundoraphia—Petrovsky and Kanshin, 1964).

Ancillary considerations involve 2 supplemental procedures, as follows:

Phrenicotomy. Crushing the left phrenic nerve has been advised as either a concomitant or a definitive procedure in the treatment of hiatal hernia, particularly of the short esophagus type. Lam (1954) showed that in the experimental animal and in a human being, mechanical or faradic stimulation of the left phrenic nerve did not cause the left crus to contract. These studies indicate that any beneficial effect of phrenicotomy would be indirect from elevation of the diaphragm rather than direct by relieving "spasm" of the hiatus. Phrenicotomy now is seldom employed as a mode of therapy for hiatal hernia. Blades and Hall (1956) prefer procaine injection of the phrenic nerve at the end of the operation, if indicated.

Displacement of the Hiatus Anterolaterally into a New Opening. This more radical method involves an anterolateral incision in the diaphragm for about 2 to 4 cm., extending from the hiatus. In making the incision in the diaphragm, care should be taken not to cut major diaphragmatic branches of the phrenic nerves (for technic to avoid these, see Merendino, Johnson, Skinner and Maguire, 1956). The esophagus then is moved to the anterolateral end of the incision, and the diaphragm is closed behind it. This technic, first advocated by Merendino, Varco and Wangensteen in 1949, is applicable to occasional large or difficult hiatal hernias in which the crural tissues are not satisfactory for suture.

SUBSIDIARY PROBLEMS IN THE FIELD OF HERNIA

Hernia in Infancy and Childhood

This involves the following 3 factors: (1) different types of hernias; (2) indications for repair; and (3) technical differences in the type of repair. Many of the congenital hernias present in infants and children are considered in the glossary at the end of this chapter (e.g., Bochdalek hernia, paraduodenal hernia, etc.). Among the groin hernias, indirect inguinal ones are more common, and femoral (Bryant, 1965), and particularly direct, hernias are much rarer in infants and children. The problem of inguinal hernia *complicated by undescended testis* also arises much more often in infants and children. Snyder and Chaffin (1955) found this combination in 7 percent of their patients at the Los Angeles Children's Hospital and concluded that such children "may have both defects safely and simultaneously operated upon without delay."

Certain misconceptions exist concerning hernia in infants:

1. "Infants are poor surgical risks."
2. "Hernias in infants and childhood may cure spontaneously."
3. "A truss may obliterate the funicular process and cure the hernia."
4. "Hernias in infancy seldom incarcerate or strangulate."
5. "Hernias in infancy are seldom bilateral." Actually, about 25 per cent (Williams, 1959) to 60 per cent (Gilmore, 1960) are bilateral, or an inguinal hernia on the opposite side develops subsequently. McLaughlin and Coe (1960) did routine exploration of the opposite side in cases of single hernia, with a finding of previously unrecognized hernia in 55 per cent. They advised: "Routine exploration of the opposite side with single primary hernia in pediatric patients under three years of age is advised if the general condition permits." In a similar study, Kiesewetter and Parenzan (1959) found a contralateral hernia in 61 per cent of cases where it had not been suspected preoperatively. In another group of cases, these Pittsburgh authors did not explore the opposite side, and 31 per cent of these patients subsequently underwent contralateral herniorrhaphy. The evidence seems to be strong that hernias in infancy are often bilateral and that treatment should be planned accordingly.

Specific indications for treatment of 2 common hernias of infancy and childhood (indirect inguinal and umbilical) have been considered under these headings. In general, the tendency is toward earlier operation. Technical differences in the type of repair likewise are treated under the discussion of these 2 last-named hernias. In infants, strangulation and particularly incarceration are recognized as being more common than was formerly thought to be the case (Potts, Riker and Lewis, 1950; Smith, 1954; Holcomb, 1956). However, one precaution in this regard should be observed; namely, in infant females one should be alert to the possibility of the presence of an ovary in a hernia thought to be strangulated.

Outpatient Herniorrhaphy in Infants and Young Children

Wheeler (1968) points out the advantages of herniorrhaphy in infants and young children, when performed in the outpatient department, assuming good anesthesia to be available. First, this avoids the risk of hospital-acquired infection. Second, such procedures avoid utilization of a hospital bed, and, third, the infant or child does not have to experience unnecessary separation from his home environment. Indeed, for most groin hernias, a general anesthetic carries a greater risk than the surgical repair, and for this reason, if the surgeon or an available anesthesiologist is skilled at local or regional anesthetics, most inguinal and femoral hernias in adult patients could also be repaired in the outpatient department.

Hernia in the Aged

Associated prostatic hypertrophy or carcinoma of the bowel must be looked for. The commonly accepted treatment in these instances is conservative. However, it must be remembered that hernias do not grow at a steady rate but may progress in size exponentially, particularly in the aged. With good anesthesia (see Chap. 13), the risk of operation for hernia in the aged is quite low in the experience at the King County Hospital, Seattle, where many such patients are treated. Local infiltration anesthesia has a definite place in the surgical treatment of hernias in the aged. Operation can be made simpler in the case of groin hernias by orchiectomy in selected cases (see "Aids to Repair") (Jesseph, 1964).

INDUSTRIAL ASPECTS OF HERNIA

The actual treatment of hernia in industry differs only in certain minor details from that in nonindustrial practice. However, there are several points that make such hernias of especial importance. Whether a hernia is congenital or has developed as a result of the occupational activities of the individual is an important consideration. The statement of a reliable industrial examiner must be given weight. Local practices in different communities may vary. Many of the industrial aspects of hernia may be subjects for litigation. If a patient with no pre-existing hernia has an "accident" during employment, after which a hernia is found, the condition usually is compensable. If a patient with a pre-existing hernia has an "accident" during employment, after which the hernia is found to be larger, the condition usually is compensable because of aggravation of the pre-existing hernia. The industrial examiner during physical examinations and the industrial surgeon at operation must pay more attention to an enlarged external ring than is the case in nonindustrial practice. (See section below on size of subcutaneous inguinal ring.) Since medical records on employed patients may be consulted by others or may appear in court, the recorder must consider not only the medical aspects of his patient but also the legal implications of the same when writing the history and the physical examination. Iason (1964) and Estes and Charnock (1964) have presented good summaries of the medico-legal and the industrial aspects of hernia.

TREATMENT BY NONSURGICAL MEANS

In infants, the truss treatment of indirect inguinal hernia is rapidly declining in popularity, while adhesive strapping of umbilical hernia is now restricted to infants less than 1 year old and preferably less than 6 months old. In healthy adults, the use of a truss would seem to the author to have little or no place in modern therapy. In some elderly individuals with reducible hernia (there is no place for the use of a truss in the treatment of irreducible hernia), especially those in whom operation is deemed to carry significant risk, a carefully fitted truss may be tried. It is the responsibility of the physician who orders the truss to see that it fits and that it is applied properly. The truss should be applied in the recumbent position with the hernia reduced. These patients should be kept under careful observation because of the constant danger of strangulation.

The injection treatment of hernia involves the introduction of a sclerosing anesthetic mixture around the sac in selected cases of reducible hernia so as to produce fibrosis and eventual fixation of the sac in the reduced position. The method has suffered a progressive decline in the last 15 years. This was influenced by several factors: (1) the method never really gained a foothold in the larger surgical centers; (2) improvements in the results of the operation made a substitute procedure less necessary; (3) the unsurgical nature of the method, combined with the difficulties produced by varying positions of the sac, made little appeal to experienced surgeons; and particularly (4) the unfavorable report of the Council on Pharmacy and Chemistry of the American Medical Association on August 17, 1940, militated against it. Lawrence (1948) published a case report concerning fatal intestinal obstruction following injection treatment of hernia; he believed the method to be unreliable and hazardous. With this opinion the author is in accord. The injection treatment is mentioned only to be condemned.

BILATERAL REPAIR AT ONE OPERATION

The question has often been raised as to whether a bilateral hernia should be repaired at a single operation or whether it is best to do the second side a week later. A decision in this regard involves 3 main factors: (1) infection, (2) recurrence, and (3) mortality in poor risk patients. So far as the first factor is concerned, it seems to the author that if adequate aseptic precautions are used, and if the operation on the first side does not take over 90 minutes, the increased risk should be insignificant. In a series of over 100 bilateral repairs, infection occurred in only one instance, and then in the wound on the side *first* repaired. If bowel is entered, or an abscess is encountered on the first side, it would seem wise to do the other side later. Otherwise it may be concluded that the danger of increased risk of infection in the second side is not a frequent contraindication to bilateral operation.

The second factor in increased recurrence rate—in this instance the supposed increase applying to *either* side because of tension on the peritoneum and the endo-abdominal fascia —may be important in certain circumstances. If the hernia is very large on one side, or if the hernia is recurrent on one side, it usually is best to do a one-sided operation and then repair the smaller hernia at a later date.

In poor risk patients, the larger or otherwise more important hernia should be repaired first. If the patient is standing the procedure well, the second side may be done at the same sitting if 2 factors apply: (1) if the second hernia needs repair (which often is not so in bedridden patients with a small second side hernia); and (2) if the increased risk of a second anesthesia exceeds the risk of prolonging the first operation. Koontz (1954) was in agreement with this policy.

The additional point should be mentioned that often a bilateral hernia exists even when it is not demonstrable, except on one side, preoperatively. Rothenburg and Barnett (1955) reported that in 100 per cent of their infants under 1 year with hernia and in 66 per cent of those from 1 to 12 years of age the lesion was bilateral. This is an additional consideration in favor of more frequent bilateral operations.

Aside from the question of *when* a bilateral hernia should be repaired at one sitting, discussed above, the problem arises as to *how* this should be done when indicated. Many surgeons advise 2 separate groin incisions. Others advise a transverse, or Pfannenstiel-type incision. And still others advise a mid-line incision with internal repair. Knott (1954) advocated a transpubic horizontal incision of the Pfannenstiel type in bilateral cases. At the same time, Knott pointed out that a "second side" hernia often is overlooked.

The Relationship Between Inguinal Hernia and Previous Appendectomy Incisions

While it is generally recognized that inguinal hernia is more common on the right than on the left, this increased frequency seems to be accentuated in patients with previous appendectomy incisions. Pitkänen (1948), in a study of 1,062 postappendectomy patients, found that the incidence of inguinal hernia on the right side was no greater in those patients in whom there had not been diffuse peritonitis, but was about 2 times the normal expected rate in patients who had had diffuse peritonitis at the time of the appendectomy. Hicks (1941) also stated:

We found that a considerable number of right inguinal hernias followed the McBurney incision for appendicitis. This is, no doubt, due to a blind tearing injury to nerves and muscle when this incision is used.

To obviate the difficulty, Hicks adopted the transverse incision for appendicitis without abscess.

The different but related problem of concomitant appendectomy with herniorrhaphy is important. No hard-and-fast rule can be laid down. In general, if the appendicitis is acute and the hernia is large (hence apt to recur), the appendectomy should be done through a separate incision. On the other hand, an interval appendectomy is permissible through a herniorrhaphy incision when the hernia is small, the appendix presents itself in the wound, and the surgeon is experienced. If these criteria are not all met, coincident interval appendectomy with herniorrhaphy should be avoided.

Choice of Suture Material

This choice always has been a matter of debate. Since 1939 the author has used nonabsorbable sutures (generally silk; although when cotton was used in a few cases at hospitals which did not regularly use silk, cotton seemed to work equally as well). During the years 1931 to 1938 he used catgut. While it is true that the catgut available in the thirties was not as good as that now on the market, it is the author's opinion that silk is preferable to catgut for the repair of hernias. At the same time, it must be admitted that an improperly performed silk repair is not as good as a properly performed catgut repair. The surgeon using steel wire more and more in place of silk, may have difficulty in tying it square in the deep wound where the conjoined tendon is sutured to Cooper's ligament, so that silk is still preferred for this deep layer. Silk (and steel even more so) seems to give rise to less frequent "seroma" development, wound infection and recurrence of the hernia (see Chap. 2, Wound Healing). Even in the rare instance in which wound infection has required that the incision be laid wide open and the silk removed, recurrence has not resulted. The one objection to silk—extrusion of sutures or sinuses down to them requiring their removal ("silkosis")—rarely applies if care is taken to use aseptic technic and avoid too heavy sutures, sutures too near the skin or continuous silk sutures.

Disposal of Distal Portion of the Indirect Sac

In many clinics great care is taken, after dividing a long indirect sac not only to close the proximal end but also to excise the remaining distal segment because of fear of developing a hydrocele. We believe that while high ligation of the proximal stump of the sac is the most important step in the repair of hernia, in most instances it is preferable to leave the distal portion of the sac in place. In cases of congenital hernia, generally we do not even do a bottle type of operation in the absence of a pre-existing hydrocele. The rationale behind this mode of treatment is that the almost certain danger of hematoma (from sac excision) is more to be feared than the more remote possibility of a subsequent hydrocele. Larsen (1949), speaking of hernias in infancy and in childhood, also emphasized that the distal portion of the sac should be disregarded. Griffith (1959), on the other hand, advised removal of the sac in most instances.

Size of the Subcutaneous Inguinal Ring

In physical examinations much is made of the size of the subcutaneous or external inguinal ring as an indication of both potential and actual inguinal hernia. In an excellent review, Chassin (1947) found less correlation than would be expected between these factors. A study was made of 3,199 soldiers between 18 and 36 years of age to determine the range of sizes of subcutaneous or external inguinal rings in large numbers of healthy young men. It was found that 78.1 per cent of these men had external rings sufficiently large to admit the index finger, almost half being from 1.4 to 1.9 cm. This does not agree with the previous statements of many authorities, and it indicates that normal external rings vary widely in size, and that the average is appreciably larger than was formerly believed to be the case. In 724 men with asymmetric rings, the larger occurred on the left side in 57.5 per cent, but 58.3 per cent of inguinal hernias discovered during this study occurred on the right side. There was no convincing evidence to indicate that a large subcutaneous ring was abnormal or that it predisposed to future herniation. No correlation could be demonstrated between the size of the subcutaneous ring and the weight or the height of the subject. (See also Knott, 1964.)

Errors and Safeguards in the Repair of Hernia

Two of the chief errors are committed during the preoperative phase: (1) overlooking a strangulated hernia; and (2) delaying operation on a hernia in an older individual until not only is the hernia much bigger, but also the patient is much older than when first seen, hence less able to withstand operation. At operation many errors can occur. One of the chief of these is a diagnostic blunder, already referred to in the section on femoral hernia, which involves the omission of finger exploration from within of Hesselbach's triangle and the femoral region for associated direct inguinal or femoral hernia when repairing an indirect inguinal hernia. In making the incision care should be taken not to cut the ilioinguinal or the iliohypogastric nerves. Similarly, in freeing the cord, the vascular supply must be preserved, and the vas (the location of which is noted by its hard feel on palpation) should not be cut. An indirect inguinal sac may not be ligated high enough, or it may be overlooked entirely. In performing a Bassini type of operation for inguinal hernia, care must be taken to see that the needle that sutures the conjoined tendon to Poupart's ligament does not penetrate the underlying femoral vein. In performing a Cooper's ligament repair the same error can be avoided more easily, but still this requires retraction of the femoral vein under direct vision during the placing of the most lateral sutures. There are many other errors and safeguards, but a final one that should not be overlooked involves the selection of operation for the particular patient at hand. Thus, even the advocates of a Bassini repair would admit that it is not adequate for a large direct hernia. On the other hand, a Cooper's ligament repair involves too much alteration of normal structures to be necessary for the repair of an indirect inguinal hernia in an infant.

AIDS TO REPAIR

The previous discussion in the main body of this chapter includes that of the procedures ordinarily used in the repair of the common types of hernia. When the hernia is unusually large or difficult, certain additional "aids" should be available in the armamentarium of the surgeon. Some of these may have frequent application; others may be needed only rarely; still others (denoted by an asterisk) are applicable so seldom that the author never used them, even though they are popular with others. Before considering any of these individually, it should be emphasized that an aid is like a crutch: it should be used only if absolutely necessary. The aim should be always to get the fascial edges together. While certain aids may help in accomplishing this, those that consist of a type of patch (cutis, whole skin, tantalum mesh, etc., see p. 1242) generally should be reserved for reinforcement of a suture line between fascial layers rather than for bridging a gap. Thus, Moyer (1960) states: "The use of prostheses is practically never necessary, even for the largest hernias." The aids may be classified as follows:

PREOPERATIVE AND OPERATIVE TECHNICS FOR FACILITATION OF SURGERY OF MASSIVE HERNIAS

In certain instances a hernia may be so large that the bowel contents may be said to have lost their "right of domain" within the abdominal cavity. Aside from the general careful preparation of the patient, which in such instances may include weight reduction and studies of cardiac and pulmonary function, 3 specific methods of preparation are available:

1. **Pneumoperitoneum.** This method, used especially in large ventral hernias, was introduced by Goñi Moreno (1940), of Buenos Aires, and has been used chiefly in certain South American clinics since that time. The technic includes a series of 4 to 6 intraperitoneal air injections at intervals of from 2 to 5 days (Goñi Moreno, 1964; Moyer and Butcher, 1964). Connolly and Perri (1969) have recently reported their favorable experience with pneumoperitoneum, a procedure that may be quite useful in some cases.

It is surprising how relaxed the margins of the hernial ring are at operation and how undistended the bowel appears to be. Moyer (1960), on the basis of an experience with the method in over 30 cases, most often for the secondary repair of omphalocele, agrees that the bowel actually becomes smaller in diameter and also that even if the abdominal wall stretches, the hernia usually does not increase in size. This latter point may be because the hernia is the one portion of the abdominal wall circumference that contains scar tissue. In the case of hernias, in the repair of which it would ordinarily be difficult to get the edges together, after a course of pneumoperitoneum preparation the edges often can be imbricated liberally. The author used this technic in a few selected cases since the autumn of 1949 with uniformly good results. Among the best references to the technic in the American literature are those of Koontz and Graves (1954) and Mason (1956). These authors use a 19-gauge lumbar puncture needle, which is usually inserted in the linea semilunaris, well away from the hernia to avoid adhesions. Air is injected (in Goñi Moreno's original report he advocated the use of oxygen, but since then he has switched to the use of air) until the patient begins to have slight respiratory distress (usually after 500-1,500 cc.). Subsequent injections at 2- to 5-day intervals may be as much as several liters at 1 sitting and are continued until "the abdominal cavity has become enlarged enough to accommodate the contents of the hernial sac." An abdominal binder is worn to prevent the air simply from becoming captive in the hernial sac and not enlarging the peritoneal cavity. From 10 to 20 days should be sufficient time for preparation for operation. Koontz and Graves (and the author) have kept the patients in the hospital during this period, but this may not always be necessary. In 4 cases, Koontz and Graves injected totals of 1,700, 7,000, 5,000 and 6,700 cc. of air in series of 2, 7, 2 and 4 injections respectively.

2. **Phrenic Crush.*** Touroff (1954) recommended a "phrenicectomy," left-sided in his case report, to be done a few days before herniorrhaphy to relax the diaphragm and better to accommodate the contents of the hernia within the abdomen. Most certainly, if such a procedure is to be done, a simple phrenic crush, which is rarely permanent, is preferable to a phrenicectomy, which almost always is permanent. A phrenic crush is something that can be done at the time of operation if necessary and takes only 5 to 10 minutes of extra operating time. It would seem that, generally, pneumoperitoneum is preferable to phrenic crush. Pneumoperitoneum is over with as soon as the operation, hence it does not impair the patient's recovery during the postoperative period. Furthermore, if respiratory embarrassment occurs, pneumoperitoneum always can be decompressed, while the effects of the phrenic crush cannot be reversed at will.

3. **Long Intestinal Tube.** Preoperative threading of the bowel on a long intestinal tube for decompression and keeping it down for 2 to 4 days after operation not only may make the operative reduction of a large hernia easier but may be a lifesaving procedure during the postoperative period. A corollary of this method is the use of physostigmine to permit closure of the abdomen at the time of operation and to keep down postoperative distention. Even if a long tube is not used, in large hernias a regimen involving preoperative liquid diet, castor oil and enemas the day before operation and gastric aspiration for 12 hours before, is advisable.

Three other technics, which are utilizable at the time of operation rather than preoperatively, are as follows:

1. **Bowel Resection.** The temptation to do a bowel resection for mechanical reasons only to reduce the volume of bowel content to be replaced is an ever-present one, but it should be resisted, just like the temptation to do a gastroenterostomy in the presence of apparent obstruction of the duodenum after simple closure of a perforated peptic ulcer. Bowel resection is seldom necessary for the reason of reducing bowel content of the peritoneal cavity in experienced hands; it increases the chances of infection, not only of the wound, but also of the main peritoneal cavity.

2. **Relaxing Incisions.** These are of 4 types, 2 applicable to ventral hernias and 2 to groin hernias. The first 2 involve a longitudinal incision in the anterior rectus sheath either with or without turning the medial flap over medialward (Wilkie maneuver) to reinforce the suture line. It is important not to place these relaxing incisions where there is no muscle beneath them. The other 2 involve the relaxing incision already described in the Cooper's ligament repair, either with or without turning the lower flap downward.

3. **Two-Stage Wound Closure.*** Gross, of Boston, recommended 2-stage wound closure, especially for infants with large hernias of the foramen of Bochdalek, in which the intestine has lost the "right of domain" in the abdominal cavity. At the 1st stage only the skin is closed, and then 6 days later the entire wound is closed in layers as a 2nd stage. This method is not so readily applicable to adults because of poorer blood supply in the abdominal wall. Even in infants Gross has not found it necessary since 1945. In omphalocele, the 2-stage method is becoming increasingly popular (see "Rarer Hernias"). Ziffren and Womack (1950) have described a modification of this technic for use in adults with gigantic hernias, which they applied successfully to a male with a right inguinal hernia which reached to just below the knees and at repair was found to be irreducible because of loss of "right of domain." Therefore, a long transverse incision was made in the upper abdomen down to the peritoneum. The latter was allowed to bulge into the wound, the skin was closed, and the space thus created permitted reduction of the inguinal hernia. The upper abdominal "new hernia" was easily repaired 12 days later when the patient had adjusted himself to the newly increased abdominal contents.

METHODS TO FACILITATE CLOSURE OF THE INTERNAL RING IN A DIFFICULT INGUINAL HERNIA REPAIR

Often it has been said that the repair of inguinal hernia in males would be much simpler if one were permitted to close the internal ring entirely rather than to have to strike the delicate balance of closing it just

---

* See page 1239 for explanation.

tight enough to prevent recurrence, yet not so tight as to strangulate the cord. In large repeatedly recurrent or otherwise difficult hernias the following 2 methods are available to obviate this difficulty, generally in elderly males only:

1. Cord Division With Orchiectomy. This should be done only with the full understanding of the patient and his wife and with their written consent. It permits a complete closure of the internal ring. Fowler and Stephens (1959) pointed out the importance of a knowledge of testicular vascular anatomy in operations of this type. Careful hemostasis, especially in the loose tissues within the scrotum, to prevent hematoma formation and insertion of a small Penrose drain for a few days may be indicated but is not always necessary. Hagan and Rhoads (1953) noted in their series that recurrence rates in males, when concomitant orchiectomy was done, and in females were much lower than in other patients. They concluded that these observations support the "argument that adequate closure of the internal ring is of particular importance, and suggests that in difficult or recurrent hernias in older patients orchiectomy may be justified."

2. Cord Division Without Orchiectomy. This method, first advocated by Burdick and Higinbotham (1935), has the advantage that if the testis does not atrophy, a better cosmetic result is obtained.

These authors gave the following indications for the procedure (these would also apply to cord division *with* orchiectomy):

1. Recurrent hernias which have had one or more unsuccessful attempts at a radical cure in individuals past 50 in whom the opposite testicle apparently is normal

2. Recurrent hernias in younger subjects who are incapacitated from their usual occupation and have an apparently normal testicle on the opposite side, especially when more than one attempt at repair has been made previously

3. Large scrotal hernias in the aged, which are either irreducible or cannot be retained satisfactorily by a truss

4. Large sliding hernia

When cord division is performed in cases of scrotal hernia, the distal sac never should be removed, nor should the testicle be delivered intentionally into the wound for fear of damaging the anastomotic blood supply. Burdick and Higinbotham advocated elevating the scrotum on a bridge for a few days postoperatively. They stated that there is "always considerable swelling accompanied by redness of the skin and edema of the scrotum. . . . Gangrene did occur in four. . . . Many of the testicles atrophy, in fact some almost completely disappear, but it is surprising how many do not." Two hundred such cord divisions were performed, and, of 169 cases followed, there were notes as to the condition of the testicle available in 64. The testicle was normal in 42 cases (including all bilateral cord divisions), slightly atrophied in 11, and atrophied to one half or less of normal size in 11. These figures do not include the 4 cases with gangrene necessitating orchiectomy.

Heifetz and Goldfarb (1952) reported 23 cases with cord divisions with the following results: 6 without postoperative swelling or atrophy and 17 with postoperative swelling (of these 4 became atrophic, 2 slightly atrophic, 1 had to be removed because of chronic infection, and the remaining 10 were normal when last seen). In dog experiments these same workers reported no gangrene or necrosis of the testicle after division of the spermatic cord at various levels, although there was some degeneration of the tubules and the spermatic cells. Paradoxically, when the ductus deferens and its artery were preserved after division of the rest of the cord structures in the dog, the testes atrophied completely.

In patients in whom retention of the internal secretions of the testicles or a single remaining testicle is important, or in whom the psychic effect of testicular absence is important, this method should be considered in the light of its possible complications in preference to orchiectomy.

METHODS OF SUTURE REINFORCEMENT

These include the following:

1. Attached Fascial Suture (McArthur, 1901). These are often called living fascial sutures, and if viable they do have an advantage. Often the circulation is deficient, and they are not viable. These sutures can be obtained only from contiguous structures, usually the external oblique aponeurosis, and this practical consideration limits their length, strength and size.

2. **Free Fascial Sutures** (Gallie and Le Mesurier, 1921). Such sutures can be obtained of satisfactory size from the tensor fascia lata tendon (iliotibial tract) using a fascial stripper. The objections to them are that of necessity they make large needle holes in the tissue being sutured and also may become infected. However, they are strong and, even though inserted loosely, fill in weak spaces quite adequately.

3. **Darning and Filigree Technics.*** Such methods are especially popular in Great Britain, where faith in the classic Bassini operation is beginning to falter, and reliance has not yet been widely placed in the Cooper's ligament technic. Such technics have been used by Cole (1941), Moloney, Gill and Barclay (1948), Doran (1964) and Moloney (1964).

PATCHES

These are becoming more popular and include fascia lata (Strode, 1964), cutis grafts, whole skin grafts,* tantalum mesh, steel-wire mesh, Vitallium plate, Ivalon (polyvinyl alcohol sponge, used by Schofield, 1955) other plastics and cartilage (for repair of large ventral hernias, Satinsky and Kron, 1953). Of these, tantalum mesh (Koontz, 1955; Koontz and Kimberly, 1950; Smith, 1954, 1959, 1964) and cutis grafts (Cannaday, 1942; Swenson and Harkins, 1943b; Harkins, 1945; Swenson, 1950; and Ali, 1954) are most popular, although Mair, in Scotland, has used whole-thickness skin-graft patches in several hundred instances of repair of hernia with reportedly good results. Theoretically, Vinyon "N" cloth could be used as a patch. It should be re-emphasized that almost always such patches should be used to *reinforce* rather than to *supplant* a layer-to-layer closure. Furthermore, it should be emphasized that these patches complicate the operation and lead to additional complications, and they do not eliminate recurrences.

Tantalum Mesh. Lam, Szilagyi and Puppendahl (1948) studied the effects of implantation of tantalum (a biologically inert metallic element) in the form of gauze as implanted in dogs with favorable results. In 24 large postoperative ventral hernias these authors also reported good results. Throckmorton (1948) in 16 cases, Koontz (1948, 1955a, 1964) in several reports and a large series of 139 cases, Smith (1954) in 43 cases, and Guy, Werelius and Bell (1955) in 302 cases have all reported their experiences with the method. Smith (1954) and Erwald and Rieger (1960) pointed out that the fragmentation of the mesh may be disadvantageous in the upper abdomen. Experience by the author of this chapter would indicate that if tantalum mesh is used, tantalum sutures should be utilized to suture it in place. The experience of Guy *et al.* is based on the use of largely tantalum mesh in 302 of 1,073 total hernia operations. Only 37 of the 302 were ventral hernias, the rest being groin hernias. Even though mesh was used in the more difficult hernias, so far as inguinal hernias are concerned the recurrence rate was 3.0 per cent without mesh and 1.9 per cent with mesh. The experience of Allen (1955) with tantalum mesh is less encouraging. In his clinic 7 of 10 cases had to have the tantalum removed in 2 months to 3 years. Infection was not always the dominant factor. The tantalum was fragmented and uncomfortable. In the majority of cases it was utilized above the umbilicus; hence, a warning should be voiced against its use in the upper abdomen.

Steel-wire mesh is cheaper and does not fragment as much as tantalum mesh. However, its adoption is slow despite its availability. The experimental observations of Koontz and Kimberly (1950) indicating the superiority of tantalum as compared with steel-wire mesh partly explain this reluctance to adopt the latter.

Cutis Grafts. Cutis may be defined as the deeper layers of the skin which have been stripped of their epidermal covering. Anatomically, this includes approximately the deeper three quarters of the thickness of the skin, the entire skin averaging about 1 mm., or 40/1,000 inch, in depth. Histologically, cutis comprises the dermal layer with no epidermal covering, but with sebaceous and sudoriferous glands and occasional hair follicles, as well as some of the underlying subdermal fat.

Since Loewe's report, in 1913, cutis grafts have been adopted sporadically for 2 purposes: (1) in the field of plastic surgery when the cutis is utilized to fill in tissue defects; and (2) in the operative treatment of hernia

---

* See page 1239 for explanation.

when patches of cutis are applied to strengthen the repair.

Cannaday (1942) was the first writer in this country to report the use of cutis in hernial repair work; he presented 14 such cases. Two years later he had increased the size of his hernia series to 56 and reported good results. In 1945, Harkins reported experimental studies in dogs and the clinical use of cutis in 11 cases of large ventral or incisional hernias. In the animal experiments cyst formation was noted, while in the clinical cases the results seemed excellent, so that the wounds remained healed. Swenson (1950) is one of the chief workers in this field at present.

Whole Skin. This procedure is more radical than the introduction of cutis grafts. The method was introduced by Mair (1945, 1948). Mair's technic was controlled by careful animal experiments. In 2 cases in which the skin implant was examined later in human subjects, it was found to be converted into stout fibrous tissue. Mair (1948) stated:

> In my own practice I have repaired 140 indirect inguinal herniae with the whole skin graft technique and with a recurrence rate of 0.71 per cent after a follow-up of 1 year. I have also repaired 40 direct inguinal herniae by the same technique without a recurrence at the end of 3 years. This is associated with a morbidity rate, both immediate and remote, which compares well with figures from both my own practice and results from other clinics for other methods. These figures embrace those repairs performed with skin only over a short period.
>
> So far I have found no contra-indication to the routine use of the operation where sound repair is indicated, but insist on an adequate pre-operative skin preparation as being essential to elimination of sepsis as a complication.

West and Hicks (1948) have also reported favorably on the use of whole skin grafts in the repair of inguinal hernia, particularly recurrent cases, and femoral hernia. The method has been also used successfully at the University of Tennessee (Wilson, 1948), by Zavaleta and Uriburu (1950) in 211 cases and Strahan (1951) in 413 cases.

The use of plastic materials is becoming more common. Rigid plastic implants should be avoided (Fitzgerald and Mehigan, 1959). Nylon (Smith, 1959); Teflon (Adler and Firme, 1959); and Marlex meshes (Usher, Ochsner and Tuttle, 1958; Ponka, Wylie, Chäikof, Sergeant and Brush, 1959; Usher, 1959; Usher Fries, Ochsner and Tuttle, 1959; and Usher and Gannon, 1959) have all been tried. It should be re-emphasized that while these supports are very useful when indicated, for the vast majority of hernia repairs they are entirely superfluous.

RARER HERNIAS: TREATMENT AND GLOSSARY OF TERMS

Bochdalek (Foramen of) Hernia. Hernias in posterolateral region of the diaphragm, along the old pleuroperitoneal canal (foramen of Bochdalek), are the most common among congenital hernias of the diaphragm (90% of all cases at the Boston Children's Hospital). They are 5 times as common on the left as on the right. In most instances no sac exists, and the absence of adhesions to the parietal pleura is also noteworthy. Associated malrotation of the intestine is often present. Treatment includes immediate operation, preferably during the first 48 hours of life before the intestines are distended. Most surgeons (Harrington, 1951; Gross, 1953) prefer an abdominal approach, although some use a thoracic one. On the right side it is usually preferable to replace the liver last, and on the left side to replace the stomach first. The ring is closed with interrupted silk-mattress sutures, with imbrication if possible. The abdominal wound should be closed in layers, although if the intestine truly has lost the "right of domain," skin closure with later repair of the entire wound is an available method (see section on "Aids to Repair").

Cloquet's Hernia (see "Pectineal Hernia").

Congenital Hernia. This includes any hernia which results from either abnormal persistence of a normally present opening (e.g., indirect inguinal hernia) or the presence of an abnormal opening (e.g., paraduodenal hernia, see p. 1246).

Cooper's Hernia (see "Femoral Hernia With Multilocular Sacs").

Epigastric Hernia (hernia of the linea alba above the umbilicus). Since hernia of the linea alba below the umbilicus is so rare, "epigastric" hernia is the term commonly used. The symptomatology of epigastric hernia is important; such hernias may mimic peptic ulcer, cholecystitis, acute pancreatitis, etc. The pain may be worse when the patient lies down, due to the pull on the omentum by gravity. Some of the most symptomatic epigastric hernias are so small as not to be visible. Such hernias comprise about 1 per cent of all hernias. They may occur anywhere between the xiphoid and the umbilicus, but they are most common immediately above the latter structure. The initial defect which predisposes to these hernias is most likely the aperture for a perforating blood vessel. Because of these blood vessels, in doing a repair when the herniated lobule of fat is excised, its base should be secured with a suture ligature. A closure of the fascial defect is usually done transversely, fastening the upper flap over the lower as in an umbilical hernia and utilizing relaxing incisions similar to those described under the repair of umbilical hernia.

Eventration of the Diaphragm. This is often classified as a type of diaphragmatic hernia, but actually it consists by definition merely in elevation into the thorax of one or both leaves of the diaphragm associated with defective muscular action, similar to that which follows the surgical procedure of crushing one or both phrenic nerves. Also it may occur following pneumoperitoneum, or it may be of idiopathic origin. Neuman, Ellis and Andersen (1955) advise operation more often than has been done in the past. Plication and strengthening with fascia, etc., have been used to lower the thinned-out diaphragm in cases in which symptoms of respiratory embarrassment exist.

External Femoral Hernia (Hesselbach's Hernia). First described by Hesselbach (1806) and almost always associated with an indirect inguinal hernia on the same side, this type of hernia passes into the thigh below the inguinal ligament and the iliopubic tract, but lateral to the femoral and the deeper epigastric arteries.

Femoral Hernia With Multilocular Sacs. Also called "Cooper's hernia," this type has a main sac which follows the femoral canal but with subsidiary loculi into the scrotum or the labium majus and toward the obturator foramen (Aird, 1957).

Hesselbach's Hernia (see "External Femoral Hernia").

Incarcerated Hernia (syn.: **Irreducible Hernia**). According to another definition, there is, in addition to irreducibility, obstruction to the flow of intestinal contents in any intestinal loop which may be present but in which, unlike a *strangulated hernia*, the blood flow and the lymph drainage remain intact. According to our definition, this type of hernia is an *obstructed hernia*. The term *incarceration* usually is used to denote an irreducible hernia without obstruction or strangulation.

Internal Hernia. Such hernias are of 3 main types: (1) congenital in origin, of which paraduodenal hernia (q.v.) is the most common type; (2) due to adhesive bands—congenital (e.g., attached Meckel's diverticulum), inflammatory (e.g., after appendictis with perforation) or iatrogenic (e.g., from talcum implantation at the time of previous operation); and (3) due to volvulus around colostomies, etc. Strangulation is frequent, and careful observation with prompt laparotomy in indicated cases is mandatory. Prophylactic measures include the general abandonment of the use of talcum on gloves (about 1950). The starch powder now used is much less noxious than talcum in this regard (see Chap. 2, Wound Healing), but, like any foreign body, starch is not entirely innocuous. It should be washed off the gloves *carefully* before any abdominal operation and care should be taken in closing the lateral peritoneal gutter adjacent to laterally placed colostomies or ileostomies.

Interparietal Hernia. Lower and Hicken (1931) classified interparietal hernias into 3 anatomic types, as follows:

(1) Properitoneal hernia, that type in which the hernial sac lies between the peritoneum and the transversalis fascia; (2) interstitial hernia, in which the sac lies between the transversalis fascia and the transversalis, internal oblique, or external oblique muscles; and (3) superficial hernia, in which the sac is situated between the aponeurosis of the external oblique and the integument.

Of these 3 types, the interstitial is the most common and is described below:

Interstitial Hernia. A hernia that lies in one of the planes of the abdominal wall, e.g., between the internal and the external oblique aponeuroses. This type of hernia, first described by Bartholin in 1661, has many subvarieties. While most interstitial hernias are also inguinal hernias, this is not always true (Koontz and Stafford, 1955). Interstitial hernia may be very large. It is over 3 times as common in males as in females. Its treatment is essentially that of the type of hernia it represents, independent of its burrowing propensities. (See "Interparietal Hernia" above.)

Irreducible Hernia. The opposite of *reducible hernia*.

Lacunar Ligament Hernia (see "Laugier's Hernia").

Laugier's Hernia (hernia ligamenti lacunaris gimbernati, hernie de Laugier, hernie interne de Velpeau, medical femoral hernia). This hernia was first described by Laugier in 1833. Since such hernias pass through the fibrous plate of Gimbernat's ligament, reduction may require incision into the lateral border of the ring as advocated by Priesching (1956).

Lipoma of the Cord. A soft lobulated fatty projection from the retroperitoneal space, coming out usually at the lateral margin of the internal ring. Its importance is that it may be confused with a simple indirect hernia. When seen at operation, it should always be removed to prevent a future possible misdiagnosis and unnecessary secondary operation.

Littré Hernia. A hernia of Meckel's diverticulum through a hernial opening (Littré, 1700). This type of hernia is found most frequently in adult males. Among 143 cases collected by Watson, 109 were on the right and only 34 on the left. Treatment includes that of the hernia itself plus, if possible, excision of the Meckel's diverticulum. When Meckel's diverticulitis is present—and this may have drawn the patient's attention to the hernia—resection is mandatory, possibly through a separate abdominal incision (see Davis, 1954).

Lumbar Hernia (also called **Petit's Triangle Hernia**). While such hernias may occur in any part of the lumbar region, they are particularly prone to protrude through Petit's triangle (bounded by the iliac crest below, the external oblique in front, and the latissimus dorsi behind; the floor is made up by the internal oblique). Petit's triangle is also known as the inferior lumbar triangle. About 2 in. above and slightly anterior to it is the superior lumbar triangle of Grynfelt-Lesshaft. This superior triangle represents the bare space where there is neither external nor internal oblique. It has no muscular floor but has the latissimus dorsi for a roof or an outer covering. It is larger and more constant than Petit's triangle, but herniation through it is rarer. Watson collected reports of 146 lumbar hernias from the literature; of those in which the sex was stated, 103 were males and 39 were females. They occurred at all ages but were rare in young children and common in older persons. Nine per cent were strangulated. Usually there is a sac. Treatment usually is accomplished by pushing in on the sac and by overlapping muscular and aponeurotic layers over the defect. Swartz (1954) advocated free fascial sutures for the repair of these hernias, but in most instances silk or steel wire is adequate.

While primary lumbar hernias are the third rarest of the main types of hernia according to Koontz (1955b) (the 5 rare hernias being in the order of frequency, beginning with the rarest: sciatic, perineal, lumbar, obturator and internal), incisional lumbar hernias are more common. These usually follow kidney operations. Koontz described an operation used successfully in 5 cases. This involved (1) the freeing of the sac, (2) inversion and plication of the sac with interrupted mattress sutures, (3) reflection of a flap of fascia lata upward to cover the anterior portion of the defect, and (4) reflection forward of a flap of lumbar fascia to cover the posterior portion of the defect.

Mesenteric Defect Hernias (Winterscheid, 1964). Such hernias go through a rent in the mesentery, most often that of the ileum, and represent the most common intra-abdominal hernia in the childhood period (cf. paraduodenal hernia, which is the second most common hernia of this type).

Morgagni (Foramen of) Hernia. A type of diaphragmatic hernia involving the anterior and parasternal region (space of Larrey). These hernias (which also are called subcostosternal, retrocostoxiphoid, parasternal, or retrosternal) may be congenital or acquired, and a sac is present. At the Boston Children's Hospital, hernias of the foramen of Morgagni constituted 5 per cent of congenital hernias of the diaphragm. In his thorough review of this particular type of hernia, Harrington (1940) stated that they constituted 1.5 per cent (4 cases) of his entire series of diaphragmatic hernias. Helsby and Wells (1954) collected 24 operated cases from the literature. Strangulation is more frequent than with hernias of the esophageal hiatus. The colon is present in the sac in about two thirds of the cases. Lateral roentgen examination may help in the diagnosis of these hernias, as indicated by De Nicola and Vracin (1950). As Denisart (1951) has shown, closure of the neck of the sac followed by fascial closure of the foramen is the essential feature of operative repair. Occasionally, the sac can be peeled out of the mediastinum, but such a traumatic procedure may lead to hematoma or injury to the heart of the pleura. The abdominal approach is preferable. In most cases the operation is simple, and the results are excellent.

Obturator Hernia. Such a hernia passes through the obturator foramen or canal in the os inominatum. Watson collected 442 cases from the literature. In the cases in which the sex was given, females outnumbered males 5 to 1. It is of interest, as Anson, McCormack and Cleveland (1950) pointed out, that in a relatively restricted zone in the abdominopelvic wall, 4 areas of potential herniation occur. The upper 2 are inguinal (indirect and direct), the intermediate is femoral, and the lower is obturator. These follow an almost vertical line approximately 2 inches in height. Because the diagnosis of obturator hernia is difficult, treatment usually is applied only in late or complicated cases. Also, because of the unyielding nature of the internal opening of the canal, the strangulation rate in treated cases is extremely high. The combination in elderly women who have lost weight of generalized abdominal pain and rigidity, together with pain down the inner side of the thigh to the knee (Howship-Romberg sign), pain on movement of the hip and palpation of a mass on rectal examination, is characteristic of a strangulated obturator hernia (Rogers, 1964; Anson, 1964).

Surgical treatment is advised and can be by several routes:

1. The abdominal route with inversion of the sac. Muraro (1959) reported a successful operation for strangulated obturator hernia in a 73-year-old woman by this approach.

2. The obturator route, using a vertical incision beginning in the femoral region with the thigh flexed and retracting the pectineus muscle outward and the adductor longus inward. After inversion or ligation of the sac, aponeurotic flaps are utilized to close the defect.

3. A combined obturator-abdominal route.

4. An inguinal approach, which is recommended only for the nonstrangulated variety because it does not give enough room to deal with gangrenous bowel.

5. The anterior preperitoneal approach. (We used this in one case with good exposure resulting.)

The 2 chief features of obturator hernia are that diagnosis is very difficult before the onset of strangulation (and often misleading then), and that operative treatment is technically difficult.

Omphalocele (Umbilical Eventration). This congenital defect is a herniation of abdominal viscera into the base of the umbilical cord. The pouch is a thin translucent structure consisting only of peritoneum and amniotic membrane. Unlike its less severe counterpart, umbilical hernia, it has no skin covering. The average omphalocele is 6 to 8 cm. in diameter; the size makes considerable difference as to the prognosis. The underlying fascial opening is usually 4 to 5 cm. in diameter. The small intestine is included in the contents of almost all omphaloceles, although portions of the stomach, the spleen, the pancreas or the urinary bladder may also be included. The transverse colon participates in a third of the cases and the liver in half. Since the membrane is essentially avascular (except that the 3 umbilical vessels traverse its dome), it soon becomes infected, even if not ruptured, and prompt repair is mandatory.

The repair of omphaloceles is considered in Chapter 50, Pediatric Surgery.

Paraduodenal (Mesentericoparietal) Hernia. These congenital hernias have their orifices just below the ligament of Treitz. The hernia involves the space behind the mesentery, particularly the mesocolon. The sac may go to the right or the left, behind the ascending or the descending colon, respectively. In the case of left mesentericoparietal hernia, the inferior mesenteric arteries and veins course along the neck of the sac. In the case of right mesentericoparietal hernia, the superior mesenteric vessels do likewise. Hence, the neck of the sac cannot be split in either instance when reducing the hernia.

Pectineal Hernia (Cloquet's Hernia). This variety of femoral hernia was first described by Callisen (1777) and later in more detail by Cloquet (1817) and then by Fasano (1910), who collected 16 cases from the literature. It supposedly first enters the femoral canal and then perforates the aponeurosis of the pectineus muscle, rather than protruding through the saphenous opening as does the usual femoral hernia.

Peritoneoscopial Hernia. This is a late complication of peritoneoscopy (Levy, 1967). Similar hernias have been observed following stab wound drainage of the abdomen. Infection generally is a contributing factor.

Perineal Hernia. A perineal hernia is a protrusion of abdominal viscera through the muscles and the fascia of the outlet of the pelvis. Such hernias occur most frequently between the ages of 40 and 60 years. Anterior perineal hernias protrude anterior to the transverse perinei muscles and posterior perineal hernias posterior to the same. Anterior perineal hernias start as a defect in the levator ani, they usually contain bladder, and almost always they are found in women. Posterior perineal hernias start as a defect in the levator ani or in a gap between this muscle and the coccygeus, they usually contain ileum, and, while they may occur in men, they are 5 times as common in women. A third type is complete rectal prolapse (see Chap. 41, Anorectum; also see Chap. 51, Gynecology, regarding enterocele). Unlike obturator hernia, perineal hernia is usually reducible, and strangulation is infrequent. However, the condition is progressive, and operation, usually by the abdominal route, with sac inversion and ligation, is advised.

A perineal hernia (also called sacral) may occur following an abdominal perineal resection for rectal cancer. Its treatment, when indicated, is the reapproximation of the levator ani muscles, using a double row of interrupted suture material, one approximating the endofascia and exo-fascia (Bach-Nielson, 1967).

Posterolateral Hernia. This is a foramen of Bochdalek hernia.

Prevascular Hernia. This is a rare type of femoral hernia which is situated within the femoral sheath and anterior to the femoral vessels (Burton, 1950, 1953; Harkins, 1964b). Only when the neck of the sac extends laterally across the front of the iliac and the femoral vessels should the hernia be designated as prevascular. A hernia in which the neck traverses the femoral canal, the sac of which then deviates laterally across the femoral vessels, is a femoral hernia with lateral deviation. Turner (1953) reported a case of prevascular femoral hernia treated by means of a Cooper's ligament repair.

Reducible Hernia. One in which the sac contents can be put back into the cavity from which they originally protruded.

Retroanastomotic Hernia. A true "iatrogenic" condition, this complication may follow almost any anastomosis, but especially gastrojejunostomy. It can be stated—albeit tritely—that if all gastric anastomoses were performed *ad modum* Billroth I, there would be far fewer of these hernias.

Retrovascular Hernia. First described by Serafini in 1917, this is also called "Serafini's hernia." It is the exact opposite of a prevascular hernia (q.v.).

Richter's Hernia (partial enterocele, lateral pinching of the intestine, sometimes incorrectly called Littré's hernia). This is a strangulated hernia in which only a part of the circumference of the intestine is caught in the constricting ring. Since the original report by Richter in 1785, Orr (1950) reported that 126 cases have been described in the literature. The vast majority are femoral in location, with right-sided involvement being more frequent than left. Of all femoral hernias, only 0.7 per cent are of the Richter type. External perforation with fistula formation may result. Butters (1948) reported an incidence of 7 out of 45 *strangulated* femoral hernias (16%) as being of the Richter type. Hagan and Rhoads (1953) observed Richter's hernia in 0.65 per cent of their entire series or groin hernias. Of these 5 were femoral and 2 indirect inguinal hernias. Their figure for the over-all incidence of Richter's hernia agrees quite closely with that of Orr. Richter's hernia is particularly dangerous because intestinal obstruction is incomplete, even though strangulation of the outpouched bowel may be complete. Thus, signs and symptoms are slow in developing. The incidence is at least 5 per cent of strangulated hernias. Treatment is similar to that of other strangulated hernias, except that even greater care than usual must be exercised in preventing escape of the involved segment of bowel into the peritoneal cavity before the extent of necrosis can be assessed. If doubt as to bowel viability exists, the involved segment should be resected. In other respects the repair is similar to that of other femoral (or inguinal) hernias.

Sacrosciatic Hernia. A sciatic hernia.

Sciatic Hernia. A sciatic hernia is one that makes its exit through the greater or the lesser sacrosciatic foramen. Watson stated that it was the rarest of all hernias, and he was able to find only 35 cases reported in the literature. Such hernias involve all ages and both sexes almost equally. The protrusion is usually posterior below the fold of the buttock. While operation can be either by the abdominal or the sciatic approach (occasionally the combined approach is used), the former is preferable with inversion and ligation of the sac (Thomas, 1964).

Serafini's Hernia (see "Retrovascular Hernia").

Sliding Hernia (Hernia-en-glissade). These are inguinal hernias in which a portion of the wall is formed by a viscus that in its normal position is only partly covered by peritoneum (Walton, 1913). Moyer (1955) defines it as "an inguinal hernia containing retroperitoneal bowel." Usually the posterior wall consists of the cecum on the right, or of the sigmoid on the left. Thus, a sliding hernia involves the prolapse of a retroperitoneal or partially retroperitoneal structure (Figs. 42-23 to 42-25). Ryan (1956) divided sliding hernias into 3 types: (1) *intrasaccular*, in which the sliding component is free except for its mesentery, the peritoneum of which is continuous with that of the sac; (2) *parasaccular* (*intramural*), in which the sliding component lies in the wall of the sac, the peritoneum of the sac being in intimate contact with it so that the two cannot be separated without danger of injury to the sliding organ; and (3) *extrasaccular*, in

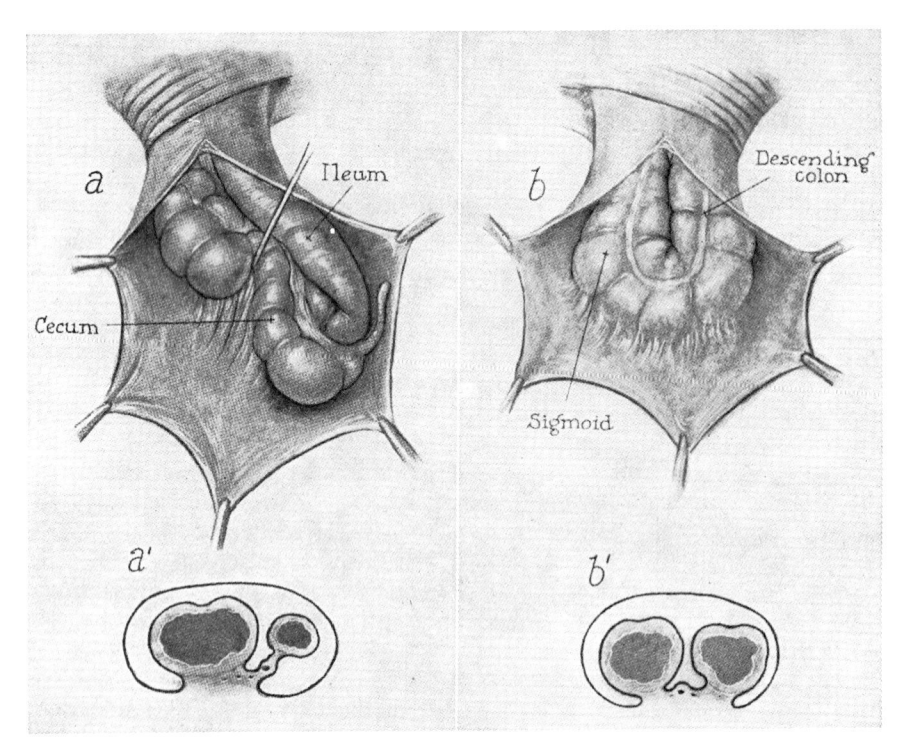

(*Left*) Fig. 42-23. Cross section of sliding hernia of cecum and ascending colon.
(*Right*) Fig. 42-24. Cross section of sliding hernia of descending colon and sigmoid.
(Bevan, A. D.: Ann. Surg., 92:754)

which the sliding element can be readily separated or may be distinctly separate from the sac, or there may be even no sac at all, the so-called sacless type. There is some doubt that Ryan's first type is a true sliding hernia, but this may be true in certain instances. In his series of 313 consecutive cases of sliding hernia, over 95 per cent were of the second (parasaccular) type, there being only one sacless sliding hernia.

Sliding hernia generally increases in incidence with advancing years. Males are more often affected, and in Ryan's series all 313 cases were in males. The incidence of sliding hernias relative to inguinal hernias is shown in Table 42-8.

The diagnosis of sliding hernia is difficult (large size, irreducibility, and difficulty in freeing the sac should alert one to be on the lookout for this complication) so that Bevan (1930), who had a large experience with the condition, stated that he could not remember making a diagnosis of sliding hernia before operation. A true sliding hernia must be differentiated at operation from a mere adhesion, as is often present when a supposed sliding hernia involves the small bowel. A sliding hernia is usually an indirect inguinal hernia and involves an actual downward prolapse of the viscus (cecum, sigmoid or bladder) with attached mesentery and posterior parietal peritoneum. Preoperative barium enema may show sigmoid (left) or cecum (right) in an irreducible hernia, indicating the probability of sliding.

Repair is more difficult than in a hernia of similar size without true "sliding." By one simple technic (Bevan, 1930) the first step consists of cutting the peritoneum along both sides of the mesenteric attachment. The blood supply of the colon should be carefully preserved. The second step consists of longitudinal suture of the diamond-shaped defect

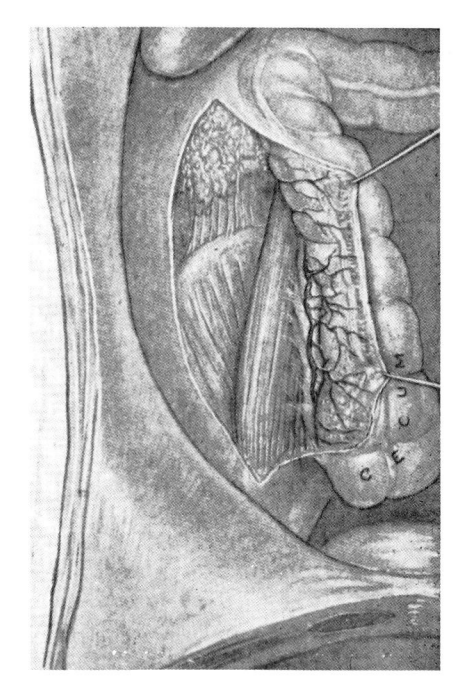

FIG. 42-25. Blood supply of sliding hernias on the right and the left, with incisions necessary to mobilize the bowel safely by dividing the outer avascular layer of the mesocolon. (Bevan, A. D.: Ann. Surg., 92:755)

produced (Fig. 42-26), utilizing essentially the Heineke-Mikulicz principle of transverse closure of a longitudinal defect. With careful attention to the principles of closure of the peritoneal defect, these hernias should not be attended by the high recurrence rate that they apparently have. Since high ligation of all hernial sacs is the first step in repair, and since this is difficult to do without freeing the prolapsed cecum or sigmoid first, this incidence of high recurrence rate is probably due largely to inadequate high sac ligation. Thus,

TABLE 42-8. INCIDENCE OF SLIDING HERNIA

AUTHOR	PERCENTAGE INCIDENCE	TYPE OF HERNIA CONSIDERED
Zimmerman and Anson (1953)	3.0	Indirect inguinal
Ryan (1956)	6.8	Indirect inguinal
Bevan (1930)	1.0	Inguinal
Burton and Blotner (1942)	1.0–2.0	Inguinal
Sensenig and Nichols (1955)	4.9	Inguinal
Ryan (1956)	5.1	Inguinal

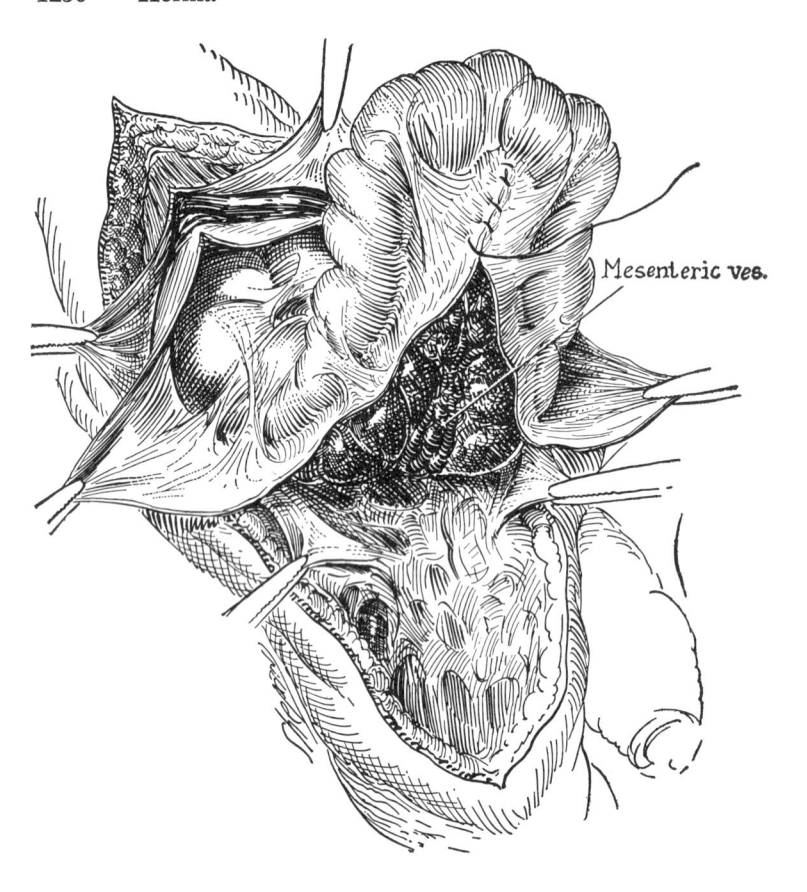

FIG. 42-26. Operation for sliding hernia of the large intestine. The intestinal loop and its mesentery have been freed and the sac trimmed along either side of the bowel as high as the neck of the sac. The peritoneal edges of the trimmed sac are being sutured together behind the bowel to form a new mesocolon. (Watson, L. F.: Hernia. ed. 3. St. Louis, C. V. Mosby)

indirect sliding hernias should not be reduced en bloc.

The simple Bevan technic by an inguinal approach outlined above is applicable to smaller sliding hernias, particularly on the right side. The Lyter method, also by an inguinal approach, of dealing with larger sliding hernias is as follows:

After opening the sac and determining that a sliding hernia is present, the cecum or mesosigmoid is separated from the vas deferens and the internal spermatic vessels to expose the iliacus (endo-abdominal) fascia covering the iliopsoas muscle. This is done through the already dilated internal ring, sometimes facilitated by a lateralward incision from the ring through the internal oblique and transversus muscles. In very difficult cases a second abdominal incision with traction on the prolapsed bowel may be advisable. Because of the high incidence of 55 per cent recurrence rate following the repair of 15 sliding hernias by the inguinal route alone, Hagan and Rhoads (1953) and Rhoads and Mackie (1964) stated that they now managed all such hernias by the combined inguino-abdominal approach. Moyer (1955) also advocated a laparotomy wound in these cases. The hernia then is reduced, and the retroperitoneal aspect of the cecum or mesosigmoid (or sigmoid itself) is carefully sutured to the iliacus fascia. Next, the anteromedial edge of the sac is sutured high to the lateral edge behind the cecum or sigmoid to close the peritoneum. The internal ring, including any lateral extension incision of its margin, is closed, and the inguinal floor is repaired in the usual manner.

The abdominal (La Roque) approach is also useful (Williams, 1947, 1964). The author of this chapter advocates a preperitoneal suprapubic approach for repairing the hernia with intraperitoneal handling of the bowel through the opened sac. Sensenig and Nichols (1955) reported only 13 per cent recurrence using the inguinal approach in 53 cases of sliding hernia, and preferred this to the combined approach. Ryan (1956) also preferred the inguinal approach, reporting a 1 per cent recurrence rate.

Sliding direct or (even more seldom) femoral hernias containing the bladder are rare, but they do occur. As mentioned in the section on direct hernias, reduction of a direct hernia en bloc without opening the direct sac is considered preferable in either the simple or the sliding variety.

Spigelian Hernia (Lateral Ventral Hernia, Hernia of the Linea Semilunaris). The fold of Douglas (linea semicircularis Douglasii) is a transverse fold somewhat below the umbilicus. Above, a portion of the internal oblique and all of the transversus abdominis aponeuroses lie deep to the rectus muscle; below, all the aponeuroses lie anterior to the rectus. The transition makes the fold. More laterally, the fold turns downward from its transverse direction near the mid-line, and fibers from it descend as pillars to insert on the pubis. The fold of Douglas has considerable surgical importance aside from the connotation regarding hernia. Above the fold, closure of medial abdominal incisions is different from that below the fold, because of the different arrangement of the aponeuroses.

The 2 lineae semilunaris Spigelii (named after the Flemish anatomist Adrian van der Spigelius, 1578-1625) are just lateral to the rectus. Each is vertical, but slightly convex outward, and extends from the cartilage of the 9th rib to the pubic spine. Each represents the transition of the internal oblique and the transversus abdominis muscles laterally to aponeuroses medially (Gould).

The crossing of the transverse fold of Douglas by the linea semilunaris on each side presents a weak point, the inadequacy of which may be compounded by the fact that the inferior deep epigastric vessels in their ascending course turn medially near or at this point to go behind the rectus muscle but superficial to the fold of Douglas. This crossroads of the two lines plus the penetration of the vessels is the site of spigelian hernias. Thus, these hernias are lateral to the rectus, medial to the muscular portion of the transversus, and below the fold of Douglas. Pull by the accessory slip of internal oblique (Chouke, 1938) may help to widen the opening.

Diagnosis should be made by palpating the area in question, which usually presents the chief complaints of tenderness and possibly a mass, with the patient supine and with the head off the pillow. In this way the abdominal wall is tense, and visceral tenderness can be excluded. Strangulation is frequent. The condition usually occurs in adults (River, 1942), but Hurwitt and Borow (1955) reported a case in an 8-year-old boy. Treatment involves inversion of the sac, aponeurotic suture and often a patch of tantalum mesh or cutis because of the weak aponeurotic structures in some patients with these hernias. There should be no hesitation about doubly ligating and dividing the deep epigastric vessels so that the hole may be sutured tightly. McVay (1954) stated that fine silk sutures were adequate, and that while the diagnosis was difficult, repair was easy and "there should be no recurrence."

Parenthetically, it should be pointed out that the medial variety of direct hernia represents a type of lateral ventral hernia, even though not spigelian in location.

Strangulated Hernia. One in which there is not only incarceration (syn.: *obstructed hernia*) but also either partial or complete occlusion of the blood supply and lymph drainage. Tardy or incorrect treatment of strangulated hernia is the major cause of death in this type of surgery. (See section on femoral hernia earlier in this chapter.)

Supravesical Hernia. This type of hernia was first described by Sir Astley Cooper in 1804. Further subdivisions of this rare entity into internal and external varieties are best understood by consulting Keynes (1964).

Traumatic Hernia of the Diaphragm. Such hernias are a common result of automobile accidents (Schneider, 1956); the tear may be at any point, although usually it is on the dome or posterior part of the left half of the diaphragm (69 out of 71 cases were on the left, Harrington, 1950); associated injuries are common; and repair is difficult because of pleural adhesions (cf. lack of adhesions in foramen of Bochdalek hernia). The condition is a common one and represented 13 per cent of a total of 435 diaphragmatic hernias repaired by Harrington (1950). This high figure is all the more remarkable when it is remembered that the Mayo Clinic does not have a large emergency service. The diagnosis usually is relatively simple. The decision as to time of operation (and operative approach) often depends on the associated injury, but generally it should be as early as possible. The approach preferably is thoracic (Schneider, 1964), especially on the right, thoracoabdominal if the reposition of the viscera is difficult or possibly abdominal on the left as advocated by Harrington. The repair should be with interrupted nonabsorbable sutures.

Velpeau's Hernia (see "Lacunar Ligament or Laugier's Hernia").

BIBLIOGRAPHY

MONOGRAPHS

There are several selected classic monographs on hernia which are available to the student of the subject. Watson (1948) and Zimmerman and Anson (1953) are good reference works, while McVay (1954) presents a good brief summary of up-to-date methods in atlas form. Some others are of historical interest or cover special aspects of the field. Among the monographs on hernia, the following are listed chronologically:

Richter, A. G.: Abhandlung von den Bruchen. Göttingen, Dieterich, 1785 (cited by Watson).
Marcy, Henry O.: The Anatomy and Surgical Treatment of Hernia. New York, Appleton, 1892.
Ferguson, Alexander H.: The Technic of Modern Operations for Hernia, Chicago, Cleveland Press, 1907.
Iason, Alfred H.: Hernia. Philadelphia, Blakiston, 1941.
Mair, George B.: The Surgery of Abdominal Hernia. Baltimore, Williams & Wilkins, 1948; London, Arnold, 1948.
Watson, Leigh F.: Hernia: Anatomy, Etiology, Symptoms, Diagnosis, Differential Diagnosis, Prognosis, and Treatment. ed. 3. St. Louis, C. V. Mosby, 1948.
Iason, Alfred H.: Synopsis of Hernia. New York, Grune & Stratton, 1949.
Vogeler, Karl: Chirurgie der Hernien. Berlin, de Gruyter, 1951.
Zimmerman, Leo M., and Anson, Barry J.: Anatomy and Surgery of Hernia. Baltimore, Williams & Wilkins, 1953.
McVay, Chester B.: Hernia: The Pathologic Anatomy of the More Common Hernias and Their Anatomic Repair. Springfield, Ill., Charles C Thomas, 1954.
Ogilvie, H.: Hernia. Baltimore, Williams & Wilkins, 1959.
Nissen, R., and Rossetti, M.: Die Behandlung von Hiatushernien und Refluxosophagitis mit Gastropexie und Fundoplicatio: Indikation, Technik und Ergebnisse. Stuttgart, Thieme, 1959.
Ravitch, M. M., and Hitzrot, J. M.: The Operations for Inguinal Hernia. St. Louis, C. V. Mosby, 1960.
Koontz, A. R.: Hernia. New York, Appleton, 1963.
Nyhus, L. M., and Harkins, H. N.: Hernia. Philadelphia, J. B. Lippincott, 1964.

JOURNAL AND OTHER REFERENCES

Journal references on the subject of hernia are also numerous. According to Watson, nearly 2 centuries ago, Georges Arnaud, the Parisian surgeon, published his treatise on hernia, and, in his preface, remarked that he planned a work embracing all that had been written on hernia. In the libraries of Paris alone, he transcribed 4,000 pages of writings on hernia before he abandoned his ambitious plan. The following references are selected because they represent classic contributions, in the case of some of the older ones, or are pertinent to present-day thought, in the case of some of the recent ones. All are referred to in the text.

Adler, R. H., and Firme, C. N.: Use of pliable synthetic mesh in the repair of hernias and tissue defects. Surg., Gynec. Obstet., 108:199-206, 1959.
Aird, I.: A Companion in Surgical Studies. ed. 2. pp. 653-654. Baltimore, Williams & Wilkins, 1957.
Ali, Munawar: Cutis strip and patch repair of large inguinal hernias. New Eng. J. Med., 251:932-934, 1954.
Allen, J. G.: Personal communication. April 30, 1955.
Allison, P. R.: Reflux esophagitis, sliding hiatal hernia, and the anatomy of repair. Surg., Gynec. Obstet., 92:419-431, 1951.
Andrews, E.: Personal communication. 1933.
Andrews, E., and Bissell, A. D.: Direct hernia: a record of surgical failures. Surg., Gynec. Obstet., 58:753-761, 1934.
Andrews, E. W.: Imbrication or lap joint method: a plastic operation for hernia. Chicago M. Rec., 9:67-77, 1895. Cited by Watson (see reference below), 1948.
Annandale, T.: Case in which a reducible oblique and direct inguinal and femoral hernia existed on the same side, and were successfully treated by operation. Edinburgh, M. J., 21:1087-1091, 1876.
Anson, B. J.: Anatomy of obturator hernia. In: Nyhus and Harkins (1964), op. cit.
Anson, B. J., McCormack, L. J., and Cleveland, H. C.: The anatomy of the hernial regions; III. obturator hernia and general considerations. Surg., Gynec. Obstet., 90:31-38, 1950.
Anson, B. J., Morgan, E. H., and McVay, C. B.: The anatomy of the hernial regions; I. inguinal hernia. Surg., Gynec. Obstet., 89:417-423, 1949.
Babcock, W. W.: The ideal in herniorrhaphy: a new method efficient for direct and indirect inguinal hernia. Surg., Gynec. Obstet., 45:534-540, 1927.
Bach-Nielsen, P.: New surgical method of repair of sacral hernia following abdominoperitoneal excision of the rectum. Acta chir. scand., 133:67-68, 1967.
Baritell, A. L. M.: A review of our experience with hernioplastic procedures. Permanente Found. M. Bull., 2:114-120, 1944.

Barrett, N. R.: Chronic peptic ulcer of the oesophagus and "oesophagitis." Brit. J. Surg., 38:175-182, 1950.

Bassini, E. (1888): Cited by Watson (see reference below), 1948.

———: Nuovo metodo operativo per la cura radicale dell'ernia crurale. Padua, Draghi, 1893. Cited by Spivack (see reference below), 1938.

Beardsley, J. M.: Esophageal hiatus hernia: repair from below. New Eng. J. Med., 254:409-412, 1956.

———: Transabdominal repair of esophageal hiatus hernia. Chap. 29. In: Nyhus and Harkins (1964), op. cit.

Berne, C. J.: Selective vagotomy and cardiofundoplasty for peptic esophagitis with hiatal hernia. In: Nyhus and Harkins (1964), op. cit.

Berry, W. C., Holbrook, J. P., Langdon, E. A., and Mathewson, C. W.: A study of hiatal hernias using pneumoperitoneum. U. S. Armed Forces M. J., 6:1715-1720, 1955; also Arch. Surg., 72: 1014-1017, 1956.

Bevan, A. D.: Sliding hernias of the ascending colon and cecum, the descending colon and sigmoid, and of the bladder. Ann. Surg., 92:754-760, 1930.

Birt, A. B.: Some views on femoral hernia and its treatment. Practitioner 159:362-368, 1947.

Blades, B., and Hall, E. R.: The consequences of neglected hiatal hernias. Ann. Surg., 143:822-832, 1956.

Boerema, I.: Fixation of reduced esophageal hiatus hernia by suturing the lesser curvature to the anterior geniculata). Abstr. J.A.M.A., 161:281-282, 1956.

———: Hiatal hernia: gastropexia anterior geniculata. Chap. 31. In: Nyhus and Harkins (1964), op. cit.

Boerema, I., and Germs, R.: Anterior geniculate gastropexy for hiatal hernia of the diaphragm. Zbl. Chir., 80:1585, 1955.

Borgström, S.: Recurrence rates of lateral inguinal hernia in adults. Acta chir. scand., 101:429-443, 1951.

Braasch, J. W., and Ellis, F. H., Jr.: The gastroesophageal sphincter mechanism: an experimental study. Surgery, 39:901-905, 1956.

Brown, R. K.: Umbilical hernia repair by layer closure of posterior and anterior rectus sheaths. Surg., Gynec. Obstet., 110:381-382, 1960.

Brown, R. K., and Galletti, G.: Bassini's contribution to our understanding of inguinal hernia. Surgery, 47:631-635, 1960.

Bryant, J. F.: Femoral hernias in infants and young children: Case report. Am. Surg., 31:200-201, 1965.

Burdick, C. G., and Higinbotham, N. L.: Division of the spermatic cord as an aid in operating on selected types of inguinal hernia. Ann. Surg., 102: 863-874, 1935.

Burton, C. C.: Hernias of the supravesical, inguinal, and lateral pelvic fossae: their diagnosis, classification, and relationship. Internat. Abstr. Surg., 91:1-16, 1950.

———: A suggested terminology for ligaments of the groin: their clinical and surgical application in repair of hernia. Surgery, 31:562-574, 1952.

———: Inguinopectineal hernias—a classification and correlation. Internat. Abstr. Surg., 97:417-431, 1953.

———: The combined Cooper's ligament and inguinal ligament hernia repair. Surg., Gynec. Obstet., 98:153-160, 1954.

———: The critical point of Cooper's ligament hernia repair. Am. J. Surg., 91:215-226, 1956.

Burton, C. C., and Blotner, C.: Sliding and other large bowel herniae: development, classification and operative management. Ann. Surg., 116:394-404, 1942.

Butters, A. G.: A review of femoral herniae with special reference to the recurrence rate of the low operation. Brit. M. J., 2:743-745, 1948.

Callisen, H.: Herniorum rariorum biga acta societatis medicae hafniae. Hanniae, 2:321, 1777. Cited by Watson (see reference below), 1948.

Cannaday, J. E.: The use of the cutis graft in the repair of certain types of incisional herniae and other conditions. Ann. Surg., 115:775-781, 1942.

Carey, J. M., and Hollinshead, W. H.: An anatomic study of the esophageal hiatus. Surg., Gynec. Obstet., 100:196:200, 1955a.

———: Anatomy of the esophageal hiatus related to repair of hiatal hernia. Proc. Mayo Clin., 30: 223-226, 1955b.

Carlson, R. I.: The historical development of the surgical treatment of inguinal hernia. Surgery, 39:1031-1046, 1956.

Carter, B. N., and Giuseffi, J.: Strangulated diaphragmatic hernia. Ann. Surg., 128:210-225, 1948.

Chassin, J. L.: The subcutaneous inguinal ring: a clinical study. Surgery, 22:540-544, 1947.

Cheatle, G. L.: An operation for the radical cure of inguinal and femoral hernia. Brit. M. J., 2:68-69, 1920.

———: An operation for inguinal hernia. Brit. M. J., 2:1025-1026, 1921.

Cherney, L. S.: Intestinal stenosis following strangulated hernia. Ann. Surg., 148:991-993, 1958.

Chouke, K. S. (1938): Cited by River, L. P. (see reference below), 1942.

Clark, J. H., and Hashimoto, E. I.: Utilization of Henle's ligament iliopubic tract, aponeurosis transversus abdominis and Cooper's ligament in inguinal herniorrhaphy: a report of 162 consecutive cases. Surg., Gynec. Obstet., 82:480-484, 1946.

Clatworthy, H. W., Jr., and Thompson, A. G.: Incarcerated and strangulated inguinal hernia in infants: a preventable risk. J.A.M.A., 154:123-126, 1954.

Clear, J. J.: Ten year statistical study of inguinal hernias. Arch. Surg., 62:70-78, 1951.

Cloquet, J.: Recherches anatomiques sur les hernies de l'abdomen. p. 225, Thése, Paris, 1817. Cited by Cox, R.: Aust. N. Zeal. J. Surg., 31:318-321, 1962.

Cole, P. P.: The filigree operation for inguinal hernia. Brit. J. Surg., 29:168-181, 1941.

Collins, J. D.: A method of disposal of the sac in operations for oblique inguinal hernia. Ann. Surg., 115:761-767, 1942.

Condon, R. E.: The anatomy of the inguinal region

and its relationship to groin hernias. Chap. 2. *In*: Nyhus and Harkins (1964), *op. cit.*

Connolly, D. P., and Perri, F. R.: Giant hernias managed by pneumoperitoneum. J.A.M.A., 209: 771-774, July 7, 1969.

Cooper, A.: The Anatomy and Surgical Treatment of Inguinal and Congenital Hernia. ed. 1. London, Longman & Co., 1804.

Council, A.M.A., Report of: Present status of injection treatment of hernia. J.A.M.A., 115:533-534, 1940.

Davis, C. E., Jr.: Littré's hernia. Ann. Surg., 139: 370, 1954.

DeNicola, R. R., and Vracin, D. J.: Diaphragmatic hernia through the foramen of Morgagni. J. Pediat., 36:100-104, 1950.

Denisart, P.: De la variété rétro-costo-xiphoïdienne des hernies diaphragmatiques. J. chir., 67:407-427, 1951.

Dennis, C., and Enquist, I. F.: Strangulating external hernia. Chap. 17. *In*: Nyhus and Harkins (1964), *op. cit.*

Dennis, C., and Varco, R. L.: Femoral hernia with gangrenous bowel. Surgery, 22:312-323, 1947.

DeVito, R. V., Listerud, M. B., Nyhus, L. M., Merendino, K. A., and Harkins, H. N.: Hemorrhage as a complication of reflux esophagitis. Am. J. Surg., 98:657-663, 1959.

Dillard, D. H.: Mechanism of sphincteric failure in sliding hiatal hernia. *In*: Nyhus and Harkins (1964), *op. cit.*

Donald, D. C.: The value derived from utilizing the component parts of the transversalis fascia and Cooper's ligament in the repair of large indirect and direct inguinal hernia: a group of cases. Surgery, 24:662-676, 1948.

Doran, F. S. A.: Inguinal herniorrhaphy. Lancet, 2:1307-1314, 1955.

———: Nylon net in the treatment of inguinal hernias. Chap. 52. *In*: Nyhus and Harkins (1964), *op. cit.*

Doran, F. S. A., and Lonsdale, W. H.: A simple experimental method of evaluation for the Bassini and allied types of herniorrhaphy. Brit. J. Surg., 36:339-345, 1949.

Easton, E. R.: The incidence of femoral hernia following repair of inguinal hernia—ectopic recurrence: a proposed operation of external and internal herniorrhaphy. J.A.M.A., 100:1741-1744, 1933.

Elman, R.: Editorial: the hernia problem. Arch. Surg., 65:807-808, 1952.

Enquist, I. F., and Dennis, C.: The management of strangulating external hernias. S. Clin. N. Am., 35:429-439, 1955.

Erwald, R., and Rieger, A.: Tantalum mesh in hernial repair. Acta chir. scand., 119:55-59, 1960.

Estes, W. L., Jr., and Charnock, M. P.: Industrial hernia. Chap. 55. *In*: Nyhus and Harkins (1964), *op. cit.*

Fallis, L. S.: Recurrent inguinal hernia: an analysis of 200 operations. Ann. Surg., 106:363-372, 1937.

———: Direct inguinal hernia. Ann. Surg., 107:572-581, 1938.

Farris, J. M.: Umbilical hernia. Chap. 20. *In*: Nyhus and Harkins (1964), *op. cit.*

Fasano, M.: Dell'ernia crurale pettinea del Cloquet. Clin. chir., 18:883-898, 1910.

Ferguson, A. H.: Oblique inguinal hernia: typical operation for its radical cure. J.A.M.A., 33:6-14, 1899.

Fisher, H. C.: The surgical repair of inguinal hernia in infants and children. Rocky Mountain M. J., 48:424-426, 1951.

Fitzgerald, P., and Mehigan, J. E.: A complication resulting from the use of a rigid inlay in the repair of an inguinal hernia. Brit. J. Surg., 46:422, 1959.

Fowler, R., Jr., and Stephens, F. D.: The role of testicular vascular anatomy in the salvage of high undescended testes. Aust. N. Zeal. J. Surg., 29: 92-106, 1959.

Galletti, G., and Brown, R. K.: Halsted's operation for inguinal hernia. Exactly what is it? Surgery, 47:633-635, 1960.

Gallie, W. E., and Le Mesurier, A. B.: The use of living sutures in operative surgery. Canad. M.A.J., 11:504-513, 1921.

Gilmore, W. E.: A technical aid in bilateral inguinal herniorrhaphy in infants and children. Surg., Gynec. Obstet., 110:501-502, 1960.

Ginzburg, L., and Freund, S.: Hernias of supravesical fossa presenting externally through the conjoined tendon. Surg., Gynec. Obstet., 99:295-300, 1954.

Goñi Moreno, I.: XII Congreso Argentino de Cirurgia, pp. 85-87, 1940. Cited by Koontz and Graves (see reference below), 1954.

———: The rational treatment of hernia and voluminous chronic eventrations: preparation with progressive pneumoperitoneum. Chap. 47. *In*: Nyhus and Harkins (1964), *op. cit.*

Graham, E.: Editorial comment: diaphragmatic hernia through esophageal hiatus. *In*: Year Book of General Surgery, 1954. Chicago, Year Book Pub., 1954.

Griffith, C. A.: Inguinal hernia: an anatomic-surgical correlation. S. Clin. N. Am., 39:531-556, 1959.

Gross, R. E.: The Surgery of Infancy and Childhood: Its Principles and Techniques. Philadelphia, W. B. Saunders, 1953.

Guy, C. C., Werelius, C. Y., and Bell, L. B., Jr.: Five years' experience with tantalum mesh in hernia repair. S. Clin. N. Am., 35:175-188, 1955.

Hagan, W. H., and Rhoads, J. E.: Inguinal and femoral hernias. Surg., Gynec. Obstet., 96:226-232, 1953.

Halsted, W. S.: The radical cure of hernia. Bull. Johns Hopkins Hosp., 1:12, 1889.

———: The cure of the more difficult as well as the simpler inguinal ruptures. Bull. Johns Hopkins Hosp., 14:208-214, 1903.

———: The radical cure of inguinal hernia in the male. Bull. Johns Hopkins Hosp., 4:17-24, 1893.

Harkins, H. N.: A Cooper's ligament herniotomy; clinical experience in 322 consecutive cases. S. Clin. N. Am., 23:1279-1297, 1943.

———: Cutis grafts: clinical and experimental studies on their use as a reinforcing patch in the

repair of large ventral and incisional herniae. Ann. Surg., 122:996-1015, 1945.
———: The repair of groin hernias: progress in the past decade. S. Clin. N. Am., 29:1457-1482, 1949.
———: Recent advances in the treatment of hernia. Ann. West. Med. Surg., 6:221-225, 1952.
———: The Cooper's ligament repair of direct inguinal hernia. Chap. 10. *In*: Nyhus and Harkins (1964), *op. cit.* (a).
———: Prevascular and other special varieties of femoral hernia. Chap. 15. *In*: Nyhus and Harkins (1964), *op. cit.* (b).
Harkins, H. N., and Schug, R. H.: Hernial repair using Cooper's ligament: follow-up studies on 367 operations. Arch. Surg., 55:689-708, 1947.
Harkins, H. N., Szilagyi, D. E., Brush, B. E., and Williams, R.: Clinical experiences with the McVay herniotomy. Surgery, 12:364-377, 1942.
Harrington, S. W.: Subcostosternal diaphragmatic hernias (foramen of Morgagni). Tr. West. S. A., pp. 332-356, 1940.
———: Diaphragmatic hernia. *In*: Cyclopedia of Medicine, Surgery and Specialties. Philadelphia, F. A. Davis, 1950.
———: Clinical manifestations and surgical treatment of congenital types of diaphragmatic hernia. Rev. Gastroenterol., 18:243-256, 1951.
———: Esophageal hiatal diaphragmatic hernia. Surg., Gynec. Obstet., 100:277-292, 1955.
———: Discussion of paper by Blades and Hall. Ann. Surg., 143:831-832, 1956.
———: Early experiences with diaphragmatic hernia. *In*: Nyhus and Harkins (1964), *op. cit.*
Hayward, J.: Sliding esophageal hiatus hernia. Chap. 27. *In*: Nyhus and Harkins (1964), *op. cit.*
Heifetz, C. J.: Inguinal hernias: management of these hernias of infancy and childhood. M. Times, 81:238-243, 1953.
Heifetz, C. J., and Goldfarb, A.: Division of the spermatic cord as an aid in the repair of recurrent and other difficult inguinal hernias. J. Internat. Coll. Surgeons, 28:498-512, 1952.
Helsby, R., and Wells, C.: Subcosternal hernia (hernia through the formamen of Morgagni): report of a case. Brit. J. Surg., 42:274-275, 1954.
Henry, A. K.: Operation for femoral hernia by a midline extraperitoneal approach: with a preliminary note on the use of this route for reducible inguinal hernia. Lancet: 1:531-533, 1936.
———: The extraperitoneal approach in femoral hernia. *In*: Nyhus and Harkins (1964, *op. cit.*
Herrington, J. L., Jr., Edwards, W. H., and Sawyers, J. L.: A physiologic and anatomic approach to the surgical treatment of sliding esophageal hiatus hernia. J. Tenn. M. A., 56:465-469, 1963.
Hesselbach, F. K: Anatomisch—chirurgische Abhandlung über den Ursprung der Leistenbrüche. Würzburg, Baumgärtner, 1806.
Hey Groves, E. W.: A note on the operation for the radical cure of femoral hernia. Brit. J. Surg., 10:529-531, 1923.
Hicks, E. S.: Inguinal hernia. Canad. M.A.J., 45:134-136, 1941.
Hillemand, P., and Watteblede: Une affection fréquente et trop méconnue: la hernie diaphragmatique de l'hiatus oesophagien. Presse méd., 61:886, 1953.
Hoguet, J. P.: Direct inguinal hernia. Ann. Surg.. 72:671-674, 1920.
Holcomb, G. W.: Incarcerated inguinal hernia in infants and children: a preventable condition. J. Tenn. M.A., 49:37, 1956.
Hurwitt, E. S., and Borow, M.: Bilateral spigelian hernias in childhood. Surgery, 37:963-968, 1955.
Iason, A. H.: Medicolegal aspects of hernia. Chap. 54. *In*: Nyhus and Harkins (1964), *op. cit.*
Jesseph, J. E.: Hernia in the aged. Chap. 18. *In*: Nyhus and Harkins (1964) *op. cit.*
Keynes, W. M.: Supravesical hernia. Chap. 41. *In*: Nyhus and Harkins (1964), *op. cit.*
Kiesewetter, W. B., and Parenzan, L.: When should hernia in the infant be treated bilaterally? J.A.M.A., 171:287-290, 1959.
Knott, J. I.: The second side inguinal hernia and routine transpubic exposure. Am. J. Surg., 87:97-100, 1954.
———: The enlarged inguinal ring and its significance. *In*: Nyhus and Harkins (1964), *op. cit.*
Kohli, D. R., and Pearson, C. C.: A study of hiatus hernia. Gastroenterology, 23:294-300, 1953.
Koontz, A. R.: Preliminary report on the use of tantalum mesh in the repair of ventral hernias. Ann. Surg., 127:1079-1085, 1948.
———: Some common fallacies and confusions with regard to repair of inguinal hernia. J.A.M.A., 141:366-369, 1949.
———: The inguinal hernia problem. Mil. Surgeon, 115:93-100, 1954.
———: Failure with tantalum gauze in ventral hernia repair. Arch. Surg., 70:123-127, 1955a.
———: An operation for massive incisional lumbar hernia. Surg., Gynec. Obstet., 101:119-121, 1955b.
———: Views on the choice of operation for inguinal hernia repair. Ann. Surg., 143:868-880, 1956.
———: Historical analysis of femoral hernia. Surgery, 53:551, 1963.
———: Tantalum mesh in hernia repair. Chap. 50. *In*: Nyhus and Harkins (1964), *op. cit.*
Koontz, A. R., and Graves, J. W.: Preoperative pneumoperitoneum as an aid in the handling of gigantic hernias. Ann. Surg., 140:759-762, 1954.
Koontz, A. R., and Kimberly, R. C.: Tissue reactions to tantalum mesh and wire. Ann. Surg., 131:666-686, 1950.
Koontz, A. R., and Stafford, E. S.: Unusual types of interparietal hernia. Arch. Surg., 71:723-726, 1955.
Laimer, E.: Beitrag zur Anatomie des Oesophagus. Med. Jahrb. Wien., pp. 333-338, 1883.
Lam, C. R.: Personal communication. November 16, 1954.
Lam, C. R., and Kenney, L. J.: The problem of the hiatus hernia of diaphragm. J. Thoracic Surg., 27:1-12, 1954.
Lam, C. R., Szilagyi, D. E., and Puppendahl, M.: Tantalum gauze in the repair of large postoperative ventral hernias. Arch. Surg., 57:234-244, 1948.
La Roque, G. P.: The permanent cure of inguinal and femoral hernia: a modification of the standard

operative procedures. Surg., Gynec. Obstet., 29:507-510, 1919.

———: The intra-abdominal operation for femoral hernia. Ann. Surg., 75:110-112, 1922.

Larsen, R. M.: Inguinal hernia in infancy and early childhood. Surgery: 25:307-328, 1949.

Laugier, M. (1883): Cited by Priesching (see reference below), 1956.

Lawrence, K. B.: Fatal intestinal obstruction following injection treatment of an inguinal hernia. New Eng. J. Med., 238:397-398, 1948.

Lendrum, F. C.: Anatomic features of the cardiac orifice of the stomach, with special reference to cardiospasm. Arch. Int. Med., 59:474-511, 1937.

Levy, A. H., Wren, R. S., and Friedman, M. N.: Complications and recurrences following inguinal hernia repair. Ann. Surg., 133:533-539, 1951.

Levy, M.: A late complication of peritoneoscopy. Gastroint. Endosc., 14:117-119, 1967.

Listerud, M. B., and Harkins, H. N.: Anatomy of the esophageal hiatus. Arch. Surg., 76:835-842, 1958.

———: Variations in the muscular anatomy of the esophageal hiatus: based on dissections of two hundred and four fresh cadavers. West. J. Surg., 67:110-113, 1959.

Littré (1700): Cited by Watson (see reference below), 1948.

Loewe, O.: Über Hautimplantation an Stelle der Freien Faszienplastik. München. med. Wschr., 60: 1320-1321, 1913.

Lotheissen, G.: Zur Radikaloperation der Schenkelhernien. Zbl. Chir., 25:548-550, 1898.

Low, A.: A note on the crura of the diaphragm and the muscle of Treitz. J. Anat. Physiol., 42: 93-96, 1907.

Lower, W. E., and Hicken, N. F.: Interparietal hernias. Ann. Surg., 94:1070-1087, 1931.

Lucas-Championnière, J. (1892): Cited by Koontz (see reference above), 1949.

Lyter, C. S.: Cited by Griffith (see reference above), 1959.

Lytle, W. J.: A history of hernia. Med. Press. Vol. 232. No. 6034, Dec., 1954.

McArthur, L. L.: Autoplastic suture in hernia and other diseases; preliminary report. J.A.M.A., 37: 1162-1165, 1901.

McClure, R. D., and Fallis, L. S.: Femoral hernia; report of 90 operations. Ann. Surg., 109:987-1000, 1939.

McEvedy, P. G.: Femoral hernia. Ann. Roy. Coll. Surgeons, 7:484-496, 1950.

MacGregor, W. W.: The demonstration of a true internal sphincter and its etiologic role in hernia. Surg., Gynec. Obstet., 49:510-515, 1929.

———: The fundamental operative treatment of inguinal hernia. Surg., Gynec. Obstet., 50:438-440, 1930.

———: Observations on the surgical treatment of hernia. Ann. Surg., 122:878-884, 1945.

———: Surgical repair of inguinal hernia based upon closure of internal inguinal sphincter. Grace Hosp. Bull., 117:125, 1949.

MacKenzie, W. C.: Why do inguinal hernias recur? Paper given before the Annual Meeting, Washington State Medical Association, Seattle, Sept. 13, 1955.

McLaughlin, C. W., Jr., and Coe, J. D.: Inguinal hernia in pediatric patients. Am. J. Surg., 99:45-47, 1960.

McVay, C. B.: An anatomic error in current methods of inguinal herniorrhaphy. Ann. Surg., 113:1111-1112, 1941.

———: Personal communication. February 21, 1947.

———: Inguinal and femoral hernioplasty. Minnesota Med., 32:599-607, 1949.

———: Femoral hernioplasty: the inguinal approach. Chap. 14. In: Nyhus and Harkins (1964), op. cit.

McVay, C. B., and Anson, B. J.: A fundamental error in current methods of inguinal herniorrhaphy. Surg., Gynec. Obstet., 74:746-750, 1942.

———: Inguinal and femoral hernioplasty. Surg., Gynec. Obstet., 88:473-485, 1949.

McVay, C. B., and Savage, L. E.: The relaxing incision in inguinal hernioplasty. Chap. 12. In: Nyhus and Harkins (1964), op. cit.

Madden, J. L.: Anatomic and technical considerations in the treatment of esophageal hiatal hernia. Surg., Gynec. Obstet., 102:187-194, 1956.

Mair, G. B.: The use of whole skin grafts as a substitute for fascial sutures in the treatment of hernias: preliminary report. Am. J. Surg., 69:352-365, 1945.

Marshall, S. B.: Indirect inguinal hernia and the internal ring. U.S. Armed Forces M. J., 11:191-198, 1960.

Mason, E. A.: Pneumoperitoneum in the management of giant hernia. Surgery, 39:143-151, 1956.

Merendino, K. A., Johnson, R. J., Skinner, H. H., and Maguire, R. X.: The intradiaphragmatic distribution of the phrenic nerve with particular reference to the placement of diaphragmatic incisions and controlled segmental paralysis. Surgery, 39: 189-198, 1956.

Merendino, K. A., Varco, R. L., and Wangensteen, O. H.: Displacement of the esophagus into a new diaphragmatic orifice in the repair of paraesophageal and esophageal hiatus hernia. Ann. Surg., 129:185-197, 1949.

Mikkelsen, W. P., and Berne, C. J.: Femoral hernioplasty: suprapubic extraperitoneal (Cheatle-Henry) approach. Surgery, 35:743-748, 1954.

Moloney, G. E.: Nylon yarn in hernia repair, Chap. 51. In: Nyhus and Harkins (1964), op. cit.

Moloney, G. E., Gill, W. G., and Barclay, R. C.: Operations for hernia: technique of nylon darn. Lancet, 2:45-48, 1948.

Monro, A. K.: Strangulated femoral hernia. In: Maingot, Rodney: Techniques in British Surgery, Philadelphia, W. B. Saunders, 1950a.

———: The treatment of inguinal hernia. In: Maingot, Rodney: Techniques in British Surgery. Philadelphia, W. B. Saunders, 1950.

———: Femoral hernia: the lower approach. Chap. 13. In: Nyhus and Harkins (1964), op. cit.

Morris, K. N.: Gastric mucosa within the oesophagus. Aust. N. Zeal. J. Surg., 25:24-30, 1955.

Moschcowitz, A. V.: Femoral hernia: a new operation for the radical cure. New York J. Med., 7:396-400, 1907.

Moyer, C. A.: Personal communication. January 23, 1955.
———: Personal communication. July 13, 1960.
Moyer, C. A., and Butcher, H. R., Jr.: Experiences with pneumoperitoneum for massive ventral hernias. In: Nyhus and Harkins (1964), op. cit.
Muller, C. J. B.: Hiatus hernia, diverticula and gall stones: Saint's triad. South African M.J., 22:376-382, 1948.
Muraro, U.: Strangulated obturator hernia. Riforma med., 73:332-336, 1959; Abstr. J.A.M.A., 170:1852, 1959.
Nauta, J.: En studie van het afsluitingsmechanisme tussen slokdarm en maag. Leiden, H. E. Stenfert Kroese N. V., 1955.
———: Movements of the lower oesophageal segment: the cardiac mechanism. Bull. Soc. Int. Chir., 15:97-110, 1956.
Nelson, T. Y.: Hiatus hernia in infants and children. Aust. N. Zeal. J. Surg., 22:192-197, 1953.
Neuman, H. W., Ellis, F. H., Jr., and Andersen, H. A.: Eventration of the diaphragm. Proc. Staff Meet. Mayo Clin., 30:310-318, 1955.
Nissen, R.: Die Gastropexie als alleiniger Eingriff bei Hiatushernien. Deutsch. med. Wschr., 81:185, 1956.
———: The treatment of hiatal hernia and esophageal reflux by fundoplication. Chap. 30. In: Nyhus and Harkins (1964), op. cit.
Nyhus, L. M.: An anatomic reappraisal of the posterior inguinal wall: Special considerations of the iliopubic tract and its relation to groin hernias. S. Clin. N. Am., 44:1305-1313, 1964a.
———: The preperitoneal approach and iliopubic tract repair of all groin hernias. Chap. 19. In: Nyhus and Harkins (1964), op. cit. (b).
Nyhus, L. M., Condon, R. E., and Harkins, H. N.: Clinical experiences with the preperitoneal hernia repair for all types of groin hernia: with particular reference to the importance of transversalis fascia analogues. Am. J. Surg., 100:234-244, 1960.
O'Connor, F. J., and Ritvo, M.: Diagnosis of hiatus hernia on plain roentgenograms of thorax and abdomen. J.A.M.A., 157:113-117, 1955.
Ogilvie, W. H.: Hernia in Maingot, R.: Postgraduate Surgery. Vol. 3, p. 3637. New York, Appleton, 1937.
Olch, P. D., and Harkins, H. N.: Historical survey of the treatment of inguinal hernia. Chap. 1. In: Nyhus and Harkins (1964), op. cit.
Olson, H. H., Kanar, E. A., and Harkins, H. N.: The use of wire markers in Cooper's ligament hernia repairs with roentgenologic studies; report of 72 hernioplasties. Surgery, 36:270-277, 1954.
Orr, T. G., Jr.: Richter's hernia. Surg., Gynec. Obstet., 91:705-708, 1950.
Owen, H. W., Kirklin, J. W., and DuShane, J. W.: Femoral hernias in infants and young children. Surgery, 36:283-285, 1954.
Packard, G. B., and McLauthlin, C. H.: Treatment of inguinal hernia in infancy and childhood. Surg., Gynec. Obstet., 97:603-607, 1953.
Palmer, E. D.: Saint's triad: hiatus hernia, diverticulosis coli and gallstones. Am. J. Digest. Dis., 18:240-241, 1951.
Palumbo, L. T., and Mighell, S. J.: Primary direct inguinal hernioplasty. Surgery, 36:278-282, 1954.

Petrovsky, B. V., and Kanshin, N. N.: The problem of the surgical treatment of sliding hiatus hernias and a shortened esophagus. Chap. 32. In: Nyhus and Harkins (1964), op. cit.
Phetteplace, C. H.: The intra-abdominal (La Roque) approach to hernioplasty. West. J. Surg., 63:490-496, 1955.
Pitkänen, A.: The relation of incisional and inguinal herniae as well as of mechanical intestinal disturbances to previous operations for appendicitis with peritonitis. Acta chir. scand. (Supp. 138), 96:1-166, 1948.
Ponka, J. L., Wylie, J. H., Chäikof, L., Sergeant, C., and Brush, B. E.: Marlex mesh—a new plastic mesh for the repair of hernia. Henry Ford Hosp. M. Bull., 7:278-280, 1959.
Potts, W. J., Riker, W. L., and Lewis, J. E.: The treatment of inguinal hernia in infants and children. Ann. Surg., 132:566-576, 1950.
Priesching, A.: Laugerische Hernia. Arch. klin. Chir., 281:411-419, 1956.
Querna, M. H.: Reduction of hernia en masse: a cause of intestinal obstruction. Paper presented before Annual Meeting, North Pacific Surgical Association, Portland, Ore., Nov. 18, 1955.
Ravitch, M.: The great Boston hernia controversy concerning the permanent cure of reducible hernia or rupture. Bull. N.Y. Acad. Med., 45:767-798, 1969.
Rhoads, J. E., and Mackie, J. A.: Sliding inguinal hernia. In: Nyhus and Harkins (1964), op. cit.
Rienhoff, W. F.: The use of the rectus fascia for closure of the lower or critical angle of the wound in the repair of inguinal hernia. Surgery, 8:326-339, 1940.
Ritchey, J. O., and Winsauer, H. J.: Anemia and its relation in diaphragmatic hernia. Am. J. Med. Sci., 214:476-482, 1947.
River, L. P.: Spigelian hernia: spontaneous lateral ventral hernia through the semilunar line. Ann. Surg., 116:405-411, 1942.
Rogers, F. A.: Strangulated femoral hernia: a review of 170 cases. Ann. Surg., 149:9-20, 1959.
———: Strangulated obturator hernia: Chap. 42. In: Nyhus and Harkins (1964), op. cit.
Rothenburg, R. E., and Barnett, T.: Bilateral herniotomy in infants and children. Surgery, 37:947-950, 1955.
Ruggi, G. (1892): Cited by Koontz, A. R. (see reference above), 1956.
Ryan, E. A.: Recurrent hernias: an analysis of 369 consecutive cases of recurrent inguinal and femoral hernias. Surg., Gynec. Obstet., 96:343-354, 1953.
———: An analysis of 313 consecutive cases of indirect sliding inguinal hernias. Surg., Gynec. Obstet., 102:45-58, 1956.
Satinsky, V. P., and Kron, S. D.: Transposition of cartilage for repair of large ventral hernia. J. Albert Einstein M. Center, 1:109-113, 1953.
Schneider, C. F.: Traumatic diaphragmatic hernia. Am. J. Surg., 91:290-297, 1956.
———: Traumatic hernia of the diaphragm. Chap. 36. In: Nyhus and Harkins (1964), op. cit.
Schofield, T. L.: Polyvinyl alcohol sponge: an inert

plastic for use as a prosthesis in the repair of large hernias. Brit. J. Surg., 42:618-621, 1955.

Sensenig, D. M., and Nichols, J. B.: Sliding hernias: a follow-up study. Arch. Surg., 71:756-760, 1955.

Serafini, G.: Sulle varietà dell'ernia crurale e particolarmente sull'ernia crurale retrovascolare intravaginale e sull'ernia pettina. Policlinico sez. chir. 24:230, 264, 273, 1917.

Smith, G. A., Moore, J. R., and Perry, J. F., Jr.: Intestinal obstructions due to external hernia. Arch. Surg., 71:260-264, 1955.

Smith, I.: Irreducible inguinal herniae in children: gangrenous bowel in a 25-day-old infant. Brit. J. Surg., 42:271-274, 1954.

Smith, R. S.: The uses of tantalum mesh in hernia repair. West. J. Surg., 62:1-6, 1954.

———: Adjuncts in hernial repair. Arch. Surg., 78: 868-877, 1959.

———: The use of adjuncts in hernia repair. Basic principles, Chap. 48. In: Nyhus and Harkins (1964), op. cit.

Snyder, W. H., Jr., and Chaffin, L.: Inguinal hernia complicated by undescended testis. Am. J. Surg., 90:325-330, 1955.

Spivack, J.: The Surgical Technic of Abdominal Operations. Chicago, Debour, 1938.

Stensrud, N.: Hiatus hernias. Acta chir. scand., 107: 57-71, 1954.

Strahan, A. W. B.: Hernial repair by whole-skin graft with report on 413 cases. Brit. J. Surg., 38: 276-284, 1951.

Strode, J. E.: The use of fascia lata grafts in inguinal hernia repair. Chap. 49. In: Nyhus and Harkins (1964), op. cit.

Swartz, W. T.: Lumbar hernias. J. Kentucky M. A., 52:673-678, 1954.

Sweet, R. H.: Esophageal hiatus hernia of the diaphragm: the anatomical characteristics, technic of repair, and results of treatment in 111 consecutive cases. Ann. Surg., 135:1-13, 1952.

Swenson, S. A., Jr.: Cutis grafts: clinical and experimental observations. Arch. Surg., 61:881-889, 1950.

Swenson, S. A., Jr., and Harkins, H. N.: Cutis grafts; application of the dermatome-flap method: its use in a case of recurrent incisional hernia. Arch. Surg., 47:564-570, 1943a.

———: The surgical treatment of recurrent inguinal hernia with special reference to a Cooper's ligament herniotomy and the use of free fascial grafts. Surgery, 14:807-818, 1943b.

Tanner, N.: A "slide" operation for inguinal and femoral hernia. Brit. J. Surg., 29:285-289, 1942.

———: Personal communication. July, 1955b.

———: Treatment of oesophageal hiatus hernia. Lancet, 2:1050-1055, 1955b.

Thomas, G. I.: Sciatic hernia. Chap. 43. In: Nyhus and Harkins (1964), op. cit.

Throckmorton, T. D.: Tantalum gauze in the repair of hernias complicated by tissue deficiency: a preliminary report. Surgery, 23:32-46, 1948.

Touroff, A. S. W.: Phrenicectomy as aid to repair of large abdominal hernias. J.A.M.A., 154:330-332, 1954.

Turner, D. P. B.: Prevascular femoral hernia. Brit. J. Surg., 41:77-78, 1953.

Usher, F. C.: A new plastic prosthesis for repairing tissue defects of the chest and abdominal wall. Am. J. Surg., 97:629-633, 1959.

Usher, F. C., Fries, J. G., Ochsner, J. L., and Tuttle, L. L. D., Jr.: Marlex mesh, a new plastic mesh for replacing tissue defects. II. Clinical studies. Arch. Surg., 78:138-145, 1959.

Usher, F. C., and Gannon, J. P.: Marlex mesh, a new plastic mesh for replacing tissue defects. I. Experimental studies. Arch. Surg., 78:131-137, 1959.

Usher, F. C., Ochsner, J., and Tuttle, L. L. D., Jr.: Use of Marlex mesh in the repair of incisional hernias. Am. Surg., 24:969-974, 1958.

Walton, A. J.: Extrasaccular hernia. Ann. Surg., 57: 86-105, 1913.

Wangensteen, O. H.: Discussion of paper by McVay (see reference above), 1949.

Waugh, R. L., and Hausfeld, K. F.: Femoral hernia; a simple operation with report of cases. Am. J. Surg., 58:73-78, 1942.

West, W. T., and Hicks, E. S.: Skin as a supporting graft in repair of herniae. Canad. M.A.J., 58:178-180, 1948.

Wheeler, W. E.: Outpatient herniography in infants. J.A.M.A., 205:300, 1968.

Williams, C.: Repair of sliding inguinal hernia through the abdominal (LaRoque) approach. Ann. Surg., 126:612-623, 1947.

———: The abdominal (LaRoque) approach in the repair of sliding inguinal hernia. In: Nyhus and Harkins (1964), op. cit.

Williams, C., Jr.: Inguinal hernia in infants and children. Virginia M. Month, 86:314-318, 1959.

Wilson, H.: Personal communication. January 28, 1948.

Winterscheid, L. C.: Mesenteric hernia. Chap. 38. In: Nyhus and Harkins (1964), op. cit.

Zavaleta, D. E., and Uriburu, J. V., Jr.: Whole thickness skin grafts in the treatment of hernias; analysis of 211 cases. Surg., Gynec. Obstet., 91:157-172, 1950.

Zawacki, S., and Thieme, E. T.: Study of the types of recurrence following inguinal herniorrhaphy. Arch. Surg., 63:505-510, 1951.

Zieman, S. A.: The diagnosis of hernia. J.A.M.A., 115: 1873-1874, 1940.

Ziffren, S. E., and Womack, N. A.: An operative approach to the treatment of gigantic hernias. Surg., Gynec. Obstet. 91:709-710, 1950.

Ziperman, H. H.: Hiatus hernia repair by intraperitoneal gastric fixation. In: Nyhus and Harkins (1964), op. cit.

CHAPTER 43

JULIAN JOHNSON, M.D.

Cardiac Surgery

Congenital Heart Lesions
Acquired Heart Disease
Open Cardiac Surgery Under Direct Vision
Cardiac Resuscitation

In days of old the brain was considered to be the source of the intellect; the heart, the seat of the soul. This general concept may have played some part in the fact that only relatively recently has the surgeon attempted to operate upon the heart. No doubt, the problems of the physiologic changes that occur when the thorax is opened have been important in delaying the development of cardiac surgery, as well as thoracic surgery, in general.

In recent years, thoracic surgical procedures have become commonplace, and rapid advances have been made in cardiac surgery. Initially, attention was turned to various cardiac lesions that could be corrected or improved physiologically by operations outside the heart. Later, operative procedures were carried out inside the heart by palpation without interrupting the blood flow through the heart. More recently, the heart has been opened, and intracardiac defects have been repaired under direct vision. This was first done by taking advantage of the fact that the circulation can be stopped for short periods if the patient's body temperature is lowered.

For the past several years the attention of the cardiac world has been focused on the heart-lung machine which allows the surgeon to bypass the heart and the lungs completely, so that he may open the heart and repair various defects under direct vision with deliberation. The advantage of this method was demonstrated very rapidly, and its usefulness has been conceded by all who are interested in this field. At present several varieties of heart-lung machines are being used successfully, and a major effort is being made to improve them further and perhaps simplify them. A great many advances have already been made, using this technic, and the possibilities which lie ahead seem to be almost limitless. It is evident, therefore, that much of what is recorded here may rapidly become outdated. Insofar as possible, an effort has been made to indicate the procedures that have been accepted generally at the present time and to state when the procedure is simply one for use until something better is available.

CONGENITAL CARDIAC LESIONS

The Acyanotic Group

Patent Ductus Arteriosus

The surgical correction of a patent ductus arteriosus was first performed successfully by Gross in 1938 (Gross, 1939). Since that time this lesion has been operated upon all over the world with a low mortality.

The ductus arteriosus is a vessel connecting the pulmonary artery with the aorta, usually at a point just distal to the left subclavian artery. In normal circumstances this vessel becomes obliterated at or shortly after birth. In unusual circumstances, it remains patent.

Pathologic Physiology. In embryonal life the blood flow through the ductus arteriosus is from the pulmonary artery to the aorta, so that in embryo, as well as shortly after birth, the right ventricle is the predominant ventricle. At the time of birth, with the expansion of the lungs the pulmonary arterial resistance in the lungs is reduced greatly, and the blood flow through the lungs is increased greatly. With the fall in pressure in the pulmonary artery and the rise in pressure in the aorta, the direction of flow is changed in the patent ductus arteriosus and becomes a left-to-

1260 Cardiac Surgery

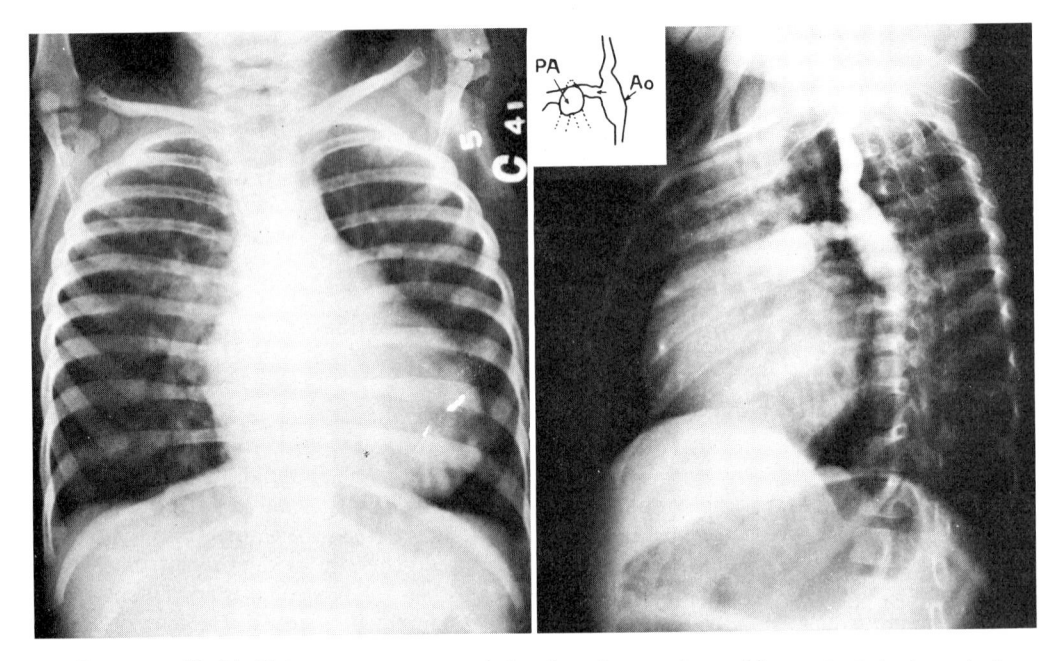

FIG. 43-1. (*Left*) Plain roentgenogram of the chest in a patient with a patent ductus arteriosus. Note the prominence of the pulmonary conus producing a convex border to the heart. Also note the prominent vascular markings especially shown in the right lung. (*Right*) Aortogram performed by injecting the contrast medium through the left subclavian artery. The contrast medium fills the aorta and passes through the patent ductus arteriosus into the pulmonary artery.

right shunt; that is, from the aorta to the pulmonary artery. In normal circumstances for the patent ductus arterious, the diastolic pressure in the aorta is higher than the systolic pressure in the pulmonary artery, so that there is a continuous flow of blood from the aorta to the pulmonary artery through the patent ductus arteriosus. In unusual circumstances secondary changes may occur in the arterioles in the lung and increase resistance to blood flow, with the consequent rise in pressure in the pulmonary artery. In such event the pulmonary artery pressure may equal the aortic pressure, except during systole, so that the flow from the aorta to the pulmonary artery is no longer continuous but is intermittent and occurs only during systole. In the presence of extreme pulmonary resistance the pulmonary artery pressure may become higher than that in the aorta, so that actually there is a right-to-left shunt through the patent ductus arteriosus; that is, from the pulmonary artery to the aorta. This produces some peripheral cyanosis with a decrease in the arterial oxygen content, particularly to the lower part of the body, since the patent ductus arteriosus usually joins the aorta distal to the left subclavian artery. It should be emphasized that this is an unusual happening, and it occurs very rarely in this disease.

Signs and Symptoms. In most instances the child with the patent ductus arteriosus will not be aware of it until the diagnosis is made at the time of a routine physical examination. The child's color is normal, since the flow, except in rare cases, is continuously from left to right, and the child may live a perfectly normal existence with little or no decrease in exercise tolerance, particularly if the patent ductus arteriosus is a small one. If, on the other hand, the patent ductus arteriosus is a large one, the child may develop dyspnea on exertion, and it is not uncommon to find such children considerably underdeveloped physically. In extreme instances, when the patent ductus arteriosus is very large, the patient may go into cardiac failure during infancy within the first few months of life.

The patient may be cyanotic in very exceptional cases, and then under only one of two conditions: either the patient is in cardiac failure and the cyanosis is caused by pulmonary edema and inadequate oxygenation of the blood that passes through the lungs, or there is a reversal of blood flow through the patent ductus arteriosus with blood flowing from the pulmonary artery into the aorta and bringing about the cyanosis. With few exceptions, however, the color of the patient is normal.

The characteristic *physical finding* is a continuous "machinerylike" murmur heard most readily in the second interspace to the left of the sternum anteriorly. In some patients a thrill can be felt on palpation, in addition to the continuous murmur on auscultation. Because of the large runoff from the aorta through the patent ductus arteriosus, the diastolic blood pressure is apt to be low, with a resulting widening of the pulse pressure. A roentgen examination of the patient usually will reveal a fullness in the area of the pulmonary conus with evidence of more than normal blood flow in the pulmonary vascular bed. On fluoroscopic examination there is apt to be an increased pulsation in the hilar vessels, particularly in those patients with an increased pulse pressure.

In some instances the continuous murmur may not be present, and the patient may have only a systolic murmur. This is apt to be present in those who have an increase in the pulmonary artery pressure. In those rare cases in which the aortic and pulmonary artery pressures are approximately the same throughout the cardiac cycle, no murmur will be heard. Not infrequently it is difficult to hear a continuous murmur in infants.

Diagnosis. In the vast majority of cases the diagnosis of the patent ductus arteriosus can be made on the clinical examination alone, without any special studies. The presence of the continuous murmur usually is diagnostic in itself. The two conditions in which there may be a continuous murmur not due to a patent ductus arteriosus are very uncommon: (1) an aortic window and (2) a ruptured sinus of Valsalva. In these instances the murmur is apt to be at a different location, so that the variation may be suggested. When a continuous murmur cannot be heard and only a systolic murmur is present, the diagnosis of the patent ductus arteriosus may be more difficult. This is especially important in the infant, since not infrequently the patient may be close to extremis from cardiac failure, and a failure to make the diagnosis of a patent ductus arteriosus may result in a preventable death.

There are several methods by which the diagnosis of patent ductus arteriosus may be confirmed by special studies. In the infant, if a contrast medium is injected into the brachial artery quite rapidly, an aortogram may be obtained that will afford a good visualization of the aorta. If a patent ductus arteriosus is present, the contrast medium will run off through the patent ductus arteriosus into the pulmonary artery, pass through the lungs and reappear in the left atrium. In questionable cases this is perhaps the simplest method of obtaining the diagnosis of patent ductus arteriosus in the infant. In the adult a catheter is usually passed through a needle in the femoral artery to the arch of the aorta and the opaque injected with a power injector.

The diagnosis of patent ductus arteriosus may also be definitely confirmed by cardiac catheterization. If there is an increase in the arterial oxygen in the pulmonary artery as opposed to the right ventricle, a patent ductus arteriosus is very likely to be present. A rise in the pressure in the same area may be indicative of a patent ductus, and, in some instances, the catheter may pass directly through the patent ductus arteriosus and go down the descending aorta.

Treatment. Surgical obliteration of the patent ductus arteriosus is the treatment of choice. This treatment is advocated as a matter of election because of the poor prognosis for the patient if the lesion is not obliterated surgically. There is little, if any, chance that the patent ductus arteriosus will become obliterated spontaneously, and, according to the figures of Maud Abbott (Abbott, 1920), the average life expectancy in the patient with patent ductus arteriosus is about 33 years. Although these figures were collected before the advent of antibiotics, nevertheless, much of the mortality associated with patent ductus arteriosus is on the basis of vascular complications, and, furthermore, the antibiotics have not relieved us completely of the dangers and the fears of subacute bacterial endarteritis

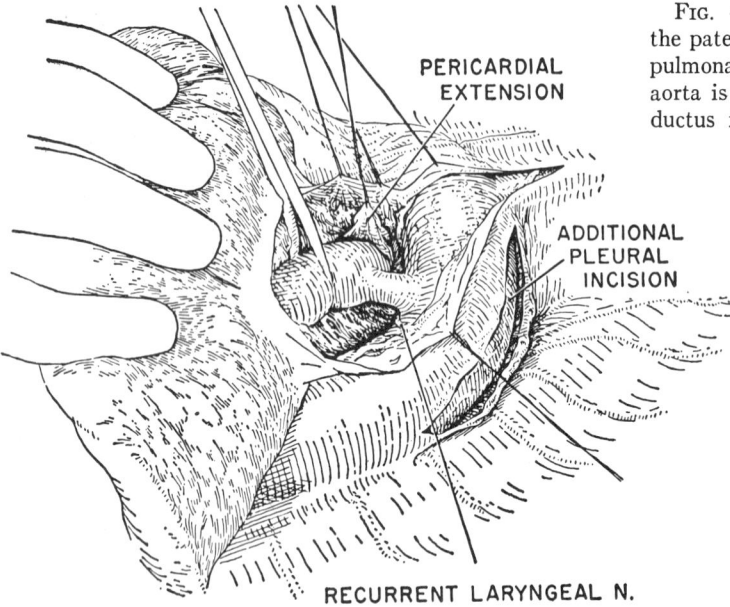

FIG. 43-2. Operative exposure of the patent ductus arteriosus. The left pulmonary artery is on the left, the aorta is on the right, and the patent ductus is seen going between them just proximal to the recurrent laryngeal nerve which passes around the aorta. The parietal pleura has been opened over the aorta so that the aorta may be occluded temporarily in the event that the patent ductus should be torn. (Johnson, J., and Kirby, C.: Surgery of the Chest. Chicago, Year Book Publishers)

and endocarditis that are engrafted so frequently upon the patent ductus arteriosus if it is left alone.

The method of obliteration of a patent ductus arteriosus probably is not important so long as it is successful. Gross (1952) and many others advocate the complete division of the ductus with closure of the two ends by suture in all cases. We, on the other hand, have felt that if the ductus is fairly long, triple ligation with silk is a satisfactory method of closure. As far as we are aware, we have had only one recurrence or persistence of a patent ductus arteriosus following this method of closure in about 400 operations. However, when the patent ductus arteriosus is short and broad, we obliterate it by division and suture as a matter of preference. This applies routinely in adults. It is our belief that in those instances in which there apparently has been a recurrence of the patent ductus arteriosus following the ligation technic, the ligature, in fact, has not been tied tightly enough, or such heavy ligature material has been used that it binds upon itself and does not allow complete obliteration of the ductus.

In the vast majority of instances when the diagnosis of a patent ductus arteriosus is made, the surgeon can proceed with its obliteration without further concern. However, there are two situations that require some comment. In an occasional patient there is some other congenital abnormality, and the patent ductus arteriosus may be acting as a compensatory factor. For example, if the patient has tetralogy of Fallot, the patent ductus arteriosus may be keeping the patient alive. Therefore, if there is any suggestion of another congenital abnormality, particularly of the cyanotic type, the patient should be studied very carefully before a closure of the ductus is considered. The second situation in which the surgeon should go slowly is when there is reason to suspect a reversal of flow through the ductus from right to left, causing partial unsaturation of the arterial oxygen content of the peripheral blood. Now, generally, it is thought that if there is a continuous right-to-left flow, the chances are that the ductus cannot be obliterated safely. On the other hand, if the right-to-left flow is only intermittent, the secondary changes in the lung may be reversible and the patient returned to normal after obliteration of the ductus.

If the preoperative studies do not preclude completely the possibility of exploration, the surgeon may undertake to find out what happens when the ductus is occluded temporarily. If pulmonary hypertension is present, the surgeon always should be hesitant about a hasty

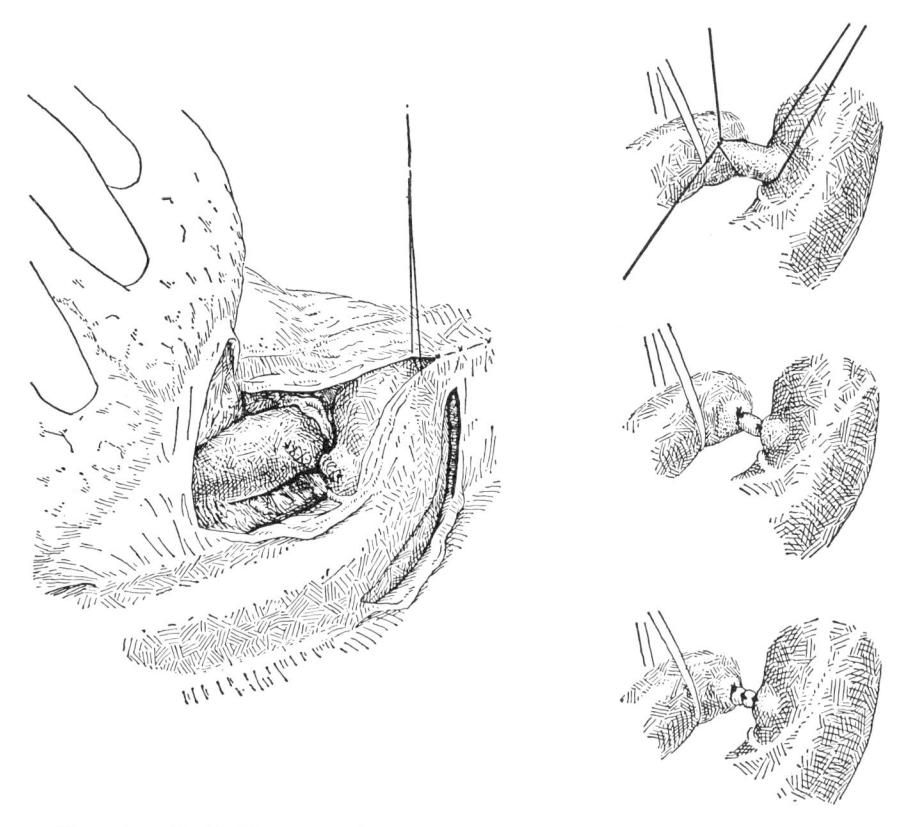

Fig. 43-3. (*Left*) The patent ductus in this view has been divided and the 2 ends sutured with fine silk sutures. (*Right*) This view shows the obliteration of the patent ductus arteriosus by 3 ligatures. This method of closure of the patent ductus arteriosus is satisfactory when the ductus is long enough to allow the ligatures to be placed in this manner. (Johnson, J., and Kirby, C.: Surgery of the Chest. Chicago, Year Book Publishers)

occlusion of the ductus. If the pressure in the pulmonary artery as measured at operation or before operation is lower than that in the aorta, the chances are that the occlusion of the ductus will be successful. If it is higher than that in the aorta at all times, the chances are that it will be unsuccessful.

It is now common practice for the surgeon to measure the pressure before and after temporary occlusion of the ductus. If the pulmonary artery pressure decreases with temporary occlusion of the ductus, then permanent occlusion of the ductus would seem to be indicated. If the pulmonary artery pressure remains the same, it may also be indicated. If, however, the pulmonary artery pressure increases after a temporary occlusion of the ductus, it probably is wisest not to attempt to make the occlusion permanent for fear that the patient will die because of the inability of the right heart to force blood through the lungs satisfactorily.

Results and Prognosis. The mortality rate for the operation of patent ductus arteriosus in most of the large hospitals is in the neighborhood of 1 per cent. It is felt now that there is little reason to delay operation once the diagnosis of patent ductus arteriosus is made, and that its obliteration may be carried out at almost any age. Whereas formerly we waited electively until the child was 4 or 5 years of age, we now have abandoned that practice and are apt to operate upon the patient whenever the diagnosis is made. On the other hand, if the heart is not enlarged and the child is not having any difficulty, there is no reason why one should not wait until the age of 2 or 3 for the operative procedure. However, if the heart is somewhat enlarged, it would seem wiser and safer to proceed with the operation without further delay, regardless of the age.

Aortic Window

The term *aortic window* is applied to a condition in which there is an opening between the aorta and the pulmonary artery just above the heart. It is apt to give the signs and symptoms of a patent ductus arteriosus, although the continuous murmur is more likely to be situated somewhat lower. Fairly frequently the opening may be quite large, and only a systolic murmur may be heard. It is a fairly uncommon lesion, and probably it cannot be differentiated from the patent ductus arteriosus on the basis of clinical grounds alone. The diagnosis can be confirmed by injecting opaque in the base of the aorta by way of a catheter passed retrogradely from the femoral artery and making a cineangiogram. It is best to operate upon the lesion using cardiopulmonary bypass. The separation of the two vessels and their careful closure may be carried out. In some instances, when the defect is large, it is wise to open one of the vessels and close the defect with a patch.

Coarctation of the Aorta

Coarctation of the aorta is a congenital lesion that is manifested by stenosis or complete occlusion of the aorta, usually at or about the level of the ligamentum arteriosum. Rarely, the coarctation involves some other portion of the thoracic or abdominal aorta.

When the constriction occurs at the usual level, the ductus arteriosus may or may not remain patent, but it is seldom a prominent factor in the distorted physiology. Any flow through the patent ductus arteriosus is from left to right. A marked collateral circulation develops round the site of constriction in the aorta and keeps the lower part of the body alive.

In rare instances the aortic constriction is above the ductus arteriosus, and the ductus arteriosus remains patent. In those cases the blood-flow is apt to pass from the pulmonary artery into the descending aorta, and relatively small amounts of blood-flow pass from the arch of the aorta into the descending aorta. Because of the large amount of blood-flow going from the patent ductus into the descending aorta, the usual collateral circulation has not been highly developed. This uncommon condition usually is referred to as the infantile type of coarctation of the aorta, because of the fact that these patients seldom live beyond infancy.

The physiologic response to coarctation of the aorta is an extremely interesting one. The patient develops hypertension in the upper part of the body, and, most frequently, the cause of death is associated with this hypertension. The hypertension certainly must be helpful in producing the collateral circulation, and the blood-flow into the descending aorta may occur by the reverse flow of blood through the large intercostal arteries distal to the constriction. The cause of the development of hypertension is not entirely certain. In some way it is related to the kidney, since it can be produced experimentally by performing a coarctation proximal to the kidney. The hypertension so produced can be relieved by transplanting the kidney to an area above the coarctation. It is not entirely a mechanical problem, as demonstrated by the fact that the blood pressure may not return to normal for several days or weeks following the correction of coarctation of the aorta. In man a few cases of coarctation of the abdominal aorta with partial occlusion of only one renal artery have been reported. The hypertension in these patients has been relieved immediately by nephrectomy or a splenorenal shunt. These observations confirm the animal experiments —that the hypertension is renovascular in origin.

One other point in the physiologic response to the constriction of the aorta is the dilatation that frequently occurs distal to the constriction. This phenomenon is referred to as "post-stenotic dilatation," and it has been emphasized by many writers, notably Halsted (1916) and Holman (1954). The mechanism that brings this about is not precisely known, but it is thought to be related to the turbulence of the blood stream distal to the constriction.

Signs and Symptoms. The patient with coarctation of the aorta may be unaware of being abnormal, and the diagnosis may be made accidentally on a routine physical examination.

In many instances, however, the upper extremities and the upper part of the body are apt to be more developed than the lower. When the patient's attention is called to it, it is found that the blood-flow to the lower part of his body is reduced somewhat, and that his feet are unusually cold in many circumstances. The symptoms that are most likely to direct the patient's attention to coarctation of the aorta are those associated with the hypertension.

The common causes of death are cerebral hemorrhage or rupture of an aneurysm, or factors of that type. According to Maud Abbott's survey (1920), the average life expectancy is about 35 years.

Not infrequently, a patient will be found with coarctation of the aorta who does not have hypertension to any marked degree at rest, and yet, with exercise, hypertension will be unusually severe and much beyond the usual response to such exercise. The physical findings in the patient with coarctation usually are characteristic if the diagnosis is suspected. Usually, a systolic murmur is heard not only in front but also in back on the posterior aspect of the chest. Frequently, evidence of the collateral circulation can be felt by palpating vessels between the scapulae posteriorly, and the murmur can be heard to be transmitted in this area. With coarctations of the abdominal aorta the physical signs may be lacking except for hypertension.

A most important observation is the absence of pulses in the lower part of the body or the decrease in blood pressure in this area. In normal circumstances, as the blood pressure is taken with the sphygmomanometer the systolic blood pressure should be higher than that obtained in the upper extremities. In many instances, however, in coarctation of the aorta, a blood pressure cannot be obtained in the lower extremities, and, when it is obtained, it will be considerably lower than in the upper extremities. It should be pointed out that when the collateral circulation is very good, pulses and blood pressure may be obtained in the lower extremities, although the blood pressure will usually not be so high as that in the upper.

Frequently a diagnosis of coarctation may be suspected on the basis of the ordinary roentgen film of the chest in which the aortic arch is much less prominent than usual and evidences of collateral circulation may be seen by the notching of the inferior borders of the ribs caused by the enlarged intercostal arteries. Rib notching may be less evident early in the course of the disease in infants and in young children.

Diagnosis. As a general rule, a diagnosis of coarctation of the aorta may be made on a clinical basis, and exact information need not be obtained before the time of thoracotomy. With very few exceptions, the site of the coarctation of the aorta will be found to be just below the subclavian artery on the left, so that, for practical purposes, actual demonstration is not necessary before the time of operation. It can be readily shown, however, particularly in infancy and childhood, by means of the angiocardiogram as administered through the right side of the heart, and, not only can the location of the coarctation of the aorta be determined, but also its configuration can be seen with considerable accuracy. In the adult, particularly the heavily built individual, the angiocardiogram is not entirely reliable, but an

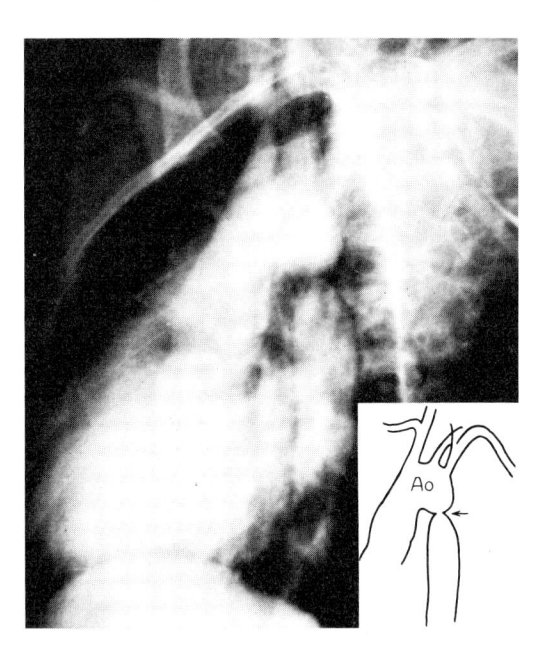

FIG. 43-4. Angiocardiogram, showing a coarctation of the aorta. While the visualization is adequate in this particular patient, this method does not always show the lesion as satisfactorily as this, particularly in an adult.

1266   Cardiac Surgery

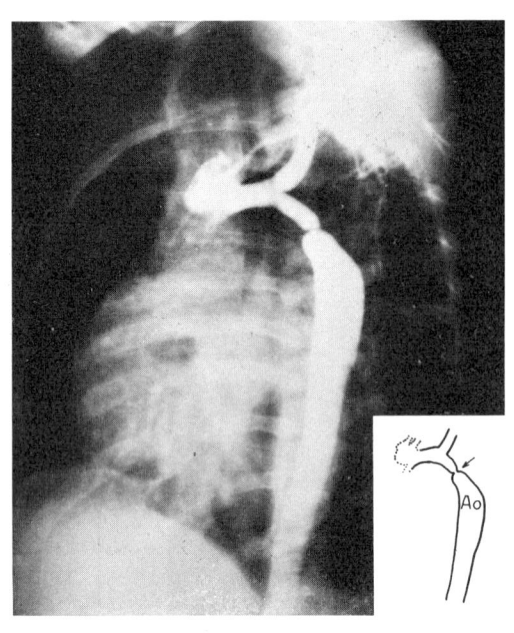

FIG. 43-5. An aortogram, showing a coarctation of the aorta in a child. The exact anatomic structure is shown much more vividly than with the angiocardiogram as seen in Figure 43-4.

With coarctation of the thoracic aorta the clinical diagnosis of coarctation can be relied upon. Now that vascular prostheses are readily available in the event that one is necessary, it is not important to delineate the exact anatomic relationships preoperatively.

Treatment. The treatment of choice for coarctation of the aorta is excision of the constricted area with end-to-end anastomosis. This was first performed successfully in 1944 by Crafoord (1945). The surgeon, naturally, is interested in the physiologic response to total occlusion of the aorta during the surgical correction of the coarctation. If the aorta has been completely occluded, obviously nothing further is done when the aorta is clamped. If the coarctation was not complete, the clamping of the aorta might add something that was not present formerly. It is common practice, however, to put noncrushing clamps across the aorta above and below the coarctation for long periods of time while the constricted area is excised and the ends are sutured, and there have been few, if any, instances of paraplegia resulting from it. The collateral blood-flow has been adequate for long periods of time. If, on the other hand, the opening in the coarctation is unusually large, and the collateral circulation appears to be small, the distal aorta may collapse appreciably when the aorta is clamped. In this situation it may be wise to reduce the patient's temperature before resecting the coarctation or utilize some type of bypass during the procedure. It is probable that paraplegia will seldom occur with less

aortogram may outline the defect if this is desired. Actually, there seems to be very little point in carrying out this study for thoracic coarctations. However, aortography should be used when an abdominal coarctation is suspected. It is important to ascertain the exact extent of the lesion and the status of the renal arteries.

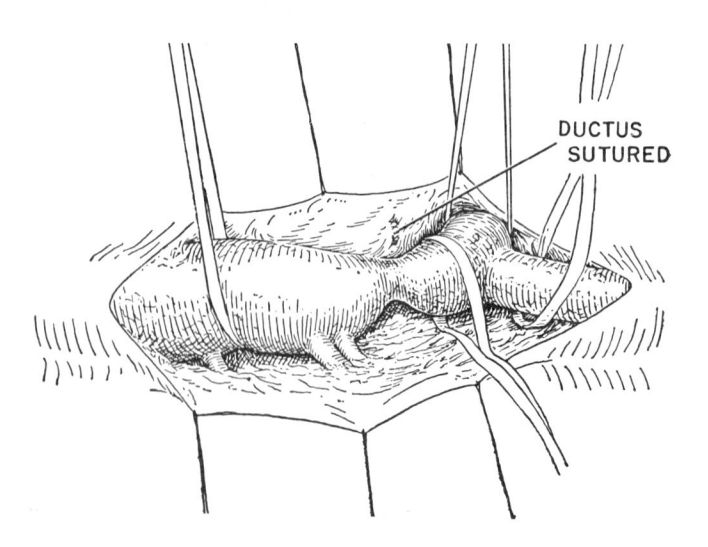

FIG. 43-6. Operative exposure of a coarctation of the aorta. The patent ductus arteriosus has already been divided and sutured. Hernia tapes have been placed around the proximal and distal aorta and the subclavian artery. (Johnson, J., and Kirby, C.: Surgery of the Chest. Chicago, Year Book Publishers)

FIG. 43-7. (*Top*) Noncrushing clamps are placed across the aorta above and below the coarctation. (*Bottom*) The constricted segment is cut out and the 2 ends are sewed together with fine silk sutures. (Johnson, J., and Kirby, C.: Surgery of the Chest. Chicago, Year Book Publishers)

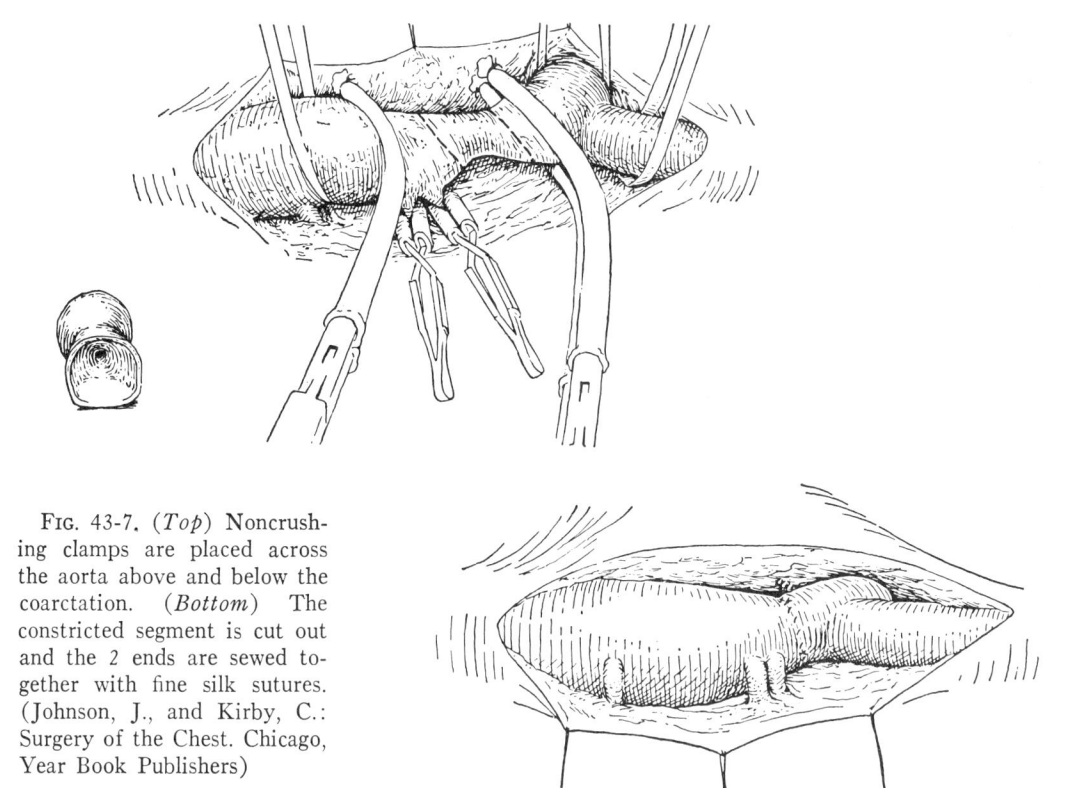

than 20 minutes' occlusion of the normal aorta.

The ideal treatment for coarctation is an end-to-end anastomosis. In some circumstances, however, the aorta may be tapered to a degree that may not allow an opening of adequate size without cutting away an undue portion of the aorta. In the past it was common practice to turn down the subclavian artery in some of these patients. In those instances in which the subclavian artery was unusually large this gave a good result, with return of the blood pressure to normal. In about half of the patients, however, the subclavian artery apparently was not sufficiently large, and a satisfactory drop in blood pressure did not occur. This procedure, therefore, has been practically abandoned in favor of aorta grafts when a satisfactory opening cannot be obtained by an end-to-end anastomosis. Aorta grafts used experimentally by Carrel (1908) as early as 1906 and adapted for clinical use by Gross (1951) some 40 years later were widely accepted at one time. More recently, plastic grafts have been used. Since even the aortic grafts do not grow, the grafts should be used in infancy and childhood only in dire circumstances. A satisfactory lumen can usually be obtained by some type of plastic procedure. A longitudinal strip graft enlarging the lumen of the subclavian is preferable to a circumferential graft, since the subclavian artery will continue to grow in circumference.

The time of election for operation for the patient with coarctation of the aorta has not been established. In general, it seems that from 4 to 12 years of age is a satisfactory period. At that time the vessels are pliable and easily brought together. Therefore, the chances of having to use a graft at this age are reduced greatly, and almost always some type of plastic procedure can be performed to give a satisfactory opening. There is probably no upper age limit for operating upon patients with coarctation of the aorta now that grafts are available and can be put into position, reducing all tension on the suture line. There may well be no age limit in the lower ages for coarctation of the aorta, for several patients

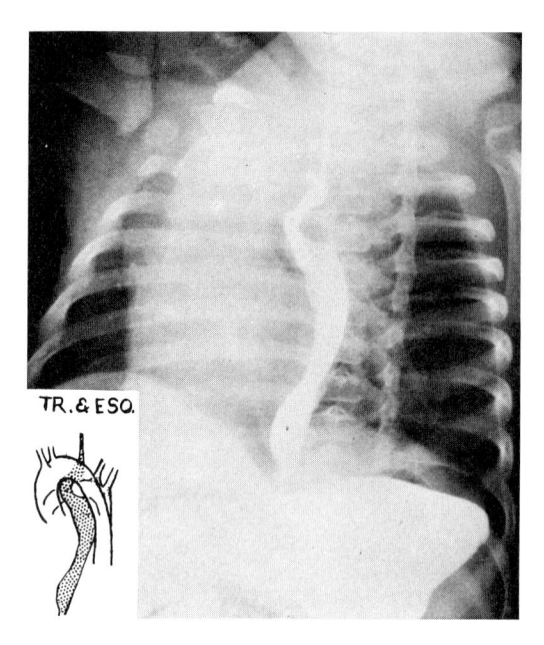

FIG. 43-8. Esophagogram of a patient with a double aortic arch. The esophagus is displaced forward at one point by the posterior arch and constricted anteriorly by the anterior arch.

have been operated upon successfully in infancy. In general, the author has preferred to attempt to carry newborn infants along, if necessary, by digitalization if cardiac failure occurs, until they reach about 2 years of age.

Results and Prognosis. The results of the operation for coarctation of the aorta of the adult type have been excellent. The mortality has been in the neighborhood of 5 per cent or below. The blood-pressure response usually has returned toward normal, depending upon the surgeon's ability to obtain a sufficiently large opening at the site of the anastomosis. If the blood pressure in the lower extremities is higher than that in the upper extremities, the surgeon can be content that he has obtained a satisfactory opening, and, if hypertension persists, it is on some other basis. In the majority of instances, however, the blood pressure will return to normal or nearly normal, and it is anticipated that such patients will have a normal life expectancy. When it is necessary to use a graft, the longevity is uncertain, primarily for the lack of long-term evidence at the present time.

Only a few attempts have been made to repair the infantile type of coarctation of the aorta, and the mortality up to the present time has been high.

Vascular Rings

The congenital anomalies that occur in the aortic arch may show great variation. In themselves, they are unimportant and place no stress on the cardiocirculatory system. They are important when a vascular ring persists around the esophagus and the trachea and therefore may cause compression of these structures.

In embryo there are 2 aortic arches. Usually, the right disappears, and the left persists. Occasionally, the left disappears, and the right persists. When both vessels persist, there is a double aortic arch, one in front and one behind the trachea and the esophagus. The difficulty involved in this condition arises from the compression of these latter structures.

Similar compression from a vascular ring may occur with a right aortic arch, where the ductus arteriosus and the left subclavian artery arise from a common diverticulum on the right descending aorta to pass to the left behind the esophagus. There are many possible types of vascular rings. When the ring is incomplete, symptoms are less likely to develop, as when the right subclavian artery arises from a left descending aorta and passes to the right behind the esophagus.

The symptoms of a vascular ring usually develop in infancy and consist of a wheeze on respiration and frequent respiratory infection. Difficulty in swallowing may be noted in rather severe cases. The diagnosis should be considered in any infant with respiratory distress.

The diagnosis can be made by a careful roentgenographic examination. Compression of the trachea may be noted on a proper chest film. An esophagogram should reveal an indentation of the esophagus from behind at the level of the aortic arch.

The treatment is the division of the smaller of the two vessels forming the vascular ring. When there is a double aortic arch, usually one is small, and this is the one that should be divided. The left thoracic approach is commonly preferred. In some instances, when the vascular ring is divided, the vessels tend to maintain their position. In such cases the pressure must be removed from the trachea and the esophagus by displacing the involved vessels by suturing them to surrounding structures. When the constriction is caused by the ligamentum arteriosum or the subclavian behind the esophagus, these structures may be divided. In any event, great care should be taken to remove all pressure from the esophagus and the trachea.

The preoperative and postoperative care of these infants is of the greatest importance. They should be made as free as possible of respiratory infection preoperatively and watched very closely postoperatively. When diligence is exercised in providing adequate room for the trachea and the esophagus, and more than usual care is given in the postoperative period, the mortality is low and the results excellent.

Isolated Pulmonary Stenosis

The term *isolated pulmonary stenosis* refers to the congenital cardiac condition in which only the pulmonary valve is stenotic and no other congenital abnormalities are present. The stenosis usually is valvular in type. As a general rule, the valve is cone-shaped, and the small opening in the valve is at the apex of the cone, very much as a reversed megaphone. There is a great deal of variation, however, and in some instances the stenosis is infundibular in type; that is, a muscular constriction within the right ventricular outflow tract.

Since there is no communication between the two sides of the heart in this lesion, the patient is not cyanotic. All the blood that circulates through the heart goes through the lungs and is oxygenated, and for that reason the patient's peripheral arterial oxygen saturation is normal. The only inconvenience occasioned by the constriction of the pulmonary valve is that the right ventricle has to work harder in order to force the blood through such a small opening. For that reason, the cardiac output is apt to be reduced, even though the right ventricle may become hypertrophied and the right ventricular pressure increased greatly.

The symptoms that these patients are apt to experience are dyspnea and fatigue, particularly on exertion. As the heart begins to fail, the patient may have all the signs and symptoms of right heart failure. The electrocardiogram will show a right axis deviation because of the hypertrophy of the right ventricle. There is a harsh systolic murmur with a thrill over the pulmonary area to the left of the sternum in the second interspace anteriorly. There is apt to be post-stenotic dilatation of the pulmonary artery, frequently giving a false impression during roentgenologic studies of increased blood-flow through that vessel.

Frequently, the diagnosis of pulmonary stenosis can be made on a clinical basis by the murmur and the thrill and an apparent decrease in the amount of blood in the lungs. Cardiac catheterization, however, is essential for proper evaluation and accurate diagnosis of the condition, even though it may be suspected on the clinical examination. When the catheter is placed in the right side of the heart, there are no changes in the arterial oxygen saturation of the blood, indicating no shunts. However, the pressure in the pulmonary artery is low, and that in the right ventricle is high. If the catheter is first placed in the pulmonary artery and withdrawn slowly into the right ventricle at a time when a recording of the pressure curves is being made, a differentiation between valvular stenosis and infundibular stenosis usually is possible. In valvular stenosis there is a sudden transition from the low pulmonary artery pressure to the high

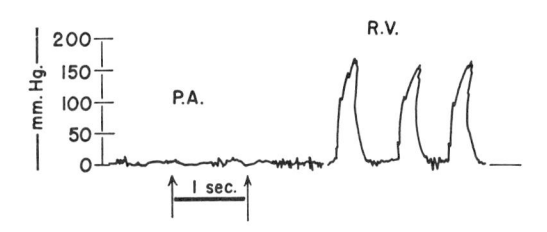

FIG. 43-9. Curves obtained on cardiac catheterization in a patient with an isolated pulmonary stenosis. First, the catheter was advanced into the pulmonary artery. The pressure curves shown were recorded as the catheter was withdrawn from the pulmonary artery into the right ventricle. The pressure in the pulmonary artery above the valve was approximately 10 mm. Hg systolic, whereas that in the right ventricle below the valve was approximately 160 mm. Hg systolic.

right ventricular pressure. In the event of infundibular stenosis, an intermediate pressure usually is recorded as the catheter passes through the infundibular chamber.

Treatment. If the patient has a mild degree of pulmonary stenosis that does not raise the pressure in the right ventricle unduly, there probably is no indication for any surgical therapy. On the other hand, it is perfectly obvious that if these patients are to be operated upon, the operation should be carried out before the patient is in desperate condition from cardiac failure. The question arises, therefore, as to how high the right ventricular pressure should go before the operation should be done as a matter of election. The consensus at the present time is that if the pressure is as much as 100 mm. of mercury systolic in the right ventricle, operation as an elective procedure is justifiable. Some surgeons feel that 75 mm. of mercury is a proper figure to choose. Few, if any, feel that the operation should be advocated if the pressure is below 75 mm. of mercury in the right ventricle and the patient is asymptomatic.

Several methods have been employed in the surgical treatment of pulmonary stenosis. Brock (1948) in 1947, was the first to advocate operation upon this lesion. He inserted an especially designed knife into the right ventricle that cut the valve open as it was passed out into the pulmonary artery. The same procedure has been accomplished by a cutting type instrument inserted through the wall of the pulmonary artery.

There was a fair amount of dissatisfaction with these procedures because of the feeling that the valve may be sufficiently elastic to stretch over the knife blade and not be opened completely by this maneuver. In many instances, although the patients have been improved vastly, pressures in the right ventricle have not returned to normal but perhaps only halfway to normal. If the operation is to be done blindly, the guillotine type of knife is probably the most satisfactory for opening the valve completely.

However, most surgeons are now operating upon this lesion under direct vision, using either hypothermia or cardiopulmonary bypass. If the stenosis is entirely valvular in type, hypothermia with an approach through the pulmonary artery has been successful for most surgeons. Nevertheless, many surgeons, along with the author, prefer to use cardiopulmonary bypass because of the possibility of finding some infundibular stenosis in addition to the pulmonary stenosis. Some authors feel that the infundibular stenosis may be the result of hypertrophy of the musculature of the right ventricle and will disappear in time after the relief of the valvular stenosis. However, the author prefers to relieve the pulmonary stenosis at the time of operation. In the case of infundibular stenosis, this means the excision of the muscular obstruction in the outflow tract of the right ventricle. Although this has been carried out as a blind procedure in the past (Brock, 1950), it is now seldom done except under direct vision, utilizing cardiopulmonary bypass.

To date, the results of the operation on

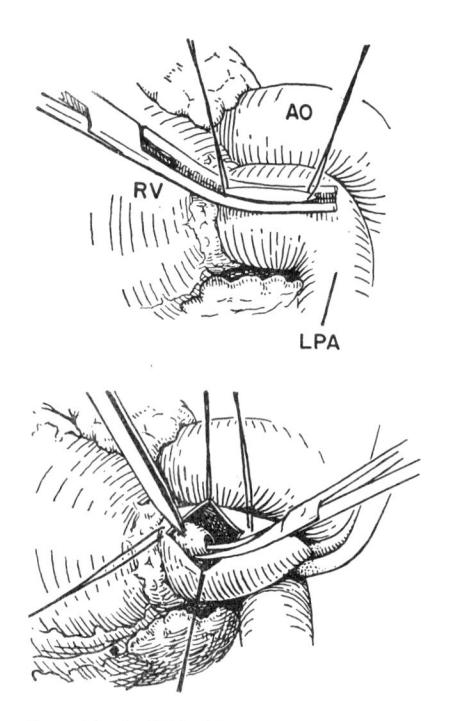

FIG. 43-10. This illustrates one method of correcting valvular pulmonary stenosis under direct vision. Utilizing moderate hypothermia, the valve may be visualized through an incision in the pulmonary artery. Cardiopulmonary bypass should be used if a right ventriculotomy is contemplated for the relief of infundibular stenosis. (Johnson, J., and Kirby, C.: Surgery of the Chest. Chicago, Year Book Publishers)

patients with pulmonary stenosis have been excellent as to mortality and morbidity, there being a very low mortality associated with the operation, particularly if it is valvular in type. In many instances in the past the stenosis has not been removed completely, and it may be that in the future some of these patients may have to be operated upon again. At the present time, however, the valvular stenosis would appear to be correctable to a nearly normal state, utilizing cardiopulmonary bypass and direct vision.

Pulmonary Stenosis With Ventricular Septal Defect

If an acyanotic patient has pulmonary stenosis plus a ventricular septal defect, the condition is often referred to as an "acyanotic tetralogy." In this condition the pulmonary stenosis is not sufficiently severe to cause a right-to-left shunt through the ventricular defect. There may be little or no shunt in either direction, or there may be a left-to-right shunt if the pulmonary stenosis is not severe.

Should the ventricular septal defect be undiagnosed and the pulmonary valvular stenosis corrected completely, the patient would suffer all the problems of a ventricular septal defect. This procedure has been carried out in the past and may be done unwittingly even now. However, if the correct diagnosis is made, all would now agree to the use of cardiopulmonary bypass for the closure of the ventricular septal defect and the relief of the pulmonary stenosis as one procedure.

The possibility of the presence of an unsuspected ventricular septal defect along with a pulmonary valvular stenosis is one reason for advocating operation upon that lesion by the right ventricular approach.

Atrial Septal Defect

An atrial septal defect should not be confused with a patent foramen ovale. In many instances there is a patent foramen ovale in which the flaplike valve over the opening is kept closed functionally by a slightly higher pressure in the left atrium. However, when a real atrial septal defect is present, there is a flow from left to right because of the higher pressures in the left atrium. The location of the atrial septal defect may be greatly varied. In general, there are two types—the so-called septum secundum, which is located high in the septum, and the septum primum, which extends low to include the area between the mitral and the tricuspid valves. In extreme cases, the defect may go on down and include the upper portion of the ventricular septum. This is called a persistent atrioventricular canal.

Pathologic Physiology. The blood-flow is from the left to right through the atrial septal defect, so that some of the blood that has just arrived in the left atrium passes back through the defect into the right atrium, through the right ventricle, and into the lungs again. Thus, in this instance, the blood is going round and round through the lungs and the right heart in a manner somewhat similar to the patent ductus arteriosus, where the blood is going round and round through the lungs and the left heart. With the atrial septal defect the total cardiac output of the left heart will be considerably lower than that of the right heart, so that the pulmonary artery may become enormous and the aorta may be very small. It is not uncommon, for example, for the output of the right heart to be 4 or 5 times higher than that of the left heart.

As times go on, secondary obliterative vascular changes are apt to occur in the lungs, and resistance to the flow of blood is increased. Therefore, the pulmonary artery pressure will increase, and, if this process is carried to the extreme, the pressure may rise in the right ventricle and the right atrium so that the left-to-right shunt may disappear. In such circumstances, there usually is some mixing of the blood between the right and the left atria through the large defect, and the patient's systemic arterial oxygen saturation will be below normal. In such instances the right-to-left shunt and the left-to-right shunt may be approximately equal or a little bit in excess in either direction.

The symptoms of the atrial septal defect may be insignificant early in life, particularly if the defect is small. As a general rule, when the symptoms have been insignificant in early life and later develop to a significant degree, the defect is apt to be small, and surgical repair is relatively easy. If the defect has produced symptoms early, it is more likely to be a large one. The symptoms of the atrial septal defect are those of cardiac failure.

1272   Cardiac Surgery

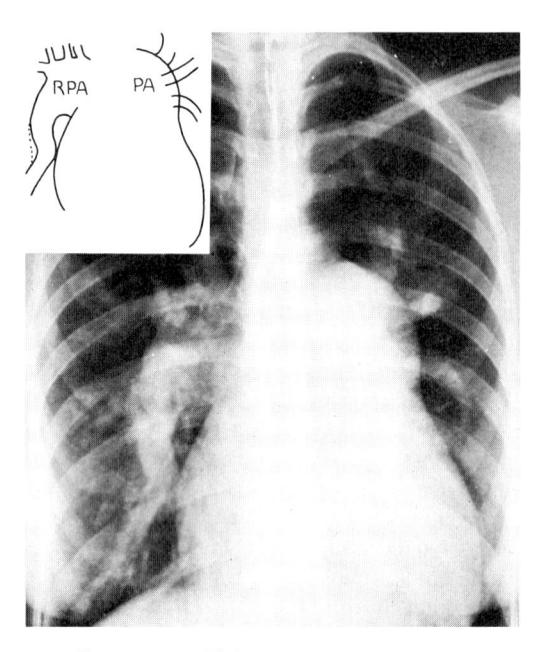

FIG. 43-11. Plain roentgenogram of the chest of a patient with an atrioseptal defect. Note the enlarged heart and the tremendously enlarged pulmonary conus, as well as the enlarged pulmonary arteries in the lung, visualized in this film, particularly in the right side.

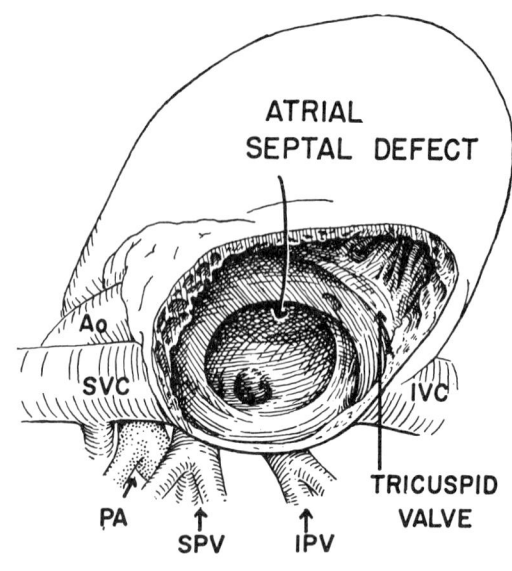

FIG. 43-12. Diagrammatic view of an atrioseptal defect of the secundum type. The opening of the right-sided pulmonary veins where they enter the left auricle can be seen through the septal defect. The opening of the coronary sinus can be seen inferior to the septal defect and superior to the opening of the inferior vena cava. Such a defect can be closed very easily under direct vision. Also it could be closed readily by various technics noted in the text.

When cardiac failure occurs in infancy, the lesion is apt to be a persistent atrioventricular canal.

The signs of atrial septal defect are those of an excess amount of blood-flow through the lungs and the right heart. A large pulmonary artery and an excessive amount of blood in the lungs can be demonstrated readily on fluoroscopy and roentgen examination. It may be difficult to distinguish between an atrial septal defect and a ventricular septal defect on a clinical basis, but a lead in this direction is given by the nature of the murmur.

The definitive diagnosis of atrial septal defects is made by cardiac catheterization. When the catheter passes from the vena cava into the right atrium, there is an immediate increase in the arterial oxygen saturation, and in many instances the catheter may pass through the septal defect into the left atrium. After the catheter enters the right ventricle or passes into the pulmonary artery, there is no further increase in the arterial oxygen saturation. Also, the systolic pressure in the pulmonary artery and the right ventricle should be the same.

Treatment. The method first used extensively to close the atrial septal defect was that of inverting the atrial wall against the defect and suturing it in place, as suggested by Cohn (1947) and popularized by Bailey (1952). By inserting the finger into the right atrium, the size of the defect was ascertained, and some method of closure could usually be worked out in the secundum type defect. Bjork and Crafoord (1953) recommend a circumferential suture around the atrial septum, and this was successful in many instances. Another method which was used successfully was that of suturing a patch over the defect by working through a rubber well attached to the wall of the right atrium (Gross, 1952).

In recent years all of the "blind" methods for the closure of these defects have given way to the use of direct vision, either under hypothermia or with cardiopulmonary bypass. The use of hypothermia has been highly successful in large series of patients (Lewis, 1955; Swan, 1955). However, it does place a premium on speed in the closure of the defect. At a temperature of about 30° C. the circulation can be occluded safely for 4 or 5 minutes. Additional time for suture can be obtained by using 2 or 3 such periods if necessary (Johnson, 1959) or by perfusing the coronary arteries during the inflow occlusion (Mahoney, 1959). However, the use of cardiopulmonary bypass allows the surgeon all the time that he may need for the deliberate closure of the defect. For this reason, and the fact that cardiopulmonary bypass is now so widely utilized, it has become practically the only method used for the repair of atrial septal defects.

Ventricular Septal Defect

In the patient with a ventricular septal defect, the flow is from left to right because of the higher pressure in the left ventricle. The patient is not cyanotic, since oxygenated blood, which has just arrived in the left ventricle from the lungs, passes into the right ventricle, out the pulmonary artery, through the lungs and the left atrium and back into the left ventricle again. Thus, a goodly portion of the blood goes round and round through the lungs and the left heart without going to the systemic circulation in the same manner as it does in a patent ductus arteriosus.

The symptoms of a ventricular septal defect are those of heart failure when the disease is advanced. Before that time, they are apt to be few and inconsequential. The physical examination of a patient with a ventricular septal defect reveals a loud systolic murmur over the area of the base of the heart and the pulmonary artery, and fluoroscopic examination and roentgenograms show a large pulmonary artery with prominent vascular shadows in the lung fields. As a rule, the diagnosis can be made with certainty only by cardiac catheterization. As the catheter passes from the right atrium into the right ventricle, the systolic pressures increase abnormally, and the arterial oxygen saturation increases. Upon occasion, the catheter actually may pass through the septal defect.

Treatment. The surgical closure of ventricular septal defects using cardiopulmonary bypass has now been accomplished in large series of patients (Kirklin, 1960), with a low mortality. When the pulmonary artery pressure is normal or only moderately elevated, the risk should be no more than 5 per cent. As the pulmonary artery pressure rises, the risk increases. If the increased pressure is due to the increased flow, the patient is still a satisfactory risk. However, if the pressure in the pulmonary artery is roughly equivalent to that in the aorta due to abnormally high vascular resistance in the lung, and there is very little left-to-right shunt, the risk of operation is high.

The technical feat of obtaining a secure closure of the defect without injury to the bundle of His is the greatest problem facing the surgeon. At the same time it is advantageous to make as small a wound in the right ventricle as possible in order to reduce the efficiency of the right ventricle as little as possible during the postoperative period.

The use of a transverse incision in the right ventricle seems to decrease its efficiency less than a perpendicular one and should be used if possible when the vascular resistance in the lungs is high. Some surgeons use a patch to close the ventricular septal defect most of the time, while others use one rarely. Now that most surgeons recognize the importance of placing the sutures on the right side of the septum in the area of the conductive bundle, heart block is rare.

THE CYANOTIC GROUP

Tetralogy of Fallot

The congenital heart which includes the 4 anomalies described by Fallot (1888) generally is referred to as the tetralogy of Fallot. Such a heart has a pulmonary stenosis, a ventricular septal defect, an overriding of the aorta and hypertrophy of the right ventricle. In those instances in which an atrial defect is added to this tetralogy, the term *pentalogy* sometimes has been used.

The exact pathologic anatomy present in the tetralogy of Fallot may vary tremendously. In the vast majority of instances the pulmonary stenosis is infundibular rather than valvular in type. The size of the ventricular septal defect may vary considerably from a small defect to the presence of a common ventricle. The amount of overriding of the aorta

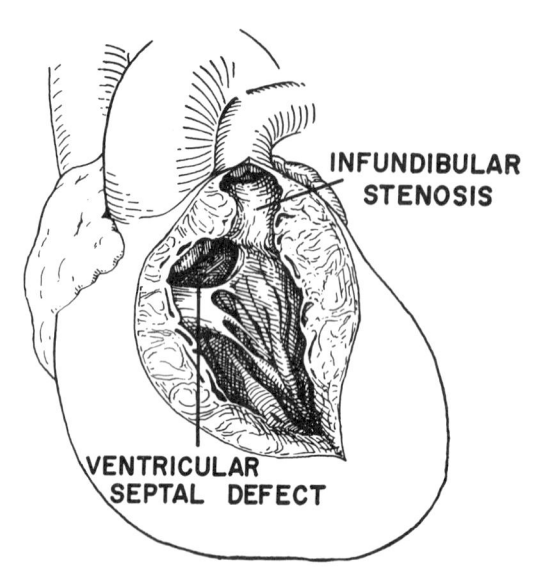

Fig. 43-13. Diagrammatic sketch of the tetralogy of Fallot. Note the muscular type of infundibular stenosis in the outlet of the right ventricle proximal to the normal pulmonary valve. Also, note the ventricular septal defect through which some of the blood from the right ventricle flows into the left ventricle and out through the aorta.

also may vary tremendously—to the extent, in fact, that the aorta apparently may arise completely from the right ventricle.

The physiologic derangement of the heart with the tetralogy of Fallot is primarily that of a right-to-left shunt—that is, the shunting of blood from the right ventricle out through the aorta rather than having it pass through the lungs. This may be accomplished because the aorta partially overrides the right ventricle, and this shunting is increased by the stenosis that interferes with the flow of blood into the lungs through the pulmonary artery. As a result of the great right-to-left shunt, an inadequate amount of blood passes through the lungs, so that the peripheral arterial oxygen saturation may be quite low, and the patient suffers from severe oxygen deficiency and cyanosis. Incident to this tissue hypoxia, the patient may develop clubbing of the fingers and the toes and severe polycythemia.

Primarily, the symptoms of the tetralogy of Fallot are cyanosis with dyspnea on exertion. If the patient survives to childhood, he is apt to be found characteristically in the squatting position in an effort to increase his ease in breathing. If the right-to-left shunt is severe, the patient may die in infancy; if less severe, he may live into childhood. Few of these patients live past their teens without some type of surgical intervention.

Physical examination will reveal varying degrees of cyanosis, depending upon the severity of the lesion. There will be a systolic murmur over the pulmonary artery area, and the blood count will reveal a polycythemia, although the hemoglobin may not be high if the infant is malnourished. When the polycythemia becomes severe, the danger of vascular thrombosis is increased greatly, and it is not uncommon for these patients to suffer strokes in infancy or in childhood. Fluoroscopic and roentgenographic examinations reveal characteristically a "boot-shaped" heart with a concavity at the pulmonary conus area and evidence of a decreased amount of blood in the lungs, as indicated by unusually clear lung fields.

Diagnosis. The diagnosis of the tetralogy of Fallot can be made on a clinical basis with considerable accuracy, but special studies may be necessary to make it with certainty. When the angiocardiogram is done by using a rapid cassette changer or cineangiography, the dye passes from the right atrium into the right ventricle and from the right ventricle into both the aorta and the pulmonary artery. This gives a positive diagnosis of an overriding aorta, or at least a ventricular septal defect, and one can feel reasonably certain of the diagnosis of the tetralogy of Fallot, although in some instances a common ventricle cannot be ruled out. If the cassette changer used is not a rapid one, there may be some fear that some of the dye may have passed from the right to the left atrium, into the left ventricle and out through the aorta, so that the aorta may be visualized at the same time as is the pulmonary artery. With a fairly rapid cassette changer or a cineangiogram, however, this mistaken diagnosis is not likely to be made.

A definitive diagnosis of the tetralogy of Fallot also may be made by cardiac catheterization. If the catheter passes from the right ventricle into the pulmonary artery and a low pressure is recorded in the pulmonary artery as compared with the right ventricle, the diagnosis of pulmonary stenosis can be made. If, then, the catheter can be passed out through the aorta, the overriding aorta, or at least a ventricular septal defect, can be assumed. This, along with the cyanosis, makes a diagnosis of tetralogy of Fallot reasonably certain.

Treatment. The first successful efforts at the surgical treatment of the tetralogy of Fallot were carried out in 1944 by Blalock (1945). On the basis that methods were not available actually to correct the anatomic defects inside the heart, he and Taussig worked out a method of overcoming the physiologic inconvenience of the tetralogy of Fallot by surgical procedures outside the heart. Since the fundamental difficulty with the patient's heart in the tetralogy of Fallot is a right-to-left shunt, with inadequate amounts of blood going to the lungs, the Blalock operation was designed to shunt blood from the systemic circulation to the pulmonary circulation. Thus, it provides a left-to-right shunt outside the heart to compensate for the right-to-left shunt inside the heart. This is accomplished by turning down the subclavian artery and anastomosing it end-to-side to the pulmonary artery. There can be no doubt that this operation has been highly successful in many clinics throughout the world. The operation is usually performed on the right side, using the subclavian branch of the innominate artery, because the angle at which the subclavian artery comes off the innominate is a favorable one. However, other surgeons have preferred to use the subclavian branch of the aorta and have done so successfully. In some instances there is kinking at the angle as the subclavian is turned down from the aorta.

A side-to-side anastomosis of the descending aorta to the pulmonary artery on the left side, as suggested by Potts (1946), accomplishes the same result of a left-to-right shunt. For several years it was preferred by most surgeons when the anastomosis had to be done during early infancy, since the subclavian artery in the infant was apt to be small. In recent years an anastomosis between the ascending aorta and the right pulmonary artery, as described by Waterston (1962), has replaced the Potts operation, since it is easier to perform and easier to take down if a corrective procedure can be done at a later date. It is especially useful in infants, giving a lower mortality than the other procedures. Wald-

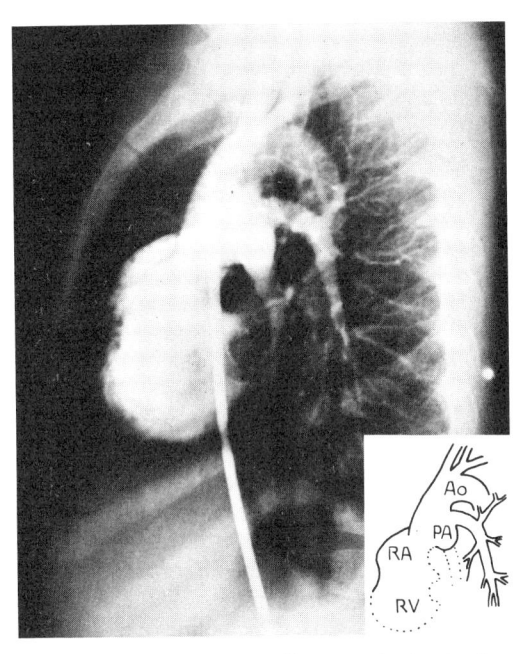

Fig. 43-14. Angiocardiogram obtained of a patient with the tetralogy of Fallot by placing a catheter up through the femoral vein into the vena cava in order to inject the contrast medium. The right side of the heart is visualized, and the aorta and the pulmonary artery are visualized simultaneously before the contrast medium has entered the left side of the heart.

hausen (1968) has reported 12 per cent, in infants in the first year of life.

A direct attack upon the pulmonary stenosis in the tetralogy of Fallot was advocated by Brock (1948). In most instances this required the removal of some muscle from the outflow tract of the right ventricle, since the stenosis was usually infundibular rather than valvular. Although Brock and a few other surgeons obtained good palliative results by this procedure, it was never widely accepted.

By the use of cardiopulmonary bypass it is now possible to do corrective surgery for the tetralogy of Fallot by closing the ventricular septal defect and removing the pulmonary stenosis. Those surgeons who have had the most experience in this field now use this technic almost exclusively. The greatest difficulty has been encountered in infants and small children, especially when the patient is severely cyanotic. The author and many other surgeons are still doing shunt procedures on infants and small children and reserving the direct approach for the older children and adults. Success depends upon the ability to get an adequate outflow tract from the right ventricle without jeopardizing the efficiency of the right ventricle to too great a degree.

Results. Patients with the tetralogy of Fallot who have been operated upon by the shunting type procedures of Blalock, Potts or Waterston have been improved vastly by the procedure. By and large, the mortality has been below 15 per cent. In general, the mortality has been higher in infants and in the older age group. An ideal time for the operation, from the standpoint of low mortality, probably is from 4 to 8 years of age. However, many children will not live to this age; therefore, in such cases, the operation must be done of necessity before that time. In general, the author now uses the Waterston operation in infants and the Blalock operation in children. There has been some difficulty due to unusual enlargement of the heart in the postoperative period following the Potts operation, probably as a result of having made the anastomosis too large, and this may be a problem with the Waterston procedure. In the Blalock operation, the size of the anastomosis is limited by the size of the subclavian artery, but, even so, some large hearts develop after this procedure.

The vast majority of patients who are operated upon, either by the shunting type procedure or the Brock procedure, are much improved following the operation. Even though they do not have a normal heart again, their cyanosis will be decreased greatly and their exercise tolerance increased greatly. The polycythemia likewise will decrease. While there can be no doubt that most of the patients have been vastly improved, nevertheless these operations are palliative ones, and an increasing number of patients get into trouble as time goes on.

The results of the total correction of the tetralogy of Fallot, utilizing cardiopulmonary bypass, has improved greatly in the recent past. In the hands of those surgeons who have had the greatest experience, the immediate mortality now compares favorably with that of the shunt procedures, and it is hoped and assumed that the long-term results following a successful operation will be far superior. The execution of this procedure in infants is still hazardous in the hands of most surgeons.

Pulmonary Stenosis with Atrial Septal Defect or Patent Foramen Ovale

Frequently, this congenital defect is referred to incorrectly under the term *isolated pulmonary stenosis*, although obviously two defects are present. These patients are cyanotic because the resistance to blood-flow caused by the pulmonary stenosis increases the pressure in the right ventricle, which, in turn, increases the pressure in the right atrium, and blood flows through the atrial septal defect from right to left. Therefore, the systemic arterial oxygen saturation is decreased, and the patient is cyanotic.

The symptoms of these patients are apt to be similar to those of the tetralogy of Fallot. On physical examination the findings may be

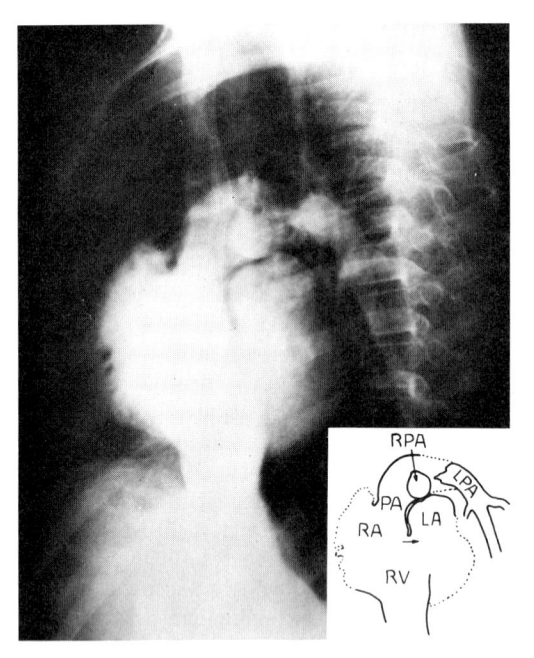

FIG. 43-15. Angiocardiogram of a patient with a valvular type of pulmonary stenosis and an atrioseptal defect. The contrast medium can be seen to have filled the right side of the heart and has passed through the atrioseptal defect into the left atrium but has not yet reached the left ventricle. The tremendously dilated pulmonary artery (post-stenotic dilation) is also visualized.

very similar, but the cardiac configuration is somewhat different, and the diagnosis usually can be suspected on a clinical basis. It is very important that this condition be differentiated from the tetralogy of Fallot, since the direct attack upon the pulmonary stenosis gives a much better result than an anastomosis type procedure in this lesion.

On physical examination the systolic thrill over the pulmonary area is present, and there is right preponderance on the electrocardiogram, as there is in the tetralogy of Fallot. On fluoroscopic and roentgenographic examinations, the lung fields are apt to be clear also, but there is likely to be post-stenotic dilatation of the pulmonary artery, giving some prominence of the pulmonary conus rather than the concavity, as seen frequently in the tetralogy of Fallot. Therefore, the general cardiac configuration is helpful in making the suspected diagnosis. The diagnosis usually is confirmed, however, on the basis of the angiocardiogram, since, as a rule, the dye can be seen to pass from the right to the left atrium and into the left ventricle before appearing in the aorta. The diagnosis also can be made with reasonable certainty on cardiac catheterization if the catheter passes through the atrial septal defect, but, even so, it would be difficult to distinguish this condition from a "pentalogy" unless the catheter passed through the ventricular septal defect. The presence of a right-to-left shunt at the ventricular level may be ruled out by dye curves following a right ventricular injection of the dye.

Treatment. If the surgeon plans to make a direct attack upon the pulmonary stenosis, whether it is associated with a ventricular or an atrial septal defect, it is not important to make a differential diagnosis before operation. However, the anastomosis type procedure should not be done for this condition. If the surgeon is one who uses the anastomosis procedure for the tetralogy of Fallot, obviously it is important that a definitive diagnosis be made before operation. The treatment of the patient with pulmonary stenosis and an atrial septal defect always should be made by the direct attack. It is essentially the same as that described under isolated pulmonary stenosis above. Once the pulmonary stenosis is relieved, the atrial septal defect, which is usu-

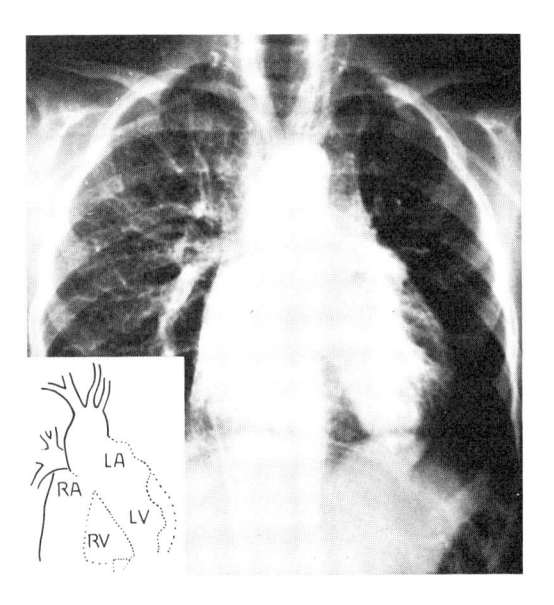

Fig. 43-16. Angiocardiogram of a patient with tricuspid atresia. The contrast medium is seen in the right atrium and in the left atrium, and partially fills the left ventricle so that the aorta and the pulmonary arteries are also shown. The contrast medium does not fill the right ventricle, a circumstance which is diagnostic of tricuspid atresia.

ally a patent foramen ovale, closes and is apt to be no longer of clinical physiologic significance. However, the presence of a real atrial defect should be ruled out, and if one is found to be present it should be closed.

The results obtained in this lesion have been excellent, and the mortality has been low.

Tricuspid Atresia

This lesion must be associated with an atrial septal defect or it is incompatible with life. Even so, a patient with tricuspid atresia is apt to get into difficulty as a very young infant. There are various degrees of tricuspid stenosis, going on to complete atresia, but complete or almost complete atresia is the most common. Usually, the diagnosis can be made or strongly suspected clinically on the configuration of the heart on roentgenographic and fluoroscopic examinations, upon the cyanosis and the polycythemia and the left axis deviation on the electrocardiogram.

The diagnosis can be made with consider-

1278 Cardiac Surgery

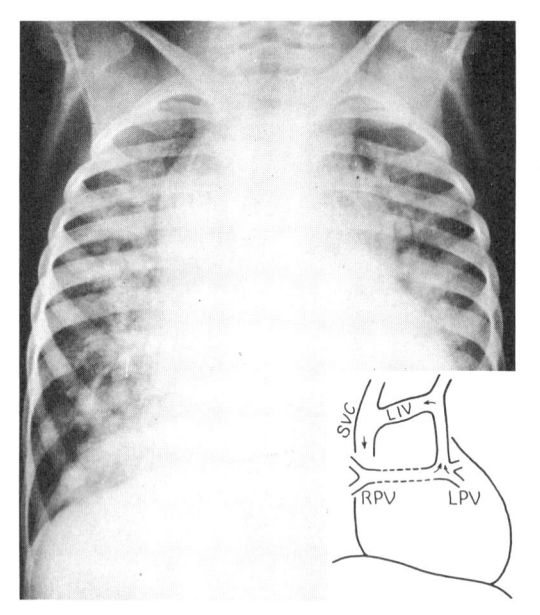

FIG. 43-17. Plain roentgenogram of the chest of a patient with abnormal venous drainage of the type illustrated in the inset. The shape of the heart on the plain roentgenogram and the tremendous engorgement of the pulmonary vessels are diagnostic in many instances. As shown in the inset, the pulmonary veins join, and the blood flows into the left innominate vein, on to the superior vena cava and back into the right atrium. The patient is kept alive by virtue of an atrioseptal defect. See text for corrective surgical procedure.

able certainty on the basis of the cineangiocardiogram. The dye passes into the right atrium, then into the left atrium, into the left ventricle and out through the aorta. The pulmonary artery may receive some blood from the left ventricle, but in inadequate amounts. Often the lungs may get their major bloodflow through a patent ductus arteriosus. On the angiocardiogram, the absence of dye in the right ventricle is diagnostic.

Treatment. To date, no method has been developed whereby this lesion can be totally corrected. The surgical therapy so far has been directed toward getting an increased flow of blood to the lungs. A left-to-right shunt, produced either by a Blalock or a Waterston operation is now the common method of attack. Blalock (1948) has suggested making a larger atrial septal defect to avoid the possibility of partial closure of a patent foramen ovale by the increased venous return to the left atrium. If this is necessary it can now be done by the balloon technic described by Rashkind (1966).

In the recent past the "Glenn" operation (Glenn, 1958) has been advocated for this condition and appears to have considerable advantage over the other types of anastomoses. In this procedure a side-to-end anastomosis is made between the superior vena cava and the right pulmonary artery, shunting the superior vena caval blood directly to the right lung without passing through the left heart. The work load of the left heart is thus less than it would be with either of the arterial shunts.

Abnormal Drainage of the Great Veins

The abnormal drainage of the great veins is fairly uncommon, and there may be considerable variation. Perhaps the most common type of abnormality is that of the right-sided pulmonary veins entering the right atrium in association with an atrial septal defect.

The more serious type of abnormal drainage of the great veins is that in which not only the right but also the left pulmonary veins enter the right atrium. This may occur in a number of ways. In some patients (Fig. 41-17) the veins from both lungs may join on the left side to drain into a vein called the "vertical vein," from which the blood flows through the left innominate vein and on to the right atrium. In other instances, all the branches of the left pulmonary vein may join and pass inferiorly to a vein entering the inferior vena cava. In addition to the abnormal drainage of the great veins, there is an atrial septal defect, and thereby blood gets across to the left side of the heart. Therefore, these patients are cyanotic because of the mixing of the blood of the pulmonary veins and the vena cavae and its getting into the left side of the heart. Their signs and symptoms are those of tissue anoxia.

The diagnosis can be suspected on the basis of the cardiac configuration. A definitive diagnosis can be made at times by cardiac catheterization and angiocardiography, but it is difficult to be entirely certain of the complete diagnosis unless one is fortunate enough to have one of the cardiac catheters go out through the various veins and show their course with certainty.

Surgical correction of the abnormal drainage of the pulmonary veins is obviously indicated. When only the right-sided pulmonary veins enter the right atrium in association with an atrial septal defect, the correction can be carried out fairly simply by suturing the septum in front of the right-sided veins, shunting their flow into the left atrium.

When the two pulmonary veins join to drain into the right atrium by the route shown in Figure 41-17, the operation must be done utilizing cardiopulmonary bypass. A large anastomosis is made between the left atrium and the vein passing behind the heart. Then the vertical vein may be ligated and the atrial defect closed either by suture or by a patch.

Occasionally, the right pulmonary vein drains directly into the superior vena cava, usually associated with an atrial septal defect. It is usually possible to devise some means by suture or by means of a patch to have the superior vena cava blood continue to flow into the right atrium while shunting the superior pulmonary vein blood into the left atrium.

Transposition of the Great Arteries

The congenital transposition of the great arteries, so that the aorta arises from the right ventricle and the pulmonary artery arises from the left ventricle, is a very serious congenital abnormality.

The patient usually is quite cyanotic, and in most instances, these patients die in early infancy. As a rule, the diagnosis is easily suspected because of the configuration of the heart, particularly when the aorta is seen to arise from the anterior position on the lateral view. If there is any doubt as to the diagnosis, it may be ascertained on angiocardiogram, which shows the dye to go from the right ventricle out through the aorta without appearing in the pulmonary artery until much later.

Patients who do not die at birth are kept alive by virtue of some communication between the right and the left circulations. This may be due to a ventricular septal defect, an atrial septal defect and/or a patent ductus arteriosus.

The problem would seem to be a simple surgical one of dividing the two vessels and

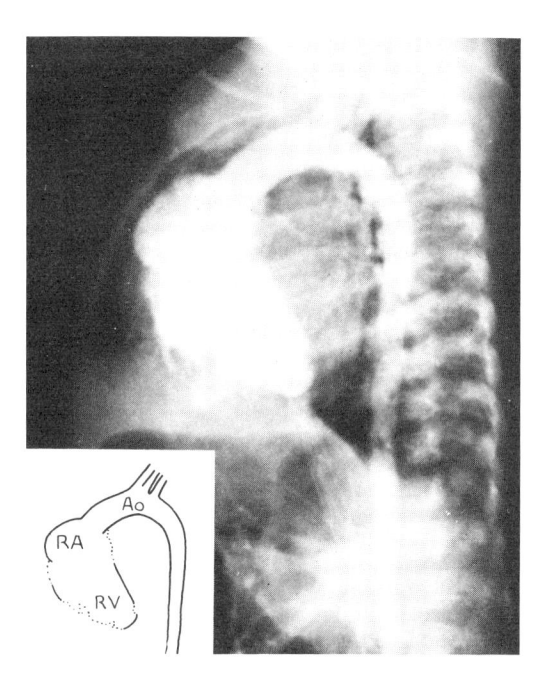

FIG. 43-18. Angiocardiogram in a patient with transposition of the great arteries. The right side of the heart is visualized with the contrast medium, and the aorta is seen to arise from the right heart and is brilliantly visualized. The contrast medium has not yet entered the left side of the heart or the pulmonary circulation.

reanastomosing in the opposite manner. However, this maneuver has not been successful as yet. It would appear that in addition to transplanting the great arteries, the coronary arteries would have to go with the aorta so as to obtain oxygenated blood from the left ventricle. This has not been carried out successfully to date, but it would appear to be feasible. In view of the failure of the efforts to transplant the great arteries, efforts have turned to transplanting the great veins. Some success has been experienced with a partitioning of the atria to reroute the blood to the opposite ventricle (Senning, 1959). Baffes (1960) had some success with the palliative operation of shunting blood from the inferior vena cava to the left atrium by means of a graft, and shunting the blood from the right lung into the right atrium by direct anastomosis. Also, considerable palliation was achieved by producing a common atrium as suggested by Blalock and Hanlon (1950).

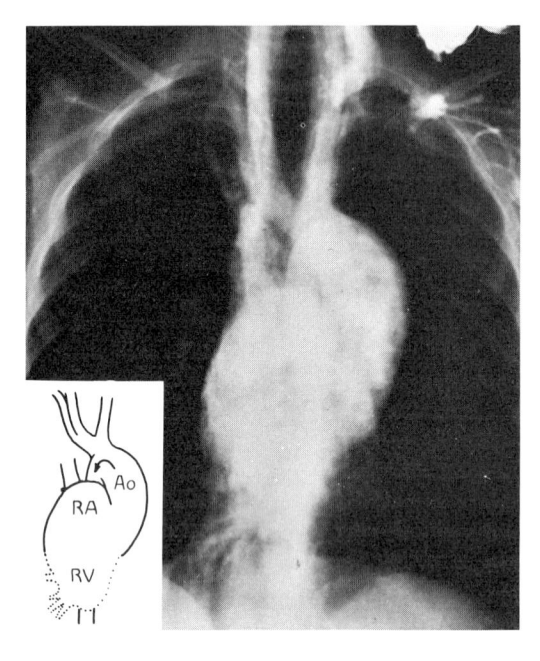

FIG. 43-19. Angiocardiogram of a patient with a truncus arteriosus. In this patient the blood flow to the lungs apparently was dependent entirely upon collateral circulation arriving from the systemic circulation.

In recent years this has been accomplished by Rashkind (1966) by a nonoperative approach. A balloon-tipped catheter is passed from the right atrium into the left atrium. The balloon is inflated and pulled back, tearing open the atrial septum.

Following the creation of a larger atrial septal defect, the child may improve sufficiently to survive to 2 or 3 years of age. Then the atrium may be partitioned with a graft to—in effect—transpose the great veins as suggested by Mustard (1964). If pulmonary hypertension is present at the beginning, banding of the pulmonary artery may be done early to prevent the development of severe pulmonary vascular resistance. If a ventricular septal defect is present, it should be closed at the time of the Mustard operation.

Truncus Arteriosus

There is one variety of truncus arteriosus in which a single vessel arises from the ventricle and there is no pulmonary artery, the lung thereby receiving all the blood-flow through collateral circulation. This diagnosis can be suspected clinically on the basis of the configuration of the heart, and it can be suspected on angiocardiography because of the large single vessel and the absence of typical pulmonary arteries. The only method of surgical treatment that may be of some value to these patients is an effort to increase the collateral circulation to the lungs. In general, if the patient is doing reasonably well and the diagnosis is made preoperatively, operation is not advised. If the patient is doing poorly, however, or if the diagnosis is arrived at when the chest is opened, the parietal pleura is removed, and talc is sprinkled over the surface of the lung in the hope of increasing the blood-flow to the lungs. This maneuver is used also in some patients with the tetralogy of Fallot when the anastomosis procedure cannot be accomplished. In the author's opinion, there is very little doubt that some of the tetralogy patients have been improved by this maneuver.

There is another type of truncus arteriosus in which a single artery coming from the heart divides very shortly into the aorta and the pulmonary artery. The cyanosis is not apt to be severe. In this situation, the pulmonary artery pressure is high, so that a continuous murmur will not be heard. In other respects, it may be difficult to differentiate between this type of truncus arterious and the patient with an aortic window. It is difficult to make this diagnosis with certainty except at autopsy, although it may be suspected. If the diagnosis were established, the only method of treatment at present available would be the production of pulmonary stenosis, as suggested by Muller and Dammann (personal communication), for the patient with a ventricular septal defect and high pulmonary artery pressure.

Eisenmenger's Complex

Eisenmenger's complex is the term applied to a congenital defect somewhat similar to the tetralogy of Fallot except that the right-to-left shunt through the ventricular sepal defect is brought about by pulmonary hypertension due to vascular resistance to blood flow through the lungs rather than to a pulmonary stenosis. Sometimes this condition is present in infancy and childhood. Not infrequently, however, the child starts out with a ventricular septal defect and a left-to-right shunt, only to develop cyanosis as the years go by, due to vascular changes in the lung, increasing vascular resistance, increasing pulmonary hypertension and a reversal of the shunt to a right-to-left one. At the present time it is the objective of cardiac surgeons to repair ventricular septal defects before the above process occurs. If a considerable degree of right-to-left shunt is already present, the surgeon has little hope to offer the patient. However, Muller and Dammann (personal communication) have suggested that the vascular changes in the lungs may be reversed by surgically producing pulmonary stenosis as the first stage of a corrective operation. A most difficult question at the present time is how severe the pulmonary hypertension may be and how small the left-to-right shunt may be and still give hope of success in the closure of a ventricular septal defect.

Pulmonary Arteriovenous Fistula

In the presence of a pulmonary arteriovenous fistula, blood is shunted directly from the pulmonary artery to the pulmonary vein without having passed through the capillaries of the lungs to undergo oxygenation. Therefore, such a fistula would amount to the same as a right-to-left shunt inside the heart, and the patient is cyanotic. Along with the cyanosis, polycythemia develops, and in severe degrees of the condition the patient is dyspneic on exertion. In favorable circumstances a continuous murmur may be heard over a pulmonary arteriovenous fistula.

Pulmonary arteriovenous fistulae are considered to be congenital in origin, and several individuals in the same family may be afflicted with the condition. Such fistulae may be progressive, and they may not be detected until adult life. It is not uncommon to have cutaneous manifestations of telangiectasis, but this is not always present.

The patient's signs and symptoms are primarily cyanosis and polycythemia associated with dyspnea, particularly on exertion, when the size of the fistula is large. If the fistula is unusually large, there will be a right axis deviation on the electrocardiogram, and the right side of the heart may be larger than the left.

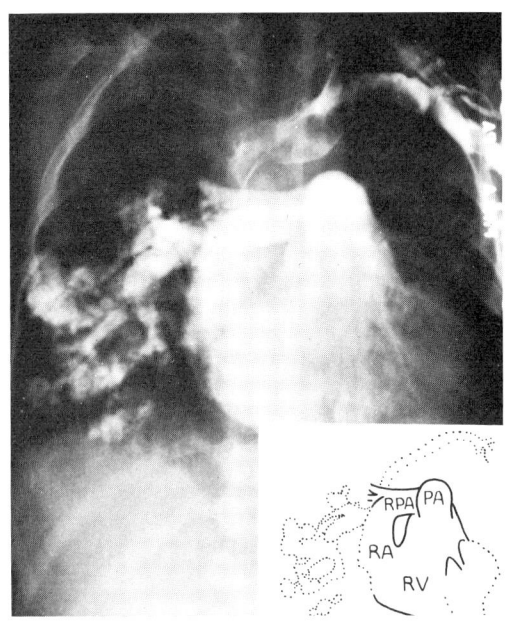

FIG. 43-20. Angiocardiogram of a 4-year-old child with a large pulmonary arteriovenous fistula. The fistula apparently was confined to the right lower lobe. It was estimated that 84 per cent of the right heart output went through this fistula. The child was severely cyanotic. Following the removal of the right lower lobe the cyanosis disappeared completely.

Unlike the peripheral arteriovenous fistula, the pulmonary arteriovenous fistula is not associated commonly with cardiac enlargement.

The diagnosis of pulmonary arteriovenous fistula can be suspected on the basis of the clinical examination. Roentgenographic and fluoroscopic examinations actually may reveal the large arteriovenous communications in the lung. If these communications are large, they can be shown beautifully on an angiocardiogram.

If the pulmonary arteriovenous fistula is confined to one lobe or one lung, the resection of the area involved will bring about a tremendous improvement in the patient. Great care should be exercised to determine the extent of the arteriovenous fistula before operation, since it is not uncommon to have multiple small ones throughout the remaining portion of the lungs that may be overlooked. There is also some danger that after the re-

TABLE 43-1. RIGHT HEART CATHETERIZATION

Blood-Oxygen Saturations and Pressures in the Heart and the Great Vessels in Cardiac Abnormalities

Cardiac Abnormality	Vena Cava O$_2$ Sat.	Vena Cava Pressure	Right Atrium O$_2$ Sat.	Right Atrium Pressure	Right Ventricle O$_2$ Sat.	Right Ventricle Pressure	Pulmonary Artery O$_2$ Sat.	Pulmonary Artery Pressure	Systemic Artery O$_2$ Sat.	Systemic Artery Pressure	Remarks
Normal	75%	5/0	75%	5/0	75%	30/0	75%	30/0	96%	120/90	Approximate values
Interatrial septal defect	Normal		>V.C.	Normal or high	Same as R.A.	Normal or high	Same as R.A.	Normal or high		Normal	O$_2$ saturation in R.A. greater than V.C., catheter may pass into the L. A.
Ventricular septal defect	Normal or low		Normal or high	Same as V.C.	Normal or high	>R.A. High	Same as R.V.	High		Normal	R. V. O$_2$ saturation is higher than R.A. or V.C., catheter may pass R.V. to L.V. and aorta.
Pulmonary stenosis	Normal		Normal or high	Same as V.C.	Normal or high	Same as V.C.	High	Same as V.C.	Low		Normal	R.V. pressures are much higher than P.A. pressures
Tetralogy of Fallot	Low		Normal or high	Same as V.C.	Normal or high	Same as V.C.	High	Same as V.C.	Low	Low	Normal	Pulmonary stenosis with systemic arterial saturation and catheter passing through ventricular septal defect overriding aorta.
Eisenmenger's complex	Low		Normal or high	Same as V.C.	Normal or high	Same as V.C.	High	Same as V.C.	High	Low	Normal	No pulmonary stenosis with overriding aorta. O$_2$ saturation of P.A. and systemic arterial blood may vary.
Patent Ductus	Normal		Normal or high	Same as V.C.	Normal or high	Same as V.C.	Normal or high	>R.V.	Normal or high	Normal	Increased pulse pressure	P.A. O$_2$ saturation greater than R.V., R.A. and V.C. catheter may pass into aorta.

V.C.: Vena cava
R.A.: Right atrium
R.V.: Right ventricle
L.V.: Left ventricle
P.A.: Pulmonary artery
L.A.: Left atrium
>: Greater than

moval of the one arteriovenous fistula, other smaller ones may increase in size as the years go on. This of course does not militate against the surgical removal of the more serious arteriovenous fistula, particularly if the patient has gone on to severe polycythemia.

ACQUIRED HEART DISEASE

Surgery of the Pericardium

Constrictive Pericarditis

Constrictive pericarditis is a condition in which the heart is compressed by a thickened, diseased pericardium, so that it cannot expand to its normal size during diastole.

Frequently, the etiology cannot be ascertained. Many authors are inclined to think that it is almost always on a tuberculous basis, while others feel that a viral infection is the most likely etiologic factor in those instances in which the diagnosis cannot be established by microscopy.

Usually, the surgeon sees the patient with constrictive pericarditis at a time when the process appears to be a healed lesion from the pathologic standpoint. The pericardium is thick and scarred, and areas of calcification are frequently present. As a rule, the areas of calcification do not extend into the myocardium, but they may do so occasionally.

From the physiologic standpoint, constrictive pericarditis may be thought of as a constricting lesion involving the heart as a whole and preventing it from filling adequately during diastole. As a result of inadequate filling the total cardiac output is reduced, and the blood is apt to back up in the great veins. The venous pressure will be increased. As a result, enlargement of the liver with secondary ascites occurs in many instances. Passive

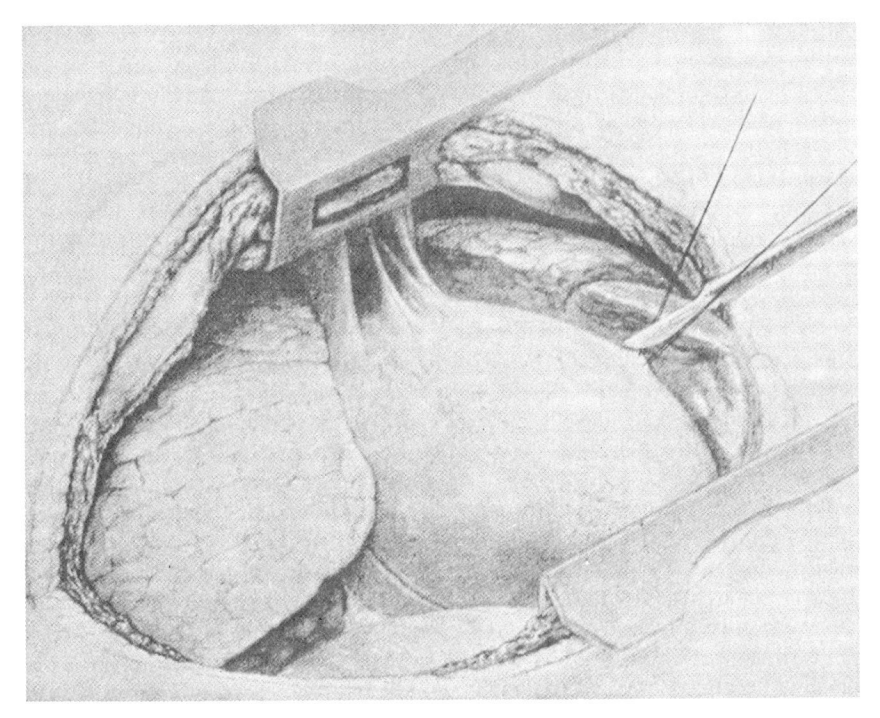

FIG. 43-21. Operative view of an operation for constrictive pericarditis. By making a trans-sternal incision from the anterior axillary line on one side to the anterior axillary line on the other in about the fourth interspace, it is possible to remove the pericardium from the hilum of one lung to the hilum of the other with excellent exposure. This type of exposure is also useful in a good many other procedures employing open cardiac surgery. (Johnson, J., and Kirby, C.: Surgery of the Chest. Chicago, Year Book Publishers)

congestion in the portal system may bring about an enlargement of the spleen with secondary hypersplenism in long-standing cases. Because of the constricting nature of the pericardium, the heart is apt to be smaller than it would be otherwise, and the effectiveness of its impulse is decreased, in respect to both palpation and auscultation.

The signs and symptoms of constrictive pericarditis on the basis of the above physiologic findings are those of cardiac failure. The diagnosis is suspected easily if the roentgenographic examination reveals calcification in the pericardium. However, when this is not the case, it may be very difficult to be certain that one is dealing with a patient with constrictive pericarditis rather than simple heart failure. The diagnostic triad suggested by Beck (1937) is that of a small quiet heart, increased venous pressure and ascites. This differs from the usual patient with cardiac failure only in that the heart usually is large and more active in the latter type of patient. However, there may be many borderline situations in which it is extremely difficult to make a differential diagnosis between the two conditions. Not infrequently, the condition may be misdiagnosed as being due to primary cirrhosis of the liver.

Treatment. The treatment of constrictive pericarditis is the removal of the pericardium so as to allow the heart to expand and fill normally. In the vast majority of instances, the pericardium constricts the heart as a whole rather than any one particular area, so that, if a major portion of the pericardium is removed over a convenient area, the heart may expand, and the patient will be cured. If, for example, the pericardium can be removed from about the hilum of the lung on one side to the same area on the other side, then the heart can expand satisfactorily.

There has been some question in the surgical literature as to how decortication of the heart may be accomplished most readily. When the patient is very sick and has been allowed to reach the stage of desperation before being subjected to surgery, the greatest skill on the part of the anesthetist and the surgeon may be required to get the patient through an operative procedure.

The preoperative care is of the greatest importance. The patient should be dehydrated and made as free of excess fluid as possible before operation, and great care should be taken not to overhydrate the patient during the immediate postoperative period.

The operation itself may be performed in a number of ways. Some surgeons go through the left chest and remove the major portion of the pericardium from the left side of the heart. If a large enough area of the pericardium is removed, this undoubtedly is satisfactory in most instances unless there is actual constriction of a localized area. Occasionally one encounters a patient in whom there is constriction of the venous inlet to the right atrium and one in whom there is a constriction of the venous inlet to the left atrium. However, these are the exceptions. The author has felt that a wider decortication than can be accomplished through a left pleural cavity incision probably is desirable in most patients, and he has accomplished this by a transsternal incision in the fourth or the fifth interspace, decorticating the heart from the hilum of the lung on one side to the hilum of the lung on the other. Other surgeons have accomplished essentially the same type of operation by an incision splitting the sternum from above downward. When the patient is in desperate condition, probably it is safer to do a simple left-sided thoracotomy with a decortication of the left side of the heart, with the thought of going back and doing more later if it should become necessary. In our own experience, such a secondary procedure has not been necessary if the left side of the pericardium was removed adequately.

The results of decortication of the heart in the cases of constrictive pericarditis have been excellent. When the patient goes to operation before the terminal stage, the mortality is low. Following decortication of the heart, it is the consensus at the present time that the patient should be carried along a little bit more slowly than the average patient following an operative procedure. Since the myocardium has been constricted for a long time, it may take a considerable period for it to recover from this period of constriction. It is probably wise, therefore, to advise the patient to avoid even moderate exertion for a period up to 6 months.

Recurrent Acute Pericarditis

In recent years a syndrome has been recognized (Zinsser, 1959) in which the patient may have recurrent bouts of acute pericarditis. The patient's fever and malaise may subside at rest, only to flare up again when he returns to work. The patient may have repeated attacks extending over a period of many months. Even in the absence of constriction of the pericardium, the patient may suffer considerable disability due to the recurrent nature of the disease. In recent years such patients have been subjected to pericardiectomy with excellent results. The operation is technically simple, since the pericardium usually is not tightly adherent to the heart.

PERICARDIAL EFFUSION

The patient with a pericardial effusion, particularly a tuberculous one, may present a considerable problem to the surgeon. The question always arises as to whether one is dealing with a large heart or whether an effusion actually is present. The cardiologist usually can have some opinion on this subject, but in some instances it is exceedingly difficult for him to be certain.

The ultimate diagnosis of pericardial effusion is the removal of some of the fluid by needle aspiration. When the fluid is clear and obviously from the pericardial area, the diagnosis is established. After the removal of some of the fluid, a small quantity of air may be injected and roentgenographic films taken to delineate the size of the heart. Upon occasion, the fluid in the pericardial sac may be grossly bloody, and the question may arise as to whether the needle is in the cardiac cavity or in the pericardial sac. In most instances, if a hemoglobin determination is made of the fluid removed, it will be found that it is not so high as that in the blood stream. Sometimes, however, there may be some real question in the mind of the person who is doing the pericardicentesis. If air were injected into the cardiac cavity, the result might be catastrophic. An easy method of determining whether the needle is in the pericardial space with grossly bloody fluid or whether it is in the cardiac cavity is to inject some Decholin. If the patient tastes it immediately, then one can be sure that the needle is in the cardiac cavity. If the patient does not taste it, then air can be injected and a film taken to delineate the size of the heart.

The treatment of the patient with pericardial effusion depends to a considerable extent upon the etiology of the effusion. The most common variety is incident to heart failure, and the treatment depends fundamentally upon relief of that condition. In patients with either tuberculous pericarditis and effusion or with bloody pericardial effusion of uncertain etiology, a more direct attack may be worth while. If the diagnosis of tuberculosis can be established, probably the patient should be treated with antitubercular drugs for a matter of 6 months, if possible, and then undergo a resection of the pericardium. However, we have seen an occasional patient with bloody pericardial effusion in whom a diagnosis of tuberculosis could not be established and have operated without delay with resection of the pericardium. In some instances the pericardial effusion has turned out to be on the basis of metastatic malignancy, but undoubtedly there are some instances in which the etiologic agent is not determined.

In the absence of a diagnosis, we feel that operation through the left chest with removal of a large segment of the pericardium is advisable. This will prevent further accumulation of fluid in the pericardial cavity and also allow a generous biopsy for diagnostic purposes.

Acute Pyogenic Pericarditis

Acute pyogenic pericarditis was a not uncommon occurrence before the advent of antibiotics. Frequently, it was a terminal event in patients dying from various types of pneumonia. At the present time the surgeon seldom is called upon to treat a patient with acute pyogenic pericarditis. Most commonly now it is the result of trauma. However, the pericardium may be drained through the mediastinum without entering the pleural cavity should the necessity arise.

Pericarditis incident to uremia or rheumatic fever seldom is confused with pyogenic pericarditis.

SURGERY OF THE MYOCARDIUM

Stab Wounds of the Heart

The suture of stab wounds of the heart was perhaps the first operation performed upon the heart itself. It was first done successfully by Rehn in 1896 (Rehn, 1897). The patient with a wound of the heart who survives to reach the hospital is likely to have been stabbed with a knife or an ice pick rather than to have received a gunshot wound.

The patient who dies of a stab wound of the heart is apt to do so for two reasons: one is the loss of blood from the circulation; the other—and perhaps the more frequent cause—is the filling of the pericardial sac with blood, causing tamponade of the heart. For that reason, the heart cannot fill and cannot maintain an effective cardiac output.

The diagnosis of a stab wound of the heart should be suspected in any instance in which there is a stab wound anywhere within the general neighborhood of the heart, even though the patient may not be in extremis when seen. If the patient is in shock and pulseless, the diagnosis will be suspected, of course, but, when the patient is in relatively good condition, the unwary clinician is apt to overlook the possibility of the heart wound. One of the most helpful maneuvers in the diagnosis of cardiac tamponade is fluoroscopy, the cardiac impulse being barely demonstrable. If there has been very little blood loss, the pressure in the venous side may be increased, but in most instances total blood loss has been sufficient, so that the venous pressure is not increased.

The treatment of stab wounds of the heart falls into two categories: (1) the conservative treatment in which pericardial aspiration is used; and (2) the operative treatment in which the heart is exposed and the wound in the heart sutured.

The advocates of the conservative form of treatment have come to the conclusion that in most instances the actual bleeding from the cardiac cavity will be overcome fairly early following the trauma, and that the major problem will center in the cardiac tamponade preventing effective cardiac filling. They also feel that most of the patients can be brought through satisfactorily on conservative therapy, and that only those patients who do not respond to this method of treatment should be operated upon.

The advocates of operative therapy have felt that it is better to open the pericardial sac to suture the wound in the heart and at the same time decompress the pericardium completely. The author has advocated the operative treatment in these patients largely on the theoretic basis that, if the proper operating team is available, the patient who could survive the conservative treatment would also survive the operative treatment, and that an occasional patient might be brought through by operating immediately, whereas he might have died had conservative therapy been used originally.

There can be no doubt, however, that those individuals who have had the greatest experience with stab wounds of the heart have depended more and more on conservative therapy and have had excellent results by that means. So long as the patient is watched carefully and an operating team can stand by ready to open the chest if necessary, it may well be that it is worth while to try the conservative approach. Whether treatment is operative or nonoperative, the liberal use of transfusions is most important.

Myocardial Ischemia

Undoubtedly, obliterative disease of the coronary arteries is the greatest problem facing those investigators interested in the heart. In normal circumstances, when a coronary artery becomes occluded or nearly so in one or more areas, a collateral blood-flow is apt to develop to keep the myocardium alive. If an acute area of occlusion occurs over too large an area, the patient dies. The desire of the surgeon has been to produce some means of increasing the blood-flow to the myocardium when the coronary arterial flow is inadequate.

Many procedures have been advocated in the hope of increasing the myocardial blood-flow, but, as yet, none of them has been accepted universally. The simplest of these procedures is that of putting an irritating substance into the pericardial sac, such as talcum powder or powdered bone, with the thought that the irritating substance will cause adhesions between the myocardium and the pericardium, and that a new blood supply will grow in from the surrounding structures to supply the myocardium.

Other methods of bringing a blood supply to the myocardium have included the transplantation of muscles, skin or omentum directly to the myocardium. Beck (1955), who has been the most persistent investigator in the field, has attempted to bring a new blood supply to the heart by an arterial graft from the aorta to the coronary sinus. Removal of the obstruction in the coronary artery by endarterectomy has been employed with and without the aid of the heart lung machine (Dilley, 1965) (Effler, 1967). None of these procedures has been widely used. Transplantation of the internal mammary artery into the myocardium as utilized by Vineberg (1955) has become popular in the recent past, since the cineangiograms by Sones (1962) have shown blood going to the myocardium by this technic.

The advocates of these various procedures have felt that many patients have been improved by them. However, the greatest difficulty in evaluating these operative procedures has been the fact that many of these patients improve as they develop their own collateral circulation, and they may go on for years without any type of operative procedure.

SURGERY OF ACQUIRED VALVULAR DISEASE

Mitral Stenosis

Almost always, mitral stenosis is incident to rheumatic heart disease, which usually occurs in childhood or the early teens. During the healing process of acute rheumatic fever with valvular involvement, the opening in the mitral valve may decrease gradually.

Pathology. At times the disease may be minimal, and mitral stenosis is produced by simple fusion of the leaflets at the commissures. In some instances, the disease is severe, causing great thickening of the leaflets with fusion of the leaflets at the commissures, and there may also be shortening and fusing of the chordae tendineae and the papillary muscles. When there is necrosis of the leaflet with scarring and contraction, the edges may no longer be able to meet, and regurgitation as well as stenosis occurs. In the healing process of severe acute disease, extensive calcification may occur.

The reduced size of the opening in the mitral valve may remain relatively constant for a number of years. It is believed that, whereas the patient's heart may be able to force blood through the small opening at a satisfactory rate during the early years, following recovery from the acute disease, as time goes on the heart may fail and no longer be able to do so. The pressure in the left atrium increases gradually, and this increase in pressure is transmitted to the vascular bed in the lungs. Over a period of time there may be hemoptysis as a result of hemorrhages into the alveoli in the lungs. With the pouring out of exudate and the organization of this exudate, there may be actual vascular constriction in the arterioles in the lungs. As a result, the pulmonary artery pressure increases in order to force the blood through the lungs. As time progresses, the patient may go into right heart failure because of the increased effort needed to push blood through the narrowed vascular bed of the lung. In many instances, the patient may do reasonably well, so long as the cardiac rhythm remains normal. However, frequently, with the onset of auricular fibrillation, which causes a loss of an effective left atrial beat, acute symptoms may develop as the result of a decreased cardiac output.

Diagnosis. The diagnosis of mitral stenosis usually is not difficult for the trained cardiologist. The presystolic rumble at the apex is fairly characteristic, and, on fluoroscopy and orthodiagram, the heart will assume a typical so-called mitral configuration with enlargement of the left atrium. The lung fields will be congested with blood in many instances, and the pulmonary artery may be increased in size. Occasionally, however, the murmur may be insignificant or absent, and the diagnosis may be a real problem. More commonly, the diagnostic problem is one of distinguishing

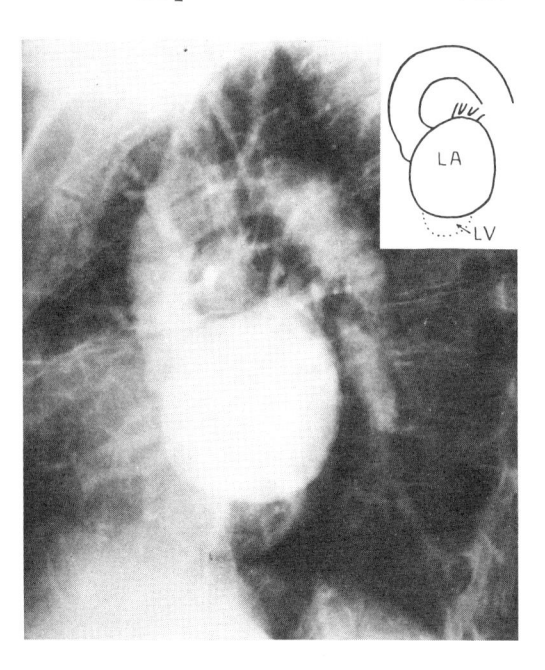

FIG. 43-22. Angiocardiogram of a patient with mitral stenosis. Note the intense opacification of the left atrium and the relatively poor visualization of the left ventricle. This represents a hang-up of the contrast medium at the level of the mitral valve.

between the relative severity of mitral stenosis and mitral regurgitation.

There are several methods by which some conclusion can be reached regarding this problem. Angiocardiography is a valuable one (Zinsser, 1953). When the mitral stenosis is severe, the contrast medium is held up in the left atrium for a considerable period of time, with the contrast medium showing poorly in the small left ventricle. When the regurgitation (insufficiency) is the predominant factor, the medium will flow back and forth between the left atrium and the left ventricle, and the two cavities will be visualized to approximately the same extent. In recent years this method for evaluating the amount of mitral regurgitation has been replaced largely by left heart catheterization. A movie is taken as opaque is injected into the left ventricle through a catheter passed retrograde from the femoral artery through the aortic valve. The amount of regurgitation may be visualized directly.

In expert hands the ultrasound technic has

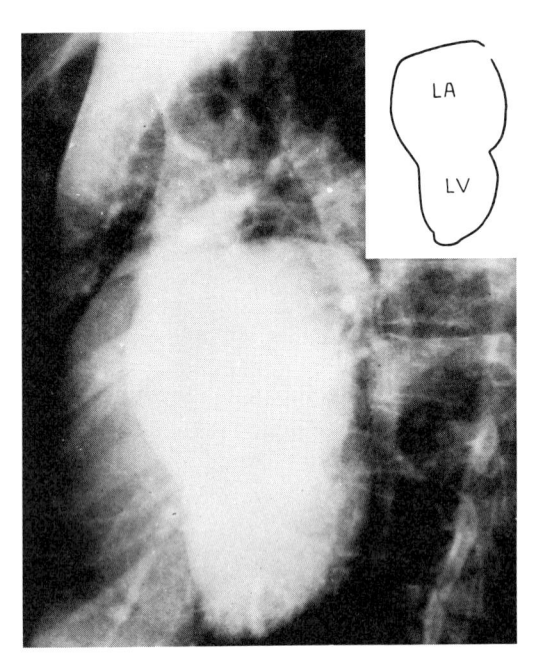

FIG. 43-23. Angiocardiogram of a patient with mitral regurgitation. The large left atrium and the large left ventricle are opacified to about the same extent by the contrast medium. This suggests that the contrast medium is going back and forth between the two cavities because of regurgitation at the mitral valve. This is shown in contrast with the angiocardiogram in a patient with pure mitral stenosis as shown in Figure 43-22.

been very helpful in determining the severity of the mitral stenosis. It also has been quite accurate in determining the condition of the mitral leaflets and is relied upon heavily in the selection of patients for the closed operation on the mitral valve (Joyner, 1963).

Treatment. Mitral commissurotomy for the patient with mitral stenosis was first performed apparently by Souttar in 1925, and more recently revived by Bailey (1949) and by Harken (1948). Cutler and Beck (1924) did a great deal of work on the problem of mitral stenosis in the 1920's, but abandoned the procedure because most of their work was directed toward increasing the mitral opening by cutting away a portion of the mitral valve. The amount of regurgitation obtained by this method was not tolerated by the heart. The concept of opening the fused commissures, as originally practiced by Souttar (1925), however, was designed to obtain an increase in the size of the opening without increasing the regurgitation.

The likelihood of performing a successful mitral commissurotomy in the patient with mitral stenosis will depend to a considerable degree upon the type of valve present. In some instances, the valve leaflets are thin and pliable, and fused only at the commissures, so that they may be separated to function essentially normally again, and the patient's condition may return to normal. In other instances, however, the valve may be so severely calcified that it is difficult or impossible to

FIG. 43-24. Pressure curves obtained on left heart catheterization on two different patients, one with mitral stenosis on the right and one with mitral insufficiency on the left. In the patient with mitral stenosis note the high level of the left auricular pressure which is maintained throughout the cardiac cycle and not influenced materially by ventricular systole.

In mitral insufficiency the left auricular pressure curve is similar in contour to that of the left ventricle with a peak during ventricular systole, although of course the peak does not go nearly so high.

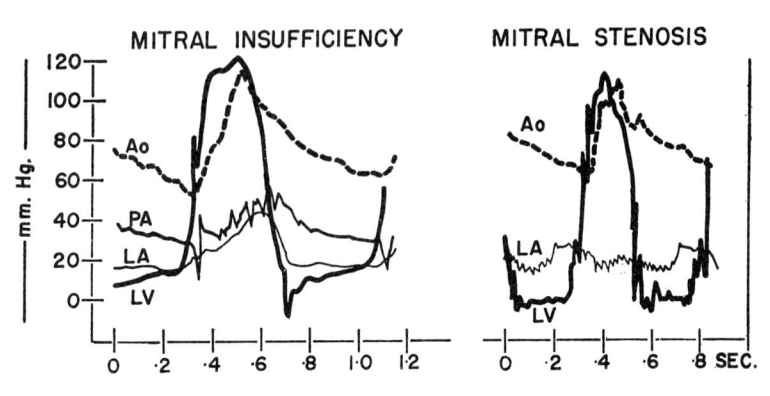

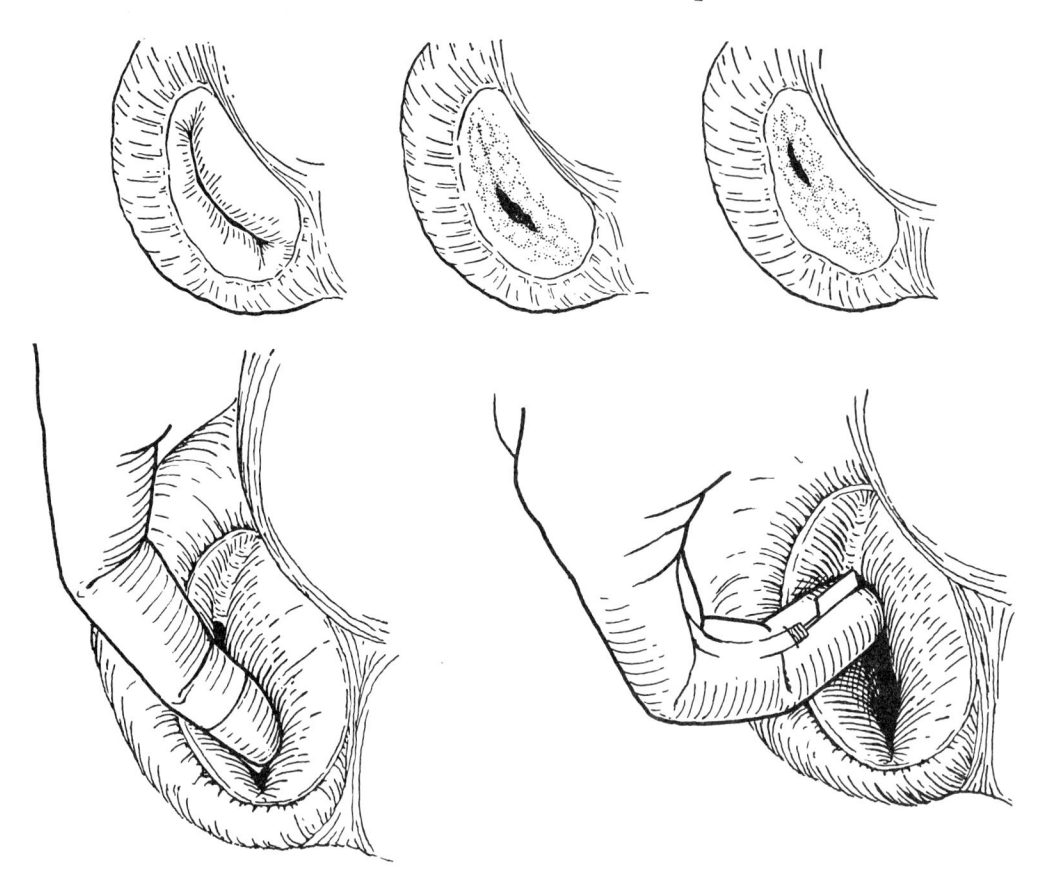

Fig. 43-25. (*Top*) The mitral valve is shown in a diagrammatic sketch. The valve on the left is a normal valve. The other two show fusion of the commissures in various locations. Both of the stenotic valves shown are relatively favorable ones for commissurotomy. (*Bottom*) Illustrating commissurotomy of a stenotic mitral valve. In many instances it is possible to open both the anterior and posterior commissures by means of finger fracture. When it is not possible to do this, some type of knife is commonly used. (*Left*) The posterior commissure is being opened by finger fracture, utilizing the fingernail to help tear open the posterior commissure. (*Right*) The knife shown in opening the anterior commissure is that designed by Brock. (Johnson, J., and Kirby, C.: Surgery of the Chest. Chicago, Year Book Publishers)

obtain a reasonably functioning valve, regardless of the operative procedure employed.

Mitral commissurotomy was carried out for many years by inserting the finger through the left atrial appendage and opening the valve by finger fracture. Various types of knives were used at times. Later, a dilator was inserted through the left ventricular wall and guided into position by the finger in the left atrium, to separate the fused leaflets.

As the use of cardiopulmonary bypass has become more and more widespread, and confidence in this method has increased, most surgeons are doing an increasing number of these operations by the open technic. The ultrasound technic has been very helpful in picking out the patients whose valves may be opened satisfactorily by the closed method.

The risk of closed commissurotomy in the patient with mitral stenosis centers in the possibility of some unexpected catastrophic hemorrhage, upon the possibility of a cerebral embolus (either a clot from the left atrium or some calcium from the valve), the inadvertent production of significant regurgitation, or of operating upon a patient who already has reached the end stages of the disease. The operative mortality among unselected patients should not exceed 10 per cent, and in selected groups, when the favorable valves are selected by ultrasound for the closed method, the mortality should approach zero.

At the present time most surgeons operate upon the patient with simple mitral stenosis by the closed technic. If the patient has had a previous embolism, or there is a fear of clots in the left atrium because of atrial fibrillation, or there is a calcified valve, raising the likelihood of an embolism at operation, the author prefers to operate under direct vision, reserving the closed method for the patients with thin, pliable leaflets as shown by ultrasound.

The postoperative management of the good-risk patient with mitral stenosis may be similar to that of any other thoracic patient. In the poor risk patient or when the valve cannot be opened satisfactorily, great care must be exercised in the patient's postoperative care. In general, the measures taken in preparing the patient for operation must be repeated, namely, low salt intake, mercurial diuretics, digitalis and careful attention to fluid balance.

When there is a high pulmonary artery pressure and the lungs are stiff it is often helpful to do a tracheostomy and use a ventilator for a while postoperatively in the poor-risk patient.

Mitral Regurgitation

There can be no question that mitral regurgitation places a severe limitation on the heart as a pump. It is obviously desirable to overcome this valvular deficiency. The various methods not requiring cardiopulmonary bypass which have been used in the past have been successful occasionally, but the over-all results have left much to be desired.

At the present time all of these operations are done under direct vision utilizing the heart-lung machine. In some patients the leaflets appear to be relatively normal but allow regurgitation because of a dilated annulus. By placing sutures in the annulus, it may be possible to shorten it so that the leaflets meet. In some patients apparently operated upon successfully, the regurgitation has recurred within a few months to a year, apparently due to the sutures pulling through. In many patients there is a deficiency of the valve at the posterior commissure and also fusion of the leaflets anteriorly. After the leaflets are separated, getting rid of the stenosis, it has been possible to overcome the regurgitation by annuloplasty. Various plastic procedures have also been used on the valves in an effort to overcome regurgitation. When a heavily calcified stenotic valve is opened and an important degree of regurgitation is produced, it is very difficult to make a good valve out of it by annuloplasty. For this reason, most surgeons have gone over to the artificial valve. Some use it almost exclusively. The ball or disc type valve prostheses are now widely used. The valve functions satisfactorily from a physiologic standpoint. The biggest hazard of the valve is the tendency for clotting to occur. For this reason, most patients are carried on permanent anticoagulant therapy. It is hoped that further improvements in the design of the prosthetic valves may solve this problem.

Aortic Stenosis

Pathologic Physiology. In most instances, the etiology of aortic stenosis is rheumatic heart disease. Frequently the aortic valve is involved at the same time as the mitral valve, but aortic stenosis may occur as an isolated lesion. When the aortic valve alone is involved, it is apt to be very extensively diseased, and frequently it is severely calcified by the time the patient sees the surgeon. In some instances the aortic valve becomes stenotic by simple fusion of the commissures, in which event one still can ascertain where the commissures were located. In other instances, however, the aortic valve is completely calcified and the previous location of the commissures is not detectable by palpation alone.

As the result of aortic stenosis, the left ventricle becomes hypertrophied and the myocardium very thick in order to force the blood through the small opening. The left ventricular cavity will be small, and the patient may do quite well so long as the myocardium can overcome the obstruction at the aortic valve. However, once the patient with aortic stenosis develops heart failure, the ventricular cavity enlarges, and then his prognosis is apt to be very bad. Whereas a patient with mitral stenosis may go in and out of failure on a number

Acquired Heart Disease

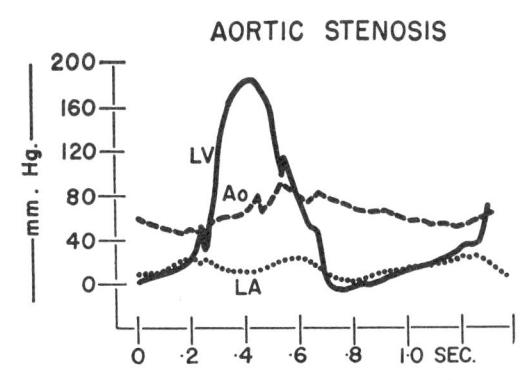

FIG. 43-26. Pressure curves obtained on left heart catheterization in a patient with aortic stenosis. Note that the peak of the pressure in the left ventricle is about 185 at a time when the peak of the pressure in the aorta is only about 90. The pressure curve in the left auricle indicates that the mitral valve is normal.

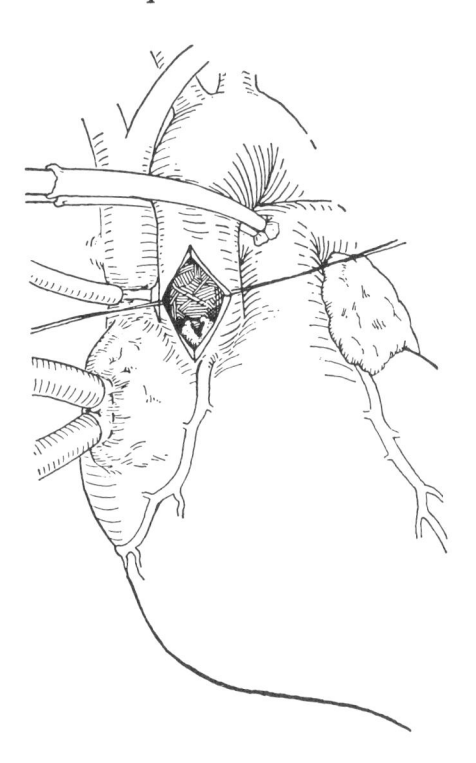

FIG. 43-27. In the past the greatest number of operations for acquired aortic stenosis were done using a dilator inserted through the left ventricle. In recent years there has been a trend toward performing the operation under direct vision utilizing cardiopulmonary bypass. The cannulae for perfusion of the coronary arteries are not shown in the diagram, but this adjunct gives the surgeon adequate time to work on the valve. (Johnson, J., and Kirby, C.: Surgery of the Chest. Chicago, Year Book Publishers)

of occasions and still recover, the patient with aortic stenosis is not nearly so likely to do so.

When the aortic stenosis is congenital in origin, the lesion is most commonly valvular. Less frequently there is subvalvular stenosis in the outflow tract of the left ventricle, while rarely there is supravalvular stenosis of the aortic wall. When the valvular stenosis is severe, operation may be necessary in childhood. The valve is often bicuspid. Frequently, the stenosis, even though valvular, is not severe enough to require operation until the leaflets become partially calcified in later life, apparently due to long-standing trauma.

Diagnosis. The diagnosis of aortic stenosis can be made readily. From the standpoint of symptoms, the patient may have periods of syncope. Anginal pain is frequently associated with it. The systolic murmur over the aortic area is often characteristic, and, as a general rule, the systolic blood pressure is low, as is the pulse pressure.

The most exact diagnostic procedure that can be used is left heart catheterization, so that a pressure tracing may be taken from the left ventricle as well as the base of the aorta. With aortic stenosis, the systolic pressure in the left ventricle will be considerably higher than that in the aorta during systole, and the pressure curves will be characteristic.

Treatment. In congenital aortic stenosis the valvular type is the type most commonly requiring operation in infancy or childhood. The fused leaflets must be opened with great care to avoid prolapse and subsequent regurgitation. When the valve is bicuspid, the opening can usually be greatly improved even though the surgeon cannot make a tricuspid valve of it. The supravalvular type usually requires a patch of the aortic wall. The subvalvular stenosis of the membranous type may be easily corrected through the aortic valve opening in late childhood and adult life. The muscular hypertrophy type is not well understood, but has been handled by a simple incision through the hypertrophied muscle (Morrow, 1961) and by muscular excision (Julian, 1964).

The early attempts to correct acquired aortic stenosis consisted of efforts to break open the commissures of the valve blindly by means of a dilator inserted through the left ventricle. The lowest mortality was attained with this approach when the heart was put partially at rest by means of left heart bypass (Johnson, 1961). Also, efforts were made to open the valve digitally from above through a diverticulum sutured on the ascending aorta. The efforts by either of these methods were occasionally strikingly successful, at least for a while. The greatest success at dilatation was in the cases without severe calcification of the valve and with simple fusion of the leaflets.

The first efforts to operate upon acquired aortic stenosis under direct vision consisted of attempts to open the commissures and to remove enough of the calcium when it was present to allow better mobility of the leaflets. When it became apparent that it frequently was not possible to reconstruct a calcified cusp, one or more cusps were replaced with various types of plastic cloth cusps, usually made of Teflon. Then it became apparent that an aortic valve from which the calcium had been removed frequently would become calcified again within a few years, and indeed that prosthetic leaflets would become rigid and stenosed and occasionally rupture. In recent years most surgeons have adopted the use of the ball-type aortic valve. Clotting on the valve is not as frequent as when the valve is in the mitral position, but it still constitutes a problem. Bits of endothelium may also break off to form emboli. The completely cloth-covered valve may overcome this problem. Homograft valves are not likely to produce emboli but have not been more widely accepted to date for fear that they will not hold up over a long period of time.

Aortic Regurgitation

Marked aortic regurgitation produces a severe handicap upon the pumping mechanism of the heart. However, mild degrees of regurgitation may be tolerated for many years. The diagnosis is usually easily established by the diastolic murmur extending from the base of the heart to the apex and by the wide pulse pressure. It may be difficult to distinguish from regurgitation at the pulmonary valve under some circumstances. Definitive studies can be carried out most easily using cineangiography by injecting opaque into the root of the aorta, usually by way of a catheter passed from the femoral artery. If aortic regurgitation is present, the opaque will be seen to pass into the left ventricle. The severity of the regurgitation can also be estimated.

There are several types of aortic valves in which regurgitation is present. There may be sufficient deformity associated with calcific disease to produce both stenosis and regurgitation; there may be destruction of one or more leaflets by bacterial endocarditis; and there may be dilatation of the aortic root with or without shortening of the leaflets to produce regurgitation but without calcification.

None of the early efforts to correct aortic regurgitation without the use of cardiopulmonary bypass was of much use. The early efforts to relieve aortic regurgitation by the open technic involved attempts to elongate individual cusps or to replace one or more cusps with various artificial cusps when dealing with calcific disease, and attempts to produce a competent bicuspid valve by obliterating the noncoronary cusp when dealing with relatively normal leaflets but a dilated aortic root. The latter of these procedures appears to hold up fairly well in some instances if properly executed. However, most surgeons have now adopted the use of the ball or disc type prosthesis or homografts. The immediate results with these methods have been satisfactory. It is too early to know the long term results.

Mitral and Aortic Stenosis

When both the aortic and the mitral valves are involved, the operation is now done by the open technic almost exclusively. In the early experience the surgeon was apt to try to correct the worst of the two valves, feeling that the risk would be increased by operating upon both. More recently it has become the consensus that the patient's best chance lies in giving him the best possible valvular function at all valves.

Tricuspid Stenosis and Regurgitation

Tricuspid stenosis is usually the result of rheumatic fever, and most often it occurs in association with involvement of the mitral

FIG. 43-28. This is a diagrammatic sketch of an aneurysm in the descending aorta distal to the left subclavian artery which has been excised and replaced by homograft. This may be carried out by utilizing partial left heart bypass. Blood is pumped from the left atrium to the left femoral artery. This method is probably safer than using hypothermia alone. Plastic grafts have now largely replaced homografts for this purpose.

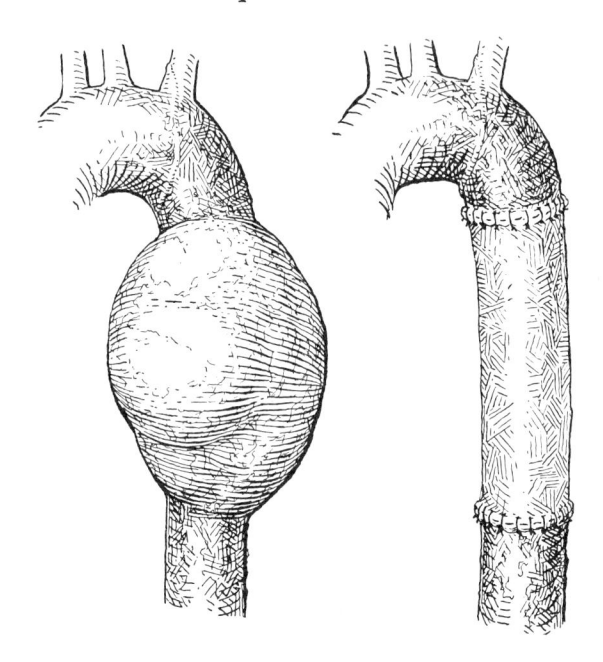

and/or the aortic valve. The most important problem is the danger of overlooking the diagnosis when tricuspid stenosis is present in association with other valve involvement. It is apt to occur in about 10 per cent of the patients who have involvement of both the mitral and the aortic valves, even though it may not be diagnosed preoperatively. Theoretically, the diagnosis of tricuspid stenosis should be ascertainable by right heart catheterization, by placing catheters in the right atrium and the right ventricle and taking simultaneous pressure curves. The fact that this has been done so infrequently to date is probably the result of the difficulty in suspecting the diagnosis clinically.

Severe tricuspid regurgitation may be associated with long-standing mitral stenosis resulting in dilation of the right heart. At the time of operation on the mitral valve, an annuloplasty on the tricuspid valve will usually correct the regurgitation. When tricuspid stenosis is present, the valve will often require replacement.

Aneurysm of the Thoracic Aorta

Aneurysms of the thoracic aorta usually are due to weakening of the aortic wall incident to syphilis or arteriosclerosis, followed by dilatation. In most instances, the symptoms produced by aortic aneurysms are due to the compression of surrounding structures. When the arch of the aorta is involved, the trachea is most commonly compressed. When the aneurysm is large, it may cause erosion of the sternum or the trachea, and death due to rupture of the aneurysm is common. Aneurysms of the descending aorta are apt to erode the spine and cause back pain.

The diagnosis of an aortic aneurysm usually is not difficult. However, it may be confused with a mediastinal tumor, since it is difficult to differentiate between the expansile pulsation of an aneurysm and the transmitted pulsation of a mediastinal tumor lying close to the heart or the aorta. When there is doubt, frequently the diagnosis can be confirmed by an angiocardiogram or an aortogram. It is possible, of course, that such studies would not be helpful if the aneurysm were filled with blood clot. In the dissecting aneurysm the double lumen of the aorta will usually be visualized.

The surgical treatment of aneurysm of the thoracic aorta is the resection of the aneurysm and repair of the defect, usually by a graft. Not very long ago it was common practice, when dealing with an aneurysm protruding from one side of the aorta, to attempt to clamp it at its neck and suture it at that point after resection of the aneurysm. That technic has been abandoned now, due to the fear of displacing old blood clots.

In aneurysms distal to the left carotid artery, the aorta may be clamped proximal and distal to the aneurysm, the aneurysm resected and replaced with a graft. Aortic homografts were used in the early experience with this technic, but at the present time plastic grafts are considered to be superior and are obtained much more easily. During the period while the aorta is clamped, partial left heart bypass is used to provide blood flow to the lower part of the body. Blood is pumped from the left atrium to the left common femoral artery at the rate of roughly half the estimated resting cardiac output. This technic is superior to the hypothermia technic formerly used. With that technic it was hoped that the oxygen requirements of the spinal cord and the kidneys would be reduced sufficiently so that the aorta could be clamped long enough to do the operation and still not injure the spinal cord or kidneys. Another objection to that technic was that with the clamping of the aorta, the cold heart might be overloaded by suddenly having to pump all of the blood against the resistance of the vascular bed supplied by the innominate and the left carotid arteries only.

When the aneurysm is located proximal to the left common carotid artery, the partial left heart bypass technic is not applicable. When the ascending aorta close to the coronary arteries is involved, total cardiopulmonary bypass is necessary during the period that the aorta is clamped. If the aneurysm is sufficiently distal to the coronary arteries, it is probably best not to use cardiopulmonary bypass since the heparinization required causes more bleeding. If enough aorta is available proximal to the aneurysm, a bypass plastic graft is first placed from the ascending aorta to the descending aorta. This serves as the new arch of the aorta. Side arms are then attached to it and then to the innominate and the left carotid arteries. Having thus established an alternate pathway for the blood to leave the heart, the arch of the aorta may be clamped on either side of the aneurysm, the innominate and the left carotid clamped proximal to the grafts, the aneurysm resected, and the free ends closed. The technical problems involved in replacing the arch of the aorta are obviously greater, and the risk is higher than when dealing with the descending aorta alone.

In a dissecting aneurysm of the aorta, the diseased intima and internal layers of the media usually have ruptured, allowing the blood from the aortic lumen to dissect out between the layers of aorta, producing a double lumen. In some instances the second lumen appears to have been due to hemorrhage from the vasa vasorum. If the second lumen extends downward, it may shut off the various branches of the aorta as the dissection proceeds, producing such phenomenon as cord paralysis, anuria, and ischemia of the legs. When the point of rupture is situated where it can be resected and a graft inserted, that should be done. If not, some palliation may be provided by dividing the descending aorta, suturing the intima to the media and the adventitia below, to prevent further downward dissection, and reuniting the aorta, leaving a point of re-entry to the main channel from the secondary lumen proximally.

When a definitive study can be carried out and the site of the dissection determined, the operation can be planned more intelligently. Now that more definitive studies are being done, it has been found that the dissection often starts at the ascending aorta. When this can be determined, the patient should be placed on cardiopulmonary bypass and the coronary arteries perfused as the ascending aorta is replaced.

OPEN CARDIAC SURGERY UNDER DIRECT VISION

The development of a technic by which intracardiac surgery could be done under direct vision was the dream of all cardiac surgeons for many years. It has now been used successfully more or less routinely in a large number of hospitals throughout the world.

Because of difficulties in the development of a satisfactory heart-lung machine, the first "open heart" operations were done with the aid of hypothermia. Swan (1955) and Lewis (1955) were among the first to operate on a large number of patients with atrial septal defects, utilizing this technic. The method has now been used quite widely and successfully for that lesion, as well as for operations on patients with the valvular type of pulmonary stenosis. However, most surgeons were unhappy with the limitation as to time imposed by moderate hypothermia and were desirous of a heart-lung machine which would allow the surgeon unlimited operating time.

In the development of the heart-lung machine, Gibbon was perhaps the most persistent investigator over the years (Miller, 1953). It is his machine, with modifications by many other workers, which is perhaps the best one available today. It utilizes a screen-type oxygenator. However, its use has been limited by the cost of its production. The bubble-type oxygenator is the least expensive to produce and has been used with real success in many clinics. The disk-type oxygenator offers a compromise as to cost and safety. It would appear that the membrane-type oxygenator would most closely simulate the action of the human lungs, but it has not been widely used. Further development in method is required, since successful prolonged perfusion is not possible with any of the present machines.

CARDIAC RESUSCITATION

Cardiac arrest is a term that includes ventricular asystole and ventricular fibrillation; it simply indicates that the effective pumping mechanism of the heart has stopped. It is a catastrophe that is apt to occur once or twice a year on any busy surgical service. The incidence in patients not undergoing cardiac surgery has been about 1 in 6,000 operations at the Hospital of the University of Pennsylvania.

It has been demonstrated that these patients may be revived if the diagnosis is made and treatment is instituted within about 4 minutes (Johnson, 1954). If the patient's pulse and blood pressure disappear suddenly and unexpectedly, the anesthetist should report it promptly to the surgeon. Unless the surgeon is in a position to deny the presence of cardiac arrest by feeling the heart or a pulsating artery, he should institute closed-chest cardiac massage at once. In the past it was customary to open the chest and compress the heart directly, but it has now been amply demonstrated that closed-chest cardiac compression is satisfactory (Kouwenhoven, 1960). If the compression is effective, a peripheral pulse will be palpable at each compression, and the patient's color should return toward normal. If the heart has stopped due to an overdose of the anesthetic, the vagovagal reflex, or hypoxia, it should start up again after a short period of artificial circulation and respiration. If the heart is found to be in ventricular fibrillation, it can be returned to a normal rhythm most effectively by electric shock. This too can be done by a shock through the closed chest. However, the shock should not be instituted until the patient has been gotten out of the state of anoxia by artificial ventilation and circulation. Of course, an external defibrillator as opposed to an internal defibrillator is required. A stronger current (100-300 watt seconds) is required. A direct current is also superior to the old method of using alternating current.

Once the heart has recovered from asystole or ventricular fibrillation, some drugs may be helpful in maintaining a useful heart beat. Epinephrine may speed up the heart beat and increase its effectiveness. It also increases the risk of ventricular fibrillation. Calcium chloride also has at times apparently increased the forcefulness of the heart beat. Molar sodium lactate has been helpful in certain situations by correcting the chemical disturbances brought about by metabolic changes in the myocardium. Norepinephrine has also been very helpful at times by raising the blood pressure and thereby supplying more blood to the myocardium, as well as by being a direct stimulant to the myocardium perhaps.

While electric shock was originally used only to stop ventricular fibrillation, it has recently been widely used to revert the heart in atrial fibrillation to a normal rhythm. This has been most useful to date in the postoperative period after surgery of the mitral valve. It has also been useful occasionally in the reversion of other arrythmias.

REFERENCES

Abbott, M. E.: Congenital cardiac disease. *In*: Nelson's Loose Leaf Medicine. New York, 1920.

Baffes, T. G., Lev, M., Paul, M. H., Miller, R. A., Riker, W. L., DeBoer, A., and Potts, W. J.: Surgical correction of transposition of the great vessels—a five-year survey. Read before the American Association for Thoracic Surgery, May, 1960. J. Thorac. Cardio. Surg., 40:298, 1960.

Bailey, C. P.: Surgery of the Heart. Philadelphia, Lea & Febiger, 1955.

———: Surgical treatment of mitral stenosis. Dis. Chest, 15:377, 1949.
Bailey, C. P., Downing, D. F., Geckeler, G. D., Likoff, W., Goldberg, H., Scott, J. C., Jantoni, O., and Redondo-Ramirez, H. P.: Congential interatrial communications: clinical and surgical considerations with a description of a new surgical technic: atrio-septo-pexy. Ann. Int. Med., 37:888, 1952.
Beck, C. S.: Acute and chronic compression of the heart. Am. Heart J., 14:515, 1937.
Beck, C. S., and Leighninger, D. S.: Scientific basis for the surgical treatment of coronary artery disease. J.A.M.A., 159:1264, 1955.
Blalock, A., and Hanlon, C. R.: Interatrial septal defect—its experimental production under direct vision without interruption of the circulation. Surg., Gynec., Obstet., 87:183, 1948.
———: The surgical treatment of complete transposition of the aorta and the pulmonary artery. Surg., Gynec., Obstet., 90:1, 1950.
Blalock, A., and Taussig, H. B.: The surgical treatment of malformation of the heart in which there is pulmonary stenosis or pulmonary atresia. J.A.M.A., 128:189, 1945.
Bjork, V. O., Blakemore, W. S., and Malmstrom, G.: Left ventricular pressure measurements in man; a new method. Am. Heart J., 48:197, 1954.
Bjork, V. O., and Crafoord, C.: The surgical closure of interauricular septal defects. J. Thoracic Surg., 26:300, 1953.
Brock, R. C.: Infundibular resection or dilatation for infundibular stenosis. Brit. Heart J., 12:403, 1950.
———: Pulmonary valvulotomy for relief of congenital pulmonary stenosis. Brit. Med. J., 1:1121, 1948.
Carrel, A.: Results of the transplantation of blood vessels, organs and limbs. J.A.M.A., 51:1662, 1908.
Cohn, R.: An experimental method for the closure of interauricular septal defects in dogs. Am. Heart J., 30:453, 1947.
Crafoord, C., and Nylin, G.: Congenital coarctation of the aorta and its surgical treatment. J. Thoracic Surg., 14:347, 1945.
Cutler, E. C., Levine, S. A., and Beck, C. S.: Surgical treatment of mitral stenosis. Arch. Surg., 9:689, 1924.
Dilley, R. B., Cannon, J. A., Kattus, A. A., MacAlpin, R. N., and Longmire, W. P., Jr.: The treatment of coronary occlusive disease by endarterectomy. J. Thor. Cardiov. Surg., 50:511, 1965.
Effler, D. B., Groves, L. K., Suarez, E. L., and Favaloro, R. G.: Direct coronary artery surgery with endarterotomy and patch-graft reconstruction. J. Thor. Cardiov. Surg., 53:93, 1967.
Fallot, A.: Contribution à l'anatomic pathologique de la maladie bleue. Marseille med., 25:77, 138, 207, 270, 341, 403, 1888.
Gibbon, J. H., Jr.: Artificial maintenance of the circulation during experimental occlusion of the pulmonary artery. Arch. Surg., 34:1105, 1937.
Glenn, W. W.: Circulatory bypass of the right side of the heart. IV. Shunt between superior vena cava and distal right pulmonary artery; report of clinical application. New Eng. J. Med., 259:117, 1958.

Gordon, A. S., Meyer, B. W., and Jones, J. C.: Open heart surgery using deep hypothermia without an oxygenator. Read before the American Association for Thoracic Surgery, May, 1960. J. Thorac. Cardiov. Surg., 40:787, 1960.
Gross, R. E.: Patent ductus arteriosus. Am. J. Med., 12:472, 1952.
———: Treatment of certain aortic coarctations by homologous grafts. Ann. Surg., 134:753, 1951.
Gross, R. E., and Hubbard, J. P.: Surgical ligation of patent ductus arteriosus. J.A.M.A., 112:729, 1939.
Gross, R. E., Pomeranz, A. A., Watkins, E., Jr., and Goldsmith, E. I.: Surgical closure of defects of the interauricular septum by use of the atrial wall. New Eng. J. Med., 247:455, 1952.
Halsted, W. S., and Reid, M. R.: An experimental study of circumscribed dilatation of an artery immediately distal to a partially occluding band. J. Exp. Med., 24:271, 1916.
Harken, D. E., Ellis, H. B., Ware, P. F., and Norman, L. R.: Surgical treatment of mitral stenosis. 1. Valvuloplasty. New Eng. J. Med., 239:801, 1948.
Holman, E.: The obscure physiology of poststenotic dilatation. J. Thoracic Surg., 28:109, 1954.
Hufnagel, C. A., and Harvey, W. P.: The surgical correction of aortic regurgitation. Bull. Georgetown Univ. M. Center, 6:60, 1953.
Johnson, J., and Kirby, C. K.: Prevention and treatment of cardiac arrest. J.A.M.A., 154:291, 1954.
Johnson, J., Kirby, C. K., and Blakemore, W. S.: Physiologic considerations in cardiac surgery, S. Clin. N. Am., 35:1729, 1955.
Johnson, J., Kirby, C. K., Blakemore, W. S., and Zinsser, H. F.: Intermittent inflow occlusion for the direct visual repair of atrial septal defect. J. Thoracic Surg., 37:314, 1959.
Johnson, J., Kirby, C. K., and Horn, R. C., Jr.: The growth of preserved aorta homografts. Surgery, 31:141, 1952.
Johnson, J., Kirby, C. K., Blakemore, W. S., Joyner, C. R., Helwig, J., Jr., and Zinsser, H. F.: Left heart bypass as an aid to transventricular aortic valvulotomy. J. Thorac. Cardiov. Surg., 41:787, 1961.
Joyner, C. R., Jr., Reid, J. M., and Bond, J. P.: Reflected ultrasound in the assessment of mitral valve disease. Circulation, 27:503, 1963.
Julian, O. C., Dye, W. S., Javid, H., Hunter, J. A., Muenster, J. J., and Najafi, H.: Apical left ventriculotomy in subaortic stenosis due to fibromuscular hypertrophy. Circulation, 31:44. 1964.
Kirklin, J. W., McGoon, D. C., and DuShane, J. W.: The results of surgical treatment for ventricular septal defect. Read before the American Assocation for Thoracic Surgery, May, 1960. J. Thorac. Cardiov. Surg., 40:763, 1960.
Kouwenhoven, W. B., Jude, J. R., and Knickerbocker, G. G.: Closed-chest cardiac massage. J.A.M.A., 173:1064, 1960.
Lewis, F. J., Taufic, M., Varco, R. L., and Niazi, S.: The surgical anatomy of atrial septal defects: experience with repair under direct vision. Ann. Surg., 142:401, 1955.
Lillehei, C. W., Cohen, M., Warden, H. E., Read, R. C., Aust, J. B., DeWall, R. A., and Varco, R.

L.: Direct vision intracardiac surgical correction of the tetralogy of Fallot, pentalogy of Sallot and pulmonary atresia defects. Ann. Surg., 142:418, 1955.

Mahoney, E. B., Manning, J. A., DeWeese, J. A., and Schwartz, S. I.: Clinical results of correction under hypothermia of atrial septal defects and pulmonary valvular stenosis. J. Thorac. Cardiov. Surg., 38:292, 1959.

Miller, B. J., Gibbon, J. H., Jr., and Fineberg, C.: An improved mechanical heart-lung apparatus. M. Clin. N. Am., 37:1603, 1953.

Moffitt, G. R., Zinsser, H. F., Jr., Kuo, P. T., Johnson, J., and Schnabel, T. G., Jr.: Pulmonary stenosis with left to right intracardiac shunts. Am. J. Med., 16:521, 1954.

Morrow, A. G., and Brockenbrough, E. C.: Surgical treatment of idiopathic hypertrophic subaortic stenosis: Technique and hemodynamic results of subaortic ventriculotomy. Ann. Surg., 154:181, 1961.

Muller, W. H., and Dammann, F.: Results following the creation of pulmonary stenosis (personal communication).

Mustard, W. T.: Successful two-stage correction of transposition of the great vessels. Surgery, 55:469, 1964.

Potts, W. T., Smith, S., and Gibson, S., Anastomosis of the aorta to a pulmonary artery. J.A.M.A., 132:627, 1946.

Rashkind, W. J., and Miller, W. W.: Creation of an atrial septal defect without thoracotomy. Palliative approach to complete transposition of the great arteries. J.A.M.A., 196:991, 1966.

Rehn, L.: Ueber penetrierende Herzwunuden und Herznaht. Arch. klin. Chir., 55:315, 1897.

Scott, H. W., Jr., and Bahnson, H. T.: Evidence for a renal factor in the hypertension of experimental coarctation of the aorta. Surgery, 30:206, 1951.

Scott, H. W., Jr., and Sabiston, D. C., Jr.: Surgical treatment for congenital aorticopulmonary fistula. J. Thoracic Surg., 25:26, 1953.

Senning, A.: Surgical correction of transposition of the great vessels. Surgery, 45:966, 1959.

Sones, F. M., Jr., and Shirey, E. K.: Cine Coronary Arteriography. Mod. Concepts Cardiovas. Dis., 31:725, 1962.

Souttar, H. S.: Surgical treatment of mitral stenosis. Brit. Med. J., 2:603, 1925.

Swan, H., Virtue, R. W., Blount, S. G., Jr., and Kircher, L. T., Jr.: Hypothermia in surgery: analysis of 100 clinical cases. Ann. Surg., 142:382, 1955.

Taussig, H. B.: Congenital Malformations of the Heart. New York, Commonwealth Fund, 1947.

Vineberg, A., Munro, D. D., Cohen, H., and Buller, W.: Four years' clinical experience with internal mammary artery implantation in human coronary insufficiency. J. Thoracic Surg., 29:1, 1955.

Waldhausen, J. A., Friedman, S., Tyers, G. F. O., Rashkind, W. J., Petry, E., and Miller, W. W.: Ascending aorta–right pulmonary artery anastomosis. Circulation, 3:463, 1968.

Waterston, D. J.: Treatment of Fallot's tetralogy in children under 1 year of age. Rozhledy v Chirurgii (Praha), 41:181, 1962.

Zinsser, H. F., Jr., and Johnson, J.: The use of angiocardiography in the selection of patients for mitral valvular surgery. Ann. Int. Med., 39:1200, 1953.

Zinsser, H. F., Blakemore, W. S., Kirby, C. K., and Johnson, J.: Invalidism due to recurrent idiopathic pericarditis with recovery after pericardiectomy. J.A.M.A., 171:274, 1959.

CHAPTER 44

ORMAND C. JULIAN, M.D., AND WILLIAM S. DYE, M.D.

Peripheral Vascular Surgery

Arterial Surgery
  Introduction
  Acute Arterial Occlusion
  Arterial Trauma
  Chronic Occlusive Arterial Disease
  Renal Artery Disease
  Arterial Insufficiency Affecting the Brain
  Visceral Arteriosclerosis
  Buerger's Disease

Angiospastic Conditions
Arterial Aneurysm
Surgery of the Venous System
  Introduction
  Varicose Veins
  Thrombophlebitis
  Syndrome of Superior Vena Cava Obstruction
  Acute Thrombosis of the Subclavian Vein

Arterial Surgery

INTRODUCTION

Much of the groundwork for the development of vascular surgery was laid when Alexis Carrel developed a simple direct method of vascular suture in 1905 (Carrel, 1907). Surgery of the arteries, up until that time, had been confined largely to the treatment of aneurysms which had progressed from the ligation technics of Antyllus and Hunter to the endoaneurysmorrhaphy of Matas. Interest was directed even earlier to the repair of arterial injuries by suture, and a few blood vessel grafts were used in this period successfully to restore circulation in trauma and disease. Carrel also suggested and demonstrated that vessels could be preserved for use as transplants.

It is remarkable that widespread application of these principles waited for 30 years. Perhaps the best reasons for the great recent impetus to the field lie in the availability of the anticoagulant, heparin, and the development of roentgen technics for arterial visualization. Roentgenograms have provided much of the information that many vascular lesions, even in diffuse arteriosclerosis, are localized and because of the more nearly normal character of the adjacent vessel, susceptible to direct repair.

Fundamental knowledge of arterial pathology from the standpoint of pathogenesis of disease and etiology has had little recent impetus. Study of arterial disease from the time it chiefly concerned the anatomy and the structure of aneurysms has consisted of a gradual accumulation of data and impressions concerning arteriosclerosis, punctuated by the descriptions by Raynaud (1862) and Buerger (1908), of the conditions bearing their names. Almost everything remains to be discovered. The chemical changes which cause arteriosclerosis, the etiologies of the entities which constitute Buerger's disease, the very existence of which has been questioned by some, and the meanings of the slightly different arteritides—periarteritis and panarteritis—are outstanding challenges.

ACUTE ARTERIAL OCCLUSION

Other than by external violence or compression, an arterial channel may become acutely occluded through 2 mechanisms—arterial embolism and arterial thrombosis. An *embolus* is a bolus of material which has traveled through the artery to become lodged at the point at which the vessel size becomes too small to pass it. The composition of the embolus may be a mass of bacteria, a foreign body, or a thrombus which has become detached from its site of origin. Lodgment of a bacterial mass as an arterial embolus produces a very special kind of condition and is known as a *mycotic embolus*. A foreign-body embolus is, as one might suppose, a rarity. Usually it has been a bullet or other small missile, although the extremely rare tumor embolus arising in a lung tumor or a cardiac tumor might be added. A detached clot or portion of clot is the common type of arterial embolus and of particular interest.

Primary *thrombosis* of an otherwise normal artery is rare. Severe debilitating disease, such as intractable diarrhea of ulcerative colitis, has been known to lead to this complication. The increased tendency to intravascular thrombosis which accompanies polycythemia vera more frequently produces venous thrombosis but may affect an artery. The polycythemia of cyanotic congenital heart disease carries the same hazard. The more common mechanism of arterial thrombosis is an underlying arterial disease, arteriosclerosis.

Severe dehydration and periods of hypotension following surgery are factors which increase the danger of arterial thrombosis in patients with or without arteriosclerosis.

ARTERIAL EMBOLISM

Etiology. Most arterial emboli arise from thrombi which develop within the heart chambers. Two cardiac conditions are outstandingly responsible for the initial origin of the intracardiac clot. The *arrhythmia of auricular fibrillation* produces a significant degree of stasis within the 2 atria because of the failure of the chambers to empty themselves forcefully while in the abnormal rhythm. Stasis allows for the formation and the growth of a blood clot (Fig. 44-1A) and, although the thrombus certainly is attached to the endothelium or to trabeculae within the chamber, there is increasing likelihood of a portion being dislodged by the blood stream as it grows. Pulmonary artery emboli result when the thrombus detaches from the right atrium, but this is very rare compared to the peripheral arterial emboli arising from thrombi within the left side of the heart. The condition underlying the auricular fibrillation may be arteriosclerotic heart disease, hyperthyroidism, or rheumatic heart disease. If the element of mitral stenosis is added to the fibrillation in a rheumatic heart the incidence of peripheral emboli is multiplied because the stasis is increased by the stenosis. One of the common complications of long-standing mitral stenosis is peripheral arterial embolism.

The second common cardiac condition likely to produce peripheral embolism is *myocardial infarction secondary to coronary artery occlusion*. The stimulus to the development of the intracardiac thrombus in this condition is the necrotic area of heart muscle which lies beneath the endocardium. A thrombus, called a *mural* thrombus because of its location against the wall, develops over this area. Not all such thrombi detach to form emboli. Many undoubtedly remain securely attached and take part in the healing of the infarct. Detachment, when it happens, is likely to take place on the 5th to the 12th day after the original infarct (Fig. 44-1A).

In addition to their development in these two conditions, *intracardiac thrombi* may be laid down without demonstrable reason. The source of emboli has been demonstrated within the ventricle of hearts not otherwise abnormal in patients dying of the embolism. The absence of a cardiac lesion of the usual type does not rule out the heart as the source in cases of acute arterial occlusion due to embolus.

An extracardiac source of emboli to the extremities exists in patients with *advanced arteriosclerosis of the aorta*. The roughening and even ulceration which develops in the intimal lining of the diseased vessel results in the deposition of thrombus on its wall which may break loose and become emboli (Fig. 44-1D). Another source of emboli is the ulcerated lesion at the carotid bifurcation (Julian, 1963) (Fig. 44-1C).

When a clot detaches from any of these sites it travels in the arterial blood stream, its final lodgment determined by chance and by its size. It may enter the carotid and cerebral circulation to lodge in the brain, enter the subclavian system and enter an arm, or proceed down the aorta to lodge in the aortic bifurcation or continue into one of the lower extremities. In either the arm or the leg it most often stops at a major bifurcation. The reason for this seems quite clearly to be that arterial caliber remains almost constant between origins of major branches of the main channel.

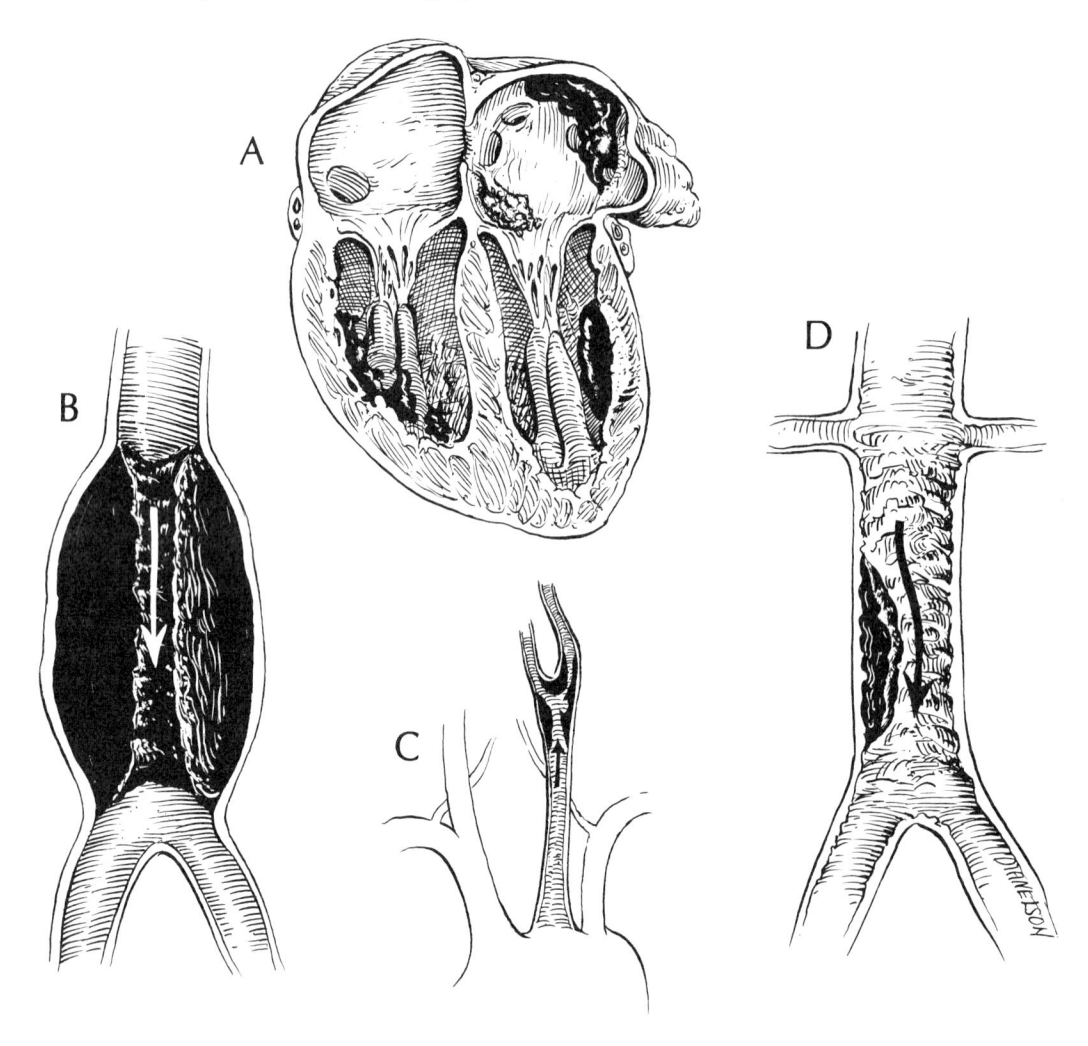

FIG. 44-1. Common sources of peripheral emboli. (A) Composite showing sources of emboli within the heart. (B) Aneurysm with mural thrombus as source of emboli. (C) Carotid artery bifurcation with arteriosclerotic narrowing and ulceration. (D) Arteriosclerotic plaque with thrombus formation in aorta.

The common sites of embolism in the upper extremity are the innominate bifurcation on the right and the circumflex scapular branch of either axillary artery, the profunda brachii branch of the brachial artery and the brachial bifurcation at the elbow. In the lower extremity the common sites of lodgment are the aortic and the iliac artery bifurcations, the origin of the profunda femoris branch of the femoral and the bifurcation of the popliteal artery.

The forceful nature of lodgment of an embolus is evidenced by the expansion of the artery at the point of occlusion and the observation that the clot extrudes under pressure when an incision is made over it during surgical removal. This impact and expansion causes a vasoconstrictor reflex. The impulse arises at the point of stimulus and is carried by afferent and efferent sympathetic fibers to return to a large area of the adjacent arterial tree.

This reflex vasoconstriction multiplies the occlusive effect of the embolism, which now becomes not only a matter of mechanical block but also one of vascular constriction serving to diminish sharply the effectiveness of the collateral arterial channels which should be used to bypass the obstruction (Miles, Dacus, and Booth, 1968).

Symptoms. The symptoms of an acute arterial occlusion due to embolism are pain and loss of function. Pain is most often severe, acute and continuous. It is of a sharp constricting type. A most surprising fact is that pain may be slight or entirely absent in a small proportion of patients with major arterial embolism. Freedom from pain may result from a particularly severe ischemia of the peripheral nerves which renders them functionless rather acutely. Loss of function is both motor and sensory. The patient observes that he is unable to move the toes or the fingers within a few minutes of the onset. The sensory element is interpreted as numbness by the patient and is independent of the presence or the absence of pain. Paralysis and loss of sensation are never absent in embolism of a major artery.

Signs. The signs exhibited by a patient who has sustained embolism of a major artery in an extremity are those of muscular paralysis and cutaneous anesthesia, pallor and coldness. These develop rapidly. Their extent depends on the site of lodgment of the embolus and the severity of the resultant reflex arterial spasm. Paralysis of the small muscles of hand or foot is almost always observed, and if the occlusion is high enough, the muscles of calf or forearm will be affected. Involvement of thigh or arm muscles is rarely observed in embolism. Loss of perception of light touch and pain (pin prick) is usually complete in hand or foot but rarely extends above the elbow in embolism involving the subclavian or the brachial arteries and, in the legs, extends above the knee only in aortic bifurcation embolism. Extension to a higher level of the neurologic signs accompanying acute arterial occlusion in the lower extremities raises the suspicion of an etiology other than embolism. The principal cause to be suspected is dissecting aneurysm of the thoracoabdominal aorta (see p. 1344). The skin color depends on the blood present within the skin capillaries which very soon loses its oxygen and very naturally diminishes in amount. Therefore, the color changes of pallor and cyanosis are present from the distal end of the part upward for a variable distance. The appearance becomes progressively more waxy white during the early period of occlusion. The skin temperature falls rapidly after the occlusion. The extent of the zone of coldness roughly corresponds to the zone of color change.

The final characteristic signs of acute occlusion concern the changes in the pulses of the extremity as determined by palpation. Pulses cannot be palpated at their normal locations distal to the obstruction. Immediately proximal to the embolism the arterial pulse may be slightly exaggerated in comparison to the other side because of the greater lateral pressure exerted as the blood meets the block and is thrown into eddies and cross currents. This observation is made most clearly on palpation of the common femoral artery when an embolus has lodged at the femoral bifurcation. The oscillometer may be of value in determining the level of obstruction. Likewise, arteriography may be used to determine the site of obstruction. In most cases, however, the diagnosis is obvious and the level of the obstruction easily determined by palpation of the pulses.

Course. The course following the embolic occlusion is widely variable. Its severity depends not only on the site of the occlusion but also on the intensity and the duration of the reflex arterial spasm, and the extent of development of progressive thrombosis of the arterial lumen above and below the embolus. If spasm is unremitting and the development of progressive thrombosis rapid and extensive, the extremity will remain severely ischemic and become moribund in 8 to 10 hours. In other instances the extremity may begin to show return of motor function and sensation within a few minutes or hours of the embolism and recover without loss of tissue.

Treatment. Treatment of embolism is directed to the removal of the obstruction by surgery in almost every case. In the past, attempts have been made in many cases to relieve the arterial spasm by sympathetic nerve block prior to surgery. However, in present day management the general plan is to take the patient immediately to the operating room and remove the embolus without doing any regional or sympathetic nerve blocks.

The most important step in the surgical treatment of emboli is its immediate application (Dye *et al.*, 1955). Although in some cases of embolism the collateral circulation is adequate to allow tissues to remain viable, in

1302   Peripheral Vascular Surgery

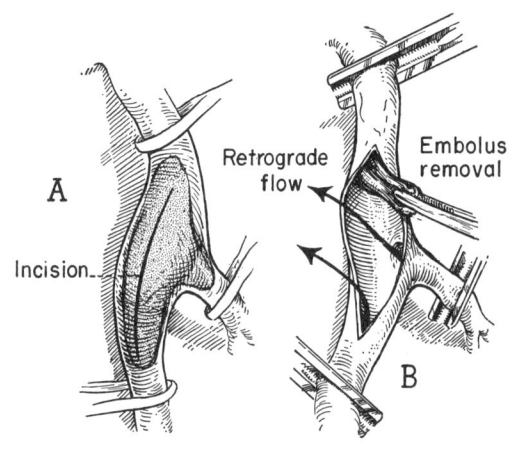

FIG. 44-2. General steps in embolectomy. (A) Control tapes are placed above and below the site of lodgment, and the incision is made directly over the embolus and slightly below its superior limits. (B) Distal and proximal removal of clot is done with the Fogarty catheter (see Fig. 44-3).

general, immediate surgery is the treatment of choice. Even though some limbs will survive, due to the adequate collateral circulation, in their subsequent course arterial insufficiency of this extremity will appear when it is used. An early sign of non-viability in the extremity is the development of rigidity in the muscles of the leg or the forearm. Likewise, the presence of paralysis is a grave sign. Thrombosis of the venous side has received more attention recently. Although embolectomy should be done within 8 hours or so of the incident, delayed embolectomy has been reported (Olwin, *et al.*, 1953). This is possible in patients who have survived the initial insult of the embolus and whose collateral circulation has allowed viability of the part.

Surgery is performed most of the time under local anesthesia. Heparinization of the patient is done at the time of surgery. The artery is explored at the site of the embolus and following removal of the embolus, the Fogarty catheter is then passed distally and all of the

FIG. 44-3. The Fogarty catheter with the inflatable balloon at its tip may be used through the femoral or popliteal arterotomy for removal of thrombotic material.

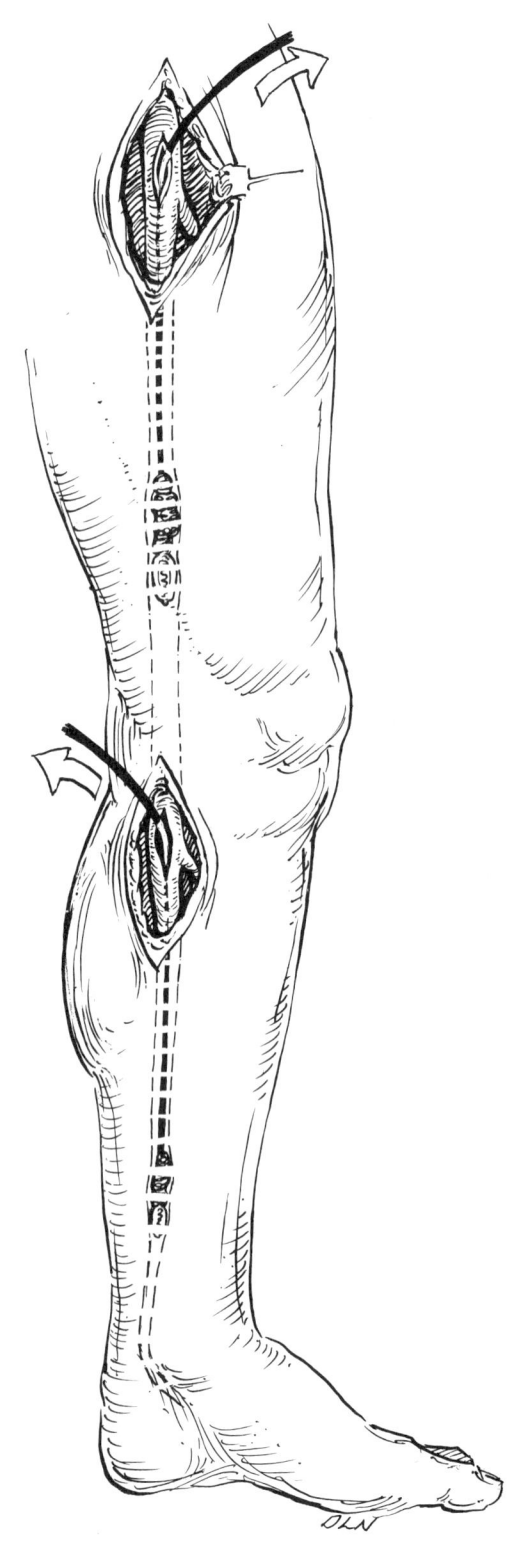

distal propagating thrombus is removed (Fogarty et al., 1963a). At times it is necessary to pass it proximally to remove embolus and proximal thrombosis above. If, for example, the embolus is at the femoral region and the Fogarty catheter does not pass well into the calf of the leg, it may then be necessary to expose the popliteal artery bifurcation, reenter the artery there and pass the Fogarty catheters proximally and distally (Fig. 44-3). The arterial lumens are irrigated well with heparinized saline. The arterotomy wounds are closed with 5-0 silk or 5-0 Teflon and Dacron sutures. Prior to closure of the wounds it is accurately determined whether pulses have been restored to the distal part of the extremity (Darling, 1967; Javid, 1967).

If an embolus at the aortic bifurcation resists removal from below, the site of lodgment must be exposed through an abdominal incision. This requires the addition of a general anesthesia, increasing the risk to the patient who is often ill with the cardiac lesion etiologic to the embolus. However, the surgical indication is greatest of all in cases of aortic bifurcation embolism, because the mortality from this accident is very high, probably 90 per cent, if the embolus is not removed. The operation virtually becomes lifesaving and should be tried (Fig. 44-4).

Postoperatively, motion of the extremity is encouraged to avoid stasis, and the anticoagulant therapy may be continued with careful use of heparin. This last is done not only to prevent thrombosis of the operated artery but also to diminish development of more thrombi at the original source of the embolus. It may be continued for long periods after an embolus has occurred, and in this case the anticoagulant drug is changed in an orderly fashion from heparin to Dicumarol.

Treatment of the underlying condition must not be lost sight of, and careful follow-up of these patients is required to determine which might require active therapy. This would pertain particularly to patients with rheumatic heart disease who may need a mitral commissurotomy to relieve stasis in the left atrium, as well as a possible open-heart procedure to evacuate clots from within the left atrium at the same time that the mitral valve is relieved of its stenosis.

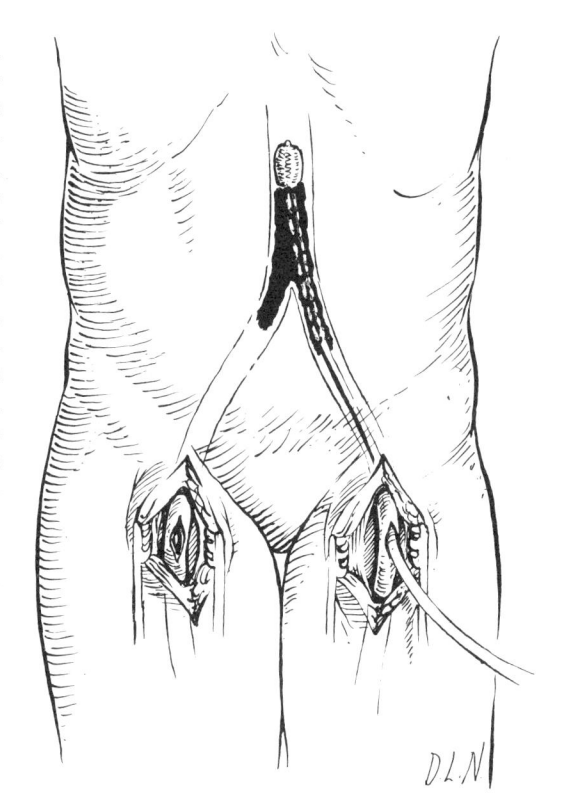

FIG. 44-4. Aortic bifurcation embolectomy may be done from below through femoral incisions and the retrograde use of Fogarty catheters.

Arterial Thrombosis

Etiology. The usual underlying arterial disease leading to arterial thrombosis is arteriosclerosis. In the presence of this degenerative condition the factors leading to development of a thrombus in the lumen are the narrowing of the lumen and roughening of the lining.

Symptoms. The symptoms at the onset of an arterial thrombosis superimposed on chronic arterial disease are not necessarily very severe. The reason for this is that the preexisting arteriosclerosis has slowly developed a certain degree of chronic obstruction. During this time collateral arterial routes have widened. When the final acute occlusion of the diseased point in the artery occurs, the resulting sudden fall in blood flow is less than is the case when a normal artery is obstructed. This mechanism may be so prominent that no acute episode is registered by the patient. This is demonstrated to be so by the fact that specimens of segments of chronic arterial occlusion removed at the operating table for replacement with vascular grafts frequently show thrombotic occlusion of the narrowed lumen in patients whose course has been gradual and without an acute episode. However, when the final thrombosis occurs in a relatively wide open, diseased artery, a variable symptomatology will result.

In the acute phase there is a lesser degree of arterial spasm than accompanies arterial embolism. The pain is distinctly less than that observed in severe forms of embolism. However, since pain can be absent in either condition, this is a poor point in differentiation. On the basis of history some indication of the preexisting arterial disease may be recognized. Intermittent claudication, the earliest symptom of chronic arterial occlusion, is most likely to be discovered as a previous complaint. The presence of a cardiac arrhythmia or disease likely to produce an embolus is helpful in differentiating arterial thrombosis from arterial embolism but is not necessarily accurate. The cardiac status of the patient can be misleading in those instances of embolism already mentioned in which the heart is not demonstrably abnormal.

The presence of a heart condition likely to cause embolism does not rule out thrombosis, particularly if a phase of the cardiac disease has been productive of a depressed blood pressure. Although arterial hypotension can develop in the course of a condition producing auricular fibrillation, the more important condition is coronary occlusion. A frequent manifestation of myocardial infarction due to coronary occlusion is hypotension. During the period of depressed blood pressure there is the additional factor of reduced peripheral arterial flow to encourage the development of peripheral arterial thrombosis. Since coronary occlusion is usually a manifestation of degenerative arterial disease, it is frequent that the same patients have some degree of similar change in the peripheral arteries.

Therefore, a 3-fold relationship can be seen to exist between coronary occlusion and peripheral arterial obstruction of the acute type. An understanding of the problem is much more than academic in its importance. The first element is the incidence of arterial embolism in patients having myocardial infarcts. It has been mentioned that this complication occurs most often from the 5th to the 12th day. The second point is the tendency to thrombosis in arteriosclerotic vessels of the extremities during the period of hypotension, most frequently present during the initial hours of an acute myocardial infarct. The third facet, which has not been discussed so far, is the effect of hypotension of an acute coronary attack on the appearance of extremities of a patient who has chronic arterial obstruction due to arteriosclerosis but has *not* developed an arterial thrombosis. Cold skin, small pulses and a pale cyanotic color are frequently seen in this stage of the heart attack. If significant arterial disease is present the appearance can very closely mimic an acute occlusion. If the patient responds to cardiac management and heart action improves, the signs of acute peripheral arterial occlusion disappear.

In the presence of a myocardial infarct, therefore, the clinical appearance of acute peripheral arterial occlusion may denote an arterial embolus, a thrombosis of a diseased segment of peripheral artery, or a simple augmentation of a chronic arterial insufficiency due to the depressed blood pressure without additional occlusion. The treatment of arterial embolism has already been pointed out to be the removal of the obstructing embolus wherever possible and has been described in some detail. The treatment of an arterial thrombosis has the same purpose but is affected very much by the state of the patient's cardiovascular system in general and the cardiac status and blood pressure specifically.

Treatment of an arterial thrombosis offers a greater challenge to the surgeon than does treatment of arterial embolism. The fact that the obstructed segment is the site of a degenerative condition is responsible for the technical difficulties which are involved. The removal of the obstruction usually does not consist of simple removal of the clot but demands that the arteriosclerotic segment either be cleared of its atheromatous lesions or be bypassed or replaced by a graft. The elements of these procedures are discussed later in relation to treatment of chronic occlusive lesions of arteriosclerosis. However, if the best of these methods are applied in a patient who has developed the thrombosis in a period of hypotension and remains in the hypotensive state, the result will be the almost immediate recurrence of thrombosis. Therefore, the initial requirement in deciding to intervene directly in arterial thrombosis is the restoration of the patient's arterial blood pressure. The inability to do so contraindicates surgery on the artery. This contraindication has the additional effect of preventing surgical approach to a supposed arterial occlusion when the signs are produced by the hypotensive state without arterial obstruction.

ARTERIAL TRAUMA

Improved technics and dissemination of knowledge of how to perform surgical procedures on the arteries has distinctly improved the prognosis in cases of arterial trauma. This is due in part to experience gained during World War II, De Bakey et al. (1946). However, much more was learned in the postwar period because of the surgical correction of arterial damage sustained during the war but corrected months and years later (Freeman, 1946; Shumacker, 1948). Application of these technics in the acute cases occurring during the Korean conflict led to a much higher proportion of immediate restoration of damaged arteries during that period than had occurred in World War II (Jahnke and Seeley, 1953; Seeley et al., 1952; Ziperman, 1954). More recent reports from Viet Nam have demonstrated an even greater salvage by the immediate application of restorative procedures (Jones, Peters and Gasior, 1968). It has been learned that systematic handling is imperative, and the immediate surgical emergency which exists with an arterial injury has come to be appreciated more thoroughly. With proper handling correction of major arterial wounds is well within the realm of possibility (Dye, 1963a, 1963b; Javid, 1963; Julian and Hunter, 1963; Spencer and Tompkins, 1960; Hughes, 1958).

Classification

A classification of the types of arterial injuries is important in order to develop a scheme of treatment which will be widely applicable. The division of arterial injuries into incision or laceration, perforation and contu-

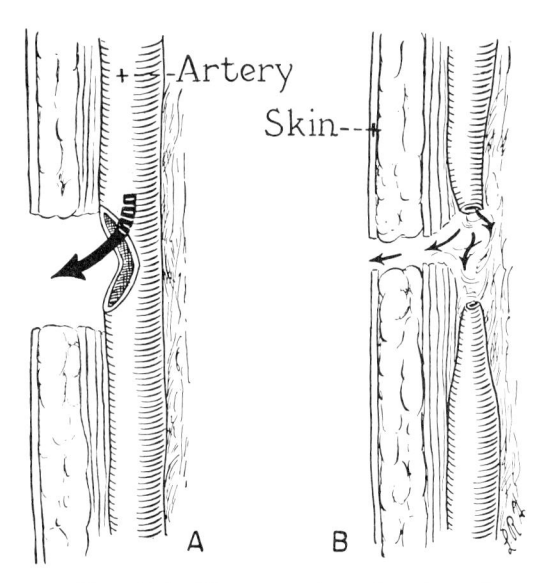

FIG. 44-5. Diagrammatic explanation of the tendency of a partial laceration of an artery (A) to bleed more profusely and longer than a complete transection (B). The retraction of the artery ends into adjacent tissue, and constriction of the cut ends minimize the bleeding in (B).

sion is not simply a didactic matter but is one of technical importance.

Incision or Laceration. An artery which is subjected to damage by a sharp instrument may be partially or completely transected. An incision or laceration without transection results in a gaping opening in the wall of the artery which is held open by the retraction of the vessel wall adjacent to the hole. A completely transected artery, on the other hand, is drawn back into the tissues by its elasticity. The surrounding tissues tend to close over the ends. There is also a distinct tendency for the transected ends to constrict, due to the circular coats of muscular and elastic tissue. Both of these actions aid in stopping hemorrhage, and for these reasons a partially severed artery is productive of more blood loss than is one which is completely divided (Fig. 44-5).

Perforations of an artery occur when a high velocity missile of small size or a small sharp instrument, such as an ice pick or a thin knife, pass through the vessel. These injuries are accompanied by a minimal amount of surrounding tissue damage and a small opening on the body surface. Usually little outside

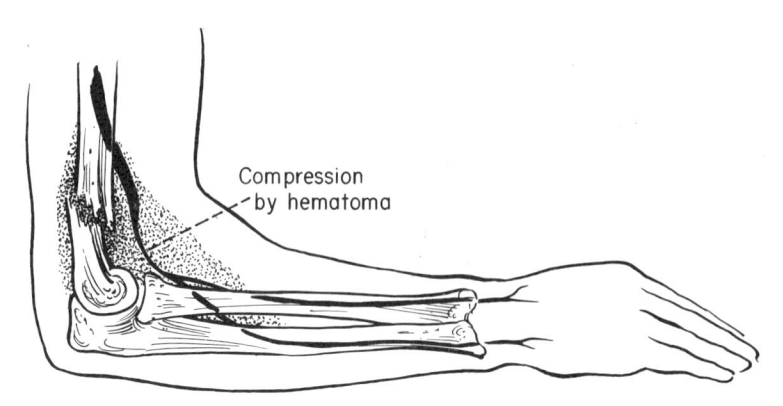

FIG. 44-6. Supracondylar fracture of humerus with severe hematoma producing compression and spasm of brachial artery.

bleeding occurs. Injuries of this type may be followed by specific lesions such as pulsating hematoma and arteriovenous fistula which will be described later.

A **contusion** of an artery is caused by a broad, crushing or grinding force or missile (Edwards and Lyons, 1954; Lord, 1950). A large, relatively slow missile may produce this kind of lesion, as will very high velocity missiles passing through tissue near the wall of an artery. The impingement of a fractured bone against the artery, as in fractures of the lower end of the femur, can injure the vessel in this manner. It should be emphasized that contusion of an artery may be caused by a sudden blow to an extremity without there being an associated fracture or wound (Fig. 44-6). This lesion has been met with most frequently in the brachial artery in patients who have hooked their arm over some structure in order to break a fall, and in the lower thigh at about the femoral-popliteal artery junction in patients who have been struck obliquely from behind by the bumper of an automobile (Fig. 44-7).

The lesion can also be described as an intramural hematoma of the artery. The crushing force produces damage within the coats of the vessel in such a way that bleeding occurs between the various layers. As the hematoma grows, it compresses the lumen of the vessel and produces obstruction (Fig. 44-8).

The thoracic aorta is subject to quite a different type of damage of the general contusion type (Alley et al., 1961; Eiseman and Rainer, 1958; Jahnke et al., 1964; Parmley et al., 1958; Spencer et al., 1961a; Strassman, 1947; Bennett and Cherry, 1967). This occurs most frequently in the portion of the descending aorta within 1 or 2 inches of the left subclavian artery. A heavy blow to the chest, either directly depressing the sternum or applied laterally in such a way as to fracture some of the ribs in the left chest, may produce a tear in the intima and the internal layers of the media of the aorta at this area. Horizontal deceleration, such as occurs in head-on auto accidents or in airplane accidents, is the most frequent mechanism of this injury, the explanation being that the arch of the aorta is more fixed than the descending aorta, and the greatest stress is in the region of the subclavian artery. Vertical deceleration probably produces injury in the ascending aorta more frequently. The tear in the internal layers is usually transverse to the long axis of the aorta and may involve a portion or the entire circumference. Continuity of blood flow is maintained because of the resistance of the overlying pleura supporting the remaining layers of the vessel. This type of contusion

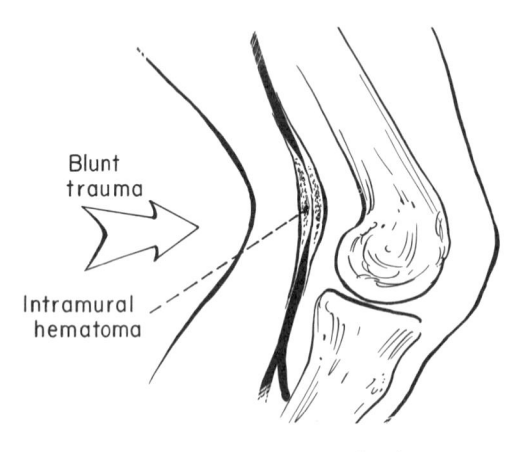

FIG. 44-7. Contusion of popliteal artery produced by blunt trauma such as a "bumper injury."

leads to the development of a traumatic aneurysm of the descending aorta, rather than an obstruction of the intramural hematoma type (Fig. 44-9). Often, patients with this injury die immediately. If they survive, the diagnosis may not be made for some time. Ultimately, these aneurysms increase in size and may rupture. For this reason they should all be resected.

DIAGNOSIS

The hemorrhage from arterial injury is variable. It may dissect into tissue spaces or into body cavities or viscera. The wound may coincidentally involve the adjacent vein and permit hemorrhage to occur from the artery into the vein. Finally, in cases of arterial contusion or intramural hematoma, hemorrhage may be absent. Therefore, the diagnosis of an arterial injury cannot depend primarily on the presence and the character of the bleeding. Diagnostic features other than that of hemorrhage must be sought. If bleeding is free to occur from the arterial injury to the outside, the pulsatile character of the escaping blood will make the diagnosis obvious. Hemorrhage from an arterial injury into a closed tissue space produces a pulsating swelling.

If the artery and the vein are injured simultaneously in such a way as to allow blood loss from artery into vein a permanent fistulous communication can be established immediately or develop later if the communication is at first blocked by a thrombus. The initial sign which is diagnostic of an arteriovenous communication is the continuous "machinerylike" murmur, audible with the stethoscope over the region of the injury and sometimes palpable as a thrill.

Intramural hematoma is a type of arterial injury which may escape detection with disastrous results unless other specific signs are looked for carefully. Such an injury produces an acute occlusion of the artery involved. Acute arterial occlusions tend to produce pain in the region of the body that is deprived of its blood supply. However, the injuries to other tissues may also be painful, and pain alone is not pathognomonic of arterial occlusion. If a major vessel to an extremity is bruised and closed, the distal part of the extremity may appear pale immediately because of lack of blood supply and soon thereafter becomes paralyzed and anesthetic. These signs, together

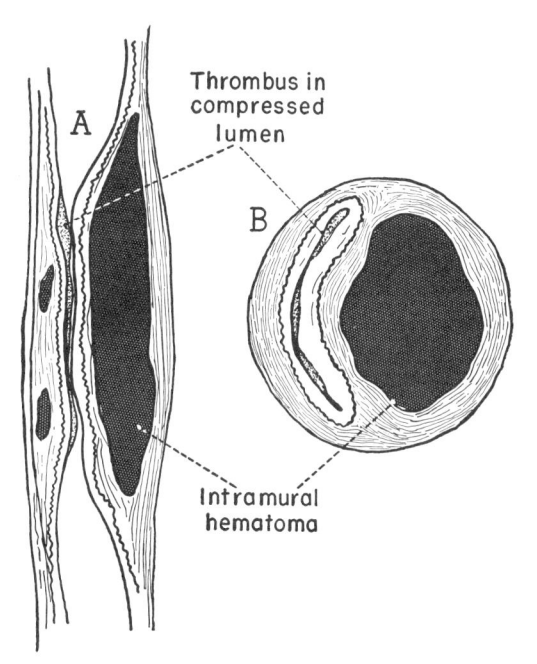

FIG. 44-8. Traumatic occlusion of an artery without blood loss occurs following a contusion. The longitudinal (A) and cross-section (B) of the artery shows compression of the lumen by the intramural hematoma plus thrombus formation in the lumen.

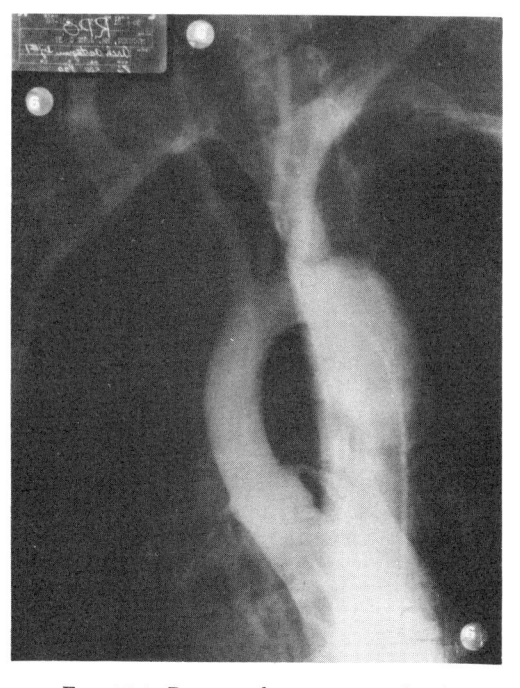

FIG. 44-9. Retrograde aortogram showing a traumatic aneurysm in the first part of the descending thoracic aorta.

with the loss of pulses in the region in which they are normally palpable distal to the obstruction, indicates the presence of a traumatic occlusion.

Differential Diagnosis. The presence of an intramural hematoma must be differentiated from an acute intense arterial spasm secondary to an injury not actually involving an artery at all. Such severe spasm of the vessels of an injured extremity is a common occurrence and usually attributed to a reflex which is elaborated through the sympathetic nervous system. Rarely does reflex vasospasm attain the intensity or last long enough to produce numbness and paralysis of the distal part of the involved extremity. Failure of these specific signs to appear is an aid in differentiating the two conditions. Also, spasm can make the pulses distal to the injury temporarily impalpable. Final distinction between these two conditions may depend upon interrupting the sympathetic nervous system reflex responsible for spasm by the injection of procaine into the appropriate part of the sympathetic nervous system. Sympathetic blocks, the technic of which will be described elsewhere, may be done simply and quickly.

Further accuracy of diagnosis of the traumatic arterial obstruction may be obtained by the injection of contrast media into the artery proximal to the injury. These iodine-containing substances are opaque to x-rays, and if an exposure is made as the medium is being transported by the artery, an accurate picture is obtained of the vessel lumen showing obstruction if it is present. Arteriography is not often required in the diagnosis of an injury but may be of value in difficult cases (Fig. 44-10).

The differentiation of arterial hemorrhage from venous bleeding is seldom of much practical importance. The difference may be immediately obvious on the basis of the color of the blood being lost. Most venous bleeding and many instances of arterial bleeding can be controlled by moderate pressure over the region of the vascular injury. If severe bleeding which cannot be controlled by this method is present, adequate surgical exposure for the control of hemorrhage is required, and appropriate management of the vein or artery lesion accomplished.

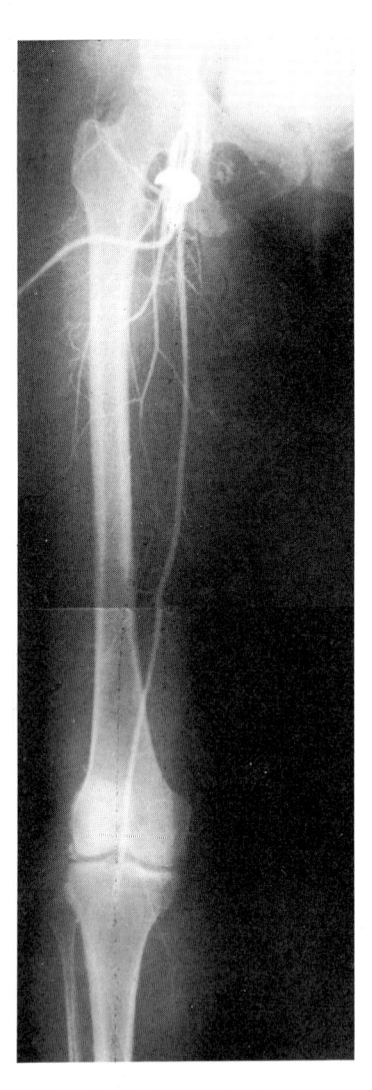

FIG. 44-10. Femoral arteriogram showing occlusion of popliteal artery produced by blunt trauma to the posterior aspect of the knee.

TREATMENT

Three Phases. The treatment of an arterial injury may be divided into 3 phases.

1. In the initial phase it deals with the control of hemorrhage. As is noted above, there are very few instances in which pressure or tourniquet application will fail to control bleeding from the extremities. Arterial injuries high in the groin, deep in the axilla or the base of the neck, as well as within the abdomen and the thorax, present problems which cannot always be treated adequately except in a well-equipped operating room. Injuries

such as these, if they are so located and formed as to allow free hemorrhage, often will be productive of deep shock which the patient will not survive. Rapid transfusion combined with immediate surgery to control the hemorrhage is, in severe cases, the only practical means of treatment of the injury.

2. The second phase in treatment consists of restoration of the blood volume by blood transfusion until the blood pressure returns to normal and is maintained. Blood is the fluid of choice in restoring the blood volume but may be substituted in part by various solutions, such as plasma, dextran or, in a limited degree, by rapid infusion of electrolyte solution should no other fluid be immediately available (see Chap. 7, Shock, and Chap. 8, Blood Transfusion).

3. The third phase involves definitive treatment of the arterial lesion. This should include, under all possible circumstances, a repair of the damaged vessel adequate to restore normal circulation to the part. Repair is undertaken as an emergency measure but should be carried out under the same optimum conditions as would accompany an elective surgical procedure on an artery (Jahnke, 1958).

In locations where adequate facilities or personnel for arterial repair are lacking, consideration should be given to transferring the patient. This may be done if control of hemorrhage and replacement of blood loss have been accomplished and associated injuries do not contraindicate moving the patient. Time becomes a most important factor if the injury has produced ischemia of the part.

The general plan of operation upon an artery for an injury or, indeed, the general plan of operation upon any artery for any reason follows a very definite sequence. Adequate anesthesia is used without the requirement of deep muscular relaxation. Because of the specific danger of disruption of a suture line in an artery if infection results from the operation, meticulous care is taken in the preparation of the skin.

The primary task in operating upon an artery is to expose the vessel sufficiently proximal to the lesion to be able to isolate a segment of it without disturbing the damaged area. This process is known as gaining proximal control of the artery. A length of cotton tape is passed about the artery so that it may be pulled up to be constricted against the finger or to apply suitable blood vessel clamps for stopping blood flow through the vessel. The second step of the procedure consists of gaining the same sort of control beyond the lesion. Following this, the dissection of the artery is carried out in both directions toward the actual site of operation, and finally, with the vessel constricted above and below, the repair is done.

Repair may consist of a simple *suture* of a laceration or an end-to-end anastomosis of a transected vessel. In treating high-velocity puncture wounds of large arteries, it is important to remember that the hidden damage to the inner portion of the wall is often much more extensive than the visible damage to the outer portion of the wall. This may lead to secondary blowouts if the puncture wound is merely closed by suture. Such wounds should be débrided with removal of an adequate margin of the adjacent wall or it may be best to excise the injured segment and to bring the vessel together again by end-to-end suture. Complicated lacerations which defy reconstructive suture directly along the incised edges are treated by removal of that portion of the artery which is damaged and, wherever possible, advantage is taken of the elasticity of the artery, bringing the 2 ends together for simple anastomosis. When the amount of vessel lost is too great to bring the ends together without undue tension, the defect which is produced by its removal is replaced by the insertion of a vessel graft. In a person with normal arteries a surprising amount of lost vessel length may be compensated for by stretching.

A variety of technics of blood vessel suture is currently in use. Simple laceration of an artery is repaired with a suture of very fine silk swedged onto a fine needle, applied in an over-and-over fashion. The suture is placed 1 mm. from the edge of the vessel and the adjacent sutures are 1 mm. apart (Fig. 44-11 and 44-12). When carefully done, it will be almost water tight and always will be impervious to blood because of blood's greater viscosity and early fibrin deposits. An anastomosis between the ends of a severed vessel or between the vessel end and a graft may be made in this same over-and-over fashion (Fig. 44-11 C and D) or may be done so as to bring

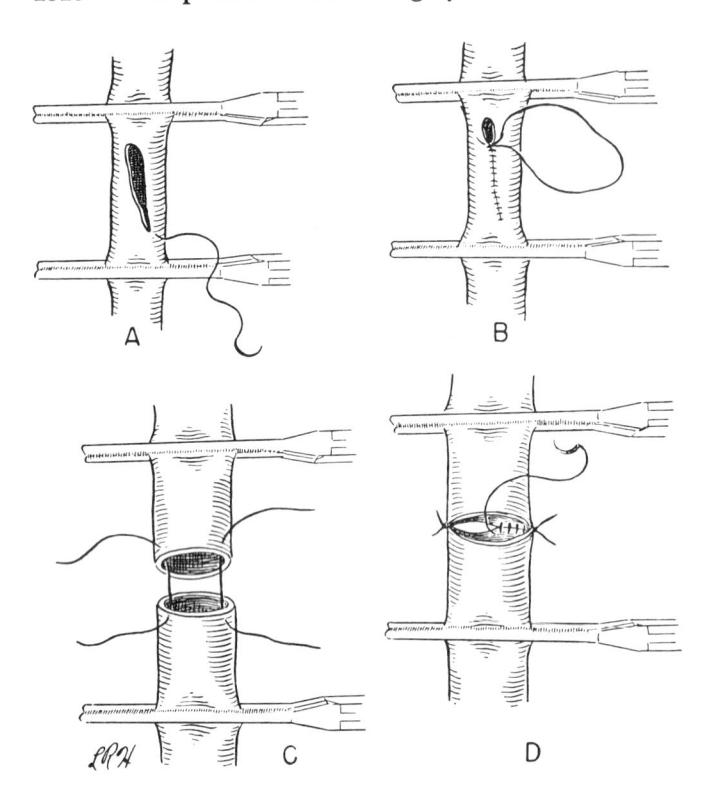

FIG. 44-11. Repair of a simple linear laceration of an artery may be accomplished by anatomic suture (A and B). If the laceration is more extensive, the damaged area is removed, and closure is done by approximating the ends by traction on the atraumatic vascular clamps and reanastomosing by one of two technics. The use of a simple over-and-over suture is diagrammed (C and D).

the inner lining, the intima, of the vessel ends into apposition. An everting mattress suture employs the same material, and the placement is in the same dimensions as described for an over-and-over suture (Fig. 44-12).

The choice of grafts in the repair of a vascular injury is dictated by availability of materials and by the diameter and the length of the arterial segment which needs replacing (Fig. 44-13). Vascular tissue taken from the patient himself makes the best material, strictly on the basis of acceptance of the tissue in its new site. For this reason, a vein graft is usually selected for repair of the medium-sized vessels of the extremities. The vein often used is the patient's own long saphe-

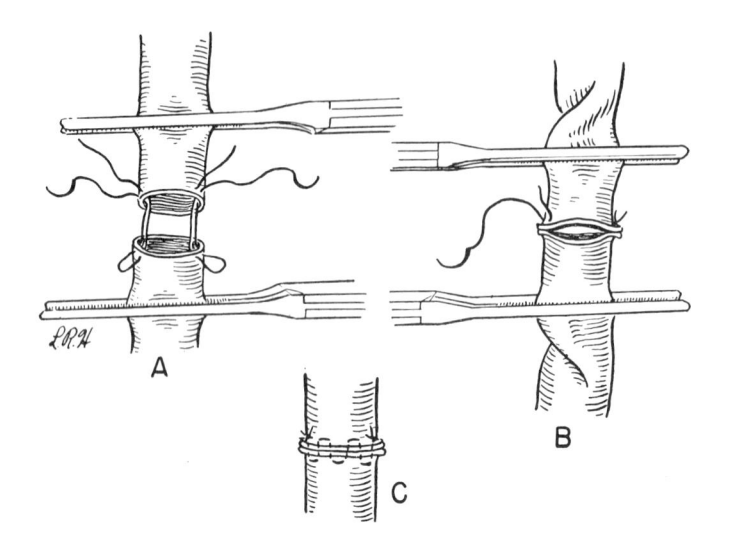

FIG. 44-12. The alternate method of performing an arterial anastomosis is an everting mattress suture. This may be done as a continuous suture, illustrated here, or as an interrupted suture. The technic is simplified by rotating the vessel with the clamps to expose the posterior aspect of the anastomosis (B).

FIG. 44-13. When resection of contused segment is necessary, the defect is bridged by a synthetic or autogenous vein graft.

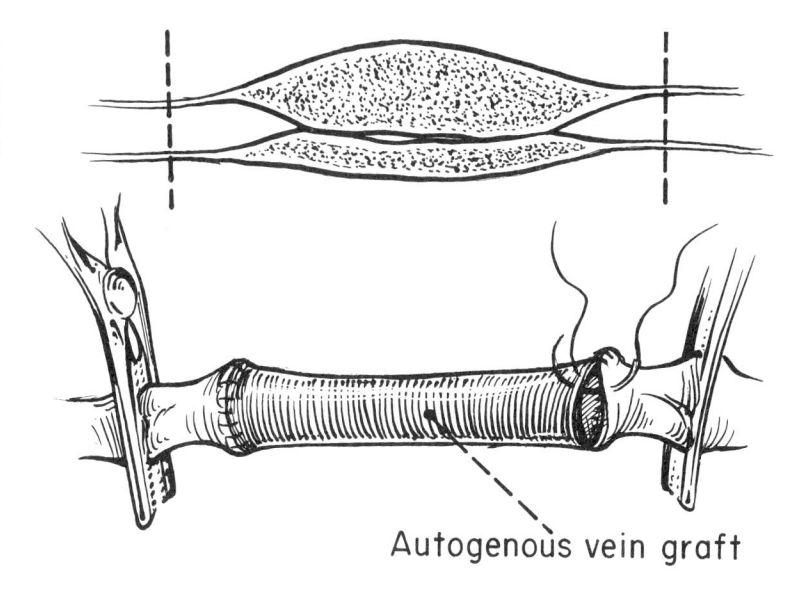

Autogenous vein graft

nous vein. It can be readily spared in any patient and is a relatively muscular vein which substitutes well for most extremity arteries. A point of great importance in the implantation of a vein graft is to remember to orient the vein graft end-to-end in such a way that the valves do not obstruct the flow of arterial blood. Arterial prostheses of woven plastic yarn are available in a wide range of sizes corresponding to the size of all vessels from the small brachial artery to the large aorta. They are reliable, and their availability without the necessity of additional surgical maneuvers, such as are necessary to obtain a vein graft, is in favor of their use. Arterial homografts are no longer used, because degeneration ultimately occurs.

Pulsating Hematoma (False Aneurysm)

Perforation of an artery by a sharp instrument or a high-speed, small-size missile often produces a pulsating hematoma or false aneurysm. If the tissues of the point of injury are sufficiently resistant, the pressure in the pool of blood lost into the area soon builds up to the mean arterial pressure. Thereafter some blood extravasates through the vessel opening into the tissue space during systole, and some returns to the artery during diastole (Fig. 44-14). The accumulation of blood pulsates within the tissues. In many such cases the blood flow distal to the injury is maintained, and a pulsating hematoma frequently is tolerated for a long time before it is repaired. Fibrosis occurs in the wall, and in time the sac becomes endothelialized.

Indirect trauma sometimes causes a pulsating hematoma. Abrupt stretching of the femoral artery in a fall in which the thighs are abducted suddenly and forcefully, or of

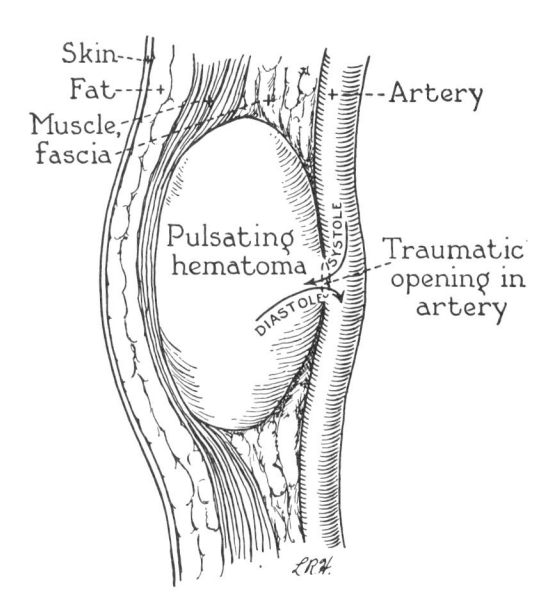

FIG. 44-14. Diagram of false aneurysm or pulsating hematoma. The directions of flow through the opening during diastole and systole are indicated by the arrows.

the popliteal artery if the knee is hyperextended, tears the vessel wall and allows this lesion to form. This is most likely to occur when the vessel is previously the site of some such disease as arteriosclerosis and therefore is weak and inelastic.

The clinical signs of a pulsating hematoma are the palpable pulsation of the mass and the sounds which are audible with the stethoscope as the blood leaves and enters the hematoma. The sound produced usually is confined to systole but may be heard also during the diastolic phase. When heard in both systole and diastole the murmur is not continuous. This is because blood flow ceases momentarily at the end of systole and again at the end of diastole as the pressures within the sac and the artery equalize and the direction of flow through the arterial opening prepares to reverse. This interrupted character differentiates it from the murmur of arteriovenous fistula which is continuous. The location and the extent of such a lesion may be determined exactly by an arteriogram.

Treatment. Where facilities are available, surgical repair of a pulsating hematoma is indicated immediately upon making the diagnosis of the arterial injury. Formerly, it had been general practice to delay treatment of such a lesion for several months. The reason for this is that a false aneurysm to some degree produces a partial occlusion of the artery which has been damaged. This is caused by the turbulence of flow within the artery developed by the exit and the return of blood through the opening, and also by the compression of the artery resulting simply from the mass of the adjacent hematoma. Chronic occlusion stimulates the branches of the artery above and below the lesion to dilate and, by enlarging their natural communications, to form a collateral arterial bed. This may become sufficient in a moderate period of time to protect the part, usually an extremity, from gangrene if the segment of artery bearing the lesion is simply doubly ligated and removed. At the present time such ligation and excision is no longer practiced by choice but rather direct anastomosis or interposition of a vessel graft is done. In applying the principle of waiting for collateral arteries to be stimulated, operation sometimes becomes necessary before the optimum period has passed because of changes which go on in the region of the pulsating hematoma. The hematoma itself may become intimately attached to the skin overlying it and by pressure and associated inflammation thin out the skin and threaten to rupture, particularly at the point of the healing skin wound which was produced by the penetrating object. Pain of compression of the adjacent nerves and other structures in the region of the pulsating hematoma may necessitate early operation. Finally, the mass of the pulsating hematoma can produce ischemia of the tissues distal to the lesion by compression of the collateral arteries and by pressure on the injured vessel itself. Such pain and ischemia make waiting the optimum period impossible. Then the operation may be required during the period of 6 to 9 days following the initial injury. At exactly this time the softening and the edema of the artery wall adjacent to the injury are at their maximum, and the least desirable condition of the vessel will be found at operation for the necessary repair. These factors, together with the relative ease with which operation can be done at the time of the injury, make immediate treatment more desirable.

The actual operation to be carried out upon the lesion, whether it is done immediately as is recommended above or as a delayed procedure after the pulsating hematoma has been present for weeks, months or years, varies, depending upon the size and the importance of the vessel concerned and the extent of damage to the vessel. A very small unimportant artery injured such a way as to produce a pulsating hematoma is simply ligated at points above and below the traumatic opening in the vessel, and the lesion is removed. Larger vessels are preserved by excision of the segment of vessel which has been damaged, followed either by direct repair of the artery by end-to-end anastomosis or by the interposition of a graft, depending upon the length of segment lost and the elasticity of the adjacent artery. This, of course, varies in no way from the repair of an arterial injury of any type. When the delayed method of repair has been planned, and when the symptoms of compression, ischemia or threatening rupture necessitate emergency operation, it will be necessary to resect the segment of the damaged vessel because of the arterial softening.

TRAUMATIC ARTERIOVENOUS FISTULA

Etiology. An arteriovenous fistula occurs as the result of a trauma involving adjacent arteries and veins. Usually it is produced by a high-speed missile or a stab wound but also may occur because of rupture of an arteriosclerotic aneurysm into the adjacent vein to which it has gradually become adherent and into which it has finally eroded. Arteriovenous fistulae on the basis of congenital malformation are discussed elsewhere. In the traumatic type of arteriovenous fistula there is often not much external hemorrhage. The fistula which is produced by the trauma sometimes becomes active immediately after the injury. However, the actual establishment of the fistula can be delayed until there is some organization of the adjacent wounds and absorption of a thrombus which happens to occupy the opening between the 2 vessels. Sometimes fistulae are caused by surgical trauma. This occurs most frequently in thyroidectomies or in nephrectomies when the artery and the vein of the superior pole of the thyroid or of the renal pedicle are ligated together (Elkin, 1948). The ligature erodes through the 2 vessels in such a way as to establish a communication. Surgically produced fistulae are also known to develop when vessels not being ligated are damaged inadvertently. Fistulae have appeared between the aorta or the right common iliac artery and the inferior vena cava when these vessels have been damaged by an instrument passing between the lumbar vertebral bodies during surgery for removal of a herniated intervertebral disk (Linton and White, 1945).

Diagnosis. The presence of an arteriovenous fistula is diagnosed on the basis of the characteristic auscultatory finding of a continuous machinerylike murmur. This continuous murmur is produced by the continuous flow of blood from the artery into the vein where the jet produces turbulence and vibration of the vein wall. The machinerylike character of the continuous murmur is due to the fact that the velocity of this shunt and therefore the pitch of the murmur is increased during the systolic phase of the pulse. The flow of blood is not a to-and-fro action as in pulsating hematoma but is always from the artery into

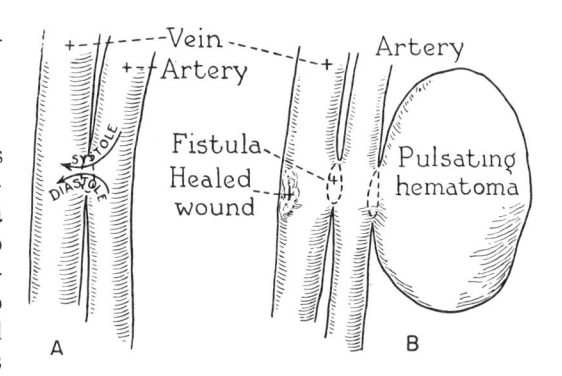

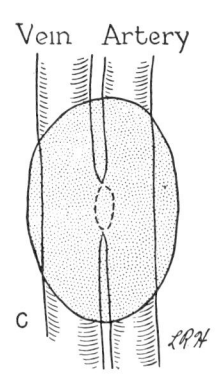

FIG. 44-15. Common forms of arteriovenous fistulae resulting from trauma. The direction of flow through the fistula during diastole and systole is indicated by the arrows (A). Combinations of pulsating hematoma with arteriovenous fistulae are diagrammed (B and C).

the vein. Such a murmur is often associated with a palpable thrill. Anatomically, an arteriovenous fistula produced by a stab wound or a missile is often a compound lesion, consisting of the fistula between the 2 vessels and a pulsating hematoma on the opposite surface of the artery. This compounding of the lesion is due to the fact that the damage to the artery, whether it be missile or stab, enters and leaves the artery, producing 2 openings. The apposed holes produce the fistula; the wound in the free surface of the artery forms the false aneurysm. For this reason there is a pulsating mass palpable in the immediate region of an arteriovenous fistula (Fig. 44-15).

Arteriography in cases of arteriovenous fistula confirms the diagnosis and provides accurate localization to guide the surgeon in repair (Fig. 44-16).

1314 Peripheral Vascular Surgery

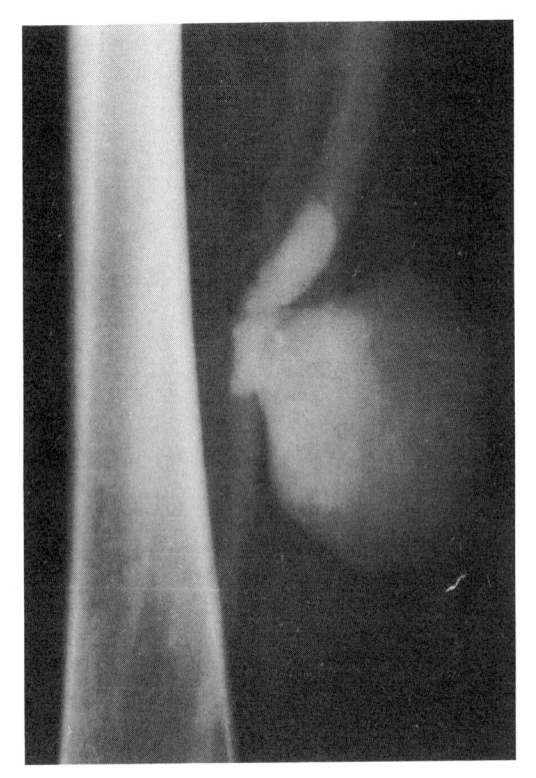

FIG. 44-16. Reproduction of an arteriogram in a patient who developed a superficial femoral artery-vein fistula and a pulsating hematoma after a bullet wound of the lower thigh. The artery feeding the fistula is enlarged, while the artery leaving the fistulous point is diminished in size. The superficial femoral vein proximal to the fistula is seen in the arteriogram less densely filled with dye than is the artery.

Further points in the diagnosis depend upon a series of physiologic disturbances which are produced by the abnormality (Elkin and Warren, 1947; Holman, 1937).

When it is established, the shunt immediately increases the venous return to the heart; velocity, pressure and minute flow into the right atrium are raised. Ventricular filling time is shortened, and the pulse rate is accelerated. An important clinical sign is made possible by this sequence of events. If the artery proximal to or directly over the fistula is compressed manually to stop flow through the fistula, the pulse rate will drop immediately. This phenomenon is called the Branham-Nicoladoni sign (Branham, 1890; Nicoladoni,

1875). It is almost universally present in arteriovenous fistulae so located that the maneuver can be accomplished.

The abnormal flow and pressure in the venous system in the region of the fistula causes a visible venous dilatation. There is a greater volume of blood in the tissues in the region of the fistula due to massive engorgement of the veins and increased flow. This produces a warming of the skin in the region of the fistula. For some distance beyond the lesion the skin also is warmer than on the contralateral side. When the arteriovenous fistula involves the major vessel of the thigh, the skin of the thigh will be warm, but the skin of the foot will be cooler than the opposite normal foot. This cooling distally is the result of diminished head of pressure in the artery beyond the shunt and lower arterial circulation from that point onward. Other physiologic results of the fistula are an increased cardiac output and an increase in blood volume. The arterial blood pressure is diminished by an arteriovenous fistula. Both systolic and diastolic pressures fall. Later, however, the systolic pressure rises to its former level or higher, whereas the diastolic remains lower, producing an increase in pulse pressure.

The increased cardiac output, increased blood volume, and the rapid pulse secondary to the accelerated venous return to the heart distinctly produce a strain upon the heart. Evidence of this strain is the almost constant cardiac enlargement in those patients who have a fistula for a significant length of time.

TABLE 44-1. PREOPERATIVE AND POSTOPERATIVE DATA AT REST OF A 32-YEAR-OLD PATIENT WITH ARTERIOVENOUS FISTULA OF 18 YEARS' DURATION*

	PREOPERATIVE	POSTOPERATIVE
Cardiac output (L./min. × 100)	5.36	2.16
Oxygen consumption (ml.)		
Stroke index (ml./beat/M^2)	140	77
Heart rate (beats/min.)	61	55
Systemic pressure (mm. Hg) Mean	69	93
Total blood volume (ml.)	6789	4835

* From Cardiopulmonary Laboratory, Division of Medicine, Presbyterian-St. Luke's Hospital, Chicago, Dr. John Graettinger, Director.

The strain is infrequently a cause of heart failure in patients with normal hearts. However, patients who have valvular heart disease, even mild, as a result of healed rheumatic fever, or have arteriosclerotic heart disease, often will go into heart failure when an arteriovenous fistula has been established.

Treatment. Treatment of an arteriovenous fistula is entirely surgical unless some degree of heart failure has occurred. In the latter case maximum competency of the myocardium should be obtained by proper treatment before surgery.

As in pulsating hematoma, arteriovenous fistulae were managed formerly by delaying the operative procedure for the purpose of development of arterial collaterals. This was for the reason that until recently the method of surgical treatment of a fistula of this type was the excision of the fistula after ligation of the 2 arterial and the 2 venous limbs. With the application of technics of vascular suture, anastomosis and grafting, the optimum treatment now consists of removal of the fistula and re-establishment of the circulation. In subjects with otherwise normal vessels this procedure is sufficiently dependable that the waiting period for development of collaterals can be abandoned and surgery done as soon as the diagnosis is made. Actually, if early operation in all forms of arterial damage becomes routine, the development of arteriovenous fistula will be a rarity.

Various types of surgical procedures were done long before the 2 modern technics of quadrilateral ligation and excision and of excision with re-establishment of the circulation were developed. These technics and the changes which resulted from them are of interest from a physiologic point of view.

Proximal ligation of the artery alone produces immediate severe ischemia of the extremity distal to the fistula. This, of course, is because all the blood that enters the artery from collaterals distal to the fistula drains backward through the fistula into the vein, disastrously reducing the head of pressure in the vascular bed supplying the tissues.

Distal ligation of the artery also has a most unsatisfactory result. Ligation at this point alone immediately and sharply increases the amount of blood which is shunted into the vein. The degree of heart strain is increased, and heart failure results. Theoretically, proximal and distal ligation of both the artery and the vein would seem to result in a cure of the fistula. However, some recurrences come about through the fact that relatively small arterial branches between the ligatures are overlooked, later to re-establish arterial circulation into the occluded segment, reactivating the fistula.

Simple ligation of the 4 ends was soon abandoned in favor of excising the area after ligating the vessels. This operation seldom, if ever, produces ischemic necrosis of the tissues distal to the fistula if it is delayed 3 months or more because by this time collateral arterial supply has become adequate. However, after this type of repair, the patients are limited in their ability to exercise, because the collateral bed upon which their limb depends cannot increase the blood flow to the extremity adequately to meet the needs of exercise. It has been not only the incidence of gangrene that has led to the procedures re-establishing arterial flow, but also the symptoms which result during exercise in a limb that has been treated by the ligation methods (Hughes and Jahnke, 1958).

CHRONIC OCCLUSIVE ARTERIAL DISEASE

General

The pathologic states productive of chronic arterial occlusion fall into 2 distinct groups: the degenerative arterial diseases, and a group of inflammatory arterial changes which are represented by the example of Buerger's disease.

Chronic occlusion of arteries may involve any organ or part of the body. Most by far of such occlusions are caused by degenerative arterial diseases. The symptoms produced depend on the organ or the body part involved, such as cerebral ischemia secondary to carotid artery involvement, hypertension secondary to renal artery involvement, abdominal angina secondary to mesenteric artery obstruction, angina caused by coronary artery obstruction, and a characteristic symptom complex caused by arterial occlusions in the extremities. The clinical picture which results from occlusive arterial disease will be considered in some detail as it involves the extremities. The effects of occlusion of the arteries to the brain, the intestines and the kidney will be discussed under these particular sections.

Symptomatology. INTERMITTENT CLAUDICATION. Chronic occlusion of the arterial supply to the extremities produces symptoms of essentially the same type, independent of the underlying pathology of the obstructing lesion. The earliest symptom is met with in the lower extremities during the work of the calf muscle groups in walking, running, or climbing stairs. The symptom develops initially during such exercise because, although the arterial supply may be quite adequate to meet all the needs of the part during rest, it cannot meet the increased demand of exercise. The symptom produced is a severe cramping pain in the muscle groups which are inadequately supplied with blood. Resting of the muscle by standing still or sitting down relieves the pain as soon as the metabolites are removed and an adequate ratio of work to blood supply is restored. This symptom is termed "intermittent claudication." It is not reproduced accurately by conditions other than those which restrict muscle blood supply during exercise.

Certain *characteristics of intermittent claudication* tend to distinguish it from other types of pain. One important characteristic is its independence of the general fatigue of the patient. The repeated reproducibility of the pain after the same amount of exercise and the constancy of the length of rest needed for relief in the same subject are also distinguishing characteristics of intermittent claudication. The afflicted patient has his cramping pain after walking a certain distance at a given rate of speed, and when the pain occurs he requires a definite rest period for relief. After this period of rest he is able to duplicate the exercise, and again the pain returns. The distance he can walk or the number of stairs he can climb before pain starts is the same in the morning as it is in the evening, even though the patient is tired after a day's work. No pain at all results in these patients when they walk a shorter distance than that required to produce claudication. Therefore, in walking about the home or the place of work the patient is perfectly comfortable.

Intermittent claudication particularly differs from the pain of hypertrophic arthritis in that the arthritic pain begins almost immediately at the beginning of exercise. It is worse when the patient gets up in the morning, relieved somewhat during the day as he loosens up, and increases again at night during fatigue. Much attention is paid to this symptom of intermittent claudication because it is the outstanding one, almost the hallmark, of chronic arterial occlusion.

REST PAIN. As the degree of arterial obstruction increases and intermittent claudication requires less exercise for its production and more rest for its relief, other symptoms appear. A sense of coldness in the distal part of the extremity is often the next symptom. Muscle pain of a cramping nature during rest and sleep becomes disturbing as the disease progresses. This symptom which is termed "rest pain" is, in effect, an intermittent claudication though in reverse. It is a result of the continued muscle work of normal tonus going on during the reduced circulation of repose. The patient actually finds that he may relieve the pain by stirring about or walking which increases cardiac output and local blood supply.

ISCHEMIA. The ischemia that results from chronic occlusive disease produces its most disturbing symptom by the direct effect of the lack of circulation on the peripheral nerves. The neuritic pain of ischemia differs from intermittent claudication and rest pain in that it is constant once it has become established. The pain is burning and compressing in quality and comes on relatively late in the course of the disease. It has one very distinctive characteristic. The patient so afflicted finds it difficult or impossible to elevate his legs or even to allow them to remain on a level with the rest of his body. When they are in any position other than hanging down as the patient sits, the pain is markedly exaggerated. This characteristic of the ischemic neuritis may account for some of the *edema of the feet and the ankles* which occurs in advanced arterial disease. The swelling itself is a very damaging factor in the arterial insufficiency because it renders the small vessel circulation in the part even more inefficient. The tendency to develop a *gangrenous ulcer* because of ischemic necrosis of the edematous tissue is markedly increased.

Whenever the ischemia progresses to the

point at which blood supply is inadequate for tissue life, *ischemic ulcers* develop. At any time in the course of the disease ulcers may be precipitated by minor trauma or blister formation because the demand for increased metabolism of healing cannot be met. The pain of ulceration is usually severe, although the ischemic neuritis which often has preceded it may have produced enough nerve damage to reduce the pain sensation.

These common symptoms including intermittent claudication, a sense of coldness, rest pain, ischemic neuritis, and the pain of ulceration are shared by various types of chronic occlusive arterial disease, although they appear in different degrees in the various conditions.

Physical Examination. In every general physical examination, whether arterial pathology has been suggested by the history or not, the peripheral pulses should be sought for in their normal locations and compared with those of the opposite side. The pulses which are normally palpable are the femoral, the popliteal, the dorsalis pedis and the posterior tibial arteries in the lower extremities; the subclavian, the axillary, the brachial, the radial and the ulnar in the upper extremities. Not only is the loss of palpability important, but also the comparative fullness of the pulse between the two sides should be noted and recorded. At the ankle the more important pulse is the posterior tibial because of the occasional congenital absence of the dorsalis pedis artery. This infrequent anomaly is probably always bilateral. The ulnar arterial pulse may be difficult to palpate but is demonstrable by a simple maneuver described by Allen (1929).

In addition to noting the presence or the absence of pulses and comparing the fullness and the strength of the pulses on the two sides, the character of the blood vessel wall should be observed. Thickening, stiffness and calcification of the vessel wall can be palpated, particularly at the femoral, the brachial, the ankle and the wrist levels.

Auscultation over various arteries during physical examination provides very important information. Under normal circumstances, one hears only faint crisp sounds, roughly corresponding in time to the first and the second heart tones, over large vessels. In addition to characteristic abnormal sounds produced by aortic stenosis and aortic valvular insufficiency, intrinsic changes in the blood vessels proximal to the point at which auscultation is carried out may produce very characteristic abnormal sounds. Roughening of the lining of a blood vessel, or changes in its caliber, particularly in the direction of stenosis, causes the appearance of a systolic *bruit*. The character of the sound, whether it be soft or coarse or pitched high or low is determined by the character of abnormality in the vessel wall, but changes in these characters cannot be ascribed directly to different kinds of lesions. The commonest cause of a harsh bruit over a vessel is stenosis of the vessel proximal to the area. The stenosis is caused by the development of an elevated atheroma or degenerated and calcified lesion in the vessel intruding on its lumen. Much attention must be paid to the bruit and its interpretation. The bruit is absent distal to a complete occlusion of an artery, even though a small pulse may be palpable in the artery due to the fact that the collateral arterial circulation is very well developed. Therefore, if a patient exhibits pulses at both femoral levels with that on the left being stronger than that on the right, and with a bruit over the stronger left femoral pulse and none over the weaker right femoral pulse, the interpretation would be that there is a stenosis in the iliofemoral system on the left and a complete occlusion on the right with good collateral development, at least on the right side (Javid, Dye, and Cagle, 1964).

The objective skin temperature is an important observation rendered somewhat unreliable because of its strong vasomotor control. Coldness of the skin of the hands and the feet may indicate a physiologic response to an unfamiliar situation rather than arterial insufficiency. However, when skin temperature is diminished on one side, the finding has greater meaning.

The skin color which is observed during the examination is also of importance but is also affected by vasomotor stimuli. If the abnormal color is asymmetrical it has meaning, and its extension above the portions of the extremities which have a heavy vasomotor control also gives it importance.

Skin color changes in relation to changes in posture of the extremities can be characteristic for chronic arterial occlusion. The

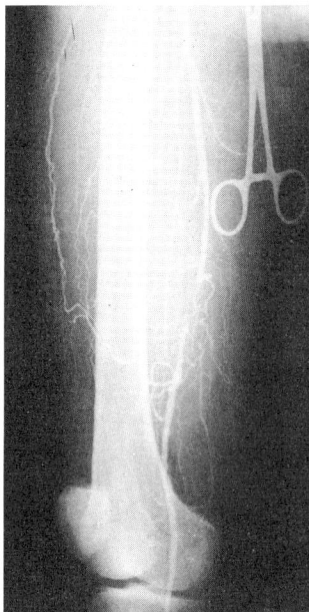

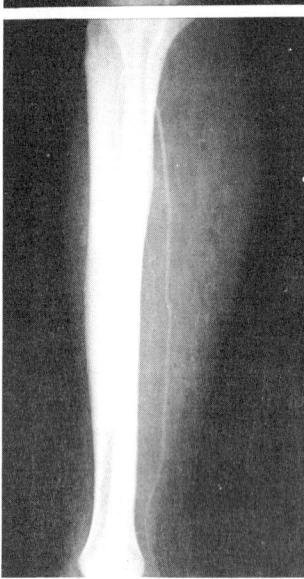

Fig. 44-17. Femoral arteriogram produced by injection of opaque iodine solution into the common femoral artery. A short segment of the superficial femoral artery at the level of the adductor tendon is shown to be completely obstructed. Many collaterals are visualized, and the artery above and below the obstruction is relatively normal.

normal extremity blanches perceptibly during elevation. This can be demonstrated in any normal subject. Following elevation, acute dependency of the part produces a brief flushing of the skin with a quick return to normal. In arterial disease the blanching that occurs during elevation is increased, and the time required for the appearance of the heightened color following dependency is lengthened. When color does appear in the arterial-insufficient extremity, it is deeper and more intense than in the normal. It is also more lasting and in severe cases may not return to normal during the period of observation unless the extremity is brought up to the horizontal position. This phenomenon is termed *"reactive hyperemia."* It is thought to be based upon a relative ischemia and anoxia of the skin capillary walls during elevation. The vessels are then in maximum caliber as the new fill of arterial blood slowly comes into the skin when the extremity is lowered. The degree of ischemia during elevation governs the length of time it takes for the artery to regain its normal tone.

At the same time that the limb is brought into dependency after elevation to observe reactive hyperemia, one measures the length of time necessary for normal veins in the skin of the extremity to fill. In the normal subject without varicose veins or arterial insufficiency the so-called *"venous filling time"* is approximately 5 to 6 seconds. In arterial insufficiency this venous filling time is prolonged. If varicose veins are present, the retrograde flow of blood in the veins themselves renders this observation unreliable.

OSCILLOMETER AND PLETHYSMOGRAPH. Certain mechanical aids in the diagnosis of arterial insufficiency are useful. The oscillometer and the plethysmograph are respectively crude and very delicate methods of recording the changes in volume in a part coincident with the heart action. The oscillometer is a manometer attached to a blood pressure cuff and records the swing of the differences in pressure of the tissue contained within the cuff due to heart action at various pressures of inflation of the cuff. The plethysmograph records the changes in volume in a portion of the extremity, usually a portion of toe or finger, which is enclosed in a container having an air-tight seal around the tissues. Plethysmography is rarely used except in specialized examinations. The oscillometer is a valuable practical instrument to record the relative pulse volume. It is used to demonstrate the approximate level of an arterial occlusion by making readings up and down the extremity, showing the point at which the oscillometric index is diminished. It is of utmost value to compare one limb to the other. The oscillometer readings are recorded as an oscillometric index of millimeters of mercury fluctuation at various pressures. The plethysmograph reading is recorded as the number of cubic millimeters change in volume per cubic centimeter of tissue that occurs during the cardiac cycle.

Angiography. Visualization of the arterial system by x-rays has been mentioned already in relation to arterial trauma. However, its essential use is in the evaluation of chronic occlusion in arterial disease.

Much of our present knowledge concerning the typical segmental distribution of arteriosclerosis, its method of progression, the production of partial occlusion of the vessel by atherosclerotic plaques, and the development of collaterals, comes from x-ray visualization of the lumens of the blood vessels. The technic of visualizing the vascular system by x-rays is known as angiography and constitutes the greatest single aid in the evaluation of chronic arterial occlusions. Typical patterns of filling defects in occlusions are demonstrated by angiography, and the extent of the disease may be mapped out accurately when this is thought to be a necessary prerequisite to surgical treatment. The trend, as experience is gained in the evaluation of a patient by physical examination, is to carry out x-ray examination somewhat less frequently.

In studying the arterial system several methods of angiography are available. Most commonly used is the peripheral *arteriogram*. A peripheral arteriogram is made by introducing a suitable iodine-containing solution into the artery through a needle inserted into its lumen and making one or several rapid x-ray exposures as the dye progresses through the arteries (Fig. 44-17). In the femoral artery the needle can be introduced under local anesthesia through the skin. However, in case of the brachial artery, the many adjacent major nerves make this percutaneous method hazardous, and more frequently the artery is exposed through a small incision, in order that the needle may be introduced without endangering these other structures. In actual practice arteriography of the upper extremity is rarely done except for proximal lesions of the sub-

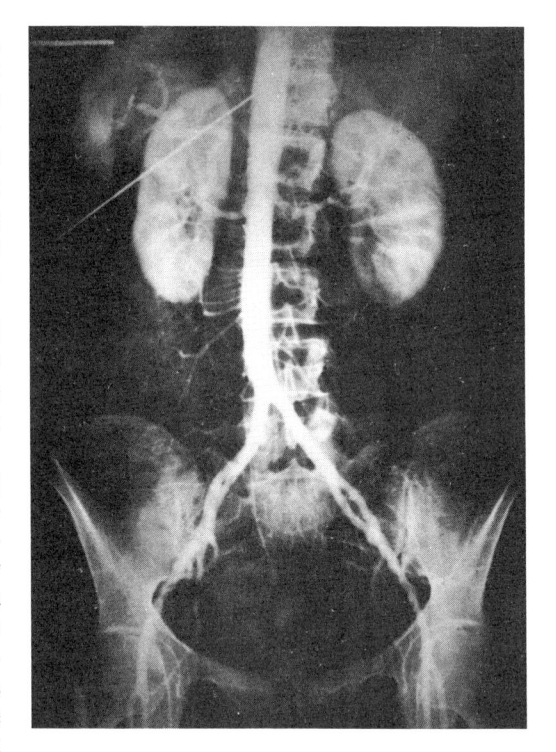

FIG. 44-18. Abdominal aortogram produced by the injection of opaque iodine solution into the aorta at the level of the 1st lumbar vertebra. The needle has been introduced through the lumbar region while the patient is under general anesthesia in the prone position. The resulting picture visualized the splenic artery, the renal arteries and several lumbar arteries as well as the aorta and the iliofemoral systems below. Mild arteriosclerotic changes in the vessels are indicated by the slight elongation of the lumbar aorta and the irregularity of the internal and the external iliac arteries.

clavian. In the femoral region, percutaneous introduction of the needle is routine except when the artery seems to be seriously hardened by arteriosclerosis at the site of the proposed puncture. In such instances a short incision may be made under local anesthesia so that the needle can be introduced in as atraumatic a manner as possible.

Visualization of the abdominal aorta rather than of the femoral system is indicated when decreased or absent femoral pulses and the symptoms which are present indicate that the occlusive lesion is at iliac artery level or

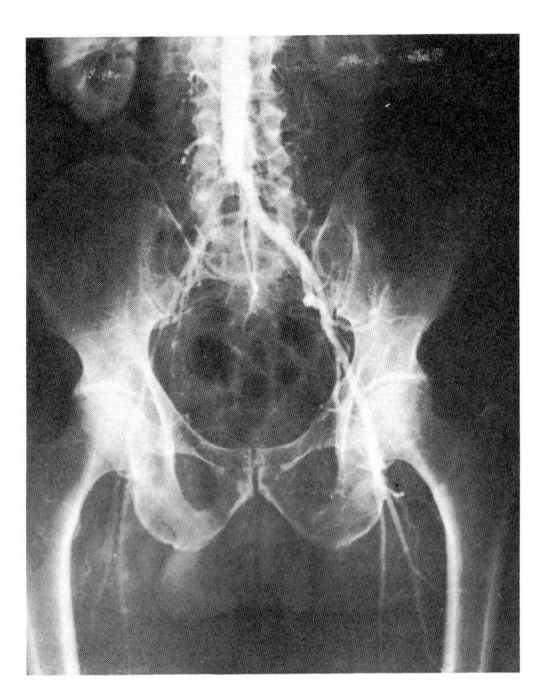

FIG. 44-19. Abdominal aortogram showing complete obstruction of left common iliac with delayed filling of that iliofemoral system.

higher. In order to produce an *aortogram*, a long, relatively large-bore needle is introduced through the left lumbar area directly into the aorta at the level of the first lumbar vertebra with the patient in the prone position. From 5 to 8 ml. of the contrast medium is injected, and a scout film is made. This is for the purpose of determining that the tip of the needle is completely within the lumen of the aorta, rather than partially buried within its wall, or in a branch. The aortogram is made by exposing the film just at the conclusion of the rapid injection of 20 to 40 ml. of the radiopaque substance. The use of a 36-inch x-ray film cassette makes it possible to visualize not only the aorta but also a good portion of the upper part of the femoral system (Figs. 44-18 and 19).

There is a very small incidence of complication with aortography which must be accepted in those cases in which the information to be obtained is important. Direct injection into the renal artery or into the superior mesenteric artery may be damaging to the tissues supplied by these vessels. An intramural injection in the wall of the aorta causes damage to the wall with some hemorrhage into the layers of the vessel. This has been known to be sufficiently extensive as to occlude an important vessel, such as a renal artery. The introduction of the needle may of itself cause dislodgment of an arteriosclerotic plaque or a clot lying against the wall of the aorta and produce an acute arterial occlusion of some smaller distal vessel.

Visualization of the thoracic aorta may be done by one of two means. A catheter introduced through one of the arteries in the arm or the leg is passed up to the arch of the aorta and the dye injected through it (Fig. 44-20). The retrograde technic through the femoral arteries is now used commonly for selective angiography of visceral vessels as well as the aorta itself (see Fig. 44-9). The second method of visualizing the thoracic aorta and its branches is by means of contrast medium injected very rapidly into a vein of the arm. The rapid injection causes this material to travel through the right side of the heart and the lungs, back to the left ventricle, without too much dilution. Then it travels on into the aorta in sufficient concentration to outline it in x-ray films made at that time. If films are made as the dye passes through the cardiac chambers, an angiocardiogram results. If the exposures are made at the time the dye traverses the thoracic aorta, the visualization is termed a transvenous thoracic aortogram.

By use of the aortogram and the peripheral arteriogram, diffuse and segmental forms of arteriosclerosis obliterans and aneurysms may be studied. The dorsal aortogram produced by angiocardiography or aortogram per catheter delineates such lesions of the descending aorta as coarctation of the aorta, aneurysms of the arch or thoracic aorta wherever they may occur, and dissecting aneurysm of the dorsal aorta.

ARTERIOSCLEROSIS OBLITERANS

Arteriosclerosis undoubtedly is the commonest pathologic condition of man. Its almost universal appearance during advancing age is evidence of the part played in its production by wear, tear and degeneration. However, the etiology of arteriosclerosis is understood only in broad terms, which include the factors of aging and of disturbed metabolism. Evidence of the latter is shown most strongly by the early appearance and the rapid advance of arteriosclerosis in some diabetics.

Pathology. The arterial lesion in arteriosclerosis may be described in terms of its effect on the various layers of the arterial wall. The intima, the subintimal layer, the elastic lamina, the media and the adventitia are involved to varying degrees, and on the basis of the degree to which each is involved, types of arteriosclerosis have been subdivided.

The earliest change observed in arteriosclerosis is the deposition of lipoid material in the subendothelial layer. This primary lesion is called an *atheroma*. This type of change is accelerated in diabetics, but it is often exaggerated and occurs early in certain individuals who are not diabetic. A satisfactory explanation of this tendency is lacking. However, there is suggestive evidence that it is familial, much as is diabetes, and that the primary disturbance is an abnormality in lipid metabolism.

The findings in the media characteristic of arteriosclerosis include fibrosis, fragmentation of the elastic fibers, necrosis of areas of the media, hemorrhage, and later calcification of the necrotic or hemorrhagic areas. At present these changes are explained best on the basis of aging and wear. When the intimal and the subintimal layer changes are predominant, producing large plaques, yellow in color, the disease has been termed *atherosclerosis*. The medial change predominates in some patients, producing the pathologic picture of medial sclerosis and calcification. These vessels have a pipestem characteristic. They retain patency of the lumen for a surprising length of time. This is known as *Mönckeburg's medial sclerosis*.

Most commonly, the intimal and the medial changes go on together after initial preponderance of one or the other. The building up of the intima and the thickening of the media result in progressive narrowing of the vascular lumen. This finally leads to thrombosis. Another factor accentuating the effect of the narrowing of the lumen is the roughening and actual ulceration of the vessel lining.

It would be a mistake to consider that these lesions occur diffusely and evenly throughout the arterial system in any one patient. Rather,

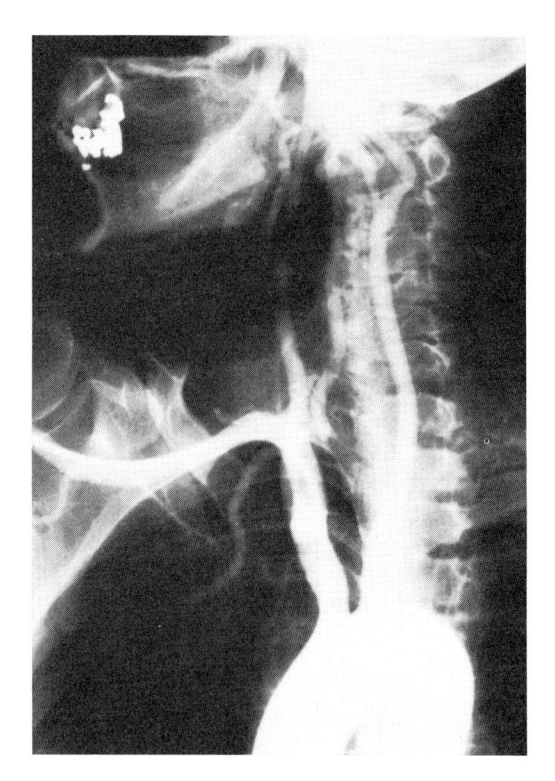

FIG. 44-20. Retrograde angiogram of brachiocephalic vessels via right brachial artery. Complete occlusion of left subclavian artery, filling of right vertebral, and adequate visualization of left carotid bifurcation are noted.

they develop to various degrees and stages and are distributed in irregular fashion. Severe degeneration in one segment of artery will be adjacent to other segments having moderate or insignificant pathology. The disease of arteriosclerosis obliterans shows a very definite tendency to be segmental and to involve primarily specific areas of the arterial tree. The commonest areas to be involved include the aortic bifurcation (producing the Leriche syndrome, described later), the iliac arteries immediately at the aortic bifurcation, and the superficial femoral artery at two points, one being just below the common femoral bifurcation, and the other at the adductor hiatus. The popliteal bifurcation, the coronary arteries, renal, carotid and origins of the celiac and superior mesenteric arteries are other points at which segments of occlusion occur.

Course. The clinical characteristics of the

FIG. 44-21. Femoral arteriogram of a 58-year-old man, showing moderate ischemic changes in the foot. The needle has been introduced into the common femoral artery. The superficial femoral artery is completely occluded from the bifurcation down to the level of the adductor tendon. At this point it is seen to be patent and to contain dye which has been brought to it through collaterals from the profunda femoris branch. The most proximal collateral entering this distal segment is about to be pinched off by the advancing disease. Progressive obstruction of collateral branches above and below an occluded segment is the manner in which arteriosclerosis advances.

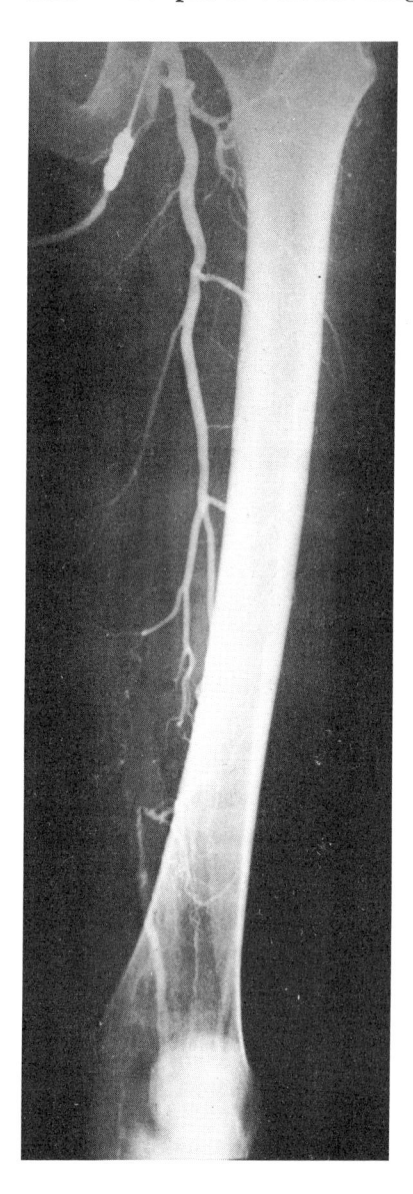

disease and its progression are connected intimately to the tendency for segmental occurrence of the individual lesions. The early symptom of claudication becomes disturbing when a significant degree of local obstruction has developed. During the course of development of total occlusion, the progression is usually slow, allowing time for the development of the available collateral circulation. Nutrition of the involved part may not be disturbed at all if the collateral circulation keeps up with the progressing obstruction, so that the distal part of the extremity retains its normal color and resists atrophy of either the muscles or the skin. From this stage, which is usually encountered when a single occlusion has occurred, progression results from upward or downward extension of the obstructing thrombus, progressively obstructing the orifices of the collateral arteries (Fig. 44-21). As these are obstructed in sequence, a greater severity of symptoms occurs, and finally, when enough collateral has been blocked, the blood flow becomes inadequate to support tissue metabolism, and ischemic necrosis develops.

The level of the occlusion determines the location of the symptoms. In the lower extremities, superficial femoral and popliteal arterial occlusion produces intermittent claudication of the foot and the calf, while iliac and lower aortic obstruction may produce thigh and hip claudication as well. A form of claudication also occurs in the upper extremities as a result of occlusion of the subclavian or the axillary arteries. In this condition the patient suffers pain in the muscles of hand, forearm and arm during prolonged activity and is particularly unable to work with the hands raised up over his head.

Attention was drawn to a clinical syndrome typically produced by chronic arteriosclerotic occlusion of the aortic bifurcation by Leriche (1934; 1940). This syndrome, which has been further clarified by others (Elkin and Cooper, 1949; Oudot and Beaconsfield, 1953), consists of intermittent claudication of the lower extremities, loss of pulses everywhere in the lower extremities, impotence in male patients and the notable point that the nutrition of the feet remains good over a relatively long period of the disease.

With the exception of the impotence, which probably is due to the diminished arterial pressure within the pelvis, the same type of syndrome is produced also by unilateral or bilateral segmental arteriosclerosis of the iliac arteries or the superficial femoral arteries.

Treatment. GENERAL MANAGEMENT. Curative treatment of the arteriosclerosis is totally lacking. Any study of the histologic picture of well-established arterial lesions convinces one that the changes observed are irreversible. Perhaps at some early stage in which the initial lesion of atheromata is the only manifestation of the disease, some method of alteration of metabolism might in the future be effective. It is clear that the advance which must be sought in the general problem of arteriosclerosis is one of prevention. On the basis of information now available concerning the part played by ingested fats and lipids, some rigid regimen of a dietary nature started very early in life might succeed in producing individuals more free of arteriosclerosis than the average. For obvious reasons a major clinical work in this direction has not been done. Many patients with mild involvement require only general management, while another large group with very advanced disease is seen at a time at which only general management can be applied.

In the peripheral arteries the relief sought generally will be for symptoms of the lower extremities. The first step in treatment of a patient with symptoms in the lower extremities due to arteriosclerosis is a reduction in the work that must be done by the legs. Weight reduction to accomplish this is of prime importance in general management.

It has been amply demonstrated experimentally and clinically that smoking plays a part in the general efficiency of the peripheral arterial circulation. In relation to arteriosclerosis it does so largely through the fact that smoking increases the general vasomotor tone. When a patient with early symptoms of arteriosclerosis, such as intermittent claudication, stops smoking, improvement is frequent.

The third item of general management consists of careful instructions as to foot hygiene and protection from injury. This is important because the reduced arterial supply diminishes the ability of the tissues of the feet to heal traumatic lesions and infections. Even minor skin conditions, such as intertrigo or fungus infection, may lead to disaster and must be avoided.

DRUGS. The class of drugs which seems most likely to aid in the relief of symptoms in arteriosclerosis is the vasodilator group. A wide choice of vasodilators has been offered, and new ones are being added constantly. Their effectiveness can hardly be predicted in individual cases without trial, but most frequently they are disappointing. The principal defect in the use of vasodilator drugs is that they produce a dilatation of all the arteries in the body which are capable of dilating. They are ineffective on the diseased vessels which have become rigid, and the collateral arteries in the area of disease, although dilated, fail to benefit very much because of the general increase of the vascular bed caused by the drug throughout the body.

Substances which diminish the coagulability of the blood are indicated in chronic arterial insufficiency when the pathologic change in the blood vessels is arteriosclerosis. The phenomenon leading to final obstruction of an arterial lumen narrowed by arteriosclerosis is thrombosis. It is doubtful that anticoagulants prevent total occlusion, but there is good reason to believe that the rate of obstruction is slowed. When rapid and temporary alteration in coagulation is desired, heparin is used. For chronic depression of the coagulation system, one of the prothrombin depressing drugs is indicated.

INDIRECT SURGICAL TREATMENT. Symptomatic improvement in arteriosclerosis may be obtained by indirect surgical means in properly selected cases by removal of an appropriate portion of the sympathetic nervous system (Coller *et al.*, 1949; DeBakey *et al.*, 1950; Julian and Shabart, 1950). Other indirect means which have been used are excision of diseased portions of the artery, supposedly to reduce vasomotor reflexes (Leriche *et al.*, 1934), and inactivation of the group of muscles most commonly involved in intermittent claudication, by cutting the Achilles tendon (Boyd *et al.*, 1949). Achilles tenotomy and the operation of simple arteriectomy are not now in use, and their effectiveness must be said to be in question but they are of historical interest, indicating the scope of past surgical attacks on the problem. When properly selected patients with arteriosclerosis are subjected to sympathectomy, the majority will benefit.

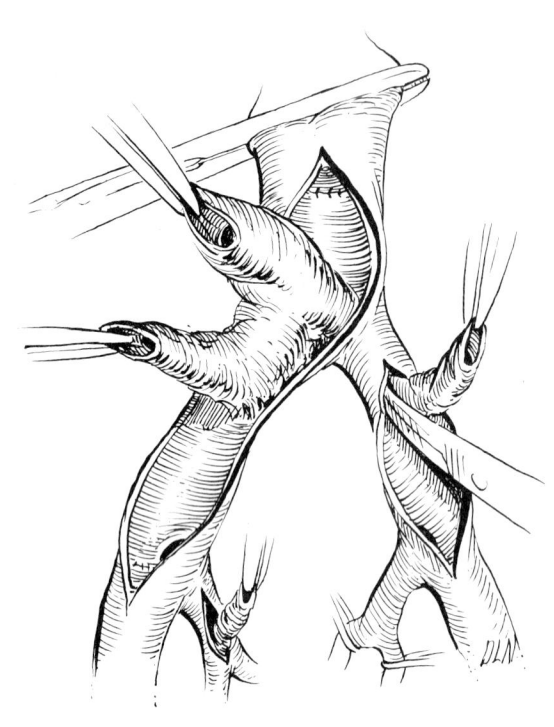

FIG. 44-22. Endarterectomy of the bifurcation of aorta. Separate endarterectomy of right internal iliac artery.

SYMPATHECTOMY. On the basis of experimental evidence surgical ablation of the sympathetic nervous system in the lumbar region for arterial insufficiency of a lower extremity and in the dorsal region for an upper extremity principally improves the circulation of the skin of the part (May et al., 1963; White et al., 1952). However, numerous clinical studies indicate that the operation also provides a significant degree of relief from intermittent claudication (Berry et al., 1955; Blain et al., 1963; de Takats et al., 1950; Kirtley et al., 1953). It is apparent that there is a very real tendency for a sympathectomy in the lumbar region to increase the rate of development of collateral arterial circulation in the lower extremity (Hermann et al., 1954). In selecting patients for lumbar sympathectomy, use is made of the fact that the sympathetic system controls the blood flow through the skin. A temporary sympathetic paralysis is produced by introducing procaine into the region directly about the lumbar sympathetic chain. Carefully measuring the resulting changes in skin temperature is helpful.

Three types of skin temperature responses occur. In a patient who has a normal arterial system the elevation in skin temperature may vary between 12° and 15° C. In a patient with arterial insufficiency of an organic type which will probably benefit by doing a lumbar sympathectomy, the elevation of temperature may be between 2° and 5°. The third type of response is a fall in the skin temperature in response to sympathetic block. This is observed in advanced cases of arterial insufficiency and is usually taken to contraindicate a lumbar sympathectomy. The test is relatively unreliable unless the observations are made in a comfortable, cool room of stable temperature and humidity. Other observations, such as testing the patient's ability to walk without pain after a procaine sympathetic block has been done, are not generally considered as reliable because the procaine may diffuse to interrupt somatic sensory fibers of the adjacent nerve roots and relieve pain by this mechanism.

DIRECT SURGICAL APPROACH. A large proportion of patients with arteriosclerosis obliterans, particularly of the lower end of the aorta and of the major vessels of the thighs, have a segmental form of the disease. This does not mean that the disease appears in one part of the vessels while the artery above and below the area is normal, but rather that certain areas are found to be in a far more advanced state than the adjacent areas at any given time. By the use of arteriography an estimate can be made of the state of the disease above and below the advanced segment. Three methods of direct surgical approach are now available for use in these cases which provide for more definitive treatment than can be gained by the indirect technics (Julian, 1960; Julian et al., 1959a).

Thrombo-endarterectomy. This type of direct surgery in arteriosclerosis consists of exposure of the segmentally obstructed portion of the artery and removal of the diseased inner coats of the vessel by one technic or another (Fig. 44-22). Thereafter, repair of the more normal muscular layers, usually consisting of about half of the media and the adventitia, is done with fine silk sutures. The opening in the artery through which the diseased portions are removed may be made longitudinally throughout the section of disease or the artery may be opened above and below the segment and the diseased tissue removed with special instruments. After the procedure, the resulting rough lining of the vessel becomes smooth, either by condensation of fibrous tissue or by the direct growth of intima from each end (Barker and Cannon, 1959; Bazy, 1948; Brittain and Earley, 1963; Cannon and Barker, 1955; Cannon et al., 1961; dos Santos, 1947; Edwards, 1962; Julian and Dye, 1952; Leriche and Kunlin, 1947; Reboul and Huguier, 1949; Wylie, 1952; Wylie et al., 1951; Thompson et al., 1966; Sawyer et al., 1967).

RESTORATION WITH VASCULAR GRAFTS. Grafts are used to restore the circulation in the presence of segmental occlusion of an artery. Sometimes they are implanted after complete excision of the segment, during which the ends of the artery above and below the area of disease are prepared for anastomosis to the grafts in an end-to-end fashion. Much more frequently, grafts are implanted as *bypass* grafts (Fig. 44-23). In this type of graft, the graft is installed simply by connecting it end-to-side to the diseased blood vessel above and below the area of obstruction (Crawford et al., 1955; Julian et al., 1962; Kunlin, 1951; Linton, 1955; Wesolowski et al., 1962; Whitman and McGoon, 1962; Garrett and De Bakey, 1966; Darling et al., 1967b; Dale, 1966; DeWeese et al., 1966; Tyson and DeLaurentis, 1966; Julian, 1967; Kouchoukos et al.,

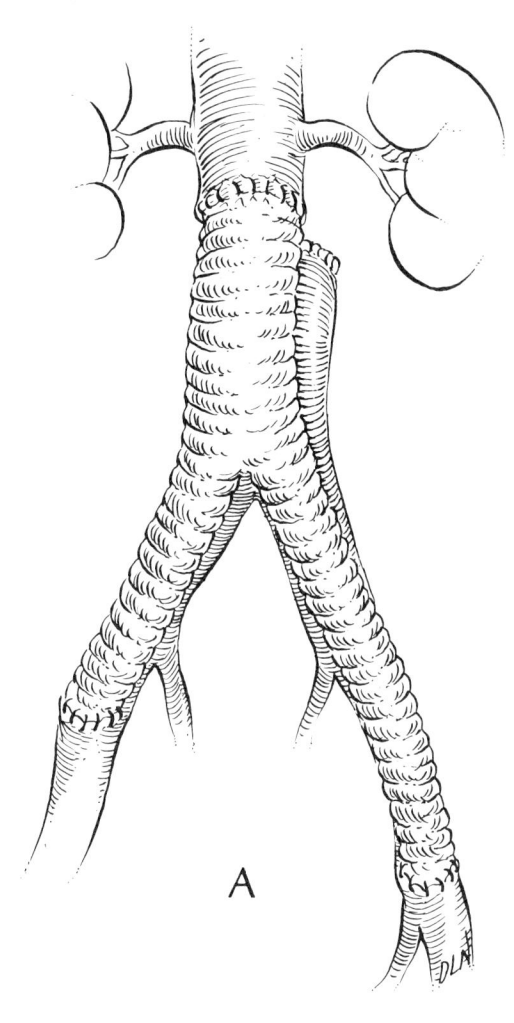

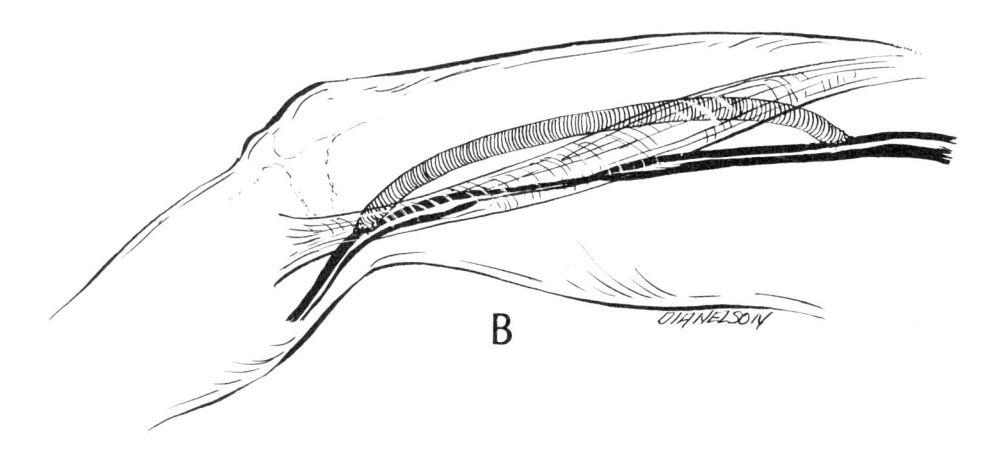

FIG. 44-23. (A) Bifurcation graft end-to-end to aorta above, end-to-side right external iliac and end-to-side left common femoral. (B) Femoral-popliteal bypass graft—obstruction in adductor canal.

1968; Barner et al., 1968; Moore et al., 1968; Ehrenfeld et al., 1968).

The bypass method of installation of a graft has the great advantage of reducing the amount of surgical trauma, because it is not necessary to remove the obstructed segment of artery. The collateral arteries which remain open are preserved by this method.

For either method of implantation, the grafts in common use are autogenous vein grafts, usually the saphenous vein, and prosthetic appliances woven of synthetic fiber yarns, such as Dacron and Teflon. Homologous grafts consisting of human aortic bifurcations were the type first used in treatment of abdominal aortic aneurysms and of obstructions of the bifurcation of the aorta when these lesions were initially successfully subjected to curative surgery. The convenience and the high degree of reliability of prosthetic materials has caused them virtually to replace the use of homologous arteries (Julian et al., 1959). The autogenous vein grafts which were the first type of graft used for reconstruction of the femoral artery have continued to be a favored material, having the specific disadvantage that the saphenous vein of a certain proportion of patients is unsuitable in length or diameter for this purpose (Hardin, 1962; Linton, 1962).

SELECTION OF PATIENT FOR ARTERIAL RECONSTRUCTION. There is great variability in the rate at which progression of symptoms occurs in different patients with arteriosclerotic involvement of the lower extremities. In some a mildly limiting degree of claudication will remain stationary for 5 to 15 years, while in others rest pain, ischemic neuritis, and necrosis will ensue within a few months of onset of claudication. For this reason careful individual evaluation must be the basis upon which patients are selected for surgery.

An objective evaluation of the results of arterial surgery in arteriosclerosis shows a proportion of failures, many of which leave the patient with more symptoms than were present before surgery. This fact increases the necessity for individual evaluation and completely negates any tendency to advise surgical correction of every chronic arteriosclerotic occlusion.

These two facts dominate the application of surgical judgment in arteriosclerosis of the lower extremities. Another point or two in relation to each makes it possible to evolve a reasonable broad approach. The variability in progression of symptoms cannot be applied to patients who have rest pain, neuritic pain, or even a very severe, easily produced claudication. The prognosis in such persons is uniformly bad, and a strong indication exists for surgery. Further, there are certain lesions the repair of which has been demonstrated to be remarkably dependable and lasting. These are occlusion of the aorto-iliac region between the renal artery level and the inguinal ligament and limited lesions of the femoral-popliteal region, the repair of which requires reconstruction by graft or endarterectomy 3 to 5 inches in length.

Three general statements may be made on the basis of these considerations: (1) reconstruction is indicated when an aorto-iliac occlusion or a short femoral or popliteal occlusion is demonstrated; (2) extensive reconstructions are indicated only when the claudication they cause is of a grade which limits the patient's ability to accomplish *necessary* activities, when rest pain and ischemic neuritis are present, or when necrosis has appeared or is impending; (3) unless there is destruction of function of the foot by ischemia, an amputation should not be done until a major attempt has been made to restore circulation with a reconstructive procedure on the arteries.

LIMB SALVAGE. The attempt to restore adequate circulation to an extremity which otherwise is irretrievably lost results in salvage in a worthwhile proportion of cases attempted. These operations are done in the presence of extensive aorto-iliac and femoral artery involvement. Some of the procedures are simply extensions of the bypass graft or endarterectomy technics already described. An aortic bifurcation graft may be extended on one or both sides down to the popliteal area, or a graft from the common femoral level may be carried to the proximal segment of the posterior tibial artery. Another form of extension of a more ordinary procedure is to endarterectomize the branches of the popliteal artery to a point far below the knee, closing the arterial incision with a strip of autogenous vein wall to enlarge the small artery. The penalty for failure of this procedure is severe, limiting its application to that of salvage.

Among a variety of unusual salvage procedures the *femoro-femoral bypass* and *profunda revascularization* are most useful. The former consists of connection of the femoral artery of the severely affected limb to the contralateral femoral artery. The connection is by way of a graft which traverses a subcutaneous tunnel across the suprapubic region of the lower abdomen. The latter procedure takes advantage of a tendency of the profunda femoris artery and its collateral extensions to remain relatively free of disease. When femoral and popliteal artery disease is so severe that their reconstruction seems not to be feasible, the proximal portion of the profunda branch is exposed. It is then cleared of atheroma so that it may again receive blood flow from the common femoral. If ilio-femoral disease is also present, a source of strong flow to the profunda is obtained from above with a bypass graft from the aorta or common iliac artery.

The two procedures are sometimes combined and a femoro-femoral graft is used to bring blood from the opposite side to the profunda femoris system of the severely affected limb. Additional salvage procedures that may be used are the axillary-femoral bypass and the long femoral to posterior tibial vein graft (Garrett and De Bakey, 1966). Also bypass grafts have been used from the profunda femoris to the anterior tibial artery (Royster and Reiss, 1968).

RENAL ARTERY DISEASE

Disturbances of the blood supply of the kidney are produced by a variety of arterial lesions, some of which have surgical importance. In the investigation of patients for the cause of hypertension or renal insufficiency it is of great practical importance to differentiate surgically correctable arterial lesions from arterial and arteriolar disease not treatable by mechanical means and from primary parenchymal lesions as well as from conditions involving the urinary tract (renal pelvis, ureters, bladder and urethra).

There is a definite relationship between renal blood flow and the systemic blood pressure (Janeway, 1909). The experimental background was provided by the valuable work of Goldblatt (Goldblatt *et al.*, 1934) in showing that arterial hypertension resulted from experimentally induced stenosis of the renal artery in dogs. The analogous relationship occurs spontaneously in man in a variety of abnormal situations.

Etiology. Disturbances of renal arterial blood flow resulting in arterial hypertension in man arise from either congenital or acquired lesions.

The congenital narrowing may be as far proximal to the renal artery as the thoracic aorta where a "coarctation" produces elevated blood pressure at least in part because it changes the character of renal arterial inflow. Coarctation of the abdominal aorta above the renal arteries, also occurring as a congenital lesion, similarly causes hypertension. Parenthetically, it should be noted that complete occlusion of the aorta below the renal arteries does not per se cause hypertension. Congenital narrowing of one or both renal arteries causes hypertension and, in contrast with thoracic and abdominal aortic coarctation, the elevation of blood pressure is present in the lower extremities as well as in the upper (Hunter *et al.*, 1963b; Varco *et al.*, 1962).

The renal arteries themselves are more commonly affected by acquired lesions than by congenital ones. Two forms are presently recognized. One consists of a typical atheroma of the renal artery, usually close to the origin of the vessel but sometimes seen at other points in the renal artery or its main branches (Perloff *et al.*, 1961). The second lesion consists of a hypertrophy of the media of the artery which results in a localized stenosis (Wylie *et al.*, 1962).

Pathophysiology. These arterial lesions are found on one or both sides. In either event they rarely fail to cause a sustained systolic and diastolic hypertension probably because the kidney is stimulated to produce abnormal amounts of vasopressor substances. Suppression of renal function need not be of such a degree as to cause nitrogen retention even in bilateral lesions. Disturbances in filtration are detected by clearance studies. This provides clear evidence when only one renal artery is involved and is more difficult to interpret when both sides are affected. In unilateral disease, the lesion tends to protect the involved kidney from arteriolar damage by the blood pressure elevation that it has produced. In unilateral renal artery stenosis the involved kidney be-

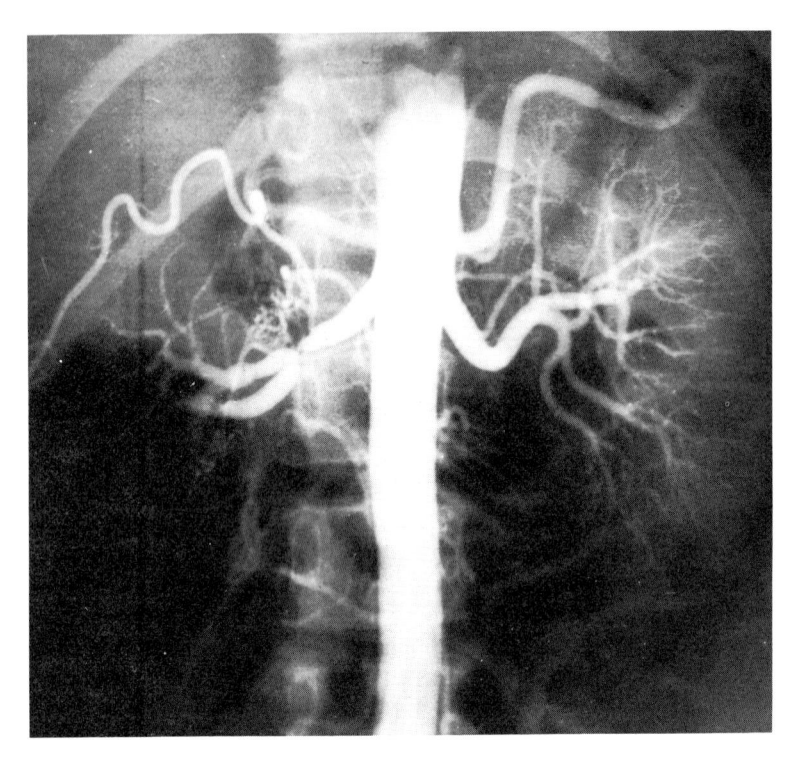

FIG. 44-24. Stenosis of right renal artery near its bifurcation in 18-year-old female with hypertension. Surgical relief of the stenosis was not effective in lowering the blood pressure, but subsequent nephrectomy was curative.

comes smaller while the normally supplied kidney hypertrophies. There is a tendency for arteriolar changes to occur in the parenchyma of the uninvolved kidney. It is not clear whether or not these are due to the obviously possible mechanism of the hypertension caused by the contralateral arterial stenosis.

The frequency of renal artery stenosis as a cause of hypertension in comparison with parenchymal renal disease or intrarenal arterial disease is not clearly known. Its frequency in any given series of hypertensive patients is proportional to the amount of effort expended in looking for it.

Diagnosis. The finding of a bruit over the kidney area may suggest renal artery stenosis. The absolute diagnosis depends on its demonstration by roentgenograms. Renal arteriograms may be made by injection of contrast medium into the suprarenal aorta through a needle introduced by the translumbar route or through a catheter passed upward to the renal level of the aorta from the femoral artery below (Figs. 44-24 and 44-25). By either route, this examination is somewhat imposing as to time, discomfort and possible dangers. Therefore, other tests are used to screen hypertensive patients before renal arteriograms are done.

None of the "screening" tests is of certain reliability, and either new methods or improvements are needed. History of onset of the hypertension, age and presence of atherosclerotic lesions elsewhere are of little value. Asymmetry of kidney size as seen in a plain roentgenogram of the abdomen suggests stenosis on the side of the smaller kidney but may also be a normal congenital variation or due to unilateral pyelonephritis.

Differential renal function studies often provide a strong lead in unilateral disease. An excretory urogram (intravenous pyelogram) in which additional x-ray exposures are made $\frac{1}{2}$, 1 and 2 minutes after injection of the dye is a simple form of differential renal function test. When one kidney is affected by an arterial stenosis the pyelogram on that side will be delayed. The early pictures are required to detect this delay. The excretory urogram is considered the most reliable screening test.

Other methods of obtaining information of the function of each kidney entail the catheterization of the ureters in such a way as to collect all of the urine excreted from each

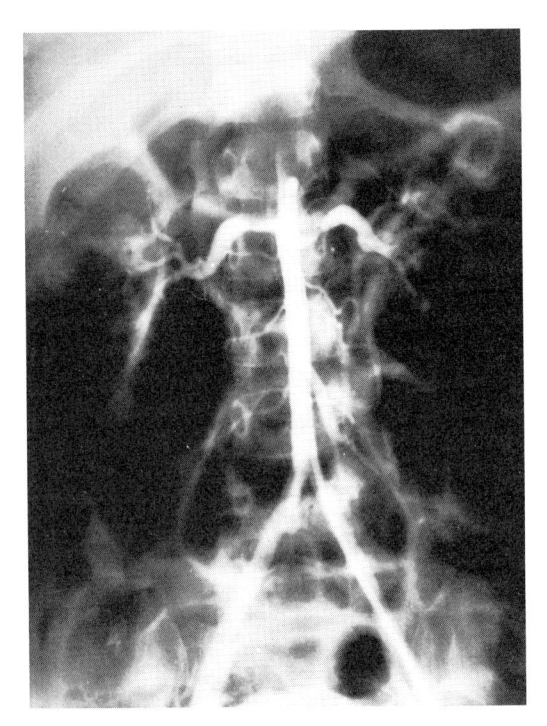

FIG. 44-25. Retrograde aortogram showing bilateral renal artery stenosis in a 6-year-old child with severe hypertension. Surgical correction of the stenosis resulted in relief of the hypertension.

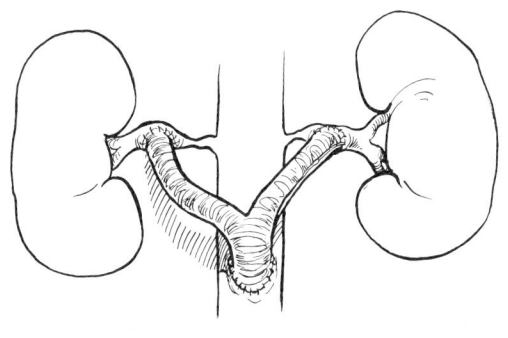

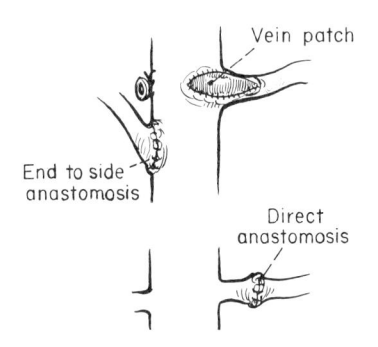

FIG. 44-26. Various methods of renal artery reconstruction. Bypass graft, vein patch and endarterectomy, re-implantation and resection with end-to-end anastomosis.

during test periods. Total urine volume, sodium content, and various clearances are determined during these "split-function" tests.

A *radioactive hippuran renogram* provides information which helps in detecting unilateral and, sometimes, bilateral renal artery disease. The hippuran, which is selectively excreted by the kidney, is tagged radioactively and injected intravenously. The appearance and the progressive concentration in each renal area is recorded by a radiation pickup placed over each renal area.

The examination of specimens taken by needle biopsies of the kidneys shows renal changes possibly etiologic of the hypertension. These may be characteristic of glomerulonephritis, pyelonephritis or nephrosclerosis, or they may suggest the sole presence of renal artery stenosis.

The detection of abnormal amounts of vasopressor substances in blood drawn from each renal vein through a catheter introduced into each from below by way of femoral vein puncture offers hope of the most direct diagnosis. This depends presently on highly critical bioassay which must be standardized before there can be general clinical use.

Since an encouraging proportion of the surgical procedures which correct the renal artery lesion result in a return of the blood pressure to normal levels, the management of each patient with hypertension should include a consideration of the possible presence of such a lesion. The excretory urogram, differential function tests and the aortogram are the three most valuable tests.

Treatment requires reconstruction of the renal artery in order to eliminate the stenosis. A variety of technics is available; some are shown in Figure 44-26. Thromboendarterectomy, bypass graft and reimplantation of the artery into the aorta are commonly done (De Bakey *et al.*, 1961b; DeCamp and Birchell, 1958; Hunter and Julian, 1968; Hunter *et al.*, 1963a; Luke and Levitan, 1959; Morris *et al.*, 1960; Poutasse *et al.*, 1961; Spencer *et al.*, 1961b; Stewart *et al.*, 1962;

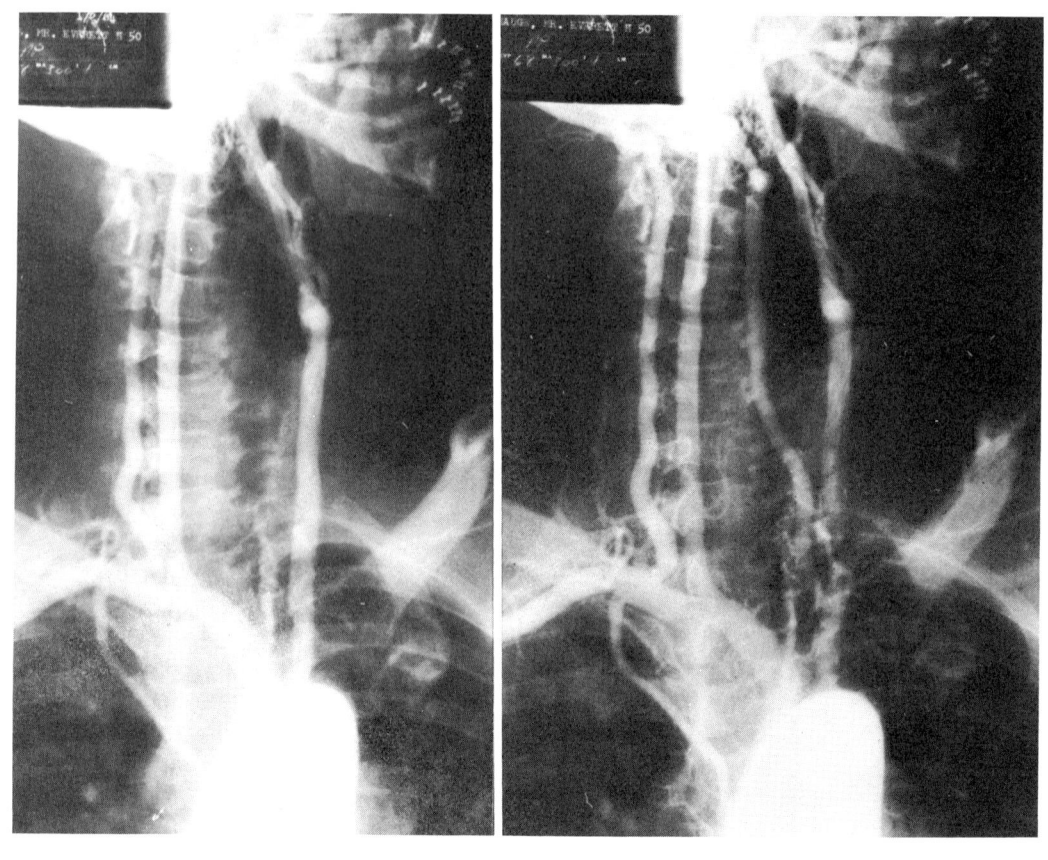

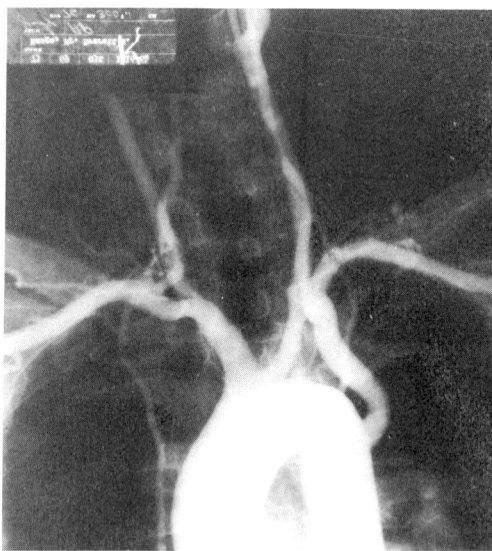

FIG. 44-27. (*Top, left*) Initial injection of arch of aorta opacifies left common carotid, right common carotid and vertebral; left vertebral and left subclavian are not seen. (*Top, right*) Later pictures show the left vertebral entering the subclavian. Blood is flowing from the brain in a retrograde fashion via the vertebral artery. (*Bottom*) Postoperative angiogram in same patient, showing a bypass graft from the aorta to the left subclavian artery with immediate visualization of left vertebral artery superimposed on left common carotid.

Trippel, 1960; Foster *et al.*, 1966; Morris *et al.*, 1966b; Smith *et al.*, 1968; Hunter *et al.*, 1967). Anastomosis of the splenic artery to the renal artery has been carried out with success. The most common procedure is a bypass graft from the aorta to the renal artery. If the aorta itself is replaced, 8 mm. side-arms can be sewed to the graft and then anastomosed to the renal artery.

ARTERIAL INSUFFICIENCY AFFECTING THE BRAIN

The technics of restorative vascular surgery are applicable to obstructing lesion of the arteries supplying the brain. The principal lesion affecting the cerebral circulation is arteriosclerosis.

Blood supply of the brain is vulnerable to arteriosclerotic lesions in both the extracranial and the intracranial portions of the arteries involved. The extracranial vessels in which obstructions can be relieved by surgery are the paired internal carotid arteries and the vertebral arteries. Internal carotid blood flow can be impeded by lesions of the vessel itself between the common carotid bifurcation and the skull, or by any lesion of the common carotid artery proximal to its bifurcation (Davis et al., 1956; Fisher, 1951; Hunt, 1914; Siekert et al., 1960). The arteries of this system are accessible to surgical repair in all parts of their extracranial course. The vertebral arterial flow can be interfered with at any point in the artery itself or by lesions of the subclavian artery proximal to the vertebral origin.

In this latter instance where the subclavian artery is obstructed proximal to the vertebral orifice, the flow of blood in the vertebral artery may be in a reverse direction and there may actually be a draining off of the blood from the brain, producing the so-called vertebral or subclavian steal. This may in itself produce a reduced blood flow to the brain and result in symptoms (Mannick et al., 1962; Killen et al., 1966) (Fig. 44-27).

Surgical repair of these vessels must be done before irreversible brain damage has resulted from ischemia. In a general way, patients with cerebral ischemia can be divided into groups which are related to the selection of individuals for surgical treatment. Group I consists of patients who suffer transient episodes of cerebral ischemia. These episodes are manifested by a great variety of symptoms, common among which are dizziness or fainting, visual disturbances, aphasia and muscular weakness or lack of co-ordination. Between attacks, these patients are essentially normal. In general, the lesion responsible for attacks of this type is a partial occlusion or stenosis of one of the arteries. Group II consists of patients who show the gradual development of a neurologic deficit which does not prove to be transient. Actually, these patients are those who are seen in the early stages of an arterial occlusion which, if not relieved, will lead to a brain infarct. These patients must have relief of the obstruction early in order for surgery to be useful. In later stages, relief of the obstruction which is almost invariably a total one does not affect the irreversible brain damage. The third group of patients are those with multiple bilateral cerebral deficiencies. These patients may have multiple lesions of the carotid and the vertebral systems, some of the lesions being intracranial and relief of partial occlusions of the extracranial vessels may be of some benefit.

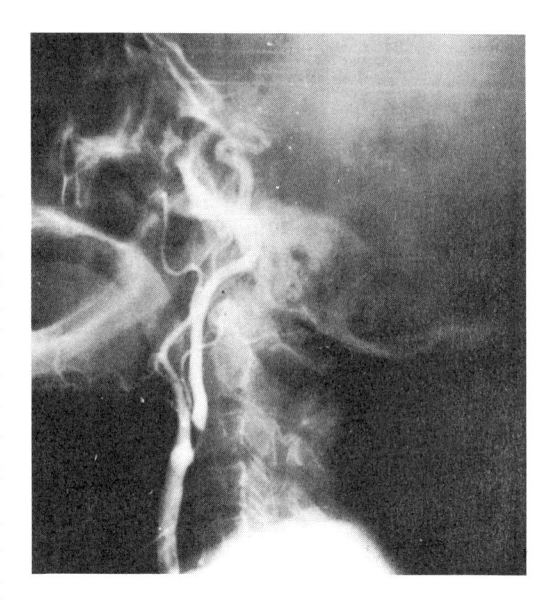

FIG. 44-28. Severe stenosis of the origin of the internal carotid artery. Patient had symptoms of contralateral weakness and numbness of the arm and the leg. Endarterectomy restored normal flow, with relief of symptoms.

Diagnosis. The diagnosis of an arteriosclerotic lesion in the carotid or vertebral artery can often be made on history and physical examination alone. The history of various symptoms related to the carotid-vertebral systems as pointed out in prior paragraphs may suggest a lesion involving one or both of these arteries. Physical examination revealing bruits over the stenosed vessel, such as the bifurcation of the carotid artery, or striking differences in amplitude of the carotid pulse strongly supports the suspicion. This bruit may also be heard at the base of the neck in instances of stenosis of the origin of the vertebral artery.

The most frequent site of arteriosclerotic stenosis is the common carotid bifurcation. A majority of the patients with this lesion exhibit a palpable enlargement of the bifurcation area. This is firm in consistency and represents the atheroma.

Impedence of flow through one carotid artery may be demonstrated by digital compression for a few seconds of the contralateral carotid. A positive result is the precipitation of a cerebral episode usually like those experienced previously by the patient. However, the episode may be far more severe and actually dangerous. Therefore, the so-called *contralateral compression* test is to be avoided.

The definitive diagnosis is provided by arteriograms which show the various portions of the carotid and vertebral systems. By far the most frequent lesion is an atheroma of the common carotid bifurcation which interferes with internal carotid flow. This lesion is best visualized by the percutaneous introduction under local anesthesia of a needle into the common carotid artery and manual injection of contrast medium (Fig. 44-28). It is desirable to take multiple rapid exposures in two planes. To visualize the vertebral arteries in addition, one of several technics is employed. Retrograde catheterization of each subclavian, forceful injection of contrast solution through the brachial arteries, and retrograde passage of a catheter into the arch from the femoral artery are some of these methods.

Treatment. After a stenosing lesion has been amply localized by physical examination and arteriography, the obstruction to blood flow may be relieved by one of several different technics. The most common locations of stenosing lesions are the proximal portions of the internal carotid artery and of the vertebral artery. In carotid artery stenosis, endarterectomy is generally successful in restoring circulation (Crawford *et al.*, 1962; Javid and Julian, 1962; Julian *et al.*, 1963; Najafi *et al.*, 1964; De Bakey *et al.*, 1965; Yashon *et al.*, 1966; Garamella *et al.*, 1966; Javid and Julian, 1967; Bloodwell *et al.*, 1968). During the period of total occlusion of the circulation through the vessel which is being operated upon, a small plastic tube is used as a temporary shunt to avoid the possibility of damage to the brain (Wells *et al.*, 1963) (Fig. 44-29). The ostium of the vertebral artery is approached through a longitudinal incision in the subclavian artery, and endarterectomy is carried out up into the vessel. When the first part of the left subclavian artery is obstructed and a vertebral steal exists, then restoration of flow into the vertebral artery in the proper direction is accomplished by endarterectomy of the subclavian artery or, more frequently, a bypass graft from the aorta to the subclavian artery (see Fig. 44-27, p. 1330). In poor risk patients or where there is a combination of carotid and subclavian lesions, a vein graft between the common carotid and subclavian may be used. When long segments of obstruction are present in the carotid system, and when the carotid obstruction is at the origin of the innominate artery or the left carotid artery from the aortic arch, a bypass graft may be used. In such a case, this graft must extend from the aorta to the common carotid artery or the internal carotid artery, by-passing all of the disease in that system (De Bakey *et al.*, 1958; Javid, 1960; Lin *et al.*, 1956; Lyons and Galbraith, 1957; Rob and Wheeler, 1967).

The results of such surgery are best in patients with partial obstructing lesions. In such persons, recovery is usually complete and very gratifying. These patients are not only relieved of their attacks of intermittent cerebral ischemia, but they are also relieved of the imminent day-to-day danger of complete thrombosis of the stenosed arterial segment which would be likely to cause a major stroke and a brain infarct.

VISCERAL ARTERIOSCLEROSIS

Arteriosclerosis at the origin of the celiac axis and superior mesenteric artery is another manifestation of generalized arteriosclerosis. It may, however, be an isolated finding, as is true of lesions in other areas of the body. The disease usually involves the proximal 1 to 2 cm. of the celiac or superior mesenteric arteries. With disease of both of these arteries, the inferior mesenteric artery may become markedly enlarged and serve as the major collateral to the intestines. Visceral angina or intestinal claudication occurs when the collateral supply is insufficient to provide proper function of the bowel. Abdominal distress follows soon after eating. Diarrhea with explosive bowel movements, malabsorption and weight loss are

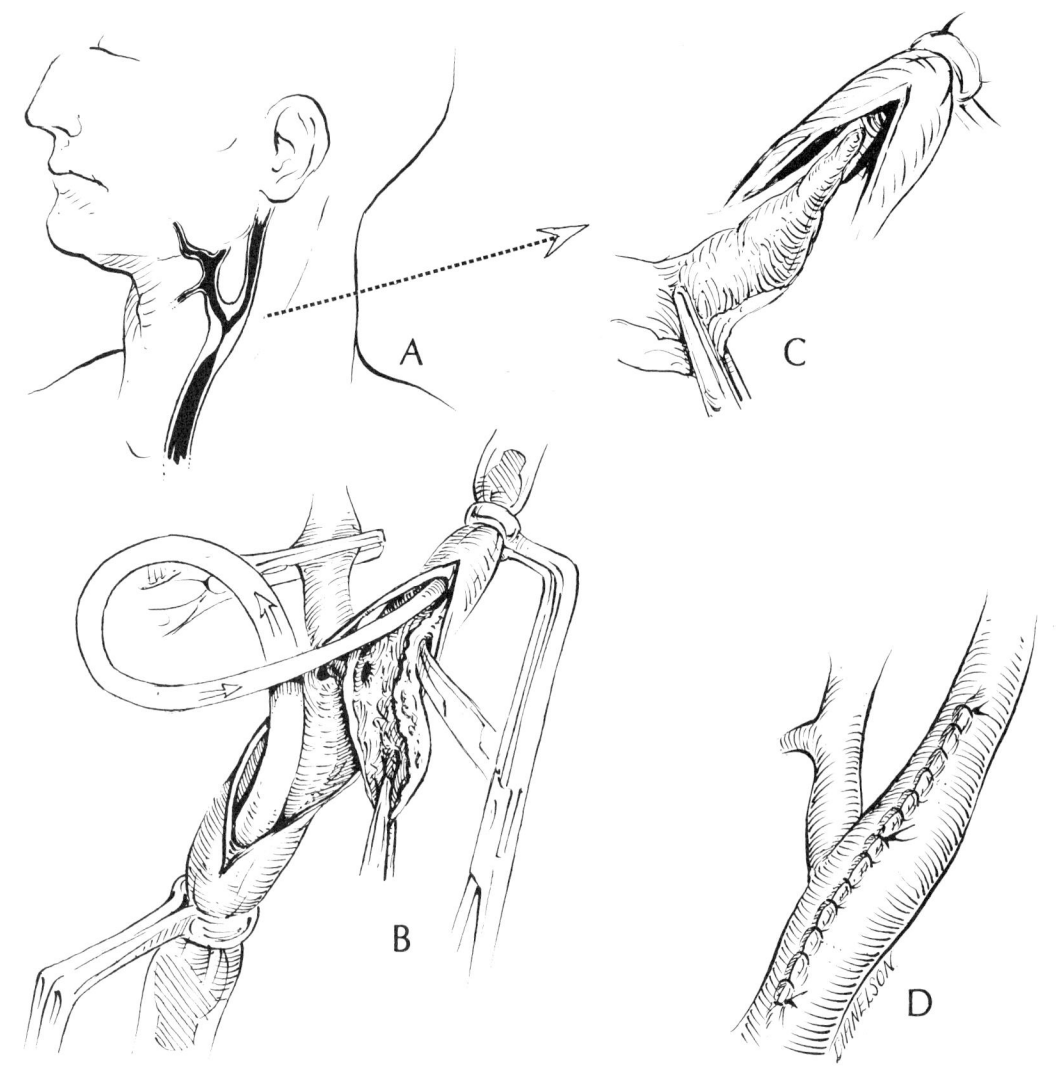

Fig. 44-29. Carotid endarterectomy. (A) Diagrammatic outline of stenosis carotid bifurcation. (B) Endarterectomy using a shunt. (C) Lesion "peels out" superiorly into essentially normal internal carotid artery. (D) Arterotomy closed—a vein patch may be used.

all part of the syndrome. The patient's pain at times may be almost continuous. Weight loss is a universal finding. A variation of this syndrome may be seen after extensive surgery on the abdominal aorta with interruption of collaterals or, as has been suggested, the creation of a steal syndrome. Of utmost significance are the prodromal symptoms prior to total ischemia of the bowel. The diagnosis at this stage may prevent the catastrophic gangrene of the bowel that may ensue. The incidence of chronic symptomatic cases reported in the literature is small. Awareness of the possibility of the diagnosis as well as aortograms to specifically outline these vessels provide the important information. Lateral aortography is necessary and selective angiography in a retrograde fashion is the best method. Abdominal bruits may be heard on physical examination but are difficult to interpret because of associated bruits often originating from the abdominal aorta. Bypass graft from the aorta to the affected artery is the treatment of choice (Stoney and Wylie, 1966;

Morris, De Bakey and Bernhard, 1966; Rob, 1966; Vye, 1963; Dye and Hunter, 1967).

An unusual cause of ischemia is from a diaphragmatic band (Marable, 1966). A high takeoff of the celiac axis may result in compression of the origin of the celiac axis by the fibers of the cruciate ligament of the diaphragm. This may produce an anterior indentation of the origin of the celiac artery axis, which produces the symptoms. Relief is obtained by sectioning this band. Another unusual cause of intestinal ischemia may result from methysergide maleate (Sansert). Angiograms in these cases show multiple areas of stenosis. These areas are reversible, however, on cessation of the medication (Buenger and Hunter, 1967).

BUERGER'S DISEASE—THROMBOANGIITIS OBLITERANS

Thromboangiitis obliterans is an inflammatory disease of unknown etiology of arteries and veins and of the adjacent nerves. Its inflammatory nature contrasts sharply with the degenerative, metabolic nature of arteriosclerosis. The terms "thromboangiitis obliterans" and "Buerger's disease" are used interchangeably. The condition occurs most often in young men and has its onset between the ages of 20 and 35. It involves the extremities predominantly and is more frequent in the lower extremities than in the upper. It is seen occasionally in the vessels of the viscera, such as the heart, the brain and the mesenteric vessels. It is characteristically a disease of medium-sized arteries, such as the posterior tibial, the anterior tibial, the ulnar and the radial arteries.

Leo Buerger's name (1879-1943) is applied to the condition because of his classical description of the disease (Buerger, 1908). This was not the first description of the condition, the first being by von Winiwarter (Winiwarter, 1879). Buerger's description was based on a study of 11 amputated limbs showing chronic arterial occlusion of this type.

Etiology. The specific etiology is not known. Secondary etiologic features which have a positive effect on the disease include age, sex, race, heredity and tobacco. Sex and age have been mentioned already. Heredity is an uncertain factor included because of the occasional occurrence of more than one case of Buerger's disease in a family. The higher incidence in Jewish people, as was assumed by Buerger, does not exist. However, the condition is rare among Negroes, but one instance of the disease has appeared in our series in a Negro woman. Tobacco is the strongest secondary etiologic factor in the disease. Buerger's disease has rarely been described in nonsmokers, and all attempts at alleviating the condition fail in patients who continue to smoke. The etiologies of bacteria or virus, fungus and sensitivity to fungus have been suggested and explored, but none has been substantiated.

The suspicion must be entertained that thromboangiitis obliterans is not etiologically a single condition. It may be a common entity with many etiologies brought together by similar clinical features and pathologic appearances.

Symptoms. The symptoms in Buerger's disease are those which arise from the arterial occlusion, those which depend upon the inflammatory nature of the lesions, and those resulting from the breakdown of the tissues rendered ischemic by the arterial occlusion.

The symptoms of arterial insufficiency depend upon the area involved and the caliber of the vessels primarily attacked. Intermittent claudication occurs but is less frequent than in arteriosclerosis obliterans because, instead of attacking such major channels as the femoral artery, producing ischemia of the gastrocnemius group of muscles, the disease occurs in the smaller vessels named earlier, producing extensive tissue damage in many instances without there ever having been claudication.

The symptoms which result from the inflammatory nature of the condition are those of direct irritation of the adjacent sensory nerves producing intense pain and those resulting from the associated thrombophlebitis as the disease affects the vein. The symptoms produced by the involvement of the veins are not in any way characteristic, but the habit of the disease to affect short segments of superficial veins is a striking feature. Such superficial phlebitis occurs in short segments and in a migratory manner. Red, painful lumps appear under the skin, progressively heal and then occur in other areas over a variable length of time. The favorite sites for these segments of segmental thrombophlebitis are over the lower extremities, although they have been seen in many areas of the body, including the upper extremity. The presence of migrating phlebitis, in the absence of obvious local cause, should raise the question of Buerger's disease.

Pathology. The lesions of superficial phlebitis may precede or accompany the acute stage of the disease and have often been biopsied. The microscopic picture found in these lesions may or may not show the histologic changes which are thought to be characteristic of the acute stage as it occurs in arteries. In the early stage the arteries show a panarteritis in which all of the layers of the artery are involved in an inflammatory reaction with a relatively sparse distribution of chronic inflammatory cells. A characteristic part of the picture is the early appearance of a diffuse sprinkling of multinucleated giant cells. Thickening of the intima progresses rapidly, and thrombosis of the lumen occurs. Organization and fibrosis of the entire artery proceeds, and in the subsided stage the vessels which have been involved are represented by fibrous cords containing a large number of small vascular channels. These vascular channels are discontinuous and do not represent an efficient recanalization of the artery. At any time in an individual active case of Buerger's disease, various stages of acute, subsiding and healed lesions are present. There are inflammation and thrombosis of the concomitant veins. This dual involvement is the basis of the name thromboangiitis obliterans rather than thromboarteritis obliterans. The accompanying perivascular inflammation involves the entire neurovascular bundle, producing a dual type of pain from involvement of sensory nerves as well as from ischemia of tissues below the vascular obstruction.

Clinical Course. The most characteristic feature of the acute stage is an appearance of pain and erythema with a co-existing coolness of the skin which is due to mechanical obstruction of the vessels and to some degree of vasospasm. A tenacity of the acute stage is often observed because new segments of the medium-sized arteries of an extremity are progressively involved with the lesion and, although healing of the initial lesions may have occurred, the new ones keep the process alive. This part of the course is completely unpredictable. Even under the best management it may be self-sustaining and be terminated only by the appearance of gangrene extensive enough to require amputation. In other instances the acute process dies out, and the patient is left with some degree of arterial insufficiency. Symptoms during the subsided stage of the disease depend upon how much arterial occlusion has occurred during the acute process.

Treatment. The relationship between superficial phlebitis of the migratory type and Buerger's disease is strong enough to suspect the disease in any patient displaying it and even to call this lesion a part of the premonitory stage of the disease. Suspicion of this disease is the signal for complete abstinence from tobacco and the institution of a variety of other supportive measures, none of which is nearly so specific. These include the eradication of areas of infection about the body, avoidance of exposure to cold, maintenance of good hydration and a regimen of sufficient rest and adequate diet, to bring the patient into the maximum possible state of health.

During the acute stage bed rest with sedation is absolutely required because of the pain. All measures should be aimed at the prevention and the reduction of swelling of the affected part. A very frequent characteristic of the pain suffered is that it becomes worse when the extremity is kept in an elevated position. Therefore, dependency is insisted upon by the patient, edema results, and the atmosphere for healing or combating of the inflammation is made less favorable by the increased intercellular fluid. Antibiotics do not seem to be indicated except in those cases in which a skin lesion goes on to the point of ulceration. Then antibiotics may be used to combat the secondary invaders. Heat is contraindicated as a direct application to the affected part but may be helpful when it is applied elsewhere to the body to produce reflex vasodilatation in the extremity. This does not appear to be too important because it is obvious from examination of the skin color that much vasodilatation is already present in response to the inflammation. During the acute stage, however, the extremity may show a tendency to become sensitive to the vasoconstrictor stimuli, such as environmental coolness and emotional upset. Then, vasodilators and heat to the abdomen particularly may be indicated. All efforts should be spent on bringing the patient through the acute stage of the disease with the minimum of tissue damage and loss. Sometimes amputation will be required in acute patients whose pain cannot be relieved otherwise.

After the acute process has subsided, the degree of arterial insufficiency with which the patient has been left is estimated. Sympathectomy and amputations are done then as they are indicated and necessary. Sympathectomy is applied when the patient is left with a cold, temperature-sensitive foot or hand. Peripheral gangrenous ulcers are indications for sympathectomy. More extensive ischemic necrosis requires amputation.

ANGIOSPASTIC CONDITIONS

The vascular system, and particularly the capillary bed, constantly fluctuates in its caliber in response to needs for blood flow, heat loss or preservation, or of secretory activity. Portions of the body principally affected by this constant change are the various mucosal surfaces and the skin of the hands and the feet. The effective stimuli other than actual physiologic need are the external application of heat and cold and emotional experience. The simplest form of derangement of this normal vasomotor mechanism is seen in persons who chronically have an increased vasomotor tonus in the hands and the feet so that these parts are always cold. This is sometimes distinctly uncomfortable but not necessarily a pathologic state.

The system is subject to pathologic states in which there is an abnormal sensitivity to the vasoconstrictor influence of exposure to cold and emotional disturbances. These responses occur largely where the density of vasomotor control is greatest, primarily in the skin of the hands and the feet. The most severe pathologic vasomotor phenomena follow a routine set of changes. In sequence, the skin color rapidly becomes white, due to arteriolar and capillary spasm, and then goes through stages of a blue cyanotic color, rubor, finally returning to normal. This progression of changes occurs as a result of a variety of underlying causes so as to suggest that the exaggerated response to a vasoconstrictor stimulus is in some way self-limited. It is not difficult to theorize a sequence of events beginning with diffuse arteriolar spasm producing the dead white appearance, which, causing an ischemic paralysis of the arteriolar muscle, leads to a stage of wide dilatation. Since the capillary-venule end of the system is most severely subject to hypoxia, it dilates first, allowing a back-filling of the gradually opening capillaries and producing a cyanotic skin color. As arterial blood is finally admitted by anoxic paralysis of the arterial end of the capillary loop, the dilated capillaries are flushed with red blood, and rubor results. In a few moments the arteriolar and capillary walls are oxygenated, and normal tonus is re-established.

The name of Raynaud's phenomenon is given to these changes on the basis of the classical description by Raynaud (1862). His thesis was entitled "On the Local Asphyxia and Symmetrical Gangrene of the Extremities." He considered the condition to be a pathologic entity. His theory based the defect on a fault in the vasomotor nerves supplying the part of the body which is affected without there being any arterial lesion per se.

The original report of Raynaud contained not only the cases which actually consisted of a functional vasomotor disturbance but also a number in which he did not recognize that arterial disease was present. We now classify patients who show this form of vasoconstrictor response into 3 groups: (1) those in whom there is apparently no primary arterial pathology; (2) those having an underlying arterial disease; and (3) a group presenting this vasomotor response because of trauma, scleroderma, certain nerve lesions and poisonings with ergot or such metals as lead. In recent years the 1st group has retained the name of Raynaud's disease. The 2nd and the 3rd groups are said to exhibit "Raynaud's phenomenon" attributable to an arterial disease or to the other etiologic agents.

Raynaud's Disease. The group remaining under the name of Raynaud's disease shows age and sex preponderance. More than three quarters of the patients presenting this complaint are women. The onset of the condition is usually between the ages of 15 and 35 years. The patients frequently are emotionally immature or inadequate. The earlier symptoms of the condition occur in the most highly innervated parts of the body in response to strong vasomotor constrictor stimuli. This results in the hands being the common primary site of the reaction and the response first occurring during local exposure to very cold water or ice or during a severe emotional upset. Later the response is noted in wider areas, that is to say, spreading from one finger to all the fingers and then to other less innervated parts, such as the feet. The reaction is caused by progressively lesser stimuli. The color changes described earlier vary in individual severity but all are present in most patients.

The disease is strongly bilateral and symmetrical. There is usually some numbness associated with the stage of pallor, particularly if it lasts very long, but pain is not present. The parts involved are quite normal between the attacks until the condition has been present for a long time. Ischemic necrosis is not observed frequently, and when it is present after years of affliction, the areas of necrosis are very small; they occur on the fingertips, heal rapidly and leave pinhead-size depressed scars. Pain occurs in Raynaud's disease while these ischemic necrotic areas are present. It is characteristic that the pulses of the extremities remain undisturbed.

Severe cases of Raynaud's disease lead to varying degrees of handicap due to the frequency of attacks and the repeated occurrence of small painful ulcers. After a long course of the disease, the skin of the fingers and the hands becomes thickened, and there is an excessive dryness. The soft tissues of the distal parts of the fingers become atrophied, and the characteristic tapered appearance of late Raynaud's disease becomes manifest.

TREATMENT. The general management which immediately suggests itself in the treatment of Raynaud's disease is the protection of the subject from the stimuli which cause the vasomotor response. Reassurance and avoidance of cold exposure are important. Therapy with drugs is relatively difficult because of the long, chronic course of the condition. Vasodilator drugs which may be taken frequently over a long period of time would be indicated. The results obtained with the best available drugs are usually disappointing.

Surgical removal of the controlling region of the sympathetic nervous system, which ought to be completely curative if the lesion were simply an abnormal vasomotor reflex, produces only comparative relief of the symptoms in reducing the frequency of the attacks and increasing the stimulus required for production. The fact that the attacks are not completely relieved by sympathectomy indicates that there is a local vascular sensitivity in effect which, in part, produces the condition. It is the opinion of most that sympathectomy should be reserved for severe cases and particularly applied in those cases showing the minute areas of necrosis characteristic of the disease.

Consistent reconsideration of the diagnosis in order to pick up an underlying organic pathologic condition is important.

Raynaud's Phenomenon. The same type of color reaction in response to cold and emotion is seen in a group of patients in whom a distinct underlying cause is present. The underlying conditions responsible are fairly diverse. This lends weight to the idea that the vasoconstrictor phenomenon which is observed is a fundamental pathologic response.

Intrinsic vascular disease, particularly in the upper extremity, of both the degenerative and the inflammatory types, is frequently a cause of Raynaud's phenomenon. The suspicion of an underlying arterial disease as a cause should be aroused when an individual patient diverges from the pattern of the condition typical to Raynaud's disease. An asymmetrical appearance of the disturbance should raise suspicion of an arterial disease. Raynaud's phenomenon developing in a patient beyond the age of 35 suggests arteriosclerosis, and the occurrence in a male indicates the possibility very strongly. Loss of pulses or more extensive gangrene than that described is further evidence of arterial disease. When pain is an important symptom in an individual case, the indication is that an underlying pathologic state exists.

Raynaud's phenomenon is also frequently associated with the early stages of *scleroderma*. Some confusion in its relation to scleroderma results from the fact that in the very late stages of Raynaud's disease the fibrosis, atrophy and stiffening of the skin

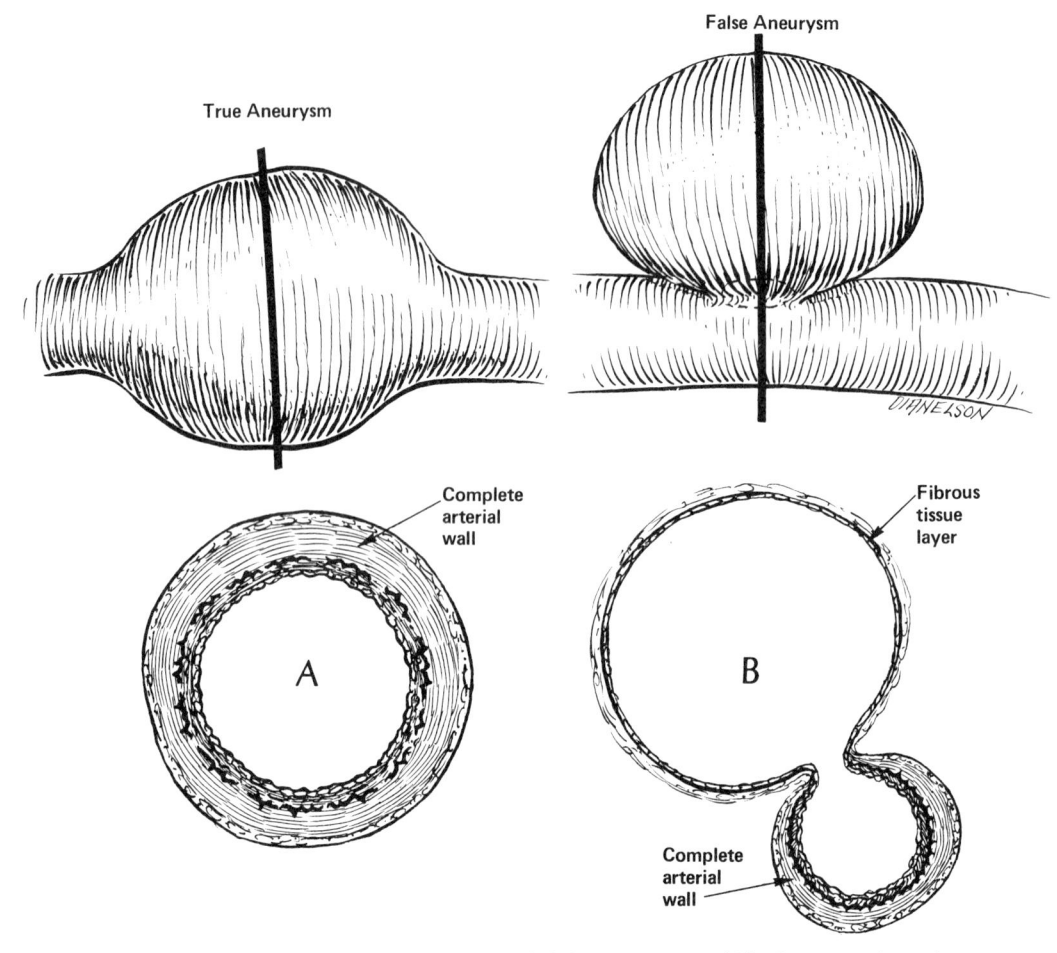

FIG. 44-30. Differentiation between true and false aneurysm. (A) Cross section of a true aneurysm showing all layers of wall present. (B) The only vascular layer present in the pulsating hematoma is the endothelial lining which is present if the lesion has been in existence long enough.

resembles scleroderma. However, the sequence of events under both circumstances should be fairly clear. Raynaud's phenomenon occurs early in scleroderma, before and during the edematous stage. On the other hand, sclerodermatoid change in Raynaud's disease is a late feature after a long progressive course. Furthermore, scleroderma associated with Raynaud's phenomenon may be generalized; on the other hand, sclerodermatous changes in Raynaud's disease are localized to the involved portions of the extremity.

Scalenus anticus syndrome, cervical ribs, herniated cervical disk, chronic lead poisoning, ergotism or trauma to the extremity of a type which produces a post-traumatic sympathetic dystrophy, all occasionally bring about the vasomotor discharges of Raynaud's phenomenon.

The importance of designating a definite pathologic condition as the cause of any case of Raynaud's phenomenon leads to the constant search for new signs in patients thought to have Raynaud's disease. In every such instance the proper treatment of the patient will be directed against the underlying condition, if such therapy is available, rather than against the phenomenon.

ARTERIAL ANEURYSM

A true arterial aneurysm may be defined as the area of enlargement that develops when an artery dilates beyond its normal anatomic size as a result of a loss of elastic property of the vessel wall caused by a disease process. This loss of elasticity, which is the fundamental cause of stretching, renders the wall unable to return to its unexpanded size following each distending force of the systolic thrust of the blood stream. Progressive enlargement is the rule. A true arterial aneurysm is to be differentiated from a false aneurysm or pulsating hematoma resulting from trauma, which has been described on page 1311 (Fig. 44-30).

Another form of aneurysm, which might be said to occupy a position as to definition somewhat between true aneurysm and false aneurysm, is the dissecting aneurysm or dissecting hematoma. This lesion develops when, as a result of a tear in the internal coats of the artery, blood dissects under pressure in a plane between layers of the arterial wall, expanding the outer layers to aneurysmal proportions. The size to which the area expands is determined in part by the depth to which the tear admits the flow of blood, and the thickness of wall, therefore, that remains as the outer retaining tube. Degenerative changes in the medial coats of the vessel of congenital or acquired origin predispose to this lesion, as does arteriosclerotic ulceration.

CLASSIFICATION

Arterial aneurysms may be classified according to their location, shape and etiology. The location of the aneurysm has a self-evident meaning and is usually included in the descriptive diagnosis of each individual lesion. Classification as to shape has little practical value, but has been widely used for a long time because most aneurysms do tend to be either fusiform in shape, or to develop as saccular projections from the vessel.

A *fusiform aneurysm* is one in which the dilatation is diffuse in the segment of vessel involved and results in the development of a spindle-shaped expansion. The *saccular aneurysm* is a bulbous expansion of a portion of the circumference of the arterial wall. This results from a more localized change in the vessel so that a relatively small area of the vessel wall expands.

To this classic anatomic classification should be added the *dissecting aneurysm* as a separate type, even though this lesion usually causes a more or less fusiform enlargement of the involved artery.

This method of classification should probably be considered of secondary value, although there is a certain etiologic reference, in that most saccular aneurysms are syphilitic in origin. The term saccular is also useful in considering one form of surgical treatment, the lateral aneurysmectomy, which takes advantage of the occasional presence of a relatively small defect in the artery wall.

Etiologic. Aneurysms are classified in terms other than anatomic on the basis of the disease which produced the original injury to the arterial wall. Certain of these are very well known. Arteriosclerosis, syphilis and pyogenic infections comprise the list of known acquired diseases. Congenital deficiencies of the elastic properties of an artery occur but are less well recognized than the medial weakness which is the arterial component of Marfan's syndrome. True aneurysm is recognized to develop in patients with Marfan's syndrome and in individuals not showing other stigmata of the syndrome who are members of Marfan families. This is much less frequent than the dissecting aneurysm which is the much better known arterial lesion in these patients. A further type of aneurysm which is etiologically distinct develops in an artery just distal to an area of constriction. The phenomenon of *post-stenotic dilatation* is very frequently observed in moderate degree distal to a point of partial obstruction of an artery. This is caused by the increase in lateral pressure against the wall of the vessel in this area of turbulence. Post-stenotic dilatation of such magnitude as to deserve the term aneurysm is sometimes seen distal to a coarctation of the aorta or in the subclavian artery just beyond the anterior scalene muscle is long-standing scalenus anticus syndrome.

Finally, it is theoretically possible for a true aneurysm to be produced by trauma to a normal artery. This would occur if a moderate crushing injury or high-speed missile damaged the arterial wall without opening the vessel or occluding it, the blood pressure later expanding the damaged area.

CLINICAL FEATURES OF ARTERIAL ANEURYSM

Once an aneurysm has appeared, its continued enlargement is a certainty. This growth continues until the aneurysm wall tears and rupture occurs, or it erodes into an adjacent structure, or the aneurysm totally thromboses. Another limiting possibility is death of the patient due to compression by the aneurysm of an adjacent structure, disturbing a vital function. Although the rate of this inexorable growth cannot be predicted, the fact that it will occur must be accepted as the most important consideration in the treatment of aneurysm wherever it occurs.

The symptoms of an arterial aneurysm principally result from compression of adjacent structures and from interference with blood flow. Many aneurysms can grow to quite large size without producing symptoms unless they are in such a location that the patient can recognize the presence of a mass which pulsates. Most aneurysms do not produce spontaneous pain within themselves, and tenderness is not a significant feature. The mycotic aneurysm is an outstanding exception, as will be noted later. This lesion is intensely inflammatory and is both painful and tender. A dissecting aneurysm produces severe pain in most cases at the time of onset. Later, however, when it stabilizes, as it sometimes does, pain is absent.

Further specific features of the clinical course and of methods available for treatment of aneurysms will be considered under the headings of Thoracic Aortic Aneurysm, Abdominal Aortic Aneurysm, Visceral Aneurysm and Peripheral Aneurysm. Separate consideration will be given to Dissecting Aneurysm because of the many special features of this condition, in spite of the fact that the thoracic and abdominal aorta is the site of involvement. Similarly, Mycotic Aneurysm will be dealt with separately, even though the areas of involvement coincide with visceral and peripheral lesions.

THORACIC AORTIC ANEURYSMS

Either arteriosclerosis or syphilis can be the etiology of a thoracic aneurysm. Both types of change are sometimes involved in a single lesion because an old arrested syphilitic aortitis leads to a seemingly much exaggerated tendency for arteriosclerotic degeneration to take place. There is a difference in the mechanism by which syphilis and arteriosclerosis lead to stretching of the vessel wall. In syphilis, the healing of the original aortitis results in a replacement of muscle and elastic tissue to some degree by a fibrous tissue scar. This scar tissue lacks the ability of the original tissue to withstand the internally applied blood pressure and it stretches. The scar of the healed disease is often well localized and the most easily stretched portion may actually involve less than the circumference of the vessel, and be, in effect, a patch. When this is so, the stage is set for a very local expansion producing the saccular aneurysm, a form which is probably never seen in arteriosclerosis. If the syphilitic scar is more diffuse and entirely circumferential, the tendency for the resulting lesion to be saccular is much less pronounced. Arteriosclerosis, on the other hand, weakens the wall of the vessel diffusely by destruction of the elastic laminae and degeneration of the muscle of the media. The tendency of arteriosclerosis to produce aneurysms fusiform in shape is explained by this diffuse change. However, a resulting lesion is seldom symmetrical and smoothly spindle shaped. Elongation of the aorta accompanies its enlargement in circumference, while at the same time the adjacent firm rib cage and spine also distort the lesion.

Syphilitic aneurysms have a definite tendency to involve the ascending and transverse arch portions of the thoracic aorta and arteriosclerosis to produce aneurysms of the descending aorta. This tendency is not by any means entirely exclusive. There is little practical value in considering the relative incidence of aneurysm of the two etiologies within the chest. This certainly depends far more on the amount of endemic syphilis in the geographic area than on anything else. In general, most thoracic aneurysms are arteriosclerotic in nature.

Symptoms. A thoracic aneurysm disturbs the patient almost entirely by the effect it has on surrounding structures. Chest pain and a feeling of tightness are frequent only after the lesion has developed considerable size. Before this, symptoms are usually entirely absent unless the aneurysm presses on a specific structure. Cough and difficulty in breathing are the result of compression of the trachea or a bronchus. These are sometimes exaggerated when the patient lies down and easier when he is propped up or sitting. This respiratory difficulty must not be confused with the orthopnea of cardiac disease. Hoarseness and stridor develop when a recurrent laryngeal nerve is compressed, inactivating a vocal cord, more frequently the left than the right. Compression on the esophagus produces pain on swallowing or dysphagia. Impingement upon the superior vena cava produces venous congestion in the upper extremities and the head and the neck. Distended neck veins and the development of enlarged subcutaneous venous channels in the shoulder girdle are observed as a result of such compression.

Signs. There may be no positive evidence on physical examination of the presence of even quite a large thoracic aneurysm. Evidence of widening of the superior mediastinum is looked for by percussion of the anterior chest. Abnormal pulsation is sought by palpation of the intercostal spaces, particularly along the upper right sternal border, as well as in the sternal notch and the thoracic inlet. The trachea may be deviated, or the pulsation of the aneurysm be transmitted into the trachea so that it can be felt as a distinct downward tug with each heartbeat. The pulses in the upper extremities and the carotid pulses in the neck are rarely disturbed and remain symmetrical. Auscultation rarely contributes anything of value, such as an arterial bruit resulting from abnormal flow caused by the aneurysm. A Horner's syndrome may be present because of the impingement of the aneurysm on the upper dorsal sympathetic ganglia.

X-ray Examination. The mediastinal mass seen in the chest roentgenogram of a patient with a thoracic aneurysm must always be differentiated from a mediastinal or lung tumor, and this differentiation may not always be conclusive on the basis of this examination alone. Fluoroscopic examination does not always help. The pulsatile nature of an aneurysm may be observed, but inasmuch as the wall of the aneurysm is inelastic, almost by definition, it is much less than might be expected and may be entirely absent. The definitive x-ray diagnosis is made by visualization of the aorta with contrast media. The dye is introduced into the aorta either directly through a catheter which is passed in a retrograde fashion from a brachial artery or femoral artery, or it may be passed to the aorta after injection per catheter into the right atrium, the right ventricle or the pulmonary artery. The thoracic aortogram is almost essential as the most valuable means of planning surgical correction of the abnormality.

Treatment. There is no effective conservative treatment of a thoracic aneurysm. Surgical therapy is indicated because of the known

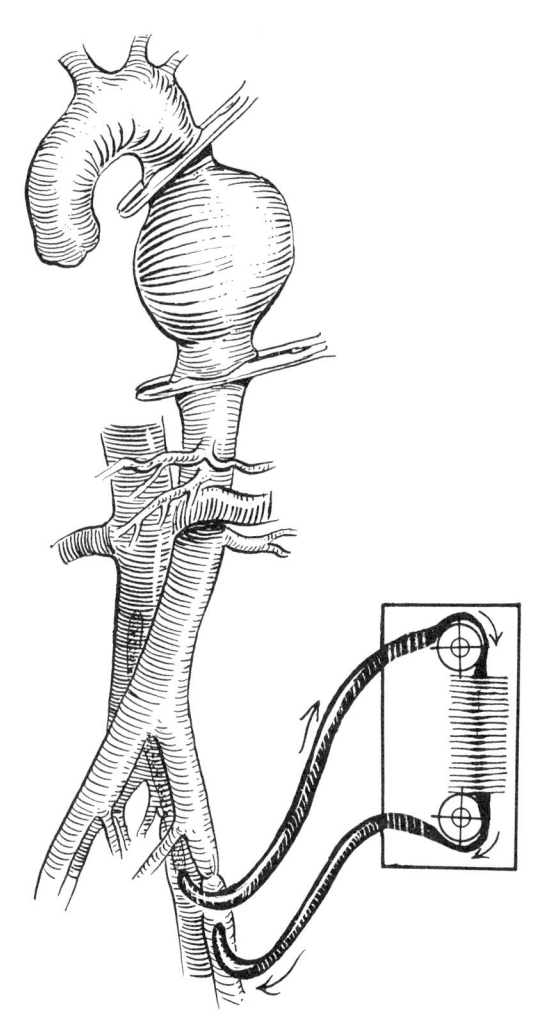

FIG. 44-31. Resection of aneurysm of descending thoracic aorta. Femoral vein–femoral artery partial bypass is used during resection of the aneurysm.

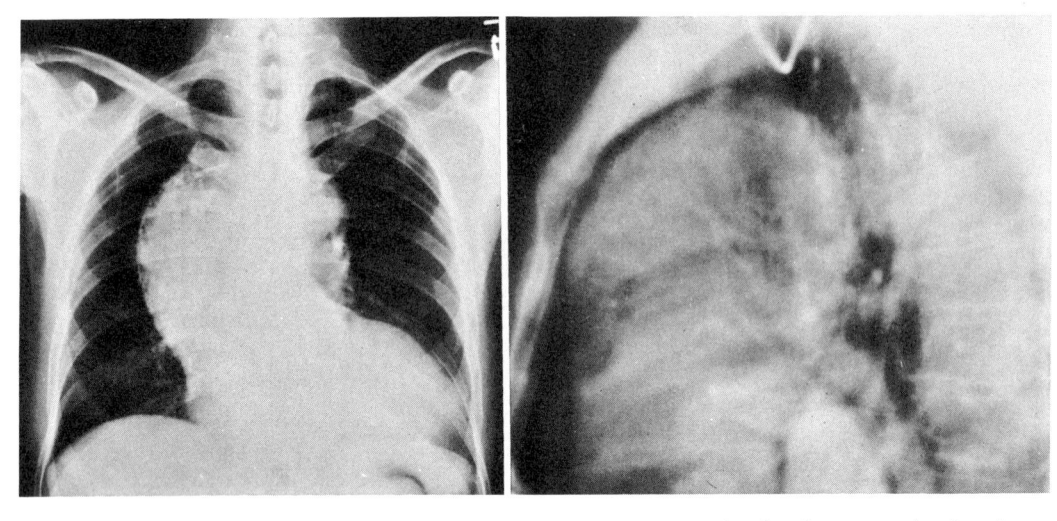

FIG. 44-32. Posteroanterior and lateral chest roentgenograms showing large arteriosclerotic aneurysm of ascending aorta.

progressive nature of the lesion. It is withheld only in the presence of associated conditions which increase the risk of surgery to a serious degree.

In the past palliative surgery has been applied, consisting of division of the sternum or excision of a portion of the sternum overlying the aneurysm in order to give more space and relieve compression of the trachea or the esophagus. The relief obtained by such treatment is always temporary, because the aneurysm continues to grow and fills the new space made available to it. Stimulation of the development of a thrombus within the aneurysm by threading coils of tightly wound wire into its lumen was done frequently in the past with meager results in truly large, symptomatic aneurysms.

Reconstructive Surgery. More direct surgical therapy consisting of resection of the lesion and re-establishment of continuity of the aorta offers the most in these patients. This usually involves removal of a significant portion of the aorta, and the magnitude of the surgical problem depends on the location, whether it be in the ascending arch or the descending portions of the thoracic aorta (Mulder, Dilley, and Joseph, 1966).

Occasionally a saccular aneurysm has a sufficiently confined neck that a *lateral aneurysmectomy* (Bahnson, 1953) may be done. This operation consists of removal of the lateral expanded wall of the saccular aneurysm by clamping the neck at its base and oversewing the edges left by the resection. At times, following the removal of a small saccular aneurysm the defect may be replaced with a patch. *Resection and grafting* consists of removal of the entire length of the involved aorta and replacing the defect with a graft (De Bakey and Cooley, 1953a). The grafts used for this purpose are of tightly woven Dacron or Teflon formed as tubes, 1 to 1¼ inches in diameter, and permanently crimped in an accordionlike manner.

Resection of an aneurysm of the descending thoracic aorta presents the least surgical problem (Lam and Aram, 1951). Although formerly the aorta was cross clamped, either using hypothermia or chemical means of reducing blood pressure, at present more sophisticated methods are used. In the authors' experience, a femoral vein-femoral artery partial bypass through the pump oxygenator provides reduction of blood returning to the heart, thereby keeping the pressure in the upper part of the body at a normal level and, at the same time, furnishing blood supply to the lower part of the body (Fig. 44-31).

Other methods of avoiding difficulties during resection of a descending thoracic aorta consist of the implantation of a plastic tube as a temporary bypass between the left subclavian artery and the femoral artery. Heart

Arterial Surgery: Arterial Aneurysm 1343

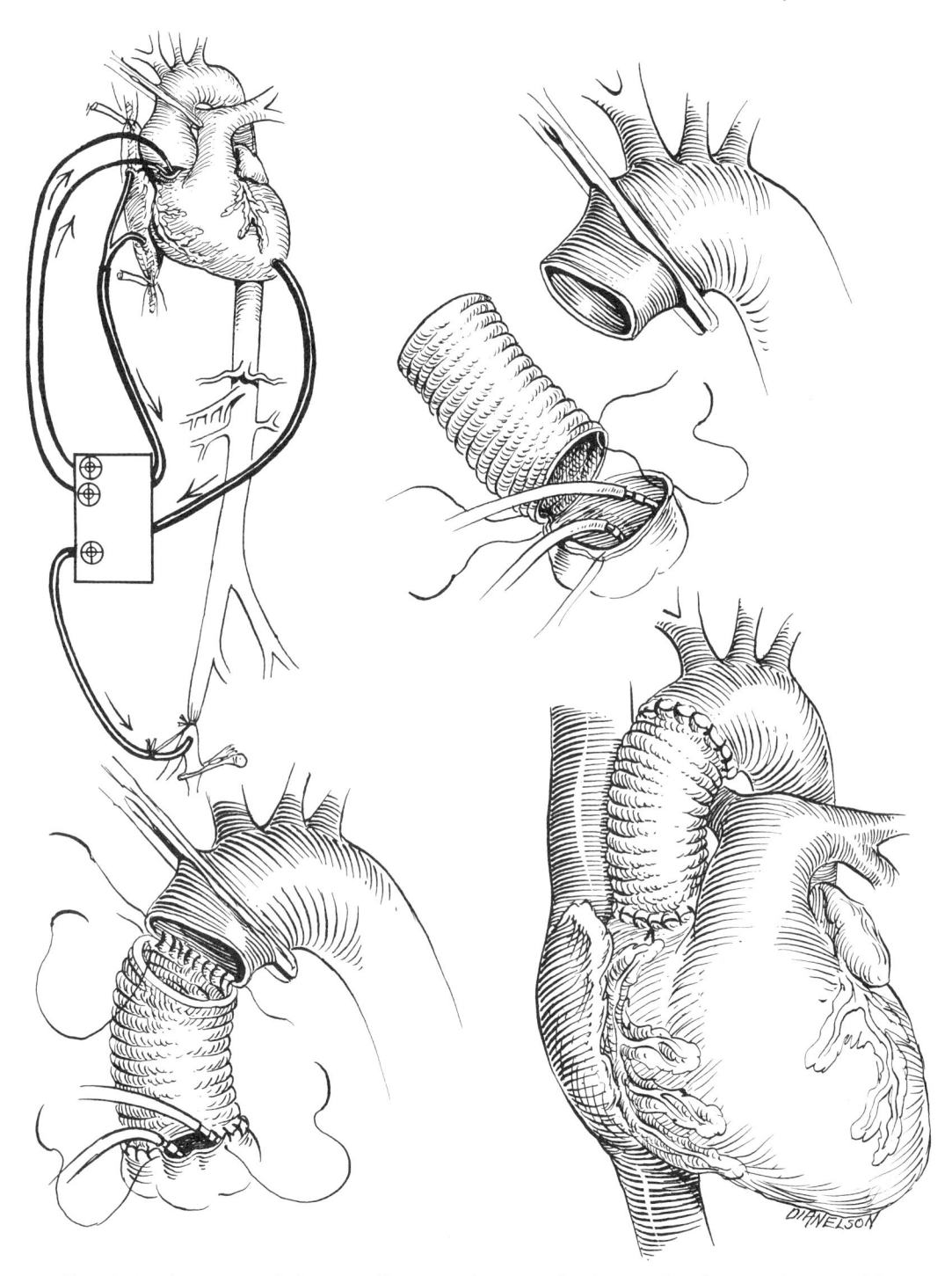

Fig. 44-33. Aneurysm of the ascending aorta is resected using cardiopulmonary bypass with coronary perfusion during graft replacement.

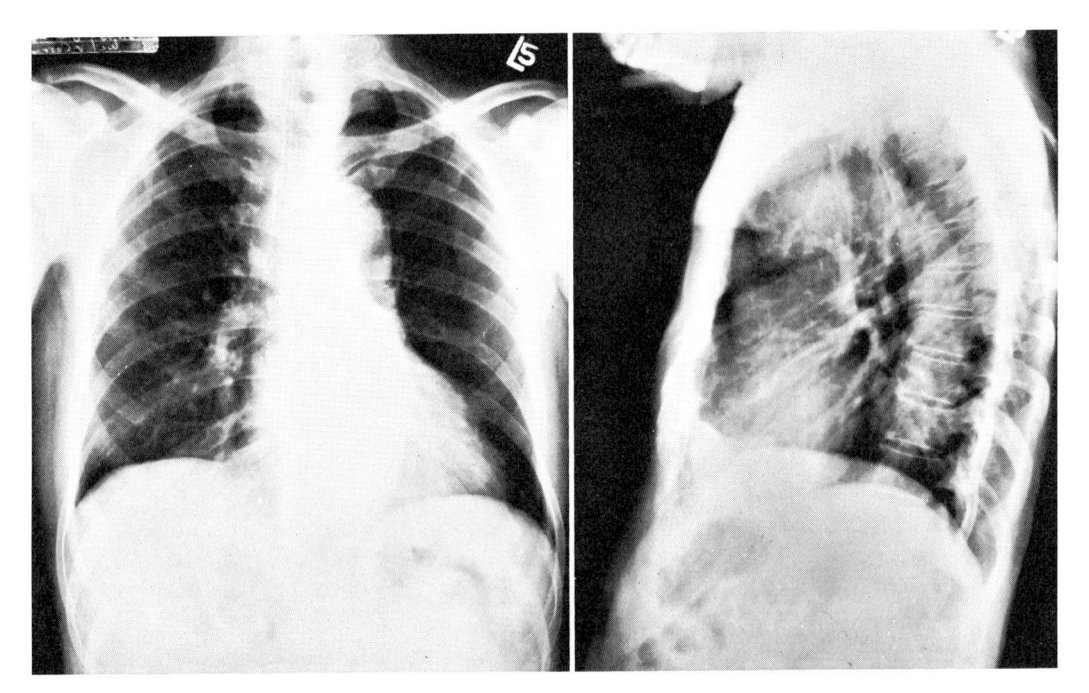

FIG. 44-34. Postoperative chest roentgenogram after resection of ascending aortic aneurysm and replacement by graft. Posteroanterior and lateral views. Same patient as shown in Figures 44-32 and 44-33.

action alone is used to cause circulation through this tube. Another method involves bypass from the left atrium to the femoral artery. In this case, a pump must be placed in the circuit. In both methods the patient's clotting mechanism is totally inactivated by the administration of heparin in a dose of approximately 3 mg. per kilogram of body weight.

In aneurysms involving the arch of the aorta, or the ascending portion, much more elaborate technics are required in order to maintain cerebral circulation, and, sometimes, coronary artery circulation during the period of resection and replacement. These requirements are accomplished by the use of the heart-lung machine. Blood is drained to the equipment from the inferior vena cava which is cannulated through a femoral vein and after passing through an oxygenator it is pumped back to the patient by several routes. A femoral artery is cannulated to return blood to the lower part of the body. Other branches from the arterial return from the heart-lung machine are provided for leads to the carotid arteries and, when necessary, to the coronary arteries (Bahnson and Spencer 1960) (Figs. 44-32, 33 and 34).

In spite of the imposing nature of the surgical procedures required, the indication for surgical removal of a thoracic aneurysm is virtually absolute (Javid, 1961). This is because growth, although often slow, always occurs. Death due to erosion and rupture follows after a course, the severity and the symptom characteristics of which depend on the direction of pressure by the mass. The rupture which terminates the illness may be into a pleural cavity, lung tissue, bronchus or the trachea, esophagus, superior vena cava, or to the outside by actual erosion of the chest wall.

DISSECTING ANEURYSM

A lesion termed a *dissecting aneurysm* (or sometimes a dissecting hematoma) is established in an artery when a defect develops in the intima and the subintimal layers of the media through which the circulating blood gains access to a layer within the wall of the vessel. Once having entered a plane between

FIG. 44-35. Schematic representation of dissecting aneurysm of the thoracic aorta. (A) Dissection starting in proximal ascending aorta and extending into abdominal aorta. Dissection may be limited to ascending aorta. (B and C) Variations of dissection originating distal to left subclavian.

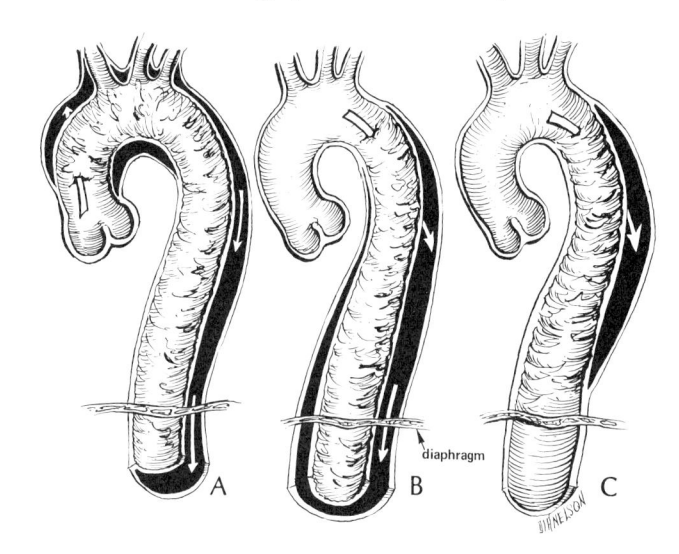

layers of the vessel wall, the blood forces its way distalward and to a limited extent in a proximal direction. The thoracic aorta is the only commonly involved artery, although it is quite possible that a similar mechanism may play some part in acute occlusions occurring in smaller, more peripheral vessels.

Etiology. The basic cause of this condition is believed to be a defect of the media or some form of cystic medial necrosis. Mucoid material appears in the media with degenerative changes of the elastic and muscle tissues. In a certain smaller percentage of dissecting aneurysms, arteriosclerosis, syphilis or other types of medial degeneration may be a cause (Burchell, 1955; Hirst, Johns, and Kime, 1958).

The influence of some inherited factor is exhibited by aortic dissection occurring in patients with Marfan's syndrome (arachnodactyly) (McKusick, 1955), or in cases of spinal deformity such as kyphosclerosis, and also coarctation of the aorta. Aortic dissection has been associated with pregnancy (Schnitker and Bayer, 1944). It is commonly and most frequently associated with severe hypertension.

There may be a more rare relationship of aortic dissection to dietary deficiency, as observed in experimental work in which dissection was produced in growing rats by feeding them a sweet-pea meal (amino-nitrites) (Bean and Ponseti, 1955).

Pathology. Separation of the layers of the aorta by rupture of the vasa vasorum into the degenerative medial layer is thought to be the primary pathology in many cases. Other explanations are that the actual intimal tear allows the entrance of blood into the medial layer and further produces separation. Cases have been observed in which there is dissection without intimal tear, but it is very likely that the actual tear with entrance of blood is a factor in most cases. Dissection may take place in a dilated aneurysmal aorta and the tear may be in the neighborhood of an arteriosclerotic plaque, or the dissection may be in a normal size aorta.

The lesion varies in its extent and also its point of origin. The intimal tear often arises in the ascending aorta just distal to the aortic valve and involves usually a portion of the circumference of the aorta. It may proceed both proximally and distally and progress throughout the thoracic aorta to the bifurcation of the abdominal aorta. Any number of the branches may be involved along the course of the dissection, while in certain situations the dissection is limited to the ascending aorta and may proceed in a retrograde fashion into the heart, producing incompetence of the aortic valve as well as dissection of the coronary arteries. The other common site of tear is just distal to the subclavian artery (Fig. 44-35 B and C). Dissection here may be limited to the thoracic aorta or extend into the abdominal aorta. Re-entry may occur distally and produce so-called "self cures" if the dissecting lumen becomes a second channel preserving the vital branches. More frequently, however, the lesion progresses proximally and ruptures into the pericardium causing tamponade. Direct rupture is also seen into the pleural space despite the barrier of the parietal pleura.

Clinical Evaluation. The clinical picture of the patient with dissecting aneurysm is variable. Classically the patient presents with a severe, excruciating chest pain radiating into the back and the neck and shows progression of these symptoms downward as the dissection proceeds. One may see changes in the pulses in the upper and the lower extremities, depending on the particular branches affected by the dissection. The patient is usually hypertensive, and often the diagnosis is confused with acute coronary occlusion. Men are affected more frequently than women. After the initial severe pain there may be a quiescent period, or the dissection may progress to rupture into the pericardial sac with signs of cardiac tamponade. At times the dissection may present as an acute occlusion of a peripheral artery, and the underlying pathology may be overlooked. This is particularly true in those patients who have had very little pain associated with the dissection. If the dissection is extensive and affects the blood supply to the spinal cord, one may see the clinical picture of what appears to be an arterial occlusion of the lower extremities with total anesthesia of the extremities. However, close examination will reveal that the level of anesthesia extends to a much higher level than can be accounted for on the basis of level of arterial occlusion. Renal artery involvement may produce oliguria and anuria with subsequent renal failure. Prognosis in general is grave and, as has been noted in one study, 21 per cent of the patients died within 24 hours, 44 per cent within 3 days, 74 per cent within 14 days, and by 6 months 91 per cent had died (Hirst, Johns and Kime, 1958; McCloy, Spittell and McGoon, 1965).

The definitive diagnosis can often be made on the clinical picture alone. Roentgenogram of the chest may help in showing widening of the aorta as compared with previous roentgenograms. An electrocardiogram is done to rule out coronary occlusion. The appearance of a diastolic murmur of aortic incompetence may verify extension of the dissection into the region of the aortic valve. Definitive diagnosis by x-ray studies depends on appropriate angiograms, since at times the size of the aortic shadow on roentgenograms is normal. Venous angiocardiogram if properly done with multiple exposures and appropriate lateral views will demonstrate the dissection in most cases (Fig. 44-36 A to C). On rare occasions the diagnosis has been made indirectly by abdominal aortogram studies which were being done for the mistaken diagnosis of peripheral arterial occlusion. In these cases the arterial occlusion is demonstrated to be due to the dissecting lumen occluding the vessel (Gurin, Bulmer and Derby, 1935).

Surgical treatment of dissecting aneurysm has improved greatly with the advent of cardiopulmonary bypass (De Bakey, Cooley and Creech, 1955; De Bakey et al., 1961a; Hume and Porter, 1963; Rohman, Goetz and State, 1963; Shaw, 1955). The surgical approach depends on the location and the extent of the dissection. When the dissection starts in the ascending aorta, surgical treatment is aimed at transecting the ascending aorta, suturing the two layers of the aorta together and obliterating the false lumen, and then reanastomosing the transected aorta. At times a portion of the ascending aorta may have to be resected. This is particularly true where there is aneurysm formation and weakness of the wall, as in Marfan's syndrome (Dillard et al., 1962). Aortic incompetence produced by proximal dissection and lack of support of the aortic valves is corrected by approximation of the inner and the outer layers of the dissecting process, which brings the aortic valves into proper position. Those patients having dissection originating just distal to the left subclavian artery are most amenable to surgical treatment, and here part or all of the descending thoracic aorta is resected and replaced by a graft. Mortality associated with procedures involving the ascending aorta is still significant but should decrease progressively. Aneurysms starting at the left subclavian artery carry a relatively low surgical mortality.

Recent work has shown that in very extensive dissections from the ascending aorta to the abdominal aorta, medical therapy of the hypertension may be of value. This is particularly true in the dissections that have stabilized and become free of pain (Wheat, 1966; Harris et al., 1967).

ARTERIOSCLEROTIC ANEURYSM OF THE
ABDOMINAL AORTA

Abdominal aortic aneurysms are almost without demonstrated exception degenerative or arteriosclerotic in etiology. They consistently arise at a point 1 to 5 cm. below the origins of the renal arteries, but may infrequently involve the abdominal aorta up to the diaphragm and sometimes are continuous with a lower thoracic aneurysm. The process of loss of elasticity and dilatation commonly extends down to include the aortic bifurcation and often proceeds into the common iliac arteries.

FIG. 44-36. (A, *top*) Case of a 54-year-old hypertensive male with dissecting aneurysm of the thoracic aorta originating at left subclavian artery. Posteroanterior film of chest showing dilated thoracic aorta and enlarged heart. (B, *bottom, left*) Venous angiocardiogram showing ascending aorta with narrow true lumen in descending thoracic aorta. (C, *bottom, right*) Lateral view showing dye-filled narrow true lumen and wide false lumen of descending thoracic aorta.

Symptoms. The patient having an abdominal aortic aneurysm may remain asymptomatic even while the aneurysm grows to sizes up to 10 and 15 cm. in diameter. This is un-

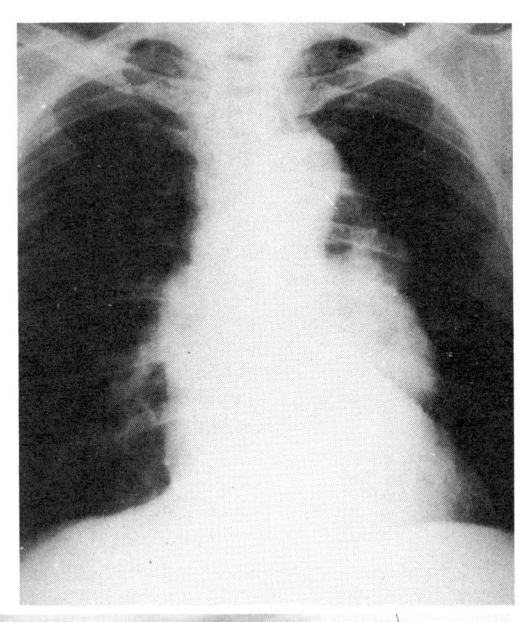

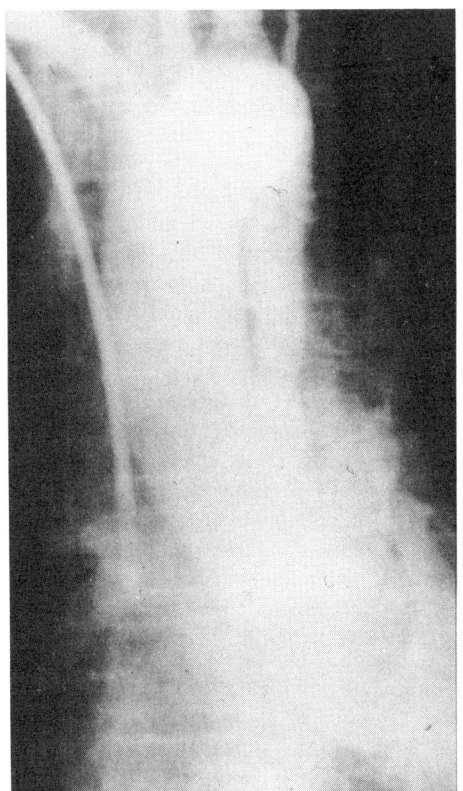

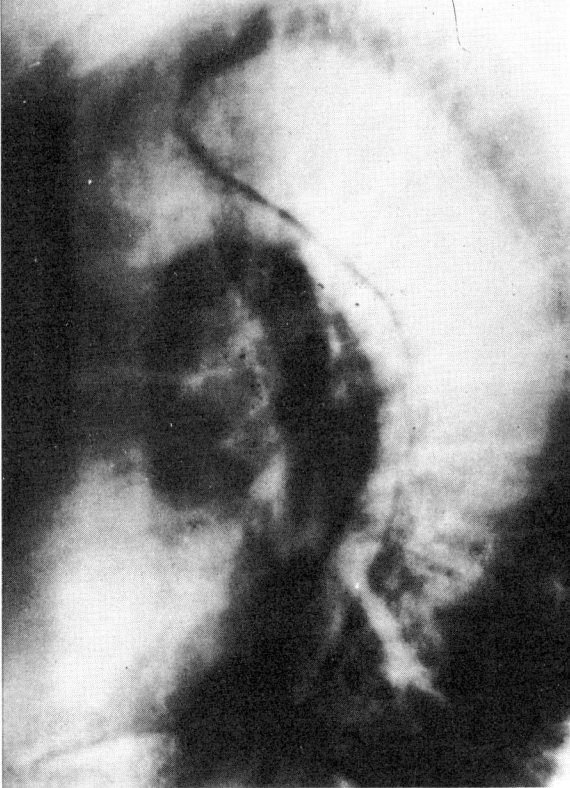

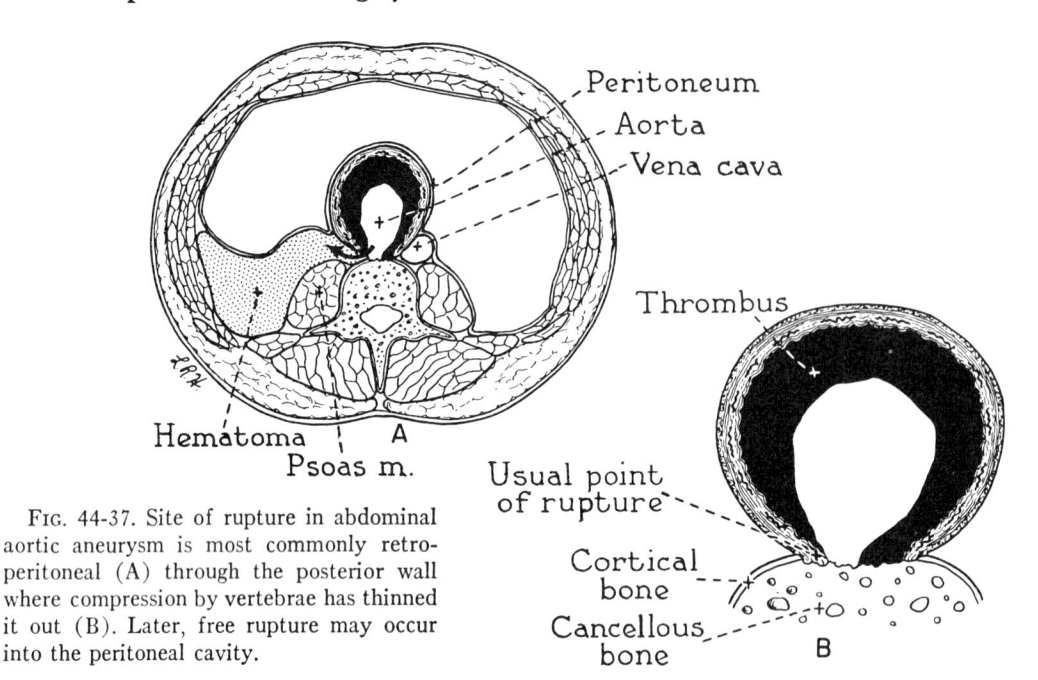

FIG. 44-37. Site of rupture in abdominal aortic aneurysm is most commonly retroperitoneal (A) through the posterior wall where compression by vertebrae has thinned it out (B). Later, free rupture may occur into the peritoneal cavity.

doubtedly because of the availability of space within the abdomen among the hollow viscera. More frequently, symptoms are produced as a result of compression of the surrounding structures. Intermittent claudication is present occasionally, due to the relative obstruction to the blood flow produced by the aneurysm. Pressure on the bodies of the vertebrae, which are frequently eroded by the pulsating mass, causes back pain. When the aneurysm extends to the side of the spine, radiating pain is produced by pressure on the lumbar nerve roots. Distention of the small intestine mesentery into which the aneurysm expands may produce abdominal pain and digestive disturbances such as attacks of ileus and distention. Obstruction to the third portion of the duodenum occasionally results when the aneurysm distends upward against the duodenum held by the ligament of Treitz at the duodenaljejunal junction. Such patients have nausea and vomiting, which may be either intermittent or progressive until the aneurysm is removed or until it ruptures.

Course. Occasionally, an abdominal aortic aneurysm will follow a long and benign course. Aside from the production of symptoms by compressing the spine or involving the gastrointestinal tract, the common complication of abdominal aortic aneurysm is rupture. Reviews of collected cases by several investigators have disclosed the true, rather grave prognosis in patients with aneurysm when it is asymptomatic and the more serious prognosis when symptoms have developed (Estes, 1950). Rupture is into the retroperitoneal space most commonly but also may be into any adjacent viscus of the gastrointestinal tract or into the vena cava. When the retroperitoneal rupture occurs, free rupture into the peritoneal cavity almost always follows unless death occurs from the retroperitoneal blood loss (Fig. 44-37). Rare resolution of the retroperitoneal hematoma with temporary stabilization of the wall of the aneurysm may occur, but in the overwhelming majority of patients rupture leads progressively to a fatal outcome. Death by hemorrhage ensues rapidly when free abdominal cavity bleeding develops or when the aneurysm ruptures into the gastrointestinal tract. The progression to death by hemorrhage is sometimes delayed for hours or days in patients with a retroperitoneal rupture. These patients show the development of a wide pulsating mass in the abdomen extending into the flanks and the lower abdomen above Poupart's ligament. Signs of hemorrhage such as increased pulse rate, falling blood pressure, and particularly a drop in the red blood count, together with such a pulsating growing

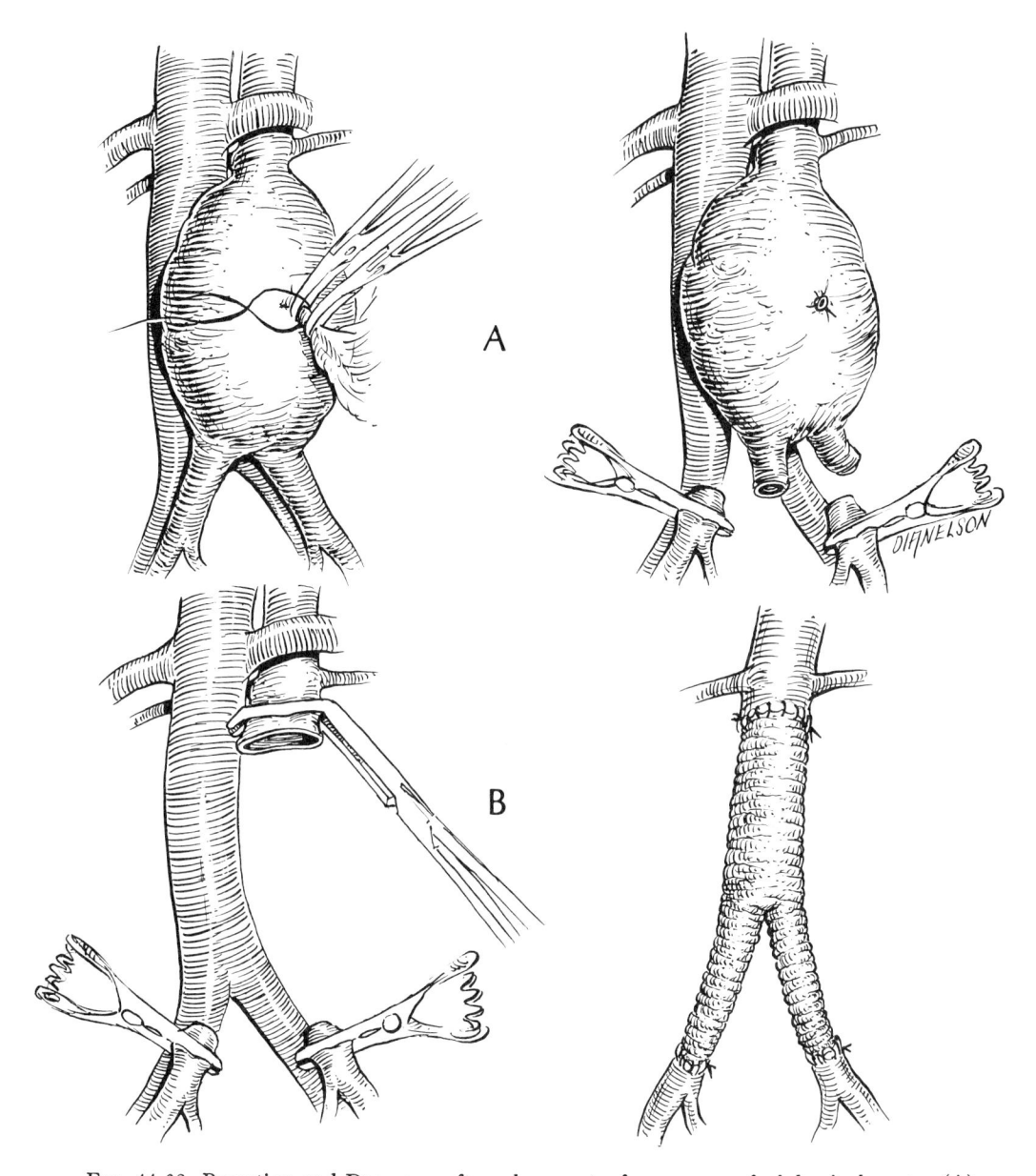

FIG. 44-38. Resection and Dacron graft replacement of aneurysm of abdominal aorta. (A) Resection of aneurysm of bifurcation of aorta coming off below renal arteries. (B) Dacron bifurcation graft sutured in place.

mass, are diagnostic of ruptured aneurysm. Another much less common complication of abdominal aneurysm is acute thrombosis. This was seen in 2 of the first 300 cases in the authors' series.

With rare exception all abdominal aneurysms should be treated surgically. Reference has been made to the course and prognosis of untreated abdominal aneurysms as compared to surgically treated ones (Bernstein, Fisher and Varco, 1967; Klippel and Butcher, 1966). Most series that have been analyzed carefully show a significant difference in survival between the surgically and the nonsurgically treated aneurysms (Szilagyi *et al.*, 1966; De Bakey *et al.*, 1964).

Treatment of abdominal aortic aneurysm had been entirely palliative until recent years when more definitive curative surgery has become well established. An early form of treatment consisted of ligation of the abdominal aorta above the aneurysm (Morton and Scott, 1944). When this ligation was carried to the point of occlusion of the aorta the pulsations within the aneurysm ceased. However, hemorrhage frequently resulted from the ligature cutting through, and there was a discouraging incidence of gangrene of both lower extremities. Stimulation of the development of a large clot within the aneurysm by the introduction of wire has been practiced similar to that used in thoracic aneurysms (Blakemore, 1953; Linton, 1951). Gradual occlusion of the aorta proximal to an aneurysm at the bifurcation can be accomplished by wrapping the vessel in this region with a cuff of polyethylene film containing a sizing compound, dicetyl phosphate (de Takats and Marshall, 1952). This substance stimulates development of scar tissue which shrinks and gradually shuts off the blood flow. At their best, when successful, these methods provide only a temporary cessation in growth of the aneurysm or relief of symptoms.

Real help to these patients, developed during 1952 (Du Bost *et al.*, 1952; Schafer and Hardin, 1952) and used progressively more widely since (Brock, 1953; De Bakey and Cooley, 1953b; Julian *et al.*, 1954; Kirklin *et al.*, 1953; MacVaugh and Roberts, 1961; May *et al.*, 1968), consists of the total removal of the lower abdominal aorta and its bifurcation, and a variable amount of the iliac systems, with subsequent replacement of the defect with an aortic bifurcation graft (Fig. 44-38). The grafts used in earliest work were human aortic bifurcations salvaged at autopsies. Woven Dacron prostheses have completely displaced this homologous material because of better strength, sterility and lasting qualities.

While these surgical procedures are ideally applied electively when the diagnosis of abdominal aneurysm is made, they are also available in cases of ruptured aneurysm. This is successful in about one half of those patients who survive to reach the operating room. The best chance is afforded the patient when plans for rapid action have been made and rehearsed in anticipation that such cases will appear.

Peripheral Arterial Aneurysms

Virtually all peripheral arterial aneurysms are arteriosclerotic. These have been known to involve almost all branches of the aorta. In the intra-abdominal viscera they develop in the mesenteric, the splenic, the renal and the hepatic arteries. More peripherally, femoral and popliteal arteries are common sites.

In each of the peripheral locations, the aneurysm threatens the well-being of the patient because of a degree of interference with blood supply through the artery involved and by the likelihood of acute thrombosis or rupture of the lesion. The diagnosis of an aneurysm in a peripheral site available to direct examination is based on the demonstration of a usually quite obvious pulsating mass. Attention may be directed toward an aneurysm within the thoracic or the abdominal cavity by accident, as in finding a shadow later proved to be a subclavian artery aneurysm in a routine chest roentgenogram, or an unexplained curvilinear shadow of aneurysm wall in a roentgenogram of the abdomen. A renal artery aneurysm may be brought to light in the evaluation by aortography of the renal arteries in a patient whose hypertension is suspected to be renovascular in origin.

The most frequent of the peripheral arteriosclerotic aneurysms is that of the popliteal artery. Here the lesion is usually brought to the patient's attention by his discovery of a pulsating area or pulsating mass behind the knee. He often experiences some discomfort and annoyance when he crosses his legs in sitting. This aneurysm usually produces some obstruction to the flow of blood because it disturbs the smooth pattern of blood flow which otherwise exists in a normal artery. The elongation of the vessel which accompanies the dilatation also causes obstruction (Fig. 44-39). Therefore, there is usually some degree of intermittent claudication involving the calf muscles when the patient walks. In this location growth of the aneurysm often causes pain by compression of adjacent nerves and can produce swelling of the leg below the knee because it compresses the popliteal veins. The patient begins to experience difficulty in extending the knee, and a form of flexion contracture develops, simply because of the mass in the popliteal space. In about one third of

FIG. 44-39. Popliteal aneurysm illustrating the elongation which occurs along with the dilatation. This serves to obstruct the branches of the artery, particularly the anterior tibial as shown in (B), and is one of the mechanisms by which popliteal aneurysm causes chronic arterial obstruction.

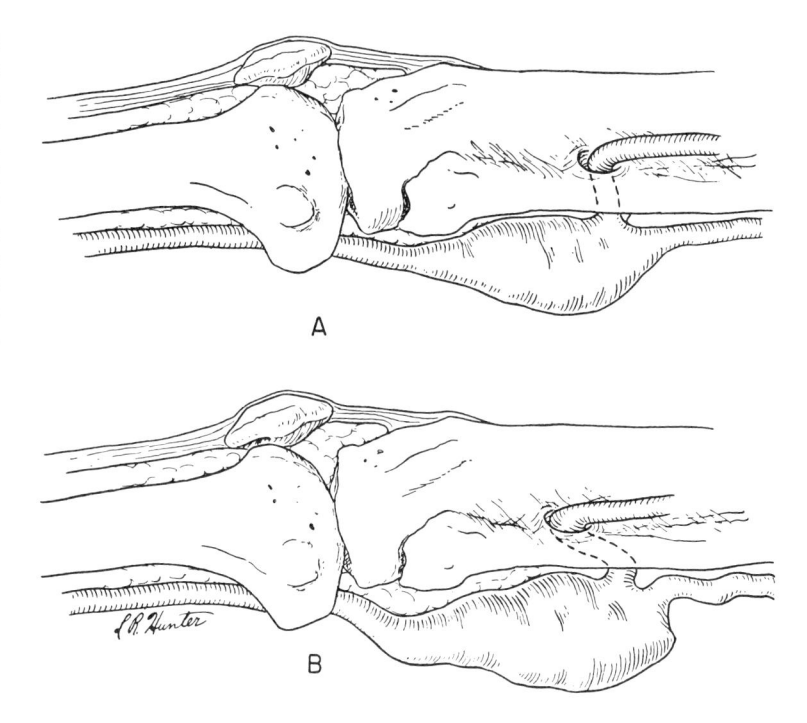

patients with popliteal aneurysms the lesion exists on both sides.

Two complications of popliteal aneurysm are frequent. These are acute thrombosis of the aneurysm and rupture. It is notable that thrombosis is far more frequent a complication of popliteal aneurysm than is rupture, whereas in arteriosclerotic aneurysms of the abdominal aorta the reverse is true. Acute thrombosis causes a sudden ischemia of the extremity and may be followed by gangrene unless treatment is successful. Rupture of a popliteal aneurysm results in a massive increase in the pulsating tumor in the popliteal space because of blood loss into the tissues. This dissects its way up through Hunter's canal to fill the fascial compartments of the thigh and downward into the calf where the limited available space usually prevents very much blood loss in this direction. Exsanguination does not occur, and the maximum effect of a ruptured popliteal aneurysm is rapidly progressive deterioration of the blood supply to the leg, leading to gangrene.

Because of its peripheral location and usually obvious diagnosis, popliteal aneurysms received very early surgical attention. The earliest rational surgical treatment of popliteal aneurysm was the surgical ligation of the femoral-popliteal segment of the artery above the lesion. This operation has been explained best as a part of the work of Hunter in a description by one of his students. The ligation did not always result in gangrene of the leg, depending upon the effectiveness of the collateral circulation which had developed about the knee in response to the long-standing presence of the aneurysm.

A far better technic of taking care of popliteal aneurysm was introduced by Rudolph Matas (1920) who opened directly into the aneurysm, evacuated the clots which were within it and then, without further dissection which might damage the collateral arteries, sutured the orifices of the artery entering and leaving the aneurysm from the inside of the aneurysmal sac. Much of the remaining sac was then sutured in upon the aneurysm cavity, portions of the redundant wall being resected. This operation, known as *endo-aneurysmorrhaphy*, results in about 10 per cent incidence of gangrene of the leg. In addition to this obliterative type of operation, Matas also used a technic which restored arterial continuity. He folded down the trimmed aneurysmal wall, suturing it in place to leave a lumen. Further improvement in the treatment consisted of *combining complete resection of the aneurysm with a lumbar sympathectomy.* The lumbar sympathectomy was depended upon to improve the efficiency of the collateral circulation and to prevent spasm of the arteries adjacent to the operative site. In the hands of surgeons who have reported on this operation the incidence of gangrene has been essentially zero (James and Ivens, 1951; Linton, 1949).

The most definitive and reparative type of surgery for this lesion consists of *removal of the aneurysm followed by the implantation of a suitable vein, artery or prosthetic graft* sutured to the carefully prepared ends of the popliteal artery above and below the lesion. Although this grafting was done very early by Pringle (1913), only sporadic use has been made of this technic until recently (Julian et al., 1955). Blakemore of New York used a slightly different method of implantation, opening the aneurysm and suturing the graft ends from within to the internal proximal and distal openings (Blakemore, 1947). The advantage of restoring the circulation through the artery at the knee level lies in the fact that these patients are not only protected from having gangrene of any part of the extremity but, after the operation, having a normal blood supply to the calf, they are not subject to intermittent claudication or other symptoms of arterial insufficiency (Crawford et al., 1961; Friesen et al., 1962; Hunter et al., 1961; Baird et al., 1966; Crichlow and Roberts, 1966; Edmunds, Darling and Linton, 1965).

Mycotic Aneurysms

A rare but distinctive form of aneurysm occurs in cases of subacute bacterial endocarditis. The arterial wall at some point in the body is weakened by a bacterial infection carried to it by small emboli arising from the vegetations on the heart valve involved with the endocarditis. It is supposed that the embolus is quite small and implants itself in the vessel wall by entering one of the vasovasorum. It is equally likely that the embolus lodges in a small branch of the major artery and the infection involves the arterial wall by spreading along the periarterial tissues. These emboli would be the same type that produce the intensely tender fingertips by lodging in the digital vessels in patients with endocarditis. The acute episode of lodgment of the embolus is apparently entirely asymptomatic in many cases, and the first evidence of an arterial lesion is the appearance and the rather rapid development of a pulsating swelling. Mycotic aneurysms have been observed in many locations in the lower extremities. The brachial artery is the point of most frequent site in the upper extremity. They have been seen in the mesenteric arteries. The symptomatology produced by the aneurysm includes pain almost from the beginning of development. Why these aneurysms should be more painful than those of arteriosclerosis or syphilis probably depends on the acute inflammatory nature of the lesion. The inflammation causes them to attach themselves very quickly to surrounding structures or to the undersurface of the skin. Therefore, they may dissect through adjacent structures and rupture. The other frequent complication of mycotic aneurysm is early thrombosis.

In our experience the aneurysm continues to grow after subacute bacterial endocarditis and the blood stream infection which is associated with it have been arrested by chemotherapy. Therefore, though antibiotics are indicated in the treatment of mycotic aneurysm they probably do not reverse the tendency for the aneurysm to enlarge because the wall already has been weakened by the inflammatory reaction.

Treatment consists of resection and restoration of the blood flow by the implantation of a vein or artery graft if a major channel is involved. This operation obviously should be deferred until the causative infection has been overcome. However, ideal timing cannot always be accomplished because the extremely painful expanding lesion may require earlier operation simply because of the pain, because of threatened rupture, or because thrombosis has led to a serious degree of ischemia in an extremity or in a viscus.

Surgery of the Venous System

INTRODUCTION

The pathologic processes involving the venous system are limited in number. The principal ones are dilatation and elongation, intrinsic occlusion by thrombosis and inflammation, and pathologic processes not inherent to the veins which cause extrinsic venous occlusion. Additional, but rare, processes include suppurative inflammation, intrinsic occlusion by the invasion of the vein lumen by tumor, and degenerative lesions.

Dilatation and elongation of the vein occur because of chronic increased pressure within the vein or overloading of the venous system concerned. As is the case with arteries, veins are so constructed that when they are forcibly expanded the expansion occurs both in circumference and in length. Elongation and dilatation aside from the varices of the legs is seen in varicosities of the veins of the submucosal area of the esophagus in portal vein obstruction and liver disease, and hemorrhoids and the venous enlargement which accompanies arteriovenous fistulae in any location.

Occlusion by inflammation and thrombosis is termed *thrombophlebitis*. The clinical manifestations of the thrombophlebitis are very diverse, depending upon the severity of the acute inflammation and later on the residual vein damage. The complications of thrombophlebitis reflect this damage to the veins, particularly in the lower extremities. Another complication is pulmonary artery embolism which occurs when the thrombus within the vein lumen breaks loose and travels to the lungs.

Extrinsic occlusion of a vein may be due to compression by tumor or pregnant uterus, or as a result of an adjacent chronic fibrosing inflammation. One very important clinical manifestation of this latter form of extrinsic occlusion is superior vena caval syndrome. The clinical features produced by compression of a vein by tumor are variable according to region and will not be described.

VARICOSE VEINS OF THE LOWER EXTREMITY

Structure. Varices of the lower extremities are the result of dilatation of the subcutaneous venous channels to a degree which renders the valves incompetent because they are no longer capable of coapting across the enlarged vein area (Fig. 44-40). This loss of valve competence is the feature displayed in common by varicose veins of any etiology.

Certain features of the structure of the venous systems involved are important in order to understand the development of the condition and the rationale of its treatment. The veins affected are the long saphenous vein and the short saphenous vein, together with their tributaries. Both of these systems lie beneath the superficial fascia and superficial to the deep fascia throughout the major portion of their course in the thighs and the legs.

The *long saphenous vein* arises in superficial veins on the dorsum and the medial aspects of the foot. These form a channel at the level of the medial malleolus which courses directly upward along the calf medial to the tibia. At the level of the knee the course becomes somewhat more posterior, and the vein continues up the medial and then the anteromedial surface of the thigh to enter the common femoral vein high in the groin. The point of entrance into the femoral vein is approximately 2 cm. distal to Poupart's ligament. The vein gains entrance into the deep compartment of the thigh through the deep fascia by way of an oval opening, the fossa ovalis. At or near the point

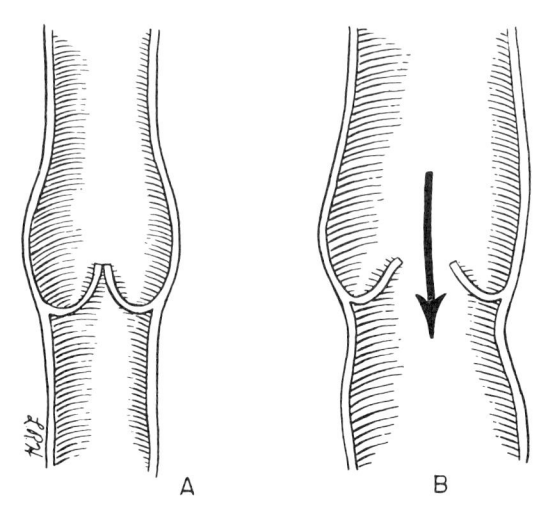

FIG. 44-40. Diagrammatic representation of vein dilatation in producing valvular incompetence.

of entrance into the common femoral vein the saphenous vein receives tributaries which are exceedingly important from the standpoint of treatment. These tributaries are the superficial circumflex iliac, entering laterally, the superficial epigastric, entering superiorly, and the superficial pudendal entering medially. In addition the accessory saphenous veins, medial and lateral, enter the long saphenous vein a short distance below the saphenofemoral junction, or right at the junction, or they may even enter the femoral vein directly. Normally, only one of the accessory saphenous veins is prominent.

Throughout its course the long saphenous vein receives tributaries which drain the skin and the subcutaneous tissue of the thigh and the medial aspect of the leg and the foot. It communicates frequently with the deep veins of the extremities through branches which penetrate the deep fascia of the leg and the thigh.

The entire course of the saphenous vein is protected by valves occurring at intervals of 4 to 8 inches which are so positioned as to permit only cephalad flow of blood. The perforating branches of the saphenous vein which communicate with the deep venous system also contain valves. These direct flow from the saphenous to the deep veins.

The *short saphenous vein* drains the posterior and the lateral aspects of the leg. It arises posterior to the lateral malleolus from superficial veins on the lateral aspect of the foot and then takes its course upward approximately in the midline of the calf to penetrate the deep fascia and enter the popliteal vein. The point of penetration of the fascia varies in individuals from the level of the Achilles tendon to the popliteal space. Communications with the deep system are not plentiful. The lesser saphenous vein usually communicates through a large branch with the greater saphenous vein. The position of this vessel is variable. It may leave the short saphenous vein at almost any point in the leg, entering the greater or long saphenous at the ankle level or above.

Pathology. No intrinsic pathologic change is seen as the cause of the dilatation. The primary lesion in the involved vein is simply the dilatation which renders the valves incompetent. However, after the process has been present for a long time, fibrosis and thickening of the vein wall are present. There is also at an early stage a distinct hypertrophy of the muscularis of the vein.

Several factors are identifiable as predisposing to the development of varicose veins. On the basis of these predisposing causes varicose veins are divided into two classes—primary and secondary. Primary varicose veins are those which arise because of intrinsic weakness of the vein walls, because of occupational stress, or due to pregnancy.

There is little doubt that the unexplained and sometimes very early development of varicose veins in certain individuals is due to a deficiency in the elastic and muscular layers of the vein wall. It is probable, also, that this is congenital rather than acquired. The generally held impression that it is also familial is not supported by any very good evidence.

Pregnancy is an etiologic factor principally because of the humoral mechanisms which effect a general relaxation of smooth muscle and, perhaps, changes in elastic tissue. There is also some effect of the increased vascularity in the pelvis and of the pressure exerted on pelvic veins by the enlarged uterus.

Occupations requiring long periods of standing, as opposed to walking or sitting, potentiate any tendency to varicose vein development. However, this effect of an occupation should probably not be considered a primary factor in the etiology of the varices in such individuals.

Secondary varicose veins are those varicose veins that develop as a part of the tremendous venous collateral growth which is stimulated by thrombophlebitic occlusion of the deep venous system of the lower extremities.

Primary Varicose Veins. Local dilatation of a segment of the saphenous vein provides the beginning of structural failure of the entire system. The primary enlargement in circumference renders the valve or valves in the segment incompetent. This brings a longer blood column to rest on the subjacent valve. As the dilatation continues the valves of the perforating branches are rendered incompetent, allowing flow in a retrograde direction in these veins from the deep to the superficial systems. The blood thus escaping into the saphenous system from the deep veins flows in a retrograde direction unhampered by the valves already incompetent. It re-enters the deep system at whatever point of leg or ankle its pressure in relation to deep vein pressure permits it to do so. It then resumes its flow upward.

SYMPTOMS. Uncomplicated varicose veins are seldom productive of severe symptoms, and frequently there are none at all. Increased fatigue, some aching of the legs at night, slight edema, and moderate pain and tenderness over the distended veins are the usual symptoms when any are present. Complaints of severe pain or disability in patients exhibiting varicose veins is a strong suggestion to search for some other cause of the symptoms, such as arthritis of the hip, the knee or the lower back, or for arterial insufficiency.

COMPLICATIONS of varicose veins of the lower extremities are productive of a more symptomatic course. The unphysiologic level of the back pressure in the local venous drainage results in a disturbance of skin nutrition, causing changes in the skin and, to some degree, in the cutaneous nerves. Paresthesias of the skin of the leg, eczematoid dermatitis, pigmentation, fibrosis and finally ulceration may occur. The appearance of edema of the ankle or the dorsum of the foot is rare except perhaps in a very mild degree as a complication of varicose veins alone. The amount of back flow and the height of the column of blood in the superficial veins ordinarily is handled quite well by an entirely normal deep venous system. Therefore, the presence of edema is suggestive of concomitant deep vein pathology or of cardiac or renal insufficiency.

A second complication is acute inflammation with thrombosis of a segment of the dilated tortuous vein. This produces pain, tenderness and local heat of a magnitude which depends on the size of the varix involved.

EXAMINATION. The physical examination of the patient with varicose veins must be complete. The general portion of such an examination determines the presence of any pathologic process which might have a causal relation with the varices or might alter the treatment of the veins. The local examination determines the extent and the severity of the dilatation. It points out the presence and the location of incompetent valves in the saphenous system and in the perforating veins communicating between saphenous and deep circulation. The presence of complications of the varicose veins is sought for, and the deep venous circulation is evaluated.

The initial observation is made with the patient standing relaxed, allowing time for the veins to fill to a maximum extent. This is carried out best in an oblique light, and palpation of the channels will reveal pathologically dilated veins which are invisible because of obesity. Palpation should be done by a percussing movement with the fingers, delineating veins by the ballottement of the contained blood. This percussion is done with firm, brisk strokes of one hand while the other hand is placed over the course of the vein, either above or below. The pressure wave can be felt transmitted through the column of blood. The point in local examination most frequently overlooked is an evaluation of the short saphenous vein. In its classically normal anatomic form, the short saphenous vein is subcutaneous from the popliteal space to the ankle. However, it frequently lies beneath the deep fascia along the posterior surface of the calf down to a point as low as the development of the Achilles tendon before it emerges as a dilated channel. When this is true the pathologic state in the short saphenous vein may be missed. Dilatation of veins under the skin of the lateral aspect of the ankle or dermatitis in this region are indicative of a varicose short saphenous vein.

The incompetence of the valves in the saphenous channels may be demonstrated by a test which allows the varicose veins to fill from above. The classical test was described first by Brodie (1846) and later by Trendelenburg (1890) and is known by the names of both men. To perform this maneuver, first the veins are emptied of blood by elevating the legs. A tourniquet is applied at thigh level, and the patient stands. With the tourniquet in place the veins tend to remain empty, filling gradually from below. If the tourniquet is removed quickly with the veins unfilled, the blood from above drops immediately into the dilated system below. This response indicates competent valves in the perforating veins and incompetent valves in the saphenous vein. If the veins are seen to fill rapidly with the tourniquet in place high on the thigh the test is interpreted to mean that the perforating vein valves are incompetent. The level of incompetence of valves in the perforating veins may be demonstrated by an extension of the maneuver which was described by Ochsner and Mahorner (1938). When filling occurs from above with a tourniquet in place at the mid-thigh level, it may be assumed that an incompetent perforating vein exists some place below the tourniquet. By repeating the test with the tourniquet at progressively lower points on the thigh and the calf, the level of the most distal incompetent perforator may be demonstrated. This actually can be done with only one change of position by putting 4 tourniquets at various levels down the thigh and the leg with the leg elevated and then, with the patient standing, removing them progressively from below until rapid filling occurs.

The ability of the deep venous system to drain off the blood collected in the varicose veins may be demonstrated by the *Perthes test* which is done by occluding with a tourniquet the subcutaneous veins at the knee or thigh level (Perthes, 1895). The tourniquet must be at or distal to the lowest significant incompetent perforator. The tourniquet will prevent all downward filling from above this level, and, as the patient walks, the normal pumping action of the muscles exerted on the deep veins drains the dilated varices. Failure of the veins to empty may mean that the tourniquet is above a large incompetent perforating vein which allows flow out into the varices. Also it may mean that the deep veins have been damaged by an inflammatory process so that their function is disturbed. Formerly, the latter conclusion from the test was considered as a contraindication to surgical therapy of the varicose veins. As will be discussed in the management of secondary varicose veins, the contraindication no longer is considered valid, and such veins are given definitive surgical treatment.

Secondary Varicose Veins. These are the superficial components of the general massive development of venous collaterals which results from deep vein damage due to thrombophlebitis. The differentiation between primary and secondary veins depends on the history of an attack of thrombophlebitis and the presence of other signs of deep venous insufficiency. If other complications of previous deep-vein disease are present, the varicose veins must be considered only as a part of the stasis syndrome.

A rare cause of varicosities of the superficial veins is the presence of arteriovenous fistulae, usually of the congenital type. In this condition the extremity is usually the site of congenital hemangiomata of the skin and increased warmth and skin color. Sometimes a bruit is heard in the congenital fistulae and is always present in the acquired type. Finally, the abnormal filling of the veins from the arteries is manifested by increased oxygen in the venous blood which can be measured and by increased pressure in the varices. Sometimes the pressure is great enough to delay or prevent emptying of the varicose veins when the extremity is elevated.

Indications for surgery in varicose veins vary. The presence of small superficial and asymptomatic veins is not in itself a strong indication for their removal. Symptoms from varicosities must be evaluated carefully, and other causes of leg discomfort should be ruled out. Large and tortuous varicosities should be removed because of possible future phlebitis as well as for the relief of symptoms. Varicosities occurring during pregnancy present a problem. These patients with few exceptions are carried to term on conservative management. Elastic support and periods of bed rest with elevation of the extremities are used. Surgery is done after delivery with the reservation that recurrences are usual with further pregnancies. Injection therapy is seldom used as a primary treatment. It may be of value in controlling the remaining small ones following surgical removal of the major veins.

TREATMENT. The surgical treatment of varicose veins consists of removal of the long or short saphenous veins or both, together with their affected tributaries. At the same time the incompetent perforating veins must be ligated or otherwise inactivated. The ligation of the main saphenous trunk accurately at its point of entrance into the deep vein into which it would normally drain is fundamental to the surgical procedure. This is at the junction of the common femoral vein in the case of the long saphenous, and the popliteal vein in the case of the short saphenous.

The saphenous channel is then removed by withdrawing it with a long wire stripper, passed through the length of the vein from

FIG. 44-41. Ligation and stripping of the great and the small saphenous veins. (A) The tributaries of the saphenous vein have been ligated, and the saphenous vein has been ligated at the saphenofemoral junction. Vein stripper has been inserted from the ankle superiorly to the groin. (B) The vein is stripped from above downward. A number of alternate incisions may be needed to remove separate varicose masses. (C) The small saphenous vein is stripped from its junction with the popliteal vein to a point posterior to the lateral malleolus.

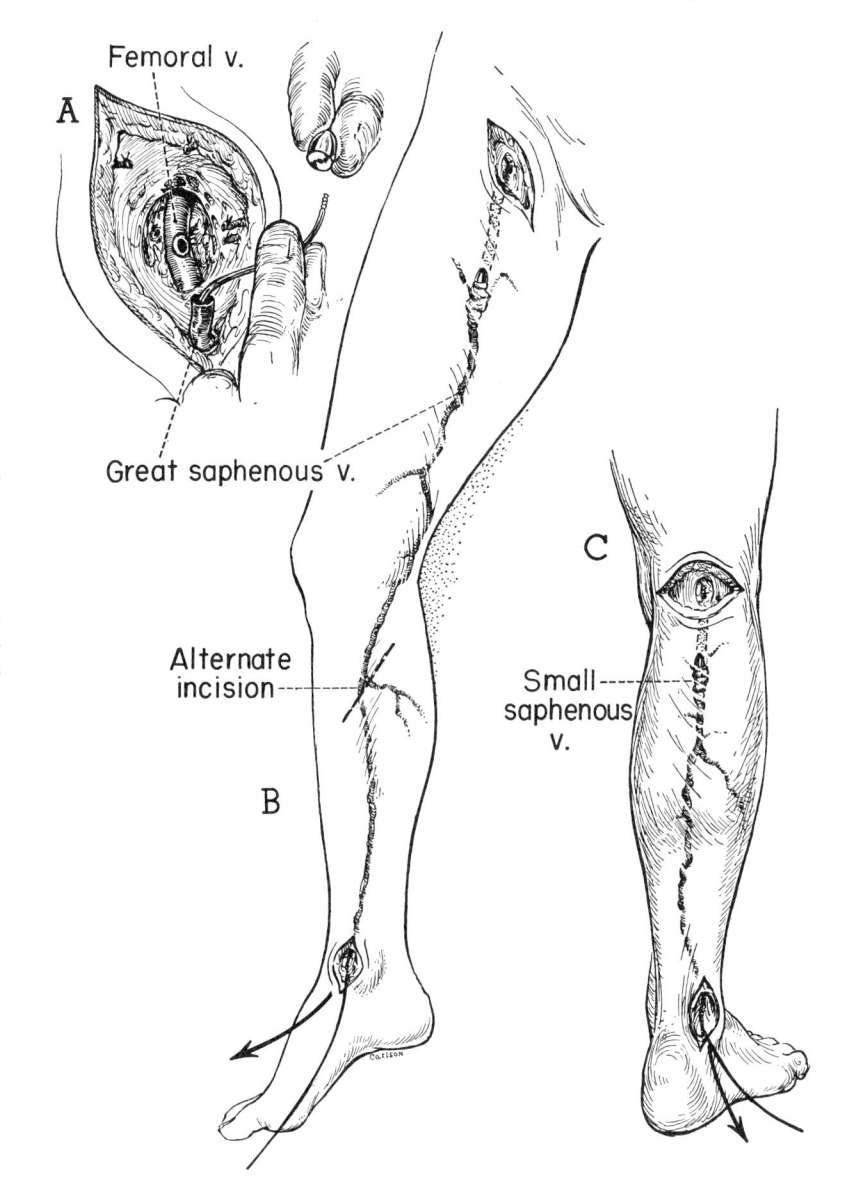

groin or popliteal space to ankle. Varicose tributaries are excised through accessory incisions if they are large or, if small, they are treated with direct injection of sclerosing solutions at a later date. Particular attention should be paid to large tributaries of the long saphenous channel because of the fact that perforator veins may communicate with these tributaries rather than with the channel itself. If they are left behind, local recurrence of the varicose condition will develop on the basis of the remaining perforating veins (Fig. 44-41).

Emphasis has been placed in the past on an evaluation of the deep venous function as a guide to choice of therapy, particularly surgical, in secondary varicose veins. The varices were considered to be a valuable part of the collateral bed. Actually, this is rarely true. In the great majority of cases the varicose veins serve not as a collateral venous route but, because of complete loss of their valve function, lack of fascial support and their inability to be affected by muscle-pumping action, they carry blood downward. This actually increases the load to be carried by the deep venous collaterals which do serve more or less effectively. In most present-day experience complete removal of the incompetent superficial veins has been beneficial rather than detrimental to the total venous drainage of a lower extremity. Therefore, the various tests for deep vein damage are not of practical use in deciding whether extirpation of secondary varicose veins should be done. The decision as to choice of therapy depends more on the presence and the severity of the other complications of deep venous obstruction. In the absence of significant edema secondary varicose veins should be eradicated by ligation and stripping as in the case of primary varices. The presence of cutaneous ulcers and eczema reinforces the insistence on complete removal. However, if edema is present, as will be discussed in the next section, the primary therapeutic attack should be toward the control of the swelling by general management.

THROMBOPHLEBITIS

Definition. Thrombophlebitis is an inflammatory disease of the vein wall and the surrounding tissue, including lymphatics, accompanied by thrombosis in the lumen of the vessel. It may involve the superficial veins (superficial phlebitis) or the deep veins (deep phlebitis). The severity of the inflammation varies widely. In some it is very mild, producing minor febrile reaction and only slight pain. In others all features of an acute inflammation—heat, redness, tenderness and fever—are marked. This variation in the severity of the inflammatory aspect of thrombophlebitis led Ochsner (1939) to make a purely artificial subdivision of inflammatory deep vein disease into two groups.

Classification. The first group, *thrombophlebitis*, consists of those cases in which the inflammatory reaction is severe. In the second group, *phlebothrombosis*, the presence of the thrombus is the most important aspect. It is practical to use this subdivision, although fundamentally the two conditions have one identity. Morphologically, the elements are the same, merging from one to another, and both can be present in the same extremity simultaneously. Individual patients are frequently observed to enter the phase of thrombophlebitis after first exhibiting signs of the milder state for some time.

Complications. The major complications are pulmonary embolism during the early stage and stasis disease later. Pulmonary embolism results when a portion of the intraluminal clot detaches from its site of origin, travels through the venous system and the heart and lodges in a branch of the pulmonary artery. Pulmonary embolism occurs much more frequently in the milder form of the disease, namely, phlebothrombosis. Late stasis disease is the manifestation of damage to the venous drainage and to the surrounding lymphatics by the inflammation. This is more frequent after the greater destruction which occurs in the inflammation of thrombophlebitis.

Phlebothrombosis. This bland form occurs as a complication of surgery, any acute illness, unusual activity such as a long hike by an ordinarily sedentary person, or unusual inactivity such as sitting long periods in a boat while fishing. It also occurs without any determinable deviation from normal activity.

SYMPTOMS. The symptoms consist of mild pain and stiffness in the calf of the leg on active motion and a duplication of these symptoms on passive dorsiflexion of the ankle. This discomfort is accompanied by mild or moderate swelling with or without a low-grade fever and tachycardia. The course of the condition may be very benign, the fever and symptoms disappearing in a few days on bed rest. In other cases the originally bland phlebothrombosis may go on to display a picture of acute thrombophlebitis.

The clinical importance of the illness is the complication of pulmonary embolism, which sometimes occurs before the local symptoms are very manifest.

PROPHYLAXIS. Much attention has been paid to the prevention of phlebothrombosis as a complication of surgery. The factors in its production in the postoperative patient are probably 3-fold. Changes in the coagulation mechanism, hemoconcentration, and stasis resulting from bed rest and infrequent changes of position probably all contribute. Modern fluid and electrolyte management of the surgical patient, early ambulation and the prophylactic administration of the anticoagulants Dicumarol and heparin have all been emphasized in prevention of phlebothrombosis. The incidence remains significant in spite of preventive therapy (De Bakey, 1954).

DIAGNOSIS. Individuals developing phlebothrombosis usually have very mild symptoms. These consist of stiffness and aching of the calf and of a limp because of pain when they walk. Body temperature elevation is mild when present. The first sign of phlebothrombosis may be a pulmonary embolism, whether the patient has been well preceding the illness or it overtakes him in the hospital after surgery.

The serious nature of pulmonary embolism and its habit of occurring as a sudden unexpected complication of other disease or surgery makes the constant search for signs of phlebothrombosis in hospitalized patients mandatory (Gorham, 1961). The daily inspection of the temperature chart and of the patient's lower extremities is a habit to be developed by all physicians. An early diagnosis and immediate institution of treatment will diminish the chances of embolism.

An unexplained mild simultaneous rise in pulse and temperature is one of the danger signals of phlebothrombosis (Donaldson, 1947). Inspection of the extremities includes looking for mild edema, dilatations of the veins over the anterior tibia, congestion of the calf muscles, and a positive Homans' sign. This consists of a feeling of tightness and discomfort when the ankle is passively dorsiflexed (Homans, 1928).

TREATMENT. Therapy has two purposes. One is to limit the course of the local condition, and the second is to prevent pulmonary embolism. The local treatment is not complicated. It consists of bed rest with elevation of the lower extremities. The patient is allowed good mobility in bed but massage of the legs or active exercise of the lower extremities is forbidden. Local heat is useful in increasing comfort. It should be in the form of a heat cradle at not more than 115° F. rather than

TABLE 44-2. ANTICOAGULANT REGIMENS

INDICATION	PURPOSE	HEPARIN	DICUMAROL
Arterial Embolism (Peripheral and Aortic)	Rapid, temporary prolongation of clotting time to limit growth of intra-arterial clot	75-100 mg. i.v. Followed by 50 mg. i.v. every 3 hours until embolectomy	None
Phlebothrombosis Therapeutic	Rapid, continued depression of clotting activity to diminish growth of thrombus in involved vein and diminish incidence of pulmonary embolism	A. Heparin Alone 30-50 mg. deep subcut. (not intramuscular) every 3 to 4 hrs. to prolong clotting time to approx. 3 times normal	None
Prophylactic	Depression of clotting activity effective 4-6 hrs. after surgery to diminish tendency to develop phlebothrombosis in patients thought to be likely to develop it	—or— B. Heparin plus Dicumarol 30-50 mg. heparin subcut. every 3-4 hrs. until Dicumarol becomes effective	100 mg. by mouth every 6 hrs. for 5 doses then 25-100 mg. per day to maintain 25-40% clotting activity
Thrombophlebitis	Prolonged depression of clotting activity to: (1) diminish propagation of intraluminal venous clots to limit extent of damage to system; and (2) diminish incidence of pulmonary embolism	Either method outlined for use in phlebothrombosis	

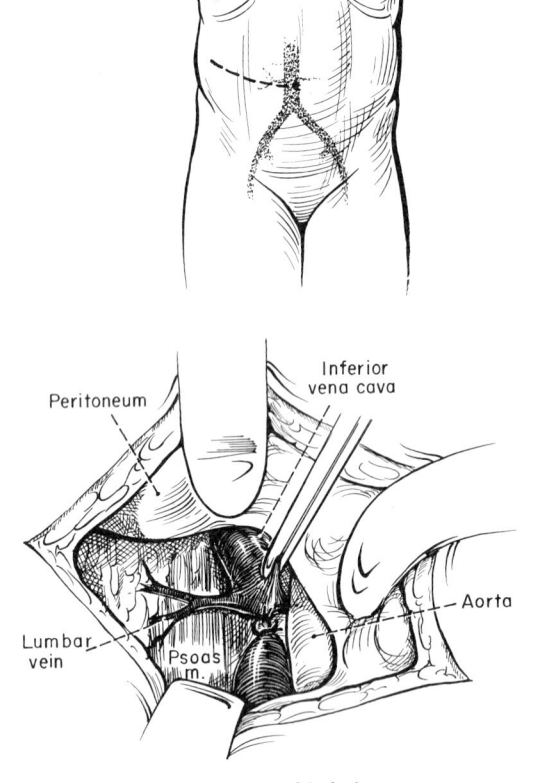

FIG. 44-42. Ligation of inferior vena cava through an extraperitoneal exposure.

hot, wet foments, which necessarily produce complete immobilization.

Good hydration must be obtained and the fluid management directed to avoid or correct dehydration. Data obtained through culture of the clots removed from involved veins indicate that bacterial agents probably are not responsible. Therefore, antibiotics such as penicillin or streptomycin are not required. The anticoagulant agents heparin and Dicumarol produce an effect which is beneficial both in the local management and in the prevention of emboli (Table 44-2. See also Chap. 15, p. 324, Arterial Occlusive Edema).

The period of local therapy is hard to determine. Ambulation may be permitted gradually after all local signs have been gone 1 or 2 days. As the patient is allowed up it is important to watch for a recurrence. The anticoagulant therapy should be kept up for longer periods. The duration of this varies in the opinions of authorities from 10 days to several months. The purpose of maintaining the depression in coagulation is to prevent upward growth in the involved vein of a nonadherent segment of thrombus which might break loose even after a week or two. Since very few emboli have occurred more than 2 weeks after subsidence of local signs, this has been taken by many surgeons as the period of anticoagulant therapy after subsidence of symptoms and signs.

PREVENTION of pulmonary embolism in cases of phlebothrombosis may also be obtained by *interrupting surgically the involved vein above the process*. This operation was originally applied at the proximal superficial femoral vein level. This site has virtually been abandoned in favor of one on the vena cava below the renal veins. The cava is conveniently exposed retroperitoneally through a right flank muscle-splitting incision. The vein is sometimes simply ligated but more often it is plicated by sutures or compressed by a special clip, either of which technics compartment the caval lumen into 3 lumens that are too small to permit passage of a significant clot (Fig. 44-42). Plication and clipping are designed to allow continued flow of blood. However, even complete ligation probably causes little if any more residual venous insufficiency than would have resulted from the thrombophlebitis for which it was done (DeWeese and Hunter, 1963; Spencer et al., 1962; Wheeler et al., 1966; Taber et al., 1966; Leather et al., 1968) (Fig. 44-42).

Massive pulmonary embolism may now be treated successfully utilizing cardiopulmonary bypass with direct exposure and removal of the clot in the pulmonary artery (Cooley and Beall, 1961; Sharp, 1962).

Thrombectomy may be tried as a primary treatment of deep venous thrombosis. The thrombus is aspirated in the early stages of the disease. The vein is closed or ligated, and anticoagulants are continued (Haller, 1961; Fogarty et al., 1966).

For several reasons *anticoagulant therapy* is preferred to vein interruption for the prevention of pulmonary embolism, except when a contraindication exists or in areas where facilities to control the anticoagulants are not available, or in patients sustaining pulmonary embolism despite good anticoagulant therapy. Statistical evaluation favors anticoagulant therapy slightly in the prevention of embolism. It is also possible that late venous stasis is intensified by mechanical block by ligation of the veins. Finally, it is quite evident that the substitution of an equally effective medical therapy for one involving an operative procedure is desirable. However, it must be remembered that caval interruption is an effective form of therapy and that the administration of anticoagulants is not without its complications. Therefore, ligation may easily be resorted to when difficulty is encountered either in the patient's response to anticoagulants or in the facilities for its management.

Acute Thrombophlebitis

Although acute thrombophlebitis is considered to be less dangerous in regard to production of pulmonary embolism, it is more incapacitating than is phlebothrombosis in point of causing persistent trouble in the legs. The onset of thrombophlebitis usually is rapid, the first symptom being pain and stiffness in the foot and the calf or the thigh. There is some indication that much of the initial pain is due to reflex arterial spasm in that a procaine block of the lumbar sympathetic ganglia may afford relief at times. Further, many cases of thrombophlebitis, if observed early, will be seen to pass through a stage of arterial spasm in which pallor of arterial insufficiency precedes the plethora of venous occlusion. This so-called "white stage" can be sufficiently prolonged and intense as to produce superficial ischemic necrosis in the distal part of the extremity. This forms a subgroup of thrombophlebitis called *phlegmasia cerulea dolens* (Fogarty et al., 1963b; Stallworth et al., 1965).

As the white stage, which is usually fleeting, passes, the signs of inflammation and venous occlusion develop. Fever, swelling, redness and an aching pain less intense than the earlier pain of spasm develop.

A significant degree of lymphatic obstruction occurs by direct extension of the inflammation from the adjacent veins. This obstruction is manifested early by peau d'orange type of edema of the skin.

While the inflammation is present the edema persists in spite of elevation of the extremity. Complete subsidence leaves the venous and lymphatic drainage with a variable degree of obstruction. The degree is determined by the anatomic extent of the thrombophlebitis as well as its severity. Involvement may be limited to the veins of the calf or extend up through the iliac system to attack a major portion of the vena cava. Restoration of the venous drainage develops through 2 mechanisms. One is recanalization of the major vein and the second is development of collaterals. Tributaries of the major veins lying beneath the deep fascia of the limbs and those in the superficial layers all are forced to dilate. The former provide relatively efficient collaterals; the latter do not. Even when a significant-sized lumen is restored in a healed vein, such as the superficial femoral vein, the channel is functionally deficient in that the valves cannot be restored. Back flow or a tendency for back flow to occur is then present. This may be demonstrated by retrograde filling of the vein with Diodrast, if this solution is injected into the common femoral vein with the patient in a nearly vertical position on the x-ray table.

The course of the patient who has healed his acute phlebitis and is not managed adequately leads to continued morbidity. The complications are development of fibrosis in the skin and the subcutaneous tissues, pigmentation and the development of hypersensitivity of the skin leading to dermatitis and finally to ulceration.

Treatment. The treatment of thrombophlebitis of the lower extremities is aimed at the limitation and the early resolution of the acute phase and at the prevention of late sequelae.

Rest and elevation of the involved extremity with local application of heat, either by fomentation or carefully controlled heat cradle, is insisted upon until signs of inflammation have subsided. This simple treatment is often all that is required when only the superficial veins are involved. However, when the thrombus extends superiorly toward the foramen ovale, ligation of the great saphenous vein may be necessary. Heparin therapy is instituted with the aim of helping to limit the extent of vein occlusion by thrombus and possibly to limit fibrin deposition and organization of the intercellular edema fluid. Antibiotic therapy usually is applied, but the indication for its use must be questioned. The occasional bacteriologic studies which have been done on clots and tissues removed from thrombophlebitis have been negative.

The elevation of the extremity is continued after the acute process has subsided until the edema of the extremity is entirely gone. Then ambulation of the patient is conducted on a gradually increasing regimen, using elastic support with bandages and stockings. At no time should the period of ambulation be long enough to cause the development of swelling, and at the same time the increase in activity should be as rapid as possible within this limit. Such a regimen is often very time-consuming and will be tolerated by the patient only if he understands the purpose is to prevent the even more time-consuming late sequelae of his condition. Management for many months is often necessary but, in the majority, gainful occupations may be resumed early if periods of recumbency with elevation can be arranged during the working hours.

Complications of late stasis disease—dermatitis, fibrosis, pigmentation, secondary varicose veins, and ulceration—are frequently met with because the need of a careful regimen was not recognized at the beginning. The successful treatment of these complications again depends upon the complete management of the continued daily swelling (Luke, 1953).

It is fundamental to the surgical treatment of late stasis disease that edema be entirely controlled before operation and that the patient's long-term postoperative regimen be directed to prevent recurrence of swelling.

The actual operative treatment consists of total removal of the varicose veins, resection of the entire fibrotic and ulcerated area, and restoration of the skin defect by a skin graft (Julian, Dye and Schneewind, 1954; Moyer and Butcher, 1955). When the changes in the skin and the subcutaneous tissue are less advanced, operation may consist of exposure and ligation of the incompetent perforating veins in the region. This is accomplished by raising a flap of the tissues in the stasis area, exposing these veins at the deep fascial level (Linton, 1938). For chronic iliofemoral vein occlusion, cross-over vein grafts have been used (Dale, 1966; Dale and Harris, 1968).

SYNDROME OF SUPERIOR VENA CAVA OBSTRUCTION

The superior vena cava, formed by the confluence of the two innominate veins, runs a course of only 4 or 5 cm. before it enters the right atrium. Its only tributary, the azygos vein, enters in its upper half. The cava is vulnerable to obstruction, which usually causes a significant clinical problem because it is poorly compensated for by the collateral venous system available. The collateral route is long and circuitous, carrying venous blood from head, neck, upper extremities and shoulder girdle down and around to drain into the inferior vena cava. The syndrome which develops from superior caval occlusion is usually unremitting.

The elements of the clinical picture are due to the high venous pressure in the superior caval drainage bed and to the development of collateral veins. The venous stasis produces distention of the neck veins and a plethoric appearance of the face. The distention increases markedly when the patient bends over or lies down. Edema of his face develops during recumbency at night and may be so severe that the puffed-up eyelids cannot be opened in the morning. He learns to sleep with trunk elevated to minimize this. Dizziness and even fainting may result from stooping or bending forward too long.

The collateral veins first appear beneath the skin of the upper chest and progressively become prominent downward over the trunk. They are usually most pronounced anteriorly and the skin may be virtually covered with the plexus of enlarged veins. More effective collateral circulation is probably provided by the similarly enlarged veins at the level of the deep fascia of the chest and by the azygos system which connects the intercostal vessels with lumbar veins leading to the inferior vena cava.

Esophageal veins have been demonstrated by x-ray examination to be enlarged. Bleeding from such veins has been reported by Otto (1964).

Pathology. The occluding lesion is exterior to the vein almost without exception. Benign and malignant tumors in the superior mediastinal structures, aneurysms of the aortic arch or its branches, and inflammatory lesions of the superior mediastinum are the common causes.

Of these the tumors and aneurysms are visible on roentgenograms, which also serves to some extent to differentiate between them. The inflammatory lesions produce caval obstruction by formation of contracting scar tissue and do not always produce an x-ray visible mass. In some instances healed tuberculosis is demonstrated in tissues removed at surgery. In others the fibrous tissue is nonspecific on microscopic examination. It is likely that the inflammation responsible originally involved a mediastinal lymph node, whether tuberculous or pyogenic. In the latter instance it seems reasonable to suggest that an upper respiratory infection of the past had involved the mediastinal node.

Treatment. In instances displaying a superior mediastinal mass by roentgenography the management is dictated by the character of the tumor. Curative resection of a malignant lesion which has occluded the cava is not likely to be possible. Roentgen therapy offers the most to the patient if the lesion is a lymphoma. Resection of a benign tumor which may occasionally compress the vessel will be curative.

The problem of relief of the venous engorgement in chronic superior vena caval syndrome has proved to be a difficult one. Most attempts to do so involve the use of grafts bridging the occluded segment (Deterling, 1955). Homologous artery and prosthetic vascular grafts usually fail to remain open (Whiffen, 1965). An autogenous vein graft constructed from segments of the patient's femoral or jugular vein offers a better chance of continued patency. The discrepancy in caliber is overcome by incising longitudinally two segments of the selected graft and suturing them together to form one graft of double the original circumference (Fraser et al., 1968).

The difficulties encountered in overcoming this problem, pointed out by Effler (1962) and Templeton (1962), illustrate the general need for methods of replacing or restoring diseased venous channels in any location.

ACUTE THROMBOSIS OF THE SUBCLAVIAN VEIN (EFFORT THROMBOSIS)

The subclavian and the axillary veins are subject to acute thrombosis probably secondary to an intimal tear or to sustained compression by surrounding muscles. The fact that this may occur during or just after an activity involving prolonged or unusual use of the arms or sudden effort with the involved arm suggests the term "effort thrombosis."

The *onset* is acute and is characterized by the rapid development of edema of the extremity which often becomes severe. The pain which accompanies the swelling varies in intensity but is seldom severe. Pallor, cyanosis, and coolness of the hand and forearm are seen in the period of onset, but very soon the extremity becomes warmer than the uninvolved one.

Distention of the veins of the extremity itself may be hidden by the edema, but the subcutaneous veins about the shoulder which dilate to act as collateral channels become visible very soon after onset. The axillary vein is palpable as a firm cord, and if the thrombosis extends peripherally the brachial vein may also be palpable.

Prognosis. The prognosis is excellent. Venous drainage of the extremity becomes adequate in 1 to 4 weeks, either by collateral vein development or by eventual recanalization of the subclavian-axillary channel. Pulmonary emboli due to detachment of a portion of the thrombus are rare. Recurrences after complete recovery are infrequent.

Management usually requires only bed rest with elevation of the extremity. External application of heat or cold is not useful, and a compression dressing may be harmful. The effect of anticoagulant drugs has not been evaluated, but the lack of frequent evidence of progression of the thrombus is against their use.

In the infrequent instance of recurrences, changes in the patient's occupation or method of working are useful and surgical efforts to enlarge the muscular route through which the subclavian vein passes may be required.

Thrombectomy may be useful if done very

early before the thrombus is adherent to the vein. It is usually performed through a longitudinal incision in the subclavian vein exposed after transection of the pectoralis minor muscle near its insertion.

REFERENCES

Allen, E. W.: Thromboangiitis obliterans: methods of diagnosis of chronic occlusive arterial lesions distal to the wrist with illustrative cases. Am. J. Med. Sci., 178:237, 1929.

Alley, R. D., Van Meirop, L. H. S., Li, E. Y., Kausel, H. W., and Stranahan, A.: Traumatic aortic aneurysm, graftless excision and anastomosis. Arch. Surg., 83:158, 1961.

Atlas, L. N.: Lumbar sympathectomy in the treatment of selected cases of peripheral arteriosclerotic disease. Am. Heart J., 22:75-85, 1941.

Bahnson, H. T.: Considerations in the excision of aortic aneurysms. Ann Surg., 138:377, 1953.

Bahnson, H. T., and Spencer, F. C.: Excision of aneurysm of the ascending aorta with prosthetic replacement during cardiopulmonary bypass. Ann. Surg., 151:879, 1960.

Baird, R. J., Sivasankar, R., Hayward, R., and Wilson, D. R.: Popliteal aneurysms: review and analysis of 61 cases. Surgery, 59:911, 1966.

Barker, W. F., and Cannon, J. A.: Technic of endarterectomy. Am. Surgeon, 25:912-918, 1959.

Barner, H. B., Judd, D. R., Kaiser, G. C., William, V. L., and Hanlon, C. R.: Blood flow in femoropopliteal bypass vein grafts. Arch. Surg., 96:619, 1968.

Bazy, L.: A propos du procès-verbel sur l'endarteriectomie désobliterante. Mém. Acad. chir., 74:109, 1948.

Bean, W. B., and Ponseti, I. V.: Dissecting aneurysm produced by diet. Circulation, 12:185, 1955.

Bennett, D., and Cherry, J. K.: The natural history of traumatic aneurysms of the aorta. Surgery, 61:516, 1967.

Bernstein, E. F., Fisher, J. C., and Varco, R. L.: Is excision the optimum treatment for all abdominal aortic aneurysms? Surgery, 61:83, 1967.

Berry, R. E. L., Flotte, C. T., and Coller, F. A.: A critical evaluation of lumbar sympathectomy for peripheral arteriosclerotic vascular disease. Surgery, 37:115-129, 1955.

Blain, A., III, Zadeh, A. T., Teves, M. L., and Bing, R. J.: Lumbar sympathectomy for arteriosclerosis obliterans. Surgery, 53:164-172, 1963.

Blakemore, A. H.: Progressive, constrictive occlusion of the aorta with wiring and electrothermic coagulation for the treatment of arteriosclerotic aneurysms of the abdominal aorta. Ann. Surg., 137:760, 1953.

―――: Restorative endoaneurysmorrhaphy by vein graft inlay. Ann. Surg., 126:841, 1947.

Bloodwell, R. D., Hallman, G. L., Keats, A. S., and Cooley, D. A.: Carotid endarterectomy without a shunt. Arch. Surg., 96:644, 1968.

Boyd, A. M., Ratcliffe, A. H., Jepson, R. P., and James, G. W. H.: Intermittent claudication: a clinical study. J. Bone Joint Surg., 31-13:325-355, 1949.

Branham, H. H.: Aneurysmal varix of the femoral artery and vein following a gunshot wound. Internat. J. Surg., 3:250-251, 1890.

Brittain, R. S., and Earley, T. K.: Emergency thromboendarterectomy of the superior mesenteric artery: report of four cases. Ann Surg., 158:138-143, 1963.

Brock, R. C.: Discussion on reconstructive arterial surgery. Proc. Roy. Soc. Med., 46:115, 1953.

Brock, Russell: Late arterial embolectomy. J. Cardiov. Surg., 3:39-47, 1962.

Brodie, B. C.: Lectures Illustrative of Various Subjects in Pathology and Surgery. London, Longmans, 1846.

Buenger, R. E., and Hunter, J. A.: Reversible mesenteric artery stenoses due to methysergide maleate. J.A.M.A., 198:144, 1966.

Buerger, Leo: Thromboangiitis obliterans: a study of the vascular lesions leading to presenile spontaneous gangrene. Am. J. Med. Sci., 136:567-580, 1908.

Burchell, H. B.: Aortic dissection (dissecting hematoma; dissecting aneurysm of the aorta. Circulation, 12:1068, 1955.

Cannon, J. A., and Barker, W. F.: Successful management of obstructive femoral arteriosclerosis by endarterectomy. Surgery, 38:48-60, 1955.

Callon, J. A., Kawakami, I. G., and Barker, W. F.: Present status of aortoiliac endarterectomy for obliterative atherosclerosis. Arch. Surg., 82:813-825, 1961.

Carrel, A.: The surgery of the blood vessels. Bull. Johns Hopkins Hosp., 17:1907.

Coller, F. A., Campbell, K. N., Harris, B. M., and Berry, R. E. L.: The early results of sympathectomy in far advanced arteriosclerotic peripheral vascular disease. Surgery, 26:30-40, 1949.

Cooley, D. A., and Beall, A. C., Jr.: Technic of pulmonary embolectomy using temporary cardiopulmonary bypass: clinical and experimental considerations. J. Cardiov. Surg., 2:469-476, 1961.

Cooley, D. A., and De Bakey, M. E.: Ruptured aneurysms of abdominal aorta, excision and homograft replacement. Postgrad. Med., 16:334, 1954.

Coran, A. G., and Warren, R.: Arteriographic changes in femoropopliteal arteriosclerosis obliterans: five-year follow-up study. New Eng. J. Med., 274:643, 1966.

Crawford, E. S., Creech, O., Cooley, D. A., and De Bakey, M. E.: Treatment of arteriosclerotic occlusive disease of the lower extremities by excision and graft replacement or bypass. Surgery, 38:981-992, 1955.

Crawford, E. S., Edwards, W. H., De Bakey, M. E., Cooley, D. A., and Morris, G. C., Jr.: Peripheral arteriosclerotic aneurysm. J. Am. Geriat. Soc., 9:1-15, 1961.

Crawford, E. S., De Bakey, M. E., Morris, G. C., Jr., and Cooley, D. A.: Thromboobliterative disease of great vessels arising from aortic arch. J. Thorac. Cardiov. Surg., 43:38-53, 1962.

Crichlow, R. W., and Roberts, Brooke: Treatment

of popliteal aneurysms by restoration of continuity: review of 48 cases. Ann. Surg., 163:417, 1966.
Dale, W. A.: Autogenous vein grafts for femoropopliteal arterial repair. Surg., Gynec. Obstet., 123: 1282, 1966.
———: Chronic iliofemoral venous occlusion including seven cases of crossover vein grafting. Surgery, 59:117, 1966.
Dale, W. A., and Harris, J.: Cross-over vein grafts for iliac and femoral venous occlusion. Ann. Surg., 168:319, 1968.
Darling, R. C., Austen, W. G., and Linton, R. R.: Arterial embolism. Surg., Gynec. Obstet., 124:106, 1967.
Darling, R. C., Linton, R. R., and Razzuk, M. A.: Saphenous vein bypass grafts for femoropopliteal occlusive disease: reappraisal. Surgery, 61:31, 1967.
Davis, J. B., Grove, W. J., and Julian, O. C.: Thrombotic occlusion of the branches of the aortic arch, Martorell's syndrome: report of a case treated surgically. Ann. Surg., 144:124, 1956.
De Bakey, M. E.: A critical evaluation of the problem of thromboembolism. Surg., Gynec. Obstet., (Internat. Abstr. Surg.), 98:1-27, 1954.
De Bakey, M. E., and Cooley, D. A.: Successful resection of aneurysm of thoracic aorta and replacement by graft. J.A.M.A., 152:673, 1953a.
———: Surgical treatment of aneurysm of abdominal aorta by resection and restoration of continuity with homograft. Surg., Gynec. Obstet., 97:257, 1953b.
De Bakey, M. E., Cooley, D. A., and Creech, O., Jr.: Surgical considerations of dissecting aneurysms of the aorta. Ann. Surg., 142:586, 1955.
DeBakey, M. E., Crawford, E. S., Cooley, D. A., Morris, G. C., Jr., Garrett, H. E., and Fields, W. S.: Cerebral arterial insufficiency: 1-11 year results following arterial reconstructive operation. Ann. Surg., 161:921, 1965.
De Bakey, M. E., Crawford, E. S., Cooley, D. A., Morris, G. C., Jr., Royster, T. S., and Abbott, W. P.: Aneurysm of the abdominal aorta: analysis of results of graft replacement therapy one to eleven years after operation. Ann. Surg., 160:622, 1964.
De Bakey, M. E., Creech, O., and Woodhall, J. P.: Evaluation of sympathectomy in arteriosclerotic peripheral vascular disease. J.A.M.A., 144:1227-1231, 1950.
De Bakey, M. E., Henly, W. S., Cooley, D. A., Crawford, E. S., and Morris, G. C., Jr.: Surgical treatment of dissecting aneurysm of the aorta: analysis of 72 cases. Circulation, 24:290, 1961a.
De Bakey, M. E., Morris, G. C., Jr., Crawford, E. S., and Cooley, D. A.: Surgical considerations of renal hypertension. J. Cardiov. Surg., 2:435-448, 1961b.
De Bakey, M. E., Morris, G. C., Jr., Jordan, G. L., Jr., and Cooley, D. A.: Segmental thromboobliterative disease of branches of aortic arch. J.A.M.A., 166:998, 1958.
De Bakey, M. E., and Simeone, F. A.: Battle injuries of the arteries in World War II. Ann. Surg., 123:534-579, 1946.

DeCamp, P. T., and Birchell, R.: Recognition and treatment of renal arterial stenosis associated with hypertension. Surgery, 43:134, 1958.
de Takats, G., Fowler, E. F., Jordan, P., and Risley, T. C.: Sympathectomy in the treatment of peripheral vascular sclerosis. J.A.M.A., 144:1227-1231, 1950.
de Takats, G., and Marshall, M. R.: Surgical treatment of arteriosclerotic aneurysms of the abdominal aorta. Arch. Surg., 64:307, 1952.
Deterling, R. A., and Bhonslay, S. B.: An evaluation of synthetic materials and fabrics suitable for blood vessel replacement. Surgery, 38:71-91, 1955.
———: Use of vessel grafts and plastic prostheses for relief of superior vena caval obstruction. Surgery, 38:1008, 1955.
Deterling, R. A., Jr., Vargas, L. L., and McAllister, F. F.: Follow-up studies of patients with embolic occlusion of aortic bifurcation. Ann. Surg., 155: 383-391, 1962.
DeWeese, J. A., Barner, H. B., Mahoney, E. B., and Rob, C. G.: Autogenous venous bypass grafts and thromboendarterectomies for atherosclerotic lesions of femoropopliteal arteries. Ann. Surg., 163:205, 1966.
DeWeese, M. S., and Hunter, D. C., Jr.: Vena cava filter for prevention of pulmonary embolism: five-year clinical experience. Arch. Surg., 86:852-868, 1963.
Dillard, D. H., Vetto, R. R., Bruce, R. A., and Merendino, K. A.: Correction of aneurysm of the ascending aorta and of aortic insufficiency in Marfan's syndrome. Am. J. Surg., 104:337, 1962.
Donaldson, G. A.: The therapy and prophylaxis of venous thrombosis and pulmonary embolism. S. Clin. N. Am., 27:1037-1051, 1947.
dos Santos, J. C.: Sur la désobstruction des thromboses artérielles anciennes. Mém. Acad. chir., 73: 409-411, 1947.
Dubost, C., Allary, M.; and Deconomas, N.: Resection of an aneurysm of the abdominal aorta. Arch. Surg., 64:405, 1952.
Dye, W. S.: Recognition and treatment of acute vascular injuries associated with orthopedic problems. Chicago Medicine, 1963a.
———: Technics in arterial repair. Clin. Orthop., 28:38-43, 1963b.
Dye, W. S., and Hunter, J. A.: Reconstructive arterial surgery: local treatment for a generalized disease. Med. Clin. N. Am., 51:215, 1967.
Dye, W. S., Julian, O. C., Javid, H., and Hunter, J. A.: Surgical treatment of arteriosclerosis obliterans. Presented at the Middle East Medical Assembly, May, 1961. Official Publication of Transactions of Middle East Medical Assembly.
Dye, W. S., Olwin, J. H., Javid, H., and Julian, O. C.: Arterial embolectomy. Arch. Surg., 70:715-722, 1955.
Edmunds, L. H., Jr., Darling, R. C., and Linton, R. R.: Surgical management of popliteal aneurysms. Circulation, 32:517, 1965.
Edwards, W. S.: Composite reconstruction of small leg arteries after endarterectomy. Surgery, 51:58-61, 1962.
Edwards, W. S., and Lyons, C.: Traumatic arterial

spasm and thrombosis. Ann. Surg., 140:319-323, 1954.
Edwards, W. S., and Tapp, J. S.: Chemically treated nylon tubes as arterial grafts. Surgery, 38:61-70, 1955.
Effler, D. B., and Groves, L. K.: Superior vena caval obstruction, J. Thorac. Cardiov. Surg., 43:574-584, 1962.
Ehrenfeld, W. K., Levin, S. M., and Wylie, E. J.: Venous crossover bypass grafts for arterial insufficiency. Ann. Surg., 167:287, 1968.
Eiseman, B., and Rainer, W. G.: Clinical management of post-traumatic rupture of the thoracic aorta. J. Thoracic Surg., 35:347, 1958.
Elkin, D. C.: Aneurysm following surgical procedure. Ann. Surg., 127:769, 1948.
Elkin, D. C., and Cooper, F. W.: Surgical treatment of insidious thrombosis of aorta. Ann. Surg., 130: 417, 1949.
Elkin, D. C., and Warren, J. V.: Arteriovenous fistulae: their effect on the circulation. J.A.M.A., 134:1524-1528, 1947.
Estes, J. E., Jr.: Abdominal aortic aneurysms; a study of 102 cases. Circulation, 2:258, 1950.
Fisher, M.: Occlusion of the internal carotid artery. Arch. Neurol. Psychiat., 65:346, 1951.
Fogarty, T. J., Cranley, J. J., Krause, R. J., Strasser, E. S., and Hafner, C. D.: A method for extraction of arterial emboli and thrombi. Surg., Gynec. Obstet., 116:241, 1963a.
Fogarty, T. J., Cranley, J. J., Krause, R. J., Strasser, E. S., and Hafner, C. D.: Surgical management of phlegmasia cerulea dolens. Arch. Surg., 86:256-263, 1963b.
Fogarty, T. J., Dennis, D., and Krippaehne, W. W.: Surgical management of iliofemoral venous thrombosis. Am. J. Surg., 112:211, 1966.
Fontaine, R.: Remarks concerning venous thrombosis and its sequelae. Surgery, 41:6-24, 1957.
Fontaine, R., Buck, P., Riveaux, R., Kim, M., and Hubinot, J.: Treatment of arterial occlusion, comparative value of thrombectomy, trromboendarterectomy, arteriovenous shunt, and vascular grafts: fresh venous autografts. Lyon chir., 46:73, 1951.
Foster, J. H., Oates, J. A., Rhamy, R. K.. Klatte, E. C., Pettinger. W. A., Burko, H., Younger, R. K., and Scott, H. W., Jr.: Detection and treatment of patients with renovascular hypertension Surgery, 60:240, 1966.
Fraser, R. E., Halseth, W. L., Johnson, B., and Paton, B. C.: Experimental replacement of the superior vena cava. Arch. Surg., 96:328, 1968.
Freeman, N. E.: Arterial repair in the treatment of aneurysms and arteriovenous fistulae: a report of 18 successful restorations. Ann. Surg., 124:888-919, 1946.
Friesen, G., Ivins, J. C., and Janes, J. M.: Popliteal aneurysms. Surgery, 51:90-98, 1962.
Garamella, J. J., Lynch, M. F., Jensen, N. K., Sterns, L. P., and Schmidt, W. R.: Endarterectomy and thrombectomy for totally occluded extracranial internal carotid artery: use of Fogarty balloon catheters. Ann. Surg., 164:325, 1966.
Garrett, H. E., and De Bakey, M. E.: Distal posterior tibial artery bypass with autogenous vein graft: report of three cases. Surgery, 60:283, 1966.
Gifford, R. W., Jr., Tarkin, T. W., and Janes, J. M.: Atherosclerotic popliteal aneurysm in a man 35 years old. Circulation, 9:363, 1954.
Goldblatt, H., Lynch, J., Hanjal, R. F., and Summerville, W. W.: Studies on experimental hypertension: production of persistent elevation of systolic blood pressure by means of renal ischemia. J. Exp. Med., 59:347, 1934.
Gorham, L. W.: Pulmonary embolism. I. Clinicopathologic investigation of 100 cases of massive embolism of pulmonary artery; diagnosis by physical signs and differentiation from acute myocardial infarction. Arch. Int. Med., 108:8-22, 1961.
Gurin, D., Bulmer, J. W., and Derby, R.: Dissecting aneurysm of aorta: diagnosis and operative relief of acute arterial obstruction due to this cause. N. Y. J. Med., 35:1200, 1935.
Haller, J. A., Jr.: Thrombectomy for acute iliofemoral venous thrombosis in postpartum period. Surg., Gynec. Obstet., 112:75, 1961.
Hardin, C. A.: Bypass saphenous grafts for relief of venous obstruction of extremity. Surg., Gynec. Obstet., 115:709-712, 1962.
Harris, E. J.: Patency after thrombectomy for iliofemoral thrombosis. Ann. Surg., 167:91, 1968.
Harris, P. D., Malm, J. R., Bigger, J. T., Jr., and Bowman, F. O., Jr.: Follow-up studies of acute dissecting aortic aneurysms managed with antihypertensive agents. Circulation (Supp. 1), 35 & 36:183-187, 1967.
Hermann, L. G., Cranley, J. J., and Prenninger, R. M.: Importance of collateral circulation in obliterative arterial disease of lower extremities. Geriatrics, 9:1-7, 1954.
Hirst, A. E., Jr., Johns, V. J., Jr., and Kime, S. W., Jr.: Dissecting aneurysm of the aorta: A review of 505 cases. Medicine, 37:217, 1958.
Holden, W. D.: Reconstruction of the femoral artery for arteriosclerotic thrombosis. Surgery, 27: 417-422, 1950.
Holman, E.: Arteriovenous Aneurysm: Abnormal Communications Between the Arterial and Venous Circulations. p. 244. New York, Macmillan, 1937.
Homans, J.: Thrombophlebitis of lower extremities. Ann. Surg., 87:461, 1928.
Hufnagel, C. A., and Conrad, P. W.: Dissecting aneurysms of the ascending aorta: Direct approach to repair. Surgery, 51:84, 1962.
Hufnagel, C. A.: The use of rigid and flexible plastic prostheses for arterial replacement. Surgery, 37: 165-174, 1955.
Hughes, C. W.: Arterial repair during the Korean War. Ann. Surg., 147:555, 1958.
Hughes, C. W., Jahnke, E. J.: Surgery of traumatic arteriovenous fistulas and aneurysms: five year follow-up study of 215 lesions. Ann. Surg., 148: 790-797, 1958.
Hume, D. M., and Porter, R. R.: Acute dissecting aortic aneurysms. Surgery, 53:122, 1963.
Hunt, J. R.: The role of the carotid arteries in the causation of vascular lesions of the brain, with remarks on certain special features of the symptomatology. Am. J. Med. Sci., 147:704, 1914.

Hunter, J. A., and Julian, O. C.: The surgical correction of hypertension of renovascular origin. *In*: Luisada, A. A. (ed.): Cardiology and the Encyclopedia of the Cardiovascular System. Supplement No. 1. Chap. 10. pp. 43-49. New York, McGraw-Hill, 1962.

Hunter, J. A., Julian, O. C., Dye, W. S., and Javid, H.: Hypertension of renal vascular origin. M. Bull. Presbyterian-St. Luke's Hosp., 2:113-122, 1963a.

Hunter, J. A., Julian, O. C., Dye, W. S., Javid, H., Feinhandler, E., and Emanuel, B.: Hypertension in a child relieved by bilateral renal arterioplasty. Am. J. Surg., 106:43-48, 1963b.

Hunter, J. A., Julian, O. C., Javid, H., and Dye, W. S.: Arteriosclerotic aneurysms of the popliteal artery. J. Cardiov. Surg., 2:404, 1961.

Hunter, J. A., Wilcox, H. G., and Kark, R. M.: Problems in the management of renovascular hypertension. Surg. Clin. N. Am., 47:91, 1967.

Jahnke, E. J., Jr.: Late structural and functional results of arterial injuries primarily repaired: study of 115 cases. Surgery, 43:175-183, 1958.

Jahnke, E. J., Jr., Fisher, G. W., and Jones, R. C.: Acute traumatic rupture of the thoracic aorta. Report of six consecutive cases of successful early repair, J. Thorac. Cardiov. Surg., 48:63-77, 1964.

Jahnke, E. J., and Seeley, S. F.: Acute vascular injuries in the Korean War: an analysis of 77 consecutive cases. Ann. Surg., 138:158, 1953.

Janes, J. M., and Ivens, J. C.: A method of dealing with arteriosclerotic popliteal aneurysms. Surgery, 29:398, 1951.

Janeway, T. C.: Note on the blood pressure changes following reduction of the renal artery circulation. Proc. Soc. Exp. Biol. Med., 6:109, 1909.

Javid, H.: Surgical management of cerebral vascular insufficiency. Arch. Surg., 80:883-889, 1960.

———: Surgical therapy of the aorta—aneurysms and related problems. Chicago Medicine, 1961.

———: Vascular injuries of the neck. Clin. Orthop., 28:70-78, 1963.

———: Surgical treatment of arterial emergencies. Modern Treatment, 4:405, 1967.

Javid, H., Dye, W. S., and Cagle, J. E.: Importance of vascular evaluation in surgical patients. S. Clin. North Am., 44:25-33, 1964.

Javid, H., Dye, W. S., Grove, W. J., and Julian, O. C.: Resection of ruptured aneurysms of the abdominal aorta. Ann. Surg., 142:613-623, 1955.

Javid, H., and Julian, O. C.: Surgical management of internal carotid occlusion. Am. Heart Bull., 11: 84-88, 1962.

———: Prevention of stroke by carotid and vertebral surgery. Med. Clin. N. Am., 51:113, 1967.

Johnson, J., Kirby, C. K., Greifenstein, F. E., and Castillo, A.: The experimental and clinical use of vein grafts to replace defects of large arteries. Surgery, 26:945-956, 1949.

Jones, E. L., Peters, A. F., and Gasior, R. M.: Early management of battle casualties in Vietnam. Arch. Surg., 97:1-15, 1968.

Julian, O. C.: Surgical treatment of chronic aortoiliac and femoral arterial disorders. Modern Treatment, 4:386, 1967.

———: Chronic occlusion of the aorta and iliac arteries. S. Clin. North Am. 40:139-151, 1960.

Julian, O. C., Deterling, R. A., Jr., Dye, W. S., Bhonslay, S., Grove, W. J., Lopez-Belio, M., and Javid, H.: Dacron tube and bifurcation arterial prostheses produced to specification. II. Continued clinical use and the addition of microcrimping. Arch. Surg., 78:260-270, 1959a.

Julian, O. C., and Dye, W. S.: Treatment of peripheral vascular disease: modern concepts. S. Clin. North Am., 32:263-285, 1952.

Julian, O. C., Dye, W. S., Javid, H., and Grove, W. J.: The use of vessel grafts in the treatment of popliteal aneurysms. Surgery, 38:970-980, 1955.

Julian, O. C., Dye, W. S., Javid, H., and Hunter, J. A.: Handbook of Cardiovascular Surgery. Chicago, Year Book Publishers, 1962.

———: Ulcerative lesions of the carotid artery bifurcation. Arch. Surg., 86:803-809, 1963.

Julian, O. C., and Hunter, J. A.: Vascular injuries occurring in relation to bone and joint trauma. Clin. Orthop., 28:14-20, 1963.

Julian, O. C., Dye, W. S., Olwin, J. H., and Jordan, P. M.: Direct surgery of arteriosclerosis. Ann. Surg., 136:459-474, 1952.

Julian, O. C., Dye, W. S., and Schneewind, J.: Surgical management of ulcerative stasis disease of the lower extremities. Arch. Surg., 68:757-768, 1954.

Julian, O. C., Grove, W. J., Dye, W. S., Javid, H., and Sadove, M. S.: New methods of surgical treatment of degenerative diseases of the abdominal aorta. Ann. Int. Med., 41:36-49, 1954.

Julian, O. C., Grove, W. J., Dye, W. S., Olwin, J. H., and Sadove, M. S.: Direct surgery of arteriosclerosis: resection of abdominal aorta with homologous aortic graft replacement Ann. Surg., 138: 387-403, 1953.

Julian, O. C., Javid, H., Dye, W. S., and El Issa, S.: Diagnosis and surgical approach to aorticoiliac arterial disease. Am. J. Cardiol., 4:622-631, 1959b.

Julian, O. C., and Shabart, E. J.: Lumbar sympathectomy in peripheral vascular disease. Arch. Surg., 61:804-809, 1950.

Key, Einar: Embolectomy in the treatment of circulatory disturbances in the extremities. Surg., Gynec. Obstet., 36:309-316, 1923.

Killen, D. A., Foster, J. H., Gobbel, W. G., Jr., Stephenson, S. E., Jr., Collins, H. A., Billings, F. T., and Scott, H. W., Jr.: Subclavian steal syndrome J. Thorac. & Cardiov. Surg., 51:539, 1966.

Kirklin, J. W., Waugh, J. M., Grindlay, J. H., Openshaw, C. R., and Allen, E. V.: Surgical treatment of arteriosclerotic aneurysms of the abdominal aorta. Arch. Surg., 67:632-644, 1953.

Kirtley, J. A., Jr., Garrett, S. Y., and Martin, R. S., Jr.: An evaluation of lumbar sympathectomy in 200 consecutive cases of peripheral vascular disorders. Surgery, 33:256-267, 1953.

Klippel, A. P., and Butcher, H. R.: The unoperated abdominal aortic aneurysm. Am. J. Surg., 111: 629, 1966.

Kouchoukos, N. T., Levy, J. F., Balfour, J. F., and Butcher, H. R.: Operative therapy for aortoiliac arterial occlusive disease. Arch. Surg., 96:628, 1968.

Kunlin, J.: Le traitment de l'ischémie artérique par la graffe veineuse longue. Rev. chir., 70:206, 1951.

———: Venous grafts in therapy of endarteritis obliterans. Arch. mal. coeur, 42:371, 1949.

Lam, C. R., and Aram, H. H.: Resection of the descending thoracic aorta for aneurysm; a report of the use of a homograft in a case and an experimental study. Ann. Surg., 134: 743-752, 1951.

Leather, R. P., Clark, W. R., Powers, S. R., Parker, F. B., Bernard, H. R., and Eckert, C.: Five year experience with the Moretz vena caval clip in 62 patients. Arch. Surg., 97:357, 1968.

Leriche, R.: De la résection du carrefour aortico-iliaque avec double sympathectomie lombaire pour thrombose artéritique de l'aorte; le syndrome de l'oblitération termino-aortique pour artérite. Presse méd., 48:601-604, 1940.

Leriche, R., Froment, R., and Vacton, A.: Artérectomie pour embolie de l'artère fémorale superficielle: rétrocession de tous les terribles. Lyon méd., 154:416-422, 1934.

Leriche, R., and Kunlin, J.: Essais de désobstruction des artères thromboses suivant la technique de J. Cid dos Santos. Lyon chir., 42:675, 1947.

Lin, P. M., Javid, H., and Doyle, E. J.: Partial internal carotid artery occlusion treated by primary resection and vein graft: report of a case. J. Neurosurg., 13:650, 1956.

Linton, R. R.: The arteriosclerotic aneurysm: a report of 14 patients treated by preliminary lumbar sympathetic ganglionectomy and aneurysmectomy. Surgery, 26:41, 1949.

———: Intrasaccular wiring of abdominal arteriosclerotic aortic aneurysms by the "pack" method. Angiology, 2:458, 1951.

———: A new surgical technique for the treatment of postphlebitic varicose ulcers of the lower leg. New Eng. J. Med., 219:367, 1938.

———: Some practical considerations in the surgery of blood vessel grafts. Surgery, 38:817-834, 1955.

Linton, R. R., and Darling, R. C.: Autogenous saphenous vein bypass grafts in femoropopliteal obliterative arterial disease. Surgery, 51:62-73, 1962.

Linton, R. R., and White, P. D.: Arteriovenous fistula between the right common iliac artery and the inferior vena cava: report of a case of its occurrence following an operation for a ruptured intervertebral disc, with cure by operation. Arch. Surg., 50:6-13, 1945.

Lord, J. W.: Traumatic lesions of arteries, S. Clin. N. Am., 30:377-386, 1950.

Luke, J. C.: The sequelae of thrombophlebitis. Angiology, 4:413, 1953.

Luke, J. C., and Levitan, B. A.: Revascularization of kidney in hypertension due to renal artery stenosis. Arch. Surg., 79:269-275, 1959.

Lyons, C., and Galbraith, G.: Surgical treatment of atherosclerotic occlusion of internal carotid artery. Ann. Surg., 146:487, 1957.

McCloy, R. M., Spittell, J. A., Jr., and McGoon, D. C.; Prognosis in aortic dissection (dissecting aortic hematoma or aneurysm). Circulation, 31: 665, 1965.

McKusick, V. A.: Cardiovascular aspects of Marfan's syndrome: a heritable disorder of connective tissue. Circulation, 11:321, 1955.

MacVaugh, Horace, III, and Roberts, Brooke: Results of resection of abdominal aortic aneurysm. Surg., Gynec. Obstet., 113: 17-23, 1961.

Mahorner, H. R., and Ochsner, A.: A new test for evaluating circulation in the venous system of the lower extremity affected by varicosities. Arch. Surg., 33:479, 1938.

Mannick, J. A., Suter, C. G., and Hume, D. M.: "Subclavian steal" syndrome: further documentation. J.A.M.A., 182:254-258, 1962.

Matas, R.: Endoaneurysmorrhaphy. Surg., Gynec. Obstet., 30:456, 1920.

May, A. G., De Weese, J. A., and Rob, C. G.: Effect of sympathectomy on blood flow in arterial stenosis. Ann. Surg., 158:182-188, 1963.

May, A. G., DeWeese, J. A., Frank, I., Mahoney, E. B., and Rob, C. G.: Surgical treatment of abdominal aortic aneurysms. Surgery, 63:711, 1968.

Miles, R. M., Dacus, D., and Booth, J. L.: The dynamics of peripheral arterial embolism. Ann. Surg., 167:801, 1968.

Moore, W. S., Cofferata, H. T., Hall, A. D., and Blaisdell, F. W.: In defense of grafts across the inguinal ligament: an evaluation of early and late results of aorto-femoral bypass grafts. Ann. Surg., 168:207, 1968.

Morris, G. C., Jr., De Bakey, M. E., and Bernhard, V.: Abdominal angina. S. Clin. N. A., 46:919, 1966.

Morris, G. C., Jr., De Bakey, M. E., Crawford, E. S., Cooley, D. A., and Zanger, L. C. C.: Late results of surgical treatment for renovascular hypertension. Surg., Gynec. Obstet., 122:1-7, 1966.

Morris, G. C., Jr., De Bakey, M. E., Cooley, D. A., and Crawford, E. S.: Surgical treatment of renal hypertension. Ann. Surg., 151:854-66, 1960.

Morton, J. J., and Scott, W. J. N.: Ligation of the abdominal aorta for aneurysm. Ann. Surg., 119: 457-467, 1944.

Moyer, C. A., and Butcher, H. R., Jr.: Stasis ulcers; an evaluation of the effectiveness of 3 methods of therapy and the implication of obliterative cutaneous lymphangitis as a credible etiologic factor. Ann. Surg., 141:577, 1955.

Mulder, D. G., Dilley, R. B., and Joseph, W. L.: Surgical management of aneurysms of the thoracic aorta. Surgery, 60:142, 1966.

Najafi, Hassan: Aortic root aneurysm: diagnosis and treatment. J.A.M.A., 197:133, 1966.

Najafi, H., Javid, H., Dye, W. S., Hunter, J. A., and Julian, O. C.: Kinked internal carotid artery: clinical evaluation and surgical correction. Arch. Surg., 89:134-143, 1964.

Nicoladoni, C.: Phlebarteriectasie der rechten oberen Extremität. Arch. klin. Chir., 18:252-274, 1875.

Ochsner, A., and De Bakey, M. E.: Thrombophlebitis and phlebothrombosis. South Surgeon, 8:269-290, 1939.

Olwin, J. H., Dye, W. S., and Julian, O. C.: Late peripheral arterial embolectomy. Arch. Surg., 66: 480-487, 1953.

Otto, D. L., and Kurtzman, R. S.: Esophageal varices in superior vena cava obstruction. Am. Roentgenol., 92:1000, 1964.

Oudot, J., and Beaconsfield, P.: Thrombosis of the aortic bifurcation treated by resection and homograft replacement: report of 5 cases. Arch. Surg., 66:365, 1953.

Parmley, L. F., Mattingly, T. W., Manion, W. C., and Jahnke, E. J.: Non-penetrating traumatic injury of the aorta. Circulation, 17:1086, 1958.

Perloff, D., Sokolow, M., Wylie, E. J., Smith, D. R., and Palubinskas, A. J.: Hypertension secondary to renal artery occlusive disease. Circulation, 24:1286, 1961.

Perthes, G.: Ueber die Operation der Unterschenkelvaricen nach Trendelenburg. Deutsche med. Wschr., 1:253-357, 1895.

Poutasse, E. F.: Surgical treatment for renal hypertension: results in patients with occlusive disease of renal arteries. J. Urol., 82:403, 1959.

Poutasse, E. F., Dustan, H., and Page, I. H.: Surgical treatment of hypertension due to renal vascular lesions. M. Clin. N. Am., 45:479-486, 1961.

Price, D. J.: Subclavian steal. GP, 28:112-117, 1963.

Pringle, J. H.: Two cases of vein grafting for the maintenance of direct arterial circulation. Lancet, 1:1795-1796, 1913.

Rasmussen, J. A., Potter, S. E., and Best, R. R.: Management of acute massive venous occlusion. Surgery, 40:387-390, 1956.

Raynaud, A. G. M.: De l'asphyxie locale et de la gangrène symétrique des extrémités. p. 6. Paris, Rignoux, 1862.

Reboul, H., and Huguier, J.: Endarteriectomie aortico-iliaque gauche datant de 16 mois. Mém. Acad. chir., 75:318, 1949.

Rob, Charles: Surgical diseases of celiac and mesenteric arteries. Arch. Surg., 93:21, 1966.

Rob, C., and Wheeler, E. B.: Thrombosis of internal carotid artery treated by arterial surgery. Brit. Med. J., 2:264-266, 1957.

Rohman, M., Goetz, R. H., and State, D.: Surgical treatment of dissecting aneurysms of the aorta with cardiac tamponade. J. Thorac. Cardiov. Surg., 46:498, 1963.

Royster, T. S., and Reiss, I.: Bypass grafting from the profunda femoris to the distal anterior tibial artery. Arch. Surg., 97:521, 1968.

Sawyer, P. N., Kaplitt, M. J., Sobel, S., and DiMaio, D.: Application of gas endarterectomy to atherosclerotic peripheral vessels and coronary arteries: clinical and experimental results. Circulation (supp. 1), 35-36:163-168, 1967.

Schafer, P. W., and Hardin, C. A.: The use of temporary polyethylene shunts to permit occlusion, resection, and frozen homologous graft replacement of vital vessel segments. Surgery, 31:186, 1952.

Schnitker, M. A., and Bayer, C. A.: Dissecting aneurysms of the aorta in young individuals, particularly in association with pregnancy: with report of a case. Ann. Int. Med., 20:486, 1944.

Seeley, S. F., Hughes, C. W., and Jahnke, E. J.: Direct anastomosis versus ligation and excision in traumatic arteriovenous fistulae and aneurysms: experience with 150 consecutive Korean wounds. S. Forum, 152:154, 1952.

Sharp, E. H.: Pulmonary embolectomy: successful removal of massive pulmonary embolus with support of cardiopulmonary bypass: case report. Ann. Surg., 156:1-4, 1962.

Shaw, R. S.: Acute dissecting aortic aneurysm: treatment by fenestration of the internal wall of the aneurysm. New Eng. J. Med., 253:331, 1955.

Shumacker, H. B., Jr.: The problem of maintaining the continuity of the artery in the surgery of aneurysms and arteriovenous fistulae. Ann. Surg., 127:207-230, 1948.

Shumacker, H. B., Jr., Harris, E. J., and Siderys, H.: Pliable plastic tubes as aortic substitutes. Surgery, 37:80-93, 1955.

Shumacker, H. B., Jr., and Mandelbaum, I.: Management of arterial embolism. Am. J. Surg., 28:199-205, 1962.

Siekert, R. G., Whisnant, J. P., Baker, H. L., Jr., Bernatz, P. E., Ellis, H. F., and Millikan, C. H.: Symposium on surgical treatment of extracranial occlusive cerebrovascular disease. Proc. Staff Meet. Mayo Clin., 35:473-502, 1960.

Smith, G. W., Muller, W. H., and Beckwith, J. R.: Surgical results and the diagnostic evaluation of renovascular hypertension. Ann. Surg., 167:669, 1968.

Spencer, F. C., and Blake, H.: A report of the successful surgical treatment of aortic regurgitation from a dissecting aortic aneurysm in a patient with the Marfan syndrome. J. Thorac. Cardiov. Surg., 44:238, 1962.

Spencer, F. C., Guerin, P. F., Blake, H. A., and Bahnson, H. T.: Report of 15 patients with traumatic rupture of the thoracic aorta. J. Thorac. Cardiov. Surg., 41:1, 1961.

Spencer, F. C., Quattlebaum, J. K., Quattlebaum, J. K., Jr., Sharp, E. H., and Jude, J. R.: Plication of inferior vena cava for pulmonary embolism: report of 20 cases. Ann. Surg., 155:827-837, 1962.

Spencer, F. C. Stamey, T. A., Bahnson, H. T., and Cohen, A.: Diagnosis and treatment of hypertension due to occlusive disease of renal artery. Ann. Surg., 154:674-697, 1961.

Spencer, F. C., and Tompkins, R. K.: Management of acute arterial injuries. Postgrad. Med., 28:476-481, 1960.

Stallworth, J. M., Bradham, G. B., Kletke, R. R., and Price, R. G., Jr.: Phlegmasia cerulea dolens: 10-year review. Ann. Surg., 161:801, 1965.

Stewart, B. H., DeWeese, M. S., Conway, J., and Corea, R. J., Jr.: Renal hypertension: appraisal of diagnostic studies and of direct operative treatment. Arch. Surg., 85:617-636, 1962.

Stoney, R. J., and Wylie, E. J.: Recognition and surgical management of visceral ischemic syndromes. Ann. Surg., 164:714, 1966.

Strassman, G.: Traumatic rupture of aorta. Am. Heart J., 33:508, 1947.

Swan, H., Maaske, C., Johnson, N., and Grover, R.: Arterial homografts: II. Resection of thoracic aortic aneurysm using a stored human arterial transplant. Arch. Surg., 61:732, 1950.

Szilagyi, D. E., Smith, R. F., DeRusso, E. J., Elliott, J. P., and Sherrin, F. W.: Contribution of abdominal aortic aneurysmectomy to prolongation of life. Ann. Surg., 164:678, 1966.

Szilagyi, D. E., Smith, R. F., Macksood, A. J., and

Whitcomb, J. G.: Expanding and ruptured abdominal aortic aneurysms: problems of diagnosis and treatment. Arch. Surg., 83:395-408, 1961.

Taber, R. E., Zikria, E., Hershey, E. A., and Lam, C. R.: Prevention of pulmonary emboli with a vena caval clip. J.A.M.A., 195:889, 1966.

Templeton, J. Y., III: Endvenectomy for relief of obstruction of the superior vena cava. Am. J. Surg., 104:70-76, 1962.

Thompson, J. E., Kartchner, M. M., Austin, D. J., Wheeler, C. G., and Patman, R. D.: Carotid endarterectomy for cerebrovascular insufficiency (stroke): follow-up of 359 cases. Ann. Surg., 163:751, 1966.

Trendelenburg, F.: Ueber die Unterbindung der Vena Saphena Magna bei Unterschenkelvaricen. Beitr. Z. Klin. Chir., 7:195, 1890.

Trippel, O. H.: Surgical management of hypertension due to renal artery occlusion. S. Clin. N. Am., 40:177-189, 1960.

Tyson, R. R., and DeLaurentis, D. A.: Femoropopliteal bypass. Circulation, 33-34 (Suppl. 1): 183, 1966.

Varco, R. L., Doberneck, R. C., and Funke, J. L.: Hypertension secondary to congenital stenosis of renal artery. Lancet, 82:76-79, 1962.

Veal, J. R., and Dugan, T. J.: Peripheral arterial embolism. Ann. Surg., 133:603-609, 1951.

Voorhees, A. B., Jaretzki, A., III, and Blakemore, A. H.: The use of tubes constructed from vinyon "N" cloth in bridging arterial defects. Ann. Surg., 135:332, 1952.

Vye, W. J., and Craft, R. O.: Visceral angina. Surg. Gynec. Obstet., 117:417, 1963.

Wells, B. A., Keats, A. S., and Cooley, D. A.: Increased tolerance to cerebral ischemia produced by general anesthesia during temporary carotid occlusion. Surgery, 54:216-223, 1963.

Wesolowski, S. A., Fries, C. C., Liebig, W. J., Sawyer, P. N., and Deterling, R. A., Jr.: Synthetic vascular graft: new concepts: new materials. Arch. Surg., 84:56-72, 1962.

Wheat, M. W., Jr., Palmer, R. F., Bartley, T. D., and Seelman, R. C.: Treatment of dissecting aneurysms of the aorta without surgery. J. Thorac. Cardiov. Surg., 50:364, 1965.

Wheeler, C. G., Thompson, J. E., Austin, D. J., Patman, R. D., and Stockton, R. L.: Interruption of inferior vena cava for thromboembolism: comparison of ligation and plication. Ann. Surg., 163:199, 1966.

Whiffen, J. D., and Gott, V. L.: Prosthetic thoracic vena cava grafts. J. Thorac. Cardiov. Surg., 50:31, 1965.

White, J. C., Smithwick, R. H., and Simeone, F. A.: The Autonomic Nervous System. p. 569. New York, Macmillan, 1952.

Whitman, E. J., and McGoon, D. C.: Surgical management of aortoiliac occlusive vascular disease. J.A.M.A., 179:923-929, 1962.

Willman, V. L., and Hanlon, C. R.: Safer operation in aortic saddle embolism: four consecutive successful embolectomies via the fmoral arteries under local anesthesia. Ann. Surg., 150:568-574, 1959.

Winiwarter, Felix von: Ueber eine eigenthümliche Form von Endarteriitis und Endophlebitis mit Gangrän des Fusse. Arch. klin. Chir., 23:202-226, 1879.

Wylie, E. J.: Thromboendarterectomy for arteriosclerotic thrombosis of major arteries. Surgery, 32:275-292, 1952.

Wylie, E. J., Kerr, E., and Davies, O.: Experimental and clinical experiences with the use of fascia lata applied as a graft about major arteries after thrombo-endarterectomy and aneurysmorrhaphy. Surg., Gynec. Obstet., 93:257, 1951.

Wylie, E. J., Perloff, D., and Wellington, J. S.: Fibromuscular hyperplasia of renal arteries. Ann. Surg., 156:592-607, 1962.

Yashon, D., Jane, J. A., and Javid, H.: Long-term results of carotid bifurcation endarterectomy. Surg., Gynec. Obstet., 122:517, 1966.

Ziperman, H. H.: Acute arterial injuries in the Korean War. Ann. Surg., 139:1, 1954.

CHAPTER 45

K. ALVIN MERENDINO, M.D.

Lung

There are three wicks you know to the lamp of a man's life: brain, blood, and breath. Press the brain a little; its light goes out, followed by both the others. Stop the heart a minute and out go all three wicks. Choke the air out of the lungs, and presently the fluid ceases to supply the other centers of flame, and all is stagnation, cold, and darkness.
Oliver Wendell Holmes (1809-1894), *Professor at the Breakfast Table*, XI

O! that sad breath his spongy lungs bestowed ...
William Shakespeare (1564-1616)
A Lover's Complaint, L. 326

Anatomic Considerations
Physiologic Considerations
Thoracic Trauma
Lung Abscess
Bronchiectasis
Empyema
Certain Fungal Diseases
Trachea

ANATOMIC CONSIDERATIONS

The pulmonary arteries carry venous blood from the right ventricle to the lungs; they accompany the bronchial tubes and terminate in a dense capillary network about the alveoli. The pulmonary veins begin in the pulmonary capillaries and, coalescing with larger branches, eventually reach the hilum of the lung. Thence they convey the oxygenated blood into the left atrium for distribution to the remainder of the body.

The bronchial arteries are derived directly from the thoracic aorta or the upper intercostal arteries and are distributed to the bronchial glands, the larger bronchial tubes, the visceral pleura and the coats of the pulmonary vessels. The bronchial arteries supply oxygenated blood for the nutrition of the lung. The bronchial veins in general correspond to the branches of the arteries. On the right side they end in the azygos vein, and on the left either the highest intercostal or the accessory hemiazygos vein.

The sympathetic and the vagus nerves form anterior and posterior pulmonary plexuses which supply efferent fibers to the bronchial muscle and afferent fibers to the bronchial mucous membrane.

The lymphatic vessels of the lung originate in 2 plexuses: the superficial and the deep. The superficial plexus is immediately beneath the pleura. The deep follows the pulmonary vessels and bronchi. Little or no anastomosis occurs between these 2 sets of lymphatics except in the hilum. The superficial set empties into the hilar glands; the deep, into the tracheobronchial glands.[15]

It is recognized that the 2 lungs are composed of 5 lobes: 3 on the right and 2 on the left. Individual lobes may be subdivided into segments: on the right, a total of 10 segments, and 8 in the left lung (Fig. 45-1).[19]

The anatomic unit of pulmonary resection has been progressively reduced as shown by the shift from pneumonectomy to lobectomy and now to segmental resection. The technic of excision of an entire lung originally was performed by mass ligation of all hilar structures. Present-day technics involve the method of ligation of individual component elements. The major anatomic structures that must be ligated incident to a pneumonectomy are the pulmo-

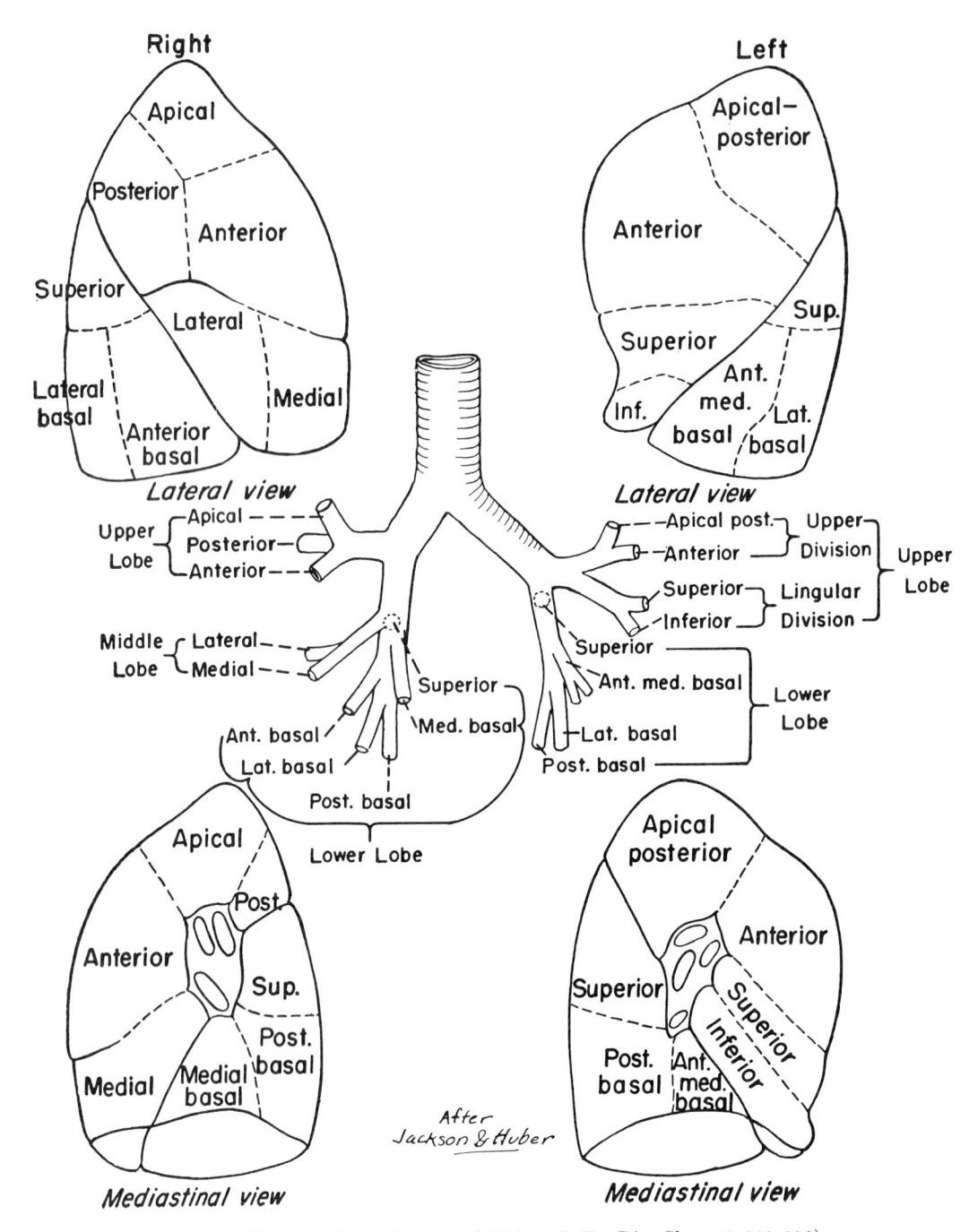

FIG. 45-1. (After Jackson, C. L., and Huber, J. F.: Dis. Chest, 9:319-326)

nary artery, the superior and the inferior pulmonary veins and the main stem bronchus. It is apparent that the performance of a lobectomy or a segmental resection requires a considerable knowledge of detailed pulmonary anatomy. Actually, until rather recently, a hiatus in precise anatomic knowledge existed. Because of the desire of the surgeon to excise only diseased tissue with the simultaneous preservation of as much normally functioning lung as possible, the need for the clarification of more detailed anatomic relationships became apparent. Through the combined efforts of anatomists and surgeons, this area of deficit has been eliminated. Consequently, the lung segments are recognized as both anatomic and surgical units which may be excised separately from the individual lobes.

While the lung segments have been considered to be bronchovascular units, they represent essentially a bronchial distribution with intersegmental planes that may be crossed by arteries from adjacent segments and contain veins draining contiguous segments. The most stable element in segmental patterns is the bronchus, next the arteries. The veins are the most variable. In general, however, the arteries follow the peripheral distribution of the bronchi, while the veins assume an intersegmental or intersubsegmental position.[3]

It has been implied that segmental resection may be carried out with facility in all instances. Of course, there are exceptions, dependent upon anatomic variations and the specific disease process present.[4,5] However, it is not amiss to profile those areas which may be the site of the greatest number of anatomic variants.

The following generalities seem to be warranted: From the standpoint of the relationship of segmental arteries to bronchi, the most variable segments appear to be the apical and the posterior segments of the right upper lobe and those of the middle lobe. Usually, in the middle lobe, the medial segmental artery tends to supply the lateral segmental bronchus. Consequently, from the practical viewpoint, the variations in the segmental anatomy of the middle lobe indicate that a clean lobectomy is preferable in situations where only the medial or the lateral segment is diseased. In the left upper lobe, it is usually advisable to resect both lingular segments together. Historically, lingulectomy constituted the first segmental resection.[9]

In each of the lower lobes, essentially 5 segments are present. Here, it is best to consider resection of the superior segment only with preservation of the 4 basal segments or excision of the basal segments with preservation of the superior segment. Because of important variations in the venous patterns of the basal segments of the lower lobes, it seems unwise to attempt to remove individual segments. There is general agreement, if more than one basal segment must be excised, that all basal segments should be sacrificed as a unit. Successes have been reported with individual basal segmental resection; nonetheless, it is difficult, if not impossible, to determine the actual venous pattern, except with deep dissection which negates any advantage in most instances. Likewise, in superior segmental resection, care must be taken to avoid the arterial supply to the middle lobe as well as the ascending artery, frequently present in this area, which supplies the posterior segment of the upper lobe. Consequently, from the surgical viewpoint, essentially 2 units of excision exist in the lower lobes. It is apparent that the segmental resection of certain areas may be gross in terms of the arterial and the venous patterns. In short, it is possible to destroy unknowingly the arterial supply to an area left behind, or the venous channels to an insitu element may be obstructed. While dire consequences may not result, these circumstances should be avoided if at all possible. Therefore, the properly equipped surgeon must be familiar with the usual arrangements in each segment as well as the variations that may be encountered.

As a consequence, while segmental resection is correctly considered the anatomic unit of surgical excision, the anatomic situation may preclude its use. Likewise, the extent of the disease process may indicate the need for a larger unit of resection. The disease process actually conditions the unit of resection, e.g., in general, pneumonectomy is utilized in bronchogenic carcinoma or for a totally destroyed lung for any reason; lobectomy usually is performed for lung abscess; segmental resections are used most frequently in bronchiectasis, tuberculosis and isolated solitary lesions. In addition, solitary lesions are sometimes removed by "wedge" excision, which essentially represents a wedge-shaped removal of lung between clamps without particular regard to anatomic units.

PHYSIOLOGIC CONSIDERATIONS

The control of ventilation is mainly through both central (medullary) and peripheral receptors which are affected by chemical, pressure and temperature changes. The respiratory center is rhythmically active. Stretch receptors in the lung (Hering-Breuer reflex) may affect the rhythmicity or modify it and change the characteristics of breathing. In addition, within limits, the respiratory center is stimulated when the pCO_2 or the hydrogen ion concentration is raised. A reduced pO_2 usually depresses the center and especially during anesthesia. On the other hand, peripheral receptors in the carotid and the aortic bodies are more sensitive to decreases in pO_2 than changes in pCO_2 and hydrogen ion. Receptors in the carotid bulb and the aortic arch stimulate respiration when blood pressure falls. A sneeze or a cough results from reflex stimulation of the centers; by swallowing they are inhibited.[16]

Pulmonary function per se consists of 2 components: (1) ventilatory function and (2) gas exchange. Ventilation is a term used to denote the actual mechanism of breathing in and out. Ventilatory function is dependent upon the intactness and the mobility of the thoracic cage and diaphragm, the elasticity and the distensibility of the lung, an intact pleura and a clear airway. These may be interrelated, and each facet is dependent on many other factors. Gaseous exchange is dependent upon the pressure gradient of gas between alveolar air and blood, the availability of gas and blood to the membrane surface, and the rate of the transport of blood and gas to and from the alveoli, the effective area of the membrane, and the permeability of the tissue barrier between the blood and the air.

An important function of the lung that is little emphasized is its role in the excretion of the chief acid waste product of metabolism. Daily the lungs excrete 14,000 mEq. of carbonic acid with no cation. This is equivalent to the excretion of 1.5 liters of C.P. hydrochloric acid. This contrasts sharply with the relatively small daily average of 100 mEq. ($\cong$ 10 ml. C.P. HCl) of free acid metabolites excreted without cations by the kidneys. Consequently, the lungs are most important organs in the regulation of acid-base balance. Any disease, acute or chronic, which interferes with the ability of the lungs to rid the body of carbonic acid, will result in respiratory acidosis.

It is apparent that any disease that affects those factors upon which ventilatory function and gaseous exchange are dependent will affect pulmonary function adversely. Many tests have been devised to study these 2 subdivisions of pulmonary function. They are utilized in research activities designed to further our knowledge of respiratory physiology, to evaluate alterations in function created by certain thoracic surgical procedures, and on occasion to determine whether a given patient is capable of tolerating a specific operative procedure. This latter item is of considerable importance to the surgeon. Of the many tests available, the most helpful in determining pulmonary function for the surgical needs are fluoroscopy, the timed vital capacity, maximum breathing capacity and differential bronchospirometry. As will be pointed out later, specialized tests such as these are needed only in occasional situations but are of particular value where excisional pulmonary surgery is contemplated in patients with bilateral disease, such as bronchiectasis, tuberculosis, emphysema or fibrosis.

Space does not permit a detailed description of the normal variations and the limitations in the interpretation of these tests, and the reader is referred to specialized sources of such information.[10] The normal, predicted values are based upon age, sex, etc., and in the final analysis in certain instances the results may not be conclusive in themselves. The results of such tests must be considered together with the physician's knowledge of all aspects of the patient's health status. However, it is apropos to consider briefly the fields in which these tests give valuable information.

By fluoroscopy one may ascertain the mobility of the chest wall and, particularly, the movement of the diaphragm in maximal inspiration and expiration. Lateral as well as anteroposterior views are important. This aids in determining the efficiency of the mechanics of breathing and gives insight into the volume exchange of which the lungs are capable. This in turn gives information concerning lung elasticity and mobility of the important structures. Thus, information concerning the presence of emphysema and fibrosis of the lung is gathered.

The vital capacity is the total amount of air in cubic centimeters or liters which can be expired after a maximum inspiration. This, actually, is only a measure of lung volume and does not give much information regarding function. For example, a patient with emphysema may have a large vital capacity, yet the gas exchange in his lung is poor. More important is the timed vital capacity which introduces a time factor. In short, it is important to know how rapidly one is able to expel the vital capacity. This gives information regarding the dynamics of respiration. A more reliable test of ventilatory capacity is the maximum breathing capacity. With the patient breathing as deeply and rapidly as possible over a 15-second period, one measures the maximum volume of gas breathed per minute. The ability of a patient to breathe at a sustained high velocity depends on many factors: the muscular force available, the resiliency of the lungs and the thorax, the patency of the airway, and tissue resistance.

Differential bronchospirometry is a method for obtaining separate measurements of the individual function of each lung. This is obtained by endobronchial catheterization of the patient by a double lumen tube surrounded by inflatable cuffs. This permits the collection of gas from each lung and the determination of the tidal volume, vital capacity, maximum breathing capacity and O_2 consumption of the right and the left lungs, separately. Whereas the pulmonary function of both lungs measured together may be within normal limits, conceivably one lung could be practically functionless. Thus, the advantage of differential bronchospirometry becomes apparent. This is of primary importance when a pulmonary resection is contemplated in the presence of bilateral disease.

Normally, the right lung accounts for 55 per cent of the minute ventilation and 55 per cent of the O_2 consumption, and the left lung the remainder. This congruity of ventilation and oxygen absorption is very important. For example, if by bronchospirometry the right lung was found to be responsible for 55 per cent of the ventilation and only 10 per cent of the O_2 consumption while the left was effecting 45 per cent of the ventilation and 90 per cent of the total O_2 absorbed, the conclusion is drawn that in the right lung there exists a marked impairment of diffusion of O_2 across the alveolar membrane, or a reduction in pulmonary blood flow, or both. It is apparent that if there were a reason for it, the right lung could be removed without significant loss to O_2 consumption, and with improvement of the respiratory capacity of the patient by virtue of the reduction of the dead space of the poorly absorbing right lung. As a corollary, the removal of the left lung would be contraindicated because therein resides almost the entire oxygen absorptive function of both lungs. While this gross example is clean cut, there are gradations of pulmonary insufficiency of the right and the left lungs which often make the decision more difficult.

These tests do not make a diagnosis of the disease present; they measure pulmonary function. Neither can pulmonary function tests tell the surgeon which patient will tolerate major surgery and survive. In the borderline case, the information obtained will indicate under circumstances of clean surgery without complication that the patient's function is adequate to tolerate the removal of a designated area of the lung and, if he survives, he will not be a respiratory cripple. Be mindful that pulmonary function tests must be considered as measurements of one facet of the patient's total physical assets and liabilities.

As implied earlier, special tests of pulmonary function are unnecessary except in relatively few patients. Therefore, one must be concerned with practical means of evaluating pulmonary function, using clinical methods mainly. The history and the physical examination are important, not only in assaying pulmonary function but also for selecting those patients who may require special tests. If the patient has no difficulty in meeting everyday activities without dyspnea, pulmonary function is adequate for ordinary operations. If dyspnea is present at times, this can be grossly quantitated by further questioning, e.g., how far can you walk at an average pace without shortness of breath; do hills bother you; how many stairs can you climb before becoming short of breath, etc.? If dyspnea is present, cardiac dyspnea must be differentiated from pulmonary dyspnea. A proper decision usually can be made by quantitating the patient's disability and the magnitude of the operation contemplated, tempered by sound clinical judgment based on experience.

Under similar circumstances, a knowledge of the behavior of certain pulmonary diseases is essential when the removal of lung parenchyma is contemplated. Furthermore, consideration must be given to the status of the lung to be removed. If the lung is destroyed by disease and obviously nonfunctioning, and if the patient is not short of breath, it is apparent that one may remove the diseased tissue by a segmental resection, lobectomy or pneumonectomy, without reducing pulmonary function much. In short, an anatomic removal of pulmonary tissue can be accomplished without loss of pulmonary function. Actually, after the removal of a functionless lung in the absence of inflammatory pleural complications, an improvement in pulmonary function may result. By the removal of such tissue it is obligatory for all unoxygenated blood to circulate through the remaining normal lung tissue. The removal of such a lung closes a right-to-left cardiac shunt. Even if an entire lung has been destroyed, dyspnea may be improved by its removal for this reason. Removal of a destroyed lung may reduce the workload of the heart and be additionally helpful. It has been shown that in a destroyed lung, particularly the bronchiectatic variety, the normal communications between the bronchial and the pulmonary arteries may become enlarged and constitute sizable arteriovenous shunts, increasing the workload for the left ventricle.[26]

When pulmonary resection of a normal-appearing and presumably normal-functioning lung is considered, the problem may be more complex. However, in general, an individual who exhibits normal activity without dyspnea will tolerate pneumonectomy of a functioning lung or any component thereof without much difficulty. This situation arises most frequently in bronchogenic carcinoma. On the other hand, an individual with dyspnea at rest with normal-appearing lung fields ordinarily would not be considered a candidate for pulmonary resection, because the removal of any pulmonary tissue would render him more dyspneic. Of course, one cannot always assay the function of the lung by the x-ray appearance of the lung field. However, from the x-ray appearance combined with the history, physical examination and fluoroscopy, usually a good estimate of pulmonary function can be made. In patients with dyspnea and normal-appearing lung fields the specialized pulmonary function tests find their greatest usefulness and give valuable information in this group and in those patients with bilateral disease.

In the evaluation of a patient with borderline pulmonary function, it must be remembered that the most dangerous period in terms of survival is immediately postoperative, because the extensive thoracic incision of itself inactivates certain neuromuscular components of the chest wall and reduces the capacity to breathe. Postoperative pain will temporarily limit chest excursion and thereby decrease ventilation. In addition, clearing the tracheobronchial tree of secretions is hampered because coughing is painful. Consequently, consideration must be given to the patient's ability to weather these troubles as well as the eventual result in terms of pulmonary function.

THORACIC TRAUMA

A chest injury may represent the only area involved or be one aspect of a more generalized injury. One must keep in mind the structures contained within and protected by the thoracic wall. Besides the thoracic cage, consisting of both hard and soft tissues, there is, in addition, the respiratory tract, the heart and the major vessels, the esophagus and the thoracic duct. Because of injuries to them a chest injury may have far-reaching and widespread general effects.

At times it is difficult to assess properly the total injury. Frequently, even in the absence of abdominal trauma, there may be abdominal signs and symptoms. This is due to the fact that the intercostal nerves also supply the abdominal wall. When they are damaged by trauma to the chest, they may give rise to severe referred abdominal spasm and pain. In addition, ileus and acute gastric dilatation may accompany "pure" thoracic injuries.

Thoracic injuries may be effected from within through the esophagus or the bronchus or from without. Esophagoscopy, gastroscopy and bronchoscopy infrequently lead to thoracic complications. With gastroscopy, rupture of the esophagus may take place. The posterior esophageal wall is thin and may be penetrated by the gastroscope, although it is a pliable instrument. For this reason, gastroscopy is contraindicated in the presence of esophageal disease, severe kyphosis and aneurysms of the thoracic aorta.

Esophagoscopy also carries a minor risk in experienced hands. The esophagoscope is a rigid instrument, and the danger of esophageal perforation is real. With partial or complete obstructions of the esophagus, the proximal esophagus may become saccularily dilated and present pouches which may be mistaken for the esophageal channel. Although the walls of such esophagi may be hypertrophied, they are usually edematous and friable. Esophageal perforations may occur posteriorly into the mediastinum or laterally into the pleural cavities. Occasional complications attend bronchoscopy. During bronchoscopic biopsy, a full thickness of the cartilaginous ring may be removed accidentally, leading to mediastinitis or pneumothorax.[1]

The wounds from without may be penetrating or contusional. Penetrating wounds are usually produced by knives or bullets. Contusional injury follows the application of a force directly to the thoracic wall. This force may be of short duration as in a fall, or prolonged as in a crush injury. Indirect injury to the contents of the chest may occur from any cause which results in increased intrapulmonic pressure such as an abdominal blow, blast or severe coughing.

All trauma to the chest, whether from within or without, may produce rupture of the thoracic duct, the esophagus, the aorta or the tracheobronchial tree. In general, thoracic duct injuries are treated by merely aspirating the chyle from the chest. Occasionally, ligation is necessary. Esophageal rupture should be treated by immediate operation and closure of the rent and closed drainage of the chest. If the tracheobronchial openings are small, they may be treated conservatively, or if severe, by surgical suture. Aortic rupture usually results in immediate death. On occasion, delayed rupture occurs. In some instances immediate operation with direct suture or the insertion of an aortic graft will be possible. Although this is feasible, the issue is often clouded by a lack of certainty in the diagnosis and the poor condition of the patient.

Most frequently, in civilian practice, one encounters hemothorax, pneumothorax, pulmonary contusion and/or laceration, rib fractures, or any combination thereof. In general, these are treated by conservative means. The major indications for exploratory thoracotomy are (1) continuing intrathoracic hemorrhage and (2) continuing air leak from the lung or the tracheobronchial tree, which cannot be controlled by the usual means. Large thoracic defects also are an indication but rarely are seen in civilian practice.

The proper management of chest injuries is rapidly becoming more important. Chest injuries are second only to head injuries as the most common cause of death in car accidents. This section is not meant to be all-inclusive with regard to the management of chest injuries (see Chap. 25, Military Surgery); however, a more detailed account of 2 injuries which are not uncommonly encountered in civilian practice are included because of the severe alterations in pulmonary function which they create. If recognized and properly treated, death often can be prevented.

Tension Pneumothorax

Tension pneumothorax exists when the pressure in the pleural cavity is atmospheric or above. Various degrees of pneumothorax may occur following spontaneous rupture of an emphysematous bleb, cyst, or in the presence of apparently normal lung. Likewise, in the presence of an intact thorax, sharp fragments of fractured ribs may lacerate the lung surface with a similar result. In order for air to enter the pleural cavity from without, a communication between the atmosphere and the pleural space must exist. Often this is secondary to penetrating wounds, e.g., knife, bullet, etc. With a penetrating wound air may reach the pleural cavity also from the lung, if injury of the latter simultaneously occurs.

Minor degrees of pneumothorax may not create much difficulty. Severe alterations occur in so-called tension pneumothorax. In order for tension pneumothorax to develop, there must exist a valvular mechanism, created usually by soft tissue adjoining the air leak, which allows air to enter the pleural cavity during inspiration more readily than it permits it to escape during expiration. Consequently, the valvular mechanism is similar to the mechanics of a one-way flutter valve.

Pathologic Physiology. Due to the presence of elastic fibers in the lung substance, the lung removed from the body tends to collapse. In its normal position, the lung is maintained in various degrees of expansion by the nega-

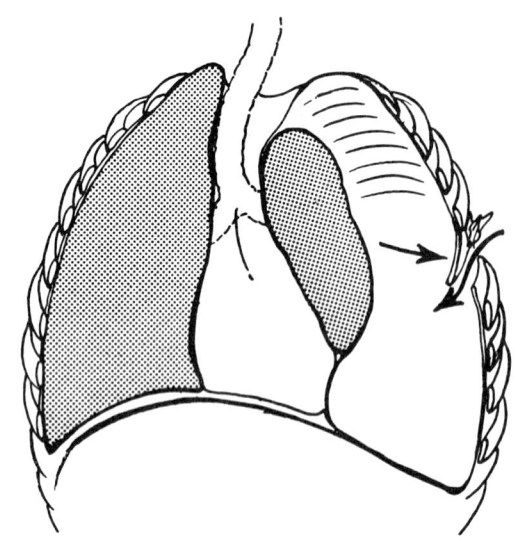

FIG. 45-2. Tension pneumothorax. Here is indicated the "flutter valve" mechanism necessary for the development of a tension pneumothorax. During inspiration, the active phase of respiration, the chest wall expands, the intercostal spaces widen, and the negativity of the pleural cavity increases. Consequently, air enters the pleural cavity. On expiration, the thorax relaxes, and the tissues surrounding the injury partially or completely prevent the escape of pleural air. It is apparent that a similar mechanism may exist in air leaks from the lung or in certain cases of bronchial or tracheal injuries with pleural communications.

tive pressure in the pleural cavity. The degree of expansion is dependent upon the phases of ventilation which varies the degree of negative pressure in the pleural space. With pneumothorax, the degree of negativity is altered toward the positive side. As this occurs, the lung of the involved side begins to collapse (Fig. 45-2). The amount of collapse will be dependent upon the interplay of 2 factors, namely, the inherent elasticity of the lung in one direction and the pull created by the degree of negative pleural pressure in the opposite direction. If the lung is exposed to atmospheric pressure by means of a large communication to the outside, the pressure in the pleural cavity is atmospheric. Therefore, the position of the lung is one of maximum collapse. The degree of collapse is dependent upon the inherent elasticity of the lung itself. The presence of any disease which affects lung elasticity, the presence of visceroparietal pleural adhesions, etc., will affect the degree of collapse.

In tension pneumothorax, the increments of trapped air in the pleural cavity result in an increased positive pleural pressure. The adverse effects are multiple. In addition to the loss of function due to collapsed lung, as the tension increases, the mediastinum, if pliable, is displaced toward the uninvolved side. This decreases the effective expansion of the uninvolved lung. In addition to the pain due to the irritative effects of pleural air, the patient attempts to compensate for this loss by an increased respiratory rate. In addition, the circulation is affected adversely on 2 scores. Normally, the venous return via the superior and the inferior venae cavae is aided by the periodic changes in negative pressure of the pleural cavity incident to ventilation. Not only is this action ablated, but positive pleural pressure actually may hamper venous return. Because, by location, the venae cavae are more a part of the right hemithorax, it would be expected that right pneumothorax would affect venous return more severely than one on the left side. With mediastinal shift, angulation of the heart occurs. The heart may be likened to a cherry hanging by a stem. The stem consists of the major vessels by which the heart is actually suspended. When torsion of the heart occurs, the major vessels may become angulated. The aorta is thick-walled and carries a high intraluminal pressure and bends like a sapling. The cavae are thin-walled and have low intraluminal pressures and, consequently, tend to kink. When this occurs, venous return is further reduced, with a resultant diminished cardiac stroke output. In order to compensate for this, tachycardia develops, which may result in a further decrease of cardiac output. Thus, a vicious cycle is set up. It is apparent that tension pneumothorax may rapidly result in death unless proper therapy is instituted.

Diagnosis. Tension pneumothorax is characterized by chest pain (if due to spontaneous pneumothorax, this is of sudden onset and frequently without history of precipitating factors), rapid short respiration, tachycardia, cyanosis, anxiety and apprehension. On physical examination, in severe cases, the signs and

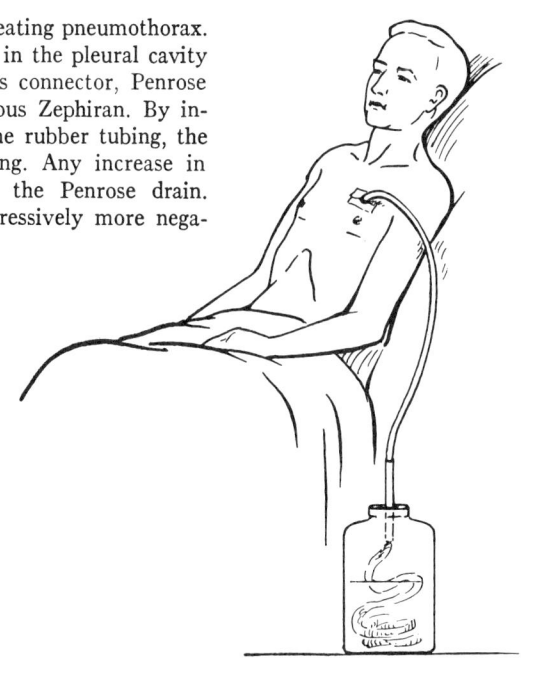

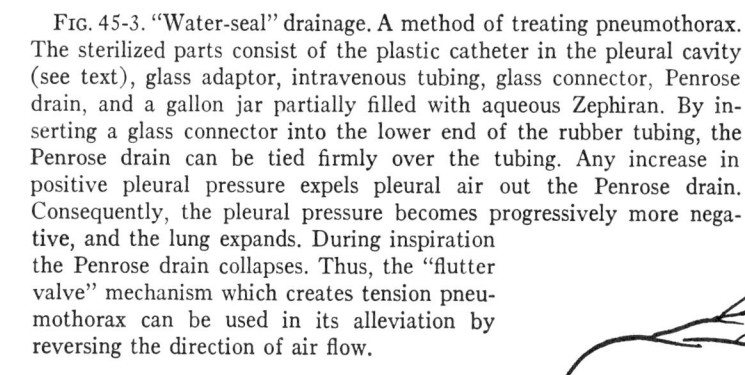

Fig. 45-3. "Water-seal" drainage. A method of treating pneumothorax. The sterilized parts consist of the plastic catheter in the pleural cavity (see text), glass adaptor, intravenous tubing, glass connector, Penrose drain, and a gallon jar partially filled with aqueous Zephiran. By inserting a glass connector into the lower end of the rubber tubing, the Penrose drain can be tied firmly over the tubing. Any increase in positive pleural pressure expels pleural air out the Penrose drain. Consequently, the pleural pressure becomes progressively more negative, and the lung expands. During inspiration the Penrose drain collapses. Thus, the "flutter valve" mechanism which creates tension pneumothorax can be used in its alleviation by reversing the direction of air flow.

symptoms of shock will be obvious; venous distention may or may not be present. Inspection reveals a full immobile hemithorax exhibiting little excursion with ventilation. The use of the ancillary muscles of respiration may be prominent with intercostal retraction on inspiration of the uninvolved side. Percussion reveals tympany of the involved side, and on auscultation bronchovesicular breath sounds are absent. X-ray examination demonstrates a collapsed lung, with air clearly evident in the pleural cavity, a flattened diaphragm, widening of the intercostal spaces and mediastinal shift. Pulmonary disease may be apparent in the opposite lung, which may give a clue to etiology in the spontaneous form. If the pneumothorax is due to trauma, there may be additional x-ray findings. Severe abdominal pain with marked rigidity of the abdominal wall sometimes occurs and may confuse the diagnosis.

Treatment. Rarely, tension pneumothorax must be treated on an emergency basis outside the confines of the hospital. In the absence of any obvious penetrating injury of the chest wall, the most expedient manner of treatment is the insertion of an ordinary intravenous needle, the larger the better, into the pleural space. This is accompanied by an audible rush of air to the outside. In a desperate situation, an entry into the pleural cavity may be imperative with any instrument at hand. The wound must be maintained open by the insertion of any reasonably clean implement into the newly created wound. If a chest wound is present, it should be maintained open by any means available. By these emergency measures one creates an open communication with the atmosphere and an open pneumothorax. While the lung will not expand, the damaging effects of mediastinal shift are obviated. This situation is compatible with life and transport of the patient.

In the hospital, tension pneumothorax of the spontaneous type may be treated by multiple aspirations but preferably by a plastic catheter inserted through a No. 13 gauge needle introduced into the pleural space through the second intercostal space anteriorly. After the plastic catheter is passed into the pleural cavity a short distance, the needle is withdrawn. Then the catheter may be connected to a water-seal drainage or to a negative pressure system to aid in rapid expansion (Fig. 45-3). The catheter should not be inserted low in the chest and it should have several perforations in its intrapleural portion. A small serous effusion accompanies most pneumothoraces. If the catheter is inserted into the lower chest it is apt to become plugged by fibrin. The presence of such a catheter may give one a false sense of security. Unless it is patent it is useless; consequently, the patency of the system should be checked periodically.

If there is a penetrating wound of the chest wall, debridement should be done. Rarely, in the presence of lung injury, it may be impossible to keep abreast of the air loss into the

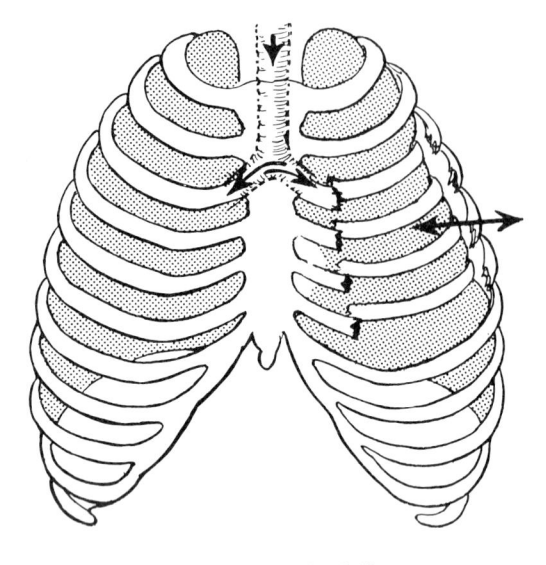

FIG. 45-4. Flail chest. The flail area moves in response to changes in intrapleural pressure. The movement of air down the trachea is mainly dependent on the degree of negative pressure created by the volume enlargement of the pleural cavity during inspiration. Because of the inward movement of the flail segment, normal expansion of the pleural cavity is reduced; consequently, the effective flow of air via the trachea to the involved lung is diminished. During expiration, as the flail segment moves outward, the expired air from the uninvolved side is not only expelled out the trachea but also into the bronchus of the involved side. With the next inspiration, the lung of the normal side receives fresh air via the trachea but also "rebreathes" air previously shunted into the opposite bronchus. Thus, the effective dead space is increased. Stabilization of the segment and tracheotomy are important measures in combating these alterations.

pleural cavity. In this situation exploratory thoracotomy is indicated, in order to close the point of air loss.

FLAIL CHEST

A portion of the thoracic wall becomes "flail" when one or more ribs are fractured in at least 2 spatially separated areas. This portion of the thoracic cage becomes excessively mobile, and its direction of movements will be dependent upon the pressure relationships within the pleural cavity.

Pathologic Physiology. With inspiration the lower ribs flare outward, the sternum is elevated, and there is a descent of the diaphragm. These factors increase the volume of the thoracic cavity, which in turn creates greater negative pressure in the closed pleural space. The lung expands in response to this increased negativity of the pleural cavity. When a segment of the chest wall is flail, with inspiration the increased negative pleural pressure sucks in the flail portion of the chest. If the size and the mobility of this area is large, the negative pleural pressure is dissipated. Consequently, the lung does not expand completely, and the air movement down the trachea is diminished. With expiration, as pleural pressure moves toward the more positive side, the flail area is pushed outward. These movements of this mobile segment are in opposite direction of the remainder of the chest wall during both phases of ventilation. These abnormal motions of the flail portion of the chest are referred to as paradoxical movements.

In addition, ventilation is affected adversely by the to-and-fro movement of air at the carinal level (Fig. 45-4). The limited excursion of the lung secondary to the alterations in the pleural pressure is inadequate to move air completely in and out of the tracheal dead space; and, in fact, the to-and-fro movement of air between the 2 lungs further increases the effective dead space.

It becomes apparent that with such an injury significant pain is present. Because of pain, the involved side is splinted voluntarily. In addition, involuntary splinting due to spasm occurs secondary to the local trauma. As a consequence, aeration of the involved lung is incomplete, and coughing is inhibited. Furthermore, thoracic trauma is accompanied by increased bronchial secretion and retention. This has resulted in the term traumatic "wet lung."[7] Consequently, the stage is set for atelectasis and its sequelae. By the retention of secretions the exchange of O_2 and CO_2 may be interfered with across the alveolar membrane.

The cough is an extremely important defense mechanism, particularly in chest injuries. It is apparent that in order to clear the respiratory tract of secretions, an explosive cough is necessary. However, an explosive cough is impossible unless air is built up behind the material to be expelled. Decreased aeration of the involved side precludes this. Furthermore, with cough the closed epiglottis builds up a positive pleural pressure. However, the positive pressure build-up is dissipated because the flail segment moves outward as the remainder of chest wall actively contracts downward. Pain also is a serious deterrent to an effective cough by the patient.

Treatment. Immobilization of the flail chest is mandatory. The flail segment may be stabilized by strapping a sandbag over it or by grasping one of the involved ribs by a sterile towel clip which is connetced to a weight by means of an overhead traction system; only a small incision is necessary. The former method usually suffices. Of almost equal importance is the alleviation of pain. Periodic intercostal nerve block is most effective. One should block not only the nerves of the involved ribs but 2 intercostal spaces above and below as well. By these maneuvers, immobilization of the chest wall is aided, and pain is practically abolished. As a result, paradoxical motion is obviated to a great degree, and splinting is lessened with the result that better aeration of the lung on the involved side occurs. An effective cough may now result.

If the raising of secretions becomes a problem, tracheal aspiration, bronchoscopy and tracheotomy should be resorted to in that order. Nasal oxygen may be necessary. The advantages of tracheotomy in a severe case are 2-fold. Not only does it serve as a readily available vent for tracheal aspiration, but it also reduces the respiratory dead space. If oxygen is required with tracheotomy, it is possible by this means to deliver O_2 under slightly positive pressure. In addition, respiratory acidosis may be avoided by washing out CO_2.

Respirators, such as the Bird and the Bennett types, are effective and life-saving when the patient is unable to ventilate adequately. This occurs in crush injuries where the involvement is massive unilaterally or severe bilaterally. Observation is of assistance in deciding the need for tracheotomy and positive-pressure assistors. However, the degree of the ventilatory inadequacy is not always appreciated. Cyanosis may be only equivocal; however, anxiety and restlessness sometimes attributed to a possible associated head injury may be the key to a severely desaturated patient. This can be confirmed by studies of the arterial pO_2. When a low pO_2 exists, the need for tracheotomy and assistors is obvious. Periodic checks on arterial pO_2 and pCO_2 are invaluable in management. Once mental symptoms are present because of a low pO_2, it may take 48 hours before these signs disappear. Obviously, severe states are best anticipated and proper treatment initiated before these more flagrant signs of respiratory insufficiency occur.

LUNG ABSCESS

Nontuberculous lung abscess occurs as a solitary unilocular or multilocular cavity. Multiple lung abscesses occur secondary to septicemia or pyemia. The latter types frequently are associated with a serious medical problem; consequently, they may fall in the province of the internist. Lung abscess is more frequent in the male than in the female; no age group is immune. The peak of incidence occurs in the 3rd, the 4th and the 5th decades. The mechanism of development is mainly aspirational; however, some abscesses are of hematogenous or embolic origin.

CLINICAL ETIOLOGY

One third of all lung abscesses occur postoperatively or postanesthetically. An equal number are of undetermined etiology. The remaining cases of lung abscess are secondary to primary respiratory infections, bronchogenic carcinoma, bronchiectasis, foreign body aspiration, pulmonary infarct, infection of congenital cysts and coma with presumed aspiration. The coma may be alcoholic, epileptic or due to trauma, brain tumor or excessive morphine sedation.

In the postoperative-anesthetic group, most abscesses follow operations on the upper respiratory tract; tonsillectomy and dental extractions are the worst offenders. Following tonsillectomy, blood in the trachea and the bronchi is a common finding after all bleeding is controlled. The Trendelenburg or Rose position during tonsillectomy offers excellent prophylaxis against this complication. Consequently, aspiration seems to be the logical explanation in the majority of cases. A similar mechanism occurs following the extraction of teeth. The unilateral dulling of the pharyngeal reflex affected by the commonly employed nerve blocks, particularly of the inferior dental and the anterior palatine nerves, allows easy access to the lower respiratory tract for the entry of infected material. Lung abscess has been known to follow anesthesia without operation and operation without anesthesia.

Of those cases classified as having an undetermined etiology, the insidious onset of symptoms defies attempts to establish the definite date of onset. Many cases in this category formerly were considered to be secondary to an atypical pneumonia. In the older literature, lung abscess frequently was diagnosed following a respiratory illness. It is probable that many cases were primary abscess with a surrounding pneumonitis. Oral sepsis is present so frequently in this group of patients that its etiologic portent cannot be overlooked.[27]

ANATOMIC LOCATION

The right lung is involved more frequently than the left in the ratio of 2:1. The right lower lobe is the most frequent site of lung abscess due to the dependent position of its bronchus, the less acute angle which the right main bronchus forms with the trachea, and its larger size. While this pertains where aspiration may have occurred in the upright position, the most dependent portion of the lung is altered by changes in position of the patient. Consequently, in the supine position the dorsal segment of the lower lobes may be involved. In the lateral recumbent position the posterior segment or the lateral (axillary) division of the anterior segment of the upper lobes become the most dependent portions of the lung.[6] Embolic abscess occurs most commonly in the lower lobes; the right lung again is involved more frequently than the left.

DIAGNOSIS AND LOCALIZATION

The history is the most important diagnostic aid and is within the reach of every physician. Cough with expectoration is the most common complaint, with pleuritic chest pain, fever, malaise, headache, asthenia, hemoptysis and weight loss following in that order. The sputum is usually foul, yellow, green or dark mucopurulent material. Pleuritic chest pain is of aid in localization. The localization of pleuritic pain identifies the site of pleural adhesions. Circumscribed tenderness to pressure is often associated with pleuritic pain. Such pain is usually absent with either central or upper lobe abscesses. While hemoptyses are usually small, exsanguinating hemorrhages can occur.

On physical examination there are no pathognomonic signs of pulmonary abscess. Cavitary signs are distinctly unusual. Consolidation with or without friction rib is present in half the cases. Pneumonitis without consolidation is frequently present; 10 per cent of the patients will have a negative physical examination or reveal the presence of a complication such as pleural effusion, empyema or bronchopleural fistula. Clubbing of the fingers and the toes, when present, may be marked. This sign may be present as early as the 4th week after onset and completely disappears after cure. If there is persistence of clubbing, one should suspect an undrained focus or bronchiectasis.

LABORATORY STUDIES

In acute cases, a high leukocyte count may indicate a good prognosis. In the chronic phase, a mild normocytic anemia with slight

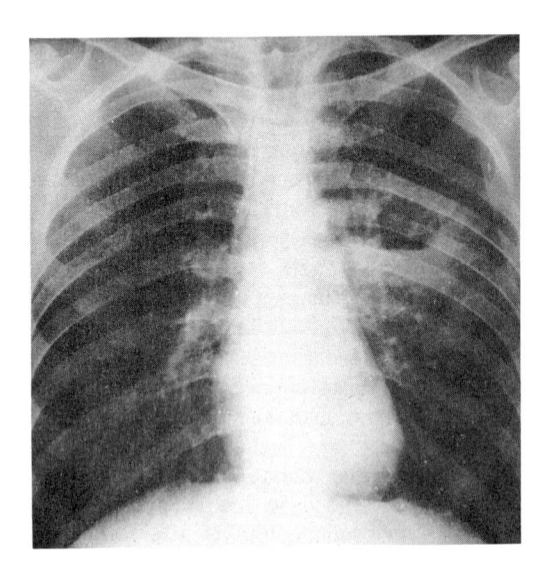

FIG. 45-5. Typical acute, thin-walled lung abscess with fluid level and surrounding pneumonitis. This lesion completely resolved under antibiotic therapy.

leukocytosis is present. At this stage of the illness a high leukocyte count may indicate a complication. The bacteriologic findings are extremely complex; however, streptococcus viridans is found frequently. Anaerobic streptococcus is the most common of the strictly anaerobic microorganisms. Pneumococci, staphylococci, fusiform bacilli and spirochetes frequently are present.

X-ray studies are important in the diagnosis and the localization of the lesion (Fig. 45-5). A cavity with a fluid level is diagnostic. Bronchograms with Lipiodol or water-soluble contrast media are sometimes essential in the differential diagnosis of lung abscess and bronchiectasis. It is difficult to fill the abscess cavity with opaque material. When filling occurs there can be no question of the diagnosis. More commonly there is an inability to fill the bronchus draining the abscess. Thus, the exact segmental localization may be made indirectly. Diagnostic bronchoscopy is indicated in all cases to establish the presence or the absence of bronchial tumor or a foreign body. A biopsy of suspected tissue is always taken, and washings are made for Papanicolaou stains. Serial roentgenograms are necessary in evaluating the progress of therapy.

TREATMENT

Medical. The use of antibiotics has reduced markedly the incidence of lung abscess. Similarly, in the subacute phase the judicious use of antibiotics, based upon the sensitivity of the organisms cultured, frequently results in cure. It is important to remember that the treatment of a lung abscess, as with abscesses anywhere in the body, entails adequate drainage. Therefore, postural drainage and, occasionally, bronchoscopy for the removal of granulation tissue remain important measures in management. In addition, supportive measures, including high protein and high vitamin diets and transfusions, are important. Significant protein loss may occur when the sputum volume is large.

Surgical. MINOR SURGICAL PROCEDURE. These include phrenic crush and pneumothorax. The success of phrenic crush is difficult to evaluate. Pneumothorax frequently results in pyopneumothorax and metastatic brain abscess. For these reasons, neither procedure warrants consideration in therapy. They are mentioned only to be condemned.

MAJOR SURGICAL PROCEDURE. If for any reason the patient shows little or no improvement in 4 to 6 weeks of adequate medical management, a major surgical procedure should be considered.

Incision and Drainage. The usefulness of external drainage of a lung abscess is determined by the relative accessibility of the cavity. A short rib resection frequently is necessary. The agglutination of visceral and parietal pleura must be adequate, otherwise a pneumothorax is produced which tends to uncap the pus pocket, resulting in pleural infection or bronchopleural fistula. If there is firm adherence between the visceral and the parietal pleura, the abscess may be drained in one stage. Otherwise, the procedure must be staged, first creating an irritation between the 2 pleural membranes by packing iodoform gauze immediately against the outside of the parietal pleura with drainage of the abscess 5 to 7 days later. External incision and drainage are utilized mainly for those patients who for any reason cannot tolerate a major thoracotomy. Some surgeons have utilized incision and drainage in the acute phase with excellent results.[21]

Excision. The excision of chronic abscess cavities has become the procedure of choice. While occasionally a wedge excision or a segmental resection may be done, the infiltrative pneumonitis surrounding the lung abscess pocket usually extends beyond the segmental confines. For this reason, frequently lobectomy must be employed in the treatment of lung abscess, except where a combination of segments (e.g., basal segments) may be removed as a unit. Because lung abscess is usually a once-in-a-lifetime occurrence, the removal of a single lobe is well tolerated. It is accomplished with low morbidity and mortality and is almost always curative.

BRONCHIECTASIS

The term implies merely a dilated bronchus. Without sputum it is considered a dry type. However, chronic infection together with an increased secretion of mucus from the bronchial epithelium are present so frequently that the wet type must be considered as comprising the more characteristic clinical picture. The wet type is more frequently of surgical interest. Local anatomic changes in the bronchus and the bronchioles may be minimal or extensive. Cylindrical forms represent early changes, and the saccular the most severe.

Etiology

Despite considerable investigation and much speculation, the true cause of bronchial dilatation remains unknown. The main theories advanced involve the following: nutritional changes in the bronchial walls, derangement of the neuromuscular mechanism of the bronchial walls, increased fibrous tissue of the lung substance and congenital deformity of the bronchi. Whatever the fundamental causes of bronchiectasis are, the precipitating factors are not always the same. Some cases follow the aspiration of foreign bodies or infected material from the stomach and the upper respiratory tract. Others occur as a sequel to pneumonia or a lung segment which has been collapsed for any reason. Many develop as a gradual accompaniment of repeated upper respiratory infections. The association of chronic sinusitis is common and may have etiologic importance.

Pathology

Early pathologic changes are seldom confined to the ectasia of the bronchi but almost always involve the bronchial mucosa and submucosa. Chronic inflammatory changes in these layers develop and progress to a state of extensive and progressive fibrosis of the area involved. Eventually, areas of normal mucosa are destroyed and replaced by chronically infected granulation tissue. Elastic fibers and muscle bundles may become replaced partially or largely with fibrosis, and occasionally there is destruction of portions of the cartilaginous structures. Weakening of the bronchial wall is inevitable. Finally, progressive shrinkage and contraction of involved segments results. Accompanying the chronic inflammatory changes, the bronchial wall may stenose, with the retention of infected secretions. Consequently, the weakened, diseased bronchi become further dilated distal to this narrowing. These factors when combined bring about the saccular type of bronchiectasis seen as an end-stage. The bacteriologic picture is complex, and no etiologic significance can be ascribed to any single organism.

An additional change occurs in the hemodynamics of bronchial-pulmonary arterial communications (see section on Physiology).

Prognosis

When the disease begins in early childhood, few survive beyond the age of 40 when untreated or treated by nonsurgical methods. Considerable impairment in the physical development begins in childhood, and chronic invalidism continues throughout life. Because of the presence of a productive cough with foul-smelling sputum, social ostracism frequently results. Eventually, many children develop psychological changes, varying in degree from mild depression to actual psychopathic personalities. Therefore, it has become apparent that untreated and medically treated bronchiectasis is attended with a high mortality, a relatively short life expectancy and a devastating morbidity on both a physical and a psychological basis.[8]

Pattern of Involvement

Bronchiectasis may involve all lobes of the lung. However, it rarely involves all segments of the lung. There is a typical distribution in that the left lung is involved more frequently than the right. In 30 to 50 per cent of cases the disease is bilateral. The lower lobes are involved more frequently than any other lobes of the lung. More specifically, one or all of the basal segments of either lower lobe may be involved. Characteristically, the superior segments of the lower lobes are free of disease. When the left basal segments are involved, the lingula is likewise diseased in 60 to 80 per cent of cases.[9] Similarly, if the basal segments of the right lung are diseased, from 45 to 60 per cent of patients have disease in the middle lobe.

Diagnosis

Dilatation of the bronchi, so-called dry bronchiectasis, gives rise to no symptoms except hemoptyses. In many patients so-called dry bronchiectasis is converted to wet types when bronchial infection supervenes. Wet bronchiectasis gives rise to the chief symptoms of cough and purulent sputum. Hemoptyses and sputum are frequently worse in the morning, purulent secretions having accumulated during sleep. The sputum is characteristically foul. If bronchiectasis is extensive with considerable destruction of lung tissue, emphysema supervenes with dyspnea, particularly on exertion.

On physical examination, clubbing of fingers may be present, and rales may be detected over the involved lung. A roentgenogram of the chest often shows a honeycombed appearance of the affected lung fields. There may be areas of atelectasis and cavitation. The actual diagnosis of bronchiectasis rests on the demonstration of dilated bronchi on x-ray study after the intrabronchial instillation of Lipiodol or a water-soluble opaque medium (Fig. 45-6). It is of importance to map out the entire lung, both right and left, in order to determine the extent of bronchiectasis present. Particularly is this important where surgical therapy is considered, for the removal of a portion of the infected areas without removal of all bronchiectatic segments results in incomplete cure.

Pseudobronchiectasis is a term used for bronchial changes observed after atypical pneumonia (viral). These changes are reversible and should not cause any difficulty in diagnosis.[2]

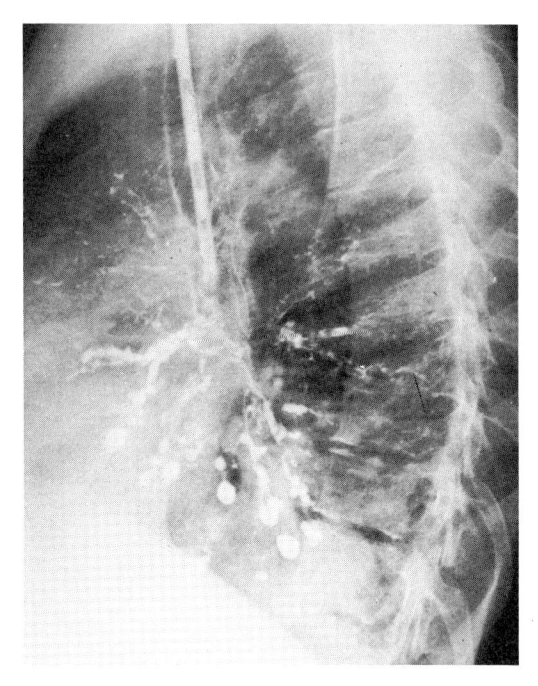

FIG. 45-6. Saccular bronchiectasis of the basal segments of the lower lobe with normal appearing superior segment.

COMPLICATIONS

Recurrent attacks of atypical pneumonia are common. Bronchiectasis not only gives rise to secondary lung abscess but also may develop as a complication of lung abscess. Metastatic brain abscess is an uncommon complication most frequently affecting the right frontal lobe. Empyema and pyopneumothorax do occur. Amyloid disease may follow long-standing cases with extensive involvement.

TREATMENT

Once the anatomic changes characteristic of bronchiectasis are observed, they are irreversible. Consequently, bronchiectasis is a surgical disease. Medical measures are reserved only for those cases so extensive that surgical therapy is not feasible or for patients who refuse therapy or are unable for other reasons to tolerate thoracotomy. These measures consist of rest, postural drainage and bronchoscopy. Broad-spectrum antibiotics are of value in reducing sputum, thus obtaining symptomatic relief and aborting acute respiratory infections. Intermittent usage is advocated to avoid the development of resistant strains of organisms.

Surgical therapy is directed toward the removal of all diseased tissue with the sparing of all healthy, functioning lung parenchyma. Pulmonary function studies are particularly important when there is extensive involvement or when other pulmonary changes are present which indicate borderline pulmonary function. Bronchiectasis lends itself well to segmental resection.[22]

When there is unilateral involvement, it is customary to remove all diseased segments of the entire lung on that side at one operation. If the disease is bilateral, usually the most seriously involved side is operated upon first. To avoid spill-over of secretions into the noninvolved lung, endobronchial intubation and positioning of the patient with the operated side dependent are important maneuvers. Recently, it has been shown that bilateral disease may be attacked simultaneously at the same operation, either by 2 separate incisions of the posterolateral type or a single anterior transsternal incision. Except for unusual indications, this approach would appear to be unwise.

When the basal segments are incompletely involved, it is considered inadvisable to leave behind less than 2 segments though they may be normal. Ordinarily, a left basal segmental resection is done with sparing of the superior segment of the lower lobe with resection of the lingula if involved; on the right side, basal segmental resection is combined with right middle-lobe lobectomy in case of its involvement.

Bronchiectasis is a surgically curable disease when all diseased segments are removed. The value of surgery in bronchiectasis has been reconfirmed in a collective review of over 800 cases. An average cure rate of 43 per cent can be anticipated, while an additional 43 per cent will be improved. Thus, 86 per cent of patients treated surgically will be benefited and capable of normal activity. Surgical treatment fails in 6 per cent of cases. This includes patients with a continued productive cough or physical limitation preventing gainful employment. While the complication rate of 23 per cent is high, the mortality rate is less than 1 per cent.[17] Recently, it has been shown that with resection of the lower lobe for bronchiectasis, the anterior segment of the upper lobe may be realigned in the chest so that it may reside in a dependent position. Subsequently, it may become involved in the bronchiectatic process. In such instances it is difficult to know whether bronchiectasis existed in the anterior segment prior to operation.

In addition to the surgical aspects of the lung itself, one must clear up any infectious disease in the upper respiratory tract with particular attention to the nasal sinuses.

EMPYEMA

Empyema, or the occurrence of pus in the pleural cavity, is usually secondary to pulmonary infections (pneumococcal, streptococcal) but may follow trauma or pulmonary surgery. With the advent of antibiotics this complication is seen less frequently. Surgical management consists of (1) closed thoracotomy drainage, (2) open thoracotomy and (3) excision or decortication of the empyema pocket.

ACUTE AND SUBACUTE EMPYEMA

Closed Thoracotomy Drainage. This term is derived from the fact that the cavity is subjected to a negative pressure in a closed system. First, an intercostal catheter is inserted into the empyema pocket and connected to a Y tube. One limb is connected to a collection bottle subjected to a constant negative pressure. The other limb is connected to an irrigation bottle. Consequently, the cavity can be irrigated periodically. At all other times, the cavity is exposed to negative pressure (Fig. 45-7).

The procedure is used primarily in acute and subacute empyema. However, a more conservative method has partially supplanted closed thoracotomy technics. This consists of the intermittent aspiration and installation of antibiotics combined with enzymatic debridement agents (streptokinase and streptodornase, trypsin). While this method is effective in the early stages of empyema, occasionally a sterilized empyema persists. When this occurs, it must be drained or excised, for an empyema, though sterile, still may result in a pleurocutaneous or bronchopleural fistula.

CHRONIC EMPYEMA

Open Thoracotomy Drainage. By this method the empyema cavity is opened to atmospheric pressure. A short rib segment is removed *at the most dependent portion of the empyema cavity*. A large drainage tube then is inserted into the empyema pocket (Fig. 45-8). Because the cavity is exposed to atmospheric pressure, one must be certain that the empyema is adequately sealed from the remainder of the pleural cavity. Otherwise, a pneumothorax will result with the development of a total empyema. Ordinarily, from 14 to 21 days after onset, the empyema is adequately sealed. Another empirical method for determining the safe period for open thoracotomy is by the observation of the percentage of the aspirate which is sediment. First, the pocket is aspirated; the material is placed in a test tube and taped to the bed of the patient. In 24 hours it will be noted that a considerable cellular debris has settled in the bottom of the tube. Above it is a clear liquid. By periodic aspiration additional samples are obtained. The amount of sediment

Fig. 45-7. Closed thoracotomy drainage. The Stedman pump generates negative pressure for the entire system. The 1st bottle is merely for the collection of aspirate; the purpose of the 3rd bottle is to protect the pump from being damaged in the event that the middle bottle is inadvertently upset. The long tube in the middle bottle is open to the atmosphere. The amount of negative pressure is dependent upon the depth of the lower end of this tube below the water level. Consequently, by adjusting the depth of the tube, the water level, or both, the degree of negative pressure can be controlled. When the negative pressure generated by the motor is greater than desired, atmospheric air is pulled in from the outside through the middle tubing. Consequently, when bubbling occurs, the negative pressure is stabilized at the desired level. This system is similar in principle to any "break-over" type manometer. This apparatus can be applied also in treating pneumothorax.

In empyema, saline solution is an excellent agent for irrigation. By the application of a clamp on the tubing to the 1st bottle and release of the forceps depicted, the irrigating fluid is instilled into the cavity. This tubing is reclamped, and clamps on the tubing to the drainage bottle are reopened. At all times, except for periods of irrigation, negative pressure is maintained in the empyema cavity (see text). Usually the cavity is irrigated every 4 hours with a volume approximately half of the size of the cavity. The size of the cavity can be measured easily by allowing fluid to run in until there is no further flow or the patient complains of discomfort.

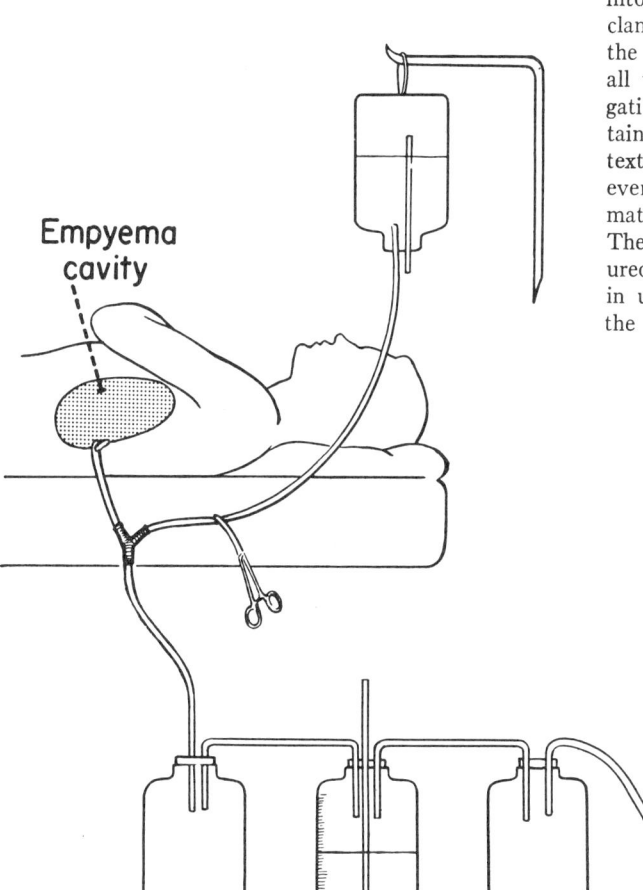

increases as the empyema matures. When the aspirate consists of approximately 80 to 85 per cent sediment, the empyema can be safely drained by open thoracotomy (Fig. 45-9).

The relationship of the etiologic organism and therapy can be credited to Dr. E. A. Graham and the U. S. Army Empyema Commission (1918) which he headed. This commission was established because of the frightening mortality of empyema treated in the military by open thoracotomy drainage during the "influenza" epidemic, due to hemolytic streptococcus. It was demonstrated clearly that empyema due to streptococci accompanied the active pneumonia, and open thoracotomy was performed while the exudate was thin

1388   Lung

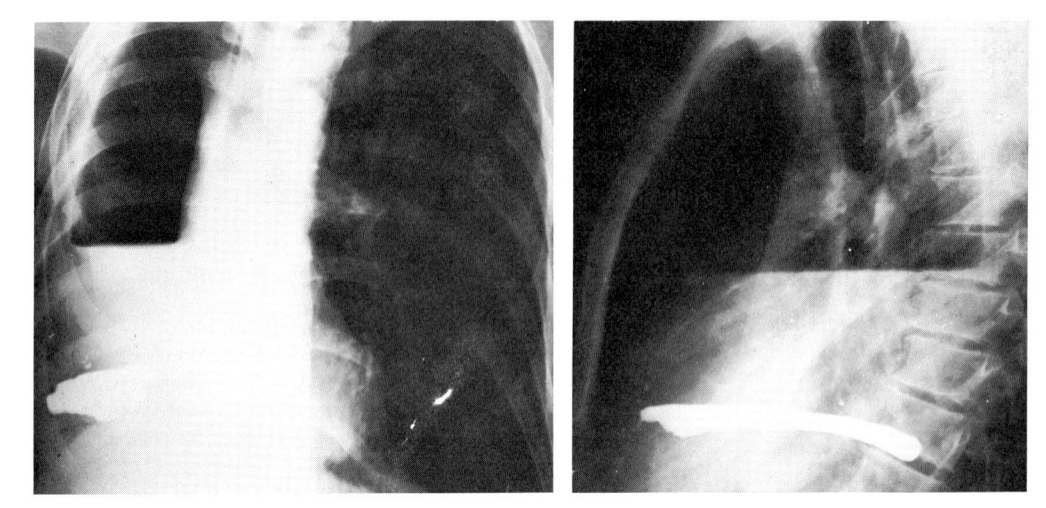

FIG. 45-8. Empyema following pneumonectomy. The instillation of Lipiodol into an empyema cavity is an excellent method to determine its lowermost level and the rib segment which should be removed for dependent drainage. First, the empyema pocket is located by the aspiration of pus, and 10 ml. of Lipiodol is instilled. The patient should remain upright for approximately 10 minutes. Since Lipiodol is heavier than the contents of the cavity, it gravitates to the bottom. Overexposed roentgenograms of the anterior and the lateral views are usually sufficient.

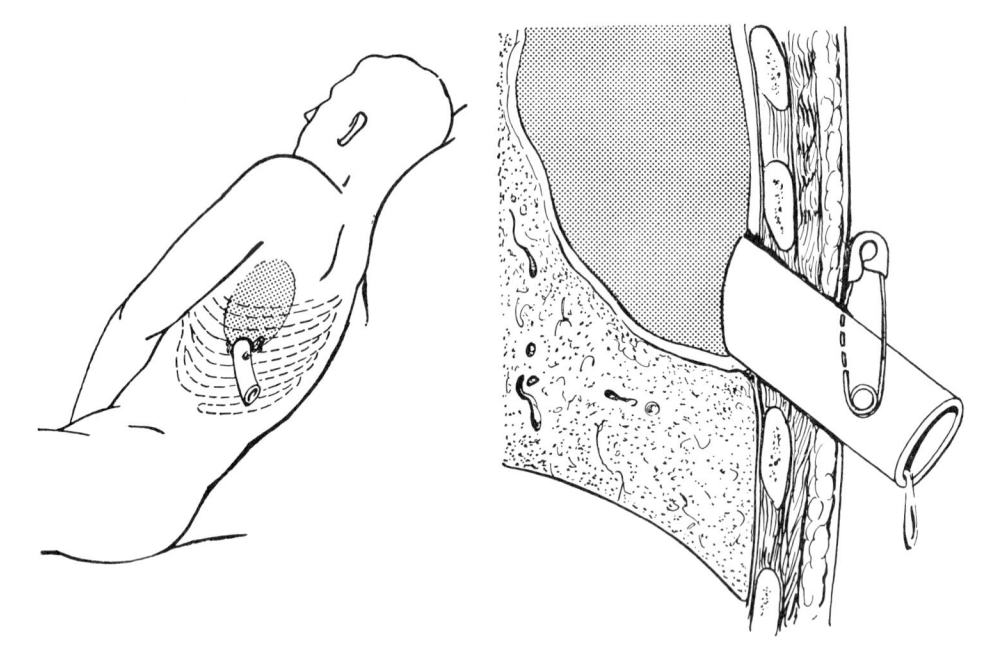

FIG. 45-9. Open thoracotomy drainage (see text). In order for this method to be effective it is essential that the thoracotomy tube be at the most dependent portion of the empyema pocket. The tube should be flush with the parietal pleura. It should be noted that the inner end of the tube has been tailored obliquely so that no lip of the tubing is above the fluid. Consequently, no puddling of undrained pus results. The safety pin is inserted through the tubing and held to the skin by adhesive tape.

and watery. Thus many patients died of asphyxia resulting from an open pneumothorax. On the other hand, empyema in association with pneumococcal pneumonia (a common civilian entity) was a postpneumonic phenomenon, and drainage by open thoracotomy was done when the empyema contained frank pus and during a period when the mediastinum was stabilized by edema and adhesions. These concepts still form the basis for present-day therapy. Early in the course of empyema, regardless of the organism, periodic aspiration is carried out, with the instillation of antibiotics into the pleural cavity. If open thoracotomy is resorted to, frank pus must be present which ensures a localized empyema cavity and mediastinal stability.

This method is effective in curing empyema. Drainage may be prolonged, but the patient need not be hospitalized during this period. Open and closed methods require only local anesthesia.

Excision or Decortication. This procedure may be used as an alternative to open thoracotomy drainage or, in the event of a failure to cure—following open thoracotomy. Excision of all walls of the empyema is preferred by some; however, decortication of the inflammatory membrane or "peel" only over the visceral pleura allows re-expansion of the lung with ablation of the cavity. The thickening of the parietal pleura is due mainly to edema. When the empyema cavity is obliterated, the parietal pleura recedes in thickness and becomes practically normal. Unfortunately, in empyema the visceral peel is very adherent to the visceral pleura. Thus, it can be removed only piecemeal and with considerable trauma to the underlying lung. Negative pressure exerted through a chest catheter is necessary to obtain immediate and continued local pulmonary expansion. Mediastinal empyema is treated best in this fashion. Excision of the empyema pocket, if extensive, carries some risk in younger children. In the ordinary case, many prefer open thoracotomy first. A disadvantage of excision or decortication is the need for a general anesthesia and the postoperative discomfort, for considerable force may be necessary to gain exposure due to the local fixation of the chest wall involved with infection and edema. However, it is an effective and definitive form of therapy and it reduces the duration of the illness sharply.

CERTAIN FUNGAL DISEASES

Coccidioidomycosis

Coccidioidomycosis is an endemic disease peculiar to the San Joaquin valley and the Southwest portion of the United States. *Coccidioides immitis* is the causative fungus. This fungus is diphasic and thus similar to *Histoplasma capsulatum*. In its vegetative phase it consists of long, thin mycelia which segment and form chlamydospores. These chlamydospores are highly infective. It is this form which occurs in nature and has been isolated from the soil and airborne dust in endemic areas.[23]

The initial infection is almost always respiratory and is incurred by the inhalation of fungus in contaminated dust. It is localized in the lungs and usually subsides spontaneously and without sequelae. A history of a patient having visited or traveled through the endemic areas, who, in addition, exhibits a positive coccidioidin skin test, suggests the diagnosis. Hematogenous disseminated forms of the disease occur but are uncommon. In the disseminated forms, the mortality is approximately 50 per cent.

If the disease is localized or the patient survives the disseminated type of illness, lesions in the lung are found. Such lesions are seen in approximately 10 per cent of such patients. These lesions may be solid, discrete, soft granulomatous areas, or cavitation may be present. These findings are usually revealed only by roentgenogram and are unaccompanied by any constitutional symptom.

Amphotericin B is the only agent of proven value for the control of this disease.[29] Surgical treatment is utilized infrequently. Cavitary lesions usually require no therapy. Some will close spontaneously. However, if hemoptyses or recurrent localized pneumonitis occurs, excision is advised (Fig. 45-10). Usually, lobectomy is the procedure of choice because of the frequent presence of satellite granulomas undiagnosed by roentgenograms. Lobectomy, for what appears to be contained disease, should not be regarded as curative. One should entertain the same reservations as in the

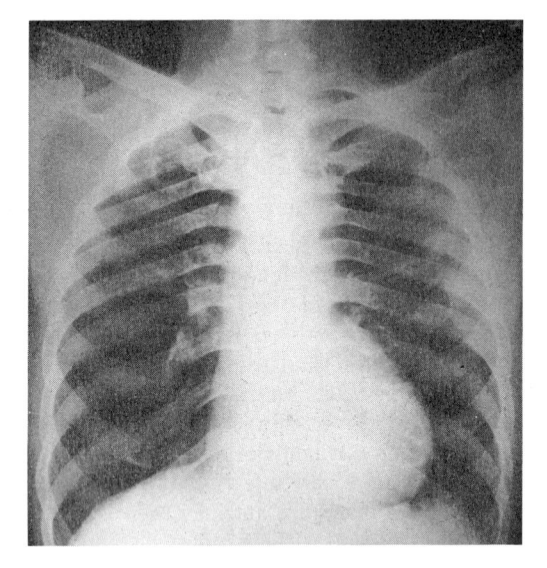

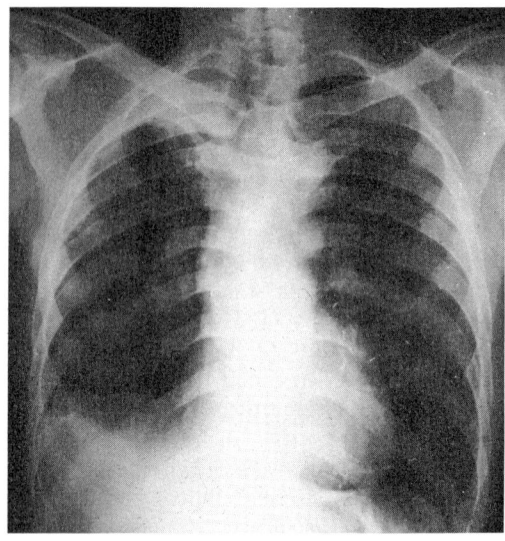

FIG. 45-10. Pulmonary coccidioidomycosis with cavity. Ordinarily, such a cavity is not considered as an indication for surgery. However, this patient had suffered 2 episodes of severe hemoptysis. (*Left*) The cavity is present in the right upper lobe. (*Right*) A right upper lobectomy has been performed. A lobectomy was indicated because of satellite areas of involvement.

tuberculous patient. Solid discrete pulmonary granulomas are quite common. Consequently, the excision of all "coin" lesions becomes impractical in endemic areas. Such lesions must be followed periodically by roentgenograms in these areas whereas in nonendemic portions of the country usually they are excised incidental to establishing an accurate diagnosis.

HISTOPLASMOSIS

Histoplasmosis is caused by the fungus *Histoplasma capsulatum*. The fungus has 2 phases in its life cycle: the yeastlike or parasitic phase and the mycelial or saprophytic phase. Formerly, it was considered to be a disseminated disease and often fatal. This form of the disease actually is rare. Now it is recognized as a relatively benign disease which is widely prevalent. The disease is endemic in the Mississippi Valley. About 70 per cent of adults in this area are histoplasmin positive.[20] However, due to the travel characteristics of the American population and the shunting of military personnel throughout the country, histoplasmosis has been uncovered in practically all parts of the United States.

The organism is a parasite of the reticuloendothelial system and therefore is found in places where these cells are most numerous. In most fatal cases, the organism is disseminated throughout the body and can be isolated in cultures from almost every organ. The pathologic response is a granulomatous reaction which is characterized by epithelioid, giant cells and necrosis. These lesions often calcify. With pulmonary calcific deposits, a positive histoplasmin test in the presence of a negative tuberculin test would allow the diagnosis to be made. Of course, it is possible that both diseases may coexist.

How man acquires an infection with *Histoplasma capsulatum* is not clearly understood. The spores have been found in the soil in endemic areas and in the air. The inhalation of histoplasma spores is the only plausible explanation for the high incidence of positive skin tests in endemic areas. The available epidemiologic and experimental evidence strongly supports the view that the respiratory tract is the port-of-entry of the fungus, regardless of the type of illness it provokes. In the great majority of instances the inhalation of spores results in a nonfatal illness which often remains clinically unrecognized.

The pathologic response to the fungus makes it apparent that sometime following the subacute phase of infection, isolated pulmonary granulomas may result with or without calcifications; or cavitation may be present. Such lesions may be confused with chronic lung abscess, tuberculoma, or primary pulmonary carcinoma. Consequently, in the absence of skin testing or the fear of a more serious coexisting lesion, the surgeon occasionally removes a "coin" lesion by wedge resection, which proves to be histoplasmosis granuloma.[13] Undoubtedly, in endemic areas considerable judgment is required concerning the decision to explore patients exhibiting so-called "coin" lesions. Likewise, on occasion, a lobectomy is performed for cavitation secondary to histoplasmosis.[18] It has been suggested recently that the presence of a cavitary lesion due to histoplasmosis localized to a lobe or even one lung constitutes ample indication for excisional therapy. Such aggressive therapy seems justified at times because cavitary disease is usually progressive and has been observed to produce eventual death from pulmonary insufficiency or disseminated infection. Such lesions can be excised with relative safety.[12] Usually, exploration is incidental to establishing an accurate histologic diagnosis of a pulmonary lesion of undetermined etiology.

Newer, more effective antifungal agents may alter surgical attitudes. Recent experiences with amphotericin B indicate that it is the treatment of choice for chronic pulmonary histoplasmosis with active pulmonary lesions and sputum cultures positive for the organism.[28] It appears to be effective in lowering the mortality and decreasing progression of the disease in the chronic pulmonary type.[14]

Actinomycosis

Actinomycosis is a chronic suppurative or granulomatous disease caused by a specific organism, *Actinomyces bovis*. This organism is in an intermediate position between the "higher" bacteria and fungi. From the clinical viewpoint, it may be considered as a type of pathogenic fungus.[24] The disease is characterized by multiple abscesses, draining sinuses, excess granulation tissue, dense fibrous tissue and by the appearance of mycelial masses (sulfur granules) in the discharges from involved tissue.

The thorax is involved in approximately 20 per cent of cases. Actinomycetes may reach the lung by several routes. Primary infection may occur by aspiration of saliva containing pathogenic actinomyces. Secondary infection may result from downward spread of established cervical infection or by the extension of abdominal infection through or behind the diaphragm. In the past, thoracic involvement carried a grave prognosis; however, the advent of sulfonamides and penicillin have altered the prognosis considerably.

Medical therapy is of prime importance (see Chap. 4, Surgical Infections). Surgery is reserved for the drainage of loculated pus and the excision of destroyed pulmonary tissue or thoracic wall.[11, 25] Surgical therapy is usually considered as an adjunct to chemotherapy and antibiotic therapy with the penicillins.

TRACHEA

Foreign bodies, tumors and diverticula constitute the main items of interest. The diverticula are congenital and presumably represent arrested development of supernumerary lung buds. These are rare and usually have no surgical implications. Foreign bodies occur frequently in children. When large, these may be impacted in the glottis or the trachea with acute suffocation. Sharp objects may lacerate or perforate the trachea. Most foreign bodies are held in place by the surrounding inflammatory process and seldom are coughed out spontaneously. Immediate removal by bronchoscopic methods is indicated; at times, tracheotomy is necessary for their removal. (See Chap. 47 for additional details concerning tumors of the trachea.)

REFERENCES

1. Abbott, O. A., and deOliveira, H. R.: Spontaneous pneumothoraces in patients undergoing peroral endoscopy. J. Thoracic Surg., 14:453-460, 1945.
2. Blades, B., and Dugan, D. J.: Pseudobronchiectasis. J. Thoracic Surg., 13:40-48, 1944.
3. Boyden, E. A.: The intrahilar and related segmental anatomy of the lung. Surgery, 18:706-731, 1945.
4. ———: Segmental Anatomy of the Lungs. New York, McGraw-Hill, 1955.
5. Brock, R. C.: The Anatomy of the Bronchial Tree. ed. 2, London, Oxford University Press, 1954.
6. Brock, R. C., Hodgkiss, F., and Jones, H. O.:

Bronchial embolism and posture in relation to lung abscess. Guy's Hosp. Rep. 91:131-139, 1942.
7. Burford, T. H., and Burbank, B.: Traumatic wet lung: observations on certain physiologic fundamentals of thoracic trauma. J. Thoracic Surg., 14:415-424, 1945.
8. Churchill, E. D.: Bronchiectasis: physical and psychological manifestations. New Eng. J. Med., 218:97-101, 1938.
9. Churchill, E. D., and Belsey, R.: Segmental pneumonectomy in bronchiectasis: the lingula segment of the left upper lobe. Ann. Surg., 109: 481-499, 1939.
10. Comroe, J. H., Forster, R. E., II, Dubois, A. B., Briscoe, W. A., and Carlson, E.: The Lung: Clinical Physiology and Pulmonary Function Tests. Chicago, Year Book Publishers, 1955.
11. Decker, H. R.: The treatment of thoracic actinomycosis by penicillin and sulfonamide drugs. J. Thoracic Surg., 15:430-440, 1946.
12. Diveley, W., McCracken, R., Stoney, W., Guest, J., and McConnell, V.: Surgical treatments of cavitary pulmonary histoplasmosis. J. Thorac. Cardiov. Surg., 45:101, 1963.
13. Forsee, J. H., and Pfotenhauer, M.: Surgical management of focalized pulmonary histoplasmosis. J.A.M.A., 173:878-883, 1960.
14. Furcolow, M. L.: The use of amphotericin B in blastomycosis, cryptococcosis and histoplasmosis. Med. Clin. N. Am., 47:1119-1130, 1963.
15. Goss, C. M. (ed.): Gray's Anatomy. ed. 28. Philadelphia, Lea & Febiger, 1966.
16. Gray, J. S.: Pulmonary Ventilation and Its Physiological Regulation. Springfield, Ill., Charles C Thomas, 1950.
17. Hewlett, T. H., and Ziperman, H. H.: Bronchiectasis: results of pulmonary resection. J. Thorac Cardiov. Surg., 40:71-78, 1960.
18. Hodgson, C. H., Weed, L. A., and Clagett, O. T.: Pulmonary histoplasmosis: summary of data on reported cases and a report on two patients treated by lobectomy. J.A.M.A., 145:807-810, 1951.
19. Jackson, C. L., and Huber, J. F.: Correlated applied anatomy of the bronchial tree and lungs with a system of nomenclature. Dis. Chest., 9: 319-326, 1943.
20. Loosli, C. G.: Histoplasmosis: some clinical epidemiological and laboratory aspects. M. Clin. N. Am., 39:171-199, 1955.
21. Neuhof, H.: The surgical treatment of acute pulmonary abscess. Dis. Chest., 7:74-79, 1941.
22. Overholt, R. H., and Langer, L.: A new technique for pulmonary segmental resection; its application in the treatment of bronchiectasis. Surg. Gynec., Obstet., 84:257-268, 1947.
23. Peterson, J. C., Mapes, R., and Furcolow, M. L.: Round table discussion: systemic mycoses, coccidioidomycosis and histoplasmosis. Pediatrics, 2:709-721, 1948.
24. Pittman, H. S., and Kane, L. W.: Fungus infections of the lungs. M. Clin. N. Am., 35:1323-1331, 1951.
25. Poppe, J. K.: Treatment of pulmonary actinomycosis, with a report of severe arrested cases. J. Thoracic Surg., 15:118-126, 1946.
26. Shedd, D. P., Alley, R. D., and Lindskog, G. E.: Observations on the hemodynamics of bronchialpulmonary vascular communications. J. Thoracic Surg., 22:537-548, 1951.
27. Stern, L.: Etiologic factors in the pathogenesis of putrid abscess of the lung. J. Thoracic Surg., 6:202-211, 1936.
28. Sutliff, W. D.: Histoplasmosis cooperative study II. Chronic pulmonary histoplasmosis treated with and without amphotericin B. Am. Rev. Resp. Dis., 89:641-650, 1964.
29. Winn, W. A.: Coccidioidomycosis and amphotericin B. Med. Clin. N. Am., 47:1131-1148, 1963.

CHAPTER 46

W. E. ADAMS, M.D.

Pulmonary Tuberculosis

Pathology
General Considerations
Indications for Surgical Therapy
Operative Procedures
Results of Surgery

Although pulmonary tuberculosis in the United States has become greatly decreased in incidence during the past two decades and has a much lower associated mortality, surgical therapy continues to be indicated in selective patients. The future outlook for complete control of this disease continues to brighten. However, it is likely that surgical treatment will play a useful role in its overall management for some years to come.

This area of thoracic surgery had its development at the beginning of the present century. However, progress was slow until rather recently. A number of factors have contributed to the rapid acceleration of progress in this field during recent years. Chief among these factors has been the discovery of antimicrobial agents which are effective against the tubercle bacillus. These agents include streptomycin (Schatz and Waksman, 1944), para-aminosalicylic acid (P.A.S.) (Lehmann, 1946), isonicotinic and hydrazide (Isoniazid) (Robitzek, 1952), viomycin (Finley, 1951) and, more recently, pyrazinamide (Yeager, 1952), cycloserine (Jones, 1956), kanamycin (Hok, 1964), ethionamide (Lees, 1964), capreomycin (Schless, 1966) and ethambutol (Oka, 1965). These drugs administered alone or more often in combination, along with bed rest and other supportive measures, improve the status of the pathologic process prior to surgery, thus reducing the magnitude of the operation as well as preserving a greater percentage of pulmonary function. They also greatly reduce the risk of operative procedures and contribute materially in increasing the percentage of arrested cases following surgery. These drugs have been largely responsible for the present marked reduction in mortality following resection of the lung as compared with that existing before their discovery.

A second factor of considerable significance which has contributed to the rapid acceleration of improvement during the past few years has been the development of technics for pulmonary resection and their application in the management of pulmonary tuberculosis. Although these procedures had been evolved previously and applied in the treatment of other pulmonary lesions, their application in the field of pulmonary tuberculosis was relatively unsafe until chemotherapeutic agents became available.

Another factor of considerable importance has been the development of reliable tests for the evaluation of pulmonary function. As judged by present-day standards, tests available for this purpose were of relatively little help prior to the last decade. Although our present methods leave something to be desired and no doubt will continue to be improved, much information can now be obtained which, when correlated with roentgenologic films and other available information, aid materially in the choice of operative procedures as well as the selection of the optimum time for instituting surgical therapy. The decision as to the type of surgical management of the disease process often depends mainly upon clinical evaluation of pulmonary function studies.

A fourth factor contributing to this accelerated progress has been the improvement in methods of collapse therapy. A number of technics have been developed in recent years, all based on a common principle, namely, a selective type of complete collapse of the involved lung, produced by a 1-stage operation, and with preservation of maximum pulmonary function. These procedures consist of a modified type of thoracoplasty with the removal of few or no ribs, and the use of a prosthesis for maintaining the collapse. The objectives of these newer technics have been (1) a higher percentage of arrested cases following the operation, (2) a 1-stage operative procedure, (3) avoidance of postoperative deformity and (4) preservation of maximal lung function. All 4 of these objectives have been accomplished by these procedures without increasing the risk of operation or the frequency of complications.

Since antimicrobial therapy does not always render the sputum free of *Mycobacterium tuberculosis*, the use of collapse therapy in the form of thoracoplasty preceding resection of the diseased lung tissue will reduce the incidence of complications and increase the safety of surgery. This is especially true when more than an upper lobe or an entire lung needs resection. Also, in the case of smaller upper lobe lesions in poor-risk patients, an effective localized collapse by thoracoplasty may be enough to arrest the disease and free the sputum of bacteria.

PATHOLOGY

In the surgical treatment of pulmonary tuberculosis, the time as well as the type of therapy is dictated by the pathologic status of the disease. This is determined largely by (among other things) the virulence of the organism and the resistance of the host. With progressive disease, one or more cavities usually develop and are accompanied by some bronchogenic spread of the infection to the same or opposite side, or to both sides. The size, the location and the distribution of cavities, as well as the presence of the bronchogenic dissemination, will determine if and when surgical therapy is indicated, as well as the type of management best suited for the patient.

The amount of pulmonary destruction with reduction in pulmonary reserve will have a direct bearing upon therapy. X-ray appearance of the lung may be very misleading, both as to the amount of pulmonary destruction as well as the status of pulmonary reserve. The nature of a bronchial communication with a pulmonary cavity may have considerable influence on the over-all pathologic picture presented. If the bronchus shows evidence of stenosis with partial obstruction, one of the following may develop: (1) a persistent or expanding cavity, (2) atelectasis of the obstructed lung, (3) a "closed cavity" filled with inspissated caseous material, or (4) development of tension cavity. When a tuberculous process involves a lower lobe near the hilum, tuberculous bronchiectasis is apt to develop due to partial obstruction of the bronchial outlet. In such patients symptoms usually are due to a combination of tuberculosis and nontuberculous inflammatory processes and atelectasis.

When the tuberculous process is near the periphery of the lung, involvement of the pleura, either in the form of a fibrous pleurisy or a pleural effusion, may result. This fluid may become contaminated with *Mycobacterium tuberculosis*, resulting in the formation of empyema of the pleural space. If pyogenic organisms are also present, the lesion is known as a mixed tuberculous empyema. This usually occurs only when a direct communication between a bronchus and the pleural cavity, viz., a bronchopleural fistula, develops. The management of these various pathologic processes will be discussed under subsequent headings.

In the surgical therapy of pulmonary tuberculosis, the principal objectives may be defined as: (1) permanent arrest of the disease, (2) preservation of function of the uninvolved lung, (3) prevention of complications in surgical management, (4) early return to useful activity and (5) rendering the person incapable of transmitting the disease to others. Thus, as previously noted, the character and the distribution of pathologic lesions will largely determine whether these objectives may be secured. Likewise, the status and the course of the disease at the time of surgery will play a major role in this regard. A third factor of importance is the method of surgical management.

One of the most important considerations in surgical treatment of pulmonary tuberculosis is proper selection of patients for operation. In the evaluation of tuberculous patients for surgery, a number of factors concerned with the status of the disease must be taken into consideration. These factors consist of (1) the entire duration of the disease, (2) duration of the present problem presented by the patient, (3) status of the activity of the disease, (4) distribution of the lesion (unilateral or bilateral and the amount of lung involved), (5) type and status of nonsurgical therapy, (6) presence and extent of extrapulmonary disease, (7) physical factors, such as obstructed cavity, and (8) consideraton of the patient's resistance.

These factors will have a direct bearing not only on the time of operative intervention but also on the type of surgical procedure indicated. In the evaluation of a patient for surgery, not only should the history, the physical findings and the laboratory examination be scrutinized carefully but, in addition, various tests to determine the status of cardiopulmonary reserve should be made in order to have a complete evaluation of the problem.

GENERAL CONSIDERATIONS

Preparation of the Patient for Operation

Primary consideration must be given to the proper preparation of patients for surgery in order to avoid serious complications. The nutritional condition of the individual and the status of the blood regarding hemoglobin concentration and cell volume, as well as protein content, are important. Preparation of the patient for surgery always should be preceded by the use of chemotherapy both for pyogenic as well as acid-fast organisms, the length of time of such medication varying according to the status of the disease. The use of special x-ray examinations, such as planigrams, as well as oblique views, aids materially in accurate localization of the lesion in order to plan definitive surgery. All patients should be examined by bronchoscopy prior to surgery, to determine the presence or the absence of tuberculous bronchitis or stenosis of the bronchus. This is particularly indicated where excisional therapy is planned but is also of value in collapse therapy. Since most patients with bilateral pulmonary tuberculosis develop some reduction in the size of the lesser circulatory bed and pulmonary arteriovenous shunt, a careful check for evidence of cardiac strain is important before operation. Finally, in order to evaluate the pulmonary reserve, pulmonary function studies should be made to aid in planning the type of surgery, as well as to prognose the outcome following therapy.

Anesthesia

Since deep muscular relaxation is unnecessary in thoracic surgery, a light anesthesia making use of simpler methods and mixtures of anesthetic agents has much to be recommended. Ether-oxygen has gained greater favor because of its wide range of safety and the absence of depression of the respiratory center. Induction with a gas-oxygen mixture that is not depressing to respiration or circulation is advantageous. Constant adequate ventilation should be assured and oxygen administered in adequate amounts.

INDICATIONS FOR SURGICAL THERAPY

In spite of adequate antimicrobial therapy, persistent cavitary lesions associated with either a negative or positive sputum continue to present problems. In the case of the former, continuation of drug therapy for a period of months or even years is frequently justified if complete cooperation of the patient can be obtained. However, in patients who give a history of alcoholism or other drug addictions, dependability is still uncertain. Again, cavitary lesions in certain groups, such as school teachers, food handlers, or people with similar occupations, present a hazard not only to themselves but to others as well and therefore prolonged drug therapy should be avoided. Furthermore, pulmonary tuberculosis coexisting with other diseases, such as diabetes, makes early complete control by surgical excision desirable even in open negative cavities.

Open positive cavities in patients with drug-resistant organisms present a special problem. Here the risk of excisional surgery is much greater from the standpoint of complications, as well as mortality following surgery.

The general principles governing all surgical management of pulmonary tuberculosis are: (1) preoperative determination of pulmonary reserve; (2) the use of anesthesia which assures adequate circulation and oxygenation during operation; (3) employment of a surgical approach which provides adequate exposure; (4) maintenance of normal blood volume, (normovolemia) during surgery by replacement of blood loss; and (5) postoperative care which provides for adequate oxygenation of the vital tissues and for control of infection.

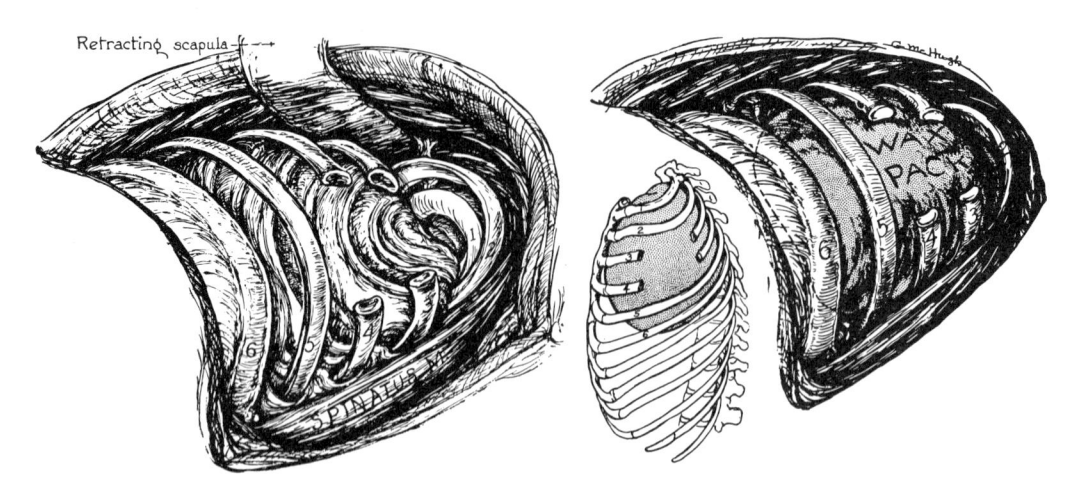

FIG. 46-1. (*Left*) Drawing to illustrate the appearance of the collapsed area following freeing of the periosteum and the intercostal structures from the first 5 ribs in the treatment of pulmonary tuberculosis. Note that the structures are depressed from beneath these ribs and that only short segments of the 3rd and the 4th ribs were removed. (*Right*) Appearance of chest with the wax prosthesis placed beneath the ribs from which the soft parts have been mobilized. Note the selective nature of the collapse. By resecting only short segments of 1 or 2 ribs no scoliosis results, and the wax is well maintained in position.

OPERATIVE PROCEDURES

It is universally agreed that in 75 per cent or more of patients needing surgery, excisional therapy is the procedure of choice. Paralysis and elevation of the diaphragm by phrenic nerve crush introduced by Sauerbruch (1913) is now used only in patients with a lower lobe lesion with persistent positive sputum in spite of drug therapy or as a pleural space-reducing mechanism.

Extrapleural Paravertebral Thoracoplasty

This operative procedure was one of the earliest used in the surgical treatment of pulmonary tuberculosis. It was first designed by Cerenville in 1885 and has been modified by a number of workers in this field. In order to obtain greater effectiveness and reduced surgical risk, Sauerbruch (1920) developed a procedure termed extrapleural paravertebral thoracoplasty which was used for many years. The conventional present-day thoracoplasty is patterned somewhat after the Brauer (1909) type of operation with the exception that it is performed in 2 or more stages in order to reduce the risk of the procedure.

Indications. Since more prompt and effective care is now available for most patients with pulmonary tuberculosis, the indications for thoracoplasty are much less frequent than in the past. They include: (1) fibrocavernous lesions at the apex of the lung, especially in the presence of bilaterally active disease and where the organisms are no longer sensitive to antimicrobial drugs; (2) as a preliminary procedure to resection in some bilateral cavitary lesions; (3) where pulmonary function is inadequate for safe excisional therapy; and (4) where the extent and the character of the disease or the presence of extrapulmonary lesions make resection hazardous.

It is difficult to compare accurately the results of various types of surgical therapy in the treatment of pulmonary tuberculosis. However, when various advantages, disadvantages and risks are considered, it may be said that for far-advanced fibrocavitary lesions, thoracoplasty will carry less risk than resection but will not yield as high a percentage of arrested cases.

Thoracoplasty With Extrafascial and Extraperiosteal Paraffin Prosthesis

Because of the several deficiencies in the conventional type of thoracoplasty, attempts have been made to produce a more selective

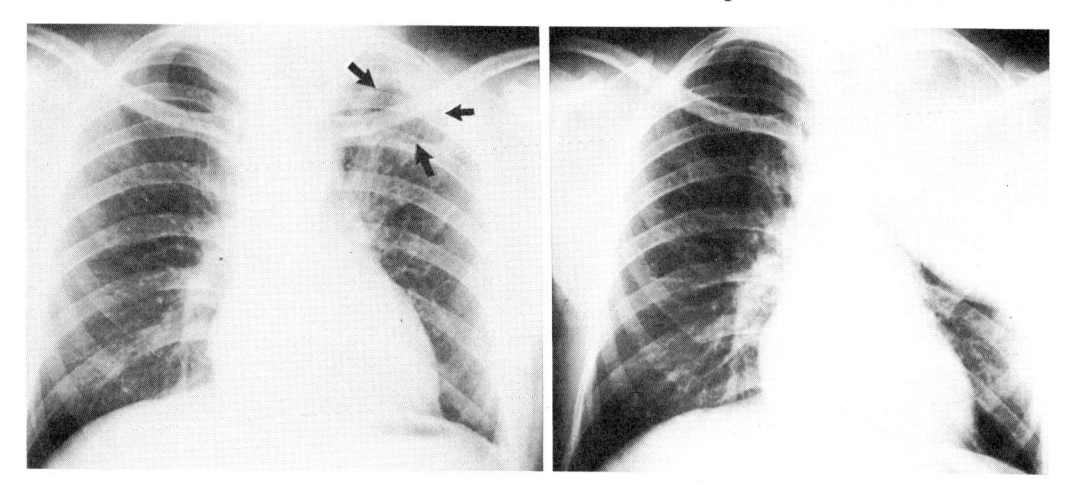

FIG. 46-2. (*Left*) Roentgenogram of a 27-year-old East Indian student who had had pulmonary tuberculosis for several years. The patient improved temporarily and then his condition remained stationary. The tubercle bacilli became insensitive to all chemotherapeutic agents. Note large cavity in the left apex. This patient had had bilateral involvement, although, at the time of surgery, the disease in the right lung was stationary. A collapse of the upper portion of the chest wall prior to resection of that portion of lung was thought to be indicated in order to reduce the risk of resectional therapy. (*Right*) X-ray appearance of the chest approximately 7 weeks following a single-stage modified thoracoplasty with subscapular extrafascial paraffin prosthesis. Note the selective nature of collapse with preservation of aerated lung tissue below. The patient's sputum was converted following operation, and he was completely relieved of symptoms. In view of the size of the cavitary lesion it was concluded that complete healing was very unlikely. Therefore, a resection of the upper lobe was made a few months following the operation. The patient has made a good recovery and has had no further trouble since operation. A. P. views.

type of collapse by a 1-stage procedure. The operation was developed in 1947 (Adams) and entails the mobilization of the periosteum and the intercostal structures from the ribs and the use of an extrafascial prosthesis of a suitable plastic material placed in the collapse area. It is a 1-stage procedure which produces a selective type of collapse of the lung tissue beneath as many as 8 ribs. A short segment of approximately 2 inches of only 1 rib, usually the 3rd, is resected (Fig. 46-1).

Advantages of this procedure include: (1) increased percentage of arrested cases (approximately 90%), (2) a single-stage operation, (3) obviation of scoliosis and resultant deformity, thus minimizing reduction in pulmonary function, (4) lessened surgical expense (Figs. 46-2 and 46-3) and (5) when used preceding resection in persistently positive cases, considerable reduction in both morbidity and mortality. Complications observed following the use of this procedure have been minimal (Ortega, 1954).

RESECTION THERAPY

This type of surgical management was first suggested by Forlanini approximately 70 years ago and was attempted by Ruggi in 1884 and by Tuffier in 1897. However, due to the delay in advancement of ancillary therapy this type of operative management did not become practical until during the past 20 years. Factors which contribute to the present success of resectional therapy include: (1) alteration in character and decrease in extent of the disease by the use of chemotherapy prior to surgery; (2) development of surgical technics which permit the safe excision of varying amounts of pulmonary tissue; and (3) development of tests of pulmonary function which more accurately reveal the status of cardiopulmonary reserve prior to surgery.

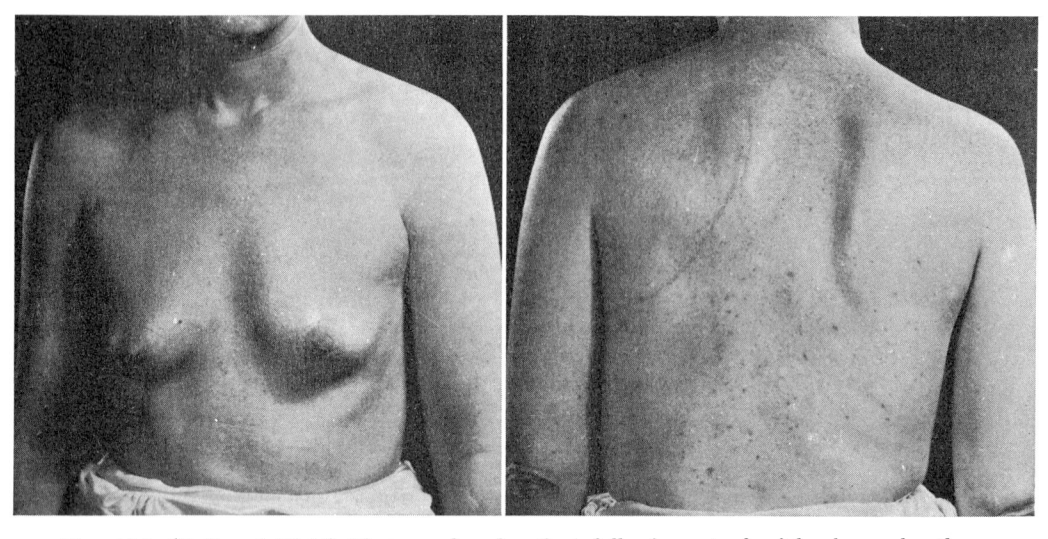

FIG. 46-3. (*Left* and *Right*) Photographs of patient following extrafascial subscapular thoracoplasty with wax prosthesis in which collapse of the lung beneath the first 6 ribs was carried out. Note complete lack of deformity.

Indications. Because of the safety of operation and the high percentage of successful results, the value of pulmonary resection is established.

At present the principal indications for this operation in the treatment of pulmonary tuberculosis are: (1) thoracoplasty failure; (2) lower lobe lesions, particularly cavities in the superior segment, or secondary bronchiectasis; (3) destroyed lung; (4) closed (active) tuberculous lesions; (5) when malignancy cannot be excluded; (6) small cavitary lesions which do not heal completely with antimicrobial therapy; and (7) very large cavities.

Excisional therapy has a number of advantages over the conventional thoracoplasty where smaller isolated lesions are present: (1) it is selective in type and is more conservative of pulmonary function; (2) only one operation is required; and (3) little or no postoperative deformity occurs (the last two advantages do not apply to extrafascial-extraperiosteal thoracoplasty with paraffin or plastic prosthesis).

Contraindication. The principal contraindication to excisional therapy is the presence of advanced bilateral fibrocavernous lesions of considerable magnitude in patients having poor host resistance, and with tubercle bacilli no longer sensitive to chemotherapy.

Mortality and morbidity following excisional therapy have been reduced markedly by the use of chemotherapy. However, when lesions of considerable magnitude are accepted for resection, complications may occur. Those most commonly observed are (1) bronchial obstruction with atelectasis of the remaining lung tissues; (2) contralateral or ipsilateral spread of the infection; (3) bronchopleural fistula with tuberculous or mixed empyema and spread of the infection; and (4) spread of the tuberculous infection to extrapulmonary tissues such as the mediastinum and the pericardium. Of these complications, the one most commonly seen is spread of the disease within the lungs. However, the complication which more often contributes to the mortality of the operation is the development of a bronchopleural fistula accompanied by a tuberculous or a mixed empyema. This complication is almost always accompanied by an additional spread of infection to the contralateral or ipsilateral lung. These serious complications are observed more often after pneumonectomy or lobectomy rather than following segmental resection.

Operations. Four types of procedures are employed: (1) pneumonectomy, (2) lobectomy, (3) segmental resection (Churchill, 1939), (Blades, 1940), (Björk, 1959), and

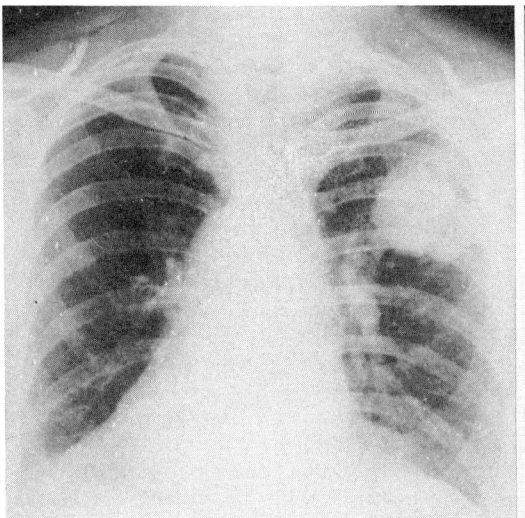

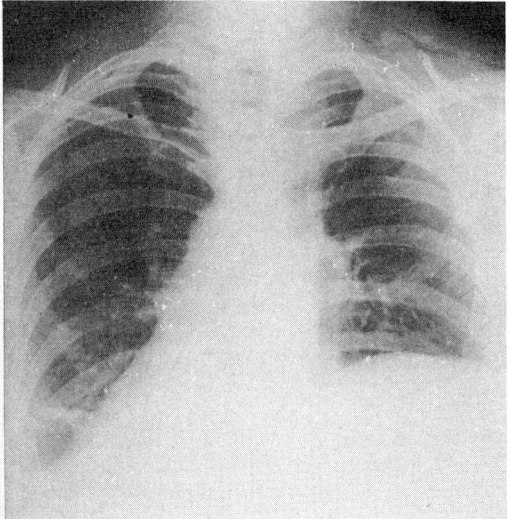

FIG. 46-4. This patient was a 62-year-old white female having had a nonproductive cough of several months' duration. She had lost no weight and was in good general condition. (*Left*) P. A. view of the thorax, showing a circumscribed opacity in the right upper lung lobe. Differential diagnosis included pulmonary tuberculosis and carcinoma of the lung. (*Right*) P. A. view of the chest following extirpation of the right upper lung lobe. The lesion was found to be a closed tuberculous abscess with evidence of activity. Note expansion of the right middle and lower lobes to fill the right thorax completely. Partial collapse of the chest wall following resection of the lung is unnecessary when the remaining portion is normal.

(4) local excision. The choice of these operations is determined by the location and the extent of the lesion as well as the cardiopulmonary reserve of the patient. Temporary paralysis of the diaphragm is helpful at times in reducing the size of the pleural space following surgery (Fig. 46-4). Since tuberculous lesions are frequently considerably reduced in size with the use of antimicrobial therapy, segmental resection has been more frequently employed (Fig. 46-5, A to C) (Webb, 1960).

RESULTS OF SURGERY

As stated earlier, the results of surgery for the treatment of pulmonary tuberculosis will vary considerably according to the status of the pathologic process, virulence of the organisms, host resistance, and selection of patients for operation. For this reason proper evaluation of reported statistics in this regard is quite difficult. It may be stated, however, that when various operative procedures are not pushed beyond their limitations, satisfactory results may be obtained in a high percentage of patients (90 to 95%). In the collapse type of operation the risk of surgery is somewhat less, reduction of pulmonary function may be somewhat greater, and arrest of the disease may be anticipated in between 85 to 90 per cent of patients. Excisional therapy must be used where a collapsing operation has failed. The mortality risk of lobectomy and pneumonectomy will average approximately 5 and 8 per cent respectively. The risk to life of segmental resection is much less, being approximately 1 or 2 per cent (Mendenhall, 1960). Arrest of the disease may be anticipated in 85 to 95 per cent of patients in whom a lobectomy or a pneumonectomy is required. This figure will be somewhat higher in patients following segmental resections for smaller lesions (Chamberlain, 1950), (Overholt, 1950). These results are much better than those of a decade ago. With a gradual diminution of the number of patients with

1400 Pulmonary Tuberculosis

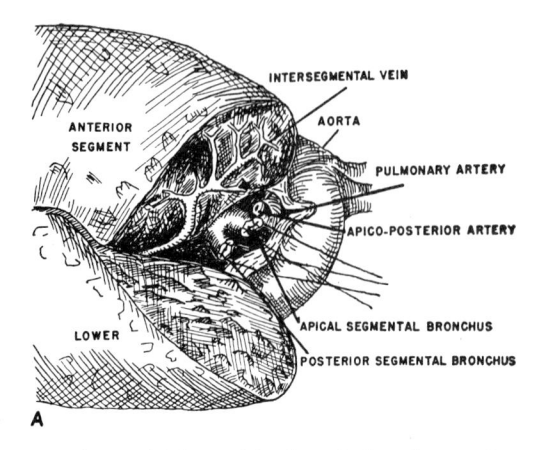

FIG. 46-5. (A) Drawing to show appearance of the left hilum following resection of the apical posterior segment of the left upper lung lobe. The apical posterior bronchi are closed by interrupted sutures. No attempt is made to close or pleuralize the raw surface following segmental resection. This patient was a 43-year-old female who presented a symptomless lesion in the left apex. This shadow was discovered by her physician on routine x-ray examination. Sputum examinations were positive for acid-fast bacilli. (B) P. A. view of the chest of another patient showing an ill-defined opacity at the level of the right clavicle. (C, *inset*) Laminogram demonstrating multiple cavities in apical and posterior segments of right upper lobe. (D) P. A. view of the chest taken 3 months following resection of the right apical and posterior segments. Note complete filling of the right chest by the remaining pulmonary tissue. This patient has been followed for over 7 years after operation and has had no evidence of activity.

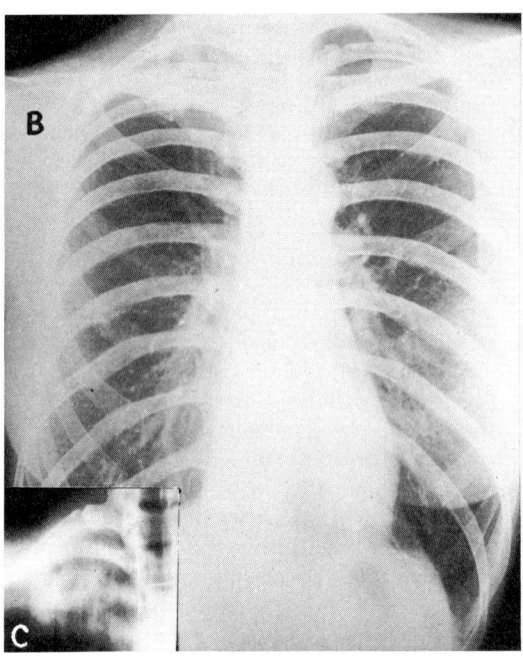

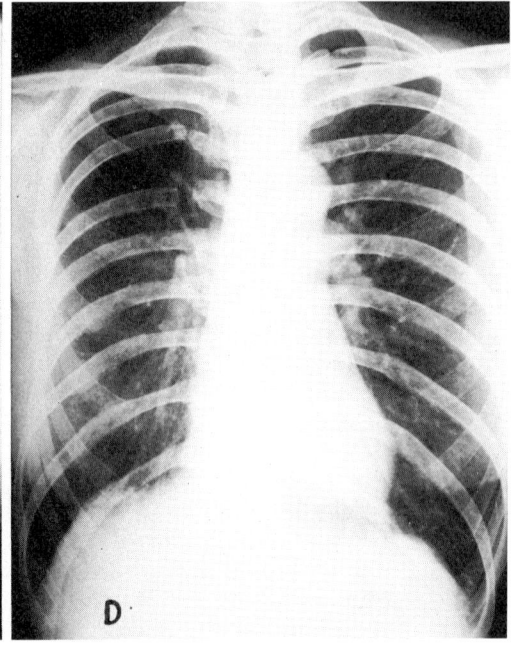

severe and advanced lesions, the outlook for further improvement in these statistics is quite good.

REFERENCES

Adams, W. E., Lees, W. M., and Fritz, J. M.: Subcapsular paraffin pack as a supplement to thoracoplasty in the treatment of pulmonary tuberculosis. Thoracic Surg., 22:375, 1951.

Baer, G.: Ueber extrapleurale Pneumolyse mit sofortiger Plombierung bei Lungentuberkulose. München med. Wschr., 60:1587, 1913.

Björk, V. O.: Segmental resection for pulmonary tuberculosis. J. Thoracic Surg., 37:135, 1959.

Blades, B., and Kent, E. M.: Individual ligation technique for lower lobe lobectomy. J. Thoracic Surg., 10:84, 1940.

Brauer, L.: Erfahrungen und Überlegungen zur Lungenkollapstherapie: I. Die ausgedehnte extrapleurale Thorakoplastik. Beitr. klin. Tuberk., 12:49, 1909.

Chamberlain, J. M., and Ryan, T. C.: Segmental

resection in pulmonary diseases. J. Thoracic Surg., 19:199, 1950.

Churchill, E. D., and Belsey, R.: Segmental pneumonectomy in bronchiectasis; the lingual segment of the left upper lobe. Ann. Surg., 109:481, 1939.

Finley, A. C., Hobby, G. L., Hochstein, F., Lees, T. M., Lenert, T. F., Means, J. A., P'an, S. Y., Regna, P. P., Routien, J. B., Sobin, B. A., Tate, K. B., and Kane, J. H.: Viomycin, a new antibiotic active against mycobacteria. Am. Rev. Tuberc., 63:1, 1951.

Hok, T. T.: A comparative study of the susceptibility to streptomycin, cycloserine, viomycin and kanamycin of tubercle bacilli from 100 patients never treated with cycloserine, viomycin or kanamycin. Am. Rev. Resp. Dis., 90:961, 1964.

Jones, L. R.: Calorimetric determination of cycloserine, a new antibiotic. Ann. Chem., 28:39, 1956.

Lees, A. W.: Ethionamide and isoniazid in previously untreated cases of pulmonary tuberculosis. Dis. Chest., 45:247, 1964.

Lehmann, J.: Para-aminosalicylic acid in the treatment of tuberculosis. Lancet, 1:15, 1946.

Mendenhall, J. T., Cree, E., Rasmussen, H. K., Bauer, H., and Curtis, J. K.: Studies of pulmonary function before and after pulmonary resection in 450 tuberculous patients. II. Case analysis of patients with large loss of vital capacity and maximum breathing capacity. J. Thoracic Surg., 39:189, 1960.

Oka, S., Konno, K., and Kudo, S.: Clinical studies on ethambutal. Am. Rev. Resp. Dis., 91:762, 1965.

Ortega, Flores, Lopez-Belio, M., Adams, W. E., Fox, R., and Lees, W. M.: La parafina como coadyuvante colapsoterapica dela toracoplastia; Estudio de 400 casos tratados por este método. Presented at Decima tercera Conferencia Internacional de la Lucha contra la Tuberculosis, Madrid, Spain, September, 1954.

Overholt, R. H., Woods, F. M., and Ramsay, B. H.: Segmental pulmonary resection: details of technique and results. J. Thoracic Surg., 19:207, 1950.

Robitzek, E. H., Selikoff, I. J., and Ornstein, G. G.: Chemotherapy of human tuberculosis with hydrazine derivatives of isonicotinic acid. Quart. Bull. Sea View Hosp., 13:25, 1952.

Ruggi, G.: La tecnica della pneumectoma nell'uomo. Bologna, 1884.

Sauerbruch, F.: Die Beeinflussung von Lungenerkrankungen durch künstliche Lahmung des Zwerchfells (Phrenikotomie). München med. Wschr. 60:625, 1913.

———: Die chirurgie der Brustorgane. Berlin, Springer, 1920.

Schatz, A., and Waksman, S. A.: Effect of streptomycin and other antibiotic substances upon mycobacterium tuberculosis and related organisms. Proc. Soc. Exp. Biol. Med., 57:244, 1944.

Schless, J. M., Allison, R. F., and Inglis, R. M.: Capreomycin-ethionamide as a retreatment regimen for pulmonary tuberculosis. Ann. N.Y. Acad. Sci., 135:1085, Apr. 20, 1966.

Tuffier, T.: Chirurgie du poumon, en particulier dans les cavernes tuberculeuses et la gangrene pulmonaire. p. 31, Paris, Masson, 1897.

———: Collapsthérapie par décollement pleuropariétal pour tuberculose limitée au sommet du poumon, greffe d'un fragment de tissu adipeux dans l'espace décollé. Bull. et mém. Soc. chirurgiens Paris, 49:1249, 1923.

Webb, W. R., Wofford, J. K., and Stauss, H.: Resectional therapy for residual noninfectious cavitary tuberculous lesions. Am. Rev. Resp. Dis., 81:850, 1960.

Yeager, R. L., Munroe, W. G. C. and Dessau, F. I.: Pyrazinamide (Aldinomide). Am. Rev. Tub., 65:523, 1952

CHAPTER 47

JOHN H. GIBBON, JR., M.D., AND THOMAS F. NEALON, JR., M.D.

Carcinoma of the Lung and Tumors of the Thorax

Tumors of the Lung
Tumors of the Mediastinum
Tumors of the Thoracic Wall

The widespread utilization of chest x-ray surveys in recent years has brought to light many intrathoracic tumors. These lesions have proved to be much commoner than had been realized formerly. The discovery of previously unrecognized lesions and the apparent absolute increase in cancer of the lung has made the thorax a region of great surgical significance. Thoracic tumors will be considered under 3 headings according to the site of origin: (1) tumors of the lung, (2) tumors of the mediastinum, (3) tumors of the thoracic wall.

TUMORS OF THE LUNG

Tumors of the lung are by far the largest group of thoracic tumors because of the great prevalence of cancer of the lung. They will be considered under the headings of: malignant tumors (primary and metastatic) and benign tumors (adenoma and hamartoma).

Primary Malignant Tumors

Bronchogenic carcinoma is the commonest primary malignant tumor of the lung, and it is rapidly fatal if untreated. It is predominantly a disease of the male sex, about 90 per cent of all tumors occurring in men. In this sex it is the commonest cause of death from cancer (Fig. 47-1). During 1964 in the United States 45,838 persons died of carcinoma of the lung (U.S.P.H.S., 1966). Approximately 95 per cent of all cases occur between the ages of 40 and 70.

Etiology. Much has been written concerning possible predisposing causes of cancer of the lung, but little is definitely known. The incidence of carcinoma has been reported to be unusually high among workers in chromate, uranium, arsenic, certain nickel and copper ores in which arsenic occurs as an impurity and in asbestos. Apparently all types of dust cannot be incriminated because the incidence is not higher in miners with anthrocosilicosis.

The relationship of smoking to cancer of the lung has been widely discussed not only in medical journals but also in the lay press. Wynder and Graham (1950) in this country and Doll and Hill (1950) in England reported a higher incidence of cancer of the lung among heavy cigarette smokers. Shortly after this, Hammond and Horn (1954), working with large population samples, showed that both the incidence of, and the death rate from, cancer of the lung were higher among heavy cigarettes smokers. Thus, there appears to be a definite relationship between cigarette smoking and cancer of the lung. The Advisory Committee to the Surgeon General of the Public Health Service, U. S. Department of Health, Education and Welfare, came to the conclusion that epidemiological evidence concerning cigarette smoking and lung cancers has confirmed positive relationships with increasing numbers of cigarettes smoked, with increasing duration, and with decreasing age of initiation of habit. Male cigarette smokers of less than one pack a day have mortality ratios as high as 10 and smokers of more than one pack a day have mortality ratios as high as 30 (Public Health Service Publication No. 1996).

Pathology. The 3 main histologic types of bronchogenic carcinoma in order of frequency are the epidermoid, the anaplastic and the adenocarcinomas. In any cancer of the lung, all 3 cell types usually may be found if mul-

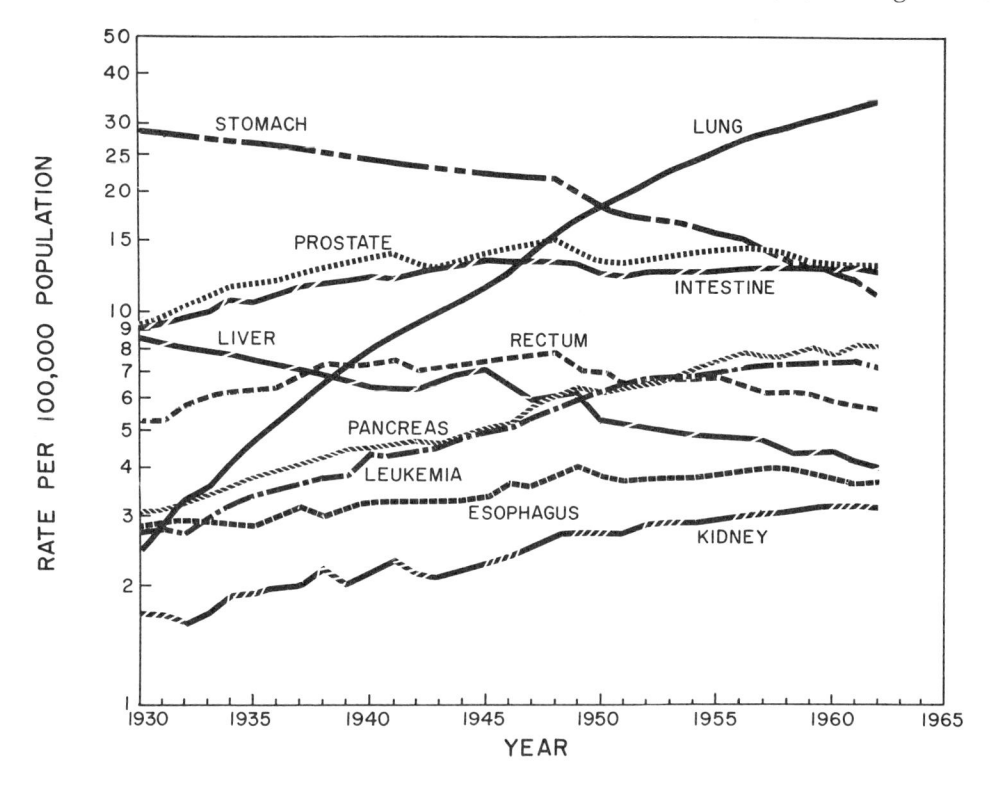

FIG. 47-1. Male cancer death rates by site, United States, 1930-1962. The rates for the male population are standardized for age on the 1940 population of the United States. (Graph prepared by the American Cancer Society from data obtained from the National Office of Vital Statistics and the Bureau of the Census, U.S.)

tiple sections are taken. Nevertheless, tumors are classified according to the predominant cell type. The epidermoid, or squamous cell, carcinoma is the commonest type and accounts for about half the lesions. The epidermoid carcinoma usually originates in the segmental bronchi and extends into the lobar bronchi. It may produce a polypoid tumor projecting into the bronchus or a cicatricial narrowing of the bronchus. This cell type tends to invade the bronchial mucosa adjacent to the gross tumor mass. Cavitary carcinomas of the lung (Fig. 47-2) are most frequently squamous. This cavitation results from excavation of the cornified epithelium which forms in the center of the mass of squamous cells.

About 20 per cent of cancers of the lung are adenocarcinomas. Usually they are circumscribed peripheral lesions, although they may involve larger bronchi. This type is relatively uncommon in men but comprises approximately half of the carcinomas of the lung in women. The remaining 30 per cent are undifferentiated tumors. These tumors most frequently occur in the larger bronchi and often are characterized by massive extrabronchial involvement. Often the extrabronchial involvement is so marked as to suggest a mediastinal tumor in the roentgenogram.

Finally, there is a rare type of cancer of the lung called alveolar cell carcinoma. Bronchiolar carcinoma is probably a better term, as the cells apparently arise from the epithelium of the terminal bronchioles. These tumors generally appear as ill-defined masses in the parenchyma of the lung and do not produce symptoms early.

Sarcomas may arise from the connective tissue elements in the lung but are very rare. Unless a bronchoscopic biopsy is obtained, the lesion cannot be distinguished from a carcinoma before operation. Involvement of the mediastinal lymph nodes is less common than in bronchogenic carcinoma.

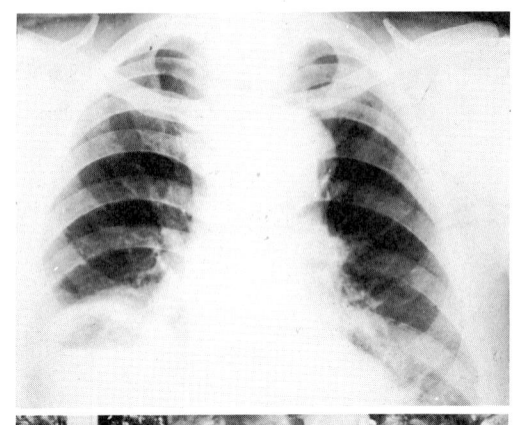

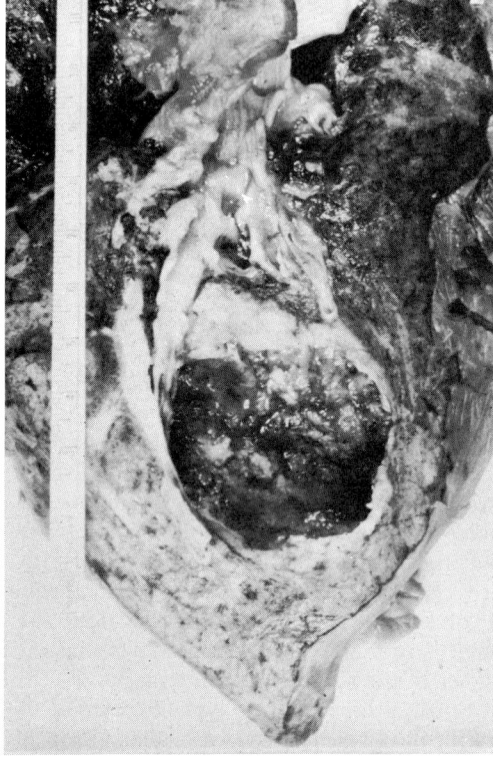

FIG. 47-2. (*Top*) Roentgenogram of a cavitary lesion with a fluid level in the right lower lobe. (*Bottom*) At operation this proved to be an epidermoid carcinoma with a large central area of cavitation.

Cell type affects the prognosis (Kirklin, 1955). The epidermoid carcinoma probably has the best prognosis. The adenocarcinomas occupy an intermediate position. The anaplastic, or undifferentiated, carcinoma is the most malignant. Regardless of cell type, if metastasis to the mediastinal lymph nodes or invasion of the chest wall has occurred the prognosis is poor.

Invasion of contiguous structures is a characteristic of bronchogenic carcinomas. The trachea or the opposite bronchus, the main pulmonary artery or the pulmonary veins up to the left atrium may be invaded. Invasion of the parietal pericardium is common. Peripheral tumors may extend into the chest wall, necessitating resection of the overlying ribs and intercostal structures in continuity. The prognosis for patients with chest wall involvement is very poor.

Metastasis may occur by the lymphatics or the blood stream. Hilar tumors generally metastasize by the lymphatics, while peripheral lesions are more prone to spread by the blood stream. However, cancers in either location may spread by either route. The lymphatic route is to the carinal and the paratracheal lymph nodes and then to the para-esophageal and cervical chain, particularly the supraclavicular group. The axillary nodes are less often involved by spread across the pleural space via adhesions to the chest wall or by lymphatic connections with the cervical and the mediastinal lymphatics. Hematogenous metastases appear most frequently in the liver, the adrenal glands, the brain and the bodies of the vertebrae but may occur in any part of the body. In view of the frequent finding of cancer cells in the sputum and the bronchial secretions, it is surprising that endobronchial metastasis is rare.

Symptoms. Cough is the first symptom noted by more than half the patients with cancer of the lung, and over 90 per cent have a cough by the time the diagnosis is established. In the early stages the cough is dry but later tends to become productive. The frequency and the intensity of the cough usually are out of proportion to the sputum produced. Most men who are heavy cigarette smokers have a chronic cough. When such individuals develop bronchogenic carcinoma, the cough usually becomes worse. About half the patients with cancer of the lung have expectorated blood-streaked sputum on one or more occasions. Severe bleeding is rare. Unfortunately, hemoptysis is rarely a first symptom. If it were, more patients undoubtedly would seek professional help earlier.

Many patients complain of vague discomfort in the chest. Actual pain is a bad prognostic sign. It usually indicates invasion of the chest wall or the vertebrae by the tumor. More than half of the patients with resectable lesions have lost weight prior to operation. Loss of appetite and interference with normal sleep by constant cough and expectoration are probably responsible. Excessive weight loss, more than 15 lbs., is usually a bad prognostic sign. Shortness of breath, while not an early symptom, is usually present by the time a physician is consulted. The dyspnea is probably due to interference with normal aeration of all or part of the lung by the tumor.

Febrile episodes are common and are often the first indication of the cancer. The fever results from infection of the lung distal to a partial or complete obstruction of a bronchus by the tumor. Frequently, the pneumonitis is diagnosed as a viral pneumonia. Yet antibiotics usually are administered by the attending physician and often temporarily control the infection. This not infrequently results in further delay in diagnosis. The indiscriminate use of antibiotics without a definite diagnosis has deprived many patients with cancer of the lung of an opportunity to be cured.

Unilateral wheezing, due to partial obstruction of a bronchus, is an important diagnostic sign. Hoarseness may occur from involvement of the left recurrent laryngeal nerve at the level of the aortic arch by a tumor originating in the left upper lobe or left hilar region. Involvement of the right recurrent laryngeal nerve is very rare, due to its high position in the thorax as it passes around the right subclavian artery. Paralysis of a vocal cord is a generally accepted indication of inoperability. We have yet to explore a patient with a left recurrent laryngeal nerve paralysis in whom we were able to remove the cancer.

The physical signs which may be elicited depend on the size, the site and the complications of the growth. Often physical signs are lacking. Special attention should be paid in the physical examination to the common areas of metastasis. The commonest site of extrathoracic metastasis is the supraclavicular lymph nodes. The axillary lymph nodes are infrequently involved. Any enlarged supraclavicular node should be excised and examined histologically. The entire surface of the

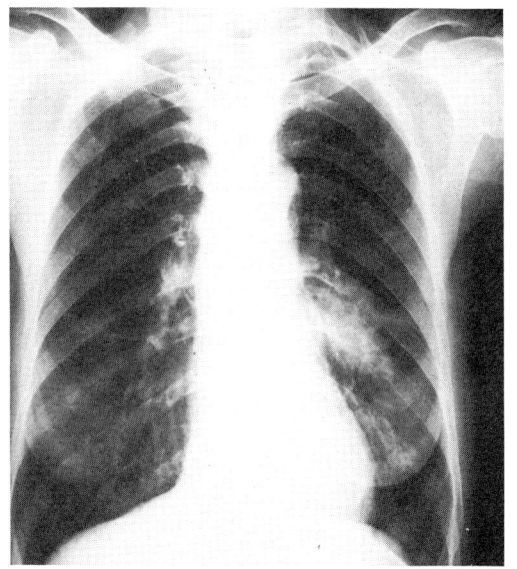

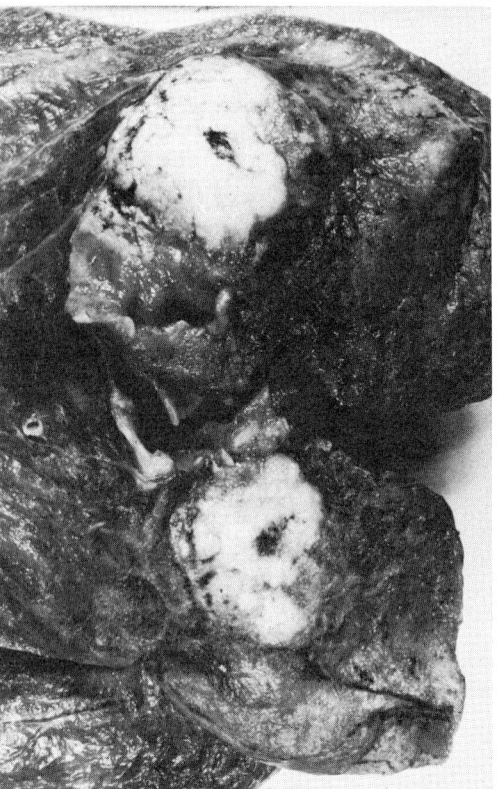

FIG. 47-3. (*Top*) Roentgenogram of a bronchogenic carcinoma of the superior segment of the left lower lobe. The x-ray density in this instance is due almost entirely to the mass of the tumor itself, as shown (*bottom*) by the photograph of the lesion.

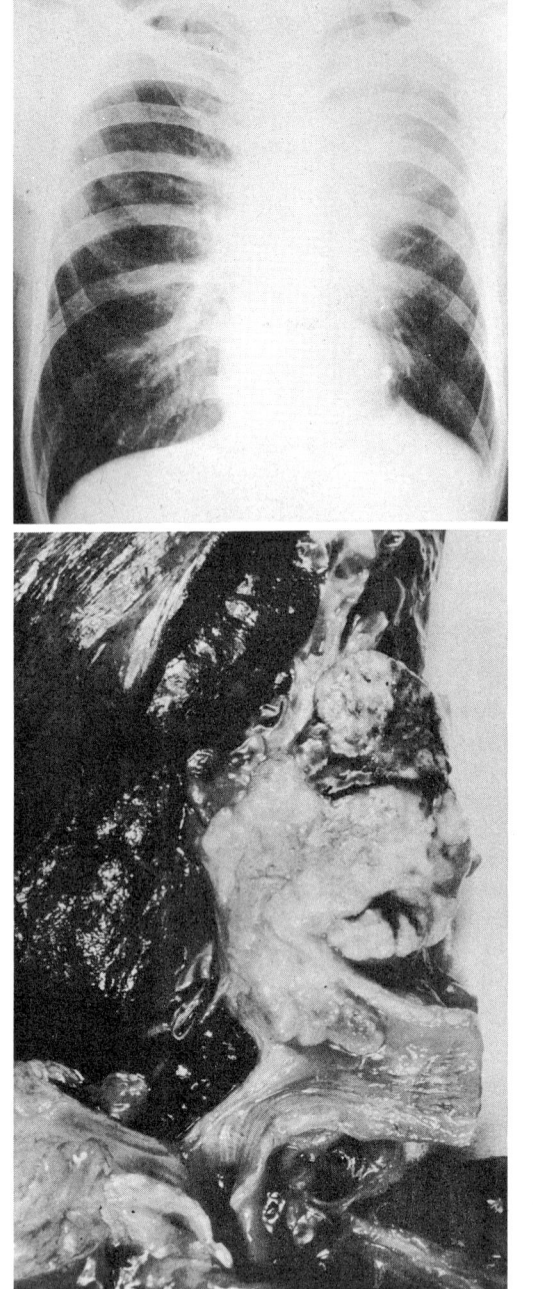

Fig. 47-4. (*Top*) Roentgenogram showing opacification of the left upper lobe. (*Bottom*) Photograph of the carcinoma completely occluding the left upper lobe bronchus with retained secretions and atelectasis distal to the tumor.

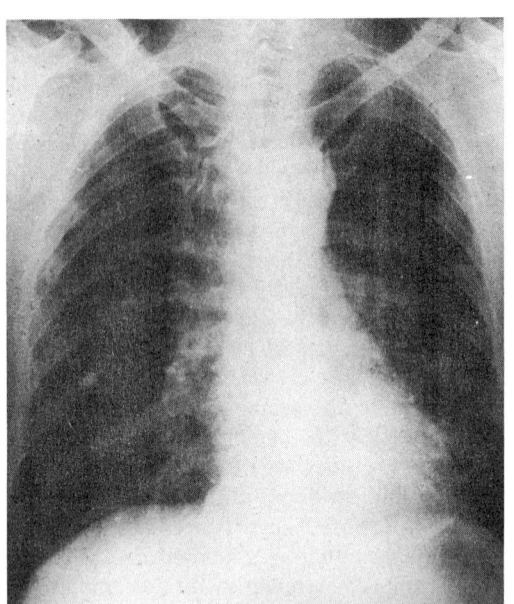

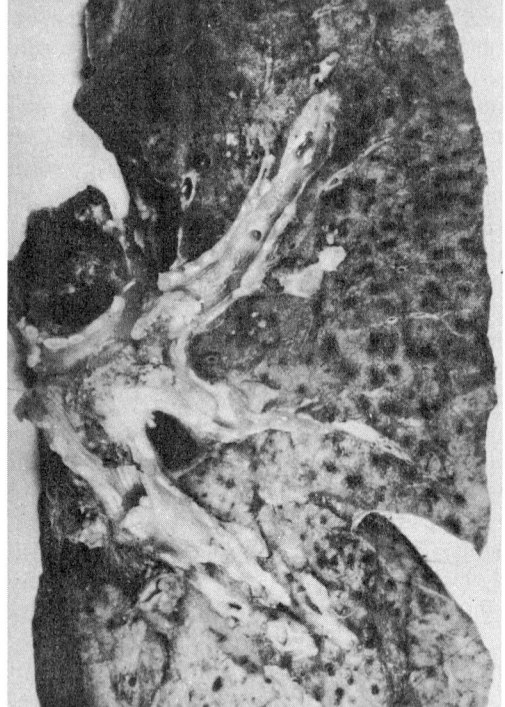

Fig. 47-5. (*Top*) Roentgenogram of the chest, revealing only a Ghon tubercle in the right lower midlung field. The patient had cough and hemoptysis. Bronchoscopic biopsy of a mass protruding from the left upper lobe revealed epidermoid carcinoma. (*Bottom*) Photograph of specimen, showing tumor almost occluding the bronchus.

body should be examined for subcutaneous hematogenous metastases. Neurologic symptoms may indicate metastasis to the central nervous system. Pain in the back, the pelvis or the extremities should be investigated by x-ray examination for osseous metastasis.

Diagnosis. X-ray examination of the chest is by far the most important diagnostic procedure. The radiolucency of normal pulmonary tissue provides an ideal background for the detection of densities produced by solid tumors and their complications. Thus carcinoma of the lung is the most easily detectable of all cancers of internal organs. There is some abnormality in the roentgenogram of the chest in 97 per cent of cases. In intermediate and peripheral tumors some, if not all, of the density on the film is due to the actual tumor itself (Fig. 47-3). In small cancers centrally located, the area of abnormal density may be due solely to bronchial obstruction with resultant atelectasis (Fig. 47-4). In approximately 3 per cent of cases, the usual posterior-anterior roentgenogram will not reveal any abnormality. This is due to the fact that the tumor is either within the shadow of the mediastinum or behind the heart, or is small and has not yet obstructed a bronchus (Fig. 47-5). Therefore, patients with a history and symptoms compatible with cancer of the lung should be studied completely, even though roentgenograms of the chest are normal.

Asymptomatic cancers of the lung discovered by a routine chest roentgenogram have a better prognosis than lesions which have reached the stage where they produce symptoms. Overholt (1950) reported that all such cancers seen by him could be removed, and that in over two thirds the cancer had not spread beyond the lung. Special x-ray examinations such as planography, angiography and bronchography are of only occasional value. Periodic roentgenograms to detect change in the size of a lesion should never be used because time may be lost during which an operable cancer may become inoperable. X-ray therapy as a diagnostic measure is mentioned only to be condemned.

An x-ray diagnosis of cancer of the lung is only presumptive. All patients with such a diagnosis should be examined with a bronchoscope. In approximately 25 per cent of patients with cancer of the lung, it is possible

BRONCHO-SCOPIC BIOPSY	NEOPLASTIC CELLS NO BIOPSY	CLINICAL SYMPTOMS AND X-RAY ALONE
28%	33%	39%

Fig. 47-6. Basis of the preoperative diagnosis in authors' series of 912 patients operated upon for cancer of the lung.

to obtain a bronchoscopic biopsy. This means that 25 per cent of cancers of the lung occur in, or project into, the main bronchus or the upper part of the lower lobe bronchus. An additional 33 per cent can be diagnosed preoperatively by finding cancer cells in the secretions, or saline washings, from the suspected bronchus. Failure to find neoplastic cells does not rule out the diagnosis of cancer. On the other hand, positive identification of cancer cells in the sputum or the bronchial secretions by an experienced cytologist is rarely erroneous. About one third of our patients have been operated upon without a positive cell, or tissue, diagnosis (Fig. 47-6). A presumptive diagnosis of cancer of the lung was made in these patients on the basis of the history and the x-ray findings.

Needle aspiration biopsy of undiagnosed pulmonary lesions should not be performed because of the danger of implantation of tumor cells in the chest wall (Allbritten, 1952). However, needle biopsy is justified to establish a tissue diagnosis in lesions which are obviously inoperable. When pleural fluid is present, it should be aspirated and examined. If the fluid contains neoplastic cells, the lesion is inoperable. We have found needle biopsy of the pleura in patients with effusion an effective means of establishing a diagnosis. Mediastinoscopy is advocated by Carlens (1959) and Pearson (1968) to rule out metastases in the superior mediastinum.

Treatment. The proper treatment of cancer of the lung is total extirpation of the lesion together with the regional lymph nodes (Churchill, 1950; Gibbon, 1955; Graham,

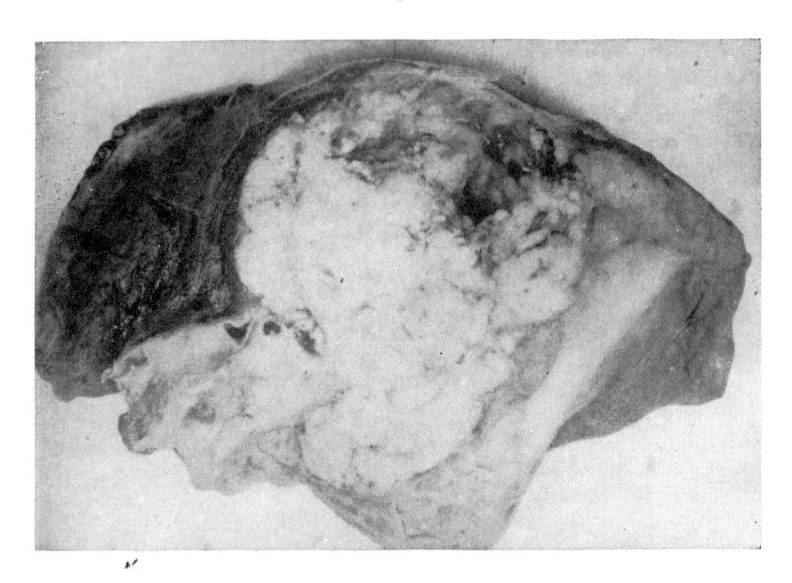

1408 Carcinoma of the Lung and Tumors of the Thorax

FIG. 47-7. Some cancers of the lung may grow to a considerable size and still be curable. This large epidermoid carcinoma of the lung was removed Oct. 15, 1946. Thirteen years later the patient was well and working, without evidence of metastasis.

1933). In all hilar cancers this requires a pneumonectomy and removal of all the mediastinal lymph nodes. Lobectomy with removal of the adjacent mediastinal lymph nodes, should be performed when it is considered that the patient's cardiovascular status would seriously augment the risk of pneumonectomy. Similarly, a small, solitary pulmonary nodule that proves to be cancer on frozen section may be adequately treated by lobectomy with removal of the adjacent lymph nodes. Patients with peripheral lesions requiring resection of the chest wall, because of direct extension, also fall into this group.

X-ray therapy is helpful in alleviating the pain of chest wall invasion or the symptoms of superior caval obstruction. However, it does not appear to prolong life, with very rare exceptions. The dyspnea accompanying persistent pleura effusion may be relieved by producing pleural symphysis by talc poudrage (Camishion, 1962; Chambers, 1958; Haupt, 1960). This has proved to be more effective than the injection of radioactive gold. Cytotoxic chemicals, such as Cytoxan, nitrogen mustard, methotrexate and 5-fluorouracil, are being evaluated in the treatment of inoperable cancer of the lung. Conclusive results are not yet available, except that Cytoxan has given some encouraging results in patients with anaplastic cancer.

In reported series of patients with cancer of the lung (Churchill, 1950; Gibbon, 1953; Mason, 1949; Ochsner, 1952) the cancer was excised in 15 to 40 per cent. Approximately one fourth of these patients were alive without evidence of recurrence 5 years later (Fig. 47-7). The prognosis is poorer if the cancer has spread beyond the lung by either direct extension or lymph node metastasis. If the tumor is confined to the lung, approximately 40 per cent of patients will be alive after 5 years, while the figure drops to about 10 per cent if the tumor has spread beyond the lung. If the tumor cannot be removed, over 80 per

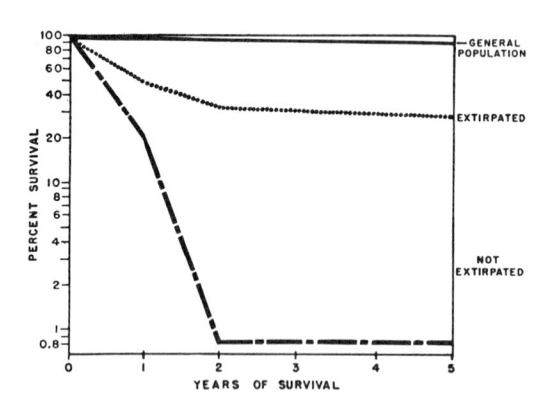

FIG. 47-8. Survival rates of patients with cancer of the lung compared with the general population (adjusted for age and sex). The patients with cancer of the lung are further subdivided with respect to whether or not the cancer was removed. (Semilogarithmic scale) (Based on 617 cases)

cent of patients will be dead within 1 year, and less than 1 per cent live more than 2 years (Fig. 47-8).

METASTATIC MALIGNANT TUMORS

Cancer cell emboli, with the exception of those in the portal venous system, will lodge in the lungs if the clump of cells is large enough to obstruct a pulmonary capillary. These metastatic deposits in the lungs are usually multiple and more frequently involve the lower than the upper lobes. These metastatic growths, because they rarely involve bronchi, do not produce symptoms early. A solitary pulmonary metastasis, as from a hypernephroma, an ovarian or colonic carcinoma, or a sarcoma, should be excised if there is no evidence of any other metastasis and if the primary lesion was completely eradicated at least 2 years before (Wilkins, 1961).

Differential Diagnosis. Tuberculosis, pneumoconiosis and lipoid pneumonitis at times may be difficult to distinguish from bronchogenic carcinoma. Sarcoidosis and histoplasmosis and the other fungus infections of the lung such as actinomycosis, nocardiosis, coccidioidomycosis, etc., are confused with bronchogenic carcinoma far less frequently. Pneumoconiosis, tuberculosis and sarcoidosis usually appear in a disseminated form which will not be confused with primary bronchogenic carcinoma. However, all 3 of these lesions occasionally produce a conglomerate mass from coalescence of adjacent nodules. If such a mass is solitary, it may be difficult or impossible to distinguish preoperatively from bronchogenic carcinoma.

Pneumoconiosis results from prolonged exposure to an irritant dust. A gradually increasing pulmonary fibrosis occurs with its attendant dyspnea. Fibrotic nodules may coalesce to produce a larger mass. Hemoptysis may occur. Such a lesion is difficult to distinguish from a bronchogenic carcinoma. Disseminated fibrosis in other portions of the lung, if present, gives a clue to the diagnosis. Tuberculosis in the healed form of a fibrous nodule may be impossible to distinguish by x-ray from a bronchogenic carcinoma. A ring of calcium in the nodule almost certainly indicates a tuberculoma, whereas small areas of density which appear to be calcium may be seen in either cancer or tuberculosis. The failure of a tuberculoma to increase in size on periodic x-ray examination in contrast with a bronchogenic carcinoma is, of course, an improper way of making the differential diagnosis, as mentioned above. It should be remembered that bronchogenic carcinoma may coexist with either tuberculosis or pneumoconiosis.

Sarcoidosis and the various fungal infections are not as likely to be confused with bronchogenic carcinoma. Nevertheless, solitary masses may appear and abscesses form which resemble a rapidly growing bronchogenic carcinoma with necrosis in its center. The detection of eosinophilia in the circulating blood, examination of the sputum for fungi, and specific skin tests will aid in the differential diagnosis of these conditions.

Lipoid pneumonitis is usually the result of prolonged use of mineral oil for constipation, or of oily preparations to shrink the nasal mucous membranes. Some of the oil passes through the larynx and reaches the pulmonary parenchyma. A localized granulomatous reaction may occur. The resulting mass may bear a close resemblance to cancer of the lung on x-ray examination. The granuloma frequently causes hemoptysis. The demonstration of lipoid material in the sputum and the history of the use of oil may help in the differential diagnosis. In any of the diseases discussed above, if bronchogenic carcinoma cannot be ruled out, the proper procedure is an exploratory thoracotomy and a wedge excision of the suspicious lesion, with immediate histologic examination of a frozen section.

Bronchial Adenoma. Although most of these tumors may be considered as benign, some of them do metastasize after many years. Bronchial adenomas are relatively rare tumors. In our experience, they constitute from 2 to 3 per cent of all pulmonary neoplasms. These adenomas appear equally in the male and the female sexes in contrast with the strong predilection of bronchogenic carcinoma for the male sex. The tumors usually become manifest between the ages of 20 and 40 in contrast with the prevalence of bronchogenic carcinoma in the age range of 40 to 70. Eighty-five per cent of the bronchial adenomas are of the carcinoid type. The remaining 15 per cent are cylindromas. The histologic distinction between the carcinoid tumors and the cylindromas is quite clear-cut, but the symptoms and the clinical course of these pathologic types is quite similar. Bronchial adenomas generally occur in the larger bronchi and produce symptoms from obstruction and from erosion of their surface. The common symptoms are cough, hemoptysis and dyspnea. Hemoptysis is a much more frequent symptom than in carcinoma of the lung. The dyspnea is generally related to obstruction of the bronchus which, when complete, produces atelectasis.

The diagnosis is almost invariably made by bronchoscopic biopsy. The histologic appearance of the lesion is quite characteristic. Formerly, the treatment of these lesions was endoscopic removal. Recurrence was almost invariable with this treatment because of failure to excise the growth completely. The modern treatment is transthoracic excision of the tumor, together with that portion of the lung distal to the involved bronchus. A lobectomy is the usual operation. Pneumonectomy is necessary only when the adenoma involves the main bronchus. The prognosis is excellent after surgical excision.

Hamartoma. This term is applied to tumors consisting of an abnormal arrangement of normal components of an organ. Hamartomas of the lung may be made up of one or all components of pulmonary tissue. Usually, pulmonary hamartomas consist mainly of cartilage and therefore are sometimes referred to as chondromas. Hamartomas of the lung are relatively uncommon. They are apt to occur in the peripheral portion of the lungs. They rarely produce symptoms and usually are discovered on routine x-ray films of the chest. As it is generally impossible to differentiate them from a bronchogenic carcinoma, a thoracotomy with a local excision of the tumor mass should be done, and the diagnosis established by frozen section.

Tumors of the Trachea

Tumors of the trachea are rare. However, both bronchial adenomas and bronchogenic carcinomas may be primary in the trachea in any position from the bifurcation to the larynx. The symptoms are similar to those produced by tumors of the major bronchi. The treatment is local excision with plastic repair of the trachea by an autogenous graft, or a foreign material, which will prevent collapse of the tracheal wall.

TUMORS OF THE MEDIASTINUM

The mediastinum is bounded posteriorly by the vertebral bodies and anteriorly by the sternum. The lateral boundaries are the lungs; the caudad limit is the diaphragm; and the cephalad limit is at the level of the suprasternal notch. This region is occupied chiefly by the heart, the great vessels, the esophagus and the trachea. The thymus gland lies in the anterosuperior portion of the mediastinum. The phrenic nerves and the vagus nerves and their branches traverse the mediastinum. The remainder of the space is occupied by fibrous connective tissue, fat and lymph nodes. Obviously, a wide variety of tumors can arise from these structures. Tumors of the trachea and the major bronchi have been considered already, and tumors of the esophagus are discussed in another chapter.

The symptoms produced by mediastinal tumor masses are related to their effect upon important contiguous structures. Thus, projection or growth of the tumor mass laterally, compressing the lung on either side, may permit the tumor to become of considerable size without producing symptoms. On the other hand, in the region of the superior mediastinum, symptoms of dyspnea, dysphagia, and congestion of the head, the neck and the upper extremities may occur from compression of trachea, esophagus or superior vena cava, respectively. If a tumor is of large size, a widening of the upper mediastinum may be noted by percussing the chest anteriorly. Usually, however, physical signs are absent, and the tumor mass is recognized by rounded projection from, or widening of, the usual mediastinal density on a postero-anterior roentgenogram of the chest. The more common types of mediastinal tumors will be discussed below, and then lesions that must be differentiated from true tumors will be considered.

Thymoma

Thymomas are relatively rare tumors. They vary considerably in their histologic characteristics. They tend to grow slowly, and it may be many years before they attain a large size. They rarely, if ever, metastasize and usually run a benign course for many years. If malignant change develops, it is apt to be of the locally invasive type rather than spread by lymphatic or hematogenous channels. Approximately three fourths of all thymomas are associated with myasthenia gravis. Removal of a thymoma usually will alleviate the symptoms of a coexisting myasthenia gravis and reduce the amount of Prostigmin required by the patient (Blalock, 1944). The treatment of a thymoma is surgical excision, either through a median sternotomy or through the conventional posterolateral approach for tumors presenting more predominantly on one side.

Teratoma

The mediastinum is a common site for these interesting tumors. A teratoid tumor may be either benign or malignant. The benign teratomas are often called dermoids. These tumors are composed chiefly of ectodermal elements. Dermoid cysts are lined with squamous epithelium and contain hair and sebaceous material. However, derivatives from both endoderm and mesoderm also may be present. Teratoid tumors generally have rounded margins and project beyond the mediastinum into one or the other lung field. If a teratoid tumor ruptures into a bronchus, the diagnosis may be obvious from the expectoration of hair or sebaceous material. The x-ray finding of structures resembling bone or teeth in the tumor mass may reveal the diagnosis. When the diagnosis is established, the treatment is complete surgical excision. Preferably, these tumors should be excised before the complications of infection, fistula formation, or hemorrhage have occurred.

Tumors of Lymphoid Origin

The benign tumors of lymphoid origin in the mediastinum are the cystic lymphangiomas. These are cystic lymphoid structures, mutilocular in character, which may communicate with a similar tumor mass presenting in the neck, especially in children. These tumor masses, presumably because of their softness, are usually asymptomatic. They are benign in character but have a tendency toward local recurrence if not completely excised.

Malignant lymphatic tumors comprise Hodgkin's disease, the lymphocytic lymphomas, the leukemias and lymphosarcoma. None of these lesions is amenable to surgical treatment in the mediastinum. Malignant lymphatic tumors are frequently associated with enlarged cervical or axillary lymph nodes. The leukemias and the malignant lymphomas may be associated with enlargement of the liver or spleen. Low-grade fever is often present. The diagnosis should be established by biopsy. Treatment of the lymphosarcomas and Hodgkin's disease by radiation therapy will often lead to palliation of symptoms arising from compression of normal structures by these bulky masses.

Differential Diagnosis

It is often difficult to differentiate between true tumors of the mediastinum and masses which are not neoplastic in nature. Perhaps the commonest cause of an enlarged mediastinal shadow in a posterior-anterior roentgenogram is an intrathoracic extension of the thyroid gland. This usually occurs in the anterior mediastinum, but it may present in the posterior mediastinum. Most of these intrathoracic extensions of goiters can be dealt with through the usual cervical approach, as their blood supply arises from the inferior thyroid arteries. Occasionally, it may be necessary to approach these lesions through the thorax. Adenomas of the inferior parathyroid bodies producing hyperparathyroidism also may be found occasionally in the superior mediastinum. These adenomas are too small to be recognized by physical signs or x-ray enlargement of the superior mediastinal density. The diagnosis of hyperparathyroidism is a biochemical one; once it has been made, if the adenoma cannot be found in the cervical region, then the upper mediastinum should be explored. (See Chap. 28 on the parathyroid.)

At times it may be difficult to differentiate aneurysms of the arch of the aorta from true mediastinal tumors, especially if they are filled with laminated clot and fail to show expansile pulsation on fluoroscopic examination. A history of syphilis or a positive Wassermann or Kahn test will be helpful in these cases. An angiocardiogram will succeed in making the distinction in practically all cases. Enterogenous, bronchogenic, or pericardial cysts also may at times be difficult to distinguish from true tumors arising in the mediastinum. Bronchogenic and enterogenous cysts are elements arising from the primitive foregut in the embryo and persisting as isolated cystic structures. If these structures are lined with pseudostratified ciliated epithelium, they are referred to as bronchogenic cysts. If they are lined with squamous epithelium, or gastric or intestinal epithelium, they are referred to as enterogenous cysts. The latter may be actual reduplications of portions of the esophagus or the gastrointestinal tract. If they communicate with the lumen of the gut, their cystic nature will be evident from the presence of air and fluid levels. Hemorrhage or infection in these cysts is not uncommon, but malignant change is very rare. Symptoms may or may not be present, depending upon the size and the location of the cyst and the presence of complications. The treatment is always surgical excision. In the inferior mediastinum, herniation of the abdominal contents through the foramen of Morgagni may simulate a true tumor of the inferior mediastinum. (See Chap. 42, Hernia.) The nature of the density on the x-ray examination should be suspected if a lateral roentgenogram shows the mass to be anterior. If intestines are present in the hernia, air and fluid levels may be apparent and, of course, a gastrointestinal x-ray with barium will confirm the diagnosis.

TUMORS OF THE THORACIC WALL

Pleural Tumors

Metastatic tumors of the parietal pleura are not uncommon. They usually are accompanied by a pleural effusion that is serosanguineous. As these metastatic malignant nodules grow, they may invade the contiguous ribs or the intercostal nerves and produce pain. Usually, however, the only symptom is dyspnea from the pleural effusion which will be relieved by aspiration of the fluid. The diagnosis is often apparent on posterior-anterior and oblique x-ray views of the thorax. A nodular wavy density replacing the normal straight smooth lining of the thoracic cage beneath the ribs is characteristic. Aspiration needle biopsy of such metastatic malignant tumors of the pleura is quite justifiable. The only treatment is palliative. The most effective palliation for the pleural effusion is the production of pleural symphysis by talc poudrage (Camishion et al., 1962; Chambers, 1958; Haupt et al., 1960). Pain from involvement of ribs can be treated adequately by local x-ray therapy. If the pain is due to involvement of an intercostal nerve, the nerve may be sectioned proximal to the point of invasion.

Mesothelioma of the Pleura

In the past benign mesotheliomas of the pleura have been given the misnomer of "giant sarcoma of the pleura." However, these tumors are not malignant. Regardless of the exact origin of the cells composing these tumors, they run a characteristically slow, benign clinical course. They may arise from any portion of the pleural surface, either parietal or visceral. They grow slowly over a period of many years and adapt themselves in shape to conform to surrounding rigid structures. Generally, they produce a globular mass. They are almost invariably symptomless until they reach a considerable size; then they may produce symptoms from compression of the lung. Frequently, they are discovered on a routine x-ray film of the chest. The treatment is complete surgical excision which will be curative. These tumors do not metastasize.

Malignant mesotheliomas of the pleura are always multiple and do not attain the large size of the solitary benign lesions. These tumors are highly malignant and cause massive pleural effusion. Chest pain is often present. They are incurable.

Neurogenic Tumors

Neurogenic tumors are discussed under "Tumors of the Thoracic Wall" because most of them are quite distinct and separate from the mediastinum itself. Aside from bronchogenic carcinomas and lymphoid tumors of the mediastinum, neurogenic tumors are the commonest thoracic neoplasms. The 3 main pathologic types are the ganglioneuromas which arise in the ganglia of the thoracic sympathetic chain, the neurilemmomas, and the neurofibromas which may arise in the sympathetic trunks but more commonly originate in the intercostal nerves. If a neurilemmoma or a neurofibroma arises near the origin of an intercostal nerve, it may extend through the intervertebral foramen in an hourglass fashion and produce compression of the spinal cord.

Most of these tumors, when they have reached any size, may be easily recognized from their paravertebral position in the posterior-anterior and lateral roentgenograms of the chest. These neurogenic tumors are apt to be slow-growing and encapsulated, but they have the potentiality of undergoing malignant change (Blades, 1946). Therefore, they should be excised surgically when first recognized. The ganglioneuromas are almost always symptomless and usually are discovered in a routine chest x-ray. The neurilemmomas and the neurofibromas are apt to produce pain from involvement of the intercostal nerves. If they are of the dumbbell-shape type growing through the intervertebral foramen, in addition they may produce symptoms of spinal cord compression. Malignant degeneration will be evident from erosion of bone and severe pain. The characteristic paravertebral position of the vast majority of these tumors makes a presumtive diagnosis easy, and surgical excision through a posterolateral thoracic incision is always indicated. Complete excision will result in cure if malignant change has not occurred. If a tumor has grown through an intervertebral foramen, a laminectomy to remove the intraspinal portion of the growth should precede thoracotomy for removal of the intrathoracic portion.

Tumors of Ribs and Cartilages

Chondromas and chondrosarcomas are the commonest primary tumors of the ribs and the cartilages. A bony component is present not infrequently, and such tumors should be referred to as osteochondromas or osteochondrosarcomas. The benign chondromas or osteochondromas are prone to appear at the anterior ends of the ribs where they join the costal cartilages. They may involve the sternum in this region or the clavicle. Benign tumors are not apt to produce symptoms but are usually recognized first by the presence of a globular firm swelling. Malignant tumors are more common in the posterior portions of the ribs near their junctions with the vertebrae. The lesions grow fairly rapidly and produce pain from involvement of the intercostal nerves and erosion of the ribs and the vertebrae. The presence of a lesion involving the ribs can be established by roentgenograms, but it is not always possible to distinguish these primary neoplasms from metastatic or other lesions of bone. The treatment is excision of the involved rib or cartilage, leaving a considerable margin of normal bone or cartilage attached to the tumor mass. The periosteum, or perichondrium, and attached intercostal muscles should be removed with the tumor.

Eosinophilic granulomas of the rib are found not uncommonly in young adults. They produce localized rarefaction of the rib which may be difficult to distinguish from a primary tumor. A solitary plasmacytoma produces an expanding lesion of the rib which gives an appearance somewhat similar to the eosinophilic granuloma. Ewing's endothelioma is also occasionally primary in a rib. The diagnosis should be established in all these cases by complete excision of the lesion and histologic examination.

The ribs and the sternum are frequently invaded by metastatic carcinoma. Such secondary metastases to ribs, vertebrae, or sternum commonly arise from primary carcinomas of the breast, the kidney, the prostate, the thyroid gland and the lungs. Pathologic fractures of ribs with metastatic carcinoma may occur on the slightest exertion, sometimes calling first attention to the lesion. If the lesion is obviously metastatic carcinoma, the proper therapy is local radiation which frequently will relieve the pain promptly and result in healing of the pathologic fracture. If there is any question of the lesion's being a primary tumor, then complete local excision should be practiced.

REFERENCES

Allbritten, F. F., Jr., Nealon, T. F., Jr., Gibbon, J. H., Jr., and Templeton, J. Y., III: The diagnosis of lung cancer. S. Clin. N. Am., 32:1657, 1952.

Blades, B.: Mediastinal tumors. Ann. Surg., 123:749, 1946.

Blalock, A.: Thymectomy in the treatment of myasthenia gravis, J. Thoracic Surg., 13:316, 1944.

Camishion, R. C., Gibbon, J. H., Jr., and Nealon, T. F., Jr.: Talc poudrage in the treatment of pleural effusion due to cancer, S. Clin. N. Am., 42:1521, 1962.

Carlens, E.: Mediastinoscopy: A method for inspection and tissue biopsy in the superior mediastinum. Dis. Chest., 36:343, 1959.

Chambers, J. S.: Palliative treatment of neoplastic pleural effusion with intercostal intubation and talc instillation West. J. Surg., 66:26, 1958.

Churchill, E. D., Sweet, R. H., Soutter, L., and

Scannell, J. S.: The surgical management of carcinoma of the lung: a study of the cases treated at the Massachusetts General Hospital from 1930 to 1950. J. Thoracic Surg., 20:349, 1950.

Crafoord, C.: On the Technique of Pneumonectomy in Man. Stockholm, Tryckeri Aktiebolaget Thule, 1938.

Doll, R., and Hill, A. B.: Smoking and carcinoma of the lung. Brit. Med. J., 2:739, 1950.

Gibbon, J. H., Jr., Allbritten, F. F., Jr., Templeton, J. Y., III and Nealon, T. F., Jr.: Carcinoma of the lung: an analysis of 532 consecutive cases. Ann. Surg., 138:489, 1953.

Gibbon, J. H., Jr., Stokes, T. L., and McKeown, J. J., Jr.: The surgical treatment of carcinoma of the lung. Am. J. Surg., 89:484, 1955.

Graham, E. A., and Singer, J. J.: Successful removal of an entire lung for carcinoma of the bronchus. J.A.M.A., 101:1371, 1933.

Hammond, E. C., and Horn, P.: The relationship between human smoking habits and death rates. J.A.M.A., 155:1316, 1954.

Haupt, G. J., Camishion, R. C., Templeton, J. Y., III, and Gibbon, J. H., Jr.: Treatment of malignant pleural effusions by talc poudrage. J.A.M.A., 172:918, 1960.

Kirklin, J. W., McDonald, J. R., Clagett, O. T., Moerschand, H. J., and Gage, R. P.: Bronchogenic carcinoma: cell type and other factors relating to prognosis. Surg., Gynec., Obstet., 100:429, 1955.

Mason, G. A.: Cancer of the lung: review of a thousand cases. Lancet, 2:587, 1949.

Ochsner, A., DeCamp, P. A., DeBakey, M. E., and Ray, C. J.: Bronchogenic carcinoma; its frequency, diagnosis and early treatment. J.A.M.A., 148:691, 1952.

Overholt, R. H.: Cancer detected in surveys. Am. Rev. Tuberc., 62:491, 1950.

Pearson, F. G.: An evaluation of mediastinoscopy in the management of presumably operable bronchial carcinoma. J. Thorac. Cardiov. Surg., 55:617, 1968.

U. S. Public Health Service, National Center for Health Statistics: Mortality from diseases associated with smoking: United States, 1950-64. Washington, U.S. Department of Health, Education and Welfare, Vital and Health Statistics Series 20, No. 4. Public Health Service Publication No. 1000, October 1966.

Wilkins, E. W., Jr., Burke, J. F., and Head, J. M.: The surgical management of metastatic neoplasms in the lung. J. Thoracic. Cardiov. Surg., 42:298, 1961.

Wynder, E. L., and Graham, E. A.: Tobacco smoking as a possible etiologic factor in bronchogenic carcinoma; study of 684 proved cases. J.A.M.A., 143:329, 1950.

CHAPTER 48

ERLE PEACOCK, JR., M.D.

Tumors of the Head and the Neck

Although tumors in the head and neck region usually are presented together because of their anatomic proximity—and as a matter of editorial convenience—there is often so little similarity in the biologic behavior of malignant neoplasms arising above the clavicle that such a classification may not seem justified on first analysis. Even within a single organ such as the tongue, the problems of diagnosis, treatment and prognosis of cancer are so different in the anterior two thirds as compared with the posterior third that the condition should be considered as two separate diseases. Epidermoid cancer of the lip has a most favorable prognosis, while epidermoid carcinoma of the tonsil or antrum, a few centimeters away, is one of the most deadly of human neoplasms. As a group, however, tumors in the head and neck region show one important biologic characteristic in common —they metastasize to organs below the clavicle relatively infrequently. It has been thought that such tumors almost never metastasize below the clavicle but, recently, complete autopsy and follow-up examinations have revealed a definite, although low (less than 20%), incidence of pulmonary metastases, particularly in highly invasive tumors such as cancer of the posterior tongue and tonsil.

The apparent relatively low incidence and long delay before distant metastasis occurs is both a blessing and a curse to the clinician. On the one hand it seems beneficial to have malignant cells restricted to a relatively small area which may be surgically or radiologically accessible; on the other hand, failure of these lesions to invade distant organs promises death by inanition and asphyxiation, or mercifully, in some cases, sudden exansinguination. Moreover, during periods of uncontrolled growth, the tumor and its secondary complications such as infection, necrosis, nerve involvement, etc., are easily palpable and plainly visible. Perhaps no other group of malignant tumors, therefore, requires more skill and knowledge for eradication when possible, or palliation when eradication is not possible, than neoplasms in the head and neck area. Here, more than in any other area of the body, the understandably strong urge not to mutilate must be controlled by the application of sound knowledge of tumor behavior and the peculiarities of the region in which the tumor develops. But, the head and neck region also is an area where overzealous, injudicious surgery or radiation therapy may make the last days of an incurable patient indescribably more miserable. Hence, intensive study of the biology of tumors in this region is important to general physicians and specialists alike.

EYELIDS

Benign Tumors

One of the most common lesions of the eyelids is the whitish-yellow oval patch or streak, usually located first on an upper lid in one of the canthal regions, called xanthalasma or xanthoma. It is a collection of histiocytes containing lipid and probably represents an area of localized altered lipid metabolism frequently seen in patients with diabetes and arteriosclerosis. The lesion has only cosmetic significance and may be excised to improve appearance. Papillomas occurring in a lid margin, and warty keratoses further back from the lid margin, are of importance only in that they may be confused with basal cell carcinoma. Electrodesiccation of such lesions is probably not wise unless there is no doubt as to the diagnosis. Keratoses usually require only removing excess keratin and keeping the surface lightly lubricated with a water-soluble emollient such as cold cream. Papillomas,

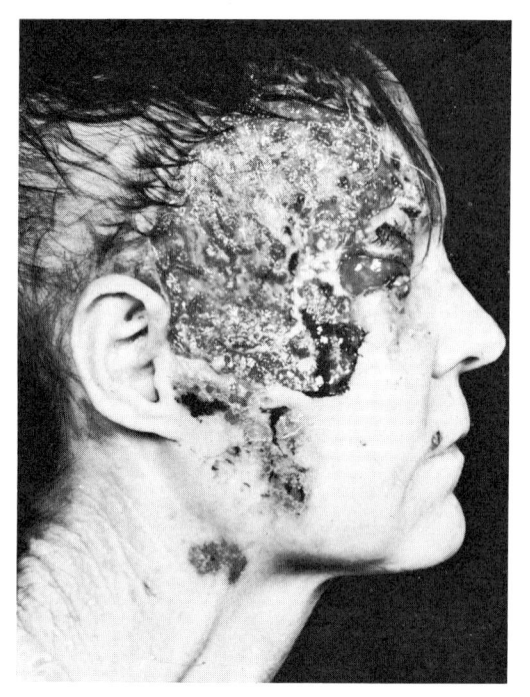

FIG. 48-1. Extensive destruction of right orbit and face from basal cell carcinoma beginning in the outer canthus. Note keratinization, pigmentation, and multiple sites of origin.

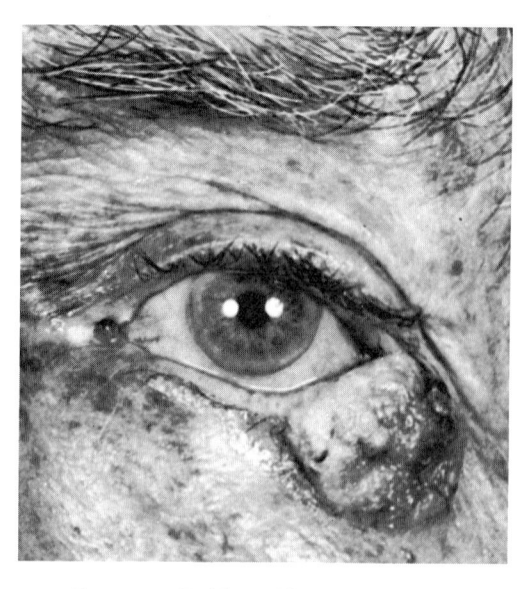

FIG. 48-2. Epidermoid carcinoma beginning on conjunctival margin of lower eyelid. Full-thickness excision of lateral half of lid necessary for cure by surgery.

identifiable by their corrugated surface, can be excised under local anesthesia. Small cysts at the lid margin are usually due to obstruction of a gland of Moll and can be cured by merely unroofing the cyst; large cysts may have to be excised. Cysts at the lateral margin of the upper lid frequently are dermoids, which should be excised for cosmetic purposes and to prevent dangerous abscess formation. A chalazion (Greek name for hailstone) is not a true cyst but is more properly considered as a granuloma of a meibomian gland. Occlusion of the duct of the gland, followed by infiltration of sebaceous material into surrounding soft tissue, produces a chemical irritation with neutrophilic response and the accumulation of giant cells. The lesion is round or oval, and the overlying skin is movable. The conjunctival side reveals the true inflammatory nature of the lesion, since the conjunctiva directly overlying the tumor is usually inflamed. Spontaneous rupture on the conjunctival side does not result in cure as with a cyst of a gland of Moll. Complete excision through a skin incision, or curettage through the conjunctiva (as practiced by some ophthalmologists) is necessary for eradication.

MALIGNANT TUMORS

Malignant tumors are most often basal cell carcinomas which affect predominantly the inner canthal regions. Squamous cell carcinomas, which occur less frequently, are located primarily at the mucocutaneous junction where they show hard, irregular edges and a bleeding base, and may metastasize to regional lymph nodes. The inner canthal region is one of the worst areas in the head and neck region for basal cell carcinomas because of their propensity to extend into foramina of the skull. Although metastasizing extremely rarely, basal cell carcinoma of the inner canthus is a dangerous disease, often requiring exenteration of the orbit for control, or causing death by invasion of the cranial cavity. Wide excision usually is the preferred treatment; skillfully administered radiation therapy produces excellent results; radiation, however, is most often indicated for tumors farther out on the lids rather than in the canthal regions where the depth of the tumor may be uncertain. On the lids proper, basal cell carcinomas occur either in nodular or indolent ulcer form and may be so superficial that simple excision of an ellipse of skin is sufficient; when tarsal plate and conjunctiva are involved, the entire thickness of the lid must be excised. Reconstruction is primarily a problem of finding enough conjunctiva; this is accomplished by mobilizing conjunctiva off the globe, transferring flaps from the other lid, or occasionally resorting to free grafts. Skin is readily obtainable by free grafts or rotation flaps. An entire lid can be reconstructed if enough conjunctiva can be mobilized to line it. When only a portion of the lid is absent, it can often be replaced by a composite tissue graft from the other lid.

EAR

Benign Tumors

Any cystic swelling or sinus high in the neck or in the immediate vicinity of the ear canal should be suspect as an anomaly of the first branchial cleft; ear discharge without a ruptured drum or middle ear infection may help to confirm the diagnosis. The tract may extend from the external auditory canal into the neck by passing medial or lateral to the cervical branches of the facial nerve. They are usually lined with stratified squamous epithelium and may contain hair follicles and sebaceous glands, thus establishing their origin from ectodermal tissue. For cure, complete excision of the sinus tract from external auditory canal to point of termination in the lower face or the upper neck is mandatory. Two small transverse incisions (one in the face and one in the neck) often are needed for adequate exposure.

Fibromas, papillomas, lipomas and chondromas are seen infrequently. Osteomas or exostoses are more common and are usually found in the region of the auditory canal. The external ear is a frequent site for hemangiomas in infants, and the lobule is often the site of a massive keloid when a crudely performed puncture wound for ear-rings develops secondary infection.

Malignant Tumors

Both epidermal and basal cell carcinomas occur in the external ear, with epidermoid carcinoma the more frequent. The posterior superior portion of the pinna is most involved in males, while the concha is most frequently involved in females. Both tumors are usually ulcerating in type and seldom attain large size because of their prominent position and the pain which secondary inflammation causes. They usually grow slowly and metastasize late —the greatest danger being direct extension into the auditory meatus. Carcinoma which has invaded the temporal bone is extremely difficult to eradicate; once these tumors invade bone, they have a tendency to involve the cranial cavity with resulting temporal lobe infarction and abscess.

Because the skin is so thin over cartilage and because the skin of the ear may already show changes from actinic exposure, radiation treatment of external ear carcinoma is usually not so satisfactory as surgical excision. Relatively large tumors on the posterior surface of the ear near the junction with the scalp can be excised and the defect closed by merely setting the ear back a little farther. Most carcinomas involve perichondrium, and these lesions in the midportion of the ear usually must be excised as a disk of tumor including cartilage and, occasionally, the skin of the opposite side. The defect produced by this procedure can be closed by setting in a postauricular skin flap turned on itself to provide anterior and posterior ectodermal surfaces. Three weeks later the flap is detached and set in permanently. Tumors on the helix frequently are excised as a wedge, and the triangular defect is closed primarily. However, it should be remembered that this maneuver tends to make the ear more concave on the anterior surface, and that the spring of the cartilage must be broken all the way to the skull for best results.

FACE

Benign tumors of the face, for the most part, represent focal areas of maldevelopment and include soft-tissue lesions such as hemangioma, lymphangioma and plexiform neurofibroma, and osseous lesions such as giant cell granuloma and fibrous dysplasia. Around the cheeks and the eyelids, large hemangiomas and lymphangiomas seldom are found in pure form, although one cell type may predominate histologically. Almost invariably, scattered elements of neurofibroma will be

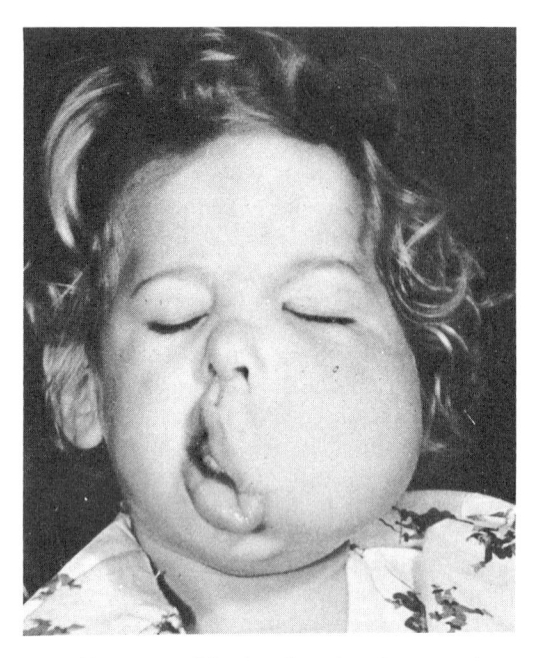

FIG. 48-3. Massive lymphangioma with scattered elements of neurofibroma of left side of face; lesion present at birth. There are no muscles of facial expression or lower facial nerve branches on the affected side. Fibrous dysplasia on left facial bones is present also.

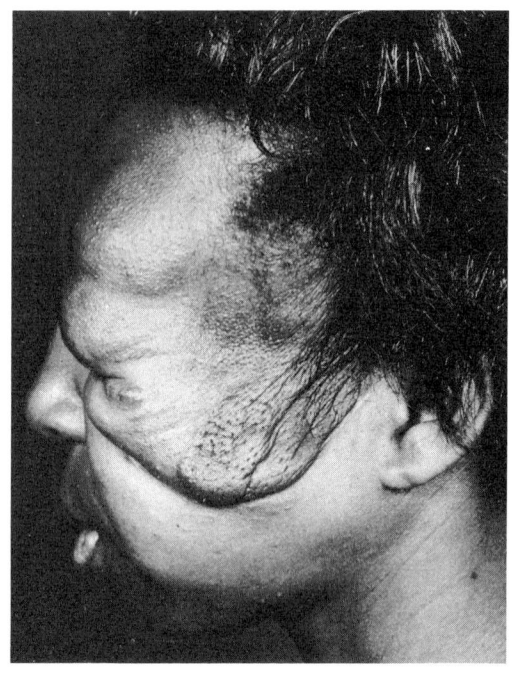

FIG. 48-4. Massive neurofibroma of left side of face and eyelids. The sheer weight of the lesion stretches the skin into dependent folds. Note nodularity and pigmentation. The upper eyelid contains some lymphangioma.

found in hemangiomas and lymphangiomas, and some of these compound lesions may attain massive size, occupying the entire side of the face. There may be no facial nerve, no muscles of facial expression, and the overlying skin may be pigmented or contain small areas of cutaneous hemangioma or nodules of lymphangioma. These findings strongly suggest a failure of organization of developing mesodermal and ectodermal structures as the primary defect during development of the facial structures. Although the reported incidence of malignant changes in neurofibromas runs as high as 5 per cent, such transformations are usually seen in deeply situated tumors in the extremities or the buttocks and are rare in the facial area. Repeated piecemeal excision of large tumors is often necessary; portions of skin and subcutaneous tumor may be used to reconstruct the defect produced by partial excision of the main tumor mass. Distortion of facial symmetry is often made worse by overgrowth of the underlying maxillary bone. This has been thought to be due to increased blood supply, but it more often appears to result from some type of fibrous dysplasia, perhaps signifying still another developmental defect in the organization of mesodermal tissue. As in the case of the overlying soft tissue mass, excision of bone is primarily for cosmetic reasons.

Monostotic or polyostotic fibrous dysplasia of maxillary and zygomatic bone occurs most often in young females. This condition is essentially the same as ossifying fibroma or osteofibroma. It does not become malignant, although the more cellular forms occasionally may be mistaken for osteogenic sarcoma. When bone formation is predominant, roentgenograms may show opacity; when a cyst is present, radiolucence is characteristic. In the maxillary region, it is often possible to excise completely monostotic fibrous dysplasia,

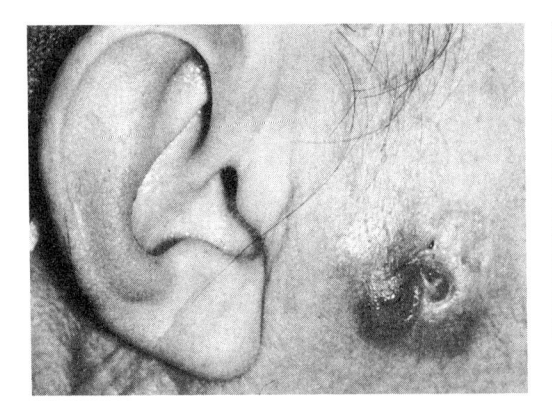

FIG. 48-5. Sweat gland carcinoma in skin of cheek. Ulceration is small; first appearance was that of a purplish umbilicated nodule. Early metastasis is frequent.

leaving no evidence of external deformity. In the malar area, or where involvement of the maxilla is too extensive to permit complete removal of the involved bone without producing facial deformity, shaving the distorted surface down to the dimensions of the opposite side through an incision in the buccoalveolar sulcus produces a satisfactory cosmetic result.

Among malignant tumors in the facial area, sweat gland carcinoma should be remembered especially, because of the potential danger of early metastasis. The tumors frequently appear as purplish-red elevated nodules, and they should be excised widely as soon as possible. Prophylactic neck dissection is usually not performed, but patients who have had sweat gland carcinomas excised should be followed very closely for local and distant recurrence. Blood vessel invasion and metastasis have been reported.

NOSE, PARANASAL SINUSES AND NASOPHARYNX

EXTERNAL NOSE

In the glabellar region, cystic protuberances are usually dermoids which can be excised easily. The possibility that a cyst in this area is an encephalocele or a frontonasal glioma should always be excluded by obtaining roentgenograms to show any developmental defect in the cribriform plate. When such defects

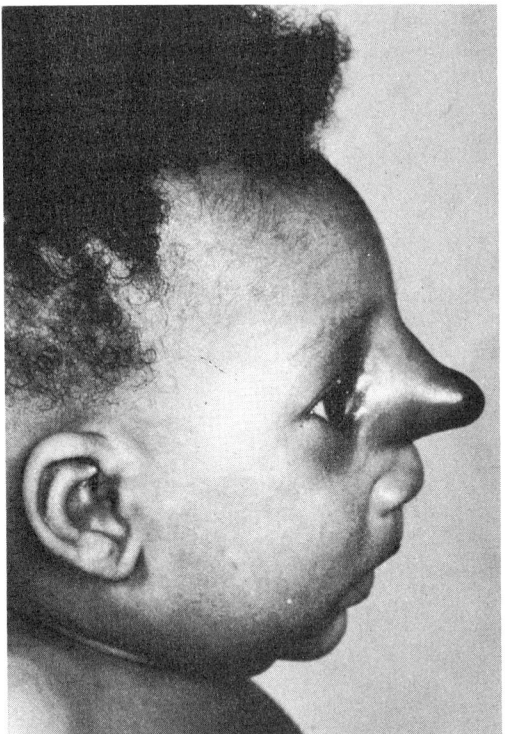

FIG. 48-6. Meningo-encephalocele caused by a congenital defect in cribriform plate. Repaired by combined anterior cranial fossa and external approach.

appear, the deformity should be corrected by combination external and anterior cranial fossa exploration with restoration of the dura by fascia lata grafting if necessary. Rhinophyma, the result of acne rosacea, is characterized by nodular hypertrophy of the skin of the nose, particularly in the region of the nostrils. The skin often has a characteristic violet hue. Histologically, there is tremendous hypertrophy and hyperplasia of sebaceous glands. Dermal scarring and inflammatory cell infiltration—and occasionally squamous metaplasia in glands—may lead to a mistaken diagnosis of epidermoid carcinoma. Although a few cases of basal cell carcinoma have been reported in rhinophyma, malignancy is rare, and the condition can be treated best by shaving the skin to normal thickness and allowing epithelization to occur.

Malignant tumors of the external nose are primarily basal cell and epidermoid carci-

1420 Tumors of the Head and the Neck

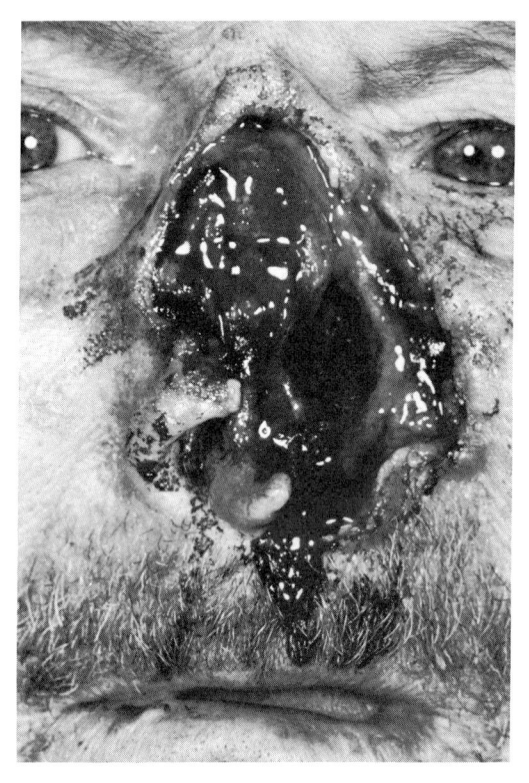

FIG. 48-7. Complete destruction of external nose by inadequately treated basal cell carcinoma arising in the skin of the tip of the nose. Both maxillary sinuses are involved by direct extension of the tumor in submucous tissue.

nomas. These tumors are often treated inadequately in prominent people because of the reluctance of surgeons and radiologists to produce cosmetic defects in such individuals. An entire composite tissue section of any portion of the nose can be removed and replaced with a composite tissue graft from the ear or with a lined forehead or cheek flap with excellent cosmetic results.

INTERNAL NOSE AND PARANASAL SINUSES

Tumors of the nasal passages and sinuses produce symptoms of obstruction, infection, hemorrhage, pain and external deformity, in that order; and in many instances, a year may elapse before a tumor is suspected. Roentgenograms may show only obstruction of an air passage, displacement of a facial bone, or erosion of the facial skeleton. Without good anesthesia and an experienced operator positive biopsies may be difficult to obtain.

Benign tumors include vestibular cysts, osteomas, chondromas, fibromas, polyps and hemangiomas. Other than polyps, osteomas and fibromas are the most frequent; they occur most often in children but are seen in all age groups. Surgical excision may be difficult because of extensive vascularity of fibromas, so severe in some instances that they are classified as juvenile angiofibromas. Biopsy of these lesions also may be hazardous; in some patients it is necessary to resect part of the maxilla to get rid of them. Interstitial radiation may be the treatment of choice in extremely vascular lesions.

Malignant tumors are usually squamous cell carcinomas arising in areas of metaplasia in chronically inflamed mucous membrane. Fortunately, the disease accounts for only 0.2 per cent of human cancer. Presently there are no known initiating causes of cancer in this area, although chronic sinusitis and nasal obstruction with polyp formation may be promoting influences, since internal nasal and sinus cancer is most often found in individuals in the 5th and the 6th decades who have a history of chronic inflammation in the upper respiratory passages. Malignant tumors of the upper respiratory passages in children are most often angiosarcomas. Because diagnosis is dependent upon late complications such as obstruction of an air passage or invasion and destruction of facial bones, most of these tumors usually kill by invasion of the cranial vault. A certain diagnosis can be made only by biopsy, frequently involving a major operation such as a Caldwell-Luc approach to the antrum or direct exposure of the ethmoid air cells through a transnasal approach. In many patients there is such destruction and extensive involvement of contiguous structures that the actual site of first involvement is unimportant. It is significant in the maxillary region, however, to know whether an antral tumor arose primarily in the mucous membrane of the sinus or began as an intra-oral tumor of the alveolar ridge, which extended into the antrum. The outlook is much more favorable for alveolar ridge caricnoma than for neoplasms beginning within the antrum.

For years, radiation was the preferred treatment for sinus and intranasal cancer even though ignorance of the extent of the tumor, extensive involvement of bone, and the persistence of pain and hemorrhage kept it from being ideal therapy for most patients. The operative inaccessibility of a portion of the area, hesitance to mutilate facial features, and the ever-present hazard of severe hemorrhage and exposure of vital structures militated against surgery in this area. Presently, the author prefers a combination of surgery and radiation for lesions which are not confined to a single, anatomically intact and resectable bone, such as the maxilla. Indications for surgery have been enlarged by the realization that the cribriform plate can be removed by combined fronto-intracranial approach, and modern technics of skin grafting of denuded cavities have encouraged development of surgical technics in this area. A careful dissection of the center one third of the face, in which all of the involved bone possible is removed to prepare the area for radiation and to obtain accurate information on the extent of the tumor, may be helpful at times. This maneuver may be of value not only from the standpoint of possible eradication of the tumor but also to remove necrotic and bleeding tissue so that an accessible cavity is produced for direct examination and the introduction of radiation by external or intercavitary sources. Frazell has reported a 5-year survival rate of 35 per cent following combined treatment of this type, more than double the 15 per cent 5-year survival rate usually reported for cancer in this area.

Nasopharynx

Although hemangiomas, neurofibromas and osteomas arise in the nasopharynx, the most common benign tumor is the nasopharyngeal fibroma, usually found in children. It may protrude down into the soft palate, causing dysphagia, but most often is suspected because of hemorrhage and obstruction. Biopsy should be done as a hospital procedure because severe hemorrhage may require packing. Surgical removal is almost always required; radiation therapy has not been successful. Chordomas, which appear similar to fibromas on inspection, are a collection of connective tissue embryonal cells which may be extremely dangerous because of extension into the skull and the dura.

Carcinoma of the nasopharynx is one of the most malignant growths of the upper respiratory passage; there is usually delay in diagnosis because of anatomic inaccessibility. Occurring at any age, it affects children and young adults more than any other malignant tumor of the upper respiratory passage. Regional lymph node dissemination is early, and nodes low in the posterior cervical chain may be involved before upper cervical nodes are palpable. About 15 per cent of these tumors appear to be of the transitional cell type. Because these tumors often contain lymphoid elements, they are often called lympho-epitheliomas. Early involvement of the cavernous sinus accounts for cranial nerve palsy of the upper cranial nerves; direct extension into the retroparotid and upper cervical area accounts for involvement of the lower cranial nerves. Treatment is entirely by radiotherapy; presently, supervoltage external therapy through multiple ports, occasionally combined with intracavitary radium, is used. Long survival is rare, and the prognosis is worse in young people than in adults.

LIPS

Benign tumors of the lips include verrucae, papillomas, mucoceles, hemangiomas, sebaceous cysts, aberrant salivary gland tumors, and chancres. Verrucae (warts) should be removed surgically for tissue diagnosis and should have their base fulgurated lightly to destroy the virus particles. Papillomas and mucoceles should be excised. Hemangiomas should be treated as described under Plastic Surgery, except those small hemangiomas, occasionally appearing on the lips of pregnant women, which disappear spontaneously after delivery. Tiny sebaceous cysts (milia) are small pear-like nodules which can be cured by merely removing the surface epithelium and curetting out the sebaceous inclusion. The chancre of syphilis is diagnosed by appropriate bacteriologic and serologic tests. Aberrant salivary gland tumors are occasionally found in the lips where they appear as small, discrete, hard nodules deep within the substance of the lip. Complete excision is required for cure.

Malignant tumors of the vermilion of the lip are almost always epidermoid carcinoma

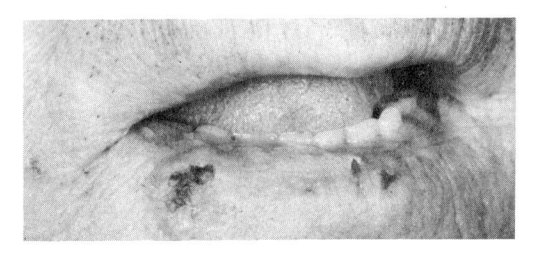

FIG. 48-8. Carcinoma of right side of lip. Note leukoplakia, keratoses and thin epithelium over rest of vermilion.

except for an occasional basal cell lesion which starts in the skin of the lip and spreads onto the vermilion. Carcinoma affects men 30:1 over women and is most likely to be found in a 50 to 60-year-old man with fair complexion and dry skin who has been exposed to wind and sun for most of his life. Smoking has long been linked to carcinoma of the lip, but there does not seem to be any good evidence that a cause and effect relation exists, with the possible exception of the inveterate pipe smoker who habitually holds the stem of his pipe on the same place.

More significant in the etiology of lip cancer is a tendency for cancer to occur upon lips afflicted with hyperkeratoses and leukoplakia. In most cases of lip cancer other areas of the lip are affected with leukoplakia, or show a thin, bluish, scaling mucous membrane typical of exposure keratitis. Because cancer occurs predominantly on the lower lip (upper lip in shade) and occurs infrequently in women (possibly because women are not exposed as much as men to the elements, and have some protection afforded by lipstick), development of lip cancer would seem to be the result of solar radiation. The radiation lesions appear to progress from keratosis to leukoplakia to chronic ulceration and inflammation, and finally to epidermoid carcinoma. Such a sequence means that carcinoma of the lip is probably a preventable disease. If physicians are on the lookout for premalignant changes in the lip, the change to carcinoma can be anticipated and prevented by simple excision of the entire vermilion and reconstruction of a new vermilion by advancement of undamaged mucous membrane from the inside of the lip. This procedure is easily performed under local anesthesia and gives the lip a "retread" good for many more years. In addition to its use in preventing carcinoma, resurfacing the vermilion should also be done in conjunction with surgical treatment of cancer because the remainder of the lip may be progressing through premalignant changes near the area which had developed invasive cancer.

A typical carcinoma of the lip is a painless indurated ulcer with raised edges. It may be cornified and have the appearance of a hard wart. Diagnosis is made by biopsy. Any ulcer of the lip which does not heal in 3 weeks should be biopsied. For a lesion that is in plain view of patient and physician there is no excuse for letting a carcinoma of the lip grow larger than 1 cm. in diameter before the diagnosis is made by biopsy.

The primary lesion can be treated equally satisfactorily by surgical excision or radiotherapy, despite claims by surgeons and radiologists extolling the cure rate of one type of treatment over another. In expert hands, over 90 per cent of lower lip cancer should be cured by excising the lesion or by administering approximately 5,000 r of soft external radiation or the equivalent amount of interstitial radiation. The major advantage of radiation therapy over surgical excision is that, expertly administered, radiant energy will not significantly injure normal lip tissue,

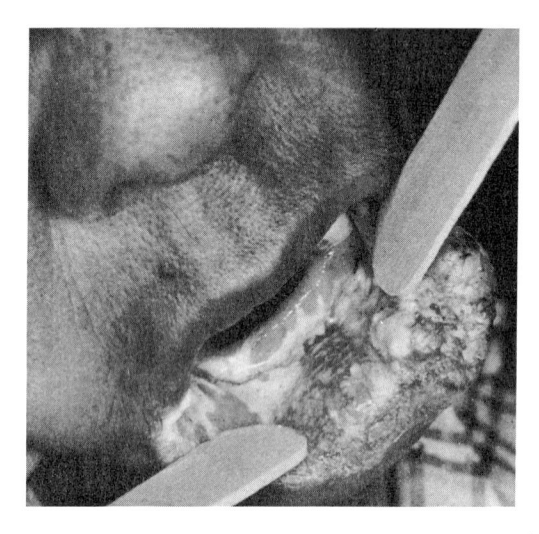

FIG. 48-9. Extensive leukoplakia of inferior labial sulcus and invasive carcinoma of the left side of the lip.

while the surgeon must remove a full-thickness segment of normal lip at least 1 cm. surrounding the apparent margins of the tumor. With small lesions, this is not important because little deformity of the lip is produced; but in large lesions involving more than one third of the lip, the mutilation factor must be considered.

Surgical excision has several advantages. It provides an excisional biopsy specimen for study, expedites treatment, removes precancerous adjacent lesions, and does not add further radiant energy damage to surrounding tissue which may already be damaged to some extent by solar and cosmic radiation. In summary, because the rate of cure of cancers of the lip is the same following radiation and surgery, the author is of the opinion that size of the lesion is the most important single criterion for selection of therapy for the primary lesion. Small lesions (less than one third of the lip) should be excised, while lesions which would require sacrifice of more than one third of the lip are usually treated best by radiotherapy. Lip cannot be purchased for any amount of time or money, and the superior cosmetic results obtained by radiation of large lesions is significant. Of course, the all-important consideration is cure, and the above analysis holds only when expert radiation and surgical therapy are available. Given inexpert radiotherapy and expert surgery, surgery would be the choice every time. However, given expert radiotherapy and poor surgery, the reverse is true.

Spread of lip cancer is by lymphatic dissemination through superficial collecting lymphatics which pierce the platysma and superficial fascia entering the lingual, the sublingual and the submaxillary lymph nodes. A few channels may enter the alveolar foramen and thus provide direct admission for cancer to the medullary canal of the mandible. Fortunately, only about 10 to 15 per cent of lip cancers ever metastasize. However, highly invasive lesions may involve the mandible and the floor of the mouth by direct extension. Such lesions require extensive local resection for cure. If lymph nodes are clinically involved, a complete neck dissection on one or both sides (if the tumor is in the middle of the lip) must be performed. The question of whether a neck dissection should be done if nodes are not palpable has been argued a great deal. Because only about 1 in 15 dissections performed without clinical evidence of metastasis ever shows tumor in the regional nodes, and because, even if cancer should be found later in nodes not palpable at the time of primary treatment, it is usually found only in the submental area where neck dssection is still effective, most surgeons do not believe that precautionary neck dissections for carcinoma of the lip should be performed. Statistically speaking, this judgment appears wise; an operation which has an operative mortality rate of 1 to 2 per cent usually should not be performed if it can help a maximum of only 1 out of 15 people.

ORAL CAVITY AND TONGUE

Benign tumors of the oral cavity and the tongue are relatively rare. Syphilis may be found in the form of a primary chancre, a secondary mucous patch or a tertiary gumma. Tuberculosis is secondary to pulmonary tuberculosis and occurs as a painful nodular ulcer

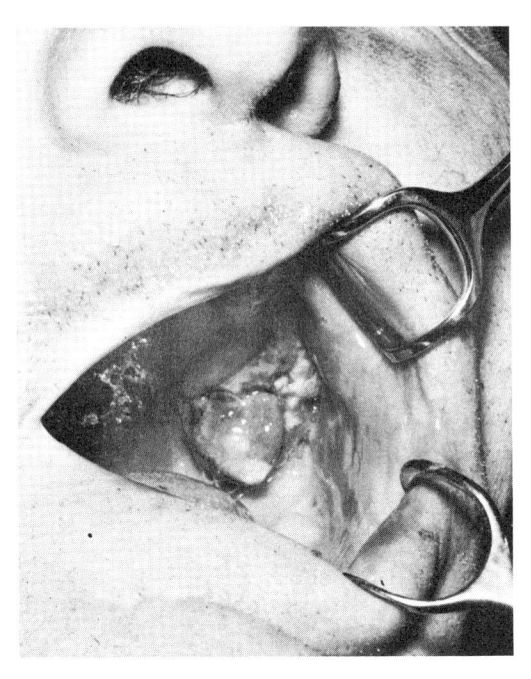

FIG. 48-10. Epidermoid carcinoma of left upper posterior alveolar ridge. Carcinoma this far posterior spreading onto anterior pillar is more serious than more anterior located lesions.

1424   Tumors of the Head and the Neck

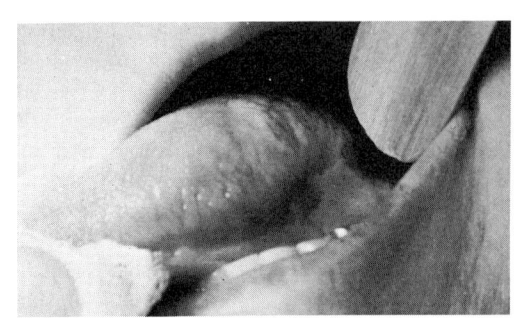

FIG. 48-11. Superficially ulcerated plaque of epidermoid carcinoma of tongue. Note leukoplakia in lingual sulcus. There is a high incidence of carcinoma of the tongue exactly in this site.

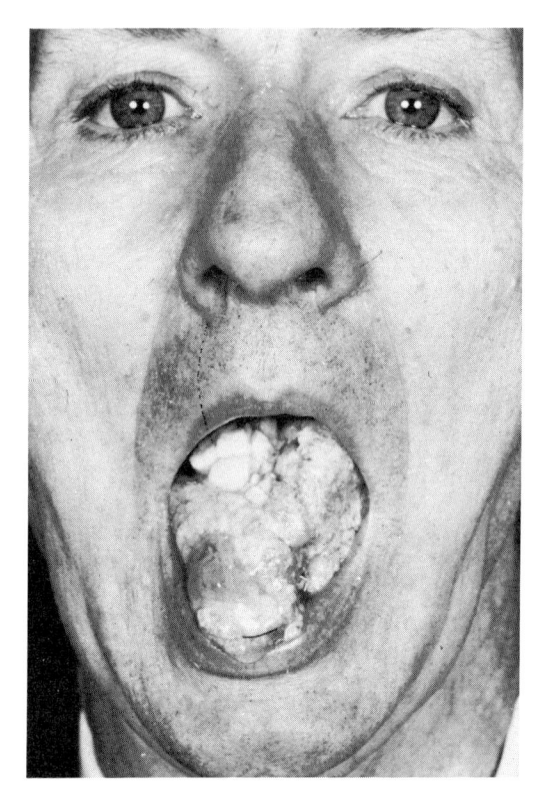

FIG. 48-12. Extensive carcinoma involving and destroying entire tongue. Note enlarged mass of lymph nodes in right digastric region and just above the collar on the left side. Only palliative treatment is indicated.

or fissure. Papillomas of the tip of the tongue are pedunculated and usually not ulcerated. Mucoceles are found anywhere mucus-secreting glands are located. Cystic enlargement of the entire floor of the mouth from obstruction of the sublingual gland or the submaxillary duct is called ranula. Mesodermal tumors, such as fibromas, lipomas, angiomas and neurogenic tumors as well as mixed tumors of anlage salivary gland, may be found occasionally as discrete nodules in the submucous tissue of the oral cavity. Local excision of these lesions is curative.

Malignant tumors of the oral cavity are usually epidermoid carcinoma. It is unnecessary to delineate carcinoma located in the floor of the mouth from carcinoma of the anterior two thirds of the tongue, for one arising in one or the other locus almost always involves the other by direct extension, and the therapy and prognosis are similar. However, carcinoma of the posterior tongue is a much more dangerous disease than carcinoma of the anterior tongue or the floor of the mouth, and for this reason should be considered apart from the rest of oral cancer. Buccal surface cancer ranks intermediate between lip cancer and anterior tongue cancer in prognosis. Although the prognoses for all oral cancers are frequently considered as a whole in textbooks, there are differences in the degree of seriousness of the various lesions. Carcinoma of the lip is one of the most favorable cancers in the human body while cancer of the posterior tongue and tonsil is one of the worst. More than 90 per cent of lip cancer can be cured, in contrast to cancer of the posterior tongue which is curable in less than 10 per cent of individuals.

Oral cancer accounts for about 3 per cent of human cancer in the United States and as much as 40 per cent in South India. This marked difference raises many interesting questions concerning etiology. Males in the 5th, the 6th and the 7th decades are most frequently affected, but an increase in the incidence in women has been noted in recent years. Previously, the life-long habit of some Asian people of holding areca nut and betel leaf in the buccal cavity was thought to be important, but more attention has been directed lately to the concomitant use of tobacco and unslaked lime. Experimentally, it has not been possible to produce a carcinoma in laboratory animals by the use of tobacco, areca nut, or betel leaf, alone or combined with nonspecific irritants. Although there are many reports of the use of tobacco (burned and unburned) in as high as 75 to 80 per cent of patients with oral cancer, the best that can be said now is that nonspecific irritants such as tobacco, betel leaf, areca nut, jagged teeth, and poor dental hygiene are only promoting—not definitely proved initiating—factors.

That leukoplakia in the oral cavity is a premalignant lesion is much more definite. From the first white flakes which characteristically appear in the lower dental sulcus to the thick, white, exophytic, verrucous cancer of the buccal cavity, there seems to be a definite progression of *some* leukoplakias through a carcinoma-in-situ stage to invasive epidermoid cancer. All leukoplakia is not destined to become cancer, and most leukoplakia varies in its appearance from time to time in the same individuals. The important factor in assessing a patient with leukoplakia is to determine what the over-all progress of the disease has been. Extensive leukoplakia which is quiescent in that it is not becoming thicker, more nodular, inflamed or ulcerated can be watched carefully without the need for radical excision of all areas. Areas which are thick, or contain chronically inflamed plaques which ulcerate, must be excised if invasive cancer is to be prevented.

The treatment of buccal cavity carcinoma depends upon the size, the duration, the microscopic appearance and the location of the lesion. Lesions so posterior that they encroach on tonsil or posterior alveolar ridge are more dangerous than anterior lesions. Verrucous lesions are usually large, soft, fungating growths with a distinctive morphology, seemingly having evolved from leukoplakia. Verrucous lesions may be locally destructive but seldom metastasize. Wide local excision, resurfacing the defect with skin or mucous membrane grafts, is adequate for cure. Precautionary neck dissection should not be done for verrucous carcinoma. Invasive ulcerative epidermoid carcinoma of the buccal mucous membrane must be widely excised; neck dissection should be done, particularly if the biopsy showed lymphatic invasion or if the lesion was large and had been present for a long time. Most buccal carcinoma also responds favorably to radiation.

Carcinomas of the anterior two thirds of the tongue and the floor of the mouth are most likely to occur on the undersurface or lateral surface of the anterior portion of the tongue. Any hard, plaquelike, or ulcerated area which does not heal spontaneously, or disappear within 3 weeks should be biopsied regardless of the age or sex of the patient. Treatment of carcinoma can be either by radiation or surgery, depending upon the expertness and the availability of each, the position of the lesion, and other factors such as general health of the patient, associated dental disease, etc. Because approximately 50 per cent of patients with tongue carcinoma will have metastasis in regional lymph nodes in the extremely critical jugulodigastric area where attachment to the internal carotid artery may make dissection without resection of the artery impossible by the time nodes are palpable, precautionary neck dissection is advisable in most cases. Recently a 5-year cure rate of about 35 per cent from anterior tongue and floor of mouth carcinomas has been reported.

Radiation prior to surgical extirpation of an oral carcinoma is advocated in some clinics. Although there are reports which suggest that cure rate by surgery can be increased by use of preoperative radiation, data to support this hypothesis are lacking. Soft-tissue complications following radiation, such as delayed wound healing and necrosis are well known.

There is probably no more dangerous or capricious cancer than carcinoma of the posterior tongue and tonsil. The posterior tongue is not seen by the patient and is seldom visualized by the physician during a routine physical examination. Many lesions can only be suspected by palpating a hard area in the substance of the tongue; therefore, palpation of the tongue should be done as a routine part of oral examination. Deviation of the tongue (inability to stretch affected muscle on one side) may be seen in some cases, but the usual initial symptom is the tragic finding of a mass in the neck caused by metastasis into a jugulodigastric lymph node. Delay in diagnosis, rich lymphatic supply, constant muscular pumping action, and direct communication with the lymphatics around the internal carotid artery and associated lymph nodes make this lesion rank with the worst of human neoplasms so far as prognosis is concerned. If the truth were known (and it is not because

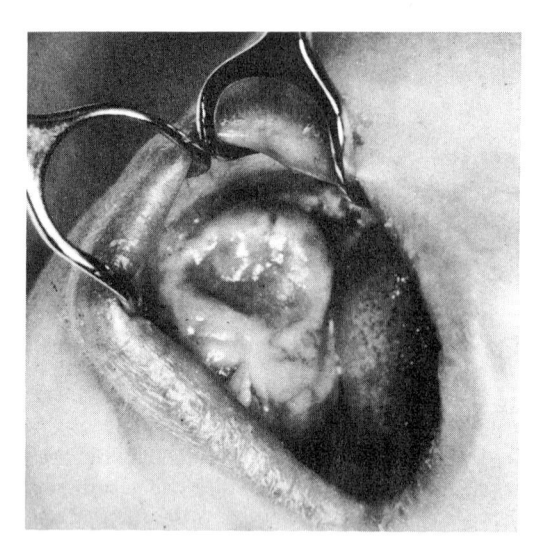

FIG. 48-13. Expansion of mandible by giant cell tumor in symphysis area. Umbilication of surface and paper-thin cortex are seen, but ulceration has not occurred.

of wide diversity of reporting), the 5-year survival rate of posterior tongue carcinoma is probably no better than 10 per cent, if that good.

Treatment of the primary lesion by radiation is difficult because the posterior tongue is surrounded by bone, making external irradiation (except by supervoltage) unsatisfactory. Moreover, the consistency and the motion of the tongue, as well as its anatomic inaccessibility, make interstitial radiaton extremely difficult. Surgical excision is possible when the lesion is located on one side, such as a tonsil carcinoma extending onto the tongue, but often the lesion is so extensive before diagnosis has been made that, for all practical purposes, total glossectomy is necessary for eradication. Although technically possible, total glossectomy is so mutilating from a functional standpoint that many experienced surgeons feel it should not be done. Thus, there is no completely satisfactory method for treating most primary lesions of the posterior tongue, and secondary metastases frequently involve structures which cannot be removed. Carcinoma of the posterior tongue remains, therefore, one of the most difficult problems confronting surgeon and radiologist alike.

MANDIBLE

BENIGN TUMORS

Benign tumors of the mandible are usually cystic. However, some solid tumors such as exostoses of the mandible (torus mandibularis) are encountered and are of importance when artificial dentures are needed and cannot be fitted accurately to the alveolar ridge because of surface irregularities. Giant cell tumors of the mandible are similar to giant cell tumors elsewhere in that they probably should be considered as a form of fibrous dysplasia characterized by giant cell preponderance, osteoclastic activity, and cyst formation. Such tumors cannot be distinguished clinically or histologically from the characteristic lesions seen in hyperparathyroidism; the presence of such a lesion, therefore, is an indication for careful study of calcium and phosphorus metabolism.

Of the frankly cystic lesions of the mandible, traumatic or hemorrhagic cysts and three types of cysts of dental origin are the most common. Hemorrhagic cysts may be found in the area of an empty socket following extraction of a tooth or after some other type of trauma. They are unlined cavities, appearing as radiolucent areas roentgenologically, and containing brown fluid after hemolysis has occurred. They may expand and destroy bone if not uncovered and their contents evacuated. It is tragic to mistake these lesions for an ameloblastoma and resect them with part of the mandible, because the walls of traumatic cysts show areas of intramembranous bone formation and the cavity of a traumatic or hemorrhagic cyst will always fill in with normal bone if the cysts are unroofed and the fluid withdrawn.

Radicular cysts are similar to hemorrhagic cysts in that they are the result of destruction of bone secondary to a collection of fluid. Characteristically they are the result of an infected tooth root and often contain granulation tissue surrounded by a thin cortex of compressed bone. When found in edentulous areas, they are usually the result of not being recognized at the time of extraction of a tooth. Unroofing the cyst and curetting the cavity is all that is required after the source of infection has been eliminated. Follicular or primordial cysts are simple cysts which occur most often in the molar region and are due to cyst formation during tooth development. Teeth are not present in these cysts, and fistula formation with discharge of fluid into the mouth often is a late symptom. Painless expansion of the jaw is the first symptom, and unlike dentigerous cysts, a normal number of teeth will be present in the alveolar ridge. Unroofing the cyst and curetting the cavity will stop enlargement and result in restoration of the structure of the mandible by new bone formation.

Dentigerous cysts, one of the most common mandibular cysts, are usually found as an expanding lesion of the mandible about a tooth that has failed to erupt. The wall of the cyst may be so thin that it may give a crackling feeling when compressed, and x-ray examination shows a perfectly developed tooth crown—often with good root structure attached. The entombed tooth is usually pushed away from the alveolar ridge by expansion of the cyst; squamous epithelium lining the cyst must be removed with the tooth for cure. It is easy to miss fragments of epithelium during curettage and, for this reason, it is the practice of some surgeons to pack the cyst cavity with a mild irritant such as iodoform gauze for about 1 week before removing it. The inflammation produced by this maneuver renders the epithelium hypertrophic and easier to identify and remove completely.

Cystic odontoma is a conglomeration of developmental defects which (unlike a dentigerous cyst which involves only one tooth) may involve several teeth in one area. The tumor may be the result of a fusion of several germ layer elements, and by x-ray it appears of varying consistency, as would be expected in a dysontogenetic growth. Complete excision is necessary for cure.

Ameloblastoma (adamantinoma), as the term suggests, is a tumor which takes origin from the enamel organ or ameloblast. Considered as such, it would seem impossible to find a tooth or even a tooth crown in these tumors, but occasionally a tooth is found in an otherwise typical ameloblastoma. The most likely explanation for such an occurrence is that the ameloblastoma developed in the wall of a dentigerous cyst. Ameloblastomas are cystic tumors and usually multiloculated, thus giving a soap bubble appearance, on x-ray;

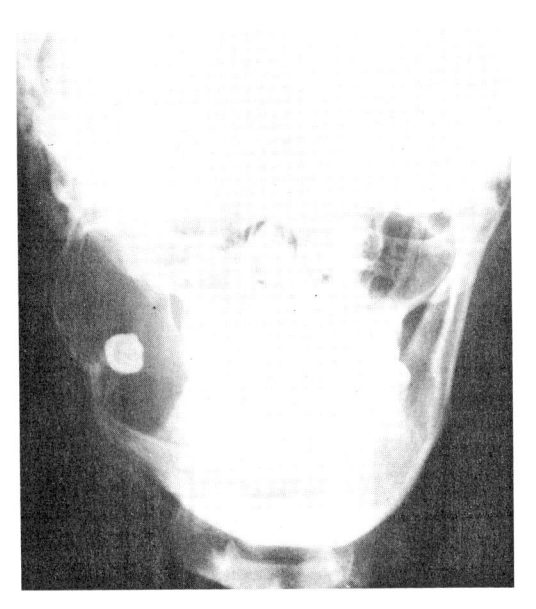

FIG. 48-14. Large dentigerous cyst arising in molar area and expanding most of body and ramus of right side of mandible. Note unilocular cavity and aberrant tooth.

they may expand the jaw to unbelievable proportions in untreated cases. The tumors are irregular in shape and often will show marked crepitation on palpation; growth is slow and overlying ulceration is rare. The question of whether carcinoma develops in ameloblastomas or whether these tumors can metastasize is often discussed. There have been a few reported cases where carcinoma and distant metastasis appeared following inadequate excision of an ameloblastoma. However, the same

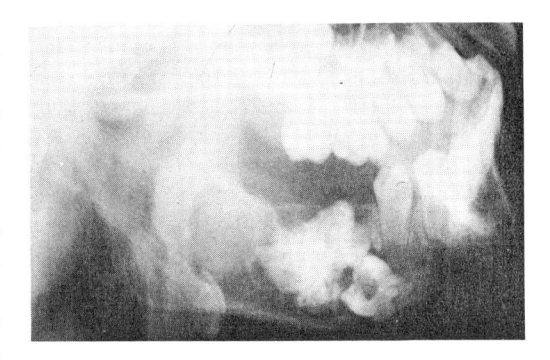

FIG. 48-15. Mixed odontoma involving more than one tooth bud and multiple embryonic germ layers.

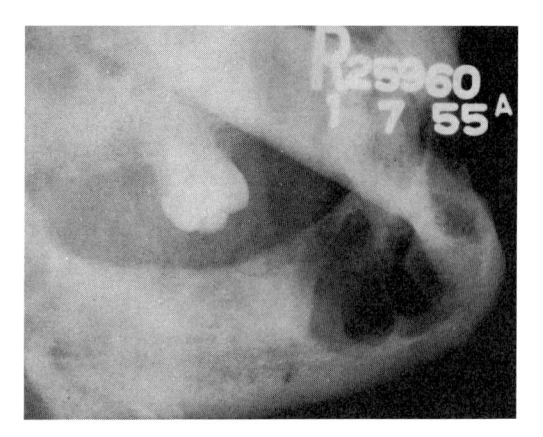

FIG. 48-16. Ameloblastoma of mandible. Note "soap bubble" appearance in symphysis area.

cases have been repeated in surgical literature so frequently that the possibility of malignant change in ameloblastomas is probably overestimated at this time. While possible, it certainly is not a usual or even a probable occurrence, and the main reason for advocating wide excision of ameloblastomas by partial or segmental mandibulectomy is that incision and curettage alone is followed by almost certain recurrence with increased local destruction of bone. Excision of the portion of the mandible involved, followed by replacement with an autogenous bone graft, cures the lesion and produces an excellent cosmetic result.

Malignant Tumors

Carcinoma of the alveolar ridge usually appears as a deep ulcer in a tooth socket or along the gingival margin. Because of the presence of subperiosteal lymphatics, excision of the lesion without removing some underlying bone is inadequate treatment. Even when there is no x-ray evidence of invasion of bone and the duration of the lesion is short, making it seem unlikely that bone has been involved, some bone should be excised in order to perform an adequate excision of the soft tissue. How much bone should be removed is a problem of clinical judgment; the important aspect of the question relates to the involvement of the medullary canal. Because the perineural and perivascular lymphatics in the spongy tissue of the canal offer virtually no resistance to the spread of cancer, most surgeons recommend hemimandibulectomy if the neural canal is involved. In edentulous patients, there is frequently such marked atrophy of the body of the mandible that the neural canal will be almost on the alveolar surface; consequently, any cancer in this area has almost free access into the medullary canal. Hemimandibulectomy will, therefore, be more often necessary in carcinoma of the alveolar ridge in edentulous patients than in the dentulous in whom a full centimeter of bone may be present between the tumor and the canal. In patients who have teeth on either side of the tumor, segmental resection to ensure adequate soft tissue removal is all that is necessary. It is common practice to stabilize the mandible following segmental resection by inserting a metal strut between the cut ends of the mandible to prevent soft tissue collapse. After the oral soft tissue has healed, a free autogenous bone graft can be inserted through an external approach with excellent reconstructive results. Neck dissection is usually indicated in carcinoma of the alveolar ridge. Radiotherapy is not recommended for this lesion because its proximity to and frequent involvement of bone make necrosis of the mandible a predictable complication of radiotherapy.

SALIVARY GLANDS

Some of the most capricious, difficult to diagnose, and difficult to classify tumors in the human body are located within the major salivary glands. Most mesenchymal tumors are probably dysontogenetic growths; in an organ where two germ layers exert an organizer influence upon each other, it is not surprising that this is true. Mixed tumor, one of the most common tumors of the salivary glands, is an example of how almost any type of mesodermal- or ectodermal-derived tissue can be found at the same time in a single neoplasm. Most of these tumors occur in the parotid gland, where there would be no problem in therapy, regardless of the nature of the tumor, except for one important factor—the intimate relationship of the 7th cranial nerve to the parotid gland. The division of the facial nerve (pes anserinus) into its many ramifications is almost completely within the substance of the gland and, with the exception of some tumors in the lower pole, it is impossible for a tumor in the parotid gland to become large enough to be discernible clinically without contacting one or more branches of the motor nerve to the face. Furthermore, there probably is no other tumor which is easier to spread by local implantation of cells than mixed tumors. At least one fourth of parotid tumors are malignant; thus the surgeon is faced with the complex problem of an undiagnosed tumor with a known incidence of 25 per cent malignancy lying in juxtaposition to an important cranial nerve. In addition, benign or malignant, he must completely excise the tumor the first time or it will be seeded throughout a relatively large wound and, for all practical purposes, be difficult or impossible to eradicate because of wide local dissemination.

Experienced surgeons can remove a benign parotid tumor by simultaneous nerve-tumor dissection without seeding the tumor or damaging the nerve. If tissue examination reveals invasive carcinoma, however, the patient will have been done a distinct disservice in that an inadequate operation (dissecting tissue from a malignant lesion) may result in spreading dangerous tumor throughout the side of the face. Cure of a malignant tumor of the parotid area requires excision of the entire parotid gland and the facial nerve. Thus one needs to know the exact nature of the tumor before any operative procedure is performed.

Incisional biopsy through a small incision placed so that it can be excised subsequently if need be is both dangerous and inadequate. Thirty per cent of tumors in the parotid gland lie deep to the facial nerve, and some damage to the facial nerve is almost inevitable if the nerve is not positively identified before performing a biopsy. Moreover, fear of damaging the nerve may lead to a "fat plucking" type of biopsy which fails to obtain a representative section of the tumor while still running the risk of damaging the nerve and seeding the neoplasm. Needle biopsy also has been disappointing. In the first place, both benign and malignant tumors have been shown to be spread along the needle tract. Secondly, parotid tumors are usually mixed tumors and there is no assurance that a needle will do anything more than strike a cystic area, producing only a few nonrepresentative cells, while the nearby invasive cancer is unsampled. Total parotidectomy, advised by some for all tumors

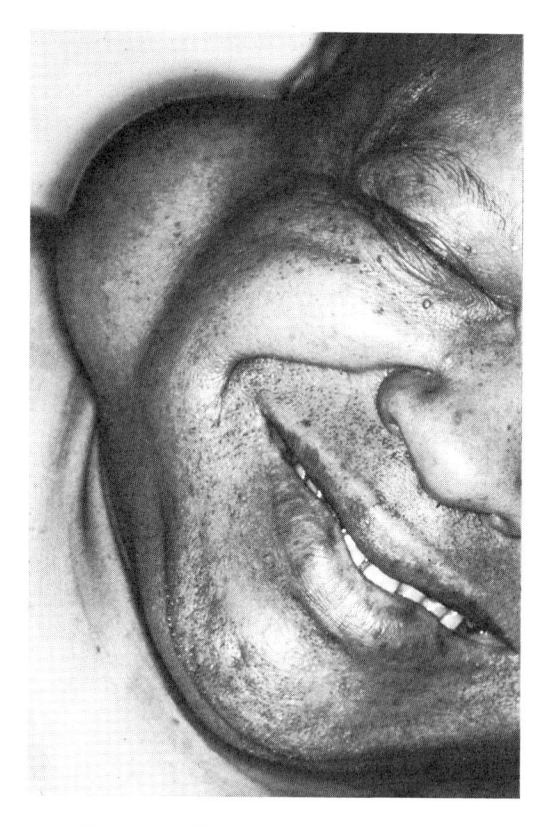

Fig. 48-17. Large benign mixed tumor in deep lobe of right parotid salivary gland. Note absence of facial nerve palsy in spite of severe stretching of nerve.

in the parotid area, is also unsatisfactory, in the opinion of the author. Total parotidectomy, except in a piecemeal fashion, is impossible without sacrificing the facial nerve. To do this for every parotid tumor in order to anticipate the 25 per cent of lesions which are malignant is unthinkable in view of the mutilation suffered by the 75 per cent who do not need such an operation. Removing the gland in a piecemeal fashion to preserve the facial nerve would seem to violate every principle of good cancer surgery and would therefore not be of much value in cases where malignancy is present.

Although no completely satisfactory solution to the dilemma has evolved, in cases showing no sign of paresis of any part of the facial nerve, complete local excision of the tumor by simultaneous nerve-tumor dissection to protect the nerve and without performing any

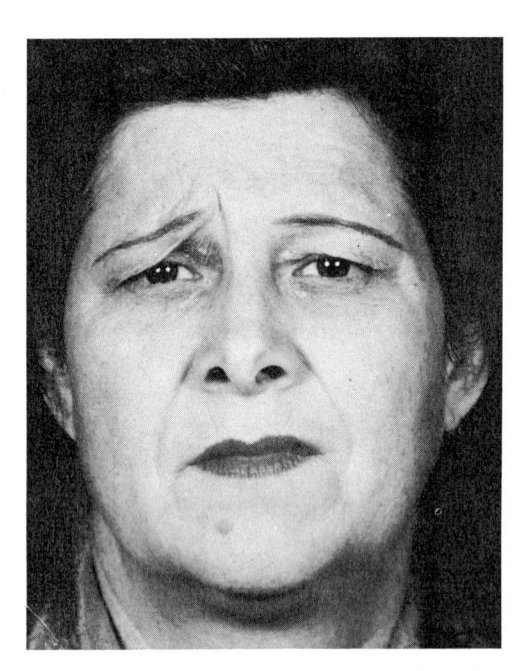

FIG. 48-18. Facial nerve palsy (upper) produced by small malignant mixed tumor of left lobe of parotid gland (just below lobe of left ear).

preliminary incisional biopsy appears to be the best solution for the author. Seventy-five per cent of all tumors of the parotid gland are benign tumors which include angiomas, lymph nodes, Warthin's tumors (bilateral in 10 per cent of cases) and benign mixed tumors. Benign mixed tumors produce paresis of the facial nerve rarely, if at all. Thus, excisional biopsy with preservation of the nerve will be the correct treatment for at least 75 per cent of the patients. Of the remaining 25 per cent, paresis of part or all branches of the facial nerve will exist in half (approximately 13 per cent of patients) and consequently these patients will be reasonably certain of having a malignant tumor. All will not agree with this statement because there are many reports of facial nerve palsy caused by benign tumors. In the author's experience, however, this is extremely rare. Only where a peripheral nerve is trapped within a bony canal, such as a lumbar or sacral nerve root trapped between the vertebral column and an intervertebral disk protrusion, does a benign lesion cause motor palsy. Even though the facial nerve may be splayed into almost unrecognizable tiny flat filaments by an enormous tumor such as an ameloblastoma or a benign mixed tumor, there is usually not even a suggestion of facial nerve palsy. In soft tissues, motor palsy almost invariably means perineural invasion by a malignant tumor. Although the possibility of facial nerve palsy without invasion of the nerve by tumor must be recognized, such an occurrence is so rare that unquestionable facial nerve palsy can be regarded as one of the best signs of malignancy in the parotid area. When facial nerve palsy is certain, many surgeons do not hesitate to perform a radical excision of the parotid area without subjecting the patient to the danger of excisional biopsy. In some cases where the history of the lesion and the history of the facial palsy leave doubt as to the cause and effect relation, excisional biopsy is performed through an incision in the line of contemplated future incisions should the lesion be malignant. The risk of seeding the tumor in these cases must be taken in order to guard against performing an unnecessarily radical operation.

In the 10 to 15 per cent of patients having a malignant tumor in whom facial paralysis is not present and a local excision of the tumor has been done, all may not be lost. Mucoepidermoid carcinomas of the salivary glands occur in all grades of malignancy, and these lesions account for about 5 per cent of tumors of the parotid area. A type of adenocarcinoma comprising another 5 per cent of tumors has been erroneously called cylindroma because of its microscopic appearance. These tumors are relatively radiosensitive and seem to retain radiosensitivity for a long time. Also, some of the malignant tumors of lower grade may be cured by local excision, particularly if they are located in the lower lobe of the gland or very superficially in the superficial lobe. In such cases, nothing other than the excisional biopsy is required unless there is recurrence. If the tumor persists, or if the microscopic sections and position of the tumor are such that immediate aggressive therapy is mandatory, immediate re-excision of the entire parotid area, resection of the facial nerve, and simultaneous neck dissection should be performed. Even so, there will be tumors (perhaps not more than 1-2%) which will become incurable because an excisional biopsy instead of a primary resection of the entire side of the face was performed first. However, it does not seem justifiable to subject patients to the risk of facial nerve damage on inaccurate information, or to perform a procedure so mutilating as sacrifice of the facial nerve in all patients in order to obviate the risk of performing a noncurative operation in the 1 to 2 per cent of patients with unsuspected cancer in the parotid area.

In the submaxillary gland all tumors are potentially more dangerous than in the parotid gland, and complete excision of all tumors in this unimportant area is indicated.

LARYNX

Benign tumors of the larynx rarely are true neoplasms. Many laryngeal lesions which appear to be tumors by direct laryngoscopy are actually the result of infection or voice strain, the most common example of which is a hematoma. Hematomas are usually the result of extensive and very forceful use of the vocal cords. On laryngoscopy, they look like hematomas elsewhere; a reddish-brown or purple enlargement on the margin of the cord which keeps it from meeting normally with the opposite side is usual. Although some hematomas may disappear spontaneously, there is a danger of fibrous organization which leaves the cord with an uneven margin; removal by direct laryngoscopy is curative. Polyps and vocal nodules are other examples of benign tumors of vocal cords often traceable to acute or chronic laryngeal strain. Both can be removed during indirect laryngoscopy, but the need for extremely accurate excision without damaging the underlying cord is so essential that all but the most experienced otolaryngologists advise removal by direct exposure through a laryngoscope. Laryngeal cysts are usually congenital in origin and are confined to the area of the ventricular appendix. Such cysts, often called laryngoceles, may cause symptoms of dyspnea and cough from internal protrusion or, when filled with air, they protrude externally in the area of the thyrohyoid membrane. External protrusion is usually the result of paroxysms of coughing. In addition to direct and indirect laryngoscopy, diagnosis of laryngoceles can be aided by the use of planigram roentgenograms. Small cysts may not require any treatment; large ones should be excised.

Specific granulomas such as tuberculosis and syphilis, and nonspecific granulomas developing in contact ulcers or other areas of chronic irritation, are diagnosed by appropriate bacteriologic, immunologic and direct biopsy technics. Keratoses and leukoplakia should be treated by excision when possible. Keratoses recur frequently but seldom become malignant; leukoplakia, as elsewhere, is important because of the danger of progression to epidermoid carcinoma.

The most frequent symptom of benign tumors of the larynx is hoarseness. Cough, dyspnea (intermittent if the lesion is pedunculated), hemoptysis, the feeling of a lump in the throat, and dysphagia can result at different stages in the development of a tumor of the larynx. Therefore, any of these symptoms must be investigated by visualization of the larynx by an expert in this field.

Malignant tumors of all types occur in the larynx, but all except carcinoma are rare. Because the larynx is mostly enclosed by cartilage with relatively few lymphatics, and because laryngeal cancer frequently involves a vocal cord producing early hoarseness, the prospect for cure of cancer of the larynx is better than for most oral cavity carcinomas. This is especially true when intelligent patients consult alert physicians at the first symptom—hoarseness lasting longer than 2 weeks. Persistent hoarseness must be thoroughly investigated by a physician acquainted with the anatomy and the physiology of the larynx, and technically competent to perform and interpret specialized endoscopic and radiologic examinations. Cancer of the larynx usually occurs in the 5th or 6th decade but can occur at any age. Men are affected 5 times more often than women, which raises the question of the use of tobacco, voice strain, etc., as possible promoting causes.

Treatment of carcinoma of the larynx is by radiation and surgery, but before any plan for therapy is decided upon, an extremely precise determination of the extent of the lesion is required. Small carcinomas of the central one third of one cord can be removed during laryngoscopy, but most such lesions are best removed by exposing them through a cartilage-splitting incision (commonly referred to as laryngo-fissure). In addition to visual inspection of the extent of the lesion, it is also important to determine whether the affected vocal cord moves freely. An immovable cord must be considered as a cord in which cancer has extended into the cricoarytenoid joint even if inspection suggests the tumor to be confined to one margin of the cord. Patients who have fixation of a vocal cord or who have visible extension of carcinoma into the anterior commissure must have a total wide field laryngectomy rather than any type of subtotal procedure. Radiation therapy for lesions involving one cord, when the cord is normally mobile, has produced excellent results (90% 5-year survivals). In addition, patients treated with irradiation have a practically normal voice as contrasted with those who have had a portion or all of one vocal cord removed. However, radiation therapy is not recommended when the tumor has extended out of the cord; in such cases wide field excision of the larynx and radical neck dissection should be done. Most surgeons recommend that a neck dissection be performed on the same side as the lesion even though no lymph nodes are palpable. Approximately 35 per cent of the patients without palpable lymph nodes are found to have metastasis in the cervical lymph nodes. In the author's opinion, neck dissection does not increase the risk of the operation so much that it is contraindicated in most cases. A more difficult problem is the decision of when to perform a bilateral neck dissection should the carcinoma involve mid-line structures or both vocal cords. Simultaneous total laryngectomy and bilateral neck dissection, though more hazardous than total laryngectomy and unilateral neck dissection, can be done with a respectable mortality and morbidity, and should be performed whenever the tumor cannot be shown to have extended out of the neck or to involve unresectable structures. Preoperative irradiation is advised by most surgeons at present, although conclusive data to support the hypothesis that surgical cure rates are increased by combined therapy are not available.

Total laryngectomy, with or without accompanying neck dissection, requires a permanent tracheostomy and results in loss of normal voice. Esophageal speech can be learned rapidly by some patients so that adequate conversation is possible. For those who cannot master the technic of pulling air into the esophagus and expelling it during speech, a number of ingenious electronic devices are available for producing sound which can be modified by teeth, lips and tongue to produce intelligible speech.

Permanent tracheostomy involves the need for special care of the tracheostome to prevent crusting of the tracheal and bronchial mucosa from excessively dry air. Tracheostomy patients learn to keep a moist fabric of some type over the tracheostomy site, to sleep with a humidifier close by, and to use some type of topical enzyme preparation such as papain to keep crusts from forming. Crusts are easier to prevent than to treat once they begin to form.

NECK

All of the soft tissue tumors discussed previously may be found as primary tumors of the soft tissues in the neck. In addition, a peculiar type of lymphangiomatous malformation known as cystic hygroma (Hygroma colli) is seen in the area of major lymphatic channels in the root of the neck and the upper medias-

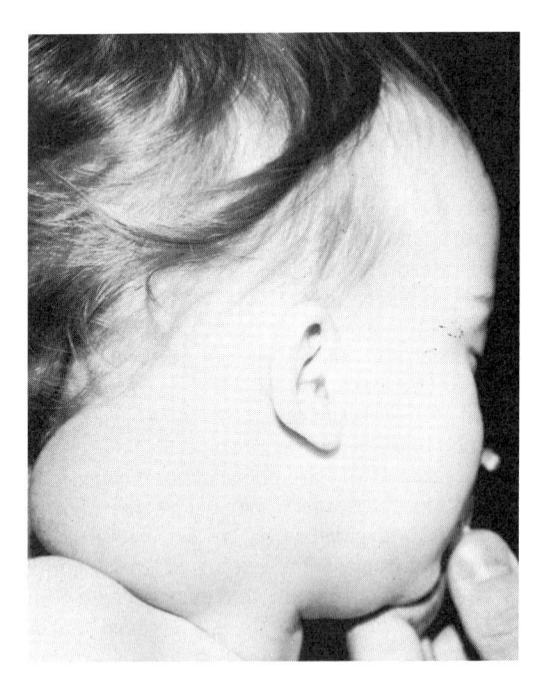

FIG. 48-19. Cystic hygroma in the base of the right side of the neck in a young infant. Lesions of similar size located more anteriorly can cause respiratory difficulty.

tinum. This lesion differs from lymphangioma in that it is primarily a cystic lesion in infants in which the multiloculated cyst walls are extremely thin and contain many intercommunications. About 75 per cent of hygromas are present at birth; a few may be so large as to produce respiratory or deglutitory embarrassment. Only surgical excision is successful, and this may be an extremely formidable procedure because the cysts give the appearance of having been "shot through the side of the neck" and do not shell out cleanly. Operation should always be delayed as long as possible unless respiratory distress is evident. When respiration is embarrassed, the cyst should be opened, the part which is easy to get out removed, and the rest converted into a single cyst cavity into which a drain or small pack soaked in 5 per cent sodium morrhuate may be inserted. Complete excision should await further growth of the neck.

A thyroglossal duct cyst or sinus seemingly arises from a disorganized part of the tract of descent of the thyroid gland from the base of the tongue into the neck. Characteristically, it is located in the anterior midline of the neck, inferior to the hyoid bone. It is more or less attached to the pyramidal lobe of the thyroid inferiorly. Superiorly, it frequently passes into the base of the tongue as a narrow thin-walled tube piercing and notching the hyoid bone.

Patients having such a cyst often do not seek a physician's care until it becomes infected or painful, or until it becomes obviously disfiguring; usually no symptoms attend these cysts except when infected. The treatment consists of excision of the uninfected cyst in its superior tract through a transverse incision. A central segment of the hyoid bone must be removed with the duct in order to ensure complete excision without fear of disturbing speech or swallowing. Infected cysts are simply drained; the excision is performed after the wound heals and all signs of infection disappear. Unless the superior tract is removed completely, they are likely to recur. They have no neoplastic propensity. Before removing what appears to be a thyroglossal duct cyst, a scintigram of the thyroid should be performed in order not to remove a centrally located normal thyroid gland—an avoidable surgical error.

Branchial cleft cysts presumably originate

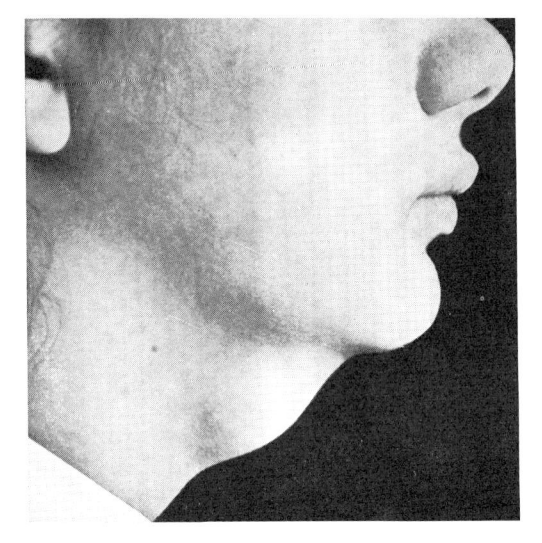

FIG. 48-20. A typically located thyroglossal duct cyst in a child.

from unobliterated remnants of the fetal branchial clefts. Like thyroglossal duct cysts, they rarely produce symptoms unless infected. They appear as swellings mainly along the anterior border of the sternocleidomastoid

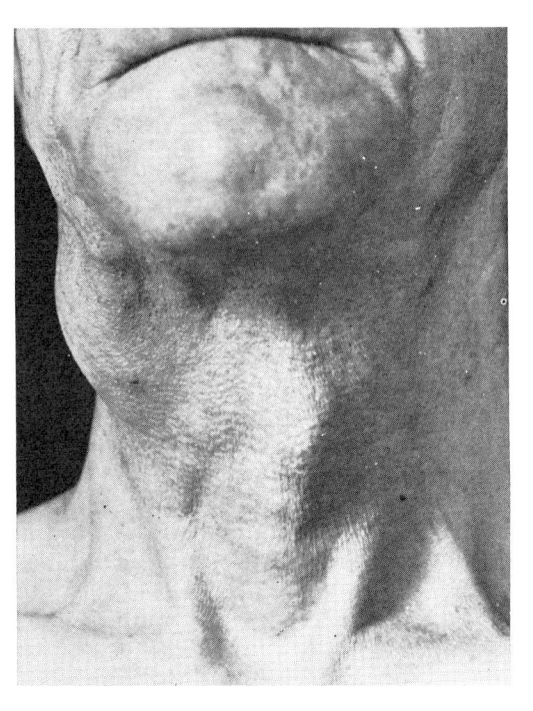

FIG. 48-21. A typically located branchial cleft cyst in an adult.

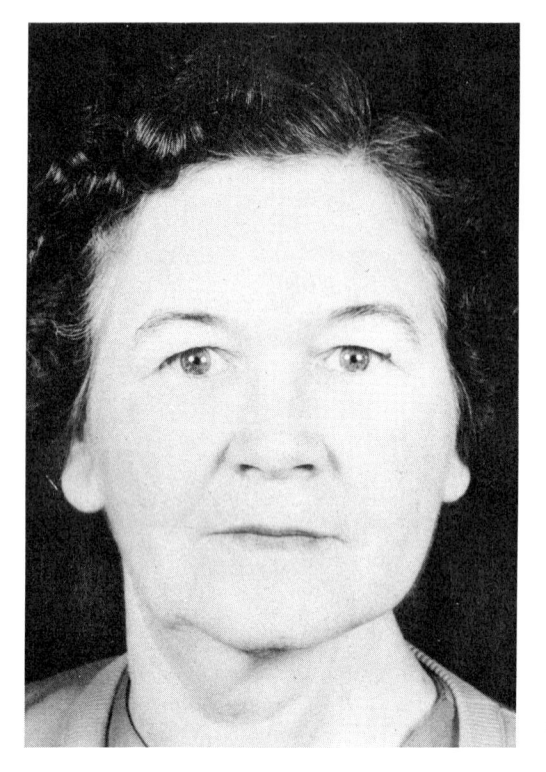

FIG. 48-22. Postoperative appearance after left radical neck dissection. Note flatness of left side of neck and sharp outline of anterior border of trapezius muscle secondary to excision of sternocleidomastoid muscle and contents of anterior triangle.

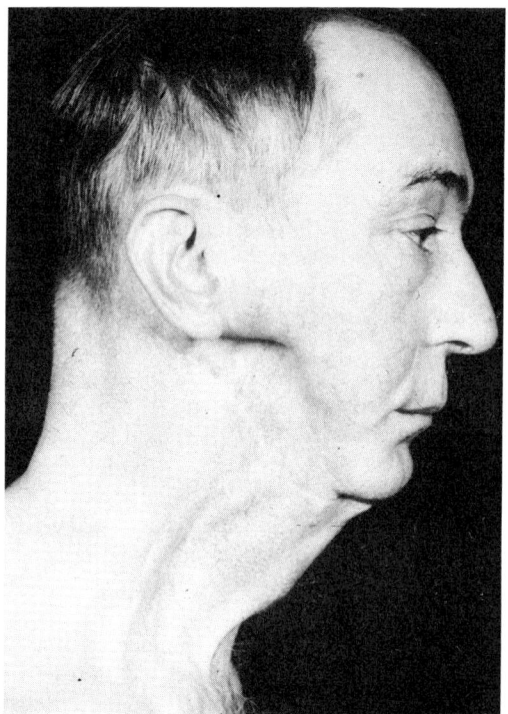

FIG. 48-23. Appearance after combination right neck dissection and segmental resection of mandible for right alveolar ridge carcinoma. Wire spacer holds symphysis forward and in midline. Contour can be re-established by removing spacer and inserting an iliac bone graft.

muscle from the level of the mastoid process to the sternum, although they are usually located above the level of the thyroid cartilage. For all practical purposes, it can be said that cancer does not arise within a branchial cleft cyst, but cystic swellings that contain cancer in areas often occupied by branchial cleft cysts are not uncommon and usually represent metastatic cancer within lymph nodes.

Treatment consists of drainage when they are infected and excision when they are not infected.

Carotid body tumors (nonchromaffin paraganglia) lie in the crotch of the bifurcation of the common carotid artery. They may be moved from side to side during physical examination but cannot be moved in a vertical direction. They do not produce epinephrinelike substances, but surgical removal may be hazardous because of their close attachment to the carotid vessels. These tumors have a very low incidence of malignancy and when large should be removed completely only in cases where excision can be accomplished without risk of damaging the internal carotid artery.

The most important malignant tumors in the neck are metastatic carcinoma in cervical lymph nodes and primary tumors of lymph nodes such as Hodgkins' disease and other types of lymphosarcoma. When complete evaluation of the patient indicates that a lymphosarcoma is limited to a single node or a group of nodes confined to one region in the neck, it is the opinion of most surgeons that radical excision of the area should be performed, followed by external irradiation. Such an approach appears entirely logical, and, yet, it must be pointed out that evidence is not available to support the notion that lymphosarcoma is a localized disease, curable by excision of the one obviously involved area. Review of the life history of the disease reveals that approximately 16 per cent of all patients affected by lymphosarcoma will survive 5 years without any treatment, whereas only about 25 per cent of patients will survive with any type or combination of types of treatment (Stout).

Metastatic tumors in lymph nodes are treated by radical neck dissection which includes excision of the contents of the anterior triangle of the neck, including all lymph nodes, the sternocleidomastoid muscle, omohyoid and other strap muscles, jugular vein, and subcutaneous tissue in an area usually bordered by the clavicle inferiorly, the trapezius muscle posteriorly, the mandible superiorly, and the midline of the neck anteriorly. The procedure can be done in conjunction with glossectomy, mandibulectomy, thyroidectomy or laryngectomy in an operation designed to remove all of the primary tumor and regional lymphatics as a single surgical specimen. Dissection may be extended posteriorly to include the posterior cervical fascia and muscles in cases of parotid or occipital lesions and may be performed concomitantly on the other side of the neck when bilateral metastases are present. Bilateral neck dissections have a higher mortality and morbidity than do unilateral operations. For this reason, in many patients, it may be wiser to stage the procedures than to do both neck dissections at the same time. Cancer involvement of the vertebral column, subclavicular tissue, the internal carotid artery, or the base of the skull is a contraindication to radical neck dissection.

PALLIATIVE CARE

Because only about 30 per cent of patients with malignant disease of the head and neck region (exclusive of lip and skin) will return from a treatment center cured of their disease, physicians are confronted with the extremely sobering knowledge that about 70 per cent of such patients are going to require palliative and terminal care. Therefore, skillful palliative and terminal care is one of the most important things to be learned, yet it is often overlooked in the excitement of mastering technical details aimed at the cure of cancer. Of course there is only one objective in the treatment of cancer —eradication of every single cancer cell—until it is obvious that this objective is impossible. The physician will be the first to realize when this objective is no longer possible. The instant he becomes aware that this is true, another objective—the relief of pain and the preservation of some degree of tranquility—takes its place. Whereas any reasonable amount of mutilation, discomfort, or expense may be permissible as long as complete eradication of the tumor is possible, the converse becomes true when unmistakable evidence of inability to remove or destroy every cancer cell is at hand. Not only must patients be protected from useless further mutilation, operative pain and mounting expense, but a detailed plan should be made for assuring that whatever time the patient may have left is as comfortable as possible. This type of care requires unusual skill and experience, even more than that required to perform a radical neck dissection, but a few principles can be stated here.

The single most important principle of good palliative care is to always have something to do for the patient. More than anything else, this attitude, backed up by action which may be no more than having the patient come in daily for cleansing and applying a local anesthetic pack to a necrotic ulcer, will often prevent the terrible despair which sweeps over patients who feel that they may have to go the rest of the way alone. With modern, skillful use of judiciously administered, palliative radiation, with the use of regional and systemic chemotherapeutic agents, with neurosurgical interruption of cranial nerve pathways in carefully selected patients, and—terminally—with proper use of the most effective analgesic drugs, the average patient can be helped to live the remainder of his life in a pain-free, odor-free, and cosmetically presentable condition.

As long as patients are sufficiently free from pain to engage in any productive occupational or social endeavor, narcotics, depressants and strong tranquilizers should be avoided. Repeated chemotherapy and palliative radiation can be very effective in controlling pain and local tumor growth in many patients.

Gastrostomies and tracheostomies in patients with neck metastasis usually should not be done. Some type of swallowing can be preserved by skillful alterations of the diet in most instances. A tracheostomy wound with cancer growing out of it is no brilliant achievement, and when anoxia is present as indicated by air hunger, restlessness, extreme anxiety, or the use of extra respiratory muscles, the use of morphine to allay apprehension and develop peaceful euphoria is, at last, indicated. Space does not permit detailed description of the many useful technics which good doctors have developed to carry patients through a period of useful palliative and dignified terminal care. It must be emphasized, however, that the majority of patients who have neoplasms of the head and neck area at this time will require palliative care of this type and that the acquisition of skill in this important area must not be overlooked while preparing to serve those unfortunate individuals who fall victim to cancer in the head and neck region.

BIBLIOGRAPHY

Arant, J. B.: Juvenile fibromas of the nasopharynx. Arch. Otol., 62:277, 1955.

Backus, L. H.: Five year end results in epidermoid carcinoma of the lip with indications for neck dissection. Plast. Reconstr. Surg., 17:58, 1956.

Brown, J. B., and Fryer, M. P.: Tumors in the parotid region, direct surgical approach and preservation of seventh nerve in benign tumors—description of radical operation for malignant tumors. Ann. Surg., 18:880, 1952.

Byars, L. T.: Extent of mandibular resection required for treatment of oral cancer. Arch. Surg., 70:914, 1955.

Byars, L. T., and Anderson, R.: Anomalies of the first branchial cleft. Surg., Gynec., Obstet., 93:755, 1951.

Byars, L. T., and Sarnat, B. G.: Surgery of the mandible: the ameloblastoma. Surg., Gynec., Obstet., 81:575, 1945.

Catlin, D.: Surgery for head and neck lymphomas. Surgery, 60:1160, 1966.

Conley, J. J.: The management of carotid body tumors. Surg., Gynec., Obstet., 117:722, 1963.

Fletcher, G. H., and Lindberg, R. D.: Squamous cell carcinomas of the tonsillar area and palatine arch. Am. J. Roentgen., 96:574, 1966.

Frazelle, E. L., and Lewis, J. S.: Cancer of the nasal cavity and accessory sinuses. A report of the management of 416 patients. Cancer, 16:1293, 1963.

Frazelle, E. L., and Lucas, J. C.: Cancer of the tongue. Report of management of 1,554 patients. Cancer, 15:1085, 1956.

Hedrick, J. W.: Treatment of cancer of the nasal cavity and paranasal sinuses. Surg., Gynec., Obstet., 102:322, 1956.

Hilton, G., and Sutton, P. M.: Classification, prognosis, and treatment of malignant lymphomas. Lancet, 282:7224, 1962.

Jacobson, Y. G.: Metastasizing sweat gland carcinoma. Arch. Surg., 78:574, 1959.

Kinsey, D. L., and James, A. G.: Evaluation of failures in the treatment of lingual carcinoma. Arch. Surg., 84:670, 1962.

Kostrubala, J. G.: Cancer of the palate. Am. J. Surg., 92:885, 1956.

Kragh, L. V., Soule, E. H., and Masson, J. K.: Benign and malignant neurilemmomas of the head and neck. Surg., Gynec., Obstet., 111:211, 1960.

Lampe, I.: The place of radiation therapy in the treatment of carcinoma of the lower lip. Plast. Reconstr. Surg., 24:34, 1959.

MacFee, W. F.: Carcinoma of the floor of the mouth. Clinical observations and surgical treatment. Ann. Surg., 149:172, 1959.

Marchetta, F. C., Maxwell, W. T., Riegler, H. C., and Schobinger, R.: Carcinoma of the intrinsic larynx. Surg., Gynec., Obstet., 104:401, 1957.

Marchetta, F. C., Riegler, H. C., and Maxwell, W. T.: Carcinoma of the extrinsic larynx. Surg., Gynec., Obstet., 107:429, 1958.

Modlin, John: Neck dissections in cancer of the lower lip. Surgery, 28:404, 1950.

Murray, J. E., Lawrence, K., Kingsbury, P., and Friedman, P.: Critical surgical problems in the treatment of oral and laryngopharyngeal cancer. New Eng. J. Med., 270:650, 1964.

Nydell, C. C., and Masson, J. K.: Dermoid cysts of the nose: a review of 39 cases. Ann. Surg., 150:1007, 1959.

Peacock, E. E., and Byars, L. T.: Management of tumors of the parotid salivary glands. N. C. Med. J., 19:1, 1958.

Peacock, E. E., Greenberg, B. G., and Brawley, B. W.: The effect of snuff and tobacco on the production of oral carcinoma: an experimental and epidemiological study. Ann. Surg., 151:542, 1960.

Pemberton, J., and Stalker, L. K.: Cysts, sinuses and fistulae of thyroglossal duct: results in two hundred and ninety-three surgical cases. Ann. Surg., 111:950, 1940.

Perry, H., Florence, C. H., Chu, T. K., Glicksman, A. S., and Nickson, J. J.: Clinical evaluation of the treatment of advanced head and neck cancers with high energy electron beams. Cancer, 19:1081, 1966.

Pollack, R. S.: Carcinoma of the maxillary sinus. Ann. Surg., 145:68, 1957.

Proctor, B.: Lateral vestigial cysts and fistulas of the neck. Laryngoscope, 65:355, 1955.

Putney, F. J.: Elective versus delayed neck dissection in cancer of the larynx. Surg., Gynec., Obstet., 112:736, 1961.

Rufino, C. D., and MacComb, W. S.: Bilateral neck dissection. Cancer, 19:1503, 1966.

Sistrunk, W. E.: Technique of removal of cysts and sinuses of thyroglossal duct. Surg., Gynec., Obstet., 46:109, 1928.

Sonesson, A.: Odontogenic cysts and cystic tumours of the jaws. Acta radiol., 81:1, 1950.

Stewart, F. W., Foote, F. W., and Becker, W. F.: Micro epidermoid tumors of salivary glands. Ann. Surg., 122:820, 1945.

Thoma, K. B., and Goldman, H. M.: Odontogenic tumors. Am. J. Path., 22:433, 1946.

Vieta, L. J., and Guraieb, S. R.: Fibrous dysplasia of the maxilla. Arch. Otolaryng., 78:94, 1963.

CHAPTER 49

JAMES BARRETT BROWN, M.D., AND MINOT P. FRYER, M.D.

Principles of General Plastic Surgery

Skin Grafting, Burns and Radiation Injury
Cleft Lip and Cleft Palate
Deformities and Inflammatory Diseases of the Jaws
Reconstruction of the Jaw
Compound Facial Injuries
Facial Paralysis
Deformities of the Ear
Deformities of the Eyelids
Salivary Glands
Congenital Wryneck
Industrial and Farm Injuries
Hypospadias
Repair of Surface Defects of the Feet
Use of Silicone, Teflon, Polyvinyl Alcohol and Di-isocyanate as Prostheses in Reconstructive Surgery

SKIN GRAFTING AND DEEP BURNS

Treatment of the local burned areas, with burns of thermal, chemical or electrical origin or irradiation effect, is discussed. Depth and extent of the burns are considered because of their pertinence to the treatment and prognosis.

Fluid balance, nutrition and general care of the burned patient are covered elsewhere but are considered a part of this section and both should be studied by the student.

The 4 phases in the care of deep, extensive burns are (1) control of shock and primary local care, (2) postmortem homograft coverage as biologic dressings when needed, (3) flat surface grafting with the patient's own skin for permanent healing and holding distortion to a minimum, (4) the repair of contractures and dysfunction and the reconstruction of features by procedures in reconstructive surgery.

See Chapter 17, Burns and Cold Injury, for classification and treatment of burns.

Healing Time

Superficial burns should be healed in 10 to 14 days and less extensive deep burns in a month.

Skin Grafting

Extensive deep burns should be ready for coverage with skin grafts in 3 weeks. Excision of the eschar and grafting in 2 weeks' time is done in some places, but usually this is not applicable to the face, the hands and the feet until the depth of the burn is known and this often takes more than 2 weeks.

Split skin grafts give the most satisfactory permanent coverage to extensive raw areas.[30] This graft contains from one third to three fourths the thickness of the skin and of course includes an appreciable pad of derma. This pad of derma is very important functionally.

Split-thickness skin grafts are cut with a long skin graft knife from areas that can be flattened by pressure or stretched into a diaphragm in the simplest way. Suction retractors aid in providing a diaphragm of skin in taking the grafts. Various mechanical, electrical or vacuum dermatomes are available and are useful in cutting split grafts from some areas.

Application of split-thickness or full-thickness grafts requires fixation and steady, even pressure for an assurance of take. Fixation may be by suture around the graft or by tying the sutures over fine mesh grease gauze and a bulk of mechanic's waste or other medium. Or the graft may be "snubbed" into place, which is accomplished by carefully rolling fine mesh grease gauze over the graft to fix it firmly, and then firmly fixing the rest of the bulk of the dressing with soft gauze rolls, being

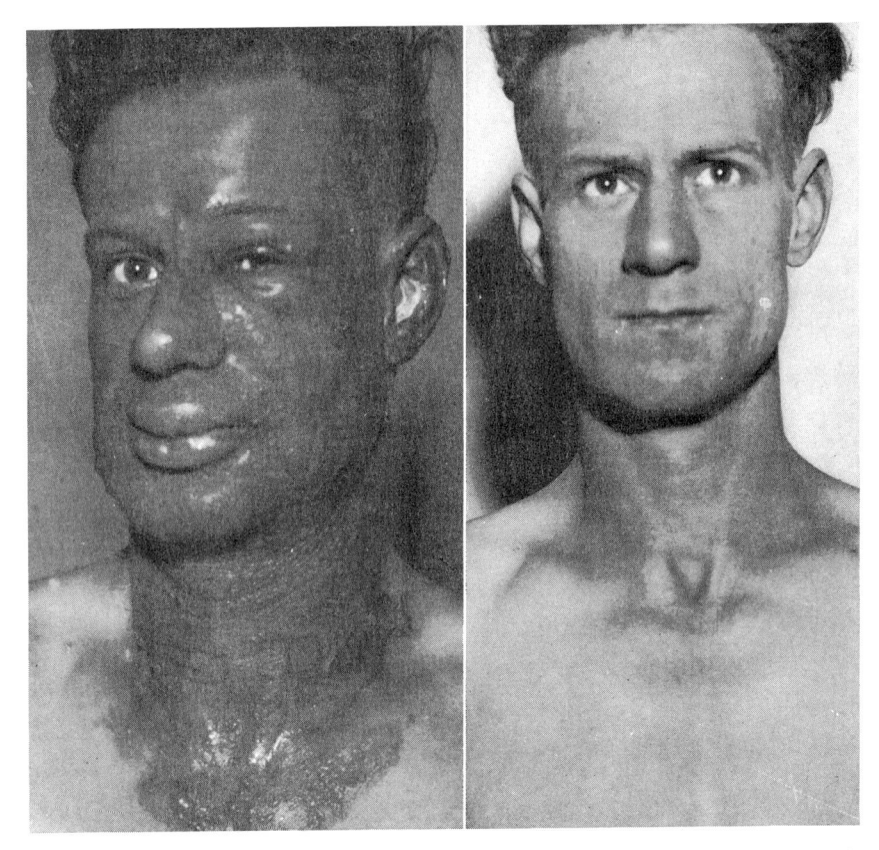

FIG. 49-1. (*Left*) Painful acute superficial burn of face and neck 24 hours following injury. Superficial blistering, weeping, generally uncomfortable. (*Right*) Immediate healing, comfort and prevention of infection promoted by pressure, fine mesh grease gauze dressing. Initial dressing left in place for 6 days. No other treatment necessary. Primary healing possible because this was a superficial burn. Comfort, promptness of healing, avoidance of infection, treatment as an outpatient made possible by dressing. (Brown, J. B., and Fryer, M. P.: J. Missouri M. A., 48:973-981)

careful not to slip the graft out of place. This is often used on extremities.

Donor site dressings aim at protection of the fresh wound from chemical, bacterial and mechanical trauma and consist of fine mesh grease gauze fixed with overlying gauze pads, held with adhesive to prevent local slipping and then gauze rolls and bandage in turn held with adhesive. Fixation of the part and the adjacent joints with steady, even pressure invites healing. Healing should be complete in 2 weeks' time. Variation can be done in dressing technic or no dressing may be applied to the grafted area or the donor site, but as yet these alternatives have not been proved better than the dressing described above. The healing of a donor site is comparable with a superficial burn. If the delicate exposed surface is protected, it will heal in 10 to 12 days; if not, and it is traumatized, a full-thickness loss of the remaining epidermal structures may result, with subsequent scarring and distortion.

Epithelial healing of donor sites of split grafts gives one of the most interesting studies of wound healing. The deep epithelial cells in the derma, finding themselves without a normal epidermal covering, "dedifferentiate" into squamous epithelium and resurface the area in as little as 6 days' time and give solid enough healing to omit dressings after 12 days.

Skin Grafting and Deep Burns 1439

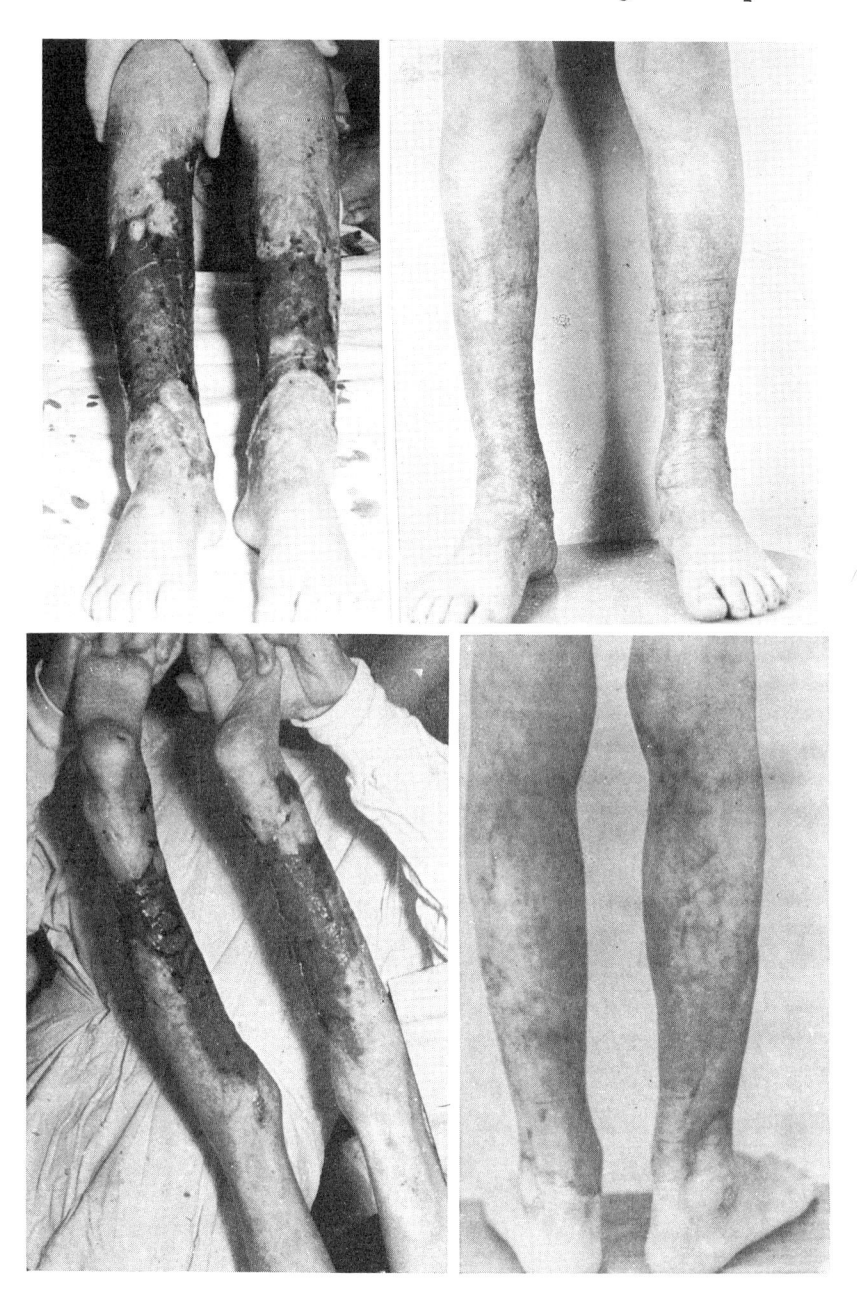

FIG. 49-2. (*Left, top and bottom*) Circular full-thickness loss of the skin of both legs resulting from deep burn when clothes caught on fire. Open areas prepared for grafting with frequent fine mesh (pressure) grease gauze dressing, done in the ward dressing room or the operating room under sterile conditions. (*Right, top and bottom*) Appearance several months following coverage of open areas with thick split-thickness grafts transferred from the back. Permanent repair in one operation. (Brown, J. B., and Fryer, M. P.: J. Missouri M. A., 48:973-981)

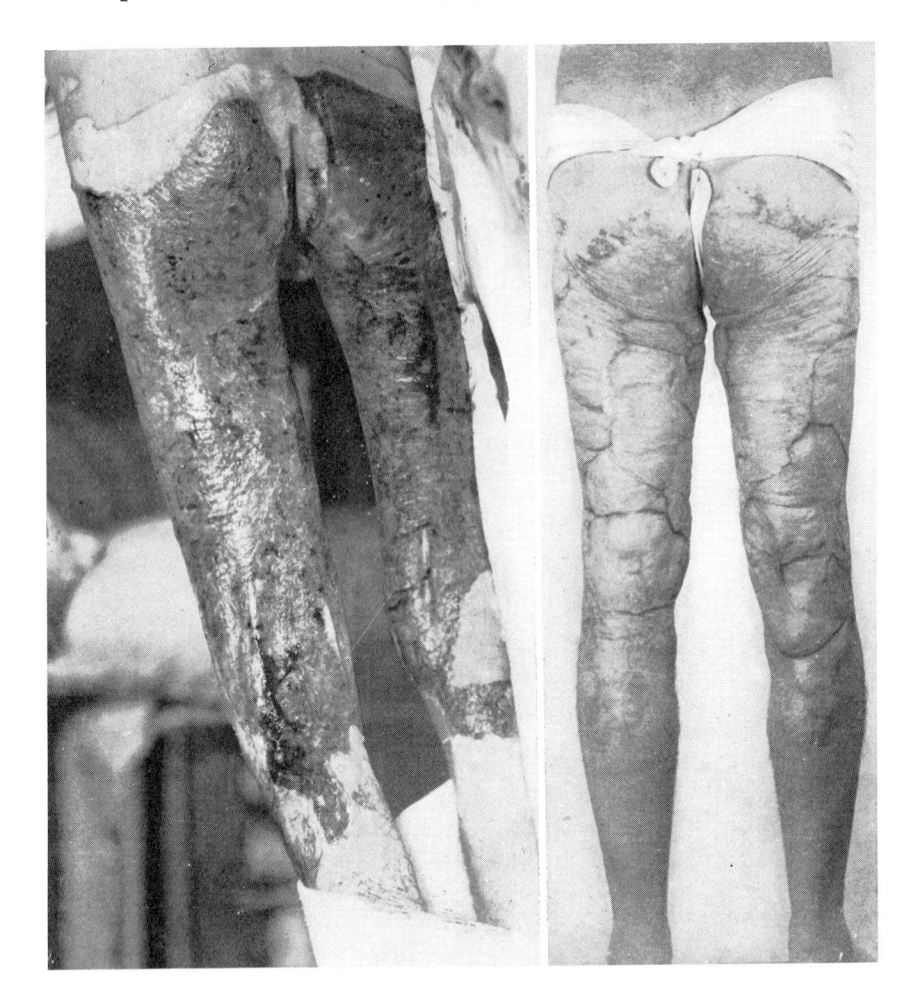

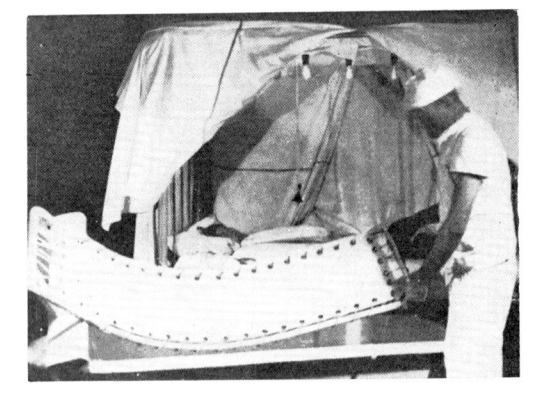

1440   Principles of General Plastic Surgery

Fig. 49-3. (*Top, left*) Full-thickness loss of skin over most of both thighs and buttocks following burn with gasoline. Taken care of elsewhere for several months. Appearance after several dressings consisting of washing with soap and water, then applying fine mesh grease gauze pressure dressing. At this length of time following a burn these open areas become so painful that often general anesthesia is necessary for adequate cleansing. (*Top, right*) Appearance 1 year later following resurfacing of the open areas on the thighs with long, wide, thick split-thickness grafts cut from the back with the knife and suction box. (Brown, J. B., and Fryer, M. P.: J. Missouri M. A., 48:973-981)

(*Bottom*) Frame, tub and bed used in preparing this burn and other deep burns for rapid coverage with skin.

This is considered the reverse of the formation of cancer, in which surface cells grow down and lose their differentiation.

Homografts are often important for the emergency, though temporary, coverage of extensive burns after the removal of the eschar, particularly in the very young or old.[21] Homografts are to be thought of as biologic dressings for large open wounds. They serve to prevent the excessive vaporization of water that takes place upon the cutaneously denuded surface and thereby to reduce the loss of heat from the body and the hypermetabolism characteristically associated with large burns (see Chap. 17). In addition, the number of the bacteria on the surface of the burn is very quickly reduced to the vanishing point when the wound is covered with a living homograft, just as it is when the wound is covered by a living autograft. Consequently, the living homograft constitutes an important means of aiding in the control of infections in burn wounds. Their use may be considered as the *second phase* in the local treatment of extensive burns.

Often the extensively burned patient is deemed unable to stand the operation required for transference of his own skin to his open areas, or none of his own skin is available. Then the application of homografts stops the "leaks" of vital body fluids and may serve to carry the patient over this critical period. Covering an open wound with them also gives respite from pain and obviates the need for dressings; the patient literally walks around in another's skin. The speed with which the application of a graft abolishes the pain and the tenderness of an open wound is remarkable; all pain and tenderness disappear within a minute or two.

For one extensively burned patient, the taking of homografts from living donors requires a large number of donors, who must be anesthetized, operated upon and have their wounds cared for afterward. However, *postmortem homografts* have been proved to have the same general properties as homografts taken from living donors and by using them one avoids the need of taking homografts from live donors. Postmortem grafts are removed from the clothed areas of patients who have just died. The grafts are usually taken from the cadaver in the operating room under sterile conditions after obtaining written consent from the donor's relatives. Permission for a general postmortem examination is not necessary if proper permission for the taking of the skin is obtained. The donor should not have carcinoma, a blood dyscrasia or a transmissible disease. Using these grafts immediately obviates the need for storage. Because the skin lives for a number of hours after the heart stops, living homografts may be obtained from a cadaver for some time after death. There is no reason for not using them in place of homografts cumbersomely taken from living donors. The use of postmortem grafts has been considered for many years. We used them first in 1927 and sporadically up to 1951. Since 1951 they have been employed regularly whenever homografting was needed.[15, 25, 27, 28] It is our belief that the temporary coverage of large cutaneously denuded surfaces with homografts may have effected a reduction in the death rate from very extensive burns (larger than 50 per cent of body surface) which has remained about the same for 100 years, despite the great improvement in control of shock and general care.

It is important to remember that, at the present time, homografts do not survive indefinitely. From 3 to 12 weeks after their application they are rejected by the recipient. Much investigative work is being done in attempting to effect the permanent take of homografts.

A skin bank was developed and thoroughly explored as an adjunct for the use of postmortem homografts because it was thought they would be needed when suitable postmortem donors are not available. The results of these studies are given below.

Skin grafts may be stored alive in a number of ways. The simplest, most practical and suitable way is their moist storage in an ordinary household refrigerator at temperatures of $+3°$ to $+5°$ C. After removing the grafts from the body, they are rolled in fine meshed gauze and kept moist in a jar with saline in the refrigerator for as long as 3 weeks. The period of viability can be lengthened somewhat by the addition of 10 per cent serum and antibiotics to the saline. It may be prolonged further by soaking them in glycerol and then freezing and storing at $-40°$ and $-80°$ C. Recently postmortem grafts have been frozen

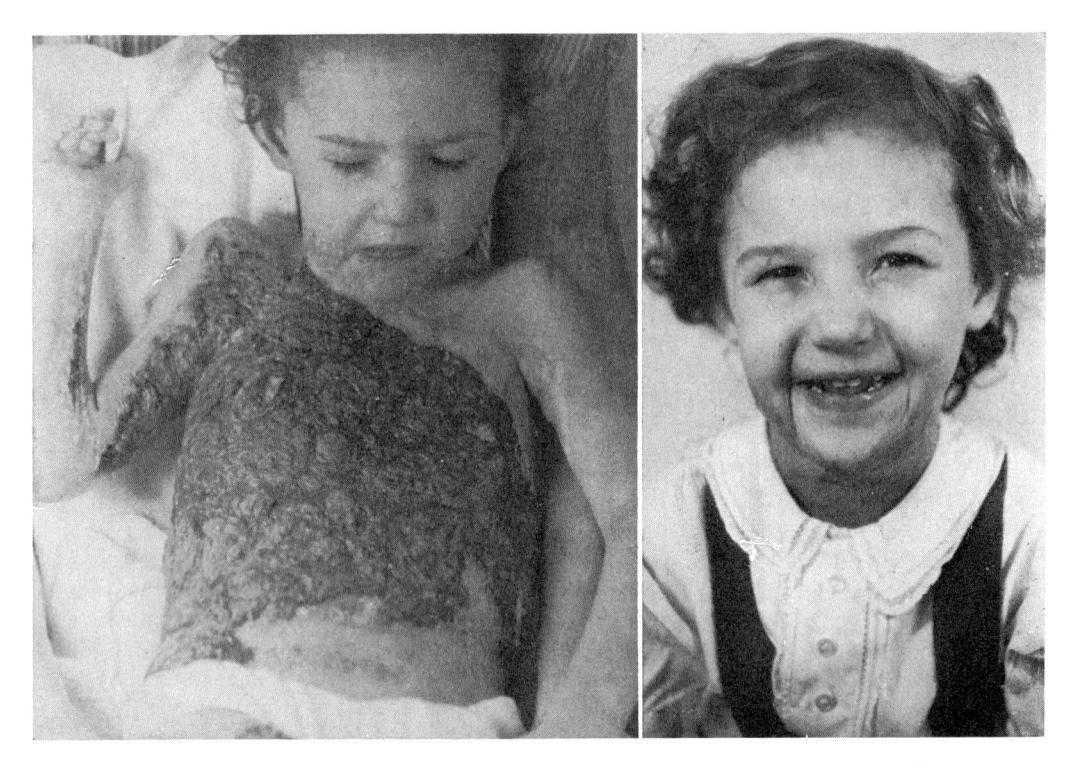

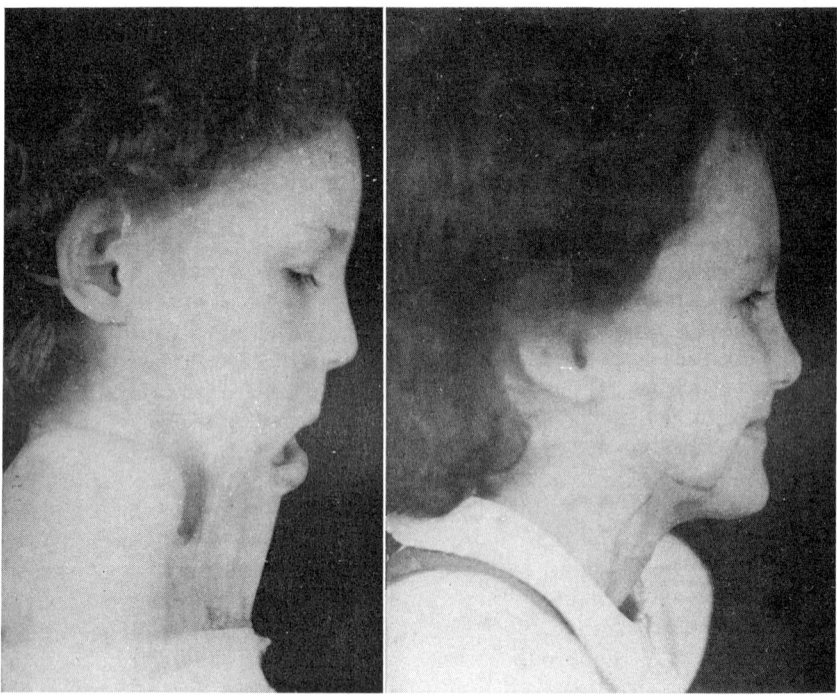

Fig. 49-4. (*Left, top*) Deep burn of abdomen, chest, neck, shoulder and arm in a child, with deformity resulting from the spontaneous healing (*left, bottom*) in flexion areas. In spite of uncomfortable position of head, chief complaint was of loss of "watertight mouth." (*Right, top and bottom*) One operation has restored the "watertight mouth" and the normal neck angle. Smoothing out around the edges of the graft can be done subsequently.

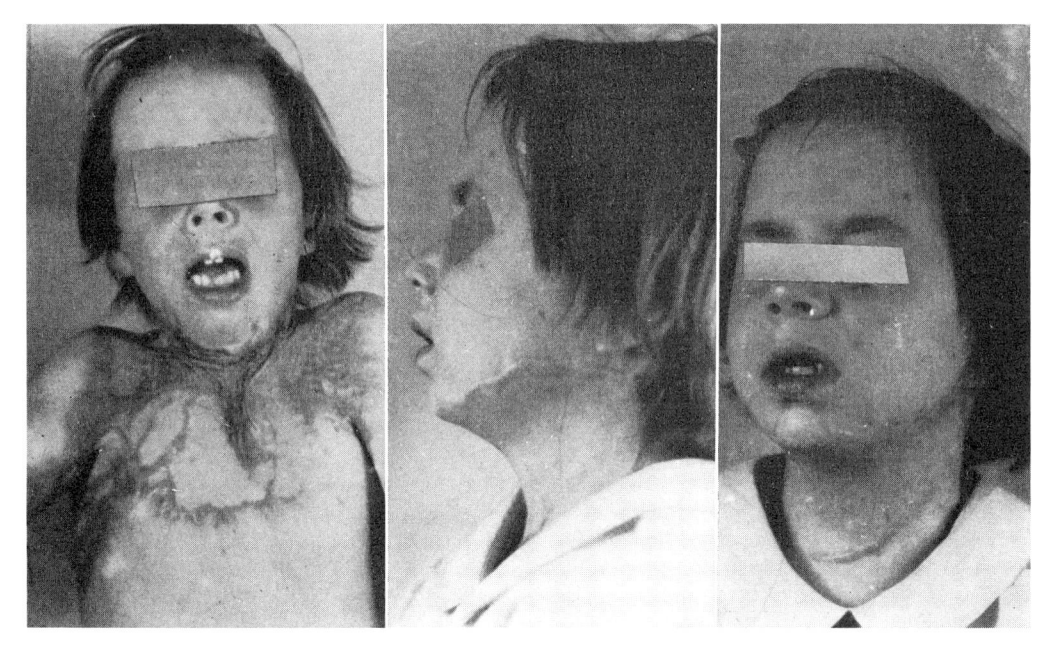

FIG. 49-5. (*Left*) Severe contracture of the neck following deep burn. (*Center and right*) Result possible by release of chin and excision of deep scar and chronically infected sinuses. Free, thick, split-thickness graft used to cover defect at same operation, which has created normal neck angle and allowed normal growth. (Brown, J. B., and Fryer, M. P.: J. Missouri M. A., 48:973-981)

and vacuum dried (freeze-dried). This is the easiest way to store nonviable grafts. Nonviable freeze-dried grafts serve well as temporary biologic dressings, although they are not as long lasting as fresh postmortem homografts and consequently not as good for the temporary coverage of open areas.[15, 25, 27, 28] The source of postmortem homografts in a large medical center is beyond expectations, and an active skin bank is unnecessary under such circumstances.

Homografts taken from one of *identical twins* and applied to the other survive permanently. We first effected such a transfer in 1937. Since then this demonstration has served as the basis for the transfer of organs from one identical twin to another.

Autografts. The third stage (or phase) of treatment of an extensive deep burn is the covering of the denuded areas with autografts and is carried out by using grafts from the patient as soon as he is judged capable of standing the procedure. The early coverage of flat surfaces with autografts and the securing of complete healing hold to a minimum contracture, deformity and dysfunction and, in many instances, are all that is needed for the complete rehabilitation of the patient.

Final Phase of Treatment. The final (fourth) phase in the treatment of the severely burned patient is the release and repair of contractures, the restoration of articular function and the reconstruction of features. Frequently, the healing of raw surfaces in flexion areas is attended by contractures, requiring release of the contracture for the restoration of function and appearance. Eyelids, axilla, neck, hand or fingers are especially prone to be so affected. Excision of this contracting scar leaves a raw surface which usually can be covered best by a split-thickness graft. Local flaps and webs may be utilized when they are available, but further addition of skin grafts is almost always needed. Cumbersome distant flaps are unnecessary in most burn repairs, and this is a point that seems to be missed frequently. One patient with a burn contraction of the neck was seen on whom a

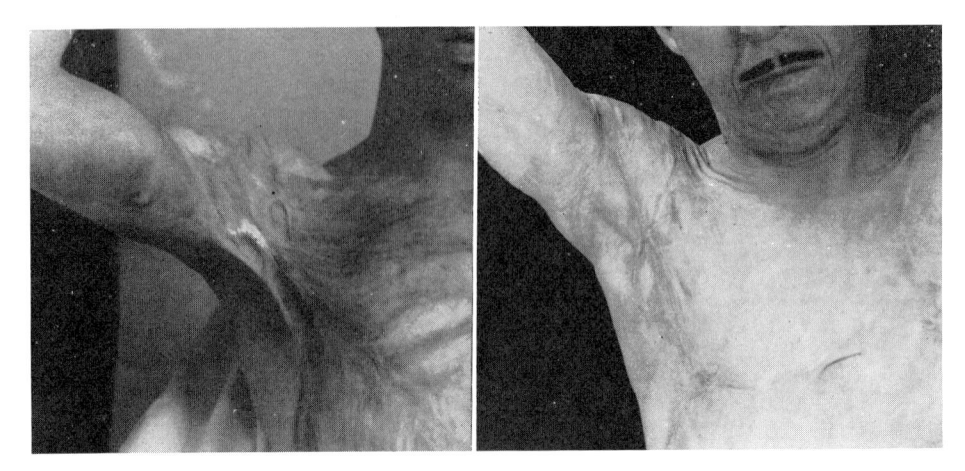

FIG. 49-6. (*Left*) Contracture of axilla resulting from spontaneous healing of a deep burn. Part of natural healing process of an open wound is contraction of the edges which, when it occurs in the neck, the axilla or other such place, pulls that part toward the heavier side or fixed part. The patient is unable to abduct the arm fully. (*Right*) Twenty years later: permanent restoration of function and improvement in appearance by one operation. This consisted of the release of the contracture and excision of the deep scar, resurfacing the open area with a free graft. (Brown, J. B., and Fryer, M. P.: J. Missouri M. A., 48:973-981)

large back flap was used and 100 operative procedures performed before we saw the case. Usually the whole front of the neck can be repaired in 1 to 4 operations with free skin grafts, and the functional result will be much better than with a heavy, cumbersome flap.

DISTORTION OR LOSS OF A FEATURE. This presents one of the most difficult problems in repair. Loss of the alar border, the tip of the nose or the columella can best be substituted for by a free *composite graft* from the ear in one operation.[9] This graft includes both surfaces of skin and the supporting cartilaginous framework, and the resulting repair is superior to any other method.

Full-thickness skin grafts consist of the entire thickness of the skin, as the name intimates. The use of this type of graft requires antecedent closure or coverage with a split-thickness skin graft for healing before the full-thickness graft is put in place. Full-thickness skin grafts are used in small specialized areas, as about the face, the eyelids or the hands.

Full-thickness grafts from the neck give the best results in the repair of limited defects about the face because of color match and kinetic possibilities. Healing of burns of the face often is followed by eyelid contractures which leave the globe exposed, inviting irritation and ulceration, and consequently necessitate early repair in order to save the eye. The repair of eyelid contracture consists of release of the contracture, meticulous excision of the deep scar and coverage with a soft full-thickness graft from the neck. Elsewhere on the face release of contracting scars of limited size and repair with a graft from the supraclavicular region often results in a repair indistinguishable from the normal.

Burns of the hands, of some extent, are usually seen accompanying burns of other areas of the body and often are the most important parts to be treated. Resurfacing of the hand is an important part of plastic surgery in general and will be outlined here for completeness. Repair of the deeper structures and treatment of infections of the hand are considered elsewhere in this text. Also a short description will be given here of the first recorded burns of the hands from atomic irradiation.

SUPERFICIAL BURNS of the hands are treated, in general, in the same manner as are superficial burns elsewhere in the body. Flash burns not even deep enough to cause superficial blistering are often extremely painful. Placing the hand in cold water usually relieves the pain,

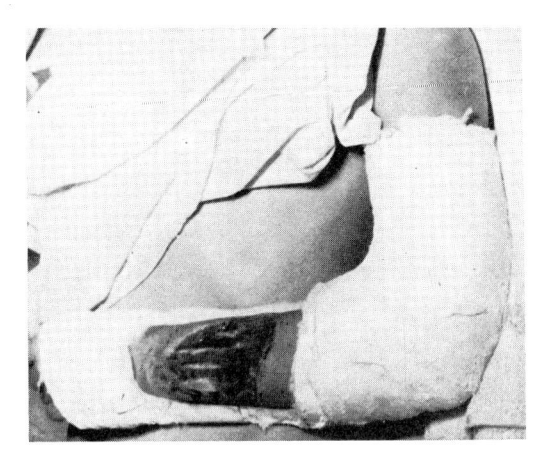

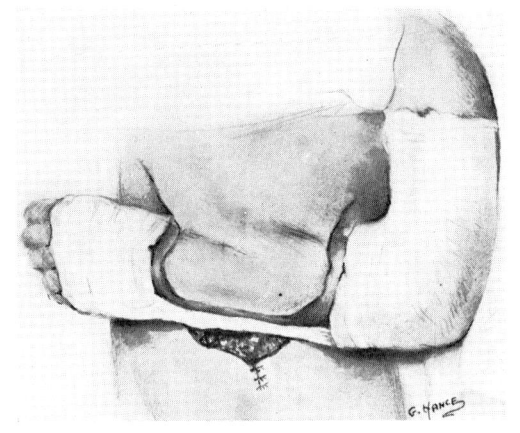

Fig. 49-7. (*Top, left*) Deep injury from gunshot wound of forearm. (*Top, right*) Drawing showing short broad-base pedicle flap from abdomen applied directly to defect in forearm. Delay of flap unnecessary. (*Bottom*) Normal function restored. Bone graft unnecessary.

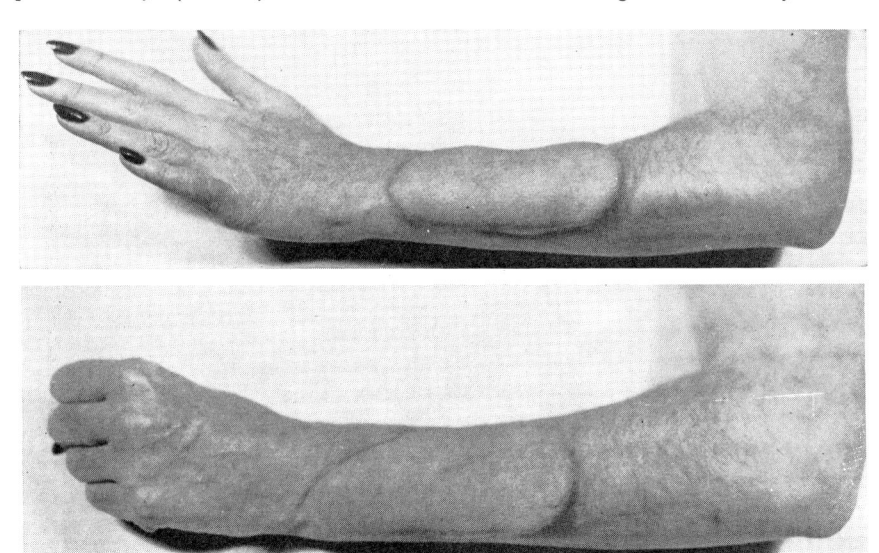

but this may have to be persisted in for several hours. Following this relief of pain a light coverage with grease gives the most comfort in cases of very superficial burns of the hand.

DEEP BURNS of the hands should be cleansed and the eschar excised as soon as the depth of deep burns can be recognized, and the wound covered with grafts as soon as possible to prevent deep infection and fixation of tendons and joints. It is generally agreed that dressings with open surgical drainage, fingers apart and with the hand in the position of function is the method of choice from the onset of treatment.

Early mobilization of burned hands is not difficult if prompt healing is secured, and this is encouraged by active motion in soapy water at the time of each dressing.

Deep burns of the dorsum of the hand are usually worse than those of the palm because frequently the midportion of the extensor sleeve over the middle interphalangeal joints is destroyed. The lateral slips of these extensor tendons then slip volarward when extension is attempted, flexing the joint instead of extending it and giving a characteristic and, for the most part, permanent functional loss.

Late deformities of the hand resulting from deep burns are minimized by their early

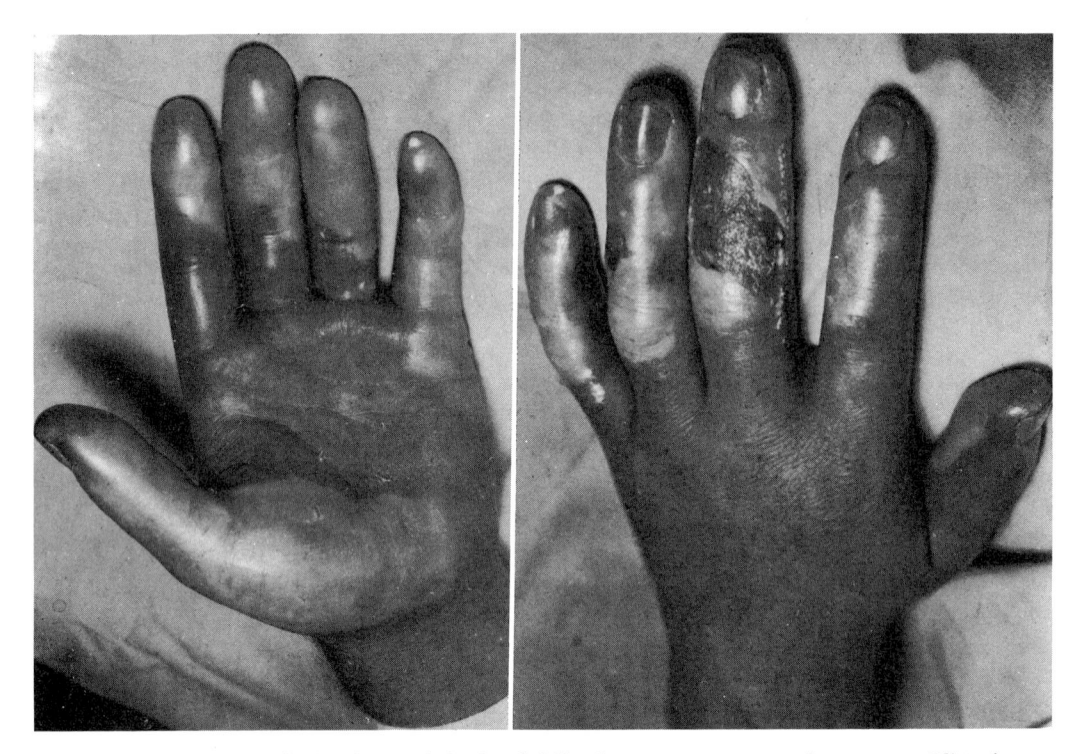

FIG. 49-8. Acute radiation burn of the hand following overexposure to fluoroscope. Blistering and deep slough. Intense pain required 3 to 5 grains of morphine a day. Received general supportive treatment and conservative management of local areas. Resection of involved skin as it definitely declared itself, with immediate coverage by free split-thickness grafts. Amputation avoided.

coverage with free grafts. Early healing up to necrotic tendon or bone usually can be obtained by early coverage of adjacent granulating areas with free grafts. This may save function in the remainder of the hand which otherwise may be lost by waiting for complete separation of dead tissue and later total flap replacement. Contractures require careful opening, avoiding wide exposure of tendons, and coverage with free grafts or flaps if the destruction is of enough depth to require the latter. The usual flap is a direct one from the inguinal region of the abdominal wall. The direct flap was developed and used hundreds of times at Valley Forge General Hospital during World War II, more for gunshot injuries than for burns.[8] Because of the change from the tubed pedicle to a short, broad pedicle, the time element was cut from several months to days, with a tremendous saving in patient hospital days.

A DIRECT FLAP is raised and applied immediately to the recipient area with a broad, short base allowing an adequate blood supply.[8]

A DELAYED FLAP is one having a single pedicle raised in stages, progressively inducing the blood supply to enter from the attached end. The delayed flap is rarely needed because more rapid application of a flap is possible by use of a direct flap which lessens scar formation in the flap itself and saves parts that might be lost during the delay of preparation of a delayed flap graft.

TUBED PEDICLE FLAPS require even longer periods of preparation and are indicated only rarely for use on the hand.

PHYSIOTHERAPY is usually unnecessary in children, but older patients require it, depending on the depth of the burn and the rapidity of healing, and on the patient's own ideas and desires for his rehabilitation. Often in hands the setting of the joints is the most serious drawback to useful function and can occur even if the surface is restored. The sooner the

Skin Grafting and Deep Burns   1447

surface *is* restored, however, the less joint fixation may be expected.

Irradiation burns occur frequently and often are seen in their late stages.[35, 37] They may result from recent single heavy exposure to irradiation, or from multiple smaller doses sustained years before (see Chap. 18).

THE ACUTE IRRADIATION INJURY often in-

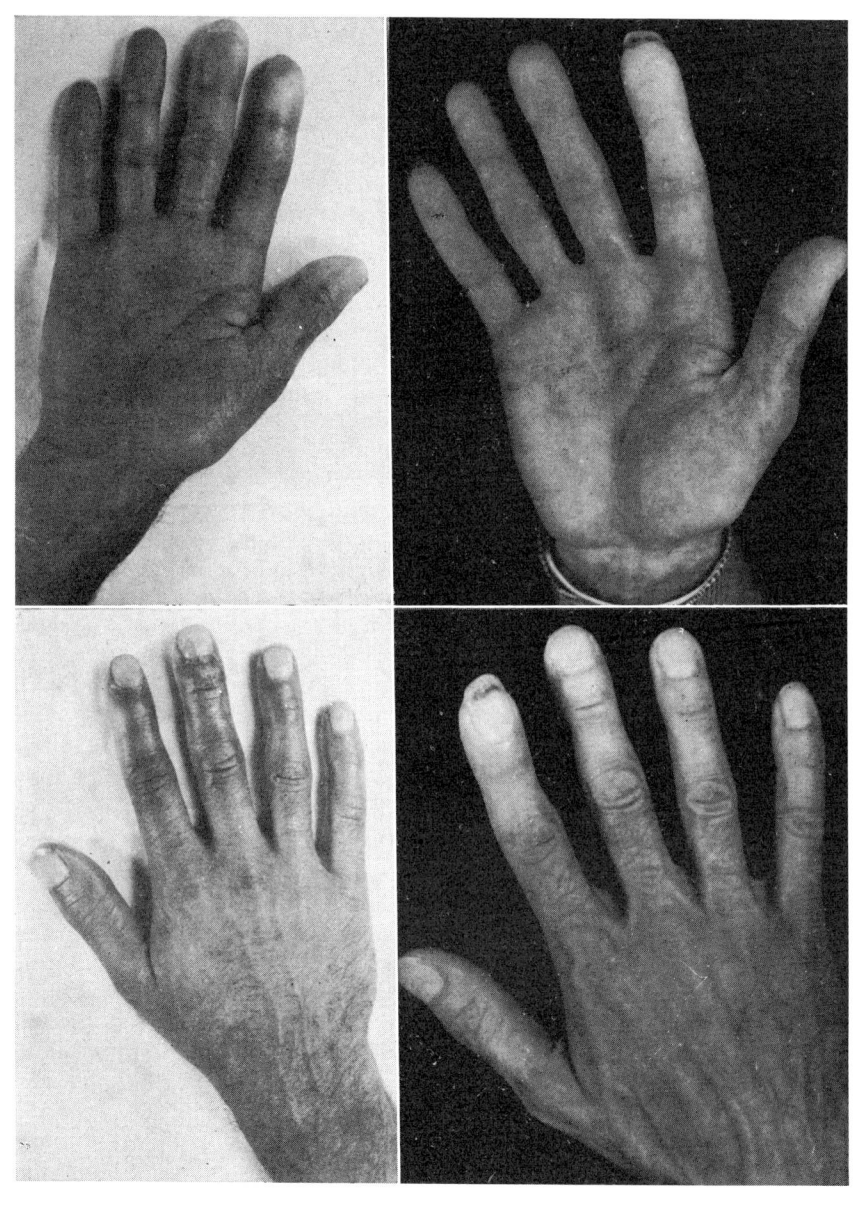

FIG. 49-9. (*Left, top and bottom*) Acute irradiation burn from cyclotron. Redness, pain and blistering following exposure to cyclotron neutron beam. Received conservative treatment to involved part with at least temporary avoidance of operation. (*Right, top and bottom*) Hand healed but result of even mild trauma to irradiated tissue seen at end of index finger. Open ulcer which looked as though it would require shortening of the finger. Again conservative care encouraged complete healing. Patient being seen at intervals with plan to excise definite, declared involvement before breakdown of the injured skin occurs.

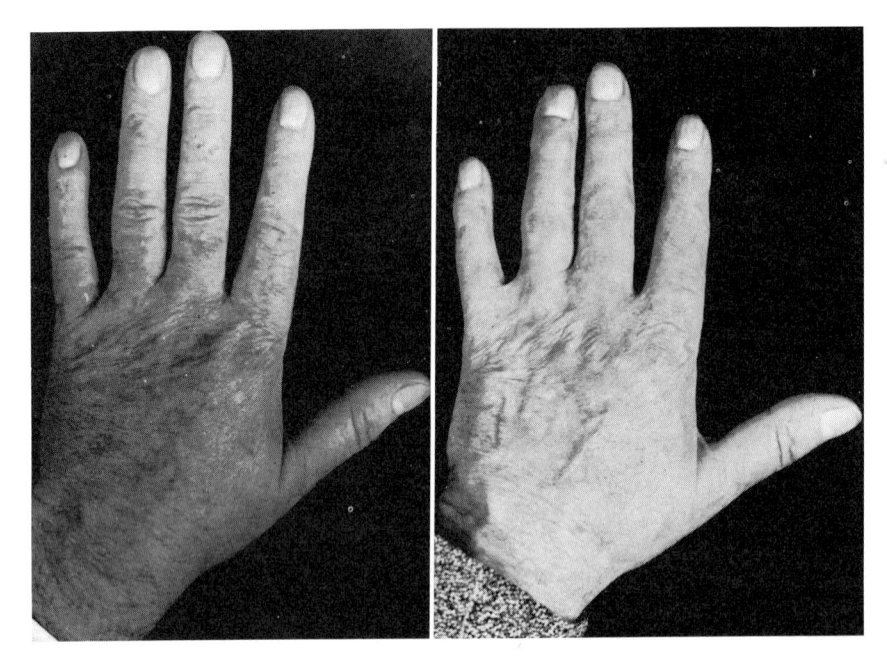

FIG. 49-10. Chronic irradiation burn of the hand. (*Left*) All the signs of chronic irradiation present, with telangiectasis, "coal spots," atrophy, keratosis, ulceration and carcinoma. Due to repeated exposure to x-rays, a physician incurred these burns while taking care of others. (*Right*) Entire back of hand and the fingers was excised, and the open area was covered with split-thickness graft. One operation. Normal function. Progression to carcinoma in an irradiation burn assured if the patient lives long enough. (Brown, J. B., and Fryer, M. P.: J. Missouri M. A., 48:973-981)

volves the hands, and the severe, steady, almost unbearable pain is unforgettable. Not unlike thermal burns, redness, blistering and deep slough follow the severe injuries. Resection and graft replacement of irreparably damaged skin is performed as its delimitations become clear, and the pain is relieved almost miraculously. Immediate coverage with free grafts has saved hands that appeared to be lost.

Chronic irradiation dermatitis follows a definite predictable progression through atrophy, telangiectasis, keratosis and ulceration to ultimate carcinoma formation. Pain and itching are prominent symptoms which are relieved immediately, and carcinoma is prevented by excision of the affected areas and replacement with a free graft from other areas on the body. Usually this is done in one operation, and function is restored.

A PERMANENT PEDICLE BLOOD-CARRYING FLAP has been developed to use in the repair of some deep avascular areas resulting from irradiation.[22] Use of this type of flap actually permanently increases the vascularity of previously vascularly deficient irradiated areas which the usual pedicle flap that has to be detached from its source cannot do.

By early replacement of skin damaged by radiation, serious sequelae can be avoided, and the usefulness of irradiation therapy in general could be extended if this concept of early removal and repair were adopted.

BURNS DUE TO ATOMIC IRRADIATION are discussed because of the possible imminence of large numbers and the personal experience already obtained in the treatment of the only recorded burns of this origin.[12] In the acute phase the treatment should be the same as for any severe burn. Grease gauze pressure dressings have proved to be most satisfactory. Burns of atomic origin differ from other irradiation burns only in that local symptoms begin sooner after exposure and progress more rapidly to the chronic phase. There is local redness in a few hours, blistering begins in about

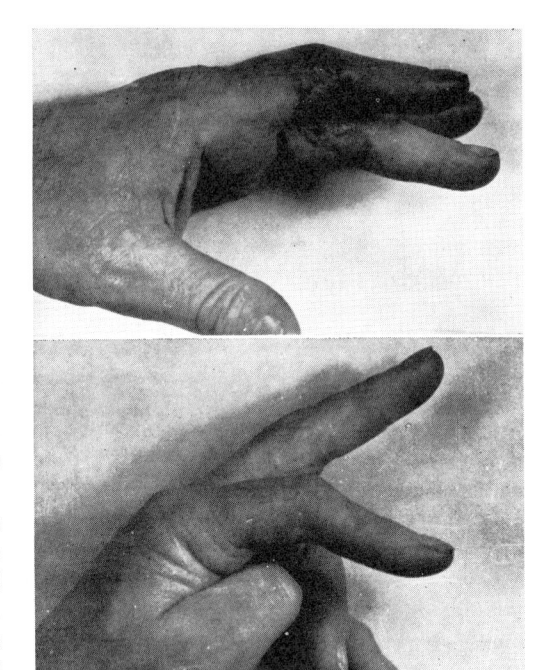

Skin Grafting and Deep Burns 1449

Fig. 49-11. Chronic irradiation burn of a dentist's fingers. (*Top*) Same signs as in Figure 49-9 but had not yet proceeded to carcinoma. (*Bottom*) Involved area excised and covered immediately with free graft. One operation. Normal function. Amputation avoided.

a week, and the injury has either progressed to an open wound or has healed in a month. In cases of open sores early free split graft coverage is indicated. Subsequently, all injuries showing chronic irradiation effect should be resected and covered with split-thickness grafts.

It may be pointed out that at this date the only pure radiation burns of atomic origin that have been recorded have been resected and grafted without the loss of any fingers. From this first experience with such burns there is some hope offered for the control of atomic radiation damage. The only hitch is that if the whole body received such a quantity of atomic radiation as to destroy skin, life would be lost. However, when the exposure has been limited to the hand, there has been little if any systemic effect and the local repair has sufficed for good rehabilitation.

Electrical burns are considered separately because they are usually deeper but more con-

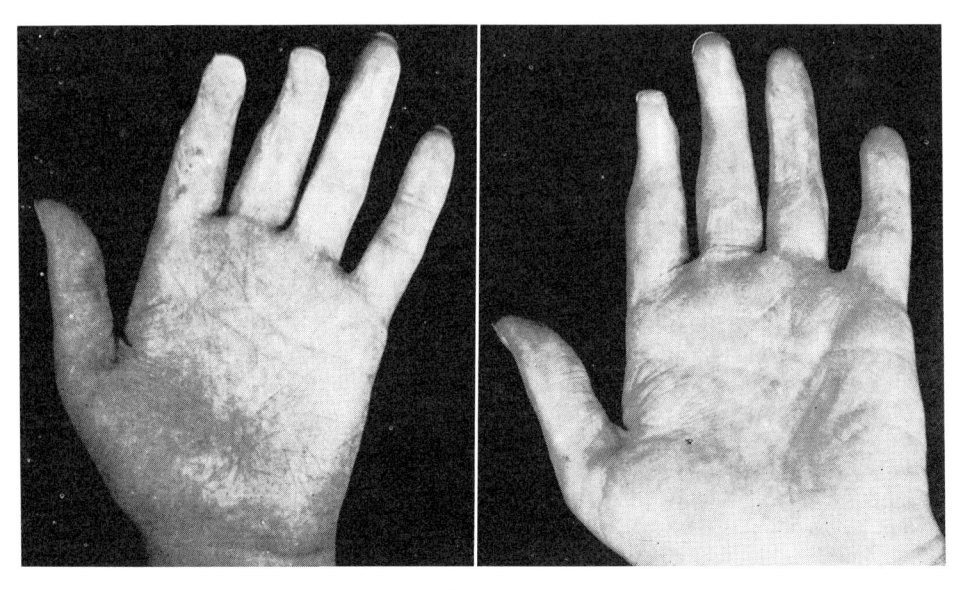

Fig. 49-12. Atomic burn of the hand. (*Left*) Rapid progression of changes to those characteristic of chronic irradiation effect, namely: atrophy, telangiectasis, "coal spots," and ulcers. (*Right*) The same hand following excision of badly damaged skin and immediate resurfacing with split-thickness grafts. The function of the hand is good. Should the excision not have been done relatively early, carcinoma would almost certainly have occurred in the damaged skin and then amputation would probably have been required.

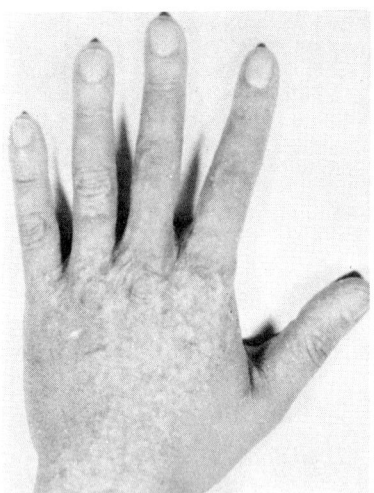

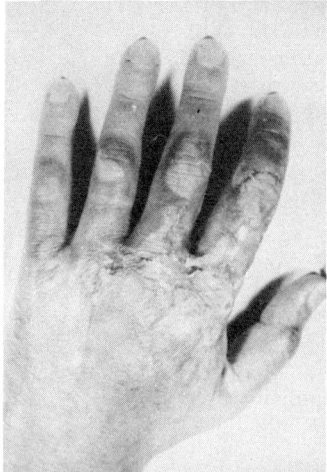

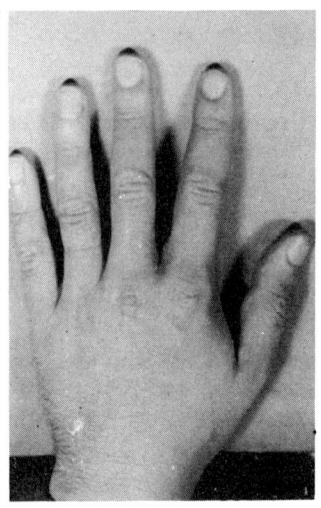

FIG. 49-13. Cathode-ray burn from heavy electron beam of an industrial machine, in research. (*Left*) Slight erythema and edema when first seen 2 weeks after exposure. (*Center*) Two weeks later, 4 weeks after exposure, blistering of dorsum of hand which was healing under conservative management. (*Right*) Three years after burn. Chronic changes noted in burned area required resection and repair with thick split graft over whole dorsum of forearm, hand and fingers. This is believed to be the first cathode-ray machine burn recorded. (Preliminary Report, Ann. Surg., 146: No. 3, 1957)

fined than those of thermal origin. However, there may be dangerous damage to large blood vessels between the point where the electric current enters the body and its place of exit. Shock, and associated injuries, such as fractures from falling, may accompany electrical burns and require recognition and treatment. Primary or early excision and coverage of the burned areas is often possible in this type of burn. Also, a thicker type of coverage is more often necessary than that afforded by a free graft. The direct abdominal flap is of particular use in the primary repair of electrical burns to the arms and the hand and the permanent pedicle blood-carrying flaps are especially useful for the coverage of electrical burns to other parts of the body.

Cathode-ray machine burns are like those resulting from other sources of irradiation. They are mentioned because their use is becoming much more common in industry. Some industrial uses of these investigative rays are to determine the purity of solids and the effects of certain rays on plastics and solids. The effect on human tissue with the acute burn progressing to chronic breakdown requires the same treatment described for other irradiation burns. It is most important to recognize the rapidity of disease progress, as is demonstrated in Figure 49-13, of high energy electron injury from accelerator machines.

CLEFT LIP AND CLEFT PALATE

Cleft lip and cleft palate occur singly or in combination, at a rate of about 1 in 900 live births. The combination of cleft lip and cleft palate is slightly more common in male infants, but incomplete cleft of the palate is seen a little more often in girls. However, the ratio between sexes is almost the same, as is the side on which the cleft occurs. Double clefts of the lip and the palate are less than half as frequent as single clefts. Deformities of other parts of the body may be associated with cleft lip and palate.

Etiology of cleft lip and palate is unknown, except that it is a failure of fusion of the 3 primary segments of the face or the palate. Understanding this process, which occurs before the 2nd month of pregnancy, permits explanation for any deformity of the lip or the palate. In the face failure of fusion of the glabellar or central process with one or both

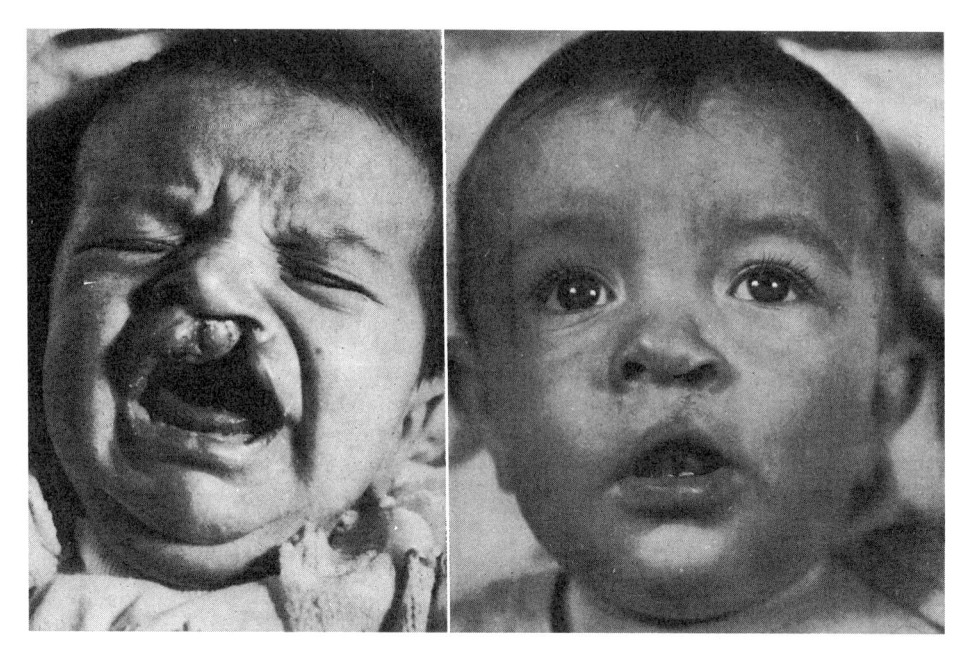

Fig. 49-14. (*Left*) Single complete cleft with the usual flat nostril. (*Right*) Repaired lip and nose in one operation, using the markings illustrated in Figure 49-15. Palate to be closed later.

lateral facial processes results in single or double cleft lip. Similarly, in the palate, when the central process does not fuse with one lateral palatine body, a single cleft of the palate results, or a double cleft of the palate follows failure on both sides.

Diagnosis of cleft lip or palate is obvious on inspection.

Deformity of the nose is usually as marked as the lip and in some instances makes acceptable repair difficult.

Scholastic standing in school by the child with a cleft lip or palate is usually above average, possibly due to greater effort or superior intelligence. Progress through life is easier now that stigma is no longer attached to this deformity. The old term of "harelip" should not be used, as it was a stigma visited on the patient because of insufficiencies of surgery and anesthesia.

Superior initial surgical repair is in a large measure responsible for the improved chance in life for these patients. Repair, when coupled with love and understanding at home, is all that is necessary to ensure a successful, happy, full life. Surgical repair is so important that some of the principles are outlined here.

CLEFT LIP REPAIR

At the initial operation prevention of deformity is sought by constructing: (1) a good alar level and direction; (2) a good nostril floor; (3) a good curve to the nostril; (4) a straight columella; (5) a full upper lip in advance of the lower lip; (6) a full vermilion; (7) if possible, a flexion crease in the lip. Widely placed sutures are avoided, as they leave "ladder" scars which are often impossible to remove without making the lip too long.[31]

Time for repair of a single cleft lip is any time after birth that it is thought safe for the child, but the sooner the better. The technical difficulties of repair for the surgeon should not influence this decision. It is advantageous to have the child leave the hospital with the mother, around 10 days after birth, and this is usually possible only if repair is done during the first few days of life. If the infant is jaundiced or losing weight, operation can be postponed for a few days. There is no doubt that the operation is easier to do after some weeks, and the third month has been advocated by some. Double cleft lips are not closed as soon as single clefts are. The closure is usually de-

1452   Principles of General Plastic Surgery

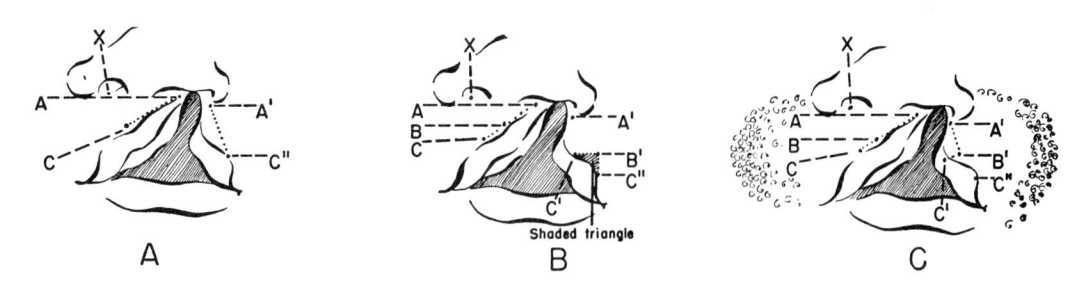

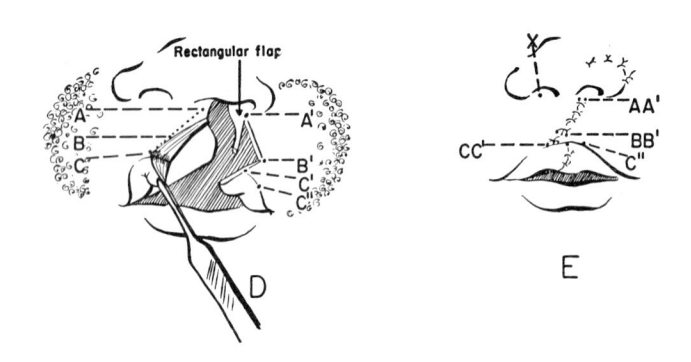

FIG. 49-15. Design for repair of single cleft lip. (A) The V-excision operation. While the columella is held over straight, A is marked at the junction of the skin and the vermilion border at the level of the base of the columella. X is in the same relation to the columella on the sound side. A' bears the same relation to the ala on the cleft side that X bears to the ala on the normal side. C" is on the *mucocutaneous junction* at the point where the vermilion border first begins to thin out. C is on the *mucocutaneous junction*, the same distance from A' that C is from A. To perform the V-excision operation A' is brought over to A, and C" to C, after excision of the edges of the cleft.

(B) The flap operation. The V-excision operation is marked out first. C' is on the mucocutaneous junction at the most medial point of good full vermilion border. B' is on the line A'-C", equidistant from C' and C". The incision is A'-B'-C', saving the amount of lip indicated by the shaded isosceles triangle. B is on the mucocutaneous junction, the same distance from C that B' is from C'.

(C) The lines A-B-C and A'-B'-C' are incised lightly with a knife. The incision is carried upward from C' on the mucocutaneous junction to separate the vermilion border from the skin. This is done on the other side also at A, to keep any vermilion border out of the nostril floor. The triangle (see B) is to be undermined at the next step.

(D) The lightly incised lines A-B-C and A'-B'-C' are cut completely through the lip with a stab blade, with care to keep the knife exactly perpendicular to the lip. All angles should be opened completely. The vermilion border is inspected, and any attached skin is removed with a stab blade. The rectangular flap freed from A'-B'-C' must be loose enough to be rotated up 180° into the nostril floor. Dotted stippling indicates areas of soft parts undermined.

(E) C and C' are united, and the vermilion flaps are interdigitated in a zigzag fashion, fitting them so that they lie naturally together without any pull or stretching. Then suturing is continued on around the vermilion border and up the inside to the fornix. The little flap in the nostril is trimmed to fit with the one from the opposite side, and they are sutured together to form the floor. A few key mattress sutures are placed through the ala to unite the lining and the covering (which were separated during the undermining). Then the mucosa inside the lip is closed.

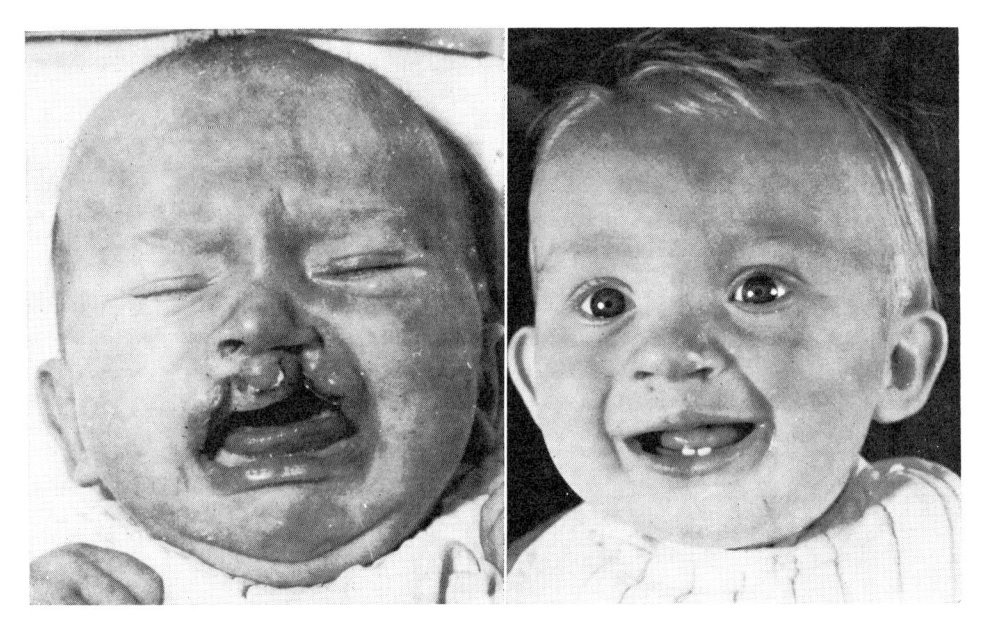

Fig. 49-16. (*Left*) Double cleft of lip with incomplete cleft on one side and the complete cleft on other. (*Right*) Repaired in one operation. Palate closed later.

layed until the infant has gained in weight or a month after birth has passed because of the longer operative time required.

The method of surgical repair of a single cleft lip summarized in Figure 49-15 is fundamentally simple and definite and permits the method of repair to fit the deformity rather than attempting the reverse. This method of marking and repair has been used for 20 years with predictably superior results.

Repair of double cleft lips is more than twice as difficult as single clefts; unfortunately, the results are usually only about half as good.[32] Notching of the vermilion is hard to avoid if full-thickness of the lip is not used in the repair, but then it is equally difficult not to make the lip too long. Repair of double cleft lips is summarized in Figure 49-17.

Secondary repair of a cleft lip or associated deformity of the nose may be necessary in spite of the best possible primary repair. When possible, tissue, available in the area of the defect is readjusted. This may require flaps from the buccal fornix to advance the lip, and usually osteoplastic reconstruction of the nose, including septal resection. In extreme deformities a flap of lower lip may be set into the upper lip for proper balance between the two; "L"-shaped cartilaginous support may be added to the nose through a columellar incision; most double clefts with the usual deficient columella require elongation to get the tip of the nose up as illustrated in the drawings in Figure 49-19. An associated "recessive ramisection" of the mandible may be necessary for proper balance between the lower jaw and the middle third of the face.

CLEFT PALATE REPAIR

Speech is a very complicated action, involving the interrelationship between thought processes and a neuro-anatomic mechanism. Children with a cleft palate may have deficiencies in any or all parts of the interacting setup. Anatomic deformities of the palate are repaired surgically as a routine procedure for perfect physiologic function. Although this does not guarantee perfect speech, because there may be a deficiency in other elements of this action, it should be done at as early an age as other factors will allow. *Time* for closure of a cleft palate is decided for each individual patient on the basis of growth of the maxilla which is complete enough at 4 years not to be hindered; repeated attacks of otitis media, resulting from open communication of the mid-

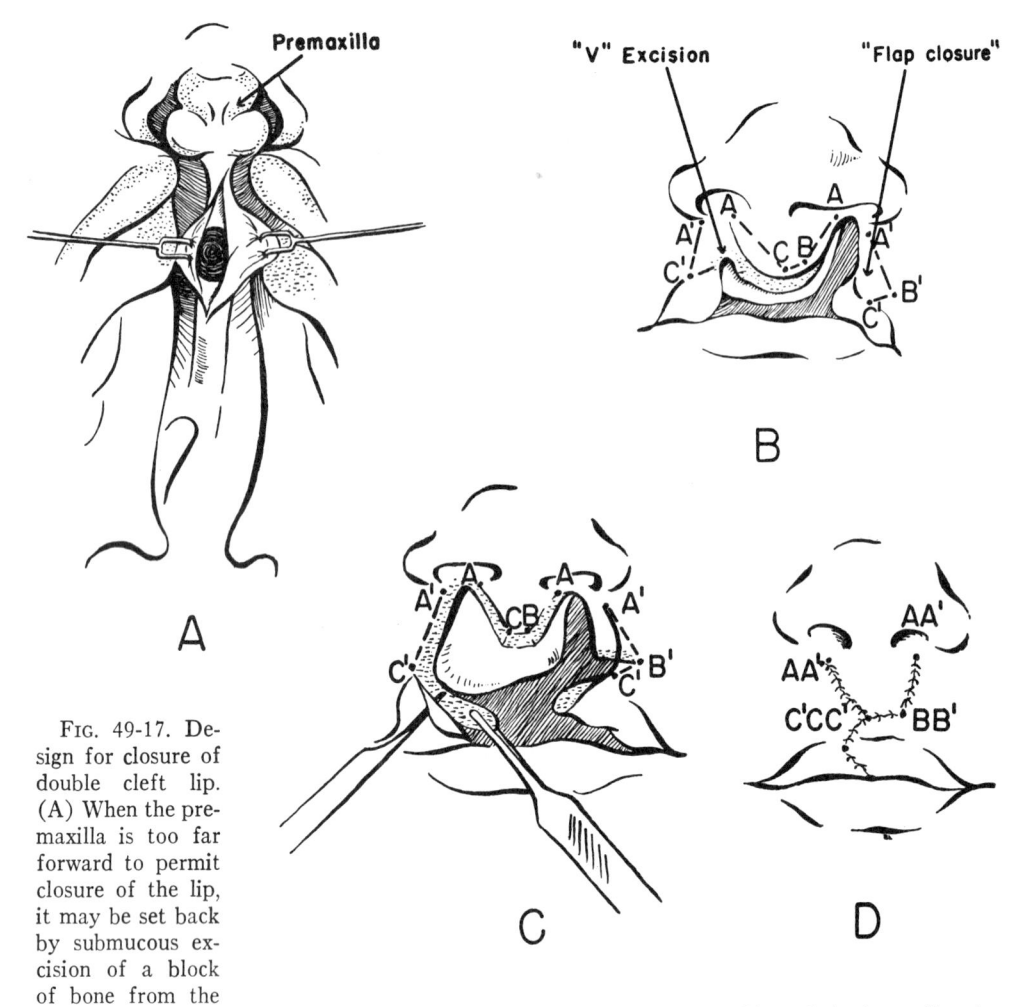

1454   Principles of General Plastic Surgery

FIG. 49-17. Design for closure of double cleft lip. (A) When the premaxilla is too far forward to permit closure of the lip, it may be set back by submucous excision of a block of bone from the vomer. This removal of a block, rather than a wedge, permits the pushing of the bone directly back like closing a drawer, rather than tilting it back. This factor is of some advantage, as the finished lip should slant forward in the profile view from above downward. (B) Flap closure is done on the total side, and a V-excision operation on the partial side. (C) Both sides of the lip are opened up, going completely through the lip with a stab blade knife and using a perpendicular sawing motion. Any skin remnants are sliced off of the vermilion flaps. The vermilion border of the prolabium is cut loose from the skin and turned back all around. (D) The closure is done with many fine silk sutures, put in not more than 1 to 2 mm. from the wound edges and about as far apart. Any stay sutures are put in from the inside and are not visible. The lip is closed by interdigitating small flaps.

dle ear with the mouth through a cleft palate, have caused deafness in some instances and necessitated early closure of the palate. The development of faulty speech habits with an open cleft also may dictate that an earlier closure than usual be done. When necessary the palate usually can be closed in the second or the third year.

The drawings in Figure 49-20 illustrate the method used to close a complete cleft of the palate.

CONGENITAL INSUFFICIENCY OF THE PALATE

Congenital insufficiency of the palate, wherein there is no cleft as such but a short palate with an open nasopharynx, requires

Cleft Lip and Cleft Palate 1455

Fig. 49-18. Profile before and after elongation of columella from upper lip as illustrated in diagram Figure 49-19. (*Left*) Before and (*right*) after operation of total reconstruction of the columella from upper lip, getting tip of nose up out of lip and creating proper angle between the nose and the lip.

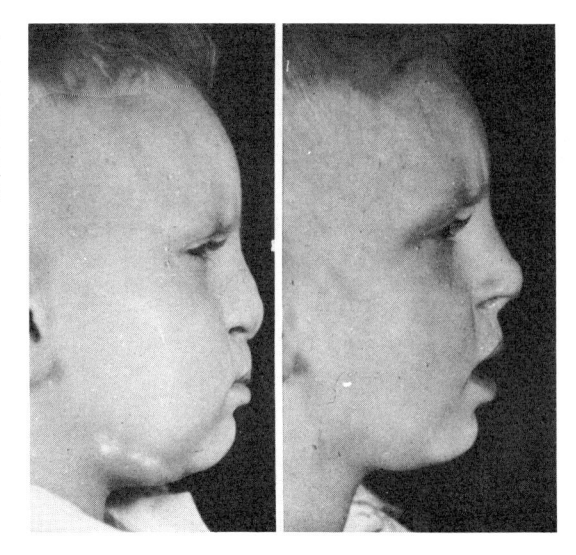

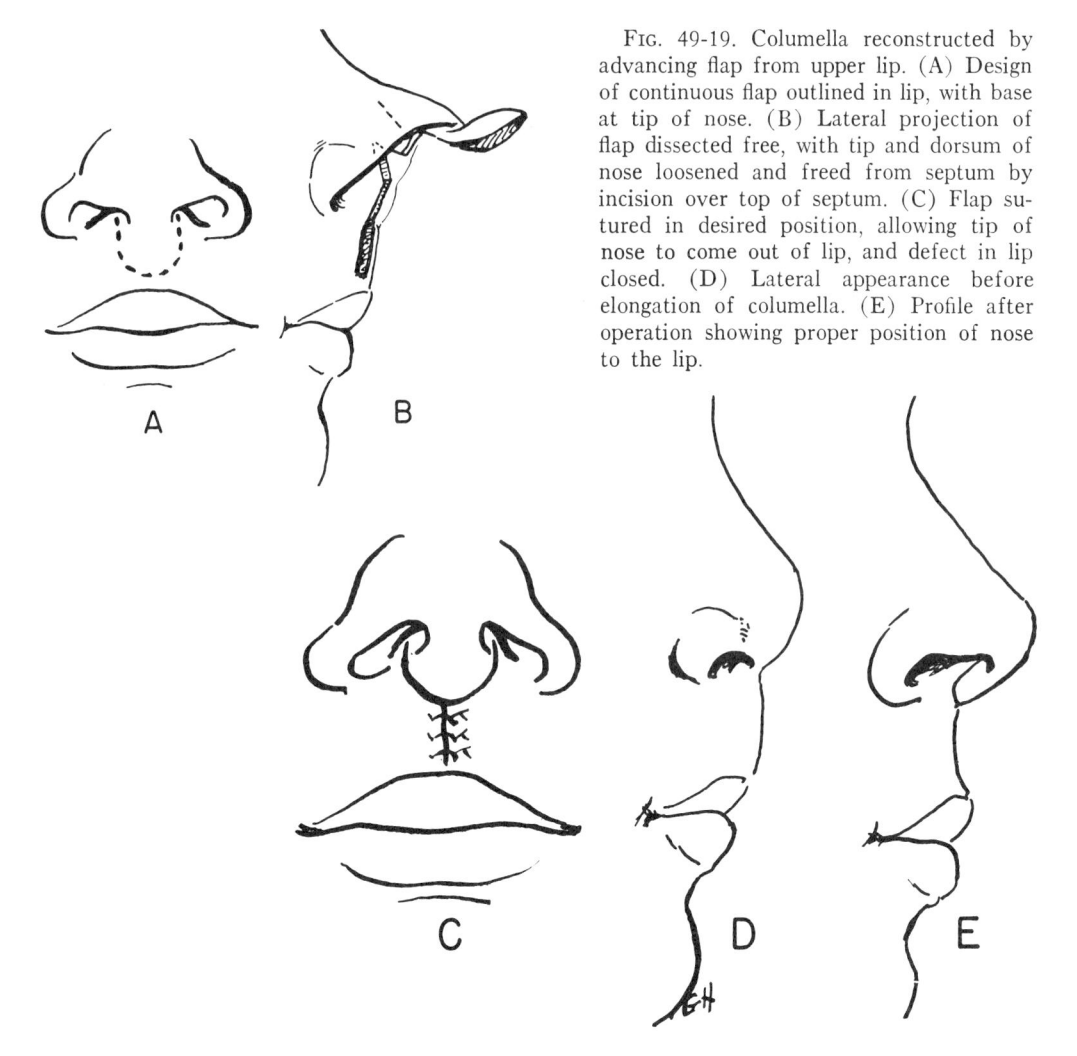

Fig. 49-19. Columella reconstructed by advancing flap from upper lip. (A) Design of continuous flap outlined in lip, with base at tip of nose. (B) Lateral projection of flap dissected free, with tip and dorsum of nose loosened and freed from septum by incision over top of septum. (C) Flap sutured in desired position, allowing tip of nose to come out of lip, and defect in lip closed. (D) Lateral appearance before elongation of columella. (E) Profile after operation showing proper position of nose to the lip.

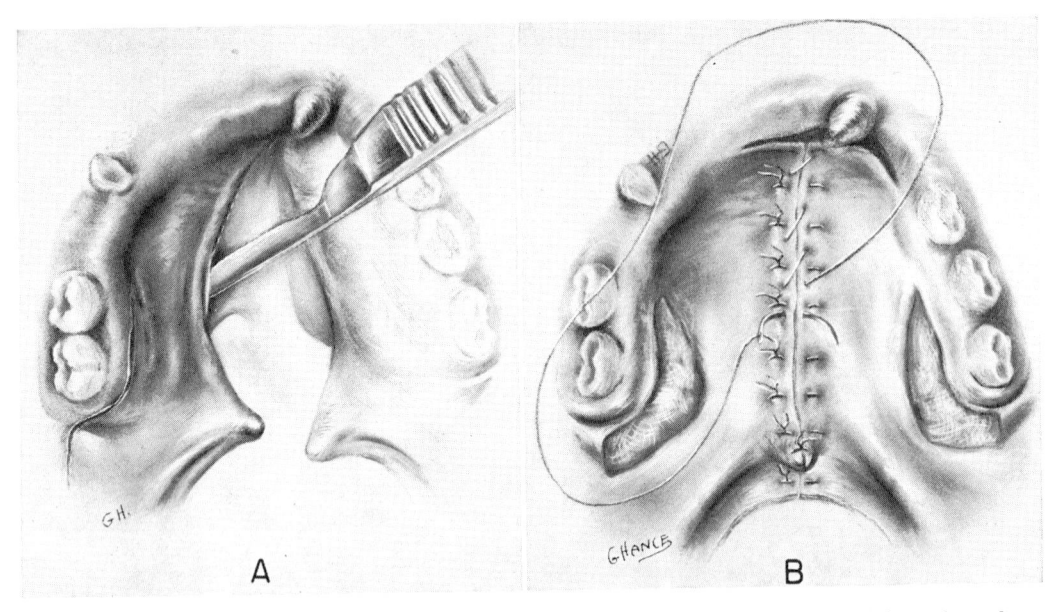

Fig. 49-20. Closure of cleft palate. (*Left*) Elevation of mucoperiosteal flaps is done through lateral incisions, including the major palatine artery, and followed by opening of medial margin. (*Right*) The medial margins of the mucoperiosteal flaps are approximated and sutured with vertical sutures. Packs in lateral incisions are removed in 48 hours.

elongation of the palate. Usually this can be done in one operation if there is also an incomplete cleft or if the palate actually can be split and elongated. The drawings in Figure 49-21 illustrate closure and elongation.

Careful surgical closure of a cleft palate in one operation most closely secures the approximation of the normal palatal anatomy and action. Occasionally, prosthetic appliances may be necessary to secure a degree of palatal function in swallowing and speaking if the closure has been done unsatisfactorily. These palatal prostheses are in essence a partial denture with a solid plug of plastic material attached to occlude the nasopharynx. Such an appliance cannot possibly approximate the physiologic action normally expected of a palate that has been repaired surgically in one operation.

DEFORMITIES AND INFLAMMATORY DISEASES OF THE JAWS

The common deformities of the mandible requiring surgery are micrognathia and macrognathia (mandibular underdevelopment and overgrowth, respectively).

MICROGNATHIA

Micrognathia, which is a short underdeveloped mandible, may be associated with a short incomplete cleft of the palate. The infant with this deformity may have considerable difficulty breathing shortly after birth and requires careful nursing care to survive. Forward fixation of the tongue to the lip to pull the tongue forward so that it does not occlude the upper airway or even tracheotomy may be necessary at this time. Both of these procedures are to be avoided as long as breathing and feeding can be developed satisfactorily with meticulous nursing care.

Treatment. The surgical treatment of micrognathia is first directed toward effecting the immediate survival of the infant by securing a safely open airway by fixation of the tongue to the lip or tracheotomy. Surgical efforts to increase the rate of growth of the jaw have not been successful. Later orthodontic procedures may be very useful, especially if the jaw itself can be moved forward rather than only slanting the teeth forward. At any rate, by orthodontia the occlusion of the teeth should be achieved to the point where they will be as normal as possible. After maximal

FIG. 49-21. Closure and elongation of partially cleft palate in one operation. (A) Incision is made as shown, and the entire palate is elevated as a mucoperiosteal flap. (B) Soft tissue separated and major palatine artery brought out of canal. (C) Edge of flap being sutured to band of nasal mucosa. (D) Medial margin of palatal defect opened. (E) Palate has been closed and elongated in one operation. Defect in hard palate has healed in 1 month. (Brown, J. B.: Surg., Gynec., Obstet., 63:768)

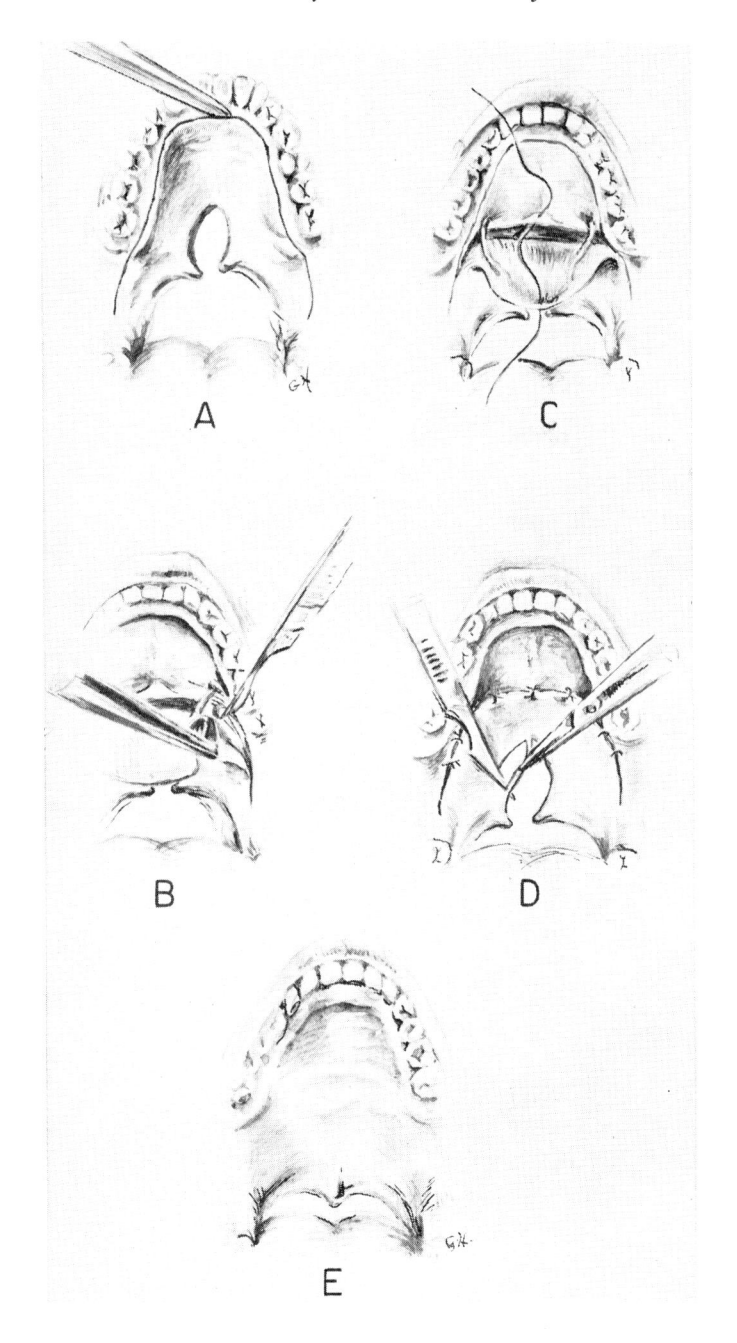

growth in the mandible has been attained, the type of treatment is decided on the basis of function and appearance. If the occlusion is relatively normal or is functional, the receding chin can be built up by adding bone or cartilage to the outer surface of the mandible beneath the periosteum without disturbing the relationship of the upper and the lower teeth.

This operation is done through a small incision beneath the chin or near the angle of the jaw through which cartilage or bone is built up on the mandible by inserting it beneath the elevated periosteum in order to get the closest contact. Synthetics or bank cartilage may be employed.

If the occlusion is poor, with the upper teeth

1458   Principles of General Plastic Surgery

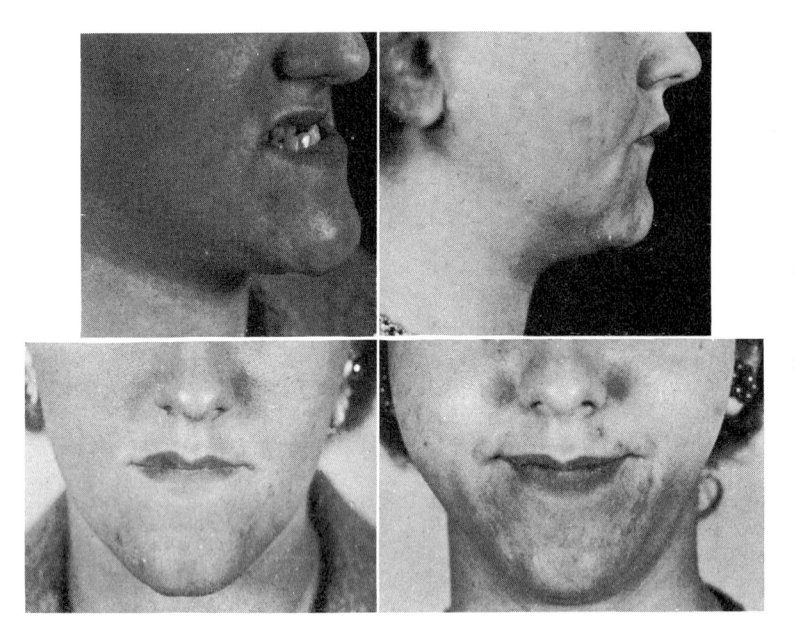

FIG. 49-22. Prognathism. Before and after views of results of recessive ramisection of lower jaw as shown in diagram Figure 49-23. (*Top, left*) Profile showing imbalance between upper and lower jaws and impossible occlusion and (*top, right*) proper balance of face and good occlusion after operation. (*Bottom, left*) Front view before operation with marked improvement (*bottom, right*) as in profile.

so far anterior to the lower that even proper mastication may be impossible, they can be placed in better relationship by displacing the mandible forward after section through the rami. The technic of ramisection is illustrated in Figure 49-23 where it is used to correct macrognathia. In the case of micrognathia the jaw is moved forward instead of backward.

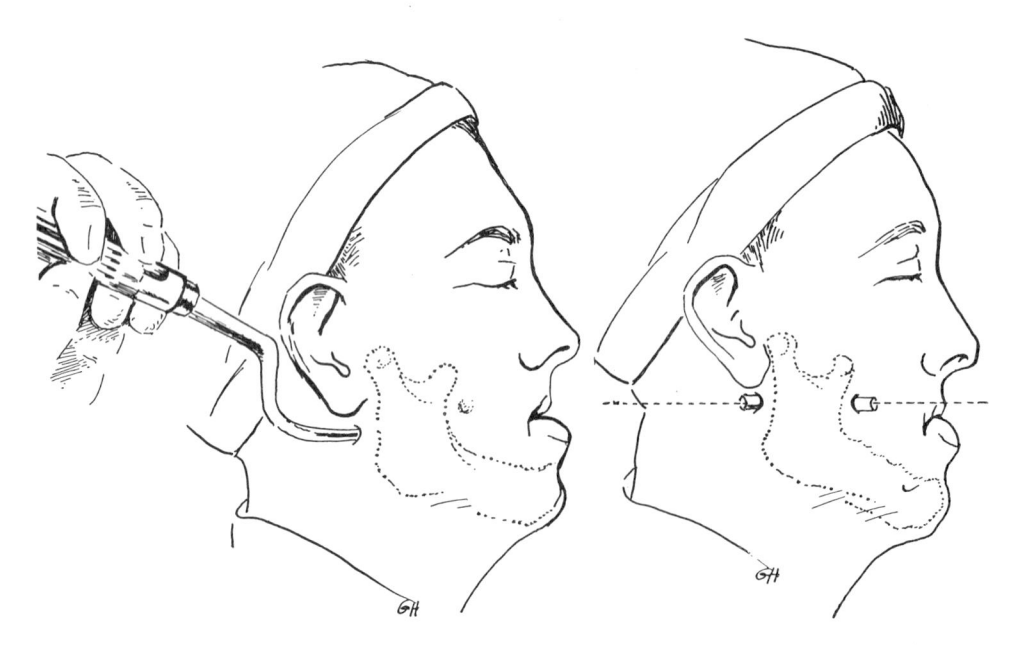

FIG. 49-23. Correction of prognathism by closed ramisection of the mandible. (*Left*) Large jaw needle passed closely behind the ascending ramus of the mandible through 1-cm. skin incisions placed at anterior and posterior borders of jaw, avoiding facial nerve and entrance into mouth. Then a Gigli saw is attached to the end of the jaw needle so that by withdrawing the needle, the saw is in position on the inside of the jaw.

Fixation of the jaw in its new position is maintained with interdental wires for up to 12 weeks.

MACROGNATHIA

Macrognathia attends overgrowth of the mandible and is the opposite of micrognathia. Often the lower teeth are displaced more anteriorly relative to their upper counterparts.

Diagnosis of macrognathia is obvious on inspection alone.

Treatment depends on the position of the teeth. If the occlusion is relatively normal and does not need correction, the enlarged portion of the mandible may be removed locally by simply cutting off bone subperiosteally from the external surface. If the occlusion of the teeth is not satisfactory, the entire mandible may be set back in one operation after section through the rami has been done, as illustrated in Figure 49-23. Fixation with interdental wiring up to 12 weeks results in permanent normal relationship between the upper and the lower teeth.

In these rearrangements of the dental occlusion dental consultation is necessary, and casts of the teeth are required. In addition, cutting down of certain of the teeth is often necessary.

Other surgical methods involve resection of the body of the ramus at a high level for prognathism, and forward positioning in the body of the jaw for micrognathia.

ARTHRITIS OF THE JAW

Arthritis commonly occurs at the temporomandibular joint, and the complaint is of pain in the joint, limitation of opening, cracking, locking, with occasional progress to fixation in the joint. Roentgenograms may show erosion of the joint or narrowing.

Treatment of arthritis consists of putting the joint at rest by the patient's own efforts with foods and the gentlest uses, or by bandaging from chin to vertex. Interdental wiring may be required. Reefing of the capsule has been suggested, as well as several local procedures of fixation. Resection of the joint disk should be resorted to only in very occasional instances.

INFLAMMATORY DISEASES OF THE JAWS

Osteomyelitis usually includes all inflammatory diseases of the jaw, but division can be made on the basis of etiologic agent, osteomyelitis being an inflammatory process in the bone due to staphylococcus or streptococcus, tuberculosis, actinomycosis, syphilis, metals, heat, irradiation, and trauma.[36]

The anatomy of the jaws is important, as it influences the inflammatory process, and the teeth are the most important difference between the jaws and other bones, since their normal poisition in the jaws establishes a path for deep infection. Where the spongiosum is thicker in the maxilla, as in the incisor, canine and tubercle regions, infection is most severe. In the mandible the thickest areas are around the angle extending forward and up, and infection here is most persistent.

Osteomyelitis usually is caused by staphylococci and streptococci, and often they are found in the smear and the culture with the other usual mouth organisms. Anaerobic culture often grows out melanogenicum. This organism may account for the foul odor of the purulent drainage. Other anaerobic organisms may also be present.

ETIOLOGY. *Affected teeth* are the commonest cause of osteomyelitis of the jaws. A periapical abscess is a localized osteomyelitis which may spread, should the tooth be extracted during the acute phase. Pericoronitis is an inflammatory process in the soft tissue pocket around a partially erupted third molar or wisdom tooth. This infection can also spread to the jaw, the mouth and the neck upon the extraction of the affected tooth during the acute phase.

Fractures of the jaw are the second most common cause of osteomyelitis because breaks of the jaw are so often associated with lacerations of the mucosa around the teeth. These mucosal breaks set up avenues for infection of the bone in the zone of fracture.

Draining cysts, blood stream infections, injuries to the mucosa around the teeth, the metastasis from osteomyelitis elsewhere are other causes of osteomyelitis but are rarely seen and then practically only in debilitated patients. The nasal cavity and sinuses are additional sources of osteomyelitis in the upper jaw.

DIAGNOSIS. *Acute osteomyelitis* is diagnosed on the history of severe pain and diffuse swelling of the jaw with the general signs of infection as fever, leukocytosis and general malaise, usually starting after the extraction

1460   Principles of General Plastic Surgery

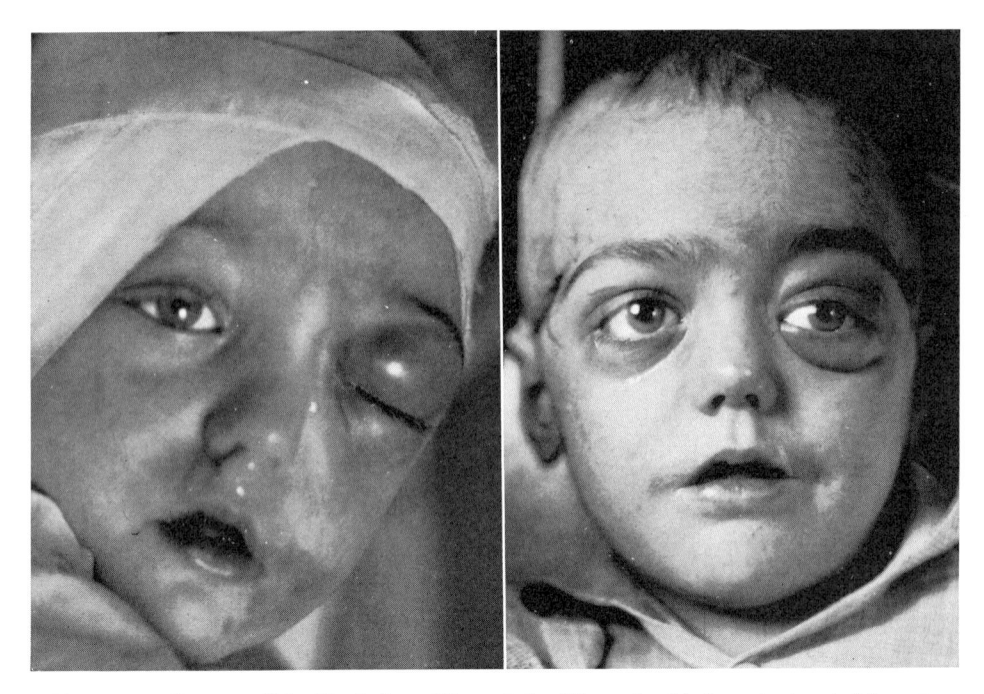

FIG. 49-24. Osteomyelitis. Typical swelling of the lids and orbital content noted in osteomyelitis of the upper jaw and the zygoma. This lesion occurred in the course of a general osteomyelitis and also occurred in the right side, as shown by the scar in the temporal region in view at right 2½ months later. (Brown, J. B., and Fryer, M. P.: The Cyclopedia of Medicine, Surgery and Specialties. Vol. 7. Pp. 553-562. Philadelphia, F. A. Davis)

of an acutely infected tooth or following a fracture. Periorbital edema may be the most prominent sign of osteomyelitis in the upper jaw. Roentgenograms at this early stage usually fail to demonstrate signs of a destructive inflammatory process, but within 10 days an extension of the cavity left by the extracted tooth or dissolution of bone around the fracture may be demonstrable roentgenographically. *Chronic osteomyelitis* is diagnosed by a history of recurrent flare-ups, multiple sinus tracts and the draining of purulent material

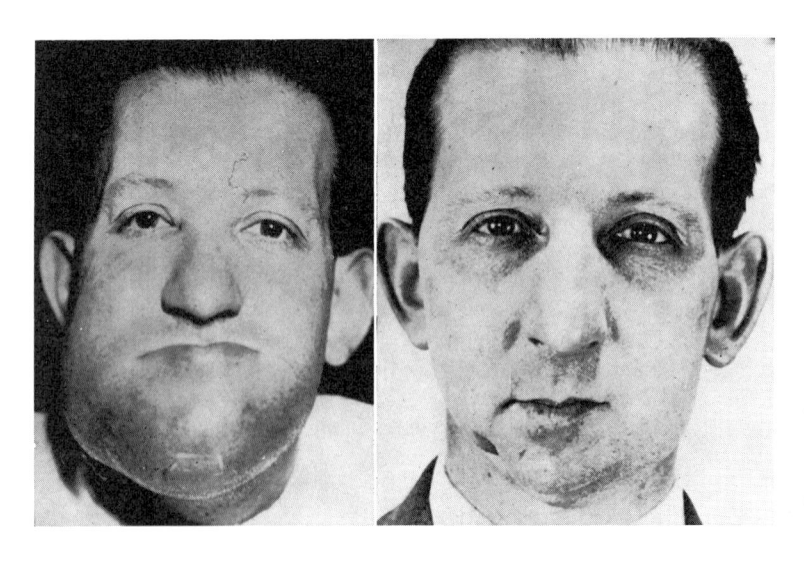

FIG. 49-25. Actinomycosis of lower jaw. (*Left*) Brawny swelling of lower jaw treated by multiple drainage operations and sequestrectomies.(*Right*) Major portion of lower jaw saved and infection cured.

FIG. 49-26. Actinomycosis, showing multiple draining in later stages of infection than that illustrated in Figure 49-25.

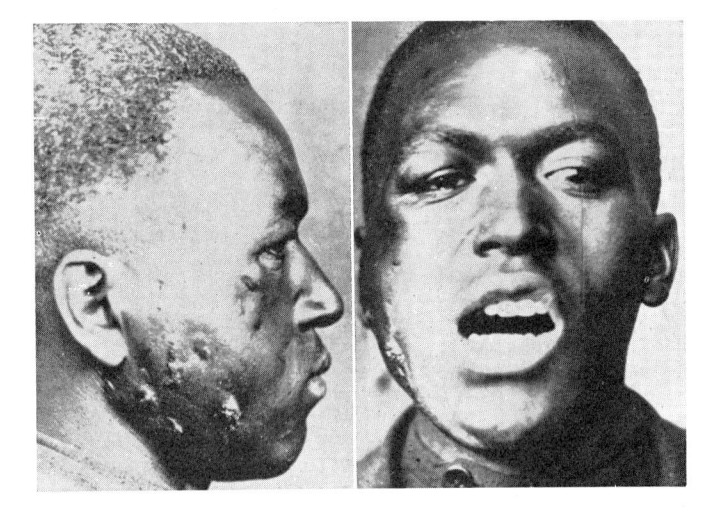

and pieces of bone. Roentgenograms show sequestra, cavities and later the formation of an involucrum.

TREATMENT of osteomyelitis is primarily prevention. This consists of postponing the extraction of the acutely inflamed tooth, and the routine drainage of the fractured jaw. Surgical drainage of acute periapical abscesses is done gently alongside the tooth over the swollen area. Large doses of antibiotics have been effective in avoiding osteomyelitis and preventing the spread if already present. Acute osteomyelitis is treated conservatively; drainage of the affected bone through soft tissues is established with the least possible operative trauma. In the chronic stage fluctuant areas are opened, but sequestra are not removed until adequate involucrum has developed to support the jaw. Tooth buds are not removed indiscriminately.

Tuberculosis. Tuberculosis infection of the jaw is seen occasionally with pulmonary involvement. Diagnosis is made on the history of a slightly painful swelling over the jaw which may be fluctuant. Later a fistula may form. Roentgenograms may show spotty areas of necrosis. Final proof of diagnosis rests upon the identification of tubercle bacilli by culture methods. Treatment may be started with repeated aspiration of pus but should this, together with streptomycin, not effect a cure, excision of the affected bone is necessary. To the present, streptomycin has been the most useful antibiotic for tuberculous osteomyelitis.

Actinomycosis often follows the extraction of a tooth. Its first signs appear several days after the extraction as a slightly tender swelling over the jaw. Later the swelling extends into the neck, and still later multiple cutaneous fistulae develop. Roentgenograms may show multiple sites of decreased density in the jaw. The finding of "sulfur granules" in the drainage material and cultural identification of the organism complete the diagnosis. Treatment consists of drainage and the use of antibiotics (sulfadiazine 4 Gm. daily with penicillin 50,000 to 100,000 units daily). Radical excision of the afflicted area may be necessary later should the treatment outlined above fail.

Irradiation necrosis is probably the most painful of the inflammatory processes involving the jaw. Usually the lesion is widespread. Radical débridement of bone and soft tissue may be necessary to relieve the pain. The reconstruction necessary is usually equally difficult because the healing of heavily irradiated tissues is slow.

Ankylosis of the jaw may follow an inflammatory process in the temporomandibular region or a gunshot wound.[40] Soft tissue scarring may require removal and replacement, along with excision of a block of bone to create a false joint. The mouth should be "blocked open" following resection. Ankylosis on both sides is extremely serious. Bilateral operation should rarely be carried out because of excessive retraction, crippling and loss of normal contour that attend it. Although arthroplasty or replacement is not uniformly successful,

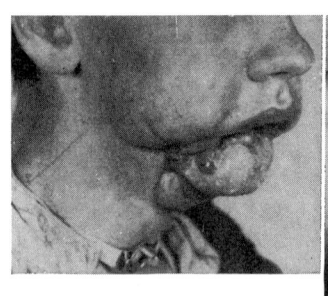

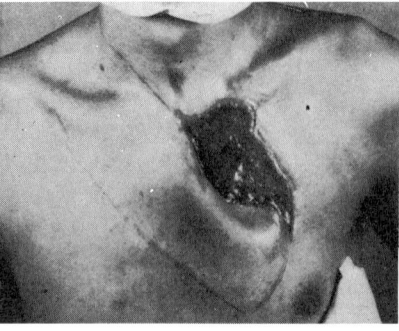

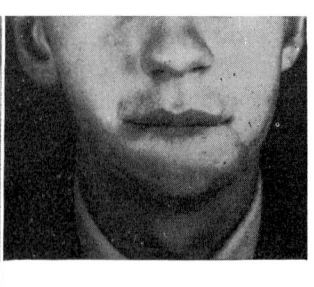

FIG. 49-27. (*Left*) Gunshot loss lower third of face with large defect in mandible. (*Center*) Delayed flat flap from chest with a side flap turned in from above to line the flap and form the lining of the inside of the mouth. Flap made mouth watertight and prevented further flow of saliva on the chest. Defect in chest covered with free graft. (*Right*) Flap has covered soft tissue defect in lower third of face and permitted bone graft to be placed between ends of the mandible. Soft tissue coverage was necessary before bone graft could be done. Jaw is solid. (Brown, J. B., and Fryer, M. P.: Am. J. Surg., 85:401-406)

very careful evaluation and effort should be put forth before considering a bilateral resection of both mandibular joints.

RECONSTRUCTION OF THE JAW

Restitution of a function arch is the aim following loss of the jaw by any means. Resection of hard, contracting scar in the mouth and on the outside and replacement with soft viable tissue may be necessary before a bone graft can be placed between the remaining ends of the jaw. Autografts of rib or ilium should be used because these defects must be bridged by living solid bone. For this reason nonviable bone from a bank is not used to repair jaw defects. However, appearance may be improved, following loss of the jaw bone, by preserved cartilage placed on the remaining misshapen bone beneath its periosteum. This may have to be put upon the intact hemimandible because the intact side collapses toward the side of loss, thereby flattening out the side of the face opposite the loss and making a bulge on the damaged side.

COMPOUND FACIAL INJURIES

Compound facial injury connotes simultaneous injury to the soft parts and the bones of the face.[10] The term "compound" is outmoded for other fractures, but when the nose, the eyelids, the lacrimal duct, or other features or systems are involved, it is a compound injury by virtue of its complexity. This term emphasizes the importance of recognizing facial fractures that may be masked initially by soft tissue laceration, contusion and swelling. If bony displacement is overlooked, healing occurs, and reduction later may be impossible, though the deformity becomes obvious after the soft tissue injury has healed. Severe trauma recognizes no anatomic boundaries; separation here is only for purposes of description.

EMERGENCY CARE

Emergency care of compound facial injuries includes the provision of an airway, the control of bleeding, and splinting of the injured parts. Patients with fractures of the mandible that loosen the support of the tongue or with severe intra-oral or cervical bleeding may require tracheotomy for survival. However, positioning and anchoring most mandible fractures is sufficient to secure an open airway. Bleeding from large neck muscles requires ligation of individual vessels near or at the point of discontinuity. Neck vessel ligation for facial or mouth hemorrhage at points distant from the site of injury is practically useless and may add further trouble. Support of a loose jaw or torn soft parts with a Barton type bandage may increase comfort and avoid the

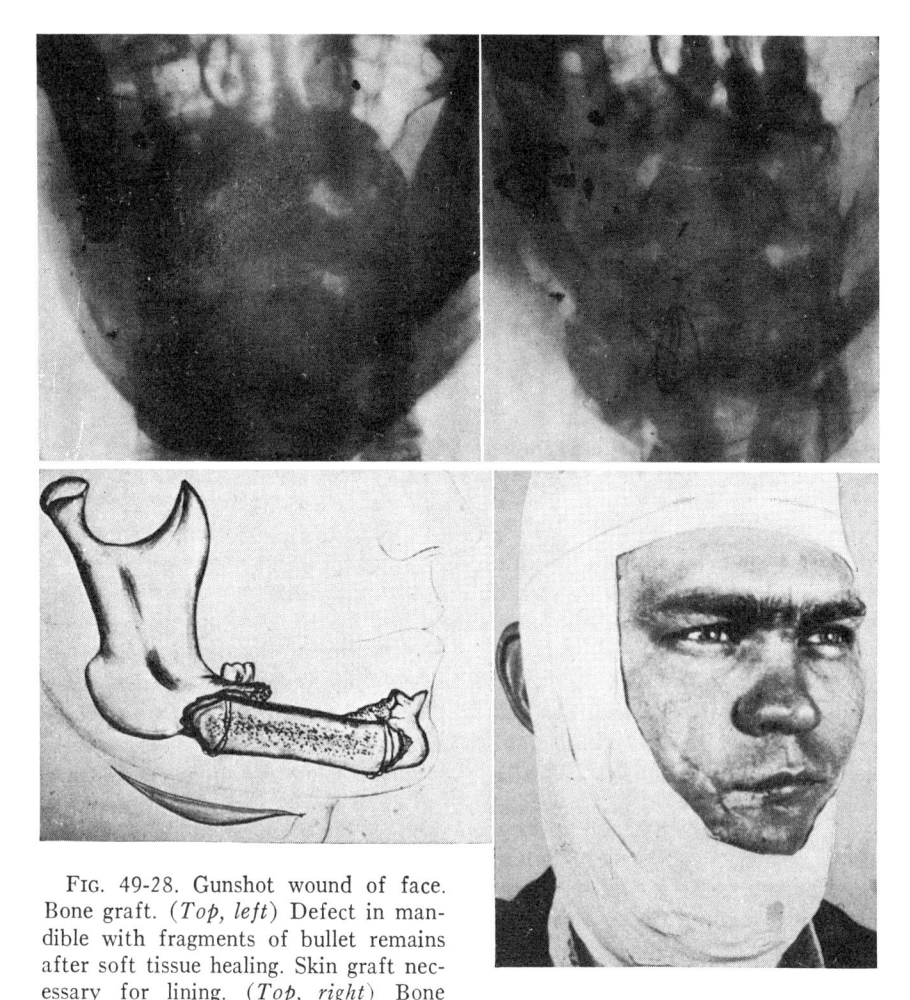

FIG. 49-28. Gunshot wound of face. Bone graft. (*Top, left*) Defect in mandible with fragments of bullet remains after soft tissue healing. Skin graft necessary for lining. (*Top, right*) Bone graft in place held with wire to ends of bone acting as its own splint. Rib graft was used in this instance. (*Bottom, left*) Diagram of bone graft held to bone with wires. (*Bottom, right*) Firm pressure dressing aids fixation of jaw and promotes healing. (Brown, J. B., and Fryer, M. P.: Postgrad. Med., 4:420-434)

use of sedatives and analgesics that might compromise breathing.

Repair

The time to repair a compound facial injury is as soon as the patient's general condition permits. Shock, brain damage, dangerous cervical spine fractures, or intoxication are contraindications to early operation. However, by virtue of the fact that bony fragments become permanently fixed out of position if reduction is not done in 10 to 14 days, the reduction needs be effected within that time limit after injury.

Roentgenograms of the face, the skull and the cervical spine are important parts of the examination of all severe facial injuries, though it may be impossible to obtain all wanted views before definitive repair is undertaken.

General condition of the patient is considered after a careful physical examination and consultation with other specialists. The presence of brain or peripheral nerve damage is tested for routinely, and fractures of other bones and abdominal injury are to be suspected and sought after. It is especially important to record the function of the 2nd, the

1464 Principles of General Plastic Surgery

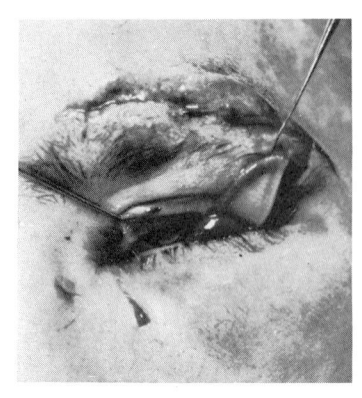

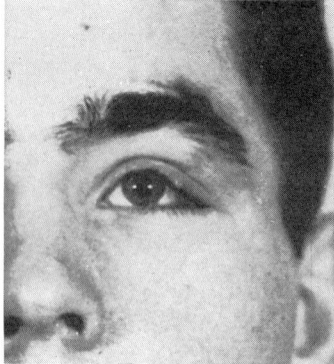

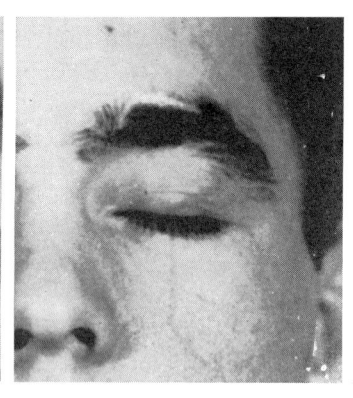

FIG. 49-29. Through-and-through laceration of upper eyelid. (*Left*) Primarily repaired in one operation, maintaining protection of eye and obviating necessity of secondary reconstruction of eyelid (*center and right*).

5th and the 7th nerves before any operation upon the injured face. *Shock* is often present, and when it is it requires treatment before repairing the facial injury. However, as stated in Chapter 7, Shock, operative intervention for the control of hemorrhage is a most important therapeutic measure in treating shock in an actively bleeding patient. Consequently, delaying the operation in order to treat shock should be practiced only in those cases in which rapid bleeding has stopped. Tetanus protection is given routinely, and antibiotics are used as indicated. (See Chap. 4, Surgical Infections.)

The repair of facial injuries, excepting the simple superficial ones, should be done in an operating room. All facilities and assistance should be used for the best possible repair.

Anesthesia. Local block is used in small lacerations and can be used in extensive repairs, but general anesthesia is often necessary. If general anesthesia is used, an airway must be provided with an endotracheal tube.

Soft Tissue Repair

Simple Lacerations

Simple lacerations are closed carefully with adequate anesthesia secured by infiltrating the wound margins with ½ to 1 per cent procaine

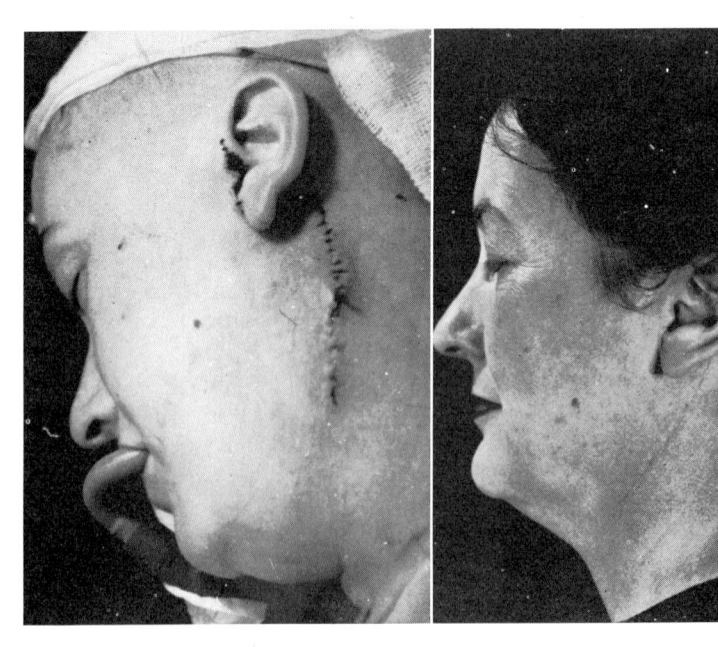

FIG. 49-30. (*Left*) Small, fine sutures placed near the edge of an incision or laceration closed the wound without adding scar. (*Right*) Wound healed. This also illustrates the author's method of approaching the parotid.

or lidocaine. Facial wounds never are packed open. In closing a facial laceration, known or recognizable normal coaptation points are first approximated with fine suture material placed in the subcutaneous tissue, then the remainder of the separation is closed by suturing the skin by progressively bisecting the distances between sutures until the wound is closely coapted in its entirety. Before the skin is closed bleeding points are ligated individually, and hematomas are evacuated. Fine silk sutures placed close to the wound margins prevent slippage of the wound margins by each other. Widely placed sutures which permit slippage leave permanent "ladder type" scars that upon the face are remarkably disfiguring because they may never be removed by any number of secondary operations. If one cannot place stitches closely it is preferable to permit a facial wound to heal spontaneously by leaving it open without packing than to leave widely placed sutures in an attempt to effect partial closure. The residual scarring is less with the wound left open than closed with widely placed sutures. If the wound must be closed under some tension, sutures may be tied over the dressing, as illustrated in Figure 49-31.

Primary repair may require a free graft for closure, but local or distant flaps are rarely required at this stage. Innumerable secondary procedures may be avoided by a careful painstaking initial repair. The *dressing* applied should fix the wound and apply steady, even pressure. The dressing is a most important part of the repair. Adhesive strapping gives adequate fixation, and a gauze bandage wound around the part over fine mesh grease gauze and sterile mechanics waste secures pressure, invites healing and prevents pain. Cutaneous sutures in the face are removed after 4 or 5 days, but the fixation of the wound by adhesive strapping and pressure bandaging is maintained for several days.

FRACTURES OF THE MANDIBLE

Mandibular fractures are reduced and fixed in the simplest direct method available until union results.

Diagnosis of a fractured jaw is made by palpation which will usually elicit point tenderness, and by roentgenograms in the postero-anterior and both lateral views. Swelling is usually diffuse, but the presence of a

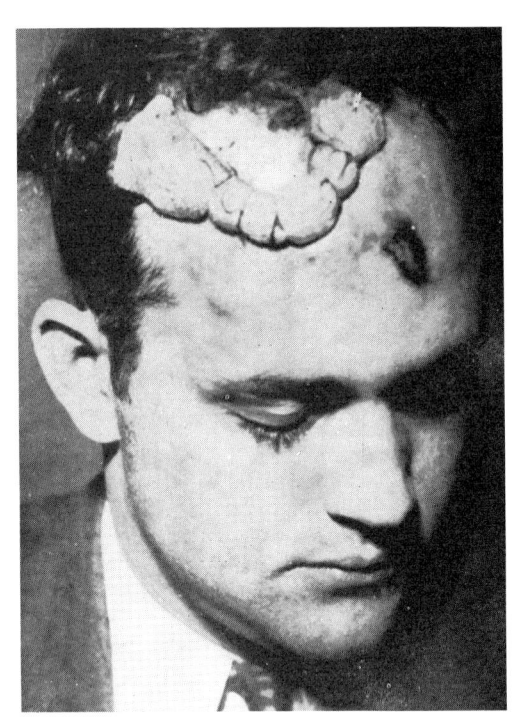

FIG. 49-31. Method of wound closure by sutures tied over roll of gauze, avoiding stay suture marks.

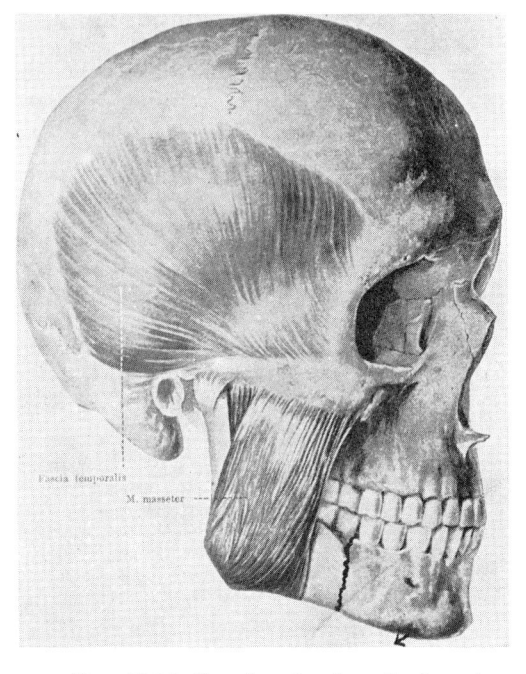

FIG. 49-32. Drawing showing attachment of muscles on angle of jaw and ascending ramus which may determine position of fragments in this area following fracture.

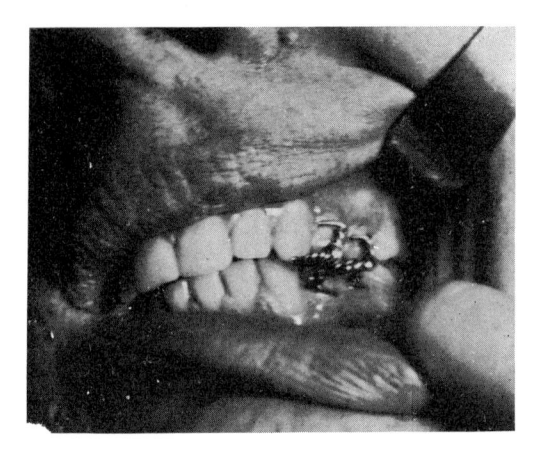

FIG. 49-33. Interdental wiring. Simple fixation of lower jaw to upper jaw by No. 24 steel wires placed around bicuspids, using upper jaw as splint for fractured mandible.

laceration in the mouth may indicate the point of fracture.

Full reduction is judged to have been accomplished when the teeth in the maxilla and the mandible are in the patient's normal occlusion. Fractures of the edentulous mandible are palpated readily, and their reduction is determined by touch.

Drainage is established routinely from the point of mandibular fracture to the outside whenever the oral mucosa has been disrupted by placing a small incision beneath the jaw in the neck, taking care to avoid the mandibular branch of the facial nerve and vessels.

Fixation after reduction is done most simply with interdental wiring, using No. 26 or 24 steel wire, between apposing bicuspids, as illustrated in Figure 49-33. A *twisted wire arch* may give fixation in another plane by being closed around a lower molar tooth on each side and brought together in front with individual wires to other teeth as necessary. Solid union usually requires from 6 to 8 weeks of fixation.

Internal wire-pin fixation of a fractured mandible is necessary when proper teeth are not available in all fragments or the jaw is completely edentulous. They are also indicated when a prolonged period of time has elapsed before reduction and fixation; with extensive comminution; when a large soft tissue defect opening into the mouth is present; and when the fracture is in an area with a known tendency to nonunion such as the symphysis mentis.[16] Kirschner wires, .045 or .062 size, are driven across the fracture site with a power drill and may be used alone or in conjunction with interdental or direct bone wiring. The use of these wire pins often allows relatively normal eating during the period of healing. As many pins are used as the type of fracture requires.

Condylar fractures may require an open operation for reduction. However, satisfactory function usually can be obtained by fixation of the jaw in the patient's normal occlusion for 3 weeks with interdental wiring.

Middle Third Facial Fractures

Fracture-Dislocation of the Zygoma

This is one of the commonest types of facial bone fractures. The natural position of this facial bone predisposes it to this injury—the zygoma is somewhat analogous to the bumper on an automobile. Usually the force of the trauma dislocates, rather than fractures, the bone from all of its attachments, crushing the surrounding thinner facial bones such as those of the antral walls or the orbital floor. Diplopia often follows a fracture-dislocation of the zygoma when the orbital floor is displaced. Anesthesia over the distribution of the infra-orbital nerve may be present also. Fail-

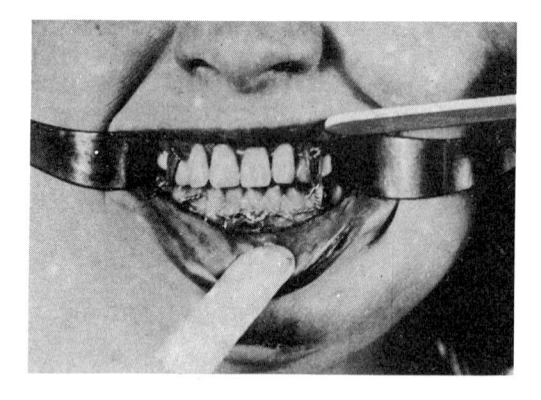

FIG. 49-34. Interdental wire and elastic fixation for fractured mandible. Elastic bands placed over twisted ends of No. 26 steel wire applied to opposing teeth in patient's normal occlusion. Continuous lower wire arch shown around lower teeth gives further fixation.

ure to bring the displaced zygoma back into normal position flattens that side of the face. *Diagnosis* usually can be made by palpation of the zygoma, even though there may be considerable swelling. Roentgenograms of the facial bones in the posterior-anterior or modified Waters positions to show the orbital borders are taken rountinely and are very valuable diagnostically and as means of determining adequacy of reduction in some cases.

Reduction of a fracture-dislocation of the zygoma may be done through the outside of the face with a *large jaw hook*, as shown in Figure 49-37. If the fragments become impacted during reduction, nothing further is required. However, if reduction is not maintained spontaneously, the zygoma may be supported by placing a pack in the antrum. A *wire pin* driven through the loose zygoma across the face through the opposite zygoma can give cantilever support adequate for the maintenance of reduction and the securing of solid union.[11]

Extensive comminution of the antral walls and the orbital floor by a displaced or fractured zygoma requires accurate replacement of the multiple small fragments. Entrance into the antrum is made through buccal mucosa and then through the fracture line, and after reduction of the zygoma with an elevator or a Kelly clamp in the antrum, the fragments are "mulched" or pressed into place and held in place with an iodoform pack into which balsam of Peru has been incorporated. The pack serves as an internal splint holding the zygoma, the antrum and the orbital floor in proper relationship until primary tissue fixation occurs. Obviously, it can be removed from 12 to 14 days after the reduction.

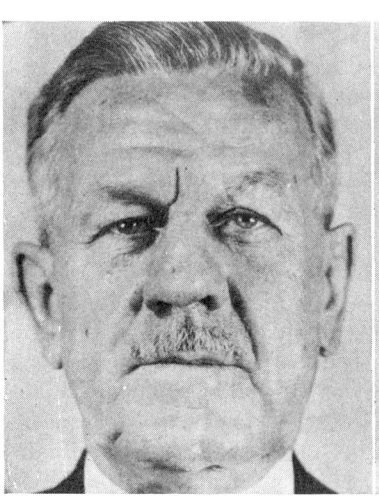

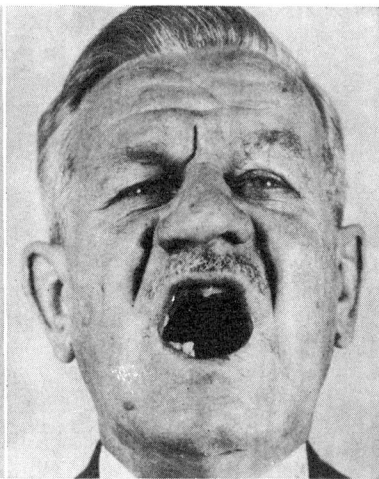

Fig. 49-35. Severe, splintered, locally infected lower jaw widely compounded by anterior fragment being driven into the mouth, reduced and held immobilized until union was solid, by combination of internal wires, circumferential wire and arch constructed of twisted No. 24 steel wires. Normal opening action and ingestion of soft food possible during comfortable convalescence and on complete healing.(Brown, J. B., Fryer, M. P., and McDowell, F.: Plast. Reconstruct. Surg., 4:30-35)

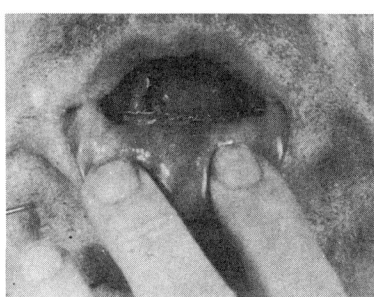

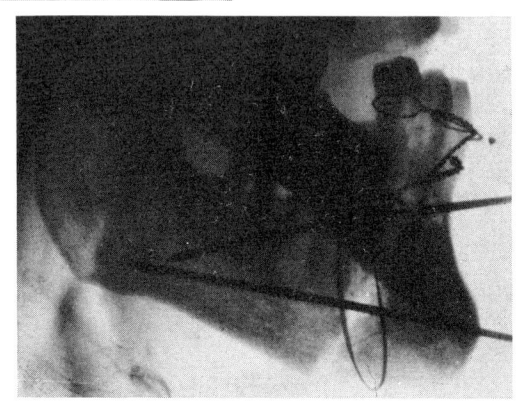

1468   Principles of General Plastic Surgery

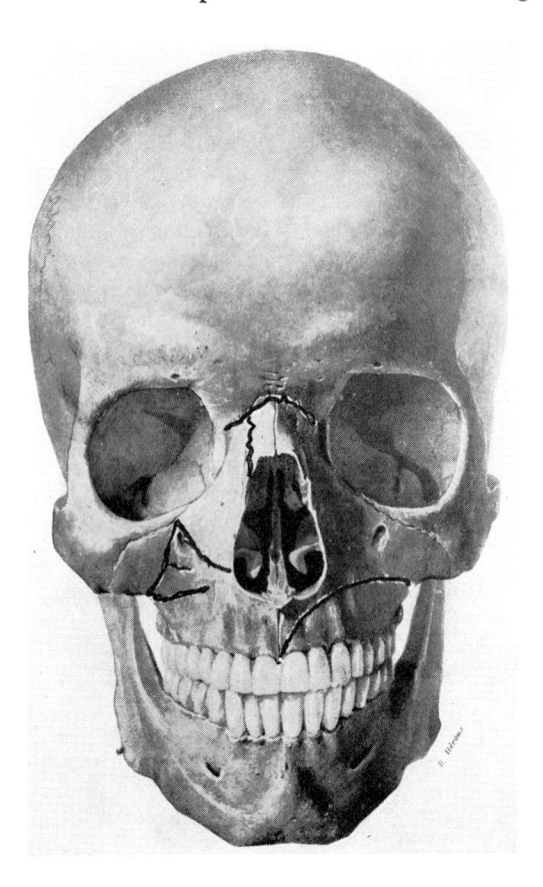

FIG. 49-36. Drawing illustrating major potential lines of separation in middle third facial fractures. One or all may be present. Comminution of smaller bones usually occurs in conjunction with displacement of larger bone elements.

Transverse facial fractures may involve the alveolus above or extend up across the pyriform space into either or both zygomas. At a higher level the transverse fracture tends to extend through both orbits so as to effect a complete detachment of the entire face from the skull. A roentgenogram may show little, but an adequate examination readily shows the extent of the injury. *Alveolar fractures* after reduction may be stabilized by a wire arch with interdental wires, using the lower jaw as a splint for the upper. However, internal wire pin fixation may be used alone or in combination with dental wiring. Other *transverse facial fractures* are reduced and then stabilized by interdental wiring in combination with internal wire pins.[21] Reduction of transverse fractures involves applying a force in the direction opposite to the force that caused the displacement. In many instances the displacing force has been applied in an upward as well as a backward direction and has pushed the upper jaw up as well as back. External traction-fixation devices actually tend to increase rather than decrease the deformity in such fractures.

Fractures of the Nose

Fractures of the nose are the most frequently seen facial fractures. They should be reduced and stabilized as in the case of any other fracture. Bleeding from the nose following trauma to the outside indicates that the lining of the nose has been lacerated by a fractured bone or cartilage.[30] Consequently, direct examination of the nasal passages and roentgenograms always should be made in order to establish the cause of the bleeding and the extent and the nature of the fracture. Nasal fractures are a particular problem in children because many remain displaced, with progressive deformation of the nose until growth stops; in addition, even though the initial reduction has been good, growth deformity may occur. After reduction, fractures of the nose usually can be stabilized properly with an external aluminum splint and nasal packing. Badly depressed comminuted nasal fractures may require the passage of wires beneath the nose and their anchorage to lead plates on the sides in order to maintain proper position. In cases of residual nasal deformity in children, *secondary reconstruction* usually is done after nasal growth is complete. Marked distortion of the nose can be improved and the dorsum built up with preserved cartilage transplants after growth has been attained, as shown in Figure 49-40. Recently, plastic materials seem to have some advantage as a subcutaneous prosthesis. Dimethyl siloxanes, halogenated carbons and polyvinyl alcohol are being used as supports.[38]

The use of silicone rubber for secondary reconstruction of the nose after severe trauma is shown in Figure 49-48.

Severe Facial Crushes

Severe facial crushes involving many facial bones usually require multiple means of sta-

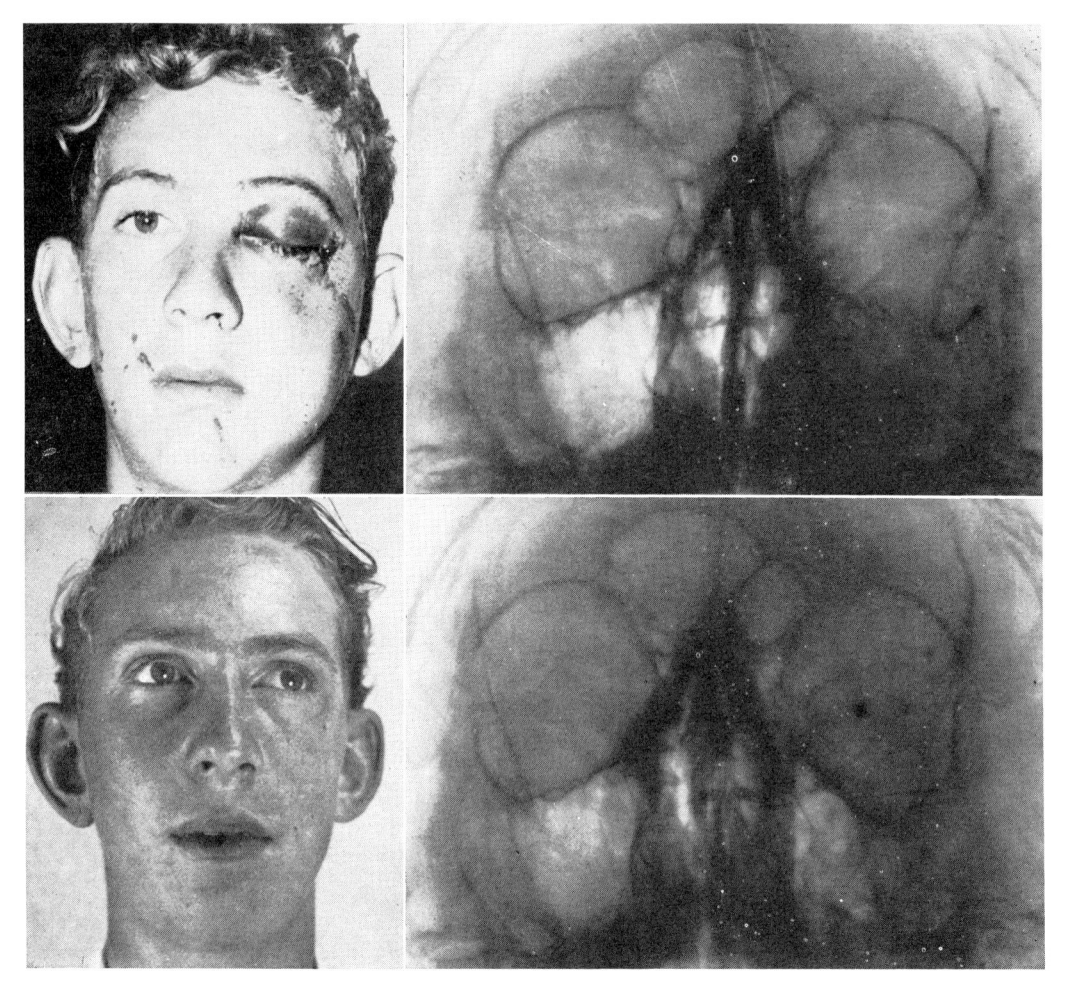

Fig. 49-37. (*Top, left*) Fracture-dislocation of the zygomatic bone with crumbling in of the antral wall and dropping of the orbital border. (*Top, right*) Appearance when first seen with contusion of eyelid, laceration and flatness of zygomatic region. (*Bottom, left*) Appearance 6 months following reduction. (*Bottom, right*) Result 6 weeks following immediate reduction by direct approach through the buccal fornix into antrum. (Brown, J. B., and Fryer, M. P.: Postgrad. Med., 6:400-406)

bilizing the multiple fragments. *Internal wire pins* can be used to hold both zygomas securely enough for union to occur, and in addition be made to serve as a base for the fixation of other fractures of the face.[16] Both antra can be held by loose packs introduced as superimposed folds through openings made in the buccal fornix. Direct bone wiring may be used wherever applicable. Alveolar and other transverse fractures can be held with internal wires driven obliquely, using the zygoma for cantilever support. External traction apparatus is expensive, cumbersome and unnecessary for the treatment of even severe facial crushes.

FACIAL PARALYSIS

The paralyzed face, whatever its cause, need not be suffered without treatment. The paralyzed face can be supported and some degree of animation secured by anchoring loops of fascia lata between the corners of the mouth and the temporalis muscle.

1470   Principles of General Plastic Surgery

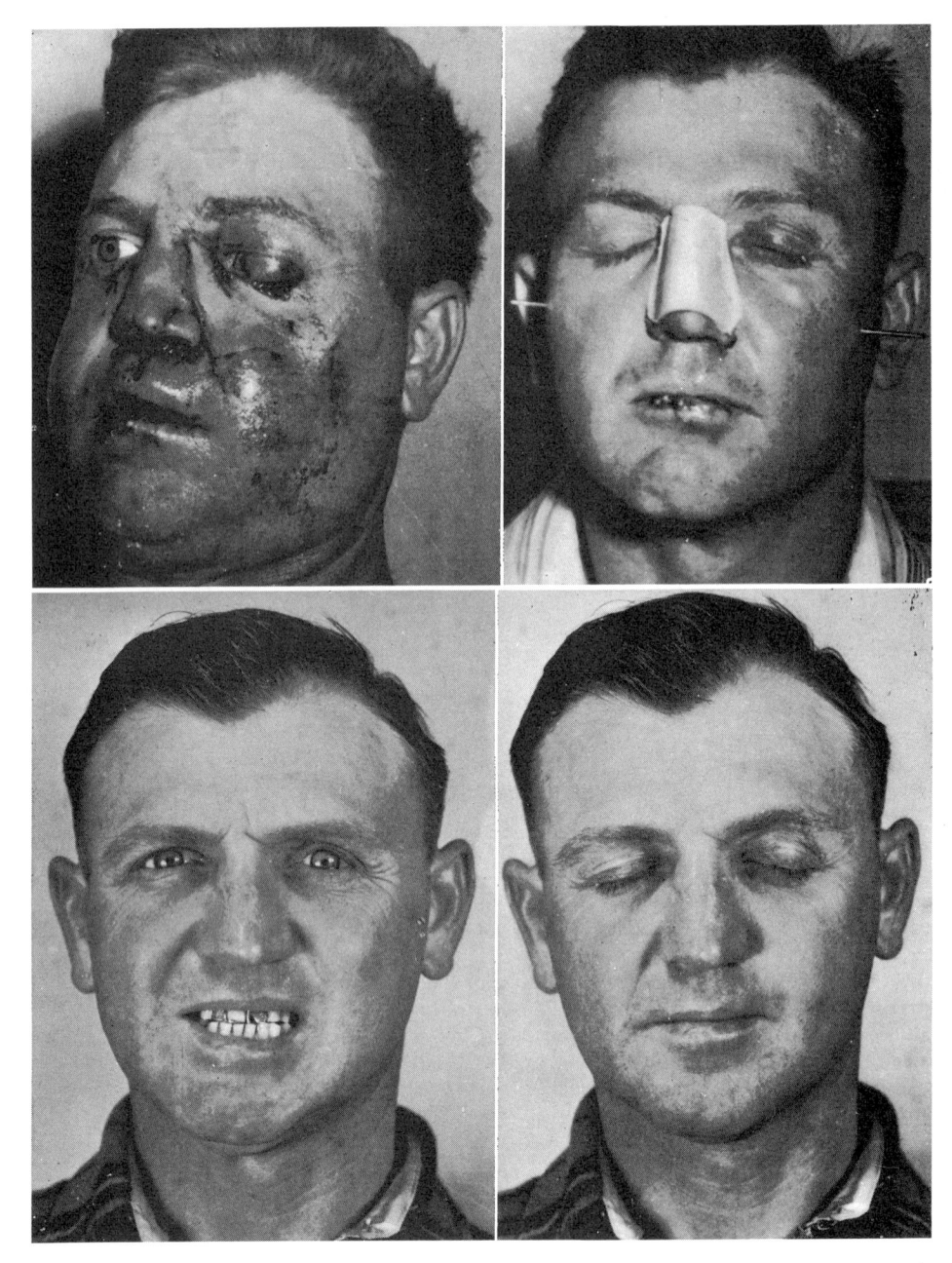

FIG. 49-38. Extensive crushing injury and soft tissue damage in farm accident. Not much stable bone was left, and practically no shape to the nose, which was torn loose and inverted into the face. Operation was performed within 12 hours under intratracheal anesthesia. The reverse of what the accident did was carried out in "unfolding" the nose and the face, elevating the left orbit and fixing the parts with cross wires and aluminum splint for the nose and with one internal wire for the shattered pyramidal fracture and the left zygomatic displacement. (*Fig. 49-38 continues on facing page*)

Fig. 49-38 (*Cont.*) Roentgenogram shows pin in place and the zygoma restored along with the orbital border. The left eyelid is torn completely open so that the eye looks through the rent. This case is an excellent example of the necessity of early operation. To wait 10 days, as has been advised elsewhere, would result in possible eye damage and the need of multiple operations. This patient has had full restoration and rehabilitation in one operation. No further work is necessary. (Brown, J. B., Fryer, M. P., and McDowell, F.: Surg., Gynec. Obstet., 93:676-681)

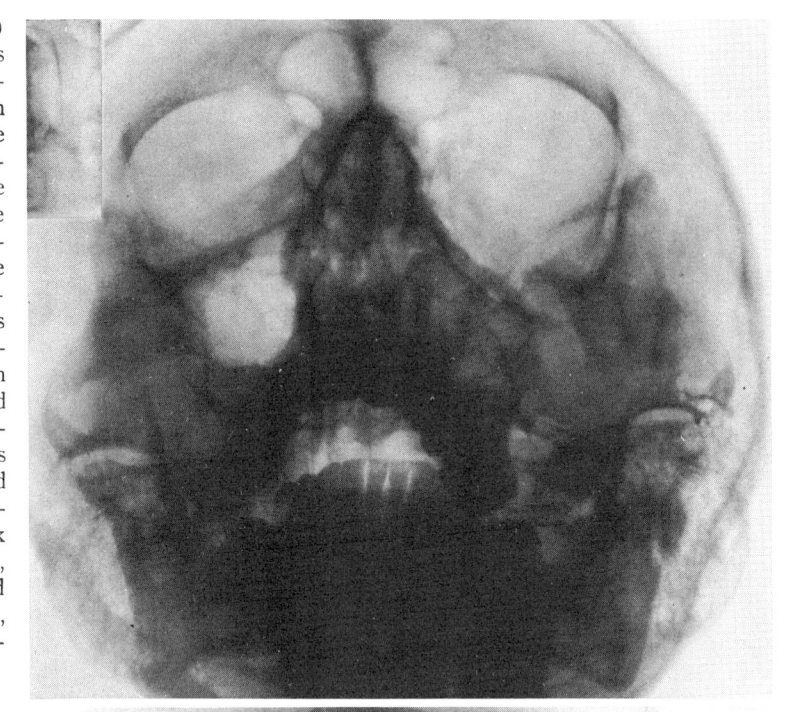

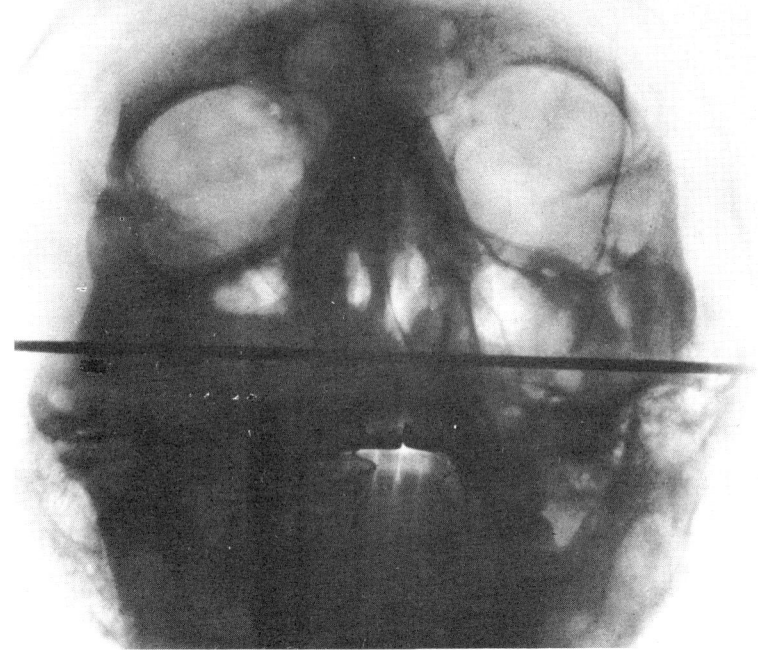

ETIOLOGY

Paralysis of the facial nerve may have as its origin congenital defects, infections, trauma (operative and other) and neoplastic invasion.

Congenital facial paralysis may be central or peripheral, unilateral or bilateral, complete or incomplete with involvement of any or all branches or divisions.

Infection involving the facial nerve, directly or indirectly by pressure, may induce partial

1472 Principles of General Plastic Surgery

paralysis when it involves a peripheral branch or complete paralysis when it affects the nerve in the parotid gland, or in the facial canal. The degree or extent of paralysis is dependent on where along the course of the nerve the inflammation, trauma or cancer impinges.

Operative paralysis of the facial nerve is usually the result of operations on the mastoid

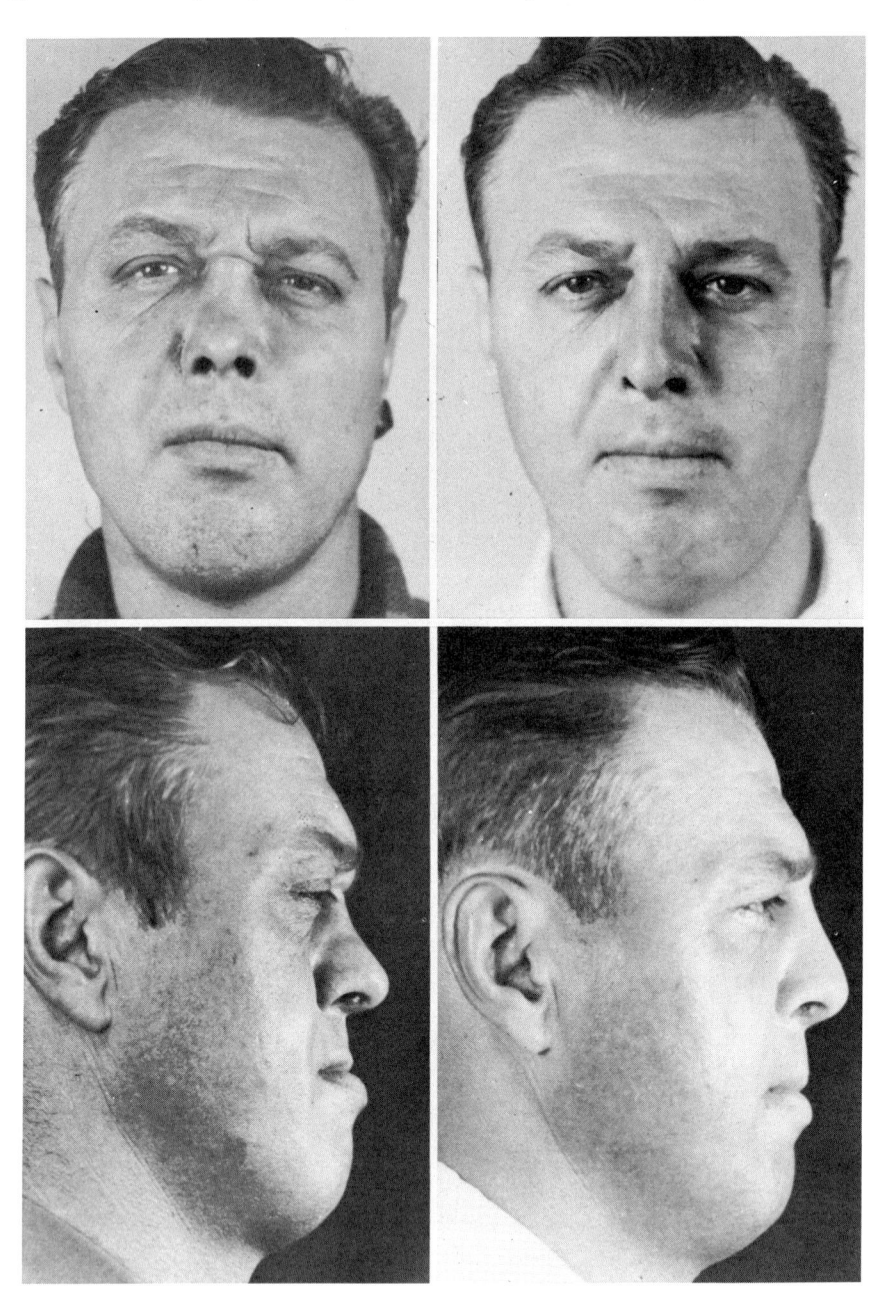

FIG. 49-39. The whole face and the nose were pushed back or caved in, from a traffic accident. The patient was seen late when bones were firm in depressed position. The whole face built forward with 4 cartilage transplants, both orbital borders, across under nose and side to side, and L-shaped transplant for dorsum of nose and columella. (Brown, J. B., and Fryer, M. P.: Postgrad. Med., 4:420-434)

Facial Paralysis 1473

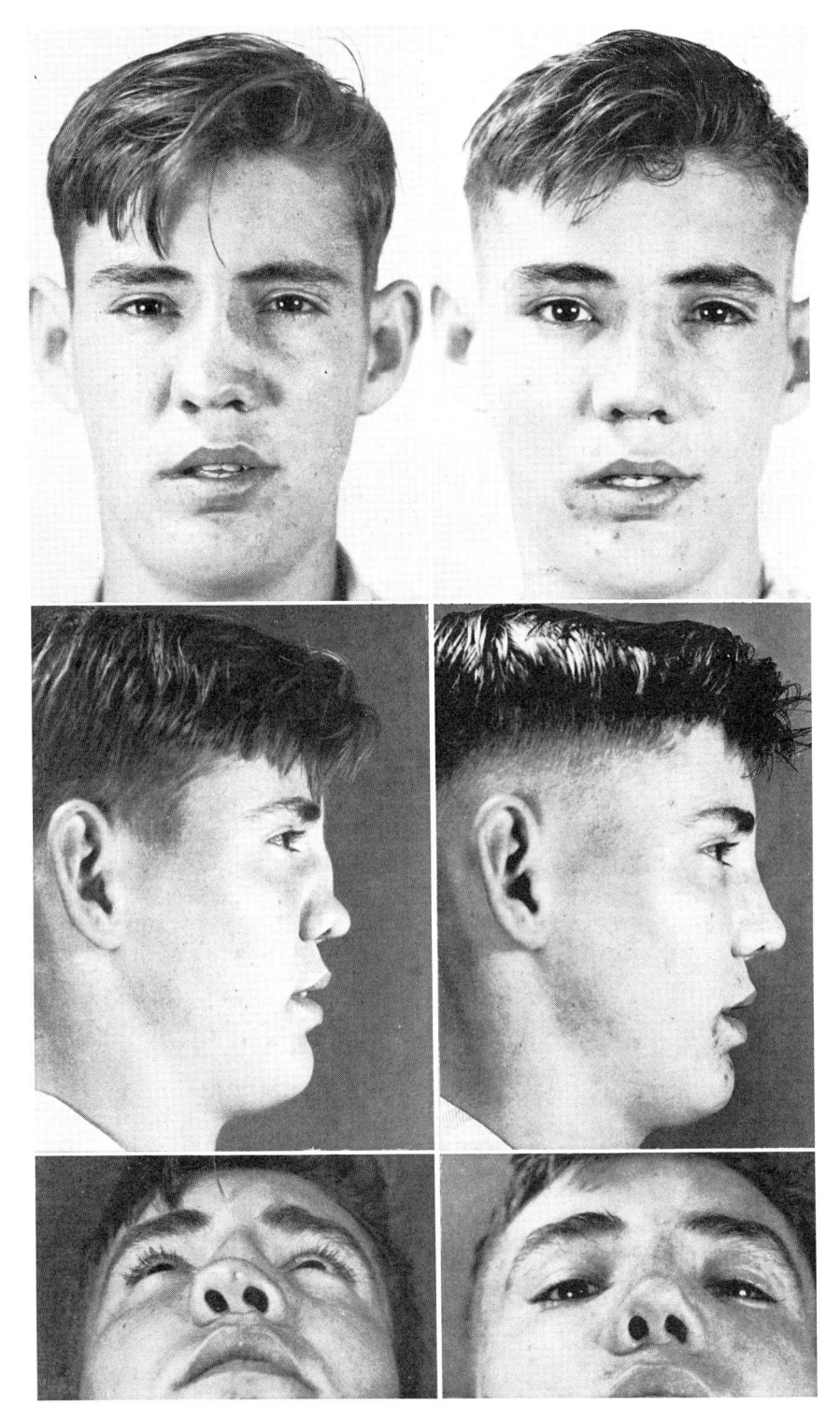

FIG. 49-40. (*Left*) Result of childhood fracture. (*Right*) Elevation and reconstruction of supports of nose done in one operation.

or the parotid gland. However, parotid tumors can be removed safely without damage to the facial nerve.[13]

Benign tumors in the parotid gland do not cause facial paralysis, even though very large. The facial nerve has been found flattened to a ribbon by pressure from a large benign tumor without any demonstrable evidence of distal paralysis. To the contrary, malignant tumors within the parotid gland are associated with facial nerve paralysis to a remarkably high degree, so much so that one can be fairly certain that a neoplasm within the parotid is malignant when facial paralysis and tumor coexist.

DIAGNOSIS

The diagnosis of facial paralysis is usually obvious, even with the face at rest. The face is flat and drooped, and the lid slit is widened. The degree of involvement may be judged fairly accurately by having the patient actively move all parts of the face. With acute complete paralysis, eating and talking may be very difficult.

TREATMENT

Musculofascial active support of the paralyzed face and some degree of animation can be secured by inserting loops of fascia lata beneath the skin from the corners of the mouth and anchoring them in the temporalis muscle near its tendon. By this maneuver a muscle innervated by the 5th cranial nerve is made to perform a function previously attended to by ones supplied by the 7th.

Occasionally fascial nerve anastomosis and substitution may be used to restore facial nerve function, but even if such a procedure is indicated and contemplated, overstretching of the face should be avoided by support of the face with fascial loops while nerve regeneration is awaited.

The fascial strip repair is effected by removing strips of fascia lata over 1 cm. wide and 25 to 30 cm. long with a stripper of the Masson type.[14] These strips are passed through an incision above the hairline in the temple region to the upper and the lower lips and looped back up and anchored in the temporalis muscle near the tendon. This placement near the tendon makes for the maximum movement, as illustrated in Figure 49-41. The

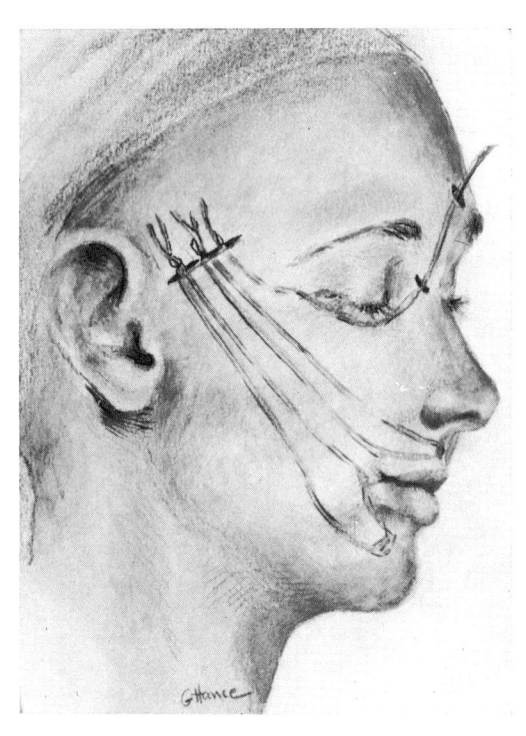

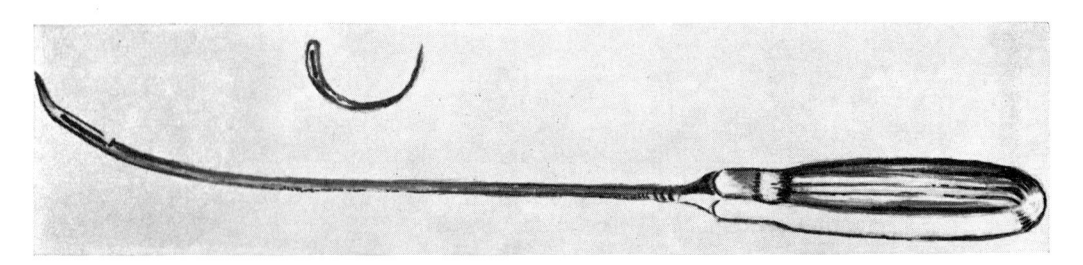

FIG. 49-41. (*Top*) Autogenous fascia lata strips looped to elevate paralyzed face, fixed in temporal muscle and tendon. Lost 7th nerve action is substituted for by 5th nerve temporal muscle action. Upper separate loop through the lower eyelid helps to hold it in contact with the globe, along with external canthoplasty. (*Bottom*) Fascia needles.

Facial Paralysis

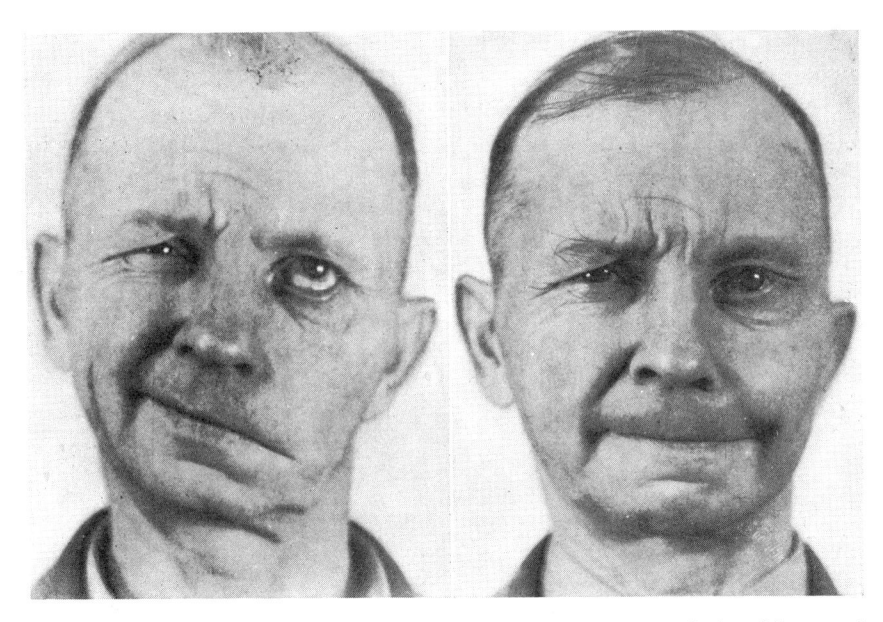

FIG. 49-42. (*Left*) Complete unilateral peripheral facial paralysis with sagged face and eyelid. (*Right*) Result of one operation one month later with face supported by loops of fascia lata anchored to temporalis tendon combined with external canthoplasty. Normal lid aperture and nasolabial fold. Comfortable and expressive movement is possible. (Brown, J. B., and Fryer, M. P.: Plastic surgery for severe facial paralysis in elderly patients. J. Am. Geriatrics Soc., 2:820-825)

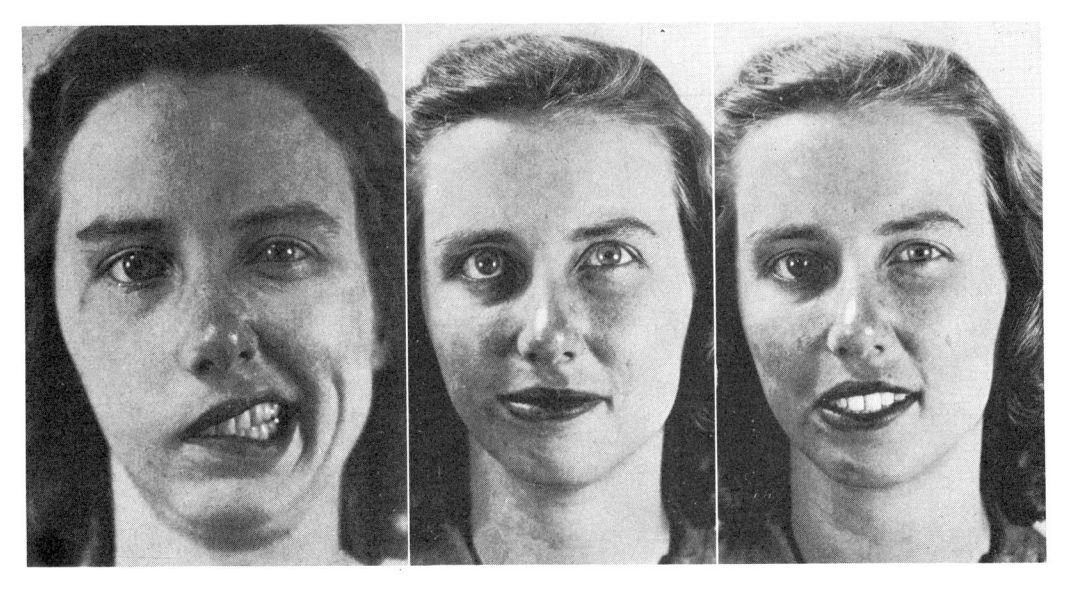

FIG. 49-43. Facial paralysis. (*Left*) From malignant parotid tumor necessitating radical operation. (*Center*) Face supported by loops of fascia lata in face anchored to temporalis muscle and fascia. (*Right*) Balanced emotional expression possible by substituting 5th cranial nerve action for lost 7th cranial nerve. No further addition of scars in the face by this operation. (Brown, J. B., McDowell, F., and Fryer, M. P.: Direct operative removal of benign mixed tumors of anlage origin in the parotid region. Surg., Gynec., Obstet., 90:257-268)

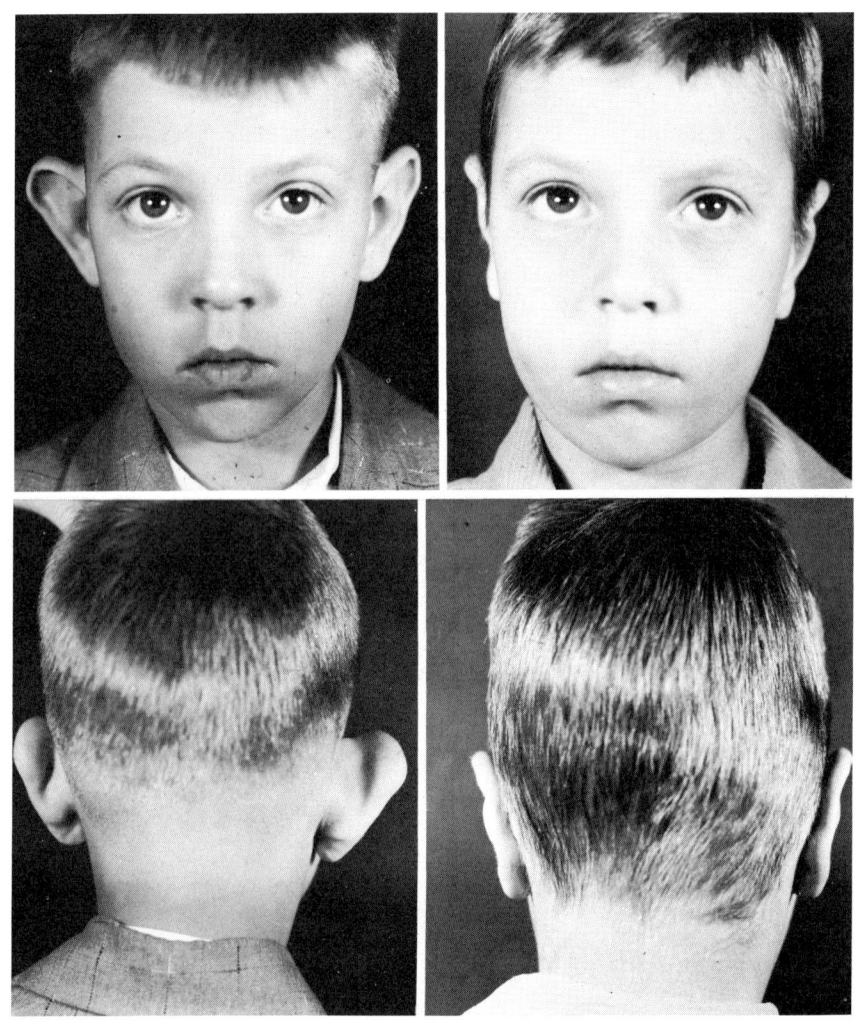

FIG. 49-44. (*Left*) Prominent ears set back in one operation through posterior incision. (*Right*) Early postoperative photograph.

long fascial needle used to pass the fascia is drawn in the lower part of Figure 49-41. The smaller curved needle is used to implant the fascia in the temporalis muscle.

Support of the face by this method permits the construction of a flexion crease in the nasolabial region. The loss of this crease is the most noticeable deformity attendant upon facial paralysis, even with the face in repose.

In a somewhat similar way the drooped lower eyelid can be supported by a loop of fascia passed from the temporal region through the eyelid to the frontalis region. In addition, the eye can be made more comfortable and the exposure of the cornea reduced without disturbing the eyelashes with a lateral canthoplasty.

Actually, even after complete facial paralysis of long duration, eating, speaking, normal appearance, and maintenance of watertight integrity of the mouth can be practically fully restored with this fascial support method. The degree of animation is unpredictable but can be developed by minor exercises.

DEFORMITIES OF THE EAR

Ear deformities may be congenital or traumatic. Congenital deformities may be of any degree and involve one or both ears. Traumatic loss of ears may follow an automobile or industrial accident but more often is the consequence of burns of the face and the ears. With burn denudation the cartilage is exposed to infection, resulting in a deformity that is more unsightly than is the actual loss of an ear.

Ears widely placed from the head or flop ears are usually of congenital origin. They can be corrected usually in one operation through an incision that is hidden behind the ear. During the operation the cartilaginous support to the ear is opened to permit permanent repositioning and the construction of normal markings.

Total construction of an absent ear can be done in 3 fundamental stages without the addition of scars in the neck or elsewhere. Vestigial remnants are smoothed out or placed in the proper direction in the first stage. The cartilaginous support for the future ear is placed in its proper position beneath the scalp in a subcutaneous pocket at the second operation. Cartilage and other materials such as dimethyl siloxanes, halogenated carbons and polyvinyl alcohol have been used to construct the support to the ear.[38] If the patient is large enough to have sufficient available cartilage, it can be used; however, fresh homografts from other members of the patient's family may be relied on; otherwise, preserved cartilage from the cartilage bank may be used. This avoids an unpleasant operation on another member of the family. At the third stage, usually done from 3 to 6 months after implantation of the support, the skin covered cartilage is raised forward from the scalp, and its posterior surface and the defect in the scalp are covered with a free split graft. Acceptable ear outlines may be made in these 3 stages and are preferred by most patients to artificial prostheses. Additional adjustments and addition of a round helix with a small tubed flap from the neck may be required after the basic procedures have been completed.

There are many suggestions as to various more laborious procedures for ear reconstruction, for which reference to specific texts is necessary if details are desired.

Traumatic loss of an ear requires essentially the same stages for reconstruction as those for the congenitally absent one.

With deep burns of the face ears are often burned off or so deformed as to require practically total reconstruction. In such cases the outer surface of the ear and the cartilage is usually so infected, wrinkled and scarred as to require total replacement.

DEFORMITIES OF THE EYELIDS

Ptosis (the inability to elevate the upper lid properly), deformities about the canthus and absence of a part of an eyelid, such as coloboma palpebrale, are the most common congenital deformities seen about the eye requiring repair. However, traumatic destruction and surgical removal constitute the most frequent causes of deformities of the eyelids.

PTOSIS

Because of the difficulty in elevating the lid above the pupil, the skin of the forehead is arched, and the head is held back so the patient may see beneath his drooped eyelids. The correction of ptosis requires elevation of the eyelid. If any levator palpebrae action remains, the tendon of this muscle may be shortened, thereby elevating the lid. However, usually there is no function remaining in this muscle, and another technic must be used. The superior tarsal plate may be shortened and brought up to the region of the frontalis muscle, or a tendon can be constructed from fascia lata and this looped down to the tarsal border and then attached to the frontalis muscle. This in effect substitutes a muscle innervated by the 7th nerve for the missing one innervated by the 3rd. Both of these technics permit the raising of the lid when the skin over the forehead is lifted. This the patient learns to do soon after operation. Postoperatively, there may be some difficulty in effecting normal closure of the eyes, especially during sleep. Should this occur, usually it can be cared for with a small piece of adhesive tape.

The operation described above is extraorbital and does not restore normal intraorbital elevation of the lid. To obtain intraorbital elevation the use of the superior rectus muscle is required in the repair. This is an ophthalmologic operation. All patients having ptosis should be examined by an ophthalmologist and the type of operation selected for a given patient on a consultative basis.

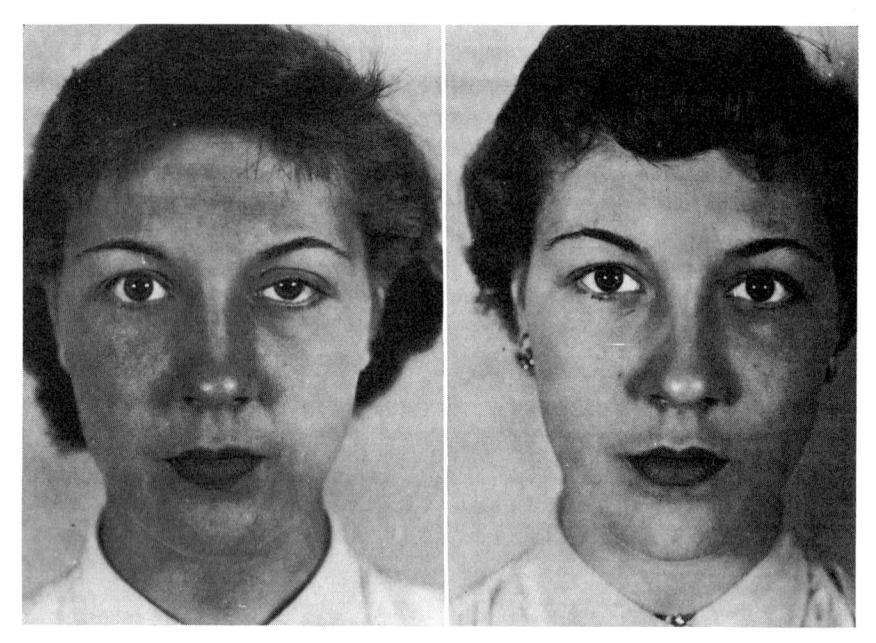

FIG. 49-45. (*Left*) Ptosis of patient's left upper eyelid repaired in one operation. (*Right*) Two weeks after repair.

Conditions Requiring Reconstruction of an Eyelid

Congenital absence of an eyelid, coloboma palpebrale (a slit in the lid) or loss due to trauma or operative removal are alike in that the defect requires reconstruction of an eyelid to protect the cornea. Total eyelid reconstruction requires the formation of a mucosal lining, as well as an outer layer of skin. Protection of the exposed cornea is extremely important to the maintenance of sight; consequently, its covering may be a real emergency. Often coloboma palpebrale can be repaired in one operation by rotating the lining of the adjacent segments of the lid and utilizing local flaps for closure. This principle may be used even for the total reconstruction of lids lost from any cause. Cross-lid flaps may be used in some instances, but it is best to avoid damage to a normal lid whenever possible. However, parts of a normal companion lid must be used occasionally in order to provide a lining mucosa because skin is not tolerated by the bulbar conjunctiva.

Spontaneous reconstitution of an eyelid after its excision for carcinoma may completely obviate the necessity for secondary reconstruction, although this process may be prolonged and require the exposure of bulbar conjunctiva. However, the functional result may be more satisfactory than that which follows an attempt at primary surgical reconstruction.

Spontaneous reconstitution of the eyelid after the resection of a neoplasm of the lid is effected by the surgical coaptation of any remaining part of the resected lid to its normal partner. This may effect a spontaneous generation of mucosa and skin from the surrounding area and the adjacent lid so as to permit separation of the adherent lids later with the securance of adequate corneal coverage with little or no addition of skin such as free full-thickness grafts from the ear or the neck, or as a small local flap.

Ectropion

Spontaneously healing deep burns of the eyelids heal with contracture and eversion of the conjunctiva of the eyelid (ectropion). This exposes the cornea with the possible result of corneal ulceration and loss of sight. The treatment consists of excising the deep scar from the eyelids while taking care to preserve all possible muscle function. This excision of scar releases the contracture and allows the lid to come in contact with the globe. The excisional defects are readily resurfaced with free full-thickness skin grafts taken from behind an ear, from the supraclavicular region or the inguinal region. Innumerable eyes of burned persons have been saved by prompt release of ectropion and immediate coverage with a skin graft.

SALIVARY GLANDS

The usual disorders of the submaxillary and the parotid glands are ductal obstruction, infection, trauma and tumors. The parotid glands are the most common sites of tumors, and the submaxillary gland ducts are the more frequent site of obstructions (see Chap. 48).

OBSTRUCTION

Calculi. The origin of salivary stones may be related to partial ductal obstruction and infection. The calculi usually found in the ducts may be multiple. Ductal calculi characteristically produce intermittent obstructions with swelling of the obstructed gland.

Diagnosis of salivary duct obstruction is made on the basis of acute swelling of the gland following the secretory stimulation of eating or chewing gum. Pain and swelling over the gland follows. Occasionally, fever and general malaise attend it, particularly if there is infection. When the infection occurs behind a ductal obstruction, often pus may be expressed from the duct. Simple roentgenograms may show the stones. However, sialograms may be required to demonstrate obstruction of the duct by stenosis, etc. The treatment of calculous obstruction is the removal of the calculi. Often this can be done rather easily by extracting it from the duct in the mouth, or enlarging the orifice of the duct, allowing the stone to pass spontaneously. The repeated recurrence of symptoms and calculi may require removal of the gland to cure the trouble.

Congenital narrowing of salivary ducts usually occurs at their orifices in the mouth. The signs and symptoms of congenital stenotic obstructions are the same as those caused by a calculus. Relief is afforded by enlarging the orifice in the mouth.

Infection in the salivary ducts usually is related to obstruction which, when corrected, may cure the infection. However, antibiotics are given routinely in most instances of obstruction before and for a time after its correction because some infection within the ducts is usually present by the time the patient seeks relief.

Infection in the salivary glands themselves is often secondary to obstruction or infection in the ducts. The general reaction is usually more severe than when it is confined to the ducts, but the signs of obstruction are predominant. Infection in salivary glands may occur without demonstrable obstructions of their ducts coming from infection elsewhere in the body. Surgical mumps or *parotitis* (non-obstructive parotitis) was seen more frequently in the past in markedly debilitated patients with poor mouth care who were taking little by mouth; it was in general a symptom of some other disease process. Occasionally, all salivary glands were affected simultaneously, but the parotids alone most often. The treatment of surgical mumps is stimulation of salivary flow with chewing and mouth washes, antibiotics and care of the general debilitation. Opening of the parenchyma of the glands to the outside through multiple incisions is often necessary for the cure of parenchyma suppuration, especially when the infection is staphylococcal. Infection in a major salivary gland not apparently related to obstruction may eventually necessitate removal of the gland, but the use of light inflammatory doses of x-rays, antibiotics and salivary stimulation may avoid it.

Trauma to the salivary system is usually the result of glass cuts from automobile accidents, knife cuts or surgical exploration. Lacerations of the gland usually can be closed, and healing follows. Fistulas communicating with the intraglandular ducts usually close spontaneously. However, if a major duct has been cut, careful approximation of the two ends always should be done, or if in the mouth, the duct may be short-circuited by anastomosing the proximal end to the buccal mucosa. If neither an anastomosis nor shortening is done, persistant fistulae are prone to develop, and subsequent repair or short-circuiting is made more difficult. Secondary scarring following trauma may cause obstruction to the ducts, in which case resection of scar and reanastomosis or short-circuiting may be tried.

CONGENITAL WRYNECK

Congenital wryneck probably is seen most often by the plastic surgeon because of its related deformities of the jaw or the face.[34]

The etiology has always been indeterminate. Presumptively, it has been related to injury at birth. The microscopic appearance of the lesion is important because of its importance to the treatment. In most instances the normal structure of the sternocleidomastoid muscle is incompletely replaced by scar, grossly and microscopically. This scar is probably the result of fibrosis secondary to a hematoma or the tearing of the muscle. However, other theories of cause have been advanced. The mass in the muscle generally is noticed about 2 weeks after birth. It may disappear spontaneously, leaving very little deformity.

Congenital wryneck is not to be confused with spasmotic torticollis, which is an entirely different entity and cannot be relieved by removal of muscle.

Diagnosis of congenital torticollis can be made upon noting the position of the ear and the mastoid region. They are pulled down to the shoulder of the affected side while the chin points toward the normal side. The patient cannot bend the head to the normal side. In addition, a solid mass may be felt in the sternocleidomastoid muscle during infancy. Later the mass becomes less apparent, but the mastoid process remains approximated to the clavicle by the palpably tight band of fibrous tissue representing the sternocleidomastoid muscle bundle. Roentgenograms of the cervical spine are needed to rule out congenital deformities of the cervical spine which superficially mimic congenital wryneck. Failure to correct the deformity during early childhood ultimately causes deformity of the jaw and the head on the affected side.

Treatment consists of complete excision of the scarred muscle band through a low collar incision. If the lesion is of relatively long duration, the cervical fascia overlying the fibrous muscle remnant may be shortened and require opening. Casts or braces are not required after the excision if total excision of the contracting mass is done. Because spontaneous subsidence of the entire process occasionally occurs, the operation is deferred until the 6th to the 8th month of age. Should the deformity remain at this age it is looked upon as a permanent one, and operative correction should be undertaken.

INDUSTRIAL AND FARM INJURIES

Some injuries from farm and industrial machines are sufficiently peculiar to warrant their separate consideration. Tractor power take-off injuries are one of these.

TRACTOR POWER TAKE-OFF GENITAL INJURIES

These injuries attend the catching of trousers and the dragging of the leg and the lower torso over the revolving power take-off. This tears the skin of the perineum, the penis and the scrotum, and the lower abdomen and the back, from the body, often completely denuding the penis and leaving the testes attached only by the cords. When the skin of the back and the abdomen is torn off, often the underlying muscles are exposed and torn.

Emergency care is directed toward the prevention and the control of shock. The prompt use of whole blood may prevent shock. However, often these patients are alone in the field when the accident occurs, and therefore treatment is often delayed. When it is, a large volume of whole blood has been necessary to save life.

These patients should be brought to the operating room as soon as possible and individual bleeding points ligated. The poor general condition of the person may permit only cleansing with saline irrigation after controlling hemorrhage and the application of a firm comfortable fine-mesh grease gauze pressure dressing. In other words, cutaneous reconstruction is delayed. Tetanus protection with 25,000 units or more of tetanus antitoxin in cases not actively immunized with toxoid, or a booster of toxoid to those who are, and large doses of antibiotics are given.

Repair. The first steps in definitive repair of the damaged area are done when shock has been treated and the general condition permits. These steps consist of

(1) Débridement of nonviable tissue and the cleansing of open areas.

(2) Protection of the testes by implanting them beneath the skin of the thighs. A subcutaneous tunnel is made from the torn perineum into the thigh, and the testes are anchored in it. Also, temporary protection can be provided by encasing them in saline-moistened gauze packs. This will suffice for protection during immediate transportation.

After inserting the testes into the pockets, often the perineum may be closed, and this can be done safely, provided that drainage is assured. Insertion of the testes into the inner thigh tunnels may be followed by the natural withdrawal of the testes toward the midline, effecting the spontaneous appearance of a small bifid scrotum. During the early reconstructive period there seems to be no necessity of attempting to construct a scrotum with local flaps. One young man who had both testes buried beneath the skin of the thighs later developed a new bifid scrotum spontaneously and begot children.

(3) Re-covering the penis usually can be accomplished with free autografts. This is done at the time of primary repair of the other damaged areas. The split-thickness graft is taken with a knife and suction retractors from the thigh and is wrapped around the penis and held in place with sutures and/or a carefully applied dressing. If a plastic surgeon is not available the penis may be temporarily buried subcutaneously with an indwelling catheter in place.

(4) Bare areas on the abdomen or the back, after cleansing and débridement, are covered by split-thickness grafts held in place by sutures and the dressing.

Subsequent care of these newly covered areas is the same as that described for any graft.

Primary definitive repair of tractor power take-off injuries is usually all that is necessary for permanent function. Rarely is complex plastic surgery necessary if the primary repair is conducted as described.

HYPOSPADIAS

Hypospadias is a congenital penile defect in which the ventral surface is foreshortened and the urethral meatus is on the ventral surface often close to the penile-scrotal junction. The ventral curvature is exaggerated by erection. Repair consists of correction of the curvature and building a tube from the opening of the short urethra to the end of the penis. This usually requires 2 or 3 operations. *Circumcision should not be done.* The repair is performed when there is sufficient tissue available, usually by the 4th or the 5th year.

Release of the curvature is the first operation. The curvature is released by dissecting the urethra free, permitting it to drop back toward the scrotum and excising the tight bands under the corpora cavernosum. The defect left by these dissections is covered by interdigitated local penile flaps, utilizing the prepuce when needed. This step may be performed before the second birthday.

Construction of the tube from the urethra to the end of the penis can be done after release of the curvature. The entire tube can be constructed and connected to the end of the short urethra in one operation if preliminary diversion of the urinary stream is done through a perineal urethrostomy. Otherwise, the tube is constructed at one operation and connected to the urethra later. Numerous methods are available for construction of the tube, but the most satisfactory method in the author's experience has been the incision of a strip of skin on the ventral surface wide enough to circumscribe a No. 10 catheter at least and the careful approximation of the edges of this strip over a catheter with multiple sutures. The tube lined by skin but uncovered by skin is covered over by interdigitating skin flaps from the remaining normally outward-facing penile skin. The same method is used to connect the newly constructed tube to the urethra.

A firm pressure dressing encourages healing and avoids bleeding after correction of the curvature and the building of the tube.

REPAIR OF SURFACE DEFECTS OF THE FEET

Surface defects of the feet may follow removal of tumors or result from circulatory deficiency, infection or trauma. Repair may be difficult because the plantar surface, like the palm of the hand, is a specialized type of skin which cannot be reconstituted but at best can only be substituted for.

Primary closure is the simplest means of

covering a defect if sufficient skin is available for closure or the resultant scar is not over a weight-bearing surface of the foot.

Coverage with a free graft can be done for larger defects if there is an adequate soft tissue pad upon which to place the graft. Skin from elsewhere on the body constitutes only a substitute type of coverage for normal plantar skin and must be protected constantly because it cannot stand the pressures of walking and standing that the original plantar skin could.

Local flaps may be necessary if the defect covers the heads of the 1st and the 5th metatarsals or the heel. The open area left by rotation of a flap from a nonweight-bearing surface of the foot to the above locations can be covered by a free graft.

Distant flaps may be necessary to cover larger deep losses of skin of the foot. Their use requires preparation in stages. The opposite thigh is used most often as a donor site. These flaps are raised in stages, training the blood supply to come in from the desired direction, and then are applied to the foot. Detachment of the flap from the thigh usually is possible within 3 weeks after its attachment to the foot. The cutaneous defect left upon the thigh is covered with a free graft.

Short, broad flaps are used whenever possible in order to avoid the delay of staging, such as in abdominal flap repair of deep injuries of the arm and the hand.

Flaps covering defects of the foot require the same permanent protection as split or free full-thickness grafts do because they, too, cannot take the pounding that the original skin could.

The preceding discussion of principles and methods in plastic surgery has been taken from the original articles listed under "References," and these can be consulted for details.

USE OF SILICONE, TEFLON, POLYVINYL ALCOHOL AND DI-ISOCYANATE AS PROSTHESES IN RECONSTRUCTIVE SURGERY

The use of plastic materials as subcutaneous prostheses may be the most significant recent development in reconstructive surgery, particularly about the face. Laboratory studies and clinical uses of these materials have been recorded,[1-3, 5, 6, 19, 20, 23, 24, 26, 41-43] and the student is referred to these sources for completeness.

Reconstructive surgeons have searched for years for substitutes for fresh homotransplants, and the list of materials is a long one; efforts still are being made to try to arrive at final decision and proof as to consistent success with such foreign-body implantations. The most frequent work of plastic surgery about the face and the jaws really is not comparable with orthopedic surgery deep in the tissues where rigidly held metal, or synthetic, prostheses have a good chance of retention and of giving function; the same is true of blood vessel and heart work where deeply placed and well-covered substitutes have a better chance of being retained. This may prove to be true also in some neurologic work with synthetic conduits now used in the therapy of hydrocephalus.

But in plastic surgery with defects close to the surface and with little covering tissue, there is a more difficult problem of getting such a foreign body to be retained, and this problem is still greater if there is movement of the prosthesis or of the tissues around it. In the field of plastic surgery, the breast offers a fairly deep place for implantation, but even here the prosthesis is without the rigid fixation that is readily obtained with a bone prosthesis.

The quality of inertness naturally gives the best chance for a foreign body, including a prosthesis, to be retained subcutaneously, and there are many instances of long-term accidental retentions of foreign bodies such as metal.

Synthetic materials have been developed with attributes of inertness and stability that make them theoretically suitable for subcutaneous implantation. A synthetic that after implantation changes its chemical structure or loses any element cannot be used. Celluloid is such a substance; it has been tried many times but with no documented series of its successful implantation in lower animals or man. This material, for example, has the odor of camphor, and if such a molecule were lost into the tissue, it could be toxic.

An acceptable synthetic subcutaneous prosthesis should be inert, should not cause inflammation, should not constitute a bacterial culture medium, and should not cause neoplasm. Its physical properties—elasticity, hardness, mass, etc.—should be similar to the replaced tissue. Because different tissues have different physical properties such as degrees of resilience and flexibility, different synthetics are needed for the replacement of various tissues. Fortunately, today the chemistry of polymers is well advanced and the chemical industry has been and is cooperating actively with the development of suitable plastics for prostheses.

Silicones have a basic dimethyl siloxane radical, which may be highly polymerized, so that the material ranges from a liquid to a resin:

$$CH_3-\underset{\underset{CH_3}{|}}{\overset{\overset{CH_3}{|}}{Si}}-O\left[-\underset{\underset{CH_3}{|}}{\overset{\overset{CH_3}{|}}{Si}}-O\right]\rightarrow$$

The end-group may be a methyl or hydroxy radical. Even though polymerized to a resinous state, the material still behaves as a liquid in that it slowly changes its shape; consequently, its clinical application is limited. However, experimental work with it proved it to be inert and demonstrated that it is retained in living tissue with no reaction to it, and in our work with it in animals no tumors were caused by it.

Silicone rubber is a clear amber resilient substance with the appearance of organic rubber. It is stable from $-54°$ to $+540°$ C. It is not affected by acids or alkalies; it is free of any soluble or leachable material; it has a specific gravity of 1.13; and it is easily sculptured into any shape with a sharp blade.

A silicone sponge, medical grade, has also been made by Dow Corning from the dimethyl siloxane. It is nonreactive and is not invaded by the host tissues and consequently does not produce as much scar as other sponge materials. This may lead to its wider use in the future. A few CH_3 groups are reduced to CH_2 to make change to solid rubber.

Halogenated Carbons. Tetrafluorocarbon and Teflon (Du Pont) are long-chain polymers with the following basic formula:

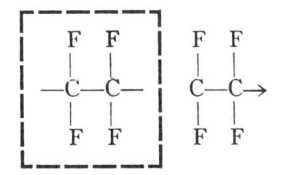

$$\left[-\underset{\underset{F}{|}}{\overset{\overset{F}{|}}{C}}-\underset{\underset{F}{|}}{\overset{\overset{F}{|}}{C}}-\right]\underset{\underset{F}{|}}{\overset{\overset{F}{|}}{C}}-\underset{\underset{F}{|}}{\overset{\overset{F}{|}}{C}}\rightarrow$$

This is made by polymerization of tetrafluoro-ethylene gas at high temperature and pressure. These fluorocarbons are chemically inert, being insoluble in all general solvents. They are thermostable from $-195°$ to $+326°$ C. We have studied and used the Du Pont product, Teflon, available in blocks, sheets, rods, linters, and sponge. The block material is hard and shows the least surrounding tissue reaction to it. We have seen no tumors develop from it in laboratory animals or after its clinical use.

A similar product, polytrifluoromonochlorethylene (Kel F, Minnesota Mining and Manufacturing Company), has one chlorine in place of fluorine in the tetra group and has properties the same as Teflon. Both Teflon and Kel F probably can be annealed at $270°$ C. to retain a form memory so that the prostheses constructed from them will not change their shapes after implantation.

Polyvinyl alcohol sponge, Ivalon, is so well known at this time that little discussion is indicated. It has its basic molecule in long chains as the other polymers.

$$-CH_2-\underset{\underset{OH}{|}}{CH}-CH_2-\underset{\underset{OH}{|}}{CH}-CH_2-\underset{\underset{OH}{|}}{CH}-CH_2$$

It is prepared in a white sponge that is soft and pliable when wet, and hard when dry. It has a continuous sponge structure into which the cells of fibrous and vascular tissue grow freely, making it a real part of the tissue about it. In this way it is comparable to living tissue. This would seem to be an ideal foreign implant, but if it is supplementing soft resilient tissue, as in the breast, the hardness of the sponge itself is abnormal in comparison with normal breast. Furthermore, should infections occur, it spreads through sponge, making it difficult to deal with and often resulting in the necessity of its removal. In spite of these objections, it is satisfactory for the filling in of depressed areas and for building up atrophic

1484 Principles of General Plastic Surgery

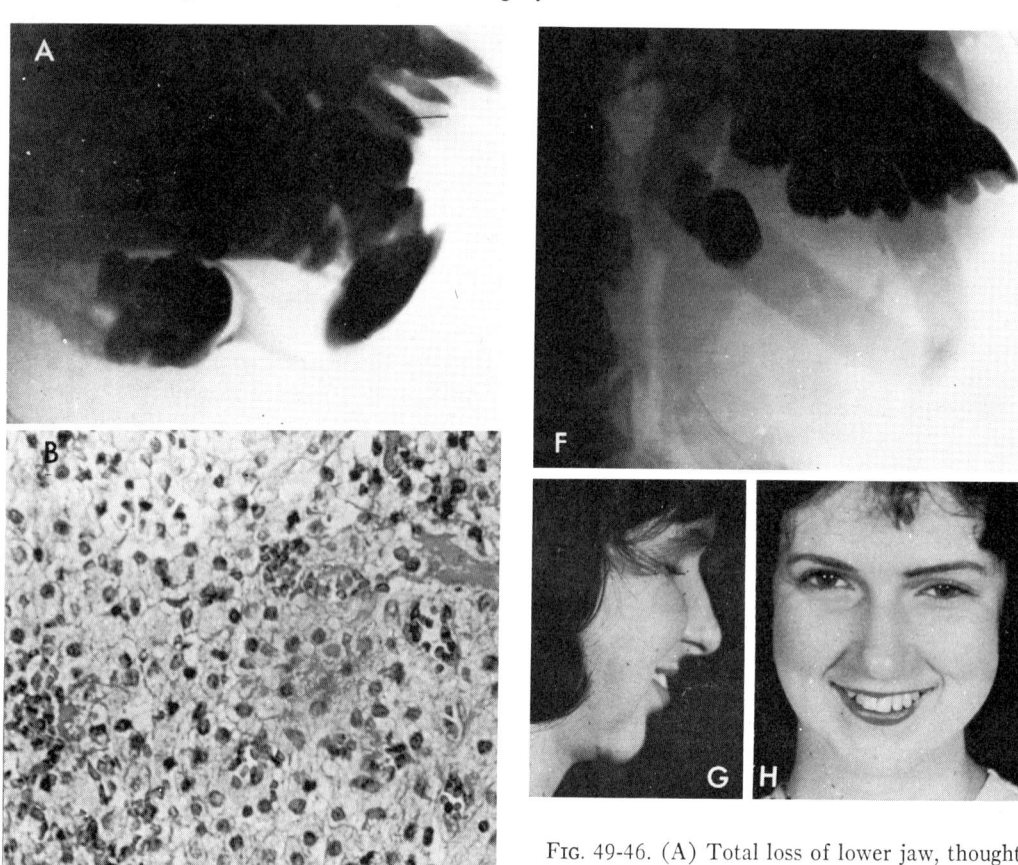

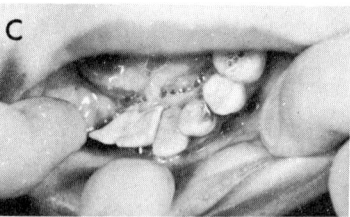

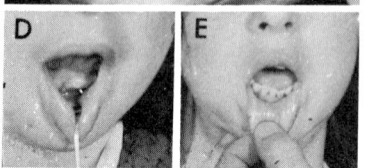

FIG. 49-46. (A) Total loss of lower jaw, thought to be from Hand-Schüller-Christian or related disease and associated infection. No regeneration of the jaw took place. Only 1 molar tooth retained in mouth. (B) Giant cells, histiocytes with lipids and eosinophils in a biopsy specimen taken during absorption of the jaw. (C) Toward final stage of loss of jaw bone and teeth. (D) Total loss of bone and teeth. (E) Useful dental prosthesis fitted over subcutaneous prosthesis of Teflon. (F) Teflon substitution for total loss of jaw, fortunately placed so as to provide functional muscle action (able to eat even potato chips). Total loss of jaw without any osseous regeneration. (G and H) Form and function restoration with Teflon substitution for total loss of jaw (3 years). (Brown, J. B., et al.: Silicone and Teflon prostheses. Ann. Surg., 157:932-943)

areas. This makes it valuable for the relief of many patients.

Laboratory approach to these plastic implants has been followed. Tumor investigation in animals, though not a final answer, has been pursued. During a 16-year period, 600 animals have been implanted with these materials, and no tumors have been noted, other than 1 fibroma reported in 1952 adjacent to a polyvinyl alcohol implant. Microscopic examination has been made of a great many implants and the surrounding tissue and gross examination of all. Knowing that any substance that might be used clinically is nontumorgenic is mandatory before it is put in human beings. What can be done with plastic materials today is illustrated by a number of cases.

Teflon substitution for total loss of the lower jaw is a clinical demonstration of the use of one of these materials. The patient

FIG. 49-47. (*Left, top* and *bottom*) Solid ankylosis from early infancy. No motion. No development of chin area. (*Right, top* and *bottom*) Ankylosis relieved by wide bone resection and temporary silicone rubber implant to separate the jaw from the skull. Chin area built out with silicone sponge. Patient rehabilitated to normal life—educational, social, physical and emotional. Able to chew for the first time in his life. Now has a career in music. (Brown, J. B., and Fryer, M. P.: Ankylosis of the jaw, Am. Surg., 27:11-13)

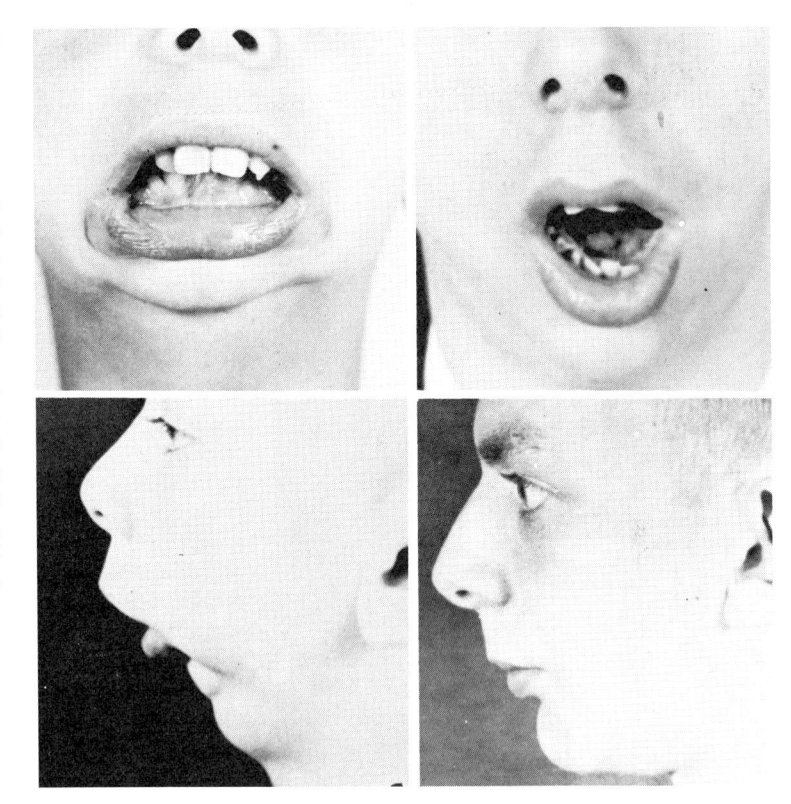

shown in Figure 49-46 had complete loss of the lower jaw, throughout its full extent with no bony elements left and with no regeneration. Substitution for the totally absent jaw has been made with a bar of Teflon annealed into the proper curve and implanted through the front of the neck. This implant has been in place 4 years; the patient had a functioning dental prosthesis made and uses it quite well.

The diagnosis of this lesion was thought to be Hand-Schüller-Christian or a related disease (Fig. 49-46, and A and B), with complete loss of all osseous elements in the lower jaw, and with some destruction in the skull. She has outgrown this tendency, or retrogression has occurred with x-ray treatment. During the time of activity some pieces of bone were lost from infection. She has remained well under close observation, has married and has one child.

The problem of reconstructive surgery was to get an armature throughout the area and to try to engage the muscles of the jaw without a completely open dissection. There were no bone elements left to give attachment with any bone implant or with any processed animal bone material.

The excellent Teflon replacement, as shown in Figure 49-46, F, G and H, is considered fortunate and might not be duplicated routinely. The total absence of jaw bone can be noted in Figure 49-46 F in the roentgenogram of the Teflon implant. The loss of the teeth was gradual, as shown near its final stage in Figure 49-46 C. The edentulous outcome is seen in Figure 49-46 D, and the replacement with the denture, as made by Dr. Templeton, being retained over the Teflon implant in Figure 49-46 E.

This probably is the first such synthetic substitution that has been made for total loss of the jaw. It is, necessarily, a floating implant with no connection with the skull, but with a fortunate implantation having been done within the muscle action, somewhat blindly, but very carefully. It is of importance that the sensory nerves in the area have been maintained, presumably due to the slow degeneration and absorption and rejection of her own natural jaw bone.

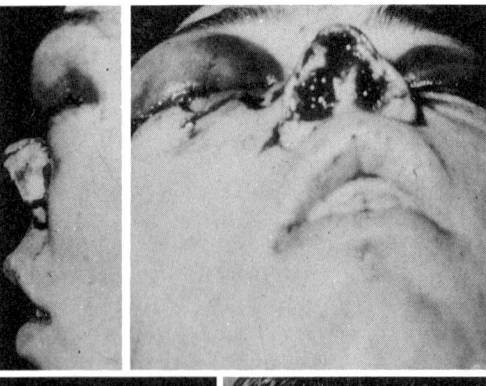

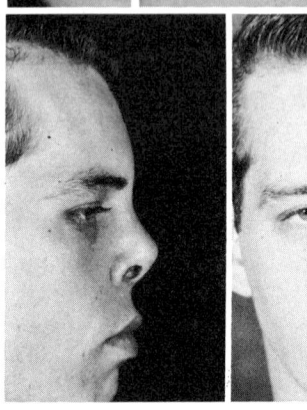

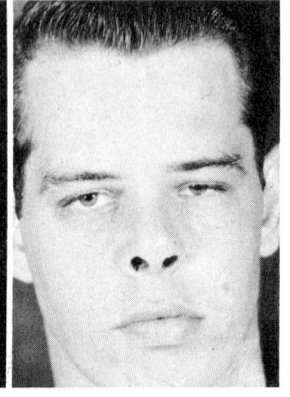

FIG. 49-48. (*Top*) Loss and destruction of most of the bony support of nose, maxilla, and lacrimal, nasal and frontal bones. Nose driven up between the eyes with many small fractures. (*Bottom*) Restoration of function, airways and contour with careful sorting and saving of all possible bone and soft tissues. Secondary support with large triangle of silicone rubber with base up in area of greatest loss (2 years). (Brown, J. B., et al.: Silicone and Teflon prostheses. Ann. Surg., 157:932-943)

We believe this to be an extremely worthwhile restoration of, or substitution for, feature, function and bone, shown after 3 years in Figure 49-46 G and H. The fact that it is so well tolerated and retained is one of the best expressions of our hope, from the start, that such inert synthetic materials might be retained as subcutaneous prostheses. A needed element for success was that the patient was cooperative and appreciative of all efforts made for her.

Silicones have been extended in use; an important one is shown in Figure 49-47. This patient had solid bony ankylosis of both temporomandibular joints from infancy, with no jaw movement at all and no forward progression of the chin. Here again, important elements of success have been the patient's desire to be relieved, along with full cooperation of the parents.

These solid joint areas were resected, from the rami to deep under the skull because of the excessive hypertrophy. This is an extensive and difficult procedure, with large blood loss; most careful attention of the anesthetist and of all concerned with the patient's care is required. One of the main concerns was protection of the 7th nerve, which was done successfully on both sides.

Resection was carried out to get empty spaces of about a cubic inch on each side. To maintain this resected ramus away from the glenoid area, a large block of silicone rubber was inserted into each cavity. Movement was encouraged after 2 weeks; excellent function has developed and the patient can chew for the first time in his life.

An important point of consideration is that motion of an implant, or around the implant, is apt to cause rejection of it. Both of these implants were removed after several months, but their long stay in place successfully held the joint space open, so that function of the jaw has remained excellent over a 2½-year period and continues to be so.

Persistence of function and contour has occurred in a few other instances of build-up of soft tissues with implants in which the stretch and the realignment of the soft tissues is such that even though the implant may be rejected or removed, the defect has remained in satisfactory contour and surface anatomy.

Silicone sponge has been used, in addition to the silicone rubber, in this patient to build the chin forward after a pocket had been prepared in front of the retruded bone, and, again, with preservation of both motor and sensory nerves. This restoration is of 2½ years' duration, with every sign of continuing.

This patient, who was greatly handicapped from lack of function and lack of the fourth function of the face, that of looking normal, is now able to go ahead with musical studies and with great promise (Fig. 49-47).

Secondary corrections of traumatic facial deformities with synthetic implants are shown

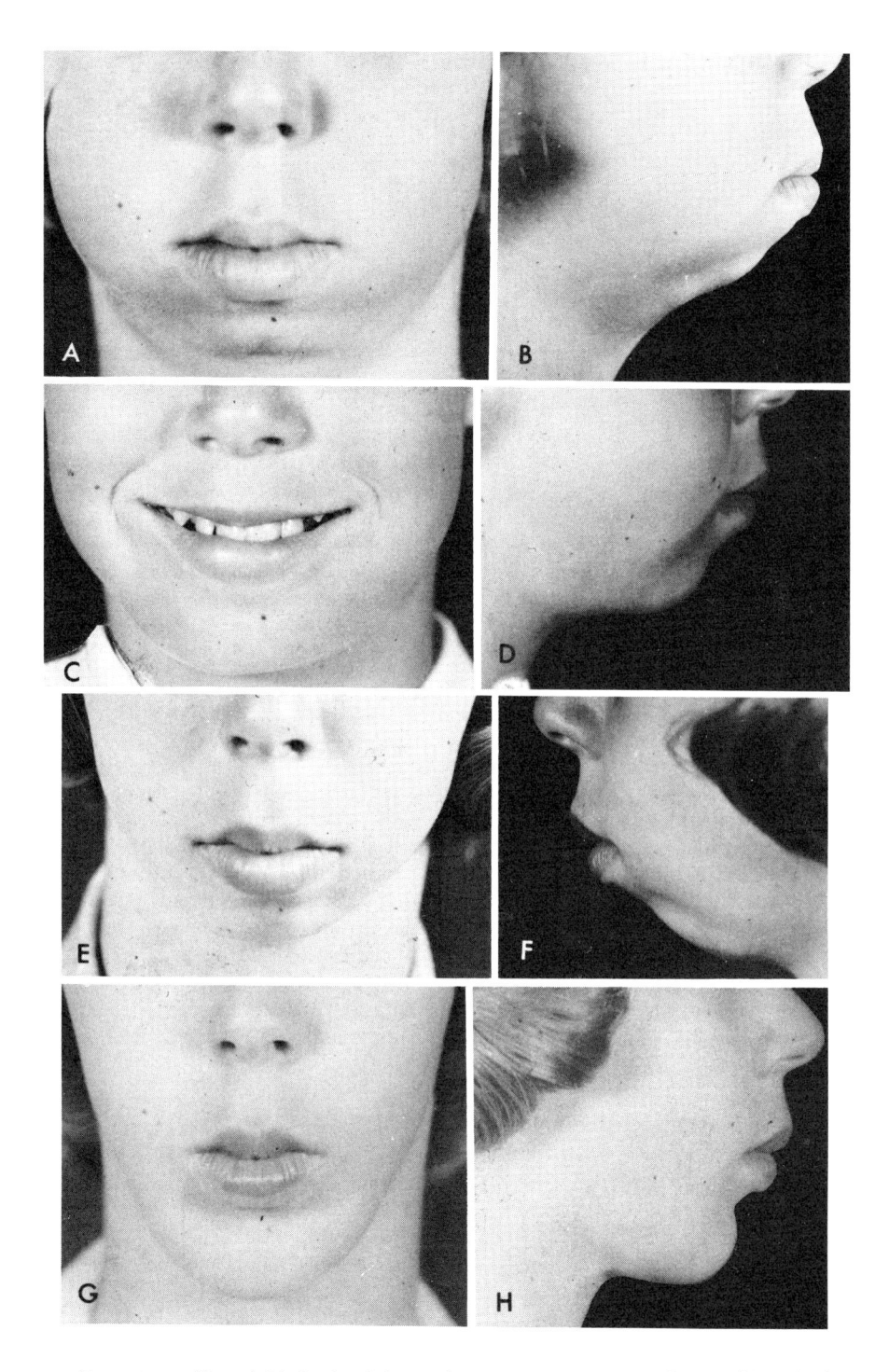

FIG. 49-49. (A and B) Lack of forward progression of jaw and chin. (C and D) Building out of jaw and chin in early childhood to normal contour with bank cartilage. (E and F) Absorption of cartilage implant several years later. This should be expected when cartilage is implanted beneath soft tissues, although many remain permanently. (G and H) Final restoration of function and contour, with silicone implant put under the skin in one operation. The patient now has fine features and normal function (3 years). (Brown, J. B., et al.: Silicone and Teflon prostheses. Ann. Surg., 157:932-943)

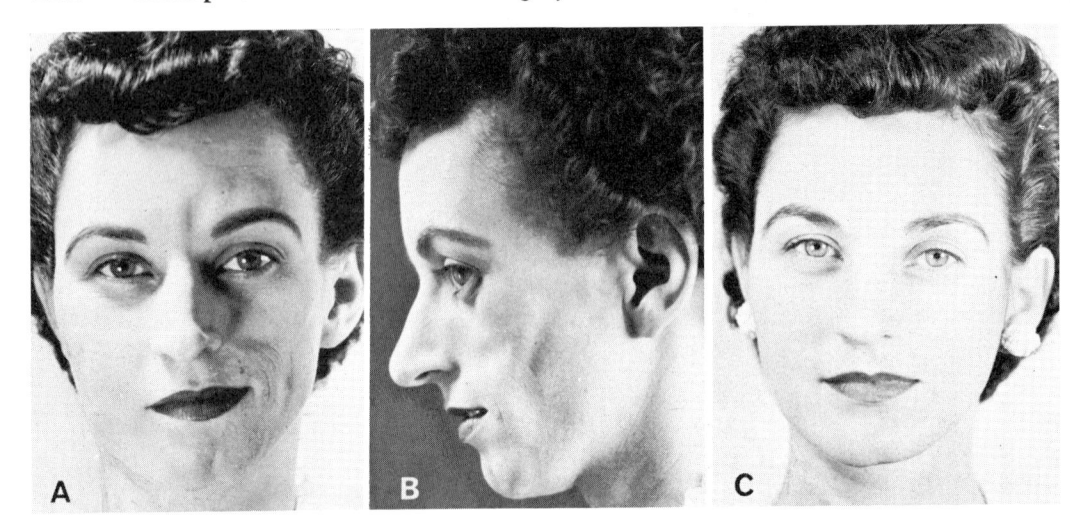

Fig. 49-50. (A and B) Hemiatrophy of face. (C) Face filled out with polyvinyl alcohol synthetic before surface foreshortening was too marked to be relieved. Soft tissues were built out. Realignment of defect with restoration of features, contour and function, and preservation of motor and sensory nerves in spite of necessarily wide undermining. (Brown, J. B., *et al.*: Silicone and Teflon prostheses. Ann. Surg., 157:932-943)

in Figure 49-48. There was a large loss of bone in the maxilla, the nose and the middle third of the face. This defect has been filled in secondarily with a triangular block of silicone rubber with its base upward, because the great loss was above. This has been maintained 3½ years without trouble.

Congenital deficiencies. The application of synthetics in this field has been extended, as in the patient shown in Figure 49-49. Agenesis of the chin region produces a disturbing deformity and upsets a child's progress in many ways. During childhood this patient has had her chin area built out with bank cartilage to a successful degree, as noted from her pleasant features, and the normal smile (Fig. 49-49, C and D).

Homocartilage such as used in this case, both fresh and preserved, may be absorbed, as it was in this patient after several years.

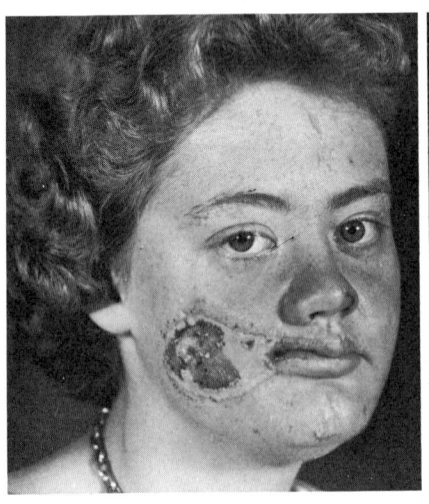

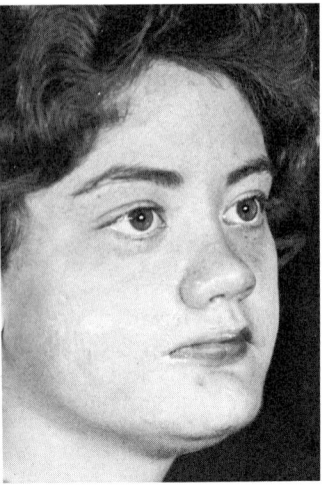

Fig. 49-51. (*Left*) Distortion and loss of facial tissue and contour resulting from traffic accident. (*Right*) Resurfacing with free skin grafts across lip and cheek. Filling of cheek depression with soft synthetic Etheron. Normal function and contour (2 years). (Brown, J. B., *et al.*: Silicone and Teflon prostheses. Ann. Surg., 157:932-943)

This was evidenced by the reappearance of deformity (Fig. 49-49, E and F). By this time the patient was large enough to use her own bone or cartilage. However, in cases such as this, satisfactory support and correction of deformity can be obtained with synthetics and thus save the patient from removal of a rib or a piece of ischium. The correction illustrated in Figure 49-49, G and H, was with silicone, and the correction is good after $3\frac{1}{2}$ years and facial development is normal. Both sensory and motor nerve functions were preserved. This patient and her parents were extremely cooperative, and this was very important to the outcome.

Facial hemiatrophy, a developmental deficiency, also has been further corrected by implantation of *soft synthetics*. The face of the patient shown in Figure 49-50 has been built up during two procedures. As a result, she has become a different individual with a practically normal appearance. The material used for such corrections could be any of the soft synthetics; in this instance it was polyvinyl alcohol sponge, which stays soft when wet and when implanted.

Etheron (di-isocyanate) is a soft white spongy material that has been used for augmentation of soft tissues, such as the face and the breast (Fig. 49-51). At this time Etheron is thought to be superior to polyvinyl alcohol.

REFERENCES

1. Arons, M. S., Sabesin, S. M., and Smith, R. R.: Experimental studies with Etheron sponge. Effect of implantation in tumor-bearing animals. Plast. Reconstr. Surg., 28:72, 1961.
2. Brown, J. B.: Homografting of skin with report of success in identical twins. Surgery, 1:559, 1937.
3. ———: Preserved and fresh homotransplants of cartilage. Surg., Gynec. Obstet., 70:1079, 1940.
4. ———: *In* Womack, N.: On Burns. Springfield, Ill., Charles C Thomas, 1953.
5. ———: Studies of silicones and Teflon as subcutaneous prostheses (Editorial). Plast. Reconstr. Surg., 28:86, 1961.
6. Brown, J. B., *et al.*: Establishing a preserved cartilage bank. Plast. Reconstr. Surg., 3:283, 1948.
7. Brown, J. B., and Cannon, B.: Composite free grafts of skin and cartilage from the ear. Surg., Gynec. Obstet., 82:253-255, 1946.
8. Brown, J. B., Cannon, B., Graham, W., Lischer, C., Scarborough, C., Davis, W., and Moore, A.: Direct flap repair of defects of the arm and hand: preparation of gunshot wounds for repair of nerves, bones and tendons. Ann. Surg., 122:706-715, 1945.
9. Brown, J. B., Cannon, B., Lischer, C., and Davis, W.: Composite free grafts of skin and cartilage from the ear. J.A.M.A., 134:1295-1296, 1947.
10. Brown, J. B., and Fryer, M. P.: Management of compound facial injuries. Am. J. Surg., 76:625-630, 1948.
11. ———: Fracture-dislocation of the zygoma and orbit. Postgrad. Med., 6:400-406, 1949.
12. ———: Treatment of burns: general condition, early definitive care of the local area, and repair of the sequelae; a plan for care of the survivors of an atomic attack or any mass disaster. J. Missouri M.A., 48:973-981, 1951.
13. ———: Tumors in the parotid region: direct surgical approach and preservation of seventh nerve in benign tumors; description of radical operation for malignant tumors. Am. Surgeon, 18:880-890, 1952.
14. ———: Plastic surgery for severe facial paralysis in elderly patients. J. Am. Geriatrics Soc., 11:820-825, 1954.
15. ———: Postmortem homografts to reduce mortality in extensive burns. J.A.M.A., 156:1163-1166, 1954.
16. ———: Multiple internal wire fixation of facial fractures. Am. J. Surg., 89:814-818, 1955.
17. ———: Repair of industrial electrical burns. Plast. Reconstr. Surg., 18:177-184, 1956.
18. ———: Plastic surgical principles in farm, industrial and traffic accidents. A.M.A. Arch. Surg., 72:780-787, 1956.
19. ———: Postmortem Homografts. Springfield, Ill., Charles C Thomas, 1960.
20. Brown, J. B., Fryer, M. P., Kollias, P., Ohlwiler, D. A., and Templeton, J. B.: Silicone and Teflon prostheses, including full jaw substitution: laboratory and clinical studies of Etheron. Ann. Surg., 157:932, 1963.
21. Brown, J. B., Fryer, M. P., and McDowell, F.: Internal wire-pin stabilization for middle third facial fractures. Surg., Gynec. Obstet., 93:676-681, 1951.
22. ———: Permanent pedicle blood-carrying flaps for repairing defects in avascular areas. Ann. Surg., 134:486-494, 1951.
23. Brown, J. B., Fryer, M. P., and Ohlwiler, D. A.: Study and use of synthetic materials, such as silicones and Teflon, as subcutaneous prostheses. Plast. Reconstr. Surg., 26:264, 1960.
24. Brown, J. B., Fryer, M. P., Ohlwiler, D. A., and Kollias, P.: Dimethylsiloxane and halogenated carbons as subcutaneous prostheses. Am. Surg., 28:146, 1962.
25. Brown, J. B., Fryer, M. P., Randall, P., and Lu, M.: Postmortem homografts as "biological dressings" for extensive burns and denuded areas. Ann. Surg., 138:618-630, 1953.
26. ———: Silicones in Plastic Surgery. Plast. Reconstr. Surg., 12:374, 1953.

27. Brown, J. B., Fryer, M. P., Zaydon, T. J.: Establishing a skin bank; use and various methods of preservation of postmortem homografts. Plast. Reconstr. Surg., 16:337-351, 1955.
28. ———: A skin bank for postmortem homografts. Surg., Gynec. Obstet., 101:401-412, 1955.
29. Brown, J. B., and McDowell, F.: Neck Dissection (Am. Lecture Series). Springfield, Ill., Charles C Thomas, 1954.
30. ———: Plastic Surgery of the Nose. St. Louis, C. V. Mosby, 1951.
31. ———: Simplified design for repair of single cleft lips. Surg., Gynec. Obstet., 80:12-26, 1945.
32. ———: Skin Grafting. St. Louis, C. V. Mosby, 1949; Skin Grafting. ed. 3. Philadelphia, J. B. Lippincott, 1958.
33. Brown, J. B., McDowell, F., and Byars, L. T.: Double clefts of the lip. Surg., Gynec. Obstet., 85:20-29, 1947.
34. Brown, J. B., McDowell, F., and Fryer, M. P.: Facial distortion in wryneck prevented by early resection of the fibrosed sternomastoid muscle. Plast. Reconstr. Surg., 5:301-309, 1950.
35. ———: Radiation burns, including vocational and atomic exposures; treatment and surgical prevention of chronic lesions. Ann. Surg., 130:593-607, 1949.
36. ———: Surgery of the Face, Mouth and Jaws. St. Louis, C. V. Mosby, 1954.
37. ———: Surgical treatment of radiation burns. Surg., Gynec. Obstet., 88:609-622, 1949.
38. Brown, J. B., Ohlwiler, D., and Fryer, M. P.: Investigation of and use of dimethyl siloxanes, halogenated carbons and polyvinyl alcohol as subcutaneous prostheses. Am. Surg., 152:534-547, 1960.
39. ———: Study and use of synthetic materials such as silicones and Teflon as subcutaneous prostheses. Plast. Reconstr. Surg., 26:264-279, 1960.
40. Brown, J. B., Peterson, L., Cannon, B., and Lischer, C.: Ankylosis of the coronoid process of the mandible (and associated scar limitation of jaw function). Plast. Reconstr. Surg., 1:277-283, 1946.
41. Fryer, M. P., and Brown, J. B.: Repair of atomic, cathode-ray, cyclotron and x-ray burns of the hand. Long-term follow-up examinations and microscopic studies. Am. J. Surg., 103:688, 1962.
42. Moore, A. M., and Brown, J. B.: Investigation of polyvinyl compounds for use as subcutaneous prostheses. Plast. Reconstr. Surg., 10:453, 1952.
43. Murray, J. F., Merrill, J. P., and Harrison, J. H.: Kidney transplantation in identical twins. Ann. Surg., 148:343, 1958.

BIBLIOGRAPHY

Brown, J. B.: Burns—A Symposium. 2 Chaps. and 3 discussions. Goldman and Gardner, Thomas, Jan. '65.

Brown, J. B., and Fryer, M. P.: Report of surgical repair in the first group of atomic radiation injuries. Surg., Gynec., Obstet., 103:1-6, 1956.

———: Reconstruction of electrical injuries with preliminary report of cathode ray burns. Ann. Surg., 146:Sept., 1957.

———: Hypospadias—complete construction of penis, establishment of proper sex status. Postgrad. Med., 22:489-491, 1957.

———: Peno-scrotal skin losses, repaired by implantation and free skin grafting. Ann. Surg., 145:656-664, 1957.

———: Ankylosis of jaw for 22 years: restoration of function in one operation. Am. Surg., 11-13, 27 Jan. '61.

———: Correction of hypospadias with mistaken sex identity and transvestism resulting in normal marriage and parenthood. Surg., Gynec., Obstet., 118:45-46, 1964.

———: High energy electron injury; radiation injury of chest wall; 17 year follow up on atomic burns. Ann. Surg., 162:426-436, 1965.

Brown, J. B., Fryer, M. P., Ohlwiler, D., and Kollias, P.: Synthetic Replacement for Total Loss of Jaw, etc. Proceedings of Third International Congress of Plastic Surgery, Series No. 66, pp. 745-751, Oct. '63, Amsterdam.

Brown, J. B., McDowell, F., and Fryer, M. P.: Direct operative removal of parotid tumor (facial paralysis). Surg., Gynec., Obstet., 90:1-12, 1950.

Brown, J. B., and Zaydon, T. J.: Early Treatment of Facial Injuries. Lea & Febiger, 1964.

Moyer, C. A., Brentano, L., Gravens, D. S., Margraf, H. W., and Monafo, W. W., Jr.: The treatment of large human burns with dressings continuously wet with a 0.5 per cent aqueous solution of silver nitrate. Arch. Surg., 90:779-867, 1965.

CHAPTER 50

MARK M. RAVITCH, M.D.

Pediatric Surgery

General Considerations
Head and Neck
Thorax
Gastrointestinal Tract
Sacrococcygeal Teratoma and Other Pelvic Tumors

GENERAL CONSIDERATIONS

The inclusion of a chapter on pediatric surgery in a textbook of surgery, initiated in the first edition of this book, and now common practice, is recognition of the growth of interest in this special field and of the significance of the recent accomplishments in it. Certain subjects of pediatric surgical interest are omitted from the present discussion for considerations of space or because they are treated adequately in other chapters. The surgical problems of infancy and childhood differ from those of later life in several ways:

Newborn infants present certain conditions, the continued existence of which, uncorrected, is incompatible with life and which therefore are not seen except by those dealing with infants.

Infants and children are subject to almost all of the conditions seen in later life, but the incidence of these conditions is so different in childhood as to require a rearrangement of the clinical approach to differential diagnosis.

The physical and emotional reactions of infants and children to illness and metabolic derangements frequently differ both qualitatively and quantitatively from the response of adults to the same stimuli. This often calls for a different set of values in the evaluation of symptomatic and objective responses to illness.

In drug therapy, while infants may be more susceptible to the effects of some drugs, they have rather enormous tolerance for others when needed, such as digitalis and the barbiturates.

TIME OF OPERATION

The decision as to when an infant is to undergo an essential surgical procedure, and whether it is to be definitive or temporizing, is no longer widely discussed. It is well understood that infants and children can stand operations of any magnitude, if properly conceived, and executed with appropriate preparation and after-care. There is less tendency to delay operation until the child is older or has reached some token milestone. At the same time the tendency is to make the initial operation definitely corrective rather than a means of preserving the baby until it is "large enough" to be operated upon. Tumors, benign and malignant, should be treated definitively when discovered. Malignant processes are now the leading cause of in-hospital deaths in children (Ariel and Pack, 1960). Far from being considered an unlikely possibility in the presence of a solid mass in an infant or a child, a malignant tumor is the most likely possibility, even at birth. Immediate, thorough, radical operations offer a rewarding percentage of cures, the opportunity for which may be lost by temporizing delays for "study" and "observation."

With congenital anomalies, the aim is to restore the child to as normal a state as possible, as soon as possible, and in as few steps as possible. The condition of the child—as in premature babies with esophageal atresia and tracheo-esophageal fistula—or technical factors imposed by our limitations in dealing with small structures, as in complicated anorectal anomalies, may counsel staged procedures. The not yet overcome technical problems of intracardiac operations in the tiny patient lead to preliminary palliative procedures and postponement of the definitive correction, as in transposition of the great vessels, or large ventricular septal defects. In general, the tendency in pediatric surgery is for the proper operation for a given lesion to be performed whenever the necessity for it is apparent. Small size of the patient and of the structures to be dealt with tends not to be a serious limiting factor in most procedures. Scar tissue, as in intestinal and vascular anastomoses, tends to grow as the anastomosed structures grow, and little difficulty need be anticipated. In plastic reconstructive surgical procedures, as on the nose and the ear, it may be necessary to wait until the feature has attained its final shape and most of its size. New approaches modify old attitudes. The importance of preserving the function of the levator sling in high rectal atresias now counsels a staged operation in the view of many (Stephens, 1963). The development of the Duhamel operation for Hirschsprung's disease has encouraged some to earlier operation for this disease (Steichen, et al., 1968).

Psychologically, it is obvious that the sooner a child is like his fellows in appearance, in deglutition, defecation and urination, in vigor and general stamina, the better he is in every way.

PREPARATION FOR OPERATION

Shortly before the event, to avoid needlessly prolonged anticipation, any child old enough to talk should know that he is coming to a hospital for an operation and that he will be put to sleep. He should be given a brief description of the anesthesia technic, and told that he will be made better and then return home. Hospitalization and operation on a well-ordered service need not be upsetting to a child. It is a "traumatic experience" chiefly to children from homes overcharged with tensions. While I invite mothers to sleep in their children's rooms, I am accustomed to point out that the most painful feature of leaving a child in the hospital is the discovery that he gets along so well. So far as possible, deceptions and misstatements should be avoided. Necessary examinations and treatments should be explained and then performed. Painful procedures should not be heralded as painless. The confidence of a child is too valuable an asset to the physician to be lost for momentary expediency, and once lost is not easily regained.

PREMEDICATION

A drowsy, sedated child is a better candidate for anesthesia than one alarmed and struggling. Children, a year of age or older, may be transported to the operating room drowsy or asleep with 3 to 4 mg. of Nembutal/Kg. body weight given intramuscularly 1 or 1½ hours before operation, together with scopolamine or atropine. The tranquilizer drugs have a place in premedication and particularly in the preparation of the child for uncomfortable or alarming examinations or treatments for which general anesthesia is not required. They are never used on my service for any other purpose. Restlessness, anxiety, nausea are frequently important symptoms, not to be obscured.

Morphine and barbiturates should be avoided in the first 6 months of life, because of the respiratory depression induced by them. Atropine is most important to keep a dry airway, but overdosage in children should be avoided, and the drug is dangerous in hyperpyrexia, dehydration and the presence of high ambient temperatures. If a very rapid pulse, fever, or marked flushing occur following atropine, operation should be postponed. Scopolamine is perhaps a little less likely to give such reactions. In older children, morphine sulfate is given in doses of 1 mg. for each 5 Kg. of body weight. The dosage of atropine is 0.05 mg. *total dose* in the first year of life, 0.2 to 0.3 mg. in the next 2 years, 0.2 to 0.4 mg. thereafter, increasing to the adult dose of 0.6 mg. with large adolescents. Scopolamine is given in slightly lower dosages than atropine.

ANESTHESIA

Anesthetic choices will vary with local experience and preferences. In general, local anesthesia has little place in major pediatric surgery. The struggling of an infant tied to the operating table, straining, expelling intestines through the wound, causes more harm and danger than a skillful inhalation anesthesia. Spinal anesthesia has had a vogue in some clinics but is psychologically a severe trial to older children. We have with satisfaction used caudal anesthesia for inguinal herniorrhaphy in infants. Intravenous barbiturates are useful but considerably more hazardous in children than in adults. The choice is therefore mainly one of inhalant agents and technics. Open drop ether, although providing a wide margin of safety, is not commonly used today. The halogenated hydrocarbons and cyclopropane are widely and satisfactorily used in nonrebreathing systems. Intratracheal anesthesia through an orotracheal tube, appropriately sized and expertly introduced, is invaluable. If intubation has been traumatic, or too large a tube employed, laryngeal injury and edema may result and demand close attention in a moist atmosphere after operation. Infrequently, tracheostomy may be required.

In all pediatric anesthesia, except for the briefest surgical procedures the child is placed on a temperature regulating mattress and the body temperature taken by rectal thermocouple is constantly monitored. Newborn infants, particularly, do not tolerate hypothermia very well: it may be necessary to warm them and it is generally advisable to wrap their limbs with glazed cotton to help preserve body heat. In older children, there is as much risk of hyperthermia as of hypothermia, and probably more hazard from hyperthermia, which is prevented by running cold water through the mattress.

Administration of Blood and Parenteral Fluids

Any parenteral fluid required is given intravenously. With the modern, fine scalp needles attached to plastic tubing, babies can be maintained for considerable periods of time on total intravenous support for hydration and nutrition. "Cut downs" are required only for infants in collapse or those undergoing large operative procedures. In such cases we insert a polyethylene catheter, preferably into the basilic vein, passing it, if possible, to the superior vena cava to obtain the advantage of monitoring the central venous pressure. If the infant is one in whom major fluid or blood losses are expected so that the monitoring of central venous pressure is of particular importance, the catheter is inserted in the external jugular vein (Talbert and Haller, 1966). There is no objection to the use of the saphenous vein just anterior to the internal malleolus. In any of these sites a competent house officer requires no more than a 1-cm. incision. The longer the catheter remains in place, the more likely is phlebitis to occur, with fever, tenderness, redness or induration. Removal of the catheter and application of compresses bring relief. Septic thrombophlebitis is an occasional but rare complication, curable by interruption of the vein proximal to the needle or catheter site (Rush and Ravitch, 1960). The use of rigid aseptic technic in insertion of the catheter, whether by open venoclysis (probably preferable) or percutaneously, and the protection of the catheter-skin junction with Neosporin ointment, reapplied every few days under an occlusive dressing, has recently allowed us to prolong the use of a single venoclysis for weeks or months. The use of a silastic catheter still further prolongs the life of the vein.

There has been a general awareness in recent years that it is safer to carry infant surgical patients "on the dry side," that is, less than fully hydrated, although this should not be carried to excess. Infants will do well in the immediate postoperative period when receiving 75 to 100 ml. of fluid/Kg. body weight/day intravenously, apart from replacement of any special fluid losses. In the neonatal period the lower figures should be used. In recent years a great fetish has been made of "precise" calculations of fluid requirements based on a body surface formula, which is itself an imprecise approximation. We continue to agree with Wilson (Oliver, Graham and Wilson, 1958) that this pretends an accuracy beyond the precision of the method. The sodium requirement may be taken as 1 to 2 mEq./Kg./day. Glucose, 10 per cent, in distilled water serves as the constant intravenous infusion with 0.45 per cent NaCl added as required.

While potassium has great usefulness in patients who have had grave electrolyte losses from vomiting or diarrhea, it is dangerous, and in infants a miscalculation in dosage may be fatal. There is a tendency today to use potassium on almost all patients receiving intravenous therapy. Actually, it need be used only in instances of severe loss of intestinal fluids, the basic requirement being 2 to 3 mEq./Kg./day. In the case of sodium, the pendulum has swung from the old mistake of excessive dosage to the current practice of frequently inadequate dosage leading to sodium depletion. About one quarter of the intravenous fluid may be 0.9 per cent saline, and intestinal drainage should be replaced by 0.45 per cent saline in 10 per cent glucose, volume for volume, over and above the daily requirements. The volume and the specific gravity of the urine are the practical guides to intravenous electrolyte therapy. In infants fluid intake and output should be totaled and evaluated either every 6 or every 8 hours. The adhesive-ring connected urine collectors are invaluable.

Blood, plasma, or human serum albumin for anemia or hypoproteinemia are given in single infusions of 10 to 20 ml./Kg. body weight. Because of the danger of acute cardiac dilatation and pulmonary edema that occasionally attend the rapid infusion of concentrated solutions of human albumin, caution must be taken as to the rate of the intravenous infusion of concentrated albumin solution, especially in infants with cardiac distress and any degree of dehydration. During operation blood must be administered to replace blood loss, volume for volume. In the polycythemic newborn, if blood loss is not excessive, plasma may be used instead of whole blood.

In infants requiring prolonged intravenous alimentation, protein balance becomes a serious problem. For this purpose the protein hydrolysates in 5 per cent solutions may be used in volumes up to a third of the daily fluid requirement. It has now become apparent (Dudrick, Wilmore, Vars and Rhoads, 1968) that, with the use of a central venous catheter, 20 per cent glucose can be administered for long periods of time, allowing adequate caloric intake and this, together with protein hydrolysates and appropriate additions of minerals and of vitamins, will allow an infant to grow, gain weight and develop essentially normally on purely intravenous alimentation. Human serum albumin has some limited nutritional value. On the basis of canine experiments, whole plasma can meet the entire protein requirement if supplemented with sufficient carbohydrate and fat. The small size of the younger pediatric patients makes this approach feasible in the unusual situation in which prolonged parenteral alimentation is necessary. If plasma is to be used, room temperature storage to reduce the chance of transmitting hepatitis virus is recommended (see Chap. 8, Blood Transfusions). Preparations of fat emulsions, suitable for intravenous use, are available and provide a high caloric intake but are still not free from undesirable effects.

Antibiotics

Penicillin remains the most widely applicable and the safest of the antibiotics. Nothing replaces the precise knowledge of the bacterial agent to be combated. Even the preliminary information that the organism is gram positive or gram negative can be enormously useful. It should be automatic to smear pus, sputum, discharge, etc. to obtain this immediate information, without waiting for the culture report from the laboratory (see Chapter on Applied Surgical Bacteriology).

Dressings

For some years now, first in pediatric surgery, and then in adult surgery, we have dispensed with conventional dressings. A layer of flexible collodion, or one of the aerosol plastic sprays, provides a neat covering, protecting the wound from saliva, urine or feces —if any such protection is required. The small patient then is examined more readily and without the necessity for removing adhesive tape and bandage. Buried subcuticular sutures spare surgeon and child the ordeal of suture removal and are employed whenever appropriate.

Activity

In general, within the restricting confines of a hospital, a child who is doing well may be permitted as much activity as he wishes.

HEAD AND NECK

Impetigo and the other troublesome pyodermas of childhood are extremely contagious because of the abundance of bacteria-laden discharge and the susceptibility of the skin of small children. Impetigo contagiosa is a staphylococcic infection of the derma. The lesions occasionally respond to gentle washing with soap and protection of the surrounding skin from constant exposure to pus. For this purpose a soap containing hexachlorophene is preferable. In stubbornly resistant cases, or in instances with sepsis, the appropriate antibiotics should be used systemically; antibiotic ointments are to be avoided, in general. As in pyogenic infections elsewhere, regional lymphadenitis usually becomes manifest while the primary lesion is still acutely inflamed.

Adenitis. Occasionally, adenitis does not appear until after the primary infection has receded, or even healed and been forgotten. In the presence of numerous small shotty nodes in the occipital area and in the posterior triangle of the neck, one should make careful search of the scalp for small crusted lesions which might escape a casual examination. Acute cervical adenitis in the anterior triangle of the neck, particularly under the angle of the mandible, is more likely to have resulted from a pharyngeal infection—not uncommonly a week or two after its subsidence. While lymphadenitis, early in its course, will yield to systemic administration of antibiotics, once suppuration has occurred, incision and drainage is required, as in adults. There is no difficulty in determining that a superficial node, fixed to the skin, red, tender, edematous and fluctuant, is ready for incision. In a deep-lying node, fixation and a brawny elasticity are the early signs of suppuration. Superficially, there develop what ordinarily would be taken as signs of cellulitis—edema, induration, tenderness and a faint violaceous erythema. In general, in deep cervical adenitis, necrosis and liquefaction have occurred well before physical signs are unequivocal. If the old surgical technic of John Hilton is followed—of incising only the skin and finding the pus by blunt dissection with a hemostat—injury to the nerves and the blood vessels need not be feared.

Tuberculous cervical adenitis may be difficult to distinguish from adenitis due to pyogenic bacteria. Either may present as a single node, or as a group of nodes, as a relatively indolent, nontender mass, or as an acute, red, tender, inflammatory process. Chronicity, indolence and extensiveness suggest tuberculosis, apart from the history of exposure, and a positive tuberculin test. Forty or 50 years ago, radical resection of the cervical nodes, the jugular vein and the sternocleiodomastoid muscle was the standard treatment for cervical tuberculosis. Its proved inefficacy and lack of demonstrable advantage finally brought the operation into disuse in favor of rest, vitamins, ultraviolet light treatment and, for liquefied nodes, aspiration (Charcot's *aspiration à distance*, through an oblique tract commencing in healthy skin to avoid formation of a sinus tract).

The advent of streptomycin and an increasing number of other effective antituberculous drugs has altered our approach to tuberculous adenitis which is, in any case, less common than formerly. Early processes will respond to specific drug therapy. The hazard of excisional biopsy for histologic confirmation of the diagnosis has been reduced considerably; and incision and drainage of a broken-down tuberculous process, under the mistaken impression that it is pyogenic, is no longer so deplorable an error. A mass of tuberculous nodes not responding or disappearing under antimycobacterial therapy may be relatively safely excised. The surgeon is warned that seemingly localized masses of tuberculous lymph nodes will prove to be surrounded in all directions by other involved nodes that logically should be removed, and that an apparently movable mass may be found fixed to the jugular vein and the spinal accessory or other nerves, so that frequently a major dissection is required for what was intended as a limited resection. Atypical acid fast bacilli are beginning to appear as an increasingly common cause of chronic cervical adenitis, particularly in Australia.

B.C.G. Adenitis. Prophylaxis against tuberculosis, by inoculation with the bovine tubercle bacillus results in adenitis, axillary or cervical, in 5 per cent of infants, occasionally to an impressive degree. The disease is usually self-limited, occasionally generalized and rarely fatal (Horwitz, 1957).

Lymphosarcoma, Hodgkin's disease and other malignant processes as well as Letterer-Siwe's form of lipoid histiocytosis, may produce masses of enlarged cervical lymph nodes as their first manifestation. If the remainder of the clinical picture does not make the diagnosis, local physical examination is not likely to, although in Hodgkin's disease the swelling is most likely to be unilateral and in Letterer-Siwe's least likely. Biopsy is required to establish the diagnosis. Radical operative procedures for lymphosarcoma and Hodgkin's disease, when apparently localized, are advocated by some and have been practiced from time to time. The firm, discrete, nontender enlarged lymph node is better biopsied than neglected.

The new knowledge of the classification of the forms of Hodgkin's disease (Lukes and Butler, 1966) and the effectiveness of extensive, well-planned irradiation (Kaplan and Rosenberg, 1966) have transformed the prognosis of this disease.

Sternocleidomastoid tumor in newborn babies presents as a firm nontender tumor, usually in the mid-portion of the muscle. The cause is unknown (Jones, 1968). The resultant torticollis or wryneck, with the head tilted toward the shoulder of the affected side, is alarming to parents who can be reassured that disappearance of the tumor and recovery of full and normal motion is the rule. The use of sandbags to hold the head straight while the baby sleeps may be of more benefit to the parents than to the baby. Excision of the tumor, counseled by some, may be postponed for 6 to 8 months, awaiting spontaneous relief. (See Chap. 49, Principles of General Plastic Surgery.)

Dermoid cysts about the supra-orbital ridge and the margins of the glabella are small, tense, hard, round and unattached to the skin. The frontal bone at operation will be found to be scooped out to hold the cyst, and occasionally preliminary roentgenograms will show a circular defect in the frontal bone. The cysts, even in such cases, are readily removed and have no intimate attachment to the intracranial tissues. Meningoceles in the same position are softer but become tense when the child cries.

Preauricular pits (fistula auris congenita) represent one of the curious hereditary defects (Stiles, 1945) associated with the embryonic branchial clefts and arches in a fashion still disputed. They occur in the tragus, in front of it or in the ascending portion of the helix and occasionally in the lobe of the ear. They may safely be ignored except for those few which become infected. At the time of infection the edema may obscure a tiny external orifice so that the source of infection is obscure, since patients and parents are commonly unaware of the existence of these pits. At operation, once the infection has subsided, the orifice is circumscribed and sinus and the cyst from which it comes are removed intact.

The more complicated anomaly of the first pranchial cleft consists of a fistula open at one end inside the external auditory canal and at the other below the angle of the mandible (Byars, 1951).

The parotid gland may be the site of inflammatory processes other than the virus parotitis of mumps. In the newborn, purulent parotitis occurs (Sanford, 1954), with high fever, parotid swelling and pus expressible from Stensen's duct, with the *Staphylococcus aureus* as the usual organism. In older children, mild, recurrent parotitis with pus in the duct and no demonstrable stones may produce a puzzling picture. Division of the sphincter of the duct and irrigation of the duct give relief. Tumors of the parotid gland in children occur in all the varieties seen in adults (Howard, 1950), and some, such as hemangiomas and lymphangiomas, occur principally in children. Sarcomas, mixed salivary gland tumor, papillary cystadenoma lymphomatosum and carcinoma, both of the slower growing cylindroma type and of the more malignant muco-epidermoid type, all occur in children. Once more the liability of children to malignant tumors must be borne in mind and therapy instituted appropriate to the lesion rather than some inadequate modification urged out of mistaken consideration for the tender age of the patient and the disbelief that one so young could harbor so malignant a tumor.

Oral Tumors. In the mouth, cysts of the mucous glands, on the lip, the tongue, the floor of the mouth, hemangiomas and lymphangiomas may all give smooth, rounded painless cystic tumors, inconvenient because of their location but readily excised. More diffuse hemangiomas, at times invasive, are more serious lesions but sometimes respond well to irradiation (see Chap. 18, Radiation Injury, for necessity of careful shielding). Diffuse lymphangiomatous tumors of tongue and lip, one cause of macroglossia (Ward, 1950) and macrocheilia, are deforming lesions, vexingly difficult to treat. Carefully planned repeated partial excisions may succeed in instances in which the process has not extended to invade neighboring tissues.

Epignathus. A bizarre variety of oral lesions has been reported in the newborn, epignathus, mucous cysts at the base of tongue, often causing difficulty in respiration or nursing.

Pierre Robin Syndrome. Mandibular retrusion or underdevelopment, often associated with cleft palate, in essence provides a mouth too small for the tongue, which falls back to obstruct the pharynx, making feeding difficult and causing dangerous respiratory obstruction. Suture traction on tongue or mandible is an unpleasant measure and is difficult to maintain, except as a temporary expedient. Advancing the tongue by incision and resuture in the floor of the mouth satisfactorily relieves the obstruction. Tracheostomy is a seemingly obvious first measure but can and should be avoided. A tracheostomy inserted in the neonatal period is too often extraordinarily difficult to abandon. Gavage feedings may tide the infant over the first few weeks until he is able to hold his jaw forward. (See also Chap. 49.) Dennison (1967) points out that an infant can be satisfactorily managed by tube feedings prone and the head held extended with stockinette-cap traction.

Choanal Atresia. Occasionally, the choanae are occluded by a bony block, covered over with unbroken mucosa so that no communication exists between the nares and the nasopharynx. Newborn infants find difficulty in breathing through the mouth and may literally suffocate before the diagnosis of choanal atresia is made, or, unable to master the technic of alternate swallowing and breathing, may starve. Associated deformities of eyes or the nasal passages, or excessive nasal discharge, and rhinorrhea of tears during crying suggest the diagnosis. Relief is afforded by transpalatine construction of an epithelium-lined nasopharyngeal passage (McKillin, 1957).

Ranula, a retention cyst of the sublingual or submaxillary salivary gland ducts, presents in the floor of the mouth as a thin-walled, softly fluctuant cyst. The cause for its development, although not settled is presumably an inflammatory obstruction. Treatment is by complete excision, or by an unroofing procedure in which the mucous membrane of the floor of the mouth and the underlying superficial wall of the cyst are removed, allowing the deep wall of the cyst to form the new oral mucosa.

Cystic hygroma (hygroma cysticum colli, cervical lymph hygroma), although occasionally seen in adults without previous history of a cervical swelling, is a characteristic lesion of infancy and childhood, usually present and recognized at birth. The swelling is rounded, extremely soft, fluctuant, usually lobulated and often transilluminates well. Characteristically, it originates in the posterior cervical triangle but may extend into the anterior triangle, the axilla or the mediastinum, or may be limited largely to one of these. The tumor is composed of a very thin-walled endothelial sac, usually multilocular (Gross and Hurwitt, 1948; Ravitch, 1969). The several large locules, both communicating and noncommunicating, generally have attached processes of tissue honeycombed by tiny cysts containing the same clear, slightly yellowish fluid, and ramifying between muscles, around vessels and nerves, often enveloping these. Hygromas occur at the time when the lymphatic system forms in the embryo from the venous system. Large hygromas cause the head to be held to the opposite side. In the anterior triangle, large hygromas, especially those suddenly increasing in size from hemorrhage within them, may cause pharyngeal compression and respiratory obstruction. Infection in the cysts, usually in association with a pharyngitis, produces severe symptoms. Antibiotic treatment should be given before decision as to incision and drainage. The uncomeliness of the swelling, the inconvenience it causes, its likelihood to infection, its tendency to growth and extension, all constitute reasons for the removal of these cysts. Irradiation, often employed, is ineffective. Operation may be undertaken as soon after birth as the patient presents himself. The delicacy of the cysts, and the difficulty of the dissection if the cysts rupture, require a painstaking dissection in the course of which the major deep structures of the neck will be exposed. If all the major cyst walls are removed and as much as possible of the tongues and extensions of watery lymphangiomatous tissue in areas not permitting block excision, recurrence is rare. Lymphangiomas in the parotid area are usually superficial to the gland but may surround the facial nerve which must be preserved. About the head and the neck and elsewhere, lymphangiomas, particularly those associated with hemangiomas and classified at times as "mixed angiomas," may infiltrate tissues to such a degree as to require radical excision. In such angiomas, repeated re-recurrence is not at all uncommon (Harkins and Sabiston, 1960, 1951; Bill, 1969). (See also Chap. 26.)

Lateral branchial cleft cysts, derived from the 3rd and the 4th branchial clefts, appear characteristically along the anterior border of the sternocleidomastoid muscle. They are thick-walled, unilocular cysts, occasionally with open communications to the skin or the pharynx. The lining is ciliated columnar epithelium, occasionally squamous, with prominent submucosal lymphoid tissue. Diagnostic aspiration shows cholesterol crystals in the thin yellow fluid. The cysts may become infected and very rarely, late in life, may be the site of a carcinoma. Operative removal is curative and, except in those with an internal pharyngeal communication, is technically simple.

The thyroid, in the newborn, is the seat of **cellular hemangiomas, teratomata and colloid goiters.** These have in common the production of respiratory obstruction by laryngeal, tracheal and pharyngeal compression. Operation for relief of the obstruction by resection of the tumor or splitting of the thyroid isthmus in goiters should be undertaken at once, with tracheotomy being resorted to instead if facilities for intratracheal anesthesia and definitive surgery are lacking. In general, it may be said that whenever the advisability of tracheotomy or intubation is being considered, the procedure is already overdue. Neonatal goiters may occur in babies born of mothers treated with thiourea drugs or with cobalt or other goitrogens during gestation.

Ectopic thyroid tissue presents as a lingual goiter or median subhyoid thyroid. In either case this is usually the only thyroid tissue in the body and removal requires lifelong substitution therapy. Median, subhyoid thyroid may be split and the two halves, with blood supply intact, placed in the tracheo-esophageal sulcus on either side (Ravitch and Rush, 1969).

Acute thyroiditis produces a painful, tender, modestly enlarged thyroid, usually self-limited, in association with an upper respiratory infection. Chronic lymphocytic thyroiditis of the Hashimoto type is being diagnosed with increasing frequency as a result of the availability of tests for antithyroglobulins and the observation that there appears a diagnostic disparity in the protein-bound iodine and butanol-extractable-iodine values of the serum (Winter, Eberlein and Bongiovanni, 1966).

Carcinoma of the thyroid occurs in children and forms a far higher proportion of childhood thyroid nodules than of adult thyroid nodules, so that all thyroid nodules in children should be removed with the possibility of cancer and a radical operation in mind (Tawes and de Lorimier, 1968; Winship and Rosvall, 1961). It has been generally held that whereas malignant neoplasms in most of the body appear to grow more rapidly and kill more quickly in younger patients, thyroid cancers represent an exception and are more benign in children than in adults. At least one publication (Winship and Chase, 1955) tends to cast doubt on this assertion, claiming from careful analysis of published material that cancer of the thyroid, type for type, is no more and no less malignant and no different in distribution in children than in adults. The relationship of thyroid cancer to previous— even low dosage—irradiation of the neck is well established (Hagler, Rosenblum and Rosenblum, 1966). The nature, the prognosis and proper treatment of thyroid carcinoma in general continues to be in hot dispute (cf. Chap. 28, p. 721) (Klopp *et al.*, 1967). I favor resection of the entire involved lobe and ipsilateral glands of the neck and lifelong thyroid hormone administration. Most clinicians have felt that any relative melioration of prognosis in childhood thyroid cancer is explained by a greater frequency of papillary carcinoma of the kind associated with the indolent metastases once thought to be lateral aberrant thyroid tissue.

Goiter. Diffuse goiters of the colloid type in children usually will respond to treatment with desiccated thyroid or iodides. Diffuse toxic goiter occurs in children. Although nonoperative treatment is usually followed, the course is prolonged and the outcome uncertain, so that a good case can be made, specifically in children, for primary operative treatment (Ravitch and Rush, 1969).

The thymus may falter in its embryologic descent into the thorax from the 3rd pharyngeal pouch. There may result a persistent cervical or cervicomediastinal thymus, causing pressure on the trachea and presenting as a cervical mass made more conspicuous by coughing or crying. The mass may be so soft as to suggest a hygroma. Removal of the thymus, in these uncommon instances, is curative (Arnheim, 1950). Irradiation in this area is to be avoided because of a 1 to 2 per cent incidence of thyroid carcinoma developing later in childhood.

FIG. 50-1. Pectus excavatum. A 6-year-old girl with marked pectus excavatum. Before operation (*left*) note the retraction of the sternum and protrusion of the abdomen. (*Right*) 9 months after operation the chest expanded normally, with deep inspiration, and the abdomen no longer protruded.

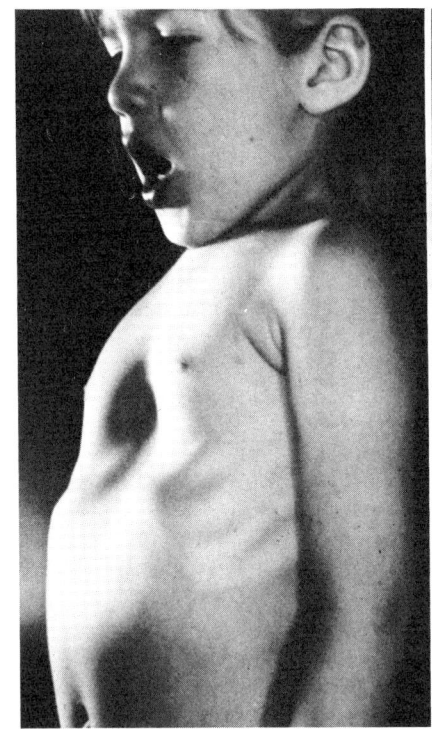

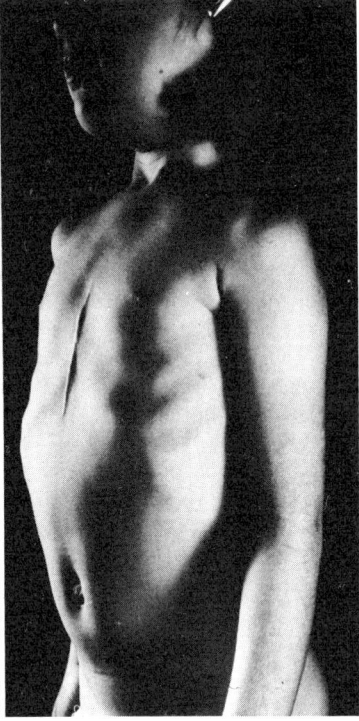

Later cervical tumors of childhood include teratomas (Ravitch and McGoon, 1960), carotid body tumors, tumors of spinal nerves, tumors of the cranial nerves, tumors of the sympathetic nerve trunks and ganglia, and even of the ganglion nodosum of the vagus nerve (Clay, 1950).

THORAX

CHEST WALL

Anomalies. A variety of deformities of the chest wall are seen in infants (Ravitch, 1969). In the mid-line there may be sternal defects varying from an incomplete cleft to a wide separation of the embryologically paired sternal halves. The heart, covered by thin skin or only by a transparent membranous tissue, may protrude through such a defect, in the anomaly known as *thoracic ectopia cordis*. With clefts of the upper sternum, the heart seems to be in the neck; hence the misnomer *cervical ectopia cordis*. With clefts of the lower sternum (*thoracoabdominal ectopia cordis*), a syndrome is recognized with a pentalogy of defects—distal sternal cleft, ventral abdominal defect, anterior diaphragmatic defect, pericardial defect and interventricular septal defect or diverticulum of the ventricle (Cantrell, Haller and Ravitch, 1958). Separation of the sternal halves is readily corrected by simple suture in the neonatal period when the chest wall is maximally flexible. In older children, plastic procedures are required. Major degrees of ectopia cordis have seldom been corrected successfully, in part because severe associated cardiac anomalies usually are present.

Pectus Excavatum. The sternum may be either depressed or abnormally prominent. In *pectus excavatum* (funnel breast, trichterbrust) there is a dorsal displacement of the sternum, forming a concavity from above downward and from side to side. The costal cartilages, from the 3rd or the 4th to the costal margin, are sharply depressed toward the sunken sternum. The deformity is congenital, often familial, and usually progressive during childhood. The children exhibit paradoxical retraction of the sternum and protrusion of the abdomen during deep inspiration. Poor posture—kyphosis, rounded shoulders, forward thrust neck—is characteristic. The heart is usually displaced to the left and rotated. Murmurs and minor degrees of electrocardiographic change indicative of rotation are common. Arrhythmias are frequent. Symptoms rarely appear before adolescence, when easy fatigability may be noticed. Mild dysphagia is not rare in infants, and in three babies we have seen severe inspiratory stridor, relieved by operation. In a few individuals, severe cardiac distress ultimately occurs. The deformity is easily corrected (Fig. 50-1). Indications and technics among surgeons vary (Welch, 1958; Peters and Johnson, 1963; Morris, 1961). The writer of this chapter feels that the corrective operation should be performed in all infants or children with pronounced or progressive defects, in the absence of serious associated anomalies of overriding importance. Our preference is for subperichondrial resection of all of the deformed cartilages, division of the intercostal bundles, xiphisternal disarticulation, transverse osteotomy of the posterior cortex of the sternum above the cephalic extremity of the defect, elevation of the sternum and maintenance in corrected position by heavy silk sutures across the sternal osteotomy in which a chock-block of rib bone has been wedged. In well over 250 such procedures, symptoms have been relieved in all patients who had them; gain in weight and vigor has been extremely common, and the reconstruction has usually been excellent. Morbidity is low, and mortality almost nonexistent. External fixation is never employed, and internal fixation is not used often.

In pigeon breast (pectus carinatum) the sternum buckles forward, to the accompaniment of deep lateral depression of the costal cartilages on either side. Much less common than funnel chest, this deformity is also congenital. The lateral depressions may compress the heart or significantly decrease lung volume. Operation to elevate the lateral runnels produces a gratifying result.

Absence of Ribs or Costal Cartilages. A bizarre variety of absence or deformities of ribs occurs. Associated hemivertebrae, predisposing to scoliosis, may be more significant than the rib anomalies. A syndrome is seen of absence of the costal portion of the pectoralis major, absence of the pectoralis minor, hypoplasia of breast and subcutaneous tissue and absence of costal cartilages II, III and IV. Appropriate plastic reconstruction with rib grafts supporting a Teflon felt prosthesis fills out and bridges over these defects (Ravitch, 1966).

Harrison's groove, a transverse groove on either side at the line of diaphragmatic insertion, above the costal margin which is thus made to flare, is one of the most common thoracic deformities. It may be associated with rickets. It does not appear to be surgically remediable.

Asymmetry of Thorax. The plastic, growing chest wall of a child is readily influenced by pressures from within, and thoracic asymmetries must not be dismissed as idiopathic without study to be sure that the space requirements of an enormous but slow-growing dermoid or other tumor or of a hypertrophied heart or the changes associated with a congenitally absent lung are not the cause of a striking difference in the shape of one side of the chest or the other.

Tumors of the chest wall occur so early in infancy as to make it probable, despite their frequently malignant nature, that they have been present from birth. *Chondromas of ribs and sternum* occur, may reach great size and after any but radical excision tend to recur, with ultimately fatal outcome. *Sarcomas of the chest wall* occur and a wide variety of tumors of neural origin—*neurofibromas, ganglioneuromas* and *paragangliomas* of the sympathetic chain. *Ewing's tumor* may manifest itself in a rib. Whenever possible, in dealing with chest wall tumors, wide, en bloc dissection of full thickness of chest wall should be employed, except for the essentially intrathoracic nerve tumors (Ravitch, 1969).

MEDIASTINUM

(See also Chap. 47, Carcinoma of the Lung and Tumors of the Thorax.)

Tumors. In the anterior mediastinum, 2 principal types of tumors occur in childhood —dermoids-teratomas and lymphomas (Ravitch and Sabiston, 1969; Heimburger and Battersby, 1965). The dermoids and the teratomas are the same tumor with different manifestations. The characteristic dermoid is made up of ectodermal derivatives and shows keratinizing squamous epithelium, sweat and sebaceous glands, hair and teeth—any or all of these. Almost invariably, if sufficient care is taken, an area will be found in the wall of the cyst in which there are abnormal tissues from other germ layers. The teratomata are characteristically more obviously derived from all three germ layers, as often solid as cystic, and show various types of abnormal appearing secretory epithelium, respiratory epithelium, glial tissue characteristically, bone and cartilage and, in fact, tissue of all types (Ravitch and McGoon, 1963). *Dermoids* rarely become malignant but may reach enormous size, compress and displace the thoracic structures, become infected and rupture into pleural cavity, pericardium or bronchus. Sudden increase in size or symptoms from an anterior mediastinal tumor, suggesting the malignant transformation of one element in a teratoma, is a frequent occurrence. Dermoids and teratomata should be removed before complications occur. The diagnosis of any mediastinal tumor is likely to be uncertain in advance of operation, and the position usually taken, when such a tumor is demonstrated by x-ray studies, is that operation is the only safe course with any mediastinal tumor. If lymphosarcoma or Hodgkin's disease is discovered, operation will have given a definitive histologic diagnosis on which to base chemotherapy and roentgenotherapy, and local extirpation itself may have some value.

The pericardium itself is, rarely, the site of a dermoid or other tumor, and occasionally a defect in the pericardium is continuous with a defect in the diaphragm so that herniation of the abdominal viscera takes place into the pericardial sac, producing a radiologic appearance suggestive of an intrapericardial tumor (Thomsen *et al.*, 1954).

Tumors of the posterior mediastinum are particularly those of the neural elements—*neurofibroma, ganglioneuroma, paraganglioma*. These are slow-growing and become malignant in an uncertain but probably high percentage of cases (Kent *et al.*, 1944). The roentgenographic appearance is of a dense, rounded, discrete, posteriorly placed lesion. The tumors, particularly the ganglioneuromas, are occasionally of enormous size and then may produce pressure symptoms. The neurofibromata, which always should be looked for here in patients with von Recklinghausen's neurofibromatosis, occasionally may show a dumbbell shape with extension through the vertebral foramina into the vertebral canal. Neuroblastomata, malignant and rapidly growing, may require combinations of operative therapy, irradiation and chemotherapy for maximal benefit.

The esophagus, in the posterior mediastinum, is a source of a number of lesions peculiar to infancy and childhood.

Esophageal Atresia

One of the most gratifying chapters in the history of pediatric surgery deals with the development of the operation for the correction of esophageal atresia with tracheo-esophageal fistula (Fig. 50-2) (Holder and Ashcraft, 1966). The condition in over 90 per cent of cases consists of a blind, proximal esophageal segment, dilated and hypertrophied as the result of obstruction to fetal deglutition, and ending at the level of the 3rd to the 5th dorsal vertebra. A few strands of muscle connect it to the distal segment which communicates openly with the trachea. In the other cases, both ends may have a fistulous communication to the trachea, or neither end, or solely the proximal end, or the distal esophagus may be altogether rudimentary (Haight, 1969). First treated as an anatomic curiosity beyond correction and invariably fatal, atresia was then attacked in laborious multistage operations designed to establish drainage of the proximal esophagus to the exterior, close the tracheo-esophageal fistula, open the distal esophagus or stomach to the exterior, and finally to link the esophageal and gastric fistulae by a tube of skin or intestine, thus restoring deglutition and completing the operation. Leven, in 1938, and Ladd, 24 hours later, each saved the life of the first of a series of infants operated upon by this complicated scheme. In 1941, Cameron Haight of Ann Arbor, after the unsuccessful experiences of Lanman, Sampson and Shaw, performed the first successful 1-stage division and closure of a tracheo-esophageal fistula and end-to-end anastomosis of the esophageal segments. Haight's operation was performed through an extrapleural exposure of the posterior mediastinum from the left side. The right-sided extrapleural approach, which avoids the aorta, became standard soon after. A number of surgeons (Gross, 1953; Potts and Idriss, 1960) prefer the technically more attractive right transpleural approach. The increased ease of achieving a perfect anastomosis is almost precisely offset by the increased hazard of an

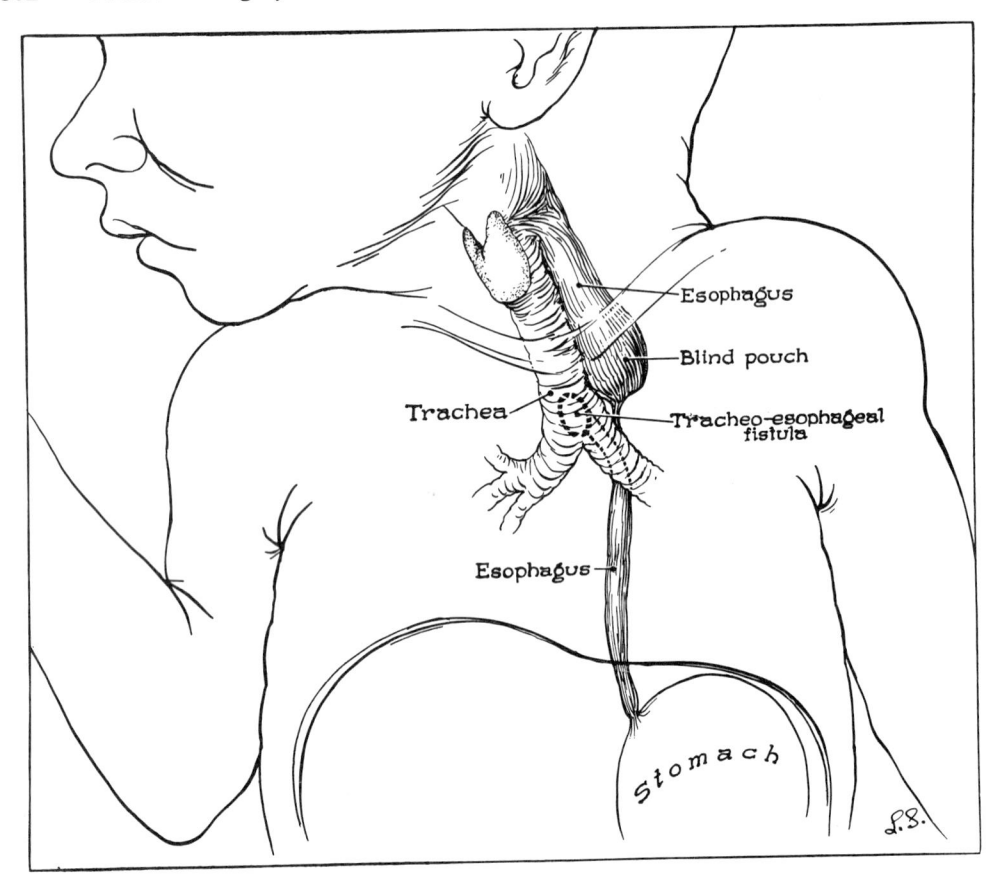

FIG. 50-2. Esophageal atresia with tracheo-esophageal fistula. In over 90 per cent of the cases of esophageal atresia, the anomalies are found as pictured here. The proximal, blind esophagus is dilated and hypertrophied from the obstruction of fetal swallowing. A few strands of muscle attach it to the slender distal segment. The fistulous communication with the distal segment is to the trachea just above the carina. Aspiration of regurgitated saliva from the obstructed esophageal pouch and of gastric juice directly into the trachea through the fistula leads to atelectasis and pneumonia. The operation consists of division of the fistulous tract, closure of the tracheal opening and anastomosis of the esophageal segments. (Ravitch, M. M.: S. Clin. N. Am., 29:1541)

anastomotic leak when it is intrapleural (Holder, 1964).

The condition is to be suspected in an infant, often premature, who bubbles spittle and chokes and becomes cyanotic when nursing. Attempted passage of a firm radiopaque rubber catheter under fluoroscopic control confirms the diagnosis. A cubic centimeter of Diontosil may be injected in the catheter which has been seen to meet an obstruction and turn back on itself. After a roentgenogram has been taken the radiopaque material is withdrawn. Pneumonia commonly of the right upper lobe, from gastric juice regurgitated into the trachea through the fistula, and from overflow from the blind esophageal pouch into the pharynx, with reflux, or aspiration into the trachea, presents the greatest hazard in these infants. Preoperative treatment consists of tracheal aspiration, constant suction of the esophageal pouch, with the head of the crib elevated so that the pooled saliva is aspirated readily as it accumulates in the pouch, correction of dehydration, and administration of antibiotics. The operation is not an emergency procedure but undertaken when the baby has been evaluated and the aspiration pneumonia overcome. If there is to be a delay, gastrostomy will prevent gastric reflux into the trachea. For prematures, in babies with other anomalies, or in babies with severe pulmonary infection, a staged operation is performed (Holder, 1966). At the first stage the fistula is closed and a gastrostomy performed. The esophageal ends are anastomosed when the initial problems have been overcome, care being taken to keep the pharyngeal pouch aspirated in the interim. In full-term babies in good condition a one-stage reconstruction is performed. Gastrostomy need not be routinely performed. Postoperative strictures are not rare and may be dilated fairly readily. If the anastomosis fails or is impossible, the surgeon may resort to a swifter version of the old multi-staged operations. Esophageal reconstruction with a transpleural colonic loop lying behind the lung root is presently the simplest and most satisfactory type (Waterston, 1969).

As in all neonatal surgery, the two factors contributing most to increased mortality are prematurity and the existence of associated anomalies. In full-term babies without other anomalies a salvage of 90 to 95 per cent should be achieved, whereas in premature infants who also have other anomalies, the salvage may be only 40 to 46 per cent (Waterston, Carter and Aberdeen, 1962).

Esophageal Strictures

Congenital strictures of the esophagus are much more rare than atresias. At birth, the child appears to be able to swallow, but gradually the retention above the stricture leads to stasis and edema and complete occlusion of the esophagus days or weeks after birth. Immediate gastrostomy, pharyngeal suction and subsequent dilatation on a swallowed string have been regularly curative in our hands. Resection, or plastic reconstruction of the stenotic area, is feasible but rarely necessary (Sandblom, 1948).

Hiatus hernia in the newborn is manifested by regurgitation and malnutrition. The vomiting may be forceful enough to suggest pyloric stenosis. At times peptic esophagitis and stricture result. In most cases the condition responds if the infant is maintained constantly in the erect position. Occasionally operation is required to repair the hernia (Waterston, 1969). Currently we prefer the Nissen procedure of intra-abdominal fundiplication together with closure of the hiatus (Ravitch, Rowe and Halperin, 1968).

Acquired strictures, from the ingestion of escharotics—usually lye—are better prevented than corrected. In all children thought to have swallowed lye, immediate esophagoscopy is performed to avoid the necessity for treatment of the majority in whom no burn of the esophagus will be found. If burns of the esophagus are found, then our preference is now for combined therapy with prednisone and penicillin for at least 6 weeks, with periodic bouginage for calibration of the esophagus during this period and for several months thereafter to detect any incipient stricture formation (Ray and Morgan, 1956; Schobel, 1959). If the strictures form, dilatation, with or without temporary gastrostomy, will restore deglutition in most cases (Gellis and Holt, 1942; Gross, 1953). In severe or neglected cases, the esophageal channel may be so tortuous that success cannot be achieved, or the lumen actually may be entirely obliterated. In such instances, esophageal substitution is made, preferably today with a loop of colon brought through the pleural cavity to connect the cervical esophagus and the stomach. The ingestion of chlorine-liberating bleaches is now common. They usually do not cause esophageal injury, but can do so (Weeks and Ravitch, 1969).

Mediastinal cysts of foregut origin, the so-called duplications of the esophagus (Fallon, Gordon and Hendrun, 1954; Ladd and Scott, 1944), like enteric cysts associated with any other part of the alimentary canal, are thick-walled, muscular structures lined by gastric, intestinal or colonic epithelium, and filled with thin mucoid secretion. Usually they are united so closely to the wall of the esophagus as to be fused to it. A communication with the esophageal lumen is rare. Spinal deformities are frequently associated. The cysts tend to be large, swelling out into the pleural cavity, more often the right. Symptoms are caused by compression of the esophagus, the trachea or the bronchus. In many instances, the cyst is lined by gastric mucosa, secreting acid, and eroding into the lung, the bronchus or the esophagus, with bleeding as a prominent symptom. Treatment consists of removal of the cyst or the cyst lining. Anastomosis of the cyst to the esophagus is acceptable treatment for those cysts not lined by gastric mucosa.

PLEURA

Chylothorax is seen in the neonatal period, presumably from rupture of the thoracic duct as a result of venous distention and back pressure during the birth process, or from congenital fistulae, and at any age from trauma or from obstruction by tumors or tuberculosis, and rarely from no apparent cause. Today surgical trauma during thoracic, particularly cardiovascular, procedures is probably the most common cause. In the neonatal instances, dyspnea and signs of fluid lead to thoracentesis and discovery of a milky fluid (Randolph and Gross, 1957). If dyspnea is relieved by thoracenteses or catheter drainage, the accumulation of chyle will presently cease in most instances, although successful ligation of the thoracic duct on both sides of a leak usually can be achieved if aspiration therapy fails after an adequate trial. Before ligation is attempted, 3 to 4 days of intravenous alimentation with *nothing* being given orally, and constant intercostal catheter drainage, may permit spontaneous closure. Chyle—intestinal lymph—is not formed in quantity unless food or drink is ingested.

Empyema. Once almost the only commonly treated thoracic condition in pediatric surgery, postpneumonic empyema is now almost a clinical rarity. It occurs relatively earlier in the course of the disease than in adults, and the susceptibility of the small bronchi to necrosis leads to frequent occurrence of pyopneumothorax. While persistent and continued attempts at aspiration of pus and instillation of antibiotics may result in an appreciable percentage of recoveries, early trochar thoracotomy and tube drainage will promptly cure most childhood empyemas at the cost of the single manipulation. Delay in healing, as evidenced by persistence of fever or tachycardia or arrest in the decrease of the volume of the empyema cavity, should raise the question of rib resection and open drainage (see Chap. 46, Surgery of the Lung) or decortication.

Streptococcal and influenza pneumonia and empyema have disappeared. Pneumococcal empyema is uncommon. Staphylococcal empyema in infancy reached epidemic proportions about 1954 to 1956, but has since undergone a sharp decrease in incidence, although it is still commoner than any other form (Ravitch and Fein, 1961). Characteristic of staphylococcal pneumonia is the appearance of air sacs or pneumatoceles. These result from bronchial necrosis and escape of air into the parenchyma. Great enlargement of the cysts may cause dyspnea, and rupture of the cysts may cause tension pneumothorax. Earlier in the course of staphylococcal pneumonia massive effusions may cause severe dyspnea. Catheter suction drainage is required for empyema, massive effusions, pneumothorax and for rapidly expanding pneumatoceles (Sabiston, Hopkins, Cooke and Bennett, 1961).

LUNGS

Agenesis of the lung may occur in several forms. There may be true aplasia of lung and bronchus with no trace of either, aplasia of the lung with the bronchus represented by a blind pouch or by a nodule of cartilage and fibrous tissue, or extreme hypoplasia of the lung in which the main bronchus appears to be normal but ends in a fleshy rudiment of lung. In some instances, the anomaly is little more than a physical and roentgenographic curiosity—one half of the thorax or more being occupied by the one good lung, the other containing the much-displaced heart. In other instances, in infancy, extreme respiratory difficulty and death occur (Maier and Gould, 1953). It is not clear why the absence of one lung should produce fatal respiratory difficulty. Maier suggests that the single pulmonary artery in its abnormal course may compress the trachea or the single bronchus, causing a fatal respiratory obstruction.

Neonatal Atelectasis, Aspiration and Pneumothorax. In the newborn, failure of areas of the lung to expand, obstruction by excessive aspiration of amniotic fluid, or hyaline membrane disease may be suspected in the cyanotic infant with difficult respirations. Congenital pneumonia seems to be more frequent than was realized previously. Physical examination may show areas of decreased aeration and roentgenograms usually will show opaque areas in the lungs. Infants with congenital cerebral defects or brain damage may fail to breathe well enough to expand normal alveoli. In very premature infants, the pulmonary tissue may not be capable of expansion.

Excessive aspiration of amniotic fluid leads to grave difficulties or death. Skillful bronchoscopic aspiration may produce dramatic improvement. Infants with extensive areas of unexpanded lung and making forceful (and frequently mechanically assisted) respiratory efforts may overdistend inflated segments of lung with rupture of alveoli and production of pneumothorax. Prompt aspiration of the pleural air and insertion of a catheter into the pleural cavity for under-water drainage with negative pressure are lifesaving. *A roentgenogram of the entire infant* should be taken whenever respiratory distress or cyanosis is noted. Physical signs are not to be depended on for evidence of pneumothorax, atelectasis, diaphragmatic hernia or other lesions causing respiratory difficulty.

Congenital Cystic Disease of the Lungs. Cysts of the lungs may be single giant air-filled cysts or multiple smaller cysts containing air and/or liquid. In distribution, they may be unilobar, multilobar or, rarely, involve all lobes (Ravitch, 1969). Air in the cysts, anthracotic pigment in their lining or entrance of contrast material on bronchography, demonstrate communication with the bronchial tree in all cases. The cysts are lined by tall, ciliated columnar epithelium and may contain cartilage in their walls. The commonest presenting clinical picture results from infection of the cysts. Such infected cysts have been mistaken for lung abscesses and for empyemas with pyopneumothorax. Single large cysts, with a flap-valve type of bronchial communication, may distend with air under tension and cause severe respiratory distress. The repeated infections result from the presence of large, ill-drained spaces connected to the bronchial tree, and excision of the cyst or involved pulmonary lobes or segments is the only effective treatment. After diagnosis, early operation is indicated. Infants tolerate pulmonary resection very well, and such procedures have been performed successfully even on the first day of life (Minnis, 1962).

The term "sequestration of the lung" we owe to Pryce, who impugned traction upon the lung by abnormal vessels from the aorta as the causative mechanism for both totally detached "accessory lungs" and for cysts ("intralobar sequestration"). The term sequestration implies a mechanism which is, at best, unproved (Pryce, 1946; Pryce, Sellors and Blair, 1947; Ravitch, 1969). While with cystic disease we have seen such associated systemic arteries, trilobed left lungs and other anomalies, some otherwise typical instances of congenital cystic disease of the lung seem to be innocent of such stigmata of "sequestration." Cysts are to be distinguished from bronchiectatic cavities and lung abscess, in which treatment would be similar, and, in the newborn, from diaphragmatic hernia with multiple intestinal fluid levels in the chest. Infants with pneumonia, particularly that due to stapyhlococci, are particularly prone to develop bronchiolar necrosis and intrapulmonary pneumatoceles strongly simulating cysts with infection (Almkov and Hatoff, 1946; Brock, 1952; Potts and Riker, 1950; Sabiston, Hopkins, Cooke and Bennett, 1961). Inspiratory trapping of air by mucus in the bronchi also may be responsible for such pneumatocele formation. If the true nature of pneumatoceles is appreciated, they may be watched as they slowly disappear over a course of weeks.

Lobar emphysema, huge overdistention of a lobe or lobes, in the newborn may cause acute respiratory distress by compression of the remaining lung and displacement of the mediastinum. Inspiratory obstruction by aspirated curds, or a collapsed defective bronchial wall has been blamed. Immediate lobectomy is required (Szöts and Jakab, 1964; Leape and Longino, 1964).

With tension pneumothorax, the roentgenograms show mediastinal displacement, the collapsed lung is visible against the mediastinum and the radiolucency follows the contours of chest wall and diaphragm. With a distended lung cyst the radiolucency is confined, no lung markings are seen in it and the upper lobe is unlikely to be involved. In lobar emphysema the radiolucency is confined, lung markings can be seen and the upper lobe is the most likely to be involved.

Pulmonary Arteriovenous Fistulae. These are single or multiple areas of communication in the pulmonary substance between pulmonary arteries and veins. They may form one or several masses, centimeters in diameter, or scores of minute almost telangiectatic communications. Cyanosis, polycythemia and clubbing of the fingers are characteristic. Violent hemoptyses may occur. The heart is normal. The lesions are demonstrable, if large enough, on ordinary roentgenograms, laminograms and by angiocardiography. Many of the reported cases are familial. Resection is the treatment of choice. Since the lesions may be multiple and the apparently uninvolved lobe or lobes may contain small communications which subsequently will enlarge, it is important to excise the vascuar lesion or lesions rather than the containing lobe or segment (Sloan and Cooley, 1953; Yater, Finnegan and Griffin, 1949). (See also Chap. 43, Cardiac Surgery.)

Lung Tumors. Every sort of lung tumor occurring in adults occurs also in children, and treatment, as in adults, is by resection. Once more, the frequent occurrence of malignant tumors in childhood must be borne in mind. Bronchial adenoma (Ward, Bradshaw and Prince, 1954) is a slowly growing malignant tumor giving early symptoms because of its intrabronchial growth and tendency to bleed or cause bronchial obstruction. If it is resected properly, the results are excellent. Carcinoma of the lung in children is rare but not unknown (Cayley, Caez and Mersheimer, 1951) and has been described even in infants.

GASTROINTESTINAL TRACT

Neonatal Intestinal Obstruction

Atresias and Stenosis. Atresia (absence of an opening) and stenosis (a narrowing) may affect any portion of the intestinal tract. The standard attribution of atresia is to a failure of coalescence of vacuoles in the epithelial mass which fills the embryonic intestine. This does not explain the instances of atresia in which one or several segments of bowel are represented by little more than fibrous cord, nor the instances in which segments of the mesentery are missing, together with the segments of bowel. Cornified squamous epithelium and lanugal hairs have been found in the rectal plugs of infants with intestinal atresia, proving the presence of a patent alimentary canal fairly late in development. Atresias have been reported in which histologic study has shown unequivocal evidence of an intra-uterine intussusception with necrosis, scarring and obliteration of the lumen (Parkkulainen, 1958). It seems probable that vascular insufficiency, ischemia and necrosis by one mechanism or another is the cause of many of the forms of atresia of the intestine (Louw, 1959). The epithelial mass mechanism may be operative chiefly in the duodenum and the proximal jejunum, and it is here chiefly that occasionally one sees an atresia due solely to a mucosal diaphragm. An incomplete diaphragm may result in a stenosis. Other stenoses appear as narrowed areas of thickened bowel. The ileum is the commonest site of atresia and stenosis, the duodenum and the jejunum following. Atresia on the gastric side of the pylorus has been reported a few times. Atresia of the duodenum, proximal to the ampulla of Vater, is a rarity.

The frequency with which atresias of the intestine are associated with hydramnios is recognized, and Apgar has demonstrated brilliantly the utility of immediate gastric aspiration in the newborn. Accumulations of more than 25 ml. of fluid in the infant's stomach are pathologic and suggest obstruction (Santulli, 1960).

Vomiting, the cardinal symptom of intestinal atresia, begins within a day of birth, is unremitting and usually contains bile. Newborn babies do not normally vomit or regurgitate more than a portion of their feedings. Any excessive regurgitation, any vomiting and certainly the appearance of bile in the returned material should suggest the possibility of intestinal obstruction. In duodenal atresia, vomiting often will be effective in preventing the appearance of distention, although at times the stomach and the duodenum may be dilated tremendously and visibly.

A plain x-ray film of the chest and the abdomen is so extremely informative that it should be taken at the first suspicion of obstruction. Distention of stomach and duodenum and the two fluid levels of the "double bubble" sign with absence of air in the remainder of the abdomen indicates a duodenal atresia. Down's syndrome (mongolism) occurs in 15 per cent or more of such cases. Dilated loops of small bowel with no gas visible in the colon are evidence of obstruction in the ileum or jejunum (Fig. 50-3). Other causes for such obstruction must be differentiated. In meconium ileus, the opaque loops of small bowel may show a granular shadow; and in meconium peritonitis, spotty calcification may be seen in some of the opaque areas. An enema with Gastrografin will demonstrate whether the colon is in normal position or not; in meconium ileus, and in meconium plug in which inspissated meconium simply fails to be evacuated, the enema may be curative in itself. Such an enema may temporarily relieve the functional obstruction in Hirschsprung's disease and may show the pathognomonic distal narrowing. While the meconium in infants with intestinal atresia (whose intestines, at operation, distal to the obstruction are incredibly tiny coils, relatively thick walled and empty) is generally scanty, drier and grayer than normal, it may appear surprisingly unremarkable.

Nothing is said about roentgenograms with ingested barium or Lipiodol, because these rarely give any more information than the plain film and even may obscure it. Barium, given to a newborn who is vomiting, may be regurgitated and aspirated. That which remains in the intestine may prove to be embarrassing. Insufflation of the stomach with air has been recommended as a safe method of obtaining contrast roentgenograms and may be useful. The water-miscible contrast media (e.g., Gastrografin) are not as objectionable as barium or Lipiodol but are not often required except in instances of suspected partial obstruction. They are hypertonic solutions and may cause a significant loss of fluid into the bowel whether given by mouth or by rectum.

Treatment is directed to the establishment of a high probability of the existence of obstruction, which constitutes the indication for operation, and to immediate institution of gastric suction so that further swallowing of air will not increase distention. Preparation for operation includes the insertion of a polyethylene intravenous catheter, administration of glucose and electrolytes and matching of blood for transfusion. For all the causes of neonatal obstruction, the treatment is prompt operation (Benson, 1969; Louw, 1966). In the newborn, a transverse incision, which rarely disrupts, made just above the umbilicus, will give access to the entire abdomen, so that no time need be lost in the intellectual exercise of pinpointing the nature and the location of the obstruction. Stenoses and mucosal diaphragm atresias are relatively more common in the duodenum than elsewhere. At operation, in duodenal obstructions, duodenoduodenostomy

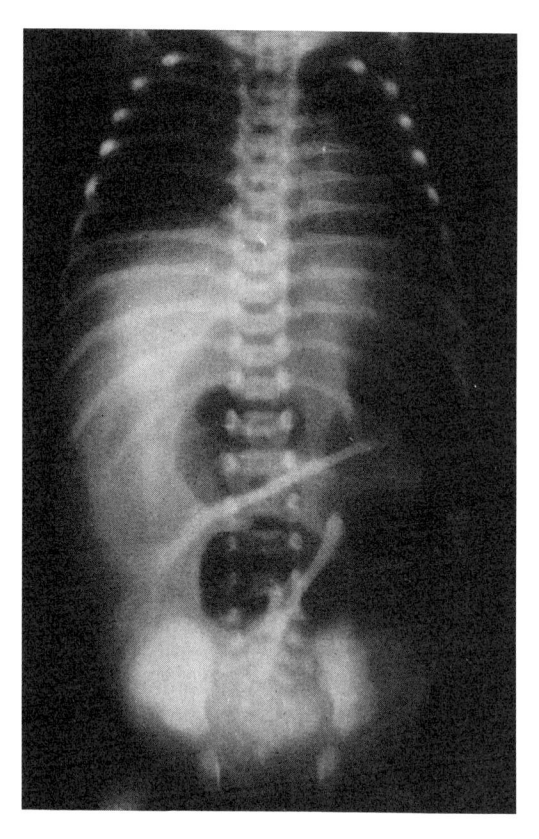

FIG. 50-3. Atresia of ileum. Roentgenogram of infant 36 hours old with great dilatation of small bowel loops and no air recognizable in the colon.

or duodenojejunostomy, around the obstruction, is most satisfactory. Gastrojejunostomy lays the basis for a future anastomotic ulcer (Marshall, 1953) although it is easier technically. Diaphragm obstructions may be excised and the longitudinal incision in the bowel closed transversely by the Heineke-Mikulicz procedure. In the jejunum and the ileum, the massively distended proximal bowel is best resected and an end-to-end anastomosis performed. If an end-to-end anastomosis is not performed, we prefer a side-to-end, bringing the remaining open end out the wound as a vent which will close spontaneously, and in the interim allows for a feeding tube into the distal loop and a suction tube to compress the dilated proximal loop. Double-barreled ileostomies are favored by Gross, but require a second operation. Gastrostomy for aspiration and decompression, and subsequently for feeding, has

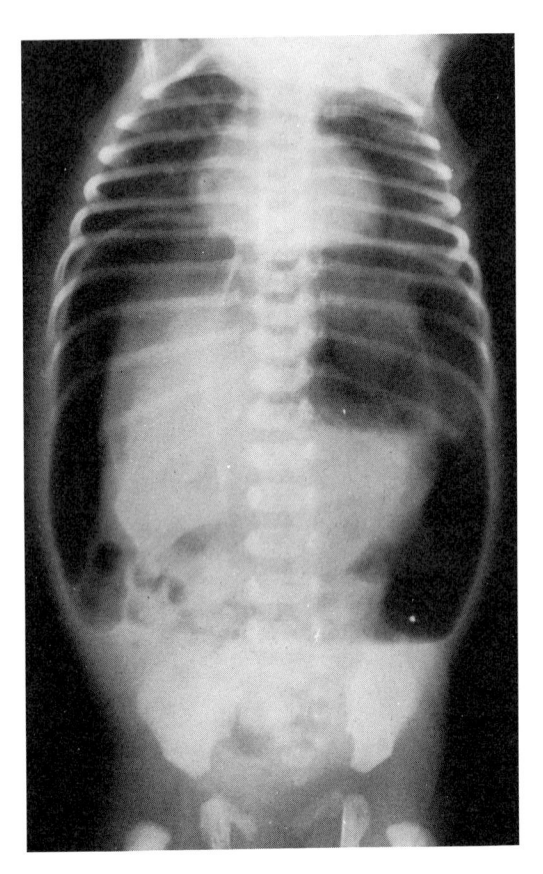

FIG. 50-4. Neonatal gastrointestinal perforation. Massive pneumoperitoneum in a 3-day-old infant who had vomited a little, begun to refuse feedings and had become massively distended and quiet. At operation a prepyloric gastric perforation was found. It would have been less remarkable to have found a duodenal perforation or a linear fundal tear in an area of apparent muscular deficiency. The infant survived operative closure of the perforation.

become deservedly popular. Atresias may be multiple so that the few seconds required to inject saline solution and see it pass the full length of an infant's intestinal tract are well spent. Atresias of the colon, excluding rectum and anus, do occur but are very rare.

Malrotation of the Intestine. For an understanding of the anomalies of rotation and the principles of their treatment, an outline of the embryologic development of the bowel must be borne in mind. From the 5th through the 10th week, most of the midgut—the small intestine and the proximal large intestine—lies outside the body cavity in the communicating exocoelomic space at the base of the umbilical cord. If the intestine fails to return to the abdominal cavity, the condition known as an *amniotic hernia* (exomphalos, omphalocele) results. The intestine will be found in the primitive, nonrotated position. As the intestine grows and enters the cord and then returns to the abdomen, the simple straight tube suspended on its dorsal mesentery, begins to coil. The duodenojejunal loop is bulged out and then passes behind the stalk of the superior mesenteric artery. At the same time as the cecum moves back into the abdomen on the left, it moves upward and across to the right, anterior to the superior mesenteric artery, finally reaching the right lower quadrant. One more event is of clinical importance—the fusion of the duodenojejunal loop, ascending and descending colon, and the base of the mesentery of the small bowel, to the posterior parietal peritoneum. Failure of rotation usually is associated with failure of normal fusion and with abnormal peritoneal bands passing from the colon in the left upper quadrant, across the duodenum, to the posterior parietal peritoneum in the right upper quadrant. The failure of peritoneal fusion, with the entire small intestine hanging from the stalk of the superior mesenteric vessels, predisposes to volvulus of the entire small bowel on this stalk. The peritoneal bands from colon to right upper quadrant across the duodenum lead to compression of the duodenum and duodenal obstruction. It was Ladd, the father of pediatric surgery, who, in 1932, pointed out the necessity for dividing these avascular peritoneal folds. In some instances, symptoms are present at birth, suggesting the volvulus existed in utero. Symptoms tend to be insidious and misleading. With a volvulus of the entire small intestine and the additional duodenal compression, vomiting begins early, and distention appears late if at all. The obstruction may be incomplete, and meconium and flatus, and later on, curds are passed intermittently. Whereas vascular obstruction and gangrene appear early in some infants, the twist in others is apparently loose enough, despite a 360° or greater anticlockwise rotation, to allow an adequate circulation in the bowel. The vomitus usually contains bile, the roentgenogram shows dilatation of stomach and the first portion of the duodenum and usually some gas in the intestines. Roentgenograms of an enema with contrast material may show an interesting picture of incompletely rotated colon.

In the newborn, then, the picture is similar to that in atresia or stenosis, and promptness in operating is even more important because of the threat of massive infarction of the intestine. Fever, leukocytosis, distention and discoloration of the abdominal wall suggest that the bowel is already gangrenous. The duodenal obstruction, without volvulus, may lead to chronic vomiting, malnutrition and bouts of abdominal pain for years. In some cases, malrotation of the intestine is entirely asymptomatic.

Recurrence of volvulus after operation is rare. Snyder and Chaffin (1954) and Gardner (1950) suggest that this is due to the careful operative mobilization of the duodenojejunal loop which comes to lie in the right peritoneal gutter. Gross (1953) suggests that it is due to fixation by postoperative adhesions. It seems at least as reasonable to suppose that the volvulus develops in the fetus to become symptomatic at birth or sometimes later, and that once derotated, a volvulus will rarely develop anew.

Neonatal Perforation of the Gastrointestinal Tract. In a number of situations a neonate feeds poorly, may vomit, or becomes strikingly distended and tympanitic. Roentgenograms (Fig. 50-4) show a massive pneumoperitoneum. This may result from rupture of the stomach (Linkner and Benson, 1959), usually at the proximal end, perhaps due to overdistention and bursting, or from a perforated duodenal or gastric ulcer, or from overdistention proximal to an area of atresia. Perforation of the colon also occurs—for unknown reasons in some instances, or in others, in the bowel proximal to the obstruction in Hirschsprung's disease. Treatment is operative closure of gastric and duodenal perforations, correction of atresia, or, in the colon, usually a colostomy exteriorizing the perforation (Soper and Opitz, 1962).

Meconium ileus has come to be recognized as the neonatal manifestation of the systemic disease known as fibrocystic disease of the pancreas or mucoviscidosis. The clinical picture is one of complete intestinal obstruction

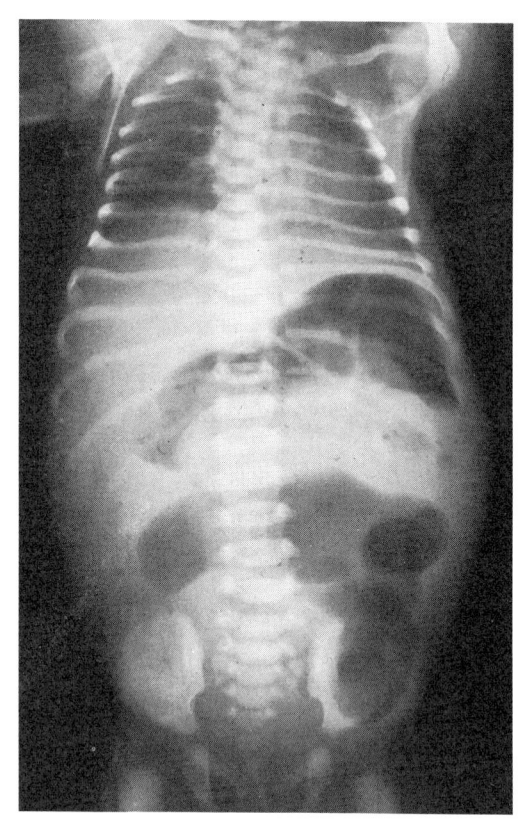

Fig. 50-5. Meconium ileus. Infant 48 hours old. Numerous loops of small bowel are dilated. Opaque, meconium-filled loops are not distinguishable in this instance, but the previous occurrence of meconium ileus in a sibling permitted the correct diagnosis to be made before operation.

from birth. Vomiting and distention attract attention to a baby who has passed no meconium or only a plug of dry, slate-gray material. Roentgenograms (Fig. 50-5) demonstrate many dilated loops of small bowel and may show granular shadows of retained meconium. At operation, the distal ileum is found distended with thick, blackish, tarry, tenacious material which adheres to gloves and instruments and equally well to the mucosa of the bowel. The material can be removed only with the greatest difficulty by milking and saline washing through one or several enterostomies. Hiatt (1948) published the first series of operative successes in this condition by this method. The results of Gross, with a simple resection of the "tar"-filled loop and tempo-

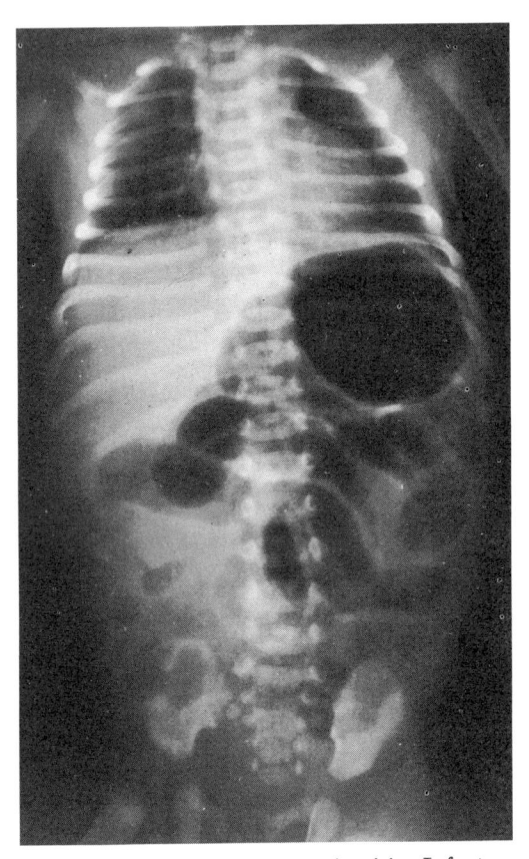

FIG. 50-6. Meconium peritonitis. Infant 48 hours old. The stomach and many loops of small bowel are distended with air. There may be some air in the colon. The generally opaque area on the right side of the abdomen contains a number of denser areas indicative of calcification and pathognomonic of meconium peritonitis. The point of perforation had sealed off and was not demonstrable at operation. A lateral anastomosis about a kink in the small bowel, probably at the site of a marked stenosis, relieved the obstruction which had been responsible for the intrauterine perforation. While there are differences in these roentgenograms (Figs. 50-3 to 50-6) which indicate the nature of the underlying lesion, all required immediate operation, and the same midabdominal transverse incision will give access to any lesion which may be found.

rary double-barreled ileostomy, are spectacular—15 of the 19 treated were relieved of their obstruction. Acetylcysteine, or detergents such as Tween 80, either instilled in the bowel at laparotomy, or given by mouth or enema with and, sometimes, without operation, may detach and liquefy the inspissated meconium. The grim aftermath lies in the subsequent course of many of these patients. In a total group of 22 infants with meconium ileus successfully relieved by operation, 8 died of other consequences of mucoviscidosis, such as nutritional disturbances and overwhelming pulmonary infection. The condition of the survivors is said to be satisfactory. The postoperative treatment includes high caloric diet, high vitamin intake, protein hydrolysate feedings, or added pancreatic enzyme. Antibiotics are given indefinitely to ward off respiratory infections (Gross, 1953). Occasionally older children develop a syndrome of intestinal obstruction termed a "meconium ileus equivalent" (Cordonnier and Izant, 1963).

Meconium peritonitis is the result of intrauterine intestinal perforation with leakage of meconium into the fetal peritoneal cavity. An intense foreign body inflammatory reaction occurs, the result of which is neonatal intestinal obstruction (Lorimer and Ellis, 1966). Roentgenograms show distended loops of bowel. Spotty calcification, in the abdomen, presumably as a result of fat necrosis associated with the peritonitis, is pathognomonic (Fig. 50-6). The perforation may occur proximal to an area of atresia or stenosis, or proximal to an ileum obstructed with the glutinous meconium of meconium ileus. In almost half the cases, no cause for the perforation has been found. At operation, the adherent intestinal loops must be dissected away painstakingly and the primary condition dealt with. In most instances, the perforation itself will have healed over.

DUPLICATIONS AND ENTEROGENOUS CYSTS

At any point along the entire length of the alimentary tract there may occur intimately attached to its wall cystic structures formed of smooth muscle and lined by mucous membrane like that of some portion of the intestinal tract. A number of embryologic explanations are offered—that embryonic diverticula are pinched off to persist as cysts or that vacuoles forming in the dissolution of the stage of epithelial plugging of the bowel fail to coalesce, hence remain as cysts. Many of these enterogenous cysts are explained inadequately by such mechanisms, particularly the instances in which an entire segment of bowel is paralleled by a second and similar channel. For this reason, Ladd and Gross (1940) preferred the term duplication, implying an attempt at doubling of the bowel. There is certainly a group of cases of duplication of anus, rectum and colon and external and internal genitalia which appear to be true doubling and have been interpreted as due to incomplete caudal twinning (Ravitch, 1953). The older term of enterogenous cyst, which makes no pretense to a developmental explanation that cannot be supported strongly, probably is best retained for the more frequently occurring localized cysts. A curious feature is that the cysts may be lined by mucosa of a segment of intestine remote from that of the location of the cyst. Most of the cysts do not communicate with the lumen of the attached bowel. Symptoms are: a mass, occasionally large enough to distend the abdomen of an infant; pain from the tenseness of the mass; obstruction of the bowel to which it is attached; bleeding from necrosis of the bowel by pressure, or from erosion by the strongly acid secretion of cysts lined by gastric mucous membrane. In two instances we have seen a small enteric cyst at the ileocecal valve cause an intussusception. The treatment is operative. Because the muscular walls of the cyst and the bowel are fused, clean excision of the cyst is not often possible. Either the adjacent bowel is resected with the cyst, or the bulk of the cyst is excised and its mucosa stripped from the common muscular wall of cyst and bowel, or the cyst is widely anastomosed to the bowel (Gardner and Hart, 1935) in locations in which more definite treatment presents too great hazard.

Mesenteric cysts are usually lymphatic cysts, frequently chylous. They tend to be thin-walled and soft and are rarely palpable through the abdominal wall. Arising usually between the leaves of the mesentery, they may form very large sacs extending through the mesentery in dumbbell fashion and stretching the bowel over them. Intestinal obstruction, with a history of repeated attacks, and volvulus are the most common sequelae, but acute inflammation may occur in the apparent absence of obstruction (Handelsman and Ravitch, 1954). Resection usually entails resection of the associated bowel. Omental cysts, lymphatic or angiomatous, are found occasionally.

Torsion and infarction produce acute abdominal symptoms. Very large cysts may produce vague symptoms. Mesenteric cysts and omental cysts may be so soft as to defy palpation through the intact abdominal wall.

STOMACH AND DUODENUM

Peptic Ulcer in Infancy and Childhood. Peptic ulcers associated with burns (Curling's ulcer) are well known, as are ulcers associated with manifest or occult lesions of the central nervous system (Cushing's ulcers) (Sale, 1956), and what we have come to know as stress ulcers, not rare after open heart operations (Gilbert and Morrow, 1960). There is now a considerable experience with peptic ulcer, largely duodenal, in infants and children without any such obvious precursor (Fig. 50-7). In newborn infants, even in the first day of life, ulcers may bleed or perforate, or both (Lyday, Markarian and Rhoads, 1959; Plummer and Stabins, 1953). Ulcers causing intractable pain or leading to stenosis are less likely to be seen in infancy than later in childhood, and the younger infants are the ones most likely to bleed. Perforation, of course, demands immediate operation, and bleeding may be massive and cause death from exsanguination. At times death has resulted from vomiting, rejection of food and cachexia without perforation or hemorrhage. In infants with bleeding duodenal ulcer, simple excision of the ulcer or duodenotomy and transfixion of the bleeding vessels is all that is required.

Chronic peptic ulcer occurring in childhood and adolescence is indicative of a particularly strong ulcer diathesis, and with this in mind it is probably reasonable to apply operative therapy sooner to a child than to an adult (Leix and Greaney, 1963; Johnston and Snyder, 1968). Our choice is vagectomy and pyloroplasty, the procedure least likely to interfere with growth and nutrition (Boley et al., 1965). We have performed a vagotomy and a drainage operation five times in the last $2\frac{1}{2}$ years in children ages $3\frac{1}{2}$ years to 14 years for symptoms of pain or bleeding or obstruction. In children with chronic peptic ulcers, endocrine abnormalities should be especially sought out, such as islet cell tumors of the pancreas, hyperparathyroidism, and tumors of the adrenal or the pituitary glands.

Pyloric Stenosis. Infantile hypertrophic

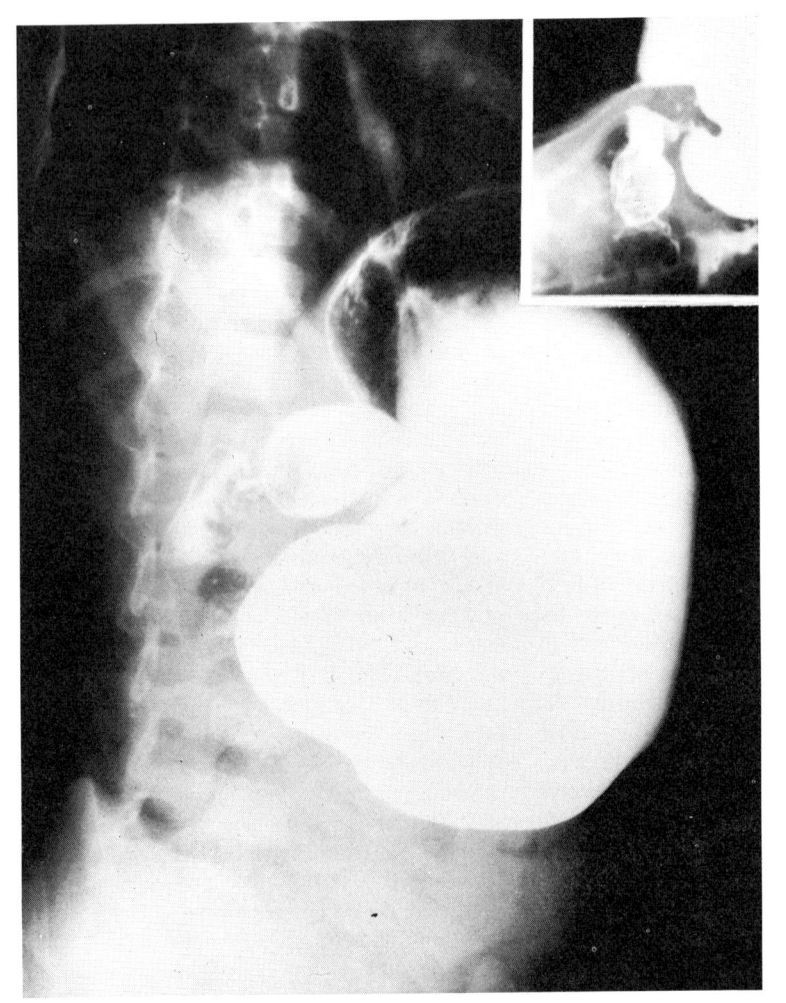

FIG. 50-7. Duodenal ulcer in a 3-year-old boy who had had 3 severe hemorrhages in the previous 18 months, requiring transfusion each time. He has been well for 4 years after pyloroplasty and vagotomy, certainly the procedure of choice in a child.

pyloric stenosis is certainly the commonest condition requiring laparotomy in infancy. It consists of a great hypertrophy of the muscle fibers of the pyloric sphincter, such that the mass usually is large enough to be palpated through the abdominal wall and bulges inward on the lumen as well, reducing it to a threadlike channel. Males are affected more commonly than females in the proportion of 4 to 1. Classically, a vigorous and apparently normal infant begins to vomit in the 3rd week of life, although characteristic tumors have been found at operation in rare instances in the 1st week of life and occasionally symptoms do not appear until the baby is several months old. Vomiting increases rapidly in severity until the infant empties his stomach after every feeding by a forceful emesis accurately described as projectile. As a rule, the vomitus is free of bile, but with violent effort may be blood-streaked. Immediately preceding the vomiting, the outline of the distended stomach is visible, and peristaltic waves may be seen to traverse it from left to right. The olive-shaped tumor, to the right of the right rectus muscle, can be felt in almost every instance. Its presence is pathognomonic. Failure of experienced clinicians to feel the mass should lead to consideration of other conditions. Vomiting occurs in cerebral injuries but is seldom so consistent. Infants with hiatus hernia have symptoms which may simulate pyloric stenosis. In atresias of the intestinal tract the vomitus appears at once and usually contains bile. The radiologic picture of pyloric stenosis—delayed and incomplete emptying, threadlike pylorus with no peristalsis across it, is characteristic (Runstrom, 1939), but only rarely will it be necessary to resort to roentgenography for diagnosis.

In such a common disease, it is remarkable not only that the cause remains unknown but also that it is not certain whether it ever has been observed in a stillborn infant. Wallgren, in Sweden (1946), studied 1,000 male newborn infants roentgenographically. All showed pyloric canals normal in caliber and function. Five subsequently developed vomiting, typical symptoms of pyloric stenosis, and the classical roentgenographic picture. This may mean that the hypertrophy is not congenital but appears only after birth or, on the other hand, that while it may be congenital, a second factor—spasm, edema in response to gastric work—is required to produce obstruction and the roentgenographic picture. In some instances, symptoms do not develop for several months. Apparently the tumor persists indefinitely, unless a pyloromyotomy is performed.

In the United States, the operation of Fredet (1910) and Rammstedt (1912) is generally accepted as the standard treatment. Performed electively, after deliberate rehydration and transfusion of the dry, hypochloremic, alkalotic infants (who usually show acetonuria as well), it results in cure and in discharge from the hospital in less than a week in over 99 per cent of the infants. The operation, performed preferably through a small transverse or gridiron right upper quadrant incision, consists in splitting the heavy muscular tumor, from normal stomach, where it tapers off, to normal duodenum, where it ends abruptly. Glistening submucosa should bulge into the cleft in the white, gristly avascular tumor. Operative perforation of the duodenum occasionally occurs, but is of no consequence if it is recognized and repaired with fine arterial sutures. Rarely, an inadequate operation demands a second procedure. When one surgeon can report 143 consecutive operations without a death 30 years ago (Donovan, 1937), and Gross and his colleagues (1953) 642 cases in 6 years (1946-1952) with 5 deaths, 2 of them in babies with serious congenital anomalies requiring operative correction, the mortality can be seen to be extremely low. Although with great effort, and much longer intensive medical care (Wallgren, 1940), many infants can be carried along nonoperatively, the risk of prolonged malnutrition and the frequent necessity for long hospitalization would appear to make the mere avoidance of an operation a questionable triumph.

Biliary Tract

Atresia of the Extrahepatic Bile Ducts. Newborn infants who soon become jaundiced, in whom the jaundice is intense and progressive, associated with hepatomegaly and acholic stools, may be presumed to have a mechanical obstruction of the biliary tract. Icterus neonatorum is usually milder and clears more rapidly. Hepatitis may occur in the newborn, and inclusion disease affecting the liver may cause jaundice. The icterus gravis of erythroblastosis can be anticipated in many instances before birth and diagnosed, in any event, on clinical and hematologic grounds.

The nature of biliary atresia is in dispute. It is certainly suggestive that it results from a pathologic process in the intrauterine life which widely injures the liver and its ducts. It is not associated with other anomalies—and, obviously, for the liver, formed from an outpouching of the gut, to be present, the duct must have once existed and been destroyed. Thus far analysis of liver function, stool, urine and even liver biopsy do not reliably indicate the nature of the lesion causing jaundice (except in cytomegalic inclusion disease) nor whether the jaundice is due to obstruction or to parenchymal disease. Unfortunately in most cases the atresia is total and irremediable and no biliary ducts can be found, but rarely, a stubby common duct or hepatic duct can be found for anastomosis to the intestine with good recovery. In a similar number of cases, the ducts appear to be normal, apparently are plugged with thickened bile and can be induced to open up by operative or nonoperative "flushing" of the ducts.

Operation should be undertaken early before marked cirrhosis has occurred. Operative cholangiography by injection of contrast material into the gallbladder may spare the patient a detailed exploration if a patent extrahepatic biliary apparatus is demonstrated. The first successful operation was performed by Ladd in 1927. Direct anastomosis of the proximal blind end of the bile duct to duodenum, over a polyethylene catheter, is the procedure of choice. Finding the proximal end may be difficult. In a number of instances a proximal end, which escaped detection at a first operation, has been found at a reoperation dilated into a structure easily anastomosed to the duodenum. When the extrabiliary ducts are entirely absent the intrahepatic architecture seems to be similarly deranged, for dilated intrahepatic ducts do not appear. When no bile duct is present, death is inevitable. Unfortunately, it is frequently delayed for 2 or 3 years and occasionally for 5 or 6 (Redo, 1954). However, almost as many children have ultimately survived to live normal lives in whom the operative report was of complete absence of extrahepatic ducts, as have been salvaged by effective anastomoses (Krovetz, 1960). Obviously, adequate ducts were present but missed in the first group so that even when no ducts are found, great care should be taken to avoid rough handling of the surrounding tissues.

Choledochal cyst is a curious anomaly in which the distal end of the common duct is dilated to form a cyst, sometimes of great size. The proximal common duct, or hepatic ducts, are not always dilated, and the thick-walled cyst is in essence a great aneurysmal dilatation of the common duct. Obstructions in the distal common duct due to valve formation or stenosis have not been reported regularly in association with choledochal cysts, and the portion of common duct beyond the cyst may be normal or in some instances dilated (Alonso-Lej, Rever and Pessagno, 1959). The clinical picture is that of chronic and intermittent pain and jaundice with a palpable mass, which may vary in size and tenseness. The attacks of pain in some cases seem to have been due to bouts of acute pancreatitis (Ravitch and Snyder, 1958).

The cyst lies against and partly under the duodenum, and a direct anastomosis between cyst and duodenum provides a simple and effective treatment in the smaller cysts. With large cysts, the generally more preferable Roux-en-Y anastomosis with the jejunum is feasible and becomes the procedure of choice. Resection of the cyst is seldom feasible.

Cholelithiasis and Cholecystitis. In association with some hemolytic diseases the formation of bile pigment stones in the gallbladder is common in children. This is particularly true and important in congenital spherocytosis (congenital hemolytic icterus) and in sickle-cell anemia (Weens, 1945). The abdominal crises in these conditions are not unlike attacks of biliary colic or cholecystitis, and alertness is required to discover the superimposed biliary disease. Splenectomy is curative for familial hemolytic icterus, and abdominal "crises" occurring after splenectomy should be investigated for evidence of cholelithiasis. It is our practice at the time of splenectomy in patients with spherocytic familial icterus to examine the gallbladder and to remove it through a transverse extension of the subcostal splenectomy incision if calculi are felt.

Acute cholecystitis may occur as a feature of a systemic bacterial infection or apparently independently. It differs from cholecystitis in adults in the frequent occurrence of jaundice in the absence of stones. Treatment is, of course, cholecystectomy. A child with one attack of gallbadder disease can look forward to repeated distress unless cholecystectomy is performed, and even in children the complications of cholecystitis and cholelithiasis do occur (Glenn and Hill, 1954; Ulin, Nosal and Martin, 1952).

Liver tumors, both malignant and benign, occur in childhood (Fraumeni et al., 1968). One form of neuroblastoma appears as a disseminated tumor causing enormous hepatomegaly with no evidence of a primary tumor elsewhere. Primary carcinoma of the liver is another cause of hepatic enlargement not often susceptible to treatment and manifested at first solely by the hepatomegaly. Hemangiomas of a number of varieties, cysts and other benign tumors tend to be softer and cause more localized hepatic enlargement. Resection of either lobe of the liver is feasible and has been tolerated well by children (Alpert et al., 1967). One cannot be certain without operation that a liver tumor is benign. Hemangiomas can cause fatal hemorrhage; some tumors may be present for several years before demonstrating rapid growth.

PANCREAS

Annular and Ectopic Pancreas (see also Chap. 34, Pancreas). The pancreas arises from a dorsal and a ventral anlage and at times fusion of the two encircles the duodenum with a band of pancreatic tissue. Curiously enough, symptoms are characteristically produced late in life—duodenal obstruction and a more than coincidental occurrence of duodenal ulcer.

Neonatal duodenal obstruction due to annular pancreas does occur. The obstruction—except in cases with associated duodenal atresia—is not complete. The roentgenogram shows a smooth, sharp obstruction in the 3rd part of the duodenum. Division of the pancreatic band is difficult in an infant and may result in pancreatitis or pancreatic fistula; duodenojejunostomy is the procedure of choice (Ravitch and Woods, 1950).

Nodules of ectopic pancreatic tissue may occur anywhere along the gastrointestinal tract. The most frequent locations are in a Meckel's diverticulum. The ectopic tissue may initiate an intussusception, or may be the site of acute pancreatitis. It has been found also in association with intestinal bleeding, and in a prolapsing gastric polyp has caused pyloric obstruction (Collett, 1946). However, most such foci are asymptomatic and appear as incidental findings.

Spleen

Splenectomy in children (Welch, 1969) is most frequently required in association with rupture of the spleen. Other indications for this operation are discussed in Chapter 34, Spleen.

Congenital absence of the spleen may be suspected in a child with repeated serious infections and a congenital cardiac defect. Associated may be situs inversus and other visceral anomalies, polycythemia with increased target cells, Howell-Jolly bodies, normoblastemia and decreased osmotic fragility of the red cells (Gilbert, Nishimura and Wedum, 1958).

Umbilicus and Associated Structures

Omphalitis, a pyogenic infection, can be particularly hazardous because of transmission of inflammation along the umbilical vein to cause portal vein thrombosis. Portal hypertension with cavernomatous transformation of the portal vein may result from a neonatal omphalitis with ascending thrombophlebitis. Neonatal exchange transfusions may similarly produce umbilical vein thrombophlebitis and ultimate portal thrombosis and cavernomatous transformation (Oski, Allen and Diamond, 1963). Happily, modern hygiene has made serious omphalitis, and the tetanus that was formerly seen with it, quite rare except in parts of India and Africa where they are still common.

Umbilical granuloma, a tuft of granulation tissue on the uncicatrized umbilical stump is a common and annoying lesion. Amputation of the granuloma with a ligature or crushing hemostat usually will permit the stump to heal over. From time to time histologic examination will discover an apparent granuloma to be a mucosal remnant of the omphalomesenteric or vitelline duct.

Anomalies Associated with the Omphalomesenteric Duct

This duct represents a patent communication between midgut and yolk sac from the 3rd week of embryonic life to the 6th. Any portion of the duct, or all of it, may persist (Figs. 50-8 and 50-9). If all of it persists, there is found a muscular tube lined by intestinal mucosa leading from an umbilical opening to a point in the distal ileum. The tube and its external opening may be as large as the bowel so that a fecal discharge issues from the opening, or the bowel may evert itself through it. Treatment is excision of the umbilicus and the persistent duct and closure of the intestine. At the external end, cysts lined by intestinal mucosa may appear in the umbilical cord at a distance from the umbilicus and may be amputated with the cord. A rosy tuft of mucosa on the umbilicus may suggest a granuloma in appearance. A cyst may persist in or under the abdominal wall, with or without communication with the skin. The obliterated omphalomesenteric vessels, persisting as a strand from ileum to umbilicus, may cause intestinal obstruction or volvulus. An intestinal cyst may persist in the middle of such a cord. Meckel's diverticulum is the result of persistence of the intestinal end of the vitelline or omphalomesenteric duct. It shows great variation in size, shape and position but usually is found within 2 or 3 feet of the ileocecal valve, occurs on the antimesenteric surface of the bowel and is marked by a characteristic vessel with accompanying fat running to its tip from the mesentery of the bowel. The diverticulum, if long and narrow, is subject to an acute inflammatory process clinically indistinguishable from appendicitis. In operating for appendicitis, if the appendix is normal, search always is made for a Meckel's diverticulum. Ectopic tissue—pancreatic or gastric—is commonly found in

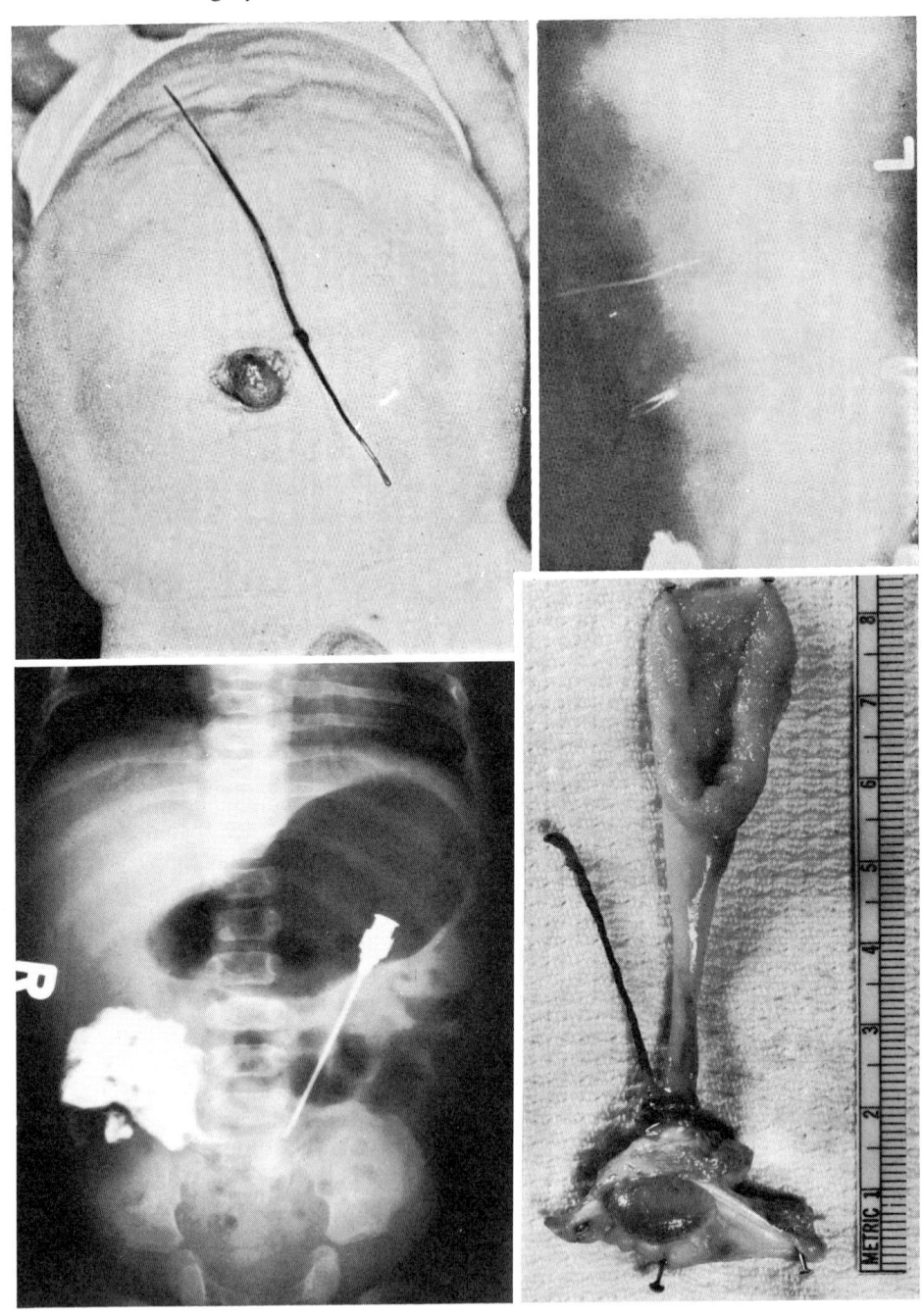

FIG. 50-8. Three-month-old male with pouting umbilical tumor obviously covered by intestinal mucosa (*top, left*). The silver probe passes deeply into the abdomen through the relatively large opening in the mucosa as seen in the lateral roentgenogram (*top, right*). Injection of Lipiodol into the sinus through a polyethylene catheter fitted to a needle shows the free communication with the intestine (*bottom, left*). The specimen (*bottom, right*) removed at operation shows the umbilicus, the tubelike patent omphalomesenteric duct, and, at its flared end, a portion of the wall of the ileum with which it connected widely. Despite the widely patent communication, only mucus discharged from the umbilicus. In some of these patients, feces or flatus may escape from the umbilical fistula.

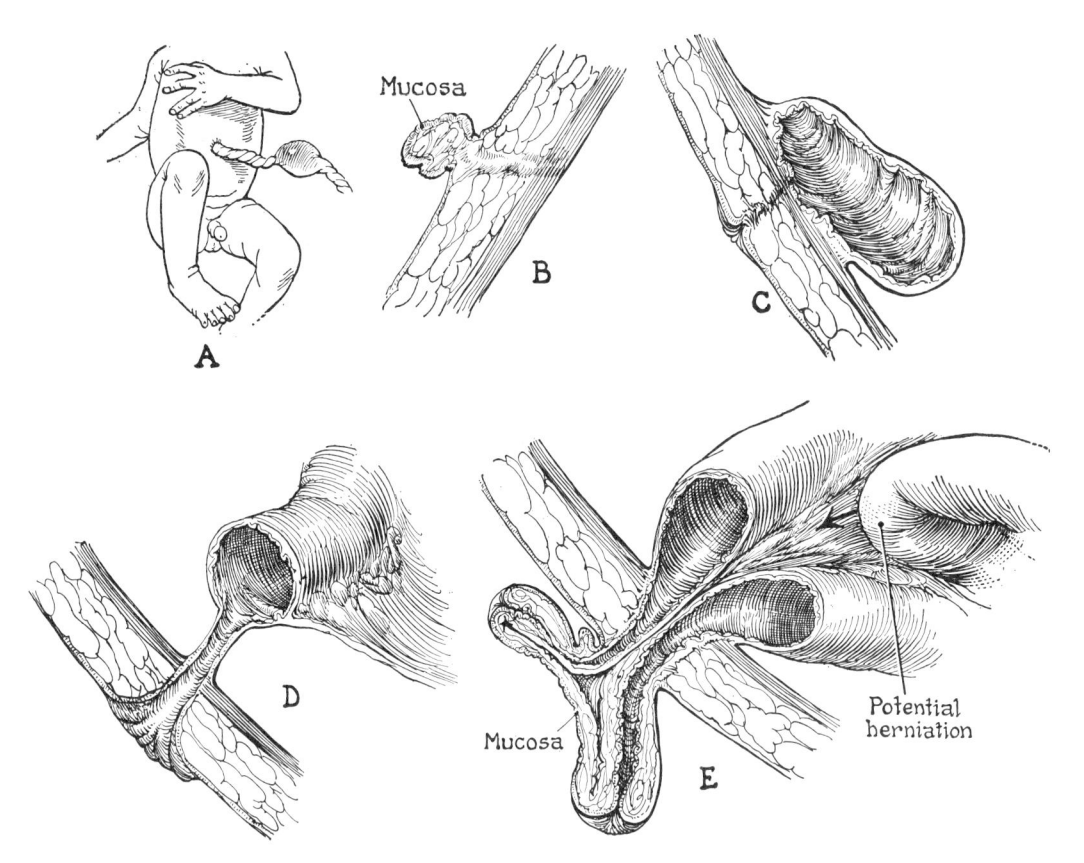

FIG. 50-9. Omphalomesenteric duct (vitelline duct) remnants. Clinical manifestations of persistence of various portions of the duct.

A. A mucosa-lined cyst exists in the umbilical cord, distant from the umbilicus. Removed when the cord is divided, it is no more than a pathologic curiosity.

B. The umbilicus is partially or completely covered with a pouting tuft of red, easily recognized intestinal mucosa, which may dip down into the abdominal wall. Sometimes small tufts are mistaken for umbilical granulomas.

C. A mucosa-lined cyst with muscular wall lies beneath the umbilicus, properitoneally, and may extend upward through the umbilicus to the skin.

D. An enteric tube forms a widely patent communication between the ileum and the umbilicus. The tube of intestine is generally much longer than shown. Gas and feces are discharged through the opening.

E. In the presence of the complete persistence of the omphalomesenteric duct, shown in D, particularly if it is wide, the proximal and distal loops may prolapse out through it, as when both loops prolapse in some tangential colostomies. A serosa-lined cavity, or hernial sac, is formed, into which another loop of bowel may herniate.

(Continued on next page)

Meckel's diverticula. Peptic ulcers in the normal ileal mucosa of the diverticulum or the adjacent bowel are not rare in association with such ectopic gastric mucosa. Like peptic ulcers elsewhere, they may bleed, or perforate, or both. The bleeding is characteristically painless; it may be so slow as to produce dark stools and a profound chronic anemia, or so massive as to produce bright red blood and shock. Meckel's diverticulum with a peptic ulcer is an important cause of occult intestinal bleeding (Kittle, Jenkins and Dragstedt, 1947; Rutherford and Akers, 1966). In the small minority of intussusceptions associated with

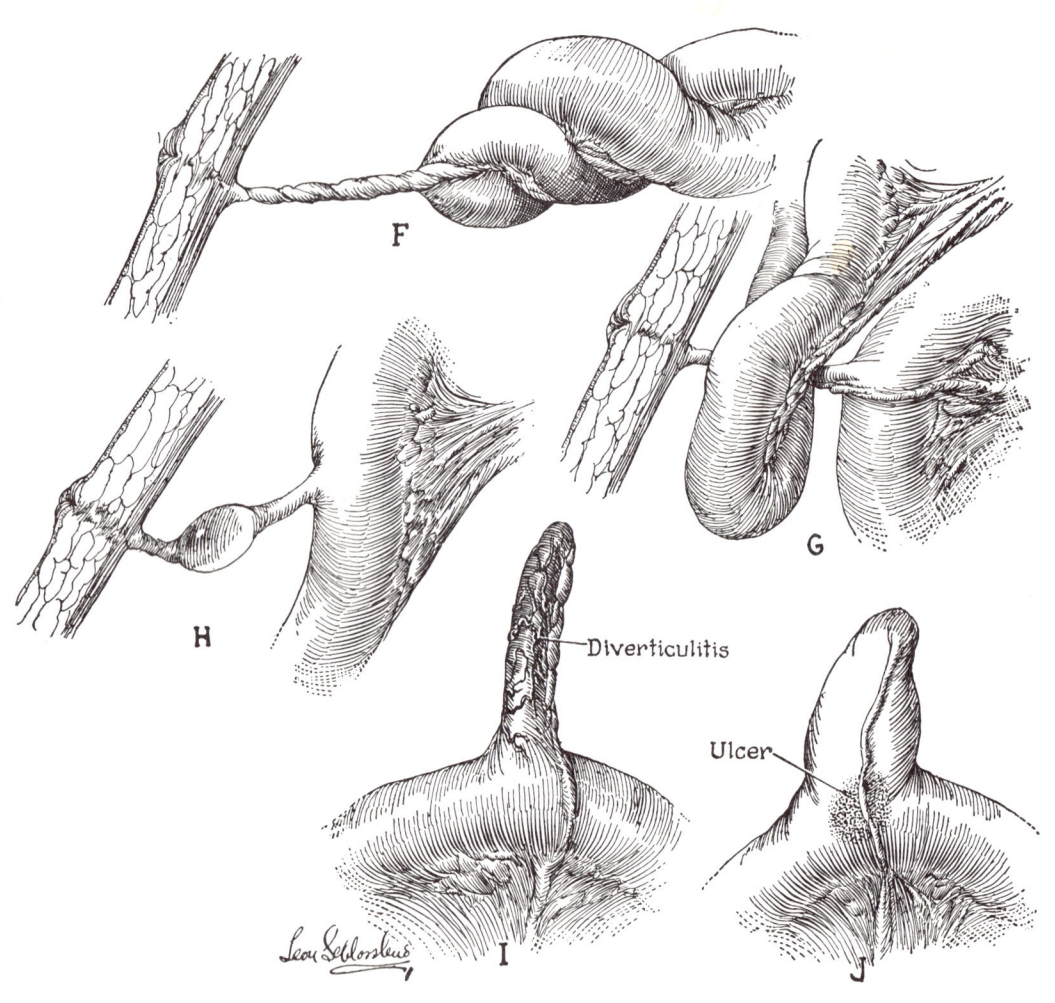

Fig. 50-9. (*Continued*)

F. The obliterated omphalomesenteric vessels persist, attaching the ileum to the abdominal wall, and creating the fixed point about which a volvulus may form.

G. A knuckle of bowel may be caught across such an obliterated omphalomesenteric artery, causing intestinal obstruction in this manner.

H. The cord of the obliterated omphalomesenteric vessels may contain in its mid-portion a mucosa-lined, smooth-muscle walled cyst, as a persistence of the mid-portion of the duct.

I & J. The intestinal end of the omphalomesenteric duct persists—the diverticulum of Meckel. If it is slender and vermiform it may be the seat of diverticulitis, indistinguishable clinically from appendicitis. Most omphalomesenteric duct remnants contain gastric mucosa. The result, in Meckel's diverticulum, is frequently a peptic ulcer of the ileum, or of the ileal mucosa in the diverticulum. Massive, painless intestinal bleeding is the only symptom in most cases. Perforation occurs occasionally.

specific lesions, Meckel's diverticula are prominent. Meckel's diverticula causing symptoms are resected, depending on the anatomic situation, like an appendix, or with a segment of bowel. Since 1 to 2 per cent of the population have such diverticula and most of them remain asymptomatic for a lifetime, the decision with respect to a diverticulum incidentally found at operation will depend on the nature of the primary operation.

Anomalies Associated With the Urachus. The urachus is the fetal structure connecting allantois and bladder and derived uncertainly from either or both. At birth it persists as a mid-line cord between bladder and umbilicus. In fully a third of normal individuals, a fine probe demonstrates a connection between bladder and a short urachal sinus. In most individuals, section of the urachal cord will show scattered epithelial persistences (Begg, 1930). Like the vitelline duct, any portion of the urachus or the entire structure may persist. If the urachus persists as a patent communication between bladder and umbilicus, a urinary fistula occurs. At times a small weeping cyst or sinus at the umbilicus represents a urachal persistence in the umbilicus. The most common lesion is a cyst on the under side of the abdominal wall, in the midline and extraperitoneal, which causes symptoms either from its size, which may be very great, or from infection. Infected lesions are drained and subsequently, like uninfected ones, excised, care being taken to avoid injury to the bladder.

Omphalocele (amniotic hernia, exomphalos) results when the intestines fail to return to the abdomen, and remain in the exocoelomic cavity of the umbilical cord, covered only by amniotic membrane. The defect in the abdominal wall may be small, 1 or 2 centimeters, or enormous, almost from flank to flank (Fig. 50-10), but the loss is only of skin and fat; the muscles are intact but widely separated in the midline. The contents may be only a few loops of small bowel, or liver, spleen, stomach, and almost the entire intestinal tract. The covering membrane is avascular and will ordinarily dry, crack, lead to infection and death. The common, small herniae through small defects are easily repaired immediately after birth. The method of Gross (1948) for dealing with the massive herniae—undermining the surrounding skin and closing it over the intact sac—is being replaced by the treatment of Grob (1967), or a modification thereof. This involves long hospitalization while the sac is painted daily with one or another mild antiseptic until it is finally covered by epithelium growing in from the edges. The cicatrizing effect seems actually to decrease the size of the hernia. Intestinal atresia is a frequent concomitant of omphalocele. Intra-uterine rupture of an omphalocele results in the coating of the exposed intestines with a thick yellow-green layer of

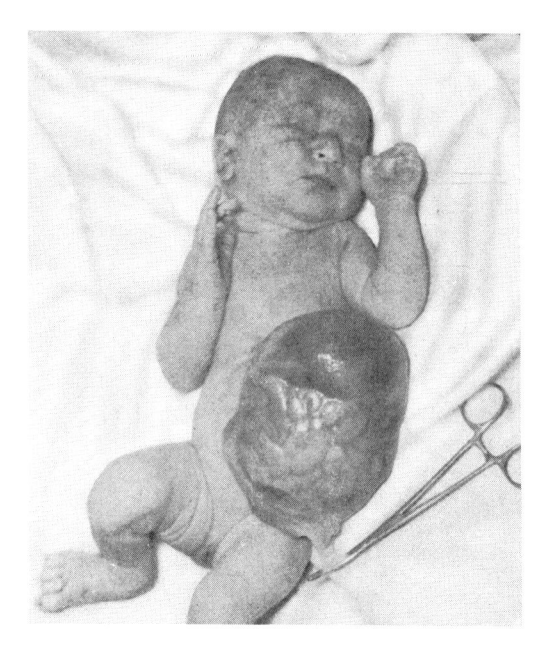

FIG. 50-10. Omphalocele. Newborn infant with massive omphalocele containing liver, spleen, stomach and intestines. The translucent sac of amniotic membrane was carefully preserved, the skin widely undermined and brought over the membrane, by the method of Gross. A series of complicated procedures ultimately repaired the resultant ventral hernia. Recently we have employed pneumoperitoneum in preparation for second-stage operations in such cases (Ravitch, 1963). The general adoption of the Grob technic of nonoperative treatment of massive omphaloceles may reduce the necessity for special measures at the time of secondary repair.

fibrin, forming a mass difficult to replace in the abdomen (Riemensnyder, 1963).

Gastroschisis is a condition similar to omphalocele but the herniation is through a defect in the abdominal wall near, but not at the umbilicus, usually to the right. The intestines are imbedded in a mass of gelatinous matrix uncovered by any sac. Formerly considered hopeless, it is now treatable with success (Cordero et al., 1969).

Congenital absence of the abdominal muscles is a curious condition in which the ventral musculature is represented by only a few scattered strands of abnormal muscle fibers. The skin of the mid-line frequently appears scarred as if by a burn or an operation

(Fig. 50-11). The thin abdominal wall bulges in any direction, and the presence of numerous wrinkles is characteristic. The defect occurs almost exclusively in males. Unopposed pull of the diaphragm frequently results in a pigeon chest with a pronounced Harrison's groove. Of greatest importance is the almost unfailing concomitant occurrence of cryptorchidism and urinary tract anomalies—megacystica, megaureter and hydronephrosis. Some cases have shown mechanical obstruction, but Nunn and Stephens (1961) have demonstrated the basic lesion to be muscular deficiency in the wall of the bladder and ureter. Malrotations of the intestine also occur commonly in these patients. Various types of plastic procedures on the urinary tract have permitted some of these patients to survive. Plastic operations upon the abdominal wall, since all the parietal muscles

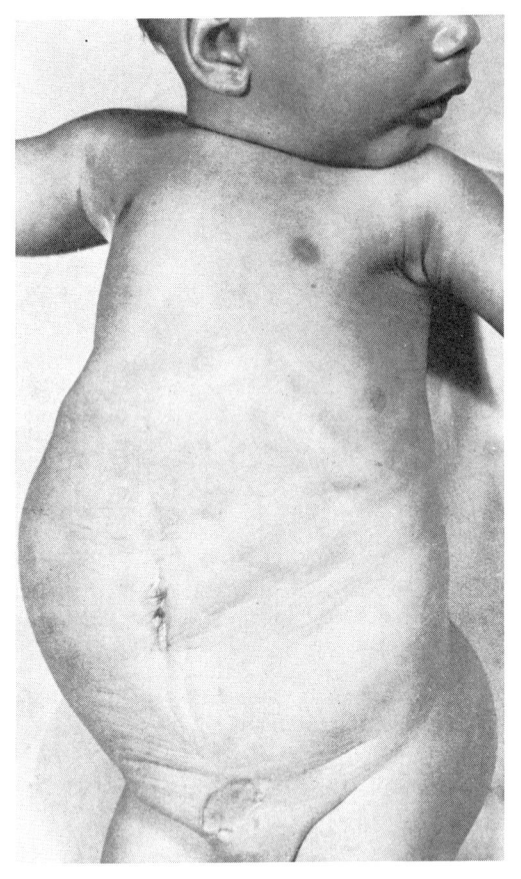

FIG. 50-11. Congenital absence of abdominal musculature. A 7-month-old male with absence of abdominal musculature. Note (*left*) the bulging of the contents through the flabby abdominal wall and the visible intestinal patterns. The curious mid-line scars are congenital stigmata. Retrograde pyelogram (*bottom*) shows an extensive hydronephrosis on the left. The left ureter is colossally dilated and tortuous, and there is a massively enlarged bladder. The nonfunctioning right kidney was removed, and a left nephrostomy has permitted the child to survive several years in good vigor. A convincing vesical neck obstruction was not demonstrated in this instance.

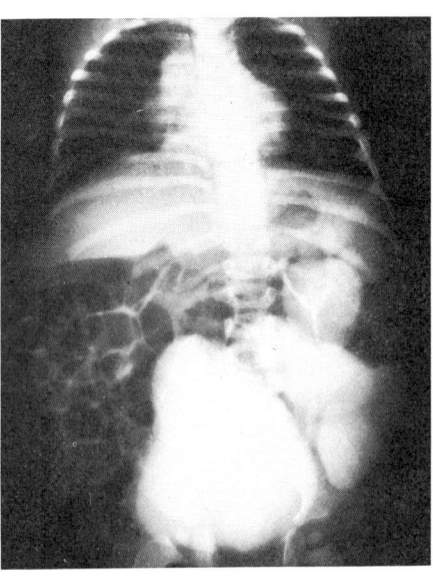

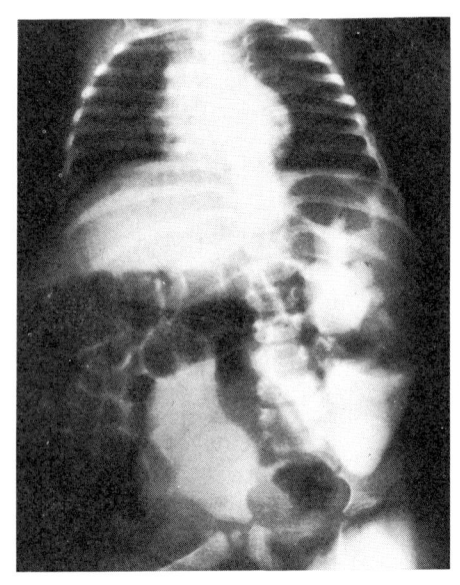

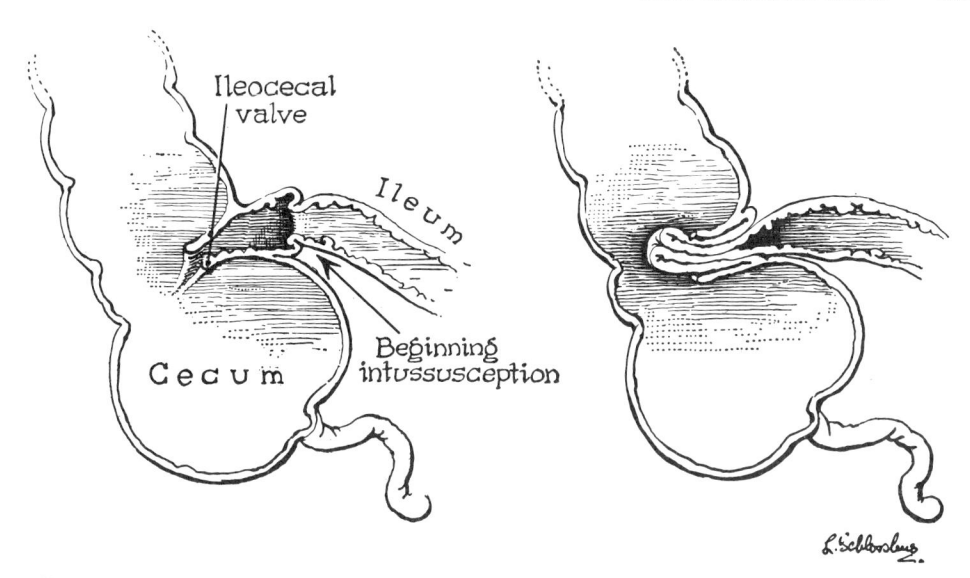

Fig. 50-12. The vast majority of intussusceptions begin at or near the ileocecal valve (*left*). In some, the ileum protrudes through the valve; in others, the valve is pushed before it. In most cases, as soon as the intussusception commences, intestinal obstruction occurs (*right*), although the condition should be recognized and the intussusception relieved before distention develops. (Ravitch, *In* Barnett, H. L.: Pediatrics. ed. 14. New York, Appleton.)

are not absent, achieve some success (Fitch and Denman, 1958).

Intestine and Colon

Intussusception consists in the invagination of one portion of the intestine into another. Characteristically, it affects infants in the first 2 years of life, the peak of incidence being in the 7th, the 8th and the 9th months. Males are affected more frequently than females in the ratio of 3:2, and the victims are characteristically well nourished, breast fed, vigorous and well, up to the onset. The condition is commoner in Northern Europe than in the U.S., and extremely common in Nigeria, Taiwan, and China. In most instances the intussusception begins at or near the ileocecal valve (Fig. 50-12). In less than 10 per cent of the cases, and in only 2.5 per cent of the patients under the age of 2 years, is a polyp, a Meckel's diverticulum or a nodule of ectopic pancreas or other local lesion such as extreme lymphoid hyperplasia in the terminal ileum seen as the obvious inciting cause. It has been pointed out that in infancy the disproportion between the caliber of the cecum and the ileum is greater than in later life, facilitating the occurrence of intussusception, and that in infancy there is great enlargement of the lymphoid patches in the bowel, perhaps arousing expulsive efforts.

Once an intussusception forms, the leading point is constant, and the increase in length occurs at the expense of the receiving loop, the intussuscipiens (Fig. 50-13). Compression of the mesenteric vessels between the 2 inner layers and the "U"-shaped angulation of these vessels at either end of the intussusception lead to venous stasis, engorgement, edema, exudation, further vascular compression and ultimately gangrene. Discharge of blood is one of the first results, and the early evacuation of mucus is correlated with the appearance of great numbers of goblet cells in the mucosa of the intussusceptum. The tension of the mesentery on the intussusceptum tends to arch the bowel in a curve around the mesenteric root, producing the characteristic sausage-shaped mass. Edema and compression produce intestinal obstruction, although most patients should be relieved of their intussusception before they have come to suffer from ileus. The rapidity of development of gangrene is highly variable, as Jonathan Hutchinson pointed out in 1873 when he reported the first successful operative reduction of intussusception in an infant.

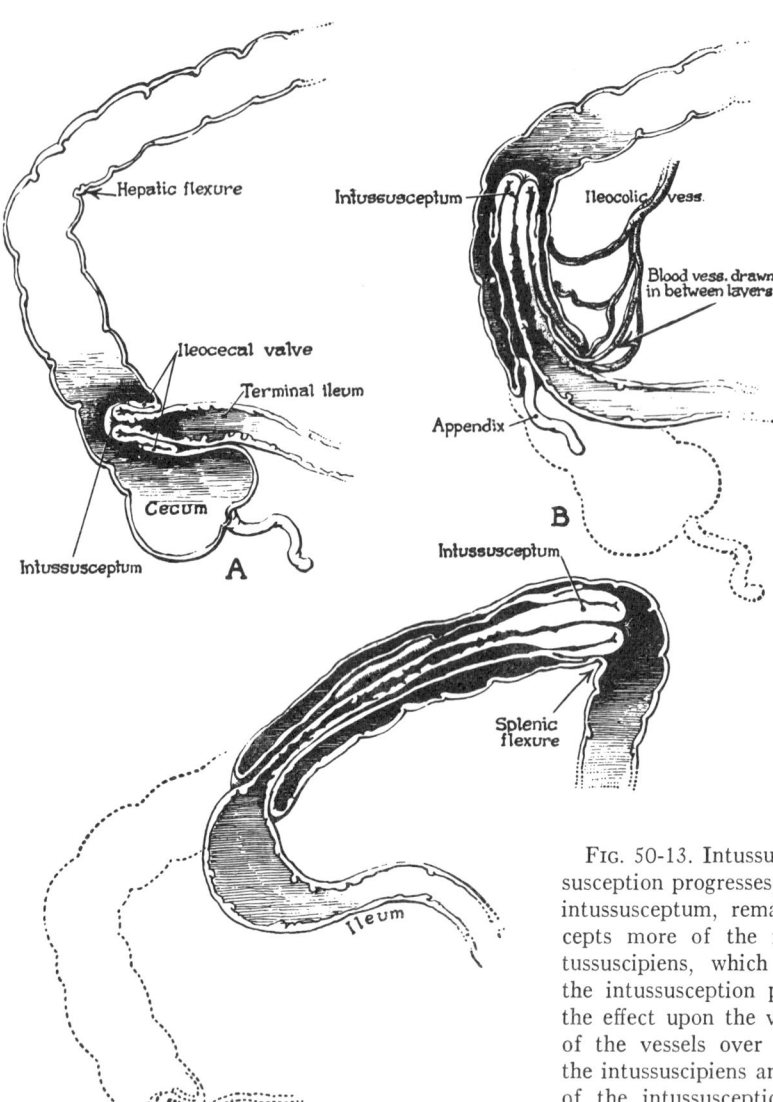

FIG. 50-13. Intussusception. As the intussusception progresses, the leading point, the intussusceptum, remains constant, and accepts more of the receiving loop, or intussuscipiens, which invaginates more as the intussusception progresses. Note in B the effect upon the vessels. The angulation of the vessels over the proximal edge of the intussuscipiens and at the leading point of the intussusception, together with the compression between the invaginated bowel and its sheath, all lead to vascular obstruction. As venous obstruction leads to exudation of fluid and edema, the pressure upon the vessels increases until the venous outflow is unable to accept the arterial blood which is being pumped in and the distended venules literally drip blood through the mucosa. At the same time, in the edematous bowel, the mucosal epithelium is transformed until all of its cells are goblet cells, secreting mucus. The mixture of blood and mucus produces the characteristic currant jelly stools. Finally, the tissue pressure obstructs the circulation of the bowel to the point at which infarction and gangrene appear. This affects first the outer layer of the intussusceptum. The inner layer of intussusceptum becomes affected next. The outer layer of bowel remains viable. (Ravitch, In: Barnett, H. L.: Holt Pediatrics. ed. 14. New York, Appleton)

The clinical picture of acute intussusception is so striking and characteristic that once seen it should be recognized regularly thereafter. A well-nourished infant in apparent good health suddenly cries out with obvious colic, and vomits. The attacks of colic recur regularly and with some increase in frequency. In the intervals the infant is flaccid or prostrated, although in rare instances seemingly normal and playful. There is usually one normal stool, evacuating the colonic contents. Thereafter, there is passed only thin blood or bloody mucus, the currant jelly stool of medical lore.

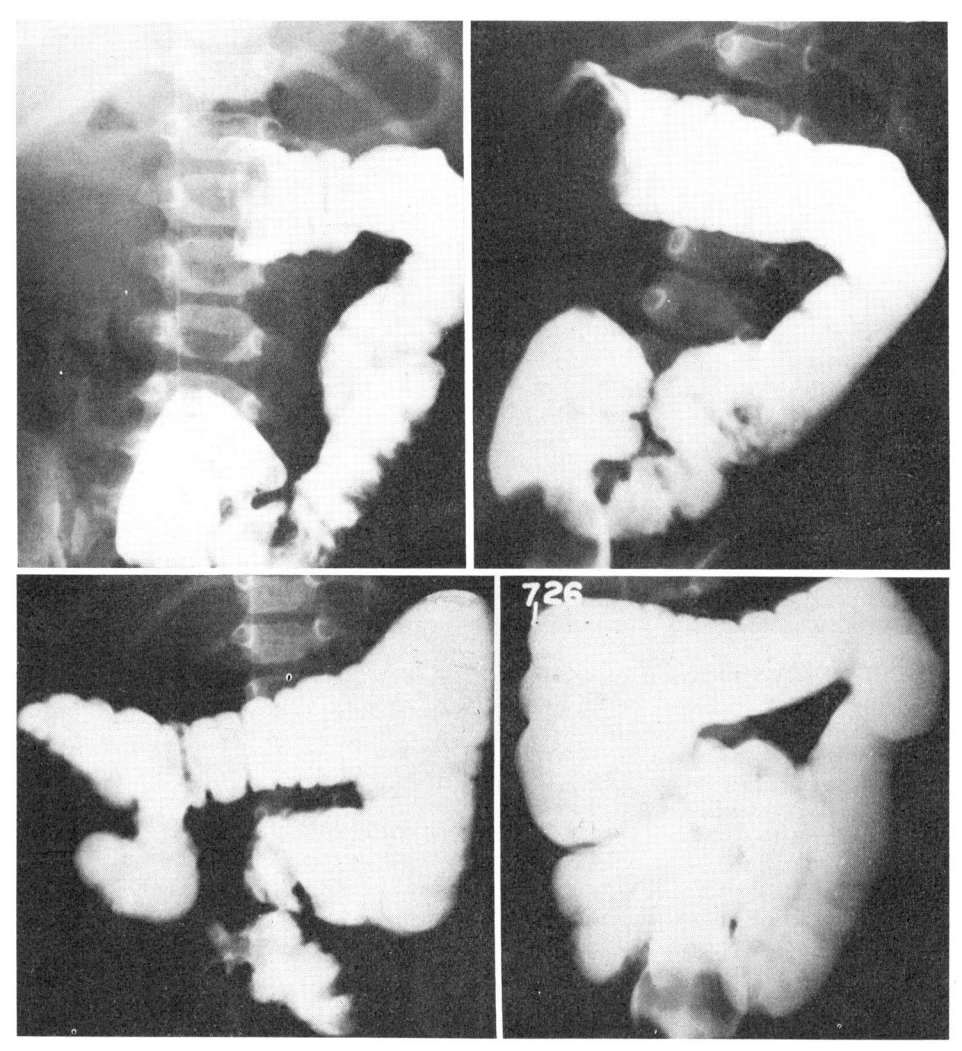

Fig. 50-14. Intussusception. Reduction by barium enema, administered under hydrostatic pressure of 3½ feet to a 9-month-old infant with characteristic history of intussusception of 29 hours' duration. (*Top, left*) Barium encounters the intussusceptum in the midtransverse colon. The concave, meniscoid appearance at the head of the barium column is typical. (*Top, right*) The intussusception is reduced by the pressure of the column of barium and has reached the hepatic flexure. (*Bottom, left*) The cecum is now filling, but no barium has yet entered the ileum. (*Bottom, right*) As the cecum distends, the intussusception is reduced through the ileocecal valve, and there is a sudden rush of barium into many loops of ileum. Free filling of these ileal loops indicates complete reduction.

Lassitude increases, and collapse ensues. The abdomen is relaxed, soft and nontender, except at times over the palpable intussusception. Signs of ileus—distention, vomiting, tachycardia—gradually supervene. Fever and leukocytosis are common. In almost 90 per cent of cases, a mass is palpable abdominally or rectally. Occasionally, the intussusception presents through the anus.

TREATMENT. In a few cases, without treatment the intussusception reduces spontaneously, or the gangrenous intussusceptum sloughs before the child has succumbed, leaving an intact intestinal canal behind. Reduc-

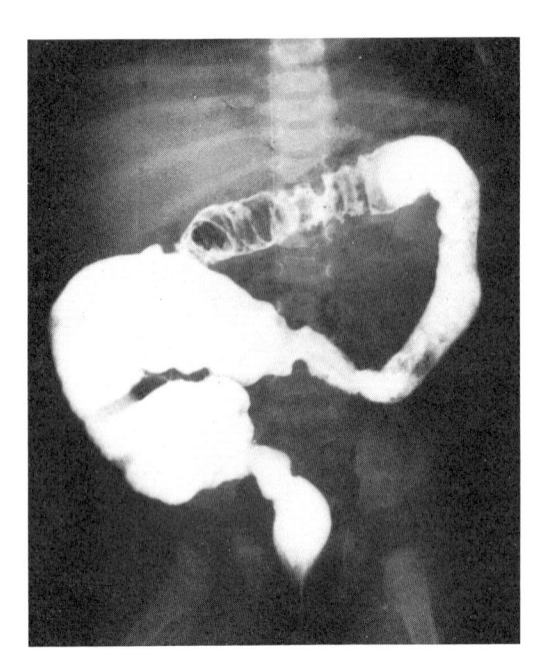

FIG. 50-15. Hirschsprung's disease. Barium enema in a 4-month-old infant with history of constipation from birth. The relatively normal-appearing distal segment is the aganglionic segment which is at fault. The grossly dilated bowel proximal to this is structurally normal. This child had severe melena, an occasional finding in infants with Hirschsprung's disease. The resected specimen showed extensive ulceration in much of the dilated, redundant sigmoid in this infant. A low anastomosis, performed by the Swenson technic, restored normal bowel evacuation and the melena gradually disappeared.

tion by enema, first practiced in antiquity, was systematized by Hirschsprung (1905) and his successors (Monrad, 1926). Hipsley (1926), in Australia, and others accumulated a massive experience with enema reduction of intussusception. Barium enema reduction under fluoroscopic control was added by Olsson and Pallin (1927) in Sweden and Retan (1927) in the United States. More recently others (Ravitch, 1959, 1969) have accumulated a large experience with reduction of intussusception by barium enema (Fig. 50-14). For 70 years after Hutchinson's first operative triumph, the hydrostatic pressure method gave superior results in terms of mortality. Today there is little to choose from in mortality statistics. In hospitals accustomed to care for sick infants no child should die of intussusception regardless of the therapy employed, except for infants already moribund upon admission. However, since in 70 to 75 per cent of infants treated primarily by barium enema, no anesthesia and no incision are required, the morbidity inevitably must be lower and the hospital stay shorter. Resection appears to be necessary much less frequently in the barium enema series. This leads to the suspicion that in some instances it is operative trauma or mistaken assumption of nonviability that necessitates bowel resection.

If operation is undertaken, it is important to prepare the infant by intravenous hydration and blood transfusion and by gastric lavage. At operation the intestine is milked back as gently as possible. Resection and anastomosis may be required for irreducible or gangrenous bowel. If barium enema is to be performed, the operating room should be prepared in any case, administration of intravenous fluids or blood begun and the stomach emptied by a tube. Through a securely taped balloon catheter, barium is run into the rectum from a height of 3 to $3\frac{1}{2}$ feet. The flow is uninterrupted and unassisted. The abdomen is never manipulated. The intussusception is outlined like a cervix in the vagina. It is reduced, sometimes haltingly, sometimes swiftly. In over 70 per cent of the cases, the operating room is notified that the operation is cancelled. With this technic, gangrenous bowel will not be reduced, and there appears to be little or no risk of perforation. The fluoroscoping surgeon makes the diagnosis of a complete reduction by (1) complete filling of many loops of ileum, (2) disappearance of the mass, (3) passage of feces or flatus and (4) abrupt and striking improvement in the child's condition.

For further confirmation, charcoal is instilled in the stomach and recovered by enema, on the ward, in 6 hours. Operation through a simple McBurney incision is undertaken if reduction is incomplete (when the intussusception is almost always found at the cecum), or if it is not certain that it is complete.

Hirschsprung's Disease (Megacolon) (Hirschsprung, 1888). This is a condition in which obstinate constipation occurs from birth. In true Hirschsprung's disease if an accurate history of the period in the obstetric nursery

FIG. 50-16. Hirschsprung's disease, gross specimen. Note the remarkable difference between the narrow distal aganglionic section and the enormously hypertrophied, greatly dilated normally ganglionic proximal segment. The sutures show the site of incisions made for biopsies. There were no ganglion cells in the junction between dilated and narrow bowel. There were ganglion cells in the biopsy taken in the middle of resected portion of dilated bowel.

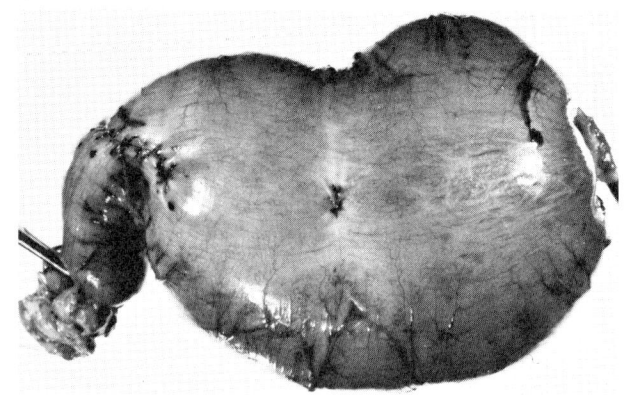

is available the baby will invariably be found to have had neonatal difficulty in evacuation. Repeated enemata may be required, severe distention may be frequent, and in infants death may occur from respiratory insufficiency due to elevation of the diaphragm by the massively distended intestine or from intestinal obstruction due to fecal impaction, or from perforation of the cecum, or from volvulus of the redundant sigmoid, occasionally, for unexplained reasons following an enema, or in the course of repeated bouts of enterocolitis, a severe fluid-losing, dehydrating, bacterially nonspecific malady associated with distention (Jewett, Leahy and Jamison, 1959). The colon gradually distends to an enormous size and becomes strikingly thickened and hypertrophied (Fig. 50-15). The rectum and the distal sigmoid are small. Fecal masses are felt in the abdomen. Digital rectal examination usually shows an empty ampulla. Incontinence is not a feature of this disease, and the presence of incontinence should suggest psychogenic constipation (Ravitch, 1958). If the children survive, it is with preposterous "potbellies," flared costal margins, malnutrition and underdevelopment. In time, careful dietary habits and a regular enema regimen can effect a tolerable modus vivendi. After childhood, the symptoms tend to be less troublesome, perhaps because this is then easier to achieve. Nevertheless, we have operated upon a man of 54, gravely troubled with Hirschsprung's disease with which he had struggled from birth.

Early in infancy, before the radiologic changes are marked, there may be substantial difficulty in establishing a diagnosis, and, in such cases, a transanal biopsy of the rectal musculature will show the characteristic absence of the ganglion cells of the myenteric plexus (Swenson, Fisher and Gherardi, 1959).

The history of the discovery of the etiology of the disease is the history of repeated obstinate failure to appreciate the reported observations that the ganglion cells of the myenteric plexus are lacking. This is all the more remarkable in that most pediatricians and surgeons for half a century had felt that the disease had a neurogenic basis. Even when the evidence accumulated in the reports of Robertson and Kernohan (1938) and of Zuelzer and Wilson (1948), it was neglected with equanimity. Finally, Swenson (1948), demonstrating that in most cases of Hirschsprung's disease the distal rectal segment is narrowed, concluded that it was this segment which was at fault. In a nice adaptation of Maunsell's 19th-century operative procedure, he resected this narrowed distal segment, heretofore largely neglected by clinicians who had concentrated on the obvious, dilated colon above. Bodian (1949), in the specimens resected according to Swenson's principles by Stephens at Great Ormond Street, conclusively demonstrated that in cases of megacolon (true Hirschsprung's disease) with a narrowed distal segment of rectum or rectum and sigmoid, the ganglion cells of the myenteric plexuses were absent in the narrowed—apparently normal—distal bowel and appeared in normal numbers in the dilated and hypertrophied proximal bowel (Fig. 50-16). Whereas in Hirschsprung's disease the ganglion cells of the myenteric plexus are absent, the nerve fibers are actually more abundant and more conspicuous than usual. Thus the proximal dilatation and hypertrophy were seen to be due to obstruction in the narrow, improperly fuctioning aganglionic distal bowel. Sympathectomy and management with parasympathomimetic drugs were abandoned, and the resections which some surgeons had long performed were now given a sound basis and direction. The Swenson procedure, slightly modified, consists in telescoping the dissected rectum and sigmoid out through the anus, amputating close to the anus the huge prolapse thus produced and effecting an effortless 2-layer anastomosis outside the anus, then permitting the suture line to retract just inside the sphincters. The requisite upper limit of resection may be determined by frozen section identification of ganglion cells. The results in the relief of megacolon are excellent, and the mortality low. Fecal and urinary incontinence and sexual impotence in males are theoretical hazards. The latter two should not be met if pelvic dissection is held close to the bowel. The first is avoided if, in addition, resection is not too low (Swenson, 1957).

In rare instances the entire colon is aganglionic, creating a condition extremely difficult to treat even if the diagnosis is made (Swenson and Fisher, 1955).

Because some children have shown incontinence after the Swenson procedure; because it is, perhaps, technically demanding in the smallest infants; because a "re-do" after a previously inadequate resection is extremely difficult; and because attacks of serious enterocolitis may occur even after operation, some surgeons (Beardmore, 1964; Ehrenpreis, 1961) have been dissatisfied. Duhamel (1960), adapting the old Gersuny operation (for use of the isolated rectum as a new urinary bladder), devised a procedure which is now receiving wide trial. His method consists in dividing and closing over the rectum at the peritoneal reflection, resecting the remainder of the aganglionic segment, and bringing the normal bowel posterior to the rectum to emerge through an opening in the posterior rectal wall, just inside the sphincter. The posterior wall of the rectum and the anterior wall of the normal bowel are cut through, opening the space between the two segments and creating a new rectum, the anterior wall of which retains the sensory portion of the defecatory reflex arc and the posterior wall of which has normal motor function. This operation and Swenson's are both undergoing modification, and the last word has not been said. We have used both with satisfaction (Steichen et al., 1968). Soave (1964) modified an old endorectal pull-through technic, bringing the proximal bowel through the rectum denuded of mucosa and suturing the normal ganglionated bowel to the anus. The operation is being widely employed and initial reports are good.

Atresia or stenosis of the colon is rare. Surgeons unacquainted with the appearance of the tiny, empty colon found distal to atresias of the small bowel frequently comment on microcolon and question the ability of such a colon to receive the fecal stream. In most of these cases the colon is merely collapsed because it never has been distended with meconium, but is anatomically normal.

Lymphosarcoma of the intestine is the commonest malignant intestinal tumor in childhood. Remarkable is its capacity for involving extensive segments of small bowel, the wall of which is replaced by a thick, rigid tumor mass, without any striking gastrointestinal symptoms. In the cecum, a chronic, nonstrangulating, nonobstructing intussusception is strongly suggestive of lymphosarcoma. The mesenteric glands are almost always widely involved, and while resection of the involved intestine may be of some benefit, ultimate recovery has been rare. The newer chemotherapeutic agents may affect this picture but are not known to result in permanent cure at the present time.

Carcinoma of the colon does occur in childhood and tends to be more insidious than in adults, perhaps because little heed is given to such a possibility. The tumor is frequently inoperable by virtue of metastases, before operation is undertaken (Williams, 1954).

Intestinal polyposis occurs in a wide variety of forms in infants and children. The polyps in stomach and colon may cause anemia from chronic blood loss. In the small bowel, polyps are prone to cause intussusception. In the colon, polyps may lead to or attend the development of carcinoma.

Polyps may involve the entire gastrointestinal tract (Ravitch, 1948), may be familial or sporadic, may occur in the small bowel alone in familial form, may occur in association with the telltale melanin pigmentation of the lips, the palms and the soles known as Hutchinson's spots (Yeghers, McKusick and Katz, 1949) (Peutz-Jeghers' Syndrome, see Chap. 40), may occur in association with sexual infantilism (Bensaude, Hillemand and Augier, 1932), or with multiple sebaceous cysts (Oldfield, 1954) and osteomas (Gardner's syndrome). Multiple polyposis of the colon—sporadic or familial—may cause constant bloody diarrhea, serious protein loss and malnutrition and inevitably leads to death from cancer of the rectum or the colon. The only certain preventive is total colectomy (Ravitch and Handelsman, 1951).

Juvenile polyps of the rectum, unlike adenomatous polyps, are smoothly rounded, covered with normal mucosa and have a loose fibrous stroma with large mucus spaces. These polyps are self-limited, never malignant, may bleed or prolapse, frequently slough spontaneously, and can usually be removed endoscopically (Todd, 1964).

Fissure in ano is common in infants and manifested by the infant's obvious reluctance to defecate, and by pain and discomfort during the act. If the little sentinel pile is clipped away, the sphincter carefully dilated with one finger and massaged daily, and measures taken to avoid costive stools, relief can be expected. In rare cases the anal ulcer is so indurated as to require excision.

Perianal abscesses and fistula in ano occur in children and are treated exactly as in adults (see Chap. 41, Anorectum).

Rectal prolapse is commonly encountered in pediatric practice. Firm pressure will reduce the prolapse. Reduction may then be maintained for several days by the unsanitary but effective measure of strapping the buttocks together and allowing the child to defecate at will. Occasionally, a 2nd or a 3rd prolapse occurs before the measure is permanently effective. Operation is almost never required. In 2 particularly severe instances, we have performed a Mikulicz excision of the long sigmoid and the upper rectum and subsequently closed the colostomy extraperitoneally, the bowel remaining adherent to the abdominal wall.

IMPERFORATE ANUS

The complicated embryologic derivation of the rectum and anus and bladder resulting from the differentiation of the cloaca affords wide opportunity for the development of malformations. The contributions of Stephens (1963) have been widely accepted (Louw, 1965). A few relatively minor anomalies are readily diagnosable by inspection. The anal opening may be covered over by a translucent membrane against which meconium bulges when the baby strains. This membrane need only be punctured. In males the anus may appear covered over, but a tiny blue meconium-filled tract is found ascending in the median raphe toward the scrotum. This is a covered anus and responds to excision of the tract and opening of the anus. In either sex, but particularly in females, an apparently normal-appearing anus with contracting sphincter and furrowed mucosa may lie somewhat anterior to its normal position. This is an ectopic anus, functions normally and need not be disturbed. In the female an ectopic anus surrounded by dry skin for at least its posterior half will be continent. If the opening is entirely in the vestibule near the fourchette and surrounded by moist pink epithelium, we are dealing with a vestibular anus. This will be found usually to connect to a rectum that extends behind it to the site of the normal anal dimple. The "cut-back" operation of Dennis Browne (1951) is all that need be done. In the vast majority of all children with an imperforate anus there is some type of fistulous external communication: in the higher lesions, it is with the posterior urethra, in males, and with the vagina, in females. X-ray of the child in the upside-down position (Wangensteen and Rice, 1930), in the lateral view, will demonstrate the level to which air has passed in the rectum. Stephens has pointed out that the significant level is the line between the pubis and the first coccygeal segment, the pubococcygeal line. When the rectum ends above this line, it is above the pubo-rectalis portion of the levator sling apparatus, which is the prime consideration in continence. In such instances a colostomy should be done on the newborn infant and the definitive operation delayed for 6 to 8 months.

An infant can tolerate an imperforate anus for 24 to 48 hours with little hazard in most instances. In the past, innumerable infants have come to grief through hasty attempts to bring the rectum down considerable distances to the anal skin. Even when the operation appeared to be achieved, Stephens has demonstrated that the bowel was usually brought down behind the pubo-rectalis sling and incontinence inevitably resulted. Rhoads (1948) introduced the simultaneous abdominoperineal

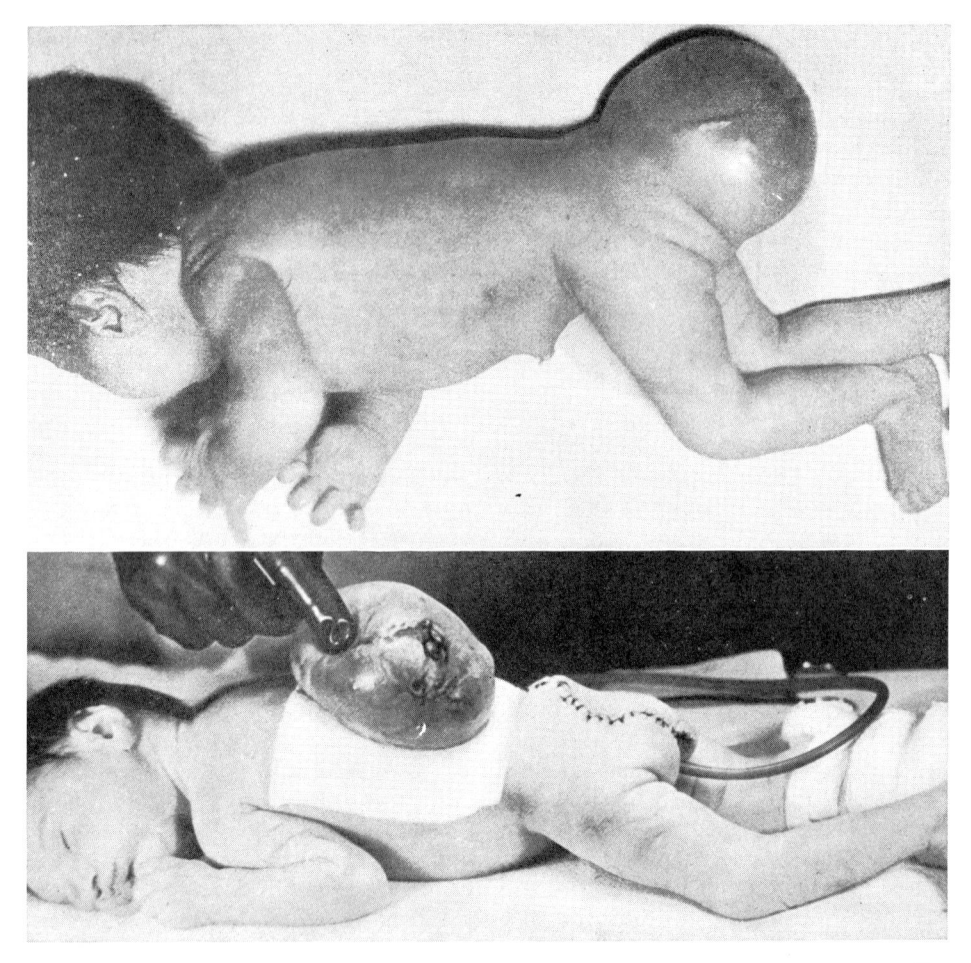

FIG. 50-17. Sacrococcygeal teratoma. (*Top*) A 10-day-old infant with a large teratoma distending the skin over it so markedly as to produce necrosis and ulceration. There was a large intrapelvic component. Such tumors may become malignant and metastasize, may ulcerate and become infected, by pressure may obstruct the rectum, the urethra or the ureters. (*Bottom*) The tumor is readily excised, with a large area of superfluous skin, leaving a posterior mid-line incision. A balloon-catheter distends the rectum and facilitates the separation of the tumor from it in the dissection.

procedure. Stephens has now pointed out the importance of bringing the rectum down through the levator sling when this sling is large enough to be identified and the necessity for doing this through a posterior, sacral approach combined with a perineal trap-door incision. For the higher lesions an abdominal approach is required as well, to deliver the bowel. Stephens tends to employ the sacral approach even for distal rectovaginal fistulae but most surgeons (Santulli, 1969) core out the rectovaginal fistulous tract and bring it down through the anal sphincter ring. Fibers of the external sphincter are frequently present, but, in any case, in most of these children continence is dependent upon the function of the levator.

One occasionally sees girls or women who are disclosed to have ectopically abnormal anal openings in the perineum or even at or just below the fourchette, are continent and lead normal lives. Obviously, no operation should be undertaken in these.

With all repairs of imperforate anus, the after-care and gentle, persistent and long continued anal dilatation and massage are important if a satisfactory percentage of good results is to be achieved. These babies rarely afford the surgeon more than a single opportunity for a good result. The operation is never an emergency. If there is any doubt as to the procedure to be followed, a colostomy is always a safe choice, and operation can be postponed until the most favorable auspices exist. Reoperations are difficult and unsatisfactory and too much emphasis cannot be placed upon the importance of proper performance of a good procedure at the first operation.

SACROCOCCYGEAL TERATOMA AND OTHER PELVIC TUMORS

A variety of pelvic tumors occurs—neuroblastomas, sarcomas, anterior meningoceles, dermoids, chordomas, enterogenous cysts of the rectum—but perhaps the most interesting are the sacrococcygeal tumors (Gross, Clatworthy and Meeker, 1951); (Ravitch and Smith, 1951). These teratomas may be entirely external (Fig. 50-17), like great coccygeal appendages, or largely internal and not visible from without, or, most commonly, both intrapelvic (occasionally intra-abdominal) and external. The tumors are often large enough to ulcerate the overlying skin with resultant infection. They may obstruct rectum, urethra, or ureters, and finally some 25 per cent of them are or become malignant. Regardless of their great size and intrapelvic and intra-abdominal extension, they can be totally removed from behind, the coccyx being excised and the rectum dissected away. Once a malignant teratoma has invaded the surrounding tissues, cure is unlikely.

REFERENCES

Almklov, J. R., and Hatoff, A.: Pneumatocele during the course of pneumonia in children. Am. J. Dis. Child., 72:521-528, 1946.
Alonso-Lej, F., Rever, W. B., and Pessagno, D. J.: A study of the congenital choledochal cyst with a report of two patients and an analysis of 94 cases. Surg., Gynec. Obstet., Internat. Abstr. Surg., 108:1, 1959.
Alpert, S., Metcalf, W., Vreede, A. A., and Meng, C. H.: Right hepatectomy for hamartoma in an eleven month old infant. Ann. Surg., 165, 286-292, 1967.
Ariel, I. M., and Pack, G. T.: Tumors of infancy and childhood: a general appraisal. *In*: Cancer and Allied Diseases of Infancy and Childhood. pp. 3-4. Boston, Little, Brown & Co., 1960.
Arnheim, E. E., and Gemson, B. L.: Persistent cervical thymus gland: thymectomy. Surgery, 27:603-608, 1950.
Beahrs, O. H., Devine, K. D., and Hayles, A. B.: Tumors of the head and neck. *In*: Cancer and Allied Diseases of Infancy and Childhood. pp. 62-65. Boston, Little, Brown & Co., 1960.
Beardmore, H. E.: An evaluation of the present status of the operations for Hirschsprung's disease. Proc. 1963 Ross Conference, 1964.
Begg, R. C.: Urachus, its anatomy, histology, and development. J. Anat. 64:170-183, 1930.
Bensaude, R., Hillemand, P., and Augier, P.: Polypose intestinale et infantilisme, Bull. et mém. Soc. méd. hôp. Paris, 48:251-257, 1932.
Benson, C. D.: Intestinal stenosis and atresia. *In*: Mustard, Ravitch, Snyder, Welch and Benson: Pediatric Surgery. Ed. 2. Chicago, Yearbook Publishers, 1969.
Bill, A. H.: Branchiogenic cysts and sinuses. *In*: Mustard, Ravitch, Snyder, Welch and Benson: Pediatric Surgery. Ed. 2. Chicago, Yearbook Publishers, 1969.
Bill, A. H., Jr., and Johnson, R. S.: Congenital median band of the anus. Surg., Gynec. Obstet., 97:307-311, 1953.
Bodian, M., Stephens, F. D., and Ward, B. C. H.: Hirschsprung's disease and idiopathic megacolon. Lancet 1:6-11, 1949.
Boley, J. S., Krieger, H., Schwartz, S. S., Harandian, B. and Pearlman, B.: The effect of operations for peptic ulcer on growth and nutrition of puppies. Surgery, 57, 441-447, 1965.
Brock, R. C.: Lung Abscess. p. 86. Oxford, Blackwell Scientific Publications, 1952.
Browne, D.: Some congenital deformities of the rectum, anus, vagina and urethra. Ann. Roy. Coll. Surg., 8:173-192, 1951.
Burnett, W. E., and Caswell, H. T.: Lobectomy for pulmonary cysts in a 15 day old infant with recovery. Surgery, 23:84-91, 1948.
Byars, L. T., and Anderson, R.: Anomalies of the first branchial cleft. Surg., Gynec. Obstet. 93:755-758, 1951.
Cantrell, J. R., Haller, J. A., and Ravitch, M. M.: A syndrome of congenital defects involving the abdominal wall, sternum, diaphragm, pericardium and heart. Surg., Gynec. Obstet., 107:602-610, 1958.
Cayley, C. K., Caez, H. J., and Mersheimer, W.: Primary bronchogenic carcinoma of the lung in children. Am. J. Dis. Child., 82:49-60, 1951.
Clay, R. C.: Ganglioneuroma of nodose ganglion of vagus. Ann. Surg., 132:147-152, 1950.
Collett, R. W.: Prepyloric polypus in stomach of child diagnosed histologically as aberrant pancreatic tissue. Am. J. Dis. Child., 72:545-551, 1946.
Cordero, L., Touloukian, R. J., and Pickett, L. J.: Staged repair of gastroschisis with silastic sheeting. Surg., 65:676-682, 1969.
Cordonnier, J. K. and Izant, R. J., Jr.: Meconium ileus equivalent. Surgery, 54:667-672, 1963.

Dennison, W.: Surgery in Infancy and childhood. Edinburgh, E. & S. Livingstone, 1967.
Donovan, E. J.: Congenital hypertrophic pyloric stenosis in infancy. J.A.M.A., 109:558-561, 1937.
Dudrick, S. J., Wilmore, D. W., Vars, H. M., and Rhoads, J. E.: Long-term total parenteral nutrition with growth, development, and positive nitrogen balance. Surgery, 64:134-142, 1968.
Duhamel, B.: A new operation for the treatment of Hirschsprung's disease. Arch. Dis. Child., 35:38, 1960.
Ehrenpreis, T.: Longterm results of rectosigmoidectomy for Hirschsprung's disease, with a note on Duhamel's operation. Surgery, 49:701-706, 1961.
Fallon, M., Gordon, A. R. G., and Lendrum, A. C.: Mediastinal cysts of foregut origin associated with vertebral anomalies. Brit. J. Surg., 41:520-533, 1954.
Fitch, E. A., and Denman, F. R.: Congenital deficiencies of abdominal musculature (a syndrome): a surgical repair. Am. Surgeon, 24:371-376, 1958.
Fraumeni, J. F., Jr., Miller, R. W., and Hill, J. D.: Primary carcinoma of the liver in childhood—an epidemiologic study. J. Nat. Cancer Inst., 40:1087, 1968.
Fredet, P., and Guillemot, L.: La sténose du pylore par hypertrophie musculaire chez les nourrissons. Ann. Gynec. Obstet., 7:504-629, 1910.
Gardner, C. E.: The surgical significance of anomalies of intestinal rotation. Ann. Surg., 131:879-898, 1950.
Gardner, C. E., and Hart, D.: Enterogenous cysts of duodenum; report of case and review of literature. J.A.M.A., 104:1809-1812, 1935.
Gellis, S. S., and Holt, L. E.: The treatment of lye strictures by the Salzer method. Ann. Otol., 51: 1086-1088, 1942.
Gilbert, J. W., and Morrow, A. G.: Gastrointestinal bleeding after cardiovascular operations in children. Surgery, 47:685-690, 1960.
Gilbert, E. F., Nishimura, K., and Wedum, B. G.: Congenital malformation of the heart associated with splenic agenesis. Circulation, 17:72-86, 1958.
Glenn, F., and Hill, M. R.: Primary gallbladder disease in children. Ann. Surg., 139:302-311, 1954.
Glover, D. M., and Barry, F. M.: Intestinal obstruction in the newborn. Ann. Surg., 130:480-511, 1949.
Grob, M.: Lehrbuch der Kinderchirurgie. pp. 311-315. Stuttgart, Georg Thieme, 1957.
———: Intestinal obstruction in the newborn infant. Arch. Dis. Child., 35:40, 1960.
Gross, R. E.: A new method for surgical treatment of large omphaloceles. Surgery, 24:277-292, 1948.
———: The Surgery of Infancy and Childhood. Philadelphia, W. B. Saunders, 1953.
Gross, R. E., Clatworthy, H. W., and Meeker, I. A.: Sacrocygeal teratomas in infants and children. Surg., Gynec. Obstet., 92:341-354, 1951.
Gross, R. E., and Goeringer, C. F.: Cystic hygroma of the neck. Surg., Gynec. Obstet., 69:48-60, 1939.
Gross, R. E., and Hurwitt, E. S.: Cervicomediastinal and mediastinal cystic hygromas. Surg., Gynec. Obstet., 87:599-610, 1948.

Hagler, S., Rosenblum, P. and Rosenblum, H.: Carcinoma of the thyroid in children and young adults, iatrogenic relation to previous irradiation. Pediatrics, 38:77-81, 1966.
Haight, C.: Congenital esophageal atresia and tracheo esophageal fistula. In: Mustard, Ravitch, Welch, Synder and Benson. Pediatric Surgery. Ed. 2. Chicago, Year Book Publishers, 1969.
Haight, C., and Towsley, H. A.: Congenital atresia of the esophagus with tracheoesophageal fistula. Surg., Gynec. Obstet., 76:672-688, 1943.
Handelsman, J. C., and Ravitch, M. M.: Chylous cysts of the mesentery in children. Ann. Surg., 140:185-193, 1954.
Harkins, G. A., and Sabiston, D. C.: Lymphangioma in infancy and childhood. Surgery, 47:811-822, 1960.
Heimburger, I. L., and Battersby, J. S.: Primary mediastinal tumors of childhood. J. Thorac. Cardiov. Surg., 50:92-103.
Hiatt, R. B., and Wilson, P. E.: Celiac syndrome: VII. Therapy of meconium ileus; report of 8 cases with a review of the literature. Surg., Gynec. Obstet. 87:317-327, 1948.
Hipsley, P. L.: Intussusception and its treatment by hydrostatic pressure based on analysis of 100 consecutive cases so treated. M. J. Australia, 2:201-206, 1926.
Hirschsprung, H.: Hundertundsieben Fälle von Darminvagination bei Kindern behandelt im Königin Louisen-Kinderhospital in Kopenhagen während der Jahre 1871-1904, kurze tabellarische Darstellung. Mitt. Grenzgeb. Med. u. Chir., 14:555-574, 1905.
———: Stuhlträgheit Neugeborener in Folge von Dilatation und Hypertrophie des Colons. Jahrb. Kinderh., 27:1-7, 1888.
Holder, T. M.: Esophageal atresia and tracheoesophageal fistula, A survey of its members by the Surgical Section of the American Academy of Pediatrics. Pediatrics, 34:542, 1964.
Holder, T. M., and Ashcraft, K. W.: Esophageal atresia and tracheo-esophageal fistula. Cur. Prob. Surg., August, 1966.
Holder, T. M., McDonald, V. G., Jr., and Woolley, M. M.: The premature or critically ill infant with esophageal atresia; increased success with a staged approach. J. Thorac. Cardio. Surg., 44:344, 1962.
Holinger, P. H., Johnston, K. C., Potts, W. J., and da Cunha, F.: The conservative and surgical management of benign strictures of the esophagus. J. Thoracic Surg., 28:345-366, 1954.
Horwitz, O., and Meyer, J.: The safety record of BCG vaccination and untoward reactions observed after vaccination. Adv. Tuberc. Res., 8:245-271, 1957.
Howard, J. M., Rawson, A. J., Koop, C. E., Horn, R. C., and Royster, H. P.: Parotid tumors in children. Surg., Gynec. Obstet., 90:307-315, 1950.
Hutchinson, J.: A successful case of abdominal section for intussusception; with remarks on this and other methods of treatment. Medico-Chir. Tr., 57: 31-76, 1874.
Jeghers, H., McKusick, V. A., and Katz, K. H.:

Generalized intestinal polyposis and melanin spots of the oral mucosa, lips, and digits. New Eng. J. Med., 241:993-1036, 1949.

Jewett, T. C., Leahy, L. J., and Jamison, J.: Hirschsprung's disease in infants. Arch. Surg., 79:455-458, 1959.

Johnston, P. W., and Snyder, W. H., Jr.: Vagotomy and pyloroplasty in infancy and childhood. J. Pediat. Surg., 2:238-245, 1968.

Jolleys, A.: Micrognathos: A review of 38 cases treated in the newborn period. J. Pediat. Surg., 1:460-465, 1966.

Jones, P.: Torticollis in infancy and childhood. Springfield, Ill., Charles C Thomas, 1968.

Kaplan, H. S., and Rosenberg, S. A.: The treatment of Hodgkin's disease. Med. Clin. N. Am., 50:1591-1610, 1966.

Kent, E. M., Blades, B., Valle, A. R., and Graham, E. A.: Intrathoracic neurogenic tumors. J. Thoracic Surg., 13:116-161, 1944.

Kittle, C. F., Jenkins, H. P., and Dragstedt, L. R.: Patent omphalomesenteric duct and its relations to the diverticulum of Meckel. Arch. Surg., 54:10-36, 1947.

Klopp, C. J., Rosvall, R. V., and Winship, T.: Is destructive surgery ever necessary for treatment of thyroid cancer in children? Ann. Surg., 165:750, 1967.

Krovetz, J. L.: Congenital biliary atresia. I. Analysis of thirty cases with particular reference to diagnosis. Surgery, 47:453-467, 1960.

——: Congenital biliary atresia. II. Analysis of the therapeutic problem. Surgery, 47:468-489, 1960.

Ladd, W. E.: Congenital atresia and stenosis of the bile ducts. J.A.M.A., 91:1082-1085, 1928.

——. Congenital obstructions of the duodenum in children. New Eng. J. Med., 206:277, 1932.

——: The surgical treatment of esophageal atresia and tracheo-esophageal fistulas. New Eng. J. Med., 230:625-637, 1944.

Ladd, W. E., and Gross, R. E.: Surgical treatment of duplications of the alimentary tract. Surg. Gynec. Obstet., 70:295-307, 1940.

Ladd, W. E., and Scott, H. W., Jr.: Esophageal duplications or mediastinal cysts of enteric origin. Surgery, 16:815, 1944.

Leape, L. L., and Longino, L. A.: Infantile lobar emphysema. Pediatrics, 34:241-255, 1964.

Leix, F., and Greaney, E. M.: Surgical experience with peptic ulcer in infancy and childhood. Am. J. Surg., 106:173-184, 1963.

Leven, N. L.: Congenital atresia of esophagus with tracheoesophageal fistula. J. Thoracic Surg., 10:648, 1941.

Linker, L. M., and Benson, C. D.: Spontaneous perforation of the stomach in the newborn. Ann. Surg., 149:525-533, 1959.

Lorimer, W. S., and Ellis, D. B.: Meconium peritonitis. Surgery, 60:470-475, 1966.

Louw, J. H.: Congenital intestinal atresia and stenosis in the newborn. Ann. Roy. Coll. Surg., 25:209-34, 1959.

——: Congenital abnormalities of the rectum and anus, Curr. Probl. Surg., May, 1965.

——: Jejunoileal atresia and stenosis, J. Pediat. Surg., 1:8-23, 1966.

Lukes, R. J., and Butler, J. J.: The pathology and nomenclature of Hodgkin's disease. Cancer Res., 26:1063-1083, 1966.

Lyday, J. E., Markarian, M., and Rhoads, J. E.: Perforated duodenal ulcer in a 2100 Gm. female infant with survival. Am. J. Surg., 97:346-349, 1959.

McKibben, B. G.: Congenital atresia of the nasal choanae. Laryngoscope, 67:731-755, 1957.

Maier, H. C., and Gould, W. S.: Agenesis of the lung with vascular compression of the tracheobronchial tree. J. Pediat., 43:38, 1953.

Marshall, J. M.: Gastrojejunal ulcers in children. Arch. Surg., 67:490-492, 1953.

Minnis, J. F.: Congenital cystic disease of the lung in infancy. J. Thorac. Cardiov. Surg., 43:262-266, 1962.

Monrad, S.: Acute invagination of the intestine in small children. Acta paediat., 6:31-52, 1926.

Morris, J. D.: Surgical correction of pectus excavatum. Surg. Clin. N. Am., 41:1271-1279, 1961.

Nunn, I. N., and Stephens, F. D.: The triad syndrome: A composite anomaly of the abdominal wall, urinary system and testes. J. Urol., 86:782-794, 1961.

Oldfield, M. C.: The association of familial polyposis of the colon with multiple sebaceous cysts. Brit. J. Surg., 41:534, 1954.

Oliver, W. J., Graham, B. D., and Wilson, H. L.: Lack of scientific validity of body surface as basis for parenteral fluid dosage. J.A.M.A. 167:1212-1218, 1958.

Oski, F. A., Allen, D. M., and Diamond, L. K.: Portal hypertension—a complication of umbilical vein catheterization. Pediatrics, 31:297-302, 1963.

Parkkulainen, K. V.: Intrauterine intussusception as a cause of intestinal atresia. Surgery, 44:1106-1111, 1958.

Peters, R. M., and Johnson, G.: Stabilization of pectus excavatum with wire strut. J. Thorac. Cardiov. Surg., 47:814-816, 1964.

Plummer, G. W., and Stabins, S. J.: Bleeding duodenal ulcer in infancy: a surgical problem. J. Pediat., 37:899-904, 1950.

Potts, W. J.: Surgical treatment of congenital pulmonary stenosis. Ann. Surg., 130:342-362, 1949.

Potts, W. J., and Idriss, F.: Review of our experience with atresia of the esophagus with and without complicating fistulae. Maryland M. J., 9:528-37, 1960.

Potts, W. J., and Riker, W. L.: Differentiation of congenital cysts of the lung and those following staphylococcal pneumonia. Arch. Surg., 61:684-695, 1950.

Pryce, D. M.: Lower accessory pulmonary artery with intralobar sequestration of lung: a report of 7 cases. J. Path. Bact., 58:457-467, 1946.

Pryce, D. M., Sellors, T. H., and Blair, L. G.: Intralobar sequestration of lung associated with an abnormal pulmonary artery. Brit. J. Surg., 35:18-29, 1947.

Rammstedt, C.: Zur Operation der angeborenen Pylorusstenose. Med. Klin., 8:1702-1705, 1912.

Randolph, J. G., and Gross, R. E.: Congenital chylothorax. Arch. Surg., 74:405-419, 1957.

Ravitch, M. M.: Polypoid adenomatosis of the entire gastrointestinal tract. Ann. Surg., 128:283-297, 1948.

———: Radical treatment of massive mixed angiomas (hemolymphangiomas) in infants and children. Ann. Surg., 134:228-243, 1951.

———: Hindgut duplication—doubling of colon and of the genital and lower urinary tracts. Ann. Surg., 137:588-601, 1953.

———: Pseudo Hirschsprung's disease. Ann. Surg., 147:781-795, 1958.

———: Intussusception in Infants and Children. Springfield, Ill., Charles C Thomas, 1959.

———: Giant omphalocele: second stage repair with the aid of pneumoperitoneum. J.A.M.A., 185:122-124, 1963.

———: Atypical deformities of the chest wall—absence and deformities of the ribs and costal cartilages. Surgery, 59:438-449, 1966.

———: Congenital deformities of the chest wall. In: Mustard, Ravitch, Welch, Snyder and Benson: Pediatric Surgery, ed. 2. Chicago, Year Book Publishers, 1969.

———: Congenital cystic disease of the lung. In: Mustard, Ravitch, Welch, Snyder and Benson: Pediatric Surgery. ed. 2. Chicago, Year Book Publishers, 1969.

———: Cystic hygroma. In: Mustard, Ravitch, Snyder, Welch and Benson: Pediatric Surgery. ed. 2. Chicago Yearbook Publishers, 1969.

Ravitch, M. M., and Fein, R.: The changing picture of pneumonia and empyema in infants and children. A review of the experience at the Harriet Lane Home from 1934 through 1958. J.A.M.A., 175:1039-1044, 1961.

Ravitch, M. M., and Handelsman, J. C.: One stage resection of the entire colon and rectum for ulcerative colitis and polypoid adenomatosis. Bull. Johns Hopkins Hosp., 88:59-82, 1951.

Ravitch, M. M., and McGoon, D. C.: Teratoid tumors and dermoid cysts. In: Cancer and Allied Diseases of Infancy and Childhood. pp. 249-273, Boston, Little, Brown & Co., 1960.

Ravitch, M. M., Rowe, M. I., and Halperin, D. C.: Hernia of the esophageal hiatus in infants. Illinois Med. J., 134:269-273, 1968.

Ravitch, M. M., and Rush, B. F., Jr.: The thyroid. In: Mustard, Ravitch, Snyder, Welch and Benson: Pediatric Surgery. ed. 2. Chicago, Year Book Publishers, 1969.

Ravitch, M. M., and Sabiston, D. C.: Mediastinal cysts and tumors. In: Mustard, Ravitch, Welch, Snyder and Benson: Pediatric Surgery. ed. 2. Chicago, Year Book Publishers, 1969.

Ravitch, M. M., and Smith, E. I.: Sacrococcygeal teratoma in infants and children. Surgery, 30:733-762, 1951.

Ravitch, M. M., and Snyder, G. B.: Congenital cystic dilatation of the common bile duct. Surgery, 44:752-765, 1958.

Ravitch, M. M., and Woods, A. C.: Annular pancreas. Ann. Surg., 132:1116-1127, 1950.

Ray, E. J., and Morgan, D. L.: Cortisone therapy of lye burns of the esophagus. J. Pediat., 49:394, 1956.

Redo, S. F.: Congenital atresia of extrahepatic ducts. Arch. Surg., 69:886-897, 1954.

Retan, G. M.: Non-operative treatment of intussusception. Am. J. Dis. Child., 33:765-770, 1927.

Rhoads, J. E., Pipes, R. L., and Perlingieró-Randall, J.: A simultaneous abdominal and perineal approach in operations for imperforate anus with atresia of the rectum and rectosigmoid. Ann. Surg., 127:552-556, 1948.

Riemensnyder, J. P.: Intrauterine rupture of omphalocele. Surgery, 54:681-686, 1963.

Robertson, H. E., and Kernohan, J. W.: Myenteric plexus in congenital megacolon. Proc. Mayo Clin., 13:123-125, 1938.

Runström, G.: On Roentgen-anatomical appearance of congenital pyloric stenosis during and after manifest stage of disease. Acta paediat., 26:383-433, 1939.

Rush, B. F., Jr., and Ravitch, M. M.: Septic thrombophlebitis due to a species of achromobacter in a four-year-old boy. J.A.M.A., 173:253-254, 1960.

Rutherford, R. B., and Akers, D. R.: Meckel's diverticulum—a review of 148 pediatric patients with special reference to the pattern of bleeding and to mesodiverticular vascular bands. Surgery, 59:618-626, 1966.

Sabiston, D. C., Hopkins, E. H., Cooke, R. E., and Bennett, I. L.: The surgical management of complications of staphylococcal pneumonia in infancy and childhood, J. Thorac. Cardiov. Surg., 38:421-434, 1959.

Sale, T. A.: Successful treatment of a perforated Rokitansky-Cushing ulcer. Arch. Dis. Child., 31:233-235, 1956.

Sandblom, P.: Plastic repair of congenital esophageal stenosis. Acta chir. scand., 97:35-41, 1948.

Sanford, H. N., and Shmigelsky, I. H.: Purulent parotitis in the newborn. J. Pediat., 26:149-154, 1954.

Santulli, T. V.: Management of surgical conditions of the alimentary tract in infancy. Bull. N. Y. Acad. Med., 36:185, 1960.

———: Imperforate anus. In: Mustard, Ravitch, Snyder, Welch and Benson: Pediatric Surgery. ed. 2. Chicago, Yearbook Publishers, 1969.

Schobel, H.: Zur Therapie der akuten Speiseröhrenverätzungen und der besonderen Berücksichtigung der Hormon Behandlung. Z. Hals-, Nas.- u. Ohrenheilk., 7:193, 1959.

Sloan, R. D., and Cooley, R. N.: Congenital pulmonary arteriovenous aneurysm. Am. J. Roentgenol., 70:183-210, 1953.

Snyder, W. H., Jr., and Chaffin, L.: Embryology and pathology of the intestinal tract: presentation of 40 cases of malrotation. Ann. Surg., 140:368-380, 1954.

Soave, F.: A new surgical technique for treatment of Hirschsprung's disease. Surgery, 56:1007-1014, 1964.

Soper, R. T., and Opitz, J. M.: Neonatal pneumoperitoneum and Hirschsprung's disease. Surgery, 51:527-533, 1962.

Steichen, F. M., Talbert, J. L., and Ravitch, M. M.: Primary side-to-side colorectal anastomosis in the the Duhamel operation for Hirschsprung's Disease. Surgery, 64:475-484, 1968.

Stephens, E. D.: Congenital Malformations of the Rectum, Anus and Genitourinary Tracts. Edinburgh, E. S. Livingstone, 1963.

Stiles, K. A.: The inheritance of pitted ear. J. Hered., 36:53-61, 1945.

Swenson, O.: Follow-up on 200 patients treated for Hirschsprung's disease during a ten year period. Ann. Surg., 146:706-714, 1957.

———: Pediatric Surgery. pp. 155-172, New York, Appleton-Century-Crofts, 1958.

Swenson, O., and Bill, A. H., Jr.: Resection of rectum and rectosigmoid with preservation of the sphincter for benign spastic lesions producing megacolon. Surgery, 24:212-220, 1948.

Swenson, O., and Fisher, J. H.: Treatment of Hirschsprung's disease with entire colon involved in aganglionic defect. Arch. Surg., 70:535-538, 1955.

Swenson, O., Fisher, J. H., and Gherardi, G. J.: Rectal biopsy in the diagnosis of Hirschsprung's disease. Surgery, 45:690-695, 1959.

Szöts, I., and Jakab, T.: Indications for urgent operation in pulmonary tension disorders in childhood. Arch. Dis. Child., 39:172-176, 1964.

Talbert, J. L., and Haller, J. A.: The optimal site for central venous measurement in newborn infants. J. Surg. Res., 6:168-170, 1966.

Tawes, R. L., and deLorimier, A. A.: Thyroid carcinoma during youth. J. Pediat. Surg., 3:210-218, 1966.

Thomsen, G., Vesterdal, J., and Winkel-Smith, C. C.: Diaphragmatic hernia into the pericardium. Acta paediat., 43:485-492, 1954.

Todd, I. P.: Juvenile polyps. Arch. Dis. Child., 39: 166-168, 1964.

Ulin, A. W., Nosal, J. L., and Martin, W. L.: Cholecystitis in childhood; associated obstructive jaundice. Surgery, 31:312, 1952.

Wallgren, A.: Lingual application of eumydrin in the treatment of congenital pyloric stenosis. Arch. Dis. Child., 15:103, 1940.

———: Preclinical stage of infantile hypertrophic pyloric stenosis. Am. J. Dis. Child., 72:371-376, 1946.

Wangensteen, O. H., and Rice, C. O.: Imperforate anus—a method of determining the surgical approach. Ann. Surg., 92:77, 1930.

Ward, D. E., Jr., Bradshaw, H. H., and Prince, J. C.: Bronchial adenoma in children. J. Thoracic Surg., 27:295-299, 1954.

Ward, G. E., and Hendrick, J. W.: Diagnosis and Treatment of Tumors of the Head and Neck. p. 232. Baltimore, Williams & Wilkins, 1950.

Waterston, D.: Hiatus hernia. In: Mustard, Ravitch, Welch, Snyder, and Benson: Pediatric Surgery. ed. 2. Chicago, Year Book Publishers, 1969.

———: Reconstruction of the esophagus. In: Mustard, Ravitch, Snyder, Welch and Benson: Pediatric Surgery. ed. 2. Chicago, Yearbook Publishers, 1969.

Waterston, D. J., Carter, R. E., and Aberdeen, E.: Oesophageal atresia: tracheo-oesophageal fistula. A study of survival in 218 infants. Lancet, 1:819-822, 1962.

Weeks, R. S., and Ravitch, M. M.: Esophageal injury by liquid chlorine bleach: experimental study. J. Pediat., 74:911-916, 1969.

Weens, H. S.: Cholelithiasis in sickle cell anemia. Ann. Int. Med., 22:182-191, 1945.

Welch, K. J.: Satisfactory surgical correction of pectus excavatum deformity in childhood; a limited opportunity. J. Thoracic Surg., 36:697-713, 1958.

———: Traumatic lesions of the abdomen. In: Mustard, Ravitch, Snyder, Welch and Benson: Pediatric Surgery. ed. 2. Chicago, Yearbook Publishers, 1969.

Williams, C., Jr.: Carcinoma of the colon in childhood. Ann. Surg., 139:816-825, 1954.

Winship, T., and Chase, W. W.: Thyroid carcinoma in children. Surg., Gynec. Obstet., 101:217-224, 1955.

Winship, T., and Rosvall, R. V.: Childhood thyroid carcinoma. Cancer, 14:734, 1961.

Winter, J., Eberlein, W. R., and Bongiovanni, A. M.: The relationship of juvenile hypothyroidism to chronic lymphocytic thyroiditis. J. Pediat., 69:709-718, 1966.

Yater, W., Finnegan, S., and Griffin, H. M.: Pulmonary arteriovenous fistula; review of the literature and report of 2 cases. J.A.M.A., 141:581-589, 1949.

Zuelzer, W. W., and Wilson, J. L.: Functional intestinal obstruction on a congenital neurogenic basis in infancy. Am. J. Dis. Child., 75:40-64, 1948.

CHAPTER 51

MICHAEL NEWTON, M.D.

Gynecology

There are three main requirements for the surgeon who concerns himself with diseases of the female genital tract. (1) He must be thoroughly familiar with the reproductive physiology and psychology of women, including the wide variations within the normal range. (2) He must be aware of the changes of the obstetrical cycle. (3) He must be mindful that the majority of common gynecologic conditions are managed best by nonsurgical means, and that when surgery is indicated in the premenopausal woman, preservation of her reproductive function is of paramount importance.

HISTORY AND EXAMINATION

History

This includes:
1. History of the present illness.
2. Detailed menstrual history. Specifically, this includes the age of onset or cessation of menstruation, length of cycle, duration and amount of flow, date of last 2 menstrual periods. Recent menstrual changes, bleeding between the periods, pain at the time of menstruation, and amount and type of vaginal discharge should also be noted.
3. Detailed obstetric history. This includes number of children, date of last delivery, number and causes, if known, of abortions, and any complications of pregnancy, delivery or abortion.
4. Brief systemic review with special reference to the urinary and the lower intestinal tracts.
5. Past medical history, particularly with regard to gynecologic procedures.
6. Evaluation of psychological, social and environmental factors. These are of great importance in gynecology. The patient should be given an opportunity to talk about her husband, parents, children and her daily life, and the feelings that she expresses about them should be noted. Careful listening will also give information about her attitude toward her female functions. Disgust or fear about menstruation, pregnancy, childbirth, breast feeding, motherhood or sexual intercourse are frequently related to medical problems (Newton). The fear of growing old and the fear of cancer may be very real problems to the female patient.

Examination

A brief but thorough general physical examination should be performed. It should include examination of the breasts, since these organs are frequently closely concerned with gynecologic disorders.

Pelvic and rectal examinations are disagreeable but not painful to the average woman. They should be conducted quietly, gently and without haste. The patient frequently finds it easier to relax during these examinations if she is encouraged to breathe slowly and deeply, concentrating on expiration. An attendant should be present during the examination both from the medicolegal standpoint and to give reassurance to the patient.

The examination of female infants and children often presents special problems in management. These are summarized by Schauffler.

Examination should not be postponed because a patient is apparently menstruating. Often observation of the site of the bleeding is a great help in diagnosis.

Equipment for an adequate gynecologic examination need not be elaborate. A full list is given by Greenhill. The basic requirements are: an examining table with a drop leaf at the bottom and stirrups, drapes, a small stool for the examiner, a good light either of the gooseneck or spotlight variety, a waste receptacle and a small movable table containing appropriate instruments. These instruments should include specula—medium Graves type or Pederson specula are suitable for most gynecologic examinations—long forceps, malleable uterine sounds, uterine dressing forceps, tenacula, cotton swabs and lubricant. A good biopsy forceps and cotton tampons to control minor bleeding are useful. Equipment for obtaining cytologic studies should be readily available—suction pipette, cotton-tip applicator, Ayre spatula, clean slides and a bottle containing fixative.

It is helpful to develop a definite routine of examination so that important areas will not be missed. Sterilized gloves should be used. Inspection and palpation of the external genitalia is followed by a speculum examination of the cervix. In children, a Kelly urethroscope, nasal speculum or lighted vaginoscope may be used. Next follows the vaginoabdominal examination in which the cervix, the uterine fundus, the tubes and the ovaries are palpated. The dominant hand is best used for the abdominal part of the examination and one or, preferably, two fingers of the less dominant hand for the vaginal part. Finally, a rectovaginoabdominal examination is performed, usually with the middle finger in the rectum and the index finger in the vagina and the dominant hand again on the abdomen: by this means the paracervical tissue, the cul-de-sac and the rectovaginal septum may be palpated.

CONGENITAL ABNORMALITIES

The abnormalities of congenital origin found in the female genital tract are most easily understood by reference to their embryologic development. The 3 structures concerned are the wolffian body or mesonephros, the müllerian ducts, and the urogenital sinus. The wolffian body forms the ovary; the unfused müllerian ducts, the tubes; the fused müllerian ducts, the uterus, the cervix and the upper vagina; and the urogenital sinus forms the lower vagina and the squamous epithelium of the vagina and the cervix.

Abnormalities of the ovary are rare and consist of the failure of descent of the ovary into the true pelvis or aplasia of one or both ovaries. Supernumerary ovaries have also been reported rarely. Aplasia, atresia and duplication of the tubes are very uncommon.

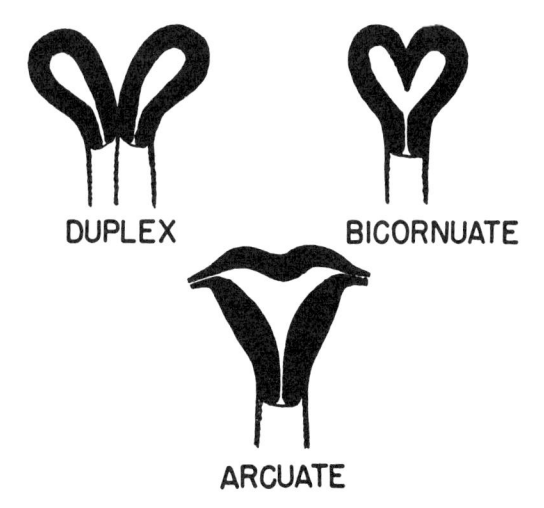

FIG. 51-1. Congenital anomalies of the uterus. Effects of failure of fusion of müllerian ducts.

Failure of one or both müllerian ducts to develop or fuse accounts for abnormalities of the uterus (see Fig. 51-1). Failure of development leads to absence of the uterus. Incomplete development with normal fusion may give rise to hypoplasia of the uterus. Failure of fusion may take various forms. They may range from complete duplication of uterus and cervix down to minor septa or indentations of the top of the uterus. These anomalies may have varying clinical significance, particularly in regard to obstetrics (Semmens).

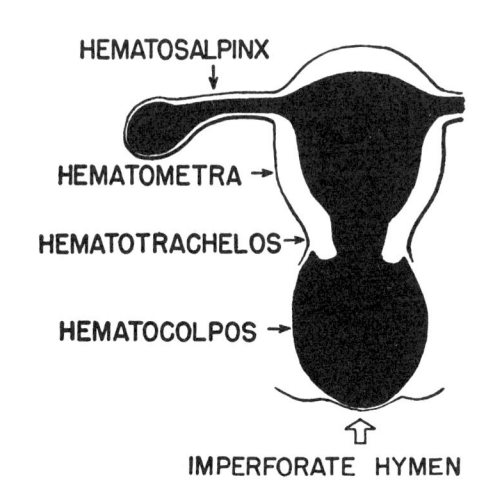

FIG. 51-2. Effects of retention of menstrual flow with imperforate hymen.

Failure of fusion of the müllerian ducts may also lead to a vagina which is completely duplicated or has a partial septum. Complete failure of development in this area may lead to partial or complete absence of the vagina.

The most important abnormality of the external genitalia is imperforate hymen (see Fig. 51-2). Double vulva or hypospadias due to failure of development of the septum between vagina and urethra may be seen.

Other congenital anomalies of the upper and lower genital tract may be associated with intersex conditions such as male and female pseudohermaphroditism and true hermaphroditism. Anomalies of other organ systems, especially of the urinary tract, are frequently found in association with those of the genital tract.

CLINICAL FEATURES AND TREATMENT

In infancy or early childhood two congenital anomalies may be seen: hydrocolpos (or hydrometrocolpos), and intersex conditions, resulting in confusion of gender. However, most anomalies are not recognized until after the normal age for the onset of menstruation. Where there is obstruction to the flow of menstrual blood, symptoms usually occur. The absence of normal menstruation in a girl who has reached the age of 16 should lead to a careful examination of the genital system. Many minor uterine abnormalities may not give rise to symptoms and may be discovered only incidentally during later life.

There are 3 main types of clinical picture due to congenital abnormalities.

1. **Retention of Menstrual Discharge.** Imperforate hymen is the most common cause, but partial absence of the vagina may also be responsible. The retained blood causes successively distention of the vagina (hematocolpos), cervix (hematotrachelos), uterine cavity (hematometra) and tubes (hematosalpinx). With each menstrual period the patient experiences increasing pain and discomfort. Distention of the lower abdomen may occur and difficulty on urination may be noted. Sometimes the symptoms may suggest an acute abdominal condition. Diagnosis in the case of imperforate hymen is easily made by examination; the bulging blue hymen is readily seen. Treatment is by cruciate incision or excision of the hymen. Infection is a not uncommon sequel of hematocolpos, and if treatment is delayed there may be permanent effects upon the reproductive capacity of the patient. When part of the vagina is aplastic, management is usually along the lines of that suggested below for complete agenesis.

2. **Inability to Have Marital Relations.** If the absence of menstruation is not investigated, a girl may begin to consider marriage without being aware of a congenital absence of the vagina. This usually means that the whole of the lower genital tract is absent, although there may be a rudimentary vaginal pouch. Construction of an artificial vagina is possible in certain instances and should be attempted if the patient is anxious to have normal marital relations and is willing to cooperate fully. The most satisfactory method is by the artificial formation of a tract by dissection between the rectum and the urethra and maintenance of the tract by means of a light (usually plastic) obturator covered with a skin graft. It may be best to perform the operation soon after diagnosis (provided that the patient is at least adolescent), so that she may consider herself more truly a woman. Before operation the patient should understand that the best she can expect will be a functioning vagina. It requires determination on her part to continue wearing the obturator for many months, since contraction of the artificial vagina is prone to occur. Good anatomic results may be expected in 60 to 70 per cent, although good function, i.e., sexual satisfaction, may be higher than this (Evans).

3. **Abnormalities of Pregnancy and Delivery.** Not infrequently the first symptoms of an abnormality of the uterus may be discovered when the patient presents a sterility problem, has repeated abortions or has some difficulty with labor and delivery. In such cases, in addition to the usual methods of examination, hysterography is valuable. Unfortunately, treatment is practical in only a few instances. For example, Strassman reports good results in selected cases by plastic unification of a double uterus.

DISPLACEMENTS OF THE UTERUS AND PELVIC RELAXATION

NORMAL POSITION AND SUPPORT OF THE PELVIC ORGANS

The uterus normally lies between the rectum and the bladder with its long axis almost in

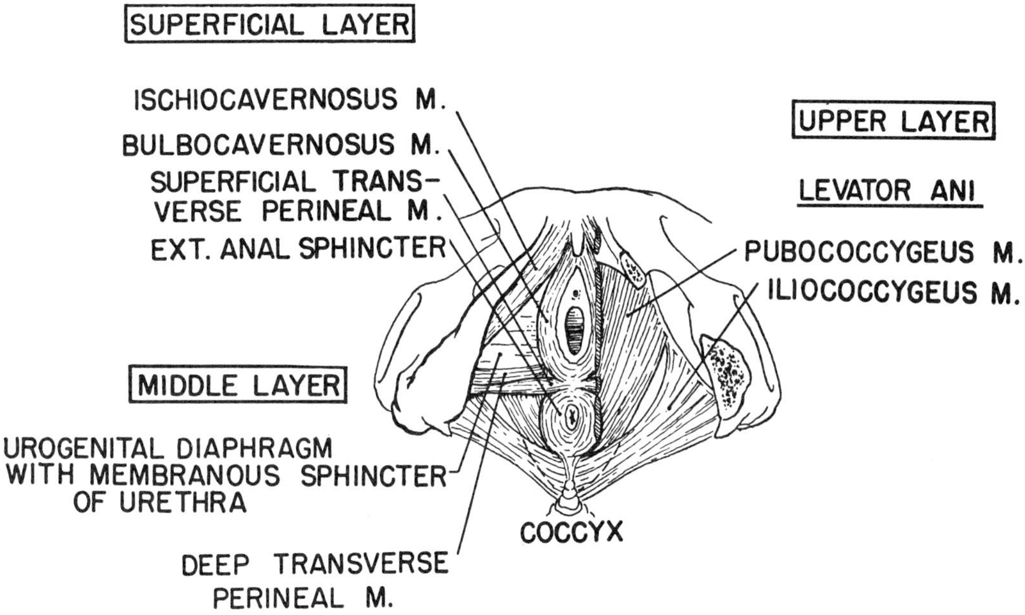

FIG. 51-3. Fascia and muscles of the pelvic floor (seen from below).

the horizontal plane so that it covers the top of the empty bladder. In this situation the cervix points almost directly backward, and the corpus bends forward slightly from the cervix. The uterus is held in this position by (1) the fascial planes of the pelvic floor (Fig. 51-3), (2) the uterine ligaments and (3) the pressure of the abdominal contents. The fascial planes of the pelvic floor consist of an area of fibromuscular thickening concentrated around the base of the broad ligament; this is variously called the cardinal or Mackenrodt's ligament. The ligaments of the uterus act as guy ropes to keep the organ in position. The broad ligaments hold it in the middle of the pelvis and keep it up. The uterosacral ligaments pull the cervix back. The round ligaments may exert some effect on holding the fundus forward, but the weight of the abdominal contents is probably of most importance in this regard.

The pelvic organs, including the bladder, the urethra and the rectum, are also supported by the muscles and the fascia of the pelvic floor. These consist of 3 layers: (1) the upper pelvic diaphragm of the levator ani muscles, (2) the triangular ligament, extending forward from the deep transverse perinei muscles at the base, (3) the superficial pelvic diaphragm, consisting of the superficial transverse perinei, the bulbocavernosus and ischiocavernosus muscles.

Childbirth and age normally result in changes in the position of the pelvic organs. Some weakening of the ligaments may be expected to follow vaginal delivery, with consequent slight descent of the uterus and increased relaxation of the walls of the vagina. After the menopause the fundus of the uterus commonly loses its forward inclination and lies in the mid-position so that it extends straight upward from the cervix.

DISPLACEMENTS OF THE UTERUS

Anterior and lateral displacements of the uterus occur occasionally, but they are usually the result of an enlarging tumor or abscess and are not of clinical importance in themselves.

Posterior displacements of the uterus are of more significance, though not as much as was thought 30 years ago. They may be divided into 3 types (Fig. 51-4): (1) retrocession, where the whole uterus is displaced toward the back of the pelvis; (2) retroversion, where the cervix is tilted forward so as to point anteriorly on vaginal examination but retains its relationship with the corpus; (3) retroflexion, where the corpus is bent backward on the cervix. The most important displacement is retro-

RETROCESSION   RETROVERSION

RETROFLEXION

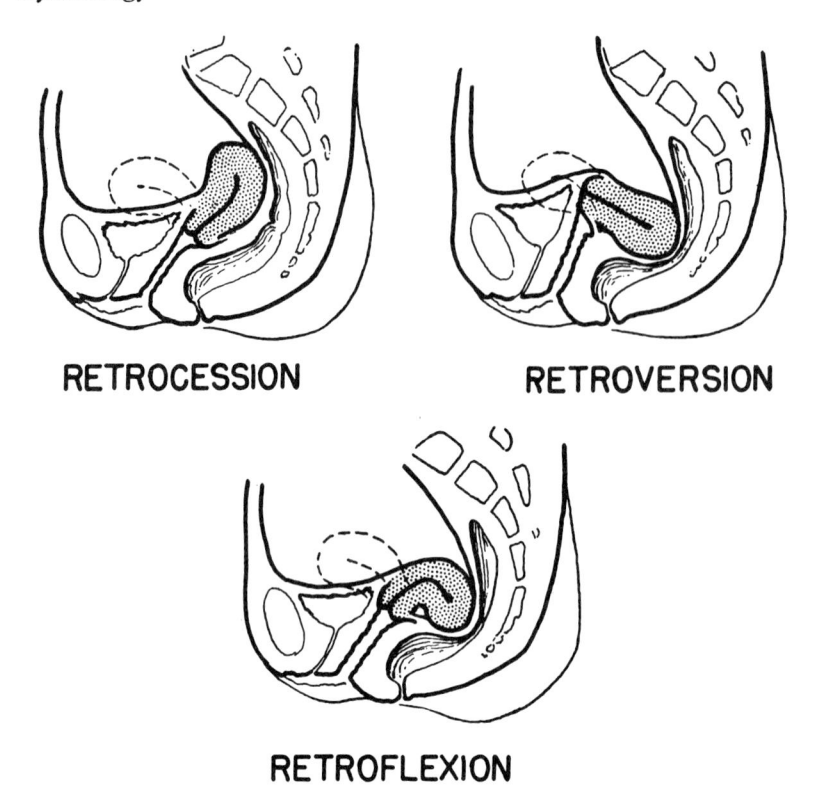

FIG. 51-4. Retrodisplacements of the uterus.

flexion but all 3 may be found together or separately and may be of varying degrees.

Cause. About 20 per cent of retrodisplacements are congenital in origin. The remainder are acquired. These may be due to: (1) childbirth, (2) age, (3) adnexal inflammation or endometriosis and (4) tumors and cysts of the uterus or the adnexa. Previously, it had been thought that trauma was a factor, but except for childbirth it is difficult to see how this could be severe enough to be important.

Clinical Features. Simple uncomplicated retrodisplacements frequently give no symptoms. However, the following may occur:

1. BACKACHE. This is characteristically of a dull aching nature and is felt in the sacral or lumbosacral area. It is commonly worse before and during menstruation.

2. DYSPAREUNIA, especially just before menstruation.

3. MENSTRUAL DISORDERS. Dysmenorrhea with occasional slowness in starting the flow may be noted.

4. STERILITY AND ABORTION. Relative infertility may result from the cervix being displaced anteriorly out of the apex of the vagina where the semen is pooled. Abortions may occur more frequently in patients with retrodisplacements of the uterus than in normal women. This may be due to congestion of the uterus, an unfavorable location for nidation or incarceration of the enlarging retroflexed uterus.

Diagnosis. This is made readily on pelvic examination, unless the patient is very obese or holds herself very tense. Sometimes it may be made more difficult by the presence of a myoma on the anterior surface of the uterus or by an adnexal mass which lies behind the uterus and simulates the retroflexed corpus.

Treatment. In general, if there are no symptoms, no treatment is needed. The only possible exception to this is the retroflexion which commonly follows pregnancy. Some authorities feel that this should be treated. However, many such uteri may be found later to have reverted to the anterior position without treatment.

It is important to attempt to ascertain whether the symptoms complained of are due to the retrodisplacement rather than to the associated conditions which commonly accompany acquired retrodisplacements. This is frequently difficult. In doubtful cases it may be well to treat the retrodisplacement and see if the symptoms are improved. If they are, and then return after treatment has been discontinued, one can assume that the retrodisplacement was responsible—provided that the effect of suggestion has been discounted.

If the uterus is movable, first it is replaced in the anterior position. The cervix is pushed backward toward the sacrum, and the fundus is pushed up by the fingers in the posterior fornix of the vagina. Then the fundus is grasped by the external hand and pushed further forward while the cervix is again pushed toward the back of the vagina. Sometimes traction on the cervix by means of a tenaculum will help the maneuver. The use of intrauterine sounds to turn the fundus up may be successful in expert hands but is attended with the risk of perforation of the uterus.

Once the uterus is in the anterior position it may stay there of its own accord, aided by the pressure of the abdominal contents. The anterior position may be encouraged and maintained by knee-chest exercises practiced 3 or 4 times a day for 10 minutes (see Fig. 51-5).

Usually it is wise to maintain the uterus in the anterior position by means of a pessary. The best types for use in retrodisplacements are the Hodge or Smith pessaries. Insertion is relatively easy and painless. A well-fitting pessary should not cause any discomfort. The only care needed by the patient is to take a douche every day or every other day because the presence of the pessary causes a certain amount of vaginal irritation and discharge. Once a pessary has been inserted it should be removed every 6 to 8 weeks, cleaned and replaced. At this time the vaginal wall should be inspected carefully to see if any ulceration has occurred.

After the pessary has been left in place through at least 2 menstrual cycles and then is removed, the uterus may stay in the anterior position of its own accord. If it reverts to the posterior position, then the pessary may be replaced.

Operation should be advised for uncomplicated retrodisplacement only as a last resort. If symptoms are relieved by a pessary and return when the pessary is removed and are

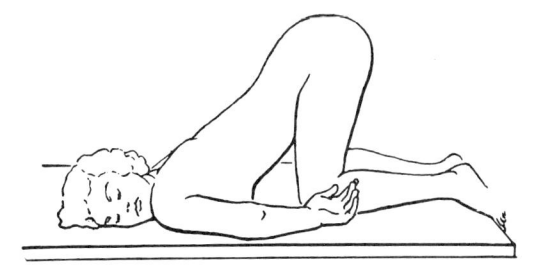

FIG. 51-5. Knee-chest position.

distressing enough so that the patient is incapacitated, then some type of operative fixation of the uterus should be considered. The principles of operative treatment are: (1) shortening of the round ligaments and changing the direction of their pull by attaching them to the back of the uterus (Baldy-Webster); (2) shortening the round ligaments by attaching them to the abdominal wall (Gilliam).

If the uterus is fixed in the posterior position, treatment is usually more difficult. However, in this case the retrodisplacement itself is less likely to be causing the patient's symptoms than the associated disease. Therefore, management may resolve itself into the treatment of the underlying condition. Manual replacement is not usually possible, though sometimes knee-chest exercises may return the uterus to the anterior position. Replacement under anesthesia may sometimes be possible under these circumstances, although if great difficulty is encountered it should not be persisted in, owing to the possibility of injury. If one is considering freeing the adhesions by laparotomy and replacing the uterus, one should be sure that there are other indications for operation besides the retrodisplacement; e.g., endometriosis. Notoriously difficult to manage are the retrodisplacements associated with chronic pelvic inflammatory disease, since the mass of adhesions in the pelvis at the time of operation tends to lead to more radical surgery than would be necessary solely for the retrodisplacement.

PELVIC RELAXATION

Pelvic relaxation includes the following conditions: they may occur together or separately.
1. Prolapse of the uterus (descensus uteri)
2. Prolapse of the intestine into the pouch of Douglas (enterocele)

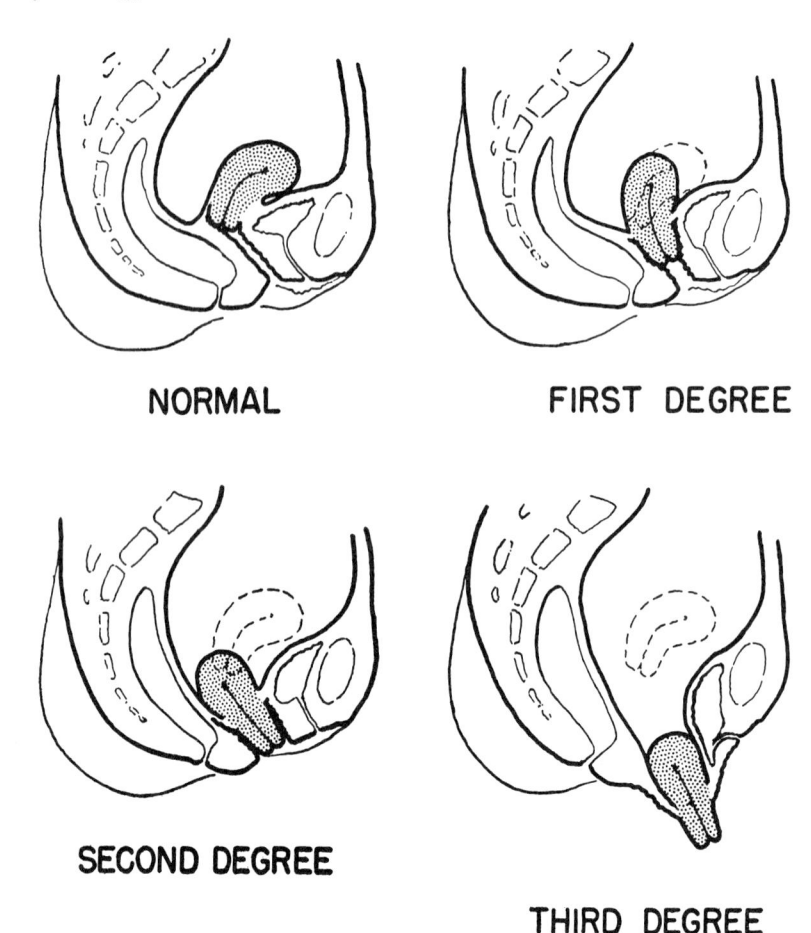

NORMAL **FIRST DEGREE** **SECOND DEGREE** **THIRD DEGREE**

FIG. 51-6. Degrees of prolapse of the uterus.

3. Prolapse of the bladder into the anterior vaginal wall (cystocele)
4. Prolapse of the urethra into the anterior vaginal wall (urethrocele)
5. Prolapse of the rectum into the posterior vaginal wall (rectocele)
6. Weakness of the perineum (relaxed vaginal outlet)

Cause. These conditions occur most commonly, but not invariably, in parous and older women. Primarily, they are due to an exaggeration of the normal relaxation of the pelvic ligaments and support which occurs during childbirth and after the menopause. A contributing factor may be traumatic prolonged labor, although the importance of this is difficult to estimate.

Clinical Features. Prolapse of the uterus may be divided conveniently into 3 stages (see Fig. 51-6): (1) First-degree prolapse occurs when the cervix descends below its normal position in the vaginal canal. (2) In second-degree prolapse, the cervix reaches the introitus. (3) In third-degree the cervix is outside the introitus. The term *procidentia* may be used when the whole uterus protrudes. The exact degree of prolapse of the uterus may not be realized upon examination unless the patient is asked to stand or strain down vigorously: straining may be reproduced by pulling the cervix down with a tenaculum. The descent of the cervix may be felt by the patient as a lump in the vagina, which is noticed on prolonged standing or straining. If the cervix becomes irritated or eroded as a result of its descent, vaginal discharge or bleeding may be noted.

Enterocele, in addition to accompanying

other types of prolapse, may occur by itself following vaginal hysterectomy. It usually does not cause symptoms until it is felt as a protruding mass. Incarceration occurs only very rarely.

Cystocele and urethrocele are frequently associated. They may be asymptomatic, but since they predispose to the retention of urine, infection commonly occurs. In the case of urethrocele this leads to burning and frequency of urination. On occasion a urethral diverticulum may develop. In the case of cystocele, frequency and urgency of urination, together with suprapubic pain, occur. Infection is commonly recurrent and eventually may lead to upper urinary tract infection. If marked cystocele is associated with prolapse of the uterus, obstruction of the lower ureter may occur with resulting hydronephrosis and uremia.

Minor degrees of rectocele do not normally cause symptoms. If the rectocele is large, fecal material may be retained in it, and the patient may have trouble expelling it unless she manually pushes the rectocele back.

Weakness of the perineum is due to damage to the smaller muscles, such as may occur during childbirth. By itself it usually causes no symptoms, except perhaps for a sensation of gaping at the introitus. Occasionally, however, it may involve division of the fibers of the anal sphincter. This may cause incontinence of feces, especially if the bowel movements are loose.

Involuntary discharge of urine on straining, coughing, laughing or sneezing (stress incontinence) is a common concomitant of pelvic relaxation. Much investigation has been devoted to elucidating its cause. That it is not necessarily the result of age or parity is shown by the study of Nemir and Middleton, who found that 52 per cent of 1,327 college women reported some degree of stress incontinence and that in 5 per cent this was severe. Present explanations are well summarized by Green.

Diagnosis. Usually the diagnosis is made readily on examination. The anterior vaginal wall may be observed by having the patient strain down while pushing the posterior wall backward. The posterior wall may be observed by having the patient strain down while pushing the anterior wall forward. Stress incontinence can be observed by having the patient

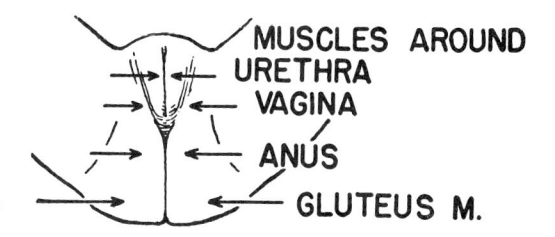

FIG. 51-7. Direction of muscle contraction in perineal exercises.

strain down with a full bladder and noting the escape of urine from the urethra. If the base of the bladder is elevated and leakage occurs, a guide to operative treatment is obtained. It may be helpful to use the propped or standing position for complete examination. The condition of the perineal body and the anal sphincter is evaluated best by rectal examination.

Treatment. Prophylaxis of pelvic relaxation by good obstetric practice is very important. During the second stage of labor the fascial supports of the uterus, the bladder and the rectum and the small muscles of the perineum are greatly stretched and may even tear. Any technic that prevents these fibers rupturing or stretching beyond their capacity to return to normal is of value. In the past 2 or 3 decades it has been felt by obstetricians in this country that shortening of the second stage of labor by performing an episiotomy and extracting the baby by forceps applied at the pelvic outlet would achieve this objective. A logical approach in most normal women would seem to be by antepartal perineal muscle exercises (Bushnell) (see Fig. 51-7). If these are combined with adequate preparation of the patient for the second stage of labor, and gradual delivery is allowed, good perineal muscle tone may be restored postpartally. Of course, this does not preclude the use of forceps if the second stage is abnormally prolonged or if the patient is unable to take advantage of such exercises.

In line with the prophylaxis of pelvic relaxation, the primary treatment for minor or moderate relaxation, especially in women of childbearing age, should be by nonoperative measures. This involves the patient's learning to contract the pubococcygei and the other perineal muscles effectively. She can conveniently be asked to stop the flow of urine each time she voids or, alternatively, to contract and draw in the perineal muscles 8 to 10 times in succession 3 times daily. Kegel noted improvement in the strength of the perineal muscles by this type of exercise in 69 per cent of patients. He utilized a perineometer to measure this, although if the patient is simply asked to contract the muscles on the examining hand, a good indication of their strength may be obtained. Perineal exercises are particularly valuable when the patient has some stress incontinence and may be useful in improving sexual responsiveness.

Where the anatomic changes are very marked, or where nonoperative treatment has not produced improvement, operation is indicated. Before this is done any urinary tract infection should be investigated and treated. Vaginal infection also should be treated, and in the postmenopausal woman improvement of the condition of the vaginal mucosa may be obtained by the use of estrogens orally or as a vaginal cream before operation.

Operative procedures for pelvic relaxation are reviewed by TeLinde. Repair of the prolapsed uterus is often best handled by vaginal hysterectomy, when childbearing is no longer desired or marked prolapse is present. Lesser procedures, such as amputation of the cervix and fixation of the lower part of the parametria to the cervix (Manchester-Fothergill operation), may occasionally be useful in the younger patient.

In the older debilitated patient who is a poor operative risk, prolapse occasionally may be treated satisfactorily by occlusion of the vagina (LeFort procedure—colpocleisis). This involves denudation and approximation of the anterior and the posterior vaginal walls, leaving lateral channels for drainage when the uterus is still present. Local anesthesia can be used, and the procedure may not be as traumatic as the other procedures described above.

When operation cannot be performed for any reason, relief of symptoms may be obtained by the use of a pessary of the ring or Menge type. They act by distending the vagina and suspending the cervix at a higher level than before and work best if perineal relaxation is minimal. The care of these pessaries is the same as for the Smith or Hodge types, except that vaginal ulceration must be watched for even more carefully in the older patient.

Repair of a cystocele and urethrocele (anterior colporrhaphy) or a rectocele (posterior colporrhaphy) consists of excising the excess vaginal mucosa over the organ concerned, plicating the fascia and resuturing the vagina. Repair of a rectocele usually should be combined with repair of the perineum with some narrowing of the introitus. Francis and Jeffcoate point out that unnecessarily tight posterior perineorrhaphies may lead to postoperative dyspareunia. Repair of the anal sphincter can be combined with a perineorrhaphy by identifying the divided ends of the muscle and suturing them together.

Special problems in vaginal repair occur with enterocele or where stress incontinence is marked. As with the repair of any hernia, the sac of the enterocele must be dissected out and the peritoneum securely closed. Frequently, it is difficult to add any support to the repair from below since the uterosacral ligaments are attenuated. In the primary repair of an enterocele an attempt should be made to close these as well as possible (McCall). However, in recurrent enterocele, obliteration of the posterior cul-de-sac from the abdominal approach may be indicated (Moschcowitz procedure).

Stress incontinence occasionally presents great difficulty in treatment. When the associated anatomic deformity is great, or conservative management has failed, operation is indicated, provided that neurologic disorders have been excluded. Careful preoperative evaluation, including a metallic bead-chain urethrocystogram, may indicate the best procedure. When the main problem is straightening of the posterior urethrovesical angle, a repair of the anterior vaginal wall (with or without vaginal hysterectomy) is appropriate. When, in addition, the angle of the urethral axis to the vertical is greatly increased, a suprapubic urethrovesical suspension is indicated. Even so, many different procedures have ben advocated, indicating that no one is entirely satisfactory.

DISEASES OF THE LOWER GENITAL TRACT

Anatomically, the lower genital tract consists of the vulva and the lower half of the vagina. Its arterial supply comes from the branches of the internal pudendal artery, and its lymphatics go primarily to the superficial inguinal nodes. Functionally, the upper vagina and the cervix up to the external os must also be considered as a part of the lower genital tract, since their squamous epithelium is derived from the urogenital sinus. However, the Müllerian origin of the vaginal tube has resulted in its arterial supply coming from the internal iliac arteries and its lymphatics going primarily to the nodes surrounding these vessels. Thus, this area has to be considered somewhat as a separate entity as well as being a part of the lower genital tract.

Physiologic changes occur with age in the lower genital tract, especially in the thickness of the epithelium and in the acidity of the vaginal fluid. Thus, in the newborn infant, owing to the maternal estrogens which have passed through the placenta, the vaginal epithelium is thick, and the pH is low. Soon afterward it reverts to the childhood type, consisting only of a basal layer of cells and having a higher pH. At puberty the epithelium becomes thicker and undergoes cyclical changes. Greater cornification is noted in the proliferative phase of the cycle. The pH is generally in the range of 4.5 to 5.0, although it is somewhat higher just after menstruation. After the menopause the epithelium reverts to the childhood type.

Disorders Caused by Trauma

Direct trauma to the lower genital tract is rare. It may consist of forcible rupture of the hymen with occasional troublesome bleeding, perforation by instruments, or damage due to the retention of foreign bodies. Recognition of these injuries depends upon a careful history and thorough examination. Treatment depends upon the type of injury.

Indirect trauma is more frequent and consists chiefly of vaginal fistulae. The common ones are: (1) vesicovaginal, (2) urethrovaginal, (3) ureterovaginal and (4) rectovaginal. They may be due to childbirth, operative injury, radiation or tumor.

Vesicovaginal Fistula. Clinical Features. There is a constant discharge of urine from the vagina with irritation and infection of the vulva and the perineal skin.

Diagnosis. When the fistula is large it is usually obvious on pelvic examination. When it is small, insertion of methylene blue into the bladder and subsequent observation of it in the vagina may be conclusive.

Treatment. Since these fistulae do not tend to heal spontaneously, treatment is usually surgical. They may be closed from the vaginal or transvesical or from a combined approach. The first is usually preferable. The primary object is to close separately the bladder mucosa, the fascia between bladder and vagina and the vaginal mucosa. The repair of large and complicated fistulae is discussed by Moir. Where the cervix has been removed, colpocleisis of the upper vagina, as suggested by Falk and Bunkin, may succeed. When the fistula is very large and follows pelvic radiation, the shortening and the scarring of the anterior vaginal wall may be so extensive that repair is impossible. In such instances diversion of the urinary stream into an isolated loop of ileum, brought out as an ileostomy in the right lower quadrant of the abdomen, may greatly increase the patient's comfort and prolong her life (Fig. 51-8).

Urethrovaginal Fistula. This is a rare condition. If it is small and continence is maintained, symptoms may consist only of misdirection of the urinary stream. Provided that some urethral wall remains, repair over a catheter is satisfactory. Large fistulae present problems similar to those of large vesicovaginal fistulae.

Ureterovaginal Fistula. This type of fistula has become more common following the

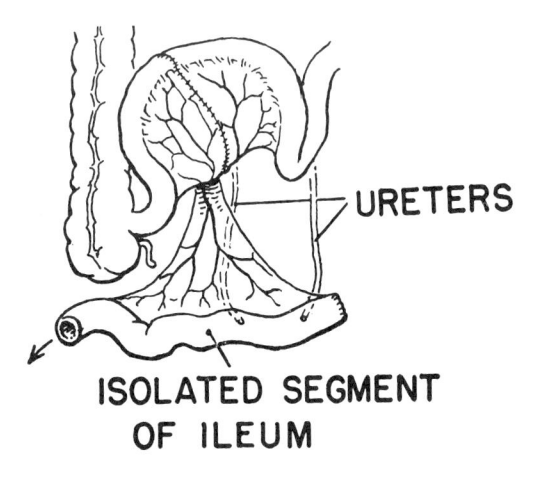

Fig. 51-8. Uretero-ileostomy.

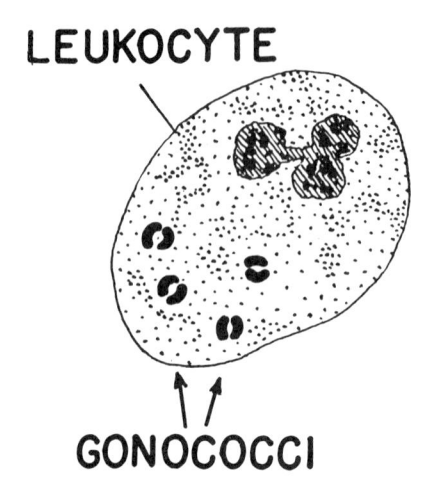

FIG. 51-9. Gonococci within a leukocyte.

more radical surgical procedures used recently in the treatment of pelvic malignancy. Although some close spontaneously, kidney function may be lost and operative repair is usually indicated. This is discussed in the section on urology.

Rectovaginal Fistula. CLINICAL FEATURES. Discharge of feces through the vagina is the chief symptom. When the fistula is small, this may be intermittent, occuring only when the patient has diarrhea. Vaginal, vulvar and perineal infections may follow.

TREATMENT. Although a small rectovaginal fistula may occasionally close spontaneously, surgical repair is usually the only possible treatment. It follows the same principles as for repair of a vesicovaginal fistula: it may be performed from the vaginal approach, or if the fistula is high a combined abdominoperineal or pull-through type of procedure may be done. It is frequently advisable to divert the fecal stream by means of a loop sigmoid or transverse colostomy before proceeding to the repair.

VENEREAL INFECTIONS OF THE LOWER GENITAL TRACT

Gonorrhea is the most common venereal disease in women. It is caused by the diplococcus Neisseriae, which is identified by the fact that it is intracellular, gram-negative and oxidase-positive on culture. It is transmitted primarily by sexual intercourse, although occasional infection may occur by contact with an infected towel, toilet seat or douche nozzle.

Gonorrhea affects primarily the lower genital tract. Squamous epithelium is resistant, but the organism flourishes in the glands of the urethra (Skene's glands), the vulva (Bartholin's glands) and the cervix. Secondary invasion of the uterus and the tubes by the surface route and spread to distant parts of the body may occur, especially at the time of menstruation. These serious consequences will be considered among the diseases of the upper genital tract.

CLINICAL FEATURES. The acute stage is relatively mild and may not be noticed by the patient. Within a few days after infection dryness and irritation of the vagina are noticed. There may be some urinary frequency and burning on urination. A small amount of discharge appears. These symptoms may become more marked or may pass away. Upon examination the vagina and the vulva appear reddened, and there may be more or less purulent discharge.

Spontaneous cure of the acute infection may occur, but it is likely to become subacute and chronic. In this case the organism is maintained in the cervical glands, Bartholin's glands and Skene's glands. The clinical appearance is one of continuous purulent discharge and irritation of the vagina and the vulva from the pus, associated with urethritis. From both the acute and the chronic stages infection of the upper genital tract may result, and this remains a constant hazard while the infection is untreated.

In children the organism affects primarily the vaginal and the vulva. A persistent purulent vaginal discharge occurs. There is usually no spread to the upper genital tract.

DIAGNOSIS. The diagnosis can be made positively only by culture of the organism. In acute cases a smear of the discharge stained by Gram's method may be helpful (Fig. 51-9).

TREATMENT. The advent of the sulfonamide drugs and antibiotics has revolutionized the treatment of gonorrhea. Penicillin is effective. An initial dose of 1.2 million units is given, followed by a similar dose 3 days later. Where the infection appears to be resistant to penicillin, other antibiotics or sulfonamide drugs may be used. Local treatment in the acute stage should be confined to rest, local washing with soap and warm water, and careful attention to avoid infecting other persons: this latter involves avoidance of intercourse as well as sterilization and disposal of infected linen, until cure is established. The tracing and the treatment of contacts is also important.

It is frequently difficult to be sure that cure of the infection has actually occurred. Ideally, at least 2 negative cultures should be obtained. It is best to take at least one of these immediately after menstruation when the infection commonly becomes active again.

In chronic cases both diagnosis and treatment are more difficult. Eradication of the foci of infection in Skene's, Bartholin's and the cervical glands may be necessary. Such treatment, especially in the cervix, is not without danger of infection of the upper genital tract.

In children antibiotics are the best method of treatment, but in resistant cases it may be advisable to attempt to convert the vaginal epithelium to the adult type by the administration of estrogens.

Other Venereal Infections. Syphilis, chancroid, granuloma inguinale and lymphopathia venereum may also affect the lower genital tract. These are identified by the demonstration of the specific organism involved or, in the case of lymphopathia, by the Frei test. As a rule they do not spread to involve the upper genital tract.

OTHER INFECTIONS

Trichomoniasis is caused by the flagellated protozoan, *Trichomonas vaginalis*. The organism is quite common, particularly among women with poor personal hygiene. It may exist for long periods in the vagina without causing symptoms. It has also been found in the upper genital tract, in urine and in the blood stream. In males it has been found in the urine, the prostatic secretion and the semen. Thus while the infection is primarily vaginal, it may also be generalized. How a quiescent is changed into an active infection is not well understood, although psychosomatic factors may be important.

CLINICAL FEATURES. The patient complains of a profuse irritating vaginal discharge which frequently has a foul odor. Frequency and burning of urination are commonly noted. On examination a foamy yellow discharge is seen

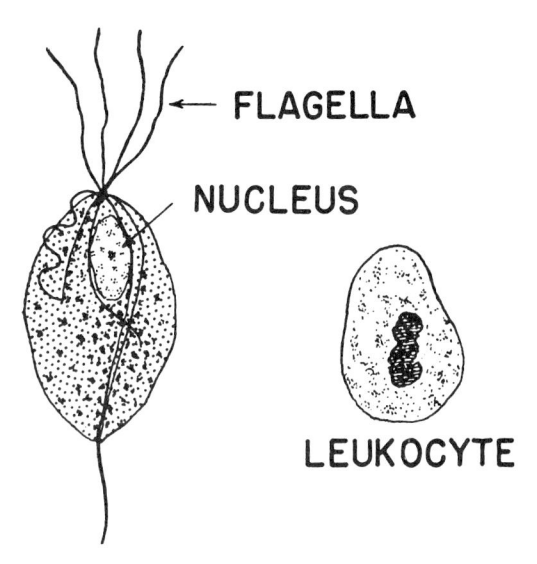

FIG. 51-10. *Trichomonas vaginalis*.

in the vagina. The vagina itself is reddened and may show punctate red spots. The cervix also may be involved.

DIAGNOSIS. The motile organism may be detected by microscopic examination of a small amount of discharge mixed with warm saline (Fig. 51-10). The use of lubricant for examination may destroy the motility of the organism and make diagnosis more difficult. A large number of pus cells compared with epithelial cells may indicate a more severe and resistant infection (Donald).

TREATMENT. The preferred method is to use the oral trichomonacide, metranidazole, in doses of 250 mg. 3 times daily for 10 days. Cure rates of 90 per cent or better may be expected with metranidazole. When there is evidence that the husband is a source of reinfection, he should also be treated in the same manner. The local use of douches of white vinegar (3 to 4 tablespoonfuls to 1 quart of warm water) twice daily may also be helpful in conjunction with metranidazole. Metranidazole and other protozoicides are also available for intravaginal application.

Moniliasis. Infection by *Candida albicans* or other fungi is relatively common especially in pregnancy. Some increase in incidence has been noted with the use of oral contraceptive pills, especially of the combined estrogen-progestin type.

CLINICAL FEATURES. Itching of the vulva

1546   Gynecology

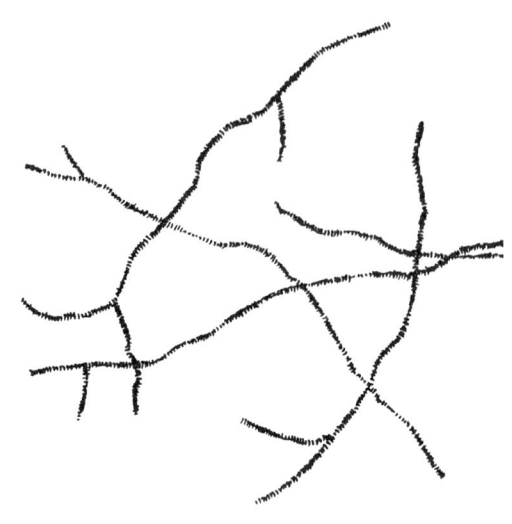

FIG. 51-11. Monilia.

usually is more prominent than discharge. The vagina and the vulva may appear inflamed on examination, and patches of white cheesy material are seen clinging to the epithelium.

DIAGNOSIS. A small amount of discharge may be mixed with 10 per cent potassium hydroxide (to obliterate the cellular elements) and examined microscopically. The fungi are seen as fine branching and budding threads (Fig. 51-11). In doubtful cases culture on Nickerson's medium may be helpful.

TREATMENT. The most effective remedy available is the intravaginal application of nystatin tablets twice daily for 12 days, combined with the use of nystatin ointment externally to relieve itching. Candicidin also may be effective. If these fail (as they may do, especially in pregnancy), painting the area with 1 or 2 per cent gentian violet, or the intravaginal application of gentian violet jelly may be useful. Other preparations such as propionic acid jelly are occasionally of value.

Nonspecific Infections. Frequently no specific cause can be found for the discharge of which the patient complains, and culture reveals only a mixed group of organisms. In this connection it is well to remember that vaginal discharge is frequently a symptom of psychosomatic disturbance and attention to these factors, particularly in relation to the patient's sexual feelings, may be curative. Local treatment may consist of intravaginal application of bacteriostatic sulfa creams and attempts to restore the normal acidity of the vagina by acid jellies or by vinegar douches.

OTHER DISEASES OF THE LOWER
GENITAL TRACT

Atrophic Vaginitis. This condition is found in postmenopausal women, and in premenopausal women who have lost ovarian function. It is due primarily to lack of estrogens. Clinically it is characterized by a thin irritating vaginal discharge, which at times may be bloody. On examination the vaginal mucosa is reddened and presents many petechiae. Provided that cancer of the upper and the lower genital tracts and leukoplakia have been excluded, treatment with oral estrogens or intravaginal applications of estrogenic cream usually is helpful.

Leukoplakia and Related Conditions. The vulvar skin may respond in a variety of ways to different adverse factors. These reactions may take the form of leukoplakia (white patches of thickened skin occurring around the introitus), kraurosis (excessive shrinkage and thinning of the skin), lichen sclerosus et atrophicus and other conditions. A useful inclusive term for these disorders is chronic epithelial dystrophy, as suggested by Jeffcoate and Woodcock.

PATHOLOGIC FEATURES. These include hypertrophic changes with hyperkeratosis and parakeratosis, round-cell infiltration in the superficial part of the dermis and also atrophy of the epithelium with loss of subepithelial elastic fibers. On occasion, atypical cellular activity, especially of the basal layers, may be seen, and it is this rather than the clinical entity or other pathologic findings which may represent a true precancerous lesion.

CLINICAL FEATURES. In almost all instances of chronic epithelial dystrophy the patient complains of persistent itching and burning of the vulva. Increasing pain on coitus may be noted. Examination may show the skin to be thin and inelastic with white patches situated anywhere on the labia majora or minora. Cracks and inflammation in the skin may appear as a result of the scratching.

DIAGNOSIS. It is important to determine whether atypical epithelial changes are present. Therefore, it is essential to take one or more biopsies of representative areas of the vulva. Specific infections should be excluded and, since many patients with vulvitis show abnormal glucose metabolism, a glucose tolerance test should be performed.

TREATMENT. When biopsy clearly shows atypical cellular changes in the epithelium, but not intra-epithelial or invasive carcinoma, local excision or, preferably, simple vulvectomy, is usually advisable to forestall the development of frank cancer. If atypical changes are not found, excision should generally be avoided, since the lesions tend to recur. Various conservative measures can be used after treatment of specific infections or control of any diabetes which may be present. It is important to discontinue the use of substances which may cause irritation, such as harsh soaps or detergents used in washing, contraceptives or home remedies. Tight clothing and pads should be avoided. Cotton underwear should be worn. The area should be washed only with plain water. Compresses of 1:10,000 potassium permanganate or aluminum acetate solution (diluted 1:20) and the local application of witch hazel or a simple dusting powder may help to control the itching. Ointments or creams containing analgesics or cortisone may be helpful. Adequate diet and supplementary vitamins, especially high doses of vitamin A, have been used with success.

Pruritus Vulvae. Itching is a common concomitant of vulvitis, vaginitis and atrophic conditions of the vulva. The term pruritus has become limited conventionally to those cases where itching is the primary complaint, without clear evidence of associated disease. Frequently, it is accompanied by itching around the anus and the inner thighs. The skin in these areas eventually may become thick, fissured and inflamed. Every attempt should be made to exclude a specific cause for the itching. Many of these patients show abnormal glucose metabolism. Therefore, a glucose tolerance test should be performed routinely.

Treatment consists first in eradicating any obvious cause for the itching. Where no cause is found management may be extremely difficult. Local applications to relieve itching, dietary advice, and attention to psychological factors, which are commonly present, are important. As a last resort, surgical undermining of the skin (Mering) or injection of long-acting anesthetic agents to remove sensory stimulation have been reported to be of help (Reich and Nechtow).

BENIGN CYSTS AND TUMORS OF THE LOWER GENITAL TRACT

Condylomata Acuminata. These lesions are microscopically papillomata. They are frequently multiple and are situated anywhere on the external genitalia. They may grow to a large size during pregnancy. They are due to a chronic irritating vaginal discharge of any sort. A satisfactory method of treatment is by application of 25 per cent podophyllin in tincture of benzoin or mineral oil. Larger or resistant growths may require cauterization or surgical removal. Any infection present in the lower genital tract should also be treated.

Urethral Caruncle. Caruncle is the term given to a small red growth which develops just at or inside the external urinary meatus. Pathologically, these have the appearance of granulomata, although in some there may be evidence of papilloma formation. They are not true tumors and in general do not become malignant. Clinically, they may give no symptoms at all, or the patient may notice pain in the area, burning on urination or bleeding. They appear as small (1-2 mm. up to more than 1 cm. in diameter) red growths in the region of the urinary meatus. Care should be taken to avoid confusion in diagnosis with eversion of the mucosa of the urethra, which is common, or carcinoma of the urethra, which is very rare. Treatment, if indicated, is by excision or cauterization: for both of these adequate anesthesia, usually general, is needed.

Cysts and Abscesses of Bartholin's Glands. Obstruction of the duct of Bartholin's gland is common. This leads to retention of secretions (cyst) or pus (abscess). Abscess is a common sequel of gonorrheal infection but may be due to nonspecific causes.

CLINICAL FEATURES. A cyst may cause no symptoms except the sensation of a mass in the vulvar region. Abscess formation is accompanied by pain, redness, tenderness and fever. Tender inguinal nodes are often palpable.

DIAGNOSIS. A Bartholin's cyst lies at the posterior end of the introitus as contrasted with other labial cysts which lie more an-

1548   Gynecology

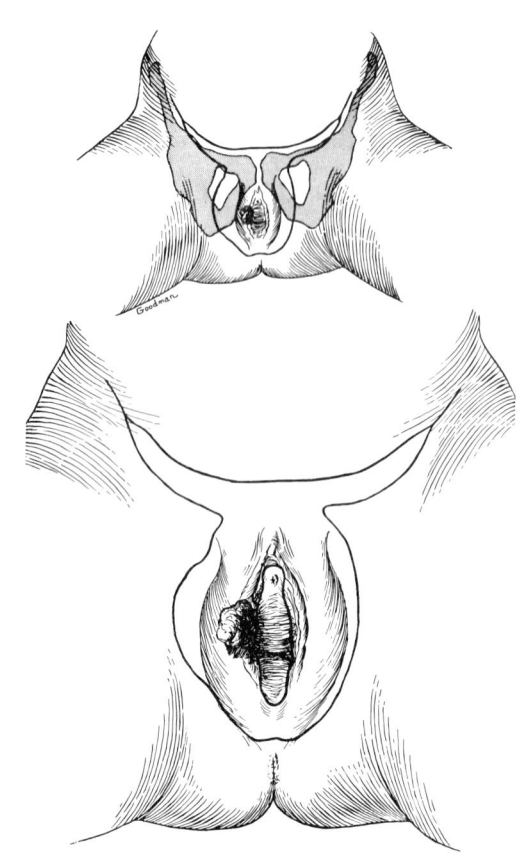

FIG. 51-12. Skin incision for radical vulvectomy and bilateral inguinal node dissection.

teriorly and laterally, and with abscesses resulting from perianal infections which are felt more posteriorly.

TREATMENT. An abscess should be opened widely and antibiotics given. A permanent cure may be attempted even in the acute case by suturing the margins of the abscess to the adjacent skin. This type of management by marsupialization is most satisfactory for the definitive treatment of Bartholin's cysts and is simpler than excision.

Other Cysts and Tumors. A wide variety of cysts and tumors are seen in this area. The most common are vaginal inclusion cysts, cysts of wolffian duct remnants, or tumors arising from the skin of the vulva, especially fibromata and hydroadenomata. Simple surgical excision is the treatment of choice.

MALIGNANT TUMORS OF THE LOWER GENITAL TRACT

Cancer of Vulva and Surrounding Structures. Cancer of the vulva comprises between 3 and 4 per cent of all cancers of the female genital tract. By far the greatest number (over 95%) are squamous cell carcinomata, although melanomata, adenocarcinomata of Bartholin's gland, and basal cell carcinomata are found occasionally. The lesion may start anywhere on the external genitalia. Multiple origins are not uncommon. From the initial point the disease may extend backward to the rectum, anteriorly into the urethra or upward into the vagina. Metastasis takes place to the inguinal nodes, often to the opposite side or bilaterally, and thence to the femoral and the deep pelvic nodes. Nodal spread was found by Way to have occurred in 60 of 143 operative cases (42%); in 23 of the 60 cases, the deep pelvic nodes were involved.

CLINICAL FEATURES. The symptoms of cancer of the vulva are few in the early stages. It is primarily a disease of older women, the average age being at least 60 years. Frequently, there is a history of some chronic epithelial dystrophy, especially leukoplakia. Slight itching or burning of the vulva may be noted, with bleeding only rarely being observed. Often the feeling of a hard lump in this region may be the only thing to bring the patient to a physician. Examination reveals one or more suspiciously hard nodules, parts of which may be ulcerated and may bleed easily. Inguinal nodes are frequently palpable, but this may be due to inflammation rather than metastatic tumor, unless they are very hard and fixed.

DIAGNOSIS. This usually can be suspected on examination but always should be confirmed by adequate biopsy before definitive treatment is started.

TREATMENT. Surgery provides the best treatment available at present. The most logical approach, and one which conforms to accepted standards of cancer surgery, is that originally recommended by Way. The inguinal nodes, the tissue between the inguinal region and the vulva and the vulva itself are removed en bloc in one procedure. (See Fig. 51-12.) Extraperitoneal removal of the nodes above the inguinal ligament (up to the bifurcation of the aorta) is advocated as a routine procedure by some. Others recommend it if the primary lesion is large or Cloquet's node shows cancer on frozen section. The success of operative treatment is indicated by reports of 5-year survival rates of 61 per cent (Green, Ulfelder and Meigs) and 54 per cent (Way). The procedure is a formidable one, since many of the patients are old, debilitated and affected by intercurrent disease. Even in the best hands these wounds do not heal well, and later postoperative swelling of the legs is common, although usually temporary. In some poor-risk patients it may be well to stage the procedure, though this sacrifices the principle of removal of the cancer and metastatic nodes in continuity. In patients who are considered to be too poor risks to stand any surgical procedure or in recurrent disease, radiation may be of palliative and possibly of curative value; it is used best in the form of implantation of radium needles with or without external irradiation.

The above type of procedure is applicable to most invasive vulvar carcinomas. In the rare instance where the anus is involved it may be necessary to perform an abdominoperineal resection of the rectum. It may be noted that it is quite practical to remove up to half of the urethra without the patient's becoming incontinent, and a large portion of the vagina also may be removed from below without difficulty. When intra-epithelial carcinoma of the vulva is present, radical vulvectomy alone without node dissection is sufficient therapy.

A basal cell carcinoma of the vulva does not need extensive vulvectomy, and a wide local excision is sufficient.

Cancer of the Vagina. Primary cancer of the vagina is rare, comprising from 1 to 2 per cent of all cancers of the female genital tract. Metastatic cancer of the vagina may occur from cervix, endometrium, ovary or other organs. Primary cancer is almost always of the squamous cell type. It tends to grow in the long axis of the vagina, and because of its proximity to the rectum on the posterior wall and to the bladder on the anterior wall it may involve either of these organs at an early stage. It also spreads laterally to the paravaginal and paracervical tissues. Metastases may pass to both iliac and inguinal nodes. Carcinoma of the urethra, usually of the transitional cell type, is often difficult to distinguish from primary carcinoma of the vagina.

CLINICAL FEATURES. Painless vaginal bleeding or discharge are usually the first symptoms, although pain and particularly dyspareunia are not uncommon. Usually it is found in the postmenopausal woman but it may occur at an earlier age. Examination reveals a hard nodule infiltrating the vaginal wall. Ulceration and a tendency to bleed easily on manipulation are common.

DIAGNOSIS. This is made on the basis of clinical examination and biopsy.

TREATMENT. The proximity of the bladder and rectum impedes treatment by radiotherapy or surgery. Intravaginal application of radium with or without external therapy is preferable in many instances. Occasionally radical surgery may be indicated: this may involve anterior, posterior or even total exenteration with the possible addition of inguinal lymphadenectomy. However, the over-all five year survival rate of 28 per cent in 256 collected cases, as reported by Latourette and Lourie, certainly leaves room for improvement. The importance of individualizing treatment is emphasized by Rutledge.

DISEASE OF THE CERVIX

INFECTIONS OF THE CERVIX

Acute Cervicitis. This condition is usually part of a generalized infection of the lower genital tract. Specific symptoms are not usually present. The diagnosis is made by inspection of the cervix, which appears red and inflamed; there is a profuse discharge. Treatment is primarily that of the specific infection involved and is described above. Instrumentation of the cervical canal and local applications to the cervix should be avoided for fear of spreading infection to the upper genital tract.

Chronic Cervicitis. This disease is found in at least one third of the adult female population. Frequently, it is associated with erosions, lacerations and cysts, and these 4 conditions have to be considered together. Infection itself may play a major part, such as in trichomoniasis or gonorrhea, or it may be secondary to the other disorders.

Erosions represent extension of the columnar epithelium of the endocervix outward on the external surface of the cervix. They may be congenital or acquired. The congenital type may be present in as many as one third of newborn girls. It commonly extends in a circular fashion around the external os and in the nulliparous woman may not be accompanied by infection. Acquired erosions occur in association with lacerations, cysts and infections and commonly are irregular in appearance.

Lacerations result from childbirth and usually occur at 3 and 9 o'clock, giving the typical fish-mouth appearance to the parous cervix.

Cysts occur as the result of blockage of the mouth of the cervical glands by infection or trauma.

CLINICAL FEATURES. Chronic cervicitis may cause no symptoms and may be discovered only on routine pelvic examination. If symptoms are present they usually consist of mild to moderate vaginal discharge, and slight vaginal bleeding occurring following intercourse or douches. Usually pain is not noted unless inflammation involves the paracervical tissues.

Lacerations and cysts are easily visible on examination. Infection may produce a slight irregular reddening of the cervix. Erosions appear as granular and sometimes papillary red areas extending outward from the external os.

DIAGNOSIS. The most important consideration is to exclude cancer. Cytologic studies are a valuable screening device. Material can be obtained by aspiration of the vaginal vault or endocervix, by applying a cotton-tipped applicator to the cervical canal or by scraping the ectocervix with an Ayre spatula. The material is spread on slides and fixed in a 50-50 mixture of ether and 95 per cent alcohol. The slides are stained by Papanicolaou's method or modifications thereof. According to the Papanicolaou classification 5 classes of smears are recognized—(I) normal, (II) slightly abnormal, possibly due to inflammatory changes, (III) suspicious, (IV) occasional malignant cells, and (V) many malignant cells. In addition to cytologic studies, punch biopsy of any obvious lesion of the cervix may be performed. Negative smears and punch biopsies serve, in general, to rule out cancer, and specific treatment for chronic cervicitis can then be instituted. When the cytologic study is reported as Class III, IV or V and no obvious lesion is seen grossly on the cervix, colposcopy is very useful. Magnification of the surface of the cervix 10 or 20 times enables areas suspicious for malignant change to be clearly identified and spot biopsies to be taken (Bolten). The final diagnostic tool is the cold-knife conization with pathologic study of semiserial sections of the cervix. However, this requires hospitalization and anesthesia and has occasional complications in the form of delayed bleeding and cervical stenosis. Application of all possible preliminary diagnostic studies with emphasis on colposcopy may avoid the necessity of conization in selected cases.

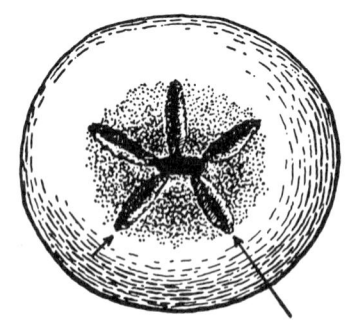

TREATMENT. Because of the likelihood, presumed though not proved, that chronic cervicitis predisposes to the development of cancer, treatment should be given to all cases where symptoms occur and to all women over 30 even if they are asymptomatic. Treatment of chronic cervicitis in the woman who is under 30 years of age and has no symptoms is usually but not always advisable.

Where nonspecific infection appears to be the main problem, restoration of the vaginal acidity by acid douches or intravaginal application of acid jelly is helpful. Sulfonamide creams used intravaginally are useful. Erosions may be treated in the office by radial cauterization with the electric cautery; following this the squamous epithelium usually will regenerate over the eroded area (Fig. 51-13). Cervical cysts can be punctured with a needle-point cautery. If the area of infection, erosion and laceration is very large, then more extensive cauterization may be per-

FIG. 51-13. Radial cauterization of the cervix.

formed as a hospital procedure. Alternatively, the whole area may be coned out with the electric wire and the external os reconstructed by means of a Sturmdorf or other type of inverting suture. Cryosurgical treatment of chronic cervicitis offers an interesting new approach, but has not yet been fully evaluated.

Any procedure involving cauterization or conization should be followed by careful and regular examinations including postmenstrual sounding of the cervical canal at least once to avoid the development of stenosis.

Cervical Polyps

Cervical polyps are small pedunculated growths which arise from the endocervix or more rarely from the external surface of the cervix. They are often multiple. They are composed of a connective tissue stroma covered by columnar epithelium, which is thrown into many folds. Inflammatory changes are common, and frequently the tip is congested. Squamous metaplasia of the epithelium is common, but malignant change occurs in less than 1 per cent.

Clinical Features. There may be no symptoms, or the patient may notice slight vaginal bleeding or discharge. Examination of the cervix usually will show the lesion. Polyps are soft and sometimes may be missed on palpation.

Diagnosis. The important conditions to be distinguished from cervical polyps are endometrial polyps, pedunculated submucous myomata and cancer of the cervix. Other benign tumors are occasionally seen in the cervix (Farrar and Nedoss).

Treatment. If irregular vaginal bleeding has occurred, particularly in the postmenopausal woman, a D. and C. should be performed to exclude intra-uterine causes. The polyp itself may be twisted off and the base cauterized to control bleeding. All polyps should be examined microscopically to rule out malignant changes.

Cancer of the Cervix

Cancer of the cervix comprises more than 50 per cent of all cancers of the female genital tract. Next to cancer of the breast it is the commonest malignant tumor in women. Thus the problem of early diagnosis and adequate treatment of this disease is of major importance. Considerable strides have been made in this area as a result of the use of cytologic screening methods, as evidenced by the work of Fidler et al.

Cause. The present-day ignorance of the exact mechanism which causes cells to become malignant applies to cancer of the cervix. Several contributory factors have been thought to be of importance. Hereditary patterns have been postulated but never proved. Early age of first coitus and of marriage and circumcision of the sexual partner may be of importance (Wynder et al., 1954). Support for these theories is obtained from the lower incidence of cervical cancer in nuns and in Jewish women. Considerable evidence has been advanced for progressive changes in the cervical epithelium, leading eventually to cancer. Thus, dysplasia (the most satisfactory name for epithelial disorders) may progress to intraepithelial carcinoma (carcinoma in situ) and then to invasive carcinoma. But the point at which this progression becomes irreversible and the factors responsible for this are unknown.

Pathologic Features. Ninety five per cent of cervical cancers are of the squamous cell type. About 5 per cent are glandular (adenocarcinoma).

The cellular changes characteristic of dysplasia include: (1) lack of cellular differentiation; (2) lack of cellular polarity; (3) numerous and sometimes atypical mitotic figures; (4) pleomorphism of cells with variably enlarged hyperchromatic nuclei; (5) an intact basement membrane. The extent to which the epithelium is involved leads many pathologists to classify dysplasia as mild, moderate or severe. Intraepithelial carcinoma then implies that the whole of the epithelium has undergone these changes. However, the interpretation of these precise histologic differences is often debatable. (See Fig. 51-14.)

When invasive cancer is present the basement membrane is broken, and nests of tumor cells may be seen beneath it. They may have no definite arrangement, or they may show considerable differentiation with formation of epithelial pearls. Since there are presumably degrees of invasion, considerable interest has recently been shown in micro-invasive carcinoma where the basement membrane appears to be broken in a small area, for example, in only one place and to a depth of not more than 3 mm. It is possible that metastases to lymph nodes may be less likely than with more extensive invasion, but the condition remains difficult to define pathologically and clinically.

Spread. Cervical cancer spreads locally in the first instance through the cervix and into the paracervical tissues. Extension to the uterine cavity and to the vagina may occur early. Lymphatic spread occurs primarily to the hypogastric, obturator, common iliac and external iliac nodes. The incidence of such spread, according to data collected from the literature by Morton et al., is 16.5 per cent for Stage I disease, 31.9 per cent for Stage II and 56.7 per cent for Stage III. Distant metastases are found most commonly in the liver, the lungs and the bones.

Grading and Staging. Attempts to gauge the malignant potentiality of a particular tumor, based on the degree of cell differentiation seen in biopsy or excised specimens, have not so far been very satisfactory. Of interest are attempts to foretell the success of treatment from the examination of serial biopsies or cytologic studies.

Clinical staging of the disease has been of great value in prognosis and in comparing the results of treatment from different centers. The most commonly used classification is that of the International Federation of Gynaecology and Obstetrics, which is based on the older League of Nations classification (International classification). This is as follows:

Stage O. Carcinoma in situ: also known as intramucosal carcinoma, preinvasive carcinoma, intra-epithelial carcinoma, and similar conditions.

Stage I. The carcinoma is confined strictly to the cervix (extension to the corpus should be disregarded).

Stage II. The carcinoma extends beyond the cervix but has not reached the pelvic wall. The carcinoma involves the vagina but not the lower third.

Stage III. The carcinoma has reached the pelvic wall or involves the lower third of the vagina.

Stage IV. The carcinoma involves the bladder or the rectum or both or has extended beyond the limits previously described.

Various minor modifications of these stages have been described: they are of value in indicating specific treatment and, in some instances, prognosis.

It has been found that experienced clinicians usually will agree on the staging of a particular lesion. However, such staging depends only on examination and does not take into account the malignant potentialities of the tumor or its spread to lymph nodes, both of which greatly affect the outcome.

Clinical Features. About 75 per cent of patients with intra-epithelial and perhaps one third of those with Stage I carcinoma of the cervix have no symptoms. In fact, many far advanced lesions frequently give the unsuspicious patient little cause for concern. When symptoms occur they almost always consist of irregular bleeding which is intermenstrual in the woman of childbearing age and frequently follows coitus or other trauma such as douching. Discharge sometimes occurs. With involvement of the bladder or the rectum symptoms may be referable to these organs. If the disease extends to the pelvic wall, pain in the back or pain down the legs may be noted. It is to be noted that these symptoms are due occasionally to associated inflammatory changes in the paracervical tissues and not primarily to the cancer.

Diagnosis. The diagnosis of cervical cancer is made by the scrupulous use of all the diagnostic technics described above (Newton and Bolten). A positive cytologic report (Fig. 51-14) must be confirmed by microscopic examination of a biopsy specimen. It is important to be sure whether one is dealing with an intra-epithelial or an invasive lesion. If the distinction cannot be made from a punch biopsy, then conization should be performed. Treatment should not be begun without a definite diagnosis.

The detection of early curable lesions is made more likely by regular yearly pelvic examinations and cytologic studies of women over 25 years of age and of married women whatever their age. Constant awareness of the problem by both patient and physician is essential.

Treatment. INTRA-EPITHELIAL CANCER. Since it is assumed that preinvasive cancer eventually will become invasive, treatment is indicated. In the postmenopausal women or in the premenopausal woman who does not desire further children, a simple total hysterectomy

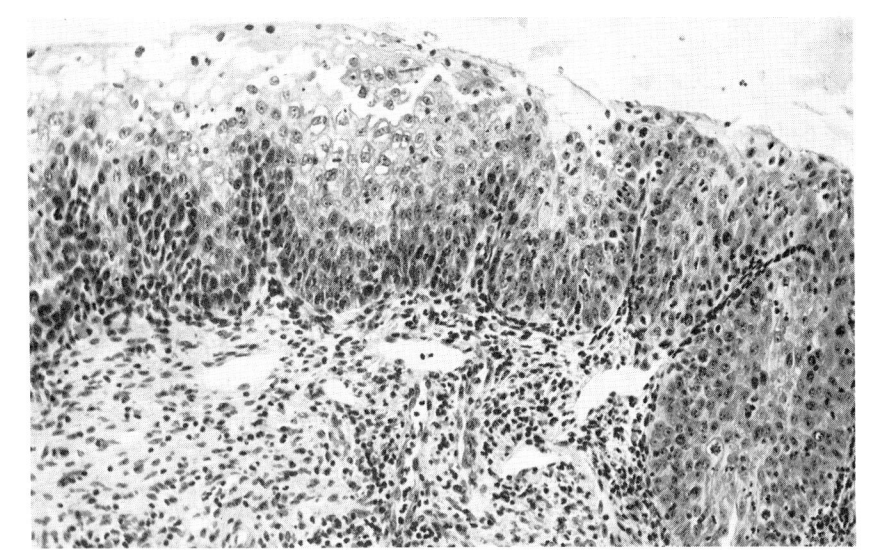

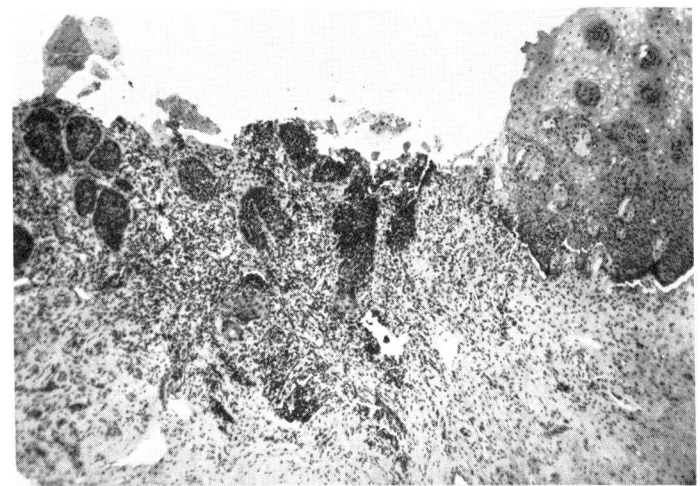

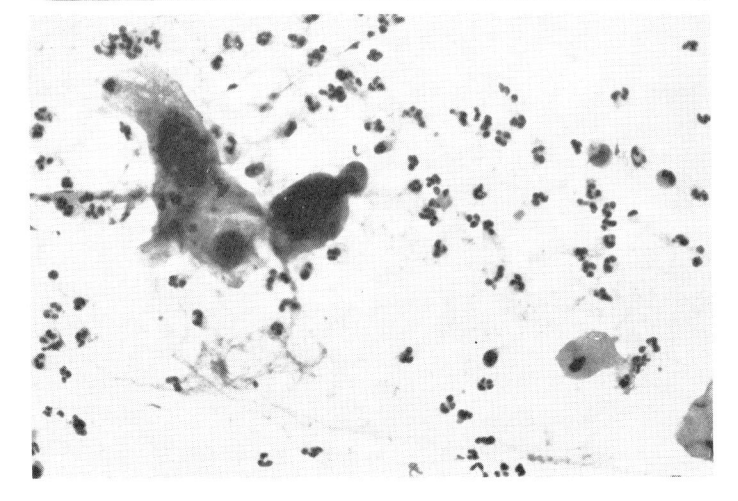

FIG. 51-14. Epithelium of the cervix, showing transition from normal stratified squamous type to intra-epithelial carcinoma (*top*) and to invasive carcinoma (*center*). (*Bottom*) Cervical smear showing malignant cells with large, irregular, dark-staining nuclei.

without oophorectomy (unless the ovaries are diseased) and with resection of a 1 to 2 cm. vaginal cuff is sufficient. In the woman who wants to have more children, a wide conization of the cervix, either by the knife or electrical wire, may be performed. In this case, however, it is important to be reasonably sure that all the lesion has been removed. Careful follow-up, with cytologic studies and biopsy when appropriate, should be carried out at 6-month intervals.

The management of dysplasia has to be considered along with that of intraepithelial carcinoma. Mild and moderate dysplasia can be managed as described above for chronic cervicitis. Since severe dysplasia is difficult to distinguish histologically from intraepithelial carcinoma, it may be advisable to treat it as the latter in many instances, particularly if the patient has already had the children she desires.

INVASIVE CANCER. Best results are obtained if invasive cancer is treated in centers staffed by a cooperating team of gynecologists and radiotherapists experienced in its management (Graham and Paloucek). Adequate study, especially of the urinary tract, should be performed before treatment is begun. Facilities for follow-up and consultation are essential.

At the present time 2 general methods of treatment are available—surgery or radiation. In the early 1900's the only possible treatment was surgical, and operative technics were described by Clark, Rumpf, Ries and Wertheim, using the abdominal route (Kimbrough). Schauta used the vaginal approach. These procedures were attended with great risk to the patient, and the results were poor, largely because of the lack of adequate supportive therapy such as antibiotics, prolonged anesthesia and blood transfusions. With the discovery of the radiosensitivity of cervical cancer and better methods of using radiation, the surgical approach fell into disuse in the United States. In the past 2 decades interest in surgery has increased again, and large series of cases treated surgically have been reported (Liu and Meigs, Yagi, Parker et al.). Along with this has been the recognition that radiation, while initially a safe procedure so far as the patient's life is concerned, does carry the danger of crippling complications when used in cancerocidal doses.

Adequate surgical treatment consists of a radical hysterectomy with wide excision of the parametrial and the paracervical tissues and the upper vagina with removal of the pelvic lymph nodes. Although this is a major surgical procedure, the operative mortality in good hands has been from 1 to 2.5 per cent. The main complication to be feared is fistula formation. In particular, ureterovaginal fistula has been reported to occur following 2 to 9 per cent of operations.

Treatment by radiation involves the use of external radiation by means of x-rays, together with the application of radium to the cervix by means of one of a number of different applicators. Radium may be given in single or divided doses and may be either preceded or followed by external radiation. Whatever the technic used the amount of radiation delivered to the cervix and to the surrounding structures (rectum, bladder and ureters) should be calculated as accurately as possible in terms of rads. The use of fixed points in the pelvis to calculate and compare dosage has been of great advantage. Two commonly used points of reference are Point A, which lies 2 cm. above the external os and 2 cm. lateral to the center of the cervical canal, and Point B, which lies 2 cm. above the external os and 5 cm. lateral to the center of the cervical canal. A suggested cancerocidal dose to Point A is 7,500 to 9,500 r and to Point B 5,000 to 6,000 r delivered in 40 days or less (Newton, Hickman and Bolten, 1961). Variations in dosage may be necessary, depending on the individual lesions and on the dose delivered to neighboring organs.

Decision as to the best type of treatment for a particular case involves 3 considerations: (1) the stage of the patient's disease, (2) the general physical condition and age of the patient and (3) the type of treatment available in a particular center.

For patients with a Stage III or IV lesion surgical treatment would require excision of either bladder or rectum as well as the uterus and the cervix, in order to remove the lesion adequately. The high mortality of these procedures and the permanent stomata which result outweigh the possible slight improvement in survival. Even such an improvement is theoretical only.

For patients with Stage II lesions which

involve the parametria, surgery is probably contraindicated, since it may again be difficult to excise the tumor completely. The value of surgery in patients with early Stage II lesions (involving the upper vagina) is debatable.

When a patient has a Stage I lesion (and possibly an early Stage II), is relatively young and is in good general health, the choice of treatment may depend on which method is readily available. A good program of radiation will achieve better success than inadequate surgery and vice versa. Surgery may have some advantage for these patients, since the cervix can be removed with no chance of local recurrence, the lymph nodes, for which radiation is perhaps 50 per cent effective, can be excised, and the patient's treatment is completed at one time, rather than being continued over a 6-week period. In a randomized series (Newton, Hickman and Bolten, 1964) the results of both types of therapy appear to date to be similar.

Various combinations of radiation and surgical treatment have been reported. Where surgical treatment unexpectedly turns out to be inadequate, there would seem to be good reason for administering postoperative radiation. However, it is of questionable value to give full radiation first and follow this by radical surgery. Radiation alters the tissues in the pelvis, so that dissection is made more difficult, and healing is impeded. The value of the application of less than full doses of radiation prior to surgery is uncertain.

The management of microcarcinoma is still under debate. Because the chance of lymph node metastases is relatively small, radical vaginal hysterectomy, or possibly even lesser procedures, have been suggested. However, pending more data, it is probably best in most instances to treat microcarcinoma as if it were Stage I. On the other hand, if the pathologist describes invasion as questionable, it is best to treat the patient as if she had intra-epithelial disease.

When invasive carcinoma of the cervix is discovered in a pregnant patient, it should be managed without regard to the pregnancy unless, by preserving the pregnancy for a few more weeks, a viable infant can be obtained. Results of treatment during pregnancy do not differ greatly from those in the nonpregnant woman. If intraepithelial carcinoma is discovered during pregnancy, and invasion is excluded, radical treatment is not indicated. The pregnancy should be allowed to proceed to term and vaginal delivery to occur. Further investigation should then be carried out 6 to 8 weeks postpartum.

Adenocarcinoma responds to radiation in a way similar to squamous cell carcinoma, and the same considerations as to treatment apply to it.

The results of treatment of cancer of the cervix vary according to different authors. In general, provided that a patient receives adequate treatment, one may expect a 5-year survival rate of about 75 per cent for Stage I, 50 per cent for Stage II, 25 per cent for Stage III and 5 per cent or less for Stage IV lesions. Intra-epithelial cancer should be virtually 100 per cent curable.

Recurrent and Radioresistant Cancer of the Cervix

Close follow-up of patients is important during and after therapy. After operation cytologic studies of the vagina should be obtained regularly. These are less valuable in the first 12 months after radiotherapy, although they may be helpful later. Here, clinical examination, biopsy of the cervix or vagina or of the parametrium (using a Vim-Silverman or similar needle) have to suffice.

Whether continued active growth of cancer is due to resistance or recurrence makes little difference. Where an adequate course of radiation has been given this type of treatment can offer little more, except perhaps in areas where little therapy has been given (e.g., pelvic nodes), and even here palliation is all that can be expected. Chemotherapy has at present nothing to offer in this situation. However, the development of more radical surgical procedures during the past decade has made it possible to offer selected patients among this previously doomed group a chance of survival. These procedures involve anterior exenteration (removal of uterus and bladder), posterior exenteration (removal of rectum and uterus), and complete pelvic exenteration. The operative mortality is high—10 to 30 per cent—and the early and late complications of operation are 44 per cent and 39 per cent, respectively, according to Kiselow *et al.* Moreover, the patient is left with a considerable permanent disability owing to the artificial stomata. Therefore, such operations should not be performed unless actively growing cancer is present, the patient has received all possible treatment by other means, and finally unless there is a chance of cure. Furthermore, the patient must have the emotional stamina and the home circumstances to cope with the stomata involved. Under these conditions it would seem worthwhile to offer the patient what represents her only chance of survival.

Even if no curative surgical procedure can be offered the patient with recurrent cancer of the cervix, much can be done surgically, medically and psychologically to prolong her life and decrease her suffering. The management of the patient under these circumstances presents a real challenge.

THE UPPER GENITAL TRACT

INFECTIONS

Infections of the upper genital tract may affect the uterus (endometritis), tubes (salpingitis), ovaries (oophoritis) or the structures lying beside the uterus (parametritis). Frequently, all the pelvic organs are involved to a greater or less degree. The general term —pelvic inflammatory disease—is used commonly for this type of infection.

Infection usually reaches the upper genital tract from the vagina or the cervix. The following conditions may help to break down the normal barrier of the internal os of the cervix and cause the ascent of infection: (1) pregnancy and delivery, including abortion; (2) menstruation; (3) sexual intercourse; (4) instrumentation of the cervical canal. More rarely, infection may occur from the blood stream or may be spread from neighboring intra-abdominal organs.

Four common types of infection occur:

1. *Puerperal.* This usually is due to an anaerobic streptococcus and occurs following abortion or normal delivery. Spread occurs through the parametria, forming a pelvic cellulitis.

2. *Gonococcal.* This follows acute or chronic infection of the lower genital tract. Spread in this instance occurs along the surface of the uterus and along the tubes.

3. *Nonspecific.* This may be due to a variety of organisms of which the most important lie in the *E. coli* group.

4. *Tuberculous.* This is due to the *M. tuberculosis* and commonly involves the tubes first. It is usually chronic in nature and may be associated with tuberculosis elsewhere in the body.

Acute Pelvic Inflammatory Disease. CLINICAL FEATURES. A history of some existing cause (see above) is frequently obtainable. The symptoms consist of:

1. *Abdominal pain.* This is usually in the lower abdomen and bilateral, although it may be unilateral or generalized. In gonorrhea it may be very severe.

2. *Vaginal discharge*

3. *Malaise and fever*

4. *Nausea, vomiting and abdominal distention* may occur if the infection has spread widely through the peritoneal cavity.

Examination of the abdomen may show lower abdominal tenderness, rigidity and rebound tenderness or possibly signs of peritonitis such as distention and diminished peristalsis. Pelvic examination confirms the presence of discharge. The uterus may be enlarged and soft if the patient has been pregnant. The cervix is acutely tender on motion. If the adnexal areas can be adequately examined, acute tenderness in the region of one or both tubes will be noted. In the puerperal type an area of tender brawny induration may be felt extending out from the uterus on one or both sides.

DIAGNOSIS. Smear and culture from the cervix should be taken as soon as possible. Where abortion is likely, the presence of gram-positive rods in the smear may be significant. The culture should include study of anaerobic organisms and Neisseria as well as the more common types. The common conditions to be considered in the differential diagnosis are:

1. *Appendicitis.* Pain is commonly localized in the right lower quadrant, the temperature is lower and intestinal symptoms are more prominent.

2. *Tubal pregnancy.* Fever is absent, and symptoms and signs of pregnancy are present. The pregnancy test may be positive. If the tubal pregnancy has ruptured, culdocentesis may be productive of nonclotting blood.

3. *Accident occurring in an ovarian cyst or*

uterine tumor. Palpation of the mass may be possible.

4. *Renal tract disease,* such as pyelitis or stone. The symptoms and signs are usually unilateral, and the urine shows white or red blood cells.

5. *Diverticulitis.* Pain is usually on the left side, unless rupture has occurred. Fever may be less. Pelvic findings are minimal.

TREATMENT. Conservative treatment is usually in order. Rest in bed is important, and adequate doses of antibiotics should be given. Penicillin is usually effective against gonococci. Broad-spectrum antibiotics are valuable in other types of infection. Supportive therapy in the form of intravenous fluids, gastric suction or blood transfusion may be indicated.

Operative treatment is not primarily indicated, and any sort of instrumentation of the uterus is to be avoided. On occasions it may be impossible to differentiate pelvic inflammation from an acute intra-abdominal condition such as appendicitis. In this case it is safer to explore the patient; but if salpingitis is found, nothing should be done. Evacuation of the uterus may be advisable in postabortal infections.

Chronic Pelvic Inflammatory Disease. This is a troublesome condition both to diagnose and to treat. It is important to avoid labeling a patient as having chronic gonorrheal pelvic inflammatory disease without sufficient proof of the cause.

PATHOLOGIC FEATURES. The following pathologic changes commonly occur in the course of the disease.

1. *Recurrent attacks of infection*—acute or subacute—in tubes, ovaries or parametria, with persistent chronic inflammation between the attacks.

2. *Development of adhesions* between the pelvic organs themselves, or between the pelvic and other intra-abdominal organs.

3. *Closure of the cornual and fimbriated ends of the tube* with formation of a serous (hydrosalpinx) or purulent (pyosalpinx) collection within the tube.

4. *Involvement of both tube and ovary in a tubo-ovarian abscess.*

5. *Rupture of a hydrosalpinx, pyosalpinx or tubo-ovarian abscess into the peritoneal cavity.*

CLINICAL FEATURES. A history of one or more attacks of acute inflammation is suggestive.

The patient with uncomplicated chronic pelvic inflammatory disease or with pelvic adhesions resulting from the disease may complain of:

1. *Chronic vaginal discharge*
2. *Pelvic pain and backache*
3. *Menstrual irregularities and secondary dysmenorrhea*
4. *Generalized weakness and tiredness*

Examination may disclose slight fever. Some lower abdominal tenderness is frequently present. Pelvic examination confirms the presence of a purulent vaginal discharge and lower genital tract infection. The cervix may be tender on motion. Thickness of the adnexal areas may be noted with a sense of adherence in the pelvis. The uterus may be fixed in retroflexion.

The presence of a hydrosalpinx, a pyosalpinx or a tubo-ovarian abscess may cause the patient to notice a tender mass in the lower abdomen, and this may be palpable on pelvic examination.

Closure of the tubes, from previous infection, may result in involuntary sterility.

Rupture of a pelvic abscess presents an acute picture of shock with low blood pressure and rapid weak pulse. The abdomen is rigid with generalized tenderness and diminished or absent peristalsis.

DIAGNOSIS. Uncomplicated chronic pelvic inflammatory disease and adhesions have to be distinguished from endometriosis, disease of the lower intestinal tract, and disease of the bladder.

Adnexal masses due to inflammatory disease may be confused with tubal pregnancy, tumors of the ovary or the uterus and extragenital conditions such as diverticulitis or tumors of the colon or the retroperitoneal space.

Rupture of a pelvic abscess may give symptoms similar to those produced by rupture of any other intra-abdominal organs, such as a tubal pregnancy, the appendix or a peptic ulcer.

TREATMENT. *Conservative.* The treatment of uncomplicated chronic pelvic inflammatory disease is primarily conservative. This is important, since many of these patients are young; and surgery, to be effective, usually involves sacrifice of childbearing function. The following measures are of value:

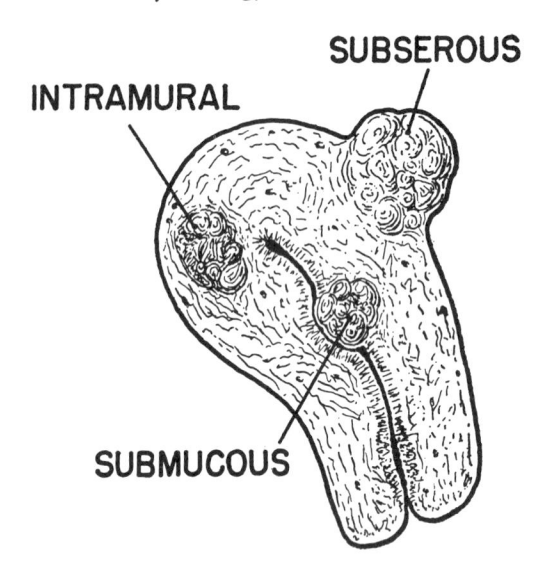

FIG. 51-15. Sites of myomata in uterus.

1. *Antibiotics.* These are of most value in acute inflammation but may be given a trial in chronic disease.
2. *Local heat* by means of hot vinegar douches, heating pads to the abdomen or short or microwave diathermy.
3. *Abstinence from intercourse or douching at the time of menstruation.*
4. *Adequate rest and emphasis on superior diet with supplemental administration of vitamins and iron.*
5. *Local treatment of disease of the lower genital tract.* It should be remembered that procedures on the cervix are likely to cause a flare-up of upper genital tract infection. They should be performed only when the disease is quiescent.

Surgical treatment is indicated in the following instances:

1. *Abscess presenting vaginally or rectally.* Drainage may be performed by opening the posterior cul-de-sac between the uterosacral ligaments, breaking up loculations with the finger and inserting a drainage tube.
2. *Rupture of a pelvic abscess.* Immediate laparotomy may be lifesaving (Lardaro). If the patient's condition permits, hysterectomy with bilateral salpingo-oophorectomy should be strongly considered. Otherwise, excision of the abscess or simple drainage is indicated.
3. *Adnexal mass.* Any adnexal mass over 6 cm. in size requires operation and excision.

It is never possible to be entirely sure on clinical examination that one is dealing with an abscess and not an ovarian tumor. If localized disease is found on one side in a young woman, local excision may be possible. However, more radical procedures are frequently necessary.

4. *Severe disability* due to recurrent disease or persistent inflammation which has not responded to conservative measures. Surgery should be resorted to only after careful deliberation, since such procedures in order to be curative usually mean removal of both tubes and ovaries and the uterus.
5. *Sterility due to closed tubes* (see under sterility).

Tuberculosis. While the picture of pelvic inflammation produced by tuberculosis is frequently indistinguishable from that found with other types of infection, it does present certain particular features. For example, the infection is commonly a descending one from the tubes to the uterus and often is associated with tuberculosis elsewhere in the body. It may give no symptoms, or the patient's only complaints may be of menstrual irregularity or sterility.

DIAGNOSIS is frequently impossible preoperatively. Where the diagnosis is suspected, cultures of menstrual blood or of curettings are valuable.

TREATMENT is primarily by the use of antibiotics, such as streptomycin, para-aminosalicylic acid and isoniazid, together with the commonly accepted measures for the treatment of the disease as a whole; i.e., rest and superior diet. Surgery may be indicated if the pelvic masses cause acute symptoms or if they do not respond to antibiotics. In any case the patient should be protected by antibiotics before and after operation.

TUMORS OF THE UPPER GENITAL TRACT

BENIGN TUMORS OF THE BODY OF THE UTERUS

Myoma. Myomata are the most common tumors of the female genital tract. They are present in fully 20 per cent of women over the age of 35. They are more common in nulliparous than in parous women, and in Negro than in white patients. Their etiology is unknown. Hormonal imbalance may play a part in their development, since they grow during the late years of a woman's reproductive life and decrease in size after the menopause.

PATHOLOGIC FEATURES. Although the short term myoma(ta) is acceptable, leiomyomata most accurately describes these tumors, since they are composed of interlacing bundles of smooth muscle fibers with a varying admixture of fibrous tissue. They are frequently multiple and may grow to a very large size. They may be located underneath the peritoneal covering of the uterus (subserosal), within the uterine wall (intramural) or just beneath the endometrium (submucous) (Fig. 51-15). They may be found also in the cervix, and both the subserosal and the submucous types may become pedunculated. In this case the myoma may begin to receive some of its blood supply from the omentum or other organs and may eventually become detached from the uterus (parasitic myoma). Myomata may also develop from smooth muscle tissue in the genital tract which is located outside the uterus.

Secondary changes are common and consist of:

1. *Hyalinization.* This is very common but of little practical importance.

2. *Cyst formation.* This is common in large myomata and is due to lack of blood supply in the center.

3. *Calcification.* This is a common change in myomata of long duration.

4. *Necrosis* may occur in the center of the tumor or on the surface as in submucous myomata.

5. *Sarcomatous change* occurs in well under 1 per cent of all myomata.

CLINICAL FEATURES. Myomata may give no symptoms until they attain a large size. When symptoms occur they may be divided into the following groups.

1. *Menstrual Disturbances.* Menorrhagia, dysmenorrhea and intermenstrual bleeding may occur. The last is most common with submucous tumors.

2. *Pressure Symptoms.* These may consist of a vague sense of pressure in the lower abdomen or the back, or of bladder irritability or constipation.

3. *General Effects.* Tiredness, weakness and malaise are common.

4. *Acute Accidents.* Necrosis, or twisting of the pedicle of a pedunculated tumor may cause acute lower abdominal pain, with fever and leukocytosis. Minor symptoms of this sort are common in myomata associated with pregnancy.

If the tumor is large, abdominal examination will reveal a hard, nodular mass arising from the pelvis. Pelvic examination will show the uterus to be irregularly enlarged and firm. Anemia is commonly present even in the absence of menorrhagia.

DIAGNOSIS. Myomata which project to the side of the uterus may be confused with adnexal masses. Acute accidents in myomata have to be distinguished from pelvic inflammatory disease, accidents in ovarian tumors, endometriosis, tubal pregnancy and other intra-abdominal disorders such as acute appendicitis or diverticulitis. The possibility of pregnancy or pregnancy associated with a myoma always must be kept in mind.

TREATMENT. Myomata can be cured only by surgical excision. No hormonal or medical treatment known at the present time will cause them to shrink or disappear. However, they are frequently small and asymptomatic: the chance of malignant change occurring is small, and spontaneous regression in size occurs after the menopause. For these reasons continued observation with examination every 6 months in the premenopausal years and every 12 months postmenopausally is advisable in the vast majority of patients with myomata. Surgery should be performed only on the following indications:

1. *Size.* Any tumor larger in size than a 3-month pregnancy generally should be removed. A sudden increase in size on repeated examinations is also an indication for operation.

2. *Pressure.* Evidence by x-rays of pressure on ureters or colon makes operation advisable.

3. *Symptoms.* It is important to be sure that the symptoms complained of really are due to myomata.

4. *Acute accidents,* such as twisting of the pedicle of a pedunculated myoma.

5. *Sterility or repeated abortions.*

The importance of investigating any abnormal bleeding that is reported in association with myomata, so as to exclude cancer, cannot be overemphasized. This may include cytologic studies, appropriate biopsy of the cervix and dilatation and curettage.

Myomectomy. This procedure is of value where preservation of reproductive function is of importance. Even in the case of tumors that are of considerable size and are numerous, the persistent surgeon can restore the uterus to a remarkably normal appearance. Bleeding may be quite severe, although it can be controlled by temporary compression of the uterine arteries or by the intra-uterine injection of vasopressin. Complications in the form of adhesions are more likely than with a hysterectomy. However, the preservation of normal menstrual function and the possibility of retaining or increasing the patient's ability to have children are strong recommendations in favor of myomectomy.

Hysterectomy. This is the operation of choice in the woman who has finished having her family or where the tumor is too large or too adherent to the surrounding structures to make myomectomy practical. Both corpus and cervix should be removed (total hysterectomy) (Fig. 51-16). If the patient's condition is not good enough to permit of the extra dissection required to remove the cervix, the corpus alone may be excised (supracervical hysterectomy). When the cervix is not removed, regular postoperative examinations must be performed to watch for the possible development of cancer in the stump.

It is generally desirable to leave in both ovaries at the time of hysterectomy, provided that they appear to be normal.

Endometrial Polyps. These common growths are made up of endometrium, which may undergo cyclical changes, or more commonly of an unripe type of epithelium. They may occur in premenopausal and postmenopausal women and may be multiple. Sometimes they project down into the cervical canal on a pedicle. They may be associated with adenocarcinoma in another area of the uterine cavity.

The importance of endometrial polyps is that they may cause slight irregular bleeding which has to be distinguished from that due to cancer. Frequently, however, they may cause no symptoms.

Treatment is by division or avulsion of the pedicle and thorough curettage to remove the base. Sometimes polyps may be missed on routine curettage, unless the uterine cavity is explored with placental forceps in addition to the usual curette.

Malignant Tumors of the Body of the Uterus

Adenocarcinoma is by far the commonest tumor of the body of the uterus. It is the second most frequent type of cancer in the female genital tract. An interesting variant of this tumor is the adeno-acanthoma in which squamous metaplasia of the endometrial elements occurs. This comprises up to 25 per cent of cases of adenocarcinoma of the body of the uterus.

Cause. The development of endometrial adenocarcinoma has long been linked to an endocrinologic imbalance, with particular re-

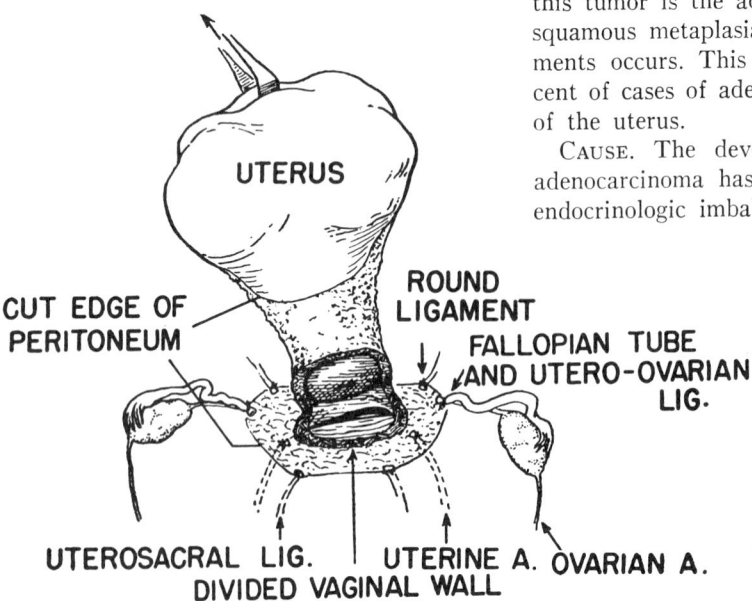

Fig. 51-16. Hysterectomy, showing upper vagina divided and uterus about to be removed.

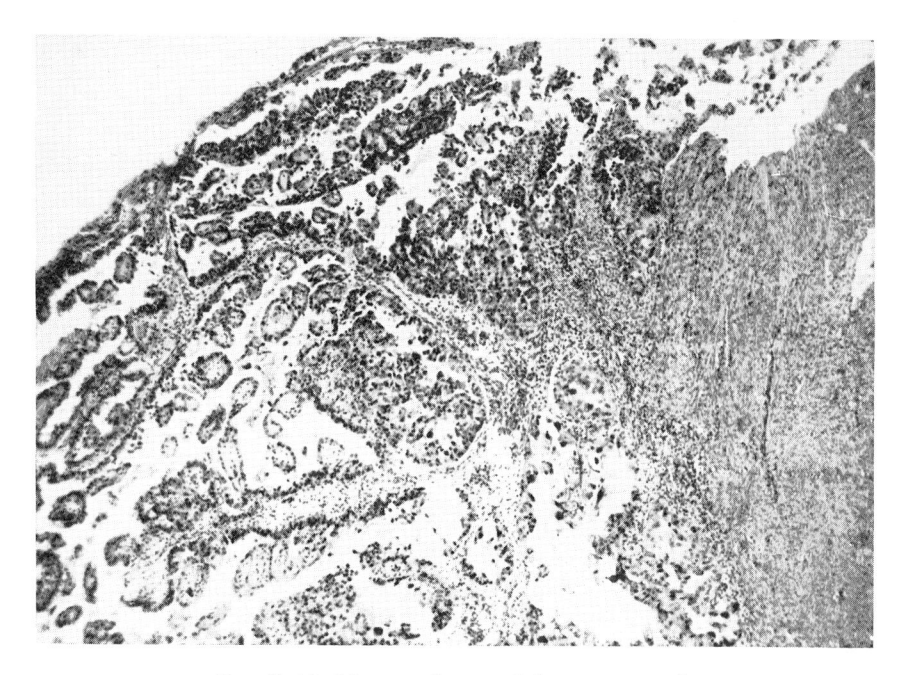

FIG. 51-17. Adenocarcinoma of the corpus uteri.

gard to estrogens. There is an increased incidence of obesity and tallness among women with endometrial cancer (Wynder et al., 1966). An increase in hypertension and elevated blood sugar has also been found, but this relationship needs to be more clearly defined. Estrogens are more specifically implicated by the observations that these women are more commonly nulliparous and give histories of menstrual abnormalities and late menopause. Endometrial cancer is also occasionally associated with functioning tumors of the ovary such as granulosa cell tumors or thecomas.

The relationship of endometrial cancer to endometrial hyperplasia is a debatable point, although there is some evidence that the two conditions are part of the same process. It seems likely that the so-called atypical hyperplasia, with excess proliferation of cells lining the glands and many mitoses, is a precancerous lesion, whereas the typical "Swiss-cheese hyperplasia" seen in premenopausal women does not predispose to cancer.

PATHOLOGIC FEATURES. Characteristically, the microscopic picture is one of abnormal endometrial glands invading the stroma (see Fig. 51-17). These glands are of irregular shape and size and commonly appear back to back with the epithelium of one directly touching the epithelium of another. The cell nuclei are large, irregular in size and hyperchromatic. An intra-epithelial type has been identified, in which the cells appear to be malignant, but no invasion is present. Histologic grading of the tumor may be a useful guide to treatment and prognosis. Well differentiated lesions (Grades I and II) offer a better outlook than those that are poorly differentiated (Grades III and IV).

Adenocarcinoma of the body of the uterus spreads into the myometrium, down into the cervix and the vagina and into the parametrial tissues. Local metastases to tubes and ovaries are common, but distant metastases to lungs and liver occur late in the course of the disease. Metastases to pelvic lymph nodes, according to data derived from operative cases, occur in 10 to 40 per cent, being lower when the disease is confined to the uterus (Rickford).

CLINICAL FEATURES. The average age is about 57 years. Intermenstrual or irregular postmenopausal bleeding is the most common symptom. Abnormal discharge may also occur. Pain, general weakness and debility are

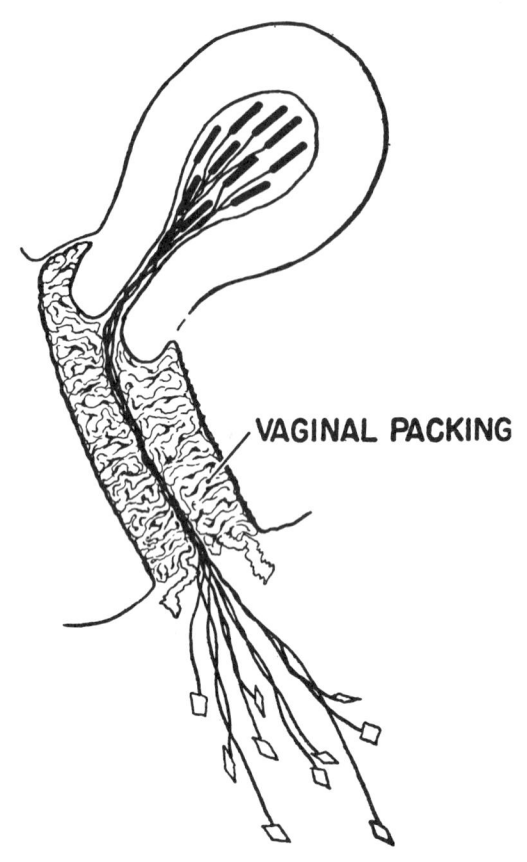

FIG. 51-18. Intra-uterine application of radium.

Clinical staging of the extent of the disease has not been as reliable nor as widely used as in carcinoma of the cervix. The International Classification, accepted by the International Federation of Gynaecology and Obstetrics, is as follows:

Stage I—Carcinoma confined to the corpus.
Stage II—Corpus plus cervix involvement.
Stage III—Extension outside the uterus but not outside the pelvis.
Stage IV—Carcinoma involves the bladder or rectum or extends outside the pelvis.

This classification does not, however, take into account the differentiation of the tumor, nor the size of the uterus, both of which may be important. On the basis of his experience, Gusberg has suggested modifications of this classification which may be more realistic and useful.

TREATMENT. Definitive treatment should not be begun without first establishing a positive diagnosis, staging the extent of the lesion and performing a pretreatment work-up similar to that used prior to treatment of cervical cancer. Diagnosis by gross inspection of curettings is often misleading. Histologic examination of frozen sections may be helpful, but should be used in conjunction with the overall evaluation of the patient.

There is increasing recognition of the need to individualize treatment according to the extent of the lesion. Thus, in Stage I, when the uterus is relatively normal in size and the tumor well differentiated, total hysterectomy and bilateral salpingo-oophorectomy is appropriate. Because of the danger of recurrence at the apex of the vagina, 1 to 2 cm. of vaginal cuff should be removed and, in addition, a radium plaque should be inserted 2 to 3 weeks postoperatively. When the tumor is poorly differentiated or the uterus large, radium may first be applied to the uterine cavity. This is best done by the multiple source packing technic of Heyman (Fig. 51-18). Four to six weeks later total hysterectomy and bilateral salpingo-oophorectomy is performed with removal of 1 to 2 cm. of vaginal cuff. Again radium is applied to the vaginal cuff postoperatively. If the cervix or the parametrium (Stages II and III) are involved, radium is applied to the cervix as well as to the endometrial cavity prior to hysterectomy. In these instances, a radical hysterectomy may be indi-

late symptoms. Examination in the early stages may be entirely negative, or the uterus may be somewhat enlarged, soft and irregular in shape.

DIAGNOSIS. Since endometrial cancer may cause as much as 30 to 40 per cent of all postmenopausal bleeding, both gynecologist and patient must be alert to this symptom. Routine cytologic studies of material from the vagina or the cervix are not completely reliable, since positive smears are obtained in only about 70 per cent of patients with endometrial cancer. Endometrial biopsies, taken with a suction curette, may be useful if positive. Basically, the diagnosis rests on obtaining adequate material for study by means of a diagnostic curettage. This should be done even if there is another obvious cause for the bleeding, such as a cervical polyp. In performing this curettage, it is important, when possible, to obtain tissue from the endocervix as well as the endometrium (fractional curettage).

cated if the patient is a good operative risk. In Stage IV, localized radiotherapy to relieve symptoms or chemotherapy (see below) is all that can be offered. When it is not possible to remove all the cancer at operation, postoperative external radiotherapy may be given. If the patient is a very poor operative risk, she can be treated by application of radium and external radiotherapy with limited chance of success.

Over-all five year survival rates of 60 to 70 per cent may be expected with adequate treatment in adenocarcinoma of the corpus uteri. Results are considerably better (80-90%) when the tumor is confined to a small uterus and is well differentiated, but are much worse when extension has occurred. With adenoacanthoma the results are similar.

Recurrent adenocarcinoma of the uterus presents a difficult problem in management. Although the occasional case can be treated by exenterative surgery, this is not usually practical because of the extent of the disease and the patient's poor general condition. Local recurrence in the vagina, a common site, may be treated by the application of radium, and external radiotherapy may be of some value in pelvic recurrence. Recently, the use of the synthetic progestins, given in large doses, has appeared to give remissions in 20 to 30 per cent of patients with extensive recurrent disease. The maximum duration of the response is probably about 2 years. Other chemotherapeutic agents are as yet of little value.

Sarcoma of the Uterus. Leiomyosarcoma is the commonest type. It may arise in a preexisting myoma (less than 1%) or independently in the uterine muscle. Symptoms are similar to those for endometrial carcinoma in general, although they may arise later in the course of the disease. Treatment is primarily surgical, by means of total hysterectomy. The addition of bilateral salpingo-oophorectomy or more radical procedures probably does not improve survival rates. If leiomyosarcoma is discovered in the operative specimen and has not extended outside the uterus, the prognosis is good. If the diagnosis has been made preoperatively or extension is found outside the uterus, the prognosis is very poor. The degree of malignancy, as seen histologically, has not been shown clearly to be related to prognosis. When the disease is widespread or recurs after treatment, both radiotherapy and chemotherapy with various agents have been used. Neither method has proved to be particularly effective.

Malignant mixed müllerian neoplasms (mixed mesodermal tumors) represent a rare but important type of sarcoma of the uterus. Because of the difficulty of the clinical and the pathologic identification of these tumors, it is possible that lesions, described as sarcoma botryoides and carcinosarcoma, actually fall into the group of mixed mesodermal tumors. Characteristically, carcinomatous as well as sarcomatous structures seem to develop without sharp transition from the primitive stromal background, often in several areas. The disease is almost uniformly fatal, Krupp *et al.* reporting no survivals for more than 1 year in a group of 51 patients, in spite of various types of treatment.

Tumors of the Fallopian Tube. Tumors of any sort in the fallopian tube are rare. The most important are the malignant ones—papillary carcinoma and sarcoma. Usually they are discovered accidentally during laparotomy. Surgical removal of the uterus and both tubes and ovaries is the best treatment.

TUMORS OF THE OVARY

Classification. The ovary has the potentiality of developing many different kinds of cysts and tumors. The following is a classification of the more common ones.

1. NON-NEOPLASTIC CYSTS. These comprise follicle cysts and corpus luteum cysts. They are extremely common and usually of small size.

2. NEOPLASTIC CYSTS:

A. *Pseudomucinous Cysts.* These may grow to a very large size. They often are multilocular and contain a clear, viscid fluid. Microscopically, they are lined by a single layer of columnar epithelium, with basal nuclei. Goblet cells are common (Fig. 51-19).

B. *Serous Cysts.* These are slightly less common than the pseudomucinous cysts and usually are not so large. Microscopically, they are lined by flatter epithelium, which is frequently ciliated and bears a close resemblance to the epithelium of the tube (Fig. 51-20).

C. *Dermoid Cysts (Cystic Teratomata).* These tumors are derived from embryonal tissue and often show derivatives of all three germ layers although ectodermal elements pre-

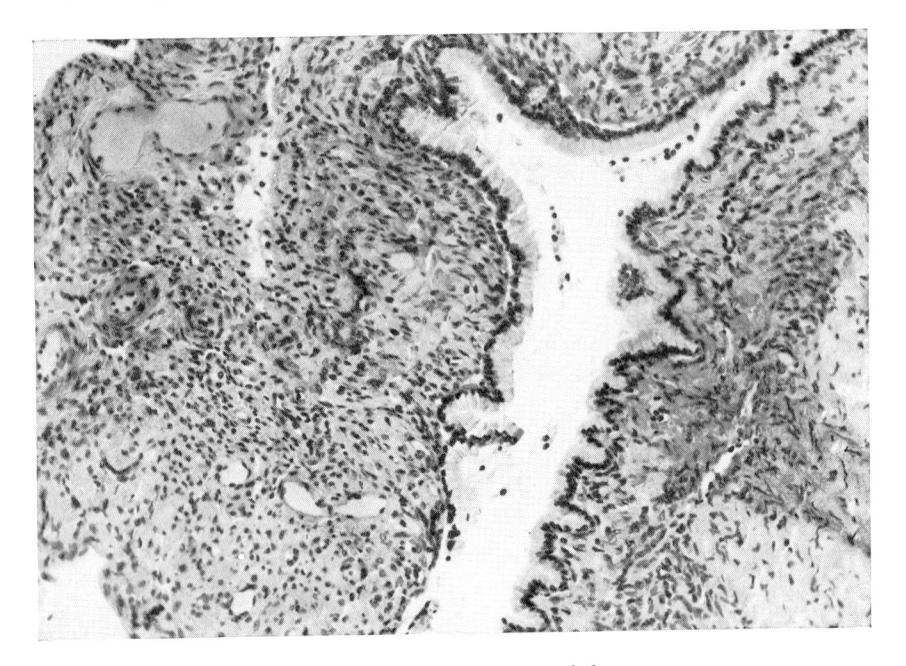

FIG. 51-19. Pseudomucinous cyst of the ovary.

dominate. They comprise 11 per cent of all ovarian tumors and are bilateral in 12 per cent of cases (Peterson *et al.*). Grossly, dermoid cysts present a thick white capsule and characteristically contain a large amount of thick, yellow sebaceous material. Microscopically, they are lined by squamous epithelium; skin appendages, such as hairs, sebaceous glands and sweat glands, are usually present. Cartilage, ciliated epithelium lining small ducts,

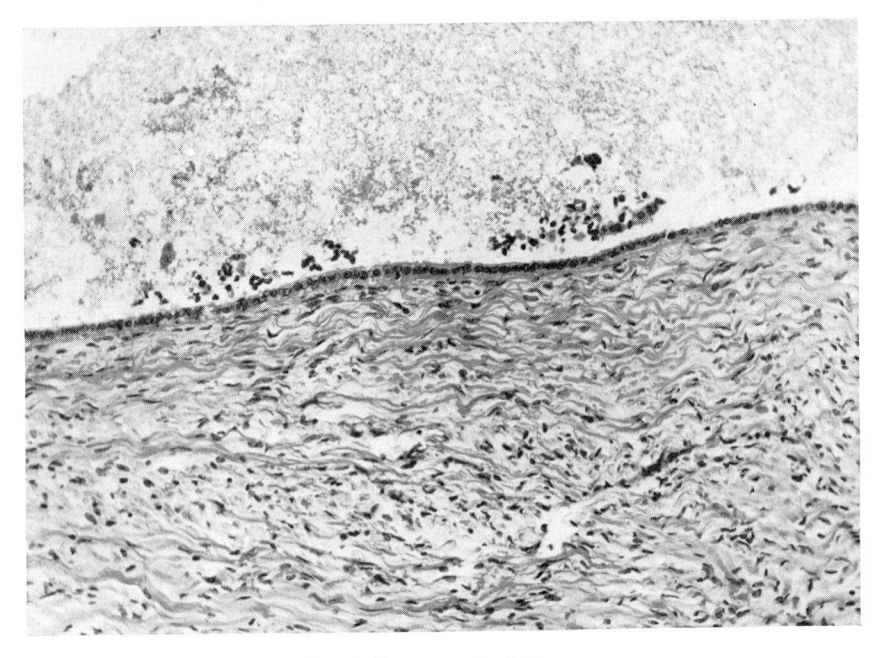

FIG. 51-20. Serous cyst of the ovary.

thyroid tissue and other embryonic remnants may be seen. Calcification is commonly present, and well-developed teeth may occur. This feature, combined with the radiolucency produced in some instances by the sebaceous material in the cyst, may enable the diagnosis to be made preoperatively by roentgenography. Malignant change, usually squamous cell carcinoma, is found in less than 1 per cent of dermoid cysts.

3. BENIGN SOLID TUMORS:

A. *Fibromata*. These are usually small asymptomatic tumors, although occasionally they may grow to a large size. Sometimes they are associated with ascites and hydrothorax (Meigs's syndrome). The cause of this phenomenon is obscure, but the accumulation of fluid usually disappears on removal of the fibroma.

B. *Brenner Tumors*. These probably arise from the so-called Walthard cell rests which are found anywhere on the ovaries, the tubes or the surrounding ligaments. Microscopically, Brenner tumors are composed of fibrous tissue in which are situated nests of epithelial cells of a uniform type. Cyst formation is not uncommon.

4. PRIMARY MALIGNANT TUMORS. These tumors of the ovary form the third largest group of malignant tumors in the female genital tract, comprising about 10 per cent of the total. They occur most commonly between the ages of 45 and 65, and more than 50 per cent are bilateral. Malignant tumors make up about 20 per cent of all ovarian tumors. Frequently, they are associated with benign lesions in the same or the other ovary.

Adenocarcinoma and papillary carcinoma are the most common pathologic types. Sarcoma forms from 2 to 5 per cent of the total and is most often of the spindle cell or round cell variety. Teratomata are not uncommon. Among these, various cell types may predominate. In this group the tumor in which thyroid tissue predominates (struma ovarii) is an example of the remarkable potentialities of ovarian tissue.

5. SEX-CELL TUMORS. These may or may not be malignant, and in any case are not common. They consist of:

A. *Functioning Tumors*. These may cause feminization—granulosa cell tumor, thecal cell tumor (thecoma), and lutein cell tumor (luteoma); or masculinization—arrhenoblastoma, hilar cell tumor or adrenal rest tumor.

B. *Nonfunctioning Tumors*. Dysgerminoma is the main example of this group and appears to be composed of undifferentiated sex cells.

6. METASTATIC TUMORS. Metastases to the ovary can occur from tumors of the endometrium, the intestinal tract, the breast and elsewhere in the body. The most noteworthy type is the so-called Krukenberg tumor, of which the primary tumor arises in the stomach or elsewhere in the intestinal tract. In this the ovarian metastases are frequently the most impressive part of the malignancy.

Clinical Features. Simple ovarian cysts and tumors frequently give only minor symptoms. The patient may notice a mass, a sensation of weight and pressure in the pelvis, some bladder irritability, constipation or menstrual disturbance. Feminizing tumors may cause abnormal vaginal bleeding and precocious puberty in the young girl or irregular bleeding in the older woman. Masculinizing tumors may cause defeminization and then masculinization with amenorrhea, breast atrophy, hirsutism, deepening of the voice and development of masculine secondary sexual characteristics. Functioning non-neoplastic cysts may also give some specific symptoms. For example, a corpus luteum cyst may be accompanied by delayed menstruation, while polycystic ovaries, in which the capsules are greatly thickened, resulting in the retention of many follicle cysts, may lead to amenorrhea, sterility and even masculinizing changes such as hirsutism (Stein-Leventhal syndrome). On examination a cystic mass may be palpable in the lower abdomen: this is confirmed on pelvic and rectal examination when a cystic mobile mass which is usually close to the lateral pelvic wall can be felt.

Diagnosis. The diagnosis of an uncomplicated cyst or tumor is often difficult to make from the history and depends on the finding of an adnexal mass on pelvic examination. Occasionally, roentgen study of the abdomen is helpful, particularly in the case of dermoids: sometimes, the intraperitoneal injection of carbon dioxide may be helpful. Hormonal studies of the function of the pituitary (follicle-stimulating hormone), thyroid (protein-bound iodine) or adrenal cortex (17 keto-steroids, pregnanetriol) materially assist in the diagnosis of a functioning tumor. By means of culdoscopy, or possibly laparoscopy, the ovaries can be visualized directly in doubtful cases.

Other conditions which may be confused with ovarian cysts and tumors are: myomata, especially subserous pedunculated myomata, hydrosalpinx, pyosalpinx, tubo-ovarian abscess, endometriosis and extragenital masses, such as tumors of the colon, pelvic kidney and retroperitoneal tumors.

Complications. The following complications of ovarian cysts and tumors occur frequently and are of importance because they change the clinical picture of a simple cyst and add further diagnostic problems.

1. *Size.* Ovarian cysts may grow to an enormous size and then may cause marked abdominal distention with intestinal symptoms and interference with respiration. Large cysts may be confused with a distended bladder, pregnancy, other intra-abdominal tumors and distention due to ascites.

2. *Torsion.* Many cysts and tumors are pedunculated, and the pedicle may become twisted with subsequent interference with the blood supply and necrosis and gangrene of the tumor. The patient may notice sudden or gradual onset of pain, and on examination tenderness over a cystic mass, fever and leukocytosis are commonly found. The clinical picture is very similar to that found in myomata with twisted pedicles, tubo-ovarian abscess or ectopic pregnancy.

3. *Hemorrhage* is common in or from cysts. Occasionally it may be so severe as to cause shock similar to that found with ruptured ectopic pregnancy.

4. *Rupture* may occur spontaneously or as a result of injury or examination. Signs of peritoneal irritation occur similar to those found with any ruptured viscus, although evidence of infection and hemorrhage is usually absent.

5. *Infection* occasionally occurs in ovarian cysts, especially dermoids, either from local ascending infection or from the blood stream.

6. *Malignant Change.* It is frequently impossible to determine whether a given ovarian cyst or tumor is malignant until after careful pathologic study. However, certain symptoms suggest that one is dealing either with a primary malignant tumor or with a tumor that has undergone malignant change. The patient may notice sudden increase in the size of her abdomen: she may have lost weight and give the appearance of generalized chronic disease. Examination may show ascites, a common concomitant of ovarian cancer, and on pelvic examination the ovarian mass may feel solid or may contain soft and firm areas. Bilateral masses may be present, and additional nodules may be felt in the cul-de-sac.

Treatment. At present surgery provides the only satisfactory treatment. Therefore, the problem is, when to operate. As a general rule ovarian cysts or tumors which are causing symptoms or are asymptomatic and have an estimated diameter of over 6 cm. should be removed. In a young woman of under 30 years of age observation of an asymptomatic cyst of this size for 3 or even 6 months is justifiable, since it may disappear spontaneously. In the menopausal or postmenopausal woman the discovery of a cyst even smaller than 6 cm. in diameter, especially if it has not been noted on a previous examination, may be an indication for removal. Aspiration of ovarian cysts through the abdominal wall or the vagina is not advisable. Ovarian masses which are definitely felt to be solid should usually be removed, even if less than 6 cm. in diameter, in the woman who is over 30 years of age; in the younger woman if observation is chosen it should probably last no longer than 6 to 8 weeks.

Frequently, it is extremely difficult to determine at the operating table whether a given ovarian cyst or tumor is benign or malignant. Evidence of ascites, peritoneal metastases, or papillary projections from the wall of the cyst are suggestive of malignancy. A frozen section may be helpful.

If the cyst is clearly benign and the patient is young, the cyst alone should be removed where possible. When cysts are likely to be bilateral, as with dermoids, the opposite ovary should usually be bisected to exclude a small dermoid within it.

Where the diagnosis is in doubt at operation, it is probably best in a younger woman to do the minimum procedure, whereas with an older woman the tumor should be treated as though it were malignant.

OVARIAN CANCER. If the cyst or tumor is clearly malignant, a bilateral salpingo-oophorectomy and total hysterectomy should be performed. Because the lymphatic drainage of the ovary follows the ovarian vessels, pelvic node dissection is of no value. Removal of the greater omentum is usually indicated, since this is a common site of metastases. Care should be taken to avoid rupturing a potentially malignant tumor during removal, since this disseminates malignant cells through the peritoneal cavity. Even if the whole tumor mass cannot be removed, there is some advantage in excising as much as possible. Any peritoneal fluid should be removed and the cells in it studied, so as to determine the need for additional treatment. If there is no intraperitoneal fluid, the peritoneal cavity should be irrigated with saline and the fluid examined for the presence of malignant cells.

A classification of the stages of ovarian cancer has been approved by the International Federation of Gynaecology and Obstetrics. In contrast to those for carcinoma of the cervix and corpus uteri this takes into account operative as well as clinical findings. It is as follows:

Stage I—Growth limited to the ovaries.

Stage Ia—Growth limited to one ovary: no ascites.

Stage Ib—Growth limited to both ovaries: no ascites.

Stage Ic—Growth limited to one or both ovaries: ascites present with malignant cells in the fluid.

Stage II—Growth involving one or both ovaries with pelvic extension.

Stage IIa—Extension and/or metastases to the uterus and/or tubes only.

Stage IIb—Extension to other pelvic tissue.

Stage III—Growth involving one or both ovaries with widespread intraperitoneal metastases to the abdomen (omentum, small intestine and its mesentery).

Stage IV—Growth involving one or both ovaries with distant metastases outside the peritoneal cavity.

Special Category: Unexplored cases which are thought to be ovarian carcinoma (surgery, exploratory or therapeutic, not having been performed). The presence of ascites will not influence the staging for Stages II, III and IV.

Staging of ovarian cancer may be of help in prognosis and in guiding treatment subsequent to operation. If the lesion has been completely removed, if there is no evidence of spread and the peritoneal washings are negative, the patient has the best chance for survival. Although postoperative radiotherapy has been suggested in these cases, it is doubtful whether it is of benefit. Intraperitoneal instillation of radioactive material, such as radioactive gold or radioactive phosphorus, is relatively innocuous and may be of prophylactic value. If the tumor has been completely removed, but some spillage has occurred during operation, or if the peritoneal fluid is doubtful or positive for malignant cells, further treatment is indicated. In this case, again, the intraperitoneal instillation of radioactive materials may be appropriate, since their limit of penetration is only 2 to 3 mm., and they would be most likely to be effective where only a few cancer cells are present. Radiotherapy has some disadvantages, in that it is difficult to administer a cancerocidal dose over a large area of the abdominal cavity without causing considerable radiation reaction. On the other hand, some reports indicate that external radiotherapy given to the lower abdomen alone may be beneficial in these circumstances. If obvious metastases are noted at operation, which are larger than 0.5 cm. in diameter, if the tumor has been incompletely removed or if it has been possible merely to biopsy the lesion, further treatment is likely to be palliative only. The same situation occurs when recurrence is noted after primary therapy. Radiotherapy may offer some temporary relief under these circumstances. Some success has been recently achieved with chemotherapy. Many of the drugs now available have been used with some effect. Alkylating agents appear to be the most helpful. Chlorambucil is at present the drug of choice, since it can be given orally and its toxicity is relatively low. Good palliation was obtained in 44 per cent of 95 patients given chlorambucil by Parker and Shingleton. Thiotepa has also been found effective to a similar degree. When ascites is a problem, intraperitoneal radioactive gold or nitrogen mustard may be effective in controlling it.

The prognosis of cancer of the ovary depends on the type of tumor, the evidence of spread beyond the ovary and upon the histologic grading of malignancy. Specific survival rates are difficult to assess because of the rarity of many ovarian tumors. In the relatively common serous cystadenocarcinoma the over-all figures indicate that from 20 to 40 per cent of patients survive more than 5 years. Long-continued observation is necessary in this disease, since late recurrences may occur.

MENSTRUAL DISORDERS

The Normal Menstrual Cycle

Menstruation may be defined as the periodic discharge of bloody fluid from the uterus, occurring during the reproductive phase of a woman's life.

The mean length of the menstrual cycle, as calculated from the first day of one menstruation to the first day of the next, is about 28 days. Variations from 24 to 35 days are common. Variability is greatest up to age 25, declines to a minimum between ages 35 and 39 and increases again slightly from 40 to 44 (Chiazze et al.).

The usual duration of the flow is from 2 to 7 days. The mean amount of blood lost is reported to be 25 to 50 cc. There is considerable variation between women but some consistency for each woman (Hallberg and Nilsson). It is often difficult both for the woman and her physician to estimate accurately the actual amount of flow.

In the healthy woman the menstrual flow varies at different periods of her life and may be affected by many factors, both physiological and psychological. The latter are of interest. Motherly women tend to menstruate more copiously and/or more frequently than less motherly women. Anxiety and elation can cause increased flow: depression may be accompanied by decreased flow. Sudden emotional shock, such as imprisonment, change in environment or fear of pregnancy, can stop menstruation completely. Frequently, the menstrual cycle can be influenced by hypnosis, simple suggestion, administration of placebos or by superficial psychotherapy (Newton).

The events of the menstrual cycle are governed by a complex hormonal control involving primarily the pituitary and the ovaries. In addition, other endocrine organs such as the thyroid and the adrenal glands as well as nutritional and other factors are concerned with the menstrual cycle. Further details are discussed by Israel. It must be remembered that the evidence for many of the details, such as the exact mechanism of ovulation and of the onset of bleeding, is not complete. Menstruation is also associated with many systemic changes. These involve almost all organs of the body, and are probably related to the basic endocrinologic changes. They are discussed in detail by Southam and Gonzaga.

Menarche

The first menstruation occurs from 10 to 16 years of age (menarche). A regular rhythm is not usually established for several months or years. There is a high proportion of anovulatory cycles at this time, and lowered fertility exists as compared with that 3 or 4 years later.

Menarche is a time of great emotional changes and instability in the adolescent girl. Preparation for and understanding of this by parents and school authorities can make the transition to adulthood easier. Certainly, no attempt should be made to adjust the early irregular cycles with hormones, and detailed investigation should be undertaken only if excessive bleeding occurs. Provided that skeletal growth is occurring and that the child is normal, there should be no great concern about amenorrhea until the age of 16 is reached.

Menopause

Cessation of menstruation (menopause) occurs at about 49 years of age. In the latter part of a woman's reproductive life, anovulatory cycles (lack of progesterone) again become more common. Then estrogen secretion decreases and menstruation ceases. Concurrently there is a rise in pituitary gonadotrophins. As a result of the hormonal changes the secondary sexual characteristics gradually atrophy. The ovary continues to produce some estrogens for a varying time, and some are also produced by the adrenal cortex.

Clinical Features. About 20 per cent of women pass through the menopause with virtually no symptoms, 60 per cent have mild to moderate symptoms and 20 per cent have considerable difficulty. The symptoms are as follows.

Menstrual Alterations. Typically there is a decrease in flow, shorter menstrual periods and a longer cycle. Rarely (1 in 10 women) menstruation stops suddenly. In some women excessive and possibly irregular bleeding may occur.

VASOMOTOR PHENOMENA. The hot flash is the chief cause of distress at the menopause. It is probably due to the hormonal imbalance. Characteristically, the patient experiences a sensation of warmth, often in the shoulders, the neck and the face which is associated with blushing and followed by perspiration. The number and the severity of the flashes varies greatly.

OTHER SYMPTOMS. Varying degrees of nervousness, tension, headache, insomnia and depression may be reported. Libido probably does not change markedly.

Treatment. Although the symptoms are very real to the menopausal patient, they are interwoven with psychosomatic factors. These include feelings of uselessness, boredom or unhappiness. Therefore, an adequate social history is essential in evaluating the menopausal patient. Also of great importance is a thorough study of any menstrual irregularities, particularly if there has been excessive or irregular flow. In addition, if a woman has had a year without menstruation, any bleeding should be regarded as suspicious of malignancy. In these cases appropriate investigation should be undertaken.

Assuming that no organic changes are found, the principles of treatment should include (1) reassurance, (2) encouragement of participation in social and other activities including physical exercise, (3) provision of adequate diet and supplementary vitamins and (4) specific therapy. Mild sedatives may be sufficient. If, however, the patient has marked disability from hot flashes, hormonal substitution therapy is appropriate. The exact indications for the use of hormones, the length of time they should be given and the types to be employed are debated. Some recommend continuous use during and after the menopause on the grounds that this prevents premature osteoporosis and arteriosclerosis. A more cautious view is to give them when symptoms warrant it, since much remains to be learned about their long-term use. Under these circumstances administration until past the time of normal menopause and then gradual reduction of dosage and discontinuation is appropriate: further therapy can be given if symptoms justify it. The best drug is estrogen, given daily in the smallest effective dose. Intermittent therapy (20 days each month) may also be used. Simulation of a regular menstrual cycle, by giving estrogen followed by estrogen and progesterone, is probably not advisable. This, as well as larger doses of estrogen, may give rise to irregular bleeding which will require proper investigation. Any patient taking hormones in this manner should receive regular general and pelvic examinations with at least annual cytologic studies of the cervix and vagina.

PREMENSTRUAL TENSION

Many women suffer from this condition. In few is it severe enough to cause them to seek medical aid. The cause of it is not entirely established, but probably it is due in large part to retention of excess fluid just before menstruation. This causes a sensation of being bloated, nervous irritability and insomnia. In addition, increased emotional instability and decreased aptitude for mechanical and intellectual tasks may be noted at this time. Provided that a thorough gynecologic examination discloses no abnormalities, treatment is essentially symptomatic. It consists of attempts to remove excess water by laxatives and diuretics, dietary advice (especially vitamin B complex) and mild sedatives or tranquilizers. In severe cases temporary suppression of ovulation by oral administration of hormones may be necessary.

DYSMENORRHEA

About 50 per cent of all women have some pain during menstruation, usually on the first day. In perhaps 15 per cent it is severe enough to cause them to go to bed. Clinically, it is convenient to divide the condition into primary dysmenorrhea, which has been present since the menarche, and secondary dysmenorrhea, which develops later in the reproductive life.

Cause. Primary dysmenorrhea probably is chiefly of psychological origin, although cervical stenosis and retroflexion of the uterus are sometimes responsible. Nutritional factors play a part, and the importance of hormones is shown by the fact that anovulatory cycle is usually not accompanied by dysmenorrhea. Secondary dysmenorrhea may be due to many factors, such as myomata, pelvic inflammatory disease and endometriosis.

Diagnosis. Complete pelvic evaluation is important in every case. This should include postmenstrual sounding of the uterus to exclude cervical stenosis.

Treatment. In primary dysmenorrhea, where no organic cause can be demonstrated, simple explanation of the physiology of menstruation, psychological support and symptomatic treatment can be of great value. The last consists of advice regarding nutrition and hygiene, sedatives or tranquilizers, antispasmodics and analgesics. Suppression of ovulation for 2 to 3 months by means of estrogens or a combination of estrogen and progestin is often helpful. Frequently, patience and understanding are required to arrive at a satisfactory plan of treatment. In secondary dysmenorrhea, the treatment of any associated disease is of first importance.

Menstrual Disorders

During the reproductive life any bleeding other than regular menstruation must be considered as abnormal. Occasional women do note a slight amount of vaginal bleeding at the time of ovulation: this may be due to the sudden drop of estrogens at this time and may not be abnormal for that particular woman. In the prepubertal girl and in the postmenopausal woman any bleeding at all is abnormal.

Bleeding abnormalities may be divided into those which occur at the time of menstruation and those which occur between or without regular menstruation. Various symptomatic terms have been applied to the former, such as amenorrhea (absence of menstruation), oligomenorrhea (scanty menstruation), polymenorrhea (frequent menstruation), or hypermenorrhea or menorrhagia (excessive menstrual flow). The latter is known as intermenstrual bleeding, metrorrhagia (bleeding between menstruation), prepubertal bleeding or postmenopausal bleeding.

Causes. The following causes can be applied to most types of menstrual disorder, whether characterized by irregular or excessive bleeding or by amenorrhea:
1. Specific causes
   A. Constitutional causes
      a. Blood dyscrasias
      b. Systemic diseases such as tuberculosis, nephritis
   B. Diseases of the vagina
      a. Trauma
      b. Foreign body
      c. Vaginitis
      d. Tumors, benign and malignant
   C. Diseases of the cervix
      a. Infections and erosions
      b. Polyps
      c. Tumors, benign and malignant
   D. Diseases of the uterus
      a. Infections
      b. Polyps
      c. Adenomyosis
      d. Myoma
      e. Other tumors, benign and malignant
   E. Diseases of the tubes and ovaries
      a. Infections
      b. Ovarian cysts
      c. Ovarian tumors, benign and malignant
   F. Complications of early pregnancy
      a. Ectopic pregnancy
      b. Abortions
      c. Hydatidiform mole and chorioepithelioma
2. General causes
   A. Endocrine factors (congenital or acquired)
      a. Ovarian dysfunction, e.g., ovarian dysgenesis, failure of ovulation
      b. Adrenal cortical dysfunction or tumor
      c. Thyroid disorder
      d. Pituitary dysfunction or tumor
   B. Emotional factors
      a. Anxiety states
      b. Emotional shock
      c. Deeper psychological causes
   C. Nutritional factors

Diagnosis. It is of fundamental importance to discover the cause of the abnormal bleeding before proceeding to treatment, and particularly before performing an exploratory operation which might lead to removal of any pelvic organs.

A thorough history and physical examination as outlined on pages 1534-1535 is essential, particularly in regard to problems of congenital or endocrine origin.

Additional diagnostic measures which are of value are as follows:

1. *Examination under anesthesia* is helpful where the findings on pelvic examination are indeterminate because of the patient's age, resistance or obesity.

2. *Diagnostic curettage* is a relatively simple procedure, requiring dilatation of the cervix under general or, perhaps, local anesthesia (Hegar or Goodell dilators) (Fig. 51-21), scraping the endometrial cavity thoroughly with a blunt or sharp curette, and careful pathologic examination of the tissue obtained. However, it does carry some risk due both to the anesthesia and also to the possibility of perforating the uterus (especially where pregnancy has occurred); it should not be considered too lightly. Curettage should generally be accompanied by appropriate studies of the cervix.

3. *More detailed psychological information,* particularly in regard to emotional shocks or problems which flared up around the time when the menstrual difficulty became manifest.

4. *Endometrial biopsy.* This office procedure can give valuable information on the state of the endometrium. However, it is not usually possible to obtain enough tissue to exclude some intrauterine lesions.

5. *Additional tests of endocrine function.* These include thyroid studies (protein-bound iodine or basal metabolic rate), assays of follicle-stimulating hormone excretion by the pituitary or determination of adrenal function by means of 17-ketosteroids or other studies.

6. *Genetic studies.* In certain instances, especially where congenital abnormalities are suspected, studies of genetic sex by buccal smear or chromosome analysis may be important.

It is often difficult to determine whether extensive investigation should be undertaken for menstrual disorders. Although the use of hormones as a therapeutic trial may give some indication regarding an intrinsic deficiency, the temptation to persist with this method of management should be resisted, since it is particularly important, especially in the woman who is over 35 years of age, to exclude the presence of cancer and also to determine the exact cause of the disorder so that specific treatment can be initiated.

Treatment should be directed to the specific cause of the irregularity if this can be determined. Attention to general nutrition and psychological problems may be of help. Diagnostic curettage itself is sometimes curative. Endocrine therapy by estrogens or progesterone or combinations of both may be of value. Ovulation can be induced in selected cases by clomiphene or human chorionic gonadotrophin. Where adrenal hyperplasia is demonstrated, cortisone or its derivatives may be effective, while the use of thyroid extract, when specifically indicated, may be of help.

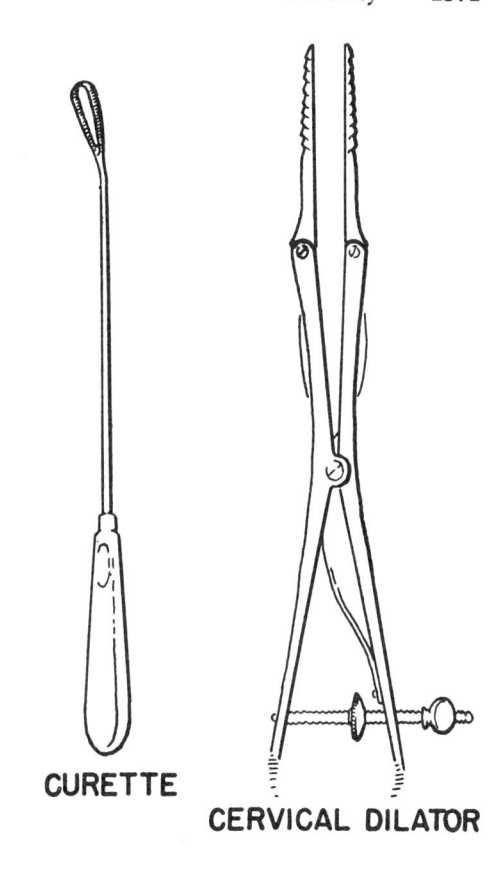

FIG. 51-21. Uterine curette and Goodell cervical dilator.

FERTILITY

Contraception. A problem commonly encountered by the gynecologic surgeon is a request for help in controlling fertility and spacing children. Even if the patient does not raise this question herself it should be part of the regular history taken for every married woman and for many who are unmarried.

The effectiveness of contraception has been greatly increased by the discovery of the oral contraceptives and of the plastic intrauterine devices. However, it is important to be familiar with all methods so that the patient can be given advice most suited to her as an individual.

With each contraceptive technic there are certain disadvantages which contribute significantly to the failure rate, in part because the couple fail to use the method properly or continuously. Thus, the rhythm method (Hartman), either by using a formula such as those of Kraus or Ogino or by abstaining until three days after the midcycle temperature rise, requires a regular menstrual cycle and considerable determination for success. Mechanical and chemical methods such as the condom, diaphragm or vaginal foam or jelly, may interfere with the spontaneity of coitus. The intrauterine devices may be expelled or may cause symptoms such as menorrhagia which necessitate removal. Lastly, the oral contraceptive pills, whether combined or sequential, have to be taken regularly and are contraindicated in the presence or with a history of thromboembolic disease and other conditions.

The provision of adequate contraceptive advice requires a complete pelvic examination and cytologic studies, as well as thorough discussion with the patient. Regular follow-up is essential.

Sterilization. Permanent interruption of fertility may be indicated in certain women. This operation may be done shortly after delivery but may also be advisable in the nonpregnant patient. Since the procedure involves not only the woman but also her husband, proper permission from both must be obtained and legal requirements satisfied. It is appropriate that specific indications for sterilization be developed by the hospital medical staff on the advice of the qualified members of the department of obstetrics and gynecology. They do not usually apply when sterilization is an inevitable concomitant of surgery for specific pelvic disease.

Procedures for sterilization include hysterectomy and tubal ligation. There is little indication for the former unless other conditions are present or tubal ligation has failed. Tubal ligation is most commonly performed by excising a segment of both tubes between catgut ligatures (Pomeroy operation) or by excising segments and burying the proximal ends in the broad ligament (Irving operation). It may be done abdominally or vaginally. Complications are rare. Failures may occur and their incidence is about 1 per cent (Eastman and Prystowsky).

INFERTILITY

Involuntary sterility occurs in about 12 per cent of all marriages in the United States (Weir and Weir). Study of a particular problem involves a consideration of all the possible factors concerned, and the application of a plan of investigation and treatment which includes both husband and wife. When no contraceptives are used, 70 per cent of married couples conceive in 6 months and half of the remainder will conceive within 2 years. Therefore, 1 year without a pregnancy is an appropriate time after which a young couple should seek help. It may be advisable for an older couple to seek help after 6 months of infertile marriage.

Causes

The mechanism of fertilization in humans is still virtually unknown. Recent interest has centered around methods of transport of spermatozoa to the outer third of the tube where fertilization is presumed to take place (Hartman) and with the actual union of the spermatozoon and the ovum. Clinically, certain barriers to conception can be identified, some obvious and some more subtle.

Specific Genitourinary Tract Disorders. Any factor which may prevent the production or transport of the sperm or the ovum or prevent the meeting of the two for fertilization may be a cause of sterility. In the male this means defective spermatogenesis, obstruction of the vas deferens or urethra by trauma or infection, or inability to deposit the sperm in the vagina. In the female this involves deformities of the vagina which may prevent penetration, diseases of the cervix or the uterus, obstruction of the tubes or defective oogenesis.

General Factors. The general health of both partners is important. Debilitating disease in either husband or wife, even such mild infections as a cold, may be a barrier to conception. Nutritional factors also may be important. Recently, it has been established that certain women develop antibodies to their husband's sperm (Franklin and Dukes). When fully elucidated these findings are likely to be of great help in management.

Psychological Factors. Sterile women with no abnormality of the genital tract more frequently suffer from psychosexual disorders, such as failure to have orgasm, lack of sexual feeling or presence of pain during intercourse, as compared with fertile women (Wittkower and Wilson). In this study the sterile women frequently gave histories of ailing, timid, or unsociable childhoods, while as adults the vast majority of such sterile women showed unusual self-centeredness in their relationships with family and acquaintances. Possible psychophysiologic mechanisms are reviewed by Heiman. Impotence in the male and faulty technics of intercourse, each of which may prevent deposition of the semen near the cervix, frequently have psychological origins. Valuable data on coital physiology and relationships have been obtained by Masters and Johnson.

Investigation

The study of sterility should be accomplished within a reasonable period of time. The steps which should be taken are discussed in detail by Davis.

History and Examination. This usually starts with the wife, since it is most often she who comes first to her physician for study. The usual gynecologic history should be taken, and special emphasis should be placed on her general condition, details of her marital and general relationship with her husband and possible psychological factors. This is followed by a general physical examination and a pelvic examination. The husband also should undergo a general physical examination with special attention being paid to the genitalia and to psychological factors. Additional study in both partners should include blood count, urinalysis, chest roentgenogram, serology, tests of thyroid function and nutritional evaluation. The last should include actual calculation of average daily intake of proteins and certain key vitamins and minerals, in comparison with the standards recommended by the National Research Council.

Examination of Sperm. This may be done by a semen analysis or by the Huhner (postcoital) test. Semen analysis is done best on a specimen produced by masturbation into an open-mouthed bottle. Analysis should include estimation of volume (normal—2.5 to 5 ml.), motility (60-70% immediately and 25-40% after 6 to 8 hours at room temperature), cell count (more than 60 million per ml.), and morphology (80% or more of normal forms). Since masturbation is distasteful to some men on religious or other grounds, the Huhner test may be used as a substitute for this. It does not give a true picture of the sperm count. However, if the mucus taken from inside the cervical canal within 6 hours after coitus contains 5 to 20 spermatozoa per high-power field with 50 per cent motility and few abnormal forms when examined microscopically, the husband is likely to be fertile. Additional information given by the postcoital test is that if active spermatozoa are seen there may be assumed to be no obvious hostility of the cervical mucus to the sperm.

Determination of Ovulation. Apart from the rather indefinite symptom of pain felt by some women at this time, ovulation can be detected only by indirect methods. These depend on the presence of a functioning corpus luteum and include: (1) absence of the "ferning" pattern when cervical mucus is spread on a slide, allowed to dry and examined microscopically; (2) decrease in the number of cornified cells seen in a cervical or vaginal smear; (3) a rise in the basal body temperature (see Fig. 51-22); and (4) the finding of secretory endometrium in an endometrial biopsy taken just before or preferably immediately after the onset of menstruation.

Tests of Tubal Patency. This may be determined by insufflation of CO_2 (Rubin test) or by hysterosalpingography. The Rubin test is performed as an office procedure, within a week after the end of menstruation. Any one of various apparatuses may be used, and the test is safe if performed with care. If the Rubin test is equivocal or if it shows closed tubes, then hysterosalpingography should be performed. In addition to showing the site of any obstruction of the tubes, this test may also reveal any congenital abnormalities within the uterine cavity which might be acting as a barrier to fertility.

Special Endocrinologic Tests. These may be required at a later date to determine endocrine function in both partners.

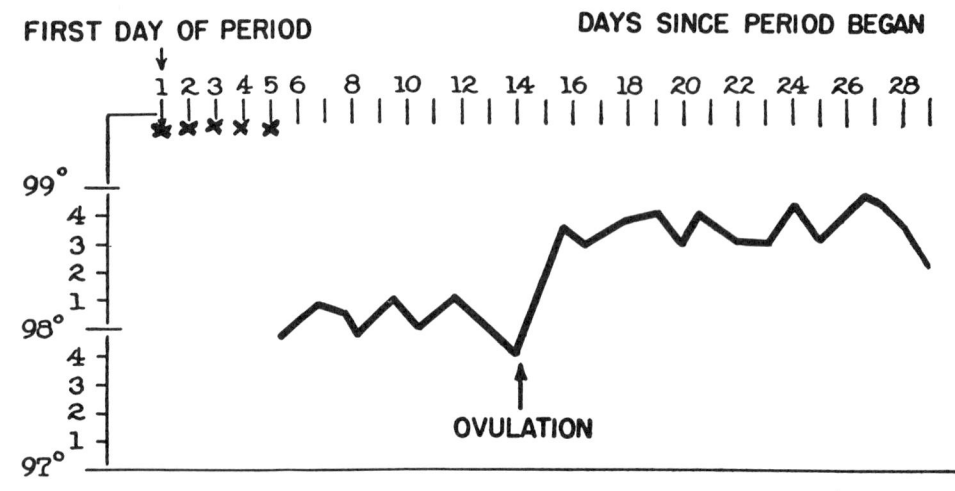

FIG. 51-22. Basal temperature chart showing postovulatory temperature rise.

TREATMENT

General Treatment. The high spontaneous cure rate in sterility has been emphasized by Bender. Of 700 sterile couples studied at Liverpool, England, from 1934 to 1949, pregnancy occurred in 46.3 per cent. In only half of these was it possible to ascribe conception to medical treatment, the remainder being due to time and chance. This emphasizes the fact that discussion of the problem and the progress of investigation with both husband and wife is the first step in treatment. This should be combined with simple explanations about the mechanism of intercourse, conception and timing of intercourse, and detailed nutritional advice.

Specific Treatment for Husband. Oligospermia or azoospermia may be extremely difficult to treat, and the husband should be referred to a competent urologist. Even when the sperm count is very low the couple should not be discouraged. In Bender's series 33 per cent of wives whose husbands had a sperm count of under 10 million conceived.

Specific Treatment for Wife. Conditions which can be managed conservatively should be handled first. These include infections of the lower genital tract, diseases of the cervix, and minor disorders of the upper genital tract. Anovulation may be treated as described above for menstrual disorders. Major surgical procedures such as myomectomy and plastic reconstruction of the tubes should be adopted only as a last resort, if it seems that nothing else will help the couple. The best that can be expected with salpingoplasty is about 20 per cent success as measured by subsequent pregnancy. Tubal patency is obtained in a larger number of cases.

Later Management. If, after adequate investigation has been completed, no specific causes for a couple's sterility have been found, the patients should be informed of this. Either no further treatment is advisable—and the couple has a certain statistical chance of achieving a pregnancy under these circumstances—or the possibilities of artificial insemination by the husband or a donor may be considered. Finally, adoption may be suggested through an appropriate adoption agency.

ENDOMETRIOSIS

Endometriosis is a disease produced by the growth of ectopic islands of endometrial glands and/or stroma. It may be divided into internal and external types. In the former, which is commonly termed adenomyosis, the islands are found in the myometrium; in the latter they appear on ovaries, tubes, uterine ligaments, cervix, peritoneum and even as far away from the uterine cavity as umbilicus, appendix, intestine, vagina and vulva. Distant locations such as the lungs and the skin of the arm and the thigh have been reported.

Endometriosis occurs during the reproductive life, between the ages of 25 and 45, and

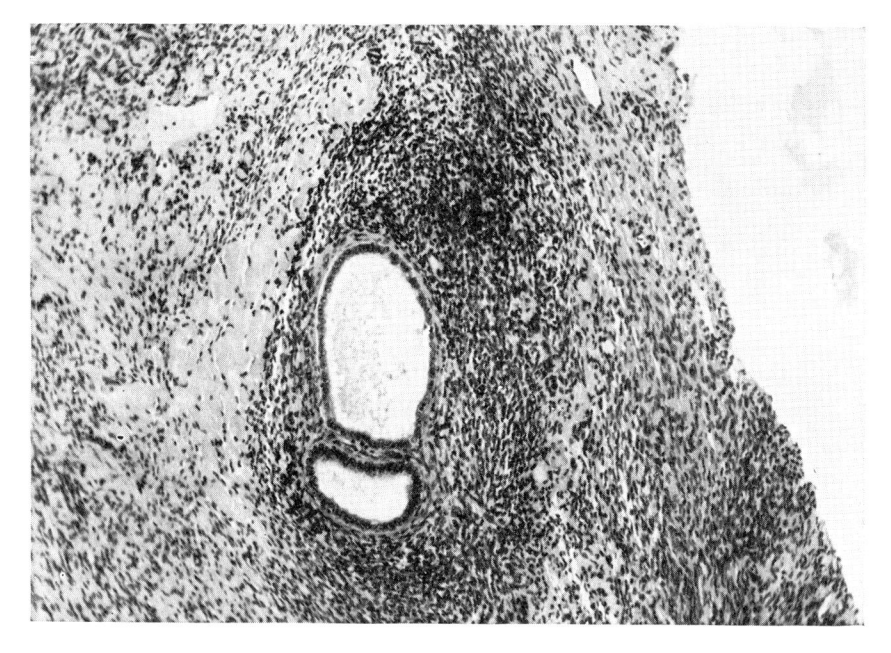

FIG. 51-23. Endometriosis of the ovary.

rarely in the postmenopausal woman. It is more frequent among the higher socioeconomic groups and in white rather than Negro patients.

CAUSE

The exact cause of endometriosis has not been determined. Three main theories have been used to explain the ectopic location of the endometrial tissue: (1) transtubal regurgitation of menstrual blood and endometrial particles, (2) lymphatic dissemination and (3) metaplasia of embryonic celomic epithelium. There is little concrete evidence to support the third theory. The first, which was advanced originally by Sampson in 1921, has received recent support from the work of Scott *et al.*, and Allen *et al.* These investigators have produced experimental endometriosis in monkeys by causing the menstrual flow to be directed into the peritoneal cavity. The idea of lymphatic dissemination has received some support from the finding of endometriosis in a considerable proportion of pelvic nodes removed during the course of radical pelvic surgery (Javert). Sampson's theory is the most attractive but does not explain all cases, and it may be that more than one mechanism is responsible. Hormonal and psychological factors have also been implicated, but it is uncertain how they act.

PATHOLOGIC FEATURES

The ectopic endometrial tissue undergoes cyclical changes, as does normal endometrium. Blood-filled (chocolate) cysts may form, or the tissue may rupture into the surrounding peritoneum or other tissues, resulting in acute symptoms or in the formation of adhesions, which may be particularly dense (Fig. 51-23).

CLINICAL FEATURES

Internal endometriosis usually produces secondary and increasing dysmenorrhea with menstrual irregularities. On examination the uterus may be found to be symmetrically enlarged, firm and especially tender during the premenstrual and menstrual phases of the cycle.

External endometriosis is commonly associated with internal endometriosis but may exist by itself. In addition to the symptoms of internal endometriosis the patient may complain of persistent backache, especially premenstrually but also throughout the cycle. Dyspareunia is common. Sterility may result from blockage of the tubes and from pelvic adhesions. Examination will commonly show the uterus to be retroflexed and fixed. Nodules may be palpable on the uterosacral ligaments or elsewhere in the pelvis. The ovaries may be enlarged and tender. Involvement of the intestine may rarely give rise to symptoms and signs of intestinal obstruction. Thus endometriosis should be considered in the differential diagnosis of carcinoma of the colon and the rectum and of diverticulitis.

Diagnosis

Examination in the premenstrual phase of the cycle is important, since enlargement of the endometrial nodules usually occurs premenstrually. Chronic pelvic inflammatory disease with pelvic adhesions is the most common source of confusion in diagnosis. Ovarian cysts due to endometriosis have to be distinguished from other ovarian cysts and tumors; the latter are frequently not tender. Culdoscopy may be very useful.

Treatment

It must be remembered that endometriosis is practically always a disease of the childbearing age. Many patients are anxious to have children. Therefore, whenever possible, attempts should be made to preserve this function. Treatment may be divided into: (1) no treatment, (2) endocrine and symptomatic treatment, (3) conservative operation and (4) radical operation.

In some cases endometriosis may be discovered on routine examination and may be symptomless. No treatment is advisable in such instances, but repeated regular examinations are essential.

Where symptoms are mild, and no cysts large enough to necessitate laparotomy are found, conservative treatment should be tried. Symptomatic relief of dysmenorrhea may be offered by any one of a number of measures, such as analgesics, mild sedation, diuretics, attention to diet, and local application of heat to the abdomen. Both male and female hormones have been used with success. In part the action of both appears to be by the suppression of ovulation, although particularly with androgens smaller doses than would be required normally for this may cause symptomatic relief. Recently, the effective use of drugs containing an estrogen and a progestin, which presumably produce their effect by inhibiting ovulation, has been reported. These may be given cyclically or continuously: in the latter instance increasing dosage is required to prevent breakthrough bleeding; treatment should be continued for 9 to 12 months. The side effects of these drugs make these regimens difficult for the patient to follow.

If conservative therapy does not help, or if the patient has an ovarian mass of significant size, laparotomy should be performed. In a young woman who is anxious to have children, only as much tissue as is necessary should be removed. This frequently consists of removing the cyst, or one tube and ovary, and cauterizing or excising any endometrial implants which may be found. Adhesions are freed, and suspension of a retrodisplaced uterus is advisable. Division of the pelvic nerves at the brim of the pelvis can also be performed to relieve menstrual distress and backache. The use of a progestin before and after operation may be advisable.

Radical operation consists of bilateral salpingo-oophorectomy and total hysterectomy. It should be reserved for older women who have had a conservative surgical procedure done or have no desire for more children, or rarely for those younger women in whom it is impossible to save any pelvic organ because of extensive involvement and adhesions.

ECTOPIC PREGNANCY

This is a most important condition, since it is potentially a major threat to the patient's life and because it can be confused with many other gynecologic disorders. The exact incidence of ectopic pregnancy is difficult to determine, since many cases may go unrecognized. Its most common site is in the tube, but it may occur on the ovary, the cervix, the uterine ligaments or in the abdominal cavity (Fig. 51-24).

Cause

The mechanism by which the fertilized ovum implants in the tube rather than the uterus is uncertain. Iffy suggests that conception may occur from an ovulation in the latter part of the menstrual cycle and that the products of conception are swept into the tube by retrograde menstrual flow. However this may be, conditions which cause partial blockage of the tube may predispose to tubal pregnancy. Such are pelvic inflammatory disease, and adhesions or tumors arising within or outside the tubal lumen. Patients with sterility problems due to tubal factors are more likely to have tubal pregnancies (1.7%, Bender).

Pathologic Features

Tubal pregnancies may be located in the lateral part of the tube (ampullar), middle (isthmial) or medial part (interstitial). Very few ectopic pregnancies reach full development, although these have been reported. They may either rupture or undergo spontaneous degeneration. Rupture may occur into the peritoneal cavity or into the uterus. Occasionally, rupture and secondary implantation on another abdominal organ may occur. Rupture occurs later with the ampullar type and is usually earlier and attended with greater hemorrhage in the interstitial type.

Clinical Features

In a typical case the patient presents the symptoms of early pregnancy; e.g., amenorrhea, breast fullness, frequency of urination, constipation, nausea. She may also notice some slight vaginal bleeding and lower abdominal pain which is persistent and unilateral. On examination the cervix may be blue and the uterus soft and enlarged, although perhaps not to the degree expected from the length of amenorrhea. An acutely tender adnexal mass is noted.

Rupture into the uterus gives moderate to marked vaginal bleeding and intermittent lower abdominal and back pain. The picture is similar to that of abortion of an intra-uterine pregnancy.

Rupture into the peritoneal cavity causes sudden lower abdominal pain which soon becomes generalized and may spread to the shoulder. Examination may show evidence of shock with a low blood pressure and a weak and rapid pulse. The abdomen may be tender and present generalized rebound tenderness and rigidity with diminished or absent peristalsis. Pelvic examination is often difficult because of the abdominal tenderness, but an adnexal mass may be felt, and a semisolid hematoma may be palpable in the cul-de-sac.

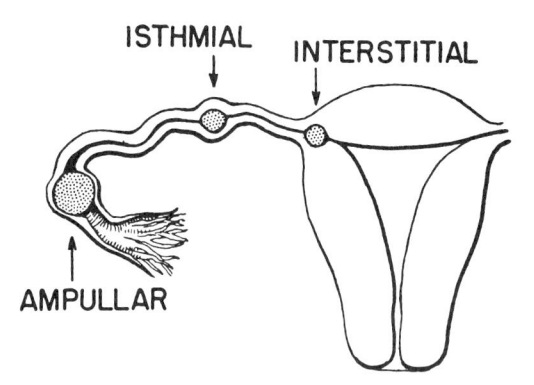

Fig. 51-24. Sites of tubal pregnancies.

Spontaneous degeneration may cause little except a regression of the previous symptoms and signs.

Diagnosis

The typical picture of either unruptured or ruptured ectopic pregnancy is relatively clearcut. Unfortunately, not all cases are typical. In an unruptured ectopic pregnancy, a pregnancy test may be of help, and culdoscopy, in the hands of those experienced in its use, may be of considerable value. Conditions to be considered in the differential diagnosis include:

1. Intra-uterine pregnancy with a large corpus luteum
2. Abortion
3. Pelvic inflammation with a hydrosalpinx or pyosalpinx or tubo-ovarian abscess
4. Myoma
5. Ovarian cyst or tumor

For the characteristic symptoms and signs of these conditions the reader is referred to the specific sections above.

In a ruptured ectopic pregnancy, culdocentesis is a valuable diagnostic procedure. The posterior cul-de-sac is punctured with a 15 to 18 gauge needle attached to a syringe. Aspiration of nonclotting blood indicates intraperitoneal hemorrhage and, when associated with appropriate symptoms and signs, is strongly suggestive of ruptured ectopic pregnancy. Other intra-abdominal emergencies may be confused with ruptured ectopic pregnancy. These include ruptured ovarian cyst or pelvic abscess, ruptured appendix or perforated ulcer.

TREATMENT

Since the danger of rupture is ever-present, there is no place for expectant treatment. Once the diagnosis of ectopic pregnancy has been established the patient should be operated upon promptly. If shock is present, blood transfusion should be started as soon as possible, but it is not wise to wait until shock has been controlled completely before starting the operation because that time may never come, and control of the hemorrhage is vital. It is of the utmost importance to have suitable blood available for transfusion and preferably running by the time the operation is begun.

The simplest operative procedure necessary to control the bleeding and remove the pregnancy should be done. This usually involves removal of the tube, with, if possible, preservation of the ovary. A wedge of the uterine horn should be removed to prevent the chance of a subsequent pregnancy developing in the remnant of the tube. Reconstruction of the involved tube is generally not advisable, since pregnancy can occur in the other tube. However, it may be attempted when one tube has already been removed or is occluded, and the patient is very anxious to become pregnant. The area should be reperitonealized as well as possible, and excess blood removed from the peritoneal cavity.

In the rare instance where an advanced abdominal pregnancy has occurred, it may be well to wait until the infant is viable before performing laparotomy, since living children have been obtained by this procedure. If the placenta can be removed easily, this should be done. However, it may be adherent to many organs and, in this case, should be left in situ, since catastrophic bleeding may occur during attempts at removal. If the placenta is left in place, it may eventually be absorbed. Equally likely is the persistence of a mass, often cystic, for which a secondary operation may be required.

BIBLIOGRAPHY

Allen, E., Peterson, L. F., and Campbell, Z. B.: Clinical and experimental endometriosis. Am. J. Obstet. Gynec., 68:56, 1954.

Bender, S.: End results in primary sterility. Brit. Med. J., 2:409, 1952.

Bolten, K. A.: Introduction to Colposcopy. New York, Grune & Stratton, 1960.

Bushnell, L. F.: Physiologic prevention of postpartal relaxation of genital muscles. West. J. Surg., 58:66, 1950.

Chiazze, L., Jr., Brayer, F. T., Macisco, J. J., Jr., Parker, M. P., and Duffy, B. J.: The length and variability of the human menstrual cycle. J.A.M.A., 203:377, 1968.

Davis, M. E.: Management of infertility. J.A.M.A., 201:1030, 1967.

Donald, I.: Etiology and investigation of vaginal discharge. Brit. Med. J., 2:1223, 1952.

Evans, T. N.: The artificial vagina. Am. J. Obstet. Gynecol., 99:944, 1967.

Falk, H. C., and Bunkin, I. A.: The management of vesicovaginal fistula following abdominal total hysterectomy. Surg., Gynec., Obstet., 93:404, 1951.

Farrar, H. K., Jr., and Nedoss, B. R.: Benign tumors of the uterine cervix. Am J. Obstet. Gynec., 81:124, 1961.

Fidler, H. K., Boyes, D. A., and Wort, A. J.: Cervical cancer detection in British Columbia: A progress report. J. Obstet. Gynaec. Brit. Comm., 75:392, 1968.

Franklin, R. R., and Dukes, C. D.: Antispermatozoal antibody and unexplained infertility. Am. J. Obstet. Gynec., 89:6, 1964.

Graham, J. B., and Paloucek, F. P.: Where should cancer of the cervix be treated? Am. J. Obstet. Gynec., 87:405, 1963.

Green, T. H., Jr.: The problem of urinary stress incontinence in the female. Obstet. Gynec. Survey, 23:603, 1968.

Green, T. H., Jr., Ulfelder, H., and Meigs, J. V.: Epidermoid carcinoma of the vulva: an analysis of 238 cases. Am. J. Obstet. Gynec., 75:834, 1958.

Greenhill, J. P.: Office Gynecology. ed. 8. Chicago, Year Book Publishers, 1965.

Gusberg, S. B.: The problem of staging endometrial cancer. Obstet. Gynec., 28:305, 1966.

Hallberg, L., and Nilsson, L.: Constancy of individual menstrual blood loss. Acta. obstet. gynec. scand., 43:352, 1965.

Hartman, C. G.: Science and the Safe Period. Baltimore, Williams & Wilkins, 1962.

———: How do sperms get into the uterus? Fertil. Steril., 8:403, 1957.

Heiman, M.: Reproduction: emotions and the hypothalamic-pituitary function. Fertil. Steril., 10:162, 1959.

Iffy, L.: The role of premenstrual, post-mid-cycle conception in the aetiology of ectopic gestation. J. Obst. Gynaec. Brit. Comm., 70:966, 1963.

Israel, S. L.: Diagnosis and Treatment of Menstrual Disorders and Sterility. ed. 5. New York, Paul B. Hoeber, 1967.

Javert, C. T.: The spread of benign and malignant endometrium in the lymphatic system with a note on coexisting vascular involvement. Am. J. Obstet. Gynec., 64:780, 1952.

Javert, C. T., and Douglas, R. G.: Treatment of endometrial adenocarcinoma. Am. J. Roentgenol., 75:508, 1956.

Jeffcoate, T. N. A., and Woodcock, A. S.: Premalignant conditions of the vulva, with particular reference to chronic epithelial dystrophies. Brit. Med. J., 2:127, 1961.

Kegel, A. H.: Physiologic therapy for urinary stress incontinence. J.A.M.A., 146:915, 1951.

Kimbrough, R. A.: An evaluation of treatment of invasive cervical carcinoma. Obstet. Gynec., 20: 901, 1962.

Kiselow, M., Butcher, H. M., Jr., and Bricker, E. M.: Results of the radical surgical treatment of advanced pelvic cancer. Ann. Surg., 166:428, 1968.

Krupp, P. J., Sternberg, W. H., Clark, W. H., St. Romain, M. J., Jr., and Smith, R. C.: Malignant mixed müllerian neoplasms (mixed mesodermal tumors). Am. J. Obstet. Gynec., 81:959, 1961.

Lardaro, H. H.: Spontaneous rupture of tubo-ovarial abscess into the free peritoneal cavity. J.A.M.A., 156:699, 1954.

Latourette, H. B., and Lourie, W.: End results of treatment of cancer of the vagina. Ann. N.Y. Acad. Sci., 114:1020, 1964.

Masters, W. H., and Johnson, V. E.: Human Sexual Response. Boston, Little, Brown & Co., 1965.

McCall, M. L.: Posterior culdeplasty. Obstet. Gynec., 10:595, 1957.

Mering, J. H.: A surgical approach to intractable pruritus vulvae. Am. J. Obstet. Gynec., 64:619, 1952.

Moir, J. C.: The Vesico-vaginal Fistula. ed. 2. London, Bailliere, Tindall and Cassell, 1967.

Morton, D. G., Lagasse, L. D., Moore, J. G., Jacobs, M., and Amromin, G. D.: Pelvice lymphnodectomy following radiation in cervical carcinoma. Am. J. Obstet. Gynec., 88:932, 1964.

Nemir, A., and Middleton, R. P.: Stress incontinence in young nulliparous women. Am. J. Obstet. Gynec., 68:1166, 1954.

Newton, M., and Bolten, K. A.: Carcinoma of the cervix: diagnosis and evaluation. J. Mississippi M. A., 2:239, 1961.

Newton, M., Hickman, B. T., and Bolten, K. A.: Carcinoma of the cervix: treatment and follow-up. J. Mississippi M. A., 2:279, 1961.

———: Radical hysterectomy versus radiotherapy in Stage I cervical cancer: preliminary results. Obstet. Gynec., 24:563, 1964.

Newton, N.: Maternal Emotions. New York, Paul B. Hoeber, 1955.

Parker, R. T., and Shingleton, W. W.: Chemotherapy in genital cancer: systemic therapy and regional perfusion. Am. J. Obstet. Gynec., 83:981, 1962.

Parker, R. T., Wilbanks, G. D., Yowell, R. K., and Carter, F. B.: Radical hysterectomy and pelvic lymphadenectomy with and without preoperative radiotherapy for cervical cancer. J. Obstet. Gynec., 99:933, 1967.

Peterson, W. F., Prevost, E. C., Edmunds, F. T., Hundley, J. M., Jr., and Morris, F. K.: Benign cystic teratomas of the ovary—a clinico-statistical study of 1,007 cases with a review of the literature. Am. J. Obstet. Gynec., 70:368, 1955.

Prystowsky, H., and Eastman, N. J.: Puerperal tubal sterilization: report of 1830 cases. J.A.M.A., 158: 463, 1955.

Reich, W. J., and Nechtow, M. J.: A ten year study of treatment and its results in intractable pruritus vulvae. Am. J. Obstet. Gynec., 69:94, 1955.

Rickford, R. B. K.: Involvement of pelvic lymph nodes in carcinoma of the endometrium. J. Obstet. Gynaec. Brit. Comm., 75:580, 1968.

Rutledge, F.: Cancer of the vagina. Am. J. Obstet. Gynec., 97:635, 1967

Schauffler, G. C.: Pediatric Gynecology. ed. 4. Chicago, Year Book Publishers. 1958.

Scott, R. B., Te Linde, R. W., and Wharton, L. R.: Further studies on experimental endometriosis, Am. J. Obstet. Gynec., 66:1082, 1953.

Semmens, J. P.: Congenital anomalies of the female genital tract. Obstet. Gynec., 19:328, 1962.

Southam, A. L., and Gonzaga, F. P.: Systemic changes during the menstrual cycle. Am. J. Obstet. Gynec., 91:142, 1965.

Strassman, E. O.: Plastic unification of double uterus. Am. J. Obstet. Gynec., 64:25, 1952.

Te Linde, R. W.: Prolapse of the uterus and allied conditions. Am. J. Obstet. Gynec., 94:444, 1966.

Way, S.: Carcinoma of the vulva. Am. J. Obstet. Gynec., 79:692, 1960.

Weir, W. C., and Weir, D. R.: The natural history of infertility. Fertil. Steril., 12:443, 1961.

Wittkower, E., and Wilson, A. T. M.: Dysmenorrhea and sterility. Personality studies. Brit. Med. J., 2:586, 1940.

Wynder, E. L., Cornfield, J., Schroff, P. D., and Doraiswami, K. R.: A study of environmental factors in carcinoma of the cervix. Am. J. Obstet. Gynec., 68:1016, 1954.

Wynder, E. L., Escher, G. C., and Mantel, N.: An epidemiological investigation of cancer of the endometrium. Cancer, 19:489, 1966.

Yagi, H.: Extended abdominal hysterectomy with pelvic lymphadenectomy for carcinoma of the cervix. Am. J. Obstet. Gynec., 69:33, 1955.

CHAPTER 52

J. LAPIDES, M.D. AND KARL F. SCHROEDER, M.D.

Urology

Introduction
Renal Physiology
Diuretics
Renal Function Tests
Renal Function in Disease
Acute Renal Failure
Chronic Renal Failure
Hypertension
Obstructive Urinary Tract Disease
Urinary Tract Infections
Neoplasms of the Genitourinary Tract
Calculous Disease
Traumatic Lesions
Physiology of Urinary Transport and Micturition
Congenital Anomalies

INTRODUCTION

Urology is that branch of surgery which concerns itself with the male and the female urinary tracts and the male genital organs. Therefore, the urologist deals with the following: kidney, ureter, bladder, urethra, penis, scrotum, epididymis, testis, spermatic cord, seminal vesicle and prostate, and occasionally with abnormalities of the adrenal gland.

Diagnosis

Endoscopy. Urologic diagnosis is precise because methods are available for viewing the entire urinary tract directly or indirectly. The urethra, the lumen of the bladder and ureteral orifices may be viewed through instruments embodying illumination and lens systems. Through such an instrument, the cystoscope, tissue may be taken for biopsy, catheters may be passed into the ureters, and ureteral or vesical calculi may be removed. The cystoscope cannot be used for viewing the urethra because its lens system affords only right-angle vision. However, the use of the panendoscope, which provides for seeing things ahead and to the side of it (for oblique vision) permits visualization of the urethra.

Roentgenography[2, 3, 6] is requisite to determine the condition of the ureters and the kidneys. A radiopaque material (various iodine compounds such as Cystokon, Diodrast, sodium iodide and Neo-Iopax) is used to fill the hollow portion of the urinary tract, and then roentgenograms are taken. The ureters, the renal pelves and the calyces can be filled by injecting opaque material through ureteral catheters which have been passed up the ureters into the renal pelves. This type of urography has been designated *retrograde pyelography* (Fig. 52-1). Another form, *intravenous pyelography*, involves the intravenous administration of radiopaque material which is cleared from the blood stream by renal excretion. If renal function is 25 per cent or more of normal, the kidneys will excrete enough radiopaque medium (e.g., Diodrast) per unit of time to outline the upper urinary tract (Fig. 52-2). This not only serves to visualize the urinary tract but also gives a gross estimation of renal function. However, extremely high concentrations of radiopaque material, such as 90 per cent Hypaque, may outline the urinary tract when renal function is less than 25 per cent of normal. Contrast material administered in a large volume of fluid by means of a fast intravenous drip may help visualize kidneys with extremely poor function.[14]

Nephrotomography utilizes the special radiologic technic of laminography.[5] The x-ray source and the cassette are moved in opposite directions, spatially creating a focal plane. The structures that are on this plane are seen clearly, but those structures that are not on the plane are excluded by blurring. In this

FIG. 52-1. Retrograde pyelogram, demonstrating calyces, infundibula, pelves and ureters of both kidneys. Observe the ureteral catheters through which radiopaque sodium iodide has been injected.

technic the renal parenchyma is rendered of greater radiodensity than the surrounding structures by the infusion of excretory pyelographic contrast media before and during the exposures. The renal outlines can be seen with greater clarity, and on occasion this technic allows for the differentiation of hollow and solid expanding lesions.

Angiography during the past several years has been developed to such a degree that it now is being used extensively as an aid in the diagnosis of renal hypertension (Fig. 52-3), renal neoplasms, renal cysts, arteriovenous fistulas of the kidney, renal aneurysms, acute renal trauma and acute occlusion of the kidney artery. The Seldinger technic[15] involves introducing a radiopaque polyethylene catheter percutaneously into the femoral artery and, by means of image intensification, guiding the

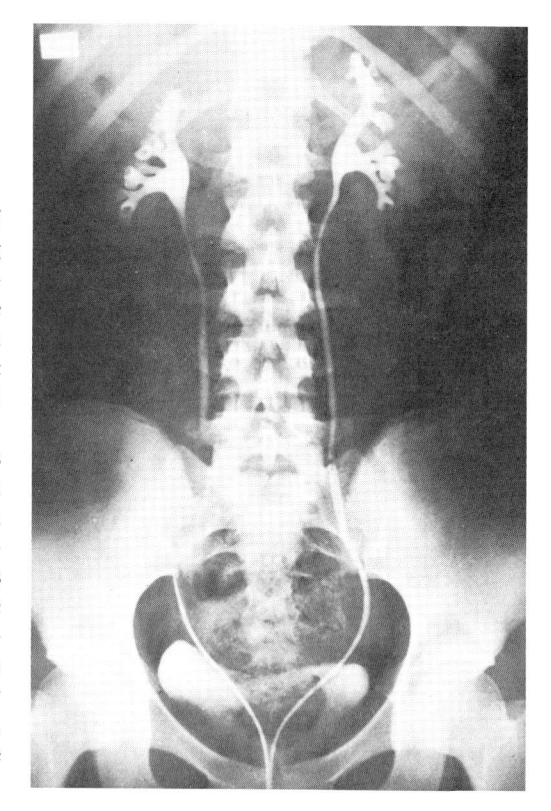

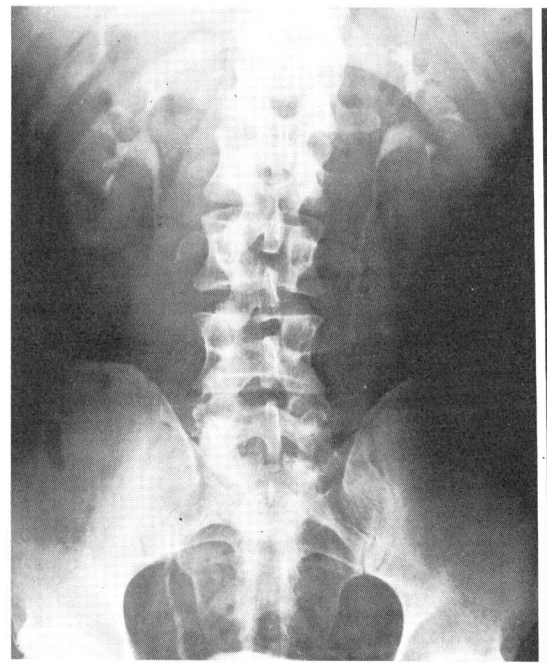

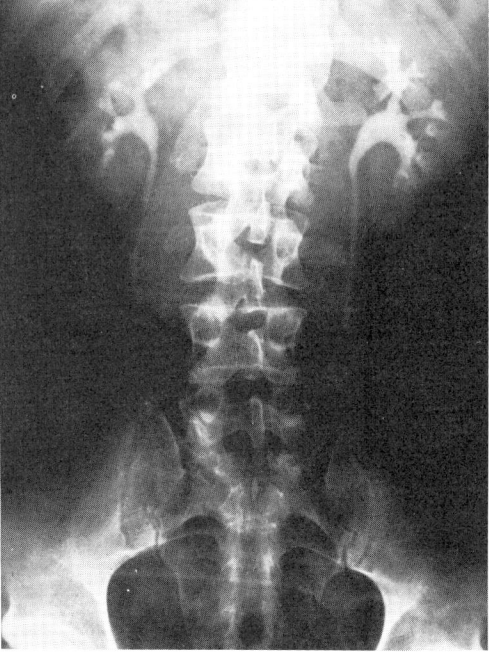

FIG. 52-2. Intravenous or excretory pyelograms made by administering radiopaque material intravenously and then obtaining roentgenograms of the kidneys, the ureters and the bladder after the material has been excreted by the nephrons into the collecting system.

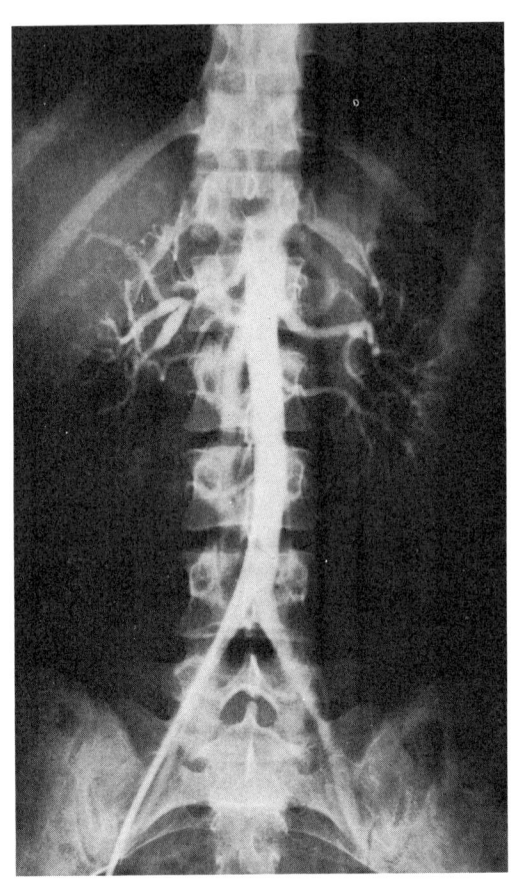

FIG. 52-3. Arteriogram depicting the renal arteries and their branches in addition to the aorta, the splenic, the hepatic, the mesenteric and the iliac vessels. Observe the stenosis of the right renal artery and the poststenotic dilation of its two main branches.

catheter up the aorta into the artery desired. Radiographs are made by injecting small amounts of contrast material. Recently, venous angiography has been employed to localize adenomas of the adrenal gland in patients with primary aldosteronism.[11] Presacral or perirenal gas insufflation (Fig. 52-4) is employed in detecting adrenal and renal neoplasms. Unlike perirenal air insufflation, which occasionally causes air embolus, carbon dioxide is safe.[1] Acute renal failure, transverse myelitis, infarction of the bowel and aortic dissection may follow aortography in rare instances.[7] Persistent renal functional impairment also may follow aortography.

None of the special methods for investigation of the urinary tract is used until a medical history, a physical examination and urinalysis have been completed and evaluated.

SIGNS AND SYMPTOMS

Changes in Micturition. When eliciting symptoms and signs referable to the genitourinary tract, special attention is paid to the act of micturition, the gross characteristics of the urine, masses in the flank, the abdomen and the scrotum, and pain. Normal urination is a painless function which occurs 3 to 4 times daily and occasionally once at night. The normal individual can inhibit micturition until a suitable time and place are available. On volition, a forceful urinary stream is initiable within 1 to 2 seconds; normally, the stream is continuous and uninterrupted until the bladder is emptied.

Increased frequency of urination, urgency

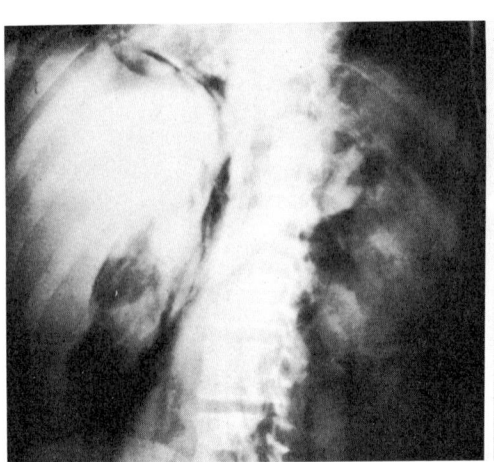

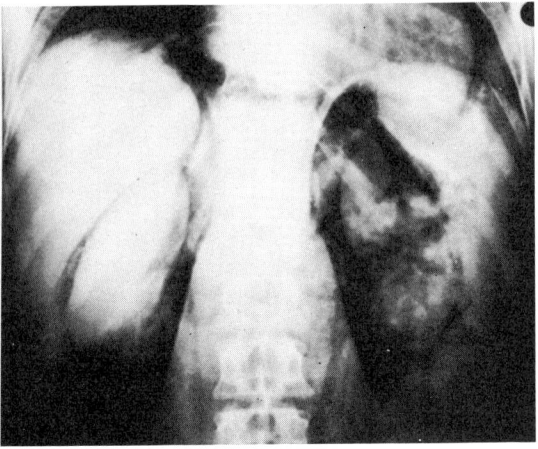

FIG. 52-4. Retroperitoneal pneumogram.

(inability to hold urine after the sensation of bladder filling is initiated) and dysuria (painful or difficult urination) are to be observed in such conditions as inflammatory cystitis, vesical calculi, renal tuberculosis, prostatism, urethral stricture, etc. Hesitancy in starting urination, a decrease in size and force of the urinary stream, abdominal straining and an interrupted stream should lead the physician to suspect an obstruction of the urethral channel by scar tissue contraction at the vesical neck, an enlarged prostate or a stricture of the urethra, although such symptoms may be psychic in origin. Urinary incontinence is abnormal except in infancy and early childhood.[9] Incontinence associated with urgency and frequency, occurring at intervals during the day and especially at night, may be a manifestation of disease involving the central nervous system, e.g., multiple sclerosis, cerebrovascular accidents, or spinal cord tumor. In the female the involuntary loss of urine when coughing, straining or sneezing is suggestive of stretching or tearing of the ligaments holding the bladder neck in place; this condition is called stress incontinence. The continuous involuntary dribbling of urine may be associated with urinary retention of the overflow type, sometimes called paradoxical incontinence because although the patient is continually losing urine, he still has a bladder distended with urine. The continuous leaking of urine also may be associated with an empty bladder in persons who have suffered injury to the sphincter mechanisms following prostatectomy or trauma.

Hematuria is a danger signal and indicates the likely presence of cancer of the genitourinary tract. Hematuria may be associated also with renal tuberculosis, urinary tract calculi, prostatism, acute cystitis and trauma. Far too many patients with cancer of the urinary tract are seen belatedly by the urologist because the importance of hematuria is not recognized by the physician who first sees the individual. Only one episode of gross hematuria is sufficient to demand a complete investigation of the urinary tract and this must include an endoscopic examination of the entire urethra and the bladder, as well as a roentgenographic examination of the ureters and the kidneys. From 2 to 3 red blood cells observed in the urine of a patient on more than one occasion is as much of a danger signal as gross hematuria.

Pneumaturia, or air in the urine is associated with entero-urinary tract fistulae and very rarely with infections caused by *B. aerogenes, E. coli* and certain yeasts, the latter especially in diabetes. Fecaluria associated with pneumaturia is pathognomonic of a connection between the intestinal and the urinary systems.

Pain. Diseases of the kidney may cause characteristic pain or they may give rise solely to a discomfort or pain suggestive of disease in some other organ. Typical renal colic originates in the flank and may radiate anteriorly to the epigastrium; it is an intermittent, sharp, excruciating type of pain often associated with nausea, vomiting and hypotension. Nonobstructive calculous disease of the kidney may produce a dull boring discomfort in the epigastrium which is interpreted frequently as evidence of a peptic ulcer or cholecystic disease. Ureteral colic can be characterized as an intermittent, sharp pain radiating along the course of the ureter into the scrotum or the labium majus. This type of pain may be produced by the passage of a calculus down the ureter. On the right side it is mistaken occasionally for acute appendicitis.

The pain associated with disease of the bladder may be a vague and generalized suprapubic discomfort as in complete urinary retention and subacute cystitis, or it can be a sharp, localized suprapubic one as in interstitial cystitis. Irritation at the bladder neck is often associated with a pain at the urethral meatus.

Inflammatory swelling of the epididymis or the testis will cause severe nonradiating pain in the scrotal region. Infections involving the vas deferens may produce discomfort in the upper scrotum and along the inguinal canal.

Acute prostatitis and prostatic abscess may be associated with pain in the rectum and the perineal region.

Physical Examination

Palpation. Obviously, every patient should have a complete physical investigation. However, in this discussion the examination will be limited to the genitourinary tract. In examining a patient for urinary tract disease one first palpates the abdomen and the flank areas. The kidneys may or may not be palpable, depending upon the patient's body build. The slender asthenic type of person will often have readily palpable, highly mobile normal kidneys. In examining the kidney one hand should be placed with the fingers in the costovertebral angle area and pressure applied there in order to ascertain tenderness. Renal disease may produce tenderness in this region. Should tenderness be elicited in this area, it frequently signifies renal disease. Pain produced by pressure to areas adjacent to the costovertebral angle area, e.g., sacrospinalis muscle, 12th rib, etc., does not signify renal disease.

With one hand in the costovertebral angle region and the other hand in the lower anterior abdominal quadrant, the examiner palpates for any unusual masses. The hand on the abdomen should be moved gradually up toward the lower costal margins in order to avoid missing the lower border of a large mass. The normal kidney moves with respiration and may be palpable during inspiration. Retroperitoneal structures such as the kidney may be differentiated from masses in the peritoneal cavity by the use of ballottement, i.e., pushing on the kidney with one hand in the costovertebral angle region will cause the kidney to be felt by the other hand pressing against the abdomen. A mass in the peritoneal cavity, e.g., liver, spleen, bowel neoplasm, usually cannot be ballotted with one hand in the costovertebral angle region and the other on the abdomen.

A bruit or murmur may be detected by auscultation of the abdomen when there is turbulent flow in one or more of the large arteries of the abdomen including the renal arteries. This bruit may be highly localized and may not be present at all times.

Percussion and palpation are most useful procedures for ascertaining the presence of a distended bladder and other suprapubic masses. In examining the penis the foreskin is retracted first, and the urethral meatus, the glans and the coronal sulcus are inspected closely for the presence of abnormalities. Then the shaft of the penis is palpated for induration and nodules.

The scrotum and its contents are next in the order of examination. The spermatic cord is palpated, first high in the scrotum for the presence of varicocele, spermatocele, beaded vas deferens or nodules. Then the testis and the epididymis are felt carefully for unusual firmness, nodularity or large masses. If a large mass is palpated in the scrotum, then a flashlight is employed in an attempt to transilluminate the mass. If it transilluminates, it may be a spermatocele or a hydrocele. If it does not, it may be a testicular neoplasm, epididymitis, torsion of the testis or hernia. All hydroceles and spermatoceles should be aspirated because occasionally they are superimposed upon testicular cancer which cannot be felt until the overlying fluid has been withdrawn. This step may be omitted in those cases in which an operation is planned.

The rectal examination is used to determine the status of the prostate gland, the seminal vesicles and the rectum. The normal prostate is a slightly tender, elastic and firm body felt through the anterior rectal wall. Three longitudinal grooves or sulci may be palpated on the posterior aspect of the prostate, two laterally and one centrally. The seminal vesicles lie above and lateral to the prostate and are felt as bands, beginning at the base of the prostate and running superolaterally from the prostate at an angle of about 45°. A stony hard nodular prostate suggests carcinoma, tuberculosis or calculi. A smooth hard prostate with obliteration of the sulci is indicative of infiltrating prostatic neoplasm. Early carcinoma may manifest itself as an isolated circumscribed small nodule. Marked tenderness of the prostate can be caused by acute prostatitis, while an extremely tender, bulging, tense prostate suggests abscess. A tense, exquisitely painful seminal vesicle indicates seminal vesiculitis.

While performing the rectal examination one should test for integrity of the sacral spinal cord by attempting to elicit the bulbocavernosus reflex[10] and sensory changes in the saddle area. The observations made with these examinations may be extremely helpful in determining the presence of neurologic deficits responsible for abnormalities in urination and continence.

Urinalysis. The examination of the urine is one of the most important aspects of the urologic investigation. In many instances it alone determines the need for detailed expensive urologic procedures entailing hospitalization. Persistent microscopic hematuria suggests the same diseases as gross hematuria and necessitates endoscopy and pyelography. A urinary tract infection should be investigated with endoscopy and pyelography, since pyuria may be produced by neoplasms, tuberculosis, calculous disease, hydronephrosis or pyogenic bacteria. In addition to ascertaining the presence of hematuria, pyuria and bacteriuria, the routine urinalysis may lead to the suspicion of impaired renal function.

RENAL PHYSIOLOGY[22, 23]

The purpose of the urinary tract[16, 21] is to aid in maintaining an optimal environment for the efficient functioning of the body cells. When the kidneys do not perform their functions in a normal fashion, either because of intrinsic disease or involvement of other components of the urinary system, illness follows. Anemia, malaise, nausea, vomiting, disorientation, coma, convulsions, weakness, paralysis and cardiac abnormalities are some of the manifestations of the general cellular dysfunction[77] at times associated with renal disease. The renal cells per se also are influenced by the results of their activities, e.g., inability of the kidneys to maintain a proper environment for all of the body means an improper environment for the renal cells also. Many of the diseases of the genitourinary tract are of prime importance because they interfere with the homeostatic function of the kidneys.

A 70-kilo adult contains approximately 45 L. of water; 30 L. are in the cells (of which 3 are in the blood cells) and 15 L. are extracellular. Of the 15 extracellular liters of water, 11 L. are intercellular, or between the cells, and 4 L. are in the cardiovascular system as plasma.

The cells of the body carry on metabolic activities continuously and need the transport of material to them for anabolism and away from them so as to remove their catabolic products. The blood is the vehicle for the transport of these substances. The exchange of material between blood and cells is indirect in that it must pass into the intercellular fluid first. The forces accomplishing the exchange of material between blood and intercellular fluid through the capillary wall are diffusionary forces that account for 99 per cent of the movement and the intravascular protein osmotic and intravascular hydrostatic pressures. Secondary forces are tissue pressure and a small amount of protein osmotic pressure in the intercellular space.

Essentially, intravascular hydrostatic and tissue protein osmotic pressure tend to promote the movement of water and crystalloids from the blood into the intercellular space, while the intravascular protein osmotic pressure and tissue pressure tend to cause material to go from the intercellular fluid into the capillary. Thus on the arterial side of the capillary the sum (35 mm. Hg) of the intravascular hydrostatic (30 mm. Hg) and tissue protein osmotic (5 mm. Hg) pressures is greater than the sum (30 mm. Hg) of the intravascular osmotic (20 mm. Hg) and tissue hydrostatic (10 mm. Hg) pressure; therefore, material will tend here to go slightly more rapidly from the capillary into the intercellular fluid. The intravascular hydrostatic pressure drops from 30 to 15 mm. Hg on going from the arterial end of the capillary to the venous portion. Since the other pressures remain approximately constant, material here will move a little more rapidly from the intercellular space into the capillary; intravascular osmotic (20 mm. Hg) and tissue hydrostatic (10 mm. Hg) pressures now exceed intravascular hydrostatic (15 mm. Hg) and tissue protein osmotic (5 mm. Hg) pressures.

In the normal adult approximately 1,000 ml. of blood is pumped through both kidneys in 1 minute; this is about one fifth of the cardiac output. The human kidney is a tremendously vascular organ.

ANATOMY[16, 21]

Each kidney is composed of about 1,000,000 units, the nephrons. Each nephron consists of a glomerulus, a proximal convoluted tubule, an elongated segment (loop of Henle) and a distal convoluted tubule (Fig. 52-5). The nephron is the functional unit of the kidney; its product, urine, passes into the collecting tubule. The collecting tubule in turn empties its contents into the calyx. The calyx propels the urine through the infundibulum into the pelvis. Then the urine is transported down

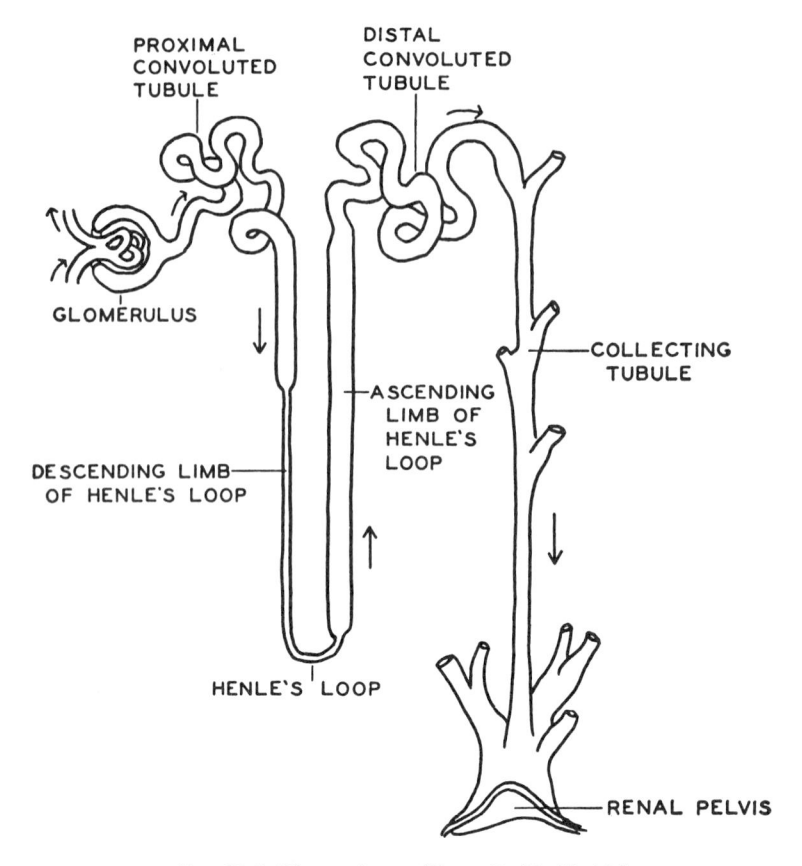

Fig. 52-5. The nephron. (From R. M. Nesbit)

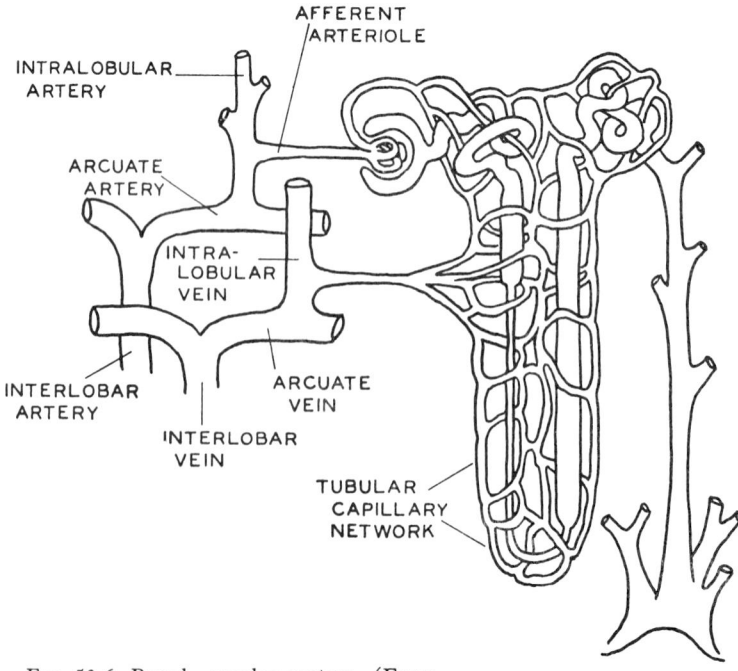

Fig. 52-6. Renal vascular system. (From R. M. Nesbit)

the ureter into the bladder. The urine is collected in the bladder, which is emptied voluntarily at intervals through the urethra into the external environment. The nephron and the urinary collecting system are actually parts of one long conduit; therefore, an abnormality of a distal part such as the urethra may affect directly the proximal functioning unit.

The cortex of the kidney contains the glomeruli and convoluted tubules; the medulla, the portion adjacent to the pelvis, consists of elongated tubular segments (Henle's loops) and the collecting tubules. The renal artery is a short, large caliber vessel springing directly from the aorta and dividing into an anterior and a posterior branch as it enters the renal parenchyma. The branches next divide into the interlobar arteries (Fig. 52-6), which course through the medulla. At the corticomedullary junction the interlobar vessels give off the arcuate arteries which branch further to give rise to the intralobular arteries in the cortex. The afferent arteriole comes from the intralobular artery and gives off the capillaries of the glomerulus which empty into the efferent arteriole. The efferent arteriole then branches and forms the peritubular arterial capillary network which empties into the venous portion of the network. From the venous capillaries blood flows into the intralobular, arcuate, interlobar and renal veins and finally into the inferior vena cava.

The flow of blood through the glomerular capillaries is regulated, in part, by the afferent and efferent arterioles. Concomitant vasoconstriction of the afferent arteriole and vasodilation of the efferent arteriole will result in a decreased blood flow and a decreased glomerular hydrostatic pressure.

GLOMERULAR FILTRATION

As has been stated previously, 1,000 ml. of blood or about 600 ml. of plasma flows through the kidneys in 1 minute. Approximately 120 ml. of the plasma is filtered through the 2,000,000 glomeruli in 1 minute. Glomerular filtration is essentially a passive phenomenon and is very similar to the process whereby material moves from capillary into the intercellular space. In the glomerular capillary the intravascular hydrostatic pressure is 75 mm. Hg instead of 3 mm. Hg as in capillaries elsewhere in the body. This force of 75 mm. Hg together with diffusional forces tends to promote filtration of plasma through the glomerular membrane. Opposing filtration are the intratubular hydrostatic pressure (10 mm. Hg), the interstitial pressure without tubular pressure (10 mm. Hg) and the intravascular protein osmotic pressure (20 mm. Hg)—a total opposing pressure of 40 mm. Hg. The effective glomerular filtration pressure, 35 mm. Hg, is the algebraic sum of these opposing forces. Knowing these things one need not be surprised that oliguria or anuria attend shock: a drop in systemic blood pressure sufficient to lower the pressure in the glomerular capillary by 35 mm. of Hg may abolish glomerular filtration.

So too is the suppression of urine associated with prostatic urinary retention understandable. With acute urinary retention due to prostatism, the intravesical pressure increases as does the intra-ureteral, the intrapelvic and the *intratubular hydrostatic pressures*. Since the intratubular hydrostatic pressure opposes filtration, a rise in this pressure will decrease glomerular filtration, and urinary suppression follows. Swelling of the renal parenchyma itself can impair glomerular filtration by raising the interstitial pressure; this may attend acute pyelonephritis, which is associated with filtration of the interstitial spaces with leukocytes. Acute inflammation of the glomerular membrane will result in impaired filtration as will vascular disease compromising the lumen of the glomerular capillary or the renal artery.

The glomerular filtrate is essentially protein-free plasma; the blood cellular elements and most of the protein are not filtered.[20] The pH of the filtrate is 7.4, specific gravity 1.010, glucose 80 mg. per 100 ml., urea nitrogen 15 mg. per 100 ml., sodium 142 mEq./L., chloride 103 mEq./L., bicarbonate 27 mEq./L. and potassium 4.5 mEq./L.

THE FUNCTION OF THE TUBULE AND THE COLLECTING DUCT

Before delving into function of the tubule, it would be useful to redefine its various segments and limits. The tubule begins with Bowman's capsule, which is the expanded, thinned out portion surrounding the glomerular tuft. Proceeding distally from Bowman's capsule, the segments are, in order: *the proximal segment* which includes the proximal convolution and its terminal portion, the thick descending limb of the loop of Henle; *the thin segment* which incorporates not only the thin descending portion of the loop of Henle of the cortical nephron but includes the thin part of the descending limb, the hairpin turn and the thin part of the ascending limb of the juxtamedullary nephron; *the distal segment* which consists of the thick ascending limb of Henle's loop and the distal convoluted tubule; and *the collecting tubule* incorporating the cortical collecting tubule, the collecting tubule and the papillary or Bellini's duct. The papillary duct drains urine into the calyx.

Tubular function includes all the processes that convert extracellular fluid (minus protein) into urine. Richards[56] and Oliver[51] have shown that the glomerulus presents to the tubule a filtrate that is essentially free of protein and cellular elements, has a pH of 7.4, specific gravity of 1.010, glucose 80 mg. per 100 ml., urea nitrogen 15 mg. per 100 ml., sodium 142 mEq./L., chloride 103 mEq./L., bicarbonate 27 mEq./L., and potassium 4.5 mEq./L. To comprehend some of the functions of the tubular portion (including ducts) of the nephron, one need only compare the urine with the glomerular filtrate. The normal individual will excrete during 24 hours about 1,500 ml. of urine having a pH of 5.5, a specific gravity of 1.020, no glucose, 0.5 to 1.0 per cent of the filtered sodium and urea nitrogen concentrated 70 times above its blood level.

Normally the kidneys with their 2 million nephrons and blood flow of 1,000 ml./min., form a combined glomerular filtrate of 120 ml. per minute. If the tubules were absolutely inert, a person would theoretically void 172,800 ml. in 24 hours. Since the total extracellular fluid is approximately 15,000 ml., it is obvious that an individual would expire in a very short time if the tubules were not functioning. Since the average 24-hour output of urine is approximately 1,440 ml. and there are 1,440 minutes per day, it is apparent that the kidneys excrete 1 ml. of urine per minute and reabsorb the remaining 119 ml. of glomerular filtrate water.

The renal nephron performs its homeostatic function through three processes involving glomerular filtration, tubular excretion and tubular reabsorption. Practically all of the unwanted substances are excreted from the body through glomerular filtration. Water and solute essential for normal body cellular activity are taken back into the body through tubular reabsorption. Tubular excretion plays a part in ridding the body of unwanted substances by excreting such native solutes as potassium, creatinine, hydrogen ion, ammonia, and such foreign solutes as phenol red, paraminohippurate, contrast material (Diodrast, Hypaque, Cystokon, Neo-Iopax, etc.), penicillin, sulfonamides, glucuronides, ethereal sulfates and the secondary, tertiary and quaternary amines. Thus, glomerular filtration and tubular excretion are concerned with disposal of materials from the body; tubular reabsorption is needed for conservation of water and essential solutes.

Reabsorption and Excretion in the Proximal Tubule

Tubular reabsorption has been divided into active and passive types.[61] The active type of tubular reabsorption requires metabolic energy, takes place from a lower to higher concentration, can be abolished by inhibitors, cooling or anoxia, and may have a limited transport capacity. Passive tubular reabsorption does not require direct metabolic energy, is usually caused by physical forces such as differences of concentration, electrical potential or friction, and takes place along a downward gradient.

Active Tubular Reabsorption—Glucose.[51] The reabsorption of glucose is an excellent example of the active type, since all of the filtered glucose is gradually reabsorbed in the proximal tubule, starting from a concentration equal to that in the blood, until in the tubular lumen the concentration is reduced to zero. Glucose is transported from the tubular fluid to the renal interstitial fluid, theoretically, by a carrier system which involves coupling and uncoupling glucose by an enzymatic process. This complex process, which requires metabolic energy, is carried out by the cells of the proximal convoluted tubule. The maximum amount of glucose that can be reabsorbed by this carrier system varies between 250 and 350 mg. per minute. The question is frequently raised that if the kidneys can reabsorb 350 mg. of filtered glucose per minute, why does the diabetic spill sugar into the urine when the blood level is only 160 to 170 mg. per cent. Part of the answer lies in the fact that the 160 to 170 mg. per cent figure relates to venous blood, whereas the arterial blood delivered to the glomerulus in the same patient would show a level of 200 mg. per cent. With a glomerular filtration rate of 120 ml./min. and an arterial blood level of 200 mg. per cent, the amount of glucose delivered to the tubules in 1 minute is 240 mg., which still is much less than the 350 mg. capacity of many normal individuals. It has been suggested that the discrepancy may be due to a difference in the capacity of the individual nephrons to reabsorb glucose. Some nephrons may be loaded to capacity when the blood sugar level is 160 mg. per cent, while other nephrons may be only half loaded. The patient shows glycosuria because of the low-capacity nephrons despite the fact that when the patient's blood sugar is raised much higher, the total capacity of both high and low capacity nephrons shows an ability to reabsorb 450 mg. of glucose per minute.

Thus in uncontrolled diabetes mellitus sugar is found in the urine because of the abnormally large amount of glucose in the blood and hence in the glomerular filtrate. The tubules are functioning normally, but the work capacity of some of the nephrons is exceeded when the glucose in the glomerular filtrate is greater than normal.

Glycosuria may also occur in individuals with normal blood sugar levels but with abnormal renal tubules; in these people the tubules are incapable of transporting the normal amount of glucose per unit of time. The tubules may have a congenital defect of the glucose carrier system, as in renal glycosuria, or there may be specific injury to the carrier system as in phlorizin glycosuria, in which phlorizin is the toxic agent. Glycosuria is observed infrequently in glomerulonephritis, a condition in which both tubule and glomerular membrane are diseased. Glycosuria does not occur despite the tubule's decreased capacity to transport glucose because less glucose is presented to the tubule per unit of time by virtue of a decreased glomerular filtration rate. It is interesting to note that patients with high blood sugar and in severe diabetic acidosis may not demonstrate glycosuria because of marked dehydration and associated decreased glomerular filtration rate.

Amino acids, uric acid, phosphate, sulfate, creatinine, lactate, citrate, ascorbic acid and other organic compounds are reabsorbed in the proximal tubule by an active process similar to that described for glucose.[36] Structurally similar amino acids are absorbed by the same transport mechanism, and thus there are several transport mechanisms for amino acids.[58] Arginine, histidine and lysine are dibasic amino acids and are reabsorbed by one transport mechanism; leucine and isoleucine, monoamino-monocarboxylic acids, compete for another transport system; glycine, proline and hydroxyproline utilize a third reabsorptive system.

Although reports have suggested that phosphates may be excreted by the tubule, most of the available evidence supports the concept that phosphates are reabsorbed by an active process in the proximal tubule[54] which is influenced by the parathyroid hormone and vitamin D.

It is believed that most of the filtered uric acid and urates are reabsorbed actively in the proximal tubule and that the amount excreted in the urine is by virtue of distal tubular secretion.[34]

Sodium and Chloride. The bulk of the solute reabsorbed in the proximal tubule is sodium and chloride. In addition, almost all of the potassium in the glomerular filtrate is reabsorbed in the proximal tubule. Despite the reabsorption of all the previously mentioned solutes by the proximal tubule into the interstitial space, the solution remaining in the tubular lumen is isotonic. This means that a large proportion of the glomerular filtrate water is reabsorbed along with the solutes. In fact, 100 ml. or 83 per cent of the 120 ml. of filtered plasma is reabsorbed during its passage through the proximal tubule (secondary to the reabsorption of the solutes) in order to maintain osmotic equilibrium. Thus the reabsorption of the major portion of the water of the glomerular filtrate is passive and has been termed "obligatory" by Homer Smith.

As water and solute are reabsorbed in the proximal tubule, some of the substances not reabsorbed or not reabsorbed as rapidly as water increase in concentration because 80 per cent of the solvent has been reabsorbed. Thus such substances as urea and creatinine are concentrated. However, the tubular fluid leaving the proximal segment is still isotonic because the remaining sodium salts still provide the major portion of its osmotic pressure and the loss of glucose and amino acids is equalized by the urea and creatinine.

As the urea concentration in the proximal tubule begins to rise with the loss of water through tubular reabsorption, a concentration gradient is established between the urea in the tubule and the urea in the interstitial space; and urea then begins to move from the tubular lumen into the interstitial space (through a permeable cell membrane). This movement is "passive reabsorption," and its rate varies with diuresis and antidiuresis.

At this point it would be well to summarize briefly and generally the effect of proximal tubular activity upon the glomerular filtrate. The proximal tubular segment withdraws from the glomerular filtrate and returns to the corporeal circulation an isotonic solution containing most of the filtered sodium, potassium, glucose, amino acids and other solutes of the filtrate essential to normal body cellular function.

The reabsorption of sodium in the proximal tubule probably takes place under influence of several stimuli. It has been demonstrated that the excretion of hydrogen ions starts in the proximal tubule and probably takes place all along the nephron rather than being confined only to the distal convoluted tubule.[41] The carbon dioxide tension or partial pressure of carbon dioxide regulates the rate of hydrogen ion excretion.[55] In the renal tubular cell, water and carbon dioxide combine under the influence of carbonic anhydrase to form carbonic acid, which then dissociates or ionizes to form hydrogen and bicarbonate ions. The hydrogen ion traverses the cellular membrane into the tubular lumen and exchanges positions with the sodium of the filtered sodium bicarbonate. Thus the hydrogen ion combines with the bicarbonate ion in the lumen to form carbonic acid which is then slowly decomposed into water and carbon dioxide. Simultaneously, sodium is transported into the cell to combine with the dangling bicarbonate ion to form sodium bicarbonate. This ion-exchange mechanism in the proximal tubule serves to return to the body all of the sodium previously combined with filtered bicarbonate. Functionally, the process is equivalent to the reabsorption of all of the filtered sodium bicarbonate. Insofar as the body economy is concerned, one of the primary buffer materials, $NaHCO_3$ has been returned to the body and, in the process, excess hydrogen ions (produced by formation of strong nonvolatile acids, (e.g., phosphoric, sulfuric) and organic acids and weak volatile acids during metabolism) have been excreted. As the glomerular filtrate is pushed down the proximal tubule its pH does not change until all of the bicarbonate in the lumen is decomposed.

Another stimulus for the reabsorption of sodium in the proximal tubule is provided by aldosterone, an adrenocortical hormone.[33, 38] The secretion of aldosterone is influenced by extracellular fluid volume and potassium blood levels. A decrease in ECF volume stimulates increased secretion of aldosterone with a resultant increase in tubular reabsorption of sodium, much of it in the form of sodium chloride. Recent evidence suggests that aldosterone is secreted in response to angiotensin which is formed from renin, a substance secreted by the juxtaglomerular apparatus of the kidney into the blood stream.[60]

A third stimulus which may play a part in the reabsorption of sodium as sodium chloride in the proximal tubule relates to a passive mechanism. Malvin and associates[48] feel that water is reabsorbed from lumen of the proximal tubule primarily because of the increased colloid osmotic pressure of the fluid in the peritubular capillary network (resulting from concentration of protein in the blood of the efferent arteriole after removal of water through glomerular filtration). Following the shifting of fluid from the tubule into the cells and the capillaries, there is also a diffusion of sodium and chloride in the same direction in order to maintain isotonicity.

Function of the Nephron Distal to the Proximal Segment

As stated previously, the proximal segment of the nephron removes an isotonic solution from the glomerular filtrate. In the normal individual this solution contains practically all of the filtered glucose, amino acids, bicarbonate, uric acid and other essential organic constituents of the extracellular fluid. In addition, 80 per cent of the filtered electrolytes and water are reabsorbed by the proximal tubule. All of the potassium and most of the sodium and chloride are removed. Some hydrogen ions have been added to the glomerular filtrate by tubular excretion. The tubular fluid entering the loop of Henle amounts to 20 ml. volume in 1 minute, contains about 1/6 of the filtered electrolytes, has a pH of 7.4 and a specific gravity of 1.010 or an osmolality of 290 m Osm.

To a great extent the processes occurring in the proximal tubule are constant and not too directly related to variations in body function. In contrast the various activities of the cells of the distal nephron are attuned to the momentary needs of the cells of the body and will add hydrogen ions, potassium ions and uric acid to the tubular fluid or extract from the tubular lumen sodium ions, chloride ions and water in accord with the needs of the organism relative to extracellular fluid volume, pH of the extracellular fluid, serum potassium level, etc. Thus, depending on the needs for homeostasis, the distal nephron may excrete few hydrogen ions and result in a urine with a pH of 7.4, as in cases of alkalosis; or, conversely, as in acidosis, the distal nephron may excrete many hydrogen ions and result in a urine of pH 4.5. Similarly, if the individual is dehydrated and there is an increase in osmolality of the ECF, the distal nephron may resorb most of the 20 ml. of water coming from the proximal segment so that only 0.3 ml. of urine is excreted per minute with an osmolality of 1,000 m Osm. On the other hand, if the individual is overhydrated, the distal nephron may permit most of the 20 ml. of tubular water to be excreted into the bladder.

Maintenance of a normal pH of the blood and extracellular fluid and indirectly of the cellular contents is provided by several buffer systems, the lungs and the kidneys. The nephrons contribute their share by excreting part of the formed volatile carbonic acid (the rest being excreted by the lungs as CO_2 and water) and the strong nonvolatile acids such as chloride, sulfuric, phosphoric and organic acids. Sulfuric acid is derived from the oxidation of the sulfur-containing amino acids, cysteine and methionine; phosphoric acid results from the metabolism of phospholipid and amino acid containing phosphorus.

In order to maintain a pH of 7.4 the body must neutralize these strong acids produced by metabolism or ingestion. The primary buffering occurs by reaction of the strong acid with sodium bicarbonate to produce the weak, volatile, carbonic acid and the sodium salt of the strong acid, e.g., $NaHCO_3 + H_2SO_4 \rightleftarrows Na_2SO_4 + H_2CO_3$. The H_2CO_3 then decomposes to H_2O and CO_2 which can be excreted by the lungs. The sodium sulfate is excreted from the body by the kidneys.

If the nephron excreted unchanged the sodium sulfate and other sodium salts of the strong acids, the body would soon be depleted of its sodium and its primary buffer, sodium bicarbonate, for metabolism is continuous in the living organism and waste-product acids are being formed constantly. The renal tubule has an elegant mechanism for excreting the unwanted acid, retaining the sodium ion and replenishing the bicarbonate anions. As mentioned in the section on "Reabsorption and Excretion in the Proximal Tubule" the cells of the renal tubule can manufacture the hydrogen and bicarbonate ions from cellular carbon dioxide and water with the aid of the enzyme carbonic anhydrase. The hydrogen ion is excreted into the tubular lumen by the cell while the bicarbonate ion remains in the cell. The hydrogen ion exchanges places with the sodium ion of a strong acid salt in the tubular lumen so that the sodium ion enters the cell and combines with the bicarbonate to return to the extracellular fluid sodium bicarbonate—a buffer again available for neutralizing metabolic acids.

In the discussion on the function of the proximal tubule it was mentioned that hydrogen ion exchange started in the proximal tubule. The main function of the exchange in this part of the nephron is to conserve the sodium ions of the sodium bicarbonate filtered through the glomerulus. It is believed that the filtered sodium bicarbonate per se is not reabsorbed by the proximal renal tubule. The pH of the glomerular filtrate begins to decrease as it moves from the proximal segment into the loop of Henle. This is due to the decomposition of most of the filtered bicarbonate and the continued excretion of hydrogen ions by the tubular cells.

In the distal and the collecting tubule segments of the nephron, hydrogen ions continue to be excreted into the tubular fluid and the bicarbonate buffer continues to diffuse from the renal tubular cell into the blood stream. The hydrogen ion is excreted in the distal nephron by two mechanisms. One method involves the process described previously for the proximal tubule; the other mechanism utilizes the formation of ammonia from deamination of the amino acid glutamine primarily and, to a lesser extent, amino acids such as glycine, alanine, aspartic acid, etc.[52] The deamination of glutamine into glutamic acid and NH_3 is promoted by the enzyme glutaminase. The ammonia which is produced in the renal tubular cell diffuses into the lumen of the tubule where it combines with excreted hydrogen ion to form the ammonium ion. The ammonium ion then exchanges for the sodium ion of the strong acid salt to form the ammonium salt; the sodium ion returns to the cell to form the buffer sodium bicarbonate which is taken back into the blood stream. The ammonium ion mechanism permits the body to excrete large amounts of hydrogen ion without making the urine too acid.

Factors other than pCO_2 or carbon dioxide tension influence the excretion of hydrogen ions and the replenishment of the bicarbonate buffer. The potassium ion and the hydrogen ion in the tubular cell compete for the sodium ion in the tubular lumen. Thus when there is potassium depletion, excretion of hydrogen ions into the tubular fluid is increased, with a resultant increase in plasma bicarbonate level. On the other hand, an increase in the blood level of potassium leads to depression of hydrogen ion secretion and resultant alkalinity of the urine. Inhibition of the enzyme carbonic anhydrase leads to decreased secretion of hydrogen ions with resultant loss of bicarbonate buffer and sodium ions in the urine. Over a period of time this process leads to hyperchloremic acidosis, hypokalemia and an alkaline urine.

A decrease in the glomerular filtration of the buffers sodium bicarbonate and disodium phosphate also affects hydrogen ion excretion, since sodium ions must be present in the tubular fluid in order to effect an exchange between hydrogen ion and sodium ion.

Potassium Excretion[37]

Most of the filtered potassium is reabsorbed in the proximal tubule, and the potassium eventually excreted in the urine is the result of secretion by cells in the distal tubule. The potassium is secreted in exchange for sodium ions in the tubular fluid. The rate of potassium secretion is influenced by the amount of potassium in the tubular cell, the amount of hydrogen ion in the tubular cell and the amount of sodium ion in the tubular fluid.

As has been stated previously, the hydrogen ion and the potassium ion in the tubular cell compete for the sodium ion in the tubular fluid. Thus potassium ion excretion is augmented in hyperkalemia, alkalosis, aldosteronism and hypernatremia. Conversely, systemic acidosis, Addison's disease, dehydration, hyponatremia and mercurial diuretics decrease potassium excretion.

Maintenance of normal tonicity or osmolality of cellular and extracellular body fluid is accomplished by a complex process occurring in the medulla of the kidney, and involving the loop of Henle, the distal tubule, the collecting tubule, the vasa recta and the antidiuretic hormone.[42] When an individual ingests a large amount of water and begins to dilute the body fluids, the kidneys assume their homeostatic role and excrete the excess water by forming an increased volume of dilute urine. On the other hand, if an individual loses an excess amount of water from the body by virtue of sweating, inadequate intake of fluid, vomiting or diarrhea, the nephrons will protect the organism by forming a small amount of highly concentrated urine in order to conserve water and minimize abnormal hypertonicity of the body fluids.

It will be recalled that 80 per cent of the water filtered through the glomerulus is reabsorbed passively in the proximal tubule secondary to the active reabsorption of organic and inorganic solute. Thus, in a minute, 100 ml. of the 120 ml. of water filtered by the glomeruli is reabsorbed by the *proximal tubule*. The fate of the remaining 20 ml. of fluid depends on the osmolality and perhaps the volume of body fluids. In general it can be stated that water is never secreted into the renal nephron; all of the fluid reaches the tubule via glomerular filtration. Thus the amount of water excreted by the kidney is directly related to reabsorption. A urine more dilute than plasma can be formed only by increased absorption of solute relative to water reabsorption; a concentrated urine can result only if water reabsorption is increased relative to solute reabsorption. This selective reabsorption of water is called the facultative phase of water reabsorption because it is in direct accord with the immediate needs of the body for fluid; *and this phase takes place in the distal convoluted and collecting tubules.*

COUNTER-CURRENT MECHANISMS

Before discussing the fate of the water leaving the proximal tubule and entering the descending limb of the loop of Henle, it would be well to consider certain anatomic and physiologic differences between the cortex and the medulla of the kidney. It has been shown that the fluids and the tissues in the renal cortex are for the most part isotonic, i.e., the blood in the cortical vessels, the interstitial tissue and the fluid in the proximal tubule. On the other hand, the blood in the vasa recta of the medulla, the interstitial fluid in the loop of Henle and in certain instances the fluid in the collecting tubule are markedly hypertonic. The hypertonicity in the medulla is produced primarily by the increased concentration of sodium and urea in the area. It should be noted that most of the large blood vessels are in the cortex of the kidney; smaller vessels are situated in the medulla. Thus blood flow (measured in ml./Gm. of tissue) is approximately 20 times as high through the cortex as compared with the medulla. In addition, the effectiveness of blood flow through the medulla is less than through the cortex even considering the difference in the size of the vessels because of the hairpin or looping arrangement of the vasa recta. The blood in the vasa recta is in contact with a given portion of the medulla over a much longer period of time because it traverses the same tissue in both the descending and the ascending limbs of the blood vessel. Contrast this arrangement with the cortical blood vessel which courses through a tissue only once! Not only do the blood vessels in the medulla have the looping arrangement but also that portion of the nephron called the loop of Henle. Again it will be quite obvious that the contents in the lumen of the loop of Henle will be in contact with adjacent medulla and vasa recta over a much longer period of time than would be possible if the loop arrangement were not present. In brief, the arrangement and the size of the blood vessels and the arrangement of the loops of Henle in the medulla predispose to stasis and thus increasing concentrations of materials, e.g., sodium and urea, being transported and diffused into the interstitial fluid and blood in the area.

The previously described medullary blood flow is in the manner of a counter-current exchanger and serves to reduce the effectiveness of blood flow in removing solute from the medulla. The principle of any counter-current exchanger, whether it be in animate or inanimate objects, involves interaction between the medium flowing in one direction in one limb of a conduit and the same medium flowing in the opposite direction in another limb of the same conduit. In order for the principle to work, the walls of the conduit must permit transport of the entity in question—such as heat, oxygen or sodium—and the limbs of the conduit must be close enough to each other to permit equilibration within a common interspace.

The increased concentration of sodium, chloride and urea in the renal medulla is due in part to decreased effective blood flow on the basis of a counter-current exchanger mechanism, and in part to the activity of the loop of Henle as a counter-current multiplier system in building up the concentration of sodium and chloride in the medulla. The hypertonicity of the medulla has been found to increase in a linear fashion starting with the corticomedullary area having the least hypertonicity and gradually increasing the osmolality as the papilla is approached. At any particular level of medulla the hypertonicity is the same in all of the fluids at that level, including blood, fluid in the descending limb and the ascending limbs of the loop of Henle and in the interstitial fluid. These findings strongly suggest that the loop of Henle does actually function as a counter-current multiplier system. It is believed that as tubular fluid flows down through the descending limb of the loop of Henle, water is lost to the interstitium in excess of salt so that the tubular fluid tends to become increasingly hypertonic as it approaches the papillary region of the medulla. When the hypertonic fluid begins to flow back toward the cortex through the ascending limb of the loop of Henle, sodium is pumped into the interstitium but essentially no water traverses the wall of the ascending limb of the loop of Henle. Thus the fluid in the loop becomes progressively more dilute as it ascends through the medulla toward the cortex. This system produces a maximally concentrated solution at the turn of the loop of Henle by multiplying the effect of transfer of small amounts of water from the lumen of the descending limb of the loop of Henle to the interstitial space all along the surface of the descending limb. In each transfer the expenditure of energy is small because only a small gradient must be overcome. As the concentrated solution ascends the loop small amounts of sodium are pumped into the interstitium at each level. The transfer again is against a small gradient at each level. Thus by multiplying the small exchanges of water and electrolyte along the length of both limbs of the loop of Henle the depths of the medulla become hypertonic and the fluid leaving the loop of Henle is hypotonic. For a more detailed description of the counter-current exchanger and counter-current multiplier principles, the reader is referred to pertinent articles in the bibliography.

Renal Concentration and Dilution Mechanisms

As a result of counter-current mechanisms in the medulla the isotonic proximal tubular fluid becomes increasingly hypertonic as it traverses the descending limb of the loop of Henle into the depths of the medulla and then gradually becomes hypotonic as it travels upward through the ascending limb in approaching the cortex of the kidney. It might be mentioned that the walls of the proximal tubule and the descending limb of the loop of Henle are relatively permeable to water, whereas the lining of the ascending limb, the distal convoluted tubule and the collecting tubule are relatively impermeable to water except under the influence of the antidiuretic hormone. Irrespective of the state of hydration or osmolality of the extracellular fluid, the glomerular filtrate participates in all of the processes described thus far as it is pushed through the proximal nephron into the distal convoluted tubule. Thus the fluid leaving the ascending limb of the loop of Henle and entering the distal tubule is always hypotonic. *However, the osmolality or tonicity of the fluid as it flows through the distal and collecting tubules will vary in accord with the needs of the body for water.*

Verney has demonstrated that the osmolality or tonicity of extracellular fluid is monitored continuously by vesicular cells in the supraoptic nuclei. These cells act as osmometers, swelling when the osmolality of fluid bathing them is decreased and losing fluid to their surroundings and shrinking when the extracellular fluid osmolality is increased. It is the shrinking response of the osmoreceptors to hypertonicity that stimulates the posterior pituitary to release antidiuretic hormone. The antidiuretic hormone is carried to the kidney where it acts upon the cells of the distal and the collecting tubules to increase their permeability to water and result in increased absorption of water. The secretion of antidiuretic hormone with resultant increased reabsorption of water by the kidney and formation of a scant concentrated urine continues until enough water has been ingested to dilute the extracellular fluid and decrease its osmolality. With the decrease in effective osmotic pressure of the fluid surrounding the osmoreceptors, the vesicular cells swell and stop stimulating the posterior pituitary to secrete ADH. A decrease in circulating ADH results in resumption of impermeability of the membranes lining the distal and the collecting tubules, and less water will be reabsorbed by the kidney with formation of a copious, dilute urine.

The antidiuretic hormone, an octapeptide, is formed by the cells of the hypothalamic supraoptic and paraventricular nuclei. After being formed by these neurons it migrates along the axons to be stored at nerve endings applied to capillary blood vessels in the neural lobe of the pituitary.

The exact relationship between the hypertonic interstitium of the medulla, the collecting tubule and the antidiuretic hormone must now be correlated. It will be recalled that the collecting tubule traverses the medulla in close proximity to the loop of Henle and the vasa recta, and passes through the areas of hypertonicity in the medulla. The proximal tubule and the descending limb of the loop of Henle are freely permeable to water; the remainder of the tubule including the ascending limb of the loop of Henle, the distal tubule and the collecting tubule are quite impermeable to water. However, under the influence of the antidiuretic hormone the distal tubule and the collecting tubule can become quite permeable to water.

A few years ago it was believed that water was absorbed by the distal tubule solely through the effect of ADH in stimulating the cells of the distal tubule to actively resorb the water against a marked gradient. Studies later demonstrated that it was impossible for the cells of the distal tubule to accomplish this activity in view of the high energy requirements. Subsequently it was learned that the force primarily responsible for reabsorption of water in the collecting tubule was derived from the high osmotic pressure in the medullary tissue surrounding the collecting tubule; and the hyperosmolality resulted from the counter-current mechanisms previously described.

Urine Concentration. If the body is dehydrated and there is an increase in ECF osmolality, the osmoreceptors stimulate the pituitary to secrete antidiuretic hormone. The ADH can affect only the membranes of the distal convoluted tubule and the collecting ducts to increase their permeability to water. Thus the hypotonic tubular fluid from the ascending limb of the loop of Henle, as it enters the distal tubule, begins to lose water through the wall of the tubule into the cortex surrounding it. Water diffuses from the distal tubule into the cortex because (1) the osmolality of the interstitial fluid in the cortex is the same as plasma or isosmotic, while the fluid in the tubule is initially hypo-osmolar and so osmotic pressure tends to attract water from tubule into cortex and (2) the antidiuretic hormone has acted upon the membrane of the distal tubule, converting it from a membrane impermeable to water to one that permits the water in the distal tubule to respond to the osmotic pressure difference and move into the cortex. Since the osmolality of the cortical interstitial fluid is isosmolar, the tonicity or osmolality of the fluid in the distal tubule will never exceed isotonicity. When the tubular fluid has traversed the length of the distal tubule, approximately 18 ml. (of the 20 ml. of water leaving the proximal tubule and entering the loop of Henle) of water has been reabsorbed into the cortex. Thus 2 ml. of the original hypotonic fluid remains now as isotonic fluid to enter the collecting tubule.

It will be quite obvious at this point that a urine with an osmolality greater than plasma must be formed from a volume of urine less than 2 ml./minute. It is for this reason that no one has ever encountered an individual who can excrete a concentrated urine in amounts greater than several liters. As the tubular fluid is pushed down the collecting tubule from cortex to calyx, additional amounts of water are withdrawn from the tubule into the interstitial fluid of the medulla. Again the transfer of water requires an osmotic pressure difference between tubular fluid and medullary interstitial fluid, and the antidiuretic hormone to render the collecting tubule wall permeable to water. Since the renal medulla becomes increasingly hypertonic from corticomedullary junction to renal papilla, so the fluid in the collecting tubule becomes increasingly hypertonic as it flows down through the depths of the medulla. Thus the urine may enter the calyx at the rate of 0.3 ml./minute or 432 ml./24 hours with an osmotic pressure equal to 4 times that of plasma or about 1,160 m Osm. The high osmolality of urine is made possible by the marked hypertonicity of the medulla which in turn is created by the counter-current mechanisms in the medulla.

Urine Dilution. If a patient is given a large amount of water orally, the fluid is absorbed from the gut into the blood stream and lowers the osmotic pressure of the plasma and the extracellular fluid. Water then diffuses from the extracellular fluid into the osmoreceptors and causes them to distend. The distention inhibits the stimulating effect of osmoreceptors upon the pituitary, and the secretion of ADH stops. With the fall in the blood level of ADH the membranes of the distal convoluted tubule and the collecting tubule regain their impermeability to water. As a consequence the hypotonic fluid emerging from the ascending limb of the loop of Henle (which has become hypotonic because sodium has been pumped from the ascending limb into the medullary interstitium without accompanying water) at a rate of 20 ml./minute remains hypotonic, despite the isotonicity of cortical tissue surrounding the distal tubule and the hypertonicity of medullary tissue surrounding the collecting tubule. The hypotonic fluid in the distal tubule may become more hypotonic as it flows toward the collecting tubule and the calyx because additional sodium may be reabsorbed actively by the now waterproof membranes of the distal and the collecting tubules.

From the preceding discussion it is apparent that in diabetes insipidus, a syndrome related to lack of secretion of antidiuretic hormone, the individual cannot excrete more than 20 ml. of urine per minute, 1.2 liters per hour or 28.8 liters per 24 hours. When renal disease involves the tubules, a copious dilute urine results because the membranes may lose their responsiveness to the antidiuretic hormone; and, more important, the counter-current mechanisms may be so affected by disease that the medulla loses its hypertonicity.

A bit of reflection upon the preceding discussion involving maintenance of isomolality of the extracellular fluid by the kidneys reveals the following pertinent points: (1) The active transport of sodium by the renal cells serves as the basic mechanism for either excreting a large amount of water in the urine or reabsorbing most of it and excreting a small amount. The active pumping of sodium out of the ascending limb of the loop of Henle is the start of making the urine hypotonic, and this hypotonicity may increase as more sodium is actively transported across water-impermeable membranes of the distal and the collecting tubules. Reabsorption of large amounts of fluid and the excretion of small amounts of urine is made possible, again by the pumping of sodium from the ascending limb of the loop of Henle into the medulla, and producing a hypertonicity which withdraws fluid through the membranes of the distal and the collecting tubules made permeable by antidiuretic hormone. (2) A dilute urine always has its origin in the ascending limb of the loop of Henle. (3) A concentrated urine can be formed only in the collecting tubule.

UREA EXCRETION

In the individual with normal kidneys it will be noted that urea is one of the major solutes in urine. It is rather remarkable that this occurs in view of the fact that urea is so diffusible and that its reabsorption is a passive phenomenon in contrast with glucose and amino acids. The urea filtered by the glomerulus begins to diffuse back through the membrane of the proximal tubule as soon as its concentration has been raised by virtue of the reabsorption of water accompanying the reabsorption of glucose, amino acids and sodium chloride. Under ordinary circumstances about 40 per cent of the filtered urea is reabsorbed through the wall of the proximal tubule.

In the collecting tubule urea reaches a concentration some 70 times that in blood. In order to attain this level it is necessary for the renal medulla surrounding the collecting tubule to have a markedly high urea concentration, since urea always diffuses from a higher concentration to a lower one. It is postulated that the high concentration of urea in the medulla is attained by a recirculation phenomenon of urea. As urea diffuses from the collecting tubule it tends to accumulate in the medullary interstitial fluid and to re-enter the tubules by diffusion into the descending limb of the loop of Henle. In this manner there is more urea entering the collecting tubule than can be found in the fluid coming from the proximal tubule.

Because of the low blood flow in the medulla and its counter-current exchanger configuration, most of the urea diffusing from the collecting duct into the medulla stays in the medulla and leaves only by reentering the descending limb of the loop of Henle; very little is carried away by the blood. Thus a high concentration of urea can be obtained in the medulla with only a small amount of urea diffusing back from the collecting duct.

Since under ordinary circumstances 30 to 40 per cent of the filtered urea is reabsorbed in the proximal tubule and since reabsorption of urea is dependent upon water reabsorption, it follows that in water diuresis little urea is reabsorbed in the distal tubule and thus 60 to 70 per cent of the filtered urea is excreted in the urine. On the other hand, in dehydration much water is reabsorbed in the distal and the collecting tubules; therefore much urea also is reabsorbed (both because of its increased concentration and the action of ADH), and only 40 to 50 per cent of the filtered urea may be excreted into the urine.

DIURETICS[64]

Diuretic agents promote the increased excretion of urine by acting upon the kidney in one fashion or another.

A physiologic diuretic is water. As previously described, the administration of large amounts of water to an individual produces, initially, hypotonicity of the extracellular fluid. The hypotonicity of the extracellular fluid causes movement of water into the osmoreceptor, resulting in swelling of the osmoreceptors and cessation of stimulation of ADH secretion. Decreased circulating ADH causes resumption of the impermeable state of the membranes of the distal and the collecting tubules. Thus a large amount of the 20 ml. of hypotonic fluid emerging from the ascending limb of the loop of Henle passes on into the renal pelvis and causes an increased excretion of urine. It is well to remember that physiologic diuresis results in no net loss of either water or salt from the body. Also, the increased excretion of water starts in the distal convoluted tubule.

An osmotic diuretic is a solute that is filtered by the glomerulus and is found in the tubule in concentrated amounts because of (1) unusual concentration in the blood, or (2) decreased or no reabsorption by the tubules, or (3) both of these factors. In diabetes mellitus there is an increased amount of glucose in the glomerular filtrate because of the high blood sugar. In phlorizin or renal glycosuria there is an increased amount of sugar in the tubules because of decreased tubular resorption. In uremia or azotemia there is an increased amount of urea in the tubule because of high blood concentrations. Mannitol is an osmotic diuretic because it is not reabsorbed at all by the renal tubule.

The osmotic diuretic opposes the reabsorption of water by the tubule through its osmotic activity. In turn the increased retained water in the tubule inhibits sodium reabsorption because the gradient against which the sodium must be transported is limited and eventually becomes too great as some sodium is reabsorbed and the concentration drops. Thus not only increased amounts of water are presented to the distal tubule but also increased amounts of sodium. It should be noted that unlike physiologic water diuresis, osmotic diuresis brings an increased amount of water to the loop of Henle and the distal tubule. The increased flow of fluid through the structures in the medulla tends to cause more water to move into the interstices of the medulla, wash out the medulla and reduce the hypertonicity of the medulla. Thus in osmotic diuresis the concentration of the urine always tends to approach that of plasma. In contrast with water diuresis, osmotic diuresis produces a net loss of water and salt from the extracellular space.

Diuretics Used Clinically. Most of these act by inhibiting the reabsorption of sodium. It will be recalled that sodium is reabsorbed by the renal tubule under the influence of (1) aldosterone in an effort to maintain normal extracellular fluid volume and (2) pCO_2 in an effort to maintain a pH of 7.4 of the extracellular fluid. The mercurial diuretics inhibit the reabsorption of sodium and chloride to cause increased excretion of sodium, chloride and water. The mercurials probably act on the cells of the proximal tubule to produce their effect. A typical mercurial diuretic is mercuhydrin.

The carbonic anhydrase inhibitors act as diuretics by preventing the formation of $H·HCO_3$ from H_2O and CO_2. Decrease in hydrogen ion production will lead to (1) decreased exchange of sodium ion for the hydrogen ion and also ammonium ion, (2) decreased absorption of sodium as sodium bicarbonate, and (3) increased excretion of potassium in exchange for the sodium ion. The net result of the inhibition is an increased urinary excretion of sodium, potassium and bicarbonate, and a decreased excretion of ammonium ion and titratable acids. Chloride excretion is not affected. Diamox, a sulfanilamide derivative, is a compound producing diuresis by inhibition of carbonic anhydrase.

Chlorothiazide (Diuril)[65] and its derivatives are diuretics that produce their effects by inhibiting carbonic anhydrase activity and also by inhibiting the reabsorption of chloride. Thus Diuril acts like a combination of mercurial and acetazolamide. It promotes the excretion of sodium, potassium, chloride and bicarbonate. If a mercurial is given in combination with Diuril, there is an enhanced excretion of sodium and chloride over that with either diuretic alone. When Diamox is given in conjunction with Diuril, the excretion of bicarbonate and potassium is markedly enhanced.

The xanthine derivatives (such as aminophylline) act as diuretics by affecting tubular reabsorption of sodium and, in cardiac patients, by also improving myocardial function directly and thus indirectly increasing glomerular filtration.

An acidifying agent such as ammonium chloride can produce diuresis by virtue of the fact that after it is absorbed into the blood stream, the ammonium portion is converted into urea and the chloride ion is made available to combine with the sodium of the sodium bicarbonate buffer. A metabolic acidosis results. Initially much sodium is excreted into the urine with the chloride. However, after several days the ammonium ion mechanism of the kidney is so stimulated by the acidosis that it produces enough ammonium ions to exchange for the sodium ions being lost in urine with the chloride ions of the original HN_4Cl. Thus when additional sodium is no longer excreted, no diuresis results; the individual has become refractory to ammonium chloride diuresis.

Diuresis can be produced by aldosterone antagonists such as the spirolactones.[67] These compounds inhibit the action of aldosterone and cause decreased reabsorption of sodium and decreased excretion of potassium by the tubule. This results in increased sodium excretion in the urine.

Drugs believed to diminish sodium reabsorption in the region of the loop of Henle have been found to be effective diuretics. Furosemide (Lasix) and ethacrynic acid (Esedrix) are two such agents.

RENAL FUNCTION TESTS

QUALITATIVE TESTS

A gross estimation of renal function may be obtained by routine urinalysis. Albumin and casts indicate damage to the glomerulus. In the absence of diabetes mellitus, a high specific gravity of the urine indicates good tubular function. No conclusions can be drawn if the specific gravity is low and the pH neutral or alkaline, because these may be the results of dietary peculiarities and overhydration.

Intravenous or excretory pyelography is a gross test of renal function when a moderate amount (30 to 50 ml.) of 30 to 50 per cent concentration of radiopaque medium is used; under these conditions the renal collecting systems will not be visualized if more than 75 per cent of the total renal parenchyma is functionally inactive.

Determination of blood urea nitrogen or nonprotein nitrogen will afford a gross estimate of renal function. The blood levels of these substances become elevated above normal when more than 75 per cent of total kidney tissue is damaged. With lesser damage these determinations give the physician no idea of the renal status. Other factors such as dehydration, gastrointestinal hemorrhage and excessive catabolism may cause an elevation in the blood nonprotein and urea nitrogen levels, the so-called prerenal azotemia.

QUANTITATIVE TESTS

The clearance tests provide a fairly accurate estimate of renal function. The urea and creatinine clearance tests[72] provide an estimate of glomerular filtration. The normal urea clearance[71] varies between 70 to 120 per cent of average normal, while the normal creatinine clearance value is about 140 L. per 24 hours. The onset of uremia may occur when the urea clearance drops below 25 per cent of normal or the creatinine clearance below 35 to 45 liters/24 hours.

The serum creatinine concentration has been correlated with the creatinine clearance, and it can be said that there is a linear relationship between these two quantities.[69] The difficulty of obtaining strictly accurate urine collections and the additional time and expense of the clearance study make the simple serum creatinine more valuable. A serum creatinine level of 1.0 mg. per cent is correlated with 100 per cent normal creatinine clearance. When the clearance falls to 25 per cent of normal the serum creatinine is 2.0 mg. per cent. As this relationship is linear, 7.5 per cent decrease in glomerular filtration may be equated to each 0.1 mg. per cent of serum creatinine above 1.0 mg. per cent.

The phenolsulfonphthalein or PSP test[70] and the concentration test estimate tubular function. The PSP determination measures the ability of the renal tubules to excrete 6 mg. of parenterally administered phenolsulfonphthalein. Normal kidneys will excrete 33 per cent of the dye in 15 minutes. The 15-minute PSP test is also a measure of glomerular status in that it has been shown that the glomerular function can rarely be more impaired than tubular function.[70] Thus, the PSP determination, in addition to giving an estimation of tubular efficiency, also provides an index of the minimal glomerular function compatible with that degree of tubular function. *The 15-minute PSP determination is the best routine clinical quantitative test of renal function.*

The concentration test can be performed in a number of ways. The urinary specific gravity obtained with it depends on the length of the period of dehydration. The concentration test is not particularly good because: (1) it cannot follow progressive impairment of renal function after the specific gravity of the urine becomes fixed; and (2) 12 to 16 hours of dehydration may endanger the life of the patient with poor renal function.

In many situations the urologist finds it necessary to ascertain the function of each kidney separately. This knowledge is especially important in suspected cases of renal hypertension or when nephrectomy is contemplated. The performance of a nephrectomy in the presence of a contralateral poorly or nonfunctioning kidney is a catastrophe. Separate determinations of the function of each kidney (split-functions) are obtained by inserting catheters up the ureters into the renal pelves. Then, the PSP test, creatinine clearance, sodium excretion, fluid volume output or urine osmolality may be determined for each kidney.

RENAL FUNCTION IN DISEASE

Obviously, the renal tubule has many functions while the glomerulus apparently has only one. Therefore, renal abnormalities may manifest themselves in as many different ways as there are tubular functions; for example, glycosuria, cystinuria, renal rickets, etc. The more common renal diseases such as pyelonephritis,[76] hydronephrosis, glomerulotubular nephritis[74] and hypertensive renal disease tend to present the same clinical and laboratory findings when renal deterioration becomes advanced.

Impairment of glomerular filtration, whether due to increased intratubular hydrostatic pressure as in hydronephrosis, structural change in the glomerular membrane as in glomerular nephritis and intercapillary glomerular sclerosis or inflammatory involvement as in pyelonephritis, will lead to an accumulation of all metabolic end products destined to be excreted from the body primarily by the kidneys. Particularly, the products of protein metabolism, such as phosphates, sulfates, urea and uric acid, will accumulate and produce uremia when filtration is sufficiently impaired because they are excreted primarily by the kidneys. Clinically, uremia is attended by nausea, vomiting, diarrhea, malaise, dyspnea on slight exertion, hyperpnea, twitching, anemia, ease of fatigue, and occasionally by acute abdominal pain and tenderness. Blood chemical studies show elevated blood urea and nonprotein nitrogen levels, a decreased serum bicarbonate or carbon dioxide combining power, and increased phosphate and sulfate concentrations. The serum potassium level tends to rise above 5 mEq./L. As the blood level of phosphate rises that of calcium falls. The ionized calcium may remain normal if the concomitant acidosis is sufficiently great.

ACUTE RENAL FAILURE

Etiology. Acute renal failure, for a time called the lower nephron syndrome, has been observed in patients poisoned with carbon tetrachloride, bichloride of mercury, uranium nitrate, phosphorus, bismuth, etc., and in patients in shock caused by severe dehydration, Addison's disease, hemorrhage and trauma. In other words, acute renal failure can be caused by (1) *nephrotoxins* and (2) any condition which leads to a prolonged period of *renal ischemia*.

Pathology. The kidneys of most patients dying with acute renal failure are swollen, have cortical pallor and a dark blue medulla. Microscopically, 2 types of lesions[94] are found: a generalized proximal tubular cellular (nephrotoxic) necrosis down to the basement membrane but not including it; and a randomly distributed patchy tubular necrosis, involving the basement membrane (tubulorhexic). The former is believed to be produced by toxic substances, the latter by ischemia.

Patients with acute renal insufficiency who have increased catabolism due to breakdown of traumatized tissue and fever deteriorate much more rapidly than the patient who is afebrile and has no tissue necrosis.

Death may occur at any time during the

period of oliguria or during the first few days of recovery. Pulmonary or cerebral edema incident to the administration of too much fluid may be the cause of death during the first few days.

Diagnosis. Acute renal failure must be distinguished from acute urinary obstruction and from severe dehydration. The history often helps in differentiation. A urinary specific gravity of 1.020 or greater suggests dehydration. A specific gravity of about 1.010 suggests acute renal failure but is not absolutely diagnostic, because dehydrated patients with previous renal disease may exhibit a urinary specific gravity of 1.010. Anuria as distinguished from oliguria is seen in complete urinary obstruction but rarely in acute renal failure. Acute ureteral obstruction can be determined readily by retrograde pyelographic methods.

The therapy of oliguria depends upon the cause. Obstructive anuria or oliguria demands alleviation of the obstruction. Dehydrational oliguria requires the administration of appropriate fluids. Nephrotoxic and tubulorhexic oliguria requires the careful adjustment of diet and fluid administration. An error in diagnosis of the cause of anuria may rapidly lead to an untimely death.

Mechanism of Production of Oliguria or Anuria. An abnormal decrease in urinary output may attend a decreased blood flow through the nephrons,[85] or a complete diffusion of glomerular filtrate back through the damaged tubular wall, acting as an inert membrane.

Clinical Picture. During the early phase the 24-hour output usually will be less than 400 ml. but rarely zero. Examination of the urine may show a specific gravity between 1.010 and 1.015, a pH hovering around 7.0 albumin 1 to 2+, pigment casts, and red and white blood cells. Initially, the blood-chemistry studies may be normal.

As time passes (5 to 7 days) the blood pressure may rise to hypertensive levels, the pulse becomes rapid, the sensorium is dulled, breathing may become rapid and deeper, and vomiting may occur. As these signs of illness develop the concentrations of creatinine, urea nitrogen, polypeptide nitrogen, potassium, phosphate and sulfate increase and that of serum bicarbonate decreases. The sodium and chloride levels, although they may be increased or decreased, are frequently found to be within normal limits. Often anemia will be present. Presumably this is caused by hemolysis and depressed erythropoiesis.

After the passage of 5 to 10 days the urinary output may suddenly increase. However, usually little or no clinical or chemical improvement will attend this change for 2 to 3 days, and then improvement occurs gradually.

Therapy. Because death from acute renal failure is often attributable to hyperkalemia or the giving of excessive fluids, therapy should be directed toward alleviating processes causing hyperpotassemia, inorganic acidosis and toward maintaining proper hydration.

To decrease protein catabolism with its production of sulfate, phosphate and urea, and to decrease the formation of ketone bodies from fat, 100 Gm. of carbohydrate per day in the form of rock candy orally or 15 per cent glucose in water parenterally need be given. This amount of carbohydrate will decrease the rate of rise in nitrogen, potassium and acids. Some fatty substances may be given also to supply additional calories without nitrogen, sulfate, phosphate, or potassium. However, the giving of fat usually complicates the picture because it aggravates the nausea already present and often induces vomiting, thereby depriving the body of fluids and electrolytes. Giving much more than 100 Gm. of carbohydrate will not further decrease protein breakdown. By adhering strictly to glucose or rock candy as foodstuff, there will be no opportunity for other foods containing protein and potassium to be given to the patient inadvertently.

Unless the blood volume is below normal or the hemoglobin concentration is below 10 Gm. per 100 ml., blood transfusions should not be given during the period of oliguria because they may trigger the onset of pulmonary congestion and cardiac failure.[92] Furthermore, a mild transfusion reaction which would not endanger normal kidneys could well tip the scales against recovery in these patients. Similarly, the giving of alkaline electrolyte solutions (sodium lactate or bicarbonate) as treatment for acidosis is contraindicated unless hyperpnea due to uncompensated acidosis is present. In most cases of acute renal failure neither the anemia nor the acidosis is of sufficient severity to warrant the use of remedial measures, the side effects of which may cause death.

The daily water requirements of any patient can be calculated roughly by considering the water lost and the water gained by the body. If an individual be starved, the body will be provided approximately 300 ml. of water each day from the water of oxidation of carbohydrate, protein and fat, and from the water of solution (water holding protein and carbohydrate in solution in cells); this is water gained from within the body. The body loses water under normal conditions through the skin, the lungs, the urinary tract and the bowel. Water vapor loss through the skin and the lungs is called insensible loss and under average conditions of temperature and humidity amounts to about 600 to 800 ml. per 24 hours. Insensible loss increases with fever and hyperpnea. Unless the patient has diarrhea, water loss in the feces is negligible. Thus a patient with an oliguria of 100 ml. per 24 hours, loses 800 ml. of water by insensible loss, 100 ml. of water in the urine and gains 300 ml. of water from oxidation and water of solution. Subtracting 300 from 900 ml. leaves a 24-hour net loss of 600 ml. of water from the body. Thus fluid replacement should be 600 ml. of a 10 or 15 per cent solution of glucose in water if it is given intravenously or 600 ml. of water containing 100 Gm. of carbohydrate if it is given orally. If urinary output increases, additional water equal to urinary flow (within limits) should be added to insensible loss. Any losses through vomiting or diarrhea should be replaced *with appropriate electrolyte solutions*. (See Chap. 5, Fluids and Electrolytes.)

It is well to start a patient on rectal ion-exchange resins as soon as the diagnosis of acute renal failure is made, for hyperkalemia is inevitable. Serum potassium levels can be kept within normal range very readily with the use of sulfonate resins. Emergency measures such as intravenous insulin and glucose or one sixth molar sodium lactate may be necessary to reduce rapidly the near-lethal serum potassium levels in patients just admitted to the hospital.

Using the therapeutic regimen just outlined, pulmonary and cardiac complications will be minimized; and as the kidneys recover, the extent of the diuresis will be limited. Some of the patients with acute renal failure will recover completely using the therapeutic regimen just outlined. However, those patients with increased catabolism due to extensive ecchymoses, massive hemorrhage into body cavities or the gastrointestinal tract, marked soft tissue trauma, high fever, active delirium and infections, demonstrate rapidly rising levels of end products of protein metabolism with associated clouding of the sensorium. In this situation it is imperative to utilize some form of dialysis in order to save the patient's life. Intermittent irrigation of the peritoneal cavity[90] and hemodialysis[92] are the two methods most commonly used at the present time. We employ the Kolff coil type of artificial kidney at the University of Michigan Medical Center and have found it to be extremely satisfactory from all aspects, including compactness, the time necessary to prepare the unit for use and efficiency of dialysis.

Some practitioners are using a small artificial kidney to dialyze the patient daily in an effort to prevent the onset of uremia.[95]

Formerly, it was believed that persons recovering from acute renal failure pass through a phase characterized by a tremendous urinary output, up to 12 L. per day. However, evidence indicates that, when seen, the "recovery" diuresis is usually iatrogenic,[92] i.e., diuresis occurs mainly in those patients who have received an excessive volume of fluids during the period of oliguria or anuria. Consequently, if recovery diuresis occurs, volume for volume replacement with an electrolyte solution should not be practiced unless incontrovertible signs of dehydration attend it. The patient should be given only enough water to compensate for the insensible loss and to provide for a urinary output of about 2,000 ml.: a total of about 2,700 ml. Occasionally, an excessive urinary loss of fluid requires replacement; but in these instances replacement will be indicated by physical evidences of dehydration (see Chap. 5, Fluid and Electrolytes). During the recovery phase it is well to check the output of sodium and chloride in the urine, for occasionally it becomes excessive and should be replaced. A good replacement solution contains sodium, chloride and lactate or bicarbonate.

CHRONIC RENAL FAILURE

Until relatively recently patients dying from advanced renal disease had no hope for recovery. Now renal transplantation[100] and chronic hemodialysis[98] have permitted the survival of these people for a number of years. Many problems are still present in the use of both methods but these are gradually being solved. It is anticipated that an ever-increasing number of those dying from renal failure will be restored to a useful, productive status in society in the future. (See Chap. 19, Transplantation.)

HYPERTENSION

All physicians should be concerned with the recognition of curable hypertension, i.e., secondary or nonessential hypertension. This may result from thyrotoxicosis, Cushing's syndrome, primary aldosteronism, pheochromocytoma or renal artery stenosis. The urologist is intimately involved in the investigation and the treatment of patients suspected of having secondary hypertension. Thyrotoxicosis is a rare but frequently overlooked cause of hypertension and will not be discussed further here.

ADRENAL CAUSES

Cushing's syndrome is an infrequent cause of hypertension but one that can be treated readily by removing the adrenal source of the excess cortical steroids. Fortunately, those patients with significant hypertension of this etiology usually have florid hypercorticism and all the clinical and laboratory abnormalities that result from functioning adrenal cortical hyperplasia, adenoma or carcinoma.

Primary aldosteronism[104] is a much more subtle cause of hypertension. These patients do not appear hypercorticoid, may be asymptomatic (except for occasional periods of weakness, resulting from hypokalemia), but eventually develop chemical abnormalities of reduced serum potassium and increased sodium concentration, alkalosis, and persistently alkaline urine. It has been suggested that the hypertension may antedate the chemical abnormalities by months or years.[102, 105] Primary aldosteronism generally results from a small adenoma of the adrenal cortex but may be associated with hyperplasia or carcinoma.

The suppression of renin formation by excessive aldosterone has led to the development of a laboratory test that distinguishes primary aldosteronism from other causes of hypertension associated with secondarily increased aldosterone formation.[103]

In both renal ischemia and primary aldosteronism the aldosterone output is increased. However, the renin level in aldosteronism is very low, whereas in renal ischemia it is quite high.

Diagnosis and localization of adrenal adenoma have been facilitated by percutaneous selective adrenal venography.[105]

Treatment involves partial or complete adrenalectomy.[114, 115]

Pheochromocytoma results from a functioning tumor of the adrenal medulla or other chromaffin tissue which produces norepinephrine and/or epinephrine. This hypertension usually occurs in paroxysms accompanied by sweating, palpitation and anxiety but may result in sustained hypertension on occasion. Pharmacologic tests (Regitine and histamine) or chemical tests (catecholamine or VMA analysis of urine) are available but may be falsely positive or negative. Treatment of these lesions is adrenal exploration and adrenalectomy. Excretory pyelograms and retroperitoneal CO_2 studies may be helpful, but the adrenal neoplasms are usually too small to detect by these methods. Occasionally very large neoplasms, which are usually malignant, can be detected by these means.

RENAL ARTERY STENOSIS

More than 30 years ago Dr. Goldblatt demonstrated that hypertension could be produced by constriction of the renal artery in dogs. It is apparent now that not all unilateral renal disease and not even all renal artery stenosis produces hypertension in man.[110, 113, 118, 119] The urologist is intimately involved in the recognition of renal artery lesions producing hypertension and in the treatment of these lesions with conservation of as much functioning renal tissue as possible. The mechanism that produces hypertension in renal artery stenosis has not been completely elucidated but it has been observed that high-grade obstruction of the renal artery (with greater than 40 mm. Hg gradient by direct measurement) produces decreased renal blood flow or decreased renal pulse pressure, decreased glomerular filtration and slow progress of the glomerular filtrate through the tubule with excessive reabsorption of water and sodium and resultant hyperconcentration of those substances that cannot be reabsorbed (creatinine, PSP, PAH and contrast media).[120] The theory has been advanced that increased renin production by the juxtaglomerular cells results in increase of angiotensin and aldosterone.[109] Renin is the enzyme that catalyzes the reaction producing angiotensin, a potent pressor agent and a stimulus for aldosterone secretion.

In the investigation of the patient with hypertension the history and the physical examination are of great importance. Patients with renal hypertension usually have sustained significant hypertension and few evidences of damage to target organs (retinopathy, cardiomegaly or reduced renal function). An abdominal bruit may be present due to the turbulent flow past the stenosis. Other evidences of vascular disease may be present. The hypertension is usually of recent onset or has recently undergone exacerbation. There is no family history of hypertension such as is common in the patients with essential hypertension. There is often no history of antecedent urinary tract disease. Patients are usually less than 40 years of age or more than 55 years of age, whereas those with essential hypertension are in the middle years.

When there is evidence for renal hypertension in the history and the physical examination, special excretory pyelography is indicated. The contrast medium is injected rapidly and exposures are made at 30 sec., 2 min., 3 min., 5 min., 10 min., 15 min., and 30 min.[108] Significant pyelographic signs include decrease in renal size on the ischemic side with delayed initial visualization and late hyperconcentration on that side. Ureteral notching due to pressure on the upper ureter by collateral vessels may be seen. When there has been renal infarction or segmental artery disease, irregularity of the renal outline may be observed. The "routine" pyelogram may be perfectly normal in renal hypertension. A positive pyelogram or strongly positive history and physical examination should lead to arteriography by the route most suited to the patient. Generally, transfemoral percutaneous retrograde renal arteriography will give the most satisfactory results.

When a significant abnormality is seen on the arteriogram, separate renal function studies [107, 117, 121] will help to determine the functional significance of an anatomic lesion. If there are bilateral lesions, the more important side may be revealed. The separate function studies are based on the phenomenon of excessive water and sodium reabsorption occurring on the ischemic side with hyperconcentration of those substances not reabsorbed. Therefore, when measured by direct ureteral catheterization, there is a decreased urine volume with lower sodium concentration and higher creatinine or PAH concentration on the ischemic side. The ^{131}I renogram and the Hg renoscan may be helpful in selected cases and in following the treated patient but generally cannot be relied upon as a single screening study.[122]

Treatment consists of the operation most appropriate for the specific lesion.[123] Nephrectomy, heminephrectomy, specific treatment of other renal pathology, and revascularization by various technics have been utilized with a cure rate of 67 per cent in correctly selected cases. These procedures are of fair magnitude and some thought should be given to the risk involved for the individual patient before embarking upon an elaborate program of studies, for it may be clear from the outset that the patient cannot tolerate operative treatment if a correctable lesion is found. The degree to which nephrosclerosis from the effects of sustained elevated blood pressure on the contralateral side may prevent cure by nephrectomy or revascularization has not been completely evaluated. However, the fact that sustained hypertension may produce irreversible nephrosclerosis and other vascular changes may be an indication for an earlier diagnosis and more vigorous treatment.[124, 125]

OBSTRUCTIVE URINARY TRACT DISEASE

General Physiopathology

Interference with the normal orderly propulsion of urine anywhere along the urinary tract will lead to functional and structural changes in the urinary tract proximal to the

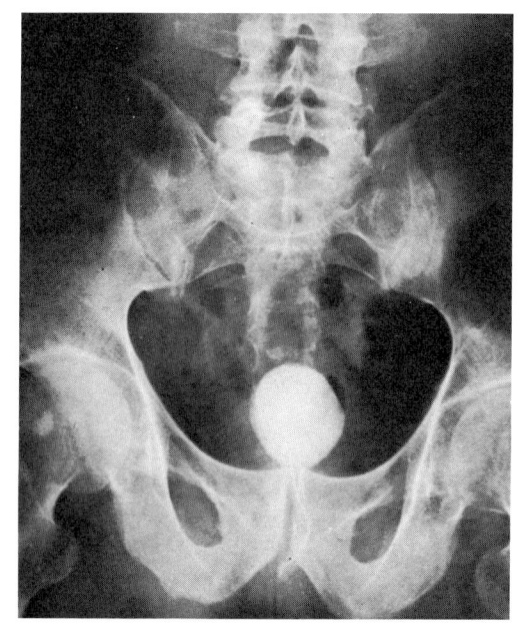

FIG. 52-7. (*Top, left*) Cystogram of a normal bladder. (*Top, right*) Cystogram of a bladder with trabeculation, cellules and small diverticula. (*Bottom*) Cystogram of a bladder with several diverticula.

obstruction. For example, a stricture of the urethral meatus impedes urinary expulsion and, after a time, in a child will be attended by dilation of the urethra proximal to the stricture,* the bladder hypertrophies and becomes trabeculated. Later, outpouching cellules consisting of mucosa not covered by muscle develop; these are called diverticula. Cystoscopically, the interior of the trabeculated bladder looks like a lattice. Figure 52-7 (*Top, left*) is the cystogram of a normal bladder made by taking a roentgenogram of the bladder filled with a solution of sodium iodide; its outline is smooth. In Figure 52-7 (*Top, right and bottom*) the irregular serrated outline indicates trabeculation, cellule and diverticulum formation.

Bladder diverticula are either acquired or congenital. A congenital diverticulum consists of muscle, mucosa and serosa, whereas the acquired type lacks the muscular coat. Small completely evacuable diverticula require no treatment; large incompletely emptying ones

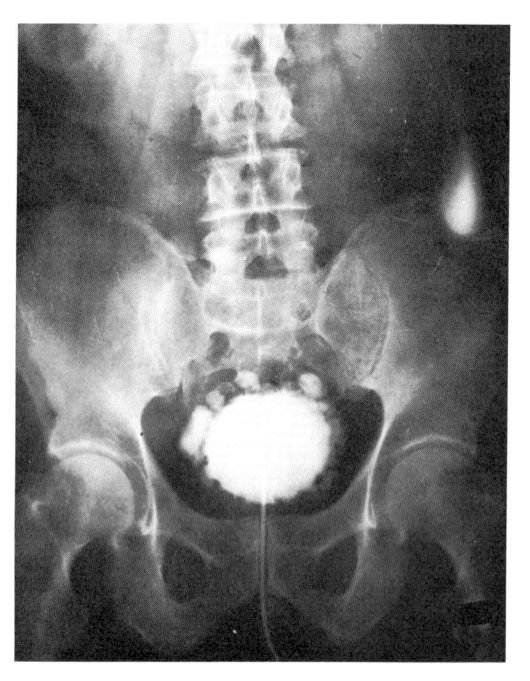

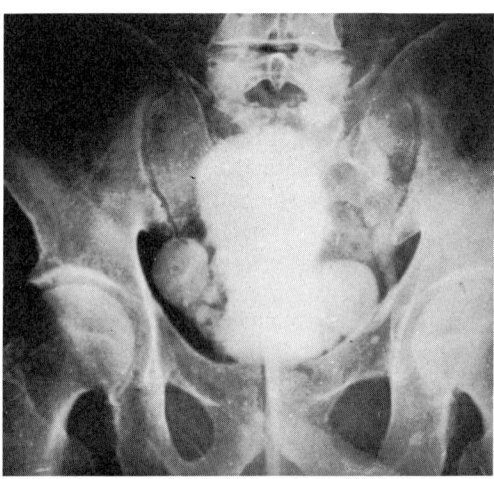

* This does not occur in the adult urethra.

do. Excision through a suprapubic approach is the only means of eradicating those requiring treatment. Occasionally, neoplasms arise in bladder diverticula.

Continuance of urethral obstruction results eventually in decompensation and atonicity of the bladder and urinary retention. Occasionally, as the bladder decompensates the valvular mechanism at the ureterovesical junction becomes incompetent and allows reflux of urine up the ureters (illustrated in the cystogram shown in Figure 52-8). Ureteral reflux does not occur from normal bladders. However, even though reflux may not occur in the face of urethral obstruction, nevertheless vesical obstruction with dilatation and atonicity of the bladder is attended by hypertrophy of the ureteral musculature and later by dilatation and elongation of the ureter. A similar process occurs within the pelvis and calyces producing hydro-ureter and hydronephrosis (Fig. 52-9).

As hydro-ureter and hydronephrosis develop the hydrostatic pressure within the renal pelvis and calyces increases and impairs glomerular filtration and tubular function[126, 128, 129, 131] (as discussed in Renal Physiology and Renal Function in Disease). Tubular function is impaired by 2 processes: by direct pressure atrophy and by compression of the peritubular capillary network. Both the direct pressure upon the renal tubules and the compression of the peritubular capillaries ultimately destroy the renal parenchyma.[127]

In brief, the effects of obstruction of the distal urinary tract are: (1) dilatation of the urethra in children (meatal obstruction); (2) hypertrophy, trabeculation, and the formation of cellules and diverticula of the bladder; (3) atonicity of the bladder; (4) ureteral reflux; (5) hydro-ureter, hydronephrosis and renal atrophy; (6) temporary or permanent loss of renal function incident to impaired glomerular filtration and tubular function, and (7) urinary tract infection. The role of obstructive uropathy in urinary tract infection has only recently been recognized.[128] It has been suggested that obstruction causes increased intraluminal pressure proximal to the impediment which, in turn, decreases blood flow through the wall of the organ and renders it susceptible to hematogenous or lymphogenous invasion by pathogenic organisms.

GENERAL THERAPY

The treatment of any obstruction of a tubular organ consists of the removal or the short-circuiting of the obstruction. If the patient is very sick, a simple diversion or short-circuiting of the urinary stream is necessary. Depending upon the site of the obstruction, the diversion may be effected with an inlying urethral catheter, a perineal urethrostomy, a suprapubic cystostomy, a ureterostomy or a nephrostomy. The site of diversion needs to be proximal to the obstruction. Urinary diversion permits the urinary tract and the kidneys to

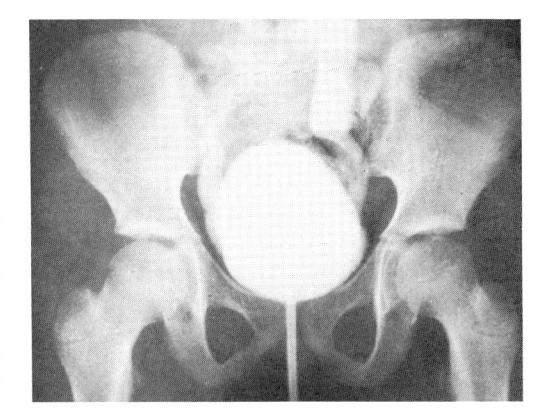

FIG. 52-8. Cystogram of a bladder with bilateral ureteral reflux.

recover by relieving back-pressure upon them. In some cases the diversion of the urine for 3 or 4 days is attended by a fall of NPN to normal, alleviation of the acidosis and relief from anorexia, nausea and vomiting. In others a urinary diversion for several months may be required to restore renal function adequately. A few patients require diversion permanently because it is not possible to restore adequate function of the urinary tract. The extent of renal impairment obtaining with an obstruction is directly related to the length of time it has

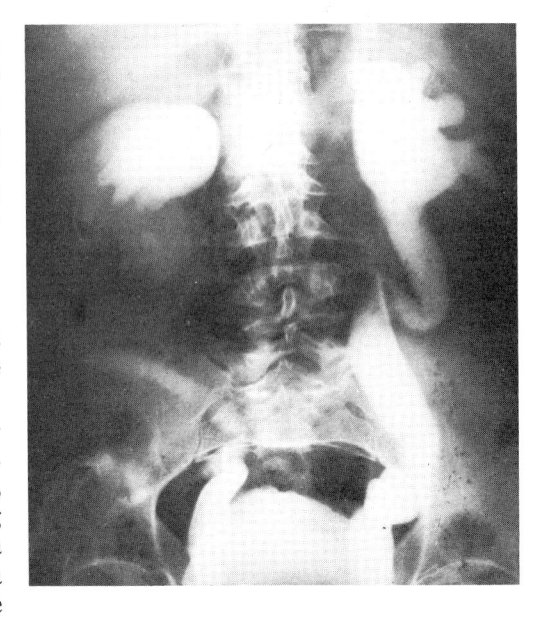

FIG. 52-9. Bilateral hydro-ureter and hydronephrosis.

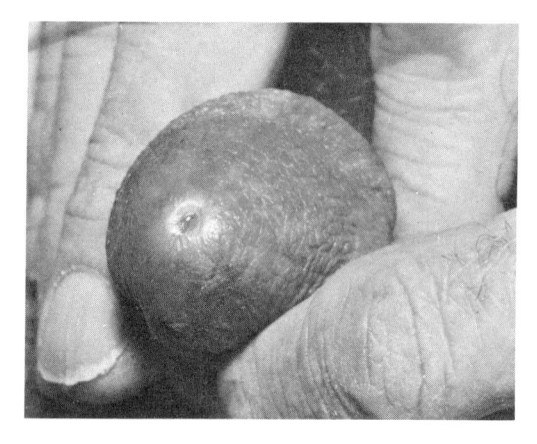

FIG. 52-10. Congenital narrowing of the urethral meatus.

existed and the completeness of the obstruction.

SPECIFIC OBSTRUCTIONAL UROGENITAL DISEASES

Congenital. URETHRA. A congenital pinpoint narrowing of the urethral meatus[144] occurs occasionally in male infants (Fig. 52-10). It may manifest itself as a needlelike stream when the child voids or as a continuous wetting of the diaper with subsequent excoriation of the perineum and the lower abdomen when overflow incontinence occurs. Occasionally, the symptoms and signs of uremia may constitute the first indications of a urethral obstruction. The diagnosis is made upon physical examination and urethral calibration. The performance of a simple urethral meatotomy saves not only the entire urinary tract from destruction, but the baby as well.

URETHRAL VALVES.[147] These occur primarily in boys and are mucosal folds extending from the verumontanum laterally toward the vesical neck so as to form a V on the floor of the prostatic urethra (Fig. 52-11). As the bladder empties, the flowing urine balloons out the mucosal folds, and these then act as valvelike structures to obstruct the urinary flow. Bed-wetting, overflow incontinence and a poor stream in males are the primary signs of this entity in childhood. Every mother, when taking the newborn male child home, should be instructed to observe the character of the urinary stream when the child urinates while lying on his back unclothed. A high stream is normal, a low stream under 1 foot in height should bring him to a urologist.

The diagnosis is made with the use of voiding urethrocystography and urethroscopy. The urogram usually shows a constriction in the region of the membraneous urethra and a marked enlargement of the prostatic urethra (Fig. 52-12). Transurethral transection or resection of the mucosal folds is the easiest and most effective form of therapy.

Occasionally urethral valves may be found in female children[147] and are diagnosed and treated in much the same fashion as the male posterior urethral valve.

PENIS. Occasionally the preputial opening is so small that obstruction to urination occurs. This is called phimosis.[138] The symptoms and signs are similar to those of urethral meatal stricture. On inspection an apparent enlargement of the penis is evident, which when palpated is discovered to be a preputial sac distended with urine. The treatment is circumcision.

BLADDER. *Vesical outlet obstruction*[143, 145] may be caused by fibrosis and narrowing of the vesicourethral junction or by a large redundant mucosal fold. More often, increased resistance to urinary outflow is produced by rigidity of the urethrovesical junction. The decreased mobility can be caused by fibrosis or by muscular hypertrophy at the vesical outlet. Although the vesical outlet appears adequate on urethroscopy, it cannot be pulled open during urination as it is in the normal individual. This entity is observed rarely in young girls with histories of persistent or recurrent urinary tract infections.

The cause of urinary obstruction and the extent of damage to the upper urinary tracts can be demonstrated with appropriate diagnostic procedures: cystometric examination, pyelography, voiding cystourography, renal function tests, and endoscopy including urethral calibration with bougie à boule. Treatment consists of (1) excision of the mucosal fold or (2) the plastic revision of the vesical neck to increase its mobility during micturition.

Neurogenic disturbances of the bladder are prone to occur in children suffering from myelodysplasia associated with such entities as spina bifida, myelomeningocele, etc. The signs and symptoms are those met in patients

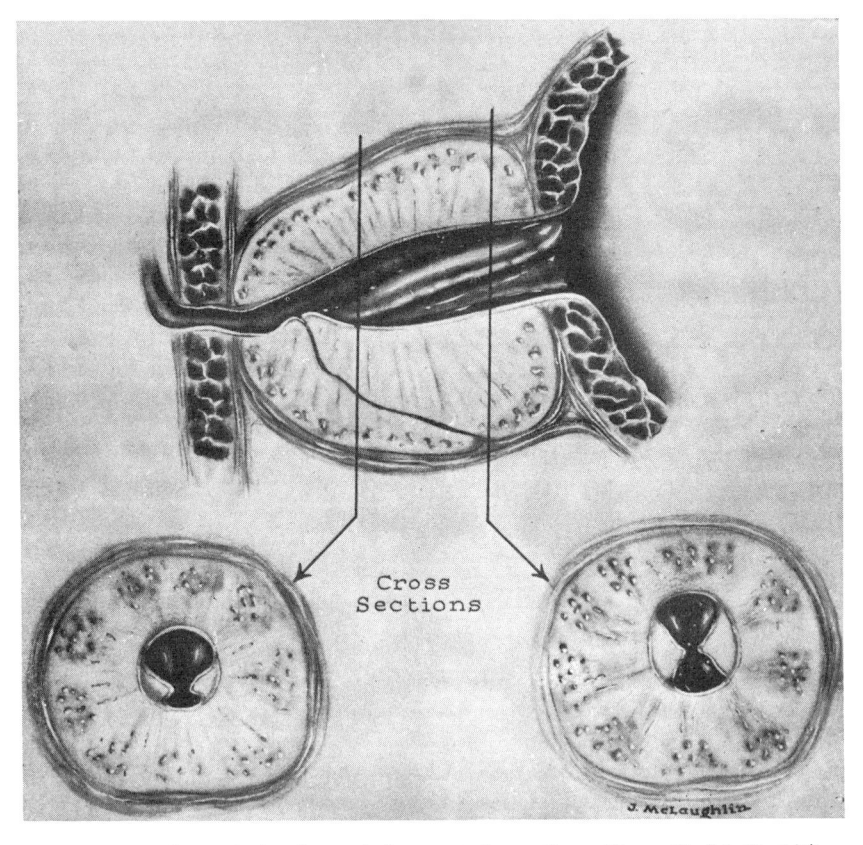

FIG. 52-11. Congenital valves of the prostatic urethra. (From R. M. Nesbit)

with partial or complete motor paralysis of the bladder.[305] In addition to incontinence, excoriation and increased frequency of urination, one of the characteristic signs of a congenital neurogenic bladder is the inability to void a continuous stream. Such children often void only by applying abdominal pressure. The diagnosis is made by cystometric examination and endoscopy. The treatment will vary with the ability of the patient to empty the bladder. It may involve transurethral resection or plastic revision of the vesical neck if the patient carries a large residual urine. The treatment of choice in children with neurogenic bladders due to sacral spinal cord disease is anastomosis of the ureters to an ileal conduit. Recently, the formation of a permanent vesicocutaneous fistula to drain the bladder constantly into a collecting device appears to be superior to the ileal conduit.[139]

URETER. *Ureterocele* (Fig. 52-13) is an

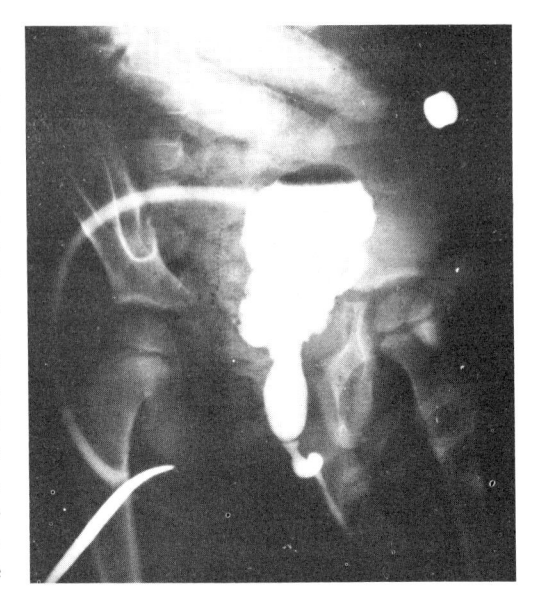

FIG. 52-12. Urethral valves.

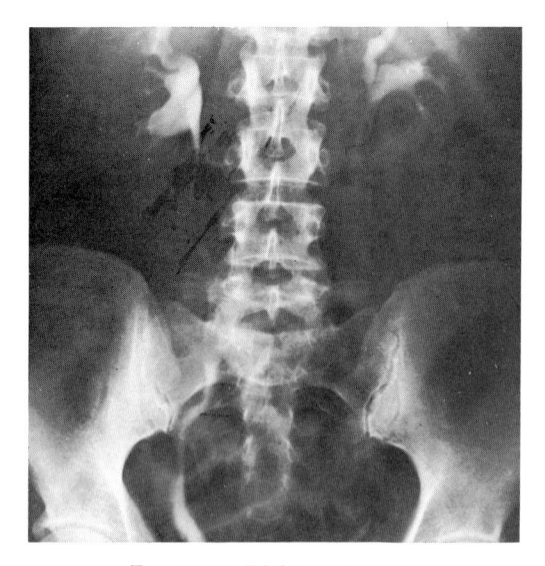

FIG. 52-13. Right ureterocele.

abnormality of the distal end of the ureter characterized by a cystic enlargement of the ureter protruding into the bladder lumen. It is thought to be caused by a narrowing of the ureteral meatus with resultant dilatation of the intravesical portion of the ureter.[133] The ureterocele may be small, unilateral and associated with mild hydronephrosis or it may be so large that it obstructs the bladder-outlet. A ureterocele obstructing the vesical outlet causes bilateral hydro-ureter, hydronephrosis and decompensation of the bladder. The patient may be asymptomatic if the ureterocele is small. If the ureterocele obstructs micturition at the vesical neck, overflow incontinence, dysuria, increased frequency of urination and a small weak stream will attend it. Diagnosis is made by cystoscopy. The treatment consists of the transurethral enlargement of the ureteral meatus in the case of small ureteroceles or its suprapubic excision if large and obstructing.

Congenital megalo-ureter is a condition in which unilateral or bilateral dilatation of the ureters occurs without any apparent evidence of organic obstruction distal to the hydro-ureter. Most of the cases that appear to be congenital megalo-ureter are found, upon meticulous examination, to be related to unrecognized neurogenic bladder, obstruction, abnormal voiding habits (particularly in the female[141, 142] and defects in the musculature of the distal ureter[134]).

Persistent pyuria and ureteral reflux are the most common manifestations of the disease. Other symptoms that attend it may be due to uremia, e.g., anorexia, malaise, anemia, delayed growth, etc. The diagnosis is made by pyelography and cysto-urethrography after organic obstructive entities have been excluded by endoscopy, cystometrography, and, perhaps, surgical exploration of the vesical outlet.

No completely satisfactory treatment is known for this disease.[134, 146] Therapy may involve excision of the distal end of the ureter and reimplantation of the ureter into the bladder.[149]

Ureteropelvic obstruction may be caused by a congenital narrowing of the upper ureter, a congenital high insertion of the ureter into the renal pelvis, compression of the ureter by anomalous renal vessels or defective development of the musculature of the proximal ureter.

Hydronephrosis and impaired renal function follow ureteropelvic obstruction. If the obstruction is unilateral, the patient may not be at all ill and carries only a ballotable mass in the flank. If infection occurs, a persistent pyuria, recurrent episodes of chills, fever and flank pain may be the predominant manifestations. A diagnosis of obstruction at the ureteropelvic junction can be made only with pyelography which shows a hydronephrosis coupled with a normal ureter (Fig. 52-14). If the hydronephrosis is far-advanced and the disease is limited to one side while the other kidney is normal, a nephrectomy is the best treatment. Plastic surgical procedures[135, 136] are requisite to correct the ureteropelvic obstruction if the kidney is worth saving or the disease is bilateral.

SPECIFIC DISEASES

Acquired. URETHRA. Strictures of the pendulous and bulbous portions of the urethra may follow urethral trauma or infection. The most common infection is still gonorrhea. Occasionally, other pyogenic organisms and the tubercle bacillus may be the cause of chronic urethritis and an inflammatory stricture.

Trauma to the urethra from straddle injuries, auto accidents and urethral instrumentation with sounds, catheters or resectoscopes may, after healing, cause severe narrowing of the urethra.

The patient with a urethral stricture may complain of a decrease in size and force of stream, hesitancy in starting urination, dysuria, increased frequency of urination and a feeling of incomplete emptying of the bladder. When complete urinary retention occurs, paradoxic incontinence may ensue. Often the patient with a urethral stricture presents himself to the physician solely with complaints referable to uremia, i.e., fatigue, malaise, anorexia and weight loss, no difficulty in urination having been experienced.

In addition to the usual structural and functional abnormalities produced by obstructive uropathy, a urethral stricture may cause changes peculiar to itself. Strictures are usually associated with *infection and inflammation* of the urethra proximal to the stricture. This, with the high intra-urethral pressure exerted in attempting to void, will frequently disrupt the urethra so that urine will escape through its wall. The escape may be slow and attended by small communicating abscesses. These erode the skin and perforate the skin of the penis, the scrotum or the perineum, forming urethrocutaneous *fistulae*. Numerous urethrocutaneous fistulae opening into the perineum constitute the entity of the "watering-pot" perineum (see Chap. 41, Anorectum).

Should the escape of urine through the wall of the urethra be sudden and massive, the urine extravasates widely along fascial planes. A perforation through the urethral mucosa but within Buck's fascia produces swelling of the penis (not including the glans) and the perineum. An extravasation through Buck's fascia but still contained within Colles' fascial layer tends to give rise to swelling of the penis, the scrotum, the perineum and the anterior abdominal wall. The relationships of the pertinent structures and fascial layers are illustrated in Figure 52-15. Because Colles' fascia is limited laterally by its attachment to the fascia lata and posteriorly by its attachment to the urogenital diaphragm, the only routes for a urinary extravasation contained within this fascia to follow are the abdominoscrotal openings and along the anterior abdominal wall just beneath Camper's and Scarpa's fasciae. These fasciae are continuous with Colles' fascia.

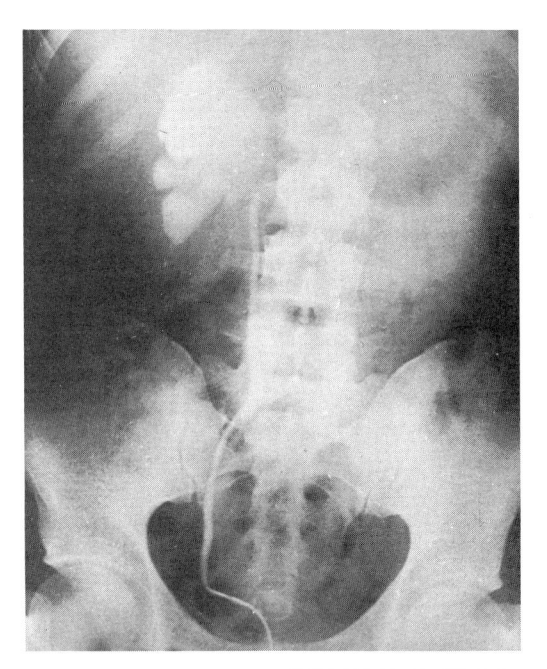

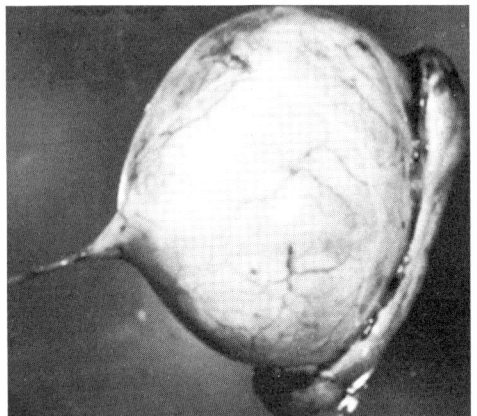

FIG. 52-14. (*Top*) Right hydronephrosis due to ureteropelvic obstruction. Ureter is normal in caliber except at UP junction. (*Bottom*) Actual specimen of a hydronephrotic kidney due to congenital narrowing of the ureter at the ureteropelvic junction. The pelvis is tremendously dilated with a relatively small cap of parenchyma.

The *diagnosis of stricture* of the urethra is made by calibration, i.e., the passage of various bougies or sounds of increasing diameters up the urethra and through the stricture to determine the diameter and the location of the urethral narrowings. Urethroscopy and urethrography[154] may aid in the diagnosis.

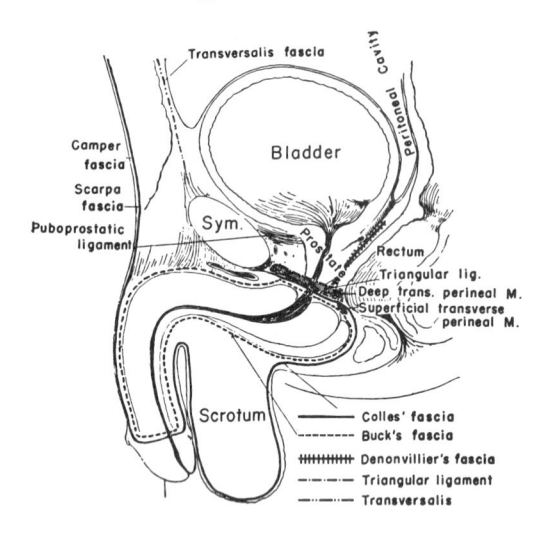

FIG. 52-15. Diagram of fascia of urogenital region concerned in urinary extravasation.

The *prophylactic therapy* of urethral strictures includes (1) the prompt treatment of neisserian and nonspecific pyogenic urethral infections with appropriate antibiotics; (2) the recognition and the splinting of ruptured urethrae;[151, 155, 156] (3) gentleness and care in urethral instrumentation; and (4) the avoidance of prolonged urethral catheter drainage.

Until recently the only therapy available for established urethral strictures was their dilatation at intervals, frequently for the rest of the patient's life. Urethroplasty[152, 153, 157] now may be employed to correct them.

Urethrocutaneous fistulae are treated best by excision of the tracts and elimination of the stricture. Urinary extravasation demands the immediate incision and drainage of all areas in which urine has appeared and the diversion of the urinary stream by suprapubic cystostomy. After recovery from the acute phase, definitive procedures such as the Johanson urethroplasty are employed to remove the urethral stricture—the cause of all the difficulty.

PROSTATE. *Benign prostatic hypertrophy, fibrosis of the prostate* and *carcinoma of the prostate* are the 3 most common prostatic abnormalities causing prostatism. Prostatism must not be confused with prostatitis which refers to inflammation of the prostate gland. *Prostatism* is a term used to describe any or all of the pathologic and clinical manifestations of urinary obstruction caused by the prostate gland.

A knowledge of the anatomy and the physiology of the prostate is necessary to the understanding of the ways by which disease of this gland impedes the passage of urine.

Physiology. The prostate is a part of the male genital system which undergoes a remarkable pubertal development, provided that the anterior pituitary and the testes are normal. Pubertal enlargement of the prostate and the formation of the prostatic secretion are

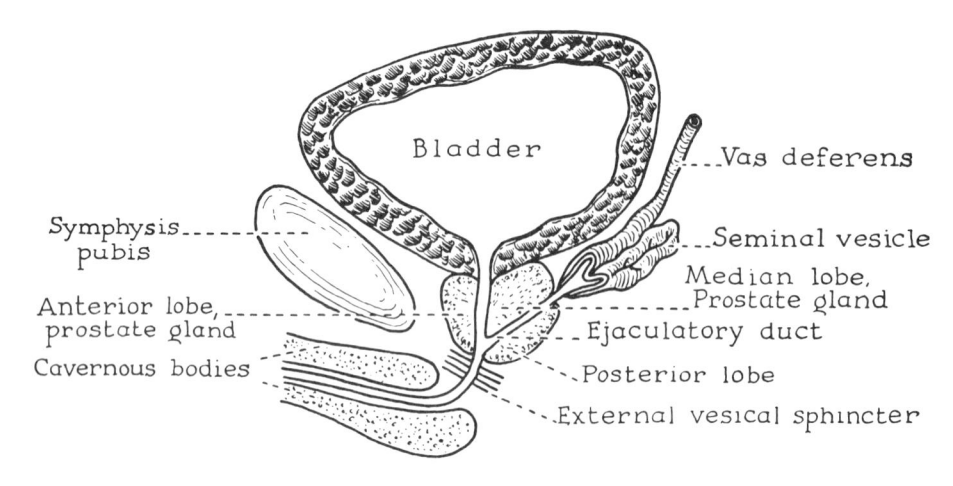

Sagittal Section of Urogenital Tract

FIG. 52-16. Relationships of prostate to its adjacent structures. (R. M. Nesbit)

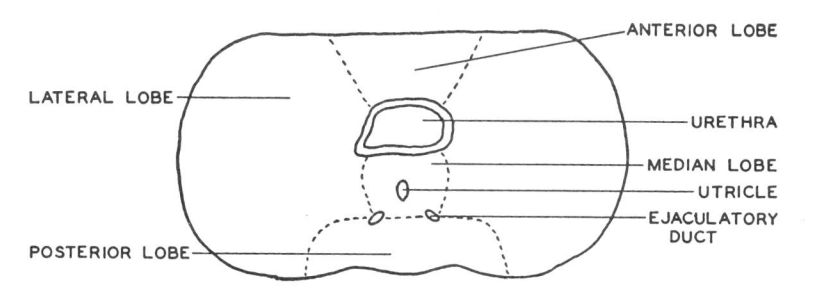

FIG. 52-17. Cross section of the prostate.

dependent upon the elaboration of a hormone from the testicular cells of Leydig. In the adult the function of the prostate is the secretion of a fluid forming a part of the ejaculate and providing a transport vehicle and a nutritional medium for the spermatozoa.

Anatomy. The relationships of the prostate to its adjacent structures are illustrated in Figure 52-16. The bladder rests upon the prostate, and the vesical outlet and the proximal urethra are surrounded by it. The ejaculatory ducts from the seminal vesicles traverse the prostate and open into the urethra on either side of the utricle. The ducts of the prostate open into the urethra on each side of the verumontanum. Figure 52-17, a cross section of the prostate, shows it to be composed of 5 lobes: 1 anterior, 2 lateral, 1 median and 1 posterior. Note how they surround the urethra! The entire gland is enclosed in a strong fibrous capsule and anteriorly is fixed to the symphysis by the puboprostatic ligaments.

Benign Prostatic Hypertrophy. After the age of 45 to 50 the submucosal glands and the smooth muscle of the prostatic urethra undergo glandular and leiomyomatous hyperplasia.[158, 159] This growth presses the normal prostatic tissue against the fibrous capsule and forms a so-called surgical capsule—the compressed normal prostatic tissue.

Primary idiopathic prostatic hypertrophy affects primarily the median and the lateral lobes; the anterior and the posterior lobes are not affected.

As the prostate enlarges, it may expand posteriorly and is readily palpated rectally. This type of enlargement may not encroach upon the vesical neck or the urethra, and consequently there may be no symptoms referable to prostatism even though the prostate may be very large. On the other hand, most or all of the hypertrophy may be toward the lumen of the urethra or upward into the bladder through the vesical outlet. In such a case great difficulty in urination occurs, while no prostatic enlargement is discernible upon rectal digital examination. Clearly, the rectal examination of the prostate gland cannot provide any estimate of the degree of urinary obstruction that may be caused by the gland. However, the rectal examination of the prostate is very important for the determination of the presence or the absence of prostatic carcinoma; in the case of obstructive prostatic hypertrophy it provides the surgeon with a basis for the selection of the appropriate operative procedure.

Vesical Neck Contracture. Increased rigidity of the urethrovesical junction by virtue of hypertrophy of smooth muscle or fibrosis is, in our experience, by far the most common cause of prostatism. It may coexist with prostatic hyperplasia. The fibrosis may be the result of prostatitis. Frequently, strictures of the urethra are associated with it because the inflammatory process may involve both the urethra and the prostate. Prostatic carcinomatous narrowing of the urethra and the vesical neck also cause prostatism. Carcinomas of the prostate usually originate in the posterior lobe and grow infiltratively into the other prostatic lobes, the seminal vesicles and the bladder (see section on Neoplasms for complete discussion).

Clinical Manifestations of Prostatism. The earliest symptoms indicative of prostatism may be associated with recurrent urinary infection or noninfectious irritation of the bladder: they consist mainly of abnormal frequency of urination and dysuria. As the obstruction progresses there occur the complaints of difficulty in starting the urinary stream (hesitancy), a decrease in size and force of stream, an interrupted stream and abdominal straining, which may be so intense as to be associated with the passing of flatus, distention of neck veins and protrusion of the eyeballs. At last comes partial or complete urinary retention with its characteristic functional and structural change of obstructive uropathy.

Diagnosis of prostatism is based upon the history, the physical examination, cystometrography and endoscopy. All of these are necessary because urethral strictures, neurogenic bladders, bladder calculi and acute cystitis, having essentially the same signs and symptoms as prostatism, cannot be differentiated from prostatic hypertrophy, fibrosis, or cancer without them.

Treatment of prostatism varies with the cause of the obstruction, the severity of the obstruction and the condition of the patient. Prostatism with only mild symptoms of nocturia and dysuria sometimes can be treated satisfactorily with elixir of hyoscyamus, tincture of belladonna and hot sitz baths.

The patient with recurrent urinary infection or a weak dribbling stream without residual urine or carrying more than 60 ml. of residual urine requires some form of prostatectomy, provided that he is not gravely ill from another disease.

Should the person be very ill because of uremia, cardiovascular disease, etc., and judged incapable of recovering from a prostatectomy, urinary diversion by suprapubic cystostomy or perineal urethrostomy are performed first to permit improvement in the general health before the prostatectomy. A vasectomy is performed in such cases to reduce the incidence of epididymitis. An inlying urethral catheter is a dangerous form of urinary diversion when practiced for more than a week or two because it predisposes to urethritis, prostatitis, epididymitis, pyelonephritis, urethral strictures and urethrocutaneous fistulae.

Vesical neck contractures are usually remedied by transurethral resection of the prostate. Resection of only the urethrovesical junction may lead to recurrence of the contracture because an incomplete resection predisposes to partially devitalized tissue and chronic infection. On occasion it may be necessary to expose the vesical neck contracture transabdominally, resect a wedge of fibrous tissue and alleviate the rigidity of the vesical neck with a plastic procedure involving the insertion of a flap of mobile bladder wall into the perimeter of the vesical outlet.

The type of prostatectomy performed should be suited to the particular patient's needs. Transurethral prostatectomy[162] is well suited to the palliative treatment of advanced infiltrating prostatic carcinoma and the definitive care of the majority of patients with benign prostatic hypertrophy. The enucleative procedures such as the suprapubic, retropubic[160] or perineal prostatectomy are more suitable for the removal of very large benign hypertrophic prostates. The various enucleative procedures differ in the way the prostate is reached, but once the plane between the surgical capsule and the adenomatous tissue is found, the procedure is the same. With all types of prostatectomy the prostatic urethra is removed; it regenerates in 4 to 6 weeks. The true capsule is not removed excepting with the performance of the radical perineal or retropubic prostatectomy. This is the only known means of curing an early prostatic carcinoma. The presence of bladder calculi or diverticula in addition to an enlarged prostate may influence the surgeon to use the suprapubic or retropubic approach to the prostate. Fixation of the hip joints so that the lithotomy position, requisite for the transurethral approach, cannot be obtained, necessitates the suprapubic or retropubic approach.

BLADDER. *Vesical calculi* (Fig. 52-18) occur

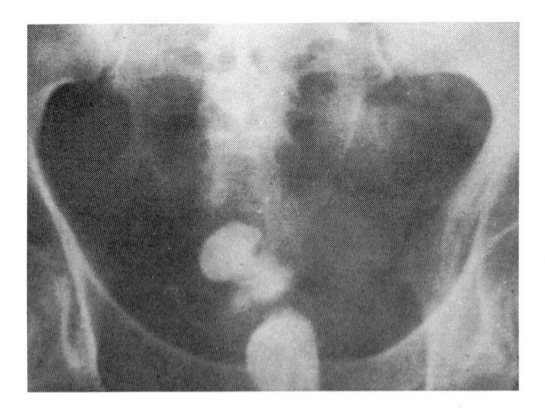

FIG. 52-18. Flat film of the pelvis showing two vesical calculi; one is dumbbell in shape; the other appears to be wedged into the prostatic urethra.

most frequently as a complication of prostatism, though they may form about a foreign body or in conjunction with urinary tract infections or in the presence of a residual urine due to causes other than prostatism. The symptoms and signs of vesical lithiasis may be similar to those of prostatism. However, certain symptoms are pathognomonic of a calculus in the bladder, e.g., the patient may complain of difficulty in voiding in the upright position but have no trouble in the supine position. The diagnosis can be made readily with endoscopy or roentgenography. The treatment involves their removal. This can be accomplished in several ways: (1) usually they can be crushed with a lithotrite transurethrally and the fragments evacuated (litholapaxy) or (2) when very large, removed unbroken by opening the bladder suprapubically (cystolithotomy).

Vesical neoplasms may obstruct the bladder neck or the ureteral orifices.

URETER. *Ureteral stones, neoplasms and strictures* obstruct the ureter and give rise to hydro-ureter and hydronephrosis. Involvement of the ureter by an adjacent neoplasm, e.g., carcinoma of the cervix or the rectosigmoid, may produce ureteral obstruction.

Pregnancy, in most cases, is associated with some degree of hydro-ureter and hydronephrosis. Formerly it was believed that the dilatation of the ureters was due mainly to the elaboration of progesterone[166] and, to a lesser extent, to the pressure of the fetus upon the lower ureteral segments.[164] However, recent evidence suggests that the pressure factor is mainly responsible for the enlargement of the ureters. Ureteral and renal pelvic dilatation begin about the 3rd month of pregnancy and disappear completely 6 to 8 weeks postpartum. The hydronephrosis of pregnancy is a normal physiologic phenomenon (Fig. 52-19).

Intermittent hydronephrosis and hydroureter is a syndrome characterized by recurrent episodes of dilatation of the renal pelvis and the proximal ureter, associated with attacks of pain in the costovertebral angle area and accompanied by nausea, vomiting, tachycardia, and hypotension (sometimes called Dietl's crisis). Often, the onset of pain is associated with excessive diuresis following drinking of beer, "soda pop" or large amounts of water. Sometimes the pain occurs when the person lies in a certain position upon the right side, the left side, or the back) and disappears when the position is changed. e.g., to the erect position. The entity is suspected from the history and may be confirmed by pyelography.[167] Excretory pyelograms, taken when the patient has pain and is lying in the position inducing it, demonstrate hydronephrosis; those performed after the pain has disappeared with position change may show a normal collecting system. Kinking of the ureter over an anomalous renal vessel or fascial band when the kidney shifts with change in position of the body is the cause for the intermittent hydronephrosis associated with change in body position. Treatment consists of relieving pain during the acute attack by change in position or by opiates. Occasionally ureteral catheterization may be required for relief.

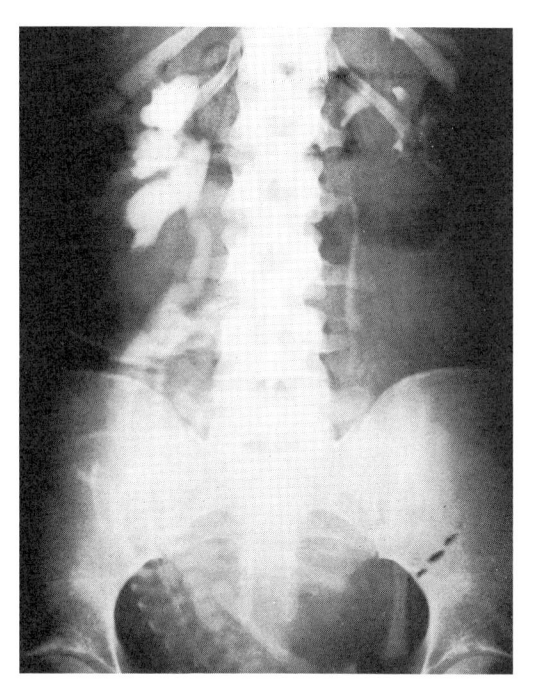

FIG. 52-19. Hydronephrosis of pregnancy.

The cause of intermittent hydronephrosis occurring with excessive hydration is a defective segment of proximal ureter which, under conditions of normal body hydration, evacuates urine from the kidney at a rate sufficient to prevent abnormal distention of the renal pelvis. However, when rate of urine formation becomes high, the proximal ureter cannot cope with it; the renal pelvis gradually becomes overdistended with urine and pain occurs. The defective ureteral segment may function abnormally because of stricture, unusual smooth muscle disposition, hypertrophy or atrophy. Permanent relief from attacks requires surgical excision of the defective ureteral segment and reanastomosis of normal ureter to pelvis. The operative technic includes sparing of aberrant renal vessels in order to avoid infarction of a portion of kidney, with its complications.

For many years, a number of operations have been devised and used for the fixation of the highly mobile kidney—renal ptosis. All normal kidneys move downward when a person stands. Excretory pyelograms taken in both the upright and the supine positions show that normal kidneys always move downward when the person stands up. The distance of descent upon standing varies widely; it may be as little as 1 cm. or as much as 8 to 10 cm. Nevertheless, in all cases it should be considered normal, just as pulse rates varying from 60 to 90 per minute may be normal. *Renal mobility is pathologic only when it can be demonstrated objectively that it is associated with hydronephrosis.* The performance of a nephropexy for a nonhydronephrotic mobile kidney is unwarranted excepting in rare instances.

URINARY TRACT INFECTIONS

Nontuberculous Infections

Gonorrhea. Etiology. A neisserian infection[172] is a venereal disease in adults. The offending organism, the gonococcus, is a nonmotile, gram-negative, intracellular diplococcus.

Pathology. In the male the anterior urethra is invaded first by the organisms. They travel upward along the mucous membrane and in about half of the cases invade the prostatic urethra and prostate. This in some persons ultimately produces a fibrotic contracture of the vesical neck and obstructive uropathy. In addition, the acute infection may penetrate through the mucosa of the urethra into the corpus spongiosum. The inflammatory process in the corpus spongiosum may give rise to a urethral stricture which may not become evident until many years after the attack of gonorrhea. The most common sites of urethral strictures in gonorrhea are the bulbous and pendulous portions of the urethra.

Symptoms and Signs. From 3 to 5 days after exposure to the gonococcus, swelling, redness and pouting of the urethral meatus appear and are associated with the dripping of a greenish-white pus through the urethral meatus. Urination is painful, and painful nocturnal erections are frequent. These occasionally are associated with a downward curvature of the erect penis called chordee. The relative inelasticity of the inferiorly placed inflamed urethra causes the downward curvature.

As the posterior urethra becomes inflamed, the frequency of urination and the dysuria increase, and strangury, the slow, painful passage of urine, may occur.

Diagnosis. The impression of urethral gonorrhea is obtained from the history and the physical examination. A positive diagnosis is made by smearing the urethral discharge and demonstrating the presence of gram-negative intracellular diplococci with stains and is further confirmed by culture.

Treatment. Penicillin is highly effective and inexpensive. As little as one intramuscular dose of 400,000 units may cure gonorrhea.[171] In case of an allergic sensitivity to penicillin, erythromycin, oxytetracycline, chloromycetin, cephalothin or Colymycin may be used. If the organisms are resistant to penicillin, ampicillin in addition to the previously mentioned drugs) has been found to be effective. A cure is judged to have been effected when 1 week after antibiotic therapy no gonococci are grown from cultures of the urethral discharge.

Nongonorrheal Infections.[128, 175, 177, 178] Bacterial invasion of the urinary tract is a very serious matter. It causes discomfort, pain and on occasion, sepsis. It predisposes to calculus formation and strictures. Should bacterial nephritis occur, pyelonephritis may destroy the kidney, jeopardizing the person's life with renal insufficiency or renal hypertensive cardiovascular disease.

Etiology. The occurrence of infection anywhere in the body depends upon the virulence of the microorganisms and the resistance of the patient. Although bacteria are present constantly in the mouth, gut, skin, vagina and urethra and intermittently in the blood stream, invasion of tissues by bacteria occurs relatively infrequently because of the defense mechanisms of the body. It is believed that normal, healthy people are constantly being subjected to transient bacteremias from carious teeth, furuncles and the gut but suffer no ill effects because the organisms are rapidly destroyed by antibodies, etc. In general, most of the antibacterial factors either are present in the blood stream or depend on normal circulation for their activity, as with local tissue immunity. Thus, infection occurs more readily in persons with leukopenia, agammaglobulinemia and anemia or in tissues and organs with disruption of structural integrity or decreased blood supply.

In the urinary tract, stones, neoplasms, parasites, foreign bodies and instrumentation may so traumatize or impair tissue integrity that a urethritis, cystitis, ureteritis or pyelonephritis may result from direct invasion of organisms in the blood stream. Blood supply to the organs of the urinary tract may be diminished by disease involving blood vessels, such as diabetes mellitus and severe arteriosclerosis. More commonly reduction of blood supply to the tissues of the urinary tract involves increase in intraluminal pressure or overdistention of the organ so that its blood vessels are compressed.[181]

The bacteria invading the urinary tract originate from the patient's own intestinal tract and belong to the gram negative bacillary group, *E. coli* being the most common. The bacilli reach the tissue of decreased resistance primarily by way of the blood or lymphatic streams.

In the male it is primarily the obstructive abnormalities such as stricture, prostatism or urethral valves, and neurogenic bladder disease that compromise blood flow; in the female poor or abnormal voiding habits[182, 183] account for more than 80 per cent of the recurrent upper and lower urinary tract infections. It has been demonstrated that infrequent urination leading to overdistention of the bladder is associated with 66 per cent of recurrent urinary infection in adult females and 30 per cent in girls. Persistence of the infantile or uninhibited neurogenic bladder beyond 2 to 3 years of age may result in abnormally high intravesical pressures if the individual withholds urination after an intensive desire to micturate is perceived. This mechanism has been found to present in 60 per cent of female children and 17 per cent of adult females with recurrent urinary infection.

It should be emphasized that nearly all urinary tract infections are related to an abnormality in function or structure of the genitourinary system and that, in order to treat such an infection appropriately, it is necessary to correct the abnormality of the urinary tract as well as use antibacterial medication. Another important point is that many cases of bacterial pyelonephritis are secondary to lower urinary tract infection (e.g., cystitis, urethritis).

Occasionally, the kidney is involved by an acute staphylococcal infection. This infection is so different from the others that it will be discussed as a separate entity under perinephric abscess.

PATHOLOGY. Acute cystitis and urethritis frequently occur without involvement of the upper urinary tract. With these entities the bladder and the urethra are erythematous, edematous and congested. Acute pyelonephritis[176] is an inflammation of the renal pelvis, the tubules and the interstitial tissue. Acute pyelitis is a misnomer, since it is only part of the generalized process of pyelonephritis.

A chronic infection of the bladder frequently may cause hyperplastic cystitis, e.g., cystitis glandularis and cystitis cystica. If the infection is caused by an organism that splits urea, with formation of ammonia, the interior of the bladder may be coated with encrustations of mineral salt—the so-called ammoniacal encrustive cystitis. Cystic change (ureteritis cystica, Figs. 52-20, 52-21) may occur in the chronically infected ureter as it does in the bladder.

Renal parenchymal suppuration may attend acute pyelonephritis. These abscesses tend to break out into the perinephric tissue and produce perinephritis and perinephritic abscesses. Occasionally, the kidney is functionally destroyed. If the pyelonephritis is mild and subsides completely, the kidney may show no demonstrable injury. However, severe pyelonephritis always leaves residua, such as atrophy, fibrosis and cellular infiltration of the renal parenchyma and sclerosis of the renal vessels. The kidney may be smaller than nor-

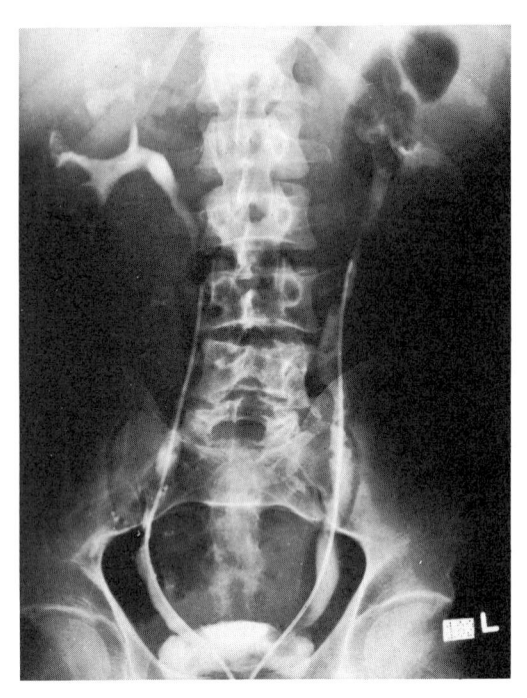

FIG. 52-20. Retrograde ureterogram, illustrating ureteritis cystica.

mal, with narrowed infundibula and hydrocalyces (Figs. 52-22 and 52-23).

Acute pyelonephritis may clear up completely but all too often it only simmers down and smolders and becomes chronic active pye-

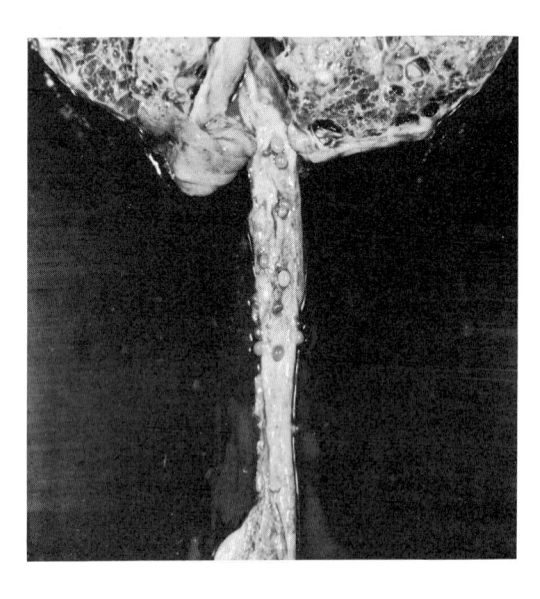

FIG. 52-21. Ureteritis cystica.

lonephritis. Chronic active pyelonephritis is an active inflammatory process of the kidney and its pelvis superimposed upon fibrosis and contracture, etc. This ultimately leads to complete destruction of the kidney and its function, an autonephrectomy.

SIGNS AND SYMPTOMS. Should the infection be limited to the lower tract, an increased frequency of urination, dysuria, urgency, pyuria and occasional hematuria are the predominant signs and symptoms. Should pyelonephritis become superimposed upon cystitis, additional signs and symptoms appear: chills and fever, pain and tenderness in the costovertebral area, nausea, vomiting and prostration.

DIAGNOSIS. The presence of pathogenic bacteria and leukocytes in catheterized urine associated with the above signs and symptoms establishes the diagnosis of a urinary tract infection. Urinalysis including microscopic examination of the stained urinary sediment is the most efficient method for determining the presence of infection;[181] culture and sensitivity studies are reserved as an aid in selecting appropriate medication. Calyceal contractures and abnormalities characteristic of chronic active pyelonephritis may be demonstrated by intravenous pyelography. Retrograde ureteral catheterization may be necessary to confirm the presence and the extent of chronic active pyelonephritis.

THERAPY. Because infection of the urinary tract is believed to be secondary to a functional or structural abnormality of the genitourinary system, it is necessary to seek the cause for the infection and eradicate it before treating the patient with antibacterial medication. This implies the use of diagnostic examinations such as excretory urography, voiding cystourethrography, cystoscopy, urethroscopy, urethral calibration with the bougie à boule and cystometry. If the patient is found to have prostatism, prostatectomy is performed; bladder calculus, cystolithotomy or litholapaxy; neoplasm, excision of tumor; infrequent voider, regimen of frequent voiding; urethral meatal stenosis, meatotomy: vesicorectal fistula, fistulectomy; etc. When the contributing cause is removed, appropriate antibacterial medication is then instituted. Culture and sensitivity studies will help the physician in determining the drugs to be used. Fortunately, many effective antibiotic and chemo-

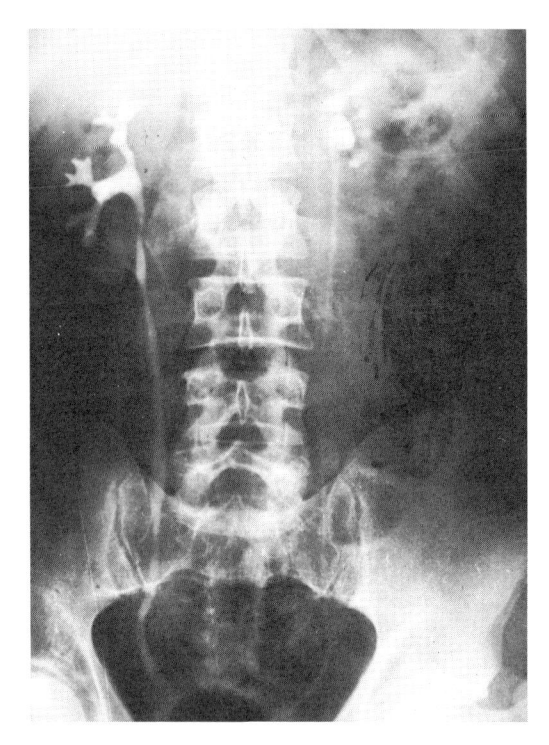

Fig. 52-22. Contracted left kidney, due to chronic pyelonephritis.

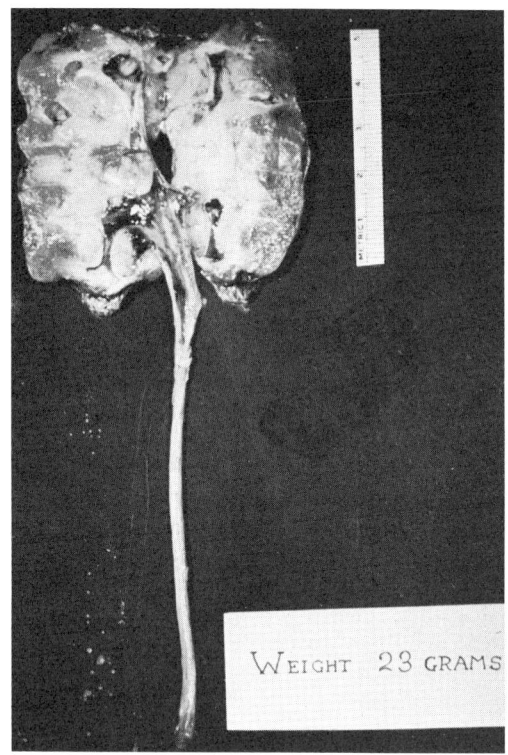

Fig. 52-23. Far-advanced chronic pyelonephritis with secondary contraction of the kidney.

therapeutic drugs are available such as kanamycin, cephalothin, colistin, chloromycetin, penicillin, erythromycin, Furadantin, nalidixic acid, ampicillin, sulfa preparations, etc.

Patients who exhibit sepsis associated with acute cystitis and/or pyelonephritis on their initial visit to the physician are not subjected to the regimen just described but are immediately hospitalized and empirically placed on a course of intramuscular kanamycin and massive doses of intravenous penicillin. After the patient has become afebrile for several days, he is subjected to the series of diagnostic studies.

The practice of treating recurrent urinary tract infection with various drugs and not investigating the genitourinary tract is to be condemned, because the causes of a recurrent or persisting infection may be neoplasm, tuberculosis, calculus disease, hydronephrosis, prostatism, etc.

Perinephric Abscess. Bacillary pyelonephritis, tuberculous pyelonephritis, traumatic rupture of the kidney and acute staphylococcal infections may lead to perinephric suppuration,[184] i.e., pus situated about the kidney but lying without the renal capsule.

ETIOLOGY. Infection may reach the perinephric space and tissues by direct extension from a cortical abscess, by lymphatic extension from a renal lesion or by the hematogenous route from an extra-urinary tract infection.

PATHOLOGY. Usually the perinephric infection begins within Gerota's fascia. From there it may spread downward inside the periureteral fascia and ultimately point in the floor of the bladder; it may extend through Gerota's fascia and pass superiorly to involve the diaphragm and the adjacent pleura; occasionally, it will penetrate the lung and drain into a bronchus,[186] forming a bronchoperinephric fistula; it may pass downward in the retroperitoneal space to point at Petit's triangle or to present itself in the perineum via the ischiorectal fossa.

SIGNS AND SYMPTOMS. The clinical manifestations of perinephric abscess are varied, depending upon the severity of the process and its chronicity. An acute fulminating infection is characterized by an abrupt onset with high fever to 105° F., chills, severe pain and tenderness in the costovertebral area; swelling, redness and increased warmth in the flank area; and nausea, vomiting, anorexia and prostration. The urine may contain leukocytes and bacilli if a bacillary pyelonephritis is present, or it may contain only cocci and be without leukocytes for a day or so if a staphylococcal infection is the etiologic agent. Generally, a leukocytosis exists. When the perinephric abscess is subdiaphragmatic, there may be rales, absent breath sounds and dullness to percussion in the lower lung field adjacent to the perinephric abscess.

If the perinephric abscess has been present for months, the patient may exhibit generalized debility, cachexia, anemia, low-grade fever, chronic discomfort in the flank area, infected urine and slightly elevated white count. Occasionally, these abscesses produce no signs other than fever and leukocytosis. In fact, perinephric abscesses constitute one of the important causes of "pyrexia of unknown origin."

DIAGNOSIS. In addition to the signs and symptoms, both needle aspiration of the fluctuant area through a large short-beveled needle and pyelography may aid in diagnosis. Typical x-ray findings of a perinephric abscess are: (1) absence of the psoas shadow on the involved side—this sign attends the collection of fluid in the retroperitoneal space; (2) lateral deviation of the spine with the concavity or hollow toward the abscess; and (3) fixation of the kidney on the affected side—the fibrosis and the adhesions produced by the inflammatory process immobilize the kidney. Fixation of the kidney is demonstrated by taking a pyelographic film while the patient is breathing (the renal shadow will be clear on the side of fixity and indefinite on the side of the mobile kidney) or by comparing films made in the supine and the erect positions.

TREATMENT. Prompt incision and drainage of the abscess is the treatment. Antibacterial therapy is appropriate only if high fever persists after the abscess is drained. If the kidney has been severely damaged or destroyed by calculus pyonephrosis, pyelonephritis, etc., and the other kidney is sufficiently functional, a nephrectomy is performed after the patient has recovered fully from the ravages of the perinephric abscess.

Staphylococcal Kidney. Staphylococcal infections of the kidney[185] are peculiar in that the organism almost invariably reaches the renal cortex by way of the blood stream. Furuncles and carbuncles of the skin and upper respiratory infections are common origins for the organism.

PATHOLOGY. Abscesses are produced in the renal cortex by the staphylococcus. The abscesses may heal spontaneously with practically no residua or they may coalesce to form large abscesses of the kidney, the so-called renal carbuncle.[179] The infection may extend to the perinephric tissue, with a resultant perinephric abscess.

SIGNS AND SYMPTOMS. Fever, chills, costovertebral tenderness, and pain are the usual manifestations of staphylococcal kidney. Early in the illness urinalysis demonstrates cocci but no leukocytes. No symptoms of cystitis occur unless there is secondary invasion of the urinary tract by the colon bacilli; this phenomenon occurs in about one half of the cases of staphylococcal kidney during the 2nd week of the disease.

THERAPY. Appropriate antibiotics administered parenterally constitute an effective form of treatment, provided that neither destruction of the kidney nor a perinephric abscess exists (see Chap. 3, Applied Surgical Bacteriology, for specific management of staphylococcal infections).

TUBERCULOUS INFECTIONS

Tuberculosis of the genitourinary system is always secondary to tuberculosis elsewhere in the body. The primary origin may be in the lung or infected lymph nodes. Many cases of urinary tract tuberculosis occur in individuals with no apparent evidence of active tuberculosis. The tubercle bacilli reach the cortex of the kidney through the blood stream; therefore, the infection tends to be bilateral. The primary renal tuberculous lesions may heal spontaneously[193] and remain unsuspected until demonstrated at autopsy.

Pathology. The initial lesion of renal tuberculosis[192] occurs in the glomerulus. From there it may break into the tubule and from the tubule extend into the peritubular tissue, as well as down the tubule, involving the mucosa and the submucosa of the renal pelvis. Having affected the renal pelvis, it may spread back into another portion of the kidney. It may attack the ureter and the bladder by direct mucosal or submucosal spread. Ulceration, caseating necrosis and fibrosis occur in the involved area, and these in turn give rise to strictures of the infundibula, the renal pelvis and the ureter and contraction of the bladder. In addition, the fibrosis and the stenosis may result in hydrocalycosis and even complete obliteration of the ureteral lumen with resultant autonephrectomy.

Tuberculous involvement of the prostate, the seminal vesicles and the epididymides occurs in 75 per cent of males having renal tuberculosis. A small number of male patients have genital tuberculosis without apparent renal tuberculosis; the infection in these cases is believed to be hematogenous in origin.

Signs and Symptoms. The usual symptoms are those of severe bladder irritation associated with pyuria, microscopic hematuria and the absence of bacteria when the usual staining technics are used alone.

Diagnosis. A history of persistent pyuria, recurrent urinary tract infections and/or marked bladder irritability should make the clinician suspicious of tuberculosis and lead to the performance of endoscopy, retrograde pyelograms and the collection of urine specimens from each kidney and the staining and culturing of these urines for *Myobacterium tuberculosis.*

Tuberculous ulceration of the bladder mucosa may be seen through the cystoscope, and often the pyelograms will demonstrate irregular, moth-eaten-appearing calyces (Figs. 52-24 and 52-25). The ureters may be irregularly dilated and stenosed.

Positive diagnosis of tuberculosis is made after tubercle bacilli have been demonstrated in the urine by culture and guinea pig inoculation.

Treatment. The present therapy of genitourinary tuberculosis involves: (1) a minimal period of hospitalization and rest, (2) prolonged use of multiple-drug regimens,[190] and (3) surgical procedures.[189] The drugs employed include isoniazid, para-aminosalicylic

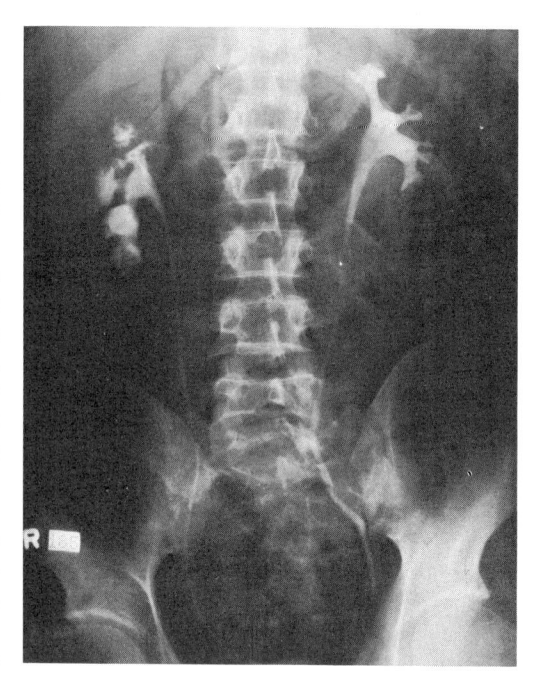

FIG. 52-24. Right renal and ureteral tuberculosis.

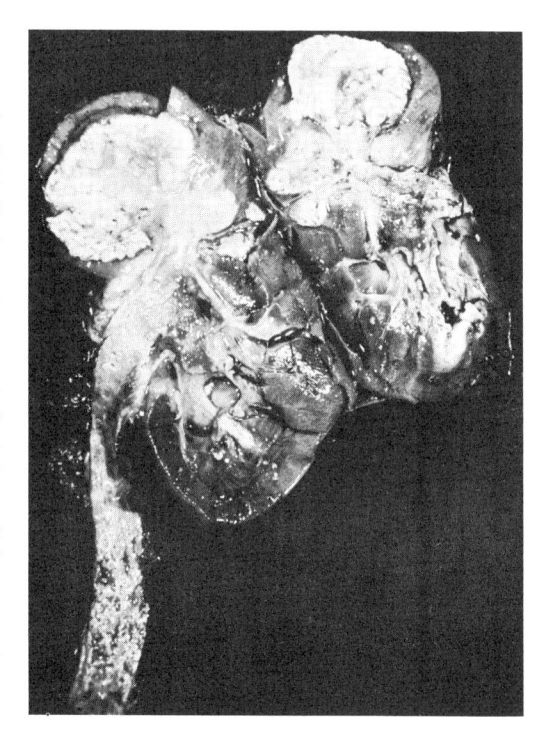

FIG. 52-25. Tuberculosis involvement of the kidney and the ureter.

acid, streptomycin, cycloserine, ethionamide, ethambutal, pyrozinamide and kanamycin in various combinations. These agents are given for a period of 2 years.

Nephrectomy is performed rarely at present for renal tuberculosis and then only in cases of extensive unilateral renal tuberculosis that does not respond well to drug therapy. Kerr[189] believes that some tuberculous kidneys can be saved from partial destruction or complete autonephrectomy by using appropriate operative procedures to alleviate scarring with obstruction of the urinary conduits. All operative procedures dealing with tuberculous organs are preceded by at least several weeks of specific drug therapy. The antituberculous drugs are continued postoperatively for a period of 1 to 2 years.

Prognosis. The present-day antituberculous regimens have definitely improved the prognosis of genitourinary tuberculosis. Available statistics suggest an over-all arrest rate of 70 to 80 per cent for renal tuberculosis.

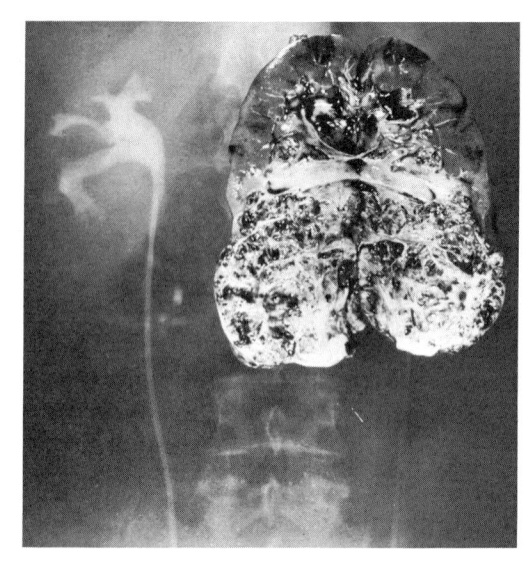

FIG. 52-26. Right retrograde pyelogram demonstrates a tumor deformity. Bivalved kidney specimen shows a hypernephroma involving the lower half of the kidney and accounting for the pyelographic abnormality.

NEOPLASMS OF THE GENITOURINARY TRACT

KIDNEY

Wilms's Tumor. Tumors of the kidney in children demonstrate both epithelial and connective tissue structures and have been called adenosarcoma, adenorhabdomyosarcoma, etc. The etiology is unknown.

SIGNS AND SYMPTOMS. The most common manifestation of Wilms's tumor is an abdominal mass, usually first noticed by the mother when bathing or caring for the child. Other symptoms and signs may be fever, malaise, loss of weight and anemia; these occur when the neoplasm is very large or has metastasized.

DIAGNOSIS. The suggestion of renal neoplasm on physical examination is usually confirmable by pyelography. Renal arteriography and venacavography are distinct aids in defining the diagnosis and outlining the extent of the lesion in order to facilitate the operative procedure.

TREATMENT. A combination of nephrectomy, irradiation and dactinomycin therapy is considered to be the most effective form of treatment at present. Radiotherapy is usually instituted postoperatively but may be used preoperatively to shrink large neoplasms and make them easier to remove. The dactinomycin is started on the day of operation and then is given intermittently over a period of 15 months.[205, 206]

PROGNOSIS. Recent reports suggest that the addition of chemotherapy to radiation plus operation has raised the 2-year survival level from 40 to 80 per cent and that metastases have been prevented in almost all patients.

Hypernephroma.[196] The most common malignant renal tumor in the adult is the renal cell carcinoma which arises from the renal tubule.

PATHOLOGY. Grossly, the tumor is well encapsulated, vascular and composed of yellowish-white lobules. Microscopically, the neoplastic cellular population contains large clear polygonal cells and small dark granular cells. The neoplasm grows into the renal venules and may block the renal veins. In the male this often gives rise to varicocele on the left side, because the left spermatic vein empties into the left renal vein. This does not happen with right renal tumors, because the right spermatic vein enters the vena cava. Consequently, these tumors metastasize frequently via the renal vein. Metastases to the lung are very common. Hypernephroma is one of the neoplasms with special predilection to bone metastases. Bilateral hypernephromas are not uncommon.

SIGNS AND SYMPTOMS. Gross hematuria is the most common sign of this primary renal parenchymal neoplasm. Some of the patients bearing it may have palpable abdominal masses as well as fever and an anemia of unknown origin.

DIAGNOSIS. Pyelography demonstrates the characteristic features of a neoplasm of the renal parenchyma, namely, distortion and elongation of the infundibula and the calyces, flattening of the collecting system and enlargement or segmental bulging of the renal outline (Fig. 52-26). Selective renal angiography,[198] percutaneous aspiration of the mass,[197] nephrotomography and venacavography have been tremendous aids in differentiating cyst from solid lesions, in determining the type of therapy (including necessity for operation and kind of operation); and in differentiating the vascular hypernephroma from the avascular metastatic lesions to the kidney and the avascular supporting tissue tumors—e.g., sarcomas, hamartomas, etc. Percutaneous aspiration of the mass provides a sample not only of the fluid within the mass but also of cells for cytological study. In addition, after aspiration one can inject contrast material through the needle into the mass to outline the cavity.

TREATMENT. Unless the patient cannot tolerate an operative procedure or has a solitary kidney or massive metastatic involvement, radical nephrectomy[203] is indicated for renal cell carcinoma. This implies lymph node dissection and excision of local metastases including vena caval involvement. Data indicate that irradiation improves the 5-year survival rate; a national cooperative study involving irradiation is in progress. Drug therapy for advanced renal carcinoma has not been particularly beneficial[207]; testosterone and medroxyprogesterone offer some hope.

PROGNOSIS. In some series the 10-year survival rate has been increased from 25 to 50 per cent with the use of radical nephrectomy and the 5-year rate 30 to 49 per cent with irradiation plus simple nephrectomy. Perhaps the use of radical nephrectomy in addition to irradiation may further improve the prognosis.

Neoplasms of the Collecting System. The most common cancer of the renal pelvis is the transitional cell papillary carcinoma. Other less common neoplasms are adenocarcinoma and squamous cell carcinoma. Over 50 per cent of the squamous cell carcinomata occur in association with calculi in the renal pelvis.

SIGNS AND SYMPTOMS. Compared with hypernephromas, tumors of the renal pelvis,[201] give rise to episodes of gross total hematuria relatively early. The reason is obvious. The pelvic neoplasm is located in the collecting system, and any bleeding erosion thereof will be attended by the appearance of blood in the urine immediately, whereas, before the hypernephroma causes gross hematuria, it must grow extensively and break into the collecting system, and this takes time.

Other clinical evidence of renal pelvic tumors may be pain and tenderness in the costovertebral area, fever, malaise, anemia and occasional renal and ureteral colic attendant upon the passage of blood clots.

DIAGNOSIS. Pyelography will demonstrate a filling defect in the renal pelvis. Other causes for filling defects of the renal pelvis are blood clots and nonopaque calculi. Repeat pyelograms in 5 to 7 days will rule out blood clots, since clots in the pelvis tend to disappear within a week. Occasionally, cystoscopy is an aid in making the diagnosis, for one may see a papillary growth protruding through the ureteral orifice or surrounding the ureteral orifice.

TREATMENT. Nephrectomy is indicated for squamous cell carcinoma and adenocarcinoma of the renal pelvis. Nephro-ureterectomy with excision of a small cuff of bladder around the ureteral orifice is the treatment for papillary neoplasm of the renal pelvis. This extensive excision of ureter and uretervesical structure is necessary because the urothelium on the same side as the neoplasm is predisposed to formation of other papillary cancers should it not be removed.

URETER

Incidence. Primary ureteral neoplasms[210] are relatively rare. The most common type of tumor is the transitional cell papilloma and papillary carcinoma. Neoplastic growths in the ureter are more frequently metastases from carcinomas primary in the cervix, the rectum, the prostate and the bladder than they are carcinomas primary in the ureter.

Signs and Symptoms. Gross hematuria is the most common presenting symptom and sign by virtue of the erosion of the neoplasm. Neoplastic obstruction to the flow of urine through the ureter ultimately gives rise to ureteral colic, dull flank pain, costovertebral tenderness, fever and chills.

Diagnosis. A filling defect in the ureter is readily demonstrated pyelographically, and upon cytoscopy blood may be seen spurting from the ureteral orifice.

Treatment. Nephrecto-ureterectomy is indicated (provided that the opposite kidney is adequately functional).

BLADDER

Incidence. Tumors of the bladder[211, 218] are similar to those of the renal pelvis and the ureter. The most common neoplasms are the transitional cell papilloma and papillary carcinoma; the less common tumors are the squamous cell carcinoma and the adenocarcinoma. Sarcoma is very rare, very malignant and has a poor prognosis.

Pathology. Grossly, tumors of the bladder may appear flat (sessile), polypoid or papilliferous. The neoplasm may involve only the mucosa but it ultimately extends into or through any or all of the layers of the bladder. It may be anywhere in the bladder and cover areas of all sizes. It can occlude the ureteral orifices as well as the vesical neck.

Etiology. Most of the causes of neoplasm of the bladder epithelium in the human are unknown. Suspected factors include chemicals, body metabolites, chronic irritation and tobacco tar. Certain aniline dyes and bilharziasis are known to contribute to the genesis of bladder cancer.

Signs and Symptoms. Hematuria is the most common and constant finding in patients having bladder neoplasms. Persistent and recurrent urinary tract infections are also frequent manifestations. Other symptoms are urgency, increased frequency of urination and dysuria.

Diagnosis. Cystoscopy and biopsy of the bladder lesion provide a positive diagnosis. The extent of the lesion can be estimated grossly by bimanual examination under anesthesia.[214] The Papanicolaou method for studying cells shed from the bladder wall is being evaluated at the present time relative to its place in diagnostic urology. It now appears that exfoliative cytology will not replace cystoscopy as the primary method for making a diagnosis. However, it may be the most important procedure for making a diagnosis in cases of sessile, infiltrating neoplasms of bladders with generalized vesical inflammation.

Prognosis depends somewhat upon the characteristics of the tumor. The prognosis is poorer for infiltrating than for noninfiltrating types. The growth of a tumor more than halfway through the muscularis reduces the prospect for 5 years or more of life almost to the vanishing point.

Treatment. The ideal treatment for *all bladder neoplasms* would be complete cystectomy and transplantation of the ureters into the bowel. Unfortunately, uretero-intestinal transplantation has led in the past to many troubles with ascending pyelonephritis and renal failure.[213] Therefore, cystectomy has not been adopted as the best way to treat carcinomas of the bladder. Recent experience with the implantation of the ureters into ileal segments suggest that this type of urinary diversion may obviate some of the complications seen previously with uretero-intestinal anastomoses. However, more conservative measures still are being used, e.g., transurethral resection, segmental resection of the bladder and fulguration. Without a doubt, cystectomy is indicated for multiple papillomata and superficially infiltrating lesions not amenable to less extensive procedures.

Uretero-intestinal transplantation without cystectomy is a valuable operation for patients with inoperable bladder neoplasms who have strangury and intermittent vesical obstruction by blood clots. Transplantation does not, however, stop hemorrhage from the vesical cancer but may reduce it.

External irradiation of the bladder[212] is widely used at the present time for definitive as well as palliative therapy for transitional neoplasm. The results have been so good that some consider it preferable to total cystectomy for lesions extending into detrusor and not amenable to transurethral excision.

A patient having a vesical neoplasm treated by a modality other than total cystectomy must return for periodic examination of the bladder for the rest of his natural life, because persistent growth as well as new growths are common.

Prostate Gland

Incidence. Carcinoma of the prostate occurs in 15 to 30 per cent of all males past the age of 50 years who have testes. Prostatic neoplasms do not occur in eunuchs.

Etiology is unknown.

Pathology. Adenocarcinoma usually originates in the posterior lobe of the prostate and spreads by local infiltration into the remainder of the gland, the seminal vesicles and the bladder. It may invade the lymphatics and the vertebral veins[220] and has a marked predilection for spread to the bones of the pelvis and the lumbosacral vertebrae. Terminally prostatic carcinoma may be found in practically all of the organs of the body.

Signs and Symptoms. All of the symptoms of prostatism attend the neoplastic obstruction of the prostatic urethra, osseous pain attends osseous metastases, and no symptoms are experienced so long as the lesion has neither obstructed the flow of urine nor metastasized. Rectal palpation may disclose a stony-hard, nodular prostate, or a hard, smooth prostate with obliterated lateral and median sulci.

Diagnosis. Early isolated carcinomatous nodules can be detected only by digital rectal examination of the prostate. Metastatic neoplasm often can be discovered by roentgenography of the pelvis, and the determination of serum acid phosphatase. Ultimately, carcinoma of the prostate causes metastases in most patients. When this occurs the serum acid phosphatase rises above normal in approximately 60 per cent of patients.[227] Many prostatic carcinomas are physiologically similar to normal prostatic tissue in that they produce enzymes, e.g., acid phosphatase and fibrinolysins.[229] Consequently, when they metastasize into bone, lymphatics or blood vessels the concentration of fibrinolysin and acid phosphatase in the blood rises. Normally, acid phosphatase and fibrinolysin are found in the seminal fluid.

Treatment. Radical removal of the prostate and the seminal vesicles by the retropubic or perineal approach is the only method by which cure can be obtained. Radical prostatectomy is indicated only if there are no obvious signs of metastases.

Transurethral prostatectomy is utilized for the relief of obstructions due to infiltrating neoplastic glands.

Bilateral orchiectomy and stilbestrol, 1 mg. per day, are indicated for glands not amenable to radical removal, as soon as the diagnosis is made. This treatment is based on the work of Huggins and others[223] who demonstrated that the growth and the hormonal stimulation of prostatic cancer are partially dependent upon androgens elaborated by the testes and the adrenals. Suppression of the androgens by orchiectomy and stilbestrol temporarily inhibits the growth of many prostatic cancers.[226] However, the prostatic neoplasm eventually adapts itself and grows rapidly again.

Relapses after orchiectomy and stilbestrol have been treated with high doses of cortisone, hypophysectomy, stilbestrol diphosphate and radioactive phosphorus. In many cases these forms of therapy afford a further period of comfortable existence. None is curative.

Flocks[222] used intraprostatic injections of radioactive gold to control the growth of prostatic neoplasm not confined entirely to the gland.

External cobalt irradiation for prostatic carcinoma has been reintroduced and is being tried for all types of neoplasm. Although further experience is needed to delineate its role, it is possible that irradiation plus simple prostatectomy may supplant radical prostatectomy.

Urethra

Incidence. Neoplasm of the urethra are rare in both men and women.[230] In the male, carcinoma of the urethra[231] occurs in association with stricture in 50 per cent of the cases.

Pathologically, most of the neoplasms are squamous cell in type and arise from the distal portion of the urethra which is lined by stratified squamous epithelium.

Clinical manifestations of urethral neoplasms may be bleeding from the urethra, difficulty in voiding and dysuria.

Diagnosis is made by urethroscopy and biopsy of the lesions. Condyloma accuminata and, in women, urethral caruncle may be difficult to distinguish from urethral meatal carcinoma.

Treatment of a localized urethral neoplasm is the radical excision of the urethra. However, most urethral neoplasms have infiltrated beyond the walls of the urethra when seen by the physician and are amenable only to palliative therapy. This consists of either internal or external irradiation and suprapubic urinary diversion. The prognosis of urethral carcinoma is poor.

PENIS

Incidence. Carcinoma of the penis is relatively common among uncircumcised men and rare among the circumcised.

Etiology.[236] Smegma has been demonstrated to contain material that is carcinogenic for animals. It is probable that the retention of smegma is intimately concerned with the formation of penile cancer among the uncircumcised.

Pathology. Neoplasms of the penis are squamous cell in type. Precancerous lesions are erythroplasia, leukoplakia and condylomata.[235] The penile neoplasms metastasize to the superficial and deep inguinal as well as to the external iliac lymph nodes.

Diagnosis. Carcinoma of the penis may involve the prepuce, the glans and the shaft. Inspection and palpation of the penis will suggest neoplasm which is confirmed by biopsy.

Treatment. Partial[233] or radical amputation of the penis and bilateral inguinofemoral node dissection is the therapy of choice. Radical amputation and perineal urethrotomy are done when anticipated excision of the involved penis plus 1 cm. of normal tissue will leave an inadequate stump of urethra for urination, i.e., the patient would soil his scrotum and perineum when voiding. Prophylactic treatment[232] consists of circumcision, preferably shortly after birth.

Prognosis. Cancer of the penis is relatively slow-growing and thus bears a favorable outlook if discovered early. Death in patients with far advanced cancer of the penis may ultimately result from exsanguination caused by erosion of the iliac or the femoral blood vessels.

SCROTUM

Squamous cell carcinoma of the scrotum[238] may be caused by skin irritants such as soot and petroleum products. It is seen infrequently today. The diagnosis is made by biopsy. Therapy consists of local excision with a wide margin of normal skin.

TESTIS

Incidence. Several of the most malignant neoplasms arise in the testicle. Although they may appear at any age, they occur most commonly during the 2nd and the 3rd decades of life. Testicular cancer is insidious and metastasizes early. Statistics suggest that it is 22 times more frequent in the cryptorchid than in the normally descended testis, and this relationship pertains in both the uncorrected and the corrected cryptorchids.

Etiology. Two theories[214] in regard to the origin of testicular neoplasms have been advanced: one proposes that they arise from cell rests; the other, that testicular neoplasms arise from the germinal tissue of an identical twin in the testicle.

Pathology. The types of testicular neoplasm are teratoma, seminoma, embryonal carcinoma, chorio-epithelioma, teratocarcinoma and interstitial cell neoplasm. When a testicular tumor metastasizes, it does so usually by the lymphatic route and to a lesser degree through the blood vessels; chorioepithelioma differs from the rest in that it invades and metastasizes through blood vessels early. Since the lymphatics closely follow the route of the internal spermatic vessels that supply the testes, the first lymphatic nodes to be involved usually are the retroperitoneal nodes in the region of the renal pedicles. Spread from these nodes involves the preaortic nodes.

Signs and Symptoms. Most of the testicular neoplasms are asymptomatic and cause only slight enlargement of the testis. Occasionally, some of the neoplasms secrete estrogens, making gynecomastia an early sign. Testicular pain occurs frequently.

Fever, anemia, dyspnea and mid-line abdominal masses are late manifestations of metastatic testicular neoplasms.

Diagnosis. Since neoplasms of the testicle are so malignant, a scrotal mass should be presumed to be a cancer of the testicle until proved to be benign. A "red herring" frequently placed in the diagnostic pathway is the history of trauma. *In the author's experience, scrotal swelling due to trauma is seen less frequently than any other scrotal enlargement.* Scrotal masses may be due to acute or chronic epididymitis, hydrocele, spermatocele, hernia, torsion of the testis and testicular granulomata. Transillumination and needle aspiration (if the mass transilluminates) will establish the diagnosis of spermatocele and hydrocele. Palpation of the testis always should be done again after aspiration, because occasionally a testicular neoplasm occurs in conjunction with a hydrocele. Epididymitis is a frequent cause of scrotal swelling and is associated usually with urinary tract infections.

If there is the slightest doubt in the mind of the examiner as to the diagnosis of the scrotal swelling, the contents of the scrotum should be exposed surgically and examined without spreading tumor cells.

The Aschheim-Zondek test for chorionic gonadotropin[247] in the urine is used as an aid in diagnosis as well as prognosis. Some patients have testicular tumors that elaborate chorionic gonadotropin, and their urine gives a positive A-Z test. The A-Z test becomes negative after complete excision of the tumor. Recurrence of the neoplasm is indicated by a positive A-Z test after an initial postoperative negative test.

Chest roentgenogram and intravenous pyelograms are obtained for determination of metastases. The findings on chest roentgenograms are obvious; on pyelography massive metastatic involvement of the retroperitoneal lymph nodes often is seen to displace the upper two thirds of the ureters laterally.

Treatment. Radical orchiectomy and removal of retroperitoneal lymph nodes followed by external irradiation is the modern form of therapy for all malignant testicular neoplasms. If obvious metastases to the lungs or the retroperitoneal nodes are present, palliative irradiation and chemotherapy may be used.

Prognosis. The survival rate depends upon the type of testicular neoplasm. Seminomas offer the best prognosis because they are very radiosensitive. The outlook for chorio-epitheliomas is very poor. Most patients with persistent testicular neoplasms die within 2 years after the diagnosis is made.

Early diagnosis, radical lymphadenectomy,[246] effective radiation and modern chemotherapy regimens have improved the survival rate markedly and it is anticipated there will be much more optimism in regard to the outlook for cure than there has been in the recent past. Evidence from a number of sources[241, 243] indicates that appropriate chemotherapy regimens are capable of inducing complete or partial regression of widespread metastases from testicular neoplasms. Some investigators feel that they have actually effected cures with chemotherapy.

CALCULOUS DISEASE[262]

The cause of stones in the urinary tract is unknown in at least 50 per cent of the cases.[259] Often, the normal urine is supersaturated with salts which are held in solution by chelating compounds such as amino acids, colloids, citric acid, etc. When the solute status of supersaturated urine is changed, the salts may precipitate and form calculi. Factors that may upset the solute status are: (1) a change in urinary pH, (2) a decrease in urinary chelating compounds, (3) an increase in urinary salts and (4) the presence of a nidus.

Etiology. When urine becomes highly alkaline, i.e., pH above 7.0, calcium phosphate tends to precipitate. This occurs among patients on a Sippy regimen, which not only alkalinizes the urine but tends to cause hypercalciuria. Renal tubular acidosis,[248] resulting from impairment of the base-saving mechanism in the distal tubule, also gives rise to an alkaline urine and hypercalcinuria. Infections of the urine with urea-splitting ammonia-forming organisms[251] (*Pseudomonas aeruginosa, Proteus vulgaris,* etc.) alkalinizes the urine and promotes the formation of stones containing calcium, magnesium, ammonium and phosphate. It is believed that the most common cause for uric acid stones is a persistently acid urine rather than the excretion of excessive quantities of uric acid.[254]

Little is known about the role of urinary chelating compounds in the formation of urinary calculi.

Urinary salts precipitate upon foreign bodies and may even precipitate upon small areas of the renal papillae. The nidus may be a catheter, a hairpin, a piece of wire, desquamated epithelial cells (especially in vitamin A deficiency), necrotic tissue with pyelonephritis or neoplasm and clumps of bacteria. All urinary calculi are believed to have an organic matrix composed of mucoid material.[249]

The excessive excretion of urinary crystalloids is frequently the cause of urinary calculi. Patients with cystinuria[253] are notorious stone formers. Uric acid stones[256] may form in persons having gout. Any patient with hypercalciuria is prone to form stones. Hypercalciuria occurs with hyperparathyroidism, the excessive ingestion of vitamin D, acidosis, extensive bone disease, immobilization of the patient in casts, bed or frame and in idiopathic increased absorption of calcium by the gut.[250]

All patients with renal or ureteral calculi should be studied to determine the possible causes of their stones prior to any operative procedure for removal of the calculi, unless the patient's condition is so serious that immediate operative intervention is indicated. The reasoning behind this involves the possibility of recurrent stone formation during the postoperative period if the etiologic factor is not removed first. Diagnostic studies should include repeated determinations of serum calcium, phosphorus, sodium, potassium, chloride, bicarbonate, protein, uric acid, BUN and creatinine levels, urinary calcium, phosphorus and creatinine concentrations, and the pH of the urine. The serum calcium, phosphorus and creatinine, and the urinary calcium, phosphorus and creatinine levels are obtained with the patient on a normal diet and then on a low calcium phosphorus intake. With these studies one can search for hyperparathyroidism,[252] renal tubular acidosis, persistently alkaline or acid urine, etc.

Pathology. Calculi may obstruct the urinary tract anywhere and produce obstructive uropathy with renal or ureteral colic, hydro-ureter, hydronephrosis, renal atrophy and uremia. Sharp stones may lodge in the ureter and induce ulceration, erosion, perforation, urinary extravasation and stricture. Stones in the urinary tract predispose the person bearing them to urinary tract infections.

Types of Stones. In North America the most common component of the first stone is *calcium oxalate*. Calcium oxalate is radiopaque. *Calcium phosphate*, also radiopaque, is the primary constituent of recurrent calculi. *Uric acid stones* are *not* radiopaque and occur less frequently than phosphate and oxalate stones. *Cystine stones* are radiopaque but less dense than calcium stones, occur as a familial inborn error of metabolism, and are very infrequent.

Signs and Symptoms. Renal calculi may be silent, producing no symptoms, or, when in the renal pelvis, may be associated with constant dull flank pain or sharp, excruciating pain in the costovertebral region and flank. At times the pain of renal calculus origin may simulate closely the pain of peptic ulcer or obstruction of the biliary tract. The passage of a calculus down the ureter is associated at times with excruciating pain, characterized by intermittency, radiation from the flank area anteriorly down the course of the ureter, ending in the scrotum or the labium majus and at times down the leg. Prostration is frequent, and hypotension may occur.

A vesical calculus usually is attended by frequency, urgency, hematuria and dysuria. Occasionally, it obstructs the vesical outlet during upright voiding but not while voiding in the supine position; this is pathognomonic of a bladder stone.

Fever and chills may accompany the pain. Anuria occurs occasionally with ureteral calculus obstruction and the more frequently in persons having only one kidney.

Diagnosis. A history characteristic of renal or ureteral colic or vesical obstruction by stone and the presence of red blood cells in the urine are suggestive of urinary calculus. Should the stone be opaque, a plain roentgenogram covering the renal, the ureteral and the vesicular areas may demonstrate an opacity. In the case of nonopaque stone, excretory pyelograms may show only the existence of a hydro-ureter, hydronephrosis or a delayed excretion of the contrast medium on the involved side. Endoscopy permits direct confirmation of the presence of bladder calculi, and retrograde catheterization that of ureteral calculus. Oblique films with the catheter in the ureter aid in differentiating ureteral calculi from extra-urinary tract opacities such as phleboliths, calcified lymph nodes and gallstones.

An erroneous diagnosis of appendicitis or cholecystitis is made occasionally in cases of right ureteral calculus. All cases of suspected appendicitis should have a urinalysis, and if erythrocytes or numerous white cells are found, excretory pyelograms should be made.

Treatment. Renal and ureteral colic may be relieved by using analgesics or vasospasmolytics.[257] Morphine is an adequate analgesic, and intravenous Banthine an effective vasospasmolytic. Occasionally, the passage of a ureteral catheter beyond the stone is needed to relieve the pain when other methods fail.

Large vesical calculi can be removed by suprapubic cystolithotomy or transurethral crushing (litholapaxy).

Ureteral calculi smaller than 1 cm. in diameter are treated by watchful waiting. Unless the stone causes constant pain or gives rise to hydro-ureter, hydronephrosis or anuria, time is permitted for it to pass spontaneously. Stones larger than 1 cm., or smaller stones coupled with complications or renal enlargement, are removed by ureterolithotomy. If the stone is small and in the most distal portion of the ureter its transurethral removal may be attempted with the Balkus loop, the Levant basket, the Dormia basket, or the Dourmashkin bag.[260]

Large calculi in the renal pelvis are removable only by pyelolithotomy or nephrolithotomy. In elderly patients it is often best to leave renal stones alone unless they cause persistent or intense pain or recurrent bouts of chills and fever.

After the removal of calculi from the urinary tract, measures should be instituted to prevent their recurrence. This may consist solely of treating a urinary tract infection; the repair of any condition leading to urinary stasis, such as a malpositioned blood vessel, positional ureteral kinking, etc.; instituting physical activity; discontinuance of the Sippy regimen, etc. Diluting the urine by the forced drinking of water is to be employed after the removal of all types of stones. The Shorr regimen is being employed[258] widely to prevent the formation of calcium phosphate calculi. This consists of a low calcium, low phosphorus diet and the ingestion of aluminum gel. In the intestine the aluminum gel forms insoluble aluminum phosphate and thereby prevents absorption of phosphorus. In this manner the urinary excretion of calcium and phosphorus is diminished. There is evidence that the Shorr regimen is effective in reducing the frequency of recurrent nephrolithiasis. Patients who have formed urinary tract stones should be investigated for possible hyperparathyroidism (see Chap. 28, Thyroid, Thymus and Parathyroids).

If the patient shows unusual absorption of calcium by the intestine, sodium phytate[250] can be used. Howard[255] has advocated the use of oral phosphates to increase the solubility of calcium in the urine.

Renal tubular acidosis is treated with the oral administration of a mixture of sodium citrate and citric acid, calcium gluconate, vitamin D and potassium salts.

The occurrence of uric acid, calculi and persistently acid urine is an indication for the oral administration of alkali.

Recurrent calculi in patients with cystinuria can be prevented with a regimen consisting of high 24-hour urinary output and alkali intake to maintain urinary pH above 7.5. Penicillamine is being used to control urinary excretion of cystine and has been found to be quite effective. However, recent reports suggest that the beneficial effects of the drug may be countered by nephrotoxic effects.

TRAUMATIC LESIONS

KIDNEY

Incidence. Automobile accidents and boxing now injure the kidney more often than other forms of trauma. In the case of renal trauma sustained in automobile accidents and boxing the kidney may be crushed by the blunt force or torn from its bed by sudden deceleration of the body. Also, it is readily injured directly by penetrating objects such as knives, bullets, shell fragments, etc.[267]

Pathology. Minor renal injuries are frequent and consist solely of the rupture of small vessels, producing hematomas and hematuria. The severe renal injuries include tears or incisions through the parenchyma, the pelvis, the calyces or the renal pedicle. Hemorrhage into the collecting system and about the kidney follows such tears or cuts. It is limited by Gerota's fascia unless that too is torn or cut. Should Gerota's fascia be discontinuous, the hemorrhage extends retroperitoneally, obliterating the psoas shadow, and with it urine extravasates into the retroperitoneal space, especially after fragmentation of the kidney. Should the hematoma or the urinary extravasation become infected, a perinephric abscess may ensue.

Thrombosis and infarction without any other obvious renal injury may follow renal trauma.

Signs and Symptoms. Pain in the costovertebral area, gross or microscopic hematuria, and swelling in the flank are characteristic signs of renal injury; any or all of them may exist. Shock follows renal injuries attended by extensive retroperitoneal hemorrhage or a fulminant infection of the hematoma or urinary extravasation. Associated injuries, including rib fracture on either side and splenic rupture on the left, are frequent.

Diagnosis. All cases with serious abdominal trauma should have preliminary screening of a catheterized urine specimen, in order to look for the presence of gross or microscopic blood. Intravenous pyelography is very helpful in establishing a diagnosis of renal injury. The preliminary plain film demonstrates an enlarged renal shadow should the hemorrhage be confined within Gerota's fascia; should the hemorrhage be retroperitoneal, the psoas shadow is obscured, and lateral deviation of the spine with the concavity toward the side of injury occurs. The injured kidney may not be visualized with excretory pyelography. In cases with visualization, distortion of the collecting system and extravasation of the dye may occur. Renal angiography is used if excretory pyelography is unsatisfactory for diagnostic purposes or incidentally when arteriography is being used to determine vascular leaks elsewhere in the abdominal cavity.

Treatment. Most renal injuries do not require operative intervention, and their treatment[264] consists of the treatment of hemorrhagic shock, the control of pain and rest in bed. *Special diagnostic studies should not be done while shock exists.*

Signs of continuing or life-endangering hemorrhages, such as a bulging mass in the flank and recurrent hypotension despite large blood transfusions, constitute indications for surgical intervention. The operation consists of repairing the kidney when possible, hemostasis, and evacuation of blood clots. Nephrectomy may be necessary in cases of renal avulsion or extreme fragmentation, but it should not be performed until the presence of a functioning opposite kidney has been ascertained. Necessary treatment of associated injuries such as ruptured spleen, bowel, liver, etc., should not be overlooked (see Chap. 34, Spleen, and Chap. 39, Small Bowel and Colon).

Surgical procedures are also required in cases of injury attended by very extensive urinary extravasations or perinephric abscesses.

Prognosis. A severely traumatized kidney may live but later atrophy, and then hypertension may occur. All persons having experienced severe renal injury should be checked regularly, looking for high blood pressure. Should hypertension follow a severe renal injury, a nephrectomy should be performed, but only after ascertaining the injured kidney's function and that of its mate, employing split-function studies.

URETER

Incidence. Injuries to the ureter are practically always iatrogenic.[269] Radical surgery for cancer of the uterus and the rectosigmoid, instrumental manipulation of the ureter for calculi, and vesical diverticulectomy and segmental resection of the bladder constitute the commonest hazards to the ureter.

The most frequent type of ureteral injury is its accidental ligation. Other forms of injury include instrumental crushing, transection, tearing, excision and puncture.[270]

Pathology. Ureteral ligation is followed by hydro-ureter, hydronephrosis and eventual autonephrectomy if the ligature is nonabsorbable. A break in ureteral continuity is followed by the extravasation of urine, periureteral abscesses and entero-ureteral and cutaneous-ureteral fistula. Extensive periureteral scarring often follows transection or contusions, producing strictures with hydroureter and hydronephrosis above them.

Signs and Symptoms. Ligation of one ureter may cause no overt pain and especially so if the ligation has been performed during anesthesia. Obviously, anuria immediately follows the ligation of both ureters.

The extravasation of urine from an opening in the ureter may cause severe flank pain, abdominal distention and sepsis and at other times be attended by no symptoms. Presumptively, should the urine be of neutral pH, be nearly isotonic and not contain organisms, it should cause no more pain than saline injected beneath the skin or into the peritoneal cavity. The seeping of urine from the surgical wound or from the vagina after a ureteral injury usually requires a day or more for its appearance. It is a pathognomonic of a uretero-cutaneous or ureterovaginal fistula.

Diagnosis. Retrograde pyelography with ureteral catheterization will demonstrate the obstruction if the ureter has been tied. Excretory pyelography is to be used first in cases of suspected ureteral tears or transection in order to obviate the danger associated with retrograde pyelography of introducing pathogenic organisms into the injury. If visualization is not obtained with the intravenous pyelogram, then retrograde pyelography is performed. Antegrade pyelography by the percutaneous route may be quite helpful in delineating the status of the lesion on occasion.

Treatment. Most surgical injuries to the ureter are preventable. Constant cognizance of the ease of ureteral injury during operations upon pelvic and posterior abdominal organs and the placing of catheters in the ureters through the urethra before beginning large pelvic operations will serve to prevent most of the surgical ureteral injuries. Every general surgeon or gynecologist should be prepared to repair a divided ureter on the spot when this accident is discovered. A useful method is to place a catheter upward through an incision in the ureter from below the point of division. The catheter passes through the division line which in turn is resutured end-to-end with a single row of fine interrupted catgut sutures. The distal end of the catheter is then brought out through the flank. Obstructive ligatures, even though they may be absorbable, should be removed as soon as possible. Should the accident remain undetected for a long time and the patient be uremic or very ill for other reasons, nephrostomy rather than deligation is performed first. After the patient's renal function recovers, corrective procedures to restore ureteral patency and continuity are carried out.

When urinary extravasation occurs through a transected or injured ureter, incisional drainage of the urine may be indicated in addition to nephrostomy. After a suitable time interval of drainage, definitive ureteral plastic procedures to establish continuity and patency of the ureter are done. Frequently, nephrectomy must be substituted for ureteral plastic procedures, because the ureter has been so injured as to be beyond repair.

BLADDER

Rupture of the bladder occurs quite frequently with pelvic fractures. Automobile accidents and falls are the predominant causes of vesical rupture.[274] Openings through the bladder are made occasionally during transurethral resection of the prostate or of vesical neoplasms. After rupture of the bladder, urine may extravasate into the perivesical space or the peritoneal cavity, or both.

Signs and Symptoms. If the urinary extravasation is extraperitoneal, pain is suffered suprapubically, with tenderness and dullness evident suprapubically and infra-umbilically. Signs of peritonitis, such as ileus, boardlike rigidity, etc., often attend intraperitoneal urinary extravasation. Attempts to void may bring the passage of a little blood and no urine. Occasionally, the rupture of the bladder with the free flow of urine into the peritoneal cavity is unattended by pain or signs of peritonitis. In such cases the pathognomonic signs of the accident are ascites, oliguria or anuria, and uremia.

When the bladder is ruptured during transurethral resection, low abdominal pain and shock attend it, and the abdomen is distended and cold—the cold irrigating fluid introduced into it having cooled the abdominal wall.

Diagnosis. In all cases of pelvic or lower abdominal trauma a catheterized urine specimen should be obtained for the detection of microscopic red cells. Unequivocal evidence of a ruptured bladder can be obtained by introducing 200 ml. of a 10 per cent solution

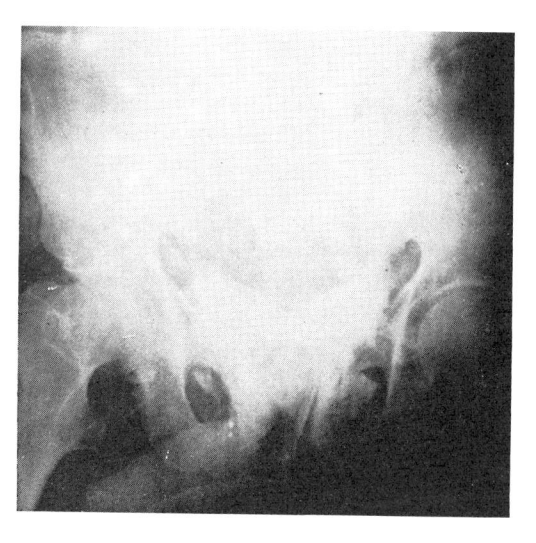

FIG. 52-27. Marked extravasation of sodium iodide beyond confines of the bladder confirms the diagnosis of ruptured bladder.

of sodium iodide, Urokon, Diodrast, Neoiopax or Hyopaque through the urethral catheter and then taking a roentgenogram. Figure 52-27 shows the extravasation of contrast material in a case of ruptured bladder.

Treatment. Through a suprapubic incision the extravasated urine and blood are evacuated, and the rent is débrided and closed. Then a suprapubic cystostomy is done, and multiple drains are placed in the perivesical space, and the wound is closed over them. The drains and the suprapubic tube are removed after drainage through and about them has stopped and the bladder has healed.

URETHRA

Trauma to the urethra may tear it posteriorly and anteriorly. The injury may be inflicted by intra-urethral instrumentation and manipulation or by the application of external force to the para-urethral area. The common causes of intra-urethral trauma are the forceful passage of steel sounds, fiber bougies and other foreign bodies.[276] Occasionally, an irrational patient bearing a Foley catheter will pull it out while the balloon is inflated and sustain an extensive tear of the urethra. Straddle injuries caused by falling astride bars, fences, etc., crush the bulbous urethra. Sharp bony fragments from pelvic fractures may rupture the prostatic and membranous portions of the urethra.[278] Sudden arrest of the momentum of a person with a full bladder in an automobile accident may shear the membranous urethra clear across. This is possible because the bladder and the prostatic urethra are mobile, while the membranous urethra is fixed by the urogenital diaphragm. In the female such a shear is more apt to occur at the bladder neck.

Pathology. When a break in the continuity of the urethra occurs, hemorrhage follows, and urine extravasates if the patient attempts to force urine down the ruptured urethra or if the injury is at the vesical neck.

If the rupture in the urethra is distal to the urogenital diaphragm and does not involve Buck's fascia, the urinary extravasation will be limited by Buck's fascia, and swelling will occur along the shaft of the penis and along the perineal urethra. When the injury perforates Buck's fascia, the extravasation will be limited by Colles' fascia, and the extravasated urine will swell the shaft of the penis, the scrotum, the perineum and the anterior abdominal wall. A urethral tear proximal to the urogenital diaphragm permits extraperitoneal and perivesical extravasation.

A fibrous stricture of the urethra may follow all types of traumatic lesions of the urethra.

Signs and Symptoms. The signs of an injury to the anterior urethra are pain in the region of the injury, bleeding from the urethral meatus not associated with urination, and difficulty in voiding. Straddle injury often makes a large hematoma in the perineum. If urinary extravasation occurs, swelling will take place as previously described. Posterior urethral injuries are characterized by hematuria, little urethral bleeding, suprapubic pain, tenderness and inability to void, and a hematomatous swelling in the region of the triangular ligament and displacement of the prostate discernible upon digital rectal examination.

Diagnosis. The history and the physical findings alone suffice to establish the diagnosis in many cases. A urethrocystogram readily confirms the diagnosis and aids in locating the position of the tear.

Treatment. Urinary diversion and establishment of urethral continuity are the primary therapeutic aims. If urinary extravasation has occurred, incision and drainage of the involved parts are also necessary. Urinary diversion is accomplished by suprapubic cystostomy. With prostatic and membranous urethral injuries, continuity is reestablished by splinting the urethra over a urethral catheter passed throught the site of injury into the bladder. Some surgeons[279] have been using a transpubic approach in order to perform a primary anastomosis of the ruptured posterior urethra. Anterior urethral injuries are amenable to débridement and primary anastomosis of the severed parts.

POST-TRAUMATIC URETHRAL STRICTURES

Trauma as well as neisserian infections of the urethra may be followed by fibrotic narrowing [281] of the urethral lumen.

Pathology. The urethra becomes occluded by contracture of the scar about it and gives rise to obstructive uropathy. In addition, periurethral abscesses, urinary extravasations and formation of urethrocutaneous fistulae may complicate the stricture. The breaks in the continuity of the strictured urethra which give rise to these complications occur just proximal to the stricture. Through the break a small amount of urine escapes, and a localized abscess forms which may burrow its way to the skin to form a urethrocutaneous fistula. Should a large amount of bacteria laden urine escape and spread rapidly along fascial planes a life-endangering urinary phlegmon is formed.

Signs and Symptoms. The individual clinical picture varies widely, one being partial obstruction with hesitancy, decrease in size and force of stream and increased frequency; another, uremia; still another, urinary extravasation with periurethral abscesses, phlegmon, or "watering pot" perineum.

Treatment. Uncomplicated strictures generally can be managed by periodic urethral dilatations. These must be carried on from time to time for the rest of the patient's life. If the stricture is very stiff and does not respond to dilatations, internal and external urethrotomy are often performed, and these are followed by dilatation ad infinitum. A plastic procedure devised by Johanson completely eradicates the stricture and effects reconstitution of the urethra with little scar. This may obviate the necessity of repeated dilatation. On occasion, especially after severe trauma to the bony pelvis and the posterior urethra, impassable calcified urethral strictures may develop. The author has treated this type of case by creating an abdominal neourethra from a flap of bladder wall. The patients have been able to void voluntarily through the abdominal wall and to remain continent. The physiologic basis for this operative procedure was elucidated during experimental studies on the urinary sphincter.[275]

The complications of urinary retention, uremia and urinary extravasation are treated according to the principles previously outlined.

PENIS

Trauma to the penis may consist of denudation, amputation or transection, strangulation, or fracture.

Denudation[286] usually is effected by being caught in machinery. The early use of scrotal or free skin grafts or, in selected cases, the replacement of the penile skin is the treatment of choice. *Traumatic amputation or transection*[285] is the handiwork of psychotics or of irate wives and mistresses or husbands. In cases of such amputation or transection, the transected segment should be anastomosed to the base, even though it may have been severed for an hour or more. *Strangulation*[287] of the penis usually is a manifestation of abnormal auto-eroticism; wedding rings, washers, rubber bands and circular erection aids are the usual etiologic agents. Therapy involves the early removal of the constricting object. *Fracture* results from trauma to the organ when in the erect state. Splinting of a torn urethra, or incision and drainage of a secondary thrombosis of the corpora cavernosa may be necessary items in the treatment.

Peyronie's Disease. This condition of the penis is characterized by induration of the tunica albuginea of the corpora cavernosa and/or the intercavernous septum. The cause for the induration is not known. It occurs primarily in middle-age males.

It may produce symptoms consisting of abnormal bending of the penis on erection associated with pain during intercourse. The curvature of the penis may be so great that sexual intercourse cannot be accomplished. On physical examination a hard plaque or cord may be palpated along the dorsal or the lateral aspects of the penile shaft; the urethra and the corpus spongiosum are not involved.

Numerous remedies have been used to treat symptomatic Peyronie's disease, but none has been completely successful. Some of the more recent therapeutic measures include cortisone,[347] vitamin E[346] and para-aminobenzoate.[289]

SCROTUM

Avulsion of scrotal skin is the most common type of scrotal trauma. The treatment[290, 291] depends upon the amount of skin lost. In any case, whenever possible, the testes should be re-covered with remaining scrotal skin, and when this is not possible skin grafts should be applied or the testis placed subcutaneously on the medial aspect of the thigh or over the anterior lower abdomen. The blood supply of the testis is independent of the scrotum; therefore, the testes usually remain viable even though all the scrotal skin is gone, and their surfaces readily accept thick split-thickness skin grafts.

BENIGN SCROTAL ENLARGEMENTS. Hydrocele, one of the most common masses occurring in the scrotum, is characterized by an accumulation of clear, straw-colored fluid within the tunica vaginalis. The hydrocele may be acute and associated with testicular tumor, epididymitis, orchitis or trauma (including herniorrhaphy, orchiopexy and varicocelectomy); most frequently the cystic enlargement of the tunica vaginalis is chronic in character and idiopathic in origin.

Acute hydroceles may be painful. The chronic hydrocele is usually asymptomatic unless it is very large, in which case the patient may complain of a heavy dragging sensation in the groin associated with difficulty in crossing the legs.

The diagnosis of hydrocele is suggested by the history of a scrotal swelling which on examination appears cystic and transilluminates. Needle aspiration of serous yellow fluid from the mass confirms the diagnosis.

Treatment includes (1) simple aspiration of the hydrocele, (2) aspiration and injection of a sclerosing solution or (3) surgical obliteration of the sac. Hydroceles in infants should not be treated by an open operation because, in most instances, the cyst will disappear spontaneously or following simple aspiration. Excision or eversion of the hydrocele sac[350] is the treatment of choice for all chronic *symptomatic* hydroceles.

Spermatocele is a cyst within the scrotum which is attached most commonly to the epididymis or the rete testis. It is relatively rare and usually quite small in size.

It produces no symptoms unless it becomes very large and causes a heavy, dragging sensation.

The spermatocele is similar to the hydrocele in that it feels cystic and transilluminates. It differs from the hydrocele in that it usually is connected to the epididymis or the vas deferens, and its fluid, when aspirated will be found to be white and opalescent and to contain numerous spermatozoa.

No therapy except reassurance is indicated for most spermatocele. If the spermatocele is extremely large, simple excision will suffice.

Varicocele refers to venous varicosities of the vessels of the spermatic cord or the pampiniform plexus. On physical examination it feels like a mass of worms and does not transilluminate.

Varicocele may be idiopathic in origin or it may be caused by obstruction of the internal spermatic vein by retroperitoneal masses such as sarcoma, neuroblastoma or renal neoplasm. Metastases from a left renal tumor into the left renal vein will obstruct the left spermatic vein which empties into the left renal vein and cause a left varicocele.

The idiopathic varicocele is differentiated from the type caused by neoplastic obstruction in that the veins of the idiopathic type empty themselves when the patient is placed in the supine position. No change will be observed in the varicocele caused by obstruction of the internal spermatic vein when the patient is lying flat.

If the idiopathic varicocele is symptomatic, a psychotherapeutic approach is indicated. Surgical treatment is notoriously unsuccessful because most of the symptoms associated with varicocele are psychoneurotic in origin.

TESTIS

Injuries to the testis are rare. Any swelling of the testis not due to obvious inflammation (mumps orchitis) should not be attributed to injury but should be explored for the possibility of neoplasm or torsion. Torsion of the testis is a rotation of the testis and the spermatic cord. When sufficiently twisted, the blood flow to the testis stops and then is attended by testicular infarction or gangrene.

Etiology. Developmental abnormalities of the testis and the adjacent structures predispose to torsion.[292, 293] Absence of the gubernaculum and lack of attachment between epididymis and tunica vaginalis permit the testis, the epididymis and a portion of the spermatic cord to hang free in the surrounding envelope of the tunica vaginalis. Under such circumstances the cord and the testis become twisted more readily. Factors initiating torsion are not known.

Signs and Symptoms. Torsion of the testis may occur at any time but usually during physical exertion or sleep. Sudden excruciating testicular pain associated with nausea and vomiting occurs. Soon after torsion has occurred, the testis will be found high in the scrotum having been raised by the shortened twisted cord. After the passage of hours, edema, erythema and tenderness of the scrotum appear, and pain decreases. Then the scrotum and its contents become difficult to examine.

Treatment. Surgical exploration should be performed as soon as presumptive diagnosis of torsion has been made. The testis may be saved, even though much time has passed. The operation consists of untwisting the cord. If after untwisting the cord, the testis appears to be viable it is attached to the inner layers of the scrotum with several silk sutures taken through the tunica albuginea. In the case of testicular gangrene, orchiectomy is required. The other testis also should be anchored, because the developmental anomaly is usually bilateral; therefore, both testes are subject to torsion.

PHYSIOLOGY OF URINARY TRANSPORT AND MICTURITION

After urine enters the calyceal system it is propelled by coordinated segmented smooth muscle contractions into the infundibulum, the pelvis and down the ureter. The ureter propels the urine from the renal pelvis into the bladder where it collects for varying periods of time, depending somewhat upon the desire of the individual.

URETER

Sympathetic fibers to the ureter control its vascular elements but have no recordable effect upon ureteral peristalsis. The ureter is autonomous in that its peristalsis proceeds normally, even though the nerves to it are rendered nonconductive. The normal stimulus for ureteral peristalsis appears to be the pressure of urine high in the renal calyces.[298] The contraction of the ureter is superimposed upon a high-tensional quiescent state, the contraction is followed by relaxation and the fall of intra-ureteral pressure to a level below that existing during rest. When urine output is low, ureteral peristaltic waves are infrequent. During diuresis peristaltic waves are very frequent, and their amplitudes are so shallow as to make the ureter appear to be a rigid tube.

Ureteral contractions increase in amplitude and frequency when the intravesical or intra-ureteral pressures are raised. Traumatic irritation of the ureter by catheters or calculi can produce large irregular muscular contractions which are not related to urine volume or intravesical pressure. Portions of ureter can be excised and an anastomosis accomplished without impairing ureteral contractions, excepting for a temporary delay in conduction at the anastomotic site, provided that little fibrous tissue appears at the anastomotic site.

Human ureteral muscular tonicity and peristalsis are not affected by therapeutic doses of drugs.[297] Morphine does not cause spasm of the ureter and therefore is an effective analgesic for alleviating ureteral colic.

BLADDER

The normal individual voids 3 or 4 times during the day and occasionally once during the night. On volition the urinary stream is started within 1 to 2 seconds, and it can be stopped quickly at will. The urinary stream is continuous until terminally when efforts to evacuate the urethra interrupt the stream. Abdominal muscular contractions are not requisite for micturition[304] However, should they be instituted they put pressure upon the bladder and increase the force of the urinary stream once it has been started. Experimental data is subject to voluntary control and that micturition can be started or stopped voluntarily without the contraction or relaxation of the striated muscle of the sphincter. However, in the absence of the sphincteric striated muscle the urinary stream cannot be stopped as rapidly; instead of the normal stopping time of 1 to 2 seconds, from 6 to 10 seconds are needed.

Micturition is actually a simple process governed by the higher centers in the normal individual. The bladder consists not only of a globular portion called the fundus but also of a tubular part commonly known as the urethra. The muscular layer of the urethra is a continuation of the muscle in the wall of the bladder[313, 318] and is innervated by the same parasympathetic fibers. The smooth muscle of the bladder possesses the qualities of tonicity and accommodation that are inherent in the smooth muscle and independent of motor impulses from the central nervous system. Tonicity refers to the ability of smooth muscle to maintain continuous tension; accommodation is that property of bladder that permits

URETHROVESICAL DYNAMICS

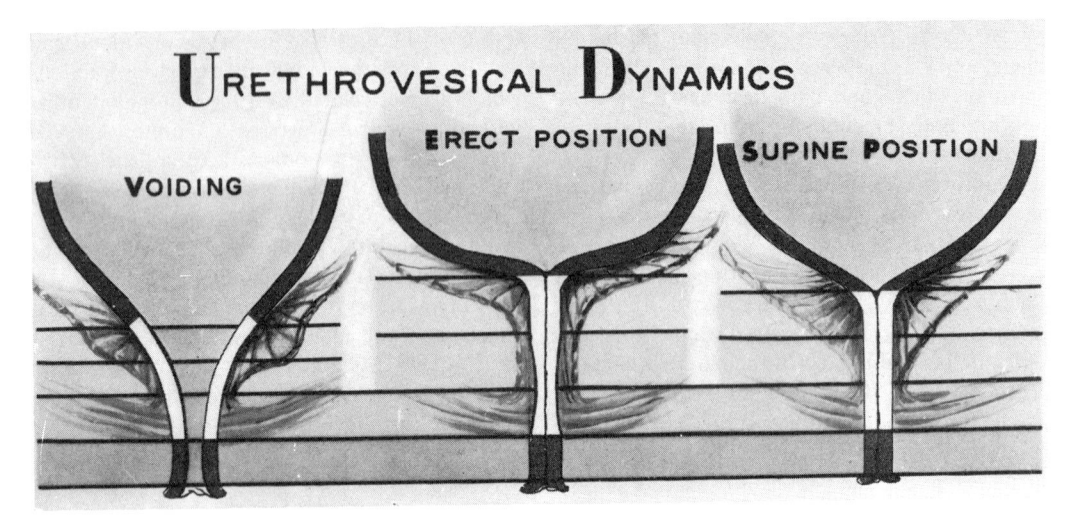

FIG. 52-28. Role of the urinary sphincter in urethrovesical dynamics.

it to maintain a constant low intravesical pressure in the face of increasing volumes of fluid. Smooth muscle does not depend upon the central nervous system for its tonicity, whereas skeletal muscle does. Therefore, an atonic flaccid bladder is one that has been overdistended with urine, regardless of the cause of the retention. Bladder muscle is not weakened or rendered flaccid by cutting nerves to it.[314] A flaccid distended bladder may be rendered hypertonic and small by frequent voidings or by keeping the bladder empty through constant catheter or suprapubic cystotomy drainage, regardless of the neurologic state of the individual.

NEUROANATOMY

The fundus or globular portion of the bladder receives urine continually from the ureters and stores it at relatively low pressures until capacity is reached. The urine is prevented from flowing out of the bladder during the period of storage by the urinary sphincter (Fig. 52-28). The urinary sphincter has been found to be a tubular structure synonymous with the promixal three fourths of the female urethra or the prostatic and membranous portions of the male urethra; in both male and female these segments of urethra are actually the true bladder necks.[307, 309] The wall of the urethra contains much elastic tissue in addition to smooth muscle.[318] The urinary sphincter maintains continence by virtue of the resistance its apposing walls present to fluid pressure. The elastic and muscle fibers in the urethral wall keep the lumen of the urethra narrow without the aid of motor impulses from the central nervous system. Thus, the storage of urine by the bladder (fundus and neck) is a very efficient process in that it is performed in an autonomous, tireless fashion with a negligible expenditure of energy.

When intravesical pressure is markedly elevated by exertion, urethral resistance must be increased to prevent urinary incontinence. In the normal human male or female this is accomplished by the 2-fold action of the striated muscle of the urogenital diaphragm and the pelvic floor.[309] These muscles compress the urethra or urinary sphincter circumferentially as well as elongate it by pulling it cephalad toward the fundus (Fig. 52-28). The net result of the striped muscle activity is to decrease the caliber of the urethral lumen, to increase the tension of the urethral walls against its lumen and to increase the length of the urethra—all factors that increase the resistance of the urinary sphincter to the flow of fluid through it. The levator ani and muscle of the urogenital diaphragm can be contracted or relaxed voluntarily. They can contract reflexly also as in standing, coughing, sneezing, etc. These muscles are essential for the abrupt termination of urination.[302, 303]

The motor nerves to bladder muscle are

FIG. 52-29. Neuroanatomy of the bladder: sites of action of Banthine.

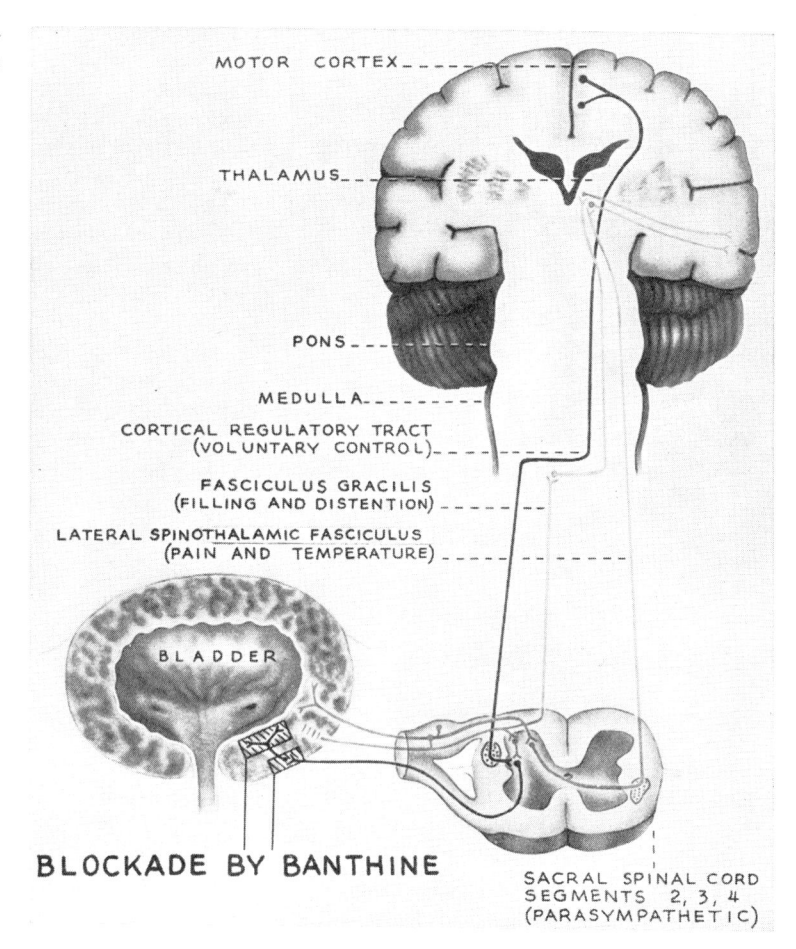

quiescent when urination is not occurring. The efferent nerves conducting motor impulses to the bladder are from the craniosacral or parasympathetic nervous system and from part of the pelvic nerve. The sympathetic nervous system plays no part in the process of micturition in man. Most of the sensory nerve fibers carrying exteroceptive and proprioceptive sensations from the bladder to the central nervous system accompany the parasympathetic motor fibers in the pelvic nerve. The exteroceptive sensations include pain and temperature; the proprioceptive endings give rise to the feeling of bladder fullness and to the desire to void.

The motor neurons supplying the bladder musculature lie in the lateral horns of the sacral spinal cord at the levels of S2, S3 and S4. The motor fibers extend from the motor neuron to the wall of the bladder where ganglionic synapses and postganglionic fibers are situated (Fig. 52-29).

An intact spinal reflex arc and a normal vesical musculature are requisites for complete emptying of the bladder. As the bladder fills with urine, the proprioceptive endings are stretched, and sensory impulses are carried to the spinal cord. In the spinal cord the afferent impulses bombard and, eventually, cause a discharge of the lower motor neurons. The impulses arising in the motor neurons travel over the efferent parasympathetic fibers, ganglionic synapses and nueromuscular endings to stimulate contraction of the bladder fundus and neck. The bladder fundus contracts down upon the bolus of urine and simultaneously pulls open the tubular bladder neck to expel the urine.[307, 318]

If the muscles of the pelvic floor and the urogenital diaphragm are in a state of contraction prior to urination, they must be relaxed in order for urine to transverse the urethra. These muscles are striated, and their

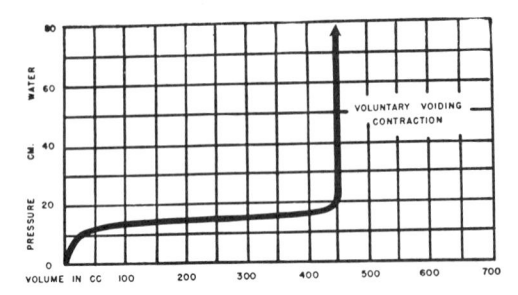

EXTEROCEPTIVE SENSATION
- HEAT - PRESENT
- COLD - PRESENT

PROPRIOCEPTIVE SENSATION
- FIRST DESIRE - PRESENT AT 175 CC. VOL.
- FULLNESS - PRESENT AT 450 CC. VOL.

CAPACITY - 500 CC. VOL.

UNINHIBITED CONTRACTIONS - NONE

VOIDING STREAM - UNINTERRUPTED

RESIDUAL - 0 CC.

FIG. 52-30. Cystometrograph of a normal bladder.

motor neurons lie in the anterior horn of sacral spinal segments 2, 3 and 4.

The spinal reflex arc concerned with urination functions without voluntary control in the infant. As the child grows, the long spinal nerve tracts linking the higher centers to the lower reflex arcs begin to operate. Pain and temperature sensations are carried to the higher centers by the lateral spinothalamic tract, and proprioceptive impulses ascend by way of the fasciculus gracilis. The lower reflex arc is brought under the control of the higher centers through the descending cortico-regulatory tracts (Fig. 52-29). The cortico-regulatory tract can initiate as well as inhibit voiding contractions of the bladder by directly influencing the lower motor neurons to the bladder—a direct cortical control over smooth muscle.[313]

Cystometry. Bladder function can be evaluated by the cystometric examination,[306] which is conducted as follows:

1. The person is requested to void. The character of micturition is observed, noting especially the time taken to initiate micturition, the size and the caliber of stream, the continuity of stream and the relationship of abdominal straining to micturition.

2. After voiding, a catheter is passed, and the volume of the residual urine is recorded. Through the catheter 60 ml. of cold and then 60 ml. of warm water are instilled to test exteroceptive perception.

3. The urethral catheter is then connected to a water manometric cystometer, and water is instilled into the bladder at the rate of 60 drops per minute. The person is requested to tell the examiner when he becomes conscious of the desire to micturate and again when the bladder feels full. The intravesical pressures and volumes are plotted on a cystometrographic sheet.

4. When the patient's bladder is full, the catheter is withdrawn, and the patient is requested to void. Again observations similar to those outlined in Step 1 are made. A typical normal cystometrograph is shown in Fig. 52-30.

Denervation Supersensitivity. Investigations have demonstrated that the intrinsic stretch reaction of the chronically denervated human bladder responds in an exaggerated manner to the parasympathomimetic drug Urecholine.[311] This phenomenon is the basis for the development of a specific, objective test for the motor and the sensory paralytic types of bladder. The examination is now used routinely as part of the cystometric procedure and is performed as follows: (1) The usual cystometric test is conducted as previously described. (2) With the patient attached to the cystometric apparatus and the rate of flow from the reservoir adjusted to a slow stream (1 ml./sec.), fluid is permitted to flow into the bladder. When the volume instilled into the bladder reaches 100 ml., the intravesical pressure is recorded and the flow then stopped. (3) The adult patient is administered 2.5 mg. of Urecholine subcutaneously. The stretch response test described in Step 2 is repeated 10, 20, and 30 minutes after the Urecholine injection.

A patient with a normal bladder will demonstrate a rise in intravesical pressure of no greater than 15 cm. of water over that of the control run, in response to the Urecholine. In contrast, the patient with a motor or sensory paralytic bladder will exhibit an increase in intravesical pressure greater than 15 cm. of water pressure; usually the response is in the range of 30 to 60 cm. of water pressure.

When the usual cystometric examination indicates uninhibited contractions, or if the Urecholine evokes uncontrolled voiding contractions of the bladder, then it is necessary to repeat the Urecholine test on another day, for it is important to delineate the lesions of the lower reflex arc from upper motor neuron dysfunctions by repeating the Urecholine test after spinal anesthesia or ganglion blockade with Arfonad.

A normal response to Urecholine has been designated arbitrarily as a *negative Urecholine test*, while the supersensitive response is called a *positive Urecholine test*.

Neurogenic Bladder. Lesions of one or more of the nerve tracts concerned with urination produce dysfunction of the bladder. Bladders so affected are called neurogenic bladders and can be one of several different types or combinations thereof.

THE UNINHIBITED NEUROGENIC BLADDER.[305] This is caused by a lesion of the corticoregulatory tract and is characterized by difficulty in controlling urination. The patient complains of hesitancy, increased frequency of urination, urgency and incontinence. The sensation of filling is not disturbed, and urine is not retained in the bladder after voiding. The residual urine is within normal limits. A cystometrograph (Fig. 52-31) demonstrates uninhibited contractions of the bladder musculature. Multiple sclerosis, paresis and cerebrovascular accidents are prone to be attended by the uninhibited neurogenic bladder. Therapeutic efforts are directed toward the improvement of the control of micturition by blocking aberrant motor impulses at the terminal ganglia and nerve endings with drugs such as Banthine[257] and belladonna. The dosage of these drugs is adjusted to provide good control of micturition while maintaining the bladder's capacity to empty itself completely.

THE REFLEX NEUROGENIC BLADDER.[299, 303] This type occurs in transverse myelitis in which both the sensory and the motor tracts to and from the higher centers are interrupted above the level of sacral spinal segments 2, 3 and 4. The patient has neither exteroceptive

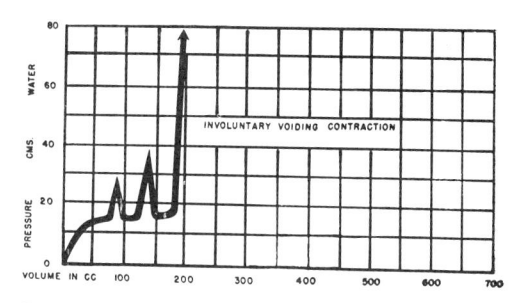

EXTEROCEPTIVE SENSATION
   HEAT - PRESENT
   COLD - PRESENT

PROPRIOCEPTIVE SENSATION
   FIRST DESIRE - PRESENT AT 75 CC. VOL.
   FULLNESS - PRESENT AT 175 CC VOL

CAPACITY - 175 CC. VOL.

UNINHIBITED CONTRACTIONS - PRESENT

VOIDING STREAM - UNINTERRUPTED

RESIDUAL - 0 CC.

Urecholine Test - Negative

FIG. 52-31. Cystometrograph of an uninhibited neurogenic bladder.

sensation or the capacity to start or stop micturition volitionally in a normal way. The person responds as does a baby before urinary continence is acquired. The cystometrograph (Fig. 52-32) demonstrates uninhibited contractions, no sensation and frequently an abnormally high residual urine. Vesical neck contracture, a weak reflex voiding contraction or spasm of the periurethral striated muscle[300] are the possible causes for the carrying of a larger urinary residuum.

During the period of spinal shock, the bladder is exactly the same as that observed in the patient subjected to spinal anesthesia. There is no sensation and no evidence whatsoever of any voiding contractions of the detrusor. *However, bladder tonicity and accommodation are perfectly normal*, provided that the bladder is drained soon after urinary retention develops. It is quite obvious then that all patients in spinal shock should be catheterized as soon as possible. If drainage is not instituted immediately, the patient's bladder will

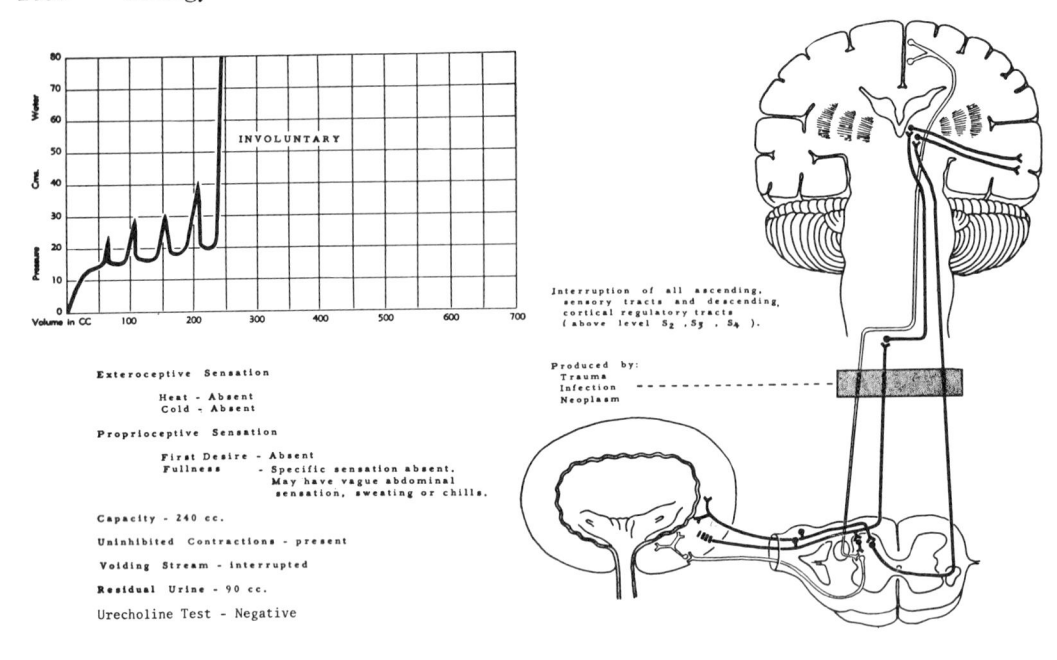

FIG. 52-32. Cystometrograph of a reflex neurogenic bladder and illustration of the involved nerve tracts.

become overdistended by retained urine, and atonicity will occur. It is our belief that in all cases of spinal cord injury not recovering normal function within a week or two after trauma a cutaneous vesicostomy[310] should be performed. This is an operative procedure designated to create an abdominal vesicocutaneous fistula that will not stricture and will drain the bladder continuously. The patient is kept dry by means of a suitable device applied to the abdominal wall.

Cutaneous vesicostomy may appear to be radical therapy, but our recommendation of its use is based on 20 years of experience dealing with the urologic problems of the paraplegic and 12 years of experience with cutaneous vesicostomy. A large proportion of paraplegics, irrespective of their ability to empty their bladders, eventually develop kidney disease, such as pyelonephritis, hydronephrosis and nephrolithiasis. Many of them will also demonstrate lesions related to the urethra, such as diverticula, periurethral abscesses and urethrocutaneous fistulas. In addition, nearly every true paraplegic must wear a device to prevent soiling from urinary incontinence. Thus the patient with the cutaneous vesicostomy contends with no more than the individual without the fistula insofar as the incontinence device is concerned, and our observations in over 200 patients indicate that vesicostomy can prevent the renal and the urethral complications in paraplegia.

THE AUTONOMOUS NEUROGENIC BLADDER. This type characteristically attends the destruction of the sacral segment of the spinal cord and is a trouble borne by patients with myelomeningocele, spina bifida and other lesions causing destruction of the sacral spinal cord. In these patients the lower reflex arc is interrupted, and all sensations of vesical origin are absent, and no voiding contractions, voluntary or involuntary, occur (Fig. 52-33). The periurethral striated muscle is flaccid, the bulbocavernous reflex is absent, and there is saddle anesthesia. The exertion of pressure upon the bladder, either manually (Credé) or by abdominal straining, is the only means of effecting interval micturition. If these maneuvers are not performed, overflow urination keeps the patients wet. Typically, micturition in these patients is characterized by

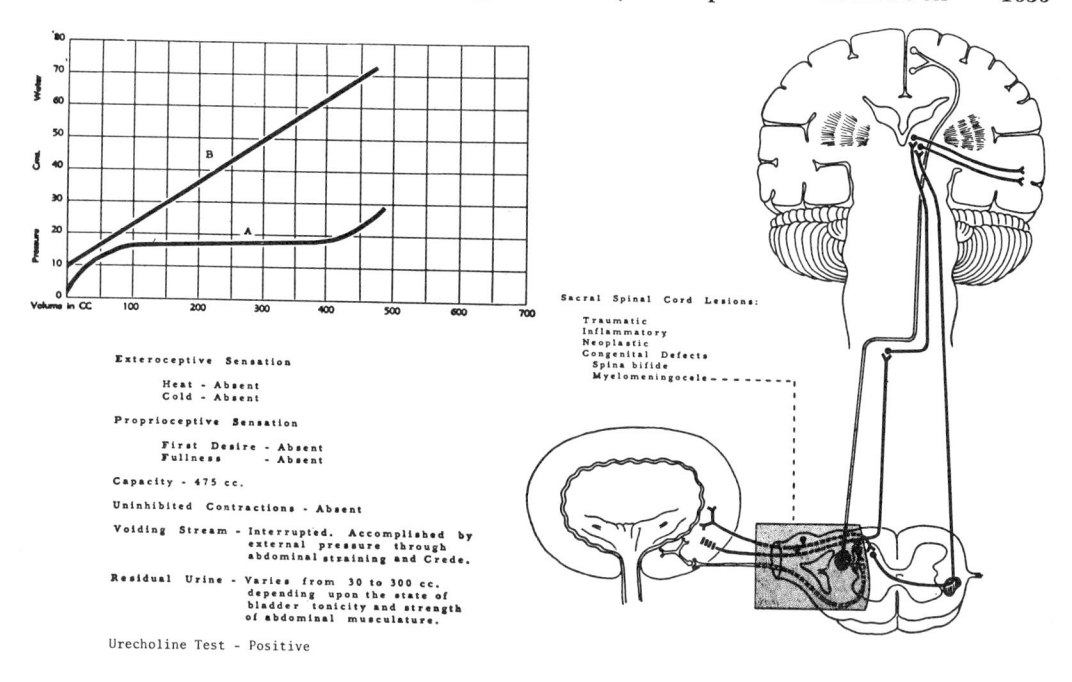

Fig. 52-33. Cystometrograph of an autonomous neurogenic bladder and its associated nerve tract lesion.

inhaling deeply and then straining. Urine is expelled during the strain but stops as soon as the forced expiration against the closed glottis ceases. The residual urine may be within normal limits.

Cystometric examination in these individuals reveals absent sensation and lack of any voiding contractions of the detrusor muscle (Fig. 52-33). The bladder exhibits a supersensitive stretch response to a minimal dose of Urecholine. Curve A represents the test response of patients who have been on catheter drainage and whose bladder capacity has been maintained within normal limits; Curve B, that of patients who have been evacuating their bladders by Credé or abdominal straining over a period of months.

Since most of these patients eventually develop recurrent episodes of pyelonephritis, hydronephrosis and, in some cases, periurethral abscesses, it is best to place these patients on permanent suprapubic drainage by means of the cutaneous vesicostomy; this is a primary and definitive procedure.

MOTOR PARALYTIC BLADDER. This is encountered most frequently in patients with poliomyelitis and polyradiculoneuritis (Fig. 52-34). Usually the patient suffers from complete urinary retention incidental to paralysis of the lower motor neurons but has perfectly normal sensation. In the case of poliomyelitis treatment consists of catheter drainage until the paralysis disappears. This is usually a period of 7 to 10 days in length. Permanent paralysis of lower motor neurons may require cutaneous vesicostomy. The detrusor muscle of the chronic motor paralytic bladder is supersensitive to Urecholine.

SENSORY PARALYTIC BLADDER. This type occurs with locomotor ataxia. The proprioceptive sense of fullness is lost, and consequently the musculature of the bladder becomes overdistended and as a result is atonic and decompensated (Fig. 52-35). Treatment is directed toward correcting the atonicity and preventing its recurrence. Continuous Urecholine has been found to be extremely effective in restoring the tonicity of the tabetic bladder.[308] A 1- to 3-week course of treatment is used, beginning with a 3-day regimen of 7.5 to 10 mg. of Urecholine subcutaneously every 4

1640   Urology

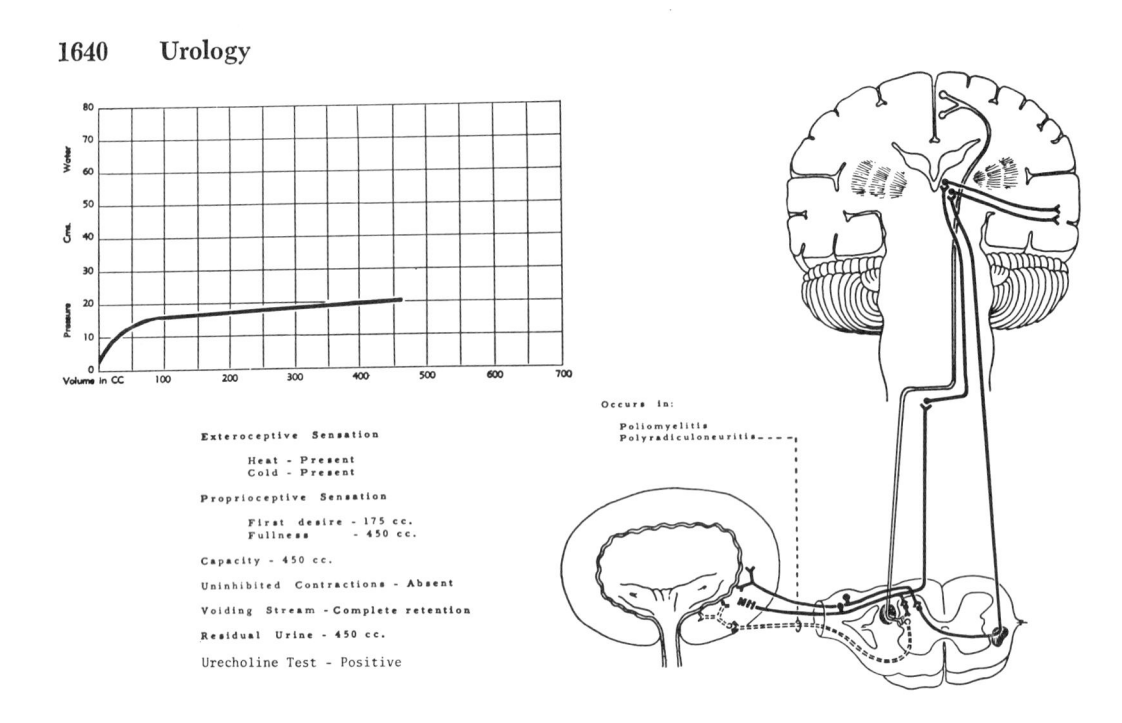

FIG. 52-34. Cystometrograph of motor paralytic bladder and its neuropathology.

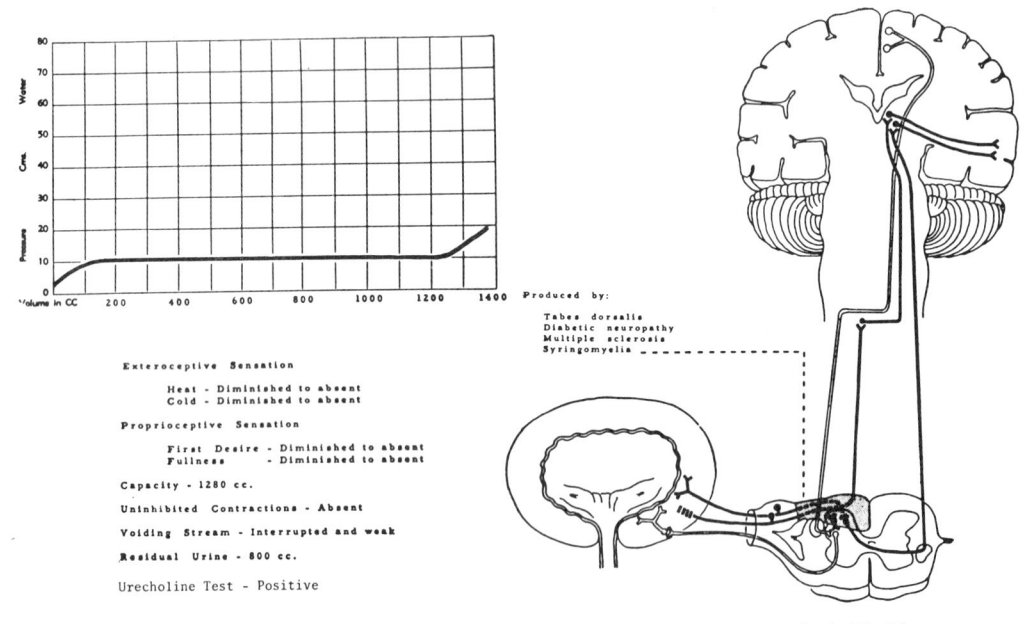

FIG. 52-35. Cystometrograph and neuropathology of the sensory paralytic bladder.

hours and continuing with an oral dosage of 50 to 100 mg. every 4 hours. In order to forestall overdistention, the sensory paralytic bladder must be emptied at normal intervals, e.g., every 3 hours, irrespective of bladder sensation. The optic nerves and the clock must become substitutes for the impaired bladder sensory tracts.

TYPES OF URINARY INCONTINENCE[319]

The error most commonly made in the diagnosis and treatment of urinary incontinence in children is the assumption that most of the cases observed are psychogenic. Experience indicates that a large number of children with urinary incontinence suffer from obstructive uropathy, sacral spinal cord lesions, upper motor neuron defects, and developmental anomalies of the urinary tract. It is obvious that urinary incontinence of the "physiologic type" does not alarm the physician or the parents until the child is about 3 years old. At this age one expects most children to be toilet-trained; complete urologic investigation is necessary if incontinence persists beyond the age of three.

Urinary incontinence of a type other than the "physiologic" should be studied as soon as possible, irrespective of the age of the child. The incontinence may be indicative of a progressive process that is endangering the life of the individual as, for example, in obstructive uropathy.

The most frequent mistake in diagnosis of enuresis in the adult female is the presumption that all cases are stress urinary incontinence, and the most common error in therapy is the idea that most of the cases can be cured by anterior colporrhaphy or the Marshall-Marchetti procedure.

Paradoxical or Overflow Incontinence. When the bladder is unable to empty itself and becomes overdistended, the intravesical pressure increases and eventually overcomes the resistance of the urinary sphincter. The patient leaks urine constantly from the urethra and is unable to initiate and maintain a good urinary stream. Examination of the abdomen reveals a distended bladder.

The inability of the bladder to empty may be due to obstruction to the outflow of urine or to an impaired voiding contraction of the bladder. The exact diagnosis requires endoscopy, cystometry, pyelography, voiding cystourethrography, urethral calibration with the bougie à boule and measurement of urethral length in the female. Incidentally, *this diagnostic armamentarium must be employed in virtually every case of urinary incontinence in order to identify accurately the type and the etiology of enuresis.*

The treatment of the patient with overflow incontinence varies with the cause. In the individual with obstructive uropathy it is necessary to remove impediments to urinary outflow such as stricture of the urethra and its meatus, urethral valves, prostatic hyperplasia, vesical neck contracture, carcinoma of the prostrate, etc. When the voiding contraction of the bladder is impaired by a partial lesion of the sacral spinal cord or the cauda equina, Urecholine may be helpful in emptying the bladder.[308] If there is involvement of all the lower motor neurons, urinary diversion by cutaneous vesicostomy is the treatment of choice.[310]

Ectopic Ureter.[328] Continual leaking of urine may be encountered in the female with an ectopic ureteral orifice opening into the distal urethra or outside the urinary sphincter such as the vestibule or the vagina. When the ureteral orifice opens into the distal portion of urethra, incontinence is present because the resistance in the distal urethra to urinary flow is much less than the resistance of the midportion of the urethra. The male with an ectopic ureter is usually continent because the ectopic ureteral orifice opens into the prostatic urethra which presents less resistance to urinary flow than the membranous portion of the urethra; thus, the urine flows back into the bladder rather than through the distal urethra.

The female patient with urinary incontinence due to an ectopic ureter will relate that since infancy she has had constant leaking of urine which is present day and night. In addition the patient will state that she voids normal amounts of urine at regular intervals.

The diagnostic armamentarium reveals duplication anomalies of the ureter and the renal collecting system and an ectopic ureteral orifice.

Treatment depends on the condition of the ectopic ureter and its associated renal segment. If the renal segment and the ureter are in good shape, reimplantation of the ureter into the bladder is indicated; a badly damaged kidney necessitates nephro-ureterectomy.

Total Incompetence of the Urinary Sphincter. When the proximal three fourths of the urethra in the female or the prostatic and the membranous portions in the male are compromised, a constant dripping type of incontinence will result. In the child, congenital failure of the urethra to close (epispadias) may result in continuous leakage of urine. In the female adult, trauma during parturition may produce a defect in the urethral musculature along its entire length and result in enuresis. A similar type of defect may be created iatrogenically during repair of procidentia, cystocele, urethral diverticulum, vaginal hysterectomy and transurethral resection of the urethra.

In the male, radical prostatectomy and at times simple prostatectomy may be associated with disruption of the integrity of the urinary sphincter remaining in the region of the membranous urethra, with resultant dripping incontinence.[320] Whenever incontinence ensues after a transurethral prostatectomy, the surgeon can be fairly certain that he has gone beyond the confines of the prostatic fossa and resected part of the wall of the membranous urethra—not the periurethral striated muscle.

In contrast with the patients with parodoxical incontinence who have dripping of urine with distended bladders, the individuals with total incompetence of the urinary sphincter have very little urine in their bladders. Occasionally the patient with a myelomeningocele may exhibit incontinence of the dripping type with a nearly empty bladder and possess an intact urethra. This occurs when the bladder has become spastic because of cystitis, the urethra has become dilated because of constant high pressure applied to it by the paralyzed spastic bladder, and the periurethral striated muscle mass is ineffective because of flaccid paralysis.

A continual dripping type of incontinence without bladder distention and intact urethra may also be observed in the rare female in whom stress incontinence has deteriorated into the dripping type. The mechanism for this will be discussed later under stress incontinence.

Treatment of the patient with total incompetence of the urinary sphincter varies with the etiologic mechanism. Obviously, the entire diagnostic armamentarium must be employed to delineate the exact cause of a dripping type of urinary incontinence.

The principle upon which therapy is based in the case of the partially damaged urethra involves reconstruction of the urethra.[321] In the case of epispadias this implies closure of the urethra to form a muscular tube. When there is a defect along the floor of the urethra, excision of the defect and reapproximation of the separated muscle layer are indicated.[322] At the present time there is no satisfactory method for treating the female whose urethra is completely destroyed or the male with post-prostatectomy incontinence. Neo-urethras constructed from bladder muscle have been used but have been unsatisfactory in the dependent subpubic position.

Partial Incompetence of the Urinary Sphincter—Stress Incontinence.[323] Urinary incontinence on coughing, straining, flexing, lifting, etc., has been designated stress incontinence. It is seen infrequently in males following prostatectomy and in paralysis of the periurethral striated muscles and is a common occurrence in females.

The basic defect in this group of patients is a partial reduction in the length of effective urinary sphincter. Most of the women with stress incontinence exhibit a total urethral length of less than 3.0 cm. in the standing position in contrast with continent women who demonstrate urethral lengths greater than 3.0 cm. The urinary sphincter shortens in these patients because the urethrovesical junction is not maintained in its normal position in the upright position. As the length of the urethra is decreased, the less the resistance or pressure it presents to counteract intravesical pressure. Thus it takes less and less intravesical pressure to produce incontinence as the urethra collapses to a greater and greater degree. Eventually the point may be reached where the patient who began with loss of urine only on marked exertion, will deteriorate into a constant dripping type of enuresis.

The exact treatment for this type of stress incontinence is to lengthen the urethra to normal proportions and fix it in this position so that it will not collapse in the erect position. This is accomplished most efficiently by the anterior urethropexy procedure.[323]

On occasion the patient may have scar tissue replacing a portion of the normal muscular and elastic tissue of the urethral wall. Urethral length in these patients may be within normal limits in both the supine and the standing positions but the individual may still exhibit stress incontinence. Under these circumstances the actual length of the urethra or sphincter is normal but the functional length has been decreased by the dimensions of the segment of scar tissue; adequate tension of the urethral wall requires normal muscle and elastic tissue around the entire circumference of the urethra. Fibrous tissue formation has been produced by electroresection of the urethra, inadequate repair of urethrovaginal fistulas and iatrogenic trauma to the urethral floor during transvaginal operative procedures.

Adequate therapy for the urethra with scar tissue in its wall is to excise the scar tissue either transvaginally or suprapubically and reestablish normal muscle and epithelial layers around the entire circumference of the urethra.

Urinary Fistulas in the Female. The complaint of leaking of urine from the vagina is common to all members of this group. The dripping of urine may be constant, or it may occur at intervals not associated as well as associated with micturition. The fistulous tract may be ureterovaginal, vesicovaginal, urethrovaginal or any combination thereof. Therapy involves excision of the fistulous tract and reestablishment of integrity of the involved organs of the urinary tract.

The suprapubic approach is preferable in handling vesicovaginal and ureterovaginal fistulas; the transvaginal approach is adequate for most urethrovaginal fistulas. In the young child and in some adults the suprapubic approach is necessary for repair of urethrovaginal fistulas.

Uninhibited Neurogenic Bladder. (See p. 1637.)

Psychogenic Incontinence. Some cases of incontinence in children and adults arise as the result of conflicts in the relationship between patient and environment. The patient develops urinary incontinence in an attempt to solve some difficult problems.

The urinary incontinence is usually of an intermittent type and manifests itself primarily by bed-wetting and soiling of clothes with urine. There are no symptoms of urgency or pollakiuria. The entire examination may be negative except for the history, which may uncover obvious evidence of an unfavorable home environment.

The patient with a presumptive diagnosis of psychogenic incontinence should be referred to the psychiatrist for examination, advice and treatment.

Mixed Types of Incontinence. Not all cases of incontinence are strictly of one pure type; many different combinations can occur. In children one may encounter enuresis which may be both uninhibited and psychogenic in type. In the elderly male overflow incontinence due to obstruction and an uninhibited neurogenic bladder due to an upper motor neuron lesion may be present simultaneously. The female with stress incontinence may also be plagued by an uninhibited neurogenic bladder.

The diagnosis of a mixed type of urinary incontinence can be made without too much difficulty provided that a complete examination is performed. For alleviation of the incontinence one must treat each of the types involved.

CONGENITAL ANOMALIES

KIDNEY

Embryology. The nephrons are derived from mesodermal renal blastema, whereas the excretory system, including the collecting tubules, the calyces, the infundibula, the pelvis and the ureter, is derived from the entoderm of the hindgut. In the normal course of development the two systems become one when the secretory tubules of the nephrons join the collecting tubules of the excretory system.

As the embryo develops the kidneys ascend from the region of the pelvic cavity to their adult lumbar position. In the pelvic cavity the kidney lies with its medulla and pelvis facing anteriorly and the cortical and the cortical convex border facing posteriorly. As the kidney ascends, it turns through 90° so that its pelvis faces medially and the cortex laterally. While the embryonic kidney lies in the pelvis the calyces point posteriorly; after attainment of the lumbar position, they point laterally.

Renal Agenesis. During the development of some embryos, abnormalities arise in the formation of the kidneys and the ureters. Both kidneys may be absent, and the fetus consequently nonviable, or one kidney and ureter may fail to develop. This is called renal agenesis.

Duplication of the pelvis and the ureter is the most common renal anomaly. As a general rule, the ureter originating from the higher part of the kidney inserts lower into the bladder or other organ. The double ureter may be partial or complete. When two completely separate ureters exist unilaterally, there are

2 ureteral orifices on the same side of the ureteral ridge.

Ectopic Ureter. Occasionally, the ureter from the upper pelvis opens into the urethra, the vagina or the seminal vesicle and is called an ectopic ureter.

Ectopic Kidney. A pelvic ectopic kidney is one that fails to ascend and remains in the pelvis. This anomaly in a woman may interfere with normal pregnancy and delivery. Frequently, the kidney ascends but fails to rotate.

Horseshoe Kidney. The kidneys may join one another at their lower poles before ascending from the pelvis, forming a fused kidney. The fusion tissue may be parenchymal or fibrous. When the joined kidneys ascend into the lumbar region while each kidney attains its normal paravertebral position, the fused kidney is called a horseshoe kidney.

Crossed Renal Ectopia. If the fused kidney is located entirely to one side of the spine it is designated as crossed renal ectopia.

Aberrant Lower Pole Vessels. Abnormal blood vessels to the kidney include accessory arteries and veins to either the upper or the lower poles. The aberrant lower pole vessels may cross the ureter and compress it, giving rise to ureteral narrowing and intermittent or continuous hydronephrosis. Sometimes it may be the cause of Dietl's crises or hypertension of the Goldblatt type.

Polycystic disease of the kidney is a most interesting congenital anomaly. It is hereditary and frequently lethal, either at birth or during middle age. The polycystic kidneys of infants succumbing shortly after birth demonstrate the failure of union of the nephron tubule with the collecting tubule. Adults with polycystic disease demonstrate union between secretory and collecting tubules but show diverticula of the tubules. The adult type of polycystic kidney is thus capable of adequate functioning until the enlarging diverticula, or cysts, destroy most of the renal tissue by pressure atrophy.[326, 327]

The polycystic kidney is markedly enlarged and composed primarily of cysts of varying size. Polycystic kidneys are usually bilateral and palpable because of their size. They may be asymptomatic or give rise to pain, hematuria, urinary infection, hypertension and progressive renal failure. They may be associated with cystic changes in other organs, especially the liver, the pancreas and the lungs.

DIAGNOSIS can be made by pyelography which demonstrates relatively enormous collecting systems with multiple cystic deformities of the calyces and infundibula.

TREATMENT is palliative and includes measures directed toward delaying progression of renal failure.

URETER

There is a considerable variety of developmental anomalies of the ureter, but only a few are clinically important. Ureteral ectopia[328] and duplication have been mentioned before.

An ectopic ureter may be the cause of a constantly dripping incontinence when its opening enters the urogenital tract below the vesical sphincter. This happens most often in the female. The *diagnosis* is readily made by finding the ectopic ureteral orifice and this is not difficult. *Treatment* involves ureterectomy and segmental resection of the part of the kidney it drained.

Ureterocele. Congenital obstructions of the ureteral meatus lead to intravesical ureteral dilatation just proximal to the stenosis. This produces a cystlike structure inside the bladder. This ureteral cyst or ureterocele[330] may be small, or it may be so large as to obstruct the vesical outlet and thereby lead to bilateral hydronephrosis. The *diagnosis* is made upon cystoscopy. The *treatment* consists solely of its transurethral or suprapubic excision.

Congenital megalo-ureter is a hydroureter having no discernibly organic obstruction as its cause. The *diagnosis* is made by exclusion. The *etiology* is unknown. Its *treatment* is still an unsolved problem.[329]

BLADDER

The most common bladder anomalies are congenital diverticula, patent urachus and exstrophy.

A congenital diverticulum[334] is an outpouching of a segment of bladder wall unassociated with obstructive uropathy. It differs from an acquired diverticulum in that it contains muscle, whereas the acquired type does not. When the diverticula are large they may retain urine; they predispose to cystitis, calculus formation and difficulty in micturition. The *diagnosis* is readily made upon cystoscopy and cystography. If the diverticula are large and troublesome they should be removed.

The urachus[331] is a fetal canal which connects the bladder with the allantois. After birth the urachus loses its connection with the umbilicus and becomes a cord—the middle umbilical ligament. In some people partial or complete patency of the urachus persists after birth. Complete patency is associated with leaking of urine through the umbilicus. Obliteration at the distal and the proximal ends of the urachus while the remainder is patent gives rise to cysts or abscesses beneath the anterior abdominal wall below the umbilicus. Should the umbilical end close while the vesical connection remains open, stones or neoplasms may form in it. The *diagnosis* can be made by cystoscopy and injection of the urachus with a radiopaque medium, if the urachus communicates with the bladder. Similarly, the probing or the injection of a radiopaque medium at the umbilical end of the tract, should it open there, may serve to make the diagnosis and delineate the tract. Another method of diagnosis, though rarely applicable, is the finding of a dye in the urine immediately after its injection into the tract. The *treatment* involves the complete excision of the urachus.

Exstrophy of the bladder[335] is a rather rare anomaly occurring in both the male and the female. It is said to be due to a mesodermal deficiency. It is characterized by absence of (1) the anterior wall of the bladder, (2) that portion of the anterior abdominal wall that overlies the bladder, (3) the symphysis pubis, and (4) the dorsal portion of the urethra in males. Because of these defects the posterior wall of the bladder and the trigone with its ureteral orifices form the lower anterior abdominal wall, thereby exposing the mucosa of the bladder and the ureteral orifices to view. The sufferer is a social outcast because he or she constantly emanates the odor of urine and wets his pants or skirt. The abnormal development of the pelvic bones leads to a waddling gait.

TREATMENT[332, 333] until the past several years consisted primarily of excision of the bladder, supravesical urinary diversion (ileal conduit, ureterosigmoid transplantation) and repair of the epispadias. Recently, many surgeons were attempting to close the bladder and the urethra so that normally functioning organs would result. Preliminary results of such reconstructive efforts seemed to indicate that the motor supply to many of the reconstructed bladders is defective. If this is the case, procedures to close the bladder primarily again may have to be abandoned, and many surgeons have abandoned primary closure of the bladder.

PROGNOSIS. Unless patients are treated successfully during infancy, they will soon develop hydro-ureter, hydronephrosis and ascending pyelonephritis. The exposed, infected and irritated bladder mucosa is apt to undergo malignant degeneration during the adult years, should survival be that long.

URETHRA AND PENIS

Posterior urethral valves[339] are a common cause of urinary obstruction in the male infant. They are believed to be remnants of the urogenital membrane and are found in the prostatic urethra. The valves are delicate membranes, usually extending laterally from the verumontanum toward the bladder neck. The membranes appear as folds on the floor of the urethra during endoscopy. Urinary incontinence, including bedwetting, is one of the most common manifestations of this disease. The *diagnosis* can be made at the time of urethroscopy when the valves are seen; however the voiding cystourethrogram is the best single method for diagnosing urethral valves. The roentgenogram will demonstrate apparent tiny indentations of the urethra in the region of the valves and marked dilation of the prostrate urethra. Treatment involves transection of the folds of tissue so that the valve will not billow out when urination occurs. This is best accomplished transurethrally with the resectoscope or Bugbee electrode.

Stricture of the urethral meatus or pinpoint meatus is seen occasionally in male infants. If not treated promptly by simple incision, it will give rise to severe obstructive uropathy in early childhood.

Epispadias[337, 338] has been mentioned during the discussion of bladder exstrophy. Most cases of epispadias are associated with bladder exstrophy, but they may occur alone. The dorsal wall of the urethra is absent, and the corpora cavernosa lie ventral to the posterior wall of the urethra. The treatment consists of the plastic closure of the urethra and its transposition to the normal ventral position.

Hypospadias is a congenital abnormality of the urethra incident to failure of closure of the distal urethral groove. The urethral meatus is not found in its normal position on the glans but anywhere between the perineum and the corona. In addition, the prepuce is present only dorsally. The penis is curved ventrally (chordee) because the corpus spongiosum is absent and is replaced by fibrous tissue. The ventral curvature is exaggerated during erection. This condition should be corrected during childhood; otherwise, it may cause mental and emotional disturbances. Children having this defect frequently find it necessary to void in the sitting position because of the location of the urethral meatus. Therefore, they feel inferior to their companions who urinate while standing. In the adult phase of life the patient with untreated hypospadias cannot participate satisfactorily in sexual intercourse. The *treatment*[336] is carried out in several stages. Initially, the penis is straightened by the excision of the ventral scar tissue. At a later date a new urethra is formed from skin so that the urethral meatus comes to lie near its normal glandular position.

Phimosis is the most common congenital anomaly of the penis and is characterized by the inability to retract the prepuce over the glans. This situation predisposes to collection of smegma beneath the foreskin with resultant possibility of carcinoma of the penis in later life. Wynder recommends that all males should be circumcised during infancy and calls attention to the lower incidence of carcinoma of the cervix in wives of circumcised men. The circumcision should completely remove the prepuce, because a residual cuff of prepuce borne by an unhygienic individual predisposes the person to penile cancer.

TESTIS

Cryptorchism in the strict sense is a developmental defect in which the testes remain in the peritoneal cavity. However, it is often used as being synonymous with incomplete descent of one or both testes. In the normal male infant the testes are in the scrotum at birth. In some boys the testes are arrested in their descent. Because the testes are derived from the genital fold in the region where the kidneys come to lie eventually, undescended testes may be located anywhere from the inguinal canal up to the level of the renal pedicle.

ETIOLOGY. Bilateral undescended testes are believed to be caused by a deficiency of chorionic gonadotropin.[340] Unilateral cryptorchism is usually the result of some obstructing factor such as fascial bands, scar tissue, hernia, etc. The unilateral undescended testis must have had the same amount of hormone acting upon it as did its mate which is in its normal position.

DIAGNOSIS. In young children the testicles often ascend into the inguinal canal during play, excitement and cold. Should the physician not be aware of this, an erroneous diagnosis of cryptorchism may be readily made. Examination of the child's genitalia should be done only after the boy has been kept quiet and warm for a time.

COMPLICATIONS OF UNTREATED CRYPTORCHIDS. Moore[343] demonstrated conclusively that an undescended testis manifests aspermatogenesis because of the abnormally high temperature present in the abdomen. A testis remaining in the abdomen after puberty is aspermatogenic. Data have been accumulated regarding testicular tumors, indicating that undescended testes are 22 times as prone to develop carcinoma as are normal testes. This holds true regardless of the degree of testicular reposition attained by any means.

Treatment. The ultimate purpose of any therapy for cryptorchism is to place the testis in its normal position in the scrotum. The reason for attempting it is to avoid aspermatogenesis and the development of undetectable testicular neoplasms. The treatment may be hormonal, surgical or a combination of both. If the patient has unilateral cryptorchism, a surgical procedure should be employed to bring the testis into the scrotum no later than the age of 6 years. If both testes are undescended, hormone therapy should be instituted at the age of 6 for a short period of time. Engle[344] recommends that from 4,000 to 5,000 units of chorionic gonadotropin be given daily for 3 days: should there be no demonstrable descent of the testes within a week, operative correction is indicated.

The giving of large doses of gonadotropin for a short period of time avoids the precocious sexual development and the bone changes that occur when small doses of gonadotropin are given for a longer period of time.

Normal growth of an undescended testis is unlikely unless it is fixed in the scrotum by the age of 5 or 7 years.

REFERENCES

Diagnosis

1. Blakemore, W. S., Murphy, J. J., Pendergrass, H. P., and Greening, R. R.: Carbon dioxide as contrast medium in roentgenography. J.A.M.A., 167:310, 1958.
2. Braasch, W. F., and Emmett, J. L.: Clinical Urography. Philadelphia, W. B. Saunders, 1951.
3. Bunge, R. G.: Further observations with delayed cystograms. J. Urol., 71:427, 1954.
4. Dustan, H. P., Page, I. H., and Poutasse, E. F.: Renal hypertension. New Eng. J. Med., 261:647, 1959.
5. Emmett, J. L.: Clinical Urography. ed. 2. Philadelphia, W. B. Saunders, 1964.
6. Kerr, D. H., and Gillies, C. L.: The Urinary Tract; A Handbook of Roentgen Diagnosis. Chicago, Year Book Pub., 1944.
7. Kincaid, O. W., and Davis, G. D.: Abdominal aortography. New Eng. J. Med., 259:1067, 1958.
8. Lalli, A. F.: Essentials of Urography. Springfield, Ill., Charles C Thomas, 1967.
9. Lapides, J.: Urinary incontinence. Med. Clin. N. Am., 43:1629, 1959.
10. Lapides, J., and Bobbitt, J. M.: Diagnostic value of bulbocavernosus reflex. J.A.M.A., 162:971, 1956.
11. Melby, J. C., Spark, R. F., Dale, S. L., Egdahl, R. H., and Kahn, P. C.: Diagnosis and localization of aldosterone-producing adenomas by adrenal–vein catheterization. New Eng. J. Med., 277:1050, 1967.
12. Nesbit, R. M.: Dangers of perirenal air insufflation. Urologists' Correspondence Club Newsletter, August, 1953. (Quoted in Year Book of Urology 1953-1954, p. 32, Chicago, Year Book Pub., 1954.)
13. Olsson, O., Jonsson, G., Lindblom, K., and Romanus, R.: Diagnostic Radiology. In: Handbuch für Urologie. Vol. V. nr. 1, pp. 1-476, Berlin, Springer-Verlag, 1962.
14. Schencker, B.: Drip infusion pyelography: indications and applications in urologic roentgen diagnosis. Radiology, 83:12, 1964.
15. Seldinger, S. I.: Catheter replacement of the needle in percutaneous arteriography. Acta Radiol., 39:368, 1953.

Renal Physiology

16. Black, D. A. K.: Renal Disease. Philadelphia, F. A. Davis, 1962.
17. Earle, D. P.: Introduction to the study of renal function. Am. J. Med., 9:78, 1950.
18. Gamble, J. L.: Chemical Anatomy, Physiology and Pathology of Extracellular Fluid (A Lecture Syllabus). Cambridge, Mass., Harvard Univ. Press, 1947.
19. Oliver, J.: An essay toward a dynamic morphology of the mammalian nephron. Am. J. Med., 9:88, 1950.
20. Smith, H. W.: The Kidney. New York, Oxford Univ. Press, 1951.
21. Strauss, M. B., and Welt, L. G.: Diseases of the Kidney. Boston, Little, Brown and Co., 1963.
22. Symposium Physiology and pathology of the kidney. Brit. M. Bull., 13:1, 1957.
23. Symposium on renal physiology. Am. J. Med., 24:659, 1958.
24. Taggart, J. V.: Mechanisms of renal tubular transport. Am. J. Med., 24:774, 1958.
25. Wesson, L. G., Jr.: Physiology of the human kidney. New York, Grune and Stratton, 1969.

Glomerular Function

26. Bott, P. A., and Richards, A. N.: The passage of protein molecules through the glomerular membrane. J. Biol. Chem., 141:291, 1941.
27. Hayman, J. M.: Estimations of afferent arteriole and glomerular capillary pressures in the frog kidney. Am. J. Physiol., 79:389, 1927.
28. Hinshaw, L. B., Day, S. B., and Carlson, C. H.: Tissue pressure as a causal factor in the autoregulation of blood in the isolated perfused kidney. Am. J. Physiol., 197:309, 1959.
29. Smith, H. W., Chasis, H., Goldring, W., and Ranges, H. A.: Glomerular dynamics in the normal human kidney. J. Clin. Invest., 19:751, 1940.
30. Wallenius, G.: Renal Clearance of Dextran as a Measure of Glomerular Permeability. Uppsala, Almquist and Wilsells, 1954.
31. Waugh, W. H., and Shanks, R. G.: Cause of genuine autoregulation of the renal circulation. Circulation Res., 8:871, 1960.
32. Wearn, J. T., and Richards, A. W.: Observations on the composition of glomerular urine with particular reference to the problem of reabsorption in the tubules. Am. J. Physiol., 71:209, 1924.

Tubular Function

33. August, J. T., Nelson, D. H., and Thorn, G. W.: Aldosterone. New Eng. J. Med., 259:917, 1958.
34. Berliner, R. W., Hilton, J. G., Yii, T. F., and Kennedy, T. J., Jr.: The renal mechanism for urate excretion in man. J. Clin. Invest., 29:396, 1950.
35. Berliner, R. W., Levinsky, N. G., Davidson, D. G., and Eden, M.: Dilution and concentration of the urine and the action of antidiuretic hormone. Am. J. Med., 24:730, 1958.
36. Beyer, K. H., Wright, L. D., Skeggs, H. R., Russo, H. F., and Shaner, G. A.: Renal clearance of essential amino acids; their competition for reabsorption by the renal tubules. Am. J. Physiol., 151:202, 1947.

37. Black, D. A. K., and Emery, E. W.: Tubular secretion of potassium. Brit. M. Bull., 13:7, 1957.
38. Conn, J. W.: Presidential Address: 1. Painting background; 2. Primary aldosteronism, a new clinical syndrome. J. Lab. Clin. Med., 45:3, 1955.
39. Ford, R. V., and Rochelle, J. B.: The differing mechanisms of action of mercurials, carbonic anhydrase inhibitors, and chlorothiazide as diuretic agents. J. Lab. Clin. Med., 53:53, 1959.
40. Gilman, A.: The mechanism of the diuretic action of the carbonic anhydrase inhibitors. Ann. N. Y. Acad. Sci., 71:355, 1958.
41. Gottschalk, C. W., Lassiter, W. E., and Mylle, M.: Localization of urine acidification in the mammalian kidney. Am. J. Physiol., 198:581, 1960.
42. Lamdin, E.: Mechanisms of urinary concentrations and dilution. Arch. Int. Med., 103:644, 1959.
43. Lassen, N. A.: Munck, O., and Thaysen, J. H.: Oxygen consumption and sodium reabsorption in the kidney. Acta physiol scand., 51:371, 1961.
44. Levinsky, N. G., and Berliner, R. W.: The role of urea in the urine concentrating mechanism. J. Clin. Invest., 38:741, 1959.
45. Malvin, R. L.: The renal concentrating mechanism: counter-current multiplier system. Univ. Michigan M. Bull., 26:45, 1960.
46. Malvin, R. L., and Wilde, W. S.: Washout of renal counter-current sodium gradient by osmotic diuresis. Am. J. Physiol., 197:177, 1959.
47. Malvin, R. L., Wilde, W. S., and Sullivan, L. P.: Localization of nephron transport by stop flow analysis. Am. J. Physiol., 194:135, 1958.
48. Malvin, R. L., Wilde, W. S., Vander, A. J., and Sullivan, L. P.: Localization and characterization of sodium transport along the renal tubule. Am. J. Physiol., 195:549, 1958.
49. Murdaugh, H. V., Jr., Schmidt-Nielsen, B., Doyle, E. M., and O'Dell, R.: Renal tubular regulation of urea excretion in man. J. Appl. Physiol., 13:263, 1958.
50. Newbergh, L. H.: Renal tubule work; its significance for the clinician. Bull. N. Y. Acad. Med., 24:137, 1948.
51. Oliver, J., and MacDowell, M.: The structural and functional aspects of the handling of glucose by the nephrons and the kidney and their correlation by means of structural-functional equivalents. J. Clin. Invest., 40:1093, 1961.
52. Orloff, J., and Berliner, R. W.: The mechanism of the excretion of ammonia in the dog. J. Clin. Invest., 35:223, 1956.
53. Pitts, R. F.: Some reflections on mechanisms of action of diuretics. Am. J. Med., 24:745, 1958.
54. Pitts, R. F., Gurd, R. S., Kessler, R. H., and Hierholzer, K.: Localization of acidification of urine, potassium and ammonia secretion and phosphate reabsorption in the nephron of the dog. Am. J. Physiol., 194:125, 1958.
55. Relman, A. S., Etsten, B., and Schwartz, W. B.: The regulation of renal bicarbonate reabsorption by plasma carbon dioxide tension. J. Clin. Invest., 32:972, 1953.
56. Richards, A. N.: Processes of urine formation. Croonian Lecture. Proc. Roy. Soc. London [B], 126:398, 1939.
57. Schmidt-Nielsen, B.: Urea excretion in mammals. Physiol. Rev., 38:139, 1958.
58. Scriver, C. R., Schafer, I. A., and Efron, M. L.: Evidence for a renal tubular amino acid transport system common to glycine, L-proline and hydroxy-L-proline, J. Clin. Invest., 40:1080, 1961.
59. Smith, H. W.: The fate of sodium and water in the renal tubule, Bull. N. Y. Acad. Med., 35:293, 1959.
60. Tobian, L.: Sodium, renal arterial distention and juxtaglomerular apparatus, Canad. M. A. J., 90:160, 1964.
61. Ussing, H. H.: The distinction by means of tracers between active transport and diffusion. Acta physiol. scand., 19:43, 1949.
62. Verney, E. B.: The antidiuretic hormone and the factors which determine its release, Proc. Roy. Soc., London, s. B. 135:25, 1947.
63. Walker, A. M., and Oliver, J.: Methods for the collection of fluid from single glomeruli and tubules of the mammalian kidney, Am. J. Physiol., 134:562, 1941.

Diuretics

64. Earley, L. E.: Diuretics. New Eng. J. Med., 276:966, 1023, 1967.
65. Earley, L. E., and Orloff, J.: Thiazide diuretics. Ann. Rev. Med., 15:149, 1964.
66. Laragh, J. H., Cannon, P. J., Stason, W. B., and Heinemann, H. O.: Physiologic and clinical observations on furosemide and ethacrynic acid. Ann. N. Y. Acad. Sci., 139:453, 1966.
67. Liddle, G. W.: Aldosterone antagonists and triamterene. Ann. N. Y. Acad. Sci., 139:466, 1966.

Renal Function Tests

68. Chasis, H., Redish, J., Goldring, W., Ranges, H., and Smith, H.: The use of sodium-p-aminohippurate for the functional evaluation of the human kidney. J. Clin. Invest., 24:583, 1945.
69. Lapides, J.: Use of renal function tests in surgical practice. J.M.A. Georgia, 51:210, 1962.
70. Lapides, J., and Bobbitt, J. M.: Preoperative estimation of renal function. J.A.M.A., 166:866, 1958.
71. Miller, E., McIntosh, J. F., and Van Slyke, D. D.: Studies in urea excretion. J. Clin. Invest., 6:427, 1928.
72. Steinitz, K., and Türkand, H.: The determination of the glomerular filtration by the endogenous creatinine clearance. J. Clin. Invest., 19:285, 1940.

73. Weller, J. M., and Cottier, P. T.: Clinical evaluation of renal function. Univ. Michigan M. Bull., 26:36, 1960.

RENAL FUNCTION DISEASE

74. Addis, T.: Glomerular Nephritis: Diagnosis and Treatment. New York, Macmillan, 1948.
75. Albright, F., Consolazio, W. V., Coombs, F. S., Sulkowitch, H. W., and Talbot, J. H.: Metabolic studies and therapy in a case of nephrocalcinosis with rickets and dwarfism. Bull. Johns Hopkins Hosp., 66:7, 1940.
76. Boyd, W.: Changing concepts of pyelonephritis. Canad. M.A.J., 47:128, 1942.
77. Bradley, S. E., Bradley, G. P., Tyson, C. J., Curry, J. J., and Blake, W. D.: Renal function in renal disease. Am. J. Med., 9:766, 1951.
78. Bricker, N. S., Morrin, P. A. F., and Kime, S. W., Jr.: The pathologic physiology of chronic Bright's disease. Am. J. Med., 28:77, 1960.
79. Mudge, G. H.: Clinical patterns of tubular dysfunction. Am. J. Med., 24:785, 1958.
80. Waring, A. J., Kajdi, L., and Tappan, V.: A congenital defect of water metabolism. Am. J. Dis. Child., 69:323, 1945.

ACUTE RENAL FAILURE

81. Balslov, J. T., and Jorgensen, H. E.: Survey of 499 patients with acute anuric renal insufficiency; causes, treatment, complications and mortality. Am. J. Med., 34:753, 1963.
82. Burns, R. O., Henderson, L. W., Hager, E. B., and Merrill, J. P.: Peritoneal dialysis. New Eng. J. Med., 267:1060, 1962.
83. Finckh, E. S., Jeremy, D., and Whyte, H. M.: Structural renal damage and its relation to clinical features in acute oliguric renal failure. Quart. J. Med., 55:429, 1962.
84. Flynn, R. B., Merrill, J. P., and Welzant, W. R.: The treatment of the oliguric patient with a new sodium exchange resin and sorbitol. New Eng. J. Med., 264:111, 1961.
85. Franklin, S. S., and Merrill, J. P.: Acute renal failure. New Eng. J. Med., 262:711, 761, 1960.
86. Gillenwater, J. Y., and Westervelt, F. B., Jr.: Current concepts in the pathogenesis and management of acute renal failure. J. Urol., 101:433, 1969.
87. Holmes, J. H., and Taylor, E. S.: Acute renal failure requiring hemodialysis. Am. J. Obst. Gynec., 87:109, 1963.
88. Kiley, J. E., Powers, S. R., Jr., and Beebe, R. T.: Acute renal failure; 80 cases of renal tubular necrosis. New Eng. J. Med., 262:481, 1960.
89. Kountz, S. L., Tuttle, K. L., Cohn, L. H., Eschelman, L. T., and Cohn, R.: Factors responsible for acute tubular necrosis following lower aortic surgery. J.A.M.A., 183:447, 1963.
90. Maxwell, M. H., Rockney, R. E., Kleeman, C. R., and Twiss, M. R.: Peritoneal dialysis. J.A.M.A., 170:917, 1959.
91. Merrill, J. P.: Consideration in the patient with diminished renal function. Am. J. Cardiol., 13:640, 1963.
92. ———: The Treatment of Renal Failure: Therapeutic Principles in Management of Acute and Chronic Uremia. New York, Grune & Stratton, 1955.
93. ———: The Treatment of Renal Failure. ed. 2. Grune and Stratton, 1965.
94. Oliver, J., MacDowell, M., and Tracy, A.: The pathogenesis of acute renal failure associated with traumatic and toxic injury: renal ischemia, nephrotoxic damage and the ischemuric episode. J. Clin. Invest., 30:1307, 1951.
95. Teschan, P. E., Baxter, C. R., O'Brien, T. F., Freyhof, J. N., and Hall, W. H.: Prophylactic hemodialysis in the treatment of acute renal failure. Ann. Int. Med., 53:992, 1960.
96. Vertel, R. M., and Knochel, J. P.: Non-oliguric acute renal failure, J.A.M.A., 200:598, 1967.

CHRONIC RENAL FAILURE

97. Hampers, C. L., and Merrill, J. P.: Hemodialysis in the home—13 months experience. Ann. Int. Med., 64:276, 1966.
98. Rae, A. I., Marr, T. A., Steury, R. E., Gothberg, L. A., and Davidson, R. C.: Hemodialysis in the home. J.A.M.A., 206:92, 1968.
99. Rapoport, F.: Human transplantation. New York, Grune & Stratton, 1967.
100. Straffon, R. A., Kiser, W. S., Stewart, B. H., Hewitt, C. B., Gifford, R. W., Jr., and Nakamoto, S.: Four years clinical experience with 138 kidney transplants. J. Urol., 99:479, 1968.

HYPERTENSION

101. Bookstein, J. J.: Segmental renal artery stenosis in renovascular hypertension. Radiology, 90:1073, 1968.
102. Conn, J. W.: Plasma renin activity in primary aldosteronism. J.A.M.A., 190:222, 1964.
103. Conn, J. W., Cohen, E. L., and Rovner, D. R.: Suppression of plasma renin activity in primary aldosteronism. J.A.M.A., 190:213, 1964.
104. Conn, J. W., Knopf, R. F., and Nesbit, R. M.: Clinical characteristics of primary aldosteronism from an analysis of 145 cases. Am. J. Surg., 107:159, 1964.
105. Conn, J. W., Rovner, D. R., Cohen, E. L., Bookstein, J. J., Cerny, J. C., and Lucas, C. P.: Preoperative diagnosis of primary aldosteronism. Arch. Int. Med., 123:113, 1969.
106. Conn, J. W., Rovner, D. R., Cohen, E. L., and Nesbit, R. M.: Normokalemic primary aldosteronism. J.A.M.A., 195:21, 1966.
107. Connor, T. B., Berthrong, M., Thomas, W. C., Jr., and Howard, J. F.: Hypertension due to unilateral renal disease with a report on a functional test helpful in diagnosis. Bull. Johns Hopkins Hosp., 100:241, 1957.
108. Correa, R. J., Jr., Stewart, B. H., and Boblitt, D. E.: Intravenous pyelogram as a screening test in renal hypertension. Am. J. Roentgenol., 88:1135, 1962.

109. Crocker, D. W., Newton, R. A., Mahoney, E. M., and Harrison, J. H.: Hypertension due to primary renal ischemia: a correlation of juxtaglomerular cell counts with clinicopathological findings in 25 cases. New Eng. J. Med., 267:794, 1962.
110. Dustan, H. P., Humphries, A. W., deWolfe, V. G., and Page, I. H.: Normal arterial pressure in patients with renal artery stenosis.
111. Egdahl, R. H.: Surgery of the adrenal gland. New Eng. J. Med., 278:939, 1968.
112. Haber, E.: Recent developments in pathophysiologic studies of the renin-angiotensin system. New Eng. J. Med., 280:148, 1969.
113. Holley, K. E., Hunt, J. C., Brown, A. L., Kincaid, O. W., and Sheps, S. G.: Renal artery stenosis: acclinical-pathologic study in normotensive and hypertensive patients. Am. J. Med., 37:14, 1964.
114. Kirkendall, W. M., Fitz, A. E., and Lawrence, M. S.: Renal hypertension: diagnosis and surgical treatment. New Eng. J. Med., 276:480, 1967.
115. Nesbit, R. M.: Primary aldosteronism: its diagnosis and surgical management. J. Urol., 97:404, 1967.
116. Maxwell, M. H.: Diagnosis and treatment of renovascular hypertension. The Kidney. 1:1, 1968.
117. Rapoport, A.: Modification of the "Howard test" for the detection of renal artery obstruction. New Eng. J. Med., 263:1159, 1960.
118. Smith, H. W.: Hypertension and urologic disease. Am. J. Med., 4:724, 1948.
119. ———: Unilateral nephrectomy in hypertensive disease. J. Urol., 76:685, 1956.
120. Stamey, T. A.: Renovascular Hypertension. Baltimore, Williams & Wilkins, 1963.
121. Stamey, T. A., Nudelman, I. J., Good, P. H., Schwentker, F. N., and Hendricks, F.: Functional characteristics of renovascular hypertension. Medicine, 40:347, 1961.
122. Stewart, B. H., and Haynie, T. P.: Critical appraisal of the renogram in renal vascular disease. J.A.M.A., 180:454, 1962.
123. Stewart, B. H., DeWeese, M. S., Conway, J., and Correa, R. J.: Renal hypertension: an appraisal of diagnostic studies and of direct operative treatment. Arch. Surg., 85:617, 1962.
124. Vertes, V. Gravel, J. A., and Goldblatt, H.: Renal angiography, separate renal function studies and renal biopsy in human hypertension. New Eng. J. Med., 270:656, 1964.
125. ———: Studies of patients with renal hypertension undergoing vascular surgery. New Eng. J. Med., 272:186, 1965.

Obstructive Uropathy

General Physiopathology and Therapy

126. Finkle, A. L., Karg, S. J., and Smith, D. K.: Parameters of renal functional capacity in reversible hydroureteronephrosis in dogs. Invest. Urol., 6:26, 1968.
127. Hinman, F.: The pathogenesis of hydronephrosis. Surg., Gynec. Obstet., 58:356, 1934.
128. Lapides, J.: Role of hydrostatic pressure and distension in urinary tract infection. *In*: Progress in Pyelonephritis. Philadelphia, F. A. Davis, 1965.
129. Murphy, G. P., Johnston, G. S., van Zyl, J. J. W., and DeKlerk, J. N.: Renal functional response to ureteral occlusion during isolated bloodless perfusion of baboon kidneys with helium or oxygen gas. Invest. Urol., 6:134, 1968.
130. Pilcher, F., Jr., Bollman, J. L., and Mann, F. C.: The effect of increased intra-ureteral pressure on renal function. J. Urol., 38:202, 1937.
131. Selkurt, E. E.: Effect of ureteral blockade on renal blood flow and urinary concentrating ability. Am. J. Physiol., 205:286, 1963.
132. Smith, H. W., Chasis, H., Goldring, W., and Ranges, H. A.: Glomerular dynamics in the normal human kidney. J. Clin. Invest., 19:751, 1940.

Congenital Specific Diseases

133. Campbell, M. F.: Ureterocele. Surg., Gynec. Obstet. 93:703, 1951.
134. Creevy, C. D.: The atonic distal ureteral segment (ureteral achalasia). J. Urol., 97:457, 1967.
135. Dorsey, J. W.: Pyeloplasty by modified ureteronepyelostomy. J. Urol., 100:353, 1968.
136. Gibson, T. E.: Classification and plastic repair of ureteropelvic obstructions. Surg., Gynec. Obstet., 80:485, 1945.
137. Grantham, W. L., and Bunts, R. C.: Congenital obstruction of the bladder neck. South. M.J., 33:939, 1940.
138. Jones, F. W.: The development and malformations of glans and prepuce, Brit. M.J., 1:137, 1910.
139. Karafin, L., and Kendall, A. R.: Vesicostomy in the management of neurogenic bladder disease secondary to myelomeningocele in children. J. Urol., 96:723, 1966.
140. Lapides, J., Anderson, E. C., and Petrone, A. F.: Urinary-tract infection in children. J.A.M.A., 195:248, 1966.
141. Lapides, J., Costello, R. T., Jr., Zierdt, D. K., and Stone, T. E.: Primary cause and treatment of recurrent urinary infection in women: preliminary report. J. Urol., 100:552, 1968.
142. Lapides, J., and Costello, R. T., Jr. Uninhibited neurogenic bladder: a common cause for recurrent urinary infection in normal women. J. Urol., 101:539, 1969.
143. Leadbetter, G. W., Jr., and Leadbetter, W. F.: Diagnosis and treatment of congenital bladder neck obstruction in children. New Eng. J. Med., 260:633, 1959.
144. Lloyd, E. I.: Treatment of congenital stenosis of the urinary meatus. Lancet, 2:1252, 1927.
145. Nesbit, R. M., and Baum, W. C.: Diagnosis and surgical management of obstructive uropa-

thy in childhood. A.M.A. Am. J. Dis., Child., 88:239, 1954.
146. Nesbit, R. M., and Labardini, M. M.: Urethral valves in the male child. J. Urol., 96:218, 1966.
147. Nesbit, R. M., McDonald, H. P., Jr., and Busby, S.: Obstructing valves in the female urethra. Trans. Am. Assoc. Genito-Urinary Surg., 56:20, 1964.
148. Nesbit, R. M., and Withycombe, J. F.: The problem of primary megaloureter. J. Urol., 72:162, 1954.
149. Politano, V. A., and Leadbetter, W. F.: Operative technique for correction of vesicoureteral reflux. J. Urol., 79:932, 1958.

Acquired Specific Diseases

Urethral Stricture

150. Harrison, J. H.: The treatment of rupture of the urethra, especially when accompanying fractures of the pelvic bones. Surg., Gynec. Obstet., 72:622, 1941.
151. Hornaday, W. R.: Care of traumatic injuries of the male urethra. J.A.M.A., 114:303, 1940.
152. Johanson, B.: Die Rekonstruktion der männlichen Urethra bei Strikturen. Z. Urol., 46:361, 1953.
153. Lapides, J.: Simplified modification of Johanson urethroplasty for strictures of deep bulbous urethra. J. Urol., 82:115, 1959.
154. Lapides, J., and Stone, T. E.: Usefulness of retrograde urethrography in diagnosing strictures of the anterior urethra. J. Urol., 100:747, 1968.
155. Pierce, J. M., Jr.: Exposure of the membranous and posterior urethra by total pubectomy. J. Urol., 88:256, 1962.
156. Ragde, H., and McInnes, G. F.: Transpubic repair of the severed prostatomembranous urethra. J. Urol., 101:335, 1968.
157. Turner-Warwick, R.: The repair of urethral strictures in the region of the membranous urethra. J. Urol., 100:303, 1968.

Benign Prostatic Hypertrophy

158. Deming, C. L.: The development of prostatic hyperplasias. Surg., Gynec. Obstet., 70:588, 1940.
159. Huggins, C.: The etiology of benign prostatic hypertrophy. Bull. N. Y. Acad. Med., 23:696, 1947.
160. Millin, T.: Retropubic Urinary Surgery. Edinburgh, Livingstone, 1947.
161. Moore, R. A.: Benign hypertrophy of the prostate; a morphological study. J. Urol., 50:680, 1943.
162. Nesbit, R. M.: Transurethral Prostatectomy. Springfield, Ill., Charles C Thomas, 1943.
163. Young, H.: Some problems in surgical treatment of the prostate. J.A.M.A., 110:280, 1938.

Hydronephrosis of Pregnancy

164. Crabtree, E. C.: Urological Disease of Pregnancy. Boston, Little Brown & Co., 1942.
165. Harrow, B. R., Sloane, J. A., and Salhanick, L.: Etiology of the hydronephrosis of pregnancy. Surg., Gynec. Obstet., 119:1042, 1964.
166. Wagener, van, G., and Jenkins, R. H.: Experimental examination of factors causing ureteral dilation of pregnancy. J. Urol., 42:1010, 1939.

INTERMITTENT HYDRONEPHROSIS

167. Nesbit, R. M.: Diagnosis of intermittent hydronephrosis: importance of pyelography during episodes of pain. J. Urol., 75:767, 1956.
168. Kendall, A. R., and Karafin, L.: Intermittent hydronephrosis; hydration pyelography. J. Urol., 98:653, 1968.

URINARY TRACT INFECTIONS

Nontuberculous Infections

Gonorrheal

169. Blumberg, N.: Penicillin-resistant gonorrhea. J. Urol., 101:106, 1969.
170. Fromer, S., Cutler, J. C., and Levitan, S.: Masking of early syphilis by penicillin therapy in gonorrhea. J. Ven. Dis. Inform., 27:174, 1946.
171. Heller, J. R., Jr.: The adequate treatment of gonorrhea. J. Ven. Dis. Inform., 27:225, 1946.
172. Pelouze, P. S.: Gonorrhea in the Male and Female. ed. 2. Philadelphia, Saunders, 1931.

Nongonorrheal

173. Allen, A. C.: The Kidney: Medical and Surgical Diseases. New York, Grune & Stratton, 1951.
174. Beer, E.: Coccal infections of the kidney. J.A.M.A., 106:163, 1936.
175. Beeson, P. B.: Factors in the pathogenesis of pyelonephritis. Yale J. Biol. Med., 28:81, 1955.
176. Braasch, W. F.: Pyelonephritis and its treatment. Surg., Gynec. Obstet., 68:534, 1939.
177. Cabot, H., and Crabtree, E. G.: The etiology and pathology of nontuberculous renal infections. Surg., Gynec. Obstet., 23:495, 1916.
178. Cox, C. E., and Hinman, F., Jr.: Experiments with induced bacteriuria, vesical emptying and bacterial growth on the mechanism of bladder defense to infection. J. Urol., 86:739, 1961.
179. Graves, R. C., and Parkins, L. E.: Carbuncle of the kidney. Tr. Am. A. A. Genito-Urin. Surgeons. 28:41, 1935.
180. Heaney, N. S., and Kretschmer, H. L.: Pyelitis of pregnancy. J.A.M.A., 128:407, 1945.
181. Lapides, J., and Alkema, H. D.: Culture versus urinalysis in diagnosing urinary infection. Invest. Urol., 4:485, 1967.
182. Lapides, J., and Costello, R. T., Jr.: Uninhibited neurogenic bladder: a common cause for recurrent urinary infection in normal women. J. Urol., 101:539, 1969.
183. Lapides, J. Costello, R. T., Jr., Zierdt, D. K., and Stone, T. E.: Primary cause and treatment of recurrent urinary infection in women: preliminary report. J. Urol., 100:552, 1968.
184. Mathe, C. P.: Diagnosis and treatment of perinephric abscess. Am. J. Surg., 37:35, 1937.

185. Nesbit, R. M., and Dick, V. S.: Acute staphylococcal infections of the kidney. J. Urol., 43:623, 1940.
186. ———: Pulmonary complications of acute renal and perirenal suppuration. Am. J. Roentgenol., 44:161, 1940.

Tuberculous Infections

187. Borthwick, W. M.: Renal tuberculosis: its pathogenesis and management in patients with extraurogenital disease. Edinburgh M. J., 59:583, 1952.
188. Borthwick, U. M.: Genito-urinary tuberculosis. Tubercle, 37:120, 1956.
189. Kerr, W. K., Gale, G. L., and Peterson, K. S. S.: Reconstructive surgery for genitourinary tuberculosis. J. Urol., 101:254, 1969.
190. Lattimer, J. K., and Spirito, A. L.: The current status of the chemotherapy of renal tuberculosis. J. Urol., 75:375, 1956.
191. Lattimer, J. K., Wechsler, H., Ehrlich, R. M., and Fukushima, K.: Current treatment for renal tuberculosis. J. Urol., 102:2, 1969.
192. Lieberthal, F.: Renal tuberculosis: the development of the renal lesion. Surg., Gynec. Obstet., 67:26, 1938.
193. Medlar, E. M., Spain, D. M., and Holliday, R. W.: Postmortem compared with clinical diagnosis of genito-urinary tuberculosis in adult males. J. Urol., 61:1078, 1949.
194. Rich, A. R.: The Pathogenesis of Tuberculosis. ed. 2. Springfield, Ill., Charles C Thomas, 1951.

Neoplasms of the Genitourinary Tract

Kidney

195. Bloom, H. J., and Wallace, D. M.: Hormones and the kidney: possible therapeutic role of testosterone in a patient with regression of metastases from renal adenocarcinoma. Brit. Med. J., 2:476, 1964.
196. Carter, R. L., Evans, J., Grabstald, H., Riches, E., and Rubin, P.: Cancer of the urogenital tract: kidney. J.A.M.A., 204:219, 1968.
197. Lalli, A. F.: Percutaneous aspiration of renal masses. Am. J. Roentgen., 101:700, 1967.
198. Meany, T. F., and Stewart, B. H.: Selective renal angiography: an integral part of the management of renal mass lesions. J. Urol., 96:644, 1966.
199. Melicow, M. M.: Classification of renal tumors: a clinical and pathological study based on 199 cases. J. Urol., 51:333, 1944.
200. Nelson, O. A., and Mousel, L. H.: Renal tumors. J.A.M.A., 148:171, 1952.
201. O'Conor, V. J., Cannon, A. H., Laipply, T. C., Sokol, K., and Barth, E. L.: Renal tumors. Radiology, 85:830, 1952.
202. Papanicolaou, G. N.: Cytology of the urinary sediment in neoplasms of the urinary tract. Tr. Am. A. Genito-Urin. Surgeons, 38:147, 1947.
203. Robson, C. J., Churchill, B. M., and Anderson, W.: The results of radical nephrectomy for renal cell carcinoma. J. Urol., 101:297, 1969.
204. Smith, P. G., Rush, T. W., and Evans, A. T.: An evaluation of translumbar arteriography. J. Urol., 65:911, 1951.
205. Sutow, W. W.: Effective chemotherapy in children with Wilms' tumor. South Med. J., 60:254, 1967.
206. Wolff, J. A., Krivit, W. Newton, W. A., Jr., and D'Angio, G. J.: Single versus multiple-dose dactinomycin therapy of Wilms' tumor. New Eng. J. Med., 279:290, 1968.
207. Woodruff, M. W., Wagle, D., Gailani, S. D., and Jones, R., Jr.: The current status of chemotherapy for advanced renal carcinoma. J. Urol., 97:611, 1967.

Ureter

208. Mortensen, H. J., and Murphy, L.: Primary epithelial tumors of the ureter. Brit. J. Urol., 22:103, 1950.
209. Newman, D. M., Allen, L. E., Wishard, W. N., Jr., Nourse, M. H., and Mertz, J. H. O.: Transitional cell carcinoma of the upper urinary tract. J. Urol., 98:322, 1967.
210. Senger, F. L., and Furey, C. A., Jr.: Primary ureteral tumors with a review of the literature since 1943. J. Urol., 69:243, 1953.

Bladder

211. Ash, J. E.: Epithelial tumors of the bladder. J. Urol., 44:135, 1940.
212. Buschke, F., and Jack, G.: Twenty-five years experience with supervoltage therapy in the treatment of transitional cell carcinoma of the bladder. Am. J. Roentgen., 99:387, 1967.
213. Editorial: Hyperchloremic acidosis following ureterosigmoidostomy. J.A.M.A., 152:334, 1953.
214. Jewett, H. J.: Conservative treatment vs. radical surgery for superficial cancer of the bladder. J.A.M.A., 206:2720, 1968.
215. McDonald, D. F.: Carcinogens and chemical causes. J.A.M.A., 206:1774, 1968.
216. Price, J. M., Wear, J. B., Brown, R. R., Satter, E. J., and Olson, C.: Studies on etiology of carcinoma of urinary bladder. J. Urol., 83:376, 1960.
217. Thompson, G. J.: Treatment of cancer of urinary bladder with particular reference to choice of operation. J. Missouri M.A., 49:813, 1952.
218. Wallace, D. M.: Tumours of the Bladder. Edinburgh, Livingstone, 1959.
219. Whitmore, W. F., Jr.: Combined radiotherapy and surgical treatment. J.A.M.A., 207:349, 1969.

Prostate

220. Batson, O. V.: The function of the vertebral veins and their role in the spread of metastases. Ann. Surg., 112:138, 1940.
221. Dykehuizen, R. F., Sargent, C. R., George, F. W., and Kurahara, S. S.: Use of cobalt-60 teletherapy in the treatment of prostatic carcinoma. J. Urol., 100:333, 1968.
222. Flocks, R. H.: Carcinoma of the prostate. J.A.M.A., 163:709, 1957.

223. Huggins, C. B., and Hodges, C. V.: Studies on prostatic cancer: I. The effect of castration, of estrogen and androgen injection on serum acid phosphatases in metastatic carcinoma of the prostate. Cancer Res., 1:293, 1941; II. Effects of castration on advanced cancer of prostate gland. Arch. Surg., 43:209, 1941.
224. Jewett, H. J., Bridge, R. W., Gray, G. F., Jr. and Shelley, W. M.: Palpable nodule of prostatic cancer: results 15 years after radical excision. J.A.M.A., 203:403, 1968.
225. Miller, G. M., and Hinman, F., Jr.: Cortisone treatment in advanced carcinoma of the prostate. J. Urol., 72:485, 1954.
226. Nesbit, R. M., and Baum, W. C.: Endocrine control of prostatic carcinoma. J.A.M.A., 143:1317, 1950.
227. ———: Serum phosphatase determinations in diagnosis of prostatic cancer. J.A.M.A., 145:1321, 1951.
228. Presti, J. C.: Carcinoma of prostate: diagnosis and treatment. California Med., 78:440, 1953.
229. Tagnon, H. J., Whitmore, W. F., Jr., Schulman, P., and Kravitz, S. C.: Significance of fibrinolysis occurring in patients with metastatic cancer of the prostate. Cancer, 6:63, 1953.

Urethra

230. Grabstald, H., Hilaris, B., Henschke, U., and Whitmore, W. F., Jr.: Cancer of female urethra. J.A.M.A., 197:835, 1966.
231. Kaplan, G. W., Bulkley, G. J., and Grayhack, J. T.: Carcinoma of the male urethra. J. Urol., 98:365, 1967.

Penis

232. Bleich, A. R.: Prophylaxis of penile carcinoma. J.A.M.A., 143:1054, 1950.
233. Dean, A. L.: Conservative amputation of penis for carcinoma. J. Urol., 68:374, 1952.
234. Lynch, K. M., Jr.: Carcinoma of penis. J. South Carolina M.A., 48:298, 1952.
235. Melicow, M. M., and Ganem, E. J.: Cancerous and precancerous lesions of the penis. J. Urol., 55:486, 1946.
236. Schrek, R., and Lenowitz, H.: Etiologic factors in carcinoma of the penis. Cancer Res., 7:180, 1947.

Scrotum

237. Butlin, H.: Cancer of the scrotum in chimney-sweeps and others. Brit. M. J., 1:1341, 1892.
238. Graves, R. C., and Flo, S.: Carcinoma of the scrotum. J. Urol., 43:309, 1940.
239. Wilson, S. R.: Cancer in cotton-mule spinners. Brit. M. J., 2:993, 1927.

Testis

240. Beilby, J. S., Kurland, I., and Jacob, M.: Hormone excretion and bioassay of extirpated tumor in teratoma. Endocrinology, 26:965, 1940.
241. Mackenzie, A. R.: Chemotherapy of metastatic testis cancer: results in 154 patients. Cancer, 19:1369, 1966.
242. Maier, J. G., Van Buskirk, K. E., Sulak, M. H., Perry, R. H., and Schamber, D. T.: An evaluation of lymphadenectomy in the treatment of malignant testicular germ cell neoplasms. J. Urol., 101:356, 1969.
243. Moore, C. A.: Triple chemotherapy in the treatment of metastatic testicular neoplasms. J. Urol., 100:527, 1968.
244. Melicow, M. M.: Embryoma of testis. J. Urol., 44:333, 1940.
245. Pierce, G. B., Jr.: Ultrastructure of human testicular tumors. Cancer, 19:1963, 1966.
246. Stanbitz, W. J., Magoss, I. V., Grace, J. T. and Schenk, W. G.: Surgical management of testis tumors. J. Urol., 101:350, 1969.
247. Vermooten, V., and Hettler, W. F.: The significance of gonadotropic hormones in the urine of patients with testicular tumors. J. Urol., 61:519, 1948.

Calculous Disease

248. Albright, F., Burnett, C. H., Parson, W., Reifenstein, E. C., Jr., and Roos, A.: Osteomalacia and late rickets. Medicine, 25:399, 1946.
249. Boyce, W. H., and King, S. J., Jr.: Crystal-matrix interrelation in calculi. J. Urol., 81:351, 1959.
250. Boyce, W. H., Garvey, F. K., and Goven, C. E.: Abnormalities of calcium metabolism in patients with "idiopathic" urinary calculi. J.A.M.A., 166:1577, 1958.
251. Carroll, G., and Brennan, R. V.: Urea-splitting organisms in formation of urinary calculi. J. Internat. Coll. Surgeons., 17:809, 1952.
252. Chambers, E. K., Gordan, G. S., Goldman, L., and Reifenstein, E. C., Jr.: Tests for hyperparathyroidism: tubular reabsorption of phosphate, phosphate deprivation and calcium infusion. J. Clin. Endocrinol., 16:1507, 1956.
253. Dent, C. E., and Senior, B.: Studies on treatment of cystinuria. Brit. J. Urol., 27:317, 1955.
254. Henneman, P. H., Wallach, S., and Dempsey, E. F.: Metabolic defect responsible for uric acid renal stone formation. J. Clin. Invest., 37:901, 1958.
255. Howard, J. E.: Clinical and laboratory research concerning mechanisms of formation and control of calculous disease by the kidney. J. Urol., 72:999, 1954.
256. Kittredge, W. E., and Docons, R.: Role of gout in formation of urinary calculi. J. Urol., 67:841, 1952.
257. Lapides, J., and Dodson, A. J., Jr.: Observations on effect of methantheline (Banthine) bromide in urological disturbances. A.M.A. Arch. Surg., 66:1, 1953.
258. Marshall, V. F., and Green, J. L.: Aluminum gels with constant phosphorus intake for control of renal phosphatic calculi. J. Urol., 67:611, 1952.
259. Melick, R. A., and Henneman, P. H.: Clinical and laboratory studies of 207 consecutive pa-

tients in a kidney-stone clinic. New Eng. J. Med., 259:307, 1958.
260. Nesbit, R. M. (Moderator): Panel discussion on urolithiasis. Urol. Survey, 4:2, 1954.
261. Nesbit, R. M., Lapides, J., and Baum, W. C.: Fundamentals of Urology. Ann Arbor, Mich., Edwards, 1953.
262. Smith, L. H., Jr.: Symposium on stones. Am. J. Med., 45:649, 1968.
263. Suby, H. I.: Medical management of patients with urinary calculi. M. Clin. N. Amer., 32:1315, 1948.

Traumatic Lesions

Kidney

264. Cheetham, J. G.: Clinical management of kidney injuries. Internat. Abstr. Surg., 72:573, 1941.
265. Heller, E.: War injuries of the upper urinary tract. J. Urol., 72:149, 1954.
266. Prather, G. C.: Traumatic conditions of the kidney. J.A.M.A., 114:207, 1940.
267. Scott, R., Jr., Carlton, C. E., Jr., and Goldman, M.: Penetrating injuries of the kidney: an analysis of 181 patients. J. Urol., 101:247, 1969.
268. Waterhouse, K., and Gross, M.: Trauma to the genitourinary tract: a 5-year experience with 251 cases. J. Urol., 101:241, 1969.

Ureter

269. Aschner, P. W.: Accidental injury to ureters and bladder in pelvic surgery. J. Urol., 69:774, 1953.
270. Rusche, C., and Morrow, J. W.: Injury to the ureter. In: M. F. Campbell (ed.): Urology Vol. 1, p. 834, Philadelphia, W. B. Saunders, 1963.
271. St. Martin, E. C., Trichel, B. E., Campbell, J. N. and Locke, C. M.: Ureteral injuries in gynecologic surgery. J. Urol. 70:51, 1953.
272. Stickel, D. L., and Howse, R. M.: Injuries of the ureter due to external violence: a review of the literature and report of two cases. Ann. Surg., 154:137, 1961.
273. Flaherty, J. F., Kelley, R., Burnett, B., Bucy, J., Surrian, M., Schildkraut, D., and Clarke, B. G.: Relationship of pelvic bone fracture patterns to injuries of urethra and bladder. J. Urol., 99:297, 1968.

Bladder

274. Prather, G. C.: Bladder injuries: treatment, past and present. New York J. Med., 53:318, 1953.

Urethra

275. Lapides, J.: Structure and function of the internal vesical sphincter. J. Urol., 80:341, 1958.
276. Laury, R. B.: Diagnosis and treatment in traumatic injuries of bladder and urethra. New York J. Med., 52:187, 1952.
277. O'Conor, V. J.: Repair of rupture of the male urethra. Surg., Gynec. Obstet., 63:198, 1936.
278. Ormond, J. K., and Fairey, P. W.: Urethral rupture at apex of prostate. J.A.M.A., 149:15, 1952.
279. Ragde, H., and McInnes, G. F.: Transpubic repair of the severed prostatomembranous urethra. J. Urol., 101:335, 1969.

Urethral Strictures

280. Ainsworth-Davis, J. C.: Prevention and treatment of strictures of inflammatory origin. Brit. J. Urol., 5:1, 1933.
281. Ballenger, E. G., and Edder, O. F.: Notes on urethral strictures. Am. J. Surg., 34:340, 1920.
282. Dodson, A. I.: Urological Surgery. p. 554, St. Louis, C. V. Mosby, 1944.
283. Johanson, B.: Die Rekonstruktion der männlichen Urethra bei Strikturen. Z. Urol., 46:361, 1953.
284. Turner-Warwick, R.: The repair of urethral strictures in the region of the membranous urethra. J. Urol., 100:303, 1968.

Penis

285. Adams, J. P.: Mutilations of the penis. Delaware M. J., 18:41, 1946.
286. Douglas, P.: One-stage reconstruction for traumatic denudation of the male external genitalia. Ann. Surg., 133:889, 1951.
287. Hoffman, H. A., and Colby, F. H.: Incarceration of the penis. J. Urol., 62:391, 1945.
288. Kenyon, H. R., and Hyman, R. M.: Total autoemasculation. J.A.M.A., 151:207, 1953.
289. Zarafonetis, C. J. D., and Horrax, T. M.: Treatment of Peyronie's disease with potassium para-aminobenzoate (Potaba). J. Urol., 81:770, 1959.

Scrotum

290. Ewell, G. H., Bruskewitz, H. W., and Steeper, J. R.: Traumatic avulsion of skin of penis and scrotum. J. Internat. Coll. Surg., 29:207, 1953.
291. Whelan, E. P.: Repair of an avulsed scrotum. Surg., Gynec. Obstet., 73:649, 1944.

Testis

292. Ormond, J. K.: Torsion of the testicle. J.A.M.A., 111:1910, 1938.
293. Riba, L. W., and Schmidlapp, C. J.: Torsion of the spermatic cord. Surg., Gynec. Obstet., 63:163, 1946.

Physiology of Urinary Transport and Micturition

Ureter

294. Baker, R., and Huffer, J.: Ureteral electromyography. J. Urol., 70:974, 1953.
295. Bozler, E.: The response of smooth muscle to stretch. Am. J. Physiol., 149:299, 1947.

296. Johnson, T. H.: Peristalsis of the upper urinary tract as demonstrated by a new x-ray technique. New York J. Med., 52:189, 1952.
297. Lapides, J.: Physiology of the intact human ureter. J. Urol., 59:501, 1948.
298. Narath, P. A.: The hydromechanics of the calyx renalis. J. Urol., 43:145, 1950.

Bladder

299. Bors, E.: Bladder disturbances and the management of patients with injury to the spinal cord. J. Internat. Coll. Surg., 21:513, 1954.
300. ———: Urological aspects of rehabilitation of spinal cord injuries. J.A.M.A., 146:225, 1951.
301. Boyarsky, S.: The neurogenic bladder. Baltimore, Williams & Wilkins, 1967.
302. Caine, M., and Edwards, D.: Peripheral control of micturition: a cineradiographic study. Brit. J. Urol., 30:34, 1958.
303. Denny-Brown, D., and Robertson, E. G.: The state of the bladder and its sphincters in complete transverse lesions of the spinal cord and cauda equina. Brain, 56:397, 1933.
304. Langworthy, O. R., Kolb, L. C., and Lewis, L. G.: Physiology of Micturition. Baltimore, Williams & Wilkins, 1940.
305. Lapides, J.: Observations on normal and abnormal bladder physiology. J. Urol., 70:74, 1953.
306. ———: Cystometry. J.A.M.A., 201:618, 1967.
307. ———: Structure and function of the internal vesical sphincter. J. Urol., 80:341, 1958.
308. ———: Urecholine regimen for rehabilitating the atonic bladder. J. Urol., 91:658, 1964.
309. Lapides, J., Ajemian, E. P., Stewart, B. H., and Lichtwardt, J. R.: Urethrovesical dynamics in the normal human. Surg. Forum, 10:896, 1959.
310. Lapides, J., Bourne, R. B., and Lanning, R. J.: Present status of cutaneous vesicostomy. Tr. Am. Assoc. Genito-Urin. Surg., 56:78, 1964.
311. Lapides, J., Friend, C. R., Ajemian, E. P., and Reus, W. F.: A new test for neurogenic bladder. J. Urol., 88:245, 1962.
312. Lapides, J., Hodgson, N. B., Boyd, R. E., Shook, E. L., and Lichtwardt, J. R.: Further observations on pharmacologic reactions of the bladder. J. Urol., 79:707, 1958.
313. Lapides, J., Sweet, R. B., and Lewis, L. W.: Role of striated muscle in urination. J. Urol., 77:247, 1957.
314. McClellan, F. C.: The Neurogenic Bladder. Springfield, Ill., Charles C Thomas, 1939.
315. Nesbit, R. M., Lapides, J., et al.: Effects of blockade of the autonomic ganglia on the urinary bladder in man. J. Urol., 57:242, 1947.
316. Nesbit, R. M., and Lapides, J.: Tonus of the bladder during spinal shock. Arch. Surg., 56:139, 1948.
317. Prather, G. C.: Spinal cord injuries: care of the bladder. J. Urol., 57:15, 1947.
318. Woodburne, R. T.: Structure and function of the urinary bladder. J. Urol., 84:79, 1960.

Urinary Incontinence

319. Lapides, J.: Urinary incontinence. Med. Clin. N. Amer., 43:1629, 1959.
320. ———: Urinary incontinence in the male. South. M.J., 55:965, 1962.
321. ———: Reconstruction of damaged urinary sphincter in a female child. J. Urol., 91:58, 1964.
322. ———: Problems in diagnosis and treatment of stress incontinence in the female. Surg. Clin. N. Amer., 41:1401, 1961.
323. Lapides, J., Ajemian, E. P., Stewart, B. H., Lichtwardt, J. R., and Breakey, B. A.: Physiopathology of stress incontinence. Surg., Gynec. Obstet., 111:224, 1960.

Congenital Anomalies

324. Arey, L. B.: Developmental Anatomy. ed. 7. Philadelphia, W. B. Saunders, 1965.
325. Patten, B. M.: Human Embryology. ed. 8. New York, Blakiston-Div. McGraw-Hill, 1953.

Kidney

326. Braasch, W. F., and Schacht, F. W.: Pathological and clinical data concerning polycystic kidney. Surg., Gynec. Obstet., 57:467, 1933.
327. Lambert, P. P.: Polycystic disease of the kidney. Arch. Path., 44:34, 1947.

Ureter

328. Moore, T.: Ectopic openings of the ureter. Brit. J. Urol., 24:3, 1952.
329. Nesbit, R. M., and Withycombe, J. F.: The problem of primary megaloureter. J. Urol., 72:162, 1954.
330. Thompson, G. J., and Greene, L. F.: Ureterocele. J. Urol., 47:800, 1952.

Bladder

331. Begg, R. C.: The urachus, its anatomy, histology and development. J. Anat., 64:170, 1930.
332. Harvard, B. M., and Thompson, G. J.: Congenital exstrophy of the urinary bladder: late results of the Coffey-Mayo method of ureterointestinal anastomosis. J. Urol., 65:223, 1951.
333. Higgins, C. C.: Exstrophy of the bladder. J. Urol., 63:852, 1950.
334. Kretschmer, H. L.: Diverticula of the urinary bladder. Surg., Gynec. Obstet., 71:491, 1940.
335. Patten, B. M.: The possible embryological mechanisms involved in the genesis of exstrophy of the bladder and epispadias. Anat. Rec., 109:334, 1951.

Urethra and Penis

336. Burns, E., and Beckman, G. E., Jr.: Evaluation of operations for hypospadias. J. Urol., 67:1000, 1952.
337. Campbell, M.: Epispadias. Tr. Am. A. Genito-Urin. Surgeons, 43:154, 1951.
338. Gross, R. E., and Cresson, S. L.: Treatment of epispadias. J. Urol., 68:477, 1952.

339. Nesbit, R. M., Thirlby, R. L., and Raper, F. P.: Diagnosis and treatment of congenital urethral valves. J. Michigan M. Soc., 50: 1244, 1951.

Testis

340. Aberle, S. B. P., and Jenkins, R. H.: Undescended testes in man and Rhesus monkey; treated with the anterior pituitary-like principle from the urine of pregnancy. J.A.M.A., 103:314, 1934.
341. Deming, C. L.: The evaluation of hormonal therapy in cryptorchidism. J. Urol., 68:354, 1952.
342. Grove, J. S.: The cryptorchid problem. J. Urol., 71:735, 1954.
343. Moore, C. R.: The influence of hormones on the development of the reproductive system. J. Urol., 45:869, 1941.
344. Robinson, J. N., and Engle, E. T.: Some observations on the cryptorchid testis. J. Urol., 71:726, 1954.
345. Torek, F.: Orchidopexy for undescended testicle. Ann. Surg., 94:97, 1931.

Peyronie's Disease

346. Dahl, O.: Treatment of plastic induration of penis. Acta radiol., 41:290, 1954.
347. Teasley, G. H.: Peyronie's disease: a new approach. J. Urol., 71:611, 1954.

Interstitial Cystitis

348. Hand, J. R.: Interstitial cystitis: report of 223 cases. J. Urol., 61:291, 1949.
349. Pool, T. L., and Crenshaw, J. L.: Treatment of interstitial cystitis with silver nitrate. Proc. Mayo Clin. 16:718, 1941.

Hydrocele

350. Dodson, A. I.: Urological Surgery. St. Louis, C. V. Mosby, 1944.

CHAPTER 53

FRED C. REYNOLDS, M.D., LAWRENCE
M. HAAS, M.D., AND
STANLEY F. KATZ, M.D.

Orthopedics (Nontraumatic)

Development of the Skeleton
Composition of Bone
Composition of Cartilage
Metabolism of Bone and Cartilage
Response of Bone to Injury
The Fate of Bone Grafts
Deossification of the Skeleton
    Osteoporosis
    Osteomalacia and Rickets
Scurvy
Other Metabolic Diseases of Bone
Inborn Errors of Metabolism
Developmental Abnormalities
    Congenital Dysplasia and Dislocation of the Hip
    Club Foot and Other Developmental Abnormalities
    Developmental Abnormalities of the Upper and Lower Extremities
    Slipped Capital Femoral Epiphysis
    Osteochondroses
Orthopedic Treatment of Paralytic Disorders
Cerebral Palsy
Myelodysplasia
Scoliosis
Infection in Bones
Degenerative Disease of Joints
Arthritis
Upper Extremity Pain
Tumors of Bone and Soft Tissue
Common Foot Problems
Low Back Pain

DEVELOPMENT OF THE SKELETON

The skeleton may be looked upon as a calcified connective tissue and closely related to other tissues of mesodermal origin. In the mammalian embryo the mesenchymal cells which are to create the skeleton differentiate into two structures, a cartilaginous mold of the future skeleton and the perichondrium, a membrane that surrounds the cartilage and later becomes the periosteum. Zones of segmentation develop in this primary cartilage. These are the sites of future joints.

Once started, differentiation of the primitive mesenchymal cells into segmented cartilage with its covering perichondrium continues in an orderly way with the cells of embryologic cartilage uniformly and rapidly changing from a primitive to a relatively mature type. According to Luck (1950), a thin sheath of bone begins to form beneath the perichondrium about the 9th week of intrauterine life. At the time bone begins to form blood vessels are seen growing into the approximate center of what is eventually to be the diaphysis of the bone. Budding of capillaries beneath the perichondrium and into the area of the middle of the diaphysis of the cartilaginous mold is accompanied by calcification of the cartilage cells in this vascularized area. Subsequently, calcification of the cartilage cells spreads from the centers to the ends of the primordial osseous anlagen. Only the zones of primitive cartilage that are destined to be the epiphyseal cartilage plate escape calcification. After calcification has taken place, cartilage is reabsorbed by a vascular granulation-like tissue and replaced with an immature type of cancellous bone.

Endochondral ossification is the name applied to the maturation and the calcification of the primitive cartilage, its destruction by a vascular granulation tissue, and its final replacement with cancellous bone. All the bones of the body except the skull, some face bones and the clavicle are formed in this way. In the case of the skull, the bones of the face and the clavicle the actual form of the bone develops as plates of primitive mesenchymal tissue. This tissue does not become cartilage before ossification takes place. Ossification simply involves metaplasia of the mesenchymal tissue to osseous tissue. This process is known as *intramembranous ossification*.

During endochondral ossification the primitive cartilage is not destroyed and replaced in the zones destined to be the epiphyseal plates. Here the cartilage remains as layers of primitive cartilage cells, separating the epiphyses from the metaphyses. Proliferation of cartilage within the epiphyseal plate and its subsequent conversion to bone accounts for the growth in the length of bones. Within the epiphyseal plate columns of cartilage cells grow, mature, calcify and are destroyed and replaced by bone. The calcific zone of the epiphyseal cartilage is known as the zone of provisional calcification. After having been laid down in juxtaposition to the epiphysis the osteoid trabeculae are modified so as to conform to the inherited characteristics of the bone and the stresses and strains put upon it.

Five enzymes important to carbohydrate metabolism have been measured at 4 stages of endochondral bone formation in the growing dog. Lactic dehydrogenase, phosphoglucoisomerase, malic dehydrogenase, glucose-6-phosphate dehydrogenase and alkaline phosphatase have been determined quantitatively. Enzymes mediating metabolism through aerobic pathways are more prominent in areas closest to invading blood vessels, whereas enzymes more important to anaerobic glycolysis are more active in the more avascular areas of endochondral bone formation. The enzyme content of the epiphyseal plate indicates that endochondral bone formation derives energy and synthetic intermediates from an enzymatically regulated metabolic sequence (Kuhlman, 1960).

An increased rate of bone growth as manifested by an increase in length can be brought about by altering the circulation to the part. The creation of an arteriovenous fistula in an extremity results in an increase in bone length and an alteration of the blood supply to the bone (McKibbin, 1967). The creation of an arteriovenous fistula significantly alters the normal relationship of intramedullary blood pressure in the epiphysis and the diaphysis. When the fistula is functioning the epiphyseal pressure is elevated (Kelly et al., 1959; Koskinen et al., 1967; Stein et al., 1959).

Using various radioisotopes a number of investigators have attempted to determine the resting blood flow in bone in different laboratory animals (Risser, 1958; Weinman et al., 1963; Shim, 1968; Shim et al., 1968). White et al., (1964) developed a technic utilizing ^{15}Cr-tagged red cells in the intact rabbit. Their comparative figures are:

Whole bone	0.16 ml./Gm./minute
Skin	0.54 ml./Gm./minute
Skeletal muscle	0.27 ml./Gm./minute
Tendon	0.10 ml./Gm./minute

Growth in thickness of bone occurs by the appositional formation of new bone beneath the periosteum and from the endochondral surfaces. The appositional formation and destruction of bone occurs throughout the life of the individual. In normal healthy adults the rates of bone formation and bone destruction are about equal. This causes the bones of adults to appear to be changeless structures; however, bone is not static. It is highly active metabolically; consequently the amount and the character of bone is readily altered throughout life should the individual's metabolism change. Many of the changes that take place in the life history of bone are unknown. Even the exact composition of the bone crystal is unknown. The solution of many problems in orthopedic surgery awaits the discovery of what occurs when bone is formed and what may be done to control this process.

COMPOSITION OF BONE

Although the exact organic composition of the crystal of bone is not clearly understood, it is known that bone contains approximately 25 per cent water, 30 per cent organic substances and 45 per cent inorganic substances (Luck, 1950). There is evidence that the water and the organic components decrease while the inorganic salt components increase as bone ages. Bone has an important organic matrix composed of cells called osteocytes and extracellular substances. The inorganic compounds of calcium, phosphorus, magnesium and carbon are the major bone salts, these are laid down upon and about the extracellular matrix and the cells. Besides the above salts small amounts of the salts of sodium, potassium, chloride and fluoride are found in bone. Magnesium has the ability to substitute or replace calcium in the apatite crystal and may have a regulatory effect on the rate of deposition of bone. Small amounts of copper and zinc also are present and probably are important enzyme regulators. The inorganic salts, bound with protein, form a crystal structure resembling an apatite. This has been demonstrated by x-ray refraction studies, as well as by chemical analysis. Roseberry, Hastings and Morse (1931) concluded that bone is a dahlite with the probable formula of $CaC_3NCO_3(PO_4)_2$. However, others disagree with them and believe that it closely resembles a hydroxyapatite. Armstrong's table of the mineral constituents of bone based upon the work of Dallemagne and Carter is as follows (Armstrong, 1950):

	Per Cent
Alpha tricalcium phosphate	74.6
Calcium carbonate	10.4
Calcium citrate	2.0
Trimagnesium phosphate	0.9
Magnesium carbonate	1.0
Disodium phosphate	2.4
Ca^{--} PO_4^{++} } Protein	8.7

Employing electron microscopy, Robinson (1952) showed that bone crystals are rectangular, having the dimensions 500 × 250 × 100 angstroms, that such crystals have a surface area of about 103 square meters per gram, and that the crystals are embedded in a cement substance covering the collagen fibers, the crystals being arranged along the long axis of the collagen fiber. More recently, Glimcher has shown that the crystals are actually formed within the collagen fibers.

COMPOSITION OF CARTILAGE

Cartilage is composed of chondrocytes embedded in an extracellular matrix containing collagen fibers and ground substance. The cells and ground substance appear to be functionally interdependent. The morphology varies with the type (hyaline, elastic or fibro cartilage), the anatomic site, the depth of the section in question, and the age of the individual. Cartilage demonstrates histologic and biochemical signs of regression in both aging and degenerative joint disease. Aging cartilage shows reduced number of nuclei and loss of normal matrix staining. In osteoarthritis cartilage becomes fibrillar and ground substance degenerate. The ultrastructure of cartilage demonstrates typical findings in both normal, aging, and degenerative states and is discussed in detail elsewhere (Meachim, 1967; Weiss et al., 1968). The water–solid content of articular cartilage has been determined in puppies as follows (Eichelberger et al., 1958).

Extracellular water	52.2%
Extracellular solids	16.1%
Chondrocyte water	26.3%
Chondrocyte solids	5.4%

Water content decreases with aging from 80 to 75 per cent. Chondroitin sulfate decreases and connective tissue increases. Denervation is followed by a decrease in solids and an increase in total water content.

The extracellular solids are mainly collagen and some of the connective tissue polysaccharides: chondroitin-4-sulfate, chondroitin-6-sulfate, and keratosulfate. These polysaccharides comprise as much as 40 per cent of the dry weight and are bound to protein.

THE METABOLISM OF BONE AND CARTILAGE

Present knowledge concerning bone and cartilage metabolism is far from complete. These tissues require energy derived from glucose and other substrates to maintain cell integrity. Energy may also be needed to perform specialized functions which might include the following (Krane et al., 1967):

1. Secretion of extracellular components, such as protein polysaccharides and collagen
2. Modification of the matrix to render it calcifiable (e.g., phosphorylation)
3. Production of metabolic compounds which may influence initial mineralization and subsequent inorganic crystal growth (two such compounds are citrate and pyrophosphate)
4. Secretion of enzymes and metabolic products involved in the resorption of protein polysaccharides and collagen in the process of remodeling

Cartilage, unlike bone, has an anaerobic type of metabolic pattern. It normally has poor vascular supply. Cartilage consumes little oxygen and produces increased lactate from glucose (anaerobically). Bone, however, has a more aerobic pattern and requires more oxygen.

Bone metabolism is being increasingly studied with radioisotope technics, particularly autoradiography. With matrix production, increasing sulfur-35 is incorporated indicating production of sulfated mucopolysaccharides (Duthie, 1961; Duthie and Barker, 1955). Just prior to calcification large amounts of phosphorus-32 in incorporated, probably signifying matrix phosphorylation (Solheim, 1965). In addition, zinc-65 can be localized at these sites because of its presence in zinc metallo-enzymes, such as alkaline phosphatase and SGOT, which may play a role in calcification (Pories *et al.*, 1967). Calcium-25 uptake increases with bone formation (LeMain, 1966).

The interaction of vitamins and hormones is important, but unclear. Vitamin A may function in remodeling cell maturation (Udupa, 1966). Androgens may increase matrix formation (Kolar, 1965). Estrogens can increase calcification and experimentally block bone resorption (Koskinen, 1965). In higher doses, estrogen can suppress bone formation (Tapp, 1966). Growth hormone and thyrotropin may have an anabolic effect (Koskinen, 1963) but have not been shown to accelerate osteogenesis. There is probably an important interaction between parathyroid hormone, Vitamin D_3 and thyrocalcitonin (Pechet *et al.*, 1967). The destruction of bone collagen and dissolution of bone mineral induced by parathyroid hormone can be blocked by thyrocalcitonin. The bone resorption effect of Vitamin D_3, which requires small amounts of parathyroid hormone, can also be blocked by thyrocalcitonin. In addition, thyrocalcitonin may stimulate osteoblastic activity.

Bone dynamics have been found to vary with disease states (Frost, 1966). Bone formation is decreased in postmenopausal osteoporosis, Cushing's syndrome, and rickets. It is increased in acromegaly, Paget's disease and osteomalacia. (See Table 53-1).

RESPONSE OF BONE TO INJURY

Fracture healing is one of the most complex and interesting of all biologic phenomena. A fracture is disruption of bone and vessels—and sometimes of muscle, nerves and even skin. The healing of a fracture is similar to the healing of any wound except that, in normal fracture healing, osteogenesis occurs and bone continuity is established.

BASIC MECHANISMS OF FRACTURE HEALING

Differentiation (Young 1962, 1967) suggested the following mechanism for cell specialization in bone from mesenchymal tissue (related to the hypothesis of Jacob and Monod, 1963): The sequence of 4 different nucleo-

TABLE 53-1

TYPE OF DISTURBANCE	SERUM Ca.	P	Alkaline Phosphatase	Serum Protein	URINE Ca	P	TISSUE
Osteoporosis	N	N	N	N-L	N	N	Normal-appearing but slender bone trabeculae
Osteomalacia	N-L	N-L	H	N	N-L	N-L	Marked increase in osteoid formation about all trabeculae
Hyperparathyroidism	H	L	H	N	H	H	Very active bone formation and destruction—osteoblasts, osteoclasts prominent
Osteogenesis Imperfecta	N	N	N	N	N	N	Normal-appearing but slender bone trabeculae
Myeloma	N-H	N-H	N	H	Bence Jones prot.		Tumor cells
Paget's Disease	N	N	H	N	N	N	Active bone formation with mosaic pattern

tides in DNA in groups of three in combination with certain genes record the potential of the cell. A *structural gene* linked with DNA determines the type of messenger RNA released into the cytoplasm. Messenger RNA controls the organization of ribosomes and therefore the type of secretion or differentiation. However, *regulator genes*, unless they are inactivated by environmental stimuli such as hormones, vitamins, mechanical stimuli, pH, peptides or changes in oxygen tension, may repress these systems. Therefore, cellular differentiation or secretion may take place under multiple stimuli.

A multipotential fibroblast can differentiate into chondroblasts, osteoblasts, osteoclasts or osteocytes, depending on the type of stimulus, and each of these cells has varied functions, secretions, enzymes and metabolism. Chondroblasts, when transplanted into a fracture gap, appear to have osteogenetic potential, whereas mature chondrocytes have lost this ability (Lawrence and Smith, 1968).

Secretion is important in osteogenesis and chondrogenesis, and involves the triple mechanism of synthesis, storage and transport. (Godman (1960) and Tonna (1965a) investigated secretion by autoradiography.) Two pertinent examples are mucoprotein and collagen.

Mucoprotein is found in chondroid and osteoid and is a protein bound covalently to carbohydrate. Synthesis begins when messenger RNA, released from the nucleolus into the cytoplasm, organizes the ribosomes to produce the protein moiety. This protein is carried through the rough endoplasmic reticulum to the Golgi apparatus where it is bound to carbohydrate and may be sulfated. These molecules (chondromucoprotein for example) are stored in the cytoplasm and transported across the cell wall into the extracellular space.

Collagen, a sclero-protein, 30 per cent of total body protein (Sjoerdsma, 1965). Normally it is a polymer of 3 left-handed polypeptide chains wound in a right-handed helix. Peacock (1967) described tropocollagen as the basic macromolecule with a molecular weight of over 300,000 and diameters of 10Å × 2800Å. The manufacture of collagen is a analogous to that of mucoprotein, but 100 ribosomes are needed to assemble this giant molecule. The process begins by hydroxylation of proline. The final content is hydroxyproline 10 to 14 per cent, glycine 33 per cent, hydroxylysine 0.5 per cent, and minute quantities of tryptophan and tyrosine. The arrangement of the ribosomes directs the assembly of these hydroxyproline amino acid radicals into the giant molecule tropocollagen. Tropocollagen is transported across the cell wall and polymerization into the super helix occurs in the extracellular space. At this time, binding of mucoproteins (Highberger, 1951), seeding of hydroxy apatite crystals, cross linking, or collagenolysis (Grillo, 1967) may occur.

Collagen molecules are assembled in stepwise fashion with $\frac{1}{4}$ overlap into collagen fibrils, which are arranged into primitive fibers. The site of overlap can be identified by electron microscopy as banding at 640Å intervals. Cross linking of fibrils occurs at the fifth amino acid from the end by aldehyde-lysine combination. Lathyrism is a defect in cross linking produced by administering beta amino proprionitrile, and Marfan's syndrome may be a genetic counterpart to this. Scleroderma may be a defect in collagen with excessive cross linking.

Berliner (1967) reported that fibroblasts treated with cortisone have a dilated endoplasmic reticulum and decreased mature collagen. Kirchheimer (1965) stated that ascorbic-acid-deficient fibroblasts demonstrate disruption of ribosomes and markedly altered endoplasmic reticulum, resulting in little collagen production and excess accumulation of hydroxyproline.

The organic matrix, which is synthesized by the osteoblasts and chondroblasts (Cameron, 1963) is an important part of osseous tissue. It contains collagen and minute but important amounts of enzymes, substrates and metabolites, but its general composition is (approximately) water 10 per cent, noncollagenous protein 30 per cent and mucopolysaccharide 60 per cent (Eastloe, 1956; Shatton, 1954). Meyer (1956) listed the mucopolysaccharides of connective tissue as follows: (1) hyaluronic acid, (2) chondroitin, (3) keratosulfate, (4) heparitin sulfate, (5) chondroitin sulfate B, (6) chondroitin sulfate A, and (7) chondroitin sulfate C. Of these, osseous tissue contains principally the latter two. In cartilage, chondroitin sulfates A and C are bound to protein, but before cartilage calcifies this bond is disrupted, possibly by release of lysosomal enzymes, and chondroitin sulfate may then interact with either collagen or inorganic components during the ossification process (Sobel, 1954). The mechanism for this is unknown. Mucoproteins play an important but ill-defined role in ossification. It has been demonstrated that all biologic systems that calcify, including systems in sand dollars, oysters and man, require a mucoprotein that can bind calcium. The binding of calcium by a mucoprotein has been associated, in man, with not only osteogenesis, but also the formation of gallstones, kidney stones, salivary gland stones and dental plaques (Sognnaes, 1960). In addition, Huggins and McCarroll (1936) and others (Anspach, 1964, Kagawa, 1965) have shown that living urinary bladder or gallbladder mucosa, when transplanted near living fibroblasts, result in bone formation. Osteogenesis may occur because the bladder cells secrete a mucoprotein, perhaps analogous to osteoid, that alters the local milieu or binds calcium so that surrounding fibroblasts manufacture calcifiable collagen. Bladder mucosa experimentally increased osteogenesis in fracture gaps (Copher, 1934; Makin, 1962), whereas the placing of calcium in the gap failed to induce osteogenesis (Key, 1934).

The role of mucoprotein in deossification is not well understood. When Vitamin D_3 or parathyroid hormone was administered experimentally, mucoprotein levels in blood and urine were elevated (Engel, 1952). This also suggests the close relationship of mucoproteins to calcified tissues.

Calcification (Bachra, 1967; Blackwood, 1964; Howell, 1963; Richelle, 1965; Urist, 1966). The first and, perhaps the most important part of calcification is the formation of a calcifiable matrix (Weidman, 1963), which is composed of three important parts: (1) sulfated mucopolysaccharides, (2) a matrix which is phosphorylated, and (3) native collagen fibers. The energy source for this matrix production is adenosine triphosphate (ATP). Subsequent steps in calcification may be as follows:

1. Uptake of calcium, possibly by binding to mucoprotein
2. Uptake of phosphorus, possibly by ion association
3. Reduction of barriers to nucleation, possibly by enzymatic action
4. Efflux of water or protein from collagen to allow space for crystal growth
5. Formation of a protein-calcium-phosphorus complex at nucleation sites
6. Nucleation at the collagen sites by hydroxyapatite crystals
7. Crystal growth

There is much debate about the order and importance of the above steps. The contributing roles of pyrophosphate, pyrophosphatase, ATPase, cellular lysosomes, acid hydrolases, peptides and trace metals are unclear.

Robinson (1955) demonstrated that hydroxyapatite crystals are deposited directly on the 640Å banding regions of the collagen fiber. Glimcher (1959, 1968) showed that, of the multiple types of collagen, only the 640Å repeat or native collagen will calcify and nucleate with hydroxyapatite crystals. Therefore, collagen of skin, muscle, tendon, or any other type, will calcify if first depolymerized and then repolymerized into 640Å repeat collagen, possibly because nucleation barriers are removed. If assembled into collagen of any other type, calcification will not occur. Glimcher also showed that crystals deposit at the 640Å bands of native collagen and that crystal growth continues from these nucleation sites. Hydroxyapatite crystals are actually present inside and outside of collagen fibrils. It appears that crystals replace water in "holes" formed at overlap intervals of collagen molecules. These holes are present at 640Å intervals.

Factors in bone production which could direct multipotential tissue to form bone include (1) induction (2) inhibition, and (3) environmental stimuli.

INDUCTION of bone (Burwell, 1966; Moss, 1960; Urist, 1965) is not a well defined occurrence. Urist (1967) stated that HCl-decalcified bone, if protected properly, will consistently induce bone in experimental animals. The inducing ability of this decalcified bone may be antigen dependent. It is transmitted short distances, possibly across Millipore, and it can be destroyed by heat, cold, radiation and poisons that denature proteins. When implanted, the preparation alters surrounding fibroblasts to become swollen "inducing cells," which results in adjacent fibroblasts becoming "responding cells." The responding cells secrete osteoid and bone is formed. These observations are potentially of importance, but they may not be entirely correct. This matrix may contain an inhibitor that results in osteogenesis or, alternatively, the HCl treatment may remove inhibitors of calcification.

INHIBITION. For many years research has disclosed substances that can inhibit calcification (Fleisch, 1963; Harris, S., 1967; Miller, Z. B., 1952; Perkins, 1968; Urist, 1966). These compounds fall into the categories listed in Table 53-2.

TABLE 53-2. INHIBITORS OF CALCIFICATION

1. Compounds (and other factors) that Denature Proteins
   Heat shrinkage
   Dinitrofluorobenzene
   Ethyl alcohol
   N ethyl maleimide
2. Compounds that Block Nucleation Sites
   $CuCl_2$
   $SrCl_2$
   Protamine
   Toluidine blue
3. Compounds that Interfere With Crystal Growth or Bind Calcium
   Pyrophosphate
   Alizarin red
   Tetracycline
4. Anticoagulants
5. Natural Blocking Compounds (See text)

None of the first four types has ever been found in physiologic quantity sufficient to block calcification. Howard (1967) reported the presence in man of a peptide in urine and serum which, in minute quantities, inhibits calcification. This may explain why all collagen does not calcify. Perhaps bone collagen calcifies because something inhibits this inhibitor.

ENVIRONMENTAL STIMULI that control osteogenesis are numerous. Bassett (1962, 1965) showed that *anoxia* of tissue culture fibroblasts resulted in differentiation into chondroblasts, while compression and increased oxygen tension produced osteoblasts. Distraction or rotation of tissue culture cells results in fibrous tissue formation. This may explain why rotation and distraction are harmful to fracture healing. Various oxygen tensions also alter the amount and type of bone collagen (Stern, 1966), and 20 per cent oxygen apparently is the best concentration (Ketenjian, 1968).

Bioelectric effects may affect bone growth, development, and perhaps fracture healing. Bassett (1965) and colleagues (Bassett and Becker, 1962) demonstrated that dead or alive bone, dry or moist, when stressed, develops a negative potential along the stressed segment This may be a result of PN junction diode (Becker, 1967) or piezo-electric effects. Tropocollagen molecules can be organized by an electric current perpendicular to an electric field and near the anode (Becker et al., 1964). Amphibian red cells are dedifferentiated into fibroblast-like cells by a negative current, and various potentials are found in the fracture hematoma (Becker and Murray, 1967). Increased bone production can be produced by a battery placed in a dog femur (Bassett et al., 1964). Positive charges are present when stressed bone is released (Cochran, 1968), and there is marked variation in the charge distribution of loaded bone (McElhaney, 1967). Similar studies may some day explain the control of bone growth.

Numerous other local, regional and systemic factors affect fracture healing. The interaction of these multiple factors in fracture healing is not completely understood. Eagleson (1967) found that elevating the medullary canal temperature 2° C. increased fracture callus. Pearse (1930) and others reported that venous stasis may stimulate osteogenesis. Tonna (1965) has discussed skeletal cell aging and its effects on osteogenesis.

Local systemic supplements have been administered in an attempt to increase healing rates. Goldsmith (1967) reported a beneficial effect of phosphates on fracture healing, and Pories (1967) described the acceleration of healing in skin wounds with oral zinc sulfate. Prudden (1957, 1967) showed acceleration of wound healing with cartilage preparations. The effect of elements such as magnesium, copper or iron on fracture healing is poorly understood.

Vitamins and hormones also have been used in an attempt to improve osteogenesis. Ewald (1967) states that thyrocalcitonin inhibits bone resorption and increases the amount of callus in fractured humeri. Harrison (1967) observed interaction of vitamin D and parathyroid hormone on calcium, phosphorus and magnesium homeostasis in the rat. Kolar (1965) felt that androgens had a beneficial effect on matrix formation in fractures in rats. Steier (1967) reported that increased callus was noted when vitamin D_2 and fluorides, were given together, although separately each had no beneficial effect on fracture healing in rats. Zadek (1967) reviewed the effect of growth hormone on the healing of experimental defects in long bones. The improved prognosis of children's fractures may be partly the effect of growth hormone or the absence of androgens. Other factors that may affect fracture healing are metabolic or disease states, drugs (especially anticoagulants), nerve supply, blood supply and muscle function.

FRACTURE HEALING

The Closed Fracture

Components of the Closed Undisplaced Fracture. Some degree of bone death occurs in every fracture, and this may be a major stimulus for bone production. The important components of the fractured limb are: (1) skin, (2) soft tissue, (3) surrounding muscle, (4) fracture hematoma, (5) periosteum and its circulation, (6) fracture fragments, and (7) the endosteum and its circulation. In the closed fracture, the periosteum, the endosteum and the fracture hematoma contribute to callus formation, but these play varying roles with different types of fractures and fracture treatment.

Bassett (1961) and Hurley (1959) studied the role of soft tissues in osteogenesis and feel that they are an important source of nutrition. Long bone defects and spine fusions were separated from adjacent soft tissues with Millipore filters and silastic sheets. In the Millipore group, osteogenesis and little chondrogenesis occurred, possibly because Millipore allowed metabolite exchange, whereas the silastic group allowed no exchange and demonstrated chondrogenesis and nonunion.

The role of the fracture hematoma is a matter of dispute. The hematoma begins at the moment of the fracture and stops growing when vasoconstriction and thrombosis occur. Aegerter (1968) feels that the hematoma is beneficial because its fibrin meshwork is organized into a significant portion of the callus. The hematoma might also be helpful because it may prevent soft tissue interposition. Geist and Spencer (1964), Heiple and Herndon (1965), Post et al., (1966) and Ham and Harris (1956) feel that the hematoma is harmful because it impedes the progress of fracture healing and appears to be "in the way." Excess hematoma may delay revascularization of bone grafts. However, attempts at increasing or decreasing the hematoma by suction have not proved it to be harmful. At present, the role is still undefined.

Cellular Response. There are many descriptions of the healing fracture and the following paragraph is a composite of several sources (Aho, 1966; Duthie, 1967; Enneking, 1948; Levenson, 1966; Pritchard, 1963; Robinson, 1967; Tonna, 1961, 1966; Urist, 1943).

Immediately after the hematoma forms, the fracture begins to show the cellular response to injury, as does any wound. Various chemical substances are released as a result of cell death and stress. Proteases, plasmin and globulins are present. Polypeptides, such as leukotaxin and bradykinin, attract phagocytes and other cells. Amines, such as histamine, cause vasodilatation. 5-Hydroxy tryptamine may stimulate phagocytosis. Epinephrine, norepinephrine and steroids may have local effects because of their release in the stress reaction. In the first 12 hours after the fracture a steady leakage of tissue fluid and lymph into the wound occurs. The earliest vasodilatation is a result of histamine, and can be blocked by antihistamines, but after 2 hours this leak is resistant to antihistamines and is probably due to capillary permeability and drainage from the flaplike valves of small lymphatics which remain open until tissue osmotic pressure equilibrium occurs. Mast cells are present and may release mucopolysaccharides; plasma cells produce nucleoproteins and gamma globulin; lymphocytes produce histones, and macrophages begin active phagocytosis. Periosteal cells and endosteal cells, blood monocytes, tissue fibroblasts, and perivascular connective cells are present and are termed osteoprogenitor cells, since they may be incorporated into the callus. After 24 to 36 hours phagocytosis is usually complete. Osteocytes deprived of nutrition die, but the bone usually remains. Osteoprogenitor cells begin to multiply rapidly. In the child the periosteum is as many as 9 cell layers thick and can respond much better than in the adult but it is an important source of cells in both groups. By the third day, marked capillary budding has occurred from existing vessels and by the fifth to the seventh day the fracture hematoma is a mass of organizing granulation tissue. It takes approximately 5 to 10 days for collagen and matrix formation to begin, and by 10 to 14 days, chondroid, collagen and osteoid are usually present in moderate quantity. The earliest calcification of the matrix usually occurs at between 14 and 17 days and continues until the fracture unites. The control mechanism for these phenomena is unclear, and there is great variation in this time sequence. If much motion is present or if blood supply is poor, marked cartilagenous callus is produced, which acts as "nature's splint" and then undergoes endochondral ossification. If the fracture is immobilized and blood supply is good, direct bone formation with little cartilagenous callus occurs. Variations in this pattern occur with various fracture types. Fiber bone undergoes remodeling under the possible stimuli of collagenolysis (Grillo, 1967), deossification and bioelectric effects and mature bone is formed.

Biochemistry. The sequence that can be observed in the healing fracture includes histologic and biochemical events, as well as gross changes. There is great variation between subjects studied and between types of fractures or even sites of fractures. The following description of changes occurring within the fracture is a composite of several sources (Balogh, 1966; Balogh and Hajeh, 1965; Bourne, 1956; Duthie, 1961; Duthie and Barker, 1955b; LeMain, 1966; Meyer, K., et al., 1956; Paff, 1948; Solheim, 1965, 1966; Swenson, 1946; Wray, 1965).

Days 1 through 5 are termed the period of the hematoma, although the hematoma may begin early organization at 24 to 36 hours. Multiple fibroblasts and new capillaries are present. Day 10 through day 15 may be called the matrix period when multiple cells of the osteoprogenitor type produce new collagen and organic matrix. Day 15 through day 30 is titled the osteogenesis period, with multiple osteoblasts, chondroblasts, and osteoclasts. These cells are also present in the final period of remodeling, which lasts from 30 to 60 days. There is much variation of this arbitrary assignment.

Many enzyme systems are active in the healing fracture (Balogh, 1965, 1966), only a few of which will be discussed. Their exact function is unclear. Isocitric dehydrogenase and glucose-6-phosphate dehydrogenase are found in chondroblasts. TPNH dehydrogenase, LDH, esterases and alkaline phosphatase are present in osteoblasts. Amino peptides, succinic dehydrogenase, pyrophosphatase and acid phosphatase are prominent in osteoclasts. The levels of these enzymes rise with cellular activity and peak with the phosphorylation of the matrix at 7 to 10 days. Following this, activity decreases steadily. Alkaline phosphatase is associated with osteoblastic activity but has no proven function in osteogenesis. The greatest rise in level occurs by day 10; then the level remains elevated and continues to rise with osteogenic activity. Just prior to the period of calcification of the matrix, at about 15 days, there is a peak of chondroitin sulfate, sulfur uptake by the matrix, and collagen. These levels steadily decrease until the termination of osteogenesis (Duthie, 1961; Solheim, 1966). Hydroxyproline is one of the major building blocks of collagen and rises to high levels before peak collagen production, reaching its peak at approximately day 5 and remaining elevated until the termination of collagenesis. Calcium is present at low levels initially and these levels rise proportionally to osteogenesis (LeMain, 1966; Soliman, 1964). The early low level is due to the binding of calcium in the matrix, after 15 days the rise in level is due to the massive quantities of calcium salts as hydroxyapatite. The levels of phosphate are similar to those of calcium in their pattern of increase. Phosphorus is present in the fracture hematoma (Solheim, 1965; Swenson, 1946) and reaches its peak levels in the hematoma in 2 to 3 days. The level decreases to its lowest point at day 5 to day 7 and then increases with osteogenesis. The uptake of radioactive phosphorus increases to a peak at day 7 to day 10, which marks the phosphorylation of the matrix. Phosphorus uptake then steadily decreases and is minimal at the completion of fracture healing. The pH of the early fracture is acid (as low as 5.7) and rises to neutral at day 7 to day 10. Thereafter, the pH often becomes slightly alkaline until the termination of fracture healing. This low pH may be caused by increased levels of lactate in the fracture hematoma secondary to anaerobic metabolism. Low pH's were reported to have increased the amount of bone growth in tissue culture experiments (Paff, 1948). The water content of early callus is 90 per cent and decreases with maturation of callus and bone formation until it is approximately 10 per cent at the completion of the healing process. Much work is needed to assemble this biochemical picture into a more understandable pattern, but even now it is apparent that with present knowledge the diagnosis of delayed or nonunion could be made much earlier biochemically than radiographically or clinically.

Later Stages. After active osteogenesis has begun, bone remodeling and resorption of larger devitalized fragments occurs and new bone is laid down along lines of stress.

OTHER FRACTURE TYPES

The preceding pattern of healing holds true for most closed fractures, but there is great variation with different types of fractures. For example, a varying degree of trauma alters osteogenesis. Breaks in the skin allow entrance of foreign bodies and bacteria. Loss of muscle or subcutaneous tissue removes the soft tissue source of nutrition. The loss of cancellous bone increases the time required for healing. The loss of the periosteal or endosteal blood supply removes an important source of new bone. Large bony gaps may not unite unless the patient is a child with an intact periosteal tube (Macnab, 1954, Zadek, 1967). Key (1934) demonstrated that a gap larger than $1\frac{1}{2}$ times the diameter of the long bone consistently results in nonunion. Attempts at bridging the gap with polyethylene tubes (Linghorne, 1960) or Millipore tubes (Rabhan, 1969) have been only partly successful. The open fracture carries less favorable prognosis, not only because of tissue trauma, but also because of the risk of infection, with resulting thrombosis of vessels and bone death (Boyd, 1960). As many as 50 per cent of nonunions in tibial fractures were found to have been related to previous osteomyelitis (Errico, 1967). The pattern of fracture healing also may be altered by delayed open reduction, early mobilization of the patient, compression fixation, metal implants (Bechtol et al., 1959) and bone grafts (Chase, 1955).

Fixation. Osteogenesis is altered with the type of fracture and the type of fixation utilized. The following examples are taken in part from studies, pioneered by Reynolds (1954) and subsequently repeated by Anderson (1965), of fracture healing in dog femurs. The results of microangiographic studies by Trueta (1960, 1963) and Rhinelander (1962) will be correlated with these healing patterns.

With no fixation and marked displacement the fracture hematoma is large and contributes a major part to fracture healing, since the medullary canal and the periosteum are too displaced for bridging callus to develop. Organization of the fracture hematoma followed by cartilage formation and endochondral ossification beginning at the periphery is the mechanism for the healing of this fracture. Healing is often prolonged and there is a high incidence of nonunion. With loose intramedullary nails a moderate quantity of cartilagenous callus is produced because of motion and the relatively large hematoma. The nail causes obliteration of the endosteal circulation, but there usually is compensatory hyperemia of the periosteal circulation. Because of the moderate amount of motion, more time is required for organization and remodeling, and some portions of the bone ends often are resorbed. There is increased incidence of nonunion. Tight intramedullary nailing often results in excellent and sometimes early union. Although the endosteal circulation is obliterated, periosteal direct bone formation is abundant and there is little cartilagenous callus. Conventional screw and plate fixation usually only partly damages the endosteal circulation. With rigid fixation, circulation across the fracture gap often can be re-established within one week. Endosteal direct bone formation and cartilagenous callus usually are abundant and the fracture unites by an endosteal plug of bone. The periosteum does not contribute a major portion of the callus, since it is removed with the operative procedure. If plate and screw fixation is not rigid, nonunion is common because the medullary callus cannot unite. Compression plate fixation probably has an advantage because it provides more rigid fixation. Another advantage may be that the fracture gap is smaller. Bony union is not more rapid or solid, but histologic observations demonstrate probably less cartilage production and more direct bone formation across the medullary canal. This pattern of healing is nearly identical with regular plate and screw fixation.

There is no evidence that compression accelerates fracture healing. In nearly all of these studies, the bone ends were not resorbed and the avascular portions remained to maintain the length of the bone until long after the fracture was united. In fractures where one fragment is completely devascularized, such as in experimental fractures of the femoral neck with the ligamentum teres avulsed, union can occur if rigid fixation is employed to allow revascularization of dead fragment. Without rigid fixation, nonunion is common. Banks (1965) has shown that intra-articular fractures cannot heal by periosteal bone or organization of the fracture hematoma, but must heal by direct fiber bone formation across the fracture gap. Therefore, good fixation is essential in most intra-articular fractures. The role of increased intra-capsular pressure or venous stasis is unclear in these fractures.

THE FATE OF BONE GRAFTS

Improved methods in storage of bone have stimulated a considerable interest in the use of preserved bones as grafts and also in the study of the fate of these grafts in the host. It has long been known that fixation and replacement of the graft by living bone is more rapid with cancellous grafts than with cortical grafts (Abbott *et al.,* 1947). Likewise, much of an autogenous bone graft dies and must be replaced with living bone by action of the host tissue (Chase and Herndon, 1955).

There has been a question as to whether any elements of an autogenous graft survive transplantation and assist in the incorporation of the graft into the recipient part. It has now been established that some of the cells of connective tissue derivation do survive in autogenous transplants and are capable of growth. How important the presence of these viable cells of the transplant are in the process of fixation and replacement is not known. We do know that freshly taken undenatured autogenous transplants are incorporated more rapidly and more surely than any other type of graft such as fresh or preserved homografts or heterografts.

Preservation of bone by any method tends in time to kill all elements of the bone. However, Ray (1963) has been able to demonstrate growth in tissue culture of bone preserved by freezing for as long as 90 days.

For the most part, the preserved graft should be considered to be dead. Utilization of the graft must be primarily the function of the host. Experimental studies comparing the effect of autogenous and various dead grafts under favorable conditions reveal few visible differences between them in the basic processes of fixation and replacement. However, replacement of the graft is more rapid with autogenous bone, and fewer are resorbed or sequestered and walled off by connective tissue. At present there is evidence that these differences may be due to unfavorable host response to the graft rather than to the state of viability of transplant. Recently Ray and Sabet (1963) using tritiated thymidine have demonstrated that new bone formation about an isograft may be derived both from the graft and from the host. New bone formation resulting from a homograft in the time interval of their experiment when present came only from the graft. At present, however, we feel that autogenous grafts are always preferred if it is possible to obtain them. An excellent review of bone grafting is that of Chase and Herndon (1955; Heiple, Chase and Herndon, 1963).

DEOSSIFICATION OF THE SKELETON

As stated previously, bone absorption and reconstruction go on continuously throughout life. Anything that alters the rate of absorption and reconstruction tends to lead to alteration of the skeleton. Osteoporosis is the most common consequence of altered rates of absorption and reconstruction. A rate of bone absorption more rapid than the rate of new bone formation leads to osteoporosis. Rapid destruction of bone of the type seen with hyperparathyroidism and with certain types of renal insufficiency usually leads to osteitis fibrosa cystica, while less rapid destruction results in generalized wasting and atrophy of bone without cystic changes (see Chap. 28, Thyroid, Thymus and Parathyroids).

When the roentgenographic picture of decalcification of the skeleton presents itself the initial problem is to differentiate between the basic physiologic disturbances—osteoporosis,

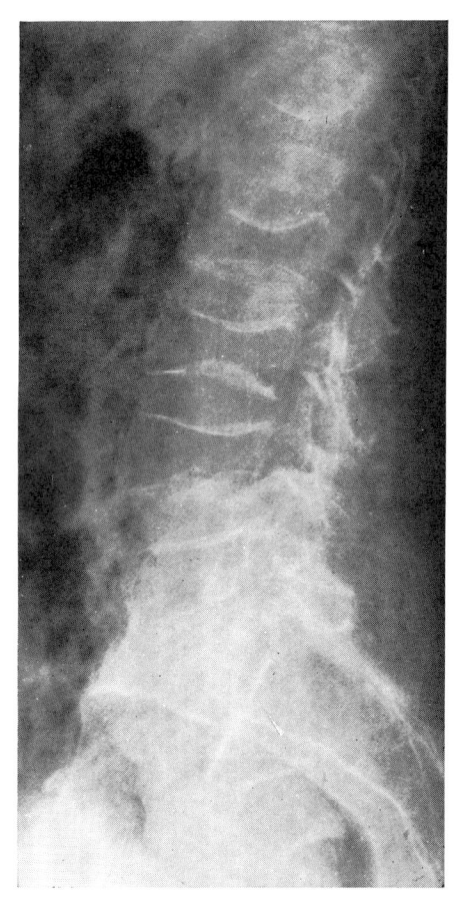

FIG. 53-1. Osteoporosis. At first glance the disk spaces may be mistaken for the vertebral bodies.

osteomalacia or hyperparathyroidism. This differentiation can usually be established by means of blood chemistries and bone biopsy. In Table 53-1 the usual chemical relationships are indicated. Included are the findings in osteogenesis imperfecta, myeloma and Paget's disease which at times may be confused with osteoporosis, osteomalacia and hyperparathyroidism.

OSTEOPOROSIS

When the diagnosis of osteoporosis has been made the etiologic factor must be determined in order to institute effective therapy.

Failure of formation of a proper osteoid matrix which leads to osteoporosis may attend the faulty protein metabolism seen in starvation, Cushing's syndrome and the postmenopausal period. Albright (1948) differentiates between postmenopausal osteoporosis and senile osteoporosis, because in the former the skull and the extremities are somewhat less involved in the demineralization process, and the lamina dura of the teeth remain normal, while in senile osteoporosis changes involve all of the bones.

Osteoporosis also results from disuse. This osteoporosis of disuse is to be distinguished from the localized acute bone destruction which occurs in Sudeck's atrophy. Osteoporosis of disuse is almost always demonstrable roentgenographically in the bones of a limb long contained in a cast. With osteoporosis secondary to a deficient matrix formation, the serum calcium, phosphorus and phosphatase are within normal limits. However, disuse osteoporosis associated with immobilization in body casts and traction apparatus is associated with slight hypercalcemia and a pronounced hypercalciuria. The latter predisposes the person to renal lithiasis.

The picture of postmenopausal osteoporosis is one of lessening stature, rounded shoulders, a painful back with restricted motions and tenderness over the spinous processes. Compression fracture of osteoporotic vertebral bodies occurs frequently after slight injuries and lifting. The x-ray examination may show extensive deossification of the vertebral bodies. The disk spaces are widened, producing a "codfish" type of vertebrae. Prolapse of the disk material into the weakened vertebral bodies may take place. At times decalcification is so severe and the destruction so advanced that the vertebral bodies are difficult to distinguish on the roentgenogram (Fig. 53-1). The serum calcium, phosphorus and phosphatase in these individuals is usually within normal limits. However, the total serum protein is usually low. In women with severe senile decalcification the sedimentation rate is often elevated.

Treatment of an uncomplicated but painful compression fracture in an osteoporotic patient usually consists of bed rest and the control of pain with analgesics. However, the period of bed rest should be as short as possible and limited to the period of severe pain. The stress and strain of muscular activity conserves and improves the general condition of the patient and prevents the superimposition of disuse osteoporosis upon the postmenopausal syndrome. Adequate bracing of the spine is fairly effective. Although this form of treatment may be effective in relieving symptoms, it does not result in visible x-ray evidence of recalcification. Biopsy studies before and after hormonal therapy have been done by Levine, Gitman and Balker (1955). Bone samples were taken from the pelvis. These revealed no change in the character or amout of bone. X-ray therapy in small doses over the painful spine may be helpful in relief of severe pain.

A review of some concepts of osteoporosis is found in the August, 1962 issue of the *Journal of Bone and Joint Surgery* (Atkinson et al.; Casuccio; Fraser; Little and Kelly; Urist et al.).

OSTEOMALACIA

Osteomalacia is a disturbance in the proper deposition of bone salt in the osteoid matrix. Histologically, bone trabeculae are thickened by layers of osteoid formation, but calcification of the osteoid is strikingly absent. Osteoblasts are in abundance (Fig. 53-2).

Albright (1948) feels that any condition which produces this histologic change should be classified as rickets or osteomalacia, depending upon the age of the patient—rickets in children and osteomalacia in adults. An inadequate intake of vitamin D or the deficient absorption of this vitamin from the intestinal tract consequent to such diseases as sprue, celiac disease, chronic pancreatitis or steatorrhea may lead to rickets ond osteomalacia. The pathologic process consists of a reduction of calcification at the zone of provisional calcification prefixed to the epiphyseal plate.

As the child grows the deficient calcification within the zone of provisional calcification leads to improper calcification and ossification of the cartilaginous trabeculae, extending irregularly into the metaphyseal regions of the bone. These alterations are manifest in the x-ray picture as a widened cone-shaped epiphyseal plate with widening of the epiphysis and sclerosis of this structure along its metaphyseal margin. The epiphysis is less firmly attached to the metaphysis, allowing easier dislocation of the epiphysis among rachitic children. The serum calcium is usually normal, but the inorganic phosphate of the blood is lower than normal, and the alkaline phos-

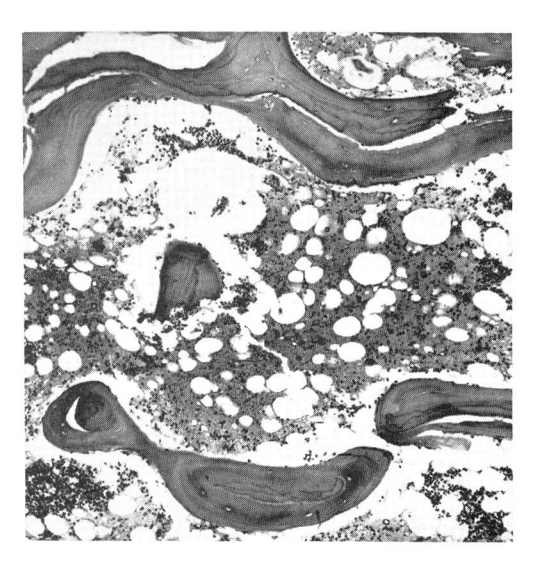

FIG. 53-2. Photomicrograph of bone from the iliac crest of a patient with osteomalacia. The symmetrical deposition of osteoid about each bone trabecula is the characteristic histological feature. The classical chemical findings of a high alkaline phosphatase, low serum phosphorus and normal serum calcium led to the biopsy which confirmed the diagnosis. The cause of osteomalacia in this patient (a 50-year-old woman) was faulty phosphate reabsorption.

phatase may be increased 100 per cent or more. Calcium and phosphorus balances are less positive than normal.

Osteomalacia in the adult may be due to a variety of etiologic factors. When the diagnosis of osteomalacia has been established, the defect in calcium-phosphorus metabolism must be identified in order to institute correct therapy. Simple vitamin D lack, resistance to vitamin D, steatorrhea, renal acidosis, Fanconi syndrome, idiopathic hypercalcemia, lactation and failure of renal phosphate resorption can all produce the clinical and histologic picture of osteomalacia. However, the osseous and clinical manifestations differ somewhat from those of rickets. Decalcification of the skeleton is generalized, the epiphyseal changes are lacking because the epiphyseal plates have disappeared, the bones are softer than with rickets and deform readily, the acetabula approach one another, misshaping the pelvis. The serum calcium level is lower than normal, and hypocalcemic tetany may occur. The calcium

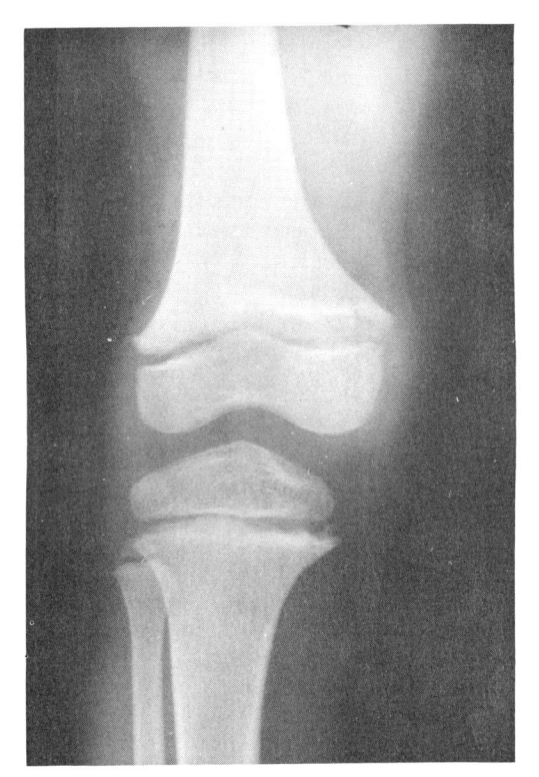

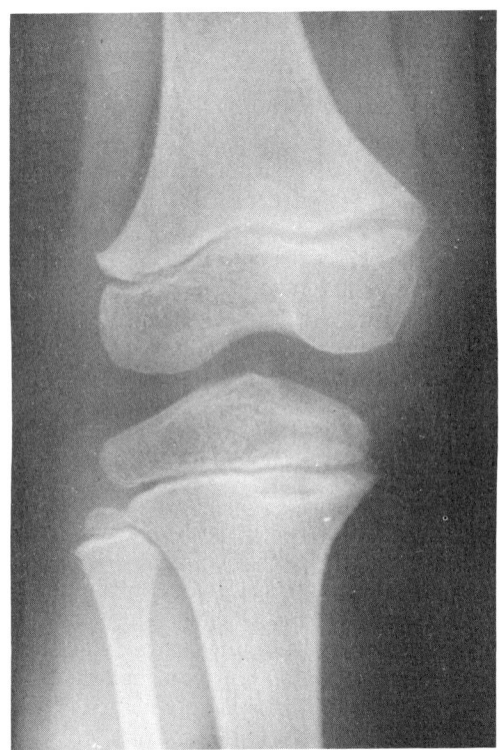

Fig. 53-3. (*Left*) Vitamin-D-resistant rickets in a 6-year-old girl. The distal femoral and proximal tibial metaphyses are wide. The zone of provisional calcification is indistinct. Serum phosphorus was 2.1 mg. per cent; Serum calcium was 10.0 mg. per cent. (*Right*) The same patient after 3 months of massive doses (100,000 u. per day) of vitamin D. The ephiphyseal line has narrowed and the zone of provisional calcification has reappeared. Serum phosphorus was 3.5 mg. per cent; serum calcium was 12.0 mg. per cent.

balance is negative, and the phosphorus is near normal. The combination of a diet low in calcium and deficient in vitamin D, with an indoor life, is usually requisite to the development of osteomalacia.

A predisposition to spontaneous fractures of the posterior ribs associated with pseudofractures of the femurs and the axillary border of the scapula should lead one to suspect a diagnosis of osteomalacia. Severe deformities of the pelvis are likely to interfere seriously with childbirth.

Albright (1948) considers the syndrome described by Milkman (1934), characterized by symmetrical fractures starting in the cortex, to be identical with osteomalacia. Rarely, cases of rickets seem to have a familial tendency (Fig. 53-3, *left*). These cases are resistant to vitamin D therapy, showing no clinical response to normal amounts of vitamin D intake. Albright, Butler and Bloomsberg (1937) described 6 cases and demonstrated that the pathologic process was exactly the same as in rickets, and that the only difference was the resistance to vitamin D therapy (Fig. 53-4). However, they found that giving very large doses of vitamin D would result eventually in healing (Fig. 53-3, *right*). They termed these cases *vitamin-D-resistant rickets*. Pedersen and McCarroll (1951) presented a large series of such patients, pointing out that the diagnosis is commonly missed, and that these individuals were subjected to repeated surgical procedures for correction of osseous deformities, only to have the deformity recur until proper diagnosis was made and treatment was instituted. The main problem presented by these cases is that the enormous vitamin D dosage required to control the disease closely approximates the toxic level and requires very careful observation during therapy (Stamp et al., 1964).

This disease must be differentiated from other chondrodystrophies, particularly metaphyseal dysastosis tarda (Rubin, 1964) in which blood chemistry is normal. Vitamin-D-resistant rickets is inherited as an X-linked dominant. It most likely is a defect in the ability to convert vitamin D to its more active metabolite, vitamin D-3. When the active form of this vitamin becomes available, this disease may be completely controlled (Avioli*).

SCURVY

Except for the epiphyseal changes, the clinical and pathologic conditions are similar in both the child and the adult. It has been well established that a 6-month deficit of vitamin C is usually necessary before symptoms of scurvy appear. The classical pathologic changes are found in tissues of mesodermal origin. Periosteal hemorrhage, decreased osteoblastic activity in the epiphyseal regions, replacement of the myelogenous elements of the bone marrow by fibrous tissue, increased brittleness of the teeth, gingival hemorrhage, and a secondary anemia are the classic pathologic changes seen in scurvy. Severe pain in the legs is frequently the first symptom of scurvy and is the direct result of the sub-

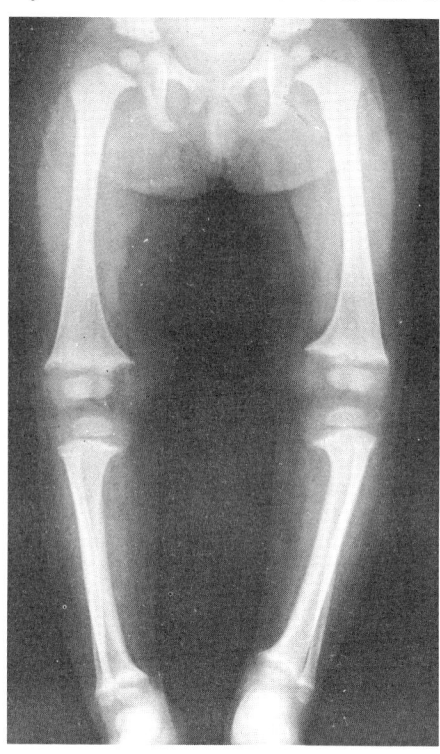

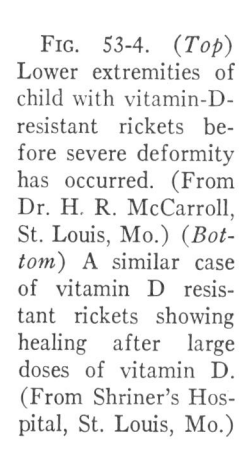

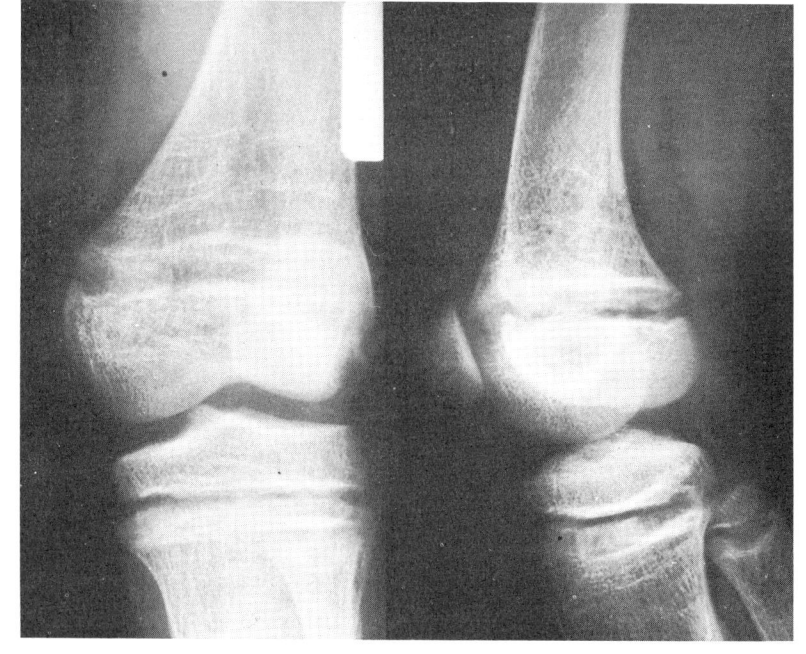

*Personal communication.

Fig. 53-4. (Top) Lower extremities of child with vitamin-D-resistant rickets before severe deformity has occurred. (From Dr. H. R. McCarroll, St. Louis, Mo.) (Bottom) A similar case of vitamin D resistant rickets showing healing after large doses of vitamin D. (From Shriner's Hospital, St. Louis, Mo.)

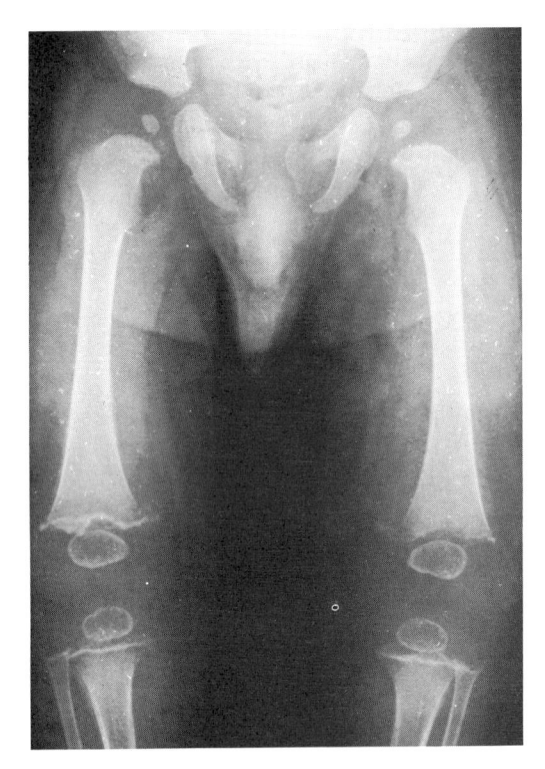

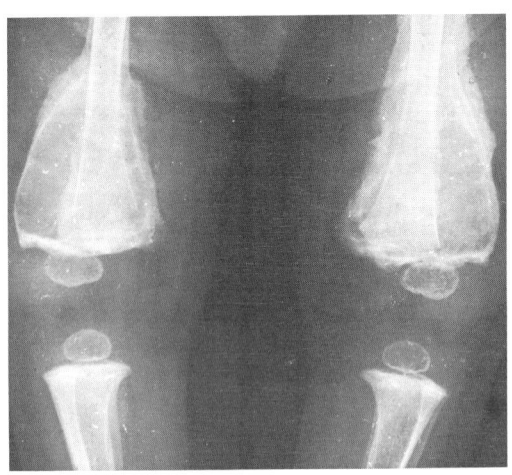

FIG. 53-5. (*Left*) Roentgenogram of childhood scurvy showing alteration of the epiphyseal lines and early subperiosteal new bone formation. The apparent increased density of the margins of the epiphyses at the knee, producing a ring appearance, is typical of this condition. (*Right*) Later stage of the disease with calcification and ossification of the large subperiosteal hematoma. The distal femoral epiphysis seems to have shifted on both sides. (From Shriner's Hospital, St. Louis, Mo.)

periosteal hemorrhage (Fig. 53-5). Swollen, bleeding gums, loose teeth, and hemorrhagic lesions of the skin are other common findings. Epiphyseal separations and metaphyseal fractures are frequently seen in children. Due to the generalized deossification of the skeleton in late adult scurvy, pathologic fractures through the diaphyseal region of the long bones may also occur.

The classic x-ray changes are broad irregular zones in the provisional area of calcification of the growing epiphyseal plate. Ringing of the epiphysis itself, periosteal calcification and ossification, and a ground-glass translucency of the bones are also changes typical of scurvy.

If the condition remains untreated, death occurs within a few months. Pneumonia has been reported as the leading cause of death. The response to vitamin C therapy is prompt and curative. Pain and tenderness from subperiosteal hemorrhage is often relieved in 24 to 36 hours. Endochondral ossification is resumed, and frequently the ossified subperiosteal hematoma may disappear entirely.

The roentgenographic changes about the epiphysis must not be confused with the changes seen in lead poisoning. The finding of increased radiodensity of the calcified portion of the epiphyseal plate should cause a search for the other stigmata of plumbism (history of lead exposure, anemia, radial palsy, colic, increased lead level in the serum, increased urinary excretion of lead, and stippling of the red cells) (Fig. 53-7). Phosphorus and bismuth intoxication may produce roentgenographic changes similar to those found in plumbism.

OTHER METABOLIC DISEASES OF BONE

Seemingly, Paget's disease is a metabolic disease of bone. Moehlig and Abbott (1947) believe it to be the result of a disturbance of carbohydrate metabolism. However, the etiology of Paget's disease remains unknown and no effective treatment has been devised. Paget's disease almost always occurs in persons past the age of 40 and in advanced stages is char-

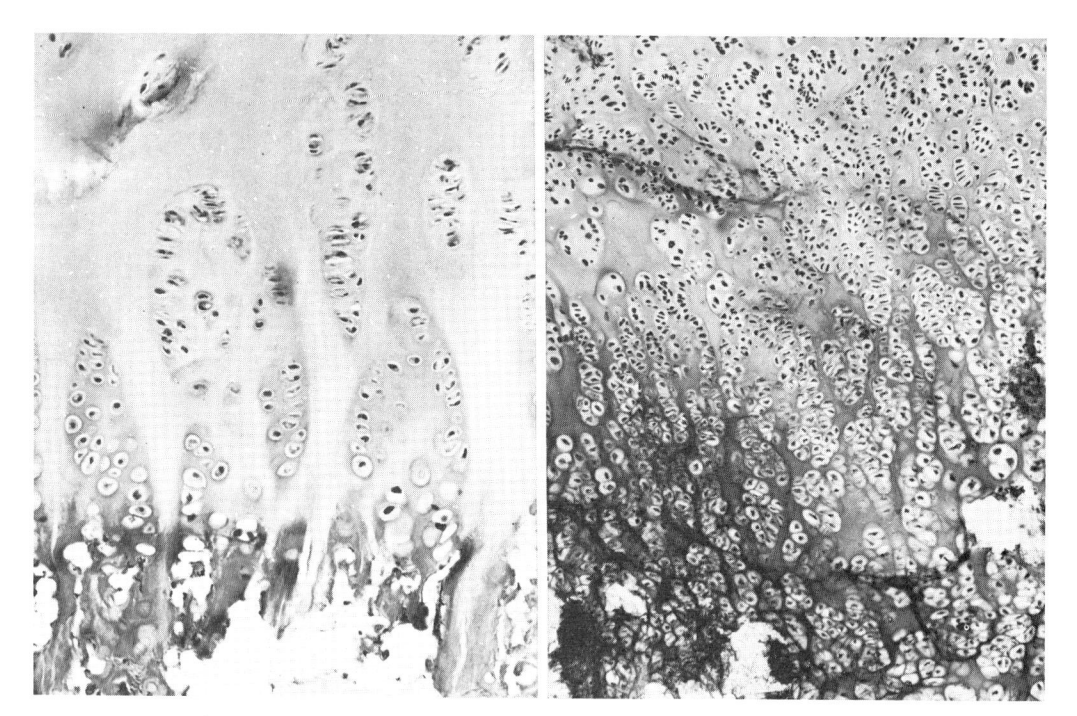

FIG. 53-6. (*Left*) Photomicrograph of a normal epiphyseal plate, demonstrating the orderly arrangement of the cartilage cells as they progress through the proliferative to the hypertrophic stage. (H & E, original magnification × 130) (*Right*) Photomicrograph of a rachitic epiphyseal plate, demonstrating the markedly widened and disrupted proliferating and hypertrophic cell areas. (H & E, original magnification × 55)

acterized by an increase in size of the skull (often requiring a change in hat size in men), curvature and shortening of the extremities and kyphosis. However, the disease may appear first in only one bone, all the rest of the skeleton remaining normal. When it does it is called *monostotic Paget's disease* (Fig. 53-8, *top*). Pain, thickening of the bone, increased heat and tenderness in the region of the lesion constitute the clinical signs of the monostotic form. Roentgenograms may show an irregular or fusiform lytic cavity in the bone, which may readily be confused with fibrous dysplasia.

Whether the disease is monostotic or generalized, the parts of the skeleton most commonly affected are the skull, the pelvis, the spine, the tibia and the small bones of the hands (Fig. 53-8, *bottom*). The feet and the ribs are rarely affected. There is an increased blood flow in the bone about the lesions in Paget's disease. The blood chemical studies may be within normal limits with the monostotic form; at times a positive diagnosis is made only from biopsy study. When the disease is more widespread, the differential diagnosis seldom offers any difficulty. With Paget's disease progressive active bone destruction, simultaneously attended by a rapid overcompensating new bone formation, produces bones of greatly increased size. However, because of failure of proper orientation of the newly formed bone to lines of force there is decreased strength.

Fracture of the long bones is frequently found at the junction of the normal and the pathologic bone. The affected skull cap grows larger, and the progessive destruction of normal bone and the rapid overproduction results in the so-called "cottonwool" texture of the skull seen on roentgenograms. In the extremities the process results in broad irregular trabeculae lacking a definite pattern of arrangement.

The histologic examination of tissue taken from an active lesion shows active new bone formation and bone destruction going on in

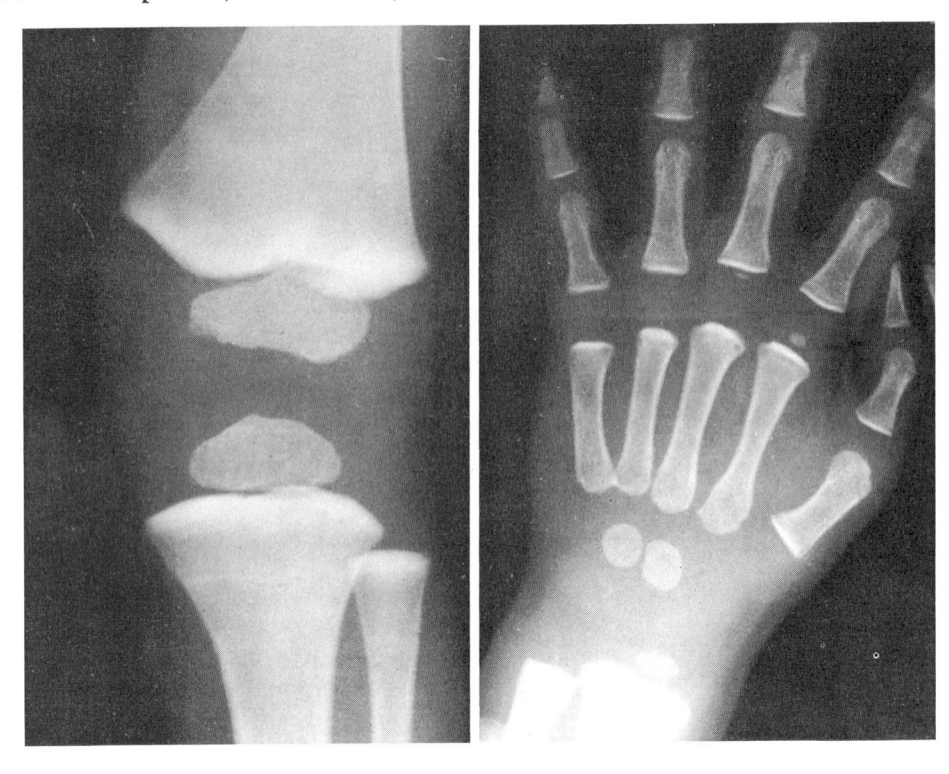

FIG. 53-7. Roentgenogram of the knee and hand of a child with lead poisoning. The increased density of metaphysis adjacent to the epiphyseal plate is characteristic. Toxic blood levels of lead and increased lead excretion in the urine confirmed the diagnosis.

the same area; broad irregular trabeculae with many cement lines produce a mosaic pattern (Fig. 53-9).

Chemical studies in Paget's disease show that the serum calcium and inorganic phosphorus content are usually within normal limits and that the calcium output in the urine is within normal limits. However, the alkaline phosphatase is increased and may be as much as 20 or 30 times normal.

The complications of Paget's disease are: (1) pathologic fracture; (2) compression fracture of the spine, at times with spinal cord pressure; (3) deafness; (4) degenerative changes of joints secondary to incongruities and irregularities from pressure molding of the soft bone contiguous with them; (5) pain (Nicholas, 1965) found that heavy doses of steroids for a 7- to 10-day period may provide temporary relief of pain in cases where other therapy fails), and (6) the development of osteogenic sarcoma, which occurs in 5 to 10 per cent of the cases. The incidence of sarcoma in Paget's disease seems to occur in about 3 per cent of 600 cases of osteogenic sarcoma (Dahlin, 1967).

INBORN ERRORS OF METABOLISM

A number of skeletal dysplasias may confront the orthopedic surgeon. Only those in which the inheritance pattern and the biochemical defect are known will be discussed. For a complete description of the skeletal dysplasias the reader is referred to Rubin (1964) and McKusick (1960).

The Mucopolysaccharidoses

Six distinct entities have been identified and differentiated by combined clinical, genetic, and biochemical studies, and are more or less arbitrarily designated MPS I (Hurler syndrome), MPS II (Hunter syndrome), MPS III (Sanfilippo syndrome), MPS IV (Morquio syndrome), MPS V (Scheie syndrome), and MPS VI (Maroteaux-Lamy syndrome). Apparently, a genetic aberration results in failure of normal metabolic maturation of fibroblasts, causing them to elaborate abnormal quantities of mucopolysaccharides. Probably because of the excess amounts, these substances are stored in the cells of various systems and secreted in the urine. Storage of excessively large quantities interferes with normal growth of cartilage cells and function of the reticuloendothelial system and the brain.

The clinical, genetic and biochemical characteristics of the six syndromes are given in Table 53-3.

Diagnosis. The amount of mucopolysac-

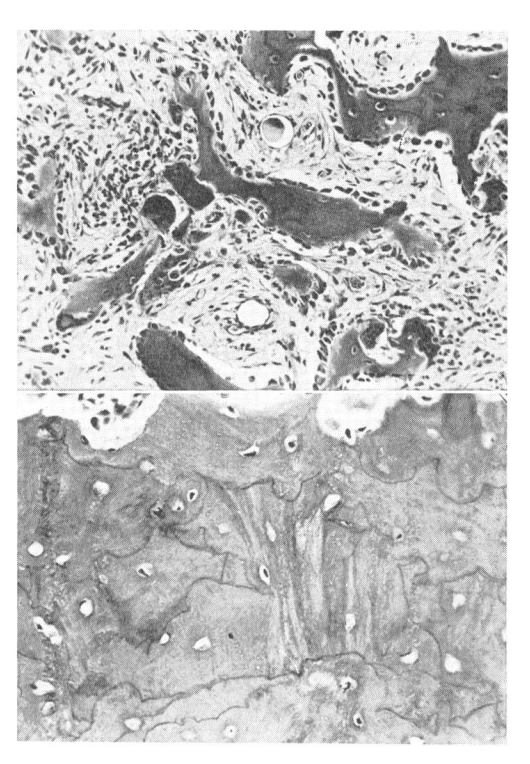

FIG. 53-9. (*Top*) Photomicrograph showing active new bone formation and bone destruction going on in a vascular fibrous stroma. (*Bottom*) Specimen from a somewhat older portion of the diseased bone showing irregular cement lines in greatly thickened bone trabeculae resulting in a mosaic pattern.

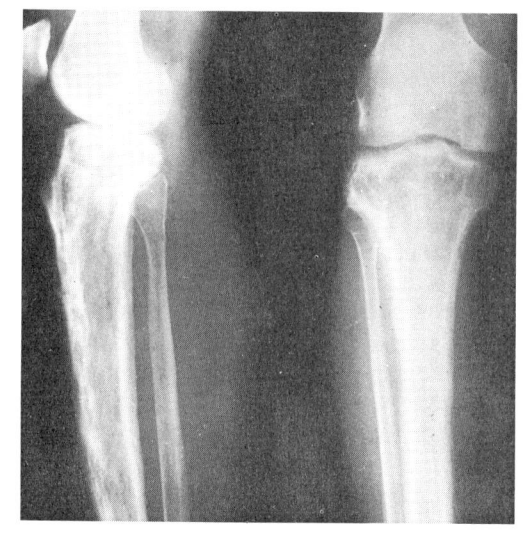

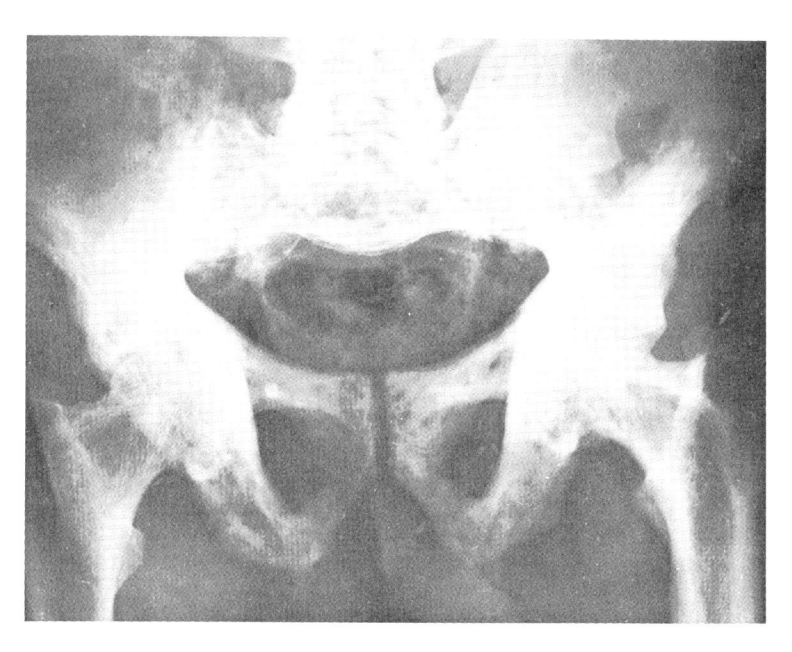

FIG. 53-8. (*Top*) Advanced changes in the tibia from Paget's disease. Note cortical thickening, coarse trabeculation. Transverse fissures in the anterior cortex represent the pathologic fractures of a type similar to Looser's. There are no other roentgenologic evidences of Paget's disease in this patient. (*Bottom*) Advanced Paget's disease, involving the lower lumbar spine, the sacrum, both innominate bones and the left femur. This patient presented himself because of painful hips, the diagnosis not having been made previously.

TABLE 53-3. THE MUCOPOLYSACCHARIDOSES*

MPS	EPONYM	CLINICAL FEATURES	GENETICS	BIOCHEMICAL FINDINGS (IN URINE)
I	Hurler Syndrome	Evident in childhood or early infancy Death earliest of the 6 types, secondary to cardiorespiratory failure Early corneal clouding, mental retardation, hydrocephalus Spinal gibbus, long bone diaphyseal changes Hepatosplenomegaly, dwarfism, stiff joints	autosomal recessive	chondroitin sulfate B heparitin sulfate
II	Hunter Syndrome	Less severe than MPS I No corneal clouding, no gibbus Mental deterioration slower in onset Progressive deafness Hepatosplenomegaly, dwarfism, stiff joints	X-linked recessive	chondroitin sulfate B heparitin sulfate
III	Sanfilippo Syndrome	Severe mental retardation, dwarfism No corneal clouding, mild joint stiffness Minimal hepatosplenomegaly	autosomal recessive	heparitin sulfate
IV	Morquio Syndrome	Severely dwarfed; death before age 20 Flat vertebrae, osteoporosis, no stiff joints Slowly progressive corneal clouding Aortic regurgitation, short neck Barrel chest, short nose, broad mouth, prominent maxilla	autosomal recessive	keratosulfate
V	Scheie Syndrome	Minimal CNS changes Stiff joints, claw hand, corneal clouding Normal- to low-normal stature Aortic regurgitation, carpal tunnel syndrome	autosomal recessive	chondroitin sulfate B
VI	Maroteaux-Lamy Syndrome	Normal intellect Corneal clouding, deafness Stunting of limb and trunk (severe) Hepatosplenomegaly	autosomal recessive	chondroitin sulfate B

* Modified after McKusick (1960).

charides excreted in the urine ranges from 3 to 15 mg. per 24 hours. Chondroitin sulfate A comprises about 80 per cent of the excreted mucopolysaccharide, with chondroitin sulfate B and heparitin sulfate accounting in equal parts for the remainder. These substances are not excreted in the urine of normal persons. However, mucopolysaccharide excretion may normally be greater early in life.

Metachromatic granules have been reported in lymphocytes of all types except in MPS IV and MPS V. Its appearance in neutrophils is inconsistently positive.

Why some clinical features occur in some and not in others of the six mucopolysaccharidoses is not known. The relation between heparitin sulfate and mental retardation is most suggestive of a clinical-chemical correlation. McKusick found heparitin sulfate to be absent in MPS V and MPS VI (in which mental retardation is mild at the most) and excreted in large amounts in MPS III (in which the clinical picture is dominated by mental retardation). This finding has not been supported by other investigators. Many questions still remain unanswered. It is probable that future accounts will report still other variations.

HOMOCYSTINURIA

An inborn error of metabolism has been discovered that simulates the Marfan syndrome in several respects. Homocystinuria results from a defect in the enzyme cystathionine synthetase. The diagnosis is made by the cyanide-nitroprusside screening test. In the screening of over 600 families with one or more cases of ectopia lentis, homocystinuria was found in 31 families (58 affected persons). About 5 per cent of nontraumatic ectopia lentis is due to homocystinuria. A comparison of the two syndromes is given in Table 53-4 (McKusick, 1960).

TABLE 53-4

	HOMOCYSTINURIA	MARFAN SYNDROME
Inheritance	recessive	dominant
Basic defect	deficiency in enzyme cystathionine synthetase	not known
Ectopia lentis	present	present
Pectus deformity tall, scoliosis long limbs	often present	usually present
Osteoporosis	present	absent
Loose jointed	inconsistently present	present almost always
Mental retardation	60%	absent
Cardiac complications	venous and arterial thrombosis	aortic aneurysm
Malar flush	present	absent
Treatment	diet low in methionine and cystine	not known

At one time the reticuloendothelioses were comprised of six different entities. Chemical analysis of the tissues of diseased individuals resulted in their being grouped as follows: (1) those in which the dominant lipid is cholesterol (Hand-Schüller-Christian disease, Letterer-Siwe disease, and eosinophilic granuloma); (2) that in which a cerebroside is the offending agent (Gaucher's disease), and (3) those in which the cells contain various phosphosphingosides (Niemann-Pick and Tay-Sachs disease).

Eosinophilic granuloma, Letterer-Siwe disease, and Hand-Schüller-Christian disease probably should be grouped under the term histiocytosis X after Lichtenstein (1964).

LETTERER-SIWE DISEASE

This condition is characterized by granulomatous lesions made up of collections of histiocytes (macrophages) without lipid occurring in them. These lesions occur especially in bones, spleen and other parenchymatous organs. It usually appears in children under the age of 1 year.

The clinical signs are cutaneous ecchymoses at times combined with superficial ulcerations, low-grade fever, a large liver and spleen, enlarged lymph nodes and a chronic progressive anemia. The osseous lesions destroy the bone and most commonly are found in the skull. This condition was formerly considered a universally fatal disease. In recent years because of its infectionlike characteristics, these patients have been treated with antibiotics, and many have recovered. Bierman *et al.* (1952) isolated the Arizona type of salmonella organism from a case of Letterer-Siwe disease. Antibiotic therapy was successful in arresting the lesions.

Theoretically, a patient with Letterer-Siwe disease who survives would slowly develop the clinical picture of Hand-Schüller-Christian disease. We have never seen these possibly closely related abnormalities change from one to the other (see Chap. 34).

HAND-SCHÜLLER-CHRISTIAN DISEASE

This disease is characterized by the proliferation of fibrous tissue in which are nests of histiocytes containing esters of cholesterol. Clinically, the syndrome is characterized by multiple round defects in the skull, exophthalmos, diabetes insipidus and some signs of infantilism. As no demonstrable disturbance or abnormality of cholesterol metabolism has been demonstrated, it seems likely that the collection of cholesterol in the histiocytes is not related to a generalized disturbance of cholesterol metabolism but is merely the local

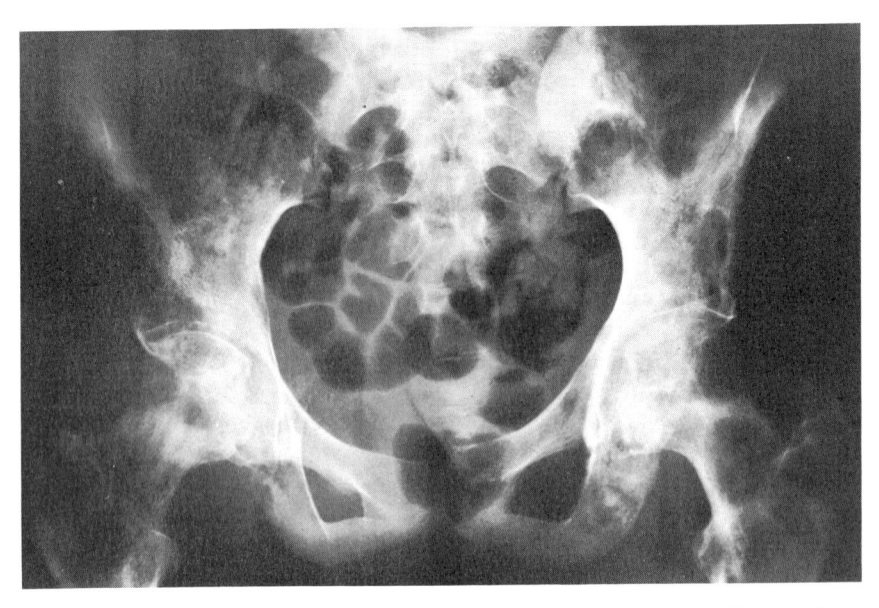

FIG. 53-10. The roentgenogram reveals multiple destruction areas in bone without new bone formation. A biopsy of one of these lesions was compatible with the diagnosis of Hand-Schüller-Christian disease.

collection of cholesterol by the granuloma cells (Fig. 53-10).

EOSINOPHILIC GRANULOMA

The eosinophilic granuloma of Jaffe and Lichtenstein (1940) seems to be closely related to the preceding 2 diseases. It occurs primarily in young persons and has not been seen in a patient over 45 years of age. Histologically, the eosinophilic granuloma is a mixture of histiocytes and eosinophils. The bone lesions are common in the skull, the pelvis, the ribs, the vertebrae, the humerus and the femur and are more common in the diaphysis than the metaphyseal or epiphyseal regions (Fig. 53-11). Although the majority of the osseous eosinophilic granulomas are solitary, occasionally they are multiple. Green and Farber (1942) reported that in some eosinophilic granulomas as maturity of the individual is approached deposition of lipid materials occurs, and the eosinophils tend to disappear. However, Jaffe and Lichtenstein (1940) feel that the eosinophilic granuloma does not necessarily become a lipid granuloma before healing but may heal through simple resolution.

Mallory (1942) tentatively expressed the relationship between these 3 conditions to be as follows: (1) Letterer-Siwe disease usually occurs in infancy and early childhood and is rapidly fatal. The histiocytic proliferations are widely scattered throughout the soft tissue, especially the lymphoid tissue and the skull. (2) Hand-Schüller-Christian's disease occurs in both children and adults and is more chronic in character. The histiocytic lesions undergo lipidization in about one third of the patients. The prognosis is grave because of damage to heart, lungs, brain and the pituitary gland. (3) Eosinophilic granuloma occurs in children and young adults. It is comparatively benign and is largely localized in the skeleton and usually to only one bone, although rarely the lesions are multiple. As a rule it heals readily after curetting with or without x-ray therapy. According to McGavran and Spady (1960) these lesions all heal regardless of treatment.

GAUCHER'S DISEASE

This is also a disease of lipid metabolism. The histiocytes and the reticular cells in the spleen, the liver and the bone marrow become filled with a gluco-galactoside kerasin. Kerasin contains nitrogen but no phosphorus. It is

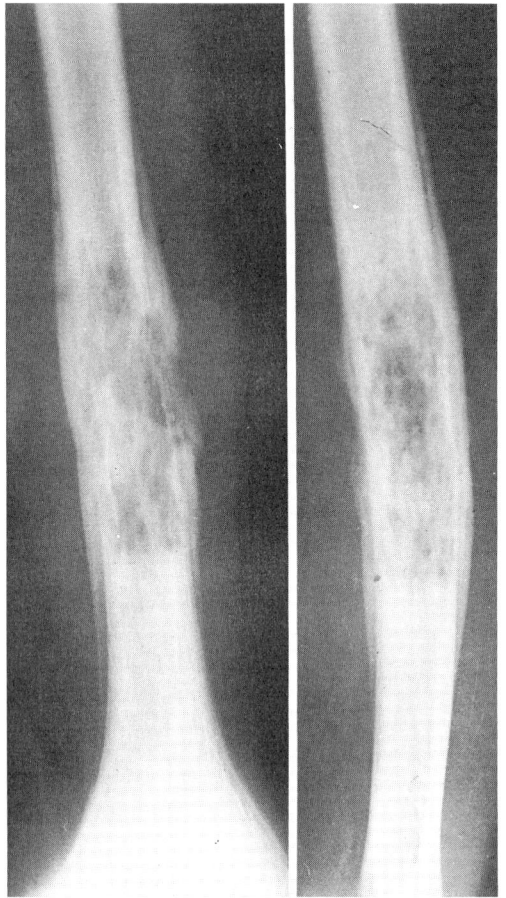

Inborn Errors of Metabolism 1679

FIG. 53-11. (*Right*) This teen-aged boy presented himself with pain and swelling of the arm of about 6-weeks' duration. Examination revealed a hard, brawny, tender enlargement of the arm with marked increase in local heat. The roentgenogram revealed a mottled, irregular area of bone destruction in the shaft of the humerus at the middle and the lower thirds with periosteal new bone formation. This, plus fever and leukocytosis suggested a clinical diagnosis of Ewing's sarcoma. However, the microscopical picture (*below*) was that of eosinophilic granuloma. Unfortunately, the eosinophils do not show without color.

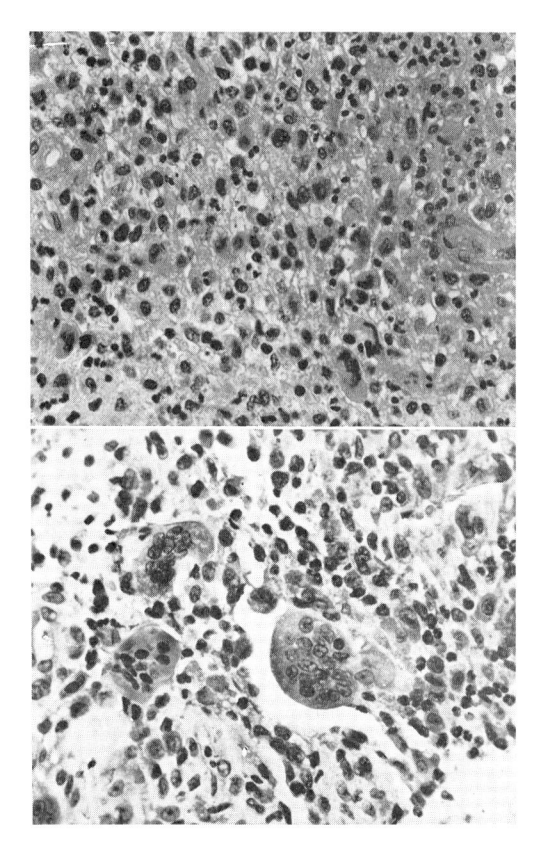

nant. The bone lesions may be widespread; the lower end of the femur is a common site. The roentgenogram presents a mottled motheaten appearance with little evidence of new bone formation. The articular cartilage is not invaded by the Gaucher cells, although aseptic necrosis and crumbling of the epiphysis or articular surface may occur. As the bone marrow contains a large number of the Gaucher cells, sternal puncture is effective in establishing a diagnosis. Splenectomy often helps the anemia and thrombocytopenia.

chemically inactive and is not stainable with the usual lipid stains. However, it can be stained with Mallory's aniline blue orange G stain. Gaucher's disease is characterized by progressive hepatic and splenic enlargement, starting early in life. Anemia, leukopenia and thrombocytopenia are frequently observed. The disease is usually familial (Snapper, 1949). The inheritance is autosomal domi-

NIEMANN-PICK DISEASE

This is a rather rare, strongly familial disease characterized by the collection of abnormal deposits of phospholipids and cholesterol in the reticuloendothelial tissues with a seeming predilection for the Jewish people. The predominant lipid is sphingomyelin, with some lethicin. The disease occurs most frequently in infants of less than 18 months and runs a short course; it is usually fatal within a year of onset. The reticulum of the bone marrow is always involved; however, a diffuse osteoporosis may be the only manifestation of bone involvement. The cherry-red spot on the macula may be present. There is no known effective treatment.

Tay-Sachs disease (amaurotic familial idiocy) is frequently associated with Niemann-Pick disease. Analysis has shown a predominance of lecithin rather than sphingomyelin in the nerve tissue. When the brain is involved, both the cherry-red macula and mental deterioration are to be expected. The mode of inheritance is autosomal recessive. Usually, the child is blind and regresses to complete idiocy. Death usually occurs by three years of age. There is no known treatment.

Skin-fibroblast cultures can be used for both genetic and metabolic studies of human inborn errors of metabolism. Cellular metachromasia has been used to detect cellular abnormalities in skin fibroblasts in the genetic mucopolysaccharidises, Gaucher's disease and, recently, in juvenile amaurotic familial idiocy (Spielmeyer-Vogt disease) (Danes and Bearn, 1968).

DEVELOPMENTAL ABNORMALITIES

Introduction

The term "congenital abnormality" cannot be applied strictly to the broad group of pathologic changes that are manifest as aberrations of normal development of the early growing individual. Although the majority of these abnormalities are present at birth (congenital), some of them may be incipient at the time of birth and become increasingly manifest with postnatal growth and development.

The pathogenesis of developmental abnormalities is incompletely understood, although several different factors appear to be important and may be divided into 2 groups: extrinsic and intrinsic. Congenital furrows and bands as well as some congenital amputations have been thought to be due to amniotic adhesions and are examples of extrinsic influences on the developing fetus, such as the drug thalidomide. Faulty intra-uterine position is undoubtedly important in some cases.

Intrinsic factors such as primary germ plasm variation, with and without hereditary linkage, must be considered. Experimentally, various degrees and types of abnormalities may be produced by environmental alterations applied to the embryo and the fetus. These include mechanical, thermal and x-ray injury, maternal nutritional deficiencies, maternal infections, metabolic and hormonal disorders, and drugs. Duraiswami (1952) has published an excellent review on this subject, including brilliant experimental studies. The different malformations that have been recorded are too numerous to be described here, and only those more commonly encountered and of orthopedic significance will be considered.

Congenital Dysplasia and Dislocation of the Hip

If congenital dysplasia and dislocation of the hip are diagnosed and treated in infancy, results will be satisfactory in greater than 90 per cent of cases. Without early treatment, a high percentage of patients will develop premature disabling degenerative arthritis of the hip.

Etiology and Pathogenesis

Experimental studies suggest, but do not prove, that dislocation may originate in utero, at birth, or during the first month of life (Ponseti, 1966). The underlying abnormality may be ligamentous laxity of the hip joint capsule, possibly resulting from hormonal effects. Various forces, particularly adduction and extension, may dislocate such a hip. These forces could be produced by intra-uterine position, breach presentation, or postnatal positions that maintain the hip in extension and adduction (Salter, 1968). Acetabular dysplasia and other abnormalities may occur secondary to dislocation. Some authorities, however, feel that dysplasia may be a separate entity that is a precursor to subluxation and dislocation (Coleman, 1965; McCarroll, 1965). Subluxation is a less severe degree of dysplasia in which the femoral head is in an abnormal position, but not dislocated.

Incidence

Congenital dislocation has been estimated to occur in from one to three infants per 1,000 live births (Salter, 1968; Weissman, 1966). The condition occurs in females in 85

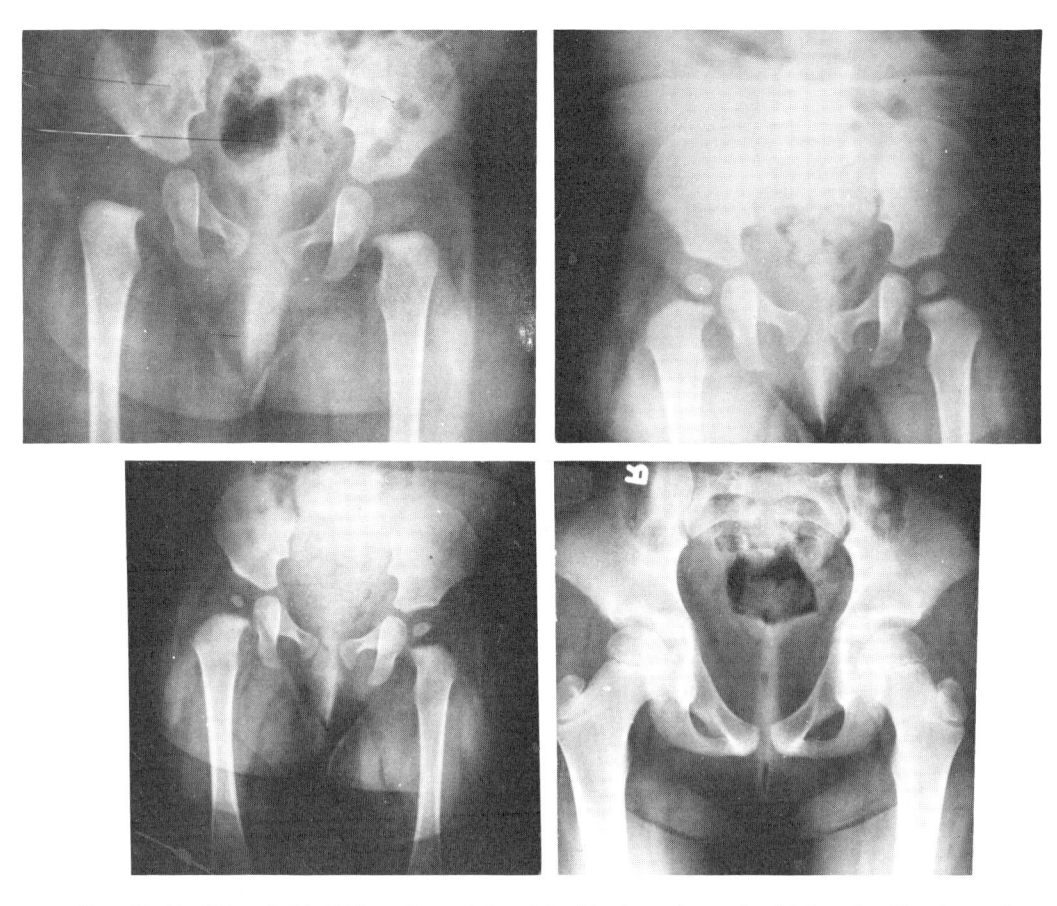

Fig. 53-12. (*Top, left*) Dislocation of the right hip in a 5-month old female. The femoral head, which has not yet developed an ossification center, lies superior and lateral to the normal contralateral hip. The acetabulum is shallow. (*Bottom, left*) The same patient 3 months after closed reduction and maintenance of reduction with a bilateral hip spica cast. The femoral head is in a normal position, but its ossification center is delayed. The acetabulum is still shallow. (*Top, right*) Same patient, age 11 months, after 6 months of treatment. Ossification is still delayed, but the slope of the acetabulum is normal. Cast treatment discontinued. (*Bottom, right*) Same patient, age 7 years. The hip is normal radiographically and by physical examination. (From Dr. H. R. McCarroll, St. Louis, Mo.)

per cent of cases, and is unilateral in 75 per cent. Incidence is higher in winter and among Northern Italians, North American Indians, West Germans, and Northern Scandinavians, and ten times higher than the average in breech presentations. Hip dislocation is rare in the Negro. There is a genetic factor in its distribution, but the mode of inheritance is unclear.

Signs and Symptoms

In children under age one (not walking) the earliest physical findings are: (1) manual displaceability of the hip and (2) limitation of abduction. If the hip is completely dislocated, there may be (3) deepening or an increase in the number of skin creases of the thigh or buttock, (4) shortening of the involved extremity, and (5) telescoping of the femur. The last-mentioned sign is demonstrated by a pistonlike mobility of the femur that attends the pushing and pulling of the thigh while the pelvis is fixed by a hand. This is done with the child supine and the hip and the knee flexed to 90°. An additional finding in a subluxatable or relocatable hip may be (6) the Ortolani Sign, a palpable click that is heard or felt during abduction of the hip.

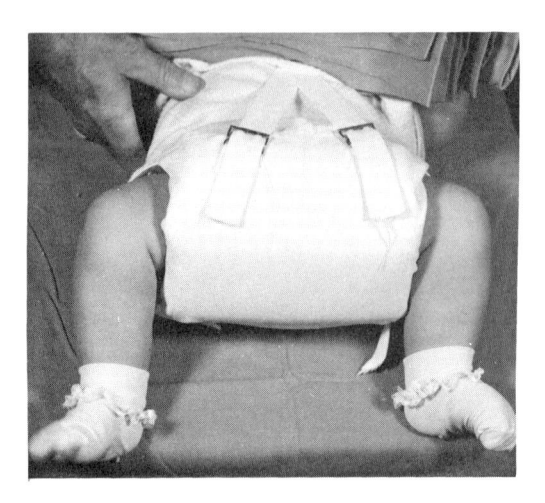

FIG. 53-13. Pillow splint (Frejka type) used to maintain the "frog-leg" position in a young infant with a subluxating or dislocatable hip. If the femoral heads can be maintained in the reduced position, normal acetabular development can proceed. (From Dr. H. R. McCarroll, St. Louis, Mo.)

This click occurs as the femoral head slips over the posterior rim of the acetabulum, the so-called "click of entry."

In the child over age one, the same signs are present but they are more obvious and the child demonstrates a waddling gait.

Dislocation

Diagnosis of Dislocation. Presence, or suspicion of the presence, of any of the signs described above should lead to a careful x-ray examination. The x-ray signs are: (1) delayed ossification of both femoral and acetabular components of the hip joint; (2) increased obliquity of the angle made by the roof of the acetabulum with the horizontal line drawn through the "Y" cartilages (Fig. 53-12) in an infant the upper limit of normal is 28° to 30°; (3) dislocation of the developing head of the femur if the epiphysis is present or of the proximal femoral shaft if the epiphysis is not present; (4) increased antiversion of the neck of the femur, demonstrated by comparing (a) an anteroposterior view of the pelvis with the hip in neutral position (knee pointing to the ceiling) and (b) with the hip held in forced internal rotation. If abnormally antiverted the hip will appear to have a valgus deformity in neutral position but will appear normal when forcibly internally rotated.

Pathology of Dislocation. The characteristic abnormalities of a complete dislocation include: elongation of the joint capsule which may be associated with an hourglass constriction of the capsule located between the head of the femur and the acetabulum; a shallow acetabulum; a groove on the superior acetabular rim secondary to pressure from the head of the femur; the filling of the acetabular fossa with the inverted fibrocartilaginous rim attached to the superior rim of the acetabulum (the so-called *limbus*) and the filling of the deep acetabular fossa with fibrous tissue representing a hypertrophied "haversian gland" (Somerville, 1953). Secondary contracture of the joint capsule, muscles, nerves and vessels also occurs. The femoral neck is antiverted.

Treatment. The treatment of congenital dislocation of the hip is a disputed subject, but general principles can be presented (Crego, 1948; McCarroll, 1948; 1965; Ryder, 1966). In a child less than one year of age a gentle closed reduction under general anesthesia should be attempted. Preliminary traction may be helpful to relax tight structures. Forceful reduction may damage the femoral capital epiphysis. Occasionally, a subcutaneous release of tight adductor or superficial flexor muscles is necessary to allow reduction. After the hip is reduced, the child is placed in a spica cast in the most stable hip position, which is usually one of flexion, abduction, and external rotation (the "frog-leg" position). With serial cast changes, the hips are gradually brought into the position of abduction, extension, and internal rotation over a period of from 6 to 9 months. Occasionally, a night abduction brace is subsequently used.

In young infants whose hips are easily relocatable, a small pad or pillow splint placed between the legs to maintain abduction is usually successful, and therefore, casts may not be needed (Fig. 53-13). This is especially true for the newborn where contractures have not developed.

The Dysplastic Hip

Signs and Symptoms of the Dysplastic Hip. This diagnosis depends a great deal on

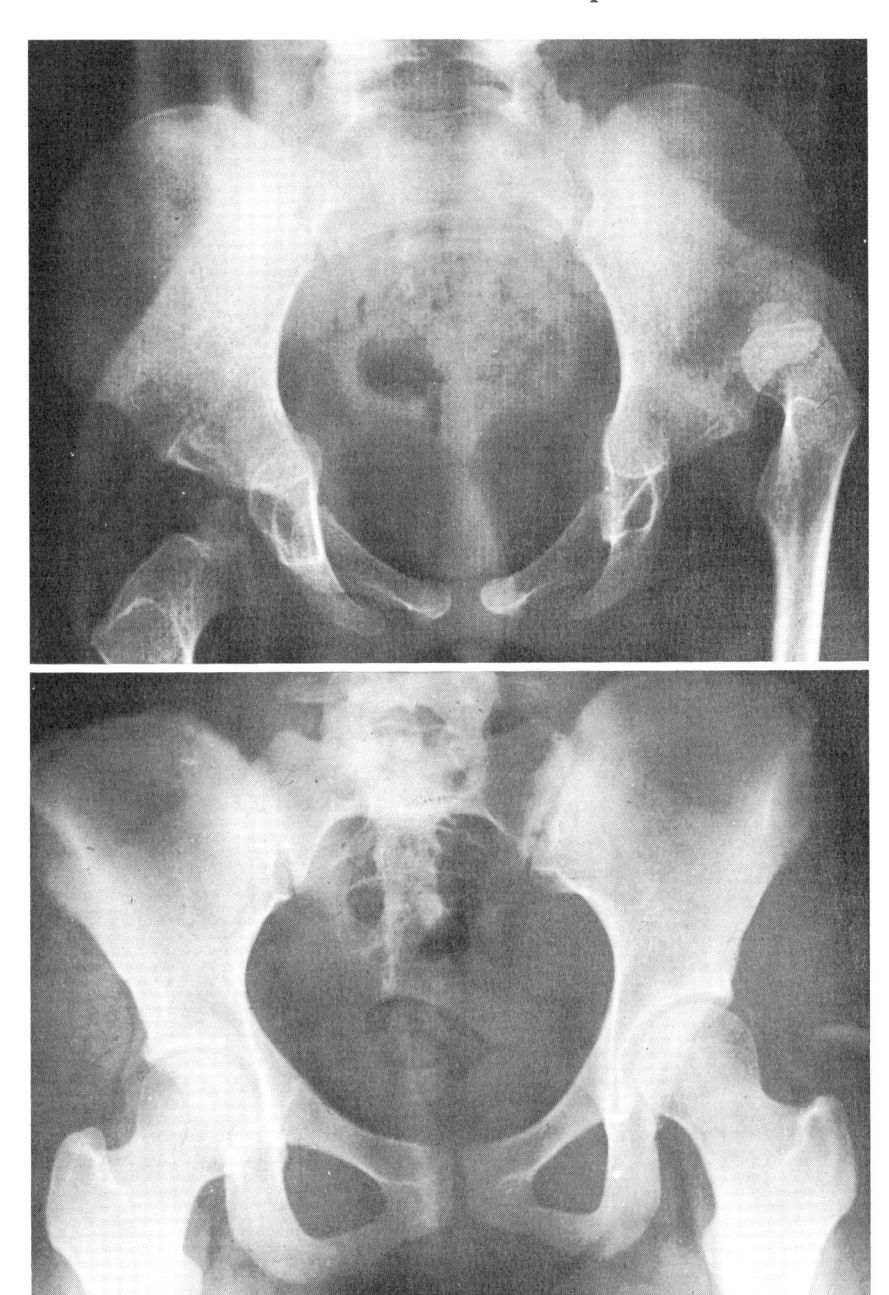

Fig. 53-14. (*Top*) Appearance of a typical congenital dislocation of the hip in an older child prior to treatment. (*Bottom*) Same patient. A very satisfactory result 14 years after adequate treatment. (From Shriner's Hospital, St. Louis, Mo.)

intuition. The detection of slight limitation of abduction or a little instability of the child's hip when the telescoping test is performed may be the main tips. A family history of congenital dislocation of the hip or another congenital anomaly such as club feet should make one at least suspicious that a dysplasia may exist. If a subluxation is present the Ortolani sign may be positive, and an extra skin fold may be present. Instability of the

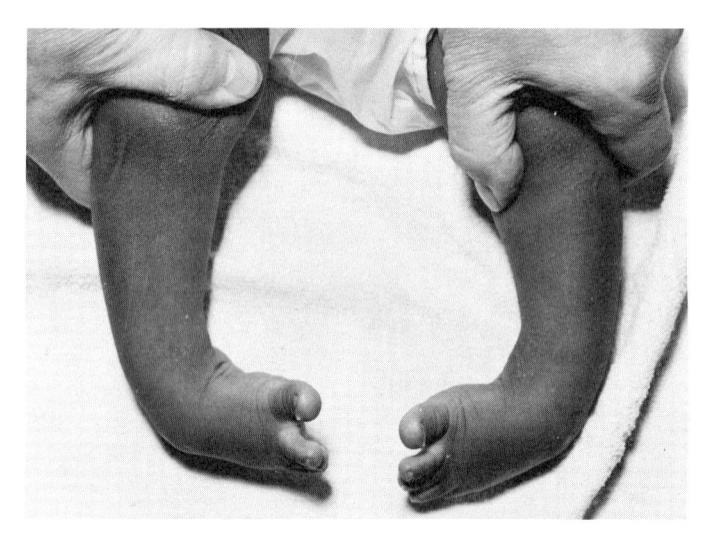

FIG. 53-15. Bilateral talipes equinovarus (clubfeet) in an infant prior to any cast correction. The photographs demonstrate the 3 components of the deformity: (*Top*) Forefoot varus. (*Center*) Hindfoot varus. (*Bottom*) Equinus.

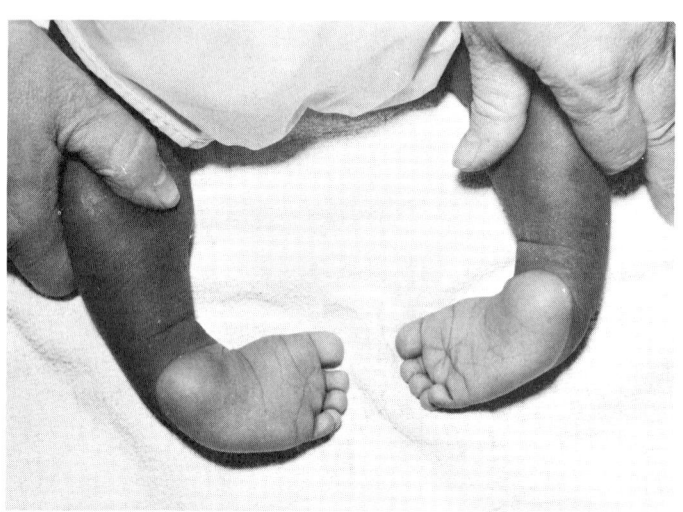

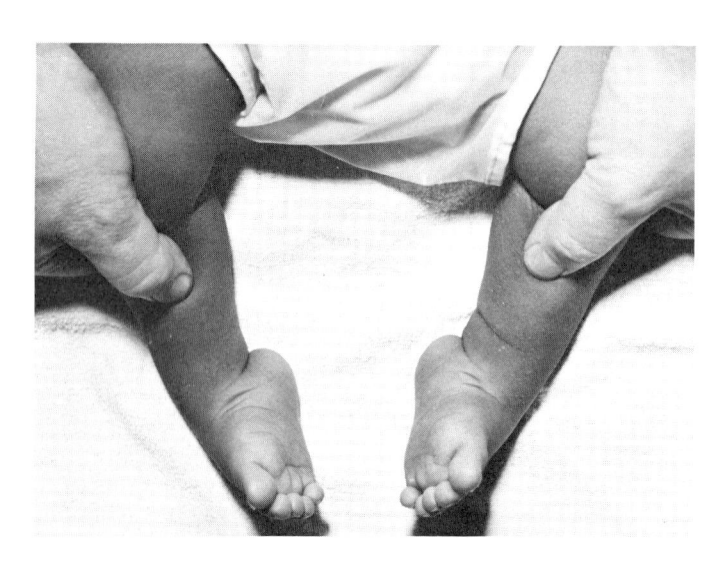

hip will be noted on the telescoping test, but the diagnosis will be made only by an examiner who is looking for or thinking about a dislocation of the hip.

Diagnosis. The diagnosis rests upon the roentgenographic detection of (1) delayed ossification; (2) a shallow acetabulum; (3) and lateral displacement of the femoral epiphysis.

Treatment of the Dysplastic and Subluxated Hip. One may maintain constant reduction of the hip while at the same time permitting active motion of the extremity by applying a Frejka pillow splint. This consists of a firm pillow placed between the knees and holding the legs in a "frog-leg" position. The Ilfeld splint (Ilfeld, 1957) is as effective, but with it excessive pressure may be placed on the epiphysis by the forcible abduction. In those children who cannot be controlled in a pillow splint, a plaster cast may be necessary. Usually, from 3 to 6 months of fixation of the thigh by one means or another will permit the acetabulum to develop and thereby cure the affliction if the apparatus be applied early in life.

Equinovarus Clubfoot

There are several forms of clubfoot, of which the equinovarus form (talipes equinovarus) is the most common. This condition has three separate components of deformity: adduction of the forefoot in relation to the hindfoot, varus of the entire foot, primarily of the subtalar joint, and equinus of the foot with contracture of the heel cord (Fig. 53-15, A, B, C). Internal torsion of the tibia is frequently associated.

Etiology. The cause in most cases is unknown, but it is probably related to contracture of muscle or tendon units. This may be a result of abnormal muscle or tendon development, congenital neurogenic defects, or deformities resulting from abnormal intrauterine position or amniotic bands. Clubfoot may also be a result of congenital abnormalities, such as arthrogryposis (Alberman, 1965; Hersh, 1917) or abnormal cartilaginous anlage of the foot. Distribution of some cases shows a definite genetic influence, and this disorder can be inherited as an autosomal dominant with variable penetrance (Palmer, 1964; Wynne Davies, 1964).

Pathology. Dissections of stillborn infants with clubfeet have revealed varied deformities. Irani and Sherman (1963) reported abnormalities in the cartilaginous anlage of the anterior talus and calcaneus. Attenborough (1966) described small and shortened muscle bellies. There may also be abnormal muscle insertions and tendon sheaths.

Prognosis. Usually at birth there is no bony deformity and, if the condition is corrected

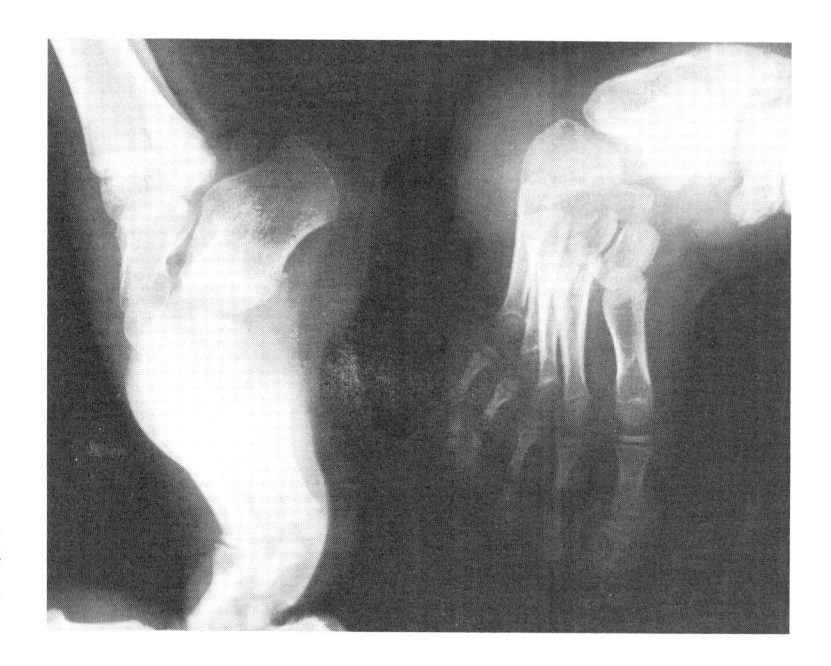

Fig. 53-16. Typical x-ray appearance of uncorrected clubfoot in an older child.

properly, an essentially normal foot can be obtained. If neglected, the deformity becomes worse and more resistant to correction and actual bony deformity develops consequent to abnormal function (Fig. 53-16).

Diagnosis. Diagnosis is made by inspection of the attitude of the feet and by testing the range of active and passive movement. (See Fig. 53-15). Radiographic evidence of forefoot and hindfoot varus and equinus is also diagnostic.

Treatment. Ideally, treatment should begin as soon as the diagnosis is made. If proper management is instituted in the first few days of life, not only is correction more certain but the surgeon's task is easier.

CONSERVATIVE. The method of choice in most of these cases is the use of wedging plaster casts, as described by Kite (1935, 1939, 1963). A plaster boot is used to hold and, by wedging, to correct gradually the three components of the deformity. It is of utmost importance to correct the adduction and the varus before starting to correct the equinus. The casts are usually wedged or changed at intervals of 1 week. Correction is obtained when the foot is in a position representing the normal extent of passive abduction, valgus and dorsiflexion. Depending on the extent and flexibility of the deformity, correction usually can be obtained in from a few weeks to 3 or 4 months. Once full correction is obtained (see Fig. 53-17, *right*) a final cast is used to hold this position for 4 to 6 weeks. In the very mild cases, correction may be obtained by frequent daily passive stretching of the contracted soft parts by the mother. Such manipulation usually is done after plaster correction to restrain the tendency to recurrence. Other forms of nonoperative treatment include the Dennis-Browne splint, with various modifications, and adhesive strapping and these have their advocates.

SURGICAL. Surgery is indicated when a resistant or recurrent clubfoot (Fig. 53-17, *left*) fails to respond to conservative measures (Hersh, 1917). Persistent equinus in an infant may respond to a heel cord tenotomy (Ponseti, 1963), whereas older children may require a posterior capsulotomy, heel cord lengthening or, sometimes, a radical release of all tight structures. Persistent forefoot and hindfoot deformities may require capsulotomy (Heyman, 1959), osteomotomies or removal of wedges of bone. Recurrent deformities are often due to muscle imbalance and may respond to transfer of the tibialis anterior (Garceau, 1967) or the tibialis posterior tendon (Fig. 53-17, *right*) (Gartland, 1964). In older children in whom deformity persists, a triple arthrodesis is often indicated.

METATARSUS ADDUCTUS

A more commonly encountered anomaly of the foot is a metatarsus adductus which is frequently and incorrectly called metatarsus varus. In this condition the forefoot is turned medialward in relation to the hindfoot. This deformity usually is associated with some degree of internal tibial torsion. The forefoot adduction responds well to plaster cast correction if done in the first year, and the tibial torsion will be corrected spontaneously if not too marked or may require the use of some type of splint to hold the extremity in full external rotation during the sleeping hours. A variety of satisfactory appliances which attach to shoes are available for this purpose.

FLATFOOT

So-called "flatfoot" will be considered here, although many cases are in no way true developmental abnormalities. The development of longitudinal and transverse arches usually is delayed until the child has walked for a sufficient time to permit the muscles supporting these arches to develop in strength. It is quite common to see flatfeet in children who have just started to walk and to have this deformity disappear in a few weeks or months. This tendency to flatfeet may be accentuated by obesity, serious illness or malnutrition. These forms of flatfeet in small children require only a good corrective shoe and time to permit attainment of a foot normal in function and appearance.

There is a hereditary form of flatfoot that has a strong racial preponderance (Negro) that is not influenced by treatment. Fortunately, these individuals usually do not have significant disability.

There is an extreme degree of flatfoot produced by an anomaly of the talus in which the head of this bone is directed into the plantar aspect of the foot instead of forward toward the forefoot. This usually is disabling and can

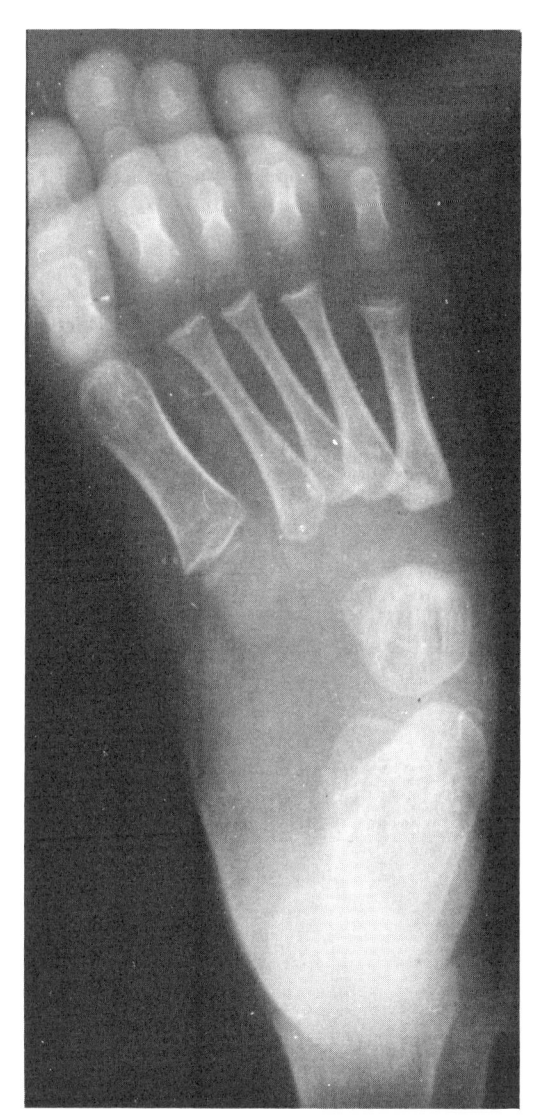

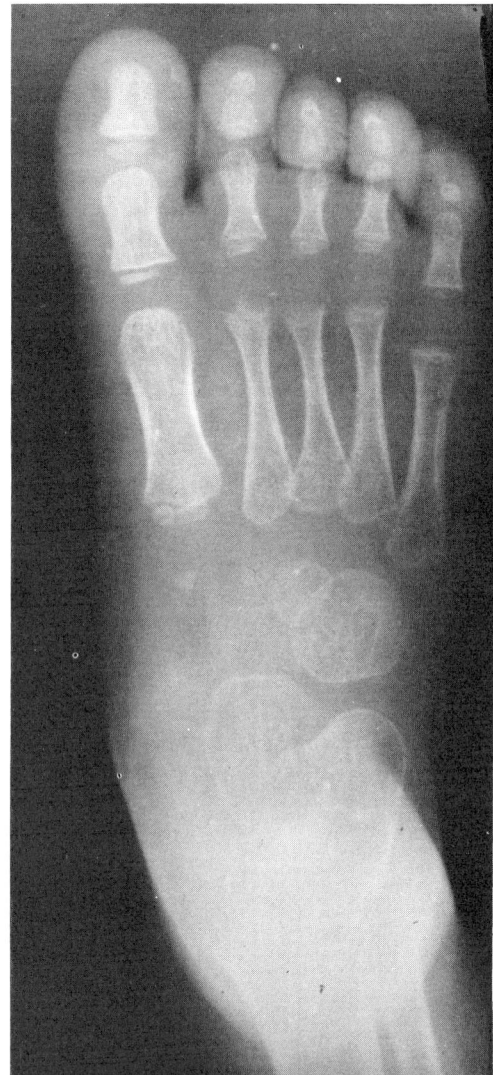

FIG. 53-17. (*Left*) Clubfoot in a 3-year-old boy, which recurred after complete correction. The recurrence was believed to be due to muscle imbalance. Note the varus of the forefoot and hindfoot. (*Right*) Same patient 3 months after weekly corrective cast changes. There is nearly complete correction. Transfer of the tibialis anterior tendon to the lateral tarsus was performed to prevent recurrence.

be corrected only by stabilization of the foot. This has been called a *"diving duck" talus* or vertical talus because of its x-ray appearance.

The so-called *spastic flatfoot* (Silk, 1968), is considered to be the result of altered subtalar function with or without anomalous bars is not common in children. Frequently, it may be treated adequately by manipulation and cast.

A common cause of painful spastic flatfoot is talocalcaneal and/or calcaneonavicular bars, either bony or cartilaginous (Fig. 53-18). When fibrous or cartilaginous it may be impossible to establish the diagnosis prior to sur-

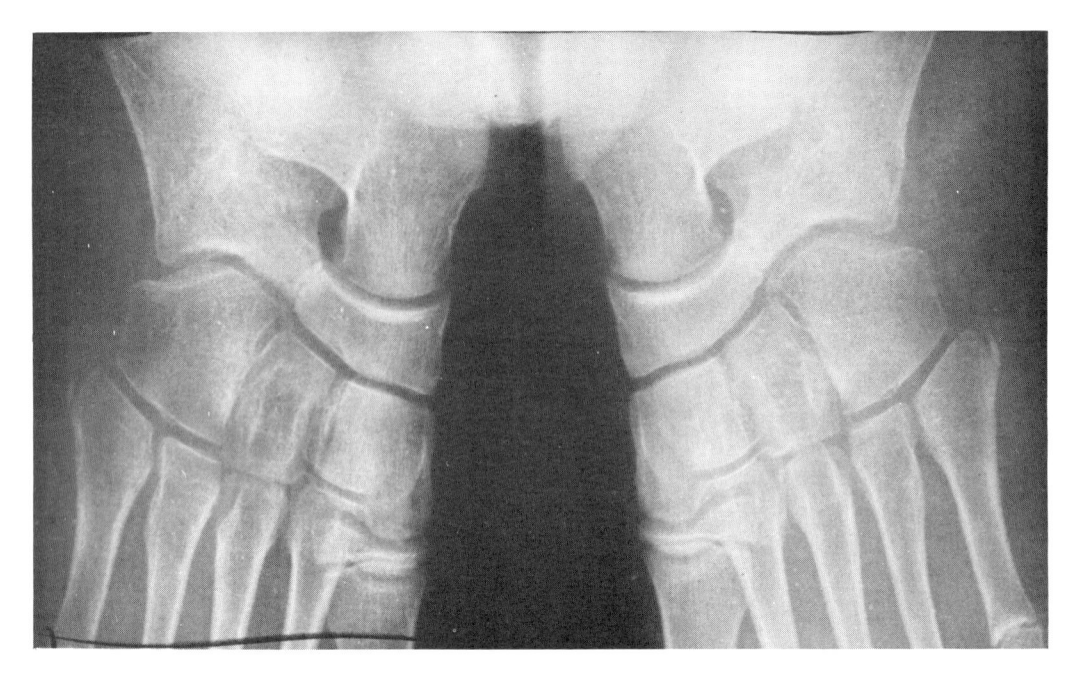

Fig. 53-18. Bilateral incomplete calcaneonavicular coalition in a 12-year-old male whose sister had a similar abnormality.

gery. When bony there is no difficulty in making the diagnosis, provided that oblique roentgenograms are obtained.

Treatment may require triple arthrodesis as recommended by Harris and Beath (1947). We prefer to resect the bar, particularly in young children. Resection has been successful in over half the cases, arthrodesis being reserved for those not relieved.

Developmental Abnormalities of the Hand and the Forearm

Only the more common abnormalities will be mentioned.

Syndactylism, or webbing of the fingers, is most frequent in this group (see Chap. 24, Principles of Hand Surgery).

Congenital absence of tendons may occur in any muscle but more frequently affects the common extensors of the fingers and results in a flexion deformity. Tendon transpositions or grafts may be useful to restore function.

The so-called "thumb clutched hand" is one of the common thumb deformities of the newborn infant. The thumb is held in the acutely flexed position and may be due to either a stenosis of the flexor tendon sheath at the metacarpophalangeal joint or a congenital absence of the extensor pollicis brevis tendon. Section of the flexor tendon sheath may be necessary in the former condition, and tendon transfer in the latter situation.

Congenital absence of digits or whole finger rays is encountered and present problems of surgical closure of clefts, pollicization of fingers when the thumb is absent, and other plastic procedures (see Chap. 24).

Congenital absence (partial or total) of the radius is seen occasionally and produces a "club hand" in which the hand is fixed in radial deviation and the thumb may be absent or deformed. The function in these extremities is sometimes surprisingly good, and the surgeon should be particularly careful not to do anything to give it a better cosmetic appearance at the expense of function.

In congenital absence of the radius or the ulna a severe bowing of the forearm may result and require operative correction. The absent bone usually has a fibrous band in its place. The failure of the fibrous band to grow at the rate of the bone present results in severe curving. The student is referred to Riordan (1959) for a discussion of the surgical management of

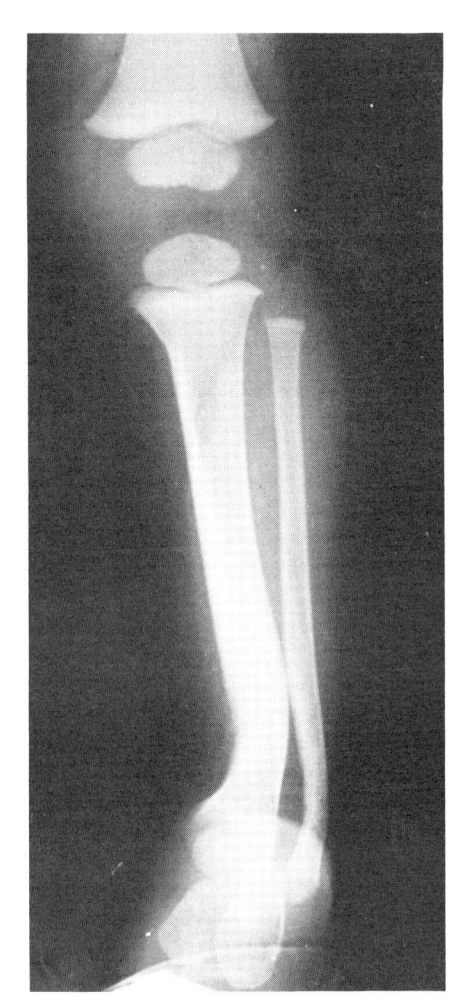

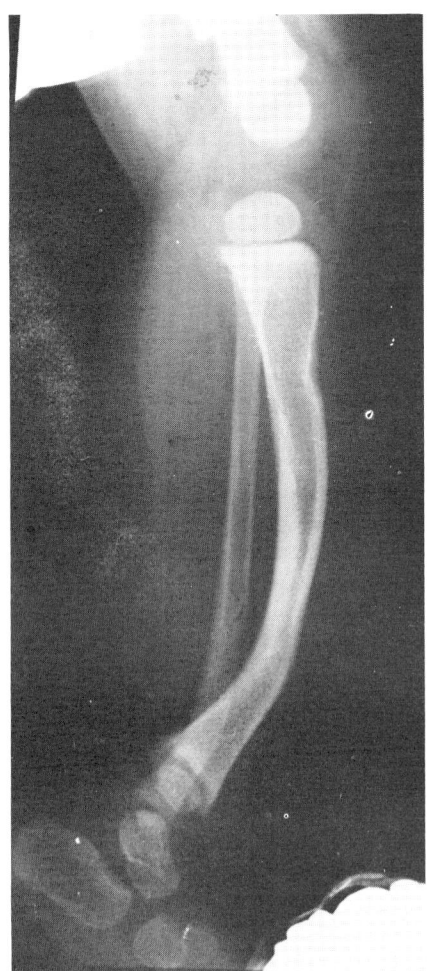

Fig. 53-19. Pseudoarthrosis of the tibia. There is marked anterior bowing of the tibia. The cortex is sclerotic and the medullary canal is narrow. This stage is often termed a "pre-pseudoarthrosis." Fracture in the area of the bow will likely result in nonunion. Bracing and/or posterior bone graft is the treatment of choice.

these problems. Stretching of the soft tissue contracture by plaster casts as soon after birth as possible is indicated. Later surgical release of contracted bands, repositioning of the carpus and a bone graft to replace the missing radius are steps that have been used to improve the deformity. Riordan advocates early operation (about 6 months). Relocation of the carpus on the ulna is done early with the end result being a single-bone forearm.

Congenital fusion of carpal bones usually is nondisabling and requires no treatment.

Congenital amputation of part or all of one or more extremities is seen and presents a problem of prosthesis-fitting and stump-revision. The use of a prosthesis in the young child of 2 or 3 is worthwhile. The prosthesis is used as a helping hand surprisingly well.

Congenital Polydactylism. An additional number of partial or complete digits may be present on the hands or the feet. Such deformities are usually bilaterally symmetrical and often appear in several members of the same family. Removal of the extra digit is indicated only after the surgeon has ascertained which digit is the abnormal one.

Congenital pseudarthrosis of the tibia and the fibula with marked deformity has been a particularly difficult surgical problem for years, with a high incidence of failure of bone grafting. Reports indicate that excision of the entire area of pseudarthrosis scar prior to bone graft and internal fixation improves the chance of success (Fig. 53-19). However, after multiple attempts have failed, one may of necessity resort to the Symes amputation (van Nes, 1966).

There are many generalized afflictions of bone that are presumed to be developmental anomalies. They are rare and usually are not amenable to surgical attack; the student is referred to Fairbank's (1952) treatise for detailed description of this interesting group of afflictions.

Congenital Absence (Partial or Total) of the Fibula. The fibula is the long bone most commonly congenitally absent, followed in order of frequency by the radius, the femur, the tibia, the ulna, and the humerus (Coventry, 1959). This syndrome in its classic form consists of: (1) complete or partial absence of the fibula; (2) congenital shortening of the extremity; (3) anterior bowing of the middle and lower parts of the fibula, and (4) deformity of the foot (plano-valgus or equino-valgus position of the foot, and complete or partial dislocation of the talo-tibial joint, associated with the absence of the lateral malleolus).

The deformity increases with age, secondary to a fibrous replacement of the fibula, shortened peroneal muscles and lateral transposition of the extensor tendons of the foot (Serafin, 1967).

Various procedures have been attempted with very limited success. We now feel that the Symes amputation is the procedure of choice when severe shortening can be predicted and when a poorly formed foot cannot be maintained in weight-bearing position (Wood, 1965).

Congenital coxa vara, although rare, appears to be due to failure of development of the neck of the femur. When treated early with fixation of the neck and the capital epiphysis and the varus deformity corrected by a subtrochanteric osteotomy of the rotational type, very satisfactory hips can be obtained. Late cases with severe deformity and nonunion may be improved, but the end results are disappointing.

SLIPPING OF THE CAPITAL FEMORAL EPIPHYSIS

Incidence. A gradual displacement of the upper femoral epiphysis is a condition frequently encountered in adolescence. Most of the cases are seen between the ages of 12 and 14; however, the condition may be found in individuals varying from 8 to 19 years of age. It is commonly stated that this most frequently occurs in an individual who is overweight and has a body configuration similar to that which is associated with Fröhlich's syndrome. However, the condition not infrequently is seen also in the tall slender individual during a period of rapid growth. The incidence is slightly higher in males.

Etiology of the slipped capital femoral epiphysis remains unclear. However, it is probably related to excessive growth hormone (Wilson, 1965). Although trauma may be associated with an acute slipping of the epiphysis, more frequently the trauma that is related to the onset of symptoms is actually of a rather trivial nature. Endocrine imbalance also has been incriminated as an etiologic factor, particularly in those individuals who present the appearance of body habitus associated with Fröhlich's syndrome.

It is possible that rapid growth or hormonal imbalance may loosen the perichondrium, the attachment of the epiphysis. Shear stresses produced by low-grade forces, such as sitting, may produce slipping (Alexander, 1966). Negroes with this disorder were found to have a poorer prognosis than Caucasians, but the reason is unknown (Orofino, 1960).

It has been found that rats fed on a diet containing aminoproprionitrile, which may interfere with crosslinking of collagen, develop slipping of the epiphysis in the region of the

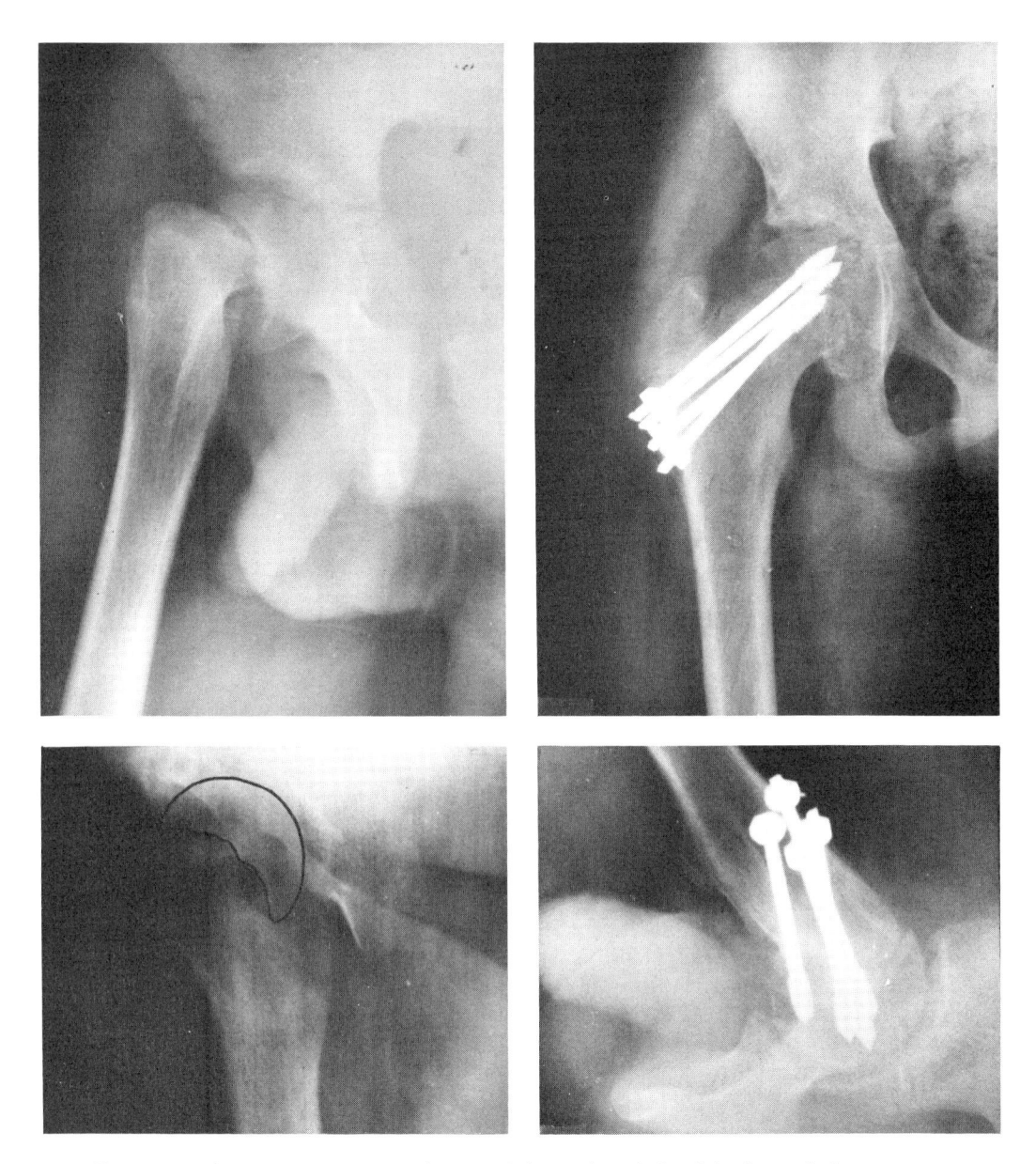

FIG. 53-20. (*Left, top and bottom*) Slipped femoral capital epiphysis, typical x-ray appearance. Note the inferior-posterior displacement of the femoral head, with demineralization of bone about the epiphyseal plate. The patient was a 14-year-old boy who had been limping for 7-8 weeks. (*Right, top and bottom*) Same hip, following reduction with skeletal traction and fixation with multiple threaded pins.

knees and the shoulder (Ponseti, 1954). In these animals it has been reported that there is a disintegration between the zone of proliferating cells and the calcified cartilage of the epiphysis. Slipping of the epiphysis occurred along this line of diminished resistance, with the periosteum being detached at the metaphysis.

Diagnosis of a slipped femoral epiphysis must be entertained in any adolescent who complains of either pain in the hip or is walking with a limp. It must always be remembered that the pain may be referred along the path of the obturator nerve, and not infrequently the chief complaint may be pain at the inner aspect of the knee. In the early stages—the so-called preslipping stage—physical examination may be essentially normal. However, as actual slipping of the epiphysis progresses, limitation of flexion and an external rotational deformity will become increasingly apparent. In cases that have gone unrecognized there may be thigh and calf atrophy on the affected side, and limitation of abduction is a common finding in the more acute phases.

X-ray examination of both hips in the anteroposterior and lateral views will almost always confirm the diagnosis. The early changes seen on the roentgenogram are a slight roughening and widening of the epiphyseal line of the affected side. When displacement occurs, the epiphysis displaces posteriorly and inferiorly. In the anteroposterior view the varus deformity is clearly evident (Fig. 53-20, *left, top*), but the posterior displacement is recognized most readily in the lateral view (Fig. 53-20, *left,* bottom).

Treatment. In the natural course of this disease, displacement is finally stabilized by solid bony fusion of the epiphysis, and the symptoms may subside until the onset of the traumatic arthritis, which may come years after the slipping has occurred. It is generally agreed that when the diagnosis has been established, operative fixation to prevent further slipping is the best treatment. This fixation is probably best accomplished by means of multiple threaded pins (Fig. 53-20, *right, top and bottom*). In older cases where the displacement has been more than one third the diameter of the neck of the femur, restoration of the anatomic relationships should be done. In such cases osteotomy of the femoral neck followed by internal fixation is often employed. However, the end results may be disappointing, for aseptic necrosis of the epiphysis or an early onset of degenerative arthritis not infrequently is a complication of this procedure. Separation through the epiphyseal plate, followed by repositioning of the epiphysis with internal fixation, may be the most successful method of management in severe displacement. Subtrochanteric osteotomy has been used successfully at times to correct the varus and rotational deformity and has the advantage of being less likely to produce an aseptic necrosis of the epiphysis (Southwick, 1967; Wilson et al., 1965). However, incongruity of the hip remains and degenerative arthritis may be expected in later life.

During the postoperative period weight-bearing of the affected side must be forbidden for 4 to 6 months or until bone has bridged the epiphysis. The opposite hip must be watched carefully, for in some series of cases it has been reported that as high as 40 per cent of individuals have developed slipping of the capital femoral epiphysis on the other side (Badgley et al., 1948; Ferguson, 1931; Klein et al., 1952; Speed, 1963).

OSTEOCHONDROSES

There is a group of localized bone afflictions that have been grouped together under this term because of a pathologic similarity. The common finding is avascular necrosis of bone that cannot be attributed to trauma. These cases occur almost entirely in children and adolescents, and there is accumulating evidence that disease of epiphyseal cartilage may precede the avascular necrosis; however, the etiology is undetermined. Avascular necrosis is characterized by the typical x-ray finding of a relative increased density of the necrotic part in the middle stages of the disease, because atrophy of disuse of the surrounding viable bone leads to demineralization, while the dead bone remains unchanged because of lack of blood supply.

Coxa Plana (Legg-Calvé-Perthes' Disease). The most important of these conditions, known variously as coxa plana, osteochondritis deformans juveniles or Legg-Perthes' disease, involves the capital femoral epiphysis. It is bilateral in approximately 10 per cent of cases. It was described independently around 1909-1910 by Calvé, Legg and Perthes, and by Waldenstrom (1936). The condition is more common in boys than in girls, usually beginning between the ages of 4 and 10 years. The initial sign is a slightly painful limp which becomes worse with activity; the pain is referred to hip, thigh or knee. There is usually a history of no trauma. Physical findings are limited to slight atrophy of the musculature of the involved side, slight limitation of the hip motions, particularly extension and abduction, and discomfort at the extremes of motion.

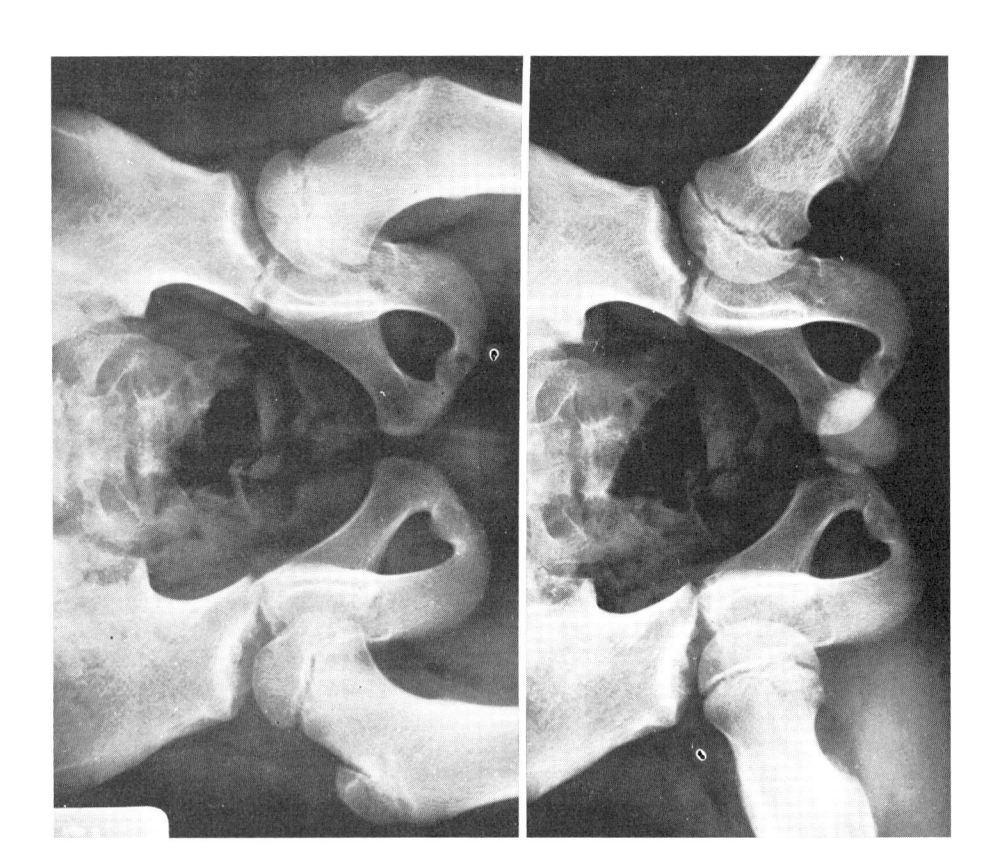

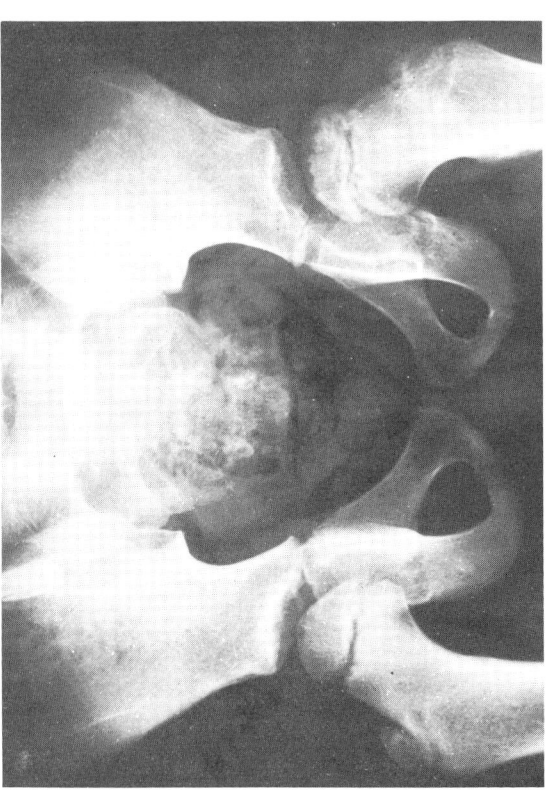

FIG. 53-21. (*Left*) Anteroposterior films of both hips of a 6-year-old child with moderately early changes in the left hip. (*Right*) Same case 18 months later, showing almost complete regeneration of the capital epiphysis.

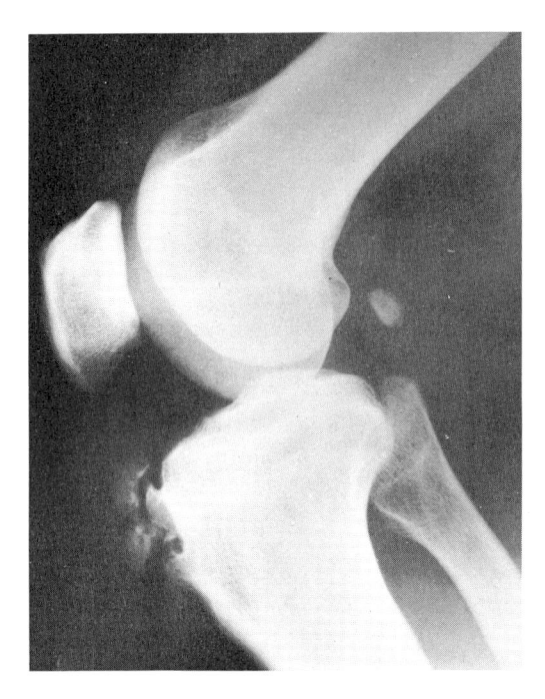

FIG. 53-22. Lateral roentgenogram of the knee in a 30-year-old white man who had Osgood-Schlatter's disease as a boy. Large fragments of the tibial tubercle failed to unite, and they remain as loose bodies. Pain eventually led to the removal of these loose pieces of bone. The pain disappeared after the loose pieces of bone were removed.

Rarely, there may be more acute pain and disability, but this will subside with rest.

The very early roentgenogram may show only slight decreased density of the upper metaphysis of the femur or only minimal changes in the epiphysis. Diagnosis at this stage may be quite difficult. Tuberculosis is the most common differential diagnostic condition. Later there is irregular sclerosis of the epiphysis leading to fragmentation (Fig. 53-21). The course of the disease may run from 2 to 4 or 5 years, which includes the time for onset of symptoms to eventual resorption of necrotic bone and replacement with new viable bone sufficient to support full, active weight-bearing.

This condition may occasionally be simulated by one of the epiphyseal dysplasias. An excellent classification of bone dysplasias is given by Rubin (1964).

We feel that some form of non-weight bearing during the active course of the disease will result in a better hip than would occur if unrestricted weight bearing were permitted (Harrison, M., and Menon, 1966; Stamp et al., 1964). The simplest way to institute non-weight bearing in a cooperative child is the use of crutches with a sling-strap holding the shoe or the ankle to the belt with the knee at 90°. An ischial weight-bearing brace may also be satisfactory at times. In the occasionally encountered bilateral case, bed rest at home with skin traction is advocated.

The use of abduction casts or braces has been recently advocated to contain the femoral head more completely within the acetabulum. Ambulation with the aid of crutches can be allowed with the use of these casts. Abduction cast has a great advantage in that it permits ambulation in cases with bilateral involvement when formerly these patients were confined to a bed or wheelchair. Long-term results of ambulatory treatment with abduction casts have not been completely evaluated and this method will require several years of follow-up before it is accepted as the best method of treatment.

Osgood-Schlatter's Disease. The next most important disease in this group is Osgood-Schlatter's disease. Clinically, there is a painful enlargement of the tibial tubercle in an adolescent, usually a male, and the symptom is aggravated by physical activity and relieved by rest. A roentgenogram may show a variety of types of fragmentation of the epiphysis of the tuberosity and frequently will show some separation of the epiphysis from the shaft, due, apparently, to the pull of the patellar tendon. The majority of cases do well with rest and protection and do not have any permanent sequelae, except for enlargement of the tibial tubercle. Surgical intervention during the early stages is absolutely unwarranted in our opinion. Occasionally, fragmentation is such that all the fragments do not solidify with healing so that a detached piece of bone remains. This may be painful on kneeling. Simple excision at this stage relieves the pain (Fig. 53-22). Rarely, the enlargement is such that it is unsightly in the female, and excision for cosmetic reasons is worthwhile.

There are several other conditions having localized bone necrosis that may or may not be etiologically similar to Legg-Perthes' and

Osgood-Schlatter's disease. They are less common, less serious and usually self-limiting, responding to conservative treatment. They are commonly referred to by the names of men responsible for their early description and are so listed here:

Avascular necrosis of secondary ossification center of os calcis (Sever and Haglund)

Avascular necrosis, tarsal scaphoid (Köhler)

Avascular necrosis, carpal lunate (Kienböck)

Avascular necrosis of second metatarsal head (Freiberg's infraction)

Epiphysitis of vertebrae (Scheuermann)

Avascular necrosis of patella (Sinding-Larsen; Johannson; Köhler)

Avascular necrosis of capitellum humeri (Panner)

Avascular necrosis with collapse of vertebra (Vertebra plana; Calvé's disease). Recently eosinophilic granuloma has been noted as an etiologic factor; this may not be an avascular necrosis (Compere et al., 1954).

ORTHOPEDIC TREATMENT OF PARALYTIC DISORDERS

In former years, the majority of paralytic disorders treated by the orthopedic surgeon were the result of poliomyelitis. It appears that new cases of poliomyelitis are being almost entirely prevented with the use of the vaccine. However, there is a tremendous reservoir of paralytic cases that will require orthopedic attention for many years. Many of the same principles involved in the management of the paralytic residua of poliomyelitis are today used to treat the musculoskeletal abnormalities in patients with spina bifida, cerebral palsy, muscle disease, spinal cord injury, cerebral vascular disease, and miscellaneous neurologic diseases. The orthopedist should begin his management as early as possible and end only when the maximum degree of rehabilitation has been accomplished. The following paragraphs, written for the management of poliomyelitis are still quite applicable to the many types of paralytic disorders seen by orthopedic surgeon.

APPLIANCES

Mention should be made of the use of various appliances such as braces, splints and corsets. Their use serves 2 primary purposes: (1) prevention of deformity by holding the part in the functional position and (2) permitting functional use of a part that otherwise would be useless because of paralysis and instability. For example, a patient with complete paralysis of the quadriceps and the peroneal muscles in one lower extremity might be unable to bear full weight on the leg because the knee would buckle and give way and probably would develop a varus deformity of the foot. A long leg brace with a knee-lock would permit full weight-bearing, and the proper shoe attachment to the brace would tend to prevent the foot deformity.

OPERATIVE PROCEDURES

The operative procedures may be properly divided into those on the upper and those on the lower extremities, on the basis that the aims differ in respect to these members. In the upper extremity the primary concern is either directly to improve hand function or to improve arm function so that the hand may be better used. In the lower extremity, we are concerned with weight-bearing, stability and ambulation. With these aims in mind we can better understand the purpose of some of the procedures.

Upper Extremity. In the upper extremity any procedure must be considered in the light of whether or not it serves to improve the use of the hand. In the presence of a totally useless hand that cannot be rehabilitated in any way, obviously it is absurd to consider any reconstructive work on the remainder of the arm or the shoulder, except in rare instances in which the shoulder and the arm can be made adequate for the operation of a prosthesis. At the shoulder it is not uncommon to have a deltoid paralysis associated with good scapular musculature; in such cases with satisfactory hand function, an arthrodesis of the shoulder may be preferable to muscle transposition. Fusion may give active and stable abduction to 90° and flexion to 60° and still permit the arm to be carried at the side. Tendon transposition to replace lost deltoid power has been advocated by some, but such procedures have not gained wide acceptance. Muscle transposition may be satisfactory.

PARALYSIS OF THE TRICEPS. This condition is not badly disabling, since gravity will extend the elbow in situations not requiring force, but a paralyzed biceps and brachialis can prevent the hand from being brought to the mouth and the face. If the forearm flexor muscles are of good power, transposition of the common flexor origin from the medial epicondyle up the humerus 2 or more inches as described by Steindler (1963) may produce fairly satisfactory flexion without disturbing the function of the finger and the wrist flexors (Kettlekamp and Larson, 1963).

WRISTDROP due to the paralysis of wrist extensors commonly is treated by arthrodesis of the wrist in a position of mild dorsiflexion. The efficiency of such an operation may be easily tested preoperatively by applying a cast or a splint to immobilize the wrist and leave the fingers free. Then the patient can tell by actual trial in exactly what manner his disability will be altered by the arthrodesis. In a few cases of wristdrop, the wrist may be stabilized by transportation of wrist flexor tendons or the pronator teres into the wrist extensors. Frequently, however, with loss of wrist extension there is also loss of finger extension, in which case the wrist flexors are needed to motivate finger extensors after the wrist is stabilized by an arthrodesis. In the severely damaged arm and hand tenodesis may give a much better functional result, because it allows motion not possible with an arthrodesis. However, function resulting from tenodesis of finger flexor tendons is completely dependent upon powerful active wrist extension.

Opposition of Thumb. One of the most common of the serious disabilities in the hand that can be corrected surgically is loss of opposition of the thumb. The loss of opposition is due to paralysis of the abductor pollicis brevis muscle. This may be treated by one of several tendon transpositions, using a variety of muscles for the motor power, or by putting a bone graft across the space between the first and the second metacarpals to hold the thumb in a position of opposition (Thompson, 1942). The choice of procedure depends upon available active muscle power and also on performance requirements and can be made only on detailed study of the individual case.

Lower Extremity. In the lower extremity, with weight-bearing, stability and ambulation as the prime objectives, we desire stable joints, freedom from deformity, maximum use of remaining muscle strength and equal leg length.

In order to be justified, surgical procedures should accomplish one or more of these aims (Sideman, 1965).

STABILIZATION OF THE FOOT. The most commonly indicated surgical procedure in the surgical reconstruction of the lower extremity involved with paralytic poliomyelitis is the stabilization of the foot, or "triple arthrodesis." This procedure is designed to correct deformity of the foot as well as accomplish stability for weight-bearing. Regardless of the type of deformity, which may vary greatly, depending on the type of muscle imbalance around the foot, this operation can restore the position of the foot to the normal standing position by variations in technic. In essence, the procedure consists of excising the talocalcaneal, the talonavicular and the calcaneocuboid joints and allowing arthrodesis of the involved bones to occur by immobilization in a plaster cast. By taking wedges of bone with the joint excision almost any deformity may be corrected. For example, a peroneal paralysis may permit a varus or inversion deformity to occur; in stabilizing such a foot, sufficient bone is removed at the calcaneocuboid and the lateral side of the talocalcaneal joints to permit the foot to be straightened out of the varus position.

The average child does not have sufficient bone in the foot to do the stabilization until the age of 8 to 10 years; in marginal cases, a roentgenogram should be made to determine if enough bone is present. Stabilization of the foot sacrifices the motions of inversion and eversion, which has the disadvantage of making it difficult to walk on irregular surfaces. It also shortens the foot and usually increases the discrepancy of foot size. Furthermore, it may not correct a flatfoot deformity. For these reasons, plus the fact that it may be performed at an earlier age, the Grice (1952) operation (extra-articular fusion between the astragalus and the calcaneus) has a very definite place and the advantage of releasing the anterior and the posterior tibial and peroneal muscles, whichever are of significant muscle strength, for transference to aid in dorsiflexion or plantar flexion. The general principal of treating the paralytic foot is to stabilize the hindfoot in order to prevent inversion and eversion. After the hindfoot has been stabilized, the tendons of the remaining and available functioning muscles may be shifted toward the mid-line to serve as dorsi- and plantar flexors at the ankle. The anterior tibial and peroneal tendons work well as dorsiflexors when transposed to the midtarsus anteriorly, and the posterior tibial and peroneal tendons work well as plantar flexors when transposed to the os calcis in the mid-line posteriorly. Anterior tibial transfer to the os calcis may work well in many instances. Thus, no remaining functioning muscle need be wasted. It must be remembered that no stabilization procedure will be successful unless muscle imbalance is also corrected.

It is not uncommon to have loss of dorsiflexors of the foot with unparalyzed dorsiflexors of the toes, so that a cockup deformity of the toes, particularly the great toe, develops as a result of the attempt to use the toe extensors to raise the foot. A very satisfactory procedure is the transposition of the great toe extensor insertion from the distal phalanx to the first metatarsal so that the muscle will dorsiflex the foot without first hyperextending the toe. This is the *Jones suspension operation*.

The stabilization procedure preserves the ankle motion, but with a completely flail leg and foot it may be necessary to do some type of bone block to prevent the foot from dropping into full plantar flexion. The *Campbell bone block* (Speed and Knight, 1963) is such a procedure and consists of elevating a flap of bone from the posterior aspect of the tuberosity of the calcaneus so that this will impinge on the posterior tibia as the foot drops down beyond a right angle. The motion of dorsiflexion is preserved by such a procedure. This operation is not always successful, but has given more satisfactory results than those obtained by a Lambrinudi type of arthrodesis (Lambrinudi, 1927).

STABILIZATION OF THE KNEE. The knee joint may offer a problem of instability due to quadriceps paralysis. In some cases with good hamstring function and partial quadriceps power a very satisfactory result may accrue from transposition of the tendons of the biceps femoris and the semi-tendinosus to the patella to aid extension (Caldwell, 1955). In absence of any quadriceps power or poor hamstring power, consideration must be given to an arthrodesis of the knee; some patients prefer to wear a long leg brace with a knee lock rather than to have an arthrodesis. This is an example of a situation that occurs commonly in reconstructive orthopedics, in which the patient must choose between alternative plans after careful explanation of the advantages and the disadvantages of each by the surgeon. Popliteal dissection with lengthening of hamstring tendons, release of gastrocnemius origins, and posterior capsulotomy of the knee may be necessary at times to correct flexion deformity. This is frequently associated with flexion deformity of the hip, which also may have to be corrected by surgical release of contracted soft tissue and usually is seen in neglected patients. Genu recurvatum is occasionally a disabling occurrence associated with gastrocnemius and hamstring weakness. It may be treated by constructing a check ligament or performing an osteotomy of the tibia (Heyman, 1962).

STABILIZATION OF THE HIP (Parson and Seddon, 1968). About the hip, the most common disability is abductor weakness; this permits a downward sag of the opposite side of the pelvis during the standing phase of the gait, called a "positive" Trendelenburg sign. The normal or "negative" Trendelenburg sign refers to the ability of the abductors to maintain the opposite side of the pelvis elevated during the standing phase of the gait. Several operative procedures have been designed to transpose muscle power to abduction; none has been sufficiently proved to gain wide usage. Instability about the hip sufficient to produce serious disability probably is best corrected by arthrodesis; such a procedure produces less disability than most people would think when done in childhood. However, in certain instances the transfer of the iliopsoas after the method of Mustard (1959) will provide functional stabilization of the hip and obviate arthrodesis.

DEFORMITIES OF LONG BONE (Sharp *et al.*, 1964). Osteotomy to correct deformities of long bones, particularly rotational deformities, is frequently indicated. The necessary correction is carried out under direct vision of the surgically exposed bone, and the fracture thus created is treated by immobilization in plaster.

It must be kept in mind that the indications for various of the aforementioned procedures may have to be reconsidered in light of other disabilities in the same or other extremities.

That is to say, one always should consider the effect of any given surgical procedure on the whole patient.

EQUALIZATION OF LEG LENGTH. This procedure will be considered at this point because it is most frequently a problem related to poliomyelitis. The principles of its correction may be applied to other conditions that may produce a significant leg length discrepancy. As a rule, a discrepancy of leg length of 1 inch or less in an average-sized adult is usually asymptomatic and requires no treatment, other than a simple elevation of the heel of the shoe. Discrepancies of between 1¼ and 5 inches produce an ungainly limp and can and should be corrected in most cases if possible. Discrepancies of more than 5 inches usually are uncorrectable by the ordinary means and require some other management.

The group under consideration is the discrepancy of between 1¼ and 5 inches. The surgeon has a choice of: (1) operative lengthening of the shortened extremity, (2) operative shortening of the long extremity and (3) some type of epiphyseal arrest of the long extremity in childhood. The first is very seldom indicated because of technical difficulties and hazards. Suitable technics with special apparatus have been described for use in special circumstances (Abbott and Crego, 1928). The second is not particularly difficult or hazardous but is usually indicated only after bone growth has ceased. Epiphyseal arrest of the distal femur and/or the proximal tibia of the long extremity is the easiest method available, although applicable only in children. Permanent closure of the epiphysis by the method described by Phemister (1930) or temporary closure by use of staples advocated by Blount and Clarke (1949) may be carried out. With the permanent closure methods, the correct time of closing must be chosen with care so as to obtain as nearly as possible to correct amount of shortening. Several methods are available to aid the surgeon in deciding when such closures should be done. The interested student should seek further information on this subject (Green and Anderson, 1947). The use of stapling to close an epiphyseal plate temporarily has the theoretical advantage that growth may be resumed by removal of the staple before closure of the plate. Either of these methods will be successful if properly employed. The most common cause of failure is to delay the operation too long, so that the anticipated amount of growth restriction does not occur.

Ideally, equalization of leg length would be accomplished best by some form of stimulation of the epiphysis or epiphyses of the short side. This problem has been and is being pursued by many investigators. So far all the published and the unpublished results have revealed failure of the various methods to produce a suitable degree of increased length. In a few instances the creation of an arteriovenous fistula between the femoral artery and vein has resulted in a significant increase in length of a shortened extremity (Janes and Musgrave, 1950; Cooley et al., 1960). The possibility of severe cardiovascular changes exists in this approach to leg-length equalization, and further experience is required before the method can be employed in other than very selected cases. However, further study in experimental animals may yet result in a satisfactory method of epiphyseal stimulation (Harris and McDonald, 1936); Pease, 1952; Green and Anderson, 1947; Blount, 1960).

CEREBRAL PALSY

The term *cerebral palsy* is used to cover a variety of clinical syndromes caused by brain damage. This damage may be the result of a developmental defect, direct trauma or anoxia incident to the birth process, or even some post-partum disease affecting the central nervous system. Depending on the portion of the brain affected, an extremely wide range of clinical pictures may exist. Spasticity, rigidity or athetosis may be present, singly or in combination. Monoplegia, paraplegia, hemiplegia or quadriplegia may exist. Mental deficiency commonly exists. Potentially average or above average mentality may escape detection because of lack of opportunity of development or ability to detect it; thus, careful evaluation of mentality is indicated in the over-all treatment of the patient.

Numerous surgical procedures have been described to benefit victims of these conditions. Only about 25 per cent of these patients meet the criteria of suitability for surgery. It must be drawn to the attention of the families of these patients that the surgical procedure is directed at the results of the disease, e.g., flexion deformity, and not at correction of the disease itself.

A number of operations have been advocated for management of certain specific disabilities resulting from cerebral palsy, chiefly those found in spastic paralysis. Only those that have been well-established and accepted as beneficial will be mentioned. It should be pointed out that surgery may be used to improve active function of the extremity and thereby lessen physical disability or, at times, may be done merely to increase the ease of handling a severely crippled individual.

UPPER EXTREMITY

Contracture of the adductors and the internal rotators of the shoulder because of abnormal tonus may develop. Surgical severance of the contracted insertions of the pectoralis major and the subscapularis with immobilization for several weeks in a position of external rotation and abduction, as described by Sever (1918) is very beneficial when a good hand is present. Also, osteotomy of the humerus to correct rotational deformity has been useful in older children.

There are several procedures to choose from for correction of pronation and flexion deformities of the forearm. A satisfactory one is section of the pronator teres or release of the flexor pronator origin (Inglis and Cooper, 1966).

Flexion deformity of the wrist is handled best either by arthrodesis of this joint in a position of slight dorsiflexion or by transfer of the flexor carpi unaris to the extensor carpi radialis (Green and Banks, 1962). This operation must be done only in those patients who have the capacity voluntarily to release the grasp when held in the position of proposed arthrodesis. It is wise to immobilize the wrist in a cast prior to arthrodesis to be certain that hand function will be improved.

The hand is so intricate that serious spasticity or rigidity or athetosis of its muscles cannot be helped significantly by surgical procedures (Goldner, 1961). Sections of adductors of the thumb to prevent premature flexion and adduction of the thumb into the palm on closure of the fist may be useful (Keats, 1965). Fusion by bone graft of the 1st and the 2nd metacarpals to hold the thumb in a position of opposition is indicated occasionally (Thompson, 1942).

LOWER EXTREMITY

At the hip, spasticity produces flexion adduction and internal rotation contractures. Adductor spasm may be handled adequately by detachment of the adductor muscles from their origin of the pubis and/or obturator nerve neurectomy. Internal rotation caused by adductor tightness will be relieved by these procedures while internal rotation caused by hip flexion contractures will be improved by surgical release of hip flexors (Anthonsen, 1966). Knee and hip flexion resulting from hamstring spasm may be reduced by transposition of the hamstring tendons from the tibia to the distal femur (Eggers, 1952).

At the knee, flexion contracture is common and may be corrected by advancement of the patellar tendon insertion, if active but not passive full extension of the knee has been lost (Chandler, 1933, 1947; Pollock et al., 1967). Where there is fixed flexion contracture, this must be corrected by wedging casts or popliteal dissection and then a hamstring transplant done to prevent recurrence.

Equinus deformity of the foot producing a toe-to-heel gait may be corrected readily by a neurectomy of nerves supplying the gastrocnemius in mild cases without structural shortening of the heel cord or by heel cord lengthening in more severe cases.

Various foot deformities may occur (Baker and Hill, 1964). They may require tendon subluxations, tendon transfers, or arthrodeses.

It should be emphasized that corrective surgery will probably not succeed in any child that does not have enough balance to stand or walk along before surgical correction. Surgery may also fail if the patient has insufficient intelligence to be trainable.

It is surprising how well a child with severe deformity will be able to get around if there is a good sense of balance. Procedures requiring postoperative recumbency for several weeks should be avoided in children who just recently have learned to walk alone, because such recumbency will "set back" the developing sense of balance so that such a child may take months relearning to walk (Stamp, 1962).

One of the great challenges to the orthopedic surgeon is the management of the family

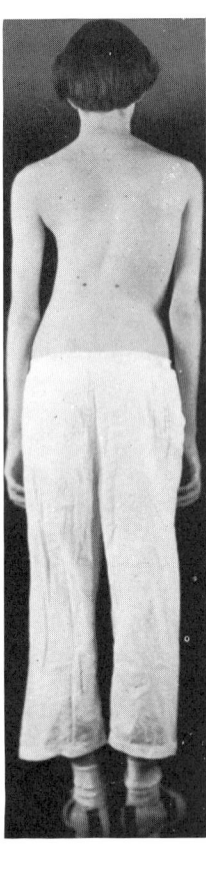

FIG. 53-23. The typical appearance of a girl with idiopathic scoliosis.

of the patient with cerebral palsy so that they may have maximum legitimate hopefulness and as true an understanding as possible of the limitations of medical treatment.

Recurrent deformities can be prevented by bracing and physical therapy. Family cooperation and understanding is mandatory for optimum results in patients with cerebral palsy.

MYELODYSPLASIA

The term *myelodysplasia* is used to describe a variety of clinical syndromes that include a developmental defect in the spinal cord associated with a peripheral neurologic deficit involving the thoracic, the lumbar, or the lumbosacral region (Hayes et al., 1964). The incidence of this disorder has been estimated at two or three per thousand live births. The defect results from a partial or complete failure of the neuroectodermal elements to fuse between the 21st and 29th days of gestation, but the etiology is unknown. Degree of involvement varies from a minimal spina bifida with minor sensory motor changes in the feet to a massive thoracolumbar myelomeningocele with paraplegia, bladder and bowel incontinence, and hydrocephalus. In infants who might be rehabilitated, immediate attention by the pediatrician, neurosurgeon, urologist, and orthopedic surgeon is indicated (Swinyard, 1966). The myelomeningocele must be closed soon after birth and hydrocephalus must be controlled. The genitourinary tract should be carefully managed to minimize renal damage by infection and retention. The orthopedic care of the child with myelodysplasia includes: (1) the prevention of trophic ulcers over anesthetic areas, (2) the prevention of deformity with physical therapy and bracing, and (3) the correction of deformities by nonoperative and surgical means. Although types of deformities and their management cannot be discussed in detail here, it may be mentioned that the degree of involvement varies with the neurologic level. The involvement may vary from clawtoes and foot deformities to dislocated hip, scoliosis, and totally flail lower extremities. Treatment will vary accordingly—from bracing, cast correction, and tendon transfers, to major reconstructive and stabilization procedures. All of these patients require careful and long-term follow-up because of the high incidence of recurrent problems.

SCOLIOSIS

Scoliosis refers to a lateral and rotary deviation of the spine beyond normal and, in most cases, develops in the growing spine (Fig. 53-23). Less than 20 per cent of patients who are seen with this condition have some recognizable underlying etiology; this group includes cases of poliomyelitis with asymmetrical paresis of paraspinal, thoracic or abdominal musculature, patients with vertebral anomalies, neurofibromatosis, myopathies, myelodysplasia, spinal tumors, inequality of leg length, chest disease, and many others. The remainder of cases are referred to as idiopathic scoliosis. It is likely that the majority of these constitute a real disease entity, the cause of which is unknown. Idiopathic scoliosis is seen most commonly in females between the ages of 10 and 15 years; it develops insidiously, it is usually asymptomatic and is first noticed by someone other than the patient. Although several

FIG. 53-24. The Milwaukee Brace for scoliosis. The majority of flexible or partly flexible idiopathic curves can be controlled by a well fitted and properly used brace. Normal physical activity may be permitted. Deforming curves that do not repond to the brace may require spinal fusion.

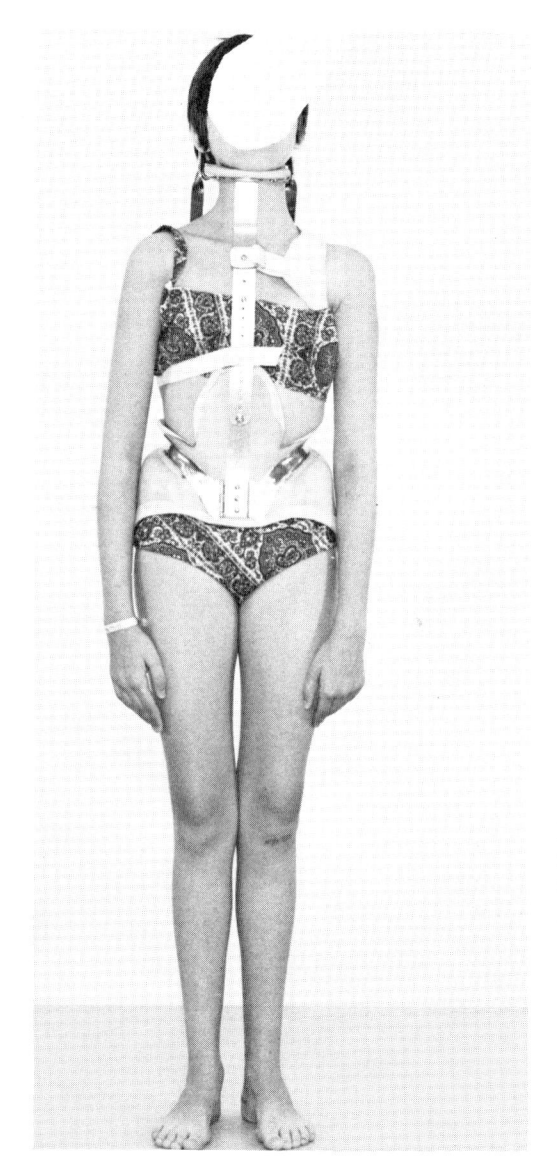

different types of curves are seen, the most common is right dorsal and left lumbar "S"-shaped scoliosis. As the curve develops in progressive cases there also develops associated rib cage deformity of a degree comparable with the spine deformity (Gucker, 1962).

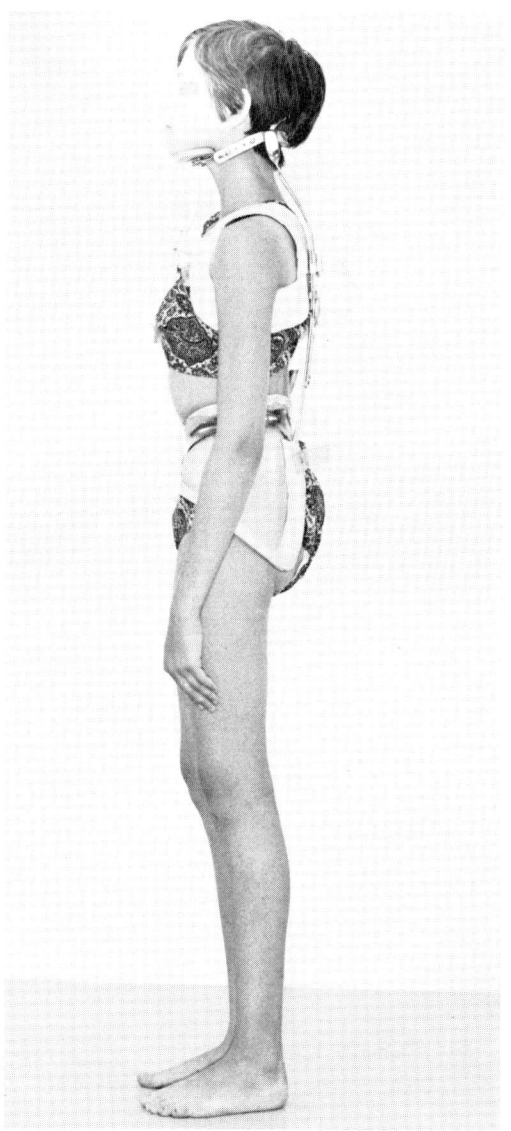

Since a wide range of severity of deformity occurs, it may be difficult to decide initially whether bracing or surgery will be required. In the past all too many of these adolescents have been observed over a period of years while their deformity increased to grotesque proportions. Prolonged conservative treatment, with improper bracing and neglect of alternate procedures, can, in these cases, carry a graver risk than surgery.

The physician should attempt to determine the etiology by means of careful examination.

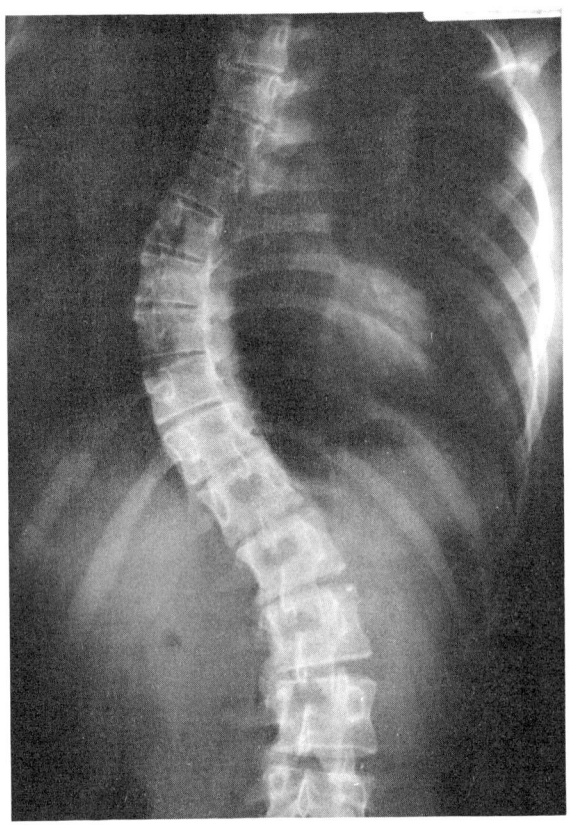

Fig. 53-25. (*Top*) Idiopathic scoliosis in a 15-year-old girl. The roentgenogram reveals a prominent right dorsal curve, which measured 50°. In this patient the correction of the curve could not be maintained with a Milwaukee Brace. Spinal fusion was therefore indicated. (*Right*) Same patient, 6 months after spinal fusion and Harrington rod instrumentation. The longer rod (*right*) supplies a distraction force and purchases on the facet of T-5 and the lamina of L-2. The shorter rod (*left*) supplies a compression force. The hooks are applied to the transverse processes. The curve now measures 20°.

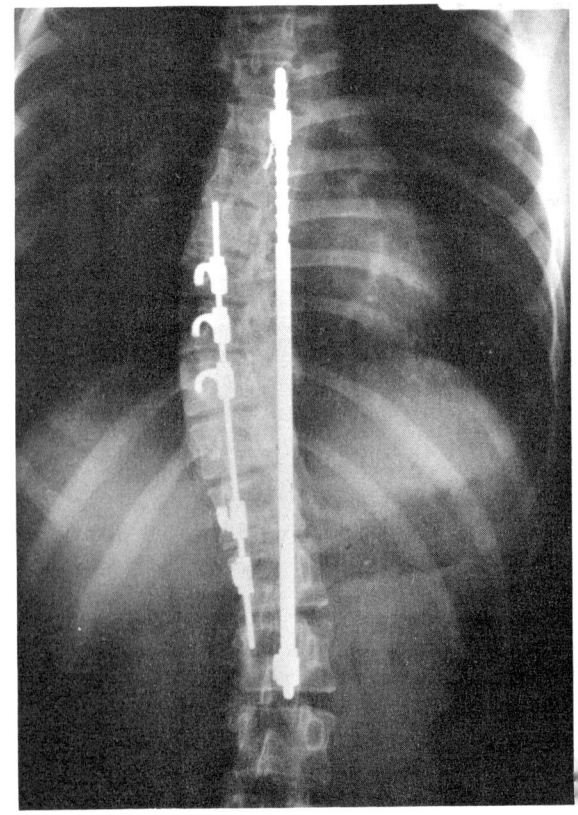

However, most curves are idiopathic, and the following comments in regard to management pertain principally to this type. Curves are best followed by regular roentgenographic examinations. The minimal (10 to 20°) non-progressive curve can be safely followed by cautious observation. Curves that are larger or progressive, but flexible, should be treated with the Milwaukee Brace (Blount, 1968). (See Fig. 53-24.) In the small to moderate flexible curves discovered during growth years, a Milwaukee Brace has no peer (Moe, 1969). Since untreated curves may progress rapidly during growth, the use of the Brace until bone maturity may prevent progression. In the early years of childhood, every effort should be made to control the curve by non-operative means, but sometimes surgery is necessary. In the older child whose curve becomes progressively deforming and inflexible in spite of the brace, correction to the best possible position, instrumentation and fusion are indicated (Fig. 53-25). Inflexible deforming curves do not respond to brace treatment and require early spinal fusion (Moe and Gustillo, 1964). The flexible versus the structural, or inflexible) component of the curve may be improved preoperatively with the use of corrective body casts (Goldstein, 1966; Moe, 1958; Risser and Norquist, 1958). A valuable adjunct to spinal fusion is the use of distraction and compression rods designed by Harrington (1963) (Tamborino et al., 1964). These implants provide good internal fixation and increase and maintain correction if used properly. Postoperative casts to protect the fusion until it is solid (6 to 9 months) are needed. Pseudarthroses may require refusion. A good cosmetic result at time, may be obtained, particularly where the rotational deformity and, thus, the rib cage prominence are corrected. However, even with excellent correction some increase in the curve can be expected, since the living bone of a quite solid spinal fusion is subjected to the same stresses that produced the curves.

Considerable deformity may be compatible with good health, but a prominent curve may seriously impair a child's social development. There also is an increased tendency for scoliotic spines to develop symptomatic degenerative changes in later life. In addition, cardiopulmonary function may be impaired (Manken, 1964). Patients with severe uncontrolled curves (between 100 and 180°) may die of pulmonary infection and right heart failure. Such curves can be prevented by early recognition and treatment.

INFECTION IN BONE

Osteomyelitis

Definition. Pyogenic osteomyelitis is an inflammation of any portion of the bone, produced by one of the pyogenic organisms in contradistinction to such agents as tuberculosis, syphilis and fungi. The development of pyogenic inflammation of bone must be preceded by the deposition of the causative organisms, most commonly the staphylococcus and the streptococcus, in a suitable bed in the bone structure.

This may occur (1) by the organisms being carried to the bone by the circulation, (2) by direct extension from a nearby abscess or infection and (3) by a communicating wound, such as an open fracture. There seems to be little evidence that infection of the bone can occur through the lymphatic system.

Pathogenesis. Although acute osteomyelitis may be initiated by introduction of bacteria from the outside through a wound or through continuity with a neighboring soft tissue infection, hematogenous spread from a pre-existing focus is by far the most common route of infection. A septicemia or bacteremia is invariably present. An infective embolus enters the nutrient artery and is trapped in the vessel of small caliber. Most of the small end arteries and capillaries are located in the metaphysis adjacent to the epiphyseal plate. This satisfactorily explains the predilection of the metaphysis to infection. The predisposition to infection in the metaphysis of a long bone is in direct proportion to the rate of growth at that area and to the size of the bone. The longer and larger the bone, the more susceptible it is to acute osteomyelitis, particularly at its more rapidly growing end. Thus the upper metaphysis of the tibia is more likely to become infected than the lower. Other explanations advanced for the predilection of the metaphysis include: (1) slowing of the circulating blood in the sinusoids, (2) the fact that the epiphyseal arteries are end arteries, allowing blood to accumulate in the sinusoid areas, and

Orthopedics (Nontraumatic)

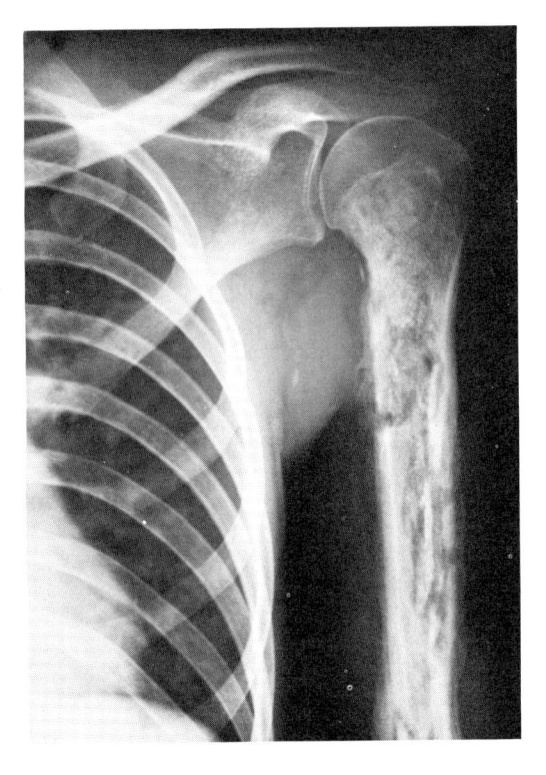

FIG. 53-26. Chronic osteomyelitis. Note the multiple sequestra of dead bone, surrounded by a large involucrum in which there are multiple cloacae. There is gross destruction of the humeral diaphysis.

(3) defective phagocytosis. Initially there is acute exudative inflammation with increased vascularity, edema, and polymorphonuclear leukocytes. Within two to three days, thrombosis and obliteration of the vessels through increased intramedullary pressure produce ischemia and bone necrosis. An intramedullary abscess forms, and edema fluid and purulent exudate are forced through the Haversian and the Volkmann's canals, stripping the periosteum from the bone. This isolates the cortical bone from its blood supply, and produces more dead bone. The pus, following the path of least resistance, may then re-enter the medullary canal through the cortex at a distance, or may perforate the periosteum and enter soft tissues or extend into the neighboring joint. The progression from acute to chronic osteomyelitis is subtle, for once pus accumulates under pressure, causing bone ischemia and forcing bacteria into the vascular channels, the stage is set for the chronic process.

In children the epiphyseal cartilage plate acts as a barrier to infection, delaying extension into the epiphyseal end of the bone and then into the joint. When the metaphyseal area is intracapsular, however, infection may spread quickly into the joint. An important example is the hip joint. Osteomyelitis of the neck of the femur may lead very quickly to the serious complication of septic arthritis of the hip. Often the joints develop a secondary synovitis before they become actually infected.

With the accumulation of pus beneath the periosteum, new bone is laid down on its inner surface, forming an involucrum. In this new bone numerous openings, or cloacae, for the discharge of pus and bone debris appear. Certain areas of bone may become ischemic from the stripping up of periosteum and the thrombosis of cortical capillaries. These areas become necrotic and separate, forming sequestra. Small sequestra may be extruded from the involucra through cloacae into sinuses draining upon the skin surface (Fig. 53-26). It is impossible, however, for the larger sequestra to be extruded, and they may have to be removed surgically. Sequestra may become surrounded by granulation tissue and gradually disintegrated and absorbed by the action of proteolytic ferments liberated in the purulent exudate.

In extensive osteomyelitic involvement of the shaft of a long bone, pathologic fracture occasionally occurs. This is particularly likely to happen if stress is placed upon the bone before sufficiently mature involucrum has restored its strength.

Not all pyogenic osteomyelitis is accompanied by the formation of sequestra. Atypical infections from relatively avirulent organisms are not uncommon. The defenses of the body, especially when supplemented by antibiotics, may early overcome the infection, which then completely subsides. Osteomyelitis in infancy rarely results in gross sequestration.

Osteomyelitis of a long bone in children frequently produces a slight overgrowth in length.

The x-ray manifestations of suppurative osteomyelitis are related to the destruction of bone, to the formation of new bone as a reaction to infection and to the presence of devitalized bone. Radiographic examination reveals no abnormalities early in the course of the process, and changes are not apparent until there is macroscopic evidence of bone destruction or of new bone formation, usually seven to ten days after the onset of the infection. The early administration of antibacterial agents further modifies the radiographic manifestations, so that with mild infections there may be no radiographic evidence of the disease or with more severe infection there may be a marked delay in the radiographic manifestations of the process. Because osseous changes are dependent on destruction of bone or new bone formation, the first evidence of an underlying osteomyelitis may be the presence of soft tissue swelling adjacent to the infected bone. Usually recognizable is edema, which results in obliteration of fat between groups of muscles, a regular opacity of subcutaneous fatty tissue and an increase in the size of muscle.

The lesion, by its nature, tends to wall off pockets of infection, which may lie dormant for long periods and then, under exacerbation, may flare up actively. Thus chronic sinuses are formed that eventually reach the surface and drain. They suppurate until the infection becomes static, then the channels are plugged with granulation and remain closed until the pressure of the pus within builds up to the point of reopening the sinuses or establishing new ones. The process may continue in this manner over a period of many years, and the bone may become so riddled and useless that amputation is imperative. In a small percentage the sinus tract opening onto the skin becomes lined by stratified squamous epithelium growing down from the surface. Constant inflammation of these lining cells may induce cancerous change. The resulting neoplasm behaves in all respects like an ordinary squamous cell carcinoma.

Although epidermoid carcinoma is a rare complication of chronic osteomyelitis, it must be kept in mind when patients with draining sinuses are being treated. Complication can be prevented by aggressive treatment of the infection. Biopsy is a most important diagnostic procedure. If biopsy shows only chronic osteomyelitis or benign epithelial hyperplasia, every effort must be made to heal the sinus. Epidermoid carcinoma in chronic osteomyelitis should be treated by amputation, at an adequate level for malignant lesions.

Etiology. Key (1954) reported the staphylococcus as the causative agent in about 90 per cent of the cases. Most of his strains were hemolytic *Staphylococcus aureus* (in 52 cases), and he encountered the streptococcus in 5 cases and the pneumococcus in 1, in a total of 58 cases.

In a more recent series by Clawson and Dunn (1967), of 118 patients with osteomyelitis the cause, in 65 patients, was *Staphylococcus aureus* alone and, in 19 patients, *S. aureus* and other micro-organisms. Other causes listed were proteus, pseudomonas, etc. It is frequently stated that in infants under 2 years of age, the causative organism is more apt to be the streptococcus, and that in those over 2 years of age the staphylococcus predominates; however, in very young infants colon bacillus osteomyelitis is not uncommon. The disease produced by each of these various infectious organisms is somewhat different in that the streptococcus toxin does not seem to have the same destructive influence on bone that is present with the staphylococcus. Even in untreated cases in which recovery occurs in spite of considerable involvement of the bone, the bone lesion often heals with little, if any, sequestration. On the other hand, with the staphylococcus there is almost always a large amount of bone killed, with sequestra of various sizes resulting. In addition to the necrotizing effect of the staphylococcus toxin, the amount of nonviable bone is also somewhat dependent upon the extent of the subperiosteal abscess.

Another group of micro-organisms, the salmonella, may produce suppurative osteomyelitis but this is much less common than the disease caused by staphylococci. Almost without exception these infections have been found in patients with sickle cell anemia. The reason for the association of the two conditions is not clear. It has been suggested that the anemia plus the autosplenectomy may lower the resistance to the salmonella organisms. It also has been suggested that the minute infarctions of the intestinal wall induced by poor oxygen-carrying capacity of the erythrocytes promote the diffusion of the organisms. Recently it has been shown that the frequency of multiple infarctions of bone is relatively high in patients with sickle cell anemia and those with hemoglobin S-C disease. In most cases these infarcts are aseptic. It appears probable that these areas of aseptic necrosis provide a locus of inadequate resistance that allows the organisms to flourish, so that the disease can occur only in patients whose red cells contain hemoglobin S or hemoglobin C and who develop a salmonella septicemia.

This condition occurs more commonly in children than in adults, although persons of any age may be affected. The foci of infection usually are multiple, apparently conforming to the multiple areas of infarction. The disease is much more serious than ordinary staphylococcic osteomyelitis: the many foci of infection plus the sickle cell anemia may lead to a fatal outcome.

Radiographically, salmonella osteomyelitis in patients with sickle cell anemia usually involves more than one bone. Characteristically there are multiple destructive lesions through the diaphysis, extensive periosteal new bone formation and irregular sclerosis (Ebrahim and Grech, 1966).

Treatment. SURGICAL. The special ability of the staphylococcus toxins to kill bone, plus the damage to the circulation, led surgeons to advocate early operation in these cases, in the hope that if the lesion could be opened and drained to the outside the amount of bone destroyed would be reduced considerably. A great effort was put forth to make a diagnosis in these cases very early in the course of the disease, long before there was x-ray evidence of bone damage, and to drain the infected area immediately as an emergency procedure. The result was to submit a critically ill child, most often dehydrated, to a surgical procedure. The mortality was rather high. Furthermore, it never was clearly shown that early operation and drainage materially limited the amount of bone destroyed; in fact, there are instances in which there was some question as to whether or not the early operation actually contributed to the spread of infection or caused damage to the epiphysis.

Orr (1927) introduced an entirely new principle in the treatment of osteomyelitis, namely, surgical drainage combined with rest. He reported many cases of acute hematogenous osteomyelitis in which the infected area was opened early, and the wound packed open with petrolatum gauze and immobilized in a plaster cast. Many of the wounds treated by this method healed without difficulty and without extensive loss of bone. This method was more generally applicable to the subacute and the chronic cases of osteomyelitis and constituted one of the greatest advances in the treatment of this condition.

CHEMOTHERAPY AND ANTIBIOTICS. The development and use of the chemotherapeutic and antibiotic agents not only revolutionized the treatment of acute hematogenous osteomyelitis but also practically eradicated the disease itself. It is rare indeed now to see a case of acute hematogenous osteomyelitis. Indeed, when such a case does appear, appropriate antibiotic therapy has completely altered the course of the disease—to such an extent that it is unusual for a case to come under the observation of an orthopedic surgeon.

In the treatment of osteomyelitis with an antimicrobial agent a bactericidal antibiotic is preferable to a bacteriostatic one. A microbiostatic (suppressive) antibiotic slows cell division of the pathogen, and host defense mechanisms must eradicate the organisms. Bactericidal and bacteriostatic antibiotics should not be used concurrently. Bactericidal antibiotics destroy organisms by preventing the formation of new cell-wall material as the bacteria divide. If cell division is stopped by a bacteriostatic antibiotic, the bactericidal one cannot act. For *Staphylococcus aureus*, a non-penicillinase-producing organism, the following antimicrobial agents are preferred: penicillin G, penicillin V, phenethicillin, cephalothin, or vancomycin. For penicillinase-producing *Staphylococcus aureus*, the use of cloxacillin, methicillin, cephalothin, or vancomycin is satisfactory. For aerobacter infections, colistin, kanamycin, or cephalothin is satisfactory. The most effective antibiotic for pseudomonas is colistin. Penicillin, of course, is the effective agent for streptococcus. The use of tetracycline, a bacteriostatic antibiotic, in the treatment of osteomyelitis seems to be suggested by its concentration in bone. However, it is localized in areas in which osteoid is being calcified and, therefore, would not be particularly effective, because these are not areas in which the bacteria are concentrated (Clawson and Dunn, 1967; Meyer et al., 1965).

The treatment of acute hematogenous osteomyelitis, if the prognosis is to be good, must be early and effective. Hall and Silverstein

(1963) successfully treated 87 per cent of their cases; Harris and Kirkaldy-Willis (1965) reported only one relapse in 24 patients treated within the first three days of the illness as contrasted with twelve relapses in 21 patients treated after three days. A bacteriologic diagnosis is essential. As soon as the diagnosis is suspected, blood should be obtained for culture and studies of antibiotic sensitivity. The blood culture yields a positive result in more than 50 per cent of patients with acute hematogenous osteomyelitis. Because of the frequency of *Staphylococcus aureus* as the offending organism intravenous administration of methicillin (ampicillin) should be started.

Operative treatment is not necessary if effective medical treatment is instituted within 72 hours of onset of the disease. If antibiotic treatment is begun later than this, early decompression may be indicated. Often fluid and electrolyte balance must be restored, and transfusions may be required to correct anemia.

In the treatment of chronic osteomyelitis one must realize that the underlying process is the ischemia rather than the infection. Organisms thrive in avascular bone and scar tissue, and frequently the surrounding scar acts as an impenetrable barrier to antibiotic therapy. Therefore, effective treatment must accomplish (1) excision of all dead bone and scar tissue; (2) provision of effective antibiotic therapy; and (3) elimination of dead space when the wound is closed (Clawson, 1965; Clawson and Stevenson, 1965). At the time of operation all scar tissue, including the sinus tract and dead bone, must be removed.

The technic of primary closure with irrigation and suction has reduced considerably the duration of hospitalization and disability, has almost eliminated secondary bacterial infection, and has yielded extremely encouraging results to the present time (Compere *et al.*, 1967). In this method of treatment a pair of multiperforated polyethelene tubes are placed in the cavity created by débridement, and the nonperforated ends are brought out through normal tissue as far away from the wound edges as possible. A solution for irrigation contains a nontoxic detergent as well as one or more antibiotics. The detergent has several effects. It inhibits or prevents the formation of penicillinase, so that penicillin used with the detergent becomes effective against resistant bacterial strains. The detergent also breaks up pus, mucus, and necrotic tissue, permitting the antibiotics to reach bacteria that might otherwise be inaccessible.

At the present time the greatest difficulty with this form of treatment is that there is a tendency on the part of those handling these cases to fail to recognize spread of the infection to one of the adjacent joints. Although we are not called upon to see and treat many cases of extensive local abscesses with large sequestra, we do see all too often a case of osteomyelitis in which—while being well managed from the bone standpoint—the spread of infection into the adjacent joint was not recognized until irreparable damage to that joint had occurred. This is particularly true of the hip joint, in which so often the osteomyelitis is intra-articular almost from the start. Therefore, in spite of the great advances that have been made in the management of this condition (and of its almost total eradication from the general population), it still behooves those who are treating the occasional case to be on constant guard for involvement of the joints, so that early drainage of the joint may be provided. Preferably, this is accomplished by aspiration and instillation of an appropriate antibiotic agent, but if this is not immediately successful in combating the infection, the joint should be opened and drained. Otherwise, permanent damage or total loss of the joint probably will occur.

Brodie's Abscess

Brodie's abscess is a localized infection of bone originally described by B. C. Brodie (1832). Usually it is found in the metaphyseal area of the long bones and is characterized by a roughly spherical area of bone destruction, forming a cavity which may be filled with pus or, in an old abscess, filled with connective tissue only. The bone surrounding this cavity is hard and eburnated and has an x-ray appearance of a sclerotic rim (Fig. 53-27). Sequestra have been reported in the cavity. The causative organism is most commonly the *Staphylococcus aureus*, and the most frequent symptom is pain, which may be more severe while resting than with activity. Local or systemic antibiotic therapy may not be sufficient to cure the condition or to relieve the pain. Sur-

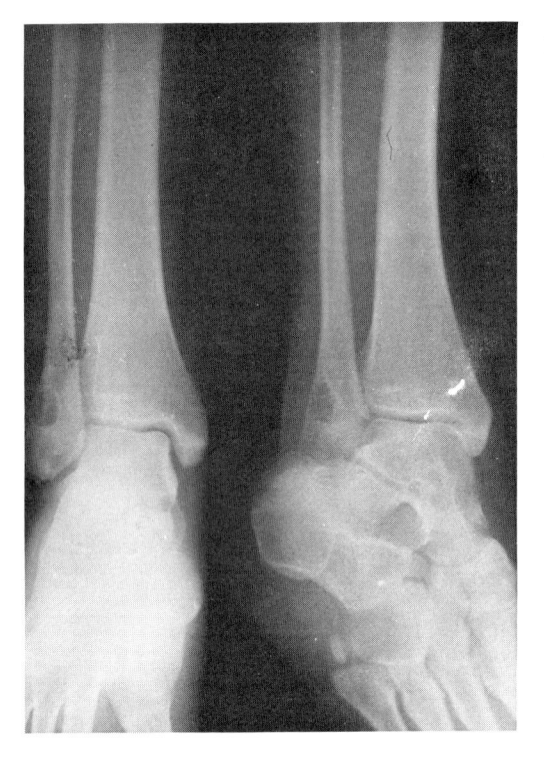

FIG. 53-27. Roentgenograms of the distal fibula with a spherical area of bone destruction forming a cavity which may be filled with pus—or, if the infection is entirely burned out, with connective tissue only. There is a sclerotic medial border. This picture may mimic a metaphyseal fibrous defect roentgenographically. However, this patient complained of pain, which is not characteristic of metaphyseal fibrous defect.

gical intervention is indicated in those cases producing symptoms. Recommended surgical procedures are of 3 types: (1) to open the abscess, unroof the abscess cavity, wash out the contents, curette the walls and close the wound. This method was successful in a majority of cases reported by Wagner and Hanby (1938). (2) In Campbell's *Operative Surgery* (Speed and Knight, 1963) it is suggested that if the abscess contains a considerable quantity of purulent material it may be best to pack the wound open and close it secondarily. The authors recommend giving antibiotics preoperatively and postoperatively. (3) It has been suggested that in purulent cases of Brodie's abscess the wound may be closed loosely, with a tube left into the cavity through which antibiotic solutions may be instilled at regular intervals.

In the majority of cases, the first of the above methods is most satisfactory. The extremity is immobilized during the period of primary wound healing. Since a number of cases fail to heal by this method, we think that in those cases in which the cavity is filled with pus the second method should be utilized and the wound packed open with glycerin gauze pack. At the end of 5 to 7 days the gauze is removed in the operating room with aseptic precautions, the wound is inspected, and, if it appears to be clean, the cavity may be filled with cancellous bone chips and final skin closure effected at this time. However, if the cavity does not appear to be clean, the best form of treatment is to pack it with glycerin gauze, immobilize the extremity and let it fill in from the bottom after the method described by Orr (1927).

PYOGENIC ARTHRITIS

Pyogenic arthritis, like osteomyelitis, is most commonly of blood-borne origin—although, of course, it may result from spread of local or nearby infection or from penetrating wounds into a joint. It often occurs as a complication of osteomyelitis and, like osteomyelitis, it is not nearly so common as it was before the antibiotic age. It is more apt to occur in children, and, although any joint may be involved, the knee and the hip joints are involved most frequently. Any of the pyogenic organisms may be responsible, but the staphylococcus and the streptococcus are found more frequently.

Reports of septic—or preferably, bacterial—arthritis of the hip in adults recently have appeared in the literature (Bulmer, 1966; Kelly et al., 1965). Perhaps bacterial arthritis of the hip is too often considered a disease of infants and children. The possibility of bacterial infection must always be considered in the adult who has a painful hip. In adults, acute hematogenous pyogenic arthritis presents a variable pattern, sometimes with migrating polyarthralgia followed by definite septic involvement of one or more joints. In the infant less than one year of age, articular infection may be manifested by irritability, apprehension, failure to feed well and to gain weight-bearing portions are susceptible to at-

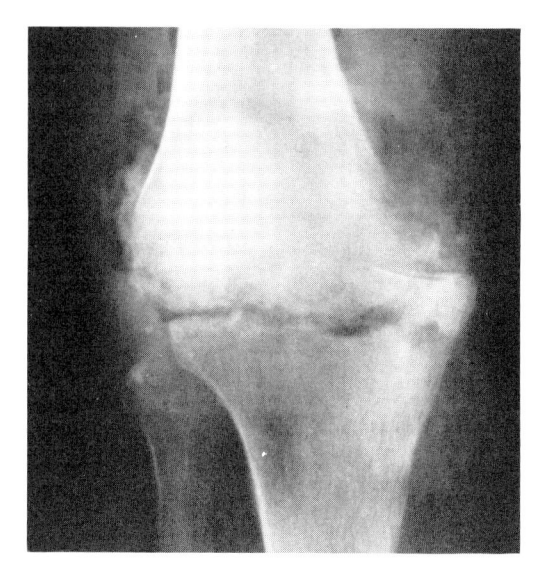

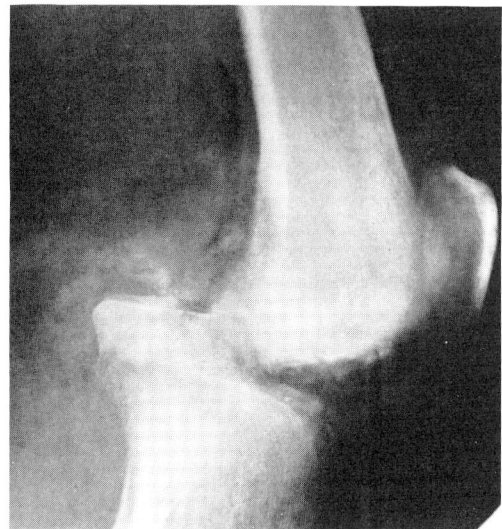

FIG. 53-28. Chronic suppurative arthritis. There is gross destruction of the articular cartilage, with posterior subluxation of the tibia. Note the air within the joint.

elevated pulse rate, or anemia. The only manifestation of severe involvement of the hip joint may be the tendency to maintain the hip in the froglike position. Any of the pyogenic organisms may be responsible, but the *Staphylococcus aureus* is the etiologic agent in 40 to 60 per cent of these patients, with streptococcus next in frequency (Borella et al., 1963). In infants and small children who are suffering from inflammatory diseases, the possibility of a septic joint should be kept in mind whenever the infectious process seems to flare up. There is an elevation of the pulse and the temperature, with increased irritability, a limp if the child is old enough to walk, or a splinting or refusal to use the affected extremity in younger children and bed patients. Increased local heat and swelling develop rapidly. In the superficial joints evidence of infections of the joints almost always is recognized early, but in the hip joint infection not infrequently may be overlooked for some days after its inception. It is particularly important to make the diagnosis at the earliest possible time, because the articular cartilage does not withstand either the toxins of the organisms or the proteolytic enzymes liberated from dead leukocytes, and the periarticular structure is damaged by the acute inflammatory process (Curtiss and Klein, 1965 a, b) (Fig. 53-28). Partial or complete ankylosis may result (Fig. 53-29). In the superficial joints the physical findings are: restricted motion, pain on active or passive motion, increased local heat and evidence of effusion into the joint.

Treatment. The diseased joint should be aspirated with a large bore needle and then irrigated thoroughly with saline solution. The synovium should be distended in order to facilitate cleansing of all surfaces and breaking up of the fibrin clots. It has been demonstrated experimentally that intra-articular instillation of antibiotic produces sterility of the joint more rapidly than does intramuscular administration (Bardenheier et al., 1966; Rapp et al., 1966). At the time the joint is aspirated, culture should be taken for sensitivity tests, and one gram of methicillin and one gram of ampicillin instilled into the synovial cavity. Immobilization is obtained by splinting or skeletal traction. The joint is aspirated and irrigated and the antibiotic instilled as often as effusion recurs. Failure of the infection to begin to subside promptly indicates walled off collections of pus, and operation should be performed without delay. In those cases requiring drainage some permanent loss of function almost always results (Morgan et al., 1963).

Gonococcal Arthritis. Infection of joints

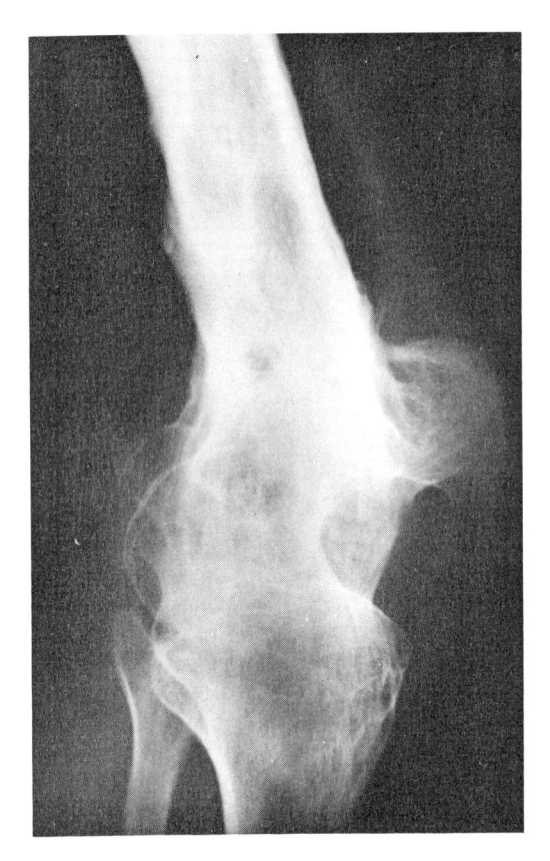

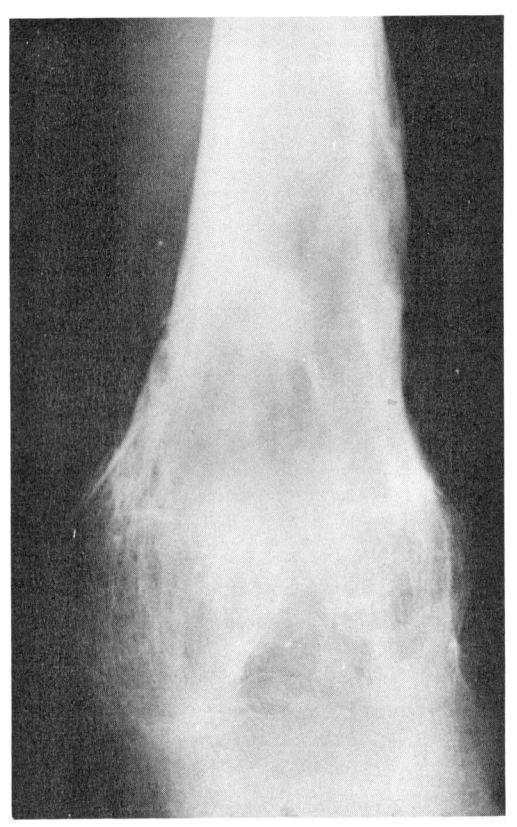

FIG. 53-29. Roentgenograms showing bony ankylosis of the knee following a suppurative arthritis.

with *Neisseria gonorrhea* is rare. When gonococcal arthritis does develop, many joints are affected with migratory arthralgia in most cases. Usually, effusion develops in only one or two joints. In newborn babies gonorrheal arthritis becomes manifest from the fifth day to the fifth week after birth, but generally the infection becomes overt within two weeks. A history of recent gonorrhea or positive prostatic, cervical or urethral culture lends strong support to a diagnosis of gonococcal arthritis; genitourinary symptoms are elicited in only 50 per cent of the patients. Gonococcal arthritis must be differentiated from Reiter's syndrome, in which there is associated conjunctivitis as well as urethritis. It is often difficult to demonstrate the gram-negative diplococci on a smear of the articular fluid. Therefore, the aspirated fluid should be planted on warm chocolate agar medium and cultured in an atmosphere containing 3 to 5 per cent carbon dioxide (Clawson and Dunn, 1967). Gonococcal arthritis will usually respond to penicillin.

VERTEBRAL OSTEOMYELITIS

Osteomyelitis of the spine deserves special comment. Tuberculosis once accounted for more than 90 per cent of infections of the spine; now it is rare in the United States. The pyogenic causes are: (1) idiopathic intervertebral disk space infection of childhood; (2) hematogenous osteomyelitis of the adult; and (3) postoperative infection of the vertebra or disk space.

Idiopathic infection of the intervertebral disk space in children can occur at any age but it is most common between the ages of two and five years. Infants with this condition usually are seen by the physician because of refusal to walk, whereas the older child may complain of vague pain in the back and hips. Scoliosis and tightness of the hamstring muscles are found on physical examination. Blood cultures are usually negative, and roentgenography of the spine shows no abnormality for the first two or three weeks. Thereafter, gradual narrowing of the disk space involved is noted. Erosion and subsequent sclerosis of the vertebral end-plates are seen. The levels from the 12th thoracic space to the 5th lumbar vertebra are affected most commonly. A bacteriologic diagnosis often is difficult to obtain. Staphylococcus appears to be most commonly the offending organism. In all reported cases satisfactory healing without suppuration has occurred. Spontaneous fusion is unlikely. The recommended treatment includes antibiotics, as prescribed for acute hemotogenous infections of bone, and immobilization in a body cast for 10 to 12 weeks.

The clinical manifestations of osteomyelitis of the vertebra in adults are similar to those seen in childhood osteomyelitis. Acute osteomyelitis of the spine is caused most frequently by staphylococcus, but sometimes by *Escherichia coli,* pseudomonas, proteus, or salmonella as well. The lumbar spine is involved most often but any part of the spine may be affected. The infection usually remains localized and tends to heal spontaneously. If a neural arch is involved, the disease may recur, with neurologic symptoms of an epidural abscess or meningitis. When the disease is diagnosed and treated early, conservative measures consisting of bed rest, a cast or brace, and antibiotics are usually effective. When treatment is late, incision and drainage of an abscess or sequestrectomy is usually necessary. In osteomyelitis of the lumber spine an abscess usually forms in the paravertebral area, in Petit's triangle, or in the inguinal region. Often the spine fuses spontaneously and may become stable enough to make arthrodesis unnecessary. A persistent draining sinus is rare. In a series involving 60 patients, the diagnosis of vertebral osteomyelitis was not made before the third month in every case (Young and Owens, 1966). When the cause of a destructive lesion of the vertebra and an associated disk is elusive, a needle biopsy of the vertebra for histologic examination and culture will usually establish a definite diagnosis (Schajowicz and Derqui, 1968).

Osteomyelitis of the spine may also occur secondary to diagnostic or operative procedures. Batson demonstrated that blood from the pelvic veins flows retrograde into the vertebral veins when intra-abdominal pressure is increased. Thus, because there is a sinusoidal venus system within the cancellous part of the vertebra, metastatic spread of an infection from the genitourinary system to the vertebra is easily understood. Lumbar puncture and diskography, as well as laminectomy and spine fusion, may be complicated by osteomyelitis (Thibodeau, 1968). Eliason and Dunlap (1965) reported that osteomyelitis of the spine has been noted following needle biopsy of the prostate.

Actinomycosis

This disease is caused by the fungus *Actinomyces israelii*. The fungus affects the soft tissues more than bone and the latter usually is involved by extension of the primary infection. Actinomycosis usually involves the soft tissues of the head and neck and may spread to the mandible, the lungs (involving the ribs or dorsal vertebrae) or the appendiceal region, and extend to the pelvic bones. If the organisms gain access to bone they form multiple abscesses that are connected by sinuses. The fungus has a powerful lytic action on all tissues and the sinuses are formed by liquefaction necrosis with a wall of granulomatous inflammatory tissue. Colonies of the fungi removed in the pus may appear as amorphous yellow granules which are referred to as sulfur granules. Actinomycosis is a chronic infection and when it involves bone it is difficult to eradicate. Most of the reported cases have responded favorably to large doses of penicillin.

Mendelsohn (1965) has described actinomycosis of the metacarpal bone of the hand. It is thought that actinomycosis of the metacarpal usually is secondary to an injury on the teeth of an opponent. The author's recommended treatment was potassium iodide, beginning with small doses and working up to several hundred grains daily, and drainage of abscesses.

Coccidioidomycosis

Infection caused by the fungus *Coccidioides immitis* occurs in an endemic area that includes the San Joaquin Valley in California, southern Arizona, southern New Mexico, southwestern

Texas, and southeastern Colorado. It has been stated that, in approximately 20 per cent of the patients with disseminated disease, involvement of bones and joints occurs. This is usually in the form of multiple lesions, with some predilection for cancellous bone: the lesion occurs more commonly in the ends of long bones, the vertebral bodies and the pelvis. An occasional monoarticular involvement has been reported. Primary involvement of joints is very rare; the joints are involved through direct extension through the bone and the articular cartilage or adjacent bone lesions. Coccidioidal synovitis of the knee has been reported by Pollock et al. (1967). There also seems to be some predilection for the bony prominences, such as the tibial tubercle, the malleoli, the humeral condyles, the olecranon processes, and the radial styloid.

The outlook is poor in the disseminated type. On the other hand, when a single focus exists, such as in the bone, cure is quite possible with resection of the osseous lesion. Extensive involvement of a part may justify amputation. Amphotericin B has been found effective against this organism.

Syphilis

The incidence of skeletal lesions in newborn infants with syphilis is high. The spirochete characteristically attacks the epiphyseal areas in skeletal syphilis of the unborn. Any or all cylindrical bones may be involved. The normal metaphyseal tissues are replaced by syphilitic granulation. The infection prevents the emergence of the osteoblasts from the capillary lining or the fibroblasts pool, and, consequently, osteoid production is inhibited or prevented. Because the epiphyseal cartilage is avascular the organisms are unable to gain access to this region, and, therefore, the chondroid scaffolding is usually produced. Because osteoid production is inhibited, there is a paucity of cancellous bone in the subchondral area, which produces a zone of abnormal translucency. The lack of spongiosa causes the area to be weakened, and fractures through this site are common. The periosteal reaction is like that of postnatally acquired syphilis. A proliferative reaction most often predominates. The tibia is most often affected and the subperiosteal apposition of bone to the anterior cortical surface produces a forward bowing and sharpening of the anterior margin—the saber shin of congenital syphilis (Aegerter and Kirkpatrick, 1968).

There may be luetic dactylitis of the hands and feet that resembles spina ventosa of tuberculosis, but the involvement is always bilaterally symmetrical and may be thus distinguished.

Acquired syphilis of bones and joints is primarily a periostitis. Both long and flat bones may be involved, predominantly the large bones of the lower leg and the bones of the skull.

Tuberculosis

Bone and joint tuberculosis, like hematogenous osteomyelitis, is a blood-borne disease which of necessity must spread from infection somewhere else in the body, either from the lung or the gastrointestinal tract. In areas where pasteurization of milk is not practical there is a high incidence of bovine tuberculosis. At the time of the onset or the time of diagnosis of bone or joint tuberculosis, there may be no other evidence of tuberculosis, except a primary complex. On the other hand, there may be extensive systemic tuberculosis associated with the bone and joint lesions. Bone and joint tuberculosis is encountered more often in young individuals. Most commonly the spine is involved, with the hip, the knee and the ankle next most commonly involved and in that order. The small bones of the feet, and the shoulder and upper extremity joints are affected much less commonly. Still more rare is the involvement of tendon sheaths and bursae. The involvement may be single or multiple, but more commonly only a single lesion is present. In the extremities a single lesion is more common, but in the spine multiple vertebrae are apt to be involved. Multiple joint lesions are said to occur in about 15 per cent of the cases, although in our experience it has been much less than this.

The "physiologic" relationship between the subchondral cancellous tissue of the metaphysis and the soft tissues that constitute the joint has been pointed out in several instances. In rheumatoid arthritis, when biopsy material is taken from the metaphysis contiguous to the affected joint, an exudative reaction similar to that of the soft tissues is found. Apparently the lymphatic channels of the joint capsule serve as the pathways by which organisms in one area gain access to the other. With tuberculosis, when there is involvement of the metaphyseal area, in most instances there also is a related tuberculous arthritis, and it is impossible to state whether the infection begins within the joint or the cancellous tissue of the metaphysis. Therefore it is not remarkable that tuberculosis often involves both sites. It is remarkable that tumors and suppurative arthritis so rarely do the same.

The lodging of the tubercle bacilli in the bone or joint initially produces vasodilatation, with the inflowing of small round cells; soon this is followed by a fibroblastic response, with the formation of a tubercle, a varying number of giant cells and thrombosis of the small vessels in the neighborhood, so that a necrotic caseous mass is formed (both by action of death of phagocytic cells and the interference with the blood supply in the area of the tubercle).

The x-ray manifestations of tuberculosis of bone are those of slowly progressive bone destruction, which usually is associated with a minimum of bone reaction and little or no formation of sequestra. In cases in which a joint is affected, the destruction of articular cartilage is much slower than is the case with suppurative infections because proteolytic enzymes are not present in the exudate. Tuberculosis of a joint in a child is often associated with enlargement of participating epiphyses.

Tuberculosis of the Spine (Pott's Disease). This disease, like tuberculosis elsewhere, is usually of insidious onset. Often not until the development of a "bump" on the patient's back or even of a secondary psoas abscess is the patient taken to the doctor. The site of the infection is usually the anterior portion of the body of the vetebra at its inferior or superior margin. As a rule it is a destructive lesion resulting in atrophy and bone destruction, without evidence of new bone formation or reaction about it. The intervertebral disk seems to be destroyed early and rapidly when the infection originates at the periphery of the vertebra (Figs. 53-30, 53-31); but if the onset is within the body, there may be considerable destruction without x-ray evidence of involvement of the disk. Occasionally, the host response is such that there is increased density revealed on the roentgenogram.

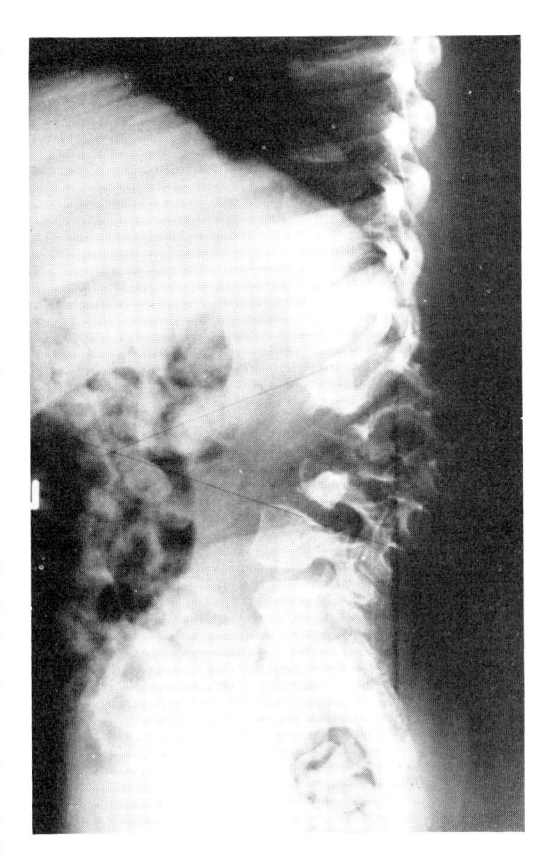

Fig. 53-30. Lateral roentgenogram of the thoracolumbar spine, showing extensive tuberculous destruction of the lumbar vertebrae and early gibbus formation in a child.

In almost all cases of spinal tuberculosis a paravertebral abscess develops which is usually fusiform in nature and is helpful in establishing a diagnosis (Fig. 53-32). The disease is usually more extensive than is demonstrated in the roentgenogram, as pointed out by Cleveland et al. (1958). The paravertebral abscess may form and rupture in the paravertebral area posteriorly (rarely), or (commonly) it may form a psoas abscess which presents at a point in the thigh below the inguinal ligament. Rarely, they may involve the mediastinum. The differential diagnosis is usually not difficult, although the Mantoux test may be negative early in the disease. There have been cases of proved tuberculosis of bones and joints with a negative Mantoux in children. Pyogenic secondary infection or tumor may obscure the diagnosis, and if an accurate diag-

1714   Orthopedics (Nontraumatic)

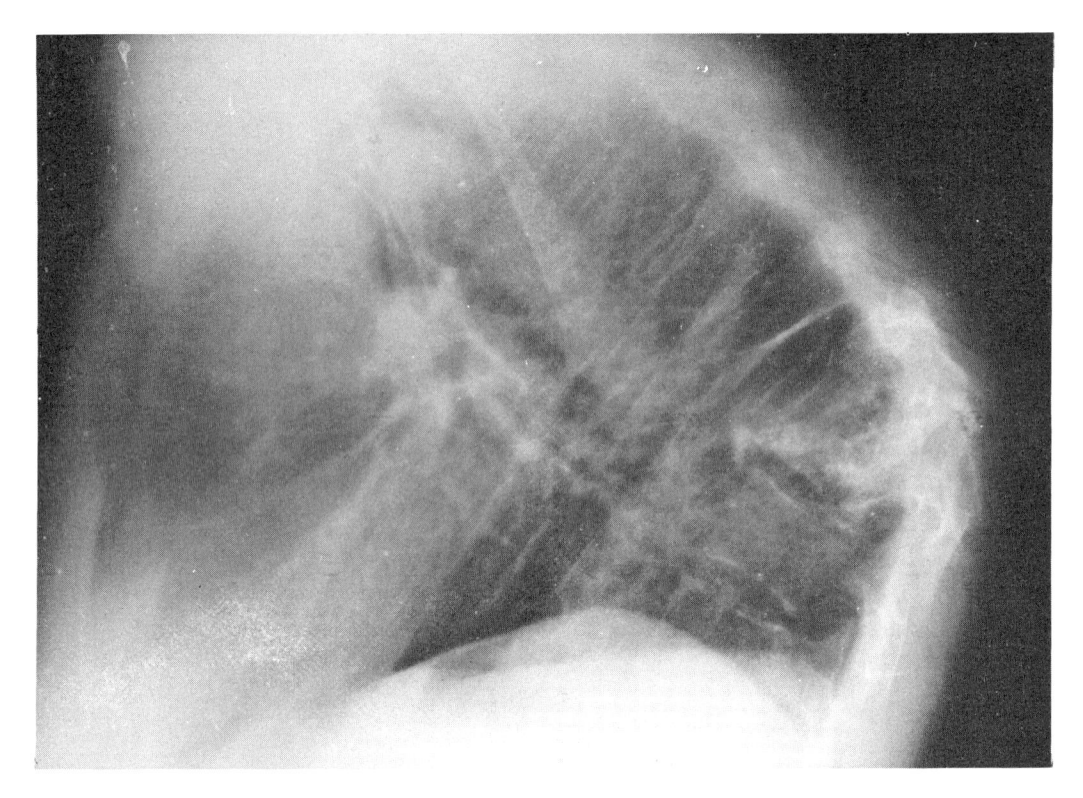

FIG. 53-31. Lateral view, showing extensive destruction of vertebrae and gibbus formation secondary to tuberculosis in an adult.

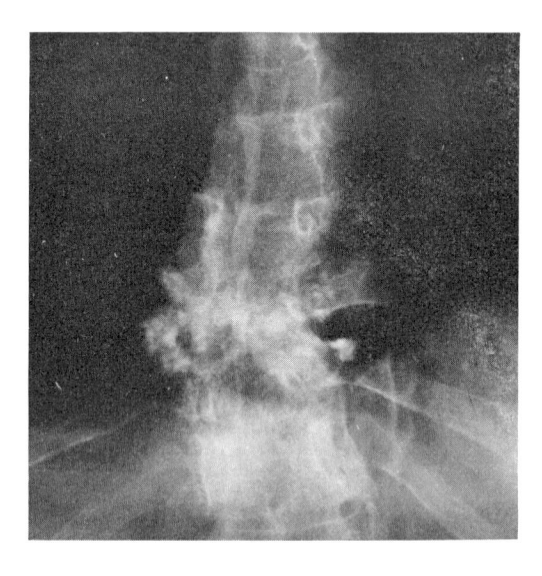

FIG. 53-32. Roentgenogram showing calcified paravertebral tuberculous abscess.

nosis cannot be assured from the usual clinical method, biopsy should be undertaken.

In a series of 64 patients with tuberculosis of the spine, 63 patients had the usual forms of tuberculosis spondylitis with involvement of the vertebral body. In the one exception, the disease was localized in the posterior portion of the vertebral body and in the pedicles, but without neurologic involvement. The thoracolumbar segment of the vertebral column was the most frequently involved site, the lumbosacral region being the second most common site of infection. In this same series of 64 patients, paralysis complicated the course of 8 patients. In each instance paralysis presented during the active stage of the vertebral tuberculosis (Friedman, 1966). The paraplegia is most commonly secondary to a granuloma. However, it also can occur secondary to an old abscess or from extension of the tuberculous infection through the coverings of the spinal cord, presenting at autopsy as tuberculous granulation tissue (Hodgson and Stock, 1960; Hodgson et al., 1967).

Treatment of Tuberculosis of the Spine.
CHEMOTHERAPY. Understanding of the chemotherapy of tuberculosis requires consideration of how the tubercle bacillus is affected by antibacterial agents; the pathology of the process being treated; and the defense mechanisms, or the response of the host to tuberculous infection. At the present time, no antimycobacterial agent or combination of agents is capable of eliminating all tubercle bacilli regularly from infected tissue even when such therapy is prolonged. A number of factors account for this: (1) Tubercle bacilli that are not multiplying are not significantly affected by present day chemotherapy. (2) Some of these bacteria become resistant to the antibacterial drugs to which they are exposed. (3) Many tubercle bacilli are not free in body fluids but exist intracellularly. Streptomycin and para-aminosalicylic acid penetrate phagocytes inadequately and, therefore, suppress growth only of extracellular tubercle bacilli.

In addition, the acidic reaction in areas of caseation necrosis inhibits streptomycin activity, and nucleic acids bind streptomycin, rendering it inert. Para-aminosalicylic acid is inactivated by para-aminobenzoic acid, which is found in purulent exudate. Isoniazid is effective against both intra- and extracellular organisms; however, pyruvic acid, a normal metabolite, suppresses the action of isoniazid (Hollander, 1966).

It is generally agreed that a combination of agents is preferable to single drug therapy, in order to take advantage of synergistic action and to delay or prevent the emergence of drug-resistant bacilli. When two agents are used, some of the bacteria will be resistant to one drug and some to the other. However, the number of mutants that are simultaneously resistant to both drugs is extremely low or almost negligible. If an organism becomes resistant to one of the drugs, the other agent present should overcome it as it multiplies. The use of all three antituberculous drugs simultaneously has not been shown to be superior to the use of two, and with three used together toxicity is increased (Badger, 1959). There is no unanimity in regard to a preferable schedule, but any regimen containing isoniazid is superior to all others. The experience in bone and joint tuberculosis has been chiefly with streptomycin combined with either PAS or INH. Both regimens have been highly effective; however, on the basis of the present experience in skeletal tuberculosis, isoniazid with streptomycin is the preferable combination. Intra-articular streptomycin may be used in addition to parenteral administration but, since the drug passes readily into joint fluids when given intramuscularly, this is not necessary.

SPINAL FUSION. Although the chemotherapeutic agents are very valuable, some form of immobilization for the spine remains the basis of treatment. Bed rest and plaster cast and fixation alone may be helpful, but the best method of putting the spine to rest and immobilizing it is spinal fusion. It is the opinion of some orthopedic surgeons with experience in the field of skeletal tuberculosis that posterior spine fusion, by rigidly immobilizing such a segment, can prevent the development of a deforming kyphosis that might occur either from the stress of weight bearing or from the destruction of vertebral bodies by the disease (Cleveland et al., 1958). It is difficult to determine to what extent posterior spine fusion prevents the development of deformity, since kyphosis does not occur in all patients with spinal tuberculosis; in a recent series of tuberculosis of the spine, an angulation of 10 degrees or greater developed in only one fourth of the 64 patients (Friedman, 1966). Of these patients, slightly less than half already had the maximum kyphosis before they became ambulatory. Bakalim (1960) reported on 59 patients with Pott's disease treated with modified Albee spine fusion; some were given the antituberculous drugs; others had been treated before these drugs came into use. He reported that in 44 per cent a kyphosis greater than 10 degrees developed.

Most authors have concluded that solid fusion may not prevent increasing spinal deformity because of the amount of deformity was found to be directly proportional to the degree of destruction of the vertebral bodies. In the majority of reported cases of patients treated with spinal fusion, the fusion did not hold the diseased vertebrae apart for long.

Stabilization by anterior fusion has been gaining in popularity over the past few years (Kirkaldy-Willis, 1965). It is reported to be an effective means of preventing kyphosis. Hodgson and Stock (1960) stated that only one instance of increasing deformity followed their 100 anterior spine fusions, and this in a patient in whom chip grafts were used.

The treatment of spinal tuberculosis in the elderly poses special problems. In general, old people are unwilling to stay in the hospital for long periods of time. They tolerate immobilization in plaster casts or plaster beds poorly and frequently discontinue treatment too early, only to return later in worse condition. In a recent series (Arct, 1968), 72 patients over the age of 60 years were treated by operative excision of the diseased bone, bone grafts, and local and systemic antituberculous drugs. These patients were compared to a series of 61 patients over 60 years of age who were treated by conservative therapy alone. In the latter group the patients were quite unhappy and often uncooperative, and the rate of recurrence was found to be 31 per cent. The average hospital stay was 16 months for the patients treated conservatively and 5 months for the patients treated by surgery.

It must be remembered that a fusion of the spine is merely the best way to put the spine at rest; it does not cure the tuberculous process but merely affords the host a better chance to control the disease process.

Paraplegia in a patient with tuberculosis of the spine is a very serious complication. Laminectomy usually is advocated although it does not attack the site of the disease. Costotransversectomy or anterolateral decompression appears to be a more rational operation for decompression of the spinal cord in a patient with paraplegia due to tuberculous spondylitis. There is still disagreement whether a thoracotomy or lateral rhachotomy (anterolateral decompression) should be used to expose a thoracic vertebral body. It was felt that, whenever possible, a transpleural approach (thoracotomy) should be used because it is simpler and easier and gives more exposure and, hence, permits the performance of a better surgical procedure (Kirkaldy-Willis, 1965).

Articular Tuberculosis. Joint tuberculosis may involve the periarticular soft tissues, the synovium, the cartilage, the bone, or all four. Most joint tuberculosis starts in the synovium at the point of its reflection from the articular cartilage or the epiphyseal plate.

After the involvement of the synovium, lesions may spread along the articular cartilage from the periphery by direct extension from the synovial reflection and invade and destroy the cartilage, with pannus formation. In children tuberculous granulation tissue may invade the subcondylar plate or attack the epiphysis distal to the epiphyseal line, depriving a large segment of bone of its blood flow and nutrition and thus killing it. In articular tuberculosis, the weight-bearing portion of the articular cartilage tends to be preserved, while the periphery and the non-weight-bearing portions are susceptible to attack and destruction. This is in contrast with the pyogenic arthritic joint in which the weight-bearing surfaces are destroyed first. At times in tuberculous arthritis the weight-bearing surfaces are well preserved while a large amount of the cartilaginous bone is undermined by the fibrous granulation tissue, and as a consequence a large section of the articular surface may be deprived of support and sequestrate. Such sequestration on both sides of the joint constitutes the so-called "kissing sequestrae."

Treatment of Extravertebral Tuberculosis. The use of streptomycin and isonicotinic acid (INH) or para-aminosalicylic acid (PAS) has radically changed the treatment and improved the outlook in tuberculous arthritis. If the infection is recognized early, before necrosis and walling off of the process with caseation and abscess formation have developed, drug therapy combined with the usual conservative measures—rest, splinting of the lesion, and proper diet—often results in healing of the lesions. If walling off, necrosis and caseation have occurred, surgical intervention is necessary to control the infection. When possible, total excision is preferred; if excision is not possible, débridement of all necrotic and caseous tissue and open packing of the wound, to be closed with delayed suture. Surgery should be undertaken as early as possible, before resistance to the drugs has a chance to develop.

If significant destruction of joint surfaces has taken place, complete healing is unlikely to occur without surgical fusion. In non-weight-bearing joints, arthrodesis may be postponed until conservative measures alone have been tried. In weight-bearing joints, arrest of the disease is most rapidly attained and secured, by drug therapy combined with early solid fusion of the joint, which has been first débrided of all caseous and necrotic tissue. Drug therapy should be continued for a minimum of 1 year, preferably for 18 months. It must be remembered that tuberculous arthritis is almost always a metastatic infection, and great care must be taken to seek the primary focus and other possible metastatic lesions (Hollander, 1966). A 10-year follow-up study of combined drug therapy and early fusion in bone and joint tuberculosis found that solid fusion with normal cancellous trabeculation occurred in all patients. Arthrodesis of the peripheral joints was advocated because much greater destruction of the articulation was found on exploration than was evident on the roentgenograms. None of the patients had reactivation of their tuberculosis even though they received triple drug therapy for a relatively short time (only one for longer than 1 year), and drug therapy was not continued after discharge (Allen and Stevenson, 1967).

Other Forms of Synovial Tuberculosis. Tuberculosis of Bursae. This is not rare. It should be treated by radical excision en bloc.

Tendon sheaths are not uncommonly involved. The process varies from a chronic, relatively mild tenosynovitis to an enormous distention of the sheath, with a granulomatous mass and rice bodies and with matting together of neighboring tendons. The best treatment of this condition has not been clearly established. Key (1954) in a general survey of this problem from a number of orthopedic centers, found a lack of uniformity of opinion. Our experience suggests that surgical débridement of the lesion so that the sheath is completely opened, washing away of the pus and the necrotic debris, closure of the wound, immobilization and chemotherapy offer an excellent chance of cure.

DEGENERATIVE DISEASE OF JOINTS

Degenerative Arthritis

The etiology of the degenerative changes that commonly occur in joints as individuals age is very poorly understood. Because many patients who develop this disease early are overweight, theories suggesting endocrine or metabolic dysfunction have been formulated. Systemic infections and climatic conditions have largely been discarded as the causes. Some believe there may be hereditary developmental weakness of the articular cartilage that predisposes it to damage and early degeneration. However, these theories fail to explain the histopathologic changes that occur.

In many instances the underlying cause of degeneration is insult to the joint surfaces of a mechanical nature, i.e., (1) fractures into a joint surface with resultant irregular joint surfaces; (2) abnormal motion due to injury to ligaments and supporting structures; (3) direct damage to the articular cartilage from (a) pyogenic arthritis or (b) atrophic arthritis; (4) impaired circulation of the subchondral bone secondary to injury, and (5) developmental anomalies of the joint, resulting in incongruity of the articular surface.

Because many of the known causes of degenerative arthritis are of a mechanical nature, it seems likely that this may be the most important cause in all instances of the disease.

In studying degenerative changes of the hip joint, Harrison, Schajawiez and Trueta (1953) found that without exception the initiation of the osteoarthritic process took place in the articular cartilage. There was softening, fibrillation, necrosis and frictional erosion of the cartilage. Harrison *et al.* (1953) found that the histochemical change was a reduction of metachromasia of the cartilage and that the area of the joint in which the degenerative process started was the non-weight-bearing portion. Some of these changes were present in all the joints of persons examined who were over 14 years of age.

Hyperemia, irregular calcification of the deeper layers of cartilage, and sclerosis and thickening of the subchondral line in which both bone destruction and new bone formation is active occurs.

Exostoses around the edges of the joint surfaces are well known characteristics of osteoarthritis. They occur only at joints in which an osteoarthritic pattern of reaction constitutes the major pathologic feature. Their presence is not essential to the diagnosis of osteoarthritis and they are relatively late mani-

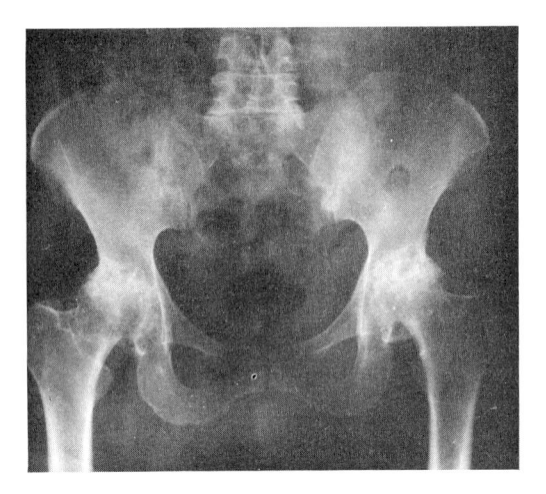

FIG. 53-33. Roentgenogram of the pelvis, showing advanced osteoarthritis of both hips, with osteophyte formation, multiple subchondral cysts, sclerosis and almost complete obliteration of the joint line.

festations. Osteophytes always indicate the presence of advanced cartilage destruction in the more central parts of the articulation on which they appear. Unlike most exostoses arising from bone shafts, intra-articular osteophytes are not formed in the insertion of ligaments and tendons, and their tips, covered only by a smooth fibrous or fibrocartilagenous sheet, reach out into the synovial cavity. The direction of growth of marginal osteophytes usually continues the contour of the surface from which they project. The effect of all osteophytes is, therefore, to exaggerate the shape of the bone end and the contour of the articular surface. In the later stages of the disease the marginal osteophytes fuse to form continuous blocks of new bone on either side of the joint. A good example of this may be seen in the "mushroom deformity" of the femoral head, with the correspondingly deepened acetabulum (Collins, 1949).

Cysts filled with fluid, fibrous tissue or fibrocartilage are commonly found in juxtaposition to the articular weight-bearing area of the subchondral bone. They connect with the joint cavity and may be surrounded by a rich vascular bed. The process of functional erosion of the articular cartilage is progressive, and ultimately the subchondral bone may be completely denuded of cartilage. By this time the bone has become dense and eburnated, cortical bone having replaced the lost cancellous structure of normal subchondral bone (Fig. 53-33).

Calcified loose bodies are occasionally seen in advanced osteoarthritis; their origin is obscure. In the condition known as synovial chondromatosis, multiple small chondro-osseous bodies arise by metaplasia in synovial villi. Many bodies thought to be loose are in fact still attached by a thin pedicle to the synovial tissues, and, when these are removed, sections show blood filled vessels. Detached bodies show necrotic bone surrounded by living but avascular cartilage. Fragments of detached articular cartilage are occasionally found, but they do not persist indefinitely nor, of course, are they visible on the x-ray film.

In some cases the synovial cells proliferate, and the synovium becomes hyperplastic, forming villi. In others the synovium and the capsule contract and become fibrotic.

Once these degenerative changes have started, they tend to be progressive and may result in complete disorganization of the joint. The rate of progression varies a great deal from case to case, yet, given enough time, the end result will be about the same in all. There are no known means of reversing the process, although the rate of progression and the symptoms may be retarded by remedial exercises.

Although marked restriction of joint motion results, bony ankylosis does not occur. The dense eburnated, relatively avascular bone surfaces opposed to each other and the absence of vascular granulation tissue account for the failure of union at the two joint surfaces by bone. In fact, arthrodesis of the joint cannot be produced unless the avascular ends are excited to bring more vascular cancellous surfaces into contact. However, vertebral bodies may fuse by marginal osteophytic bridging (Lewin, 1964). A similar process does not occur in the major articulations of any extremities.

Because it has not been found possible to restore the degenerative arthritic joint to normal, treatment is necessarily directed toward relief of pain and retardation of the rate of progression. With advanced disease, treatment is directed again to the relief of pain and restoring as much function as possible. Surgery is indicated only after conservative measures have failed.

The surgical procedures available include proximal femoral osteotomies (Crellin and Simorda, 1965; Ferguson, 1964); total replacement of the hip joint (McKee, 1966); replacement of the femoral head, using an Austin Moore prosthesis (Heywood-Waddington, 1966; McDonough et al., 1967), or the use of a metal cup (McDonough, 1967). Degenerative arthritis of the knee may be treated by patellectomy, proximal tibial osteotomy (Coventry, 1965; Torgerson, 1965) and, more recently, the use of a hinged metal knee prosthesis (Girzadas et al., 1968; Young, 1963).

Rheumatoid Arthritis

Although the actual cause of rheumatoid arthritis remains unknown, in recent years great strides have been taken toward better understanding of the basic nature of the disease and its pathogenesis. Perhaps since the earliest days of bacteriology, it was suspected that rheumatoid disease was an infectious disorder, and the organism most suspect was the tubercle bacillus. Allergic, nutritional, endocrine, and hereditary factors have claimed—and in some cases still enjoy—their share of the spotlight. It is also now well recognized that rheumatoid arthritis has important psychosomatic aspects.

The concept of autoimmunity implies that an organism under certain conditions may produce antibodies against its own cells or tissues, which act as antigens. That some alteration of the immune mechanism seems to exist in rheumatoid arthritis is supported by the discovery of rheumatoid factor. This protein is a high molecular weight macroglobulin that can be demonstrated in the serum of a large percentage of patients with rheumatoid arthritis. Two questions that still remain unanswered are: (1) What induces the patient's own protein to suddenly become antigenic? and (2) Do these complexes of antigen and antibody have anything to do with the induction of the disease, or are they only immunologic by-products unrelated to pathogenesis?

The current concepts of the pathogenesis of joint inflammation and rheumatoid arthritis are discussed in an article by Zvaifler (1965). The American Rheumatism Association (1959) has set forth certain diagnostic criteria for rheumatoid arthritis. These include morning sickness, pain in one joint, swelling of one joint, swelling of a second joint, symmetrical swelling, subcutaneous nodules, typical x-ray changes, rheumatoid factor, a poor mucin clot, characteristic synovial histology and characteristic nodule histology. Classification of rheumatoid arthritis as classic, definite, probable, or possible depends on the number of the above-mentioned criteria that are met. Rheumatoid nodules, if proved histologically, are practically pathognomonic for rheumatoid arthritis. However, pseudorheumatoid nodules have been described in patients without rheumatoid arthritis (Mesara et al., 1966). The rheumatoid factor is present in approximately 70 per cent of cases, but it is present in approximately 5 per cent of normal persons also.

Rheumatoid arthritis is in many respects similar in nature in both children and adults; however, there are certain distinguishing features. The high fever and rash are seen in approximately 25 to 30 per cent of the juvenile form and in approximately 1 to 5 per cent of the adult. Absence of joint pain, which is highly unusual in the adult form, may be noted in approximately 25 per cent of the juvenile form. The symptoms may present in a single joint in the juvenile form in about 30 per cent of cases; in the adult form this is a rather unusual finding. Subcutaneous nodules are approximately four times as prevalent in the adult form of arthritis, compared with the juvenile form. The test for rheumatoid factor is positive in approximately 10 to 20 per cent of the juvenile form and in approximately 65 to 85 per cent of the adult form.

The so-called RA cell was first described in 1964 by Hollander (1966). This cell is an ordinary leukocyte that is present in the synovial fluid and contains inclusion bodies appearing as dark spots in the cytoplasm. In some studies RA cells have been found in more than 75 per cent of rheumatoid fluids. However, morphologically indistinguishable intra-leukocytic inclusions were identified in more than 50 per cent of samples of nonrheumatoid inflammatory fluids, such as occur with gout, septic joints, etc. (Sones, 1968).

A peculiar form of rheumatoid arthritis is rheumatoid spondylitis, which occurs 10 times more commonly among men than women and involves the sacroiliac joints and the small apophyseal joints of the spine, with calcifica-

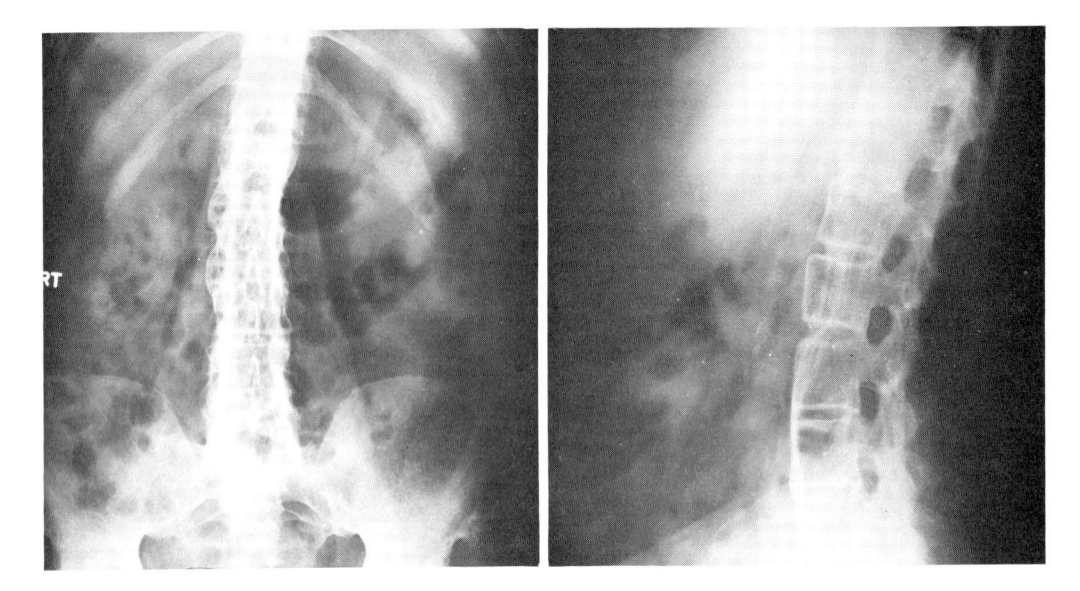

Fig. 53-34. Roentgenograms illustrating extensive bony ankylosis of the entire spine, in a patient with rheumatoid spondylitis. The vertebral bodies are squared off, with calcification of the anterior longitudinal ligament. The result is a "bamboo" spine.

tion of the spinous ligaments (Fig. 53-34). It does not involve the intervertebral disks. Cases of rheumatoid spondylitis do not have the high titers of agglutinins to hemolytic streptococci that are found with peripheral involvement, and pain is often relieved by small doses of deep x-ray therapy, but the course of the disease is not altered by x-ray therapy. The pathology in both conditions is essentially the same. Bennett et al. (1942) found that the earliest changes in atrophic arthritis were hyperemia, with lymphocyte and plasma cell infiltration of the subsynovia, showing a tendency for these cells to collect into follicles. Ghormley and Deacon (1936) pointed out the diagnostic value of this round cell collection and demonstrated that they were not perivascular. The synovium becomes edematous and proliferative, with the development of a vascular pannus which spreads over the articular cartilage, destroying and replacing the joint cartilage. There is an associated proliferation of connective tissue in the marrow spaces beneath the subchondral plate, with destruction of bone and cartilage, thinning of the bone trabeculae and cortex, and effusion into the joint.

Synovial biopsies and excision of rheumatoid nodules may be helpful in the diagnosis of rheumatoid arthritis. The usefulness of synovial biopsy is limited by the fact, that, in early stages of the disease when diagnosis may prove most challenging, the synovitis is often quite nonspecific.

The medical treatment of rheumatoid arthritis includes: (1) A program of rest, physical therapy and salicylate therapy; (2) intra-articular medication, including steroids; (3) orthopedic appliances; and (4) supplementary medication, which includes gold, systemic steroids, phenylbutazone, and indomethacin. It should be emphasized that approximately two thirds of the patients who have rheumatoid arthritis will respond satisfactorily to nonsurgical measures and thus are not candidates for operation.

In evaluating the role that surgery should take in the over-all treatment program, one must consider both what procedures are available and practicable and what one is trying to accomplish with them. The goals one hopes to achieve include: relief of pain; prevention of destruction of cartilage or tendon; and improvement of over-all joint function—by increasing or decreasing joint motion, by correction of deformities, by increasing stability, by improving effective muscle forces, or by some combination of these measures.

Everyone is concerned primarily with preventive surgery—for example, synovectomy—rather than reconstructive surgery. Of major importance in planning synovectomy is the timing of the procedure. Ideally, this operation should be performed when the features of chronic reactive synovitis are present and before significant destruction of cartilage has taken place.

Considerable relief may be obtained by reconstructive procedures on both the upper and the lower extremities. In a patient with early rheumatoid involvement of the knee, synovectomy is the procedure of choice, and in the patient with great involvement, joint débridement, patelloplasty, patellectomy, arthroplasty, proximal tibial osteotomy and, finally, arthrodesis should be considered (Peterson, 1968).

In the management of rheumatoid arthritis at the hip, results are not as successful as with degenerative joint disease, and frequent revisions are probable.

In the rheumatoid foot, surgery on the fore part of the foot involves bone stabilization by arthrodesis. Flexion deformities of the toes are easily corrected.

Similar procedures are used in upper extremity joints. In the shoulder joint, pain can be controlled by periodic intra-articular injections of steroids. Synovectomy has seldom been indicated but can be accomplished. The basic program of aspirin, heat, massage, and range-of-motion exercises has in general been sufficient for the shoulder without surgical intervention.

Synovectomy of the elbow is indicated when x-rays reveal severe proliferative synovitis, ligamentous instability, and erosive changes of the joint. Subcutaneous nodules are common over the olecranon and the subcutaneous surface of the ulnar and, when excised, periosteum beneath the nodule as well as the nodule itself should be excised.

Proliferative rheumatoid synovitis affects the tendon sheaths as well as the multiple small joints of the hand and wrist. Synovectomy of the involved tendon sheath is indicated before tendon rupture occurs. If tendon rupture has occurred, tendon transfer or tendon grafting should be done at the time of synovectomy. Occasionally tenosynovitis on the volar aspect of the wrist may result in the carpal tunnel syndrome. This will necessitate excision of the synovium around the flexor tendons.

Rheumatoid arthritis involving the wrist may necessitate a synovectomy, or, if the distal portion of the radio-ulnar joint is badly destroyed, the resection of the distal end of the ulnar. If the wrist joint is severely destroyed or satisfactory reconstruction is not possible, an arthrodesis should be performed (Fig. 53-35).

Rheumatoid involvement of the hand may necessitate a synovectomy, correction of ulnar drift, interphalangeal arthrodesis or a combination of any of these procedures (Linscheid, 1968).

Often flexion contractures may be corrected by wedging casts and traction. Osteotomy is a useful operation in selected cases, particularly of the spine (Goel, 1968; Smith-Petersen et al., 1945). Smith and Kaplan (1967) have written an excellent article describing the rheumatoid deformities at the metacarpo-phalangeal joints of the fingers.

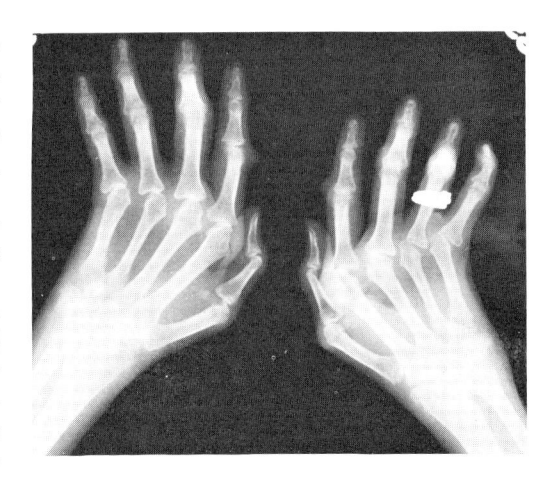

FIG. 53-35. Severe rheumatoid arthritis. There are narrowing of the proximal interphalangeal joints, ulnar drift and subluxation at the metacarpophalangeal joints, and marked destruction of the carpal bones.

NEUROPATHIC JOINT DISEASE (CHARCOT JOINT)

Neuropathic joint disease—formerly called chronic progressive degenerative arthropathy—affects one or more peripheral and/or vertebral articulations and develops as a result of a disturbance in normal sensory innervation of the joints. Charcot joints occur more often in

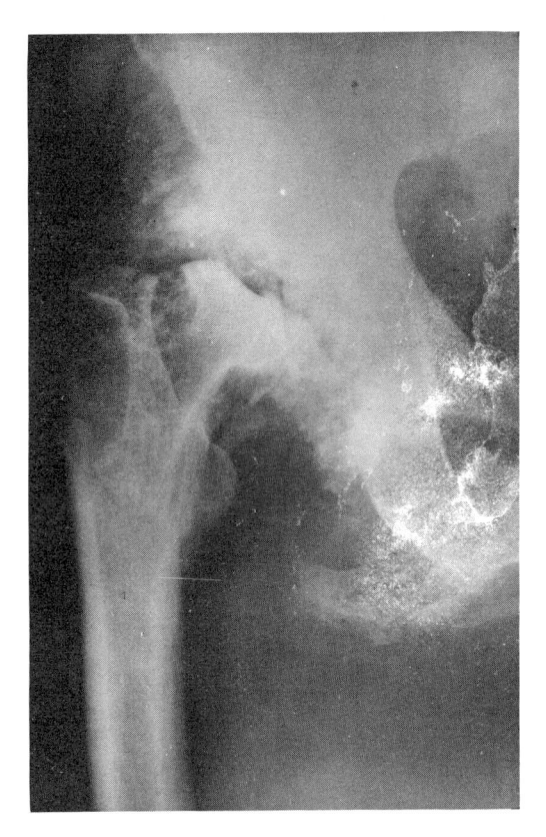

FIG. 53-36. Neurogenic arthropathy. There is massive destruction of the femoral head, with evidence of moderate new bone formation and extensive disorganization of the joint.

men than women and, if pediatric cases are excluded, usually develop past the age of 40. Historically Charcot neuropathy is associated with tabes dorsalis, yet only 5 to 10 per cent of tabetic patients have bone and joint changes. These occur primarily in active individuals who often are ataxic and show a propensity for injury. For many years recognition of this arthropathy was limited almost solely to its occurrence in patients with syphilitic tabes dorsalis. However, neuropathic arthropathy may have other causes: diabetic neuropathy, syringomyelia, myelomeningocele, congenital insensitivity to pain and arthropathy following intra-articular injection of corticosteroids.

The proprioceptive loss apparently allows the joint to be subjected to multiple injuries. The main feature that all these conditions producing Charcot joint have in common is absence or depression of pain sensation in the presence of continued physical activity. By contrast, absence of pain combined with severe physical disability, as in paraplegia, is associated with marked osteoporosis and limited activity. The various neurologic disorders resulting in a Charcot-like joint do not all affect the same joints. Syphilitic tabes dorsalis affects the knee, the hip, the ankle, and the lumbar and lower dorsal vertebrae. Diabetic neuropathy constitutes an increasingly frequent basis for Charcot joint disease and now ranks a close second to, if not the equal of tabes dorsalis in this respect. The tarsus, tarsometatarsal and metatarsophalangeal joint are usually affected. Syringomyelia commonly affects the shoulder, the elbow, and the cervical vertebrae. Neuropathic joint disease is said to occur in approximately one fourth of the patients with syringomyelia (Hollander, 1966). Myelomeningocele commonly affects the ankle and the tarsus. This is the most frequent basis of neuropathic arthropathy in childhood. Congenital insensitivity to pain (an entity recently identified) also affects commonly the tarsus and the ankle joints. A number of reports have described rapid deterioration of the hip or knee following repeated intra-articular injection of hydrocortisone, with clinical and roentgenographic findings similar to those of neuropathic arthropathy (Evelagos et al., 1966; Miller and Restifo, 1956; Salter et al., 1967). It has been suggested that the relief of pain provided by such treatment permits excessive weight bearing and mobility and interferes with normal protective processes, thereby accelerating the progress of the underlying joint disease (usually rheumatoid arthritis or osteoarthritis). However, the question of a neuropathic basis for these joint changes remains a controversial matter, since patients treated with steroids retain normal sensibility to pain.

The pathogenesis and end result of neurogenic arthropathy are those of a greatly exaggerated and fulminant degenerative joint disease. The onset is insidious but the pace of the degenerative process, particularly if the patient remains active, is much more rapid than is found in osteoarthritis. One of the most important early features of the disease, and one that is more often than not overlooked, is loss of stability of the joint. This is probably due to early decrease in tendon and ligament tone. The involved tissues attempt to compensate for this loss by a remarkable peripheral growth of cartilage, which matures to form bone. Thus, long struts and bizarre craggy masses of bone are produced in the joint space, the joint capsule, about the joint and extending far beyond the joint along muscle planes, sometimes to attach to the adjoining bone member (Fig. 53-36).

Mechanical injury to the synovium is probably the most important cause of the effusion that plays such an important role in the Charcot joint. Although the effusion causes less pain than might be expected, it may nonetheless be the most prominent and most complained of feature for many months of the early phase of the disease.

The current concepts of the treatment of neuropathic joints are reviewed in an excellent article by Johnson (1967). Essentially it consists in bracing the joints, but, with the progressive nature of the disease, arthrodesis may ultimately be required.

Arthropathy following radiation was recently described by Kolar and Vrabec (1967).

UPPER EXTREMITY PAIN

In office orthopedics, one of the most common of the patient complaints is a painful neck, shoulder or arm. At times it may be difficult to identify the responsible pathologic process. Pain in the shoulder may be caused by (1) calcified tendinitis of a segment of the "rotator cuff," (2) so-called bursitis without calcification; (3) degenerative changes in the joint or affecting the tendon of the long head of the biceps; (4) tumor, either primary or secondary, of any element of the scapulohumeral articulation; (5) degeneration or dislocation of the acromioclavicular joint; (6) rupture of a component of the rotator cuff; (7) atrophic or degenerative arthritis of the scapulohumeral joint; or it may be (8) referred pain, from a lesion of the cervical spine, compression of a nerve root due to narrowing of the intervertebral foramen, by spur or degenerative changes and spinal cord tumor; referred pain from neurovascular irritation or compression at the base of the neck (scalenus anticus syndrome); pain from a tumor of the apex of the lung; or (9) referred pain from gallbladder or a cardiac condition.

CALCIFIED TENDINITIS

The etiology of this condition is unknown. Theories that postulate repeated trauma of the tendons of the rotator cuff, with subsequent degeneration of a portion allowing calcification, are most popular; however, they do not answer all the questions, because (1) there is no evidence of necrotic or degenerative tendon on microscopic study, and (2) the condition occurs most commonly in middle life and is rarely seen in old age, whereas degeneration or spontaneous rupture of the rotator cuff is frequently found in the aged when calcification is seldom encountered.

Single trauma probably plays no part, as the x-ray evidence of a calcium deposit suggests its presence prior to the injury. Furthermore, the vast majority of sufferers report no injury or other known cause.

Calcium and phosphorus metabolism in all cases studied has been normal. However, since calcium deposits could not be expected in normal tendon, some changes of a chemical nature must take place in the tendon to allow deposition of this material. McCarroll (1957) found that in the early "acute shoulder" without roentgenographic evidence of calcification a white liquid could be aspirated that had the appearance of a calcium suspension; however, on study it proved to have very little calcium and contained for the most part white blood cells. Later, calcification took place and reached a high degree of concentration. These findings suggest that an acute inflammatory change occurs which is followed rather rapidly with calcium deposition. The deposits are found initially in the tendon and work their way to the surface, eventually rupturing into the bursa.

Bosworth (1941) found calcifications in one or both shoulders in 2.7 per cent of 6,061 supposedly normal people. Thus, the deposits may be asymptomatic and x-rays should be obtained of both shoulders.

Pain and restriction of motion may be severe and acute, or subacute or chronic. Pain is usually about the shoulder and referred to the deltoid insertion on the humerus with an ache in the arm, the forearm and the hand. Pain may radiate to the base of the neck, although neck motions are not restricted, nor does motion of the neck produce arm pain. However, there may be tenderness over the body of the

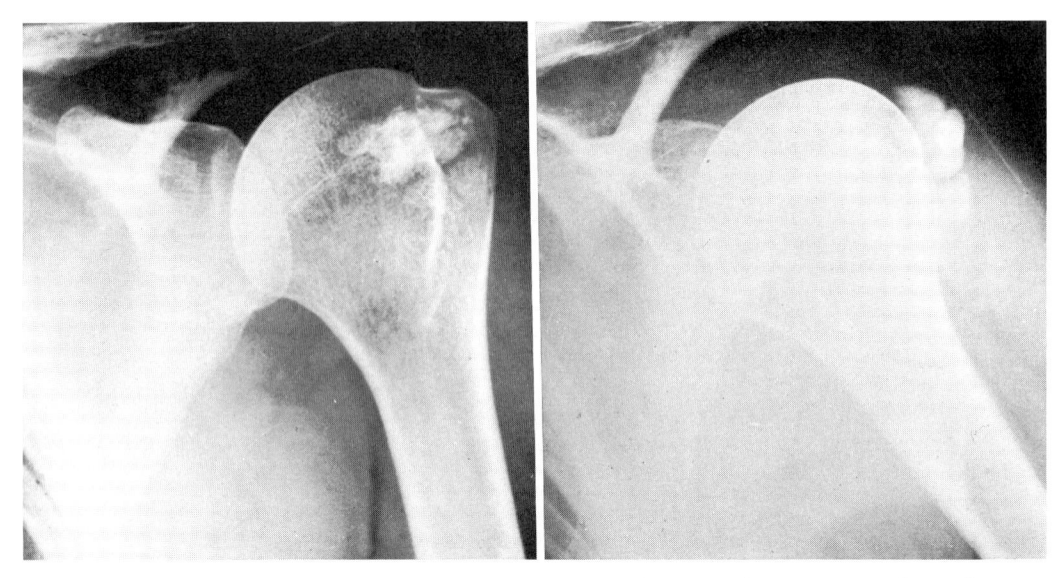

FIG. 53-37. External and internal rotational views of the upper humerus, revealing a large multilocular calcium deposit in the rotator cuff.

muscle of the involved tendon (i.e., supraspinatus (Moseley, 1963).

In most cases the roentgenogram will reveal a calcium deposit, usually a faint irregular shadow. Occasionally, there is also a dense smooth deposit in addition that represents an old calcification. In some, the calcification is so fluid that a shadow is not made out and may never show if the inflammatory process is severe enough to result in rapid absorption. We know this is true as we have been able on occasion to wash out a milky solution which we have assumed to be calcium from these shoulders presenting a picture of acute tendinitis but with a negative roentgenogram.

Treatment by irrigation with procaine by the single needle technic and instillation of hydrocortisone has given dramatic relief of symptoms (Quigley, 1963). On the other hand, even repeated injection has not been effective in some patients. In many, deep x-ray therapy is successful in relieving pain, but occasionally all measures fail to control pain, so that surgical excision of as much of the calcium deposit as possible is required (McLoughlin, 1963). None of these measures will remove all the deposit. Often the calcification will disappear with the subsidence of symptoms. This is dependent on the inflammatory responses rather than the therapy. More often a portion remains even after complete relief of symptoms. This old deposit becomes walled off and does not produce symptoms. Recurrence of pain months or years later is usually the result of a new deposit, but is uncommon.

The complication of this condition is restriction of motion of the shoulder—the so-called frozen shoulder, or adhesive periarthritis. After pain subsides, exercise usually will restore function. Occasionally, there is so much restriction that manipulation under anesthesia is helpful in starting recovery of function (Quigley, 1963). However, the life history of the condition is such that if untreated even the severely painful and stiff shoulder may be expected to recover completely in time.

Bursitis without calcification is seldom so acute; it is more common in the female and may have a high psychogenic element. Pain and tenderness are more diffuse, and restriction of motion less marked. These are often resistant to all forms of therapy but usually can be relieved by combined psychotherapy and physical measures, such as x-ray therapy, hydrocortisone injections and appropriate psychosomatic adjustment.

A painful, swollen and often stiff hand associated with a painful shoulder which may also have considerable restriction of motion is encountered occasionally. This so-called shoulder-hand syndrome perhaps occurs more often in cardiac cases. The hand is usually warm, moist and more deeply colored than the opposite one. Frequently, sensation is increased without segmental distribution. Pain is described as a burning ache, and at times the patient will state that it feels as though a band were fixed tightly about the hand or the wrist. To complete the syndrome there is restriction of motion of the shoulder because of pain in the early stages and adhesions about the joint later on. There is diffuse pain about the shoulder with radiation down the arm, and there also may be diffuse or localized tenderness. The x-ray findings are always negative except for evidence of atrophy in long-standing cases.

As the primary condition seems to be a reflex dystrophy, treatment includes (1) sympathetic block of the stellate ganglion with procaine, (2) cortisone to control pain and (3) physiotherapy or (4) manipulation. Late cases always have some residual impairment of function of the hand.

BICIPITAL TENOSYNOVITIS

This problem is often overlooked by some and not considered a clinical entity by others. The problem occurs where the tendon of the long head of the biceps muscle glides through the bicipital groove in the proximal humerus. Here, although covered by synovium, the tendon is intra-articular but extrasynovial. In a series of 89 patients the etiology was considered traumatic in 31 per cent, secondary to other shoulder lesions in 40 per cent, and was unknown in 43 per cent (Crenshaw and Kilgore, 1966). The pain is localized over the anterior lateral aspect of the shoulder and referred along the anterior surface of the arm. It is aggravated by motion, relieved by rest. Physical examination reveals tenderness directly over the biceps tendon in its groove anteriorly. X-rays are usually negative. Conservative therapy consists in rest until the pain subsides, then gentle motion until a full range of motion is restored. Chronic involvement usually results in adhesive fibrosis and surgical intervention is often necessary.

TENNIS ELBOW

The term tennis elbow is a catch-all phrase used to designate one or more of several conditions, some well defined and some vague, which cause pain and tenderness in the lateral side of the elbow. The tenderness is usually marked and quite localized over the origin of the extensor carpi radialis brevis, and any action such as dorsiflexion of the wrist or strong grasp accentuates the pain. It is often self-limited and usually can be relieved by rest and local injection of hydrocortisone to the painful area. The x-ray findings are usually negative. Occasionally a small flake of bone anterior to the upper condyle suggests an avulsion, or the surface of the upper condyle may be roughened as an indication of periostitis. In a series of 150 tennis elbows, 5 (3.3%) failed to respond satisfactorily to conservative treatment, and Z-elongation of the extensor carpi radialis brevis tendon was performed. The results thus far have been very satisfactory (Singer, 1964). In another operation that was described by Bosworth (1955), the pain and tenderness was relieved by sectioning of the orbicular ligament of the upper radioulnar joint.

DEQUERVAIN'S DISEASE
(STENOSING TENOSYNOVITIS)

Stenosing tenosynovitis of the abductor pollicis longus and extensor pollicis brevis tendons occurs typically between ages of 30 and 50 years. Women are affected 10 times more frequently than men. The cause is frequently occupational but may be associated with rheumatoid arthritis. It is most frequently found in manual workers, particularly those who pinch while moving the wrist. At the styloid process of the radius these tendons are subject to an unusual degree of sharp angulation in the various motions of the wrist. Presenting symptoms usually are pain and tenderness at the radial styloid. Sometimes a thickening of the fibrous sheet is palpable. Finkelstein's test (Finkelstein, 1930) is usually positive. Conservative treatment consists of immobilizing the hand in a splint with an injection of hydrocortisone into the sheath of the two tendons. This is most successful when tried within the first 6 weeks after the onset of the symptoms. However, when the pain persists, surgery is the treatment of choice. Two things are important to remember in the surgical treatment of this disease: (1) to avoid the superficial branches of the radial nerve and (2) to be aware of the possibility of aberrant tendons of the abductor pollicis longus, for if all of the tendinous slips are not decompressed the patient may continue to have pain postoperatively. Various studies have reported approximately 50 to 75 per cent of the wrists examined revealed at least one aberrant tendon (Woods, 1964).

CARPAL TUNNEL SYNDROME

This syndrome, also known as Tardy median nerve palsy, results from compression of the median nerve within the carpal tunnel. Because there may be variations in the volume of the contents of the canal and because the capacity of the canal can vary with the position of the wrist in relation to the axis of the forearm, the periods of compression may be inconsistent and the resultant symptoms thus tend to fluctuate. Any condition that crowds or reduces the capacity of the carpal tunnel may initiate the symptoms, with malaligned Colles fracture and edema from infection or trauma among the more obvious. The cause is obscure in some patients, hence the term spontaneous median nerve neuropathy.

Hypoethesia over the sensory distribution of the median nerve is the most frequent symptom; it occurs more often in women past 40 years of age, particularly at night. Tinel's sign may also be demonstrated in as high as 80 per cent of patients by percussing median nerve at the wrist. Atrophy to some degree of the thenar muscles has been reported as high as 41 per cent of patients. Acute flexion of the wrist for sixty seconds or strenuous use of the hand increases the hypoesthesia; in one series this wrist flexion test was positive in approximately 75 per cent of the hands tested (Phalen, 1964). Ischemia results in a latency of transmission of electrical impulses, thus permitting diagnosis by the nerve conduction test. Motor latency of 5 to 8 milliseconds is an indication for surgical intervention. The sensory or large size nerve fibers are the first to be affected, and this may account for the early appearance of paresthesia.

Many systemic diseases or conditions are associated with the carpal tunnel syndrome. In a series of 318 patients, rheumatoid arthritis accounted for 93 cases, myxedema accounted for 77, diabetes mellitus for 69 and pregnancy for 20 cases (Yamaguchi, 1965). Conditions that produce radiculitis and may simulate the carpal tunnel syndrome include: (1) cervical disk protrusion, (2) syringomyelia, (3) cervical rib syndrome, (4) scalenus anticus syndrome, (5) neuropathies, (6) supracondylar process of the humerus (Kessel, 1966, and (7) abnormal anastamoses of the median and ulnar nerves in the forearm.

Treatment should be complete section of the transverse carpal ligament. Usually a neurolysis of the median nerve is carried out and in some cases resection of the palmaris longus tendon also is done. At the time of operation the median nerve may be noted to be abnormal or flattened and constricted; increased perineural fibrosis is noted at the point of constriction. Proximally there is apt to be a fusiform enlargement of the nerve. In a series of 313 patients, with an average follow-up of 3 years, satisfactory results were obtained in 81 per cent of the patients (Cseuz, et al., 1966). In decompressing the carpal tunnel the surgeon must be sure that the entire transverse carpal ligament is sectioned and that care is taken to avoid the recurrent motor branch of the median nerve.

TRIGGER FINGER

The most common cause of the trigger phenomenon, or sudden snapping movement of the finger, is direct trauma (single or multiple) usually incurred in grasping, and the middle and the ring fingers mainly are affected. The ligamentous sheath and the flexor tendon are pinched between the object and the head of the metacarpal until, as a result of local tenosynovitis, a thickening forms in the sheath with local swelling in the tendons. Commonly, the chronic inflammation is of a rheumatoid nature, although the biopsy may show only nonspecific inflammation. When the finger is two-thirds flexed, the motion is held up until, on more force, the nodule pulls through and the finger snaps into the palm in flexion. A similar phenomenon occurs at the same place on extending the finger; however, the finger usually locks in flexion. A nodule moving with the tendon can be felt under the examining finger. With increased irritation, the nodule no longer slips through the constriction, and the finger is caught in either extension or flexion. If the distal joint is extended first, the thickenings of two tendons will not coincide, thus allowing the tendon to slip through. It should be noted that, while the constriction is over the metacarpal head, it is the distal joint that locks or snaps. Treatment consists in incising the ligamentous sheath of the flexor tendons (Boyes, 1964).

Ganglia

Ganglia are the most common of the tumors seen in the hand and occur principally at one of three sites: (1) The dorsum of the wrist, arising from the scaphoid-lunate ligament, where they present to the surface between the common digital extensor tendons and the long extensor of the thumb; (2) the volar radial aspect of the wrist, arising from the ligamentous structures joining the distal radius to the greater multangular; and (3) in the tendon sheath over the flexor tendons at the proximal crease of the finger. These usually arise from the ligamentous structures comprising the pulley mechanism of the flexor tendons. Ganglia have been noted arising from the wrist joint and extending into the carpal tunnel, where they cause symptoms of median nerve compression, or from the ulnar size of the carpus, where they follow the course of the deep motor branch of the ulnar nerve and result in paralysis of the ulnar intrinsics. In other cases ganglia have arisen from the distal radio-ulnar joint region and compressed the dorsal sensory branches of the ulnar nerve.

Ganglia arise within the connective tissue near the joints or tendon sheaths but do not communicate with the synovial spaces. They may be single and large, or multiple and small, or a combination, with many minute areas of cystic degeneration near the base of the tumor. There is no special cell lining the cavity, and the contents are clear, colorless, and of jelly-like consistency. There are no inflammatory changes and malignant changes have not been reported in true ganglia.

The common dorsal carpal ganglia may be without symptoms except the local swelling, though usually there is the complaint of some weakness and occasional pain. Paradoxically, the small, barely palpable tumor may produce more discomfort than the large protruding type. Usually, the diagnosis is made by noting the location and the typical appearance. Aspiration of the clear contents with the consistency of jelly will verify the diagnosis. The ganglia arising on the flexor surface of the fingers are more tender, quite firm to palpation, discrete and do not move with the tendon.

Sometimes a ganglion disappears spontaneously, but usually a surgical excision is necessary to eliminate it. Many forms of nonoperative treatment have been tried, and periodically reports appear extolling the results of local injection of material into the cyst cavity (Derbyshire, 1966). Rupture by external force and injection of sclerosing agents, such as iodine or carbolic acid, have been discarded. Most authors agree that complete excision is the best treatment, but recurrence is frequent. If operative excision is done under the ischemia of a tourniquet, with complete removal of the ligamentous tissue comprising the base, recurrences will be rare. Since the common dorsal ganglion arises from the scaphoid-lunate ligament, a complete excision necessarily entails arthrotomy of the wrist joint for adequate exposure and excision. Opening the wrist joint is not a procedure to be undertaken under local anesthesia (Boyes, 1964).

A small cyst on the flexor tendon sheath can be incised with a sharp needle (Brunner, 1963).

Dupuytren's Contracture

This condition appears predominantly in Caucasian males of North European stock. In 60 per cent of one series the onset was between 40 and 60 years of age. The youngest patient reported was 11 years of age. The male to female ratio is approximately 9 to 1. All of the digits may be affected, the ring and little fingers most often (Skoog, 1967). It appears bilaterally in 40 per cent of patients, and "handedness" is not a factor. This condition is more prevalent in people who do not use their hands for manual work than it is in manual workers.

The etiology of Dupuytren's contracture is still unknown, although many theories have been advanced. The disease is definitely hereditary, there being numerous instances of many in one family being afflicted with the condition and of its having cropped out in as many as four to seven consecutive generations. In a recent article it was concluded that Dupuytren's contracture is probably a spontaneous disturbed-tolerance autoimmune disease. It is a disease probably initiated by four random, dependent-type autosomal somatic gene mutations in a stem cell of the lymphoid system. The target tissue primarily attacked by the "forbidden" lymphocyte is unknown, although proliferating fibroblasts are evidently a consequence of the autoimmune attack (Burch, 1966).

Certain diseases, such as gout, rheumatic tendency and diabetes, have been associated with Dupuytren's contracture more frequently than have others. A high percentage (42%) of patients with epilepsy were found to have Dupuytren's contractures (Skoog, 1967). The condition is often bilateral, rarely symmetrical, and may be associated with contracture of ligamentous bands elsewhere. There may be thickening and contracture of the connective tissue septum between the two corpi cavernosum of the penis (Peyronie's disease) in about 3 per cent of cases. In 5 per cent of cases a similar condition is found in the plantar fascia of the foot (Boyes, 1964).

Symptoms from Dupuytren's contracture are not great and often the contracture may be well established without producing any pain or discomfort. The usual symptoms complained of are a dull ache in the palm and numb feeling or tingling. The progression of the contracture may be rapid or slow. Usually, first the ring finger commences to flex in its proximal joint. This may soon be followed by flexion contracture of the proximal joints of either one or both of the adjoining fingers, in which case subcutaneous bands of thickened palmar fascia may be felt running to one side or the other of the finger. Rarely does the distal joint contract; often it hyperextends. When the fingers remain strongly flexed, the deep folds of the skin macerate and the deep funnel-like puckering of the skin of the palm may become infected. In a series of 2,612 hands, the frequency of involvement of the various digits were: ring (62%), little (53%), middle (22%), index (5.5%) and thumb (4%) (Boyes, 1964). A recent study showed that there was a high incidence of circulatory impairment and abnormality of the ulnar artery, with associated impairment of sensation over areas supplied by the ulnar nerve.

Treatment is symptomatic in the sense that the cause of the disease is unknown and its progress often slow (Hueston, 1965). The aim is to provide sufficient relief of the symptoms and the flexion contracture, to allow the hand to open well for grasp and not to jeopardize its more important function of closing around objects. Subcutaneous fasciotomy, combined with partial local excision, limited excision, and radical fasciectomy are the surgical procedures available to the surgeon (Davis, 1965; McFarlan, 1966; Skoog, 1967). Uncommonly, amputation of the digit may be necessary (Tubiana, 1964; Weckesser, 1964).

BONE TUMORS

The difficulties the pathologist may encounter in the diagnosis of some bone tumors may stem from several sources: Since neoplasms of bone are rare, opportunities for diagnoses may be limited to a few cases unless the pathologist is an authority in the field or is associated with a specialized institution; many biopsies of bone tumors submitted for study are inadequate; and histologic preparation of bone is difficult.

Anyone concerned with bone tumors should attempt to achieve what one may call a tridimensional view of them—that is, the surgeon, the radiologist and the pathologist, individually, should be able to view the diagnostic problem not only from his own angle but from that of the other two specialties as well.

Classification of bone tumors is often difficult and seldom worthwhile insofar as any particular lesion is concerned. However, in order to have a clear picture of the various kinds of tumors, a classification is helpful (Table 53-5).

When presented with a skeletal lesion it is mandatory of course to arrive at an accurate diagnosis as early as possible. Such a diagnosis seldom can be made with any degree of certainty from roentgenologic examination alone. The possible exception to this is the osteoid osteoma and metaphyseal fibrous defects (Fig. 53-38), and even these rather characteristic lesions may have such an unusual picture as to cast doubt on the x-ray interpretation. It is imperative that a careful history and physical examination and pertinent laboratory studies be available for proper understanding of the x-ray picture. With this information an experienced radiologist or orthopedic surgeon may come reasonably close to the correct answer much of the time. Definite therapy should not be undertaken on the basis of this information alone except with regard to a few quite

TABLE 53-5. CLASSIFICATION OF PRIMARY TUMORS OF BONE*

HISTOLOGIC TYPE	BENIGN	MALIGNANT
Hematopoietic		Myeloma
		Reticulum cell sarcoma
		Acute and chronic leukemias
		Malignant lymphoma
		Lymphosarcoma
		Hodgkin's disease
Chondrogenic	Osteochondroma	Primary chondrosarcoma
	Chondroma	Secondary chondrosarcoma
	Chondroblastoma	Mesenchymal chondrosarcoma
	Chondromyxoid fibroma	
Osteogenic	Osteoid osteoma	Osteogenic sarcoma
	Benign osteoblastoma	Parosteal osteogenic sarcoma
Unknown origin	Giant cell tumor	Ewing's tumor
		Malignant giant cell tumor
		Adamantinoma
Fibrogenic	Fibroma	Fibrosarcoma
	Desmoplastic fibroma	
Notochordal		Chordoma
Vascular	Hemangioma	Hemangio-endothelioma
	Hemangiopericytoma	Malignant hemangiopericytoma
Lipogenic	Lipoma	Liposarcoma
Neurogenic	Neurilemmoma	Malignant schwannoma
	Neurofibroma	

* Lichtenstein's classification, slightly modified.

characteristic lesions, i.e., osteoid osteoma, metaphyseal fibrous defect and exostoses (Fig. 53-39). In all other instances microscopic study of representative tissue from the lesion must be obtained before intelligently directed treatment can be instituted. There is some danger of seeding malignant cells or even spreading malignant tissue from the trauma of biopsy. The danger of tumor spread from this procedure is minor compared with the error of unnecessary amputation as a result of treatment without the knowledge gained from tissue study.

Biopsy should be done at the treatment center that is going to be responsible for the complete care of the patient. All too often we are faced with the problem of receiving a patient with a skeletal lesion who has already had a biopsy performed, in which one or all of the following circumstances exist: (1) wound infection of the biopsy site, which in some cases has profoundly influenced the course of the patient and made more difficult the proper care; (2) the slides, which may accompany the patient, may be of such poor quality that proper interpretation is not possible; (3) the original block is lost or not available for further study; (4) the biopsy material may not be diagnostic, because the surgeon failed to get it from a representative area of the lesion.

The biopsy should be regarded as a final diagnostic procedure and should not be undertaken lightly, as a mere shortcut to diagnosis. Finally, a biopsy should be done, if possible, when radiation is to be the therapeutic procedure, to avoid the danger of radiating a lesion for which that form of treatment is not indicated, or for which surgery would be more appropriate.

The decision to do an open vs. a needle biopsy is still controversial. If one is to do an open biopsy, it should be carried out in such a way that surgical trauma is minimal and that it will in no way compromise the definitive procedure. If the tumor is a malignant one, an unduly traumatic biopsy may encourage metastatic spread. Then there is the matter of deciding if the diagnosis should be made on the basis of a frozen section of the biopsy specimen, or whether the wound should

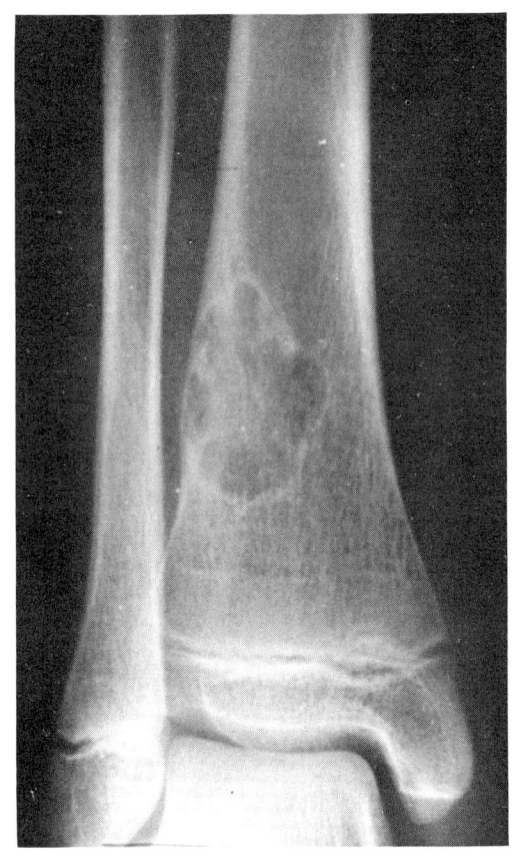

FIG. 53-38. Distal tibia in a 15-year-old female. The eccentrically located loculated lesion is typical of a metaphyseal fibrous defect (a benign lesion). The majority of these lesions tend to undergo spontaneous regression.

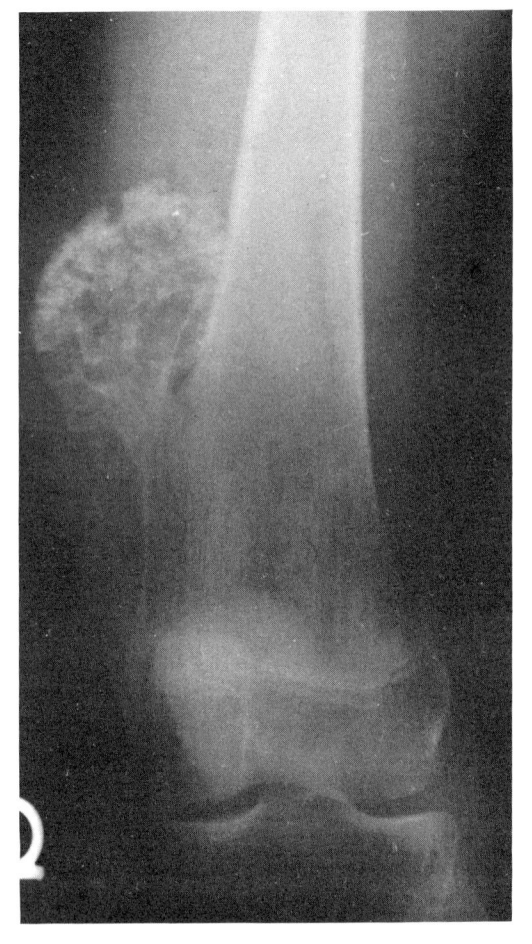

FIG. 53-39. A typical benign osteochondroma of the distal end of the femur. This was removed for cosmetic reasons.

be closed and the diagnosis and decision about further treatment postponed until after paraffin sections have been prepared. This depends largely on the kind of tissue yielded by the biopsy. If the tissue is not calcified or ossified, an experienced pathologist will be able to make the diagnosis. In the case of cartilage tumor, however, it is better to await the paraffin section for evaluation of benignity or malignancy.

On the other hand, a lesion in an accessible site lends itself particularly well to needle biopsy. The obvious advantage is that it constitutes a limited intervention that disturbs the lesion only slightly and causes little morbidity to the patient. In a series of over 4,000 puncture biopsies of bone, joint and soft tissue, positive results were obtained in 76 per cent (Schajowicz, 1968). Included in this series were more than 900 biopsies of the vertebrae. However, it is not a simple procedure, and should be performed only by one versed in its use.

The biopsy material must be properly handled. Then a pathologist experienced in the study of bone lesions usually is able to make an accurate diagnosis, but the tissue examination does not stand alone as an exact science. The pathologist must take into consideration the history, the physical findings and the laboratory studies, including the roentgenograms, and even with all information at hand it is sometimes impossible to be sure of the exact nature of the lesion.

Laboratory studies are of little aid in the diagnosis of the average bone tumor. Myeloma, with its sometimes practically pathognomonic alterations of proteins in serum or urine, is a notable exception. Alkaline phosphatase levels may be elevated in osteoid-producing neoplasms, either primary or metastatic. Elevated levels of acid phosphatase point to metastatic prostatic carcinoma. The ominous nature of rapidly growing sarcomas, such as Ewing's tumor, may be suggested by systemic evidence that includes fever, anemia, and rapid sedimentation rate.

Arteriography has been a useful adjunct in the diagnosis of bone and soft tissue tumors (Dos Santos, 1956; Halpern, 1965). However, with many tumors it is often difficult to make precise histologic identification from their arteriographic appearance. If the tumor shows clearcut arteriographic evidence of malignancy, it is certain that the lesion will contain malignant cells. Arteriographically, a malignant tumor shows a number of irregular pools from which contrast material is rapidly shunted into the venous side. These irregular spaces and vessels are lined by tumor cells rather than endothelium. Benign lesions, such as the giant cell tumor, aneurysmal bone cyst (Fig. 53-40), and osteitis fibrosis cystica of hyperparathyroidism, may be very vascular during the venous phase but the arterial phase does not show "laking."

A biopsy interpretation of benignity in the face of clearcut malignant arteriographic findings should be highly suspect and a more extensive biopsy should be made. Since malignant tumors may also be avascular, the benign arteriographic appearance of a lesion is unreliable and biopsy is the only dependable means of identification (Staple et al., 1968).

Pre-biopsy arteriography will demonstrate the areas of greatest vascularity. These areas are the most fruitful for obtaining a representative biopsy (Lagergren, 1962). Demonstration of satellite nodules, the extent of the tumor, and evidence of recurrence are useful in treatment and prognosis. The history, physical examination and plain film findings must all be used in the accurate interpretation of the arteriographic examination.

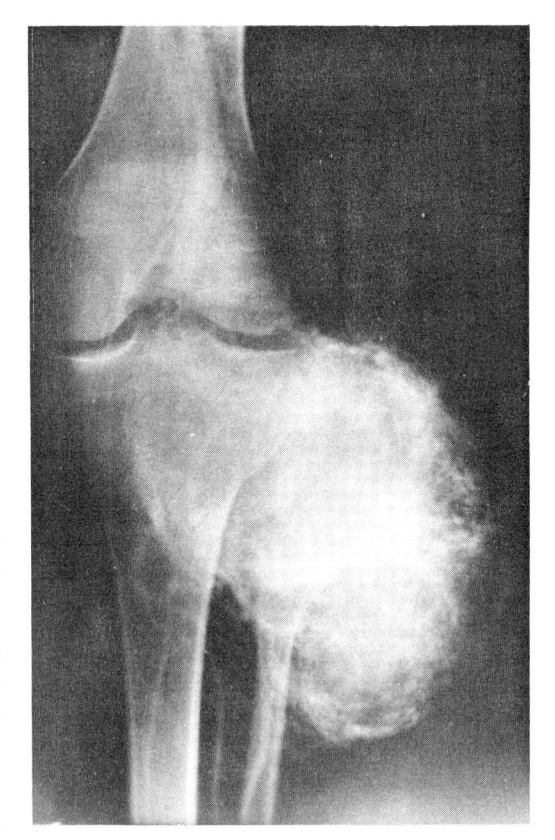

Fig. 53-40. Arteriogram showing typical flush in a benign aneurysmal bone cyst of the fibula. The tumor was excised en bloc.

Photoscanning with Strontium 85 and 87 is a valuable aid to detection of early lesions in bone before they are visualized on the x-rays (Charkes et al., 1966) (Fig. 53-41). The scan becomes positive in some patients many months before observable x-ray changes are visualized, since the calcium content must be decreased by about 30 per cent to 50 per cent before visible changes occur. Vertebral lesions must be about 1 cm. to 1.5 cm. in diameter before they can be seen on x-rays. Thus, earlier diagnosis is possible and treatment can be begun before the lesions become obvious, saving the patient months of suffering. Deposition of strontium in bone is a nonspecific process, so that other diseases (Paget's disease, osteomyelitis, fracture or benign tumors) also have a positive scan. False negative scans are rare.

Radioactive isotopes of calcium as well as Fluorine 18 has been utilized in an effort to

Orthopedics (Nontraumatic)

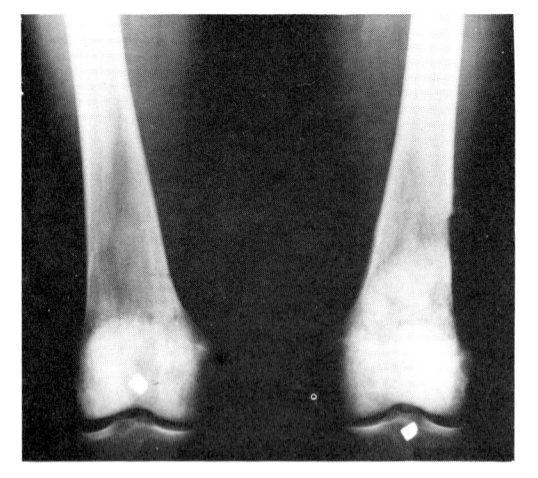

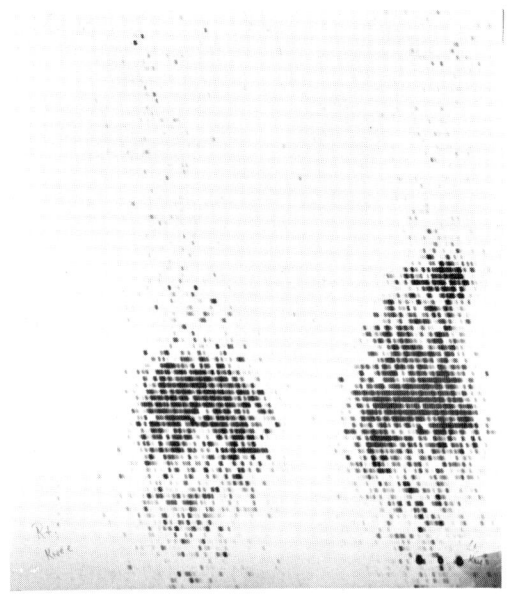

FIG. 53-41. (*Left*) X-ray evidence of *unilateral* involvement by reticulum cell sarcoma. Note the cortical destruction and moth-eaten appearance of the distal femur on the right. (*Right*) Strontium scan in the same patient reveals involvement of *both* femora with reticulum cell sarcoma.

outline the extent of neoplastic lesions (Blau et al., 1962).

Both normal and neoplastic cells possess a wide variety of enzymes, some restricted to certain types of cells, others more widespread in their distribution. Bone tumors have been found to contain varying levels of certain measurable enzymes (Jeffree and Price, 1965). This may eventually lead to a more sophisticated classification of bone tumors.

When a complete study of the patient, together with his bone lesion, has been accomplished, then and only then should definite treatment be carried out.

Treatment will be considered here only briefly; for a more detailed study the reader is referred to the works of Lichtenstein (1965), Ackerman (1968), and Jaffe (1964).

Benign tumors for the most part are not radiosensitive, with the possible exception of benign giant cell tumors. Not enough information is available to be sure how effective radiation in this group of tumors really is, so at present we prefer excision of benign lesions, with replacement of bone to fill surgically created defects or gaps in the involved bone where indicated because of structural weakness.

The frequent recurrence of primary tumors of bone emphasizes the need for a fresh approach to their management. The misnomer "local recurrence" is really a euphemism for surgical failure that has left behind growing tumor cells to become manifest later. Curettement cannot remove all neoplastic cells filling minute crevices in the wall of the tumor. Therefore, the entire area should be removed en bloc with total excision and replaced with bone grafts. This has been applied successfully only for giant cell tumor, parosteal osteosarcoma, chondrosarcoma developing from a central chondroma and benign lesions that could recur if treated with curettement alone (Parrish, 1966).

Malignant bone tumors fall into 2 groups: primary and metastatic. Operation is indicated in metastatic lesions with pathologic fractures for the purpose of relief of pain and improving function by means of internal fixation or, more rarely, prosthetic replacement. Occasionally, amputation may be advisable to relieve the patient of a painful fungating mass. In other metastatic lesions palliative radiation should be employed (Fig. 53-42).

The appearance of a solitary pulmonary

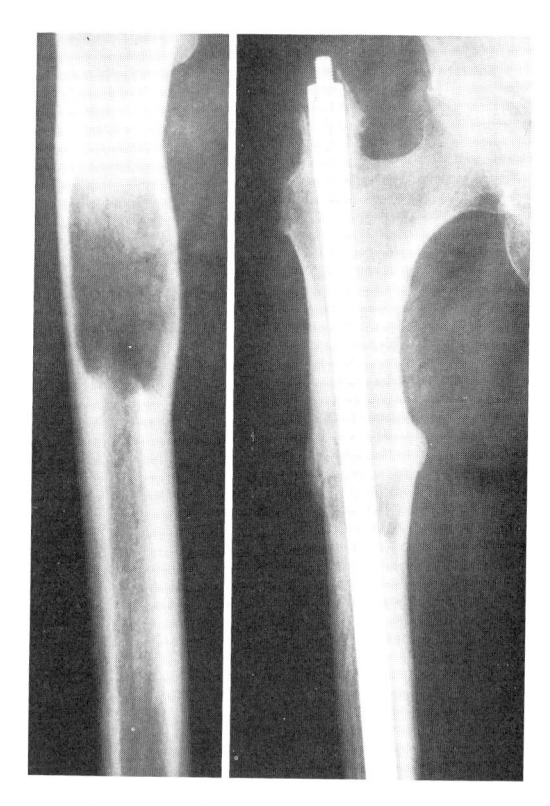

Fig. 53-42. (*Left*) This large lesion within the femur is a metastasis from a carcinoma of the breast. A pathologic fracture impends. (*Right*) A femoral nail, used to support the fragile femur, and x-ray therapy to the lesion have preserved a useful and painless extremity for 18 months.

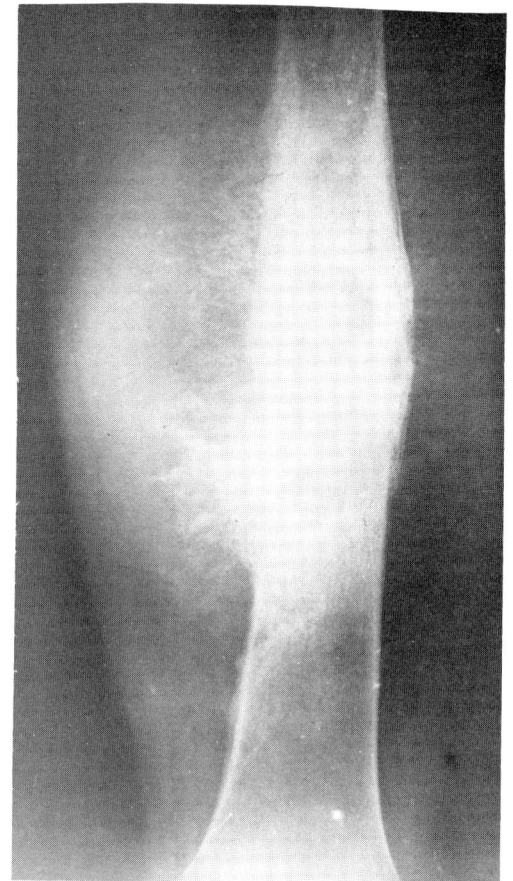

Fig. 53-43. Roentgenogram illustrating Codman's triangle and the "sunburst" appearance in Ewing's sarcoma of the femoral diaphysis. Codman's triangle is the triangular area in which the elevated periosteum rejoins the cortex. The "sunburst" appearance results from the formation of reactive or neoplastic bone, which is laid down perpendicular to the shaft along vessels passing from the periosteum to the cortex.

metastasis from a primary bone tumor must no longer be regarded as inevitably fatal. Although reported series are small, partial or complete pulmonary resections of a solitary metastatic focus has prolonged the survival time in some instances (Sweetman and Ross, 1967). This was also noted in another series of 14 patients with pulmonary metastases (Dahlin and Coventry, 1967).

Primary malignant bone tumors remain an unsolved therapeutic problem. The state of our present knowledge indicates that the only chance of survival is sterilization, or ablation of the lesion before spreading occurs. In some very radiosensitive tumors this occasionally occurs with x-ray alone, as in Ewing's tumor (Fig. 53-43). However, the authors' experience until very recently was that, in all patients with Ewing's sarcoma and the other quite radiosensitive lesions, such as reticulum cell sarcoma, the lesion proved fatal regardless of type of therapy—(1) radiation alone; (2) radiation followed by amputation (even when microscopic examination of the amputated extremity has failed to reveal any remaining malignant cell), and (3) amputation and subsequent roentgenography of regional nodes.

The combination of radiotherapy and chem-

1734 Orthopedics (Nontraumatic)

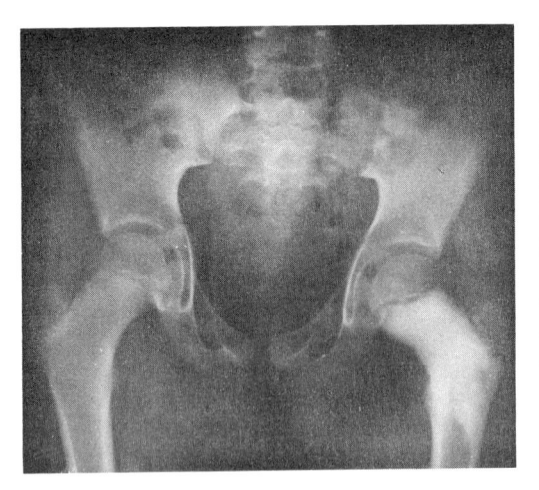

FIG. 53-44. Osteogenic sarcoma of the proximal femur in a 13-year-old boy. The patient complained of pain 2 to 4 weeks prior to the initial x-ray. He was treated by hemipelvectomy.

otherapy, using nitrogen mustard, has somewhat proved the outlook for Ewing's sarcoma. In a recent series, 13 of 39 patients treated with 3,000 to 4,000 r and with mechlorethamine (nitrogen mustard) were alive 5 years after the diagnosis was made (Phillips and Higinbotham, 1967). Husto *et al.* (1968) reported a series of 5 patients treated with 4,700 to 5,000 r and intravenous vincristine and cyclophosphamide who demonstrated regression of the disease in 4 weeks and are alive 3 years after diagnosis. A favorable response to chemotherapy was also reported by Samuels and Howe (1967).

Other malignant bone tumors have a small chance of cure with early adequate surgical removal of the tumor (Fig. 53-44). So long as all the tumor cells are removed from the body it matters little what method is employed. Ideally, this would be a local resection so that some function of the extremity could be main-

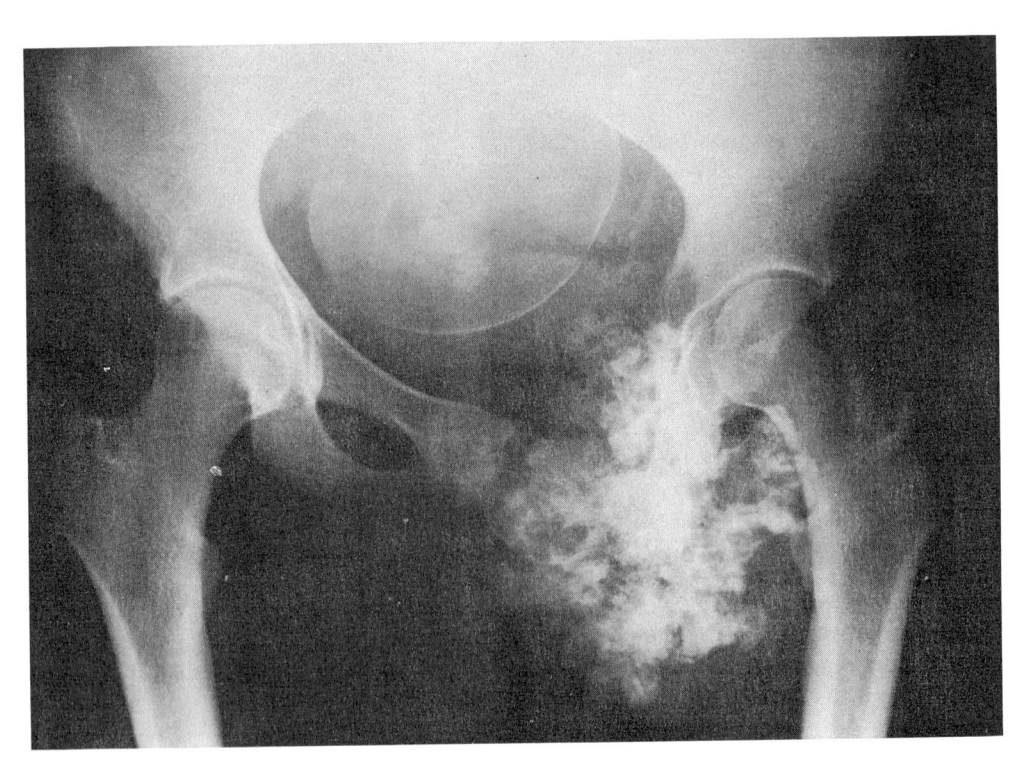

FIG. 53-45. A huge chondrosarcoma of the pelvis discovered in an 18-year-old woman seven months pregnant. The large lobulated tumor mass with areas of calcification in it is a typical chondrosarcoma. Several weeks following cesarean section, wide local resection of the tumor and all pubic rami was done.

tained. However, it is seldom possible to carry out complete eradication of the malignant growth and maintain function, so that amputation gives the best functional result at the least cost to the patient, in regard to both money and pain. Furthermore, there is a tendency for these tumors to spread up the medullary canal of the affected bone and they may even jump areas of apparently normal marrow, so that resection may not be successful in getting around the tumor (O'Hara et al., 1968). The value of postoperative x-ray therapy is still open to question, unless tumor cells were spilled out at the time of surgery. The place of preoperative radiation is also not clearly defined.

The author would like to suggest that chondrosarcoma has been taken too lightly (Fig. 53-45). This rather slow-growing tumor, tending to mestastasize late is a very formidable one. One can hardly point with pride when a patient, who has had a surgical resection or local excision of this tumor and remains free of trouble for a number of years, dies of recurrence and metastases, whereas radical removal of all the diseased tissue perhaps would have saved the patient's life.

There is never any justification for enucleating or curetting a potentially malignant cartilage tumor. The 5-year survival rate is more favorable with amputation, where this is possible, than with resection. In the case of tumors involving the pelvis, the first surgical procedure often offers the only chance of curing the patient (McKenna et al., 1966). Normally, this procedure must be sufficiently radical to ensure complete eradication of all tumor cells. Often this will require hemipelvectomy.

TUMORS OF THE SOFT TISSUE

If we exclude tumors of skin structures and lymph nodes, all neoplasms develop from either the mesoderm or the neuroectodermal tissues of the peripheral nervous system. If the various tumors developing from these tissues reproduced their prototypic tissues in pure form, even in various stages of differentiation, recognition would be relatively simple. However, this is not always the case and it is the aberrations that are difficult to recognize. Also, neoplasms tend to form multiple tissues, so that one tumor may consist of several more or less differentiated tissues without the predominance of any one type. Therefore, histologic diagnosis may require not only the usual hematoxylin and eosin stains, but special stains for lipoid, mucoid, melanin, elastic tissue and amyloid substances as well as for nerve fibers. As with bone tumors, arteriograms also may be a diagnostic aid. It is not yet clear whether electron microscopy will be useful in the more nearly exact classification of soft tissue tumors. Where available, tissue cultures may permit recognition of specific neoplastic growths.

If one is quite similar with the usual distribution, relative frequency and gross growth characteristics of the soft tissue tumor, it is sometimes possible to make an accurate diagnosis on physical examination alone.

An excellent discussion of soft tissue tumors as well as their classification may be found in a recent publication by the Armed Forces Institute of Pathology (Stout and Lattes, 1967).

COMMON FOOT PROBLEMS

Corns (Heloma Durum). A corn is a simple localized hyperkeratosis produced by pressure from within and pressure from without. The pressure from within is usually from an osseous condyle and that from without from the shoe. Not infrequently, a corn on the foot of a child is the result of either an ill-fitting shoe or an abnormal gait pattern, such as external rotation or pronation. In middle aged patients, predominantly women, a corn frequently results from pressure of a shoe or an irregular surface within the shoe, such as a seam. In older patients, the condyles enlarge and the increased pressure causes corn formation. The usual sites are on the lesser toes, principally the fifth toe, the bursa and bony prominence of which have come to be known as a bunionette. This has also been referred to as tailor's bunion. The corn may occur over the joints, especially if the toes are contracted or flexed abnormally, as in mallet toe or hammer toe deformity. Corns may be treated either by palliative measures, which include removal of the hyperkeratosis or the use of protective shields or pads, or by surgical removal of the prominent condyle (Kelikian, 1965).

Soft Corns (Tyloma Molle). The soft corn is extremely painful and usually occurs between the fourth and fifth toes or in the web spaces. The lesion usually results from pressure and friction exerted on the skin and soft tissues by the head of the promixal phalanx of the fifth toe and the lateral condyle of the base of the proximal phalanx of the fourth toe. It is soft and the skin is often eroded because of constant moisture between the toes. A soft corn can be treated by excision of only the lateral condyle of the base of the proximal phalanx of the fourth toe; in more severe long-standing cases the head and neck of the proximal phalanx of the little toe are also excised. This procedure eliminates the two areas of pressure responsible for the original corn and precludes possible future development of another corn (Margo, 1967).

Plantar Hyperkeratosis (Calluses). The common cause of plantar calluses is abnormal local pressure on the plantar surface of the foot under one or more of the metatarsal heads. The callosities may be widespread or they may be localized beneath each of the metatarsal heads. The condition frequently is diagnosed incorrectly as a plantar verruca or wart, and the consequent improper treatment may produce a lesion not unlike plantar hyperkeratosis. Because of the risk of permanent damage to the skin on the plantar surface of the foot, the seriousness of improper use of caustics, keratolytic agents and x-ray therapy cannot be overemphasized. These agents cause atrophy and increase the probability of painful lesions on the plantar surface. The treatment of these lesions consists in palliative removal of the hyperkeratosis, proper use of pads or supports to shift the pressure or balance weight bearing, or, finally, surgical removal of that portion of the metatarsal that is causing pressure in the sole of the foot (Brahms, 1967).

Verruca Plantaris (Wart). A verruca is a common lesion found on the plantar surface of the foot. Differential diagnosis of a verruca from a callus is difficult at times. In general, pressure keratoses occur in older persons with established forefoot deformities, the most obvious being hallux valgus and hammer or claw toes. As mentioned previously, the skin may be involved under all five metatarsal heads. More often it is confined to the region under one or two metatarsal heads. In most instances the thickened skin does not contain a central core and the callus as a whole is not acutely tender to pressure. Verruca plantaris occurs more prominently in children and young adults with soft, moist skin and pliable feet, and on retracted or malformed toes. These warts are most painful in the morning when one is starting to walk, in contrast to the pressure keratoses, which are painful after the patient has been on his feet for some time. Verrucae may be multiple or solitary. Verruca do not occur under the metatarsal heads but are found proximal or distal to them. Each wart contains a central core which is surrounded by a definite ring of reactive dermis. The core is dark brown in color, often specked with black spots. The core is exquisitely tender, both on direct pressure and when an attempt is made to move it sideways. It bleeds even when shaved superficially. Some plantar warts tend to disappear spontaneously, and with a few exceptions they are radiosensitive.

Of the many methods of treating plantar verruca, the simple way is to use a small curette and attempt to skirt the lesion by finding a proper plane of separation. By doing so, the verruca may be enucleated, much as a pea from a pod. Simple elliptical excision may also result in a satisfactory cure. The author has personally seen a Syme's amputation as a result of a nonhealing ulcer of the plantar surface of the foot secondary to radiation therapy for plantar warts (see also Brahms, 1967; Kelikian, 1965).

Perineural Fibrosis (Morton's Neuroma). Perineural fibrosis always must be considered as a cause of pain in the fore part of the foot. Failure to keep this condition in mind results in failure in diagnosis. The condition occurs more often in women than men and frequently is associated with pain that comes on after walking, especially in high heels. Thick soled shoes usually tend to minimize the discomfort. The pain is confined to the region between the third and fourth toes usually, rarely the more medial digits. The pain is paroxysmal. It is described as being knifelike, stabbing or burning. Pressure in the web space between the involved toes or slightly proximal may elicit pain. Occasionally, a tumor mass is palpable. Rarely, the location of the lesion causing the sensation along the contiguous surfaces of the third and fourth metatarsal heads may be open to question, because the third common digital nerve from the medial plantar receives a branch from the lateral plantar nerve. Complete and permanent relief of pain results from surgical extirpation (Kelikian, 1965).

Hammer Toe Deformities. Hammer toe, a cockup deformity of the proximal interphalangeal joint, may occur singularly or involve all of the toes. The single toe type generally is associated with a painful hard corn over the dorsal aspect of the proximal interphalangeal joint. Rarely the distal interphalangeal joint is involved.

Pressure is produced by hyperflexion of the proximal interphalangeal joint and extension of the distal interphalangeal joint. An extension contracture at the metatarsophalangeal joint is also associated with hammer toe. The deformity may be treated by padding to reduce discomfort, or surgically, by performing an arthroplasty or fusion of the proximal interphalangeal joint.

Ingrowing Toenails. Ingrowing toenail and onychogryposis (long hooked toenail) cause much disability and discomfort. Pain with inflammation or sepsis is a presenting symptom of ingrowing toenail, and the disease is common in adolescence and young adults.

Onychogryposis causes pain but is seldom associated with sepsis. In one series all patients requiring surgical ablation underwent the Zadik operation, in which the distal half of the nail is left and no bone is removed (Townsend, 1966). However, in many patients with sepsis, avulsion only of the nail is performed, the more radical procedure being deferred until the toe is healed. In performing the radical operation the plane of dissection is subcutaneous. The nail is avulsed, the proximal nail bed is removed and the two halves of the distail nail bed are dissected down to bone. It is usually necessary to dissect off some fibrous tissues on the lateral surface of the phalanx so as to leave no soft tissue over the bone. Laterally the nail folds are excised with similar care and the flap is sutured to the distal nail bed. This procedure has given satisfactory results in 89 per cent of the cases.

Posterior Tibial Tenosynovitis. Frequently when there is no apparent traumatic factor or common problem associated with metatarsal dysfunction and the heel can be ruled out as a cause of pain, the attention should be focused on the posterior tibial tendon. A tenosynovitis of posterior tibial tendon may occur in association with a planovalgus decompensation or acute foot strain. The point of maximum tenderness may be located plantar to the talonavicular joint where the posterior tibial tendon passes. Persons with an enlarged or an accessory navicular, with severe flat foot deformity or with peroneal spastic flat foot almost always have pain in this region. The posterior tibial tendon sheath may become thickened, and a synovial enlargement, not unlike a ganglion, may develop. Treatment designed either to relieve the stress or decrease inflammation in the area is beneficial. If an injection of a small amount of local anesthetic agent relieves the pain, the diagnosis is made. Injection of a combination of a local anesthetic and corticosteroids has been efficacious. Ultimate success of treatment will depend on the maintenance of a balanced distribution of weight. In some cases local resection of a thickened tendon sheath should be considered (Brahms, 1967).

Heel Tuberosities. Dickinson et al (1966), coined the term "pump bump" to designate enlargements on the heel in the region of the attachment of the tendo Achillis, a condition usually seen in young women and frequently associated with the wearing of pumps or shoes with high heels. The condition is a result of a prominent posterosuperior margin of the calcaneus and the wearing of shoes with a closely contoured heel counter. Either a painless callus forms on the heel or painful bursitis develops over the Achilles tendon. Dickinson et al. (1966) reported that they have successfully treated, in 21 patients, 40 involved heels by resection of the posterior prominence of the calcaneus. The amount of bone excised must be generous, enough so that no bony prominence can be felt anterior to the heel cord at the side of the bump when the posterior aspect of the heel is palpated. In our hands, surgical intervention has seldom proved to be necessary. Relief has been attained by removing shoe pressure.

Heel Bursitis. Pain in the plantar surface of the foot is not an uncommon complaint of people who do a considerable amount of walking or standing. These patients are afflicted with pain on the bottom of the heel in the region of the plantar attachment of the plantar ligament. The use of a hollow heel pad, a

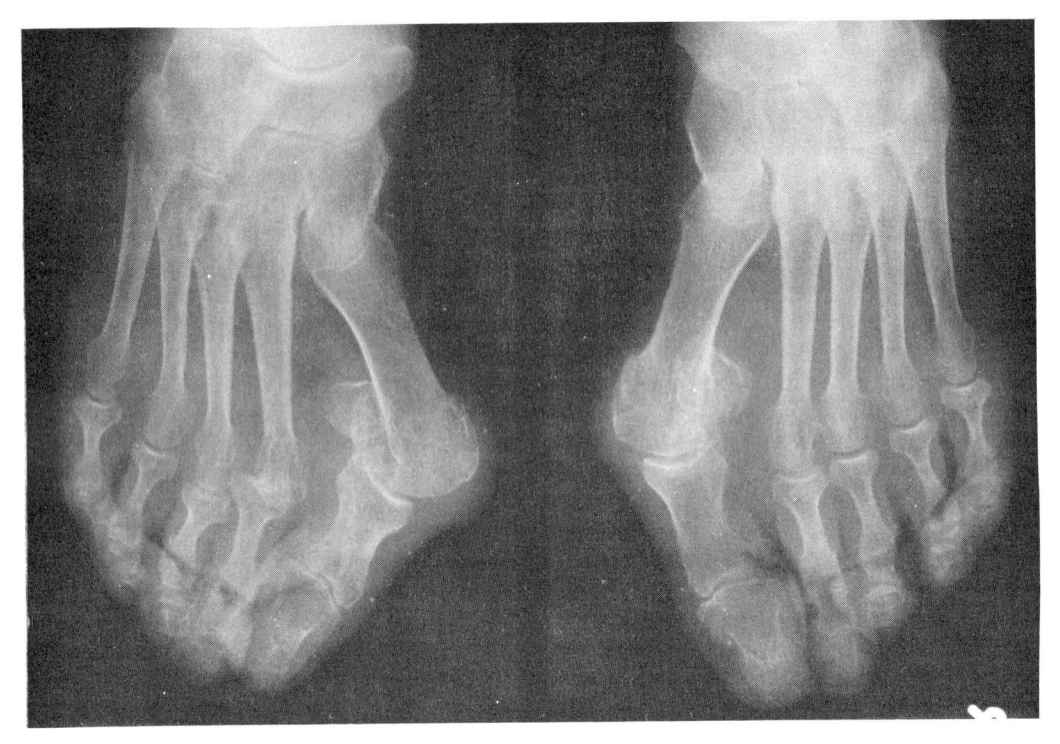

FIG. 53-46. Typical bilateral hallux valgus, metatarsus primus varus and bunions in a 60-year-old woman. Note the overlapping of the great toe and the exostosis formation on the head of the 1st metatarsal.

comma shaped pad, or proper arch supports may afford some relief, and injections of hydrocortisone and procaine preparations into the tender area may produce total relief. If these measures prove inadequate, surgical excision of the calcaneal spur may be necessary.

Freiberg's Disease, a type of osteochondritis, usually involves the head of the second metatarsal, and less commonly involves the third, fourth, and fifth metatarsal heads. The patient generally complains of pain and stiffness in the involved area. Clinically, motion of the metatarsophalangeal joint is markedly limited and there is thickening about the metatarsal head. Roentgenograms reveal marked irregularity, with hypertrophy of the head of the metatarsal and, usually, irregularity of the base of the corresponding proximal phalanx. Relief may be afforded by a well placed metatarsal pad and modification of the shoe; surgical correction is seldom required.

Hallux Rigidus. This condition is a limitation of plantar or dorsal flexion of the great toe, usually resulting from bony proliferation at the margins of the metatarsophalangeal joints. This condition greatly interferes with the push-off function of the toes in walking and occasionally is associated with hallux valgus. Permanent subjective relief may be obtained in early cases by a properly made shoe with pads, supports, and a metatarsal bar. A stiff sole or a long arch support will at times relieve symptoms. Surgical procedures include shaving any unusual prominence from the head of the first metatarsal and excision of a good portion of the base of the proximal phalanx (Keller bunionectomy). An alternative procedure is fusion of the metatarsophalangeal joint but the resulting stiffness of the great toe may impair walking (Margo, 1967).

Hallux Valgus. In this condition the great toe is adducted so that it lies on top of or under the other toes. Associated with this is a marked prominence of the first metatarsophalangeal joint, with bony enlargement of the medial side of the first metatarsal head, over which a bursa may form (due to pressure from the shoe). This bursa is commonly called a bunion (Fig. 53-46). Inflammation may occur in the bursa, occasionally with suppuration. Hallux valgus may be present without the formation of a bunion and without marked discomfort even in the presence of marked deformity. Short, narrow, pointed shoes may be a cause of hallux valgus. A congenital metatarsus varus may precede this condition.

In mild cases with slight discomfort, relief may be obtained by the use of proper shoes, insertion of a pad between the first and second toes, and proper arch supports and exercises. Severe deformity of hallux valgus and hallux rigidus can be corrected usually by removal of the exostoses from the metatarsal heads and excision of a small portion of the proximal phalanx (Hollander, 1966). There are numerous surgical procedures for correction of this deformity (Kelikian, 1965).

Overriding Fifth Toe. The dorsally adducted 5th toe is a common familiar deformity which causes disability in half of the affected patients. The phalanges of the 5th toe are laterally rotated and the capsule of the metatarsophalangeal joint is contracted on the dorsal aspect. The toe has an extended, adducted, lateral rotation deformity at the metatarsophalangeal joint. Treatment includes either extensor tenotomy and dorsal capsulotomy of the metatarsophalangeal joint or syndactylization of the 4th and 5th toes (Leonard and Rising, 1965).

LOW BACK PAIN

It has been estimated that from 25 to 50 per cent of all patients treated by the orthopedist have as a presenting complaint low back pain with or without sciatica. Backache, like headache, may result from a variety of abnormal conditions. It is essential, therefore, to establish an accurate pathologic diagnosis. But the desire to make such a diagnosis must be tempered with judgment so that each patient seen with low back pain is not subjected routinely to all possible diagnostic tests. The vast majority of patients can be managed satisfactorily as outpatients, with conservative treatment such as low back supports, rest, local heat and drugs for relief of pain, and exercise. The more common causes of back pain with or without sciatica are (1) acute strain, (2) abnormality of the intervertebral disk, (3) degenerative arthritis, (4) defect of the pars interarticularis, (5) pelvic disease, (6) rheumatoid arthritis affecting the spine, (7) senile osteoporosis, (8) tumors, both primary and metastatic, (9) infection of spine, (10) psychoneurosis, (11) pathologic fracture, (12) disk space infection, (13) multiple myeloma, (14) Paget's disease, and others. Postural backache, although quite frequent, is seldom of such severity that the sufferer seeks medical advice.

It is apparent that a rather complete history and physical examination must be carried out for the physician to begin to grasp the patient's problem. At times the cause is quite obvious, and at other times considerable time and effort is expended before the source of trouble comes to light. These patients may be divided readily into those with a history of injury and those who cannot remember an injury.

Of those with history of injury the effort-strain type is the most common. A number of years ago one of us reviewed a large series of cases with a history of this type of injury. These patients were more or less disabled and had restriction of motion, local tenderness in the low back or below, and many had radiation of pain in the legs. Of these patients, 96 per cent responded rapidly to rest and local heat and were able to return to work in less than 4 weeks. It appears that about this percentage recovers from these strains or sprains regardless of treatment. The remaining 4 per cent who did not recover in this period were found on further study to have a ruptured disk, defect of pars interarticularis, tumors or infections, with the greatest number having a ruptured disk.

Of the group having a history of back injury by a direct blow many have hematomas and muscle damage or fractures of one or more transverse processes of the lumbar vertebrae. In spite of the history and the physical evidence of a direct blow, it is generally believed that the transverse processes are fractured only by muscle pull of the quadratus lumborum muscle.

The various fractures of the spine are discussed in Chapter 23, Fractures and Dislocations of Spine, Pelvis, Sternum and Ribs.

Disease and Injury of the Intervertebral Disk

Approximately 50 per cent of the patients in whom a diagnosis of a symptomatic degenerative disk condition with or without rupture of the nucleus pulposus is made give a history of trauma. A detailed description of sciatica was made by Momenico Contugno in 1764; he originated the term. Further clinical description was made by Lasegue (1864). Virchow (1857) described a fracture of the disk. Protrusion of disk material was reported by von Luschka (1858) as well as details of anatomy of the disk. Fick (1911), Brown (1922), Beadle (1931), Keyes and Compere (1932), Coventry, Ghormley and Kernohan (1945, a, b, c) have contributed to knowledge of anatomic characteristics of disks. Keyes and Compere determined physiologic function of the disk and carried out experimental investigations and reviewed the literature. Virchow described the nuclear cells of the disk as large cells with eccentric nuclei with clear zones. He called these physaliferous cells and thought that they were of notochordal origin. He also described cartilaginous masses of protruded disk material and called them physaliferous enchondromas. Dandy (1929) reported 2 cases of cartilaginous enchondroma compressing the cord.

Although a number of men were close to the proper understanding of the role of the disk in producing low back pain and sciatica, the placing of this in proper clinical perspective was the work of Mixter and Barr (1934), who described the clinical picture, proved the existence of disk rupture with nerve root compression and demonstrated relief of symptoms by surgical removal of the protruded portion of the disk.

Puschel (1930) found that the nucleus pulposus contained 88 per cent water in newborns and that there was gradual loss of water with aging so that there was 66 per cent water at age 77. Keyes and Compere substantiated these findings. DePusky (1935) noted that there was increased length of the spine after resting and a decrease with standing. The extension of blood vessels into the disk substance through the cartilaginous plates has been described to about age 30. After this age none are found. Roofe (1940) found nerve fibers extending to the posterior portion of the annulus fibrosus. Jackson *et al*. (1966), and Hirsch (1965) found nerve endings in the vertebral end plates and facet joints. The ligament flava were relatively free of nerve elements. Adult supraspinal and intraspinal ligaments had very few nerve endings. Only in the outer zones of the annulus fibrosis and thin lamina of the disk surfaces were nerve fibers seen. No nerve fibers were seen in the body of the disk nor in the nucleus pulposus.

The disk contributes 25 per cent of the length of the vertebral column above the sacrum. The lumbar disks account for 30 to 36 per cent of the length of the lumbar spine (Hollingshead, 1965).

In childhood the nucleus is well demarcated from the annulus fibrosus, while in the 2nd decade the cells become fewer and the demarcation not so clear, and in the 3rd decade cavities appear, as do also cartilage cells. Dehydration is accompanied by a change to fibrocartilage with an associated loss of elasticity of the annulus fibrosus. All investigators have agreed that at an early age evidence of alteration of the nucleus and the annulus fibrosus of a degenerative nature is evident. These alterations reduce the elasticity of the annulus, and it appears that damage to the annulus with cracks and fissure formation is the important alteration, as the elastic nature of the disk results from function of the annulus and not the nucleus pulposus.

The intra-diskal pressure is about 30 pounds per square inch when the spine is non-weight-bearing, and it is generally reported that pressures of 200 or 300 pounds per square inch or more may be exerted in the lumbosacral disk when the back is used as a lever during lifting (Hollingshead, 1965). Nachemson, (1966) has published a study of the load on the lumbar disks in different positions of the body.

There is evidence that low back pain or low back pain and sciatica may be caused by degeneration of the disk with alteration of the physiologic function as well as by nerve root compression when there is posterior protrusion of disk material.

Ghormley (1933) has described the facet syndrome. However, there is very little evidence that alterations of the apophyseal joints are primary factors in low back pain with or without sciatica except in rheumatoid arthritis or fracture. Changes in the apophyseal joints are for the most part secondary to alterations of disk function. The correlation of ruptured lumbar disk with heavy labor was borne out by the findings of a study made of a series of over 400 patients (Goodsell, 1967).

Therefore, it appears that the most common cause of unexplained low back pain with or without sciatica must be due to disturbance in the disk. Whether or not the cases usually grouped under acute strains are due to slight alteration of the disk remains to be proved. So far there is no available pathologic evidence of damage to ligaments and muscles, as these cases that respond readily to treatment are not explored.

With impairment of function of the disk mechanism spine motions are altered permanently. The normal repair process is sclerosis of the adjacent vertebral borders, narrowing of the disk space, osteophyte formation and, in time, even bony ankylosis of the involved segment or segments. Rupture of disk material with nerve root compression in the aged is quite rare. Therefore, treatment is directed to the relief of pain. Conservative measures are usually successful in all cases but those with massive posterior rupture of disk material into the spinal canal and even in these instances nonoperative treatment may successfully carry a patient through several acute episodes. Such treatment may include rest, support, rehabilitation exercises, and manipulation. Manipulation, if properly carried out in patients without contraindications (i.e., pedicle defects, marked motor weakness, spondylolisthesis, or spinal osteoporosis), can give gratifying results (Mensor, 1955). Those patients with recurrent severe episodes usually can be relieved by operation and removal of the protruding disk material. However, many do well on conservative treatment, with only an occasional mild recurrence.

Whether improvement is due to (1) a shift of the tissue away from the nerve, (2) desiccation or absorption of the protruded material, or (3) the nerve root becoming insensitive we do not know. However, with a large protrusion and nerve root compression the chances of relief of low back pain and sciatica are small. It is true that in time pain may be relieved, but there may be permanent nerve damage reflected in atrophy of the involved muscles, sensory loss and at times changes in the circulation.

The neurologic symptoms and signs produced by the herniated intervertebral disk are usually those of compression of a single lumbar nerve root. The history of intermittent back pain followed by sciatic radiation of pain is common. About 75 per cent of patients have the pain accentuated by coughing and sneezing. About half of them have a list or "sciatic" scoliosis which is usually away from the affected side. About 50 per cent of disk herniations occur at the L4-L5 interspace, 45 per cent at the L5-S interspace, and 5 per cent at the L3-L4 interspace. The neurologic signs depend on the level of the lesion.

Herniation of the disk at the L4-L5 interspace usually involves the 5th lumbar root. Radiation of pain is often to the great toe and the medial side of the foot, and hypesthesia in this area is frequent. Weakness of the long extensor of the great toe is also frequent, and 10 to 15 per cent will have a diminished knee jerk. Pain in the back on straight leg raising is almost always present. Local tenderness at the L4-L5 interspace is common.

Herniation of the disk at the L5-S interspace usually compresses the first sacral root, and the radiation of pain is to the lateral side of the foot. Hypesthesia over the lateral side of the foot, a diminished or absent ankle jerk, positive straight leg raising test and tenderness at the L5-S interspace are the common signs of herniation of the lumbosacral disk.

When the signs indicate that more than a single nerve root is compressed, the possibility exists that more than one herniation has occurred, or that there is a tumor of the spinal cord or a granuloma in the spinal canal. Rarely, a massive protrusion of a disk in the mid-line may result in severe neurologic abnormalities such as bilateral drop foot, quadriceps paralysis and loss of bowel and bladder control. Cases have been reported of bladder paralysis secondary to cauda equina lesions from disk prolapse (Scott, 1965). Herniated intervertebral disks have been reported in teenage children, occurring in approximately 0.5 per cent of 560 patients (Day, 1967; Epstein, 1964; Rugtveit, 1966). Low back pain and sciatica in the elderly are generly treated conservatively (Reccitelli, 1965),

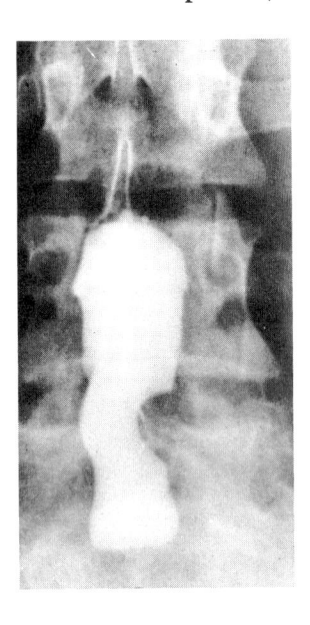

FIG. 53-47. Myelogram showing a large defect at the L4-L5 disk level. The defect is the result of a completely extruded nucleus pulposus. The myelogram is performed by injecting ethyl iodophenylundecylate (Pantopaque) into the subarachnoid space. This hyperbaric material can then be made to flow up and down the subarachnoid space by tilting the patient and clearly delineating such space-filling lesions. Spinal fluid for protein and other chemical determinations should be removed before injecting the contrast material. About half of the patients with a herniated nucleus pulposus will have a slight elevation (50-75 mgm. %) of spinal fluid protein; elevation of the spinal fluid protein greater than this is more likely due to a cord tumor than to a herniated disk.

although surgery has been performed in the aged with good results (Simon et al., 1965).

Treatment. We feel that all patients who do not respond to conservative therapy in a reasonable period of time (1 to 4 months), depending on the severity of symptoms and the character of the physical findings, should have further diagnostic studies made, including myelograms and EMGs (Fig. 53-47), followed by operation if the diagnosis is confirmed. The only patients not submitted to myelography are those presenting an acute and severe picture in which the localizing neurologic signs leave little doubt as to the location of the protruding mass and in whom it is felt that, because of the severity of the clinical picture, further conservative treatment will be worthless. The only indications for early operation are profound neurologic changes when the case is first seen or a rapidly progressing neurologic deficit.

Myelography, although it is useful, is not 100 per cent accurate. The percentages in the literature vary from 50 to 100 per cent, the true accuracy being about 85 per cent (Lansche and Ford, 1960). Intradiskal injection of dye (diskography) has been used in an attempt to improve diagnostic accuracy. Because of the high percentage of false positives, lumbar diskography is unreliable as a diagnostic test at the present time (Holt, 1968). A more recent diagnostic procedure is the use of intraosseous **vertebral** venography.

Its accuracy in localizing disk disease was reported as 83 per cent in a series of 42 patients. It may be useful in those patients in whom myelography is contraindicated (Amsler and Wilbert, 1967).

The extradural approach to the disk (Love, 1937) has greatly simplified the operative technic. Furthermore, we have at times used local anesthesia for further simplification.

The question still remains whether or not a spinal fusion also should be done at the time of removal of the protruded disk. As the removal of the protruded disk material only relieves nerve root compression and does not correct the altered mechanics of the spine resulting from degeneration of the disk, there remains a chance for continued low back pain and even sciatica. Froning and Frohman (1968) have recently shown that those patients who had a successful laminectomy and disk removal demonstrated restriction of flexion and extension, while persistence of mobility was found in patients judged to have poor results. Perhaps it is these patients who would benefit from the additional spinal fusion.

In our experience, approximately 50 per cent of the patients with simple disk excision remain completely free of pain. There is evidence that combining disk excision with a spinal fusion will increase the over-all per cent of good results by about 10 to 15 per cent. Spinal fusion increases the operative risk and the postoperative convalescent period. It appears that local fusion is desirable, and we feel sure that when a satisfactory and simple method of obtaining fusion following disk surgery is evolved it will be employed in a larger number of cases. However, a solid spinal fusion does not ensure relief of pain; it may be that following fusion of the involved area extra stress is placed on other degenerating disks, either above or below the operated one. In spite of the theoretical and clinical evidence that the end result would be improved by the combined operation of disk removal and spinal fusion (Hoover, 1968), we seldom carry out this procedure because we have felt that the results do not justify the additional surgery.

At times an unstable degenerative disk without posterior protrusion may continue to cause disabling low back pain in spite of continued conservative measures, and spinal fusion may be required.

Smith and Brown (1967) investigated the possibility of removing intervertebral disks chemically using chymopapain, a proteolytic enzyme. The results were stressed as good in 68 of 75 patients. This is said to be a safe, effective means of relieving sciatic and low back pain in selected cases; its use is being tested in a number of centers.

COMPLICATIONS. Visceral injuries involving the ureter, bladder, ileum and appendix have been reported. However, vascular injuries are more common. Arteriovenous fistula was reported in approximately 25 per cent of all published cases of vessel injuries (Staple and Friedenberg, 1968). The largest comprehensive series was published by DeSaussure, (1959), reporting on 106 cases. The most frequent site of injury was the common iliac artery, usually occurring with operations on the 4th or 5th lumbar disk. Diagnosis may be made by the finding of a palpable thrill or an audible bruit or symptoms of progressive cardiac failure. Immediate signs are those of shock secondary to blood loss. The over-all mortality rate from vascular injury has been reported to be as high as 50 per cent (Holscher, 1968; Stokes, 1968). Complications such as may be seen after any major surgery and unrelated to surgical technics include gastric dilatation, paralytic ileus, urinary retention and venous thrombosis. Although uncommon, closed disk space infections may occur (Ford and Key, 1955; Thibodeau, 1968). Neural complications include direct injury to a nerve root or injury to the cauda equina secondary to a large extruded disk fragment or excessive traction (Morgan, 1968). Postoperatively the patient may develop meningeal pseudocysts from incomplete repair of dural tears (Ford, 1968; Miller and Elder, 1968).

In summary, of patients with low back pain and sciatica due to degenerative disk disease with or without protrusion, only about 10 per cent require surgery. Of this group the cases without nerve root compression who fail to respond to conservative treatment may be treated by spinal fusion. Those with nerve root compression are treated by simple disk excision, and unless there is considerable instability fusion is not done.

DEGENERATIVE ARTHRITIS OF THE SPINE

The evidence of hypertrophic changes seen in the roentgenogram and commonly called degenerative arthritis are all probably secondary to alteration of disk function or to major trauma to the vertebra. These changes in themselves do not as a rule cause pain. However, at times a nerve root will be encroached upon in the vertebral foramen by a hypertrophic spur, with resultant (and often severe) pain.

Pelvic disease of various types has been blamed for low back pain and at times neuritis of the sciatic nerve. Spread of cancer from the pelvic organs, particularly in the female, may produce low back pain and sciatica from direct involvement of the components of the sciatic nerve within the pelvis. At times the diagnosis may be difficult, but the neurologic findings usually become marked and progressive, and a negative myelogram plus the evidence of pelvic neoplasm should readily suggest the diagnosis. However, we are aware of more than one such case that had exploration for a ruptured disk. On the other hand, a considerable number of women have had pelvic operations for low back pain due to disk degeneration. It appears that tumors and chronic infections of the female pelvis may cause some back pain, but we suggest that hysterectomy not be done for back pain alone.

The roentgenogram, coupled with a good history and a physical examination, should be adequate in separating defects of the pars interarticularis, infections, tumors, senile osteoporosis and rheumatoid arthritis from cases of disk rupture. However, repeated examination and time may occasionally be required to distinguish a case of rheumatoid arthritis.

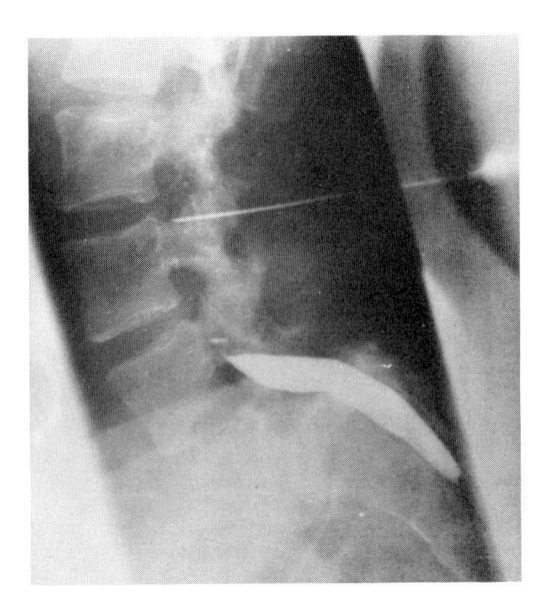

FIG. 53-48. Spondylolisthesis, grade III. Myelogram, demonstrating forward displacement of the 5th lumbar vertebra on the first sacral segment. The needle is in the interspace between the 2nd and the 3rd lumbar vertebrae.

Rarely, tuberculosis and slow-growing tumors present difficult diagnostic problems.

Some doubt has been cast on the proper treatment of defects of the pars interarticularis (Fig. 53-48). Gill *et al.* and Bosworth *et al.* (1955) indicated that resection of the loose posterior element, together with complete decompression of the roots, results in relief of pain. Bosworth follows this with spinal fusion. In a more recent series (Henderson, 1966) the best results were obtained by iliac fusion, with concurrent removal of the loose dorsal element. Removal of the dorsal elements appeared to have no adverse effect on the ratio of successful fusion.

We continue to believe that spinal fusion is the treatment of choice. In the presence of sciatica the involved root should be decompressed at operation, but the posterior element is not removed unless this is required to obtain adequate decompression of a root. The bone of the loose posterior element is viable, and we feel that it aids in obtaining fusion. Furthermore, Bosworth *et al.* (1955) has shown that the retained posterior element helps to prevent further forward displacement of the vertebral body. For both of these reasons we see no excuse for removal of the posterior element except in the rare case where adequate exposure of the root cannot be obtained without it.

BIBLIOGRAPHY

Abbott, L. C.: The operative lengthening of the tibia and fibula. J. Bone Joint Surg., 9:128, 1927.

Abbott, L. C., and Crego, C. H.: Operative lengthening of the femur. South. M. J., 21:823, 1928.

Abbott, L. C., Schottstaedt, E. R., Saunders, J. B. de C. M., and Bost, F. C.: The evaluation of cortical and cancellous bone as grafting material: a clinical and experimental study. J. Bone Joint Surg., 29:381, 1947.

Ackerman, L. V.: Surgical Pathology. St. Louis, C. V. Mosby, 1968.

Aegerter, E., and Kirkpatrick, J. A.: Orthopedic Diseases. Chap. 10. Philadelphia, W. B. Saunders, 1968.

Aho, A. S.: Electron microscopy and histological observations in fracture repair in young and old rats. Acta path. Microbiol. scand. (suppl.) 184:1-95, 1966.

Alberman, E. D.: Causes of congenital clubfoot. Arch. Dis. Child. 40:548, 1965.

Albright, F. Butler, A. M., and Bloomsberg, F.: Rickets resistant to vitamin D therapy. Am. J. Dis. Child., 54:629, 1937.

Albright, Fuller, and Reifenstein, E. C., Jr.: The Parathyroid Glands and Metabolic Bone Disease. Baltimore, Williams & Wilkins, 1948.

Alexander, C.: The etiology of femoral epiphyseal slipping. J. Bone Joint Surg., 48-B:299, 1966.

Allen, A., and Stevenson, A.: A ten year follow-up of combined drug therapy and early fusion in bone tuberculosis. J. Bone Joint Surg., 49-A:1001, 1967.

American Rheumatism Association: Primary on the rheumatoid diseases. Part I. J.A.M.A., 17:1205, 1959.

Amsler, F. R., and Wilbert, M. C.: Intraosseous vertebral venography as a diagnostic aid in evaluating intervertebral disc disease of the lumbar spine. J. Bone Joint Surg., 49-A:703, 1967.

Anderson, L. D.: Compression plate fixation. J. Bone Joint Surg., 47-A:191, 1965.

Anspach, W. E.: Bone formation by epithelium of the urinary bladder. Arch. Surg., 89:446, 1964.

Anthonsen, W.: Treatment of hip flexor contracture in cerebral palsy. Acta orthop. scand., 37:387, 1966.

Arct, M. W.: Operative treatment of tuberculosis of the spine in old people. J. Bone Joint Surg., 50-A: 255, 1968.

Armstrong, W. D.: Composition and crystal structure of the bone salt. In:Tr. 2nd Conf. on Metabolic Interrelations. New York, Macy, 1950.

Atkinson, P. J., Weatherell, J. A., and Weidmann, S. M.: Changes in density of the human femoral cortex with age. J. Bone Joint Surg., 44-B:496, 1962.

Attenborough, G. G.: Severe congenital talipes equinovarus. J. Bone Joint Surg., 48-B:31, 1966.

Bachra, B.: Molecular aspects of tissue calcification. Clin. Orth. Rel. Res., 51:199, 1967.

Badger, T. L.: Tuberculosis. New Eng. J. Med., 261: 30, 74, 1959.

Badgley, C. E., Isaacson, A. S., Walgamot, J. C., and Miller, J. W.: Operative therapy for slipped upper femoral epiphysis: an end result study. J. Bone Joint Surg., 30:19-28, 1948.

Bakalim, G.: Tuberculosis spondylitis. A clinical study with special reference to the significance of spinal fusion and chemotherapy. Acta orthop. scand. (Suppl. 47:1-111, 1960.

Baker, L., and Hill, L. M.: Foot alignment in the CP patient. J. Bone Joint Surg., 46-A:1-15, 1964.

Balogh, K.: Enzymes in mineralized tissues. Clin. Orth. Rel. Res., 48:285, 1966.

Balogh, K., and Hajeh, J. U.: Oxidative enzymes of intermediary metabolism in healing bone fractures. Am. J. Anat., 116:429, 1965.

Banks, H. H.: The healing of intra-articular fractures. Clin. Orth. Rel. Res., 40:17, 1965.

Bardenheier, J. A., III, Morgan, H. C., and Stamp, W. G.: Treatment and sequelae of experimentally produced septic arthritis. Surg., Gynec. Obstet., 122:249, 1966.

Bassett, C. A. L.: Current concept of bone formation. J. Bone Joint Surg., 44-A:1217, 1962.

———: Electrical effects in bone. Sci. Am., 213:18, 1965.

———: Environmental and cellular factors regulating osteogenesis. In: Frost, H.: Bone Biodynamics. Boston, Little, Brown & Co., 1964.

Bassett, C. A. L., et al.: Contribution of endosteum, cortex, and soft tissues to osteogenesis. Surg. Gynec. Obstet., 112:145, 1961.

Bassett, C. A. L., and Becker, R. O.: Generation of electric potentials by bone in response to mechanical stress. Science, 137:1063, 1962.

Bassett. C. A. L., Pawluh, R. J., and Becker, R. O.: Effects of electric currents on bone in vivo. Nature, 204:652, 1964.

Batson, O. V.: The vertebral vein system as a mechanism for the spread of metastases. Am. J. Roentgen, 48:715,1942.

Beadle, O. A.: The intervertebral discs; observations on their normal and morbid anatomy in relation to certain spinal deformities. Rep. Med. Res. Counc., (London) 161:1-79, 1931.

Bechtol, C. O., Ferguson, B., and Laing, P. G.: Metals and Engineering in Bone and Joint Surgery. Baltimore, Williams and Wilkins, 1959.

Becker, R. O.: The electrical control of growth. Med. Times, 95:657, 1967.

Becker, R. O., Bassett, C. A. L., and Bachman, C. H.: Bioelectrical factors controlling bone structure. In: Frost, H. M.: Bone Dynamics. Boston, Little, Brown & Co., 1964.

Becker, R. O., and Murray, D. G.: A method for producing cellular dedifferentiation by means of very small electrical current. Paper presented at New York Acad. Sci. February 14, 1967.

Bennett, G. A., Waine, H., and Bauer, W.: Changes in knee joint at various ages, with particular reference to the nature and development of degenerative joint disease. New York, Commonwealth Fund, 1942.

Berliner, D.: Ultrastructure of fibroblasts following topical corticosteroid therapy. Endocrinology, 81: 461, 1967.

Bierman, H. R., Lanman, J. T., Dod, K. S., Kelly, K. H., Miller, E. R., and Shimkin, M. D.: The amelioratic effect of antibiotics on nonlipoid reticuloendotheliosis (Leterer-Siwe disease) in identical twins. J. Pediat., 40:269, 1952.

Blackwood, H. J. (ed.): Bone and Tooth Symposium. New York, Macmillan, 1964.

Blau, M., Nagler, W., and Bender, M. A.: Fluorine-18, a new isotope for bone scanning. J. Nucl. Med., 3:332, 1962.

Blount, W. P.: The non-operative treatment of scoliosis. In: Symposium on the spine, Amer. Acad. Orthop. Surg. pp. 188-195. St. Louis, C. V. Mosby, 1969.

———: Unequal leg length. Instructional Course Lectures, Am. Acad. Orthop. Surg., 17:218, 1960.

Blount, W. P., and Clark, G. R.: Control of bone growth by epiphyseal stapling. J. Bone Joint 31-A:464, 1949.

Borella, L., Goobar, J. E., Summitt, R. L., and Clark, G. M.: Septic arthritis in childhood. J. Pediat., 62:742, 1963.

Bosworth, D. M.: The role of the orbicular ligament in tennis elbow. J. Bone Joint Surg., 37-A:527, 1955.

———: Supraspinatus syndrome, symptomatology, pathology, and repair. J.A.M.A., 117:422, 1941.

Bosworth, D. M., Fielding, J. W., Demarest, L., and Bonaquist, M.: Spondylolisthesis; a critical review of a consecutive series of cases treated by arthrodesis. J. Bone Joint Surg., 37-A:767, 1955.

Bourne, G. H.: The biochemistry and physiology of bone. New York, Academic Press, 1956.

Boyce, W. H., Garvey, F. H., and Norfleet, C. M.: Ion binding properties of electrophoretically homogeneous mucoproteins of the urine in normal subjects with renal calculus disease. J. Urol., 72:1019, 1954.

Boyd, H. B.: Cause and treatment of non-union in long bones. Instr. Course Lectures, 17:165, 1960.

Boyes, J.: Bunnell's Surgery of the Hand. 4th ed. Philadelphia, J. B. Lippincott, 1964.

Brahms, M. A.: Common foot problems. J. Bone Joint Surg., 49-A:1653, 1967.

Briggs, R. C.: Detection of osseous metastases. Cancer, 20:392, 1967.

Brodie, B. C.: An account of some cases of chronic disease of the tibia. Medico-Chir. Tr., 17:239, 1832.

Brown, L. T.: Beef bone in stabilizing operations of the spine. J. Bone Joint Surg., 20:711, 1922.

Brunner, J. M.: Treatment of "sesamoid" synovial ganglia of hand by needle rupture. J. Bone Joint Surg., 45-A:1689, 1963.

Bulmer, J. H.: Septic arthritis of the hip in adults. J. Bone Joint Surg., 48-B:289, 1966.

Burch, P. R. S.: Dupuytren's contracture, an autoimmune disease? J. Bone Joint Surg., 48-B:31 1966.

Burwell, R. G.: Biological mechanism in foreign bone transplantation. *In*: Modern Trends in Orthopaedics. 4. The Science of Fractures. Washington, D.C., Butterworth, 1964.

———: Studies in the transplantation of bone. 8. Treated composite homograft-autografts of cancellous bone, an analysis of inductive mechanisms in bone transplanting. J. Bone Joint Surg., 48-B:532, 1966.

Caldwell, G. D.: Transplantation of the biceps femoris to the patella by the medial route in poliomyelitic quadriceps paralysis. J. Bone Joint Surg., 37-A:347, 1955.

Cameron, D. A.: The fine structure of bone and calcified cartilage. Clin. Orthop., 26:199, 1963.

Casuccio, C.: Concerning osteoporosis. J. Bone Joint Surg., 44-B:453, 1962.

Chandler, F. A.: Patellar advancement operation; a revised technique. Paper Presented at Internat. Coll. Surg. Meet., Chicago, Jan. 1947.

———: Re-establishment of normal leverage of the patella in knee flexion deformity in spastic paralysis. Surg., Gynec. Obstet., 57:523, 1933.

Charkes, N. D., Skarloff, D. M. and Young, I.: Critical analysis of strontium bone scanning for detection of metastatic cancer. Am. J. Roentgeno, 96:647, 1966.

Chase, S. W., and Herndon, C. H.: The fate of autogenous and homogenous bone grafts, a historical review. J. Bone Joint Surg., 37-A:809, 1955.

Clark, J. M. P.: Modern Trends in Orthopedics. 4. The Science of Fractures. Washington, D.C., Butterworth, 1964.

Clawson, D. K.: Common bacterial infections of bone. G. P., 32:125, 1965.

Clawson, D. K., and Dunn, A. W.: Management of common bacterial infections of bone and joints. J. Bone Joint Surg., 49-A:164, 1967.

Clawson, D. K., and Stevenson, J. K.: Treatment of chronic osteomyelitis. Surg., Gynec. Obstet., 120:59, 1965.

Cleveland, M., and Bosworth, D. M.: Pathology of tuberculosis of the spine. J. Bone Joint Surg., 24:527, 1942.

Cleveland, M., Bosworth, D. M., Fielding, J. W., and Smyrnis, P.: Fusion of the spine for tuberculosis in children. A long range follow-up study. J. Bone Joint Surg., 40-A:91, 1958.

Cochran, G.: Electromechanical characteristics of moist bone. Paper given at American Acad. Orthop. Surg., Chicago, Jan. 20, 1968.

Cockin, J.: Butler's operation for an over-riding 5th toe. J. Bone Joint Surg., 50-B:78, 1968.

Coleman, S.: Treatment of congenital dislocation of the hip in the infant. J. Bone Joint Surg., 47-A:590, 1965.

Collins, D. H.: The pathology of articular and spinal diseases. London, Edward Arnold & Co., 1949.

Compere, E. L., Johnson, W. E., and Coventry, M. B.: Vertebra plana (Calve's disease) due to eosinophilic granuloma. J. Bone Joint Surg., 36:969, 1954.

Compere, E. L., Metzger, W. I., and Mitra, R. N.: The treatment of pyogenic bone and joint infections by closed irrigation (circulation) with a non-toxic detergent and one or more antibiotics. J. Bone Joint Surg., 49-A:614, 1967.

Cooley, J. C., Mussey, R. D., and Rogers, J. C. T.: Femoral arteriovenous fistula creation in the treatment of the short leg. Arch. Surg., 80:838, 1960.

Copeland, M: Early detection of bone radioactive strontium. Cancer, 20:734, 1967.

Copher, G. H., and Key, J. A.: Influence of bladder transplants on the healing of defects of bone. Arch. Surg., 29:64, 1934.

Coventry, M.: Osteotomy of upper portion of tibia for degenerative arthritis of the knee. Preliminary report. J. Bone Joint Surg., 47-A:984, 1965.

Coventry, M. B., Ghormley, R. K., and Kernohan, J. W.: The intervertebral disc: its anatomy and pathology. Part I Anatomy, development and physiology. J. Bone Joint Surg., 27:105, 1945.

———: The intervertebral disc: its microscopic anatomy and pathology; 2. Changes in the intervertebral disc concomitant with age. J. Bone Joint Surg., 27:233, 1945b.

———: The intervertebral disc: its microscopic anatomy and pathology; 3. Pathological changes in the intervertebral disc. J. Bone Joint Surg., 27:460., 1945c.

Coventry, M. B., and Johnson, E. W.: Congenital absence of the fibula. Clin. Orthop., 14:20, 1959.

Crego, C. H., Jr., and Schwartzman, J. R.: Followup study of the early treatment of congenital dislocation of the hip. J. Bone Joint Surg., 30:428, 1948.

Crellin, R. Q., and Simorda, M. A.: Intertrochanteric osteotomy of the femur for osteoarthritis of the hip. A follow-up study. Brit. J. Surg., 52:437, 1965.

Crenshaw, A. H.: Campbell's Operative Orthopedics. 4th ed. p. 1144. St. Louis, C. V. Mosby, 1963.

Crenshaw, A. H., and Kilgore, W.: Surgical treatment of bicipital tenosynovitis. J. Bone Joint Surg., 48-A:1496, 1966.

Cseuz, K. A., Thomas, J. E., Lambert, E. H., Love, J. G., and Lipscomb, P. R.: Long-term results of operation for carpal tunnel syndrome. Mayo Clin. Proc., 41:232, 1966.

Curtiss, P. H., and Klein, L.: Destruction of articular cartilage in septic arthritis. I. *In vitro* studies. J. Bone Joint Surg., 45A:797, 1963.

———: Destruction of articular cartilage in septic arthritis: II. *In vivo* studies. J. Bone Joint Surg., 47-A:1595, 1965.

Dahlin, D. C.: Bone Tumors. 2nd ed. Springfield, Ill. Charles C Thomas, 1967.

Dahlin, D., and Coventry, M.: Osteogenic sarcoma. J. Bone Joint Surg., 49-A:101, 1967.

Dandy, W. E.: Loose cartilage from intervertebral disc simulating tumor of spinal cord. Arch. Surg., 19:567, 1929.

Danes, B. S., and Bearn, A. G.: Metachromasia and skin fibroblast cultures in juvenile familial amaurotic idiocy. Lancet, 2:855, 1968.

Davis, J. E.: On surgery of Dupuytren's contracture. Plast. Reconstr. Surg., 36:277, 1965.

Day, P. L.: Teenage disc syndromes. South. M. J., 60:247, 1967.

DePusky: The physiological oscillation of the length of the body. Acta orthop. scand., 6:338, 1935.

Derbyshire, R. C.: Observations on treatment of ganglion: with report on hydrocortisone injection. Am. J. Surg., 112:635, 1966.

DeSaussure, R. L.: Vascular injury coincident to disc surgery. J. Neurosurg., 16:222, 1959.

Dickinson, P. H., Coutts, M. B., Woodward, E. P., and Handler, D.: Tendo-achillis bursitis: report of 21 cases. J. Bone Joint Surg., 48-A:77, 1966.

Dos Santos, R.: Arteriography in bone tumors. J. Bone Joint Surg. 32-B:17, 1956.

Duraiswami, P. K.: Experimental causation of congenital skeletal defects and its significance in orthopedic surgery. J. Bone Joint Surg., 34:646, 1952.

Duthie, R. B.: The possible role of mast cells in tissue injury and their presence in fracture sites. In: Robinson, R. A. (ed.): Healing of Osseous Tissue. Nat. Acad. Sci. Nat. Res. Council, Washington, D.C., 1967.

———: 35-S-Sulphate in bone repair of rats. In: Lacroix and Budy (eds.): Radioisotopes and Bone. Oxford, Blackwell Scientific Publications, 1961.

Duthie, R. B., and Barker, A. N.: An autoradiographic study of mucopolysaccharide and phosphate complexes in bone growth and repair. J. Bone Joint Surg., 37-B:304, 1955.

———: The histochemistry of the pre-osseous stage of bone repair studied by autoradiography. J. Bone Joint Surg., 37-B:691, 1955.

Eagleson, W.: Effect of heat on the healing of fractures. Canad. M. A. J., 97:274, 1967.

Eastloe, J. E.: The organic matrix of bone. In: Bourne, G. (ed.): The Biochemistry and Physiology of Bone. New York, Academic Press, 1956.

Ebrahim, G. J., and Grech, P.: Salmonella osteomyelitis in infants. J. Bone Joint Surg., 48-B:350, 1966.

Eggers, G. W.: Transplantation of hamstring tendons to femoral condyles in order to improve hip extension and to decrease knee flexion in cerebral spastic paralysis. J. Bone Joint Surg., 34-A:827, 1952.

Eichelberger, L., Akeson, W. H., and Ronia, M.: Biochemical studies of articular cartilage. J. Bone Joint Surg., 40-A:142, 1958.

Eisenstein, R., and Groff, W. A.: Experimental hypervitaminosis D, hypercalcemia, hypermucoproteinemia. Proc. Soc. Exp. Biol. Med., 95:341, 1959.

Eliason, O., and Dunlap, D.: Osteomyelitis of spine following needle biopsy of prostate. J. Urol., 94:271, 1965.

Engel, M. B.: Mobilization of mucoprotein extract. Arch. Path., 53:339, 1952.

Enneking, W.: The repair of complete fractures in rat tibia. Anat. Rec., 101:515, 1948.

Epstein, J. A., and Lavine, L. S. Herniated lumbar intervertebral disc in teenage children. J. Neurosurg., 21:1070, 1964.

Errico, M. J.: Incidence of osteomyelitis in nonunion of fractures of the shaft of the tibia. J. Trauma, 7:838, 1967.

Evelagos, E., Leidholt, J. D., Smith, C., and Priest, R: Arthropathy associated with steroid treatment. Ann. Int. Med., 64:759, 1966.

Ewald, F., and Tachdjian, M.: The effect of thyrocalcitonin on fractured humeri. Surg., Gynec. Obstet. 125:1075, 1967.

Fairbank, T. H.: Atlas of General Affections of the Skeleton. Baltimore, Williams and Wilkins, 1952.

Ferguson, A. B., Jr.: High intertrochanteric osteotomy for osteoarthritis of the hip: A procedure to streamline the defective joints. J. Bone Joint Surg., 46-A:1159, 1964.

Ferguson, A. B., and Howorth, M. B.: Slipping of the upper femoral epiphysis. J.A.M.A., 97:1867, 1931.

Fick, R.: Handb. Anat. und Mech. d. Gelenke, 1911.

Finkelstein, H.: Stenosing tendovaginitis at the radial styloid process. J. Bone Joint Surg., 30:509, 1930.

Fleisch, H., and Bisay, S: Isolating from urine of pyrophosphate, a calcification inhibitor. Am. J. Physiol., 203:671, 1963.

Ford, L. T.: Local complications of disc surgery. J. Bone Joint Surg., 50-A:418, 1968.

Ford, L. T., and Key, J. A.: Postoperative infection of the intervertebral disc space. South, M. J., 48:1295, 1955.

Fraser, R.: The problem of osteoporosis. J. Bone Joint Surg., 44-B:485, 1962.

Friedman, B.: Chemotherapy of tuberculosis of the spine. J. Bone Joint Surg., 48-A:451, 1966.

Froning, E. C., and Frohman, B.: Motion of the lumbosacral spine after laminectomy and spine fusion. J. Bone Joint Surg., 50-A:897, 1968.

Frost, H. M.: Bone dynamics in metabolic bone disease. J. Bone Joint Surg., 40-A:1192, 1966.

Garceau, G. J., and Palmer, R. M.: Transfer of the anterior tibial tendon for recurrent clubfoot. J. Bone Joint Surg., 49-A:207, 1967.

Gardner, R. S.: Tennis elbow. J. Bone Joint Surg., 43-B:100, 1961.

Gartland, J. J.: Posterior tibial transplant in surgical treatment of recurrent clubfoot: A preliminary report, J. Bone Joint Surg. 46-A:1217, 1964.

Geist, H. J., Spencer, G. E., Chase, S. W., and Herndon, C. H.: The effect of continuous suction of the fracture on fracture healing in dogs. Surg., Gynec. Obstet., 118:972, 1964.

Ghormley, R. K.: Low back pain, with special reference to the articular facets with presentation of an operative procedure. J.A.M.A., 101:1773, 1933.

Ghormley, R. K., and Deacon, A. E.: Synovial membranes in various types of arthritis. Am. J. Roentgen., 35:740, 1936.

Gill, G. G., Manning, J. G., and White, H. L.: Surgical treatment of spondylolisthesis without spine fusion. J. Bone Joint Surg., 37-A:493, 1955.

Girzadas, D., Geens, S., Clayton, M., and Leidholt, J.: Performance of a hinged metal knee prosthesis. J. Bone Joint Surg., 50-A:355, 1968.

Glimcher, M.: Molecular biology of mineralized tissue with particular reference to bone. Rev. Mod. Phys., 3:359, 1959.

———: Structure and organization of bone. 2. Collagen and apatite crystal, the mechanism of calcification. Am. Acad. Orth. Surg. Instruct. Course, Chicago, Jan. 22, 1968.

Godman, G. C., and Porter, K. R.: Chondrogenesis studied with the electron microscope. J. Biophys. Biochem. Cytol., 8:719, 1960.

Goel, M. K.: Vertebral osteotomy for correction of fixed flexion deformity of the spine. J. Bone Joint Surg., 50-A:287, 1968.

Goldner, J. L.: Upper extremity reconstructive surgery in cerebral palsy or similar conditions. Instruct. Course Lect. Am. Acad. Orthop. Surg., 18:169, 1961.

Goldsmith, R. S., Woodhouse, C. F., and Ingbar, S. H.: Effect of phosphate supplements in patients with fractures. Lancet, 1:687, 1967.

Goldstein, L. A.: Surgical management of scoliosis. J. Bone Joint Surg., 48-A:167, 1966.

Goodsell, J. O.: Correlation of ruptured lumbar disc with occupation. Clin. Orthop., 50:225, 1967.

Green, W. T., and Anderson, M.: Experiences with epiphyseal arrest in correcting discrepancies in length of the lower extremities in infantile paralysis; a method of predicting the effect. J. Bone Joint Surg., 29:659, 1947.

———: Skeletal age and the control of bone growth. Instruct. Course Lect. Am. Acad. Orthop. Surg., 17:199, 1960.

Green, W. T., and Banks, H. H.: Flexor carpi ulnaris transplant and its use in cerebral palsy. J. Bone Joint Surg., 44-A:1343, 1962.

Green, W. T., and Farber, S: Eosinophilic or solitary granuloma of bone. J. Bone Joint Surg., 30:499, 1942.

Grice, D. S.: An extra-articular arthrodesis of the subastragalar joint for the correction of paralytic flat feet in children. J. Bone Joint Surg., 34-A:927, 1952.

Grillo, H. C., and Gross, J.: Collagenolytic activity during mammalian development. Biol., 15:300, 1967.

Gucker, T.: Changes in vital capacity in scoliosis. J. Bone Joint Surg., 44-A:469, 1962.

Hall, J. E., and Silverstein, E. A.: Acute hematogenous osteomyelitis. Pediatrics, 31:1033, 1963.

Halpern, M., and Freiberger, R. H.: Arteriography in orthopedics. Am. J. Roentgen., 44:194, 1965.

Ham, A. W., and Harris, W. R.: Repair and transplantation of bone. In: Bourne, G.: Biochemistry and Physiology of Bone. New York, Academic Press, 1956.

Harrington, P. R.: The management of scoliosis by spine instrumentation; an evaluation of more than 200 cases. South. M. J., 56:1367, 1963.

Harris, N. H., and Kirkaldy-Willis, W. H.: Primary subacute pyogenic osteomyelitis. J. Bone Joint Surg., 47-B:526, 1965.

Harris, R. I., and McDonald, J. L.: The effect of lumbar sympathectomy upon the growth of legs paralyzed by anterior poliomyelitis. J. Bone Joint Surg., 18:35, 1936.

Harris, R. T., and Beath, T.: Army Foot Survey. Ottawa, Nat. Res. Council, 1947.

Harris, S: The in vivo inhibition of bone formation by Alizarin Red., J. Bone Joint Surg., 46-A:493, 1967.

Harrison, H. E.: The integration of vit. D, parathyroid hormone on Ca, phos, Mg hemostasis in the rat. Metabolism, 13:952, 1967.

Harrison, M. H. M., and Menon, M. P. A.: Legg-Calvé-Perthes Disease. J. Bone Joint Surg., 48-A:1301, 1966.

Harrison, M. H., Schajawiez, F., and Trueta, J.: Osteoarthritis of the hip; a study of the nature and evolution of the disease. J. Bone Joint Surg., 35-B:598, 1953.

Hayes, J. T., Gross, H. P., and Dow, S.: Surgery for paralytic defects secondary to myelomeningocele and myelodysplasia. J. Bone Joint Surg., 46-A:1577, 1964.

Heiple, K. G., Chase, S. W., and Herndon, C. H.: A comparative study of the healing process following different types of bone transplantation. J. Bone Joint Surg., 45-A: 1593, 1963.

Heiple, K., and Herndon, C: The pathologic physiology of non union. Clin. Orthop., 43:11, 1965.

Henderson, F. D.: Results of surgical treatment of spondylolisthesis. J. Bone Joint Surg., 48-A:619, 1966.

Herndon, C. H., Heyman, C. H., and Bell, D. M.: Treatment of slipped capital femoral epiphysis by epiphysiodesis and osteoplasty of the femoral neck. J. Bone Joint Surg., 45-A:999, 1963.

Hersh, A: The role of surgery in the treatment of club feet. J. Bone Joint Surg., 49-A:1684, 1917.

Heyman, C. H.: Operative treatment of paralytic genu recurvatum. J. Bone Joint Surg., 44-A:1246, 1962.

———: The surgical release of fibrous tissue structures resisting correction of congenital club-foot and metatarsus varus. Am. Acad. Orthop. Surg. Lect, 16:100, 1959.

Heywood-Waddington, M. B.: Use of the Austin Moore prosthesis for advanced osteoarthritis of the hip. J. Bone Joint Surg., 48-B:236, 1966.

Highberger, J. H., Gross, J., and Schmidt, F. O.: The interaction of mucoprotein with soluble collagen: An electron microscopic study. Proc. Nat. Acad. Sci., 37:286, 1951.

Hirsch, C.: Efficiency of surgery in low back disorders. J. Bone Joint Surg., 47-A:991, 1965.

Hodgson, A. R., Skinsnes, O. K., and Leong, C. Y.: The pathogenesis of Pott's paraplegia. J. Bone Joint Surg., 49-A:1147, 1967.

Hodgson, A. R., and Stock, F. E.: Anterior spine fusion for the treatment of tuberculosis of the spine. The operative findings, and results of treatment in the first 100 cases. J. Bone Joint Surg., 42-A:295, 1960.

Hollander, J. L.: Arthritis and Allied Conditions. Ed. 7. p. 1020. Philadelphia, Lea and Febiger, 1966.

Hollingshead, W. H.: Anatomy of the spine: points of interest to orthopedic surgeons. J. Bone Joint Surg., 47-A:212, 1965.

Holscher, E. C.: Vascular and visceral injuries during lumbar disc surgery. J. Bone Joint Surg., 50-A:383, 1968.

Holt, E. P.: The question of lumbar discography. J. Bone Joint Surg., 50-A:720, 1968.

Hoover, N. W.: Indications for fusion at time of removal of intervertebral disc. J. Bone Joint Surg., 50-A:189, 1968.

Howard, J. E., et al.: The recognition and isolation from urine and serum of a peptide inhibitor to calcification. Johns Hopkins Med. J., 120:119, 1967.

Howell, D. S.: Concepts of calcification. Arthritis, Rheum., 6:736, 1963.

Hueston, J. T.: Dupuytren's contracture: trend to conservatism. Ann. Roy. Coll. Surg., 36:134, 1965.

Huggins, C. B., and McCarroll, H. R.: Experiments on the theory of osteogenesis. Arch. Surg., 32:915, 1936.

Hurley, L. A., Stinchfield, F. E., Bassett, C. A. L., and Lyon, W. H.: The role of soft tissue in osteogenesis. J. Bone Joint Surg., 41-A:1243, 1959.

Husto, H., Hulton, C., James, D., Jr., and Pinkel, D.: Treatment of Ewing's sarcoma with concurrent radiotherapy and chemotherapy. J. Pediat., 73:249, 1968.

Ilfeld, F. W.: The management of congenital dislocation of the hip by means of a special splint. J. Bone Joint Surg., 39-A:99, 1957.

Inglis, A. E., and Cooper, W.: Release of the flexor-pronator origin for flexion deformity of the hand and wrist in spastic paralysis. J. Bone Joint Surg., 48-A:847, 1966.

Irani, R. N., and Sherman, M. S.: The pathological anatomy of club foot. J. Bone Joint Surg., 45-A: 45, 1963.

Jackson, H. C., II, Winklemann, R. K., and Bickel, W. H.: Nerve endings in human lumbar spinal column and related structures. J. Bone Joint Surg., 48-A:1272, 1966.

Jacob, F., and Monod, J.: Genetic repression, allosteric inhibition and cellular differentiation. In: Michael Locke. (ed.): Cytodifferentiation and Macromolecular Synthesis. pp. 30-64. New York, Academic Press, 1963.

Jaffe, H.: Tumors and Tumorous Conditions of the Bones and Joints. Philadelphia, Lea and Febiger, 1964.

Jaffe, H. L., and Lichtenstein, L:. Eosinophilic granuloma of bone. Am. Path., 16:595, 1940.

Janes, J. M., and Musgrave, J. E.: Effect of arteriovenous fistula on the growth of bone: experimental study. Surg. Clin. N. Am., 30:1191, 1950.

Jeffree, G. M., and Price, C. H. G.: Bone tumors and their enzymes. J. Bone Joint Surg., 47-B:120, 1965.

Johnson, J. T. H.: Neuropathic fractures and joint injuries. J. Bone Joint Surg., 49-A:1, 1967.

Johnson, L. L., and Kempson, R. L.: Epidermoid carcinoma in chronic osteomyelitis: diagnostic problems and management; report of ten cases. J. Bone Joint Surg., 47-A:223, 1965.

Kagawa, S.: Enzyme histochemistry of bone induced by urinary bladder epithelium. J. Histochem. Cytochem., 13:255, 1965.

Kane, W. J.: Fundamental concepts in bone blood flow studies. J. Bone Joint Surg., 50-A:801, 1968.

Keats, Sidney: Surgical treatment of the hand in cerebral palsy: correction of thumb in palm and other deformity. J. Bone Joint Surg., 47-A:274, 1965.

Kelikian, H.: Hallux Valgus, Allied Deformities of the Forefoot and Metatarsalgia. Philadelphia, W. B. Saunders, 1965.

Kelly, P.: Anatomy, physiology and pathology of the blood supply of bones. J. Bone Joint Surg., 50-A: 766, 1968.

Kelly, P. J., Janes, J. M., and Peterson, L. F. A.: The effect of arteriovenous fistulae on the vascular pattern of the femur of immature dogs. J. Bone Joint Surg., 41-A:1101, 1959.

Kelly, P. J., Martin, W. J., and Coventry, M. B.: Bacterial arthritis of the hip in the adult. J. Bone Joint Surg., 47-A:1005, 1965.

Kessel, L.: Supracondylar spur at the humerus. J. Bone Joint Surg., 48-B:765, 1966.

Ketenjian, M. D., and Bassett, C. A. L.: Effect of varying concentrations of oxygen upon collagen biosynthesis in vitro. Paper given at Orthop. Res. Soc., Chicago, Jan. 19, 1968.

Kettelkamp, D. B., and Larson, C. B.: Evaluation of the Steindler flexorplasty. J. Bone Joint Surg., 45-A:513, 1963.

Key, J. A.: Effect of a local calcium deposit on osteogenesis and healing of fractures. J. Bone Joint Surg., 16:176, 1934.

———: Osteomyelitis. In: Lewis' Practice of Surgery. vol. 2, pp. 1-95. Hagerstown, Md., Prior, 1954.

Keyes, D. C., and Compere, D. C.: The normal and pathological physiology of the nucleus pulposus of the intervertebral disc. J. Bone Joint Surg., 14: 897, 1932.

Kirchheimer, G.: Vitamin C deficiency and connective tissue. Acta rheum. scand., 11:185, 1965.

Kirkaldy-Willis, W. H., and Thomas, G.: Anterior approaches in the diagnosis and treatment of infections of the vertebral bodies. J. Bone Joint Surg., 47-A:87, 1965.

Kite, J. H.: Principles involved in the treatment of congenital clubfoot. J. Bone Joint Surg., 21:595, 1939.

———: Some suggestions on the treatment of club foot by casts. J. Bone Joint Surg., 45-A:406, 1963.

———: The treatment of congenital clubfoot. Surg., Gynec. Obstet., 61:190, 1935.

Klein, A., Joplin, R. J., Reidy, J. A., and Hanelin, J.: Slipped capital femoral epiphysis. J. Bone Joint Surg., 34:233, 1952.

Kolar, J.: Effect of androgenic steroid on the formation of skeletal matrix in rats with fractures. Nature, 206:941, 1965.

Kolar, J., and Vrabec, R.: Arthropathies after radiation. J. Bone Joint Surg., 49-A:1157, 1967.

Koskinen, E. V. S.: The effect of growth hormone and thyrotropin on human fracture healing. Acta orthop. scand., Suppl. 62, 1963.

———: Influence of hormonal treatment and orchiectomy, oophorectomy and thyroidectomy on experimental fractures. Acta orthop. scand. 36:supp. 80, 1965.

Koskinen, E. V. S., Pekka, T., and Siltanen, P.: The effect of massive arteriovenous fistula on hemodynamics and on bar growth. Clin. Orthop., 50:309, 1967.

Krane, S. M., Parsons, V., and Kunin, A. S.: Studies on the metabolism of epiphyseal cartilage; In: Cartilage: degradation and Repair. Nat. Acad. Sci., Nat. Res. Council, Washington, D.C., 1967.

Kuhlman, R. E.: A microchemical study of the developing epiphyseal plate. J. Bone Joint Surg., 42-A:457, 1960.

Lagergren, C., Lindbloom, A., and Soderberg, C.:

Angiography of peripheral tumors. Radiology, 79: 371, 1962.

Lambrinudi, C.: A new operation on drop foot. Brit. J. Surg., 15:193, 1927.

Lansche, W. E., and Ford, L. T.: Correlations of the myelogram with clinical and operative findings in lumber disc lesions. J. Bone Joint Surg., 42-A:193, 1960.

Lasegue, C.: Considerations sur la sciatique. Arch. gen. med., 2:558, 1864.

Lawrence, M., and Smith, A.: Effect on union of fractures of homografting isolated chondrocytes. Paper given at Orthop. Res. Soc., Chicago, Jan. 19, 1968.

LeMain, R. G.: Calcium metabolism in fracture healing. J. Bone Joint Surg., 48:1156, 1966.

Leonard, M. H., and Rising, E. E.: Syndactylization to maintain correction of overlapping 5th toe. Clin. Orthop., 43:241, 1965.

Levenson, S. M.: Proceedings, Workshop on Wound Healing. Nat. Acad. Sci., Nat. Res. Council, Washington, D.C., 1966.

Levine, J., Gitman, L., and Balker, H.: Histological study of treated and untreated cases of osteoporosis in humans. J. Bone Joint Surg., 37:624, 1955.

Lewin, T.: Osteoarthritis in lumbar synovial joints: morphologic study. Acta orthop. Scan., Supp. 73, 1964.

Lichtenstein, L.: Bone Tumors. ed. 3. St. Louis, C. V. Mosby, 1965.

———: Histiocytosis X (eosinophilic granuloma of bone, Letterer-Siwe disease, and Schuller-Christian disease). J. Bone Joint Surg., 46-A:76, 1964.

Linghorne, W. J.: The sequence of events in osteogenesis as studied in polyethylene tubes. Ann. N.Y. Acad. Sci., 85:445, 1960.

Linscheid, R. L.: Surgery for rheumatoid arthritis—timing and techniques:the upper extremity. J. Bone Joint Surg., 50-A:605, 1968.

Little, K., and Kelly, M.: Studies on bone matrix in normal and osteoporotic bone. J. Bone Joint Surg., 44-B:503, 1962.

Love, R.: The role of intervertebral discs in the production of chronic low back and sciatic pain. Proc. Mayo Clin. 12:369, 1937.

Luck, J. V.: Bone and Joint Disease. Springfield, Ill., Charles C Thomas, 1950.

Macnab, I.: Fractures of the shaft of the tibia. Am. J. Surg., 97:543, 1954.

Makin, M.: Osteogenesis induced by vesical mucosa transplant in the guinea pig. J. Bone Joint Surg., 44-B:165, 1962.

Mallory, T. B.: Disease of bone. New Eng. J. Med., 227:955, 1942.

Manken, H. J.: Cardiopulmonary function in mild and moderate idiopathic scoliosis. J. Bone Joint Surg., 46-A:53, 1964.

Margo, M. K.: Surgical treatment of the foot. J. Bone Joint Surg., 49-A:1665, 1967.

McCarroll, H. R.: Diagnosis and treatment of congenital sublaxation (dysplane) and dislocation of the hip in infancy. J. Bone Joint Surg., 47-A:612, 1965.

———: Early management of congenital dislocation of the hip. In: Lectures on regional orthopedic surgery and fundamental orthopedic problems. 21:125, Ann Arbor, Edwards, 1948.

———: Some clinical observations in problems of soft tissue calcification. Arch. Surg., 74:578, 1957.

McClean, F. D., and Urist, M. R.: Bone. University of Chicago Press, 1961.

McDonough, J. M., Brandfass, W. T., and Stinchfield, F. E.: Idiopathic osteoarthritis of the hip. J. Bone Joint Surg., 49-A:625, 1967.

McElhaney, J. H.: The charge distribution on the human femur due to load. J. Bone Joint Surg., 49-A:1561, 1967.

McFarlan, R. M., and Jamieson, W. G.: Dupuytren's contracture: management of 100 patients. J. Bone Joint Surg., 48-A:1095, 1966.

McGavran, M. H., and Spady, H. A.: Eosinophilic granuloma of bone. J. Bone Joint Surg., 42-A:979, 1960.

McKee, G. W., and Watson-Farrar, J.: Replacement of arthritic hips by McKee-Farrar prosthesis. J. Bone Joint Surg., 48-B:245, 1966.

McKenna, R. J., Schwinn, C. P., Soong, K. Y., and Higinbotham, M. D.: Sarcomata of the osteogenic series (osteosarcoma, fibrosarcoma, parosteal osteogenic sarcoma, and sarcomata arising in abnormal bone). J. Bone Joint Surg., 48-A:1, 1966.

McKibbin, B., and Ray, R. D.: Experimental study of peripheral circulation and bone growth. part 1. Clin. Orthop., 53:175, 1967.

McKusick, V. A.: Heritable Disorders of Connective Tissue. ed. 3. St. Louis, C. V. Mosby, 1960.

McLoughlin, H. L.: Selection of calcium deposits for operation: technique and results of operation. S. Clin. N. Am., 43:1501, 1963.

Meachim, G.: The histology and ultra structure of cartilage. In: Bassett, C. A. L. (ed.): Cartilage: Degradation and Regeneration. Nat. Acad. Sci., Res. Council, Washington, D.C. 1967.

Mendelsohn, B. G.: Actinomycosis of a metacarpal bone. J. Bone Joint Surg., 47-B:739, 1965.

Mensor, M.: Non-operative treatment including manipulation for lumbar intervertebral disc syndrome. J. Bone Joint Surg., 37-A:295, 1955.

Mesara, B. W., Brody, G. L., and Oberman, H. A.: "Pseudo rheumatoid" subcutaneous nodules. Am. J. Clin. Path., 45:684, 1966.

Meyer, K., et al.: The acid mucopolysaccharides of connective tissue. Biochem. biophys. acta, 21:506, 1956.

Meyer, T. L., Kieger, A. B., and Smith, W. S.: Antibiotic management of staphylococcal osteomyelitis. J. Bone Joint Surg., 47-A:285, 1965.

Milkman, L. A.: Multiple spontaneous idiopathic symmetrical fracture. Am. J. Roentgen, 32:623, 1934.

Miller, P. R., and Elder, F. W.: Meningeal pseudocysts (meningocele spurius) following laminectomy. J. Bone Joint Surg., 50-A:268, 1968.

Miller, W. T., and Restifo, R. A.: Steroid arthropathy. Radiology, 86:652, 1956.

Miller, Z. B., et al.: The effect of dyes on the calcification of hypertrophic rachitic cartilage in vitro. J. Exp., Med., 95:497, 1952.

Mixter, W., and Barr, J.: Rupture of the intervertebral disc with involvement of spinal canal. New Eng. J. Med., 211:210, 1934.

Moe, J. H.: A critical analysis of method of fusion for scoliosis. J. Bone Joint Surg., 40-A:529, 1958.

———: Methods and technique of evaluating idiopathic scoliosis. In: Symposium on the spine, Amer. Acad. Orthop. Surg. pp. 196-240. St. Louis, C. V. Mosby, 1969.

Moe, J. H., and Gustillo, R. B.: Treatment of scoliosis: results in 196 patients treated by cast correction or fusion. J. Bone Joint Surg., 46-A:293, 1964.

Moehlig, R. C., and Abbott, H. L.: Carbohydrate metabolism in osteitis deformans or Paget's disease. J.A.M.A., 134:1521, 1947.

Morgan, H. C.: Neural complications of disc surgery. J. Bone Joint Surg., 50-A:411, 1968.

Morgan, H. C., Hertel, R. C., and Stamp, W. G.: Quantitative barrier of synovium to penicillin. Arch. Surg., 87:450, 1963.

Moseley, H. F.: Natural history and clinical syndromes produced by calcified deposits within the rotator cuff. S. Clin. N. Am., 43:1489, 1963.

Moss, M. D.: Experimental induction of osteogenesis In: Sogannaes, R. F. (ed.): Calcification in Biological Systems. Am. Ass. Adv. Sci., Washington, D.C., 1960.

Mustard, W. T.: A follow-up study of iliopsoas transfer for hip instability. J. Bone Joint Surg., 41-B:289, 1959.

Nachemson, A.: The load on lumbar discs in different positions of the body. Clin. Orthop., 45:107, 1966.

Nicholas, J. A., and Killoran, P.: Fracture of the femur in patients with Paget's disease. Results of treatment in twenty-three cases. J. Bone Joint Surg., 47-A:450, 1965.

O'Hara, J. M., Hutter, R. V. P., Foote, F. W., Miller, T., and Woodard, H.: An analysis of thirty patients surviving longer than ten years after treatment for osteogenic sarcoma. J. Bone Joint Surg., 50-A:335, 1968.

Orofino, C., Innis, J. J., and Lowrey, C. W.: Slipped capital femoral epiphysis in Negroes. A study of 95 cases. J. Bone Joint Surg., 42-A:1079, 1960.

Orr, H. W.: The treatment of acute osteomyelitis by drainage and rest. J. Bone Joint Surg., 9:733, 1927.

Paff, G. H.: Influence of pH on growth of bone in tissue culture. Proc. Soc. Exp. Biol. Med., 68:288, 1948.

Palmer, R. M.: The genetics of talipes equinovarus. J. Bone Joint Surg., 46-A:542, 1964.

Parrish, F.: Treatment of bone tumors by total excision and replacement with massive autologous and homologous grafts. J. Bone Joint Surg., 48-A:968, 1966.

Parson, D. W., and Seddon, H. J.: The results of operation for disorders of the hip caused by poliomyelitis. J. Bone Joint Surg., 50-B:266, 1968.

Peacock, E., Jr.: Dynamic aspects of collagen biology. J. Surg. Res., 7:9-10, 1967.

Pearse, H. E., and Morton, W.: The stimulation of bone growth by venous stasis. J. Bone Joint Surg., 12:97, 1930.

Pease, C. N.: Local stimulation of growth of long bones; a preliminary report. J. Bone Joint Surg., 34:1, 1952.

Pechet, M. M., Bobadilla, E., Carroll, E. L., and Hesse, R. H.: Regulation of bone resorption and formation. Am. J. Med., 43:696, 1967.

Pedersen, H. E., and McCarroll, H. R.: Vitamin D-resitant rickets J. Bone Joint Surg., 33:203, 1951.

Perkins, H. R., and Walker, P. C.: The occurrence of prophosphate in bone. J. Bone Joint Surg., 40-B:333, 1968.

Peterson, L. F.: Surgery for rheumatoid arthritis—timing and techniques: the lower extremity. J. Bone Joint Surg., 50-A:587, 1968.

Phalen, G. S.: Carpal tunnel syndrome, 17 years experience in diagnosis and treatment of 654 hands. J. Bone Joint Surg., 48-A:211, 1966.

Phemister, D. B.: Repair of bone in presence of aseptic necrosis resulting from fractures, transplantation and vascular obstruction. J. Bone Joint Surg., 12:769, 1930.

Phillips, R. F., and Higinbotham, N. L.: The curability of Ewing's endothelioma of bone in children. J. Pediat., 70:391, 1967.

Pollock, S., Morris, J. and Murray, W.: Coccidioidal synovitis of the knee. J. Bone Joint Surg., 49-A:1397, 1967.

Ponseti, I. V.: Lesions of the skeleton and of other mesodermal tissues in rats fed sweet pea. J. Bone Joint Surg., 36:1031, 1954.

———: Nonsurgical treatment of congenital dislocation of the hip. J. Bone Joint Surg., 48-A:1392, 1966.

Ponseti, I. V., and Smoley, E. N.: Congenital club foot: the results of treatment. J. Bone Joint Surg., 45-A:261, 1963.

Pories, W. J., et al.: Acceleration of healing with zinc sulfate. Ann. Surg., 165:432, 1967.

Post, R. H., Heiple, K. G., Chase, S. W., and Herndon, C. H.: Bone grafts in diffusion chambers (millipore). Clin. Orthop., 44:265, 1966.

Pritchard, J. J.: Bone healing. In: Scientific Basis of Medicine Annual Reviews. pp. 288-301, 1963.

Prudden, J. F.: The acceleration of wound healing with cartilage. Surg., Gynec. Obstet., 105:283, 1957.

———: The reversal of inhibition of wound healing by cartilage. Surg., Gynec. Obstet., 124:109, 1967.

Puschel, J.: Der Wassergehalt normaler und degenerierter Zwischenwirbelscheiben. Betr. Path. Anat., 84:123, 1930.

Quigley, T. B.: Non-operative treatment of symptomatic calcareous deposits in the shoulder. S. Clin. N. Am. 43:1495, 1963.

———: Indications for manipulation and corticosteroids in treatment of stiff shoulders. S. Clin. N. Am., 43:1715, 1963.

Rabhan, W., and Haas, L. M.: The role of the fracture hematoma in the union of long bones. Paper presented at the American Academy of Orthopedic Surgeons Meeting N.Y., N.Y., Jan. 22, 1969.

Rapp, G. F., Griffith, R. S., and Hebble, W.: The permeability of traumatically inflamed synovial

membrane to commonly used antibiotics. J. Bone Joint Surg., 48-A:1534, 1966.
Ray, R. D., Aovad, R., and Kawabata, M.: Experimental study of peripheral circulation and bone growth. 1. Clin. Orthop., 52:221, 1967.
Ray, R. D., and Sabet, T. Y.: Bone grafts: cellular survival versus induction. J. Bone Joint Surg., 45-A:337, 1963.
Reccitelli, M. L.: Low back pain and sciatica in elderly patients. J. Am. Geriat. Soc., 13:80, 1965.
Reynolds, F. C., and Key, J. A.: Fracture healing after fixation with standard plates, contact splints, and medullary nails. J. Bone Joint Surg., 36-A:557, 1954.
Rhinelander, F. W., and Baragry, R. A.: Micro angiography in bone healing: 1. Undisplaced closed fracture. J. Bone Joint Surg., 44-A:1273, 1962.
Richelle, L. J. (ed.): Calcified Tissues. New York, Stechert-Hafner, 1965.
Riordan, D. C.: Congenital absence of the radius. J. Bone Joint Surg. 37-A:1129, 1959.
Risser, J. C., and Norquist, D. M.: A follow-up study of the treatment of scoliosis, J. Bone Joint Surg., 40-A:555, 1958.
Robinson, R. A.: An electron microscopic study of the crystalline inorganic component of bone and its relationship to the organic matrix. J. Bone Joint Surg., 34:389, 1952.
———: The healing of osseous tissue. Nat. Acad. Sci., Nat. Res. Council, Washington, D.C., 1967.
Robinson, R. A., and Watson, M. D.: Crystal collagen relationships in bone as observed in the electron microscope. Ann. N.Y. Acad. Sci., 60:596, 1955.
Roofe, P. G.: Innervation of the annulus fibrosus and the posterior longitudinal ligament. Arch. Neurol. Psychiat., 44:100, 1940.
Roseberry, H. H., Hastings, A. B., and Morse, J. K.: X-ray analysis of bone and teeth. J. Biol. Chem., 90:395, 1931.
Rosenthal, S.: Acceleration of primary wound healing by insulin. Arch. Surg., 96:53, 1968.
Rubin, P.: Dynamic classification of bone dysplasias. Chicago, Year Book Medical Publishers, 1964.
Rugtveit, A: Juvenile lumbar disc herniations. Acta orthop. Scand., 37:348, 1966.
Ryder, C. T.: CDH in the older child: surgical treatment. J. Bone Joint Surg., 48-A:1404, 1966.
Salter, R. B.: Etiology, pathogenesis, and possible prevention of congenital dislocation of the hip. Canad. M. A. J., 98:933, 1968.
Salter, R., Gross, A., and Hall, J. H.: Hydrocortisone arthropathy: experimental investigation. Canad. M. A. J., 97:374, 1967.
Samuels, M. L., and Howe, C. D.: Cyclophosphamide in management of Ewing's sarcoma. Cancer, 20:961, 1967.
Schajowicz, F., and Derqui, J. C.: Puncture biopsy in lesions of the locomotor system. Cancer, 21:531, 1968.
Schilling, J. A.: Wound healing. Physiol. Rev., 48:374, 1968.
Scott, P. J.: Bladder paralysis in cauda equina lesions from disc prolapse. J. Bone Joint Surg., 47-B:224, 1965.

Serafin, J.: A new operation for congenital absence of the fibula. J. Bone Joint Surg., 49-B:59, 1967.
Sever, J. W.: The results of a new operation for Obstetrical paralysis. Am. J. Orthop. Surg., 16:248, 1918.
Sharp, N., Guhl, J. F., Sorenson, R. I., and Vashell, A. F.: Hip fusion in poliomyelitis in children: preliminary report. J. Bone Joint Surg., 46-A:121, 1964.
Shatton, J., and Schubert, M.: Isolation of mucoprotein from cartilage. J. Biol. Chem., 211:565, 1954.
Shim, S. S.: The effect of epinephrine on blood flow in dogs and rabbits. M. Bone Soc. Internat. Chir. Orthop. Traumatol. 1:6-9, 1963.
———: Physiology of blood circulation of bone. J. Bone Joint Surg., 50-A:812, 1968.
Shim, S. S., Copp, D. H., and Patterson, F. P.: Measurement of the rate and distribution of the nutrient and other arterial blood supply in long bones of the rabbit. J. Bone Joint Surg., 50-B, 1968.
Sideman, S.: Surgery of poliomyelitis of lower extremity. S. Clin. N. Am., 45:175, 1965.
Silk, F. F., and Wainwright, D.: The recognition and treatment of congenital flat foot in infancy. J. Bone Joint Surg., 49-B:628, 1968.
Simon, S. D., Silver, C. M., and Litchman, H. M.: Lumbar disc surgery in the elderly (over the age of 60). Clin. Orthop., 41:157, 1965.
Singer, M.: Tennis elbow. S. Afr. Med. J., 38:896, 1964.
Sjoerdsma, A.: Hydroxyproline and collagen metabolism: Clinical implication. Ann. Int. Med., 63:672, 1965.
Skoog, T.: Dupuytren's contracture: Pathogenesis and surgical treatment. S. Clin. N. Am., 47:433, 1967.
Smith, L., and Brown, J. E.: Treatment of lumbar intervertebral disk lesions by direct injection of chymopapain. J. Bone Joint Surg., 49-B:502, 1967.
Smith, R., and Kaplan, E.: Rheumatoid deformities at the metacarpo-phalangeal joints of the fingers. J. Bone Joint Surg., 49-A:31, 1967.
Smith-Petersen, M. N., Larsen, C. R., and Aufranc, O. E.: Osteotomy of the spine for correction of flexion deformity in rheumatoid arthritis. J. Bone Joint Surg., 27:1-11, 1945.
Snapper, I: Medical Clinics on Bone Diseases. ed. 2. New York, Interscience Publishers, 1949.
Sobel, A.: Role of chondroitin sulfate in calcification. Proc. Soc. Exp. Biol. Med., 87:7, 1954.
Sognnaes, R. F.: Calcification in Biological Systems. Am. Ass. Adv. Sci., Washington, D.C., 1960.
Solheim, K.: Distribution of glycosaminoglycans, hydroxyproline and calcium in healing fractures. Acta soc. med. Upsal., 71:1-13, 1966; J. Oslo City Hosp. 16:17, 1966.
———: Fracture healing in rats studied with radioactive phosphorus. Acta chir. scand. 129:131, 1965.
Soliman, F. A., and Hassan, S. Y.: Serum calcium and phosphorus in rabbits during fracture healing. Nature, 204:693, 1964.
Somerville, E. W.: Development of congenital dis-

location of the hip. J. Bone Joint Surg., 35-B:568, 1953.
Sones, D. A.: Surgery for rheumatoid arthritis—timing and techniques: general and medical aspects. J. Bone Joint Surg., 58:576, 1968.
Southwick, W. O.: Osteotomy through the lesser trochanter for slipped capital femoral epiphysis. J. Bone Joint Surg., 49-A:807, 1967.
Speed, J. S., and Knight, R. A. (eds.): Campbell's Operative Orthopedics. ed. 4. vols. 1 and 2. St. Louis, C. V. Mosby, 1963.
Stamp, W. G.: Bracing in cerebral palsy. J. Bone Joint Surg., 44-A:1457, 1962.
Stamp, W. G., Canales, G., and Odell, R. D.: Late results in osteochondrosis of capital epiphysis of femur (Legg-Calvé-Perthes disease). J.A.M.A., 169: 1443, 1959.
Stamp, W. G., Whitesides, T. E., Fields, M., and Scheer, G. E.: Treatment of vitamin D resistant rickets. J. Bone Joint Surg., 46-A:965, 1964.
Staple, T. W., and Friedenberg, M. J.: Ilio-iliac arteriovenous fistula following intervertebral disc surgery. Clin. Radiol. 16:248, 1965.
Staple, T. W., Evans, R. G., and Stein, Jr., A. H.: Arteriography in orthopedics. Arch. Surg., 97:682, 1968.
Steier, A., et al.: Effect of Vitamin D_2 and fluoride on experimental bone fracture healing in rats. J. Dent. Res., 46:675, 1967.
Stein, A. H., Morgan, H. C., and Porras, R.: The effect of an arteriovenous fistula on intramedullary bone pressure. Surg., Gynec. Obstet., 109:287, 1959.
Steindler, A.: Transference of flexor muscles of forearm at elbow. In: Campbell's Operative Orthopedics. vol. 2. St. Louis, C. V. Mosby, 1963.
Stern, B: The effect of various oxygen tensions on the synthesis and degradation of bone collagen in tissue culture. Proc. Soc. Exp. Biol. Med., 121: 869, 1966.
Stern, I. J., and Smith, L.: Dissolution by chymopapain *in vitro* of tissue from normal or prolapsed intervertebral discs. Clin. Orthop., 50:269, 1967.
Stokes, J. M.: Vascular complications of disc surgery. J. Bone Joint Surg., 50-A:394, 1968.
Stout, A. P., and Lattes, R.: Tumors of the Soft Tissues. Armed Forces Institutes of Pathology, 1967, second series, Fascicle I, 1967.
Sweetman, R., and Ross, K.: Surgical treatment of pulmonary metastases from primary tumors of bone. J. Bone Joint Surg., 49-B:74, 1967.
Swenson, O.: Biochemical changes in the fracture hematoma. J. Bone Joint Surg., 28:288, 1946.
Swinyard, C. A.: Comprehensive Care of the Child with Spina Bifida Manifesta. Rehabilitation Monograph 31. Institute of Rehabilitation Medicine, N.Y. Univ. Med. Center, 1966.
Tamborino, J. M., Armbrust, E. N., and Moe, J. H.: Harrington instrumentation in correction of scoliosis: comparison with cast correction. J. Bone Joint Surg., 46-A:313, 1964.
Tapp, E.: Effects of hormones on bone in growing rats. J. Bone Joint Surg., 48-B:526, 1966.
Thibodeau, A. A.: Closed space infection following removal of lumbar intervertebral disc. J. Bone Joint Surg., 50-A:400, 1968.
Thompson, C. F.: Fusion of the metacarpals of the thumb and index fingers to maintain functional position of the thumb. J. Bone Joint Surg., 24: 907, 1942.
Thyrocalcitonin. A Symposium. Am. J. Med., 43: 1967.
Tonna, E. A.: Protein synthesis and cells of the skeletal system. In: Leblond, C. P., and Warren, K. B. (eds.): Use of Radioautography in Investigating Protein Synthesis. vol. 4, New York, Academic Press, 1965.
———: Skeletal aging and its effect on osteogenesis. Clin. Orthop., 40:57, 1965b.
———: Response of the cellular phase of the skeleton to trauma. Periodontics, 4:105, 1966.
Tonna, E. A., and Cronkite, E. P.: Cellular response to fracture studied with tritiated thymidine. J. Bone Joint Surg., 43-A:352, 1961.
Torgerson, W.: Tibial osteotomy of the treatment of osteoarthritis of the knee. Surg. Clin. N. Am., 45: 779, 1965.
Townsend, A. C., and Scott, P. J.: Ingrowing toenails and onychogryposis. J. Bone Joint Surg., 48-B:354, 1966.
Trueta, J.: The role of the vessels in osteogenesis. J. Bone Joint Surg., 45-B:402, 1963.
Trueta, J., and Morgan, J. D.: The vascular contribution to osteogenesis: studies by the injection method. J. Bone Joint Surg., 42-B:97, 1960.
Tubiana, R.: Limited and extensive operations in Dupuytren's contracture. S. Clin. N. Am. 44:1071, 1964.
Udupa, K. N.: The role of vitamin A in the repair of the fracture. Indian J. Med. Res., 54:1122, 1966.
Urist, M. R.: Bone formation by auto-induction. Science, 12:150, 893, 1965.
———: The bone induction principle. Clin. Orthop., 53:243, 1967.
———: The healing of fractures in man under clinical conditions. J. Bone Joint Surg., 25:375, 1943.
———: Origins of current ideas about calcification. Clin. Orthop., 44:13, 1966.
Urist, M. R., and Adams, J. M.: Effects of various blocking reagents upon local mechanism of calcification. Arch. Path. 81:325, 1966.
Urist, M. R., Zaccalini, P. S., MacDonald, N. S., and Skoog, W. A.: New approaches to the problem of osteoporosis. J. Bone Joint Surg., 44-B:464, 1962.
van Nes, C. P.: Congenital pseudoarthrosis of the leg. J. Bone Joint Surg., 48-A:1467, 1966.
Virchow, R. L.: Ueber die Entwicklung des Schädelgrundes (cited by Waris, Berlin, 1857).
von Luschka, H.: Die Halbgelenke des menschlichen Körpers. Berlin, Reimer, 1858.
Wagner, L. C., and Hanby, J. E.: Brodie's abscess, pain distribution: occurrence and diagnosis. Am. J. Surg., 39:135, 1938.
Waldenstrom, H.: The first stages of coxa plana. J. Bone Joint Surg., 20:559, 1936.
Weckesser, E. C.: Results of wide excision of palmar fascia for Dupuytren's contracture: special refer-

ence to factors which adversely affect prognosis. Ann. Surg., 160:1007, 1964.

Weidman, S. M.: Calcification of skeletal tissue. Int. Rev. Connect. Tissue Res., 1:339, 1963.

Weinman, D. D., Kelly, P. J., Owen, C. A., and Orvis, A. L.: Skeletal clearance of CA^{47} and Sr^{85} and skeletal blood flow in dogs. Proc. Mayo Clin., 38:559, 1963.

Weiss, C., Rosenberg, L., and Helfet, A. J.: An ultrastructural study of normal young adult human articular cartilage. J. Bone Joint Surg., 50-A:663, 1968.

Weissman, S. L., and Salama, R.: Treatment of congenital dislocation of the hip in the newborn infant. J. Bone Joint Surg., 48A:1319, 1966.

White, N. B., Ter-Pogossian, M. M., and Stein, A. H.: A method to determine the rate of blood flow in long bone and selected soft tissue. Surg., Gynec. Obstet., 119: 535, 1964.

Wilson, P. D., Jacobs, B., and Schecter, L.: Slipped capital femoral epiphysis: an end result study. J. Bone Joint Surg., 47A:1128-1145, 1965.

Wood, W., and Zlotsky, N.: Congenital absence of the fibula. J. Bone Joint Surg., 47-A:1159, 1965.

Woods, T. H. E.: DeQuervain's disease: plea for early operation. Brit. J. Surg., 61:358, 1964.

Wound Healing (Editorial). Brit. Med. J., 3:567, 1967.

Wray, J. B.: Glucose uptake by fractured and immobilized limbs in the dog. Surg., Gynec. Obstet., 120:45, 1965.

Wyley, A. M.: Reconstruction of osteoarthritic knee by high tibial osteotomy and joint clearance. Canad. J. Surg., 10:28, 1967.

Wynne Davies, R.: Family studies and the cause of congenital club foot. J. Bone Joint Surg., 46-B: 445, 1964.

Yamaguchi, D. M., Lipscomb, P. R., and Soule, E. H.: Carpal tunnel syndrome. Minn. Med., 48:22, 1965.

Young, H. H.: Use of a hinged Vitallium prosthesis for arthroplasty of the knee: a preliminary report. J. Bone Joint Surg., 45-A:1627, 1963.

Young, H., and Owens, N.: Yearbook of Orthopedics, Traumatic and Plastic Surgery. Chicago, Yearbook Medical Publishers, 1965-1966.

Young, R. W.: Cell proliferation and specialization during endochondral osteogenesis in young rats. J. Cell. Biol., 1:14:357, 1962.

———: The control of cell specialization in bone. *In*: Robinson, R. A. (ed.): The Healing of Osseous Tissue. Nat. Acad. Sci., Nat. Res. Council, Washington, D.C., 1967.

Zadek, R. E., and Robinson, R. A.: The effect of growth hormone on healing of an experimental long bone defect. J. Bone Joint Surg., 43-A:1261, 1961.

———: The healing of an osteal-periosteal discontinuity of standard length in skeletally mature and immature canine radii. *In*: The Healing of Osseous Tissue. Robinson, R. A., (ed.): Nat. Acad. Sci., Nat. Res. Council, Washington, D.C., 1967.

Zvaifler, N. J.: A speculation on the pathogenesis of joint inflammation and rheumatoid arthritis. Arthritis Rheum., 8:289, 1965.

CHAPTER 54

WILLIAM H. SWEET, M.D.

Surgery of the Nervous System

Diseases Affecting the Central Nervous System
  Lesions with Surgical Implications, Intracranial
  Lesions with Surgical Implications, Intraspinal
Diseases Affecting Peripheral Nervous System
Neurosurgical Operations on Normal Tissues to Relieve Disease Elsewhere
Diseases Affecting Autonomic Nervous System
Conclusion

DISEASES AFFECTING THE CENTRAL NERVOUS SYSTEM

Although the feasibility and the fruitfulness of operations on the central nervous system have been established for over 70 years, the crucial importance and the delicacy of many of the structures still limit sharply the scope of surgery here. Early recognition of disease advancing in brain or cord is especially important because of the absence of regeneration either in nerve cells or fiber tracts, as well as the vulnerability of the tissue. Hence, we shall devote our attention mainly to the symptoms, signs and simple diagnostic tests of the disorders usefully managed neurosurgically, so that the general physician or surgeon may spot them more promptly. Horsley, Krause, Cushing and Dandy, the principal pioneers, did most of their work on tumors and on relief of pain, fields which continue to present challenging problems. We begin by considering the localized intracranial lesions which the surgeon may attack profitably.

Lesions with Surgical Implications, Intracranial

Symptoms and Signs

Neoplasms, infections, hematomas, trauma, aneurysms, arteriovenous malformations, congenital malformations, scars and adhesions, pseudotumor cerebri and, much more rarely, parasitic and other cysts, as well as tuberculous, syphilitic or other granulomata, comprise the lesions to be discussed. They become manifest either by (1) *generalized effects* of (A) increase in intracranial pressure, or (B) changes produced in the cerebrospinal fluid (CSF), or by (2) the *local effects* of (A) excess or (B) diminution of function.

Increased Intracranial Pressure. CHRONIC INCREASE. Chronic increase in intracranial pressure, either constant or intermittent, ensues when the lesion progresses slowly. The deleterious associated effects commonly attributed thereto may be headache, vomiting, papilledema, diplopia and enlargement of the head.

1. *Headache.* In the early stages, pain may not be severe, and its relief by aspirin or cold packs to the head may give patients and physicians a false impression that the cause is inconsequential. Often the pain appears the first thing in the morning, immediately upon awakening—an unusual time for headache of less ominous etiology (if one excludes that from alcoholic imbibing the night before). Coughing, sneezing or straining raise intracranial pressure and often worsen the headache due thereto. Reference to only a portion of the head does not necessarily indicate that a mass lies just beneath, but if the pain is occipital, and especially if it is accompanied by nuchal rigidity, this is a warning that the primary lesion may be in the posterior cranial fossa or, more urgently, that the cerebellar tonsils are being crowded down into the foramen magnum against the lower medulla oblongata. Bursts of cephalic pain of agonizing intensity also warn the physician that an emergency is at hand. When there is no papilledema, the headache due to a brain tumor is referred over or near the tumor in about two thirds of these

patients. Such pain probably is due to localized rather than generalized pressure.

2. *Vomiting* is usually not so violent as to fit the term "projectile" but it may be. Virtual absence of nausea preceding the vomiting may occur, and this precipitate urge provides a clue that the cause is intracranial. In children the focal insignia of intracranial masses tend to be less conspicuous, so that headache and vomiting assume special importance, and unless they are acted on promptly, the child may be left blind despite otherwise successful treatment. Consequently, in this age group, continuing and otherwise unexplained vomiting should lead to early investigation of a primary intracranial cause.

3. *Papilledema*—elevation of the optic disks or blurring of the disk margins, often accompanied by hemorrhages and/or exudates —is the sign of a visual impairment that can lead to blindness. The hemorrhages usually occur in or near the disks; they lie along the radially disposed fibers in the nerve fiber layer of the retina and hence tend to be thin and splinter- or flame-shaped. Even though useful vision may still be present when the mass is removed, further damage and loss of more sight may follow subsidence of a severe papilledema. The associated visual field is constricted concentrically, and the blind spot is enlarged, but central visual acuity—the function of the macula—may be preserved. In the presence of gross papilledema, the whole visual field may suddenly become dim or even black entirely for seconds to minutes with spontaneous recovery. This is another important symptom of emergency, i.e., that mechanisms compensating for the increased pressure in the head are about to fail; one must be careful not to pass it off as a hysterical symptom.

4. *Diplopia*. The 2 images are side by side and parallel, and the image seen by the abducting eye is the more lateral when an abducens paresis is present. Such weakness of the 6th cranial nerve on one or both sides may be caused by generalized increased intracranial pressure without focal lesion. This is the least frequent of the 5 manifestations of such pressure. Cushing showed this to be due to notching of the nerve from behind by any transversely directed branch of the basilar artery which shifts forward. In most instances the diagnosis should have been made before papilledema or abducens palsy appear.

5. *Enlargement of Head*. Before the cranial sutures close at roughly 15 years of age, an expanding intracranial mass will spring the sutures apart and a "cracked-pot" note (Macewen's sign) may be heard on percussion. In infancy and early childhood, this may provoke an abnormally rapid increase in the circumference of the head with bulging fontanelles. For the range of normal sizes at various ages, see Matson's monograph.

ACUTE INCREASE. An acute increase in intracranial pressure, when accompanied by acute deterioration of cerebral function, evokes different responses:

1. *Headache*. This may be of extreme intensity for a few moments before the patient becomes unresponsive, as when an aneurysm at the base of the brain bursts wide open. Usually, however, the most important change with a less acute increase in intracranial pressure is:

2. *Increasing lethargy progressing to coma*, often without subjective complaint. This crucial sign should not be obscured by injudicious sedation in a patient initially restless.

3. Classically, the *4 vital signs alter:* (1) the systolic arterial pressure mounts while the diastolic pressure falls or stays the same; (2) the pulse becomes slower, and because of a rise in pulse pressure, fuller as well; (3) the breathing is slower, at times deeper, or irregular or of Cheyne-Stokes type; (4) the body temperature rises. However, even when increased intracranial pressure has nearly killed the patient, some or all of the vital signs may remain normal.

DECREASE IN RESPONSIVENESS OF THE PATIENT is the principal criterion of worsening in the presence of hemorrhage within the brain or into the subdural or extradural spaces, or in the later evolution of a more slowly expanding mass. An enlarging supratentorial mass soon or late pushes the ipsilateral temporal lobe's uncus and hippocampal gyrus downward and medially through the tentorial notch against the midbrain. This produces the so-called *tentorial pressure cone* (Fig. 54-1). The 3rd (oculomotor) cranial nerve is depressed, and its fibers to the constrictor pupillae muscle are usually the most affected by the external pressure. The unopposed sympathetic dilator fibers produce a widely dilated pupil ipsilaterally, which becomes fixed to light. The temporal lobe may even push the

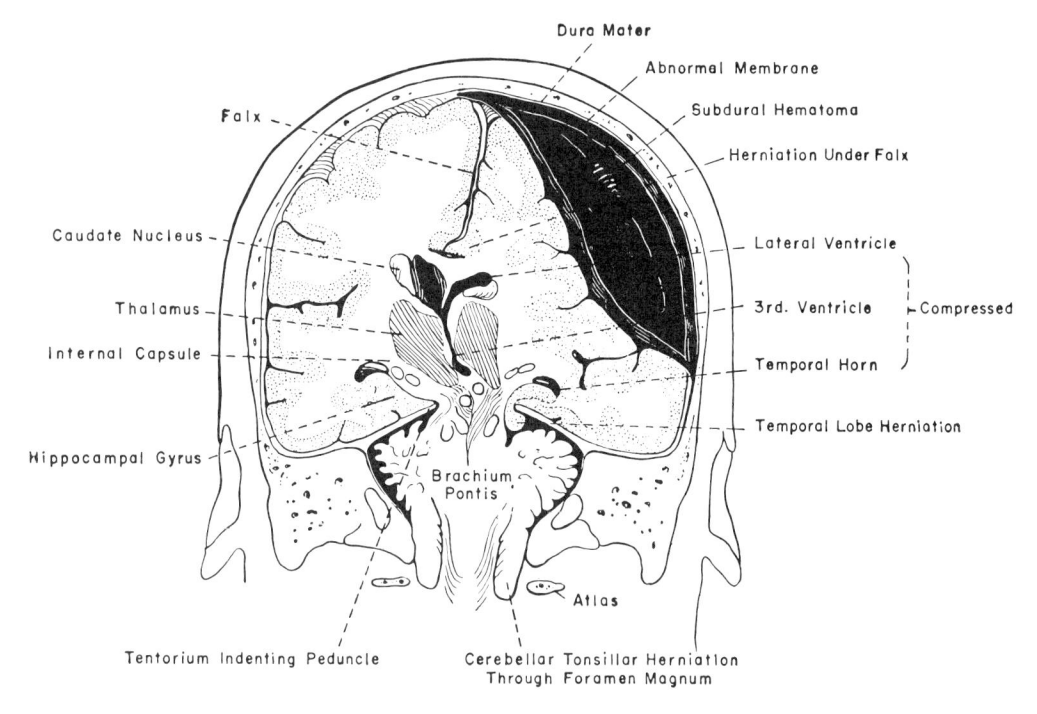

Fig. 54-1. Temporal and cerebellar tonsillar herniations—notching of cerebral peduncle. The medial herniation of the hippocampal gyrus and the downward movement of the cerebellar tonsils are also referred to respectively as tentorial and cerebellar tonsillar pressure cones.

midbrain against the medial free edge of the tentorium *on the other side,* so as to indent that cerebral peduncle and thereby cause a hemiplegia on the same side as the expanding lesion. A hemiplegia of intracranial etiology usually is caused by a primary lesion on the side of the brain opposite the weakness, since the pyramidal tracts decussate in the lowermost medulla oblongata. Hence, the weakness ipsilateral to the primary lesion brought on by the tentorial pressure cone may be confusing. The intracranial mass is likely to be on the side of the dilated fixed pupil. The lateralizing value of this sign may not persist, however, because in this parlous state the opposite 3rd nerve may also shortly become compressed and the other pupil dilate. A patient whose condition is deteriorating rapidly may pass briskly through the state of anisocoria, and the one-sided dilated pupil escape careless observation. Deepening stupor and a dilating pupil reacting sluggishly to light are then the heralds of a tentorial pressure cone; this critical state leads promptly to death unless effective surgical treatment is carried out at once.

That fibrous barrier, the tentorium cerebelli, may also cause the superior portion of the cerebellum to squeeze the midbrain in a lethal embrace if an expanding lesion in the posterior fossa pushes cerebellum upwards, a "reversed tentorial pressure cone." Finally, intracranial masses may kill by forcing the cerebellar tonsils against the medulla, in which situation the respiration at first may be more compromised than the circulation, by the *cerebellar tonsillar pressure cone* (Fig. 54-1).

In general, space-taking masses give rise to increased intracranial pressure not only by virtue of their own volume but also because they tend to impede circulation and absorption of CSF. There appears in man to be a net formation of around 100 to 150 ml. of this fluid per day in the ventricles over and above the amount reabsorbed back into the blood through the ventricular walls. As shown by Dandy, the excess fluid must be able to flow from one ventricle to another, out of the lower end of the 4th ventricle, and in the subarachnoid space back up through the tentorial notch to reach the surface of the cere-

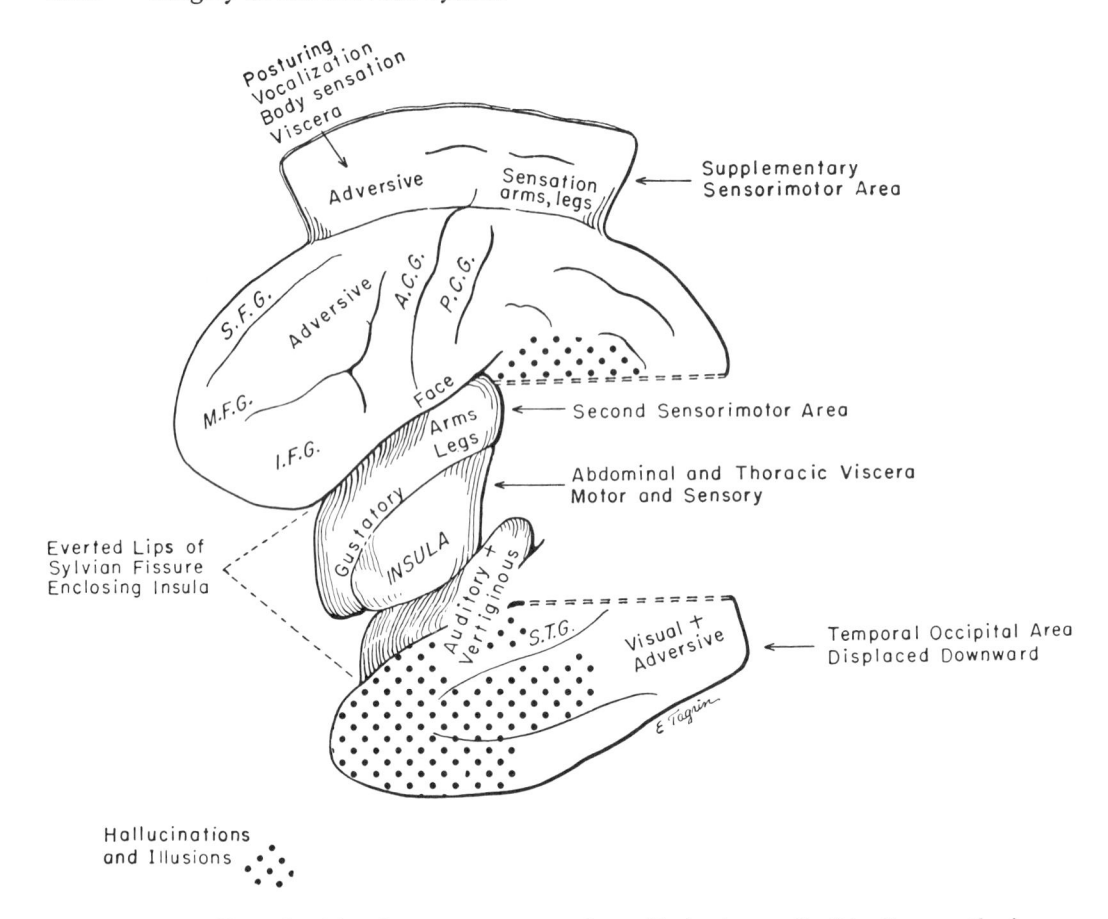

FIG. 54-2. Sites of origin of motor, sensory and psychical seizures. In this diagram, the inferior part of the brain has been displaced downward; the superior and the inferior lips of the sylvian fissure are represented as though everted with the insula between them; the central part of the medial surface of the hemisphere is drawn as though reflected upward. The main or primary sensorimotor cortex lies on either side of the rolandic fissure on the lateral surface of the hemisphere and extends slightly onto the medial surface. The second sensorimotor area, continuous with the primary area, begins on the lateral surface just above the sylvian fissure and extends onto the hidden superior lip of this fissure. A third or supplementary sensorimotor area lies on the medial surface of the hemisphere surrounding the medial end of the primary area.

S.F.G.—Superior frontal gyrus
M.F.G.—Middle frontal gyrus
I.F.G.—Inferior frontal gyrus
A.C.G.—Anterior central gyrus
P.C.G.—Posterior central gyrus
S.T.G.—Superior temporal gyrus

bral hemispheres, the locus of most of the absorbing arachnoidal villi. A mass while still small, if strategically placed near ventricular foramina, or in general in the posterior cranial fossa, may slow the flow of CSF and give ominous symptoms and signs of increased intracranial pressure. A complete obstruction can produce an acute dangerous increase in this pressure within hours. A tap into a lateral ventricle proximal to the block temporarily relieves the emergency. Slow-growing or static lesions obstructing flow of CSF may be treated merely by restoring the balance of CSF formation and absorption.

Symptoms and Signs Due to Abnormal Cerebrospinal Fluid (CSF). Bleeding into the CSF in any quantity increases the pressure in the fluid, but even if the pressure is normal, the red cells are likely to cause nuchal pain, nuchal rigidity or even opisthotonos, along with a positive Kernig sign—meningismus, in short. A major increase in the number of

Fig. 54-3. Diagrammatic coronal section of brain through precentral gyrus. Localization of function in cerebrum.

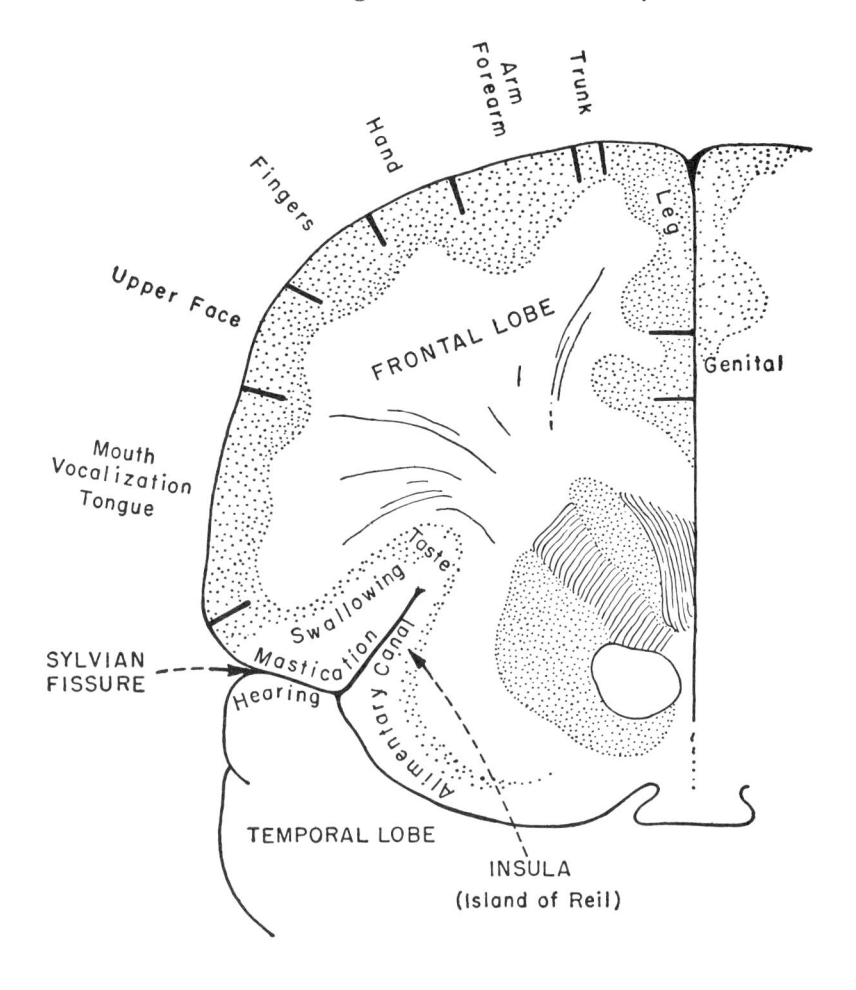

white cells, which occurs in meningitis or when an abscess ruptures into the CSF, causes similar signs; an increased white cell count in the CSF may also follow as a reaction to subarachnoid hemorrhage.

Localizing Symptoms and Signs of Hyperactivity of the Brain. These arise from irritation of a particular part of the brain and cause any of the protean manifestations of a focal or generalized seizure. Following the lead of Penfield and associates, who have made the most important contributions to our knowledge in this field, we classify focal cerebral seizures as motor, sensory, autonomic and psychical. Figures 54-2 and 54-3 indicate the portions of the brain, stimulation of which gives rise to these specific types of seizure. Reference to these figures will aid understanding of the following description.

MOTOR SEIZURES. To the casual observer, the manifestations most obviously cerebral in origin are those in which a clonic jerky or a tonic maintained contraction of muscles begins at some one part, usually in face, hand or foot because of the relatively large portion of the motor cortex representing these areas. From the starting point, there may be a progression, or, as Hughlings Jackson put it, a march, to other parts of the body on the same side, which occurs in the sequence dictated by localization of function indicated in Figure 54-3.

Vocalization, commonly a long-drawn-out cry, may start a seizure which then usually becomes rapidly generalized. The "cry" may occur upon stimulus within the face area or in the supplementary motor area.

An adversive seizure, consisting of *conjugate turning of the eyes* and often of the head, usually to the side opposite the lesion, occurs on irritation of the precentral gyrus, the posterior part of the middle frontal gyrus, the supplementary sensorimotor cortex or the occipital lobe. It is a symptom of a focal lesion which is of great importance because it usually results from discharge starting in the cortex of the prerolandic frontal or the occipital lobes —regions which are surgically resectable with minimal deficit. If the origin is anterior frontal, the patient loses consciousness before turning; if midfrontal, he may remember the turning. In the former case, only another alert observer will be able to give the crucial history of lateralizing behavior.

Mastication and *swallowing* are provoked by discharge deep in the sylvian fissure over the insula.

Aphasic arrest, i.e., an attack of inability to speak or to understand the speech of others, occurs when one of the speech areas of the dominant hemisphere is discharging.

Rhythmic movements or *adoption of a posture* involving limbs of both sides and the body as well may occur when the supplementary sensorimotor area becomes activated. For example, in one patient the first such seizure began with slow elevation and dropping of the right arm as though she were wielding an old farm pump handle. When a friend held this arm, the other arm began such movements. These were interpreted erroneously as hysterical; actually the irritant was a small tumor.

Discharges in the midbrain produce *"decerebrate seizures"* in which all 4 limbs move into rigid extension with hyperpronation of forearms and plantar flexion of the feet. Opisthotonos—backward arching or stiffness of neck and back—may be associated. These are threatening signs of severe mesencephalic malfunction.

SENSORY SEIZURES. When a primary sensorimotor gyrus on either side of the rolandic fissure is discharging, the first experience of the patient may be of somatic sensory type, beginning in one restricted area of the opposite side of the face, torso or limbs. Tingling, numbness, a peculiar "absence of all sensation," a sense of movement of a part when none is actually occurring, or, rarely, pain, heat or cold, are the feelings that may be evoked. Activity of the second sensorimotor area in the lowermost central gyri and adjoining upper lip of the sylvian fissure or in the supplementary sensorimotor area on the medial surface of the hemisphere (Fig. 54-2) brings on more diffuse sensations in the *opposite or in both sides* of the patient. Discharge in the second sensorimotor area often evokes sensations in the terminal portions of one or more limbs.

SEIZURES INVOLVING SPECIAL SENSES. *Visual seizures,* of positive type with the seeing of lights or of inhibitory nature with darkness or blindness, occur not only from discharges in the calcarine cortex of the occipital lobe but also in the neighboring Brodmann's areas 18 and 19 which occupy the rest of this lobe. This light or the darkness appears usually to be straight ahead but may be in the contralateral or even in the ipsilateral visual field. Likewise, in *auditory seizures* there may be a positive ringing or buzzing, or an inhibitory partial deafness. The sound usually is referred to the opposite ear but may be referred to both ears. The affected area lies in the lower lip of the sylvian fissure and the nearby superior temporal gyrus. Activity of virtually the same area may also bring on a *vertiginous seizure,* a feeling of rotation, bodily displacement or dizziness. *Olfactory seizures* occur upon stimulation of the uncus, and *gustatory attacks* probably are referable to the depths of the sylvian fissure above the insula.

Both motor and sensory seizures may be followed for hours or even a few days by impairment of function of the discharging area of cortex. The commonest form is the postictal weakness of a convulsing part, a so-called Todd's paralysis.

VISCERAL AND AUTONOMIC SEIZURES. Abdominal or thoracic sensations referred within the torso occur often as the aura of a focal seizure; a sensation in the epigastrium rising toward the head is one of the commonest of these. They suggest a discharge deep within the sylvian fissure or in the frontal lobe. Autonomic manifestations may include any or many of the following: localized or generalized flushing or sweating, lacrimation, salivation, pilo-erection, yawning, vomiting, borborygmus, abdominal cramp, defecation, urination, priapism, change in pupillary size, shivering, hiccuping, and a rise, a fall or an irregularity in rate or level of the vital signs—pulse, respiration, blood pressure or temperature. If many such features are present, the lesion probably involves thalamus or hypothalamus. Because of widespread cerebral representation of many of these functions, a few such symptoms may occur in attacks along with the cerebral somatic motor or the sensory phenomena already described.

PSYCHICAL SEIZURES AND AUTOMATISMS. Discharges in temporal lobe and inferior parietal lobule may cause attacks of altered mental or emotional attitude, classifiable as illusions, emotions or hallucinations. Thus the patient may have illusions in which objects look abnormal, e.g., too small or too large, or in which sounds seem too loud, or in which objects are abnormally placed in space. Or suddenly the environment may seem falsely familiar as though he were reliving a previous experience (the *déjà vu* phenomenon), or contrariwise it may seem absurd, strange or remote. The illusion also may have an emotional component of fear, sadness or loneliness. More complex experiences, hallucinations independent of the environment, occur and resemble dreams in which, e.g., the patient sees scenes or hears conversations or songs. In all of these psychical seizures, he is able to relate the experience later.

Distinct from these are the episodes of automatism in which the patient carries out actions of greater or lesser complexity and cannot recall them later. If the movements are irrelevant or stereotyped or the patient seems confused, his associates may recognize an abnormality, but at times the patient may move for minutes or even hours in an apparently purposive fashion so that those about him are unaware of any "attack." Although automatic movements for which there is a later amnesia may occur in a variety of circumstances, lesions in the inferomedial temporal lobe are an important cause.

Paroxysmal irritative manifestations, i.e., seizures, do not occur from neuronal discharge in the cerebellum. The term "cerebellar fits" has been applied sometimes to midbrain seizures because a cerebellar mass may evoke them by irritation of the midbrain.

Any of the foregoing manifestations of localized activity of the brain may pass off within minutes, may persist for hours as an *epilepsia partialis continua,* or may extend to neighboring ipsilateral, deep, or contralateral parts. They may end as a generalized tonic-clonic seizure with any of the diffuse manifestations thereof, such as unconsciousness, tongue biting, salivation, urinary or fecal incontinence and stertorous breathing with cyanosis. Should the point of irritation lie in a "silent" area of the brain whose activity evokes no apparent change in behavior, the cerebral excitation spreading from this region may reach the whole sensorimotor areas of both hemispheres or deeper motor structures at about the same time, producing a seizure generalized at onset and indistinguishable clinically from those often seen with epilepsy of unknown cause. *It is especially important that such patients with generalized seizures be studied carefully,* because even gliomatous tumor in a silent area may be removable in toto along with a safe margin of normal brain and yet leave a functionally normal individual. Unfortunately, such patients are often treated with anticonvulsant drugs without full and repeated special diagnostic studies. The initial seizure caused by a space-taking mass may not be followed by another for weeks or even years.

ENDOCRINE HYPERFUNCTION. The overactivity of endocrine glands may arise by overstimulation from the controlling neural centers or from pituitary neoplasms producing an excess of hormone.

In the former category are the rare lesions, including among other causes, neoplasms or hamartomas, which produce sexual precocity in boys. The causative lesion affects the posterior hypothalamus just behind the infundibular recess of the floor of the 3rd ventricle. The eosinophilic tumors of the anterior pituitary gland produce an excess of growth hormone, leading to gigantism in the young and to acromegaly in the adult. In about one fifth of the active acromegalics the lesion turns out to be a chromophobe adenoma. More rarely, this general tumor type may, via the mammotropic hormone, cause galactorrhea, and in Cushing's disease both before and after adrenalectomy, chromophobe adenomas may develop which may produce ACTH and the melanocyte-stimulating hormone, MSH. A variety of disorders including diffuse intracranial trauma or infection may provoke an inappropriate secretion of antidiuretic hormone, ADH, leading to serum hypo-osmolarity and worsening the cerebral edema that already tends to be present.

Localizing Symptoms and Signs of Intracranial Hypoactivity. Proceeding as we did with the irritative features, we may consider the motor, sensory, autonomic, psychical and endocrine phenomena encountered.

MOTOR. In the initial phases of a juxtarolandic cerebral mass, and in cerebellar tumors also, clumsiness, slight weakness, terminal tremor on precise movement, and slowing of rapid alternating movement occur—contralateral to a cerebral mass, ipsilaterally in the case of the cerebellum. As a cerebral lesion progresses, the weakness dominates the disability, and abnormal resistance to passive movement appears. The increased tonus is often of lead pipe or cogwheel type in deep lesions involving the basal ganglia or the diencephalon. It is usually of a spastic or clasp-knife type in more superficial lesions of the hemisphere. Often the tendon jerks are increased in the contralateral limbs, along with forced grasping, and superficial reflex changes such as the positive Hoffmann, Babinski, and Rossolimo signs, with absence of abdominal and cremasteric reflexes on the affected side. Any facial weakness affects the contralateral *lower* facial muscles much more than those in the forehead and usually is incomplete because of bilateral representation in each hemisphere. This *upper motor neuronal paresis* is thus distinguished from the *lower motor neuronal involvement* of the facial nucleus in the brain stem or the emergent facial nerve. Here the weakness affects about equally and usually severely all the facial muscle on the ipsilateral side.

When a cerebellar hemisphere is involved, there may be past pointing and deviation of gait toward the side of the lesion, with hypotonia, the rebound phenomenon, overshooting on precise motion, slight weakness and pendular tendon jerks in the ipsilateral limbs. The arm is usually worse than the leg. Horizontal nystagmus on lateral gaze to either side occurs; the quick component of the eye movement is in the direction of gaze with a slower return toward the central point; the movements are slower and coarser when the patient looks toward the side of the lesion. When the cerebellar vermis only is injured, a symmetrical unsteadiness of gait is likely without nystagmus or specific motor signs on testing an individual limb. As the lesion advances in the cerebellum, compensatory assumption of its function by other areas occurs; hence, the signs of a huge slow-growing mass in the cerebellum may be slight, and removal of cortex and subcortical white matter of an entire cerebellar hemisphere happily leaves a minimal permanent deficit. The incoordination, lateral deviation and hypotonia become severe only when the lesion invades or compresses a cerebellar peduncle or the brain stem.

SOMATIC SENSORY. Involvement of the cerebral pathways leading to the somatic sensory areas in one parietal lobe produces a contralateral defect in discriminative capacities. Tests likely to show impairment are those for stereognosis, for determining the distance of separation of two points on the skin requisite for perception as a dual stimulus, for recognition of numbers written on the skin, for localizing the spot touched, for distinguishing textures of cloth or weights, and for proprioception. Any major decrease in acuity of appreciation of the basic modalities of touch, pain, heat or cold points to a lesion encroaching on thalamus, posterior limb of internal capsule or some lower level.

SPECIAL SENSES. Hyposmia or anosmia is a symptom which the patient usually ignores; when the examiner finds it and can exclude disease in the upper air passages as the cause, it points to affection of the olfactory bulb or tract, an inferomedial frontal lesion. Impairment in the sense of taste is rarely observed clinically and only when the primary afferent pathway in the entering 7th nerve or brain stem is involved. The same applies to the sense of hearing and the 8th nerve; auditory pathways in the brain are so diffuse that lesions therein are rarely extensive enough to cause deafness, although this does occur if both inferior colliculi of the midbrain are afflicted. Tumor in the cerebellopontine angle, the commonest type being the 8th nerve's acoustic neuroma, produces ipsilateral deafness usually preceded by tinnitus. This involvement of the cochlear division of the nerve often appears years before any other sign. The clinical insignia of malfunction of the vestibular component of the 8th nerve consist of whirling vertigo or of less definite giddiness. A tendency to fall on abrupt turning of the head without subjective warning of unsteadiness also occurs. Audiometric measurements quantitate the hearing loss at each frequency tested; caloric testing yields a semiquantitative measure of equilibratory dysfunction. A unilateral nerve type deafness may be caused by pressure on the cochlear components of the 8th nerve as by a cerebellopontine angle tumor or by disorder of the organ of Corti as in Ménière's syndrome. Early differentiation of these two causes with diagnosis of a tumor before it becomes embedded in the side of the brain stem is now possible by use of a battery of audiologic tests for (1) loudness recruitment, (2) word discrimination, (3) pathologic auditory adaptation and (4) the more elaborate tests devised by the Nobel prize-winning efforts of von Békesy.

A diligent examination of the visual functions is one of the most important means for detecting and localizing intracranial lesions at an early, or indeed, any stage. The intracranial visual pathways extend anteriorly from the optic foramina back to the cells of the lateral geniculate bodies; fibers from these nuclei pass into the optic radiations, expanding widely in the temporal and inferior parietal region to reach cortical visual areas as far back as the tip of the occipital lobe. So, many intracranial masses may encroach on this sensitive apparatus at some point. Focal pressure directly on the optic nerve causes primary atrophy of the disk on that side. Painstaking charting of the visual fields permits quantitative assessments, and serial studies may enable one to establish the slight worsening of a lesion so suggestive of tumor. Superior or inferior altitudinal defects point respectively to pressure from below or from above against the optic nerve. Bitemporal defects indicate a chiasmal lesion; homonymous defects go with unilateral encroachment on optic tract, optic radiations or calcarine cortex. An upper quadrantic homonymous defect usually implicates the inferior or temporal portion of the optic radiations, whereas the superior or parietal radiations are correlated with the lower quadrants of the fields. Hughes' *The Visual Fields* documents beautifully the great scope of the deductions feasible from such studies.

AUTONOMIC AND METABOLIC EFFECTS. Recognizable autonomic effects are confined largely to the irritative sphere, already discussed, or to lesions in the descending pathway in the medulla. A striking example of this is the vasodilatation, Horner's sign and reduction in sweating often seen on the side of a thrombosis of the posterior-inferior cerebellar artery. Lesions in the posterior parasagittal part of either frontal lobe may bring on involuntary micturition, perhaps by impairing inhibitory mechanisms. One metabolic effect of a disturbance in the hypothalamus is obesity. Other metabolic features of involvement of the hypothalamic-pituitary mechanism are considered below. Associated with many of the autonomic centers in the hypothalamus are those concerned with arousal. Depression of these causes drowsiness, stupor or excessive requirement of sleep.

PSYCHICAL CHANGES. Subtle changes in personality may be the first clue to disease in the so-called "silent areas" of the cerebrum. Thus a patient of Cushing with a bilateral inferior frontal meningioma made such an obviously unsuitable marriage that her friends were dumbfounded. After Cushing had removed her tumor, her mental recovery was accompanied by mystification equalling that of her friends at her choice of a husband, and she terminated the marriage. Decreases in energy and ambition, impaired memory, inattention to the courtesies of conversational intercourse, carelessness in personal habits, poor business judgment, or deviations in sexual mores may be the first symptoms of a brain tumor but are rarely recognized as such. An astute examiner usually must acquire data from an observant close associate of the patient before such symptoms lead to intensive diagnostic study.

With more serious involvement, defects in memory, especially for recent events, disorientation, indifference, apathy and drowsiness become obvious. There may be a stage of euphoria with a tendency to make silly jokes. Lesions in the frontal lobes or the corpus callosum or those causing high intracranial pressure are among the commonest to produce this picture.

Disturbances in the sphere of understanding and expressing language, called *aphasias*, have specific localizing value—in a right-handed person to some portion of the left cerebral hemisphere. In a left-handed person the language dominance of one hemisphere is not likely to be so pronounced. The related *apraxia* is an inability to carry out acts with a specific purpose, despite adequate strength and coordination in the necessary part, and *agnosia* refers to the inability to appreciate the significance of stimuli that are perceived. An aphasia may be largely *expressive* or *motor* in type in that the patient may know what he wishes to say, to repeat, or to read aloud but is unable to do so. This oral expressive aphasia is likely to be associated with a lesion in the posterior part of the inferior frontal gyrus of the dominant hemisphere. A lesion just above this in the posterior part of the middle frontal gyrus may produce inability to write or print words despite adequate strength in the hand and the fingers, an *agraphia*.

The lesions causing the *receptive* or *sensory* aphasias lie in general posteriorly in the dominant hemisphere. There may be loss of ability to read (a visual agnosia for words, word-blindness or *alexia*) seen especially in lesions of the dominant angular gyrus, which surrounds the upturned posterior end of the superior temporal sulcus (Fig. 54-2). If the lesion involves much of the occipital lobe behind this but spares the striate or calcarine cortex, the visual agnosia may be more severe, with inability to identify many sorts of objects which, however, the patient sees clearly enough. Lesions in the posterior half of the dominant superior temporal gyrus cause an auditory receptive aphasia or word deafness. Although the patient can hear, he cannot understand the words and may even be unable to repeat what he hears. Inability of the patient to understand his own spoken words may result in senseless speech or even gibberish—paraphasia or jargon aphasia. A more extensive lesion in this area produces a more severe auditory agnosia with incomprehension of the cause of such simple sounds as the rattling of coins. *Amnesic aphasia, nominal aphasia* and *anomia* are the terms applied to the inability to think of nouns even though the patient understands the concept embodied in a noun or name. Thus, when shown a pencil he may not be able to think of the word "pencil," describes the object as "something you write with" but usually can select the proper word from a series presented for his choice. Lesions in the dominant posterior temporal region and those around the posterior part of the sylvian fissure may produce this picture, or it may occur with diffuse lesions of the subcortical association pathways between the various language areas already described.

In most aphasic patients there is a mixture of a number of the above features, because the lesion involves either a correspondingly extensive area of cortex or the subcortical connecting fibers between them. Especially likely to be implicated are those deep to the insula and the inferior parietal lobule. There may be even a total loss of the appreciation and the expression of language, a global aphasia. Perseveration, i.e., inappropriate repetition of a syllable, a word or a phrase, is common in many types of aphasia.

ENDOCRINE HYPOFUNCTION. The thyroid, the adrenal cortex, the gonads and possibly the breasts are all under control of specific trophic hormones secreted by the anterior pituitary gland. In addition, there is the anterior pituitary growth hormone which does not act via another gland. The antidiuretic hormone is secreted by certain hypothalamic nuclei and then passes down within the fibers of the hypophyseal stalk to the posterior lobe of the pituitary gland for storage and appropriate release into the blood stream.

Tumors which encroach on the sellar area before puberty tend to produce dwarfism plus incomplete or absent sexual development and a varying degree of polyuria and polydipsia (diabetes insipidus). Decrease in gonadotrophic hormone is nearly always the first evidence of hypofunction in the adult. Cessation of menses is the common early sign in women, and both men and women may be sterile. Libido as well as other primary and secondary sexual characteristics deteriorate. Next comes decreased production of thyrotrophic and finally of adrenocorticotrophic hormones (TSH and ACTH) to produce symptoms similar to those of myxedema and Addison's disease, respectively. Other manifestations of hypopituitarism are an easy fatigability, progressing to apathy associated with anorexia and weight loss. The skin is pale from loss of its melanin as well as from a mild normocytic anemia which develops. In addition, the skin is likely to be delicate, finely wrinkled and hairless. Vascular hypotension, a fasting hypoglycemia, a flat oral glucose tolerance curve and a lowered basal metabolic rate, a low protein-bound iodine in the blood and decreased radioiodine uptake are all likely to be found in study of more advanced patients with compression of the normal pituitary gland.

Accessory Diagnostic Tests

Lumbar Puncture. With the patient recumbent and fully relaxed, any initial pressure greater than 200 mm. of CSF is abnormally high. If papilledema, lethargy or agonizing headache already point to marked elevation of this pressure, and especially if there is a mass in the temporal lobe or the posterior cranial fossa, the withdrawal of lumbar fluid may provoke a dangerous temporal (tentorial) or

Fig. 54-4. Lateral roentgenogram of the skull: generalized increased intracranial pressure shown by: (1) separation of coronal and lambdoidal sutures; (2) increased convolutional markings (beaten silver appearance) especially in frontal areas; and (3) partial decalcification of dorsum sellae.

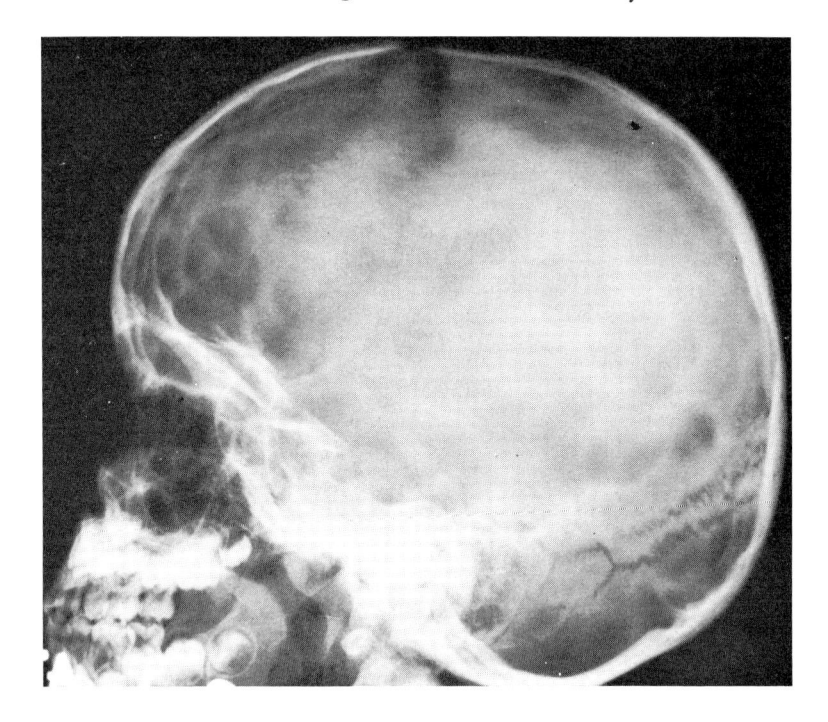

cerebellar tonsillar movement against the brain stem. Deaths from this cause remain unfortunately frequent. Hence, in the above circumstances lumbar puncture should be carried out cautiously with a fine-bore needle, if at all, and when gross elevation of pressure is found, usually it is good judgment to remove only the contents of the manometer (enough for a cell count). When an intracranial mass is strongly suspected, but a sample of CSF is needed to aid diagnosis, often it is better judgment to have a neurosurgeon secure this via ventricular tap. An atraumatic lumbar tap which yields more than a few hundred red cells/cu. mm. indicates a spontaneous subarachnoid hemorrhage. The commonest causes are a rupture into the CSF of an aneurysm, an arteriovenous malformation, an intracerebral hematoma, or a vessel in a tumor.

Extra white blood cells, usually lymphocytes, in the lumbar CSF, and especially an elevation of the total protein may occur if a mass lies next to a ventricle or a subarachnoid space. Meningiomas and in particular acoustic neuromas commonly are accompanied by a lumbar CSF total protein greater than 100 mg. %. Polymorphonuclear leukocytes, even a few, suggest the presence of an abscess or a granuloma. Cells that resemble lymphocytes, but are actually tumor cells, may be found when the tumor invades the meninges.

Plain Roentgenograms of the Skull. The following roentgenographic signs of generalized increased intracranial pressure occur: (1) decalcification in the dorsum sellae or floor of the sella turcica, (2) dilatation of the foramina through which pass occipital emissary veins, (3 & 4) in children, diastasis of the as yet unclosed cranial sutures, and increased convolutional markings in the inner table of the skull, the "beaten silver" appearance. (Fig. 54-4)

These are some of the roentgenologic signs of *focal intracranial disease*: The sella turcica may be symmetrically expanded beyond its maximal normal roentgenographic measurements of 17 mm. length and 13 mm. depth by an intrasellar, i.e., pituitary, tumor. More recently we have appreciated the importance of measuring the width of the sella in sagittal projections (normal 9-18 mm.) and computing sellar volume which should not exceed 1,100 cu. mm. An enlarged sella can also be produced by any obstructive lesion which raises intraventricular pressure, dilating the lateral and the third ventricles. Tumors or aneurysms contiguous to the sella can sometimes give the same appearance, but more often

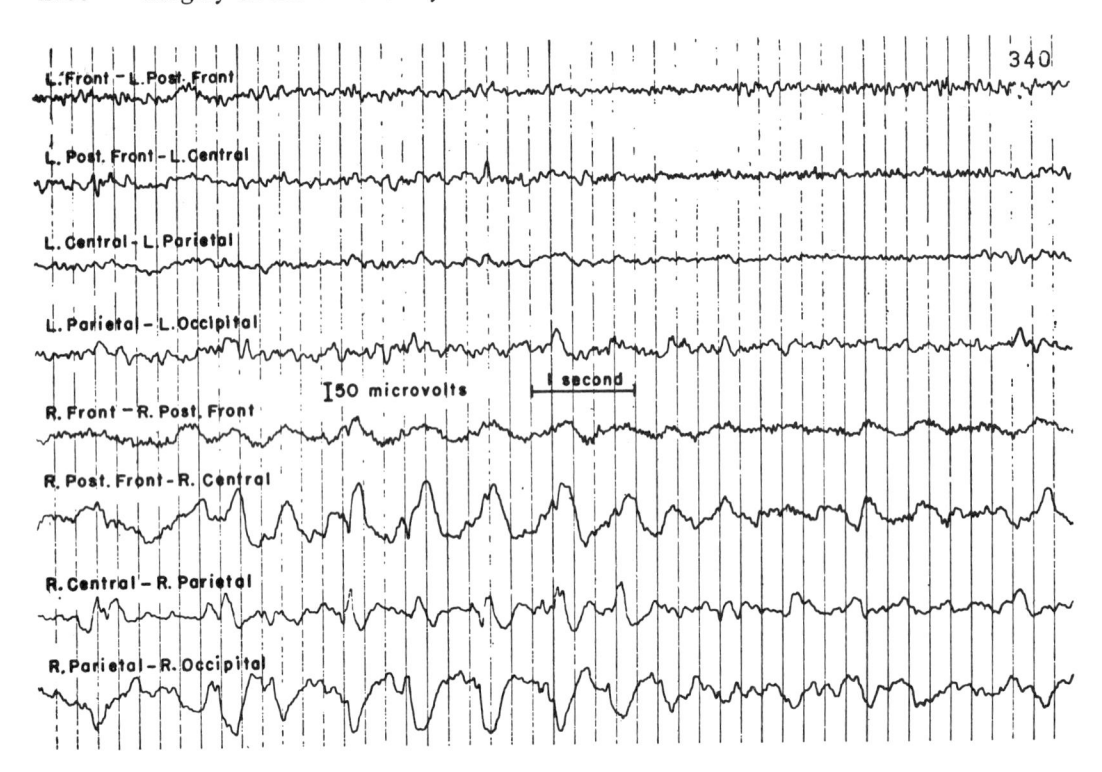

FIG. 54-5. Electroencephalogram—right parietal hemorrhage. This 10-second sample of a 1-hour tracing shows a burst of high voltage delta waves in the right-sided leads. These deflections are in opposite directions—i.e., show a reversal of phase—between the 2 posterior tracings. The electrode common to these is in the parietal region, which places the origin of the abnormal waves nearest to this electrode. (Interpretation of Dr. John Abbott)

they produce an asymmetrical or parasellar erosion at the point of most direct pressure. Any other part of the skull may be eroded by neoplasm, by a benign eosinophilic granuloma or by lipoid storage disease. There is enough calcification in the pineal gland to permit its roentgenographic identification in about 60 per cent of adults, and a lateral shift of greater than 2 mm. from the mid-sagittal plane is seen frequently—away from a space-taking mass, or toward an atrophic cerebral hemisphere. Abnormal intracranial calcification may occur in the slower growing gliomas, meningiomas, tumors arising from congenital rests, such as craniopharyngiomas, and in the walls of old hematomas and aneurysms. Such deposits may be so delicate that stereoscopic views, an essential in cranial work are required for their identification. Abnormal thickening of the cranial bone adjoining a meningioma occurs either in the floor or the vault of the skull in the so-called hyperostosing types. A similar roentgenogram is given by the benign slowly growing osteoma composed only of bone cells. Extensive new bone formation, usually around the orbit, is also provoked in fibrous dysplasia, a benign disorder in which the overgrowth may require operative decompression of the optic nerve and of the orbit. Asymmetrically broad and numerous vascular markings in one area of the skull suggest the presence of an underlying vascular meningioma. Special views of the foramina for passage of the cranial nerves out of the skull may reveal enlargement on one side indicative of tumor of that nerve, most frequently of the optic or the acoustic nerves.

Electroencephalography, the EEG. Following Grey Walter's pioneer studies, this innocuous procedure has been developed into a great aid in distinguishing focal organic from other forms of cerebral disease. Painstaking technics that blanket the scalp with numerous electrodes and include simultaneous recording from many channels are likely to disclose localizable abnormal potentials. These include single or multiple waves or irregular deflections at 1 to 4 per second, called delta waves, and waves at 4 to 7 per second, classed as theta waves. The abnormal waves, present over large and varied extents of the patient's brain, may reach a maximum voltage and be the slowest in the vicinity of the tumor. One seeks to find the point or points at which these waves show reversal of phase—since this provides the most accurate localization of the origin of the abnormal potential (Fig. 54-5). A small amount of theta rhythm may be present symmetrically in the normal record; it becomes pathologic when its amplitude exceeds by > 50 per cent that of the normal 9-11/second alpha rhythm. In general, the main criterion of focal abnormality is any asymmetry of electrical activity. An exception is that the voltage and the amount of the posterior alpha rhythm (8-13/second) may normally be mildly asymmetrical. Episodic sharp waves or spikes lasting 1/10 to 1/50 of a second are also found infrequently in the neighborhood of most focal lesions, but are commoner as the electrical insignia of such lesions when they are epileptogenic. All of the local electrographic changes may occur with localized trauma, atrophy, inflammation or vascular accident as well as with a space-taking mass. The method may give only a rough clue as to the precise location of the lesion since (1) it is the brain itself and not the mass that is giving rise to the abnormal discharges; (2) the most striking abnormal potentials may arise at some distance from the main lesion, e.g., in edematous brain or because of neuronal conduction; (3) the abnormal features may occur at irregular intervals and may be missed in the sample obtained on the tracing; (4) tactics for judging the depth of the lesion are inadequate. However, a roughly correct localization is achieved in about 75 per cent of supratentorial space-taking masses; accuracy is less in posterior fossa neoplasms, dropping to about 40 per cent.

Radioactive Isotopes. There is a formidable barrier phenomenon between blood and normal brain, by virtue of which many substances in the blood stream gain delayed or meager access to the brain. This barrier is much less effective between blood and the tissue in most neoplasms, abscesses, granulomata and traumatized brain as well as in many ischemic infarcts. Hence, radioactively tagged, gamma-emitting isotopes, which concentrate differentially in these lesions as compared with the normal brain, may be injected intravenously and the zone of increased isotopic uptake plotted with appropriate apparatus to detect the gamma ray photons emerging through the skull. Since gamma rays scatter markedly as they traverse solid matter, the image outside the head of an intracranial area with moderate increase in isotopic uptake tends to blur into the background and may escape detection. Rejection of the scattered gamma rays from the recorded image is achieved in one of two ways. So-called pulse height spectroscopy may be applied to the individual rays. When the original gamma ray photon is scattered, i.e., deflected from its original course by collision with a subnuclear particle, it loses some of its original energy. The electronic detector can be designed to ignore these weaker, "degraded" gamma rays, and this tactic is usefully combined with a focusing collimator consisting of a number of tapered apertures in a metal shield coming to a focus at the detector. ^{131}I human serum albumin (RISA) and ^{197}Hg neohydrin, the first gamma sources used with this system, have been replaced in many centers by ^{99m}Tc (techentium) pertechnetate. This isotope with a half-life of only 6 hours and a gamma emission of but 140 Kev yields diagnostic scans at low doses of radiation and at a low financial cost.

Rejection of the scattered gamma rays is also possible if one uses positron-emitting isotopes coupled with coincidence counting. A positron, once it is given off, undergoes within a tiny fraction of a second an "annihilation" collision with an electron. The mass of the two particles appears as the energy of a pair of gamma rays which leave the site of the collision back to back, i.e., they move in precisely opposite directions. A pair of detectors—one on either side of the head—is connected to circuits which tally a count only when each member of the pair of annihilation gamma rays reaches its detector. If one or both of these rays scatter, no count ensues. The detectors move continuously, and their coincidence counts are recorded automatically as marks on paper, so that a slow motion televisionlike

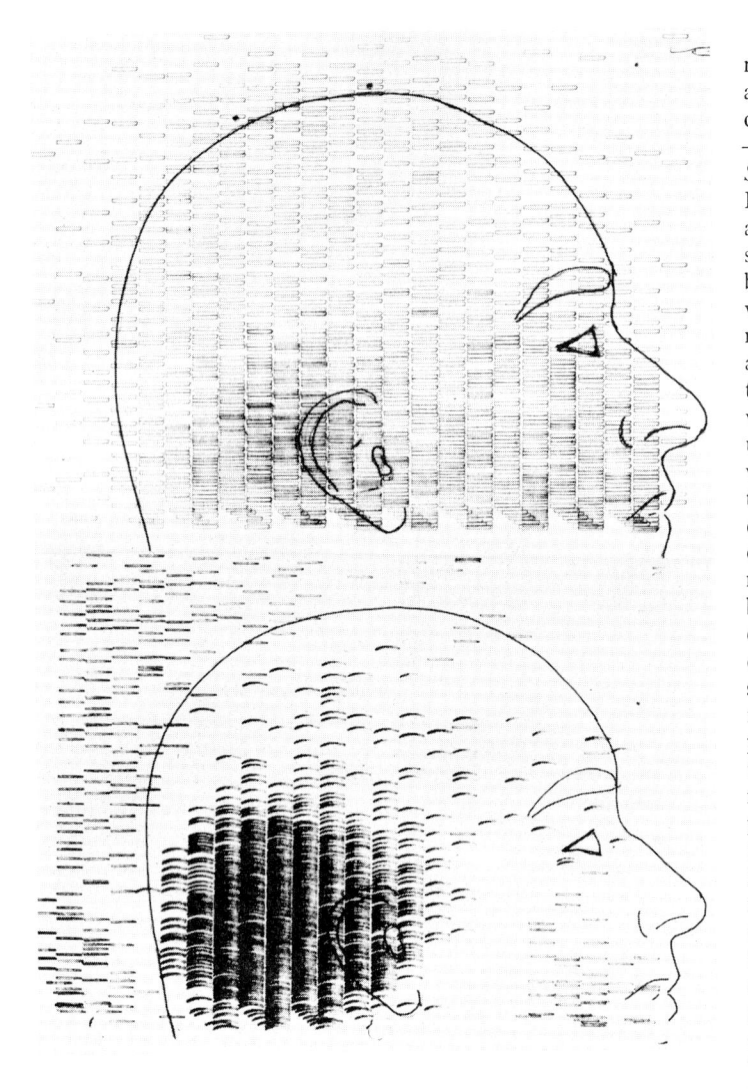

FIG. 54-6. Radioactive scanning with positron-emitting arsenic. (*Top*) PCG—positrocephalogram. (*Bottom*) AGG—Asymmetrogammagram. *Case Summary:* 39-year-old female. For 4 years before entry, brief attacks of suboccipital pressure sensation. L > R. Three years before entry, an episode of severe headache, vomiting, dizziness and unsteady gait, apathy and disorientation with spontaneous recovery after several weeks in hospital. For 2 years unsteady gait, progressively worse with tendency to deviate to right; for 1 year progressive clumsiness in right hand and deafness in right ear; for 6 months dysphagia; recently blurring of vision on right lateral gaze. Abnormal findings confirmed symptoms plus slightly diminished sensation right cornea, face and soft palate. Loudness recruitment test: no recruitment in the nearly deaf right ear. Lumbar puncture: pressure 210 mm. CSF; total protein 23 mg. %. Roentgenograms of skull normal. Radioarsenic scan: PCG—area of marked increase in isotopic uptake just behind right ear; ACG—extreme right-sided asymmetry in this zone indicated by dense concentration of ⌒ marks; unequivocal diagnosis of tumor. Suboccipital craniectomy with total removal of large meningioma arising from right sigmoid sinus. Discharged 12th postoperative day free of symptoms and signs except for deafness, a lucky result because the severe temporary neurologic illness 3 years before entry with full recovery led to erroneous diagnosis of multiple sclerosis or vascular lesion, and growth of a huge tumor.

scan of the head appears. This picture, called a *positrocephalogram* or *PCG* (Fig. 54-6, *top*), shows the precise projection in the lateral view of the area of increased uptake of isotope but does not indicate its side or its depth. The nearer the mass is to one detector, i.e., the farther it is from the mid-line, the higher the total gamma count at the nearer detector, because of the inverse square effect of increasing distance. Therefore, one can usefully obtain simultaneously with the PCG another record of the degree of side-to-side asymmetry of the total gamma counts. This *asymmetrogammagram* or *AGG* (Fig. 54-6, *bottom*), indicates the side and the depth of the lesion. A sagittal PCG, i.e., a scan with the detectors looking at the front and the back of the head, likewise indicates the side and the depth of the abnormal uptake. ^{72}As and ^{74}As as a mixture of arsenate

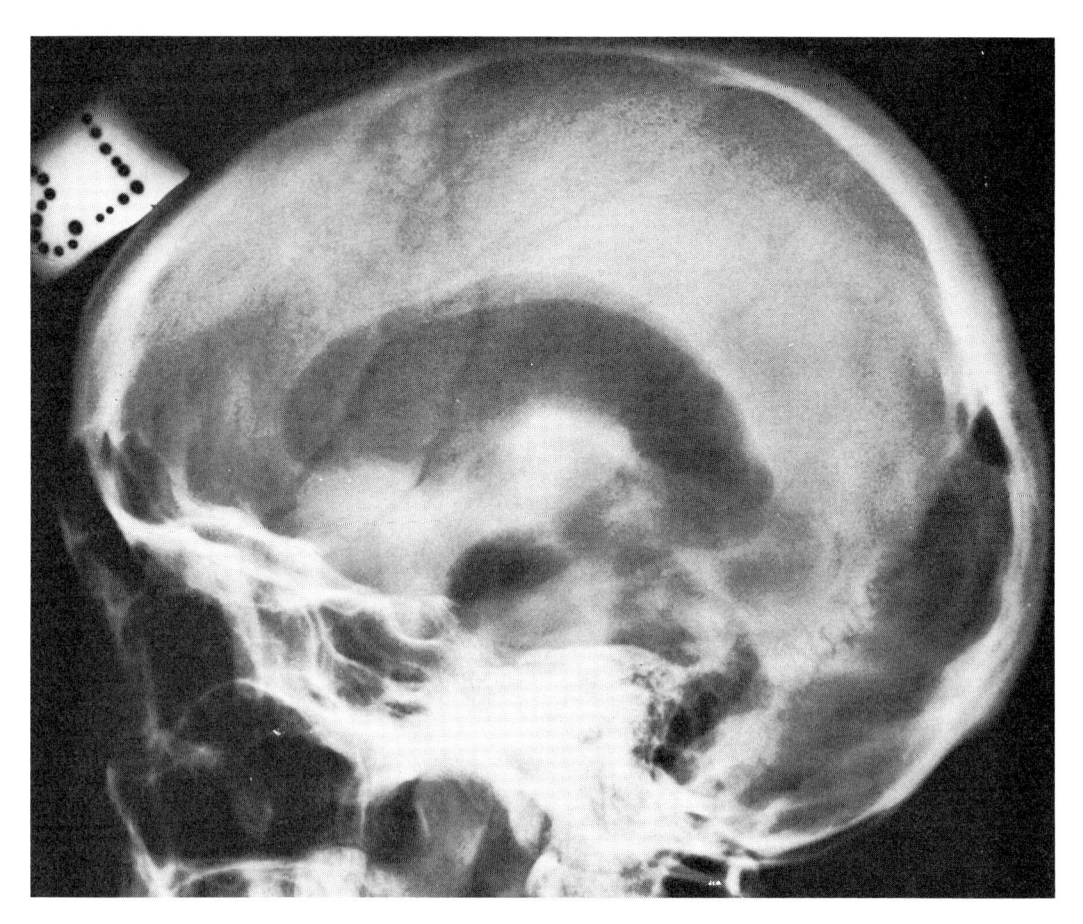

FIG. 54-7. A. Ventriculogram. Enlargement of all ventricles. Patient: 22-year-old female. History: frontal and occipital headache for 5 weeks. Vomiting, 2 weeks. Unsteady gait, nystagmus on lateral gaze, 1 week. Findings: drowsiness; tendency to veer equally to each side in walking, coarse horizontal nystagmus, incoordination on heel-shin and finger-nose tests. No papilledema. Ventriculogram: symmetrical enlargement of all ventricles to over 2 times normal size; extremely marked in 4th ventricle. Absence of air in basal cisternae and sulci points to block at outlets of 4th ventricle. Operation: suboccipital craniectomy; fibrous veil obliterating foramen of Magendie was removed with complete permanent recovery.

and arsenite, ^{64}Cu or ^{68}Ga as a chelate are the principal positron emitters in current use.

There are various methods of displaying the information to heighten the contrast: (1) a succession of changes in color of the stamp marks for stepwise increases in the count rate; (2) technics of "background erase," i.e., failure to record any counts until a certain background is exceeded; (3) photoscanning types of intensification. All 3 tactics are applicable to both pulse height and positron detection systems. Gamma ray cameras which will look at the entire head at once will yield a major increase in resolution of the study and decrease

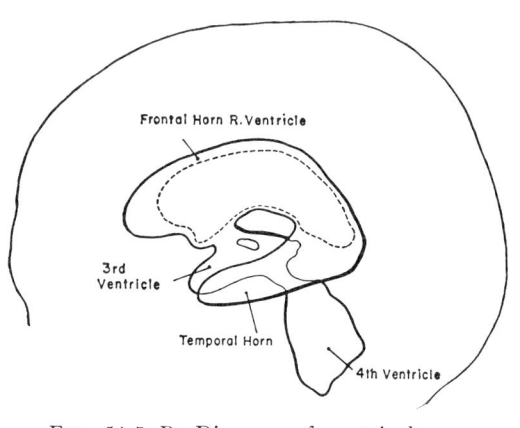

FIG. 54-7 B. Diagram of ventriculogram.

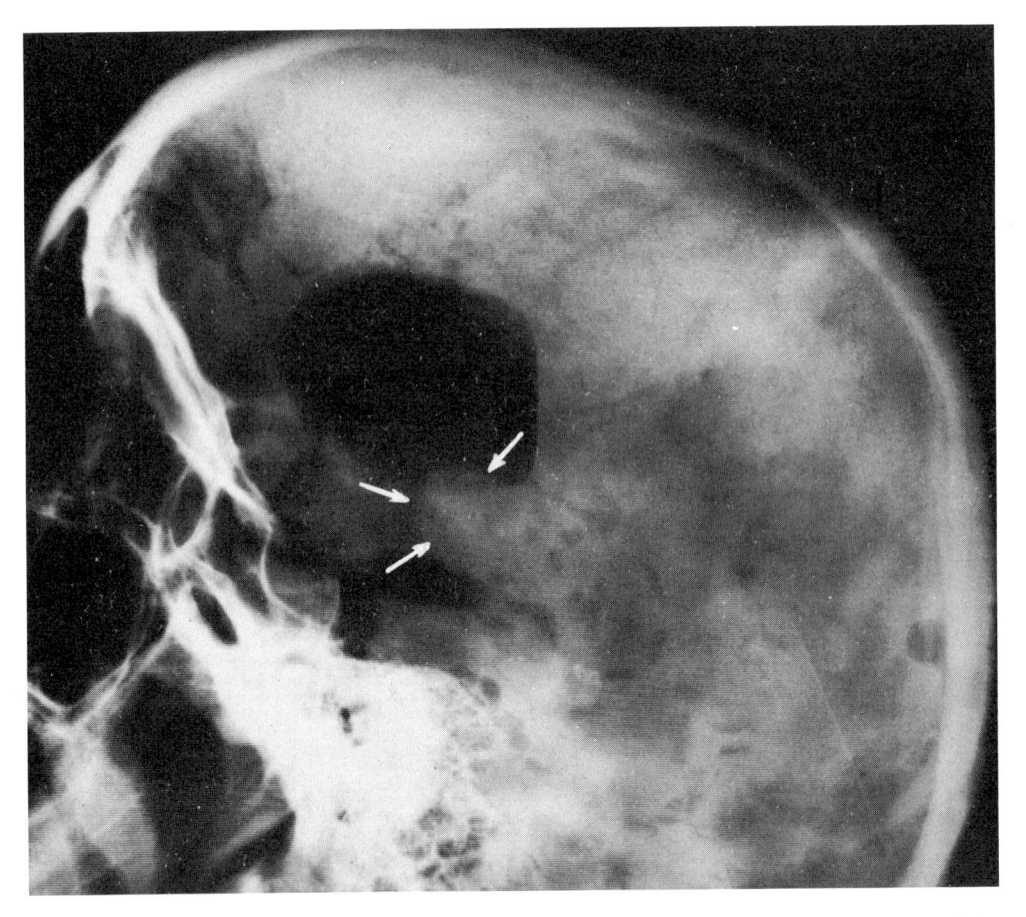

FIG. 54-8. Ventriculogram—colloid cyst, third ventricle. *Case Summary*: 41-year-old female. Brief attacks of frontal headache and vomiting when she became "carsick." For 6 months infrequent and transient incoordination of left limbs; for 3 weeks right frontotemporal headaches with screaming and vomiting for which she was amnesic—duration only 2 to 3 minutes, suggesting lesion with ball-valve action on flow of CSF. Neurologic examination, roentgenograms of skull, radioarsenic scans—all normal. Ventricular puncture: initial pressure, 180 mm. CSF; total protein, 10 mg. %. Ventriculogram: arrows indicate a cherry-sized filling defect in anterior part of third ventricle with dilated lateral ventricles—a striking picture even though lesion producing it is small. Operation: removal of colloid cyst. Slow but satisfactory recovery.

in time required for it. Several types are now on trial.

In general the current standard methods all yield similar results. Supratentorial meningiomas, glioblastomas and malignant metastases encroaching on the cerebral gray mantle or underlying white matter are demonstrated in over 90 per cent of the patients. Since these are readily accessible to the surgeon and small lesions here are those most frequently missed with pneumography or angiography, radioisotopic methods are an important adjunct to diagnosis and early therapy. The scans achieve their highest percentage of accuracy in the meningioma—a benign tumor often difficult to diagnose clinically at an early stage, yet revealed early by the radioisotopic study. Unfortunately the scan is still likely to miss at this stage the slow-growing gliomas.

This study has, like the EEG, the additional advantage of being painless, harmless and, in the case of most isotopes, repeatable at will. However, this does not distinguish between an infarct and such space-taking masses as tumor,

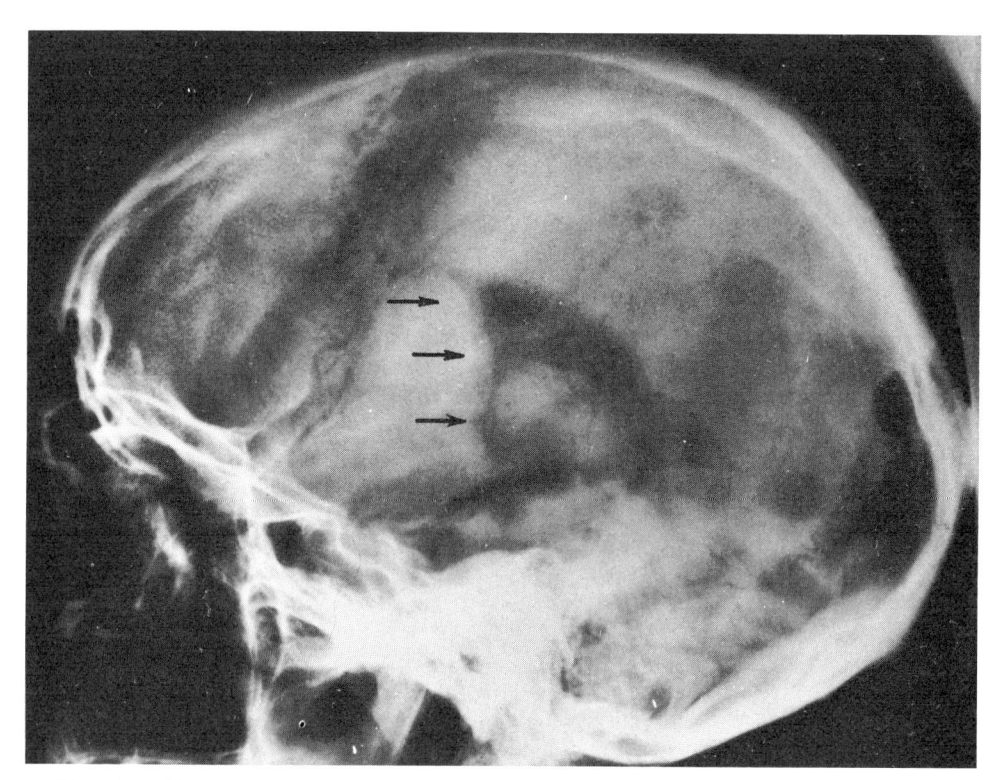

Fig. 54-9. Ventriculogram—right frontal tumor. *Case Summary*: 47-year-old male. Intermittent bilateral frontal headache and poor memory for 1 month—progressively worse. Vomiting for 1 week. Abnormal findings: unable to give consistent history, apathetic, long delays in replies to questions; diminished left abdominal reflexes. Roentgenograms of skull: normal with no pineal shift. Lumbar puncture: initial pressure 160 mm. CSF. Total protein 276 mg. %. EEG: bilateral frontal 1½/second, high voltage waves. Radioarsenic scan: PCG —inferior frontal concentration; AGC—slight right-sided asymmetry. Ventriculogram: irregular cutoff of anterior part of body right lateral ventricle (indicated by arrows). Operation: right frontal lobectomy with only partial removal of glioblastoma invading basal ganglia and other hemisphere via corpus callosum. Death 11th postoperative day.

abscess or hemorrhage. Nevertheless, the site of increased uptake guides the surgeon's aspirating needle to the right spot and thereby helps him to distinguish a lesion requiring surgical removal from an area of softening.

When one uses the positron emitting isotopes ^{72}As and ^{74}As injected as a mixture of arsenate and arsenite, one can see in the radioactive scan an abnormal concentration corresponding well with the locus of the neoplasm or abscess in about 80 per cent of such verified lesions. An abnormal uptake of arsenic occurs in only about 60 per cent of patients with a major cerebral hemorrhage or infarct.

Pneumography. *Pneumo-encephalography* (roentgenography of the head after injection of air or other gas into the lumbar or cisternal CSF) and *ventriculography* (similar films after the air is introduced directly into one or both lateral ventricles) have played a major role in the final diagnosis and the definitive location of intracranial masses ever since the tactic was introduced by Dandy in 1918. Subsequent refinements from many quarters enable one to spot over 90 per cent of intracranial tumors by this method. In most clinics the air is introduced into the subarachnoid space only when the intracranial pressure is normal. Even then, if the films demonstrate a space-taking mass, operation the same day is advisable because abrupt severe worsening in the patient's condition may occur following the dynamic upset involved in the instillation of air whether it is added to or exchanged for CSF. When the

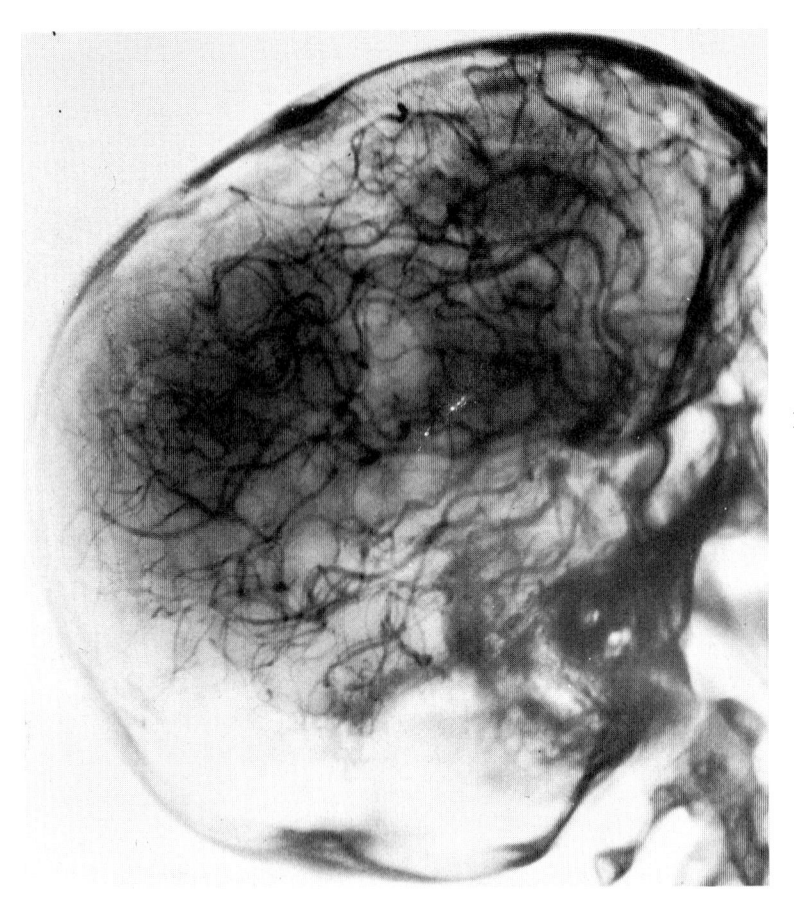

FIG. 54-10. Normal arteriogram. (A) Injection of a single carotid usually fills carotid branches on one side only. Occlusion in neck of opposite carotid during the injection often permits simultaneous filling of the opposite anterior and middle cerebral arteries. Filling as well of the basilar artery and its posterior cerebral and superior cerebellar branches as occurred here is rare.

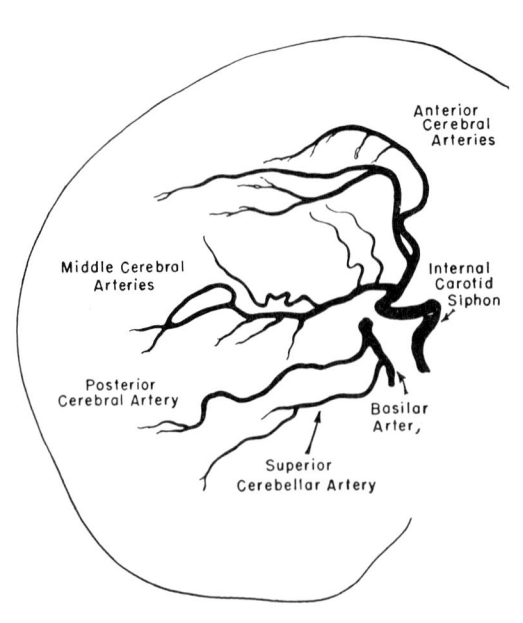

FIG. 54-10 B. Diagram of lateral view. (*Continued on facing page*)

intracranial pressure is elevated, it is advisable to do a ventriculogram and follow it with a craniotomy as soon as the locus of the mass is clear. By displacement of, enlargement of, or filling defects in ventricles, basal cisternae or cerebral sulci, the position of the mass is inferred. In Figure 54-7 one sees how a sheet of adhesions blocking outflow from the 4th ventricle led to enlargement of all 4 ventricles. The photograph permits one to pinpoint precisely the tiny lesion. Figures 54-8 and 54-9 demonstrate the clarity with which tumors may be shown. Infrequently, the ventricular needle encounters a cyst, or the wall thereof may rupture into the CSF pathways, so that the cyst itself fills and is displayed directly.

Angiography, introduced a decade later by Moniz, has steadily gained favor. Injection of the carotid in the neck on each side and of one vertebral artery is usually necessary if nearly all of the vascular supply to the head is to be shown. Puncture of the desired artery through

Fig. 54-10 (*Cont.*).
(C) Normal arteriogram. Sagittal view.

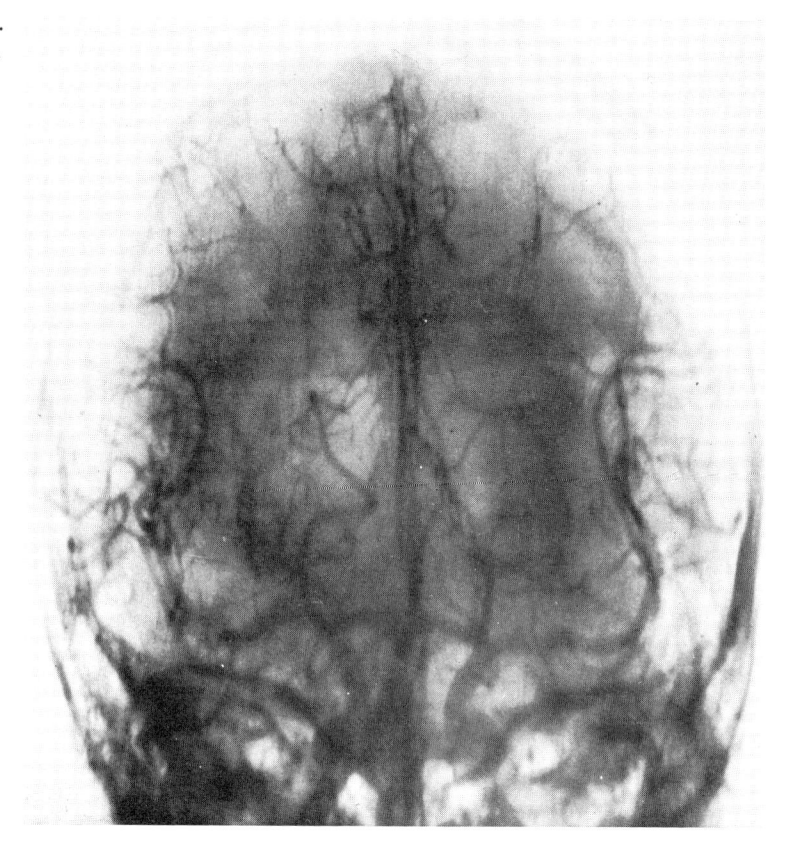

the intact skin is nearly always successful, and open exposure is rarely required. In Figure 54-10 one sees an extraordinarily complete filling following injection of one carotid artery. Rapid serial films following a single injection show arterial, capillary and venous phases of the circulation and not only reveal displacement of the normal vessels but also may demonstrate a total absence of vessels, in the zone occupied by an avascular mass (Fig. 54-11).

This technic may also depict the abnormal vessels in a highly vascularized tumor or an arteriovenous malformation, i.e., a positive demonstration of the lesion. Moreover, following the demonstration of a tumor, there is no dynamic change which makes immediate craniotomy mandatory. Precise delineation of the feeding arteries and the draining veins in a highly vascular lesion may be especially helpful to guide the surgeon's attack. The paucity of clinical localizing features of arteriovenous malformations and aneurysms, the usual absence of displacement of CSF channels or even normal arteries by these lesions, and the nor-

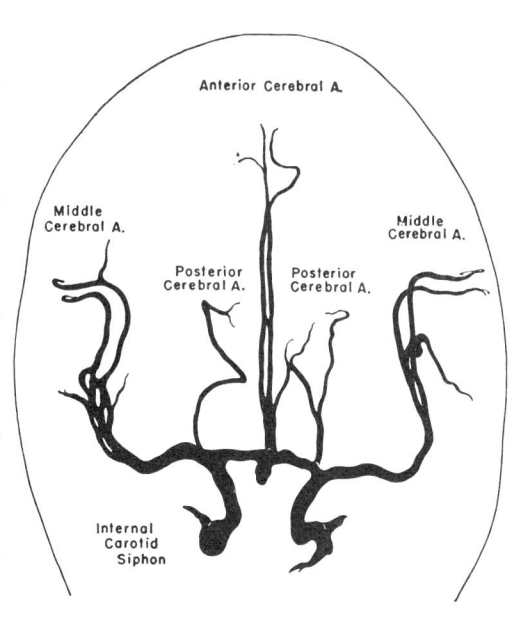

Fig. 54-10 D. Diagram of sagittal view.

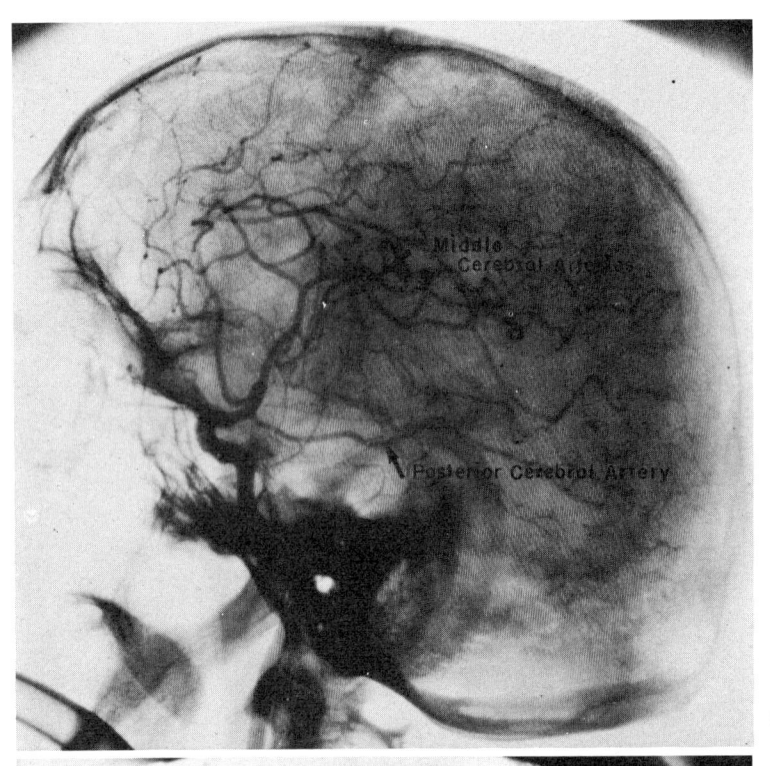

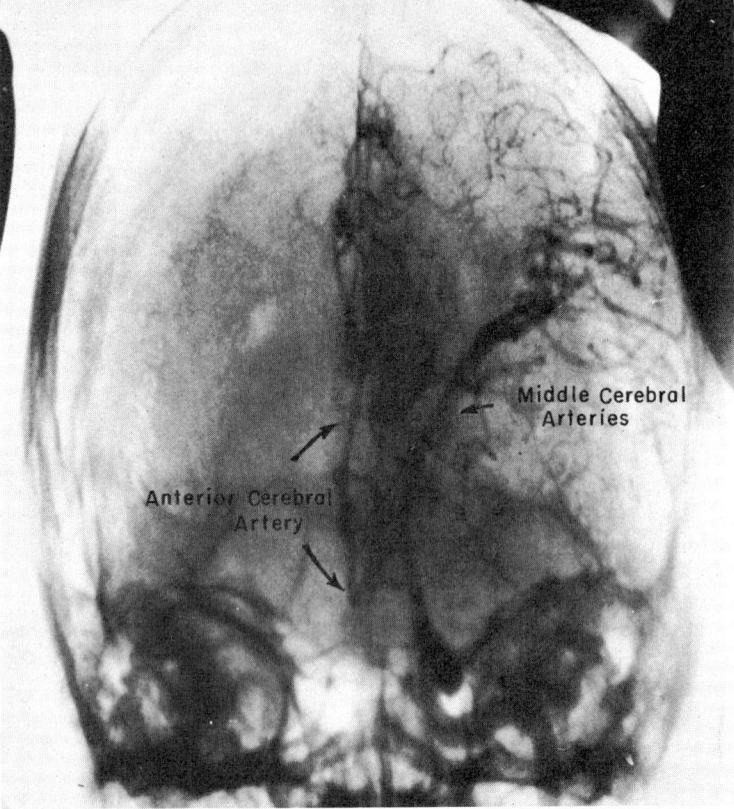

Fig. 54-11. Sagittal and lateral right carotid arteriograms: sphenoidal wing meningioma. *Case Summary*: 37-year-old male. In previous 6 months, a few attacks of right temporal pounding headache, each lasting "a few minutes," relieved promptly by aspirin. Five weeks previously, awoke in middle of night, smelling peculiar odor of "rotten damp dirt" for few seconds only. Two weeks previously, a seizure beginning with illusion that a lamp in front of him was whirling clockwise in horizontal plane; shortly, the same olfactory aura recurred, followed by violent shaking of both upper limbs, whereupon he pitched forward and remembers no more. A generalized seizure ensued. On entry, general physical and neurologic examinations were normal. Lumbar puncture: initial pressure only 75 mm. CSF: total protein, 265 mg. %. EEG: spike focus, right temporal. Arsenic scan: PCG gross increase in isotopic concentration temporal and posterior inferior frontal area, suggesting meningioma; AGG marked right-sided asymmetry in same area. Right carotid arteriogram: extreme upward and medial displacement right middle cerebral artery and slight displacement to left of anterior cerebral artery, indicated by arrows. Operation: total removal of massive meningioma arising from right sphenoidal wing. Discharged 13 days later with no abnormal signs.

mal EEG's and radioactive scans accompanying them, make angiography indispensable in their detailed diagnosis and management (see Fig. 54-14).

Continuing improvements in injection media and injection technic have reduced the risk to almost insignificant proportions in competent hands. The diatrizoates of sodium or methyl glucamine or the tri-iodothalamate of methylglucamine (Conray 60%) are currently the least irritant of the agents available and also are unlikely to induce arterial constriction so that even intracranial arterial occlusive disease may be studied with relative safety.

Neoplasms

The majority of the primary intracranial tumors arise either from the glial connective tissue or from the meninges, i.e., are either gliomas or meningiomas. We owe our basic knowledge regarding the behavior within these two groups mainly to Bailey and Cushing.

Gliomas. All gliomas infiltrate the brain. Those with the most differentiated type of cell may be composed mainly of slow-growing astrocytes or of oligodendroglia, and patients with astrocytomas or oligodendrogliomas have average survival times of over 5 years. The most favorable of all of the gliomas for a cure is the astrocytoma which occurs typically in childhood in a cerebellar hemisphere and is often predominantly cystic. Extirpation of cyst wall, as well as of the neoplastic mural nodule and a safe margin of cerebellum, is usually possible without permanent neurologic deficit and with a postoperative mortality of around 5 per cent. In general, the presence of a largely cystic content improves the prognosis in such tumors as gliomas, hemangioblastomas or acoustic neuromas. More rapidly growing gliomas are the astroblastoma, the polar spongioblastoma and the ependymoma, with average survival times of 2 to 3 years. The polar spongioblastoma is one of the commoner tumors of the brain stem. Despite the proximity to aqueduct and 4th ventricle, oddly enough, neoplasms here do not cause increased intracranial pressure until late in their evolution; instead, both lower cranial nerve and long tract signs predominate. Ependymomas arise from the ependyma of any of the ventricles, those in the 4th ventricle occurring much more commonly in children. The highly malignant gliomas, unfortunately the commonest, are the glioblastoma multiforme, seen mainly in the cerebral hemispheres of adults, and the medulloblastomas, which usually arise in the posterior cranial fossa and are about 4 times as common in children as in adults. There are almost no recorded cures of either of these 2 vicious lesions.

Meningiomas. The meningiomas, on the other hand, present an encouraging challenge to the surgeon; these encapsulated tumors are usually benign, grow slowly and may even attain large size before any symptoms appear. Then intracranial compensatory mechanisms may fail rapidly, leading to the erroneous impression of a rapidly growing tumor. Meningiomas usually lie on the surface of the brain, but so do the arteries nourishing the cerebral cortex; hence, early operation gives the best chance of saving the nutrient vessels of the brain. The vascularity of these tumors may be formidable and require the surgeon to employ not only multiple transfusions but also ganglionic blocking agents to lower the blood pressure during the operation. In patients with normal cerebral blood vessels the systolic pressure may be carried safely at 85 to 95 mm. Hg while the tumor is being extirpated in order to reduce the blood loss. Under these circumstances it is especially important that blood replacement keep pace with the actual loss which occurs. The total removal of the dural origin of the tumor required for cure can be achieved in the majority, but even if this is not attainable, subtotal extirpation often results in remission of symptoms for many years. Dr. Cushing's practice of having these and other patients report annually following tumor operations is an important routine to aid in the early detection of a recurrence.

Metastatic Tumors. Metastatic intracranial tumors are not necessarily hopeless problems. Solitary metastases to cerebellum or a resectable portion of cerebrum occur so often that a previous history of malignant tumor elsewhere should not lead to incomplete study when the next symptoms of a mass lesion point to the brain. Those individuals with carcinomas which are usually slower growing, such as the ones of renal origin, or those amenable to some control by hormones, e.g., the cancers of the breast, may be particularly propitious candidates for surgery. This may consist of removal of the metastases, usually technically easy, or in extensive cranial decompression to control headache. A bronchogenic carcinoma is often clinically silent until its cerebral metastasis speaks. Hence, such a lesion should always be sought in roentgenograms of the chest of any patient at or beyond middle age whose clinical picture intimates a rapidly growing intracranial mass.

Tumors from Congenital Rests. The tumors arising from congenital rests occur mainly in regions where there is complex folding of ectoderm for skin and nerve along with mesodermal elements, principally in the midline in the neighborhood of the 3rd and the 4th ventricles. The commonest, the *craniopharyngioma*, arises from squamous epithelial remnants of the craniopharyngeal duct, from which the anterior lobe of the hypophysis forms. It lies above and/or within the sella turcica and usually contains one or more cysts. Its symptoms usually begin in childhood. Evacuation of the cystic fluid and removal of some of the solid portion of these tumors were rarely more than temporarily palliative in children and usually disappointing in adults as well. But the tumor's often intimate association with the vital structures around the 3rd ventricle used to cause frequent postoperative fatality if complete removal was carried out. Now, however, semimicromanipulation during surgery and vigilant correction of metabolic imbalances after operation permit total extirpation of these lesions in all children and many adults with an acceptably low operative mortality. Other congenital rest tumors in order of increasing complexity in their tissue content are *epidermoid, dermoid, teratoid* and *teratomatous* tumors. The epidermoids are usually filled with a white, scaly, totally avascular debris, which is readily ladled out of otherwise inoperable loci. Remnants of the notochord in sellar and prepontine regions may give rise to a *chordoma*.

Glandular Tumors. Those of the anterior lobe of the hypophysis are usually *chromophobe adenomas*, rarely develop before the 3rd decade, and give signs of endocrine deficiency along with the visual field defects of lesions pressing on optic nerve or chiasm.

Rotational x-ray or proton beam radiation therapy centered on the sella turcica are vying with transphenoidal or transfrontal operative approaches in the management of these lesions.

The *eosinophil adenomas*, producing gigantism before puberty and acromegaly thereafter are not held in check by rotational or other tactics involving gamma radiation. Regression of the acromegalic deformities and lowering of the grossly elevated plasma levels of growth hormone do ensue upon total removal of the pituitary gland plus associated tumor—now a low-risk procedure in the hands of Ray and others. Even safer and apparently as effective is Kjellberg's recently developed method of concentrating the terminal or Bragg peak of a proton beam within the expanded sella turcica. The 6 month interval required for the radiation effect is not a serious drawback in this disorder and a huge series of 94 patients in a few years attests to its success.

Pinealomas and *congenital rest tumors*, which press downward on the superior colliculi and thereby cause paresis of upward gaze as their most striking localizing sign, are the commonest cause of a ventriculographic filling defect in the posterior part of the 3rd ventricle. The preferred treatment is ventriculocisternostomy or ventriculovascular shunt combined with x-ray therapy and often gives long remissions; direct removal has a discouraging high mortality.

Acoustic Neuromas. Tumors of nerve sheaths within the cranial cavity rarely occur on any but the 8th nerve. The acoustic neuromas give the syndrome of a mass in the cerebellopontine angle. This includes, initially, (1) disturbance of hearing and equilibrium; then a progressive involvement of (2) the trigeminal nerve with ipsilateral reduction of corneal reflex, facial paresthesias and later numbness, (3) the facial nerve with ipsilateral facial weakness and loss of taste, (4) the cerebellar hemisphere with signs as mentioned earlier, (5) the lower 4 cranial nerves with dysphagia, dysarthria and hoarseness, and (6) the abducens nerve with external rectus paresis. Skillful surgeons can usually achieve a total removal of these benign encapsulated tumors. Early diagnosis by special audiologic and vestibular tests (see p. 1762) is now made more frequently, especially since the otologist who performs the tests often joins with the neurosurgeon at the operation. Laminagraphs of the petrous bone and iophenyldate (Pantopaque) studies of the cerebellopontine angle confirm the diagnosis. The otologic surgeon, via a translabyrinthine approach, removes that part of the tumor in and neighboring the internal auditory canal. At the same stage or a later one the neurosurgeon is usually able to complete the removal, including the critical dissection of capsule from the side of the brain stem. In the most capable hands the postoperative mortality has dropped to under 5 per cent; over 80 per cent of the survivors are able to return to their original work. These striking improvements are attributable to early operation aided by the Zeiss microscope.

Miscellaneous Tumors of Mesodermal Origin. A variety of intracranial neoplasms arise from other connective tissue. These include the *hemangioblastoma*, a cystic tumor with a mural nodule of compact blood vessels, found nearly always in the cerebellum of adults. An as yet mysterious association with polycythemia vera often occurs. The lesion may be a part of the complex known as Lindau's disease. In this hereditary disorder, multiple tumors are present, of which the easiest to see is a capillary hemangioma of the retina (von Hippel's disease). Multiple cysts or tumors in pancreas, kidneys or epididymis also occur. Regardless of the presence or the absence of other features of Lindau's disease, the total or subtotal removal of the cerebellar hemangioblastoma is usually a fruitful procedure. Sarcomas, melanomas and even lipomas occur in the intracranial cavity.

Papillomas arising from the choroid plexus in any ventricle and *colloid cysts* in the anterior end of the 3rd ventricle are other benign tumors whose critical locus calls for special judgment and care in removal. Adherence to vital portions of ventricular walls may dictate leaving a remnant of the tumor or the cyst in order to leave a functional patient.

Orbital Tumors and Exophthalmos. Retrobulbar tumors and some other lesions provoking protrusion of the eyeball, such as the ill-understood proptosis accompanying thyrotoxicosis, are best approached surgically by a transfrontal exposure. When CSF is evacuated via a lumbar puncture needle, the frontal lobe with its dura literally falls away from the orbit. Removal of its bony roof and if necessary of the lateral and posterior wall gives easy access to the area behind the eyeball and the best chance to preserve that structure and vision if the type of lesion does not make mandatory an exenteration of the orbit. Proptosis, at times with displacement of the eyeball out of its central axis, loss of visual acuity, a field defect, weakness of extraocular muscles with diplopia and strabismus, impaired pupillary reactions, and papilledema or optic atrophy may all occur. Over a score of different types of space-taking pathologic processes— no one of them common—may be responsible for this clinical picture.

Infections

This type of lesion has become less common and presents a less stereotyped clinical picture since the antibiotics have come into use. Intensive use of the agent or agents to which the patient's organism is sensitive remains a major part of the treatment when the bacteria settle in the skull or the brain. Local instillation at the site of the pus after its removal permits a high concentration at the right spot and properly supplements high parenteral dosage. The principal available avenue of attack may be local when one uses such drugs as bacitracin, with which systemic levels effective against staphylococci threaten renal function. Those agents which do not enter CSF readily from the blood should be injected directly into ventricle or lumbar region if there is any suspicion of meningitis, but penicillin may not be so used in high concentration because of its convulsant effect.

Brain Abscess. Focal infection almost never begins in the brain in the absence of direct open trauma or operation. The primary source may be infections of the accessory nasal or mastoid air sinuses, which may lead by direct extension or by infected venous emboli to abscess within the brain. Usually bacteria in the nasal sinuses spread to the frontal lobe, while those from the mastoid go to the temporal lobe or the cerebellar hemisphere, but such relations are not always found. Bacteria starting from any part of the body and reaching the arterial blood may lodge in any part of the brain. Children with congenital cardiac lesions involving a right-left shunt and patients of any age with pulmonary infection are especially likely to develop a brain abscess. The systemic reactions to infection of fever, chills and leukocytosis are usually completely absent in the brain abscesses; despite this, they may evolve in devastating fashion with extensive edema or "cerebritis." *Development of any intracranial symptoms or signs in the presence* *either of infection elsewhere or in patients with congenital heart disease producing cyanosis should lead to an emergency analysis and full study*, even though the primary lesion may be smoldering or subsiding. The surgical portion of the treatment may consist of aspiration, or open drainage of the pus via a small bony opening, of a total excision of abscess plus capsule at a craniotomy, or a combination of these maneuvers. Aspiration, especially of a deep abscess, is properly followed by Kahn's tactic of injecting a small amount of Thorotrast which is phagocytized by the capsule and enables roentgenograms to show the locus and the course of the lesion as a guide to therapy. In cerebral lesions, convulsions during treatment should be forestalled with anticonvulsant therapy. Convulsions as a sequel to the disease from the residual scar in the brain are less likely to occur if the entire abscess capsule is removed. Moreover, the abscess may be multilocular so that aspiration or open drainage fail to eradicate the infection. Hence, total extirpation is the procedure of choice if the lesion can be removed via a relatively "silent" area of the brain. Late seizures are not a problem when the abscess is in the cerebellum.

Subdural Abscess. When pus spreads in the subdural space, the source is usually a severe nasal sinusitis, and the clinical picture is often fulminant with coma succeeding rapidly upon focal neurologic signs such as adversive seizures and hemiparesis. Pus spreads along the medial and inferior as well as the superolateral surfaces of one or both cerebral hemispheres. Catheter irrigation and drainage via multiple burr holes at all of these sites are necessary.

Cranial Osteomyelitis. Cranial osteomyelitis now occurs rarely. Antibiotic therapy, en block excision of the infected sector of the cranial vault, and cranioplastic repair after many months represent the therapeutic sequence.

Hematoma, Intracerebral

This may arise from (1) trauma (see below), (2) rupture of diseased vessels as seen in arteriosclerosis and hypertension, vascular malformations, aneurysms and tumors, and (3) systemic hemorrhagic diathesis. In the absence of trauma, abrupt evolution of focal symptoms and signs, especially with the finding of blood in the CSF, should lead to suspicion of this diagnosis. The fact that in many patients the hemorrhage does not lie in a deep-seated inoperable area makes it incumbent to study each of them critically and urgently. Often the patient's parlous clinical condition precludes his giving the examiner much assistance in diagnosis, and there may be time to place a burr opening in the skull over the most likely site of hemorrhage and to tap into the brain with a blunt ventricular needle in the hope of striking clot which can be aspirated. This may relieve acute embarrassment of vital functions enough to permit a full exposure via craniotomy with evacuation of all the clot and management of the causative lesion under direct vision.

Craniocerebral Trauma

The rising number of traffic accidents in which head injuries present acute problems makes a basic knowledge of this subject a must for most physicians. Whenever there is any question of cerebral injury, *opiates such as morphine or methadone should be avoided*, even though they effectively control pain and restlessness. These drugs tend to aggravate a rising intracranial pressure, to depress already impaired respiratory functions to a lethal low and, by causing pupillary constriction, to obscure the important lateralizing sign of unilateral pupillary dilation. The profuse bleeding from a scalp laceration may be controlled by digital compression along the scalp margins until hemostats can be applied to the galea and reflected backward to evert this layer, which closes the vessels and makes direct ligation of most of the bleeders unnecessary. If a depressed fracture can be seen, either directly or in roentgenograms, or can be palpated with a gloved finger, the wound should be repaired as soon as traumatic shock has been treated. It is important to remove indriven bone fragments lest they form a nidus for later development of a brain abscess. A thorough, gentle débridement, including discrete removal of necrotic brain, is needed not only to promote primary healing but also to minimize post-traumatic convulsive seizures, which occur in a high percentage of penetrating cerebral wounds. The dura should be closed tightly, if necessary, with a fascial or pericranial graft, in order to prevent a progressive outward herniation or cerebral fungus of edematous, injured brain. This must be done even in the presence of probable bacterial contamination. Otherwise, cerebral veins on the surface of and draining the herniating gyri are compressed by the dural edge, whereas the arteries continue to pour in blood, and a vicious circle of steadily increasing herniation develops.

Signs of Focal Hemorrhage. A major initial task in assaying an acute head injury is the detection of intracranial hemorrhage or pulpified hemorrhagic brain. In Figure 54-12 are shown the sites of predilection for the occurrence of extradural, subdural and intracerebral hematomas. The most important indication of such a lesion is progressive decrease in responsiveness. This may follow a period of normal behavior after the injury, the so-called lucid interval. Alternatively, the patient may decline steadily from a state of decreased responsiveness to a deep coma. In such a patient a surgically removable lesion is so likely that the search for a focal clot or area of pulpification should be pursued exhaustively by every diagnostic means available. The faster the deterioration, the more urgent the indication for surgery. Increasing intracranial pressure is also likely to produce an elevation in systolic and pulse pressures, a rising temperature, bradycardia, and slow, irregular breathing. However, these warning signs may all be absent, and the lumbar CSF pressure even be normal or subnormal in the presence of a huge intracranial clot.

The side of supratentorial bleeding is shown most reliably, but not with certainty by an ipsilateral dilating pupil unresponsive to light. In patients with even minor head injuries, the size of the pupils should be checked regularly for at least 24 hours, as anisocoria may warn of an impending tentorial pressure cone before lethargy becomes severe. Its presence should lead to efforts to rouse an apparently sleeping patient; the sleep may prove to be a coma! Decerebrate rigidity, even bilaterally, may be evoked by a unilateral supratentorial hematoma in the temporal region; the primary causative lesion need not necessarily lie within the midbrain; if removed promptly, recovery may follow. A stiff neck, cerebral or bulbar signs, or a fracture entering the foramen magnum suggest the possibility of bleeding in the posterior cranial fossa.

Extradural Hematoma. In general, a frac-

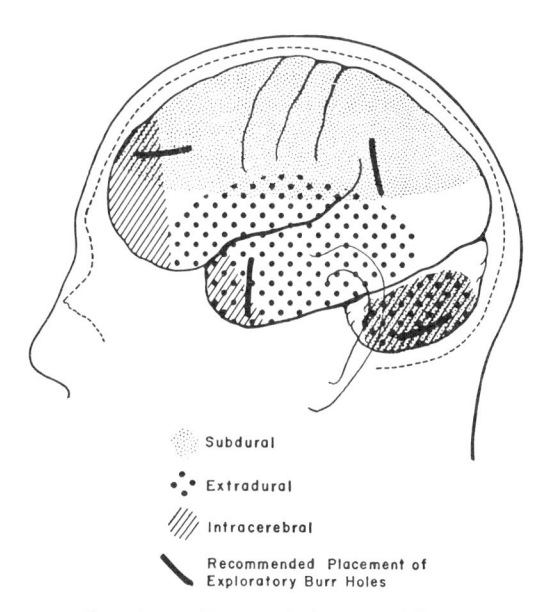

FIG. 54-12. Traumatic intracranial hematoma. Sites of predilection for the occurrence of various types.

ture line which crosses one of the grooves for the middle meningeal vessels or the venous sinuses should lead to suspicion of an extradural hematoma underlying the crossing—X marks the spot. When the clinical signs are in agreement, this is the first place to look. If the patient's downhill course is extremely rapid, extradural arterial bleeding from a main middle meningeal vessel is a likely and the most remediable cause. To check for this, an opening may be made (even through unshaved scalp with any unsterile drill in a grave emergency) just above and in front of the ear. Provision of space for the blood clot to spout out or be aspirated through a hole in the skull, thereby relieving acute high pressure against the brain, is even more important than securing the bleeding point, which is of course the next order of business. If an experienced surgeon is not at hand, an inexperienced doctor may find himself obligated to carry out these dramatic life-saving gestures.

Subdural Hematoma. This lesion often presents a picture of subacute or chronic illness because it usually arises from a tiny tear in a vein from the cerebrum bridging this space to enter a venous sinus—most commonly the superior sagittal sinus. A minimal blow in the long axis of the head, so minor as to appear negligible, may provoke such bleeding, especially in an older person or an alcoholic. In the subdural space a striking semipermeable membrane forms around the clot which not only precludes its absorption after the bleeding stops but actually results in a slow increase in the size of the mass. This "growth" is attributed to increasing osmolar concentration from splitting of protein molecules and consequent net entry of more water into the sac. Symptoms may be indistinguishable from those of neoplasm; headache and mental changes are prominent; fluctuation in symptoms, especially in the level of responsiveness, is often seen. This disorder is treated so simply and effectively, frequently requiring only drainage of the brownish fluid content of the sac through one or two burr holes, that often the lesion should be sought even when the chance of finding it seems to be small.

Subdural Hematoma in Infancy. This presents a special picture in which one may note at first only irritability, failure to gain weight and vomiting. Later, the head and the facies suggest the development of hydrocephalus, and convulsions and retinal hemorrhages may be present. Puncture at the lateral aspect of one or both sides of the anterior fontanelle yields yellow fluid. Repeated aspiration or drainage may eliminate the abnormal fluid or it may prove necessary to turn down a bone flap and remove the abnormal membranes.

Intracerebral Hematoma. Recognition of the peculiar torsion movements often undergone by the brain within the skull when the head is struck has led to realization that one or both temporal or frontal poles may become contused and hemorrhagic, even when the blow is delivered elsewhere (Fig. 54-12). Especially since one or more of these areas may be sacrificed without permanent deficit, the internal decompression of the remainder of the brain purchased by removal of such destroyed zones is beneficial at small cost. Much less often, occipital poles or cerebellar hemisphere become contused and hemorrhagic. If a hematoma is found in the occipital lobe above the transverse sinus, it is often advisable to seek one below it in the cerebellum and vice versa.

As indicated in Figure 54-12, exploration by as many as 4 burr holes on each side may be advisable in searching for a removable hemorrhage. If none is found and the brain continues to bulge at the openings, ventriculography or angiography may be necessary.

Cerebrospinal Rhinorrhea and Otorrhea. Leakage of CSF from nose or ear occurs in about 2 per cent of patients following a closed head injury. A fistulous pathway for the fluid is created by a fracture plus dural and mucosal tears. A spontaneous rhinorrhea may also develop. In either case the communication permits infection from the upper respiratory passages to gain direct access to the subarachnoid space and the brain, at times with a rapidly fatal result. The hazard of such infection is much less in otorrhea than in rhinorrhea because a fracture in the petrous bone tends to close promptly and effectively. The blood from nose or ear at the time of the original injury should be collected; if it does not clot, probably it is mixed with some CSF. Usually the fistula is not suspected until water-clear fluid drips from the nose later on. A collected sample of nasal fluid does indeed contain CSF if its glucose or chloride concentrations approach those in the patient's lumbar CSF and differ thereby from blood samples obtained at the same time. If the sample is water-clear, the presence of even a few milligrams per cent of glucose establishes it as CSF and not the secretion of vasomotor rhinitis. Even if the leak stops spontaneously, as it usually does, the possibility of direct infection into the intracranial cavity persists. One or more attacks of meningitis with such a mechanism may appear even as late as a decade after the injury. Formerly, the rhinorrhea was treated merely by urging the patient not to blow his nose or sniff up; operative repair was advised only if the leak did not stop in a week or two. However, long-term follow-up of patients with a CSF rhinorrhea reveals that about one fourth of them develop a later meningitis which is of a fulminant fatal type in about half of those affected. Consequently, we now advise prophylactic administration of antibiotics and, early after recovery from the original injury, a transfrontal craniotomy with repair of the dural tear. This relatively minor operation has a mortality of less than 2 per cent when done electively.

Aneurysms

These are usually saccular out-pouchings on any of the larger intracranial arteries and are principally of congenital or arteriosclerotic origin. They may rarely have a traumatic, mycotic or syphilitic cause. In another type, a fusiform dilation and tortuosity of one of the major arterial trunks at the base of the brain occurs. These lesions may give rise initially to focal signs whose nature depends on their locus; oculomotor, trigeminal or optic nerves are those most frequently indented by the expanded vessel. But a spontaneous subarachnoid hemorrhage commonly provokes the first symptoms; the converse of this, that an aneurysm is the commonest cause of such hemorrhage, is also true. The rupture of the aneurysm is signaled by the abrupt onset of severe pain in the head, often occipital, but occurring anywhere. This is followed by pain and rigidity in the nuchal region and on down the spine —promptly in major bleeding, but not for some hours if the hemorrhage is smaller. Unconsciousness may come on almost at once if bleeding is severe; in other patients recurrent bouts of leakage of blood may lead to such mistaken diagnoses as "sinusitus," especially if intense pain is preceded by duller headache. Careful questioning may elicit a history of brief focal motor or sensory symptoms at the onset or later. Retinal and/or more massive subhyaloid hemorrhages appear shortly in about 10 per cent of the patients; papilledema may come on later. The diagnosis of a spontaneous subarachnoid hemorrhage is confirmed by lumbar puncture. Persistent neurologic deficit suggests that a hematoma remains around the affected cranial nerve or within the brain.

About 60 per cent of the patients who survive the initial hemorrhage ictus will bleed again within a month. On the conservative management of bed rest, roughly half of all the patients will survive the initial and any subsequent hemorrhages without crippling neurologic deficit. Neurosurgeons are improving on this figure and are treating many unruptured lesions as well. Recurrent hemorrhage and death, a great risk at first, become less likely with the passage of each successive week after the initial episode. The sooner one operates the less the likelihood of a fatal recurrent hemorrhage; but the more serious the original ictus, the greater the arterial spasm and cerebral damage, and the more dangerous is early surgery.

Angiography not only pinpoints the lesion but also shows the degree of local and generalized arterial spasm and, by displacement of vessels from their normal position, indicates the presence of a hematoma. Figure 54-13 illustrates these points. Since over 80 per cent of the aneurysms are on one or both carotid arterial trees and the lesions are multiple in about 20 per cent of cases, bilateral carotid angiography has become routine in most clinics. Perfecting of the technics for percutaneous injection both of these and of the vertebral arteries has reduced the mortality plus permanent significant morbidity to well under 1 per cent in experienced hands. Because of (1) increasing success in operations for posterior fossa aneurysms and (2) demonstration of an increasing percentage of patients with multiple aneurysms, vertebral angiography is being performed routinely in more and more clinics even when the carotid injections have already shown one or more aneurysms.

Appraisal of the results of early and later operation has not yet reached a point at which even tentative rules of surgical conduct can be suggested. It is clear, however, that angiography is virtually indispensable to proper management. Figure 54-13 indicates how striking the lesion may be.

Surgical treatment may consist of (1) carotid occlusion in the neck, or of intracranial approach with (2) proximal occlusion of the vessel bearing the aneurysm, (3) "trapping" of the lesion between proximal and distal clips on the parent vessel, (4) occlusion of the neck of the aneurysm, (5) application of plastic and/or other supportive substance around the lesion, or (6) removal of the aneurysm and repair of the parent vessel. The least dangerous of these is occlusion of the cervical carotid. The intra-arterial systolic pressure in the neck distal to occlusion of the internal carotid falls to an average of about one half and the pulse pressure to about one third of that with the flow free. This degree of residual pressure usually suffices to prevent dangerous cerebral ischemia. However, the collateral inflow varies tremendously in different patients, and it is advisable to carry out a measurement in each. The percentage drop in pressure found in the cervical internal carotid is the same in all parts of that carotid's larger arterial branches, so that the location of the aneurysm on the tree would appear by this criterion to be immaterial in determining the value of carotid closure. If

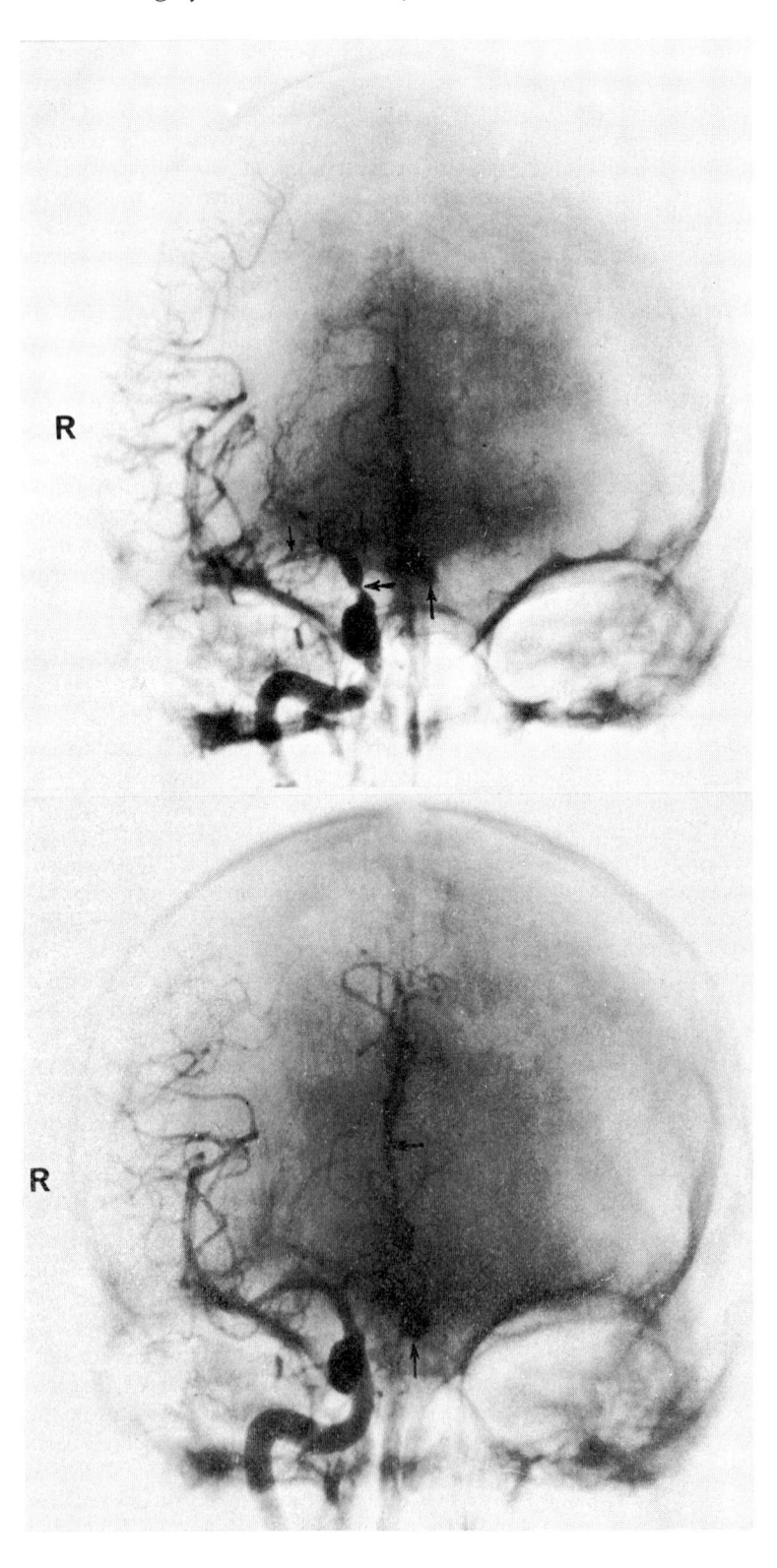

FIG. 54-13. Aneurysm of anterior communicating artery. *Case Summary:* 45-year-old female. Abrupt onset of bifrontal headache; then nausea, vomiting and momentary blackout. Walked without weakness, but fell gently; was briefly unconscious and incontinent of feces. Mental confusion the only neurologic deficit. Lumbar puncture: initial pressure 160 mm. of grossly bloody CSF. Ten days later increased obtundation, positive left Babinski; transferred to Massachusetts General Hospital. (*Top*) Serial right carotid angiogram, 5-26-64. Film 2 of series: slow filling of arteries with focal spasm of internal carotid (←), and entire anterior and middle cerebral trunks (↓↓↓↓); bilobed aneurysm (↑). No arterial displacement. Operation deferred pending improvement of serious memory deficit. This occurring, when on 6-17-64 vomiting came after another subarachnoid hemorrhage. (*Bottom*) Serial right carotid angiogram, 6-22-64. Film 1 of series: normal rate of arterial filling, spasm gone, but a third even larger lobe of aneurysm now present (↑) and midline vessels displaced to right (←). Bilateral frontal craniotomy under hypothermia at 29° C. and after tapes around innominate, left common carotid and left vertebral arteries low in neck. Wrapping of aneurysm in fine mesh gauze plus Handa's mixture of 3 plastics. Edema, not hematoma, explained midline arterial shift. Two months required for recovery.

the drop in pressure is small or, contrariwise, is excessive, a direct intracranial approach may be advisable. However, in the case of marked drop in pressure or the development of signs of cerebral ischemia during a period of trial occlusion under local anesthesia, a fractional staged closure, leading finally to full shutoff, may be tolerated.

In the randomized series of McKissock, Walsh and Richardson the mortality was 10 per cent in the 50 per cent of the cases treated by cervical carotid closure for ruptured aneurysm of the intracranial internal carotid, whereas in the conservatively managed half of the group treated by 6 weeks of bed rest 38 per cent died. The value of intra-arterial pressure measurements to assess in a particular patient the fruitfulness of carotid closure was demonstrated in the series of Wright and Sweet; of 8 patients whose internal carotid pressure distal to the site of full occlusion was greater than 100 mm. Hg, 7 later bled again, whereas of 85 patients in whom that pressure was under 85 mm. Hg only 8 did so.

The intracranial operations at present carry a higher immediate mortality but are receiving a thorough trial because they permit a curative attack on the lesion, whereas later and fatal hemorrhages still occur in a few patients after arterial ligations proximal to the aneurysm. Cerebral metabolism drops $\frac{1}{4}$ to $\frac{1}{3}$ normal levels when the patient is deliberately cooled to 25° C., and at this hypothermic level a temporary clamping of both carotid and both vertebral vessels can be maintained for a succession of 10- to 15-minute periods without permanent ischemic damage. Shorter periods of occlusion and somewhat higher body temperature usually suffice when hypothermia is used in intracranial operations.

Lower body temperatures with cardiac arrest and a pump oxygenator to maintain the circulation are being tried but are probably not as important here as in cardiac surgery, since a field dry enough for critically precise repair of the lesion is nearly always obtainable by temporary closure of the carotid and the vertebral arteries in the neck.

A ganglionic blocking agent such as Arfonad to produce hypotension may also be used here, as one does in vascular tumors, to reduce hemorrhage, and such use may be combined with hypothermia.

Logue has presented evidence that aneurysms of the vertebral arterial tree may be treated effectively by proximal ligation of the ipsilateral vertebral artery. However, there is no fall in pressure just distal to such ligation if the other vertebral artery is in the normal range of size. So the objective basis for the therapy of occlusion, namely the pronounced pressure drop seen typically after carotid occlusion, is lacking here.

Arteriovenous Fistulas

Rupture of the intracranial carotid artery in its subclinoid, intracavernous portion permits the blood to pass directly into the cavernous sinus, thereby creating a carotid cavernous fistula. This may occur spontaneously, but usually cephalic trauma is its cause. A striking picture develops within hours to weeks, characterized by pulsating exophthalmos on the side of the lesion with chemosis and redness of the conjunctiva, impaired vision, weakness of the extra-ocular muscles and a loud bruit often heard by the patient himself or even by a person standing near him.

The recommended methods of treatment are: (1) 1-stage closure of the intracranial internal carotid, the ophthalmic and the cervical carotid arteries or (2) the foregoing combined with the introduction of a muscle embolus into the fistulous carotid segment after the intracranial carotid closure, but before the cervical carotid is occluded. The embolus will then be driven into the intracavernous portion of the carotid and seal off the small collateral channels tending to keep the fistula open. Although cervical carotid ligation alone has sufficed to control the symptoms in some patients, it fails so often that the more thorough measures described above seems preferable.

Arteriovenous Malformations

Small or massive remnants of the embryonic vascular networks in the brain may persist and enlarge to form arteriovenous malformations. The 3 commonest manifestations of this disorder are: (1) focal convulsive seizures, (2) spontaneous subarachnoid and/or intracerebral hemorrhage and (3) headaches, often migrainous in type. A bruit occurs in a minority of the patients. The fistulous shunts are rarely large enough to provoke cardiac hypertrophy. A pneumogram may show focal or

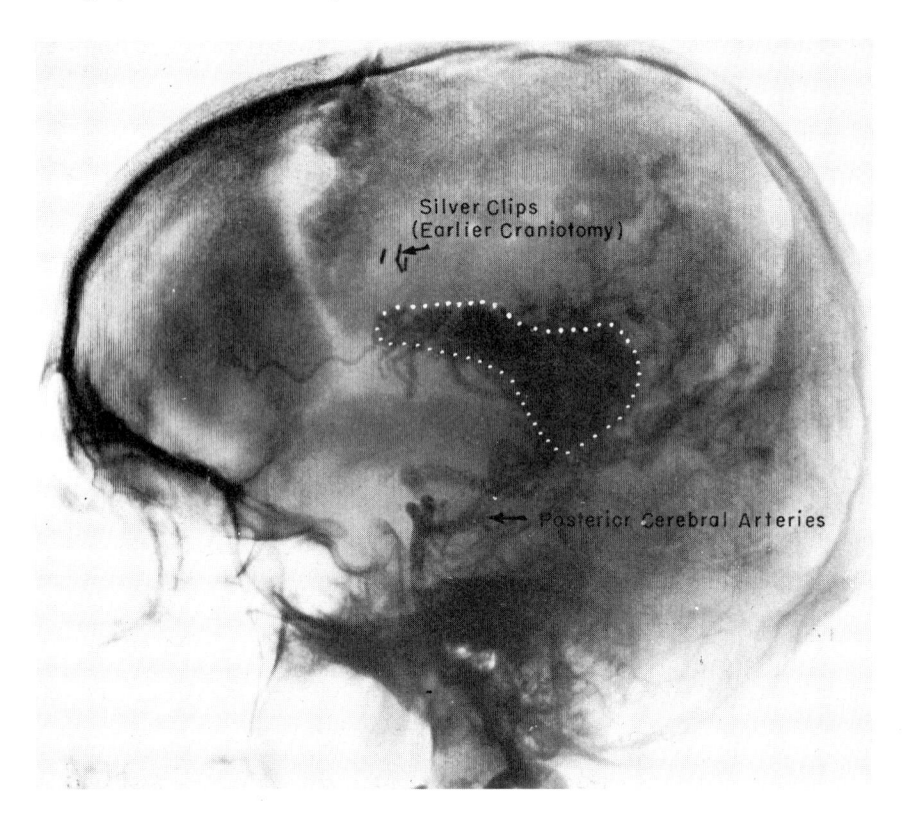

FIG. 54-14. Arteriovenous malformation. Vertebral angiograms. *Case Summary:* 17-year-old male. Bouts of spontaneous subarachnoid hemorrhage from malformation filling from both carotid and both vertebral arteries. In illustrations dotted lines enclose the main mass of lesion below corpus callosum, above midbrain and between thalami. Arrow points to metal clips applied at earlier operation to both anterior cerebral arteries feeding the lesion. Neither this operation nor clipping of right posterior cerebral and posterior communicating arteries stopped the hemorrhages. Under hypothermia at 25° C. the lesion itself was exposed, and the immediate feeding arteries were occluded. To aid this, both carotid and both vertebral arteries were closed for a total of 47 min. over a 2-hr. period; longest single period of closure was 14½ min., the first such deliberate procedure in man. Probable maximal tolerable period of such closure *at normal temperature* is 3 to 5 min. Good postoperative recovery, but death 5 days later from thrombosis of right vertebral artery, propagating from site of temporary occlusions in neck. We now carry out these occlusions so as to minimize local injury.

generalized cerebral atrophy, which perhaps occurs because of significant diversion of the brain's blood directly to the veins. The sovereign aid to diagnosis and planning of treatment is angiography (Fig. 54-14). These lesions usually have so little normal brain between their tangle of vessels that their total extirpation will not increase neurologic deficit, if trauma during control of bleeding can be avoided. The problem of knowing where to seek the feeding arteries is solved by the angiogram, and many of these lesions in the cerebral hemispheres are now removed readily, provided that one divides the feeding arteries *before* the draining veins. If total removal is not feasible, occlusion of as many feeding arteries as possible and evacuation of any intracerebral hematoma may still be rewarding. Luessenhop's tactic of releasing artificial emboli of critical size into the internal carotid circulation is of proven value for the huge lesions with feeding arteries larger than those nour-

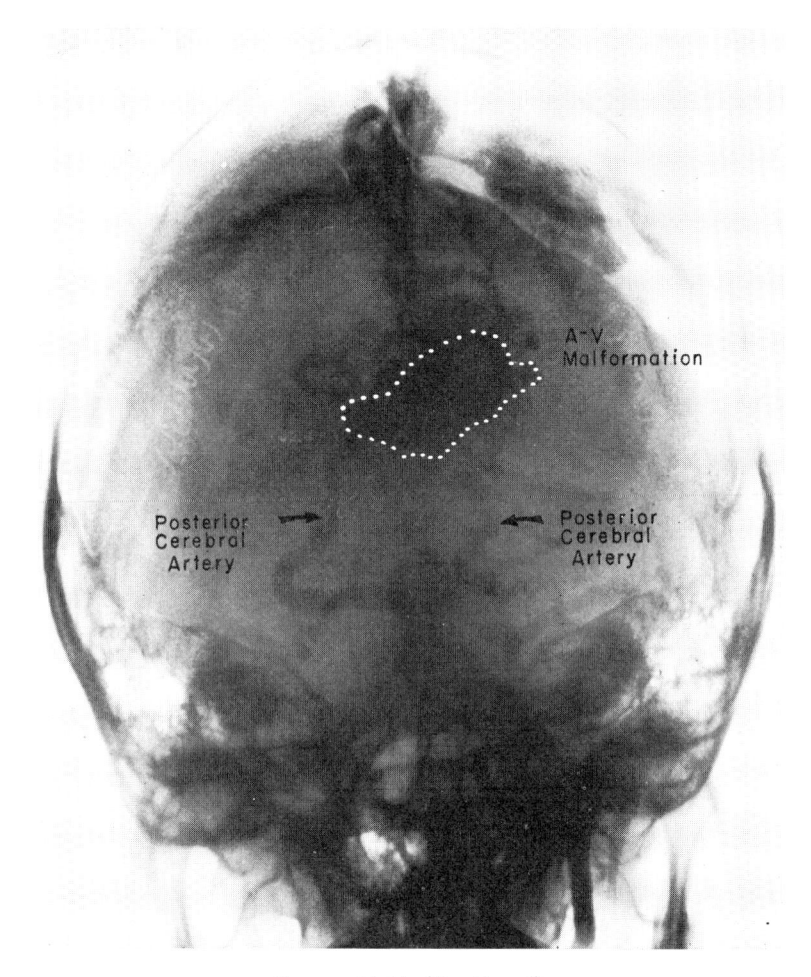

Diseases Affecting the Central Nervous System   1785

FIGURE 54-14. (*Continued*)

ishing the brain proper. The large embolus almost invariably takes the course into the artery feeding the lesion. Hence, such therapy is not a form of internal Russian roulette (as it might seem to be at first glance).

Congenital Malformations

Hydrocephalus. Overproduction of the CSF by a papilloma of the choroid plexus, overwhelming normal absorptive mechanism and producing dilated cerebral ventricles, has been recorded but is an extreme rarity. Some CSF is absorbed throughout the chambers containing it, but the excess must attain the subarachnoid space over the cerebral hemispheres for final absorption. The usual cause of hydrocephalus is a lesion interfering with the essential flow or absorption of that excess. When this occurs in infancy without other major cerebral hypogenesis, the baby usually looks relatively normal at birth. However, within a few months, a frankly hydrocephalic infant with enlarged head, prominent cranial bosses, bulging fontanelles and apathetic expression is readily recognized. When this diagnosis is suspected, in order to confirm it before the stage of excessive pressure atrophy of the brain has been reached, the physician should measure the occipitofrontal circumference of the head several times a week in order to establish that an abnormal rate of increase is present. When the lesion prevents dye injected into the lateral ventricles from reaching a needle in the lumbar spinal canal, one speaks of obstructive hydrocephalus. When the lesion does not prevent such flow of the dye, the hydrocephalus is of the "communicating" type. Although tumors are the commonest cause of an obstruction to the outflow of CSF from the ventricles, congenital stenosis of the aqueduct of Sylvius or at the outflow foramina of Magendie and Luschka in the 4th ventricle may cause dilation of all ventricles rostral to the obstruction and evidence of increased intracranial pressure. The block is by-passed by a shunting tube from lateral ventricle to upper cervical spinal canal rather than cisterna magna, because the latter structure is too tiny in early childhood. In infants under 6 months a ventriculovenous shunt, as described below, has proved to be preferable.

The site of obstruction in congenital communicating hydrocephalus may be at the foramen magnum and be produced by the Arnold-Chiari malformation or may lie in closure of or failure of development of the subarachnoid channels. Myelomeningoceles are nearly always associated with the Arnold-Chiari deformity, which consists of a downward displacement and often a folding of the medulla through the foramen magnum along with crowding of the cerebellar tonsils into this small space. Because of this caudal position of the medulla, CSF may flow from the 4th ventricle directly into the spinal canal and be unable to pass up through the foramen magnum into the cerebral subarachnoid space. Hence hydrocephalus often develops in association with a myelomeningocele, and a decompressive enlargement of the foramen magnum with upper cervical laminectomy may aid in the treatment. However, for the vast majority of children with communicating hydrocephalus, no direct therapy of the lesion is feasible. Then one may attack the problem of excess CSF by decreasing its rate of formation. Electrocoagulation of the choroid plexuses of the lateral ventricles has achieved this with some success, but drainage of the excess CSF into some other area of the body is simpler. Catheters placed with one end in the subarachnoid space and the other in the distal ureter after nephrectomy, or in some part of the peritoneal cavity, the pleural cavity, a fallopian tube or a vein have all been tried. This predominantly mechanical problem probably is solved best by placement in a lateral ventricle of a plastic catheter which leads to a pair of one-way valves lying subcutaneously behind the ear or in the uppermost neck. Caudally, a silicone tube passes into the internal jugular, thence into the innominate vein, the superior vena cava or the uppermost right atrium. The subcutaneous position of crucial portions of the system makes them readily available for checking. The placement of the caudal tip of the shunting tube in a turbulent portion of the circulation, along with occasional digital pressure on the tube between the 2 valves, has solved the problem of occlusion of the lower end of the tube by clot. Since the fluid is taken from the lateral ventricle, the method applies to both communicating and obstructive types of hydrocephalus.

Cranium Bifidum and Encephalocele. Failure of tissues overlying the brain to develop properly usually occurs somewhere along the mid-line from the bridge of the nose back to the nuchal region. The outward herniation of brain at this site may be accompanied by other more serious intracranial anomalies. In only about one third of the patients does surgical repair yield a relatively normal child.

Craniosynostosis. The reverse type of defect occurs in which one or more of the cranial sutures closes prematurely. If the coronal suture is involved, the head is too short and wide; if the sagittal suture is affected, the head is too long and narrow. If all of the sutures are involved the brain bulges up at the fontanelles and down into the orbits. Mental retardation will follow unless the brain is given enough room for growth. The successful treatment consists of removal of 2 strips of bone parallel to and on each side of the closed sagittal suture and of a single strip of bone through the closed coronal or lambdoidal sutures. One then lines the bone edges with strips of a plastic such as polyethylene to prevent bony regrowth and closure, which is a very active process in infants.

Anomalies at the Craniovertebral Junction. A variety of skeletal lesions in this region may produce neurologic malfunction or be accompanied by neurologic malformation. The commonest of the bony disorders has been called *platybasia* or, perhaps better, *basilar impression*. The latter term describes the nature of the lesion in which the anterior part of the cervical spine becomes invaginated or impressed upward into the base of the occiput, encroaching on the foramen magnum from in front. Compression of the ventral aspect of the pons, the medulla and the emergent lower cranial nerves with crowding of the cerebellum occurs. An enormous variety of clinical pictures ensues, depending upon which of these regions bears the brunt of the pressure. Long tracts moving into the cord, local bulbar nuclei, cranial nerves from V to XII, sensory pain fibers to the occiput and the neck, the cerebellum, or pathways for CSF flow may be involved singly or in combination. Symptoms rarely appear before adolescent or adult life, usually progress slowly, perhaps with remissions. An erroneous diagnosis of some intrinsic disease of the nervous system such as syringomyelia or multiple sclerosis is often made. Roentgenograms may reveal: (1) an elevation of the tip of the odontoid process more than 6 mm. above "Chamberlain's line" (drawn on a lateral view of the skull to join the dorsal surface of the hard palate and the dorsal lip of the foramen magnum). Or (2) the films may show an angle of 13° or more between the plane of the hard palate and the plane of the atlas vertebra. Normally, these two planes are nearly parallel. Although such abnormal findings may occur in some asymptomatic people, their presence in company with advancing local neurologic signs suggests that decompressive craniectomy and laminectomy will provide more space for the cramped nervous structures and may permit them to perform properly. Basilar impression may also occur as an acquired disorder in any condition which produces softening of the base of the skull; the commonest such cause is Paget's disease.

Scars and Adhesions

The residual scar in the cerebrum following trauma, infection, vascular lesions or operation may give rise to convulsive seizures which in turn may provoke some mental deterioration. If the seizures are not controlled by nontoxic doses of anticonvulsant agents, operative removal of the abnormal tissue and of the nearby abnormally discharging cerebral cortex is advisable. Recognition that small scars and other lesions in the temporal lobe are a frequent cause of paroxysmal behavior disorders or seizures has come recently. Ischemic or other damage to the medial aspect of the temporal lobe at birth appears to occur and to cause seizures at a much later date. The seizures of temporal lobe origin, the automatisms or "psychomotor" seizures, have been especially refractory to medication and are among the commonest to require surgical treatment. Evidence is accumulating that those subject to dangerous bouts of rage may have such focal temporal lesions even in the absence of frank psychomotor seizures.

Adhesions in the subarachnoid space following upon meningitis or severe subarachnoid hemorrhages may interfere with the absorption of CSF. The communicating hydrocephalus which ensues is to be treated as indicated in the discussion of the congenital form of this disorder.

Pseudotumor Cerebri
(Benign Intracranial Hypertension)

A benign, self-limited disorder occurs in which increased intracranial pressure with the appropriate symptoms and signs thereof is caused by a disturbance in the input-output balance of CSF with normal constituents. Normal ventricles and no space-taking mass are seen in intracranial air studies. The disease may come on in patients with extensive thrombosis or occlusion of (1) cerebral veins, (2) a dural venous sinus, or (3) cervical veins. The probable mechanism of the rise in CSF pressure in this group seems to be impaired absorption of CSF. However, in most of the patients, who are often obese women, aged 20 to 40, there is no evidence of venous obstruction, and the mechanism is obscure. Typically the patient seems unusually well for the degree of papilledema she has. The disorder usually subsides within a few weeks or months with repeated drainage of CSF and/or repeated use of cerebral dehydrating agents (see under cerebral edema). But visual deficit may worsen rapidly and require prompt subtemporal decompression or ventriculovenous shunt.

Granulomatous and Parasitic Cysts

In the United States, tuberculomas and syphilitic gummas are now rarely seen in the brain because of the effectiveness with which these infections are controlled by prophylactic measures and at their primary sites. Parasitic invasions by echinococcus and cysticercus are also rare in the United States. One sees them most often in patients who come from other quarters of the world where the dog is infested with the echinococcus tapeworm or, in cysticercosis, where food is contaminated with ova in the excreta of carriers of the tapeworm *Taenia solium*. The first three types of lesions present clinically and are treated surgically as one would a neoplasm, with special care to avoid contamination of the brain by the infection or the cystic fluid. Cysticerci in the brain usually cause numerous small calcified spheres which may provoke epilepsy treatable by anticonvulsants. The cysts may also block the CSF flow, requiring either a surgical removal in the case of the solitary cysts or an appropriate type of shunt when the cysts are racemose or multilocular and hence dangerous to remove.

Palliative Intracranial Surgery

When an intracranial mass is completely or partially irremovable, additional useful life for the patient may be obtained by extensive removal of cranial vault—a "decompression" which encourages the neoplasm to grow outward away from the brain. The tumor or its remnants are often deep and block outflow of CSF from the ventricular system. The many symptoms caused by the back pressure from this CSF can be relieved by short-circuiting the fluid by the operation of Torkildsen. This is a ventriculocisternostomy in which a catheter is placed to connect one or both lateral ventricles with the subarachnoid space at the cisterna magna just below the cerebellum. If the mass tends to block the upward flow of CSF at the tentorial notch or diffusely invades the cerebral subarachnoid spaces preventing its absorption, then the shunt must be directly from the lateral ventricle to a point outside the head, preferably into the right common facial vein and, thence, virtually straight down via internal jugular and innominate veins to the junction of superior vena cava and right atrium. This same type of operation is required when adhesions form in the cerebral subarachnoid spaces after meningitis or subarachnoid hemorrhage. The fluid in dangerously placed cystic tumors may be aspirated and partially replaced with a fluid containing a β-emitting isotope in order to retard growth and reaccumulation of cystic fluid. Such isotopic or roentgen or proton beam may be directed at an inoperable tumor or at the remnants of one partially removed surgically. Tumors in and near the sella turcica are especially favorable targets for one of the above 3 forms of radiation or for drainage of their cystic content continuously into the sphenoid sinus and the nasopharynx by removal of the anterior bony wall and the floor of the sella and the contiguous tumor wall.

Normal Pressure Hydrocephalus

It was recently recognized that impaired flow or absorption of CSF can occur without a chronic rise in intracranial pressure above the accepted upper limit of normal of 190 to 200 mm. of CSF, and with no previous history of infection or hemorrhage. The principal symptoms—a decline in mentation and in gait, occurring in an older adult and presenting as a presenile dementia—prove to be associated with dilated ventricles. Such dilatation is due to a block, which prevents the flow of CSF in the normal direction anywhere along its intraventricular or extracerebral course. The commonest site is in the cerebral sulci, as shown by their failure to fill with air at encephalography or with ^{131}I serum albumin. Treatment by ventriculo-caval shunt is remarkably successful.

Supportive Aspects of Treatment After Intracranial Injuries, Hemorrhages or Operations

The airway requires special attention in the unconscious patient with a lesion in the brain who tends to have excessive secretions in the respiratory tract and inadequate expulsion thereof by coughing. Careful positioning *on the side* with the head low encourages postural drainage. But if cephalic venous congestion or possible intracranial bleeding are problems, these dictate elevation of the head. The lateral position is still needed to keep the tongue from falling back and obstructing the oral pharynx. A plastic oral airway may be required. The use of oxygen by nasal catheter may permit adequate exchange in the lungs. But if tracheobronchial secretions are profuse, neither drugs nor oral suction will suffice, and a tracheotomy should be done promptly. Gentle sterile suctioning via the tracheotomy tube, not exceeding a vacuum of 4 lb./sq. in., along with input of a proper mixture of humidified air or oxygen, may play a major role in the patient's recovery. Swelling of the brain is increased by even mild hypoxia, so that every effort to avoid this is rewarding. Suction with a greater vacuum, or even a bronchoscopy, may become mandatory to remove tenacious bronchial plugs of mucus.

Hyperthermia as a consequence of impaired central regulation of temperature, formerly a major threat to patients with severe cerebral lesions, is now avoided by prompt administration of aspirin, alcohol sponging or the exposure of the unclothed patient to a cool atmosphere, such as that conveniently provided by a refrigerated oxygen tent. The more drastic measures used to produce deep hypothermia should be invoked without delay if necessary. External cooling by plastic bags filled with ice cubes should be used if special cooling units are not available. Chlorpromazine or meperidine (Demerol) may be required to prevent shivering as well as to make the intense cold tolerable to the patient.

Convulsive seizures increase cerebral edema or bleeding; one seeks to prevent their initial appearance by prophylactic use of diphenylhydantoin (Dilantin) 100 mg., or phenobarbital, 100 mg., 3 or 4 times per day —intramuscularly in the unconscious patient. If seizures do occur, one must use parenteral anticonvulsants intensively, changing to another drug promptly if the first is ineffective. One need not hesitate to use intravenous Pentothal Sodium or Valium.

Restlessness. Moderate restlessness to wild thrashing about may be a problem, especially in young men. Barbiturates may make the patient even less controllable; morphine and related alkaloids are contraindicated; paraldehyde is perhaps the most satisfactory sedative and Demerol the best analgesic agent in conjunction with such tranquilizers as chlorpromazine. Straining at stool may be dangerous, and easy bowel movements must be assured by cathartics or enemas.

Cerebral edema is the unsolved problem in many comatose patients. We know that overhydration, especially if NaCl is given, will worsen this and kill them, but excessive dehydration in an effort to reduce edema may cause elevated levels of serum electrolytes, producing a lethargy and coma clinically indistinguishable from that associated with cerebral edema. It is standard practice to give a daily intake to adults of 1,500 ml. of fluid for the first several days with frequent measurements of hemoglobin, hematocrit and urinary output to guide daily intake. If coma continues beyond 2 or 3 days, fluids, drugs and high caloric mixtures should be given via a long tube extending from the nose to the stomach. If the edema or injury to the brain is not too severe, it is possible differentially to abstract water from the brain by injecting into the blood substances which enter rapidly nearly all extracellular areas but that of the brain. The hyperosmolarity of the blood serum vis-à-vis brain then results in a net transfer of water from brain to blood. Urea, 30 per cent, in doses of 1 Gm. per Kg. of body weight, or mannitol, 25 per cent, 2 Gm. per Kg., have replaced all previous agents used for this purpose. They must be excreted by the kidney. The more recently introduced glycerol may be given either orally (50%, 2 Gm. per Kg.) or intravenously (30%, 1 Gm. per Kg.) and is at least partially metabolized as a food.

Another type of agent for control of cerebral edema is the group of high potency cortisonelike synthetic compounds exemplified by dexamethasone and methylprednisolone. They diminish the entry of water into traumatized brain when given at the massive dose rate of, e.g., 4 mg. of dexamethasone every 6 hours; this dose should be tapered down rapidly after a few days. The complications of such therapy include a heightened tendency to wound and other infection, poor wound healing, psychotic manifestations, gastrointestinal bleeding and masking of intracranial bleeding, but used with proper vigilance these drugs are valuable both prophylactically and therapeutically against cerebral edema.

When the ventricles are large, increased intracranial pressure is relieved effectively by tapping these cavities, and if necessary by maintaining continuous catheter drainage to a sterile reservoir at a level that will maintain roughly normal pressure.

Metabolic disturbances of varying types, all potentially leading to coma, may occur. The intake and the urinary excretion both of water and of sodium and the metabolism of protein and carbohydrate are controlled precisely by a group of mechanisms including osmolar and volume receptors situated partially within the central cerebral and pituitary area. Injury to or near these may precipitate an acute problem requiring urgent determination and correction of the imbalance. In one category hypernatremia and hyperchloremia are seen and occur in 3 primary groups of disorder.

1. Patients with normal osmolar and volume receptors but often stuporous from their brain lesion. Such patients may have abnormally high water requirements because of: (1) hyperthermia with excessive evaporation from the skin, (2) hyperpnea with increased water loss from the lungs, (3) profuse sweating and (4) large amounts of nonprotein nitrogen. For this load of NPN to be excreted by the kidney a substantial loss of water is also necessary. Such load may arise by virtue of: (1) inadequate food intake so that endogenous protein catabolism makes up the deficit, (2) the increased protein breakdown related by as yet obscure mechanisms to the cerebral lesion, (3) major gastrointestinal bleeding due to a lesion near the cerebral midline with reabsorption into the blood stream of the nitrogenous breakdown products of the hemorrhage, or (4) too high a protein content of nasogastric tube feedings. Less commonly, a hyperglycemia may add to the obligatory renal loss of water. The renal tubules diminish the water loss by maximally reabsorbing the sodium and chloride, permitting extreme rises of these in the blood in preference to further loss of water. If the increased aldosterone secretion promoting this retention has been having its usual effect of increasing renal loss of potassium, hypokalemia may ensue. However, in situations otherwise similar hyperkalemia occurs and one must measure serum potassium to see what is happening. A water deficit may also arise from impairment of the thirst mechanism or from physical inability to drink. The hypernatremic tendency as part of the normal metabolic response to surgery may be exacerbated by an excess of exogenous or endogenous aldosterone. All of these patients excrete urine of normal or high specific gravity but with very low sodium and chloride content.

2. Patients with defects in the osmolar and/or volume receptors, on the other hand, will not show low urinary excretion of sodium and chloride. Minor defects of water balance remain uncompensated; hypernatremia and hyperchloremia develop as well, and greater vigilance is required to prevent major imbalances.

In both of these groups of patients, peritoneal dialysis may be the fastest, safest way to correct an extreme hyperosmolar state. If sodium chloride and NPN must be cleared, one instills into the peritoneal cavity of an adult 2 liters of isotonic glucose, and re-collects it by gravity drainage after 1 hour, continuing this process if necessary for 6 to 12 hours. If azotemia is the main threat, normal concentrations of serum electrolytes can be in the dialyzing fluid; this fluid should of course contain no potassium if hyperkalemia is present. If an artificial kidney is available, its use to achieve extracorporeal hemodialysis is ideal. In less critical states one may energetically rehydrate with 4,000 or more ml. of water per day, via nasogastric tube to avoid overshoot to cerebral edema, giving enough carbohydrate and emulsified fat down the tube to minimize endogenous protein catabolism, and potassium in amounts guided by its plasma levels.

3. Patients with reduced antidiuretic hormone, ADH, excrete large volumes of urine of low specific gravity and tend to go into a hypovolemic as well as a hyperosmolar state. These patients with severe diabetes insipidus and 5 or more liters of urine per day should have intake and output recorded hourly; intake per hour must keep pace with output to avoid hypovolemic shock. This, plus cautious administration of pitressin tannate in oil replacing the ADH deficit, is the proper regimen. One must avoid a cumulative action of pitressin throwing the patient over into water intoxication.

In the other category are those with hyponatremia and hypochloremia, the *"cerebral salt waters"* who excrete increased amounts of sodium and chloride in the urine. When the serum sodium drops to levels of 100 to 120 mEq./L., the clinical picture of nausea, vomiting, mental confusion or delirium, worsening of focal cerebral signs already present, lethargy and coma is similar to that seen with hyperosmolarity. The chemical laboratory is crucial to the differential diagnosis. Normally ADH is no longer released when serum tonicity drops below 280 milliosmols per Kg. of water. More water is then excreted to correct the dilution of body water. But in one group of "cerebral salt waters" ADH secretion continues despite hemodilution. This further increases the volume of blood and extracellular fluid, and a corrective increased glomerular filtration rate and decreased aldosterone secretion ensue, both of which increase renal loss of sodium. In this disorder correction simply requires limitation of fluid intake, whereupon blood volume and salt excretion return to normal. In a second group of "cerebral salt wasters" there is a defect in the reabsorption of salt by the proximal convoluted tubule. In addition to rehydration, these patients must have a constant daily supplement of salt to replace the continuing abnormal losses.

Blood bicarbonate and glucose must be checked because even a latent or mild diabetic may slip into acidosis under the stress of serious cerebral disease. Moreover, parasellar disorders with or without diabetes may provoke a hypoglycemic coma. The blood volume, also subject to cerebral regulation, must be watched, because the patient may slip into hypovolemic shock in the absence of occult bleeding.

We are only at the threshold of our efforts to understand how to help the injured brain regulate metabolism of the body as a whole and of the local lesion—a challenging task, since we know that much of the damage in edematous brain is reversible.

Cranioplasty to repair major skull defects is a much later step in the management of these patients. Plates utilizing tantalum or acrylic resins or the patient's own ribs or ilium are the favored materials.

LESIONS WITH SURGICAL IMPLICATIONS, INTRASPINAL

Symptoms and Signs

Protrusions of intervertebral disks, neoplasms, abscesses, traumatic disorders, vascular malformations and congenital malformations are the main lesions encountered. Although CSF circulates around the spinal cord, neither increased pressure in nor block to the outflow of this fluid is a significant cause of disturbed function of the cord. So the symptoms arise from local effects of the lesion producing (1) *stimulation* or (2) *diminution* of function.

Stimulation of Function. The spectacular variety of responses of the brain upon irritation is absent in the cord. Pain and paresthesias, muscle spasm and excessive autonomic discharge are the main clinical manifestations of excessive neural activity seen with disease in the spinal canal.

PAIN OR PARESTHESIAS. Three different types of pain or paresthesias occur: (1) Local pain in the back at the level of the lesion comes from stimuli to small neighboring nerves and nerve endings. (2) Segmental pain or paresthesia lies in the distribution of one or more posterior nerve roots affected by the lesion. This is referred along a limb when the affected roots enter the brachial or lumbosacral plexuses, and often in a girdle fashion in the case of the thoracic roots. But at other times when pain arising from the thoracic posterior roots is referred to various local areas in the torso, one tends to think first of some commoner disease affecting that thoracic or abdominal viscus nearest the site of reference of pain. (3) Pain is also produced by irritation of the specific pain pathways in the cord itself. Because of the compactness of this bundle of fibers, a small lesion on one side may cause pain referred over wide areas of the opposite side.

The following features are characteristic of pain of intraspinal origin: (1) exacerbation upon maneuvers which raise CSF pressure, such as coughing, sneezing or straining. Such activities also raise pressure within the chest or the abdomen, but if one compresses both internal jugular veins, the subsequent rise in pressure will be confined to the head and the spinal canal. If this provokes the patient's pain in torso or limbs, the hyperirritable focus almost certainly lies in the spinal canal. (2) Worsening during motions of the spine, or relieved only in certain positions of the spine or the legs. (3) Tendency to waken the patient out of sleep. Tonic muscular activity splinting the diseased area probably is decreased in sleep, and when the patient then turns, his nerves are more likely to be pinched.

Spasms of localized muscle groups occur—ordinary cramps—and intraspinal lesions are a cause to be thought of, especially if the cramps are frequent and waken the patient from sleep. Major lesions of the cord, causing severe weakness or paralysis of one or both legs, may be accompanied by bursts of painful contraction of the muscles in the affected limb, throwing it into involuntary flexion at all joints. Extensor spasms in this situation may also be seen.

Hyperactivity of autonomic fibers is seen most often in the severe chronic lesions of the cord producing muscle spasm. The patient may have episodes of high blood pressure or of excessive sweating, with chilliness and faintness spontaneously or on other autonomic activity such as urinating or defecating. Priapism may occur in acute high lesions of the cord.

Diminution of Function. Somatic motor, sensory and autonomic deficits occur, and, as in the case of intracranial lesions, when their evolution is rapid, operations for a removable cause must be carried out as an emergency measure if they are to have their best chance of success.

Lesions affecting the *lower motor neuron*, i.e., anterior horn cells or anterior rootlets, produce a weakness that is associated with (1) atrophy, (2) flaccidity, (3) diminished or absent tendon jerks, (4) normal abdominal and cremasteric reflexes and (5) no sign of Babinski. When the lesion is in the cauda equina, the motor involvement is of this type. Inasmuch as the lower end of the spinal cord lies at the first lumbar vertebra when adult stature is attained, lumbar and sacral lesions usually involve only the rootlets of the cauda equina. Visible twitching of small or larger segments of muscle, called fasciculation, occurs spontaneously or may be brought out by tapping the weak muscle when the anterior horn cell is deteriorating. In contrast, the weakness produced by involvement of the *upper motor neuron* within the white matter of the cord proper is associated with (1) little or no atrophy, (2) increased resistance to passive movement, (3) increased tendon jerks, (4) absent abdominal and cremasteric reflexes and (5) positive Babinski and Hoffmann signs.

Somatic sensory loss includes impairment of ipsilateral proprioceptive and vibratory sense when a posterior white column is affected, and of contralateral pain and temperature sense when an anterolateral white column is involved. For complete loss of touch to be present, both anterior and posterior white matter must be nonfunctional.

Insignia of autonomic hypofunction are sudomotor and vasoconstrictor inactivity with hot, dry limbs and, if the lesion is in the cervical or upper thoracic cord, vascular hypotension. These changes are pronounced in the early stage of spinal injury but tend to fade out in the later stages when, as noted above, autonomic hyperactivity may appear. A lesion of these pathways in the cord down to the T1 level also produces an ipsilateral Horner's sign. One sees bladder dysfunction (1) with an atonic detrusor and urinary retention or (2) with better detrusor activity but impaired synergism between this and the sphincters giving irregular retention and overflow incontinence. Constipation or obstipation and in males impotence or sterility also occur.

Accessory Diagnostic Measures

Spinal Puncture. Following measurement of the resting initial pressure, one checks the patency of the spinal CSF pathway whenever a spinal (not an intracranial) lesion is suspected. A high-grade block will be shown by the Queckenstedt test of bilateral jugular compression, carried out digitally or by means of a blood pressure cuff around the neck inflated to 30 mm. Hg. The increased intracranial pressure should produce a rise in the pressure at the lumbar needle. An absent or a delayed rise or a delayed fall on release indicates an almost complete block in the CSF sleeve around the cord or in the cauda equina above the needle. The CSF below the block is often yellow and contains an elevated total protein.

Plain Roentgenography of Spine. A narrowing of the interspace between the vertebral bodies (Fig. 54-15 A), often with a bony spur formation at the margins of the bodies (see Fig. 54-20 A), indicates degeneration and/or extrusion of the intervertebral disk, the commonest lesion in the spinal canal. Destruction of bone, proliferation of bone or calcification occurs in a variety of tumors. Sites vulnerable to pressure are the vertebral pedicles, which may show a widening of the interpediculate distance at one or more vertebrate or an erosion of their medial surfaces. Examination of the lateral film may show a similar widening of the canal by erosion of the lamina and the vertebral body. The foramina of emergence of the spinal nerves revealed in oblique views may show enlargement by tumor or constriction by arthritic spur or by collapse of disk.

Myelography. Intrathecal introduction of

Fig. 54-15. Ruptured intervertebral disk. (A, *Left*) Plain film, lumbosacral junction. Arrow indicates the abnormally narrow interspace at L5-S1 level associated with massive posterior protrusion of the disk. (B, *Right*) Myelogram (*Upper arrow*) Lumbar puncture needle in situ during fluoroscopy. (*Lower arrow*) Filling defect caused by medial part of huge extruded fragment.

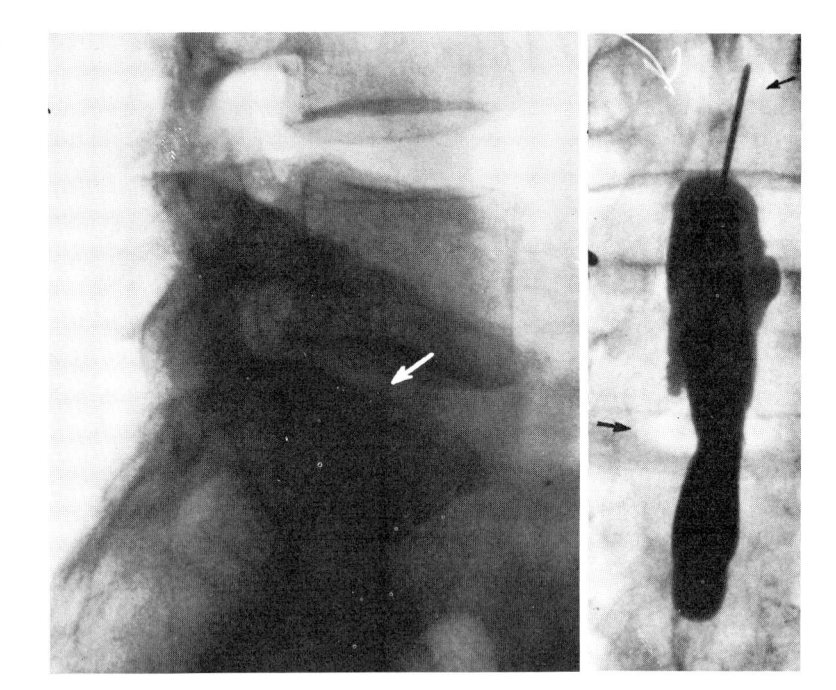

3 to 12 ml. of a radiopaque oil, Pantopaque, followed by fluoroscopy and spot films of the spinal canal, enables one to confirm the clinical suspicion of a significant space-taking intraspinal lesion in the great majority of instances, with the exception of ruptured disks placed far laterally. Not only the site but also the type of the lesion often can be foretold by the character of the filling defects. The fact that one can aspirate the opaque oil back out of the spinal canal makes the procedure almost innocuous. Cisternal puncture and introduction of contrast medium may be used to demonstrate the upper level of a complete block in the spinal canal.

Diskography. Direct injection of the intervertebral disk itself with an absorbable radiopaque agent such as Diodrast is a more recent innovation. Normally in the lumbar region the fluid stays within the disk inside its confining annulus fibrosus. If the annulus is ruptured, roentgenograms will show the site of the tear. The lowest 3 lumbar disks are those most commonly studied. In the cervical region even such small amounts of the contrast fluid as 0.2 ml. extravasate beyond the disk margin in normal individuals so that the procedure has less diagnostic value here (Fig. 54-16). However, if injection of a cervical disk reproduces the patient's clinical pain, the inference is strong that he has an abnormal protrusion at this level.

Electromyography. The action potentials in muscles give objective evidence of the functional state of the *lower motor neurons:* (1) for normality in the form of normal motor-unit

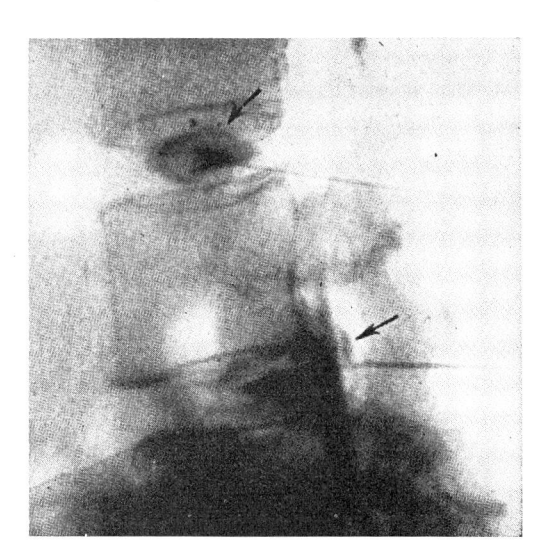

Fig. 54-16. Ruptured intervertebral disk. Diskogram. (*Upper arrow*) Ellipsoidal shadow of Diodrast in normal nucleus pulposus at lumbar 3-4 interspace. (*Lower arrow*) Diodrast shadow in ventral aspect of spinal canal; flow thence through hole in posterior annulus after injection into lumbar 4-5 disk.

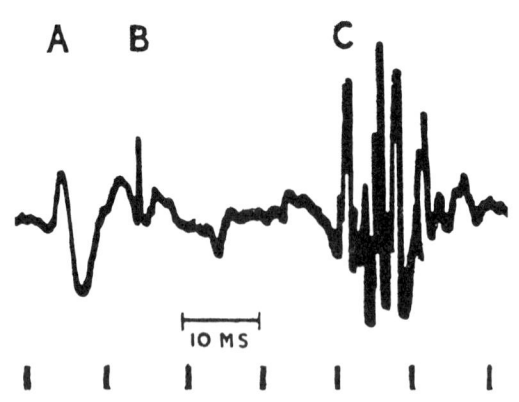

FIG. 54-17. Electromyographic recording from biceps muscle (partial denervation with recovery). (A) Normal motor unit potential. (B) Fibrillation potential. (C) Polyphasic motor unit potential (regeneration). (Richardson, A. T.: Proc. Roy. Soc. Med. 44:992-994)

action potentials (Fig. 54-17 A), (2) for neuronal *de*generation with excitable tissue present in the form of fibrillation potentials (Fig. 54-17 B), and (3) one of the earliest signs of neuronal *re*generation in the form of spike and polyphasic motor-unit potentials (Fig. 54-17 C). Thorough exploration by needle electrodes is required to find the fibrillation potentials in a slightly denervated muscle.

Protrusion of Intervertebral Disks

Most of these lesions occur at one or both of the lowest 2 intervertebral spaces in the spinal column—below the 4th or the 5th lumbar vertebra. Protrusions below lumbar 3, or below the 5th, the 6th or the 7th cervical vertebrae are the next most likely to appear. The syndromes earlier called sciatic and brachial neuritis are now known to have as their commonest cause a posterior protrusion of the intervertebral fibrocartilage into the lateral part of the spinal canal so as to press on the emergent nerve root (Fig. 54-18). Minor or major strain or injury may play a causative role but is often absent from the history.

When one or more lumbar disks are involved, attacks of low back pain with or without relation to acute or chronic strain usually usher in the syndrome. Often bed rest, a tight corset or a back brace relieve the symptoms promptly. In later attacks the pain may start in or spread to the buttock, the posterior thigh and the calf or the foot. Paresthesias and objective hypalgesia or hypesthesia in the anterolateral leg, the medial foot and the great toe, along with a diminished or normal ankle jerk, suggest that the protrusion is at the lumbar 4-5 space, whereas such sensory findings in the posterolateral leg, the lateral foot and the small toes, along with a diminished or absent ankle jerk, point to a protrusion at the L5-S1 level (Fig. 54-15 B). Careful examination may reveal weakness of the dorsiflexors of the toes and of the peronei everting the foot in lesions at either of the 2 lowest disks. Sensory findings in the anterior thigh and the medial leg and a diminished knee jerk may occur in the much less common lesions at L3-4. In lesions at the lower 2 levels, sciatic pain is provoked upon stretching that nerve by straight leg raising from the supine position; the pain is often referred only to the side of protrusion, whichever leg is raised. In lesions at lumbar disks above L4-5, pain in the anterior thigh may be started upon stretching the femoral nerve by extension of the thigh at the hip. Tenderness over or to one side of the spinous processes at the level of the lesion and decreased mobility of the lumbar spine with loss of the lordosis in this region are typical findings.

In the cervical region, an extruding disk causes pain in the back of the neck, radiating into the lateral aspect of an upper limb. Either sudden movements of head and neck or maintenance of a fixed position of these parts may

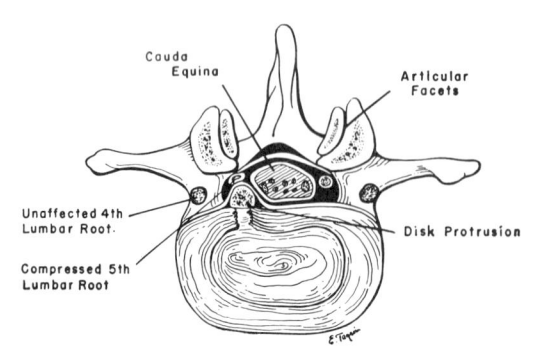

FIG. 54-18. Anatomic relations in protruded intervertebral disk. Superior view of 5th lumbar vertebra. Lesion at lumbar 4-5 interspace. Note that it usually compresses the root emerging one vertebra lower, rather than the one at the same interspace.

worsen the pain. In the hand and the fingers, numbness and paresthesia occur more often than actual pain. Over 95 per cent of the lesions occur at the C5-6 or C6-7 levels. Pressure on the 6th cervical root as it emerges between the 5th and the 6th cervical vertebrae is likely to cause these sensations in the thumb and the 1st metacarpal area, whereas pressure on the 7th cervical root tends to cause the reference of abnormal sensation mainly to the index and the middle fingers and, to a lesser degree, to the thumb. Objective sensory changes are usually slight, but demonstrable weakness, atrophy or fasciculations of the biceps or the triceps and decrease in the corresponding tendon reflex occur, respectively, with 6th or 7th root compression (Fig. 54-19). Pressure at the level of the lesion in the back of the neck and just to the painful side of the midline may produce local tenderness and radicular pain or paresthesias. The same response may be evoked by the *foraminal compression test*, which consists of tilting the head and the neck to the painful side and pounding the top of the head. Tilting head and neck to the side opposite the lesion may give relief.

Multiple disk protrusions, especially in the lumbar region, occur in perhaps 5 to 10 per cent of the patients. Myelography is especially valuable in the dual diagnosis.

Conservative management by bed rest on a firm mattress or with boards beneath the mattress may stop the pain. Appropriate traction may also be used. The wearing of a back or neck brace, depending on the site of the lesion, may permit resumption of full activity. When this is not successful, and particularly when significant weakness is present, surgical removal of the offending disk is advisable. In the lumbar region, one takes away most of the disk inside the lateral and ventral margins of the annulus fibrosus in order to avoid a later recurrent protrusion; in the cervical region, excision of the tissue between the vertebral bodies is less necessary. In the presence of a frank posterior protrusion or rupture, the yield of such surgery is a grateful patient after 80 to 95 per cent of the procedures, which have become by far the commonest of neurosurgery. However, the proliferation of surgeons in this country interested in performing this operation has exceeded the supply of patients requiring such treatment—to the detriment both of the patients and the profession. In certain patients a "fusion" or insertion of bone grafts between the lumbar vertebral bodies or behind the laminae may be required to strengthen the spine, especially if a spondylolisthesis is also present or the patient must earn his living by heavy manual labor. Late postoperative studies reveal good results in so many of the patients who have had simple disk removal that most surgeons now rarely advocate fusion as part of the primary operation, reserving it for a secondary procedure if necessary.

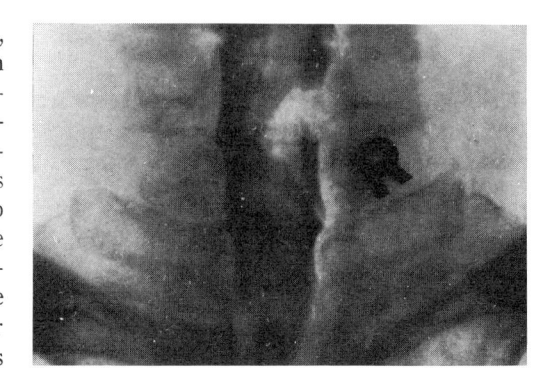

FIG. 54-19. Ruptured intervertebral disk. Cervical myelogram. Protrusion of intervertebral disk at C 6-7 interspace, right side.

In the neck, the protruding disk may lie more medially as well and press against the spinal cord, giving far more serious long tract symptoms and signs resembling those of cord tumors. A similar syndrome may result from multiple osteoarthritic bars at the level of several cervical disks, a cervical spondylosis, which typically yields the picture of slow degeneration of the upper motor neurons with little or no sensory loss. This is often mistaken for degenerative disease such as amyotrophic lateral sclerosis. A decompressive laminectomy and division of the dentate ligaments which anchor the cord to the inner surface of the dura may suffice to control the symptoms, or the more hazardous curetting away of the bars from ventral to the cord may be necessary. In some patients, centrally placed bars may combine with lateral protrusions to produce weak, stiff legs along with pain and paresthesias in one or both arms (Fig. 54-20 A, B, and C). The anterior approach to the cervical spine for

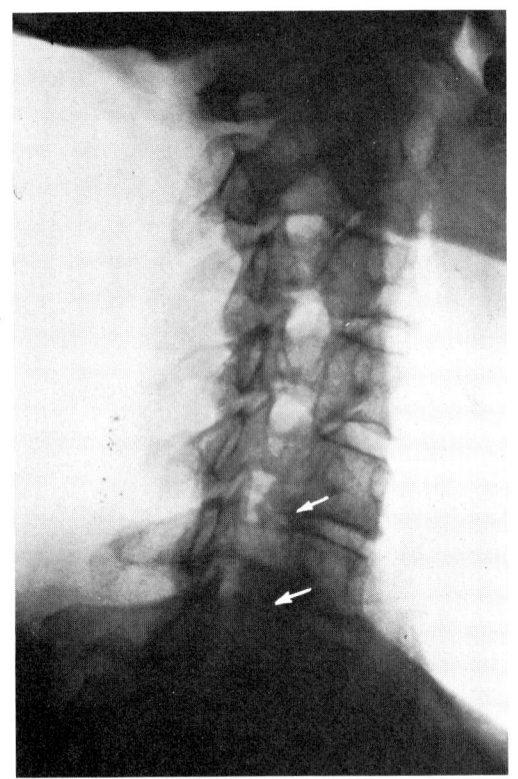

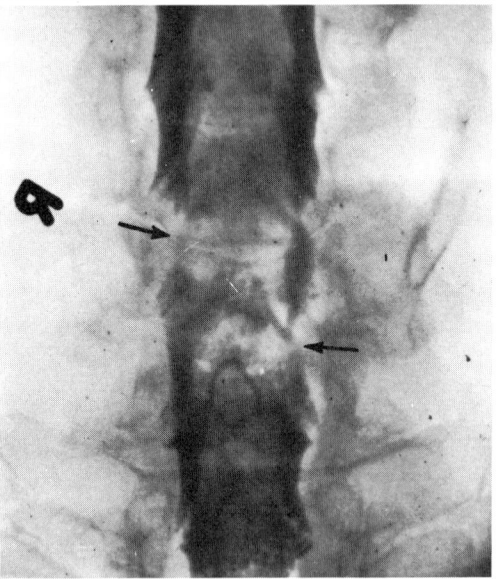

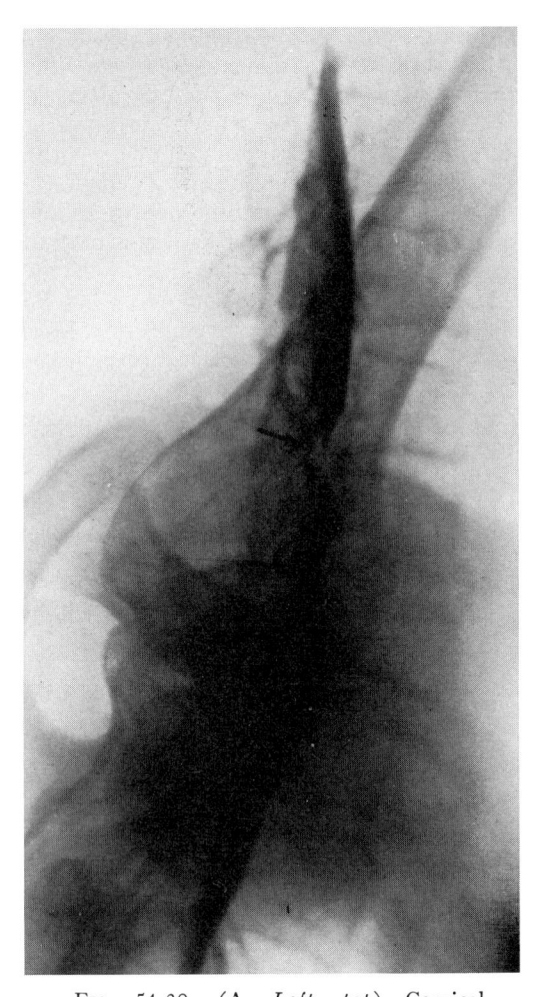

FIG. 54-20. (A, *Left, top*) Cervical spondylosis. Lateral roentgenogram, cervical spine. Arrows point to enostoses into ventral aspect of spinal canal at narrowed interspaces C 5-6 and C 6-7. (B, *Left, bottom*) Cervical myelogram, sagittal view. Arrows point to filling defects in midline and to right at C 5-6, in midline and to left at C 6-7. (C, *Right*) Cervical myelogram, lateral view. Patient's arm alongside head. Arrows point to transverse bars encroaching on spinal canal at C 5-6 and C 6-7, confirming impression from plain films. Patient: 67-year-old male with severe pain in left arm and forearm; paresthesias in left index finger; moderately weak, stiff legs.

removal of a posteriorly protruding disk or a spondylotic bar is steadily gaining favor consequent to development of the necessary instruments and technic by Cloward. The rare thoracic disk protrusions usually are not diagnosed until the cord is compressed.

Neoplasms

New growths in the spinal canal may arise primarily from any of the neural or mesodermal tissues in the neighborhood or may present secondarily after origin elsewhere. The metastatic or multiple tumors are almost always extradural, and, as would be expected, the symptoms they provoke progress rapidly. Despite their poor eventual prognosis, useful palliation is often achieved by prompt removal of laminae and the readily excisable tumor. The disconcerting speed with which a slight weakness becomes a paralysis means that many of these patients, including those with curable maladies, often must receive emergency operations if they are not to end their days with paralyzed legs, bowels and bladder. Of the remaining intradural tumors, about two thirds are happily benign and lie outside the cord, i.e., are extramedullary. The overwhelming majority grow either from a nerve rootlet as neurofibromas or from the meninges as meningiomas. Even when their slow compression has greatly deformed the cord before they are completely removed, gradual full recovery is still a probability. Intramedullary tumors are at times susceptible of total removal if careful microdissection reveals a cleavage plane between tumor and surrounding cord. They are often cystic and slow growing; drainage of the cyst or a longitudinal incision in the cord over the tumor permitting it to extrude or grow outside the cord may purchase protracted relief of symptoms. The same is true of syringomyelia a cystic disease in the spinal cord.

In children the commonest cord tumors are those arising from congenital rests and range in histologic complexity from dermoids to teratomas. Congenital bony malformations or extensive erosions often accompany them. Although they may be so attached to the cord that only subtotal removal is feasible, again a prolonged satisfactory result may be obtained. In general, in childhood the difficulty in eliciting symptoms and signs of intraspinal disease makes advisable a prompt resort to lumbar puncture as well as plain and myelographic roentgenograms of the whole spine whenever a space-taking mass is faintly suspected. In the past, many children incubated their spinal tumors to massive proportions while being treated for their "infantile paralysis." Hopefully, with the virtual disappearance of this disorder, physicians will think sooner of a cord tumor.

Abscesses

Infection in the spinal canal is usually secondary to a source elsewhere in the body and is usually in the epidural space, a locus favorable for drainage. Exceedingly prompt institution of such drainage via extensive laminectomy is vital to success, and any patient with infection elsewhere who develops severe pain plus local tenderness and rigidity in the back should be operated on at the slightest confirmatory sign on neurologic examination, lumbar puncture or myelography. A flaccid paraplegia may develop in less than 24 hours and once present will shortly prove to be irreversible.

Traumatic Disorders

Injuries to the spine and the cord occur mainly as a result of falls, vehicular accidents and dives in shallow water. The cord lesion varies from a completely and often promptly reversible concussion all the way to a total transection. A fracture or a fracture-dislocation may take place, at times with spontaneous return of the cervical vertebrae to normal position after delivery of a blow to the cord. When weakness or sensory loss abruptly follows an injury to the neck, the patient should be transported with maximal caution, utilizing traction applied to the long axis of the neck by pulling manually or via a halter applied to chin and occiput. As soon as thorough roentgenograms have indicated the site of the lesion, it may be reduced or maintained in reduction by the amazingly comfortable maneuver of skeletal traction. This consists of placing a pair of metal tongs in the skull on each side just above and in front of the ears and applying a weight of 2 to 15 Kg. to these.

The larger thoracic and lumbar vertebrae tend to hold their post-traumatic positions, and these patients may be transported with a pillow under the spine at the site of the injury or in the prone position. In order to avoid further injury, it is vital to avoid flexion of the lumbar vertebrae.

The following are usually accepted as indications for surgical exploration: (1) worsening of the neurologic deficit after injury; (2) a penetrating wound of the spine; (3) bony or foreign fragments within the spinal canal; (4) persistent gross dislocation of bone despite skull or other traction of hyperextension. Other indications are more controversial; these include a dynamic block on the Queckenstedt test at lumbar puncture, and the syndrome of injury to the anterior spinal cord comprising paralysis and severe loss of pin-prick sensation with relative preservation of touch and proprioception. A peculiarly dangerous injury is a fracture at the base of the odontoid process, often demonstrable only by roentgenograms through the open mouth. The only complaint may be of pain, tenderness and stiffness in the back of the neck, but a later sharp movement of the head may permit vertebral movements with fatal crushing of the upper cervical cord. Immediate skull traction and operative posterior fixation by bony fusion and/or appropriate wiring at this level are necessary to forestall this catastrophe.

Even when a total transverse lesion of the spinal cord persists despite early treatment, remarkable rehabilitation of the patient is still feasible. Vigilant medical and nursing care is required to avoid bedsores and to keep infection of the urinary tract at a minimum. Involuntary muscle spasms may be such a problem that extensive anterior rhizotomy may be needed before the patient can even sit in a chair. Tenotomies, peripheral neurectomies or more limited rhizotomies may suffice when spasm is less extensive. Incredible though it may seem, a person with paralyzed legs can learn to walk with crutches and braces which keep the legs straight and permit them to bear weight. Development of mighty muscles in the shoulder girdle is prerequisite to this achievement.

Vascular Malformations

A fascinating variety of such anomalies occurs within the spinal canal. When a spontaneous subarachnoid hemorrhage is superimposed on the clinical picture of a cord lesion or when the myelogram reveals large tortuous vessels, this diagnosis may be ventured preoperatively. Decompression of such lesions, clipping of the feeding arteries or, rarely, total removal may be utilized in treatment.

Congenital Malformations

Spina Bifida. Failure of the posterior vertebral bony arch to close may have no other abnormal accompaniment and occurs at the first sacral vertebra in about 25 per cent of otherwise normal people. But if signs or symptoms in legs, bowel or bladder coming on in childhood are accompanied by a *spina bifida occulta*, shown in the x-ray film, operation may disclose a lipoma or a stalk of tissue whose removal will help the patient. If the defect is larger, a dural sac may protrude back through it, reaching the surface as a flat membrane or, more commonly, blossoming out as a posterior mass called a *meningocele*.

If the sac contains spinal cord or nerves, i.e., is a *myelomeningocele*, there will be weakness, sensory loss and sphincteric disturbance, whose degree will depend on the extent of malformation. Three fourths of these lesions are in the lumbar and/or the sacral areas; the remainder are more rostral.

Most neurosurgeons feel that an operation serves no useful purpose for a baby born with such a lesion and with paralyzed legs, bowels and bladder. This is especially true when the dismal spectacle of termination of cord and nerve roots in the wall of the sac is seen.

In less severe lesions after such surgical repair as may be done, one must follow the baby carefully for signs of hydrocephalus. If this develops, the Arnold-Chiari malformation is almost certainly the cause and should be treated promptly by suboccipital craniectomy and upper cervical laminectomy, followed by a shunting operation should the decompression be ineffective in controlling the hydrocephalus.

Congenital Dermal Sinuses. A tract of persisting stratified squamous epithelium may project inward from the skin along the midline anywhere from sacrum to skull. At the skin one may see only a tiny dimple, or there may be dermal thickening, pigmentation or red coloration, and hairs may protrude from the opening. These tracts often extend to the brain or the cord and may be accompanied by small dermoid tumors beneath the skin and/or at their neural end. Roentgenographs may or may not reveal a bifid spine or the tiny hole in the occipital bone by which the tracts reach the interior. Their special importance arises from the fact that they may conduct infection from the surface to the meninges, and a fulminant meningitis may ensue, destroying a significant part of the patient's nervous system. These tracts should be recognized and removed completely along with any associated tumors, if possible before meningitis develops—and certainly after meningitis has helped draw attention to their presence.

Diastematomyelia. This lesion, whose embryologic basis is obscure, consists of a bony spike projecting backward from a vertebral body into the middle of the spinal canal and dividing the spinal cord or the cauda equina into halves. Cutaneous accompaniments in the midline of the back at the level of the lesion are similar to those seen with congenital dermal sinuses. Major neurologic deficits may be arrested or improved by removing the offending spicule. This may be seen in roentgenographs anywhere in the thoracic or the lumbar region.

DISEASES AFFECTING THE PERIPHERAL NERVOUS SYSTEM

The principal intrinsic lesions of the peripheral nerves arise as a consequence of trauma or as neoplasms. Extrinsic pressure against the nerves also produces local disease.

Intrinsic Disease

A vast number of peripheral nerve injuries occurs in wartime, largely from wounds by missiles; it is from the study of collected experiences of the two World Wars that we base our management of these lesions. From such studies has come the realization that the primary task in restoring an injured limb to action involves mainly providing optimal conditions for regeneration of the nerve. Adequate repair of other soft tissues, vascular injury and the shattered bones usually is carried out at a preliminary operation, and the nerve is sutured a month later when swelling and infection have subsided.

The rarity with which peripheral nerve injuries occur in peace time, the ease with which such injury can be recognized by a decent examination, the variation from person to person in distribution of any normal nerve, and a lack of grave urgency about definitive repair make it unnecessary to treat the subject in detail in a general text. Even in a clean cut or a stab wound of a nerve in which a prompt end-to-end suture may be feasible and advisable, there is ample time for the operator to consult detailed anatomic and surgical texts regarding the nerve in question before performing the operation. Such a practice would result in fewer sutures of a severed median or ulnar nerve to a tendon, for instance, in the course of repairing a wrist laceration by capable surgeons of broad general experience.

Birth or other traumata, in which the brachial plexus is stretched unduly, may result in actual avulsion of the nerve roots from the spinal cord, often demonstrable by myelography, the contrast medium showing an abnormal configuration. The complex possibilities in any injury of the brachial plexus make it essential to study each case in detail. As knowledge in the domain of medicine increases, it becomes progressively more imperative to select fields of information in which the student need keep very few facts constantly in mind. Peripheral nerve injuries belong in this category.

Many tumors in peripheral nerves are benign neurofibromas, which may cause local pain and tenderness. The pain radiates into the distribution of the nerve on local pressure or may be confined to the site of the pressure. Later a sensory or motor loss may develop. Even when no tumor is palpable through the skin, local exploration may reveal a neurofibroma whose removal may well be possible without division of the fibers of the nerve trunk. Occasionally, some of the many neurofibromata seen in von Recklinghausen's disease may become painful and require removal. Malignant tumors of peripheral nerves are happily an extreme rarity.

Extrinsic Disease

Only 3 examples will be given of conditions in which extrinsic pressure against peripheral nerves occurs. The *syndrome of the scalenus anterior* arises as a consequence of pinching of the lower trunk of the brachial plexus and/or the subclavian artery as they cross above the first rib between the anterior scalene muscle in front and some firm structure behind. This latter may be a bony cervical rib or other osseous anomaly visible in a roentgenograph or may be a tendinous structure or cartilaginous rib which cannot thus be visualized. Symptoms tend to come on in early adult years because of the descent at puberty of the shoulder girdle with respect to the thorax. This occurs more markedly in women, who develop the disorder more frequently. Local tenderness may be present lateral to the sternocleidomastoid just above the clavicle. Pain, paresthesias, numbness and objective sensory loss to pin, touch or temperature develop along the ulnar aspect of arm, forearm, hand or fingers, the distribution of much of the medial cord of the brachial plexus arising from the anterior primary divisions of the 8th cervical and the 1st thoracic nerves. Symptoms may be exacerbated upon stretching the plexus by forcibly snapping the head away from the shoulder while pulling downward on the arm. Atrophy and weakness may appear, especially in the intrinsic muscles of the hand supplied by the ulnar nerve. Compression of the subclavian artery by the lesion may cause generalized weakness of the limb, blanching of fingers, and a low brachial blood pressure, worsened by elevation of the arm. Progression of symptoms may necessitate thorough operative exploration and removal of the offending structures.

Late ulnar neuritis may occur months or years following a severe injury at the elbow or upon repeated minor traumata to the ulnar nerve at the olecranon groove, particularly when the nerve slips over the epicondyle each time the elbow is flexed. Symptoms are similar to those in the preceding syndrome, but the zone of focal tenderness is at the olecranon groove. There is no sensory loss above the hypothenar eminence, no worsening of the symptoms on elevation of the arm and no evidence of arterial compression. Transplantation of the ulnar nerve to a position anterior to the medial condyle of the humerus but deep to the muscles arising therefrom is the treatment of choice.

The *carpal tunnel syndrome* of compression of the median nerve at the wrist, also called tardy median palsy, occurs principally in middle-aged women, often bilaterally. Insidious onset and progression of pain, paresthesias and numbness in the distribution of the median nerve below the wrist are followed by atrophy and weakness of muscles of the thenar eminence. There is tenderness over the transverse carpal ligament at the nerve, often with tingling into the lateral fingers upon such local pressure or upon movements at the wrist. Roentgenograms may show a post-traumatic or other bony lesion but are usually normal. If immobilization of the wrist joints fails to give relief, division of all the transverse ligaments ventral to the median nerve at the carpus is likely to do so without causing other sequelae of manual disability.

NEUROSURGICAL OPERATIONS ON NORMAL TISSUES TO RELIEVE DISEASE ELSEWHERE

Tissues which are presumed to be normal may be sacrificed in order to improve symptoms in an increasing variety of situations. These include the relief of (1) pain, (2) psychiatric symptoms, (3) involuntary movements, (4) Ménière's syndrome, (5) malignant disease, and (6) diabetic retinopathy. Such a sacrifice of tissue in some of the procedures to treat hydrocephalus has been discussed already. In addition, nondestructive stimulation to potentiate normal inhibitory mechanisms for pain may be moving from the experimental to the practical clinical stage.

PAIN

The first focal lesions deliberately made in normal tissues were those for the treatment of pain of unknown or incurable etiology. Often the full extent of the pain pathways involved in any particular case is unclear, and in such a situation it is good practice to utilize for diagnosis or even treatment procaine or, in selected sites, alcohol or phenol block of the nervous pathways under suspicion.

Peripheral Neurotomy. Denervation of the area of reference of pain was first tried by *interruption of impulses in the peripheral nerves thereto*. Since most peripheral nerves have a major motor component and are capable of sensory regeneration, division of such nerves has practical value in only 2 common problems: (1) In the treatment of pain confined to the foot or a finger, such as one sees in some vascular occlusive disorders. Crushing of digital nerves to a finger or of the superficial and the deep peroneal and tibial nerves a few inches above the ankle knocks out no consequential motor fibers. By the time the sensation has returned, peripheral collateral circulation may be adequate to preclude pain. (2) In the treatment of trigeminal neuralgia. Avulsion or alcohol injection of its peripheral divisions gives the patient a trial period of several months to determine whether or not the degree of relief of pain is worth the price of the annoying facial numbness. Although the motor nerve to the masticator muscles accompanies the third trigeminal division, its unilateral loss is insignificant.

Cranial Posterior Rhizotomy. This was historically the next operation tried and remains the sovereign tactic in the treatment of idiopathic *trigeminal, nervus intermedius, glossopharyngeal and upper vagal neuralgias* (Fig. 54-21, Nos. 2 and 3). In these disorders, the patient has pain with most or all of the following characteristics: (1) it is *paroxysmal,* lasting seconds to a few minutes; (2) it is *provoked by obvious stimuli* to the face, the ear or the pharynx; (3) it is confined to the zone of the affected nerve; (4) in any one paroxysm it is unilateral; (5) it is accompanied by no objective sensory loss on routine clinical testing. The paroxysms tend to come in cycles, each lasting several weeks or months. When the trigeminal zone is afflicted, the reference of pain is to some part of the face or the mouth; when nervus intermedius, glossopharyngeal or upper vagal fibers are concerned, the paroxysms start in the throat or deep in the ear. After a cutting of all posterior root fibers, which provokes anesthesia to touch and temperature as well as pain, the denervated zone after trigeminal rhizotomy exhibits a major degree of constant peculiar unpleasant sensation in about 4 per cent of patients, but the procedure nearly always affords gratifying and permanent relief of pain which often had previously attained such agonizing intensity that the patient lived in terror of the next attack.

A "compressive massage" of the exposed rootlets and gasserian ganglion, or a percutaneous phenol block of the ganglion is less likely to produce total numbness and major paresthesias. Even more controllable and safer is the destructive heating of the ganglion and rootlets with radiofrequency current via percutaneous electrode. The protective myelin on the touch fibers often permits one to conserve this sensation while destroying the smaller fibers concerned with pain by virtue of the precision obtainable with thermister-controlled heating.

Idiopathic facial pains without the above-described features, "atypical facial neuralgias," especially when there are continuous pains unaffected by external stimuli, are unlikely to be relieved by section of trigeminal rootlets, and if this is done the postoperative paresthesias tend to be more exasperating to the sufferer.

For the control of pain associated with cephalic or facial tumors, single or multiple cranial posterior rhizotomies may be needed, at times in combination with the operation to be discussed next.

Spinal Posterior Rhizotomy. Cutting of the upper cervical posterior roots (Fig. 54-21, No. 9) often stops pain in the neck or the occiput caused by malignant tumors or trauma to the roots emerging from the spinal canal. It may be efficacious in a few other situations in which one or only a few roots are specifically involved in the disorder. In general, however, spinal posterior rhizotomy has been disappointingly inadequate, partly because of the remarkable overlap in the innervation of any zone by nerves from several somatic segments and partly because other pain fibers travel with the sympathetic nerves and enter the spinal cord many segments away from those which enter the cord directly.

Intrathecal Injection of Destructive Chemicals. Alcohol for intrathecal injection to control pain has been replaced by the less dangerous and more controllable phenol. If this is dissolved in Pantopaque, the intrathecal position of the agent can be followed at the fluoroscopic tilt table and the fluid placed over those posterior rootlets likely to be conducting the undesired pain impulses. The phenol moves into and becomes fixed in the rootlets it surrounds; the Pantopaque can be removed half an hour later. Or the phenol can be injected as a solution in glycerine; the position of shifting mild paresthesias the patient experiences as the table is tilted serves as a reliable guide to the locus of the drug. Somewhat better results have followed this seemingly less precise tactic. Useful relief is afforded in this simple way in half to two thirds of the patients. Although the procedure is more easily repeatable than open operation, poorly controllable motor loss limits its allure.

Sympathectomy. This (Fig. 54-21, No. 8) is usually effective when denervation is needed in the control of pain arising exclusively from certain abdominal viscera, from the heart, and from the limbs in the conditions called causalgia and sympathetic dystrophy. A small number of painful disorders associated with *disease confined to the biliary tree, the small intestine, the kidney and the pancreas* are managed most satisfactorily by splanchnicectomy. As shown by White, there is also a small fraction of the patients with *angina pectoris* in whom an alcohol block or surgical excision of the upper 3 or 4 thoracic sympathetic ganglia on one or both sides may be needed to stop otherwise intractable attacks of such pain. Bilateral denervation has the added advantage that myocardial performance is improved,

1802   Surgery of the Nervous System

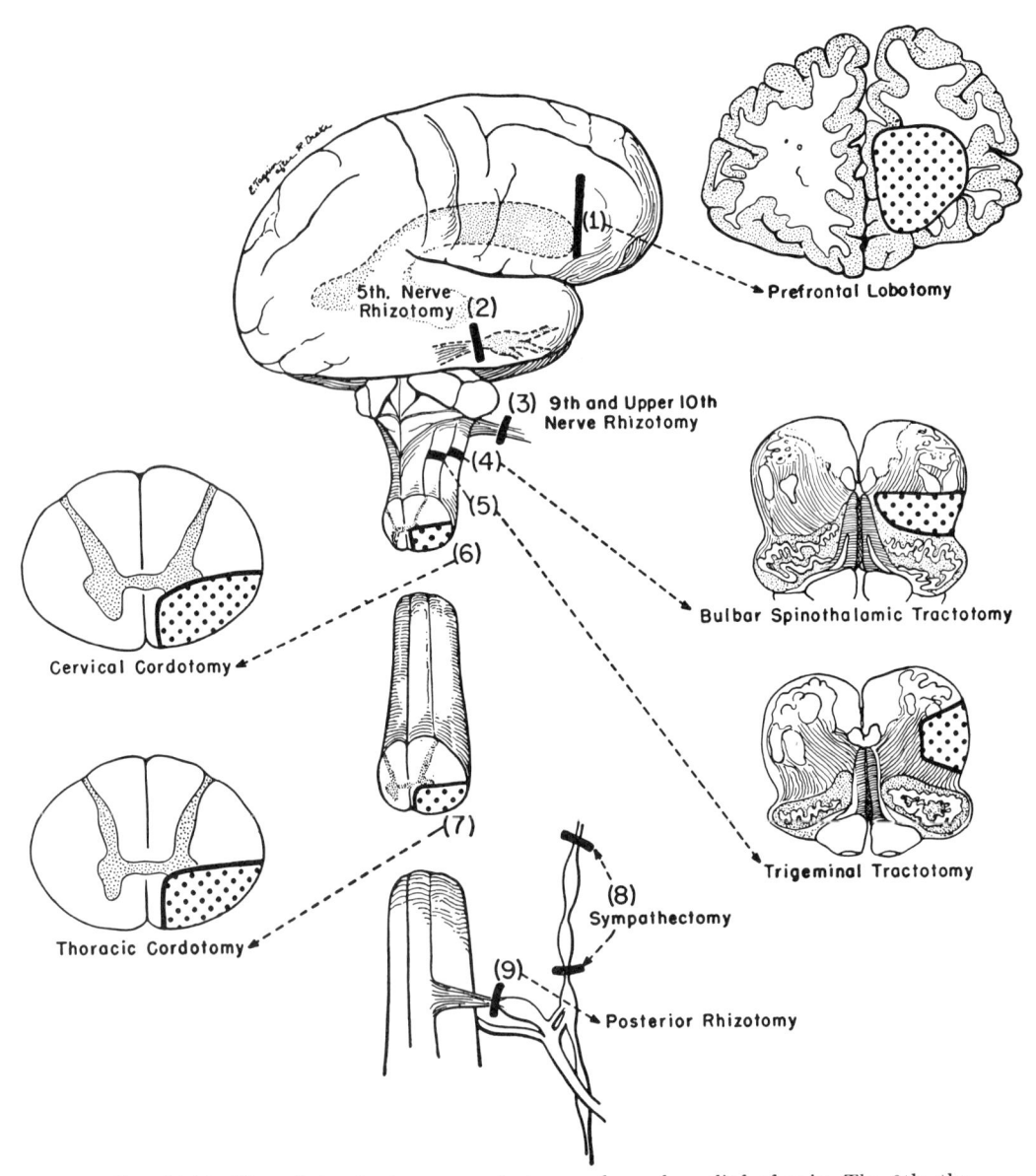

Fig. 54-21. Sites of standard neurosurgical procedures for relief of pain. The 9th, the 10th and 11th nerves leave the brain stem along a line dorsal to which lies the descending trigeminal tract (incision 5) and ventral to which lies the crossed pain pathway from the limbs and the torso (incision 4).

probably due in part to the simultaneous efferent denervation of β-sympathetic fibers. *Causalgia* may develop after a penetrating wound or other trauma which produces a partial injury of a peripheral nerve. A peculiar burning pain spreads to involve much of the whole affected limb, rather than being limited to the area of any one nerve; the patient tends to immobilize the whole extremity. A thin, shiny, smooth skin and long, uncut nails develop; there may be excessive sweating along with abnormal coolness and whiteness or heat and redness of the part. The touch of clothing, winter's cold and summer's heat, any emotional upset, even casual activity of others nearby, may provoke unbearable pain, and the patient may become a motionless recluse. A similar but less spectacular picture infrequently ensues after trauma, infection or arthritis in any portion of a limb. Sudomotor, vasomotor and trophic changes may be accompanied by a patchy osteoporosis which is most striking in roentgenographs of the affected hand or foot (Sudeck's atrophy). This picture, often called a "sympathetic dystrophy," is, like causalgia, dramatically amenable to change for the better upon repeated paravertebral chemical blocks of the sympathetic ganglia supplying the affected limb. Sympathectomy is often required to achieve a permanent cure.

Bulbar Trigeminal Tractotomy. After *the primary afferent neurons* enter the central neuraxis, those for pain and temperature split away from those for other sensory modalities. The pain and temperature fibers entering with the trigeminal, nervus intermedius, glossopharyngeal and upper vagal rootlets all move caudally in a bundle which becomes superficial in the lower medulla, the so-called descending trigeminal tract (Fig. 54-21, No. 5). This conveniently contains the pain fibers from the whole head on the ipsilateral side, and its division does not destroy the sense of touch. Hence, such an operation is of particular value when one must denervate the 1st trigeminal division in neuralgia, yet wishes to leave the protective afferent component of the corneal reflex arc intact. Preservation of the sense of touch to the cornea accomplishes this. Touch must also be left intact over at least some of the lower face when bilateral trigeminal neuralgia occurs in order to permit the patient to know the position of food in his mouth; otherwise, eating becomes a major problem.

Cordotomy. One of the most satisfactory of all of the procedures for relief of pain is a cordotomy, in which one incises the cord so as to divide the pain and temperature fibers of *the secondary afferent neuron* on their way to the brain. These fibers arise in the posterior horn of spinal gray matter, usually cross within 1 to 6 segments to the opposite side, where they ascend in the anterolateral and the anterior white matter. The pain fibers traveling with the sympathetic and those with the somatic nerves both converge into this area. This happy dispensation permits a single simple incision into the cord on one side to provide relief of nearly all types of pain referred to the opposite side of the body anywhere up to 5 or 6 segments below the level of the incision. If the pain is bilateral or is soon likely to be so because of a malignant midline tumor, one may make the incisions bilaterally, usually separating them by a few centimeters in the rostrocaudal direction.

Upper thoracic incisions (Fig. 54-21, No. 7) are commonly used for pain below the costal margin; upper cervical incisions, just caudal to the decussation of the pyramids (Fig. 54-21, No. 6), are required if pain is in the chest or arm. Bilateral thoracic incisions are followed occasionally by persisting urinary retention or incontinence or by weakness in a leg. Even when such annoying sequelae appear, the patient may consider them a small price to pay for relief from the relentless misery provoked by an advancing cancer.

Mullan has shown the feasibility of performing cordotomy by introducing percutaneously into the ventral part of the cord at the C1-C2 junction an electrode insulated except at the tip. The procedure has such simplicity and low risk that even the more emaciated, dangerously ill patients can be given pain relief.

Incurable neoplasms are the usual cause of pain sufficiently diffuse and severe to require cordotomy; recourse to this operation is advisable as soon as direct attack on the lesion by surgical, radiation or chemical therapy can no longer control the pain, and before addiction to Demerol or other habit-forming analgesics depletes still further the patient's reserves.

Other disorders in which pain in limbs or torso may lead to cordotomy, which is often followed by success, are: (1) neuralgias observed with amputation stumps, phantom limbs, after peripheral nerve injuries, other trauma or surgery and after herpes zoster; (2) intraspinal lesions such as tabes dorsalis (causing tabetic crises), chronic arachnoiditis or trauma to cauda equina. Lesions of the cord itself are less likely to be relieved by cordotomy at a higher level.

Tractotomy in Medulla. The crossed pathway for pain and temperature may also be cut conveniently and appropriately in the medulla (Fig. 54-21, No. 4) in patients whose pain extends into middle or upper cervical segments. Extensive cancer is the main disorder whose pain is so treated.

Thalamotomy. Stereotactic methods discussed below under "Involuntary Movements" are being used to guide the placement of electrical lesions both in the terminal nuclei of afferent pathways in the posterior and ventral thalamus and more anteriorly in nuclei whose functions are less clear. Inlying electrodes are used and the lesions enlarged when pain persists or the initial relief fades. Whereas there is a close correlation between relief of pain and production of objective analgesia to pin prick by surgical lesions lower in the neuraxis, Mark and Ervin have shown that complete relief may ensue following thalamic lesions giving little or no sensory loss upon neurologic examination. This may be attained without the blunting of emotional responses likely to occur after lobotomy, and the relief is gratifying, although the mechanism is at present a challenging enigma. Patients with malignant tumors of the head and the neck and those with lesions of the central nervous system causing pain are the principal candidates for such thalamotomy.

Frontal Lobotomy. The foregoing procedures have as their objective the blocking of impulses for pain before they reach the sentient areas in the brain. Another procedure, frontal lobotomy, also may eliminate suffering, not only that due to activity of specific pain fibers but also that on a psychological basis. Division of some of the frontal cerebral white matter in the coronal plane at the anterior tip of the lateral ventricles (Fig. 54-21, No. 1) produces a state in which the individual is aware of his pain but disregards it, no longer complains about it or requests medication. Cutting too many of the frontal white fibers produces an undesirable state of mental apathy; cutting too few gives inadequate relief of pain. A pair of small lesions in the infero-medial part of each frontal lobe or in the anterior part of the gyrus cinguli's supracallosal course may control the pain and suffering. If these are inadequate, or the originally satisfactory effect wears off, the area of destruction may be enlarged. The simplest way to achieve and later to increase a fractional lobotomy is by means of the radiofrequency electrode technic. After the initial making of small openings in the frontal skull and the meninges, the next and any necessary later stages are carried out in the radiologic suite, involving only freehand placement of the small electrodes with radiologic control of their positions. Not only widespread organic pain referred to any part of the patient but also mental anguish as a consequence of other symptoms and signs such as disfiguring malignant ulcers or fear of imminent death may be effectively assuaged thereby.

PSYCHIATRIC SYMPTOMS

Akin to the relief of the psychological suffering in organic disease is the relief of tension in some functional psychiatric disorders afforded by frontal lobotomy (Fig. 54-21, No. 1). Although originally proposed for this purpose and used effectively for disorders ranging in severity from obsessive compulsive neuroses to schizophrenia, frontal lobotomy's useful effects are usually but not always reproduced by drugs such as chlorpromazine and reserpine. Operative lobotomy, although largely replaced by drugs, should not be forgotten when these fail.

INVOLUNTARY MOVEMENTS

In a variety of neurologic disorders characterized by nearly constant undesired movements in the waking state, destruction of various portions of the brain has been carried out in an effort to stop the distressing tremor or other less rhythmic activity while preserving voluntary power and coordination. These efforts have culminated in the demonstration that relatively small lesions of volume 1.0 to 1.5 cc. in the neighborhood of the medial globus pallidus or of a lesser size in the lateral thalamus are likely to produce gratifying relief in a number of these disorders. To obtain the beneficial effects the adjoining fibers of the internal capsule need not be damaged, and weakness, spasticity or abnormality of limb reflexes need not—and, in nearly all the successful cases, does not ensue. In the commonest of these disorders, parkinsonism, major incapacitating features are the cogwheel or lead-pipe type of rigidity and a tremor, usually worst at rest. Both of these manifestations disappear or revert markedly toward normal on one side in about 85 per cent of patients immediately following the placement of one of the above-mentioned lesions in the opposite side of the brain. This useful effect persists for years in about two thirds of the total. The severely handicapped individual welcomes the effective use of half his limbs, and the patient with unilateral affliction resumes normal mobility. Other phenomena seen in many patients with the disorder, such as extreme paucity of movement when rigidity is small or absent (akinesia), a feeble speaking voice, and autonomic hyperactivity are not affected favorably. If mental deterioration is present, it may be worsened following operation. (Fortunately, these aspects of the disease are now often favorably affected by massive oral doses of L-dopa.) Those with cerebral atrophy or of advanced years are poor candidates for surgery; hence, careful preoperative study and selection of patients are important. After a substantial interval, presently many months rather than weeks, the opposite side of the brain is being attacked in the common bilaterally affected patient.

Other, and less frequent, types of involuntary movement in which surgery has a high degree of success are the extreme intention tremors which may be seen in such disorders as multiple sclerosis, familial tremors and cerebellar degenerative disease. The utterly incapacitating twisting movements of body and trunk in dystonia musculorum deformans and the violent, exhausting movements of hemiballismus have signally subsided with this type of surgery, and such patients have enjoyed some of the most spectacular returns from bedridden incapacitation to almost unfettered productivity. The tremor of Huntington's chorea and the disability of spasmodic torticollis have yielded to this therapy in some cases; the place of surgery here is still undecided. On the other hand, the choreoathetotic movements of cerebral palsy have tended to persist.

Technics for finding the precise site at which to make the lesion as well as the tactic for producing and controlling the destruction are still evolving but have attained great safety. In fact, the lack of more postmortem confirmation of the site of effective and inefficient lesions is holding up progress in the field, even though several thousand such operations have now been performed in the active centers concerned. New "stereotactic" methods have been developed for placing the device producing the lesion at the desired point in the depth of the brain. Most of the pioneers—Myers, Spiegel and Wycis, Leksell, Riechert, Guiot, Talairach and others—have used precision placement almost to the desired cubic millimeter in relation to radiographically identifiable points in the wall of the third ventricle, such as the anterior and the posterior commissures. The definitive lesion usually is made via electrodes passing a radiofrequency current. Cooper with great originality has sought to make a temporary lesion by brisk but less precise placement of a probe whose tip is cooled with liquid nitrogen. If the desired degree of improvement is not achieved, the probe is tried in a new position, the permanent lesion being made by increase of the cooling.

Knowledge of the neurophysiologic basis of normal movement in man, not to mention that of the neuropathologic basis of abnormal movements, is still fragmentary. The study of these deeper-seated mechanisms during therapeutic procedures in man is in its infancy.

There are at least 3 syndromes of involuntary movement limited to specific parts of the body in which production of a local flaccid paresis or paralysis may be preferable to the clinical disorder.

In *facial spasms* on one or both sides the facial muscles may be so diffusely, vigorously or frequently in contraction that, if the primary cause of the irritation cannot be found and treated, the patient may prefer facial paralysis to the incessant facial contortions. Gardner has shown that many of these patients have minor lesions irritating the nerve in the posterior cranial fossa remediable at operation without injury to the nerve. In those unrelieved, selective division of many of the fibers in each of the branches of the nerve as they emerge from the anterior border of the parotid gland may stop the movements without provoking facial deformity at rest. If movements still persist, total section of the nerve as it emerges from the stylomastoid foramen and suture of its proximal end into the cut distal end of the spinal accessory or hypoglossal nerve will give permanent relief of spasm but at the price of very little recovery of any voluntary movement.

In *spasmodic torticollis* the patient has a tonic or tonic-clonic twisting of the head to one side or, more rarely, in retrocollis directly backward. In many patients other involuntary movements in face, shoulder or limbs constitute a lesser part of the picture. Division of the 3 upper cervical anterior roots plus the spinal portion of the spinal accessory roots bilaterally usually quiets satisfactorily the head and the neck without weakening unduly the muscles holding the head up. Division of the insertion of the sternocleidomastoid muscle and of the spinal accessory nerve in the neck on the more active side may be added if necessary. In the most intractable cases division of one or both of the C4 anterior roots may be superimposed, but only if procaine block of the root demonstrates that the phrenic paresis thereby provoked is tolerated.

In *paraplegia with reflex flexor spasms in the legs*, arising from serious but not necessarily total transverse lesions of the spinal cord, the reflex withdrawal of the legs at all joints may be so severe as to preclude rehabilitative wearing of braces or even sitting in a wheel chair. Evacuation of the bladder or even of the bowel may be a part of this "mass reflex" and the slightest stimulus may bring involuntary jerking of the knees toward the chest. Under these circumstances and when it is clear that no useful motor power will return, Munro's operation of division of the anterior roots from T10 down through about S1 on both sides will help a hopeless dying invalid to achieve a useful life. It is important positively to identify the highest motor roots which cause bladder contraction by electrical stimulation during operation and observation of a manometer attached to the fluid-filled urinary bladder. All such sacral roots must be preserved in order to permit development of an automatic bladder and reflex sexual activity. For this reason the less accurate method of destruction of anterior roots by intrathecal phenol in glycerine is recommended only when these functions in the lumbosacral cord itself are already destroyed.

Malignant Disease

Total hypophysectomy is one of the procedures used to deprive the body of its normal hormones in an effort to arrest a cancer. The only tumors thus far favorably affected are cancers of the breast and possibly of the prostate. Using transfrontal operations for direct surgical removal of the gland Olivecrona and Ray in two independent series have achieved objective evidence of remission in about 50 per cent of their patients.

Transsphenoidal insertion of a beta-emitting isotope, a cryogenic probe, or a smaller probe for radiofrequency heating (the safest of the three), are the methods currently used for a controlled placement of a destroying device within the sella turcica. Concentration here of a high energy beam of protons or alpha particles is even safer because gross penetration of mucosa and bone with consequent risk of infection and cerebrospinal fluid rhinorrhea does not occur. The focal radiation methods are not applicable to those with such advanced disease that they might die before lapse of the several months required for the lethal radiation effects to appear. The freezing and the heating methods destroy the tissue at once.

A direct frontal surgical approach in the midline or obliquely via the antrum through the sphenoid sinus competes effectively in terms of safety and low morbidity with the foregoing indirect methods. The added precision obtainable with the direct operating microscope provides the greatest assurance given by any method of total destruction of the gland.

The more complete the destruction the more likely is a remission. Severe pain has often been relieved even without a measurable reduction in size of the metastases. All of these forms of hypophysectomy are both less hazardous and less annoying to the patient than bilateral adrenalectomy. Patients whose cancers have been affected favorably by hormonal treatment or ovariectomy are particularly likely to have another remission after hypophysectomy.

Diabetic Retinopathy

The hemorrhagic type of diabetic retinopathy improved markedly in a young woman after she developed panhypopituitarism consequent upon a pituitary apoplexy related to pregnancy. This clinical observation led to efforts to achieve the same improvement in a more controlled fashion by the methods described above under malignant disease and also by hypophyseal stalk section. The bad diabetic is often a worse risk for hypophysectomy than the patient with advanced cancer, but fortunately stalk section proves to be less hazardous and equally effective in treatment of the lesions related to the retinal hemorrhages. When regeneration of neural or vascular tissues at the hypophyseal stalk is precluded by interposition of a metal barrier, the long-term preservation of vision is at least as good as it is after total hypophysectomy. The improvement is due to decrease in (1) the frank retinal hemorrhages, (2) the retinal aneurysms, (3) the skeins of delicate new blood vessels, and (4) the increased vascular permeability leading to a cloudy vitreous humor. At present, operation or radiation is recommended only if progressive hemorrhages are threatening loss of vision and detailed investigations of cardiac, renal and cerebral function give at least a fair prognosis for life. Which of the pituitary hormones must be eliminated to stop the retinal hemorrhages is unknown. Indeed, the good results after stalk section alone intimate that one or more hypothalamic releasing factors or hypothalamo-hypophyseal neural pathways may be crucially implicated.

DISEASES AFFECTING THE AUTONOMIC NERVOUS SYSTEM

Neurosurgical procedures on this portion of the nervous system might well have been discussed fully under the previous heading of operations on normal structures, since there is essentially no evidence that the parasympathetic or sympathetic nerves divided are themselves abnormal. We have already considered the place of sympathectomy in the treatment of pain. In the disorders next to be discussed, as in the problems connected with pain, preliminary anesthetic blocking of the sympathetic fibers is often a valuable diagnostic procedure. A favorable response makes both the surgeon and his patient more confident of the effectiveness of the proposed denervation.

Parasympathetic System

Cranial Parasympathectomy. The only operation of established value in this area to be discussed is *denervation of the carotid sinus* in certain patients with a hypersensitive reflex arising from this structure. Such individuals on even minor movements of the head or the neck or mild pressure over the region of the bifurcation of the common carotid artery may have one of the following: (1) bradycardia or asystole, (2) arterial hypotension, (3) cerebrally induced syncope or seizures, or (4) any combination of the foregoing. No treatment except surgical denervation is effective in eliminating epileptic seizures of sinus origin. Atropine may prevent slowing of the heart rate, and vasoconstrictor agents may preclude a fall in blood pressure, but when medical management is ineffective, denervation of the afferent pathway of the hyperactive reflex arc is likely to stop the symptoms. To assure removal of the sinus nerve of Hering, the sensory portion of the reflex arc, one decorticates the common, external and internal carotid arteries for 2 cm. above and below the carotid sinus at the arterial bifurcation.

For the results of vagal denervation in the treatment of peptic ulcer see Chapter 31.

Sacral Parasympathectomy. In lesions of the spinal cord producing paraplegia, the spasm of the bladder neck which produces urinary retention may require relief by division of parasympathetic fibers to the bladder as they travel in the 2nd, the 3rd and/or the 4th pairs of sacral nerves. Thorough but unsuccessful conservative efforts to restore an "automatic bladder" and demonstration of ability to void after sacral foraminal nerve block are indispensable prerequisites to this operation.

Sympathetic System

The dividing of sudomotor and vasoconstrictor fibers which occurs in sympathectomy may control the symptoms of a number of disorders.

Hyperhidrosis. Rarely an individual has so extreme a tendency to sweat in the palms and the fingers or in the feet that he soon soaks whatever he touches or wears and finds himself under a major social or professional handicap. Effective denervation is provided by removal of the 2nd and the 3rd thoracic sympathetic ganglia for the upper limb and of the 3rd and the 4th lumbar sympathetic ganglia for the lower limb. The long-term results are excellent, since the regeneration of sudomotor fibers does not reach a troublesome degree.

Raynaud's Disease. In this peripheral vascular disorder, episodes of tonic contraction of the smaller arteries in the limbs occur. Exposure to cold and emotional stimuli are the main precipitants that evoke coldness, cyanosis and at times pain in fingers or toes, often in symmetrical areas on the 2 sides. A white asphyxia of the parts supervenes when the vasoconstriction is maximal and is succeeded by redness and painful tingling on rewarming. In between these episodes of phasic color change, the hands may be constantly cold and clammy with sweat. When the disorder is severe and chronic, the tips of the phalanges may develop dry ulcers, the skin of the digits may become shiny, hard and smooth, and the bone of the terminal phalanges be decalcified. Peripheral pulses in the main arteries of the limbs remain excellent because the abnormal constriction is distal to them. When, as is usual, vasodilator drugs fail to control the symptoms, removal of the 2nd and the 3rd lumbar sympathetic ganglia is likely to provide excellent relief if the feet are affected. When the hands are involved, the early result of removal of the upper 3 thoracic sympathetic ganglia is usually good, but a late return of the trouble has plagued many of the patients, and the inferior cervical and the 4th and the 5th thoracic ganglia may have to be removed as well (see Chap. 44).

In *acrocyanosis* the peripheral vasoconstriction tends to be present constantly. Otherwise, the disorder resembles Raynaud's disease in signs and treatment.

Occlusive Disease of Major Peripheral Vessels. The ischemia caused by thromboangiitis obliterans, arteriosclerosis, laceration, embolic occlusion or ligation of the main arteries has been partially relieved in past years by appropriate sympathectomy which promptly opens the collateral channels. When the occlusion is chronic, direct arterial grafting has now replaced the simpler operation of denervation in all but these special situations: (1) small digital ulcers in which one need only improve the circulation in the skin, (2) the presence of a cold sweaty skin as evidence of sympathetic overactivity, and (3) obstructions at and below the popliteal level, possibly because the vasoconstrictor impulses predominate in the distal vessels. The first 3 lumbar sympathetic ganglia are removed in an effort to maximize the denervation.

CONCLUSION

Many of the operations used routinely or undergoing trial by neurosurgeons depend upon detailed critical knowledge of normal neuro-anatomy and neurophysiology or of the functional pathology of a specific disease. Such information about the nervous system of man (in contrast with experimental animals) is still in an early phase of development. More and more we are coming to realize that the operative effort at therapy of a patient presents a favorable opportunity to increase our general knowledge and that such increase is likely to aid that particular patient. For example, information in regard to localization of function gained from the statements of the epileptic consequent upon stimulation of his cerebral cortex may be essential to treatment of his seizures; and knowledge of variations in site of pain pathways which may be inferred from the patient's description of pain upon stimulus within his cord or brain is of course necessary in making a lesion to stop the pain. Moreover, the explorations incident to gaining these data have yielded unexpected dividends in other new and basic knowledge. The mechanisms of disease of the nervous system and the treatment are comparatively not simple in nature, and the cream of major discoveries has not yet been skimmed. The wide-open character and the complexity of this field present a generous challenge to the finest minds.

BIBLIOGRAPHY

Baldwin, M., and Bailey, P.: Temporal Lobe Epilepsy. p. 581. Springfield, Ill. Charles C Thomas, 1958.

Brock, S. (ed.): Injuries of the Brain and Spinal Cord and Their Coverings. ed. 4. p. 739. New York, Springer, 1960.

Bushe, K. A., and Glees, P.: Chirurgie des Gehirns und Rückenmarks im Kindes- und Jugendalter. p. 1208. Stuttgart, Hippokrates, 1968.

Clinical Neurosurgery. Vols. 1-16. Proc. Congress of Neurol. Surgeons. Baltimore, Williams & Wilkins, 1954-1969.

Cushing, H., and Eisenhardt, L.: Meningiomas: Their Classification, Regional Behavior, Life History, and Surgical End Results. p. 785, Springfield, Ill., Charles C Thomas, 1933.

Dandy, W. E.: Selected Writings of Walter E. Dandy. p. 789. Springfield, Ill., Charles C Thomas, 1957.

David, M., Pourpre, H., Lepoire, J., and Dilenge, D.: Neurochirurgie. p. 973. Paris, Éditions Médicales Flammarion, 1961.

Gurdjian, E. S.: Operative Neurosurgery. ed. 2. p. 560. Baltimore, Williams & Wilkins, 1964.

Hortwitz, N. H., and Rizzoli, H. V.: Postoperative Complications in Neurosurgical Practice. p. 427. Baltimore, Williams & Wilkins, 1967.

Jefferson, G.: Selected Papers. p. 563. London, Pitman, 1960.

Kahn, E. A., Bassett, R. C., Schneider, R. C., and Crosby, C. E.: Correlative Neurosurgery. p. 413. Springfield, Ill., Charles C Thomas, 1955.

Knighton, R. S., and Dumke, P. R. (ed.): Pain: Henry Ford Hospital International Symposium, p. 587, London, Churchill, 1966.

Krayenbühl, H., Maspes, P. E., and Sweet, W. H.: Progress in Neurological Surgery. Vols. 1-3. Basel, S. Karger, 1966-1969.

Matson, D. D.: Neurosurgery of Infancy and Childhood. p. 913. Springfield, Ill., Charles C Thomas, 1969.

Olivecrona, H., and Tönnis, W. (eds.): Handbuch der Neurochirurgie. Vol. 4. Klinik und Behandlung der raumbeengenden intrakraniellen Prozesse. Part 1, p. 782, 1960; Part 2, p. 399, 1966; Part 3, p. 674, 1962; Part 4. p. 677, 1967: Vol. 6. Chirurgie der Hirnnerven und Hirnbahnen. p. 249, 1957, Berlin, Springer.

Penfield, W., and Jasper, H.: Epilepsy and the Functional Anatomy of the Human Brain. p. 896. Boston, Little, Brown & Co., 1954.

Pool, J. L., and Potts, D. G.: Aneurysms and Arteriovenous Anomalies of the Brain. p. 463. New York, Harper & Row, 1965.

Poppen, J. L.: An Atlas of Neurosurgical Techniques. p. 522. Philadelphia, W. B. Saunders, 1960.

Spiegel, E. A., and Wycis, H. T. (eds.): Advances in Stereoencephalotomy. Vol. 1. p. 232, 1963; Vol. 2. Part 1, p. 371, 1965; Vol. 2. Part 2, p. 261, 1966; Vol. 3. p. 282, 1967. Basel, S. Karger.

Taveras, J. M., and Wood, E. H.: Diagnostic Neuroradiology. p. 960. Baltimore, Williams & Wilkins, 1964.

Walker, A. E. (ed.): A History of Neurological Surgery. p. 561. Baltimore, Williams & Wilkins, 1951.

White, J. C., and Sweet, W. H.: Pain and the Neurosurgeon—A Forty Year Experience. p. 950. Springfield, Ill., Charles C Thomas, 1969.

Wilkins, R. H.: Neurosurgical Classics. p. 523. New York, Johnson Reprint Corp., 1965.

CHAPTER 55

HARVEY R. BUTCHER, JR., M.D.

Mathematical Analysis of Surgical Data

Now if I wanted to be one of those ponderous scientific people, and "let on" to prove what has occurred in the remote past by what had occurred in a given time in the recent past, or what will occur in the far future by what has occurred in late years, what an opportunity is here! ... Please observe: In the space of one hundred and seventy-six years the Lower Mississippi has shortened itself two hundred and forty-two miles. That is an average of a trifle over one mile and a third per year. Therefore, any calm person, who is not blind or idiotic, can see that in the old Oolitic Siluran Period, just a million years ago next November, the Lower Mississippi River was upward of one million three hundred thousand miles long, and stuck out over the Gulf of Mexico like a fishing-rod. And by the same token any person can see that seven hundred and forty-two years from now the Lower Mississippi will be only a mile and three-quarters long, and Cairo and New Orleans will have joined their streets together, and be plodding comfortably along under a single mayor and a mutual board of aldermen. There is something fascinating about science. One gets such wholesale returns of conjecture out of such a trifling investment of fact.—Mark Twain: *Life on the Mississippi,* Chapter 17.

The distrust often expressed by physicians toward statistical methods of analysis undoubtedly arises principally from a lack of understanding of the meaning and limits of these methods. Erroneous applications of statistical technics and the associated unjustified conclusions such as those just quoted undoubtedly have contributed to this mistrust. The fact remains that the proper analysis and interpretation of observational data require the calculation of probabilities by statistical methods. Every diagnosis made by the physician is arrived at by either a conscious or unconscious consideration of probabilities. A working knowledge of this field has become an important asset for a practicing surgeon to possess.

Actually, statistical methods of analysis of data prove nothing by themselves, A probability value is only a number arrived at by arithmetic; tests of significance measure only the probability of sameness in groups of data irrespective of the reasons for the variations between them. However, only by the proper application of methods for assessing the magnitudes of chance variations can one ever know how nearly an investigation has proved anything. The relative nature of "proof" of anything is expressed best by a mathematically calculated probability, a value permitting an assessment of the significance of the data.

What requisites must the surgeon have for the *proper* application of statistical methods to observational data encountered by him? He first must possess enough insight to permit him to avoid the pitfalls inherent in his own bias. Even the most experienced physician must constantly remind himself of the extent to which subconscious prejudices can mislead him. He must realize that the application of tests of significance to the results of a poor experiment does not make the experiment a good one. The most erudite statistical analysis of poorly collected, nonobjective data is worthless, and indeed it harms by influencing the courses of action of the uninitiated. The surgeon need not possess the theoretical knowledge of the professional statistician, but only an understanding of the meaning of tests of significance and of the proper ways for using them.[5,6]

POPULATION SAMPLING

Statistically speaking, the *population* of measurements is considered infinitely large. However, the idea of an infinite population from which samples are taken is an abstraction. In practice we deal with finite groups or aggregates of things. Random *sampling* is our only method of assessing the characteristics of these populations; all observational data may be considered such samples. Randomization of sampling is the process of choosing a portion of the population in such a way that only chance variations occur between the characteristics of the sample and the characteristics of the total population. In other words, all bias attributable to factors other than chance has been removed from the procedure of sampling.

Random sampling often is best accomplished in the study of human beings by the use of a table of random numbers (Table 55-1).[7] Tables of random numbers are constructed from ordinary digits (0 through 9) successively generated by a random physical process. One way to generate random numbers is to roll a die and at the same time toss a coin having assigned the digits 0 through 9 to each of the 10 possible combinations between the numbers 1 through 5 on the die and the two sides of the coin, ignoring the 6 on the die. In such an instance each digit has a probability of 0.1 of occurring on each trial, and each trial is entirely independent. The proper use of tables of random sampling numbers gives the best guarantee now available of obtaining a truly random sample.

Before the clinical investigator undertakes any study in which a table of random numbers should be used, he must define carefully the characteristics of the population he proposes to study. Obviously, it does not make sense to include in the group to be randomized those things (or individuals) that cannot be changed by the procedures to be studied.

How does one "take a sample" of a given population in practice? The *sample* in clinical work often consists of all the similarly ill patients seen at a hospital during a specific interval of time. Since the populations of hospitals vary widely, this sample is rarely, if ever, representative of all patients with this illness in the world. However, this fact does not prevent one from assessing the relative merits of various methods of treatment in such a group and drawing valid conclusions for that group from the endeavor if the experiment is properly controlled. By the use of controls, experiments become comparative and not merely absolute. By randomization of the sample one may establish a control and an experimental groups of persons which can be expected to be comparable in so far as the extent and the severity of the disease are concerned. Of course, there is always a probability that the control and the experimental groups are *not* the same as a result of chance alone; this probability is the smaller, the larger the numbers in the two groups. One need only to test for the sameness of the two randomly selected groups with proper statistical methods to know whether they are by chance incongruous.

DOUBLE-BLIND STUDIES

The "double-blind" technic of collecting observational data is another refinement in sampling which further eliminates bias of the investigator. The technic not only establishes a control and an experimental group by random selection but keeps the identity of these groups a secret until the end of the experi-

TABLE 55-1. RANDOM NUMBERS
(From A Table of Ten Thousand Randomly Assorted Digits[3])

54463	22662	65905	70639
15389	85205	18850	39226
85941	40756	82414	02015
61149	69440	11286	88218
05219	81619	10651	67079
41417	98326	87719	92294
28357	94070	20652	35774
17783	00015	10806	83091
40950	84820	29881	85966
82995	64157	66164	41180

ment. Double-blind studies are particularly appropriate for the evaluation of some drugs. In such instances neither the patient nor the administering and evaluating physician knows whether the patient was given a placebo or the drug in question until the results have been recorded; i.e., whether the patient is a member of the control or of the experimental group. For example, this technic was used to assess the effectiveness of "prophylactic" antibiotics.

First, the population sample was defined as all patients on the ward surgical service undergoing elective operations of a potentially contaminated nature. Other studies had shown that approximately 30 per cent of such cases became infected on the same wards in that institution. Had the expected incidence of infection been 0.1 per cent, the study would have required such a large sample as to make its collection in any one institution highly improbable.

The second step was the selection of a sequence of numbers from a table of random sampling numbers. This was done by arbitrarily selecting a number in the table as the first one in the sequence, the digits following it across the page being then listed until 120 numbers were obtained. Approximately half the numbers were odd, the remaining ones even.

Finally, the list of random numbers was given to the chief pharmacist who had prepared two solutions of identical appearance, one containing the antibiotic preparation, the other not. Subsequently, when the investigators ordered the antibiotic preparation for use before, during and immediately after a potentially contaminated operation the pharmacist dispensed either the preparation containing antibiotics or the placebo, according to whether the next number on the list of random numbers was odd or even.

Only after the patients had been discharged from the hospital and the presence or absence of postoperative infection established did the investigators know which patient received antibiotics. The code was broken only in patients who became infected and in whom the knowledge of previous antibiotic medication might influence therapy. The study was terminated after approximately 120 patients had received either the antibiotic or the placebo preparation because analysis of the data showed that the persons receiving the antibiotics had a significantly lower incidence of postoperative infections than the patients receiving the placebo (Table 55-2).

MEANS AND RATES

Knowledge of the technics used for comparing rates and means or averages of collections of clinical data is essential to a critical analysis of it. The merit of much of the professional literature the practicing surgeon reads can be assessed only by untilizing such knowledge. The *chi-square* test is used to compare frequencies or "counts" of things; the *t-test* to compare means of data collected by measurement. In other words, the chi-square test is used most often to define the degree of likeness of sets of qualitative data, while the t-test compares the means of quantitative data obtained from measurements of continuous variables such as weight, temperature and blood flow.

THE CHI-SQUARE TEST

The significance of differences in proportions or frequencies may be established with the chi-square (χ^2) test. Chi-square is defined as an index of dispersion attributable to sampling a hypothetical population. The chi-square table states the probable occurrence of certain values of this index in the process of

TABLE 55-2. THE EFFECTIVENESS OF ANTIBIOTICS IN PREVENTING INFECTION AMONG PATIENTS UNDERGOING POTENTIALLY CONTAMINATED OPERATIONS—A "DOUBLE-BLIND" STUDY

SOLUTION GIVEN	NO. OF PATIENTS	NUMBER HAVING INFECTIONS POSTOPERATIVELY	NUMBER HAVING NO INFECTION
(a) Antibiotic	55	3 (5%)	52
(b) Placebo	63	16 (25%)	47

Comparing (a) with (b)—chi-square = 7.23, probability <0.01, >.001.

TABLE 55-3. Two by Two Contingency Table

METHOD OF TREATMENT	NUMBER ALIVE 5 YEARS AFTER TREATMENT	NUMBER DEAD 5 YEARS AFTER TREATMENT	TOTAL NUMBER
Radical mastectomy	(a) 67 (52%)	(b) 62	129 (a+b)
Radical mastectomy and postoperative irradiation	(c) 37 (47%)	(d) 41	78 (c+d)
	104 (a+c)	103 (b+d)	207 (N)

sampling. When we use the chi-square test to examine the difference in the frequencies of a characteristic in two or more groups, we are determining the probability that these frequency ratios differ because of chance alone. In other words, a calculated chi-square value is used to find (in the chi-square distribution table) the probability of getting, by random sampling, another chi-square value equal to or greater than the calculated one on repeated sampling.

Because of the usefulness of the chi-square test a number of different forms for its calculation have been developed to deal with specific problems, but all are based on a comparison of expected and observed frequencies in various categories by the formula $\chi^2 = \Sigma \frac{(f - F)^2}{F}$ where f = observed frequency, F = expected frequency and Σ denotes summation. We shall illustrate two uses of the test which are quite frequently applicable to clinical data. When one wishes to determine the significance of a difference in two frequencies using the chi-square test, the data are arranged as shown in Table 55-3. This table shows data from two groups of patients arranged in what is called a 2 by 2 contingency or 4-fold table. The arithmetic used to calculate chi-square is:

This quotient may be arrived at using longhand arithmetic, a calculator or a slide rule. If care is taken to avoid errors in decimal place, the use of a slide rule results in sufficient accuracy for most situations. Having now determined that chi-square = 0.394, we enter the table of distribution of χ^2 (Table 55-4) with 1 degree of freedom* and find that the probability value is between 0.70 and 0.50. This means that the magnitude of the observed difference in the proportions surviving in Table 55-3 would occur with repeated random sampling 5 to 7 times out of 10 due to chance alone. Since the difference observed is easily attributable to chance variation in sampling, we conclude that survival from mammary cancer in this series is the same whether

* The degrees of freedom are defined as the number of groups, specimens or samples being compared minus 1 (N — 1). Degrees of freedom may be thought of as corresponding to the number of independent observations present in the data being analyzed. If the two groups we are comparing were compared to some theoretical group, then there would be 2 degrees of freedom. However, we have actually compared the two series with the sum formed by adding them. Since each series has contributed to the sums, neither series is entirely independent of the sum. When such a sum is used instead of a hypothetical group, 1 degree of freedom for variation is lost.

$$\text{Chi-square } (\chi^2) = \frac{(ad - bc)^2 N}{(a + b)(c + d)(a + c)(b + d)}$$

or

$$\chi^2 = \frac{(67 \times 41 - 62 \times 37)^2\, 207}{129 \times 78 \times 104 \times 103}$$

$$\chi^2 = \frac{(453)^2\, 207}{129 \times 78 \times 104 \times 103}$$

$$\chi^2 = 0.394$$

Mathematical Analysis of Surgical Data

TABLE 55-4. AN ABBREVIATED TABLE OF THE DISTRIBUTION OF χ^2

DEGREES OF FREEDOM	PROBABILITY					
	.70	.30	.10	.05	.01	.001
1	.148	1.074	2.706	3.841	6.635	10.827
2	.713	2.408	4.605	5.991	9.210	13.815
3	1.424	3.665	6.251	7.815	11.345	16.268
4	2.195	4.878	7.779	9.488	13.277	18.465
5	3.000	6.064	9.236	11.070	15.086	20.517

treatment be radical mastectomy alone or radical mastectomy plus postoperative irradiation. In other words, we accept the *Null hypothesis*, which, stated simply, is that the observed difference in mortality is due to chance—and not to something other than chance. It is customary in medicine and biology to *reject* the Null hypothesis when chi-square is found to be equal to or greater than 3.84, which is the value where probability becomes 0.05 or less. Actually, the probability level for rejecting a Null (no difference) hypothesis is selected by the investigator corresponding to the risk he is willing to assume of rejecting a true hypothesis.

Also of particular value to the clinical investigator is the chi-square test for homogeneity of frequency distributions. This technic tests the hypothesis that two or more frequency distributions come from the same homogeneous population. This chi-square test is particularly useful in testing the congruity of two different groups of patients by examining, for example, the likeness of their age distributions, the frequencies of different stages of disease in the two groups, or the size distributions of the primary tumors when the patients being studied are ill of cancer.

As an example of the use of the chi-square test for homogeneity,[4] the age distributions of two groups of similarly ill patients will be examined. Group A came from one hospital, Group B from another. The formula for calculating chi-square is:

$$\chi^2 = \frac{1}{\bar{p}\bar{q}} (ap - N\bar{p})$$

$$p = \frac{a}{a+a'}, \quad \bar{p} = \frac{N_1}{N_1+N_2}, \quad \bar{q} = 1.0 - \bar{p}$$

The data are arranged as follows:

Age in Years	(a') Group A	(a) Group B	$p = \dfrac{a}{a'+a}$	$ap = \dfrac{a^2}{a'+a}$
<40	30	21	21/51	$(21)^2/51 = 8.647$
40 – 49	112	61	61/173	21.509
50 – 59	101	78	78/179	33.989
60 – 69	92	118	118/210	66.305
70 +	41	85	85/126	57.341
Total	376 (N_2)	363 (N_1)	$363/739 = \bar{p}$ $\bar{p} = .491$ $\bar{q} = .509$	$Sap = 187.791$

$$\chi^2 = \frac{1}{.491 \times .509} [187.791 - (363 \times .491)]$$

$$\chi^2 = \frac{187.791 - 178.233}{.250}$$

$$\chi^2 = 38.232$$

Entering the chi-square table for 4 degrees of freedom (5 decades of age were tested), we find: $P_4 < .001$, since χ^2 for $P = .001$ with 4 degrees of freedom is equal to 18.6. In other words, the probability that chance alone, or variation in sampling is responsible for the differences in the age distributions of Groups

A and B is less than 1 in 1,000. We conclude then that some factor other than chance variation in sampling of the population makes patients in Group B more often older than patients in Group A are. The importance of such a difference in age distribution becomes evident if mortality rates of the two groups are to be compared. Since the age distributions differ, we cannot validly make such a comparison without taking into account the difference in the expected rates of dying of the two groups. This may be accomplished in some instances by applying the expected rates of dying found in the U.S. Vital Statistical Tables to each specific age group.

ANALYSIS OF MEASUREMENTS

The mean or average is an abstract concept which alone has little meaning, particularly when one is considering biologic phenomena almost all of which may be considered to have a "normal range." For an arithmetic mean to convey information it must be accompanied by knowledge of the "scatter" observed in the data about it.

THE STANDARD DEVIATION

The statistical method of describing the magnitude of variation about the mean involves the calculation of *variance* and *standard deviation*. The more convenient formulae are:

1. Variance $(s^2) = \dfrac{\Sigma(x)^2 - \dfrac{(\Sigma x)^2}{N}}{N-1}$

2. $s^2 = \dfrac{\Sigma(x - \bar{x})^2}{N - 1}$

3. $s^2 = \dfrac{(\Sigma(x^2) - \bar{x}\Sigma x)}{N - 1}$

where: s^2 = variance
s = standard deviation
$\bar{x}$ = mean of the data
Σx = sum of the observed data
$\Sigma(x)^2$ = sum of the squares of the data
$(\Sigma x)^2$ = square of the sum of the data
N = number of observations
$N - 1$ = degrees of freedom

TABLE 55-5. VARIANCE (s^2) AND STANDARD DEVIATION (s)

FIFTEEN* OBSERVED VALUES (x)	OBSERVED VALUE FROM MEAN $(x - \bar{x})$	$(x - \bar{x})^2$	x^2
36	−45	2025	1296
100	+19	361	10000
27	−54	2916	729
102	+21	441	10404
45	−36	1296	2025
94	+13	169	8836
51	−30	900	2601
71	−10	100	5041
77	−4	16	5929
92	+11	121	8464
58	−23	529	3364
141	+60	3600	19881
61	−20	400	3721
185	+104	10816	34225
75	−6	36	5625
1215	00	23726	122141
Σx	....	$\Sigma(x - \bar{x})^2$	$\Sigma(x^2)$

mean of $x = \bar{x} = \dfrac{\Sigma x}{N} = \dfrac{1215}{15} = 81$

by equation (1) $s^2 = \dfrac{(122141 - \dfrac{(1215)^2}{15})}{14} = 1696$

(2) $s^2 = \dfrac{23726}{14} = 1696$

(3) $s^2 = \dfrac{(122141 - (81 \times 1215))}{14}$
$= 1696$

Standard deviation $(s) = \sqrt{1696} = 41$

*Increases in hepatic arterial blood flow associated with diversion of the portal venous blood flow into the inferior vena cava of dogs.

The calculation of these estimates is illustrated in Table 55-5.

The standard deviation expresses the degree of "scatter" of the data about the arithmetic mean of any random sample from a homogeneous population. The mean plus or minus 2 standard deviations will include approximately 95 per cent of the data. (Actually 5% of the area beneath a normal distribution curve lies outside the mean ±1.96 times the standard deviation.

THE STANDARD ERROR OF THE MEAN

The standard error of the mean $(S\bar{x})$ is estimated from a standard deviation of a sample as:

$$S\bar{x} = \frac{s}{\sqrt{N}} \text{ or } \sqrt{\frac{s^2}{N}}$$

Whereas the standard deviation defines the magnitude of the spread of the data about a mean, the standard error of the mean expresses an estimate of the scatter of other means of repeated experiment or random sampling. For example, the averages of 4 independent samplings of the same population have a standard deviation equal to $\frac{s}{\sqrt{4}}$ or one half the standard deviation of a single sample. The true mean of the total population will lie within $\bar{x} \pm S\bar{x}$ two thirds of the time and within $\bar{x} \pm 2S\bar{x}$ 95 per cent of the time. The latter interval is called the 95 per cent confidence interval.

THE T TEST

The significance of a difference between the means of 2 samples is tested by the *t* test. The question being asked is: what is the probability that the 2 groups of data are random samples of the same population. In other words, how often would the difference observed in the 2 means be expected to occur due only to chance variation in the sampling.

The calculations for the comparison of 2 means involve combining the 2 groups of measurements so that a new or pooled variance and a new standard deviation are obtained. From these new values a standard error of the difference between the means is calculated. The value (t) is the ratio of difference between the means to the standard error of this difference. The calculations are as follows:

Observed Values

Group A		Group B	
(x)*	(x)²	(x')*	(x')²
36	1296	71	5041
100	10000	77	5929
27	729	92	8464
102	10404	58	3364
45	2025	141	19881
94	8836	61	3721
51	2601	185	34225
		75	5625
$\Sigma x = 455$	$\Sigma x^2 = 35891$	$\Sigma x' = 760$	$\Sigma (x')^2 = 86250$
$N = 7$		$N = 8$	

(mean) $\bar{x} = \frac{455}{7} = 65, \bar{x} = \frac{760}{8} = 95$

The pooled variance $= s^2_{x,x'} = \frac{\Sigma(x^2) - \bar{x}\Sigma x + \Sigma(x'^2) - \bar{x}'\Sigma x'}{N + N' - 2}$
(see similarity to equation 3)

Degrees of freedom $= (N - 1) + (N' - 1) = N + N' - 2$

Thus:

$$s^2_{x,x'} = \frac{35891 - 65 \times 455 + 86250 - 95 \times 760}{7 + 8 - 2} = 1567$$

The pooled standard deviation: $s_{x,x'} = \sqrt{1567} = 39.6$

---

* The data (x) (x') are increases in hepatic arterial blood flow associated with shunting the portal blood into the inferior vena cava of dogs (ml./min.).

TABLE 55-6. AN ABBREVIATED TABLE OF THE DISTRIBUTION OF t

DEGREES OF FREEDOM	PROBABILITY				
	.2	.1	.05	.01	.001
1	3.078	6.314	12.706	63.657	636.619
3	1.638	2.353	3.182	5.841	12.941
5	1.476	2.015	2.571	4.032	6.859
7	1.415	1.895	2.365	3.499	5.405
9	1.383	1.833	2.262	3.250	4.781
11	1.363	1.796	2.201	3.106	4.437
13	1.350	1.771	2.160	3.012	4.221
∞	1.282	1.645	1.960	2.576	3.291

Using the pooled standard deviation we now calculate the standard error of the difference between the means by one of two ways:

$$(1)\ s_D = \sqrt{\frac{s^2_{x,x'}}{N} + \frac{s^2_{x,x'}}{N'}} = \sqrt{\frac{1567}{7} + \frac{1567}{8}} = 20.5$$

$$(2)\ s_D = s_{x,x'}\sqrt{\frac{N+N'}{N \times N'}} = 39.6\sqrt{\frac{15}{56}} = 20.5$$

$$t = \frac{\bar{x} - \bar{x}'}{s_D}\ \text{or}\ \frac{65 - 95}{20.5} = 1.4634$$

Degrees of freedom = $(N - 1) + (N' - 1) = 13$

The probability value corresponding to t = 1.4634 with 13 degrees of freedom is found in the table for the distribution of t (Table 55-6.) The table shows this probability to be approximately 0.17 ($P_{.20} = 1.305$, $P_{.10} = 1.771$). We therefore conclude that a difference as large as or larger than the difference between the means of changes in flow observed in Group A and Group B (30 ml./min.) would occur due to chance alone approximately 17 per cent of the time. If we accept the usual biologic limit of 5 per cent as indicating significance we must conclude that the means of these two groups of data do not differ "significantly." The use of the t test assumes the data has somewhere near a normal distribution. If the data is obviously not normally distributed the use of the Wilcoxon rank tests may be advisable (see Snedecor[7]).

MORTALITY DATA

The rates of dying of persons ill of a lethal disease represent one of the principal methods available to the physician for the assessment of the effectiveness of therapy. The analysis of mortality rates is of particular concern to those who study the biologic behavior of cancer and search for the most effective methods of treating it. For a physician to assess the relative effectiveness of different treatments of anything, the data must be sufficient to permit an assessment of the "likeness" of the therapeutic groups. Specifically we need to know such things as the criteria for the diagnosis of cancer in the groups; the race, age and sex distributions in both groups and the distribution of patients in each group by clinical stage, pathologic stage, and microscopic grades of their cancers when applicable. Obviously, the methods of staging and grading should be the same in the various groups. In other words, the relative effectiveness of two or more methods of therapy in two or more groups of patients can be assessed validly only after congruity of the groups has been established. Obviously, the likelihood of sameness in two population samples is greater if they have been randomly selected from the same hospital population during the same interval than if not. However, persons treated for the same illness at different times and places are not *necessarily* unlike each other,

TABLE 55-7. SURVIVAL OF WOMEN AFTER EXENTERATION OF THE PELVIC ORGANS FOR POST-IRRADIATIONAL CARCINOMA OF THE CERVIX (LIFE TABLE)[2]

TIME AT RISK YEARS	NUMBER ALIVE AT BEGINNING OF INTERVAL	NUMBER DYING IN INTERVAL	LOST TO FOLLOW-UP DURING INTERVAL	WITHDRAWN ALIVE DURING INTERVAL	EFFECTIVE NUMBER AT RISK*	PROPORTION DYING	PROPORTION LIVING	ACCUMULATIVE SURVIVAL RATE %
0–1	150	37	0	12	144	.25	.75	75
1–2	101	23	3	11	94	.24	.76	57
2–3	64	10	0	6	61	.16	.84	48
3–4	48	7	1	11	42	.17	.83	40
4–5	29	3	0	0	29	.10	.90	36

* The effective number at risk is the number living at the beginning of the interval minus one half the number lost and withdrawn alive during the interval. The assumption is that these cases are lost or withdrawn randomly during the interval and that their subsequent survival will be as likely as the cases with complete follow-up. The proportion dying is calculated by dividing the number dead by the effective number at risk for the interval. The proportion living is simply 1 minus the proportion dying. The accumulative survival rate after a specific time is then determined by multiplying the product of the proportions living of each of the preceding intervals by 100.

nor are they necessarily alike. If the data outlined above are known in detail for each group being compared, it is possible to assess congruity by statistical tests. If the two groups are not comparable in respect to some factor known to affect mortality, then it is valid only to compare the mortality rates of those members of the groups who possess this factor, or to compare the mortality rates of those members who do not possess this factor.

Once the homogeneity of the two groups under consideration is known, we may attribute differences in mortality rates to a difference in the effectiveness of treatment. Such

TABLE 55-8. SURVIVAL FROM TYPES III AND IV MAMMARY CANCER TREATED BY RADICAL MASTECTOMY

YEARS AT RISK	TYPE	EFFECTIVE NUMBER AT RISK	NUMBER DYING IN INTERVAL	NUMBER LIVING THROUGH INTERVAL	ACCUMULATIVE SURVIVAL RATES	CHI-SQUARE	PROBABILITY (III = IV)
0–1	III	412	18	394	.956	3.54 2.90*	<.10, >.05
	IV	226	18	208	.920		
1–2	III	394	34	360	.874	20.2	.001
	IV	208	45	163	.722		
2–3	III	360	38	322	.781	20.0	.001
	IV	163	42	121	.535		
3–4	III	322	40	282	.683	4.77	<.05, >.02
	IV	121	25	96	.425		
4–5	III	282	25	257	.623	11.34	.001
	IV	96	21	75	.332		
Total	III	412	155	257	.623	49.8	.001
	IV	226	151	75	.332		

* With Yates correction.

an evaluation is best accomplished by comparing the mortality data of the two groups presented in "life" tables. These tables present the data arranged as in Table 55-7. The principal advantage of this method of reporting mortality from cancer is that it permits all data accumulated to be used. In other words, patients followed only 1, 2, or 3 years contribute useful information to mortality data even though they cannot be counted as part of an "absolute 5-year survival or mortality rate." In order to use the life-table method of reporting mortality data the facts about the persons in the series which must be known are the intervals from treatment (or diagnosis) to death, or to last follow-up date. It is then possible to tabulate the data as illustrated in Table 55-7.[2]

In order to determine whether or not the survival rates from one life table are significantly higher or lower than those of another life table one of three methods may be used: (1) the chi-square test applied to the specific mortality data of each interval, (2) the comparison of the standard error of the accumulative survival rates, or (3) the determination of confidence limits by analysis of the data using the method of probits. An example of the chi-square method is shown in Table 55-8 where the data for each interval have been arranged essentially in a two by two contingency table. The chi-square value for the interval 0 to 1 years is given as 3.54. However, because the frequency of dying is quite small in this interval, the Yates correction should be used. The correction is made by subtracting $\frac{1}{2}N$ from the difference (ad − bc) before squaring. In other words, for interval 0 to 1 years:

$$\chi^2 = \frac{(394 \times 18 - 208 \times 18 - \frac{638}{2})^2}{412 \times 266 \times 36 \times 602} = 2.90,$$

and the probability that the mortality rates from Type III and Type IV mammary cancers are the same for this interval still are $<.10 >.05$.

TABLE 55-9. SURVIVAL FROM TYPES III AND IV MAMMARY CANCER TREATED BY RADICAL MASTECTOMY

YEARS AT RISK	TYPE	(N) EFFECTIVE NUMBER AT RISK	(d) NUMBER DYING IN INTERVAL	(q) PROPORTION DYING IN INTERVAL	$\frac{q}{N-d}$	(P) ACCUMULATIVE SURVIVAL RATES	STANDARD ERROR* OF ACCUMULATIVE SURVIVAL RATES
0–1	III	412	18	.0437	.000111	.956	.0101
	IV	226	18	.0796	.000327	.920	.0167
1–2	III	394	34	.0863	.000239	.874	.0164
	IV	208	45	.2163	.001327	.722	.0294
2–3	III	360	38	.1056	.000328	.781	.0203
	IV	163	42	.2577	.002130	.535	.0329
3–4	III	322	40	.1240	.000440	.683	.0228
	IV	121	25	.2066	.002157	.425	.0328
4–5	III	282	25	.0887	.000345	.623	.0240
	IV	96	21	.2188	.002917	.332	.0312
Total	III				.001463		
	IV				.008853		

* See text.

The formula for calculating the *standard errors of accumulative survival rates* is:

$$(1)\ s_D = Px \sqrt{\frac{q_1}{N_1 - d_1} + \frac{q_2}{N_2 - d_2} \cdots \frac{q_x}{N_x - d_x}}$$

If the number of cases is unaffected by any being lost to follow-up or withdrawn because of lack of a long follow-up, the formula becomes:

$$(2)\ s_D = \frac{P \times Q}{N} \qquad Q = (1 - p)$$

Since the data in our example (Table 55-9) are complete (none lost or withdrawn) the standard error of the 5-years accumulative survival rates may be calculated using either formula (1) or (2). For example:

The accumulative survival rate ± 2 standard errors defines the 95 per cent confidence limits. From the calculations above we find no overlap of the 62.3% ± 4.8% and 33.2% ± 6.2% confidence limits of the 5-year accumulative survival rates from Types III and IV mammary cancer. Therefore, we conclude that the 5-year survival rate after radical mastectomy for Type III mammary cancer is significantly greater than the 5-year survival rate after radical mastectomy for Type IV cancers.

Analysis of mortality from cancer in man by the *method of probits* permits rather precise definition of time-mortality relationships for various types of metastasizing visceral neoplasms. Dying from the major types of human cancers occurs at such times after diagnosis or treatment as to constitute a log-normal

Type III cancer—(1) Standard error $= .623 \sqrt{.001463} = .024$
or
(2) Standard error $= \dfrac{.623 \times .377}{412} = .024$

Type IV cancer— (1) Standard error $= .332 \sqrt{.008853} = .031$
or
(2) Standard error $= \dfrac{.332 \times .668}{226} = .031$

Frequency Distribution of the Mortality from Mammary Cancer After Radical Mastectomy

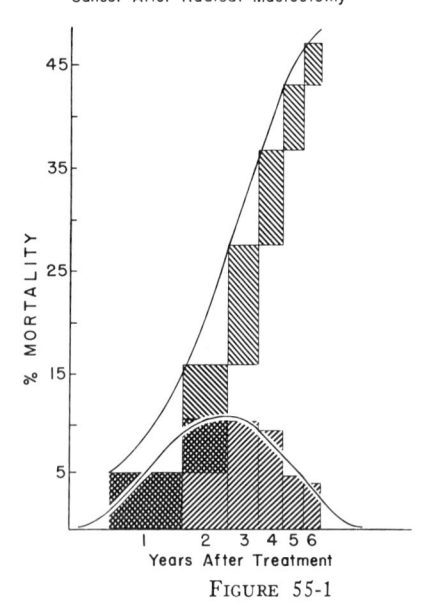

FIGURE 55-1

distribution. In other words, the rates of dying are initially low soon after therapy, increase thereafter to a maximum and finally return to rates not much higher than normal. This distribution is skewed if time is plotted linearly, but if the logarithm of time is used, the mortality data produce a roughly normal bell-shaped curve (i.e., a log-normal distribution, Fig. 55-1). If the specific interval mortalities are accumulatively summed and plotted against log-time, a sigmoid curve (ogive) results. Transforming the data to probits merely converts this ogive to a straight line which can be much more easily defined mathematically and statistically. The merit of the analysis of data by the method of probits lies in the fact that the log-normal distribution of times of dying after the onset of a disease, the administration of a poison or the diagnosis of cancer is the biologic rule. Both the biologic behaviors and the relative lethal-

TABLE 55-10. TYPE IV MAMMARY CANCER

YEARS OBSERVED	LOG-TIME (x)	NUMBER OF PATIENTS FOLLOWED (N)	PATIENTS DEAD NUMBER	%	EMPIRICAL PROBIT*	EXPECTED PROBIT† (Y)	WORKING PROBIT‡ (y)	WEIGHTING COEFFICIENT (W)§
1	0.00	226	18	7.9	3.59	3.64	3.60	.315
2	0.30	226	63	27.9	4.41	4.40	4.42	.558
3	0.48	226	105	46.5	4.91	4.83	4.91	.629
4	0.60	226	130	57.5	5.19	5.14	5.19	.631
5	0.70	226	151	66.8	5.43	5.38	5.44	.604
6	.78	226	158	69.9	5.52	5.58	5.52	.560

* Empirical probit read from table transforming percentages to probits.
† Expected probit is read from line drawn by estimation through the empirical probit points.
‡ Working probit, a correction of the expected probit obtained from appropriate tables, is used in the actual calculations (Table IV, see Finney,[3] p. 296).
§ The weighting coefficients (W) for N is found for each expected probit from the proper table.

ness of various human neoplasms are precisely defined by studying their time-mortality relationships.

The calculations for defining the linear equation best fitting the probit transformation of mortality data will be illustrated in order to clarify the technic, although computer programs now available permit such analyses without the necessity for such tedious manual work. The data are first arranged as shown in Table 55-10. Next the tabulations and the calculations shown in Table 55-11 are completed. The formulae used in the actual calculations for fitting of the weighted probit regression line are as follows:

$$\text{mean } x = \bar{x} = \frac{\Sigma nwx}{\Sigma nw} = \frac{385.9}{745.2} = .52$$

$$\text{mean } y = \bar{y} = \frac{\Sigma nwy}{\Sigma nw} = \frac{3693}{745.2} = 4.95$$

$$\text{Probit slope (b)} = \frac{\Sigma xy}{\Sigma xx} = \Sigma nw\,(x-\bar{x})(y-\bar{y}) = \frac{\Sigma nwxy + \Sigma nw\bar{x}\bar{y} - \Sigma nwx\bar{y} - \Sigma nw\bar{x}y}{\Sigma nwx^2 - 2\Sigma nwx\bar{x} + \Sigma nw\bar{x}^2}$$

Substituting $\frac{\Sigma nwx}{\Sigma nw}$ and $\frac{\Sigma nwy}{\Sigma nw}$ for $\bar{x}$ and $\bar{y}$, respectively,

$$b = \frac{\Sigma nwxy - \frac{\Sigma nwy \times \Sigma nwx}{\Sigma nw}}{\Sigma nwx^2 - \frac{(\Sigma nwx)^2}{\Sigma nw}} = \frac{\Sigma nwxy - \bar{x}\Sigma nwy}{\Sigma nwx^2 - \bar{x}\Sigma nwx}$$

(This conversion of the initial formula for probit slope simplifies the calculation.)
Substituting calculations from Table 55-11:

$$b = \frac{2011.2 - (.52 \times 3693)}{239.34 - (.52 \times 385.0)} = \frac{98.8}{39.5} = 2.5$$

Probit $Y = 4.95 + 2.5x - (2.5 \times .52)$
$Y = 2.50\,x + 3.65$ (see Fig. 55-2)

The confidence limits can now be calculated for any mortality value using formulae and tables presented by Bliss.[1] For example, at 50 per cent mortality (where $Y = 5$) the variance about the time of 50 per cent mortality =

$$Vm_1 = \frac{(S_1)^2}{N} \times E$$

(E is a constant for a given value of x' from tables by Bliss)

1822 Mathematical Analysis of Surgical Data

Probit Lines of Mortality from Mammary Cancer

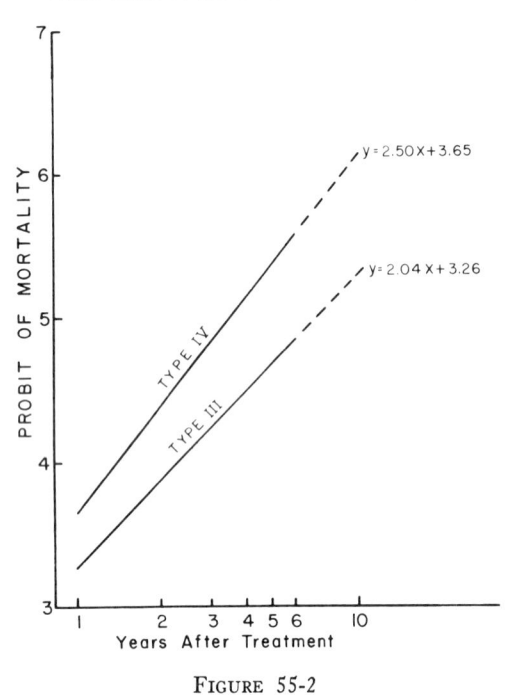

$y = 2.50x + 3.65$

$y = 2.04x + 3.26$

TYPE IV

TYPE III

Years After Treatment

FIGURE 55-2

Mortality Expectancy from Epidermoid Carcinoma of the Anus

(Probit $y = 1.62x + 2.68$) (N = 75)

Point of Truncation

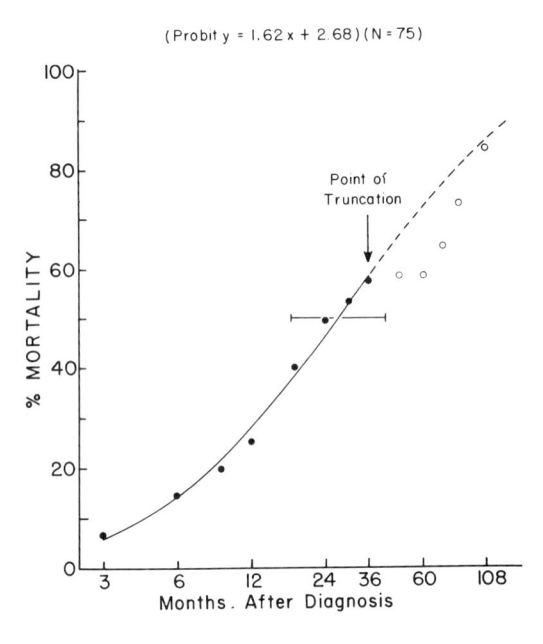

Months After Diagnosis

FIGURE 55-4

Mortality Expectancy from Mammary Cancer

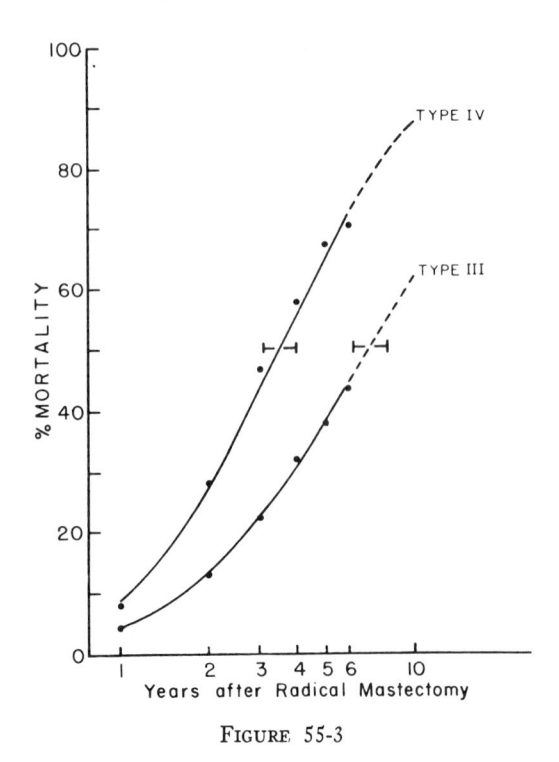

TYPE IV

TYPE III

Years after Radical Mastectomy

FIGURE 55-3

MORTALITY EXPECTANCY FROM GASTRIC CARCINOMA

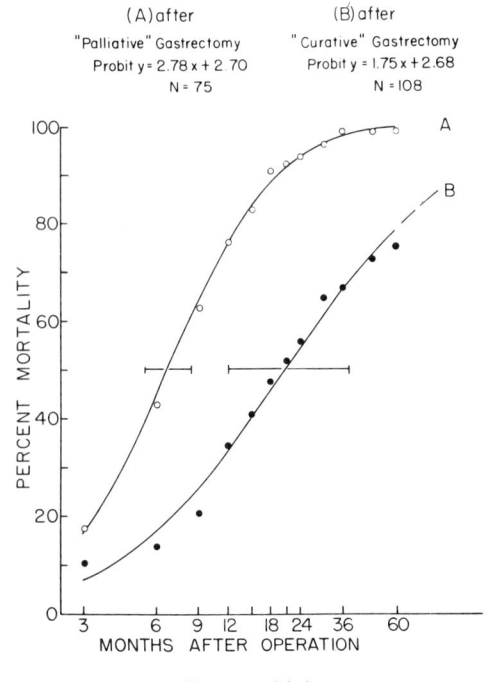

(A) after "Palliative" Gastrectomy
Probit $y = 2.78x + 2.70$
N = 75

(B) after "Curative" Gastrectomy
Probit $y = 1.75x + 2.68$
N = 108

MONTHS AFTER OPERATION

FIGURE 55-5

TABLE 55-11. CALCULATIONS FOR FITTING WEIGHTED PROBIT REGRESSION LINE

x	n	w*	nw	y	nwx	nwy	nwx²	nwxy	nwy²
.00	226	.315	71.2	3.60	0.0	256.3	0.0	0.0	922.6
.30	226	.558	126.1	4.42	37.8	557.4	11.34	167.1	2463.5
.48	226	.629	142.2	4.91	68.2	698.0	32.75	335.0	3427.1
.60	226	.631	142.6	5.19	85.6	740.1	51.34	444.1	3841.2
.70	226	.640	136.5	5.44	95.6	742.6	66.92	520.1	4039.5
.78	226	.560	126.6	5.52	98.7	698.6	76.99	544.9	3856.3
			745.2		385.9	3693.0	239.34	2011.2	18550.2
			Σnw		Σnwx	Σnwy	Σnwx²	Σnwxy	Σnwy²

* Weighting coefficient.

$$x' = \frac{t - m_1}{S_1}$$

$m_1 = x = .54$ (from $y = 5.0 - 2.5x + 3.65$)

t = point of truncation (the point in log-time where the data no longer fit the probit line derived from the rates of dying before this)

t = 0.78

S_1 = the difference in value of x when y varies by 1. When $y = 4$, $x = .14$. Therefore $S_1 = .54 - .14 = .40$

Then $x' = \frac{.78 - .54}{.40} = 0.6$, from proper table (Bliss), $E = 1.56$ when $x' = 0.6$

So $Vm_1 = \frac{(.40)^2}{226} \times 1.56 = .001104$

Standard deviation $= \sqrt{Vm_1} = .0332$

Thus the 95 per cent confidence limits about the log-time of 50 per cent mortality (0.54) from Type IV mammary cancer are 0.54 ± .065. Converting log-time to years, the time of 50 per cent mortality = 3.47 years with 95 per cent confidence limits from 2.98 to 4.03 years.

A similar application of the method of probits to the mortality data from Type III mammary cancer (Table 55-9) shows that Probit Y = 2.04x + 3.26. The time of 50 per cent mortality rate is 7.1 years, the 95 per cent confidence limits extending from 6.2 to 8.2 years. Obviously, 50 per cent of the deaths from Type IV cancer occurred significantly sooner than did 50 per cent of the deaths from Type III cancer of the breast. This is shown graphically in Figure 55-3. The confidence limits about the time of 50 per cent mortality are shown on the mortality expectancy curve derived from the fitted probit regression line. Other graphic examples of the application of the method of probits for the analysis of mortality data from cancer are shown in Figures 55-4 and 55-5.

REFERENCES

1. Bliss, C. I.: The calculation of the time mortality curve. Ann. Appl. Biol., 24:815-852, 1937.
2. Cutler, S. J., and Ederer, F.: Maximum utilization of the life table method in analyzing survival. J. Chron. Dis., 8:699-712, 1958.
3. Finney, D. J.: Probit Analysis: A Statistical Treatment of the Sigmoid Response Curve. Cambridge Univ. Press, 1952.
4. Johnson, P. O.: Statistical Methods in Research. New York, Prentice-Hall, 1949.
5. Mainland, D.: The use and misuse of statistics in medical publications. Clin. Pharm. Therap. 1:411-422, 1960.
6. ———: Elementary Medical Statistics. ed. 2. Philadelphia, W. B. Saunders, 1963.
7. Snedecor, G. W.: Statistical Methods Applied to Experiments in Agriculture and Biology. ed. 5. Ames, Iowa, Iowa State Univ. Press, 1956.

Bibliographic Index

Abbott, L. C., 1667, 1698
Abbott, M. E., 1261, 1265
Abbott, O. A., 1377
Abbott, W. O., 108
Abel, J. J., 787
Aberle, S. B. P., 1646
Abernathy, R. S., 651
Abrahamsen, A. F., 952
Aceto, T., 783
Ackerman, 661
Ackerman, L. V., 934, 1732
Ackerman, N. B., 789
Ackermann, W., 868
Adair, F. E., 679, 705
Adams, F., 947
Adams, J. P., 1631
Adams, W. E., 171, 1397
Adamsons, R. J., 16
Adler, R. H., 993, 1243
Adner, M. M., 951
Aegerter, E., 1664, 1712
Aho, A. S., 1664
Aird, I., 840, 1244
Alberman, E. D., 1685
Albers, J. H., 1108
Albert, S. N., 132
Albertini, von A., 733
Albright, F., 708, 730, 731, 778, 1625, 1668, 1669, 1670
Albright, H. L., 832
Alexander, C., 1690
Alexander, J. W., 16
Ali, M., 1242
Allbritten, F. F., Jr., 126, 1407
Allen, A., 1717
Allen, A. C., 659
Allen, A. W., 108, 909
Allen, E., 1575
Allen, E. W., 1317
Allen, J. G., 122, 174, 176, 184, 187, 188, 417, 843, 951, 1010, 1014, 1019, 1242
Allen, R. A., 864
Alley, R. D., 1306
Allison, P. R., 806, 832, 834, 1228, 1229, 1234
Almkov, J. R., 1505
Almy, T. P., 1117
Alonso-Lej, F., 1514
Alpen, E. L., 420
Alpert, S., 1514
Altemeier, W. A., 47, 135, 638, 1050, 1056, 1182, 1183
Amberg, J. R., 831, 836
Amsler, F. R., 1742

Anderson, L. D., 1666
Anderson, R. E., 432, 1184, 1194
Anderson, R. L., 801
Andresen, R. H., 28
Andrews, 1205
Andrews, E., 122, 1208, 1220
Andrews, E. W., 856
Andrews, G. A., 420
Andrews, R. P., 12
Annandale, T., 1222
Anson, B. J., 1211, 1246
Anspach, W. E., 1662
Anthonsen, W., 1699
Antopol, W., 16
Appleby, L. H., 864
Applezweig, N., 764
Arct, M. W., 1716
Arguedas, J. M., 28
Arhelger, S. W., 846, 849
Ariel, I. M., 1491
Aristotle, 149-150, 362, 947
Arminski, T. C., 1141
Armstrong, W. D., 1659
Arnheim, E. E., 1498
Arons, M. S., 1482
Aronson, A. R., 1115
Arrants, J. E., 865
Artz, C. P., 129, 616
Ascari, W. Q., 166
Asch, T., 672
Aschner, P. W., 1628
Ash, J. E., 1622
Askanazy, M., 730
Asteriadon-Samartzis, E., 115
Astwood, E. B., 714, 716, 718
Atkins, H., 708
Atkinson, M., 797
Atkinson, P. J., 1669
Attenborough, G. G., 1685
Atwater, J. S., 1141
Aub, J. C., 731
August, J. T., 1590
Ault, G. W., 1161, 1165
Austen, K. F., 439
Aylett, S. O., 1120

Babcock, W. W., 922, 1134, 1167, 1219
Bachra, B., 1662
Bacon, H. E., 1130, 1151
Baden, H., 1183
Badger, T. L., 1715
Badgley, C. E., 1692
Baffes, T. G., 1279

Bahnson, H. T., 1342, 1344
Bailey, C. P., 1272, 1288
Baird, R. J., 1352
Bakalim, G., 1715
Baker, L., 1699
Baker, W. N. W., 1054
Ballenger, E. G., 1630
Balogh, K., 1665
Banks, H. H., 1667
Banting, F. G., 926, 929
Barber, K. W., Jr., 1039
Barbosa, J. J., 942
Barclay, A. E., 820
Barclay, T. H. C., 868
Bardenheier, J. A., III, 1709
Bargen, J. A., 1152
Baritell, A. L. M., 1219
Barker, W. F., 136, 943, 1325
Barling, S., 867
Barlow, T. E., 820, 984, 988
Barner, H. B., 1326
Barnes, A. B., 1023
Barnes, D. W. H., 949
Barnes, R. B., 689
Barnes, W. A., 1083
Barnett, W. O., 127
Baronofsky, I. D., 132, 1000
Barrett, J. H., 798
Barrett, N. R., 832, 833, 834, 835, 1232
Barrington, 1044
Barron, J., 1195
Bartholin, 1244
Bartlett, M. K., 1134
Bartlett, W., 1195
Basedow, von, C. A., 716
Bassett, C. A. L., 1663, 1664
Bassini, E., 1205, 1221
Batson, O. V., 1623
Baudet, R., 961
Bauer, K. H., 820
Bauer, W., 730, 731
Baum, S., 842
Bauman, L., 934
Bayliss, W. H., 189
Bazy, L., 1325
Beadle, O. A., 1740
Beahrs, O. H., 720
Beal, J. M., 851
Bean, W. B., 1345
Beardmore, H. E., 1526
Beardsley, J. M., 1234
Beatson, G. T., 705
Beaumont, W., 4

Bechtol, C. O., 1666
Beck, C. S., 1283, 1286
Becker, R. O., 1663
Becker, V., 919
Beebe, G. W., 601
Beecher, H. K., 140, 241
Beeson, P. B., 108, 1614
Begg, R. C., 1519, 1645
Behrend, A., 862, 863
Bell, L. G., 863, 864
Beloff, A., 362
Bender, S., 1574, 1577
Bendixen, 259
Bennett, D., 1306
Bennett, G. A., 1720
Bennett, H. D., 1015
Bennett, R. C., 1187
Bensaude, R., 1527
Benson, C. D., 1507
Bentley, F. H., 820
Berard, C. W., 18
Bergkvist, A., 898
Bergman, H. C., 139
Berk, J. E., 887, 932
Berk, M., 869
Berkowitz, H. D., 884
Berkson, J., 850
Berliner, D., 1661
Berliner, R. W., 1589
Berman, E. F., 812
Berman, E. J., 840
Bernard, C., 773
Berne, C. J., 134, 845, 865, 1234
Bernstein, E. F., 1349
Berry, R. E. L., 1324
Berry, W. C., 1233
Berstein, J. E., 1015
Berti, 866
Best, R. R., 1167
Bevan, A. D., 1249
Bevan, G., 187
Beyer, K. H., 1589
Bielschowsky, F., 716
Bierman, H. R., 1007, 1027
Bierman, L. G., 994
Biggs, T. M., 1108
Bill, A. H., 1497
Bill, A. H., Jr., 1182
Billingham, R. E., 28
Bing, R. J., 128
Birt, A. B., 1222
Bisgard, J. D., 887
Biström, O., 28
Bizzozero, J., 957
Bjork, V. O., 1272, 1398
Black, D. A. K., 1585, 1592
Blackwood, H. J., 1662

Bibliographic Index

Blades, B., 1234, 1385, 1398, 1413
Blain, A., III, 1324
Blaisdell, P. C., 1197
Blakemore, A. H., 241, 1350, 1352
Blakemore, W. S., 1582
Blalock, A., 26, 27, 122, 123, 155, 728, 789, 1275, 1276, 1278, 1279, 1411
Blau, M., 1732
Blegen, H. M., 868
Bleich, A. R., 1624
Block, M. H., 955
Bloodwell, R. D., 1332
Blount, W. P., 1698, 1703
Blum, T., 429
Blumberg, B. S., 187
Blumenthal, I. S., 840
Blumgart, H. L., 723
Blundell, J., 947
Blundell, John, 152
Boas, N. F., 717
Bockus, H. L., 104, 893, 1142
Bodian, M., 1525
Boerema, I., 140, 1234
Boerhaave, H., 861, 864
Bogardus, G. M., 830, 951
Boles, E. T., 1034
Boley, J. S., 1511
Boley, S. J., 1111
Bolten, K. A., 1550
Boman, K., 860
Bombeck, C. T., 833
Bonica, J. J., 126
Bonser, G. M., 680
Booher, R. J., 862
Book, D. T., 827
Borden, F. W., 126
Borella, L., 1709
Bors, E., 1637
Bosher, L. H., Jr., 834
Bosshardt, D. K., 919
Bosworth, D. M., 1723, 1725, 1744
Bounous, G., 130, 140
Bourne, G. H., 1665
Bovie, W. T., 773
Bower, J. O., 1041, 1042
Bowers, R. F., 927
Boyce, F. F., 849, 1024, 1040, 1041
Boyce, W. H., 1625, 1626, 1627
Boyd, A. K., 219
Boyd, A. M., 1323
Boyd, G., 798
Boyd, H. B., 1666
Boyd, W., 1599
Boyden, A. M., 849, 1134
Boyden, E. A., 1373
Boyes, J., 1727, 1728
Braasch, J. W., 1228

Braasch, W. F., 1580, 1615, 1644
Brackney, E. L., 826
Bradley, S. E., 1585
Brahms, M. A., 1736, 1737
Brandborg, L. L., 836
Branham, H. H., 1314
Brant, J., 868
Brauer, L., 1396
Braunwald, N. S., 28
Brayton, D., 1182
Brennan, M. J., 230
Brenner, R. L., 868
Brent, L., 442
Breslow, L., 674, 675, 676, 700
Brittain, R. S., 1325
Brock, R. C., 1270, 1275, 1350, 1373, 1382, 1505
Brodie, B. C., 1355, 1707
Brohm, 955
Bronwell, A. S., 623
Brooke, B. N., 24, 1128
Brossy, J. J., 1187
Brown, A. L., 156
Brown, D. B., 1134
Brown, J. B., 1441, 1443, 1446, 1461, 1468, 1477, 1480, 1482
Brown, J. G., 1025
Brown, J. H. U., 748
Brown, L. T., 1740
Brown, P. M., 851
Brown, R. K., 1205, 1227
Browne, D., 1527
Bruce, J., 821
Bruce, J., Sir, 4
Brucer, M., 411
Brunner, J. M., 1727
Bruno, M. S., 861
Brunschwig, A., 219, 930, 937, 943
Bryant, J. F., 1235
Bryant, L. R., 831
Buchbinder, J. H., 962
Buckwalter, J. A., 1198
Buenger, R. E., 1334
Buerger, L., 1298, 1334
Buhl, 365
Bulmer, J. H., 1708
Bunch, G. H., 1110
Bunge, R. G., 1580
Bunker, J. P., 171, 175
Bunstock, W. H., 1197
Burch, P. R. S., 1728
Burchenal, J. H., 231
Burchell, A. R., 1005, 1015, 1016
Burchell, H. B., 1345
Burdette, W. J., 842
Burge, H. W., 855
Burgerman, A., 868
Burne, J., 1024
Burnet, M., 225, 226

Burns, E., 1646
Burrow, G. N., 432
Burt, C. A. V., 1109, 1110
Burton, C. C., 1211, 1219, 1247
Buschke, F., 1622
Bushnell, L. F., 1541
Butcher, H. R., Jr., 1163
Butler, T. J., 857
Butters, A. G., 1222, 1247
Byars, L. T., 1496
Byrd, B. F., 841
Byrne, J. J., 1099
Bystrov, N. V., 923
Bywaters, E. G. L., 129

Cabieses, F., 830
Cabot, H., 1614
Cáceres, E., 126
Cady, B., 1161
Cahan, W. G., 429
Cahill, K., 911
Caine, M., 1634
Caldwell, F. T., Jr., 377, 390
Caldwell, G. D., 1697
Calem, W. S., 994
Callaghan, P. J., 1043
Callisen, H., 1247
Calman, C., 1080
Calvé, 1692, 1695
Cameron, A. L., 917
Cameron, D. A., 1661
Camishion, R. C., 1408, 1412
Cammock, E. E., 842
Campbell, D. A., 886
Campbell, E., 618, 619
Campbell, M. F., 1608, 1645
Campbell, R. E., 864
Cannaday, J. E., 1242, 1243
Cannon, J. A., 28, 1325
Cannon, P., 103
Cannon, P. R., 1041, 1042
Cannon, W. B., 123, 124, 154
Cantor, M. O., 1093
Cantrell, J. R., 1499
Capps, J. A., 1044
Card, W. I., 821
Carey, J. M., 1228
Carlens, E., 1407
Carlson, R. I., 1205
Carpenter, G., 971
Carr, H. E., Jr., 774
Carrel, A., 26, 1267, 1298
Carroll, G., 1625
Carson, T. E., 642
Carter, B. N., 1233
Carter, R., 1059
Carter, R. L., 1620
Carver, G. M., Jr., 833

Castleman, B., 733, 734, 1142
Casuccio, C., 1669
Cattell, R. B., 931, 933, 934, 938, 941, 942
Cayley, C. K., 1506
Celestin, L. R., 812
Celsus, 11, 45
Ceppellini, R., 158
Cerenville, 1396
Chamberlain, J. M., 1399
Chambers, E. K., 1626
Chambers, J. S., 1408, 1412
Chandler, F. A., 1699
Chapman, E. M., 719
Chapman, N. D., 824, 827
Chase, S. W., 1666, 1667
Chassin, J. L., 28, 1238
Chauffard, A., 965
Cheatle, G. L., 1223
Cheetham, J. G., 1628
Cherkes, N. D., 1731
Cherney, L. S., 1209
Chiazze, L., Jr., 1568
Child, C. G., 996, 1000
Child, C. G., III, 930, 937
Chouke, K. S., 1251
Chunn, C. F., 1109
Churchill, E. D., 730, 735, 1373, 1384, 1398, 1407, 1408
Clairmont, P., 1059
Clark, C. W., 840
Clark, D. E., 412, 428
Clark, J. H., 1211
Clarke, J. S., 824, 1012
Clatworthy, H. W., Jr., 1212
Clawson, D. K., 1705, 1706, 1707, 1710
Clay, R. C., 1499
Cleveland, M., 1713, 1715
Cliffton, E. E., 932
Cloquet, J., 1247
Cloutier, C. T., 642
Cloward, 1796
Cochran, G., 1663
Code, C. F., 829
Cogan, D. G., 735
Cohen, N., 937
Cohen, P., 952
Cohen, S. N., 176, 186
Cohn, I., Jr., 708
Cohn, J. N., 133
Cohn, R., 1018, 1272
Colcock, B. P., 1120, 1154, 1159, 1168
Cole, L. J., 949
Cole, P. P., 1242
Cole, W. H., 233, 785, 909, 957, 1162, 1163
Coleman, S., 1680
Coller, F. A., 22, 79, 126, 845, 1323

Collett, R. W., 1515
Collins, D. H., 1718
Collins, J. D., 1217
Collins, V. P., 211
Collip, J. B., 730
Coman, D. R., 209
Compere, E. L., 1695, 1707, 1740
Comroe, J. H., 1374
Condon, R. E., 1223
Conn, H. O., 1015
Conn, J. W., 774, 784, 929, 1590, 1602
Connar, R. C., 856
Connell, J. F., Jr., 10
Connolly, J. E., 992
Connolly, D. P., 1239
Connor, T. B., 1603
Contugno, M., 1740
Conway, H., 18, 28, 695
Cook, G. B., 1159
Cooke, W. T., 1074
Cooley, D. A., 1360
Cooley, J. C., 1698
Coombs, R. R. A., 952, 971, 976
Cooper, A., 1251
Cooper, D. Y., 774, 884
Cooper, W. A., 886
Cope, O., 720, 725, 733, 736, 778, 779
Cope, Z., 1029, 1043
Copher, G. H., 1662
Coran, A. G., 1037
Cordero, L., 1619
Cordonnier, J. K., 1510
Cori, C. F., 776
Cormie, J., 1195
Cornes, J. S., 1191
Correa, R. J., Jr., 1603
Corry, R. J., 435
Cotlar, A. M., 962
Cottrell, J. C., 870
Counsellor, V. S., 1107
Coupal, J. F., 638
Courmelles, de F., 706
Courtiss, E. H., 19
Courvoisier, 899
Coventry, M. B., 1690, 1719, 1740
Cowley, L. L., 869
Cowley, R. A., 140
Cox, C. E., 1614
Cox, E. V., 1073
Crabtree, E. C., 1613
Crafoord, C., 1015, 1266
Crawford, E. S., 1325, 1332, 1352
Craighead, C. C., 869
Creevy, C. D., 1608
Crego, C. H., Jr., 1682
Crellin, R. Q., 1719
Crenshaw, A. H., 1725
Crichlow, R. W., 1352

Crile, G., Jr., 24, 1018
Cripps, 1148
Crocker, D. W., 1603
Crohn, B. B., 1114, 1118, 1120
Cronkite, E. P., 416, 417
Crosby, W. H., 171
Crowder, V. H., Jr., 1158
Crowell, J. W., 121, 127
Cruickshank, C. N. D., 362
Cruveilhier, J., 997
Cseuz, K. A., 1726
Curii, A. R., 764
Curling, 830
Curtis, G. M., 958
Curtiss, P. H., 1709
Cushing, H., 770, 772, 773, 774, 777, 778, 780, 781, 825, 830, 863, 1775
Cushman, G. F., 125
Cuthbertson, A. M., 10
Cuthbertson, D. P., 104, 105
Cutler, E. C., 863, 1288
Cutler, S. J., 1819

Da Costa, J. M., 932
Dahl, O., 1631
Dahlin, D., 1674, 1733
Dainko, E. A., 918
Daland, E. M., 697, 703
Dale, W. A., 1325
Dam, H., 114, 901
Dameshek, W., 952
Dandy, W. E., 1740, 1755, 1771
Danes, B. S., 1680
D'Antoni, J. S., 1112
Darbyshire, R. C., 1727
Darling, R. C., 1303, 1325
David, C., 1002
Davis, 1001
Davis, C. E., Jr., 1245
Davis, J. B., 1331
Davis, J. E., 1728
Davis, J. O., 785
Davis, M. E., 1573
Dawson, 965, 968
Day, J. J., 826
Day, P. L., 1741
Dean, A. L., 1624
Deaver, J. B., 1, 1042
De Bakey, M., 861, 1113, 1305, 1323, 1329, 1332, 1334, 1342, 1346, 1349, 1350, 1359
DeCamp, P. T., 1329
Decker, H. R., 1391
de Dombal, F. T., 1152
de Lamotte, J., 1024
Deming, C. L., 1611

Dempster, W. J., 28
DeMuth, W. E., 991, 1073, 1120
De Nicola, R. R., 1246
Denis, J. B., 152
Denisart, P., 1246
Dennis, C., 938, 1209, 1210
Dennison, W., 1497
Denny-Brown, D., 1634, 1637
Dent, C. E., 1626
Deol, J. S., 1056
DePusky, 1740
DeSaussure, R. L., 1743
Desnuelle, P., 918
de Takats, G., 1324, 1350
Deterling, R. A., 1363
Devine, H. B., 839
De Vito, R. V., 19, 833, 1233
Devitt, J. E. 679
DeWeese, M. S., 1325, 1360
Diamond, L. K. 968
Dick, A. P., 992
Dick, B. M., 924
Dickinson, P. H., 1737
Dillard, D. H., 1228, 1346
Dillard, G. H. L., 182
Dilley, R. B., 1286
DiLuzio, N. R., 885
Dionne, L., 1162
Ditzler, J. W., 126
Diveley, W., 1391
Dmochowski, L., 225
Dobbins, W. O., 864
Dobyns, B. M., 717
Dodson, A. I., 1632
Doll, R., 1402
Dollinger, M. R., 1148
Dolphin, J. A., 835
Donald, D. C., 1211
Donald, J. D., 888
Donaldson, G. A., 1359
Donhauser, J. L., 1100
Donovan, E. J., 1513
Doran, F. S. A., 1218, 1224, 1242
Dorfman, R. A., 756, 758
Dormandy, T. L., 1136
Dorsey, J. W., 1608
dos Santos, J. C., 1325
Dos Santos, R., 1731
Doubilet, H., 926
Dougherty, T. F., 727
Douglas, P., 1631
Dowidar, M. L., 961
Drabkin, D. L., 116
Dragstedt, L. R., 24, 822, 823, 825, 826, 829, 830, 831, 835, 854, 919, 1092
Drapanas, T., 933, 1002, 1072

Dreiling, D. A., 861, 919
Dresen, K-A., 1181
Drew, J. H., 121
Dripps, R. D., 244
Druckerman, L. J., 221
Drummond, D., 1018
Dubach, R., 117
Du Bost, C., 1350
Dudrick, J. J., 111
Dudrick, S. J., 1494
Duffy, B. J., Jr., 428
Duhamel, B., 1526
Dukes, C. E., 1127, 1148, 1149, 1168, 1175
Dumont, A. E., 1003
Duncan, G. W., 132
Dundee, J. W., 246
Dunlop, J., 493-495
Dunn, H. L., 840
Dunphy, J. E., 10, 924, 1161, 1167, 1168, 1183, 1190
Dupuytren, B. G., 1024, 1205
Dupuytren, G., 594
Duraiswami, P. K., 1680
Durham, M. W., 1128
Dustan, H. P., 1602
Duthie, H. L., 1178
Duthie, R. B., 1660, 1664, 1665
Du Vigneaud, R. C., 753
du Vigneaud, V., 773
Dye, W. S., 1301, 1305, 1334

Eagleson, W., 1663
Earley, L. E., 1596, 1597
Eastloe, J. E., 1661
Easton, E. R., 1221
Ebeling, W. W., 108
Ebert, R. V., 948
Ebrahim, G. J., 1706
Edelman, S., 710
Edenbuizen, M., 364, 381
Edgerton, M. T., 28, 815
Edkins, J. S., 823
Edmunds, L. H., Jr., 1352
Edsal, D. L., 108
Edsall, G., 637
Edwards, H. C., 839, 849
Edwards, L. C., 10
Edwards, W. S., 128, 1306, 1325
Effler, D. B., 1286, 1363
Egan, R. L., 688, 689
Egbert, L. D., 244
Egdahl, R. H., 970, 1022
Eggers, G. W., 1699
Ehrenfeld, W. K., 1326
Ehrenpreis, T., 1526
Eickelberger, J., 1659

Bibliographic Index

Eiseman, B., 1039, 1306
Eisenberg, H. L., 1152
Eisenhammer, S., 1175, 1180, 1181, 1187, 1188, 1189, 1190, 1191, 1192
Eker, R., 845, 866
Elias, E. G., 1026
Eliason, O. E., 1711
Elkin, D. C., 1313, 1314, 1322
Ellison, E. H., 831, 832
Elman, R., 825, 1207
Emmett, J. L., 1580
Engberg, H., 126
Engel, F. L., 386, 392
Engel, M. B., 1662
Enneking, W., 1664
Enquist, I. F., 1144, 1210
Enterline, H. T., 1142, 1143
Eppinger, H., 950
Epstein, J. A., 1741
Epstein, S. E., 786
Eraklis, A. J., 951
Erasistratus, 149
Erdheim, J., 730
Errico, M. J., 1666
Erwald, R., 679, 1242
Estabrook, R. W., 884
Estes, J. E., Jr., 1348
Estes, W. L., Jr., 1236
Evans, E. I., 371
Evans, J., 771
Evans, J. A., 898
Evans, R. S., 952, 957
Evans, T. N., 1536
Evans, W. E., 140
Evelagos, E., 1722
Everson, T. C., 839, 860, 1149
Ewald, F., 1663
Ewell, G. H., 1631

Faber, K., 1110
Fairbank, T. H., 1690
Fallis, L. S., 940, 1208, 1220
Fallon, M., 1503
Fallot, A., 1273-1277
Farhat, S. M., 16
Farmer, D. A., 827, 854
Farrar, H. K., Jr., 1551
Farrar, L. K. P., 179
Farringer, J. L., Jr., 1043
Farris, J. M., 856, 1227
Fasano, M., 1247
Faust, E. C., 1112
Feldman, M., 865
Felty, A. R., 965
Ferguson, A. B., 1692
Ferguson, A. B., Jr., 1719
Ferguson, A. H., 1205
Ferguson, J. A., 1184

Ferguson, L. K., 850, 868, 1190
Fernbach, D. J., 230
Fernel, 1024
Fevold, H. L., 765
Fick, R., 1740
Fieber, S. S., 863
Figiel, L. S., 1099, 1100
Finch, 156
Fine, J., 104, 124, 132, 1179
Finkel, A. J., 431
Finkelstein, H., 1725
Finkle, A. L., 1605
Finlay, A. C., 1393
Finn, W. F., 679
Finney, D. J., 1811
Fiorica, V., 137
Fisher, B., 28, 219
Fisher, E. R., 1074, 1162
Fisher, H. C., 1212
Fisher, J. A., 858
Fisher, M., 1331
Fitch, E. A., 1521
Fitts, W. T., 684
Fitts, W. T., Jr., 140, 902, 909
Fitz, R., 1025, 1031, 1038, 1039
Fitzgerald, P., 1243
Fitzpatrick, W. K., Jr., 967
Flatow, F. A., 965
Fleisch, H., 1663
Flerow, 1018
Fletcher, D. G., 830
Flocks, R. H., 1623
Flosdorf, E. W., 183
Floyd, C. E., 1168
Fly, O. A., Jr., 846
Fogarty, T. J., 1303, 1361
Ford, L. T., 1743
Forlanini, 1397
Foroozan, P., 1103
Forsee, J. H., 1391
Foster, G. L., 1011
Foster, J. H., 843, 1330
Fowler, G. R., 1037
Fowler, R., 1175, 1241
Fox, C. L., Jr., 136
Frank, H. A., 138
Franklin, R. R., 1572
Franklin, S. S., 1600
Franksson, C., 855
Frantz, V. K., 672
Fraser, R., 1669
Fraser, R. E., 1363
Fraumeni, J. F., Jr., 1514
Frazelle, E. L., 1421
Freckman, H. A., 705
Fredet, P., 1513
Freeman, N. E., 124, 136, 1305

Freiberg, 1695
Fretheim, B., 849
Friedell, H., 949
Friedman, B., 1714, 1715
Friesen, G., 1352
Friesen, S. R., 828
Fromer, J. L., 1185
Frommhold, W., 891
Froning, E. C., 1742
Frost, H. M., 1660
Frye, W. W., 1112
Fryer, M. P., 1482
Frykman, H. M., 1183
Funderburk, W. W., 689
Furcolow, M. L., 1391
Furth, J., 225
Fyke, F. E., Jr., 797

Gabriel, W. B., 1175, 1183, 1191
Gage, M., 922
Galante, M., 1154, 1161, 1168
Galen, 1, 149-150, 362, 947
Galletti, G., 1205
Gallie, W. E., 1242
Gans, H., 137
Garamella, J. J., 1332
Garceau, A. J., 1003, 1004
Garceau, G. J., 1686
Gardner, B., 705, 708
Gardner, C. E., 1509, 1511
Gardner, E. J., 1150
Garfinkel, D., 884
Garlock, J. H., 814, 1154, 1168
Garrett, H. E., 1325, 1327
Gartland, J. J., 1686
Gatch, W. D., 126, 887, 1091
Geist, H. J., 1664
Gelin, L-E., 138
Gell, P. G. H., 103
Gellis, S. S., 1503
Gershon-Cohen, J., 688
Gerst, P. H., 1074
Gesell, R., 128
Ghormley, R. K., 1720, 1740
Gibbon, J. H., Jr., 856, 1295, 1407, 1408
Gibson, T. E., 1608
Gilbert, E. F., 1515
Gilbert, J. A. L., 856
Gilbert, J. W., 1511
Gilbert, R. P., 137
Gilbertsen, V. A., 1154, 1161, 1168
Gilchrist, R. K., 1161

Gill, G. G., 1744
Gillespie, I. E., 827
Gillman, T., 9, 10
Gilmore, W. E., 1235
Gimbel, N. S., 191
Ginzburg, L., 1220
Girardet, R., 1046
Girzadas, D., 1719
Glaessner, C. L., 857
Glassman, J. A., 856
Glenn, F., 637, 1154, 1168, 1514
Glenn, W. W., 1278
Gley, E., 729
Glimcher, M., 1662
Glotzer, D. L., 991
Godman, G. C., 1661
Goel, M. K., 1721
Goldbeck, 1024
Goldblatt, H., 1327
Goldenberg, I. S., 705
Goldfarb, W. B., 1151
Goldgraber, M. B., 1152
Goldin, A., 228
Goldman, J. L., 798
Goldner, J. L., 1699
Goldsmith, R. S., 1663
Goldstein, L. A., 1703
Goligher, J. C., 838, 1129, 1162, 1168, 1175, 1176, 1180, 1183, 1197
Gooding, R. A., 993
Goodsall, 1191
Goodsell, J. O., 1741
Gorer, P. S., 439
Gorham, L. W., 1359
Gornel, D. L., 1007
Gorsch, R. V., 1179
Goss, C. M., 795, 1371
Gottlieb, C., 866, 867
Gottlieb, M. L., 239
Gottschalk, C. W., 1590
Grabstald, H., 1623
Grace, 999
Graham, E. A., 891, 924, 1234, 1387, 1407
Graham, J. B., 1554
Graham, J. E., 24
Graham, R., 929
Graham, R. R., 1183
Granick, S., 116, 117
Grant, R. N., 669
Grant, R. T., 615
Graves, R. C., 1618
Graves, R. J., 716, 722
Gray, H. K., 808
Gray, J. G., 440
Gray, J. S., 1374
Gray, L. A., 1148
Gray, L. H., 422
Gray, S. J., 830
Grayson, J., 988
Green, D. M., 132
Green, T. H., Jr., 1549

Bibliographic Index

Green, W. T., 1678, 1698, 1699
Greene, B. A., 133
Greengard, H., 826
Greenhill, J. P., 1534
Greenwood, M., 703
Greep, J. M., 132
Gregersen, M. I., 79, 132
Gregory, R. A., 823, 918
Grey, E., 773
Grey, S. B., 785
Grice, D. S., 1696
Griesbach, W. E., 716
Griffith, C. A., 828, 855, 1211, 1219, 1238
Griffiths, W. J., 826
Grillo, H. C., 10, 1661, 1665
Grinnel, R. S., 1154, 1165, 1168, 1198, 1199
Grob, M., 1519
Groen, J. J., 969
Gross, R. E., 132, 840, 1206, 1225, 1240, 1243, 1259, 1262, 1267, 1272, 1497, 1501, 1503, 1507, 1509, 1510, 1513, 1519, 1529, 1645
Gross, S. D., 122, 125
Grubb, R., 158
Gubler, C. J., 116, 117
Gucker, T., 1701
Guilfoil, P. H., 993
Guiss, L. W., 844, 863
Guy, C. C., 1208, 1242
Guyton, A. C., 140

Haagensen, C. D., 218, 669, 673, 691, 697
Haanes, M. L., 919
Haberer, von, H., 866
Habif, D. V., 1016
Haden, R. L., 965
Haddow, A., 705
Hadfield, G., 10
Hagan, W. H., 1207, 1208, 1209, 1222, 1224, 1241, 1247, 1250
Hagler, S., 1498
Hahn, 1011
Hahn, P. F., 117
Haight, C., 1501
Hall, 1025
Hall, J. E., 1707
Hallberg, L., 1568
Haller, J. A., Jr., 1360
Haller, J. D., 1146
Hallin, R. W., 135
Halpern, M., 1731
Halsted, W. S., 8, 20, 26, 154, 714, 1205, 1264
Ham, A. W., 1664
Hamburger, G. E., 868

Hammon, E. C., 1402
Han, S. Y., 863
Handelsman, J. C., 1511
Handley, R. S., 669, 670, 704
Hanford, J. M., 428
Hannon, R. R., 730
Hanson, A. M., 730
Hardaway, R., 616
Hardin, C. A., 1326
Hardy, J. D., 991
Hare, R., 50
Harkins, G. A., 1497
Harkins, H. N., 122, 125, 129, 823, 826, 827, 840, 853, 854, 855, 991, 1038, 1132, 1182, 1212, 1215, 1220, 1224, 1242, 1243, 1247
Harken, D. E., 1288
Harper, P. V., 770, 771, 774
Harrington, P. R., 1703
Harrington, S. W., 679, 802, 1227, 1230, 1231, 1234, 1243, 1245, 1251
Harrington, W. J., 952, 958
Harris, G. W., 716
Harris, N. H., 1707
Harris, P. D., 1346
Harris, R. I., 1698
Harris, R. T., 1688
Harris, S., 929, 1663
Harrison, H. E., 1663
Harrison, M. H., 1717
Harrison, M. H. M., 1694
Harrison, R. C., 826
Harrop, G. A., 777
Hartman, C. G., 1572
Harvard, B. M., 1645
Harvey, S. J., 8
Harvey, W., 150
Hatcher, C. H., 429
Haupt, G. J., 1408, 1412
Hawk, W. A., 1120
Hayes, J. T., 1700
Haynes, L. L., 155
Hayward, J., 1234
Heaton, L. D., 1120
Hechter, O., 139
Hedenstedt, S., 859
Heifetz, C. J., 1212, 1241
Heiman, M., 1573
Heimburger, I. L., 1500
Heiple, K., 1664, 1667
Heister, 1024
Hektoen, L., 152, 418, 949
Heller, J. R., Jr., 1614
Helsingen, N., 845
Helwig, E. B., 1141
Hempelmann, L. H., 413, 428

Henderson, F. D., 1744
Henderson, F. F., 1110
Hendrick, J. W., 672
Henegar, G. C., 132
Henley, F. A., 853, 859
Henneman, P. H., 1625
Henriques, F. C., 362
Henry, A. K., 1223
Hermann, L. G., 1324
Herrick, F. C., 1019
Herrick, J. B., 969
Herrington, J. L., Jr., 854, 1158, 1234
Hersh, A., 1685, 1686
Hershey, J. E., 924
Hershey, S. G., 140
Hertz, A. F., 856
Hertz, S., 714, 719
Hesselbach, F. K., 1244
Hewitt, J. E., 885
Hewlett, T. H., 1386
Heyman, C. H., 1686, 1697
Heywood-Waddington, M. B., 1719
Hiatt, R. B., 1509
Hicks, E. S., 1237
Higgins, C. C., 1645
Highberger, J. H., 1661
Higinbotham, 1241
Hillemand, P., 862, 1233
Hilsabeck, J. R., 1043
Hinman, F., 1605
Hinshaw, D. B., 857
Hinshaw, B., 137
Hinton, J. M., 1152
Hippocrates, 1
Hipsley, P. L., 1524
Hirsch, C., 1740
Hirschsprung, H., 1524
Hirshfeld, J. W., 104
Hirst, A. E., Jr., 1345, 1346
Hitchcock, C. R., 689
Hoag, E. W., 834
Hodgson, A. R., 1715, 1716
Hodgson, C. H., 1391
Hoerr, S. O., 846, 848, 849, 854
Hoffman, H. A., 1631
Hoffman, H. L., 1018
Hoffman, V., 857
Hogan, G. F., 671
Hoguet, J. P., 1217
Hohm, W. H., 1199
Hok, T. T., 1393
Holcomb, G. W., 1235
Holder, T. M., 1501, 1502, 1503
Holinger, P. H., 800
Hollander, J. L., 1715, 1717, 1719, 1722, 1739
Holle, F., 825

Holleran, W. M., 681
Holley, K. E., 1602
Hollingshead, W. H., 1740
Holman, C. W., 21
Holman, E., 1264, 1314
Holmes, J. H., 385
Holmes, R. H., 617
Holscher, E. C., 1743
Holt, E. P., 1742
Holt, R. L., 854
Holtz, F., 1148
Homans, J., 1359
Hoover, N. W., 10, 1743
Hornaday, W. R., 1610
Horsley, 1755
Horsley, V., 773
Horwitz, O., 1495
Hotchkiss, D., Jr., 924
Houssay, B. A., 767
Howard, J., 128, 140
Howard, J. E., 104, 105, 1627, 1663
Howard, J. M., 606, 626, 638, 881, 917, 923, 924, 925, 928, 929, 937, 942, 1496
Howell, D. S., 1662
Howell, W. H., 772, 957
Howes, E. L., 8, 28
Hubay, C. A., 28
Hueston, J. T., 1728
Huggins, C., 706, 707, 781, 1611, 1623
Huggins, C. B., 1662
Huggins, C. E., 155
Hughes, C. W., 1305, 1315
Hughes, E. S. R., 1120, 1154, 1168, 1175, 1183, 1192
Hume, A. H., 1198
Hume, H. A., 1012
Humes, D. M., 139, 1346
Hunt, J. R., 1331
Hunt, T. K., 12
Hunter, D., 730
Hunter, J. A., 4, 45, 1298, 1327, 1329, 1330, 1352
Hurley, L. A., 1664
Hurwitt, E. S., 1251
Husson, 1024
Husto, H., 1734
Hutchinson, Jr., 1521
Hyden, W. H., 17

Iason, A. H., 1236
Ilfeld, F. W., 1685
Illingworth, C. F. W., 140, 707, 771, 886
Inberg, K. R., 1183, 1194
Ingelfinger, F. J., 797
Ingle, 775
Inglis, A. E., 1699
Inouye, W. Y., 923

Bibliographic Index

Irani, R. N., 1685
Isselbacher, K. J., 1004
Iverson, P., 1010

Jackman, R. J., 1181, 1190
Jackson, A. W., 710
Jackson, C., 832
Jackson, C. L., 1371
Jackson, D. S., 10
Jackson, H. C., II, 1740
Jackson, R. G., 855
Jackson, R. H., 1034
Jacob, F., 1660
Jacob, R., 10
Jacobson, L. O., 419, 949
Jaffe, H. L., 1678, 1732
Jahnke, E. J., 1305, 1306, 1309
James, 1352
Janes, J. M., 1698
Janeway, T. C., 1327
Jankelson, I. R., 886
Janowitz, H. D., 825, 919
Javert, C. T., 1575
Javid, H., 860, 1303, 1305, 1317, 1332, 1344
Jeffcoate, T. N. A., 1546
Jeghers, H., 865
Jensen, F., 225
Jenson, C. B., 848
Jesseph, J. E., 857, 1236
Jewett, H. J., 1622
Jewett, T. C., 1525
Johannson, 1695
Johanson, B., 1610
Johnson, D. G., 136
Johnson, H. D., 133, 835
Johnson, J., 1273, 1292, 1295
Johnson, J. T. H., 1723
Johnson, L. P. 857
Johnson, P. O., 1814
Johnson, R. E., 220
Johnston, P. W., 1511
Jones, C. M., 102
Jones, E. L., 1150, 1305
Jones, F. A., 833, 835
Jones, F. W., 1606
Jones, L. R., 1393
Jones, P., 1496
Jones, R., Jr., 921
Jones, S. A., 867, 869
Jones, T. W., 826
Jordan, P. H., Jr., 826, 841
Joyner, C. R., Jr., 1288
Judd, E. S., 869
Judd, E. S., Jr., 1134
Julian, O. C., 1292, 1305, 1323, 1324, 1325, 1326, 1332, 1350, 1352, 1362

Kagawa, S., 1662

Kahan, B. D., 440
Kahil, M., 709
Kahlson, G., 10
Kamrin, B. B., 28
Kanar, E. A., 839
Kanter, I. E., 1159
Kantor, J. L., 1117
Kaplan, G. W., 1623
Kaplan, H. S., 1496
Karafin, L., 1607
Kark, A. E., 1184
Karlan, M., 1184
Kátó, L., 10, 371
Katz, R. L., 256
Kaufman, L. W., 938
Kay, G. D., 28
Kaznelson, P., 957
Keating, F. R., Jr., 736
Keats, S., 1699
Keeley, J. L., 1039
Kefalides, N. F., 384
Kelikian, H., 1735, 1736, 1736, 1739
Kelley, E. P., 1023
Kelly, H. A., 1025
Kelly, K. A., 825
Kelly, P. J., 1658, 1708
Kelly, W. D., 28, 839
Kendall, 775
Kennedy, B. J., 226, 706
Kent, E. M., 1501
Kenyon, A. T., 778
Kerr, D. H., 1580
Kerr, W. K., 1619, 1620
Kerr, W. S., Jr., 1051
Ketenjian, M. D., 1663
Kettlekamp, D. B., 1696
Kevorkian, J., 156
Key, J. A., 505, 1662, 1666, 1705, 1717
Keyes, D. C., 1740
Keynes, G., 729
Keynes, W. M., 1163, 1251
Keys, A. B., 108
Kienböck, 1695
Kiesewetter, W. B., 1182, 1235
Killen, D. A., 1331
Kimbrough, R. A., 1554
Kincaid, O. W., 1582
King, 863
Kingdom, H. S., 789
Kinney, J. M., 140
Kinsella, J. T., 801
Kirby, C. K., 907
Kirchheimer, G., 1661
Kirshbaum, J. D., 886
Kiriluk, L. B., 828
Kirkaldy-Wills, W. H., 1716
Kirkendall, W. M., 1602
Kirklin, J. W., 1273, 1350
Kirsner, J. B., 1124, 1144
Kirtley, J. A., Jr., 1324

Kiselow, M., 1555
Kitchen, H., 969
Kite, J. H., 1686
Kittle, C. F., 1517
Kittredge, W. E., 1626
Kjellberg, 1776
Klebba, A. J., 840
Kleiman, A., 857
Klein, A., 1692
Klingenberg, M., 884
Klippel, A. P., 1349
Klopp, C. J., 1498
Knisely, M. H., 138
Knott, J. I., 1237, 1238
Kocher, T., 907
Köhler, 1695
Kohli, D. R., 1233
Kolar, J., 1660, 1663, 1723
Konjetzny, G. E., 844, 862
Koontz, A. R., 1205, 1211, 1216, 1237, 1239, 1242, 1245
Korkis, F. B., 816
Koskinen, E. V. S., 1658, 1660
Kouchoukos, N. T., 1325
Kouwenhoven, W. B., 1295
Kowalewski, K., 430
Kozoll, D. D., 841
Kraissl, C. J., 16, 17, 18
Krane, S., 732
Krane, S. M., 1659
Krause, 1755
Krebs, H. A., 1011
Kretschmer, H. L., 1644
Krönlein, 1025
Krovetz, J. L., 1514
Krueger, H. C., 968
Krugman, 187
Krupp, P. J., 1563
Kuhlman, R. E., 1658
Kunlin, J., 1325
Kuo, P. T., 108, 118
Kuss, R., 435
Küttner, 962

Ladd, 1182
Ladd, W. E., 1501, 1503, 1508, 1511, 1513
Lagergren, C., 1731
Lahey, F. H., 221, 802, 849
Laimer, E., 1229
Laipply, T. C., 1115
Lalli, A. F., 1621
Lam, C. R., 1228, 1232, 1234, 1242, 1342
Lambert, P. P., 1644
Lambrinudi, C., 1697
Lamdin, E., 1592
Lamm, H., 156

Lampert, E. G., 221, 836
Landau, R. L., 705
Landelius, E., 850
Landry, R. M., 838
Landsteiner, K., 152, 156-157, 162
Langenbuch, C., 905
Langer, K., 17
Langston, H. T., 179
Langworthy, O. R., 1633
Lansche, W. E., 1742
Lapides, J., 1583, 1584, 1598, 1599, 1605, 1607, 1608, 1609, 1610, 1614, 1615, 1616, 1626, 1631, 1633, 1634, 1636, 1637, 1638, 1640, 1641, 1642
Laquer, 727
LaRoque, G. P., 1224, 1250
Lasègue, C., 1740
Larsen, R. M., 1238
Latourette, H. B., 1549
Latta, T., 76-78, 365
Lattimer, J. K., 1619
Laufman, H., 1132
Laugier, M., 1245, 1252
Laury, R. B., 1630
Lavater, 1104
Lawrence, K. B., 1236
Lawrence, M., 1661
Lawley, P. D., 228
Leadbetter, G. W., 1606
Leape, L. L., 1505
Leather, R. P., 1360
Lee, C. M., Jr., 17
Lees, A. W., 1393
Lehmann, J., 1393
Lehrfeld, J. W., 27
Leix, F., 1511
LeMain, R. G., 1660, 1665
Lemeh, C. N., 1197
LeMire, J. R., 1106
Lendrum, F. C., 1228
Leonard, M. H., 1739
Lepore, M. J., 1121
Lerche, W., 797
Leriche, R., 1322, 1323, 1325
Lesser, von, L., 365
Lester, R., 1074
Leudet, 1025
LeVeen, H. H., 132, 1069
Leven, N. L., 1501
Levene, C., 187
Levenson, S. M., 1664
Levine, J., 1669
Levinson, S. O., 183
Levy, A. H., 1215
Levy, M., 1247
Lewin, T., 1718
Lewis, A. E., 1195
Lewis, F. J., 1273, 1294
Lewis, L. A., 1073

Bibliographic Index

Lewis, R. N., 128
Lewis, T., 1044, 1045
Lewisohn, R., 827, 838
Lewison, E. F., 701
Li, C. H., 750
Lichteim, 390
Lichtenstein, L., 1677, 1732
Lichtman, H. C., 970
Liddle, G. W., 1598
Lidz, T., 717
Lieberman, Z. H., 377
Lieberthal, F., 1618
Liechty, R. D., 1154, 1168
Lillehei, C. W., 828
Lillehei, R. C., 130, 134
Lin, P. M., 1332
Lindberg, R. B., 609
Lindsey, D., 646
Linghorne, W. J., 1666
Linker, L. M., 1509
Linscheid, R. L., 1721
Linton, R. L., 241, 243
Linton, R. R., 1013, 1018, 1313, 1325, 1326, 1350, 1352
Lisco, H., 432
Lister, J. B., 4, 50, 110, 154
Listerud, M. B., 1229
Little, J. B., 432
Little, K., 1669
Littré, 1245
Liu, 1554
Lloyd, E. I., 1606
Lloyd-Davies, O. V., 1162
Lockhart-Mummery, H. E., 1115, 1148, 1149, 1175
Lockwood, A. L., 1107
Loeb, R. F., 777
Loewe, O., 1242
Lofgren, E. P., 1161
Logan, A., 816
Logan, P. B., 938
Lone, F., 1197
Longerbeam, J. K., 134, 137, 139
Longmire, W. P., Jr., 927
Looney, W. B., 429
Loosli, C. G., 1390
Lorenz, E., 949
Lorimer, W. S., 1510
Lotheissen, G., 1205, 1222
Louw, J. H., 1506, 1507, 1527
Love, R., 1742
Low, A., 1228
Lower, Richard, 151, 153
Lucas-Championnière, J., 1205
Luck, J. V., 1657, 1658
Luetscher, J. A., 777, 784, 1001

Luft, R., 707, 772
Luke, J. C., 1329, 1362
Lukens, F. D. W., 943
Lukes, R. J., 1496
Lumb, G., 1112
Lyday, J. E., 1511
Lynn, H. B., 1182
Lyons, C., 1332
Lytle, W. J., 1205

McAdams, G. B., 17
McArthur, L. L., 1031, 1032, 1038, 1205, 1241
McBurney, C., 1025, 1028, 1032, 1036, 1039
McCall, M. L., 1542
MacCallum, W. G., 729
McCance, R. A., 117
McCarroll, H. R., 1680, 1682, 1723
McCarthy, J. D., 1056
McCarthy, M. D., 136
McClellan, F. C., 1634
McCloy, R. M., 1346
McClure, R. D., 129, 1217
McCune, W. S., 862, 1134
McDermott, W. V., Jr., 902, 938, 1002, 1011, 1012
McDivitt, R. W., 680
Macdonald, J. M., 857
McDonough, J. M., 1719
McElhaney, J. H., 1663
McEvedy, P. G., 1223
McFarlan, R. M., 1728
McGavran, M. H., 1678
McGlone, F. B., 849
McGowan, G. K., 133
McGraw, J. Y., 1148
MacGregor, W. W., 1218
Machella, T. E., 107, 109
McIndoe, A. H., 961
Maciver, I. N., 830
McKee, G. W., 1719
McKenna, R. J., 1735
Mackenzie, A. R., 1625
McKenzie, I., 678
MacKenzie, R. J., 1183
McKibben, B. G., 1497, 1658
McKissock, 1783
McKittrick, L. S., 1151
McKusick, V. A., 1106, 1345, 1674, 1676, 1677
McLaughlin, C. W., Jr., 1235
McLaughlin, E. D., 167, 171
MacLean, L. D., 137, 854, 860
McLoughlin, H. L., 1724
McMahon, W. A., 1192, 1195

McMinn, R. M. H., 10
Macnab, I., 1666
McNeer, G., 845, 849
McSwain, B., 1155, 1168
MacVaugh, H., III, 1350
McVay, C. B., 1211, 1212, 1214, 1215, 1219, 1220, 1222, 1227, 1251
McWhirter, R., 679, 695
Madden, J. L., 909, 1015, 1158, 1161, 1234
Maddox, J. R., Jr., 1034
Mahoney, E. B., 1273
Mahorner, H. R., 939
Maier, H. C., 1504
Maingot, R., 1104, 1107
Mainland, D., 1811
Mair, G. B., 1242, 1243
Makin, M., 1662
Malcolm, J. A., 807
Mallam, A. S., 1146
Mallet-Guy, P., 922
Mallory, G. K., 864
Mallory, T. B., 1678
Maloney, J. V., Jr., 171
Malpighi, M., 150, 151, 947
Malt, R. A., 891
Malvin, R. L., 1590
Mandl, F., 730
Manken, H. J., 1703
Mann, F. C., 900
Mannick, J. A., 1331
Marable, 1334
Marcet, 77
March, H. C., 427
Marcucci, A., 1038
Margo, M. K., 1736, 1738
Mariani, T., 28
Marine, D., 714, 715
Marino, H., 28
Markley, K., 369
Markowitz, A. S., 28
Markowitz, J., 902
Marshak, R. H., 1112
Marshall, G. R., 1197
Marshall, J. M., 1507
Marshall, S. F., 221, 837, 866
Marshall, V. F., 1627
Marson, F. G., 966
Marston, A., 137
Martin, C. L., 1190
Martin, H. E., 421
Martinez, C., 28
Martland, H. S., 429
Marx, F. W., Jr., 1028, 1039
Mason, E. A., 1239
Mason, G. A., 1408
Masters, W. H., 1573
Matas, R., 671, 1298, 1351
Mateer, J. G., 868, 1010
Mathe, C. P., 1617

Maxwell, M. H., 1601
May, A. G., 1324, 1350
Mayo, C. H., 792
Mayo, C. W., 1149, 1167
Meachim, G., 1659
Meade, R. H., 1025
Means, J. H., 718
Meany, T. F., 1621
Meckel, J. F., 1104
Mecray, P. M., 102
Medawar, P. B., 27, 437
Medins, G., 1092
Medlar, E. M., 1618
Meeker, W., 28
Meissner, W. A., 864
Meleney, F. L., 63
Melick, R. A., 1625
Melicow, M. M., 1624
Melier, F., 1024
Mella, H., 728
Mellinkoff, S. M., 107, 1059
Melrose, D. G., 170
Meltzer, L. E., 108
Mendeloff, A. I., 1117
Mendelsohn, B. G., 1711
Mendelson, C. L., 864
Mendenhall, J. T., 1399
Menetrier, P., 865
Menkin, V., 10, 11
Menguy, R., 828
Mensor, M., 1741
Merendino, A. K., 912
Merendino, K. A., 807, 810, 812, 1016, 1234
Mersheimer, W. L., 827
Mesara, B. W., 1719
Mestivier, M., 1024
Metzger, J. T., 18
Meyer, H. W., 993
Meyer, K., 1661, 1665
Meyer, T. L., 1706
Michels, N. A., 984, 1165
Michener, W. M., 1121
Mikkelsen, W. P., 1223
Miles, R. M., 1301
Miles, W. E., 1165, 1167, 1175, 1183
Milkman, L. A., 1670
Millbourn, E., 917, 936
Miller, B. J., 108, 126, 1295
Miller, E., 1598
Miller, E. M., 957
Miller, J. R., 931
Miller, P. R., 1743
Miller, T. G., 1092
Miller, W. T., 1722
Miller, Z. B., 1663
Milligan, E. T. C., 1175
Mills, M., 624
Mills, S. D., 420
Minkowski, O., 965, 968
Minnis, J. F., 1505

Minot, A. S., 122
Mirsky, I. A., 943
Missakian, M. M., 689
Mithoefer, J., 233, 240
Mixter, W., 1740
Moe, J. H., 1703
Moehlig, R. C., 1672
Moersch, H. J., 816
Moffat, F., 821
Mollison, P. L., 155, 158
Moloney, G. E., 1242
Moltke, E., 28
Moncrief, J. A., 830
Mondor, H., 671
Money, W. L., 227, 716
Monge, J. J., 939
Monrad, S., 1524
Monro, A. K., 1221, 1222
Montgomery, P. O'B., 28
Moore, A. M., 1482
Moore, C. A., 1625
Moore, C. R., 1646
Moore, F. D., 129, 140, 708, 762
Moore, G. E., 1194
Moore, H. G., Jr., 836, 841
Moore, T., 1641, 1644
Moore, T. C., 812
Moore, W. S., 1326
Moran, T. F., 1195
Moreno, G., 1239
Morey, D. A. J., 861
Morgan, C. N., 1175, 1195
Morgan, H. C., 1709, 1743
Moritz, A. R., 362, 684
Morris, G. C., Jr., 1329, 1330, 1334
Morris, J. D., 1500
Morris, K. N., 833, 834, 1232
Morris, M. B., 951
Morrison, D. R., 815
Morrison, F. S., 158
Morrison, W., 958
Morrow, A. G., 1292
Morson, B. C., 844, 1152, 1191
Morton, D. G., 1552
Morton, J. J., 1350
Morton, T. G., 1025
Moschcowitz, A. V., 1183, 1222
Moseley, H. F., 1724
Moss, M. D., 1662
Moss, N. H., 923, 929
Motulsky, A. G., 948, 952
Mourant, A. E., 158
Moyer, C. A., 78, 124, 371, 373, 374, 377, 379, 386, 393, 398, 1183, 1206, 1232, 1239, 1248, 1250, 1362
Mozan, A. A., 940
Mueller, von, F., 719

Muir, E. G., 938, 1167
Mulder, D. G., 1342
Mullen, D. C., 807
Muller, C. J. B., 1227
Muller, W. H., 1280, 1281
Muller, W. H., Jr., 133
Munroe, D., 619
Muraro, U., 1246
Murphy, D. P., 222
Murphy, G. H., 659
Murphy, G. P., 1605
Murphy, J. B., 1036
Murray, J. F., 1482
Mustard, W. T., 1280, 1697
Muto, M., 851

Nachemson, A., 1740
Nadler, S. H., 708
Najafi, H., 1332
Nakayama, K., 815
Narath, P. A., 1633
Nardi, G. L., 920, 943
Nathanson, I. T., 697, 703
Nather, 1059
Nauta, J., 1228
Nealon, T. F. Jr., 171
Negus, D., 952
Nelson, R. M., 129
Nelson, T. Y., 1232
Nemir, A., 1541
Nemir, P., 1092
Nesbit, R. M, 1602, 1606, 1608, 1612, 1613, 1618, 1623, 1627, 1644, 1645
Neuhof, H., 1383
Neuman, H. W., 1244
Neurath, H., 918
Newbold, R. S., 1023
Newton, M., 1534, 1552, 1554, 1555, 1568
Nicholas, J. A., 1674
Nichols, 929
Nickerson, M., 136
Nicoladoni, C., 1314
Nicoloff, D. M., 843
Niemeier, O. W., 869
Nigro, N. D., 1183
Nissen, R., 835, 1234
Noer, R. J., 1092, 1132
Noon, G. P., 1050
Norris, E. H., 727, 739
North, J. P., 638
Notkin, L. J., 835
Nunn, I. N., 1520
Nusbaum, M., 842, 1159
Nyhus, L. M., 827, 839, 841, 856, 1215, 1220, 1223

Oberhelman, H. A., Jr., 823, 825, 827
O'Brien, T. G., 155

Ochsner, A., 913, 1036, 1113, 1356, 1358, 1408
O'Connor, F. J., 1233
O'Connor, V. J., 1621
Ogden, W. W., II, 990
Ogilve, W. H., 1212
Ohage, J., 905
O'Hara, J. M., 1735
Oka, S., 1393
Okochi, K., 187
Olch, P. D., 1205
Oldfield, M. C., 1527
O'Leary, C. M., 861
Oliver, C. P., 675
Oliver, J., 1588, 1599
Oliver, W. J., 1493
Olson, H. H., 1224
Olsson, 1524
Olsson, O., 836
Olwin, J. H., 1302
Opie, E. L., 917, 921
Ordahl, N. B., 838
Orloff, J., 1592
Orloff, M. J., 1000
Ormond, J. K., 1630, 1632
Orofino, C., 1690
Orr, H. W., 1706, 1708
Orr, T. G., 938, 1183, 1247
Ortega, F., 1397
Osborne, E. D., 1185
O'Shaughnessy, W. B., 76
Oski, F. A., 952, 1515
Otto, D. L., 1362
Oudot, J., 1322
Overholt, B. F., 1159
Overholt, R. H., 1385, 1399, 1407
Overton, R. C., 140
Owen, H. W., 1221
Owen, R., 729, 734
Owens, J. L., 927
Owren, P. A., 859, 966

Pack, G. T., 1198
Packard, G. B., 1212
Paff, G. H., 1665, 1666
Paget, J., 681
Paget, S., 153
Paine, J. R., 1093
Palade, G. E., 918
Palmer, E. D., 860, 863, 1227
Palmer, J. A., 1183
Palmer, R. M., 1685
Palmer, W. L., 835
Palumbo, L. T., 1220
Panke, W. F., 1016
Panner, 1695
Papanicolaou, G. M., 673
Paré, Ambroise, 8, 101, 153
Park, C. D., 937
Parker, M., 391
Parkins, W. M., 130, 131, 135, 136

Parkinson, J., 1024
Parkkulainen, K. V., 1506
Parks, A. G., 1175, 1176, 1180, 1192, 1193, 1195, 1197
Parmley, L. F., 1306
Parrish, F., 1732
Parry, C. H., 716
Parson, D. W., 1697
Parsons, E., 123
Partridge, J. P., 1182
Paschkis, K. E., 716
Patt, H. M., 419
Patten, B. M., 1645
Patton, T. B., 1004
Pauling, L., 969
Payne, J. H., 150, 158
Peacock, E., Jr., 1661
Pearce, J., 865
Pearse, H. E., 1663
Pearson, F. G., 1407
Pearson, O. H., 707, 767
Pease, C. N., 1698
Pechet, M. M., 1660
Pederson, L. F., 1670
Peer, L. A., 28
Pelouze, P. S., 1614
Peltier, L. F., 640, 642
Perkins, H. A., 191
Perkins, H. R., 1663
Perloff, D., 1327
Perrault, J., 707
Persky, L., 922
Perthes, G., 1356
Peskin, G. W., 1147
Peters, M. V., 705
Peters, R. M., 827, 1500
Peterson, J. C., 1389
Peterson, L. F., 1721
Peterson, W. F., 1564
Pettit, R. T., 638
Petrovsky, B. V., 1234
Peutz, J. L. A., 865
Phemister, D. B., 789, 1018, 1019, 1698
Phetteplace, C. H., 1224
Phillips, R. F., 1734
Pierce, J. M., Jr., 1610
Pierchalla, L., 728
Pifer, P. W., 173
Pincus, I. J., 826
Pitkänen, A., 1237
Pittman, H. S., 1391
Pitts, F. W., 23
Pitts, R. F., 1589
Plenk, H. P., 837
Plummer, G. W., 1511
Plummer, H. S., 715, 718
Politano, V. A., 1608
Polli, E., 1012
Pollock, S., 1699, 1712
Polson, R. A., 868
Pommerenke, W. T., 112
Ponka, J. L., 1132, 1159, 1243

Bibliographic Index 1833

Ponseti, I. V., 1680, 1691
Pool, 977
Pope, 717
Pope, C. E., 1187
Poppe, J. K., 1391
Pories, W. J., 13, 1660, 1663
Portis, S. A., 1071
Post, R. H., 1664
Postlethwait, R. W., 16, 1155, 1168
Poth, E. J., 825
Potts, W. J., 1212, 1235, 1501, 1505
Potts, W. T., 1275, 1276
Poutasse, E. F., 1329
Prather, G. C., 1629
Prehn, R. T., 226
Prentice, T. C., 608
Preshaw, R. M., 825
Priesching, A., 1245
Priddle, H. D., 1038
Priestley, J. R., 784
Priestly, J. T., 221
Prince, A. M., 187
Pringle, J. H., 1352
Pritchard, J. J., 1664
Probstein, J. G., 1198
Prohaska, J. V., 1137
Prudden, J. F., 13, 1663
Pryce, D. M., 1505
Pryse-Davies, J., 900
Puestow, C. B., 927
Puschel, J., 1740

Quan, S. H. Q., 1160, 1198
Querna, M. H., 1209
Quick, A. J., 901
Quigley, T. B., 1724

Rabhan, W., 1666
Radke, H. M., 17
Rae, A. I., 1602
Ragde, H., 1610, 1630
Rainer, W. G., 1195
Rains, A. J. H., 132
Ralli, E. P., 115
Rammstedt, C., 1513
Randolph, J. G., 1504
Ransom, H. K., 221, 836, 845, 850
Rapaport, F. T., 28
Rapoport, A., 1603
Rapp, G. F., 1709
Rashkind, W. J., 1278, 1280
Rasmussen, H., 762
Rasmussen, R., 707
Rasmussen, T., 771
Rath, H., 16
Ratnoff, A. D., 1004
Ravdin, I. S., 102, 103, 108, 109, 124, 129, 136, 221, 901, 903, 911, 912, 934
Raventos, A., 28
Ravitch, M., 1205
Ravitch, M. M., 1497, 1498, 1499, 1500, 1501, 1503, 1504, 1505, 1511, 1514, 1515, 1524, 1525, 1526, 1527, 1529,
Ray, 1776
Ray, B. S., 772, 927
Ray, E. J., 1503
Ray, R. D., 1667
Raynaud, A. G. M., 1298, 1336
Raynham, W. H., 1149
Reber, H. A., 919
Reboul, H., 1325
Reccitelli, M. L., 1741
Recklinghausen, von, F. D., 730, 734
Redeker, A. G., 186, 187
Redo, S. F., 806, 1514
Reemstsma, K., 446
Reeve, E. B., 948
Reeve, T. S., 132
Regester, R., 640
Rehn, L., 1285
Reichert, F. L., 1116
Reid, M. R., 22, 1042
Reinhoff, W. F., Jr., 715, 917, 926, 927, 1218
Relman, A. S., 1590
Retan, G. M., 1524
Reuter, S. R., 842
Reynolds, B. L., 10
Reynolds, F. C., 1666
Rhinelander, F. W., 1666
Rhoads, J. E., 7, 12, 103, 105, 106, 108, 111, 122, 919, 923, 925, 938, 1183, 1192, 1250, 1527
Riba, L. W., 1632
Richards, A. W., 1588
Richardson, K. C., 716, 774
Richelle, L. J., 1662
Richter, C. P., 75, 1247
Ricker, G., 390
Ricketts, H. T., 943
Rickford, R. B. K., 1561
Rider, J. A., 1141
Riegel, C., 106
Riegel, C. R., 885
Riemensnyder, J. P., 1519
Rienhoff, W. F., Jr., 1019
Riordan, D. C., 1688, 1689
Ripstein, C. B., 1183
Risholm, L., 830
Risser, J. C., 1658, 1703
Ritchey, J. O., 1233
River, L., 1135, 1136, 1251
Rob, C., 992, 1332, 1334

Robbins, L. C., 689
Roberts, B., 886
Roberts, K. E., 857
Robertson, H. E., 886, 1525
Robertson, R., 813
Robinson, A. W., 832
Robinson, J. N., 1646
Robinson, R. A., 1662, 1664
Robitzek, E. H., 1393
Robson, C. J., 1621
Rodahl, K., 646
Rogers, F. A., 1223, 1246
Rogers, H. M., 832
Rohman, M., 1346
Rokitansky, C., 830, 867
Roof, W. R., 1108
Roofe, P. G., 1740
Roseberry, H. H., 1659
Rosemond, G. P., 679
Rosenberg, J. C., 866
Rosenbloom, A. L., 771
Rosenthal, O., 109
Rosenthal, S. M., 369, 370, 385
Rosi, P. A., 1164
Ross, F. P., 1023
Ross, R., 11
Rosser, C., 1134
Roth, J. L. A., 1112
Roth, S. I., 1146
Rothchild, T. P. E., 870
Rothenburg, R. E., 1237
Rousselot, 1007
Rousselot, L. M., 1163
Rowe, C. R., Jr., 829
Rowley, D. A., 950
Roy, A. D., 1069
Royster, T. S., 1327
Rubin, C. E., 836
Rubin, E. H., 1113
Rubin, P., 1674, 1694
Ruckley, C. V., 855
Rudick, J., 855
Ruggi, G., 1222, 1397
Rugtveit, A., 1741
Ruiz-Moreno, F., 1185
Runström, G., 1513
Rusche, C., 1628
Rush, B. F., Jr., 1493
Russfield, A. B., 717
Rustad, H., 132
Rutherford, R. B., 1517
Rutledge, F., 1549
Ryan, E. A., 1208, 1248, 1250
Ryan, P., 1130
Ryder, C. T., 1682

Sabiston, D. C., 1504, 1505
Sabo, J., 13
Sachs, L. J., 863

Sainburg, F. P., 886
Sako, Y., 602
Sale, T. A., 1511
Salheim, 1660
Salter, R., 1680, 1722
Saltzstein, H. C., 132
Salzer, 1104
Samson, P. C., 800
Samuel, E., 689
Samuels, M. L., 1734
Sandblom, P., 28, 887, 1503
Sanders, R. J., 1148
Sandström, I., 729
Sanford, H. N., 1496
Santorini, 1179
Santulli, T. V., 1506, 1528
Satinsky, V. P., 1242
Sauerbruch, F., 727, 1396
Sauvage, L. R., 26, 27, 823, 824, 1182
Savlov, E. D., 28
Sawitz, W. G., 1112
Sawyer, C. D., 886
Sawyer, K. C., 867
Sawyer, P. N., 1325
Sawyer, W. A., 184
Sawyers, J. L., 855, 1198
Sborov, V. M., 640
Schaberg, A., 830
Schaetz, 1104
Schafer, P. W., 1350
Schajowicz, F., 1711, 1730
Schatten, W. E., 26
Schatz, A., 1393
Schauble, J. F., 16
Schauffler, G. C., 1534
Schayer, R. W., 137
Scheinin, T. M., 855
Schell, R. F., 844
Schencker, B., 1580
Schenk, W. G., Jr, 128
Scheuermann, 1695
Schilling, J. A., 10
Schirmer, J. F., 839
Schlagenhaufer, 730
Schlesinger, M., 721
Schless, J. M., 1393
Schlike, C. P., 1134
Schmieden, V., 865
Schneider, C. F., 1251, 1252
Schneider, C. L., 174
Schnitker, M. A., 1345
Schobel, H., 1503
Schrek, R., 1624
Schridde, H., 832
Schultz, M. O., 117
Schwab, R. S., 729
Schwartz, E., 1071
Schwartz, S. I., 191
Scott, J. E. S., 1182
Scott, P. J., 1741
Scott, R. B., 1575
Scott, R., Jr., 1627

1834 Bibliographic Index

Scriver, C. R., 1589
Seeley, S. F., 841, 1305
Seffree, 1732
Segal, G., 869
Seibert, F. B., 110
Selkert, E. E., 137, 1603, 1605
Selmonosky, C. A., 129
Seltzer, R. A., 430
Semmens, J. P., 1535
Senger, F. L., 1621
Sengstaken-Blakemore, 1014
Senning, A., 1279
Sensenig, D. M., 1250
Serafin, J., 1690
Servetus, Michael, 151
Sever, J. W., 1695, 1699
Shackelford, R. T., 1195
Shahon, D. B., 850
Shann, H., 1183
Shapira, D., 826
Sharp, E. H., 1360
Sharp, N., 1697
Shatton, H., 1661
Shaw, R. S., 991, 1346
Shedd, D. P., 1376
Shenkin, H. A., 124, 127
Shepherd, J. A., 1043
Sherlock, S., 1004
Sherman, J. L., 820
Sherman, R. T., 137
Shetlar, M. R., 10
Shim, S. S., 1658
Shimkin, M. B., 703
Shnitka, T. K., 1152
Shoemaker, W. C., 191
Shropshear, G., 1189
Shulman, N. R., 158, 951
Shumacker, H. B., Jr., 1305
Siddons, A. M. H., 1110
Sidel, V. W., 406
Sideman, S., 1696
Siekert, R. G., 1331
Sikov, M. R., 418
Silen, W., 824, 1195
Silk, F. F., 1687
Silliphant, W. M., 601, 640
Simeone, F. A., 122
Simon, G., 947
Simon, S. D., 1742
Simpson, C. L., 428
Simpson, S. A., 777
Sinding-Larsen, 1695
Singer, M., 1725
Sircus, W., 826
Sjoerdsma, A., 1661
Skipper, H. E., 228
Skoog, T., 1727, 1728
Slaney, G., 1152
Sloan, R. D., 1506
Smilow, P. C., 1146
Smith, A. U., 399

Smith, C., 1186
Smith, C. H., 970
Smith, F. H., 221
Smith, G. A., 1092, 1209
Smith, G. W., 1330
Smith, H. P., 114
Smith, H. W., 1587, 1602
Smith, L., 1743
Smith, L. H., Jr., 639, 1625
Smith, L. L., 129, 139
Smith, R., 1721
Smith, R. S., 1235, 1242, 1243
Smith, W. H., 857
Smith, W. O., 826
Smith-Petersen, M. N., 1721
Smithwick, R. H., 1134
Snapper, I., 1679
Sneierson, H., 17
Snedecor, G. W., 1811, 1817
Snoddy, W. T., 864
Snyder, W. H., Jr., 1235, 1509
Soave, F., 1526
Sobel, A., 1662
Socolow, E. L., 428
Söderlund, S., 1195
Soffer, L. J., 764
Sognnaes, R. F., 1662
Sokolov, A. P., 826
Soldant, D. Y., 957
Solheim, K., 1665
Soliman, F. A., 1665
Somerville, E. W., 1682
Sommerschild, H., 1182
Somogyi, M., 921
Sones, D. A., 1719
Sones, F. M., Jr., 1286
Soper, R. T., 1509
Southam, A. L., 1548
Southwick, W. O., 1692
Souttar, H. S., 1288
Speed, J. S., 1692, 1697, 1708
Spencer, F. C., 1305, 1306, 1329, 1360
Spink, W. W., 137
Spratt, J. S., Jr., 1142, 1144, 1145
Staley, C. J., 1136
Stallworth, J. M., 1361
Stamey, T. A., 1603
Stammers, F. A. R., 860
Stamp, W. G., 1671, 1694, 1699
Stanbitz, W. J., 1625
Staple, T. W., 1731, 1743
Starling, E. H., 182-183
Starr, K. W., 1194
Starzl, T. E., 159
State, D., 825
Stavney, L. S., 827

Stearns, M. W., Jr., 1160, 1198
Steenberg, R. W., 139
Steichen, F. M., 1492, 1526
Steier, A., 1664
Stein, A. H., 1658
Steindler, A., 1696
Steiner, D. F., 950
Steiner, P. E., 679
Steinitz, K., 1598
Stelzner, F., 1192
Stemmer, E. A., 188, 838
Stensrud, N., 1233
Stephens, E. D., 1492, 1525, 1527
Stephens, F. D., 1182
Stern, B., 1663
Stern, L., 1382
Stevenson, J. M., 15, 20
Stewart, B. H., 1329, 1603
Stewart, F. W., 680, 683
Stewart, G. D., 991
Stewart, J. D., 843
Stiles, K. A., 1496
Stobie, G. H., 962
Stock, F. E., 854
Stockman, J. M., 1182
Stokes, J. M., 1743
Stoney, R. J., 1333
Storer, E. H., 823
Storer, J. B., 419
Stout, A. P., 1735
Straffron, R. A., 1602
Strahan, A. W. B., 1243
Strassman, G., 1306
Strauss, A. A., 24, 25
Strauss, H. A., 1161
Strauss, M. B., 1585
Strawitz, J. G., 609, 630
Strax, P., 689
Strober, S., 439
Strode, J. E., 1242
Strøm, R., 831
Stroud, B. B., 1176
Sullivan, W. H., 203
Sunderland, D. A., 1150, 1151
Sutliff, W. D., 1391
Sutow, W. W., 1620
Swain, V. A. J., 1182
Swan, H., 156, 1273, 1294
Swartz, W. T., 1245
Sweet, R. H., 814, 1234
Sweetman, R., 1733
Swenson, O., 1525, 1526, 1665
Swenson, S. A., 1110, 1224, 1242, 1243
Swigart, L. L., 795
Swingle, W. W., 136, 777
Swinton, N. W., 886, 1180, 1182
Swinyard, C. A., 1700
Swynnerton, B. F., 835

Syme, J., 363
Symmers, W. St. C., 678
Szent-Gyorgi, A., 227
Szilagyi, D. E., 1349
Szöts, I., 1505

Taber, R. E., 1360
Tagnon, H. J., 1623
Takaro, T. M., 1113
Talbert, J. L., 812, 1493
Tamborino, J. M., 1703
Tanner, N. C., 835, 838, 843, 854, 862, 1019, 1218, 1234
Tapp, E., 1660
Tappeiner, von H., 85, 365, 385
Tawes, R. L., 1498
Taylor, F. H. L., 392
Teimourian, B., 1083
Te Linde, R. W., 1542
Tellem, M., 673
Templeton, F. E., 797
Templeton, J. Y., III, 1363
Tendler, M. S., 1183
Ternberg, J. L., 842
Terpstra, J. L., 993
Terry, L. L., 409, 433
Teschan, P. E., 608, 639
Thal, A. P., 835
Thein, M. P., 827
Thibodeau, A. A., 1711, 1743
Thomas, D., 1075
Thomas, E. D., 420
Thomas, G. I., 807, 1248
Thomas, H. S., 1087
Thomas, K. E., 1150
Thomford, N. R., 838
Thompson, C. F., 1696, 1699
Thompson, G. J., 1644
Thompson, J. C., 826
Thompson, J. E., 839, 1325
Thompson, W. D., 12, 103
Thompson, W. O., 717
Thomsen, G., 1501
Thorlakson, R. H., 1197
Thorn, G. W., 776
Throckmorton, T. D., 1242
Tilney, N. L., 442
Tisherman, S. E., 789
Tobian, L., 1590
Todd, I. P., 1527
Tong That Tung, N. D. Q., 924
Tonna, E. A., 1661, 1663, 1664

Bibliographic Index

Torgerson, W., 1719
Touroff, A. S. W., 1240
Townsend, A. C., 1737
Traut, H. F., 836
Travers, B., 122
Trendelenburg, F., 1355
Trier, J. S., 1067
Trimble, I. R., 936
Trippel, O. H., 1330
Trueta, J., 1666
Tubiana, R., 1728
Tucci, J. R., 772
Tuffier, T., 1397
Tullis, J. L., 155
Tumen, H. J., 1119
Turcotte, J. G., 1016
Turnbull, R. B., Jr., 1162, 1167
Turner, D. P. B., 1247
Turner-Warwick R., 1610
Turrell, R., 1142, 1181, 1185, 1194, 1198
Tyson, R. R., 1325

Udupa, K. N., 10, 11, 1660
Ulin, A. W., 901, 1132, 1514
Urban, J. A., 670, 701, 704
Urist, M. R., 1662, 1663, 1664, 1669
Usher, F., 16, 1243
Ussing, H. H., 1588

Vajrabukka, C., 1195
Valeri, C. R., 155
Valle, A. R., 620, 622
Van Buskirk, K. E., 789
van den Brenk, H. A. S., 10
Vandertoll, D. J., 1167
van Heerden, J. A., 1117
van Nes, C. P., 1690
Van Rood, 158
Van Winkle, W., Jr., 10, 12
Van Patter, W. N., 1117
Van Zwalenberg, C., 1092
Varco, R. L., 27, 28, 1327
Vargas, L. L., 865
Venable, C. S., 16
Vermooten, V., 1625
Vertes, V., 1603
Vesell, E. S., 137
Vetto, R. M., 1180
Vierordt, H., 362
Villarreal, R., 825
Vineberg, A., 1286
Vink, M., 1162
Vinson, P. P., 809

Virchow, R. L., 1148, 1740
Voltz, 1024
Von Eck, N. V., 1015
von Luschka, H., 1740
Vye, W. J., 1334

Wagener, van, G., 1613
Wagoner, J. K., 428
Wagner, L. C., 1708
Waldenstrom, H., 1692
Walder, D., 988
Waldeyer, W., 820
Waldhausen, J. A., 1275
Walker, J. C., Jr., 90
Wallace, D. M., 1622
Wallensten, S., 221, 859
Wallgren, A., 1513
Walls, E. W., 1175
Walsh, F. B., 735
Walter, L. E., 958
Walters, W., 221, 839
Walton, A. J., 1248
Wanebo, C. K., 678
Wang, C-C., 686
Wang, C. A., 743
Wangensteen, O. H., 91, 311, 806, 825, 826, 835, 842, 843, 844, 849, 854, 991, 1092, 1220, 1527
Ward, D. E., Jr., 1506
Ward, G. E., 1496
Warner, B. W., 1174
Warner, E. D., 114, 901
Warren, K. W., 930, 938, 943
Warren, R., 901
Warren, S., 427, 432, 673, 720, 1116
Wassman, 1680
Waterman, N. G., 922
Waterston, D. J., 1275, 1276, 1278, 1503
Watkins, 158
Watson, 1245, 1248
Watts, D. T., 128
Waugh, J. M., 860, 868, 1120
Waugh, R. L., 1110, 1222
Way, S., 1549
Webb, W. R., 1399
Wechsler, R. L., 843
Weckesser, E. C., 1728
Weekes, L. R., 179
Weeks, L. E., 990
Weeks, R. S., 1503
Weens, H. S., 1514
Weiber, A., 14
Weichselbaum, T. E., 370
Weidenfeld, St., 385, 393
Weidman, S. M., 1662
Weil, M. H., 140
Weinberg, 131
Weinberg, J. A., 825, 854

Weinman, D. D., 1658
Weir, W. C., 1572
Weiss, C., 1659
Welborn, J. K., 864
Welch, C. E., 1123, 1155, 1168
Welch, C. S., 1015
Welch, K. J., 1500, 1515
Wells, B. A., 1332
Wells, C., 1183
Wells, S., 948, 965, 966, 968
Werlhof, P. G., 953, 955, 957
Wesolowski, S. A., 1325
West, W. T., 1243
Wheat, M. W., Jr., 1150, 1346
Wheeler, C. G., 1360
Wheeler, W. E., 1235
Whelan, E. P., 1631
Whelton, A., 639
Whiffen, J. D., 1363
Whipple, A. O., 901, 910, 934, 936, 943, 967, 1015, 1018
Whipple, G. H., 105, 111, 1074
White, J. C., 1324
White, N. B., 1658
White, T. T., 679
Whitehead, W., 1194, 1195
Whitesell, F. B., 961
Whitman, E. J., 1325
Wiener, A. S., 160
Wilde, F. R., 1179
Wilder, R. M., 929
Wilkie, D. P. D., 867
Wilkins, E. W., Jr., 1409
Williams, C., 1224, 1235, 1250
Williams, C., Jr., 1526
Williams, J. A., 132
Williams, W. T., 126
Wilson, B., 369, 371
Wilson, H., 970, 1243
Wilson, H. L., 1493
Wilson, J. N., 133
Wilson, P. D., 1690, 1692
Wilson, T. S., 671
Windsberg, E., 1158
Winiwarter, von, F., 1334
Winkelstein, A., 805, 833
Winn, W. A., 1389
Winship, T., 1498
Winter, G., 1498
Wintrobe, M. M., 117
Wise, B. L., 17
Wise, W., 176
Witebsky, E., 158, 167
Witten, D. M., 689
Wittkower, E., 1573
Wittoesch, J. H., 1197
Wohl, M. G., 103

Wolbach, S. B., 115
Wolf, B. S., 834
Wolfer, J. A., 1099
Wolff, J. A., 1620
Wolfson, S. K., Jr., 131
Wood, L. C., 1073
Wood, W., 1690
Woodburne, R. T., 1633, 1634, 1635
Woodhall, B., 631
Woodruff, J. F., 860
Woodruff, M. W., 1621
Woods, T. H. E., 1726
Woodward, E. R., 826, 827, 859
Wray, J. B., 1665
Wright, 1783
Wright, D., 1197
Wright, J. H., 956
Wright, J. T., 840
Wright, R., 187
Wurtman, R. J., 787
Wylie, E. J., 1325, 1327
Wynder, E. L., 676, 1168, 1402, 1551, 1561
Wynne Davis, R., 1685

Yamaguchi, D. M., 1726
Yarnis, H., 865
Yashon, D., 1332
Yater, W., 1506
Yeager, R. L., 1393
Yeghers, 1526
Young, H., 1711
Young, H. M., 1181, 1197
Young, R. W., 1660, 1719
Yudin, S. S., 799

Zabinski, E. J., 961
Zadek, R. E., 1664, 1666
Zamcheck, N., 912
Zarafonetis, C. J. D., 1631
Zavaleta, D. E., 1243
Zawacki, S., 1208
Zech, R. L., 898
Zeldis, A. M., 857
Zenker, 1104
Zetzel, L., 1125
Zieman, S. A., 1206
Ziffren, S. E., 1240
Zimmerman, 943
Zinninger, M. M., 845, 868
Zinsser, H. F., 1284, 1287
Zintel, H. A., 12, 13, 940
Ziperman, H. H., 1234, 1305
Zollinger, R. M., 107, 831, 832, 854, 859, 860
Zubiran, J. M., 830
Zuelzer, W. W., 1525
Zuidema, G. D., 992
Zvaifler, N. J., 1719
Zweifach, B. W., 128

Subject Index

Abdomen, comparison of lines on male and female, 19
  greater peritoneal cavity, 1050
  gunshot wounds, 1109
  lesser peritoneal cavity, 1049
  localized tenderness, with intestinal obstruction, 1080
  muscles, congenital absence, 1519, 1520
  tenderness, after perforation of appendix, 1034
  wounds, 624
Abscess(es), 43
  amebic hepatic, 1113
  anal, 1187
  anorectal, Eisenhammer classification, 1189
    location of various types, 1188
  from appendicitis, 1040
  in brain, 1777
  of breast, 670
  intra-abdominal, 1058
  liver, drainage, 913
  of lung, 1381
  mid-abdominal, 1060
  pelvic, 1062
    drainage, 1062
  perinephric, 1617
  of spinal canal, 1797
  subdural, 1778
  subhepatic, treatment, 1060
  subphrenic, 1058
    diagnosis, 1059
    drainage, 1060
  suprahepatic, treatment, 1059
Acacia, gum, as plasma substitute, 189
Acanthosis nigrans, 667
Acetabulum, fracture, 570
Acid, gastric, neutralization, 827
  secretion, 821
    inhibiting factors, 825
Acid-base, balance, and respiration, 98
  regulation after injury, 347
Acidophils, of pituitary, 749
Acidosis, dilution, 87
  with electrolyte imbalance, 86
  hypoxic, after injury, 347
  low-flow, with hypercapnia, 355
  metabolic, 87
    in severe shock, 129
    treatment, 94
  respiratory, 86
  signs and symptoms, 87
  treatment, 87
Acne, conglobata, 649, 650
  rosacea, 649
Acrocyanosis, 1808

Acromegaly, 767
  diagnosis, 770
  organ hypertrophy, 769
  radiation therapy, 771
  skin changes, 769
  treatment, 770
  x-ray of skull, 768
ACTH, 752
  excess, pathologic changes, 764
  masking infection in wound, 301
  molecular structure, 753
  psychosis, 333
Actinomyces, 40
Actinomyces bovis, 70, 71
Actinomycin, for cancer control, 230
Actinomycosis, 70, 71, 1391
  involving bone, 1711
  of jaws, 1460, 1461
Adenocarcinoma, of colorectum, 1153
  growth rate, 211
  of lung, 1403
  of ovary, 1565
  of uterus, 1560, 1561
Adenoma(s), bronchial, 1409
  eosinophil, 1776
  eosinophil, 1776
  of parathyroids, 737
  polypoid, of colorectum, 1140
    relation to cancer, 1142
    treatment, 1144
  thyroid, 721
Adhesions, division, to relieve intestinal obstruction, 1094
  in subarachnoid space, 1787
Adenitis, B.C.G., in infants, 1495
  in children, 1495
  mesenteric, vs appendicitis, 1046
  tuberculous cervical, in children, 1495
Adrenal glands, 754-765, 774
  anatomic and surgical consideration, 774
  blood vessels, 755
  histology, 755
  nonfunctioning medullary tumors, 792
  cortex, diseases of, 777
  hyperplasia and virilism, 783
  insufficiency, diagnosis, 764
  medulla, 786
    histology, 756
    hormones, 758
Adrenal steroids, excess, 764
Adrenalectomy, bilateral, cancer of breast, 707
Adrenocortical hormones, 756
Adrenocorticotropic hormone, 752. *See also* ACTH

Adrenogenital syndromes, 781
  causes, 782
  postnatal, 783
Aerobacter aerogenes, 38
Age, effect on mortality in burns, 393
  of patient, and operative risk, 233-235
Agenesis, renal, 1643
Agglutinins, cold, 162, 168
Agnosia, 1763
Agraphia, 1764
Air embolism, 305
Airway, obstruction, 312
  in unconscious person, 1788
Albumin, effect on blood flow, 371
Alcaligenes faecalis, 39
Alcohol, psychoses, 333
Alcoholic, anesthesia for, 246
Aldosterone, increase, in ascites, 100
  response to dehydration, salt loss, and hemorrhage, 763
  as response to injury, 340
Aldosteronism, 783
  primary, 784
    as cause of hypertension, 1602
  secondary, 785
Alexia, 1764
Alimentation, intravenous, in infants, 1494
  routes of, 108
Alkalosis, 87
  after injury, 347
  postoperative, 355
  signs and symptoms, 88
  treatment, 88
Alkylating agents, for control of cancer, 228
Alpha rays, 403
Amebiasis, 1111
  intestinal, clinical pattern, 1112
Ameloblastoma, mandible, 1427, 1428
Amethopterin, for cancer control, 229
Ammonium intoxication, and hepatic disease, 1011
Amphophils, of pituitary, 750
  hypertrophic, 750
Ampulla of Vater, 881, 917
Amputations, for trauma, 635
Amputees, transportation of, 636
Amylase, serum, in pancreatitis, 921
Anabolism, post-traumatic, 343
Analgesics, in treatment of shock, 139
Analysis, of surgical data, 1810

Subject Index

Androgen, therapy, cancer of breast, 705
Anemia, acquired autohemolytic, 970
  after acute irradiation, 415
  congenital nonspherocytic, 969
  congenital spherocytic, 965
  with deep burns, 390
  and operative risk, 239
  postburn, treatment, 371
  postgastrectomy, 859
  sickle cell, 969
  sign of neoplasm, 215
  spherocytic, treatment, 968
  splenic, 970
Anesthesia, 244-274, 277
  as added insult, in combat casualties, 609
  for appendectomy, 1031
  for battle casualties, 264
  in chronic suppuration of respiratory tract, 262
  conduction, 252
  with coronary artery disease, 262
  with cyclopropane, 248
  for the drug-dependent patient, 246
  epidural, 255
  with ether, 249
  explosion hazards, 267
  fire hazards, 267
  with halothane, 249
  and hypnosis, 265
  and induced hypothermia, 265
  inhalational, 247
  in intestinal obstruction, 262
  intravenous, 251
  local, 252
  management of poor risk, 261
  with methohexital, 251
  with methoxyflurane, 250
  in mitral stenosis, 263
  muscle relaxants, 256
  with nitrous oxide, 247
  and operative risk, 241
  in pediatric surgery, 1492
  positioning of cardiac patient, 263
  premedication, 244
  recovery room, 268
  respiratory problems, 260
  special technics, 264
  spinal, 253
    complications, 254
  for splenectomy, 976
  with thiopental, 251
  with trichloroethylene, 251
  unusual complications, 266
Anesthetist, preoperative visit, 244
Aneurysm(s), 1339
  abdominal aorta, site of rupture, 1348
    resection and graft, 1349
    treatment, 1350

anterior communicating artery, 1782
arteriosclerotic, of abdominal aorta, 1347
ascending aorta, resected, 1343
clinical features, 1340
difference between true and false, 1338
dissecting, 1339, 1344
  pathology, 1345
  surgical treatment, 1346
  thoracic aorta, 1347
false, 1311
fusiform, 1339
intracranial, 1780
  treatment and results, 1781
mycotic, 1352
peripheral arterial, 1350
reconstructive surgery, 1342
saccular, 1339
of splanchnic circulation, 994
syphilitic, 1340
of thoracic aorta, 1293, 1340
  resection, 1341
  x-ray examination, 1341
Angina, intestinal, 991
Angiocardiogram, in diagnosis of tetralogy of Fallot, 1274
  mitral stenosis, 1287
  transposition of great arteries, 1279
Angiofibroma, nasopharyngeal, 656
Angiography, 1319, 1581, 1772
  for intracranial aneurysms, 1781
  in obscure abdominal pain, 992
Angiomas, 653
Angiospasm, 1336
Angiotensin, 340
Ankle, bimalleolar, fracture-dislocation, 553
  fractures and dislocations, 550-555
  fractures without displacement, 551
  trimalleolar, fracture-dislocation, 553, 554, 555
Ankylosis, of jaws, 1461
Anorectum, 1174-1203
  anatomy, 1175-1180
  blood supply, 1178
  clinical conditions, 1181
  definition, 1174
  membranes, 1176
  muscles, 1179
    and fascial septa, 1177
  physical examination, 1181
  See also Anus
Anoxia, tissue, after injury, 342
Anthrax, 72
Antibiotics, administration methods, 57
  with battle casualties, 616
  for control of cancer, 230

effective against tuberculosis, 1393
idiosyncrasy, 58
intraperitoneal, 1101
in osteomyelitis, 1706
in pancreatitis, 922
selection of, 55
surgical prophylaxis, 52
Antibodies, 46
  auto-immune, to platelets, 951
  blocking, 164
  formation, in undernourished, 103
  response, in splenectomized, 950
Anticoagulants, in chronic occlusive arterial disease, 1323
  in transfusions, 152
Anticholinergics, before anesthesia, 246
Anticholinesterases, chemical warfare, 646
Antidiuretic hormone, and diabetes insipidus, 773
Antigens, genetics and chemistry, 439
Antimetabolites, for cancer control, 229
Antisepsis, intestinal, drugs for, 1160
Antiseptics, and wound healing, 16
Antithyroid drugs, 719
Antrum, action of, 823
  criteria for retention, 824
  effects on gastric pouch secretion, 824
Anuria, maintenance of fluid balance, 97
  mechanism, 1600
  postoperative, 320
Anus, abscess, 1187
  anatomy, 1066
  atresia, classification, 1182
  carcinoma, 1197
    standard treatment, 1198
  external sphincter, 1179
  fissure, 1186
  fistula, 1190
  hygiene, 1185
  imperforate, 1182, 1527
  incontinence, 1184
  longitudinal sphincter, 1179
  stricture, 1184
  See also Anorectum
Anxiety, medication for relief, 298
Aorta, coarctation of, 1264
  double arch, 1268
  grafts, in coarctation, 1267
  occlusion, of bifurcation, 1322
  thoracic, aneurysms, 1293, 1340
  window, 1264
Aortogram, abdominal, 1319, 1320
  coarctation of aorta, 1266
  technic, 1320
Aortography, 1582

Aphasias, 1763
Appendectomy, 1031
　operative pain, 1045
　for perforative appendicitis, 1036
Appendicitis, acute, complications, 1039
　gangrenous, 1031
　nonperforative, 1028-1033
　　mortality, 1033
　　symptoms, 1028
　　treatment, 1031
　pathogenesis, 1026
　spontaneous recovery, 1031
　in the aged, 1034
　in children, 1033
　　incidence of perforation, 1034
　death from, 1042
　decreasing incidence, 1022, 1023
　differential diagnosis, 1045
　factors favoring appendectomy, 1037
　historical note, 1024
　mortality, 1041
Appendicitis, perforative, 1033
　conservative vs. operative intervention, 1037
　diagnosis, 1035
　factors favoring delayed surgery, 1038
　laboratory aids, 1035
　palpation of abdomen, 1034
　treatment, 1036
　x-ray examination, 1035
　in pregnancy, 1038
　recurrent attacks, 1030, 1039
　significance of relief of pain and tenderness, 1031
Appendix, anatomy, 1025
　locating, at operation, 1032
　perforation, 1031
　removal of normal appendix in course of other intra-abdominal operations, 1039
　stump, management, 1032
　tumors, 1043
　variety of locations, 1026
Appliances, orthopedic, 1695
Apraxia, 1763
Arctic medicine, 646
Aristotle, on movement of blood, 149
Arm, fractures and dislocations, 478-517
　upper, splinting, 462
Arrest, cardiac, 1295
Arteriogram, femoral, 1308
　peripheral, 1319
　renal, 1328
Arteriography, arteriovenous fistula, 1313
　in diagnosis of bone tumor, 1731
　for site of gastrointestinal bleeding, 842
Arteriosclerosis, obliterans, 1320
　visceral, 1332

Arteritis, with infarction of bowel, 993
Artery(ies), acute occlusion, 1298
　aneurysm, 1339
　carotid, contralateral compression test, 1332
　　endarterectomy, 1333
　　grafts, 1332
　　stenosis, endarterectomy, 1332
　chronic occlusive disease, 1315
　　course, 1321
　　pathology, 1321
　　physical examination, 1317
　　treatment, 1323
　contusion, 1306
　cystic, normal and anomalous arrangements, 882
　embolism, 1299
　end-to-end anastomosis, 1310
　femoro-femoral bypass, 1327
　gaining proximal control, 1309
　great, transposition, 1279
　hepatic, ligation, for portal hypertension, 1019
　ileocolic, 986
　iliac, injury with fracture of pelvis, 569
　inferior mesenteric, 987
　　occlusion, 993
　injuries, 630
　　with fractures, 455
　insufficiency, affecting brain, 1330
　internal carotid, stenosis, 1331
　occluded, restoration with vascular grafts, 1325
　popliteal, aneurysms, 1350, 1351
　poststenotic dilatation, 1339
　profunda revascularization, 1327
　reconstruction, selection of patient, 1326
　renal, 1582
　　lesions, 1327
　　stenosis, 1328
　　various methods of reconstruction, 1329
　right colic, 986
　right hepatic, normal and anomalous arrangements, 882
　splenic, 948
　superior hemorrhoidal, 1178
　　point of ligation, 987
　superior mesenteric, 984
　　embolic occlusion, 991
　　syndrome, 991, 1105
　　traumatic destruction, 993
　surgery of, 1298-1352
　thrombosis, 1303
　trauma, 1305
Arthritis, degenerative, 1717
　of spine, 1743
　gonococcal, 1709
　of jaw, 1459
　pyogenic, 1708, 1709
　rheumatoid, 1719

　in hand, 592
　medical treatment, 1720
　surgical treatment, 1721
Arthrodesis, triple, 1696
Artillery, wounds, 604
Aschheim-Zondek test, with testicular tumors, 1625
Ascites, associated with tumors, 1001
　chylous, and peritonitis, 1057
　pathogenesis, in portal hypertension, 1000
　protein concentration, 1002
　and suprahepatic portal hypertension, 1005
Aspergillus niger, 41
Aspiration, peritoneal, 1054
Asymmetrogammagram, 1768
Atelectasis, bronchial obstructive, 302
　treatment, 302
　compressional, 303
　congestive, 304
　neonatal, 1504
Atheroma, 1321
Atherosclerosis, and high fat diet, 107
　and cholesterol, 108
Atmosphere, control on submarines, 645
Atony, gastric, postoperative, 326
Atresia, choanal, in infants, 1497
　of colon, 1526
　esophageal, with tracheo-esophageal fistula, 1501, 1502
　of extrahepatic bile ducts, in newborn, 1513
　of intestinal tract, in newborn, 1506
Auerbach's plexus, 1068
Australia antigen, 187
Autografts, for burns, 1443
Autonomic nervous system, diseases affecting, 1807
Autotransfusions, 156, 179
Axilla, contracture after deep burn, 1444
　examination, 688

Bacilli, gram-negative, 38
Bacillus anthracis, 37, 72
　diphtheriae, 37
　pyocyaneus, 39
Bacteremia, 43
Bacteria, classification of those important in surgery, 34
　effects in surgery, 42
　incubation period, 42
　L-forms, 42
　portal of entry, 42
　primary and secondary contamination, 50
　pyogenic, 35

Bacteroides, 40
Bacteriology, applied surgical, 34-47
Bacteriophage, typing, 35
Bacteriostasis, in burns, with silver nitrate, 375
Bandages, plaster, 474
Bandaging, elastic, in thrombophlebitis, 323
Banti's syndrome, 997
Barbiturates, before anesthesia, 245
  psychoses, 333
Barbiturate-dependent, anesthesia for, 246
Barium enema, reduction of intussusception, 1524
Barrett's ulcer, 832
Bartholin's glands, cysts and abscesses, 1547
Barton's fracture, 509, 512
Basedow's disease, 717
Basophils, of pituitary, 749
Bath, continuous, for burns, 378
Benzodioxane, 791
Beta decay, 202
Beta rays, 403
Bezoars, 861
Bicarbonate, concentration in pancreatic juice, 919
Bile, 885
  duct, common, 881
    normal and anomalous arrangements, 882
    tumors, 886
  peritonitis, 1056
  salts, functions, 1074
  variations, 885
Biliary drainage, 893
Biliary tract, secondary operations, 910
Billroth I, 853
Billroth II, 853
  gastrectomies, 855
Biometry, clinical, historical landmarks, 702
Biopsy, basis for, 217
  bone tumor, 1729
  breast, 689
    technics, 690
  contralateral breast, 690
  frozen section, value, 218
  hepatic, 912, 1010
  needle, in liver, 912
  pancreatic, 933
  reliability, 218
Birthmark, 653
Bisection, gastric, for bleeding varices, 1019
Bladder, calculi, 1612
  diverticulum, congenital, 1644
  exstrophy, 1645
  external irradiation, 1622
  injury, in fractured pelvis, 569
  motor paralytic, 1639, 1640
  neuroanatomy, 1635

neurogenic, autonomous, 1638
  disturbances, 1606
  reflex, 619, 1637
  uninhibited, 1637
normal, cystogram, 1604
outlet obstruction, 1606
physiology, 1633
rupture, 1629
  diagnosis, 1629
  with fractured pelvis, 454
sensory paralytic, 1639
with trabeculation, 1604
tumors, 1622
Blalock operation, for tetralogy of Fallot, 1275
Blastomyces dermatitidis, 41
Blastomycosis, 71
  of skin, 651
Bleeding, abnormal, after transfusion, 173
  diagnostic procedures, 196
  in surgical patient, 191
  sign of neoplasm, 215
  from needle biopsy, 1011
Blind-loop syndromes, 1072
Blood, aged, as cause of hemolytic reactions, 167
  cadaver, 156
  changes, in peritonitis, 1053
  clotting, factors, 194, 195
  cold agglutinins, 162
  crossmatching, 152
  priniciples, 164
  discovery of circulation, 149
  Duffy factor, 162
  glycerolized frozen, 155
  groups, inheritance, 157
  iso-agglutinogens and iso-hemagglutinins, 157
  H substances, 157
  hazards of using type O, 165
  Kell factor, 162
  loss, combat injuries, 615
    determination of, 132
  low flow states, 353
  Lewis substance, 158
  Luther factor, 162
  minimum standards for preparation and preservation, 164
  nutritional role, 112
  and parenteral fluids, administered to infants, 1493
  peritonitis, 1056
  pH, maintenance of normal, 1591
  pressure, and shock, 128
  Rh factor, 158
  Rh-Hr types, 161
  transfusions, accidents and prevention, 162
    acidosis and cardiac arrest, 171
    allergic reactions, 172
    anticoagulants, 152
    bacterial contamination, 171
    for burn shock, 371

calcium gluconate use, 175
circulatory overload, 172
citrate intoxication, 174
first recorded, 151
fresh versus aged blood, 170
hemolytic reactions, 167
  from mismatched blood, 168
increased fibrinolytic activity, 173
practical aspects and precautions, 156
pyrogenic reactions, 172
reactions, 167
  signs and symptoms, 169
  treatment, 169
  and related problems, 149-201
safeguards, 162
in treating deep burns, 388
types, 156
typing, 152
  sources of error, 163
  minimum routine, 158
universal donor, 165
universal recipient, 166
urea nitrogen, determination, 1598
volume deficit, correction in combat casualties, 608
volume, determination of, 132
vessels, of splanchnic bed, 983
  suture methods, 27
  and wound healing, 26
Bochdalek hernia, 1243
Boerhaave syndrome, 861
Bone, absorption, 1667
  action of parathormone, 732
  cancer, after radiation, 429
  composition, 1658
  crystals, 1659
  developmental abnormalities, 1680
  grafts, 1667
    in hand reconstruction, 589
  growth in thickness, 1658
  induction, 1662
  infection, 1703
  marrow, hyperplastic, in thrombocytopenia, 967
    in idiopathic thrombocytopenic purpura, 955
  metabolism, 1659
  other metabolic diseases, 1672
  mineral constituents, 1659
  necrosis, avascular, 458, 459
    after irradiation, 426
  organic matrix, 1661
  and parathormone, 734
  response to injury, 1660
  tumors, 1728
    biopsy, 1729
    classification, 1729
    laboratory studies, 1731
    treatment, 1732
  and wound healing, 26

Subject Index 1841

Booby traps, wounds, 603
Bougies, for esophageal stricture, 799
Boutonnière deformity, 582
Bowel. See Intestines.
Bowel sounds, in appendicitis, 1029
Bowen's disease, 664
Bowman's capsule, 1587
Brachial plexus, injury during operation, 266
Brachytherapy, 206
Brain, abscess, 1777
　granulomatous and parasitic cysts, 1787
　hyperactivity, symptoms and signs, 1759
　hypoactivity, symptoms and signs, 1761
　wounds, 617
Branham-Nicoladoni sign, 1314
Breast, 668-713
　abscess, 670
　anatomy, 668
　biopsy, 689
　　technics, 690
　cancer, 674
　　by age groups, 675
　　metastatic, 683
　　operability and curability, 696
　　palliative treatment, 704
　　per cent distribution by age, 675
　　　by course of treatment, 69, 699
　　prognostic considerations, 710
　　super radical operations, 703
　　survival rates, by type of hospital, 700
　　treatment, 691
　　untreated, survival, 703
　　5-year survivals, 700, 701
　carcinoma, adenocystic, 683
　　clinical pattern, 684
　　with fibrosis, 682
　　infiltrative, lobular, 682
　　intracystic, 682
　　with lymphoid infiltration, 682
　　squamous cell, 683
　　cutaneous nerve supply, 670
　cystosarcoma, phyllodes, 683
　ectopic tissue, 679
　embryology, 668
　examination, 685
　inflammatory diseases, 670
　lymph drainage, 686
　male, 709
　　carcinoma, 710
　pain, 684
　precancerous lesions, 680
Brenner tumors, of ovary, 1565
Brodie's abscess, 1707
Bromide, excess, psychoses, 331
Bromsulphalein test, 1008, 1009
Bronchiectasis, 1383
　diagnosis, 1384
　saccular, 1385

　treatment, 1385
　tuberculous, 1394
Bronchopneumonitis, aspiration, with gastrointestinal bleeding, 1014
Bronchoscopy, for cancer of lung, 1407
Bronchospirometry, differential, 1375
Bruit, systolic, 1317
Brunner's glands, 821, 828
Bryant's traction, 533
Budd-Chiari syndrome, 998
Buerger's disease, 1334
Burns, 360-398
　associated disturbances, 385
　in atomic casualties, 644
　blood transfusions and skin grafting in treating, 388
　circulatory disturbances, 390
　classifications, 360
　continuous bath, 378
　duration of hospitalization, 382
　effect of age on mortality, 393
　electrical, 1449
　endocrine disturbances, 390
　esophageal, management, 799
　final phase of treatment, 1443
　fluid therapy, 371
　functional classification, 397
　of hand, 577, 1444
　heat loss, vaporization, 377
　hematologic disturbances, 390
　homografts, 384
　hydrational disturbances, 385
　hypo-osmolality and acidosis, 386
　immunologic disturbances, 391
　infection, 373
　irradiation, 1447
　metabolic disturbances, 386
　mortality during a century, 364
　penicillin in, 384
　physiological disturbances, 365
　principles of wound care, 373
　pulmonary edema, 391
　removal of eschar, 376
　respiratory disturbances, 391
　results of treatment, 393
　sepsis, 374
　shock, 364
　　blood transfusion, 371
　　buffered saline in treatment, 369
　　use of colloids, 370
　　vasoconstrictors and hydrocortisone, 370
　silver nitrate dressings, 374
　skin grafting, 1437
　therapy, history, 363
　　regulation, 372
　tracheostomy, 391
　use of plasma, 370
　water loss, insensible, 377

　white phosphorus, 636
Bursitis, 1724

Calcaneus, fractures, 555
Calcification, of bone, 1662
　inhibitors, 1663
Calcium, blood deficit, 88
　excretion, and parathyroids, 732
　gluconate, use in blood transfusion, 175
　metabolism, and parathormone, 732
　and parathyroids, 730
Calculus, of bladder, 1612
　of salivary glands, 1479
　in urinary tract, 1625
　etiology, 1625
Callus, in fractures, 450
Cancer, bone, after radiation, 429
　breast, 674
　　adrenalectomy, bilateral, 707
　　androgen therapy, 705
　　by age groups, 675
　　bilateral, 679
　　endocrine therapy, improvement, 706
　　estrogen therapy, 705
　　family history, 675
　　hypophysectomy, 707
　　incidence, 675
　　and irradiation, 678
　　of male, 710
　　metastatic, chemotherapy, 708
　　mortality by country, 678
　　oophorectomy, 705
　　operability and curability, 696
　　palliative treatment, 704
　　pathology, 680
　　　classification, 680
　　and pregnancy, 679
　　treatment, 691
　　untreated, survival, 703
　of cervix, 1551
　　grading and staging, 1552
　　recurrent and radioresistant, 1555
　　results of treatment, 1555
　　treatment, 1552
　in colitis, ulcerative, 1152
　of colon, age distribution, 1157
　　incidence of symptoms, 1156
　　influence of extent of disease on survival, 1168
　　location, 1154
　　obstruction, treatment, 1158
　　perforation, 1158
　　prognosis and results, 1168
　　symptoms and physical signs, 1155
　　treatment, 1160
　　x-ray therapy, 1160
　colorectum, selection of operation for various sites, 1164

1842 Subject Index

Cancer (*Cont.*)
  control, analogy with infectious disease, 224
  cytotoxic agents, 228
  deaths by site, 1154
  death rates by site, for males, 1403
  endometrial, 1561
    treatment, 1562
  etiology, 209
  head and neck, palliative care, 1435
  heredity factors, 222
  hormones for control, 226
  incidence by site and sex, 1154
  intestinal, implantation of tumor cells in anastomosis, 1162
  intramural spread, 1161
  of larynx, 1431
  of lip, spread, 1423
  of lung, diagnosis, 1407
    radioactive dust, 428
    and smoking, 1402
    survival rates, 1408
    symptoms, 1404
    treatment, 1407
  lymphatic metastases, 1161
  molecular attack on, 224-231
  operations, palliative, 219
    radical vs palliative, 218
  ovarian, classification of stages, 1567
    treatment, 1566
  pancreas, laboratory data, 934
  pancreaticoduodenal, 930
    results of treatment, 938
    symptoms and signs, 932
    treatment, 936
  from radiation, 427
  spread by direct extension, 1163
  spreading factors, 1161
  statistics, 219
  stomach, prognosis, 850
    symptoms, 849
    treatment, 849
  surgery, practical considerations, 216
    prophylactic, 220
    second look, 1161
  transperitoneal spread, 1163
  use of radioisotopes, 227
  thyroid, after radiation, 428
  of vagina, 1549
  venous spread, 1161
  virus etiology, 225
  of vulva, 1548
  See also Neoplasms.
Candida albicans, 41
Capacity, maximum breathing, 1375
  vital, 1374
    timed, 1375
Carbohydrate, 107
  metabolism, and corticoids, 776
Carbon dioxide therapy, 316

Carbonic anhydrase inhibitors, 1597
Carcinoid, of appendix, 1043
  of colorectum, 1146
  small bowel, 1137
  syndrome, 1147
Carcinoma, of ampulla of Vater, 930
  of anus, 1197
  of appendix, 1043
  breast, in situ lobular, 680
    of male, 710
    mammary ducts, 681
  bronchogenic, invasiveness, 1404
    histologic types, 1402
  buccal cavity, 1425
  cecum, lymphatic spread, 1163
    and appendicitis, 1027
  cervix, in pregnancy, 1555
    invasive, 1553, 1554
  of colon, in children, 1526
    descending, lymphatic spread, 1164
  of common duct, 931
  en cuirasse, 686
  of duodenum, 868, 931
  of esophagus, 810
  of eyelid, 1416
  gallbladder, 886
  hepatic flexure, lymphatic spread, 1163
  lip, 1422
  lung, alveolar cell, 1403
    epidermoid, 1404
  of nasopharynx, 1421
  of nose, basal cell, 1420
  pancreas, 931
    inverted-3 sign of Frostberg, 936
  pancreaticoduodenal, 5-year survivals, 939
  parathyroids, 733, 739
  penis, 1624
  prostate, 1623
    external cobalt irradiation, 1623
  rectosigmoid, lymphatic spread, 1165
  rectum, lower, lymphatic spread, 1166
  scrotum, 1624
  skin, 664
  splenic flexure, lymphatic spread, 1164
  stomach, 844
    classification, 846
    diagnosis, 848
    local spread, 844
    lymphatic spread, 845
    metastases to hilum of spleen, 845
    pathology, 844
    stages according to invasion, 848

  stages according to metastases, 847
  sweat gland, 682, 1419
  thyroid, 721
    in children, 1498
  tongue, 1425
    epidermoid, 1424
  See also Cancer
Cardiac failure, 312
Cardiofundoplasty, for esophageal hiatal hernia, 1234
Cardiospasm, 807
  hydrostatic dilatation, 809
  treatment, 809
Carotid body, tumors, 1434
Carpal tunnel syndrome, 593, 1726, 1800
Carpus, dislocations, 515, 516
  fractures, 513
Cartilage, composition, 1659
  metabolism, 1659
  semilunar, tears, 535
  types, 1659
  and wound healing, 26
Caruncle, urethral, 1547
Cast, hanging, 487, 489
  plaster, 473
    complications, 475
    cutting, 476
Casualties, atomic principles of management, 642
  in thermonuclear bomb attack, 406
Catabolism, post-traumatic, 343
Catecholamines, chemical tests, 759
  normal range, 759
  in response to injury, 340
Catheter, intratracheal, insertion, 290
  urethral, time limits, 1612
Catheterization, cardiac, aortic stenosis, 1291
  for atrial septal defects, 1272
  to diagnose pulmonary stenosis, 1269
  mitral stenosis, 1288
  for tetralogy of Fallot, 1274
  right heart, 1282
  urethral, 278
Cation abnormalities, 88
Causalgia, with fractures, 458
Cautery, as hemostatic, 153
Cavitation, of wound, by missile, 602
Cecocoloplicopexy, 1100
Cecostomy, temporary, for drainage and decompression, 1096
Cecum, carcinoma, and appendicitis, 1027
  volvulus, 1099
Cellulitis, 43
  clostridial, 65
  crepitant (nonclostridial), 65

Subject Index

Central nervous system, diseases affecting, 1755
Central venous pressure, 616
Cephalothin, and wound healing, 15
Cerebral palsy, orthopedic procedures, 1698
Cerebrospinal fluid, symptoms and signs due to abnormal, 1758
Cerebrum, residual scar, 1787
Cervicitis, acute, 1549
  chronic, 1549
  treatment, 1550
Cervix, cancer, 1551
  cauterization, 1550
  epithelium, 1553
Cesium, 413
Chalazion, 1416
Charcot, joint, 1721
Chemicals, and wound healing, 16
Chemotherapy, for metastatic cancer of breast, 708
Chest, flail, 1380
  wounds, 620, 621
Chilblains, 640
Children, fractures, 471
  surgery, preparation for operation, 1492
Chi square, calculation, 242, 243
  test, 1812
Chlorambucil, for control of cancer, 228
Chloride, exchange, across alimentary tract, 89
  with environment, 88
  excess, therapy, 95
  after injury, 344
  reabsorption in tubule of kidney, 1589
Chlorothiazide, 1597
Cholangiogram, normal, 908
Cholangiography, operative, 898
Cholecystectomy, 905
Cholecystitis, 885
  acute, 887
  vs appendicitis, 1047
  chronic calculous, 890
  noncalculous, 890
  in infants, 1514
  signs and symptoms, 887
Cholecystograms, 891-895
Cholecystojejunostomy, 909
  loop, for inoperable carcinoma of pancreas, 937
  en Y, for inoperable cancer of pancreas, 937
Cholecystostomy, 904
Choledochoduodenostomy, 909
Choledochojejunostomy, 909
Choledochostomy, 906
  indications for, 895
Cholelithiasis, 890
  in children, 1514
Cholera, O'Shaughnessy's experiments, 76

Cholesterol, ester, as liver function test, 1010
  serum, and dietary fat, 108
Cholesterosis, in gallbladder, 894
Cholografin, for visualizing gallstones, 891
Chondromas, of ribs, 1413
Chondromatosis, synovial, 1718
Chondrosarcoma, 1734, 1735
  of ribs and cartilages, 1413
Chordoma, 1776
  of nasopharynx, 1421
Chromophils, of pituitary, 749
Chylothorax, in infants, 1504
Circulation, constriction, with plaster cast, 475
Cirrhosis, alcoholic, and portal hypertension, 1004
  Laennec's, 997
  liver, 910
  principal causes, 999
Cisterna chyli, 1067
Citrate intoxication, 174
Claudication, intermittent, 1316
Clavicle, fractures, 478
  green-stick fractures, in children, 479
Clay-shoveler's fracture, 568
Cleft lip, 1450
  double, design for repair, 1454
  repair, 1451
  design, 1452
Cleft palate, repair, 1453
Cloquet's hernia, 1243
Clostridium, infections, 65
  tetani, 40
  types, 40
  welchii, 40
Clot, fibrin, formation and dissolution, 192
Clotting time, abnormal after whole-body irradiation, 416
  effect of technic, 956
Clubfoot, equinovarus, 1685
  recurrence, 1687
  treatment, 1686
  uncorrected, 1685
Coagulation, dynamics of, 192
Coarctation of aorta, 1264
  angiocardiogram, 1265
  diagnosis, 1265
  results and prognosis, 1268
  treatment, 1266
Coccidioides immitis, 41, 72
Coccidioidomycosis, 72, 1389, 1390
  involving bone, 1711
Coccyx, fractures, 569
Coin lesions, 1391
Cold injury, 398-402, 640
  types and treatment, 400-401
Colectomy, total, for familial polyposis, 1149
  for ulcerative colitis, 1127, 1153
Colic, renal, 1583

Colitis, ulcerative, and cancer, 1152
  indications for operation, 1119
  nonspecific, 1120
    age and sex distribution, 1124
    clinical course, 1123
    indications for surgery, 1127
    pathology, 1121
    personality of patient, 1125
    treatment, 1126
  and pseudopolyposis, 1152
Collagen, 1661
  in wound healing, 12, 13
Collapse, cardiovascular, after local anesthesia, 253
  respiratory, after local anesthesia, 253
  therapy, improved methods, 1393
Colles' fracture, 509-512
  reversed, fracture, 509, 512
Colloids, for burn shock, 370
Colon, atresia or stenosis, 1525
  cancer, age distribution, 1157
    incidence of symptoms, 1156
    influence of extent of disease on survival, 1168
    location, 1154
    obstruction, 1157
    prognosis and results, 1168
    symptoms and physical signs, 1155
    treatment, 1160
    x-ray therapy, 1160
  compressed air injuries, 1109
  dead and distended, surgical management, 1098
  extent of resection, after division of various arteries, 985
  intra-abdominal, 1066
  perforation, by cancer, 1158
  polyposis, familial, 1148
  polyps, 1140
  premalignant lesions, 1148-1153
  resection, and arterial supply, 987
  sigmoid, mesentery, 982
  surgery, preparation of patient, 1159
    cleansing bowel, 1160
  tumors, benign, 1146-1148
  volvulus, primary, 1099
  wounds, 627
  x-ray studies, 1159
Coloplicopexy, 1100
Coloscopy, with polypectomy, 1144
Colostomy, 1167
  of descending colon, 1095
  location, 1094
  loop, for relief of distention, 1094
  transverse, 1096
Columella, elongation, 1455

Subject Index

Coma, electrolyte imbalance, 99
  hepatic, 1011
Combat, stress, 606
Commissurotomy, mitral, 1288, 1289
Complement, 46
Complications, postoperative, prevention, 296
Concretions, in stomach, 861
Condylomata acuminata, 1174, 1547
Congestion, pulmonary, signs, 313
Contamination, of wounds caused by mines and booby traps, 603
Contingency, two by two, table, 1813
Contraception, 1571
Contractures, release and repair, 1443
Convalescence, normal, 348
Convulsions, after local anesthesia, 253
Cooley's anemia, 970
Cooling, gastric, for hemorrhage, 843
Coombs' antiglobulin test, 160
Coombs' test, direct, 161
  indirect, 161
Cooper's hernia, 1243
Cordotomy, 1803
Corns, 1735
  soft, 1735
Corn starch, as foreign body, 17
Corticoids, anti-inflammatory potencies, 786
  and carbohydrate metabolism, 776
  physiologic activity, 757
  physiologic and pharmacologic actions, 775
  and protein metabolism, 775
  and salt management, 786
  in surgical patients, 785
  in the treatment of shock, 136, 138
Corticotropin, 752
Cortisone, as immunosuppressive, 442
  psychosis, 333
  and wound healing, 785
Corynebacterium diphtheriae, 37
Cough, as defense measure, 1380
Coxa plana, 1692
Coxa vara, congenital, 1690
Craniopharyngioma, 1776
Craniosynostosis, 1786
Craniotomy, fever following, 305
Cranium bifidum, 1786
Creatinine, clearance test, 1598
Crohn's disease, 1115
Crossmatching, of blood, 152
  principles, 164
Crossmatch, high-protein, 164
Cruroraphia, for esophageal hiatal hernia, 1234

Cruveilhier-Baumgarten syndrome, 997, 1007
Cryptorchism, 1646
  complications of untreated, 1646
Crypts of Morgagni, 1066
Cuboid, fractures, 559
Cuneiform, fractures, 559
Curettage, diagnostic, 1571
Curie, 404
Curling's ulcer, 393, 830
  in infants and children, 1511
Cushing's disease, 777
  complaints of patients, 779
  pathology, 780
  treatment, 780
Cushing's syndrome, 772
  as cause of hypertension, 1602
Cushing's ulcer, 830
Cutis grafts, in hernia repair, 1242
Cyclophosphamide, in control of cancer, 229
Cyclopropane, for anesthesia, 248
Cyst, branchial cleft, 1433, 1497
  choledochal, 1514
  colloid, 1777
  dentigerous, mandible, 1427
  dermoid, in infants, 1496
  enterogenous, 1510
  of eyelid, 1416
  hemorrhagic, mandible, 1426
  inclusion, 661
  laryngeal, 1431
  of liver, 911
  of lungs, congenital, 1505
  mediastinal, in infants, 1503
  of mesentery, 990, 1511
  ovarian, treatment, 1566
    twisted, vs appendicitis, 1046
  of pancreas, 939
    signs and symptoms, 940
    treatment, 941
  pilonidal, 662
  radicular, mandible, 1426
  sebaceous, 661
  of spleen, 962
  thyroglossal duct, 1433
  vaginal inclusion, 1548
Cystadenomas, of pancreas, 940, 941
Cystic duct, 881
Cysticercosis, 1788
Cystitis, acute, 1615
Cystocele, 1541
Cystometrograph, normal bladder, 1636
Cystometry, 1636

Deafness, as sign of intracranial lesion, 1762
Death, from starvation, 342
Débridement, open fracture, 469
  of wounds, 607
Decamethonium, 256, 258
Defecation, 1069

Defect, atrial septal, 1271
  treatment, 1272
  ventricular septal, 1273
Defibrillator, external, 1295
Deficit, extracellular fluid, 78
  salt, 78
Delirium, 329
  tremens, 333
Depletion, bodily, after injury, 350
  extracellular fluid, 78
DeQuervain's disease, 1725
DeQuervain's stenosing tenosynovitis, 593
Dermatofibroma, lenticulare, 660
Dermatofibrosarcoma, protuberans, 660
Dermoid cysts, 661
  in infants, 1501
Desoxycorticosterone acetate, (DOCA), 777
Dextran, as plasma substitute, 190
Diabetes, and wound infection, 301
  in surgical patient, 113
  maintenance of fluid balance, 98
Diabetes insipidus, 1596
Dialysis, in renal failure, 1601
Diarrhea, and partial mechanical obstruction, 1079
  water loss, 90
Diastematomyelia, 1798
Dicumarol, for thrombophlebitis, 322
Diets, high fat, and atherosclerosis, 107
Digitalization, in acute postoperative heart failure, 314
Dilatation, gastric, postoperative, 326
  for esophageal stricture, 800
Diplopia, 1756
Disk, intervetebral, disease and injury, 1740
  herniated, 1741
  protrusion, 1794
  ruptured, 1793
Diskography, 1793
Dislocation, acromioclavicular, 486
  of carpus, 515, 516
  of cervical spine, 563
  definition, 449
  of elbow, 502
  of foot, 560
  general considerations, 448-477
  of hip, 524-527
  of knee, 534
  of lower extremity, 518-561
  of lunate, 516
  midcarpal, 517
  perilunar, 517
  peritalar, 560
  of shoulder, 483
  of spine, pelvis, sternum, and ribs, 562-573
  tarsometatarsal, 561

of upper extremity, 478-517
Dissections, anatomic, and wound healing, 19
Distraction, and wound healing, 15
Diuretics, 1596
  used clinically, 1597
Diverticulitis, 1130-1135
  barium enema examination, 1133
  clinical pattern and course, 1132
  differential diagnosis with cancer, 1159
  pathology, 1131
  perforation, 1134
  proctoscopic examination, 1133
  treatment, 1133
Diverticulosis, 1130
Diverticulum(a), of bladder, 1604
  of duodenum, 868
  epiphrenic, 804
  esophageal, 802
    treatment, 803
  pharyngo-esophageal, 802
  pulsion types, 802
  supradiaphragmatic, 804
  traction types, 804
Donor, blood, universal, 165
Donor organ, availability, 443
Donovania granulomatis, 72
Drain, sump, in abdominal surgery, 23
  rule for use, 23
Drainage, biliary, 893
  of infected wound, 301
  suction, alimentary, water loss, 91
  and wound healing, 21, 22
Draping, operative field, 283
Dressings, in pediatric surgery, 1494
  silver nitrate, dangers, 383
  surgical, 288
  wet, for burns, 376
    need for dry covering, 379
    thermal gradients, 381
    and wound healing, 23
Drugs, antitubercular, 1393
  depolarizing, 256
  emetic, and postoperative nausea, 327
  immunosuppressive, 442
  for intestinal antisepsis, 1160
  vasodilators, in chronic occlusive disease, 1323
Duct, common, carcinoma, 931
  obstruction, differential diagnosis, 933
  stricture, 906
  omphalomesenteric, anomalies, 1515, 1517
  of Santorini, 917
  of Wirsung, 916
Ductus arteriosus. *See* Patent ductus arteriosus
Duffy factor, 162

Dunlop's traction, for supracondylar fracture of humerus, 493, 494
Duodenitis, 869
Duodenotomy, with exploration of common duct, 907
Duodenum, 819-879
  arteriomesenteric compression syndrome, 867
  carcinoma, 868, 931
  diverticula, 868
  enterogenous cyst, 868
  fistulas, 869
  mucosa, altered resistance, 827
  peptic ulcer, 829
  perforation, traumatic, 869
  stump, methods of closure, 854
  ulcer, 838
    indications for operation, 840
  wounds, 626
Dupuytren's contracture, 594, 595, 1727
Dumping syndrome, 856
  late hypoglycemic, 859
  pathophysiology, 859
  treatment, 858
Dwarfism, pituitary, 771
Dysmenorrhea, 1569
Dysplasia, fibrous, maxillary and zygomatic bones, 1418
Dyspnea, postoperative, 312, 315

Ear, deformities, 1476
  tumors, 1417
Echinococcus cysts, 911
  in spleen, 963
Ectasia, of breast, 672
Ectropion, 1478
Edema, arterial occlusive, 324
  due to cardiac decomposition, 325
  hyposmotic, 324
  with low serum protein, 102
  of lymphadenitis, 323
  lymphatic obstructive, 324
  peripheral, with portal hypertension, 1005
  pitting, 102
  after plantaris tendon rupture, 323
  postfixation, 324
  postoperative, 102, 321
  salt-overload, 324
  traumatic myositis, 323
  venous occlusive, 321
Edrophonium, 258
Effusion, pericardial, 1284
Eisenmenger's complex, 1280
Elbow, dislocation, 502
  fractures and dislocations, 490
  splinting, 462
  tennis, 1725
Electrocardiograms, hyper- and hypokalemia, 96
Electroencephalography, 1766

Electrolytes, balance, 75-100
  abnormalities, diagnosis, 91
  in comatose patient, 99
  in infants, 1493
  maintenance, 95
  changes in shock, 129
  concentrations in plasma, 89
  in digestive secretions, 90
  and fluids, diagnoses of abnormalities, 81
Electromyography, 1793
Electron capture, 203
Electron volts, 404
Electroscope, 411
Embolectomy, aortic bifurcation, 1303
  general steps, 1302
  superior mesenteric artery, 991
Embolism, air, 305
  arterial, 1299
    symptoms, 1301
    treatment, 1301
  fat, 304
  pulmonary, 1359, 1360
Embolus(i), 1298
  common sources of peripheral, 1300
  pulmonary, 325
Emphysema, lobar, 1505
Empyema, 1386
  chronic, 1386
  excision or decortication, 1389
  following pneumonectomy, 1388
  in infants and children, 1504
  mixed tuberculous, 1394
Encephalocele, 1786
Encephalopathy, ammonia, 1012
  hepatic, 1011
Endarterectomy, of bifurcation of aorta, 1324
Endo-aneurysmorrhaphy, 1351
Endocrine glands, hyperfunction, 1761
  hypofunction, as result of intracranial lesion, 1764
  mediators between wound and response, 339
Endometriosis, 1574
  in colorectum, 1148
  of ovary, 1575
  treatment, 1576
Endoscopy, urologic, 1580
Energy, requirements after injury, 346
Enteritis, acute bacterial, vs intestinal obstruction, 1080
  regional, 1114
    vs appendicitis, 1046
    clinical pattern and course, 1116
    treatment, 1118
    x-ray examination, 1117
Enterocele, 1540
Enterocolitis, pseudomembranous, 1137

Subject Index

Enterogastrone, 826
Enuresis, diagnosis, 1641
Enzymes, of pancreatic juice, 918
Epignathus, in newborn, 1496
Epiphysis, capital femoral, slipped, 1690, 1691
  normal and rachitic, 1673
Epinephrine, adrenergic response, 759
  pharmacologic action, 787
Epispadias, 1645
Epithelioma, calcifying, of Malherke, 659
Erysipelas, 61
Erythroblastosis foetalis, 177
Erythrocyte, utilization, 960
Eschar, removed from burn, 376
Escherichia coli, 38
Esophagectomy, for cancer, 815
Esophagitis, peptic, 804
  reflux, 804
  and peptic ulceration, 833
  with stricture, 807
  treatment, 805, 806
  and sliding hiatal hernia, 833
Esophagogastrectomy, for bleeding varices, 1018
Esophagojejunostomy, in esophageal carcinoma, 813
Esophagoscopy, to detect esophageal varices, 1007
  for foriegn bodies, 798
  risks, 1377
Esophagus, 795-818
  anatomy and physiology, 795
  benign stricture, 799
  benign tumors, 816
    treatment, 817
  burns, in infants and children, 1503
  carcinoma, 810
    palliative treatment, 812
    prognosis, 812
    radical surgery, 813
  diverticula, 802
    treatment, 803
  foreign bodies, 797
  intrathoracic, anatomy, 796
  spontaneous rupture, 800, 801
  stenosis, 834
  strictures, chronic, management, 800
    in infants, 1503
  tumors, 810
  ulcer, from ectopic gastric mucosa, 832
Estrogen, therapy, cancer of breast, 705
Ether, for anesthesia, 249
Etheron, as prosthesis, 1488, 1489
Ethyl alcohol, as intravenous feeding, 110
Evacuation, of battle casualties, 610, 612
  by helicopter, 612, 613

Evans, formula for treatment of burns, 371
Eventration, of diaphragm, 1244
  umbilical, 1246
Ewing's sarcoma, 1733
Examination, gynecological, 1534
  rectal, prostate, 1584
  urological, 1583
Exercises, perineal, 1541
Exomphalos, 1519
Exostoses, of joint surfaces, 1717
Exploration, for parathyroids, 744
Explosion, hazard, in operating room, 267
  thermonuclear, effects, 406
Exstrophy, of bladder, 1645
Extremities, wounds, 628
Eye(s), injuries during anesthesia, 266
  wounds, 620
Eyelids, benign tumors, 1415
  carcinoma, basal cell, 1416
  conditions requiring reconstruction, 1478
  deformities, 1477
  ptosis, 1477
  tumors, malignant, 1416

Face, compound injuries, 1462
  severe crushing, 1468
  paralysis, 1469
    treatment, 1474
  soft tissue repair, 1464
  transverse fractures, 1468
  tumors, benign, 1417
  wounds, 619
Fallout, radiation, 408
  stratospheric, 409
Fasciitis, necrotizing, 61
  streptococcal, 62
Fat embolism, 304, 642
  with fractures, 458
Fat, after injury, 346
Fat necrosis, 656
  of breast, 671
Fat, in nutrition, 107
Fecaliths, in appendicitis, 1027
Feeding, intravenous, development of, 110
Felons, 577
Felty's syndrome, 965
Femur, epiphysis, separation, 534
  fracture, condyles, 533
    continuous balanced traction, 528
    of distal end, 533, 534
    emergency splinting, 528
    with intramedullary nail, 531
    open reduction and internal fixation, 530
    supracondylar, 533
  head, aseptic necrosis, 520
  neck, impacted fractures, 520
    unimpacted fractures, 521

  shaft, fracture, 527
    in children, 531
    comminuted, 532
  trochanter, fractures, 523
Fertility, 1571
Fever, in cancer of lung, 1405
  postcraniotomy, 305
  postoperative, 300
    from pulmonocardiac disturbances, 302
  third-day, 64
  and water loss, 351
Fibrinogen, deficiency, after blood transfusion, 174
  transfusion, 182
Fibroadenoma, of breast, 671
Fibromata, of ovary, 1565
Fibrosarcoma, 666
Fibrosis, perineural, 1736
  subepidermal nodular, 660
Fibula, congenital absence, 1690
Filling time, venous, 1318
Filtrate, glomerular, 1587
Finger, amputation, general rule, 585
  joints, 592
  replantation, 575
  skin, circumferential avulsion, 576
  snapping, 593
  trigger, 593
Fire, hazard in operating room, 267
Fissure, of anus, 1186
  in infants, 1527
Fissurectomy, 1187
Fistula, abdominal enterocutaneous, 1063
  in-ano, 1190
    and intestinal tuberculosis, 1114
  arteriovenous, common forms, 1313
    intracranial, 1783
    traumatic, 1313
    treatment, 1313
  auris congenita, 1496
  duodenobiliary, 898
  of duodenum, 869
  fecal, after appendectomy, 1041
  Goodsall's rule, 1191
  pancreatic, 928
  pulmonary arteriovenous, 1281, 1505
  rectovaginal, 1544
  ureterovaginal, 1543
  urethrocutaneous, 1609
  urethrovaginal, 1543
  urinary, in female, 1643
  vesicovaginal, 1543
  water loss, 90
Fixation, external skeletal, 466
Flail chest, 1380
  treatment, 1381
Flatfoot, 1686
  spastic, 1687

Subject Index 1847

Flechettes, wounds, 605
Fluid, balance, 75-100
  disturbances, diagnosis, 91
  in infants, 1493
  and electrolytes, diagnoses of abnormalities, 81
  losses, with malabsorption, 1073
  replacement, for shock, 137
  space, isotopic methods, 206
5-Fluorouracil, for cancer control, 229
Fogarty catheter, 1302
Folic acid, 115
  deficiency, 1073
Follicle stimulating hormone, 752
Foot, common problems, 1735
  dislocations, 560
  fractures, 555
  immersion, 398, 641, 642
  repair of surface defects, 1481
  stabilization, 1696
  wounds, combat, 635
Foraminal compression test, 1795
Forearm, of child, fractures of shafts of bones, 503, 504, 505
  fractures of the shaft of the bones, 502
  splinting, 462
Foreign bodies, in esophagus, 797
  ingested, and intestinal obstruction, 1083
  subcutaneous, 663
  and wound healing, 16
Fractures, alveolar, 1468
  apposition and alignment, 450
  at birth, 473
  of bones of foot, 555-560
  of both bones in leg, 543-548
  callus, 450
  of capitellum, 498
  of carpus, 513
  cellular response, 1664
  of cervical spine, 563
  in children, 471
    growth increased, 472
  of clavicle, 478
  closed reduction, 463
  closed undisplaced, 1664
  of coccyx, 569
  Colles', 509-512
  complications, 454
  compound, combat, 631, 632
  definitions, 448
  diagnosis, 451
  external skeletal fixation, 466
  femur, condyles, 533
    distal end, 533, 534
    shaft, 527
  of fibula, shaft, 549
  general considerations, 448-477
  healing, 450, 1664
    basic mechanisms, 1660
    biochemistry, 1665
    enzyme systems, 1665

about hip, 518-524
humerus, proximal portion, 480
  shaft, 487
  supracondylar, manipulative reduction, 491
no immobilization, 467
with intra-abdominal complications, 454
with intrathoracic complications, 455
of lateral malleolus, with dislocation of foot, 551, 552
of lower extremity, 518-561
management, methods, 463, 464
  objectives, 459
of mandible, 1465
maxims, 448
of the metatarsals, 559
of midtarsal bones, 559
Monteggia, 501
nonunion, causes, 1666
  and delayed union, 457
of navicular, 513, 514
  avascular necrosis, 515
of nose, 1468
of olecranon, 498, 499
open, 467
  débridement, 469
  reduction, 466
  splinting, 463
  treatment of wound, 468
of patella, 539
pathologic, 473, 474
of pelvis, 569
of the phalanges of the toes, 560
of radius, head and neck, 499, 500
  lower end, 507
  and ulna, 507
regulation of healing, 451
rehabilitation, 477
roentgen examination, 452
of ribs, 571
of sacrum, 568
of scapula, 479
separation of distal radial epiphysis, 512
of shaft of bones in forearm, 502
of spine, pelvis, sternum, and ribs, 562-573
splinting, emergency, 460, 461
of sternum, 571
of tibia, proximal end, 540
  shaft, 549
traction, continuous balanced, 465
types, 449
of upper extremity, 478-517
variations in healing response, 1666
Freedom, degree of, 1813
Freezing, gastric, 844
Freiberg's disease, 1738
Froment's sign, 579
Frostberg, inverted-3 sign, 936

Frostbite, 641
Fructose, for intravenous feeding, 109
Function, of combat medical service, 599

Galen, views on blood and circulation, 150
Gallamine, 258
Gallbladder, anatomy, 881
  and bile passages, 880-915
  carcinoma, 886
  with hourglass constriction, 896
  pathology, 889
  perforation, 888
    mortality, 889
  with phyrgian cap, 895
  s-shaped, 895
  standard operation, 904
  strawberry, 894
  tumors, 886
  wounds, 626
Gallstone, causing intestinal obstruction, 1087, 1088
  ileus, 888
  laminated, 891
  with layering of contrast medium, 897
  layering of nonopaque, 896
  pigmented, in spherocytic anemia, 966
  radiolucent gas pocket, 896
  on x-ray, 890
Gamma radiation, half-thickness principle of protection, 411
Gamma rays, 202, 403
Ganglion, 595, 1727
Ganglioneuromas, 1412
Gangrene, cutaneous, chronic, progressive, 63
  frost, 399
  gas, 67, 68
    statistics, 638
  hemolytic streptococcal, 61
Gardner's syndrome, 1106, 1150
Gas gangrene, battle wounds, 637
Gas therapy, postoperative, 315
Gastrectomy, proximal, 854
  subtotal, for bleeding varices, 1018
  total, 854
Gastric tube, for decompression, 1091
Gastrin, action of, 823
Gastritis, acute, 862
  atrophic, 862
  chronic, 863
  corrosive, 863
  hypertrophic, 863
  phlegmonous, 863
  postoperative, 863
  necrotizing, 863
Gastroduodenostomy, after gastric resection, 853

Gastrointestinal tract, after irradiation, 427
and wound healing, 26
Gastrojejunostomy, 853
after gastric resection, 853
types, 855
Gastromalacia, 863
Gastropexia, anterior geniculata, for esophageal hiatal hernia, 1234
Gastroschisis, 1519
Gastrostomy, 856
Gaucher's disease, 969, 1678
Geiger-Mueller counter, 203
Genital tract, diseases of lower, 1542
Genitalia, female, congenital abnormalities, 1535
Ghon tubercle, 1406
Gibbus formation, 1713, 1714
Gigantism, 767
Gliomas, 1775
Glomerulotrophin, 340
Glomerulus, filtration, 1587
Gloving, technic, self-gloving, 282
by nurse, 283
Glucose, after injury, 345
in intravenous nutrition, 109
reabsorption in tubule, 1588
Glycosuria, 1589
Goblet cells, in intestinal metaplasia, 844
Goiter, colloid, in children, 1498
exophthalmic, signs and symptoms, 717
nodular, 720
classification, 720
pathogenesis, 715
Gonococcus, 37
Gonorrhea, 1544, 1614
Gout, 663
Gown, technic, 281
Graafian follicle, vs. appendicitis, 1045
Grafts, bone, 1667
marrow, for irradiation, 420
cutis, in hernia repair, 1242
skin, delayed flap, 1446
direct flap, 1446
donor site dressings, 1438
and rejection, 438
split, 1437
vascular, with occluded artery, 1325
for repair in injury, 1310
Granuloma, amebic, 1112
annulare, 651
eosinophilic, 1678, 1679
inguinale, 72
umbilical, 1515
Grave's disease, 717
Grenades, wounds, 604
Gridiron incision, in appendectomy, 1032
Growth hormone, 750
effects, 767

Gunshot, wounds, 605
Gynecology, 1534-1579
Gynecomastia, 709

Half life, of radioisotopes, 405
Hallucinations, 330
alcoholic, 333
Hallux rigidus, 1738
valgus, 1738
Halothane, for anesthesia, 249
and hypotension, 250
Hamartoma, 1410
Hand, avulsion of tissue, 575
bones and joints, 583
burns, 1444
partial thickness, 577
radiation, 1446
compound wounds, 585
developmental abnormalities, 1688
fractures, preservation of joint motion, 583
infections, of palmar spaces, 578
of soft tissues, 577
lacerations, 575
nerves, diagnosis of sensory defect, 578
repair of peripheral, 579
principles of surgery, 574-598
reconstruction, 585
nerves, 587
rehabilitation and disability, 596
rheumatoid arthritis, 592
surgical treatment, 594
rheumatoid deformities, 592, 593
skin, radiation effect, 577
replacement, 585
soft tissue injuries, 574
splinting, 462
tendons, lacerations, 580
repair, 581-583
tumors, 595
wounds, combat, 634
Hand-Schuller-Christian disease, 1677
Hanot's cirrhosis, 910
Harrington's classification, of esophageal hiatal hernia, 1230, 1231
Harrison's groove, 1500
Hartmann's pouch, 881
Harvey, and *De Motu Cordis*, 150
Head, and neck, cancer, palliative care, 1435
normal arteriogram, 1772, 1773
tumors, 1415
Headache, from chronic increased intracranial pressure, 1755
postoperative, 327
Healing, by first intention, 8
of fractures, 450
by second intention, 8
of special tissues, 24
by third intention, 10
of wounds, 8-33
chronologic course, 9

Heart, acquired disease, 1282-1294
acquired valvular disease, surgery, 1286
atrial septal defect, 1271
congenital lesions, 1259-1282
failure, 312
rate, in shock, 127
stab wounds, 1285
surgery, 1259-1297
under direct vision, 1294
ventricular septal defect, 1273
Heat, needed to burn skin, 362
stroke, 306
in treatment of shock, 139
Heel, bursitis, 1737
tuberosities, 1737
Heidenhain pouch, 823
Heineke-Mikulicz operation, 852
Helium, for relief of partial obstructions of airway, 316
Heloma durum, 1735
Hemangioblastoma, 1777
Hemangioma, 653
cavernous, 654
of colorectum, 1148
sclerosing, 660
Hematemesis, with portal hypertension, 1004
Hematocolpos, 1536
Hematocrit, during depletion of sodium salts, 79
and rate of urine flow, in burn shock, 368
in salt and water deficits, 85
Hematoma, 663
dissecting, 1344
extradural, 1779
intracerebral, 1778, 1780
intracranial, traumatic, 1779
larynx, 1431
ossifying, with fractures, 458
pulsating, 1311
treatment, 1312
subdural, 1779
in infancy, 1780
Hematuria, 1583
Hemobilia, 886
Hemoconcentration, and shock, 126
Hemolysis, during burn, 390
after transfusion, 168
Hemoperitoneum, 1056
Hemophilia, 193
Hemophilus influenzae, 39
Hemorrhage, after acute irradiation, 416
as cause of shock, 124
as complication of fracture, 455
diagnostic procedures, 196
focal, signs, 1779
intra-abdominal, 625
management during operation, 287
massive, duodenal ulcer, indication for operation, 842
intra-abdominal, 615

water and salt loss, 91
Hemorrhoid(s), 1192-1197
  chronic internal, treatment, 1194
  differential diagnosis, 1194
  external, acutely thrombosed, 1194
  with portal hypertension, 1006
  predisposing factors, 1193
  St. Mark's Hospital operation, 1196
Hemorrhoidectomy, postoperative management, 1197
  technic, 1195
Hemostasis, clotting factors, 194, 195
  early efforts, 153
  instruments for, 154
  mechanical methods, 196
  operative, 287
  as surgical problem, 191
  and wound healing, 21
Heparin, neutralization, 181
  in thrombophlebitis, 323
Hepatic duct, common, anatomy, 881
Hepatitis, icteric serum, 183
  vs obstruction, 900
  postnecrotic, and portal hypertension, 997
  serum, attack rates, 184
    immunity, 188
    morbidity, 184
    virus inactivation, 185
  in wounded, 640
Hepatorenal syndrome, 902
Hepatectomy, partial, 912
Heredity, in cancer, 222
Hernia, 1204, 258
  in the aged, 1235
  aids to repair, 1239
  amniotic, 1519
  bilateral repair at one operation, 1236
  congenital, 1243
  definition, 1205
  diagnosis, 1205
    differential, 1206
  differentiating between direct and indirect, 1206
  differentiating between inguinal and femoral, 1206
  epigastric, 1243
  errors and safeguards in repair, 1238
  esophageal hiatal, 1227
    anatomic considerations, 1228
    complications, 1233
    diagnosis, 1233
    Harrington's classification, 1230, 1231
    incidence, 1232
    predisposing factors, 1232
    sliding type, 1231
    surgical treatment, 1233
    symptoms, 1232
  femoral, 1221
    en-glissade, 1248
    external, 1244
    with multilocular sacs, 1244
    repair, inguinal approach, 1222
      lower approach, 1221
      preperitoneal approach, 1222-1224
    tendency to strangulate, 1221
  hiatus, 807
    in newborn, 1503
    sliding, and esophagitis, 833
  historical considerations, 1205
  incarcerated, defined, 1244
    and strangulation, 1209
  industrial aspects, 1236
  in infancy and childhood, 1235
  inguinal, and cord division, 1241
    direct, 1220
    factors leading recurrence, 1224
    incidence and prognosis, 1206, 1207
    indirect, 1211
      advanced type, 1215
      infant type, 1212-1214
      intermediate type, 1215
      simple type, 1214
      steps in radical repair, 1215-1220
    methods to facilitate closure of internal ring, 1240
    recurrence rates, 1207
    recurrent, 1224
    repair, 1210-1212
  injection treatment, 1236
  internal, 1244
  interparietal, 1244
  interstitial, 1244
  intestinal tube to reduce distention, 1240
  irreducible, defined, 1244
  lacunar ligament, 1245
  lateral ventral, 1251
  lumbar, 1245
  massive, facilitation of surgery, 1239
  mesenteric defect, 1245
  mesentericoparietal, 1246
  obturator, 1246
  paraduodenal, 1246
  patches, 1242
  pectineal, 1247
  perineal, 1247
  peritoneoscopial, 1247
  posterolateral, 1247
  prevascular, 1247
  rare, 1243
  reducible, 1247
  relaxing incisions, 1240
  retroanastomotic, 1247
  retrovascular, 1247
  sacrosciatic, 1248
  sciatic, 1248
  size of subcutaneous inguinal ring, 1238
  sliding, 1248
    blood supply, 1249
    operation for, 1250
  2-stage closure, 1240
  strangulated, 1251
    reduction, 1094
  subsidiary problems, 1235
  supravesical, 1251
  suture material, 1237
  suture reinforcement, 1241
  temptation to resect bowel, 1240
  thumb test, 1206
  traumatic, of diaphragm, 1251
  treatment by nonsurgical means, 1236
  umbilical, 1225
  use of tantalum, 1242
  ventral incisional, 1225
Herniorrhaphy, in infants and young children outpatients, 1235
  prognosis, 1207
Hesselbach's hernia, 1244
Hiccough, 327
Hidradenitis suppurativa, 650
Hidradenoma, 651
Hip, dislocations, 524-527
  anterior, 526
  central, 570
  congenital, 1682, 1683
  and congenital dysplasia, 1680
  posterior, 524
    with fracture of acetabulum, 526
    with fracture of femoral head, 526
  dysplastic, 1682
  fractures, 518-524
    intracapsular, treatment, 519, 522
  joint, prosthesis, 522
  stabilization, 1697
Hirschsprung's disease, 1524, 1525
Histiocytoma, 660
Histoplasma capsulatum, 41, 73
Histoplasmosis, 73, 1390
History, gynecological, 1534
Hoarseness, as symptom of laryngeal tumor, 1431
Hodgkin's disease, in infants, 1495
Hoguet's maneuver, in hernia repair, 1216, 1217
Hollander test, for vagal function, 822
Homocystinuria, 1677
  and Marfan syndrome, 1677
Homograft(s), for burns, 384, 1441
  immunity, 27, 28
  postmortem, 1441
  and wound healing, 27
Hormone(s), of adrenal medulla, 758

1850 Subject Index

Hormone(s) (*Cont.*)
 antidiuretic, 1595
  in response to injury, 341
 in control of cancer, 226
 control mechanisms, 760
 human growth, 766
 pituitary, 750, 751
Hospital, mobile Army surgical, 613
Hot flash, 1569
Humerus, fracture, epiphyseal separation, proximal, 482
 of greater tuberosity, 482
 of lateral condyle, 495
 of lower end, in adults, 497
  in children, 490
 of medial epicondyle, 496
 medial condyle, 495
 nerve injuries, 489
 proximal portion, 480
 shaft, 487
 supracondylar and transcondylar, 490, 492, 493
Humidification, with mechanical ventilator, 272
Hunter syndrome, 1674, 1676
Hurler syndrome, 1674, 1676
Hyaline membrane disease, 1504
Hydrocele, 1632
Hydrocephalus, 1785
 communicating, 1786
 normal pressure, 1788
Hydrocolpos, 1536
Hydrocortisone, for burn shock, 370
Hydronephrosis, 1605, 1608
 intermittent, 1613
 of pregnancy, 1613
 due to ureteropelvic obstruction, 1609
Hydro-ureter, 1605
Hygroma colli, 655
Hygroma, cystic, in infants, 1497
 of neck, 1432
Hymen, imperforate, and retained menses, 1535, 1536
Hyperalimentation, intravenous, 111
Hypercalcemia, metastatic breast cancer, 708
Hypercalciuria, 1626
Hypercorticism, 777
Hyperemia, reactive, 1318
Hyperextension, of spine, 565
Hyperhidrosis, 650, 1807
Hyperkalemia, in aging blood, 170
 with burns, 385
 electrocardiogram, 96
Hyperkeratosis, plantar, 1736
Hypernatremia, in burns, 386
Hypernephroma, 1620, 1621
Hyperosmolarity, fever from, 306
Hyperparathyroidism, 730, 731
 diagnosis, 735
 pathologic calcification, 735
 roentgen aspects, 736
 treatment, 737

Hyperplasia, parathyroids, 733
Hyperpotassemia, 88
Hypersplenism, 972
Hyperthermia, in patients with severe cerebral lesions, 1789
Hyperthyroidism, 716
 psychosomatic considerations, 717, 719
 treatment, 718
Hypertension, benign intracranial, 1787
 portal, 996-1020
  anatomic causes, 997
  diagnosis, 996, 1004
  drug use, 1015
  evaluation of patients, 1007
  indications for operation and selection of patients, 1012
  location of obstruction, by x-ray, 1006
  suprahepatic, 998, 1005
  x-ray diagnosis, 1006
 due to renal artery stenosis, 1327
 secondary, etiology, 1602
Hypnosis, and anesthesia, 265
Hypocalcemia, 88
 psychic manifestations, 331
Hypocapnia, in shock, 129
Hypoglycemia, psychosis, 332
Hypokalemia, electrocardiogram, 96
 after injury, 344
Hypoparathyroidism, 731
Hypophysectomy, 770
 cancer of breast, 707
 complications, 772
 in malignant disease, 1806
Hypopituitarism, 772
Hypopotassemia, 88
Hypoproteinemia, 101
 with excess sodium salts, 86
 and gastric emptying, 103
 plasma to correct, 188
 postoperative, 353
 response to plasma, 189
 and wound healing, 103
Hyposmia, 1762
Hypospadias, 1481, 1646
Hyposthenuria, maintenance of fluid balance, 97
Hypotension, controlled (deliberate), 264
 and halothane, 250
 postoperative, treatment, 353
 preoperative, 299
 in severely wounded, 264
 with spinal anesthesia, 254
Hypothermia, 307
 generalized, 641
 induced, 265
 in open heart surgery, 1294
 with shock, 131
Hypovolemia, role in shock, 155
Hypoxia, during operation, 286
 psychosis, 332

Hysterectomy, for myomata, 1560
Hysterosalpingography, 1573

Icterus. *See* Jaundice
Idiosyncrasy, to antibiotics, 58
Ileitis, regional, x-ray, 1118
Ileostomy, 1167
 architecture, 24
 maturation, 24, 25
 early postoperative management, 1129
 technic of construction, 1128, 1129
Ileum, anatomy, 1066
 atresia of, 1507
 wounds, 627
Ileus, 1074
 adynamic, 311
  in perforative appendicitis, 1041
  with peritonitis, 1086
 complications of, 1089
 use of gastric tube, 1091
 mechanical differentiated from adynamic, 1087
  etiology, 1086
  specific treatment, 1090
 with peritonitis, 1053
 postoperative, pain, 310
 treatment, 1088
 types, 1081
 x-ray appearance, 1084
Immersion foot, 398, 641, 642
Immunity, acquired, 46
 natural, 46
 passive, 46
 specific, 46
 in transplant reaction, 437
Immunosuppression, 441
Impetigo, in children, 1494
Impression, basilar, 1786
Incapacitating agents, chemical warfare, 646
Incision, for appendectomy, 1031
 closing, 287
 skin, 283
  commonly used, 285
 and wound healing, 17
Incontinence, anal, 1184
 mixed types, 1643
 stress, 1642
 urinary, 1583
  paradoxical, 1641
  psychogenic, 1643
  types, 1640
Infants, and children, surgery for, 1491-1532
 surgery, anesthesia, 1492
  general considerations, 1491
  premedication, 1492
  preparation for operation, 1492
  time for operation, 1491
  transfusion of blood and parenteral fluids, 1493
Infarct, pulmonary, 325

Infarction, myocardial, postoperative, 311
Infection, after acute irradiation, 418
 bacillary, gram-negative, 63
  resistance of host, 44
 in bone, 1703
 in burns, 373
  in continuous baths, 378
  signs of, 374
 clostridial, 65
 as complication of fractures, 456
 in diabetics, 301
 diphtheritic, 70
 established, surgical therapy, 54
 hemolytic streptococcal, treatment, 62
 human-bite, 65
 iatrogenic, 46
 masked by ACTH, 301
 with mechanical ventilator, 273
 mixed or synergistic, 65
 mycotic, 70
 in open fractures, 468
 resistance to, hypoproteinemia, 103
 of soft tissues of hand, 577
 staphylococcal, 59
 as stimulus of metabolic change, 342
 streptococcal, 60
 surgical, 48-74
  compared with medical, 42
  methods of diagnosis, 51
  treatment, 52
 of surgical wound, 297, 300
 of upper female genital tract, 1556
 of urinary tract, 1614
 wounds, classification, 58
  factors governing, 48
 and wound healing, 15
Infertility, 1572
 investigation, 1573
Infusion, intravenous, 277
Injection, intrathecal, of destructive chemicals, 1801
Injuries, arterial, 630, 1305
 diagnosis, 1307
 incision or laceration, 1305
 perforation, 1305
 repairing with grafts, 1310
 repair by sutures, 1309
 treatment, 1308
 biochemical activity after, 341
 cardiac, 622
 catabolic response, 106
 cellular, from portal radiation, 421
 cold, 398-402, 640
 compound, facial, 1462
 craniocerebral, 1778
 endocrine activity after, 339
 energy requirements, 346
 external penetrating, colon and small bowel, 1108
 by freezing, 641
 genital, by power take-off of tractor, 1480
 industrial and farm, 1480
 intestines, penetrating from within, 1110
 kidney, 1627
 mediastinal, 622
 metabolic changes after, 342
 multiple, emergency treatment, 453
 nonpenetrating, colon and small bowel, 1106
 and pancreatitis, 928
 penis, 1631
 peripheral nerve, 631
 and potassium balance, 344
 priorities in surgical management, 453, 614
 radiation, 403-434
  symptoms, 414
 response of bone, 1660
 scrotum, 1631
 to spine, 1797
 of spinal cord, 618
 as stimulus to bodily change, 338
 testis, 1632
 thoracic, 1376
 thoraco-abdominal, 623
 ureter, 1628
 urethra, 1630
 vitamin requirements, 117
 water and salt loss, 91
 and wound healing, 15
Instrument, count, 289
Insulin, 919
 requirements, after pancreatectomy, 943
Interposition, in wound healing, 15
Interstitial cell stimulating hormone, 752
Intestine(s), absorption, 1069
 congenital disorders, of adult patients, 1103
 dead and distended, surgical management, 1098
 disruption, with obstruction, 1091
 extent of resection compatible with life, 994
 gunshot wounds, 1109
 inflammatory diseases, 1111-1135
 malrotation, 1508
 mucosa, small vessel circulation, 988
 obstruction, foreign bodies, removal, 1094
 origins of gases, 1071
 pendular or oscillating motions, 1068
 peristalsis, 1067
 postoperative mechanical obstruction, 311
 secretions, 1070
 segmental contractions, 1068
 small, anatomy, 1066
  carcinoids, 1137
  mesentery, 983
  response to direct feeding, 109
  tumors of, 1135
   ratio of benign to malignant, 1135
   malignant, 1136
   types and numbers, 1135
 strangulated, determining viability, 1097
 trauma, 1106-1111
  external penetrating, 1108
  nonpenetrating, treatment, 1108
  penetrating from within, 1110
  summary of management, 1110
 tuberculosis, 1113
Intravenous feeding, after operation, 349
 prolonged, 351
Intravenous infusion, glucose, 319
Intubation, gastric, complications, 300
 for intestinal obstruction, 1092
Intussusception, 1521
 in adults, treatment, 1098
 clinical picture, 1522
 diagnosis, 1087
 treatment, 1523
Iodine, involution of thyroid, 715
 radioactive, 205
  dangers, 412
  for hyperthyroidism, 719
Ion(s), concentrations, abnormalities, diagnosis, 92
 loss, with irrigating fluids, 91
Ionization chamber, 204
Iron, deficiency, 1073
 dietary requirements, 118
 metabolism, 117
 nutrition, 116
 radioactive, clearance from plasma, 960
 storage, 117
Irradiation, acute syndrome, 413
 as cause of cancer, 427
 erytheme, 424
 genetic effects, 432
 latent consequences, 432
 loss of skin appendages, 425
 portal, injury, 421
  systemic reactions, 422
 skin reaction, 424
 whole-body, treatment, 418
 See also Radiation
Irreversibility, of shock, 130
Ischemia, with arterial obstruction, 1316
 cerebral, peripheral vascular disease, 1331
 effect of prolonged, 608
 mesenteric arteriolar, 993
 myocardial, 1286

Ischemia (*Cont.*)
  pain of, 307
Islet cell tumors, 929
Iso-agglutinogens, in major blood groups, 157
Iso-hemagglutinins, in major blood groups, 157
Isotocin, 754
Isotopes, 202, 405, 1767
  applications, 205
  dangers in using, 204
  definition, 403
  half life, 202
  physical constants, 207
  physical properties, 202
  preparations, carrier free, 203
  radiation measurement, 203
  technics, in surgery, 202-208
  therapy, danger of excess exposure, 429
  therapeutic level, 205
  tracer, average exposure to radiation, 430
  tracer level, 204
Ivalon, for prostheses, 1483

Jaundice, 899-904
  in cholelithiasis, 890, 895
  homologous serum, 41
  liver function tests, 900
  obstructive, 899
    complications, 901
    prognostic significance, 900
  and portal hypertension, 1006
  postoperative, 321
  preparing patient for operation, 902
  transfusion, 168
Jaw(s), arthritis, 1459
  diseases, 1456
    inflammatory, 1459
  irradiation narcosis, 1461
  reconstruction, 1462
Jaw hook, for reduction of facial fractures, 1467
Jehovah's Witnesses, and transfusions, 156
Jejunostomy, as preliminary procedure in malnourished, 108
Jejunum, anatomy, 1066
  wounds, 627
Jewett brace, for hyperextension, 567
Joint(s), degenerative diseases, 1717
  of fingers, 592
  loss of motion, with fractures, 458
  neuropathic, disease, 1721
  tuberculosis, 1716
  wounds, combat, 633

Kaposi's disease, 664, 665
K-capture, 203

Kel F, for prostheses, 1483
Kell factor, 162
Keloid, 660
Keratoacanthoma, 659, 660
17-Ketosteroid urinary excretion, normal values, 779
Kidney, acute failure, 1599
  clinical picture, 1600
  treatment, 1600
  agenesis, 1643
  anatomy, 1585
  cadaver, 445
  chronic failure, 1602
  concentration and dilution mechanisms, 1594
  congenital anomalies, 1643
  counter-current mechanisms, 1593
  duplication of pelvis and ureter, 1643
  ectopic, 1644
  function in disease, 1599
  function tests, 1598
  horseshoe, 1644
  injuries, 1627
  insufficiency, after injury, 354
  mobility, 1614
  polycystic disease, 1644
  reduced output, postoperative, 320
  salt-losing, maintenance of fluid balance, 97
  staphylococcal, 1618
  stones, and hyperparathyroidism, 730
    as symptom of hyperparathyroidism, 736
  transplantation, 444
    postoperative, 445
    rejection, early signs, 445
    survival curves, 446
  tubular reabsorption, 1588
  tumors, 1620
Klebsiella pneumoniae, 39
Knee, dislocation, 534
  internal derangements, 535-539
  ligaments, collateral, tears, 537
    cruciate, tears, 537
  locked, 536
  loose bodies, 538
  stabilization, 1697
Knee-chest position, 1539
Korsakoff's psychosis, 333
Krukerberg tumor, 1565

Lacerations, of hand, 575
Lacticacidemia, after injury, 347
Lactogenic hormone, 752
Laennec's cirrhosis, 910
Laminectomy, decision to perform, 562
  in wounds of spinal canal, 618
Langer's lines, 17
Laryngoceles, 1431
Larynx, cancer, 1431

tumors, 1431
Laser-maser, radiation, 433
Latta, T., treatment of cholera, 76
Laugier's hernia, 1245
Lead, poisoning, psychoses, 331
  X-rays, distinguished from rickets, 1674
Leg, fractures and dislocations, 518-561
  length, equalization, 1698
  splinting, 462
Legg-Calvé-Perthes' disease, 1692
Leiomyomata, 1559
  of colorectum, 1146
Leishmania, and spleen, 964
Lens, sensitivity to irradiation, 425
LET, 404
Letterer-Siwe's disease, 959, 1677
  in infants, 1495
Leukemia, after irradiation, 427
Leukocyte, count, in appendicitis, 1029
  in perforative appendicitis, 1035
  grouping, 158
  typing, 441
Leukocytosis, with intestinal obstruction, 1079
Leukopenia, after acute irradiation, 415
Leukoplakia, lip, 1422
  oral cavity, 1425
  vulva, 1546
Leukotaxine, in wound healing, 10
Lewis substance, in blood, 158
Liesegang rings, and healing wounds, 12
Life, expectancy, females, 677
Ligament, middle umbilical, 1645
Ligatures, and wound healing, 20, 21
Limb salvage, 1326
Lipase, serum, in pancreatitis, 921
Lipogranuloma, of mesentery, 990
Lipoma(s), 656
  breast, 672
  colorectum, 1146
  cord, 1245
Liposarcoma, 666
Lips, tumors, 1421
Litholapaxy, 1627
Littré hernia, 1245
Liver, 880-915
  abscesses, drainage, 913
  biopsy, 912, 1010
  cirrhosis, mortality, 996
    and peptic ulcer, 1012
    and shunts, 999
  cysts, 911
  function tests, 1008, 1009
  pathology, 910
  physiology, 883
  resection, partial, 912
  reticuloendothelial cells, 884
  reversal of blood flow, 1002

in shock, 130, 902
transplanted, in ectopic position, 437
tumors, in childhood, 1514
wounds, 626, 911
Lobotomy, frontal, 1804
LSD-dependent, anesthesia for, 247
Lunate, dislocation, 516
Lung(s), 1371-1392
  abscess, 1381
    diagnosis and localization, 1382
    medical and surgical treatment, 1383
  agenesis, 1504
  anatomic considerations, 1371
  cancer, radioactive dust, 428
  irritants, chemical warfare, 646
  lobes and segments, 1371, 1372
  metastatic malignant tumors, 1409
  mechanical ventilation, 269
  physiologic considerations, 1373
  tumors, 1402
    in children, 1506
    primary malignant, 1402
Luteotropic hormone, 752
Luteotropin, 752
Luther factor, 162
Lymph, drainage, breast, 686
  spleen, 949
  flow, and ascites, 1003
  nodes, axilla, 669
    function, 45
    internal mammary chain, 669
    mesenteric, 1067
    near pancreas, 916
Lymphangiograms, 666
Lymphangiomas, 655
  face, 1418
Lymphatics, anus, 1067
  breast, 669
Lymphedema, of upper extremity, 696
Lymphocyte, mixed, culture test, 441
  normal, transfer test, 440
Lymphoma, 666
  colorectum, benign, 1148
  thyroid, 722
Lymphopathia venereum, 73
Lymphosarcoma, in infants, 1495
  of intestine, in childhood, 1526

Macewen's sign, 1756
MacGregor's maneuver, in hernia repair, 1217
Macrognathia, 1459
Magenstrasse, 820
Magnesium, deficit, 88, 1074
Malabsorption, and intentional short-circuiting operations, 1073
  syndrome, 1071
Malaria, and spleen, 964

Malformations, arteriovenous, 1783, 1784
Malleolus, lateral, fracture, with dislocation of foot, 551, 552
  medial, fractured, 551
  posterior, fractures, 553
Mallet finger, 582
Mallory-Weiss syndrome, 861, 864
Malnutrition, after appendectomy, 1041
  and operative risk, 239
Malpighi, and capillary circulation, 150
Malrotation, of intestine, 1508
Mammography, 688
Mandible, cystic lesions, 1426
  fractures, 1465
    interdental wire, 1466
  tumors, benign, 1426
    malignant, 1428
Mannitol, in renal insufficiency, 354
Mann-Williamson preparation, for experimental ulcer, 822
March fracture, 559
Maroteaux-Lamy syndrome, 1674, 1676
Masses, inflammatory, sequela of peritonitis, 1058
Mastectomy, postoperative irradiation, 695
  preoperative irradiation, 696
  radical, 691
    operative principles, 693
    skin incisions, 692
    5-year survivals, 701
  simple, 695
  super radical operations, 703
Mastitis, acute pyogenic, 670
  chronic cystic, 672
    relation to breast cancer, 673
    treatment, 674
  tuberculous, 671
Mastodynia, 674, 684
McBurney's point, 1028
Mean(s), comparison of, 1812
  standard error of, 1816
Measurements, analysis of, 1815
Meatus, urethral, stricture, 1645
Meckel's diverticulum, 1066, 1103
  in children, 1515
  diagnosis, 1104
  peptic ulcer, 840
  treatment, 1105
Meconium ileus, 1509
Meconium peritonitis, 1057
Mediastinitis, as postoperative complication, 312
Mediastinum, teratoma, 1411
  tumors, 1410
    of lymphoid origin, 1411
Megacolon, 1524, 1525
  Swenson precedure, 1526
  toxic, 1112
Mega-esophagus, 808

Megalo-ureter, congenital, 1608, 1644
Meissner's plexus, 1069
Melanocyte stimulating hormone, 753
Melanoma, 665
Menarche, 1568
Mendelson's syndrome, 864
Meningiomas, 1775
  sphenoidal wing, 1774
Menopause, 1568
Menstruation, disorders, 1570
  normal cycle, 1568
Meperidine, before anesthesia, 245
Mesentery, anatomy, 980
  colon, ascending and descending, 981
    sigmoid, 982
  cysts, 990
  diseases, 990
  lipogranuloma, 990
  panniculitis, 990
  small intestine, 980, 983
  thrombosis, 991
  tumors, 990
Mesothelioma, of pleura, 1412
Metabolism, of bone and cartilage, 1659
  changes with burns, 386
  disturbed, brain damaged, 1789
Metaplasia, intestinal, 844
Metatarsals, fractures, 559
Metatarsus adductus, 1686
Meteorism, 1078
  differentiated from intestinal obstruction, 1081
Methemoglobinemia, with silver nitrate dressings, 384
Methohexital, for anesthesia, 251
Methotrexate, for cancer control, 229
Methoxyflurane, anesthesia, 250
Microcurie, 404
Microemboli, radioactive, 206
Micrognathia, 1456
Microorganisms. See Bacteria.
Micturition, 1633
  changes in, 1582
  nerve action, 1635
Military surgery, 599-648
Miller-Abbott, tubes, 1092
Milwaukee Brace, for scoliosis, 1701, 1703
Mines, wounds caused by, 603
Minor's triangle, 1180
Mole, 652
  pigmented, 653
Molluscum contagiosum, 651
Molluscum sebaceum, 659
Mönckeburg's medial sclerosis, 1321
Mondor's syndrome, 671
Monilia albicans, 73
Moniliasis, 73, 1545
Monoxide poisoning, exchange transfusion, 177

Subject Index

Monteggia fractures, 501
Morgagni hernia, 1245
Morphine, before anesthesia, 245
  use in battle casualties, 616
Morquio syndrome, 1674, 1676
Mortars, wounds, 604
Mortality, data, 1817
  operative, 1948-1962, 232
    by anatomic site, 233
    with aneurysm and occlusive vascular disease, 241
    influence of duration of illness, 237
    influence of heart disease, 240
    influence of hypertension, 240
    influence of metabolic state, 239
    relative to age, 236
    relative to disease, 237
    relative to magnitude of procedure, 234
    relative to technic used, 240
  in thermonuclear bomb attack, 406
  of wounded in action, 609
Morton's neuroma, 1736
Motility, gastric, 829
Motivation, in rehabilitation of hand, 597
Motor, weaknesses, 1762
Mouth, care, postoperative, 328
Mucin, gastric secretion, 827
Mucocele, 1043
Mucopolysaccharidoses, 1674, 1676
Mucoprotein(s), 1661
  in ossification, 1662
Mucosa, altered resistance of gastric and duodenal, 827
Mucous membrane, wound healing, 24
Muscle(s), abdominal, congenital absence, 1519, 1520
  relaxants, 256
    antagonism, 258
    postoperative respiratory inadequacy, 259
    respiratory effects, 259
  spasm, in appendicitis, 1029
    in peritonitis, 1053
  and wound healing, 26
Myelodysplasia, 1700
Myelography, 1792
  in low back pain, 1742
Myoblastoma, granular cell, 659
Myocardium, surgery, 1285
Myoma, 1558
  treatment, 1559
Myomectomy, 1560
Myositis, clostridial, 66
  streptococcal, 63
Myxoma, 657

Nail, intramedullary, in femur, 531
Narcotic addict, anesthesia for, 247

Nasopharynx, tumors, 1421
Nausea, postoperative, 326
  and vomiting, with intestinal obstruction, 1079
Navicular, fractures, 513, 514, 559
  avascular necrosis, 515
Neck, tumors, 1432
  malignant, 1434
  wounds, 619
Necrosis, of ala nasae, 300
  in neoplasms, 214
Needle biopsy, of liver, 1010
Neisseria catarrhalis, 37
Neoplasia, of parathyroids, 733
Neoplasms, definitions, 209
  destruction of host tissue, 216
  etiology, 209
  factors that limit growth, 211
  general considerations, 209-223
  growth rate, 210
  physiologically functional, 213
  signs of, 217
  signs due to growth, 213
  signs of infiltrative growth, 215
  signs of necrosis, 214
  spread, modes of, 216
  symptoms and signs, 212
  See also Tumors.
Neostigmine, 258
Nephritis, radiation, 427
Nephron, 1585, 1586
  function distal to proximal segment, 1590
Nephrotomography, 1580
Nerve(s), defects, in reconstruction of hand, 587
  digital, anastomosis, 579
  facial, paralysis, 1430 1471
  graft, in hand reconstruction, 587
  hand, 578
  injuries during anesthesia, 266
    with fractures, 456
    with fractured humerus, 489
  long thoracic, in mastectomy, 670
  median, repair, 579
  paralysis, delayed, with fractures, 459
  sensory pathways, 1044
  thoracodorsal, in mastectomy, 670
  ulnar, repair, 579
Nervous system, and wound healing, 26
Neurilemmoma, 658, 1412
Neuritis, late ulnar, 1800
Neurofibroma, 659, 1412
  of face, 1418
Neurofibromatosis, 658
Neuroleptanesthesia, 247
Neuromas, acoustic, 1776
Neuron, lower motor, lesions affecting, 1792
Neurophyseal hormones, 753
Neurotomy, peripheral, 1800
Neutron, 404
Neutropenia, splenic, 972

Nevus, 652
  hairy, 652
Nicotinic acid, deficit, psychosis, 332
Niemann-Pick disease, 1679
Nipple, 670
  discharge, in breast cancer, 684
  Paget's disease, 681
Nitrogen, balance, and injury, 342
  and wound healing, 343
  loss, after operation, 106
    before operation, 105
    in surgical patients, 105
  mustard, for control of cancer, 228
Nitrous oxide, for anesthesia, 247
Nocardia, types, 40
Nodules, rheumatoid, 1719
Nonunion, of fractures, 457
Norepinephrine, adrenergic response, 759
  pharmacologic action, 787
Nose, external, tumors, 1419
  fractures, 1468
Nucleus pulposus, 1740
Nuclide(s), 202
  half lives, 412
Null hypothesis, 1814
Numbers, random, table of, 1811
Nurse, circulating, 279
  role in operating room, 279
  scrub, 279
Nutrients, for intravenous feeding, 109
Nutrition, 101-120

Obesity, 118
Obstipation, and intestinal obstruction, 1079
Obstruction, of airway, 312
  of common duct, differential diagnosis, 933
  duodenal ulcer, indication for operation, 841
  with herniated intestine, early signs, 1209
  intestinal, by cancer of colon, 1157
    classification, 1076
    clinical features, 1088
    diagnosis, 1074
    differential diagnosis, 1080
    mechanical, 1075, 1077
    neonatal, 1506
      treatment, 1507
    pain, 1078
    problems of anesthesia, 262
    surgical intervention for relief, 1093
    symptoms and signs, 1076
    treatment, 1092
  mechanical, in perforative appendicitis, 1041

Subject Index

respiratory, problems of anesthesia, 260
   to urinary flow, 1603
   treatment, 1605
Odontoma, cystic, mandible, 1427
Olecranon, fractures, 498, 499
Oliguria, maintenance of fluid balance, 97
   mechanism, 1600
   postoperative, 319
Omentopexy, for portal hypertension, 1018
Omentum, 980
   torsion, 990
Omphalitis, 1515
Omphalocele, 1246, 1519
Operation, abdominal, in military surgery, 625
   assessment of risks, 232-243
   catabolic response, 106
   draping operative field, 283
   exploration and management of lesion, 285
   exposure, methods to obtain, 286
   incision of skin, 283
   mortality. *See* Mortality.
   normal convalescence, 348
   orders, postoperative, 289
   orders, preoperative, 275
   patient's reaction to prospective, 293
   permit, 275
   postanesthetic observation, 268
   preoperative preparation, 275
   preparation of field, 281
   risk. *See* Risk.
   routine, 280
   suite, 276
   surgical care, 275-292
   wound management, 297
Orders, postoperative, 289
   preoperative, 275
Organ, transplantation, 435-447
Organization, of combat medical service, 599
Orthopedics, 1657-1754
Ortolani sign, 1681
Os calcis, fracture, 556
Oscillometer, 1318
Osgood-Schlatter's disease, 1694
O'Shaughnessy, W. B., experiments with treatment of cholera, 76
Osmolality, maintenance of normal, 1592
Osmotic pressure, effective colloid, 183
Ossification, endochondral, 1657
   intramembranous, 1658
Osteoarthritis, of hips, 1718
Osteochondroma, benign, 1730
Osteochondroses, 1692
Osteogenesis, 1662
   environmental factors, 1663
Osteomalacia, 1669

Osteomyelitis, 1703
   chronic, 1704
   cranial, 1778
   etiology, 1705
   jaws, 1459, 1460
   pathogenesis, 1703
   treatment, 1706
   vertebral, 1710
Osteophytes, in osteoarthritis, 1718
Osteoporosis, 1668
   causes, 1668
Otorrhea, cerebrospinal, 1780
Ovary, abnormalities, congenital, 1535
   cyst, pseudomucinous, 1564
      serous, 1564
      and tumors, complications, 1566
   tumors, 1563
Oxygen, poisoning, 316
   postoperative, 315
   in treatment of shock, 140
Oxygenation, hyperbaric, 317
   with mechanical ventilator, amount, 271
Oxypolygelatin, as plasma substitute, 190
Oxytocin, 754

Padding, plaster casts, 474
Paget's disease, 1672
   advanced changes, 1675
   complications, 1674
   of nipple, 681
Pain, abdominal, 1043-1045
   postoperative, decision to reoperate, 309
   continuous, situational, 334
   incisional, 308
   in intra-abdominal emergencies, 1048
   of ischemia, 307
   low back, 1739
      treatment, 1742
   medication for relief, 298
   neurosurgical procedures for relief, 1802
   nonincisional abdominal, 308
   operations for relief of, 1800
   parietal, 1044
   peritoneal, 1043
   with peritonitis, 1051
   postoperative, 307
   of postoperative ileus, 310
   with spinal lesions, 1791
   upper extremity, 1723
   visceral, 1044
Pancreas, 916-946
   anatomy, 916, 917
   annular, 917
      and ectopic, in infants, 1514
   biopsy, 933
   carcinoma, 931

   with calcification, 926
   and alcohol, 927
   cystadenomas, 940, 941
   cysts, 939
      treatment, 941
   function tests, 934
   heterotopia, 917, 942
   histology, 917
   juice, 918
   physiology, 917
   pseudocysts, 939
   resection, for cancer, 936, 937
      total, 937
         metabolic effects, 942
   role in peptic ulcer, 825
   solid benign tumors, 942
   tumors of islet cells, 929
   wounds, 627
   x-ray findings, 934, 935
Pancreatectomy, total, 937
   metabolic effects, 942
Pancreatic asthenia, 901
Pancreaticoduodenectomy, 910
Pancreatitis, acute, 920
   chronic, 925
      treatment, 926
   clinical picture, 920
   etiology, 921
   mortality, 923
   with parasitic infestation, 924
   postoperative, 924
   prognosis, 923
   and trauma, 928
   treatment, 922
Paneth cells, in intestinal metaplasia, 844
Panniculitis, idiopathic, 657
   of mesentery, 990
Pantothenic acid, 115
Papilla of Vater, exploration, 909
Papillae, anal, 1178
Papilledema, 1756
Papilloma(s), eyelid, 1415
   intraductal, breast, 672
Palate, congenital insufficiency, 1454
Palpation, intra-abdominal, limitations, 1095
Palsy, facial nerve, 1430
Paracentesis, as alternative to reoperation, 310
   and renal failure, 1008
Paralysis, orthopedic treatment of resulting disorders, 1695
Parasympathectomy, cranial, 1807
   sacral, 1807
Parathormone, and alkaline phosphatase activity, 733
   and bones, 734
   and calcium metabolism, 732
Parathymus gland, 741
Parathyroid glands, 729-747
   and calcium, 730
   carcinoma, 733, 739
   exploring for, 744
   hyperplasia, 733

Index

*.)

732
y, 743
.atomy, 738-744
.any, 729, 731
.ation in location, 740
.ré, care of wounds, 153
Parenteral routes, of alimentation, 109
Paresthesias, 1791
Parietal cells, 821
Paronychia, 577
Parotid gland, tumors, 1428
   surgeon's dilemma, 1429
Parotitis, purulent, in newborn, 1496
Patella, fractures, 539
Patent ductus arteriosus, 1259
   diagnosis and treatment, 1261
   operative exposure, 1262
   results and prognosis, 1263
   signs and symptoms, 1260
Patient, reaction to prospective operation, 293
Pavlov pouch, 822
Pectus excavatum, 1499
Pelvic inflammatory disease, acute, 1556
   chronic 1557
Pelvis, floor, fascia and muscles, 1537
   fractures, 569
     with dislocations of hip, 570
     splinting, 463
Penicillin, in burns, 384
Penis, carcinoma, 1624
   congenital anomalies, 1645
   injuries, 1631
   strangulation, 1631
Pepsin, gastric secretion, 827
Peptic ulcer, perforated, vs appendicitis, 1046
Perforation, of colon, by cancer, 1158
   duodenal ulcer, indication for operation, 841
   gastrointestinal, neonatal, 1508, 1509
Periarthritis, adhesive, 1724
Pericarditis, acute pyogenic, 1285
   constrictive, 1282
     operation for, 1283
   recurrent acute, 1284
Peristalsis, in esophagus, 796
   intestinal, 1067
     nervous control, 1068
   of ureter, 1633
Peripheral nervous system, diseases, 1799
Peritoneum, structure and area, 1049
Peritonitis, acute, 1050
   antibiotic sensitivity of some pathogens, 1052

auscultatory findings, 1035
bacteria and chemicals, 1050
bacteria commonly associated, 1052
bacteriology, 1051
battle wounds, 640
bile, 888
chronic, 1056
   chemical, 1057
classification of, 1050
as complication of intestinal obstruction, 1092
complications, 1058
death from, 1041
diagnosis, 1051
idiopathic chronic, 1057
meconium, 1510
mortality trends, 1042
after nonpenetrating injuries to intestines, 1107
pancreatic, 1056
from perforative appendicitis, 1040
primary and secondary, 1051
special forms, 1056
treatment, 1055
tuberculous, 1056, 1057
Permit, operative, 275
Personality, changes, as sign of intracranial lesion, 1763
Perthes test, 1356
Pessary, for retrodisplacements of uterus, 1539
Peyronie's disease, 1631
Pharmacopsychoses, 333
Phenolsufonphthalein, test, 1598
Peutz-Jeghers syndrome, 865, 1105, 1148
   15-minute test, 1599
Phenothiazines, before anesthesia, 245
Phenylalanine mustard, in control of cancer, 229
Pheochromocytoma, 789
   blood pressure changes, 791
   as cause of hypertension, 1602
   diagnosis, 790
Philosophy, surgical, 1-7
Phimosis, 1606, 1646
Phlebitis, idiopathic mammary, 671
   superficial, and Buerger's disease, 1335
Phlebothrombosis, 1358
Phlegmasia cerulea dolens, 1361
Phosphorus, excretion, and parathyroids, 732
   and parathyroids, 730
Photomultiplier tube, 204
Photoscanning, to detect bone tumors, 1731
Phrenic crush, in preparation for herniorrhaphy, 1240
Phrenicotomy, in treatment of hiatal hernia, 1234
Physiology, renal, 1585

Picocurie, 404
Pierre Robin syndrome, 1496
Pigeon breast, 1500
Pinealomas, 1776
Pitressin, to reduce portal pressure, 1015
Pits, preauricular, 1496
Pituitary dwarfism, 771
Pituitary gland, anatomic relationships, 749
   anterior lobe, 766
   cell types, 749
   controlled radiative destruction, 774
   divisions, 748
   hormones, 750, 751
   inhibition of urine, postoperative, 320
   insufficiency, diagnosis, 764
   physiology, 748-754
   posterior lobe hormones, 753
   response to body injury, 341
Pituitrin, intravenous, to reduce portal pressure, 1015
Plasma, as blood substitute, 183
   for burns, 370
     in children, 371
   electrolyte concentrations, 89
   expanders, in shock, 138
   for hypoproteinemia, 188
   hypotonic, 352
   nutritional role, 112
   protein, after injury, 345
   stability, 188
   preparation, 182
   substitutes, 189
   transfusion, 182
   volume, during depletion of sodium salts, 78
Plaster, of Paris, 473
   technic, three-way, 546
Platelets, antibodies, autoimmune, 951
   antigens, 158
   in thrombocytopenic purpura, 956
   transfusion, 181
Platybasia, 1786
Plethysmograph, 1318
Pleura, tumors, 1412
Pleurisy, 311
Pleuritis, of right diaphragm, 1047
Pneumatosis cystoides intestinorum, 1136
Pneumaturia, 1583
Pneumococcus, 36
Pneumoconiosis, differentiated from lung cancer, 1409
Pneumo-encephalography, 1771
Pneumogram, retroperitoneal, 1582
Pneumography, 1771
Pneumonia, congenital, 1504
   lobar, differential diagnosis with peritonitis, 1054
   postoperative, 304

Subject Index 1857

Pneumonitis, aspirational, prevention, 299
  after irradiation, 427
  lipoid, differentiated from lung cancer, 1409
Pneumoperitoneum, diagnosis of hiatal hernia, 1233
  to facilitate hernia repair, 1239
Pneumothorax, complicating fractured ribs, 455
  neonatal, 1504
  tension, 1377, 1378, 1505
  treatment, 1379
Polydactylism, congenital, 1690
Polyp(s), adenomatous, of colorectum, 1140
  malignant potential, 1143
  relation to cancer, 1142
  cervical, 1551
  of colon and rectum, 1140
  endometrial, 1560
  juvenile, 1146
  with malignant changes, 1143
  retention, 1145, 1146
Polypectomy, 1144
Polyposis, familial, 1142
  treatment, 1149
  intestinal, in infants and children, 1526
Polyvinylpyrrolidone, as plasma substitute, 191
Population, sampling, 1811
Portal circulation, 988
  differs from venous circulation, 989
  major branches, 986
Positrocephalogram, 1768
Positron, scanning, 202
Postgastrectomy syndrome, 856
Potassium, blood deficit, 88
  deficit, estimation of, 95
    psychosis, 330
  excess in blood, 88
  exchange across alimentary tract, 89
  exchange with environment, 88
  excretion in urine, 1592
  after injuries, 344
  intoxication, after transfusion, 170
  loss, postoperative, 355
Pott's disease, 1713
Pouch of Morison, 1058
Preconditioning, against acute irradiation, 419
Prednisone, as immunosuppressive, 442
Pregnancy, ectopic, 1576
  vs appendicitis, 1046
  diagnosis, 1577
  treatment, 1578
  sites of tubal, 1577
Premedication, for anesthesia, 244
  in pediatric surgery, 1492

Preparation, of operative field, 281
  of sterile field, for various operations, 284
Pressure, central venous, method for determining, 133
  monitoring, 133
  cone, cerebellar tonsillar, 1757
    tentorial, 1756
  intracranial, increased, acute, 1756
    increased, chronic, 1755
  paralysis, with plaster casts, 477
  sores, with plaster casts, 475
  venous, in dehydrational shock, 94
  in wound healing, 15
Priorities, in surgical management of casualties, 614
Probability, calculation of chi square, 242
Probits, method of, 1820
Procidentia, 1540
Proctosigmoidoscope, examination, 1181
Prognathism, in acromegaly, 768
  correction, 1458
Prolactin, 752
Prolapse, rectal, in children, 1527
  classification, 1182
Properdin, 46
Prophylaxis, against surgical infections, 52
Prostate, and adjacent strictures, 1610
  benign hypertrophy, 1611
  carcinoma, 1623
  cross section, 1611
  physiology, 1610
Prostatectomy, 1612
  and urinary incontinence, 1642
Prostatism, 1610
  clinical picture, 1611
  treatment, 1612
Prostheses, in reconstructive surgery, 1482
Protamine, duration of activity, 181
Protein, daily allowance, 106
  deficits, estimation of, 104
  intoxication, psychosis, 332
  for intravenous feeding, 109
  loss, postoperative, 105
    preoperative, 104
  metabolism, and corticoids, 775
  nutrition, 101
Proteus, 38
Prothrombin, activity, as test of liver function, 1010
Pruritus ani, 1184
  classification, 1184
  treatment, 1185
Pruritus vulvae, 1547
Pseudoarthrosis, of tibia and fibula, 1690

Pseudobronchiectasis, 1385
Pseudocyesis, differentiated from intestinal obstruction, 1081
Pseudocysts, of pancreas, 939
Pseudomonas aeruginosa, 39
Pseudotumor cerebri, 1787
Psychoses, due to alcohol, 333
  barbiturates, 333
  cranial trauma, 334
  endocrinopathic, 333
  Korsakoff's, 333
  metabolic, 332
  nutritional, 330
  potassium deficit, 330
  septic, 333
  sodium deficits, 331
  symptomatic, 328
    classification, 329
    treatment, 335
  treatment, 334
Ptosis, eyelids, 1477
  renal, 1614
Puborectalis "sling," 1180
Pulmonary insufficiency, after injury, 356
Pulses, peripheral, in occlusive arterial disease, 1317
Puncture, lumbar, 1764
Punji stakes, wounds, 605
Purpura, idiopathic thrombocytopenic, 952, 953, 954
  isoimmune, 950
  posttransfusion, 158
  thrombocytopenic, secondary, with splenomegaly, 958
  treatment, 957
Pus, laudable, 36
Pyelography, excretory, in renal hypertension, 1603
  intravenous, 1580
  retrograde, 1580
Pyelonephritis, 1615, 1617
Pylephlebitis, in appendicitis, 1040
Pyloromyotomy, 852
Pyloroplasty, for bleeding duodenal ulcer, 843
  Finney, 852
  types of procedures, 852

Queckenstedt test, 563
Quick test, 901

RA leukocyte, 1719
Rabies, 70
Rad, 404
Radiation, affect on spleen, 949
  energy measurement, 404
  exposure limits, 204
  fallout, 408
  injury, 403-434
    symptoms, 414

Subject Index

Radiation (Cont.)
  ionizing, 403
    measurements, 203
    and wound healing, 28, 29
  LD 50 in man, 413
  laser-maser, 433
  portal, injury, 421
    local reactioins, 422
    systemic reactions, 422
  protection guide, 409
  protection of personnel, 432
  therapeutic levels, 205, 206
    without local injury, 423
  thermonuclear, 404
  to whole body, effects, 410
    tolerance by species, 408
    treatment, 418
Radioactivity, natural, 404
Radioiodine, exposure limits, 204
Radioisotopes, 405
  in control of cancer, 227
  definition, 403
  diagnostic, radiation exposure, 430
  See also Isotopes.
Radionuclide, 403
Radiotherapy, local injury, 424
  protection of operator, 207
  successful, 423
  therapeutic levels, 206
Radius, congenital absence, 1688
  distal epiphysis, fracture-separation, 512
  fractures, of head and neck, 499, 500
    lower end, 507
    of shaft, 507
Ranula, in infants, 1497
Rates, comparison of, 1812
Raynaud's disease, 1336, 1807
Raynaud's phenomenon, 1336, 1337
RBE, 404
Reabsorption, tubular, 1588
Rebound tenderness, in appendicitis, 1029
Recovery, evolutionary aspects, 337
  room, 268
  care, 289
Rectocele, 1541
Rectum, anatomy, 1066
  cancer, abdomino-perineal resection, 1165
  perforation, 627
  polyps, 1140
  prolapse, 1182
  as a route for alimentation, 108
  tumors, benign, 1146-1148
    villous, 1199
Reflux, ureteral, 1604, 1605
Regitine, 791
  response, positive, 790
Regurgitation, aortic, 1292
  mitral, 1288, 1290
  tricuspid stenosis and, 1292
Rehabilitation, after fractures, 477

Rejection, major influences, 441
  reaction, of transplants, 436
Relaxation, pelvic, 1539
REM, 404
Renal insufficiency, post-traumatic, 608, 638
Renogram, with radioactive Hippuran, 1329
Reoperation, in presence of postoperative abdominal pain, 309
Resistance, general, to bacteria, 46
  of host to bacteria, 44
  local, to bacteria, 44
  regional, to bacteria, 45
Respiration, and acid-base balance, 98
  mechanical ventilation, 269
  paralysis, after spinal anesthesia, 254
  problems of anesthesia, 260
Respirators, in crush injuries, 1381
Rest pain, with arterial obstruction, 1316
Resuscitation, cardiac, 1295
  clinical experiences, 614
  principles, 609
Retinopathy, diabetic, 1806
Retroflexion, of uterus, 1537
Reversed Colles' fracture, 509, 512
Rh factor, in blood, 158
  comparative nomenclature, 159
  incompatibility, 159
  typing, 159
  vaccination, 166
Rh-Hr blood types, 161
Rheumatoid factor, 1719
Rhinophyma, 649, 1419
Rhinorrhea, cerebrospinal, 1780
Rhizotomy, cranial posterior, 1800
  spinal posterior, 1801
Ribs, absence of, 1500
  eosinophilic granulomas, 1413
  fractures, 571
    posterior intercostal nerve block, 572
  tumors, 1413
Richter's hernia, 1247
Rickets, 1669, 1670
  vitamin-D-resistant, 1670
Ringer's solution, lactated, in treatment of burn shock, 365
Risk, operative, according to site, 233
  by age of patient, 233-235
  and anesthesia, 241
  assessment of, 232-243
  factors, 232
  influence of suppuration, 238
  and quality of nursing, 242
  reduction through the years, 232
Roentgen unit, 404
Roentgenography, urologic, 1580
  See also X-ray

Room, operating, 280
  zones, 276
Rubin test, 1573
Rumpel-Leede test, 955
Rupture, of bladder, 1629

Saint's triad, 1131
Sacrum, fractures, 568
Salivary gland(s), 1479
  infection in ducts, 1479
  obstruction, 1479
  tumors, 1428
Salmonella typhosa, 38
Salpingitis, acute, vs appendicitis, 1046
Salt(s), depletion, with silver nitrate dressings, 383
  low, syndrome, 84
Sampling, double-blind technic, 1811
  populations, 1811
  random, 1811
Sanfilippo syndrome, 1674, 1676
Sarcoidosis, gastric, 865
Sarcoma, lung, 1403
  multiple idiopathic, hemorrhagic, 665
  osteogenic, 1734
  reticulum cell, 1732
  stomach, 866
  uterus, 1563
Scalenus anterior syndrome, 1799
Scapula, fractures, 479
Scarlet fever, surgical, 61
Scatter, expression of, 1815
Scheie syndrome, 1674, 1676
Schiller bands, and healing wounds, 12
Schistosoma, as cause of portal hypertension, 997
Sciatica, 1740
Scintigrams, and abscess of liver, 1040
Scleroderma, and Raynaud's phenomenon, 1337
Scoliosis, 1700
  idiopathic, 1700, 1702
Scrotum, benign enlargements, 1632
  carcinoma, 1624
  injuries, 1631
  masses in, 1624, 1625
Scrubbing, routine, 280
Scurvy, 1671
Sedatives, in treatment of shock, 139
Sedimentation, rate, in appendicitis, 1029
Segments, of lung, 1372, 1373
Seizures, auditory, 1760
  convulsive, avoidance, 1789
  decerebrate, 1760
  involving special senses, 1760
  motor, 1759

Subject Index 1859

olfactory, 1760
psychical, 1761
sensory, 1760
sites of origin, 1758
visceral and autonomic, 1760
Selenomethionine, radioactive, in scanning pancreas, 934
Sensitivity studies, in selection of antibiotic, 55
Sensitization, in tissue graft, 439
Septicemia, 43
Sequestra, in osteomyelitis, 1704
Serafini's hernia, 1248
Serratia marcescens, 39
Serum, for burned children, 371
Serum acid phosphatase, in carcinoma of prostate, 1623
Serum albumin, level, as test of liver function, 1008, 1010
as plasma substitute, 191
Serum, antilymphocyte, 442
Serum bilirubin, concentration test, 1008
Serum hepatitis, icteric, 183
immunity, 188
risk, 176
Servetus, and pulmonary circulation, 151
Shielding, against acute irradiation, 419
Shock, 121-148
associated with sodium deficit, 79
in atomic casualties, 644
with burns, 364
blood transfusion, 371
buffered saline in treatment, 369
use of colloids, 370
vasoconstrictors and hydrocortisone, 370
in combat injury, 615
as complication of fracture, 455
definitions, 122
diagnosis, 132
fluid replacement, 137
formulas for treatment, 371
after frostbite, 399
and hemoconcentration, 126
hemorrhagic, 125
with hypoproteinemia, 103
results of treatment, 80
history, 122
hypovolemia, role of, 155
hypovolemic, 122
accompanying pathology, 127
contraindications of epinephrine, and norepinephrine, 788
differentiated from acute heart failure, 314
etiology, 124
with nonpenetrating injuries of intestines, 1107
summary of treatment, 140
irreversibility of, 130

postoperative, 353
in relationship to hemorrhage, history, 154
septic, auxiliary treatment, 141
traumatic, 125
treatment, clinical, 137
drugs, 136, 138
experimental, 135
plasma volume expanders, 138
position of patient, 140
tests and measurements, 132
Shorr regimen, to prevent recurrent nephrolithiasis, 1627
Shoulder, dislocation, 483
acromioclavicular, 486
and fracture of greater tuberosity, 485
and fracture of neck of humerus, 485
and injury to blood vessels and nerves, 485
postreduction management, 484
recurrent, 486
reduction technic, 484
fractures and dislocations, 478
frozen, 1724
splinting, 462
Shunts, portacaval, results for control of bleeding varices, 1016
portal, 1015
for portal hypertension, late causes of death, 1017
Sicle cell trait, differentiated from sickle cell anemia, 969
Sigmoid, volvulus, 1100
Silicones, for prostheses, 1483, 1486
Silicone rubber, for prostheses, 1483
Silicone sponge, 1486
Silver nitrate, wet dressings, for burns, 374
Sinus, congenital dermal, 663, 1798
Sinusitis, association with bronchiectasis, 1384
Skeleton, deossification, 1667
development, 1657
Skin, anatomy and physiology, 361, 362
areas of parts of body, adult, 395
child, 394
bank, 1441
carcinoma, 664
care, postoperative, 328
changes in acromegaly, 769
formula for area, 361
full-thickness, in hernia repair, 1243
grafting, deep burns, 388, 1437
rejection, 438
of hand, radiation effect, 577
necrosis, after irradiation, 425
orange-peel, 686
and subcutaneous tissues, 649-667
tumors, benign, 652
malignant, 664

metastatic, 667
wound healing, 24
Skull, x-rays, 1765
Smith's fracture, 512
Smoking, and Buerger's disease, 1334
and cancer of lung, 1402
with intermittent claudication, 1323
Sodium chloride, depletion, with silver nitrate dressings, 384
Sodium citrate, as anticoagulant, 153
Sodium, concentration, clinical determination, 93
depletion, with burn shock, 365
effect on vital signs, 79
and hypometabolism, 80
physical signs, 85
psychosis, 331
translocational, therapy, 94
treatment, 85
and water deficit, 84
water in excess, 83
with water normal, 84
excess, therapy, 95
with water excess, 86
with water normal or deficit, 82
exchange across alimentary tract, 89
exchange with environment, 88
extrarenal loss, 352
after injury, 344
low, syndrome, 352
normal, with water deficit, 82
with water excess, 83
reabsorption in tubule of kidney, 1589
Sodium salts, deficits, 78
renal excretion, 86
Somatotropin, 750
Spasms, facial, 1805
Spermatocele, 1632
Sphincter, of Oddi, 881
urinary, 1634
total incompetence, 1641
treatment, 1642
Sphincterotomy, biliary surgery, 909
Spider bite, differentiated from peritonitis, 1055
Spigelian hernia, 1251
Spina bifida, 1798
Spinal canal, abscess, 1797
tumors, 1796
Spinal cord, compression, with fractured spine, 568
injury, 562, 618
with fractures, 456
Spine, arthritis, degenerative, 1743
cervical, compression fractures, 563
dislocations, 563

Spine (Cont.)
 dorsal and lumbar, fractures, 565
 fractures and dislocations, 562
 fusion, for low back pain, 1742
  for tuberculosis, 1715
 hyperextension, 565
 and immobilization, disadvantages, 566
 immobilization, in plaster jacket, 566
 injuries, 1797
 lesions with surgical implications, 1791
 plain x-ray, 1792
 puncture, 1792
 splinting, 462
 tuberculosis, 1713
  treatment, 1715
Spirochetes, 42
Spironolactone, as diuretics, 1598
Splanchnic viscera, venous return, 988
Spleen(s), 947-979
 abscess, 963
 absence, congenital, 1515
 accessory, 949, 958
 anatomy, 948
 contraction in shock, 128
 cysts, 963
 diseases, 959
 effects of radiation, 949
 function, in diseases of blood, 953
  in prenatal life, 950
 historical notes, 947
 infections, 963
 with malaria, 964
 needle biopsy, 962
 operative tears, in the normal, 962
 parasitic infestations, 964
 physiology, 949
 pulp pressure determination, 1007
 rupture, 961
  delayed traumatic, 961
  treatment, 962
 supradiaphragmatic transposition, 1018
 transplantation in classical hemophila, 977
 tuberculosis, 964
 tumors, 973
 wounds, 626
Splenectomy, anesthesia, 976
 benefiting autoimmune diseases, 953
 complications, nonhemolytic, 976
 and congenital spherocytic anemia, 965, 968
 indications and contraindications, 973
 inherited diseases benefited by, 965
 for portal hypertension, 1018
 technic, 974

 in thrombocytopenic purpura, 957
Splenomegaly, in portal hypertension, 1005
Splenoportography, 1007
Splenosis, 962
Splint, Frejka pillow, 1682, 1685
Splinting, femur, 528
 lower extremity, 462
 open fractures, 463
 pelvis, 463
 spine, 462
 upper extremity, 462
Spondylitis, rheumatoid, 1719, 1720
Spondylolisthesis, 1744
Spondylosis, cervical, 1796
Sponge, count, 287, 289
Sponging, of blood, 285
Sporothrix schenckii, 72
Sporotricha, 41
Sporotrichosis, 72
Sprain, wrist, 514
Standard deviation, 1815
Staphylococcus, infections, 59
 subgroups, 35
Starvation, death by bronchopneumonia, 342
 as factor in surgical metabolism, 342
 post-traumatic, 349
Statistics, on cancer, 219
 methods for analysing surgical data, 1810
 utility of, 243
Status thymicolymphaticus, 727
Stenosis, aortic, 1290
 esophageal, 834
  infundibular, 1270
 intestinal tract, in newborn, 1506
 isolated pulmonary, 1269
 mitral, 1286
  and aortic, 1292
 pulmonary, with atrial septal defect or patent foramen ovale, 1276
  operative treatment, 1270
  with ventricular septal defect, 1271
 pyloric, in infants, 1511
 renal artery, as cause of hypertension, 1602
 tricuspid, and regurgitation, 1292
Sterility, investigation, 1573
 treatment, 1574
Sterilization, of female, 1572
 of linens and instruments, 279
Sternum, fractures, 571
Steroid synthesis, prenatal block, 782
Stomach, 819-879
 acid, neutralization, 827
 acid secretion, inhibiting factors, 825
 anatomic divisions, 820

 arteries supplying, 820
 carcinoma, 844
  pathology, 844
  prognosis, 850
  vs ulcer, 835
 congenital malformations, 861
 cytologic studies, 836
 dilatation, acute, 862
  postoperative, 326
 diverticulum, 862
 embryology, 819
 eosinophilic granuloma, 862
 glomus tumor, 864
 histology, 821
 interrelations between phases of secretion, 827
 leiomyoma, 864
 malignancy, signs, 849
 motility, 829
 mucosa, altered resistance, 827
 operations, 852
 pepsin and mucin secretion, 827
 peptic ulcer, 829
 perforation, traumatic, 865
 polyps, 865
 prolapse of mucosa through pylorus, 865
 resections, 853
  segmental, with pyloroplasty, 853
 sarcoidosis, 865
 sarcoma, 866
 surgery, late complications, 856
 syphilis, 866
 tuberculosis, 866
 tumors, benign, 860
  lymphoid, 864
 volvulus, 866
 wounds, 626
Stone, in common duct, diagnosis, 895
 ureteral, vs appendicitis, 1046
 in urinary tract, 1625
 types, 1626
Strangulation, of hernia, 1209
 of penis, 1631
Streptococcus, infections, 60
 types, 36, 39
Stress, of combat, 606
 incontinence, 1541
  treatment, 1542
 surgical, pituitary-adrenocortical response, 762
 ulcer, 830
 and wound healing, 28
Stricture, of anus, 1184
 esophageal, benign, 799
  in infants, 1503
Stroke, heat, 306
[89]Strontium, 413
[90]Strontium, 413
Subluxation, of cervical spine, 563
Submarine, medicine, 645
Succinylcholine, 256, 258
Succus entericus, 1070

Subject Index

Suppuration, influence on operative risk, 238
Surgeon, battalion, responsibilities, 612
 as investigator, 4
 need for breadth of medical knowledge, 7
 obligations beyond patient care, 3
 opportunities for training, 5
 responsibility, 2
 as teacher, 3
Surgery, applied bacteriology, 34-47
 art of, 5
 biliary tract, instruments, 903
 for cancer, practical considerations, 216
  prophylactic, 220
 definition, 2
 effects of pathogenic bacteria, 42
 endocrine and metabolic basis of care, 337-359
 field of, 1
 historical development, 1
 infants. See Infants.
 infections, methods of diagnosis, 51
  treatment, 52
 normal convalescence, 348
 pediatric, 1491-1532
 place in society, 6
 plastic, principles, 1437-1490
 of nervous system, 1755-1809
 regional, principles, 617
 relation to medicine, 2
 on submarines, 645
 various usages of word, 2
Survival rates, accumulative, calculation of standard error, 1820
Suture, material, and wound healing, 15
 tightness, and wound healing, 20, 22
 and wound healing, 20, 21
Swan neck deformity, 593
Sweat glands, tumors, 650
Sweating, water loss, 90
Sympathectomy, 1801
 in Buerger's disease, 1336
 in chronic occlusive arterial disease, 1324
 for occlusions of major peripheral vessels, 1808
Synovectomy, 1721
 in rheumatoid arthritis, 594
Syphilis, aortic aneurysms, 1340
 skeletal lesions, 1712
 of stomach, 866
Syringomyelia, 1797
 and neuropathic joint disease, 1722

T, distribution of, table, 1817
T test, 1816
T-tube, use in biliary surgery, 907

Taeniae coli, 1066
Talcum, as foreign body, 16
Talipes equinovarus, bilateral, 1684
Talus, fractures, 558
Tamponade, esophagogastric, 1014
Tantalum, use in hernia repair, 1242
Tay-Sachs disease, 1680
Teflon, prostheses, 1483
 for total loss of lower jaw, 1484
Teletherapy, 206
Temperature, chart, basal, 1574
 in peritonitis, 1054
Tenderness, abdominal, in peritonitis, 1053
Tendinitis, calcified, 1723
Tendon, grafts, in hand reconstruction, 588
 hand, congenital absence, 1688
 lacerations, 580
 repair, 581, 582
 and wound healing, 26
Tennis elbow, 1725
Tenosynovitis, 577
 bicipital, 1725
 posterior tibial, 1737
 stenosing, 1725
Tension, premenstrual, 1569
 in wound healing, 15
Teratoma, of mediastinum, 1411
 sacrococcygeal, in infant, 1528, 1529
Terminology, of tissue transplantation, 437
Testis, congenital anomalies, 1646
 injuries, 1632
 tumors, 1624
Testosterone, 781
Tetanus, 68-70
 antitoxin, 53
 in burns, 374
 combat wounds, 637
 prophylaxis, 53
 toxoid, 54
 treatment, 69
Tetany, and parathyroids, 729, 731
Tetraiodophenolphthalein, for visualizing gallstones, 891
Tetralogy, acyanotic, 1271
 of Fallot, 1273
 treatment, 1275
Thalamotomy, 1803
Thalassemia, 970
Theater, operating, 276
Thermomammography, 689
Thiamine, 115
 deficit, psychosis, 332
Thiazide-potassium chloride, inducing small bowel lesions, 1111
Thiopental, for anesthesia, 251
ThioTEPA, for control of cancer, 228
Thiouracil, in hyperthyroidism, 718
Thomas splint, 528
Thoracic duct, 1067

Thoracoplasty, extrapleural paravertebral, for tuberculosis, 1396
 with paraffin prosthesis, 1396
Thoracotomy, closed drainage, 1386, 1387
 open drainage, for empyema, 1386, 1388
Thorax, anomalies, in infants, 1499
 asymmetry, 1500
 comparison of lines on male and female, 19
 trauma, 1376
Thromboangiitis obliterans, 1334
Thrombocytopenia, after acute irradiation, 415
 autoimmune, 951
 neonatal, 950
Thromboendarterectomy, 1324
 renal artery, 1329
Thrombophlebitis, 1358
 acute, 1361
 anticoagulant regimens, 1359
 and edema, 321
 with infections, 43
 lower extremities, treatment, 1361
 purulenta, 322
 septic, in infants and children, 1493
 signs and symptoms, 321
 treatment, 322
Thrombosis, arterial, 1303
 treatment, 1304
 of normal artery, 1299
 mesentery, 991
Thrombus, intracardiac, 1299
Thumb, amputation, subtotal, 590
 loss of opposition, 1696
 reconstruction, 590
 test, to distinguish indirect from direct hernia, 1206
Thymectomy, 729
Thymoma, 729, 1410
Thymus gland, 727-729
 and myasthenia gravis, 728
 persistent cervical or cervicomediastinal, 1498
 as seat of tumor, 728
 surgical anatomy, 727
Thyrocalcitonin, 732
Thyroid gland, 714-726
 adenomas, 721
 cancer, after radiation, 428
 carcinomas, 721
  in children, 1498
 ectopic, in infants, 1498
 examination, 723
 hyperplasia, 715
 involution with iodine, 715
 lymphoma, 722
 palpation, 724
 resection, of normal gland, 723
 technic, 726
 stimulating hormone, 752
 storm, 305
 tumors, in newborn, 1498

Subject Index

Thyroiditis, 722
  acute, in infants and children, 1498
Thyrotropin, 752
Tibia, and fibula, fractured, 543-548
  fractures, of lateral condyle, 541
    and medial condyles, 543
    of medial condyle, 542
    of proximal end, 540
  pseudoarthrosis, 1689
  spine, avulsion fractures, 541
Tilt test, 132
Tinel's sign, 580
Tissue, transplantation, 435-447
  typing for donor selection, 440
Toe(s), dislocation, 561
  fifth, overriding, 1739
  hammer, 1737
  phalanges, fractures, 560
Toenails, ingrowing, 1737
Tongue carcinoma, 1425
Tophi, 663
Torsion, of testis, 1632
Torticollis, spasmodic, 1805
Tourniquet test, 955
Trachea, 1391
  aspiration of, 302
  tumors, 1410
Tracheostomy, need for, 312
  in treatment of burns, 391
Traction, continuous balanced, 465
Tractotomy, bulbar trigeminal, 1803
  in medulla, 1803
Transaminase, values, after transfusion, 186
Transfusion(s), blood typing, minimum routine, 158
  bone marrow, for irradiation, 420
  cosmetic, 180
  direct, 177
  exchange, 176
  for extracorporeal circulation, 180
  fibrinogen, 182
  icterus, 168
  multiple portals, 615
  packed or washed red cells, 179
  plasma, 182
    for hypoproteinemia, 188
  platelet, 178, 181
  special, 176
  See also Blood transfusions
Transplantation, clinical, 443
  future, 447
  heterotopic recipient locations, 436
  kidney, 444
  rejection reaction 436
  technics, 435
  terminology, 437
  of tissue and organs, 435-447
Trauma. *See* Injury.
Tremor, operations to control, 1804
Trench foot, 398, 641
Trendelenburg test, 1355
Triage, 613

Triceps, paralysis, 1695
Trichloroethylene, for anesthesia, 251
Trichomonas vaginalis, 1545
Trichomoniasis, 1545
Tricuspid atresia, 1277
Trigger finger, 1726
Trocar, decompression of small bowel, 1097
Troncelliti procedure, for obesity, 118
Truncus arteriosus, 1280
Truss, for hernia, 1236
Tuberculosis, articular, 1716
  bone and joint, 1712
  cutaneous, 651
  extravertebral, treatment, 1716
  intestines, 1113
  jaws, 1461
  kidney and ureter, 1619
  pulmonary, 1393-1401
    indictions for surgery, 1395, 1396
    pathology, 1394
    preparation of patient for operation, 1395
    principal objectives of therapy, 1394
    resection, 1397
    complications, 1398
    surgery, anesthesia, 1395
    results, 1399
  of spine, 1713
    treatment, 1715
  spleen, 964
  stomach, 866
  synovial, other forms, 1717
  urinary tract, 1618
d-Tubocurarine, 256, 257
Tumors, appendix, 1043
  bladder, 1622
  bone, 1728
    classification, 1729
  breast, benign, 671
    malignant, 674-684
  carotid body, 1434
  chest wall, in infants, 1500
  colorectum, 1140-1173
    benign, 1146-1148
    malignant, 1153-1170
    villous, 1150
  from congenital rests, 1776
  desmoid, 657, 658
  ear, 1417
  esophagus, 810
  face, 1417
  fallopian tubes, 1563
  female genital tract, 1558
  gallbladder and bile ducts, 886
  gastric, distribution of benign and malignant, 837
  genitourinary tract, 1620
  giant cell, 596
  hand, 595
  of head and neck, 1415-1436

  malignant, palliative care, 1435
  intracranial, 1775
    glandular, 1776
    of mesodermal origin, 1777
    metastatic, 1775
  islet cell, 929
  kidney, 1620
  lips, 1421
  lung, 1402
  mandible, malignant, 1428
  mediastinum, 1410
    in children, 1500, 1501
    of lymphoid origin, 1411
  mesentery, 990
  nasopharynx, 1421
  neck, 1432
  neurogenic, 1412
  nose, 1419
    and paranasal sinuses, 1420
  oral cavity, 1423, 1424
    in infants, 1496
  orbital and exophthalmos, 1777
  of ovary, 1563
  pancreas, benign solid, 942
    non-beta cell, 920
  pleural, 1412
  renal pelvis, 1621
  ribs and cartilages, 1413
  salivary glands, 1428
  skin, benign, 652
    malignant, 664
  small bowel, 1135
  soft tissue, 1735
  spinal canal, 1796
  spleen, 973
  sternocleidomastoid, in infants, 1496
  testis, 1624
  thoracic wall, 1412
  thymus, 728
  trachea, 1410
  umbilical, 1516
  ureter, 1621
  urethra, 1623
  vascular, 653
  villous, distribution in colon, 1151
    hypersecreting, 1151
  See also Neoplasms
Tyloma molle, 1735
Typing, blood, 152
  tissue, for donor selection, 440

Ulcer, anterior hypothalamus-stimulated, 830
  duodenal, 830, 838
    indications for operation, 840
    operations, complications, 843
    mortality, 843
  from ectopic gastric mucosa, 832
  gangrenous, 1316
  gastric, 829, 835
    vs carcinoma, 835
    surgical treatment, 837

Subject Index

gastrojejunal, surgical results, 839
intractable, 831
ischemic, 1317
marginal, 838
peptic, 829
  with cirrhosis of liver, 1012
  in infancy and childhood, 1511
  of Meckel's diverticulum, 840
  types by etiology, 829
  types by location, 832
posterior hypothalamus-stimulated, 830
stomal, 838, 856
Ulna, fracture of the shaft, in adult, 506
  Monteggia fracture, 501
Union, delayed, of fractures, 457
Urachus, 1645
  anomalies, 1518
Urea, clearance test, 1598
  excretion, 1596
Urecholine, bladder test, 1636
Uremia, psychic aspects, 332
Ureter, developmental anomalies, 1644
  ectopic, 1641, 1644
  injuries, 1628
  obstructions, 1613
  peristalsis, 1633
  physiology, 1633
  reflux, 1604, 1605
  repair of divided, 1629
  tumors, 1621
Ureteritis cystica, 1616
Ureterocele, 1607, 1608, 1644
Uretero-ileostomy, 1543
Ureterolithotomy, 1627
Urethra, congenital anomalies, 1645
  congenital narrowing, 1606
  injuries, 1608, 1630
  strictures, 1608
    of meatus, 1645
    post-traumatic, 1630
  tumors, 1623
  valves, 1606, 1607
Urethritis, acute, 1615
Urethrocele, 1541
Urinalysis, 1584
Urinary tract, infections, 1614
    nongonorrheal, 1614
    treatment, 1616
  obstructive disease, 1603
  wounds, 627
Urine, concentration of, 1595
  dilution, 1595
  examination, in appendicitis, 1029
  incontinence, types, 1640
  peritonitis, 1056
  physiology of transport, 1633
  rates of excretion, 318
  reduction, postoperative, 320
  retention, postoperative, 317
Urology, 1580-1656
Uterus, anomalies, congenital, 1535
  degrees of prolapse, 1540

displacements of, 1537
normal position, 1536
retrodisplacements, treatment, 1538
sarcoma, 1563
sites of myomata, 1558
tumors of the body, benign, 1558
  malignant, 1560

Vagina, artificial, 1536
  cancer, 1549
  congenital absence, 1536
Vaginitis, atrophic, 1546
Vagotomy, 854
  with bleeding duodenal ulcer, 843
  effect on acid secretion, 821
  selective gastric, 855
Vagus, action on stomach, 822
Valve, mitral, normal and stenoses, 1289
  urethral, 1606, 1607
  posterior, 1645
Variance, and standard deviation, 1815
Varices, bleeding, causes of death, 1014
    surgical hemostasis, 1018
  bleeding, management of patient, 1014
  esophageal, visualized by x-ray, 1006
  esophagogastric, 996
    distribution, 999
    natural history, 1003
    injection with sclerosing solutions, 1015
  leg, 1353
Varicocele, 1632
Vascular rings, 1268
Vascularity, in wound healing, 14
Vasoconstriction, and shock, 128
  for burn shock, 370
Vasopressin, 754, 773
Vasotocin, 754
Vena cava, inferior, ligation, 1360
  superior, obstruction, 1362
Vein(s), coronary, 990
  dilatation and valvular incompetence, 1353
  great, abnormal drainage, 1278
  inferior mesenteric, 989
  long saphenous, use for grafts, 1310
  portal, 989, 990
    measurement of pressure, 999
    subhepatic obstruction, 997
    thrombosis, 994
  saphenous, ligation and stripping, 1357
  subclavian, acute thrombosis, 1363
  superior mesenteric, 989
  surgery of, 1353-1364

varicose, complications, 1355
  indications for surgery, 1356
  of lower extremity, 1353
  primary, 1354
  secondary, 1356
Velocity quotient, 86
Velpeau's hernia, 1252
Venesection, for posoperative cardiac failure, 313
Venoclysis, in infants and children, 1493
Venous filling time, 1318
Ventilation, inadequate, 261
  mechanical, 269
    amount, 271
    humidification, 272
    use, 272
    weaning from, 273
Ventriculocisternostomy, 1788
Ventriculogram, 1769, 1770
Ventriculography, 1771
Verruca, plantaris, 1736
Vertebrae, compression fractures, 565
  dorsal and lumbar, moderate compression fractures, 566
  severe compression fracture, 567
  spinous processes, fractures, 568
  transverse processes, fractures, 568
Vesicants, chemical warfare, 646
Vesicostomy, cutaneous, with spinal cord injury, 1638
Virchow's nodes, 1067
Virilism, 783
Virus, as cause of cancer, 225
  surgical infections, 41
Vision, defective, as sign of intracranial lesion, 1763
Vitamin, A, 113
  B_{12}, 1072
  C, 115
    deficiency, 1073
    effect on wound healing, 11
  D, 113
    and osteomalacia, 1669
  E, 114
  K, 114
    in obstructive jaundice, 901
  recommended daily allowances, 116
  for surgical patients, 113
Volkmann's ischemic contracture, 458, 493
Volume reduction, after injury, 347
Volvulus, in adults, mechanisms and treatment, 1099
  gastric, classification, 866
  of sigmoid colon, 1085
  with small bowel obstruction, 1077
  of stomach, 866

Subject Index

Vomiting, hazard in battle casualties, 616
  from intracranial pressure, 1756
  postoperative, 326
  projectile, 327
  water loss, 90
von Recklinghausen's disease, 658, 734
Vulva, cancer of, 1548

Warfare, chemical, 646
Warts, 652
  plantar, 652, 1736
Water, abnormal losses in surgical patients, 90
  balance, 75 ff
    abnormalities, diagnosis, 91
    and energy metabolism, 346
    after injury, 345
    maintenance, 95
  requirements for patients, 1601
  deficit (or excess), psychoses, 331
    with normal sodium, 82
    and sodium deficit, 84
    translocational, 94
  and electrolyte metabolism, and corticoids, 776
  excess, therapy, 95
    with sodium deficit, 83
    wtih sodium excess, 86
  exchange across alimentary tract, 89
  exchange with environment, 88
  functional volume, clinical determination, 93
  intoxication, 83
  loss, in burns, 377
    insensible, in burned patients, 380
  normal, with sodium deficit, 84
  postoperative administration, 351
  retention, with mechanical ventilator, 273
  turnover by various organs, 1070
Water-seal drainage, of thorax, 1379
Water-silk sign, in hernia, 1206
Weber-Christian disease, 657
Weight loss, after gastrectomy, 859
Werlhof syndrome, 955
Whipple's disease, 1074

Wilms's tumor, 1620
Wolff's law, 471
Wounds, abdomen, 624
  agents producing, 601
  appearance, shell fragments, 629
  ballistics, 601
  battle, 605
  brain, 617
  cavity, produced by missile, 602
  chest, 620, 621
  closure, and healing, 23
  colon, 627
  combat, bacterial contamination, 609
    blood loss, 608
    caused by specific ordnance, 603
    destruction of tissue, 607
    priorities in surgical management, 614
  contaminated, primary and secondary, 50
    with radionuclides, 430, 431
  dehiscence, causes, 289
  disruption, 308
  dressings, 288, 289
  duodenum, 626
  dynamics, 607
  of extremities, 628
  eye, 620
  face and neck, 619
  foot, 635
  gallbladder, 626
  hand, 634
  healing, 8-33
    collagen phase, 11-13
    and cortisone, 785
    general factors, 12, 14
    and hypoproteinemia, 103
    after irradiation, 425
    local factors, 14
    new developments, 27
    normal rate, 12
    physiology, 10
    relative chemical composition, 11
    substrate phase, 10
    technical factors, 17
    types, 8
  infection, appendectomy, 1041
    classification, 58

  factors governing, 48
  inflammatory phase, 10
  jejunum and ileum, 627
  joints, 633
  liver, 626, 911
  by mines, surgical management, 603
  operative, closing, 287
    management, 297
    with pelvic fractures, 628
  pancreas, 627
  penetrating spinal canal, 618
  regional distribution, 617
  spleen, 626
  stomach, 626
  treatment, in open fractures, 468
  urinary tract, 627
Wrinkle lines, and incisions, 17
  and muscles of face, 18
Wrist, fractures and dislocations, 507
  splinting, 462
  sprain vs fracture, 514
Wristdrop, orthopedic treatment, 1696
Wryneck, congenital, 1480

Xanthalasma, 1415
Xanthoma, 657, 1415
X-ray examination, appendicitis, 1030
  for cancer of lung, 1407
  colon, 1159
  diverticulitis, 1133
  intestinal obstruction, 1081
  in perforative appendicitis, 1035
  peritonitis, differential diagnosis, 1054
  portal hypertension, 1006
  regional enteritis, 1117
  slipped femoral epiphysis, 1692
X-ray therapy, in esophageal cancer, 813

Zollinger-Ellison ulcer, 831
Zones, of operating suites, 276
Zygoma, fracture-dislocation, 1466